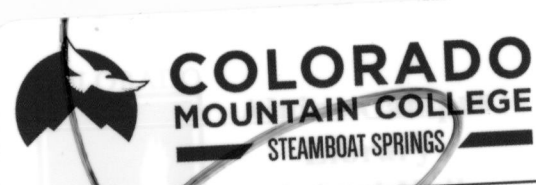

NUTRITION IN THE PREVENTION AND TREATMENT OF DISEASE

NUTRITION IN THE PREVENTION AND TREATMENT OF DISEASE

Edited by

ANN M. COULSTON
Hattner/Coulston Nutrition Associates
Palo Alto, California

CHERYL L. ROCK
Department of Family and Preventative Medicine
University of California, San Diego
La Jolla, California

ELAINE R. MONSEN
Department of Nutrition and Medicine
University of Washington
Seattle, Washington

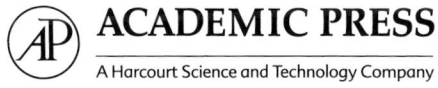

ACADEMIC PRESS

A Harcourt Science and Technology Company

San Diego   San Francisco   New York   Boston   London   Sydney   Tokyo

Academic Press
A Harcourt Science and Technology Company
525 B Street, Suite 1900, San Diego, California 92101-4495, USA
http://www.academicpress.com

Academic Press
Harcourt Place, 32 Jamestown Road, London NW1 7BY, UK
http://www.academicpress.com

Library of Congress Catalog Card Number: 00-111387

International Standard Book Number: 0-12-193155-2

PRINTED IN THE UNITED STATES OF AMERICA
01 02 03 04 05 06 EB 9 8 7 6 5 4 3 2 1

Contents

CHAPTER 45

Nutrition and Cystic Fibrosis

Philip M. Farrell and Hui-Chuan Lai

CHAPTER 46

Osteomalacia

Robert Marcus

CHAPTER 47

Nutrition and Immunodeficiency Syndromes

Jul Gerrior and Christine Wanke

G. Overall Disease Prevention

CHAPTER 48

Nutrition Guidelines to Maintain Health

Suzanne P. Murphy

Contributors

Numbers in parentheses indicate the page number(s) on which the contribution begins.

ANN ALBRIGHT, PhD, RD (429), *Sacramento, California 94234*

NANCY ANZLOVAR, RN (325), *Cleveland Clinic Foundation, Cleveland, Ohio 44195*

SUJATA ARCHER, Phd, RD (291), *Northwestern University Medical School, Chicago, Illinois 60611*

AMY BALTES, RD (291), *Northwestern University Medical School, Chicago, Illinois 60611*

PETER L. BEYER, MS, RD (577), *Department of Dietetics and Nutrition, University of Kansas Medical Center, Kansas City, Kansas 66160*

AMY BINKOSKI (279), *Department of Nutrition, Pennsylvania State University, University Park, Pennsylvania 16801*

BETTE J. CAAN, PhD (357), *Division of Research, Kaiser Foundation Research Institute, Oakland, California 94611*

LAWRENCE J. CHESKIN, MD (549), *Division of Gastroenterology, Johns Hopkins Bayview Medical Center, Baltimore, Maryland 21224*

ANN M. COULSTON, MS, RD (441), *Hattner/Coulston Nutrition Associates, Palo Alto, California 94303*

STACIE COVAL (279), *Department of Nutrition, Pennsylvania State University, University Park, Pennsylvania 16801*

DEBRA COWARD-McKENZIE (31, 69), *The University of Vermont, Burlington, Vermont 05405*

PAULA DAVIS McCALLUM, MS, RD (397), *Advantage Nutrition, Ltd., Chagrin Falls, Ohio 44023*

LINDA DELAHANTY, MS, RD (105), *Massachusetts General Hospital Diabetes Center, Boston, Massachusetts 02114*

WENDY DEMARK-WAHNEFRIED, PhD, RD (337), *Department of Surgery, Duke University Medical Center, Durham, North Carolina 27710*

ADAM DREWNOWSKI, PhD (539), *Nutritional Sciences Program, University of Washington, Seattle, Washington 98195*

BARBARA ELDRIDGE, RD (397), *University of Colorado Health Sciences Center, Denver, Colorado 80123*

PHILIP M. FARRELL, MD, PhD (715), *Medical Sciences Center, University of Wisconsin–Madison, Madison, Wisconsin 53706*

JANIS S. FISLER, PhD (183), *University of California, Davis, California 95616*

JO L. FREUDENHEIM, PhD, RD (199), *Department of Social and Preventive Medicine, State University of New York at Buffalo, Buffalo, New York 14260*

JUL GERRIOR, RD (741), *Department of Family Medicine and Nutrition Infection Unit, Tufts University School of Medicine, Boston, Massachusetts 02111*

KAREN GLANZ, PhD, MPH (83), *Cancer Research Center of Hawaii, University of Hawaii, Honolulu, Hawaii 96813*

D. JORDI GOLDSTEIN, DSc, RD (617), *IVonyx, Inc., Reno, Nevada 89509*

REJEANNE GOUGEON, PhD, RD (415), *McGill Nutrition and Food Science Centre, Crabtree Nutrition Laboratories, Royal Victoria Hospital, Montreal, Quebec, Canada H3A 1A1*

ROBERT HEANEY, MD (653), *Creighton University, Omaha, Nebraska 68178*

KARI HECKER, MS, RD (279), *Department of Nutrition, Pennsylvania State University, University Park, Pennsylvania 16801*

JOAN M. HEINS, MA, RD, CDE (105), *Washington University School of Medicine, St. Louis, Missouri 63108*

STEVE HERTZLER, PhD, RD (563), *School of Allied Medical Professions, Medical Dietetics Division, Ohio State University, Columbus, Ohio 43210*

JAMES O. HILL, PhD (465), *Center for Human Nutrition, University of Colorado Health Sciences Center, Denver, Colorado 80262*

KARRY A. JACKSON (563), *School of Consumer and Family Sciences, Purdue University, West Lafayette, Indiana 47907*

RACHEL K. JOHNSON, PhD, MPH, RD (31, 69), *The University of Vermont, Burlington, Vermont 05405*

WALTER H. KAYE, MD (685), *Western Psychiatric Institute and Clinic, University of Pittsburgh Medical Center, Pittsburgh, Pennsylvania 15213*

JANET KING, PhD (773), *USDA, Western Human Nutrition Research Center, University of California at Davis, Davis, California 95616*

LAURENCE N. KOLONEL, MD, PhD (373), *Cancer Research Center of Hawaii, University of Hawaii, Honolulu, Hawaii 98613*

PENNY KRIS-ETHERTON, PhD, RD (279), *Department of Nutrition, Pennsylvania State University, University Park, Pennsylvania 16801*

ALAN R. KRISTAL, PhD (123), *Cancer Prevention Research Program, Fred Hutchinson Cancer Research Center, Seattle, Washington 98109*

HUI-CHUAN LAI, PhD, RD (715), *Department of Biostatistics and Medical Informatics and Department of Pediatrics, Clinical Sciences Center, University of Wisconsin—Madison, Madison, Wisconsin 53792*

JOHANNA W. LAMPE, PhD, RD (139), *Cancer Prevention Research Program, Fred Hutchinson Cancer Research Center, Seattle, Washington 98109*

DAVID A. LEVITSKY, PhD (499), *Division of Nutritional Sciences, Cornell University, Ithaca, New York 14853*

PAO-HWA LIN, PhD (303), *Epidemiology & Surveillance Research, The American Cancer Society, Atlanta, Georgia 30329*

SUZANNE LUTTON, MD (325), *Diagnostic Cardiology Associates, Youngstown, Ohio 44504*

ROBERT B. LUTZ, MD (261), *Arizona Cancer Center, University of Arizona, Tucson, Arizona 85719*

LYNNE LYONS, MPH, RD, CDE (453), *Burlingame, California 94010*

ROBERT MARCUS, MD (729), *Stanford University School of Medicine, Stanford, California; and Veteran's Administration Medical Center, Palo Alto, California 94304*

LAURA MATARESE, MS, RD, LD, FADA, CNSD (245), *The Cleveland Clinic Foundation, Cleveland, Ohio 44195*

KATHLEEN E. MAYER, MS, RD, LD (229), *Ross Products Division, Abbott Laboratories, Columbus, Ohio 43215*

SUSAN T. MAYNE, PhD (387), *Department of Epidemiology and Public Health, Yale University School of Medicine, New Haven, Connecticut 06520*

MARJI McCULLOUGH, PhD, RD (303), *Epidemiology & Surveillance Research, The American Cancer Society, Atlanta, Georgia 30329*

BETH McQUISTON, MS, RD (617), *Park Ridge, Illinois 60068*

DEBRA L. MILLER, PhD (549), *Central Soya Co., Inc., Fort Wayne, Indiana 46818*

KRIS M. MOGENSEN, MS, RD, CNSD (43), *Frances Stern Nutrition Center, New England Medical Center, Boston, Massachusetts 02111*

ELAINE R. MONSEN, PhD, RD (xvii), *Department of Nutrition and Medicine, University of Washington, Seattle, Washington 98195*

SUZANNE P. MURPHY, PhD, RD (753), *Cancer Research Center of Hawaii, University of Hawaii, Honolulu, Hawaii 96813*

DIANNE NEUMARK-SZTAINER, PhD, MPH, RD (517), *Division of Epidemiology, University of Minnesota, Minneapolis, Minnesota 55454*

JOSE M. ORDOVAS (157), *USDA-HNRCA, Tufts University, Boston, Massachusetts 02111*

RUTH E. PATTERSON, PhD, RD (59), *Cancer Prevention Research Program, Fred Hutchinson Cancer Research Center, Seattle, Washington 98109-1024*

DIANE READER, RD, CDE (453), *International Diabetes Center, Minneapolis, Minnesota 55416*

SARAH H. RIGBY, MS, RD, LD (601), *Johns Hopkins Children's Center, Baltimore, Maryland 21287*

CHERYL L. ROCK, PhD, RD (139, 337, 397, 685), *Department of Family and Preventive Medicine, University of California at San Diego, La Jolla, California 92093*

EDWARD SALTZMAN, MD (43), *Tufts University and New England Medical Center, Boston, Massachusetts 02111*

JESSIE A. SATIA, PhD (123), *Cancer Prevention Research Program, Fred Hutchinson Cancer Research Center, Seattle, Washington 98109*

DENNIS SAVAIANO, PhD (563), *School of Consumer and Family Sciences, Purdue University, West Lafayette, Indiana 47907*

NANCY A. SCHONFELD-WARDEN, MD (183), *University of California, Davis, California 95616*

KATHLEEN B. SCHWARZ, MD (601), *Johns Hopkins Children's Center, Baltimore, Maryland 21287*

HELEN M. SEAGLE MS, RD (465), *Center for Human Nutrition, University of Colorado Health Sciences Center, Denver, Colorado 80262*

DENISE SHAFFER TAYLOR, MS, RD (279), *Department of Nutrition, Pennsylvania State University, University Park, Pennsylvania 16801*

NANCY E. SHERWOOD, PhD (517), *Division of Epidemiology, University of Minnesota, Minneapolis, Minnesota 55454*

MARTHA L. SLATTERY, PhD, MPH, RD (357), *Oncological Sciences/PHS, University of Utah, Salt Lake City, Utah 84108*

LINDA G. SNETSELAAR, PhD, RD, LD (95), *Department of Epidemiology, College of Medicine, University of Iowa, Iowa City, Iowa 52240*

MARCIA L. STEFANICK, PhD (481), *Department of Medicine, Stanford Center for Research in Disease Prevention, Stanford University, Palo Alto, California 94304*

MARY STORY, PhD, RD (517), *Division of Epidemiology, University of Minnesota, Minneapolis, Minnesota 55454*

FABRIZIS L. SUAREZ, MD, PhD, FACN (563), *Minneapolis Veteran's Administration Medical Center, Minneapolis, Minnesota 55417*

AMY F. SUBAR, PhD, MPH, RD (3), *National Cancer Institute, National Institutes of Health, Bethesda, Maryland 20892*

CHRISTY TANGNEY, PhD, CNS, FACN (637), *Department of Clinical Nutrition, Rush Presbyterian St. Luke's Medical Center, Chicago, Illinois 60612*

ABBA I. TERR, MD (701), *San Francisco, California 94108*

KIMBERLY THEDFORD, MS, RD (291), *Northwestern University Medical School, Chicago, Illinois 60611*

FRANCES E. THOMPSON, PhD, MPH (3), *Applied Research Program, Division of Cancer Control and Population Sciences, National Cancer Institute, Bethesda, Maryland 20892*

CYNTHIA THOMSON, PhD, RD, FADA (261), *Arizona Cancer Center, University of Arizona, Tucson, Arizona 85719*

CRISTINE M. TRAHMS, MS, RD, FADA (209), *Department of Pediatrics, University of Washington, Seattle, Washington 98195*

LINDA VAN HORN, PhD, RD (291), *Northwestern University Medical School, Chicago, Illinois 60611*

ANNE COBLE VOSS, PhD, RD (229), *Ross Products Division, Abbott Laboratories, Columbus, Ohio 43215*

CHRISTINE WANKE, MD (741), *Department of Family Medicine and Nutrition Infection Unit, Tufts University School of Medicine, Boston, Massachusetts 02111*

VICTORIA WARREN-MEARS, MS, RD (539), *Nutrition and Food Services, Harborview Medical Center and Nutritional Sciences Program, University of Washington, Seattle, Washington 98195*

HOLLY WYATT, MD (465), *Center for Human Nutrition, University of Colorado Health Sciences Center, Denver, Colorado 80262*

GUIXIANG ZHAO, MS (279), *Department of Nutrition, Pennsylvania State University, University Park, Pennsylvania 16801*

Preface

The purpose of this text is to provide an update of current knowledge in clinical nutrition and an overview of the rationale and science base of its application to practice in the treatment and prevention of disease. The text addresses basic principles and concepts that are central to the major clinical nutrition-related activities, such as nutritional assessment and monitoring, current theoretical base and knowledge of efficacious interventions, interactions between genetic and nutritional factors, and the use and interpretation of population-based or clinical epidemiological evidence. The various roles of clinical nutrition and current knowledge of nutrition in the prevention and treatment of major disease-specific conditions are also reviewed, with an emphasis on past and current scientific evidence that supports these roles. New areas of interest and study are also discussed, with the perspective that the application of the scientific method is by definition an evolutionary process.

Treatment of the disease diabetes mellitus provides an excellent and current example of treatment evolution. In the early part of the 20th century, before the discovery of insulin by F. G. Banting and C. H. Best in 1921, the treatment of choice for individuals with diabetes mellitus was morphine for pain abatement along with a very restricted, starvation diet. When insulin injections became available, dietary protocols were developed. Initially, dietary treatment was based on food exchange lists that encouraged prescribed intakes of carbohydrate, protein, and fat. Recent research from the Diabetes Control and Complications Trial and a similar research trial in the United Kingdom has been the base for the current dietary management emphasizing blood glucose monitoring throughout the day and individualized adjustment of carbohydrate ingestion and insulin injection in individuals who require insulin therapy. Nutrition intervention plays a major role in the management of the patient with diabetes mellitus and in the treatment of the disease and the prevention or delay of complications (see Part II.C).

Another essential role for nutrition intervention is in the prevention of cancer. Cancer represents a disease continuum and at all stages, from primary prevention to treatment, nutrition is a key factor. As discussed in the section highlighting nutrition and major cancer types, an explosion of new knowledge has identified nutrition as a major factor in the etiology and progression of disease (see Part II.B).

Nutrition is the process by which the human body utilizes food for the production of energy, for the maintenance of health, for growth, and for the normal functioning of every organ and tissue. Clinical nutrition is the study of nutrition and diet as related to the development and treatment of human disease. Nutrition is an interdisciplinary field of study, built on a foundation of biomedical and behavioral sciences. Clinical nutrition is the aspect of nutrition science that is related to the development, progression, or management of disease, as differentiated from the issues of normal requirements, cellular functions and activities, and various topics that must be addressed in meeting basic requirements to enable normal growth and development.

Areas of study that contribute to knowledge in clinical nutrition include the disease-relevant biochemistry, metabolism, and activities of nutrients and dietary factors within the tissues and cells; the bioavailability and utilization of nutrients from various food sources, as disease risk or diagnosis may influence these factors; the regulation and compartmentalization of nutrients in the body; the attitudes about food and the eating patterns and behaviors of the targeted individual or group; the technology of food science and specialized or modified food products; and the technology involved in providing adequate and appropriate nutrients or foods to individuals and various community-based or institutionalized groups. Other aspects of clinical nutrition include the development and evaluation of nutrition education efforts; the development of nutrition policies, guidelines, and practice standards that affect the goals and objectives of government and private health agencies, professional practice groups, and health-related organizations; and the design and implementation of individual, clinical, and community-based nutrition and diet interventions. Clinical nutrition interventions range in scope from efforts to maintain health during short-term illness, to optimization of health status in individuals at risk for or diagnosed with chronic diseases, to major nutritional and diet modifications as specific or adjuvant treatments for disease. Clinical nutrition encompasses primary, secondary, and tertiary disease prevention, in addition to management of disease.

Dietary intake or nutritional status may be altered as a result of disease or by the treatment modalities that are utilized, such as surgical treatments, or medical management strategies, such as drugs. The altered needs must be met by dietary or nutritional interventions in order to prevent malnutrition and the associated consequences, which would contribute to overall morbidity and mortality. Also, nutrition intervention can be a critical component of disease prevention, an important aspect of disease management, or the primary treatment for disease. A complicating factor is that people generally eat food, rather than nutrients, so that the practical and psychosocial aspects of diet modification and food or food product availability must be considered in any nutrition intervention, whether individual or community based, and irrespective of whether the goal is primary prevention or disease treatment.

As in any area of the biomedical sciences, the importance of science-based activities and practices cannot be understated. Clinical nutrition concepts and practices that can become popular with either the lay public or professionals are sometimes based on the type of scientific evidence that cannot truly support the rationales and practices, regardless of how standard and common they might be. Popular theories may be generated by observational epidemiological studies, case series, or anecdotal reports, all of which lack the capability of truly demonstrating a causative or efficacious role for the nutritional factor. Such studies are useful for generating hypotheses, but the apparent associations between diets and disease may be confounded by uncontrolled or unmeasured factors and other determinants of health and disease. Unproven diet therapies exist for the treatment of numerous conditions, and many aspects of common nutrition interventions are sorely in need of testing in an appropriate research design. As in any other aspect of disease prevention and treatment, the use of nutrition interventions or diet therapies should be based on a scientific rationale and sound data, not on anecdotal experience. The scientific basis for clinical nutrition needs to expand considerably in order to fully support claims for the efficacy of many of the common activities and interventions, and progress in this area is being made.

Our definitions of diseases need to further evolve to bring greater clarity and improve precision of treatment. As gene–diet interactions are scientifically delineated, laser-sharp therapies may be applied to specific individuals. For the public, however, generating and analyzing data that summarize dietary intake and its association with disease will be valuable tasks in both treating disease and developing disease prevention strategies. Well-designed focused screening will be an aid in disease detection, and well-founded medical nutrition therapies can minimize disease development and related complications. Providing scientifically sound, creative, and effective nutrition interventions can be challenging. In so doing, however, we will serve the public good.

It is our goal to update our knowledge and its application through updated editions of this text. In addition, we plan to provide online access to relevant new findings and their import to nutrition in the prevention and treatment of disease. It is our goal to raise the bar for both understanding and treatment.

Ann M. Coulston
Cheryl L. Rock
Elaine R. Monsen

Acknowledgments

We dedicate this book to all the women and men—our colleagues, teachers, and friends—who dedicated their professional lives to the pursuit of excellence in nutrition.

Your intelligence, research efforts, and perseverance brought us the scientific tools and perspective to prepare this book which brings the field of clinical nutrition into the 21st century.

Your work is truly evolutionary.

Basic Principles and Concepts

A. Examining the Relationship between Diet, Nutrition, and Disease

CHAPTER **1**

Dietary Assessment Methodology

FRANCES E. THOMPSON AND AMY F. SUBAR
National Cancer Institute, Bethesda, Maryland

I. INTRODUCTION

This chapter reviews the major dietary assessment methods, their advantages and disadvantages, and specific issues to consider when collecting these types of data. The intent is for this chapter to lead to an understanding of alternative dietary assessment methods so that the appropriate method is chosen for a particular need. This chapter updates the "Dietary Assessment Resource Manual" [1].

II. DIETARY ASSESSMENT METHODS

A. Dietary Records

For the dietary record approach, the respondent records the foods and beverages and the amounts of each consumed over 1 or more days. The amounts consumed may be measured, using a scale or household measures (such as cups, tablespoons), or estimated, using models, pictures, or no particular aid. Typically, if multiple days are recorded, they are consecutive, and no more than 3 or 4 days are included. Recording periods of more than 4 consecutive days are usually unsatisfactory, as reported intakes decrease [2] because of respondent fatigue. Theoretically, the recording is done at the time of the eating occasion, but it need not be done on paper. Dictaphones, computer recording, and self-recording scales have been used [3–5] and hold special promise for low-literacy groups and other difficult-to-assess populations because of their ease of administration and potential accuracy, although tape recording has not been shown to be useful among school-aged children [6].

To complete a dietary record, the respondent must be trained in the level of detail required to adequately describe the foods and amounts consumed, including the name of the food (brand name, if possible), preparation methods, recipes for food mixtures, and portion sizes. In some studies this is enhanced by contact and review of the report after 1 day of recording. At the end of the recording period, a trained interviewer should review the records with the respondent to clarify entries and to probe for forgotten foods. Dietary records can also be recorded by someone other than the subject. This is often done with children or institutionalized individuals.

Although intake data using dietary records are typically collected in an open-ended form, close-ended forms have also been developed [4, 7–9]. These forms consist of listings of food groups; and the respondent indicates whether that food group has been consumed. Portion size can also be asked, either in an open-ended manner or in categories. In format, these "checklist" forms resemble food frequency questionnaires (FFQs) (see Section II.C). Unlike FFQs, which generally query about intake over a specified time period such as the past year or month, they are filled out either concurrently with actual intake (for precoded records) or at the end of a day for that day's intake (daily recall).

The dietary record method has the potential to provide quantitatively accurate information on food consumed during the recording period. For this reason, food records are often regarded as the "gold standard" against which other dietary assessment methods are compared. By recording foods as they are consumed, the problem of omission is lessened and the foods are more fully described. Further, the measurement of amounts of food consumed at each occasion should provide more accurate portion sizes than if the respondents were recalling portion sizes of foods previously eaten.

A major disadvantage of dietary records is that they are subject to bias both in the selection of the sample and in the measurement of the diet. Dietary record keeping requires that respondents or respondent proxies be both motivated and literate (if done on paper), which can potentially limit the method's use in some population groups (e.g., low socioeconomic status, poorly educated, recent immigrants, children, and some elderly groups). The requirements for cooperation in keeping records can limit the generalizability of the findings from the dietary records to the broader population from which the study sample was drawn. Research indicates that there is a significant increase in incomplete records as more days of records are kept, and the validity of the collected information decreases in the later days of a 7-day recording period, in contrast to information collected in the earlier days [2]. Part of this decrease may occur because many respondents develop the practice of filling out the record at one time for a previous period.

Adapted with permission from Thompson, F. E., and Byers, T. (1994). Dietary assessment resource manual. *J. Nutr.* **124**, 2245S–2318S. © Journal of Nutrition, American Society for Nutritional Sciences.

When respondents record only once per day, the record method approaches the 24-hour recall in terms of relying on memory rather than concurrent recording. More importantly, recording foods as they are being eaten can affect both the types of food chosen and the quantities consumed [10]. The knowledge that food requires recording and the demanding task of doing it, therefore, alter the dietary behaviors the tool is intended to measure [11]. This effect is a weakness when the aim is to measure unaltered dietary behavior. However, when the aim is to enhance awareness of dietary behavior and change that behavior, as in some intervention studies, this effect can be seen as an advantage. Recording, by itself, is an effective weight loss technique [12].

As is true with all quantitative dietary information, the information collected on dietary records can be burdensome to code and can lead to high personnel costs. Dietary assessment software that allows for easier data entry using common spellings of foods can save considerable time in data coding. Even with high-quality data entry, maintaining overall quality control for dietary records can be difficult because information is often not recorded consistently from respondent to respondent.

These weaknesses may be less pronounced for the hybrid method of the "checklist" form, since checking off a food item may be easier than recording a complete description of the food, and the costs of data processing can be minimal. The checklist can be developed to assess particular "core foods," which contribute substantially to intakes of some nutrients. However, as the comprehensiveness of the nutrients to be assessed increases, the length of the form also increases, and becomes more burdensome to complete at each eating occasion. The checklist method may be most appropriate in settings with limited diets or for assessment of a limited set of foods or nutrients.

Several studies indicate that reported energy and protein intakes on diet records for selected small samples of adults are underestimated in the range of 4–37% when compared to energy expenditure as measured by doubly labeled water or protein intake as measured by urinary nitrogen [12–20]. Because of these findings, the record is considered an imperfect gold standard. A few studies suggest that low-energy reporters compared to non-low-energy reporters have intakes that are lower in absolute intake of most nutrients [21], higher in percentage of energy from protein [21, 22], and lower in percentage of energy as carbohydrate [21–23]. Underreporters may also report lower intakes of desserts and sweet baked goods, butter, and alcoholic beverages but more grains, meats, salads, and vegetables [21].

Underreporting on food records is probably a result of the combined effects of incomplete recording and the impact of the recording process on dietary choices leading to undereating [12, 20]. The highest levels of underreporting have been found among individuals with a higher body mass index (BMI) [13, 15, 16, 21, 24], particularly women [13, 15, 16, 22, 25, 26]. This effect, however, may be due, in part, to the fact that heavier individuals are more likely to be dieting on any given individual day [27]. Other research shows that demographic or psychological indices such as education, employment grade, social desirability, body image, or dietary restraint may also be important factors related to underreporting on diet records [13, 20, 22, 26, 28, 29].

B. The 24-Hour Dietary Recall

In the 24-hour dietary recall, the respondent is asked to remember and report all foods and beverages consumed in the preceding 24 hours or in the preceding day. The recall typically is conducted by personal interview or, more recently, by telephone [30, 31], either computer assisted [32] or using a paper-and-pencil form. Well-trained interviewers are crucial in administering a 24-hour recall because much of the dietary information is collected by asking probing questions. Ideally, interviewers would be dietitians with education in foods and nutrition; however, non-nutritionists who have been trained in the use of a standardized instrument can be effective. All interviewers should be knowledgeable about foods available in the marketplace and about preparation practices, including prevalent regional or ethnic foods.

The interview is often structured, usually with specific probes, to help the respondent remember all foods consumed throughout the day. One study found that respondents with interviewer probing reported 25% higher dietary intakes than did respondents without interviewer probing [33]. Probing is especially useful in collecting necessary details, such as how foods were prepared. It is also useful in recovering many items not originally reported, such as common additions to foods (e.g., butter on toast) and eating occasions not originally reported (e.g., snacks and beverage breaks). However, interviewers should be provided with standardized neutral probing questions so as to avoid leading the respondent to specific answers when the respondent really does not know or remember. National dietary surveys currently employ a multiple-pass system in which intake is reviewed more than once in an effort to retrieve forgotten eating occasions, and includes a "forgotten foods list" of foods commonly omitted in 24-hour recall reporting [34–37]. A 24-hour recall interview using the multiple-pass approach typically requires between 30 and 45 minutes.

A quality control system to minimize error and increase reliability of interviewing and coding 24-hour recalls is essential [31, 35, 38–41]. Such a system should include a detailed protocol for administration, training, and retraining sessions for interviewers, duplicate collection and coding of some of the recalls throughout the study period, and the use of a computerized database system for nutrient analysis. Data entry can be costly, but these costs can be reduced with computer software specially designed for dietary data entry.

There are many advantages to the 24-hour recall. An interviewer administers the tool and records the responses, so literacy of the respondent is not required. Because of the

immediacy of the recall period, respondents are generally able to recall most of their dietary intake. Because there is relatively little burden on the respondents, those who agree to give 24-hour dietary recalls are more likely to be representative of the population than are those who agree to keep food records. Thus, the 24-hour recall method is useful across a wide range of populations. In addition, interviewers can be trained to capture the detail necessary so that the foods eaten by any population can be researched later by the coding staff and coded appropriately. Finally, in contrast to food record methods, dietary recalls occur after the food has been consumed, so there is less potential for the assessment method to interfere with dietary behavior.

Direct coding of the foods reported during the interview is now possible with computerized software systems. The potential benefits of automated software include substantial cost reductions for processing dietary data, less missing data, and greater standardization of interviews [42]. However, a potential problem in direct coding of interview responses is the loss of the respondent's reported description of the food, in contrast to paper records of the interview, which are then available for later review and editing. If direct coding of the interview is done, methods for the interviewer to easily enter those foods not found in the system should be available and these methods should be reinforced by interviewer training and quality control procedures.

The main weakness of the 24-hour recall approach is that individuals may not report their food consumption accurately for various reasons related to memory and the interview situation. These cognitive influences are discussed in more detail in Section V.F. Because most individuals' diets vary greatly from day to day, it is not appropriate to use data from a single 24-hour recall to characterize an individual's usual diet. Neither should a single day's intake, be it a recall or food record, be used to estimate the proportion of the population that has adequate or inadequate diets (e.g., the proportion of individuals with less than 30% of energy from fat, or who are deficient in vitamin C intake) [43]. This is because the true distribution of usual diets is much narrower than is the distribution of daily diets (there is variation not only between people in usual diet, but also from day-to-day for each person). The principal use of a single 24-hour recall is to describe the average dietary intake of a group because the means are robust and unaffected by within-person variation. Multiple days of recalls or records can better assess the individual's usual intake and population distributions but require special statistical procedures designed for that purpose [44, 45].

The validity of the 24-hour dietary recall has been studied by comparing respondents' reports of intake either with intakes unobtrusively recorded/weighed by trained observers or with biological markers. In general, group mean nutrient estimates from 24-hour recalls have been found to be similar to observed intakes [2, 46], although respondents with lower observed intakes have tended to overreport, and those with higher observed intakes have tended to underreport their in-

takes [46]. Similar to findings for food records, biological markers such as doubly labeled water and urinary nitrogen show a tendency toward underreporting of energy and protein in the range of 13–24% for 24-hour dietary recalls [20, 47, 48]. One study, however, found overreporting of protein from 13–25% depending on level of BMI [49]. In national dietary surveys, data suggest that underreporting may affect up to 15% of all 24-hour recalls [41, 50]. Underreporters compared to non-underreporters tend to report fewer numbers of foods, fewer mentions of foods consumed, and smaller portion sizes across a wide range of food groups and tend to report more frequent intakes of low-fat/diet foods and less frequent intakes of fat added to foods [50]. Factors such as obesity, gender, social desirability, restrained eating, education, literacy, perceived health status, and race/ethnicity have been shown in various studies to be related to underreporting in recalls [20, 27, 28, 41, 48, 50–52].

C. Food Frequency

The food frequency approach asks respondents to report their usual frequency of consumption of each food from a list of foods for a specific period [53–55]. Information is collected on frequency and sometimes portion size, but little detail is collected on other characteristics of the foods eaten, such as the methods of cooking or the combinations of foods in meals. To estimate relative or absolute nutrient intakes, many food frequency questionnaires (FFQs) also incorporate portion size questions or specify portion sizes as part of each question. Overall nutrient intake estimates are derived by summing, over all foods, the products of the reported frequency of each food by the amount of nutrient in a specified (or assumed) serving of that food.

There are many FFQ instruments, and many continue to be adapted and developed for different populations and different purposes. Among those validated and commonly used for U. S. adults are the Health Habits and History Questionnaire (HHHQ) or Block Questionnaire [56–62], the Fred Hutchinson Cancer Research Center Food Frequency Questionnaire (a revised HHHQ) [63], and the Harvard University Food Frequency Questionnaire or Willett Questionnaire [53, 64–69]. Comparisons between the widely used Block and Willett instruments have been conducted indicating differences in estimates for some nutrients [70–72]. A new instrument, the Diet History Questionnaire, developed and in use at the National Cancer Institute, was designed with an emphasis on cognitive ease for respondents [73–75] (see http://www.dccps.ims.nci.nih.gov/ARP). Other instruments have been developed for specific populations. Two FFQs have been developed by researchers at the University of Arizona, the University of Arizona Food Frequency Questionnaire and the Southwest Food Frequency Questionnaire, to capture the diverse diets of Latinos and Native Americans [22, 76, 77]. Investigators at the University of Hawaii have developed a questionnaire for assessing the diverse diets of

Hawaiian, Japanese, Chinese, Filipino, and Caucasian ethnic groups [78, 79]. This instrument was recently adapted for use in a multiethnic cohort study conducted in Hawaii and Los Angeles [80]. In Europe, a number of FFQs have been developed within Western European countries for the European Prospective Investigation into Cancer and Nutrition (EPIC) [19, 81–86]. In addition, a few "brief" FFQs have been developed composed of shorter lists of 40–60 line items from the original 100 or so items [87–90]. Such shortened instruments may reflect distributions of usual intakes of specific nutrients/food groups or percentage of energy from macronutrients. Because of the number of FFQs available, investigators need to carefully evaluate which best suits their research needs.

The major strength of the FFQ approach is its ability to estimate the respondent's usual intake of foods over a long period of time such as one year. It can also be used to circumvent recent changes in diet (e.g., changes due to disease) by obtaining information about individuals' diets as recalled about a prior time period. Food frequency responses can be used to rank individuals according to their usual consumption of nutrients, foods, or groups of foods. Most food frequency instruments have been designed to be self-administered, require 30–60 minutes to complete depending on the instrument and the respondent, and most are optically scannable to reduce data entry costs. Because the costs of data collection and processing and the respondent burden are typically much lower for FFQs than for multiple diet records or recalls, FFQs have become a common way to estimate usual dietary intake in large epidemiological studies.

The major limitation of the food frequency method is that many details of dietary intake are not measured, and the quantification of intake is not as accurate as with recalls or records. Inaccuracies result from an incomplete listing of all possible foods and from errors in frequency and usual serving size estimations. As a result, the scale for nutrient intake estimates from a FFQ may be shifted considerably, yielding inaccurate estimates of the average intake for the group. Research suggests that longer food frequency lists may overestimate, while shorter lists may underestimate intake of fruits and vegetables [91], but it is unclear as to whether or how this applies to nutrients and other food groups. In the absence of knowledge about the true usual intake of the population, it is unknown how closely the distribution of intake estimates from FFQs reflects the distribution of true intake in that population.

Controversy has arisen over whether it is proper to use FFQs to estimate quantitative parameters of a population's dietary intake [64, 92–96] (see Chapter 4). Although some FFQs seem to produce estimates of population average intakes that are reasonable [92], different FFQs will perform in often unpredictable ways in different populations, so the levels of nutrient intakes estimated by FFQs are best regarded as only approximations [93]. FFQs are much better suited for ranking subjects according to food or nutrient intake than for estimating the levels of intake.

Serving size of foods consumed is difficult for respondents to evaluate and is thus problematic for all assessment instruments (see Section V.A). However, the inaccuracies involved in respondents attempting to estimate usual serving size in FFQs may be even greater because a respondent is asked to estimate an average for foods that may have highly variable portion sizes across eating occasions. The importance of whether or not to include portion size at all on FFQs has been widely debated. Because frequency is believed to be a greater contributor than typical serving size to the variance in intake of most foods, some prefer to use FFQs without the additional respondent burden of reporting serving sizes [53]. Others cite small improvements in the performance of FFQs that ask the respondents to report a usual serving size for each food [58, 59].

Development of the food list is crucial to the success of the food frequency method [56]. The full variability of an individual's diet, which includes many different foods, brands, and preparation practices, cannot be fully captured with a finite food list. Obtaining accurate reports for foods eaten both alone and in mixtures is particularly problematic. FFQs can ask the respondent to report either a combined frequency for a particular food eaten both alone and in mixtures, or to report separate frequencies for each food use. The first approach is cognitively complex, but the second approach may lead to double counting. Often FFQs will include similar foods in a single question (e.g., hamburger, steak, roast beef). However, such grouping can create a cognitively complex question (e.g., for someone who often eats hamburger but never eats steak). In addition, when a group of foods is asked as a single question, assumptions about the relative frequencies of intake of the foods constituting the group must be made when calculating nutrient estimates. These assumptions are often not based on information from the study population even though true eating patterns may differ considerably across population subgroups and over time.

FFQs are commonly used to rank or group study subjects for the purpose of assessing the association between dietary intake and disease risk, such as in case-control or cohort studies [97–99]. For estimating relative risks, the degree of misclassification of subjects from their correct quantile of intake is more important than is the quantitative scale on which the ranking is made [100]. Although analyses on the extent of misclassification by the food frequency method indicate that the amount of extreme misclassification (e.g., from lowest quartile to the highest) is small, even a small amount of such misclassification can create a large bias in estimates of associations [101, 102].

The definitive validity study for a food frequency-based estimate of long-term usual diet would require nonintrusive observation of the respondent's total diet over a long time. No such studies have ever been done. One feeding study,

however, with three defined 6-week feeding cycles (in which all intakes were known) showed some significant differences in known absolute nutrient intakes as compared to the Willett FFQ for several fat components, mostly in the direction of underestimation by the FFQ [103].

The most practical approach to examining the concordance of food frequency responses and usual diet is to use multiple food recalls or records over a period as an indicator of usual diet. This approach has been used in many studies examining various FFQs [5, 18, 19, 47, 53, 57, 60, 61, 63, 65, 66, 68, 80–86, 104–115]. This type of study is more properly called a "calibration study" rather than "validation study" (see Section V.H), because recalls and records themselves may not represent the time period of interest, may contain error, and may underestimate nutrient intakes [13–17, 24, 47–49, 116]. In such studies, the correlations between the methods for most foods and nutrients are in the range of 0.4–0.7. Findings from calibration studies that have incorporated biological markers, such as urinary nitrogen for protein intake or doubly labeled water for energy expenditure, have shown correlations with FFQs ranging from 0.2 to 0.7 for protein [18, 19, 47, 86, 106, 114, 117, 118] and from 0.4 to 0.5 for energy [14, 47].

Depending on characteristics of FFQs, such as length and detail of the food list, quality of the nutrient database, and method of querying portion size, the estimates of food and nutrient intake can be higher or lower than those from the more quantitative methods of the 24-hour dietary recall or food record. Given that there is measurement error in all self-reported methods of dietary assessment, various statistical methods employing measurement error models and energy adjustment are used to assess the validity of FFQs and to adjust estimates of relative risks for disease outcomes [119–129] (see Sections V.H and V.I).

In pursuit of improving the validity of the FFQ, investigators have addressed a range of questionnaire design issues such as length, closed- versus open-ended response categories, portion size, seasonality, and time frame. Frequency instruments designed to assess total diet generally list more than 100 individual line items, many with additional portion size questions, requiring 30–60 minutes to complete. This raises concern about length and its effect on response rates. Though respondent burden is a factor in obtaining reasonable response rates for studies in general, a few studies have shown this not to be a decisive factor for FFQs [74, 130–134]. Others suggest that adding more low-fat foods to the tool leads to better fat and energy estimates [135, 136]. This tension between length and specificity highlights the difficult issue of how to define a closed-ended list of foods for a food frequency instrument. Whether or not incorporating separate questions to assess some detail in portion size is necessary has been controversial given that the most important factor in estimating intakes is frequency. However, research has been conducted to determine the best ways to ask about

portion size on FFQs [73, 137, 138]. Another design issue is the time frame about which usual intake is queried. Many instruments inquire about usual intakes during the past year [56, 64], but it is possible to ask about the past week or month [139] depending on specific research situations. Even when usual intake during the past year is asked, several studies have indicated that the season in which the questionnaire is administered has an influence on reporting over the entire year [140, 141]. Finally, optically scanned instruments have necessitated the use of closed-ended response categories, forcing a loss in specificity [142].

D. Brief Dietary Assessment Methods

Many brief dietary assessment methods have been developed. These instruments can be useful in situations that do not require either assessment of the total diet or quantitative accuracy in dietary estimates. For example, a brief diet assessment might be used to triage large numbers of individuals into groups to allow more focused attention on those at greatest need for intervention or education. Measurement of dietary intake, no matter how crude, can also serve to activate interest in the respondent to facilitate nutrition education. These brief methods may, therefore, have utility in clinical settings or in situations where health promotion and health education are the goals. Brief methods have also been used to track changes in diet within an intervention setting, although there is concern that responses to questions of intake that directly evolve from intervention messages may be biased [143]. Brief methods are used often for population surveillance at the state or local level, for example, in the Centers for Disease Control and Prevention's (CDC's) Behavioral Risk Factor Surveillance System (BRFSS) (see Section III.F).

Such brief methods can be simplified FFQs or questionnaires that focus on eating behaviors other than the frequency of intake of specific foods. Complete FFQs typically must contain 100 or more food items to capture the range of foods contributing to the many different nutrients in the diet. If an investigator is interested only in estimating the intake of a single nutrient or a single type of food, however, then far fewer foods need to be included. Often, only 15–30 foods might be required to account for most of the intake of a particular nutrient in the diet of a population [144, 145].

Numerous single-exposure short questionnaires using a food frequency approach have been developed and compared with multiple days of food records, dietary recalls, and/or complete FFQs. In early work, Block selected 13 foods that accounted for most of the intake of fat in the diets of American women to develop a brief "fat screener" for use in selecting women for a dietary intervention trial; the correlation between the fat index and fat intake from multiple records was 0.58 [146]. A similar tool used in the Behavioral Risk Factor Surveillance System (BRFSS) was evaluated in five different populations relative to more extensive dietary

assessment instruments [147]. Correlations between fat scores and quantified absolute fat intakes ranged from 0.22 (in the Latino population) to 0. 60, and were lower (0.26–0.42) between fat scores and percent energy from fat. A later adaptation of the tool, tested among men and women, indicated substantial misclassification when ranking individuals for percent energy from fat, and only moderate agreement when ranking absolute fat intakes [148]. The Block fat screener, currently composed of 17 items, has been modified to ask only about versions of the food that are not low fat. Information about this tool is found at http://www. nutritionquest.com. A recently developed 16-item percent energy from fat screener correlated 0.65 with 24-hour recalls in an older U. S. population [149]. Similar sets of questions have been developed and tested by others to briefly characterize dietary fat or percent energy from fat intake [150–154]. Published validity studies of fat screeners are listed and reviewed by Yaroch *et al.* [155].

A seven-item tool developed by National Cancer Institute (NCI) staff and private grantees for the NCI "5 a Day for Better Health" effort provides an indicator of the average number of servings of fruits and vegetables consumed per day, and has been used widely in the United States. The tool is similar to one used in the BRFSS [156]. Validation studies of various brief instruments to assess fruit and vegetable intake have suggested that they underestimate actual intake [88, 157–160]. A newer tool based on cognitive interviewing methods has been developed at NCI, and its validity is currently being evaluated (see http://www.dccps.ims.nci.nih. gov/ARP). Single-nutrient FFQs have been developed for calcium [58, 161], iron [162], and isoflavones [163].

Because the cognitive processes for answering food frequency-type questions can be complex, some attempts have been made to reduce respondent burden by asking questions that require only "yes–no" answers. Kristal *et al.* [164] developed a questionnaire to assess total fat, saturated fat, fiber, and percent energy from fat which contains 44 food items for which respondents are asked whether they eat the items at a specified frequency. A simple index based on the number of "yes" responses was found to correlate well with diet as measured by 4-day records and with FFQs assessing total diet [164]. This same "yes–no" approach to questioning for a food list has also been used as a modification of the 24-hour recall [165, 166].

Often, interventions are designed to target specific food preparation or consumption behaviors rather than frequency of consuming specific foods. Examples of such behaviors might be trimming the fat from red meats, removing the skin from chicken, or choosing low-fat dairy products. Many questionnaires have been developed in different populations to measure these types of dietary behaviors, and several have been compared with more complete dietary assessments. A 9-question instrument designed to measure high-fat food consumption behaviors of Mexican Americans was shown to correspond with fat estimates from 24-hour recalls [167].

In England brief questions on high-fat behaviors correlated with fat-intake estimates from a FFQ [168] and with blood-cholesterol change [169]. The British instrument has been adapted to reflect North American eating habits; the Northwest Lipid Research Clinic Fat Intake Scale has been evaluated [170] and is available at http://depts.washington.edu/ ~nwlrc/fis.html. In rural North Carolina, an 8-item questionnaire was correlated with fat intake from 3-day food records [171]. A 33-item fat and fiber-related behavior questionnaire correlated with food frequency measures [172] among participants from a health maintenance organization in Seattle, Washington. Among white middle-class volunteers in Oregon, changes in individual responses over time to a 32-item eating behavior questionnaire were correlated with changes in lipid profiles [173].

The brevity of these methods and their correspondence with dietary intake as estimated by more extensive methods create a seductive option for investigators who would like to measure dietary intake at a low cost. Although brief methods have many applications, they have several limitations. Most measures are not quantitatively meaningful and, therefore, estimates of dietary intake for the population cannot be made. Even when measures aim at providing estimates of total intake, the estimates are not precise and have large measurement error. Generally, brief methods are only designed to capture information about a single nutrient, so the entire diet cannot be assessed. Finally, the specific dietary behaviors found to correlate with dietary intake in a particular study may not correlate similarly in another population, or even in the same population in another time period. For example, behavioral questionnaires developed and tested in middle-class, middle-aged U.S. women [174] were found to perform very differently when applied to Canadian male manual laborers [175] and to a low-income, low-education adult Canadian population [176]. Investigators should carefully consider the needs of their study and their own population's dietary patterns before choosing an "off-the-shelf" instrument designed to briefly measure either food frequency or specific dietary behaviors.

E. Diet History

The term *diet history* is used in many ways. In the most general sense, a dietary history is any dietary assessment that asks the respondent to report about past diet. Originally, as coined by Burke, the term *dietary history* referred to the collection of information not only about the frequency of intake of various foods but also about the typical makeup of meals [177, 178]. Many now imprecisely use the term *dietary history* to refer to the food frequency method of dietary assessment. However, several investigators have developed diet history methods that provide information about usual food intake patterns beyond simply food frequency data [179–182]. Some of these methods characterize foods in much more detail than is allowed in food frequency lists

(e.g., preparation methods and foods eaten in combination), and some of these methods ask about foods consumed at every meal [181, 183]. The term *diet history* is therefore probably best reserved for dietary assessment methods that are designed to ascertain a person's usual food intake in which many details about characteristics of foods as usually consumed are assessed in addition to the frequency and amount of food intake.

The Burke diet history included three elements: a detailed interview about usual patterns of eating, a food list asking for amount and frequency usually eaten, and a 3-day diet record [177, 178]. The detailed interview (which sometimes includes a 24-hour recall) is the central feature of the Burke dietary history, with the food frequency checklist and the 3-day diet record used as cross-checks of the history. The original Burke diet history has not often been exactly reproduced, because of the effort and expertise involved in capturing and coding the information if it is collected by an interviewer. However, many variations of the Burke method have been developed and used in a variety of settings [179–182, 184–186]. These variations attempt to ascertain the usual eating patterns for an extended period of time, including type, frequency, and amount of foods consumed; many include a cross-check feature [187, 188]. One such diet history has been automated, is self-administered, and eliminates the need for an interviewer to ask the questions. The software incorporates sound, orally delivered questions and dialogue, and pictures of foods to improve communication and motivation [181]. Other diet histories have been automated but still continue to be administered by an interviewer [189]. Short-term recalls or records are often used for validation or calibration rather than as a part of the tool.

The major strength of the diet history method is its assessment of meal patterns and details of food intake rather than intakes for a short period of time (as in records or recalls) or only frequency of food consumption. Details of the means of preparation of foods can be helpful in better characterizing nutrient intake (e.g., frying vs. baking), as well as exposure to other factors in foods (e.g., charcoal broiling). When the information is collected separately for each meal, analyses of the joint effects of foods eaten together is possible (e.g., effects on iron absorption of concurrent intake of tea or foods containing vitamin C). Although a meal-based approach often requires more time from the respondent than a food-based approach, it may provide more cognitive support for the recall process. For example, the respondent may be better able to report total bread consumption by reporting bread as consumed at each meal.

A weakness of the approach is that respondents are asked to make many judgments both about the usual foods and the amounts of those foods eaten. These subjective tasks may be difficult for many respondents. Burke cautioned that nutrient intakes estimated from these data should be interpreted as relative rather than absolute. All of these limitations are also shared with the food frequency method. The meal-based approach is not useful for individuals who have no particular eating pattern and may be of limited use for individuals who "graze," i.e., eat small bits throughout the day, rather than eat at defined meals. The approach, when conducted by interviewers, requires trained nutrition professionals.

The validity of diet history approaches is difficult to assess because we lack independent knowledge of the individual's usual long-term intake. Nutrient estimates from diet histories have often been found to be higher than nutrient estimates from tools that measure intakes over short periods, such as recalls or records [108, 190–194]. However, results for these types of comparisons depend on both the approach used and study characteristics. Validation studies that estimate correlations between reference data from recalls, records, or observations and diet histories are limited and show correlations in ranges similar to those for FFQs [182, 193, 195]. There are few validations of diet history questionnaires using biological markers as a basis of comparison. One study showed that, on average, 12 adults completing a diet history underreported by 12% in comparison to energy expenditure (measured by doubly labeled water) [196]; another showed that, in comparison to protein intake as measured by urinary nitrogen, 64 respondents completing a diet history questionnaire underreported by 3% [197].

Table 1 summarizes the various advantages and disadvantages of the dietary assessment instruments.

III. DIETARY ASSESSMENT IN SPECIFIC SITUATIONS

The primary research question must be clearly formed and questions of secondary interest should be recognized as such. Projects can fail to achieve their primary goal because too much attention is paid to secondary goals. The choice of the most appropriate dietary assessment tool depends on many factors. Questions that must be answered in evaluating which dietary assessment tool is most appropriate for a particular research purpose include [98]: (1) Is information needed about foods, nutrients, other food constituents or about specific dietary behaviors? (2) Is the average intake of a group or the intake of each individual needed? (3) Is absolute or relative intake needed? (4) What level of accuracy is needed? (5) What time period is of interest? (6) What are the research constraints in terms of money, time, staff, and respondent characteristics?

A. Cross-Sectional Surveys

One of the most common types of studies is the simple cross-sectional survey, a "snapshot" of the dietary practices of a population at a particular point in time. The population can be variously defined as the entire country (as in the National Health and Nutrition Examination Survey (NHANES) and Continuing Survey of Food Intakes by Individuals (CSFII)], the residents of a state (as in the BRFSS), or individuals who

TABLE 1   Advantages and Disadvantages of Dietary Assessment Instruments

Instrument	Advantages	Disadvantages
Food record	Intake quantified Could enhance self-monitoring for weight control	High investigator cost High respondent burden Extensive respondent training and motivation required Many days needed to capture individual's usual intake Affects eating behavior Intake often underreported Reports of intake decrease with time Number of days reported on decreases with time May lead to substantial sample bias
24-Hour dietary recall	Intake quantified Appropriate for most populations: low sample bias Relatively low respondent burden Does not affect eating behavior	High investigator cost Many days needed to capture individual's usual intake Intake often underreported
Food frequency questionnaire	Usual individual intake asked Information on total diet obtained Low investigator cost Does not affect eating behavior	Not quantifiably precise Difficult cognitive task for respondent Intake often misreported
Brief instruments	Usual individual intake often asked Low investigator cost Low respondent burden Does not affect eating behavior	Not quantifiably precise Assessment limited to small number of nutrients/foods Intake often misreported
Diet history	Usual individual intake asked Information on total diet obtained Information often available on foods consumed by meal Can have low investigator cost Does not affect eating behavior	Not quantifiably precise Difficult cognitive task for respondent Intake often misreported Can have high investigator burden

attend a particular facility such as a health clinic. In most dietary surveys, 24-hour recalls are used, allowing for quantitative accuracy in estimating average daily food and nutrient intake in the population studied. At least two independent days of recalls or records have to be collected from each respondent (or at least a sample of respondents) if the intent is to describe the true distribution of usual food and nutrient intake of the population. Otherwise, the prevalence of high or low intakes in the population will be overestimated. New statistical models and supporting software have been developed and are required to estimate the true distribution of nutrient intake with as few as 2 days of recall or record data [44, 45]. Food frequency instruments that are designed to measure usual individual diet also have been used in surveys, but they are limited by their lack of quantitative accuracy. Brief methods designed to measure specific diet behaviors may also be useful in some dietary surveys.

B. Case-Control (Retrospective) Studies

A case-control study design classifies individuals with regard to disease status currently (as cases or controls) and relates this to past (retrospective) exposures. For dietary ex-

posure, the period of interest could be either the recent past (e.g., the year before diagnosis) or the distant past (e.g., 10 years ago or in childhood). Because of the need for information about diet before onset of disease, dietary assessment methods that focus on current behavior, such as the 24-hour recall, are not useful in retrospective studies. The food frequency and diet history methods are well suited for assessing past diet and are therefore the only good choices for case-control (retrospective) studies.

In any food frequency or diet history interview, the respondent is not asked to call up specific memories of each eating occasion, but to respond on the basis of general perceptions of how frequently he/she ate a food. In assessing past diet, an additional requirement is to orient the respondent to the appropriate period. In case-control studies, the relevant period is often the year before diagnosis of disease or onset of symptoms, or even a time many years in the past. Cognitive factors may greatly affect the performance of this method.

Long-term reproducibility of various FFQs has been assessed in various populations by asking participants from past dietary studies to recall their diet from that earlier time [198]. Correspondence of retrospective diet reports with the

diet as measured in the original study has usually been greater than correspondence with diet reported by subjects for the current (later) period. This observation implies that if diet from years in the past is of interest, then it is probably better to ask respondents to recall it than to simply consider current diet as a proxy for past diet. The current diets of respondents may affect their retrospective reports about past diets. In particular, retrospective diet reports from seriously ill individuals may be biased by recent dietary changes [198, 199]. Studies of groups in whom diet was previously measured indicate no consistent differences in the accuracy of retrospective reporting between those who recently became ill and others [200, 201].

C. Cohort (Prospective) Studies

In a cohort study design, exposures of interest are assessed at baseline in a group (cohort) of people, and disease outcomes occurring over time (prospectively) are then related to the baseline exposure levels. In prospective dietary studies, dietary status at baseline is measured and related to later incidence of disease. In studies of many chronic diseases, large numbers of individuals need to be followed for years before enough new cases with that disease accrue for statistical analyses. A broad assessment of diet is usually desirable in prospective studies, since many dietary exposures and many disease endpoints will ultimately be investigated.

To relate diet at baseline to the eventual occurrence of disease, a measure of the usual intake of foods by study subjects is needed. Although a single 24-hour recall or a food record for a single day would not adequately characterize the usual diet of study subjects in a cohort study, such information could be later analyzed at the group level for contrasting the average dietary intakes of subsequent cases with those who did not acquire the disease. Multiple dietary recalls, records, diet histories, and food frequency methods have all been used effectively in prospective studies. Cost and logistic issues tend to favor food frequency methods, as many prospective studies require thousands of respondents.

Even in large studies using FFQs, it is desirable to include multiple recalls or records in subsamples of the population (preferably before beginning the study) to construct or modify the food frequency instrument and to calibrate it (see Section V.H). Information on the foods consumed could be used to ensure that the questionnaire includes the major food sources of key nutrients, with reasonable portion sizes. Because the diets of individuals change over time, it is desirable to measure diet throughout the follow-up period rather than just at baseline. One study showed that data from annual administrations of FFQs showed only small dietary changes over time and that repeat administrations more than 5 years apart would be acceptable to assess dietary change over time [202]. If diet is measured repeatedly over the years, repeated calibration is also desirable. Information from calibration studies can be used for three purposes: to give design information, e.g., the sample size needed [203]; to show how values from the food frequency tool (or a brief food list thus derived) relate to values from the recalls/records [96, 100]; and to determine the degree of attenuation/measurement error in the estimates of association observed in the study (e.g., between diet and disease) [122, 123, 125, 127, 129, 204–206] (see Section V.H).

D. Intervention Studies

Measurement of the dietary changes resulting from an intervention requires a valid measure of diet before, during, and after the intervention period. Very little work has been done on the development of valid methods to measure dietary change in individuals or in populations [207–210]. Measurement of specific dietary behaviors in addition to (or even in place of) dietary intake should be considered in intervention evaluations when the nature of the intervention involves education about specific behaviors. If, for instance, a community-wide campaign to choose low-fat dairy products were to be evaluated, food selection and shopping behaviors specific to choosing those items should be measured. Intentional behavior change is a complex and sequential phenomenon, however, as has been shown for tobacco cessation [211]. A complex sequence of events may also lead to dietary change [212]. The effects of educational interventions might also be assessed by measuring knowledge, attitudes, beliefs, barriers, and perceptions of readiness for dietary change, although the reliability of these types of questions has not been well assessed.

Whether an intervention is targeting individuals or the entire population, repeated measures of diet among study subjects can reflect reporting bias in the direction of the change being promoted. Even though not intending to be deceptive, respondents tend to want to tell the investigators what they think they want to hear. Though there has been little methodological research in measuring dietary change, behavioral questions and the food frequency method, because of their greater subjectivity, may be more susceptible to reporting biases than the 24-hour recall method [30, 143]. Because all subjective reports are subject to bias in the context of an intervention study, an independent assessment of dietary change should be considered. One such method useful in community-wide interventions is monitoring food sales. Often, cooperation can be obtained from food retailers [213]. Because of the large number of food items, only a small number should be monitored, and the large effects on sales of day-to-day pricing fluctuations should be carefully considered. Another method to consider is measuring changes in biomarkers of diet in the population.

E. Dietary Screening in Clinical Settings

Accurate measurement of intake is not always required in clinical settings. For some goals, a crude indication of dietary

habits to screen for probable dietary risk is adequate. The brief "fat screener" of Block *et al.* [146] was originally developed as a screening tool to crudely classify women for entry into a low-fat intervention trial. Another screening questionnaire was developed as a crude instrument intended only to identify a group of respondents who might be in need of nutritional and/or medical counseling [214, 215].

In clinical settings, the caregiver is generally interested in assessing an individual's usual dietary practices but has only limited time. Accurate information may be needed, such as for counseling on medically prescribed diets. Qualitative information about usual dietary practices and behaviors is, however, usually sufficient. Dietary recalls, diet histories, and food frequency methods are useful as methods to crudely classify ("screen") individuals in clinical settings. While 24-hour dietary recalls can provide useful quantitative information, there is a danger in interpreting yesterday's recalled diet as the individual's usual intake. Food frequency approaches may provide adequate information to qualitatively assess usual dietary practices. Brief questionnaires can serve to identify individuals who may be at dietary risk from, for example, frequent consumption of high-fat foods [146]. Short forms that measure specific dietary behaviors (e.g., choosing low-fat salad dressings or dairy products) may provide useful information about specific intervention points for counseling [164, 174, 210].

F. Dietary Surveillance or Monitoring

Nutritional surveillance is increasingly acknowledged as important at the national and state levels as an activity for problem recognition, policy making, and evaluation. In addition to assessing food and nutrient intakes in the U. S. population, the components of nutritional surveillance can include the regular monitoring of mortality, morbidity, risk factors, knowledge of information sources, and knowledge levels of the populations of interest [216]. Although it is important that the data are rapidly analyzed and reported, an important factor is that the methods for collecting data, including the sampling procedures, must be similar through time [217] to assess trends. Food composition databases must remain comparable for this purpose but also reflect true changes in actual food composition over time. The status of efforts to monitor diet in the United States is summarized in reports on the National Nutrition Monitoring and Related Research Program [218–225] and elsewhere [207, 226, 227].

Two major surveillance surveys, the National Health and Nutrition Examination Surveys (NHANES) and the Continuing Survey of Food Intakes by Individuals (CSFII), conducted by the National Center for Health Statistics (NCHS) and the U. S. Department of Agriculture (USDA), respectively, have been conducted periodically to survey the health and nutritional status of representative samples of Americans [221, 228–246]. Information about these surveys is available at their web sites: http://www.cdc.gov/nchs/nhanes.htm and http://www.barc.usda.gov/bhnrc/foodsurvey/home.htm.

National surveys of knowledge and attitudes about nutrition and health have been conducted periodically. Examples of such surveys are the Food and Drug Administration's Health and Diet Survey, and USDA's Diet and Health Knowledge Survey, which has been administered in conjunction with the CSFII [35]. Other nutrition monitoring activities sponsored by federal and state agencies are listed in *The Directory of Federal and State Nutrition Monitoring Activities* [221].

The type of information required for a surveillance or monitoring system can vary. For some purposes, quantitative estimates of intake are needed, whereas for other purposes, only qualitative estimates of intake, like food frequency or behavioral indicators, are needed. There is a particular need to monitor dietary trends at the local level. To help provide local data, the Centers for Disease Control and Prevention (CDC) has developed brief FFQs for administration on the telephone to assess the intake of dietary fat (13 questions) and fruits and vegetables (6 questions) within their Behavioral Risk Factor Surveillance System. Information about the survey is available at the CDC web site: http://www.cdc.gov/nccdphp/brfss/index.htm.

Table 2 summarizes the dietary methods commonly used in different study designs.

IV. DIETARY ASSESSMENT IN SPECIAL POPULATIONS

A. Surrogate Reporters

In many situations, respondents are unavailable or unable to report about their diets. For example, in case-control studies, surrogate reports may be obtained for cases who have died or who are too ill to interview. Although the accuracy of surrogate reports has not been examined, comparability of reports by surrogates and subjects has been studied, in hopes that surrogate information might be used interchangeably with information provided by subjects [247]. Common sense indicates that the individuals who know the most about a subject's lifestyle would make the best surrogate reporters.

TABLE 2 Dietary Assessment in Different Study Situations

Study situation	Methods commonly used
Cross-sectional	24-Hour recall; FFQ; brief methods
Case-control (retrospective)	FFQ; diet history
Cohort (prospective)	FFQ; diet history; 24-hour recall; record
Intervention	FFQ: brief methods; 24-hour recall
Clinical screening	24-Hour recall; brief methods; diet history
Surveillance	24-Hour recall; brief methods

Adult siblings provide the best information about a subject's early life, and spouses or children provide the best information about a subject's adult life. When food frequency instruments are used, the level of agreement between subject and surrogate reports of diet varies with the food and possibly with other variables such as number of shared meals, interview situation, case status, and sex of the surrogate reporter. Mean frequencies of use computed for individual foods and food groups between surrogate reporters and subject reporters tend to be similar, but agreement is much lower when detailed categories of frequency are compared. Several studies have shown that agreement is better for alcoholic beverages, coffee, and tea than for other foods.

Although subjects reporting themselves in the extremes of the distribution are seldom reported by their surrogates in the opposite extreme, many subjects who report they are in an extreme are reported by their surrogates in the middle of the distribution [248]. This may limit the usefulness of surrogate information for analyses at the individual level that rely on proper ranking. Furthermore, there may be a substantial difference in the quality of surrogate reports between spouses of deceased subjects and spouses of surviving subjects [249]. For these reasons, use of surrogate respondents should be minimized for obtaining dietary information in analytical studies. When used, analyses excluding the surrogate reports should be done to examine the sensitivity of the reported associations to possible errors or biases in the surrogate reports.

B. Ethnic Populations

Special modifications are needed in the content of dietary assessment methods when the study population is composed of individuals whose cuisine or cooking practices are not mainstream [250]. If the method requires an interview, interviewers of the same ethnic or cultural background are preferable so that dietary information can be more effectively communicated. If dietary information is to be quantified into nutrient estimates, examination of the nutrient composition database is necessary to ascertain the number of ethnic foods already included and those to be added. It is also necessary to examine the recipes and assumptions underlying the nutrient composition of certain ethnic foods. Some very different foods may be called the same name, or similar foods may be called by different names [251]. For these reasons, it may be necessary to obtain detailed recipe information for all ethnic mixtures reported. For Latino populations, the U. S. Department of Agriculture Nutrient Database for Standard Reference is a good starting point because foods reported in the Hispanic HANES have now been incorporated. Databases developed for the Hawaiian cancer studies include many foods consumed by Hawaiian natives and by Japanese, Chinese, and Polynesian groups [250].

To examine the suitability of the initial database, baseline recalls or records with accompanying interviews should be collected from individuals in the ethnic groups. These interviews should focus on all the kinds of food eaten and the ways in which foods are prepared in that culture. Recipes and alternative names of the same food should be collected, and interviewers should be familiarized with the results of these interviews. Recipes and food names that are relatively uniform should be included in the nutrient composition database. Even with these modifications, it may be preferable to collect records and recalls in the field by detailed records (not the preselected lists most common in computer-assisted methods) when special ethnic foods are common. This would prevent the detail of food choice and preparation from being lost by *a priori* coding.

Use of food lists developed for the majority population for FFQs may be inappropriate for many individuals with ethnic eating patterns. Many members of ethnic groups consume both foods common in the mainstream culture and foods that are specific to their own ethnic group. Development of the food list can be accomplished either by modifying an existing food list based on expert judgment of the diet of the target population or, preferably, by examining the frequency of reported foods in the population from a set of dietary records or recalls. Food frequency questionnaires for Navajos, Chinese Americans, and individuals in Northern India have been developed using these approaches [252–254].

Besides the food list, however, other important issues must be considered when adapting existing FFQs for use in other populations. The relative intake of different foods within a food group line item may differ, thus requiring a change in the nutrient database associated with each line item. For example, Latino populations may consume more tropical fruit nectars and less apple and grape juice than the general U. S. population and therefore would require a different nutrient composition standard for juices. In addition, the portion sizes generally used may differ. For example, rice may be consumed in larger quantities in Latino and Asian populations; the amount attributed to a large portion for the general population may be substantially lower than the amount typically consumed by Latino and Asian populations. Adaptation of an existing FFQ considering all of these factors is illustrated by Tucker *et al.* [255] for an elderly Puerto Rican population.

Performance of FFQs varies across ethnic groups [256]. Questionnaires aimed at allowing comparison of intakes across multiple cultures have been developed; however, the limited number of studies done thus far indicate that there are validity differences among the various cultural groups [255, 257–259]. Understanding these validity differences is crucial to the appropriate interpretation of study results.

C. Children

The 24-hour dietary recall, food records, and food frequency instruments have all been used to assess children's intakes, which is considered to be even more challenging than assessing the diets of adults [260–265]. Children tend to have diets that are highly variable from day to day, and their food

habits can change rapidly. Younger children are less able to recall, estimate, and cooperate in usual dietary assessment procedures, so much information by necessity has to be obtained by surrogate reporters. Adolescents, while more able to report, may be less interested in giving accurate reports. Baranowski and Domel [266] have posited a cognitive model of how children report dietary information.

For preschool-aged children, information is obtained from surrogates, usually the primary caretaker(s), who may typically be a parent or an external caregiver. If information can be obtained only from one surrogate reporter, the reports are likely to be less complete. Even for periods when the caregiver and child are together, foods tend to be underestimated [267]. A consensus recall method, in which the child and parents report as a group to give responses on a 24-hour dietary recall, has been shown to give more accurate information than a recall from either parent alone [268]. For older children, a blended instrument, the record assisted 24-hour recall (in which the children record only the names of foods and beverages consumed throughout a 24-hour period, serving as a cue for the later 24-hour recall interview), has been developed and tested. While foods were generally reported accurately, accurate reporting of portion sizes was difficult, creating only modest accuracy in overall nutrient intake estimates [269].

Adaptation of food frequency instruments originally developed for adults requires consideration of the food list and portion sizes. Food frequency instruments have been especially developed and tested for use in child and adolescent populations [8, 270]. Generally, correlations between the criterion instrument and food frequency instruments have been lower in child and adolescent populations than in adult populations.

D. Elderly

Measuring diets among the elderly can, but does not necessarily, present special problems [271, 272]. Both recall and food frequency techniques are inappropriate if memory is impaired. Direct observation in institutional care facilities or shelf inventories for elders who live at home can be useful. Even when memory is not impaired, other factors can affect the assessment of diet among the elderly. Because of the frequency of chronic illness in this age group, special diets (e.g., low sodium, low fat, high fiber) are often recommended to these individuals. Such recommendations could not only affect actual dietary intake, but could also bias reporting, as individuals may report what they should eat rather than what they do eat. Alternatively, respondents on special diets may be more aware of their diets and may more accurately report them. When dentition is poor, the interviewer should probe for foods that are prepared or consumed in different ways. Elderly individuals are also more likely to be taking multiple types of nutritional supplements, which present special problems in dietary assessment [273] (see Section V.G).

Adaptations of standard methods have been suggested and evaluated, including use of memory strategies, prior notification of a dietary interview [274], combining methods [272], and developing new methods [275]. Research suggests that under many circumstances the validity of dietary information collected from the elderly is comparable to that collected from younger adults [105].

Table 3 summarizes optimal assessment strategies for special populations.

V. SELECTED ISSUES IN DIETARY ASSESSMENT METHODS

A. Estimation of Portion Size

Research has shown that individuals have difficulty estimating portion sizes of foods, both when examining displayed foods and when reporting about foods previously consumed [276–282]. In general, consumers are not skilled at estimating the weights of foods, and there is further confusion about the term *ounces,* which is interpreted as indicating either volume or weight. Furthermore, volume amounts of foods may have limited meaning, as respondents appear to be relatively insensitive to changes made in portion size amounts shown in reference categories asked on questionnaires [283]. Portion sizes of foods that are commonly bought and/or consumed in defined units (e.g., bread by the slice, pieces of fruit, beverages in cans or bottles) may be more easily reported than irregularly shaped foods (e.g., steak, lettuce).

Portion size aids are commonly used to help respondents estimate portion size. The National Health and Nutrition Ex-

TABLE 3 Optimal Strategies for Special Populations

Special population	Optimal strategies
Surrogate reporters	Use best informed surrogate. Analyze effect of potential bias on study results.
Ethnic populations	Use interviewers of same ethnic background. Use nutrient composition database reflective of foods consumed. For FFQs, use appropriate food list and nutrient composition database.
Children	For young children, use caretakers in conjunction with child. For older children and adolescents, blended instrument and other creative ways of engagement and motivation may work best.
Elderly	Assess any special considerations, for example, memory, special diets, dentition, use of supplements, and adapt methods accordingly.

amination Surveys use an extensive set of three-dimensional models; the CSFIIs have used common household measures, such as cups and teaspoons. In one study, which compared these two approaches among men, there was little difference in the frequency of over- and underreporting [284]. However, those using the household measures had greater overestimates than did those using the food models. Studies indicate that accuracy of reporting using either models or household measures can be improved with training in that method [285, 286], but the effects of training deteriorate with time [287].

Two-dimensional and three-dimensional pictures have been developed and used in 24-hour dietary recalls, diet records, and FFQs. One study, which examined the comparability of portion size reports for the same foods using food models and equivalent two-dimensional pictures of those same models, found that although some respondents reported differently, no apparent bias in the direction of reporting was evident [288]. Another study using only photographs showed that, in general, small portion sizes were overestimated and large portion sizes underestimated, and that older subjects overestimated portion size more often than younger subjects [278].

B. Mode of Administration

One way to reduce the costs of collecting dietary information is to administer the instrument by telephone or by mail. Both telephone and mail surveys are less invasive than face-to-face interviews. The use of telephone surveys to collect dietary information has been reviewed [289]. Telephone surveys have higher response rates than do mail surveys [290], and have been used in a variety of public health research settings [291]. However, there is increasing concern about response rates in telephone surveys given increasing telemarketing and current technology, which allows for screening of calls via caller identification and message machines. For example, in the Behavioral Risk Factor Surveillance Surveys, response rates declined by approximately 10% between 1994 and 1998 (http://www.cdc.gov/nccdphp/brfss/ti-quality.htm). Nevertheless, interviews by telephone can be substantially less expensive than face-to-face interviews, but cost comparisons vary with the research setting. The difficulty of reporting serving sizes by telephone can be eased by mailing picture booklets or other portion size estimation aids to the participants prior to the telephone interview.

There is current interest in evaluating the quality of data from telephone versus in-person 24-hour dietary recall interviews. Several studies have found substantial but imperfect agreement between dietary data collected by telephone and dietary data estimated by other methods, including face-to-face interviews [31, 36, 292–294], expected intakes [295], or observed intakes [296]. Recognition of the potential economic advantages of telephone interviewing led to its adoption in the CSFII survey conducted in 1985 and 1986, and

in the Third NHANES (NHANES III), with collection of one in-person and two telephone follow-up 24-hour recalls for respondents aged 50 years and older in phase I [297]. However, some segments of the population do not have telephones, and some persons will not answer their telephones under certain circumstances. Therefore, it is important to consider a dual sampling scheme or another scheme that accounts for this concern so potential respondents who do not have telephones are included [291].

C. Multiple Days of Diet Information

When recalls or records are being used to estimate usual intake of individuals for surveillance purposes or to examine relationships between diet and disease, more than 1 day of dietary information is needed. Eating patterns vary between weekdays and weekends and across seasons, so multiple observations for individuals should include days in all parts of the week and in all seasons of the year. Nonconsecutive days are preferable to capture more of the variability in an individual's diet, since eating behaviors on consecutive days are correlated [298]. The number of days of information needed depends on which dietary parameter is being estimated, the extent of variability in the population, the research objectives, and the variability of the nutrient or food to be measured [299, 300]. For most nutrients, as many as 7–14 independent days of diet information may be necessary to characterize the individual's usual intake [298].

If the intent is only to generate a population distribution of a nutrient's intake (i.e., to separate within-person variability from total observed variability in order to estimate between-person variability), then only two days of recalls are needed on a sample. As part of an effort to estimate the distribution of usual diet in a particular population (e.g., the proportion eating diets with fewer than 30% of energy from fat), the National Center for Health Statistics collected three independent 24-hour recalls on a sample of older respondents in phase 1 of NHANES III [228]. The U. S. Department of Agriculture (USDA) has been collecting multiple days of dietary intake data since 1977. Various statistical methods to estimate the distribution of usual intakes from two or more days of dietary information have been suggested. One of these methods, developed by a National Academy of Sciences subcommittee [43], has been further developed by researchers at Iowa State University [44, 45] using computer software now available.

While studies using records or recalls often use one or the other, a combined dietary recall and record approach, in which an initial interviewer-administered 24-hour recall is followed by self-administered 2- or 3-day records, was used by USDA in its 1977–78 and 1987–88 Nationwide Food Consumption Surveys and its Continuing Survey of Food Intakes by Individuals 1989–91 [221] and by others [301].

The costs of collecting and processing additional days of information include not only increased financial costs, but

also reduced response rates as individuals tire of participating. All costs should be carefully considered relative to the benefits of collecting such information for the hypothesis of interest.

D. Choice of Nutrient Database

It is necessary to use a nutrient composition database when dietary data are to be converted to nutrient intake data. Typically, such a database includes the description of the food, a food code, and the nutrient composition per 100 g of the food. The number of foods and nutrients included varies with the database.

Some values in nutrient databases are obtained from laboratory analysis; however, because of the high cost of laboratory analyses, many values are estimated based on conversion factors or other knowledge about the food [302]. In addition, accepted analytical methods are not yet available for some nutrients of interest [303], the analytical quality of the information varies with nutrient [223, 303], and the variances or ranges of nutrient composition of individual foods are in most cases unknown [304]. Rapid growth in the food processing sector and the global nature of the food supply add further challenges to estimating the mean and variability in the nutrient composition of foods.

One of the U.S. Department of Agriculture's (USDA) primary missions is to provide nutrient composition data for foods in the U.S. food supply, accounting for various types of preparation [305]. USDA produces and maintains the *Nutrient Database for Standard Reference*, which includes information on up to 82 nutrients for 6200 foods. Interest in nutrients and food components potentially associated with diseases has led to development of databases for limited numbers of foods. These include databases for isoflavones, carotenoids, selected *trans*-fatty acids, sugar, and vitamin K. Values for selenium and vitamin D have been incorporated into the current Release 13 of the *Nutrient Database for Standard Reference.* Information regarding all of USDA's nutrient databases is available at the USDA's Nutrient Data Laboratory home page: http://www.nal.usda.gov/fnic/foodcomp. The International Network of Food Data Systems (INFOODS) [306] maintains an international directory of nutrient composition data, which is available at http://www.fao.org/infoods.

Research on nutrients (or other dietary constituents) and foods to improve current estimates is ongoing, and there is constant interest in updating current values and providing new values for a variety of dietary constituents of interest. Methods for converting dietary intake information into number of servings recommended in the U.S. Food Guide Pyramid [307] have been developed using the Minnesota Nutrition Data System [308] and the U.S. Department of Agriculture pyramid servings database [309]. One limitation in all nutrient databases, particularly for fatty acids, is the variability in the nutrient content of foods within a food category [310, 311]. For example, one study found that among 17 brands of crackers, *trans*-fatty acid content varied from 1 to 13 g per 100 g of crackers [23]. Depending on the level of detail queried on the dietary assessment instrument, the respondent's knowledge of specific brand names, and the specificity of a particular nutrient database, estimating accurate fatty acid intake can therefore be problematic. For FFQs, this problem is compounded by the collapsing of foods into categories (such as crackers) that might have highly variable nutrient content.

Many other databases are available in the United States for use in analyzing records, recalls, or FFQs, but most are based fundamentally on the USDA database, often with added foods and specific brand names. Estimates of nutrient intake from dietary recalls and records are often affected by the nutrient composition database that is used to process the data [312–314]. Differences are due to the number of food items in the database, the recency of nutrient data, and the number of missing or imputed nutrient composition values. Therefore, before choosing a nutrient composition database, a prime factor to consider is the completeness and accuracy of the data for the nutrients of interest. For some purposes, it may be useful to choose a database in which each nutrient value for each food also contains a code for the quality of the data: e.g., analytical value, calculated value, imputed value, or missing. Investigators need to be aware that a value of zero is assigned to missing values in some databases. The nutrient database should also include weight/volume equivalency information for each food item. Many foods are reported in volumetric measures (e.g., 1 cup) and must be converted to weight in grams. The number of common mixtures (e.g., spaghetti with sauce) available in the database is another important factor. If the study requires precision of nutrient estimates, then procedures for calculating the nutrients in various mixtures must be developed and incorporated into nutrient composition calculations. Another key consideration is how the database is maintained and supported.

Research or guidance on how to best compile a nutrient database for a FFQ or diet history is limited [56, 75, 315]. However, it is clear that an approach that is primarily data driven, using national or other carefully collected dietary data connected to a trustworthy nutrient database, is critical.

E. Choice of Computer Software

Current computerized data processing requires creating a data file that includes a food code and an amount consumed for each food reported. Computer software then links the nutrient composition of each food on the separate nutrient composition database file, converts the amount reported to multiples of 100 g, multiplies by that factor, stores that information, and sums across all foods for each nutrient for each individual. Many computer packages have been developed that include both a nutrient composition database and software to convert individual responses to specific foods and, ultimately, to nutrients. Information on computer software

packages can be found at the USDA's Food and Nutrition Information Center of the National Agricultural Library, which maintains a Food and Nutrition Software and Multimedia Programs database of more than 200 nutritional software programs. The programs cover dietary analysis, nutrition education, and other subjects. While the center does not loan the programs, visitors can come to the center and preview the software. Information regarding the center and other resources on computer software can be found on their web site, http://www.nal.usda.gov/fnic/software/software.html.

Software should be chosen on the basis of the research needs, the level of detail necessary, the quality of the nutrient composition database, and the hardware and software requirements [316]. If precise nutrient information is required, it is important that the system be able to expand to incorporate information about newer foods in the marketplace and to integrate detailed information about food preparation (e.g., homemade stew) by processing recipe information. Sometimes the study purpose requires analysis of dietary data to derive intake estimates not only for nutrients, but also for food groups (e.g., fruits and vegetables), food components other than standard nutrients (e.g., nitrites), or food characteristics (e.g., fried foods). These additional requirements limit the choice of acceptable software.

The automated food coding system used for the USDA CSFII and upcoming NHANES is the SURVEY NET, developed by USDA's Agricultural Research Service and the University of Texas–Houston School of Public Health [35]. SURVEY NET is a network dietary coding system that provides on-line coding, recipe modification and development, data editing and management, and nutrient analysis of dietary data with multiple-user access to manage the survey activities. It is available to government agencies and the general public only through special arrangement with USDA. However, most of the elements of SURVEY NET are available in a commercial software program called the Food Intake Analysis System available from the University of Texas at http://www.sph.uth.tmc.edu:8052/hnc/software/soft. htm.

Many diet history and food frequency instruments have also been automated. Users of these software packages should be aware of the source of information in the nutrient database and the assumptions about the nutrient content of each food item listed in the questionnaire.

F. Cognitive Research Related to Dietary Assessment

Nearly all studies using dietary information about subjects rely on the subjects' own reports of their diets. Because memory of these events is based on cognitive processes, it is important to understand and take advantage of what is known about how respondents remember dietary information and how that information is retrieved and reported to the investigator. The implications of such cognitive processes for dietary assessment have been researched and discussed by several investigators [183, 198, 266, 283, 317–319].

There is an important distinction between episodic memory and generic memory. Episodic memory relies on particular memories about episodes of eating and drinking, while generic memory relies on general knowledge about the respondent's typical diet. A 24-hour recall relies primarily on episodic memory of all actual events in the very recent past, whereas a FFQ in which the respondent is asked to report the usual frequency of eating a food during the previous year relies primarily on generic memory. As the time between the behavior and the report increases, respondents may rely more on generic memory and less on episodic memory [318].

What can the investigator do to enhance retrieval and improve reporting of diet? Research indicates that the amount of dietary information retrieved from memory can be enhanced by the context in which the instrument is administered and by use of specific memory cues and probes. For example, on a 24-hour dietary recall, foods that were not initially reported by the respondent can be recovered by interviewer probes. The effectiveness of these probes is well established and has been part of the interviewing protocols in two major national dietary surveys, the NHANES and the CSFII [34, 35]. Probes can be useful in improving generic memory, too, when subjects are asked to report their usual diets from periods in the past. Such probes can feature questions about past living situations and related eating habits.

Social scientists have long known that the way in which questions are asked affects responses. Certain characteristics of the interviewing situation may affect reporting according to social desirability for foods seen as "good" or "bad." For example, the presence of other family members during the dietary interview probably enhances biases related to social desirability, especially for certain foods like alcoholic beverages. An interview in a health setting such as a clinic may also enhance biases related to social desirability for foods tied to compliance with dietary recommendations previously made for health reasons. In all instances, interviewers should be trained to refrain from either positive or negative feedback about good or bad dietary habits and should repeatedly encourage subjects to accurately report all foods.

G. Assessment of Nutritional Supplements

It is often important or useful in dietary assessments to assess the intake of nutritional supplements, such as vitamin and mineral pills. Intake of herbal, botanical, or other biologic supplements may also be of interest [320]. Recent data from the NHANES III 1988–94 show that about 40% of the population reported taking a vitamin or mineral supplement in the past month [321]. There has yet to be a nationally representative survey specifically designed to estimate the use of nonvitamin, nonmineral supplements in the United States, but estimates range from 8 to 20%

[321–323]. In addition, there are now a wide variety of botanical products also containing vitamins and/or minerals; the array of these products and their use are changing rapidly. Their composition and bioavailability have not been documented, nor do we know how these products alter nutrient metabolism.

Supplement intake can be assessed for the past 24 hours, or for several days, by including supplement use in 24-hour dietary recalls or food records. Alternatively, the research question may require assessment of usual supplement use over a longer period of time. This requires food frequency-type supplement questions, which provide less detail and are more prone to error [324].

Of primary interest is the type of supplement taken. Hundreds of different products are available, both over the counter and by prescription. While it is possible to ask respondents to report in an open-ended manner which supplements they take, this information is difficult to code. An alternative approach is to ask close-ended questions about specific types that are of interest. Additional parameters need to be assessed for each brand of supplement taken: the amount per pill, the frequency of use, and the duration of use. A particular complexity in assessing supplement use is that many individuals take supplements inconsistently, in patterns that are hard to characterize (e.g., frequently for a while until they feel better or the bottle runs out, then not at all for a while, then irregularly). Usage can be so variable that assessment at one point in time may not reflect either long- or short-term usage [325, 326]. In many studies subjects are asked to have available all medications they take, including supplements, in order to better account for the types and amounts taken.

H. Validation/Calibration Studies

It is important and desirable that any new dietary assessment method be validated or calibrated against other more established methods [126, 127, 129, 327]. The purpose of such studies is to better understand how the method works in the particular research setting and to use that information to better interpret results from the overall study. For example, if a new food frequency questionnaire or brief assessment questionnaire is to be used in the main study, results of that questionnaire should be compared to results from another dietary assessment method, for example, 24-hour dietary recalls or a more detailed food frequency questionnaire, conducted on the same individuals, and a biological marker such as doubly labeled water or urinary nitrogen, if possible. The National Cancer Institute maintains a register of validation/calibration studies and publications on the web at http://www-davc.ims.nci.nih.gov/ [328].

Validation studies yield information about how well the new method is measuring what it is intended to measure, and calibration studies use the same information to relate (calibrate) how one method of dietary assessment compares to a reference method. Validation/calibration studies are challenging because of the difficulty and expense in collecting independent dietary information. Some researchers have used observational techniques to establish true dietary intake [52, 264, 267, 329]. Others have used laboratory measures such as the 24-hour urine collection to measure protein, sodium, and potassium intakes and the doubly labeled water technique to measure energy expenditure [13–19, 48, 49, 86, 106, 117, 118, 330]. However, the high cost of this latter technique can make it impractical for most studies. The overall validity of energy intake estimates from the dietary assessment can be roughly checked by comparing weight data to reported energy intakes, in conjunction with use of equations to estimate basal metabolic rate [16, 21–23, 26, 29, 41, 51, 330–332].

Because they are relatively expensive to conduct, validation/calibration studies are done on small samples compared to the size of the main study. However, the sample should be sufficiently large to estimate the relationship between the study instrument and a reference method with reasonable precision. Increasing the numbers of individuals sampled and decreasing the number of repeat measures per individual (e.g., two nonconsecutive 24-hour recalls on 100 people rather than four recalls on 50 people) can often help to increase precision without extra cost [299]. To the extent possible, the sample should be chosen randomly, perhaps within strata, defined by either dietary or other variables.

The resulting statistics, which quantify the relationship between the new method and the reference method, can be used for a variety of purposes. Because, in most cases, both the reference method (usually records or recalls) and the new method are imperfect and subject to bias and error, measures such as correlation coefficients may underestimate the level of agreement with the actual usual intake. This phenomenon, referred to as *attenuation bias,* can be estimated and the measure of agreement can be "corrected" to more nearly reflect the correlation between the diet measure and true diet [203, 206]. This information also gives guidance about the sample size required, because the less precise the diet measure, the more individuals will be needed to attain the desired power [203]. The estimated regression relationship between the new method and the reference method can also be used to adjust the relationships between diet and outcome as assessed in the larger study [100]. For example, the mean amounts of foods or nutrients, and their distributions, as estimated by a brief method, can be adjusted according to the calibration study results [160]. In addition, methods to adjust estimates of relationships measured in studies (e.g., relative risk estimates for disease relative to low nutrient intake) have been described [122, 123, 206, 333, 334]. Many of these adjustments require the assumption that the reference method is unbiased [122, 204]. Much evidence, however, indicates that intakes from recalls and records are underreported, violating this assumption. The possible existence of correlated person-specific biases between the reference and

test instruments requires a rethinking of measurement error models in the future [125, 129, 335, 336].

I. Energy Adjustment

Many researchers have suggested that when relationships between nutrient intakes and diseases are analyzed, nutrient intake should be adjusted for total energy intake. The rationale for this recommendation involves considering biological mechanisms, statistical confounding, and imprecision of measurements of nutrient intake. Biological mechanisms of the etiological relationship may present a compelling reason for the use of energy adjustment. Unfortunately, however, our understanding of these basic biological processes for many disease processes is limited.

In the absence of clear biological reasons, the potential for confounding is the most commonly cited reason for energy adjustment. Confounding would occur if energy intake is related both to the nutrient of interest and the outcome variable. Relationships between energy intake and various outcome variables may be unknown. However, total energy intake is related to many other dietary patterns, e.g., macronutrient intakes, meat intake, total grams of food (which might reflect exposure to contamination), and the intake of fiber, fruits, and vegetables. Because energy is derived from many nutrients, the adjustment of energy can camouflage a true nutrient effect [126]. This potential for overadjustment may be particularly important for macronutrients such as dietary fat.

Several statistical methods for incorporating energy and other nutrients in the same model have been proposed [53, 123, 124, 337, 338]. These models have been reviewed and evaluated [119, 123, 124, 128, 339, 340]. Each approach is appropriate for addressing a different study question [340, 341]. Interpretation of each of the models requires assumptions about the relative importance of other variables. Clearly, more research is needed in our understanding of when energy adjustment procedures should be used and which procedures are optimal for particular questions of interest.

References

1. Thompson, F. E., and Byers, T. (1994). Dietary assessment resource manual. *J. Nutr.* **124,** 2245S–2318S.

2. Gersovitz, M., Madden, J. P., and Smiciklas-Wright, H. (1978). Validity of the 24-hr. dietary recall and seven-day record for group comparisons. *J. Am. Diet. Assoc.* **73,** 48–55.

3. Todd, K. S., Hudes, M., and Calloway, D. H. (1983). Food intake measurement: Problems and approaches. *Am. J. Clin. Nutr.* **37,** 139–146.

4. Kretsch, M. J., and Fong, A. K. (1993). Validity and reproducibility of a new computerized dietary assessment method: Effects of gender and educational level. *Nutr. Res.* **13,** 133–146.

5. Bingham, S. A., Gill, C., Welch, A., Day, K., Cassidy, A., Khaw, K. T., Sneyd, M. J., Key, T. J., Roe, L., and Day, N. E. (1994). Comparison of dietary assessment methods in nutritional epidemiology: Weighed records v. 24 h recalls, food-frequency questionnaires and estimated-diet records [see comments]. *Br. J. Nutr.* **72,** 619–643.

6. Lindquist, C. H., Cummings, T., and Goran, M. I. (2000). Use of tape-recorded food records in assessing children's dietary intake. *Obes. Res.* **8,** 2–11.

7. Johnson, N. E., Sempos, C. T., Elmer, P. J., Allington, J. K., and Matthews, M. E. (1982). Development of a dietary intake monitoring system for nursing homes. *J. Am. Diet. Assoc.* **80,** 549–557.

8. Hammond, J., Nelson, M., Chinn, S., and Rona, R. J. (1993). Validation of a food frequency questionnaire for assessing dietary intake in a study of coronary heart disease risk factors in children. *Eur. J. Clin. Nutr.* **47,** 242–250.

9. Johnson, N. E., Nitzke, S., and VandeBerg, D. L. (1974). A reporting system for nutrition adequacy. *Home. Econ. Res. J.* **2,** 210–221.

10. Rebro, S. M., Patterson, R. E., Kristal, A. R., and Cheney, C. L. (1998). The effect of keeping food records on eating patterns. *J. Am. Diet. Assoc.* **98,** 1163–1165.

11. Vuckovic, N., Ritenbaugh, C., Taren, D. L., and Tobar, M. (2000). A qualitative study of participants' experiences with dietary assessment. *J. Am. Diet. Assoc.* **100,** 1023–1028.

12. Goris, A. H., Westerterp-Plantenga, M. S., and Westerterp, K. R. (2000). Undereating and underrecording of habitual food intake in obese men: Selective underreporting of fat intake. *Am. J. Clin. Nutr.* **71,** 130–134.

13. Taren, D. L., Tobar, M., Hill, A., Howell, W., Shisslak, C., Bell, I., and Ritenbaugh, C. (1999). The association of energy intake bias with psychological scores of women. *Eur. J. Clin. Nutr.* **53,** 570–578.

14. Sawaya, A. L., Tucker, K., Tsay, R., Willett, W., Saltzman, E., Dallal, G. E., and Roberts, S. B. (1996). Evaluation of four methods for determining energy intake in young and older women: Comparison with doubly labeled water measurements of total energy expenditure [see comments]. *Am. J. Clin. Nutr.* **63,** 491–499.

15. Black, A. E., Prentice, A. M., Goldberg, G. R., Jebb, S. A., Bingham, S. A., Livingstone, M. B., and Coward, W. A. (1993). Measurements of total energy expenditure provide insights into the validity of dietary measurements of energy intake. *J. Am. Diet. Assoc.* **93,** 572–579.

16. Black, A. E., Bingham, S. A., Johansson, G., and Coward, W. A. (1997). Validation of dietary intakes of protein and energy against 24 hour urinary N and DLW energy expenditure in middle-aged women, retired men and post-obese subjects: Comparisons with validation against presumed energy requirements. *Eur. J. Clin. Nutr.* **51,** 405–413.

17. Martin, L. J., Su, W., Jones, P. J., Lockwood, G. A., Tritchler, D. L., and Boyd, N. F. (1996). Comparison of energy intakes determined by food records and doubly labeled water in women participating in a dietary-intervention trial. *Am. J. Clin. Nutr.* **63,** 483–490.

18. Rothenberg, E. (1994). Validation of the food frequency questionnaire with the 4-day record method and analysis of 24-h urinary nitrogen. *Eur. J. Clin. Nutr.* **48,** 725–735.

19. Bingham, S. A., Gill, C., Welch, A., Cassidy, A., Runswick, S. A., Oakes, S., Lubin, R., Thurnham, D. I., Key, T. J., Roe, L., Khaw, K. T., and Day, N. E. (1997). Validation of dietary

assessment methods in the UK arm of EPIC using weighed records, and 24-hour urinary nitrogen and potassium and serum vitamin C and carotenoids as biomarkers. *Int. J. Epidemiol.* **26** (Suppl 1), S137–S151.

20. Bathalon, G. P., Tucker, K. L., Hays, N. P., Vinken, A. G., Greenberg, A. S., McCrory, M. A., and Roberts, S. B. (2000). Psychological measures of eating behavior and the accuracy of 3 common dietary assessment methods in healthy postmenopausal women. *Am. J. Clin. Nutr.* **71,** 739–745.

21. Pryer, J. A., Vrijheid, M., Nichols, R., Kiggins, M., and Elliott, P. (1997). Who are the 'low energy reporters' in the dietary and nutritional survey of British adults? *Int. J. Epidemiol.* **26,** 146–154.

22. Lafay, L., Basdevant, A., Charles, M. A., Vray, M., Balkau, B., Borys, J. M., Eschwege, E., and Romon, M. (1997). Determinants and nature of dietary underreporting in a free-living population: The Fleurbaix Laventie Ville Sante (FLVS) Study. *Int. J. Obes. Relat. Metab. Disord.* **21,** 567–573.

23. Kortzinger, I., Bierwag, A., Mast, M., and Muller, M. J. (1997). Dietary underreporting: Validity of dietary measurements of energy intake using a 7-day dietary record and a diet history in non-obese subjects. *Ann. Nutr. Metab.* **41,** 37–44.

24. Lichtman, S. W., Pisarska, K., Berman, E. R., Pestone, M., Dowling, H., Offenbacher, E., Weisel, H., Heshka, S. , Matthews, D. E., and Heymsfield, S. B. (1992). Discrepancy between self-reported and actual caloric intake and exercise in obese subjects [see comments]. *N. Engl. J. Med.* **327,** 1893–1898.

25. Johnson, R. K., Goran, M. I., and Poehlman, E. T. (1994). Correlates of over- and underreporting of energy intake in healthy older men and women. *Am. J. Clin. Nutr.* **59,** 1286–1290.

26. Hirvonen, T., Mannisto, S., Roos, E., and Pietinen, P. (1997). Increasing prevalence of underreporting does not necessarily distort dietary surveys. *Eur. J. Clin. Nutr.* **51,** 297–301.

27. Ballard-Barbash, R., Graubard, I., Krebs-Smith, S. M., Schatzkin, A., and Thompson, F. E. (1996). Contribution of dieting to the inverse association between energy intake and body mass index. *Eur. J. Clin. Nutr.* **50,** 98–106.

28. Hebert, J. R., Clemow, L., Pbert, L., Ockene, I. S., and Ockene, J. K. (1995). Social desirability bias in dietary self-report may compromise the validity of dietary intake measures [see comments]. *Int. J. Epidemiol.* **24,** 389–398.

29. Stallone, D. D., Brunner, E. J., Bingham, S. A., and Marmot, M. G. (1997). Dietary assessment in Whitehall II: the influence of reporting bias on apparent socioeconomic variation in nutrient intakes. *Eur. J. Clin. Nutr.* **51,** 815–825.

30. Buzzard, I. M., Faucett, C. L., Jeffery, R. W., McBane, L., McGovern, P., Baxter, J. S., Shapiro, A. C., Blackburn, G. L., Chlebowski, R. T., Elashoff, R. M., and Wynder, E. L. (1996). Monitoring dietary change in a low-fat diet intervention study: Advantages of using 24-hour dietary recalls vs food records. *J. Am. Diet. Assoc.* **96,** 574–579.

31. Casey, P. H., Goolsby, S. L., Lensing, S. Y., Perloff, B. P., and Bogle, M. L. (1999). The use of telephone interview methodology to obtain 24-hour dietary recalls. *J. Am. Diet. Assoc.* **99,** 1406–1411.

32. Witschi, J., Porter, D., Vogel, S., Buxbaum, R., Stare, F. J., and Slack, W. (1976). A computer-based dietary counseling system. *J. Am. Diet. Assoc.* **69,** 385–390.

33. Campbell, V. A., and Dodds, M. L. (1967). Collecting dietary information from groups of older people. *J. Am. Diet. Assoc.* **51,** 29–33.

34. Guenther, P. M., DeMaio, T. J., Ingwersen, L. A., and Berlin, M. (1996). The multiple-pass approach for the 24-h recall in the Continuing Survey of Food Intakes by Individuals, 1994–96. *FASEB. J.* **10,** a198.

35. Tippett, K. S., and Cypel, Y. S. (1997). Design and operation: The Continuing Survey of Food Intakes by Individuals and the Diet and Health Knowledge Survey, 1994–96. U.S. Department of Agriculture and Agricultural Research Service, Hyattsville, MD.

36. Moshfegh, A. M., Borrud, L. G., Perloff, P., and LaComb, R. (1999). Improved method for the 24-hour dietary recall for use in National Surveys. *FASEB. J.* **13,** A603.

37. Jonnalagadda, S. S., Mitchell, D. C., Smiciklas-Wright, H., Meaker, K. B., Van Heel, N., Karmally, W., Ershow, A. G., and Kris-Etherton, P. M. (2000). Accuracy of energy intake data estimated by a multiple-pass, 24-hour dietary recall technique. *J. Am. Diet. Assoc.* **100,** 303–308.

38. Frank, G. C., Hollatz, A. T., Webber, L. S., and Berenson, G. S. (1984). Effect of interviewer recording practices on nutrient intake—Bogalusa Heart Study. *J. Am. Diet. Assoc.* **84,** 1432–1436.

39. Dennis, B., Ernst, N., Hjortland, M., Tillotson, J., and Grambsch, V. (1980). The NHLBI nutrition data system. *J. Am. Diet. Assoc.* **77,** 641–647.

40. Tillotson, J. L., Gorder, D. D., DuChene, A. G., Grambsch, P. V., and Wenz, J. (1986). Quality control in the Multiple Risk Factor Intervention Trial Nutrition Modality. *Control. Clin. Trials* **7,** 66S–90S.

41. Briefel, R. R., McDowell, M. A., Alaimo, K., Caughman, C. R., Bischof, A. L., Carroll, M. D., and Johnson, C. L. (1995). Total energy intake of the U.S. population: The third National Health and Nutrition Examination Survey, 1988–1991. *Am. J. Clin. Nutr.* **62,** 1072S–1080S.

42. McDowell, M. A., Briefel, R. R., Warren, R. A., Buzzard, I. M., Feskanich, D., and Gardner, S. N. (1990). The dietary data collection system—An automated interview and coding system for NHANES III. *In* "Proceedings of the Fourteenth National Nutrient Databank Conference" (P. J. Stumbo, ed.), pp. 125–131. The CBORD Group, Ithaca, NY.

43. National Research Council. (1986). "Nutrient Adequacy. Assessment Using Food Consumption Surveys." National Academy Press, Washington, DC.

44. Nusser, S. M., Carriquiry, A. L., Dodd, K. W., and Fuller, W. A. (1996). A semiparametric transformation approach to estimating usual daily intake distributions. *J. Am. Stat. Assoc.* **91,** 1440–1449.

45. Department of Statistics and Center for Agricultural and Rural Development Iowa State University. (1996). "A User's Guide to C-SIDE, Software for Intake Distribution Estimation, Version 0.90." Iowa State University, Ames, Iowa.

46. Madden, J. P., Goodman, S. J., and Guthrie, H. A. (1976). Validity of the 24-hr. recall. Analysis of data obtained from elderly subjects. *J. Am. Diet. Assoc.* **68,** 143–147.

47. Kroke, A., Klipstein-Grobusch, K., Voss, S., Moseneder, J., Thielecke, F., Noack, R., and Boeing, H. (1999). Validation of a self-administered food-frequency questionnaire administered in the European Prospective Investigation into Cancer

and Nutrition (EPIC) Study: Comparison of energy, protein, and macronutrient intakes estimated with the doubly labeled water, urinary nitrogen, and repeated 24-h dietary recall methods. *Am. J. Clin. Nutr.* **70,** 439–447.

48. Johnson, R. K., Soultanakis, R. P., and Matthews, D. E. (1998). Literacy and body fatness are associated with underreporting of energy intake in U.S. low-income women using the multiple-pass 24-hour recall: A doubly labeled water study. *J. Am. Diet. Assoc.* **98,** 1136–1140.

49. Heerstrass, D. W., Ocke, M. C., Bueno-de-Mesquita, H. B., Peeters, P. H., and Seidell, J. C. (1998). Underreporting of energy, protein and potassium intake in relation to body mass index. *Int. J. Epidemiol.* **27,** 186–193.

50. Krebs-Smith, S. M., Graubard, B. I., Kahle, L. L., Subar, A. F., Cleveland, L. E., and Ballard-Barbash, R. (2000). Low energy reporters vs others: A comparison of reported food intakes. *Eur. J. Clin. Nutr.* **54,** 281–287.

51. Klesges, R. C., Eck, L. H., and Ray, J. W. (1995). Who underreports dietary intake in a dietary recall? Evidence from the Second National Health and Nutrition Examination Survey. *J. Consult. Clin. Psychol.* **63,** 438–444.

52. Poppitt, S. D., Swann, D., Black, A. E., and Prentice, A. M. (1998). Assessment of selective underreporting of food intake by both obese and non-obese women in a metabolic facility. *Int. J. Obes. Relat. Metab. Disord.* **22,** 303–311.

53. Willett, W. C. (1998). "Nutritional Epidemiology." Oxford University Press, New York.

54. Zulkifli, S. N., and Yu, S. M. (1992). The food frequency method for dietary assessment. *J. Am. Diet. Assoc.* **92,** 681–685.

55. Willett, W. C. (1994). Future directions in the development of food-frequency questionnaires. *Am. J. Clin. Nutr.* **59,** 171s–174s.

56. Block, G., Hartman, A. M., Dresser, C. M., Carroll, M. D., Gannon, J., and Gardner, L. (1986). A data-based approach to diet questionnaire design and testing. *Am. J. Epidemiol.* **124,** 453–469.

57. Block, G., Woods, M., Potosky, A. L., and Clifford, C. (1990). Validation of a self-administered diet history questionnaire using multiple diet records. *J. Clin. Epidemiol.* **43,** 1327–1335.

58. Cummings, S. R., Block, G., McHenry, K., and Baron, R. B. (1987). Evaluation of two food frequency methods of measuring dietary calcium intake. *Am. J. Epidemiol.* **126,** 796–802.

59. Sobell, J., Block, G., Koslowe, P., Tobin, J., and Andres, R. (1989). Validation of a retrospective questionnaire assessing diet 10–15 years ago. *Am. J. Epidemiol.* **130,** 173–187.

60. Block, G., Thompson, F. E., Hartman, A. M., Larkin, F. A., and Guire, K. E. (1992). Comparison of two dietary questionnaires validated against multiple dietary records collected during a 1-year period. *J. Am. Diet. Assoc.* **92,** 686–693.

61. Mares-Perlman, J. A., Klein, B. E., Klein, R., Ritter, L. L., Fisher, M. R., and Freudenheim, J. L. (1993). A diet history questionnaire ranks nutrient intakes in middle-aged and older men and women similarly to multiple food records. *J. Nutr.* **123,** 489–501.

62. Coates, R. J., Eley, J. W., Block, G., Gunter, E. W., Sowell, A. L., Grossman, C., and Greenberg, R. S. (1991). An evaluation of a food frequency questionnaire for assessing dietary intake of specific carotenoids and vitamin E among low-income black women. *Am. J. Epidemiol.* **134,** 658–671.

63. Patterson, R. E., Kristal, A. R., Tinker, L. F., Carter, R. A., Bolton, M. P., and Agurs-Collins, T. (1999). Measurement characteristics of the Women's Health Initiative food frequency questionnaire. *Ann. Epidemiol.* **9,** 178–187.

64. Rimm, E. B., Giovannucci, E. L., Stampfer, M. J., Colditz, G. A., Litin, L. B., and Willett, W. C. (1992). Reproducibility and validity of an expanded self-administered semiquantitative food frequency questionnaire among male health professionals. *Am. J. Epidemiol.* **135,** 1114–1126.

65. Willett, W. C., Sampson, L., Stampfer, M. J., Rosner, B., Bain, C., Witschi, J., Hennekens, C. H., and Speizer, F. E. (1985). Reproducibility and validity of a semiquantitative food frequency questionnaire. *Am. J. Epidemiol.* **122,** 51–65.

66. Willett, W. C., Reynolds, R. D., Cottrell-Hoehner, S., Sampson, L., and Browne, M. L. (1987). Validation of a semiquantitative food frequency questionnaire: Comparison with a 1-year diet record. *J. Am. Diet. Assoc.* **87,** 43–47.

67. Salvini, S., Hunter, D. J., Sampson, L., Stampfer, M. J., Colditz, G. A., Rosner, B., and Willett, W. C. (1989). Food based validation of a dietary questionnaire: The effects of week-to-week variation in food consumption. *Int. J. Epidemiol.* **18,** 858–867.

68. Feskanich, D., Rimm, E. B., Giovannucci, E. L., Colditz, G. A., Stampfer, M. J., Litin, L. B., and Willett, W. C. (1993). Reproducibility and validity of food intake measurements from a semiquantitative food frequency questionnaire. *J. Am. Diet. Assoc.* **93,** 790–796.

69. Suitor, C. J., Gardner, J., and Willett, W. C. (1989). A comparison of food frequency and diet recall methods in studies of nutrient intake of low-income pregnant women. *J. Am. Diet. Assoc.* **89,** 1786–1794.

70. Wirfalt, A. K. E., Jeffery, R. W., and Elmer, P. J. (1998). Comparison of food frequency questionnaires: The reduced Block and Willett questionnaires differ in ranking on nutrient intakes. *Am. J. Epidemiol.* **148,** 1148–1156.

71. Caan, B. J., Slattery, M. L., Potter, J., Quesenberry, C. P. J., Coates, A. O., and Schaffer, D. M. (1998). Comparison of the Block and the Willett self-administered semiquantitative food frequency questionnaires with an interviewer-administered dietary history [see comments]. *Am. J. Epidemiol.* **148,** 1137–1147.

72. McCann, S. E., Marshall, J. R., Trevisan, M., Russell, M., Muti, P., Markovic, N., Chan, A. W., and Freudenheim, J. L. (1999). Recent alcohol intake as estimated by the Health Habits and History Questionnaire, the Harvard Semiquantitative Food Frequency Questionnaire, and a more detailed alcohol intake questionnaire. *Am. J. Epidemiol.* **150,** 334–340.

73. Subar, A. F., Thompson, F. E., Smith, A. F., Jobe, J. B., Ziegler, R. G., Potischman, N., Schatzkin, A., Hartman, A., Swanson, C., Kruse, L., Hayes, R. B., Riedel-Lewis, D., and Harlan, L. C. (1995). Improving food frequency questionnaires: A qualitative approach using cognitive interviewing. *J. Am. Diet. Assoc.* **95,** 781–788.

74. Subar, A. F., Ziegler, R. G., Thompson, F. E., Weissfeld, J. L., Reding, D., Kavounis, K. H., and Hayes, R. B. (2000). Is shorter always better?: Relative importance of dietary questionnaire length and cognitive ease on response rates and data quality. *Am. J. Epidemiol.* **153,** 404–409.

75. Subar, A. F., Midthune, D., Kulldorff, M., Brown, C. C., Thompson, F. E., Kipnis, V., and Schatzkin, A. (2000). An evaluation of alternative approaches to assign nutrient values to food groups in food frequency questionnaires. *Am. J. Epidemiol.* **152,** 279–286.

76. Ritenbaugh, C., Aickin, M., Taren, D., Teufel, N., Graver, E., Woolf, K., and Alberts, D. S. (1997). Use of a food frequency questionnaire to screen for dietary eligibility in a randomized cancer prevention phase III trial. *Cancer Epidemiol. Biomarkers Prev.* **6,** 347–354.

77. Garcia, R. A., Taren, D., and Teufel, N. I. (2000). Factors associated with the reproducibility of specific food items from the Southwest Food Frequency Questionnaire. *Ecol. Food Nutr.* **38,** 549–561.

78. Hankin, J. H., Yoshizawa, C. N., and Kolonel, L. N. (1990). Reproducibility of a diet history in older men in Hawaii. *Nutr. Cancer* **13,** 129–140.

79. Hankin, J. H., Wilkens, L. R., Kolonel, L. N., and Yoshizawa, C. N. (1991). Validation of a quantitative diet history method in Hawaii. *Am. J. Epidemiol.* **133,** 616–628.

80. Stram, D. O., Hankin, J. H., Wilkens, L. R., Pike, M. C., Monroe, K. R., Park, S., Henderson, B. E., Nomura, A. M., Earle, M. E., Nagamine, F. S., and Kolonel, L. N. (2000). Calibration of the dietary questionnaire for a multiethnic cohort in Hawaii and Los Angeles. *Am. J. Epidemiol.* **151,** 358–370.

81. Ocke, M. C., Bueno-de-Mesquita, H. B., Goddijn, H. E., Jansen, A., Pols, M. A., van Staveren, W. A., and Kromhout, D. (1997). The Dutch EPIC food frequency questionnaire. I. Description of the questionnaire, and relative validity and reproducibility for food groups. *Int. J. Epidemiol.* **26** (Suppl 1), S37–S48.

82. Katsouyanni, K., Rimm, E. B., Gnardellis, C., Trichopoulos, D., Polychronopoulos, E., and Trichopoulou, A. (1997). Reproducibility and relative validity of an extensive semi-quantitative food frequency questionnaire using dietary records and biochemical markers among Greek schoolteachers. *Int. J. Epidemiol.* **26** (Suppl 1), S118–S127.

83. Bohlscheid-Thomas, S., Hoting, I., Boeing, H., and Wahrendorf, J. (1997). Reproducibility and relative validity of food group intake in a food frequency questionnaire developed for the German part of the EPIC project. European Prospective Investigation into Cancer and Nutrition. *Int. J. Epidemiol.* **26** (Suppl 1), S59–S70.

84. Bohlscheid-Thomas, S., Hoting, I., Boeing, H., and Wahrendorf, J. (1997). Reproducibility and relative validity of energy and macronutrient intake of a food frequency questionnaire developed for the German part of the EPIC project. European Prospective Investigation into Cancer and Nutrition. *Int. J. Epidemiol.* **26** (Suppl 1), S71–S81.

85. Riboli, E., Elmstahl, S., Saracci, R., Gullberg, B., and Lindgarde, F. (1997). The Malmo Food Study: Validity of two dietary assessment methods for measuring nutrient intake. *Int. J. Epidemiol.* **26** (Suppl 1), S161–S173.

86. Pisani, P., Faggiano, F., Krogh, V., Palli, D., Vineis, P., and Berrino, F. (1997). Relative validity and reproducibility of a food frequency dietary questionnaire for use in the Italian EPIC centres. *Int. J. Epidemiol.* **26** (Suppl 1), S152–S160.

87. Block, G., Hartman, A. M., and Naughton, D. (1990). A reduced dietary questionnaire: Development and validation. *Epidemiology* **1,** 58–64.

88. Harlan, L. C., and Block, G. (1990). Use of adjustment factors with a brief food frequency questionnaire to obtain nutrient values. *Epidemiology* **1,** 224–231.

89. Feskanich, D., Marshall, J., Rimm, E. B., Litin, L. B., and Willett, W. C. (1994). Simulated validation of a brief food frequency questionnaire [see comments]. *Ann. Epidemiol.* **4,** 181–187.

90. Potischman, N., Carroll, R. J., Iturria, S. J., Mittl, B., Curtin, J., Thompson, F. E., and Brinton, L. A. (1999). Comparison of the 60- and 100-item NCI-block questionnaires with validation data. *Nutr. Cancer* **34,** 70–75.

91. Krebs-Smith, S. M., Heimendinger, J., Subar, A. F., Patterson, B. H., and Pivonka, E. (1994). Estimating fruit and vegetable intake using food frequency questionnaires: A comparison of instruments. *Am. J. Clin. Nutr.* **59,** 283s–283s.

92. Block, G., and Subar, A. F. (1992). Estimates of nutrient intake from a food frequency questionnaire: The 1987 National Health Interview Survey. *J. Am. Diet. Assoc.* **92,** 969–977.

93. Briefel, R. R., Flegal, K. M., Winn, D. M., Loria, C. M., Johnson, C. L., and Sempos, C. T. (1992). Assessing the nation's diet: Limitations of the food frequency questionnaire. *J. Am. Diet. Assoc.* **92,** 959–962.

94. Sempos, C. T. (1992). Invited commentary: Some limitations of semiquantitative food frequency questionnaires. *Am. J. Epidemiol.* **135,** 1127–1132.

95. Rimm, E. B., Giovannucci, E. L., Stampfer, M. J., Colditz, G. A., Litin, L. B., and Willett, W. C. (1992). Authors' response to "Invited commentary: Some limitations of semiquantitative food frequency questionnaires." *Am. J. Epidemiol.* **135,** 1133–1136.

96. Carroll, R. J., Freedman, L. S., and Hartman, A. M. (1996). Use of semiquantitative food frequency questionnaires to estimate the distribution of usual intake. *Am. J. Epidemiol.* **143,** 392–404.

97. Kushi, L. H. (1994). Gaps in epidemiologic research methods: Design considerations for studies that use food-frequency questionnaires. *Am. J. Clin. Nutr.* **59,** 180s–184s.

98. Beaton, G. H. (1994). Approaches to analysis of dietary data: Relationship between planned analyses and choice of methodology. *Am. J. Clin. Nutr.* **59,** 253s–261s.

99. Sempos, C. T., Liu, K., and Ernst, N. D. (1999). Food and nutrient exposures: What to consider when evaluating epidemiologic evidence. *Am. J. Clin. Nutr.* **69,** 1330S–1338S.

100. Freedman, L. S., Schatzkin, A., and Wax, Y. (1990). The impact of dietary measurement error on planning sample size required in a cohort study [see comments]. *Am. J. Epidemiol.* **132,** 1185–1195.

101. Walker, A. M., and Blettner, M. (1985). Comparing imperfect measures of exposure. *Am. J. Epidemiol.* **121,** 783–790.

102. Liu, K. (1994). Statistical issues related to semiquantitative food-frequency questionnaires. *Am. J. Clin. Nutr.* **59,** 262s–265s.

103. Schaefer, E. J., Augustin, J. L., Schaefer, M. M., Rasmussen, H., Ordovas, J. M., Dallal, G. E., and Dwyer, J. T. (2000). Lack of efficacy of a food-frequency questionnaire in assessing dietary macronutrient intakes in subjects consuming diets of known composition. *Am. J. Clin. Nutr.* **71,** 746–751.

104. Pietinen, P., Hartman, A. M., Haapa, E., Rasanen, L., Haapakoski, J., Palmgren, J., Albanes, D., Virtamo, J., and Huttunen, J. K. (1988). Reproducibility and validity of dietary assess-

ment instruments: I. A self-administered food use question-naire with a portion size picture booklet. *Am. J. Epidemiol.* **128,** 655–666.

105. Goldbohm, R. A., von den Brandt, P. A., Brants, H. A. M., von't Veer, P. A. M., Sturmans, F., and Hermus, R. J. J. (1994). Validation of a dietary questionnaire used in a large-scale prospective cohort study on diet and cancer. *Eur. J. Clin. Nutr.* **48,** 253–265.

106. Bingham, S. A. (1997). Dietary assessments in the European prospective study of diet and cancer (EPIC). *Eur. J. Cancer Prev.* **6,** 118–124.

107. Brown, J. E., Buzzard, I. M., Jacobs, D. R. J., Hannan, P. J., Kushi, L. H., Barosso, G. M., and Schmid, L. A. (1996). A food frequency questionnaire can detect pregnancy-related changes in diet. *J. Am. Diet. Assoc.* **96,** 262–266.

108. Jain, M., Howe, G. R., and Rohan, T. (1996). Dietary assess-ment in epidemiology: Comparison of a food frequency and a diet history questionnaire with a 7-day food record. *Am. J. Epidemiol.* **143,** 953–960.

109. Bonifacj, C., Gerber, M., Scali, J., and Daures, J. P. (1997). Comparison of dietary assessment methods in a southern French population: Use of weighed records, estimated-diet records and a food-frequency questionnaire. *Eur. J. Clin. Nutr.* **51,** 217–231.

110. Martin, L. J., Lockwood, G. A., Kristal, A. R., Kriukov, V., Greenberg, C., Shatuck, A. L., and Boyd, N. F. (1997). As-sessment of a food frequency questionnaire as a screening tool for low fat intakes. *Control. Clin. Trials* **18,** 241–250.

111. Decarli, A., Franceschi, S., Ferraroni, M., Gnagnarella, P., Parpinel, M. T., La Vecchia, C., Negri, E., Salvini, S., Falcini, F., and Giacosa, A. (1996). Validation of a food-frequency questionnaire to assess dietary intakes in cancer studies in Italy. Results for specific nutrients. *Ann. Epidemiol.* **6,** 110–118.

112. Hu, F. B., Rimm, E., Smith-Warner, S. A., Feskanich, D., Stampfer, M. J., Ascherio, A., Sampson, L., and Willett, W. C. (1999). Reproducibility and validity of dietary patterns assessed with a food-frequency questionnaire. *Am. J. Clin. Nutr.* **69,** 243–249.

113. Munger, R. G., Folsom, A. R., Kushi, L. H., Kaye, S. A., and Sellers, T. A. (1992). Dietary assessment of older Iowa women with a food frequency questionnaire: Nutrient intake, reproducibility, and comparison with 24-hour dietary recall interviews. *Am. J. Epidemiol.* **136,** 192–200.

114. Ocke, M. C., Bueno-de-Mesquita, H. B., Pols, M. A., Smit, H. A., van Staveren, W. A., and Kromhout, D. (1997). The Dutch EPIC food frequency questionnaire. II. Relative valid-ity and reproducibility for nutrients. *Int. J. Epidemiol.* **26** (Suppl 1), S49–S58.

115. Boeing, H., Bohlscheid-Thomas, S., Voss, S., Schneeweiss, S., and Wahrendorf, J. (1997). The relative validity of vitamin intakes derived from a food frequency questionnaire com-pared to 24-hour recalls and biological measurements: Re-sults from the EPIC pilot study in Germany. European Prospective Investigation into Cancer and Nutrition. *Int. J. Epidemiol.* **26** Suppl 1, S82–S90.

116. Mertz, W., Tsui, J. C., Judd, J. T., Reiser, S., Hallfrisch, J., Morris, E. R., Steele, P. D., and Lashley, E. (1991). What are people really eating? The relation between energy intake de-

rived from estimated diet records and intake determined to maintain body weight. *Am. J. Clin. Nutr.* **54,** 291–295.

117. Bingham, S. A., Cassidy, A., Cole, T. J., Welch, A., Runswick, S. A., Black, A. E., Thurnham, D., Bates, C., Khaw, K. T., and Key, T. J. (1995). Validation of weighed records and other meth-ods of dietary assessment using the 24 h urine nitrogen tech-nique and other biological markers. *Br. J. Nutr.* **73,** 531–550.

118. Pijls, L. T., De Vries, H., Donker, A. J., and van Eijk, J. T. (1999). Reproducibility and biomarker-based validity and re-sponsiveness of a food frequency questionnaire to estimate protein intake. *Am. J. Epidemiol.* **150,** 987–995.

119. Bingham, S. A., and Day, N. E. (1997). Using biochemical markers to assess the validity of prospective dietary assess-ment methods and the effect of energy adjustment. *Am. J. Clin. Nutr.* **65,** 1130S–1137S.

120. Flegal, K. M. (1999). Evaluating epidemiologic evidence of the effects of food and nutrient exposures. *Am. J. Clin. Nutr.* **69,** 1339S–1344S.

121. Burack, R., and Liang, J. (1987). The early detection of can-cer in the primary-care setting: Factors associated with the acceptance and completion of recommended procedures. *Prev. Med.* **16,** 739–751.

122. Prentice, R. L. (1996). Measurement error and results from analytic epidemiology: Dietary fat and breast cancer [see comments]. *J. Natl. Cancer Inst.* **88,** 1738–1747.

123. Kipnis, V., Freedman, L. S., Brown, C. C., Hartman, A. M., Schatzkin, A., and Wacholder, S. (1997). Effect of measure-ment error on energy-adjustment models in nutritional epide-miology. *Am. J. Epidemiol.* **146,** 842–855.

124. Hu, F. B., Stampfer, M. J., Rimm, E., Ascherio, A., Rosner, B. A., Spiegelman, D., and Willett, W. C. (1999). Dietary fat and coronary heart disease: A comparison of approaches for adjusting for total energy intake and modeling repeated dietary measurements. *Am. J. Epidemiol.* **149,** 531–540.

125. Carroll, R. J., Freedman, L. S., Kipnis, V., and Li, L. (1998). A new class of measurement-error models, with applications to dietary data. *Can. J. Stat.* **26,** 467–477.

126. Kohlmeier, L., and Bellach, B. (1995). Exposure assessment error and its handling in nutritional epidemiology. *Annu. Rev. Public Health* **16,** 43–59.

127. Kaaks, R., Riboli, E., and van Staveren, W. (1995). Calibra-tion of dietary intake measurements in prospective cohort studies. *Am. J. Epidemiol.* **142,** 548–556.

128. Bellach, B., and Kohlmeier, L. (1998). Energy adjustment does not control for differential recall bias in nutritional epi-demiology. *J. Clin. Epidemiol.* **51,** 393–398.

129. Kipnis, V., Carroll, R. J., Freedman, L. S., and Li, L. (1999). Implications of a new dietary measurement error model for estimation of relative risk: Application to four calibration studies. *Am. J. Epidemiol.* **150,** 642–651.

130. Kristal, A. R., Glanz, K., Feng, Z., Hebert, J. R., Probart, C., Eriksen, M., and Heimendinger, J. (1994). Does using a short dietary questionnaire instead of a food frequency improve response rates to a health assessment survey? *J. Nutr. Educ.* **26,** 224–226.

131. Eaker, S., Bergstrom, R., Bergstrom, A., Adami, H. O., and Nyren, O. (1998). Response rate to mailed epidemiologic ques-tionnaires: A population-based randomized trial of variations in design and mailing routines. *Am. J. Epidemiol.* **147,** 74–82.

132. Morris, M. C., Colditz, G. A., and Evans, D. A. (1998). Response to a mail nutritional survey in an older bi-racial community population. *Ann. Epidemiol.* **8,** 342–346.

133. Johansson, L., Solvoll, K., Opdahl, S., Bjorneboe, G. E., and Drevon, C. A. (1997). Response rates with different distribution methods and reward, and reproducibility of a quantitative food frequency questionnaire. *Eur. J. Clin. Nutr.* **51,** 346–353.

134. Kuskowska-Wolk, A., Holte, S., Ohlander, E. M., Bruce, A., Holmberg, L., Adami, H. O., and Bergstrom, R. (1992). Effects of different designs and extension of a food frequency questionnaire on response rate, completeness of data and food frequency responses. *Int. J. Epidemiol.* **21,** 1144–1150.

135. Vandenlangenberg, G. M., Mares-Perlman, J. A., Brady, W. E., Klein, B. E., Klein, R., Palta, M., and Block, G. (1997). Incorporating fat-modified foods into a food frequency questionnaire improves classification of fat intake. *J. Am. Diet. Assoc.* **97,** 860–866.

136. Patterson, R. E., Kristal, A. R., Coates, R. J., Tylavsky, F. A., Ritenbaugh, C., Van Horn, L., Caggiula, A. W., and Snetselaar, L. (1996). Low-fat diet practices of older women: Prevalence and implicationss for dietary assessment. *J. Am. Diet. Assoc.* **96,** 670–676.

137. Kumanyika, S., Tell, G. S., Fried, L., Martel, J. K., and Chinchilli, V. M. (1996). Picture-sort method for administering a food frequency questionnaire to older adults. *J. Am. Diet. Assoc.* **96,** 137–144.

138. Kumanyika, S. K., Tell, G. S., Shemanski, L., Martel, J., and Chinchilli, V. M. (1997). Dietary assessment using a picture-sort approach. *Am. J. Clin. Nutr.* **65,** 1123S–1129S.

139. Eck, L. H., Klesges, L. M., and Klesges, R. C. (1996). Precision and estimated accuracy of two short-term food frequency questionnaires compared with recalls and records. *J. Clin. Epidemiol.* **49,** 1195–1200.

140. Subar, A. F., Frey, C. M., Harlan, L. C., and Kahle, L. (1994). Differences in reported food frequency by season of questionnaire administration: The 1987 National Health Interview Survey. *Epidemiology* **5,** 226–233.

141. Tsubono, Y., Nishino, Y., Fukao, A., Hisamichi, S., and Tsugane, S. (1995). Temporal change in the reproducibility of a self-administered food frequency questionnaire. *Am. J. Epidemiol.* **142,** 1231–1235.

142. Tylavsky, F. A., and Sharp, G. B. (1995). Misclassification of nutrient and energy intake from use of closed-ended questions in epidemiologic research. *Am. J. Epidemiol.* **142,** 342–352.

143. Kristal, A. R., Andrilla, C. H., Koepsell, T. D., Diehr, P. H., and Cheadle, A. (1998). Dietary assessment instruments are susceptible to intervention-associated response set bias. *J. Am. Diet. Assoc.* **98,** 40–43.

144. Pickle, L. W., and Hartman, A. M. (1985). Indicator foods for vitamin A assessment. *Nutr. Cancer* **7,** 3–23.

145. Byers, T., Marshall, J., Fiedler, R., Zielezny, M., and Graham, S. (1985). Assessing nutrient intake with an abbreviated dietary interview. *Am. J. Epidemiol.* **122,** 41–50.

146. Block, G., Clifford, C., Naughton, M. D., Henderson, M., and McAdams, M. (1989). A brief dietary screen for high fat intake. *J. Nutr. Educ.* **21,** 199–207.

147. Coates, R. J., Serdula, M. K., Byers, T., Mokdad, A., Jewell, S., Leonard, S. B., Ritenbaugh, C., Newcomb, P., Mares-Perlman, J., and Chavez, N. (1995). A brief, telephone-administered food frequency questionnaire can be useful for surveillance of dietary fat intakes. *J. Nutr.* **125,** 1473–1483.

148. Caan, B., Coates, A., and Schaffer, D. (1995). Variations in sensitivity, specificity, and predictive value of a dietary fat screener modified from Block *et al. J. Am. Diet. Assoc.* **95,** 564–568.

149. Thompson, F. E., Kipnis, V., Subar, A. F., Schatzkin, A., Potischman, N., Kahle, L., and McNutt, S. (1998). Performance of short instrument to estimate usual dietary intake of percent calories from fat. *Eur. J. Clin. Nutr.* **52,** 168–168 (Abstract)

150. van Assema, P., Brug, J., Kok, G., and Brants, H. (1992). The reliability and validity of a Dutch questionnaire on fat consumption as a means to rank subjects according to individual fat intake. *Eur. J. Cancer. Prev.* **1,** 375–380.

151. Ammerman, A. S., Haines, P. S., DeVellis, R. F., Strogatz, D. S., Keyserling, T. C., Simpson, R. J., Jr., and Siscovick D. S. (1991). A brief dietary assessment to guide cholesterol reduction in low-income individuals: Design and validation. *J. Am. Diet. Assoc.* **91,** 1385–1390.

152. Hopkins, P. N., Williams, R. R., Kuida, H., Stults, B. M., Hunt, S. C., Barlow, G. K., and Ash, K. O. (1989). Predictive value of a short dietary questionnaire for changes in serum lipids in high-risk Utah families. *Am. J. Clin. Nutr.* **50,** 292–300.

153. Kemppainen, T., Rosendahl, A., Nuutinen, O., Ebeling, T., Pietinen, P., and Uusitupa, M. (1993). Validation of a short dietary questionnaire and a qualitative fat index for the assessment of fat intake. *Eur. J. Clin. Nutr.* **47,** 765–775.

154. Little, P., Barnett, J., Margetts, B., Kinmonth, A. L., Gabbay, J., Thompson, R., Warm, D., Warwick, H., and Wooton, S. (1999). The validity of dietary assessment in general practice. *J. Epidemiol. Commun. Health* **53,** 165–172.

155. Yaroch, A. L., Resnicow, K., and Khan, L. K. (2000). Validity and reliability of qualitative dietary fat index questionnaires: A review. *J. Am. Diet. Assoc.* **100,** 240–244.

156. Serdula, M., Coates, R., Byers, T., Mokdad, A., Jewell, S., Chavez, N., Mares-Perlman, J., Newcomb, P., Ritenbaugh, C., Treiber, F., and Block, G. (1993). Evaluation of a brief telephone questionnaire to estimate fruit and vegetable consumption in diverse study populations. *Epidemiology* **4,** 455–463.

157. Field, A. E., Colditz, G. A., Fox, M. K., Byers, T., Serdula, M., Bosch, R. J., and Peterson, K. E. (1998). Comparison of 4 questionnaires for assessment of fruit and vegetable intake. *Am. J. Public Health* **88,** 1216–1218.

158. Baranowski, T., Smith, M., Baranowski, J., Wang, D. T., Doyle, C., Lin, L. S., Hearn, M. D., and Resnicow, K. (1997). Low validity of a seven-item fruit and vegetable food frequency questionnaire among third-grade students. *J. Amer. Diet. Assoc.* **97,** 66–68.

159. Smith-Warner, S. A., Elmer, P. J., Fosdick, L., Tharp, T. M., and Randall, B. (1997). Reliability and comparability of three dietary assessment methods for estimating fruit and vegetable intakes. *Epidemiology* **8,** 196–201.

160. Thompson, F. E., Kipnis, V., Subar, A. F., Krebs-Smith, S. M., Kahle, L. L., Midthune, D., Potischman, N., and Schatzkin, A. (2000). Evaluation of two short instruments and food frequency questionnaire to estimate daily number of servings of fruit and vegetables. *Am. J. Clin. Nutr.* **71,** 1503–1510.

161. Hertzler, A. A., and Frary, R. B. (1994). A dietary calcium rapid assessment method (RAM). *Topics Clin. Nutr.* **9,** 76–85.

162. Hertzler, A. A., and McAnge, T. R., Jr. (1986). Development of an iron checklist to guide food intake. *J. Am. Diet. Assoc.* **86,** 782–786.

163. Kirk, P., Patterson, R. E., and Lampe, J. (1999). Development of a soy food frequency questionnaire to estimate isoflavone consumption in U.S. adults. *J. Am. Diet. Assoc.* **99,** 558–563.

164. Kristal, A. R., Shattuck, A. L., Henry, H. J., and Fowler, A. S. (1989). Rapid assessment of dietary intake of fat, fiber, and saturated fat: Validity of an instrument suitable for community intervention research and nutritional surveillance. *Am. J. Health Promotion* **4,** 288–295.

165. Guthrie, H. A., and Scheer, J. C. (1981). Validity of a dietary score for assessing nutrient adequacy. *J. Am. Diet. Assoc.* **78,** 240–245.

166. Kristal, A. R., Abrams, B. F., Thornquist, M. D., Disogra, L., Croyle, R. T., Shattuck, A. L., and Henry, H. J. (1990). Development and validation of a food use checklist for evaluation of community nutrition interventions. *Am. J. Public Health* **80,** 1318–1322.

167. Knapp, J. A., Hazuda, H. P., Haffner, S. M., Young, E. A., and Stern, M. P. (1988). A saturated fat/cholesterol avoidance scale: Sex and ethnic differences in a biethnic population. *J. Am. Diet. Assoc.* **88,** 172–177.

168. Kinlay, S., Heller, R. F., and Halliday, J. A. (1991). A simple score and questionnaire to measure group changes in dietary fat intake. *Prev. Med.* **20,** 378–388.

169. Heller, R. F., Pedoe, H. D., and Rose, G. (1981). A simple method of assessing the effect of dietary advice to reduce plasma cholesterol. *Prev. Med.* **10,** 364–370.

170. Retzlaff, B. M., Dowdy, A. A., Walden, C. E., Bovbjerg, V. E., and Knopp, R. H. (1997). The Northwest Lipid Research Clinic Fat Intake Scale: Validation and utility [see comments]. *Am. J. Public Health* **87,** 181–185.

171. Beresford, S. A., Farmer, E. M., Feingold, L., Graves, K. L., Sumner, S. K., and Baker, R. M. (1992). Evaluation of a self-help dietary intervention in a primary care setting. *Am. J. Public Health* **82,** 79–84.

172. Shannon, J., Kristal, A. R., Curry, S. J., and Beresford, S. A. (1997). Application of a behavioral approach to measuring dietary change: The fat- and fiber-related diet behavior questionnaire. *Cancer Epidemiol. Biomarkers Prev.* **6,** 355–361.

173. Connor, S. L., Gustafson, J. R., Sexton, G., Becker, N., Artaud-Wild, S., and Connor, W. E. (1992). The Diet Habit Survey: A new method of dietary assessment that relates to plasma cholesterol changes. *J. Am. Diet. Assoc.* **92,** 41–47.

174. Kristal, A. R., Shattuck, A. L., and Henry, H. J. (1990). Patterns of dietary behavior associated with selecting diets low in fat: Reliability and validity of a behavioral approach to dietary assessment. *J. Am. Diet. Assoc.* **90,** 214–220.

175. Birkett, N. J., and Boulet, J. (1995). Validation of a food habits questionnaire: Poor performance in male manual laborers. *J. Am. Diet. Assoc.* **95,** 558–563.

176. Gray-Donald, K., O'Loughlin, J., Richard, L., and Paradis, G. (1997). Validation of a short telephone administered questionnaire to evaluate dietary interventions in low income communities in Montreal, Canada. *J. Epidemiol. Commun. Health* **51,** 326–331.

177. Burke, B. S. (1947). The dietary history as a tool in research. *J. Am. Diet. Assoc.* **23,** 1041–1046.

178. Burke, B. S., and Stuart, H. C. (1938). A method of diet analysis: Applications in research and pediatric practice. *J. Pediatr.* **12,** 493–503.

179. McDonald, A., Van Horn, L., Slattery, M., Hilner, J., Bragg, C., Caan, B., Jacobs, D., Jr., Liu, K., Hubert, H., and Gernhofer, N. (1991). The CARDIA dietary history: Development, implementation, and evaluation. *J. Am. Diet. Assoc.* **91,** 1104–1112.

180. Visser, M., De Groot, L. C., Deurenberg, P., and van Staveren, W. A. (1995). Validation of dietary history method in a group of elderly women using measurements of total energy expenditure. *Br. J. Nutr.* **74,** 775–785.

181. Kohlmeier, L., Mendez, M., McDuffie, J., and Miller, M. (1997). Computer-assisted self-interviewing: A multimedia approach to dietary assessment. *Am. J. Clin. Nutr.* **65,** 1275S–1281S.

182. Landig, J., Erhardt, J. G., Bode, J. C., and Bode, C. (1998). Validation and comparison of two computerized methods of obtaining a diet history. *Clin. Nutr.* **17,** 113–117.

183. Kohlmeier, L. (1994). Gaps in dietary assessment methodology: Meal vs list-based methods. *Am. J. Clin. Nutr.* **59,** 175s–179s.

184. van Staveren, W. A., de Boer, J. O., and Burema, J. (1985). Validity and reproducibility of a dietary history method estimating the usual food intake during one month. *Am. J. Clin. Nutr.* **42,** 554–559.

185. Jain, M. (1989). Diet history: Questionnaire and interview techniques used in some retrospective studies of cancer. *J. Am. Diet. Assoc.* **89,** 1647–1652.

186. Kune, S., Kune, G. A., and Watson, L. F. (1987). Observations on the reliability and validity of the design and diet history method in the Melbourne Colorectal Cancer Study. *Nutr. Cancer* **9,** 5–20.

187. van Beresteyn, E. C., van 't Hof, M. A., van der Heiden-Winkeldermaat, H. J., ten Have-Witjes, A., and Neeter, R. (1987). Evaluation of the usefulness of the cross-check dietary history method in longitudinal studies. *J. Chronic Dis.* **40,** 1051–1058.

188. Bloemberg, B. P., Kromhout, D., Obermann-De Boer, G. L., and Van Kampen-Donker, M. (1989). The reproducibility of dietary intake data assessed with the cross-check dietary history method. *Am. J. Epidemiol.* **130,** 1047–1056.

189. Slattery, M. L., Caan, B. J., Duncan, D., Berry, T. D. , Coates, A., and Kerber, R. (1994). A computerized diet history questionnaire for epidemiologic studies. *J. Am. Diet. Assoc.* **94,** 761–766.

190. Jain, M., Howe, G. R., Johnson, K. C., and Miller, A. B. (1980). Evaluation of a diet history questionnaire for epidemiologic studies. *Am. J. Epidemiol.* **111,** 212–219.

191. Nes, M., van Staveren, W. A., Zajkas, G., Inelmen, E. M., and Moreiras-Varela, O. (1991). Validity of the dietary history method in elderly subjects. Euronut SENECA investigators. *Eur. J. Clin. Nutr.* **45**(Suppl 3), 97–104.

192. EPIC Group of Spain (1997). Relative validity and reproducibility of a diet history questionnaire in Spain. I. Foods. *Int. J. Epidemiol.* **26**(Suppl 1), S91–S99.

193. EPIC Group of Spain. (1997). Relative validity and reproducibility of a diet history questionnaire in Spain. II. Nutrients. *Int. J. Epidemiol.* **26**(Suppl 1), S100–S109.

194. van Liere, M. J., Lucas, F., Clavel, F., Slimani, N., and Ville-minot, S. (1997). Relative validity and reproducibility of a French dietary history questionnaire. *Int. J. Epidemiol.* **26**(Suppl 1), S128–S136.

195. Liu, K., Slattery, M., Jacobs, D. J., Cutter, G., McDonald, A., Van Horn, L., Hilner, J. E., Caan, B., Bragg, C., and Dyer, A. (1994). A study of the reliability and comparative validity of the Cardia Dietary History. *Ethn. Dis.* **4**, 15–27.

196. Rothenberg, E., Bosaeus, I., Lernfelt, B., Landahl, S., and Steen, B. (1998). Energy intake and expenditure: Validation of a diet history by heart rate monitoring, activity diary and doubly labeled water. *Eur. J. Clin. Nutr.* **52**, 832–838.

197. EPIC Group of Spain. (1997). Relative validity and reproducibility of a diet history questionnaire in Spain. III. Biochemical markers. *Int. J. Epidemiol.* **26**(Suppl 1), S110–S117.

198. Friedenreich, C. M., Slimani, N., and Riboli, E. (1992). Measurement of past diet: Review of previous and proposed methods. *Epidemiol. Rev.* **14**, 177–196.

199. Malila, N., Virtanen, M., Pietinen, P., Virtamo, J., Albanes, D., Hartman, A. M., and Heinonen, O. P. (1998). A comparison of prospective and retrospective assessments of diet in a study of colorectal cancer. *Nutr. Cancer* **32**, 146–153.

200. Friedenreich, C. M., Howe, G. R., and Miller, A. B. (1991). An investigation of recall bias in the reporting of past food intake among breast cancer cases and controls. *Ann. Epidemiol.* **1**, 439–453.

201. Friedenreich, C. M., Howe, G. R., and Miller, A. B. (1991). The effect of recall bias on the association of calorie-providing nutrients and breast cancer. *Epidemiology* **2**, 424–429.

202. Goldbohm, R. A., van't Veer, P., Van den Brandt, P. A., van 't, H., Brants, H. A., Sturmans, F., and Hermus, R. J. (1995). Reproducibility of a food frequency questionnaire and stability of dietary habits determined from five annually repeated measurements. *Eur. J. Clin. Nutr.* **49**, 420–429.

203. Freedman, L. S., Carroll, R. J., and Wax, Y. (1991). Estimating the relation between dietary intake obtained from a food frequency questionnaire and true average intake. *Am. J. Epidemiol.* **134**, 310–320.

204. Rosner, B., Willett, W. C., and Spiegelman, D. (1989). Correction of logistic regression relative risk estimates and confidence intervals for systematic within-person measurement error. *Stat. Med.* **8**, 1051–69.

205. Kaaks, R., Plummer, M., Riboli, E., Esteve, J., and van Staveren, W. (1994). Adjustment for bias due to errors in exposure assessments in multicenter cohort studies on diet and cancer: A calibration approach. *Am. J. Clin. Nutr.* **59**, 245s–250s.

206. Carroll, R. J., Freedman, L. S., and Kipnis, V. (1998). Measurement error and dietary intake. *Adv. Exp. Med. Biol.* **445**, 139–145.

207. Briefel, R. R. (1994). Assessment of the U.S. diet in national nutrition surveys: National collaborative efforts and NHANES. *Am. J. Clin. Nutr.* **59**, 164s–167s.

208. Georgiou, C. C. (1993). Saturated fat intake of elderly women reflects perceived changes in their intake of foods high in saturated fat and complex carbohydrate. *J. Am. Diet. Assoc.* **93**, 1444–1445.

209. Srinath, U., Shacklock, F., Scott, L. W., Jaax, S., and Kris-Etherton, P. M. (1993) Development of medficts—A dietary assessment instrument for evaluating fat, saturated fat, and cholesterol intake. *J. Am. Diet. Assoc.* **Oct 28,** A105–A105 (Abstract).

210. Kristal, A. R., Beresford, S. A., and Lazovich, D. (1994). Assessing change in diet-intervention research. *Am. J. Clin. Nutr.* **59**, 185S–189S.

211. Prochaska, J. O., DiClemente, C. C., and Norcross, J. C. (1992). In search of how people change: Applications to addictive behaviors. *Am. Psychol.* **47**, 1102–1114.

212. Glanz, K., Patterson, R. E., Kristal, A. R., DiClemente, C. C., Heimendinger, J., Linnan, L., and McLerran, D. F. (1994). Stages of change in adopting healthy diets: Fat, fiber, and correlates of nutrient intake [published erratum appears in *Health Educ. Q.* **22**(2)261]. *Health Educ. Q.* **21**, 499–519.

213. Cheadle, A., Psaty, B. M., Curry, S., Wagner, E., Diehr, P., Koepsell, T., and Kristal, A. (1993). Can measures of the grocery store environment be used to track community-level dietary changes? *Prev. Med.* **22**, 361–372.

214. Posner, B. M., Jette, A. M., Smith, K. W., and Miller, D. R. (1993). Nutrition and health risks in the elderly: The nutrition screening initiative. *Am. J. Public Health* **83**, 972–978.

215. White, J. V., Dwyer, J. T., Posner, B. M., Ham, R. J., Lipschitz, D. A., and Wellman, N. S. (1992). Nutrition screening initiative: Development and implementation of the public awareness checklist and screening tools. *J. Am. Diet. Assoc.* **92**, 163–167.

216. Kohlmeier, L., Helsing, E., Kelly, A., Moeiras-Varela, O., Trichpopoulou, A., Wotecki, C. E., Buss, D. H., Callmer, E., Hermus, R. J. J., and Szajd, J. (1990). Nutritional surveillance as the backbone of national nutritional policy: Recommendations of the IUNS Committee on nutritional surveillance and program evaluation in developed countries. *Eur. J. Clin. Nutr.* **44**, 771–781.

217. Anderson, S. A. (1986). Guidelines for use of dietary intake data. Life Sciences Research Office, Federation of American Societies for Experimental Biology, Bethesda, MD.

218. U.S. Department of Health and Human Services, U.S. Department of Agriculture. (1986). Nutrition Monitoring in the United States—a Report from the Joint Nutrition Monitoring Evaluation Committee. DHHS Publication No. (PHS) 86–1255. Public Health Service, U. S. Government Printing Office, Washington, DC.

219. Life Sciences Research Office, Federation of American Societies for Experimental Biology. (1989). Nutrition monitoring in the United States—an update report on nutrition monitoring. Publication No. (PHS) 89–1255. U.S. Dept. of Health and Human Services, U.S. Department of Agriculture, Washington, DC.

220. Interagency Committee on Nutrition Monitoring. (1989). Nutrition monitoring in the United States: The Directory of Federal Nutrition Monitoring Activities. Publication No. (PHS) 89–1255–1. Department of Health and Human Services, Hyattsville, MD.

221. Interagency Board for Nutrition Monitoring and Related Research. (1992). Nutrition monitoring in the United States: The Directory of Federal and State Nutrition Monitoring Activities. Publication no. (PHS) 92–1255–1. U.S. Department of Health and Human Services, Hyattsville, MD.

222. Interagency Board for Nutrition Monitoring and Related Research. (1993). Nutrition monitoring in the United States,

chartbook I: Selected findings from the National Nutrition Monitoring and Related Research Program. Publication No. (PHS) 93–1255–2. U.S. Department of Health and Human Services, Hyattsville, MD.

223. Interagency Board for Nutrition Monitoring and Related Research. (1995). Third report on nutrition monitoring in the United States, volume 1. U.S. Government Printing Office, Washington, DC.

224. Interagency Board for Nutrition Monitoring and Related Research. (1995). Third report on nutrition monitoring in the United States, volume 2. U.S. Government Printing Office, Washington, DC.

225. Interagency Board for Nutrition Monitoring and Related Research. (1998). Nutrition monitoring in the United States. The Directory of Federal and State Nutrition Monitoring and Related Research Activities. National Center for Health Statistics, Hyattsville, MD.

226. Guenther, P. M. (1994). Research needs for dietary assessment and monitoring in the United States. *Am. J. Clin. Nutr.* **59,** 168s–170s.

227. Kuczmarski, M. F., Moshfegh, A., and Briefel, R. (1994). Update on nutrition monitoring activities in the United States. *J. Am. Diet. Assoc.* **94,** 753–760.

228. National Center for Health Statistics. (1992). Dietary methodology workshop for the Third National Health and Nutrition Examination Survey. *Vital and Health Stat.* **4**(27), Publication no. 92–1464. U.S. Department of Health and Human Services, Washington, DC.

229. National Center for Health Statistics. (1994). Plan and operation of the Third National Center for Health and Nutrition Examination Survey, 1988–1994. *Vital Health Stat.* **1**(32), Publication no. 94–1308. U.S. Department of Health and Human Services, Hyattsville, MD.

230. National Center for Health Statistics. (1985). Plan of operation of the Hispanic Health and Nutrition Examination Survey 1982–84 U. S. Dept. of Health Human Services, Hyattsville, MD.

231. U.S. Department of Agriculture, Human Nutrition Information Service. (1984). Nutrient intakes: Individuals in 48 states, year 1977–78. Nationwide Food Consumption Survey 1977–78. Report I-2. U.S. Department of Agriculture, Hyattsville, MD.

232. U.S. Department of Agriculture, Human Nutrition Information Service Consumer Nutrition Division. (1983). Food intakes: Individuals in 48 states, Year 1977–78. Nationwide Food Consumption Survey 1977–78. Report No. I-1. U.S. Department of Agriculture, Hyattsville, MD.

233. Peterkin, B. B., Rizek, R. L., and Tippett, K. S. (1988). Nationwide food consumption survey, 1987. *Nutr. Today* 18–23.

234. U.S. Department of Agriculture, Human Nurition Information Service. (1993). Food and nutrient intakes by individuals in the United States, 1 day, 1987–88: Nationwide food consumption survey 1987–88. NFCS Rep. No. 87-I-1. U.S. Department of Agriculture, Washington, DC.

235. U.S. Department of Agriculture, Human Nutrition Information Service. (1987). Nationwide Food Consumption Survey, Continuing Survey of Food Intakes by individuals. Women 19–50 years and their children 1–5 years, 1 day. CSFII Report No. 86-1. U.S. Department of Agriculture, Hyattsville, MD.

236. U.S. Department of Agriculture, Human Nutrition Information Service. (1986). Nationwide Food Consumption Survey, Continuing Survey of Food Intakes by Individuals. Women 19–50 years and their children 1–5 years, 4 days. CSFII Report No. 86–3. U.S. Department of Agriculture, Hyattsville, MD.

237. U.S. Department of Agriculture, Human Nutrition Information Service Nutrition Monitoring Division. (1985). Nationwide Food Consumption Survey, Continuing Survey of Food Intakes by Individuals: Women 19–50 years and their children 1–5 years, 1 day. CSFII Report No. 85-1. U.S. Department of Agriculture, Hyattsville, MD.

238. U.S. Department of Agriculture, Human Nutrition Information Service Nutrition Monitoring Division. (1985). Nationwide Food Consumption Survey, Continuing Survey of Food Intakes by Individuals: Low-income women 19–50 years and their children 1–5 years, 1 day. CSFII Report No. 85–2. U.S. Department of Agriculture, Hyattsville, MD.

239. U.S. Department of Agriculture, Human Nutrition Information Service Nutrition Monitoring Division. (1985). Nationwide Food Consumption Survey, Continuing Survey of Food Intakes by Individuals: Low-income women 19–50 years and their children 1–5 years, 4 days. CSFII Report No. 85-5. U.S. Department of Agriculture, Hyattsville, MD.

240. U.S. Department of Agriculture, Human Nutrition Information Service Nutrition Monitoring Division. (1986). Nationwide Food Consumption Survey, Continuing Survey of Food Intakes by Individuals: Low income women 19–50 years and their children 1–5 years, 1 day. CSFII Report No. 86-2. U.S. Department of Agriculture, Hyattsville, MD.

241. U.S. Department of Agriculture, Human Nutrition Information Service Nutrition Monitoring Division. (1986). Nationwide Food Consumption Survey, Continuing Survey of Food Intakes by Individuals: Low-income women 19–50 years and their children 1–5 years, 4 days. CSFII, Report No. 86-4. U.S. Department of Agriculture, Hyattsville, MD.

242. U.S. Department of Agriculture, Human Nutrition Information Service Nutrition Monitoring Division. (1985). Nationwide Food Consumption Survey, Continuing Survey of Food Intakes by Individuals: Men 19–50 years, 1 day. CSFII Rep. No. 85-3. U.S. Department of Agriculture, Hyattsville, MD.

243. U.S. Department of Agriculture, Human Nurition Information Service. (1993). NFCS Continuing Survey of Food Intakes by Individuals, 1989. Ascession no. PB93-500411. Computer Tape. U.S. Dept. Commerce, National Technical Information Service, Springfield, VA.

244. U.S. Department of Agriculture, Human Nurition Information Service. (1993). NFCS Continuing Survey of Food Intakes by Individuals, 1990. Ascession no. PB93-504843. Computer Tape. U.S. Department of Commerce, National Technical Information Service, Springfield, VA.

245. U.S. Department of Agriculture, Human Nurition Information Service. (1994). NFCS Continuing Survey of Food Intakes by Individuals, 1991. Ascession no. PB94-500063, Computer Tape. U.S. Dept. Commerce, National Technical Information Service, Springfield, VA.

246. U.S. Department of Agriculture, Agricultural Research Service. (1998). Food and nutrient intakes by individuals in the United States, by sex and age, 1994–96, Nationwide Food Consumption Surveys. NFS Report No. 96-2. U.S. Department of Agriculture, Hyattsville, MD.

247. Samet, J. M. (1989). Surrogate measures of dietary intake. *Am. J. Clin. Nutr.* **50,** 1139–1144.

248. Metzner, H. L., Lamphiear, D. E., Thompson, F. E., Oh, M. S., and Hawthorne, V. M. (1989). Comparison of surrogate and subject reports of dietary practices, smoking habits and weight among married couples in the Tecumseh Diet Methodology Study. *J. Clin. Epidemiol.* **42,** 367–375.

249. Hislop, T. G., Coldman, A. J., Zheng, Y. Y., Ng, V. T., and Labo, T. (1992). Reliability of dietary information from surrogate respondents. *Nutr. Cancer* **18,** 123–129.

250. Hankin, J. H., and Wilkens, L. R. (1994). Development and validation of dietary assessment methods for culturally diverse populations. *Am. J. Clin. Nutr.* **59,** 198s–200s.

251. Loria, C. M., McDowell, M. A., Johnson, C. L., and Woteki, C. E. (1991). Nutrient data for Mexican-American foods: Are current data adequate? *J. Am. Diet. Assoc.* **91,** 919–922.

252. Navajo Health and Nutrition Survey Manual. Navajo Area Indian Health Service, Nutrition and Dietetics Branch, Health Promotion/Disease Prevention Program.

253. Lee, M. M., Lee, F., Wang-Ladenla, S., and Miike, R. (1994). A semiquantitative dietary history questionnaire for Chinese Americans. *Ann. Epidemiol.* **4,** 188–197.

254. Hebert, J. R., Gupta, P. C., Bhonsle, R. B., Sinor, P. N., Mehta, H., and Mehta, F. S. (1999). Development and testing of a quantitative food frequency questionnaire for use in Gujarat, India. *Public Health Nutr.* **2,** 39–50.

255. Tucker, K. L., Bianchi, L. A., Maras, J., and Bermudez, O. I. (1998). Adaptation of a food frequency questionnaire to assess diets of Puerto Rican and non-Hispanic adults. *Am. J. Epidemiol.* **148,** 507–518.

256. Coates, R. J., and Monteilh, C. P. (1997). Assessments of food-frequency questionnaires in minority populations. *Am. J. Clin. Nutr.* **65,** 1108S–1115S.

257. Mayer-Davis, E. J., Vitolins, M. Z., Carmichael, S. L., Hemphill, S., Tsaroucha, G., Rushing, J., and Levin, S. (1999). Validity and reproducibility of a food frequency interview in a multi-cultural epidemiologic study. *Ann. Epidemiol.* **9,** 314–324.

258. Kristal, A. R., Feng, Z., Coates, R. J., Oberman, A., and George, V. (1997). Associations of race/ethnicity, education, and dietary intervention with the validity and reliability of a food frequency questionnaire: The Women's Health Trial Feasibility Study in Minority Populations [published erratum appears in *Am. J. Epidemiol.* **148**(8), 820] [see comments]. *Am. J. Epidemiol.* **146,** 856–869.

259. Baumgartner, K. B., Gilliland, F. D., Nicholson, C. S., McPherson, R. S., Hunt, W. C., Pathak, D. R., and Samet, J. M. (1998). Validity and reproducibility of a food frequency questionnaire among Hispanic and non-Hispanic white women in New Mexico. *Ethn. Dis.* **8,** 81–92.

260. Hertzler, A. A. (1990). A review of methods to research nutrition knowledge and dietary intake of preschoolers. *Topics Clin. Nutr.* **6,** 1–9.

261. Frank, G. C., Webber, L. S., Farris, R. P., and Berenson, G. S. (1986). The Dietary Databook: Quantification of Dietary Intakes for Infants, Children, and Adolescents: The Bogalusa Heart Study, 1973–1983 Louisiana State University Medical Center, New Orleans.

262. Van Horn, L. V., Stumbo, P., and Moag-Stahlberg, A. (1993). The dietary intervention study in children (DISC): Dietary assessment methods for 8 to 10 year-olds. *J. Am. Diet. Assoc.* **94,** 1396–1403.

263. Frank, G. C. (1994). Environmental influences on methods used to collect dietary data from children. *Am. J. Clin. Nutr.* **59,** 207s–211s.

264. Domel, S. B., Baranowski, T., Leonard, S. B., Davis, H., Riley, P., and Baranowski, J. (1994). Accuracy of fourth and fifth-grade students' food records compared with school-lunch observations. *Am. J. Clin. Nutr.* **59,** 218s–220s.

265. Rockett, H. R., and Colditz, G. A. (1997). Assessing diets of children and adolescents. *Am. J. Clin. Nutr.* **65,** 1116S–1122S.

266. Baranowski, T., and Domel, S. B. (1994). A cognitive model of children's reporting of food intake. *Am. J. Clin. Nutr.* **59,** 212s–217s.

267. Baranowski, T., Sprague, D., Baranowksi, J. H., and Harrison, J. A. (1991). Accuracy of maternal dietary recall for preschool children. *J. Am. Diet. Assoc.* **91,** 669–674.

268. Eck, L. H., Klesges, R. C., and Hanson, C. L. (1989). Recall of a child's intake from one meal: Are parents accurate? *J. Am. Diet. Assoc.* **89,** 784–789.

269. Lytle, L. A., Nichaman, M. Z., Obarzanek, E., Glovsky, E., Montgomery, D., Nicklas, T., Zive, M., and Feldman, H. (1993). Validation of 24-hour recalls assisted by food records in third-grade children. *J. Am. Diet. Assoc.* **93,** 1431–1436.

270. Rockett, H. R., Breitenbach, M., Frazier, A. L., Witschi, J., Wolf, A. M., Field, A. E., and Colditz, G. A. (1997). Validation of a youth/adolescent food frequency questionnaire. *Prev. Med.* **26,** 808–816.

271. McDowell, M. A., Harris, T. B., and Briefel, R. R. (1991). Dietary surveys of older persons. *Clinics Appl. Nutr.* **1,** 51–60.

272. van Staveren, W. A., de Groot, C., Blauw, Y. H., and van der Wielen, R. P. (1994). Assessing diets of elderly people: Problems and approaches. *Am. J. Clin. Nutr.* **59,** 221s–223s.

273. Block, G., Sinha, R., and Gridley, G. (1994). Collection of dietary-supplement data and implications for analysis. *Am. J. Clin. Nutr.* **59,** 232s–239s.

274. Chianetta, M. M., and Head, M. K. (1992). Effect of prior notification on accuracy of dietary recall by the elderly. *J. Am. Diet. Assoc.* **92,** 741–743.

275. Klipstein-Grobusch, K., den Breeijen, J. H., Goldbohm, R. A., Geleijnse, J. M., Hofman, A., Grobbee, D. E., and Witteman, J. C. (1998). Dietary assessment in the elderly: Validation of a semiquantitative food frequency questionnaire. *Eur. J. Clin. Nutr.* **52,** 588–596.

276. Thompson, C. H., Head, M. K., and Rodman, S. M. (1987). Factors influencing accuracy in estimating plate waste. *J. Am. Diet. Assoc.* **87,** 1219–1220.

277. Guthrie, H. A. (1984). Selection and quantification of typical food portions by young adults. *J. Am. Diet. Assoc.* **84,** 1440–1444.

278. Nelson, M., Atkinson, M., and Darbyshire, S. (1996). Food photography II: Use of food photographs for estimating portion size and the nutrient content of meals. *Br. J. Nutr.* **76,** 31–49.

279. Hebert, J. R., Gupta, P. C., Bhonsle, R., Verghese, F., Ebbeling, C., Barrow, R., Ellis, S., and Ma, Y. (1999). Determinants of accuracy in estimating the weight and volume of commonly used foods: A cross-cultural comparison. *Ecol. Food Nutr.* **37,** 475–502.

280. Young, L. R., and Nestle, M. S. (1995). Portion sizes in dietary assessment: Issues and policy implications. *Nutr. Rev.* **53,** 149–158.

281. Young, L. R., and Nestle, M. (1998). Variation in perceptions of a "medium" food portion: Implications for dietary guidance. *J. Am. Diet. Assoc.* **98,** 458–459.

282. Cypel, Y. S., Guenther, P. M., and Petot, G. J. (1997). Validity of portion-size measurement aids: A review. *J. Am. Diet. Assoc.* **97,** 289–292.

283. Smith, A. F., Jobe, J. B., and Mingay, D. J. (1991). Question-induced cognitive biases in reports of dietary intake by college men and women. *Health. Psychol.* **10,** 244–251.

284. Pao, E. M. (1987). Validation of food intake reporting by men. Research on survey methodology: Proceedings of a symposium held at the 71st annual meetings of the Federation of American Societies for Experimental Biology, April 1, 1987. Administrative Report no. 382. U.S. Department of Agriculture, Human Nutrition Information Service, U.S. Department of Agriculture, Hyattsville, MD.

285. Bolland, J. E., Yuhas, J. A., and Bolland, T. W. (1988). Estimation of food portion sizes: Effectiveness of training. *J. Am. Diet. Assoc.* **88,** 817–821.

286. Howat, P. M., Mohan, R., Champagne, C., Monlezun, C., Wozniak, P., and Bray, G. A. (1994). Validity and reliability of reported dietary intake data. *J. Am. Diet. Assoc.* **94,** 169–173.

287. Bolland, J. E., Ward, J. Y., and Bolland, T. W. (1990). Improved accuracy of estimating food quantities up to 4 weeks after training. *J. Am. Diet. Assoc.* **90,** 1402–4, 1407.

288. Posner, B. M., Smigelski, C., Duggal, A., Morgan, J. L., Cobb, J., and Cupples, L. A. (1992). Validation of two-dimensional models for estimation of portion size in nutrition research. *J. Am. Diet. Assoc.* **92,** 738–741.

289. Fox, T. A., Heimendinger, J., and Block, G. (1992). Telephone surveys as a method for obtaining dietary information: A review. *J. Am. Diet. Assoc.* **92,** 729–732.

290. Dillman, D. A. (1978). "Mail and Telephone Surveys: The Total Design Method." John Wiley & Sons, New York.

291. Marcus, A. C., and Crane, L. A. (1986). Telephone surveys in public health research. *Med. Care.* **24,** 97–112.

292. Morgan, K. J., Johnson, S. R., Rizek, R. L., Reese, R., and Stampley, G. L. (1987). Collection of food intake data: An evaluation of methods. *J. Am. Diet. Assoc.* **87,** 888–896.

293. Leighton, J., Neugut, A. I., and Block, G. (1988). A comparison of face-to-face frequency interviews and self-administered questionnaires. *Am. J. Epidemiol.* **128,** 891–891(Abstract).

294. Lyu, L. C., Hankin, J. H., Liu, L. Q., Wilkens, L. R., Lee, J. H., Goodman, M. T., and Kolonel, L. N. (1998). Telephone vs face-to-face interviews for quantitative food frequency assessment. *J. Am. Diet. Assoc.* **98,** 44–48.

295. Posner, B. M., Borman, C. L., Morgan, J. L., Borden, W. S., and Ohls, J. C. (1982). The validity of a telephone-administered 24-hour dietary recall methodology. *Am. J. Clin. Nutr.* **36,** 546–553.

296. Krantzler, N. J., Mullen, B. J., Schutz, H. G., Grivetti, L. E., Holden, C. A., and Meiselman, H. L. (1982). Validity of telephoned diet recalls and records for assessment of individual food intake. *Am. J. Clin. Nutr.* **36,** 1234–1242.

297. McDowell, M. A. (1994). The NHANES III supplemental nutrition survey of older Americans. *Am. J. Clin. Nutr.* **59,** 224s–226s.

298. Hartman, A. M., Brown, C. C., Palmgren, J., Pietinen, P., Verkasalo, M., Myer, D., and Virtamo, J. (1990). Variability in nutrient and food intakes among older middle-aged men. Implications for design of epidemiologic and validation studies using food recording. *Am. J. Epidemiol.* **132,** 999–1012.

299. Hartman, A. M., and Block, G. (1992). Dietary assessment methods for macronutrients. *In* "Macronutrients: Investigating Their Role in Cancer" (M. S. Micozzi and T. E. Moon, Eds.), pp. 87–124. Marcel Dekker, New York.

300. Wassertheil-Smoller, S., Davis, B. R., Breuer, B., Change, C. J., Oberman, A., and Blaufox, M. D. (1993). Differences in precision of dietary estimates among different population subgroups. *Ann. Epidemiol.* **3,** 619–628.

301. Larkin, F., Metzner, H., Thompson, F., Flegal, K., and Guire, K. (1989). Comparison of estimated nutrient intakes by food frequency and dietary records in adults. *J. Am. Diet. Assoc.* **89,** 215–223.

302. Schakel, S. F., Buzzard, I. M., and Gebhard, S. E. (1997). Procedures for estimating nutrient values for food composition databases. *J. Food Comp. Anal.* **10,** 102–114.

303. Beecher, G. R., and Matthews, R. H. (1990). Nutrient composition of foods. *In* "Present Knowledge in Nutrition" (M. L. Brown, Ed.), pp. 430–443. International Life Sciences Institute, Nutrition Foundation, Washington, DC.

304. Anonymous. (1997). What are the variances of food composition data? (Editorial). *J. Food Comp. Anal.* **10,** 89–89.

305. Perloff, B. P. (1989). Analysis of dietary data. *Am. J. Clin. Nutr.* **50,** 1128–1132.

306. Scrimshaw, N. S. (1997). INFOODS: The international network of food data systems. *Am. J. Clin. Nutr.* **65,** 1190S–1193S.

307. U. S. Department of Agriculture and Human Nutrition Information Service (1992). USDA's food guide pyramid. *Home Garden Bull.* 252.

308. Smith, S. A., Campbell, D. R., Elmer, P. J., Martini, M. C., Slavin, J. L., and Potter, J. D. (1995). The University of Minnesota Cancer Prevention Research Unit vegetable and fruit classification scheme (United States). *Cancer Causes Control* **6,** 292–302.

309. Cleveland, L. E., Cook, D. A., Krebs-Smith, S. M., and Friday, J. (1997). Method for assessing food intakes in terms of servings based on food guidance. *Am. J. Clin. Nutr.* **65,** 1254S–1263S.

310. Byers, T., and Gieseker, K. (1997). Issues in the design and interpretation of studies of fatty acids and cancer in humans. *Am. J. Clin. Nutr.* **66,** 1541S–1547S.

311. Innis, S. M., Green, T. J., and Halsey, T. K. (1999). Variability in the trans fatty acid content of foods within a food category: Implications for estimation of dietary trans fatty acid intakes. *J. Am. Coll. Nutr.* **18,** 255–260.

312. Jacobs, D. R., Jr., Elmer, P. J., Gorder, D., Hall, Y., and Moss, D. (1985). Comparison of nutrient calculation systems. *Am. J. Epidemiol.* **121,** 580–592.

313. Lee, R. D., Nieman, D. C., and Rainwater, M. (1995). Comparison of eight microcomputer dietary analysis programs with the USDA Nutrient Data Base for Standard Reference [see comments]. *J. Am. Diet. Assoc.* **95,** 858–867.

314. McCullough, M. L., Karanja, N. M., Lin, P. H., Obarzanek, E., Phillips, K. M., Laws, R. L., Vollmer, W. M., O'Connor, E. A., Champagne, C. M., and Windhauser, M. M. (1999). Comparison of 4 nutrient databases with chemical composition

data from the Dietary Approaches to Stop Hypertension trial. DASH Collaborative Research Group. *J. Am. Diet. Assoc.* **99,** S45–S53.

315. Kristal, A. R., Shattuck, A. L., and Williams, A. E. (1992). Current issues and concerns on the users of food composition data: Food frequency questionnaires for diet intervention research. *In* "17th National Nutrient Databank Conference Proceedings," pp. 110–125.

316. Buzzard, I. M., Price, K. S., and Warren, R. A. (1991). Considerations for selecting nutrient calculation software: Evaluation of the nutrient database (editorial). *Am. J. Clin. Nutr.* **54,** 7–9.

317. Dwyer, J. T., Krall, E. A., and Coleman, K. A. (1987). The problem of memory in nutritional epidemiology research. *J. Am. Diet. Assoc.* **87,** 1509–1512.

318. Smith, A. F., Jobe, J. B., and Mingay, D. J. (1991). Retrieval from memory of dietary information. *Appl. Cog. Psychol.* **5,** 269–296.

319. Friedenreich, C. M. (1994). Improving long-term recall in epidemiologic studies. *Epidemiology* **5,** 1–4.

320. Radimer, K. L., Subar, A. F., and Thompson, F. E. (2000). Nonvitamin, nonmineral dietary supplements: issues and findings from NHANES III *J. Am. Diet. Assoc.* **100,** 447–454.

321. Ervin, R. B., Wright, J. D., and Kennedy-Stephenson, J. (1999). Use of dietary supplements in the United States, 1988–94. *Vital Health Stat.* **11.** Publication 244 (PHS) 99–1694. National Center for Health Statistics, Hyattsville, MD.

322. Roe, B. E., Derby, B. M., and Levy A. S. (1997). Demographic, lifestyle and information use characteristics of dietary supplement user segment: Prepared for the Commission on Dietary Supplement Labeling. HFS–727. 3-12-1997. U.S. Food and Drug Administration, Center for Food Safety and Applied Nutrition, Washington, DC.

323. Wood, L. (1997). Herbal supplements attract new users. *Health Foods Busi.* **43,** 101.

324. Patterson, R. E., Kristal, A. R., Levy, L., McLerran, D., and White, E. (1998). Validity of methods used to assess vitamin and mineral supplement use. *Am. J. Epidemiol.* **148,** 643–649.

325. Patterson, R. E., Neuhouser, M. L., White, E., Kristal, A. R., and Potter, J. D. (1998). Measurement error from assessing use of vitamin supplements at one point in time. *Epidemiology* **9,** 567–569.

326. Bates, C. J., Prentice, A., van der Pols, J. C., Walmsley, C., Pentieva, K. D., Finch, S., Smithers, G., and Clarke, P. C. (1998). Estimation of the use of dietary supplements in the National Diet and Nutrition Survey: People aged 65 years and over. An observed paradox and a recommendation. *Eur. J. Clin. Nutr.* **52,** 917–923.

327. Buzzard, I. M., and Sievert, Y. A. (1994). Research priorities and recommendations for dietary assessment methodology. *Am. J. Clin. Nutr.* **59,** 275s–280s.

328. Thompson, F. E., Moler, J. E., Freedman, L. S., Clifford, C. K., Stables, G. J., and Willett, W. C. (1997). Register of dietary assessment calibration-validation studies: A status report. *Am. J. Clin. Nutr.* **65,** 1142S–1147S.

329. Baranowski, T., Dworkin, R., Henske, J. C., Clearman, D. R., Dunn, J. K., Nader, P. R., and Hooks, P. C. (1986). The accuracy of children's self-reports of diet: Family Health Project. *J. Am. Diet. Assoc.* **86,** 1381–1385.

330. Bingham, S. A. (1994). The use of 24-h urine samples and energy expenditure to validate dietary assessments. *Am. J. Clin. Nutr.* **59,** 227s–231s.

331. Samaras, K., Kelly, P. J., and Campbell, L. V. (1999). Dietary underreporting is prevalent in middle-aged British women and is not related to adiposity (percentage body fat). *Int. J. Obes. Relat. Metab. Disord.* **23,** 881–888.

332. Ajani, U. A., Willett, W. C., and Seddon, J. M. (1994). Reproducibility of a food frequency questionnaire for use in ocular research. Eye Disease Case-Control Study Group. *Invest. Ophthalmol. Vis. Sci.* **35,** 2725–2733.

333. Rosner, B., Spiegelman, D., and Willett, W. C. (1990). Correction of logistic regression relative risk estimates and confidence intervals for measurement error: The case of multiple covariates measured with error. *Am. J. Epidemiol.* **132,** 734–45.

334. Paeratakul, S., Popkin, B. M., Kohlmeier, L., Hertz-Picciotto, I., Guo, X., and Edwards, L. J. (1998). Measurement error in dietary data: implications for the epidemiologic study of the diet–disease relationship. *Eur. J. Clin. Nutr.* **52,** 722–727.

335. Plummer, M., and Clayton, D. (1993). Measurement error in dietary assessment: An investigation using covariance structure models. Part II. *Stat. Med.* **12,** 937–948.

336. Plummer, M., and Clayton, D. (1993). Measurement error in dietary assessment: An investigation using covariance structure models. Part I. *Stat. Med.* **12,** 925–935.

337. Willett, W., and Stampfer, M. J. (1986). Total energy intake: Implications for epidemiologic analyses. *Am. J. Epidemiol.* **124,** 17–27.

338. Howe, G. R. (1989). Re: "Total energy intake: Implications for epidemiologic analyses" (letter). *Am. J. Epidemiol.* **129,** 1314–1315.

339. Kipnis, V., Freedman, L. S., Brown, C. C., Hartman, A., Schatzkin, A., and Wacholder, S. (1993). Interpretation of energy adjustment models for nutritional epidemiology. *Am. J. Epidemiol.* **137,** 1376–1380.

340. Kushi, L. H., Sellers, T. A., Potter, J. D., Nelson, C. L., Munger, R. G., Kaye, S. A., and Folsom, A. R. (1992). Dietary fat and postmenopausal breast cancer [see comments]. *J. Natl. Cancer Inst.* **84,** 1092–1099.

341. Brown, C. C., Kipnis, V., Freedman, L. S., Hartman, A. M., Schatzkin, A., and Wacholder, S. (1994). Energy adjustment methods for nutritional epidemiology: The effect of categorization. *Am. J. Epidemiol.* **139,** 323–338.

CHAPTER 2

Energy Requirement Methodology

RACHEL K. JOHNSON AND DEBRA COWARD-McKENZIE
The University of Vermont, Burlington, Vermont

I. INTRODUCTION

Knowledge of energy requirements throughout the life cycle and during various physiological conditions and disease states is essential to the promotion of optimal human health. In the past, the measurement of energy intake served as an important tool from which to base energy requirements among all age groups [1]. The heavy reliance on such subjective forms of measurement, however, prompted research for more valid techniques to estimate energy needs [2]. The aim of this chapter is to familiarize the reader with contemporary techniques to measure energy expenditure. These include the highly sophisticated technique of doubly labeled water which allows nutrition scientists to accurately establish energy requirements based on the measurement of energy expenditure in free-living subjects.

II. COMPONENTS OF ENERGY EXPENDITURE

Energy is expended by the human body in the form of resting energy expenditure (REE), the thermic effect of food (TEF), and energy expended in physical activity (EEPA) [3]. These three components make up a person's daily total energy expenditure (TEE). Except in extremely active subjects, the REE constitutes the largest portion (60–75%) of the TEE [4]. The TEF represents approximately 10% of the total daily energy expenditure. The contribution of physical activity is the most variable component of TEE, which may be as low as 100 kcal/day in sedentary people or as high as 3,000 kcal/day in very active people (Fig. 1).

A. Resting Energy Expenditure

Resting energy expenditure is the energy cost of the physiological functions necessary to maintain homeostasis. These involuntary functions include respiration, cardiac output, body temperature regulation, and other functions of the sympathetic nervous system.

The term basal energy expenditure (BEE) is also used to describe this component of daily energy expenditure. BEE can be defined as the minimal amount of energy expended

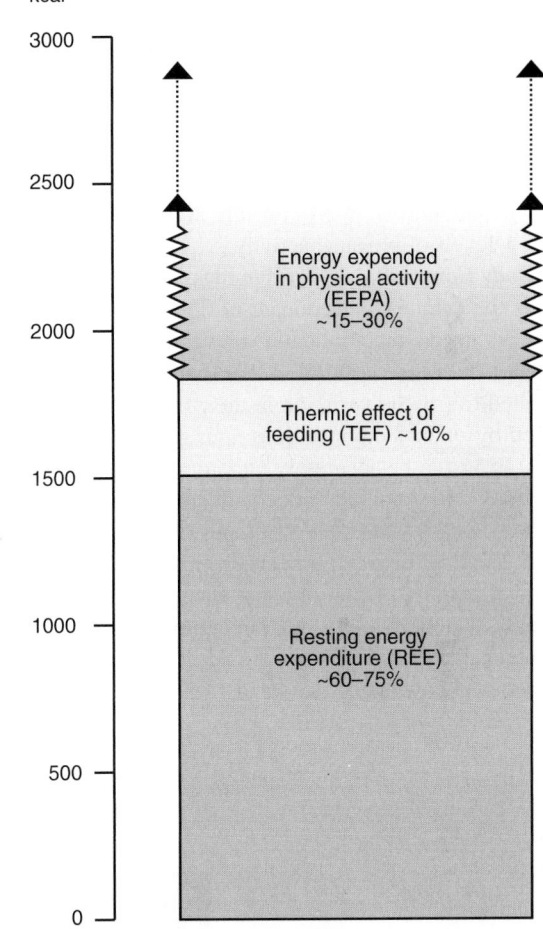

FIGURE 1 The components of total energy expenditure. [From Poehlman, E. T., and Horton, E. S. (1988). Energy needs: Assessment and requirements in humans. *In* "Modern Nutrition in Health and Disease." William & Wilkins, Baltimore, MD.]

that is compatible with life. BEE is the amount of energy used in 24 hours by a person who is lying at physical and mental rest, at least 12 hours after the last meal, in a thermoneutral environment that prevents the activation of heat-generating processes, such as shivering. Basal metabolic rate (BMR) measurements are made early in the morning, before the person has engaged in any physical activity, and with no

ingestion of tea or coffee or inhalation of nicotine-containing tobacco smoke for at least 12 hours before the measurement. If any of the conditions for BMR are not met, the energy expenditure should be termed the resting metabolic rate (RMR). For practical reasons, the BMR is rarely measured. In its place, RMR measurements are used, which in most cases, are higher than the BMR.

1. DETERMINANTS OF RESTING ENERGY EXPENDITURE

The determinants of resting energy expenditure are well established in both adults and children. The principal factors contributing to individual variation in REE include body size and composition, gender, age, physical fitness, hormonal status, and environmental influence [5–7].

a. Body Size. Larger people have higher metabolic rates than do people of smaller size. A difference in weight of 10 kg would lead to a difference in RMR of approximately 120 kcal/day in adult men or women, or a difference in total daily energy expenditure of approximately 200 kcal/day in people with low levels of physical activity.

b. Body Composition. Fat-free mass (FFM) or lean body mass is the primary determinant of TEE in all age groups [8]. FFM is the metabolically active tissue in the body. Hence, most of the variation in REE between people can be accounted for by the variation in their FFM. FFM is in turn affected by other factors such as age, gender, and physical fitness. FFM can be accurately measured using a number of techniques. These include underwater weighing, measuring total body water using stable isotopes of deuterium or oxygen-18, and dual-energy x-ray absorptiometry (DXA). DXA is a novel scanning technique that accurately estimates fat-free mass, lean body mass, and bone mineral mass. Subjects lie supine on a padded table for 20–45 minutes during which time two very low energy (6.4 and 11.2 fJ) x-ray beams are passed through the body (Fig. 2; see color plate at the back of the book). Calculation of fat mass and lean body mass using these data are discussed in detail by Svendsen *et al.* [9]. The total x-ray dose is less than 1 mrem, on the order of a single day's background radiation, for a whole-body composition analysis. Thus, DXA provides an accurate measure of lean body mass and fat mass in a short time with a minimal radiation dose. Pregnancy tests should be performed before administering the DXA to further ensure safety.

Often, due to the expense or impractical nature of research techniques for body composition, other, less accurate methods are often used in practice to estimate body composition. These include skinfold anthropometry, bioelectrical impedance, and near-infrared interactance. See Chapter 3 for a detailed description of body composition measurement techniques.

It has long been questioned whether people who are obese or at risk of developing obesity have reduced metabolic rates. Several studies have produced no evidence that children at high risk of obesity have lower metabolic rates than lean children when the measurements are adjusted for lean body mass [10, 11]. Hence, there is little evidence that a greater metabolic efficiency leads to the development of obesity.

c. Sex Sex is another factor that affects REE. The values for REE and 24-hour energy expenditure in a metabolic chamber are lower in female than in male subjects by approximately 50 kcal/day [12, 13]. The reduced energy expenditure in female subjects is not explained by the confounding effects of the menstrual cycle because the effect is consistent in postmenopausal women as well as prepubertal girls [5, 7]. Women typically have more fat in proportion to muscle (FFM) than men and in general women have metabolic rates that are 5–10% lower than men of the same weight and height.

d. Age. There is a well-documented age-related reduction in resting metabolic rate [14]. Researchers have shown that older healthy people have RMRs that are significantly lower

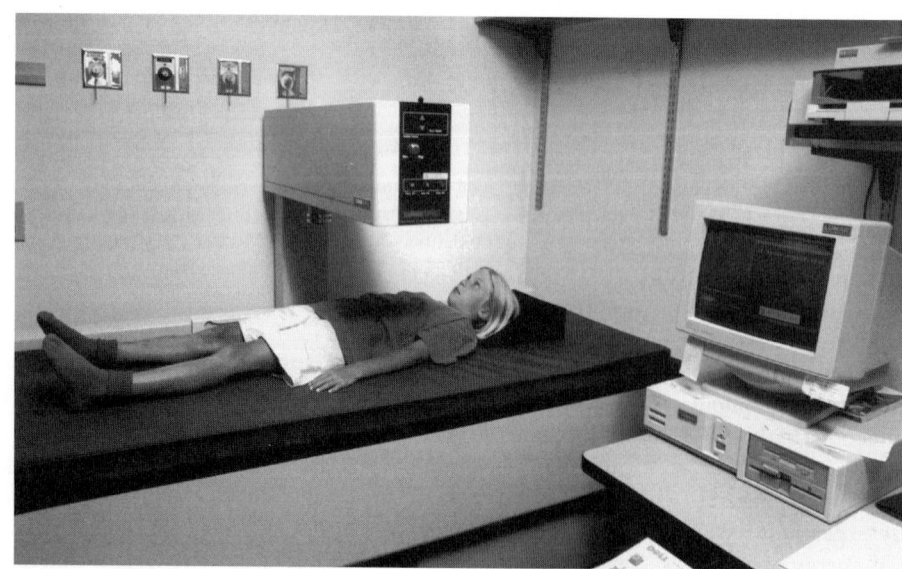

FIGURE 2 Dual-energy x-ray absorptiometry is a scanning technique that accurately estimates bone mineral, fat, and fat-free soft tissue.

than younger people, even when adjusted for differences in fat mass and fat-free mass. This decline in REE can be partly explained by a reduction in the quantity, as well as the metabolic activity, of lean body mass [14].

e. Physical Fitness. Athletes with greater muscular development show approximately a 5% increase in RMR over that in nonathletic individuals owing to their greater FFM. Habitual exercise has been shown to cause an 8–14% higher metabolic rate in men who were moderately and highly active, respectively, owing to increased FFM [15].

f. Hormonal Status. Hormonal status can impact metabolic rate, particularly in endocrine disorders, such as hyperthyroidism and hypothyroidism, when energy expenditure is increased or decreased, respectively. Stimulation of the sympathetic nervous system, such as occurs during emotional excitement or stress, increases cellular activity by the release of epinephrine, which acts directly to promote glycogenolysis. Other hormones, such as cortisol, growth hormone, and insulin, also influence metabolic rate. Researchers have shown that serum leptin concentrations are a positive determinant of RMR [16].

The metabolic rate of adult females fluctuates with the menstrual cycle. An average of 359 kcal/day difference in the BMR has been measured between its low point, about 1 week before ovulation at day 14, and its high point, just before the onset of menstruation. The mean increase in energy expenditure is about 150 kcal/day during the second half of the menstrual cycle [17]. During pregnancy, RMR decreases in the early stages, whereas later in pregnancy, the metabolic rate is increased by the processes of uterine, placental, and fetal growth and by the mother's increased cardiac work [18].

g. Environmental Influences. REE is affected by extremes in environmental temperature. People living in tropical climates usually have RMRs that are 5–20% higher than those living in a temperate area. Exercise in temperatures greater than 86°F also imposes a small additional metabolic load of about 5% owing to increased sweat gland activity. The extent to which energy metabolism increases in extremely cold environments depends on the insulation available from body fat and protective clothing.

2. MEASURING RESTING ENERGY EXPENDITURE: INDIRECT CALORIMETRY

The technique of indirect calorimetry has become the method of choice in most circumstances when a measurement of REE is needed. The term *indirect* refers to the fact that energy (heat) production is determined by measuring O_2 consumption and CO_2 production rather than directly measuring heat transfer. The equipment varies but a ventilated hood system is most commonly used. A clear plastic hood is placed over the subject's head and made airtight around the neck (Fig. 3; see color plate at the back of the book). Indirect calorimetry has the advantage of mobility and low equipment cost and is frequently used in clinical settings to assess patients' energy requirements. Indirect calorimetry also provides quantitative information about the types of substrates that are oxidized [19]. The pretesting environment impacts the measurement of RMR. Outpatient-test experimental conditions have been shown to overestimate RMR by approximately 8% compared with inpatient measurements of RMR [20]. This factor should be taken into account when results are compared between laboratories and when daily

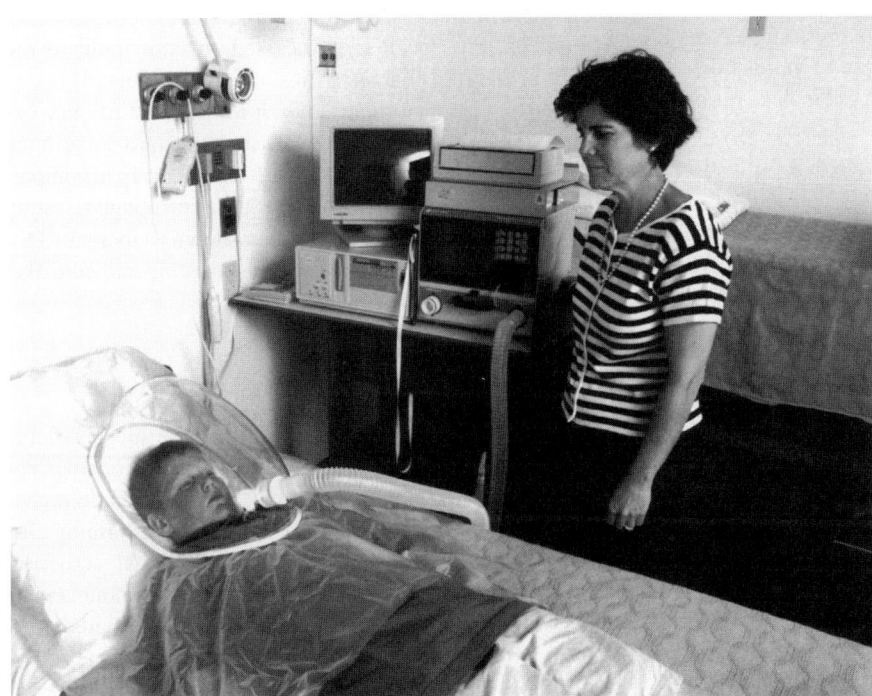

FIGURE 3   Measurement of resting metabolic rate using indirect calorimetry.

TABLE 1 Predicting Resting Energy Expenditure Using the Harris–Benedict Equations

Women:	REE (kcal/day) = 655 + 9.56 (weight) + 1.85 (height) − 4.68 (age)
	REE (kJ) = 2741 + 40 (weight) + 7.74 (height) − 28.35 (age)
	$r^2 = 0.53$, $F = 37.8$, $P < 0.001$
Men:	REE (kcal/day) = 66.5 + 13.75 (weight) + 5.0 (height) − 6.76 (age)
	REE (kJ) = 278 + 57.5 (weight) + 7.74 (height) − 19.56 (age)
	$r^2 = 0.75$, $F = 135.2$, $P < 0.001$

Source: Frankenfield, D. C., Muth, E. R., and Rowe, W. A. (1998). The Harris–Benedict studies of human basal metabolism: History and limitations. *J. Am. Diet. Assoc.* **98,** 439–445.

Note: Weight is in kilograms, height is in centimeters, and age is in years.

energy requirements based on measures of REE are being evaluated.

3. ESTIMATING RESTING ENERGY EXPENDITURE: HARRIS–BENEDICT EQUATIONS

The Harris–Benedict equations remain the most commonly used tool by clinicians when estimating people's REE. The equations are often used as a basis for prescribing energy intake for hospitalized patients and to formulate energy intake goals for weight loss. A review of the data used in the formulation of the Harris–Benedict equations in the early 1930s deduced that the methods and conclusions of Harris and Benedict appear valid but not error free [21]. Only between 50 and 75% of the variability in REE is explained by the equations, but subsequent equations have not generally improved on this level of error [21]. The equations in use today are shown in Table 1. For obese people, the Harris–Benedict equation can be applied up to a body mass index of 35–40 [21].

REE has been characterized for a variety of various disease states and physiological conditions. These include burns [22], anorexia nervosa [23], severe central nervous system impairment [24], cerebral palsy [25], pregnancy [26], and lactation [27]. In addition REE has been studied in both children [5] and the elderly [28, 29]. Clinicians should not assume that prediction equations such as the Harris–Benedict equation, which was developed in normal, healthy people, are valid in these special populations.

B. Thermic Effect of Food

The thermic effect of food (TEF) is the increase in energy expenditure associated with the consumption of food. It accounts for approximately 10% of TEE [30]. TEF is also termed *diet-induced thermogenesis.* TEF can be divided into obligatory and facultative thermogenesis. Obligatory thermogenesis is the energy needed to digest, absorb, and metabolize nutrients. Facultative thermogenesis is the excess energy expended above the obligatory thermogenesis attrib-

utable to metabolic inefficiency. TEF is not measured in clinical settings, but rather estimated as 10% of TEE. Hence, the equation:

$$TEE = (RMR + EEPA) \times 1.10$$

where TEE = total energy expenditure, RMR = resting energy expenditure, EEPA = energy expended in physical activity, and the factor of 1.10 accounts for the TEF in the equation.

1. DETERMINANTS OF THERMIC EFFECT OF FOOD

The composition of the diet affects the TEF, with TEF being greater after carbohydrate and protein consumption in comparison with fat. This is accounted for by the differences in metabolic efficiency when metabolizing carbohydrate and protein versus fat. Fat is efficiently metabolized and stored with only 4% wastage, compared with 25% inefficiency when carbohydrate is converted to fat for storage. These differences have been hypothesized to contribute to the obesity-promoting characteristics of high-fat diets [31].

Other dietary factors are known to impact TEF. For example, spicy foods such as chili and mustard have been shown to increase the metabolic rate significantly in comparison with unspiced meals. The effect was prolonged, lasting up to 3 hours [32]. Caffeine has been shown to increase TEF by 8–11% [33]. Other factors such as nicotine and cold also stimulate the TEF [34].

C. Energy Expended in Physical Activity

Energy expended in physical activity is the most variable component of total energy expenditure. EEPA includes energy expended in voluntary exercise, which include activities of daily living (bathing, feeding, and grooming, for example), sports and leisure, and occupational activities. EEPA also includes the energy expended in nonexercise activity thermogenesis (NEAT), which is associated with fidgeting, maintenance of posture, and other physical activities of daily life. The share of total energy expenditure ac-

counted for by physical activity is obviously greater for active individuals [35]. It can vary from 10% in a bedridden person to as high as 50% or more of TEE in athletes. Because of the alarmingly high rates of obesity in the United States, increasing EEPA through voluntary physical activity is being stressed as an effective way of achieving healthy weight [36].

NEAT can add significantly to a person's energy expenditure. Researchers found that when nonobese volunteers were fed 1000 kcal/day in excess of weight-maintenance requirements for 8 weeks, two-thirds of the increase in total daily energy expenditure was due to increased NEAT. Changes in NEAT accounted for 10-fold differences in fat storage that occurred and directly predicted resistance to fat gain with overfeeding. These results suggest that as humans overeat, activation of NEAT dissipates excess energy to preserve leanness and that failure to activate NEAT may result in fat gain [37].

A novel study suggested that gum chewing is sufficiently exothermic that it can lead to a meaningful increase in energy expenditure over time. Chewing gum led to a mean increase in energy expenditure of 11 ± 3 kcal/hour in seven nonobese volunteers with stable weight. The researchers speculated that if a person chewed gum during waking hours and changed no other components of energy balance, a yearly loss of more than 5 kg of body fat could be realized [38].

1. Determinants of Energy Expended in Physical Activity

Differences in EEPA are due both to patterns of activity (both voluntary and involuntary) as well as the body composition that results from that pattern of activity [39]. Hence, the level of a person's fitness will affect EEPA, due to the increased lean body mass and metabolically active tissue.

In general, EEPA declines with age. Because the decline in EEPA is often disproportionately greater than the decline in energy intake, positive energy balance results. This often leads to increased total and central body fatness, a loss of muscle mass, and a greater predisposition to comorbidities associated with obesity and physical inactivity [40]. Fortunately, it has been demonstrated that regular aerobic exercise can successfully increase EEPA in middle-aged men and hence raise the daily energy requirements for weight maintenance [41]. Thus, regular exercise may counter the age-related tendency toward obesity

2. Measuring Energy Expended in Physical Activity

Obtaining a valid and appropriate measurement of EEPA is a challenging task. There are subjective measures, such a questionnaires, which are widely used in epidemiological studies to assess physical activity in populations [35]. Objective activity assessment tools are also often used to validate the subjective activity measures. These include the doubly labeled water technique, movement counters, heart rate monitoring and graded exercise testing.

a. Objective Measures of EEPA.

i. Doubly labeled water. EEPA can be estimated by determining the difference between total daily energy expenditure as measured by doubly labeled water and resting metabolic rate and thermic effect of food measured by indirect calorimetry. The advantages of the doubly labeled water (DLW) approach are that it requires little subject cooperation, is unobtrusive, and measures free-living activity throughout a person's daily routine. Unfortunately, the high price of the isotopes, mass spectrometer instrumentation, and the need for technical expertise in sample preparation and measurement have limited its widespread application. Nevertheless, DLW has been used as a gold standard for validating other methods to measure EEPA in free-living individuals [42]. DLW measurement of total energy expenditure is discussed in detail in the TEE section of this chapter.

ii. Movement counters. Accelerometers are movement counters that can measure the occurrence of body movement and its intensity. Accelerometers cannot be used to measure the static component in exercises, like weight lifting or carrying loads. However, in normal daily life, it is assumed that the effect of static exercise on the total level of physical activity is negligible [43]. Currently, several accelerometers are available for the assessment of physical activity. The most widely available are the Caltrac (Hemokinetics, Madison, WI) and the Tritrac-R3 D accelerometer (Hemokinetics).

The Caltrac is a one-axial accelerometer for vertical movement. Energy expenditure is estimated by entering the subject's age, height, weight, and gender. Activity counts are displayed when predetermined constants are entered in place of the subject's personal data. The Caltrac was not found to be a meaningful predictor of EEPA in a group of free-living, school-aged children [44] or in older men and women [42]. The Caltrac may be useful, however, in supervised settings in which researchers want to assess children's levels of physical activity [45].

The triaxial accelerometer measures movement on three planes and possesses the ability to store extensive data within its internal computer for retrieval at a later time. The evidence to date suggests that a triaxial accelerometer provides a better estimate of usual physical activity or energy expenditure than a single-plane accelerometer. Studies have demonstrated that these instruments can be used to distinguish differences in activity levels between individuals and to assess the effect of interventions on physical activity within individuals [43].

iii. Heart rate monitoring. The use of heart rate monitoring as a proxy measure for EEPA is based on the principle that heart rate and oxygen consumption (V_{O_2}) tend to be linearly related throughout a large portion of the aerobic work range. When this relationship is known, the exercise heart rate can be used to estimate V_{O_2} [46]. Heart rate monitoring is relatively inexpensive, can assess people in a free-living

state, and has the potential for providing information on the pattern as well as the total level of energy expenditure [47]. The technique has been successfully applied in small groups of children, lactating women, normal adults, athletes, and in remote indigenous populations [46]. Wareham and colleagues have confirmed its feasibility for assessing the pattern and total level of energy expenditure in the epidemiological context [47]. However, users of the technique must be cognizant of the uncertainties and likely sources of error in its use.

b. Physical Activity Questionnaires. Physical activity questionnaires have been used in many studies because they are easy to administer to large numbers of people and do not intrude on people's everyday activities. Although questionnaires do not provide precise estimates of EEPA, they may be helpful in ranking groups of subjects from the least to the most active. The ranking can then be used to correlate activity levels with disease outcomes [37]. An accurate questionnaire is both reliable and valid. A reliable questionnaire consistently provides similar results under the same circumstances while a valid questionnaire truly measures what it was designed to measure. The validity of a physical activity questionnaire should be determined by comparing it with an objective measure of EEPA such as the doubly labeled water method. Starling and colleagues [42] found that the Yale Physical Activity Survey estimates of EEPA compared favorably with DLW on a group basis. However, its use as a proxy measure for individual EEPA is limited. In the same study, the Minnesota Leisure Time Physical Activity Questionnaire significantly underestimated EEPA in free-living older men and women [42]. This points out the importance of ascertaining the validity of a questionnaire before applying it in large epidemiological studies. The latest versions of most of the popular physical activity questionnaires, along with descriptions for their use, are available [48].

III. TOTAL ENERGY EXPENDITURE

Total energy expenditure is composed of the energy required for both unconscious and conscious activities. As already mentioned, it consists of three distinct parts: resting energy expenditure, thermic effect of food, and the energy expended in physical activity. TEE estimates energy requirements, assuming that people are in energy balance [6, 49]. The state of energy balance requires that, to maintain a specific weight, body energy stores must remain constant, that is, energy intake must match total energy expenditure. Thus, in significant weight gain or loss, when body composition is changing, metabolizable energy intake is not an accurate predictor of energy expenditure. Therefore, changes in body composition must be monitored for the accurate determination of energy expenditure.

A. Measuring Total Energy Expenditure

1. DIRECT CALORIMETRY
Direct calorimetry obtains a direct measurement of the amount of heat generated by the body within a structure large enough to permit moderate amounts of activity. These structures are called whole-room calorimeters. Direct calorimetry provides a measure of energy expended in the form of heat. The technique of direct calorimetry has several disadvantages. The structure is costly, requires complex engineering, and appropriate facilities are scarce around the world. Subjects must remain in a physically confined environment for long periods. In addition, direct calorimetry does not provide any information about the nature of substrates that are being oxidized to generate energy within the body [19].

2. DOUBLY LABELED WATER
The introduction of the DLW technique for human use in 1982 by Schoeller and van Santen [50] provided a scientific breakthrough in the measurement of TEE in free-living humans. The method was originally described by Lifson *et al.* [51] in the 1940s. It is based on the principle that carbon dioxide production can be estimated by the difference in elimination rates of body hydrogen and oxygen. Through his observations, Lifson concluded that the oxygen in expired carbon dioxide was derived from total body water [52]. This results from the equilibrium between the oxygen in body water and the oxygen in respiratory carbon dioxide [51]. With this finding, Lifson and colleagues predicted that carbon dioxide production could be indirectly measured by separately labeling both the hydrogen and oxygen pool of the body water with naturally occurring, stable isotopes. Based on the theory that the hydrogen of body water will exit as water and the oxygen of body water as carbon dioxide and water, the differential elimination rates of hydrogen and oxygen will indicate the amount of carbon dioxide expired during a given period. Carbon dioxide production can then be equated with energy expenditure under the assumption that carbon dioxide is an endproduct of substrate metabolism. Therefore, carbon dioxide production can be converted to an estimate of oxygen production using a food quotient estimated from total dietary intake.

The term *doubly labeled water* indicates that the water consists of isotopic forms of hydrogen and oxygen. Deuterium oxide (^2H_2O) is the isotope that labels the hydrogen component of body water, and oxygen–18 ($H_2^{18}O$) is the isotope that labels the oxygen component of body water. Together, these isotopes label the hydrogen and oxygen of body water and trace their path within the body during the course of the study. The levels of the isotopes can be determined by periodic sampling of body water through urine, saliva, or plasma. Before a preweighed loading dose of DLW is orally administered, a baseline measurement of body water is obtained to detect the amount of deuterium oxide and

oxygen–18 already present within the body water. After the baseline sample collection and administration of the DLW, two samples of body water are collected several days apart (usually 10–14 days) to determine the elimination rates of the isotopes. This two-point method has been shown to minimize the errors encountered from daily variations in the rate of carbon dioxide production [53].

a. Assumptions of the Doubly Labeled Water Method. As with all scientific methodology, assumptions are made that need to be understood when using the DLW technique. A few of the fundamental assumptions are examined here. First, it is assumed that there is a constant total body water pool in which the isotopes turn over. However, it is known that with certain conditions such as infancy or intense exercise, the body water pool may change because of increases or decreases in body mass. This change in body mass must be greater than 15%, however, to produce an error in the total energy expenditure measure of less than 1–2% [54].

Second, the rate of flux for carbon dioxide and water should remain constant under steady-state kinetics. However, because water intake and physical activity are episodic in nature, this rate of flux is not constant. By implementing the previously mentioned two-point sample collection method, an average carbon dioxide production rate can be obtained over the measurement period without encountering the daily fluctuations that will contribute to error [54].

Another assumption states that no carbon dioxide or water enters the body via the skin or lungs. However, when a subject is exposed to higher-than-normal levels of carbon dioxide, such as cigarette smoke, there may be an apparent increase in carbon dioxide production. Nonetheless, to produce a 3–6% error in the estimation of true carbon dioxide production, the person would have to smoke roughly three packs of cigarettes a day [54]. In addition, water vapor can

easily penetrate the lungs and skin to be directly absorbed into the body. However, Pinson and Langham [55] demonstrated that this type of exchange does not affect the calculation of carbon dioxide production, because the elimination rates of hydrogen and oxygen are proportional. Other assumptions of the method are associated with the isotopic dilution spaces and isotopic fractionations. These are beyond the scope of this chapter but are thoroughly reviewed by Schoeller [54] and Wolf [56].

b. Advantages and Disadvantages of Doubly Labeled Water. The DLW technique has numerous advantages that make it the ideal method for measuring total daily energy expenditure in a variety of populations. The advantages to the researcher and the subject are the ease of administration and the ability of the subject to engage in free-living activities during the measurement period. This is extremely advantageous in infants, young children, the elderly, and populations with disabilities that cannot be subjected to the rigorous testing involved in the measurement of oxygen consumption during various activities. The DLW technique provides the objective criterion measure necessary to validate more subjective estimates of energy expenditure such as activity logs and diet recalls. Most important, the method is accurate and has a precision of between 2 and 8% [54].

Although there are many advantages to the DLW technique, there are also drawbacks, namely, the expense of the stable isotope (approximately $500 to dose an average weight adult), periodic worldwide shortages of oxygen–18, and the expertise required to operate the highly sophisticated and costly mass spectrometer for analysis of the enrichments (Fig. 4; see color plate at the back of the book). The advantages and disadvantages of the DLW technique are highlighted in Table 2.

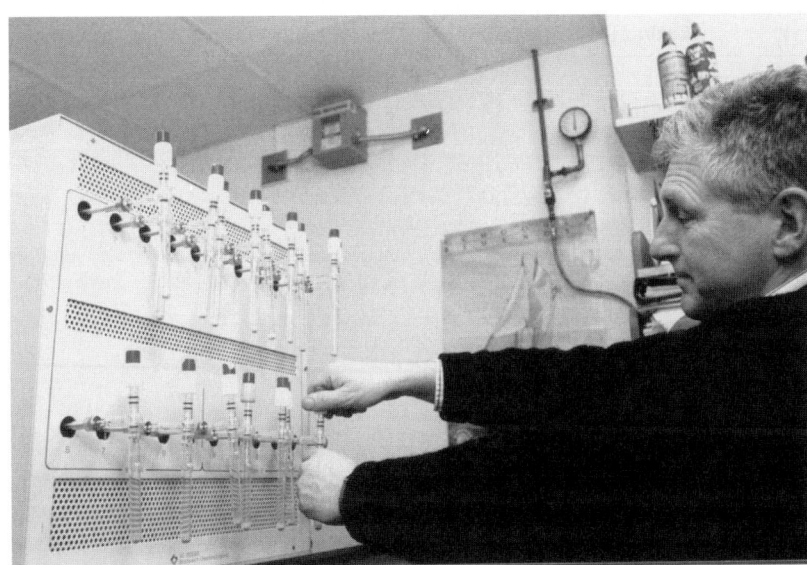

FIGURE 4 · Mass spectrometer used for the analysis of isotope enrichments in the DLW method.

TABLE 2 Advantages and Disadvantages of the Doubly Labeled Water Technique to Measure Total Energy Expenditure

Advantages	Disadvantages
Noninvasive, unobstrusive, and easily administered	Availability and expense of oxygen-18 (approximately $900 for 70-kg adult)
Measurement performed under free-living conditions over extended time period (7–14 days)	Reliance on isotope ratio mass spectrometry for analysis of samples
Accurate and precise (2–8%)	A direct measure of CO_2 production, and not energy expenditure, does not measure substrate oxidation
Can be used to estimate activity energy expenditure when combined with measurement of resting metabolic rate	Not suitable for large-scale epidemiological studies

B. Estimating Total Energy Expenditure

The introduction of the DLW technique in humans has produced a large and robust database of TEE measurements in a variety of populations. A meta-analysis of 574 DLW measurements helped to establish the average and range of habitual energy expenditures in different age and sex groups [57]. The data shown in Table 3 are compiled from healthy, free-living people aged 2–95 years. These data provide a frame of reference for energy needs in the general population and can be used to evaluate other estimates of energy expenditure. Special circumstances such as illness or enforced exertion were excluded from this database.

Due to the high cost of and small numbers of laboratories with the capacity to do DLW studies, clinicians continue to rely heavily on prediction equations to estimate energy requirements. As more measurements of TEE are conducted using doubly labeled water, increasingly accurate tools to estimate TEE should become available. In the meantime, clinicians and researchers typically use prediction equations to estimate energy requirements. The steps used to calculate total energy expenditure using prediction formulas are shown in Table 4.

C. Total Energy Expenditure in Special Populations

The number of studies using DLW to examine TEE in various disease states, physiological conditions, and across the

TABLE 3 Total Energy Expenditure across Age and Sex Groups from a Meta-Analysis of 574 Free-Living DLW Measurements

Age group (yr)	n	Age mean (yr)	TEE mean (kcal/day)	BMB mean (kcal/day)	Physical activity level factor
Females					
1–6	21	4.9	1316	861	1.57
7–12	24	9.2	1914	1148	1.68
13–17	26	14.8	2727	1603	1.73
18–29	89	24.4	2488	1483	1.70
30–39	76	33.8	2392	1435	1.68
40–64	47	51.6	2345	1388	1.69
65–74	24	69.1	2057	1268	1.62
>75	12	82.8	1459	981	1.48
Males					
1–6	29	4.7	1459	909	1.64
7–12	32	9.8	2345	1364	1.74
13–17	31	14.5	3373	1938	1.75
18–29	56	22.5	3301	1794	1.85
30–39	36	34.3	3421	1962	1.77
40–64	15	50.6	2751	1675	1.64
65–74	22	68.6	2637	1651	1.61
>75	34	80.8	2201	1435	1.54

TABLE 4   Estimating Total Energy Expenditure Using
Prediction Equations

1. Determine ideal body weight
2. Estimate resting metabolic rate (see Table 1)
3. Add factor for physical activity level (PAL)

   Factors for PAL based on doubly labeled water studies

Lifestyle and level of activity	Factor for PAL
Chair-bound or bed-bound	1.2
Seated work with no option of moving around and little or no strenuous leisure activity	1.4–1.5
Seated work with discretion and requirement to move around but little or no strenuous leisure activity	1.6–1.7
Standing work (e.g., housework, shop assistant)	1.8–1.9
Significant amounts of sport or strenuous leisure activity (30–60 minutes four to five times per week)	+0.3 (increment)
Strenuous work or highly active leisure	2.0–2.4

4. Add thermic effect of food (TEF) - 10% of RMR plus PAL
5. Sum equals the approximate total daily energy requirement

Source: Adapted from Shetty, P. S., Henry, C. J. K., Black, A. E., and Prentice, A. M. (1996). Energy requirements of adults: An update on basal metabolic rates and physical activity levels. *Eur. J. Clin. Nutr.* **50**(suppl 1), S11–S23.

life cycle have proliferated during the past decade. Hence, data are now available on energy expenditure during infancy [58], childhood [59], adolescence [60], and in the elderly [61, 62]. TEE during pregnancy and lactation has been well characterized in some elegant longitudinal studies [18, 63]. In addition TEE has been examined in adults and children with obesity [64, 65], burns [66], cerebral palsy [67], Down syndrome [68], HIV/AIDs [69], and Alzheimer's disease [70]. The effects of these various conditions on energy requirements are highlighted in Table 5.

IV. RECOMMENDED ENERGY INTAKES

Classically the Recommended Dietary Allowances (RDAs) have been used as a guide to determine energy intakes for groups of normal, healthy people. The last RDA for energy was set in 1989. RDAs for all nutrients except energy are set at levels well above those estimated to minimize the occurrence of deficiency syndromes. For energy, this obviously is not the case. Recommendations for energy have always been set as an average of energy requirements for a population group. In the past recommended energy intakes have relied heavily on data from dietary surveys that estimate energy intake. This is based on the assumption that people are in energy balance at the time of measurement and that the estimates of energy intake are valid. A large body of evidence

TABLE 5   Effects of Disease States and Physiological Conditions on Energy
Requirements: Results from Doubly Labeled Water Studies

Disease or condition	Effect on energy requirements	Explanation
Obesity	Increased	Increased fat-free mass coupled with decreased physical activity
Burned children	No change	Increased resting metabolic rate counteracts decreased physical activity
Anorexia	Increased	To counteract increased physical activity with underweight and hypometabolism
HIV/AIDS	No change	Energy expenditure not elevated, reduced energy intake causes weight loss
Cerebral palsy	Relative to individual	High interindividual variation in energy expended in physical activity; ambulation status an important predictor.
Alzheimer's	No change	Energy expenditure not elevated, low-energy intake predisposes to weight loss
Spinal cord injury	Decreased	Lower energy expended in physical activity, resting metabolic rate, and thermic effect of food
Pregnancy	Relative to individual	No prediction of metabolic response
Lactation	Increased	Energy cost of milk production partially offset by reduced physical activity

now demonstrates that self-reported estimates of food intake do not provide accurate or unbiased estimates of people's energy intake and that underreporting of food intake is pervasive in dietary studies [71]. Underreporting is discussed in detail in Chapter 5. It is anticipated that the forthcoming dietary reference intakes for energy will rely heavily on objective measurements of energy expenditure in free-living people to provide more accurate recommendations for energy intake in different age and sex groups and during various physiological conditions (e.g., pregnancy and lactation). In addition, as the prevalence of obesity has reached epidemic proportions in the United States, people's energy expended in physical activity has become so low that it may become increasingly difficult to meet micronutrient needs on the energy intakes required to keep people in energy balance. Hence, it will become increasingly imperative that emphasis be placed on increased energy expended in physical activity for the maintenance of optimal health.

References

1. World Health Organization. (1985). Energy and protein requirements. *WHO Tech. Rep. Ser.* p. 724.
2. Schoeller, D. A., and Racette, S. B. (1990). A review of field techniques for the assessment of energy expenditure. *J. Nutr.* 120:1492–1495.
3. Hildreth, H. G., and Johnson, R. K. (1995). The doubly labeled water technique for the determination of human energy requirements. *Nutr. Today* **30**, 254–260.
4. Poehlman, E. T. (1993). Regulation of energy expenditure in aging humans. *Geriatr. Biosci.* **41**, 552–559.
5. Goran, M. I., Kaskoun, M., and Johnson, R. K. (1994). Determinants of resting energy expenditure in young children. *J. Pediatr.* **125**, 362–367.
6. Poehlman, E. T. (1989). A review: Exercise and its influence on resting energy metabolism in man. *Med. Sci. Sports Exerc.* **21**, 515–525.
7. Ravussin, E., Lillioja, S., Anderson, T. E., Christin, L., and Bogardus, C. (1988). Determinants of 24-hour energy expenditure in man. *J. Clin. Invest.* **78**, 1568–1578.
8. Weinsier, R. L., Schutz, Y., and Bracco, D. (1992). Reexamination of the relationship of resting metabolic rate to fat-free mass and to the metabolically active components of fat-free mass in humans. *Am. J. Clin. Nutr.* **55**, 790–794.
9. Svendsen, O. L., Haarbo, J., Hassager, C., Christiansen, C. (1993). Accuracy of measurements of body composition by dual-energy-ray absorptiometry *in vivo. Am. J. Clin. Nutr.* **57**, 605–608.
10. Wurmser, H., Laessle, R., Jacob, K., Langhard, S., Uhl, H., Angst, A., Muller, A., and Pirke, K. M. (1998). Resting metabolic rate in preadolescent girls at high risk of obesity. *Int. J. Obes. Relat. Metab. Disord.* **22**, 793–799.
11. Goran, M. I., Nagy, T. R., Gower, B. A., Mazariegos, M., Solomons, N., Hood, V., and Johnson, R. K. (1998). Influence of sex, seasonality, ethnicity, and geographic location on the components of total energy expenditure in young children: Implications for energy requirements. *Am. J. Clin. Nutr.* **68**, 675–682.
12. Ferraro, R. T., Lillioja, S., Fontvielle, A. M., Rising, R., Bogardus, C., and Ravussin, E. (1992). Lower sedentary metabolic rate in women compared to men. *J. Clin. Invest.* **90**, 780–784.
13. Arciero, P. J., Goran, M. I., and Poehlman, E. T. (1993). Resting metabolic rate is lower in women compared to men. *J. Appl. Physiol.* **75**, 2514–2520.
14. Piers, L. S., Soare, M. J., McCormack, L. M., and O'Dea, K. (1998). Is there evidence for an age-related reduction in metabolic rate? *J. Appl. Physiol.* **85**, 2196–2204.
15. Horton, T., and Geissler, C. (1994). Effect of habitual exercise on daily energy expenditure and metabolic rate during standardized activity. *Am. J. Clin. Nutr.* **59**, 13–19.
16. Jorgensen, J. O., Vahl, N., Dall, R., and Christiansen, J. S. (1998). Resting metabolic rate in healthy adults: Relation to growth hormone status and leptin levels. *Metab. Clin. Exper.* **47**, 1134–1139.
17. Webb, P. (1986). 24-Hour energy expenditure and the menstrual cycle. *Am. J. Clin. Nutr.* **44**, 614–619.
18. Goldberg, G. R., Prentice, A. M., Coward, W. A., Davies, H. L., Murgatroyd, P. R., Sawyer, M. B., Ashford, J., and Black, A. E. (1993). Longitudinal assessment of energy expenditure in pregnancy by the doubly labeled water method. *Am. J. Clin. Nutr.* **57**, 494–505.
19. Simonson, D. C., and DeFronzo, R. A. (1990). Indirect calorimetry: Methodological and interpretative problems. *J. Appl. Physiol.* **258**, 399–411.
20. Berke, E. M., Gardner, A. W., Goran, M. I., and Poehlman, E. T. (1992). Resting metabolic rate and the influence of the pretesting environment. *Am. J. Clin. Nutr.* **55**, 626–629.
21. Frankenfield, D. C., Muth, E. R., and Rowe, W. A. (1998). The Harris–Benedict studies of human basal metabolism: History and limitations. *J. Am. Diet. Assoc.* **98**, 439–445.
22. Goran, M. I., Broemeling, L., Herndon, D. N., Peters, D. J., and Wolfe, R. R. (1991). Estimating energy requirements in burned children: A new approach derived from measurements of resting energy expenditure. *Am. J. Clin. Nutr.* **54**, 35–40.
23. Krahn, D. D., Rock, C., Dechert, R. E., Nairn, K. K., and Hasse, S. A. (1993). Changes in resting energy expenditure and body composition in anorexia nervosa patients during refeeding. *J. Am. Diet. Assoc.* **93**, 433–438.
24. Bandini, L. G., Puelzi-Quinn, H. M., Morelli, J. A., and Fukagawa, N. K. (1995). Estimation of energy requirements in persons with severe central nervous system impairment. *J. Pediatr.* **126**, 828–832.
25. Johnson, R. K., Goran, M. I., Ferrar, M. S., and Poehlman, E. T. (1996). Athetosis increases resting metabolic rate in adults with cerebral palsy. *J. Am. Diet. Assoc.* **96**, 145–148.
26. Goldberg, G. R., Prentice, A. M., Coward, W. A., Davies, H. I., Murgatroyd, P. R., Wensing, C., Black, A. E., Harding, M., and Sawyer, M. (1993). Longitudinal assessment of energy expenditure in pregnancy by the doubly labeled water method. *Am. J. Clin. Nutr.* **57**, 494–505.
27. Spaaij, C., van Raaij, J., de Groot, L., ven der Heijden, L., Boeholt, H. A., and Hautvast, J. C. (1994). Effect of lactation on resting metabolic rate and on diet- and work-induced thermogenesis. *Am. J. Clin. Nutr.* **59**, 42–47.
28. Arciero, P. J., Goran, M. I., Gardner, A. M., Ades, P. A., Tyzbir, R. S., and Poehlman, E. T. (1993). A practical equation to

predict resting metabolic rate in older females. *J. Am. Geriatr. Soc.* **41**, 389–395.

29. Arciero, P. J., Goran, M. I., Gardner, A. M., Ades, P. A., and Poehlman, E. T. (1993). A practical equation to predict resting metabolic rate in older men. *Metab. Clin. Exper.* **42**, 950–957.

30. Poehlman, E. T., and Horton, E. S. (1998). Energy need: Assessment and requirements in humans. *In* "Modern Nutrition in Health and Disease" (A. S. Bloch and M. E. Shils, Eds.). Baltimore: Williams & Wilkins.

31. Prentice, A. M. (1995). All calories are not equal. *Int. Dialogue Carbohydr.* **5**(4), 1–3.

32. McCrory, P. (1994). Energy balance, food intake and obesity. *In* "Exercise and Obesity" (A. P. Hills, M. L. Wahlqvist, Eds.). London: Smith-Gordon and Co.

33. Dulloo, A. G., Geissler, C. A., Horton, T., Collins, A., and Miller, D. S. (1989). Normal caffeine consumption: Influence on thermogenesis and daily energy expenditure in lean and post-obese human volunteers. *Am. J. Clin. Nutr.* **49**, 44–50.

34. Hofstetter, A. (1986). Increased 24-hour energy expenditure in cigarette smokers. *N. Engl. J. Med.* **314**, 79–82.

35. Kriska, A. M., and Caspersen, C. J. (1997). Introduction to a collection of physical activity questionnaires. *Med. Sci. Sports Exer.* **29**, S5–S9.

36. Pate, R. R., Prat, M., Blair, S. N., Haskell, W. L., Macera, C. A., Bouchard, C., Buchner, D., Ettinger, W., Heath, G. W., King, A. C., Kirska, A., Leon, A. S., Marcus, B. H., Morris, J., Paffenbarger, R. S., Patrick, K., Pollack, M. L., Rippe, J. M., Sallis, J., and Wilmore, J. H. (1995). Physical activity and public health—A recommendation from the Centers for Disease Control and Prevention and the American College of Sports Medicine. *J. Am. Med. Assoc.* **273**, 402–407.

37. Levine, J. A., Eberhardt, N. L., and Jensen, M. D. (1999). Role of nonexercise activity thermogenesis in resistance to fat gain in humans. *Science* 283(5399), 212–214.

38. Levine, J., Baukol, P., and Pavlidis, I. (1999). The energy expended in chewing gum. *N. Engl. J. Med.* **341**(27), 2100.

39. Food and Nutrition Board, National Research Council, National Academy of Sciences. (1989). "Recommended Dietary Allowances," 10th ed. National Academy Press, Washington, DC.

40. Poehlman, E. T. (1998). Effect of exercise on daily energy needs in older individuals. *Am. J. Clin. Nutr.* **68**, 997–998.

41. Bunyard, L. B., Katzel, L. I., Busby-Whitehead, J., Wu, Z., and Goldberg, A. P. (1998). Energy requirements of middle-aged men are modifiable by physical activity. *Am. J. Clin. Nutr.* **68**, 1136–1142.

42. Starling, R. D., Matthews, D. E., Ades, P. A., and Poehlman, E. T. (1999). Assessment of physical activity in older individuals: A doubly labeled water study. *J. Appl. Physiol.* **86**(6), 2090–2096.

43. Westerterp, K. R. (1999). Physical activity assessment with accelerometers. *Int. J. Obes.* **23**, S45–S49.

44. Johnson, R. K., Russ, J., and Goran, M. I. (1998). Physical activity related energy expenditure in children by doubly labeled water as compared with the Caltrac accelerometer. *Int. J. Obes.* **22**, 1046–1052.

45. Sallis, J. F., Buono, J. F., Roby, J. L., Carlson, D., and Nelson, J. (1989). The Caltrac accelerometer as a physical activity monitor for school-age children. *Med. Sci. Sports Exer.* **22**, 698–703.

46. Livingstone, M. B. E. (1997). Heart-rate monitoring: The answer for assessing energy expenditure and physical activity in population studies? *Br. J. Nutr.* **78**, 869–871.

47. Wareham, N. J., Hennings, S. J., Prentice, A. M., and Day, N. E. (1997). Feasibility of heart-rate monitoring to estimate total level and pattern of energy expenditure in a population-based epidemiological study: The Ely young cohort feasibility study 1994–5. *Br. J. Nutr.* **87**, 889–900.

48. Kriska, A. M., and Caspersen, C. J., Eds. (1997). A collection of physical activity questionnaires for health-related research. *Med. Sci. Sports Exer.* **29**, S3–S205.

49. Poehlman, E. T. (1992). Energy expenditure and requirements in aging humans. *J. Nutr.* **122**, 2057–2065.

50. Schoeller, D. A., and van Santen, E. (1982). Measurement of energy expenditure in humans by the doubly labeled water method. *J. Appl. Physiol.* **53**, 955–959.

51. Lifson, N., Gordon, G. B., Visscher, M. B., and Nier, A. O. (1949). The fate of utilized molecular oxygen and the source of heavy oxygen of respiratory carbon dioxide, studied with the aid of heavy oxygen. *J. Biol. Chem.* **180**, 803–811.

52. Lifson, N., Gordon, G. B., and McClintock, R. (1955). Measurement of total carbon dioxide production by means of D_2O^{18}. *J. Appl. Physiol.* **7**, 704–710.

53. Welles, S. (1990). Two-point vs. multipoint sample collection for the analysis of energy expenditure by use of the double labeled water method. *Am. J. Clin. Nutr.* **52**, 1134–1138.

54. Schoeller, D. A. (1988). Measurement of energy expenditure in free-living humans by using doubly labeled water. *J. Nutr.* **118**, 1278–1289.

55. Pinson, E. A., and Langham, W. H. (1957). Physiology and toxicology of tritium in man. *J. Appl. Physiol.* **10**, 108–126.

56. Wolf, R. R. (1992). "Radioactive and Stable Isotope Tracers in Biomedicine Principles and Practice of Kinetic Analysis," pp. 207–234. Wiley-Liss, New York.

57. Black, A. E., Coward, W. A., Cole, R. J., and Prentice, A. M. (1996). Human energy expenditure in affluent societies: An analysis of 574 doubly-labeled water measurements. *Eur. J. Clin. Nutr.* **50**, 72–92.

58. Davies, P. S. W. (1998). Energy requirements for growth and development in infancy. *Am. J. Clin. Nutr.* **68**, 939S–943S.

59. Goran, M. I., Gower, B. A., Nagy, T. R., and Johnson, R. K. (1998). Developmental changes in energy expenditure and physical activity in children: Evidence for a decline in physical activity in girls before puberty. *Pediatrics* **101**, 887–891.

60. Bratteby, L. E., Snadhagen, B., Fan, H., Enghardt, H., and Samuelson, G. (1998). Total energy expenditure and physical activity as assessed by the doubly labeled water method in Swedish adolescents in whom energy intake was underestimated by 7-d records. *Am. J. Clin. Nutr.* **67**, 905–911.

61. Goran, M. I., and Poehlman, E. T. (1992). Total energy expenditure and energy requirements in healthy elderly persons. *Metabolism* **41**, 744–753.

62. Roberts, S. B., Young, V. R., Fuss, P., Heyman, M. B., Fiatarone, M., Dallal, G. E., Cortiella, J., and Evans, W. J. (1992). What are the dietary energy needs of elderly adults? *Int. J. Obes.* **16**, 969–976.

63. Goldberg, G. R., Prentice, A. M., Coward, W. A., Davies, H. L., Murgatroyd, P. R., Wensing, C., Black, A. E., Harding, M., and Sawyer, M. (1993). Longitudinal assessment of energy

expenditure in pregnancy by the doubly labeled water method. *Am. J. Clin. Nutr.* **57,** 494–505.

64. Lichtman, S. W., Krystyna, P., Berman, E. R., Pestone, M., Dowling, H., Offenbacher, E., Weisel, H., Heshka, S., Matthews, D. E., Heymsfield, S. B. (1992). Discrepancy between self-reported and actual caloric intake and exercise in obese subjects. *N. Engl. J. Med.* **327,** 1893–1998.

65. Goran, M. I., Shewchuk, R., Bower, B. A., Nagy, T. R., Carpenter, W. H., and Johnson, R. K. (1998). Longitudinal changes in fatness in white children: No effect of childhood energy expenditure. *Am. J. Clin. Nutr.* **67,** 309–316.

66. Goran, M. I., Peters, E. J., Herndon, D. N., and Wolfe, R. R. (1990). Total energy expenditure in burned children using the doubly labeled water technique. *Am. J. Physiol.* **259**(Pt 1), E576–E585.

67. Johnson, R. K., Hildreth, H. G., Contompasis, S. H., and Goran, M. I. (1997). Total energy expenditure in adults with cerebral palsy as assessed by double labeled water. *J. Am. Diet. Assoc.* **97,** 966–970.

68. Luke, A., Roizen, N. J., Sutton, M., and Schoeller, D. A. (1994). Energy expenditure in children with Down syndrome: Correcting metabolic rate for movement. *J. Pediatr.* **125,** 829–838.

69. Macallan, D. C., Noble, C., Baldwin, C., Jebb, S. A., Prentice, A. M., and Coward A. (1995). Energy expenditure and wasting in human immunodeficiency virus infection. *N. Engl. J. Med.* **333**(2), 83–88.

70. Toth, M. J., Goran, M. I., Carpenter, W. H., Newhouse, P., Rosen, C. J., and Poehlman, E. T. (1997). Daily energy expenditure in free-living non-institutionalized Alzheimer's patients: A doubly labeled water study. *Am. Acad. Neurol.* **48,** 997–1002.

71. Johnson, R. K. (2000). What are people *really* eating? *Nutr. Today,* **35,** 40–46.

CHAPTER 3

Physical Assessment

EDWARD SALTZMAN[1,2] AND KRIS M. MOGENSEN[2]

[1]*Tufts University, Boston, Massachusetts*
[2]*New England Medical Center, Boston, Massachusetts*

I. INTRODUCTION

The purpose of clinical evaluation is to assess current health and nutritional status, to identify those nutritional and health factors that determine current status, and to provide prognostic data for risk of further nutrition-related morbidity. The mutual influence of nutrition and disease on each other is critical, and at times distinguishing between the ill effects of disease and malnutrition may be difficult or impossible.

Assessment is guided by the symptoms and signs of disease. Risk for disease and etiologic factors is often revealed by demographic, occupational, and socioeconomic conditions as well as by family histories. On a population level, or in apparently healthy persons with low risk, screening may be used in lieu of a more detailed and resource-intensive assessment. The results of screening may indicate the need for further assessment, and several screening tools have such staged approaches, as discussed later in this chapter. Individuals with existing, or at risk for, nutritional compromise or disease should undergo a more detailed assessment. Indications and tools for screening in contrast to detailed assessment have been reviewed in detail elsewhere [1].

The term *malnutrition* is often used to describe protein energy malnutrition, but micronutrient malnutrition occurs in multiple disease states and must also be assessed. Nutritional disorders of excess should also be considered malnutrition and are of increasing importance. Such disorders include obesity, diets characterized by imbalanced macronutrient intake, and micronutrient toxicity induced by food faddism or supplement use.

II. COMPONENTS OF CLINICAL ASSESSMENT

Clinical assessment of nutritional status includes the clinical and nutritional history, assessment of anthropometric parameters, physical examination, and assessment of functional status. Although some elements of the clinical evaluation are relatively insensitive or nonspecific indicators of nutritional disorders, it is these clinical observations that stimulate further confirmatory measures, such as detailed assessment of diet and appropriate diagnostic tests. Indices that combine historical, anthropometric, functional, and biochemical parameters have been developed to improve sensitivity and specificity in the diagnosis of malnutrition.

The nutritional and medical histories address details of the present complaint or illness, body weight change, and the past medical history. A review of organ systems to elicit relevant clinical factors not directly related to the present illness should also be conducted. Medication use should be reviewed, and in hospitalized patients, prehospitalization medications should also be included. The nutritional history must also address the spectrum of behaviors and physiologic functions necessary to maintain adequate nutritional status, including appetite and thirst, and the abilities to procure, prepare and ingest food. Socioeconomic and psychosocial factors may figure prominently in nutritional status and should not be neglected.

Relevant medications include prescription and over-the-counter medications, vitamin and mineral supplements, and herbal preparations. Although it is estimated that 40% of the U. S. population takes at least one vitamin or mineral supplement [2], many do not consider nutritional supplements to be medications and direct questioning may be necessary to elicit this history. Medications interfere with nutritional status by multiple mechanisms, including drug-related alterations in appetite, taste, thirst, nutrient absorption, nutrient metabolism, or excretion. Many medications induce changes in bowel function, which in turn may influence intake. Table 1 describes nutritional effects of some commonly used medications.

Physical examination may reveal etiologic factors contributing to malnutrition or may reveal manifestations of malnutrition. Unfortunately, significant physical examination findings often occur only late in the course of malnutrition. Also, many findings associated with micronutrient malnutrition such as angular stomatitis, glossitis, and dermatitis are nonspecific. The reason for this lack of specificity is twofold. First, deficiencies of several micronutrients may result in similar signs; second, micronutrient deficiencies often do not occur in isolation, such that physical findings may reflect multiple deficiencies. Use of biochemical tests can be used to diagnose specific deficiencies if indicated.

Anthropometric parameters can be used to describe the body as a whole or to subdivide the body into compartments.

TABLE 1   Common Medications and Potential Effects on Nutrient Status

Class (specific example)	Effect
Amphetamines	↓ Appetite/weight
Anorexiants	↓ Appetite/weight
Antibiotics (*N*-methylthiotetrazole sidechains)	↓ Vitamin K function
Anticonvulsants (phenytoin, phenobarbitol)	↓ calcium absorption, ↓ vitamin D, bone loss, ↓ folate levels
Antipsychotics (clozapine)	↑ Appetite/weight
Bile acid sequestrants	↓ Vitamins A, D, E, K absorption
Corticosteroids	↑ Appetite/fat mass/weight, hyperglycemia, ↓ lean mass, ↓ vitamin D, ↓ calcium, bone loss, ↓ vitamin B_6 levels (significance unclear)
Diuretics	↓ Potassium, ↓ magnesium, ↓ thiamin, ↓ sodium, ↑ calcium (thiazides)
Ethanol (abuse)	↓ Thiamin, ↓ folate, ↓ riboflavin, ↓ vitamin B_6, ↓ vitamin D, ↓ vitamin A
Insulin	↑ Appetite/weight
Isoniazid	↓ Vitamin B_6, ↓ niacin, ↓ vitamin D (significance unclear)
Lithium	↑ Appetite/weight
Methotrexate	↓ Folate
Orlistat	↓ Vitamins A, D, E, K absorption
Proton pump inhibitors	↓ Vitamin B_{12}
Selective serotonin reuptake inhibitors	↓ or ↑ Appetite/weight
Sulfasalazine	↓ Folate
Sulfonylureas	↑ Appetite/weight
Theophylline	↓ Appetite/weight
Tricyclic antidepressants	↑ Appetite/weight

Anthropometric data can be utilized directly (such as body weight) to estimate lean or fat mass, or to predict energy and protein needs.

Functional assessment, which is based on measures of strength, mobility, or function, allows semiquantitative or quantitative evaluation of processes that are indicative of current nutritional status and risk for nutritional compromise. As discussed below, functional parameters correlate with other measures of nutritional status and may predict morbidity in ill or malnourished patients.

III. ANTHROPOMETRIC ASSESSMENT

Anthropometric measurements describe or quantify basic physical characteristics, and include height, weight, circumferences of certain body parts, and skinfold thickness. Assessment of these parameters allows comparison to values in the same individual to monitor change over time, or to reference values, which can be used to classify nutritional status.

A. Height

Measurement of height is necessary to estimate ideal body weight or desirable body weight, body mass index (BMI), and is used in the calculation of body composition and energy requirements. Height should be measured when pos-

sible and is best obtained by a stadiometer. Vertical height decreases with aging as a result vertebral bone loss, vertebral compression fractures, and thinning of intervertebral discs and weight-bearing cartilage. Height begins to decline at approximately age 30 years for both men and women and accelerates with age; in one longitudinal series, between the ages of 30 and 80 years, women lost 8 cm and men lost 5 cm [3]. Loss of vertebral mass and disc compression may induce kyphosis (curvature with backward convexity of the spine), which will reduce measured height.

When height cannot be accurately measured, such as in acutely ill or immobilized patients, or in those with severe osteoporotic changes, alternatives include self-reported height, estimated height, or surrogate methods to estimate height. Self-reported heights are less accurate than measured heights, as men tend to overreport and women tend to underreport height [4]. Self-reported height is more accurate, however, than clinicians' estimates of height. Coe and coworkers [5] have reported that height tends to be overestimated by visual exam of supine patients. In this study, accuracy of visual estimation of height was better for taller patients compared to shorter patients, and the authors propose that the taller patients were closer to the length of the beds in which they were lying, thus making it easier to approximate height in those cases [5].

Arm span and knee height correlate with vertical height, but are subject to fewer age-related changes in stature and

TABLE 2   Recommended Equations for the Prediction of Stature

Group	Age	Equation	Reference
White men	18–60	1.88 (knee height) + 71.85	[92]
	17–67	2.31 (knee height) + 51.1	[93]
	60–80	2.08 (knee height) + 59.01	[9]
	17–67	2.30 (knee height) − 0.063 (age) + 54.9	[93]
	17–67	0.762 (armspan) + 40.7	[93]
Black men	18–60	1.79 (knee height) + 73.42	[92]
	60–80	1.37 (knee height) + 95.79	[9]
White women	18–60	1.87 (knee height) − 0.06 (age) + 70.25	[92]
	22–71	1.84 (knee height) + 70.2	[93]
	22–71	1.91 (knee height) − 0.098 (age) + 71.3	[93]
	60–80	1.91 (knee height) − 0.17 (age) + 75	[9]
	22–71	0.693 (armspan) + 50.3	[93]
Black women	18–60	1.86 (knee height) − 0.06 (age) + 68.1	[92]
	60–80	1.96 (knee height) + 58.72	[9]

Source: Adapted from Heymsfield, S. B. (1999). Nutritional assessment of malnutrition by anthropometric methods. *In* "Modern Nutrition in Health and Disease" M. E. Shils, J. A. Olson, M. Shike, and A. C. Ross, Eds.), pp. 903–921. Williams and Wilkins, Baltimore, MD.

are less influenced by impediments to the measurement of vertical height such as disability or frailty [6–9]. Equations to predict vertical height from measured arm span or knee height have been derived by regression analysis, and these specific formulas are available for use in several age, gender, and ethnic groups (Table 2). Arm span, which is the entire distance from the tip of the middle finger of one hand to the other, can be measured with arms stretched at right angles to the body, with the measuring tape crossing in front of the clavicles. Frail or debilitated persons may require assistance to maintain the correct position for measurement [6, 8]. Half arm span (the distance from the sternal notch to the tip of the middle finger of one hand) can also be measured and then doubled to determine arm span. Knee height is best measured with specialized calipers, and can be performed either in sitting or recumbent patients, making this useful in most ambulatory and hospital settings. Use of knee height or arm span to estimate vertical height may be useful in clinical as well as research situations [3, 7] for individuals who cannot stand, who are debilitated, or who have experienced loss of height.

B. Weight

Loss of body weight in the setting of starvation or illness is a marker of protein energy malnutrition and is associated with increased risk of morbidity and mortality [10–16]. In patients with cancer undergoing chemotherapy, loss of 5% or more of usual body weight was associated with impaired functional status and significantly decreased median survival lengths compared to patients without weight loss [11]. In

hospitalized patients with a variety of gastrointestinal, infectious, and neoplastic diseases, protein energy malnutrition at admission was associated with an approximately twofold risk of subsequent complications [17]. More than 60 years ago, Studley [12] recognized that unintentional weight loss of 20% or more of usual body weight prior to surgery for peptic ulcer significantly increased risk of postoperative mortality. Others have confirmed that protein energy malnutrition preceding surgery increases risk of postoperative complications [13, 14, 18, 19]. Patients who have lost 10–20% of initial body weight over 6 months and have associated physiological defects, or those who have lost 20% or more over 6 months, should be considered at high risk [20, 21]. Involuntary change in weight may better predict risk for protein energy malnutrition than does absolute weight [14–16, 20, 22].

Adequate store of lean and fat mass may act as buffers against chronic protein energy malnutrition, but will not prevent protein energy malnutrition in acute illness. Despite high levels of energy reserves and expanded lean body mass, obese patients still experience protein energy malnutrition when acutely ill [23]. In acutely ill obese patients, body weight may be "adjusted" or used in prediction equations to guide provision of energy and medications [23–25].

Ideally, body weight should be measured by use of calibrated beam-type or electronic scales. However, clinical situations at times dictate use of alternatives, such as a calibrated bed scale, chair scale, or wheelchair scale. To monitor changes in weight over time, use of the same scale is highly recommended given variability between scales.

TABLE 3 Classification of Weight by Body Mass Index

| | Grade | BMI (kg/m^2) | Disease risk relative to normal weight and waist circumference (inches) | |
			Men ≤40 Women ≤35	>40 >35
Underweight	III	<16		
	II	16–16.99		
	I	17–18.49		
Normal		18.5–24.9		
Overweight		25–29.9	Increased	High
Obesity	I	30–34.9	High	Very high
	II	35–39.9	Very high	Very high
	III	≥40	Extremely high	Extremely high

Source: Adapted from Ferro-Luzzi, A., Sette, S., Franklin, M., and James, W. P. (1992). A simplified approach of assessing adult chronic energy deficiency. *Eur. J. Clin. Nutr.* **46**, 173–186; and Nation Heart, Lung, and Blood Institute. (1998). Clinical guidelines on the identification, evaluation, and treatment of overweight and obesity in adults—The evidence report. *Obes. Res.* **6**(Suppl 2), 51S–209S.

Self-reported weights are often inaccurate; overweight women and men tend to underestimate weight, while men of lesser weight tend to overestimate [4]. Use of a single self-reported weight is also an insensitive measure of weight change in ill patients, because weight loss in approximately one-third of patients may be missed [26]. In cases where a person cannot be weighed, the clinician may estimate weight, an inaccurate practice that, although improving with experience [5], should be discouraged.

Gains and losses in weight should be documented, and contemporaneous factors should be sought to explain weight change. Recognizing trends in weight with intake and the behavioral or emotional determinants is essential to effect lasting change in intake patterns. Temporally demarcated gains in weight often reveal illness, psychosocial, or life changes, or may be associated with medication initiation or cessation. Precipitous changes in weight are usually due to alterations in body water due to conditions such as heart failure, cirrhosis, or renal failure. Thus, the presence of edema or ascites should be noted, as should clinically relevant data such as the presence of dehydration or volume overload.

C. Weight for Height

For comparison to population norms, weight must be expressed relative to height. Historically, ideal body weight or desirable body weight has been defined based on actuarial data of weight for height, often with adjustment for frame size. As with all predictive methods, these tables will best apply to members of the population from which the data were derived, and thus may have reduced applicability to diverse ethnic groups, older adults, or those with chronic illnesses [22, 27]. Another limitation of some of these tables is that frame size must be determined. Frame size can be determined by mea-

surement of elbow or wrist breadth or of wrist circumference, which requires use of specialized calipers or measuring tape.

Calculation of percent ideal body weight allows determination of the relative degree of over- or underweight. In practice, relative weight outside the range of 90–120% of ideal body weight is considered clinically important. Ideal body weight is also utilized in the setting of obesity or volume overload for the calculation of adjusted body weight, on which energy needs or drug dosing may be estimated.

Body weight may be expressed as a function of height and takes the general form: weight/height^x [28]. Now widely used is the body mass index (BMI) or Quetelet's index, kg/m^2. Use of the BMI to assess weight for height in individuals, with the classifications found in Table 3, is consistent with current recommendations of the National Institutes of Health [29] and World Health Organization [16].

BMI correlates with body fat [28, 30], although a linear relationship is not observed throughout the range of BMI (Fig. 1). While BMI correlates well with body fat for populations, interpretation in individuals must include consideration of clinical and other factors. For example, BMI may be elevated despite relatively low levels of body fat in those with edema or in bodybuilders. Similarly, the same low BMI may be observed in a patient who has experienced significant loss of weight and in a long-distance runner who is healthy and weight-stable.

Both low and high BMI correlate with morbidity and mortality [16, 31–33]. Low levels of BMI are also associated with lethargy and diminished work productivity [16]. The lowest survivable levels of BMI, as suggested by observations in starvation, famine, and anorexia nervosa, or by theoretical models, have been estimated to be 12–13 kg/m^2 [28, 34]. When weight loss is rapid or associated with illness, morbidity and mortality can occur at any level of BMI.

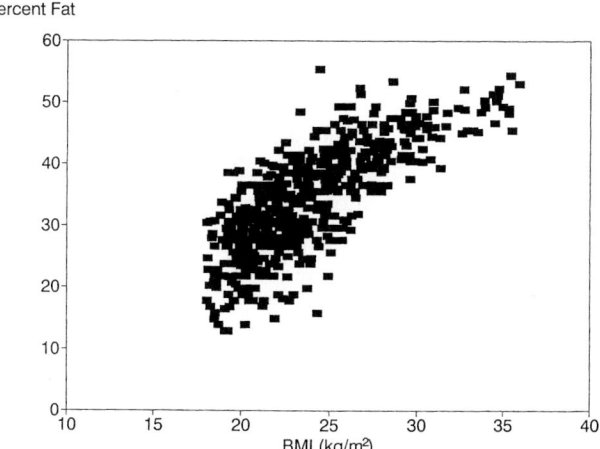

Percent Fat

FIGURE 1 Relationship between BMI and fat mass in women. [Reproduced with permission from Heysmfield, S. B., Tighe, A., and Wang, Z.-M. (1994). Nutritional assessment by anthropometric and biochemical methods. *In* "Modern Nutrition in Health and Disease" (M.E. Shils, J.A. Olson, and M. Shike, Eds.), p. 824. Lea and Febiger, Malvern, PA.]

A potential problem with use of BMI is that it does not account for body composition changes associated with aging, as body fat content may vary considerably in older and younger persons with the same BMI. Also, ethnic differences in body composition will not be reflected by BMI. Despite these potential problems, BMI remains an easily calculated and clinically useful method of classifying weight relative to height. In individuals, BMI can be used as a rough

indicator of nutritional status, and at its extreme ranges indicates nutritional compromise.

D. Circumferences and Skinfold Thickness Measurements

Measurement of circumferences of the trunk or limbs provides descriptive information about underlying lean and fat mass [28]. Skinfold measurements describe the amount of subcutaneous fat when the skin at various sites is "pinched" by specialized calipers. The sites at which these measurements are conducted are illustrated in Fig. 2. Measurements of circumference or skinfold thickness from a single body site have been used to assess protein energy status [16], but are likely to be influenced by the interindividual variability in body composition. Measurements at multiple sites reduce the potential contribution of this variability. As such, single site measurements are better used to follow trends over time in an individual than for comparison to normative standards. A number of investigators have related combinations of circumference or skinfold thickness measurements at multiple sites to other measures of body composition such as hydrodensitometry, dual energy x-ray absorptiometry (DXA), or calculated axial tomogrophy scanning to develop prediction equations for lean and fat mass for the whole body or specific segments [28, 35, 36].

Measurement of circumferences and skinfold thickness may be influenced by several factors, including age, sex, gender, ethnicity, and under- or overhydration [37]. Specific reference data for the individual or population should be

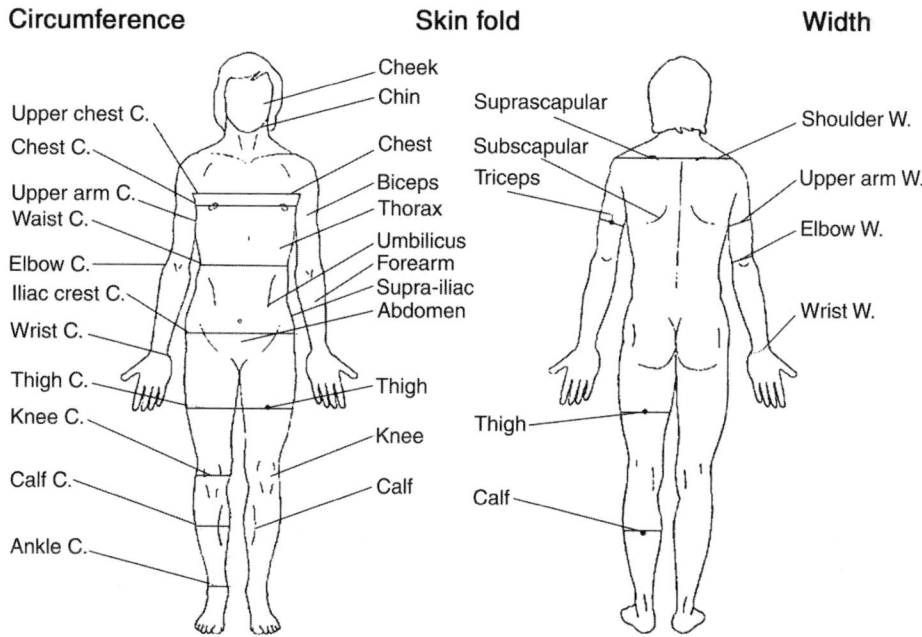

FIGURE 2 Body sites for measurement of circumferences, skinfold thickness, and widths. [From Wang, J., Thornton, J. C., Kolesnik, S., and Pierson, R. N., Jr. (2000). Anthropometry in body composition. An overview. *Ann. N.Y. Acad. Sci.* **904**, 317–326.]

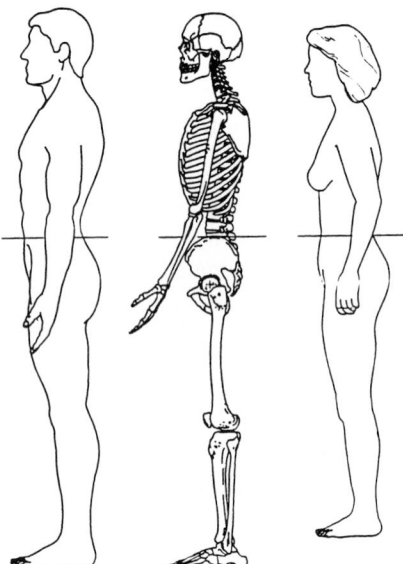

FIGURE 3 Landmarks for measurement of waist circumference. [From Nation Heart, Lung, and Blood Institute. (1998). Clinical guidelines on the identification, evaluation, and treatment of overweight and obesity in adults—The evidence report. *Obes. Res.* **6**(Suppl 2), 51S–209S.]

used when possible. Most reference data have been developed in healthy populations. Limited reference data exist for hospitalized patients; however, acute illness is associated with widely fluctuating perturbations in body water such that generalizable reference data may never be obtainable. Upper body measurements may be preferable in those individuals with evidence of edema or ascites, because the upper body is less likely to accumulate excess body water. Measurements obtained in the reduced massively obese are likely to be of diminished predictive value due to error introduced by redundant skin and other factors.

E. Body Fat Distribution

Central distribution of body fat increases risk for multiple cardiovascular risk factors such as diabetes, hypertension, and dyslipidemia [38, 39]. The traditional measure of central adiposity has been the ratio of waist to hip circumference (waist:hip ratio, WHR). However, debate exists as to the optimal landmarks to define waist and hip circumferences, a situation exacerbated by the variable geometry of the abdominal panniculus in obesity. Current guidelines suggest measurement of waist circumference only as marker of abdominal adiposity, which is measured at the level of the top of the iliac crest (Fig. 3) [29]. Use of this single measure correlates well with visceral adiposity, which is thought to contribute the risk of developing diseases associated with central fat distribution [38, 39]. Because increased waist circumference is associated with increased disease risk at all levels of BMI except extreme obesity (see Table 3), measurement of waist circumference should be performed routinely.

IV. FUNCTIONAL ASSESSMENT

Deficits in function may arise from malnutrition, predict risk for future malnutrition, and be associated with increased risk for malnutrition-related comorbidity. Functional assessment is based on the premise that protein energy malnutrition or other forms of malnutrition will be associated with impaired strength, mobility, or function [19, 21]. Tools developed for functional assessment vary in complexity from simple measures of handgrip strength or respiratory muscle strength to batteries of multistage tasks requiring complex physical and cognitive processes. Some functional assessment tools are useful for general populations, while others have been developed and validated for specific disease states or in specific groups such as the elderly, hospitalized patients, or community dwellers.

A common simple functional test is handgrip strength. Handgrip strength as measured by handgrip dynamometry has been shown to positively correlate with lean body mass and correlate negatively with protein energy malnutrition [21, 40–42]. In patients undergoing surgery, preoperative handgrip strength has also been found to predict risk of postoperative complications [43–45]. Handgrip dynamometry requires the cooperation of a conscious patient and can be hampered by factors such as neuromuscular disease or arthritis. Handgrip strength is useful in the serial assessment of an individual, but can also be used for reference to age- and sex-specific norms [44, 46]. Comparison of individual values to these norms should be approached with caution because these investigators employed different types of devices (strain-gauged vs. mechanical). Also, in the study by Bassey and Harries [46], it is interesting and of some concern that longitudinal changes in grip strength exceeded cross-sectional differences with age. Early improvement in grip strength in malnourished patients after refeeding has been observed [41, 47]. It is likely that repletion of intracellular energy, ions, and hydration contributes to this functional improvement long before significant accretion of protein [41, 47].

Non-volitional measures of muscle function have also been developed. Electric stimulation can be used to measure contraction and relaxation characteristics of the adductor pollicis muscle, and similar to handgrip strength, these measures are associated with loss of lean mass and have predicted postoperative complications [13, 19, 47]. Improvement in muscle function parameters has also been noted early in refeeding, and is likely explained by mechanisms similar to that in handgrip strength [19, 47]. Nonvolitional testing is potentially useful in those who cannot cooperate to the extent necessary for handgrip strength or other testing, such as in critically ill, comatose, or sedated individuals. However, Finn *et al.* [48] have noted that several factors may limit use of nonvolitional muscle function testing in the critically ill, such as concomitant neuromuscular blockade and illness-associated heightened sensitivity to discomfort associated with testing. Another recent report suggests that the day-to-day variability of nonvolitional muscle tests significantly ex-

ceeded that of other assessment measures such as body weight, midarm muscle circumference, triceps skinfold thickness, and handgrip strength [49].

V. CLINICAL MANIFESTATIONS IN SPECIFIC DISEASE STATES AND POPULATIONS

The following sections describe important historical, examination, anthropometric, and functional findings in specific organ systems and in populations at high risk. This chapter generally focuses on common disorders and findings, and discussion of disease-specific assessment and treatment is found later in this text and elsewhere as noted. Table 4 summarizes selected physical findings found in nutrient deficiency or excess, some of which are depicted in Fig. 4 (see color plate at the back of the book).

A. Oral and Dental Health

Dental health influences food choices and eating enjoyment [50]. Surveys in the elderly reveal a direct relationship between degree of edentulousness and measures of nutritional

TABLE 4 Signs of Nutrient Deficiency and Excess

System	Nutrient or condition	Sign
Mouth	Deficiencies of riboflavin, niacin, biotin, vitamin B_6, vitamin B_{12}, folate, iron, zinc	Glossitis
	Deficiencies of riboflavin, niacin, biotin, vitamin B_6, iron	Angular stomatitis, cheilosis
	Vitamin C deficiency	Gingivitis and gingival bleeding
	Bulimia nervosa	Parotid hyperplasia, dental erosions
Eyes	Deficiency of vitamin A	Xeropthalmia: night blindness, photophobia, xerosis, Bitot's spots, corneal ulceration, scarring
	Toxicity of vitamin A	Diplopia
	Thiamin deficiency	Nystagmus, deficit of lateral gaze
	Vitamin B_{12} deficiency	Optic nerve atrophy, blindness
	Vitamin E deficiency	Retinitis pigmentosa, visual deficits
	Copper toxicity	Kayser-Fleischer ring, sunflower cataract
Skin	Deficiencies of vitamin B_6, zinc	Seborrheic-like dermatitis
	Deficiencies of vitamin C, zinc	Impaired wound healing
	Niacin deficiency	Erythematous or scaly rash, sun exposed areas: arms, legs, neck (Casal's necklace)
	Vitamin C deficiency	Perifollicular petichiae, hemorrhage
	Vitamin K deficiency	Easy bruising
	Essential fatty acid deficiency	Dry flaky skin
	Protein-energy malnutrition	Depigmentation
	Carotenoid excess	Yellow or orange discoloration
	Deficiencies of iron, vitamin B_{12}, folate	Pallor (due to anemia)
Nails	Iron deficiency	Koilonychia (spoon-shaped nails)
	Selenium toxicity	Discolored or thickened nails
Hair	Vitamin C deficiency	Swan-neck deformity
	Protein energy malnutrition	Discoloration, dullness, easy pluckability
	Biotin deficiency	Alopecia
	Vitamin A toxicity	Alopecia
Cardiovascular	Thiamin deficiency	Congestive heart failure, rapid heart rate
	Selenium deficiency	Cardiomyopathy, heart failure
Gastrointestinal	Niacin deficiency	Stomatitis, proctitis, esophagitis
Musculoskeletal	Vitamin D deficiency	Generalized or proximal weakness, bone tenderness, fracture
	Hypophosphatemia, hypokalemia, protein energy malnutrition, hypomagnasemia	Weakness
	Protein energy malnutrition	Muscle wasting
	Hypocalcemia	Caropedal spasm
Neurologic	Deficiencies of vitamins B_6, E, thiamin; excess vitamin B_6	Peripheral neuropathy
	Vitamin B_{12} deficiency	Sensory neuropathy
	Deficiencies of thiamin, vitamins B_6, B_{12}, niacin, biotin, hypophosphatemia, hypermagnasemia	Mental status changes, delirium
	Deficiencies of vitamin B_{12}, thiamin, niacin	Dementia

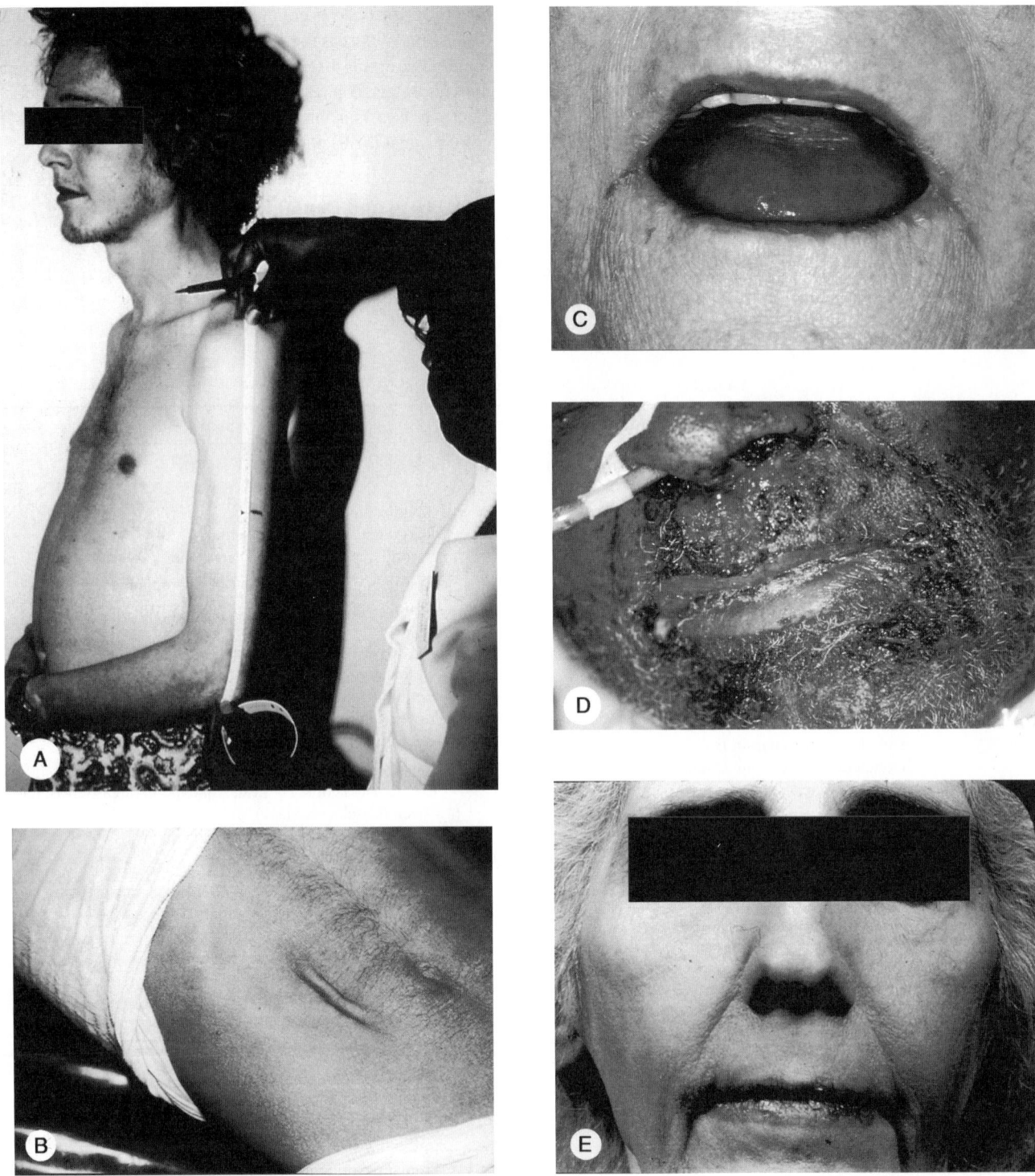

FIGURE 4   Physical signs associated with nutrient deficiencies. (A) Muscle wasting in severe protein energy malnutrition. (B) Tenting of skin in dehydration; the skin retains the tented shape after being pinched. (C) Glossitis and angular
stomatitis associated with multiple B vitamin deficiencies. (D) Dermatitis associated with zinc deficiency. (E) Cheilosis,
or vertical fissuring of the lips, associated with multiple B vitamin deficiencies. (F) Bitot's spot accompanying vitamin A
deficiency. (Photos courtesy of Dr. Robert Russell and Dr. Joel Mason.)

status or dietary intake [50, 51]. Those who are edentulous
and without dentures, or with only one denture, appear to be
at higher risk [51] than those with two dentures. Acutely ill
edentulous patients are often admitted without dentures,
which may predispose to in-hospital malnutrition by limiting
ability to chew.

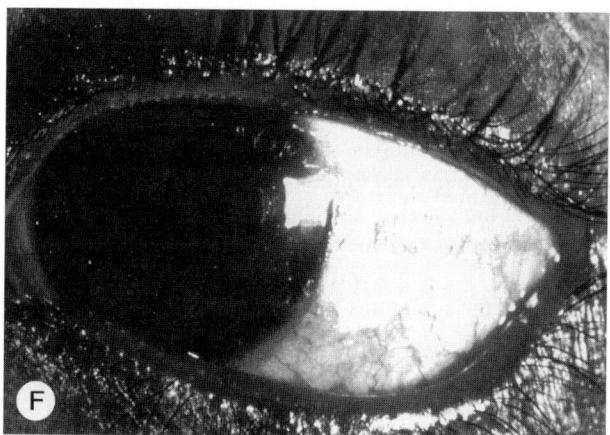

FIGURE 4 *(continued)*

Multiple deficiency states, as well as disease states and their treatments, have oropharyngeal manifestations. A sore, atrophied, red, or magenta tongue (glossitis), cracking or ulceration of the lips (cheilosis), or cracking or ulceration at the corners of the mouth (angular stomatitis) are seen in several B vitamin and other deficiencies. Bleeding from the gums may indicate coagulopathy due to vitamin K deficiency or scurvy. Cancer chemotherapy may result in pain or ulcers in the mouth and throat (mucositis), a common cause of poor intake in treated patients with cancer (see Chapter 26).

B. Skin, Hair, and Nails

Loss of subcutaneous fat is evident by simply pinching the skin. Tenting of the skin, seen with dehydration, may persist after pinching. The skin should be examined for evidence of rash or scaling, decubitus ulcer, and open wounds. Dermatitis accompanies many micronutrient deficiencies, as well as essential fatty acid deficiency (Table 4 and Fig. 4), but may only occur in advanced states of deficiency. Dermatitis herpetaformis is an itchy eruptive rash that results from gluten sensitivity. Dermatitis herpetaformis may accompany celiac sprue; thus, even if diarrhea and weight loss are absent, consideration should be made of subclinical intestinal disease and screening for vitamin deficiency. Yellow or orange discoloration of the skin may indicate carotenoid excess, which spares the sclerae and thus may be distinguished from jaundice.

C. Cardiovascular System

Cardiovascular risk factors such as dyslipidemia, hypertension, and diabetes mellitus are associated with multiple dietary factors, as well as with obesity (see Chapter 18). A newly identified risk factor for atherosclerotic disease is hyperhomocysteinemia [52], which may be elevated in inadequate intake or poor status of folate, vitamin B_{12}, and vitamin B_6 [53]. Trials are currently ongoing to assess the effect of supplementation with these nutrients on primary or secondary prevention of cardiovascular disease.

Cardiac cachexia is a syndrome associated with chronic heart failure, characterized by progressive loss of weight and lean mass, and mediated by diminished appetite and increased resting energy expenditure [54]. Loss of lean mass is likely to exacerbate symptoms because exercise tolerance will be further reduced.

Advanced thiamin deficiency may result in congestive heart failure ("wet" beriberi). High-output heart failure may occur and is characterized by rapid heart rate and pulmonary and peripheral edema.

D. Pulmonary System

Pulmonary muscle strength may be diminished in protein energy malnutrition and predisposes to respiratory complications in those with chronic pulmonary disease or in acutely ill patients. Acute respiratory failure can occur due to hypophosphatemia, which may accompany protein energy malnutrition, and alcohol abuse, and occurs during correction of diabetic ketoacidosis [55].

Chronic obstructive lung disease (COPD) is associated with protein energy malnutrition due to diminished intake and increased resting energy expenditure [56]. In patients with severe COPD, eating itself may induce dyspnea. Also, acute exacerbations or severe COPD may be accompanied by aerophagia (or swallowing air), which may cause gastric distention, abdominal bloating, and decreased intake. Chronic treatment of COPD with corticosteroids predisposes to further loss of lean mass, gains in fat mass, glucose intolerance, and bone loss.

Patients with cystic fibrosis now frequently live into adulthood, where the associated maldigestion can result in protein energy malnutrition and fat-soluble vitamin deficiencies [57, 58]. Protein energy malnutrition and these vitamin deficiencies may in turn diminish pulmonary function and increase risk for infection. Advanced cystic fibrosis may also involve the endocrine pancreas, resulting in diabetes mellitus [57].

Obesity is among the most potent risk factors for obstructive sleep apnea, characterized by disturbed sleep and daytime fatigue. Effective treatment of obstructive sleep apnea was observed to facilitate weight loss efforts [59]. Extreme obesity is also associated with other disorders including pulmonary hypertension, cor pulmonale, hypercapnea, hypoxemia, and increased risk for pulmonary embolism.

E. Gastrointestinal System

Gastrointestinal illness promotes protein energy and micronutrient malnutrition. Common diseases and mechanisms are briefly discussed below; details can be found in other chapters of this text. Dietary factors may result in gastrointestinal symptoms, some of which are uncomfortable but harmless and time limited, whereas others may progress

to serious or life-threatening disease. Included in this spectrum are lactose intolerance, consumption of osmotic cathartics such as sorbitol (in food, candy, or medications) and gluten-sensitive enteropathy (celiac disease). Following gastric resection or gastric bypass for obesity, dumping syndromes may occur in response to hyperosmolar meals [60] and are characterized by varying degrees of lightheadedness or near-syncope, nausea, diaphoresis, chest pain, and abdominal pain or cramps.

Digestive and absorptive processes may be site specific and vary by nutrient. Accordingly, the extent and location of both disease activity and resection should be noted. Inflammatory bowel disease, celiac disease, resection of the intestinal tract, and short bowel syndrome are associated with protein energy malnutrition and deficiencies of water- and fat-soluble vitamins, as well as iron, calcium, other minerals, and essential fatty acids [47, 61–64]. Recently, Geerling *et al.* [62] found that patients with Crohn's disease in remission had persistent deficiencies in several water- and fat-soluble vitamins as well as zinc. Thus the absence of current symptoms in those with chronic or remitting disease should not be taken as a guarantee of adequate nutritional status.

End-stage liver disease or cirrhosis is frequently associated with protein energy malnutrition. In the acutely ill cirrhotic individual, changes in mental status may indicate hepatic encephalopathy, which may dictate specific dietary recommendations. Chronic pancreatitis or pancreatic insufficiency may lead to maldigestion of macronutrients. In both chronic liver disease (especially cholestatic disease) and pancreatic disease, fat-soluble vitamin deficiency may occur [65]. Manifestations of deficiency states may be masked by malaise associated with chronic illness or be asymptomatic, and may only become apparent when symptoms such as night blindness, bone pain, or easy bleeding are elicited [65].

Atrophic gastritis, which predisposes to vitamin B_{12} deficiency, increases in prevalence with advancing age. Not surprisingly, more than 12% of a free-living elderly population was found to be deficient in vitamin B_{12} [66]. The common chronic use of acid-suppressing drugs (proton pump inhibitors and H2 antagonists) may also predispose to vitamin B_{12} deficiency [67].

F. Musculoskeletal

Protein energy malnutrition may result in reductions in muscular size and strength, as well as in functional changes such as diminution of work capacity or endurance. Generalized weakness is a highly nonspecific symptom and is observed in dehydration, iron deficiency (even prior to the development of significant anemia), hypophosphatemia, and in multiple vitamin deficiencies. Generalized or proximal weakness, as well as frank myopathies, due to vitamin D deficiency have recently been described [68]. Muscle wasting may be most apparent at the temporalis muscle (temporal atrophy or wasting), the shoulder girdle, and between the bones of the dorsum of the hand (interosseus wasting).

A history of fractures and bone pain may indicate metabolic bone disease or osteoporosis, and should stimulate evaluation of the skeleton, as well as of calcium and vitamin D status. Persons with diseases known to influence calcium and vitamin D metabolism (such as those with malabsorptive disorders, chronic renal failure, and the institutionalized elderly) are at high risk for metabolic bone disease, and appropriate monitoring and treatment should be undertaken.

Obesity is a potent contributor to the development of osteoarthritis, the symptoms of which may be ameliorated with weight loss.

G. Hematologic System

Classical nutritional anemias result from deficiencies of vitamin B_{12}, folate, and iron. Populations at increased risk include alcoholics (vitamin B_{12} and folate), the elderly (vitamin B_{12}), women with menometorrhagia (iron), and vegans (vitamin B_{12}). However, anemia has also been reported due to protein energy malnutrition and deficiencies of vitamin C, vitamin B_6, riboflavin, and copper [69]. The absence of anemia, or of specific findings in red and white blood cell morphology, should not be used to assess nutrient sufficiency, as deficiency states may exist without these hematologic changes.

Abnormal bleeding may be observed due to vitamin K deficiency. Most vitamin K-related bleeding usually occurs in the setting of oral anticoagulant use, which antagonizes vitamin K. Frank vitamin K deficiency with coagulopathy may be observed in alcoholics or in association with medications or starvation (see Table 1).

H. Cancer

Dietary factors that may prevent or predispose to neoplasm are beyond the scope of this chapter, but are discussed elsewhere in this text. Cancer may influence nutritional status by its effects on appetite, on energy expenditure, and on processes that are directly due to tumor burden (such as dysphagia with head and neck cancer, or bowel obstruction in advanced colon cancer) or due to pain. In addition, chemotherapy or radiation therapy may result in mucositis, nausea, vomiting, diarrhea, and alterations in taste. The implications for cancer treatment are discussed in Chapter 26.

I. Renal System

Nutritional issues in acute and chronic renal failure share common elements, but also may differ considerably depending on the etiology, the acuity and (in)stability of disease, and treatment modality. Uremia is commonly associated with anorexia and nausea, which may also occur due to conditions underlying renal failure. In addition to effects on intake, uremia-associated metabolic acidosis may perturb protein metabolism by increasing protein catabolism and limiting synthesis [70]. Nutritional issues associated with

acute renal failure include fluid management, adapting protein delivery to minimize uremia, and preventing electrolyte imbalance. Chronic renal failure and dialysis patients are at increased risk for protein energy malnutrition, and, as in other chronic diseases, an inverse relationship exists between body mass index and mortality [71]. Protein-restricted diets may be prescribed to slow progression of chronic renal disease in predialysis patients, a strategy that may require monitoring to ensure adequacy of energy and other nutrients necessary to prevent protein energy malnutrition during reduced protein intake [72]. Micronutrient issues in chronic renal failure include deficiency of vitamin D, prevention of hyperphosphatemia and related bone disease, deficiencies of several water-soluble vitamins, and toxicity of vitamin A. A newer concern is hyperhomocysteinemia, which has been observed in dialysis and renal transplant patients [73–75], and may increase risk for cardiovascular disease.

J. Neurologic and Psychiatric

Neurologic disorders, such as stroke, Parkinson's disease, and head injury, may impair ability to feed oneself or to swallow effectively (dysphagia) (see Chapter 41). A history of difficulty initiating a swallow, choking or gagging, wet cough, and retained food in the mouth are among the signs that should stimulate further evaluation for dysphagia [76]. A large number of non-neurologic conditions may also predispose to dysphagia including prolonged endotracheal intubation or absence of oral intake, as well as chronic diseases such as head and neck or esophageal cancer [76].

Anorexia nervosa, bulimia, and binge eating disorder may be suspected on the basis of eating patterns and attitudes, by low body weight or BMI, and by excessive exercise. An up-to-date clinical approach to the assessment of disordered eating is available elsewhere [77]. Signs of bulimia nervosa may include dental erosions and parotid hyperplasia. Nutritional problems associated with anorexia nervosa and bulimia nervosa include protein energy malnutrition, electrolyte abnormalities, vitamin and mineral deficiencies, and, in the longer term, osteopenia [78].

Patients suffering from advanced dementia are likely to experience malnutrition due to loss of the cognitive as well as the motor skills necessary for adequate intake. Depression may also be associated with decreased or increased intake. Medications for the treatment of depression, bipolar disease, and psychosis, as well as anticonvulsants, are often associated with changes in intake and body weight (see Table 1).

Multiple psychiatric or neurologic syndromes related to nutrient deficiency (e.g., thiamin, niacin, vitamin B_6, vitamin E, essential fatty acids) or excess have been described (Table 4). In the United States, common predisposing factors to deficiency syndromes are alcoholism and malabsorptive disorders [79, 80], as well as aging in the case of vitamin B_{12}. Of particular importance is that deficiency of vitamin B_{12} may be manifest by neurologic or psychiatric symptoms in the absence of anemia or macrocytosis [81]. Syndromes associated with micronutrient excess may result from supplementation or food faddism or may be associated with underlying diseases.

K. Infectious Disease and AIDS

Immune competence depends on adequate protein energy nutrition as well as multiple micronutrients. In hospitalized patients, the complications of protein energy malnutrition often are manifest as infection. Infectious complications are not only due to compromise of immune function per se, but also reflect other functional deficits. For example, aspiration pneumonia may be precipitated by poor ability to expectorate or cough and be facilitated by impaired ciliary clearance.

Malnutrition in acquired immunodeficiency syndrome (AIDS) may be secondary to reduced intake, malabsorption, medications, or increased nutrient needs (see Chapter 47). Reduced intake can be associated with generalized anorexia due to disease or medications, oropharyngeal or esophageal lesions, and diarrhea. The human immunodeficiency virus (HIV) wasting syndrome may result from decreased intake, increased resting energy expenditure, and HIV-induced loss of lean mass [82]. Chronic protein energy malnutrition in AIDS will likely be exacerbated by acute losses associated with infection or other complications. Multiple vitamin and mineral deficiencies have been observed in HIV infection and AIDS and have been linked to increased rates of mortality [83].

VI. PROGNOSTIC INDICATORS

Attempts have been made to improve the sensitivity and specificity in assessment of nutrition-related risk by combining various assessment parameters. Table 5 illustrates some prognostic indexes, and some popular examples are discussed below. Recent reviews of these indexes have been compiled [84, 85].

A. Prognostic Nutritional Index

The Prognostic Nutritional Index uses biochemical, anthropometric, and measures of immunocompetence to calculate an index of risk of developing postoperative complications. A prognostic nutritional index greater than 40% is indicative of presence of malnutrition, and has been predictive of in-hospital complications, sepsis, length of hospital stay, and postoperative death [84, 86, 87].

B. Subjective Global Assessment

Subjective Global Assessment combines historical elements, along with examination for edema and loss of subcutaneous fat, to stratify individuals into three categories: well nourished, moderately (or suspected of being) malnourished, or severely malnourished [88] (Table 6). Patients with a variety

TABLE 5 Selected Prognostic Index

	Equation	Interpretation
Prognostic Nutritional Index (PNI)	PNI (% risk) = 158-16.6 (albumin, g/dL) − 0.78 (triceps skinfold, mm) − 0.2 (transferrin, mg/dL) − 5.8 (DH) DH is the maximum delayed hypersensitivity to any of the three recall antigens (Candida, mumps, and streptokinase-streptodomase). Grades are 0 for nonreactive, 1 for <5-mm induration, or 2 for ≥5=mm induration.	PNI > 40% is predictive of presence of malnutrition and increased incidence of postoperative complications
Nutritional Risk Index (NRI)	NRI = (1.519 × albumin, g/L) + 41.7 (current weight/usual weight)	NRI > 100: no malnutrition NRI = 97.5–100: mild malnutrition NRI = 83.5–97.5: moderate malnutrition NRI < 83.5 = severe malnutrition
Maastrich Nutrition Index (MNI)	MNI = 20.68 − (0.24 × albumin, g/L) − (19.21 × transthyretin, g/L) − (1.86 × lymphocytes, 10^6/L) − 0.04 × IBW) IBW is ideal body weight using the Metropolitan Life Insurance Company Tables	MNI ≤ 0: no malnutrition MNI > 0: malnutrition
Prognostic Inflammatory and Nutritional Index (PINI)	PINI = $\dfrac{\text{C-reactive protein, mg/L} \times \alpha_1 \text{ glycoprotein acid, mg/L}}{\text{transthyretin, mg/L} \times \text{albumin, g/L}}$	PINI < 1: good prognosis PINI > 10: increased risk of complications

Source: Adapted from Schneider, S. M., and Hebuterne, X. (2000). Use of nutritional scores to predict outcomes in chronic diseases. *Nutr. Rev.* **58,** 31–38.

of illnesses who have been classified as moderately or severely malnourished have been shown to have greater postoperative complications, longer hospital stays, and accrued greater hospital charges compared to well-nourished patients [84]. Covinsky and colleagues [89] used Subjective Global Assessment to assess 369 hospitalized older adults (≥70 years old), and then followed patient outcomes at 3 months and 1 year. Patients classified as severely malnourished were more likely to be dependent in activities of daily living at 3 months after discharge and were more likely to have spent time in a nursing home during the year after hospitalization. Both moderately and severely malnourished patients were more likely to have died at the 3-month and 1-year follow-up after discharge compared to the well-nourished group [89].

C. Screening Tools for Older Adults

The elderly are the fastest growing segment of our population, and they are at particular risk for malnutrition because of illness, changes in body composition, diminished mobility and function, social isolation, and economic factors. Special attention to these issues is required to identify problem areas and institute early intervention [85, 90].

1. Nutrition Screening Initiative
The Nutrition Screening Initiative is a multistage screening and assessment device. The initial stage is the DETERMINE Your Nutritional Health Checklist [91], which is designed to be self-administered, but also can be administered by a care-taker. It includes 10 yes/no statements covering dietary assessment, general assessment, and social assessment. Each statement has a weighted score, which is then tallied to a final score for stratification to low, moderate, or high nutritional risk [85, 91]. Posner *et al.* [91] surveyed 749 Medicare beneficiaries using a 14-point checklist (the predecessor of the currently used checklist) and found that 24% of this population was at high nutritional risk. Of this group, 38% had dietary intakes below 75% of the recommended dietary intakes for three or more nutrients.

Those at high nutritional risk require further assessment by a health care professional by using the level 1 or level 2 screening tools. The level 1 screening tool includes information about body weight, BMI, weight change, eating habits, living environment, and functional status. The level 2 screening tool includes all of the level 1 information, but also anthropometric measurements, biochemical measurements, cognitive and emotional status assessments, medication use, and signs and symptoms of nutrient deficiencies.

2. Mini Nutritional Assessment
The Mini Nutritional Assessment was initially developed for the frail elderly, but has been validated for use in other elderly populations [90]. Designed to be administered by a health care professional, the mini nutritional assessment consists of 18 questions relating to anthropometrics (including weight loss, BMI, midarm circumference, and calf circumference), dietary intake (including change in appetite, number of meals/day, and autonomy of feeding), global assessment (including mobility, lifestyle, and medication

TABLE 6   Components of Subjective Global Assessment

Patient history:
    Weight change
        Overall loss in past 6 months
        Change in past 2 weeks (increase, stable, or decrease)
    Dietary intake change relative to normal
        No change
        Change
        Duration (number of weeks)
        Types of change
            Suboptimal solid diet
            Full liquid diet
            Hypocaloric liquids
            Starvation
    Gastrointestinal symptoms (that persisted >2 weeks)
        No symptoms
        Nausea
        Vomiting
        Diarrhea
        Anorexia
    Disease and its relation to nutritional requirements
        Primary diagnosis
        Metabolic demand (stress)
            No stress
            Mild stress
            High stress
Physical exam:
    For each trait specify: 0 = normal, 1+ = mild, 2+ = moderate, 3+ = severe
        Loss of subcutaneous fat (triceps, chest)
        Muscle wasting (quadriceps, deltoids)
        Ankle edema
        Sacral edema
        Ascites

Source: Adapted from Detsky, A. S., McLaughlin, J. R., Baker, J. P., Johnston, N., Whittaker, S., Mendelson, R. A., and Jeejeebhoy, K. N. (1987). What is subjective global assessment of nutrition status? *JPEN* **11**, 8–13.

use), and subjective assessment (self-perception of health and nutritional status). Each area of assessment receives a score, which is tallied at the end of the assessment, to a maximum score of 30. A score of 24–30 points indicates no risk of malnutrition, 17–23.5 indicates risk of malnutrition, and a score of <17 points indicates existing malnutrition [85, 90].

VII. SUMMARY

Clinical and physical assessment of nutritional status is integral to the detection of present or potential malnutrition. Because individual components may lack sensitivity or specificity, a combination of these components is recommended. Basic medical and historical data such as present illnesses, weight change, and medications, as well as anthropometric data such as height and weight, should always be collected, regardless of the clinician's perception of risk. Populations usually at increased risk include those with weight loss greater than 10% of usual weight, those with certain chronic diseases, alcoholics, and the elderly. When indicated, more detailed assessment, including use of functional parameters and prognostic indexes can then be performed.

References

1. Hensrud, D. D. (1999). Nutrition screening and assessment. *Med. Clin. N. Am.* **83**, 1525–1546.
2. Balluz, L. S., Kieszak, S. M., Philen, R. M., and Mulinare, J. (2000). Vitamin and mineral supplement use in the United States. Results from the third National Health and Nutrition Examination Survey. *Arch. Fam. Med.* **9**, 258–262.
3. Sorkin, J. D., Muller, D. C., and Andres, R. (1999). Longitudinal change in height of men and women: implications for the interpretation of the body mass index. *Am. J. Epidemiol.* **150**, 969–977.
4. Pirie, P., Jacobs, D., Jeffery, R., and Hannan, P. (1981). Distortion in self-reported height and weight. *J. Am. Diet. Assoc.* **78**, 601–606.
5. Coe, T. R., Halkes, M., Houghton, K., and Jefferson, D. (1999). The accuracy of visual estimation of weight and height in preoperative surgical patients. *Anaesthesia* **54**, 582–586.
6. Kwok, T., and Whitelaw, M. N. (1991). The use of armspan in nutritional assessment of the elderly. *J. Am. Geriatr. Soc.* **39**, 494–496.
7. Roubenoff, R., and Wilson, P. W. F. (1993). Advantage of knee height over height as an index of stature in expression of body composition in adults. *Am. J. Clin. Nutr.* **57**, 609–613.
8. Mitchell, C. O., and Lipschitz, D. A. (1982). Arm length measurement as alternative to height in nutritional assessment of the elderly. *JPEN* **6**, 226–229.
9. Chumlea, W. C., and Guo, S. (1992). Equations for predicting stature in white and black elderly individuals. *J. Gerontol.* **47**, M197–M203.
10. Reynolds, M. W., Fredman, L., Langenberg, P., and Magaziner, J. (1999). Weight, weight change, and mortality in a random sample of older community-dwelling women. *J. Am. Geriatr. Soc.* **47**, 1409–1414.
11. Dewys, W. D., Begg, C., Lavin, P. T., Band, P. R., Bennett, J. M., Bertino, J. R., Cohen, M. H., Douglass, H. O., Engstrom, P. F., Ezdinli, E. Z., Horton, J., Johnson, G. J., Moertel, C. G., Oken, M. M., Perlia, C., Rosenbaum, C., Silverstein, M. N., Skeel, R. T., Sponzo, R. W., and Tormey, D. C. (1980). Prognostic effect of weight loss prior to chemotherapy in cancer patients. *Am. J. Med.* **69**, 491–497.
12. Studley, H. O. (1936). Percentage of weight loss. A basic indicator of surgical risk in patients with chronic peptic ulcer disease. *JAMA* **106**, 458–460.
13. Windsor, J. A., and Hill, G. L. (1988). Weight loss with physiologic impairment: A basic indicator of surgical risk. *Ann. Surg.* **207**, 290–296.
14. Seltzer, M. H., Slocum, B. A., Cataldi-Bethcher, E. L., Fileti, C., and Gerson, N. (1982). Instant nutritional assessment: Absolute weight loss and surgical mortality. *JPEN* **6**, 218–221.

15. Fischer, J., and Johnson, M. A. (1990). Low body weight and weight loss in the aged. *J. Am. Diet. Assoc.* **90,** 1697–1706.

16. World Health Organization. (1995). "Physical Status: The Use and Interpretation of Anthropometry." World Health Organization, Geneva.

17. Naber, T. H., de Bree, A., Schermer, T. R., Bakkeren, J., Bar, B., de Wild, G., and Katan, M. B. (1997). Specificity of indexes of malnutrition when applied to apparently healthy people: The effect of age. *Am. J. Clin. Nutr.* **65,** 1721–1725.

18. Engelman, D. T., Adams, D. H., Byrne, J. G., Aranki, S. F., Collins, J. J., Couper, G. S., Allred, E. N., Cohn, L. H., and Rizzo, R. J. (1999). Impact of body mass index and albumin on morbidity and mortality after cardiac surgery. *J. Thorac. Cardiovasc. Surg.* **118,** 866–873.

19. Jeejeebhoy, K. N. (1998). Nutritional assessment. *Gastroenterol. Clin. N. Am.* **27,** 347–369.

20. Windsor, J. A. (1993). Underweight patients and the risks of major surgery. *World J. Surg.* **17,** 165–172.

21. Hill, G. L. (1992). Body composition research: Implications for the practice of clinical nutrition. *JPEN* **16,** 197–218.

22. Charney, P. (1995). Nutrition assessment in the 1990s: Where are we now? *Nutr. Clin. Prac.* **10,** 131–139.

23. Choban, P. S., Burge, J. C., Scales, D., and Flancbaum, L. (1997). Hypoenergetic nutrition support in hospitalized obese patients; a simplified method for clinical application. *Am. J. Clin. Nutr.* **66,** 546–550.

24. Cutts, M. E., Dowdy, R. P., Ellersieck, M. R., and Edes, T. E. (1997). Predicting energy needs in ventilator-dependent critically ill patients: Effect of adjusting for edema or adiposity. *Am. J. Clin. Nutr.* **66,** 1250–1256.

25. Wurtz, R., Itokazu, F., and Rodvold, K. (1997). Antimicrobial dosing in obese patients. *Clin. Infect. Dis.* **25,** 112–118.

26. Morgan, D. B., Hill, G. L., and Burkinshaw, L. (1980). The assessment of weight loss from a single measurement of body weight: The problems and limitations. *Am. J. Clin. Nutr.* **33,** 2101–2105.

27. Robinett-Weiss, N., Hixson, M. L., Keir, B., and Sieberg, J. (1984). The metropolitan height-weight tables: perspectives for use. *J. Am. Diet. Assoc.* **84,** 1480–1481.

28. Heymsfield, S. B. (1999). Nutritional assessment of malnutrition by anthropometric methods. *In* "Modern Nutrition in Health and Disease" (M. E. Shils, J. A. Olson, M. Shike, and A. C. Ross, Eds.), pp. 903–921. Williams and Wilkins, Baltimore.

29. National Heart, Lung, and Blood Institute. (1998). Clinical guidelines on the identification, evaluation, and treatment of overweight and obesity in adults—The evidence report. *Obes. Res.* **6** (Suppl 2), 51S–209S.

30. Livingstone, M. B. E., Prentice, A. M., Coward, W. A., Strain, J. J., Black, A. E., Davies, P. S. W., Stewart, C. M., McKenna, P. G., and Whitehead, R. G. (1992). Validation of estimates of energy intake by weighed dietary record and diet history in children and adolescents. *Am. J. Clin. Nutr.* **56,** 29–35.

31. Calle, E. E., Thun, M. J., Petrelli, J. M., Rodriguez, C., and Heath, C. W., Jr. (1999). Body-mass index and mortality in a prospective cohort of U. S. adults [see comments]. *N. Engl. J. Med.* **341,** 1097–1105.

32. Visscher, T. L. S., Seidell, J. C., Menotti, A., Blackburn, H., Nissinen, A., Feskens, E. J. M., and Kromhout, D. (2000). Underweight and overweight in relation to mortality among men aged 40–59 and 50–69. *Am. J. Epidemiol.* **151,** 660–666.

33. Landi, F., Zuccala, G., Gambassi, G., Incalzi, R. A., Manigrasso, L., Pagano, F., Carbonin, P., and Bernabei, R. (1999). Body mass index and mortality among older people living in the community. *J. Am. Geriatr. Soc.* **47,** 1072–1076.

34. Henry, C. J. (1990). Body mass index and the limits of human survival. *Eur. J. Clin. Nutr.* **44,** 329–335.

35. Jackson, A. S., and Pollock, M. L. (1978). Generalized equations for predicting body density of men. *Br. J. Nutr.* **40,** 497–504.

36. Durnin, J. V. G. A., and Womersley, J. (1974). Body fat assessed from total body density and its estimation from skinfold thickness: Measurements on 481 men and women aged from 16 to 72 years. *Br. J. Nutr.* **32,** 77–97.

37. Wang, J., Thornton, J. C., Kolesnik, S., and Pierson, R. N., Jr. (2000). Anthropometry in body composition. An overview. *Ann. NY. Acad. Sci.* **904,** 317–326.

38. Despres, J. (1998). The insulin resistance-dyslipidemic syndrome of visceral obesity: Effect on patients' risk. *Obes. Res.* **6** (Supl 1), 8S–17S.

39. Molarius, A., and Siedell, J. C. (1998). Selection of anthropometric indicators for classification of abdominal fatness—A critical review. *Int. J. Obes.* **22,** 719–727.

40. Vaz, M., Thangam, S., Prabhu, A., and Shetty, P. S. (1996). Maximal voluntary contraction as a functional indicator of adult chronic undernutrition. *Brit. J. Nutr.* **76,** 9–15.

41. Russell, D. M., Prendergast, P. J., Darby, P. L., Garfinkel, P. E., Whitwell, J., and Jeejeebhoy, K. N. (1983). A comparison between muscle function and body composition in anorexia nervosa: the effect of refeeding. *Am. J. Clin. Nutr.* **38,** 229–237.

42. Payette, H., Hanussaik, N., Boutier, V., Morais, J. A., and Gray-Donald, K. (1998). Muscle strength and functional mobility in relation to lean body mass in free-living frail elderly women. *Eur. J. Clin. Nutr.* **52,** 45–53.

43. Hunt, D. R., Rowlands, B. J., and Johnston, D. (1985). Hand grip strength—A simple prognostic indicator in surgical patients. *JPEN* **9,** 701–704.

44. Webb, A. R., Newman, L. A., Taylor, M., and Keogh, J. B. (1989). Hand grip dynamometry as a predictor of postoperative complications reappraisal using age standardized grip strengths. *JPEN* **13,** 30–33.

45. Kalfarentzos, F., Spiliotis, J., Velimezis, G., Dougenis, D., and Androulakis, J. (1989). Comparison of forearm muscle dynamometry with nutritional prognostic index, as a preoperative indicator in cancer patients. *JPEN* **13,** 34–36.

46. Bassey, E. J., and Harries, U. J. (1993). Normal values for handgrip strength in 920 men and women aged over 65 years, and longitudinal changes over 4 years in 620 survivors. *Clin. Sci.* **84,** 331–337.

47. Christie, P. M., and Hill, G. L. (1990). Effect of intravenous nutrition on nutrition and function in acute attacks of inflammatory bowel disease. *Gastroenterology* **99,** 730–736.

48. Finn, P. J., Plank, L. D., Clark, M. A., Connolly, A. B., and Hill, G. L. (1996). Assessment of involuntary muscle function in patients after critical injury or severe sepsis. *JPEN* **20,** 332–337.

49. Brooks, S. D., Gerstman, B. B., Sucher, K. P., and Kearns, P. J. (1998). The reliability of muscle function analysis using different methods of stimulation. *JPEN* **22,** 331–334.

50. Lamy, M., Mojon, P., Kalykakis, G., Legrand, R., and Butz-Jorgensen, E. (1999). Oral status and nutrition in the institutionalized elderly. *J. Dentistry* **27,** 443–448.

51. Papas, A. S., Palmer, C. A., Rounds, M. C., and Russell, R. M. (1998). The effects of denture status on nutrition. *Spec. Care Dentistry* **18**, 17–25.

52. Stein, J. H., and McBride, P. E. (1998). Hyperhomocysteinemia and atherosclerotic vascular disease: Pathophysiology, screening, and treatment. off. *Arch. Int. Med.* **158**, 1301–1306.

53. Selhub, J., Jacques, P. F., Wilson, P. W., Rush, D., and Rosenberg, I. H. (1993). Vitamin status and intake as primary determinants of homocysteinemia in an elderly population [see comments]. *JAMA* **270**, 2693–2698.

54. Poehlman, E. T., Scheffers, J., Gottlieb, S. S., Fisher, M. L., and Vaitekevicius, P. (1994). Increased resting metabolic rate in patients with congestive heart failure [see comments]. *Ann. Int. Med.* **121**, 860–862.

55. Pingleton, S. K., and Harmon, G. S. (1987). Nutritional management in acute respiratory failure. *JAMA* **257**, 3094–3099.

56. Schols, A. M., Soeters, P. B., Mostert, R., Saris, W. H., and Wouters, E. F. (1991). Energy balance in chronic obstructive pulmonary disease. *Am. Rev. Respir. Dis.* **143**, 1248–1252.

57. Dowsett, J. (1996). Nutrition in the management of cystic fibrosis. *Nutr. Rev.* **54**, 31–33.

58. Benabdeslam, H., Garcia, I., Bellon, G., Gilly, R., and Revol, A. (1998). Biochemical assessment of the nutritional status of cystic fibrosis patients treated with pancreatic enzyme extracts [see comments]. *Am. J. Clin. Nutr.* **67**, 912–918.

59. Loube, D. I., Loube, A. A., and Milton, E. K. (1997). Continuous positive airway pressure treatment results in weight loss in obese and overweight patients with obstructive sleep apnea. *J. Am. Diet. Assoc.* **97**, 896–897.

60. Vecht, J., Masclee, A. A., and Lamers, C. B. (1997). The dumping syndrome. Current insights into pathophysiology, diagnosis and treatment. *Scand. J. Gastroenterol. Suppl.* **223**, 21–27.

61. Bousvaros, A., Zurakowski, D., Duggan, C., Law, T., Rifai, N., Goldberg, N. E., and Leichtner, A. M. (1998). Vitamins A and E serum levels in children and young adults with inflammatory bowel disease: Effect of disease activity. *J. Ped. Gastroenterol. Nutr.* **26**, 129–135.

62. Geerling, B. J., Badart-Smook, A., Stockbrugger, R. W., and Brummer, R. J. (1998). Comprehensive nutritional status in patients with long-standing Crohn disease currently in remission. *Am. J. Clin. Nutr.* **67**, 919–926.

63. Purdum, P. P. III., and Kirby, D. F. (1991). Short-bowel syndrome: A review of the role of nutrition support. *JPEN* **15**, 93–101.

64. Siguel, E. N., and Lerman, R. H. (1996). Prevalence of essential fatty acid deficiency in patients with chronic gastrointestinal disorders. *Metab. Clin. Exp.* **45**, 12–23.

65. Lee, Y. M., and Kaplan, M. M. (1995). Primary sclerosing cholangitis. *N. Engl. J. Med.* **332**, 924–933.

66. Lindenbaum, J., Rosenberg, I. H., Wilson, P. W., Stabler, S. P., and Allen, R. H. (1994). Prevalence of cobalamin deficiency in the Framingham elderly population [see comments]. *Am. J. Clin. Nutr.* **60**, 2–11.

67. Marcuard, S. P., Albernaz, L., and Khazanie, P. G. (1994). Omeprazole therapy causes malabsorption of cyanocobalamin (vitamin B12) [see comments]. *Ann. Int. Med.* **120**, 211–215.

68. Prabhala, A., Garg, R., and Dandona, P. (2000). Severe myopathy associated with vitamin D deficiency in western New York. *Arch. Int. Med.* **160**, 1199–1203.

69. Chanarin, I. (1999). Nutritional aspects of hematologic disorders. *In* "Modern Nutrition in Health and Disease" (M. E. Shils, J. A. Olson, M. Shike, and A. C. Ross, Eds.), pp. 1419–1439. Williams and Wilkins, Baltimore, MD.

70. Oreopoulos, D. G. (1999). The optimization of continuous ambulatory peritoneal dialysis [clinical conference]. *Kidney Int.* **55**, 1131–1149.

71. Kopple, J. D., Zhu, X., Lew, N. L., and Lowrie, E. G. (1999). Body weight-for-height relationships predict mortality in maintenance hemodialysis patients. *Kidney Int.* **56**, 1136–1148.

72. Walser, M., Mitch, W. E., Maroni, B. J., and Kopple, J. D. (1999). Should protein intake be restricted in predialysis patients? *Kidney Int.* **55**, 771–777.

73. Bostom, A. G., Gagnon, D. R., Cupples, L. A., Wilson, P. W. F., Jenner, J. L., Ordovas, J. M., Schaefer, E. J., and Castelli, W. P. (1994). A prospective investigation of elevated lipoprotein(a) detected by electrophoresis and cardiovascular disease in women. The Framingham Heart Study. *Circulation* **90**, 1688–1695.

74. Bostom, A. G., Gohh, R. Y., Beaulieu, A. J., Nadeau, M. R., Hume, A. L., Jacques, P. F., Selhub, J., and Rosenberg, I. H. (1997). Treatment of hyperhomocysteinemia in renal transplant recipients. A randomized, placebo-controlled trial. *Ann. Int. Med.* **127**, 1089–1092.

75. Suliman, M. E., Qureshi, A. R., Barany, P., Stenvinkel, P., Filho, J. C., Anderstam, B., Heimburger, O., Lindholm, B., and Bergstrom, J. (2000). Hyperhomocysteinemia, nutritional status, and cardiovascular disease in hemodialysis patients. *Kidney Int.* **57**, 1727–1735.

76. Perlman, A. L. (1999). Dysphagia: Populations at risk and methods of diagnosis. *Nutr. Clin. Prac.* **14**, S2-S9.

77. Rock, C. L. (1999). Nutritional and medical assessment and management of eating disorders. *Nutr. Clin. Care* **2**, 332–343.

78. Becker, A. E., Grinspoon, S. K., Klibanski, A., and Herzog, D. B. (1999). Eating disorders [see comments]. *N. Engl. J. Med.* **340**, 1092–1098.

79. Cook, C. C., Hallwood, P. M., and Thomson, A. D. (1998). B vitamin deficiency and neuropsychiatric syndromes in alcohol misuse. *Alcohol & Alcoholism* **33**, 317–336.

80. Gloria, L., Cravo, M., Camilo, M. E., Resende, M., Cardoso, J. N., Oliveira, A. G., Leitao, C. N., and Mira, F. C. (1997). Nutritional deficiencies in chronic alcoholics: relation to dietary intake and alcohol consumption. *Am. J. Gastroenterol.* **92**, 485–489.

81. Lindenbaum, J., Healton, E. B., Savage, D. G., Brust, J. C., Garrett, T. J., Podell, E. R., Marcell, P. D., Stabler, S. P., and Allen, R. H. (1988). Neuropsychiatric disorders caused by cobalamin deficiency in the absence of anemia or macrocytosis. *N. Engl. J. Med.* **318**, 1720–1728.

82. Coodley, G. O., Loveless, M. O., and Merrill, T. M. (1994). The HIV wasting syndrome: a review. *J. Acq. Immun. Defic. Synd.* **7**, 681–694.

83. Baum, M. K., and Shor-Posner, G. (1998). Micronutrient status in relationship to mortality in HIV−1 disease. *Nutr. Rev.* **56**, S135–139.

84. Schneider, S. M., and Hebuterne, X. (2000). Use of nutritional scores to predict outcomes in chronic diseases. *Nutr. Rev.* **58**, 31–38.

85. Omran, M. L., and Morley, J. E. (2000). Assessment of protein energy malnutrition in older persons, part I: History, examination, body composition, and screening tools. *Nutrition* **16**, 50–63.

86. Buzby, G., Mullen, J. L., and Matthews, D. (1980). Prognostic nutritional index in gastrointestinal surgery. *Am. J. Surg.* **139,** 160–167.

87. Santoso, J. T., Canada, T., Latson, B., Aaaadi, K., Lucci, J. A., 3rd, and Coleman, R. L. (2000). Prognostic nutritional index in relation to hospital stay in women with gynecologic cancer. *Obstet. Gynecol.* **95,** 844–846.

88. Detsky, A. S., McLaughlin, J. R., Baker, J. P., Johnston, N., Whittaker, S., Mendelson, R. A., and Jeejeebhoy, K. N. (1987). What is subjective global assessment of nutrition status? *JPEN* **11,** 8–13.

89. Covinsky, K. E., Martin, G. E., Beyth, R. J., Justice, A. C., Sehgal, A. R., and Landefeld, C. S. (1999). The relationship between clinical assessments of nutritional status and adverse outcomes in older hospitalized patients. *J. Am. Geriatr. Soc.* **47,** 532–538.

90. Garry, P. J., and Vellas, B. J. (1999). Practical and validated use of the mini nutritional assessment in geriatric evaluation. *Nutr. Clin. Care* **2,** 146–154.

91. Posner, B. M., Jette, A. M., Smith, K. W., and Miller, D. R. (1993). Nutrition and health risks in the elderly: The Nutrition Screening Initiative. *Am. J. Public Health* **83,** 972–978.

92. Chumlea, W. C., Guo, S. S., and Steingaugh, M. L. (1994). Prediction of stature from knee height for black and white adults and children with application to mobility-impaired or handicapped persons. *J. Am. Diet. Assoc.* **94,** 1385–1388.

93. Han, T. S., and Lean, M. E. J. (1996). Lower leg length as an index of stature in adults. *Int. J. Obes.* **20,** 21–27.

94. Ferro-Luzzi, A., Sette, S., Franklin, M., and James, W. P. (1992). A simplified approach of assessing adult chronic energy deficiency. *Eur. J. Clin. Nutr.* **46,** 173–186.

CHAPTER **4**

Overview of Nutritional Epidemiology

RUTH E. PATTERSON

Fred Hutchinson Cancer Research Center, Seattle, Washington

I. INTRODUCTION

Nutritional epidemiology is the study of dietary intake and the occurrence of disease in human populations. One factor that distinguishes this discipline is the extraordinary challenge of the exposure assessment. In epidemiology, exposure is defined as participant characteristics or agents (e.g., food, medications, sun) with which a participant comes into contact that may be related to disease risk (see Table 1) [1]. Measuring dietary intake is unusually complicated for many different reasons. For purposes of illustration, we can compare the assessment challenges for two common exposures: cigarette smoking and diet. Because it is a single (yes/no) activity, participants usually can accurately report whether or not they smoke. Because smoking is addictive, it tends to be a consistent long-term behavior rather than one that individuals stop and start. Because it is a habit, most people smoke roughly the same number of cigarettes per day; and because of the expense, most people know how many cigarettes they smoke per day. In comparison, over the course of even 1 week, an individual can consume hundreds, even thousands of distinct food items, making it difficult for respondents to accurately report on their intake. Meals can be prepared by others (e.g., in a restaurant, by a spouse, as prepackaged food) so that the respondent is not knowledge-able about what, or how much, he is eating. Food choices typically vary with seasons and other life activities (e.g., weekends, holidays, vacations). In fact, the day-to-day variability in food intake can be so large that it is difficult to identify any underlying consistent pattern. In addition, foods themselves are often a surrogate for the exposure of interest (e.g., dietary fat), which means that investigators must rely on food composition databases to calculate the exposure variable. Given even this superficial summary of the problems inherent in assessing dietary intake, it is not surprising that it has been difficult to obtain consistent and strong evidence regarding how diet affects disease risk.

The vast majority of nutritional epidemiologic research in the past 20 years has focused on the identification of foods and/or constituents in foods (i.e., nutrients) that cause, or protect against, the occurrence of chronic diseases. Therefore, the tools and methods of nutritional epidemiology were developed to address scientific issues unique to the biology of chronic diseases. In particular, epidemiologic methods were designed to take into account the following: (1) the extensive time for disease development, (2) the multifactorial nature of chronic diseases, and (3) research conducted in human beings, which precludes direct observation of cause and effect. Below, each of these issues in relation to nutritional epidemiology is discussed.

TABLE 1   Examples of Exposures Relevant to Nutritional Epidemiologic Studies

Exposure	Diet-related example	Other example
Agent that may cause or protect from disease	Vegetable consumption may be protective for colon cancer.	Physical activity may be protective for colon cancer.
Constitutional host factors	Genetic predisposition to nutrition-related disease.	Older adults are more predisposed to chronic disease.
Other host factors	Food preferences that determine food choices.	More educated adults may have better disease screening.
Agents that may confound the association between another agent and disease	Correlation between dietary constituents (e.g., a diet high in fruits and vegetables is usually low in fat).	Smokers are less likely to engage in physical activity.
Agents that may modify effects of other agents	Fruits and vegetables may protect against lung cancer among smokers.	Alcohol results in increased risk of lung cancer from smoking.
Agents that may determine outcome of disease	Malnutrition.	Medical treatment.

A. Extensive Time for Disease Development

Chronic diseases develop over many years and even decades. This fact has important implications for the field of nutritional epidemiology. For example, the currently accepted model of colon cancer assumes that it is a multistep pathogenic pathway beginning with mutations (germline or somatic) leading to growth of polyps (preneoplastic growths), which become adenomas and progress to carcinoma [2]. Even after an adenoma finally develops, many years may elapse before it is clinically detected. Upon clinical detection of colon cancer, it is clear that a meal consumed that day, or the month before, could have no significant effect on the disease for two reasons. First, the critical period of cancer initiation and promotion occurred many years ago. Second, it is accepted that the biologically relevant exposure is the long-term or usual diet, rather than any single eating occasion. Therefore, the exposure of interest in the development of cancer (and other chronic diseases) occurred throughout the past 10–20 years.

This time lag between dietary exposure and disease occurrence presents significant difficulties in the study of diet and chronic disease. These difficulties have been addressed in two major ways. First, dietary assessment instruments described as food frequency questionnaires were developed to capture information on usual, long-term dietary intake. Second, study designs were developed that either ask about diet in a retrospective manner (e.g., case-control studies) or assess current diet and follow participants over time for the development of disease (e.g., cohort studies, intervention trials).

B. Multifactorial Nature of Chronic Diseases

In addition to dietary intake, there are many other determinants of chronic diseases, including participant constitutional factors (e.g., genetic susceptibility) and other behaviors (e.g., cigarette smoking). These other factors may "confound" our ability to find an association of dietary intake with disease risk. For example, individuals with an interest in health may eat a diet high in fruits and vegetables (which also tends to be low in fat) and have high physical activity levels. If vegetable intake is found to be associated with reduced risk of colon cancer, it can be very difficult to determine whether it is high vegetable intake or low-fat intake that is affecting disease risk. It is also possible that diet itself is not related to disease risk, but is merely serving as a marker for some other healthful behavior (such as physical activity). Statistical techniques and study designs that deal with these problems of confounding are covered in detail below.

C. Research in Human Beings

Conducting research in healthy people significantly limits the types of nutritional studies that can be performed. For example, humans cannot (knowingly) be exposed to poten-tially dangerous dietary regimes, they will not follow extremely rigid or unpalatable diets for years, and they cannot undergo hazardous procedures (e.g., liver biopsies) for purposes of providing biologic samples. For these reasons, nutritional epidemiology is a discipline that consists largely of (1) measuring an exposure (e.g., dietary intake), (2) measuring an outcome (e.g., disease occurrence), and (3) using statistical techniques to quantify the magnitude of the association between these two observations.

Epidemiology encompasses three major topic areas: (1) exposure measurement, (2) study design, and (3) interpretation of cause and effect. Below we discuss each of these in relation to nutritional epidemiology.

II. PRINCIPLES OF EXPOSURE MEASUREMENT IN NUTRITIONAL EPIDEMIOLOGY

Because chronic disease develops over many years, the biologically relevant exposure is usual or long-term diet, consumed many years prior to disease diagnosis. Therefore, assessment instruments that only capture data on current or short-term dietary intake (e.g., food records or recall) are not often useful in nutritional epidemiology. Food frequency questionnaires (FFQs) are generally regarded as the dietary assessment instrument best suited for most epidemiologic applications [3]. Although the design of FFQs can vary somewhat, they typically contain the following sections: (1) adjustment questions, (2) the food checklist, and (3) summary questions.

A. Food Frequency Questionnaires

FFQs often contain *adjustment questions* that assess the nutrient content of specific food items. For example, participants are asked what type of milk they usually drink and are given several options (e.g., whole, skim, soy), which saves space and reduces participant burden compared to asking for the frequency of consumption and usual portion sizes of many different types of milk. Adjustment questions also permit more refined analyses of fat intake by asking about food preparation practices (e. g, removing fat from red meat) and types of added fats (e.g., use of butter vs. margarine on bread).

The main section consists of a *food* or *food group checklist,* with questions on usual frequency of intake and portion size. The foods are selected to capture data on (1) major sources of energy and nutrients for most people, (2) between-person variability in food intake, and (3) major hypotheses regarding diet and disease. To allow for machine scanning of these forms, responses are typically categorized from "never or less than once per month" to "2+ per day" for foods and "6+ per day" for beverages. Portion sizes are often assessed by asking respondents to mark "small," "medium," or "large" in comparison to a given medium portion

size. However, some questionnaires only ask about the frequency of intake of a "usual" portion size (e.g., 1 cup milk). In the latter instances, respondents are asked to calculate the frequency of the amount given, rather than actual serving size consumed.

Summary questions ask about usual intake of fruits and vegetables because the long lists of these foods (needed to capture micronutrient intake) leads to overreporting of intake [4].

Note that development of a FFQ is a daunting, complex task requiring considerable understanding of exposure measurement in nutritional epidemiology, food composition knowledge, formatting and questionnaire design expertise, and programming resources.

B. Vitamin/Mineral Supplement Assessment

Considerably less attention has been paid to measuring vitamin/mineral supplement use compared to food intake. However assessing vitamin/mineral supplement use is important, because supplement use per se is an exposure of interest for the risk of several chronic diseases [5, 6]. In addition, supplements contribute a large proportion of total (diet plus supplement) micronutrient intake [7]. Epidemiologic studies typically use personal interviews or self-administered questionnaires to obtain information on three to five general classes of multiple vitamins, single supplements, the dose of single supplements, and sometimes frequency and/or duration of use.

In a validity study comparing this self-administered assessment method to label transcription among 104 supplement users, we found correlation coefficients ranging from 0.1 for iron to 0.8 for vitamin C [8]. The principal sources of error were investigator error in assigning the micronutrient composition of multiple vitamins and respondent confusion regarding the distinction between multiple vitamins and single supplements. These results suggest that commonly used epidemiologic methods of assessing supplement use may incorporate significant amounts of error in estimates of some nutrients.

In a marketplace that is becoming rapidly more complex, with vitamins, minerals, and botanical compounds combined in unusual mixtures at highly variable doses, the association of dietary supplements with disease risk is becoming increasingly difficult to assess.

C. Use of Biomarkers in Nutritional Epidemiology

Dietary biomarkers are critical to the advancement of nutritional epidemiology. Recent studies using doubly labeled water to estimate energy expenditure have found significant underreporting and person-specific biases in nutrient estimates, such as the tendency for obese women to underestimate dietary intake [9]. Identification and understanding of the effect of these person-specific biases are the major challenges now facing nutrition studies. Movement in this field, however, has been hampered by the lack of practical and available biomarkers. For example, there is no established biomarker for total fat intake. In addition, many biomakers (e.g., serum β-carotene for total fruits and vegetables) are not on the same metric as the food or nutrient being assessed and, therefore, are of limited usefulness in assessing overall or person-specific biases in self-report.

However, there is a growing awareness of the importance of biomarker substudies for the interpretation of observational nutritional epidemiologic studies. For example, the American Assocation of Retired Persons (AARP) cohort study being coordinated by the National Cancer Institute has a sizable substudy that includes doubly labeled water and urinary nitrogen assessment of protein intake [15]. These types of studies are an important step toward strengthening the reliability and interpretability of epidemiologic studies of diet and disease. Chapter 10 discusses biomarkers in more detail.

III. STUDY DESIGNS USED IN NUTRITIONAL EPIDEMIOLOGY

Epidemiologic studies can be roughly divided into two types: observational and experimental. The primary observational study designs include ecologic, cohort, and case-control studies. In studies of humans, the main experimental study design is the intervention trial, also called a randomized clinical trial. An overview of these study designs is given below in relation to nutritional epidemiology.

A. Observational Studies

1. ECOLOGIC AND MIGRANT STUDIES

Important hypothesis-generating studies have examined the relationship, between countries, of national estimates of per capita supply of foods (e.g., dietary fat) with time-lagged rates of cancer or heart disease incidence or mortality [10–13]. These correlational analyses strongly suggest that dietary fat intake is related to these major diseases. However, it must be noted that (1) the estimate of per capita intake from food disappearance data is extremely imprecise, (2) it is generally not feasible to control for other differences between the countries (e.g., differences in physical activity levels), and (3) it is unknown whether the individuals within the countries that are exposed to specific dietary factors are the same individuals experiencing the disease. Migrant studies have often shown that with a single move from Eastern to Western countries, large and significant increases occur in risk of several chronic diseases, such as breast cancer [14]. These studies point to the importance of lifestyle and environment in disease causation; however, few such studies have included pertinent dietary data [15].

2. CASE-CONTROL STUDIES

In a case-control study, individuals are identified and studied according to a single disease outcome. Specifically, individuals who have recently been diagnosed with a disease (e.g., colon cancer) are asked about their past exposure to diet and other risk factors and often provide a blood sample. A matched set of control individuals, usually drawn from the same population, is also enrolled in the study and the individuals are asked about their past exposures. The two groups (those with and without the disease) are compared for differences in dietary intake and other exposures. The major advantage of this design is that an entire study can be completed in 4 years with as few as 400 cases and 400 controls. However, this study design can only answer questions about a single disease outcome. In addition, these studies can introduce potentially serious biases.

Two major concerns with case-control studies are recall bias and selection bias. In studies of chronic disease, investigators typically ask participants to recall behavior and other exposures (e.g., dietary intake) from 5–10 years in the past. Bias can occur when cases recall exposure to potential risk factors differently than controls. Selection bias occurs when controls agree to join the study because of an interest in health and are therefore more likely to exhibit healthy behavior (e.g., eat healthful diets). The higher prevalence of healthy behavior in the controls appears to be associated with reduced risk of disease when actually it is associated with willingness to participate in a research study on health. Another problem with case-control studies is that biomarkers (e.g., serum micronutrient concentrations) are potentially affected by the disease process and therefore may not be reliable indicators of long-term status (e.g., risk) in cases.

3. COHORT STUDIES

The cohort study typically enrolls people who are free of disease, assesses baseline risk factors, and follows the participants over time to monitor disease occurrence. The major advantage of cohort studies is that exposure to potential risk factors is assessed before the development of disease. Therefore, exposures such as self-reported dietary intake or serum micronutrient concentrations cannot be influenced by the disease process. In addition, cohort studies can examine many different exposures in relation to many different disease outcomes. A cohort study is generally a large enterprise because most diseases affect only a small proportion of a population, even if the population is followed for many years. These studies typically have sample sizes exceeding 50, 000, can have a total cost in excess of $100 million, and require that the cohort be followed for 10 or more years [16].

Because of the large size of these studies, the analysis of biologic markers (e.g., serum micronutrient concentrations) for all participants is prohibitively expensive. Therefore, cohort studies often archive (e.g., bank) serum, white blood cells, DNA, or other biologic specimens for the purpose of conducting nested case-control studies in the future. In a nested case-control study, a sample of cohort participants who develop a disease such as breast cancer (e.g., cases) are matched to other individuals in the cohort who do not develop the disease (e.g., controls). Biologic samples from cases and controls are retrieved and analyses are performed to determine whether there are differences in prevalence of exposures between the cases and the controls. This can be an efficient and powerful study design that avoids many of the pitfalls of the classic case-control studies.

4. INTERVENTION TRIALS

Intervention trials prospectively examine the effect of a randomly assigned exposure, such as a low-fat diet, on an outcome such as disease occurrence, risk factor for a disease, or a biomarker. An important consideration when designing these studies is the degree of dietary control needed: controlled diet provided by the investigators vs. vitamin supplementation vs. dietary counseling. The stringency of dietary control is determined in part by the expected size of the response (e.g., change in disease risk) and the length of the treatment period required. For example, if the required dietary treatment period exceeds several months, a controlled feeding study is usually not logistically or financially viable.

In an intervention trial, the random assignment of participants to the control vs. the intervention group means that participants with predisposing conditions or unmeasured factors that might influence the outcome are equally likely to be randomized into the intervention or the control group. In addition, random allocation of the exposure eliminates the possibilities of selection bias and recall bias. However, these projects are usually expensive and labor intensive and, therefore, are only conducted for important public health questions where the observational data are suggestive, but considerable controversy remains in the scientific community.

IV. INTERPRETATION OF CAUSE AND EFFECT IN NUTRITIONAL EPIDEMIOLOGY

Given that nutritional epidemiology is the study of dietary intake and its association with disease risk, we must use scientific judgment in determining when the strength of the evidence supports a causal link between the exposure and the outcome. When assessing causality, important considerations include (1) the main measure of association used in epidemiologic studies; (2) the major alternative explanation for an observed association in observational studies, which is confounding; and (3) methods for assessing causality in studies of associations.

A. Measures of Association

The most commonly used measure of association between dietary intake and disease risk is relative risk. The relative

risk (RR) estimates the magnitude of an association between the dietary exposure and disease and indicates the likelihood of developing the disease in the exposed group relative to those who are not exposed [17]. For example, an RR of 1.0 indicates that the incidence of disease in both the exposed and nonexposed groups is the same. An RR greater than 1.0 indicates a positive association. For example, an RR of 2.0 between dietary fat and colon cancer indicates that individuals eating a high-fat diet are twice as likely to develop colon cancer as those eating a low-fat diet. RRs less than 1.0 are typically considered protective. An RR of 0.5 for the association of vegetable intake with colon cancer risk indicates that among individuals with diets high in vegetables, the risk of colon cancer is approximately half compared to those with diets low in vegetables. Often RRs are given for the highest category of intake (e.g., highest quartile of fat or vegetable intake) in comparison to the lowest category of intake.

Given the degree of error present in dietary intake estimates, RRs in nutritional epidemiology rarely exceed 3.0. RRs are typically presented with their associated confidence interval (e.g., RR 2.0, 95% confidence interval of 1.3–2.9), which provides information on the precision of the point estimate (e.g., the RR). Specifically, it is the range within which the true point estimates lies with a certain degree of assurance. Typically 95% confidence intervals (CIs) are given, which corresponds to the traditional test of statistical significant, $p < 0.05$. A 95% CI that does not include the null value (1.0) is, by definition, statistically significant at the $p = 0.05$ level. The width of the CI also provides information about the variability in the point estimate, which is a function of sample size. Therefore, the wider the CI, the more variability in the measure, the smaller the sample size, and the less confidence we can have that the observed point estimate is the true point estimate.

It is important to separate the strength of an RR from its public health significance. For example, a large RR (e.g., RR 5. 0) might be observed between a certain food and a risk of disease. However if consumption of that food is rare in a population, then its overall impact on morbidity or mortality will be minimal. Conversely, an RR of 1. 5 might be very important from a public health perspective if the dietary exposure is common. Once RR estimates are used to ascertain causality, estimates of the impact of an exposure on public health (termed population attributable risk) become important in the development of policy and allocation of resources.

B. Confounding

Confounding is the possibility that an observed association between the dietary intake and disease is actually due to other differences in the exposed vs. the nonexposed groups. Confounding is a critical concept in nutritional epidemiology because it is plausible that people who choose one behavior (e.g., healthful diets) might differ from those who did

not choose that behavior with regard to other exposures (such as physical activity).

For example, a population-based study of participant characteristics associated with supplement use among 1,449 adults confirmed that supplement users were more likely to be female, older, better educated, nonsmokers, regular exercisers, and to consume diets higher in fruits and vegetables and lower in fat [18]. We also found previously unreported associations of supplement use with cancer screening, use of other chemopreventive agents (hormone replacement therapy and aspirin), and a psychosocial factor: belief in a diet–cancer connection. These relationships could confound studies of supplement use and cancer risk in complex ways. For example, male supplement users were more likely to have had a prostate specific antigen test, which is associated with increased diagnosis of prostate cancer [19]. Therefore, supplement use could spuriously appear to be associated with increased incidence of prostate cancer. Alternatively, if early diagnosis of prostate cancer by because of a prostate specific antigen test reduces mortality, supplement users could spuriously appear to have lower prostate cancer mortality.

The observed relationship between supplement use and belief in a connection between diet and cancer is especially interesting. Health beliefs influence cancer risk through behavior such as diet and exercise. For example, in a previous prospective study, we found that belief in a connection between diet and cancer was a statistically significant predictor of changes to more healthful diets over time [20]. In cohort studies, the increasing healthfulness of supplement users' diets and other health practices over time could result in a spurious positive association between supplement use and chronic disease risk.

It is important to note that in studies in which nutrient intake is summed from foods and supplements, the intake of micronutrients in the highest exposure category often appears too high to be obtained from food alone and probably reflects supplement use [5]. Therefore, studies of nutrient intake may also be confounded by the relationship between supplement use and healthful lifestyle. In these studies, consistency of findings for the nutrient from foods and vitamin supplements separately would increase our confidence that an observed association was not confounded by supplement users' healthful lifestyles.

In theory, statistical adjustment in analyses for participant characteristics and major health-related behavior can control for some of the effects of confounding factors. However, absence of residual confounding cannot be assured, especially if other important confounding factors are unknown, not assessed, or not included in the analyses.

C. Evidence of Causality

Epidemiology is the study of associations, and statistical methods provide the means for "testing" the association.

However, it is important to note that the existence of a statistically significant association does not indicate that the observed relationship is one of cause and effect. For any observed association, the following questions should be considered:

- How likely is it that the observed association is due to chance?
- Could this association be the result of poor study design, poor implementation, or inappropriate analysis?
- How well do these results meet other criteria of causality, as given in Table 2 [17]? Specifically, is the association weak or strong? Is there a plausible biologic mechanism? Did the exposure precede the outcome? Is there a dose–response relationship?
- How well do these results fit in the context of all available evidence on this association? Causality is supported when a number of studies, conducted at different times, using different methods, among different populations, show similar results.

In a field characterized by as much uncertainty as nutritional epidemiology, it is rare for a cause-and-effect relationship to be considered unequivocal. However, lack of complete certainty does not mean that we should ignore the information that we have or postpone action that appears needed at a given time [21]. It merely means that we exercise prudence and thoughtful consideration before acting on epidemiologic evidence.

V. OBSTACLES TO FINDING ASSOCIATIONS OF DIETARY INTAKE AND DISEASE RISK

Here we review the major obstacles to epidemiologic research, including error in exposure assessment and limitations of study designs.

A. Sources of Error in Food Frequency Questionnaires

Table 3 gives a summary of the potential sources of error and bias in estimating dietary intake using an FFQ. Many of these errors are respondent based, including problems with memory, errors in frequency judgments and portion size estimation, and social desirability bias. The form itself is a major source of error because of limitations inherent in closed-ended scannable response options, the use of a limited food list (generally about 100 items) to minimize respondent burden, inadequate food composition information, and the requirement that respondents average intake over long periods of time. Finally research indicates that dietary interventions themselves introduce reporting bias toward the more desirable responses [22].

1. ASSESSING THE RELIABILITY AND VALIDITY OF FOOD FREQUENCY QUESTIONNNAIRES

Reliability is generally used to refer to reproducibility, or whether an instrument will measure an exposure (e.g., nutrient intake) in the same way twice on the same respondents. Validity, which refers to the accuracy of an instrument, is a considerably higher standard. Generally a validity study compares a practical, epidemiologic measurement method (e.g., an FFQ) with a more accurate but more burdensome method (e.g., food records). Reliability and validity are typically investigated by means of statistical measures of bias and precision.

In a reliability study, reproducibility is assessed by comparing mean intake estimates from two administrations of the FFQ in the same group of respondents. If an instrument is reliable, the mean intake estimates should not vary substantially between the two administrations. In a validity study, bias is generally assessed by comparing the mean estimates from an FFQ to those from food records or recalls in the same respondents. This comparison allows us to determine whether nutrient intake estimates from an FFQ appear to be generally under- or overreported in comparison to the criterion measure. Bias is especially important when the objective is to measure absolute intakes for comparison to dietary recommendations or some other objective criteria. For example, bias is critical when estimating how close Americans are to meeting the dietary recommendation to eat five servings of fruits and vegetables per day.

Precision is concerned with whether an FFQ accurately ranks individuals from low to high nutrient intakes, which is typically the analytic approach used to assess associations of dietary intake with risk of disease. In this situation, bias in the estimate of absolute intake is not important as long as precision is good. In a reliability study, reproducibility is assessed as the correlation coefficient between nutrient intakes estimated from two administrations of the FFQ in the same group of respondents. In a validity study, precision is the correlation coefficient between nutrient intake estimates from the FFQ in comparison to a criterion measure (usually dietary recalls or records). Often FFQ studies also assess validity by ranking nutrient intake estimates, dividing them into categories (e.g., quartiles) and comparing these to similar categories calculated from another instrument. However, classifying a continuous exposure into a small number of categories does not reduce the effects of measurement error [1] and, therefore, this analysis does not provide additional information above correlation coefficients.

It is important to know that an instrument can be reliable without being accurate. That is, it can yield the same nutrient estimates two times and be wrong (e.g., biased upward or downward) both times. Alternatively, an instrument can be very reliable and consistently yield an accurate group mean (e.g., unbiased), but have poor precision such that it does not accurately rank individuals in the group from low to high in nutrient intake. Reliability is easy to measure, and nutrient correlation coefficients between two administrations of the

TABLE 2 Criteria for Judging whether Observed Associations between Diet and Disease Risk Are Causal[a]

Criteria	
Strength of the association	The stronger the association, the less likely that it is due to effect of an unsuspected or uncontrolled confounding variable.
Biological credibility	A known or postulated biologic mechanism supports causality. However an association that does not appear biologically credible at one time may eventually prove to be so. Implausible associations may be the beginning of the advancement of knowledge regarding mechanisms.
Time sequence	The exposure of interest must precede the disease outcome by a time span consistent with known biologic mechanisms.
Dose–response	Evidence for a dose–response relationship (i.e., increased risk associated with increased exposure) is considered supportive of causality.

[a]From Ref. 17.

same FFQ are generally in the range of 0.6–0.7. Estimates of reliability give an upper bound to the accuracy of an instrument. Whereas a high reliability coefficient does not imply a high validity coefficient, a low reliability coefficient clearly means poor validity.

Studies comparing FFQs with records or recalls are often called validation studies. The theory behind this type of study is that the major sources of error associated with FFQs are independent of those associated with short-term dietary recall and recording methods, which avoids spuriously high estimates of validity resulting from correlated errors. As summarized by Willett [3], the errors associated with FFQs are the restrictions imposed by a fixed list of foods, perception of portion sizes, and the cognitive challenge of assessing

TABLE 3 Sources of Error and/or Bias in Dietary Intake Estimates from a Food Frequency Questionnaire

Source of error	Type of error	Reason for error
Participant	Memory	Unable to recall food consumption. This error increases with interval of memory required.
	Frequency judgments	Respondent has cognitive difficulty accurately providing this information. May be a particular problem in low-literacy respondents.
	Question comprehension	Respondent may not understand what foods are being asked about, understand the frequency categories, or be able to estimate portion sizes.
	Response errors	Respondent mistakenly codes incorrect frequency or skips questions.
	Portion size errors	Respondent cannot conceptualize reference portion size or his or her own portion sizes.
	Social desirability bias	Respondent unintentionally (or intentionally) misrepresents dietary intake in order to please investigators. For example, obese participants may underestimate intake.
Questionnaire (investigator)	Food list	Food list is too short or not appropriate for population being studied and therefore dietary intake data are incomplete.
	Food groups	Food groups may not appropriately group foods by nutrient composition.
	Portion sizes	The reference portion size may be too large or small for population such that they consistently over- or underestimate amounts of food consumed.
	Categorization of frequencies	Loss of information by using close-ended categories (e.g., 2–4 times/week) instead of using an open-ended format.
	Poor design	Font is too small, skip patterns are not clear, or instructions are unclear.
	Database	Database may have incorrect nutrient values, incomplete nutrient values, or be missing important exposures altogether (e.g., isoflavones).
	Data collection and programming errors	Scanning errors may occur. Nutrient analysis program may contain errors. Data from incomplete FFQs are used in analysis.
	Seasonal variation	It may not be possible to adequately report intake of foods where intake varies markedly over seasons.
	Unusual dietary patterns	Respondents with unusual eating patterns (e.g., liquid diets) may not be able to accurately report dietary patterns.
Other	Intervention-associated bias	Respondents in an intervention are more likely to report socially desirable responses.

frequency of food consumption over a broad time frame. These sources of error are only minimally shared by diet records, which are open ended, do not depend on memory, and permit measurement of portion sizes. Biases in food records result from coding errors and changes in eating habits while keeping the records. Like food records, dietary recalls are open ended. However, recalls are usually collected without advance notification. Therefore, participants cannot change what they eat retroactively and the instrument itself should not affect food intake. Bias in recalls results from estimation of portion sizes, participant memory, and coding errors. Nonetheless, it is apparent that there are correlated errors between FFQs and records or recalls. Social desirability could influence how participants record or recall food intake across all types of dietary assessment instruments [22, 23]. Participant error in estimating portion sizes could bias recall and FFQ estimates of intake in similar ways. There are also correlated errors in nutrient databases. For example, estimates of selenium intake from FFQs and food records are correlated, which is merely the result of correlated errors in the nutrient database. Finally, research using doubly labeled water to determine energy requirements has demonstrated significant underreporting of energy intakes from food records that may vary by participant characteristics [9]. (See Chapter 2.) It is important to be aware of limitations of records and recalls as criterion measures of dietary intake and to interpret cautiously results based on these measures.

A final important consideration is that an FFQ cannot, in and of itself, be validated. Only individual nutrient intake estimates can be validated by comparison of a nutrient estimate from an FFQ to a more accurate measure.

2. EFFECTS OF ERROR IN FOOD FREQUENCY QUESTIONNAIRES

Error in dietary assessment can be of two types, with markedly different consequences. Random error refers to mistakes such as inadvertently marking the wrong frequency column, skipping questions, and lapses in judgment. These errors introduce noise into nutrient estimates such that our ability to find the "signal" (e.g., an association of dietary fat and breast cancer) is masked or attenuated (biased toward no association).

Systematic error refers to under- or overreporting of intake across the population (e.g., bias), but also person-specific sources of bias. For example, studies indicate that obese women are more likely to underestimate dietary intake than normal-weight women [9]. Systematic error may result in either null associations or spurious associations. In one report, Prentice [24] used data from FFQs collected in a low-fat dietary intervention trial to simulate the effects of random and systematic error on a association of dietary fat and breast cancer, where the true RR was assumed to be 4.0. Assuming only random error exists in the estimate of fat intake, the projected (i.e., observed) RR for fat and breast cancer would be 1.4. Assuming both random error and systematic error exists, the projected RR would be 1.1, similar to that re-

ported in a recent meta-analysis on dietary fat and breast cancer [25]. These results clearly suggest that FFQs may not be adequate to detect many associations of diet with disease, even if a strong relationship exists. Therefore, it is not surprising that results from diet–disease studies are often null or conflicting, given the error in our dietary assessment methods.

B. Limitations in Research Designs

1. OBSERVATIONAL STUDIES

In studies of nutritional epidemiology, unique obstacles exist to finding clear and interpretable relationships between dietary intake and disease risk [15]. In roughly increasing order of importance, these obstacles include the following:

- Current or recent dietary intake may differ from intake over the time frame relevant to the development of disease, which will reduce our ability to find associations between diet and disease.
- Certain nutrient intakes within a population may not be highly variable. For example, energy from dietary fat in a population of postmenopausal women may only vary from 25– 40%, resulting in inadequate range of disease risk to find an association with breast cancer. This situation is akin to assessing whether smoking causes cancer by studying men who smoke 1 pack per day in comparison to men who smoke 1.5 packs per day.
- Diet is a complex mixture of foods and nutrients, including many highly correlated compounds, making it difficult to separate the effects of any one compound from other dietary factors.
- Dietary intake may relate in a complicated manner to other risk factors such as hormonal status, obesity, or hypertension. These relationships (some of which may be in the causal pathway) make it difficult to appropriately control for confounding factors.
- Measurement properties of existing dietary self-report instruments are largely unknown, although it is clear that there are many sources of random error and systematic error, both of which obscure our ability to find associations between dietary intake and disease risk.

An important point to consider is that most of the obstacles listed above will limit or attenuate our ability to find associations between dietary intake and disease. For example, as shown in Table 4, an observed association of dietary fat intake with body mass index (BMI) might appear too small to be clinically important. However, if we assume that significant measurement error exists in our estimate of fat intake (e.g., a correlation of 0.30 between our measure and "true" intake), then the real association would be 4.0 BMI points per 10 g of fat intake, which is considerably more important. Therefore, studies showing weak or no associations between dietary intake and disease (e.g., null results) need to be interpreted cautiously.

Even this cursory review of the obstacles to interpretation of observational studies of diet and disease makes it clear

TABLE 4 Estimates of the Observed Association[a] between Dietary Fat Intake (Grams Fat/10) and BMI after Adjustment for Random Measurement Error in the Measure of Dietary Fat

Correlation coefficient[b] between the FFQ estimate and "true" fat intake	Observed increase in BMI for every 10 g of fat consumed[c]
1.00 (FFQ is perfect measure of fat intake)	4.0[c]
0.70 (FFQ is a good measure of fat intake)	2.8
0.50 (FFQ is a weak measure of fat intake)	2.0
0.30 (FFQ is a poor measure of fat intake)	1.2

[a] $\beta_{observed} = \beta_{true} \times$ validity coefficient.
[b] Correlation coefficient from validity study comparing FFQ to multiple 24-hour recalls.
[c] Assume true regression coefficient from a multivariate model predicting BMI equals 4.0.

that these studies alone may not provide reliable information on the associations of dietary intake and disease, regardless of their size or duration.

2. LIMITATIONS OF CLINICAL TRIALS OF DIETARY INTAKE AND DISEASE RISK

In spite of the many desirable features of dietary intervention trials, unique obstacles are present in these types of studies [15], as summarized below.

The costs of the dietary intervention itself can be formidable. For example, the National Institutes of Health-sponsored Women's Health Initiative (WHI) is testing the impact of a "low-fat eating pattern" on the incidence of breast cancer, colorectal cancer, and coronary heart disease among 48, 837 postmenopausal women in the United States [26]. The dietary intervention requires participants to attend monthly sessions (run by specially trained nutritionists) for the first 18 months and then quarterly classes for the remainder of the trial, which will average 8.5 years. In addition, new intervention components are being added to the trial to encourage adherence. The costs of implementing this type of intervention far exceed those required for comparatively simple pill–placebo trials.

Maintenance of dietary adherence for a sufficient period of time to be able to ascertain clinical outcomes (e.g., disease risk) can be a formidable task. On one hand, the greater the difference in dietary intake between the intervention and control groups, the more likely the study will be able to detect an effect on the outcome. However, it is clearly more difficult to get participants to adhere to very strict or limited regimes, which can result in such poor adherence that the trial becomes futile.

Monitoring of dietary adherence typically requires use of self-reported dietary instruments, with their attendant weaknesses (see above).

Intervention trials can only test a specific intervention or intervention program, so that the effects of specific elements of the intervention may be unclear. For example, the WHI intervention tests a dietary pattern low in fat and high in fruits, vegetables, and grains. If this intervention is shown to

reduce risk of breast cancer, the trial itself cannot separate out the effects of these dietary exposures without relying on dietary self-report.

Given the difficulties of delivering an effective dietary intervention and assessing the degree of dietary adherence, null trial results can be ambiguous.

VI. FUTURE RESEARCH DIRECTIONS

As is apparent from this overview of nutritional epidemiology, the biggest challenge is that of addressing random, systematic, and person-specific sources of error in dietary assessment. Only when well-designed, true validity studies clarify these sources of error will we be able to markedly improve our ability to draw valid inferences from epidemiologic studies of diet and disease.

An exciting area of future research concerns diet–gene interactions in the etiology and pathogenesis of many chronic diseases [27]. Despite the vigorous investigation of environmental causes of disease, it has long been recognized that not all persons exposed to the same risk factors will develop the associated disease [28]. For example, although it is well accepted that smoking causes lung cancer, only 10–15% of smokers will be diagnosed with the disease in their lifetime [29]. More and more, we are beginning to understand the impact of differential genetic susceptibility in the etiology and pathogenesis of common diseases such as coronary heart disease and cancer. If only a subgroup of individuals is sensitive to certain dietary exposures, the effect will be diluted and the association will be undetectable when the entire population is the focus of study. Better understanding of these individual susceptibilities has the potential to bring considerable clarity to nutritional epidemiologic research. (See Chapters 11–14 on genetics and nutritional health.)

To summarize, in spite of all the historical difficulties in obtaining consistent evidence of associations between diet and chronic diseases, considerable optimism remains that nutrition offers great hope in reducing morbidity and mortality from many chronic diseases. While the elimination of

error in dietary assessment methods is probably not a realistic objective, a better understanding of these errors (based on objective biomarkers), combined with statistical methods to address these errors, may be a reachable goal. It is the combined contribution of many different study types (e.g., observational, intervention, biomarker, mechanistic feeding studies, genetic susceptibility studies) that offers the greatest potential for identification of lifestyle strategies for disease prevention.

Acknowledgment

The author thanks Ann Shattuck for her careful review and thoughtful comments on this chapter.

References

1. Armstrong, B. K., White, E., and Saracci, R. (1994). Principles of exposure measurement in epidemiology. *In* "Monographs in Epidemiology and Biostatistics" Vol. XXI, pp. 22–48. Oxford University Press, Oxford.
2. Potter, J. D. (1999). Colorectal cancer: Molecules and populations. *J. Nat. Cancer Inst.* **91,** 916–932.
3. Willett, W. (1998). "Nutritional Epidemiology, " 2nd ed. Oxford University Press, Oxford.
4. Kristal, A. R., Vizenor, N. C., Patterson, R. E., Neuhouser, M. L., and Shattuck, A. L. Validity of food frequency based measures of fruit and vegetable intakes. *Cancer Epidemiol. Biomarkers Prevent.* (in press).
5. Patterson, R. E., White, E., Kristal, A. R., Neuhouser, M. L., and Potter, J. D. (1997). Vitamin supplements and cancer risk: A review of the epidemiologic evidence. *Cancer Causes Control* **8,** 786–802.
6. Suzukawa, M., Ayaori, M., Shuge, H., Hisada, T., Ishikawa, T., and Nakamura, H. (1998). Effect of supplementation with vitamin E in LDL oxidizability and prevention of atherosclerosis. *Biofactors* **7,** 51–54.
7. Patterson, R. E., Kristal, A. R., Carter, R. A., Fels-Tinker, L., Bolton, M. P., and Agurs-Collins, T. (1999). Measurement characteristics of the Women's Health Initiative food frequency questionnaire. *Ann. Epidemiol.* **9,** 178–197.
8. Patterson, R. E., Kristal, A. R., Levy, L., McLerran, D., and White, E. (1998) Validity of methods used to assess vitamin and mineral supplement use. *Am. J. Epidemiol.* **148,** 643–649.
9. Black, A. E., Prentice, A. M., Goldberg, G. R., Jebb, S. A., Livingstone, M. B., and Coward, W. A. (1993). Measurement of total energy expenditure provide insights into the validity of dietary measurements of energy intake. *J. Am. Diet. Assoc.* **93,** 572–579.
10. Armstrong, B., and Doll, R. (1975). Environmental factors and cancer incidence and mortality in different countries with special reference to dietary practices. *Int. J. Cancer* **15,** 617–631.
11. Gray, G. E., Pike, M. C., and Henderson, B. E. (1979). Breast cancer incidence and mortality rates in different countries in relation to known risk factors and dietary practices. *Br. J. Cancer* **39,** 1–7.
12. Prentice, R. L., and Sheppard, L. (1990). Dietary fat and cancer: Consistency of the epidemiologic data and disease prevention that may follow from a practical reduction in fat consumption. *Cancer Causes Control* **1,** 81–97.
13. Roberts, D. C. (1991). Dietary factors in the fall in coronary heart disease mortality. *Prostag. Leukotr. Essent. Fatty Acids* **44,** 97–101.
14. Ziegler, R. G., Hoover, R. N., Pike, M. C., et al. (1993). Migration patterns and breast cancer risk in Asian-American women. *J. Natl. Cancer Inst.* **85,** 1819–1827.
15. Prentice, R. L. (2000). Fat and fiber and breast cancer research—where is the field going? *Breast Cancer Res.* **2,** 268–276.
16. Rothman, K. J. (1986). Types of epidemiologic studies. *In* "Modern Epidemiology." Little, Brown and Company, Boston.
17. Hennekens, C. H., and Buring, J. E. (1987). "Epidemiology in Medicine" (S. L. Mayrent, Ed.). Little, Brown and Company, Boston.
18. Patterson, R. E., Neuhouser, M L., White, E., Hunt, J. R., and Kristal, A. R. (1998) Cancer related behavior of vitamin supplement users. *Cancer Epidemiol. Biomarkers Prev.* **7,** 79–81.
19. Gann, P. H. (1997). Interpreting recent trends in prostate cancer incidence and mortality. *Epidemiology* **8,** 117–20.
20. Patterson, R. E., Kristal, A. R., and White, E. (1996). Do beliefs, knowledge, and perceived norms about diet and cancer predict dietary change? *Am. J. Public Health* **86,** 1394–1400.
21. Hill, A. B. (1965). The environment and disease: Association or causation? *Proc. R. Soc. Med.* **65,** 58–295.
22. Kristal, A. R., Andrilla, C. A. H., Koepsell, T. D., Dieht, P. H., and Cheadle, A. (1998). Dietary assessment instruments are susceptible to intervention-associated response set bias. *J. Am. Diet. Assoc.* **98,** 40–43.
23. Hebert, J. R., Clemow, L., Pbert, L., Ockene, I. S., and Ockene, J. K. (1995). Social desirability bias in dietary self-report may compromise the validity of dietary intake measures. *Int. J. Epidemiol.* **24,** 389–98.
24. Prentice, R. L. (1996). Measurement error and results from analytic epidemiology: Dietary fat and breast cancer. *J. Natl. Cancer Inst.* **88,** 1738–1747.
25. Hunter, D. J., Speigelman, D., Adami, H. O., Beeson, L., van den Brandt, P. A., Folsom, A. R., Fraser, G. E., Goldbohm, R. A., Graitam, S., Howe, G. R., Kushi, L. H., Marshall, J. R., McDermott, A., Miller, A. B., Speizer, F. E., Wolk, A., Yaun, S-S., and Willett, W. (1996). Cohort studies of fat intake and the risk of breast cancer—a pooled analysis. *N. Engl. J. Med.* **334,** 356–361.
26. Women's Health Initiative Study Group. (1998). Design of the Women's Health Initiative clinical trial and observational study. *Control. Clin. Trials* **1,** 61–109.
27. Patterson, R. E., Eaton, D. L., and Potter, J. P. (1999). The genetic revolution: Change and challenge for the profession of dietetics. *J. Am. Diet. Assoc.* **99,** 1412–1420.
28. Khoury, M. J. (1997). Genetic epidemiology. *In* "Modern Epidemiology" (K. Rothman, S. Greenland, Eds.), 2nd ed., pp. 609–621. Little, Brown and Company, Boston.
29. American Cancer Society. (1995) "Cancer Facts and Figures." American Cancer Society, Atlanta, GA.

CHAPTER **5**

Analysis, Presentation, and Interpretation of Dietary Data

DEBRA COWARD–McKENZIE AND RACHEL K. JOHNSON
The University of Vermont, Burlington, Vermont

I. INTRODUCTION

Nutritional epidemiological studies, while not an exact science, play a critical role in relating dietary intake to risk of disease. These investigations often require the gathering of dietary intake data from various samples, which must then be translated into a usable form. This chapter discusses what is done with the dietary data once they have been collected. This includes *analysis,* the examination of the dietary data to determine the nutritional composition of the subjects' diet; *presentation,* presenting the data from the research in a logical form, often done by comparing the analyzed data to a standard; and *interpretation,* the translation of the data—what do the data really tell us?

II. ANALYSIS OF DIETARY DATA

The methods most often used to obtain dietary intake information for research investigations include dietary recalls, food records or diaries, and food frequency questionnaires (FFQs). Dietary recalls and food records provide detailed descriptions of the types and amounts of food and beverages consumed throughout a specified period of time, normally 1 (24-hour recall) to 7 days. The FFQ provides a less detailed list of selected foods and the frequency of their consumption in the past. (See Chapter 1 for further description of these methods.) The data received must then be analyzed to determine the total intake of nutrients or food components consumed by each subject.

A. Computer-Based Analysis

In the past, analysis was performed manually. This process was painstakingly tedious and expensive, requiring a highly trained person to code and enter data. Coding included looking up every food in a table to find a code number to be entered. Amounts were entered by unit and a multiplier. These coding techniques required many calculations to be performed by hand, leaving numerous possibilities for error. Now, a variety of computer-based food composition data-

bases and nutrient computation systems are available in which the foods can be directly entered by name and computation of nutrient values are automated. The accuracy of the data obtained from these systems will differ, depending on several factors.

1. *Updating of the database.* New foods are constantly being added to the market, so the best databases are updated often to keep up with the changes. Most databases use the U.S. Department of Agriculture (USDA) Nutrient Database for Standard Reference (SR) as their primary source of nutrient data. The SR contains information once published in the Agriculture Handbook 8, but it is no longer available in the printed form [1]. The most recent release of the SR, number 13 [2], was issued in November 1999 and contains more than 6000 items. The USDA receives information from industry, scientific literature, government agencies, and contracted laboratories and universities [3]. Although the information is not complete, specific criteria have been established for evaluating foods to ensure the data are as accurate as possible [4]. Many databases also add information from specific food manufacturers to provide information on name brand foods not available in the SR.

2. *The number and types of food items available.* This is particularly important for recalls and food records or for FFQs containing "Write-in" sections where all foods must be given nutrient values. In regions with ethnocultural diversity, special care must be taken when selecting databases [5]. Databases that contain a variety of ethnic foods will provide greater accuracy and will require less manual entry of nutrient values for foods.

3. *The ability to add foods or nutrients.* This is most important for those investigations in areas with multiethnicity or when there is a high tendency for the subjects to include restaurant foods that may not be included in the database. The ability to adapt or add recipe information should also be available. For example, if a subject had homemade beef stew for lunch, the database should allow the coder to either add or delete ingredients from an existing recipe or add a new recipe to the file.

4. *The ease of data entry and analysis.* It is no longer necessary to code diets manually. Systems should be easy to

use to avoid unnecessary coding errors that can occur. Entry of products by name, particularly brand names, should be available. Some research databases, such as the Food Intake Analysis System [6], offer default options. These choices provide average estimations for foods for which exact information is not known. For example, if a subject had chicken breast, but was not sure of the cooking method or the serving size, the coder has the default option to choose from instead of making guesses. These options can help decrease differences in nutrient intake values caused by multiple coders or data entry technicians.

5. *The nutrients available.* Not every database contains all nutrients and some contain more accurate data for particular nutrients. Systems should be evaluated for the accuracy of the nutrient values that are being studied. Analysis should include the option of choosing nutrient calculations for each food as well as summaries for an individual meal or day.

6. *The handling of missing nutrient values.* If a specific nutrient value is unknown for a particular food, the way the database handles the missing information may affect the accuracy of the data. Some systems intelligently impute values, while others simply use a value of zero. An imputed value is almost always a better estimation [7]. However, imputing nutrient values is a labor-intensive task and requires nutritionists with knowledge of data evaluation and imputing procedures. Therefore, caution must be taken when using databases with imputed values, because few database developers have access to qualified nutrition-trained personnel required for accurately estimating values [8].

When computing nutrient intake from food consumption data, it is assumed that the nutrient quality and content of certain foods are virtually constant, and that what is consumed is available for use. However, we know that this assumption is not totally correct. There are various reasons why the actual value of a consumed nutrient may differ from the calculated value. The level of certain nutrients in foods may be affected by differences in growing and harvesting conditions (i.e., selenium [9, 10]), storage, processing, and cooking (i.e., vitamin C [11, 12]). Databases have tried to account for some of the differences by increasing the databanks to include preparation methods, cuts of meat, and specific manufacturers for processed food. For example, if chicken is entered into the database, the coder may have approximately 455 items from which to choose. This large number includes name brand foods, particular pieces of chicken available (i.e., breast or thigh), and cooking methods (i.e., baked or fried, cooked with skin on or off, skin eaten or not). Because so many choices are offered, recalls should be as detailed as possible to provide enough information to make an accurate selection.

The use of controlled feeding trials in a study, such as the Dietary Approaches to Stop Hypertension (DASH) trial [13], can help alleviate some of the differences between the calculated and actual nutrient values of food. The DASH trial was a multicenter study designed to compare the effects of dietary patterns on blood pressure. The subjects were asked to consume only foods prepared by the centers. Menu items could then be analyzed in a laboratory to obtain nutrient values [14]. Food procurement, production, and distribution guidelines were set and strictly adhered to at all sites to ensure that menus consistently met nutrient goals. For example, food items were given specific purchasing sizes, detailed descriptions, and/or defined brand names to ensure that all site recipes were of uniform composition [15]. When possible, foods can be obtained from central suppliers to further eliminate any differences in nutritional content of foods due to regional variations in a study of this type.

The diet as a whole can also affect the availability of some nutrients. For example, high-fiber diets may decrease the availability of certain nutrients, such as zinc and iron [16, 17], generally due to the binding effects of phytate. Computer-based analysis programs do not generally examine the overall diet and cannot determine how nutrient–nutrient interactions may affect availability. Iron, for example, is a mineral for which intake is not a good marker for availability. The absorption of iron is subject to many components: (1) the source of iron (heme is more easily absorbed than nonheme); (2) the iron status of the individual (decreased stores increase absorption); and (3) the overall composition of the meal. All of these components play a role in determining how much of the iron consumed is available to the body [17]. In turn, iron consumption can also affect the absorption of other nutrients, such as zinc. Nutrient–nutrient interactions can greatly determine how well a calculated nutrient value represents the actual available amount of a nutrient.

Other factors that should be taken into account are drug–nutrient interactions and those people who may be malnourished or suffer from malabsorption. The elderly, for example, have decreased ability to absorb vitamin B^{12}. This group is also at higher risk for drug–nutrient interactions because they are often prescribed many medications. Researchers must be aware of any illnesses or medications taken by subjects that could interfere with nutrient absorption.

The development of fat-blocking drugs, i.e., Orlistat [18], can decrease absorption of not only the fat, which will decrease actual fatty acids and calories absorbed, but also other fat-soluble nutrients. Orlistat is an intestinal lipase inhibitor approved for the treatment of obesity [18]. This drug has been shown to decrease absorption of fat consumed, which also reduces fat-soluble vitamins, vitamins A, D, E, and K, and other compounds.

Olestra, a sucrose esterified with fatty acids, has been approved by the U.S. Food and Drug Administration (FDA) as a fat replacer in savory snacks [19]. Studies concluded that when Olestra was eaten with foods containing fat-soluble vitamins it decreases the absorption of these nutrients. Al-

though these vitamins are added to the Olestra-containing foods, actual absorption may still be affected for constituents not fortified in olestra-containing foods such as carotenoids.

Although food composition databases are increasingly becoming more accurate and may be closer to actual values of energy intake than laboratory analysis [14], they cannot provide exact measurements for all nutrient intakes. Furthermore, even if these values are determined to be accurate, intake does not necessarily mean the nutrient is available for use. To obtain more accurate information on nutrient status, other methods, such as biomarkers (see Chapter 10), should be employed. Also, familiarity with the subjects being investigated is essential for more accurate calculations. This includes, but is not limited to, considering factors such as supplementation, medications used, specific diseases or illness, as well as special diets (i.e., vegetarian).

B. Total Diet Analysis

Because accurate measures of nutrient values based on food intake are difficult to calculate, some investigators have begun to use innovative ways to evaluate the overall diet. Although using these techniques will not provide exact numbers for specific nutrients, they will give investigators a better picture of overall diet quality and health risk. With the increasing evidence that other non-nutrient constituents, such as phytochemicals, may play a role in disease prevention [20], these indexes could prove to be very useful.

In reviewing the indexes of overall diet quality, Kant [21] found that there were three major approaches to the development of indexes: (1) derived from nutrients only, (2) based on foods or food groups, and (3) based on a combination of nutrients and foods. The definition of "diet quality" differs based on the attributes chosen by the investigators of each index [21], so the index chosen will depend on the needs of the study. Those indexes based on nutrients only tend to look at the percentage of the Recommended Daily Allowance (RDA) consumed as a marker for diet quality. Those based on foods and food groups examine the intake patterns of foods to identify patterns associated with adequacy [21].

Although numerous tools are available for examining the overall diet quality [21] those most commonly applied are based on the combination of nutrients and foods. These indexes, including the Healthy Eating Index (HEI) [22] and the Diet Quality Index (DQI) [23, 24] use the Dietary Guidelines for Americans [25] and the Food Guide Pyramid [26] to score the overall diet. These are based on the premise that if the USDA Food Guide Pyramid and guidelines are followed, including a variety of foods within each food group, the resulting diet will be adequate in nutrients and promote optimal health [27].

Patterson et al. [23] were among the first to relate diet quality to the Dietary Guidelines for Americans. The DQI included measures of eight food groups and the recommendations from the Committee on Diet and Health of the National Research Council Food and Nutrition Board, published in 1989 [28]. The index was revised by Haines et al., called the Dietary Quality Index–Revised (DQI-R) [24], to reflect the updated guidelines and Food Guide Pyramid. The DQI-R incorporates both nutrients and food components to determine diet quality. It is based on 10 components, with a 100-point scale, each component worth 10 points (Table 1).

TABLE 1 Diet Quality Index–Revised

Component	Max score criteria[a]	Min score criteria[a]
Total fat (% of energy intake)	≤30%	>40%
Saturated fat (% of energy intake)	≤10%	>13%
Dietary cholesterol	≤300 mg	>400 mg
% Recommended servings of fruit per day (2 to 4 based on energy intake)	≥100%	<50%
% Recommended servings of vegetables/day (3 to 5 based on energy intake)	≥100%	<50%
% Recommended servings of bread per day (6 to 11 based on energy intake)	≥100%	<50%
Calcium (% adequate intake for age)	≥100%	<50%
Iron intake (% 1989 RDA for age)	≥100%	<50%
Dietary diversity score	≥6	<3
Dietary moderation score	≥7	<4

Source: Adapted from Haines, P. S., Siega-Riz, A. M., and Popkin, B. M. (1999). The Diet Quality Index revised: A measurement instrument for populations. Copyright © The American Dietetic Association. Reprinted by permission from Journal of The American Dietetic Association, Vol. 99:697–704.
[a]Scoring range for each component is 0 (min) to 10 (max).

TABLE 2   Healthy Eating Index[a]

Component	Max score (10) criteria	Min score (0) criteria
Grains	6–11 servings	0 servings
Vegetables	3–5 servings	0 servings
Fruit	2–4 servings	0 servings
Milk	2–3 servings	0 servings
Meat	2–3 servings	0 servings
Total fat (% energy intake)	≤30%	≥45%
Saturated fat (% energy intake)	>10%	≥15%
Cholesterol intake	≤300 mg	≥450 mg
Sodium intake	≤2400 mg	≥4800 mg
Food variety	≥8 different items/day	≤3 different items/day

Source: Adapted from Kennedy, E. T., Ohls, J., Carlson, S., and Fleming, K. (1995). The Healthy Eating Index: Design and applications. *J. Am. Diet. Assoc.* **95,** 1103–1108.

[a]Each component has a score range of 0 to 10. The number of food group servings is based on recommended energy intake.

Components are based on total fat and saturated fat as a percentage of energy, milligrams of cholesterol consumed, recommended servings for fruit, vegetables, and grains, adequacy of calcium and iron intake, dietary diversity and dietary moderation. The dietary diversity, score was developed to show differences in intake across 23 broad food group categories including seven grain-based products, seven vegetable components, two fruit and juice categories, and seven animal-based products [24]. Dietary moderation scores added sugars, discretionary fat, sodium intake, and alcohol intake. The DQI-R was designed to monitor dietary changes in populations, but can provide an estimate of diet quality for an individual relative to the national guidelines and can note improvement or decline of diet quality with multiple calculations [24].

The HEI [22, 27] was first developed by the USDA Center for Nutrition Policy and Promotion (CNPP) to assess and monitor the dietary status of Americans using the 1989 data from the Continuing Survey of Food Intake of Individuals (CSFII) [27], and again in 1994–1996 [22]. It also uses both nutrients and food components to determine overall diet quality. Like the DQI-R, it is based on a 10-component, 100-point scale (Table 2). Components are based on recommendations of servings for fruits, vegetables, grains, milk, and meat; percentages of energy from total fat and saturated fat; cholesterol and sodium intake; and a food variety score. Dietary variety is assessed by totaling the number of different foods eaten in a day in amounts that contributed at least one-half of a serving for any food group [22].

Categorizing foods into appropriate groups, particularly combination foods, can be a problem when using these analysis techniques. Cleveland *et al.* [29] developed a method for assessing food intakes in terms of food servings. These guidelines help overcome two major obstacles when assessing food intake with respect to the dietary guidelines, including dealing with food mixtures and differing units of measurement used. Because many foods are eaten as mixtures and difficult to categorize into food groups, Cleveland *et al.* [29] developed a recipe file that helps break down food mixtures into ingredients so they can be assigned their respective groups more easily (see Fig. 1). Standard serving sizes were assigned gram weights to help overcome the units problem, allowing for the use of only one unit of measure. The 1994 USDA-CSFII database data file [30] incorporates these guidelines. Although combined foods must still be separated and coded before entering, this file does provide a more refined method for developing reproducible data [24].

III. PRESENTATION OF DATA

Once the data gathered from the dietary assessment methods have been analyzed, they must then be presented in a useful fashion. This is often done by comparing the analyzed data to a standard. These standards may include the Dietary Reference Intake (DRI) or comparison to a national average, such as the National Health and Nutrition Examination Surveys (NHANES) or the USDA (CSFII) data.

The DRIs are a set of nutrient-based reference values. This set includes an estimated average requirement (EAR), a Recommended Dietary Allowance (RDA), and an adequate intake (AI), which are defined by nutrient adequacy and may relate to the reduction of the risk of chronic disease [31]. Once the EARs have been established they are used to set the new RDAs, which should be used as a daily intake goal by healthy individuals, and should be sufficient to meet the needs of 97–98% of all healthy individuals. If

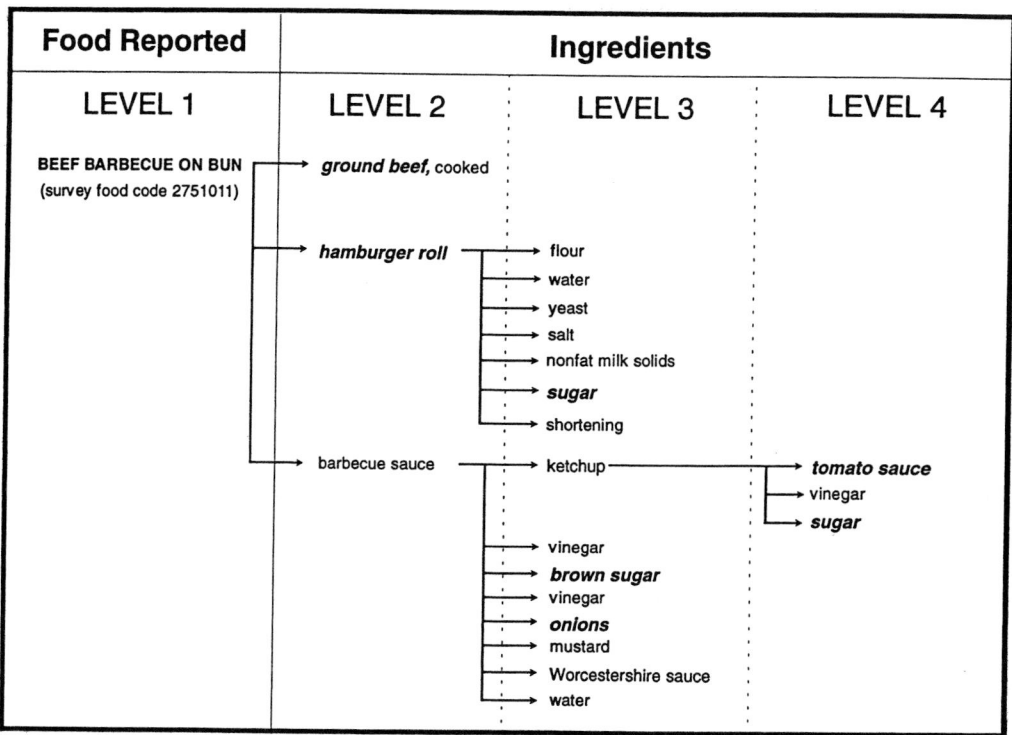

FIGURE 1   Example of a cascaded recipe file showing multiple levels of disaggregation. Italics indicates level of disaggregation required for classification according to food guidance definitions. [Reprinted with permission from Cleveland, L. E., Cook, D. A., Krebs-Smith, S. M., and Friday, J. (1997). Methods for assessing food intakes in terms of servings based on food guidance. *Am. J. Clin. Nutr.* **65**(suppl), 1254S–1263S. © *Am. J. Clin. Nutr.* American Society for Clinical Nutrition.]

there is not sufficient evidence to determine an EAR, then an AI is set, once again based on groups of healthy individuals. A tolerable upper intake level (UL) is also set where information is available as an indicator of excess for nutrients [31].

Each value has a specific goal and use [31] (Table 3). For example, the EAR is the estimate that is believed to meet the nutrient needs of half of the healthy individuals in a gender or life-stage group. When assessing nutrient intake of healthy groups, it is highly recommended that the EAR be used instead of the RDA [31]. However, because DRIs have not been set for all nutrients at this time, the old RDAs can be used for these nutrients until new guidelines have been established.

DRIs are set for specific subgroups based on age and gender. They are to be applied to healthy populations and may not be adequate for those who are or have been malnourished, or have certain diseases or conditions that increase nutrient requirements. For individuals, the RDA and AI can serve as a goal for nutrient intake.

Some researchers use national surveys as a standard when presenting dietary data. The NHANES and CSFII are both surveys that regularly collect data on the nation's nutritional status. The NHANES are conducted approximately every 5 years, while the CSFII is conducted annually. NHANES pro-

vides medical history, physical measurements, biochemical evaluation, physical signs and symptoms, and diet information from 24-hour recalls. The CSFII provides diet information based on two 24-hour recalls. Researchers may wish to compare their subjects' data to the information obtained from these surveys to determine how their sample compares to the national average. Although the data from these surveys may be applied to certain subgroups, such as specific age groups, gender, socioeconomic levels, education levels and some ethnic groups, they cannot be used as guides for others, such as malnourished or specific disease states.

Researchers who choose to use the HEI or the DQI-R report their data by using the 100-point scale. For example, the HEI scores are based on the assumption that a "good" diet has a score greater than or equal to 80, a diet that "needs improvement" has a score of 51 to 80, and those diets that score 50 or below are considered "poor" [22]. When this method was applied to the CSFII 1994–1996 data, the average mean score for the 3 years was 63 [22]. The CSFII researchers found that 70% of the population had diets that needed improvement, 12% had good diets, and 18% had poor diets. Researchers may also compare the scores from their subjects' data to the national scores for that time period, when available, to determine if their study population falls in line with the national average.

TABLE 3 Uses of Dietary Reference Intakes for Healthy Individuals and Groups

Type of Use	For the Individual	For a Group
Planning	**RDA:** aim for this intake.	**EAR:** use in conjunction with a measure of variability of the group's intake to set goals for the mean intake of a specific population.
	AI: aim for this intake. **UL:** use as a guide to limit intake; chronic intake of higher amounts may increase risk of adverse effects.	
Assessment[a]	**EAR:** use to examine the possibility of inadequacy; evaluation of true status requires clinical, biochemical, and/or anthropometric data.	**EAR:** use in the assessment of the prevalence of inadequate intakes within a group.
	UL: use to examine the possibility of overconsumption; evaluation of true status requires clinical, biochemical, and/or anthropometric data.	

Source: Standing Committee on the Scientific Evaluation of Dietary Reference Intakes; Food Nutrition Board, Institute of Medicine. (1997). "Dietary Reference Intakes for Calcium, Phosphorus, Magnesium, Vitamin D, and Fluoride." National Academy Press, Washington, DC. Reprinted with permission.

Key: EAR, estimated average requirement; RDA, recommended dietary allowance; AI, adequate intake; UL, tolerable upper intake level.

[a]Requires statistically valid approximation of usual intake.

IV. INTERPRETATION OF DATA

Once the dietary intake data have been analyzed and compared to a standard, researchers must then look at the results to determine what the data really mean. How the data are interpreted can depend on the assessment method used and the nutrient being studied, the study type, and the accuracy of the subject's responses.

A. Assessment Methods

The assessment method chosen for use in a study can determine how the data collected can be interpreted. Recalls and records gather present intake data, while FFQs provide data based on past intake. It is known that an individual's nutrient and energy intake varies not only from day to day, but season

Hierarchy of scientific evidence

From lowest to highest credibility:

Anecdotal reports
Case studies
Case–control studies
Longitudinal cohort studies
Multicenter, randomized, controlled clinical trials

FIGURE 2 Hierarchy of scientific evidence.

to season as well. So if past intake is needed, FFQs may be the better choice.

The number of days of food intake records or recalls available can also affect the interpretation of the data. If high levels of accuracy are needed for an individual's intake of a nutrient, a greater number of days will be required than if a group average could be used. Care must be taken when determining the number of days to use in a study. For example, researchers using data from a single 24-hour recall from 832 men estimated their fat intake and determined that eating saturated fat prevents strokes [32]. Because of the day-to-day variability, dietary changes or recommendations for an individual should not be based on a single day's intake. Basiotis *et al.* [33] determined the number of days of food intake data needed to estimate individual intake as well as group intake for food energy and 18 nutrients. They found that for a female, an average of 35 days is needed to determine a true average of energy intake for each individual, while 3 days of food records from each subject are required to determine a group average.

It is also important that data obtained from dietary assessment methods be utilized properly. The FFQ was developed to rank nutrient intakes from low to high. It was not intended to be used to determine and develop levels of nutrient intake to prevent disease. However, many researchers have chosen to use the FFQ for this purpose. For example, studies based on FFQ data recommended levels of vitamin E intake to prevent heart disease [34, 35]. Recently, studies have concluded that these levels may not have the effect on heart disease development as previously suggested [36]. When choosing a method for dietary assessment, care must be taken to ensure that the data are properly interpreted.

B. The Hierarchy of Scientific Evidence

To make a judgment about dietary changes, the hierarchy of scientific evidence should be kept in mind (Fig. 2). The most rigorous evaluation of a dietary hypothesis is the randomized feeding trial, which should ideally be conducted as a double-blind experiment. Large, randomized feeding trials may eventually provide definitive answers to some of the questions we have regarding the relationships between dietary factors and the major illnesses of our society. Unfortunately, these are extremely costly, and may be of long duration if the disease studied has a long latency period. For now, our

knowledge of many of these relationships has been derived mainly from cohort studies.

C. Data Validity

One major concern when interpreting dietary data is the accuracy of the information reported (see Chapter 4). Because most of the information gathered is self-reported, the reliability and validity of the data depend on the reporter's motivation, memory, ability to communicate, and awareness of the foods consumed. Most methods have been proven to be generally reliable; that is, they will provide the same estimate on different occasions. However, do the techniques gather true and accurate measurements, or valid measurements, of what people are really eating? In the past, assumptions were made that the information was indeed valid. The validity of the techniques was often verified by comparing the different methods to each other. For example, a FFQ may be "validated" by comparing results to food records. If the food records are 100% accurate, this method of validation would be fine. However, because both methods require self-reported intake, the validity of both methods should be questioned. Therefore, external independent markers of intake are needed for true validation [37].

During the 1980s, the search began for biochemical indicators that closely reflect dietary intake. These indicators, a type of biomarker, measure specific variables in body fluids or tissues to reflect intake of a food component [38]. Doubly labeled water (DLW) is the most widely used biomarker for energy intake at this time (see Chapter 2 for further details). Although this method can only determine the accuracy of a dietary intake method with respect to total energy, it is reasonable to assume that if that method is accurate (or not) for energy, it will also be so for specific macro- and micronutrients [39, 40]. Therefore, it is accepted that if group estimates of energy intake are found to be truly valid using a method such as DLW, the estimates of macro- and micronutrient intakes can also be considered valid [41].

Other biomarkers that have been used to validate nutrient intake (also discussed in Chapter 4) include fatty acid patterns in blood to reflect fatty acid intake [42], urinary nitrogen to validate protein intake [43–45], and serum carotenoids and vitamin C concentrations as markers of fruit and vegetable consumption [46, 47]. With the increased use of these biomarkers, particularly DLW, to determine the accuracy of dietary intake data in a variety of subjects, it has become clear that the traditional dietary assessment methods are not completely accurate. It is now well accepted that misreporting of food intake—over- or underreporting—is widespread and that no data gathering method is immune [37].

1. OVERREPORTING

Overreporting occurs when reported intakes are higher than the measured energy expenditure levels. Overreporting has not been found to be as big of a problem as underreporting, but still has the potential to interfere with research data. Johansson et al. [48] found that individuals who overreport tend to be younger, and with lower body mass indexes, often considered lean. The highest proportion of overreporters was found among those subjects who wanted to increase body weight. While overreporters are not common, care should be taken when obtaining data from subjects that are at highest risk.

2. UNDERREPORTING

Underreporting occurs when reported intakes are much lower than measured energy expenditure levels. These reports are often so low that basal metabolic needs could not be met and are not biologically plausible. Depending on the age, gender, and body composition of a given sample, underreporters may compose anywhere from 10–45% of the total sample. It is now understood that underreporting tends to be associated with certain groups. It is well accepted that the obese are at greatest risk of underreporting dietary intake. Many studies have shown that the obese underreport more often and to a greater degree—30–47%—than the lean [49, 50]. Women have also been found to underreport more often than men [51–53]. Other characteristics of low energy intake reporters include those associated with low-socioeconomic status, that is, low-income and low-education levels [51–53]. Table 4 provides a summary of groups who have been

TABLE 4   Summary of Underreporting

Populations most likely to underreport:	
Women	High scorers on restrained eating scales
Obese	Smokers
Low-socioeconomic status	Lower education
Foods most likely to be underreported:	
U.S. Survey[a]	
Cake/pie	Meat mixtures
Savory snacks	Regular soft drinks
Cheese	Fat-type spreads
White potatoes	Condiments
British Study[b]	
Cake	Breakfast cereal
Sugars	Milk
Fats	

[a]U.S. Survey from: Kreb-Smoth, S. M., Graubard, B., Cleveland, L., Subar, A., Ballard-Barbash, R., and Kahle, L. (1998). Low energy reporters vs others: A comparison of reported food intakes. *Eur. J. Clin. Nutr.* **52**(2), S18.

[b]British Survey from Bingham, S. A., Cassidy, A., Cole, T. J., Welch, A., Runswick, S. A., Black, A. E., Thurnham, D., Bates, C., Khaw, K. T., Key, T. J. A., Day, N. E. (1995). Validation of weighed records and other methods of dietary assessment using the 24 h urine nitrogen technique and other biological markers. *Br. J. Nutr.* **73**, 531–550.

found to be underreporters. These factors are further complicated due to the fact that they are also risk factors for many chronic diseases.

3. REASONS FOR UNDERREPORTING

Once underreporting became well accepted and documented, researchers began, and continue, to look for reasons why people underreport. We know that being obese is not the cause of underreporting, but it is most likely the psychological and behavioral characteristics associated with obesity that lead to underreporting [54, 55]. A need for social acceptance, a desire to be liked or accepted by the interviewer, may cause the subject to underreport "sinful" foods. A high level of body dissatisfaction, that is, if a person sees a leaner physique as being healthier or more desirable than their own, may cause him or her to misreport foods. Also, researchers have found that women who scored higher on restrained eating scales, those who feel they are making a conscious effort to avoid certain foods, tend to underreport as well [54, 55].

4. FOODS MOST OFTEN UNDERREPORTED

If underreporting occurred in all foods and nutrients to the same degree, the solution would be to add a correction factor to the data of the underreporters. This would bring their reported intake of all nutrients into line with that of the valid reporters. Unfortunately, it has become clear that underreporters often fail to report those foods that are seen as "bad" or "sinful" [40]. In a U. S. survey of 8334 adults, 1224 were found to be low energy reporters [56]. Some of the foods that were found to be most often underreported included cakes/pies, savory snacks, cheese, white potatoes, meat mixtures, regular soft drinks, fat-type spreads, and condiments [56]. British researchers found that little difference was seen between underreporters and normal energy reporters with regard to bread, potatoes, meat, vegetables, or fruit, but a significant difference was seen with cakes, sugars, fat, and breakfast cereal [44]. Table 4 gives a summary of underreported foods. Some researchers have found that underreporters tend to report lower intakes of fat, and higher intakes of protein and carbohydrates as a percentage of total energy [57, 58], while others show that reports of added sugar intake are significantly lower [59]. No agreement has been reached as to how much, if at all, specific macronutrients are misreported. Therefore, adding a correction factor would not be effective.

5. THE PROBLEMS WITH UNDERREPORTING

The major problem with underreporting occurs when researchers begin to classify dietary intake information to determine diet and disease associations. This is often done by ranking nutrient intakes from low to high, and then looking for any associations between nutrient intake and occurrence of disease. There is a very real danger of misclassification of subjects if this ranking is based on false or underreported intake. As pointed out earlier, those who tend to be at higher risk for underreporting are also those who are at greater risk for many chronic diseases. For example, obesity is a known risk factor for coronary heart disease as well as underreporting. Because bias in measuring dietary intake has the potential of removing as well as creating associations, it can generate misleading conclusions about the impact of diet and disease [60, 61].

Underreporting is now understood to be a very real and potentially misleading problem in nutrition research. Although the use of biomarkers can help validate and interpret dietary intake data and, ideally, should become routine in nutritional epidemiology, they cannot totally replace the collection of estimated dietary intakes. Food is made up of many components, not simply the nutrients that we are aware of and that can be found in a database. Records of foods consumed may help researchers find non-nutrient constituents that help reduce risks. More and more evidence is accumulating to support the belief that the entire food, not just specific components, leads to increased health [62, 63]. Also, there is not a biomarker for every dietary constituent that is of interest to researchers. Finally, collection methods can be performed on very large populations at a much lower cost than the use of biomarkers and requires less technology and fewer skills.

6. IDENTIFYING UNDERREPORTERS

To help identify underreporters, researchers can apply methods such as the Goldberg cutoff, extensively described by Goldberg and colleagues [64] and Black and colleagues [65]. The Goldberg cutoff identifies the most obviously implausible intake values by evaluating the energy intake against estimated energy requirements. Basal metabolic rate (BMR) can be measured using methods described in Chapter 3, or height and weight measurements can be used to predict BMR from a standard formula (the Schofield equation is recommended by Goldberg *et al.* [64]). A ratio of the estimated energy intake (EI) to measured or predicted BMR is calculated as EI/BMR. This ratio can then be compared with a study-specific cutoff value (provided in Goldberg *et al.* [64]). This cutoff represents the lowest value of EI/BMR that could reasonably reflect the energy expenditure if the person led a sedentary lifestyle. A summary of Goldberg cutoffs can be found in Table 5. Studies using the Goldberg cutoff classified 28–39% of the women and 18–27% of the men as low energy reporters [52, 57].

The Goldberg cutoff has certain limitations. Because the cutoff assumes that everyone leads a sedentary lifestyle, it tends to underestimate the underreporters. If researchers can gather information on lifestyle, occupation, leisure time, and particularly information regarding physical activity of the subjects, calculations can be more specific and improve the chances of identifying the underreporters [66].

7. HANDLING UNDERREPORTING IN DIETARY DATA

Researchers are still not sure how to handle databases containing large numbers of underreporters. Several ap-

TABLE 5   Goldberg Cutoff

The Goldberg cutoff assumes the subjects are in energy balance so,

Energy intake (EI) = energy expenditure (EE)

Therefore if EE = physical activity level (PAL) × BMR then,

EI = PAL × BMR   or   EI/BMR = PAL
where PAL = Goldberg cutoff.

The Goldberg cutoffs are factorial calculations that estimate average physical activity level based on a sedentary lifestyle.

Cutoff 1: Tests whether reported energy intake measurements can represent long-term habitual intake.

1.35 × BMR   or   EI/BMR = 1.35
where BMR is measured rather than predicted.

Cutoff 2: Is more liberal than 1 and tests whether the reported energy intakes are plausible measurements of food consumed during the measured period. It allows for day-to-day variability. Cutoff 2 limits should be determined based on the number of days of data available for each subject, the number of subjects, and the confidence level desired. Tables are provided in Goldberg *et al.* [64].

Numbers falling below the cutoff should be recognized as underreporting. If information regarding physical activity can be gathered, more accurate cutoffs can be used.

Source: Data found in Goldberg, G. R., Black, A. E., Jebb, S. A., Cole, T. J., Murgatroyd, P. R., Coward, W. A., and Prentice, A. M. (1991). Critical evaluation of energy intake data using fundamental principles of energy physiology: 1. Derivation of cut-off limits to identify under-recording. *Eur. J. Clin. Nutr.* **45,** 569–581.

proaches have been suggested, but none are ideal. One technique would be to exclude anyone who is found to report implausible energy intakes. The problem with this method is that the underreporters tend to fall into specific subgroups (i.e., obese, smokers), and as stated previously, will seriously alter the sample. Some investigators have analyzed their data with all the subjects, and then again after the underreporters have been removed [67]. If there are no significant discrepancies between the finding, this can improve the confidence in the results and conclusions.

Some have suggested that once the difference between the low reporters and valid reporters is noted, upward adjustments of all the nutrients could be made. Because underreporting does not appear to occur equally for all nutrients, this method is not advisable. Research has shown that underreporters tend to report micronutrient-rich diets when compared to valid reporters [51]. Adjusting would give a false impression of the nutrient status, and could mask possible risks of disease.

Other researchers have suggested adjusting nutrient intakes for energy intake using the regression of nutrient vs. energy [68]. This would be feasible only if portion sizes were underestimated, yet the actual foods were all reported accurately. Otherwise, this method could make the reports worse [69]. As noted earlier, it is most likely that foods are systematically omitted from recalls. So if, for example, fat-

containing foods, such as desserts, are often underreported, while vitamin A containing foods, i.e., cantaloupe, are not, energy adjustments would provide lower than actual measures of fat intake, but a higher measure of vitamin A intake. It has been recognized by many researchers that adjustments cannot eliminate bias caused by selective underreporting [70].

V. CONCLUSION

Although dietary assessment methods do not provide true nutritional intake values, it is not feasible to eliminate them from nutritional research studies. Nutritional health cannot be evaluated without also examining the total diet composition. Improving dietary intake methodology is critical to the credibility of nutrition research. Identifying underreporters and improving dietary database validity through analytical approaches should remain in the forefront of nutritional epidemiological studies until methodology improvements can be found. Researchers as well as practitioners need to keep in mind that bias does exist and should interpret dietary intake data with skepticism to prevent any misleading diet and health associations.

References

1. U.S. Department of Agriculture, Agricultural Research Service, Nutrient Data Laboratory. (1999). "About the Nutrient Data Laboratory." Available at http://www.nal.usda.gov/fnic/foodcomp/Bulletins/ndl_info.html.
2. U.S. Department of Agriculture, Agricultural Research Service. (1999). "USDA Nutrient Database for Standard Reference," Release 13. Nutrient Data Laboratory home page, http://www.nal.usda.gov/fnic/foodcomp.
3. Andrews, K. W., Cutrufelli, R., Exler, J., and Matthews, R. H. (1997). Quality assurance of analytic contract data for U.S. Department of Agriculture food-composition databases. *Am. J. Clin. Nutr.* **65**(suppl), 1331S.
4. Exler, J. (1997). Data-evaluation criteria for assessment of analytic data. *Am. J. Clin. Nutr.* **65**(suppl), 1333S.
5. Akinyele, I. O., and Aminu, F. T. (1997). Computerized database of ethnocultural foods commonly eaten in Nigeria. *Am. J. Clin. Nutr.* **65**(suppl), 1331S.
6. Food Intake Analysis System developed by The University of Texas, Health Science Center at Houston, School of Public Health and the U.S. Department of Agriculture. Human Nutrition Information Service.
7. Cowin, I., and Emmett, P. (1999). The effect of missing data in the supplements to McCance and Widdowson's food tables on calculated nutrient intakes. *Eur. J. Clin. Nutr.* **53**(11), 891–894.
8. Buzzard, I. M., Price, K. S., and Warren, R. A. (1991). Considerations for selecting nutrient-calculation software: Evaluation of the nutrient database. *Am. J. Clin. Nutr.* **54,** 7–9.
9. Diplock, A. T. (1987). Trace elements in human health with special reference to selenium. *Am. J. Clin. Nutr.* **45,** 1313–1322.

10. Levander, O. A. (1991). Scientific rationale for the 1989 Recommended Dietary Allowance for selenium. *J. Am. Diet. Assoc.* **91,** 1572–1576.

11. Sinha, R., Block, G., and Taylor, P. (1993). Problems with estimating vitamin C intakes. *Am. J. Clin. Nutr.* **57,** 547–550.

12. Snyder, P. O., and Matthews, E. (1983). Percent retention of vitamin C in whipped potatoes after pre-service holding. *J. Am. Diet. Assoc.* **83,** 454–458.

13. Vogt, T. M., Appel, L. J., Obarzanek, E., Moore, T. J., Vollmer, W. M., Svetkey, L. P., Sacks, F. M., Bray, G. A., Cutler, J. A., Windhauser, W. M., Lin, P.-H., and Karanja, N. M., for the DASH Collaborative Research Group. (1999). Dietary Approaches to Stop Hypertension: Rationale, design, and methods. *J. Am. Diet. Assoc.* **99**(suppl), S12–S18.

14. McCullough, M. L., Karanja, N. M., Lin, P.-H., Obarzanek, E., Phillips, K. M., Laws, R. L., Vollmer, W. M., O'Connor, E. A., Champagne, C. M., and Windhauser, M. M., for the DASH Collaborative Research Group. (1999). Comparison of 4 nutrient databases with chemical composition data from the Dietary Approaches to Stop Hypertension trial. *J. Am. Diet. Assoc.* **99**(suppl), S45–S53.

15. Swain, J. F., Windhauser, M. M., Hoben, K. P., Evans, M. A., McGee, B. B., and Steele, P. D., for the DASH Collaborative Research Group. (1999). Menu design and selection for multicenter controlled feeding studies: Process used in the Dietary Approaches to Stop Hypertension trial. *J. Am. Diet. Assoc.* **99**(suppl), S54–S59.

16. O'Dell, B. L. (1984). Bioavailability of trace elements. *Nutr. Rev.* **42,** 301–308.

17. Lynch, S. R. (1997). Interaction of iron with other nutrients. *Nutr. Rev.* **55,** 102–110.

18. Cahill, A., and Lean, M. E. (1999). Review article: Malnutrition and maltreatment—A comment on orlistat for the treatment of obesity. *Ailment. Pharmacol. Ther.* **13**(8), 997–1002.

19. Prince, D. M., Welschenbach, M. A. (1998). Olestra: A new food additive. *J. Am. Diet. Assoc.* **98**(5), 565–569.

20. Bloch, A., and Thomson, C. A. (1995). Position of The American Dietetic Association: Phytochemicals and functional foods. *J. Am. Diet. Assoc.* **95,** 493–496.

21. Kant, A. K. (1996). Indexes of overall diet quality: A review. *J. Am. Diet. Assoc.* **96,** 785–791.

22. Bowman, S. A., Lino, M., Gerrior, S. A., and Basiotis, P. P. (1998). The Healthy Eating Index 1994–96, CNPP-5. U.S. Department of Agriculture, Center for Nutritional Policy and Promotion, Washington, DC.

23. Patterson, R. E., Haines, P. S., and Popkin, B. M. (1994). Diet Quality Index: Capturing a multidimensional behavior. *J. Am. Diet. Assoc.* **94,** 57–64.

24. Haines, P. S., Siega-Riz, A. M., and Popkin, B. M. (1999). The Diet Quality Index Revised: A measurement instrument for populations. *J. Am. Diet. Assoc.* **99,** 697–704.

25. U.S. Department of Agriculture, Agricultural Resource Service. (2000). "Dietary Guidelines for Americans." Available at http://www.ars.usda.gov/dgac/dgacguidexp.htm.

26. U.S. Department of Agriculture. "Food Guide Pyramid." Available at http://www.nal.usda.gov:8001/py/pmap.htm.

27. Kennedy, E. T., Ohls, J., Carlson, S., and Fleming, K. (1995). The Healthy Eating Index: Design and applications. *J. Am. Diet. Assoc.* **95,** 1103–1108.

28. Food and Nutrition Board. (1989). "Diet and Health: Implications for Reducing Chronic Disease Risk." National Academy Press, Washington, DC.

29. Cleveland, L. E., Cook, D. A., Krebs-Smith, S. M., and Friday, J. (1997). Method for assessing food intakes in terms of servings based on food guidance. *Am. J. Clin. Nutr.* **65**(suppl), 1254S–1263S.

30. Food Surveys Research Group, ARS. (1994). "Continuing Survey Food Intakes by Individuals (CSFII), 1994, Recipe and Pyramid Servings" [database on CD-ROM]. Department of Agriculture, Agricultural Research Service, Washington, DC.

31. Standing Committee on the Scientific Evaluation of Dietary Reference Intakes, Food Nutrition Board, Institute of Medicine. (1997). "Dietary Reference Intakes for Calcium, Phosphorus, Magnesium, Vitamin D, and Fluoride." National Academy Press, Washington, DC.

32. Gillman, W. W., Cupples, L. A., Millen, B. E., Ellison, R. C., and Wolf, P. A. (1997). Inverse association of dietary fat with development of ischemic stroke in men. *JAMA* **278,** 2145–2150.

33. Basiotis, P. P., Welsh, S. O., Cronin, F. J., Kelsay, J. L., and Mertz, W. (1987). Number of days of food intake records required to estimate individual and group nutrient intakes with defined confidence. *J. Nutr.* **117,** 1638–1641.

34. Rimm, E. B., Stampfer, M. J., Ascherio, A., Giovannucci, E., Colditz, G. A., and Willett, W. C. (1993). Vitamin E consumption and the risk of coronary disease in women. *N. Engl. J. Med.* **328,** 1450–1456.

35. Stampfer, M. J., Hennekens, C. H., Manson, J. E., Colditz, G. A., Rosner, B., and Willett, W. C. (1993). Vitamin E consumption and the risk of coronary disease in women. *N. Engl. J. Med.* **328,** 1444–1456.

36. Yusuf, S., Dagenais, G., Pogue, J., Bosch, J., and Sleight, P. (2000). Vitamin E supplementation and cardiovascular events in high-risk patients. The Heart Outcomes Prevention Evaluation Study Investigators. *N. Engl. J. Med.* **342**(3), 154–160.

37. Black, A. E., Prentice, A. M., Goldberg, G. R., Jebb, S. A., Bingham, S. A., Livingstone, B. E., and Coward, A. W. (1993). Measurements of total energy expenditure provide insights into the validity of dietary measurements of energy intake. *J. Am. Diet. Assoc.* **33,** 572–579.

38. Katan, M. B. (1998). Biochemical indicators of dietary intake. *Eur. J. Clin. Nutr.* **52,** S5 (abstract).

39. Schoeller, D. A., and Van Santen, E. (1982). Measurement of energy expenditure in humans by the doubly labeled water method. *J. Appl. Physiol.* **53,** 955–995.

40. Mertz, W. (1992). Food intake measurements: Is there a 'gold standard'? *J. Am. Diet. Assoc.* **92,** 1463–1465.

41. Johnson, R. K., Driscoll, P., and Goran, M. I. (1996). Comparison of multiple-pass 24-hour recall estimates of energy intake with total energy expenditure determined by the doubly labeled water method in young children. *J. Am. Diet. Assoc.* **96,** 1140–1144.

42. Andersen, L. F., Solvoll, K., and Drevon, D. A. (1996). Very-long-chain n-3 fatty acids as biomarkers for intake of fish and n-3 fatty acid concentrates. *Am. J. Clin. Nutr.* **64,** 305–311.

43. Bingham, S. A., and Cummings, J. (1985). Urine nitrogen as an independent validatory measure of dietary intake: A study of nitrogen balance in individuals consuming their normal diet. *Am. J. Clin. Nutr.* **42,** 1276–1289.

44. Bingham, S. A., Cassidy, A., Cole, T. J., Welch, A., Runswick, S. A., Black, A. E., Thurnham, D., Bates, C., Khaw, K. T., Key, T. J. A., and Day, N. E. (1995). Validation of weighed records and other methods of dietary assessment using the 24 h urine nitrogen technique and other biological markers. *Br. J. Nutr.* **73,** 531–550.

45. Bingham, S. A. (1997). Dietary assessments in the European Prospective Study of diet and Cancer (EPIC). *Eur. J. Cancer Prev.* **6,** 118–124.

46. Le Marchand, L., Hankin, J. H., Carter, F. S., Essling, C., Luffey, D., Franke, A. A., Wilkens, L. R., Cooney, R. V., Kolonel, L. N. (1994). A pilot study on the use of plasma carotenoids and ascorbic acid as markers of compliance to a high fruit and vegetable dietary intervention. *Cancer Epidemiol. Biomarkers Prev.* 1994;3(3):245–51.

47. Pierce, J. P., Faerber, S., Wright, F. A., Newman, V., Flatt, S. W., Kealey, S., Rock, C. L., Hryniuk, W., and Greenberg, E. R. (1997). Feasibility of a randomized trial of a high-vegetable diet to prevent breast cancer recurrence. *Nutr. Can.* **289**(3), 282–288.

48. Johansson, L., Solvoll, K., Bjorneboe, G.-E. A., and Drevon, C. A. (1998). Under- and overreporting of energy intake related to weight status and lifestyle in a nationwide sample. *Am. J. Clin. Nutr.* **68,** 266–274.

49. Prentice, A. M., Black, A. E., Coward, W. A., Davies, H. L., Goldberg, G. R., Murgatroyd, P. R., Ashford, J., Sawyer, M., and Whitehead, R. G. (1986). High levels of energy expenditure in obese women. *Br. Med. J.* **292,** 983–987.

50. Lichtman, S. W., Pisarska, K., Berman, E. R., Pestones, M., Dowling, H., Offenbacher, E., Weisel, H., Heshka, S., Matthews, D. E., and Heymsfield, S. B. (1992). Discrepancy between self-reported and actual caloric intake and exercise in obese subjects. *N. Engl. Med. J.* **327,** 1893–1898.

51. Price, G. M., Paul, A. A., Cole, T. J., and Wadsworth, M. E. J. (1997). Characteristics of the low-energy reporters in a longitudinal national dietary survey. *Br. J. Nutr.* **77,** 833–851.

52. Pryer, J. A., Vrijheid, M., Nichols, R., Kiggins, M., and Elliot, P. (1997). Who are the 'low energy reporters' in the dietary and nutritional survey of British adults? *Int. J. Epidemiol.* **26,** 146–154.

53. Johnson, R. K., Soultanakis, R. P., and Matthews, D. E. (1998). Literacy and body fatness are associated with underreporting of energy intake in U.S. low-income women using the multiple-pass 24-hour recall: A doubly labeled water study. *J. Am. Diet. Assoc.* **98,** 1136–1140.

54. Taren, D., Tobar, M., Hill, A., Howell, W., Shisslack, C., Bell, I., and Ritenbaugh, C. (1998). The association of energy intake bias with psychological score of women. *Eur. J. Clin. Nutr.* **52,** S18.

55. Johnson, R. K., Soultanakis, R. P., and Matthews, D. E. (1999). Psychological factors and energy intake underreporting in women. *FASEB J.* **13**(5), A695.

56. Krebs-Smith, S. M., Graubard, B., Cleveland, L., Subar, A., Ballard-Barbash, R., and Kahie, L. (1998). Low energy reporters vs others: A comparison of reported food intakes. *Eur. J. Clin. Nutr.* **52**(2), S18.

57. Briefel, R. R., Sempos, C. T., McDowell, M. A., Chien, S. C. Y., and Alaimo, K. (1997). Dietary methods research in the third National Health and Nutrition Examination Survey: Underreporting of energy intake. *Am. J. Clin. Nutr.* **65**(suppl), 1203–1209S.

58. Voss, S., Kroke, A., Lipstein-Grobusch, K., and Boeing, H. (1998). Is macronutrient composition of dietary intake data affected by underreporting? Results from the EPIC-Potsdam study. *Eur. J. Clin. Nutr.* **52,** 119–126.

59. Poppitt, S. D., Swann, D., Black, A. E., and Prentice, A. M. (1998). Assessment of selective underreporting of food intake by obese and non-obese women in a metabolic facility. *Int. J. Obes.* **22,** 303–311.

60. Johnson, R. K., Black, A. E., and Cole, T. J. (1998). Letter to the editor. *N. Engl. J. Med.* **338,** 917–919.

61. Livingstone, M. B. E., Prentice, A. M., Strain, J. J., Coward, E. A., Black, A. E., Barker, M. E., McKenna, P. G., and Whitehead, R. G. (1990). Accuracy of weighed dietary records in studies of diet and health. *Br. Med. J.* **300,** 708–712.

62. Thomson, C., Bloch, A. S., and Hasler, C. M. (1999). Position of The American Dietetic Association: Functional foods. *J. Am. Diet. Assoc.* **99,** 1278–1285.

63. Craig, W. J., (1999). Health-promoting properties of common herbs. *Am. J. Clin. Nutr.* **70**(suppl), 491S–499S.

64. Goldberg, G. R., Black, A. E., Jebb, S. A., Cole, T. J., Murgatroyd, P. R., Coward, W. A., and Prentice, A. M. (1991). Critical evaluation of energy intake data using fundamental principles of energy physiology: 1. Derivation of cut-off limits to identify under-recording. *Eur. J. Clin. Nutr.* **45,** 569–581.

65. Black, A. E., Goldberg, G. R., Jebb, S. A., Livingston, M. B. E., Cole, T. J., and Prentice, A. M. (1991). Critical evaluation of energy intake data using fundamental principles of energy physiology: 2. Evaluating the results of published surveys. *Eur. J. Clin. Nutr.* **45:**583–99.

66. Black, A. E. (1998). Poor validity of dietary assessment: what have we learnt? *Eur. J. Clin. Nutr.* **52**(2), S17.

67. Munoz, K., Krebs-Smoth, S., Ballard-Barbash, R., and Cleveland, L. (1997). Food intakes of U.S. children and adolescents compared with recommendations. *Pediatrics* **100**(3), 323–329.

68. Willett, W., and Stampfer, M. J. (1986). Total energy intake: Implicationis for epidemiologic analyses. *Am. J. Epidemiol.* **124**(1), 17–26.

69. Carter, L. M., and Whiting, S. J. (1998). Underreporting of energy intake, socioeconomic status, and expression of nutrient intake. *Nutr. Rev.* **56**(6), 179–182.

70. Stallone, D. D., Brunner, E. J., Bingham, S. A., and Marmot, M. G. (1997). Dietary assessment in Whitehall II: The influence of reporting bias on apparent socioeconomic variation in nutrient intakes. *Eur. J. Clin. Nutr.* **51,** 815–825.

B. Nutrition Intervention

CHAPTER **6**

Current Theoretical Bases for Nutrition Intervention and Their Uses

KAREN GLANZ

University of Hawaii, Honolulu, Hawaii

I. INTRODUCTION

This chapter discusses contemporary theoretical bases for nutrition intervention for disease prevention and management and their applications in practice. Other chapters in this text provide specific recommendations regarding dietary advice for disease prevention and for nutritional management of patients. In this chapter we (1) introduce key concepts related to the application of theory in understanding and improving dietary behavior, (2) review behavioral issues related to healthful diets, (3) describe several current theoretical models that can be helpful in planning and conducting nutrition intervention, (4) highlight important issues and constructs that cut across theories, and (5) provide a summary of current thinking about the determinants of dietary behavior and change processes.

Nutritional intervention is a central component of disease prevention and management. Health professionals' roles in nutritional intervention are pivotal because of their centrality in health care and their credibility as patient educators [1]. Current public health recommendations in the United States give high priority to including nutrition education in all routine health care contacts [2]. People who report receiving advice about dietary change during health care visits report more health-enhancing diet changes than those who received no such advice [3].

II. IMPORTANCE OF UNDERSTANDING INFLUENCES ON DIETARY BEHAVIOR

Successful nutrition interventions take many forms. Interventions to yield desirable changes in eating patterns can be best designed with an understanding of relevant theories of dietary behavior change and the ability to use them skillfully [4]. Whereas many early reports of nutrition interventions did not cite a particular theory or model as the basis for the strategies they employ [5, 6], the application of sound behavioral science theory in nutrition interventions is becoming increasingly common [7]. Also, emerging evidence suggests that interventions developed with an explicit theo-

retical foundation are more effective than those lacking a theoretical base [8].

Six theoretical models are in current use and can be particularly useful for understanding the processes of changing eating patterns in health care and community settings: social cognitive theory, the stages of change construct from the transtheoretical model, consumer information processing, the health belief model, multiattribute utility theory, and diffusion of innovations [4, 7, 9]. The central elements of each theory and how they can be used to help formulate nutrition interventions are described in this chapter.

A. Multiple Determinants of Food Choice

Many social, cultural, and economic factors contribute to the development, maintenance, and change of dietary patterns. No single factor or set of factors has been found to adequately account for why people eat as they do. Physiologic and psychological factors, acquired food preferences, and knowledge about foods are important individual determinants of food intake. Families, social relationships, socioeconomic status, culture, and geography are also important influences on food choices. A broad understanding of some of the key factors and models for understanding food choice can provide a foundation for well-informed clinical nutrition intervention, help identify the most influential factors for a particular patient, and enable clinicians to focus on issues that are most salient for their patients.

B. Multiple Levels of Influence

Common wisdom holds that nutrition interventions are most likely to be effective if they embrace an ecological perspective for health promotion [10, 11]. That is, they should not only be targeted at individuals but should also affect interpersonal, organizational, and environmental factors influencing dietary behavior [7, 12]. This is most clearly illustrated when one thinks of the context of selecting and purchasing food. Consumers learn about foods through advertising and promotion in the media, by labels on food packages, and via product information in grocery stores, cafeterias, and

restaurants [13]. Their actual purchases are influenced by personal preferences, family habits, medical advice, availability, cost, packaging, placement, and intentional meal planning. The foods they consume may be further changed in the preparation process, either at home or while eating out. The process is complex and clearly determined not only by multiple factors but by factors at multiple levels. Still, many food choices can be represented by routines and simple, internalized rules.

Traditionally, health educators focus on intra-individual factors such as a person's beliefs, knowledge, and skills. Contemporary thinking suggests that thinking beyond the individual to the social milieu and environment can enhance the chance of successful health promotion and patient education. Health providers can and should work toward understanding the various levels of influence that affect the patient's behavior and health status. This will be discussed and illustrated with examples later in this chapter.

III. WHAT IS THEORY?

A theory is a set of interrelated concepts, definitions, and propositions that presents a systematic view of events or situations by specifying relations among variables, in order to explain and predict the events or situations. The notion of generality, or broad application, is important [14]. Even though various theoretical models of health behavior may reflect the same general ideas, each theory employs a unique vocabulary to articulate the specific factors considered to be important. Theories vary in the extent to which they have been conceptually developed and empirically tested.

Theory can help us during the various stages of planning, implementing, and evaluating interventions [4, 14]. Theories can be used to guide the search for reasons why people are or are not consuming a healthful diet or adhering to a therapeutic dietary regimen. They can help pinpoint what you need to know before working effectively with a client, group, or patient. They also help to identify what should be monitored, measured, and/or compared in evaluating the efficacy of nutrition intervention.

IV. EXPLANATORY AND CHANGE THEORIES

Theories can guide the search to understand *why* people do or do not follow medical advice, help identify *what* information is needed to design an effective intervention strategy, and provide insight into *how* to design an educational program so it is successful [14]. Thus, theories and models help *explain* behavior and also suggest how to develop more effective ways to influence and *change* behavior. These types of theory often have different emphases but are quite complementary [4]. For example, understanding why someone chooses the foods they eat is one step toward successful

nutrition management, but even the best explanations will not be enough by themselves to fully guide changes to improve health. Some type of change model will also be needed. All of the theories and models described here have some potential as both explanatory and change models, although they might be better for one or the other purpose. In particular, the health belief model was originally developed as an explanatory model, whereas in contrast the stages of change construct was conceived to help guide planned change efforts.

V. UNIQUE FEATURES OF DIETARY BEHAVIOR TO CONSIDER WHEN USING THEORY

Dietary behavior changes are most likely to be effective for preventing or managing disease when they are sustained over the long term and in people's natural environments, outside the clinical setting. To be effective in nutritional intervention, health care providers need to understand both the principles of clinical nutrition management and a variety of behavioral and educational issues [15].

Several core issues about nutritional change should be recognized. First, most diet-related risk factors are asymptomatic and do not present immediate or dramatic symptoms. Second, health-enhancing dietary changes require qualitative change, not just modification of the amount of food consumed, and cessation is not a viable option (as with smoking or other addictive behaviors). Third, both the act of making changes and self-monitoring require accurate knowledge about the nutrient composition of foods. Thus, information acquisition and processing may be more complex for dietary change than for changes in some other health behaviors, such as smoking and exercise [16]. Because of this, consumer information processing models (described below) are more important for nutrition intervention than for other types of health-related behaviors. Other important issues include long-term maintenance, the format of dietary advice, nutritional adequacy, options for initiating the change process, the changing food supply, fad diets, and special populations.

A. Long-Term Dietary Change

Because nutritional intervention leads to meaningful improvements in health only when long-term change is achieved, both providers and patients need to "look down the road" when formulating expectations and setting goals [17]. For example, for most patients who follow recommended dietary changes for cholesterol reduction, significant reductions are seen within 4–6 weeks, and cholesterol reduction goals can be reached within 3–6 months [18]. Even after goals are achieved, new dietary habits must be maintained. Thus, if it takes several weeks or even months to adjust to the new dietary regimen, patience and persistence by both physician and patient may be worthwhile in the long run. And different

skills are required to make initial changes and to maintain them over the long term, so follow-up consultations and advice should address new issues, not merely repeat or rehash old information.

B. Restrictive and Additive Recommendations: Typical Reactions

Traditionally, nutrition intervention has focused on advice to *restrict* intake of certain foods or nutrients, e.g., reduce fat and saturated fat intake, limit energy intake, or limit sodium intake. Yet the most often-mentioned obstacle to achieving a healthful diet is not wanting to give up the foods we like [19]. Basic psychological principles hold that when people are faced with a restriction, or loss of a choice, that choice or commodity becomes more attractive. In other words, focusing mainly on what *not* to eat, or on eating less of some types of foods, may evoke conscious or unconscious negativism in some people. In contrast, emphasizing *additive* recommendations, such as increasing intake of fruits and vegetables, or eating more fiber-rich foods, often appeals to people because it sanctions their doing more of something. The challenge is to make these recommendations attractive to patients, and to ensure that they are presented in the context of an overall healthful diet.

C. Implications of Counseling for Gradual Change or Very Strict Diets

Common wisdom holds that the chances of long-term dietary compliance are greater when efforts to change are guided in a gradual, stepwise manner. This might involve attempting changes within specific food groups one at a time, until the total diet comes close to recommendations. A basic principle involved is that small successes (i.e., recognition of each successful behavioral change) increase confidence and motivation for each successive change. While this is effective for many people, others become impatient or even lose their enthusiasm for changes that are minimally recognizable. An alternative is to begin with a highly restrictive diet such as a very-low-fat diet or a very-low-energy diet for weight loss. These types of programs, with very strict dietary regimens, may be useful for patients who are highly motivated, post-surgically, after a coronary incident, or for those who have not been successful in making gradual changes. In some cases, a strict diet for an initial short time period will yield visible and/or clinical changes that help motivate patients to continue adhering to a less extreme regimen. Such diets require careful supervision, however.

D. Special Populations

Ideally, each patient should be treated as an individual with unique circumstances and health history. Still, epidemiological research indicates that certain demographic subgroups differ in terms of both risk factors and diet. Understanding these population trends can help prepare a provider to work with various types of patients. Data from the National Health and Nutrition Examination Survey show that most cardiovascular disease risk factors are higher among ethnic minority women (African-American and Mexican-American) than among white women [20]. Women of lower socioeconomic status tend to have higher body mass index (BMI) than more affluent women, across all ethnic groups [20]. White women also tend to have more positive attitudes toward the impact of diet on health than African-American women, even when accounting for differences in age, education, and income [21]. Women experience gender-specific differences in cardiovascular risks related to hormones, contraceptives, and hormone replacement therapy [22]. Younger persons may feel invulnerable to coronary events, and older adults may be managing multiple chronic conditions and using both prescribed and over-the-counter medications that could interact with foods. These are just a few examples of how population subgroups may differ, and they serve as a reminder to be sensitive to group patterns, but to avoid stereotyping in the absence of firsthand evidence about an individual.

VI. IMPORTANT THEORIES AND THEIR KEY CONSTRUCTS

Several of the available and widely used models and theories of behavior change are applicable to nutrition intervention. This section describes six theoretical models that are in current use and make unique contributions to the interventionist's tool kit. They are social cognitive theory, the stages of change construct from the transtheoretical model, consumer information processing, the health belief model, multiattribute utility theory, and diffusion of innovations [4, 7, 9, 23]. The central elements of each theory and how they can be used to help formulate nutrition interventions are described in this chapter. Table 1 provides illustrative statements showing the application of each theory.

A. Social Cognitive Theory

Social cognitive theory, the cognitive formulation of social learning theory that has been best articulated by Bandura [24, 25], explains human behavior in terms of a three-way, dynamic, reciprocal model in which personal factors, environmental influences, and behavior continually interact. Social cognitive theory synthesizes concepts and processes from cognitive, behavioristic, and emotional models of behavior change, so it can be readily applied to nutritional intervention for disease prevention and management. A basic premise is that people learn not only through their own experiences, but also by observing the actions of others and the results of those actions [14]. Key constructs of social cognitive theory that are relevant to nutritional intervention

TABLE 1   Statements Representing Theoretical Approaches to Understanding and Changing Dietary Behavior

Theory	Statement(s)
Social cognitive theory	Overeating at holidays is triggered by food advertisements, store displays, and party buffets that people encounter.
Stages of change	If someone feels that the time is right and they're "ready to change," they will probably be more successful with a nutrition intervention.
Consumer information processing	The information on nutrition labels sometimes "overloads" consumers. Consumers who are concerned about nutrition tend to look at nutrient labels before deciding which food to buy.
Health belief model	After being told he has high cholesterol, a manager will avoid high-fat lunches if he thinks this will help and if there are lower fat choices available.
Multiattribute utility theory	If taste and convenience are foremost in someone's mind when deciding what to eat, a nutrition intervention that zeros in on these factors has the greatest promise of success.
Diffusion of innovations	People take up new foods more readily if they are similar to what they are already eating.

Source: Adapted in part from Glanz, K., and Rudd, J. (1993). Views of theory, research, and practice: A survey of nutrition education and consumer behavior professionals. *J. Nutr. Educ.* **25,** 269–273.

include observational learning, reinforcement, self-control, and self-efficacy [7].

Principles of behavior modification, which have often been used to promote dietary change, are derived from social cognitive theory. Some elements of behavioral dietary interventions based on social cognitive theory constructs of self-control, reinforcement, and self-efficacy include goal-setting, self-monitoring and behavioral contracting [7, 15].

Self-efficacy, or a person's confidence in his or her ability to take action and to persist in that action despite obstacles or challenges, seems to be especially important for influencing health behavior and dietary change efforts [25]. Health providers can make deliberate efforts to increase patients' self-efficacy using three types of strategies: (1) setting small, incremental, and achievable goals; (2) using formalized behavioral contracting to establish goals and specify rewards; and (3) monitoring and reinforcement, including patient self-monitoring by keeping records [14]. In group nutrition programs, it is possible to easily incorporate activities such as cooking demonstrations, problem-solving discussions, and self-monitoring that are rooted in social cognitive theory.

The key social cognitive theory construct of reciprocal determinism means that a person can be both an agent for change and a responder to change. Thus, changes in the environment, the examples of role models, and reinforcements can be used to promote healthier behavior.

B. Stages of Change

Long-term dietary change for disease prevention or risk reduction involves multiple actions and adaptations over time.

Some people may not be ready to attempt changes, while others may have already begun implementing diet modifications. The construct of "stage of change" is a key element of the transtheoretical model of behavior change, and proposes that people are at different stages of readiness to adopt healthful behaviors [26, 27]. The notion of readiness to change, or stage of change, has been examined in dietary behavior research and found useful in explaining and predicting eating habits [16, 28–32].

Stages of change is a heuristic model that describes a sequence of steps in successful behavior change: precontemplation (no recognition of need for or interest in change), contemplation (thinking about changing), preparation (planning for change), action (adopting new habits), and maintenance (ongoing practice of new, healthier behavior) [26]. People do not always move through the stages of change in a linear manner. They often recycle and repeat certain stages; for example, individuals may relapse and go back to an earlier stage depending on their level of motivation and self-efficacy.

The stages of change model can be used both to help understand why patients might not be ready to undertake dietary change and to improve the success of nutrition intervention [14, 15]. Patients can be classified according to their stage of change by asking a few simple questions: Are they interested in trying to change their eating patterns, thinking about changing their diet, ready to begin a new eating plan, already making dietary changes, or trying to sustain changes they have been following for some time? By knowing their current stage, you can help determine how much time to spend with the patient, whether to wait until he or she is more ready to attempt active changes, whether referral for

in-depth nutritional counseling is warranted, and so on. Knowledge of the patient's current stage of change can also lead to appropriate follow-up questions about past efforts to change, obstacles and challenges, and available strategies for overcoming barriers or obstacles to change [15].

C. Consumer Information Processing

People require information about how to choose nutritious foods in order to follow guidelines for healthy eating. A central premise of consumer information processing theory is that individuals can process only a limited amount of information at one time [14, 33]. People tend to seek only enough information to make a satisfactory choice. They develop heuristics, or rules of thumb, to help them make choices quickly within their limited information-processing capacity [33]. The nutrition information environment is often complex and confusing, especially when programs rely heavily on print nutrition-education materials that may be written at too sophisticated a level in terms of wording and concepts. Recently, introduction of the new food "Nutrition Facts" labels have simplified generally available nutrition information somewhat and contributed to an increase in usual label use and satisfaction with their content [34].

There are several implications of consumer information processing theory for nutrition intervention. Information that is provided should be made easily accessible, not confusing, and processable with limited effort. Messages that are food focused rather than nutrient focused may be particularly helpful [35]. Nutrition information should be tailored to the comprehension level of the audience, matched to their lifestyles and experience, and either be portable or available at or near the point of food selection [33].

Knowledge about which foods to choose and how much to consume on a therapeutic diet are the *sine qua non* of dietary adherence. However, knowledge of how to use nutrition information and the skills to choose or prepare healthful foods are not enough without motivation and support. Further, patients with low literacy skills may require more explanations and fewer printed materials, thus posing important challenges [36]. One community-based dietary fat intervention that used few print materials, emphasized interactive experiences, and was targeted to the cultural backgrounds of participants was successful in promoting desirable dietary changes [37].

D. Health Belief Model

The health belief model was one of the first models to adapt theory from the behavioral sciences to health problems, and it remains one of the most widely recognized conceptual frameworks of health behavior. It emerged in the 1950s, during a time in history when a modest number of preventive health services were available, such as flu vaccines and chest X rays for tuberculosis screening [38]. The model was based on an assumption that people fear diseases, and that health actions are motivated in relation to the degree of fear (perceived threat) and expected fear-reduction potential of actions, as long as that potential outweighs practical and psychological obstacles to taking action (net benefits) [14].

The four key constructs of the health belief model are identified as perceived susceptibility and perceived severity (two dimensions of "threat"), and perceived benefits and perceived barriers (the components of "net benefits"). More recent adaptations have added the concepts "cue to action," a stimulus to undertake behavior; and self-efficacy, or confidence in one's ability to perform an action [39]. While the health belief model was originally conceived as an explanatory model, it has some applications for planning change, as well. The most promising use of the health belief model in designing interventions is as a foundation for developing messages that may persuade individuals to make healthy decisions.

To what extent does the health belief model fit well with nutrition intervention? Does it help us understand how people view their eating habits and can it motivate them to make healthy changes? In fact, the health belief model is of limited use for *primary prevention* of chronic diseases such as cardiovascular disease and cancer. However, it can play an important role in interventions for persons with clinical nutrition-related risk factors, such as high blood cholesterol or diabetes. Such individuals are faced with the important and often overriding concern about health. For practitioners, health concerns—emphasized by applying the health belief model—are most likely to be influential when they are emphasized in a clear and specific manner, placed in the context of overall risk for diseases, and when dietary change recommendations can be linked prospectively to tangible risk reduction [15]. Symptomatic patients also tend to be more motivated [40].

E. Multiattribute Utility Theory

Both health professionals and marketers recognize that people seek the things they like and that give them pleasure, and that they take action to obtain these things. Identifying those concerns that are most important to a person's decision about performing a specific behavior can lead to the development of effective interventions and decisions aids to promote desirable behaviors [4]. Multiattribute utility theory is a form of value expectancy theory that aims to specify how people define and evaluate the elements of decision making about performing a specific behavior. Key elements of value expectancy theory are the valence, or importance, of a particular feature of a behavior or product; and the expectancy, or subjective probability, that a given consequence will occur if the behavior is performed [41].

Multiattribute utility theory is a form of value expectancy theory with particular relevance to understanding influences on food choice and changes in eating habits. Multiattribute utility theory posits that people evaluate decisions based on multiple attributes, and somehow consciously or

unconsciously weigh the alternatives before deciding what actions to take. The literature on food choice has identified several key factors that appear to be important in food selection: taste, nutrition, cost, convenience, and weight control [42]. For the general public, taste has been reported to be the most important influence on food choice, followed by cost [9]. Understanding the relative importance of various concerns to individuals can guide the design of nutrition counseling and nutrition education programs. For example, by designing and promoting a nutritious diet as tasty, an intervention might be more successful than if it is presented primarily as nutritious or inexpensive.

F. Diffusion of Innovations

The last conceptual model is the diffusion of innovations, which provides guidance both for developing successful programs and ensuring that they are optimally communicated through social environments in health care settings, homes, and the community. Diffusion concepts emphasize the macro level of social, and dietary, change [43]. A key implication of diffusion theory is that mediated information sources—that is, sources that rely on media rather than interpersonal communication (including brochures, mass media, etc.)—are most important in the early stages of adoption, such as awareness and interest building. Interpersonal communication grows more important during active evaluation, trial, and adoption of new habits [43]. Diffusion principles are consistent with social cognitive theory concepts that suggest initially creating an environment conducive to change and disseminating the program and new ideas through successful examples [24]. However, it also appears that special efforts are required to sustain the effects of nutrition interventions after an initial active period.

G. Selecting an Appropriate Theoretical Model or Models

Effective nutrition intervention depends on marshaling the most appropriate theory and practice strategies for a given situation [14]. Different theories are best suited to different individuals and situations. For example, when attempting to overcome a patient's personal barriers to changing his diet to reduce his cholesterol level, the health belief model may be useful. The stages of change model may be especially useful in developing diabetes education interventions. When trying to teach low-literacy patients how to choose and prepare healthy foods, consumer information processing may be more suitable. The choice of the most fitting theory or theories should begin with identifying the problem, goal, and units of practice [4, 14], *not* with simply selecting a theoretical framework because it is intriguing or familiar.

When it comes to practical application, theories are often judged in the context of activities of fellow practitioners. To apply the criterion of *usefulness* to a theory, most providers

are concerned with whether it is consistent with everyday observations [4]. In contrast, researchers usually make scientific judgments of how well a theory conforms to observable reality *when empirically tested.* Patient educators should review the research literature periodically to supplement their firsthand experience and that of their colleagues. A central premise in applying an understanding of the influences on health behavior to patient education is that you can gain an understanding of a patient through an interview or written assessment, and better focus on that individual's readiness, self-efficacy, knowledge level, and so on. Clearly, it is necessary to select a "short list" of factors to evaluate, and this may differ depending on clinical risk factors or a patient's history. Once there is a good understanding of that person's cognitive and/or behavioral situation, the intervention can be personalized, or tailored. Tailored messages and feedback have been found to be promising strategies for encouraging healthful behavior changes in primary care, community, and home-based settings [44–46].

The challenge of successfully applying theoretical frameworks in nutrition programs involves evaluating the frameworks and their key concepts in terms of both conceptual relevance and practical value [4]. Also, the integration of multiple theories into a comprehensive model tailored for a given individual or community group requires careful analysis of the audience and frequent reexamination during program design and implementation.

VII. FINDINGS REGARDING APPLICATIONS OF THEORY TO NUTRITIONAL BEHAVIOR

In the past 5–10 years, published research has increased in the area of applying theoretical models to the study of nutritional behavior [6, 7]. Numerous studies have examined the determinants of eating behavior using coherent theoretical frameworks and constructs [16, 31, 47]. Most of this research has been somewhat limited by the use of cross-sectional designs. There continues to be a need for more studies using longitudinal designs; studying families and changing food roles in families; and studying the relationships among various eating behaviors and not just a few nutrients or types of foods [6].

During the 1990s, a substantial increase has been seen in research applying the stages of change model to dietary behavior [16, 48, 49]. Several intervention trials have explicitly used this model to help shape their nutrition promotion programs [50–52]. Prospective intervention research examining employees' readiness to change their eating patterns has revealed "forward movement" across the stage continuum in work site nutrition studies, and shown that changes in stage of change for healthy eating are significantly associated with dietary improvements [32, 53].

Also, people's initial stage of change may influence their participation in nutritional intervention. People who are initially in the later stages of change (preparation, action, and maintenance) tend to spend more time on dietary change [32] and to report making more healthful changes in their food choices [45].

Several recent large work site nutrition programs have applied constructs from social cognitive theory [46, 51, 54]. Another multisite study, the Working Well Trial, used an intervention rooted in social cognitive theory, consumer information processing, stages of change, and the diffusion of innovations [7, 55]. Several of these nutrition interventions have been found effective when compared to a control condition, although they have done little to test the elements of social cognitive theory that might be most associated with observed changes.

A recent report used multiattribute utility theory as the framework for analyzing surveys of a national sample of 2967 adults. The study examined the relative importance of taste, nutrition, cost, convenience, and weight control on personal eating choices. Taste was reported to be the most important overall influence on food choices, followed by cost. The importance of nutrition and weight control were best predicted by respondents being within a particular health lifestyle cluster [9]. No published reports have explicitly applied multiattribute utility theory to design a nutrition intervention, but some leading nutrition professionals have suggested that professionals in the field should invest effort in designing food plans (including menus and recipes) that are good tasting and meet health guidelines [56].

There is a need for further research on diffusion of effective intervention models, because few studies have addressed how best to disseminate tested interventions [57].

VIII. CONSTRUCTS AND ISSUES ACROSS THEORIES

It is important to bear in mind that the various theories that can be used for nutrition intervention are not mutually exclusive. Not surprisingly, they share several constructs and common issues across theories. It is often challenging to sort out the key issues in various models. This section focuses on important issues and constructs across models. The first of these is that successful dietary behavior change depends on a sound understanding of the patient's, or consumer's, view of the world.

A. Patient's View of the World: Perceptions, Cognitions, Emotions, and Habits

For health professionals who work with patients and provide them with advice on health and lifestyle, adherence to treatment is often disappointingly poor, even in response to relatively simple medical advice. Such poor adherence often

arises because patients do not have the necessary behavioral skills to make changes to their diet. Following a heart attack, for example, patients might well understand the importance of adopting such changes to their lifestyle, but be unable to make those changes. In other circumstances, patients might not understand the importance of such changes, and may even believe that such changes pose an additional risk to their health. In yet other circumstances, a patient might be experiencing depression or anxiety, such that emotional dysfunction will be a major barrier to compliance.

Traditionally, it has been assumed that the relationship among knowledge, attitudes, and behavior is a simple and direct one. Indeed, over the years, many prevention and patient education programs have been based on the premise that if people understand the health consequences of a particular behavior, they will modify it accordingly. Moreover, the argument goes, if people have a negative attitude toward an existing lifestyle practice and a positive attitude toward change, they will make healthful changes. However, we now know from research conducted during the past 30 years that the relationships among knowledge, awareness of the need to change, intention to change, and an actual change in behavior are very complex indeed.

Ideally, each patient should be treated as an individual with unique circumstances and health history. Still, epidemiological research indicates that certain demographic subgroups differ in terms of risk factors and health behaviors. Understanding these population trends can help prepare a provider to work with various types of patients. For example, younger persons may feel invulnerable to coronary events, and older adults may be managing multiple chronic conditions. An active middle-aged professional may place returning to his previous level of activity above important health protective actions. These examples serve as a reminder to be sensitive to group patterns, yet to avoid stereotyping in the absence of firsthand evidence about an individual. Within this general context, various theories and models can guide the search for effective ways to reach and positively motivate patients.

B. Behavior Change as a Process

Sustained health behavior change involves multiple actions and adaptations over time. Some people may not be ready to attempt change, some may be thinking about attempting change, and others may have already begun implementing behavioral modifications. One central issue that has gained wide acceptance in recent years is the simple notion that *behavior change is a process, not an event.* Rather, it is important to think of the change process as one that occurs in stages. It is not a question of someone deciding one day to change her diet and the next day becoming a low-fat eater for life! Likewise, most people will not be able to dramatically change their eating patterns all at once. The idea that behavior change occurs in a number of steps is not

particularly new, but it has gained wider recognition in the past few years. Indeed, various multistage theories of behavior change date back more than 50 years to the work of Lewin, McGuire, Weinstein, Marlatt and Gordon, and others [4, 58–61].

The notion of readiness to change, or stage of change, has been examined in health behavior research and found useful in explaining and predicting a variety of types of behaviors. Prochaska, Velicer, DiClemente, and their colleagues have been leaders in beginning to formally identify the dynamics and structure of change that underlie both self-mediated and clinically facilitated health behavior change. The construct of stage of change (described earlier in this chapter) is a key element of their transtheoretical model of behavior change, and proposes that people are at different stages of readiness to adopt healthful behaviors [26, 27].

While the stages of change construct cuts across various circumstances of individuals who need to change or want to change, other theories also address these processes. Here we look across various models to illustrate four key concerns in understanding the process of behavior change: (1) motivation vs. intention, (2) intention vs. action, (3) changing behavior vs. maintaining behavior change, and (4) the role of biobehavioral factors.

1. Motivation vs. Intention

Behavior change is challenging for most people even if they are highly motivated to change. As has already been noted in this chapter, the relationships among knowledge, awareness of the need to change, intention to change, and an actual change in behavior are very complex indeed. For individuals who are coping with disease and illness, and who are often having to make very significant changes to their lifestyle and other aspects of their lives, this challenge is even greater. According to the transtheoretical model, people in precontemplation are neither motivated nor planning to change, those in contemplation intend to change, and those in preparation are acting on their intentions by taking specific steps toward the action of change [27].

2. Intention vs. Action

The transtheoretical model makes a clear distinction between the stages of contemplation and preparation, and that of overt action [26, 27]. A further application of this distinction comes from one of the most researched models of the relationship between cognitive-attitudinal factors and health behavior change, the health belief model. This model proposes that three constellations of factors or determinants are associated with the likelihood of change at the individual level: socioenvironmental and demographic factors, the individual's perception of the threat of disease, and the individual's perception of the potential value of treatment [39]. If all these factors point in the direction of favorably perceiving change, a person is considered "predisposed to action," or *intending* to act. It is only when a "cue to action"

sets a further process in motion that he or she actually moves into action.

3. Changing Behaviors vs. Maintaining Behavior Change

Even where there is good initial compliance to a lifestyle change program, such as changing diet, relapse is very common. It is widely recognized that many overweight persons are able to lose weight, only to regain it within a year. Thus, it has become clear to researchers and clinicians that undertaking initial behavior changes and maintaining behavior change require different types of strategies. The transtheoretical model distinction between "action" and "maintenance" stages implicitly addresses this phenomenon [26, 27]. Another model that is not described in detail here, Marlatt and Gordon's relapse prevention model, specifically focuses on strategies for dealing with maintenance of a recently changed behavior [61]. It involves developing self-management and coping strategies, and establishing new behavior patterns that emphasize perceived control, environmental management, and improved self-efficacy. These strategies are an eclectic mix drawn from social cognitive theory [24], applied behavioral analysis, and the forerunners of the stages of change model.

4. Biobehavioral Factors

The behavioral and social theories described thus far have some important limitations, many of which are only now beginning to be understood. Notably, for some health behaviors—especially addictive or addiction-like behaviors—there are other important determinants of behavior, which may be physiological and/or metabolic. Among the best known are the addictive effects of nicotine, alcohol, and some drugs. Physiologic factors increase psychological cravings and create withdrawal syndromes that may impede even highly motivated persons from changing their behaviors (e.g., quitting smoking, not consuming alcoholic beverages). Some behavior changes, for example, weight loss, also affect energy metabolism and make long-term risk factor reduction an even greater challenge than it would be if it depended on cognitive-behavioral factors alone. Research into the psychobiology of fat appetite and the role of metabolic factors, including opioid peptides, as promoters of fat and protein intake offers intriguing possibilities for understanding biobehavioral models of food intake [62].

C. Barriers to Actions, Pros and Cons, and Decisional Balance

According to social cognitive theory [24], a central determinant of behavior involves the interaction between individuals and their environments. Behavior and environment are said to continuously interact and influence one another, which is known as the principle of *reciprocal determinism*. The concept of barriers to action, or perceived barriers, can

be found in several theories of health behavior, either explicitly or as an application. It is part of social cognitive theory [24] and the health belief model [39]. An extension of the concept of barriers to action involves the net benefits of action, also referred to as the "benefits minus barriers," in the health belief model [39]. In the transtheoretical model, parallel constructs are labeled as "pros" (the benefits of change) and "cons" (the costs of change) [27]. Taken together, these constructs are known as "decisional balance," or the pros minus cons, similar to the net benefits of action in the health belief model.

The idea that individuals engage in relative weighing of the pros and cons has its origins in Janis and Mann's model of decision making, published in their seminal book more than 20 years ago [63], although the idea had emerged much earlier in social psychological discourse. Lewin's idea of force field analysis [59], the health belief model's exposition of psychological risk–benefit analysis [39], and other work on persuasion and decision counseling by Janis and Mann predated that important work. Indeed, this notion is basic to models of rational decision making, in which people intellectually think about the advantages and disadvantages, obstacles and facilitators, barriers and benefits, or pros and cons of engaging in a particular action.

D. Control over Behavior and Health: Control Beliefs and Self-Efficacy

Sometimes, "control beliefs" and self-efficacy hold people back from achieving better health. These deterrents to positive health behavior change are common, and can be found in several models of health behavior, including social cognitive theory, the health belief model, and relapse prevention. One of the most important challenges for these models—and ultimately for health professionals who apply them—is to enhance perceived behavioral control and increase self-efficacy, thereby improving patients' motivation and persistence in the face of obstacles.

IX. IMPLICATIONS AND OPPORTUNITIES

Theory and research suggest that the most effective nutrition interventions are those that use multiple strategies and aim to achieve multiple goals of awareness, information transmission, skill development, and supportive environments and policies [64]. The range of nutrition intervention tools and techniques is extensive and varied. Programs will differ based on their goals and objectives, the needs of clients, and the available resources, staff, and expertise. Nutrition programs can stand alone or be part of broader, multicomponent and multiple-focus health promotion [65] and patient education programs.

What can be expected? Program design relates closely to what one can expect in terms of results. Generally speaking,

minimally intensive intervention efforts such as one-time group education sessions can reach large audiences, but seldom lead to behavior changes. More intensive programs typically appeal to at-risk or motivated groups, cost more to offer, and can achieve relatively greater changes in knowledge, attitudes, and eating patterns.

Nutrition interventions must be sensitive to audience and contextual factors. Food selection decisions are made for many reasons other than just nutrition: taste, cost, convenience, and cultural factors all play significant roles [9]. The design and implementation of dietary change strategies must take these issues into consideration. The health promotion motto "know your audience" has a true and valuable meaning.

Further, change is incremental. Many people have practiced a lifetime of less than optimal nutrition behaviors. It is unreasonable to expect that significant and lasting changes will occur during the course of a program that lasts only a few months. Programs need to pull participants along the continuum of change, being sure to be just in front of those most ready to change with attractive, innovative offerings.

In population-focused programs, it appears to be of limited value to adopt a program solely oriented toward modifying individual choice (e.g., teaching and persuading individuals to choose low-fat dairy products). A more productive strategy would also include environmental change efforts, e.g., expanding the availability of more nutritious food choices [12]. When this is done in conjunction with individual skill training, long-lasting and meaningful changes can be achieved.

Finally, when planning interventions we should strive to be creative. Nutrition interventions should be as entertaining and engaging as the other activities with which they are competing. People will want to participate if they can have fun with the nutrition programs. Emerging communication technologies are opening up new channels for engaging people's interest in better nutrition. E-mail support and motivation systems, "Internet buddies," and interactive web-based approaches can be used creatively to promote healthful eating. The communication of nutrition information, no matter how important it is to good health, is secondary to attracting and retaining the interest and enthusiasm of the audience.

Practitioners at once benefit from and are challenged by the eclectic nature of their endeavor. For the unprepared, the choices can be overwhelming, but for those who understand the commonalities and differences among theories of health behavior, the growing knowledge base can provide a firm foundation on which to build. Theories and models can be—and *are*—useful because they enrich, inform, and complement the practical technologies of health promotion and education.

References

1, Glanz, K., and Gilboy, M. B. (1992). Physicians, preventive, care, and applied nutrition: Selected literature. *Acad. Med.* **67,** 776–781.

2. U.S. Preventive Services Task Force. (1996). "Guide to Clinical Preventive Services," 2nd ed. U. S. Department of Health and Human Services, Office of Disease Prevention and Health Promotion, Washington, DC.

3. Hunt, J. R., Kristal, A. R., White, E., Lynch, J. C., and Fries, E. (1995). Physician recommendations for dietary change: Their prevalence and impact in a population-based sample. *Am. J. Public Health* **185,** 722–726.

4. Glanz, K., Lewis, F. M., and Rimer, B. K., Eds. (1997). "Health Behavior and Health Education: Theory, Research and Practice," 2nd ed. Jossey-Bass, San Francisco.

5. Glanz, K., and Seewald-Klein, T. (1986). Nutrition at the worksite: An overview. *J. of Nutr. Educ.* **18** (Supplement), S1–S12.

6. Glanz, K., and Eriksen, M. P. (1993). Individual and community models for dietary behavior change *J. Nutr. Educ.* **25,** 80–86.

7. Glanz, K. (1997). Behavioral research contributions and needs in cancer prevention and control: Dietary change. *Prev. Med.* **26,** S43–S55.

8. Contento, I. (1995). The effectiveness of nutrition education and implications. *J. Nutr. Educ.* **27,** 279–418.

9. Glanz, K., Basil, M., Maibach, E., Goldberg, J., and Snyder, D. (1998). Why Americans eat what they do: Taste, nutrition, cost, convenience, and weight control as influences on food consumption. *J. Am. Diet. Assoc. Association,* **98,** 1118–1126.

10. McLeroy, K., Bibeau, D., Steckler, A., and Glanz, K. (1988). An ecological perspective on health promotion programs. *Health Educ. Q.* **15,** 351–377.

11. Sallis, J., and Owen, N. Ecological models. (1997). *In* "Health Behavior and Health Education: Theory, Research, and Practice," 2nd ed. (K. Glanz, F. M. Lewis, and B. K. Rimer, eds.), pp. 403–424. Jossey-Bass, San Francisco.

12. Glanz, K., Lankenau, B., Foerster, S., Temple, S., Mullis, R., and Schmid, T. (1995). Environmental and policy approaches to cardiovascular disease prevention through nutrition: Opportunities for state and local action. *Health Educ. Q.* **22,** 512–527.

13. Glanz, K., Hewitt, A. M., and Rudd, J. (1992). Consumer behavior and nutrition education: An integrative review. *J. Nutr. Educ.,* **24,** 267–277.

14. Glanz, K., and Rimer, B. K. (1995). Theory at a glance: A guide for health promotion practice, NIH Publication No. 95-3896. National Cancer Institute, Bethesda, MD.

15. Glanz, K. (1992). Nutritional intervention: A behavioral and educational perspective. *In* "Prevention of Coronary Heart Disease" (I. S. Ockene, J. K. Ockene, Eds.), pp. 231–236. Little, Brown, Boston.

16. Glanz, K., Patterson, R., Kristal, A., DiClemente, C., Heimendinger, J., Linnan, L., and McLerran, D. (1994). Stages of change in adopting healthy diets: Fat, fiber and correlates of nutrient intake. *Health Educ. Q.* **21,** 499–519.

17. Glanz, K. (1988). Patient and public education for cholesterol reduction: A review of strategies and issues. *Patient Educ. Couns.* **12,** 235–257.

18. Report of the National Cholesterol Education Program Expert Panel on Detection, Evaluation and Treatment of High Blood Cholesterol in Adults. (1988). *Arch. Int. Med.* **148,** 36–69.

19. Morreale, S. J., and Schwartz, N. E. (1995). Helping Americans eat right: Developing practical and actionable public nutrition education messages based on the ADA Survey of American Dietary Habits. *J. Am. Diet. Assoc.* **95,** 305–308.

20. Winkleby, M. A., Kraemer, H. C., Ahn, D. K., and Varady, A. N. (1998). Ethnic and socioeconomic differences in cardiovascular risk factors: Findings for women from the Third National Health and Nutrition Examination Survey, 1988–1994. *JAMA* **280,** 356–362.

21. Gates, G., and McDonald, M. (1997). Comparison of dietary risk factors for cardiovascular disease in African-American and white women. *J. Am. Diet. Assoc.* **97,** 1394–1400.

22. Rao, A. V. (1998). Coronary heart disease risk factors in women: Focus on gender differences. *J. La. State Med. Soc.* **150,** 67–72.

23. Glanz, K., and Rudd, J. (1993). Views of theory, research, and practice: A survey of nutrition education and consumer behavior professionals. *J. Nutr. Educ.* **25,** 269–273.

24. Bandura, A. (1986) "Social Foundations of Thought and Action: A Social Cognitive Theory." Prentice-Hall, Englewood Cliffs, NJ.

25. Bandura, A. (1997). "Self-Efficacy: The Exercise of Control." W. H. Freeman, New York.

26. Prochaska, J. O., DiClemente, C. C., and Norcross, J. (1992). In search of how people change: Applications to addictive behaviors. *Am. Psychol.* **47,** 1102–1114.

27. Prochaska, J. O., Redding, C., and Evers, K. (1997). The transtheoretical model of behavior change. *In* "Health Behavior and Health Education: Theory, Research, and Practice," 2nd ed. (K. Glanz, F. M. Lewis, and B. K. Rimer, Eds.), pp. 60–84. Jossey-Bass, San Francisco.

28. Curry S. J., Kristal, A. R., and Bowen D. J. (1992). An application of the stage model of behavior change to dietary fat reduction. *Health Educ. Res.* **7,** 97–105.

29. Greene, G. W., Rossi, S. R., Reed, G. R., Willey, C., and Prochaska, J. O. (1994). Stage of change for reducing dietary fat to 30% of energy or less. *J. Amer. Diet. Assoc.* **94,** 1105–1110.

30. Brug, J., Glanz, K., and Kok, G. (1997). The relationship between self-efficacy, attitudes, intake compared to others, consumption, and stages of change related to fruits and vegetables. *Am. J. Health Promotion* **12,** 25–30.

31. Glanz, K., Kristal, A. R., Tilley, B. C., and Hirst, K. (1998). Psychosocial correlates of healthful diets among male auto workers. *Cancer Epidemiology Biomarkers Prev.* **7,** 119–126.

32. Glanz, K., Patterson, R. E., Kristal, A. R., Feng, Z., Linnan, L., Heimendinger, J., and Hebert, J. R. (1998). Impact of work site health promotion on stages of dietary change: The Working Well Trial. *Health Educ. and Behav.* **25,** 448–463.

33. Rudd, J., and Glanz, K. (1990). How consumers use information for health action: Consumer information processing. *In* "Health Behavior and Health Education: Theory, Research, and Practice" (K. Glanz, F. M. Lewis, and B. K. Rimer, Eds.), pp. 115–139. Jossey-Bass, San Francisco.

34. Kristal, A., Levy, L., Patterson, R., Li, S., and White, E. (1998). Trends in food label use associated with new nutrition labeling regulations. *Am. J. Public Health,* **88,** 1212–1215.

35. Hunt, M. K, Stoddard, A. M., Glanz, K., Hebert, J. R., Probart, C., Sorensen, G., Thomson, S., Hixson, M. L., Linnan, L., and Palombo, R. (1997). Measures of food choice behavior related to intervention messages. *J. Nutr. Educ.* **29,** 3–11.

36. Macario, E., Emmons, K. M., Sorensen G., Hunt, M. K., and Rudd, R. E. (1998). Factors influencing nutrition education for patients with low literacy skills. *J. Am. Diet. Assoc.* **98,** 559–564.

37. Howard-Pitney, B., Winkleby, M., Albright, C. L., Bruce, B., and Fortmann, S. P. (1997). The Stanford Nutrition Action Program: A dietary fat intervention for low-literacy adults. *Am. J. Public Health* **87,** 1971–1976.

38. Rosenstock, I. M. (1974). Historical origins of the health belief model. *Health Educ. Monogr.* **2,** 328–335.

39. Strecher, V. J., and Rosenstock, I. M. (1997). The health belief model. *In* "Health Behavior and Health Education: Theory, Research and Practice," 2nd ed. (K. Glanz, F. Lewis, B. Rimer, eds.), pp. 41–59. Jossey-Bass, San Francisco.

40. Van Horn, L., and Kavey, R. E. (1997). Diet and cardiovascular disease prevention: What works? *Ann. Behav. Med.* **19,** 197–212.

41. Carter, W. B. (1990). Health behavior as a rational process: Theory of reasoned action and multiattribute utility theory. *In* "Health Behavior and Health Education: Theory, Research and Practice," (K. Glanz, F. Lewis, B. Rimer, Eds.), pp. 63–91. Jossey-Bass, San Francisco.

42. Food Marketing Institute. (1996). "Trends in the United States: Consumer Attitudes and the Supermarket." Food Marketing Institute, Washington, DC.

43. Rogers, E. M. (1983). "Diffusion of Innovations," 3rd ed. The Free Press, New York

44. Campbell, M. K., DeVellis, B. M., Strecher, V. J., Ammerman, A. S., DeVellis, R. F., and Sandler, R. S. (1994). Improving dietary behavior: The effectiveness of tailored messages in primary care settings. *Am. J. Public Health* **84,** 783–787.

45. Beresford, S. A., Curry, S. J., Kristal, A. R., Lazovich, D., Feng, Z., and Wagner, E. H. (1997). A dietary intervention in primary care practice: The Eating Patterns Study. *Am. J. Public Health* **87,** 610–616.

46. Brug, J., Glanz, K., Van Assema, P., Kok, G., and Van Breukelen, G. (1998). The impact of computer-tailored feedback and iterative feedback on fat, fruit, and vegetable intake. *Health Educ. Behav/* **25,** 517–531.

47. Kristal, A., Patterson R., Glanz, K., Heimendinger, J., Hebert, J., Feng, Z., and Probart, C. (1995). Psychosocial correlates of healthful diets: Baseline results from the Working Well Study. *Prev. Med.* **24,** 221–228.

48. Kristal, A., Glanz, K., Curry, S. J., and Patterson, R. E. (1999). How can stages of change be best used in dietary interventions? *J. Am. Diet. Assoc.* **99,** 679–684.

49. Campbell, M. K., Reynolds, K. D., Havas, S., Curry, S., Bishop, D., Nicklas, T., Palombo, R., Buller, D., Feldman, R., Topor, M., Johnson, C., Beresford, S., Motsinger, B., Morrill, C., and Heimendinger, J. (1999). Stages of change for increasing fruit and vegetable consumption among adults and young adults participating in the National 5 A Day for Better Health Community Studies. *Health Educ. Behav.* **26,** 513–534.

50. Sorensen, G., Thompson, B., Glanz, K., Feng, Z., Kinne, S., DiClemente, C., Emmons, K., Heimendinger, J., Probart, C., and Lichtenstein, E. (1996). Working well: Results from a worksite-based cancer prevention trial. *Am. J. Public Health,* **86,** 939–947.

51. Tilley, B., Glanz, K., Kristal, A., Hirst, K., Li, S., Vernon, S., and Myers, R. (1999). Nutrition intervention for high-risk auto workers: Results of the Next Step Trial. *Prev. Med.* **28,** 284–292.

52. Sorensen, G., Stoddard, A., and Macario, E. (1998). Social support and readiness to make dietary changes. *Health Educ. Behav.* **25,** 586–598.

53. Kristal, A., Glanz, K., Tilley, B. C., and Li, S. (2000). Mediating factors in dietary change: Understanding the impact of a worksite nutrition intervention. *Health Educ. Behav.* **27,** 112–125.

54. Sorensen, G., Hunt, M. K., Cohen, N., Stoddard, A., Stein, E., Phillips, J., Baker, F., Combe, C., Hebert, J., and Palombo, R. (1998). Worksite and family education for dietary change: The Treatwell 5 A Day Program. *Health Educ. Res.* **13,** 577–591.

55. Abrams, D., Boutwell, W. B., Grizzle, J., Heimendinger, J., Sorensen, G., and Varnes, J. (1994). Cancer control at the workplace: The Working Well Trial. *Prev. Med.* **23,** 15–27.

56. Hess, M. A. (1997). Taste: The neglected nutrition factor. *J. Am. Diet. Assoc.* **97**(suppl 2), S205–S207.

57. Sorensen, G., Emmons, K., Hunt, M. K., and Johnston, D. (1998). Implications of the results of community intervention trials. *Ann. Rev. Public Health* **19,** 379–416.

58. Weinstein, N. D. (1993). Testing four competing theories of health-protective behavior. *Health Psychol.* **12,** 324–333.

59. Lewin, K. (1935). "A Dynamic Theory of Personality." McGraw Hill, New York.

60. McGuire, W. J. (1984). Public communication as a strategy for inducing health promoting behavioral change. *Prev. Med.* **13,** 299–313.

61. Marlatt, A. G., and Gordon, J. R. (1985). "Relapse Prevention: Maintenance Strategies in the Treatment of Addictive Behaviors." The Guilford Press, New York.

62. Drewnowski, A. (1992). Nutritional perspectives on biobehavioral models of dietary change. *In* "Proceedings: Promoting Dietary Change in Communities—Applying Existing Models of Dietary Change to Population-Based Interventions" (K. K. Roos, Ed.), pp. 96–109. Fred Hutchinson Cancer Research Center, Seattle.

63. Janis, I., and Mann, L. (1977). "Decision Making: A Psychological Analysis of Conflict." Free Press, New York.

64. Glanz, K., Sorensen, G., and Farmer, A. (1996). The health impact of worksite nutrition and cholesterol programs. *Am. J. Health Promotion* **10,** 453–470.

65. Heaney, C. A., and Goetzel, R. Z. (1997). A review of health-related outcomes of multi-component worksite health promotion programs. *Am. J. Health Promotion* **11,** 290–308.

CHAPTER 7

Nutrition Intervention: Lessons from Clinical Trials

LINDA G. SNETSELAAR
University of Iowa, Iowa City, Iowa

I. INTRODUCTION

The modification of dietary patterns to the degree necessary to prevent chronic disease and to optimize management of disease has been traditionally perceived as a difficult and challenging task. However, much has been learned during the past two decades about how to successfully modify eating patterns. For example, several diet intervention studies aimed toward the prevention of cancer or cardiovascular disease have demonstrated the feasibility of reducing dietary fat intake in targeted groups, and complex dietary modifications testing the effect of diet on progression of renal disease have also been successfully achieved in clinical trials.

II. CONCEPTUAL MODELS OF MOTIVATION

A. Self-Regulation Theory

This theory, originally described by Kanfer, states that behavior is regulated by cycles that involve the monitoring of one's own status, comparing that status with expectations, and correcting the course of action when status does not match the goal or the expectancy. [1, 2] To change dietary behavior, a person seeks to increase knowledge of the discrepancy between current status and the identified goal. Two ways to accomplish this are (1) to increase the awareness of current status (e.g., through feedback such as dietary self-monitoring) or (2) to change the goal to make it more attainable. In conflict situations, when a goal is desired and yet not seen as important enough to strive to attain, ambivalence (feeling at least two different ways about something or wanting mutually exclusive goals) is a normal, key obstacle to be changed.

B. Rokeach's Value Theory

Studies in persons who have undergone sudden transformation shifts in behavior show that personality is hierarchically organized [3]. An individual's attitudes, numbering in the thousands, represent an organizational series of steps inward. More central are our beliefs and even more central are our core personal values. The most central is the sense of personal identity. The more central the shift occurs, the more sweeping is the resulting change.

C. Health Belief Model

The health belief model is a psychological model that attempts to explain and predict health behaviors by focusing on the attitudes and beliefs of individuals. The key variables of the health belief model are as follows [4]:

1. *Degree of perceived risk of a disease.* This variable includes perceived susceptibility of contracting a health condition and its perceived severity once contracted.
2. *Perceived benefits of diet adherence.* A second benefit is the believed effectiveness of dietary strategies designed to help reduce the threat of disease.
3. *Perceived barriers to diet adherence.* This variable includes potential negative consequences that may result from taking particular health actions, including physical (weight gain or loss), psychological (lack of spontaneity in food selection) and financial demands (cost of new foods).
4. *Cues to action.* Events that motivate people to take action in changing their dietary habits are crucial determinants of change.
5. *Self-efficacy.* A very important variable is the belief in being able to successfully execute the dietary behavior required to produce the desired outcomes [5, 6, 7].
6. *Other variables.* Demographic, sociopsychological, and structural variables affect an individual's perceptions of dietary change and thus indirectly influence his ability to sustain new eating behaviors.

Motivation for change depends on the presence of a sufficient degree of perceived risk in combination with sufficient self-efficacy. Perceived risk without self-efficacy tends to result in defensive cognitive coping, such as denial, rationalization, and projection, rather than behavior change. The first element of this change model can easily be converted to a

95

degree of perceived promise (for a positive goal), being the cross-product of perceived probability of obtaining the eventual reward.

D. Decisional Balance

The classic Janis and Mann decisional balance model [8] is a rational view, describing decision as a process of weighing cognitively the pros and cons of change. Change depends on the pros of change outweighing the cons.

E. Interaction

According to Miller and Rollnick [9], motivation can be thought of not as a client trait, but as an interpersonal process between nutrition counselor and participant. Rather than seeing motivational change as something the participant achieves, this process is one that is experienced by both the nutrition counselor and the participant.

III. THEORIES USED IN ACHIEVING DIETARY BEHAVIOR CHANGE IN CLINICAL TRIALS

The nutrition components of clinical trials require skills in long-term dietary maintenance. These skills go beyond educating participants, and instead involve strategies designed to reinitiate participants who no longer comply with the recommended eating plan. The studies described below provide research data collected when the theories presented above are initiated in a clinical trial setting.

A. Women's Health Initiative

The Women's Health Initiative (WHI) [10] is a randomized controlled clinical trial designed to look at prevention of cancer, heart disease and osteoporosis. The dietary arm of this study focuses on a diet with 20% energy from fat, five servings of fruits and vegetables and six servings of grain products per day.

To accomplish this change in dietary habits, nutritionists in the study use a variety of behavior change techniques based on the models discussed above. Much of the stages of change model drives efforts to increase compliance in the WHI. The Prochaska–DiClemente model includes six designated stages of change: precontemplation, contemplation, determination, action, maintenance, and relapse [11]. In an effort to simplify and accommodate different levels of adherence, WHI investigators chose to use only three levels of readiness to change: ready to change, unsure, and not ready to change. The decision to simplify levels is based on work with study participants showing that strategies to modify behavior fall within these three categories.

To test the effectiveness of using motivational strategies targeted at the above three levels of change, a small research study was devised. Results of that study show a positive change in dietary behavior following its implementation [12]. In this pilot study, researchers evaluated an intensive intervention program with diet. The basis of the program was use of motivational interviewing with participants in the WHI. The goal was to meet study nutrition goal of 20% energy from fat.

WHI dietary intervention participants ($n = 175$) from three clinical centers were randomized to intervention or control status. Those randomized to the intensive intervention program participated in three individual motivational interviewing contacts from a nutritionist, plus the usual WHI dietary intervention. Those randomized to continue continued with the usual WHI dietary management intervention. Percent energy from fat was estimated at intensive intervention program baseline and intensive intervention program follow-up (1 year later) using the WHI food frequency questionnaire (FFQ).

The change in percent energy from fat between intensive intervention program baseline and intensive intervention program 1-year follow-up was −1.2 percentage points for intensive intervention program intervention participants and +1.4 percentage points for intensive intervention program control participants. The result was an overall difference of 2.6 percentage points ($p \le .001$).

Table 1 presents summary statistics on the intensive intervention program effects comparing baseline levels of fat consumption. The changes in fat consumed varied by intensive intervention program baseline fat intake as a percentage of energy intake. Participants having the highest intensive intervention program baseline fat intake ($\ge30\%$ energy) showed the largest overall change in percent energy from fat between intensive intervention program baseline and intensive intervention program follow-up. As might be expected, the smallest change was found in participants who consumed between 25% and 30% of energy from fat at intensive intervention program baseline. These participants were closer to their goal of 20% energy from fat at baseline, allowing for less overall change.

The results of this study show that a protocol based on motivational interviewing and delivered through contacts with trained nutritionists is effective. Those subjects who participated in the intervention arm of the study further lowered their dietary fat intake to achieve study goals.

B. Diet Intervention Study in Children

A similar protocol was used in the Diet Intervention Study in Children (DISC) [13]. DISC was a randomized, multicenter clinical trial assessing the efficacy and safety of lowering dietary fat to decrease low-density lipoprotein cholesterol in children at high risk for cardiovascular disease [14, 15]. Children began this study between ages 7 and 10

TABLE 1   Effect of IIP Intervention on FFQ Percent Energy from Fat Stratified by Baseline Percent Energy from Fat[a]

	n	Baseline X (SD)	Follow-up X (SD)	Difference
% Energy from fat: <20.0				
Intervention control	23	17.75(1.8)	17.86(3.9)	0.1
	25	17.35(2.3)	19.70(4.5)	2.3
Difference[b]		−0.4	1.8	2.2
% Energy from fat: ≥20.0 and <25.0				
Intervention control	25	22.72(1.4)	21.68(4.6)	−1.0
	26	23.17(1.7)	25.29(4.8)	2.1
Difference[b]		0.5	3.6	3.1
% Energy from fat: ≥25.0 and <30.0				
Intervention control	21	27.42(1.6)	26.3(4.6)	−1.1
	15	26.94(1.2)	26.89(4.6)	0.0
Difference[b]		−0.5	0.6	1.1
% Energy from fat ≥30.0				
Intervention control	13	34.24(2.5)	30.11(6.5)	−4.1
	16	33.81(3.1)	33.82(5.0)	0.0
Difference[b]		−0.4	3.7	4.1

Source: Modified from Bowen, D., Ehret, C., Pedersen, M., Snetselaar, L., et al. (2001). Results of an adjunct dietary intervention program in the Women's Health Initiative. *J. Am. Diet. Assoc.* (in press).

[a]Participants with missing FFQ data were excluded.

[b]$p<0.05$ using paired *t*-test.

and participated in group dietary intervention programs. As they moved into adolescence (ages 13–17) and encountered added obstacles to dietary adherence and retention, researchers in the study designed and implemented an individual-level motivational intervention. The diet prescription in the DISC study required providing 28% energy from total fat, less than 8% energy from saturated fat, up to 9% energy form polyunsaturated fat, and less than 75 mg/1000 kcal/day of cholesterol. The diet met age- and sex-specific Recommended Dietary Allowance for energy, protein, and micronutrients.

Researchers used a pre- to postintervention design among a subset of the total intervention cohort ($n = 334$). The first 127 participants who appeared for regularly scheduled intervention visits after implementation of the new intervention method were considered part of the study. These participants ranged from 13 to 17 years of age with equal numbers of boys and girls. Nutrition interventionists asked all of the 127 participants to return in 4–8 weeks for a follow-up session. Initial sessions were conducted in person, and follow-up sessions were conducted either in person or by telephone.

Three 24-hour dietary recalls were collected within 2 weeks after the follow-up session. These dietary data were compared to three baseline 24-hour dietary recalls collected in the year preceding initial exposure to the motivational intervention method.

Self-reported data were also collected. At initial and follow-up intervention sessions, participants were shown "assessment rulers" (see Fig. 1) numbered 1–12, and asked to rate their adherence to dietary guidelines and their readiness to make new or additional dietary changes.

Results from the study show that the mean energy from total fat decreased from 27.7% to 25.6% ($p < 0.001$) (Table 2)

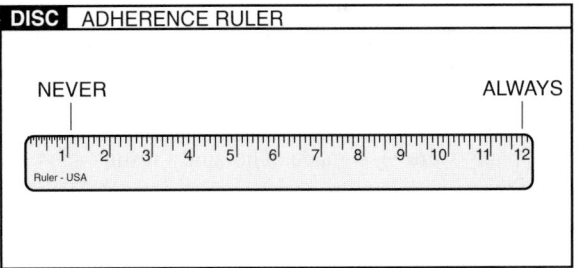

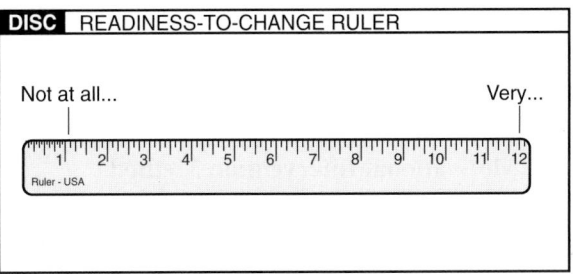

FIGURE 1   Assessment rulers. [Data from Berg-Smith, S. M., Stevens, V. J., Brown, K. M., VanHorn, L., Gernhofer, N., Peters, E., Greenberg, R., Snetselaar, L., Ahrens, L., and Smith, K., for the Dietary Intervention Study in Children (DISC) Research Group. (1999). A brief motivational intervention to improve dietary adherence in adolescents. *Health Educ. Res.* **14,** 399–410.]

TABLE 2 Changes in Total Fat Intake, Saturated Fat Intake, and Dietary Cholesterol after Two Intervention Sessions

	Mean	SD	p Level
Total fat intake			
Baseline	27.7	6.1	—
Follow-up	25.6	6.1	—
Change	−2.1	7.0	<0.001
Saturated fat intake			
Baseline	9.5	2.7	—
Follow-up	8.6	2.4	—
Change	−0.9	3.1	<0.001
Dietary cholesterol			
Baseline	182.9	97.6	—
Follow-up	157.3	87.6	—
Change	−25.6	92.3	<0.003

Source: Data from Berg-Smith, S. M., Stevens, V. J., Brown, K. M., VanHorn, L., Gernhofer, N., Peters, E., Greenberg, R., Snetselaar, L., Ahrens, L., and Smith, K., for the Dietary Intervention Study in Children (DISC) Research Group. (1999). A brief motivational intervention to improve dietary adherence in adolescents. *Health Educ. Res.* **14**, 399–410.

and the mean energy from saturated fat decreased from 9.5% to 8.6% of total energy intake ($p < 0.001$). Additionally, dietary cholesterol decreased from 182.9 to 157.3 mg/1000 kcal ($p < 0.003$). A comparison of males and females showed no differences in gender relative to study results. Note that for this preliminary test, no control group was randomly assigned or examined. Therefore, the researchers cannot predict if significant reductions in consumption of dietary fat and cholesterol are attributable to the intervention.

The self-reported adherence rating score and readiness to change score increased by approximately 1 point on a scale from 1 to 12 (both $p < 0.001$). To help accomplish goals, action plans were also made. The study results show that 94% of the participants made action plans and 89% successfully implemented them.

This study also examined counselor satisfaction. The results showed that nearly three-quarters of the nutrition counselors were satisfied or very satisfied with using the motivational intervention methods (Table 3).

C. Motivational Intervention Method

Figure 2 provides a method for establishing rapport prior to tailoring the intervention to the readiness to change level: ready to change, unsure, and not ready to change. Figure 3 provides specific strategies for each level of change.

1. First Level—Not Ready to Change

The main goal for this level of intervention is to raise awareness of the need to continue meeting goals (e.g., fat

TABLE 3 Nutrition Counselor Satisfaction with the Motivational Intervention Method

Level of satisfaction	Percent of the intervention sessions
Very satisfying	39%
Satisfying	35%
Somewhat satisfying	19%
Slightly or not satisfying	7%

Source: Data from Berg-Smith, S. M., Stevens, V. J., Brown, K. M., VanHorn, L., Gernhofer, N., Peters, E., Greenberg, R., Snetselaar, L., Ahrens, L., and Smith, K., for the Dietary Intervention Study in Children (DISC) Research Group. (1999). A brief motivational intervention to improve dietary adherence in adolescents. *Health Educ. Res.* **14**, 399–410.

grams, carbohydrate grams, energy intake). Additionally to achieve this goal it is necessary to reduce resistance and barriers to meeting goals (e.g., decreasing cues to eat high fat foods). Also, very importantly, focus is placed on increasing interest in considering behavioral steps toward meeting the goals above.

Throughout the initial interview, when working with a patient in this level, it is important to ask open-ended questions, listen reflectively, affirm, summarize, and elicit self-motivational statements. Figure 3 provides examples of questions designed to facilitate the participant's ability to make motivational statements.

a. Open-Ended Questions. Initially for a participant at this level, it is important to ask questions that require explaining or discussing. Questions focus on requiring more than one-word answers. The goal is to guide the participants to talk about their dietary change progress and difficulties. Figure 2 provides some opening questions. Other questions and statements are presented below:

"Let's discuss your experience with diet up to now. Tell me how changing your diet has been for you."

"What things would you like to discuss about your experiences with dietary change and your progress with changes? What do you like about these changes? What don't you like about these changes?"

---

b. Listen Reflectively. Listening goes beyond hearing what a person has said and acknowledging those words. Crucial in responding to a patient or participant is understanding what is meant beyond the words. Reflective listening involves a guess at what the person feels and is phrased as a statement rather than a question. Stating the feeling behind the statement serves two purposes. It allows the participant to tell you if your judgment of the feeling is on target. It also shows that you really are trying to understand more than just words and do care about feelings also. Below are some

---

ESTABLISH RAPPORT
"How's it going?"

↓

OPENING STATEMENT

"We have _____ minutes to meet. This is what I thought we might do:
- take your height and weight measurements,
- hear how the DISC diet is going for you,
- give you some information from your last diet recall and cholesterol values, and
- talk about what, if anything, you might want to change in your eating."

"How does this sound? Is there anything else you want to do?"

↓

ASSESS CURRENT EATING BEHAVIOR AND PROGRESS
- Show Adherence Ruler.

- Ask open-ended questions to explore current eating behavior and progress
* "Tell me more about the number you chose."
* "Why did you choose a 5, and not a 1?"
* "At what times do you follow the DISC diet, and at what times don't you?"
* "How are you feeling about the DISC diet?"
* "The last time we met, you were working on _____. How is that going?"

↓

GIVE FEEDBACK
- Show participant feedback graphs and forms.

- Compare participant results with normative data or other interpretive information
  * "This is where you stand compared to other teenagers."

- Elicit participant's overall response: * "What do you make of all this information?"

- Offer information about the meaning or significance of the results (only if participant asks or shows interest).
  * "For most teenagers who have cholesterol value around _____, they're more likely to _____."

↓

ASSESS READINESS TO CHANGE
- Introduce "change" ruler.
* "On a scale of 1-12 [1=not at all ready; 12=very ready], how ready are you right now to make any new changes in your life to eat foods lower in saturated fat and cholesterol?"
* Ask participant to explain choice of number.
* "What are all the reasons you chose a ___?"

↓

TAILOR INTERVENTION APPROACH

↓

CLOSE THE ENCOUNTER
- Summarize the session.
* "Did I get it all?"

- Support self-efficacy.
* "Again, I applaud your efforts and I know you can do it. If this plan doesn't work out, I'm sure there are other options that might work better."

- Arrange another time to meet.

FIGURE 2   Motivational intervention model. [From Berg-Smith, S. M., Stevens, V. J., Brown, K. M., VanHorn, L., Gernhofer, N., Peters, E., Greenberg, R., Snetselaar, L., Ahrens, L., and Smith, K., for the Dietary Intervention Study in Children (DISC) Research Group. (1999). A brief motivational intervention to improve dietary adherence in adolescents. *Health Educ. Res.* **14,** 399–410.]

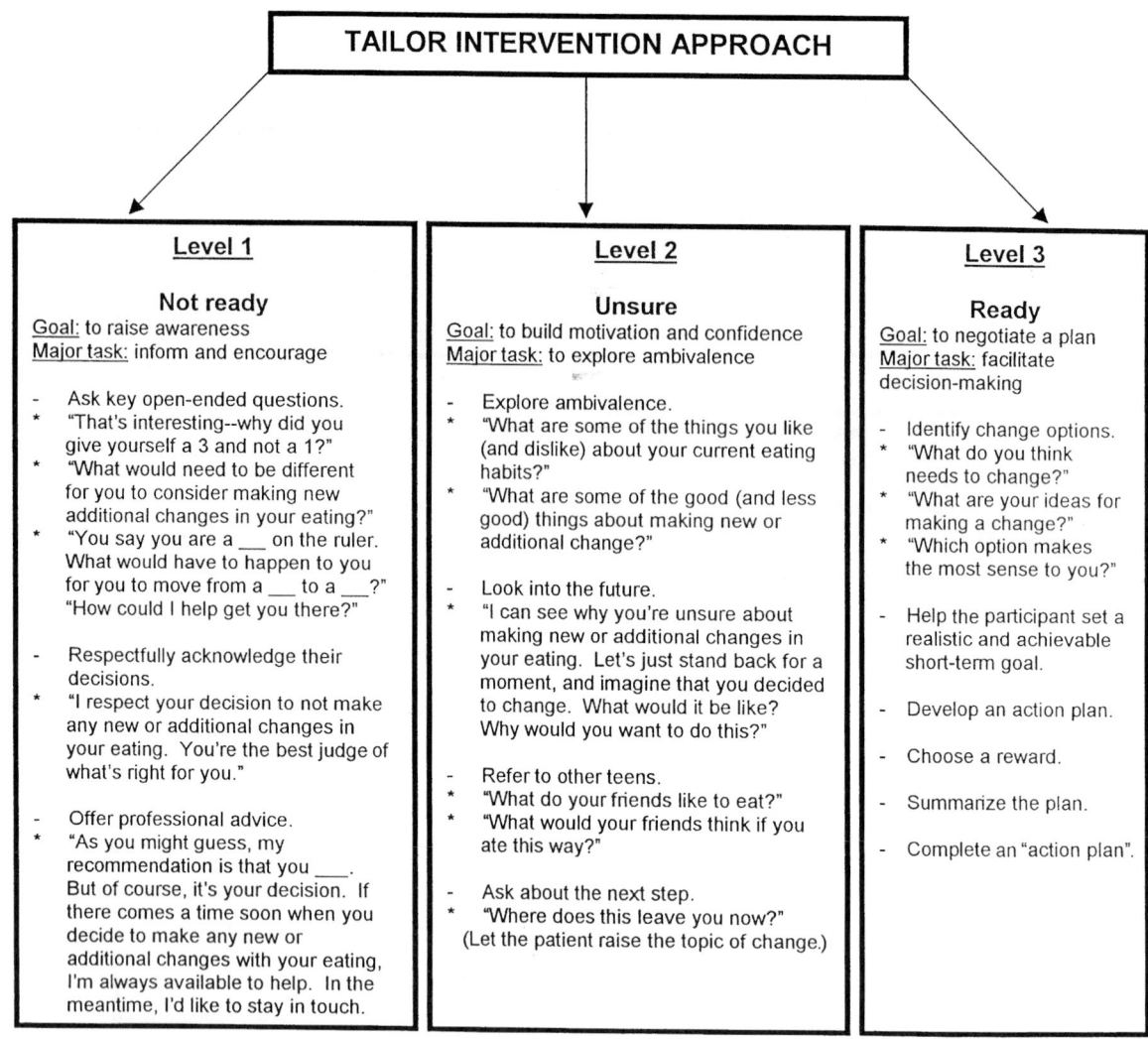

FIGURE 3   Motivational intervention components for three specific levels. [Modified from Berg-Smith, S. M., Stevens, V. J., Brown, K. M., VanHorn, L., Gernhofer, N., Peters, E., Greenberg, R., Snetselaar, L., Ahrens, L., and Smith, K., for the Dietary Intervention Study in Children (DISC) Research Group. (1999). A brief motivational intervention to improve dietary adherence in adolescents. *Health Educ. Res.* **14**, 399–410.]

participant–nutritionist interactions that illustrate reflective listening:

_____

SCENARIO 1

Participant : "There are times when I do a wonderful job of meeting my fat gram goal, but sometimes I don't do so well. I keep trying though."
Nutritionist: "You seem to feel badly that you don't always meet your fat gram goal."

SCENARIO 2

Participant: "I am so tired of trying to follow this diet. It seems that I have put hours into following it, and I have little to show for it. I certainly have not lost weight."
Nutritionist: "You feel frustrated and angry about trying so hard and still getting nowhere."

SCENARIO 3

Participant: "When I don't fill in a food diary, I am not sure that I am doing well or not."
Nutritionist: "You are worried on days when you do not fill in a food diary."

SCENARIO 4

Participant: "I really don't want to continue following this diet. I have other things that are more of a priority now."
Nutritionist: "You seem hassled by these other competing desires and feel that following a new eating pattern is getting in the way."

_____

c. Affirm. Communicating support to participants is an excellent way of letting them know that you appreciate what they are doing. Affirmations are statements that indicate

1. **Problem Recognition**
   What things make you think that this is a problem?
   What difficulties have you had in relation to your diet?
   In what ways do you think you or other people have been inconvenienced by your diet?
   In what ways has this been a problem for you?
   How has your diet stopped you from doing what you want to do?

2. **Concern**
   What is there about your diet that you or other people might see as reasons for concern?
   What worries you about your diet?
   How do you feel about your dietary problems?
   How much does that concern you?
   In what ways does this concern you?
   What do you think will happen if you don't make a change?

3. **Intention to Change**
   The fact that you're here indicates that at least a part of you thinks it's time to do something.
        What are the reasons you see for making a change?
   What makes you think that you need to make a change?
   If you were 100% successful and things worked out exactly as you would like, what would be different?
   What things make you think that you should stop following your diet? ... And
        what about the other side? What makes you think it's time for a change?
   What are you thinking about your diet at this point?
   What would be the advantages of making a change?
   I can see that you're feeling stuck at the moment. What's going to have to change?

4. **Optimism**
   What makes you think that if you decide to make a change, you could do it?
   What encourages you that you can change if you want to?
   What do you think would work for you, if you decided to change?

FIGURE 4 Examples of questions designed to elicit self-motivational statements. [Modified from Bowen, D., Ehret, C., Pedersen, M., et al. (2000). Results of an adjunct dietary intervention program in the Women's Health Initiative. *J. Am. Diet. Assoc.* (in press).]

alignment and normalization of the participant's issues. Alignment means telling participants that you understand them and are with them in their difficulties.

Normalization means telling the participants that they are perfectly within reason and "normal" to have such reactions and feelings.

Examples of affirmations include:

"It is very hard to struggle with competing priorities. You've done amazingly well."
"That is an insightful idea."
"Thank you for telling me that. It must have been hard for you to tell me."
"I can see why you would have this difficulty. Many people have the same problem."

---

d. Summarize. Periodically, and at the point when you begin to elicit self-motivational statements, summarize the content of what the participant has said. Cover key points even if they involve negative feelings. You can discuss conflicting ideas that the participant has brought up by using the strategy "on the one hand you . . . and on the other hand you. . . ." This reminds both of you about the issues and ensures clarity.

e. Elicit Self-Motivational Statements. The most important part of self-motivational statements is that they help participants realize that a problem exists, that they are concerned about the problem, that they intend to correct the problem, and that they think they can do better in the future. Figure 4 provides questions to elicit self-motivational statements. These statements fall in to four categories: problem recognition, concern, intention to change, and optimism.

It is important to respectfully acknowledge decisions that participants make. These decisions may mean that a participant has decided not to make changes immediately (see Fig. 3).

It is appropriate to offer professional advice, but still leave the actual decision to make a change up to the participant. Figure 3 provides some ideas on how to approach the participant.

Close the discussion with another summary. Concentrate on any self-motivational statements that the participant has made. End the session with the idea that both of you should think about what has been discussed and that you can revisit the issues next time.

2. SECOND LEVEL—UNSURE ABOUT CHANGE

The main goal for this intervention is to tip the balance toward working to meet the goals. Four steps are important in meeting the goals: (1) regroup, (2) ask key questions, (3) negotiate a plan, and (4) conclude the work.

a. Regroup. The first step in dealing with a participant who is unsure about changing dietary habits is regrouping to focus on the transition from not being ready to deal with the problems of change to moving toward a reinitiating of behavior adjustment. This process of regrouping can serve as a reminder of what has happened in previous sessions. Below are four ways to regroup:

1. *Summarize* the participant's perceptions of what is going on. The summary might include self-motivational statements that the participant has made.
2. *Identify* ambivalence or other conflicting issues.
3. *Review* any self-monitoring related to dietary intake.
4. *Restate intentions or plans to change or do better in the future.*

b. Ask Key Questions. Ask questions that focus on the participant's statements regarding future plans to make dietary changes. The goal is to ask open-ended questions that cause the participant to think about what you have just summarized and come to the conclusion that action is necessary. The goal is for the participant to provide a statement showing the desire to change. Here are some examples of questions that facilitate positive participant statements:

"How might we work together to proceed from here?"

"Hearing my summary of how things have gone in the past, what do you want to do?"

"How might you become more involved in dietary change? What are the good parts and the bad parts about continuing to change?"

"You are currently unsure of what to do. How might we work together to resolve the issue?"

---

c. Negotiate a Plan. There are three parts to the negotiation process. The first involves setting goals, the second, considering the options, and finally, arriving at a plan.

1. *Set goals.* Past wisdom dictated that setting goals meant being very specific and behavioral. "I will eat candy bars only one time per week on Sunday." Motivational interviewing dictates that goal setting may start out very broadly at first and then move to behavioral goals that are very specific. To elicit broadly stated goals, the following questions might be used:

"What about your diet would you like to change?"

"How would you like things to be different from how they are now?"

---

2. *Consider options.* Make a list of things that might be changed to bring the participant closer to the dietary goal. Ask the participant to choose among the options. If the first one does not work, the participant has many choices as backups.

3. *Arrive at a plan.* Ask the participant to arrive at a plan. Include in the plan the specific behavioral goals with potential problems that may serve as barriers to making these changes.

d. Conclude the Work. Always end the session with an encouraging statement and a reflection on the participant's resourcefulness in identifying the plan. Follow this statement with the idea that he is the best expert relative to behavior change. Indicate that you will stay in touch to check on how the behavior change is going.

3. THIRD LEVEL—READY TO CHANGE

The main goal for this third intervention is to reengage the participant in meeting the dietary goals.

a. Review. Cover the previous discussions with the participant. Focus on the statements made by the participant that show interest and willingness to change. Use statements that show that it was the participant's idea to meet dietary goals previously set. For example, "You said that you were interested in trying again."

b. Encourage Choices and Activities. Ask the participant what she would like to do to get reengaged. Encourage the participant to make her own choice. Collaborate and negotiate short-term, easily attained goals initially. For example, "I will drink 1% milk for a week in place of 2% milk and gradually reduce to fat-free milk."

c. Summarize. Review the discussion, the issues, and difficulties on both sides. Remind the participant to keep trying and to believe in herself.

D. Modification of Diet and Renal Disease Study (MDRD)

The Modification of Diet and Renal Disease Study (MDRD) [16] used the self-management approach to modify dietary behavior. In this population of persons diagnosed with renal disease, research nutritionists counseled participants on diets low in protein and phosphorus. Although the diets were difficult to follow, the study participants showed great motivation based on their desires to avoid renal dialysis [17]. The following strategies were used successfully in the MDRD [18]:

1. *Single-nutrient approach to dietary behavior change.* The focus in this study was on reducing protein content of the diet. With this reduction, dietary phosphorus was also reduced. When other nutrients were modified, specific food groups were identified. Even with changes in other nutrients, protein was still a primary focus.
2. *Self-monitoring.* The participant's ability to self-monitor was crucial to keeping protein intake down to goal levels. Weighing and measuring was used as a means of

matching dietary change on a daily basis with the biological marker of urinary nitrogen. Further study in self-monitoring matched with the biological marker showed that problems occur in knowing how to best represent dietary intake [19]. Often it is difficult to closely mirror the exact amount of protein in a cut of meat if that cut is not precisely specified.

3. *Staging changes.* In the MDRD, nutritionists also staged changes in dietary protein by gradually reducing the dietary protein intake. This gradual change made day-to-day modifications easier.

4. *Modeling.* Nutritionists modeled dietary changes by offering both recipes low in protein and taste-testing sessions. Group sessions were held at which a special meal was offered with food preparation techniques modeled.

E. Diabetes Control and Complications Trial (DCCT)

The Diabetes Control and Complications Trial (DCCT) [20] used techniques similar to those of the MDRD study [21]:

1. *Single-nutrient approach.* Investigators focused on carbohydrate as a single nutrient, where it was matched with insulin to achieve normalized blood glucose.

2. *Self-monitoring.* Monitoring consisted of following blood glucose concentrations and dietary intakes to verify where problems might be occurring. If dietary intake was high along with blood glucose concentrations, dietary intake and/or insulin was modified to achieve normal blood glucose levels.

3. *Staging changes.* Changes were staged by working on specific times of day that were most problematic. If lunchtimes were most often high, we focused on dietary intake modifications to alter blood glucose levels. Insulin and exercise also often played a role.

4. *Modeling.* Dietary modifications were facilitated by providing recipes, modeling, and going to restaurants to identify and anticipate blood glucose levels after eating a favorite lunch or other meals out of the home.

IV. SUMMARY

Considerable experience in clinical trials suggests that dietary modification requires a process of making changes on an individual basis with constant negotiation with the patient or participant. Working as a team, the nutritionist and participant can achieve dietary change that alters biological markers and may reduce disease risk and optimize management.

References

1. Agostinelli, G., Brown, J. M., and Miller, W. (1995). Effects of normative feedback on consumption among heavy drinking college attendants. *J. Drug Educ.* **25,** 31–40.

2. Brown, J. M., and Miller, W. R. (1993). Impact of motivational interviewing on participation in residential alcoholism treatment. *Psychol. Addict. Behav.* **7,** 211–218.

3. Rokeach, M. (1973). "The Nature of Human Values." Free Press, New York.

4. Rosenstock, I., Strecher, V., and Becker, M. (1994). The health belief model and HIV risk behavior change. *In* "Preventing AIDS: Theories and Methods of Behavioral Interventions," (R. J. DiClemente, and J. L. Peterson, Eds.), pp. 5–24. Plenum Press, New York.

5. Bandura, A. (1989). Perceived self-efficacy in the exercise of control over AIDS infection. *In* "Primary Prevention of AIDS: Psychological Approaches," pp. 128–141. Sage Publications, London.

6. Bandura, A. (1977). Self-efficacy: Toward a unifying theory of behavioral change. *Psychol. Rev.* **84,** 191–215.

7. Bandura, A. (1991). Self-efficacy mechanism in physiological activation and health-promoting behavior. *In* "Neurobiology of Learning, Emotion and Affect" (J. Madden, Ed.), pp. 229–270. Raven Press, New York.

8. Janis, J. L., and Mann, L. (1977). "Decision-Making: A Psychological Analysis of Conflict, Choice and Commitment" (Free Press, New York).

9. Miller, W. R., and Rollnick, S. (1991). "Motivational Interviewing: Preparing People to Change Addictive Behavior." Guilford Press, New York.

10. Women's Health Inititative. (1994). WHI Protocol for Clinical Trial and Observational Components, NIH Publication no. N01-WH-2-2110. Fred Hutchinson Cancer Research Center, Seattle, WA.

11. Prochaska, J., and DiClemente, C. (1982). Transtheoretical therapy: Toward a more integrative model of change. *Psychother. Theory Res. Prac.* 19:276–288.

12. Bowen, D., Ehret, C., Pedersen, M., et al. Results of an adjunct dietary intervention program in the Women's Health Initiative. *J. Am. Diet. Assoc.* (in press).

13. Berg-Smith, S. M., Stevens, V. J., Brown, K. M., VanHorn, L., Gernhofer, N., Peters, E., Greenberg, R., Snetselaar, L., Ahrens, L., and Smith, K., for the Dietary Intervention Study in Children (DISC) Research Group. (1999). A brief motivational intervention to improve dietary adherence in adolescents. *Health Educ. Res.* **14,** 399–410.

14. DISC Collaborative Research Group. (1995). Efficacy and safety of lowering dietary intake of fat and cholesterol in children with elevated low-density lipoprotein cholesterol: The Dietary Intervention Study in Children (DISC). *JAMA* **273,** 1429–1435.

15. DISC Collaborative Research Group. (1993). Dietary Intervention Study in Children (DISC) with elevated LDL cholesterol: Design and baseline characteristics. *Ann. Epidemiology* **3,** 393–402.

16. Klahr, S., Levey, A. S., Beck, G. J., Caggiula, A. W., Hunsicker, L., Kusek, J. W., and Striker, G., for the Modification of Diet in Renal Disease Study Group. (1994). The effects of dietary protein restriction and blood-pressure control on the progression of chronic renal disease. *N. Engl. J. Med.* **330,** 877–84.

17. Milas, C., Norwalk, M. P., Akpele, L., Castaldo, L., Coyne, T., Doroshenko, L., Kigawa, L., Korzec-Ramirez, D., Scherch, L., and Snetselaar, L. (1995). Factors associated with adherence to the dietary protein intervention in the modification of diet in renal disease. *J. Am. Diet. Assoc.* **95**(11), 1295–1300.

18. Snetselaar, L. (1992). Dietary compliance issues in patients with early stage renal disease. *Clin. Appl. Nutr.* **2**(3), 47–52.

19. Snetselaar, L., Chenard, C. A., Hunsicker, L. G., and Stumbo, P. J. (1995). Protein calculation from food diaries underestimates biological marker. *J. Nutr.* **125,** 2333–2340.

20. The Diabetes Control and Complications Trial Research Group. (1993). The effect of intensive treatment of diabetes on the development and progression of long-term complications in insulin-dependent diabetes mellitus. *N. Engl. J. Med.* **329,** 977–986.

21. Greene, T., Bourgorgnie, J., Hawbe, V., Kusek, J., Snetselaar, L., Soucie, J., and Yamamoto, M. (1993). Baseline characteristics in the modification of diet in renal disease study. *J. Am. Soc. Neprhol.* **3**(11), 1819–1834.

CHAPTER 8

Tools and Techniques to Facilitate Eating Behavior Change

JOAN M. HEINS[1] AND LINDA DELAHANTY[2]
[1]*Washington University School of Medicine, St. Louis, Missouri*
[2]*Massachusetts General Hospital, Boston, Massachusetts*

I. INTRODUCTION

The potential effect of medical nutrition therapy to improve health outcomes from cardiovascular, cancer, diabetes, obesity, gastrointestinal, and other health conditions is clearly described in other chapters in this text. However, the process of implementing medical nutrition therapy is not as straightforward and is based on thorough assessment of each client's lifestyle, capabilities, and motivation to change.

At a glance, one might perceive the nutrition education and counseling process to be routine, where nutrition information and recommended food choices are discussed as they pertain to particular health concerns of a client. For a patient with a high cholesterol level, teach the National Cholesterol Education Program (NCEP) Step 1 diet and possibly the NCEP Step 2 diet; for high blood pressure, teach weight loss and a Dietary Approaches to Stop Hypertension (DASH) diet; for type 2 diabetes, teach weight loss, exercise and possibly carbohydrate counting. If only changing eating behavior were that straightforward! The truth is that each person who is referred for nutrition counseling presents with varying levels of knowledge and motivation for changing eating habits. Today's nutrition counselor must draw on knowledge from the biomedical and behavioral sciences to define the nutrition prescription and design an intervention that will truly impact eating.

The traditional model for delivery of nutrition interventions has been individual consultations in health care settings. This paradigm is changing, however. Increased focus on chronic disease prevention has resulted in an enhanced need for nutrition education at a time when economic constraints in health care have led to a decline in traditional hospital-based nutrition counseling services. Thus, dietitians are providing counseling services in shopping centers, offering cholesterol education classes in health clubs, and communicating with clients via telephone and the Internet. Although individualized counseling will continue as an important component of clinical nutrition, use of alternative methods, such as group sessions or guided self-study, has been shown to be both efficient and effective. Regardless of the setting, nutrition counseling has a common goal: to help people make healthy changes in eating behaviors. This chapter will discuss tools and techniques for applying education and behavior change theories in the practice of medical nutrition therapy.

II. THE TEACHING/LEARNING PROCESS

Knowledge is not sufficient but is essential for behavior change [1]. To be effective, nutrition counselors need to understand the factors that influence learning and the different domains in which people learn.

A. Factors Influencing Learning

Learning is influenced by many factors including age, literacy, culture, and individual learner style.

1. AGE

Much of our understanding of the differences in the way adults and children learn comes from the work of Knowles [2], who identified concepts of *need to know, performance centered,* and *experiential learning* as important to the adult learner. These concepts have been expanded by the research of others who describe self-directed learning [3] and critical thinking techniques [4] as elements that enhance adult learning. A common theme that emerges across learning theories and studies of adult learning is the importance of active involvement of the individual in the learning process [5].

2. LITERACY

The term *literacy* includes not only the ability to read and write but also to process information. With the wide use of printed materials to support nutrition education, client literacy and the reading level of teaching materials are important issues. Assessing level of formal education is easy, but unfortunately not always an accurate indicator of literacy. Tests such as ABLE [6], WRAT [7], and the Cloze procedure[8] can be used to evaluate an individual's literacy level. These tests, however, take time to administer and can be fatiguing.

Their best use may be to assess reading levels in targeted groups prior to development of educational materials rather than for individual assessment in clinical practice. The steps for evaluating nutrition education materials are relatively simple and can be used by dietitians when information on the reading level of material is not provided. Methods such as the SMOG readability formula [9], Gunning's FOG Index [10], and the Fry Readability Graph [11] are described in the reading and health education literature [12–14]. These formulas use the number of words, the number of syllables, and similar criteria to assign a grade or reading level. Scoring can be done by hand or with computer programs. One of the difficulties of using readability formulas in clinical nutrition is that core words such as *calories, carbohydrate, vitamins, minerals,* and *cholesterol* contain three or more syllables and consequently raise the reading level of materials. These words may be sufficiently common, however, so that people with reading abilities lower than the assigned grade level can process and comprehend the materials based on their familiarity with the words as well as the organization of the written text [15].

3. CULTURE

Ethnicity and culture influence the way people learn. Addressing cultural difference is not simply translating educational materials into the primary language of the client. Fundamentals of values, health beliefs, and communication styles also vary by culture. The changing demographics of the American population have resulted in an increased need for nutrition education materials appropriate for a wide range of cultures. One response to this need is the *Ethnic and Regional Food Practice* series developed by the Diabetes Care and Education practice group of The American Dietetic Association [16]. The series, written for health professionals, currently includes 11 modules ranging from Jewish to Hmong cuisine. The modules discuss traditions and beliefs influencing health behaviors such as eating habits, provide nutrient analysis of foods specific to the culture, outline sample recipes, and include a reproducible master of a client teaching tool. Other sources for ethnically appropriate teaching materials include government printing agencies, volunteer health organizations, ethnic special interest groups, and vendors of health education materials. Even when specific guidelines are not available, an appreciation that food and health hold different meanings to people of different cultures can aid dietitians in counseling individuals from diverse ethnic backgrounds.

4. LEARNER STYLE

Learner style is a phrase that has been used to describe the way people cognitively process information [17] and the interaction of the individual with the learning environment [18]. Drawing from the work of Carl Jung, Osterman has identified four types of learners: *feelers, thinkers, sensors,* and *intuitors* [19]. Table 1 summarizes key characteristics that differentiate these styles. Teaching strategies can be selected to match the learning style or characteristic of the individual. When working with groups, an education session can be constructed to include components that will appeal to all learning styles [19]. Walker, in her review of adult learner characteristics [18], contrasts different environmental methods of learning, such as group vs. individual, computer vs. print vs. video, didactic vs. emotional appeal in messages, and directed learning vs. self-directed approaches. Although comparison studies of environmental methods are limited, she found that research on group vs. individual sessions for diabetes education showed some benefits for group education beyond potential cost savings. A review of research evaluating nutrition education methods found that small groups plus a follow-up telephone call were the most effective, with one-on-one sessions ranking next, followed closely by the small group (no follow-up) approach [5]. The authors concluded that in terms of cost efficiency and cost effectiveness, groups showed a clear advantage. A comparison of group vs. self-directed education for blood cholesterol reduction found that the self-directed approach was a viable alternative to group diet instruction [20]. These findings support use of alternatives to individual counseling sessions to match client learning styles as well as to provide efficient methods for serving more people.

B. Domains of Learning

Learning includes knowledge, attitude, and skill. The education literature describes these areas of learning as domains:

TABLE 1   Learning Styles

	Feelers	**Thinkers**	**Sensors**	**Intuitors**
Looks for:	Meaning, clarity	Facts and information	Practical application	Alternatives
Learns by:	Listening and sharing	Thinking through ideas	Problem solving	Trial and error
Best format:	Discussion	Lecture	Demonstration	Self-discovery
Favorite question:	Why?	What?	How?	If?

Source: Adapted from Osterman, D. N. (1984). The feedback lecture: Matching teaching and learning styles. *J. Am. Diet. Assoc.* **84,** 1221–1222.

cognitive (knowledge), affective (attitude), and psychomotor (skill) [21, 22]. Within each domain there is a range or level of learning that can be achieved.

The cognitive domain concentrates on knowledge outcome and includes six hierarchical levels: knowledge, comprehension, application, analysis, synthesis, and evaluation. The affective domain encompasses an individual's feelings or attitudes associated with a particular topic. The five levels of the affective domain progress from receiving to responding, valuing, organizing, and characterizing by a value or a value complex. The psychomotor domain looks at skill development including perception, set (prepared for learning), guided response (performance), mechanism (response more habitual), complex overt response (response is effective and routine), and adaptation (response continues in new situations.)

Detailed classification systems or taxonomies have been developed that include action verbs to define levels of learning [23, 24]. The taxonomies are used to set learning objectives. Objectives can be written for any domain, and for any level within that domain, depending on the desired outcome of the counseling session. A learning plan can be developed for an individual that systematically advances him or her from a low level to a high level of competence.

Application of the taxonomies of learning to nutrition counseling offers a framework for integrating learning and behavior change theories. Learning objectives are written in language that clearly identifies *who* will do *what, when, where,* and *how. Who* is the client, *what* is the information, *how* is the measurable behavior, and *when* and *where* define the situation. For example, a behavioral objective for a patient with hyperlipidemia, targeted at the application level of the cognitive domain, could be as follows: At the end of the counseling session (*when*), the client (*who*) will be able to identify (*how*) low-fat entrée options (*what*) from sample menus (*where*).

The value of setting behavioral objectives for nutrition interventions is well supported in the literature. A review found that programs that were more behaviorally focused were more effective [5]. This extensive review identified education and behavior change strategies that were successful in changing eating habits. Educational strategies of self-evaluation or self-assessment and active participation worked well for individual or group interventions. Effective behavioral strategies included use of a systematic behavior change process, tailoring the intervention to the specific needs of the individual, involvement of others to provide social support and an empowerment approach that enhances personal control.

In summary, for nutrition counseling to be successful, learning principles suggest that as much attention must be given to selecting the most effective way to communicate the diet to the individual as is given to assessing what would be the most effective diet for the individual. Most health professionals have strong grounding in the biological sciences, but less exposure to the behavioral sciences. For this reason, the comfort level for determining the appropriate nutrient intake is greater than for evaluating learner needs and setting behavioral objectives. The current demand in all areas of health care to measure effectiveness in terms of patient outcomes requires clinicians to look beyond the diagnosis and intervention phases of care and evaluate the ultimate results. Nutrition interventions that do not show measurable improvement in patient status are not effective. The argument that treatment failure is due to patient noncompliance does not negate the lack of effect. Dietitians and other health care providers must be adept at combining nutrition, learning, and behavior change principles in the process of nutrition education.

III. NUTRITION EDUCATION TECHNIQUES

Length of time since diagnosis, acuity of disease condition, complexity of the nutrition intervention, preferred client learning style, and readiness to change behaviors are factors to consider in developing a client's education plan. The counselor needs to assess learning needs, decide on the level of education, select an optimal method, and choose appropriate nutrition education tools.

A. Assessing Learning Needs

Assessment of learning needs should be an integral part of nutrition counseling. Table 2 provides a basic list of variables that should be assessed. Additional items are added to

TABLE 2 Nutrition Educational Assessment

Demographic	Clinical
• Age	• Medical history
• Gender	• Medication
• Occupation	• Height/weight
• Education	• Food allergies/intolerances

Social	Health Habits
• Family status	• Eating patterns
• Living environment	• Physical activity
• Social network	• Smoking status
• Cultural factors	• Alcohol intake
• Religious practices	• Health practices
• Health beliefs	• Use of health services

Learner Characteristics
• Previous health education
• Expectations for current education
• Preferred learning methods
• Learning style
• Readiness for change

gather information pertinent to the individual and the clinical condition. The amount of time spent in assessment can limit time spent in counseling. Some studies report up to 55% of a counseling session devoted to the assessment phase [25]. However, time spent on a comprehensive assessment is regained by the effectiveness of a nutrition counseling session that has been tailored to the individual's needs.

A variety of approaches can be used to reduce time spent on assessment. Before the counseling session, data can be collected from medical records, and patients can be asked to submit information. Questionnaires can be sent and received by mail, via fax, through the Internet, or completed by the client in the waiting room before the visit. If advanced data collection has not been successful, ask the patient. Although clients may not recount a comprehensive description of their referring physician's intent, their perception of what the interaction should achieve provides a basis for assessing learning needs and willingness to make behavior changes.

B. Levels of Education

Nutrition education should be planned as a continuum of learning that starts with fundamental guidelines, then incrementally adds more complex information as basic applications are mastered. The terms *initial/survival, practical,* and *continuing* have been used to differentiate three levels of education [25].

1. SURVIVAL LEVEL

The first level focuses on essential information that the client needs in order to make important fundamental adjustments in health behaviors. Ideally, initial education will occur shortly after diagnosis. The extent of information included at the survival level differs by disease condition and learner characteristics. A person with diabetes treated with insulin needs enough information to understand the association between food, activity, and insulin so that he or she can select appropriate meals to avoid hyper- and hypoglycemia. For the patient with congestive heart failure with frequent hospital admissions, the survival information would focus on the sodium content of foods and avoidance of fluid retention. Survival education needs to be simple and directive; the dietitian serves as a teacher providing concrete guidelines on what the patient should or should not do.

2. PRACTICAL LEVEL

The practical level of education can occur as follow-up to initial counseling or as a new encounter, with the patient having had initial instruction some time before. Information should expand on the fundamentals learned for survival by applying them to a variety of situations. New topics can be introduced as well. Clients often will identify "need to know" information they have found important to learn, such as how to eat in restaurants, modify recipes, and/or interpret food labels. At this level the dietitian serves as a

counselor by providing guidelines for patients to use in making decisions.

3. CONTINUING EDUCATION

Once a client has mastered the basic skills and can apply them successfully in his or her life, continuing education can be used to reinforce learning, update information, and achieve higher levels of knowledge. In-depth knowledge of the relationship between nutrition and the disease process, nutrition principles, food preparation, and eating behaviors can enable patients to "take charge" of their disease management. The dietitian at this level serves as a consultant helping the client synthesize and personalize information.

C. Educational Methods

In addition to the content of the educational intervention, the process or method offers different techniques to make nutrition education more effective. In-person individual or group sessions are the most common formats used for nutrition counseling. While decisions on group or individual counseling sessions may be made by feasibility criteria (i.e., time, money), the client's learning preference should be considered as well. Using Osterman's classification of learning styles (Table 1) *feelers* would like group sessions that have discussion opportunities, whereas *thinkers* could be frustrated by this method because they "just want the facts." *Sensors* would respond to either method as long as an application exercise is included. A combination of individual and group sessions offers practical advantages. Information presented during group sessions can be tailored to the individual in a one-on-one discussion either in-person, by telephone or e-mail.

Another method for nutrition education is the use of self-study materials. This approach has been used more often in population or community nutrition interventions than in group or individual counseling sessions. Self-study modules offer advantages in terms of convenience, pace of learning, active involvement of the individual, and economics. Modules range in size and scope. Two popular examples are the 28-page pamphlet of the Shape Up America program [26] and the 312-page Learn Program manual [27]. Self-study modules generally include self-assessment exercises, general information on the health topic, steps for identifying personal behaviors to modify, guidelines for making behavioral changes, methods for monitoring behavior change, and tips on sustaining the new behaviors in special situations (e.g., eating out, stressful days). This method of learning offers something for all learning styles, especially *intuitors* who will appreciate the opportunity for self-discovery.

A model for using patient assessment to guide selection of education methods for weight management has been developed by Caban and colleagues (Fig. 1) [28]. They use a comprehensive set of physical and psychological indicators to classify individuals by risk status, and then select inter-

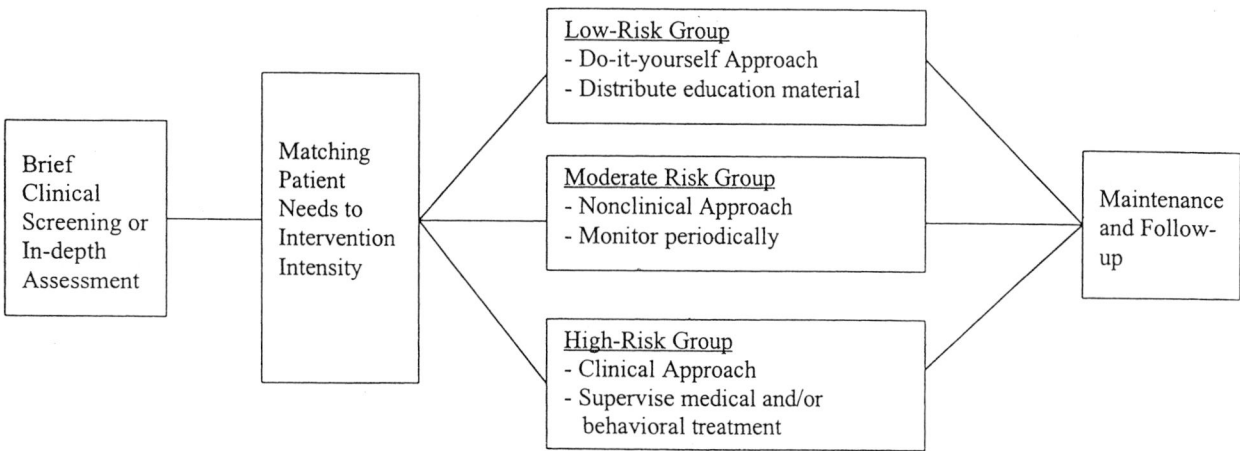

FIGURE 1   Model for individualizing treatment approaches. [Adapted with permission from Caban, A., Johnson, P., Marseille, D., and Wylie-Rosert, J. (1999). Tailoring a lifestyle change approach and resources to the patient. *Diab. Spectrum* **12**, 33–38.]

ventions with an intensity that matches individual needs. People who are in stable clinical condition, have few behaviors to change, and are highly motivated are classified as low risk and are candidates for self-directed learning methods. Those with clinical conditions targeted for improvement, several behaviors to change, and less motivation to make changes require more structure and support. Group interaction, periodic monitoring, and structured activities are appropriate for this type of client. The high-risk client, who has multiple health problems that need to be addressed, has little motivation, and requires a great deal of support, will need individualized care provided by clinicians. In their program, computers are used to access assessment data, tailor questionnaires to individual profiles, and provide feedback to the client. The authors recognize that all practice settings do not have these resources, but encourage counselors to use even a brief assessment to collect information that will determine the best type of program for the individual.

D. Nutrition Educational Tools

Nutrition counseling does not suffer from a lack of tools. Information on nutrition education materials can be found in the catalogues of publishing houses, volunteer health and professional organizations, government agencies, reviews published in professional journals, and by professional networking. Education materials also are available from companies manufacturing health products (e.g., pharmaceutical companies) and associations that promote a food or food group (e.g., National Dairy Council). Although there may not be a teaching tool that matches all aspects of a patient's learning profile, availability of educational materials is not the prominent problem. Resources for acquisition and storage are more common deterrents to dietitians and other health care providers being able to use a teaching tool tailored to a client's specific needs.

1. MEAL PLANNING TOOLS

Several formats for nutrition education tools have been applied in multiple areas of clinical nutrition. These include guidelines, menu approaches, counting methods, and exchange systems.

Guidelines, such as the Food Guide Pyramid, are a tool to provide basic information to help people make healthy food choices. They may include some information on servings and food preparation but not the specificity of nutrient information that can be found with other methods. Guidelines work well as a tool for initial education if precision in nutrient intake is not required. They may contain sufficient information for some people to be able to make eating behavior changes that reduce health risks and improve clinical indicators.

Menus are a tool to give clients specific direction on what to eat, including food type, preparation method, and serving size. For survival education, several days of menus can be written using familiar foods that ensure appropriate nutrition. The number of patients who carefully collect their tray menus during a hospital stay attests to the popularity of this approach. Menu planning tools generally rely on input from the patient so that food likes and dislikes can be taken into consideration. Menu planning can be combined with other instructional formats and used at the practical and ongoing education levels as well. Computer programs are becoming available that plan menus taking into account the nutrient prescription and individual food preferences.

Counting methods have become popular in recent years although one tool, *The Point System,* was introduced as early as 1944 [29]. Calorie counting is a standard approach for weight management. Fat gram counting is utilized in teaching materials for cholesterol reduction, cancer prevention, and weight management. Carbohydrate counting, initially considered a technique for intensive insulin therapy, is now being used with all types of diabetes for initial as well as continuing education.

Exchange approaches focus on food groups versus individual foods to teach nutrition principles. A popular example is the *Exchange Lists for Meal Planning* [30] that has been used for decades to instruct patients with diabetes. The system provides a tool for teaching patients how to select a diet that meets a macronutrient prescription. The exchange lists concept has been adapted for weight management education and is sometimes applied to nutrient information provided with recipes and manufactured food products. The Plate Model, a common teaching tool in Europe, has been used in the Diabetes Atherosclerosis Intervention Study (DIAS) [31]. The method uses a visual tool of a plate divided into three sections: one covers one-half of the plate and the other two are one-quarter sections. The guidelines place vegetables including salads in the one-half plate section, grains in one of the one-quarter sections and meat and alternatives in the other one-quarter section. Other food groups are included as side dish servings. DIAS has established target nutrient intakes for study participants that are evaluated by annual 24-hour recalls. Both the Plate Model and the more quantitative exchange lists have been used to help DIAS participants achieve the study goals.

Adaptations of the above tools for nutrition education can be found to match many idiosyncratic learner characteristics. Simplified versions appropriate for initial education or for low-literacy clients and versions that have been translated into Spanish are the most common tools. A recent trend in nutrition education materials is to provide "copy masters" for client education tools that can be photocopied without copyright infringement. Purchasing reproducible tools offers nutrition counselors an efficient way to have a wide range of teaching materials available to meet individual client needs. Even more promising is the emerging option of computer software providing nutrition education tools. Computer programs allow the provider to tailor materials to patient characteristics and to change content if it becomes obsolete.

2. SKILLS TRAINING

Meal planning tools, even those carefully selected and matched to individual learner characteristics, are not sufficient for nutrition education. People may learn what they need to do, but lack the "skill" or ability to translate knowledge into practice. Teaching an individual how to read a nutrition label provides the knowledge necessary to interpret the information. Applying that knowledge to decisions made at the point of purchase or in meal preparation requires skill. Comparison of the nutrition labels on two products requires analytical skills if the products have different serving sizes. After using the nutrition label to select a product, additional skills are required to integrate the selected food into the total diet. Tools are available in print, video, CD-ROM, and three-dimensional models for teaching clients a wide range of nutrition skills.

Some clients, however, cannot or choose not to master certain skills. Meal planning is a prime example. No matter how well educated and trained, there are some people who find meal planning a real barrier to following their diet. "Just tell me what to eat" is their common complaint. Preprinted menus offer a solution in some cases. The American Diabetes Association introduced the first of their *Month of Meals* publications in 1989 and quickly added four more editions in response to the demand [32]. Books offering low fat and/or low calorie menus are abundant, as well.

Menus, however, do not meet the needs of people who lack the skills and interest to prepare meals from menus. The Cardiovascular Risk Reduction Dietary Intervention Trial addressed the difficulty many people have in translating complex dietary recommendations into meals. The trial compared a nutritionally complete prepared meals program with (1) a diet prescribed to meet the same nutrient levels established for the prepared meals [33] and (2) usual-care dietary therapy [34]. The prepared meals program resulted in significantly greater weight loss and reduction in blood pressure than the other two interventions, and improvement in lipid and glucose levels compared with the usual-care therapy.

This "need" for more specific information that will help people choose healthy meals is not limited to clinical nutrition. The food industry, recognizing that each generation of Americans spends less time cooking, has responded with carry-out and order-in meals from restaurants, and deli, salad bar, and complete "meals to go" in supermarkets. Today's nutrition counselor must be just as adept at helping clients develop the skills to select healthy preprepared meals as teaching the fundamentals of reducing dietary fat intake.

To change eating habits, nutrition counseling needs to include more than well-selected education techniques. A review has found that many studies based on dissemination of information and teaching of skills were not effective in changing eating behavior [5]. Even studies supposedly following the knowledge, attitude, behavior communications model were not successful if the behavioral components were actually skills training (e.g., label reading, food preparation). Only in studies where participants were self-selected and already motivated were they able to show changes in eating patterns with an intervention that did not have a true behavior change technique. Unfortunately, diagnosis of a disease or health risk does not automatically result in a motivated patient, therefore, dietitians need to include behavior change techniques in their practice.

IV. BEHAVIOR CHANGE TECHNIQUES

Theories for behavior change are extensive and are described in Chapter 6. Certain theories offer techniques that are practical for use in nutrition counseling. Some techniques such as self-monitoring, behavioral contracting, and goal setting are patient focused. They allow the individual to "personalize" the nutrition intervention, to be an active participant in the process, and to receive feedback on progress made to-

ward identified goals. Other techniques such as motivational interviewing, consciousness raising, and assessing readiness for change are implemented by the counselor. The stages of change transtheoretical model [35] offers dietitians a systematic framework for applying behavior change techniques to nutrition education. While the model can be used with all education methods, the following section will describe application in nutrition counseling sessions.

A. Stages of Change

The stages of change model, discussed also in Chapter 7, was described by Prochaska & colleagues. It postulates that both cessation of high-risk behaviors and the acquisition of healthy behaviors involves progression through five stages of change: precontemplation, contemplation, preparation, action and maintenance (see Table 3) [35]. The precontemplation stage is characterized by having no intention of changing the behavior in question in the foreseeable future. People in this stage tend to be unaware that they have a problem and are resistant to efforts to modify the behavior in question. Contemplation is characterized by awareness that the particular behavior is a problem, and serious consideration about resolving the problem but having no commitment to take action in the near future. The preparation stage is the stage of decision making. The person has made a commitment to take action within the next 30 days and is already making small behavioral changes. In the action stage, clients make notable overt efforts to change. Maintenance involves working to stabilize the particular behavior change and avoid relapse for the next 6 months. People do not simply progress through the stages in a straight line; they may recycle by relapsing and repeating stage progressions and they can enter or exit at any point [36, 37]. This transtheoretical model has been shown to generalize across a broad range of problem behaviors (including diet, exercise and weight control) and populations [36].

Integral to the stages of change model is a "standard" or goal for the behavior that has been proven to produce results. For example, the goal of the NCEP Step 1 diet for a dietary fat intake of less than 30% of energy was established based on research showing associated reduction in serum cholesterol concentration. Stages of change techniques help individuals evaluate current behaviors against a defined standard then assess their readiness to change. The objective is to help patients achieve the standard for the behavior; however, incremental goals are often required. Fortunately, many nutrition interventions in clinical nutrition show benefits associated with stepwise progression to the goal.

If dietitians use the stages of change model as a basic technique for approaching nutrition counseling sessions, it often requires a modification in their teaching and counseling style [38]. The focus of attention shifts away from an agenda to merely educate the individual and shifts toward an approach that assesses the status of the individual as a basis for tailoring the counseling session. For example, instructing

a client with hypercholesterolemia who is clearly in the precontemplation stage on an NCEP Step 1 diet will be less effective than discussing the risks associated with high cholesterol levels and the benefits of reducing the fat content of the diet. While the counselor may feel an obligation to impart specific information, mismatching stages and interventions could break rapport and may lead the client to avoid further follow-up sessions.

B. Effective Use of Stages of Change Technique in Nutrition Counseling

Nutrition assessments are typically done at the initial counseling session. It is important for dietitians to use the stages of change model in each session to assess attitudes toward nutrition and health, readiness to learn, and willingness to change. Assessment of these attitudes requires proficient use of open-ended questions and listening skills.

Open-ended questions begin with what, how, why and could. The first clue about a client's stage of change is in the response to opening questions such as "How can I help you?" "What are your goals for our meeting today?" Attentive listening is an important tool to assess the client's responses to these questions. Attentive listening involves not only allowing sufficient silence to hear the client's verbal response, but also paying attention to facial expression, voice tone, and body language as the person is speaking. The nutrition counselor can use the listening technique of paraphrasing to see if he or she has accurately understood the content of the client's statements or the listening technique of reflection to find out if he or she understands the emotional feeling that the client is trying to convey [39]. It is the combination of open-ended questioning and proficient listening skills that builds rapport.

As the counselor collects assessment information in the first part of the counseling session, there are repeated opportunities to evaluate a client's stage of change through the use of open-ended questions and effective listening skills.

C. Consciousness Raising—A Technique for Precontemplators

1. A CASE OF PRECONTEMPLATION

Dietitian: "How can I help you?" "What are your goals for today's session?"

Patient: "I don't know. The doctor sent me." "I feel fine." "I already have so many problems, so why bother." (arms crossed, sitting back in the chair, stiff body posture, voice tone may display resignation, anger, upset, or denial concerning necessity for changing habits or coming to see the dietitian)

Dietitian: "Did your doctor say why he wanted you to come?" "What did your doctor tell you about your

TABLE 3 Stages of Change

Stage	Definition	Client characteristics	Expressions client may say
Precontemplation	Person is not interested in making changes within the next 6 months.	–May be unaware a problem exists. –Sees no reason or need to change. –Not interested in talking about the situation or behavior.	–It's not my problem. –I can't change. –Leave me alone. –Quit nagging me.
Contemplation	Person is thinking about making changes within the next 6 months.	–Has limited knowledge about the problem. –Weighing risks/benefits of changing a behavior. –Waiting for the "magic moment" to start. –Wishing problem behavior would solve itself.	–I'll change when the time is better—someday. –Why should I? I don't understand? –I know I should, but _____. –It takes too much effort.
Preparation	Person is planning to make changes within the next 30 days and/or has tried making some small changes, but is not consistent with new behavior yet.	–Is motivated and ready to learn. –Knows what to do, but not sure how to start. –May have tried small changes, but now ready to try more.	–I am ready to _____. –I want to _____. –How can I start? –Where can I go to learn _____?
Action	Person has changed a behavior within the past 6 months and becoming more consistent with it.	–Efforts to change are more visible to others and are more consistent. –Believes change is possible. –Started making changes in his/her environment to support the changed behavior.	–I can _____. –It's getting easier for me to _____. –I'm doing it, but sometimes _____. –I was amazed to learn that _____.
Maintenance	Person has maintained a new behavior longer than 6 months.	–Is maintaining the new behavior—the change has become a part of his/her daily routine. –Is trying to avoid slipping back into old habits. –Is confident about ability to maintain change.	–I just do it now. –It's not a problem for me to _____. –I feel good about _____. –I don't have to think about it much anymore.

Source: Reprinted with permission from HealthPartners, Inc., Bloomington, MN. © 2000. All other rights reserved. For more information, contact HealthPartners, Center for Health Promotion.

_____ (e.g., cholesterol levels/diabetes control/ blood pressure)?"

Patients in the precontemplation stage tend to focus more on the difficulties or disadvantages of changing eating behavior—the diet restriction, the inconvenience, or the expense of making healthy food choices or keeping food records. They tend to put much less emphasis on the benefits of changing eating behavior. Patients can be in the precontemplation stage for various reasons including lack of knowledge, lack of skills, lack of resources, distorted health beliefs, or competing priorities [40]. The counselor needs to explore and assess the reasons particular to each client before proceeding further with the session.

Questions to Assess Knowledge, Skills, Resources, Health Beliefs and Competing Priorities:

"What did your doctor tell you about your _____ (e.g., cholesterol level/diabetes control/blood pressure)?"

"What did your doctor tell you about your laboratory results?"

"Do you know what the goals are for _____ (cholesterol levels/hemoglobinA1c levels/blood glucose levels?"

"What are your personal goals?"

"What do you know about how your diet affects your _____ (e.g., cholesterol level/hemoglobin A1c/blood glucose patterns?"

"What do you think is most important when reading a nutrition label if you have _____ (e.g., diabetes/high cholesterol)?"

"Do you have a blood glucose meter?"

"Do you test your blood glucose levels at home?" "How often and what times of day?"

"What do you think that you would need to do to improve your _____ (e.g., cholesterol levels/hemoglobinA1c levels/blood glucose levels/activity level)?"

"Are there any factors that you feel make it difficult for you to focus on improving your _____ (e.g., cholesterol levels/hemoglobinA1c levels/blood glucose levels/activity level)?"

2. CONSCIOUSNESS RAISING

Consciousness raising is an important strategy for dietitians to use if a client presents to a session in the precontemplation stage [37]. The following steps can be used to facilitate consciousness raising (Table 4):

1. Discuss the medical problem or condition of concern.
2. Review lab results related to the condition vs. target/ normal values for the test results.
3. Review the relationship of diet, exercise, and other self-care habits to the medical condition and personal lab data.

4. Use visual aids (e.g., test tubes of fat, 1-lb or 5-lb fat models), audiovisuals, and personalized profile sheets to enhance the message.
5. Elicit feedback from the client regarding this information.

As the interaction between the counselor and the patient proceeds, the counselor can watch for changes in body language (leaning forward, changing voice tone, arms uncrossing) and in level of interaction (asking more questions). Once this information sharing process is complete, the counselor has provided the client with the information necessary to make an informed choice about changing eating behavior. The clients who are in the precontemplation stage because of lack of knowledge or skills may move toward contemplation or preparation stages once these issues are addressed. On the other hand, some clients may be fully informed about their medical condition, lab data, and the impact of eating, activity, and self-care habits on their health and still do not view changing eating habits as a priority. These clients are less likely to progress to contemplation or preparation within one session. In these cases, it is important to avoid judgment and show understanding by acknowledging their feelings and choices. For example, a client may feel too depressed to consider change at the time of the session and a competing priority may be to seek counseling and treatment for depression first. The counselor's responsibility is to provide information and then reassess the client's stage of change. It's the client's responsibility to make an informed choice.

D. Motivational Interviewing—A Technique for Contemplators

1. A CASE OF CONTEMPLATION

Dietitian: "How can I help you?" "What would you like to accomplish at our meeting today?"
Patient: "I'm not sure. I know what to do. I just need motivation." "I know that I should _____ (e.g., lose weight/eat less fat), but _____ ."

Patients in the contemplation stage view the pros and cons of changing eating, exercise or self-care habits as about equal, with the cons slightly greater than the pros. They may focus on the short-term costs of changing eating behaviors (e.g., limiting food choices, adjusting food purchases when shopping or menu selections when eating out, investing time in keeping food records or nutrition appointments) and pay less attention to the long-term health benefits [40]. Clients can be in the contemplation stage due to limited knowledge about the problem, wishing that someone else would fix the problem or that the problem would solve itself, competing priorities, or low self-efficacy regarding ability to change eating habits.

If limited knowledge is the problem, then the counselor can use the technique of consciousness raising to provide information, clarify any misconceptions, and respond to

TABLE 4 Stage Matched Counseling Techniques

Stage	Counseling strategies	Do's/don'ts that motivate/hinder change
Precontemplation	– Raise self-awareness of their behavior. – Raise awareness of health concern and implications. – Show how their behavior may affect others around them. – Encourage them to express their feelings.	Don't: – be judgmental – rush them into action – don't ignore their emotional reaction to idea of change Do: – listen and acknowledge their feelings – help them understand effects of their behavior – help them become aware a problem exists
Contemplation	– Identify and discuss their concerns, beliefs, and perceived barriers toward their behavior. – Show how benefits of change outweigh the risks of not changing. – Clarify any ambivalence felt toward changing. – Provide or suggest resources for learning more about the solution.	Don't: – ignore the potential impact the change may have on their family – nag or preach to them demanding they change – don't provide "how to" information Do: – listen to their concerns – help them identify benefits they'll receive if they decide to change a behavior – provide "facts" answering "why" questions they have
Preparation	– Help them develop a plan of action. – Teach specific "how to" skills. – Help build their self-confidence so they can form a new behavior. – Help them access educational program and obtain resources needed for change.	Don't: – recommend general behavior change—be specific – refer to small changes as "not good enough" – create new barriers for them to overcome Do: – provide specific ideas on how to change – remind them that "change" is hard work – help them realize that "any change" is better than "no change"
Action	– Reinforce their decision to change. – Provide emotional support to continue behavior change they've started. – Explain the difference between lapse vs. relapse. – Help them evaluate their progress and teach additional skills, as needed.	Don't: – nag or preach – make assumptions that they're not having lapses – overpraise so they only report successful outcomes Do: – explore their feelings about changes they've made – celebrate "milestones" big and small – compliment positive behavior changes you observe
Maintenance	– Offer ideas or ways to maintain change. – Help them build a supportive environment around them to maintain the change. – Continue teaching relapse prevention techniques. – Help validate rationale for change.	Don't: – assume that initial action means permanent change – be discouraged or disappointed when lapses happen – underestimate environmental barriers Do: – remind them of their overall progress (from the start) – review benefits they've received from changing their behavior – ask open-ended questions about how they are coping with change and feel about their changed behavior

Source: Reprinted with permission from HealthPartners, Inc., Bloomington, MN. © 2000. All other rights reserved. For more information, contact Health Partners, Center for Health Promotion.

specific questions. Before proceeding further with the session, the counselor needs to develop a clear understanding of the client's ambivalence about changing eating behavior. To do this, the counselor needs to explore the client's concerns and perceived barriers to making changes as well as the perceived benefits. This technique of exploring the pros and cons of behavior change is called *decisional balance*.

The counselor also needs to evaluate each client's self-efficacy for changing eating behavior because perceived self-efficacy influences the acquisition of new behaviors and the inhibition of existing behaviors. It also affects people's choices of behavioral settings, the amount of effort they will expend on a task, and the length of time they will persist in the face of obstacles. Finally, self-efficacy affects people's emotional reactions and thought patterns [41]." The process of using decisional balance and other techniques to increase motivation and self-efficacy is often referred to as *motivational interviewing*.

For clients to move from the contemplation stage toward the preparation stage of change, they must believe that the advantages of changing their eating behavior outweigh the disadvantages. The counselor can help reduce or minimize barriers to change by assisting the client with practical problem solving (some barriers may be related to access to treatment and resources and other barriers will be more attitudinal, such as fear of change or the results of change). It is also helpful to identify the client's positive incentives for continuing with current behaviors (i.e., the payoff for staying the same) and use strategies to decrease the perceived desirability of the behavior (e.g., increase awareness of the negative consequences of the behavior using facts and audiovisuals) [40].

Motivational interviewing is a client-centered technique designed to build commitment and reach a decision to change. It involves an interviewing process that assesses decisional balance and self-efficacy beliefs and focuses on increasing the client's intrinsic motivation to change and self-confidence in ability to do so. The following types of questions can be used to assess decisional balance [40].

2. DECISIONAL BALANCE QUESTIONS
Explore the advantages of not changing (staying the same):

Dietitian: "What are some of the positive aspects of not _____ (e.g., reducing your fat intake/losing weight)?"
Patient: "I can eat what I want and enjoy my food and not feel deprived."
Dietitian: "What else is good about it?"
Patient: "I don't have to risk failing at this again."
Dietitian: "What else?"
Patient: "Those are the main things."

Explore the disadvantages of not changing

Dietitian: "What are some of the not so good things about _____ (e.g., eating a high fat diet/maintaining your current weight)?"

Patient: " My cholesterol is too high. My clothes don't fit and I'm sluggish."
Dietitian: "Anything else?"
Patient: "I have a higher risk for a heart attack."
Dietitian: "Any other disadvantages?"
Patient: "My family worries about me."

Summarize by paraphrasing

Dietitian: "It sounds like you like to eat and enjoy your food without feeling deprived. I also get the sense that it's important to you not to feel like a failure when you try to change your eating habits. On the other hand it sounds as though there are some disadvantages to your current way of eating—your high cholesterol level, the risk for heart disease and feeling sluggish. Also, it sounds as though you think your family worries about you and your health."
Patient: "That's right."
Dietitian: "How do you feel about this now? What would you like to do about this?"
Patient: "I'm not sure."
Dietitian: "It's important to enjoy your food and not feel deprived. If we could come up with some ideas to help lower your cholesterol that are do-able and that won't make you feel deprived, would you be interested? If you'd like, we can explore some of the possibilities together."

Each client's motivation to change is influenced by two components—importance and confidence [42]. Assessing importance and confidence is a technique that dietitians can use to help decide what steps to take with patients who are in the contemplation stage of change.

3. IMPORTANCE AND CONFIDENCE TECHNIQUE*

Introduce the Discussion
"I'm not really sure how you feel about _____ (e.g., reducing your fat intake/losing weight/exercising more). Can you help me by answering two simple questions and then we can see where to go from there?"

Assess Importance and Confidence
"How do you feel *right now* about _____ (eating less fat/losing weight/exercising more)? On a scale from 0 to 10, with 0 meaning 'not important at all' and 10 meaning 'very important,' how *important* is it to you personally to _____ (eat less fat/lose weight/exercise more)?"

"If you decided *right now* to _____ (eat less fat/lose weight/exercise more), how *confident* do you feel that you

---

*This section is reprinted with permission of Allan Zuckoff, M. A., University of Pittsburgh Medical Center; adapted from S. Rollnick, P. Mason, and C. Butler (1999). "Health Behavior Change: A Guide for Practitioners." London: Churchill Livingstone.

would succeed? If 0 is 'not confident at all' and 10 is 'very confident,' what number would you give yourself?"

Summarize the answers:

Selecting the Focus
- If *importance* is low (<3), focus on *importance* first.
- If both are the same, focus on *importance* first.
- If one number is distinctly lower than the other, focus on the *lower* number first.
- If both are very low (<3), explore feelings about participating further in the session.

Exploring Importance
"This is (very/pretty/somewhat/a little bit) important to you. What made you choose _____ and not 1 or 2?"
- Reflect reasons given (self-motivational statements).
- Ask for elaboration. ("What makes that important to you?" "Tell me more about that.")
- Ask for more reasons. ("What else makes it [very/pretty/somewhat/a little] important?")
- Summarize. ("So what makes this [very/pretty/somewhat/a little] important right now is. . . ." "What would have to happen for you to move up to a _____ [score plus 3–4]?" "What stops you from being at a _____ [score plus 3–4]?")
- Reflect, ask for elaboration, ask "What else."
- Summarize. ("So what makes this [very/pretty/somewhat/a little] important is. . . ." "It would become more important to you if. . . ." "What has kept it from being more important is. . . .")

Exploring Confidence
"You feel (very/pretty/somewhat/a little) confident that you could do this if you tried. What made you choose _____ and not 1 or 2?"
- Reflect reasons given (self-motivational statements).
- Ask for elaboration. ("Tell me more about that.")
- Ask for more reasons. ("What else makes you feel [very/pretty/somewhat/a little] confident?")
- Summarize ("So what makes you [very/pretty/somewhat/a little] confident right now is. . . .") "What would help you move up to a _____ [score plus 3–4]?" "What stops you from being at a _____ [score plus 3–4]?")
- Reflect, ask for elaboration, ask "What else?"
- Summarize. (" So what makes you [very/pretty/somewhat/a little] confident is. . . ." "You would feel more confident if. . . ." "What has kept you from feeling more confident is. . . .")

The following types of questions can be used in the motivational interviewing process to reinforce confidence/self-efficacy. These types of questions are referred to as *competency–focused interviewing* [39].

Questions That Are Competency Focused and Success Oriented:

"What do you know about _____ (e.g., diabetes, high cholesterol)?"
"What kind of changes have you made in your diet so far?"
"How have you fit exercise into your schedule in the past?"
"What is the most important thing that you were able to learn?"
"What do you think you would do differently this time to enable you to _____ (lose weight/lower your cholesterol/improve your blood glucose levels?)"
"How do you think you would feel when you reach your goal?"
"What do you see as the next step?"

4. FRAMES STRATEGY
Miller and Rollnick suggest that the following specific motivational techniques can be combined to achieve an effective motivational interviewing strategy (FRAMES) [40].

1. **Feedback.** Clearly discuss the client's current health situation and risks and explain results of objective tests, share observations based on food records and weight trends. Clarify goals by comparing feedback on patient's current situation to some standard and set goals toward that standard that are realistic and attainable.
2. **Responsibility.** Emphasize that it is the client's responsibility to change.
3. **Advice.** Clearly identify the problem or risk area, explain why change is important and advocate specific change.
4. **Menu.** Offer the client a menu of alternative strategies for changing eating habits. Offering each client a range of options allows the individual to select strategies that match his or her particular situation and enhance the sense of perceived personal choice.
5. **Empathy.** Show warmth, respect, support, caring, concern, understanding, commitment, and active interest through attentive listening skills.
6. **Self-efficacy.** Reinforce the client's self-efficacy via competency-based questions and statements. Research has shown that the counselor's belief in the client's ability to change can be a significant determinant of outcome[40].

The dietitian's responsibility in counseling patients in the contemplation stage is to help the client reduce the barriers to making changes, focus more on the benefits, simplify the "to do" steps, and enhance self-efficacy. Once the dietitian has completed this process, it is the client's responsibility and choice to make a decision about changing eating habits.

E. Goal Setting—A Technique for the Preparation Stage

1. A CASE OF PREPARATION

Dietitian: "How can I help you?" "What are your goals for today's session?"

Patient: "I want to _____ (improve my blood glucose control/lower my cholesterol level/lose weight)."

Patients in the preparation stage feel that the advantages of changing their eating habits outweigh the disadvantages. They may have already tried making small changes, but are looking for more specific guidance and support. Their ambivalence may not have disappeared, however they show more interest in change by making self-motivational statements, asking more questions about change and experimenting with small changes [40]. The dietitian's responsibility is to strengthen the client's commitment to change and to assist him/her in making realistic plans to modify his/her lifestyle and eating habits. It is the client's responsibility to participate in goal setting by considering the options and selecting a strategy that provides sufficient direction to prevent floundering, but not so many goals that it undermines self-efficacy and success.

2. GOAL SETTING

For clients to move toward the action stage, they must resolve their ambivalence and establish a firm commitment to a plan of action. The counselor can use the FRAMES technique to guide the client toward a specific action plan. In addition, the counselor can ask questions and make statements that imply competency and build self-efficacy. It is important for the dietitian to accentuate and reinforce behaviors that the client is doing right and then set goals from there. Goals that are specific, realistic, positive, short term, and measurable are best. It is also important to help the client anticipate obstacles to success and problem-solve strategies to deal with those barriers (Fig. 2). Finally, the counselor can ask questions to be sure that the client has set reasonable achievable goals. If clients are not at least 80% confident in their ability to achieve their goals, it is important to help them reset their goals to a level at which they feel they can be successful.

Questions to facilitate goal setting:
"What do you think you would like to do?"

"What would you say is the first step that you need to take?"

"What other changes would you like to make?"

"What options would you consider trying?"

"What obstacles can you anticipate that might interfere with your ability to accomplish your goals?"

"How do you think you will handle these obstacles?"

"How confident are you that you will be able to accomplish your goals?"

Patient: "I'd like to start to increase my activity to improve my blood sugars."

Dietitian: "That's great! It's good that you have so many options for exercise—a treadmill, outdoor walking, an exercise bike. You've also already got a great start on increasing your activity by walking with your coworker at lunch two times per week for 20 minutes each time. If you could increase your activity minutes toward 150 minutes per week, that is a level that would be a good target. What would you say would be a reasonable next step to increase your activity?"

Patient: "I'd like to try to walk four times per week for 20 minutes at lunch."

Dietitian: "Are there any problems or roadblocks that you can anticipate that would get in the way of accomplishing this goal?"

Patient: "If it rains, we might not go out."

Dietitian: "How will you handle that situation?"

Patient: "I'll either suggest that we walk indoors or I'll make a plan to walk on my own on the weekend."

Dietitian: "Any other barriers or obstacles that you can anticipate?"

Patient: "No, not right now."

Dietitian: "Out of 100% confidence, how confident are you that you can do 80 minutes of activity in the next week?"

Patient: "I'm 80% confident."

Dietitian: "Good, because if you were less than 80% confident, that would mean that we should consider changing the goal so that you feel that the likelihood of success is fairly high."

F. Self-Management Skills Training— Techniques for Action

1. A CASE OF ACTION

Dietitian: "How can I help you?" "What would you like to accomplish in our meeting today?"

Patient: "I'm doing well with my food choices and exercise during the week, but on weekends it can be harder if I go out to eat."

Patients in the action stage have started making changes in their environment to support changes in eating habits. They need positive reinforcement for making behavioral changes and assistance strengthening self-management skills. The counselor's responsibility is to provide continued praise and support for positive behavioral changes and offer ongoing information and advice to enhance self-management skills. The client's responsibility is to actively participate in the session by sharing feelings about changes that he or she has made and discussing questions and concerns about maintaining the behavior changes.

2. SELF MANAGEMENT SKILLS TRAINING

The core techniques that dietitians can combine to help clients in the action stage to strengthen self-management skills are concrete nutrition information and advice, self-monitoring, stimulus control, and exercise [1].

1. *Concrete nutrition information and advice.* Dietitians expertise in translating nutrition recommendations into food

WEEKLY GOALS

NUTRITION /BEHAVIOR   1._____
                            2._____

EXERCISE   1._____
                            2._____

The following roadblocks could interfere with my ability to achieve these goals.
Therefore, I have devised these coping strategies.

Roadblock #1:

Plan:

_____

Roadblock #2:

Plan:

_____

Roadblock #3:

Plan:

_____

Evaluation

How did it go?_____

What did you learn?_____

Would you do anything differently next time?_____

FIGURE 2   Weekly goals form.

choices that are meaningful and satisfying is key in supporting clients in the action stage. In particular, dietitians can
assist patients in trying new recipe ideas/modifying favorite
recipes, finding healthier food choices, and suggesting new
and interesting food combinations at meals and snacks. In
this way, dietitians can help patients learn that dietary
change can occur without disrupting family food patterns or
personal enjoyment of food.

   2. *Self-monitoring.* Dietitians can encourage clients to
use self-monitoring as a tool to enhance behavior change.
When clients keep track of their eating habits by recording
the amounts and types of food eaten, they become more
aware of how their food choices affect their health outcomes (e.g., weight, cholesterol, blood sugar). Patients who
are overweight or have hypercholesterolemia may focus
on food records that track fat gram and/or energy intake,
whereas patients with diabetes may focus on self-monitoring

food, carbohydrate intake, activity, and blood sugar patterns
and then use the data to learn a problem-solving approach
for understanding food–activity–blood sugar relationships.

   3. *Stimulus control.* Dietitians can discuss with patients
how to set up their environment for success. If patients
remove problem foods from their environment and follow a
shopping list that includes only healthy food choices, then
they can create an environment conducive to successful
dietary change. Clients can also learn strategies to reduce
the temptations for undesired foods by minimizing exposure to these food items at parties or buffets.

   4. *Exercise.* Increasing exercise is a positive lifestyle
change that can improve high density lipoprotein (HDL)
cholesterol, blood glucose control, blood pressure, weight
loss and weight maintenance, self-esteem, and motivation.
Increasing physical activity therefore can enhance the impact of dietary change on health outcomes and may also

strengthen the self-esteem, self-efficacy, and motivation necessary to maintain diet behavior change.

G. Problem-Solving Skills and Coping Strategies—Techniques for Maintenance

1. A CASE OF MAINTENANCE

Dietitian: "How can I help you?" "What are your goals for today's session?"
Patient: "I feel good about the way that I'm eating now. It has become more of a habit to _____ (eat less fat/ exercise more/count carbohydrates)."

Patients in the maintenance stage have been actively working on changing eating habits for at least 6 months. Although the changes in eating habits may have become part of a patient's routine, there is still a risk of lapse or relapse. The dietitian's responsibility is to help clients plan ahead for high-risk situations and develop the problem solving and coping skills necessary to avoid relapsing. The client's responsibility is to share any feelings or concerns related to the changes that they have made, discuss the particular situations that challenge his or her ability to continue with eating behavior change and actively participate in the problem-solving process.

2. PROBLEM-SOLVING SKILLS AND COPING STRATEGIES

Some examples of the high-risk situations that can lead to lapse or relapse of eating behavior change are eating out, stress and other emotions (feeling anxious or depressed), hunger, and vacations. If clients do not develop coping strategies to deal with high-risk situations, then they are likely to interpret an experience of overeating as a failure. This can diminish self-efficacy and undermine long-term success. Alternatively, if clients can respond to high-risk situations with effective coping strategies, then the experience of managing the situation improves self-efficacy and increases the likelihood of sustaining behavior change [1].

The best way to help clients prevent relapse is to focus on both cognitive and behavioral techniques to appropriately respond to lapses. The behavioral steps to help clients include the following: (1) Anticipate and identify high-risk situations, (2) facilitate a problem-solving approach to determine possible solutions, (3) select a coping strategy, and (4) evaluate the effectiveness of the plan. The cognitive techniques that are important in preventing relapse are directed at how clients think and feel in response to a relapse. Cognitive restructuring techniques include the following: (1) Listen to self-talk associated with a lapse and evaluate if thoughts are logical, reasonable, and/or helpful; (2) counter any negative self-talk with positive statements; and (3) stay focused on the progress so far and the advantages of making changes in eating behavior [27].

In the process of discussing lapses in high-risk situations, it is important for dietitians to remind clients that lapses are normal and to ask open-ended questions about how clients feel regarding changes they have made in eating habits and respond to them with empathy not judgment [40].

Questions to Facilitate Discussion of High-Risk Situations
"How are you feeling about the changes that you have made in your eating habits so far?"

"Are there any situations that make it more challenging for you to sustain your _____ (activity level/reduced fat intake /weight loss)?"

"What strategies have you tried so far to deal with the situation?"

"How did they work?"

"Are there any other ideas that you might try?"

"Would you like to hear about some strategies that have worked for other people in the same situation?"

"If we take a moment to review the various options that we have discussed, are there any that you would like to try?" "Which ones?" (See Fig. 2.)

The problem-solving skills and coping strategies that are important for working with clients in the maintenance stage often incorporate the techniques used to help move the client forward through the stages of change. Note that patients can recycle by relapsing and repeating stage progressions, and that they can exit and reenter at any point. In fact, many new clients that dietitians see are relapsers who are coming to reenter and recycle through the eating behavior change process. In these cases, there are some important questions that the counselor can ask to assess each client's experience.

Questions to Assess Prior Experience of Relapsers
"What were your three most important reasons for _____ (losing weight/ eating less fat/ exercising more)?"

"How long did you sustain the behavior change?"

"Who supported you at that time?"

"How did you handle temptations?"

"What coping strategies did you use?"

"What was going on in your life and how were you feeling when you started slipping?"

"What did you learn from that experience?"

In sum, the stages of change model is a useful technique for approaching nutrition counseling sessions. At first glance, however, adding a new component to counseling sessions may appear difficult when allocation of time already is an issue [25]. Fisher uses a three-phase model to show that stages of change techniques can be applied in sessions as brief as 15 minutes (Fig. 3). The model expedites identification of the behavior, clarification of patient's readiness to change, and selection of stage-appropriate tools and techniques. The

1. Identify Behavior	2. Clarify Readiness
• Base on clinical need or open ended questions of patient's perception of need • Compare current situations to standard	• Questions regarding knowledge, health beliefs, motivation • Reflective listening • Pros & Cons • ➝ Staging

3. Stage-Appropriate Discussion

Not Ready	Thinking about it	Ready
Discuss: risks, rationale, priorities Correct misconceptions Communicate readiness to help	Emphasize pros Reflect progress Reassure re: addressing barriers	Inform: how to; concrete advice Discuss/review plans Offer assistance, PRN Encourage optimism Prepare for possibility of relapse

FIGURE 3 Three-phase model within 15-minute encounter. (Adapted with verbal permission from E. B. Fisher, Jr.)

time the dietitian allocates to tailor counseling to information that the patient is receptive to learning will result in a more productive session.

H. Social Support

Social support influences all stages of change. A number of studies have shown the benefit of support from family, friends, and coworkers [1, 5, 43]. When spouses or significant others understand the nutritional advice given and the importance of self-monitoring, stimulus control, and exercise in managing eating behaviors, then they are better able to provide support. Support might include cooking and shopping for appropriate food items, keeping tempting food out of sight, modeling a slower eating speed, exercising together, showing a positive attitude, and offering praise.

Support from clinical staff (e.g., nurses, dietitians) was studied in the very successful Diabetes Control and Complications Trial (DCCT) [44]. The success of the DCCT was due in part to participants in the intensively treated group being able to make multiple behavior changes that resulted in their achieving improved glycemic control [45]. A study examining the effect of diet behaviors found that adherence to meal plans and appropriate treatment of hypoglycemia were associated with better diabetes control [46]. After the close of DCCT, telephone interviews were used to ask a sample of participants about the types of staff support that helped them adhere to all aspects of their treatment plan. Nondirective types of support (suggests, willing to help but does not take over) were mentioned more often than directive types of support (tells, assumes responsibility) [43]. Studies of staff support conducted with patients with acute as well as chronic illnesses indicate that stage or phase of the patient's clinical condition may influence the type of staff

support that is most helpful [47]. Patients newly diagnosed or in an acute phase of their illness appear to appreciate directive support (gives me great solutions) while those in stable conditions value nondirective support (gives me suggestions but lets me make up my own mind). Applying type of staff support to stages of change techniques, nondirective support is most appropriate for the precontemplation, contemplation, and maintenance phases, whereas directive support would be appropriate for problem solving in the preparation and action stages.

V. CONCLUSION

The challenge in clinical nutrition is to prevent or treat disease by changing people's eating habits. Research on nutrition education is extensive but not conclusive. Although a definitive model has not been identified, a variety of strategies have shown success and can be incorporated into nutrition education programs. There is consensus on two elements: (1) Education needs to be tailored to the individual's learning needs and (2) both education and behavior change techniques are necessary. Understanding factors that influence the learning and behavior change processes enables better selection of educational tools and techniques to make counseling more effective. The stages of change model is a useful technique for tailoring education to the individual and applying behavior change strategies.

References

1. Brownell, K. D., and Cohen, L. R. (1995). Adherence to dietary regimens 2: Components of effective interventions. *Behav. Med.* **20**, 155–164.

2. Knowles, M. (1990). "The Adult Learner: A Neglected Species." Gulf Publishing Co., Houston.

3. Tough, A. (1985). How adults learn and change. *Diabetes Educator* **11**, 12–25.

4. Brookfield, S. D. (1987). "Developing Critical Thinkers: Challenging Adults to Explore Alternative Ways of Thinking and Acting." Jossey-Bass, San Francisco.

5. Contento, I., Bronner, Y. I., Paige, D. M., Gross, S. M., Bisignani, L., Lytle, L. A., Maloney, S. K., White, S. L., Olson, C. M., and Swadener, S. S. (1995). The effectiveness of nutrition education and implications for nutrition education policy, programs, and research: A review of research. *J. Nutr. Educ.* **27**, 355–364.

6. Karlsen, B., and Gardner, E. F. (1986). "Adult Basic Learning Examination Norms Booklet." Harcourt Brace, San Antonio.

7. Wilkinson, G. S. (1993). "Wide Range Achievement Test Administration Manual." Wide Range, Wilmington, DE.

8. Taylor, S. C. (1953). Cloze procedure: A new test for measuring readability. *Journalism Q.* **10**, 425–433.

9. McLaughlin, G. H. (1969). SMOG grading: A new readability formula. *J. Reading* **12**, 639–646.

10. Gunning, R. (1952). "The Technique of Clear Writing." McGraw-Hill, New York.

11. Fry, E. B. (1977). Fry's readability graph: Clarifications, validity, and extension to level 17. *J. Reading* **21**, 242–252.

12. Powers, R. D., Summer, W. A., and Kearl, B. E. (1958). A recalculation of four readability formulas. *J. Educ. Psychol.* **48**, 99–105.

13. Vaughn, J., Jr. (1976). Interpreting readability assessments. *J. Reading* **19**, 635–639.

14. Pitchert, J., Elam, P. (1985). Readability formulas may mislead you. *Patient Educ. Couns.* **7**, 181–191.

15. Nitzke, S. V. J. (1992). Overview of reading and literacy research and applications in nutrition education. *J. Nutr. Educ.* **24**, 261–265.

16. "Ethnic and Regional Food Practices: A Series (1989–1999)." The American Dietetic Association, Chicago.

17. Achterberg, C. (1988). Factors that influence learner readiness. *J. Am. Diet. Assoc.* **88**, 1426–1429.

18. Walker, E. (1999). Characteristics of the adult learner. *Diabetes Educator* **25**, 16–24.

19. Osterman, D. N. (1984). The feedback lecture: Matching teaching and learning styles. *J. Am. Diet. Assoc.* **84**, 1221–1222.

20. Johnston, J. M., Jansen, G. R., Anderson, J., and Kendell, P. (1994). Comparison of group diet instruction to a self-directed education program for cholesterol reduction. *J. Nutr. Educ.* **26**, 140–145.

21. Mager, R. F. (1975). "Preparing Instructional Objectives." Fearon, Belmont, CA.

22. Houston, C., and Haire-Joshu, D., (1995). Application of health behavior models. *In* "Management of Diabetes Mellitus: Perspectives Across the Lifespan" (D. Haire-Joshu, Ed.). Mosby-Year Book, St. Louis.

23. Bloom, B. S. (1956). "A Taxonomy of Educational Objectives. Handbook 1: Cognitive Domain." David McKay Co., New York.

24. Harrow, A. (1971). "A Taxonomy of the Psychomotor Domain." David McKay Co., New York.

25. Pichert, J. W. (1987). Teaching strategies for effective nutrition counseling. *In* "Handbook of Diabetes Nutritional Counseling" (M. A. Powers, Ed.). Aspen Publishers, Rockville, MD.

26. Glass, W. (1996). "On Your Way to Fitness." Shape Up America, Bethesda, MD.

27. Brownell, K. D. (1994). "The Learn Program for Weight Control." American Health Publishing, Dallas, TX.

28. Caban, A., Johnson, P., Marseille, D., and Wylie-Rosett, J. (1999). Tailoring a lifestyle change approach and resources to the patient. *Diab. Spectrum* **12**, 33–38.

29. Green, J. A. (1987). Meal planning approaches. *In* "Handbook of Diabetes Nutritional Counseling" (M. A. Powers, Ed.). Aspen, Rockville, MD.

30. "Exchange Lists for Meal Planning." (1995). The American Dietetic Association, Chicago, and American Diabetes Association, Alexandria, VA.

31. Camelon, K. M., Hadell, K., Jamsen, P. T., Ketonen, K. J., Kohtamaki, H. M., Makimatilla, S., Tormala, M. L., and Valve, R. H. (1998). The plate model: A visual method of teaching meal planning. *J. Am. Diet. Assoc.* **98**, 1155–1162.

32. Month of Meals series. (1989–1994). American Diabetes Association, Alexandria, VA.

33. Metz, J. A., Kris-Etherton, P. M., Morris, C. D., Mustad, V. A., Stern, J. S., Oparil S. Chait, A., Haynes, R. B., Resnick, L. M., Clark, S., Hatton, D. C., McMahon, M., Holcomb, S., Snyder, G. W., Pi-Sunyer, F. X., and McCarron, D. A. (1997). Dietary compliance and cardiovascular risk reduction with a prepared meal plan compared to a self-selected diet. *Am. J. Clin. Nutr.* **66**, 373–385.

34. Haynes, R. B., Kris-Etherton, P., McCarron, D. A., Oparil S. Chait, A., Resnick, L. M., Morris, C. D., Clark, S., Hatton, D. C., Metz, J. A., McMahon, M., Holcomb, S., Snyder, G. W., Pi-Sunyer, F. X., and Stern, J. S. (1999). Nutritionally complete prepared meal plan to reduce cardiovascular risk factors: A randomized clinical trial. *J. Am. Diet. Assoc.* **99**, 1077–1083.

35. Prochaska, J. O., and DiClementi, C. C. (1983). Stages and processes of self-change in smoking: Toward an integrative model of change. *J. Consult. Clin. Psychol.* **51**, 390–395.

36. Prochaska, J. O., Velicier, W. F., Rossi, J. S., Goldstein, M. G., Marcus, B. H., Rakowski, W., Fiore, C., Harlow, L. L., Redding, C. A., Rosenbloom, D., and Rossi, S. R. (1994). Stages of change and decisional balance for 12 problem behaviors. *Health Psychol.* **13**, 39–46.

37. Prochaska, J. O., DiClementi, C. C., and Norcross, J. C. (1993). In search of how people change: Applications to addictive behaviors. *Diab. Spectrum* **6**, 25–33.

38. Gehling, E. (1999). The next step: Changing us or changing them? *Diab. Care Educ. Newsflash* **20**, 31–33.

39. Powers, M. J. (1996). Counseling skills for improved behavior change. *In* "Handbook of Diabetes Nutritional Counseling" (M. A. Powers, Ed.). Aspen Publishers, Gaithersburg MD.

40. Miller, W. R., and Rollnick, S. (1991). "Motivational Interviewing: Preparing People to Change Addictive Behavior." The Guilford Press, New York.

41. Strecher, V. J., McEvoy Devellis, B., Becker, M. H., and Rosenstock, I. M. (1986). The role of self-efficacy in achieving health behavior change. *Health Educ. Q.* **13**, 73–91.

42. Rollnick, S., Mason, P., and Butler, C. (1999). "Health Behavior Change: A Guide for Practitioners." Churchill Livingstone, London.

43. Fisher, E. B., Jr., La Greca, A. M., Arfken, C., and Schneiderman, N. (1997). Directive and nondirective support in diabetes management. *Int. J. Behav. Med.* **4,** 131–144,

44. Davis, K., Heins, J., and Fisher, E. B., Jr. (1997). Types of social support deemed important by participants in the DCCT. *Diabetes* **46**(suppl 1), 89A.

45. The Diabetes Control and Complications Trial Research Group. (1993). The effect of intensive treatment of diabetes on the development and progression of long-term complications in insulin-dependent diabetes mellitus. *N. Engl. J. Med.* **329,** 977–994.

46. Delahanty, L. M., and Halford, B. N. (1993). The role of diet behaviors in achieving improved glycemic control in intensively treated patients in the Diabetes Control and Complications Trial. *Diab. Care* **16,** 1453–1458.

47. Fisher, E. B., Bickle, C., Harber, K., Hughes, C. R., Jeffe, D. B., Kahl, L., and LaGreca, A. M. (1997, April). Benefits of directive and nondirective support are moderated by severity of circumstances. Paper presented at the 18th Annual Scientific Sessions of the Society of Behavioral Medicine, San Francisco.

CHAPTER **9**

Evaluation of Nutrition Interventions

ALAN R. KRISTAL AND JESSIE A. SATIA
Fred Hutchinson Cancer Research Center, Seattle, Washington

I. INTRODUCTION

Nutrition interventions include a broad array of programs and activities, with many different goals. Interventions may be designed for treatment of acute or chronic disease, prevention of specific diseases, or simply improvement of nutritional status. Interventions can focus on changing an individual's dietary behavior, both directly or indirectly, or can target the composition, manufacture, and availability of food. Research in dietary intervention can be either behavioral, to test whether a dietary intervention program can promote dietary change, or clinical/epidemiological, to test whether dietary change can affect a disease endpoint or disease risk. Nutrition intervention programs can be delivered as services to individual clients, groups, or entire communities. The evaluation needs of each nutrition intervention program will differ, based on the program content, design, and goals.

The optimal way to evaluate a nutrition intervention is to complete a hypothesis-driven, randomized trial. This means that an *a priori* hypothesis should be used to evaluate whether or not the intervention was effective, an experimental design created, and careful attention paid to factors that contribute to the overall validity of a scientific experiment, such as protocol development, measurement, and statistical analysis. While expertise from many scientific disciplines is required to complete such a trial, it is important for nutritional scientists to understand the methodological issues that underlie the design of a valid intervention evaluation.

In this chapter, we give a general overview of quantitative evaluation, with an emphasis on those aspects likely to be the responsibility of a nutritional scientist. We focus on quantitative *outcome* evaluation and, in particular, on whether or not an intervention is effective in achieving change in dietary behavior.

II. OVERVIEW: TYPES OF NUTRITION INTERVENTION PROGRAM EVALUATIONS

A well-designed and clearly articulated evaluation plan is a key aspect of a successful nutrition intervention program.

An evaluation plan will require an intervention program to have clearly defined and realistic objectives. An evaluation plan can also give timely feedback at each stage of program implementation, allowing modifications to improve program effectiveness. The three types of evaluation that are most suitable for nutrition intervention programs are (1) formative evaluation, focusing on program design; (2) process evaluation, emphasizing program implementation, quality assurance, and participant reaction; and (3) outcome evaluation, measuring the achievement of program objectives.

A. Formative Evaluation

One challenge for nutrition intervention programs is matching the content of the interventions to the interests and needs of the intended audience. Nutrition information is inherently complex, and it must balance between being scientifically correct and still comprehensible and useful to the intended audience. Intervention activities should also be reasonable for the context in which they are delivered. At the stage of formative evaluation, a nutritionist assesses whether or not materials and programs are appropriately intensive, scientifically coherent, convenient, and otherwise consistent with their intended use.

B. Process Evaluation

Once in place, it is important to know if the intervention program is reaching its audience and how it is being received. There is a tendency for persons who are already interested in nutrition and motivated to change to participate in intervention trials. Thus, if an intervention is to be generalizable, it is important to ensure that program components successfully reach men, younger persons, racial and ethnic minorities, and other groups less likely to be drawn to programs in nutrition. This is also the stage at which to evaluate whether the audiences' reactions to the program are favorable, or whether changes are needed to have a broader impact.

C. Outcome Evaluation

Ultimately, the effectiveness of a nutrition intervention will be judged based on its ability to achieve program objectives.

The authors judge the specification and collection of outcome measures, and their correct analysis, to be essential to any nutrition intervention evaluation.

III. OUTCOMES OR ENDPOINTS USED TO ASSESS INTERVENTION EFFECTIVENESS

The most obvious intervention outcomes or endpoints are based on changes in nutrient intake, but for comprehensive evaluations of dietary interventions, this is too limited. Often indirect measures of intervention effectiveness, for example, changes in supermarket sales or implementation of a work site catering policy, can serve as meaningful outcomes. In addition, to understand how an intervention did or did not work, it is necessary to measure intermediate or mediating factors for dietary change, such as beliefs, attitudes, or nutrition knowledge.

Before discussing outcomes in detail, we make two overarching points. First, the single most important consideration for selecting outcomes is that they must have clear interpretations that relate directly to the intervention you are evaluating. Examples of poor evaluation outcomes include "compliance with the USDA Food Pyramid," "dietary adequacy," "compliance with the Recommendation Dietary Allowances," or even the well-characterized "Diet Quality Index" [1, 2]. These types of outcomes are not useful as evaluation endpoints, because they are too multidimensional, cannot be precisely defined, or their interpretation is too subjective. Second, if you will not measure dietary change per se, then the outcomes you select should have a known and reasonably strong relationship to dietary behavior. For example, increased nutrition knowledge or awareness of relationships between diet and disease are not sufficient in themselves as intervention endpoints, because they have low or no predictive value for dietary behavior change. Experience suggests that it is best to carefully formulate and define intervention outcomes as a part of the overall intervention design. This results in a more focused intervention program and yields evaluation data that are optimally informative.

A. Types of Outcomes or Endpoints Used to Assess Intervention Effectiveness

Outcomes can be classified most broadly into four types: (1) physiologic or biological measures, (2) behavioral measures based on self-report, (3) diet-related psychosocial measures, and (4) environmental or surrogate measures of dietary behavior.

Biological or physiologic measures are objective indicators of dietary change. For well-funded and relatively small clinical intervention trials, measures based on serologic concentration of nutrients or metabolic changes associated with dietary change are optimal approaches to evaluation. The

strength of biological measures is that they are objective and unbiased. Their weaknesses are that they do not exist for many outcomes of interest (e.g., reduced percentage of energy from fat in the diet) and they are rarely sufficiently sensitive to detect the relatively modest dietary changes one can expect from low-intensity health promotion interventions. It can also be procedurally difficult and prohibitively expensive to add biological measures to large, health-promotion intervention trials.

Self-reported dietary behavior is the most often used basis for intervention evaluation. There are two conceptually distinct types of measures based on self-reported diet. The most common measures are the intakes of specific nutrients in an individual's diet, such as percentage of energy from fat or milligrams of beta-carotene, or measures of food use, such as servings per day of fruits and vegetables. One can also characterize dietary habits, for example, removing the skin before eating chicken or using low fat instead of regular salad dressings. The primary weakness of all self-reported behavioral outcomes is that persons exposed to an intervention may bias their reports of behavior to exaggerate true behavior change. Their strengths are that they are easy to interpret and often reflect an intervention's specified goals.

Psychosocial outcomes consist of theoretical constructs that relate to diet or dietary change. These include nutrition knowledge, attitudes, and beliefs about diet, and intentions and self-efficacy to change diet. These constructs are best interpreted in the context of structured theoretical models of behavior change. For example, an intervention based on the Precede/Proceed model [3] would assess changes in predisposing, enabling and reinforcing factors for dietary change. The primary weakness of psychosocial outcomes is that they do not measure dietary change, rather they measure factors that relate, often quite weakly, to dietary behavior. Their strength is that they are often the actual target or focus of the intervention. For example, an intervention designed to increase awareness of the benefits of eating more fruits and vegetables could be evaluated by measuring changes in perceived benefits. Psychosocial measures are best considered as mediating factors for dietary change, that is, factors that explain how an intervention ultimately results in changed behavior [4–6]. Collecting information on psychosocial factors can yield valuable insights into how to improve the design and content of dietary interventions, and we believe they should be given high priority in research designs.

Environmental measures assess characteristics of communities, organizations, or the physical environment that in some way reflect dietary behavior or dietary change. Measures some researchers have used are the percentage of supermarket shelf space used for healthful versions of staple foods (e.g., low-fat milk or whole-grain breads) and percentage of foods in vending machines that are low in fat. The weakness of these measures is that there is relatively little research to support their validity as measures of dietary change, and the available evidence suggests that associations

between change in environmental measures and individual dietary behavior are modest. However, the strengths of these measures are that they are objective and unbiased, and frequently very inexpensive to collect.

Selection from among these various types of intervention outcomes is based on many criteria. However, the primary criterion is that they should be meaningful measures of the desired intervention outcome. This requires judgment and thoughtful consideration of both the goals of the intervention and of the evaluation. The following examples serve to illustrate the diversity of options available for evaluating different types of interventions. For an intensive, clinical intervention with a goal of lowering fat intake from 35% to 20% of energy, outcomes could include self-reported diet and body weight. For a work site-based intervention to increase the availability of healthful foods to workers during the work-day, outcomes could include foods offered at cafeterias and in vending machines. For a work site-based intervention designed to test different approaches to promoting healthy dietary patterns, outcomes could include self-reported diet as well as mediating psychosocial factors such as knowledge of fat in foods and stage of change to adopt a low-fat diet. For a public health campaign to increase the use of lower fat milk products, outcomes could include supermarket sales data and random digit dial surveys to assess consumption of low fat milk.

IV. DESIGN OF NUTRITION INTERVENTION EVALUATIONS

Evaluation design encompasses the protocols for participant recruitment, measuring intervention delivery and outcomes, and analyzing and presenting results. Choices made during the development of an evaluation design are primarily guided by two considerations: (1) the content, type, or design of the nutrition intervention; and (2) the purpose of the evaluation.

By type of intervention, the broadest distinctions are between *clinical* interventions and *public health* interventions. Clinical interventions target high-risk individuals and generally consist of intensive, multiple individual or group sessions that address both dietary behavior (nutrition education) and psychological support for maintaining dietary change. In contrast, public health interventions target large groups of individuals, usually not limited to persons at high risk, and generally consist of a broad range of low-intensity and low-cost components such as media messages and self-help materials. Some interventions fall between these two extremes (e.g., work site-based health promotion programs may offer a series of intensive nutrition education classes) and some may fall outside of this classification altogether (e.g., the decision to fortify cereal-grain products with folate). For purposes of evaluation, the two most important distinctions between clinical and public health interventions

are the timing and amount of expected change: Intensive clinical interventions produce rapid and dramatic change, whereas public health interventions yield slow change over long periods of time.

By purpose of the evaluation, we make a broad distinction between *research* that contributes to scientific knowledge and *documentation* that serves the needs of practitioners and administrators. Comprehensive scientific evaluations are generally beyond the financial means of any but the most well-funded research trials, because the costs of evaluation generally far exceed those for intervention design and delivery. Practitioners and administrators must assume that the interventions being delivered are at least somewhat effective, and evaluation to serve their needs is focused on evidence that the program is reaching the intended target population and is benefiting those who participate.

A. Design Components of Nutrition Intervention Evaluations

Five components characterize the design of an intervention evaluation:

1. A representative sample of persons who would be likely program participants or targets of an intervention
2. One or more measures of the evaluation outcome preintervention
3. One or more comparison groups, most often a control group not receiving an intervention
4. Randomized assignment to treatment (intervention or control) groups
5. One or more measures of the evaluation outcome postintervention.

The most robust research evaluations include all of these design characteristics. However, not all of these components need be present to have a scientifically valid design. The only necessary characteristics are that there be postintervention outcome measures and a comparison group. Intervention evaluations not based on a randomized trial can be either quasi-experimental, in which treatment is assigned in a fashion other than randomization, or observational, in which epidemiological methods are used to statistically model differences between those receiving and not receiving an intervention. Due to their complexity, nutritionists should consult with appropriate experts before choosing such design alternatives.

Administrative evaluation of program effectiveness should strive to incorporate as many of these evaluation components as feasible. In practice, however, an administrative evaluation may simply consist of documenting the number of persons receiving the intervention and measuring changes among those exposed. One improvement in this design would be to calculate participation rates, based, for example, on the number of persons offered the intervention or the number eligible. This would give administrators insight into

the acceptability and penetration of the intervention into eligible populations. Another improvement would be to document level of exposure to or participation in the intervention, and to correlate level of exposure to changes in outcome. This type of dose–response analysis can suggest whether more intensive intervention would be cost effective.

1. Representative Sample

Evaluation of a representative sample means that evaluation participants include persons from demographic and socioeconomic groups who would be targets for the intervention. Representativeness in dietary interventions is often difficult, because participation in nutrition interventions tend to be higher among women and older people [7]. However, representativeness is not always important or even desirable. If the purpose of the evaluation is to test whether an intervention can work at all (e.g., in the best of all possible circumstances), it will be preferable to recruit only highly motivated volunteers using highly selective enrollment criteria. It may even be appropriate to require participants to complete a prerandomization run-in activity, for example, completing a 4-day food record, to eliminate participants not likely to complete the trial [8]. Alternatively, if an evaluation is designed to examine how an intervention will work as it is to be delivered in practice, then participants are best recruited from representative samples from defined populations, attempting to achieve as high a recruitment rate as possible [9].

2. Preintervention Measures

Measures before intervention are desirable for two reasons. First, even in randomized experiments, there might be differences in baseline measures across treatment groups. Second, pre- and postintervention measures allow evaluators to calculate change from baseline. Basing evaluation on differences in change between treatment groups rather than simply on differences in outcome measures postintervention almost always yields superior statistical power. If possible, preintervention assessments should be completed before treatment group assignment, so that neither the evaluation staff nor the participant can be biased by knowing which intervention they will receive.

3. Comparison Group

The choice of comparison group(s) depends on the goal of the intervention. The most common design is to compare outcomes in a group receiving an intervention to one not receiving an intervention. Options include comparisons between a new and a standard intervention, or between groups receiving different levels of the same intervention. It is rarely satisfactory to have no comparison group, because it is not possible to determine whether any observed changes can be attributed to the intervention or to other factors outside of an investigator's control or not directly associated with the intervention itself.

4. Randomized Assignment to Treatment Groups

Randomization is the best way to ensure comparability between treatment groups, but it is not always possible. In this case, it may be feasible to devise an unbiased approach to assign individuals to contrasting treatments, for example, based on health care practitioner, day of the week, or hospital clinic. One entirely unacceptable design is to offer an intervention and compare results in self-selected participants to those refusing to participate. Participation in a nutrition intervention is strongly associated with characteristics that *a priori* predict dietary change, such as sex, age, and interest in nutrition and health. With this approach, comparisons between participants and nonparticipants are so strongly biased that they should be excluded from consideration for any type of evaluation design. In our judgment, examination of change among participants alone is a superior design, because no inferences can be made beyond documentation that change occurred in those who received the intervention.

5. Postintervention Assessments

It is optimal to complete two postintervention measures, one after the intervention is complete and one delayed by at least several months. The first measure assesses the immediate impact of the intervention, while the latter gives insight into whether effects are durable and whether there is continued change over time. Basing an evaluation on an early measure alone can be misleading: Some interventions may have no long-term effect, because behavior change is not sustained. Some interventions may yield continual, gradual change over time, in which case only a long-term assessment will demonstrate intervention effectiveness.

B. Analysis of Intervention Effects

Statistical analysis of nutrition interventions can pose many challenges. Below we describe some of these statistical issues and give nontechnical recommendations for the most commonly used designs and statistical models.

1. Level of Measurement and Units of Analysis

There are many choices for how outcomes are assessed and analyzed. Unit of measurement describes whether the outcomes are assessed on individual participants (e.g., self-reported diet) or on a group-level or environmental characteristic (e.g., supermarket sales or availability of fresh fruit in work site cafeterias). Unit of analysis describes whether analyses of outcomes are based on individual observations (e.g., individual changes in fat intake), on aggregated measures of individual observations (e.g., percent of population drinking low-fat milk in the previous day), or on group-level

or environmental outcomes. For clinical interventions and for public health interventions in which outcome assessments are based on measurements of individuals, the units of measurement and analysis are almost always at the individual level. For some public health interventions, especially those that target large groups or communities, there are many options for combinations of unit of measurement and unit of analysis. The most common is to aggregate measures on a sample of individuals and interpret these as measures of the community. One can also measure outcomes at the community level, such as availability of healthful foods in supermarkets and restaurants, existence of nutrition programs in the community, or media coverage of nutrition-related information.

It is of utmost importance to match the evaluation design, in particular, the randomization scheme, to the unit of analysis. In grouped randomized designs, for example, a trial randomizing work sites or schools to different intervention treatments, the analysis must be based on the unit of randomization, not the individuals participating in the intervention. Unlike individually randomized designs, the sample size for analysis of grouped randomized designs is a function both of the number of groups and the number of participants in each group. Consider an intervention trial that is evaluating whether a school nutrition curriculum can affect students' lunch choices. If 12 schools with 2000 students were each randomized such that 6 implemented the curriculum and 6 did not, the number of experimental units is 12, not 24, 000. Readers will find an excellent and nontechnical overview of these issues in reviews by Koepsell [10, 11].

2. CALCULATING THE SIMPLE INTERVENTION EFFECT

The best and most comprehensible measure of intervention effectiveness is the difference between the change in intervention group participants minus the change in control (or alternative treatment) group participants. We call this measure the *intervention effect*. As an example, in an intervention with a goal to decrease percent energy from fat the intervention effect is defined as:

$$[\text{Fat}(\%en)_b - \text{Fat}(\%en)_f]_I - [\text{Fat}(\%en)_b - \text{Fat}(\%en)_i]_c,$$

Where Fat (%en) is the percent of energy from dietary fat, subscripts b and f refer to baseline and follow-up, and subscripts I and C refer to intervention and control groups. The statistical test of whether or not the intervention effect is different from zero is based on the standard error of the intervention effect, which is defined as:

$$\sqrt{\frac{\text{var}[\text{Fat}(\%en)_b - \text{Fat}(\%en)_f]_I}{n_I} + \frac{\text{var}[\text{Fat}(\%en)_b - \text{Fat}(\%en)_f]_C}{n_C}},$$

where n_I is the sample size in the intervention group and n_C is the sample size in the control group.

Most measures of dietary intake and serum nutrient concentrations have log-normal or other non-normal distributions; however, changes in these measures are characteristically normally distributed. It is therefore rarely necessary to transform measures before analysis, and for simplicity of interpretation it should be avoided.

3. CALCULATING INTERVENTION EFFECTS ADJUSTED FOR SOCIODEMOGRAPHIC AND CONFOUNDING FACTORS

The intervention effect is best estimated after adjustment for demographic and other characteristics that are associated with dietary behavior. This is because (1) randomization may not have resulted in these characteristics being evenly divided between treatment groups and (2) there may be increased statistical power to detect a statistically significant intervention effect if variance associated with these factors is controlled for in the analyses.

Here are two approaches to calculating adjusted intervention effects, which differ depending on the scale of measurement of the outcome variable. Most outcome measures are either continuous (e.g., percent energy from fat) or ordered categories (e.g., motivation to change measured on a 1–10 scale), and thus multiple linear regression can be used to calculate adjusted intervention effects. For a simple, two-treatment randomized design, the best approach is to build a regression model as follows: The dependent variable is calculated as the change from baseline to follow-up in the outcome measure; the covariates are the baseline value of the outcome measure plus the demographic and diet-related measures you wish to control for in the analysis; the independent variable representing treatment group is an indicator variable coded 0 = control and 1 = treatment. In this model, the regression coefficient for the treatment indicator variable is the adjusted treatment effect, and the standard error of this regression coefficient is used to test the statistical significance of the adjusted intervention effect. Table 1 gives an example of how this approach is used for the primary analysis of a two-group randomized trial of a dietary intervention.

If an outcome measure is categorical, for example, whether or not a participant lost 10 pounds or more, it is then appropriate to use logistic regression models. For a simple, two-treatment design, the following model would be appropriate: The dependent variable is an indicator variable, coded 0 or 1, representing whether or not the outcome is absent or present; the covariates are variables you wish to control in the analysis; and the independent variable representing treatment group is an indicator variable coded 0 = control and 1 = treatment. The exponentiated regression coefficient of the treatment group indicator variable (e^β) is the relative odds of the outcome comparing the control to treatment group. The standard error of the regression coefficient is used to determine whether the relative odds are statistically different from 1. 0. Multiple categorical outcomes, for example, movement through stages of dietary change, pose

TABLE 1   Example of Statistical Analyses Used to Report Outcome of a Dietary
Intervention to Reduce Fat and Increase Fruit and Vegetable Intakes

	n	Baseline	Change at 3 months	Change at 12 months
Fat-related diet habits[a]				
Intervention ($x \pm$ SD)	601	2.29 ± 0.49	-0.09 ± 0.37	-0.09 ± 0.38
Control ($x \pm$ SD)	604	2.30 ± 0.49	-0.01 ± 0.36	-0.00 ± 0.40
Intervention effect ($x \pm$ SE)		Unadjusted	-0.08 ± 0.02	-0.09 ± 0.02
		Adjusted[b]	-0.09 ± 0.02	-0.10 ± 0.02
		p-Value	<0.0001	<0.0001
Fruit and vegetables (svgs/day)				
Intervention ($x \pm$ SD)	601	3.62 ± 1.49	0.41 ± 1.88	0.47 ± 1.83
Control ($x \pm$ SD)	604	3.47 ± 1.41	0.08 ± 1.63	0.14 ± 1.80
Intervention effect ($x \pm$ SE)		Unadjusted	0.33 ± 0.09	0.33 ± 0.10
		Adjusted[b]	0.39 ± 0.10	0.46 ± 0.10
		p-Value	<0.0001	<0.0001

Source: From Kristal, A., Curry, S., Shattuck, A., Feng, Z., and Li, S. (2000). A randomized trial of a
tailored, self-help dietary intervention: The Puget Sound Eating Patterns Study. *Prev. Med.* **31**, 380–389.
[a]Score from 21-item scale, scored from 1.0 (low fat) to 4.0 (high fat).
[b]Adjusted for baseline value, age, sex, race, body mass index, and income.

considerable statistical challenges [12, 13]. Consultation with a biostatistician is important in modeling these types of outcomes, and some approach to simplifying the analysis may prove to yield more interpretable and useful results.

C. Statistical Power

A final aspect of an evaluation design is to choose an appropriate sample size. This requires making a judgment on what size intervention effect is worth detecting. Even a trivially small intervention effect can be found statistically significant given a large enough sample size, and a clinically meaningful intervention effect may not reach statistical significance if the sample size is to small. For clinical interventions, it is reasonable to choose an effect size that is meaningful for an individual. For a public health intervention the effect size will be much smaller, and needs only be meaningful in terms of changes in population distributions of the outcome measure. When choosing minimum effect sizes, it is worthwhile to review what other interventions have achieved. The general recommendation is to never set a minimum detectable intervention effect larger than 1.5 times that observed in other interventions, unless there is very strong reason to believe that the new intervention being evaluated is far superior.

V. MEASUREMENT ISSUES WHEN ASSESSING DIETARY CHANGE AND OTHER INTERVENTION OUTCOMES

Once outcomes are well defined and an evaluation design is established, one must select, modify, or develop measures.

The two standard characteristics of dietary assessment methods, validity and reliability, are described in detail elsewhere in this text. Here we extend this discussion to cover measures of psychosocial factors and aspects of measurement that are relevant to measuring dietary change and, in addition, discuss practical considerations that have important implications for trial design and feasibility. Section VI describes how these measurement issues influence selection from among alternative measures of intervention outcomes.

A. Validity

Simply stated, validity is the extent to which your assessment tool measures what you want it to measure. Validity is not necessarily an intrinsic aspect of a particular tool or assessment instrument, because validity can vary as a function of method of administration, participants, or time. There are many types of validity, each having implications for intervention evaluation. Content validity is the extent to which you have sampled the domain of what you are trying to measure. For example, if your intervention goal were to lower total fat intake, high content validity would mean that you have measured all foods with meaningful amounts of fat. A limited but nevertheless important part of content validity is commonly referred to as *face validity*. Face validity is a judgment made by experts about whether or not a completed questionnaire measures what it is supposed to measure [14]. Construct validity is primarily a consideration for psychosocial measures. In this context, high construct validity means that the items used to form a scale are a good measure of some meaningful, underlying or latent construct.

An example is a scale that measures enabling factors for dietary change, consisting of six items on barriers, norms, and social support [15]. Criterion validity considers how well one measure correlates with another measure of the same construct. A type of criterion validity most important for nutrition intervention evaluations is predictive validity, which is based on whether a measure made at one time point predicts change at later point in time. For example, based on the theory of reasoned action [16], one would validate a measure of intention to eat more fruits and vegetables by examining how it predicts increased intake.

B. Reliability

Two types of reliability are important for evaluating intervention trials. Test–retest reliability measures agreement between multiple assessments. In practice, this means that a measure taken on one day would be strongly correlated with a measure taken on another day. Although no measures have perfect reliability, measures of daily nutrient intake or specific dietary behavior have particularly low reliability due to the variability in the amounts and types of foods people eat from day to day. This type of variability, termed intra-individual or within-persons variability, makes even a perfect assessment of a single day's diet not very informative for evaluating whether or not a person has changed their usual diet as a response to an intervention.

A second and entirely different type of reliability, which is relevant primarily to measures of psychosocial factors, is internal consistency reliability. Most psychosocial factors cannot be assessed directly (e.g., social support for eating low-fat foods), and they are generally measured using a set of items that taken together characterize the construct (e.g., "How much support do you get from your co-workers to select healthy foods from the cafeteria at lunch?"). The statistic called Cronbach's alpha, which ranges from 0 to 1, is a measure of how well the mean of scale items measures an underlying construct. High internal consistency reliability is a function of two factors, the average correlation among items in the scale *and* the number of items in the scale. Most scientists suggest a minimum of 0.7 for internal consistency; however, this ignores the practical problem that in applied evaluations it is not feasible to use lengthy scales. When scales are restricted to three or four items, a Cronbach's alpha of 0.50 is quite satisfactory.

C. Intervention-Associated Recall Bias

Bias is a measure of the extent to which an instrument under- or overestimates what it is attempting to measure. Ample evidence indicates that person-specific biases exist in self-reports of diet; for example, overweight persons tend to systematically underestimate energy intake [17]. If person-specific biases are constant, they will have little impact on evaluation, because analyses will be based on differences between measures assessed at baseline and follow-up. However, two unique sources of bias are introduced whenever evaluation of a dietary intervention is based on self-reported behavior. First, repeated monitoring results in changed responses to assessment instruments. For example, the number of different foods reported on a 4-day diet record decreases from day 1 to day 4, suggesting that study participants simplify their diets [18]. There is also some evidence that the quality of dietary intake data improves with repeated assessments, and this may differ by intervention treatment group [18]. Second, although well-designed dietary intervention trials randomize participants to intervention and control groups, the delivery of the behavioral intervention cannot be blinded as in conventional placebo-controlled trials. Thus, if intervention group participants report eating diets that match the goals of the intervention program rather than what they actually ate, there will be a bias toward overestimating intervention effectiveness. This bias can be substantial [20], and it appears to be larger in women then men [21–23].

D. Responsiveness

A measure only recently introduced into the nutrition literature, related specifically to measuring change, is termed *responsiveness*. Conceptually, responsiveness is a measure of whether an instrument captures information on intervention-related dietary patterns [24]. In intensive clinical interventions, in which a successful intervention results in large changes in foods consumed and food-preparation techniques, a sensitive instrument will capture information on both the most common foods and dietary practices of the sample at baseline and on new practices adopted due to the intervention. In public health interventions, in which there are only modest changes in dietary behavior, a sensitive measure will detect very small changes in behavior targeted by the intervention. Statistically, responsiveness is the ratio of the intervention effect divided by the standard deviation of the intervention effect. Responsiveness is thus a function of several aspects of a measure: (1) how well an instrument measures the intervention outcome both pre- and postintervention, (2) the magnitude of the intervention effect, and (3) the variance in the dietary or other measure used as the intervention outcome.

E. Participant Burden

If outcome assessments are too long or complicated, require biological samples, or must be repeated many times, high participant burden results. High participant burden can significantly compromise an evaluation. During recruitment, participation rates will be poor and participants will be less representative of the intervention target population. Once entered into the study, long or repeated follow-up assessments will contribute to high drop-out rates. Once recruited and

assigned to a treatment group, all participants should be included in the evaluation whether or not they complete the intervention or subsequent follow-up assessments. Thus, high drop-out rates (larger than 25%) make an evaluation suspect.

F. Instrument Complexity

Accurate assessment of nutrient intake requires complex instrumentation, regardless of whether instruments are interviewer- or self-administered. Some diet-related psychosocial factors may also require many questions with complicated skip patterns. It is important to remember that nutrition knowledge and literacy may be poor in some populations. Intervention participants may have difficulty answering detailed questions about food preparation or serving sizes, or may not be able to understand complex questions about attitudes and beliefs [25].

Complexity of analysis is an issue that is often overlooked. Before using an evaluation instrument, understand how it will be analyzed, evaluate the underlying nutrient database and associated software, and make sure that these analyses produce the variables you wish to measure. Dietary records, food frequency questionnaires, or scales to measure diet-related psychosocial factors are not useful unless there are means to transform data from these instruments into interpretable measures of the evaluation outcomes. Similarly, while it is simple to collect blood for serologic outcomes, analysis of many diet-related serologic measures is possible only in specialized research laboratories. These laboratories are primarily in academic research centers, and they are rarely capable or interested in processing the large numbers of samples required for evaluating a dietary intervention.

G. Costs

Randomized trials are expensive, and the costs of evaluating a nutrition intervention are often far greater than the costs of intervention delivery. A large proportion of evaluation cost can be attributed to outcome assessments, especially if they are based on dietary records or recalls or on serologic measures of micronutrient concentrations. Not surprisingly, the high cost of dietary assessments strongly motivates the use of alternative measures.

VI. DIETARY ASSESSMENT INSTRUMENTS AND THEIR APPLICABILITY FOR INTERVENTION EVALUATION

Most research on dietary assessment is motivated by the needs of nutritional epidemiologists, and is focused on how to best understand relationships between diet and health outcomes or on surveillance of population-level nutritional status. Dietary intervention studies have tended to use dietary assessment methods developed for other purposes, with the hope that they will serve the current intended purpose. However, as described earlier in this chapter, evaluating dietary interventions and measuring dietary change have many special nuances. Here, we review the available tools for measuring intervention effectiveness, focusing on the characteristics most relevant for outcome evaluation.

A. Anthropometric and Biochemical Measures

Many anthropometric and biochemical measures correlate with nutrient intake, but relatively few of these are useful or appropriate for the evaluation of interventions to change dietary behavior (Table 2). The exceptions will be interventions that are designed to increase intake of a specific micronutrient, for example, the fortification of cereal-grain products in the United States with folate or the fortification of sugar with vitamin A in Guatemala [26].

The most useful anthropometric measure is change in body weight, which can either be the goal of the nutritional intervention or a marker of decreased energy intake relative to expenditure, or fat intakes. Given the lack of objective markers of dietary fat reduction, this relationship with weight deserves more comment. Randomized trials of fat reduction show intervention effects for weight of about 3 kg associated with a 10 percentage point decrease in percent energy from fat [8, 27], and of about 0. 25 kg with decreases of 1 percentage point [9]. Weight loss associated with fat reduction is likely due to incomplete substitution of nonfat sources of energy in a fat-restricted diet [28].

Biochemical measures are useful for assessing changes in foods containing unique constituents that can be measured easily in blood or urine. The most often used measure is change in total serum carotenoids, which reflect usual intakes of carotenoid-containing fruits and vegetables [29–31], however total carotenoids minus lycopene is a superior measure [32] due to the low correlation of serum lycopene with other serum carotenoids. Biochemical measures are also useful to assess metabolic changes that result from dietary change. Serum cholesterol can be used as a measure of polyunsaturated and decreased saturated fatty acid intake in some target groups [33]. Because biochemical measures are expensive and require invasive collection procedures, they are impractical to use as primary outcome measures in public health interventions. An alternative is to collect biochemical measures on a small subsample of volunteers, and use these data as secondary outcomes to confirm results based on dietary self-report.

B. Self-Reported Dietary Behavior

Table 3 gives an overview of measures used to collect data on self-reported diet. Selection from among these many

TABLE 2   Anthropometric and Biochemical Measures Suitable for Intervention Evaluation

Measure	Intervention(s)	Comments [references]
Weight	Energy and/or possibly fat	[8, 27]
Serum carotenoids	Fruits and vegetables	Fasting blood samples are optimal. Control for serum cholesterol, body mass index, and smoking necessary. Confounded by beta carotene supplements. [29–32]
Urinary isoflavonoids	Soy products	Spot sample may be adequate Hidden sources of soy (e.g., processed meats) may confound measure. [90, 91]
Red cell or phospholipid Fatty acid	Fish Fat modification	Confounded by fish oil supplements. [92–94]
Plasma/urinary isothiocynates	Cruciferous vegetables	[95, 96]
Serum cholesterol	Fat modification	[97, 98]

choices requires balancing the costs and participant burden of "gold standard" measures such as multiple 24-hour dietary recalls with the practical benefits of using short, self-administered questionnaires that assess specific dietary patterns.

The primary distinctions among types of instruments are based on whether diet is measured based on foods actually consumed, foods "usually" consumed, or on patterns of food consumption. Note that there is an inherent hierarchy across these types of instruments; one can measure dietary patterns based on any dietary assessment instrument or foods usually consumed based on foods actually consumed. Measuring nutrients from foods actually consumed is a "gold standard" for intervention evaluation, because any changes in foods, portion sizes, and preparation techniques can be captured. However, because many days of foods must be assessed to characterize an individual's usual diet, any measure based on actual foods consumed will be very expensive and have high participant burden. The benefit of assessing nutrients from foods usually consumed is that only a single measure is needed at each time point, but it is not possible to

TABLE 3   Measures of
Self-reported Diet Suitable for
Intervention Evaluation

Nutrients from foods consumed
    24-hour dietary recalls
Nutrients from "usual diet"
    Food frequency questionnaires
Dietary patterns
    Diet behavior questionnaires
    Short food frequency questionnaires
    "Focused" 24-hour dietary recalls

capture details on all foods and their preparation methods in precise detail. The benefits of assessing dietary patterns alone are that it is a less burdensome task and is often a more direct measure of whether new dietary behaviors were adopted. Its limitation is that changes in dietary patterns cannot be directly interpreted as changes in nutrient intake and is thus less well accepted in the nutritional science community.

1. NUTRIENTS FROM FOODS ACTUALLY CONSUMED

The best approach to measuring nutrients from foods actually consumed are unannounced (unscheduled), interviewer-administered 24-hour dietary recalls. Unannounced recalls are administered by telephone, which in practice is facilitated by collecting information at the beginning of an evaluation on convenient days, places, and times to call. Participants can be given serving size booklets, so that they can refer to specific pictures when reporting amounts of foods consumed. The protocol or script used for collecting 24-hour recalls can also be modified to focus on assessing the intervention outcomes (e.g., for an intervention to decrease saturated fat, type of margarine will be important) and deemphasize details that are uninformative (e.g., for a fruit and vegetable intervention, probes for added salt are not relevant). Finally, it is important to consider the limitations to the accuracy of 24-hour recalls, because respondents often do not know answers to questions about food composition, preparation, or portion size.

High costs (between $35 and $55 per day) and participant burden are serious drawbacks to any study wishing to evaluate intervention effectiveness using dietary recalls. This is especially true when the evaluation is at the individual level and therefore many days of intake must be captured for each participant. For randomized designs, it may be sufficient to calculate intervention effects based on one pre- and one postintervention recall per participant. This measure of the

intervention effect will be unbiased, but there are problems due to the very low reliability of a single day's measure of nutrient intake. Most importantly, because the group-level intervention effect will have very high variance there will be low statistical power to detect differences across treatment groups. Further, it is statistically inappropriate to adjust this measure of the intervention effect for individuals' demographic characteristics or other diet-related factors (33). Intervention effects calculated from a single 24-hour recall can be used in much the same way as biochemical measures as a secondary outcome used to corroborate a more practical but less valid measure of nutrient intake.

Other methods of capturing foods actually consumed, including food records and scheduled 24-hour recalls, are inappropriate for intervention evaluation. This is because both record keeping and anticipating a dietary recall can substantially change dietary behavior. While unannounced 24-hour recalls may be subject to intervention-associated bias through differential recall of foods consumed, food records or announced recalls are much more likely to be biased due their effects on food choice.

2. NUTRIENTS FROM FOODS USUALLY CONSUMED

During the past 20 years, food frequency questionnaires (FFQs) have become a standard measure in nutritional epidemiology. They have also become quite common for intervention evaluations, because they can be self-administered, processed using mark-sense technology, and cost less than $15 per administration.

Two characteristics of any FFQ detract from their use for measuring dietary change. First, whereas FFQs are convenient for investigators, they are burdensome to participants, requiring time, high literacy, and knowledge about food. Second, the cognitive processes required to complete an FFQ might make them highly subject to intervention-associated bias. Respondents must construct answers to FFQ items using knowledge about their characteristic diet, because memory about actual eating and drinking episodes erodes after only a few days [35]. Thus, not knowing the true answer to most questions, it is likely that perceptions of behavior deemed desirable due to the intervention would bias FFQ responses [23]. Nevertheless, practical considerations often require using FFQs. For these evaluations, it is necessary to incorporate methods to minimize response burden and increase response rates, such as limiting total questionnaire length and giving incentives.

Standard FFQs developed for epidemiological studies are not necessarily good for intervention evaluation. An intervention-focused FFQ must usually collect detailed information on food choices that reflect the intervention goals. This may require any of the following: (1) regrouping foods into categories relevant to the intervention (e.g., grouping soups into "creamed," "vegetable," "bean," and "broth" to capture fat, carotenoids, and fiber); (2) assessing relatively fine distinctions between similar foods (e.g., nonfat vs. reg-

ular mayonnaise, refried vs. baked beans, or plain lettuce salads vs. mixed salads with carrots and tomatoes); (3) assessing preparation methods (e.g., chicken with or without skin, shellfish boiled or fried); and (4) collecting information on portion sizes. It is also important to examine the nutrient database and computer algorithms underlying analysis of the FFQ. Several approaches are available for assigning nutrient values to FFQ items [36, 37], and some may not produce a nutrient database that reflects substantial differences in relevant nutrients between foods targeted by the intervention. There are also different approaches in how FFQ analysis software incorporates information about types of foods (e.g., type of milk) or preparations (e.g., chicken with or without skin) when computing nutrients. It may be necessary to modify these algorithms to better reflect changes targeted by an intervention. Unfortunately, developing a new FFQ is very time consuming and complex, and most evaluations must choose wisely from among those available based on how well they capture dietary behavior of interest. Some commercially available FFQ software packages do allow minor modifications that can be helpful in developing FFQs for intervention trials [38], and some FFQs are available that were developed specifically for evaluating interventions [19, 36, 39].

3. DIETARY PATTERNS

The many practical and scientific benefits to using short, simple instruments to measure dietary patterns targeted by an intervention were described earlier in this chapter. A modest amount of research has been done in this area that has yielded four approaches to short dietary assessment: (1) short FFQs; (2) prediction equations, based on regression models; (3) diet-habits questionnaires; and (4) focused 24-hour recalls. These approaches differ substantially in their underlying statistical assumptions and their use of behavioral theory related to dietary behavior change. Understanding these differences can help nutritionists to select and modify available instruments or to develop instruments suited to the intervention under evaluation.

a. Short Food Frequency Questionnaires. These instruments typically contain between 10 and 15 FFQ items, and are designed to assess intake of a specific nutrient or frequency of eating a specific group of foods. Examples in the literature include instruments for fat [40], calcium [41], and fruits and vegetables [42–45]. For intervention evaluation, a short FFQ should be based on knowledge of dietary patterns in the sample receiving the intervention [46, 47] and the behavioral targets of the intervention. There is modest evidence that an approach based solely on statistical criteria can be valid in epidemiological studies [37], but this approach lacks face validity when evaluating an intervention. Short FFQs are appropriate for intervention evaluation only if a small number of foods is being targeted by the intervention or if the outcome is a nutrient that is concentrated in very few foods. Thus, short FFQs are best for nutrients such as

calcium or for foods groups such as fruits and vegetables, and suspect for nutrients such as fat or sodium that are spread throughout the food supply.

b. Prediction Equations. Many nutritional scientists have proposed using regression models to predict nutrient intake from a short set of questions. These models are built typically on data from FFQs, in which the frequencies of eating specific foods are entered into a stepwise linear regression model predicting the nutrient of interest. A relatively small number of foods will predict a large amount of variance in most nutrients [48], and on the surface this appears to be a useful way to simplify dietary assessment. However, these models have very poor face validity, because these prediction equations assign coefficients (weights) to food items that often have little to do with the nutrient of interest [49]. The models also have poor criterion validity, because models developed from one sample typically do not predict nutrient intake in a different, independent sample [50, 51].

A related approach is based on using factor analysis to identify patterns of association among foods on an FFQ. These patterns are given descriptive names (e.g., "junk food" or "plain home cooking") based on the interpretation of the foods in the factor, and these factors are treated as meaningful measures of an underlying dietary pattern. These patterns lack both face validity and criterion validity and are not reproducible between samples. One of the reasons both regression and factor analysis do not yield useful measures is that they are based on correlations among FFQ items in a specific sample. There is little consistency in the correlations among FFQ items across time or across samples and even less consistency if a dietary intervention changes dietary patterns. Measures based on regression models or factor analysis are entirely inappropriate for intervention evaluation.

c. Diet-Habits Questionnaires. Diet-habits questionnaires are unique because they have been developed specifically to measure intervention outcomes. These questionnaires typically contain between 15 and 30 questions, with response options that are qualitative (e.g., rarely/never to usually/always) or ordered frequency categories. The most robust of these measures is based on theoretical or at least explicit models of dietary behavior change [52, 53], and their development is facilitated by an understanding of nutrition, psychometric theory, and cognitive psychology, as well as skill in item construction and questionnaire design. There is ample evidence that these measures can be valid measures of dietary change [52–60], and they tend to have higher responsiveness than alternatives such as short FFQs, full FFQs, or repeated 24-hour recalls [7, 9, 24, 61, 62].

Diet behavior questionnaires are well suited to evaluations of public health interventions, because of their low participant burden and high sensitivity to change, and less well suited for clinical interventions requiring a measure of changes in nutrient intake. Before beginning an evaluation, it is important to pilot these measures in the target population, to make sure that the questionnaire format language and

diet patterns being measured are appropriate. Nutritionists should take the liberty of modifying existing questionnaires to better suit their target population, as long as the basic structure and content of the instrument remains intact.

d. Focused 24-Hour Recalls. A focused recall uses techniques similar to those used to collect standard 24-hour recalls, but collects only information related to the evaluation outcome. For example, if the intervention goal is to increase servings of fruits and vegetables, then the only information captured during the interview is about fruits and vegetables. The amount of detail collected can also vary. A focused recall could collect details about the type and serving size of all targeted foods, or an interviewer could simply read a list of foods and ask respondents whether of not they ate them in the previous day [63]. Focused recalls are far simpler to administer and analyze than standard 24-hour recalls, yet they share the characteristic of low bias due to reliance on episodic rather than general memory [35]. Similar to a 24-hour recall, only repeated assessments can be used to characterize behavior of an individual, but a single measure is fine for characterizing a group. For example, one could contrast the percentages of participants in intervention and control groups who drank skim milk or ate french fried potatoes on the previous day. More complex focused recalls have been developed to measure carotenoid intake [64], and more research on developing these measures is warranted. Nutritionists should consider developing instruments based on this approach when the 24-hour recalls are the desired evaluation tool but cannot be used due to costs or participant burden.

4. DIET-RELATED PSYCHOSOCIAL FACTORS

Table 4 gives an overview of psychosocial factors that can be used to assess intervention outcomes. Comprehensive behavioral models are built from many constructs [65], but in the context of an intervention evaluation it is generally both feasible and necessary to measure only those constructs that are central to the model. Thus, for each of the behavioral models used to design nutrition interventions, those psychosocial factors that are key to their evaluation are selected.

Very little research exists on the validity and responsiveness of diet-related psychosocial measures. Measures developed and validated for one behavioral domain, for example, for smoking cessation, are often adapted for dietary intervention research without consideration of their face or construct validity. For some diet-related psychosocial constructs, measurement is quite simple and little validation is necessary. For example, one could measure intention to change diet with a single item such as "In the next 6 months, how likely is it that you will change your diet to eat less fat?" Alternatively, measuring a construct such as stage of dietary change can be quite complex and requires considerable developmental research. When adopting psychosocial measures from other behavioral domains, it is important to remember

TABLE 4 Diet-Related Psychosocial Factors Suitable for Intervention Evaluation

Theoretical model	Key constructs	Reference
Utilization of health services	Predisposing (knowledge, attitudes, beliefs) Enabling (barriers, norms) Reinforcing (social support)	[99]; [70]; [100]
The theory of reasoned action	Intention	[100]; [101]; [102]
Health belief model	Perceived benefits, susceptibility, and severity	[100]; [103]; [104]
Social learning theory	Self-efficacy	[105]; [106]
Transtheoretical model	Stages of change	[68]; [107]; [108]; [109]

that dietary behavior is unique. First, dietary behavior is not a single behavior but a composite of many behaviors consisting of food choice, preparation, and frequency of consumption. Psychosocial factors related to one aspect of dietary behavior may differ from those relating to another. Second, dietary behavior is not discrete, such a smoking, rather it occurs on a continuum in which any discrete definition of desirable dietary behavior is necessarily arbitrary (e.g., <30% energy from fat). Thus, diet-related psychosocial factors related to a discrete criterion, such as eating five or more servings a day of fruits and vegetables, may not capture the intent of an intervention to simply increase servings regardless of baseline intake.

One of the most popular approaches to organizing dietary intervention programs is based on using the "stage of change" construct from the transtheoretical model [66]. Interventions are designed to move participants from preaction stages of dietary change (precontemplation, contemplation, and decision) into action and then maintenance. There is increasing evidence that interventions can move people through stages of dietary change [67], and that movement through stages of change is associated with dietary behavior change [12, 13]. However, much controversy surrounds the conceptualization of stages of change when applied to dietary behavior, and thus little agreement in the literature of how it should be assessed [67–69].

A second popular approach for organizing nutrition interventions is PRECEDE/PROCEDE, which is not a behavioral model but rather a planning model for intervention development and delivery. Practical measures of the main constructs from this model, predisposing, enabling and reinforcing factors, have been developed and validated [15, 70]. One study has demonstrated that change in these factors, in addition to stage of dietary change, explained up to 55% of the intervention effect in a large randomized trial [13].

C. Environmental and Surrogate Measures of Diet

Table 5 gives an overview of environmental indicators and other surrogate measures that can be used to assess outcomes of dietary interventions. With the exception of household food inventories, these measures are only useful to evaluate intervention outcomes at the group or community level, and thus are best suited to evaluate environmental-level interventions.

Household food inventories consist of asking a set of questions about whether or not specific foods are currently available in the household. Characteristically the list consists of 10–15 foods that relate to the intervention. Examples of foods that could be included are types of staple foods (e.g., regular vs. low-fat mayonnaise) or the types of foods available for snacks (potato chips, fresh fruit, or baby carrots). There are no studies formally evaluating household inventories as intervention outcome measures, but there is evidence that study participants can recall foods in their households accurately [71], and that the types of foods correlate with individually assessed nutrient intake [72, 73]. Due to the simplicity of this approach, further efforts to evaluate these measures are well motivated.

Monitoring food sales can be used as a direct measure of an intervention effect, but it is extraordinarily challenging [74–77]. Relating changes in supermarket sales to nutrition interventions is very difficult, and most interventions attempting this approach have failed. Reasons are many, including the complexity of the food supply, the large number of food items that are sold in typical supermarkets, business confidentiality of sales data, and poor match between the data needs for business and the needs of nutrition researchers. Very careful planning, pilot studies, and ongoing contact

TABLE 5 Surrogate and Environmental Measures Suitable for Intervention Evaluation

	References
Individual or household level Household food (pantry) inventory	[72, 75]

Group or community level
   Cafeteria plate observation
   Cafeteria sales
   Vending machine sales
   Supermarket sales
   Supermarket environment
	[110]
	[82, 83]
	[81]
	[77]

between researchers and persons responsible for data collection are necessary to make supermarket sales data useful for outcome evaluation. Monitoring sales in food services such as work site and school cafeterias or vending machines is much simpler and has been used successfully to evaluate interventions [78–83]. One good approach is to devise a simple scheme for unobtrusively observing and recording food choices as customers move through a cafeteria line [84].

Changes in the food environment, such as supermarket signage or distribution of supermarket shelf space, are also potential surrogate measures of intervention outcomes. A series of studies has shown that it is possible to reliably measure supermarket environments, that measures of shelf space correlate with community-level measures of diet, and that changes in supermarket shelf space correlate weakly with changes in community-level diet [85–89]. It is possible that changes in supermarket signage or foods offered in restaurants could reflect an effective community-level intervention, as businesses adjust to demands from consumers for information about and access to healthier foods. These are not likely to be very sensitive measures, because the supermarket environment is saturated with signage, and restaurant menus are difficult to evaluate objectively.

VII. CONCLUSIONS

Evaluations of nutrition interventions can be both scientifically and operationally challenging. Nutritionists can and should take the lead in conceptualizing and interpreting the evaluation of a nutrition intervention, but they should also seek collaborations or consultations with scientists in other disciplines to ensure that methods are optimal. When planning an evaluation, make sure that the time line allows you to test, pilot, and if necessary, refine measures and procedures, even if you are using previously developed instruments and methods. Know that your measures will have sufficient responsiveness to detect an intervention effect. Make sure that your measures assess the behaviors targeted by the intervention and that the effect sizes you expect are reasonable. These steps are often expensive and slow, but the ultimate result of using appropriate evaluation methods is that you will obtain clearly interpretable and valid results.

References

1. Haines, P., Siega-Riz, A., and Popkin, B. (1999). The Diet Quality Index revised: A measurement instrument for populations. *J. Am. Diet. Assoc.* **99**, 697–704.
2. Patterson, R., Haines, P., and Popkin, B. (1994). Diet Quality Index: Capturing a multidimensional behavior. *J. Am. Diet. Assoc.* **94**, 57–64.
3. Bandura, A. (1986). "Social Foundations of Thought and Action: A Social Cognitive Theory." Prentice-Hall, Englewood Cliffs, NJ.

4. MacKinnon, D. P., and Dwyer, J. H. (1993). Estimating mediated effects in prevention studies. *Eval. Rev.* **17**, 144–148.
5. Hansen, W. B., and McNeal, R. B. (1996). The law of maximum expected potential effect: Constraints placed on program effectiveness by mediator relationships. *Health Educ. Res.* **11**, 501–507.
6. Baranowski, T., Lin, L. S., Wetter, D. W., Resnicow, K., and Hearn, M. D. (1997). Theory as mediating variables: Why aren't community interventions working as desired. *Ann. Epidemiol.* **S7**, S89–S95.
7. Beresford, S. A., Curry, S. J., Kristal, A. R., Lazovich, D., Feng, Z., and Wagner, E. H. (1997). A dietary intervention in primary care practice: The Eating Patterns Study. *Am. J. Public Health* **87**, 610–616.
8. Kristal, A. R., Shattuck, A. L., Bowen, D. J., Sponzo, R. W., and Nixon, D. W. (1997). Feasibility of using volunteer research staff to deliver and evaluate a low-fat dietary intervention: The American Cancer Society Breast Cancer Dietary Intervention project. *Cancer Epidemiol. Biomarkers Prev.* **6**, 459–467.
9. Kristal, A., Curry, S., Shattuck, A., Feng, Z., and Li, S. (2000). A randomized trial of a tailored, self-help dietary intervention: The Puget Sound Eating Patterns Study. *Prev. Med.* **31**, 380–389.
10. Koepsell, T., Diehr, P., Cheadle, A., and Kristal, A. (1995). Invited commentary: Symposium of Community Intervention Trials. *Am. J. Epidemiol.* **142**, 594–599.
11. Koepsell, T. D., Wagner, E. H., Cheadle, A. C., Patrick, D. L., Martin, D. C., Diehr, P. H., Perrin, E. B., Kristal, A. R., Allan-Andrilla, C. H., and Dey, L. J. (1992). Selected methodological issues in evaluating community-based health promotion and disease prevention programs. *Annu. Rev. Public Health* **13**, 31–57.
12. Glanz, K., Patterson, R. E., Kristal, A. R., Feng, Z., Linnan, L., and Hebert, J. (1998). Impact of worksite health promotion on stages of dietary change: The Working Well Trial. *Health Educ. Behav.* **25**, 448–463.
13. Kristal, A. R., Glanz, K., Tilley, B. C., and Li, S. S. (2000). Mediating factors in dietary change: Understanding the impact of a worksite nutrition intervention. *Health Educ. Behav.* **27**, 112–125.
14. Nunnally, J. C., and Bernstein, I. H. (1994). Psychometric Theory. Third ed. McGraw-Hill, New York.
15. Glanz, K., Kristal, A. R., Sorensen, G., Palombo, R., Heimendinger, J., and Probart, C. (1993). Development and validation of measures of psychosocial factors influencing fat- and fiber-related dietary behavior. *Prev. Med.* **22**, 373–387.
16. Ajzen, I., and Fishbein, M. (1980). Understanding attitudes and predicting social behavior. Prentice Hall, Englewood Cliffs, NJ.
17. Johnson, R., Soultanakis, R., and Matthers, D. (1998). Literacy and body fatness are associated with underreporting of energy intake in US low-income women using the multiple-pass 24-hour recall: A doubly labeled water experiment. *J. Am. Diet. Assoc.* **98**, 1136–1140.
18. Rebro, S., Patterson, R. E., Kristal, A. R., and Cheney, C. (1998). The effect of keeping food records on eating patterns. *J. Am. Diet. Assoc.* **98**, 1163–1165.
19. Kristal, A., Feng, Z., Coates, R., Oberman, A., and George, V. (1997). Associations of race, ethnicity, education and dietary

intervention on validity and reliability of a food frequency questionnaire in the Women's Health Initiative Feasibility Study in Minority Populations. *Am. J. Epidemiol.* **146,** 856–869.

20. Forster, J., Jeffrey, R., VanNatta, M., and Pirie, P. (1990). Hypertension prevention trial: Do 24-h food records capture usual eating behavior in a dietary change study? *Am. J. Clin. Nutr.* **51,** 253–257.

21. Hebert, J., Clemow, L., Pbert, L., and Ockene, J. (1995). Social desirability bias in dietary self-report may compromise the validity of dietary intake measures. *Int. J. Epidemiol.* **24,** 389–398.

22. Hebert, J., Ma, Y., Clemow, L., Ickene, I., Saperia, G., Stanek, E., Merriam, P., and Ockene, J. (1997). Gender differences in social desirability and social approval bias in dietary self-report. *Am. J. Epidemiol.* **146,** 1046–1055.

23. Kristal, A. R., Andrilla, C. H., Koepsell, T. D., Diehr, P. H., and Cheadle, A. (1998). Dietary assessment instruments are susceptible to intervention-associated response set bias. *J. Am. Diet. Assoc.* **98,** 40–43.

24. Kristal, A. R., Beresford, S. A., and Lazovich, D. (1994). Assessing change in diet-intervention research. *Am. J. Clin. Nutr.* **59,** 185S–189S.

25. Weinrich, S., Boyd, M., and Pow, B. (1997). Tool adaptation for socioeconomically disadvantaged populations. *In* "Instruments for Clinical Health Care Research" (M. Stromburd and S. Olson, Eds.). Norwalk, CT: Jones & Bartlett, 20–29.

26. Arroyave, G., Mejia, L. A., and Aguilar, J. (1981). The effect of vitamin A fortification of sugar on the serum vitamin A levels of preschool Guatemalan children. *Am. J. Clin. Nutr.* **34,** 41–49.

27. Sheppard, L., Kristal, A. R., and Kushi, L. H. (1991). Weight loss in women participating in a randomized trial of low-fat diets. *Am. J. Clin. Nutr.* **54,** 821–8.

28. Hill, J., and Peters, J. (1998). Environmental contributions to the obesity epidemic. *Science* **280,** 1371–1374.

29. Drewnowski, A., Rock, C., Henderson, S., Shore, A., Fischler, C., Galan, P., Preziosi, P., and Hercberg, S. (1997). Serum beta-carotene and vitamin C as biomarkers of vegetable and fruit intakes in a community-based sample of French adults. *Arch. Int. Med.* **65,** 1796–1802.

30. Rock, C., Flatt, S., Wright, F., Faerber, S., Newman, S., and Pierce, J. (1997). Responsiveness of carotenoids to a high vegetable diet intervention designed to prevent breast cancer recurrence. *Cancer Epidemiol. Biomarkers Prev.* **6,** 617–623.

31. Rock, C., Thornquist, M., Kristal, A. R., Patterson, R. E., Cooper, D., Newhouser, M. L., Neumark-Sztainer, D., and Cheskin, L. (1999). Demographic, dietary and lifestyle factors differentially explain variability in serum carotenoids and fat-soluble vitamins: Baseline results from the Olestra Post-Marketing Surveillance Study. *J. Nutr.* **129,** 855–864.

32. Campbell, D., Gross, M., Martini, M., Grandits, G., Slavin, J., and Potter, J. (1994). Plasma carotenoids as biomarkers of vegetable and fruit intake. *Cancer Epidemiol. Biomarkers Prev.* **3,** 493–500.

33. Mazier, M., and Jones, P. (1999). Dietary fat saturation, but not the feeding state, modulates rates of cholesterol esterification in normolipidemic men. *Metabolism* **48,** 1210–1215.

34. Liu, K. (1988). Measurement error and its impact on partial correlation and multiple regression analyses. *Am. J. Epidemiol.* **127,** 864–874.

35. Smith, A., Jobe, J., and Mingay, D. (1991). Retrieval from memory of dietary information. *Appl. Cogn. Psychol.* **5,** 269–296.

36. Kristal, A. R., Shattuck, A. L., and Williams, A. E. (1992). Food frequency questionnaires for diet intervention research. *In 17th National Nutrient Databank Conference.* Baltimore, MD: International Life Sciences Institute, 110–125.

37. Block, G., Hartman, A., Dresser, C., Carroll, M., Gannon, J., and Gardner, L. (1986). A data-based approach to diet questionnaire design and testing. *Am. J. Epidemiol.* **124,** 453–469.

38. Block, G., Coyle, L., Hartman, A., and Scoppa, S. (1994). Revision of dietary analysis software for the Health Habits and History Questionnaire. *Am. J. Epidemiol.* **139,** 1190–1196.

39. Patterson, R. E., Kristal, A. R., Carter, R. A., Fels-Tinker, L., Bolton, M. P., and Agurs-Collins, T. (1999). Measurement characteristics of the Women's Health Initiative food frequency questionnaire. *Ann. Epidemiol.* **9,** 178–187.

40. Block, G., Clifford, C., Naughtom, M., Henderson, M., and McAdams, M. (1989). A brief dietary screen for high fat intake. *J. Nutr. Edu.* **21,** 199–207.

41. Cummings, S., Block, G., McHenry, K., and Baron, R. (1987). Evaluation of two food frequency approaches of measuring calcium intake. *Ann. Epidemiol.* **126,** 796–802.

42. Serdula, M., Coates, R., Byers, T., Mokdad, A., Jewell, S., Chavez, N., Mares-Perlman, J., Newcomb, P., Ritenbaugh, C., Treiber, F., and Block, G. (1993). Evaluation of a brief telephone questionnaire to estimate fruit and vegetable consumption in diverse study populations. *Epidemiology* **4,** 455–463.

43. Field, A. E., Colditz, G. A., Fox, M. K., Byers, T., Serdula, M., Bosch, R. J., and Peterson, K. E. (1998). Comparison of 4 questionnaires for assessment of fruit and vegetable intake. *Am. J. Public Health* **88,** 1216–1218.

44. Hunt, M. K., Stoddard, A. M., Peterson, K., Sorensen, G., Hebert, J. R., and Cohen, N. (1998). Comparison of dietary assessment measures in the Treatwell 5 A Day worksite study. *J. Am. Diet. Assoc.* **98,** 1021–1023.

45. Kristal, A., Vizenor, N., Patterson, R., Neuhouser, M., and Shattuck, A. (2000). Validity of food frequency based measures of fruit and vegetable intakes. *Cancer Epidemiol. Biomarkers Prev.* **9,** 939–944.

46. Block, G., Dresser, C., Hartman, A., and Carroll, M. (1985). Nutrient sources in the American diet: Quantitative data from the NHANES II survey. II. Macronutrients and fat. *Am. J. Epidemiol.* **122,** 27–40.

47. Block, G., Dresser, C., Hartman, A., and Carroll, M. (1985). Nutrient sources in the American diet: Quantitative data from the NHANES II survey. I. Vitamins and minerals. *Am. J. Epidemiol.* **122,** 13–26.

48. Byers, T., Marshall, J., Fielder, R., Zielezny, M., and Graham, S. (1985). Assessing nutrient intake with an abbreviated dietary interview. *Am. J. Epidemiol.* **122,** 41–50.

49. Gray, G., Paganini-Hill, A., Ross, R., and Henderson, B. (1984). Assessment of three brief methods of estimation of vitamin A and C intakes for a prospective study of cancer: Comparison with dietary history. *Am. J. Epidemiol.* **119,** 581–590.

50. Hankin, J., Messinger, H., and Stallones, R. (1968). A short dietary method for epidemiologic studies. IV. Evaluation of questionnaire. *Am. J. Epidemiol.* **91,** 562–567.

51. Hankin, J., Rawlings, V., and Nomura, A. (1978). Assessment of a short dietary method for a prospective study on cancer. *Am. J. Clin. Nutr.* **31**, 355–359.

52. Kristal, A. R., Shattuck, A. L., and Henry, H. J. (1990). Patterns of dietary behavior associated with selecting diets low in fat: Reliability and validity of a behavioral approach to dietary assessment. *J. Am. Diet. Assoc.* **90**, 214–220.

53. Shannon, J., Kristal, A. R., Curry, S. J., and Beresford, S. A. (1997). Application of a behavioral approach to measuring dietary change: The fat- and fiber-related diet behavior questionnaire. *Cancer Epidemiol. Biomarkers Prev.* **6**, 355–361.

54. Connor, S., Gustafson, J., Sexton, G., Becker, N., Artaud-Wild, S., and Conner, W. (1992). The Diet Habit Survey: A new method of dietary assessment that relates to plasma cholesterol changes. *J. Am. Diet Assoc.* **92**, 41–47.

55. Gans, K., Sundaram, S., McPhillips, J., Hixson, M., Linnan, L., and Carleson, R. (1993). Rate your plate: An eating pattern assessment and educational tool used at cholesterol screening and education programs. *J. Nutr. Edu.* **25**, 29–36.

56. Peters, J., Quiter, E., and Brekke, M. (1994). The Eating Pattern Assessment Tool: A simple instrument for assessing dietary fat and cholesterol intake. *J. Am. Diet. Assoc.* **94**, 1008–1013.

57. Kristal, A. R., White, E., Shattuck, A. L., Curry, S., Anderson, G. L., Fowler, A., and Urban, N. (1992). Long-term maintenance of a low-fat diet: Durability of fat-related dietary habits in the Women's Health Trial. *J. Am. Diet. Assoc.* **92**, 553–559.

58. Kristal, A. R., Shattuck, A. L., and Patterson, R. E. (1999). Differences in fat-related dietary patterns between black, Hispanic, and white women: Results from the Women's Health Trial Feasibility Study in Minority Populations. *Public Health Nutr.* **2**, 273–276.

59. Kinlay, S., Heller, R., and Halliday, J. (1991). A simple score and questionnaire to measure group changes in dietary fat intake. *Prev. Med.* **20**, 378–388.

60. Hartman, T., McCarthy, P., and Himes, J. (1993). Use of eating-pattern messages to evaluate changes in eating behaviors in a worksite cholesterol education program. *J. Am. Diet. Assoc.* **93**, 1119–1123.

61. Hartman, T., McCarthy, P., Park, R., Schuster, E., and Kushi, L. (1997). Results of a community-based low-literacy nutrition education program. *J. Comm. Health* **22**, 325–341.

62. Glasgow, R., Perry, J. D., Toobert, D. J., and Hollis, J. F. (1996). Brief assessments of dietary behavior in field settings. *Addict. Behav.* **21**, 239–247.

63. Kristal, A. R., Abrams, B. F., Thornquist, M. D., Disogra, L., Croyle, R. T., Shattuck, A. L., and Henry, H. J. (1990). Development and validation of a food use checklist for evaluation of community nutrition interventions. *Am. J. Public Health.* **80**, 1318–1322.

64. Neuhouser, M., Patterson, R., Kristal, A., Eldridge, A., and Vizenor, N. (2001). A brief dietary assessment instrument for assessing target foods, nutrients and eating patterns. *Public Health Nutr.* **4**, 73–78.

65. Glanz, K., Lewis, F., and Rimer, B. (1997). *Health Behavior and Health Education Theory, Research, and Practice.* 2nd ed. San Francisco: Jossey-Bass Publishers.

66. Prochaska, J. O., and Velicer, W. F. (1997). The transtheoretical model of health behavior change. *Am. J. Health Promotion* **12**, 38–48.

67. Kristal, A. R., Glanz, K., Curry, S. J., and Patterson, R. E. (1999). How can stages of change be best used in dietary interventions? *J. Am. Diet. Assoc.* **99**, 679–684.

68. Povey, R., Conner, M., Sparks, P., James, R., and Shepherd, R. (1999). A critical examination of the application of the transtheoretical model's stages of change to dietary behaviours. *Health Educ. Res.* **14**, 641–651.

69. Greene, G., Rossi, S., Rossi, J., Velicer, W., Fava, J., and Prochaska, J. (1999). Dietary applications of the stages of change model. *J. Am. Diet. Assoc.* **99**, 673–678.

70. Glanz, K., Kristal, A. R., Tilley, B. C., and Kirst, K. (1998). Psychosocial correlates of healthful diets among male auto workers. *Cancer Epidemiol. Biomarkers Prev.* **7**, 119–126.

71. Crocket, S., Potter, J., Wright, M., and Bacheller, A. (1992). Validation of a self-reported shelf inventory to measure food purchases behavior. *J. Am. Diet. Assoc.* **92**, 694–697.

72. Satia, J., Patterson, R., Kristal, A., Pineda, M., and Hislop, T. G. (in press). Use of household food inventory as an environmental indicator of dietary patterns in Chinese-Americans and Chinese-Canadians. *Public Health Nutr.*

73. Patterson, R. E., Kristal, A. R., Shannon, J., Hunt, J. R., White E. (1997). Using a brief household food inventory as an environmental indicator of individual dietary practices. *Am. J. Public Health* **87**, 272–275.

74. Shucker, R., Levy, A., Tenny, J., Mathews, O. (1992). Nutrition self-labeling and consumer purchase behavior. *J. Nutr.* **24**, 553–559.

75. Patterson, B., Kessler, L., Wax, Y., Bernstein, A., Light, L., Midthune, D., Portnoy, B., Tenny, J., and Tuckermanty, E. (1992). Evaluation of a supermarket intervention. *Eval. Res.* **16**, 464–490.

76. Kristal, A. R., Goldenhar, L., Muldoon, J., and Morton, R. F. (1997). A randomized trial of a supermarket intervention to increase consumption of fruits and vegetables. *Am. J. Health Promotion* **11**, 422–425.

77. Odenkirchen, J., Portnoy, B., Blair, J., Rodgers, A., Light, L., and Tenney, J. (1992). In-store monitoring of a supermarket nutrition intervention. *Fam. & Comm. Health* **14**, 1–9.

78. Wilbur, C., Zifferblatt, S., Pinsky, J., and Zifferblatt, S. (1981). Healthy vending: a cooperative pilot research program to stimulate good health in the marketplace. *Prev. Med.* **10**, 85–89.

79. Schmitz, M., and Fielding, J. (1986). Point-of-choice nutrition labeling: Evaluation in a worksite cafeteria. *J. Nutr. Edu.* **19**, 85–92.

80. Cincirpini, P. (1984). Changing food selections in a public cafeteria. *Behav. Modif.* **8**, 520–539.

81. Hoerr, S., and Louden, V. (1993). Can nutrition information increase sales of healthful vended snacks? *J. Sch. Health* **63**, 386–390.

82. Jeffrey, R., French, S., Raether, C., and Baxter, J. (1994). An environmental intervention to increase fruit and salad purchases in a cafeteria. *Prev. Med.* **23**, 788–792.

83. Perlmutter, C., Canter, D., and Gregoire, M. (1997). Profitability and acceptability of fat- and sodium-modified hot entrees in a worksite cafeteria. *J. Am. Diet. Assoc.* **97**, 391–395.

84. Mayer, J., Brown, T., Heins, J., and Bishop, D. (1987). A multi-component intervention for modifying food selection in a worksite cafeteria. *J. Nutr. Edu.* **6**, 277–280.

85. Cheadle, A., Psaty, B., Wagner, E., Diehr, P., Koepsell, T., Curry, S., and Von Korff, M. (1990). Evaluating community-based nutrition programs. Assessing the reliability of a survey of grocery store product displays. *Am. J. Public Health* **80,** 709–711.

86. Cheadle, A., Psaty, B., Curry, S., Wagner, E., Diehr, P., Koepsell, T., and Kristal, A. (1991). Community-level comparisons between the grocery store environment and individual dietary practices. *Prev. Med.* **20,** 250–261.

87. Cheadle, A., Wagner, E., Koepsell, T., Kristal, A., and Patrick, D. (1992). Environmental indicators: A tool for evaluating community-based health-promotion programs. *Am. J. Prev. Med.* **9,** 78–84.

88. Cheadle, A., Psaty, B., Curry, S., Wagner, E., Diehr, P., Koepsell, T., and Kristal, A. (1993). Can measures of the grocery story environment be used to track community-level dietary changes? *Prev. Med.* **22,** 361–372.

89. Cheadle, A., Psaty, B., Diehr, P., Koepsell, T., Wagner, E., Curry, S., and Kristal, A. (1995). Evaluating community-based nutrition programs: Comparing grocery store and individual-level survey measures of program impact. *Prev. Med.* **24,** 71–79.

90. Karr, S., Lampe, J., Hutchins, A., and Slavin, J. (1997). Urinary isoflavonoid excretion in humans is dose-dependent at low to moderate levels of soy protein consumption. *Am. J. Clin. Nutr.* **66,** 46–51.

91. Seow, A., Shi, C., Franke, A., Hankin, J., Lee, H., and Yu, M. (1998). Isoflavonoid levels in spot urine are associated with frequency of dietary soy intake in a population-based sample of middle-aged and older Chinese in Singapore. *Cancer Epidemiol. Biomarkers Prev.* **7,** 135–140.

92. Stanford, J. L., King, I., and Kristal, A. R. (1991). Long-term storage of red blood cells and correlations between red cell and dietary fatty acids: Results from a pilot study. *Nutr. Cancer* **16,** 183–188.

93. Agren, J., Hanninen, O., Julkunen, A., Fogelholm, L., Vidgred, H., Schwab, U., Pynnonen, O., and Uusitupa, M. (1996). Fish diet, fish oil and docosahexaeonic acid rich oil lower fasting and postrandial plasma lipid levels. *Eur. J. Clin. Nutr.* **50,** 765–771.

94. Burr, M., Fehily, A., Gilbert, J., Rogers, S., Holliday, R., Sweetnam, P., Elwood, P., and Deadman, N. (1989). Effects of changes in fat, fish, and fibre intakes on death and myocardial reinfarction: Diet and reinfarction trial (DART). *Lancet* **2,** 757–761.

95. Chung, F., Jiao, D., Getahun, S., and Yu, M. (1998). A urinary biomarker for uptake of dietary isothiocynates in humans. *Cancer Epidemiol. Biomarkers Prev.* **7,** 103–108.

96. Seow, A., Shi, C., Chung, F., Jioa, D., Hankin, J., Lee, H., Coetzee, G., and Yu, M. (1998). Urinary total isothiocynate (ITC) in a population-based sample of middle-aged and older Chinese in Singapore: Relationship with dietary total ITC and glutothione S-transferase M1/T1/P1 genotypes. *Cancer Epidemiol. Biomarkers Prev.* **7,** 775–781.

97. McDougall, J., Litzau, K., Haver, E., Saunders, V., and Spiller, G. (1995). Rapid reduction of serum cholesterol and blood pressure by a twelve-day, very low fat, strictly vegetarian diet. *J. Amer. Coll. Nutr.* **14,** 491–496.

98. Howell, W., McNamara, D., Tosca, M., Smith, B., and Gaines, J. (1997). Plasma lipid and lipoprotein responses to dietary fat and cholesterol: A meta-analysis. *Am. J. Clin. Nutr.* **65,** 1747–1764.

99. Green, L. W., and Kreuter, M. W. (1991). *Health promotion planning: an educational and environmental approach.* Mountain View, CA: Mayfield Publishing.

100. Paradis, G., O'Loughlin, J., Elliot, M., Masson, P., Renaud, L., Sacks-Silver, G., and Lampron, G. (1995). Coeur en sante St-Henri—A heart health promotion programme in a low income, low education neighborhood in Montreal, Canada: theoretical model and early field experience. *J. Epidemiol. Comm. Health* **49,** 503–512.

101. Richardson, N., Shepherd, R., and Elliman, N. (1993). Current attitudes and future influences on meat consumption in the U.K. *Appetite,* **1993,** 41–51.

102. Brewer, J., Blake, A., Rankin, S., and Douglass, L. (1999). Theory of reasoned action predicts milk consumption in women. *J. Am. Diet. Assoc.* **99,** 33–44.

103. Kloeblen, A., and Batish, S. (1999). Understanding the intention to permanently follow a high folate diet among a sample of low-income pregnant women according to the health belief model. *Health Educ. Res.* **14,** 327–338.

104. Schafer, R., Keith, P., and Schafer, E. (1995). Predicting fat in diets of marital partners using the health belief model. *J. Behav. Med.* **18,** 419–433.

105. Ling, A., and Howarth, C. (1999). Self-efficacy and consumption of fruit and vegetables: Validation of a summated scale. *Am. J. Health Promotion* **13,** 290–298.

106. Shannon, J., Kirkley, B., Ammerman, A., Keyserling, T., Kelsey, K., DeVellis, R., and Simpson, R. (1997). Self-efficacy as a predictor of dietary change in a low-socioeconomic-status southern adult population. *Health Educ. Behav.* **24,** 357–368.

107. Glanz, K., Patterson, R. E., Kristal, A. R., Di Clemente, C. C., Heimendinger, J., Linnan, L., and McLerran, D. F. (1994). Stages of change in adopting healthy diets: Fat, fiber, and correlates of nutrient intake. *Health Educ Q* **21,** 499–519.

108. Campbell, M., Symons, M., Demark-Wahnefried, W., Polhamus, B., Bernhardt, J., McClelland, J., and Washington, C. (1998). Stages of change and psychosocial correlates of fruit and vegetable consumption among rural African-American church members. *Am. J. Health Promotion* **12,** 185–191.

109. Nitzke, S., Auld, G., McNulty, J., Bock, M., Bruhn, C., Gabel, K., Lauritzen, G., Lee Y., Medeiros, D., Newman, R., Ortiz, M., Read, M., Schutz, H., and Sheehan, E. (1999). Stages of change for reducing fat and increasing fiber among dietitians and adults with a diet-related chronic disease. *J. Am. Diet. Assoc.* **99,** 728–731.

110. Graves, K., and Shannon, B. (1983). Using visual plate waste measurement to assess school lunch behavior. *J. Am. Diet. Assoc.* **83,** 163–165.

CHAPTER **10**

Biomarkers and Biological Indicators of Change

JOHANNA W. LAMPE[1] AND CHERYL L. ROCK[2]
[1]*Fred Hutchinson Cancer Research Center, Seattle, Washington*
[2]*University of California at San Diego, La Jolla, California*

I. INTRODUCTION

A biomarker or biological indicator is a characteristic that is measured and evaluated as a marker of normal biological processes, pathogenic processes, or responses to an intervention. In theory, almost any measurement that reflects a change in a biochemical process, structure, or function can be used as a biomarker. In addition, an exogenous compound that, as a result of ingestion, inhalation, or absorption, can be measured in tissues or body fluids can also be considered a biomarker.

Biomarkers can be classified broadly into markers of exposure, effect, and susceptibility and have numerous applications in nutrition. They can be used to assess dietary intakes (exposure); biochemical or physiologic responses to a dietary behavior or nutrition intervention (effect); and predisposition to a particular disease or response to treatment (genetic susceptibility).

Although certain biologic markers, such as serum cholesterol and glucose, have been used by clinicians for generations, use of biomarkers has taken on new importance with the dramatic advances in various fields of biology and desire for objective measures in large-scale, population-based descriptive and intervention nutrition research. Exquisitely sensitive laboratory techniques can detect subtle alterations in molecular processes that reflect events known or believed to occur along the continuum between health and disease.

This chapter presents the basic concepts and key issues related to the various uses of biomarkers in nutrition; it is not intended to be a comprehensive review. Identification and use of biomarkers is continuously evolving with the growing understanding of biologic processes and the improved sensitivity of laboratory assays. Consequently, our examples of existing biomarkers are mere snapshots in the greater scheme of biomarker development and application.

II. BIOMARKERS OF DIETARY INTAKE OR EXPOSURE

Biomarkers are used to monitor dietary exposure and for nutritional assessment for several reasons. One reason is to provide biochemical data on nutritional status by generating objective evidence that enables evaluation of dietary adequacy or ranking of individuals on exposure to particular nutrients or dietary constituents. Biochemical or biological measurements may also be collected to provide objective evidence of a dietary pattern, such as overall fruit and vegetable consumption, or to validate dietary assessment instruments or self-reported dietary data. Another possible purpose for obtaining these biological measures is to establish the biological link between the nutritional factor and a physiological or biochemical process, when the concentration of the micronutrient or dietary constituent is measured in a peripheral tissue.

A. Biomarkers of Nutrient Intake

Biochemical measures of nutrients can be a valuable component of nutritional assessment and monitoring. Overall, the usefulness of biochemical indicators of nutritional status or exposure is based on knowledge of the physiologic and other determinants of the measure. For several micronutrients, the concentration of the nutrient in the circulating body pool (i.e., serum) appears to be a reasonably accurate reflection of overall status for the nutrient (Table 1). In contrast, the amount of some micronutrients in the circulating pool may be homeostatically regulated when the storage pool is adequate, or may be unrelated to intake, and thus has little relationship with total body reserves or overall status. Figure 1 illustrates the relation between various compartments or body pools that may be sampled in the measurement of biological indicators.

Knowledge of the influencing nondietary factors is particularly important for accurate interpretation of the nutrient concentration in tissues. For example, tocopherols and carotenoids are transported in the circulation nonspecifically by the cholesterol-rich lipoproteins [1, 2], so higher concentrations of these lipoproteins are predictive of higher concentrations of the associated micronutrients in the circulation, independent of dietary intake or total body pool. Smoking and alcohol consumption need to be considered in the interpretation

139

TABLE 1   Biomarkers of Nutrient Intake[a]

Nutrient	Biomarkers of dietary exposure	Possible functional markers
Dietary fiber, nonstarch polysaccharides	• Fecal hemicellulose	• Fecal weight • Fecal short-chain fatty acids
Thiamin		• Erythrocyte transketolase activation
Biotin	• Urinary 3-hydroxy-isovalerate with a loading dose of leucine	• Erthrocyte pyruvate carboxylase activity
Riboflavin	• Plasma FAD • Erythrocyte FAD	• EGRAC
Niacin	• Erythrocyte NAD • Urinary metabolites of niacin	• Erythrocyte nicotinate-nucleotide: pyrophosphate phosphoribosyltransferase activity (not very responsive)
Vitamin B$_6$	• Plasma pyridoxal 5-phosphate • Urinary 4-pyridoxic acid	• Erythrocyte aspartate or alanine aminotransferase
Folate	• Plasma folate • Erythrocyte folate	• Plasma homocysteine
Vitamin B$_{12}$	• Plasma B$_{12}$	
Vitamin C	• Plasma vitamin C • Erythrocyte, lymphocyte, or platelet vitamin C	• Urinary deoxypyridinoline:total collagen cross-links • Urinary carnitine
Vitamin A	• Plasma retinol:retinol-binding protein	
Vitamin E	• α- and/or γ-tocopherol in serum or plasma, erythrocytes, lymphocytes, lipoproteins, adipose tissue, or buccal mucosal cells	• LDL oxidation • Breath pentane and ethane • Platelet adhesion and aggregation
Vitamin D	• Serum 25-hydroxyvitamin D	
Vitamin K	• Plasma vitamin K	• Plasma prothrombin concentrations
Phosphorus	• Serum inorganic phosphate	
Magnesium	• Erythrocyte or lymphocyte magnesium	
Calcium	• Calcium retention	• Bone mass • Serum osteocalcin • Serum levels of skeletal alkaline phosphatase • Urinary and serum measures of collagen turnover

(continues)

of serum and other tissue concentrations of several micronutrients, particularly compounds that may be subject to oxidation (e.g., vitamin C, tocopherols, carotenoids, folate). Knowledge of the relationship between the indicator and the risk of nutrient depletion, in addition to the responsiveness of the indicator to interventions or change, is also necessary [3]. For some nutrients, such as calcium and zinc, a specific sensitive exposure marker of diet simply has not yet been identified.

Table 1 lists examples of biochemical measures of nutrients that may serve as useful biomarkers in nutritional assessment or monitoring of dietary intake. For more details, the reader is referred to in-depth reviews addressing the use of biomarkers for assessing nutrient exposure [4–7]. Unfortunately, a static measurement (i.e., a tissue concentration) is typically not as sensitive as a functional marker in the as-

sessment of status; however, a good functional measure is still lacking in many instances.

B. Biomarkers of Other Dietary Exposures

Numerous dietary constituents, particularly of plant origin, although not recognized as essential for life, have demonstrated biologic activity and are thought to play an important role in prevention of chronic disease [8, 9]. These phytochemicals are absorbed to various degrees, often metabolized in the intestinal epithelium and liver, and excreted; thus, the metabolites can be monitored in serum or plasma and/or urine.

Some classes of compounds such as flavonoids are found in many plant foods, whereas others such as isoflavones are limited to select sources (Table 2). The isoflavones, daidzein

TABLE 1 *(continued)*

Nutrient	Biomarkers of dietary exposure	Possible functional markers
Iron		• Serum ferritin[b] • Transferrin saturation • Erythrocyte protoporphyrin • Mean corpuscular volume • Serum transferrin receptor • Hemoglobin or packed cell volume
Copper	• Platelet copper	• Erythrocyte SOD • Platelet cytochrome c oxidase activity • Serum peptidylglycine α-aminating monooxygenase activity? • Plasma diamine oxidase
Zinc		• Erythrocyte metallothionein • Erythrocyte SOD • Monocyte metallothionein mRNA • Serum thymulin activity • Plasma 5-nucleotidase activity
Manganese	• Serum manganese	• Lymphocyte Mn-SOD activity • Blood arginase activity
Molybdenum		• Urinary levels of sulfate, uric acid, sulfite, hypoxanthine, xanthine, and other sulfur-containing compounds
Iodine	• Plasma iodine • Urinary iodine	• Plasma TSH, T_4, and T_3 (total and free)
Selenium	• Plasma or whole-blood selenium • Hair or toenail selenium	• Plasma GSH peroxidase activities • Erythrocyte GSH peroxidase activities • Blood cell selenoperoxidase activities • Plasma T_4 and T_3

Key: FAD, flavin adenine dinucleotide; EGRAC, FAD-dependent erythrocyte glutatione reductase activation coefficient; NAD, nicotinamide adenine dinucleotide; LDL, low-density lipoprotein; GSH, glutathione; SOD, superoxide dismutase; TSH, thyroid-stimulating hormone; T_3, triiodothyronine; T_4, thyroxine.

[a]Direct measures of dietary exposure and nutrient-specific functional markers. This table includes both established markers and additional markers that show promise.

[b]In approximate order of increasing severity of iron shortage [104].

and genistein, are highly concentrated in soybeans and soy products [10, 11]. Urinary isoflavone excretion is associated strongly and directly with soy protein intake under con-

trolled dietary conditions [12]. In observational studies of populations that usually consume soy, soyfood intake and urinary isoflavonoid excretion also are positively correlated

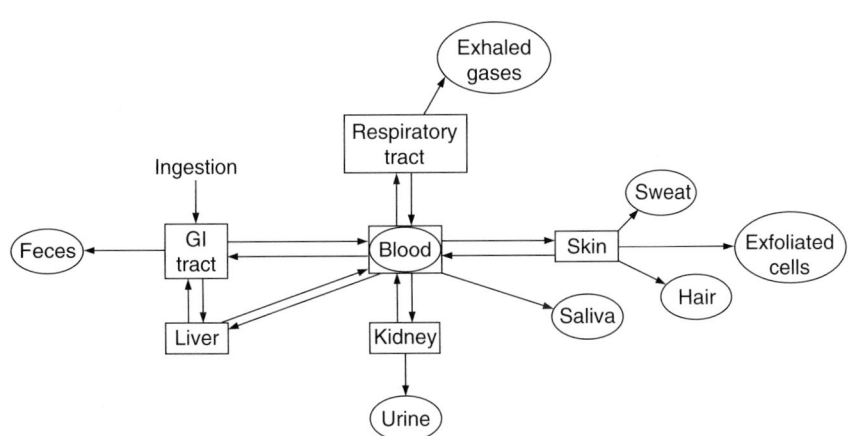

FIGURE 1 The relation between body compartments and biological specimens that can be assayed for dietary indicators.

TABLE 2 Phytochemical Content of Plant Food Families and Select Plant Foods[a]

Plant foods	Flavonoids	Isoflavones	Lignans	Carotenoids	Organosulfides	Isothiocyanates	Terpenes	Phytates
Cruciferae[b]	✓			✓	✓	✓	✓	
Rutaceae[c]	✓			✓			✓	
Alliaceae[d]	✓			✓	✓		✓	
Solanaceae[e]	✓			✓			✓	
Umbelliferae[f]	✓			✓			✓	
Curcurbitaceae[g]	✓			✓			✓	
Cereals	✓		✓				✓	✓
Soybeans	✓	✓		✓			✓	✓
Flaxseed	✓		✓					
Measurable in biological samples[h]	U, P	U, P, S	U, P, S	P	B	U	P	P, S

Source: Adapted from Caragay, A. B. (1992). Cancer-preventive foods and ingredients. *Food Technol.* **46**, 65–68; and Fahey, J. W., Clevidence, B. A., and Russell, R. M. (1999). Methods for assessing the biological effects of specific plant components. *Nutr. Rev.* **57**, S34–S40.

[a]Some phytochemicals are present in most plant foods; others are restricted to particular botanical families or even particular plant species.

[b]Cabbage family; [c]citrus; [d]onion family; [e]tomato family; [f]carrot family; [g]squash family.

[h]U, urine; P, plasma or serum; S, stool; B, breath.

[13–15]. Because the plasma half-lives of the isoflavones genistein and daidzein are short (6–8 hours) [16], intermittent soy consumption may be under- or overestimated if isoflavone exposure is monitored in plasma or spot urine specimens. Metabolism of isoflavones is also inextricably linked to the health of colonic bacterial populations, and therefore plasma and urinary levels may be influenced by the effects of diet and drugs on the colonic environment.

Dietary exposure to flavonoids and other polyphenols can be monitored by measuring parent compounds and metabolites in urine or plasma [17, 18]. Several compounds in cruciferous vegetables, such as sulforaphane and other isothiocyanates, have been of interest due to their potential chemopreventive effects. Although, with present technologies, levels of these compounds are typically too low to measure directly in plasma, dithiocarbamates (metabolites of isothiocyanates) can be quantified in urine, following extraction and measurement by high-performance liquid chromatography; these provide a measure of cruciferous vegetable exposure [19].

Biomarkers also exist for monitoring exposure to less desirable food constituents, such as mycotoxins (e.g., aflatoxin) in mold-contaminated grain products and pyrolysis products that result from cooking meat at high temperatures (e.g., heterocyclic amines). Because of the nature of these compounds, exposure to potentially carcinogenic compounds can be determined by measuring the presence of adducts—the result of covalent binding of the chemicals to proteins or to nucleic acids in DNA. The rationale for using measurements of carcinogen-DNA adducts is based on the assumption that DNA adducts formed *in vivo* are responsible for genetic alterations in genes critical for carcinogenesis and that protein adducts formed through the same processes reflect the formation of DNA adducts [20]. Because adducts represent an integration of exposure and interindividual variability in carcinogen metabolism and DNA repair, they may provide a more relevant measure of exposure, i.e., a biologically effective dose [20]. Some adducts are specific for dietary exposure; aflatoxin-albumin adducts result from ingestion of aflatoxin. Other adducts, such as benzo[a]pyrene-DNA adducts, are nonspecific because benzo[a]pyrene comes from a variety of sources besides diet, including air pollution, tobacco, and occupational exposures. Adducts can be used to monitor exposure within individuals. They can also serve as early markers of the efficacy of interventions designed to prevent exposure to genotoxic agents or to modify the metabolism of procarcinogens once exposure has occurred. An example of this latter use is an intervention to reduce aflatoxin-albumin adducts using the drug oltipraz [21].

C. Biomarkers of Energy Intake

To date, few biological measures are available that objectively monitor energy intake, and those that are available are cumbersome in free-living populations and/or expensive. Under steady-state conditions, indirect calorimetry provides an estimate of energy expenditure and some insight about intake. Indirect calorimetry estimates the rate of oxidation or energy expenditure from the rate of oxygen consumption (Vo_2) and the rate of carbon dioxide production (Vco_2). This technique is relatively inexpensive and portable, although some participant cooperation is required. These traits make the technique attractive primarily for clinical applications [22].

Energy expenditure can also be measured using a doubly labeled water technique [23], as discussed in detail in another

chapter (see Chapter 2). This method uses nonradioactive isotopes of hydrogen (^{2}H) and oxygen (^{18}O) to measure free-living total energy expenditure by monitoring urinary isotope excretion. Energy expenditures determined by room calorimetry, indirect calorimetry, and doubly labeled water measures are not significantly different within the calorimeter environment; however, in free-living subjects, doubly labeled water-derived energy expenditures are found to be 13–15% higher than those for other methods [24]. The doubly labeled water method has the distinct advantage of allowing the subjects to go about their usual activities with energy expenditure calculated after a study period of 7–14 days. Unfortunately, the ^{18}O isotope required to conduct doubly labeled water studies is expensive and is often in short supply. Although doubly labeled water methodology is suited to nutrition research aimed at quantifying total energy expenditure for specific groups, the cost for large samples limits broad use.

D. Biomarkers as General Dietary Indicators

Monitoring overall dietary patterns or changes in patterns in response to dietary interventions presents additional challenges. The goal in this case is to assess and monitor the intake of certain types of foods or food groups, rather than specific nutrients; therefore, these dietary indicators ideally should be distributed generally within certain types of foods.

Plasma carotenoids provide a good example of the use of biomarkers as a dietary indicator when the goal is to assess and monitor dietary patterns. Vegetables and fruits contribute the vast majority of carotenoids in the diet, and plasma carotenoid concentrations have been shown to be useful biomarkers of vegetable and fruit intakes in cross-sectional descriptive studies, controlled feeding studies, and clinical trials [25–28]. The consistency of this relationship across diverse groups and involving various concurrent diet manipulations (with differences in amounts of dietary factors that could alter carotenoid bioavailability) is notable, although considerable interindividual variation in the degree of response is typically observed. Also, nondietary factors that are among the determinants of plasma carotenoid concentrations (e.g., body mass, plasma cholesterol concentration) will influence the absolute concentration that is observed in response to dietary intake, so these characteristics must be used as adjustment factors.

Although vitamin C also is provided predominantly by fruits and vegetables in the diet, this measure is much less useful as a biomarker of this dietary pattern because the relationship between vitamin C intake and plasma concentration is linear only up to a certain threshold [29]. The use of vitamin C supplements (which is common in the U. S. population) often increases the intake level beyond the range in which linearity between intake and plasma concentration occurs, and thus obscures the relationship between food choices and tissue concentrations.

Lignans are a group of compounds present in high-fiber foods, particularly cereals and fruits [30]. These compounds are not found in animal products and, similar to carotenoids, may be useful markers of a plant-based diet [31]. Lignans provide an example of how using dietary constituents as biomarkers requires an understanding of the metabolism of the compounds. Lignans in plant foods are altered by intestinal microflora, so that the specific compounds, enterodiol and enterolactone, monitored in plasma or urine are actually bacterial metabolites. Because of this bacterial conversion, lignan concentrations in urine or plasma in response to a similar dietary dose will vary significantly among individuals. In addition, nondietary factors (e.g., use of oral antibiotics) will reduce enterolactone and enterodiol production [32].

As another example, the fatty acid composition of membrane phospholipids is in part determined by the omega-6 and omega-3 fatty acid composition of the diet. Thus, the fatty acid pattern of serum phospholipids or plasma aliquots has been used as a biomarker of compliance with omega-3 fatty acid supplementation in clinical trials [33, 34]. Although enzyme selectivities and other physiologic factors are also important determinants of the fatty acid composition of phospholipids, a diet high in omega-3 polyunsaturated fats will result in increased amounts of eicosapentaeneoic and docosahexaenoic acids in circulating tissue pools.

Specific fatty acids also can be associated with certain types of foods. Pentadecanoic acid (15:0) and heptadecanoic acid (17:0) are fatty acids produced by bacteria in the rumen of ruminant animals. These fatty acids, with uneven numbers of carbon atoms, are not synthesized by humans; therefore, their presence in human biologic samples can be indicative of dietary exposure to milk fat. Proportions of 15:0 and 17:0 in adipose tissue and concentrations of 15:0 in serum have been found to correlate with milk fat intake in men and women [35, 36].

III. FUNCTIONAL BIOMARKERS

If a nutrient or dietary constituent has an identified impact on physiologic, biochemical, or genetic factors, measuring markers of those functional effects can be extremely useful. Such functional indices can be classified as those which are measures of *discrete* functions of a nutritional factor and those which are measures of more *general* functions [37]. A discrete functional index often relates to the first limiting biochemical system, for example, a particular enzymatic pathway [38]. These markers can be used to identify the dosage or concentration of a nutritional factor necessary to achieve a clinically meaningful response or to define optimum nutrient status (Table 1). Unfortunately, for many nutritional factors, the first limiting biochemical system is unknown or not readily measured or accessible in humans. A general functional index is less specific, but may be more directly linked to the pathogenesis of disease or ill health.

Often a panel of markers, rather than one specific measure, provides a better picture. Examples of general functional indices or markers are oxidative stress, immune function, bone health, and cell turnover—processes that have been shown to play roles in the risk of various diseases.

For a functional index to be an effective nutritional biomarker, a cause-and-effect relationship must be established between (1) nutritional status and the functional index, (2) between the functional index and ill health, and (3) between nutrient status and ill health. Such an undertaking is a daunting and time-consuming task, but is especially important if a functional biomarker is going to be used as a proxy, or surrogate, for a clinical endpoint or disease outcome. A clinical endpoint is a characteristic or variable that measures how a patient feels, functions, or survives. A surrogate endpoint biomarker is an index whose modulation has been shown to be indicative of progression or reversal of the disease process; it is a biomarker that is intended to substitute for a clinical endpoint. In an intervention trial, the use of surrogate endpoint biomarkers (rather than the frank diagnosis of disease) requires substantially less time and fewer resources in the evaluation of efforts aimed toward reducing risk for chronic diseases such as cancer, cardiovascular disease, and osteoporosis [39].

To date, very few markers have been established as true surrogate endpoint biomarkers; i.e., they cannot accurately substitute for a clinical endpoint [40]. The evidence supporting the linkage of a biomarker to a clinical endpoint may be derived from epidemiologic studies, clinical trials, *in vitro* analyses, animal models, and simulated biologic systems. Many biomarkers have been proposed as potential surrogate endpoints, but relatively few are likely to achieve this status because of the complexity of disease mechanisms and the limited capability of a single biomarker to reflect the collective impact of multiple therapeutic effects on ultimate outcome.

A. Biomarkers of Enzyme Function

Understanding how diet influences enzyme systems is important in developing strategies for disease prevention and treatment. For example, dietary modulation of enzymes involved in carcinogen metabolism may be important in reducing cancer risk, and dietary intervention that reduces expression of rate-limiting enzymes in cholesterol synthesis may alter cardiovascular disease risk. Enzymes that require micronutrients as cofactors are also used as biomarkers of nutritional status (Table 1).

Components of diet have the capacity to modulate protein synthesis and function. An ideal discrete functional marker would be one that reflects the direct effect of a dietary constituent—for example, mRNA amount when the dietary factor regulates gene expression or level of enzyme activity when the factor acts as a competitive inhibitor of the enzyme (Fig. 2). Unfortunately, at present, monitoring at these levels

in the pathway in an intact human is not always feasible. Often, we rely primarily on a downstream marker, whose measurement may be influenced by subsequent or parallel pathways and may give a diluted signal.

Often the enzymes of interest are located primarily in tissues that are not readily accessible (e.g., liver, intestine, lung). One approach to meeting this challenge is to measure the enzymes in more accessible tissue; for example, enzymes that are present in high levels in the liver can often be measured in plasma or serum as a result of normal hepatocyte turnover. Enzyme activity of glutathione *S*-transferase (GST), a biotransformation enzyme important in carcinogen detoxification, can be measured spectrophotometrically in serum [41] or concentrations of the enzyme itself can be determined in serum by immunoassay [42]. Serum concentration of the GST isoenzyme GST-α has been shown to increase when cruciferous vegetables are added to the diet [42]. A limitation of using serum measures of a hepatic enzyme is that the assumption is made that liver function is normal. Thus, including other measures of liver function in the data collection is important to verify that no underlying hepatic disease is resulting in spurious GST values. Additionally, some enzymes are present in isoforms in various tissues. GST-μ, another GST isoenzyme, is present in lymphocytes as well as in liver; therefore, for this isoenzyme, GST activity or protein concentration can be measured in cells extracted from blood samples.

Another approach to monitor enzyme activity *in vivo* is to use a drug probe. Many of the same xenobiotic metabolizing enzymes that metabolize carcinogens also metabolize and are modulated by commonly used drugs. The metabolites of these drugs can be monitored in serum, plasma, or urine and used to determine enzyme activities. For example, caffeine metabolites measured in urine samples collected 4 hours after consumption of 500 mg caffeine allows determination of cytochrome P450 1A2, *N*-acetyltransferase, and xanthine oxidase activities [43], and urinary concentrations of the glucuronide and sulfate conjugates of acetaminophen (paracetamol) are used to measure UDP-glucuronosyltransferase and sulfotransferase activities [44]. Drugs can be administered as probes during a nutrition intervention to determine the degree of change in enzyme activity in response to diet or in population-based studies to examine gene–environment interactions [45–47].

Measurement of arachidonic acid metabolism, which involves measuring the concentration of prostaglandins or leukotrienes (metabolic products) or enzymes in the eicosanoid metabolic pathway (i.e., cyclooxygenase), provides another example. Altered arachidonic acid metabolism is among the biochemical activities of nonsteroidal anti-inflammatory agents and may also be influenced by antioxidant micronutrients, such as vitamin E [48], and quantitative changes in these products or enzymes in tissues serve as biomarkers of this activity [49]. A reasonable amount of biological evidence suggests some role for this enzymatic pathway in co-

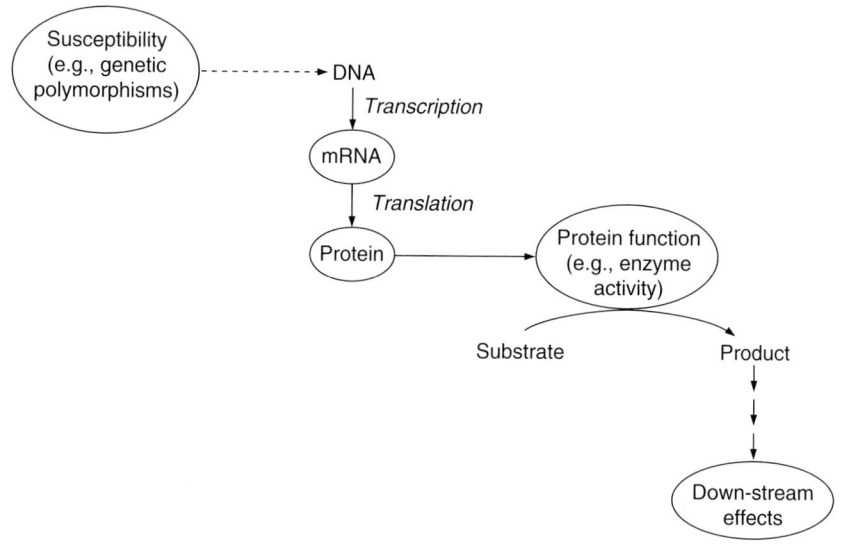

FIGURE 2   Direct functional markers of dietary exposure.

lon carcinogenesis [50], but the overall relationship with disease process is still under investigation.

Similarly, endogenous compounds can serve as probes to monitor enzyme activity. Serum concentrations of the amino acid homocysteine, compared to serum and red blood cell folate concentration, are a more sensitive systemic measure of cellular folate depletion [51, 52]. Serum concentrations of homocysteine increase with folate inadequacy because the remethylation of homocysteine requires N-5-methyltetrahydrofolate as a cosubstrate [53], which therefore provides a functional marker for folate status. Nonetheless, because homocysteine is at the intersection of two metabolic pathways, remethylation and transsulfuration, deficiencies in other nutrients in these pathways, namely, vitamin B_{12}, vitamin B_6, and possibly riboflavin, can contribute to elevated serum homocysteine concentrations [51].

B. Biomarkers of Oxidative Stress

Oxidative stress has been suggested to play a role in the pathophysiologic disease process in cancer, atherosclerotic cardiovascular disease, and many other acute and chronic conditions [54], although the specific relationship with the disease process remains to be established in most instances. Cellular damage caused by reactive oxygen species, which are generated from cellular respiration, co-oxidation during metabolism, and the activity of phagocytic cells of the immune system, is controlled by antioxidant defense mechanisms that involve several micronutrients. Oxidative stress describes the condition of oxidative damage resulting when the balance between free-radical generation and antioxidant defenses is unfavorable. Direct measurement of active oxygen and related species in biological samples is very challenging, mainly because these compounds have very short half-lives. Thus, the oxidative stress biomarkers used in human studies are typically adducts or endproducts that reflect

reactions that have occurred between free radicals and compounds such as lipids, proteins, carbohydrates, DNA, and other molecules that are potential targets [55].

One frequently described assay used as an oxidative stress biomarker is the thiobarbituric acid reactive substances (TBARS) assay. The TBARS assay basically quantifies a product of malondialdehyde, which presumably reflects lipid hydroperoxides in the sample. However, this assay has some serious limitations in specificity, and the product measured cannot be interpreted as directly reflecting lipid peroxidation *in vivo* [55]. Direct measurement of malondialdehyde in biological samples using high-performance liquid chromatography (HPLC) has also been examined as an alterative approach, although the specificity of this more direct HPLC measurement has also not been established to the level desirable.

Measurement of breath pentane is another biomarker of oxidative stress that has been utilized in human studies [56]. The approach basically involves collecting exhaled air for the measurement of the products of peroxidation of unsaturated fatty acids, a portion of which are volatile and released in the breath, using gas chromatography methods. However, the specific measurement methodologies vary a great deal and are not always reliable, and standardization of the procedure and knowledge of various influencing factors are needed to improve the usefulness of this approach [55].

Another biomarker of oxidative stress is the measurement of urinary 8-hydroxydeoxyguanosine (8OHdG) using HPLC and electrochemical detection [57]. The 8-hydroxylation of the guanine base is a frequent type of oxidative DNA damage, and 8OHdG is subsequently excreted without further metabolism in the urine after repair *in vivo* by exonucleases. In previous studies, certain demographic factors and physiologic characteristics such as gender and body mass [58] have been observed to influence urinary 8OHdG concentration, so these factors may need to be considered in interpretation.

Urinary 8OHdG is increased in association with conditions known to be characterized by increased oxidative stress, such as smoking, whole-body irradiation, and cytotoxic chemotherapy [57–59]. Urinary 8OHdG (unadjusted or adjusted for urinary creatinine) has also been observed to decline in response to a high-vegetable and fruit diet intervention in human subjects [60], which is particularly interesting because this type of diet has been suggested to promote reduced oxidative stress [8, 60, 61].

Prostaglandin-like compounds produced by nonenzymatic free-radical-catalyzed peroxidation of arachidonic acid, termed F_2 isoprostanes, are currently of great interest as useful biomarkers of oxidative damage [62]. Specific gas chromatography/mass spectrometry assays for the measurement of some of these compounds, such as iPF2a-III (also called 8-iso-$PGPF_2$) and iPF2-VI, have been developed and used to quantify the compounds in urine and blood samples. These markers have been shown to be less variable than 8OHdG [63], and elevated levels have been observed in plasma and urine samples from subjects under a wide variety of conditions of enhanced oxidative stress [64, 65].

Another approach to measuring DNA oxidative damage that appears to be useful in human nutrition research is the measurement of 5-hydroxymethyluracil levels in DNA in blood. 5-Hydroxymethyluracil is produced when DNA is exposed to oxidants, is relatively stable when compared to other oxidation products, and can be quantified with gas chromatography/mass spectrometry [66, 67]. In a small cross-sectional study, 5-hydroxymethyluracil concentration was observed to be inversely associated with cooked vegetables and directly related to beef and pork intakes in the diets of women enrolled in a low-fat diet intervention trial [68].

Oxidative damage to low-density lipoprotein (LDL) has been specifically linked to atherogenesis, and in an application of this biological activity, measurement of LDL oxidation *ex vivo* has been used in clinical studies as a biomarker of oxidative stress [69]. Basically, this process involves isolating the LDL fraction from a blood sample, exposing this fraction to oxidants such as Cu^{2+}, and measuring the lag time before oxidation. Although this biomarker might appear to be specific to cardiovascular disease risk, results from this assay have not yet been specifically linked with risk for disease, so results should be interpreted as simply another approach to the assessment of oxidative stress [55]. Also, various specific methodologies are used across laboratories, and the lack of standardization in the approaches in use constrains the ability to make comparisons across studies.

Several other approaches to measuring biomarkers of oxidative stress have been proposed and are under study, and the reader is referred to a review of this topic [55]. Because of their inherent variability, and uncertain responsiveness to dietary manipulations, clinical researchers often employ a panel of potential measures of oxidative stress, rather than relying on a single indicator [60].

C. Biomarkers of Immune Function

The human immune system is a complex and highly interactive network of cells and their products that has a central role in protecting against various external disease-promoting factors and perhaps against malignant cells. Many of the components of the immune system can serve as biomarkers and are monitored *in vivo* or *ex vivo* [70, 71]. Because of the complexity of the system, the selection of assays should be closely aligned with the research question being asked. Furthermore, multiple parameters need to be measured; one single biomarker is inadequate to monitor immune function.

Cell-mediated immune variables include the absolute amounts or ratios of various white blood cell (WBC) types (e.g., total counts, WBC differentials, T-cell subsets) and measures of T-cell function (e.g., lymphocyte proliferation, cytokine release from mitogen-stimulated cultures, cytotoxic capacities, delayed-type hypersensitivity). Both number and activity of natural killer cells (one of the cell types that plays an important role in immune surveillance) are used as biomarkers in nutrition intervention trials [72, 73]. Cytokines (e.g., the interleukins) are soluble factors released by immune cells, which control and direct the function of other immune effectors. Some of these have been used as markers of immune response in randomized trials of vitamin supplementation [73, 74].

An *in vivo* functional test, the delayed-type hypersensitivity (DTH) skin test is widely used to monitor the immune system in humans, including in studies of dietary modulation of immune function [75]. It measures the capacity of an individual's immune system to mount a response to antigenic stimulation. The DTH test typically involves the simultaneous intradermal application of one or several DTH antigens. These antigens elicit an immunologic reaction involving the release of lymphokines by antigen-sensitized T cells. These compounds, in turn, activate macrophages, which release inflammatory mediators, resulting in measurable skin induration.

D. Biomarkers of Bone Health

Bone mass measurements and biomarkers of bone turnover are used as functional indices of bone health and, to a certain extent, can also be used as markers of the adequacy of calcium intake. Measures of bone mass include bone mineral content (BMC; i.e, the amount of mineral at a particular skeletal site, such as the femoral neck, lumbar spine, or total body) and bone mineral density (BMD; i.e., bone mineral content divided by the area of the scanned region); both are strong predictors of fracture risk [76–78]. Controlled calcium intervention trials that measure change in BMD provide evidence for the intake requirement for calcium [79] (see Chapter 42 for more details).

Biochemical markers of bone turnover predict bone mass changes and fracture risk, and respond to dietary calcium

intake [79]; thus, they provide some promise for a biochemical indicator of calcium status. Unlike BMD, they reflect more subtle changes in bone metabolism. Bone turnover is the cyclical process by which the skeleton undergoes renewal by a coupled, but time-separated, sequence of bone resorption and bone formation [80]. Markers of bone turnover rely on the measurement in serum or urine of enzymes or matrix proteins synthesized by osteoblasts or osteoclasts that spill over into body fluids, or of osteoclast-generated degradation products of the bone matrix [79]. Currently, serum levels of skeletal alkaline phosphatase and osteocalcin are used as markers of bone formation, and products of collagen degradation measured in urine are used to measure bone resorption. These markers exhibit substantial short-term and long-term fluctuations related to time of day, phase of menstrual cycle, and season of the year, as well as other factors that alter bone remodeling (e.g., exercise) [81].

E. Biomarkers of Cell Turnover

Cellular markers of proliferation, differentiation, and apoptosis (i.e., programmed cell death) can be useful as biomarkers in research focused on nutritional factors and cancer, although the measured effect is a general indicator of an altered cell growth regulation effect. Use of such markers is severely restricted by the difficulty accessing the tissue of interest. Consequently, research in this area has been limited primarily to tissue available via endoscopic or fine-needle biopsy procedures, e.g., gastrointestinal tract, breast, prostate.

As a general rule, increased proliferation of undifferentiated cells defines one aspect or characteristic of carcinogenesis, and in colon cancer, this relationship has been well established. For example, cell proliferation occurs at the base of the colonic crypts, and as cells migrate from the crypts to the luminal surface, they become increasingly differentiated and mature and lose their proliferative capabilities [82]. The shift in which the proliferative zone extends to the surface, so that cells on the luminal surface retain proliferative capabilities and are immature and underdifferentiated, may be considered a field defect that sets the stage for current and future neoplastic changes [82–84]. Early work in this area relied on the incorporation of tritiated-thymidine or bromodeoxyuridine into the DNA of dividing cells during incubation of a biopsy specimen. These methods required that the tissue be freshly obtained, so the cells were viable and replicating. Often, label incorporation was incomplete. Now, with increased sensitivity in immunohistochemical techniques, proteins present in proliferating cells (e.g., proliferating cell nuclear antigen [PCNA] and Ki67) are used more widely to quantify proliferative activity in tissue specimens. Labeling indices involving tritiated thymidine and PCNA have been used to quantify the proliferative activity in colonic mucosal samples from human subjects [85] and have been used successfully as endpoints in several nutrition intervention studies to prevent colon cancer [86]. These indi-

ces are being further refined by staining for proteins present during apoptosis (e.g., Bax, Bcl–2) and in differentiated cells, in order to provide a more complete picture of cell dynamics.

Adoption of aberrant crypt foci (early morphologic changes in colonic epithelium that are considered potential precursors of adenomatous polyps) as biomarkers in humans is an example of how improvements in technology have led to the adoption of a biomarker that until recently could only be used in animal studies. Development of magnifying endoscopes with improved resolution now allows investigators to monitor aberrant crypt foci in colon tissue samples from healthy humans [87].

IV. BIOMARKERS OF GENETIC SUSCEPTIBILITY

The health of individuals and the population in general is the result of interaction between genetic and environmental factors. For the great majority of human diseases, purely genetic or purely environmental etiologies are insufficient to explain individual variability in occurrence, prognosis, or outcome [88]. This is especially the case with chronic diseases, such as heart disease and cancer. Genetically determined susceptibility factors alter disease frequency or treatment response through variations in DNA coding sequences of genes. As a result, genetically susceptible individuals produce proteins that are structurally different, or produce them in greater or lesser amounts than individuals who are not at increased risk of disease.

By genetic standards, traits with a frequency of between 1/100 and 1/10,000 in a population are considered uncommon, and rare traits are those with a frequency of less than 1/10,000 [89]. Typically, these are low-prevalence and high-penetrance genes (e.g., genes associated with familial cancers). Common genetic traits are those in which the least common allele is present in at least 1% of the population [89]. Traits with this characteristic are known as genetic polymorphisms. They include the high-prevalence, low-penetrance genes—"susceptibility genes"—thought to contribute to disease risk.

In cases where specific genetic mutations or variations may be indicative of disease risk or progression or may be modified by nutritional factors, genetic markers can also be useful biomarkers. Various molecular techniques have been developed to help characterize genetic abnormalities or differences. Genetic factors are important to consider in nutrition research for several reasons. One reason is that it is increasingly evident that genetic polymorphisms may contribute substantially to differences in the response to environmental and dietary exposures [90]. For example, genetic variations in the expression of the xenobiotic metabolizing enzymes may mediate the potentially carcinogenic effect of heterocyclic amines (obtained from meat cooked at high

temperature) [91] (see also Chapter 13). Also, results from laboratory animal studies suggest that dietary modifications can promote alterations in genetic factors [92], so that measuring genetic abnormalities may be considered an approach to demonstrating a biological link between dietary factors and disease risk.

Some polymorphic traits may only be important in the presence of a particular dietary exposure. For example, carrying the 5, 10-methylene-tetrahydrofolate reductase (MTHFR) thermal-labile variant has been shown to be a risk factor for colorectal adenomatous polyps, but only in the context of low-folate, vitamin B_{12} and vitamin B_6 intake [93].

Given that a goal of the field of nutrition is the prevention and treatment of disease, genetic markers may aid in this effort by identifying population subgroups at high risk of disease in the presence of particular dietary exposures. Genetic susceptibility markers may also strengthen our understanding of disease by focusing attention on possible pathways of disease causation and progression. There is considerable heterogeneity in disease risk within populations; thus, markers of susceptibility may also help to clarify associations between dietary exposures and diseases within population subgroups [94].

V. CRITERIA FOR SELECTING AND USING BIOMARKERS

When a candidate biomarker is identified, certain basic considerations need to be addressed before it can be adopted for use in research or in a clinical setting [95]. These considerations relate to the reliability of the laboratory assay itself, the biologic relevance of the marker, and the characteristics of the marker within a population. Whether or not a particular established marker is used also depends on the purpose the marker will serve.

Development of a biomarker usually builds on scientific knowledge from various types of laboratory studies, including tissue culture and animal studies. In the laboratory, an initial priority is to determine a marker's reliability or reproducibility. Assay performance can be evaluated using coefficients of variation [CV%; (SD/mean) x 100] to estimate within- and between-batch precision; these are measures of analytic, laboratory performance and do not reflect intra- or interindividual variation. The within-batch precision is determined by dividing single samples into multiple aliquots and analyzing them together. Between-batch precision is determined by analyzing multiple aliquots on separate days. It is difficult to generalize about acceptable numerical values for the laboratory CV% because the degree of error acceptable depends on the use of the biomarker data. For epidemiological studies, if the goal is to establish a stable estimate of the group mean, an acceptable CV% may depend on the number of samples available, the mean concentration of the biomarker, and between-individual variation [96]. If a bio-

marker is being used in a clinical setting to diagnose and monitor treatment in an individual, day-to-day quality performance of an assay is imperative. Techniques of quality control [97, 98] and statistical methodologies for managing quality control data [99] have been established and are used in clinical laboratories.

Biomarkers should be relatively easy to measure and require relatively noninvasive techniques of tissue sampling. This requires that the biologic relevance or validity—i.e., the relationship between biomarkers in tissues readily available for human monitoring (e.g., peripheral blood) to those in target tissue (e.g., lung, liver) and the relationship between the biomarker and the disease or exposure being studied—of the measure be established. One example is the use of serum ferritin as a marker of body iron stores. Serum ferritin was validated as a measure of iron stores against bone-marrow examination for stainable iron, the criterion method for—but very invasive way—of measuring iron stores [100]. As a result, serum ferritin has been adopted as a simple, quantitative biomarker of iron stores in otherwise healthy individuals.

If a particular biomarker is to be used as a measure of dietary exposure, it must be evaluated with respect to its sensitivity to that intake. Several approaches, both observational and interventional, can be used to define the relationship between long-term dietary intake and biologic levels. Investigators can rely on geographic differences in exposure: Tissue samples from areas of known nutrient deficiency of a specific nutrient can be compared with samples from average and high-exposure areas. This approach has the advantage that it can reflect the long-term intake of a settled group of individuals; however, identifying and controlling confounding factors is a major challenge [96]. Another observational approach is to establish within individuals the relation between a dietary exposure and the biochemical marker. Participants for such a study can be selected randomly or can be selected specifically in order to maximize the range of intakes. For example, in one study designed to test the use of plasma carotenoids as markers of vegetable and fruit intake, study participants were selected on the basis of their reported vegetable and fruit intake—only those who had intakes ≤2 or ≥5 of servings per day were recruited into the study [26]. Rigorous testing of the relationship between intake of the dietary factor and a biomarker under controlled dietary conditions is also valuable to establish dose–response relations; however, these trials are usually limited to weeks or months and, if they involve extensive changes to usual diet, blinding of participants may not be feasible.

Depending on the biomarker, significant variability can be seen in a biomarker. Sources of variation can be internal (e.g., age, sex, genetics, body build, biologic rhythm) or environmental (e.g., diet, season, time of day, immobilization, exercise, drugs). These can contribute to both within- and interindividual variation. Additional external sources of variation, beyond laboratory accuracy and precision, can in-

clude an individual's posture during sample collection and sample handling and storage; protocols should be established to minimize these latter sources of variability.

Selection of a biomarker is dependent in part on its use. A biologic indicator that is going to be used as a measure of a dietary exposure in an epidemiological study needs to be a valid representation of long-term intake [96]. Repeated sampling and measurement of a biomarker over time can provide some estimate of the within-individual variability and, therefore, the likelihood that the biomarker is a stable estimate of long-term intake. If repeated measures of a biochemical indicator vary substantially over time in the same individuals, then a single measure will not reflect true, long-term intake [96]. This lack of consistency may occur because diet has changed over the sampling interval or because the measure is overly sensitive to short-term influences, such as recent intake. When using dietary constituents or their metabolites as biomarkers, an understanding of the metabolism and pharmacokinetics of the compound and the frequency of exposure will help to establish the utility of the measure as a biomarker of long-term intake.

A nutritional intervention study may require a biomarker that is a short-term measure of response to treatment. A biomarker that is to serve as a short-term measure of response needs to change within the time frame of the intervention. For example, serum folate provides a measure of recent folic acid exposure; however, erythrocyte concentrations are dependent on the life span of the cells and therefore will not reflect short-term changes in dietary folate. Serum folate concentrations decline within 3 weeks after initiation of a low-folate diet, whereas erythrocyte folate concentration remains in the normal range for at least 17 weeks [101].

Additional practical considerations in the use of established biomarkers include the ability to conveniently access the body compartment for measurement, the procedures necessary to collect and process the sample, burden to study participants or patients, and the resources for laboratory analysis. For example, multiday collections of feces or urine can be a major burden for many individuals. In addition, they can result in incomplete collections, which also compromise the final results. An accurate quantification of vitamin C or folate in a circulating body pool requires processing steps that must be conducted immediately after blood collection to preserve the sample appropriately and prevent degradation that would otherwise make the resulting measurement inaccurate. These extra steps can add time and effort to the labor of blood processing. Furthermore, the complexity of an assay method can vary from the ability to analyze hundreds of samples a day at a cost of a few dollars per sample to a labor-intensive, week-long process that cost hundreds of dollars per sample.

The ability to measure particular biomarkers is also often linked to technological challenges and existing capabilities. For example, the development of HPLC in the 1970s, and improved separation and detection technologies that are currently emerging, facilitates the quantification of many micronutrients and other dietary constituents that are present in very low concentrations in biological samples. Similarly, immunoassays allow for quantitation of phytochemicals, proteins, etc. in small volumes of serum or plasma, where previous methods required substantial quantities of sample. The recent development of microarray technology has provided the ability to analyze the expression profiles for thousands of genes in parallel [102, 103]. This technique will rapidly advance knowledge regarding the mechanisms by which nutrition and diet affect disease risk; however, its application in intact humans will still be limited by access to the tissue of interest.

VI. SUMMARY

The use of biomarkers in humans is an integral component of nutrition research, as well as of nutritional care. Biochemical measurements of dietary constituents in blood or other tissues can provide a useful assessment of the intake of certain dietary factors. However, for some nutrients, functional markers, or direct functional indices, provide a better estimate of the significance of the true status for a nutrient. More general functional indices relating to processes associated with disease risk are important for establishing the relationships between diet and disease prevention and response to treatment.

The development of biomarkers continues at a rapid pace. New types of markers are being proposed constantly and analytic techniques for existing markers are improved. With this advancement comes the need to establish accuracy, reliability, and interpretability of the biomarkers; to obtain data on marker distributions within different age and sex groupings in normal populations; to determine the extent of intraindividual variation in markers with respect to tissue localization and persistence; and to assess the contribution of genetic and acquired susceptibility factors to interindividual variability.

References

1. Clevidence, B. A., and Bieri, J. G. (1993). Association of carotenoids with human plasma lipoproteins. *Methods Enzymol.* **214,** 33–46.
2. Romanchik, J. E., Morel, D. W., and Harrison, E. H. (1995). Distribution of carotenoids and a-tocopherol among lipoproteins do not change when human plasma is incubated in vitro. *J. Nutr.* **125,** 2610–2617.
3. Habicht, J. P., and Pelletier, D. L. (1990). The importance of context in choosing nutritional indicators. *J. Nutr.* **120**(suppl), 1519–1524.
4. Shils, M. E., Olson, J. A., Shike, M., and Ross, A. C., Eds. (1999). "Modern Nutrition in Health and Disease," 9th ed. Williams & Wilkins, Philadelphia, PA.

5. Ziegler, E. E., and Filer, L. J., Eds. (1996). "Present Knowledge in Nutrition," 7th ed. ILSI Press, Washington, DC.

6. Board, F. A. N. (1998). "Dietary Reference Intakes for Thiamin, Riboflavin, Niacin, Vitamin B6, Folate, Vitamin B12, Pantothenic Acid, Biotin, and Choline." National Academy Press, Washington, DC.

7. Kaaks, R., Riboli, E., and Sinha, R. (1997). Biochemical markers of dietary intake. In "Application of Biomarkers in Cancer Epidemiology" (P. Toniolo, P. Boffetta, D. E. G. Shuker, N. Rothman, B. Hulka, and N. Pearce, Eds.), pp. 103–126. International Agency for Research on Cancer, Lyon.

8. Steinmetz, K. A., and Potter, J. D. (1996). Vegetables, fruit, and cancer prevention: A review. J. Am. Diet. Assoc. 96, 1027–1039.

9. Ness, A. R., and Powles, J. W. (1997). Fruit and vegetables, and cardiovascular disease: A review. Int. J. Epidemiol. 26, 1–13.

10. Coward, L., Barnes, N., Setchell, K. D. R., and Barnes, S. (1993). Genistein, daidzein and their β-glycoside conjugates: Antitumor isoflavones in soybean foods from American and Asian diets. J. Agric. Food Chem. 41, 1961–1967.

11. Franke, A. A., Custer, L. J., Cerna, C. M., and Narala, K. (1994). Quantitation of phytoestrogens in legumes by HPLC. J. Agric. Food Chem. 42, 1905–1913.

12. Karr, S. C., Lampe, J. W., Hutchins, A. M., and Slavin, J. L. (1997). Urinary isoflavonoid excretion in humans is dose-dependent at low to moderate levels of soy protein consumption. Am. J. Clin. Nutr. 66, 46–51.

13. Adlercreutz, H., Honjo, H., Higashi, A., Fotsis, T., Hamalainen, E., Hasegawa, T., and Okada, H. (1991). Urinary excretion of lignans and isoflavonoid phytoestrogens in Japanese men and women consuming a traditional Japanese diet. Am. J. Clin. Nutr. 54, 1093–1100.

14. Franke, A. A., and Custer, L. J. (1994). High-performance liquid chromatography assay of isoflavonoids and coumestrol from human urine. J. Chromatog. 662, 47–60.

15. Maskarinec, G., Singh, S., Meng, L., and Franke, A. A. (1998). Dietary soy intake and urinary isoflavonoid excretion among women from a multiethnic population. Cancer Epidemiol. Biomarkers Prev. 7, 613–619.

16. Watanabe, S., Yamaguchi, M., Sobue, T., Takahashi, T., Miura, T., Arai, Y., Mazur, W., Wähälä, K., and Adlercreutz, H. (1998). Pharmacokinetics of soybean isoflavones in plasma, urine and feces of men after ingestion of 60 g baked soybean powder (kinako). J. Nutr. 128, 1710–1715.

17. Gross, M. D., Pfeiffer, M., Martini, M., Campbell, D., Slavin, J., and Potter, J. (1996). The quantitation of metabolites of quercetin flavonols in human urine. Cancer Epidemiol. Biomarkers Prev. , 711–720.

18. Noroozi, M., Burns, J., Crozier, A., Kelly, I. E., and Lean, M. E. J. (2000). Prediction of dietary flavonol consumption from fasting plasma concentration or urinary excretion. Eur. J. Clin. Nutr. 54, 143–149.

19. Shapiro, T. A., Fahey, J. W., Wade, K. L., Stephenson, K. K., and Talalay, P. (1998). Human metabolism and excretion of cancer protective glucosinolates and isothiocyanates of cruciferous vegetables. Cancer Epidemiol. Biomarkers Prev. 7, 1091–1100.

20. Wild, C. P., and Pisani, P. (1997). Carcinogen—DNA and carcinogen—protein adducts in molecular epidemiology. In "Application of Biomarkers in Cancer Epidemiology" (P. Toniolo, P. Boffetta, D. E. G. Shuker, N. Rothman, B. Hulka, and N. Pearce, Eds.), pp. 143–158. International Agency for Research on Cancer, Lyon.

21. Kensler, T. W., He, X., Otieno, M., Egner, P. A., Jacobson, L. P., Chen, B., Wang, J. S., Zhu, Y. R., Zhang, B. C., Wang, J. B., Wu, Y., Zhang, Q. N., Qian, G. S., Kuang, S. Y., Fang, X., Li, Y. F., Yu, L. Y., Prochaska, H. J., Davidson, N. E., Gordon, G. B., Gorman, M. B., Zarba, A., Enger, C., Munoz, A., Helzlsouer, K. J., and Groopman, J. D. (1998). Oltipraz chemoprevention trial in Qidong, People's Republic of China: Modulation of serum aflatoxin albumin adduct biomarkers. Cancer Epidemiol. Biomarkers Prev. 7, 127–134.

22. McClave, S. A., and Snider, H. L. (1992). Use of indirect calorimetry in clinical nutrition. Nutr. Clin. Prac. 7, 207–221.

23. Speakman, J. R. (1998). The history and theory of the doubly labeled water technique. Am. J. Clin. Nutr. 68(suppl), 932S–938S.

24. Seale, J. (1995). Energy expenditure measurements in relation to energy requirements. Am. J. Clin. Nutr. 62(suppl), 1042S–1046S.

25. Martini, M. C., Campbell, D. R., Gross, M. D., Grandits, G. A., Potter, J. D., and Slavin, J. L. (1995). Plasma carotenoids as biomarkers of vegetable intake: The Minnesota CPRU feeding studies. Cancer Epidemiol. Biomarkers Prev. 4, 491–496.

26. Campbell, D. R., Gross, M. D., Martini, M. C., Grandits, G. A., Slavin, J. L., and Potter, J. D. (1994). Plasma carotenoids as biomarkers of vegetable and fruit intake. Cancer Epidemiol. Biomarkers Prev. 3, 493–500.

27. Rock, C. L., Flatt, S. W., Wright, F. A., Faerber, S., Newman, V., Kealey, S., and Pierce, J. P. (1997). Responsiveness of carotenoids to a high vegetable diet intervention designed to prevent breast cancer recurrence. Cancer Epidemiol. Biomarkers Prev. 6, 617–623.

28. Le Marchand, L., Hankin, J. H., Carter, F. S., Essling, C., Luffey, D., Franke, A. A., Wilkens, L. R., Cooney, R. V., and Kolonel, L. N. (1994). A pilot study on the use of plasma carotenoids and ascorbic acid as markers of compliance to a high fruit and vegetable diet intervention. Cancer Epidemiol. Biomarkers Prev. 3, 245–251.

29. Blanchard, J., Toxer, T. N., and Rowland, M. (1997). Pharmacokinetic perspectives on megadoses of ascorbic acid. Am. J. Clin. Nutr. 66, 1165–1171.

30. Mazur, W., Fotsis, T., Wähälä, K., Ojala, S., Salakka, A., and Adlercreutz, H. (1996). Isotope dilution gas chromatographic-mass spectrometric method for the determination of isoflavonoids, coumestrol, and lignans in food samples. Anal. Biochem. 233, 169–180.

31. Lampe, J. W., Gustafson, D. R., Hutchins, A. M., Martini, M. C., Li, S., Wähälä, K., Grandits, G. A., Potter, J. D., and Slavin, J. L. (1999). Urinary isoflavonoid and lignan excretion on a Western diet: Relation to soy, vegetable, and fruit intake. Cancer Epidemiol. Biomarkers Prev. 8, 699–707.

32. Borriello, S. P., Setchell, K. D. R., Axelson, M., and Lawson, A. M. (1985). Production and metabolism of lignans by the human faecal flora. J. Appl. Bacteriol. 58, 37–43.

33. Meydani, S. N., Endres, S., Woods, M. M., Goldin, B. R., Soo, C., Morrill-Labrode, A., Dinarello, C. A., and Gorbach, S. L. (1991). Oral (n-3) fatty acid supplementation suppresses cytokine production and lymphocyte proliferation:

Comparison between young and older women. *J. Nutr.* **121,** 547–555.

34. Soyland, E., Funk, J., Rajka, G., Sandberg, M., Thune, P., Rustad, L., Hellend, S., Middefat, K., Odu, S., Falk, E. S., Solvoll, K., Bjorneboe, G. A., and Drevaon, C. A. (1993). Effect of dietary supplementation with very-long-chain n-3 fatty acids in patients with psoriasis. *N. Engl. J. Med.* **328,** 1812–1816.

35. Wolk, A., Vessby, B., Ljung, H., and Barrefors, P. (1998). Evaluation of a biologic marker for dairy fat intake. *Am. J. Clin. Nutr.* **68,** 291–295.

36. Smedman, A. E. M., Gustafsson, I. B., Berglund, L. G. T., and Vessby, B. O. H. (1999). Pentadecanoic acid in serum as a marker for intake of milk fat: Relations between intake of milk fat and metabolic risk factors. *Am. J. Clin. Nutr.* **69,** 22–29.

37. Turnlund, J. R. (1994). Future directions for establishing mineral/trace element requirements. *J. Nutr.* **124,** 1765S–1770S.

38. Strain, J. J. (1999). Optimal nutrition: An overview. *Proc. Nutr. Soc.* **58,** 395–396.

39. Kelloff, G. J., Sigman, C. C., Johnson, K. M., Boone, C. W., Greenwald, P., Crowell, J. A., Hawk, E. T., and Doody, L. A. (2000). Perspectives on surrogate end points in the development of drugs that reduce the risk of cancer. *Cancer Epidemiol. Biomarkers Prev.* **9,** 127–137.

40. Fleming, T. R., and DeMets, D. L. (1996). Surrogate end points in clinical trials: Are we being misled? *Ann. Int. Med.* **125,** 605–613.

41. Habig, W. H., Pabst, M. J., and Jakoby, W. B. (1974). Glutathione S-transferases: The first enzymatic step in mercapturic acid formation. *J. Biol. Chem.* **249,** 7130–7139.

42. Bogaards, J. J. P., Verhagen, H., Willems, M. I., van Poppel, G., and van Bladeren, P. J. (1994). Consumption of Brussels sprouts results in elevated a-class glutathione S-transferase levels in human blood plasma. *Carcinogenesis* **15,** 1073–1075.

43. Kashuba, A. D. M., Bertino, J. S., Kearns, G. L., Leeder, J. S., James, A. W., Gotschall, R., and Nafziger, A. N. (1998). Quantitation of three-month intraindividual variability and influence of sex and menstrual cycle phase on CYP1A2, N-acetyltransferase-2, and xanthine oxidase activity determined with caffeine phenotyping. *Clin. Pharmacol. Ther.* **63,** 540–551.

44. Pantuck, E. J., Pantuck, C. B., Anderson, K. E., Wattenberg, L. W., Conney, A. H., and Kappas, A. (1984). Effect of Brussels sprouts and cabbage on drug conjugation. *Clin. Pharmacol. Ther.* **35,** 161–169.

45. Sinha, R., Rothman, N., Brown, E. D., Mark, S. D., Hoover, R. N., Capraso, N. E., Levander, O. A., Knize, M. G., Lang, N. P., and Kadlubar, F. F. (1994). Pan-fried meat containing high levels of heterocyclic aromatic amines but low levels of polycyclic aromatic hydrocarbons induces cytochrome P4501A2 activity in humans. *Cancer Res.* **54,** 6154–6159.

46. Kall, M. A., O., V., and J., C. (1997). Effects of dietary broccoli on human drug metabolising activity. *Cancer Lett.* **114,** 169–170.

47. Lampe, J. W., Chen, C., Li, S., Prunty, J., Grate, M. T., Meehan, D. E., Barale, K. V., Dightman, D. A., Feng, Z., and Potter, J. D. (2000). Modulation of human glutathione S-transferases by botanically defined vegetable diets. *Cancer Epidemiol. Biomarkers Prev.* **9,** 787–793.

48. Lauritsen, K., Laursen, L. S., Bukhave, K., and Rask-Madsen, J. (1987). Does vitamin E supplementation modulate *in vivo* arachidonate metabolism in human inflammation? *Pharmacol. Toxicol.* **61,** 246–249.

49. Ruffin, M. T., Krishnan, K., Rock, C. L., Normolle, D., Vaerten, M. A., Peters-Golden, M., Crowell, J., Kelloff, G., Boland, C. R., and Brenner, D. E. (1997). Suppression of human colorectal mucosal prostaglandins: Determining the lowest effective aspirin dose. *J. Natl. Cancer Inst.* **89,** 1152–1160.

50. Krishnan, K., Ruffin, M. T., and Brenner, D. E. (1998). Clinical models of chemoprevention for colon cancer. *Hem. Onc. Clin. N. Am.* **12,** 1079–1113.

51. Selhub, J., and Miller, J. W. (1992). The pathogenesis of homocysteinemia: Interruption of the coordinate regulation by S-adenosylmethionine of the remethylation and transsulfuration of homocysteine. *Am. J. Clin. Nutr.* **55,** 131–138.

52. Kim, Y. I., Fawaz, K., Knox, T., Lee, Y. M., Norton, R., Arora, S., Paiva, L., and Mason, J. B. (1998). Colonic mucosal concentrations of folate correlate well with blood measurements of folate status in persons with colorectal polyps. *Am. J. Clin. Nutr.* **68,** 866–872.

53. Stabler, S. P., Marcell, P. D., Podell, E. R., Allen, R. H., Savage, D. G., and Lindenbaum, J. (1988). Elevation of total homocysteine in the serum of patients with cobalamin or folate deficiency detected by capillary gas chromatography-mass spectrometry. *J. Clin. Invest.* **81,** 466–474.

54. Rock, C. L., Jacob, R. A., and Bowen, P. A. (1996). Update on the biological characteristics of the antioxidant micronutrients: Vitamin C, vitamin E, and the carotenoids. *J. Am. Diet. Assoc.* **96,** 693–702.

55. Handelman, G. J., and Pryor, W. A. (1999). Evaluation of antioxidant status in humans. *In* "Antioxidant Status, Diet, Nutrition, and Health" (A. M. Papas, Ed.), pp. 37–62. CRC Press, Boca Raton, FL.

56. Lemoyne, M., Gossum, A. V., Kurian, R., Ostro, M., Azler, J., and Jeejeebhoy, K. N. (1987). Breath pentane analysis as an index of lipid peroxidation: A functional test of vitamin E status. *Am. J. Clin. Nutr.* **46,** 267–272.

57. Kasai, H., Crain, P. F., Kuchino, Y., Nishimura, S., Oostsuyama, A., and Tanooka, H. (1986). Formation of 8-hydroxyguanine moiety in cellular DNA by agents producing oxygen radicals and evidence for its repair. *Carcinogenesis* **7,** 1849–1851.

58. Loft, S., Vistisen, K., Ewertz, M., Tjonneland, A., Overvad, K., and Poulsen, H. E. (1992). Oxidative DNA damage estimated by 8-hydroxydeoxyguanosine excretion in humans: Influence of smoking, gender and body mass index. *Carcinogenesis* **13,** 2241–2247.

59. Tagesson, C., Kallberg, M., Klintenberg, C., and Starkhammar, H. (1995). Determination of urinary 8-hydroxydeoxyguanosine by automated coupled-column high performance liquid chromatography: A powerful technique for assaying *in vivo* oxidative DNA damage in cancer patients. *Eur. J. Cancer* **31A,** 934–940.

60. Thompson, H. J., Heimendinger, J., Haegele, A., Sedlacek, S. M., Gillette, C., O'Neill, C., Wolfe, P., and Conry, C. (1999). Effect of increased vegetable and fruit consumption on markers of oxidative cellular damage. *Carcinogenesis* **20,** 2261–2266.

61. Johansson, G., Holmen, A., Persson, L., Hogstedt, R., Wassen, C., Ottova, L., and Gustafsson, J. A. (1992). The effect

of a shift from a mixed diet to a lacto-vegetarian diet on human urinary and fecal mutagenic activity. *Carcinogenesis* **13**, 153–157.

62. Witztum, J. L. (1998). To E or not to E—How do we tell? *Circulation* **98**, 2785–2787.

63. Morrow, J. D., Harris, T. M., and Roberts, L. J. (1990). Non-cyclooxygenase oxidative formation of a series of novel prostaglandins: Analytical ramifications for measurement of eicosanoids. *Anal. Biochem.* **184**, 1–10.

64. Morrow, J. D., and Roberts, L. J. (1997). The isoprostanes: Unique bioactive products of lipid peroxidation. *Prog. Lipid Res.* **36**, 1–21.

65. Patrono, C., and FitzGerald, G. A. (1997). Isoprostanes: Potential markers of oxidant stress in atherothrombotic disease. *Arterioscler. Thromb. Vasc. Biol.* **17**, 2309–2315.

66. Djuric, Z., Lu, M. H., Lewis, S. M., Luongo, D. A., Chen, X. W., Heilbrun, L. K., Reading, B. A., Duffy, P. H., and Hart, R. W. (1992). Oxidative DNA damage levels in rats fed low-fat, high-fat, or calorie-restricted diets. *Toxicol. Appl. Pharmacol.* **115**, 156–160.

67. Djuric, Z., Heilbrun, L. K., Reading, B. A., Boomer, A., Valeriote, F. A., and Martino, S. (1991). Effects of a low-fat diet on levels of oxidative damage to DNA in human peripheral nucleated blood cells. *J. Natl. Cancer Inst.* **83**, 766–769.

68. Djuric, Z., Depper, J. B., Uhley, V., Smith, D., Lababidi, S., Martino, S., and Heilbrun, L. K. (1998). Oxidative DNA damage levels in blood from women at high risk for breast cancer are associated with dietary intakes of meats, vegetables, and fruits. *J. Am. Diet. Assoc.* **98**, 524–528.

69. Mosca, L., Rubenfire, M., Mandel, C., Rock, C., Tarshis, T., Tsai, A., and Pearson, T. (1997). Antioxidant nutrient supplementation reduces the susceptibility of low density lipoprotein to oxidation in patients with coronary artery disease. *J. Am. Coll. Cardiol.* **30**, 392–399.

70. Vedhara, K., Fox, J. D., and Wang, E. C. Y. (1999). The measurement of stress-related immune dysfunction in psychoneuroimmunology. *Neurosci. Biobehav. Rev.* **23**, 699–715.

71. Lourd, B., and Mazari, L. (1999). Nutrition and immunity in the elderly. *Proc. Nutr. Soc.* **58**, 685–695.

72. Murata, T., Tamai, H., Morinobu, T., M., M., Takenaka, H., Hayashi, K., and Mino, M. (1994). Effect of long-term administration of β-carotene on lymphocyte subsets in humans. *Am. J. Clin. Nutr.* **60**, 597–602.

73. Santos, M. S., Meydani, S. N., Leka, L., Wu, D., Fotouhi, N., Meydani, M., Hennekens, C. H., and Gaziano, J. M. (1996). Natural killer cell activity in elderly men is enhanced by β-carotene supplementation. *Am. J. Clin. Nutr.* **64**, 772–777.

74. Jeng, K. -C. G., Yang, C. -S., Siu, W. -Y., Tsai, Y. -S., Liao, W. -J., and Kuo, J. -S. (1996). Supplementation of vitamins C and E enhances cytokine production by peripheral blood mononuclear cells in healthy adults. *Am. J. Clin. Nutr.* **64**, 960–965.

75. Bogden, J. D., Bendich, A., Kemp, F. W., Bruening, K. S., Skurnick, J. H., Denny, T., Baker, H., and Louria, D. B. (1994). Daily micronutrient supplements enhance delayed-hypersensitivity skin test responses in older people. *Am. J. Clin. Nutr.* **60**, 437–447.

76. Black, D. M., Cummings, S. R., Genant, H. K., Nevitt, M. C., Palermo, L., and Browner, W. (1992). Axial and appendicular bone density predict fractures in older women. *J. Bone Mineral Res.* **7**, 633–638.

77. Cummings, S. R., Black, D. M., Nevitt, M. C., Browner, W., Cauley, J., Ensrud, K., Genant, H. K., Palermo, L., Scott, J., and Vogt, T. M. (1993). Bone density at various sites for prediction of hip fracture. The Study of Osteoporotic Fractures Research Group. *Lancet* **341**, 72–75.

78. Melton, L. J. I., Atkinson, E. J., O'Fallon, W. M., Wahner, H. W., and Riggs, B. L. (1993). Long-term fracture prediction by bone mineral assessed at different skeletal sites. *J. Bone Mineral Res.* **8**, 1227–1233.

79. Cashman, K. D., and Flynn, A. (1999). Optimal nutrition: Calcium, magnesium and phosphorus. *Proc. Nutr. Soc.* **58**, 477–487.

80. Kanis, J. A. (1991). Calcium requirements for optimal skeletal health in women. *Calcified Tissue Int.* **49**, S33–S41.

81. Watts, N. B. (1999). Clinical utility of biochemical markers of bone remodeling. *Clin. Chem.* **45**, 1359–1368.

82. Boland, C. R. (1993). The biology of colorectal cancer. *Cancer* **71**(suppl), 4181–4186.

83. Einspahr, J. G., Alberts, D. S., Gapstur, S. M., Bostick, R. M., Emerson, S. S., and Gerner, E. W. (1997). Surrogate end-point biomarkers as measures of colon cancer risk and their use in cancer chemoprevention trials. *Cancer Epidemiol. Biomarkers Prev.* **6**, 37–48.

84. Lipkin, M., and Newmark, H. (1985). Effect of added dietary calcium on colonic epithelial-cell proliferation in subjects at high risk for familial colonic cancer. *N. Engl. J. Med.* **313**, 1381–1384.

85. Bostick, R. M., Fosdick, L., Lillemoe, T. J., Overn, P., Wood, J. R., Grambsch, P., Elmer, P., and Potter, J. D. (1997). Methodological findings and considerations in measuring colorectal epithelial cell proliferation in humans. *Cancer Epidemiol. Biomarkers Prev.* **6**, 931–942.

86. Vargas, P. A., and Alberts, D. S. (1992). Primary prevention of colorectal cancer through dietary modification. *Cancer* **70**, 1229–1235.

87. Takayama, T., Katsuki, S., Takahashi, Y., Ohi, M., Nojiri, S., Sakamaki, S., Kato, J., Kogawa, K., Miyake, H., and Niitsu, Y. (1998). Aberrant crypt foci of the colon as precursors of adenoma and cancer. *N. Engl. J. Med.* **339**, 1277–1284.

88. Garte, S., Zocchetti, C., and Taioli, E. (1997). Gene-environment interactions in the application of biomarkers of cancer susceptiblity in epidemiology. *In* "Application of Biomarkers in Cancer Epidemiology" (P. Toniolo, P. Boffetta, D. E. G. Shuker, N. Rothman, B. Hulka, and N. Pearce, Eds.), pp. 251–264. International Agency for Research on Cancer, Lyon.

89. Murray, R. F. (1986). Tests of so-called susceptibility. *J. Occup. Med.* **28**, 1103–1107.

90. Lai, C., and Shields, P. G. (1999). The role of interindividual variation in human carcinogenesis. *J. Nutr.* **129**(suppl), 552S–555S.

91. Sinha, R., and Caporaso, N. (1999). Diet, genetic susceptibility and human cancer etiology. *J. Nutr.* **129**(suppl), 556S–559S.

92. Kim, Y. I., Pogribney, I. P., Basnakian, A. G., Miller, J. W., Selhub, J., James, S. J., and Mason, J. B. (1997). Folate deficiency in rats induces DNA strand breaks and hypomethylation within the p53 tumor suppressor gene. *Am. J. Clin. Nutr.* **65**, 46–52.

93. Ulrich, C. M., Kampman, E., Bigler, J., Schwartz, S. M., Chen, C., Bostick, R., Fosdick, L., Beresford, S. A. A., Yasui, Y., and Potter, J. D. (1999). Colorectal adenomas and the C677T *MTHFR* polymorphism: Evidence for gene–environment interaction? *Cancer Epidemiol. Biomarkers Prev.* **8,** 659–668.

94. Vine, M. F., and McFarland, L. T. (1990). Markers of susceptibility. *In* "Biological Markers in Epidemiology" (B. S. Hulka, T. C. Wilcosky, and J. D. Griffith, Eds.), pp. 196–213. Oxford University Press, New York.

95. Wilcosky, T. C. (1990). Criteria for selecting and evaluating markers. *In* "Biological Markers in Epidemiology" (B. S. Hulka, T. C. Wilcosky, and J. D. Griffith, Eds.), pp. 28–55. Oxford University Press, New York.

96. Hunter, D. (1990). Biochemical indicators of dietary intake. *In* "Nutritional Epidemiology" (W. Willett, Ed.), Vol. **15,** pp. 143–216. Oxford University Press, New York.

97. Whitehead, T. P. (1977). "Quality Control in Clinical Chemistry." John Wiley, New York.

98. Aitio, A., and Apostoli, P. (1995). Quality assurance in biomarker measurement. *Toxicol. Lett.* **77,** 195–204.

99. Westgard, J. O., Barry, P. L., Hunt, M. R., and Groth, T. (1981). A multi-rule Shewhart chart for quality control in clinical chemistry. *Clin. Chem.* **27,** 493–501.

100. Lipschitz, D. A., Cook, J. D., and Finch, C. A. (1974). A clinical evaluation of serum ferritin. *N. Engl. J. Med.* **290,** 1213–1216.

101. Herbert, V. (1987). Recommended dietary intakes (RDI) of folate in humans. *Am. J. Clin. Nutr.* **45,** 661–670.

102. Sgroi, D. C., Teng, S., Robinson, G., LeVangie, R., Hudson, J. R. J., and Elkahloun, A. G. (1999). *In vivo* gene expression profile analysis of human breast cancer progression. *Cancer Res.* **59,** 5656–5661.

103. Walker, J., and Rigley, K. (2000). Gene expression profiling in human peripheral blood mononuclear cells using high-density filter-based cDNA microarrays. *J. Immunol. Methods* **239,** 167–179.

104. Cook, J. D. (1999). Defining optimal body iron. *Proc. Nutr. Soc.* **58,** 489–495.

C. Genetic Influence on Nutritional Health

CHAPTER **11**

Genetic Influences on Blood Lipids and Cardiovascular Disease Risk

JOSE M. ORDOVAS

USDA-HNRCA, Tufts University, Boston, Massachusetts

I. INTRODUCTION

The major public health concerns in the developed world (i.e., cardiovascular disease, cancer, and diabetes) have both genetic and environmental causes. The interface between public health and genetics consists of working toward an understanding of how genes and the environment act together to cause these diseases and how the environment (e.g., diet), rather than genes, might be manipulated to help prevent or delay the onset of disease.

Cardiovascular disease (CVD), the leading cause of mortality in most industrialized countries, is a multifactorial disease that is associated with nonmodifiable risk factors, such as age, gender, and genetic background, and with modifiable risk factors, including elevated total and low-density lipoprotein (LDL) cholesterol levels, as well as reduced high-density lipoprotein (HDL) cholesterol levels. Convincing evidence shows that lowering serum lipid levels will slow the progression or even induce regression in atherosclerotic lesions [1–4]. Based on this evidence, the National Cholesterol Education Program (NCEP) has recommended that all adult Americans reduce their serum total cholesterol values to less than 5.18 mmol/L (200 mg/dL) and their LDL cholesterol values to less than 3.37 mmol/L (130 mg/dL) [5]. Although several types of drug therapies have been developed and have been shown to be highly effective in lowering serum LDL cholesterol values and CVD, the NCEP has emphasized that lifestyle modification should be the primary treatment for lowering cholesterol values, with drug therapies reserved for cases in which lifestyle modification is ineffective. The modifications advocated include dietary changes, regular aerobic exercise, and normalization of body weight. The recommended dietary changes include restriction in the amount of total fat (≤30% of energy), saturated fat (<10% of energy), and cholesterol to <300 mg/day. For individuals with elevated LDL cholesterol levels or cardiovascular disease, the saturated fat target should be much lower (<7% of energy) and the dietary cholesterol reduced to <200 mg/day. Also recommended is an increase in the consumption of carbohydrate and dietary fiber, especially water-soluble fiber. However, it is not known how many

individuals can achieve the recommended levels of serum lipids using this approach [5], one of the major reasons being our current inability to predict individual plasma lipid response to dietary changes.

Several studies demonstrated, during the first half of the 20th century, that serum cholesterol could be modified by the composition of dietary fat [6, 7], and studies by Keys *et al.* [8] and Hegsted *et al.* [9] provided the first quantitative estimates of the relative effects of the various classes of dietary fatty acids and amount of cholesterol on serum cholesterol changes. Other predictive algorithms have been developed in recent years, including predictions of response for LDL and HDL cholesterol [10–12]. These relationships between dietary changes and serum lipid changes are well founded and predictable for groups; however, a striking variability in the response of serum cholesterol to diet between subjects was reported as early as 1933 [13], and this variability has been the subject of multiple reports in recent years [12, 14–17]. In some individuals, plasma total and LDL cholesterol levels dramatically decrease following consumption of lipid-lowering diets, while they remain unchanged in others [12, 14, 15, 18]. It has been shown in elegant studies in nonhuman primates that the serum lipoprotein response to dietary manipulation has a significant genetic component [19–21]. Such genetic variability could have a significant impact on the success of public health policies and individual therapeutic interventions. At this point, the summary of a Scientific Conference on Preventive Nutrition: Pediatrics to Geriatrics, convened by The Nutrition Committee of the American Heart Association, specifically states that "theoretically, genetic differences can render a particular set of dietary conditions more harmful or beneficial in one ethnic group than in another. This is one explanation for why individuals of different ethnic groups who consume similar diets might have varying disease profiles." Moreover, the statement underscores the need to "identify specific genes and genetic variations that affect risk directly and indirectly by the way they interact with nutrients." [22]

As indicated above, we have traditionally measured the success of CVD risk-reducing strategies based on their effect on plasma lipids and, more specifically, lipoprotein levels.

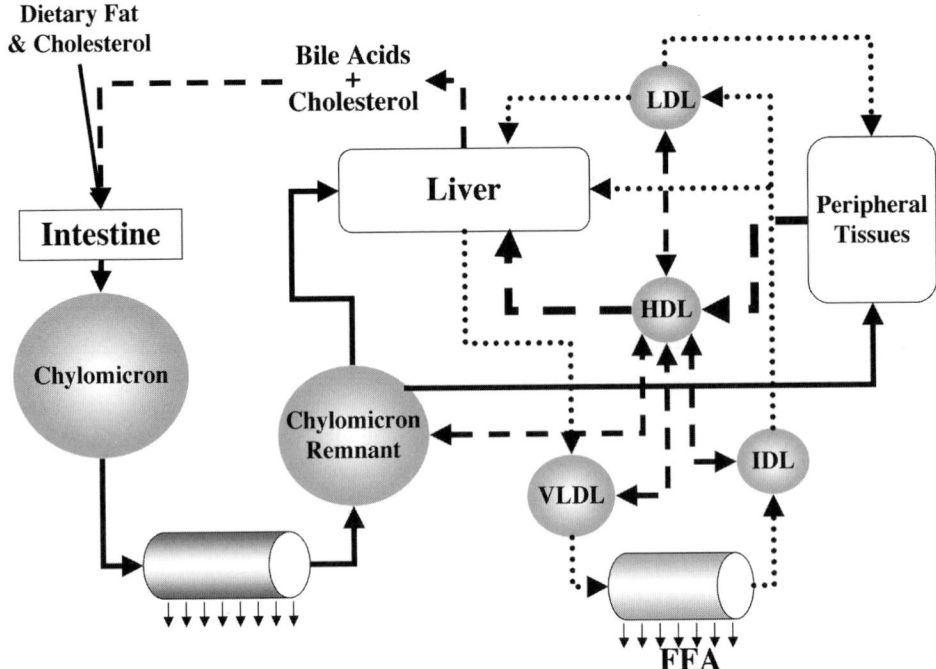

FIGURE 1   Simplified scheme of lipoprotein pathways showing the exogenous (———), endogenous (. . . . . .) and reverse cholesterol (- - - - -) pathways. Arrows indicate that following lipolysis by lipoprotein lipase, the FFA are released from the lipoproteins for utilization as a source of energy by tissues or for storage in the adipose tissue.

Lipoproteins are macromolecular complexes of lipids and proteins that originate mainly from the liver and intestine and are involved in the transport and redistribution of lipids in the body. Lipid and lipoprotein metabolism can be viewed as a complex biological pathway containing multiple steps. Lipid homeostasis is achieved by the coordinated action of a large number of nuclear factors, binding proteins, apolipoproteins, enzymes, and receptors involving hundreds of genes. Lipid metabolism is also closely linked with energy metabolism and is subjected to many hormonal controls that are essential for adjustment to environmental and internal conditions. Genetic variability has been demonstrated in humans for most of these proteins and some of these mutations can result in abnormal lipid metabolism and plasma lipoprotein profiles that may contribute to the pathogenesis of atherosclerosis. This complex picture can be dissected into three pathways (see Fig. 1). The exogenous lipoprotein pathway describes the metabolism of lipoproteins synthesized in the intestine following dietary fat intake; the endogenous pathway deals with the metabolism of lipoproteins involved in the transport of liver lipids to peripheral tissues; and finally the reverse cholesterol transport depicts the process by which excess peripheral lipids (primarily cholesterol) are transported to the liver for catabolism. Our current knowledge about how variants at candidate genes involved in each of these three interrelated processes affect dietary response and cardiovascular risk is presented below.

II. EXOGENOUS LIPOPROTEIN PATHWAY

The exogenous lipoprotein pathway has its origin in the enterocyte with the synthesis of chylomicron particles. Dietary fats absorbed in the intestine are packaged into large, triglyceride-rich chylomicrons for delivery to sites of lipid metabolism or storage. During their transit to the liver, these particles interact with lipoprotein lipase (LPL) and undergo partial lipolysis to form chylomicron remnants. These chylomicron remnants pick up apoE and cholesteryl ester from HDL, and are taken up by the liver via a process mediated by the interaction of apoE with hepatic receptors. For most people, this is a fast process and chylomicrons are not usually present in the blood after a prolonged fasting period. However, dramatic individual variability is seen in postprandial lipoprotein metabolism, which is in part determined by genetic factors and this variability could be highly relevant to achieving a more precise definition of individualized CVD risk. The most relevant candidate genes involved in this metabolic pathway and their known associations with plasma lipid levels and dietary response are described below.

A. Apolipoprotein B

ApoB is an essential protein component of intestinal chylomicron particles. In humans, the form of apoB synthesized by the intestine is apoB–48, produced by a mRNA editing

mechanism [23, 24]. However, some apoB–100 synthesis may occur also in the intestine [25, 26].

The *Apob* gene has been mapped to the region 2p24-p23 on chromosome 2 [27]. Because apoB is the major protein of chylomicrons, as well as of LDL and very low-density lipoprotein (VLDL), it is reasonable to expect that genetic variation at this locus could influence plasma cholesterol and/or triglyceride levels. More than 20 polymorphisms have been reported in this locus (http://gdbwww.gdb.org/ gdb-bin/genera/accno?accessionNum=GDB:119686). Some of these polymorphic sites have been utilized as markers in population or case-control studies in an attempt to correlate individual alleles or haplotypes with lipid levels and CVD risk. In general, the outcome of these studies has not been unanimous [28–37]. The findings and controversies associated with some of these polymorphisms are presented below.

A silent mutation causing a cytosine to thymidine (ACC→ACT) change characterizes the well-studied apoB *Xba*I restriction fragment length polymorphism (RFLP). It involves the third base of the threonine codon 2488 in exon 26 without changing the amino acid sequence [38]. This RFLP has been associated with variability in plasma lipid levels [29–31, 39, 40]. The allele lacking the *Xba*I recognition site (X−) has been associated with lower total cholesterol, LDL cholesterol, and triglyceride concentrations. Paradoxically, this same X− allele has been found to be more common among coronary artery disease cases than in controls [41–43]. It has been speculated that the causal mutation associated to the *Xba*I polymorphism might result in a structural change in apoB that affects the egression of LDL from the arterial wall [44].

The association between this polymorphism and variability in dietary response has been studied by several investigators and the results are quite controversial. Some reports show that subjects carrying the X+X+ or X+X− genotypes respond to a low-fat, low-cholesterol diet with greater reductions in plasma total cholesterol, LDL cholesterol, apoB [45, 46], and, surprisingly, HDL cholesterol levels than subjects with the X−X− genotype [45]. A recent meta-analysis suggests that this polymorphism plays a minor role in determining individual variability in response to dietary intervention [46a].

We have evaluated whether the apoB *Xba*I polymorphism is associated with the interindividual variability observed during postprandial lipemia [47]. For this purpose, we carried out an oral fat load study involving 51 healthy young male volunteers [20 X−/X− (X−), and 31 X+/X− or X+/ X+ (X+)], homozygous for the apoE3 allele. Our data showed that subjects with the X− genotype had significantly greater retinyl palmitate (RP) and apoB–48 postprandial responses on both the large and the small triglyceride-rich lipoprotein fractions compared with X+ subjects, suggesting that the X−/X− genotype is associated with greater postprandial response as compared with the X−/X+ or the X+/ X+ genotypes. These differences observed in postprandial

lipoprotein metabolism could explain some reported associations of this polymorphism to coronary artery disease risk. As indicated above, this mutation does not result in an amino acid change at the affected codon and it cannot have a direct functional effect. However, it is in strong linkage disequilibrium with the apoB Val591→Ala polymorphism (Ag al/d), which may be the functional sequence change. An alternative hypothesis relates to the position of this mutation near the apoB–48 editing site at position 2153. The mechanism of this editing involves a form of cytidine deaminase. The "mooring" sequence model for the editosome suggests that the recognition and binding sequences of nuclear factors that identify the specific site for editing and "moor" the editing activity are distal to and different from the editing site. It is possible that the *Xba*I mutation, close to the editing site, could affect these "mooring" sequences, thus modifying the editing activity on the apoB mRNA. This might result in changes on apoB–48 synthesis and intestinal triglyceride-rich lipoprotein secretion as shown in our study.

Another potentially interesting polymorphism is the three-codon (leu-ala-leu) I/D polymorphism within the apoB signal peptide [48]. This mutation has been found to be associated with variation in total and LDL cholesterol and/or triglyceride levels [37, 49] as well as CVD risk [32]; however, these effects have not been confirmed by other investigators [50, 51]. Xu *et al.* [37] reported that subjects with the I/I genotype had the highest triglyceride levels and D/D subjects had the lowest, while consuming a high-fat, high-cholesterol diet. This effect disappeared when the subjects were consuming a low-fat, low-cholesterol diet. These results were not confirmed by Boerwinkle *et al.* [52] in a study in which subjects received two levels of dietary cholesterol without modification of dietary fat. In a more recent study, the D allele was found to be associated with reduced postprandial lipid response as compared with individuals homozygous for the I allele, suggesting that this mutation in the signal peptide may affect apoB secretion during the postprandial state [53]. Moreover, this polymorphism has been reported to be involved with postprandial lipoparticles' responses [54], and with the association between free fatty acid concentrations and triglyceride-rich lipoproteins in the postprandial state [55]. A plausible mechanism to explain the observed interaction between this I/D polymorphism, postprandial free fatty acids, and triglyceride-rich lipoproteins has been proposed [55]. *In vitro* studies have shown that apoB is synthesized and then either assembled into lipoproteins and secreted or degraded intracellularly. Oleate may increase secretion by protecting intracellular apoB from degradation. Using a yeast expression system, it has been shown that the 24-amino-acid signal peptide mediates apoB translocation into the endoplasmic reticulum less efficiently than the 27-amino-acid signal peptide, which may result in reduced apoB secretion. If this mechanism held *in vivo*, then in subjects homozygous for the 27-amino-acid signal peptide, increased free fatty acids might result in increased protection

of apoB from degradation and increased VLDL production. However, in subjects carrying the 24-amino-acid signal peptide, increased free fatty acids fail to regulate VLDL production because of accelerated intracellular degradation of apoB.

The *Msp*I (CGGG→CAGC) polymorphism in exon 26 causes an adenine to guanosine change that results in an amino acid change (Arg^{3611}→Gln) [56]. We have previously found a significant association between the less common allele (M2) and the presence of premature CVD [28], with this allele being nearly twice as frequent in CVD (0.105) as in the control population (0.057). However, no associations of this allele with alterations in plasma apoB or LDL cholesterol levels in subjects with coronary artery disease were noted [28]. The association between this RFLP and variability in dietary response has been examined and the results of a recent meta-analysis suggest that this polymorphism may play a minor role as a determinant of dietary response [46a].

An *Eco*RI RFLP described in exon 29 consists of a single base pair (bp) mutation (GAA→AAA) [57], which results in an amino acid change from Gln^{4514}→Lys. This RFLP is in linkage disequilibrium with the *Msp*I described above and it should reveal similar phenotype associations.

A 3'-VNTR region approximately 300-bp distal to the 3' end of the apoB gene results in approximately 17 different alleles. Some initial reports suggested that larger number of repeats were associated with increased CVD risk [28, 41, 58]. However, other studies did not observe such association [59].

A comprehensive analysis of these polymorphisms and the Bsp 1261I RFLP in exon 4 (the second base in codon 71 causing a cytosine to thymidine change and changing threonine to isoleucine) has been recently reported by Rantala *et al.* [60]. Moreover, the authors conducted a meta-analysis on the available data. The controlled dietary intervention study was conducted in 44 healthy, middle-aged subjects, consisting of a 3-month baseline, a 1-month fat-controlled, a 1-month high-fat, and a 1-month habitual diet period. In this dietary study, the apoB *Xba*I restriction-site polymorphism affected the responsiveness to diet of the plasma LDL-cholesterol concentration, especially during the high-fat diet. The X−/X− subjects had a greater increase in LDL cholesterol (44 ± 5%) than X+/X+ (27 ± 7%) or X+/X− (40 ± 5%) subjects. The high-fat diet also induced a larger increase in plasma LDL cholesterol in subjects with the R−/R− genotype (59 ± 10%) than in those with the R+/R− (39 ± 6%) or R+/R+ (36 ± 4%) genotypes. M+/M+ subjects were also more responsive (41 ± 3% increase in LDL cholesterol) than the M+/M− subjects (27 ± 10% increase). Their meta-analysis supported the finding of the significant role of the *Eco*RI and *Msp*I polymorphisms, but not that of the *Xba*I polymorphism [60].

The results of the meta-analysis support the association between the apoB *Eco*RI and *Msp*I genotypes and responsiveness to diet. However, the percent of variability in response due to this locus is very small and this information does not yet provide enough information to be used as a clinical tool in dietary counseling.

B. Apolipoprotein A-IV

In humans, apoA-IV is synthesized primarily in the intestine as a 46-kDa glycoprotein [61]. The experimental evidence from familial apolipoprotein A-I/C-III/A-IV deficiency [62] suggests that it plays a role in dietary fat absorption and chylomicron synthesis. *In vitro* studies have shown that the activation of lipoprotein lipase by apoC-II is mediated by apoA-IV [63], and that apoA-IV can serve as an activator of lecithin cholesterol acyltransferase (LCAT) [64]. ApoA-IV-containing lipoproteins promote cholesterol efflux from cultured fibroblasts and adipose cells *in vitro,* and there is evidence that apoA-IV may be one of the ligands for the HDL receptor [65–67]. A report by Duverger *et al.* [68] demonstrated that overexpression of human apoA-IV in atherosclerosis-prone apoE-deficient mice resulted in an increased atherogenic lipid profile, with no significant effects on HDL cholesterol concentrations. Despite these findings, mice expressing human apoA-IV were more resistant to atherosclerosis. This was also true for those mice that were not knockouts for the apoE gene, but expressed the human apoA-IV. These data suggest that apoA-IV may protect against atherosclerosis by mechanisms that do not involve increased HDL cholesterol concentrations, and also may explain the absence of atherosclerosis in the apoA-I-deficient mice [69]. However, this hypothesis have been partially challenged by data generated in normocholesteroleic mice. In these animals, high plasma levels of human apoA-IV did not enhance cholesterol mobilization *in vivo* in normolipemic mice [70]. Overall, the data suggest that apoA-IV plays a role in fat absorption and reverse cholesterol transport.

It has been shown that apoA-IV expression is regulated by fat feeding and recent data provide evidence that isolated fatty acids regulate gene expression and the production of apoA-IV in the enterocyte. Specifically, in confluent Caco-2 cells incubated with 1 m*M* oleic (n–9), linoleic (n–6), alpha-linolenic (n–3), or docosahexaenoic (n–3) acids for a long-term period, both apoA-IV protein levels and *de novo* synthesis were increased. This induction resulted from the upregulation of apoA-IV mRNA transcripts. In contrast, an inhibitory effect was evident with short-term incubation. Fatty acid chain length and degree of unsaturation had little effect in altering apoA-IV transcript and biogenesis. [71].

Genetically determined isoforms of apoA-IV have been detected in humans and in other mammalian species (http://gdbwww.gdb.org/gdb-bin/genera/accno?accessionNum= GDB:119000). The most common isoform detected using isoelectric focusing is A-IV-1, with an allele frequency in Caucasians ranging from 88–95%. ApoA-IV–2 (Gln^{360} →His) is the second most common isoform with an allele frequency

in the range of 5–12% in Caucasians [72, 73]. Additional variation within these isoforms has been detected using the polymerase chain reaction (PCR). A relatively common mutation (Thr^{347} → Ser) has been documented within subjects with the apoA-IV-1 isoform. The effect of apoA-IV genetic variation on plasma lipid levels has been studied in several populations [73–77]. In some Caucasian populations, the apoA-IV-2 allele has been associated with higher levels of HDL cholesterol and/or lower triglyceride levels [72, 77, 78], but no associations have been observed in other studies [79–84].

The effect of genetic variation at this locus on dietary response has been examined [85, 86]. Our own data show that the apoA-IV-2 (Gln^{360} → His) allele (apoA-IV-2) is associated with hyporesponsiveness of LDL cholesterol to dietary therapy consisting of reduction in total fat and cholesterol intakes. McCombs et al. [86] have demonstrated that this effect may be due to the reduction in dietary cholesterol. We also observed that subjects with the apoA-IV-2 allele tended to have greater decreases in HDL cholesterol concentrations following a low-fat and low-cholesterol diet. To follow up on this observation, we have examined the effect of this polymorphism on HDL cholesterol response in 41 healthy males subjects [87]. They were fed three consecutive diets (high-saturated, low-fat and high-monounsaturated fat diets) for 4 weeks each. After consuming the high-saturated fat diet, carriers of the apoA-IV-2 allele had a greater decrease in HDL cholesterol and apoA-I. In these subjects, replacement of a high carbohydrate diet by monounsaturated fat resulted in a greater increase in HDL cholesterol and apoA-I as compared with homozygotes for the apoA-IV-1 allele. These data suggest that in apoA-IV-2 subjects, a high-carbohydrate diet may induce an apparently increased atherogenic lipid profile (LDL cholesterol does not decrease, but HDL cholesterol does decrease). Therefore, these subjects may benefit specially from a diet relatively high in monounsaturated fat.

The mechanism by which this mutation may exert the observed effect is still unknown. The apoA-IV-2 isoform binds to lipoproteins with higher affinity than apoA-IV-1, which may result in delayed hepatic clearance of chylomicron remnants, as shown in metabolic studies [88]. Given the important role that this apolipoprotein may have in lipid absorption, it is possible that mechanisms involving intestinal fat absorption and/or the metabolism of triglyceride-rich lipoproteins may be differentially affected by each isoform.

The apoa-IV-2 allele has been also studied in relation to the changes in CVD risk factors associated with urbanization in developing countries. We demonstrated in a population-based study in Costa Rica that lifestyles associated with an urban environment, such as increased smoking and saturated fat intake, elicit a more adverse plasma lipoprotein profile among subject carriers of the apoA4-IV-2 allele than in apoA-IV-1 homozygotes, which could make them more susceptible to CVD [89]. These results may be difficult to reconcile with those from the dietary metabolic studies. However, note that the changes associated with "modernization" (i.e., increased fat and cholesterol intakes, smoking, and decreased physical activity) are more complex gene–environment interactions than those taking place during a well-controlled dietary protocol carried out in a metabolic unit.

We have also examined the association between the apoA-IV(Thr^{347}→Ser) variant observed within the apoA-IV-1 allele and the LDL cholesterol response to dietary intervention [90]. Our data show that carriers of the less common Ser^{347} allele have a greater decrease in total cholesterol, LDL cholesterol and apoB concentrations when they are switched from a low-fat and cholesterol diet to a high-monounsaturated fat diet as compared with homozygous carriers of the Thr^{347} allele.

Similar studies in subjects heterozygous for familial hypercholesterolemia [91] show that the apoA-IV-2 allele was associated with lower LDL cholesterol and apoB levels independent of diet effects. No differences in total cholesterol, LDL cholesterol, HDL cholesterol, and apoB levels were observed between subjects homozygous for the apoA-IV Thr^{347} allele and those carriers of the apoA-IV Ser^{347} allele. After dietary intervention, Ser/Ser subjects showed significant reductions in plasma triglycerides and VLDL cholesterol levels, but no changes were found in carriers of the Ser allele.

The combined information for the Thr^{347}→Ser and the Gln^{360}→His suggests that the responsiveness of LDL cholesterol to changes on dietary fat could follow this pattern: 347Ser/360Gln>347Thr/360Gln>347Thr/360His. The mechanisms by which these mutations may exert the observed effects are still unknown. The apoA-IV-2 allele binds to lipoproteins with higher affinity than apoA-IV-1, which may result in delayed hepatic clearance of chylomicron remnants as shown in metabolic studies. The substitution of Ser for Thr at position 347 induces changes in the secondary structure and a slight increase in hydrophilic profile at this position, which could result in a decrease in its affinity for lipids on the triglycerite-rich lipoprotein particles. This could facilitate the exchange with apoC-II, thereby increasing LPL activity over those particles, which would in turn accelerate clearance of remnants. The increased influx of dietary cholesterol would downregulate the LDL receptors, with consequent increases in LDL cholesterol concentrations. Therefore, consumption of fat-rich diets would produce a greater increase in LDL cholesterol in Ser^{347} carriers.

C. Apolipoprotein E

ApoE in serum is associated with chylomicrons, VLDL, and HDL, and serves as a ligand for the LDL receptor and the LDL receptor-related protein [92, 93]. When apoE deficiency is present, there is marked accumulation of cholesterol-enriched lipoproteins of density <1.006 g/mL containing apoB–48 and apoA-IV, as well as apoB–100 [94]. Moreover,

in this disorder there is delayed clearance of both apoB–100 and apoB–48 within triglyceride-rich lipoproteins. Genetic variation at the apoE locus results from three common alleles in the population, E4, E3 and E2, with frequencies in Caucasian populations of approximately 15, 77, and 8%, respectively [95]. Population studies have shown that plasma cholesterol, LDL cholesterol, and apoB levels are highest in subjects carrying the apoE4 isoform, intermediate in those with the apoE3 isoform, and lowest in those with the apoE2 isoform [96, 97]. It has been suggested that apoE allelic variation may account for up to 7% of the variation in total and LDL cholesterol levels in the general population [95]. This relationship between LDL cholesterol levels and apoE genetic variation is not independent of environmental and ethnic factors. Thus, it appears that the association of the apoE4 isoform with elevated serum cholesterol levels is greater in populations consuming diets rich in saturated fat and cholesterol than in other populations. These data indicate that the higher LDL cholesterol levels observed in subjects carrying the apoE4 isoform are manifested primarily in the presence of an atherogenic diet characteristic of certain societies, and that the response to dietary saturated fat and cholesterol may differ among individuals with different apoE phenotypes. Many studies have been conducted to prove this hypothesis [98–100]. Some investigators reported greater plasma lipid responses in subjects carrying the apoE4 allele, while others failed to find significant associations between apoE genotype and plasma lipid response [101–103]. Important differences exist among these studies that could account for some of the discrepancies observed. Studies differed in subject gender, age, and baseline lipid levels, and all of these variables are known to play an important role in the variability of dietary response. Dreon *et al.* [104] have shown that the apoE-dependent mechanism may be specific for large, buoyant LDL particles. Consequently, baseline LDL particle distribution will also play a significant role on the outcome of different studies and this variable should be controlled in future studies. In addition, Lehtimäki *et al.* [105] have demonstrated that the association between serum lipids and the apoE phenotype is influenced by diet in a population based sample of free-living children and young adults.

Overall, a significant diet by apoE gene interaction has been shown in studies with men alone. In those studies including men and women, significant effects were noted only in men, suggesting a significant gene–sex interaction. Another difference between the negative studies and those reporting significant apoE gene–diet interactions related to the baseline lipid levels of the subjects. Positive findings were frequently observed in those studies reporting significant associations that included subjects who were moderately hypercholesterolemic and/or had significant differences in baseline total cholesterol and LDL cholesterol among the apoE genotype groups, suggesting that the significant gene by diet interaction is apparent only in subjects who are sus-

ceptible to hypercholesterolemia. Concerning differences in dietary interventions, significant interactions were more commonly observed among studies in which total dietary fat and cholesterol were modified. It is possible that dietary cholesterol may play a significant effect in this gene–diet interaction. Note also that some reports have shown that cholesterol absorption is related to apoE genotype.

Other less traditional dietary interventions have been also examined in terms of gene–diet interactions. Thus, Loktionov *et al.* [106] examined the effects of the apoE alleles and tea drinking on blood lipids and blood coagulation factors on healthy men and women. In this study, apoE4 subjects had significantly elevated total cholesterol, LDL cholesterol and triglyceride levels. Moreover, mean plasminogen activator inhibitor (PAI-1) activity was higher in apoE4 subjects than in E3/3 or E3/2 subjects. These findings suggest that elevated PAI-1 activity may be an additional factor involved in the increased cardiovascular risk associated with the apoE4 allele. Tea drinking was associated with significant decreases in HDL cholesterol levels of E3/3 subjects as well as decreases in triglyceride levels and PAI-1 activities of apoE2/3 subjects. These results indicate that tea drinking has a beneficial effect on plasma lipid levels and coagulation factors, especially in subjects carrying the E2 allele. Note that fruits and vegetables also contain polyphenols similar to those in tea, and high consumption of fruits and vegetables have been reported to decrease PAI-1 activity. The molecular mechanisms involved in the interaction between the apoE gene and PAI-1 are still unknown, but one possible link lies on the LDL receptor-related protein receptor, which is known to bind several ligands including apoE, tPA, and PAI-1. Per the hyperresponse observed for the apoE2 allele and triglyceride levels, it should be noted that previous studies using dietary manipulation that included type of carbohydrates and fiber rather than type and amount of dietary fat and cholesterol demonstrated that apoE2 subjects were more responsive to these dietary modifications than apoE3/3 and apoE4 subjects. Moreover, apoE2 carriers are significantly more responsive to HMG CoA reductase inhibitors than E3/3 and E4 subjects [107, 108]. However, these studies were carried out in small groups and they should be confirmed in larger studies.

After several decades of research, it is becoming evident that postprandial lipemia is a major determinant of blood lipoprotein concentrations and CVD risk [109]. The postprandial response is highly heterogeneous, and multiple factors such as age, exercise levels, body weight, fasting lipid levels, diet, and genetics have been noted to be responsible for this variability. The apoE gene has been implicated as one of the genetic factors mediating these effects. The apoE2 isoform is considered to decrease remnant clearance because of impaired affinity for the receptors. Conversely, the apoE4 isoform should induce a faster clearance. However, studies that have compared postprandial triglyceride responses across

different apoE genotypes have produced conflicting results, especially regarding the effects associated with the apoE4 allele [110–114]. Postprandial response was examined at 4 and 8 hours by Boerwinkle et al. [115] in a sample of individuals taking part in the Atherosclerosis Risk in Communities Study (ARIC), following a single high-fat meal containing vitamin A (used as a marker for intestinal lipoprotein synthesis). Postprandial plasma retinyl palmitate response was significantly different among apoE genotypes, with delayed clearance in subjects carrying the apoE2 allele, compared with E3/3 and E3/4 subjects; however, measurements of other lipid variables, such as triglyceride concentration and triglyceride-rich lipoprotein were not sensitive enough to detect these effects. Another study by Nikkilä et al. [113], carried out in CVD cases and controls, showed that in CVD patients with the apoE2/3 phenotype triglyceride levels were highest and still increasing after 7 hours, reflecting delayed chylomicron remnant clearance. The same effect was observed also in normotriglyceridemic non-insulin-dependent diabetic patients [116] and in nondiabetic normolipemic subjects [117], although in this report, the delayed chylomicron remnant was observed only on E2/2 individuals. The findings associated with the apoE4 allele have been more discordant. In an earlier report, heterozygosity for this allele was associated with lower lipemic response in relation to other phenotype groups [111]; however, in a more recent study the E4 allele was associated with prolonged postprandial responses of lipids and apolipoproteins in triglyceride-rich lipoproteins [118]. This subject has been recently revisited by Wolever et al. [119]. These investigators examined the long-term effect of soluble fiber-containing foods on postprandial fat metabolism in dyslipidemic subjects, 16 with apoE3/3 and 17 with E3/4 genotypes. These subjects consumed low-fat (20% of energy), high-fiber (> 24 g/1000 Kcal) diets for two 4-month periods separated by a 2-month washout period according to a randomized crossover design. One diet contained foods rich in insoluble fiber and the other foods rich in soluble fiber. They carried out a 1-day postprandial study during the last 2 weeks of each diet. Subjects ingested a standard, fiber-free, fatty liquid meal containing retinyl palmitate as a marker of intestinally derived lipoproteins. Blood samples were obtained at hourly intervals for 10 hours. Their results suggested that a long-term increase in dietary soluble fiber does not affect postprandial fat metabolism in subjects with the apoE4 allele; however, soluble fiber enhanced fat absorption in E3/3 subjects, which could be due to an increased bile acid pool and increased micelle formation.

Several mechanisms have been proposed to explain these apoE-related differences in individual response to dietary therapy. Some studies have shown that intestinal cholesterol absorption is related to apoE phenotype, with apoE4 carriers absorbing more cholesterol than non-apoE4 carriers. Other mechanisms, such as different distribution of apoE on the lipoprotein fractions, LDL apoB production, bile acid and cholesterol synthesis, and postprandial lipoprotein clearance, may also be involved.

D. Apolipoprotein C-III (APOC3)

Plasma apoC-III is a component of chylomicrons, VLDL, and HDL. This protein is synthesized primarily in the liver and to a lesser extent in the intestine [120]. In vitro, apoC-III inhibits LPL activity [121] and the binding of apoE-containing lipoproteins to the LDL receptor, but not to the LDL receptor-related protein [122, 123]. In agreement with the observations in vitro, the overexpression of the human apoC3 gene in transgenic mice resulted in severe hypertriglyceridemia [124]. The apoC3 gene is closely linked to the apoA1 and apoA4 genes on the long arm of chromosome 11 (region 11q13) [125]. Several RFLPs have been described at this locus. The S2 allele of the SstI RFLP (C3238G), 3' to the apoC3 gene, has been associated in some studies with hypertriglyceridemia and increased coronary artery disease risk [126–128]. A PvuII RFLP located in the first intron of the apoC3 gene has also been associated with variation in HDL cholesterol levels. In addition, several polymorphisms have been identified in the promoter region of the gene (C^{-641}→A, G^{630}→A, T^{-625} → deletion, C^{-482} → T, and T^{-455} → C) [129]. These mutations are in linkage disequilibrium with the SstI site in the 3' untranslated region [129, 130]. An insulin response element has been mapped to a 42-nucleotide-long fragment located between −490 and −449 relative to the transcription start site and in vitro studies demonstrated that transcriptional activity of the apoC3 gene was downregulated by insulin only in the construct bearing the wild-type promoter, but not in those constructs containing the C^{-482} → T, and T^{-455} →C variants [130, 131]. These results may provide the molecular basis to understand the increased levels of apoC3 found in subjects carrying the S2 allele and its association with hypertriglyceridemia. Our own studies show that following an increase in dietary monounsaturated fat intake, S1S1 subjects responded with an increase in LDL cholesterol levels, whereas S1S2 subjects experienced a significant decrease [132], suggesting that the apoC3 locus is involved in LDL cholesterol responsiveness to dietary fat. This interaction could begin to explain the different effects associated with this polymorphism that have been reported in the literature. Along those lines, Waterworth et al. [133] examined the association of the S2 allele and several other polymorphisms at this locus on postprandial lipid levels following an oral fat load test. The population consisted of young, healthy male offspring whose fathers had had a myocardial infarction before the age of 55 years, compared with age-matched controls. The apoC3 variations examined were C3238G (SstI) in the 3'-UTR, C1100T in exon 3, C-482T in the insulin response element, and T-2854G in the apo-CIII-AIV intergenic region. The postprandial response was regulated by variation at the T-2854G and C3238G sites. After

the oral fat tolerance test, carriers of the rare alleles had significantly delayed clearance of triglyceride levels; G-2854 carriers showed the largest effect on triglycerides, and G3238 carriers showed a lesser response. However, after adjustment for fasting triglyceride levels, only the effect with the T-2854G remained significant.

The reported association of the S2 allele with elevated triglyceride and cholesterol concentrations, and with high blood pressure, all of which are characteristic of an insulin-resistant state, and the presence of an insulin response element in the promoter region of the apoC3 gene, suggests that this polymorphism could also be involved in dysfunctional glucose metabolism. Therefore, we have examined the effect of the C3238G polymorphism on carbohydrate metabolism in healthy subjects. We gave 41 males three consecutive diets [134]. The first was rich in saturated fat, the second was an NCEP Step 1 diet, and the last was rich in monounsaturated fat. At the end of each dietary period, subjects received an oral glucose tolerance test. APOC3 genotype significantly affected basal glucose concentrations and insulin concentrations after the test. Carriers of the S2 allele (n = 13) had higher insulin concentrations after the test than S1/S1 subjects (n = 28) in the three periods. Multiple regression analysis showed that this polymorphism predicted the insulin response to the oral glucose tolerance test and the difference between basal insulin concentrations and insulin concentrations in response to the saturated fat-rich diet.

An association between the apoC3 locus and carbohydrate metabolism was also reported by Waterworth et al. [133] on the EARSII study. Variation at the C-482T insulin response element determined response to the oral glucose tolerance test, with carriers of the rare T-482 having significantly elevated glucose and insulin concentrations.

These data suggest that specific genetic variants at the apoC3 gene locus differentially affect postprandial lipids [133] and response to oral glucose [133, 134], which could result in reduced sensitivity to insulin, especially when persons consume diets rich in saturated fat.

E. Lipoprotein Lipase

Lipoprotein lipase is a heparin-releasable enzyme, bound to glycosaminoglycan components of the capillary endothelium. It plays a key role in lipoprotein metabolism by catalyzing the hydrolysis of 1,3 ester bonds of triglycerides in chylomicrons and VLDL. The active form of LPL is constituted by two identical subunits each of approximately 60,000 daltons, which require apoC-II as a cofactor, whereas apoC-III acts as an inhibitor. LPL is synthesized in the adipose and muscle tissue, as well as in macrophages [135]. The gene for LPL has been located to the short arm of chromosome 8 (region 8p22) [136, 137]. Several common RFLPs have been reported at this locus, including a PvuII RFLP located in the intron between exons 6 and 7 [138], a HindIII located in the

intron between exons 8 and 9 [139], and a C-to-G transversion at nucleotide 1595 of the cDNA sequence. Unlike the PvuII and HindIII RFLPs, the later mutation alters the structure of the protein and it results in the production of a truncated protein (Ser447-Stop) [140]. In population studies, these variants have been found associated with variability in plasma lipid levels and with CVD [141–143]. The HindIII RFLP has also been reported to be associated with the variability in lipid response to changing from a high saturated to a low saturated fat diet [144].

Other relatively common mutations at this locus have been recently reported to be associated with mild alteration in lipid profiles. A missense mutation (Asn291Ser) in exon 6 has been found with relative high frequency (2–4%) in Western populations, and appears to be enriched in familial combined hyperlipidemia [145, 146] and low HDL cholesterol [147]. In vivo and in vitro measurements of LPL activity indicate that this mutation is associated with approximately 50–70% of normal lipase catalytic activity. Pimstone et al. [148] have shown that normolipidemic Asn291Ser carriers exhibited a more pronounced postprandial response compared with noncarriers as shown by higher chylomicron triglyceride and retinyl palmitate peaks. It is possible that carriers of this mutation may be unable to respond to a high-fat diet by an increase in their LPL activity as normal subjects do. Thus, an oral fat challenge may unmask a hidden defect in lipolysis in these subjects that may not be evident in the fasting state. Another common variant (Asp9Asn) has been associated with elevated triglyceride levels and with increased progression of coronary atherosclerosis [149–151]; however, to date no reports have appeared regarding the response of these subjects to a fat challenge.

We have examined these LPL variants and their potential associations with lipid levels and CVD risk on the Framingham Heart Study [152, 153]. Carrier frequency of the S447X allele was 17%; in men, carrier status was associated with higher total cholesterol and HDL cholesterol, and lower triglyceride levels. Moreover, in men, the S447X allele conferred protection against CVD. These effects on lipids and CVD were not seen in women. We have also assessed in this population the effect of the D9N and N291S alleles, and we extended our study by calculating weighed means of lipids and lipoproteins in carriers and noncarriers for these mutations in patients with genetic dyslipidemias, CVD patients and healthy controls. In the Framingham Offspring sample, the D9N and N291S alleles were associated with lower HDL cholesterol and a trend towards increased triglycerides. In women, a trend toward a high triglyceride, low HDL cholesterol lipid pattern was evident. Cumulative analysis of other studies of male carriers of the D9N and N291S alleles revealed higher levels of triglycerides and lower HDL cholesterol. In females, results differed with higher triglyceride levels for the N291S and D9N carriers, and lower HDL cholesterol levels only for N291S carriers. These data provide

evidence that these LPL variants are significant modulators of lipid levels in both men and women.

F. Microsomal Triglyceride Transfer Protein

Microsomal triglyceride transfer protein (MTP) is a lipid transfer protein that is required for the assembly and secretion of VLDL by the liver and chylomicrons by the intestine. MTP is a heterodimer composed of a 55-kDa multifunctional protein, protein disulfide isomerase, and a unique large subunit with an apparent molecular weight of 88 kDa [154]. The gene has been localized to 4q22-q24. Wetterau et al. [155] demonstrated that MTP activity and the large subunit of MTP were present in intestinal biopsy samples from eight control persons but were absent in four abetalipoproteinemic subjects. They suggested that the findings proved that MTP is the site of the defect in abetalipoproteinemia and that MTP is required for lipoprotein assembly.

A common G–493T polymorphism at the MTP gene promoter has been shown to be associated with decreased plasma LDL cholesterol and apoB content of VLDL [156]. We have investigated the association of this mutation with variations in lipid and apoprotein levels, lipoprotein subclass profiles, and CVD risk in Framingham Heart Study participants [157]. In men and women, no significant association was found between the G–493T MTP polymorphism and variations of plasma levels of total cholesterol, LDL cholesterol, apoB, HDL cholesterol, apoA-I, and triglyceride. To further investigate potential relationships with variations of lipoprotein phenotypes, lipoprotein subclass profiles were measured using automated nuclear magnetic resonance (NMR) spectroscopy. Each NMR profile yielded information on lipid mass of VLDL, LDL, and HDL subclasses. In both genders, there was no significant association between the G–493T polymorphism and variability of lipoprotein subclass distributions or lipoprotein particle size. Furthermore, no significant association was found between the polymorphism of the MTP promoter and prevalence or the age of onset of CVD. Thus, our results suggest that the G–493T mutation in the MTP promoter is unlikely to have significant implications for CVD in men and women. No reports are available regarding potential associations between this locus and dietary response.

G. Intestinal Fatty Acid Binding Protein

The intestinal fatty acid binding protein (IFABP) gene (FABP2) codes for the IFABP. The IFABP is a member of a family of small (14–15 kDa) intracellular lipid binding proteins. Besides the IFABP, this family also includes the heart, epidermal, brain, and liver fatty acid binding proteins, testicular, myelin, adipocyte, and ileal lipid binding proteins, and cellular retinol and retinoic acid binding proteins [158]. The gene located in 4q28-q31[159] has the conserved 4 exons

and 3 introns characteristic of this family of genes [160, 161]. It has been found that the expression of IFABP mRNA is under dietary control [162].

IFABP plays important roles in several steps of fat absorption and transport, including uptake and trafficking of saturated and unsaturated long-chain fatty acids, targeting free fatty acids toward different metabolic pathways, protecting the cytosol from the cytotoxic effects of free fatty acids, and modulating enzyme activity involved in lipid metabolism [163, 164]. Besides free fatty acids, the IFABP may bind other ligands, such as phenolic antioxidants. The IFABP is abundant in the enterocyte and represents 2–3% of an enterocyte's cytoplasmic mass [165]. Sacchettini et al. [166] found that the fatty acid binding proteins each have 10 anti-parallel β strands, which form two orthogonal β sheets. There are two short α helices, which are connected to the first two β strands. This structure has been characterized as a β clam because it resembles a clamshell. It is hypothesized that fatty acids enter the fatty acid binding protein by passing a portal that includes three structures; the portal is comprised of one of the α helices, and two sharp turns between β strands, which include residues 54–55 and 73–74 [166, 167]. A mutation in the IFABP at any of these amino acid residues that surround the portal may alter fatty acid entry into the protein. This may result in abnormal binding of fatty acids, which can then influence lipid profiles and consequently disease risk.

Baier et al. [168] reported a new G→A mutation, which results in an amino acid substitution in IFABP at residue 54, alanine54 (wild-type)→threonine (mutant-type). This polymorphism is very common, with a thr54 allelic frequency of around 29% in most populations. To this date, the ala54thr mutation in the IFABP is the only functional mutation found in humans in a member of the cytoplasmic fatty acid binding protein family [169]. This amino acid substitution was found to be associated with elevated fasting insulin levels, insulin resistance, and increased fatty acid binding in Pima indians [168, 170]. Associations of this polymorphism with several biochemical and anthropometric variables have been subsequently carried out in Japanese, Mexican-American, Native Americans, and Caucasian populations. In general, the presence of the thr54 allele has been associated in some, but not all [171–175], studies with higher fasting insulin concentrations [168, 176] and insulin resistance. On the other hand, a study of Keewatin Inuit (Eskimos) found the thr54 allele to be associated with lower 2-hour glucose concentrations [175]. It is well known that Eskimos have large dietary intakes of omega–3 fatty acids from fish. This finding in Eskimos suggests that differences in the type of fatty acid consumed interact with the functional differences in the gene products to produce phenotypic differences.

Several studies have utilized the euglycemic, hyperinsulinemic clamp for determining insulin resistance. Using this approach, the FABP2 mutation was associated with a lower

mean insulin-stimulated glucose uptake rate in Pima indians. However, no significant findings were noted in subjects with familial combined hyperlipidemia [177] and in overweight, Finnish subjects [178]. In a separate study, Stern *et al.* [179] found that the IFABP was not significantly linked to the major gene for the age of onset for non-insulin-dependent diabetes mellitus (NIDDM) [179].

Other studies have found an association between the presence of the thr54 mutation and higher mean fat oxidation rate [168, 178] and greater fasting plasma triglycerides [180]. However, Vidgren *et al.* examined a small group of Finnish subjects after an overnight fast and found no differences in the proportion of long-chain fatty acids in serum lipids among the three genotypes.

Regarding differences in dietary response, Hegele *et al.* [182] found that the ala54thr mutation was associated with variation in the response of plasma lipoproteins to dietary fiber. Subjects with the mutant thr54 allele, compared to those homozygous for the ala54 allele, had significantly greater decreases in plasma total and LDL cholesterol and apoB when consuming a high soluble fiber diet than when consuming a high insoluble fiber diet. Moreover, Agren *et al.* [183] have shown that the triglyceride response to an oral fat load test was greater in Thr homozygotes. In addition, the classical correlation between fasting and postprandial triglyceride levels was present in Ala carriers, but not so in Thr individuals, suggesting that the delayed triglyceride-rich lipoprotein clearance may affect insulin action (or vice versa).

In vitro studies have found that the thr54 IFABP differs from the ala54 IFABP, and these studies offer a biologically plausible mechanism for thr54's role in altered lipid metabolism and disease states. Baier *et al.* [168] found, through titration microcalorimetry, that the thr54 IFABP had a two-fold greater affinity for long-chain fatty acids than the ala54 IFABP. In addition, in another study, Baier's group created permanently transfected Caco–2 cells that express the ala54 or thr54 IFABP [184]. The cells expressing the mutant thr54 protein were found to have greater transport of long-chain fatty acids and greater secretion of triglycerides than the ala54 protein. A recent study with mouse L-cells transfected with wild-type IFABP found that the increase in secretion of triglycerides over nontransfected cells was due to increased synthesis in the cell [185]. The results of these studies support Baier *et al.*'s findings in which the thr54 protein has a higher affinity for long-chain fatty acids than the ala54 protein [168, 184]. The three-dimensional structure of the wild-type IFABP has been studied by NMR and it was shown that amino acid 54 in the IFABP is important in the stabilization of the portal region, where the fatty acid enters the protein [167, 186]. Amino acid 54 interacts with α-helix II and helps to stabilize the portal region. Hodsdon and Cistola [187] hypothesize that since threonine can hydrogen bond and alanine cannot, then thr54 will be better able to interact with α-helix II and stabilize the portal, which may lead to increased binding of fatty acids [167].

In summary, the physiological function of the protein coded by this gene and the preliminary findings reported regarding the only common variant described warrant further research to assess the full impact of this locus on the interindividual variability in dietary response.

III. ENDOGENOUS LIPOPROTEIN METABOLISM

The hepatocyte synthesizes and secretes triglyceride-rich VLDL, which may be converted first to intermediate-density lipoproteins and then to LDL through lipolysis by a mechanism involving LPL, similar to that described for the exogenous lipoprotein pathway. The excess surface components are usually transferred to HDL. Some of these remnants may be taken up by the liver, whereas others are further lipolyzed to become LDL, which, in humans, contains apoB as their only apolipoprotein. This pathway shares many of the genes described already for the exogenous pathway. This section will describe briefly some of the studies related to the LDL receptor gene and coding for the LDL receptor, which has major responsibility for catabolism of the LDL particles in the liver and peripheral tissues.

A. LDL Receptor

The LDL receptor gene has been localized to the 19p13. 1 region. Mutations at this locus have been found to be responsible for familial hypercholesterolemia, an autosomal dominant disorder characterized by elevation of LDL cholesterol and premature CVD. The frequency of homozygosity is estimated to be 1 in 1 million, and the frequency of heterozygotes approximately 1 in 500. Several hundred different mutations have been already described in the LDL receptor gene and many of them have been reviewed in detail [188, 189]. In addition to those mutations associated with familial hypercholesterolemia, several highly informative (maximum heterozygosity ranging from 0.4 to 0.5) deletions [190], point mutations [191], dinucleotide repeats [192], and RFLPs [192–200] have been described in this locus.

Several lines of LDL receptor transgenics have been generated. In one of them, plasma concentrations of apoB and apoE decreased by more than 90% [201]. In another line, expression of the human LDL receptor gene in the mouse liver was able to completely obliterate the diet-induced hypercholesterolemia in these mice [202].

The targeted disruption of the LDL receptor gene resulted in hypercholesterolemia due primarily to increases in intermediate-density lipoproteins and LDL with no changes in HDL levels [203]. This LDL-receptor-deficient mouse is a good model for the human familial hypercholesterolemia, and it has been extensively used as a background to generate additional transgenic models and to test gene replacement therapy.

Although we have not directly tested the effect of different mutations at the LDL receptor locus and variability in dietary response, we have carried out several studies examining other loci in heterozygote subjects. In general, our data suggest that the strong effect of the LDL receptor mutations tend to obscure other minor effects associated with other loci in normolipemic subjects [91, 204].

B. 3-Hydroxy–3-Methylglutaryl-Coenzyme A Reductase

3-Hydroxy-3-methylglutaryl-coenzyme A reductase (HMG-CoA) catalyzes a rate-limiting step in cholesterol biosynthesis and also participates in the production of a variety of other compounds. This enzyme has been an extremely successful drug target in the form of HMG-CoA reductase inhibitors. *In situ* hybridization permitted the precise regionalization of this gene to chromosome 5. The findings from our own genome scan [205] suggest that this chromosomal region may be important in determining plasma lipid variability in this same population.

Despite its important biological role and the fact that it has been a very successful drug target, this gene has been barely examined in terms of variability in dietary response. Boucher *et al.* [206] have studied the effects of cholesterol feeding in healthy subjects on monocyte mRNA levels for the LDL receptor, HMG-CoA receptor, and LRP genes. These authors found coordinated regulation of these genes involved in the synthesis and removal of cholesterol. Briefly, during cholesterol restriction phase, LDL receptor and HMG-CoA mRNA levels increased, whereas during the cholesterol-rich phase, the levels of these mRNAs decreased significantly. Conversely the levels of LRP mRNA increased during this phase. This research demonstrates for the first time that the LRP gene is also responsive to dietary cholesterol.

IV. REVERSE CHOLESTEROL TRANSPORT

HDL is synthesized by both the liver and the intestine. Its precursor form is discoidal in shape and matures in circulation as it picks up unesterified cholesterol from cell membranes (see ATP binding cassette-1 below), other lipids (phospholipids and triglycerides), and proteins from triglyceride-rich lipoproteins as these particles undergo lipolysis. The cholesterol is esterified by the action of LCAT and the small HDL3 particle becomes a larger HDL2 particle. The esterified cholesterol is either delivered to the liver or transferred by the action of the cholesterol ester transfer protein to triglyceride-rich lipoproteins in exchange for triglyceride. The liver may then take up this cholesterol via receptors specific for these lipoproteins, or it can be delivered again to the peripheral tissues. The triglycerides received by the HDL2 are hydrolysed by hepatic lipase and the particle is converted back to HDL3, completing the HDL3 cycle in plasma. In the liver,

cholesterol can either be excreted directly into bile, converted to bile acids, or reutilized in lipoprotein production.

Some of these factors involved in reverse cholesterol transport have common genetic variants. Their associations with plasma lipid levels, CVD risk, and variability in response to diet are described below.

A. Apolipoprotein A-I (APOA1)

ApoA-I, the major protein of HDL, plays several crucial roles in the metabolism of these particles as (1) structural component, (2) activator of the enzyme LCAT [207], and (3) key component of the reverse cholesterol transport process [208]. The gene for apoA-I is clustered with the apoC-III and apoA-IV genes on the long arm of human chromosome 11 [125, 209]. This DNA region has been extensively analyzed, resulting in the identification of about 16 common RFLPs with a heterozygosity value ranging from 0.499 to 0.095. Multiple studies have examined some of these genetic variants in relation to variability in plasma lipids or CVD risk in populations. Several investigators have found statistically significant associations between some of these RFLPs and lipid abnormalities as well as increased CVD risk [127, 128, 210, 211], but others have failed to do so [212].

In addition to the common variants, more than 20 different rare genetic abnormalities have been reported within this locus (http://www3.ncbi.nlm.nih.gov/Omim/searchomim.html). Some have been associated with severe HDL deficiency and premature coronary atherosclerosis [62, 213, 214]; however, at least one of these mutations shows a protective effect despite its association with low HDL [215, 216].

The common variant most intensively studied is the one resulting from an adenine (A) to guanine (G) transition (G/A), 75-bp upstream from the apoA-I gene transcription start site. Several studies have reported that individuals with the A allele, which occurs at a frequency of 0.15–0.20 in Caucasian populations, have higher levels of HDL cholesterol than those subjects homozygous for the most common G allele. The magnitude and the gender distribution of this effect have differed among studies. These data are summarized in a recent meta-analysis [216a]. The reasons for these discrepancies are not known. Our own data [217, 218] support the notion that in well controlled dietary studies performed in normolipidemic subjects, the A allele of this G/A polymorphism appears to be associated with hyperresponse to changes in the amount and saturation of dietary fat. Moreover, other investigators have shown that the significance of the associations may depend on cigarette smoking. Therefore, these data suggest an interaction between this polymorphism and environmental factors such as dietary and smoking habits [217–219].

It is not clear whether the putative effect of this variant on HDL cholesterol levels is due to the G to A substitution per se, or to linkage disequilibrium between the A locus and

a distinct and as yet unidentified effector locus. *In vitro* analysis of the effects of this polymorphism on transcription has yielded conflicting results. Smith *et al.* [220] reported that the A allele decreased *in vitro* transcription by 30%, consistent with their own *in vivo* turnover studies that showed decreased apoA-I synthetic rates in individuals with the A allele, although plasma HDL cholesterol did not differ between GG and GA individuals. Tuteja *et al.* [221] reported that substitution of A for G decreased transcription about two-fold, and Jeenah *et al.* [222] reported a four-fold increase in transcription. Angotti *et al.* [223] reported a five- to sevenfold increase in transcription associated to the A allele, and demonstrated that this may be due to reduced binding affinity of a nuclear factor to the A allele that results in increased transcription efficiency of the apoA-I promoter. More recent research has demonstrated that the induction of apoA-I mRNA level in response to gemfibrozil is mediated at the transcriptional level and this effect is mediated by two copies of the "drug-responsive element" in the apoA-I promoter region in the same area as the -75 G/A polymorphism. These data suggest that this apoA-I variant may be a functional mutation responsible for some of the individual variability in HDL cholesterol response to gemfibrozil therapy [224].

In summary, the mechanisms responsible for the observed effect are still unknown. This mutation may have a direct effect on liver and/or intestinal apoA1 gene expression as suggested in previous studies or it may be in linkage disequilibrium with a functional mutation in either of the neighboring genes (apoC3 and apoA4). Further studies are needed to clarify these results.

B. Cholesteryl Ester Transfer Protein

Cholesteryl ester transfer protein (CETP) mediates the exchange of neutral lipid core constituents (cholesteryl ester and triglycerides) between plasma lipoproteins. The facilitation of the transfer of cholesteryl ester from HDL to triglyceride-rich lipoproteins results in a reduction in HDL cholesterol levels, but CETP may also promote the reverse cholesterol transport. Therefore, the overall effect of CETP expression on atherogenesis is uncertain. The gene has been located on chromosome 16 adjacent to the LCAT gene (16q21). A common *Taq*I polymorphism has been identified in intron 1 (*Taq*IB) [225–229]. The presence of the cutting site has been referred to as B1 and its absence as B2. The B2 allele has been shown to be associated with lower lipid transfer activity [230] and higher HDL cholesterol concentrations [231]. Fumeron *et al.* [232] found that alcohol intake modulates the effect of the *Taq*IB polymorphism on plasma HDL and the risk of myocardial infarction. They found that HDL cholesterol was increased in subjects with the B2B2 genotype only when they ingested at least 25 g alcohol per day. In that study, the cardioprotective effect of the B2B2 CETP genotype was restricted to subjects who consumed the highest amounts of alcohol.

Several reports have demonstrated a significant gene-smoking interaction associated with this RFLP, but only one study has examined the relationship between this polymorphism and dietary response. Dullaart *et al.* [233], in a study of patients with insulin-dependent diabetes, demonstrated that the ratio of VLDL cholesterol plus LDL cholesterol to HDL cholesterol fell in response to a linoleic acid-enriched, low-cholesterol diet in B1B1 homozygotes but not in B1B2 heterozygotes.

An interesting gene–drug interaction has been reported [234] in men with angiographically documented coronary atherosclerosis who were participants in a cholesterol-lowering trial designed to induce the regression of coronary atherosclerosis and were randomly assigned to treatment with either pravastatin or placebo for 2 years. The presence of the *Taq*IB polymorphism was associated with both higher plasma CETP concentrations and lower HDL cholesterol concentrations. In addition, they observed a significant association between this marker and the progression of coronary atherosclerosis in the placebo group. This association was abolished by pravastatin. Pravastatin therapy slowed the progression of coronary atherosclerosis in those homozygous for this polymorphism but not in those were homozygous for the most common allele. This common DNA variant appeared to predict whether men with coronary artery disease will benefit from treatment with pravastatin to delay the progression of coronary atherosclerosis.

The evidence of the asociation of the CETP *Taq*IB polymorphism with HDL cholesterol levels and its interaction with smoking is solid. Similar evidence for gene–diet interaction is beginning to emerge. However, the mechanism is unknown. The *Taq*IB polymorphism is within the noncoding region of the CETP, thus suggesting that the *Taq*IB may be in linkage disequilibrium with another polymorphism that may affect CETP activity and, consequently, plasma HDL cholesterol levels.

C. Hepatic Lipase

Hepatic lipase is a lipolytic enzyme that is synthesized in the hepatocytes, secreted, and bound extracellularly to the liver [235]. Hepatic lipase participates in the metabolism of intermediate density lipoproteins and large LDL to form smaller, denser LDL particles and in the conversion of HDL^2 to HDL^3. In addition, hepatic lipase can mediate the unloading of cholesterol from HDL to the plasma membrane in the liver [236]. It has also been suggested that hepatic lipase may act as a ligand protein with cell surface proteoglycans in the uptake of lipoproteins by cell surface receptors. Lipid profile of individuals with complete hepatic lipase deficiency is characterized by elevated plasma cholesterol and triglyceride levels, triglyceride enrichment of lipoprotein fractions with a density >1.006 g/Ml, the presence of a β-VLDL, and an impaired metabolism of postprandial triglyceride-rich lipoproteins [237, 238]. Four polymorphism in the 5'-flanking region of hepatic lipase gene (G → A at position -250, C →

T at −514, T → C at −710, and A → G at −763), with respect to the transcription site were observed to be in total linkage disequilibrium and were found to be associated with a lowered hepatic lipase activity and higher HDL cholesterol levels. A number of recent studies have also shown an association between low hepatic lipase activity and more buoyant, less atherogenic LDL particles and suggest that variants in the hepatic lipase promoter may contribute significantly to the prevalence of the atherogenic small, dense, LDL particle phenotype associated with an increased CVD risk [239].

In recent studies, the C−514T polymorphism in the promoter region of the hepatic lipase gene has been shown to be associated with significant variations in hepatic lipase activity, plasma HDL cholesterol levels and LDL particle size [240, 241]. We have investigated the association of this polymorphism to lipoprotein levels in the Framingham Heart Study [242]. Our data show that in men and women, carriers of the −514T allele had higher HDL cholesterol and ApoA-I concentrations compared with noncarriers. The higher HDL cholesterol levels associated with the −514T allele were due to an increase in the HDL2 cholesterol subfraction and this association was stronger in women compared with men ($P = 0.0517$ vs. 0.0043). We also measured HDL and LDL subclass profiles using automated NMR spectroscopy and gradient gel electrophoresis, respectively. The association of the −514T allele with higher HDL cholesterol levels seen in men and women was primarily due to significant increases in the large HDL subfractions (size range: 8.8–13.0 nm). In contrast, there was no relationship between hepatic lipase polymorphism at position −514 and LDL particle size distribution after adjustment for the familial relationships, age, body mass index, smoking, alcohol intake, use of beta-blockers, and ApoE genotype, and also menopausal status and estrogen therapy in women. Moreover, multiple regression analyses suggested that the C−514T polymorphism contributes significantly to the variability of HDL particle size in men and women ($P < 0.04$). Thus, our results show that the C−514T polymorphism in the hepatic lipase gene is associated with significant variations in the lipoprotein profile in men and women.

D. Cholesterol 7 Alpha-Hydroxylase

The first reaction of the catabolic pathway of cholesterol is catalyzed by CYP7 and serves as the rate-limiting step and major site of regulation of bile acid synthesis in the liver. The cholesterol catabolic pathway, exclusive to the liver, is comprised of several enzymes, which convert cholesterol into bile acids. Previous studies show that CYP7 is regulated by bile acid feedback, cholesterol, and hormonal factors [243]. In addition, dietary fats modulate the regulatory potential of dietary cholesterol on CYP7 gene expression [244]. The human CYP7 has been localized to chromosome 8q11-q12 [245]. A common A-to-C substitution at position −204 of the promoter of the CYP7 gene is associated with variations in plasma LDL cholesterol [246]. Moreover, the study of the

molecular mechanisms of the transcriptional regulation of CYP7 by sterols and bile acids has revealed that the promoter region between −432 and −220 contains several cell-specific enhancer elements whose activity is controlled, in part, by hepatocyte nuclear factor 3 [247]. Therefore, it is conceivable that the A−204C polymorphism might modulate transcription of the CYP7 gene and, consequently, the rate of cholesterol catabolism. The balance between the rates of hepatic sterol acquisition and excretion largely determines whether an individual is a hypo- or hyperresponder to dietary cholesterol. Therefore, even though there is no published evidence of the involvement of this locus in dietary response, the current evidence suggests that this should be examined in future studies [248].

E. Scavenger Receptor B Type I

Scavenger receptor B type I (SRBI) is a multilipoprotein receptor found in the liver and steroidogenic glands of mice [249] and humans [250–252]. The cDNA for human SRBI [also known as LIMPII analogous 1 (CLA-1)] was originally cloned by homology to human CD36 and rat lysosomal integral membrane protein II (LIMPII), members of a family of transmembrane proteins [253]. Another study identified the hamster homolog by its ability to mediate the binding of modified LDL, and it was also shown to bind native LDL [254]. Subsequently, murine SRBI was shown to mediate the uptake of lipid, but not apoprotein, from HDL into cells [255], a process described as selective uptake [256]. This finding established SRBI as the first HDL transmembrane receptor to be identified and cloned. Further studies of the human homolog demonstrated that it also is a multilipoprotein receptor that binds HDL, LDL, and VLDL [250, 257]. Preliminary evidence from our studies indicates that the SRBI gene plays a significant role in determining lipid concentrations and body mass index [258]. Moreover, the observation that SRBI mediates absorption of dietary cholesterol in the intestine [259] suggests that it may also play a role in the postprandial response and insulin metabolism. Our preliminary data regarding association of variants at this locus with lipid levels and anthropometric variables, as well as the differential gender effects, warrant a more detailed study of this locus.

F. ATP-Binding Cassette 1

For several decades the elucidation of the reverse pathway involving the cholesterol efflux from cells and its transport and internalization by the liver has been intensively studied. However, these mechanisms have been poorly understood. The identification of SRBI as an HDL receptor was a step forward in our understanding of reverse cholesterol transport. However the role of this receptor within the scheme of human lipoprotein metabolism is still unknown. We may have reached a breaking point in our understanding of reverse cholesterol transport with the elucidation of a biological

mystery that began almost four decades ago in the small Tangier Island located in Chesapeake Bay in the United States. Two brothers living on the island presented with orange tonsils, peripheral neuropathy and, more interesting for the present focus, deficiency of HDL cholesterol. Scores of investigators have studied families affected with this rare disease with the notion that a better understanding of this disease could provide the key to the molecular basis of reverse cholesterol transport, therefore providing with new mechanistic tools to prevent the development of atherosclerosis and the treatment of CVD.

Patients with Tangier disease are characterized by their almost complete absence of HDL and they accumulate cholesteryl esters in tissues, resulting in enlarged orange tonsils, hepatosplenomegaly, peripheral neuropathy, and deposits in the rectal mucosa [260]. After 40 years of research, several groups have reported, almost simultaneously, the gene locus and several specific mutations responsible for Tangier disease [261–263, 265] and for some forms of familial hypoalphalipoproteinemia [266]. These investigations clearly demonstrate that mutations in the ATP-binding cassette transporter 1 (ABC1) gene are responsible for the Tangier phenotype in several kindred from a variety of ethnic backgrounds. ABC1 belongs to the ABC family of genes. These genes encode for proteins involved in vectorial movement of substrates across biological membranes. The ABC1 transporter consists of two symmetric halves, each including six membrane-spanning domains and a nucleotide-binding fold. Moreover, a long charged region and a highly hydrophobic segment link these two halves of the molecule. The transporter activity depends on its interaction with ATP. This specific transporter appears to be involved in free cholesterol transport (and perhaps phospholipids), and the alteration of this important cellular function results in impaired efflux of free cellular cholesterol and onto HDL particles, thus preventing the formation of normal nascent HDL particles. Consequently, the lipid-poor HDL is quickly removed from the circulation without being able to accomplish its function. This abnormality clearly prevents normal reverse cholesterol transport and patients with Tangier disease tend to develop premature CVD, despite relatively low levels of LDL cholesterol.

It is important to remark that all these reports have found different mutations in the different kindred studied. These data support the concept that Tangier disease may be very heterogeneous, a situation similar to that of familial hypercholesterolemia, where several hundred mutations have been reported for the LDL receptor locus. This may also explain the heterogeneous phenotypic expression of this disease, with pedigrees showing a high incidence of premature CVD, whereas in other families, the risk does not appear to be much higher than in normal subjects.

These findings point toward a new physiological mechanism controlling cellular cholesterol metabolism and its efflux to HDL. However, given the rarity of Tangier disease, mutations at the ABC1 gene could have very limited impact in modulating HDL levels in the population at large. However, the findings reported by Marcil et al. [266] are of great relevance, because they demonstrate that the ABC1 locus is also responsible for a much more common HDL deficiency known as familial hypoalphalipoproteinemia that shares with Tangier's disease the low levels of HDL cholesterol but not some of the other phenotypic characteristics (such as neuropathy and orange tonsils). Familial hypoalphalipoproteinemia is one of the most common genetic abnormalities in subjects with premature CVD [267].

The identification of ABC1 as the gene for Tangier disease and for some cases of familial hypoalphalipoproteinemia opens enormous opportunities for the lipoprotein field and for CVD therapy. The metabolic pathways determined by the product of the ABC1 gene will contribute to our understanding of reverse cholesterol transport and its regulation by dietary fat and cholesterol. It remains to be elucidated whether common mutations at this locus are associated with altered HDL cholesterol levels in the population. This research is being carried out by several groups and it will determine the full impact of the ABC1 in controlling cholesterol efflux and HDL metabolism in the general population, beyond those affected by Tangier disease or familial hypoalphalipoproteinemia. This information will be applied to the genetic screening of subjects at high risk for CVD and it could provide us with new therapeutic targets thus increasing our ability to prevent and treat CVD.

V. CONCLUSION

The mechanisms involved in the regulation of plasma lipoprotein levels by dietary factors, such as intakes of cholesterol and fatty acids, have been partially elucidated during the past century, thanks to the research efforts of scores of investigators. This research has also brought up a number of candidate genes that regulate the homeostasis of blood lipids. Considering the significant effect of diet on plasma lipids, genetic variation at those loci is expected explain some of the dramatic interindividual variations in lipoprotein response to dietary change that have been shown to exist among individuals. In fact, the current evidence supports the importance of gene–diet interactions in humans. Multiple candidate genes have been examined under different experimental conditions and the major findings have been highlighted in this chapter. However, because of conflicting results, more studies will be required to increase our predictive capacity and to reconcile the multiple discordances found in the literature.

At this regard, we have to keep in mind that lipoprotein response to dietary factors is extremely complex, as illustrated by the multiple interrelated pathways and genes discussed herein. Therefore, the effects of individual gene variants can be difficult to identify. In fact, it is quite possible that the concerted action of differences in "gene families"

may be required to elicit significant interindividual differences in responsiveness to diet. Moreover, until the information generated by the Human Genome Project is available and analyzed, we currently have an incomplete list of the genes potentially involved in these processes.

We should also be cautious concerning the interpretation of studies of association between allelic variants and common phenotypes [268]. We should direct attention to the population admixture, which can cause an artificial association if a study includes genetically distinct subpopulations, one of which coincidentally displays a higher frequency of disease and allelic variants. Consideration of the ethnic backgrounds of subjects and the use of multiple, independent populations can help avoid this problem. The most robust tests involve family-based controls such as the transmission disequilibrium test. In this case, if a given allele contributes to disease, then the probability that an affected person has inherited the allele from a heterozygous parent should vary from the expected Mendelian ratio of 50:50; the association of a neutral polymorphism due to admixture displays no such deviation.

Another source of concern is multiple-hypothesis testing, which is aggravated by publication bias. Authors who test a single genetic variant for an association with a single phenotype base statistical thresholds for significance on a single hypothesis. But many laboratories search for associations using different variants. Each test represents an independent hypothesis, but only positive results are reported, leading to an overestimate of the significance of any positive associations. Statistical correction for multiple testing is possible, but the application of such thresholds results in loss of statistical power.

An additional caveat about the published literature relates to the fact that most studies were not initially designed to examine gene–diet interactions, but they are reanalysis of previously obtained data using new information from genetic analysis carried out *a posteriori*. Future studies need to be carefully designed in terms of sample size, taking into consideration the frequencies of the alleles examined. Moreover, we do not really know yet the specific dietary factors responsible for most of the effects already reported. Therefore, baseline and intervention diets should be carefully controlled in terms of dietary cholesterol, individual fatty acids, levels of fat, as well as fiber and other minor components of the diet such as phytosterols. It is also important to emphasize that some allele effects may be apparent primarily during situations of metabolic "stress," such as the postprandial state. Therefore, studies should be designed to test gene–diet interactions, both in the fasting and fed states. As indicated above, the most plausible scenario is that multiple genes will determine the response to dietary manipulation. Consequently, attention should be paid to gene–gene interactions. However, the large number of study subjects required and subsequent costs involved may make such studies infeasible. Two alternatives to examine these complex interactions in

humans are possible: One would be to select study participants based on their genetic variants; the second would be to make use of the large cohort studies for which dietary information has been collected. The latter approach would take the concept of gene–diet interactions beyond the metabolic unit into the real world.

The use of animal models will play a crucial role for mapping new genes involved in dietary responsiveness and atherogenesis. Furthermore, future studies will need to include siblings and families with the dual purpose of getting a more accurate measure of heritability and the performance of wide genome scans to search for new responsiveness loci.

Acknowledgments

This work was supported by grant HL54776 from the NHLBI and contract 53-K06–5–10 from the U.S. Department of Agriculture Research Service.

References

1. Blankenhorn, D. H., Johnson, R. L., Mack, W. J., el Zein, H. A., and Vailas, L. I. (1990). The influence of diet on the appearance of new lesions in human coronary arteries. *JAMA* **263,** 1646–1652.
2. Scandinavian Simvastatin Survival Study Group. (1994). Randomised trial of cholesterol lowering in 4444 patients with coronary heart disease: The Scandinavian Simvastatin Survival Study (4S). *Lancet* **344,** 1383–1389.
3. Sacks, F. M., Pfeffer, M. A., Moye, L. A., Rouleau, J. L., Rutherford, J. D., Cole, T. G., Brown, L., Warnica, J. W., Arnold, J. M. O., Wun, C. C., Davis, B. R., and Braunwald, E. (1996). The effect of pravastatin on coronary events after myocardial infarction in patients with average cholesterol levels. *N. Engl. J. Med.* **335,** 1001–1009.
4. Rubins, H. B., Robins, S. J., Collins, D., Fye, C. L., Anderson, J. W., Elam, M. B., Faas, F. H., Linares, E., Schaefer, E. J., Schectman, G., Wilt, T. J., and Wittes, J. (1999). Gemfibrozil for the secondary prevention of coronary heart disease in men with low levels of high-density lipoprotein cholesterol. Veterans Affairs High-Density Lipoprotein Cholesterol Intervention Trial Study Group. *N. Engl. J. Med.* **341,** 410–418.
5. Expert Panel on High Blood Cholesterol in Adults. (1993). Summary of the second report of the National Cholesterol Education Program (NCEP). Expert Panel on Detection, Evaluation, and Treatment of High Blood Cholesterol in Adults (Adult Treatment Panel II). *JAMA* **269,** 3015–3023.
6. Keys, A., Anderson, J. T., and Grande, F. (1957). "Essential" fatty acids, degree of unsaturation, and effect of corn oil on the serum cholesterol level in man. *Lancet* **1,** 66–68.
7. Ahrens, E. H. (1957). Nutritional factors and serum lipid levels. *Am. J. Med.* **23,** 928–952.
8. Keys, A., Anderson, J. T., and Grande, F. (1957). Prediction of serum cholesterol responses of man to changes in fats in the diet. *Lancet* **2,** 959–966.
9. Hegsted, D. M., McGandy, R. B., Myers, M. L., and Stare, F. J. (1965). Quantitative effects of dietary fat on serum cholesterol in man. *Am. J. Clin. Nutr.* **17,** 281–295.

10. Hegsted, D. M., Ausman, L. M., Johnson, J. A., and Dallal, G. E. (1993). Dietary fat and serum lipids: An evaluation of the experimental data. *Am. J. Clin. Nutr.* **57**, 875–883.

11. Mensink, R. P., and Katan, M. B. (1992). Effect of dietary fatty acids on serum lipids and lipoproteins: A meta-analysis of 27 trials. *Arterioscler. Thromb.* **12**, 911–919.

12. Cobb, M. M., and Teitlebaum, H. (1994). Determinants of plasma cholesterol responsiveness to diet. *Br. J. Nutr.* **71**, 271–282.

13. Okey, R. and Stewart, D. (1933). Diet and blood cholesterol in normal women. J. Biolog. Chem. **99**, 717–727.

14. Katan, M. B., Beynen, A. C., de Vries, J. H., and Nobels, A. (1986). Existence of consistent hypo- and hyperresponders to dietary cholesterol in man. Am. J. Epidemiol. **123**, 221–234.

15. Jacobs, D. R., Anderson, J. T., Hannan, P., Keys, A., and Blackburn, H. (1983). Variability in individual serum cholesterol response to change in diet. *Arteriosclerosis* **3**, 349–356.

16. Cobb, M. M., and Risch, N. (1993). Low-density lipoprotein cholesterol responsiveness to diet in normolipidemic subjects. *Metabolism* **42**, 7–13.

17. O'Hanesian, M. A., Rosner, B., Bishop, L. M., and Sacks, F. M. (1996). Effects of inherent responsiveness to diet and day-to-day diet variation on plasma lipoprotein concentrations. *Am. J. Clin. Nutr.* **64**, 53–59.

18. Schaefer, E. J., Lichtenstein, A. H., Lamon-Fava, S., Contois, J. H., Li, Z., Rasmussen, H., McNamara, J. R., and Ordovas, J. M. (1995). Efficacy of a National Cholesterol Education Program Step 2 diet in normolipidemic and hypercholesterolemic middle-aged and elderly men and women. *Arterioscler. Thromb. Vasc. Biol.* **15**, 1079–1085.

19. Rainwater, D. L. (1994). Genetic effects on dietary response of Lp(a). concentrations in baboons. *Chem. Phys. Lipids* **67–68**, 199–205.

20. Mahaney, M. C., Blangero, J., Rainwater, D. L., Mott, G. E., Comuzzie, A. G., MacCluer, J. W., and VandeBerg, J. L. (1999). Pleiotropy and genotype by diet interaction in a baboon model for atherosclerosis: A multivariate quantitative genetic analysis of HDL subfractions in two dietary environments. *Arterioscler. Thromb. Vasc. Biol.* **19**, 1134–1141.

21. Rainwater, D. L., Kammerer, C. M., Hixson, J. E., Carey, K. D., Rice, K. S., Dyke, B., VandeBerg, J. F., Slifer, S. H., Atwood, L. D., McGill, H. C., and VandeBerg, J. L. (1998). Two major loci control variation in beta-lipoprotein cholesterol and response to dietary fat and cholesterol in baboons. *Arterioscler. Thromb. Vasc. Biol.* **18**, 1061–1068.

22. Deckelbaum, R. J., Fisher, E. A., Winston, M., Kumanyika, S., Lauer, R. M., Pi-Sunyer, F. X., Schaefer, F., and Weinstein, M. C. (1999). Summary of a Scientific Conference on Preventive Nutrition: Pediatrics to Geriatrics. *Circulation* **100**, 450–456.

23. Driscoll, D. M. and Casanova, E. (1990). Characterization of the apolipoprotein B mRNA editing activity in enterocyte extracts. *J. Biolog. Chem.* **265**, 21401–21403.

24. Lau, P. P., Xiong, W., Zhu, H. -J., Chen, S. -H., and Chan, L. (1991). Apolipoprotein B mRNA editing is an intranuclear event that occurs posttranscriptionally coincident with splicing and polyadenylation. *J. Biolog. Chem.* **266**, 20550–20554.

25. Hoeg, J. M., Sviridov, D. D., Tennyson, G. E., Demosky, S. J., Jr., Meng, M. S., Bojanovski, D., Safonova, I. G., Repin, V. S., Kuberger, M. B., Smirnov, V. N., (1990). Both apolipoproteins B–48 and B–100 are synthesized and secreted by the human intestine. *J. Lipid Res.* **31**, 1761–1769.

26. Lopez-Miranda, J., Kam, N., Osada, J., Rodriguez, C., Fernandez, P., Contois, J., Schaefer, E. J., and Ordovas, J. M. (1994). Effect of fat feeding on human intestinal apolipoprotein B mRNA levels and editing. *Biochim. Biophys. Acta Lipids Lipid Metab.* **1214**, 143–147.

27. Law, S., Lackner, K. J., Hospattanakar, A. V., Anchors, J. M., Sakaguchi, A. Y., Naylor, S. L., and Brewer, H. B., Jr. (1985). Human apolipoprotein B–100: Cloning, analysis of liver mRNA, and assignment of the gene to chromosome 2. Proc. Natl. Acad. Sci. USA **82**, 8340–8344.

28. Genest, J. J., Ordovas, J. M., McNamara, J. R., Robbins, A. M., Meade, T., Cohn, S. D., Salem, D., Wilson, P. W. F., Masharani, U., Frossard, P., and Schaefer, E. J. (1990). DNA polymorphisms of the apolipoprotein B gene in patients with premature coronary artery disease. *Atherosclerosis* **82**, 7–17.

29. Law, A., Wallis, S. C., Powell, L. M., Pease, R. J., Brunt, H., Priestley, L. M., Knott, T. J., Scott, J., Altman, D. G., Miller, G. J., Rajput, J., and Miller, N. E. (1986). Common DNA polymorphism within coding sequence of apolipoprotein B gene associated with altered lipid levels. *Lancet* **1**(8493), 1301–1302.

30. Berg, K. (1986). DNA polymorphism at the apolipoprotein B locus is associated with lipoprotein level. *Clin. Genet.* **30**, 515–520.

31. Talmud, P. J., Barni, N., and Kessling, A. M. (1987). Apolipoprotein B gene variants are involved in the determination of serum cholesterol levels: A study in normo- and hyperlipidemic individuals. *Atherosclerosis* **67**, 81–89.

32. Hixson, J. E., McMahan, C. A., McGill, H. C., Jr., Strong, J. P., and PDAY Research Group (1992). Apo B insertion/deletion polymorphisms are associated with atherosclerosis in young black but not young white males. *Arterioscler. Thromb.* **12**, 1023–1029.

33. Saha, N., Tay, J. S. H., and Humphries, S. E. (1992). Apolipoprotein B-gene DNA polymorphisms (*Xba*I and *Eco*RI), serum lipids, and apolipoproteins in healthy Chinese. *Genet. Epidemiol.* **9**, 1–10.

34. Saha, N., Tay, J. S. H., and Chew, L. S. (1992). Influence of apolipoprotein B signal peptide insertion/deletion polymorphism on serum lipids and apolipoproteins in a Chinese population. *Clin. Genet.* **41**, 152–156.

35. Saha, N., Tong, M. C., Tay, J. S., Jeyaseelan, K., and Humphries, S. E. (1992). DNA polymorphisms of the apolipoprotein B gene in Chinese coronary artery disease patients. *Clin. Genet.* **42**, 164–170.

36. Xu, C. F., Nanjee, M. N., Savill, J., Talmud, P. J., Angelico, F., Del Ben, M., Antonini, R., Mazzarella, B., Miller, N., and Humphries, S. E. (1990). Variation at the apolipoprotein (apo). AI-CIII-AIV gene cluster and apo B gene loci is associated with lipoprotein and apolipoprotein levels in Italian children. Am. J. Hum. Genet. **47**, 429–439.

37. Xu, C.-F., Tikkanen, M. J., Butler, R., Huttunen, J. K., Pietinen, P., Humphries, S., and Talmud, P. (1990). Apolipoprotein B signal peptide insertion/deletion polymorphism is associated with Ag epitopes and involved in the determination of serum triglyceride levels. *J. Lipid Res.* **31**, 1255–1261.

38. Carlsson, P., Darnfors, C., Olofsson, S. O., and Bjursell, G. (1986). Analysis of the human apolipoprotein B gene: Complete structure of the B74 region. *Gene* **49**, 29–51.

39. Aalto-Setälä, K., Tikkanen, M., Taskinen, M. R., Nieminen, M., Homberg, P., and Kontula, K. (1988). XbaI and c/g polymorphism of the apolipoprotein B gene locus are associated with serum cholesterol and LDL cholesterol levels in Finland. *Atherosclerosis* **74,** 47–54.

40. Aalto-Setälä, K., Viikari, J., Åkerblom, H. K., Kuusela, V., and Kontula, K. (1991). DNA polymorphisms of the apolipoprotein B and A-I/C-III genes are associated with variations of serum low density lipoprotein cholesterol level in childhood. *J. Lipid Res.* **32,** 1477–1487.

41. Hegele, R. A., Huang, L. S., and Herbert, P. N. (1986). Apolipoprotein B gene DNA polymorphisms associated with myocardial infarction. *N. Engl. J. Med.* **315,** 1509–1515.

42. Monsalve, M. V., Young, R., Jobsis, J., Wiseman, S. A., Dhamu, S., Powell, J. T., Greenhalgh, R. M., and Humphries, S. E. (1988). DNA polymorphism of the gene for apolipoprotein B in patients with peripheral arterial disease. *Atherosclerosis* **70,** 123–129.

43. Myant, N. B., Gallagher, J., Barbir, M., Thompson, G. R., Wile, D. B., and Humphries, S. E. (1989). Restriction fragment length polymorphism in the apo B gene in relation to coronary artery disease. *Atherosclerosis* **71,** 193–201.

44. Bohn, M., and Berg, K. (1994). The XbaI polymorphism at the apolipoprotein B locus and risk of atherosclerotic disease. *Clin. Genet.* **46,** 77–79.

45. Tikkanen, M. J., Xu, C. -F., Hamalainen, T., Talmud, P., Sarna, S., Huttunen, J. K., Pietinen, P., and Humphries, S. (1990). XbaI polymorphism of the apolipoprotein B gene influences plasma lipid response to diet intervention. *Clin. Genet.* **37,** 327–334.

46. Talmud, P. J., Boerwinkle, E., Xu, C., Tikkanen, M. J., Pietinen, P., Huttunen, J. K., and Humphries, S. (1992). Dietary intake and gene variation influence the response of plasma lipids to dietary intervention. *Genet. Epidemiol.* **9,** 249–260.

46a. Rantala, M., Rantala, T. T., Savolainen, M. J., Friedlander, Y., Kesaniemi, Y. A. (2000). Apolipoprotein B gene polymorphisms and serum lipids: Meta-analysis of the role of genetic variation in responsiveness to diet. *Am. J. of Clin. Nutr.* **71,** 713–24.

47. Lopez-Miranda, J., Ordovas, J. M., Ostos, M. A., Marin, C., Jansen, S., Salas, J., Blanco-Molina, A., Jimenez-Pereperez, J. A., Lopez-Segura, F., and Perez-Jimenez, F. (1997). Dietary fat clearance in normal subjects is modulated by genetic variation at the apolipoprotein B gene locus. *Arterioscler. Thromb. Vasc. Biol.* **17,** 1765–1773.

48. Boerwinkle, E., and Chan, L. (1989). A three codon insertion/deletion polymorphism in the signal peptide region of the human apolipoprotein B gene directly typed by the polymerase chain reaction. *Nucleic Acids Res.* **17,** 4003.

49. Visvikis, S., Cambou, J. P., Arveiler, D., Evans, A. E., Parra, H. J., Aguillon, D., Fruchart, J. C., Siest, G., and Cambien, F. (1993). Apolipoprotein B signal peptide polymorphism in patients with myocardial infarction and controls. The ECTIM study. *Hum. Genet.* **90,** 561-565.

50. Peacock, R., Dunning, A., Hamsten, A., Tornvall, P., Humphries, S., and Talmud, P. (1992). Apolipoprotein B gene polymorphisms, lipoproteins and coronary atherosclerosis: A study of young myocardial infarction survivors and healthy population-based individuals. *Atherosclerosis* **92,** 151–164.

51. Bohn, M., Bakken, A., Erikssen, J., and Berg, K. (1994). The apolipoprotein B signal peptide insertion/deletion polymorphism is not associated with myocardial infarction in Norway. *Clin. Genet.* **45,** 255–259.

52. Boerwinkle, E., Brown, S. A., Rohrbach, K., Gotto, A. M., Jr., and Patsch, W. (1991). Role of apolipoprotein E and B gene variation in determining response of lipid, lipoprotein, and apolipoprotein levels to increased dietary cholesterol. *Am. J. Hum. Genet.* **49,** 1145–1154.

53. Talmud, P., Peacock, R., Karpe, F., Hamsten, A., and Humphries, S. (1996). *In* "Nutrition, Genetics and Heart Disease" (Pennington Biomedical Research Center, Ed.), pp. 366–378. LSU Press, Baton Rouge, LA.

54. Regis-Bailly, A., Visvikis, S., Steinmetz, J., Fournier, B., Gueguen, R., and Siest, G. (1996). Effects of apo B and apo E gene polymorphisms on lipid and apolipoprotein concentrations after a test meal. *Clin. Chim. Acta* **253,** 127–143.

55. Byrne, C. D., Wareham, N. J., Mistry, P. K., Phillips, D. I. W., Martensz, N. D., Halsall, D., Talmud, P. J., Humphries, S. E., and Hales, C. N. (1996). The association between free fatty acid concentrations and triglyceride-rich lipoproteins in the postprandial state is altered by a common deletion polymorphism of the apoB signal peptide. *Atherosclerosis* **127,** 35–42.

56. Huang, L. S., de Graaf, J., and Breslow, J. L. (1988). Apo B gene RFLP in exon 26 changes amino acid 3611 from Arg to Gln. *J. Lipid Res.* **29,** 63.

57. Blackhart, B. D., Ludwig, E. M., Pierotti, V. R., Caiati, L., Onasch, M. A., Powell, L., Pease, R., Knott, T. J., Chu, M. L., Mahley, R. W., Scott, J., McCarthy, B. J., and Levy-Wilson, B. (1986). Structure of the human apolipoprotein B gene. *J. Biolog. Chem.* **261,** 15364–15367.

58. Friedl, W., Ludwig, E. H., Paulweber, B., Sandhofer, F., and McCarthy, B. (1990). Hypervariability in a minisatellite 3' of the apolipoprotein B gene in patients with coronary heart disease compared with normal controls. *J. Lipid Res.* **31,** 659–665.

59. Heliö, T., Ludwig, E. H., Palotie, A., Koskinen, P., Paulweber, B., Kauppinen-Mëkelin, R., Manninen, V., Manttari, M., Frick, M. H., Ehnholm, C., and Tikkanen, M. J. (1991). Apolipoprotein B gene 3' hypervariable region polymorphism and myocardial infarction in dyslipidemic Finnish men participating in a primary prevention trial. *Nutr. Metab. Cardiovasc. Dis.* **1,** 178–182.

60. Rantala, M., Rantala, T., Savolainen, M. J., Friedlander, Y., and Kesaniemi, Y. A. (2000). Apolipoprotein B gene polymorphisms and serum lipids: Meta-analysis of the role of genetic variation in responsiveness to diet. *Am. J. Clin. Nutr.* **71,** 713–724.

61. Green, P. H., Glickman, R. M., Riley, J. W., and Quinet, E. (1980). Human apolipoprotein A-IV. Intestinal origin and distribution in plasma. J. Clin. Invest. **65,** 911–919.

62. Ordovas, J. M., Cassidy, D. K., Civeira, F., Bisgaier, C. L., and Schaefer, E. J. (1989). Familial apolipoprotein A-I, C-III, and A-IV deficiency and premature atherosclerosis due to deletion of a gene complex on chromosome 11. *J. Biolog. Chem.* **264,** 16339–16342.

63. Goldberg, I. J., Scheraldi, C. A., Yacoub, L. K., Saxena, U., and Bisgaier, C. L. (1990). Lipoprotein ApoC-II activation

of lipoprotein lipase. Modulation by apolipoprotein A-IV. *J. Biolog. Chem.* **265**, 4266–4272.

64. Steinmetz, A. and Utermann, G. (1985). Activation of lecithin:cholesterol acyltransferase by human apolipoprotein A-IV. *J. Biolog. Chem.* **260**, 2258–2264.

65. Stein, O., Stein, Y., Lefevre, M., and Roheim, P. S. (1986). The role of apolipoprotein A-IV in reverse cholesterol transport studied with cultured cells and liposomes derived from an ether analog of phosphatidylcholine. *Biochim. Biophys. Acta* **878**, 7–13.

66. Steinmetz, A., Barbaras, R., Ghalim, N., Clavey, V., Fruchart, J. C., and Ailhaud, G. (1990). Human apolipoprotein A-IV binds to apolipoprotein A-I/A-II receptor sites and promotes cholesterol efflux from adipose cells. *J. Biolog. Chem.* **265**, 7859–7863.

67. Weinberg, R. B. and Patton, C. S. (1990). Binding of human apolipoprotein A-IV to human hepatocellular plasma membranes. *Biochim. Biophys. Acta* **1044**, 255–261.

68. Duverger, N., Tremp, G., Caillaud, J. M., Emmanuel, F., Castro, G., Fruchart, J. C., Steinmetz, A., and Denéfle, P. (1996). Protection against atherogenesis in mice mediated by human apolipoprotein A-IV. *Science* **273**, 966–968.

69. Li, H., Reddick, R. L., and Maeda, N. (1993). Lack of apoA-I is not associated with increased susceptibility to atherosclerosis in mice. *Arterioscler. Thromb.* **13**, 1814–1821.

70. Stein, Y., Stein, O., Duverger, N., Halperin, G., Dabach, Y., Hollander, G., and Ben-Naim, M. (2000). Clearance of cationized LDL cholesterol from a muscle depot is not enhanced in human apolipoprotein A-IV transgenic mice. *Arterioscler. Thromb. Vasc. Biol.* **20**, 179–184.

71. Stan, S., Delvin, E. E., Seidman, E., Rouleau, T., Steinmetz, A., Bendayan, M., Yotov, W., and Levy, E. (2000). Modulation of apo A-IV transcript levels and synthesis by n−3, n−6, and n−9 fatty acids in CACO−2 cells. *J. Cell. Biochem.* **75**, 73–81.

72. Menzel, H. J., Sigurdsson, G., Boerwinkle, E., Schrangl-Will, S., Dieplinger, H., and Utermann, G. (1990). Frequency and effect of human apolipoprotein A-IV polymorphism on lipid and lipoprotein levels in an Icelandic population. *Hum. Genet.* **84**, 344–346.

73. de Knijff, P., Johansen, L. G., Rosseneu, M., Frants, R. R., Jespersen, J., and Havekes, L. M. (1992). Lipoprotein profile of a Greenland Inuit population. Influence of anthropometric variables, Apo E and A4 polymorphism, and lifestyle. *Arterioscler. Thromb.* **12**, 1371-1379.

74. Von Eckardstein, A., Funke, H., Schulte, M., Erren, M., Schulte, H., and Assmann, G. (1992). Nonsynonymous polymorphic sites in the apolipoprotein (apo). A-IV gene are associated with changes in the concentration of apo B- and apo A-I-containing lipoproteins in a normal population. *Am. J. Hum. Genet.* **50**, 1115–1128.

75. Kaprio, J., Ferrell, R. E., Kottke, B. A., Kamboh, M. I., and Sing, C. F. (1991). Effects of polymorphisms in apolipoproteins E, A-IV, and H on quantitative traits related to risk for cardiovascular disease. Arterioscler. Thromb. **11**, 1330–1348.

76. Kamboh, M. I., Hamman, R. F., Iyengar, S., Aston, C. E., and Ferrell, R. E. (1991). Apolipoprotein A-IV polymorphism, and its role in determining variation in lipoprotein-lipid, glucose and insulin levels in normal and non-insulin-dependent diabetic individuals. *Atherosclerosis* **91**, 25–34.

77. Eichner, J. E., Kuller, L. H., Ferrell, R. E., and Kamboh, M. I. (1989). Phenotypic effects of apolipoprotein structural variation on lipid profiles: II. Apolipoprotein A-IV and quantitative lipid measures in the healthy women study. *Genet. Epidemiol.* **6**, 493–499.

78. Menzel, H. J., Boerwinkle, E., Schrangl-Will, S., and Utermann, G. (1988). Human apolipoprotein A-IV polymorphism: Frequency and effect on lipid and lipoprotein levels. Hum. Genet. **79**, 368–372.

79. Kamboh, M. I., Iyengar, S., Aston, C. E., Hamman, R. F., and Ferrell, R. E. (1992). Apolipoprotein A-IV genetic polymorphism and its impact on quantitative traits in normoglycemic and non-insulin-dependent diabetic Hispanics from the San Luis Valley, Colorado. *Hum. Biol.* **64**, 605–616.

80. Bai, H., Saku, K., Liu, R., Funke, H., Von Eckardstein, A., and Arakawa, K. (1993). Polymorphic site study at codon 347 of apolipoprotein A-IV in a Japanese population. *Biochim. Biophys. Acta* **1174**, 279–281.

81. de Knijff, P., Rosseneu, M., Beisiegel, U., De Keersgieter, W., Frants, R. R., and Havekes, L. M. (1988). Apolipoprotein A-IV polymorphism and its effect on plasma lipid and apolipoprotein concentrations. *J. Lipid Res.* **29**, 1621–1627.

82. Crews, D. E., Kamboh, M. I., Mancilha-Carvalho, J. J., and Kottke, B. (1993). Population genetics of apolipoprotein A-4, E, and H polymorphisms in Yanomami Indians of northwestern Brazil: Associations with lipids, lipoproteins, and carbohydrate metabolism. *Hum. Biol.* **65**, 211–224.

83. Hanis, C. L., Douglas, T. C., and Hewett-Emmett, D. (1991). Apolipoprotein A-IV protein polymorphism: Frequency and effects on lipids, lipoproteins, and apolipoproteins among Mexican-Americans in Starr County, Texas. Hum. Genet. **86**, 323–325.

84. Zaiou, M., Visvikis, S., Gueguen, R., Parra, H. -J., Fruchart, J. C., and Siest, G. (1994). DNA polymorphisms of human apolipoprotein A-IV gene: Frequency and effects on lipid, lipoprotein and apolipoprotein levels in a French population. *Clin. Genet.* **46**, 248–254.

85. Mata, P., Ordovas, J. M., Lopez-Miranda, J., Lichtenstein, A. H., Clevidence, B., Judd, J. T., and Schaefer, E. J. (1994). ApoA-IV phenotype affects diet-induced plasma LDL cholesterol lowering. *Arterioscler. Thromb.* **14**, 884–891.

86. McCombs, R. J., Marcadis, D. E., Ellis, J., and Weinberg, R. B. (1994). Attenuated hypercholesterolemic response to a high-cholesterol diet in subjects heterozygous for the apolipoprotein A-IV-2 allele. *N. Engl. J. Med.* **331**, 706–710.

87. Jansen, S., Lopez-Miranda, J., Ordovas, J. M., Zambrana, J. L., Marin, C., Ostos, M. A., Castro, P., McPherson, R., Lopez Segura, F., Blanco, A., Jimenez Pereperez, J. A., and Perez-Jimenez, F. (1997). Effect of 360His mutation in apolipoprotein A-IV on plasma HDL-cholesterol response to dietary fat. *J. Lipid Res.* **38**, 1995–2002.

88. Rader, D. J., Schafer, J., Lohse, P., Verges, B., Kindt, M., Zech, L. A., Steinmetz, A., and Brewer, H. B., Jr. (1993). Rapid in vivo transport and catabolism of human apolipoprotein A- IV-1 and slower catabolism of the apoA-IV-2 isoprotein. *J. Clin. Invest.* **92**, 1009–1017.

89. Campos, H., Lopez-Miranda, J., Rodriguez, C., Albajar, M., Schaefer, E. J., and Ordovas, J. M. (1997). Urbanization elicits a more atherogenic lipoprotein profile in carriers of the

apolipoprotein A-IV–2 allele than in A-IV–1 homozygotes. *Arterioscler. Thromb. Vasc. Biol.* **17,** 1074–1081.

90. Jansen, S., Lopez-Miranda, J., Salas, J., Ordovas, J. M., Castro, P., Marin, C., Ostos, M. A., Lopez-Segura, F., Jimenez-Pereperez, J. A., Blanco, A., and Perez-Jimenez, F. (1997). Effect of 347-serine mutation in apoprotein A-IV on plasma LDL cholesterol response to dietary fat. *Arterioscler. Thromb. Vasc. Biol.* **17,** 1532–1538.

91. Carmena-Ramon, R. F., Ascaso, J. F., Real, J. T., Ordovas, J. M., and Carmena, R. (1998). Genetic variation at the ApoA-IV gene locus and response to diet in familial hypercholesterolemia. *Arterioscler. Thromb. Vasc. Biol.* **18,** 1266–1274.

92. Beisiegel, U., Weber, W., Ihrke, G., Herz, J., and Stanley, K. K. (1989). The LDL-receptor-related protein, LRP, is an apolipoprotein E-binding protein. *Nature (Lond.)* **341,** 162–164.

93. Mahley, R. W. (1988). Apolipoprotein E: Cholesterol transport protein with expanding role in cell biology. *Science* **240,** 622–630.

94. Schaefer, E. J., Gregg, R. E., Ghiselli, G., Forte, T. M., Ordovas, J. M., Zech, L. A., Lindgren, F. T., and Brewer, H. B., Jr. (1986). Familial apolipoprotein E deficiency. *J. Clin. Invest.* **78,** 1206–1219.

95. Davignon, J., Gregg, R. E., and Sing, C. F. (1988). Apolipoprotein E polymorphism and atherosclerosis. *Arteriosclerosis* **8,** 1–21.

96. Ordovas, J. M., Litwack-Klein, L., Wilson, P. W. F., Schaefer, M. M., and Schaefer, E. J. (1987). Apolipoprotein E isoform phenotyping methodology and population frequency with identification of apoE1 and apoE5 isoforms. *J. Lipid Res.* **28,** 371–380.

97. Schaefer, E. J., Lamon-Fava, S., Johnson, S., Ordovas, J. M., Schaefer, M. M., Castelli, W. P., and Wilson, P. W. F. (1994). Effects of gender and menopausal status on the association of apolipoprotein E phenotype with plasma lipoprotein levels: Results from the Framingham Offspring Study. *Arterioscler. Thromb.* **14,** 1105–1113.

98. Blaauwwiekel, E. E., Beusekamp, B. J., Sluiter, W. J., Hoogenberg, K., and Dullaart, R. P. F. (1998). Apolipoprotein E genotype is a determinant of low-density lipoprotein cholesterol and of its response to a low-cholesterol diet in type 1 diabetic patients with elevated urinary albumin excretion. *Diab. Med.* **15,** 1031–1035.

99. Ordovas, J. M. and Schaefer, E. J. (1999). Genes, variation of cholesterol and fat intake and serum lipids. *Curr. Opin. Lipidol.* **10,** 15–22.

100. Ordovas, J. M. (1999). The genetics of serum lipid responsiveness to dietary interventions. *Proc. Nutr. Soc.* **58,** 171–187.

101. Glatz, J. F. C., Demacker, P. N. M., Turner, P. R., and Katan, M. B. (1991). Response of serum cholesterol to dietary cholesterol in relation to apolipoprotein E phenotype. *Nutr. Metab. Cardiovasc. Dis.* **1,** 13–17.

102. Ginsberg, H. N., Karmally, W., Siddiqui, M., Holleran, S., Tall, A. R., Rumsey, S. C., Deckelbaum, R. J., Blaner, W. S., and Ramakrishnan, R. (1994). A dose-response study of the effects of dietary cholesterol on fasting and postprandial lipid and lipoprotein metabolism in healthy young men. *Arterioscler. Thromb.* **14,** 576–586.

103. Friedlander, Y., Berry, E. M., Eisenberg, S., Stein, Y., and Leitersdorf, E. (1995). Plasma lipids and lipoproteins in response to a dietary challenge: analysis of four candidate genes. *Clin. Genet.* **47,** 1–12.

104. Dreon, D. M., Fernstrom, H. A., Miller, B., and Krauss, R. M. (1995). Apolipoprotein E isoform phenotype and LDL subclass response to a reduced-fat diet. *Arterioscler. Thromb.* **15,** 105–111.

105. Lehtimäki, T., Moilanen, T., Porkka, K., Åkerblom, H. K., Rönnemaa, T., Rësënen, L., Viikari, J., Ehnholm, C., and Nikkari, T. (1995). Association between serum lipids and apolipoprotein E phenotype is influenced by diet in a population-based sample of free- living children and young adults: The Cardiovascular Risk in Young Finns Study. *J. Lipid Res.* **36,** 653–661.

106. Loktionov, A., Bingham, S. A., Vorster, H., Jerling, J. C., Runswick, S. A., and Cummings, J. H. (1998). Apolipoprotein E genotype modulates the effect of black tea drinking on blood lipids and blood coagulation factors: A pilot study. *Brit. J. Nutr.* **79,** 133-139.

107. Carmena, R., Roederer, G., Mailloux, H., Lussier-Cacan, S., and Davignon, J. (1993). The response to lovastatin treatment in patients with heterozygous familial hypercholesterolemia is modulated by apolipoprotein E polymorphism. *Metabolism* **42,** 895–901.

108. Ordovas, J. M., Lopez-Miranda, J., Perez-Jimenez, F., Rodriguez, C., Park, J. -S., Cole, T., and Schaefer, E. J. (1995). Effect of apolipoprotein E and A-IV phenotypes on the low density lipoprotein response to HMG CoA reductase inhibitor therapy. *Atherosclerosis* **113,** 157–166.

109. Dallongeville, J., and Fruchart, J. C. (1998). Postprandial dyslipidemia: A risk factor for coronary heart disease [review and 55 refs]. *Ann. Nutr. Metab.* **42,** 1–11.

110. Kesaniemi, Y. A., Ehnholm, C., and Miettinen, T. A. (1987). Intestinal cholesterol absorption efficiency in man is related to apoprotein E phenotype. *J. Clin. Invest.* **80,** 578–581.

111. Weintraub, M. S., Eisenberg, S., and Breslow, J. L. (1987). Dietary fat clearance in normal subjects is regulated by genetic variation in apolipoprotein E. *J. Clin. Invest.* **80,** 1571–1577.

112. Brown, A. J., and Roberts, D. C. K. (1991). The effect of fasting triacylglyceride concentration and apolipoprotein E polymorphism on postprandial lipemia. *Arterioscler. Thromb.* **11,** 1737–1744.

113. Nikkilä, M., Solakivi, T., Lehtimäki, T., Koivula, T., Laippala, P., and Astrom, B. (1994). Postprandial plasma lipoprotein changes in relation to apolipoprotein E phenotypes and low density lipoprotein size in men with and without coronary artery disease. *Atherosclerosis* **106,** 149–157.

114. Superko, H. R., and Haskell, W. L. (1991). The effect of apolipoprotein E isoform difference on postprandial lipoproteins in patients matched for triglycerides, LDL-cholesterol, and HDL-cholesterol. *Artery* **18,** 315–325.

115. Boerwinkle, E., Brown, S., Sharrett, A. R., Heiss, G., and Patsch, W. (1994). Apolipoprotein E polymorphism influences postprandial retinyl palmitate but not triglyceride concentrations. *Am. J. Hum. Genet.* **54,** 341–360.

116. Reznik, Y., Pousse, P., Herrou, M., Morello, R., Mahoudeau, J., Drosdowsky, M. A., and Fradin, S. (1996). Postprandial lipoprotein metabolism in normotriglyceridemic non-insulin-dependent diabetic patients: Influence of apolipoprotein E polymorphism. *Metabolism* **45,** 63-71.

117. Orth, M., Wahl, S., Hanisch, M., Friedrich, I., Wieland, H., and Luley, C. (1996). Clearance of post-prandial lipoproteins in normolipemics: Role of the apolipoprotein E phenotype. *Biochim. Biophys. Acta Lipids Lipid Metab.* **1303**, 22–30.

118. Bergeron, N., and Havel, R. J. (1996). Prolonged postprandial responses of lipids and apolipoproteins in triglyceride-rich lipoproteins of individuals expressing an apolipoprotein e4 allele. *J. Clin. Invest.* **97**, 65–72.

119. Wolever, T. M., Hegele, R. A., Connelly, P. W., Ransom, T. P., Story, J., Furumoto, E. J., and Jenkins, D. J. (1997). Long-term effect of soluble-fiber foods on postprandial fat metabolism in dyslipidemic subjects with apo E3 and apo E4 genotypes. *Am. J. Clin. Nutr.* **66**, 584–590.

120. Zannis, V. I., Cole, F. S., Jackson, C. L., Kurnit, D. M., and Karathanasis, S. K. (1985). Distribution of apolipoprotein A-I, C-II, C-III, and E mRNA in fetal human tissues. Time-dependent induction of apolipoprotein E mRNA by cultures of human monocyte-macrophages. *Biochemistry* **24**, 4450–4455.

121. Wang, C. S., McConathy, W. J., Kloer, H. U., and Alaupovic, P. (1985). Modulation of lipoprotein lipase activity by lipoproteins. Effect of apolipoprotein C-III. *J. Clin. Invest.* **75**, 384–390.

122. Weisgraber, K. H., Mahley, R. W., Kowal, R. C., Herz, J., Goldstein, J. L., and Brown, M. S. (1990). Apolipoprotein C-I modulates the interaction of apolipoprotein E with beta-migrating very low density lipoproteins and inhibits binding of beta-VLDL to low density lipoprotein receptor-related protein. *J. Biolog. Chem.* **265**, 22453–22459.

123. Kowal, R. C., Herz, J., Weisgraber, K. H., Mahley, R. W., Brown, M. S., and Goldstein, J. L. (1990). Opposing effects of apolipoprotein E and C on lipoprotein binding to low density lipoprotein receptor related protein. *J. Biolog. Chem.* **265**, 10771–10779.

124. Ito, Y., Azrolan, N., O'Connell, A., Walsh, A., and Breslow, J. L. (1990). Hypertriglyceridemia as a result of human apoCIII gene expression in transgenic mice. *Science* **249**, 790–793.

125. Bruns, G. A., Karathanasis, S. K., and Breslow, J. L. (1984). Human apolipoprotein AI-CIII gene complex is located in chromosome 11. *Arteriosclerosis* **4**, 97–104.

126. Ferns, G. A. A., Ritchie, C., Stocks, J., and Galton, D. J. (1985). Genetic polymorphisms of apolipoprotein C-III and Insulin in survivors of myocardial infarction. *Lancet*, **2**, 300–303.

127. Ordovas, J. M., Civeira, F., Garces, C., and Pocovi, M. (1991). *In* "DNA Polymorphisms as Disease Markers" (D. J. Galton, Ed.), pp. 91–105, Plenum Press, New York.

128. Ordovas, J. M., Civeira, F., Genest, J., Jr., Craig, S., Robbins, A. H., Meade, T., Pocovi, M., Frossard, P. M., Masharani, U., Wilson, P. W., Salem, D. N., Ward, R. H., and Schaefer, E. J. (1991). Restriction fragment length polymorphisms of the apolipoprotein A-I, C-III, A-IV gene locus. Relationships with lipids, apolipoproteins, and premature coronary artery disease. *Atherosclerosis* **87**, 75–86.

129. Dammerman, M., Sandkuijl, L. A., Halaas, J. L., Chung, W., and Breslow, J. L. (1993). An apolipoprotein CIII haplotype protective against hypertriglyceridemia is specified by promoter and 3' untranslated region polymorphisms. *Proc. Natl. Acad. Sci. USA* **90**, 4562–4566.

130. Li, W. W., and Leff, T. (1994). Regulation of apolipoprotein CIII gene transcription by insulin: Characterization of an insulin response element in the CIII promoter [abstract]. *Circulation* **90**, I-401.

131. Li, W. W., Dammerman, M., Smith, J. D., Metzger, S., Halaas, J. L., Breslow, J. L., and Leff, T. (1994). A common variant of the apo CIII promoter associated with hypertriglyceridemia is defective in its transcriptional response to insulin [abstract]. *Circulation* **90**, I-401.

132. Lopez-Miranda, J., Jansen, S., Ordovas, J. M., Salas, J., Marin, C., Castro, P., Ostos, M. A., Cruz, G., Lopez-Segura, F., Blanco, A., Jimenez-Pereperez, J., and Perez-Jimenez, F. (1997). Influence of the SstI polymorphism at the apolipoprotein C-III gene locus on the plasma low-density-lipoprotein-cholesterol response to dietary monounsaturated fat. *Am. J. Clin. Nutr.* **66**, 97–103.

133. Waterworth, D. M., Ribalta, J., Nicaud, V., Dallongeville, J., Humphries, S. E., and Talmud, P. (1999). ApoCIII gene variants modulate postprandial response to both glucose and fat tolerance tests. *Circulation* **99**, 1872–1877.

134. Salas, J., Jansen, S., Lopez-Miranda, J., Ordovas, J. M., Castro, P., Marin, C., Ostos, M. A., Bravo, M. D., Jimenez Pereperez, J. A., Blanco, A., Lopez-Segura, F., and Perez-Jimenez, F. (1998). The SstI polymorphism of the apolipoprotein C-III gene determines the insulin response to an oral glucose tolerance test after consumption of a diet rich in saturated fats. *Am. J. Clin. Nutr.* **68**, 396–401.

135. Nilsson-Ehle, P., Garfinkle, A. S., and Schotz, M. C. (1980). Lipolytic enzymes and plasma lipoprotein metabolism. *Annu. Rev. Biochem.* **49**, 667–693.

136. Oka, K., Tkalcevic, G. T., Wakano, T., Tucker, H., Ishimura-Oka, K., and Brown, W. V. (1990). Structure and polymorphic map of human lipoprotein lipase. *Biochim. Biophys. Acta* **1049**, 21–26.

137. Mattei, M. G., Etienne, J., Chuat, J. C., Nguyen, V. C., Brault, D., Bernheim, A., and Galibert, F. (1993). Assignment of the human lipoprotein lipase (LPL). gene to chromosome band 8p22. *Cytogenet. Cell Genet.* **63**, 45–46.

138. Fisher, L., FitzGerald, G. A., and Lawn, R. M. (1987). Two polymorphisms in the human lipoprotein lipase gene. *Nucleic Acids Res.* **15**, 7675.

139. Heinzmann, C., Ladias, J. A., Antonarakis, S. E., Kirchgessner, T., Schotz, M. C., and Lusis, A. J. (1987). RFLP for human lipoprotein lipase gene, HindIII. *Nucleic Acids Res.* **15**, 6763.

140. Stocks, J., Thorn, J. A., and Galton, D. J. (1992). Lipoprotein lipase genotypes for a common premature termination codon mutation detected by PCR-mediated site-directed mutagenesis and restriction digestion. *J. Lipid Res.* **33**, 853–857.

141. Chamberlain, J. C., Thorn, J. A., Morgan, R., Bishop, A., Stocks, J., Rees, A., Oka, K., and Galton, D. J. (1991). Genetic variation at the lipoprotein lipase gene associates with coronary arteriosclerosis. *Adv. Exp. Med. Biol.* **285**, 275–279.

142. Peacock, R. E., Hamsten, A., Nilsson-Ehle, P., and Humphries, S. E. (1992). Associations between lipoprotein lipase gene polymorphisms and plasma correlations of lipids, lipoproteins and lipase activities in young myocardial infarction survivors and age-matched healthy individuals from Sweden. *Atherosclerosis* **97**, 171–185.

143. Thorn, J. A., Chamberlain, J. C., Alcolado, J. C., Oka, K., Chan, L., Stocks, J., and Galton, D. J. (1990). Lipoprotein and hepatic lipase gene variants in coronary atherosclerosis. *Atherosclerosis* **85,** 55–60.

144. Humphries, S. E., Fisher, R., Mailly, F., Peacock, R., Talmud, P., Karpe, F., Hamsten, A., and Miller, G. J. (1996). *In* "Nutrition, Genetics and Heart Disease" (Pennington Biomedical Research Center, Ed.), pp. 279–295. LSU Press, Baton Rouge, LA.

145. Reymer, P. W., Groenemeyer, B. E., Gagne, E., Miao, L., Appelman, E. E., Seidel, J. C., Kromhout, D., Bijvoet, S. M., Van de Oever, K., Bruin, T. (1995). A frequently occurring mutation in the lipoprotein lipase gene (Asn291Ser). contributes to the expression of familial combined hyperlipidemia. *Hum. Mol. Genet.* **4,** 1543–1549.

146. Hoffer, M. J., Bredie, S. J., Boomsma, D. I., Reymer, P. W., Kastelein, J. J., Knijff, P. D., Demacker, P. N., Stalenhoef, A. F., Havekes, L. M., and Frants, R. R. (1996). The lipoprotein lipase (Asn291→Ser). mutation is associated with elevated lipid levels in families with familial combined hyperlipidaemia. *Atherosclerosis* **119,** 159–167.

147. Pimstone, S. N., Gagné, S. E., Gagné, C., Lupien, P. J., Gaudet, D., Williams, R. R., Kotze, M., Reymer, P. W. A., Defesche, J. C., Kastelein, J. J. P., Moorjani, S., and Hayden, M. R. (1995). Mutations in the gene for lipoprotein lipase—A cause for low HDL cholesterol levels in individuals heterozygous for familial hypercholesterolemia. *Arterioscler. Thromb. Vasc. Biol.* **15,** 1704–1712.

148. Pimstone, S. N., Clee, S. M., Gagné, S. E., Miao, L., Zhang, H. F., Stein, E. A., and Hayden, M. R. (1996). A frequently occurring mutation in the lipoprotein lipase gene (Asn291Ser). results in altered postprandial chylomicron triglyceride and retinyl palmitate response in normolipidemic carriers. *J. Lipid Res.* **37,** 1675–1684.

149. Jukema, J. W., Van Boven, A. J., Groenemeijer, B., Zwinderman, A. H., Reiber, J. H. C., Bruschke, A. V. G., Henneman, J. A., Molhoek, G. P., Bruin, T., Jansen, H., Gagné, E., Hayden, M. R., and Kastelein, J. J. P. (1996). The Asp9 Asn mutation in the lipoprotein lipase gene is associated with increased progression of coronary atherosclerosis. *Circulation* **94,** 1913–1918.

150. De Bruin, T. W., Mailly, F., van Barlingen, H. H., Fisher, R., Castro Cabezas, M., Talmud, P., Dallinga-Thie, G. M., and Humphries, S. E. (1996). Lipoprotein lipase gene mutations D9N and N291S in four pedigrees with familial combined hyperlipidaemia. *Eur. J. Clin. Invest.* **26,** 631–639.

151. Mailly, F., Fisher, R. M., Nicaud, V., Luong, L. A., Evans, A. E., Marques-Vidal, P., Luc, G., Arveiler, D., Bard, J. M., Poirier, O., Talmud, P. J., and Humphries, S. E. (1996). Association between the LPL-D9N mutation in the lipoprotein lipase gene and plasma lipid traits in myocardial infarction survivors from the ECTIM study. *Atherosclerosis* **122,** 21–28.

152. Gagne, S. E., Larson, M. G., Pimstone, S. N., Schaefer, E. J., Kastelein, J. J. P., Wilson, P. W. F., Ordovas, J. M., and Hayden, M. R. (1999). A common truncation variant of lipoprotein lipase (Ser447X). confers protection against coronary heart disease: the Framingham Offspring Study. *Clin. Genet.* **55,** 450–454.

153. Kastelein, J. J. P., Ordovas, J. M., Pimstone, S. N., Wilson, P. F. W., Gagne, S. E., Wittekoek, M. E., Boer, J. M. A., Gerdes, C., Schaefer, E. J., Larson, M. G., and Hayden, M. R. (1999). Two common mutations (D9N, N291S). in LPL: A cumulative analysis of their influence on plasma lipids and lipoproteins in men and women. *Clin. Genet.* **56,** 297–305.

154. Gordon, D. A., Wetterau, J. R., and Gregg, R. E. (1995). Microsomal triglyceride transfer protein: A protein complex required for the assembly of lipoprotein particles. *Trends Cell Biol.* **5,** 317–321.

155. Wetterau, J. R., Aggerbeck, L. P., Bouma, M. -E., Eisenberg, C., Munck, A., Hermier, M., Schmitz, J., Gay, G., Rader, D. J., and Gregg, R. E. (1992). Absence of microsomal triglyceride transfer protein in individuals with abetalipoproteinemia. *Science* **258,** 999–1001.

156. Karpe, F., Lundahl, B., Ehrenborg, E., Eriksson, P., and Hamsten, A. (1998). A common functional polymorphism in the promoter region of the microsomal triglyceride transfer protein gene influences plasma LDL levels. *Arterioscler. Thromb. Vasc. Biol.* **18,** 756–761.

157. Couture, P., Otvos, J. D., Cupples, L. A., Wilson, P. W. F., Schaefer, E. J., and Ordovas, J. M. (2000). Absence of association between genetic variation in the promoter of the microsomal triglyceride transfer protein gene and plasma lipoproteins in the Framingham Offspring Study. *Atherosclerosis* **148,** 337–343.

158. Banaszak, L., Winter, N., Xu, Z., Bernlohr, D. A., Cowan, S., and Jones, T. A. (1994). Lipid-binding proteins: A family of fatty acid and retinoid transport proteins. *Adv. Protein Chem.* **45,** 89–151.

159. Sweetser, D. A., Birkenmeier, E. H., Klisak, I. J., Zollman, S., Sparkes, R. S., Mohandas, T., Lusis, A. J., and Gordon, J. I. (1987). The human and rodent intestinal fatty acid binding protein genes. A comparative analysis of their structure, expression and linkage relationships. *J. Biolog. Chem.* **262,** 16060–16071.

160. Arkwright, P. D., Beilin, L. J., Vandongen, R., Rouse, I. L., and Masarei, J. R. (1984). Plasma calcium and cortisol as predisposing factors to alcohol related blood pressure elevation. *J. Hypertension* **2,** 387–392.

161. Bernlohr, D. A., Simpson, M. A., Hertzel, A. V., and Banaszak, L. (1997). Intracellular lipid-binding proteins and their genes. *Annu. Rev. Nutr.* **17,** 277–303.

162. Ockner, R. K., and Manning, J. A. (1974). Fatty acid binding protein in the small intestine: Identification, isolation and evidence for its role in cellular fatty acid binding transport. *J. Clin. Invest.* **54,** 326–338.

163. Besnard, P. (1996). Cellular and molecular aspects of fat metabolism in the small intestine. *Proc. Nutr. Soc.* **55,** 19–37.

164. Van Nieuwenhoven, F. A., Van der Vusse, G. J., and Glatz, J. F. C. (1996). Membrane-associated and cytoplasmic fatty acid-binding proteins. *Lipids* **31**(Suppl.), S223–S227.

165. Bass, N. M., Manning, J. A., Ockner, R. K., Gordon, J. I., Seethram, S., and Alpers, D. H. (1985). Regulation of the biosynthesis of two distinct fatty acid binding proteins in the rat liver and intestine. *J. Biolog. Chem.* **260,** 1432–1436.

166. Sacchettini, J. C., Gordon, J. I., and Banaszak, L. (1989). Crystal structure of rat intestinal fatty acid-binding protein.

refinement and analysis of the E. coli-derived protein with bound palmitate. *J. Mol. Biol.* **208**, 327–339.

167. Hodsdon, M. E. and Cistola, D. P. (1997). Discrete backbone disorder in the nuclear magnetic resonance structure of intestinal fatty acid-binding protein: Implications for the mechanism of ligand entry. *Biochemistry* **36**, 1450–1460.

168. Baier, L. J., Sacchettini, J. C., Knowler, W. C., Eads, J., Paolisso, G., Tataranni, P. A., Mochizuki, H., Bennett, P. H., Bogardus, C., and Prochazka, M. (1995). An amino acid substitution in the human intestinal fatty acid binding protein is associated with increased fatty acid binding, increased fat oxidation, and insulin resistance. *J. Clin. Invest.* **95**, 1281–1287.

169. Schroeder, F., Jolly, C. A., Cho, T., and Frolov, A. (1998). Fatty acid binding isoforms: Structure and function. *Chem. Phys. Lipids* **92**, 1–25.

170. Tataranni, P. A., Baier, L. J., Paolisso, G., Howard, B. V., and Ravussin, E. (1996). Role of lipids in development of noninsulin-dependent diabetes mellitus: Lessons learned from Pima Indians. *Lipids* **31**(Suppl.), S267–S270.

171. Hegele, R. A., Harris, S. B., Hanley, A. J., Sadikian, S., Connelly, P. W., and Zinman, B. (1996). Genetic variation of intestinal fatty acid binding protein associated with variation in body mass in aboriginal Canadians. *J. Clin. Endocrinol. Metab.* **81**, 4334–4337.

172. Yagi, T., Nishi, S., Hinata, S. I., Murakami, M., and Yoshima, T. (1996). A population association study of four candidate genes (hexokinase II, glucagon-like peptide–1 receptor, fatty acid binding protein–2 and apolipoprotein C-II). with type 2 diabetes and impaired glucose tolerance in Japanese subjects. *Diab. Med.* **13**, 902–907.

173. Vionnet, N., Hani, E., Lesage, A., Philippi, A., Hager, J., Varret, M., Stoffel, M., Tanizawa, Y., Chiu, K. C., Glaser, B., Permutt, M. A., Passa, P., Demenais, F., and Froguel, P. (1997). Genetics of NIDDM in France: studies with 19 candidate genes in affected sib pairs. *Diabetes* **46**, 1062–1068.

174. Saarinen, L., Pulkkinen, A., Kareinen, A., Heikkinen, S., Lehto, S., and Laakso, M. (1998). Variants of the fatty acid binding protein 2 gene are not associated with coronary heart disease in non diabetic subjects and in patients with NIDDM. *Diabetes Care* **21**, 849–850.

175. Hegele, R. A., Young, T. K., and Connelly, P. W. (1997). Are Canadian Inuit at increased genetic risk for coronary heart disease? *J. Mol. Med.* **75**, 364–370.

176. Yamada, K., Yuan, X., Ishiyama, S., Koyama, K., Ichikawa, F., Koyanagi, A., Koyama, W., and Nonaka, K. (1997). Association between Ala54Thr substitution of the fatty acid binding protein 2 gene with insulin resistance and intraabdominal fat thickness in Japanese men. *Diabetologia* **40**, 706–710.

177. Pihlajamaki, J., Rissanen, J., Heikkinen, S., Karjalainen, L., and Laakso, M. (1997). Codon 54 polymorphism of the human intestinal fatty acid binding protein 2 gene is associated with dyslipidemias but not with insulin resistance in patients with familial combined hyperlipidemia. *Arterioscler. Thromb. Vasc. Biol.* **17**, 1039–1044.

178. Rissanen, J., Pihlajamäki, J., Heikkinen, S., Kekäläinen, P., Kuusisto, J., and Laakso, M. (1997). The Ala54Thr polymorphism of the fatty acid binding protein 2 gene does not influence insulin sensitivity in Finnish nondiabetic and NIDDM subjects. *Diabetes* **46**, 711–712.

179. Stern, M. P., Mitchell, B. D., Blangero, J., Reinhart, L., Kammerer, C. M., Harrison, C. R., Shipman, P. A., O'Connell, P., Frazier, M. L., and MacCluer, J. W. (1996). Evidence for a major gene for type II diabetes and linkage analyses with selected candidate genes in Mexican-Americans. *Diabetes* **45**, 563–568.

180. Hegele, R. A., Connelly, P. W., Hanley, A. J., Sun, F., Harris, S. B., and Zinman, B. (1997). Common genomic variants associated with variation in plasma lipoproteins in young aboriginal Canadians. *Arterioscler. Thromb. Vasc. Biol.* **17**, 1060–1066.

181. Vidgren, H. M., Sipilainen, R. H., Heikkinen, S., Laakso, M., and Uusitupa, M. I. (1997). Threonine allele in codon 54 of the fatty acid binding protein 2 gene does not modify the fatty acid composition of serum lipids in obese subjects. *Eur. J. Clin. Invest.* **27**, 405–408.

182. Hegele, R. A., Wolever, T. M., Story, A., Connelly, P. W., and Jenkins, D. J. (1997). Intestinal fatty acid binding protein variation associated with variation in the response of plasma lipoproteins to dietary fibre. *Eur. J. Clin. Invest.* **27**, 857–862.

183. Agren, J. J., Valve, R., Vidgren, H., Laakso, M., and Uusitupa, M. (1998). Postprandial Lipidemic response is modified by the polymorphism at codon 54 of the fatty acid-binding protein 2 gene. *Arterioscler. Thromb. Vasc. Biol.* **18**, 1606–1610.

184. Baier, L. J., Bogardus, C., and Sacchettini, J. C. (1996). A polymorphism in the human intestinal fatty acid binding protein alters fatty acid transport across Caco–2 cells. *J. Biolog. Chem.* **271**, 10892–10896.

185. Prows, D. R., Murphy, E. J., Moncecchi, D., and Schroeder, F. (1996). Intestinal fatty acid binding protein expression stimulates fibroblast fatty acid esterification. *Chem. Phys. Lipids* **84**, 47–56.

186. Zhang, F., Lucke, C., Baier, L. J., Sacchettini, J. C., and Hamilton, J. A. (1997). Solution structure of human intestinal fatty acid binding protein: Implications for ligand entry and exit. *J. Biomol. NMR* **9**, 213–228.

187. Hodsdon, M. E., and Cistola, D. P. (1997). Ligand binding alters the backbone mobility of intestinal fatty acid binding protein as monitored by 15N NMR relaxation and 1H exchange. *Biochemistry* **36**, 2278–2290.

188. Hobbs, H. H., Russell, D. W., Brown, M. S., and Goldstein, J. L. (1990). The LDL receptor locus in familial hypercholesterolemia: Mutational analysis of a membrane protein. *Ann. Rev. Genet.* **24**, 133–170.

189. Hobbs, H. H., Brown, M. S., and Goldstein, J. L. (1992). Molecular genetics of the LDL receptor gene in familial hypercholesterolemia. *Hum. Muta.* **1**, 445–466.

190. Kass, D. H., Batzer, M. A., and Deininger, P. L. (1995). A new restriction-site polymorphism in exon 18 of the low density lipoprotein receptor (LDLR). gene. *Hum. Genet.* **95**, 363–364.

191. Warnich, L., Kotze, M. J., Langenhoven, E., and Retief, A. E. (1992). Detection of a frequent polymorphism in exon 10 of the low-density lipoprotein receptor gene. *Hum. Genet.* **89**, 362.

192. Zuliani, G., and Hobbs, H. H. (1990). Dinucleotide repeat polymorphism at the 3' end of the LDL receptor gene. *Nucleic Acids Res.* **18**, 4300.

193. Leitersdorf, E., Chakavarti, A., and Hobbs, H. H. (1989). Polymorphic DNA haplotypes at the LDL receptor locus. *Am. J. Hum. Genet.* **44**, 409–421.

194. Taylor, R., Jeenah, M., Seed, M., and Humphries, S. (1988). Four DNA polymorphisms in the LDL receptor gene: Their genetic relationship and use in the study of variation at the LDL receptor locus. *J. Med. Genet.* **25**, 653–659.

195. Kotze, M. J., Langenhoven, E., Dietzsch, E., and Retief, A. E. (1987). A RFLP associated with low density lipoprotein receptor. *Nucleic Acids Res.* **15**, 376.

196. Kotze, M. J., Langenhoven, E., Retief, A. E., Steyn, K., Marais, M. P., Grobbelaar, J. J., Oosthuizen, C. J., Weich, H. F., and Benade, A. J. (1987). Haplotype associations of three DNA polymophisms at the human low density lipoprotein receptor gene locus in familial hypercholesterolemia. *J. Med. Genet.* **24**, 750–755.

197. Funke, H., Klug, J., Frossard, P., Coleman, R., and Assmann, G. (1986). PstI RFLP close to the LDL receptor gene. *Nucleic Acids Res.* **14**, 7820.

198. Hobbs, H. H., Esser, V., and Russell, D. W. (1987). AvaII polymorphism in the human LDL receptor gene. *Nucleic Acids Res.* **15**, 379.

199. Humphries, S. E., Kessling, A. M., Horsthemke, B., Donald, J. A., Seed, M., Jowett, N., Holm, M., Galton, D. J., Wynn, V., and Williamson, R. (1985). A common DNA polymorphism of the low density lipoprotein receptor gene and its use in diagnosis. *Lancet* **1**, 1003–1005.

200. Henderson, H. E., Kotze, M. J., and Berger, G. M. (1989). Multiple mutations underlying familial hypercholesterolemia in the South African population. *Hum. Genet.* **83**, 67–70.

201. Hofmann, S. L., Russell, D. W., Brown, M. S., and Goldstein, J. L. (1988). Overexpression of low density lipoprotein receptor eliminates LDL from plasma in transgenic mice. *Science* **239**, 1277–1281.

202. Yokode, M., Hammer, R. E., Ishibashi, S., Brown, M. S., and Goldstein, J. L. (1990). Diet-induced hypercholesterolemia in mice: Prevention by overexpression of LDL receptors. *Science* **250**, 1273–1275.

203. Ishibashi, S., Brown, M. S., Goldstein, J. L., Gerard, R. D., Hammer, R. E., and Herz, J. (1993). Hypercholesterolemia in low density lipoprotein receptor knockout mice and its reversal by adenovirus-mediated gene delivery. *J. Clin. Invest.* **92**, 883–893.

204. Carmena-Ramon, R. F., Ordovas, J. M., Ascaso, J. F., Real, J., Priego, M. A., and Carmena, R. (1998). Influence of genetic variation at the apoA-I gene locus on lipid levels and response to diet in familial hypercholesterolemia. *Atherosclerosis* **139**, 107–113.

205. Shearman, A. M., Ordovas, J. M., Cupples, L. A., Schaefer, E. J., Harmon, M. D., Joost, O., DeStefano, A. L., Keen, J. D., Wilson, P. W. F., and Myers, R. H. (2001). Evidence for genes influencing TC/HDL-C ratio on chromosomes 5q14-q31 and 7q34-qter: The Framingham Study. Submitted for publication.

206. Boucher, P., De Lorgeril, M., Salen, P., Crozier, P., Delaye, J., Vallon, J. J., Geyssant, A., and Dante, R. (1998). Effect of dietary cholesterol on low density lipoprotein-receptor, 3-hydroxy–3-methylglutaryl-CoA reductase, and low density lipoprotein receptor-related protein mRNA expression in healthy humans. *Lipids* **33**, 1177–1186.

207. Fielding, C. J., Shore, V. G., and Fielding, P. E. (1972). A protein co-factor of lecithin:cholesterol acyltransferase. *Biochem. Biophys. Res. Commun.* **46**, 1493–1498.

208. Reichl, D. and Miller, N. E. (1989). Pathophysiology of reverse cholesterol transport: Insights from inherited disorders of lipoprotein metabolism. *Arteriosclerosis* **9**, 785–797.

209. Karathanasis, S. K. (1985). Apolipoprotein multigene family: Tandem organization of human apolipoprotein A-I, C-III and A-IV genes. *Proc. Natl. Acad. Sci. USA* **82**, 6374–6378.

210. Tybjærg-Hansen, A., Nordestgaard, B. G., Gerdes, L. U., Færgeman, O., and Humphries, S. E. (1993). Genetic markers in the apo AI-CIII-AIV gene cluster for combined hyperlipidemia, hypertriglyceridemia, and predisposition to atherosclerosis. *Atherosclerosis* **100**, 157–169.

211. Paul-Hayase, H., Rosseneu, M., Van Bervliet, J. P., Deslypere, J. P., and Humphries, S. E. (1992). Polymorphisms in the apolipoprotein (apo). AI-CIII-AIV gene cluster: Detection of genetic variation determining plasma apo AI, apo CIII and apo AIV concentrations. *Hum. Genet.* **88**, 439–446.

212. Marshall, H. W., Morrison, L. C., Wu, L. L., Anderson, J. L., Corneli, P. S., Stauffer, D. M., Allen, A., Karagounis, L. A., and Ward, R. H. (1994). Apolipoprotein polymorphisms fail to define risk of coronary artery disease: Results of a prospective, angiographically controlled study. *Circulation* **89**, 567–577.

213. Schaefer, E. J., Ordovas, J. M., Law, S., Ghiselli, G., Kashyap, M. L., Srivastava, L. S., Heaton, W. H., Albers, J. J., Connor, W. E., Lemeshev, Y., Segrest, J., and Brewer, H. B., Jr. (1985). Familial apolipoprotein A-I and C-III deficiency, variant II. *J. Lipid Res.* **26**, 1089–1101.

214. Karathanasis, S. K., Ferris, E., and Haddad, I. A. (1987). DNA inversion within the apolipoproteins AI/CIII/AIV-encoding gene cluster of certain patients with premature atherosclerosis. *Proc. Natl. Acad. Sci. USA* **84**, 7198–7202.

215. Weisgraber, K. H., Bersot, T. P., Mahley, R. W., Franceschini, G., and Sirtori, C. R. (1980). A-I Milano apoprotein: Isolation and characterization of a cysteine-containing variant of the A-I apoprotein from human high density lipoproteins. *J. Clin. Invest.* **66**, 901–909.

216. Franceschini, G., Sirtori, C. R., Capurso, A., Weisgraber, K. H., and Mahley, R. W. (1980). A-I(Milano) apoprotein: Decreased high density lipoprotein cholesterol levels with significant lipoprotein modifications and without clinical atherosclerosis in an Italian family. *J. Clin. Invest.* **66**, 892–900.

216a. Juo, S. H., Wyszynski, D. F., Beaty, T. H., Huang, H. Y., and Bailey-Wilson, J. E. (1999). Mild association between the A/G polymorphism in the promoter of the apolipoprotein A-I gene and apolipoprotein A-I levels: A meta-analysis. *Am. J. Med. Genet.* **82**, 235–241.

217. Lopez-Miranda, J., Ordovas, J. M., Espino, A., Marin, C., Salas, J., Lopez-Segura, F., Jimenez-Pereperez, J., and Perez-Jimenez, F. (1994). Influence of mutation in human apolipoprotein A–1 gene promoter on plasma LDL cholesterol response to dietary fat. *Lancet* **343**, 1246-1249.

218. Mata, P., Lopez-Miranda, J., Pocovi, M., Alonso, R., Lahoz, C., Marin, C., Garces, C., Cenarro, A., Perez-Jimenez, F., De Oya, M., and Ordovas, J. M. (1998). Human apolipoprotein A-I gene promoter mutation influences plasma low density lipoprotein cholesterol response to dietary fat saturation. *Atherosclerosis* **137**, 367–376.

219. Sigurdsson, G., Jr., Gudnason, V., Sigurdsson, G., and Humphries, S. E. (1992). Interaction between a polymorphism of the Apo A-I promoter region and smoking determines

plasma levels of HDL and Apo A-I. *Arterioscler. Thromb.* **12,** 1017–1022.

220. Smith, J. D., Brinton, E. A., and Breslow, J. L. (1992). Polymorphism in the human apolipoprotein A-I gene promoter region. Association of the minor allele with decreased production rate in vivo and promoter activity in vitro. *J. Clin. Invest.* **89,** 1796–1800.

221. Tuteja, R., Tuteja, N., Melo, C., Casari, G., and Baralle, F. E. (1992). Transcription efficiency of human apolipoprotein A-I promoter varies with naturally occurring A to G transition. *FEBS Lett.* **304,** 98–101.

222. Jeenah, M., Kessling, A., Miller, N., and Humphries, S. E. (1990). G to A substitution in the promoter region of the apolipoprotein AI gene is associated with elevated serum apolipoprotein AI and high density lipoprotein cholesterol concentrations. *Mol. Biol. Med.* **7,** 233–241.

223. Angotti, E., Mele, E., Costanzo, F., and Avvedimento, E. V. (1994). A polymorphism (G→A transition). in the −78 position of the apolipoprotein A-I promoter increases transcription efficiency. *J. Biolog. Chem.* **269,** 17371–17374.

224. Zhang, X., Chen, Z. Q., Wang, Z. W., Mohan, W., and Tam, S. P. (1996). Protein-DNA interactions at a drug-responsive element of the human apolipoprotein A-I gene. *J. Biolog. Chem.* **271,** 27152–27160.

225. Kondo, I., Berg, K., Drayna, D. T., and Lawn, R. M. (1989). DNA polymorphism at the locus for human cholesteryl ester transfer protein (CETP). is associated with high density lipoprotein cholesterol and apolipoprotein levels. *Clin. Genet.* **35,** 49–56.

226. Berg, K., Kondo, I., Drayna, D. T., and Lawn, R. M. (1989). "Variability gene" effect of cholesteryl ester transfer protein (CETP). genes. *Clin. Genet.* **35,** 437–445.

227. Freeman, D., Packard, C. J., Shepherd, J., and Gaffney, D. (1990). Polymorphisms in the gene coding for cholesteryl ester transfer protein are related to plasma high density lipoprotein cholesterol and transfer ester activity. *Clin. Sci.* **79,** 575–581.

228. Kessling, A., Ouellette, S., Bouffard, O., Chamberland, A., Bétard, C., Selinger, E., Xhignesse, M., Lussier-Cacan, S., and Davignon, J. (1991). Patterns of association between genetic variability in apolipoprotein (apo). B, apo AI-CIII-AIV, and cholesterol ester transfer protein gene regions and quantitative variation in lipid and lipoprotein traits: Influence of gender and exogenous hormones. *Am. J. Hum. Genet.* **50,** 92–106.

229. Kuivenhoven, J. A., de Knijff, P., Boer, J. M. A., Smalheer, H. A., Botma, G. J., Seidell, J. C., Kastelein, J. J. P., and Pritchard, P. H. (1997). Heterogeneity at the CETP gene locus—Influence on plasma CETP concentrations and HDL cholesterol levels. *Arterioscler. Thromb. Vasc. Biol.* **17,** 560–568.

230. Hannuksela, M. L., Liinamaa, M. J., Kesäniemi, Y. A., and Savolainen, M. J. (1994). Relation of polymorphisms in the cholesteryl ester transfer protein gene to transfer protein activity and plasma lipoprotein levels in alcohol drinkers. *Atherosclerosis* **110,** 35–44.

231. Freeman, D. J., Griffin, B. A., Holmes, A. P., Lindsay, G. M., Gaffney, D., Packard, C. J., and Shepherd, J. (1994). Regulation of plasma HDL cholesterol and subfraction distribution by genetic and environmental factors: Associations between the *Taq*I B RFLP in the CETP gene and smoking and obesity. *Arterioscler. Thromb.* **14,** 336–344.

232. Fumeron, F., Betoulle, D., Luc, G., Behague, I., Ricard, B., Poirier, O., Jemaa, R., Evans, A., Arveiler, D., Marques-Vidal, P., Bard, J. M., Fruchart, J. C., Ducimetière, P., Apfelbaum, M., and Cambien, F. (1995). Alcohol intake modulates the effect of a polymorphism of the cholesteryl ester transfer protein gene on plasma high density lipoprotein and the risk of myocardial infarction. *J. Clin. Invest.* **96,** 1664–1671.

233. Dullaart, R. P. F., Hoogenberg, K., Riemens, S. C., Groener, J. E. M., Van Tol, A., Sluiter, W. J., and Stulp, B. K. (1997). Cholesteryl ester transfer protein gene polymorphism is a determinant of HDL cholesterol and of the lipoprotein response to a lipid lowering diet in type I diabetes. *Diabetes* **46,** 2082–2087.

234. Kuivenhoven, J. A., Jukema, J. W., Zwinderman, A. H., de Knijff, P., McPherson, R., Bruschke, A. V., Lie, K. I., and Kastelein, J. J. (1998). The role of a common variant of the cholesteryl ester transfer protein gene in the progression of coronary atherosclerosis. The Regression Growth Evaluation Statin Study Group. *N. Engl. J. Med.* **338,** 86–93.

235. Bamberger, M., Lund-Katz, S., Phillips, M. C., and Rothblat, G. H. (1985). Mechanism of the hepatic lipase induced accumulation of high-density lipoprotein cholesterol by cells in culture. *Biochemistry* **24,** 3693–3701. 1985.

236. Johnson, W. J., Bamberger, M. J., Latta, R. A., Rapp, P. E., Phillips, M. C., and Rothblat, G. H. (1986). The bidirectional flux of cholesterol between cells and lipoproteins. Effects of phospholipid depletion of high density lipoprotein. *J. Biolog. Chem.* **261,** 5766–5776. 1986.

237. Connelly, P. W., Maguire, G. F., Lee, M., and Little, J. A. (1990). Plasma lipoproteins in familial hepatic lipase deficiency. *Arteriosclerosis* **10,** 40–48.

238. Hegele, R. A., Little, J. A., Vezina, C., Maguire, G. F., Tu, L., Wolever, T. S., Jenkins, D. J. A., and Connelly, P. W. (1993). Hepatic lipase deficiency: Clinical, biochemical, and molecular genetic characteristics. *Arterioscler. Thromb.* **13,** 720–728.

239. Jansen, H., Verhoeven, A. J., Weeks, L., Kastelein, J. J., Halley, D. J., van den Ouweland, A., Jukema, J. W., Seidell, J. C., and Birkenhager, J. C. (1997). A common C-to-T substitution at position −480 of the hepatic lipase promoter associated with a lowered lipase activity in coronary artery disease participants. *Arterioscler. Thromb. Vasc. Biol.* **17,** 2837–2842.

240. Zambon, A., Deeb, S. S., Hokanson, J. E., Brown, B. G., and Brunzell, J. D. (1998). Common variants in the promoter of the hepatic lipase gene are associated with lower levels of hepatic lipase activity, buoyant LDL, and higher HDL2 Cholesterol. *Arterioscler. Thromb. Vasc. Biol.* **18,** 1723–1729.

241. Vega, G. L., Clark, L. T., Tang, A., Marcovina, S., Grundy, S. M., and Cohen, J. C. (1998). Hepatic lipase activity is lower in African American men than in white American men: Effects of 5' flanking polymorphism in the hepatic lipase gene (LIPC). *J. Lipid Res.* **39,** 228–232.

242. Couture, P., Otvos, J. D., Cupples, L. A., Wilson, P. W. F., Schaefer, E. J., and Ordovas, J. M. (2000). Association of the C−514T polymorphism in the hepatic lipase gene with vari-

ations in lipoprotein subclass profiles: The Framingham Offspring Study. *Arterioscler. Thromb. Vasc. Biol.* **20,** 815–822.

243. Russell, D. W., and Setchell, K. D. (1992). Bile acid biosynthesis. *Biochemistry* **31,** 4737–4749.

244. Cheema, S. K., Cikaluk, D., and Agellon, L. B. (1997). Dietary fats modulate the regulatory potential of dietary cholesterol on cholesterol 7α-hydroxylase gene expression. *J. Lipid Res.* **38,** 315–323.

245. Cohen, J. C., Cali, J. J., Jelinek, D. F., Mehrabian, M., Sparkes, R. S., Lusis, A. J., Russell, D. W., and Hobbs, H. H. (1992). Cloning of the human cholesterol 7α-hydroxylase gene (*CYP7*). and localization to chromosome 8q11-q12. *Genomics* **14,** 153–161.

246. Wang, J., Freeman, D. J., Grundy, S. M., Levine, D. M., Guerra, R., and Cohen, J. C. (1998). Linkage between cholesterol 7alpha-hydroxylase and high plasma low density lipoprotein cholesterol concentrations. *J. Clin. Invest.* **101,** 1283–1291.

247. Molowa, D. T., Chen, W. S., Cimis, G. M., and Tan, C. P. (1992). Transcriptional regulation of the human cholesterol 7 alpha-hydroxylase gene. *Biochemistry* **31,** 2539–2544.

248. Schwarz, M., Russell, D. W., Dietschy, J. M., and Turley, S. D. (1998). Marked reduction in bile acid synthesis in cholesterol 7alpha-hydroxylase-deficient mice does not lead to diminished tissue cholesterol turnover or to hypercholesterolemia. *J. Lipid Res.* **39,** 1833–1843.

249. Masucci-Magoulas, L., Plump, A., Jiang, X. C., Walsh, A., Breslow, J. L., and Tall, A. R. (1996). Profound induction of hepatic cholesteryl ester transfer protein transgene expression in apolipoprotein E and low density lipoprotein receptor gene knockout mice—A novel mechanism signals changes in plasma cholesterol levels. *J. Clin. Invest.* **97,** 154–161.

250. Murao, K., Terpstra, V., Green, S. R., Kondratenko, N., Steinberg, D., and Quehenberger, O. (1997). Characterization of CLA-1, a human homologue of rodent scavenger receptor BI, as a receptor for high density lipoprotein and apoptotic thymocytes. *J. Biolog. Chem.* **272,** 33068–33076.

251. Cao, G., Garcia, C. K., Wyne, K. L., Schultz, R. A., Parker, K. L., and Hobbs, H. H. (1997). Structure and localization of the human gene encoding SR-BI/CLA-1: Evidence for transcriptional control by steroidogenic factor 1. *J. Biolog. Chem.* **272,** 33068–33076.

252. Rigotti, A., Trigatti, B., Babitt, J., Penman, M., Xu, S., and Krieger, M. (1997). Scavenger receptor BI: A cell surface receptor for high density lipoprotein. *Curr. Opin. Lipidol.* **8,** 181–188.

253. Calvo, D., and Vega, M. A. (1993). Identification, primary structure, and distribution of CLA-1, a novel member of the CD36/LIMPII gene family. *J. Biol. Chem.* **268,** 18929–18935.

254. Acton, S. L., Scherer, P. E., Lodish, H. F., and Krieger, M. (1994). Expression cloning of SR-BI, a CD36-related class B scavenger receptor. *J. Biolog. Chem.* **269,** 21003–21009.

255. Acton, S., Rigotti, A., Landschulz, K. T., Xu, S. Z., Hobbs, H. H., and Krieger, M. (1996). Identification of scavenger receptor SR-BI as a high density lipoprotein receptor. *Science* **271,** 518–520.

256. Glass, C., Pittman, R. C., Weinstein, D. B., and Steinberg, D. (1983). Dissociation of tissue uptake of cholesterol ester from that of apoprotein A-I of rat plasma high density lipo-

protein: Selective delivery of cholesterol ester to liver, adrenal, and gonad. *Proc. Natl. Acad. Sci. USA* **80,** 5435–5439.

257. Calvo, D., Gomez-Coronado, D., Lasunción, M. A., and Vega, M. A. (1997). CLA–1 is an 85-kD plasma membrane glycoprotein that acts as a high-affinity receptor for both native (HDL, LDL, and VLDL). and modified (OxLDL and AcLDL). lipoproteins. Arterioscler. Thromb. Vasc. Biol. **17,** 2341–2349.

258. Acton, S., Osgood, D., Donoghue, M., Corella, D., Pocovi, M., Cenarro, A., Mozas, P., Keilty, J., Squazzo, S., Woolf, E. A., and Ordovas, J. M. (1999). Association of polymorphisms at the SR-BI gene locus with plasma lipid levels and body mass index in a white population. *Arterioscler. Thromb. Vasc. Biol.* **19,** 1734–1743.

259. Hauser, H., Dyer, J. H., Nandy, A., Vega, M. A., Werder, M., Bieliauskaite, E., Weber, F. E., Compassi, S., Gemperli, A., Boffelli, D., Wehrli, E., Schulthess, G., and Phillips, M. C. (1998). Identification of a receptor mediating absorption of dietary cholesterol in the intestine. *Biochemistry* **37,** 17843–17850.

260. Serfary-Lacrosniere, C., Lanzberg, A., Civeira, F., Isaia, P., Berg, J., Janus, E. D., Smith, M. P., Pritchard, P. H., Frohlich, J., Lees, R. S., Ordovas, J. M., and Schaefer, E. J. (1994). Homozygous Tangier disease and cardiovascular disease. *Atherosclerosis* **107,** 85–98.

261. Brooks-Wilson, A., Marcil, M., Clee, S. M., Zhang, L. H., Roomp, K., van Dam, M., Yu, L., Brewer, C., Collins, J. A., Molhuizen, H. O. F., Loubser, O., Ouellette, B. F. F., Fichter, K., Ashbourne-Excoffon, K. J. D., Sensen, C. W., Scherer, S., Mott, S., Denis, M., Martindale, D., Frohlich, J., Morgan, K., Koop, B., Pimstone, S., Kastelein, J. J. P., Genest, J., and Hayden, M. R. (1999). Mutations in ABC1 in Tangier disease and familial high-density lipoprotein deficiency. *Nature Genet.* **22,** 336–345.

262. Bodzioch, M., Orso, E., Klucken, T., Langmann, T., Bottcher, L., Diederich, W., Drobnik, W., Barlage, S., Buchler, C., Porsch-Ozcurumez, M., Kaminski, W. E., Hahmann, H. W., Oette, K., Rothe, G., Aslanidis, C., Lackner, K. J., and Schmitz, G. (1999). The gene encoding ATP-binding cassette transporter 1 is mutated in Tangier disease. *Nature Genet.* **22,** 347–351.

263. Remaley, A. T., Rust, S., Rosier, M., Knapper, C., Naudin, L., Broccardo, C., Peterson, K. M., Koch, C., Arnould, I., Prades, C., Duverger, N., Funke, H., Assmann, G., Dinger, M., Dean, M., Chimini, G., Santamarina-Fojo, S., Fredrickson, D. S., Denefle, P., and Brewer, H. B. (1999). Human ATP-binding cassette transporter 1 (ABC1): Genomic organization and identification of the genetic defect in the original Tangier disease kindred. *Proc. Natl. Acad. Sci. USA* **96,** 12685–12690.

264. Rust, S., Rosier, M., Funke, H., Real, J., Amoura, Z., Piette, J. C., Deleuze, J. F., Brewer, H. B., Duverger, N., Denefle, P., and Assmann, G. (1999). Tangier disease is caused by mutations in the gene encoding ATP-binding cassette transporter 1. *Nature Genet.* **22,** 352-355.

265. Brousseau, M. E., Schaefer, E. J., Dupuis, J., Eustace, B., Van Eerdewegh, P., Goldkamp, A. L., Thurston, L. M., Fitzgerald, M. G., Yasek-McKenna, D., O'Neill, G., Eberhart, G. P., Weiffenbach, B., Ordovas, J. M., Freeman, M. W., Brown, R. H., Jr., and Gu, J. Z. (2000). Novel mutations in

the gene encoding ATP-binding cassette 1 in four Tangier disease kindreds. *J. Lipid Res.* **41,** 433–441.

266. Marcil, M., Brooks-Wilson, A., Clee, S. M., Roomp, K., Zhang, L. H., Yu, L., Collins, J. A., van Dam, M., Molhuizen, H. O. F., Loubster, O., Oullette, B. F. F., Sensen, C. W., Fichter, K., Mott, S., Denis, M., Boucher, B., Pimstone, S., Genest, J., Kastelein, J. J. P., and Hayden, M. R. (1999). Mutations in the ABC1 gene in familial HDL deficiency with defective cholesterol efflux. *Lancet* **354,** 1341–1346.

267. Genest, J., Jr., Bard, J. -M., Fruchart, J. -C., Ordovas, J. M., and Schaefer, E. J. (1993). Familial hypoalphalipoproteinemia in premature coronary artery disease. *Arterioscler. Thromb.* **13,** 1728–1737.

268. Altshuler, D., Kruglyak, L., and Lander, E. (1998). Genetic polymorphisms and disease. *N. Engl. J. Med.* **338,** 1626.

CHAPTER **12**

Genetics of Human Obesity

JANIS S. FISLER AND NANCY A. SCHONFELD-WARDEN
University of California, Davis, California

I. INTRODUCTION

Complex and incompletely defined interactions between environment and genetics determine each individual's height and weight, as well as many other human traits. The result is a population in which individuals vary widely for height and weight, but no one factor can be identified as controlling either trait. In humans, long-term adult weight is relatively stable, as evidenced by the difficulty of sustaining intentional weight loss and the automatic return to previous weight following brief periods of overeating. This drive to constancy of body weight is due to both behavioral and physiological alterations that accompany weight change.

Further convincing evidence of the biological basis of the regulation of body fat stores comes from the identification of single-gene mutations that result in spontaneous massive obesity or in adipose tissue atrophy. There are also Mendelian disorders in which obesity or abnormalities of fat distribution are a prominent feature and for which the chromosomal locations, but not the genes or their functions, are known.

Most human obesity, however, is not due to mutations in single genes but exhibits a complex, non-Mendelian inheritance. Obesity is usually dependent on a permissive environment. Fat deposition can occur uniformly or there can be preferential deposition of fat, for example, in the abdominal area. There are also likely to be interactions among genes such that some alleles of one gene will not cause obesity unless specific alleles of another gene are present. Although animal models clearly demonstrate that gene–gene interactions are common and can have substantial effects on many traits, technical difficulties have made it more difficult to identify such interactions in human studies. Expression of an obesity gene may also be age or gender dependent. Thus, identification of all the genes promoting human obesity is not a trivial task.

Genetics is a rapidly progressing field, and knowledge of the genetic basis for obesity is expanding exponentially. Therefore, the reader should use this chapter only as the starting point for an understanding of this exciting body of knowledge.

II. GENETIC EPIDEMIOLOGY OF HUMAN OBESITY

Genetic epidemiology of human obesity is the study of the relationships of the various factors determining the frequency and distribution of obesity in the population. Such studies of obesity are limited in that they do not examine DNA and rarely directly measure the amount or location of body fat. However, genetic epidemiology studies do provide information as to whether there is a genetic basis for the trait, whether inheritance is maternal or paternal, and whether expression of the trait is gender or age dependent.

Genetic epidemiology studies of human obesity employ a variety of designs and statistical methods, each giving somewhat different heritability estimates for obesity. For a discussion of genetic epidemiology methods employed in the study of obesity, see Bouchard et al. [1].

The heritability estimates for human obesity are derived from a large number of studies of adoptees, twins, and families. Heritability of human obesity may be as low as 10%, as estimated from some adoption studies, or as high as 80%, as estimated from some twin studies [1] (Table 1). Two studies that incorporated twins, adoptees, and nuclear families into the analyses yielded heritability estimates for obesity of approximately 25–40%. These studies indicate that familial environment has only a minor impact on obesity.

The number of genes involved in human obesity has not been estimated, primarily because such estimates are complicated by the conclusion that genes implicated in obesity have major, minor, and polygenic effects. A major gene is a single gene that has a large effect on the phenotype. Polygenic effects are due to many genes, each with a small effect on the phenotype. Segregation analyses[1] indicate that the percentage of minor gene transmission ranges from 25 to 42% and that there is a single major gene for high body mass segregating from the parents to their offspring. These data do not mean that there is only one major gene contributing to obesity in humans. Rather, the specific obesity gene may

---

[1]Segregation analysis is used to determine whether the trait is segregating in families according to Mendelian expectations.

TABLE 1   Overview of the Genetic Epidemiology of Human Body Fat/Obesity[a]

	Heritability/transmission	Maternal or paternal effect[b]	Familial environment
Nuclear families	30–50	No	Minor
Adoption studies	10–30	Mixed results	Minor
Twin studies	50–80	No	No
Combined strategies	25–40	No	Minor

Source: Reprinted from Bouchard, C., Pérusse, L., Rice, T., and Rao, D. C. (1998). The genetics of human obesity. *In* "Handbook of Obesity" (G. A. Bray, C. Bouchard, and W. P. T. James, Eds.), p. 166, by courtesy of Marcel Dekker, Inc., New York.

[a]Based on the trends in about 50 different studies. In most of the studies, the BMI was the phenotype considered. In some cases, skinfolds or estimates of percentage body fat or fat mass were used.

[b]Maternal or paternal effect indicates whether transmission through mother or father alters heritability.

vary from person to person, such that there may be several major obesity genes in the entire population. However, no major obesity genes have been identified in any population.

III. GENE–ENVIRONMENT INTERACTIONS

Why some people in modern societies become obese, despite considerable effort and expense to avoid this condition, whereas others stay lean without such effort, appears to have a genetic basis [2]. The chronic overfeeding studies by Sims and colleagues beginning in the 1960s showed interindividual differences in weight gain [3, 4]. More recently, Bouchard and colleagues determined the response to changes in energy balance by submitting pairs of monozygotic twins either to positive energy balance induced by overeating or to negative energy balance induced by exercise training. During 100 days of overfeeding by 1000 kcal/day, significant intrapair resemblance was observed for changes in body composition and was particularly striking for changes in regional fat distribution and amount of visceral fat, with six times as much variance among as within twin pairs [5]. During long-term energy deficit induced by exercise training, intrapair resemblance was observed for changes in body weight, fat mass, percent fat, and abdominal visceral fat [6]. One explanation for these differences is that some twin pairs were found to be better oxidizers of lipid, as evidenced by reduced respiratory quotient, during submaximal work than were other twin pairs [6].

An important component of the interindividual difference in response to overeating may be individual differences in spontaneous physical activity or "fidgeting" [7, 8]. A large portion of the variability in total daily energy expenditure, independent of lean body mass, is due to fidgeting, which varies by more the sevenfold among subjects [7], is a familial trait, and is a predictor of future weight gain [9]. In a very elegant study of the fate of excess energy during overfeeding, Levine *et al.* [8] again demonstrated the consid-

erable interindividual variation in susceptibility to weight gain. Two-thirds of the increases in total daily energy expenditure in nonobese subjects overfed by 1000 kcal/day for 8 weeks was due to increased spontaneous physical activity associated with fidgeting, maintenance of posture, and other daily activities of life independent of volitional exercise [8].

IV. THE OBESITY GENE MAP

A genetic map is a representation of the distribution of a set of genetic loci or markers. (For a discussion of genetic maps, see [10].) The three types of genetic maps are linkage, chromosomal, and physical maps. Genetic maps provide many kinds of information, from overall chromosomal views to more detailed molecular information, but all genetic maps place items (usually genes or clones) in an order, from top to bottom or left to right.

The Human Obesity Gene Map [11] incorporates information from all three types of maps—linkage, chromosomal, and physical. The map and its associated summary provide an overview of the data reported in peer-reviewed journals on human obesity genes and markers as well as published evidence from rodent obesity models. Five types of data were used to generate the map, all of which are represented in Fig. 1: (1) single-gene obesity mutations, e.g., *POMC*; (2) Mendelian disorders exhibiting obesity as a clinical feature, e.g., *ALMS1*; (3) quantitative trait loci (QTLs)[2] identified in linkage studies in animals, e.g., *Mob 6* and *Pfat1*, and in humans; (4) linkage studies of candidate genes in humans, e.g., *ACP1*; and (5) association studies of candidate genes, e.g., also *ACP1*. The most up-to-date compilation of obesity gene information, covering all 22 autoso-

---

[2]A quantitative trait is one that varies over a continuous range, such as body weight and height, and is generally controlled by more than one gene. A quantitative trait locus (QTL) is a chromosomal region in which alleles are linked to variation of a quantitative trait.

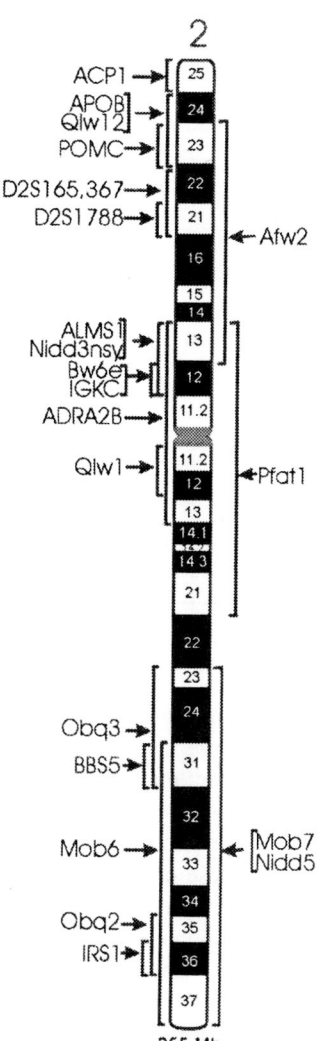

FIGURE 1   Chromosome 2 demonstrates each of the types of putative obesity loci found in the Human Obesity Gene Map. Mutation of the *POMC* gene causes single-gene obesity in humans. Mutations of *ALMS* and *BBS5* cause the rare Mendelian syndromes, Alstrom syndrome and Bardet-Beidl-5 syndrome. *IRS1*, the insulin receptor substrate-1, is a candidate gene for type 2 diabetes, obesity, and hyperinsulinemia in humans. *D2S165* is an anonymous marker linked to obesity in humans and *Obq3* is a QTL linked to adiposity in a mouse model. [Reprinted with permission from Chagnon, Y. C., Pérusse, L., Weisnagel, S. J., Rankinen, T., and Bouchard, C. (2000). The Human Obesity Gene Map: The 1999 update. *Obes. Res.* **8**, 89–117.]

mal chromosomes as well as the X and Y chromosomes, is available in the Human Obesity Gene Map, published each January in the journal *Obesity Research*. The same information is available on-line at http://www.obesity.chair.ulaval.ca/genes.html. The current update [11] of the map includes many obesity-related phenotypes, including body mass index, percent body fat, fat mass, skinfolds, abdominal fat, macronutrient intake, metabolic rate, energy expenditure, and fat-free mass.

V. SINGLE-GENE OBESITY IN HUMANS

Cloning of the rodent obesity genes,[3] *Lep^{ob}*, *Lepr^{db}*, *Cpe^{fat}*, *Tub*, and *A^y*, between 1992 and 1996 led to an explosion of knowledge, summarized below, of the genetic causes of obesity. In addition to severe obesity, most of these models are characterized by insulin resistance and infertility. The function of only one of these rodent obesity genes, *Tub*, remains unknown. The human gene, *TUB*,[4] located at 11p15.5, encodes a novel protein of unknown function, the C terminus of which is highly conserved across species. Recent papers provide hints of *Tub* function. One reports that *Tub* codes for a protein that functions in intracellular signaling by insulin [12]. The other shows that *Tub* binds to DNA and may thus influence transcription [13]. To date, no studies implicate *TUB* in human obesity or insulin resistance.

Obesity in these rodent models exhibits Mendelian segregation, indicating that the obesity is inherited as a single-gene mutation. With one exception, these mutations result in the loss of gene or protein function and are expressed only when both copies of the gene in an individual are defective. Therefore, obesity due to these mutations in humans would not be common. Although most human obesity is not believed to be due to a single-gene defect but exhibits a complex, non-Mendelian inheritance, these genes are of great interest, since subtle mutations may contribute to common forms of obesity. Also, study of these genes has identified many new pathways for investigation of the physiology of obesity and provided many therapeutic targets for new antiobesity drugs [14].

As of early 2000, five genes have been shown to cause spontaneous Mendelian obesity in humans: leptin (gene abbreviation, *LEP*), leptin receptor (*LEPR*), proopiomelanocortin (*POMC*), melanocortin-4 receptor (*MC4R*), and proprotein convertase subtilisin/kexin type 1 (*PCSK1*) (Table 2).

A. Leptin Deficiency

Cloning and characterization of the mouse *Lep^{ob}* gene identified its protein product, leptin, a hormone that is secreted from adipose tissue [15] and to a lesser extent from placenta [16] and gastric epithelium [17]. Leptin circulates in the blood [18], crosses the blood–brain barrier [19], and binds to its receptor in the hypothalamus to regulate food intake and energy expenditure. Thus, leptin functions as an afferent signal in a negative feedback loop to maintain constancy of body fat stores. Because leptin is expressed in, and secreted from, adipose tissue, circulating levels of leptin closely

---

[3]The designations *Lep^{ob}*, *Lepr^{db}*, and *Cpe^{fat}* represent mutations of the genes coding for leptin, the leptin receptor, and carboxypeptidase E that occur in the *obese* mouse, the *diabetes* mouse, and the *fat* mouse, respectively.

[4]Capital letters, e.g., *TUB*, indicate the human gene, whereas lowercase letters, e.g., *Tub*, indicate the mouse gene.

TABLE 2   Genes Known to Cause Spontaneous Mendelian Obesity in Humans

Protein product	Gene abbreviation	Location	Phenotype	Reference
Autosomal recessive inheritance				
Leptin	*LEP*	7q31.3	Severe hyperphagia and massive obesity beginning in early childhood	[29]
			Infertility due to hypothalamic-pituitary hormone insufficiency in adults	[30]
Leptin receptor	*LEPR*	1p31	Same phenotype as leptin deficiency	[35]
Proopiomelanocortin	*POMC*	2p23.3	Moderate obesity in early childhood Adrenal insufficiency, red hair	[37]
Proprotein convertase subtilisin/kexin type 1	*PCSK1*	5q15-q21	Extreme childhood obesity Abnormal glucose homeostasis, hypogonadotropic gonadism, hypocortisolism, elevated proinsulin and POMC	[38]
Autosomal dominant inheritance				
Melanocortin-4 receptor	*MC4R*	18q22	Severe hyperphagia, massive obesity from early childhood	[40, 41, 42]

match the total amount of fat stores [20] and decrease with weight loss [21]. Peripheral or central administration of leptin reduces food intake and body fat in several mouse models of obesity (those with a functional leptin receptor), while preserving lean tissue mass, although relatively high doses are required in certain models [18, 22–24]. A recent clinical trial indicates that the same is true for both lean and obese humans treated with recombinant leptin [25].

Leptin clearly has a broader physiological role than just the regulation of body fat stores. Leptin deficiency results in many of the abnormalities seen in starvation, including reduced body temperature, reduced activity, decreased immune function, and infertility. Leptin levels, for equivalent body fat mass, are higher in women than in men [20]. In prepubertal females, leptin levels are highly correlated with body fat, and the increase in serum leptin is associated with a younger age of menarche [26]. Leptin reverses the starvation-induced suppression of T cells even in the presence of continued energy deficit [27]. For a review of the physiological role of leptin see Friedman and Halaas [28].

Known mutations in leptin (Table 2) causing spontaneous massive obesity in humans are autosomal recessive and are rare in the population[5]. However, two highly consanguineous families were identified that carry mutations in *LEP*. Two severely obese children of one family have very low serum leptin levels despite massive obesity [29]. One of the children weighed 86 kg at the age of 8 years, with 57% body fat. The other child weighed 29 kg at the age of 2 years. Both children had normal birth weight but were markedly hyper-

phagic and gained weight rapidly in the early postnatal period. Four massively obese members of another family are homozygous for a different mutation in *LEP* and have very low leptin levels. Three of these individuals are adults: The females have primary amenorrhea and the male never entered puberty. Seven obese members of this pedigree, presumably also carrying the mutation in *LEP*, died of infectious diseases during childhood (no normal weight family members have died). All others in the family are either heterozygous for the mutation or homozygous for the wild-type allele and have normal body weight and serum leptin levels [30, 31]. Recombinant leptin therapy in doses sufficient to raise serum concentrations of leptin to the normal range in a 9-year-old girl with congenital leptin deficiency corrected many aspects of the obese phenotype. Over a 12-month period, this patient, with a baseline weight of 94 kg, lost 16 kg, primarily as fat mass [32].

B. Leptin Receptor Deficiency

Leptin acts through the leptin receptor, a single-transmembrane-domain receptor of the cytokine-receptor family [33]. The leptin receptor is found in many tissues in several alternatively spliced forms, raising the possibility that leptin affects many tissues in addition to the hypothalamus [34]. For additional discussion of the leptin receptor, see [28].

An autosomal recessive mutation in the human leptin receptor gene (*LEPR*) that results in a truncated leptin receptor was discovered in homozygosity in a consanguineous family. Three of nine siblings had severe hyperphagia and developed early morbid obesity despite normal birth weight [35]. Individuals homozygous for this mutation have no pubertal development and their secretion of growth hormone

---

[5]If an allele is rare and if two copies (homozygosity) of a mutation are required for the phenotype to be expressed, then homozygotes are usually found only in highly consanguineous (inbred) families.

and thyrotropin is reduced. This phenotype is similar to that seen in individuals with mutation of the leptin gene.

C. Proopiomelanocortin Deficiency

Sequential cleavage of the precursor protein proopiomelanocortin (POMC) generates the melanocortin peptides adrenocorticotrophin (ACTH), the melanocyte-stimulating hormones (α- and β-MSH), and the opioid-receptor ligand beta-endorphin. α-MSH plays a central role in the regulation of food intake by the activation of the brain melanocortin-4 receptor (Section V. E) [36]. The dual role of α-MSH in regulating food intake and influencing hair pigmentation predicts that the phenotype associated with a defect in *POMC* function would include obesity, alteration in pigmentation, and ACTH deficiency. The observations of these symptoms in two probands[6] led to the identification of three separate mutations within their *POMC* genes [37] (Fig. 2, see color plate at the back of the book). One individual is a compound heterozygote[7] for two mutations that interfere with appropriate synthesis of ACTH and α-MSH. The other patient is homozygous for a mutation that abolishes *POMC* translation. These findings define a new monogenic endocrine disorder resulting in early-onset obesity, adrenal insufficiency, and red hair pigmentation.

D. Proprotein Convertase Subtilisin/Kexin Type 1 Deficiency

A wide variety of hormones, enzymes, and receptors are initially synthesized as large inactive precursors. To release the active hormone, enzyme, or receptor, these precursors must undergo limited proteolysis by specific convertases. Examples are the conversion of proinsulin to insulin by the combined actions of proprotein convertase 1 and 2 and the clipping of *POMC* by proprotein convertase 1. A recessive mutation of carboxypeptidase E, an enzyme active in the processing and sorting of prohormones, causes obesity in the *Cpe^fat* mouse. A mutation in a homologous enzyme was found in a woman with extreme childhood obesity, abnormal glucose homeostasis, hypogonadotrophic hypogonadism, hypocortisolism, and elevated proinsulin and proopiomelanocortin concentrations but a very low insulin level [38]. This woman is a compound heterozygote for mutations in proprotein convertase subtilisin/kexin type 1 (PCSK1; also known as prohormone convertase-1), which acts proximally to carboxypeptidase E in the pathway of post-translational processing of prohormones and neuropeptides. Since the proband and the *fat* mouse share similar phenotypes, it can be inferred that molecular defects in prohormone conversion represent a generic mechanism for obesity.

[6]A proband is the index case, the person through whom the pedigree (family) was acertained.

[7]A compound heterozygote would have two different mutations in the gene, one on each chromosome.

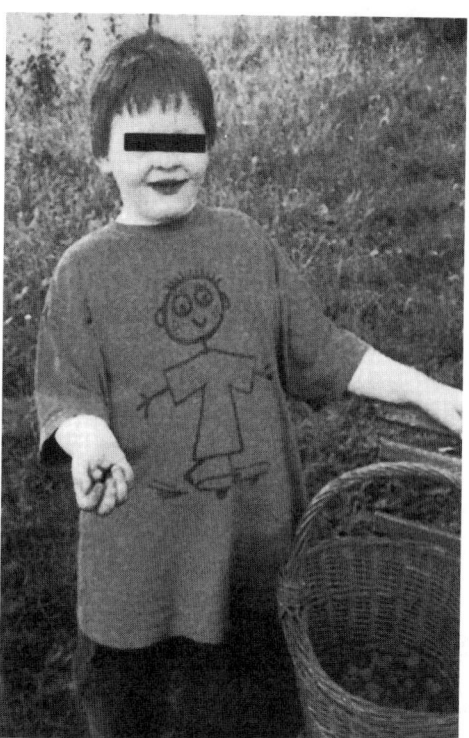

FIGURE 2 Photo of 5-year-old-boy with early-onset obesity, adrenal insufficiency, and red hair caused by mutation of the *POMC* gene. This patient had early hypoglycemia and hyponatriaemia due to ACTH deficiency. Birth weight was normal but, due to hyperphagia, obesity was apparent by 5 months of age. (See color plate.) [Reprinted with permission from Krude, H., Biebermann, H., Luck, W., Horn, R., Brabant, G., and Grüters, A. (1998). Severe early-onset obesity, adrenal insufficiency and red hair pigmentation caused by *POMC* mutations in humans. *Nature Genet.* **19**, 155–157.]

E. Mutation in the Melanocortin-4 Receptor Gene

The agouti protein, identified in the yellow obese (*A^y*) mouse, inhibits binding of α-MSH to melanocortin receptors, including Mc4r, which is located in the hypothalamus, and Mc1r, which is located in the skin. Obesity and yellow coat color in the *A^y* mouse result from expressing agouti in all tissues, not just in skin, which is the normal condition. The melanocortin-4 receptor, a G-protein-coupled receptor, is highly expressed in the hypothalamus, a region of the brain intimately involved in appetite regulation. It is a receptor for α-MSH, a product of the *POMC* gene (Section V. C), which inhibits feeding. Inactivation of *Mc4r* by gene targeting in mice results in a maturity-onset obesity syndrome associated with hyperphagia and impaired glucose tolerance [39]. Mc4r-deficient mice do not respond to a α-MSH-like agonist, suggesting that α-MSH inhibits feeding primarily by activating Mc4r [36]. Mice heterozygous for a null *Mc4r* allele exhibit phenotypes intermediate to that seen in wild-type and homozygous littermates [36].

In screening children that were severely obese from an early age, mutations in *MC4R* resulting in haploinsufficiency[8] as well as several missense[9] mutations were identified [40–43]. The functional significance of the missense mutations [42] is uncertain. The haploinsufficiency mutations were present in the heterozygous state, and other members of each family were obese in a pattern consistent with autosomal dominant inheritance. Adrenal function is not impaired in the MC4R-deficient subjects. Sexual development and fertility are normal. Affected subjects are tall, similar to the increased linear growth that occurs in heterozygous Mc4r-deficient mice. Female haploinsufficiency carriers are heavier then male carriers in their families, a pattern also seen in Mc4r-deficient mice. These data are strong evidence for dominantly inherited obesity, not associated with infertility, due to haploinsufficiency mutations in *MC4R*.

VI. SINGLE-GENE MUTATIONS RESULTING IN ADIPOSE TISSUE ATROPHY

The lipodystrophies are characterized by the absence or reduction of subcutaneous adipose tissue. Patients with familial partial lipodystrophy (FPLD) are born with normal fat distribution, but close to puberty, they experience regional adipose tissue atrophy that is often associated with insulin resistance, diabetes, and hyperlipidemia. The gene coding FPLD was mapped to 1q21. 2-q21. 3 and found to be *LMNA*, which codes for a polypeptide, lamin A, found in the nuclear lamina of the cell. Three different amino acid substitutions at one position in the lamin A polypeptide that result in heritable partial lipodystrophy were identified in a dozen families [44, 45]. Different mutations in *LMNA* result in specific muscular dystrophy and cardiomyopathy disorders as well.

VII. RARE GENETIC SYNDROMES WITH OBESITY AS A PROMINENT FEATURE

There are at least 26 rare Mendelian syndromes, in which obesity is a prominent clinical feature, described in the On-line Mendelian Interitance in Man (OMIM) database[10] [46]. Among the better known of these syndromes are the Prader-Willi syndrome, the Bardet-Biedl syndromes, and Alstrom syndrome. Currently, the pathophysiologic mechanisms leading to obesity in these syndromes are not known. The identification of the underlying genes will likely help define the mechanisms controlling appetite, satiety, and obesity. The characteristic features of these syndromes were recently reviewed [47].

With an incidence of about 1 in 25, 000 births, the most common of the Mendelian syndromes is the Prader-Willi syndrome, which results from a microdeletion of paternal chromosome 15q11-q13 or, more rarely, as a result of maternal disomy[11] of chromosome 15. In addition to obesity, the Prader-Willi syndrome is characterized by hypotonic musculature, mental retardation, hypogonadism, short stature, and small hands and feet (for review, see [48, 49]). Aberrant behavior, including hyperphagia and aggressive food seeking, makes management of these patients difficult.

Autosomal recessive Mendelian obesity syndromes include the Bardet-Biedl syndromes (BBS1–BBS5) and the Alstrom syndrome (ALMS1). The Bardet-Biedl syndromes are associated with variants on chromosomes 11q13 (BBS1), 16q21 (BBS2), 3p13-p12 (BBS3), 15q22. 3–23 (BBS4), and 2q31 (BBS5). The Bardet-Biedl syndromes are all characterized by mental retardation, pigmentary retinopathy, polydactyly, obesity, and hypogonadism. It is, therefore, apparent that mutation in at least five separate genes can result in the same phenotype. The gene on chromosome 16 coding for BBS2 may predispose males carrying only one copy of the gene to obesity and may explain approximately 3% of severely overweight males [50]. Of interest, BBS2 parents of both sexes were significantly taller than U. S. individuals of comparable age [50].

In addition to obesity, Alstrom syndrome is characterized by retinitis pigmentosa leading to blindness, insulin resistance, diabetes, and deafness, but does not involve mental retardation or polydactyly (for review, see [51, 52]). Onset of obesity is usually between 2 and 10 years of age and can range from mild to severe. The gene for Alstrom syndrome (ALMS1) was narrowed down to a small region on chromosome 2p13-p12 [53].

VIII. EVIDENCE FROM LINKAGE STUDIES OF OBESITY PHENOTYPES

A. Mapping of Loci in Animals

Animal models have been very important in the dissection of complex traits [54]. Quantitative trait locus mapping is a method for mapping Mendelian factors that underlie complex traits, in virtually any animal model, by using genetic

---

[8]Haploinsufficiency occurs when a gene, or a group of genes, is present in too few copies or too many copies. In autosomes (all but the X and Y chromosomes) one copy of each gene is inherited from each parent. The presence of extra chromosomal material or lack of chromosomal material alters gene dosage, causing abnormalities in gene function.

[9]A missense mutation is one that changes amino acid sequence, but does not produce a stop codon (nonsense mutation).

[10]The Online Mendelian Inheritance in Man (OMIM) [46] database is available at http://www3.ncbi.nlm.nih.gov/omim/. This database is a catalog of human genes and genetic disorders authored and edited by Dr. Victor A. McKusick and his colleagues at Johns Hopkins and elsewhere, and developed for the World Wide Web by the National Center for Biotechnology Information (NCBI).

[11]Maternal disomy is inheritance of an extra maternal chromosome or part thereof.

linkage maps[12] (for discussion, see [10, 54]). As of October 1999, 98 animal QTLs were linked variously to body weight, body fat, energy expenditure, food intake, leptin levels, or weight gain [11]. A number of these QTLs identified in separate crossbreeding experiments of different strains are overlapping and it is likely that the same underlying gene is responsible for these overlapping QTLs. Many of these QTLs have pleiotropic effects.[13]

B. From Mouse to Human

QTLs are valuable for identifying candidate genes to be further evaluated by gene targeting experiments in mice or by linkage studies or association studies of the candidate genes in humans. Because of the evolutionary relationship between mice and humans, many ancestral chromosomal segments have been retained where the same genes occur in the same order within discrete regions of chromosome (homology)[14] [55]. These regions of homology may include many hundreds to thousands of genes in the same orders, although some regions of homology are made more complex by chromosomal rearrangements within the region of homology. Because regions of homology between mouse and human chromosomes are well defined, the identification of a gene in the mouse frequently gives the chromosomal location of the same gene in the human. This relationship was used to map a gene for obesity to human chromosome 20 [56]. To test whether an obesity QTL on mouse chromosome 2 contributes to human obesity, linkage analysis between markers located within the homologous region on chromosome 20 and measures of obesity was performed in a large study of more than 150 French Canadian families; a locus on 20q13 that contributes to body fat and fasting insulin was found [56]. This locus was later confirmed in a second population group [57]. A polymorphism within this region in the candidate gene, adenosine deaminase (ADA), was recently associated with obesity in a population of subjects with non-insulin-dependent diabetes (NIDDM) [58] (Section IX.B).

C. Linkage Studies in Humans

Linkage studies in humans are conducted with large extended families or with nuclear families. A conceptually

simple and practical method is the nonparametric sib-pair linkage method that provides statistical evidence of linkage between a quantitative phenotype and a genetic marker [1, 59]. The method is based on the concept that siblings who share a greater number of alleles (1 or 2) identical by descent[15] at a linked marker locus should also share more alleles at the phenotypic locus of interest and should be phenotypically more similar than siblings who share fewer marker alleles (0 or 1). The method has been expanded to use data from multiple markers, allowing higher resolution mapping [60]. Linkage studies do not identify any specific gene but are useful in identifying candidate genes for further study.

A number of whole genome scans and linkage studies covering smaller chromosomal regions, published as of October 1999, identified 56 QTLs for various measures of adiposity, respiratory quotient, metabolic rate, and plasma leptin levels in humans (for details, see [11]). Many of these chromosomal loci contain candidate genes for obesity, including genes known to cause single-gene obesity (Section V). Linkage studies suggest that the LEP gene or a gene very near it on 7q31. 3 contributes to obesity in several different populations although the monogenic syndrome of leptin deficiency is rare [61–65]. One group linked both the LEPR [66] and MC4R [67] genes to multigenic obesity-related phenotypes in French Canadians. Candidate genes first identified through linkage studies include the adrenergic receptors [68, 69], UCP2/UCP3 [70], and ADA [56].

IX. ASSOCIATION STUDIES OF CANDIDATE GENES FOR OBESITY AND OBESITY-RELATED INSULIN RESISTANCE AND HYPERLIPIDEMIA

Association studies examine the correlation of a genetic variant (polymorphism) within a gene with the phenotype of interest. It is assumed that variants within a gene's coding region alter gene function, although proof of that requires gene-targeting experiments in cell or animal models. Association studies are generally carried out in unrelated individuals and are frequently designed as case-control studies. Although case-control studies remain a powerful tool in some areas, they are less powerful for genetic studies due to methodological issues that complicate analyses in complex populations such as those found in the United States. Therefore, most association studies are now conducted in isolated populations, such as occur in Finland and Quebec. A positional candidate gene is identified both by its location in a

[12]A locus is any segment of DNA that is measurable in genetic analysis. A locus may be within a gene or may be an alternative DNA sequence of no known function. A linkage map represents a set of loci on a single chromosome in which all members of the set are linked either directly or indirectly with all other members of the set. Linkage in humans refers to the cosegregation of a genetic marker and a trait together in families.

[13]Pleiotropy means that one gene has a primary effect on more than one phenotype.

[14]The Davis Human/Mouse Homology Map is a table comparing genes in homologous segments of DNA from human and mouse sources, sorted by position in each genome. A total of 1793 loci are presented, most of which are genes, in 201 homology groupings [55]. Current homology data are available at http://www.ncbi.nlm.nih.gov/Homology/.

[15]Identical by descent is in contrast to identical by state. Two siblings sharing the same allele are identical by descent if you know that it is the same allele inherited from the same parent. They are identical by state if they have the same allele, but you do not know if they are derived from the same parental haplotype.

chromosomal region that has significant linkage to obesity in family studies and because its biological functions are generally consistent with a role in body weight regulation. Forty candidate genes have been associated with varying degrees of confidence with obesity phenotypes to date [11]. The complete physical map of the human genome should be available by 2003 providing many new candidate genes for investigation.

A. Role of Single-Gene Obesity in Common Forms of Human Obesity

Several of the genes causing spontaneous massive obesity in humans have been implicated in polygenic obesity using association studies. The *LEP* gene is associated with body weight, weight loss, or leptin levels [71–73]. The *LEPR* gene is associated with obesity in three studies, including one of severe obesity in children [66, 74, 75]. Populations from the Pacific Island of Nauru have some of the highest rates of obesity and NIDDM in the world. In Nauruan males, specific combinations of alleles in the *LEP* and *LEPR* genes are associated with increased risk for development of insulin resistance [76]. *POMC* is associated with variation in leptin levels [77]. *MC4R* is associated with fat mass in one study [67]. These data suggest that mutations of the genes causing Mendelian obesity also contribute to common (polygenic) obesity in humans.

B. Candidate Genes with Variants Causing Altered Function

A number of other genes, with variants that may alter gene product function, are believed to contribute to common obesity and its comorbidities. Obesity frequently clusters with insulin resistance, hyperlipidemia, and hypertension [78]. This clustering might arise by any of several mechanisms: Obesity might promote comorbidities, comorbidities might promote obesity, or some genes might promote development of both obesity and its comorbidities. Several association studies have reported evidence for genes that influence obesity and one or more comorbidities. However, the demonstration that these variants result in single-gene obesity in any case remains to be established. The more promising candidates are described in Table 3.

Peroxisome-proliferator-activated receptor γ (PPARγ) is a member of the nuclear hormone receptor subfamily of transcription factors that includes T3 and vitamin D_3 receptors. PPARs regulate expression of genes involved in, among other things, lipid metabolism and energy balance (for review, see [79]). Due to combined effects on both fat and muscle, activation of PPARγ improves insulin sensitivity and glucose metabolism, and decreases blood triglyceride levels. Three association studies have implicated *PPARγ* in obesity and insulin resistance phenotypes. Four of 121 obese

German subjects had a missense mutation in the *PPARγ* gene compared to none in 237 normal weight individuals [80]. All of the subjects with the mutant allele were severely obese. The mutant gene was then overexpressed in mouse fibroblasts, which led to the accelerated differentiation of the cells into adipocytes with greater accumulation of triglyceride than seen with the wild-type *PPARγ* gene [80]. A different mutation of the *PPARγ* gene was identified in Finnish populations and was found to be associated with lower body mass index (BMI), lower fasting insulin levels, and greater insulin sensitivity [81].

The β-2-adrenergic receptor (ADRβ2) is a major lipolytic receptor in human adipose tissue, and, thus, plays a significant role in lipid mobilization. Several polymorphisms have been identified and their frequencies compared between lean and obese subjects. These variants were associated with body mass index and blood triglycerides in both Swedish and Japanese populations [82–84]. Swedish women with two copies of a common polymorphism, Glu27, were about 10 times more likely to be obese than those with the wild-type *ADRβ2* gene, with approximately 20 kg excess body fat and a 50% increase in fat cell size [82]. Another variant of the *ADRβ2* gene, Gly16, was associated with improved adipocyte ADRβ2 function. Thus, genetic variability in the human *ADRβ2* gene may be a significant contributor to human obesity.

The β-3-adrenergic receptor (ADRβ3) is expressed in adipose tissue and is involved in the regulation of lipolysis and thermogenesis. Disruption of the *Adrβ3* gene in mice results in moderate obesity [85]. This potential relevance to human obesity led to an initial positive report in 1995 of an association between *ADRβ3* and obesity [86] followed by numerous studies with conflicting results (for review, see [87]). A paired sibling design that aimed to detect effects of the variant by accounting for background genes examined 45 nondiabetic sibling-pairs discordant for the variant who were identical by descent at another marker that is known to be associated with obesity in this population. Presence of the variant was significantly associated with increases in BMI, fat mass, and waist circumference [88]. However, a meta-analysis[16] combining 23 studies and 7399 subjects concluded that the *ADRβ3* gene variant is not significantly associated with BMI [87]. The possible association of the variant with diabetes phenotypes was not examined in the meta-analysis. Thus, whether the *ADRβ3* gene contributes to obesity or diabetes phenotypes is still subject to debate.

Adenosine deaminase (*ADA*) was identified as a positional candidate gene for obesity by linkage studies in both mice and humans [56]. ADA is an α-adrenergic agonist with potent lipolytic and vasodilator effects that regulates both

---

[16]Meta-analysis is a statistical tool for pooling data from many studies into a single analysis, thus greatly increasing the statistical power of the analysis.

TABLE 3   Genes Associated with Obesity and Comorbidities in Humans

Protein product	Gene abbreviation	Location	Phenotypes associated with different variants	Reference
Peroxisome-proliferator-activated receptor γ	PPARγ	3p25	Severe obesity	[80]
			Lower BMI, lower fasting insulin, greater insulin sensitivity	[81]
β-2-Adrenergic receptor	ADRβ2	5q32-q34	Higher BMI and excess body fat, increased subcutaneous fat, higher blood triglycerides	[82, 83, 84]
β-3-Adrenergic receptor	ADRβ3	8p12-p11.2	Obesity, greater susceptibility to weight gain and diabetes phenotypes	[86]
			Increased BMI, fat mass and waist circumference	[88]
			No association with BMI	[87]
Adenosine deaminase	ADA	20q13.12	Obesity in subjects with non-insulin-dependent diabetes	[58]
Uncoupling protein 2	UCP2	11q13	Metabolic rate during sleep	[91]
			BMI, fasting serum leptin	[92]
Uncoupling protein 3	UCP3	11q13	Obesity, reduced capacity to oxidize fat, elevated respiratory quotient	[95]
Glucocorticoid receptor	GRL	5q31	Hyperinsulinemia	[100]
			Increased abdominal fat	[99]
			Increased insulin response to dexamethasone, increased BMI	[101]
Fatty acid-binding protein 2	FABP2	4q28-q31	Insulin resistance, increased fat oxidation	[103]
			Obesity, elevated triglycerides	[104]
			Insulin resistance, greater intra-abdominal fat	[105]
Apolipoprotein D	APOD	3q26.2-qter	NIDDM	[107]
			Obesity, elevated fasting insulin	[106]
Apolipoprotein B-100	APOB-100	2p24	Visceral obesity, dense LDL	[108, 109]
Lipoprotein lipase	LPL	8p22	Obesity, hypertriglyceridemia	[110]

lipolysis and insulin sensitivity in human adipose tissue. Thus, variants in the ADA gene could theoretically explain the effects of this locus on both energy balance and insulin levels. A recent association study of ADA reported that one ADA variant was more commonly observed in subjects with NIDDM who were obese [58].

Uncoupling proteins 2 and 3 (UCP2/UCP3) are structurally related to UCP1, a mitochondrial protein found in brown fat that plays an important role in generating heat and burning calories without the production of adenosine triphosphate. UCP1 is critical in the maintenance of body temperature of newborn humans, but is unlikely to be significantly involved in weight regulation because brown fat is normally atrophied in adult humans. UCP2 and UCP3 are recently identified genes [89, 90] located very near each other on chromosome 11 that, like UCP1, encode mitochondrial transmembrane carrier proteins. UCP2 is widely expressed in human tissues, whereas UCP3 is expressed only in skeletal muscle. In a large French Canadian study, UCP2 and UCP3 were linked with resting metabolic rate, BMI, percentage of body fat, and fat mass [70]. Several groups have, therefore, examined polymorphisms within the coding

regions of both UCP2 and UCP3. Polymorphisms in UCP2 were associated with metabolic rate during sleep in older, but not younger, Pima Indians [91]. A stronger association between a UCP2 exon variant and body mass index was found in South Indian subjects [92]. The same variant was not associated with obesity in a British population, but was correlated with fasting serum leptin concentrations in the presence of extreme obesity [92]. Two other studies failed to find a relationship between UCP2 variants and energy expenditure, obesity, or insulin resistance [93, 94]. To determine whether UCP3 mutations could contribute to human obesity, the nucleotide sequence of coding exons was determined in obese and/or diabetic Africans, African-Americans, and Caucasians. A mutation and two missense polymorphisms in the UCP3 gene were identified in two severely obese probands of African descent [95]. The gene variants were not found in the Caucasian population. The variants were transmitted in a Mendelian fashion; however, they were not consistently associated with obesity in other family members. Individuals who carried one copy of the exon 6-splice polymorphism were found to have only 50% the capacity to oxidize fat and had elevated respiratory quotients

(RQs), even though they were not obese. These data indicate that *UCP3* could alter the availability in the cell of fatty acids for oxidation, promoting fat storage. High RQ and low fat oxidation were previously identified risk factors for future weight gain in Pima Indians [96] and African-Americans [97]. Thus, *UCP3* is a potentially important obesity gene in certain population groups.

Animal models of obesity demonstrate the importance of glucocorticoid receptor (*GRL*) activity in the etiology and maintenance of the obese state. In humans, glucocorticoid excess (i.e., Cushing syndrome) results in central fat distribution. The *GRL* gene was weakly linked with BMI in a study of French obese families [98]. Therefore, polymorphisms of *GRL* were examined for association with obesity. A variant of the BC1I polymorphism of *GRL* was associated with increased abdominal fat measured by computerized tomography in middle-aged Canadians [99] and hyperinsulinemia in British Caucasian women [100]. In an elderly population in the Netherlands, 6% carried a polymorphism resulting in altered sensitivity to glucocorticoids [101]. Although healthy, these subjects had higher BMI and higher insulin response to dexamethasone suppression [101].

Intestinal fatty acid-binding protein 2 (FABP2) is thought to facilitate the uptake, intracellular metabolism, and/or transport of long-chain fatty acids. Linkage between measures of insulin action and a region on chromosome 4q near the *FABP2* locus was found in Pima Indians of Arizona [102]. Therefore, an Ala54Thr polymorphism in *FABP2* was examined in Pima Indians and in an isolated population of native Canadians. The variant was associated with insulin resistance and increased fat oxidation rate in Pima Indians [103] and obesity and higher fasting plasma triglyceride levels in the Canadians [104]. The variant was also associated with insulin resistance and greater intra-abdominal fat in Japanese men [105].

Lipoprotein function has been associated with several obesity phenotypes. Apolipoprotein D is a protein component of high-density lipoprotein (HDL). Variants of *APOD* were associated with obesity, elevated fasting insulin [106], and NIDDM [107]. Apolipoprotein B is the main apolipoprotein of chylomicrons and low-density lipoproteins (LDLs) and occurs in two main forms, apoB–48 and apoB–100. A polymorphism of the *APOB-100* gene was associated with abdominal fat and LDL particle size in obese hyperinsulinemic men [108, 109]. Lipoprotein lipase (LPL) deficiency reduces clearance of chylomicrons and other triglyceride-rich lipoproteins. *LPL* polymorphisms are associated with BMI and hypertriglyceridemia [110].

X. CLINICAL IMPLICATIONS OF THE DISCOVERY OF OBESITY GENES

The recent discoveries of human obesity genes have broad implications for clinical practice. Most human obesity genes have only been identified in the last few years. For most of the obesity gene mutations there is no information on the physiological impacts of these mutations, except for obesity. Thus, methods for their diagnosis and the implications of their discovery for treatment have not been discussed in depth. The discovery of human obesity genes will influence several areas of clinical practice including diagnosis and therapy.

A. Diagnosis of Obesity Disorders 2000

Until recently, only the rare Mendelian (single-gene) mutations, such as Prader-Willi and Bardet-Biedl syndromes, caused known heritable obesity (Section VII) [46]. These disorders are easily recognized, both by a wide spectrum of phenotypes and by the use of cytogenetics assays that are widely available. However, the new molecular Mendelian obesity disorders (Section V) are not so easily diagnosed, because obesity is often the only apparent phenotype and molecular assays for known obesity gene mutations are currently not practical. It has been estimated that 2–7% of morbidly obese patients have mutations in *MC4R* [40–43], 3% have mutations in *PPARγ* [80, 111], and an unknown, but smaller, percent have mutations in other obesity genes, including *POMC* [77]. Thus, only about 1 in 10 morbidly obese patients has a known mutation that explains the obesity, and molecular assays for the currently known Mendelian obesities would be negative in the majority of morbidly obese patients. Also, there are several known distinct mutations in each of these genes. Thus, no clinical laboratories yet provide diagnosis of these mutations, rather they have only been diagnosed by research laboratories, which are not licensed to provide patient information. However, inability to make specific molecular diagnosis does not mean that one cannot identify people with increased risk for genetic obesity, and this may influence choices or approaches to treatment.

Several criteria can be used to estimate individual risks for genetic obesity. At the present time, due to the lack of data, these estimates do not produce any quantitative values revealing individual risk that obesity is genetic.

1. The earlier the age of onset and the more extreme the obesity, the more likely that there is a genetic basis for the obesity. Extreme trait values are more likely to be genetic for many complex diseases, simply because extremes tend to result from the actions of severe mutations or from mutations in genes that have larger effects [112]. Children with single-gene obesity are normal weight at birth but severe early hyperphagia, often associated with aggressive food-seeking behavior, results in rapid weight gain, usually beginning in the first year of life.

2. Prader-Willi, Bardet-Biedl, and other Mendelian syndromes can be diagnosed by a variety of characteristic

phenotypes as well as by cytogenetic assays. Thus, one should rule out these diagnoses by phenotype determination and by absence of characteristic chromosomal abnormalities.

3. A strong family history of obesity is consistent with the presence of an obesity gene shared among family members.

4. *POMC* defects can cause red hair and obesity [37], although most red hair results from mutations in melanocortin receptor-1 (*MC1R*) [113], which does not influence obesity. Thus, red hair is only informative when red hair and obesity cosegregate within a family.

5. At present, few diagnostic tools are available for the medical evaluation of patients suspected of having Mendelian obesity. The only screening tests available are for endocrine abnormalities. Leptin should be measured. Very low or very high serum leptin levels will indicate mutation in *LEP* or *LEPR,* respectively. A subset of obese individuals has inappropriately low leptin levels for their fat mass, suggesting a less severe defect in leptin regulation [72]. ACTH and proinsulin should be measured to indicate defects in *POMC* or in prohormone processing.

B. Implications of Obesity Genes for Obesity Treatment

The recent discovery of human obesity genes may have broad future implications for diet, behavioral, and drug therapy of genetically obese humans, and perhaps of all obese people. The identification and characterization of gene products associated with obesity have provided novel pathways that can be targeted for pharmaceutical intervention. A significant new drug is the hormone leptin, which, as of this writing, is still in clinical trials. However, an early study suggests that exogenous leptin induces weight loss even in some obese subjects with elevated endogenous serum leptin levels [25]. Leptin therapy may, therefore, be effective even for obese individuals without defects in leptin production. Another potential drug target identified by the cloning of obesity genes is the melanocortin receptor. Development of safe and effective drugs such as an α-MSH-like agonist for the melanocortin receptor to inhibit food intake or stimulators of the expression of *UCP2* or *UCP3* to enhance energy expenditure are certainly goals of the pharmaceutical industry [14].

Patients with monogenic obesity will probably be more difficult to treat than those with polygenic obesity, because individuals with monogenic obesity will likely have strong food-seeking behavior and may have physiological resistance to fat loss. Certainly, the primary therapy for individuals with documented leptin deficiency is recombinant leptin. Specific pharmaceutical treatment of other single-gene obesities will have to await development of drugs targeted further along the pathway of the mutated gene. Meanwhile, lifestyle

changes that may promote weight loss and improve metabolic fitness and quality of life should be recommended. Drugs should also be considered, but whether currently available drug therapies, such as appetite suppressants (phentermine or sibutramine) or inhibitors of fat absorption (orlistat), are more or less effective in individuals with single-gene obesity than those with polygenic obesity is unknown. However, as with any severe obesity, when lifestyle changes and pharmaceutical approaches are inadequate to ameliorate morbidity, surgical treatment of the obesity may be necessary (see Chapter 31).

References

1. Bouchard, C., Pérusse, L., Rice, T., and Rao, D. C. (1998). The genetics of human obesity. *In* "Handbook of Obesity" (G. A. Bray, C. Bouchard, and W. P. T. James, Eds.), pp. 157–190. Marcel Dekker, Inc, New York.

2. Ravussin, E., and Danforth, E., Jr. (1999). Beyond sloth—physical activity and weight gain. *Science* **283,** 184–185.

3. Sims, E. A., Goldman, R. F., Gluck, C. M., Horton, E. S., Kelleher, P. C., and Rowe, D. W. (1968). Experimental obesity in man. *Trans. Assoc. Am. Physicians* **81,** 153–170.

4. Sims, E. A., Danforth, E., Jr., Horton, E. S., Bray, G. A., Glennon, J. A., and Salans, L. B. (1973). Endocrine and metabolic effects of experimental obesity in man. *Recent Prog. Horm. Res.* **29,** 457–496.

5. Bouchard, C., Tremblay, A., Després, J. P., Nadeau, A., Lupien, P. J., Thériault, G., Dussault, J., Moorjani, S., Pinault, S., and Fournier, G. (1990). The response to long-term overfeeding in identical twins. *N. Engl. J. Med.* **322,** 1477–1482.

6. Bouchard, C., Tremblay, A., Després, J. P., Thériault, G., Nadeau, A., Lupien, P. J., Moorjani, S., Prudhomme, D., and Fournier, G. (1994). The response to exercise with constant energy intake in identical twins. *Obes. Res.* **2,** 400–410.

7. Ravussin, E., Lillioja, S., Anderson, T. E., Christin, L., and Bogardus, C. (1986). Determinants of 24-hour energy expenditure in man. Methods and results using a respiratory chamber. *J. Clin. Invest.* **78,** 1568–1578.

8. Levine, J. A., Eberhardt, N. L., and Jensen, M. D. (1999). Role of nonexercise activity thermogenesis in resistance to fat gain in humans. *Science* **283,** 212–214.

9. Zurlo, F., Ferraro, R. T., Fontvielle, A. M., Rising, R., Bogardus, C., and Ravussin, E. (1992). Spontaneous physical activity and obesity: Cross-sectional and longitudinal studies in Pima Indians. *Am. J. Physiol.* **263,** E296–300.

10. Silver, L. M. (1995). "Mouse Genetics." Oxford University Press, New York.

11. Chagnon, Y. C., Pérusse, L., Weisnagel, S. J., Rankinen, T., and Bouchard, C. (2000). The Human Obesity Gene Map: The 1999 update. *Obes. Res.* **8,** 89–117.

12. Kapeller, R., Moriarty, A., Strauss, A., Stubdal, H., Theriault, K., Siebert, E., Chickering, T., Morgenstern, J. P., Tartaglia, L. A., and Lillie, J. (1999). Tyrosine phosphorylation of tub and its association with Src homology 2 domain-containing proteins implicate tub in intracellular signaling by insulin. *J. Biolog. Chem.* **274,** 24980–24986.

13. Boggon, T. J., Shan, W. S., Santagata, S., Myers, S. C., and Shapiro, L. (1999). Implication of tubby proteins as

transcription factors by structure-based functional analysis. *Science* **286**, 2119–2125.

14. Campfield, L. A., Smith, F. J., and Burn, P. (1998). Strategies and potential molecular targets for obesity treatment. *Science* **280**, 1383–1387.

15. Zhang, Y., Proenca, R., Maffei, M., Barone, M., Leopold, L., and Friedman, J. M. (1994). Positional cloning of the mouse obese gene and its human homologue. *Nature* **372**, 425–432 [erratum **374**, 479].

16. Masuzaki, H., Ogawa, Y., Sagawa, N., Hosoda, K., Matsumoto, T., Mise, H., Nishimura, H., Yoshimasa, Y., Tanaka, I., Mori, T., and Nakao, K. (1997). Nonadipose tissue production of leptin: Leptin as a novel placenta-derived hormone in humans. *Nature Med.* **3**, 1029–1033.

17. Bado, A., Levasseur, S., Attoub, S., Kermorgant, S., Laigneau, J. P., Bortoluzzi, M. N., Moizo, L., Lehy, T., Guerre-Millo, M., Le Marchand-Brustel, Y., and Lewin, M. J. (1998). The stomach is a source of leptin. *Nature (Lond.)* **394**, 790–793.

18. Halaas, J. L., Gajiwala, K. S., Maffei, M., Cohen, S. L., Chait, B. T., Rabinowitz, D., Lallone, R. L., Burley, S. K., and Friedman, J. M. (1995). Weight-reducing effects of the plasma protein encoded by the obese gene. *Science* **269**, 543–546.

19. Golden, P. L., Maccagnan, T. J., and Pardridge, W. M. (1997). Human blood-brain barrier leptin receptor. Binding and endocytosis in isolated human brain microvessels. *J. Clin. Invest.* **99**, 14–18.

20. Saad, M. F., Damani, S., Gingerich, R. L., Riad-Gabriel, M. G., Khan, A., Boyadjian, R., Jinagouda, S. D., el-Tawil, K., Rude, R. K., and Kamdar, V. (1997). Sexual dimorphism in plasma leptin concentration. *J. Clin. Endocrinol. Metab.* **82**, 579–584.

21. Maffei, M., Halaas, J., Ravussin, E., Pratley, R. E., Lee, G. H., Zhang, Y., Fei, H., Kim, S., Lallone, R., Ranganathan, S., Kern, P. A., and Friedman, J. M. (1995). Leptin levels in human and rodent: measurement of plasma leptin and ob RNA in obese and weight-reduced subjects. *Nature Med.* **1**, 1155–1161.

22. Campfield, L. A., Smith, F. J., Guisez, Y., Devos, R., and Burn, P. (1995). Recombinant mouse OB protein: Evidence for a peripheral signal linking adiposity and central neural networks. *Science* **269**, 546–549.

23. Pelleymounter, M. A., Cullen, M. J., Baker, M. B., Hecht, R., Winters, D., Boone, T., and Collins, F. (1995). Effects of the obese gene product on body weight regulation in ob/ob mice. *Science* **269**, 540–543.

24. Halaas, J. L., Boozer, C., Blair-West, J., Fidahusein, N., Denton, D. A., and Friedman, J. M. (1997). Physiological response to long-term peripheral and central leptin infusion in lean and obese mice. *Proc. Natl. Acad. Sci. USA* **94**, 8878–8883.

25. Heymsfield, S. B., Greenberg, A. S., Fujioka, K., Dixon, R. M., Kushner, R., Hunt, T., Lubina, J. A., Patane, J., Self, B., Hunt, P., and McCamish, M. (1999). Recombinant leptin for weight loss in obese and lean adults: A randomized, controlled, dose-escalation trial. *JAMA* **282**, 1568–1575.

26. Matkovic, V., Ilich, J. Z., Skugor, M., Badenhop, N. E., Goel, P., Clairmont, A., Klisovic, D., Nahhas, R. W., and Landoll, J. D. (1997). Leptin is inversely related to age at menarche in human females. *J. Clin. Endocrinol. Metab.* **82**, 3239–3245.

27. Lord, G. M., Matarese, G., Howard, J. K., Baker, R. J., Bloom, S. R., and Lechler, R. I. (1998). Leptin modulates the T-cell immune response and reverses starvation- induced immunosuppression. *Nature (Lond.)* **394**, 897–901.

28. Friedman, J. M., and Halaas, J. L. (1998). Leptin and the regulation of body weight in mammals. *Nature (Lond.)* **395**, 763–770.

29. Montague, C. T., Farooqi, I. S., Whitehead, J. P., Soos, M. A., Rau, H., Wareham, N. J., Sewter, C. P., Digby, J. E., Mohammed, S. N., Hurst, J. A., Cheetham, C. H., Earley, A. R., Barnett, A. H., Prins, J. B., and O'Rahilly, S. (1997). Congenital leptin deficiency is associated with severe early-onset obesity in humans. *Nature (Lond.)* **387**, 903–908.

30. Strobel, A., Issad, T., Camoin, L., Ozata, M., and Strosberg, A. D. (1998). A leptin missense mutation associated with hypogonadism and morbid obesity. *Nature Genet.* **18**, 213–215.

31. Ozata, M., Ozdemir, I. C., and Licinio, J. (1999). Human leptin deficiency caused by a missense mutation: Multiple endocrine defects, decreased sympathetic tone, and immune system dysfunction indicate new targets for leptin action, greater central than peripheral resistance to the effects of leptin, and spontaneous correction of leptin-mediated defects. *J. Clin. Endocrinol. Metab.* **84**, 3686–3695.

32. Farooqi, I. S., Jebb, S. A., Langmack, G., Lawrence, E., Cheetham, C. H., Prentice, A. M., Hughes, I. A., McCamish, M. A., and O'Rahilly, S. (1999). Effects of recombinant leptin therapy in a child with congenital leptin deficiency. *N. Engl. J. Med.* **341**, 879–884.

33. Tartaglia, L. A., Dembski, M., Weng, X., Deng, N., Culpepper, J., Devos, R., Richards, G. J., Campfield, L. A., Clark, F. T., Deeds, J., Muir, C., Sanker, S., Moriarty, A., Moore, K. J., Smutko, J. S., Mays, G. G., Woolf, E. A., Monroe, C. A., and Tepper, R. I. (1995). Identification and expression cloning of a leptin receptor, OB-R. *Cell* **83**, 1263–1271.

34. Lee, G. H., Proenca, R., Montez, J. M., Carroll, K. M., Darvishzadeh, J. G., Lee, J. I., and Friedman, J. M. (1996). Abnormal splicing of the leptin receptor in diabetic mice. *Nature (Lond.)* **379**, 632–635.

35. Clement, K., Vaisse, C., Lahlou, N., Cabrol, S., Pelloux, V., Cassuto, D., Gourmelen, M., Dina, C., Chambaz, J., Lacorte, J. M., Basdevant, A., Bougneres, P., Lebouc, Y., Froguel, P., and Guy-Grand, B. (1998). A mutation in the human leptin receptor gene causes obesity and pituitary dysfunction. *Nature (Lond.)* **392**, 398–401.

36. Marsh, D. J., Hollopeter, G., Huszar, D., Laufer, R., Yagaloff, K. A., Fisher, S. L., Burn, P., and Palmiter, R. D. (1999). Response of melanocortin–4 receptor-deficient mice to anorectic and orexigenic peptides. *Nature Genet.* **21**, 119–122.

37. Krude, H., Biebermann, H., Luck, W., Horn, R., Brabant, G., and Gruters, A. (1998). Severe early-onset obesity, adrenal insufficiency and red hair pigmentation caused by POMC mutations in humans. *Nature Genet.* **19**, 155–157.

38. Jackson, R. S., Creemers, J. W., Ohagi, S., Raffin-Sanson, M. L., Sanders, L., Montague, C. T., Hutton, J. C., and O'Rahilly, S. (1997). Obesity and impaired prohormone processing associated with mutations in the human prohormone convertase 1 gene. *Nature Genet.* **16**, 303–306.

39. Huszar, D., Lynch, C. A., Fairchild-Huntress, V., Dunmore, J. H., Fang, Q., Berkemeier, L. R., Gu, W., Kesterson, R. A., Boston, B. A., Cone, R. D., Smith, F. J., Campfield, L. A., Burn, P., and Lee, F. (1997). Targeted disruption of the melanocortin-4 receptor results in obesity in mice. *Cell* **88**, 131–141.

40. Yeo, G. S., Farooqi, I. S., Aminian, S., Halsall, D. J., Stanhope, R. G., and O'Rahilly, S. (1998). A frameshift mutation

in MC4R associated with dominantly inherited human obesity. *Nature Genet.* **20**, 111–112.

41. Vaisse, C., Clement, K., Guy-Grand, B., and Froguel, P. (1998). A frameshift mutation in human MC4R is associated with a dominant form of obesity. *Nature Genet.* **20**, 113–114.

42. Hinney, A., Schmidt, A., Nottebom, K., Heibult, O., Becker, I., Ziegler, A., Gerber, G., Sina, M., Gorg, T., Mayer, H., Siegfried, W., Fichter, M., Remschmidt, H., and Hebebrand, J. (1999). Several mutations in the melanocortin–4 receptor gene including a nonsense and a frameshift mutation associated with dominantly inherited obesity in humans. *J. Clin. Endocrinol. Metab.* **84**, 1483–1486.

43. Sina, M., Hinney, A., Ziegler, A., Neupert, T., Mayer, H., Siegfried, W., Blum, W. F., Remschmidt, H., and Hebebrand, J. (1999). Phenotypes in three pedigrees with autosomal dominant obesity caused by haploinsufficiency mutations in the melanocortin–4 receptor gene. *Am. J. Hum. Genet.* **65**, 1501–1507.

44. Cao, H., and Hegele, R. A. (2000). Nuclear lamin A/C R482Q mutation in Canadian kindreds with Dunnigan-type familial partial lipodystrophy. *Hum. Mol. Genet.* **9**, 109–112.

45. Shackleton, S., Lloyd, D. J., Jackson, S. N., Evans, R., Niermeijer, M. F., Singh, B. M., Schmidt, H., Brabant, G., Kumar, S., Durrington, P. N., Gregory, S., O'Rahilly, S., and Trembath, R. C. (2000). LMNA, encoding lamin A/C, is mutated in partial lipodystrophy. *Nature Genet.* **24**, 153–156.

46. McKusick, V. A. (2000). Online Mendelian Inheritance in Man, OMIM. McKusick–Nathans Institute for Genetic Medicine, John Hopkins University, Baltimore, MD, and National Center for Biotechnology Information, National Library of Medicine, Bethesda, MD. http://www.ncbi.nlm.nih.gov/omim/.

47. Bray, G. A. (1998). Classification and evaluation of the overweight patient. *In* "Handbook of Obesity" (G. A. Bray, C. Bouchard, and W. P. T. James, Eds.), pp. 831–854. Marcel Dekker, Inc., New York.

48. Couper, R. (1999). Prader-Willi syndrome. *J. Paediatr. Child Health* **35**, 331–334.

49. Khan, N. L., and Wood, N. W. (1999). Prader-Willi and Angelman syndromes: Update on genetic mechanisms and diagnostic complexities. *Curr. Opin. Neurol.* **12**, 149–154.

50. Croft, J. B., Morrell, D., Chase, C. L., and Swift, M. (1995). Obesity in heterozygous carriers of the gene for the Bardet-Biedl syndrome. *Am. J. Med. Genet.* **55**, 12–15.

51. Marshall, J. D., Ludman, M. D., Shea, S. E., Salisbury, S. R., Willi, S. M., LaRoche, R. G., and Nishina, P. M. (1997). Genealogy, natural history, and phenotype of Alstrom syndrome in a large Acadian kindred and three additional families. *Am. J. Med. Genet.* **73**, 150–161.

52. Russell-Eggitt, I. M., Clayton, P. T., Coffey, R., Kriss, A., Taylor, D. S., and Taylor, J. F. (1998). Alstrom syndrome. Report of 22 cases and literature review. *Ophthalmology* **105**, 1274–1280.

53. Collin, G. B., Marshall, J. D., Boerkoel, C. F., Levin, A. V., Weksberg, R., Greenberg, J., Michaud, J. L., Naggert, J. K., and Nishina, P. M. (1999). Alstrom syndrome: Further evidence for linkage to human chromosome 2p13. *Hum. Genet.* **105**, 474–479.

54. Warden, C. H., and Fisler, J. S. (1998). Molecular genetics of obesity. *In* "Handbook of Obesity" (G. A. Bray, C. Bouchard, and W. P. T. James, Eds.), pp. 223–242. Marcel Dekker, Inc., New York.

55. DeBry, R. W., and Seldin, M. F. (1996). Human/mouse homology relationships. *Genomics* **33**, 337–351.

56. Lembertas, A. V., Pérusse, L., Chagnon, Y. C., Fisler, J. S., Warden, C. H., Purcell-Huynh, D. A., Dionne, F. T., Gagnon, J., Nadeau, A., Lusis, A. J., and Bouchard, C. (1997). Identification of an obesity quantitative trait locus on mouse chromosome 2 and evidence of linkage to body fat and insulin on the human homologous region 20q. *J. Clin. Invest.* **100**, 1240–1247.

57. Lee, J. H., Reed, D. R., Li, W. D., Xu, W., Joo, E. J., Kilker, R. L., Nanthakumar, E., North, M., Sakul, H., Bell, C., and Price, R. A. (1999). Genome scan for human obesity and linkage to markers in 20q13. *Am. J. Hum. Genet.* **64**, 196–209.

58. Bottini, E., and Gloria-Bottini, F. (1999). Adenosine deaminase and body mass index in non-insulin-dependent diabetes mellitus. *Metabolism* **48**, 949–951.

59. Haseman, J. K., and Elston, R. C. (1972). The investigation of linkage between a quantitative trait and a marker locus. *Behav. Genet.* **2**, 3–19.

60. Kruglyak, L., and Lander, E. S. (1995). High-resolution genetic mapping of complex traits. *Am. J. Hum. Genet.* **56**, 1212–1223 [Erratum **58**(4), 920].

61. Clement, K., Garner, C., Hager, J., Philippi, A., LeDuc, C., Carey, A., Harris, T. J., Jury, C., Cardon, L. R., Basdevant, A., Demenais, F., Guy-Grand, B., North, M., and Froguel, P. (1996). Indication for linkage of the human OB gene region with extreme obesity. *Diabetes* **45**, 687–690.

62. Duggirala, R., Stern, M. P., Mitchell, B. D., Reinhart, L. J., Shipman, P. A., Uresandi, O. C., Chung, W. K., Leibel, R. L., Hales, C. N., O'Connell, P., and Blangero, J. (1996). Quantitative variation in obesity-related traits and insulin precursors linked to the OB gene region on human chromosome 7. *Am. J. Hum. Genet.* **59**, 694–703.

63. Reed, D. R., Ding, Y., Xu, W., Cather, C., Green, E. D., and Price, R. A. (1996). Extreme obesity may be linked to markers flanking the human OB gene. *Diabetes* **45**, 691–694.

64. Lapsys, N. M., Furler, S. M., Moore, K. R., Nguyen, T. V., Herzog, H., Howard, G., Samaras, K., Carey, D. G., Morrison, N. A., Eisman, J. A., and Chisholm, D. J. (1997). Relationship of a novel polymorphic marker near the human obese (OB) gene to fat mass in healthy women. *Obes. Res.* **5**, 430–433.

65. Roth, H., Hinney, A., Ziegler, A., Barth, N., Gerber, G., Stein, K., Bromel, T., Mayer, H., Siegfried, W., Schafer, H., Remschmidt, H., Grzeschik, K. H., and Hebebrand, J. (1997). Further support for linkage of extreme obesity to the obese gene in a study group of obese children and adolescents. *Exp. Clin. Endocrinol. Diabetes* **105**, 341–344.

66. Chagnon, Y. C., Chung, W. K., Pérusse, L., Chagnon, M., Leibel, R. L., and Bouchard, C. (1999). Linkages and associations between the leptin receptor (LEPR) gene and human body composition in the Quebec Family Study. *Int. J. Obes. Relat. Metab. Disord.* **23**, 278–286.

67. Chagnon, Y. C., Chen, W. J., Pérusse, L., Chagnon, M., Nadeau, A., Wilkison, W. O., and Bouchard, C. (1997). Linkage and association studies between the melanocortin receptors 4 and 5 genes and obesity-related phenotypes in the Quebec Family Study. *Mol. Med.* **3**, 663–673.

68. Oppert, J. M., Tourville, J., Chagnon, M., Mauriege, P., Dionne, F. T., Pérusse, L., and Bouchard, C. (1995). DNA polymorphisms in the alpha 2- and beta 2-adrenoceptor genes

and regional fat distribution in humans: Association and linkage studies. *Obes. Res.* **3**, 249–255.

69. Mitchell, B. D., Cole, S. A., Comuzzie, A. G., Almasy, L., Blangero, J., MacCluer, J. W., and Hixson, J. E. (1999). A quantitative trait locus influencing BMI maps to the region of the beta–3 adrenergic receptor. *Diabetes* **48**, 1863–1867.

70. Bouchard, C., Pérusse, L., Chagnon, Y. C., Warden, C., and Ricquier, D. (1997). Linkage between markers in the vicinity of the uncoupling protein 2 gene and resting metabolic rate in humans. *Hum. Mol. Genet.* **6**, 1887–1889.

71. Butler, M. G., Hedges, L., Hovis, C. L., and Feurer, I. D. (1998). Genetic variants of the human obesity (OB) gene in subjects with and without Prader-Willi syndrome: Comparison with body mass index and weight. *Clin. Genet.* **54**, 385–393.

72. Hager, J., Clement, K., Francke, S., Dina, C., Raison, J., Lahlou, N., Rich, N., Pelloux, V., Basdevant, A., Guy-Grand, B., North, M., and Froguel, P. (1998). A polymorphism in the 5' untranslated region of the human ob gene is associated with low leptin levels. *Int. J. Obes. Relat. Metab. Disord.* **22**, 200–205.

73. Mammes, O., Betoulle, D., Aubert, R., Giraud, V., Tuzet, S., Petiet, A., Colas-Linhart, N., and Fumeron, F. (1998). Novel polymorphisms in the 5' region of the LEP gene: Association with leptin levels and response to low-calorie diet in human obesity. *Diabetes* **47**, 487–489.

74. Thompson, D. B., Ravussin, E., Bennett, P. H., and Bogardus, C. (1997). Structure and sequence variation at the human leptin receptor gene in lean and obese Pima Indians. *Hum. Mol. Genet.* **6**, 675–679.

75. Roth, H., Korn, T., Rosenkranz, K., Hinney, A., Ziegler, A., Kunz, J., Siegfried, W., Mayer, H., Hebebrand, J., and Grzeschik, K. H. (1998). Transmission disequilibrium and sequence variants at the leptin receptor gene in extremely obese German children and adolescents. *Hum. Genet.* **103**, 540–546.

76. de Silva, A. M., Walder, K. R., Aitman, T. J., Gotoda, T., Goldstone, A. P., Hodge, A. M., de Courten, M. P., Zimmet, P. Z., and Collier, G. R. (1999). Combination of polymorphisms in OB-R and the OB gene associated with insulin resistance in Nauruan males. *Int. J. Obes. Relat. Metab. Disord.* **23**, 816–822.

77. Hixson, J. E., Almasy, L., Cole, S., Birnbaum, S., Mitchell, B. D., Mahaney, M. C., Stern, M. P., MacCluer, J. W., Blangero, J., and Comuzzie, A. G. (1999). Normal variation in leptin levels is associated with polymorphisms in the proopiomelanocortin gene, POMC. *J. Clin. Endocrinol. Metab.* **84**, 3187–3191.

78. Must, A., Spadano, J., Coakley, E. H., Field, A. E., Colditz, G., and Dietz, W. H. (1999). The disease burden associated with overweight and obesity. *JAMA* **282**, 1523–1529.

79. Clarke, S. D., Thuillier, P., Baillie, R. A., and Sha, X. (1999). Peroxisome proliferator-activated receptors: A family of lipid-activated transcription factors. *Am. J. Clin. Nutr.* **70**, 566–571.

80. Ristow, M., Muller-Wieland, D., Pfeiffer, A., Krone, W., and Kahn, C. R. (1998). Obesity associated with a mutation in a genetic regulator of adipocyte differentiation. *N. Engl. J. Med.* **339**, 953–959.

81. Deeb, S. S., Fajas, L., Nemoto, M., Pihlajamaki, J., Mykkanen, L., Kuusisto, J., Laakso, M., Fujimoto, W., and Auwerx, J. (1998). A Pro12Ala substitution in PPARgamma2 associ-

ated with decreased receptor activity, lower body mass index and improved insulin sensitivity. *Nature Genet.* **20**, 284–287.

82. Large, V., Hellstrom, L., Reynisdottir, S., Lonnqvist, F., Eriksson, P., Lannfelt, L., and Arner, P. (1997). Human beta-2 adrenoceptor gene polymorphisms are highly frequent in obesity and associate with altered adipocyte beta–2 adrenoceptor function. *J. Clin. Invest.* **100**, 3005—3013.

83. Ishiyama-Shigemoto, S., Yamada, K., Yuan, X., Ichikawa, F., and Nonaka, K. (1999). Association of polymorphisms in the beta2-adrenergic receptor gene with obesity, hypertriglyceridaemia, and diabetes mellitus. *Diabetologia* **42**, 98–101.

84. Mori, Y., Kim-Motoyama, H., Ito, Y., Katakura, T., Yasuda, K., Ishiyama-Shigemoto, S., Yamada, K., Akanuma, Y., Ohashi, Y., Kimura, S., Yazaki, Y., and Kadowaki, T. (1999). The Gln27Glu beta2-adrenergic receptor variant is associated with obesity due to subcutaneous fat accumulation in Japanese men. *Biochem. Biophys. Res. Commun.* **258**, 138–140.

85. Susulic, V. S., Frederich, R. C., Lawitts, J., Tozzo, E., Kahn, B. B., Harper, M. E., Himms-Hagen, J., Flier, J. S., and Lowell, B. B. (1995). Targeted disruption of the beta 3-adrenergic receptor gene. *J. Biolog. Chem.* **270**, 29483–29492.

86. Clement, K., Vaisse, C., Manning, B. S., Basdevant, A., Guy-Grand, B., Ruiz, J., Silver, K. D., Shuldiner, A. R., Froguel, P., and Strosberg, A. D. (1995). Genetic variation in the beta 3-adrenergic receptor and an increased capacity to gain weight in patients with morbid obesity. *N. Engl. J. Med.* **333**, 352–354.

87. Allison, D. B., Heo, M., Faith, M. S., and Pietrobelli, A. (1998). Meta-analysis of the association of the Trp64Arg polymorphism in the beta-3 adrenergic receptor with body mass index. *Int. J. Obes. Relat. Metab. Disord.* **22**, 559–566.

88. Mitchell, B. D., Blangero, J., Comuzzie, A. G., Almasy, L. A., Shuldiner, A. R., Silver, K., Stern, M. P., MacCluer, J. W., and Hixson, J. E. (1998). A paired sibling analysis of the beta-3 adrenergic receptor and obesity in Mexican Americans. *J. Clin. Invest.* **101**, 584–587.

89. Fleury, C., Neverova, M., Collins, S., Raimbault, S., Champigny, O., Levi-Meyrueis, C., Bouillaud, F., Seldin, M. F., Surwit, R. S., Ricquier, D., and Warden, C. H. (1997). Uncoupling protein-2: A novel gene linked to obesity and hyperinsulinemia. *Nature Genet.* **15**, 269-272.

90. Boss, O., Samec, S., Paoloni-Giacobino, A., Rossier, C., Dulloo, A., Seydoux, J., Muzzin, P., and Giacobino, J. P. (1997). Uncoupling protein-3: A new member of the mitochondrial carrier family with tissue-specific expression. *FEBS Lett.* **408**, 39–42.

91. Walder, K., Norman, R. A., Hanson, R. L., Schrauwen, P., Neverova, M., Jenkinson, C. P., Easlick, J., Warden, C. H., Pecqueur, C., Raimbault, S., Ricquier, D., Silver, M. H. K., Shuldiner, A. R., Solanes, G., Lowell, B. B., Chung, W. K., Leibel, R. L., Pratley, R., and Ravussin, E. (1998). Association between uncoupling protein polymorphisms (UCP2-UCP3) and energy metabolism/obesity in Pima Indians. *Hum. Mol. Genet.* **7**, 1431–1435.

92. Cassell, P. G., Neverova, M., Janmohamed, S., Uwakwe, N., Qureshi, A., McCarthy, M. I., Saker, P. J., Albon, L., Kopelman, P., Noonan, K., Easlick, J., Ramachandran, A., Snehalatha, C., Pecqueur, C., Ricquier, D., Warden, C., and Hitman, G. A. (1999). An uncoupling protein 2 gene variant is associated with a raised body mass index but not Type II diabetes. *Diabetologia* **42**, 688–692.

93. Urhammer, S. A., Dalgaard, L. T., Sorensen, T. I., Moller, A. M., Andersen, T., Tybjaerg-Hansen, A., Hansen, T., Clausen, J. O., Vestergaard, H., and Pedersen, O. (1997). Mutational analysis of the coding region of the uncoupling protein 2 gene in obese NIDDM patients: Impact of a common amino acid polymorphism on juvenile and maturity onset forms of obesity and insulin resistance. *Diabetologia* **40,** 1227–1230.

94. Klannemark, M., Orho, M., and Groop, L. (1998). No relationship between identified variants in the uncoupling protein 2 gene and energy expenditure. *Eur. J. Endocrinol.* **139,** 217–223.

95. Argyropoulos, G., Brown, A. M., Willi, S. M., Zhu, J., He, Y., Reitman, M., Gevao, S. M., Spruill, I., and Garvey, W. T. (1998). Effects of mutations in the human uncoupling protein 3 gene on the respiratory quotient and fat oxidation in severe obesity and type 2 diabetes. *J. Clin. Invest.* **102,** 1345–1351.

96. Ravussin, E. (1995). Metabolic differences and the development of obesity. *Metabolism* **44,** 12–14.

97. Jakicic, J. M., and Wing, R. R. (1998). Differences in resting energy expenditure in African-American vs Caucasian overweight females. *Int. J. Obes. Relat. Metab. Disord.* **22,** 236–242.

98. Clement, K., Philippi, A., Jury, C., Pividal, R., Hager, J., Demenais, F., Basdevant, A., Guy-Grand, B., and Froguel, P. (1996). Candidate gene approach of familial morbid obesity: Linkage analysis of the glucocorticoid receptor gene. *Int. J. Obes. Relat. Metab. Disord.* **20,** 507–512.

99. Buemann, B., Vohl, M. C., Chagnon, M., Chagnon, Y. C., Gagnon, J., Pérusse, L., Dionne, F., Després, J. P., Tremblay, A., Nadeau, A., and Bouchard, C. (1997). Abdominal visceral fat is associated with a BclI restriction fragment length polymorphism at the glucocorticoid receptor gene locus. *Obes. Res.* **5,** 186–192.

100. Weaver, J. U., Hitman, G. A., and Kopelman, P. G. (1992). An association between a BclI restriction fragment length polymorphism of the glucocorticoid receptor locus and hyperinsulinaemia in obese women. *J. Mol. Endocrinol.* **9,** 295–300.

101. Huizenga, N. A., Koper, J. W., De Lange, P., Pols, H. A., Stolk, R. P., Burger, H., Grobbee, D. E., Brinkmann, A. O., De Jong, F. H., and Lamberts, S. W. (1998). A polymorphism in the glucocorticoid receptor gene may be associated with and increased sensitivity to glucocorticoids in vivo. *J. Clin. Endocrinol. Metab.* **83,** 144–151.

102. Prochazka, M., Lillioja, S., Tait, J. F., Knowler, W. C., Mott, D. M., Spraul, M., Bennett, P. H., and Bogardus, C. (1993). Linkage of chromosomal markers on 4q with a putative gene determining maximal insulin action in Pima Indians. *Diabetes* **42,** 514–519.

103. Baier, L. J., Sacchettini, J. C., Knowler, W. C., Eads, J., Paolisso, G., Tataranni, P. A., Mochizuki, H., Bennett, P. H., Bogardus, C., and Prochazka, M. (1995). An amino acid substitution in the human intestinal fatty acid binding protein is associated with increased fatty acid binding, increased fat oxidation, and insulin resistance. *J. Clin. Invest.* **95,** 1281–1287.

104. Hegele, R. A., Harris, S. B., Hanley, A. J., Sadikian, S., Connelly, P. W., and Zinman, B. (1996). Genetic variation of intestinal fatty acid-binding protein associated with variation in body mass in aboriginal Canadians. *J. Clin. Endocrinol. Metab.* **81,** 4334–4337.

105. Yamada, K., Yuan, X., Ishiyama, S., Koyama, K., Ichikawa, F., Koyanagi, A., Koyama, W., and Nonaka, K. (1997). Association between Ala54Thr substitution of the fatty acid-binding protein 2 gene with insulin resistance and intra-abdominal fat thickness in Japanese men. *Diabetologia* **40,** 706–710.

106. Vijayaraghavan, S., Hitman, G. A., and Kopelman, P. G. (1994). Apolipoprotein-D polymorphism: A genetic marker for obesity and hyperinsulinemia. *J. Clin. Endocrinol. Metab.* **79,** 568–570.

107. Baker, W. A., Hitman, G. A., Hawrami, K., McCarthy, M. I., Riikonen, A., Tuomilehto-Wolf, E., Nissinen, A., Tuomilehto, J., Mohan, V., Viswanathan, M., Snehalatha, C., Ramachandran, A., Dowse, G. K., Zimmet, P., and Serjeantson, S. (1994). Apolipoprotein D gene polymorphism: A new genetic marker for type 2 diabetic subjects in Nauru and south India. *Diabet. Med.* **11,** 947–952.

108. Pouliot, M. C., Després, J. P., Dionne, F. T., Vohl, M. C., Moorjani, S., Prud'homme, D., Bouchard, C., and Lupien, P. J. (1994). ApoB-100 gene EcoRI polymorphism. Relations to plasma lipoprotein changes associated with abdominal visceral obesity. *Arterioscler. Thromb.* **14,** 527–533.

109. Vohl, M. C., Tchernof, A., Dionne, F. T., Moorjani, S., Prud'homme, D., Bouchard, C., Nadeau, A., Lupien, P. J., and Després, J. P. (1996). The apoB-100 gene EcoRI polymorphism influences the relationship between features of the insulin resistance syndrome and the hyper-apoB and dense LDL phenotype in men. *Diabetes* **45,** 1405–1411.

110. Jemaa, R., Fumeron, F., Poirier, O., Lecerf, L., Evans, A., Arveiler, D., Luc, G., Cambou, J. P., Bard, J. M., Fruchart, J. C., Apfelbaum, M., Cambien, F., and Tiret, L. (1995). Lipoprotein lipase gene polymorphisms: Associations with myocardial infarction and lipoprotein levels, the ECTIM study (Etude Cas Temoin sur l'Infarctus du Myocarde). *J. Lipid. Res.* **36,** 2141–2146.

111. Valve, R., Sivenius, K., Miettinen, R., Pihlajamaki, J., Rissanen, A., Deeb, S. S., Auwerx, J., Uusitupa, M., and Laakso, M. (1999). Two polymorphisms in the peroxisome proliferator-activated receptor-gamma gene are associated with severe overweight among obese women. *J. Clin. Endocrinol. Metab.* **84,** 3708–3712.

112. Lander, E. S., and Schork, N. J. (1994). Genetic dissection of complex traits *Science* **265,** 2037–2048 [erratum **266,** 353].

113. Palmer, J. S., Duffy, D. L., Box, N. F., Aitken, J. F., O'Gorman, L. E., Green, A. C., Hayward, N. K., Martin, N. G., and Sturm, R. A. (2000). Melanocortin-1 receptor polymorphisms and risk of melanoma: Is the association explained solely by pigmentation phenotype? *Am. J. Hum. Genet.* **66,** 176–186.

CHAPTER 13

Genetic Influence on Cancer Risk

JO L. FREUDENHEIM

State University of New York at Buffalo, Buffalo, New York

I. INTRODUCTION

Cancer leads to the death of about 5.2 million people in the world each year with more than 8 million new cases of cancer each year. In the United States alone, there are about 1 million new cases annually [1]. Therapies to cure cancer are useful but prevention is clearly a superior strategy. For most kinds of cancer, only 50% or fewer of patients survive more than 5 years after diagnosis [2]. It is generally agreed that most common cancers are caused by environmental factors with the potential to be controlled [3]. It has been estimated that about 30% of cancer cases could be eliminated with dietary changes [4]; it appears that for most kinds of cancer dietary factors play a role in etiology.

It is important to note that a cancer may have more than one cause. For example, both occupational exposures and diet could contribute to the etiology of a cancer, and either a change in the occupational exposure or a change in diet might prevent that cancer. Genetic factors likely play a role in many if not all cancers. Even when an exposure is clearly required for a particular kind of cancer, genetic factors often play a role in determining who, among exposed individuals, develops that cancer. Also for dietary risk factors, evidence is now accumulating that genetic factors may interact with diet in the etiology of the disease.

II. BACKGROUND

Cancer is a genetic disease. That is, cancer is characterized by the accumulation of changes in the structure of the DNA of the cell such that there are significant changes in the functioning of the cell. Genes are the basic unit of heredity with each gene having its own location in a particular chromosome [5]. A mutation is a structural change in the DNA [5]. *Genotype* refers to the chemical composition of the DNA, it is the nucleic acid sequence of the DNA, inherited from both parents. From knowledge of the genotype, it is possible to infer information about an individual's characteristics. That is, the genetic code can be translated into information about the amino acid sequence of a protein. From that information, it would be possible to determine, for example, whether an individual had the gene for the faster or slower version of a particular enzyme. *Phenotype,* on the other hand, refers to the appearance of the individual, the expression of the genotype [5]. Agreement between genotype and phenotype often is not perfect. A person may have the genotype for a less active enzyme, but other exposures (e.g., dietary factors) may induce a high level of expression of that enzyme. A measurement of phenotype might be based on the rate of metabolism of a particular compound, and might not be able to distinguish high activity due to genotype from that related to enzyme induction.

Penetrance of a genetic factor refers to the likelihood that those with a particular gene will exhibit a particular phenotype under particular environmental circumstances [5]. A gene with high penetrance would be one where virtually everybody with the gene has the expressed trait while a gene with low penetrance would have low likelihood of expression of the gene. The measurement of phenotype is of interest because it gives an indication as to the true level of exposure, while the measurement of genotype is of interest because it gives some indication of exposure over the lifetime and is not biased by factors such as disease and recent exposures.

Some individuals are at greater risk for certain types of cancer. This increased risk can be related to differences in exposure to cancer-inducing or -protecting agents, and/or to the individual's genetic makeup, or to a combination of these factors. Genetic factors vary widely in the magnitude of their effects. Some inherited mutations greatly increase the risk of cancer; others cause smaller increases in risk. Some mutations may only increase risk in the presence of a particular exposure. An example of an inherited mutation that causes a substantial increase in risk is the *BRCA1* gene. Particular mutations in this gene have been shown to be related to risk of breast and ovarian cancer. Current estimates are that carriers of this genetic mutation have a 50% risk of breast cancer by age 50 and an 85% risk by age 70. However, relatively few individuals in the population carry this factor (estimates range between 1 in 2000 and 1 in 500). Therefore, athough those with the gene are at high risk, only about 1–5% of women with breast cancer have this mutation [6, 7]. There are also other genetic variants that are more common and

that have weaker effects on risk. These are referred to as *genetic polymorphisms.* Genetic polymorphism means that the gene has more than one form; generally these differences entail the alteration of a single nucleic acid in the sequence or the deletion of a section of the gene. Genetic polymorphisms can be quite common; they are found in up to 50% of the population. Generally these factors have a much smaller effect on cancer risk, increasing risk two to four times. However, because they are so common, they can have a significant impact on the rate of disease in a population. Also, in general, these factors affect the response to an exposure; that is, they affect risk only when that exposure is present, referred to as a gene–environment interaction. For these types of gene–environment interactions, an understanding of both the genetic factor and the environmental exposure is important in order to understand disease etiology and prevention. In terms of diet and genetics in relation to risk of cancer, at this time it appears that the second category of genetic effects is of primary importance. Risk of cancer is affected by an interaction of commonly occurring genetic variants and diet. These interactions can occur in any of several ways.

III. MECHANISMS OF DIET–GENETIC INTERACTIONS

A. Carcinogen Metabolism

The bulk of the research on the epidemiology of gene–environment interactions at this time has focused on genetic factors that modulate the metabolism of carcinogens. These carcinogens include compounds occurring naturally in foods or contaminating foods. If an individual has a genetic variant that results in slower metabolism of a carcinogen, then they will be more affected by a given dose of that carcinogen than would someone who could metabolize and excrete the carcinogen more rapidly. The enzymes related to carcinogen metabolism and excretion are generally divided into two groups: phase I and phase II. The phase I enzymes activate the compound; phase II enzymes then attach polar groups to the activated compound so that it will be more water soluble and can be excreted in the urine. Chief among the phase I enzymes are the cytochrome P-450 family (CYP). Important phase II enzymes are glutathione-*S*-transferase (GST) and *N*-acetyltransferase (NAT). In some cases, phase I activation leads to the production of compounds with greater carcinogenic potential. Often rather than carcinogens, foods contain procarcinogens, compounds that are carcinogenic after metabolic activation. The process of metabolic activation may vary depending on genetic factors. For example, heterocyclic amines are a group of compounds found in meat cooked at high temperatures, primarily in "well-done" meat [8]. Metabolism and excretion of heterocyclic amines involve CYP1A2 and NAT2. Preliminary epidemiologic evidence indicates that intake of well-done meat may be related to risk of colorectal adenomas, and that the effect depends in part on which of the genetic variants of CYP1A2 and NAT2 is carried by an individual [9]. Figure 1 illustrates the relationships between these enzyme systems [10, 11].

B. Enzyme Induction

Another mechanism of interaction for genetic factors and diet in relation to cancer risk is that factors in foods may also induce some of the genetic factors involved in carcinogen metabolism. That is, food components may affect the activity of the enzyme related to that gene so that there is more rapid metabolism by that enzyme. For example, CYP1A2 can be induced by indole–3-carbinol found in cruciferous vegetables, by heterocyclic amines in meat, and by polycyclic aromatic hydrocarbons found in grilled meat. CYP1A2 is also inhibited by a compound found in grapefruit, naringenin [9]. Therefore, metabolism of heterocyclic amines may depend not only on the genetic variant of CYP1A2 that is carried by an individual, but also on their intake of these other food components that affect CYP1A2 induction.

C. Genetic Variation in Vitamin Pathways

A third mechanism by which genes and diet may interact in relation to risk of cancer is that there can be genetic variation in vitamin pathways. There are commonly occurring genetic differences in vitamin receptors. If a vitamin plays a role in either carcinogenesis or in cancer prevention, differences in the receptor for the vitamin could also affect the susceptibility of an individual to cancer. An example of this type of relationship is found in research on prostate cancer. There is evidence that genetic variation in the vitamin D receptor can affect prostate cancer risk [12–14].

D. Oxidative Stress

A fourth example of a mechanism for gene and dietary interaction in relation to cancer risk is with regard to oxidation. There is evidence that reactive oxygen species from both exogenous and endogenous sources affect the rate of DNA mutations. Energy consumption is correlated with the number of oxidized DNA bases [3]. Antioxidant vitamins and other enzymes affected by genetic variation are part of the body's defense against these oxidative processes. Those who have genetically weaker defense systems against oxidation may benefit more from increased intake of antioxidant vitamins, such as vitamin C and vitamin E. For example, superoxide dismutase is important in the control of endogenously produced reactive oxygen species; manganese superoxide dismutase (MnSOD2) is found in the mitochondria, an important source of oxidative species. MnSOD2 is polymorphic and there is a study suggesting that one variant of this gene may be associated with increased risk of premenopausal breast

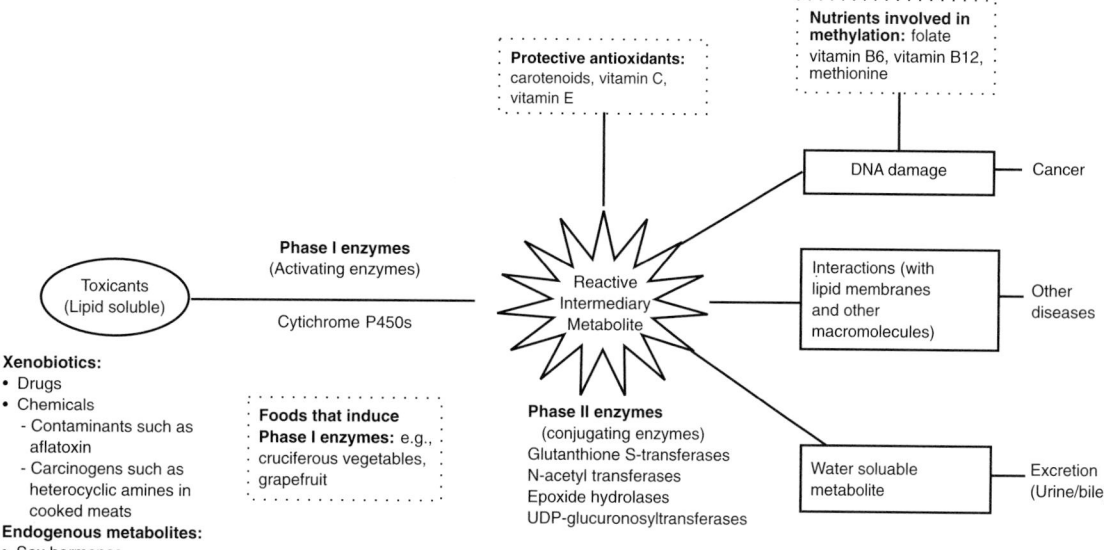

FIGURE 1   Interrelationship between the biotransformation enzyme systems. [From Patterson, R. E., Eaton, D. L., and Potter, J. D. The genetic revolution: Change and challenge for the dietetics profession. Copyright the American Dietetic Association. Reprinted by permission from *Journal of The American Dietetic Association,* vol. 99, pp. 1412–1420, 1999.]

cancer, but primarily among women with a low intake of antioxidant vitamins from fruits and vegetables [15].

Another example of a gene–environment interaction related to oxidation is evidence that relates intake of antioxidant vitamins to smoking-related DNA adducts. DNA adducts are the chemical bonding of molecules to DNA; such adducts may interfere with DNA replication and result in mutations or deletions in the DNA structure [3]. There is evidence of an inverse association between formation of these adducts and β-carotene intake among smokers. However, this association was limited to those individuals who carried homozygous deletions for the gene for glutathione *S*-transferase (*GSTM1null*) a detoxification enzyme [16]. The *GSTM1 null* genotype is found in about 50% of Caucasian populations.

E. One-Carbon Metabolism

One further mechanism for an interaction of diet and genetic factors in cancer etiology is an effect of diet on one-carbon methyl metabolism. Folate, vitamin B_{12}, vitamin B_6, and methionine are all involved in the metabolism of methyl groups. Alcohol consumption also adversely affects folate status and therefore methyl status. Methylation is important in the synthesis of purines and pyrimidines for DNA [17], and methylation of DNA can play a role in regulation of DNA transcription [18].

In animal studies, it has been shown that a diet deficient in these nutrients can lead to changes in the available nucleotides for DNA synthesis [19] and DNA strand breaks [20]. In humans, there is some evidence that hypomethylation of

DNA is a step in the carcinogenic process [18, 21, 22]. In particular, there is evidence that a diet low in one or more of these factors related to methyl metabolism may be associated with risk of colon cancer [23, 24]. Further, at least one of the enzymes in the methyl pathway, methylenetetrahydrofolate reductase (MTHFR), has been identified as polymorphic. This enzyme catalyzes the conversion of folate from the form that is most common intracellularly to the form most common in the plasma. One study showed significant differences in plasma homocysteine levels depending on the MTHFR genotype [25].

In another study, risk for colon cancer was higher for one MTHFR variant than for the other. The protective effect was less pronounced when dietary sources of methyl groups were lower, that is for higher intake of alcohol and lower intake of folate and methionine [26, 27]. It appears that these dietary factors and these genetic factors may have an interactive effect on risk of colon cancer.

The field of genetics is changing rapidly; numerous discoveries are leading to major shifts in our understanding of the role of genetic factors in cancer risk and of the interaction of environment with those genetic factors. At this time, the several pathways detailed above are the major ones identified for diet and gene interactions. However, in the next several years, other pathways of interaction may be identified and some of the ones detailed here may be determined to be of lesser importance to humans. Because much of our understanding of gene–environment interactions in relation to cancer is based on relatively new information, it is important to recognize that much of the data is subject to

reinterpretation and that an understanding of the methodologic issues involved is key.

IV. METHODOLOGIC ISSUES IN ASSESSMENT OF DIET AND GENE INTERACTIONS RELATED TO CANCER

An individual's genotype can be determined from DNA extracted from cells. The DNA is typically obtained from white blood cells, from sloughed cells in saliva, or from cells brushed from the inside of the mouth. For polymorphic genes, laboratory methods are used to identify which of the variants for a particular gene are carried by an individual based on the sequence of the DNA. Depending on the gene, one or more variants is possible. The variants may constitute the deletion of the whole gene, other mutations leading to a gene without function, or mutations leading to a change in the amino acid structure of the protein for which the gene is coding. Some variations may not affect function. For example, there may be two codes for the same amino acid, or there may be a genetic change in a part of the DNA that is not related to the function of the enzyme. Generally, epidemiologic studies should be limited to examination of polymorphisms that affect function.

An individual's phenotype may also be measured. Typically, to measure phenotype, an individual ingests a measured amount of a substance (e.g. , caffeine) and then blood or urine samples are collected for several hours or days to determine the rate of metabolism of that substance. Measurement of phenotype is advantageous in that it provides an indication of the sum of the processes involved and therefore an indication of the true level of exposure. Phenotype may depend on more than one gene; it may reflect processes involved in absorption and excretion as well as metabolism. However, when comparisons are being made of individuals with and without a disease, the phenotype may be affected by the disease state and might not be reflective of the diseased individual's lifetime exposure. In studies of this kind, a determination of phenotype may be less useful than determination of a genotype, unless it can be shown that the phenotype does not change for those with the disease.

In epidemiology, the interaction of genes and diet may be assessed in case-control studies, in nested case-control studies, or in clinical trials. In case-control studies, the cases are people with recently diagnosed disease who are compared to healthy controls from the same population. Statistical methods are used to determine whether there are systematic differences between those people who get the disease and those who do not. In a cohort study, a population of exposed and unexposed individuals is identified and their exposure status measured. Because cancer is relatively rare, these studies need to include thousands or even hundreds of thousands of individuals in order to examine diet in relation to cancer.

If blood has been collected from the study participants, it is possible to determine genotype for the participants. In a cohort study, the measurement of phenotype for metabolizing enzymes is rarely used because of the logistic difficulties. Generally, a nested case-control study is conducted for analysis of gene–environment interactions using genotype within a cohort. For this kind of study, those individuals in the cohort with incident cancer (cases) are compared to a group of controls selected from the cohort. The controls are chosen to be similar to the cases for relevant characteristics such as age, race, and gender. Genotypes are then determined, and the gene–environment interactions analyzed for this subset of the whole cohort.

For both case-control and nested case-control studies, the examination of gene–diet interactions generally involves a few steps. These include (1) the examination of the association between risk of a particular cancer and the genetic factor alone, (2) the examination of the association between risk of that cancer and the dietary factor alone, and then (3) the examination of the gene–diet interaction. The third step generally involves the analysis of the association between diet and cancer in strata defined by genotype or else the analysis of the association between gene and cancer in strata defined by level of dietary exposure. In some cases, there will be further examination of interaction with a third factor (e.g., exposure to hormone replacement therapy, body weight).

Although this is a relatively new area of research, in some clinical trials, the interaction of genes and environment are studied. The effect of a dietary intervention might be examined within groups defined by strata to determine if one group is more susceptible to the intervention.

For all of these study designs, there are some important methodological considerations. Many of these are the same considerations as for any epidemiologic study of diet and cancer [28]. A significant one is that, as in all epidemiology, conclusions about causality need to come from a synthesis of epidemiologic findings in a number of populations, animal research, and metabolic studies. No single epidemiologic study can be considered definitive and used to establish causality. In case-control and cohort studies, there is always concern that the findings may not be causal but rather the result of confounding. That is, another factor may be correlated with the exposure under study and with the disease, and may be the causative agent. If the investigators are unaware of this confounding factor or they are unable to control for it sufficiently well, it might appear that the exposure under study is associated with disease simply because it is correlated with the second factor.

For example, in a study of diet and lung cancer, if individuals who smoke are also more likely to drink alcohol, unless smoking is measured well and controlled for in analysis, one might incorrectly assess the relation of alcohol to lung cancer because of the correlation between these two behaviors. However, when studies are done in different populations in different cultures, the likelihood of confounding is diminished;

it is less likely that the same correlations exist between behaviors. Additionally, other sources of error may differ among studies making a consistent finding more believable. Only with a randomized trial can a causal link be identified with certainty. However, even among clinical trials, differences can result because of differences in participant populations, so results need to be carefully interpreted.

Because the availability of the technology to measure genotypes in large studies is relatively new, there are few hypotheses related to the interaction of diet and genetics in cancer etiology that have been examined in numerous studies. Many questions have been examined only in a single study. A large number of studies are just starting or are ongoing. With the development of this field, it will be possible to begin to identify what appear to be causal relations. At all times, it is important to examine findings critically and to look for consistent findings from well-conducted studies.

A major concern in evaluating diet and genetic interactions in relation to risk of cancer is that studies need to have large numbers of participants in order to have sufficient power to examine risk within strata defined by genotype or by diet. At the present time, stored blood and interview data from previously conducted studies are often used to examine these questions. Because these studies were designed to address other questions, the number of participants may be relatively small, and analysis of gene–environment interactions may be based on samples of 10 or fewer individuals. Even if the results are statistically significant, such findings can be unstable. That is, if the study were redone, the findings might be very different.

As more and more studies are conducted, especially to address gene–environment interactions, this problem will become less severe for studies planned with sufficient statistical power. Nonetheless, for genes with low frequencies, the number of participants required can be very large. Further, to examine the interactions of more than one gene and more than one dietary or other exposure, the number of participants required may be exceedingly large. In evaluation of any study, it is important to look at the number of participants in each cell to make a determination of the likely stability of the findings.

At this time, most of the research regarding interactions of diet and genetics focus on a single dietary factor and a single nutrient. Such a focus is of considerable interest. Nonetheless, cancer is a multifactorial disease, and it is likely that several genetic factors are of importance even within a single causative pathway. Analysis of a single polymorphism might not capture the total picture of variation in risk. Similarly, several nutrients are likely to be important even within a single causal pathway. As noted above, the examination of gene–gene and gene–environment interactions can be seriously hampered by the required sample size. Further, diet is also a complex set of exposures. A single food may include different factors with both carcinogenic and anti-carcinogenic properties. Intakes of different nutri-

ents are generally highly correlated, so that an association attributed to intake of one nutrient may in fact be the result of a causal relationship with a different nutrient. Finally, when there is evidence that a particular nutrient is related to a decrease in risk, it cannot be assumed that larger quantities of that nutrient would be even more protective. For example, while vitamin C has antioxidant properties at the level found in most foods, at higher intake levels, it may have pro-oxidant properties [29].

A final challenge in this field is in the measurement of dietary exposure. Much literature is available on the problems of measurement of diet for epidemiologic purposes [30]. Beyond those concerns, the study of gene-diet interactions in relation to cancer risk has led to an interest in a number of new dietary factors. For many of these compounds, the dietary instruments used in the past may not provide sufficient detail for assessment of intake of that compound. For example, the study of heterocyclic amines has led to the development of a questionnaire that specifically addresses the sources of these compounds, because the information regarding intake on the existing questionnaires did not include the necessary detail to assess intake of heterocyclic amines [31]. Further, nutrient composition databases may be limited and may need work in order to determine the composition for compounds that may relate to disease risk but that have not been previously analyzed.

V. DIET–GENE INTERACTIONS AND CANCER

In this section, the current information regarding diet and gene interactions for particular types of cancer is reviewed. As noted above, for most of these associations, only a few studies have been done examining a particular association. Because of the paucity of data, much of our understanding of these relationships is likely to change with further investigation. This review is provided to give some sense of the state of the field, but needs to be regarded as very preliminary. Further, only diet and gene interactions for some cancer sites will be included. Exclusion of a site does not indicate that diet and/or genetic factors do not play a role in the etiology of that disease, but rather, that there is little research at this time on any possible relations. Also, because the field is a relatively new one and because there are few studies, this review does not include studies that show no association between a diet and genetic factor. The review is limited to those studies showing some association.

A. Cancer of the Colon and Rectum

Considerable epidemiologic evidence indicates that dietary factors are associated with cancer of the colon and rectum. There is also some evidence that genetic factors modify those associations. Red meat has been found to be associated

with risk with some consistency [3]. One possible mechanism for the effect of red meat on risk is through the intake of heterocyclic amines. Heterocyclic amines are formed in the cooking of meats at high temperature; they can be activated to forms that make them mutagenic and carcinogenic. *N*-acetyltransferase is an enzyme involved in the activation of heterocyclic amines. Two forms of this enzyme are polymorphic (NAT1 and NAT2), and there is some evidence that those who are rapid acetylators are at increased risk of colorectal cancer. In a few of the studies that have been done, there is also evidence that those individuals with the highest meat consumption who are rapid acetylators are at the highest risk [32]. In a small metabolic study, individuals were fed fried meats and their urine was tested for mutagenicity. Those who were rapid acetylators, or those with the rapid NAT2 phenotype, had significantly more urinary mutagenicity than the slow acetylators over the 6 weeks of this study [33]. Further, as noted above, preliminary evidence indicates that intake of heterocyclic amines is related to risk of polyps of the colon and rectum, and that the association depends both on intake of these substances and on genetic susceptibility based on assessment of the NAT2 and CYP1A2 variants [9].

There is also evidence that a high intake of fruits and vegetables is protective for colon and rectum cancers [3]. Folate intake may explain part of this effect [23, 24]. As noted above, there is a common genetic polymorphism in the gene for MTHFR. Those with the T/T genotype have elevated levels of plasma homocysteine [25], lower levels of plasma folate in some but not all studies [25, 34], and different response to folate given as a supplement than do those with the more common C/C or C/T genotypes [34]. About 12% of Caucasians and Asians are heterozygous T/T; the prevalence is lower among African-Americans [34]. In two nested case-control studies, risk was decreased for those with the C/C genotype. For those with high alcohol intake, low methionine intake, or low plasma folate, the effect of the C/C genotype was less strong [26, 27]. All of these nutrients are involved in the one-carbon cycle that includes MTHFR.

One study looked at family history of colorectal cancer in first-degree relatives (parents, siblings, or offspring). They found that for men with a family history of colorectal cancer, the association of risk with intake of beef and alcohol was much higher than for those men who did not report a family history. No such interactions were observed for the women in the study [35]. These findings suggest that other genetic factors interact with diet in the etiology of this disease. Clearly considerable research remains to be done in this area, and our understanding of the etiology of colon cancer may change as these relationships are elucidated.

B. Breast Cancer

The evidence linking dietary factors to breast cancer is much less consistent than that for cancer of the colon and rectum. There is quite consistent evidence of a higher risk associated with alcohol intake; vegetable and fruit intake also appear to be related to lower risk [3]. Some preliminary evidence suggests that genetic factors modify both of these dietary risk factors.

As described above, manganese superoxide dismutase is an important enzyme in the modulation of oxidative stress. There is a relatively common polymorphism of the gene for this enzyme; probably about 20% of Caucasians in the United States are homozygous for the variant. One study indicates that among premenopausal women, those with the variant are at increased risk of breast cancer. Further, it appears that the increased risk is primarily for women with low intakes of fruits and vegetables, or vitamins C or E. For those women with higher intakes, there was less difference in risk by genotype. Among postmenopausal women, some increase in risk was observed with the variant genotype but little modification of risk by reported dietary intake [13].

Fairly consistent evidence links regular alcohol consumption to a modest increase in the risk of breast cancer. It may be that this increase in risk is limited to women with a particular genotype. There is a family of enzymes, the alcohol dehydrogenases (ADH), that catalyzes the rate-limiting step in the metabolism of alcohol to acetaldehyde. Acetaldehyde dehydrogenase (ALDH) catalyzes the further oxidation of acetaldehyde. Polymorphisms have been identified for two of the ADH enzymes, ADH_2 and ADH_3, and for ALDH. The frequencies of those polymorphisms vary by population. In the United States, the ADH_3 variant is relatively common among those of European descent, the ADH_2 variant is relatively common among those of African descent, and the ALDH variant is common among those of Asian descent.

In one case-control study, ADH_3 genotype was examined in relation to alcohol consumption and risk of premenopausal breast cancer. Those with the variant metabolize alcohol to acetaldehyde more rapidly; acetaldehyde has been identified as a probable carcinogen. The researchers found that women who were above the median for alcohol consumption and who were homozygous for the gene coding for the more rapid form of the enzyme were at increased risk of breast cancer. Women who drank less or who had the other genes were not at increased risk. There was also no apparent gene–alcohol effect for postmenopausal women [36].

Again, as for colorectal cancer, there is evidence that dietary risk factors may differ for individuals with a family history of breast cancer compared to those with no such history. In one study, among premenopausal women with a first degree relative with breast cancer (mother, sister and/or daughter), intake of α-tocopherol was protective, while the association was less strong for women without a family history. There was also evidence that β-carotene was more strongly related to risk among women without a family history of disease than among those reporting a family history [37]. There are most likely a number of genetic factors that are related to risk of breast cancer and that are modified by dietary intake. These factors remain to be identified. Their

identification may not only suggest interventions for women at higher risk, but also elucidate a mechanism for an effect of diet on risk of breast cancer.

C. Prostate Cancer

Prostate cancer rates are high, particularly among older men [38]. There are considerable differences in the rates of this cancer around the world, and the evidence is strong that environmental factors can explain a large part of this variation. Individuals who migrate from regions where the rate of disease is low to regions where the rate is high show higher rates of disease than their counterparts who remain in the region with a low rate [39]. There is not a great deal of evidence regarding the etiology of the disease, although among possible risk factors is vitamin D exposure [38]. Vitamin D plays a role in the control of cell division in the prostate. The vitamin D receptor has genetic variants that have been shown to have functional effects on receptor expression, and preliminary evidence suggests that these vitamin D receptor polymorphisms are related to risk of prostate cancer [12–14]. At this point, no studies have examined both vitamin D exposure and genetic variation in relation to risk.

D. Other Cancers

Alcohol and smoking have been identified as strong risk factors for oral and nasopharyngeal cancers. In general, the levels of alcohol consumption that are associated with risk are much higher than those that have been related to increased risk of breast cancer. As for breast cancer, an interaction of alcohol consumption and ADH_3 has been identified. Evidence exists that those individuals who are heavier drinkers and who have the genotype coding for the more active form of the enzyme are at increased risk [40]. Another possible interaction has also been identified. CYP2E1 is related to the metabolic activation of nitrosamines. In one study, a CYP2E1 polymorphism was shown to be associated with risk of nasopharyngeal cancer [41]. However, these researchers did not assess exposure to nitrosamines to determine if there were an interaction.

Little research has been done related to diet and gene interactions in the etiology of lung cancer. One report stated that the association between smoking and risk of lung cancer was stronger among those individuals who also had the GSTM1null genotype [42]. However, this interaction was found only among those individuals who did not take α-tocopherol supplements. Among those using α-tocopherol supplements, there was no modification of the relationship between smoking duration and lung cancer risk by *GSTM1* genotype. β-carotene supplement use did not affect the *GSTM1* and smoking interaction [42].

As another example, the foodborne mold aflatoxin has been hypothesized to be related to the etiology of cancer of the liver. Epoxide hydrolase is a polymorphic enzyme involved in the metabolic deactivation of aflatoxin. One case-control study indicates that the genetic variant of this enzyme is related to increased risk of liver cancer [43]. DNA adducts of aflatoxin have been shown to be higher in individuals with both the epoxide hydrolase variant and the *GSTM1null* genotype [43, 44]. There is also evidence of an increased risk of liver cancer associated with the ADH_2 variant in a Japanese population [45].

VI. FUTURE DIRECTIONS

This review makes it clear that this field is a very new one, and that most of the available evidence is very preliminary. However, the field is also rapidly expanding. New genotypes are being identified at a very rapid pace; many of these have implications for our understanding of the role of dietary factors in cancer etiology. Clearly, as the field progresses, extremely large studies will be needed to allow for the examination of multiple levels of interaction. As in the example given above of an effect of *GSTM1* genotype on the association between smoking and lung cancer only among men who were not receiving an α-tocopherol supplement [42], the likelihood exists that multiple layers of interaction will need to be considered to fully understand the relevant etiological pathways.

In the future, genotype is likely to be examined in metabolic studies to determine the short-term effects on intermediate outcome measures in healthy individuals. A great deal remains to be understood about the relation between genotype and phenotype of the genes that appear to be important in terms of risk. Further, we will need to understand the factors that affect gene induction and the etiologic pathways. More work is going to have to be done to identify the relevant genes that are likely to be both rate limiting and also polymorphic.

There is little doubt that a large portion of the etiology of cancer can be attributed to environmental factors. Twin studies indicate that genetic factors alone are not sufficient to explain who will get the disease and who will not [46]. Important among the likely environmental factors are dietary factors. With increased understanding of genetic susceptibility as additional risk factors, it may eventually become possible to identify individuals with higher or lower requirements for particular nutrients or to identify individuals with greater sensitivity to agents like alcohol. Further, the elucidation of genetic factors in relation to diet will help us to clarify the natural history of this disease.

References

1. Ferlay, J., Parkin, D. M., and Pisani, P. (1990). Globocan 1: Cancer incidence and mortality worldwide in 1990. International Agency for Research on Cancer, World Health Organization. Available at http://www-dep.iarc.fr/dataava/globocan/globoJava.html.

2. Berrino, F., Sant, M., Verdecchia, A., Capocaccia, R., Hakulinen, T., and Esteve, J., Eds. (1995). "Survival of Cancer patients in Europe," IARC Scientific Publ. No. 132. IARC, Lyon, France.

3. World Cancer Research Fund in association with American Institute for Cancer Research, Washington, DC (1997). "Food, Nutrition and the Prevention of Cancer: A Global Perspective."

4. Doll, R., and Peto, R. (1981). The causes of cancer. *J. Natl. Cancer Inst.* **66,** 1191–1308.

5. King, R. C., and Stansfield, W. D. (1997). "A Dictionary of Genetics." Oxford University Press, New York.

6. Easton, D. F., Ford, D., and Bishop, D. T. (1995). Breast and ovarian cancer incidence in BRCA1-mutation carriers. Breast Cancer Linkage Consortium. *Am. J. Hum. Genet.* **56,** 265–271.

7. Easton, D. F., Narod, S. A., Ford, D., and Steel, M. (1994). The genetic epidemiology of BRCA1. Breast Cancer Linkage Consortium [letter]. *Lancet* **344,** 761.

8. Sinha, R., and Caporaso, N. (1997). Heterocyclic amines, cytochrome P4501A2, and N-acetyltransferase: Issues involved in incorporating putative genetic susceptibility markers into epidemiological studies. *Ann. Epidemiol.* **7,** 350–356.

9. Sinha, R., and Caporaso, N. (1999). Diet, genetic susceptibility and human cancer etiology. *J. Nutr.* **129,** 556S–559S.

10. Patterson, R. E., Eaton, D. L., and Potter, J. D. (1999). The genetic revolution: Change and challenge for the dietetics profession. *J. Am. Diet. Assoc.* **99,** 1412–1420.

11. Rock, C. L., Lampe, J. W., and Patterson, R. E. (2000). Nutrition, genetics, and risks and cancer. *Ann. Rev. Public Health* **21,** 47–64.

12. Taylor, J. A., Hirvonen, A., Watson, M., Pittman, G., Mohler, J. L., and Bell, D. A. (1996). Association of prostate cancer with vitamin D receptor gene polymorphism. *Cancer Res.* **56,** 4108–4110.

13. Ingles, S. A., Ross, R. K., Yu, M. C., Irvine, R. A., La Pera, G., Haile, R. A., and Coetzee, G. A. (1997). Association of prostate cancer risk with genetic polymorphisms in vitamin D receptor and androgen receptor. *J. Natl. Cancer Inst.* **89,** 166–170.

14. Ingles, S. A., Coetzee, G. A., Ross, R. K., Henderson, B. E., Kolonel, L. N., Crocitto, L., Wang, W., and Haile, R. W. (1998). Association of prostate cancer with vitamin D receptor haplotypes in African-Americans. *Cancer Res.* **58,** 1620–1623.

15. Ambrosone, C. B., Freudenheim, J. L., Thompson, P. A., Bowman, E., Vena, J. E., Marshall, J. R., Graham, S., Laughlin, R., Nemoto, T., and Shields, P. G. (1999). Manganese superoxide dismutase (MnSOD) genetic polymorphisms, dietary antioxidants and risk of breast cancer. *Cancer Res.* **59,** 602–606.

16. Mooney, L. A., Bell, D. A., Santella, R. M., Van Bennekum, A. M., Ottman, R., Paik, M., Blaner, W. S., Lucier, G. W., Covey, L., Young, T. L., Cooper, T. B., Glassman, A. H., and Perera, F. P. (1997). Contribution of genetic and nutritional factors to DNA damage in heavy smokers. *Carcinogenesis* **18,** 503–509.

17. Herbert, V., and Das, K. (1994). Folic acid and vitamin B$_{12}$. *In* "Modern Nutrition in Health and Disease," (M. E. Shils, J. A. Olson, and M. Shike, Eds.) Eighth Edition, pp. 402–425. Lea and Febiger, Philadelphia, PA.

18. Robertson, K. D., and Jones, P. A. (2000). DNA methylation: Past, present and future directions. *Carcinogenesis* **21,** 461–467.

19. James, S. J., Cross, D. R., and Miller, B. J. (1992). Alterations in nucleotide pools in rats fed diets deficient in choline, methionine and/or folic acid. *Carcinogenesis* **13,** 2471–2474.

20. Pogribny, I. P., Basnakian, A. G., Miller, B. J., Lopatina, N. G., Poirier, L. A., and James, S. J. (1995). Breaks in genomic DNA and within the p53 gene are associated with hypomethylation in livers of folate/methyl-deficient rats. *Cancer Res.* **55,** 1894–1901.

21. Rogers, A. E. (1995). Methyl donors in the diet and responses to chemical carcinogens. *Am. J. Clin. Nutr.* **61**(Suppl), 659S–665S.

22. Blount, B. C., Mack, M. M., Wehr, C. M., MacGregor, J. T., Hiatt, R. A., Wang, G., Wickramasinghe, S. N., Everson, R. B., and Ames, B. N. (1997). Folate deficiency causes uracil misincorporation into human DNA and chromosome breakage: Implications for cancer and neuronal damage. *Proc. Natl. Acad. Sci. USA* **94,** 3290–3295.

23. Giovannucci, E., Rimm, E. B., Ascherio, A., Stampfer, M. J., Colditz, G. A., and Willett, W. C. (1995). Alcohol, low-methionine-low-folate diets and risk of colon cancer in men. *J. Natl. Cancer Inst.* **87,** 265–273.

24. Freudenheim, J. L., Graham, S., Marshall, J. R., Haughey, B. P., Cholewinshi, S., and Wilkinson, G. (1991). Folate intake and carcinogenesis of the colon and rectum. *Int. J. Epidemiol.* **20,** 368–374.

25. Friedman, G., Goldschmidt, N., Friedlander, Y., Ben-Yehuda, A., Selhub, J., Babaey, S., Mendel, M., Kidron, M., and Bar-On, H. (1999). A common mutation A1298C in human methylenetetrahydrofolate reductase gene: Association with plasma total homocysteine and folate concentrations. *J. Nutr.* **129,** 1656–1661.

26. Chen, J., Giovannucci, E., Kelsey, K., Rimm, E. B., Stampfer, M. J., Colditz, G. A., Spiegelman, D., Willett, W. C., and Hunter, D. J. (1996). A methylenetetrahydrofolate reductase polymorphism and the risk of colorectal cancer. *Cancer Res.* **56,** 4862–4864.

27. Ma, J., Stampfer, M. J., Giovannucci, E., Artigas, C., Hunter, D. J., Fuchs, C., Willett, W. C., Selhub, J., Hennekens, C. H., and Rozen, R. (1997). Methylenetetrahydrofolate rductase polymorphism, dietary interactions and risk of colorectal cancer. *Cancer Res.* **57,** 1098–1102.

28. Freudenheim, J. L. (1999). Study design and hypothesis testing: Issues in the evaluation of evidence from nutritional epidemiology. *Am. J. Clin. Nutr.* **69,** 1315S–1321S.

29. Panel on Dietary Antioxidants and Related Compounds, Food and Nutrition Board, Institute of Medicine. (2000). "Dietary Reference Intakes for Vitamin C, Vitamin E, Selenium and Carotenoids." National Academy Press, Washington, DC.

30. Willett, W. C. (1998). "Nutritional Epidemiology," 2nd ed. Oxford University Press, New York.

31. Sinha, R., and Rothman, N. (1997). Exposure assessment of heterocyclic amines (HCAs) in epidemiologic studies. *Muta. Res.* **376,** 195–202.

32. Gertig, D. M., and Hunter, D. J. (1998). Genes and environment in the etiology of colorectal cancer. *Semin. Cancer Biol.* **8,** 285–298.

33. DeMarini, D. M., Hastings, S. B., Brooks, L. R., Eischen, B. T., Bell, D. A., Watson, M. A., Gelton, J. S., Sandler, R., and Kohlmeier, L. (1997). Pilot study of free and conjugated urinary mutagenicity during consumption of pan-fried meats:

Possible modulation by cruciferous vegetables, glutathione S-transferase-M1 and N-acetyltransferase-2. *Mutat. Res.* **381,** 83–96.

34. Bailey, L. B., and Gregory, J. F. (1999). Polymorphisms of methylenetetrahydrofolate reductase and other enzymes: Metabolic significance, risks and impact on folate requirement. *J. Nutr.* **129,** 919–922.

35. LeMarchand, L. L., Wilkens, L. R., Hankin, J. H., Kolonel, L. N., and Lyu, L.-C. (1999). Independent and joint effects of family history and lifestyle on colorectal cancer risk: Implications for prevention. *Cancer Epidemiol. Biomarkers Prev.* **8,** 45–51.

36. Freudenheim, J. L., Ambrosone, C. B., Moysich, K. B., Vena, J. E., Graham, S., Marshall, J. R., Muti, P., Laughlin, R., Nemoto, T., Harty, L. C., Crits, G. A., Chan, A. W., and Shields, P. G. (1999). Alcohol dehydrogenase 3 genotype modification of the association of alcohol consumption with breast cancer risk. *Cancer Causes Control* **10,** 369–377.

37. Ambrosone, C. B., Marshall, J. R., Vena, J. E., Laughlin, R., Graham, S., Nemoto, T., and Freudenheim, J. L. (1995). Interaction of family history of breast cancer and dietary antioxidants with breast cancer risk (New York, United States). *Cancer Causes Control* **6,** 407–415.

38. Ekman, P. (1999). Genetic and environmental factors in prostate cancer genesis: Identifying high-risk cohorts. *Eur. Urol.* **35,** 362–369.

39. Mettlin, C. (1997). Recent developments in the epidemiology of prostate cancer. *Eur. J. Cancer* **33,** 340–347.

40. Harty, L. C., Caporaso, N. E., Hayes, R. B., Winn, D. M., Bravo-Otero, E., Blot, W. J., Kleinman, D. V., Brown, L. M., Armenian, H. K., Fraumeni, J. F., Shields, P. G. (1997). Alcohol dehydrogenase 3 genotype and risk of oral cavity and pharyngeal cancers. *J. Natl. Cancer Inst.* **89,** 1698–1705.

41. Hildesheim, A., Chen, C.-J., Caporaso, N. E., Cheng, Y.-J., Hoover, R. N., Hsu, M.-M., Levine, P. H., Chen, I.-H., Chen, Y.-Y., Daly, A. K., and Idle, J. R. (1995). Cytochrome P4502E1 genetic polymorphisms and risk of nasopharyngeal carcinoma: Results from a case-control study conducted in Taiwan. *Cancer Epidemiol. Biomarkers Prev.* **4,** 607–610.

42. Woodson, K., Stewart, C., Barrett, M., Bhat, N. K., Virtamo, J., Taylor, P. R., and Albanes, D. (1999). Effect of vitamin intervention on the relationship between GSTM1, smoking and lung cancer risk among male smokers. *Cancer Epidemiol. Biomarkers Prev. 1999* **8,** 865–970.

43. McGlynn, K. A., Rosvold, E. A., Lustbader, E. D., Hu, Y., Clapper, M. L., Zhou, T., Wild, C. P., Xia, X.-L., Bafoe-Bonnie, A., Ofori-Adjei, D., Chen, G.-C., London, W. T., Shen, F.-M., and Buetow, K. H. (1995). Susceptibility to hepatocellular carcinoma is associated with genetic variation in the enzymatic detoxification of aflatoxin B_1. *Proc. Natl. Acad. Sci. USA* **92,** 2384–2387.

44. Rebbeck, T. R. (1997). Molecular epidemiology of the human glutatione S-transferase genotypes GSTM1 and GSTT1 in cancer susceptibility. *Cancer Epidemiol. Biomarkers Prev.* **6,** 733–743.

45. Lai, C., and Shields, P. G. The role of interindividual variation in human carcinogenesis. *J. Nutr.* 552S–555S.

46. Greenwald, P. (1996). Cancer risk factors for selecting cohorts for large-scale chemoprevention trials. *J. Cell. Biochem.* **25S,** 29–36.

CHAPTER **14**

Inborn Errors of Metabolism

CRISTINE M. TRAHMS
University of Washington, Seattle, Washington

I. INTRODUCTION

Recent dramatic advances in genetics at the laboratory and clinical levels have presented opportunities for understanding and promoting health and decreasing the morbidity and mortality associated with metabolic disorders. The treatment of inborn errors of metabolism is, in fact, fairly new to medicine and nutrition. Forty years ago, some services for children with inborn errors of metabolism were offered through child development clinics; however, the children were always neurologically compromised because of late diagnosis. At that time, the diagnosis of an inborn error of metabolism was based on clinical symptoms, which often occurred after the initial neurological damage. By the late 1960s, state newborn screening programs were under way and infants were identified before neurological damage occurred. It was at this point that the impact of nutrition intervention in the treatment of inborn errors of metabolism could be appreciated and is particularly beneficial to the affected individual, family, and society.

A. Public Health Services

Although inborn errors of metabolism are individually rare, as a group they have a significant impact on the health care system. The greatest savings to health care services occurs when individuals are identified before physical and neurological damage occurs and when they are consistently treated so that damage is prevented. Thus, the backbone of an effective management program for inborn errors of metabolism is an effective newborn screening program.

Maternal and child health agencies often provide services to meet the health care needs of infants and children with metabolic disorders. Essential public health functions related to inborn errors of metabolism can be described as follows:

1. *Infrastructure planning services.* Policy development, needs assessment, evaluation of systems, quality of care, and coordination of services are functions to which health care providers for children with metabolic disorders must ascribe to ensure the best possible health outcomes.

2. *Population-based services.* Newborn screening, oral health, nutrition education, genetic counseling, and public outreach are essential components of early identification and treatment of children with metabolic disorders.

3. *Enabling services.* Care coordination, transportation, translation, and family support services are needs that many families with fragile children with metabolic disorders require.

4. *Direct health care services.* Direct provision of basic health services is mandatory if these children are to survive.

B. Definition of Inborn Errors of Metabolism

Inborn errors of metabolism make up a large group of rare disorders caused by an inherited deficiency or absence of proteins that have enzymatic, carrier, receptor, or structural roles. For many of these disorders, the molecular nature of the disorder is known and the chromosomal locus of the gene has been mapped. It is not yet possible to cure any of these disorders with gene replacement or gene repair. However, as knowledge of the pathophysiology of each disorder is more completely understood, plans of management that mitigate the effect of the disorder can be instituted.

The most frequently identified disorders are those in which the absent or defective protein serves an enzymatic function. This diverse group of disorders responds to nutritional therapy intervention and will be discussed in this chapter.

Much work has been done to improve diagnosis, nutritional intervention, and medical intervention for inborn errors of metabolism. The goal of intervention is to prevent the ravages of the missing or defective enzyme. For most disorders, a "shotgun" approach is currently available, whereas a "laser" approach to treatment is needed to completely prevent the impact of the disorder. The two discrete parts to effective intervention for inborn errors of metabolism are (1) an immediate diagnosis and initiation of treatment, which require the support of an effective newborn screening program; and (2) a long-term approach to care, in which treatment is continued to avoid symptoms of the enzyme deficiency and

to try to normalize the biochemical parameters caused by the disorder.

C. Newborn Screening Programs

The evolution of newborn screening program (mass populations screening) efforts has resulted in a more positive outcome of treatment for many metabolic disorders. Newborn screening is a preventive public health measure available to all neonates. Population-based newborn screening is a major factor in making effective nutrition intervention possible. If infants are identified in the first few days of life, the diagnostic process can be completed and treatment started before damage occurs.

The American Academy of Pediatrics recommends that a newborn screening blood sample be collected before the infant is discharged from the nursery. If the blood sample is collected before the infant is 24 hours of age, it is essential that a second screening sample be obtained [1]. A general newborn screening (NBS) timetable is shown in Table 1.

Successful newborn screening, of course, depends on reliable, valid, and timely laboratory results. Many states have established a central newborn screening laboratory, which processes a large enough number of samples to maintain quality control. A qualitative newborn screening report offers a presumptive positive result that must be quantitatively confirmed. Laboratory confirmation of diagnosis is mandatory.

An effective newborn screening program involves laboratory, education, administration, follow-up, management, and evaluation components [2, 3]. Each state has developed individual legislative newborn screening mandates. However, many commonalities are seen, as shown in Table 2. Most states provide newborn screening for phenylketonuria, congenital hypothyroidism, galactosemia, and the hemoglobinopathies. These disorders all meet the criteria for newborn screening shown in Table 3 [1].

Most newborn screening programs use a blood sample dried on filter paper to complete a bacterial inhibition assay. This type of sample requires a very small amount of blood, is easily transported to the central laboratory (after the blood has dried), and several tests can be completed on a single blood sample. Newer technologies, such as tandem mass spectrometry, have the potential to increase the number of disorders that can be effectively screened [4].

Many of the disorders included in newborn screening programs are autosomal recessive. This means each parent carries the affected gene and the incidence is 1:4 for each pregnancy. Thus affected infants identified by newborn screening usually do not have a positive family history of the disorder.

With newborn screening programs providing an opportunity for earlier diagnosis, and with recent laboratory developments and increased specificity of treatment modalities, the long-term outcome for persons with inborn errors of metabolism is brighter than in the past. The contrast between

TABLE 1   General Timetable for Collecting Newborn Screening (NBS) Samples

Day one: birth

Between day 1 and hospital discharge:
- Inform parents of NBS and their right to refuse for specific statutory reasons.
- Send sample to state lab within 24 hours of collection.
- Or   • if parents refuse, e.g., based on religious beliefs, obtain refusal signature prior to discharge.

No later than day 5:
- Draw NBS sample for infants remaining in hospital and for those born out of hospital.
- Send sample to state lab within 24 hours of collection.

Between days 7 and 14:
- Repeat NBS sample is recommended for all infants.
- Send sample to state lab within 24 hours of collection.

This is a "generic" newborn screening timetable; individual states have their own protocol. Timing of the newborn screening sample is critical to diagnosis and earliest possible intervention before the infant is irreparably damaged.

outcome without early treatment and expected outcomes with early identification and treatment is shown in Table 4. For many disorders, however, treatment is a recent development, and no long-term outcome data are available.

II. DIAGNOSIS

Although all states in the United States have a newborn screening program and screen for a variety of disorders, many disorders are not currently part of newborn screening programs. The treatment of all metabolic disorders, whether tested by newborn screening programs or not, requires a well-organized system of laboratory analysis and monitoring. There are two phases of management: (1) the initial, acute diagnostic phase, and (2) the long-term management phase.

The acute diagnostic phase requires attention to the symptoms presented by the infant. Most toxic metabolites cross the placenta and are cleared by the mother. Thus the severity of the defect and the initial feeding may affect the timing of the onset of symptoms. Depending on the disorder, the onset of symptoms can range from hours to months. If infants do not become ill in the early postnatal period, it is common for the metabolic disorder to be manifested when the child is weaned from breast milk or when high-protein solids are added to the diet.

In the newborn period, there are general, nonspecific symptoms that warrant further investigation. The most frequent signs of "trouble" are lethargy, poor feeding, and vomiting. Apnea and respiratory distress are significant symptoms that may indicate the presence of a metabolic dis-

TABLE 2 Number of States Screening for Selected Disorders in the United States

Disorder	Number of states screening[a]	Incidence per 1000 live newborns—general U.S. population
Phenylketonuria	53/53	1:10,000–1:25,000
Congenital hypothyroidism	53/53	1:3,600–1:5,000
Galactosemia	46/53	1:60,000–1:80,000
Hemoglobinopathies	45/53	1:385–1:835 (African-American) 1:40,000–1:60,000 (non-African-American)
Maple syrup urine disease	25/53	1:250,000–1:400,000
Homocystinuria	22/53	1:50,000–1:150,000
Biotinidase deficiency	21/53	1:72,000–1:126,000
Congenital adrenal hyperplasia	11/53	1:12,000
Tyrosinemia	7/53	1:120,000 (Sweden[b])
Cystic fibrosis	4/53	1:2,000 (northern European extraction)

Source: Adapted from Committee on Genetics. (1996). Newborn screening fact sheets. *Pediatrics* **98**, 473–501.
[a]Includes District of Columbia, Puerto Rico, and Virgin Islands.
[b]No current U.S. data.

order, as do jaundice and increased liver enzymes. These general symptoms usually move quickly into a more precarious situation for the infant.

Infants may frequently present with encephalopathy as a result of accumulating toxic metabolites in the central nervous system. Examples of this are organic acid disorders, urea cycle disorders, and amino acid disorders. Blood ammonia levels should be checked if the infant is lethargic, vomits, or has signs of encephalopathy. Metabolic acidosis with an increased anion gap is another sign of an infant with a metabolic disorder, as are jaundice or increased liver enzyme activity [5]

Appropriate and aggressive treatment before confirmation of the diagnosis may save the life of the infant and reduce the possibility of neurological sequelae. The first step is to remove offending metabolites. If a disorder of amino acid metabolism or protein intolerance is suspected, protein

TABLE 3 Generally Accepted Criteria for Newborn Screening for a Specific Disorder

- Symptoms usually absent in newborns.
- Disease results in developmental impairment, serious illness, or death.
- Sensitive, specific laboratory tests available on a mass population basis.
- Disease occurs frequently enough to warrant screening.
- Successful treatment procedures are available.
- Benefits of screening justify the cost.
- Follow-up and treatment programs are available.

Source: Adapted from Committee on Genetics. (1996). Newborn screening fact sheets. *Pediatrics* **98**, 473–501.

intake should immediately be discontinued. Hemodialysis may be necessary to decrease blood ammonia and/or amino acids levels [6]. The second step is to prevent catabolism. This may require administration of intravenous glucose.

III. TREATMENT: INITIATION AND MONITORING

The approach to treatment for each disorder depends on the enzyme(s) affected and the metabolic consequences of the diminished enzyme(s). The goal of treatment for inborn errors of metabolism is to strive for correction of the biochemical abnormality. Although the clinical and biochemical picture of each disorder is unique and ranges from mild to life-threatening illness, metabolic disorders can be thought of as a group in which the absence or inactivity of a specific enzyme or cofactor causes the buildup of the substrate and/or deficiency of the product. The outcome of treatment for metabolic disorders is variable and depends on early diagnosis and intensive and continuous intervention. Nutritional therapy is the primary mode of treating metabolic disorders.

In this section, the concepts, principles, and strategies of treatment of disorders of protein, carbohydrate, and fat metabolism will be discussed. A detailed approach to management of disorders amenable to treatment or a catalog of all possible disorders will not be provided. A complete discussion of diagnosis and management of the vast array of metabolic disorders can be found in Scriver *et al.* [7], McKusick [8], or the Online Mendelian Inheritance in Man (OMIM): http://www.ncbi.nlm.nih.gov/Omim/ [9]. Each disorder has been assigned a specific Mendelian Inheritance in Man (MIM)

TABLE 4 Outcome for Inborn Errors of Metabolism with and without Early Diagnosis

Disorder	Outcome without treatment	Expected outcome with early identification and treatment
Phenylketonuria	Mental retardation (IQ < 40)	Normal IQ with lifelong treatment
Maple syrup urine disease (MSUD)	Encephalopathy → death	Variable; may be cognitively compromised
Tyrosinemia, Type I	Liver failure → death	With NTBC treatment, encouraging data on preventing neurologic crises, renal and hepatic failure, rickets
Glycogen storage diseases	Hypoglycemia, liver CA → death	Typical growth, development
Galactosemia	Sepsis → severe delays, death	Often learning disabilities
Urea cycle disorders	Hyperammonemia → severe delays or death	Variable; may be cognitively compromised
Fatty acid oxidation disorders, e.g., long-chain acyl-CoA dehydrogenase deficiency (LCAD), medium-chain acyl-CoA dehydrogenase deficiency (MCAD), short-chain acyl-CoA dehydrogenase deficiency (SCAD)	Encephalopathy, hepatomegaly, often death which is attributed to SIDS	No long-term data; encouraging short-term data
Organic acidurias, e.g., methylmalonic aciduria, propionic acidemia	Metabolic acidosis → coma → death	Variable; may be cognitively compromised
Glutaric acidemia I	Impaired movement, dystonia, vomiting, seizures, coma	No long-term data
Homocystinuria	Cardiac problems, organ damage, psychiatric disturbances, death	Variable; may be physically and cognitively compromised
Isovaleriac acidemia	Metabolic acidosis → coma → death	Variable; may be cognitively compromised

number, which will be used in this chapter to differentiate similar disorders from each other and to avoid confusion. Table 5 outlines the essential components of nutritional therapy for treatment of metabolic disorders. Table 6 outlines some metabolic disorders that respond to nutritional therapy.

A. Principles of Treatment

The two major principles of treatment are (1) to mitigate the effect of the altered gene by modifying components of diet to adjust the environment at the cellular level, and (2) to provide protein, energy, and nutrients to support growth and development.

For many disorders, the treatment is determined by the identification of the missing or inactive enzyme. In an effort to modify the detrimental effect of the decreased or absent enzyme activity, the paradigm of "working around" the enzyme is used. In many cases, decreasing the substrate available for the reaction and supplementing the product to "normal" levels prevent or decrease the deleterious effects of the disorder. An example of this strategy is in the treatment of phenylketonuria (MIM 261600): Phenylalanine (substrate) is restricted because of the absence or inactivity of phenylalanine hydroxylase (enzyme), and tyrosine (product) is supplemented. In some disorders, the defective enzyme is further down the amino acid degradation pathway and may affect the metabolism of two or more amino acids [lysine

and tryptophan in glutaric acidemia (MIM 231670) or leucine, isoleucine, and valine in maple syrup urine disease (MSUD, MIM 248600)]. The amino acids in most aminoacidopathies are essential, that is, they cannot be synthesized by the body and therefore must be provided in the diet. This is critical because these essential amino acids must be provided at the requirement level so the child can grow and develop, but they must also be limited so there is no toxic build-up of amino acid(s) that cannot be metabolized.

In some disorders, the additional step of enhancing enzyme activity by supplying its co-factor can be helpful. An example of this is the provision of pharmacological doses of biotin in biotinidase deficiency (MIM 253260) [10] or of vitamin B_6, on which cystathionine β-synthase (MIM 236200) is dependent, in some forms of homocystinuria [11].

In metabolic disorders of carbohydrate metabolism, such as galactosemia (MIM 230400), the nutrient of concern,

TABLE 5 Components of Nutritional Therapy for Metabolic Disorders

- Identify precise diet appropriate to the problem.
- Provide nutritional surveillance to ensure that diet is adequate.
- Provide a mechanism for follow-up of child for symptoms of nutritional deficiency or toxicity.
- Provide emotional and educational support for child and family.

TABLE 6 Selected Metabolic Disorders That Require Nutritional Therapy

Disorder	Pathway affected	Nutritional adjustments	Composition of required specialized formula	Supplements
Amino acid disorders				
Phenylketonuria (MIM 261600)	Phenylalanine hydroxylase		Low phenylalanine, supplemented tyrosine	
Tyrosinemia, Type 1 (MIM 276700)	Fumaryl-acetoacetate hydrolase		Low phenylalanine, tyrosine	NTBC[a]
Maple syrup urine disease (MIM 248600)	Branched chain ketoacid dehydrogenase complex		Low leucine, isoleucine, valine	L-carnitine
Isovalaric acidemia (MIM 243500)	Isovaleryl-CoA dehydrogenase		Low leucine	L-carnitine, glycine
Homocystinuria (MIM 236200 and 236250)	Cystathionine-β-synthase or methyltetrahydrofolate reductase		Low methionine, supplement cystine	Folate, betaine
Glutaric acidemia, Type 1 (MIM 231670)	Glutaryl-CoA dehydrogenase		Low lysine, tryptophan	L-carnitine
Ketone utilization disorders (MIM 203750)	2-methylacetoacetyl-CoA thiolase and other ketothiolase enzymes	Low protein, avoid fasting		L-carnitine, bicitra
Organic acid disorders				
Methylmalonic aciduria (MIM 251000)	Methylmalonyl-CoA mutase or cobalamin cofactor synthesis		Low protein, isoleucine, methionine, threonine, valine	L-carnitine, sodium benzoate,[b] bicitra
Propionic acidemia (MIM 232000)	Propionyl-CoA carboxylase		Low protein, isoleucine, methionine, threonine, valine, long-chain unsaturated fatty acids	L-carnitine, sodium benzoate, biotin, bicitra
Urea cycle disorders				
Ornithine transcarbamylase deficiency (OTC) (MIM 311250)	Ornithine transcarbamylase		Low protein, supplement essential amino acids, increased energy	L-carnitine, sodium benzoate, sodium phenylbutyrate, L-citrulline
Citrullinemia (MIM 215700)	Argininosuccinate synthetase		Low protein, supplement essential amino acids, increased energy	L-carnitine, sodium benzoate, sodium phenylbutyrate, L-arginine

(continues)

TABLE 6 (*continued*)

Disorder	Pathway affected	Nutritional adjustments	Composition of required specialized formula	Supplements
Carbamyl phosphate synthetase deficiency (CPS) (MIM 114010)	Carbamyl phosphate synthetase		Low protein, supplement essential amino acids, increased energy	L-carnitine, sodium benzoate, sodium phenylbutyrate, L-citrulline
Argininosuccinic aciduria (MIM 207900)	Argininosuccinate lyase		Low protein, supplement essential amino acids, increased energy	L-carnitine, sodium benzoate, sodium phenylbutyrate, L-arginine
Arginase deficiency (MIM 207800)	Arginase		Low protein, supplement essential amino acids, increased energy	L-carnitine, sodium benzoate, sodium phenylbutyrate
Carbohydrate disorders				
Hereditary fructose intolerance (MIM 229600)	Fructose-1-phosphate aldolase B	Low sucrose, fructose		None
Galactosemia (MIM 230400)	Galactose-1-phosphate uridyl transferase	Low lactose, galactose	Soy formula	None
Glycogen storage diseases (Type Ia) (MIM 232200)	Glucose-6-phosphatase	Low lactose, fructose, sucrose, low fat, high complex carbohydrates	Soy formula	Raw cornstarch, iron and calcium supplements
Glycogen storage diseases (Type Ib) (MIM 232330)	Glucose-6-phosphatase transport	Low lactose, fructose, sucrose, low fat, high complex carbohydrates	Soy formula	Raw cornstarch, iron and calcium supplements
Glycogen storage diseases (Type III) (MIM 232400)	Amylo-1,6-glucosidase	Low lactose, fructose, sucrose, low fat, high complex carbohydrates	Soy formula	Raw cornstarch, iron and calcium supplements
Fatty acid oxidation disorders				
Long-chain acyl-CoA dehydrogenase deficiency (LCAD) (MIM 201460)	Long-chain acyl-CoA dehydrogenase	Low fat, low long-chain fatty acids, avoid fasting	Low fat or fat free	L-carnitine, medium chain triglycerides
Medium-chain acyl-CoA dehydrogenase deficiency (MCAD) (MIM 201450)	Medium-chain acyl-CoA dehydrogenase	Low fat, low medium-chain fatty acids, avoid fasting	Low fat or fat free	L-carnitine
Short-chain acyl-CoA dehydrogenase deficiency (SCAD) (MIM 201470)	Short-chain acyl-CoA dehydrogenase	Low fat, low short-chain fatty acids, avoid fasting	Low fat or fat free	L-carnitine

[a]2-(2-nitro-4-trifluoromethylbenzoyl)-1,3-cyclohexanedione that is an inhibitor of 4-hydroxy-phenylpyruvate dioxygenase.

[b]Sodium benzoate and sodium phenylbutyrate are chemicals administered to enhance waste ammonia excretion; other compounds producing the same effect are also used.

galactose, is not essential. Therefore, the goal of effective therapy is to eliminate as much of the exogenous component as possible from the diet. Other sources of nourishment need to be provided to compensate for the omitted foods and nutrients.

Disorders of fatty acid metabolism require a source of energy other than fat because fat cannot be metabolized to meet energy needs. Fatty acids of specific carbon lengths are often minimized or eliminated, depending on whether or not the fatty acid is essential for growth and development. Most fats contain a mixture of fatty acids of varying carbon lengths, making it difficult to eliminate specific fatty acids. In the cases of long-chain acyl-CoA dehydrogenase deficiency (MIM 210460) or very long chain acyl-CoA dehydrogenase deficiency (MIM 201475), shorter chain fatty acids can be metabolized [12]. Frequently, the larger problem is providing enough energy for these children to avoid oxidation of long-chain fatty acids to medium-chain derivatives. The shorter chain fatty acids are often supplemented, for example, medium-chain triglycerides as MCT oil. However, in medium-chain acyl-CoA dehydrogenase deficiency (MIM 201450), sources of medium-chain fatty acids can be eliminated without problems. Other essential components of treatment are (1) supplementation of L-carnitine, an amino acid that functions in transport of fatty acid acyl-CoA esters during mitochondrial beta-oxidation; and (2) avoidance of fasting, to reduce the accumulation of partially oxidized metabolites associated with impaired energy production [13].

In all metabolic disorders, nutritional therapy addresses the symptoms of the disorder but not the disorder itself. Perhaps when gene therapy matures as a science, this option will be available.

B. Specialized Metabolic Team

As a group, children with metabolic disorders comprise a small percentage of the pediatric population, and even the most common of these disorders is rare in the general population. However, the health care needs of these children are specific and urgent. The American Academy of Pediatrics has recommended that a team experienced in management supervise the therapy of children with metabolic disorders [1]. Effective treatment requires the expertise of a team of health care professionals, generally comprised of a geneticist, nutritionist (registered dietitian), nurse, genetic counselor, psychologist, and neurologist. This team of experts is familiar with the nuances of current treatment for metabolic disorders and will be able to incorporate new research innovations as they are deemed appropriate. The complex nutritional and medical management of these children cannot occur effectively without the follow-up and support of the community. Communication between the team at the tertiary center, the community, and the family is crucial for supporting the best possible medical, nutritional, and intellectual outcome for these children.

C. Role of the Nutritionist

The nutritionist who works with families whose children have inborn errors of metabolism must be meticulous in the understanding of metabolic disorders and should develop a collaborative support system with team members and the family.

D. Providing a Metabolic Diet

General principles of protein and energy management address the issues of biochemical control specific to the disorder. These principles also address the needs of overall nourishment: (1) The child should be provided adequate amino acids, total protein, and nitrogen to support growth; (2) the child should be provided adequate energy to support growth and prevent growth failure; (3) energy needs may be increased when L-amino acids provide the protein equivalent; (4) maintaining an adequate energy intake is essential in preventing catabolism; and (5) suppression of destructive metabolites can produce a striking biochemical and clinical improvement [14, 15].

E. Nutritional Assessment

Three components of nutritional assessment are necessary for the evaluation of children with metabolic disorders: (1) assessment of growth and comparison to appropriate guidelines, (2) assessment of nutrient intake and comparison to requirements for treatment of the specific disorder and the recommended intakes for all children, and (3) assessment of biochemical parameters specific to the disorder and those of appropriate nourishment.

F. Assessment of Growth

Normal parameters of physical growth are expected for many children with metabolic disorders, provided that all of the components of nourishment appropriate to the diagnosis are provided [16]. Optimal nutritional support is required to meet these goals. As for all children, appropriate growth reflects an adequate intake of protein, energy, vitamins, and minerals. For children with metabolic disorders, appropriate growth also reflects the achievement of metabolic balance. For growth to proceed in a normal fashion, energy and all required nutrients must be provided in adequate amounts, while the nutrients that the individual cannot effectively metabolize must be limited to the requirement level or entirely eliminated.

Growth differences are typical of children with metabolic disorders. Poor growth is often a reflection of several factors. Infants who have endured a severe neonatal illness may require an extended time of appropriate nourishment before they catch up in growth. Frequent febrile illness may interfere with achieving expected physical growth. Children with

repeated episodes of hyperammonemia or metabolic crisis are not able to grow. Slowed or altered growth patterns often reflect poor metabolic control or an inadequate protein or energy intake. However, slowed or altered growth in a child with a metabolic disorder may not be the result of noncompliance with treatment on the part of the family. Many of these children with little or no enzyme activity are medically fragile and are difficult to bring into and maintain in metabolic balance.

The disorder itself may affect growth and growth achievement. Older children with glycogen storage disease, for example, are often shorter than their age peers. Younger children with glycogen storage disease who have had the benefit of intensive treatment with cornstarch are more likely to achieve their genetic potential for physical growth. Children with galactosemia are usually shorter and lighter than their peers without galactosemia. There is no clear explanation for this altered growth pattern.

G. Growth Assessment Parameters

Gender- and age-appropriate parameters for growth assessment are weight, length or stature, weight for length or stature, skinfold measures, and increments of growth in weight and length or stature. Assessment of growth or size is the basis for many therapeutic recommendations for children with metabolic disorders. These measurements, therefore, need to be completed by someone who is properly trained to conduct them, who has a knowledge of accurate and reliable techniques, and who knows how to operate the standardized equipment [17].

H. Assessment of Nutrient Intake

The welfare of the infant or child with a metabolic disorder depends on accurate and minute adjustments of one or more dietary components. Parents are urged to provide an accurate record of food and formula intake so that, in cooperation with the metabolic nutritionist, an accurate assessment of intake of critical nutrients as well as total protein and energy intakes can be made.

I. Assessment of Biochemical Parameters

Maintaining metabolic balance for children with metabolic disorders requires frequent and intensive monitoring of biochemical parameters specific to the disorder. It also requires monitoring parameters that reflect general nutritional status. The goal of treatment for all of these disorders is to achieve biochemical levels at or near the normal range. Laboratory parameters that are frequently monitored include plasma amino acids, urine organic acids, hematologic status, protein status, electrolytes, and blood lipid and ammonia levels. A general plan for biochemical assessment is shown in Table 7.

J. Providing Adequate Nutrition

1. PROTEIN

For some disorders, total protein is not restricted, but the composition of the protein may be adjusted. The treatment of phenylketonuria, for example, requires the restriction on phenylalanine intake but not total protein. This is accomplished with the use of a specially designed semisynthetic formula. For other disorders, total protein intake is restricted. For the treatment of ketone utilization disorders (MIM 203750), for example, total protein is often restricted to 1.5 g/kg/day. Infants and children with disorders of amino acid metabolism must obtain most of their protein from specialized metabolic formulas. Natural foods seldom provide more than 25% (often 10%) of the protein requirements of infants and children with amino acid, organic acid, or urea cycle disorders. It is generally not possible to provide an adequate intake of total protein without providing an excess of the offending amino acids. Some disorders, such as the organic acidopathies, require an overall total protein restriction as well as provision of amino acids from a specialized formula. Table 8 indicates the strategies of protein restriction for infants and children with metabolic disorders.

Protein in the specialized formulas is provided as individual amino acids (excluding those amino acids, which are contraindicated for each condition). Amino acids are more readily oxidized than intact protein, thus the requirement for protein when amino acids are the protein source is greater than usual. The overall diet for the treatment of these disorders is not low in total protein, but low in specific amino acids. The infant or child will not thrive without the use of specialized formulas and the amino acids they contain. Adequate protein and energy are required to maintain an anabolic state. If adequate formula is not prescribed or consumed, a catabolic state will develop, causing both high plasma amino acids levels and clinical problems.

2. ESTABLISHING AMINO ACID REQUIREMENTS FOR THE INDIVIDUAL INFANT OR CHILD

The requirements for essential amino acids have been established [18] and are used as clinical guidelines. Frequently, these guidelines are used to establish the diet for a newly diagnosed infant or child and are adjusted as necessary to stabilize critical plasma levels. Table 9 describes situations that may arise when components of protein nutriture are adjusted inappropriately. Specialized metabolic formulas have been designed to meet the unique protein, carbohydrate, and fat needs of these infants and children. Sources of metabolic formulas are shown in Table 10.

The urea cycle disorders require the restriction of overall protein intake because excess nitrogen from any source can be toxic. However, it is also imperative to provide enough protein and energy to support growth. This fine line requires extensive collaboration between the family and the metabolic team. The formulas for the treatment of urea cycle

TABLE 7   Monitoring for Children with Metabolic Disorders
Biochemical, Growth, and Nutritional Parameters[a]

Disorder	Biochemical parameters
Aminoacidopathies	
Homocystinuria	Plasma methionine, total and free homocystine
Maple syrup urine disease	Plasma leucine, isoleucine, valine, alloisoleucine
Phenylketonuria	Plasma phenylalanine, tyrosine
Tyrosinemia	Plasma tyrosine, phenylalanine, methionine, succinate, alpha-feto-protein
Isovaleric acidemia	
Ketone utilization disorders	Urine organic acids, carnitine, electrolytes
Urea cycle disorders	
Ornithine transcarbamylase deficiency (OTC), carbamyl phosphate synthetase deficiency (CPS)	Plasma amino acids, ammonia, electrolytes, carnitine, citrulline, arginine
Argininosuccinic aciduria (ASA)	Plasma amino acids, ammonia, electrolytes, carnitine, arginine
Organic acidemias	
Methylmalonic aciduria	Methylmalonic acid, electrolytes, kidney function (BUN, creatinine), carnitine
Propionic aciduria	Urine organic acids, plasma electrolytes, carnitine, kidney function
Disorders of carbohydrate metabolism	
Glycogen storage disease	Cholesterol, triglycerides, uric acid, liver function (AST, ALT, GGT), blood glucose levels
Galactosemia	Galactose-1-phosphate

[a]The frequency of monitoring biochemical parameters depends on the age and health status of the child. Many parameters are monitored monthly if the infant or child is well; more frequently if the child is ill. Other parameters are monitored at each clinic visit. Parameters of general nutritional status may be monitored biannually or as needed.

TABLE 8   Examples of Restricted Protein Diets for the Treatment of Metabolic Disorders

Protein adjustment needed	Disorder
No restriction in protein	Fructose intolerance
Provide total protein intake at recommended level + eliminate specific protein-containing foods, e.g., all lactose, galactose containing proteins	Galactosemia
Provide total protein intake at recommended level + eliminate specific protein-containing foods, e.g., all high-fat protein foods	Glycogen storage diseases, fatty acid oxidation defects
Restrict protein intake to physiological tolerance; provide small amounts of HBV[a] proteins	Mild urea cycle and organic acid disorders, ketone utilization disorders
Restrict protein intake to physiological tolerance; provide small amounts HBV protein + specific amino acids	Severe urea cycle and organic acid disorders
Provide total protein intake at recommended level + restrict one or more amino acids to requirement level	Phenylketonuria, maple syrup urine disease, isovaleric acidemia, glutaric acidemia type I

[a]HBV, high biological value.

TABLE 9 Potential Problems with Amino Acid Prescriptions

Amino acid problem	Definition	Clinical signs	Resolution of problem
Toxicity	Adverse effects resulting from intake of large quantities of individual amino acids	Demonstrated by untreated amino acidopathies, e.g., eczema, tremors, mental retardation, poor growth	Decrease intake of offending amino acid(s)
Antagonism	Competition for transport sites between amino acids of similar structure that use the same carrier system	Depressed appetite, food intake, and growth	Readjust proportion of amino acids, use some HBV[a] protein
Imbalance	Deviation in proportion of dietary amino acids great enough to cause adverse effect	Decreased food intake and growth, fatty infiltration of liver, decreased efficiency of amino acid utilization.	Readjust proportions of amino acids, use some HBV protein
Deficiency	Intake does not meet amino acid requirement	Depressed growth and plasma amino acid concentrations	Increase intake of incriminated amino acid

[a]HBV, high biological value.

disorders have a high concentration of amino acids to ensure ready incorporation into protein. Most children with these disorders also require medications to enhance the excretion of excess nitrogen through secondary pathways other than the urea cycle. For infants and children with urea cycle disorders, catabolism from excess protein, weight loss, illness, or infection are dangers. Hyperammonemia can occur rapidly (in several hours) and can be life threatening. Effective management of children with urea cycle disorders requires frequent and intense monitoring. The total amount of protein tolerated by the individual child depends on residual enzyme activity, age, and growth rate. The proper amount of protein is determined by considering growth rate, plasma amino acids, ammonia, ketones, and urine organic acids specific to the disorder.

3. SUPPLYING RESTRICTED AMINO ACIDS

Small amounts of the "toxic" essential amino acids specific to each disorder are required for growth and development. These essential amino acids are provided to the infant by including small amounts of proprietary infant formula in the metabolic formula mixture. During infancy, adding small amounts of cow's milk or soy formula can provide an infant with these essential amino acids. In older children, the addition of fruits, vegetables, and grains can provide these amino acids.

4. BREASTFEEDING

Some infants with metabolic disorders are able to maintain low and stable plasma amino acid levels with a combination of breast and metabolic formula feedings. Many infants, however, are too metabolically fragile to maintain appropriate plasma levels with breastfeeding. Infants with phenylketonuria are most likely to be able to tolerate partial breastfeeding and maintain low plasma phenylalanine levels.

Breastfeeding is overtly contraindicated for infants with some disorders, such as galactosemia.

K. Energy

Protein and energy needs are intertwined. If sufficient energy is not provided in the diet, the body will use protein as an energy source to meet essential energy needs. When protein is used as an energy source, it is not available for incorporation into protein-containing substances such as muscle, enzymes, and hormones. Protein catabolism can have significant metabolic consequences in some metabolic disorders, such as the organic acid and urea cycle disorders where catabolism is problematic.

Infants and children with metabolic disorders have increased energy needs, often as great as 120–140 kcal/kg in infancy [14]. Energy needs vary from disorder to disorder and from child to child. Therefore, it is essential to carefully monitor growth, biochemical parameters, and nutrient intake to evaluate the adequacy of treatment.

Additional protein-free energy sources are an important adjunct to dietary management of many metabolic disorders. Foods that have been modified to be low in protein, such as flours, pastas, and baked products, are an appropriate and necessary source of energy and variety in the diet. Sources are listed in Table 10.

L. Vitamins and Minerals

Whenever a significant group of foods is eliminated or severely restricted from the diet of an infant or child, a plan for replacement of essential nutrients must be in place. For example, children whose diets are restricted in protein must eliminate muscle meats and most dairy products from their diets. Thus, they eliminate sources of vitamin B_{12}, iron, zinc, calcium, and other nutrients. Generally, the most reliable

TABLE 10 Sources of Formulas and Low Protein Foods for the
Treatment of Metabolic Disorders

Company	Contact information
Metabolic formulas	
Mead Johnson Nutritionals	http://www.meadjohnson.com/metabolics 1-800-755-4805
Ross Laboratories	http://www.ross.com/html/sitemap.cfm 1-800-986-8755
Low-protein foods	
Scientific Hospital Supply	http://www.shsna.com 1-800-365-7354
Med-Diet	http:www/med-diet.com 1-800-633-3438
Ener-G Foods	http://www2.digimktg.com/enrg/enHome1.tmpl 1-800-331-5222

method of nutrient replacement for these nutrients is from a specially formulated and supplemented formula.

M. Fats

Whenever a specific nutrient or dietary component is eliminated or severely restricted, a plan for replacement of that component must be in place. The essential fatty acids cannot be endogenously synthesized and so must be provided from external sources. Deficiency of essential fatty acids is avoided by providing 2–4% of total energy intake as linoleic acid.

N. Notes on Management Strategies

1. HYDRATION

Strict attention must be paid to fluid status, because dehydration in children with metabolic disorders can precipitate a metabolic crisis. Fluid intake and fluid requirements must be carefully monitored. Constipation can also cause metabolic imbalance for these infants and children. Both the osmolality and renal solute load of the formula mixtures should be in the safe ranges for age and health status.

2. CHILDHOOD ILLNESSES

The usual childhood illnesses often pose a medical crisis for the child with a metabolic disorder. Frequently, children require hospitalization and the administration of intravenous fluids to prevent metabolic crisis. During an illness that results in catabolism, sources of protein are often refused. Continued administration of some form of fluid and energy assists in rehabilitation.

3. FEEDING

Some children with metabolic disorders who have neurological difficulties develop oral-motor problems that inter-

fere with the intake of adequate nourishment. A hyperactive gag reflex is the most frequent problem. Some providers use nasogastric or gastrostomy tubes to support an adequate intake of nourishment and medications.

Poor appetite is not uncommon for children with metabolic disorders, especially urea cycle disorders, MSUD, and the organic acidemias. Poor appetite and poor feeding may be organic, behavioral, or both. Buildup of toxic metabolites is frequently the offender. Many children with metabolic disorders who have had acute episodes may also have a history of vomiting, which may lead to feeding avoidance. Families are fully aware that a child who does not eat may face metabolic disaster, and this stress intensifies the situation. Many families have found specialized feeding teams to be helpful.

Children who have age-appropriate oral-motor skills should be encouraged to use them. Foods should be offered that provide a variety of textures and encourage biting, chewing, and the movement of the bolus of food in the mouth.

4. ORAL HEALTH

Children with metabolic disorders may be at increased risk for dental caries and dental erosion due to the nature of their therapeutic diets. The combination of frequent intake of carbohydrates and the acidic nature of the protein formulas appear to put these children at increased risk for oral health problems [19]. It is important that oral hygiene and regular tooth brushing be an important part of everyday health management.

5. FOOD-RELATED BEHAVIORS

The requirement of the ingestion of a specialized semi-synthetic formula and accompanying food restrictions appropriately cause parents to be anxious. Parents and children may then be predisposed to the development of adverse interactions around food. A thorough knowledge of typical food patterns and the development of feeding skills and

behaviors around food will enable the nutritionist and other team members to appropriately support and guide the family as they work to provide an appropriate feeding environment for their child.

6. PARENT–CHILD INTERACTION

The rigorous requirements of nutritional therapy may place stresses on the parent–child relationship. Families should be supported as they strive to better understand the metabolic disorder in their family, to adjust personal schedules to meet the rigor of nutritional and medical therapies for the child, and to maintain a healthy family environment for all family members.

Bright Futures: Guidelines for Health Supervision of Infants, Children, and Adolescents is an important guideline for health supervision for all children. Families whose children have metabolic disorders will find these developmentally focused guidelines to be particularly helpful. The *Bright Futures* materials can be found at http://www.brightfutures.org.

IV. NEW TREATMENT DEVELOPMENTS

A. Maple Syrup Urine Disease or Branched-Chain Ketoaciduria

MSUD is an autosomal recessive disorder with a metabolic block at the decarboxylation of branched-chain alpha keto-acids derived from leucine, isoleucine, and valine. The accumulation of branched-chain amino acids (BCAA) and other compounds exerts neurotoxic effects. MSUD is heterogeneous and ranges from severe to mild. Infants with the severe manifestation usually present in the emergency room of the hospital with encephalopathy that quickly escalates to coma. If untreated, the disease is lethal. L-Alloisoleucine is the most specific and sensitive diagnostic marker for all forms of MSUD [20].

Treatment comprises dietary management, with strictly reduced quantities of protein and BCAA, as well as aggressive intervention during acute neonatal and subsequent metabolic complications. Recently, hyperalimentation solutions without the offending amino acids have been successfully used to curtail acute episodes [21].

MSUD is regarded as a metabolic disorder that has a potentially favorable outcome with carefully supervised long-term therapy. Liver replacement has been considered because of the difficulty of careful chronic supervision of dietary treatment. With successful liver transplant, patients no longer require protein restriction, and the risk of metabolic decompensation during catabolic events is eliminated. However, it is not known whether the overall risks of liver transplantation outweigh the benefits and/or if outcome is significantly different than that with dietary management [22].

B. Tyrosinemia

Tyrosinemia is an autosomal recessive disorder with a metabolic block at fumarylacetoacetate hydrolase. It is a devastating metabolic disorder that presents as severe liver disease at less than 6 months of age. If tyrosinemia is untreated, affected infants will die from liver failure within a few weeks or months after the onset of symptoms. Deficiency of fumarylacetoacetic hydrolase allows the accumulation of fumarylacetoacetate and the subsequent conversion to succinylacetone. It is believed that the accumulated succinylacetone is toxic and responsible for the liver damage.

The three treatment strategies are (1) dietary intervention that limits the precursor amino acids phenylalanine and tyrosine, and (2) metabolic inhibition of the tyrosine pathway, or (3) liver transplantation. Although dietary restriction alone slows the process of the disorder, it does not prevent liver damage. Liver transplantation has been the treatment of choice for infants and children who were healthy enough for the procedure [23]. Even with a successful transplantation procedure, succinylacetone continues to be detected in the urine. The drug 2-(2-nitro–4-trifluoromethylbenzoyl)–1, 3-cyclohexanedione (NTBC) is used to block the formation of fumarylacetoacetate and succinylacetone by inhibiting the tyrosine pathway. Currently in clinical trials, NTBC therapy plus dietary phenylalanine and tyrosine restrictions look very promising for significantly improving the outcome for these children [24].

C. Phenylketonuria

Dietary treatment of phenylketonuria is recognized as one of the first effective treatments of genetic disease. Phenylketonuria is an autosomal recessive disorder with a metabolic block at phenylalanine hydroxylase that allows the accumulation of phenylalanine and prevents the conversion to tyrosine. The abnormal metabolites phenylpyruvate and phenylacetate are produced. Infants show no signs or symptoms of metabolic derangement. Prior to newborn screening, all individuals with phenylketonuria were identified because of significant development delays at 6–9 months of age.

Phenylalanine levels of 10–20 times normal are toxic to the developing brain. There has been great debate about treatment for phenylketonuria on two counts: (1) the degree to which plasma phenylalanine levels need to be lowered to prevent neurological damage and (2) the duration of treatment. There is now consensus that (1) restricted phenylalanine therapy must be continued on a lifetime basis, and (2) plasma phenylalanine levels 1–6 times normal provide a better environment for normal intellectual development than higher levels [25–27]

Although fewer than 2% of infants with elevated phenylalanine levels will have defects in dihyropteridine reductase (MIM 261630), it is recommended that infants with elevated

phenylalanine levels be further evaluated for this disorder, which results in progressive neurological deterioration [1].

D. Galactosemia

Galactosemia is an autosomal recessive disorder with a metabolic block at galactose-1-phosphate uridyl transferase leading to a buildup of galactose and galactose-1-phosphate. Galactose-1-phosphate is believed to be the neurotoxic compound. Infants appear unaffected at birth and generally become ill during the first week of life after ingestion of galactose. Blood levels of galactose-1-phosphate are elevated and thought to be toxic to the liver, kidneys, and central nervous system. Treatment with a low-galactose diet promotes clinical improvement. However, many children develop learning disabilities. Although it is understood that endogenous production of galactose contributes significantly to blood galactose-1-phosphate levels [28], it is not understood how this contributes to clinical outcome or how stringent the dietary restriction of galactose needs to be to prevent further damage [29, 30]. Soy-based infant formula is the sole source of nourishment for the infant with galactosemia. Recent data suggest that other (nondairy) foods may also contribute dietary galactose and possibly affect plasma galactose-1-phosphate levels and outcome [31].

E. Glycogen Storage Disease

The most common types of glycogen storage disease (types Ia, MIM 232200; Ib, MIM 232330; and III, MIM 232400) are autosomal recessive disorders with metabolic blocks that prevent the utilization of glycogen for energy. The glycogen storage diseases are characterized by severe hypoglycemic episodes. Type Ia glycogen storage disease is the most severe because both gluconeogenesis and glycogenolysis are impaired. Children develop severe hepatomegaly and frequently develop liver adenoma and glomerular sclerosis [32, 33]. Glycogen storage disease type Ib is clinically and biochemically similar to type Ia. However, individuals with this disorder are susceptible to bacterial infections because of neutropenia. This impaired neutrophil function increases the mortality rate for this group of children. Glycogen storage disease type III is less severe than type I forms. Risk of cardiomyopathy increases with age [34].

Ingestion of raw cornstarch to prevent hypoglycemia and glycogen storage has improved the outcome for these children [35–37]. The treatment protocol is rigorous and requires ingestion of cornstarch at regular intervals day and night or a nasogastric tube at night. With cornstarch therapy, the growth of the children has improved, hypoglycemic episodes are prevented, and the consequent neurological damage is also prevented. Children with glycogen storage disease type Ib are now treated with granulocyte stimulating factor for neutrophil stimulation to prevent severe neutropenia

[38]. Although these recent therapies have significantly improved the short-term status of these children, limited long-term outcome data are available.

F. Homocystinuria

Homocystinuria is an autosomal recessive disorder of homocystine metabolism involving the enzyme cystathionine β-synthase or methylenetetrahydrofolate reductase (MTHFR, MIM 236250). Levels of methionine and homocystine are elevated with cystathionine β-synthase deficiency; methionine is usually not elevated with MTHFR. The elevated levels of homocystine interfere with collagen cross-linkage, and the result is dislocated lenses, osteoporosis, scoliosis, a long, thin body, and a high-arched palate. Elevated homocystine levels also interfere with the vascular epithelium and lead to thrombus formation. Many individuals with homocystinuria have behavioral or psychiatric disturbances. Recently, betaine has been added to the treatment protocol for homocystinuria [39, 40]. Betaine decreases the plasma homocystine levels and diminishes behavioral and psychiatric effects.

V. ADULT TREATMENT

Most diagnostic and treatment services are pediatric based. As diagnosis and treatment improve, persons with inherited metabolic disorders not only survive, but also thrive. Pediatric health services are inappropriate for this group of adults. However, these surviving adults, whether competent or compromised, require continued support and effective treatment to maintain their health and nutritional status.

Few, if any, adult providers are trained to meet the needs of fragile adults with metabolic disorders. These health care needs are highlighted by the need for lifelong treatment and changing service needs with age. If the precise treatments of specific metabolic disorders are not meticulously followed, biochemical status deteriorates. This leads to poor judgment and decision making and can lead to a permanent decrease in neurological function and even life-threatening illness. Young adults with inherited metabolic disorders require a specialized system of health care delivery to maintain optimal status.

A. Transition

Transition from pediatric to adult care is a major step for most families. Table 11 illustrates the differences between pediatric and adult-based care. The transition from pediatric to adult care highlights significant concerns for this group. These concerns include (1) the need for complex nutritional therapy, (2) ingestion of special metabolic formula, (3) complex schedule of medication intake, (4) the need for lifelong treatment, (5) reproductive concerns, (6) changing medical

TABLE 11 Characteristics of Pediatric- and Adult-Based Care

Pediatric care	Adult care
Parents in charge	Self-directed
Care is monitored	Self-monitored
Appointments are scheduled	Schedule own appointment
Support services offered for financial and emotional issues	Must seek support services for financial and emotional issues
Parents responsible for finances/payment	Responsible for own finances/payment
Parents have insurance	Provide own insurance
Transportation provided by parents	Provide own transportation
Parents request information on treatment	Must request own information
Parents request information on outcome	Must request own information
Specialty care program	Generic adult care
Public health nurse services	No public health nurse services
Pediatric specialty	General medicine
Team approach to services	No team approach
Interdisciplinary approach	Disciplinary approach
Usually has built-in support from parent/caregiver	Different sort of support for emotional needs
Reproduction generally not an issue	Reproductive/contraceptive decisions must be made

needs with age, and (7) monitoring of health status by providers who understand inherited metabolic disorders.

Some families need to organize specialized health care for their college-bound student, while others are struggling to find programs that support daily living skills. Regardless of the competence or status of the young adult with a metabolic disorder, transition to adult-based care is medically and socially appropriate.

1. BARRIERS

Barriers do exist, however, to effective transition from pediatric to adult-based health care. Often, pediatric health care providers feel that there are no knowledgeable providers in the adult health care system for persons with metabolic disorders. Pediatric providers may be hesitant to "let go" because they have established long-term relationships with both patient and family. Patients and their families are similarly ambivalent about transitioning out of a familiar situation. Often, adult care providers are reluctant to accept patients who have rare and chronic metabolic disorders and who often require extraordinary services from the health care system.

2. TRANSITION NEEDS

An organized approach to adult-based health care, with each step and expectation carefully outlined, is essential. Table 12 provides an example of the commitment required by family and providers to make transition a successful process.

B. Adulthood

Little is known about the natural history of those with early diagnosed and treated metabolic disorders. Two examples illustrate this point. It is clear that lifelong treatment is necessary for phenylketonuria to prevent neuropsychological problems [41]. Table 13 outlines the neuropsychological aspects of discontinued treatment for persons with phenylketonuria (PKU). However, there is no long-term outcome data to indicate how rigorous this lifelong treatment must be. In the case of tyrosinemia I (fumaryl-acetoacetate hydrolase deficiency), treatment with NTBC appears to be successful in preventing early liver failure and death.

Many disorders have secondary long-term effects. Many of these secondary effects are now being fully realized, for example, renal disease in methylmalonic aciduria [42], neuropsychological disorders in phenylketonuria [43], and ovarian failure in galactosemia [44].

C. Pregnancy

Pregnancy and its management in women with metabolic disorders have also recently been undertaken as standard care. Women with metabolic disorders face special risks to themselves and to their fetuses. There are several aspects of the impact of pregnancy on inborn errors of metabolism: (1) Maternal metabolism negatively affects the development of the fetus, e.g., maternal PKU syndrome; (2) the pregnancy poses health risks for the mother in the postpartum period,

TABLE 12   Example of Transition Services from Pediatric to
Adult Medical Services

Current status	Goal
General health monitored by pediatrician	Supervision by family practice physician
Medical supervision by pediatric geneticist	Consultation from university internal medicine and genetics
Nutritional status monitored by pediatric metabolic nutritionist	Monitored by community-based nutritionist with consultation from metabolic nutritionist
Neurological status monitored by pediatric neurologist	Neurologist
Gynecological supervision by pediatrician	Consultation by specialty gynecologist to primary care physician
Medically stable	Maintenance of medical stability
Parents supervise medications	Self-manages medications with support
In high school	Employed
Lives at home	Lives independently
Parents supervise diet	Self-manages diet with support

e.g., urea cycle disorders, and (3) the disorder diminishes reproductive capability, e.g., galactosemia.

In the case of maternal phenylketonuria, the neurotoxic effects of elevated maternal phenylalanine levels damage the fetus. There is a dose–response effect related to maternal plasma phenylalanine concentrations. The higher the maternal phenylalanine level, the greater the risks to the developing fetus for microcephaly and cardiac anomalies [45]. Some success has been reported with early, rigorous prepregnancy treatment. Although the children are young and the long-term outcome is not known, it is believed that maintaining maternal phenylalanine concentrations at near-normal phys-

TABLE 13   Phenylketonuria Outcome Data

Results of long-term neglect of management of PKU

Poor short-term memory
Deteriorating physical state
Agoraphobia
Poor judgment
Fragile emotional state
Poor impulse control that leads to loss of job, inability to maintain interpersonal relationships, and problems with the law

Results of long-term effective management of PKU and general health care

College students
Successful employment
Stable interpersonal relationships
Reliable memory
Emotional equilibrium

iological levels prior to conception and during pregnancy prevents structural and neurological damage to the fetal brain and heart [46].

Case reports of women with urea cycle disorders indicate rigorous management is needed to maintain a pregnancy. The postpartum reabsorbtion of uterine material causes an increase in ammonia levels and neurotoxic problems, which can be fatal. Case reports suggest that women who have a mild manifestation of the disorder fare better postpregnancy than those women who are severely affected. A woman with mild argininosuccinate lyase deficiency, for example, who had careful clinical and biochemical monitoring during her pregnancy is believed to have reduced the risk of maternal metabolic compensation in the perinatal period. Argininosuccinate did not appear to be teratogenic to the fetus [47].

Classic galactosemia diminishes reproductive capability. About 80% of women with galactosemia suffer ovarian failure. Those few women who successfully complete a pregnancy should be instructed about the risks of self-intoxication with galactose during breastfeeding [48, 49].

A case report of a pregnant woman with MSUD suggested that maintaining BCAA plasma levels between 100 and 300 μmol/L was compatible with the delivery of a normal infant. Careful monitoring of the mother after delivery can minimize the risk of metabolic decompensation in the postpartum period [50].

VI. SUMMARY

Progress in the diagnosis and treatment of genetic diseases has been fast paced. The goal for treatment of all disorders is to provide normal biochemical plasma concentrations.

This goal is difficult to achieve [51]. Knowledge of genetics and use of diagnostic procedures in health care have the potential to prevent symptoms and manifestations of the disorders by providing interventions at the presymptomatic stage of the disorder. At this point, treatment must await diagnosis that is based on symptoms of a metabolic disorder. There is hope that further progress in the understanding of genetic disorders will promote earlier and more effective treatment and prevent the symptomatic sequelae of metabolic disorders.

References

1. Committee on Genetics (1996). Newborn screening fact sheets. *Pediatrics* **98,** 473–501.
2. Pollitt, R. J., Green, A., McCabe, C. J., Booth, A., Cooper, N. J., Leonard, J. V., Nicholl, J., Nicholson, P., Tunaley, J. R., and Virdi, N. K. (1997). Neonatal screening for inborn errors of metabolism: cost, yield, and outcome. *Health Technol. Assess.* **1,** i–iv.
3. Thomason, M. J., Lord, J., Bain, M. D., Chalmers, R. A., Littlejohns, P., Addison, G. M., Wilcox, A. H., and Seymour, C. A. (1998). A systematic review of evidence for the appropriateness of neonatal screening programmes for inborn errors of metabolism. *J. Public Health Med.* **20,** 331–343.
4. Naylor, E. W., and Chace, D. H., (1999) Automated tandem mass spectrometry for mass newborn screening for disorders in fatty acid, organic acid and amino acid metabolism. *J. Child Neurol.* **14,** S4–S8.
5. Burton, B. K. (1998). Inborn errors of metabolism in infancy: A guide to diagnosis. *Pediatrics* **102,** 69–78.
6. Schaefer, F., Straube, E., Oh, J., Mehls, O., and Mayatepek, E. (1999). Dialysis in neonates with inborn errors of metabolism. *Nephrol. Dial. Transplant* **14,** 910–918.
7. Scriver, C. R., Beaudet, A. L., Sly, W. S., and Valle, D., Eds. (2000). "The Metabolic and Molecular Basis of Inherited Disease." McGraw-Hill, New York.
8. McKusick, V. A. (1998). "Mendelian Inheritance in Man. Catalogs of Human Genes and Genetic Disorders," 12th Ed. Johns Hopkins University Press, Baltimore, MD.
9. McKusick-Nathans Institute for Genetic Medicine, Johns Hopkins University, Baltimore, MD, and National Center for Biotechnology Information, National Library of Medicine, Bethesda, MD (2000). Online Mendelian Inheritance in Man, OMIM. Available at http://www.ncbi.nlm.nih.gov/omim/.
10. Hymes, J., and Wolf, B. (1996). Biotinidase and its roles in biotin metabolism. *Clin. Chim. Acta* **15,** 1–11.
11. Anonymous (1996). Homocystinuria. *BMJ* **313,** 1025–1026.
12. Tyni, T., and Pihko, H. (1999). Long-chain 3-hydroxyacyl-CoA dehydrogenase deficiency. *Acta Pediatr.* **88,** 237–245.
13. Saudubray, J. M., Martin, D., de Lonlay, P., Touati, G., Poggi-Travert, F., Bonnet, D., Jouvet, P., Boutron, M., Slama, A., Vianey-Saban, C., Bonnefont, J. P., Rabier, D., Kamoun, P., and Brivet, M. (1999). Recognition and management of fatty acid oxidation defects: A series of 107 patients. *J. Inher. Metab. Dis.* **22,** 488–502.
14. Acosta, P. B., and Yanicelli, S. (1993). Nutrition support of inherited disorders of amino acid metabolism: Part 1. *Topics Clin. Nutr.* **9,** 65–82.
15. Acosta, P. B., and Yanicelli, S. (1995). Nutrition support of inherited disorders of amino acid metabolism: Part 2. *Topics Clin. Nutr.* **10,** 48–72.
16. Acosta, P. B., Yannicelli, S., Marriage, B., Mantia, C., Gaffield, B., Porterfield, M., Hunt, M., McMaster, N., Bernstein, L., Parton, P., Kuehn, M., and Lewis, V. (1998). Nutrient intake and growth of infants with phenylketonuria undergoing therapy. *J. Pediatr. Gastroenterol. Nutr.* **27,** 287–91.
17. Lohmann, T. G., Roche, A. F., and Martorell, R. (1988). "Anthropometric Standardization Reference Manual." Human Kinetics Books, Champaign, IL.
18. Garza, C., Scrimshaw, N. S., and Young, V. R. (1976). Human protein requirements: The effects of variations in energy intake within the maintenance range. *Am. J. Clin. Nutr.* **29,** 280–285.
19. Kilpatrick, K. M. (1999). The implications of phenylketonuria on oral health. Pediatr. Dentistry **21,** 433–437.
20. Schadewaldt, P., Bodner-Leidecker, A., Hammen, H. W., and Wendel, U. (1999) Significance of L-alloisoleucine in plasma for diagnosis of maple syrup urine disease. *Clin. Chem.* **45,** 1734–1740.
21. Wajner, M., and Vargas, C. R. (1999). Reduction of plasma concentrations of large neutral amino acids in patients with maple syrup urine disease during crises. *Arch. Dis. Child.* **80,** 579.
22. Wendel, U., Saudubray, J. M., Bodner, A., and Schadewaldt, P. (1999). Liver transplantation in maple syrup urine disease. *Eur. J. Pediatr.* **158,** S60–S64.
23. Mohan, N., McKiernan, P., Preece, M. A., Green, A., Buckels, J., Mayer, A. D., and Kelly, D. A. (1999). Indications and outcome of liver transplantation in tyrosinaemia type 1. *Eur. J. Pediatr.* **158,** S49–S54.
24. Holme, E., and Lindstedt, S. (1998). Tyrosinemia type I and NTBC (2(2-nitro-4-trifluoromethylbenzoyl)-1, 3-cyclohexanedione). *J. Inherit. Metab. Dis.* **21,** 507–517.
25. Seashore, M. R., Wappner, R., Cho, S., and de La Cruz, F. (1999). Development of guidelines for treatment of children with phenylketonuria: Report of a meeting at the National Institute of Child Health and Human Development held August 15, 1995, National Institutes of Health, Bethesda, Maryland. *Pediatrics* **104,** 6–9.
26. Medical Research Council Working Party on Phenylketonuria (1993). Recommendations on the dietary management of phenylketonuria. *Arch. Dis. Child.* **68,** 426–427.
27. Wappner, R., Cho, S., Kronmal, R. A., Schuett, V., and Seashore, M. R. (1999). Management of phenylketonuria for optimal outcome: A review of guidelines for phenylketonuria management and a report of surveys of parents, patients, and clinic directors. *Pediatrics* **104,** 6–12.
28. Berry, G. T., Nissim, I., Lin, Z., Mazur, A. T., Gibson, J. B., and Segal, S. (1995). Endogenous synthesis of galactose in normal men and patients with hereditary galactosemia. *Lancet* **346,** 1073–1074.
29. Walter, J. H., Collins, J. E., and Leonard, J. V. (1999). Recommendations for the management of galactosemia. U.K. Galactosemia Steering Group. *Arch. Dis. Child.* **80,** 593–96.
30. Schweitzer, S., Shin, Y., Jakobs, C., and Brodehl, J. (1993). Long-term outcome in 134 patients with galactosemia. *Eur. J. Pediatr.* **152,** 36–43.

31. Gropper, S. S., Weese, J. O., West, P. A., and Gross, K. C. (2000). Free galactose content of fresh fruits and strained fruit and vegetable baby foods: More foods to consider for the galactose-restricted diet. *J. Am. Diet. Assoc.* **100,** 573–575.

32. Restaino, I., Kaplan, B. S., Stanley, C., and Baker, L. (1993). Nephrolithiasis, hypocitraturia, and a distal renal tubular acidification in type 1 glycogen storage disease. *J. Pediatr.* **122,** 392–396.

33. Wolfsdorf, J. I., Holm, I. A., and Weinstein, D. A. (1999). Glycogen storage diseases. Phenotypic, genetic, and biochemical characteristics, and therapy. *Endocrinol. Metab. Clin. N. Am.* **28,** 801–823.

34. Greene, H., L., Swift, L., L., and Knapp, H. R. (1991). Hyperlipidemia and fatty acid composition in patients treated for type 1a glycogen storage disease. *J. Pediatr.* **119,** 398–403.

35. Gremse, D. A., Bucuvalas, J. C., and Balisteri, W. F. (1990). Efficacy of cornstarch therapy in type III glycogen storage disease. *Am. J. Clin. Nutr.* **52,** 671–674.

36. Goldberg, T., and Slonim, A. E. (1993). Nutrition therapy for hepatic glycogen storage diseases. *J. Amer. Diet. Assoc.* **93,** 1423–1430.

37. Wolfsdorf, J. I., and Crigler, J. F., Jr. (1999). Effect of continuous glucose therapy begun in infancy on the long-term clinical course of patients with type 1 glycogen storage disease. *J. Pediatr. Gastroenterol. Nutr.* **29,** 136–143.

38. McCawley, L. J., Korchak, H. M., Douglas, S. D., Campbell, D. E., Thornton, P. S., Stanley, C. A., Baker, L., and Kilpatrick, L. (1994). In vitro and in vivo effects of granulocyte colony-stimulating factor on neutrophils in glycogen storage disease type Ib: Granulocyte colony-stimulating factor therapy corrects the neutropenia and the defects in respiratory burst activity and Ca^{2+} mobilization. *Pediatr. Res.* **35,** 84–90.

39. Wilcken, D. E., Wilcken, B., Dudman, N. P., and Tyrrell, P. A. (1983). Homocystinuria–The effects of betaine in the treatment of patients not responsive to pyridoxine. *N. Engl. J. Med.* **309,** 448–453.

40. Sakura, N., Ono, H., Nomura, S., Ueda, H., and Fujita, N. (1998). Betaine dose and treatment intervals in therapy for homocystinuria due to 5, 10-methylenetetrahydrofolate reductase deficiency. *J. Inherit. Metab. Dis.* **21,** 84–85.

41. Schiaffino, C. K., DiStefane, S., and Veneselli, E. (1999). Phenylketonuria: Diet for life or not? *Acta Paediatr.* **88,** 664–666.

42. Van Calcar, S. C., Harding, C. O., Lyne, P., Hogan, K., Banerjee, R., Sollinger, H., Rieselbach, R. E., and Wolff, J. A. (1998). Renal transplantation in a patient with methylmalonic acidemia. *J. Inherit. Metab. Dis.* **21,** 729–737.

43. Pietz, J., Dunckelmann, R., Rupp, A., Rating, D., Meinck, H. M., Schmidt, H., and Bremer, H. J. (1998). Neurological outcome in adult patients with early-treated phenylketonuria. *Eur. J. Pediatr.* **157,** 824–830.

44. Kaufman, F., Kogut, M. D., Donnell, G. N., Koch, H., and Goebelsmann, U. (1979) Ovarian failure in galactosemia. *Lancet* **II, Oct. 6; 2,** 737–740.

45. Rouse, B., Matalon, R., Koch, R., Azen, C., Levy, H., Hanley, W., Trefz, F., and de la Cruz, F. (2000). Maternal phenylketonuria syndrome: Congenital heart defects, microcephaly, and developmental outcomes. *J. Pediatr.* **136,** 57–61.

46. Koch, R., Friedman, E., Azen, C., Hanley, W., Levy, H., Matalon, R., Rouse, B., Trefz, F., Waisbren, S., Michals-Matalon, K., Acosta, P., Guttler, F., Ullrich, K., Platt, L., and de la Cruz, F. (1999). The International Collaborative Study of Maternal Phenylketonuria Status report 1998. *MRDD Res. Rev.* **5,** 117–121.

47. Worthington, S., Christodoulou, J., Wilcken, B., and Peat, B. (1996). Pregnancy and argininosuccinic aciduria. *J. Inherit. Metab. Dis.* **19,** 621–622.

48. Brivet, M., Raymond, J. P., Konopka, P., Odievre, M., and Lemonnier, A. (1989). Effect of lactation in a mother with galactosemia. *J. Pediatr.* **115,** 280–281.

49. DeJongh, S., Vreken, P., Ijst, L., Wanders, R. J., Jakobs, C., and Bakker, H. D. (1999). Spontaneous pregnancy in a patient with classical galactosemia. *J. Inherit. Metab. Dis.* **22,** 754–755.

50. Grunewald. S., Hinrichs, F., and Wendel, U. (1998). Pregnancy in a woman with maple syrup urine disease. *J. Inherit. Metab. Dis.* **21,** 89–90.

51. Treacy, E., Childs, B., and Scriver, C. R. (1995). Response to treatment in hereditary metabolic disease: 1993 survey and 10-year comparison. *Am. J. Hum. Genet.* **56,** 359–367.

D. Supplements and Food Replacements

CHAPTER **15**

Role of Liquid Dietary Supplements

ANNE COBLE VOSS AND KATHLEEN E. MAYER
Abbott Laboratories, Columbus, Ohio

I. MEDICAL FOODS AND NUTRITIONAL SUPPLEMENTS

Changing demographics and the current health care environment have created the opportunity for growth of medical foods and medical nutritional supplements (MNSs). Older adults are the largest consumers of health care accounting for nearly 30% of all health care expenditures. It is estimated that by 2030, adults over the age 85 will have doubled and those over the age of 65 will account for 22% of the population [1]. These consumers, the "Baby Boomers," are expected to take a very active role and interest in their health care as it relates to extending longevity and quality of life [2]. Nutrition is a modifiable, lifestyle factor that has a prominent role in the health care model of the twenty-first century.

Older adults are particularly at risk for malnutrition for a variety of reasons including functional and cognitive decline, increased nutritional needs, chronic disease conditions and co-morbidities, economic limitations, and social factors. It has been well documented in the literature that malnutrition is associated with poor outcomes such as increased morbidity and mortality [3–8], impaired immunity and wound healing [9], increased length of stay [10], decreased function [11], hospital readmissions [3], and reduced quality of life [12, 13]. Studies demonstrate that medical nutrition therapy (MNT), including supplementation with medical foods, can improve clinical and economic outcomes associated with the conditions listed in Table 1.

This chapter will address the increasing need for supplemental MNT, differentiate between medical foods and medical nutritional supplements, and provide examples of benefits and barriers to their use.

A. Prevalence of Malnutrition across the Continuum of Care

The negative impact of malnutrition has been highlighted by early classic reports such as "The Skeleton in the Hospital Closet" [14]. Since then, researchers and health care professionals have learned much more about nutritional screening and assessment, nutritional biomarkers, and the prevention and treatment of malnutrition. Despite these advances in knowledge, little has changed regarding the prevalence of

TABLE 1 Conditions in Which Medical Nutrition Therapy May Improve Outcomes

AIDS	Cancer
Cerebral vascular accident	Congestive heart failure
Chronic obstructive pulmonary disease	Dementia
Diabetes mellitus	Hip fracture
General medicine/surgery	Pneumonia
Pressure ulcers	Renal disease

malnutrition in acute care. It is estimated that malnutrition in hospital/acute care ranges from 10% to 55% [15–17] and is often dependent on diagnoses and medical procedures.

Unfortunately, malnutrition is not confined to the hospital setting. As the provision of health care has emerged into other points of service, malnutrition has been identified in these areas as well. Reports have indicated that malnutrition, or risk for malnutrition, ranges from 39% to 74% [18–20] in long-term care (LTC) facilities. In addition, LTC residents often have nutrient intakes that are less than 50% of the Recommended Dietary Allowances (RDA) [20]. Risk for malnutrition is also abundant among older adults living in the community. A study of general practice patients in England indicated that the prevalence of malnutrition was 10% [21], but a prevalence rate as high as 43% has been reported elsewhere [15]. Poor energy and nutrient intakes have also been reported among independently living older adults with studies indicating that many eat less than two-thirds of the RDA [22–24]. With increased longevity, trends indicate that more adults will remain in their homes for longer periods of time. Therefore, health care professionals will need to develop and implement ways of preventing and treating the nutritional decline that is common in the population of independently living older adults.

II. WHAT IS A MEDICAL FOOD/SUPPLEMENT?

According to the Food and Drug Administration (FDA), "A medical food is prescribed by a physician when a patient

TABLE 2   Examples of Medical Nutritional Supplements and Indicated Uses

Special need/indication	Standard examples
High protein	Ensure High Protein,[a] Promote, Promote with Fiber, Meritene, Nitro-Pro, Nubasics VHP, Replete, Sustacal, Isosource VHP, Probalance, Protain XL
High-calorie, high-protein supplements	Ensure Plus, Nubasics Plus, Nutren 1.5, Resource Plus, Restore Plus
High-fiber supplements	Ensure with Fiber,[a] Nubasics with Fiber, Nutren with Fiber, Sustacal with Fiber
High-calorie, high-nitrogen supplements	Ensure Plus HN, Two Cal HN, Comply, Entrition 1.5, Sustacal Plus, Ultra-Pro
General	Ensure, Ensure Light,[a] Nutrition, Nubasics, Resource, Restore, Sustacal, Boost
Low-fat/clear liquid	Enlive,[a] Resource[a]

Disease specific	
HIV/AIDS	Advera, Lipisorb
Liver disease (cirrhosis, encephalopathy)	Hepatic Aid
Hypermetabolic states (e.g., severe burns, trauma or sepsis)	Perative, Alitraq, Traumacal, Crucial, Impact, Peptamen, Vivonex
Diabetes	Glucerna, Ensure Glucerna OS,[a] Choice DM, Diabetasource, Glytrol, Resource Diabetic
Renal disease (e.g., chronic or acute renal failure)	Nepro, Suplena, Magnacal Renal, Amin-Aid, Renalcal Diet
Chronic obstructive pulmonary disease	Plumocare, Nutrivent, Respalor
Acute respiratory distress syndrome	Oxepa
Malabsorption	Vital HN, Alitraq, Optimental, L-Emental, L-Emental Plus, Peptamen, Lipisorb
Enteral rehydration solutions	Equalyte

Note: This list provides examples of some of the more common categories. It is not intended to be inclusive of all medical nutritional supplements available on the market.

[a]Recommended for oral consumption only.

has special nutrient needs and the patient is under the physician's ongoing care. The label must clearly state that the product is intended to be used to manage a special medical disorder or condition" [25]. Medical foods can be separated into four categories according to the FDA: (1) nutritionally complete formulas that can be used as sole-source nutrition; (2) nutritionally incomplete formulas, i.e., modular products of fat, protein, or carbohydrates; (3) oral rehydration products that are electrolyte/fluid replacements for dehydration; and (4) disease-specific nutritional formulas, which are specifically developed to help manage conditions such as phenylketonuria.

One of the specifications by the FDA definition is that a medical food must be used for special dietary needs and must be managed under the care of a physician. In recent years, oral nutritional beverages have become commercially avail-able due to increasing demand by consumers who use them as meal replacements and supplements as well as for the management of special dietary needs. However, if they are consumed without the supervision of a physician then they do not meet the FDA's definition of a medical food. This definition is important from a regulatory standpoint. For clinical application, the main question is whether a product meets an individual's medical needs. Therefore, to avoid confusion all oral nutritional beverages will be referred to as medical nutritional supplements. Table 2 provides some examples of MNSs and the indicated uses.

Clinicians often think of MNSs as a standard or disease-specific formula. Standard MNSs contain appropriate levels of carbohydrates, protein, and fat and usually at least 25% of the Recommended Dietary Intakes (RDI) for vitamins and minerals per serving. Some can be used as the sole source of

nourishment, while others can be used only as a supplement. Disease-specific, or specialized, formulas may have varying levels of macronutrients and micronutrients as appropriate for the indicated disease state. These formulas may also contain unique ingredients such as structured lipids, special fatty acid blends, prebiotics (e.g., fructooligosaccharides), peptides, protein hydrolysates, and free amino acids (e.g., L-arginine, L-glutamine).

III. PREVALENCE AND ECONOMIC IMPACT OF MEDICAL NUTRITION THERAPY

Despite increasing knowledge of the prevention and treatment of malnutrition, it remains a problem across the continuum of care. The demand for MNT is increasing as more studies indicate that MNT can reduce the costs associated with patient care by decreasing complications [4], mortality and morbidity [26], length of stay in the hospital, readmissions, and recovery time [27]. Improved outcomes result in cost reductions ranging from 35% to 75% [28]. Medical nutrition therapy has become so notably effective that managed care plans are beginning to increase and expand their coverage of MNT interventions [29]. In addition, the Institute of Medicine recently recommended that Congress expand Medicare coverage of nutrition therapy for patients in the home care setting upon referral from a physician [30]. While the significance of MNT is certainly becoming more recognized, it is important for clinicians and researchers to be cognizant of all the demonstrable outcomes of MNT. The following sections will highlight the benefits of oral supplementation in different points of service as well as different disease states.

A. Standard Medical Nutritional Supplements

1. GENERAL MEDICINE/SURGERY
Malnutrition, particularly protein energy malnutrition (PEM), is a common confounding variable in the surgical [16] and general medical patient [17] for reasons such as poor intake as a result of stress, anxiety and NPO status; elevated metabolism and increased nutrient needs required for healing; negative nitrogen balance; and limited activity [16]. Patients who are malnourished have significantly greater mortality and morbidity [5, 31] and are more likely to be readmitted to the hospital [31]. Furthermore, studies suggest that many hospitalized patients do not receive adequate dietary intake [31] and are at risk for further nutritional decline. The continued prevalence of malnutrition in this setting indicates the crucial need for MNSs as a first line of defense in combating malnutrition.

Benefits of postoperative supplementation with a high-protein MNS (1.5 kcal/mL, 0.05 g protein/mL) include improved dietary intake; less weight loss; improved hand grip

strength, which is an indicator of functional status; and fewer postoperative complications [32]. Improvements in weight and lean body mass result in improved functional status and quality of life [13]. A study by Larrson and colleagues [8] reported that the administration of MNSs twice per day to geriatric patients in the medical ward resulted in less weight loss, improved immunocompetence, and improved functional and mobility status. Patients who benefited the most were those who were well nourished at admission.

Being at nutritional risk preoperatively is also associated with poorer outcomes [33]. In a study of patients undergoing total hip replacement, presurgical albumin was an independent indicator of postoperative recovery time. Patients with serum albumin concentrations less than 3.9 g/dL were two times more likely to have longer hospitalizations. It is much easier to prevent nutritional deficiencies rather than correct them along with all of the associated sequelae. However, it is not always feasible to improve nutritional status before a major surgery. But when the surgery is an elective procedure, such as hip or total knee replacements, it is recommended that patients use high-calorie, high-protein MNSs prior to their scheduled surgery to improve outcomes such as recovery and rehabilitation time.

2. HIP FRACTURE
Hip fractures are a common consequence of osteoporosis in older adults. Patients who have had hip fractures have a higher risk of mortality, complications, and rehospitalizations [7, 34]. Hip fractures are a very costly problem for older adults and the health care industry. Protein energy malnutrition often coincides with hip fractures and is thought to contribute to the incidence and complications of hip fractures [34, 35].

Supplementation with MNSs has proven beneficial for patients who are recovering from hip fractures [35–38]. Hip fracture patients who received a daily MNS (254 kcal, 20.4 g protein) experienced a rapid improvement in protein status and had significantly fewer complications ($p<0.05$), reduced mortality ($p<0.02$) and length of stay ($p<0.02$). Research has also demonstrated that high-protein MNSs are more advantageous to this population than standard MNSs. Two studies comparing a high-protein MNS to a standard MNS reported improved laboratory indicators such as serum prealbumin and insulin-like growth factor one; increased bone mineral density; reduced complications; and reduced length of stay in the hospital and rehabilitation in the patients receiving the high-protein MNS [35, 36]. High-protein MNSs in this population improve clinical outcomes and are also cost effective.

3. CEREBRAL VASCULAR ACCIDENT
Mobility and functional and cognitive changes, as a result of a stroke, often impair an individual's ability to eat. Unosson et al. [6] reported that patients who had a recent cerebral vascular accident consumed only 72% of the food served.

Furthermore, many stroke patients often have low serum albumin and body mass index [6, 39]. Research indicates that serum albumin concentration is an independent predictor of mortality among stroke patients and is associated with a greater risk of infections and poor functional outcome [39]. Supplementation with high-protein MNSs improved nutritional intake and nutritional parameters such as albumin and hemoglobin, and also resulted in decreased length of stay and mortality in patients with a recent stroke [40]. Poor nutritional status is also related to longer length of stay in the rehabilitative setting. Malnutrition should be a primary factor addressed in this setting because it is the most likely factor that could be modified to improve functional outcomes [11].

4. LONG-TERM CARE AND HOME CARE

Medical nutritional supplements are often administered to residents in LTC in an effort to combat two of the most serious and prevalent problems: unintentional weight loss and pressure ulcers [41, 42]. It is estimated that more than 1 million individuals develop a pressure ulcer annually [43] with estimated costs as high as $1.3 billion per year to the health care industry [44]. The prevalence of pressure ulcers in LTC and home care is 2.4–23% [45, 46] and 8.7–12.9%, respectively [47]. Nutritional status is a critical factor in both the prevention and treatment of pressure ulcers [9, 20, 43, 48–50]. Low body weight, serum albumin, hemoglobin, and reduced food intake are all correlated positively with the incidence of pressure ulcers [50]. Poor nutritional status also has deleterious implications on healing times of pressure ulcers. A study by Van Rijswijk and Polansky [51] indicated that residents with a suboptimal nutritional status took 20 days longer to heal a pressure ulcer than residents who were well nourished. Many efforts have been made to improve the nutritional status of LTC residents; however, it has been demonstrated that poor intake and unintentional weight loss remain major problems. In a recent study Thomas *et al.* [52] indicated that as many as 40% of LTC residents had poor meal intake and more than 50% had unintentional weight loss.

Evidence exists to support the use of MNSs in LTC residents. Studies demonstrate that MNSs improve dietary intake [20, 22] weight gain/maintenance [20, 53], and wound healing [54]. A multicenter intervention trial demonstrated that patients who received a standard 1800-kcal diet and oral MNSs had a lower incidence of pressure ulcer development [22]. One of the most successful programs in recent years has been the Medication Pass Supplement Program (MPSP). In the MPSP, approximately 2–4 ounces of a nutrient-dense MNS (1.5–2.0 kcal/mL, 13–20 g protein) are distributed 3 times per day with the resident's medications. The consumption of MNSs is documented similar to other medications. Residents do not usually refuse the MNS because they perceive it as part of their medication distributed by their health care professional. Facilities that have implemented

this program have demonstrated weight gain or weight maintenance and reduced weight loss [55–57]. Clinicians anticipate that the MPSP can result in significant cost savings associated with the reduction of the cost of treating a pressure ulcer, savings associated with preventing a pressure ulcer, and savings associated with the minimized waste of MNSs [58].

Delivering a MNS in smaller amounts between meals in programs such as the MPSP is particularly favorable for residents who have a reduced appetite and early satiety. A MNS delivered between meals is less likely to affect the resident's meal intake, which is often a concern of dietitians and physicians in LTC facilities. Turic and colleagues [20] demonstrated that supplementation with MNSs between meals helped residents meet or exceed the RDA without replacing nutrients consumed at meals.

5. ALZHEIMER'S DISEASE

Individuals with Alzheimer's disease commonly have disturbed hunger, thirst, and satiety cues as well as altered sensory perceptions and an impaired ability to feed themselves. Because of these changes, many patients with Alzheimer's disease experience progressive weight loss [59]. Research has also demonstrated that these patients may have low serum levels of specific nutrients, such as folate and vitamin B_{12} [60]. This is significant because deficiencies of these vitamins have been associated with cognitive impairment [60]. Many patients with Alzheimer's disease are often easily distracted and have a tendency to "wander," which may result in increased energy needs and missed meals. While some of these patients are prone to hyperphagia, studies suggest that they do not typically differ in weight from patients who do not overeat, which may indicate that this subset has increased energy needs [61]. It is advantageous to provide MNSs between meals to these patients to help compensate for the dietary intake they may miss at other times. In recent years, some companies have developed alternative forms of supplements such as puddings and bars (Ensure Bars, Nubasics). These alternative forms are useful because these handheld snacks can be easily carried and eaten quickly by the patient who is likely to be distracted or wander.

6. COMMUNITY

Recent studies have indicated that independently living older adults with a body mass index (BMI) less than 22 kg/m^2 are at a much higher risk for all-cause mortality [62] and increased health care expenditures [63, 64]. Those who were at the least risk had a BMI of 24–26 kg/m^2, which is slightly higher than recommended for the general population. Researchers have also demonstrated that low BMI and inadequate dietary intake are associated with diminished functional status among older adults in the community [65, 66]. Low serum albumin has also been implicated as an independent predictor of mortality in this population [67]. In fact, albumin levels lower than 43 g/L (4.3 g/dL), a value considered

to be clinically normal, were associated with increased mortality compared to individuals who had higher albumin levels. These studies indicate that older adults living in the community may benefit from improving their nutritional status to a higher standard than what is recommended for the general public.

Many older adults are involved in meal programs that are delivered to their homes (e.g., Meals on Wheels) or served in a congregate meal setting [68]. Meals provided by such programs provide at least one-third of the RDA for energy and key nutrients. Nevertheless, as many as 33% [69] to 70% [70] of recipients of Meals on Wheels remain at nutritional risk. One way to improve the dietary and nutritional status of these recipients is to add a standard or high-calorie, high-protein MNS (250–355 kcal, 7–13 g protein) to each of the delivered meals. Studies have demonstrated that the addition of a MNS resulted in improved energy and nutrient intakes [23, 66, 71] and weight gain or stabilization [72]. One of these studies also indicated that individuals who received oral MNSs experienced fewer falls than those who did not receive MNSs [72]. This is a great benefit to a population who is at increased risk for falls and hip fractures. Beyond the nutritional benefits of the MNS-enriched meals, the interaction with other individuals provides relief from some of the loneliness and isolation experienced by older adults, both of which are additional risk factors for poor nutritional status [73].

B. Disease-Specific Medical Nutritional Supplements

Many different specialized formulas have been developed for individuals with certain dietary needs. Many of the disease-specific formulas are intended for enteral tube feeding use, however, several can be used as an oral supplement to help manage dietary needs. For some of the disease-specific MNSs, examples of outcomes will be reported from studies of enteral tube feeding.

1. HIV/AIDS

Progressive weight loss, or wasting, is very common in persons with HIV/AIDS. Malnutrition among individuals with human immunodeficiency virus/acquired immunodeficiency syndrome (HIV/AIDS) has been associated with a poor prognosis and increased hospitalizations and costs [74, 75]. The wasting associated with HIV/AIDS is multifactorial and is attributed to anorexia, altered digestion, malabsorption and metabolism, taste alterations, diarrhea and oral lesions.

Patients with HIV-related wasting lose proportionately more lean body mass than fat mass, which is associated with poor survival [75]. Studies of total parenteral nutrition (TPN) and appetite stimulation with megestrol acetate have helped patients gain weight; however, the weight gained is predominantly fat mass [76–79]. Studies have suggested that early enteral tube feeding and supplemental nutrition is beneficial

in patients with HIV/AIDS. However, because many patients suffer from nutrient malabsorption, it is possible that some standard MNSs may exacerbate bowel symptoms in the malabsorbing patient.

Elemental formulas and fat-modified formulas have been proposed as nutrition therapies for these patients. In a study using a specialized medium-chain triglyceride (MCT) formula versus dietary counseling alone, there were trends for improvement in lean body mass and hand-grip strength in the group receiving the specialized MNS [80]. A study by Salomon et al. [81] determined that an elemental formula with hydrolyzed proteins and 70% of fat from MCT was able to help manage patients' diarrhea as evidenced by reduced number of stools and fecal fat. The reduction in diarrhea had major implications on quality of life and activities of daily living.

A study by Chlebowski et al. [82] compared a standard MNS to a disease-specific MNS with hydrolyzed protein, MCT oil, and eicosapentaenoic acid. After 6 months of supplementation, the group receiving the disease-specific MNS had improved weight gain and anthropometric measurements as well as significantly fewer hospitalizations. Patients in both groups had similar dietary intakes, therefore suggesting that those who received the disease-specific MNS were able to utilize the energy and nutrients, whereas those receiving the standard MNS remained in a hypermetabolic state [82].

Each of these studies demonstrated the positive benefits of a disease-specific MNS versus a standard MNS in patients with HIV/AIDS. The malnutrition associated with HIV/AIDS has a variety of different components, and therefore not all specialized MNSs are appropriate. It is important to critically assess the primary symptoms that are responsible for the patient's weight loss and use a MNS that addresses these issues.

2. CANCER

Involuntary weight loss occurs in as many as 50–80% of patients with cancer at some stage in the course of their disease [83]. Poor nutritional status in patients with cancer is associated with increased morbidity and mortality [83, 84], reduced functional status and quality of life [85], reduced response to therapy [86–89] and increased length of stay in the hospital. Similar to HIV/AIDS, weight loss and malnutrition in patients with cancer is multifactorial and may result from diminished intake, increased losses, and altered metabolism. Weight loss in patients with cancer can be grouped into four major categories as outlined in Table 3.

A retrospective chart review of patients with head and neck cancer receiving nutrition support indicated that those who received nutrition support had enhanced immunocompetence, which was positively associated with a 2-year survival [90]. Enteral feeding has also been associated with better adherence to radiation regimens and less weight loss, according to Zogbaum and colleagues [88]. Patients who did not receive enteral supplementation in a study of patients

TABLE 3   Types and Causes of Weight Loss in Patients with Cancer

Type of weight loss	Causes
Mechanical	Due to upper or lower gastrointestinal obstruction that precludes ingestion of food or oral lesions such as stomatitis (e.g., head or neck cancer)
Diminished intake/anorexia	Due to depression, anxiety, fatigue, or pain
Treatment related	Chemotherapy and radiation therapy cause many changes, resulting in decreased food intake and increased losses
	Chemotherapy—anorexia, nausea, vomiting, diarrhea, altered taste and smell, mucositis
	Radiation therapy—anorexia, altered taste, dysphagia, mucositis, stomatitis, enteritis, constipation, fistulas/strictures
Cachexia	Anorexia, early satiety, altered metabolism, weakness

with cancer of the esophagus had significant decreases in body weight and visceral protein status, while those receiving enteral supplementation maintained their nutritional status [91]. These studies demonstrated that enteral supplementation, in patients who would otherwise have reduced or obstructed intake, improved clinical outcomes.

The clinical efficacy of standard oral MNS in the management of patients with cancer remains uncertain [82, 85, 87, 92–94]. A study by Ovesen and colleagues [85] demonstrated that aggressive dietary counseling and oral supplementation in patients with cancer improved nutritional intake but not weight gain. A study of lung and colorectal cancer patients undergoing chemotherapy and radiation reported that nutritional indicators such as serum albumin concentration, and body weight were independently associated with survival. However, there were no differences in outcomes between the groups receiving the supplement or control diet [92]. The authors suggested that the underlying metabolic abnormalities were responsible for the failure of the oral MNS to improve outcomes and that effective interventions could only be developed once the underlying mechanisms were more clearly understood and treated.

The metabolic abnormalities of cancer cachexia distinguish it from other types of weight loss associated with cancer. Due to these abnormalities, patients with cancer cachexia do not respond to standard MNS. Therefore, disease-specific MNSs that target some of the underlying mechanisms are necessary. In recent years, studies have investigated MNSs enriched with novel ingredients such as omega-3 fatty acids, protein hydrolysates, and single amino acids. Omega-3 fatty acids, such as eicosapentaenoic acid, are thought to have immunomodulating and anti-proinflammatory properties.

Cachexia is often accompanied by a prolonged acute phase protein response [95]. This response is characterized by elevated synthesis of C-reactive protein (CRP), haptoglobin, caeruloplasmin, α-1 acid glycoprotein (A1AGP) and α-1 antitrypsin (A1ATP) and decreased synthesis of albumin, prealbumin, and transferrin [94–98]. The acute phase pro-

tein response is an important part of the inflammatory response because it provides proteins that are useful in systemic immunity and tissue repair [95, 99]. Proinflammtory cytokines such as tumor necrosis factor (TNF-α), interleukin 1 (IL-1), interleukin 6 (IL-6), interleukin 8 (IL-8), and leukemia inhibitory factor (LIF) are all probable mediators of the response. In the inflammatory state, these cytokines are produced at the site of malignancy or injury and by a variety of cells throughout the body resulting in local and systemic physiological alterations. Of particular interest in cachexia, the acute phase protein response has been associated with elevated resting energy expenditure among cachectic patients with lung [100] and pancreatic [94] cancer.

Studies of ecosapentaenoic acid (EPA) supplementation have indicated an attenuation of the acute phase protein response [98], which is thought to be modulated by the proinflammatory cytokines. Studies have also shown that EPA supplementation is associated with weight stabilization in patients with pancreatic cancer [101, 102]. Additionally, omega-3 fatty acids have immunomodulatory properties, which are also potentially beneficial to patients with cancer who are undergoing surgical resection [101, 103]. Supplemental amino acids such as arginine and glutamine are thought to improve wound healing and help preserve nitrogen balance [104]. A meta-analysis by Heys *et al.* [105] indicated that a specialized enteral formula enriched with essential fatty acids, RNA, and arginine was associated with reduced infections and hospital length of stay in patients with gastrointestinal cancer, but was not associated with reduced mortality. A study by Barber *et al.* [94] indicated that an EPA-enriched MNS [1.09 g EPA, 0.46 g docosahexanoic acid (DHA)] improves markers and outcomes in cachectic patients with pancreatic cancer. Prior to diagnosis, patients lost an average of 3.2 kg/month. However, after supplementation with the EPA-enriched supplement, a mean weight gain of 1.1 kg was realized at 3 weeks and 2.5 kg at 7 weeks. Analysis of body composition by bioelectrical impedance analysis revealed that the weight gained was predominantly lean

TABLE 4 Macronutrient Compositions of Pulmonary Products

Product	% Energy from carbohydrate	% Energy from protein	% Energy from fat	Energy density (kcal/mL)
Pulmocare	28	16.7	55.2	1.5
Respalor	40	20	40	1.5
Nutrivent	27	18	55	1.5

body mass. In contrast, other cachexia therapies, such as appetite stimulation by megestrol acetate or medroxyprogesterone, increase nutrient intake and weight but the weight gain is primarily adipose tissue. An improvement in lean body mass is significant because restoration of this compartment has been associated with improved quality of life [12, 13]. Supplementation with an EPA-enriched MNS also significantly reduced resting energy expenditure and improved functional status and appetite [94]. Supplementation with EPA alone, via fish oil or pure EPA capsules, has only resulted in weight stabilization, thereby indicating that it is the combination of these factors that is effective in treating cachexia.

Similar to patients with HIV/AIDS, many standard MNSs may exacerbate some gastrointestinal symptoms or fail to address underlying mechanisms of weight loss. Novel ingredients, such as dipeptides, may be better tolerated in some patients with gastrointestinal symptoms [106]. Enteral and oral supplementation with standard MNSs can improve nutritional status if there are not underlying metabolic abnormalities. However, in cachectic patients, underlying metabolic abnormalities must be ameliorated in conjunction with supplying adequate nutrition.

3. CHRONIC OBSTRUCTIVE PULMONARY DISEASE

According to the Centers for Disease Control [107], chronic obstructive pulmonary diseases (COPD) are the fourth largest cause of death in the United States. Projections indicate that mortality from COPD will continue to rise globally over the next 20 years [108]. Malnutrition, ranging from 19% to 74% in patients with COPD, is dependent on the severity of illness and whether the patient is hospitalized [109,110]. Factors contributing to malnutrition include reduced intake due to dyspnea and early satiety and anorexia, elevated resting energy expenditure, metabolic abnormalities, and the effects of pharmacologic agents [111, 112]. Poor nutritional status in the COPD patient further compromises pulmonary structure and function. Malnutrition in COPD patients also has adverse consequences on clinical outcomes such as ventilator requirements [110, 113], intensive care unit days, decreased functional status, quality of life, and mortality [114].

Studies of nutrition support in patients with COPD have produced mixed results. A summary of studies indicated that nutrition support resulted in improved pulmonary function only in the studies where weight also improved [111]. A

study by Efthimiou et al. 115] indicated that oral supplementation resulted in weight gain and improved walking distance and dyspnea scores. Individuals who responded to nutritional support were also more likely to be weaned from ventilators sooner than those with a poorer nutritional status [116, 117].

Patients with COPD have impaired gas exchange resulting in hypercapnia, high levels of circulating CO_2 in the blood, which requires increased ventilation, or work from the lungs, to expel it. Research has demonstrated that hypermetabolism in patients with pulmonary diseases is associated with increased ventilation. Disease-specific MNSs target impaired gas exchange and try to regulate it. The composition of pulmonary disease-specific formulas are depicted in Table 4.

Disease-specific formulas for patients with COPD are typically higher in fat because fat yields the lowest respiratory quotient (RQ). Studies of both normal subjects and patients with COPD have indicated that pulmonary ventilation, VCO_2, and oxygen consumption are all elevated after a high carbohydrate load [118]. Therefore, a MNS higher in fat is more advantageous for these patients.

Comparison studies between low carbohydrate/high-fat MNSs and standard MNSs have shown improved respiratory function [119] and reduced VCO_2 and RQ [120–122], and reduced use of mechanical ventilation [123]. A study by Frankfort and associates [122] also suggested that low-carbohydrate/high-fat MNSs may help manage postprandial dyspnea, which is sometimes associated with pulmonary diseases.

In addition to the macronutrient distribution, it is also important not to overfeed patients with COPD because excessive energy intake can lead to lipogenesis, which results in large amounts of CO_2 production. A study by Talpers et al. [124] compared three isocaloric TPN formulas of varying carbohydrate content (40%, 60%, and 75% of energy) in patients with ventilators. There were no differences in CO_2 production among the three groups. In a second group of mechanically ventilated patients receiving a TPN formula providing 60% energy from carbohydrate, 20% energy from protein, and 20% energy from fat at varying caloric levels, those who received the highest caloric level (2.0 times the estimated resting energy expenditure) had the highest CO_2 production. A similar study by Van den Berg and Stam [123] demonstrated that pulmonary function parameters were

TABLE 5   Macronutrient Composition of Common Specialty Products for Diabetes

Product	% Energy from carbohydrate	% Energy from protein	% Energy from fat	% of total fat present as monounsaturated fatty acids
Glucerna	34.3	16.7	49	69.8
Diabetasource	36	20	44	65
Resource DM	36	24	40	n/a

significantly better in patients receiving enteral formulas at 1.5 times versus 2.0 times the measured resting energy expenditure. Clinical opinions vary on the most appropriate feeding regimens for patients with COPD. However, studies have demonstrated that high-fat/low-carbohydrate MNSs improve biochemical parameters in COPD patients. While similar results may be achieved by varying the caloric content, it is important to recognize that many patients with COPD are malnourished and would benefit from nutritional repletion. Therefore feeding at 1.5–2.0 times the measured resting energy expenditure is sometimes necessary.

Disease-specific pulmonary MNSs have also been beneficial for patients with cystic fibrosis (CF). Nutritional status is correlated with survival among patients with CF. A study by Kane and Hobbs [125] demonstrated that resting energy expenditure in CF patients increases as pulmonary disease progresses. In this study, the low-carbohydrate/high-fat MNS was compared to a high-carbohydrate/low-fat commercial supplement. Patients who received the low-carbohydrate/high-fat MNS experienced smaller increases in VCO_2, RQ, and minute ventilation. Similar results were also demonstrated when the disease-specific MNS was compared to a medium-carbohydrate and a high-carbohydrate MNS during nighttime enteral feedings [126]. Because patients with CF often experience pancreatic insufficiency as their disease progresses, pancreatic enzymes were provided to reduce the incidence of steatorrhea with the higher fat MNS. In addition, the higher proportion of MCT oil (20–40%) in these formulas is beneficial for more effective fat absorption in patients with CF.

4. DIABETES MELLITUS

Diabetes mellitus (DM) is the sixth leading cause of death in the United States and a major contributing factor to micro- and macrovascular conditions including cardiovascular diseases, vision problems, nerve damage, and renal disease. Diabetes is classified as either type 1, resulting from inadequate insulin production and secretion, or type 2, resulting from cellular resistance to the action of insulin. Although diabetes is a condition characterized by multiple metabolic abnormalities, results from the Diabetes Control and Complications Trial (DCCT) and the United Kingdom Prospective Diabetes Study (UKPDS) indicated that glucose control is the most important factor with respect to short- and long-term complications [127, 128]. Glucose regulation can be achieved through nutrition therapy, exercise, and medications such as oral hypoglycemic agents, antihyperglycemic agents, and insulin. Successful lifestyle modifications for patients with type 2 diabetes can delay or ameliorate the need for more expensive and complicated medical therapies including pharmaceutical treatments and interventions related to diabetes complications.

Standard MNSs administered enterally to individuals with DM can have adverse effects on glycemic control because they have rapid gastric emptying and absorption, which can lead to unpredictable glucose excursions in the patient with diabetes. Therefore, DM specialty products have been specifically designed to manage the occurrence of hyperglycemia. Characteristics of many DM-specific formulas include a reduced carbohydrate level, especially simple sugars (except fructose); high monounsaturated fatty acids (MUFA); high fiber; and elevated antioxidants. Special ingredients such as fructose, MUFAs, and fiber all reduce glycemic response and therefore help control blood glucose levels. One of the main criticisms is the high level of fat, which typically ranges from 40% to 50% of total calories (Table 5). Individuals with DM are at risk for cardiovascular diseases (CVD), therefore the concern over elevated lipid levels is justified. However, many of the products contain a high level of MUFAs, which have been demonstrated to help improve lipoprotein levels [129–132]. Furthermore, the fatty acid profiles of many of the formulas comply with the American Heart Association guidelines of ≤30% total energy from total fat and ≤10% energy from saturated fat.

The clinical benefits of DM-specialty MNSs have been demonstrated in both type 1 and type 2 DM [133–135]. These studies demonstrated controlled glucose responses and less urinary glucose loss among patients receiving the disease-specific formulas. Reduced carbohydrate formulas have also been beneficial in patients with an acute head injury who were likely to develop stress-induced hyperglycemia. The administration of a DM-specialty product helped maintain normal glucose and eliminated the need for insulin administration [136].

The DM-specific MNS has also been studied as a replacement to typical solid-food snacks served to LTC residents. In

this study the DM-specific MNS was compared to typical snacks and standard MNS. Blood glucose was much higher in the residents who received the standard MNS, but was not different between the DM-specific MNS and a typical snack [137], indicating that DM-specific MNS can be a good alternative for residents who have diminished dietary intake. The MSPS can also be implemented in patients with DM. Many of the 2.0 kcal/ ml MNSs are high in fat and actually have a similar composition to DM-specific MNSs.

Studies have been conducted to compare the clinical efficacy of the various DM-specific formulas. When the formulas were compared as enteral feedings or oral MNS, there was no difference observed between glucose or insulin curves [134, 135]. Similar results were also observed when different formulas were used for glucose tolerance tests [138]. The predominant difference in these formulas is that they vary in total fat content from 40% to 50% of energy. To determine whether the high-fat formula has any deleterious effects on serum lipid levels, a comparison was made between a standard MNS and a DM-specific MNS. There were no significant differences in the lipid levels between the two groups [139], which may be attributed to the high level of MUFA.

Until recently, none of the MNSs was designated to be specifically administered as snacks or meal replacements. Therefore, enteral supplements were often consumed as supplements. These formulas were clinically effective; however, they were not as palatable as those that have been developed for oral consumption. Recently a number of DM-specific MNSs, specifically intended for oral consumption, have become available in liquid and bar forms. The liquid MNSs have modified carbohydrate levels, are high in MUFAs, meet current guidelines for fatty acid profile, and have moderate to high levels of dietary fiber. Clinical studies indicate that these oral MNSs lower blood glucose compared with standard MNSs [140]. Bars that are specifically formulated to control postprandial blood glucose contain moderate levels of fiber and/or resistant starch. These ingredients help to delay glycemic excursions by delaying gastric emptying. Additional benefits of these bars and oral MNS include a known nutrient content and ready-to-use packaging.

The clinical efficacy of disease-specific products for individuals with DM has been demonstrated effectively in the aforementioned studies. However, limited studies have demonstrated improved outcomes, which are of much interest in the current health care environment. One study has demonstrated the clinical outcomes of a disease-specific MNS versus a standard enteral formula. Residents who received the disease-specific MNS had a reduced incidence of infections (e.g., cellulitis, pneumonia, urinary tract, pressure ulcers) and reduced utilization of insulin and oral hypoglycemic agents as well as better glucose and lipid levels [129]. More studies such as this one need to be performed to help indicate the benefit of disease-specific MNSs.

5. RENAL DISEASE

Individuals with renal disease are likely to become malnourished in the course of their disease. Similar to other disease states, malnutrition is associated with an increased risk of morbidity and mortality among these patients. Dietary modifications are often imposed to help prevent the progression of renal failure and/or manage symptoms of renal failure. Dietary modifications include high energy and protein, fluid, and electrolyte restrictions, as well as maintaining a strict balance between calcium and phosphorus intake. Renal patients often have an inadequate dietary intake [141] that may be attributed to their limited diets. Furthermore, dietary intake may be affected by symptoms of the disease such as nausea, vomiting, anorexia, and fatigue.

The goal of MNT for the renal patient is dependent on disease stage, whether they are undergoing dialysis, and which type of dialysis (hemodialysis or peritoneal dialysis). For patients with chronic renal failure, the goal is to maintain nutritional status and manage uremia without compromising renal function. Patients who are unable to meet their dietary needs may benefit from a disease-specific MNS intended for the predialysis patient. Formulas are energy dense (2.0 kcal/ mL); low in protein, fluids, and electrolytes; and have vitamin and mineral profiles specifically developed for renal patients. Patients who are receiving dialysis have a more liberalized diet with respect to protein; however, these individuals would still benefit from MNS. Formulas intended for patients on dialysis are also energy dense (2.0 kcal/mL), have a moderate level of protein, contain restricted fluids and vitamin and mineral profiles specifically for dialysis patients.

There have been very few clinical trials of enteral or oral supplementation among renal patients for several reasons including very few patients per site and a preference of the patient and physician for TPN. In one study, clinical benefits were demonstrated in patients on hemodialysis using an orally administered disease-specific formula versus a standard formula. In this study, all of the MNSs were well tolerated and there was a significant improvement in serum calcium and phosphorus with disease-specific versus standard MNSs. Hyperphosphatemia is often a limiting symptom to MNS administration. Therefore, this benefit is clinically important because it indicated a way to improve nutritional status without compromising other biochemical parameters [142]. Cockram *et al.* [143] also investigated the effects of a nutrient-dense MNS on patients with chronic renal failure (CRF) who were not undergoing dialysis. Patients were randomized to receive the disease-specific MNS or an isocaloric supplement of glucose polymers. At baseline the dietary intake was well below recommendations for patients with CRF. Supplementation with a disease-specific MNS improved energy intake by 54–58%. Food intake did not change, indicating that the MNS did not displace meal intake.

Renal MNSs have been developed to meet very specific nutrient levels within very selected ranges.

TABLE 6   Tips for Consuming Medical Nutritional Supplements

Tips	Rationale
Drink MNS with a straw and in a closed container	• Straws help direct MNS to the back of the throat for easier swallowing and may help bypass some taste receptors. • Closed containers help minimize aroma, which is helpful for patients with nausea or undergoing chemotherapy.
Freeze product and eat with a spoon	• Colder temperatures minimize aroma. • Varied texture is soothing, which is helpful for individuals with mouth lesions (from chemotherapy or radiation).
Add extracts, spices, flavorings	• Combats flavor fatigue.
Consume MNS between meals	• Less likely to affect appetite at meals.

IV. BARRIERS TO USING MEDICAL NUTRITIONAL SUPPLEMENTS

A. Cost

Cost can be a barrier to MNS; however, many individuals who require MNSs as part of their therapy can be reimbursed by third-party carriers. In the acute or LTC settings, MNSs are covered in room and board costs. Reimbursement for specialty products are even stronger under the diagnosis-related groups and the prospective payment system. Home care patients and consumers are expected to pay for MNSs as they would any other food. There are exceptions to this policy, which include patients who have special medical or financial needs. These individuals are reimbursed through local and state programs such as Medicaid.

The cost of an MNS typically varies and is dependent on whether it is a standard or disease-specific MNS. Disease-specific MNSs are typically more expensive because of specialized ingredients, and often more extensive clinical research is undertaken to validate their use. Studies referenced in this chapter have demonstrated the cost effectiveness of MNSs in terms of improved outcomes, such as decreased complications, medications (i.e., insulin, phosphate blockers), readmissions, and length of stay. Therefore, although cost is a concern for many individuals and health care plans, medical nutrition therapy should not be an area of neglect.

B. Taste

Taste is a very important consideration because it influences patient and consumer compliance with MNSs. Nutritional companies are aware of how important the taste of MNSs is and therefore strive to formulate and reformulate their products to deliver the most palatable product. In addition, many oral MNSs are available in a variety of flavors to prevent flavor fatigue, a common complaint among patients. While taste is a very important factor, some MNSs may not always be palatable to patients. Disease-specific formulas often contain unique, novel ingredients that contribute to their efficacy but may detract from their taste. As health care professionals, it is important to help patients understand that this is an important part of their therapy. Recognizing MNT as part of a therapeutic regimen helps patients adhere to their treatment because they view it as something they should be taking, similar to other medications. Table 6 contains some suggestions that may help with patient compliance.

V. SUMMARY

Medical nutritional supplements cost effectively improve outcomes across the continuum of care as well as in different disease states. Disease-specific MNSs are specifically formulated and scientifically studied to effectively help manage symptoms and improve outcomes. Concerns that MNSs displace energy and nutrients from meals have not been substantiated by the research reviewed in this chapter. Medical nutritional supplements are convenient and provide an alternative to meals when time or medical symptoms are an issue. Demonstration of improved outcomes with MNSs is an exciting area of research and can add to the health care provider's arsenal of effective disease management options.

References

1. White, J. V. (1997). "The Role of Nutrition in Chronic Disease Care." The Nutrition Screening Initiative.
2. Dychtwald, K. (1999). 'Age power': How the new-old will transform medicine in the 21st century. *Geriatrics* **54**, 22–27.
3. Sullivan, D. H. (1992). Risk factors for early hospital readmission in a select population of geriatric rehabilitation patients: The significance of nutritional status. *J. Am. Geriatr. Soc.* **40**, 792–798.
4. Woo, J., Ho, S. C., Mak, Y. T., Law, L. K., and Cheng, A. (1994). Nutritional status of elderly patients during recovery from chest infection and the role of nutritional supplementation assessed by a prospective randomized single-blind trial. *Age and Aging* **23**, 40–48.
5. Sullivan, D. H., and Walls, R. C. (1998). Protein-energy undernutrition and the risk of mortality within six years of hospital discharge. *J. Am. College Nutr.* **17**, 571–578.

6. Unosson, M., Larsson, J., Ek, A. C., and Bjurulf, P. (1992). Effects of dietary supplements on functional condition and clinical outcome measured with a modified Norton scale. *Clin. Nutr.* **11,** 134–139.

7. Wolinsky, F. D., Fitzgerald, J. F., and Stump, T. E. (1997). The effect of hip fracture on mortality, hospitalization and functional status: A prospective study. *Am. J. Public Health* **87,** 398–403.

8. Larsson, J., Unosson, M., Ek, A. C., Nilson, L., Thorslund, S., and Bjurulf, P. (1990). Effect of dietary supplement on nutritional status and clinical outcome in 501 geriatric patients—A randomized study. *Clin. Nutr.* **9,** 179–184.

9. Breslow, R. A., Hallfrisch, J., Guy, D. G., Crawley, B., and Goldberg, A. P. (1993). The importance of dietary protein in healing pressure ulcers. *J. Am. Geriatr. Soc.* **41,** 357–362.

10. Shaw-Stiffel, T. A., Zarny, L. A., Pleban, W. E., Rosman, D. D., Rudolph, R. A., and Bernstein, L. H. (1993). Effect of nutrition status and other factors on length of hospital stay after major gastrointestinal surgery. *Nutrition* **9,** 140–145.

11. Finestone, H. M., Greene-Finestone, L. S., Wilson, E. S., and Teasell, R. W. (1997). Prolonged length of stay and reduced functional improvement rate in malnourished stroke rehabilitation patients. *Arch. Phys. Med. Rehabil.* **77,** 340–345.

12. Larrson, J., Akerlind, I., Permeth, J., and Ornquist, J. O. (1994). The relation between nutritional status and quality of life in surgical patients. *Eur. J. Surg.* **160,** 329–334.

13. Jamieson, C. P., Norton, B., Lakeman, M., and Powell-Tuck, J. (1997). The quantitative effect of nutrition support on quality of life in outpatients. *Clin. Nutr.* **16,** 25–28.

14. Butterworth, C. E. (1974). The skeleton in the hospital closet. *Nutr. Today* March/April, 4–8.

15. McWhirter, J. P., Pennington, C. R. (1994). Incidence and recognition of malnutrition in hospital. *Br. Med. J.* **308,** 945–948.

16. Edington, J., Kon, P., and Martyn, C. N. (1997). Prevalence of malnutrition after major surgery. *J. Hum. Nutr. Dietet.* **10,** 111–116.

17. Naber, T. H. J., Schermer, T., de Bree, A., Nusteling, K., Eggink, L., Kruimel, J. W., Bakkeren, J., van Heereveld, H., and Katan, M. B. (1997). Prevalence of malnutrition in non-surgical hospitalized patients and its association with disease complications. *Am. J. Clin. Nutr.* **66,** 1232–1239.

18. Nelson, K. J., Coulston, A. M., Sicher, K. P., and Tseng, R. Y. (1993). Prevalence of malnutrition in the elderly admitted to long-term care facilities. *J. Am. Dietet. Assoc.* **93,** 459–461.

19. Keller, H. H. (1993). Malnutrition in institutionalized elderly: How and why? *J. Am. Geriatr. Soc.* **41,** 1212–1218.

20. Turic, A., Gordon, K. L., Craig, L. D., Ataya, D. G., and Voss, A. C. (1998). Nutrition supplementation enables elderly residents of long-term care facilities to meet or exceed RDAs without displacing intakes from meals. *J. Am. Dietet. Assoc.* **98,** 1457–1459.

21. Edington, J., Kon, P., and Martyn. C. N. (1996). Prevalence of malnutrition in patients in general practice. *Clin. Nutr.* **15,** 60–63.

22. Bourdel-Marchasson, I., Barateau, M., Rondeau, V., Dequae-Merchadou, L., Sales-Montaudon, N., Emeriau, J. P., Manciet, G., and Dartigues, J. F. (2000). A multi-center trial of the effects of oral nutritional supplementation in critically ill older inpatients. *Nutrition* **16,** 1–5.

23. Ryan A. S., Craig, L. D., and Finn, S. C. (1992). Nutrient intakes and dietary patterns of older Americans: A national study. *J. Gerontol.* **47,** M145–M150.

24. Yamaguchi, L. Y., Coulston, A. M., Lu, N. C., Dixon, L. B., and Craig, L. D. (1998). Improvement in nutrient intake by elderly meals-on-wheels participants receiving a liquid nutrition supplement. *Nutr. Today* **33,** 37–44.

25. *Federal Register* (November 29, 1996). **61,** 231.

26. Gariballa, S. E., Parker, S. G., Taub, N., and Castleden, M. (1998). Nutritional status of hospitalized acute stroke patients. *Br. J. Nutr.* **79,** 481–487.

27. The American Dietetic Association (1995). Position of the American Dietetic Association: Cost effectiveness of medical nutrition therapy. *J. Am. Dietet. Assoc.* **95,** 91–99.

28. Gallagher-Allred, C. R., Voss, A. C., Finn, S. C., and Mc-Camish, M. A. (1996). Malnutrition and clinical outcomes: The case for medical nutrition therapy. *J. Am, Dietet. Assoc.* **96,** 366–369.

29. Gilbreath, J. L., and Biesemeier, C. (1999). Medical nutrition therapy: A powerful tool in disease management. *Am. J. Managed Care* **5,** 81–86.

30. Report of the Institute of Medicine, National Academy of Sciences. (December 15, 1999). The role of nutrition in maintaining health in the nations elderly—Evaluating coverage of nutrition services for the Medicare population.

31. Sullivan, D. H., Sun, S., and Walls, R. C. (1999). Protein-energy undernutrition among elderly hospitalized patients. *JAMA* **281,** 2013–2019.

32. Keele, A. M,, Bray, M. J., Emery, P. W., Duncan, H. D., and Silk, D. B. A. (1997). Two phase randomized controlled clinical trial of postoperative oral dietary supplements in surgical patients. *Gut* **40,** 393–399.

33. Del Savio, G. C., Zelicof, S. B., Wexler, L. M., Byrne, D. W., Reddy, P. D., Fish, D., and Ende, K. A. (1996). Preoperative nutritional status and outcome of elective total hip replacement. *Clin. Orthoped. Rel. Res.* **326,** 153–161.

34. Patterson, B. M., Cornell, C. N., Carbone, B., Levine, B., and Chapman, D. (1992). Protein depletion and metabolic stress in elderly patients who have a fracture of the hip. *J. Bone Joint Surg. Inc.* **74A,** 251–260.

35. Bonjour, J. P., Rapin, C. H., Rizzoli, R., Tkatch, L., Selmi, M., Chevalley, T., Nydegger, V., Slosman, D., and Vassey, H. (1992). Hip fracture, femoral bone mineral density and protein supply in elderly patients. *Nutr. Elderly* **29,** 151–159.

36. Tkatch, L., Rapin, C. H., Rizzoli, R., Slosman, D., Nydegger, V., Vasey, H., and Bonjour, J. P. (1992). Benefits of oral protein supplementation in elderly patients with fracture of the proximal femur. *J. Am. Col. Nutr.* **11,** 515–519.

37. Schurch, M. A., Rizzoli, R., Slosman, D., Vadas, L., Vergnaud, P., and Bonjour, J. P. (1998). Protein supplements increase serum insulin-lie growth factor-I levels and attenuate proximal femur bone loss in patients with recent hip fracture. *Ann. Intern. Med.* **128,** 801–809.

38. Delmi, M., Rapin, C. H., Bengoa, J. M., Delmas, J. M., Vasey, H., and Bonjour, J. P. (1990). Dietary supplementation in elderly patients with fracture neck of the femur. *Lancet* **335,** 1013–1016.

39. Gariballa, S. E., Parker, S. G., Taub, N., and Castleden, C. M. (1998). A randomized, controlled, single-blind trial of

nutritional supplementation after acute stroke. *J. Parenteral Enteral Nutr.* **22,** 315–319.

40. Gariballa, S. E., Parker, S. G., Taub, N., and Castleden, C. M. (1998). Nutritional status of hospitalized acute stroke patients. *Brit. J. Nutr.* **79,** 481–487.

41. Kayser-Jones, J., Schell, E. S., Porter, C., Barbaccia, J. C., Steinbaugh, C., Bird, W. F., Redford, M., and Pengilly, K. (1998). A prospective study of the use of liquid oral dietary supplements in nursing homes. *J. Am. Geriatr. Soc.* **46,** 1278–1286.

42. Gilmore, S. A., Robinson, G., Posthauer, M. E., and Raymond, J. (1995). Clinical indicators associated with unintentional weight loss and pressure ulcers in elderly residents of nursing facilities. *J. Am. Diet. Assoc.* **95,** 984–992.

43. Bergstrom, N., Bennett, M. A., and Carlson, C. E. (1994). "Pressure Ulcer Treatment. Clinical Practice Guideline No. 15." AHCPR Publication No. 95-0652. U. S. Department of Health and Human Services, Public Health Service, Agency for Health Care Policy and Research. Rockville, MD.

44. Miller H., and Delozier, J. (1994). "Cost Implications of the Pressure Ulcer Treatment Guideline," Contract No. 282-91-0070. Agency for Health Care Policy and Research. Center for Health Policy Studies, Columbia, MD.

45. Peterson, N. C., and Bittman, S. (1971). The epidemiology of pressure sores. *Scand. J. Plast. Resonstr. Surg.* **5,** 62–66.

46. Langemo, D. K., Olson, B., Hunter, S., Burd, C., Hansen, D., and Cath-Silbererg, T. (1989). Incidence of pressure sores in acute care, rehabilitation, extended care, home health, and hospice in one locale. *Decubitus* **2,** 42.

47. Clarke, M., and Kadhom, H. M. (1988). The nursing prevention of pressure sores in hospital and community patients. *J. Adv. Nurs.* **13,** 365–373.

48. Olson, B., Langemo, D., Burd, C., Hanson, D., Hunter, S., amd Cathcart-Silberberg, T. (1996). Pressure ulcer incidence in an acute care setting. *Wound, Ostomo, Contin. Nurs.* **23,** 15–22.

49. Maklebust, J., and Sieggreen. M. Y. (1996). "Pressure Ulcers: Guidelines for Prevention and Nursing Management," 2nd Ed. Springhouse Corp. Springhouse, PA.

50. Breslow, R. A., Hallfrisch, J., Guy, D. G., Crawley, B., and Goldberg A. P. (1993). The importance of dietary protein in healing pressure ulcers. *J. Amer. Geriatr. Soc.* **41,** 357–362.

51. Van Risjwijk, L., and Polansky, M. (1994). Predictors of time to healing deep pressure ulcers. *Ostomy/Wound Manag.* **40,** 40–48.

52. Thomas, S., Bender, S. A., Charkey, S., and Horn, S. (1998, October). Preliminary nutrition findings from the long-term care pressure ulcer study. Poster 2627. The American Dietetic Association 81st Annual Meeting and Exhibition, Kansas City.

53. Johnson, L. E., Dooley, P. A., and Gleick, J. B. (1993). Oral nutritional supplement use in elderly nursing home patients. *J. Am. Geriatr. Soc.* **41,** 947–952.

54. Himes, D. (1997). Nutritional supplements in the treatment of pressure ulcers: Practical perspectives. *Adv. Wound Care* Jan./Feb., 30–31.

55. Robinson, G. E. (1997). Prevent weight loss . . . push calories with meds. *Qual. Manag. Outcomes Res. Prof. Pract.* **97,** 9.

56. Lewis, D. A., and Boyle, K. D. (1998). Nutritional supplements use during medication administration: Selected case studies. *J. Nutr. Elderly* **4,** 53–59.

57. Grover, L. R., Harris, L., Tubinus, P., Norman, F., and Ferraro, C. (1998). Success of a nutritional medpass program (NMP) in long term care centers. *In* "22nd ASPEN Annual Meeting" Vol. **13,** pp. 1, 53.

58. Chang, B. (1997). "The Two-Cal HN Med Pass Program: A Medically Effective Cost-Avoidance Tool for Long-Term Care Facilities in a Managed Care Era." Ross Products Division, Abbott Laboratories.

59. Finley, B. (1997). Nutrition needs of the person with Alzheimer's disease: Practical approaches to quality care. *J. Am. Dietet. Assoc.* **97,** S177–S180.

60. Renvall, M. J., Spindler, A. A., Ramsdell, J. W., and Paskvan, M. (1989). Nutritional status of free-living Alzheimer's patients. *Am. J. Med. Sci.* **298,** 20–27.

61. Smith, G., Vigen, V., Evans, J., Fleming, K., and Bohac, D. (1998). Patterns and associates of hyperphagia in patients with dementia. *Neurops. Neuropsychol. Behav. Neurol.* **11,** 97–102.

62. Allison, D. B., Gallagher, D., Heo, M., Pi-Sunyer, F. X., and Heymsfield, S. B. (1997). Body mass index and all-cause mortality among people age 70 and over: The Longitudinal Study of Aging. *Int. J. Obes.* **21,** 424–431.

63. Blaum, C., Dorris, J., Lee, J., Roehrig, C., and Voss, A. C. (1998, May). *Evaluation of body mass index and health care utilization using the longitudinal study of aging.* Poster p53. Presented at American Geriatric Society Annual Meeting, Seattle, Washington.

64. Mayer, K. E., Blaum, C., Thomas, D. R., Lee, J., Rowe, D. R., and Voss, A. C. (1999, March). *Do malnourished patients use more health care resources?* Poster 1. Presented at Annual Symposium of the American Medical Directors Association, Orlando, Florida.

65. Galanos, A. N., Pieper, C. F., Cornoni-Huntley, J. C., Bales, C. W., and Fillenbaum, G. C. (1994). Nutrition and function: Is there a relationship between body mass index and the other functional capabilities of community-dwelling elderly. *J. Am. Geriatr. Soc.* **42,** 368–373.

66. Gray-Donald, K., Payette, H., and Boutier, V. (1995). Randomized clinical trial of nutritional supplementation shows little effect on functional status among free-living frail elderly. *J. Nutr.* **125,** 2965–2971.

67. Corti, M. C., Guralnik, J. M., Salivev, M. E., and Sorkin J. D. (1994). Serum albumin level and physical disability as predictors of mortality in older persons. *JAMA* **272,** 1036–1042.

68. Weddle, D. O., Wellman, N. S., and Bates, G. M. (1997). Incorporating nutrition screening into three Older Americans Act elderly nutrition programs. *J. Nutr. Elderly* **17,** 19–37.

69. Coulston, A. M., Craig, L. D., and Voss A. C. (1996). Meals-on-Wheels applicants are a population at risk for poor nutritional status. *J. Am. Dietet. Assoc.* **96,** 570–573.

70. Stevens, D. A., Grivetti, L. E., and McDonald, R. B. (1992). Nutrient intake of urban and rural elderly receiving home delivered meals. *J. Am. Dietet. Assoc.* **92,** 714–718.

71. Lipschitz, D. A., Mitchell, C. O., Steel, R. W., and Milton, K. Y. (1985). Nutritional evaluation and supplementation of elderly subjects participating in a "Meals-on-Wheels" program. *J. Parenteral Enteral Nutro.* **9,** 343–347.

72. Gray-Donald, K., Payette, H., Boutier, V., and Page, S. (1994). Evaluation of the dietary intake of homebound elderly and the feasibility of dietary supplementation. *J. Am. Col. Nutr.* **13**(3), 277–284.

73. Walker, D., and Beauchene, R. E. (1991). The relationship of loneliness, social isolation, and physical health to dietary adequacy of independently-living elderly. *J. Am. Dietet. Assoc.* **91,** 300–304.

74. Chlebowski, R. T., Grosvenor, M. B., Bernard, N. H., Morales, L. S., and Bulcavage, L. M. (1989). Nutritional status, gastrointestinal dysfunction and survival in patients with AIDS. *Am. J. Gastroenterol.* **84,** 1288–1293.

75. Kotler, D. P., Tierney, A. R., Wang, J., and Pierson, R. N. (1989). Magnitude of body-cell-mass depletion and the timing of death from wasting in AIDS. *Am. J. Clin. Nutr.* **50,** 444–447.

76. Grunfeld, C., and Feingold, K. R. (1992). Metabolic disturbances and wasting in the acquired immunodeficiency syndrome. *N. Engl. J. Med.* **327,** 329–337.

77. Hellerstein, M. K., Wu, K., Grunfeld, C., Christiansen, M., Kaempfer, S., Kletke, C., amd Skackleton, C. H. L. (1991). Increased hepatic lipogenesis in HIV infection. Nutritional implications and relation to circulating cytokines. *Clin. Res.* **39,** 149A.

78. Oster, M. H., Enders, S. R., Samuels, S. J., Cone, L. A., Hooton, T. M., Browder, H. P., and Flynn N. M. (1994). Megestrol acetate in patients with AIDS and cachexia. *Ann. Intern. Med.* **121,** 400–408.

79. Hoh, R., Pelfini, A., Neese, R. A., Chan, M., Cello, J. P., Cope, F. O., Abbruzzese, B. C., Richards, E. W., Courtney, K., and Hellerstein, M. K. (1998). De novo lipogenesis predicts short-term body composition response by bioelectrical impedance analysis to oral nutritional supplements in HIV-wasting. *Am. J. Clin. Nutr.* **68,** 154–163.

80. Rabeneck, L., Palmer, A., Knowles, J. B., Seidehamel, R. J., Harris, C. L., Merkel, K. L., Risser, J. M. H., and Akrrabawi, S. S. (1998). A randomized controlled trial evaluating nutrition counseling with or without oral supplementation in malnourished HIV-infected patients. *J. Am. Dietet. Assoc.* **98,** 434–438.

81. Salomon, S., Jung, J., Voss, T., Suguitan, A., Rowe, B. M., and Madsen, D. (1998). An elemental diet containing medium-chain triglycerides and enzmatically hydrolyzed protein can improve gastrointestinal tolerance in people infected with HIV. *J. Am. Dietet. Assoc.* **98,** 460–462.

82. Chlebowski, R. T., Beall, G., Grosvenor, M., Lillington, L., Weintraub, N., Ambler, C., Richards, E. W., Abbruzzese, B. C., McCamish, M. A., and Cope, F. O. (1993). Long-term effects of early nutritional support with new enterotropic peptide-based formula vs. standard enteral formula in HIV-infected patients: Randomized prospective trial. *Nutrition* **9,** 507–512.

83. DeWys, W. D., Begg, C., Lavin, P. T., Band, P. R., Bennett, J. M., Bertino, J. R., Cohen, M. H., Douglass, H. O., Engstrom, P. F., Ezdinli, E. Z., Horton, J., Johnson, G. J., Moertel, C. G., Oken, M. M., Perlia, C., Rosenbaum, C., Silverstein, M. N., Skeel, R. T., Sponzo, R. W., and Tormey, D. C. (1980). Prognostic effects of weight loss prior to chemotherapy in cancer patients. *Am. J. Med.* **69,** 491–497.

84. Chlebowski, R. T., Palomares, M. R., Lillington, L., and Grosvenor, M. (1996). Recent implications of weight loss in lung cancer management. *Nutrition* **12,** S43–S47.

85. Ovesen, L., Allingstrup, L., Hannibal, J., Mortensen, E. L., and Hansen, O. P. (1993). Effect of dietary counseling on food intake, body weight, response rate, survival and quality of life in cancer patients undergoing chemotherapy: A prospective randomized study. *J. Clin. Oncol.* **11,** 2043–2049.

86. Menck, H. R., Jessup, M., Eyre, H. J., Cunningham, M. P., Fremgen, A., Murphy, G. P., and Winchester, D. P. (1997). *CA Cancer J. Clinicians* **47,** 161–170.

87. VanEys, J. (1982). Effect of nutritional status on response to therapy. *Cancer Res.* **42** (suppl.) 747–753.

88. Zogbaum, A. T., Farkas, S., and Dufy, V. B. (1996, October) *Enteral feedings are associated with improved adherence to radiation treatment prescription and weight maintenance in head and neck cancer patients.* Abstract presented at The American Dietetic Association 79th Annual Meeting and Exhibition. San Antonio, Texas. **96,** A-35.

89. Andreyev, H. J., Norman, A. R., Oates, J., and Cunningham, D. (1998). Why do patients with weight loss have a worse outcome when undergoing chemotherapy for gastrointestinal malignancies? *Eur. J. Cancer* **34** (4), 503–509.

90. Lopez, M. J., Robins, P., Madden, T., and Highbarger, T. (1994). Nutritional support and prognosis in patients with head and neck cancer. *J. Surg. Oncol.* **55,** 33–36.

91. Bozzetti, F., Cozzaglio, L., Gavazzi, C., Bidoli, P., Bonfanti, G., Montalto, F., Parra, H. S., Valente, M., and Zucali, R. (1998). Nutritional support in patients with cancer of the esophagus: Impact on nutritional status patient compliance to therapy and survival. *Tumori* **84,** 681–686.

92. Evans W. K., Nixon D. W., and Daly, J. M. (1987). A randomised study of oral nutrition support versus ad lib nutritional intake during chemotherapy for advanced colorectal and nonsmall cell lung cancer. *J. Clin. Oncol.* **5,** 113.

93. McCarter, M. D., Gentilii, O. D., Gomez, M. E., and Daly, J. M. (1998). Preoperative oral supplement with immuno-nutrients in cancer patients. *J. Parenteral Enteral Nutr.* **22,** 206–211.

94. Barber, M. D., Ross, J. A., Voss, A. C., Tisdale, M. J., and Fearon, K. C. H. (1999). The effect of an oral nutritional supplement enriched with fish oil on weight-loss in patients with pancreatic cancer. *Br. J. Cancer* **81,** 80–86.

95. Falconer, J. S., Fearon, K. C. H., Plester, C. E., Ross, J. A., and Carter, D. C. (1994). Cytokines, the acute phase protein response, and resting energy expenditure in cachectic patients with pancreatic cancer. *Ann. Sur.* **219**(4), 325–331.

96. Hyltander, A., Korner, U., and Lundholm, K. G. (1993). Elevation of mechanisms behind elevated energy expenditure in cancer patients with solid tumors. *Eur. J. Clin. Invest.* **23,** 46.

97. Fearon, K. C. H., McMillan, D. C., Preston, T., Winstanley, P., Cruickshank, A. M., and Shenkin, A. (1991). Elevated circulating interluekin-6 is associated with an acute phase response, but reduced fixed hepatic protein synthesis in patients with cancer. *Ann. Surg.* **213,** 26.

98. Wigmore, S. J., Plester, C. E., Richardson R. A., and Fearon, K. C. H. (1997). Changes in nutritional status associated with unresectable pancreatic cancer. *Br. J. Cancer* **75**(1), 106–109.

99. Falconer, J. S., Fearon, K. C. H., and Ross, J. A. (1995). Acute-phase protein response and survival duration of patients with pancreatic cancer. *Cancer* **75**(8), 2077–2082.

100. Staal-van den Brekel, A. J., Schols, A. M. W. J., ten Velde, G. P. M., Buurman, W. A., and Wouters, E. F. M. (1994). Analysis of the energy balance in lung cancer patients. *Cancer Res.* **54,** 6430–6433.

101. Wigmore, S. J., Ross, J. A., Falconer, J. S., Plester, C. E., Tisdale, M. J., Carter, D. C., and Fearon, K. C. H. (1996). The effect of polyunsaturated fatty acids on the progress of cachexia in patients with pancreatic cancer. *Nutrition* **12**, S27–S30.

102. Wigmore, S. J., Fearon, K. C. H., Maingay, J. P., and Ross, J. A. (1997). Down-regulation of the acute-phase response in patients with pancreatic cancer cachexia receiving oral eicosapentaenoic acid is mediated via suppression of interleukin-6. *Clin. Science.* **92**, 215–221.

103. Gogos, C. A., Ginopoulos, P., Slasa, B., Apostolidou, E., Zoumbos, N. C., and Kalfarentzos, F. (1998). Dietary omega-3 polyunsaturated fatty acids plus vitamin E restore immuno-deficiency and prolong survival for severely ill patients with generalised malignancy. *Cancer* **82**(2), 395–402.

104. Daly, J. M., Lieberman, M. D., Goldfine, J., Shou, J., Weintraub, F., Rosato, E. F., and Lavin, P. (1992). Enteral nutrition with supplemental arginine, RNA, and omega–3 fatty acids in patients after operation: Immunologic, metabolic, and clinical outcome. *Surgery* **112**, 56–67.

105. Heys, S. D., Walker, L. G., Smith, I., and Eremin, O. (1999). Enteral nutritional supplementation with key nutrients in patients with critical illness and cancer. *Ann. Surg.* **229**, 467–477.

106. Chlebowski, R. T., Dugan, W., Laufman, L., Whie, L., Brotherton, T., Reeves, J., Sher, H., Badolato, C., Forte, F., Sambuco, S., Courtney, K., Ceh, S., McCamish, M., Green, D., and Cope, F. (1997). *A novel peptide-based enteral formula and 5-FU/leucovorin related adverse experiences in colorectal cancer patients: An interim evaluation.* Abstract presented at American Society of Clinical Oncology Annual Meeting. p. 922.

107. National Center for Health Statistics Fact Sheet (1996). Centers for Disease Control, Fact Sheet (1996). Centers for Disease Control. Atlanta, Georgia.

108. Murray, C. J. L., and Lopez, A. D. (1997). Alternative projections of mortality and disability by cause 1990–2020: Global burden of disease study. *Lancet* **349**, 1498–1504.

109. Schols, A., Moster, R., Souters, P., Gruieve, H., Wouters, E. F. M. (1989.) Inventory of nutritional status in patients with COPD. *Chest* **96**, 247–249.

110. Laaban, J. P., Kouchakli, B., Dore, M. F., Orvoen-Frija, E., and Rochmaure, J. (1993). Nutritional status of patients with chronic obstructive pulmonary disease and acute respiratory failure. *Chest* **103**, 1362–1368.

111. Donahoe, M., and Rogers, R. M. (1990). Nutritional assessment and support in chronic obstructive pulmonary disease. *Clin. Chest Med.* **11**, 487–504.

112. Hogg, J. (1998). Wasting and chronic obstructive pulmonary disease. *Support Line* **20**, 13–18.

113. Ambrosino, N., Foglio, K., Rubini, F., Clili, E., Nava, S., and Vitracca, M. (1995). Noninvasive mechanical ventilation in acute respiratory failure due to chronic obstructive pulmonary disease: Correlates for success. *Thorax* **50**, 755–757.

114. Gray-Donald, K., Gibbons, L., Shapiro, S. H., Mackelm, P. T., and Martin, J. G. (1996). Nutritional status and mortality in chronic obstructive pulmonary disease. *Am. J. Respir. Crit. Care Med.* **153**, 961–966.

115. Efthimiou, J., Fleming, J., Gomes, C., and Spiro, S. G. (1988). The effect of supplementary oral nutrition in poorly nourished patients with chronic obstructive pulmonary disease. *Am. Rev. Respir. Dis.* **137**, 1075–1082.

116. Larca, L. and Greenbaum, D. M. (1982). Effectiveness of intensive nutritional regimen in patients who fail to wean from mechanical ventilation. *Crit. Care. Med.* **10**, 297–300.

117. Bassili, H. R. and Deitel, M. (1981). Effect of nutritional support on weaning patients off mechanical ventilators. *J. Parenteral Enteral Nutr.* **5**, 161–163.

118. Saltzman, H. A. and Salzano, J. V. (1971). Effects of carbohydrate metabolism upon respiratory gas exchange in normal men. *J. Appl. Physiol.* **30**, 228–231.

119. Garfinkle, F., Robinson, S., and Price, C. (1985). Replacing carbohydrate calories with fat calories in enteral feeding for patients with impaired respiratory function. *J. Parenteral Enteral Nutr.* **9**, 3.

120. Angelillo, V. A., Bedi, S., Durfee, D., Dahl, J., Patterson, A. J., and O'Donohue, W. J. (1985). Effects of low and high carbohydrate feedings in ambulatory patients with chronic obstructive pulmonary disease and chronic hypercapnia. *Ann. Intern. Med.* **103**, 883–885.

121. Goldstein, S., Thomashow, B., amd Askanazi, J. (1986). Functional changes during nutritional repletion in patients with lung disease. *Clin. Chest Med.* **7**, 141–151.

122. Frankfort, J. D., Fisher, C. E., Stansbury, D. W., McArthur, D. L., Brown, S. E., and Light, R. (1991). Effects of high- and low- carbohydrate meals on maximum exercise performance in chronic airflow obstruction. *Chest* **100**, 792–795.

123. Van den Berg, B., and Stam, H. (1988). Metabolic and respiratory effects of enteral nutrition in patients during mechanical ventilation. *Intens. Care Med.* **14**, 206–211.

124. Talpers, S. S., Romberger, D. J., Bunce, S. B., and Pingleton, S. K. (1992). Nutritionally associated increased carbon dioxide production. *Chest* **102**, 551–555.

125. Kane, R. E., and Hobbs, P. (1991). Energy and respiratory metabolism in cystic fibrosis: The influence of carbohydrate content of nutritional supplements. *J. Pediatr. Gastroenterol. Nutr.* **12**, 217–223.

126. Kane, R. E., Hobbs, P. J., and Black, P. G. (1990). Comparison of low, medium and high carbohydrate formulas for nighttime enteral feedings in cystic fibrosis patients. *J. Parenteral Enteral Nutr.* **14**, 47–52.

127. DCCT Research Group (1993). The effect of intensive treatment of diabetes on the development and progression of long-term complications in insulin dependent diabetes mellitus. *N. Engl. J. Med.* **329**, 977–986.

128. UK Prospective Diabetes Study (UKPDS) Group (1998). Intensive blood-glucose control with sulphonylureas or insulin compared with conventional treatment and risk of complications in patients with type 2 diabetes (UKPDS 33). *Lancet* **352**, 837–853.

129. Craig, L. D., Nicholson, S., Silverstone, F. A., and Kennedy, R. D. (1998). Use of a reduced-carbohydrate, modified-fat enteral formula for improving metabolic control and clinical outcomes in long-term care residents with type 2 diabetes: Results of a pilot trial. *Nutrition* **14**, 529–534.

130. Garg, A., Bonanome, A., Grundy, S. M., Zhang, Z., and Unger, R. (1988). Comparison of a high-carbohydrate diet with a high-monounsaturated fat diet in patients with non-insulin-dependent diabetes mellitus. *N. Engl. J. Med.* **319**, 829–834.

131. Garg, A., Grundy, S. M., and Koffler, M. (1992). Effect of high carbohydrate intake on hyperglycemia, islet function, and plasma lipoproteins in NIDDM. *Diabetes Care* **15,** 1572–1580.

132. Garg, A., Bantle, J. P., Henry, R. R., Coulston, A. M., Griver, A., Raatz, S. K., Brinkley, L., Chen, I., Grundy, S. M., Huet, B. A., and Reaven, G. M. (1994). Effects of varying carbohydrate content of diet in patients with non-insulin-dependent diabetes mellitus. *JAMA* **271,** 1421–1428.

133. Peters, A. L., Davidson, M. B., and Isaac, R. M. (1989). Lack of glucose elevation after simulated tube feeding with a low-carbohydrate, high-fat enteral formula in patients with type 1 diabetes. *Am. J. Med.* **87,** 178–182.

134. Reader, D. M., Fish, L., and Franz, M. (1996), Plasma glucose and insulin response to isocaloric quantities of three nutritional formulas in persons with non-insulin-dependent-diabetes. *Diabetes* **2** (Suppl.), 45.

135. Reader, D. M., Fish, L. H., and Franz, M. J. (1994). Response to isocaloric quantities of enteral feedings in persons with non-insulin-dependent diabetes mellitus (NIDDM) [abstract]. *J. Am. Dietet. Assoc.* **94,** A–39.

136. Grahm, T. W., Harrington, T. R., and Isaac, R. M. (1989). Low carbohydrate (CHO) with fiber enteral formula impedes development of hyperglycemia in patients with acute head injury. *Clin. Res.* **37,** 138A.

137. Galkowski, J., Silverstone, F. A., Brod, M., and Isaac, R. M. (1989). Use of a low carbohydrate with fiber enteral formula as a snack for elderly patients with type 2 diabetes. *Clin. Res.* **37,** 89A.

138. Clintec Sales Aid. Deerfield, IL, 1999.

139. McCargar, L. J., Innis, S. M., Bowron, E., Leichter, J., Toth, E., and Wall, K. (1998). Effect of enteral nutritional products differing in carbohydrate and fat on indices of carbohydrate and lipid metabolism in patients with NIDDM. *Mol. and Cell Biochem.* **188,** 81–89.

140. Kipnes, M., Shade, S., Geraghty, M., Craig, L., and Bossetti, B. (1998). Effect of a liquid nutritional designed for oral supplementation on glucose tolerance in subjects with type 2 diabetes. *Diabetes* **47,** A90.

141. Kopple, J. D. (1978). Abnormal amino acid metabolism in uremia. *Kidney Int.* **14,** 340–348.

142. Cockram, D. B., Hensley, M. K., Rodriguez, M., Agarwal, G., Wennberg, A., Ruey, P., Ashbach, D., Hebert, L.. and Kunau, R. (1998). Safety and tolerance of medical nutritional products as sole sources of nutrition in people on hemodialysis. *J. Ren. Nutr.* **8,** 25–33.

143. Cockram, D. B., Moore, L. W., and Acchiardo, S. R. (1994). Response to an oral nutritional supplement for chronic renal failure patients. *J. Ren. Nutr.* **4,** 78–85.

CHAPTER 16

Composite Foods and Formulas, Parenteral and Enteral Nutrition

LAURA MATARESE

The Cleveland Clinic Foundation, Cleveland, Ohio

I. INTRODUCTION

Oral consumption of a standard diet is the best way to meet nutrition needs. But when oral feeding with regular food is not possible, nutrients may be delivered as a supplement or as total nourishment through nonvolitional feedings. This chapter will describe composite foods and formulas, as well as the general principles of enteral and parenteral nutrition.

II. ENTERAL NUTRITION

The use of enteral feedings dates back to Egypt many centuries before Christ. The earliest recorded evidence of enteral nutrition employed the use of rectal feedings. These formulas were often composed of wine, whey, milk, and barley and were used to coat inflamed intestines and to provide nutrients. Eventually, nutrient substances were introduced into the upper gastrointestinal (GI) tract, but this was not until the 1600s. Early enteral feeding formulas were generally composed of regular foodstuffs, which were pulverized and administered with syringes. Now, sophisticated nutrient formulas are commercially available along with advanced equipment to infuse them.

The decision to feed enterally or parenterally depends on the integrity and functional status of the GI tract. If the GI tract is functional, accessible, and safe to use, enteral nutrition is always the preferred method of nutrition support. Enteral nutrition (feedings by tube) promotes comparable or better outcomes [1–3] and is less expensive [4] than parenteral nutrition. The benefits of enteral nutrition over parenteral nutrition appear to be largely due to a reduction of septic complications. It is believed that delivery of nutrients through the GI tract helps to maintain the gut mucosal barrier and prevent bacterial translocation into systemic circulation [5]. Enteral nourishment is generally considered to be safer than parenteral nutrition. But enteral nutrition therapy does possess its own set of potential complications [6].

A. Indications/Contraindications

General indications for enteral nutrition include insufficient oral intake, nutrient repletion, and support during the transi-

tion phase of parenteral nutrition. Contraindications include intractable vomiting, intestinal obstruction, upper GI tract hemorrhaging, high risk for aspiration, and severe intractable diarrhea. The decision to initiate enteral feedings begins with an assessment of GI tract function. Signs of adequate function include normal upper GI tract or small bowel X ray, flatus or bowel movement, bowel sounds, hunger, absence of vomiting, absence of obstruction or ileus, and no uncontrolled diarrhea.

B. Enteral Access

When initiating enteral feedings it is important to consider the route, access device, method of administration, and type of feeding formula [7]. The route of access is determined by the anticipated length of therapy and the risk of aspiration. Nasoenteric and oroenteric feeding tubes are used when the anticipated length of therapy is short, generally less than 4 weeks, or for interim access before the placement of a long-term feeding tube. If the risk of aspiration is low, the tip of the feeding tube can terminate in the stomach. Feeding into the stomach is more physiologic and allows feeding to be administered without a feeding pump. However, if there is an increased risk of aspiration due to mental obtundation, an incompetent lower esophageal sphincter with gastroesophageal reflux or gastroparesis, the tip of the feeding tube should be placed beyond the pylorus. This may be accomplished intraoperatively, by active bedside placement, with the use of prokinetic agents or a fluoroscope or endoscope. Spontaneous transpyloric passage of feeding tubes through peristalsis can lead to successful placement in 36–56% of weighted tubes and in 84–92% of unweighted tubes, but may take several days before feeding can be initiated [8]. Zaloga [9] has developed an active bedside technique for placing tubes transpylorically that involves careful advancement of the feeding tube while rotating it around its long axis. The rate of successful tube placement using this technique ranges from 40% to 85%. Prokinetic agents (metoclopraminde, cisapride, erythromycin) have been used to aid in tube placement [8]. In some settings (i.e., intensive care) it may be appropriate to use transpyloric feeding with simultaneous gastric decompression in order to minimize the risk

of aspiration [10]. This may be accomplished with the use of specialized tubes that perform both functions or the use of two separate tubes.

Long-term (permanent) access requires a percutaneous or surgically placed feeding enterostomy. If the risk of aspiration is low, a percutaneous endoscopic gastrostomy (PEG) can be placed [11, 12]. A surgical gastrostomy should be considered when access to the stomach is anticipated during a major abdominal procedure or when PEG placement is contraindicated. If the risk of aspiration is high, a PEG with a jejunal extension can be used [13]. Another technique for providing long-term access into the small bowel is direct endoscopic jejunostomy (DEJ) [14]. The DEJ tube is placed endoscopically, as is a PEG, except that the endoscope is passed through the duodenum, past the ligament of Treitz, into a loop of jejunum adjacent to the abdominal wall. If an endoscope cannot be passed, a surgical jejunostomy may be indicated.

C. Formula Composition: Nutrient Components

The composition and nutritional value of commercially prepared formulas vary considerably. The composition of the formula determines the use and has a tremendous bearing on patient tolerance.

1. PROTEIN

Protein generally comprises 15–20% of the total energy provided in an enteral feeding solution but may range from 8% to 25% of energy. Protein sources for enteral formulas include [1] intact protein from eggs, milk, or meat; [2] protein isolates from milk (casein, whey), soybean, or egg white; [3] hydrolyzed protein from casein, fish, meat, and soy and may contain added amino acids; [4] short-chain peptides; and [5] free amino acids. The protein source must be considered when selecting a formula for a patient, particularly when there is impaired ability to digest or absorb nutrients. The products containing hydrolyzed protein tend to be more expensive and therefore should be limited to use with patients with appropriate indications.

The quality of a protein is dependent on the amino acid composition. Casein and soy protein, which are usually the protein sources found in enteral formulas, do not have as high a biological value as albumin, and therefore more may be required to achieve positive nitrogen balance [15]. Many enteral formulas have altered amino acid composition designed to support patients in various disease states. Traditionally, a factor of 6.25 is used when converting grams of protein to grams of nitrogen. With the recent proliferation of new specialty formulas containing supplemental and altered amino acids, conversion factors ranging from 5 to 7.5 may be used depending on the amino acid and nitrogen source. This information can be obtained from the manufacturer of the specific enteral formula.

The use of short-chain peptides of varying lengths or single amino acids as the protein source in enteral feedings remains controversial. Data from animal studies suggest that peptide-based diets are associated with improved absorption, lower mortality, and decreased incidence of bacterial translocation [16–18]. Data from human studies also demonstrate more rapid and efficient absorption of peptides than for free amino acids in both the healthy and diseased gut [19–23]. However, other studies have not confirmed the beneficial effects of peptides over free amino acids or intact proteins [24–26]. It does appear that the use of peptide-containing solutions may be beneficial for those patients who have impaired digestion or absorption capabilities [27, 28].

2. CARBOHYDRATE

Carbohydrate comprises the major source of energy, generally 40–50%, but as high as 90% of total energy in an enteral formula. It also has the greatest effect on tolerance because the carbohydrate source exerts the greatest effect on the osmolality of the solution. The carbohydrate may be in the form of monosaccharides, disaccharides, oligosaccharides, or starch. Monosaccharides, such as glucose, have a greater osmotic effect than complex carbohydrates, such as starches. The use of these hyperosmolar solutions may result in abdominal discomfort, diarrhea, and dumping. However, these smaller molecules require fewer pancreatic enzymes and intestinal mucosal disaccharidases for adequate digestion and may be useful for patients with an impaired ability to digest and absorb. The predominant form of carbohydrate found in enteral formulas is from large molecules, such as glucose oligosaccharides, maltodextrin, and hydrolyzed cornstarch. Most commercially available enteral formulas are lactose free.

3. FAT

Dietary fat is necessary to supply essential fatty acids (EFA). It acts as a carrier of fat-soluble vitamins and is a concentrated energy substrate. The addition of fat to enteral formulas also enhances palatability and flavor, factors of importance when enteral formulas are used as oral supplements. The fat content of enteral formulas varies considerably in both quantity and type. In general, 30–45% of total energy is from fat but may range from 1.3% to 55% of energy. Sources of fat commonly found in enteral formulas include long-chain triglycerides (LCT) from corn, safflower, sunflower, or soybean oil. These sources are high in omega-6 fatty acids which are thought to suppress immune function [29–32].

Some formulas contain medium-chain triglycerides (MCT), which are more rapidly hydrolyzed and absorbed than LCTs. MCT oil does not require significant bile salt or lipase activity for digestion and is transported directly to the liver for metabolism by the portal circulation instead of the lymphatic system following absorption [33]. MCT oil is derived from coconut oil and does not contain essential fatty acids.

Many products now contain omega–3 fatty acids for immune enhancing properties. Recently, there has been interest in the use of structured lipids, which are formed by the ran-

dom transesterification of MCT with LCT. This compound contains both MCT and LCT on the same glycerol backbone, thus offering the advantage of enhanced absorption and EFA content [29, 34].

4. VITAMINS AND MINERALS

Vitamins, minerals, and trace elements are all included in standard tube feeding formulas. Most formulas meet the U.S. Recommended Dietary Allowances (RDA) for these nutrients in 1.5–2 L of formula. Some otherwise complete enteral formulas do not contain vitamin K. Vitamin K deficiency is rare, theoretically, because it is synthesized by bacteria in the gut. Vitamin K may also interfere with anticoagulation therapy (e.g., warfarin). Alternatively, vitamin K supplementation may be necessary for patients receiving antibiotics for prolonged periods. Some of the vitamins and minerals have been fortified beyond the RDA to meet the requirements imposed by illness and injury. Patients receiving enteral formulas for more than 6 months have been shown to have normal or high blood levels of certain vitamins [35]. Certain disease-specific formulas may not have vitamins added due to their potential toxicity in various clinical conditions.

5. FIBER

Fiber has many beneficial effects such as increasing stool bulk, serving as an energy source for colonocytes, and normalization of bowel function [36–38]. Fiber has been promoted for treating diarrhea, constipation, and blood glucose control [36, 38–40]. There are basically two types of fiber of interest in enteral nutrition: cellulosic and noncellulosic. Cellulosic fibers are of high molecular weight and are non-soluble. Examples include cellulose, and wheat bran is a rich source. These contribute to fecal mass and water content and reduce stool mean transit time. Noncellulosic fibers are more water soluble and include hemicelluose, pectin, gums, and mucilages. They are rapidly degraded by anaerobic micoflora of the cecum and colon to yield short-chain fatty acids.

6. PHYSICAL CHARACTERISTICS

The osmotic activity of an enteral formula is generally measured as osmolality, the concentration of particles (solutes) that affects the osmotic balance across a semipermeable membrane. It is expressed as mOsm/kg H_2O. Because the osmolality of an enteral formula is based on the number of dissolved particles in solution, the smaller the particle size, the greater the number of particles per unit weight of solute and the higher the osmolality. Thus, complex high molecular weight macronutrients, such as starch and proteins, contribute less to the osmolality of the solution than a lower molecular weight compound such as glucose oligosaccharides or short- chain peptides. Fats do not form a solution in water and therefore have no osmotic effect. Electrolytes added as salts, such as sodium chloride or potassium chloride, dissociate in solution and increase the osmolality of the formula.

The significance of osmolality is related to the clinical tolerance of the enteral formula. In general, the closer a formula is to isotonic concentration, the lower the potential for GI complications such as diarrhea, dumping, nausea, and vomiting. However, administration of isotonic solutions does not guarantee tolerance. Although many clinicians associate diarrhea with enteral feedings, controlled trials have failed to demonstrate this relationship [41–44].

It is common for manufacturers to report the renal solute load of the formula. This is a measure of the concentration in a feeding solution of the particles that the kidney must work to excrete. Protein, yielding urea as its endproduct, and the electrolytes sodium, potassium, and chloride are the main contributors to renal solute load. The renal solute load is of particular concern in geriatric and pediatric populations. High renal solute loads can predispose a patient to dehydration.

The hydrogen ion concentration (pH) of enteral formulas is also of interest. Gastric motility is decreased when solutions have a pH lower than 3.5. Most enteral formulas have a pH above 3.5. The pH of a formula can also contribute to tube occlusion. Most intact protein formulas coagulate when acidified to a pH of less than 5.0 [45]. However, attempts have also been made to acidify enteral feedings in order to reduce gastric colonization and the incidence of aspiration pneumonia [46]. Although acidifying enteral feedings has been shown to reduce gastric colonization in critically ill patients, larger studies are needed to examine the effect of this strategy on morbidity, such as pneumonia, and mortality.

D. Formula Classification

Enteral formulas can be divided into three major categories: polymeric, hydrolyzed, and modular and disease specific. Polymeric formulas contain intact protein generally from casein and soy protein isolates, polyscaccharides and glucose polymers, and a mixture of LCTs and MCTs in proportions that mimic a standard diet. These products tend to be relatively inexpensive and are generally well tolerated. The caloric content may vary between 1.0 and 2.0 kcal/mL; protein generally provides 15–20% of the total energy and fat provides 30–50% of energy. The osmolality of these formulas varies from 300 to 600 mOsm/kg.

Hydrolyzed formulas contain macronutrients that have been partially or completely hydrolyzed to the component oligopeptides, short-chain peptides, free amino acids, and glucose oligosaccharides. They also tend to be very low in fat. These formulas are useful for patients who have an impaired ability to digest or absorb nutrients.

Modular formulas are used to supplement individual nutrients in an existing commercial formula or to compose a specific new formula to meet the unique requirements of a particular patient. They usually consist of one or more macronutrients.

1. DISEASE-SPECIFIC FORMULAS

Renal failure formulas are generally low in protein and contain essential amino acids (EAA) or a combination of

EAA and nonessential amino acids (NEAA). The rationale for the use of these products is that urea can be recycled as a nitrogen source in the GI lumen by bacterial urease. Fragments are then reabsorbed and converted to NEAA in the liver [47]. These products may also be low in electrolytes and fat-soluble vitamins. Early studies demonstrated lowered blood urea nitrogen levels and a reduction of uremic symptoms with the use of EAA [48, 49]. Subsequent trials, however, did not demonstrate a clear benefit of EAA alone compared to a mixture [50, 51]. Now with newer dialysis techniques, the trend is to provide patients with a full complement of amino acids and then treat with dialysis. Standard amino acid formulas containing EAA and NEAA should be used during dialysis and chronic renal failure. EAA may be useful in promoting improved nutritional status in acute renal failure or to delay the initiation of treatment.

Patients with liver disease generally present in a malnourished state. Administration of protein to improve nutritional status often results in hepatic encephalopathy [52]. Patients may have abnormal plasma amino acid patterns, characterized by elevated concentrations of methionine and the aromatic amino acids (AAA), phenylalanine, tyrosine, tryptophan, and decreased levels of the branched chain amino acids (BCAA), valine, leucine, and isoleucine [53]. Hepatic failure formulas generally contain enriched levels of BCAA and low AAAs. The rationale is to normalize amino acid patterns and improve or reverse hepatic encephalopathy. The efficacy of these specialized products remains controversial [54–56]. Many of the studies involving the use of BCAAs have failed to show any benefit other than improved nitrogen balance [57–60]. Most patients with hepatic encephalopathy can tolerate low doses of standard amino acids. However, if the patient becomes encephalopathic or the encephalopathy worsens, a BCAA-enriched formula may be useful.

Patients with pulmonary disease may suffer from carbon dioxide (CO_2) retention and oxygen deprivation. This is of particular concern when attempting to wean patients off ventilators. Specialty pulmonary failure formulas tend to be high in fat. The rationale is to decrease the CO_2 production from oxidation of carbohydrate. Several studies have demonstrated lowered CO_2 production, lowered respiratory quotients, lowered $PaCO_2$, and decreased ventilatory time with the use of these products [61–64]. But most of these studies did not control for the use of sedatives and other muscle relaxants affecting mechanical ventilation. It is more important to avoid overfeeding these patients since CO_2 production seems to be more affected by the amount of energy provided than by the level of carbohydrate [65].

Metabolic stress is a phrase used to describe patients who are catabolic, hypermetabolic, and critically ill. A number of products, designed for these patients, have been enriched with BCAA, glutamine, arginine, nucleotides, and/or structured lipids. The rationale has been to blunt the hypermetabolic response and improve immune function. Products have been enriched with BCAA to stimulate protein synthesis and minimize protein degradation [66]. The profile of the BCAA for stress formulas does differ from those used in hepatic encephalopathy. The use of products enriched with BCAA for metabolically stressed patients has resulted in improvement of nitrogen retention, total lymphocyte count, and visceral protein levels [67–71]. Unfortunately none of these studies has been able to demonstrate any difference in morbidity or mortality.

Various NEAAs such as glutamine and arginine, have been added to enteral formulas designed to support patients with metabolic stress because it is hypothesized that these amino acids may be conditionally essential during these periods. Glutamine exerts a tropic effect on the bowel and stimulates nutrient absorption [72–74]. Glutamine also functions as a precursor of nucleic acids, nucleotides, amino sugars, and proteins and is the preferred fuel for rapidly proliferating cells such as enterocytes, macrophages, and lymphocytes [75]. Glutamine is an abundant amino acid and found in all enteral formulas as protein bound. It is unclear whether glutamine must be present as a free amino acid to exert a pharmacologic effect.

Arginine may also be conditionally essential during periods of metabolic stress. It has been shown to improve weight gain and increase nitrogen retention during recovery from injury in experimental animals [76]. Arginine has been shown to increase collagen deposition and improve wound healing [77, 78]. But supplemental arginine has been added to enteral formulas mostly for its reported immune-enhancing properties [79–82].

Several enteral formulas are now available that have combined supplemental levels of amino acids, omega-3 fatty acids, and enhanced vitamin levels for use in metabolically stressed patients. Many of the studies suggest promising results on various outcome parameters, such as improved immune response, better nitrogen balance, reduction in infections, decreased length of stay, and decreased days on a ventilator [83–95]. Although absolute efficacy has not been clearly demonstrated, the data suggest that these products may be helpful in reducing complications in specific patient populations.

Speciality products are available for patients with diabetes mellitus and impaired glucose tolerance. Patients with diabetes mellitus requiring long-term enteral feeding should have a formula that mimics the dietary guidelines of the American Diabetes Association [96]. Some of the specialty enteral formulas designed for use with these patients are very high in fat, providing up to 50% of energy to assist with blood glucose control. Some success has been seen with the use of these products in preventing elevation of blood glucose levels in nonhospitalized persons consuming formula by mouth [97, 98]. The fiber-containing products are useful in glucose only if fed into the stomach to delay gastric emptying.

E. Formula Selection

The clinician now has a vast array of composite foods and enteral formulas from which to choose. When choosing a

formula it is important to consider a few basic points. First, what is the patient's digestive capability? If there is any impaired ability to digest or absorb nutrients, a predigested formula may be indicated. These formulas typically have macronutrients which are present as hydrolyzed components; protein in the form of short-chain peptides or amino acids; carbohydrate in the form of glucose oligosaccharides; and fat in varying combinations of LCTs and MCTs. Secondly, does the patient have severe organ dysfunction that may benefit from a disease-specific enteral formula? Third, does the patient require a fluid restriction or have increased metabolic needs necessitating the use of a nutrient-dense formula? Finally, the feeding route should be considered. If the formula is to be administered orally, it must be palatable. If the formula is to be infused through a small-bore feeding tube, it should be of an appropriate viscosity so as to prevent occlusion of the tube.

F. Administration Techniques

The method selected for delivery of tube feeding depends on the location of the feeding tube, the emptying ability of the stomach, the risk of gastroesophageal reflux, the digestive capability of the GI tract, and patient mobility. With bolus administration, 240–400 mL of enteral formula is provided over a 20- to 30-minute period. It is easy to do and does not require the use of a pump. This method is best for gastric feedings. However, this technique may result in nausea, vomiting, and diarrhea. Many of the gastrointestinal complications associated with bolus delivery can be alleviated with the use of a timed intermittent infusion. With this technique, a similar amount of formula is delivered over 1–2 hours. This may be done by gravity or with an enteral feeding pump. Feedings may also be delivered continuously over 12–24 hours by gravity or pump. This method is generally well tolerated and is usually chosen for feedings into the small bowel [99]. Finally, patients can be cycled on tube feedings whereby the feeding is delivered over an 8- to 12-hour period. This is generally used for enteral feeding in the home setting or while transitioning patients onto oral intake.

G. Complications

Complications can be divided into three general categories: mechanical, gastrointestinal, and metabolic. Most of these problems can be avoided by using the proper technique during enteral access, administration, and close monitoring.

The frequency of mechanical complications, such as nasopharyngeal/mucosa erosion, sinusitis, and otitis media, has markedly decreased with the development of small-bore, pliable feeding tubes [100]. Tube misplacement, however, is a very serious potential complication associated with the use of these tubes. It is most likely to occur in patients who are uncooperative, obtruded, or seriously ill. The presence of an endotracheal tube does not prevent its occurrence. Because tube misplacement can lead to esophageal or pleural perfo-

ration and the inadvertent administration of feeding into the mediastinum or lung, a chest radiograph is mandatory after tube placement and prior to initiation of feeding [101, 102].

Aspiration pneumonia is a serious and potentially life-threatening complication of enteral feeding. It is important to differentiate the aspiration of tube feeding from the aspiration of oropharyngeal secretions since patients with the latter problem will aspirate while receiving any form of nutrition support [103, 104]. A decrease in the rate of gastric emptying is the most common risk factor for aspiration and is due to a wide variety of medical conditions including sepsis, trauma, head injury, electrolyte abnormalities, and anticholinergic and narcotic drugs. Gastroesophageal reflux can occur when a tube is placed through the lower esophageal sphincter; however, this risk is greatest when the patient is supine [105]. Rapid bolus feeding can lead to transient relaxation of the lower esophageal sphincter [106]. Intragastric feeding should be given with the patient's head raised 30 degrees or more, and if intermittent feeding is administered, the patient should remain in this position for at least 1 hour after the feeding [107]. The risk of aspiration can be further minimized by feeding beyond the pylorus with simultaneous gastric decompression.

Obstruction of feeding tubes is another potential mechanical complication of enteral feedings. This is generally the result of placing medications and incompletely dissolved formula through the tubes. Failure to routinely irrigate tubes will also increase the risk of tube occlusion [108–110].

Gastrointestinal intolerance is the most common complication of tube feeding. Symptoms include nausea, vomiting, diarrhea, constipation, abdominal pain, and distention. In many cases, the patient's disease or medications used to manage it contribute to these symptoms. If nausea and vomiting are due to gastric distention or gastroesophageal reflux, a slow continuous infusion of the formula may reduce these symptoms. A prokinetic agent, such as metoclopraminde or cisapride, may also be used. Diarrhea is perhaps the most common gastrointestinal complication of tube feeding. Causes of diarrhea include concomitant antibiotic treatment, *Clostridium difficile* toxin with or without pseudomembranous colitis, sorbitol-based liquid medication use, hypoalbuminemia, and magnesium content of the enteral formula [111–113]. Diarrhea can be controlled by decreasing the infusion rate and using antidiarrheal agents. In some instances, it may be necessary to change the enteral feeding formula. Fiber-containing formulas may decrease diarrhea by increasing transit time and by supplying the colon with fermentable fiber, which produces short-chain fatty acids, the primary fuel of the colon [114].

Patients receiving enteral feedings may also experience a variety of metabolic complications ranging from glucose intolerance, hyperkalemia, hypokalemia, hyponatremia, hypernatremia, hypophosphatemia, and dehydration [115]. Electrolytes can be repleted by supplementing the tube feeding or by providing them parenterally. Oral potassium salts can cause gastrointestinal upset while magnesium and phosphate

salts can result in diarrhea. Although metabolic complications are relatively uncommon in association with enteral feeding, patients should be monitored carefully, especially at the beginning of therapy.

III. PARENTERAL NUTRITION

The infusion of nutrients via the parenteral route is a fairly recent technique. During the 1960s when techniques became available to access central circulation, people began to infuse concentrated forms of dextrose into patients. Finally in 1968, a child was supported by nutrients exclusively by vein. Since that time, this area has seen tremendous growth, with sophisticated techniques and specialized nutrient formulas that have saved many lives.

When the GI tract is not functional and nutrition support is indicated, nutrients can be delivered via the parenteral route. Parenteral nutrition supplies protein in the form of amino acids, carbohydrate as dextrose, fat, vitamins, and minerals. It may be infused through peripheral or central veins. The exact route will depend of the length of therapy, availability of intravenous access, fluid status, nutritional requirements, goal of nutrition therapy, and severity of illness.

A. Indications/Contraindications

In general, parenteral nutrition is indicated for patients who are malnourished and do not have a functional GI tract [54]. More specific indications include perioperative support, inflammatory bowel disease, short bowel syndrome, severe pancreatitis, mechanical intestinal obstruction or pseudo-obstruction, severe malabsorption, and hyperemesis gravidarum. Parenteral nutrition is not indicated when the GI tract is functional, when the patient's prognosis is not consistent with aggressive nutrition support, or when the risks of parenteral nutrition outweigh the benefits.

B. Parenteral Access

The composition of the parenteral nutrition solution is dependent on the location of the vein in which it is delivered. Peripheral parenteral nutrition (PPN) is usually reserved for patients requiring short-term therapy who are not markedly hypermetabolic or fluid restricted and have adequate peripheral venous access. Hypertonic solutions may contribute to phlebitis; therefore, the osmolarity of the parenteral nutrition solution should be less than 900 mOsm/L [116]. This generally necessitates the use of a three-in-one or total nutrient admixture (TNA), where the amino acids, dextrose, and intravenous lipid emulsion are compounded in one container.

Central parenteral nutrition is indicated for patients requiring long-term parenteral nutrition who have increased nutritional and metabolic requirements and/or are fluid restricted. Because the parenteral nutrition solution is delivered centrally, where there is high and rapid blood flow, osmolarity is not a consideration. The solutions may be dextrose based (dextrose and amino acids) or TNA.

C. Parenteral Macronutrients

Protein is provided in the form of synthetic crystalline amino acids. The standard amino acid solutions contain the eight EAAs plus histidine and six NEAAs. Commercial amino acid solutions are available in concentrations ranging from 3.5% to 15% (w/vol). Most pharmacies use a 10% solution to compound parenteral nutrition. Parenteral amino acids provide 4.0 kcal/g.

As with enteral formulas, disease-specific parenteral formulas are available. The modifications are generally in the protein component. Amino acid solutions designed for renal failure contain the eight EEAs plus histidine [51]. It is indicated for short-term use only in patients with acute renal failure who are not on dialysis. Patients with acute renal failure who have been started on dialysis should use the standard amino acid preparation. Amino acid solutions designed for hepatic failure contain higher levels of the BCAAs and lower levels of the AAAs. These solutions are indicated during periods of grade III and IV hepatic encephalopathy after a trial of standard medical treatment fails [117, 118].

Dextrose is the most commonly used energy substrate. Intravenous dextrose is available in the monohydrate form, which provides 3.4 kcal/g. Dextrose solutions are available in concentrations ranging from 2.5% to 70% (w/vol). Minimum requirements are estimated to be 1 mg/kg/minute or approximately 100 g/day for a 70-kg man. The maximal amount of carbohydrate tolerated is approximated 5–7 mg/kg/minute [119]. When glucose oxidation rates are exceeded, fat synthesis will occur. This may also result in excess CO_2 production. In stressed and septic patients, ability to tolerate glucose is likely to be impaired. A carbohydrate intake of less than 5 mg/kg/minute may be necessary in the critically ill patient.

Parenteral lipid emulsions are administered as a source of EFA and calories. They contain soybean or a combination of soybean and safflower oil as a source of polyunsaturated fatty acids, egg phospholipid as an emulsifier, and water. Glycerol is added to make the emulsion isotonic. A 10% lipid emulsion provides 1.1 kcal/mL, a 20% emulsion provides 2.0 kcal/mL, and a 30% emulsion provides 3.0 kcal/mL. These emulsions have a pH range of 5.5–8.0 and an osmolarity range of 260–300 mOsm/L. The emulsified fat particles range from 0.1 to 0.5 μm in diameter. Two to 4% of total calories should come from linoleic acid to prevent EFA deficiency. This translates into 500 mL of a 10% lipid emulsion or 250 mL of a 20% lipid emulsion administered 3 times a week. The lipids should be administered slowly, generally over 8–10 hours to avoid reduced lipid clearance and impaired reticuloendothelial function and pulmonary gas exchange [120].

TABLE 1 Daily Electrolyte Requirements in Patients with Adequate Renal Function Receiving Parenteral Nutrition

Electrolyte	Usual adult daily IV dose	RDA adult (oral)
Sodium	100–150 mEq	22 mEq[a]
Potassium	60–120 mEq	40–50 mEq[a]
Chloride	100–150 mEq	22 mEq[a]
Calcium	9–22 mEq	20–30 mEq
Magnesium	8–24 mEq	11.5–14.4 mEq
Phosphorus	15–30 mM	26–39 mEq

[a]Minimum requirements of healthy persons.

TABLE 2 Electrolyte Composition of Common Intravenous Fluids (mEq/L)

Solution	Na	K	Cl	HCO$_3$
½ Normal saline	77	0	77	0
Normal saline	154	0	154	0
3% Saline	513	0	513	0
5% Saline	855	0	855	0
Dextrose 5%, ¼ saline	39	0	39	0
Dextrose 5%, normal saline	154	0	154	0
Lactose Ringer's	130	4	109	28
Dextrose 5%, lactose Ringer's	130	4	109	28

D. Fluid and Electrolytes

Once tolerance to the macronutrients has been established, the day-to-day management of parenteral nutrition evolves around fluid and electrolytes (Table 1). Fluid needs can be estimated from the sum of urine output, gastrointestinal losses, and insensible water losses from the skin and respiratory tract (approximately 500 mL). In general, young adults need 30–40 mL/kg/day and the elderly require 30 mL/ kg/day. When starting a patient on parenteral nutrition it is often helpful to note the maintenance IV solution the patient had been receiving and use this as a guide to prescribe the parenteral nutrition formula (Table 2). Patients administered parenteral nutrition should have strict intake and output records. It is important to note losses through urine, stool, and nasogastric tubes and other drains. Body fluids contain elec-

trolytes that should be replaced in the parenteral nutrition [121, 122] (Table 3).

Calcium, an extracellular cation is usually added to parenteral nutrition solutions in dosages of 9–22 mEq/day. This is generally added as calcium gluconate, which yields 4.65 mEq/g. Parenteral nutrition causes no real deficiency in calcium due to the buffering capacity of bone. However, supplemental calcium is required with phosphate administration to maintain serum calcium levels and avoid hypocalcemic tetany.

Magnesium functions in enzyme reactions, such as glycolysis, and in all reactions involving adenosine triphosphate. As parenteral nutrition is initiated, serum magnesium levels may decrease as the patient becomes anabolic. Hypomagnesemia

TABLE 3 Approximate Electrolyte Composition of Various Body Fluids

Source	Volume (mL/day)	Electrolytes (mEq/L)			
		Na	K	HCO$_3$	Cl
Saliva	500–2000	2–10	20–30	30	8–18
Gastric	2000–2500 pH<4	60	10	—	90
	pH>4	100	10	—	100
Pancreatic	1000	140	5	90	75
Bile	1500	140	5	35	100
Small bowel	3500	100	15	25	100
Colonic	—	60	30	—	75
Diarrhea	1000–4000	60	30	45	45
Urine	1500	40	0	—	20
Sweat	1500	50	5	—	55

Sources: Data from Farber, M. D., Schmidt, R. J., Bear, R. A., and Narins, R. G. (1987). Management of fluid, electrolyte, and acid–base disorders in surgical patients. *In* "Clinical Disorders of Fluid and Electrolyte Metabolism," 5th ed. (R. G. Naris, Ed.), pp. 1407–1436. McGraw-Hill, New York; and Grant, J. P. (1992). "Handbook of Total Parenteral Nutrition," 2nd ed., p. 174. W. B. Saunders Co., Philadelphia, PA.

TABLE 4   Evaluation and Treatment of Hyponatremia in Parenteral Nutrition Patients

	Osmolality	Etiology	Treatment
High	(>285 mOsm)	Hyperproteinemia	Underlying condition
Normal	(280–285 mOsm)	Hyperlipidemia	
		Hyperglycemia	
Low	(<280 mOsm)	H₂O intoxication	Restrict H₂O
	Isovolemic	Syndrome of antidiuretic hormone	
	or		
	Hypervolemic	Renal failure	
		Cardiac failure	
		Cirrhosis	
	Hypovolemic	GI losses	Isotonic saline
		Third space losses	
		Renal losses	

Source: Reprinted with permission from Matarese, L. E. (Ed.). (1997). "Nutrition Support Handbook," p. 77. The Cleveland Clinic Foundation, Cleveland, OH.

causes an increase in central nervous system and neuromuscular hyperactivity and has a significant effect on potassium, calcium, and phosphorus metabolism. Magnesium deficiencies are common in patients with GI diseases, protein energy malnutrition, and prolonged intravenous fluid therapy. Magnesium is added to parenteral nutrition solutions in the form of magnesium sulfate in dosages of 8–24 mEq/day. Magnesium sulfate yields 8.12 mEq/day.

Phosphorus is a major intracellular anion and functions in the metabolism of carbohydrate, fat, and protein. Phosphorus is also a constituent of nucleic acids, phospholipid membranes, and nucleoproteins. The usual dose of phosphorus is 15–30 mM/day and is generally supplied as either potassium or sodium. A 1 mEq potassium phosphate injection provides 0.68 mM of phosphate or 21 mg of elemental phosphorus. A 1 mEq sodium phosphate injection provides 0.75 mM of phosphate or 23 mg of elemental phosphorus.

Potassium is the major cation of intracellular fluid with 75% of body potassium located within muscle mass. The usual adult daily dosage of potassium for patients receiving parenteral nutrition is 60–120 mEq/day. Potassium is supplied as either chloride or acetate depending on acid-base balance. Potassium losses are in a fixed ratio with nitrogen losses. For every 1 g of nitrogen lost, a deficiency of 3.5 mEq of potassium exists. Hypokalemia may result from the use of diuretics, amphotericin B, nasogastric suction, or vomiting. Acute deficits of potassium should be corrected outside of the parenteral nutrition solution.

Sodium is a major extracellular ion and functions in the maintenance of osmotic pressure and in acid–base balance. Maintenance sodium requirements range from 100 to 150 mEq/day. Adjustments may be required for patients with re-

nal and cardiac disease, patients with ascites and liver disease, and patients with altered fluid status. A low serum sodium may result from high blood glucose, generalized sodium deficiency, or water excess. Each increase of 100 mg/dL serum glucose above the normal value of 100 results in a decrease of serum sodium of 1.6–2 mEq/L. Hyponatremia generally results from fluid overload and not a sodium deficit (Table 4).

Chloride is a major extracellular anion and functions in the maintenance of osmotic pressure and acid–base balance. Sodium and chloride are generally added in a one-to-one molar ratio to prevent hyperchloremic acidosis, although some patients may need a higher concentration of acetate. Chloride is added to parenteral nutrition solutions as sodium or potassium salts. Additionally, some of the amino acid solutions contain chloride.

Acetate salts should be included to prevent metabolic acidosis from amino acid metabolism. Acetate is rapidly converted to bicarbonate in the liver. Sodium bicarbonate is not used and should never be added to parenteral nutrition solutions because this product is incompatible with other additives. For example, the addition of sodium bicarbonate to a parenteral nutrition solution containing the parenteral equivalent of the RDA for elemental calcium readily forms insoluble calcium carbonate.

E. Parenteral Micronutrients

The addition of vitamins to the parenteral nutrition solution is essential to the utilization of the nutrient components. Deficiencies of the water-soluble vitamins can occur rapidly. When vitamins are given via the intravenous route there is a

TABLE 5 Daily Parenteral Vitamin Supplementation

Vitamin	RDA adult range	IV multivitamin formulation
A (IU)	2667–3333	3300
D (IU)	200	200
E (IU)	11–14	10
Ascorbic acid (mg)	60	100
Folic acid (mcg)	180–200	400
Niacin (mg)	13–20	40
Riboflavin (mg)	1.2–1.8	3.6
Thiamin (mg)	1.0–1.5	3.0
B_6 (mg)	1.6–2.0	4.0
B_{12} (mcg)	2.0	5.0
Pantothenic acid (mg)	4–7	15
Biotin (mcg)	30–100	60

greater amount of elimination through the kidney. Therefore, though exact requirements of intravenous vitamins are unknown, a higher dose, generally 2 to 3 times the RDA, is recommended for water-soluble vitamins [123]. Fat-soluble vitamins are also a component of the multivitamin injections. Vitamin K is not present in the multivitamin injections and must be added separately (Table 5).

Intravenous trace element injections are available that contain zinc, copper, chromium, selenium, and manganese [124]. These should be added to the parenteral nutrition solution on a daily basis (Table 6).

F. Medications and Other Additives

Very few medications are added to parenteral nutrition solutions due to potential incompatibilities. Additionally, if the parenteral nutrition solution should have to be suddenly discontinued for any reason, the medication is discontinued as well. The few exceptions are noted: Heparin is sometimes added to help prevent subclavian vein thrombosis and to decrease thrombus formation at the catheter tip. It is also added to peripheral parenteral nutrition solutions to improve peripheral vein tolerance to the solution. Regular insulin is added to parenteral nutrition solutions for blood glucose control. Histamine H_2 antagonists such as famotidine, ranitidine, or cimetidine are used to decrease gastric output, particularly in patients with massive small bowel resection or to prevent stress ulcers. Octreotide is a somatostatin analog that is used to decrease gastric and other intestinal secretions and has been shown to decrease the time needed for gastrointestinal fistula closure [125, 126]. Intravenous methylprednisolone can be added to parenteral nutrition solutions for those patients who need long-term corticosteroid therapy and cannot take oral corticosteroids.

G. Methods of Administration

Parenteral nutrition is generally administered continuously over 24 hours for most hospitalized patients. However, some patients, particularly those receiving parenteral nutrition at home, may cycle the parenteral nutrition so that it infuses over 10–16 hours. This allows a patient to be free of the infusion for a period of time during the day. Cycling also reverses hepatic steatosis and liver enzyme changes associated with continuous infusion [127].

H. Complications

Although parenteral nutrition has been a life-saving therapy, it is not totally benign and carries with it an extensive set of potential complications. Recognition, prevention, and treatment of the potential metabolic complications are imperative. These complications can be divided into four main categories: technical, septic, metabolic, and gastrointestinal.

1. TECHNICAL

Most of the technical complications associated with parenteral nutrition center around the placement of the catheter. Central venous access can be obtained via subclavian, jugular vein, or peripherally inserted central catheters. Hickman or Broviac catheters or implantable ports are used for long-term access. Mechanical complications of catheter insertion may include pneumothorax, hydrothorax, and vessel injury

TABLE 6 Daily Parenteral Trace Element Supplementation

Element	Stable adult	Adult with intestinal losses	1 mL of multiple trace element
Chromium	10–15 mcg	20 mcg	10 mcg
Copper	0.5–1.5 mg	—	1 mg
Manganese	150–800 mcg	—	500 mcg
Selenium	50–120 mcg	Up to 200 mcg	0–60 mcg
Zinc	2.5–4.0 mg +2 mg if catabolic	12 mg/kg small bowel fluid lost; 17 mg/kg of stool or ileostomy output	5 mg

TABLE 7   Osmolarity Calculations for Parenteral Nutrition

Grams of amino acids/L × 10 =	_____ mOsm
Grams of dextrose/L × 5 =	_____ mOsm
Grams of lipid/L × 1.5 =	_____ mOsm
Total mEq of electrolytes and minerals/L × 2.0 =	_____ mOsm
Osmolarity of parenteral nutrition = sum of all components.	

[128]. These risks are minimized when catheters are placed by experienced personnel. A chest X ray to verify venous placement should be obtained before infusing central parenteral nutrition formulas. The maximum osmolarity tolerated by a peripheral vein is 900 mOsm/L in order to prevent phlebitis . Therefore, these solutions must be carefully calculated (Table 7). Femoral lines are generally considered to be central lines. However, when administering parenteral nutrition solutions it is best to keep the concentration the same as a peripheral formula because the blood flow in the femoral vein is less than that of the subclavian or jugular. Solutions are therefore not diluted as quickly.

2. SEPSIS

Infectious complications associated with parenteral nutrition can be life threatening. Many hospitalized patients receiving parenteral nutrition have multiple other reasons for elevations in temperature and sepsis. However, a sudden change in the patient's usual temperature may be an indication of possible catheter sepsis. Sudden increases in blood glucose concentration in a patient who was previously normoglycemic may be an early indication of sepsis. The parenteral nutrition catheter can be seeded by a remote source or it can be the primary source of infection. Blood cultures should be drawn, the catheter changed over a guidewire, and the tip sent for culture. If there is obvious exudate coming from the catheter exit site, the catheter should be removed and a new one placed on the opposite side. If the catheter tip removed by a guidewire change is infected, the new catheter should be removed and another catheter placed on the opposite side [129].

3. METABOLIC

Several hepatobiliary and GI complications have been associated with parenteral nutrition. Abnormalities in liver function tests, namely, SGOT, SGPT, bilirubin, or alkaline phosphatase, have been associated with the infusion of parenteral nutrition [130]. The etiology of these changes is unclear, but the changes are transient and generally not associated with adverse clinical sequelae in adults. Hepatic steatosis has also been associated with the use of parenteral nutrition as exhibited by elevation of serum aminotransferase values, alkaline phosphatase, and bilirubin levels. But this, too, is a benign, transient, reversible phenomenon in patients on short-term parenteral nutrition and generally resolves in 10–15 days. The parenteral nutrition solution should be tailored to the individual patient's energy require-

ments and in some cases it may be necessary to provide a solution that contains dextrose, amino acids, and lipids. Intrahepatic cholestasis can occur within 2–6 weeks of initiation of parenteral nutrition. This may be manifested by a progressive increase in the total bilirubin and an elevation of serum alkaline phosphatase. The lack of intraluminal nutrients to stimulate hepatic bile flow by cholecystokinin is thought to lead to cholestasis [131]. Ursodeoxycholic acid has been used as therapy for patients with cholestasis [132]. The risk can be further reduced with the use of cyclic parenteral nutrition, restriction of dextrose, avoidance of overfeeding, and early enteral stimulation when feasible. The lack of enteral stimulation is also associated with villus hypoplasia, colonic mucosal atrophy, decreased gastric function, impaired gastrointestinal immunity, bacterial overgrowth, and bacterial translocation in experimental models [133]. Therapy should be aimed at providing some enteral nutrition as soon as possible whenever feasible.

Parenteral nutrition has also been associated with various macronutrient-related complications. There are risks associated with over- and underfeeding. Providing calories, especially in the form of hypertonic dextrose, above requirements, can result in hyperglycemia, hepatic abnormalities from fatty infiltration, potential respiratory acidosis from increased CO_2 production, and difficulty in weaning from ventilators. Minimum requirements for dextrose are estimated to be 1 mg/kg/minute or approximately 100 g/day for a 70-kg man. The maximal amount of dextrose tolerated is approximately 5–7 mg/kg/minute [119]. Underfeeding may result in depressed ventilatory drive, decreased respiratory muscle function, impaired immune function, and increased infection. Thus, it is important to tailor the parenteral nutrition prescription to the patient's needs.

Hyperglycemia is the most common complication associated with the administration of parenteral nutrition. Patients receiving parenteral nutrition often have numerous reasons for elevated blood glucose such as sepsis or administration of steroids. Serum glucose concentration should be maintained below 200 mg/dL. This may be achieved with the addition of insulin and/or substitution of lipid for dextrose. Hypoglycemia may occur from excess insulin administration, either in the parenteral nutrition solution or subcutaneously. Treatment may include initiation of a 10% dextrose infusion or administration of D_{50}.

The delivery of calories, particularly in the form of dextrose, may induce refeeding syndrome in a patient who has

TABLE 8 Dosing and Intravenous Replacement of Minerals in Adult Patients Receiving Parenteral Nutrition

Mineral	RDA oral (minimum)	Usual adult IV dose for parenteral nutrition (range)	Techniques of IV replacement
Calcium	800–1200 mg (20–30 mEq)	9–22 mEq	7–14 mEq not to exceed 0.7–1.8 mEq/minute
Phosphorus	800–1200 mg (26–39 mM)	15–30[a] mM	0.08–0.2 mM/kg over 6 hours[b]
Magnesium	280–350 mg (11.5–14.4 mEq)	8–24 mEq	24 mEq over 4–6 hours

Source: Adapted from Matarese, L. E. (Ed.). (1997). "Nutrition Support Handbook," p. 76. The Cleveland Clinic Foundation, Cleveland, OH.

[a]22–44 mEq of potassium phosphate or 20–40 mEq of sodium phosphate.

[b]1 mEq of potassium phosphate = 0.68 mM phosphorus; 1 mEq of sodium phosphate = 0.75 mM phosphorus.

been chronically starved or is extremely cachectic. Refeeding syndrome refers to the intracellular shift of electrolytes and minerals, especially phosphorus, magnesium, and potassium, as a result of aggressive nutrition support [134, 135]. This is a direct result of increased plasma insulin concentration when dextrose is administered. This shift of electrolytes and minerals can result in life-threatening low serum values. Thus, for patients who are at risk for refeeding, calories should be administered at 20 kcal/kg/day and advanced slowly.

The crystalline amino acid solutions used in parenteral nutrition are generally well tolerated in patients with normal hepatic and renal function. The amino acids should be adjusted according to the patient's tolerance, clinical response and monitoring of visceral protein status, nitrogen balance, blood urea nitrogen, and creatinine.

Intravenous lipid emulsion is administered as a source of essential fatty acids and calories. Hyperlipidemia may result with excess or rapid administration. Serum triglyceride levels should be checked in any patient with a known history of hyperlipidemia prior to infusion of intravenous lipid emul-

sion. Acceptable serum triglyceride levels are less than 250 mg/dL 4 hours after lipid infusion for piggybacked lipids, and less than 400 mg/dL for continuous lipid infusion.

Electrolyte and mineral imbalances may occur in severely stressed patients both before and after parenteral nutrition infusion begins. It is best to correct any electrolyte abnormalities before parenteral nutrition is initiated. Once parenteral nutrition is initiated, it is important to monitor electrolytes, particularly magnesium, potassium, and phosphorus, carefully. Abnormally low values of electrolytes should be corrected promptly with intravenous replacements to avoid serious complications such as seizures, arrhythmias, or even death (Tables 8 and 9).

Dehydration and fluid overload are also potential complications of parenteral nutrition. In general, fluid requirements can be estimated at 30–35 mL/kg/day. Patients who are dehydrated may have fluid requirements as high as 40–50 mL/kg/day. The problem can be further exacerbated by excessive losses from nasogastric tubes, surgical drains, high output ostomies, and diarrhea. The volume can be increased in the

TABLE 9 Dosing and Intravenous Replacement of Electrolytes in Adult Patients Receiving Parenteral Nutrition

Electrolyte	RDA[a] oral	Usual adult IV dose	Calculation of deficit	Technique of IV replacement
Sodium (Na)	500 mg (21.7 mEq)	100–150 mEq	Na deficit (mEq) = 0.6 (wt in kg) × (140 − Na) + (140) × (volume deficit in L)	Replace ½ deficit over 24 hours and repeat serum Na.
Potassium (K)	2000 mg (51 mEq)	60–120 mEq	K deficit (mEq) = 100–200 mEq if serum K 3.0–3.5	Replace ½ deficit in 12–24 hours with replacements of 20 mEq KCl in 100 mL D₅W over 1–2 hours. Recheck K level 1 hour after replacement. Continue replacement if necessary.
Chloride (Cl)	750 mg (21 mEq)	100–150 mEq	Cl deficit (mEq) = 0.5 (wt in kg) × (103 − measured Cl)	Replace ½ deficit over 24 hours.

Source: Adapted from Matarese, L. E. (Ed.). (1997). "Nutrition Support Handbook," p. 79. The Cleveland Clinic Foundation, Cleveland, OH.

[a]Minimum requirements of healthy persons.

parenteral nutrition formula to accommodate these needs and/or separate supplemental intravenous fluids can be employed. Fluid overload, edema, and anasarca may be present in critically ill patients and in patients with renal or hepatic failure, congestive heart failure, and hypoalbuminemia. In these situations, it is best to concentrate the parenteral nutrition solution.

IV. CONCLUSION

Enteral and parenteral nutrition are effective methods of providing nutrients to patients who cannot or will not eat. But both of these therapies have unique potential complications, some of which can be life threatening. When knowledgeable health care professionals provide these therapies, the complications can be minimized. Nutrition support, both enteral and parenteral therapies, have become standard, life-saving therapies across the continuum of care.

References

1. Moore, F. A., Moore, E. E., Jones, T. N., McCroskey, B. L., and Peterson, V. M. (1989). TEN versus TPN following major abdominal trauma-reduced septic morbidity. *J. Trauma* **29**, 916–922.
2. Kudsk, K. A., Croce, M. A., Fabian, T. C., Minard, G., Tolley, E. A., Poret, H. A., Kuhn, M. R., and Brown, R. O. (1992). Enteral versus parenteral feeding: Effects on septic morbidity after blunt and penetrating abdominal trauma. *Ann. Surg.* **215**, 503–513.
3. Moore, E. E., and Jones, T. N. (1986). Benefits of immediate jejunostomy feeding after major abdominal trauma: A prospective randomized study. *J. Trauma* **26**, 874–881.
4. Bower, R. H., Talamini, M. A., Sax, H. C., Hamilton, F., and Fischer, J. E. (1986). Postoperative enteral vs parenteral nutrition. A randomized, controlled trial. *Arch. Surg.* **121**, 1040–1045.
5. Kudsk, K. A., Carpenter, G., Petersen, S., and Sheldon, G. F. (1981). Effect of enteral and parenteral feeding in malnourished rats with E. coli-hemoglobin adjuvant peritonitis. *J. Surg. Res.* **31**, 105–110.
6. Beyer, P. L. (1998). Complications of enteral nutrition. *In* "Contemporary Nutrition Support Practice" (L. E. Matarese and M. M. Gottschlich, Eds.), pp. 216–226. W. B. Saunders Co., Philadelphia, PA.
7. DeChicco, R. S., and Matarese, L. E. (1998). Determining the nutrition support regimen. *In* "Contemporary Nutrition Support Practice" (L. E. Matarese and M. M. Gottschlich, Eds.), pp. 185–191. W. B. Saunders Co., Philadelphia, PA.
8. Lord, L. M., Weiser-Maimone, A., Pulhamus, M., and Sax, H. C. (1993). Comparison of weighted vs unweighted enteral feeding tubes for efficacy of transpyloric intubation. *J. Parenteral Enteral Nutr.* **17**, 271–273.
9. Zaloga, G. P. (1991). Bedside method for placing small bowel feeding tubes in critically ill patients: A prospective study. *Chest* **100**, 1643–1646.
10. Montecalvo, M. A., Steger, K. A., Farber, H. W., Smith, B. F., Dennis, R. C., Fitzpatrick, G. F., Pollack, S. D., Korsberg, T. Z., Birkett, D. H., and Hirsh, E. F. (1992). Nutritional outcome and pneumonia in critical care patients randomized to gastric versus jejunal tube feedings. *Crit. Care Med.* **20**, 1377–1378.
11. Larson, D. E., Burton, D. D., Schroeder, K. W., and DiMagno, E. P. (1987). Percutaneous endoscopic gastrostomy. *Gastroenterology* **93**, 48–52.
12. Kirby, D. F., Craig, R. M., Tsang, T., and Plotnick, B. H. (1986). Percutaneous endoscopic gastrostomies: A prospective evaluation and review of the literature. *J. Parenteral Enteral Nutr.* **10**, 155–159.
13. Ponsky, J. L., Gauderer, M. W. L., Stellato, T. A., and Aszodi, A. (1984). Percutaneous approaches to enteral alimentation. *Am. J. Surg.* **149**, 102–105.
14. Shike, M., Wallach, C., and Likier, H. (1991). Direct percutaneous endoscopic jejunostomies. *Gastrointest. Endos.* **37**, 62–65.
15. Bricker, M., Mitchell, H. H., and Kinsman, G. M. (1945). The protein requirements of adult human subjects in terms of the protein contained in individual food and food combinations. *J. Nutr.* **30**, 269–283.
16. Brinson, R. R., Hanumanthu, S. K., and Pitts, W. M. (1989). A reappraisal of the peptide-based enteral formulas: Clinical applications. *Nutr. Clin. Prac.* **4**, 211–217.
17. Trocki, O., Mochizuki, H., Dominioni, L., and Alexander, J. W. (1986). Intact protein versus free amino acids in the nutritional support of thermally injured animals. *J. Parenteral Enteral Nutr.* **10**, 139–145.
18. Zaloga, G. P. (1990). Physiologic effects of peptide-based enteral formulas. *Nutr. Clin. Prac.* **5**, 231–237.
19. Adibi, S., and Phillips, E. (1968). Evidence for greater absorption of amino acid from peptide than from free form in human intestine. *Clin. Res.* **16**, 446.
20. Brinson, R., and Kolts, B. (1988). Diarrhea associated with sever hypoalbuminemia: A comparison of a peptide-based chemically defined and standard enteral alimentation. *Crit. Care Med.* **16**, 130–136.
21. Craft, I. L., Geddes, D., Hyde, C. W., Wise, I. J., and Matthews, D. M. (1968). Absorption and malabsorption of glycine and glycine peptides in man. *Gut* **9**, 425.
22. Meredith, J. W., Ditescheim, J. A., and Zaloga, G. P. (1990). Visceral protein levels in trauma patients are greater with peptide diet than with intact protein diet. *J. Trauma* **30**, 825–829.
23. Silk, D. B. A., Fairclough, P. D., and Clark, M. L. (1980). Use of peptide rather than free amino acid and nitrogen source in chemically defined elemental diets. *J. Parenteral Enteral Nutr.* **4**, 548–553.
24. McIntyre, P. B., Fitchew, M., and Lennard-Jones, J. E. (1986). Patients with a high ileostomy do not need a special diet. *Gastroenterology* **91**, 25–33.
25. Mowatt-Larssen, C. A., Brown, R. O., Wojtysiak, S. L., and Kudsk, K. A. (1992). Comparison of tolerance and nutritional outcome between a peptide and a standard enteral formula in critically ill hypoalbuminemic patients. *J. Parenteral Enteral Nutr.* **16**, 20–24.
26. Rees, R. G., Payne-James, J. J., Grimble, G. K., and Silk, D. B. A. (1988). Requirement of peptide versus whole protein in patients with impaired gastrointestinal function: A

double-blind controlled trial. *J. Parenteral Enteral Nutr.* **12**(Suppl.), 12S.

27. Royall, D., Jeejeebhoy, K. N., Baker, J. P., Allard, J. P., Habal, F. M., Cunnane, S. C., and Greenberg, G. R. (1994). Comparison of amino acid v. peptide based enteral diets in active Crohn's disease: Clinical and nutritional outcome. *Gut* **35**, 783–787.

28. Heimburger, D. C. (1990). Peptides in clinical practice. *Nutr. Clin. Prac.* **5**, 225–226.

29. Bell, S. J., Mascioli, E. A., Bistrian, B. R., Babayan, V. K., and Blackburn, G. L. (1991). Alternative lipid sources for enteral and parenteral nutrition: Long- and medium-chain triglycerides, structured triglycerides and fish oils. *J. Am. Dietet. Assoc.* **91**, 74–78.

30. Cerra, F. B., Alden, P. A., Negro, F., Billiar, T., Svingen, B. A., Licari, J., Johnson, S. B., and Holman, R. T. (1988). Sepsis and exogenous lipid modulation. *J. Parenteral Enteral Nutr.* **12**(6 Suppl.), 63S–68S.

31. Kinsella, J. E., and Lokesh, B. (1990). Dietary lipids, eicosanoids and immune function system. *Crit. Care Med.* **18**, S94.

32. Wan, J. F., Teo, T. C., Babayan, V. K., and Blackburn, G. L. (1988). Invited comment: Lipids and the development of immune dysfunction and infection. *J. Parenteral Enteral Nutr.* **12**, 435.

33. Isselbacher, K. J. (1966). Biochemical aspects of fat absorption. *Gastroenterology* **50**, 78.

34. Gottschlich, M. M. (1992). Selection of optimal lipid sources in enteral and parenteral nutrition. *Nutr. Clin. Prac.* **7**, 152.

35. Berner, Y., Morse, R., Frank, O., Baker, H., and Shike, M. (1989). Vitamin plasma levels in long-term enteral feeding patients. *J. Parenteral Enteral Nutr.* **13**, 525.

36. Evans, M. A., and Shronts, E. P. (1992). Intestinal fuels: Glutamine, short-chain fatty acids, and dietary fiber. *J. Am. Dietet. Assoc.* **92**, 1239–1246.

37. Scheppach, W., Burghardt, W., Bartram, P., and Kasper, H. (1990). Addition of dietary fiber to liquid formula diets: The pros and cons. *J. Parenteral Enteral Nutr.* **14**, 204–209.

38. Palacio, J. C., and Rombeau, J. L. (1990). Dietary fiber: A brief review and potential application to enteral nutrition. *Nutr. Clin. Prac.* **5**, 99–106.

39. Frankenfield, D. C., and Beyer, P. L. (1989). Soy-polysaccharide fiber: Effect on diarrhea in tube-fed head-injured patients. *Am. J. Clin. Nutr.* **50**, 533–538.

40. Shorey, R. L., Day, P. L., Willis, R. A., Lo, G. S., and Steinke, F. H. (1985). Effects of soybean polysaccharide on plasma lipids. *J. Am. Dietet. Assoc.* **85**, 1461–1465.

41. Gottschlich, M. M., Warden, G. D., Michel, M., Havens, P., Kopcha, R., Jenkins, M., and Alexander, J. W. (1988). Diarrhea in tube-fed burn patients: Incidence, etiology, nutritional impact and prevention. *J. Parenteral Enteral Nutr.* **12**, 338–345.

42. Keohane, P. P., Attrill, H., Love, M., Frost, P., and Silk, D. B. (1984). Relation between osmolality of diet and gastrointestinal side effects in enteral nutrition. *Br. Med. J.* **288**, 678.

43. Pesola, G. R., Hogg, J. E., Eissa, N., Matthews, D. E., and Carlon, G. C. (1990). Hypertonic nasogastric tube feedings: Do they cause diarrhea? *Crit. Care Med.* **18**, 1378.

44. Zarling, E. J., Parmar, J. R., Mobarhan, S., and Clapper, M. (1986). Effect of enteral formula infusion rate, osmolality, and chemical composition upon clinical tolerance and carbohydrate absorption in normal subjects. *J. Parenteral Enteral Nutr.* **10**, 588.

45. Powell, S. K., Marcuard, S. P., Farrior, E. S., and Gallagher, M. L. (1993). Aspirating gastric residuals causes occlusion of small-bore feeding tubes. *J. Parenteral Enteral Nutr.* **17**, 243–246.

46. Heyland, D. K., Cook, D. J., Schoenfeld, P. S., Frietag, A., Varon, J., and Wood, G. (1999). The effect of acidified enteral feeds on gastric colonization in critically ill patients: Results of a multicenter randomized trial. *Crit. Care Med.* **27**, 2399–2406.

47. Mirtallo, J., Kudsk, K., and Ebbert, M. (1984). Nutritional support of patients with renal disease. *Clin. Pharm.* **3**, 253–263.

48. Giordano, C. (1963). Use of exogenous and endogenous urea for protein synthesis in normal and uremic subjects. *J. Lab. Clin. Med.* **62**, 231–246.

49. Giovannetti, S., and Maggiore, Q. (1964). A low nitrogen diet with protein of high biological value for severe chronic uremia. *Lancet* **1**, 1000–1003.

50. Feinstein, I., Blumenkrantz, M. J., Healy, M., Koffler, A., Silberman, H., Massry, S. G., and Kopple, J. D. (1981). Clinical and metabolic responses to parenteral nutrition in acute renal failure. A controlled double-blind study. *Medicine* **60**, 124–137.

51. Mirtallo, J. M., Schneider, P. J., Mavko, K., Ruberg, R. L., and Fabri, P. J. (1982). A comparison of essential and general amino acid infusions in the nutritional support of patients with compromised renal function. *J. Parenteral Enteral Nutr.* **6**, 109–113.

52. Fisher, J. E. (1990). Branched-chain-enriched amino acid solutions in patients with liver failure: An early example of nutritional pharmacology. *J. Parenteral Enteral Nutr.* **14**, 249S–256S.

53. Fischer, J. E., Funovics, J. M., Aguirre, A., James, J. H., Keane, J. M., Wesdorp, R. I., Yoshimura, N., and Westman, T. (1975). The role of plasma amino acids in hepatic encephalopathy. *Surgery* **78**, 276–290.

54. ASPEN Board of Directors (1993). Guidelines for the use of parenteral and enteral nutrition in adult and pediatric patients. *J. Parenteral Enteral Nutr.* **17**, 1SA–52SA.

55. Brennan, M. F., Cerra, F., Daly, J. M., Fischer, J. E., Moldower, L. L., Smith, R. J., Vinnars, E., Wannemacher, R., and Young, V. R. (1986). Report of a research workshop: Branched-chain amino acids in stress and injury. *J. Parenteral Enteral Nutr.* **10**, 446–452.

56. Talbot, J. M. (1993). Guidelines for the scientific review of enteral food products for special medical purposes. *J. Parenteral Enteral Nutr.* **15**, 99S–174S.

57. Eriksson, L. S., Persson, A., and Wahren, J. (1982). Branched-chain amino acids in the treatment of chronic hepatic encephalopathy. *Gut* **23**, 801–806.

58. McGhee, A., Henderson, J. M., Millikan, W. J., Bleier, J. C., Vogel, R., Kassouny, M., and Rudman, D. (1983). Comparison of the effects of hepatic-aid and a case in modular diet on encephalopathy, plasma amino acids and nitrogen balance in cirrhotic patients. *Ann. Surg.* **197**, 288–293.

59. Schafer, K., Winther, M. B., Ukida, M., Leweling, H., Reiter, H. J., and Bode, J. C. (1981). Influence of an orally administered protein mixture enriched in branched-chain amino acids

on the chronic hepatic encephalopathy (CHE). of patients with liver cirrhosis. *Gastroenterology* **19**, 356–362.

60. Horst, D., Grace, N. D., Conn, H. O., Schiff, E., Schenker, S., Viteri, A., Law, D., and Atterbury, C. E. (1984). Comparison of dietary protein with an oral branched-chain amino acid supplement in chronic portal-systemic encephalopathy: A randomized, controlled trial. *Hepatology* **4**, 279–287.

61. Al-Saady, N. M., Blakemore, C. M., and Bennett, E. D. (1989). High fat, low carbohydrate, enteral feeding lowers Paco₂ and reduces the period of ventilation in artificially ventilated patients. *Intens. Care Med.* **15**, 290–295.

62. Angelillo, V. A., Bedi, S., Durfee, D., Dahl, J., Patterson, A. J., and O'Donohue, W. J., Jr. (1985). Effects of low and high carbohydrate feedings in ambulatory patients with chronic obstructive pulmonary disease and chronic hypercapnia. *Ann. Intern. Med.* **103**, 883–885.

63. Goldstein, S. A., Askanazi, J., Elwyn, D. H., Thomashow, B., Milic-Emili, J., Kvetan, V., Weissman, C., and Kinney, J. M. (1989). Submaximal exercise in emphysema and malnutrition at two levels of carbohydrate and fat intake. *J. Appl. Physiol.* **67**, 1048–1055.

64. Goldstein, S. A., Thomashow, B., and Askanazi, J. (1986). Functional changes during nutritional repletion in patients with lung disease. *Clin. Chest Med.* **7**, 141–151.

65. Talpers, S. S., Romberger, D. J., Bunce, S. B., and Pingleton, S. K. (1992). Nutritionally associated increased carbon dioxide production: Excess total calories vs high proportion of carbohydrate calories. *Chest* **102**, 551–555.

66. Buse, M. G., and Reid, S. S. (1975). Leucine: A possible regulator of protein turnover in muscle. *J. Clin. Invest.* **56**, 1250–1261.

67. Cerra, F. B., Mazuski, J., Chute, E., Nuwer, N., Teasley, K., Lysne, J., Shronts, E. P., and Konstantindes, F. N. (1984). Branched-chain metabolic support: A prospective randomized, double-blind trial in surgical stress. *Ann. Surg.* **199**, 286–291.

68. Bower, R. H., Muggia-Sullan, M., Vallgren, S., Hurst, J. M., Kern, K. A., LaFrance, R., and Fischer, J. E. (1986). Branched-chain amino acid-enriched solutions in the septic patient. A randomized, prospective trial. *Ann. Surg.* **203**, 13–20.

69. Chiarla, C., Siegel, J., Kidd, S., Coleman, B., Mora, R., Tacchino, R., Placko, R., Gum, M., Wiles, C. E., III, and Belzberg, H. (1988). Inhibition of post-traumatic septic proteolysis and ureagenesis and stimulation of hepatic acute-phase protein production by branched-chain amino acid TPN. *J. Trauma* **28**, 1145–1172.

70. Kuhl, D. A., Brown, R. O., Vehe, K. L., Boucher, B. A., Luther, R. W., and Kudsk, K. A. (1990). Use of selected visceral protein measurements in the comparison of branched-chain amino acids with standard amino acids in parenteral nutrition support of injured patients. *Surgery* **107**, 503–510.

71. Cerra, F. B., Shronts, E. P., Konstantinides, N. N., Thoele, S., Konstantinides, F. N., Teasley, K., and Lysne, J. (1985). Enteral feeding in sepsis: A prospective, randomized, double-blind trial. *Surgery* **98**, 632–639.

72. Gardemann, A., Wantanbe, Y., Grosse, V., Hesse, S., and Jungermann, K. (1992). Increases in intestinal glucose absorption and hepatic glucose uptake elicited by luminal but not vascular glutamine in the jointly perfused small intestine and liver of the rat. *Biochemistry* **283**, 795–765.

73. Rhoads, J. M., Keku, E. O., Quinn, J., Woosely, J., and Lecce, J. G. (1991). L-glutamine stimulates jejunal sodium and chloride absorption in pig rotavirus enteritis. *Gastroenterology* **100**, 683–691.

74. Tamada, H., Nezu, R., Matsu, Y., Imanura, I., Takagi, Y., and Okada, A. (1993). Alanyl glutamine-enriched total parenteral nutrition restores intestinal adaptation after either proximal or distal massive resection in rats. *J. Parenteral Enteral Nutr.* **27**, 236–242.

75. Lacey, J. M., and Wilmore, D. W. (1990). Is glutamine a conditionally essential amino acid? *Nutr. Rev.* **48**, 297–309.

76. Sitren, H. S., and Fisher, H. (1977). Nitrogen retention in rats fed on diets enriched with arginine and glycine. I. Improved N retention after trauma. *Br. J. Nutr.* **37**, 195–208.

77. Barbul, A., Rettura, G., Levenson, S. M., and Seifter, E. (1981). Wound healing and thymotropic effects of arginine: A pituitary mechanism of action. *Am. J. Clin. Nutr.* **37**, 786–794.

78. Nirgiotis, J. G., Hennessey, P. J., and Andrassy, R. J. (1991). The effects of arginine-free enteral diet on wound healing and immune function in the postsurgical rat. *J. Pediatr. Surg.* **26**, 936–941.

79. Barbul, A., Wasserkrug, H. L., Yoshimura, N., Tao, R., and Efron, G. (1984). High arginine levels in intravenous hyperalimentation abrogate post-traumatic immune suppression. *J. Surg. Res.* **36**, 620–624.

80. Barbul, A., Sisto, D. A., Wasserkrug, H. L., and Efon, G. (1981). Arginine stimulates lymphocyte immune response in healthy human beings. *Surgery* **90**, 244–251.

81. Saito, H., Trocki, O., Wang, S. L., Gonce, S. J., Joffe, S. N., and Alexander, J. W. (1987). Metabolic and immune effects of dietary arginine supplementation after burn. *Arch. Surg.* **122**, 784–789.

82. Daly, J. M., Reynolds, J. V., Thom, A., Kinsley, L., Dietrick-Gallagher, M., Shou, J., and Ruggieri, B. (1988). Immune and metabolic effects of arginine in the surgical patient. *Ann. Surg.* **208**, 512–523.

83. Atkinson, S., Sieffert, E., and Bihari, D. (1998). A prospective randomized double-blind clinical trial of enteral immunonutrition in the critically ill. *Crit. Care Med.* **26**, 1164–1172.

84. Bower, R. H., Cerra, F. B., Bershadsky, B., Licari, J. J., Hoyt, D. B., Jensen, G. L., VanBuren, C. T., Rothkopf, M. M., Daly, J. M., and Adelsberg, B. R. (1995). Early enteral administration of a formula (IMPACT). supplemented with arginine, nucleotides, and fish oil in intensive care unit patients: Results of a multicenter, prospective, randomized clinical trial. *Crit. Care Med.* **23**, 436–449.

85. Galban, C., Celaya, S., Marco, P., Mesejo, A., Montejo, J. C., Sanchez-Segura, J. M., Santiago, C. H. U. S., Clinico Zaragoza, H., Aranzazu San Sebastian, N. S., and Clinico Valencia, H. (1998). An immune-enhancing enteral diet reduces mortality and episodes of bacteremia in septic ICU patients [abstract]. *J. Parenteral Enteral Nutr.* **22**, S13.

86. Senkal, M., Mumme, A., Eickhoff, U., Geier, B., Spath, G., Wulfert, D., Joosten, V., and Frei, A. (1997). Early postoperative enteral immunonutrition: Clinical outcome and cost-comparison analysis in surgical patients. *Crit. Care Med.* **25**, 1489–1496.

87. Braga, M., Gianotti, L., Vignali, A., and DiCarlo, V. (1998). Artificial nutrition after major abdominal surgery: Impact of

route of administration and composition of the diet. *Crit. Care Med.* **26,** 24–30.

88. Moore, F. A., Moore, E. E., Kudsk, K. A., Brown, R. O., Bower, R. H., Koruda, M. J., Baker, C. C., and Barbul, A. (1994). Clinical benefits of an immune-enhancing diet for early postinjury enteral feeding. *J. Trauma* **37,** 607–615.

89. Daly, J. M., Lieberman, M. D., Goldfine, J., Shou, J., Weintraub, F., Rosato, E. F., and Lavin, P. (1992). Enteral nutrition with supplemental arginine, RNA, omega-3 fatty acids in patients after operation: Immunologic, metabolic, and clinical outcome. *Surgery* **112,** 56–67.

90. Daly, J. M., Weintraub, F. N., Shou, J., Rosato, E. F., and Lucia, M. (1995). Enteral nutrition during multimodality therapy in upper gastrointestinal cancer patients. *Ann. Surg.* **221,** 327–338.

91. Kudsk, K. A., Minard, G., Croce, M. A., Brown, R. O., Lowrey, T. S., Pritchard, F. E., Dickerson, R. N., and Fabian, T. C. (1996). A randomized trial of isonitrogenous enteral diets after severe trauma: An immune enhancing diet reduces septic complications. *Ann. Surg.* **224,** 531–540.

92. Weimann, A., Bastian, L., Grotz, M., Hansel, M., Lotz, T., Trautwein, C., Tusch, G., Schlitt, H. J., and Regel, G. (1998). The influence of an immune-enhanced enteral diet on systemic inflammatory response syndrome in patients with severe multiple injury. *Nutrition* **14**(2), 165–172.

93. Cerra, F. B., Lehman, S., Konstantinides, N., Konstantinides, F., Shronts, E. P., and Holman, R. (1990). Effect of enteral nutrient on in vitro tests of immune function in ICU patients: A preliminary report. *Nutrition* **6,** 84–87.

94. Schilling, J., Vranjes, N., Fierz, W., Joller, H., Gyurech, D., Ludwig, E., Marathias, K., and Geroulanos, S. (1996). Clinical outcome and immunology of postoperative arginine, omega-3 fatty acids, and nucleotide-enriched enteral feeding: A randomized prospective comparison with standard enteral and low calorie/low fat IV solutions. *Nutrition* **12,** 423–429.

95. Beale, R. J., Bryg, D. J., and Bihari, D. J. (1999). Immunonutrition in the critically ill: A systematic review of clinical outcome. *Crit. Care Med.* **27,** 2799–2805.

96. American Diabetes Association (1994). Nutritional recommendations and principles for people with diabetes mellitus. *Diabetes Care* **17,** 519–522.

97. Peters, A. L., and Davidson, M. B. (1992). Effects of various enteral feeding products on postprandial blood glucose in patients with type I diabetes. *J. Parenteral Enteral Nutr.* **16,** 69–74.

98. Peters, A. L., Davidson, M. B., and Isaac, R. M. (1989). Lack of glucose elevation after simulated tube feeding with a low-carbohydrate, high fat enteral formula in patients with type I diabetes. *Am. J. Med.* **87,** 178–182.

99. Heibert, J. M., Brown, A., Anderson, R. G., Halfacre, S., Rodeheaver, G. T., and Edlich, R. F. (1981). Comparison of continuous vs intermittent tube feedings in adult burn patients. *J. Parenteral Enteral Nutr.* **5,** 73–75.

100. Silk, D. B. A., Rees, R. G. P., Keohane, P. P., and Attrill, H. (1987). Clinical efficacy and design changes of "fine-bore" nasogastric feeding tubes: A seven-year experience involving 809 intubations in 403 patients. *J. Parenteral Enteral Nutr.* **11,** 378–383.

101. Caufield, K. A., Page, C. P., and Pestana C. (1991). Technique for intraduodenal placement of transnasal enteral feeding catheters. *Nutr. Clin. Prac.* **6,** 23–26.

102. Metheny, N. (1992). Minimizing respiratory complications of nasogastric tube feedings: State of the science. *Heart Lung* **22,** 213–223.

103. Kadakia, S. C., Sullivan, H. O., and Starnes, H. O. (1992). Percutaneous endoscopic gastrostomy or jejunostomy and the incidence of aspiration in 79 patients. *Am. J. Surg.* **164,** 114–118.

104. Fay, D. E., Poplausky, M., Gruber M., and Lance, P. (1991). Long-term enteral feeding: A retrospective comparison of delivery via percutaneous endoscopic gastrostomy and naso-enteric tubes. *Am. J. Gastroenterol.* **86,** 1604–1609.

105. Singh, S., and Richter, J. E. (1992). Effects of a pH electrode across the lower esophageal sphincter. *Dig. Dis. Sci.* **37,** 667–672.

106. Coben, R. M., Weintraub, A., DiMartino, A. J., Jr., and Cohen, S. (1994). Gastroesophageal reflux during gastrostomy feeding. *Gastroenterology* **106,** 13–18.

107. Ibanez, J., Penafiel, A., Raurich, J. M., and Mata, F. (1992). Gastroesophageal reflux in intubated patients receiving enteral nutrition: Effect of supine and semirecumbent positions. *J. Parenteral Enteral Nutr.* **16,** 419–422.

108. Barclay, B. A., and Litchford, M. D. (1991). Incidence of nasoduodenal tube occlusion and patient removal of tubes: A prospective study. *J. Am. Dietet. Assoc.* **91,** 220–222.

109. Benson, D. W., Griggs, B. A., Hamilton, F., Hiyama, D. T., and Bower, R. H. (1990). Clogging of feeding tubes: A randomized trial of a newly designed tube. *Nutr. Clin. Prac.* **5,** 107–110.

110. Cutie, A. J., Altman, E., and Lenkel, L. (1983). Compatibility of enteral products with commonly employed drug additives. *J. Parenteral Enteral Nutr.* **7,** 186–191.

111. Keohane, P. P., Attrill, H., Love, M., Frost, P., and Silk, D. B. (1984). Relation between osmolality of diet and gastrointestinal side effects in enteral nutrition. *Br. Med. J.* **288,** 678–681.

112. Edes, T. E., Walk, B. E., and Austin, J. L. (1990). Diarrhea in tube-fed patients: Feeding formula not necessarily the cause. *Am. J. Med.* **88,** 91–93.

113. Eisenber, P. G. (1993). Causes of diarrhea in tube-fed patients: A comprehensive approach to diagnosis and management. *Nutr. Clin. Prac.* **8,** 119–123.

114. Clausen, M. R., Bonnan, H., Tvede, M., and Mortensen, P. B. (1991). Colonic fermentation to short-chain fatty acids is decreased in antibiotic-associated diarrhea. *Gastroenterology* **101,** 1497–1504.

115. Vanlandingham, S., Simpson, S., Daniel, P., and Newmark, S. R. (1981). Metabolic abnormalities in patients supported with enteral tube feeding. *J. Parenteral Enteral Nutr.* **5,** 322–324.

116. Skipper, A. (1998). Principles of parenteral nutrition. *In* "Contemporary Nutrition Support Practice" (L. E. Matarese and M. M. Gottschlich, Eds.), pp. 227–242. W. B. Saunders Co., Philadelphia, PA.

117. Freund, H., Dienstag, J., Lehrich, J., Yoshimura, N., Bradford, R. R., Rosen, H., Atamian, S., Slemmer, E., Holroyde, J., and Fischer, J. E. (1982). Infusion of branched-chain enriched amino acid solution in patients with hepatic encephalopathy. *Ann. Surg.* **196,** 209–219.

118. Naylor, C. D., O'Rourke, K., Detsky, A., and Baker, J. P. (1989). Parenteral nutrition with branched-chain amino acids in hepatic encephalopathy. A meta-analysis. *Gastroenterology* **97,** 1033–1042.

119. Wolfe, R. R., O'Donnell, T. F., Jr., Stone, M. D., Richmand, D. A., and Burke, J. F. (1980). Investigation of factors determining the optimal glucose infusion rate in total parenteral nutrition. *Metabolism* **29,** 892–900.

120. Seidner, D. L., Mascioli, E. A., Istfan, N. W., Porter, K. A., Selleck, K., Blackburn, G. L., and Bistrian, B. R. (1989). Effects of long-chain triglyceride emulsions on reticuloendothelial system function in humans. *J. Parenteral Enteral Nutr.* **13,** 614–619.

121. Farber, M. D., Schmidt, R. J., Bear, R. A., and Narins, R. G. (1987). Management of fluid, electrolyte, and acid–base disorders in surgical patients. *In* "Clinical Disorders of Fluid and Electrolyte Metabolism," 5th ed. (R. G. Naris, Ed.), pp. 1407–1436. McGraw-Hill, New York.

122. Grant, J. P. (1992). *In* "Handbook of Total Parenteral Nutrition," 2nd ed., p. 174. W. B. Saunders Co., Philadelphia, PA.

123. American Medical Association Department of Foods and Nutrition (1979). Multivitamin preparations for parenteral use. A statement by the Nutrition Advisory Group. *J. Parenteral Enteral Nutr.* **3,** 258–262.

124. AMA Department of Foods and Nutrition (1979). Guidelines for essential trace element preparations for parenteral use: A statement by an expert panel. *J. Am. Med. Assoc.* **241,** 2052–2054.

125. Lembycke, B., Creutzfeldt, W., Schleser, S., Ebert, R., Shaw, C., and Koop, I. (1987). Effect of the somatostatin analogue sandostatin SMS 201-995 on gastrointestinal, pancreatic, and biliary function and hormone release in man. *Digestion* **36,** 108–124.

126. Torres, A. J., Landa, J. I., Moreno-Azcoita, M., Arguello, J. M., Silecchia, G., Gastro, J., Hernandez-Merlof, F., Jover, J. M., Moreno-Gonzales, E., and Balibrea, J. Z. (1992). Somatostatin in the management of gastrointestinal fistulas. *Arch. Surg.* **127,** 97–99.

127. Maini, B., Blackburn, G. L., Bistrian, B. R., Flatt, J. P., Page, J. G., Bothe, A., Benotti, P., and Rienhoff, H. Y. (1976). Cyclic hyperalimentation: An optimal technique for preservation of visceral proteins. *J. Surg. Res.* **20,** 515–525.

128. Fuhrman, M. P. (1998). Management of complications of parenteral nutrition. *In* "Contemporary Nutrition Support Practice" (L. E. Matarese and M. M. Gottschlich, Eds.), pp. 243–263. W. B. Saunders Co., Philadelphia, PA.

129. Bozzetti, F., Terno, G., Bonfanti, G., Scarpa, D., Scotti, A., Ammatuna, M., and Bonalumi, M. G. (1983). Prevention and treatment of central venous catheter sepsis by exchange via a guidewire. *Ann. Surg.* **198,** 48–52.

130. Clarke, P. J., Ball, M. J., and Kettlewell, M. G. (1991). Liver function tests in patients receiving parenteral nutrition. *J. Parenteral Enteral Nutr.* **15,** 54–59.

131. Quigley, E. M. M., Marsh, M. N., Shaffer, J. L., and Markin, R. S. (1993). Hepatobiliary complications of total parenteral nutrition. *Gastroenterology* **104,** 286–301.

132. Beau, P., Labat-Labourdette, J., Ingrand, P., and Beauchant, M. (1994). Is ursodeoxycholic acid an effective therapy for total parenteral nutrition-related liver disease? *J. Hepatol.* **20,** 240–244.

133. Illig, K. A., Ryan, C. K., Hardy, D. J., Rhodes, J., Locke, W., and Sax, H. C. (1992). Total parenteral nutrition-induced changes in gut mucosal function: Atrophy alone is not the issue. *Surgery* **112,** 631–637.

134. Sacks, G. S., Walker, J., Dickersons, R. N., Kudsk, K. A., and Brown, R. O. (1994). Observations of hypophosphatemia and its management in nutrition support. *Nutr. Clin. Prac.* **9,** 105–108.

135. Brooks, M. J., and Melnik, G. (1995). The refeeding syndrome: An approach to understanding its complications and preventing its occurrence. *Pharmacotherapy* **12,** 713–726.

CHAPTER 17

Herbs and Botanical Supplements: Principles and Concepts

CYNTHIA THOMSON AND ROBERT B. LUTZ
University of Arizona, Tucson, Arizona

I. INTRODUCTION: HISTORY OF BOTANICAL MEDICINE

A. Historical Background

The use of herbal and botanical products to prevent or treat disease has been in existence for thousands of years. Asians and Native Indian tribes throughout the world have been acknowledged for their contribution to botanical medicine. It is estimated that more than 30,000 herbs and botanicals have been studied for medicinal qualities, but fewer than 300 are currently used in Western medicine. The use of botanicals to prevent or treat disease is likely innate. Given a world without prescription medications, humans explored their surroundings to find the answers to ailments. Documentation of the virtues of herbs is available as early as the eighth century B.C. through the writings of Hesiod and Hippocrates who described their usage in the fourth century B.C. [1]. The National Institute of Medical Herbalists, established in 1864, provided the first professional identity for the study of botanical medicine.

B. Definitions and Related Terminology

The study of botanical medicine warrants an understanding of the terminology used by herbal medicine practitioners. It is clear that this is an area of medicine for which consensus has generally not yet been established and legal and practical definitions vary. Table 1 provides a list of definitions of the terms commonly used. An understanding of the selected terminology is the foundation for studying any science—new or old—and is essential to the advancement of the science. Yet, with botanical medicine, there remain inconsistencies in defining the terminology, which may at least partially contribute to the unease most scientists have with the use of these products. To begin, even the word *herb* is difficult to define. Botanists would define any herb as a nonwoody, seed-producing plant that regresses to its root structure after each growing season and is generally administered as a whole plant [2]. Botanicals, in contrast to herbs, include all trees and shrubs as well as herbs, including those that thrive year round [3]. Most practitioners of botanical medicine de-

scribe herbs and botanicals based on the medicinal qualities or the ability of the plant to induce a pharmacological effect in humans. Herbs are generally administered as whole plants, while botanicals may be derived from parts of plants such as the root, stem, or leaf. Varro Tyler [4], a recognized expert in the field of botanical medicine, has defined herbs as "crude drugs of vegetable origin utilized for the treatment of disease states, often of a chronic nature, or to attain or maintain a condition of improved health." The Food and Drug Administration uses the term *botanical* in its legal definition of an herb [5].

Although the exact definition may seem a trite issue, it is in fact an issue of significant relevance in that the definition selected may determine whether botanicals are drugs or food. If the product is used to treat or mitigate a disease, it should be considered a drug. However, if the herb/botanical is used as a food flavoring or dietary component it would be considered a food [6]. The confusion evolves as more and more food products are used for multiple purposes and cross the line between food and drug. Examples include garlic, used to treat hypertension and to flavor Italian food; cranberry, used to prevent or treat urinary tract infections and a base for juice; or peppermint, used to relax smooth muscle in patients with irritable bowel syndrome and as a flavoring agent. The line between food and drug becomes even more obscure when foods are enhanced with botanicals with the intent to augment the health-promoting value of the food. These foods are generally referred to as functional foods [7]. Examples of functional foods include soups with added echinacea, snack chips with kava kava, and beverages with added ginseng.

II. USE OF HERBS AND BOTANICALS

A. Reported Use

Although there are no universally accepted statistics on herbal and botanical use in the United States, several surveys have been completed by private industries during the past several years that provide insight into the trends in herb and

TABLE 1 Botanical Medicine Terminology

Term	Definition
Botanicals	Herbs, trees, and shrubs or components thereof that exert a pharmacologic effect on the body
Elixir	Hydroalcoholic combination extract sweetened with sugar or glycerol
Ethnobotanist	Person who studies the use of plants as food and medicine in a variety of cultures throughout the world
Extract	Concentrated (1:1 dilution) ground herb that has been treated with alcohol and heat until 1 mL is equivalent to 1 g of herb powder
Functional food	Any modified food or food ingredient that may provide a health benefit beyond the traditional nutrients it contains
Guaranteed potency herb (GPH)	Herbal product tested throughout the manufacturing and harvesting processes to ensure that the endproduct has the proper percentage of active ingredient
Herb	"Crude drugs" of vegetable origin utilized for the treatment of disease states, often of a chronic nature, or to attain or maintain a condition of improved health
Herbalism	Use of crude plant-based products to treat or prevent disease
Herbal medicinal	Product derived from plants or parts of plants that elicits a pharmacological effect
Phytopharmaceuticals	Plant-based medicines that have been standardized based on the pharmacologically active constituent(s)
Standardized	Use of a particular or selected chemical or active constituent as an indicator or marker of biological activity/effectiveness
Synergy	Influence or effect that occurs when constituents of a botanical act together in biological systems to elicit an effect that is greater biologically than the effect obtained by ingestion of any of the individual constituents alone
Tincture	Less concentrated (1:3, 1:5, 1:10) liquid botanical remedy that contains alcohol and water solvents
Tonic	Agent that restores the activity of an organ or organ system within the body
Phytotherapy	Used in European literature to describe herbalism that uses only standardized products

botanical use. What is clear is that the use of botanical remedies in the United States has risen significantly during the past decade with 1500–1800 products currently on the U.S. market [8]. Internationally, it has been estimated that 80% of adults use herbal remedies [9]. A recent survey published by Aarts [10] estimated that dietary supplement sales were $12 billion annually with approximately 34% of Americans consuming herbal supplements. Specifically, U.S. expenditures for herbal supplements ranged from $2 billion in 1996 to an estimated $5 billion in 2000 [11]. This reflects a 15% annual growth rate with no clear plateau in sales in sight.

Recently, the National Institutes of Health Office of Dietary Supplements and the U. S. Department of Agriculture reported plans to expand the National Health and Nutrition Examination Survey to include more specific data regarding dietary supplement use [12]. This is an essential first step to more clearly ascertain the depth and breadth of herbal and botanical use among Americans. Secondly, there is growing interest in establishing dietary supplement databases, which allow for more accurate scientific investigation into the safety and efficacy of these products. Several reports on the use of alternative medicine, including herbal product use,

have been published in recent years [13–16] and indicate that the use of herbal product is one of the leading forms of alternative medicine selected by patients. Most recently, Eisenberg et al. [13] cited a 380% increase in botanical use among Americans.

B. Factors Associated with Increased Use of Botanicals

Several factors have been identified as contributing to the increase in botanical use [17]. First, America's population is aging and thus looking for cost-effective, convenient, and low-risk ways to reduce risk for chronic disease. In the case of those experiencing chronic disease, the goal is to reduce symptoms and improve quality of life. In addition, Americans are taking a greater responsibility for their health and are less satisfied with conventional medicine. Many believe herbals are a more natural and, therefore, less risky approach to treating disease.

In recent years, the National Institutes of Health established the National Center for Complementary and Alternative Medicine and the Office of Dietary Supplements. These

TABLE 2 Assessment of Botanical Supplement Use

1. What supplements are you currently taking? Include over-the-counter, self-selected, and those prescribed by a health care practitioner.
2. Dose and frequency
   - Regularity
   - With meals or other supplements?
   - What compound or formulation?
   - What route of administration?
3. Why?
   - Perceived benefits
   - Prevention or treatment
   - Label claims
4. Patient education
   - Potential/proven benefits
   - Interactions with medications, other nutrients, or botanicals
   - Appropriate dosage
   - Duration of use
   - Reliable resources
5. Documentation
   - Product, dose, frequency
   - Clinical application
   - Efficacy
   - Education provided and patient understanding
   - Expected adherence

offices have provided new financial and research support for this area of practice, resulting in expanded interest in this growing area of health care. Finally, the computer age has significantly increased access to information on the potential benefits of botanicals, leading to increased supply and demand. Certainly, the etiology of the recent emergence of botanical medicine is multifactorial and complex but its expansion cannot be overlooked.

C. Assessing Patient Use of Botanical Medicines

One challenge facing health care professionals is developing and maintaining open communication with patients concerning the use of botanical supplements [18]. Research by Eisenberg and others [13, 19, 20] indicates that patients are reluctant to share information regarding alternative medicine including botanical supplement use or adverse effects with their physicians. Clearly, this information is essential to providing optimal patient care. Table 2 lists the patient interview process for assessing and implementing appropriate botanical (and other) supplement use.

III. EVIDENCE FOR SAFETY AND EFFICACY

Many consumers of herbal medicines believe that herbs are safer, more effective and more "natural" than pharmaceutical medications [21]. The long history of herbal/botanical

use serves to substantiate the safety of these products. Yet, modern usage of herbs and botanicals differs from traditional use in that botanicals are consumed in an extracted form, at higher dosage and in higher frequency, and with the expectation of an almost immediate response. Safety and efficacy, particularly under the current circumstances for consumption, are not a "given," and both should be adequately studied for each botanical product before standards for safety and efficacy are established.

A. Safety

Although historical evidence would support that botanical products are generally safe, a lack of consistent report mechanisms for adverse effects makes it difficult to reach this conclusion. Certainly, dosage is central to safety, including both absolute dose and frequency. For a large percentage of the currently available botanical supplements, dosage recommendations may not be available or vary considerably depending on the disease or symptom under treatment and the form of botanical selected. Normal adult dosage is based on a standard 70-kg male and is generally divided into three equal doses spread throughout the waking hours. There is considerable variation to this dosage approach, but it is not unlike that used for conventional, over-the-counter medications. In addition, even if the label provides dosage standards, many consumers either fail to adhere to the recommendations or decide that more can only be better and, therefore, consume quantities beyond those recommended.

Prerequisite to dosage determinations is the issue of quality regarding content of active ingredients and absence of contaminants. A Canadian study, analyzing the active component in North American feverfew, reported that none of the products analyzed contained the required amount of active ingredient to achieve therapeutic efficacy, despite quality claims of label information [22]. A study by Liberti and DerMarderosian [23], using spectrodensitromic thin-layer chromotography, showed that there was considerable variation in the active constituents of panax ginseng, with tablet formulations containing no detectable panaxosides. Clearly, more stringent guidelines for dosage and integrity in quality labeling of dosage are needed to ensure safety and efficacy for botanical supplements.

B. Efficacy

As with safety, efficacy of botanical products will depend on the presence of active constituents, dosage, adherence to the recommended dosage regime, product formulation, bioavailability, and biological activity of the botanical product. Botanical products are uniquely different from pharmaceutical agents in that they are comprised of a variety of plant constituents combined in a single plant. This makes application of the scientific process to identify the biologically active ingredient that is associated with improved health

outcome more complex and difficult. In fact, ethobotanists would argue that it is the synergy among constituents that naturally occurs in the whole plant that provides the health-promoting attributes of the botanical. Thus, establishing bioavailability standards may be difficult. However, even complex botanical medicinals can be subjected to the scrutiny of well-designed research in order to "prove" the efficacy for the treatment of a specific disease or symptom.

C. The Scientific Process

The scientific process is well described in the chemoprevention literature [24]. The randomized, controlled clinical trial remains the gold standard for testing efficacy. Prior to clinical trials, products undergo phase I and II testing to determine toxicity and efficacy standards for use in clinical trials. Phase I studies are considered after epidemiological and experimental data are available. In the case of botanicals, one could consider their historical use as "epidemiological evidence"; however, this should not preclude the establishment of *in vitro* evidence. Once historical and *in vitro* data have been collected, phase I studies can be performed to establish an appropriate dosage for clinical use. The objective of phase I studies is to establish the highest dose (and frequency) that can be administered without toxicity. This is the risk:benefit ratio. The lower the risk:benefit ratio, the more desirable the treatment. Generally, botanicals are considered to have a low risk:benefit ratio; however, few have undergone well-controlled phase I trials.

Once phase I data have been collected, the dosage can be established for use in Phase II trials. Phase II studies should be randomized, double-blind, placebo-controlled studies. Phase II studies provide an opportunity to refine toxicity data in a larger population, document side effects, establish appropriate biomarkers of clinical efficacy, and study the pharmacokinetics of the botanical. Because botanicals are comprised of multiple bioactive constituents, establishing pharmacokinetics properties for each active ingredient could become quite burdensome. The phase II study would be appropriately employed to study the efficacy of a botanical to reduce clinical symptoms in studies of moderate sample size; for example, for the study of garlic as an agent to reduce cholesterol levels or ginger as an antiemetic for patients undergoing chemotherapy.

Finally, with the completion of adequate phase I and II research, the scientific community can initiate phase III clinical intervention trials. These trials are large, randomized, placebo-controlled studies that generally last several years. The primary endpoint is reduction in the incidence of a given disease. Multiple botanicals and dosages may be included in a multi-factorial study design. This type of study would be warranted for the investigation of botanicals as potential agents for chemoprevention or cardiovascular disease prevention.

To date, only a small percentage of currently available botanical products have under gone such rigorous scientific

testing. This accounts for the reluctance by many health care professionals to employ botanicals in medical practice. However, many have been investigated in controlled, clinical trials and may warrant consideration for use clinically.

Table 3 provides a listing of select herb/botanical products and their proposed health benefits, side effects, and contradictions. The scientific evidence for these select botanicals is variable [25].

D. Botanicals Use Supported by Scientific Evidence

As discussed above, the effectiveness of botanical and herbal remedies can be evaluated according to pharmacological principles and the scientific methodology. In particular, the use of randomized, controlled clinical trials allows for evidence-based outcome assessment to establish the efficacy of herbal/botanical products. A brief review of the evidence for eight commonly used botanicals is presented here.

1. ST. JOHN'S WORT FOR THE TREATMENT OF DEPRESSION

St. John's wort or *Hypericum perforatum* is licensed in Germany for the treatment of anxiety, mild to moderate depression and sleep disorders. Biologically active ingredients include naphthodianthroms, flavonoids, xanthose, and bioflavonoids [26]. A phase II study to determine the effect of St. John's wort on neurophysiological function demonstrated that the two extracts studied were able to induce electrochemical changes consistent with improved mentation [27]. A randomized controlled clinical trial conducted in Germany of 260 patients with mild to moderate depression showed St. John's wort to be equivalent to standard drug therapy in clinical efficacy [28]. Additional randomized trials by Vorbach *et al.* [29] and also by Wheatley and colleagues [30] also demonstrated clinical effectiveness. A recent meta-analysis of 1757 patients conducted by Linde et al. [31] established that *Hypericum* extracts were 33. 2% more effective than placebo or prescription medications for treating depression. A recent study of drug interaction revealed that the use of St. John's wort with indinavir reduces expected plasma drug levels. It may be that St. John's wort induces cytochromes P-450 so that all drugs metabolized by this route are affected [32].

2. ECHINACEA FOR RESPIRATORY AND INFLUENZA

Echinacea or *Echinacea purpurea* is extracted from the juice of the purple coneflower and has been widely used and studied throughout Europe for the past century. *In vitro* and animal studies have shown that the arabinogalactan-containing glycoproteins and chichoric acid are capable of inducing B-lymphocyte and macrophage proliferation, TNF-α, and interleukin 1 [33–35]. Recent randomized, controlled clinical trials, one by Melchart et al. [36] and another by Barnes [37] were unable to demonstrate the efficacy of echinacea to reduce upper respiratory tract infections. How-

TABLE 3 Common Botanicals: Purported Uses, Contraindications, and Resource Information

Botanical	Latin name	Source information WHO[a]	USPNF[b]	German Comm E[c]	Purported uses	Contraindications
Aloe	*Aloe barbadensis; Aloe ferox*	X		X	Accelerates wound healing when applied to skin; cathartic when taken internally	Not to be taken internally by women and children or used externally on surgical wounds
Astragalus	*Astragalus menbranaceus; Astragalus gummifer*	X			Antiviral; improves general strength; laxative; increases cardiac contractility	Not to be taken with immunosuppressive drugs; contraindicated with any bowel disease
Black cohosh	*Cimicifuga racemosa*	X		X	Relieves menopausal ailments; premenstrual and dysmenorrheic neurovegetative disorders	No known with proper dosage
Cat's claw	*Uticania tomenisoa*	X		X	Folkloric use as a wound healer and for treating intestinal ailments; may have some anticancer, anti-inflammatory and immunostimulant properties	No known
Chamomile	*Chamaemelum nobile*				Sedative effects; antispasmodic and antibacterial effects; promotes wound healing	No known
Cranberry	*Vaccinium macrocarpon*	X	X		Prevention of urinary tract infections	No known
Echinacea	*Echinacea angustifolia*	X		X	Used topically for wound-healing action and internally to stimulate immune system	Contraindicated in infectious and autoimmune diseases such as tuberculosis, leukosis, collagenosis, multiple sclerosis, AIDS, and lupus; caution in patients allergic to sunflower family of plants; unknown use in pregnancy and lactation
Evening primrose	*Oenothera biennis*	X			Arthritis; anti-inflammatory; atopic eczema; PMS; diabetic neuropathy	Contraindicated in people taking immunosuppressive medications
Feverfew	*Tanacetum parthenium*	X	X		Prophylactic treatment for migraine headaches; relieve menstrual pain, asthma, dermatitis, and arthritis	Should not be used by pregnant or lactating women or children under the age of 2
Garlic	*Allium sativum*	X	X	X	Arteriosclerosis; HTN; antithrombotic; antioxidants; antiviral; antifungal	No known contraindications but the potential for serious interactions with antiplatelet drugs should be kept in mind; also caution in pregnancy and diabetes
Ginger	*Zingiber officinale*	X	X	X	Antiemetic/antinausea	No good evidence regarding the safety of ingesting large amounts of ginger by pregnant women
Ginkgo	*Ginkgo biloba*	X	X	X	Treatment for cerebral insufficiency, dementia, circulatory disorders such as Raynaud's disease; neuroprotective effects; reduces platelet aggregation	Should be avoided by pregnant and lactating women and children under the age of 2; may interact with garlic, ginger, vitamin E, warfarin, aspirin, or other drugs with antiplatelet or anticoagulant effects; may potentiate MAOI; should not be used with aspirin therapy

(continues)

TABLE 3 *(continued)*

Botanical	Latin name	Source information			Purported uses	Contraindications
		WHO[a]	USPNF[b]	German Comm E[c]		
Ginseng	*Panax ginseng* (Asian); *Panax quinquefolium*	X	X	X	Protective agent; raises mental and physical capacity	Should be used with caution for people with diabetes mellitus as hypoglycemic effect has been documented; may interact with warfarin and phenelzine; avoid with stimulants including excess caffeine; avoid with steroid use
Gotu kola	*Centella asiatica*	X			*Internal:* improves memory and circulation; alleviates stress *External:* used to treat ulcers, eczema, wounds, scars	Contact dermatitis in sensitive individuals; not recommended for use during pregnancy
Hawthorne	*Crataegus oxyancantha; Cratargi folium*	X	X		Treatment of either high or low blood pressure, tachycardia, or arrhythmias	Use only under a physician's supervision; potential interaction with other cardiac drugs and blood pressure altering agents
Kava	*Piper methysticum*	X		X	Sedative and antianxiety; treatment of inflammation of the uterus, headaches, colds, rheumatisms; promotion of wound healing	Toxicity is increased with ethanol consumption, so may be useful for the management of alcohol abuse
Milk thistle	*Silybum marianum; Carduus marianus* seeds	X	X	X	Used to treat liver disorders, jaundice, gall stones, peritonitis, hemorrhage, bronchitis	No known
Saw palmetto	*Serenoa repens*	X	X	X	Prostatic enlargement (BPH); management of genitourinary problems	Contraindicated in pregnant women or those of childbearing potential because of potential hormonal effects
Stinging nettle leaf	*Urticae folium/herba*	X		X	Acute allergy treatment; rheumatism	Contraindicated in patients retaining fluid as a result of reduced cardiac or renal activity
St. John's wort	*Hypericum perforatum*	X	X	X	Depression; antiviral effects	Alters response to protease inhibitors (indinavir, oral contraceptives, anticoagulants); contraindicated in pregnant women and patients taking MAOIs and other antidepressants as excessive doses may potentiate existing MAOI therapy or other medications used for depression
Thyme	*Thymus vulgaris*	X		X	Bronchitis and whooping cough; antibacterial	No known
Tumeric	*Curcuma longa*	X		X	Anti-inflammatory; liver and gallbladder complaints; anorexia	No known
Valerian	*Valeriana officinalis*	X	X	X	Sedative	May potentiate sedative effect of barbiturates, benzodiazepines, or opiates

Source: Developed by Laswell, A., and Thomson, C. (1999). American Dietetic Association Physician Nutrition Education Project.
[a]WHO, World Health Organization.
[b]USPNF, United States Pharmacopea nonprescription formulary.
[c]German Comm E, "The Complete German Commission E Monographs: Therapeutic Guide to Herbal Medicines (Blumenthal, M., *et al.*, Eds.). German Federal Institute for Herbal Medicine, American Botanical Councils, Austin, TX, 1999.

ever, the majority of randomized controlled trials, as well as an earlier review of 26 clinical trials conducted by Barrett, have supported the use of echinacea to reduce the symptoms or duration of upper respiratory tract infections (38–44) with minimal adverse effects (33, 45). Nonetheless, results from the recent studies showing no benefit need to be considered [36, 37].

3. GARLIC FOR HYPERLIPIDEMIA OR HYPERTENSION

Garlic or *Allium sativum* has been studied for a variety of potential health benefits, based on activities ranging from antiviral to anticoagulant. Epidemiological evidence from more than 20 studies worldwide supports the potential for garlic (and onion) as a chemopreventive agent against gastrointestinal cancers [46]. The strongest scientific evidence is for the use of garlic as a lipid-lowering or antihypertensive agent [47]. Animal data demonstrate the hypotensive effects of garlic (48–50). Controlled clinical trials have shown reductions in systolic blood pressure of between 5.5% and 21% [51, 52]. Studies have shown reductions in cholesterol and triglycerides to range from 10% to 15% [53]. Other double-blind, controlled clinical trials have failed to demonstrate the efficacy of garlic for the treatment of hyperlipidemia [54–57]. However, two meta-analyses support the use of garlic as a lipid-lowering agent and an antihypertensive [53, 58, 59]. Poor study design and few subjects is a significant concern in the literature in this area [60]. Studies conducted using garlic are difficult to blind and have a relatively high frequency of side effects, such as gastrointestinal upset, dermatitis, and allergic reactions [61].

4. GINGER FOR NAUSEA OR EMESIS

Ginger or *Zingiber officinalis* as been extensively used as an antiemetic and antispasmodic for more than 2500 years in China. Although *in vitro* research appears to be lacking, randomized, controlled clinical trials have shown efficacy for motion sickness [62–64] although negative results have also been published [64, 65]. Ginger has been demonstrated to reduce postoperative nausea in gynecological patients [66] and ambulatory surgery patients [67]. One other study was unable to confirm this effect [68]. Ginger is one of the few botanicals prescribed for pregnant women because it has been shown to be efficacious for the treatment of hyperemesis gravidarum [69]. However, data supporting the safety of consumption and appropriate dosage during pregnancy are lacking [70], especially considering the potential for ginger to inhibit thromboxane synthetase, thus prolonging bleeding time [71].

5. GINKGO FOR DEMENTIA

Gingko or *Ginkgo biloba* is among the most popular herbs used by Americans. It has been approved for the treatment of dementia in Germany where prescriptions now exceed 5 million [72]. Bioactive components, including flavonoids, terpenoids, ginkgolides, and organic acids, have been iso-

lated from the ginkgo plant and are thought to contribute to its antioxidant and antiplatelet activity. *In vitro* data documenting the biological activity are available and have led to an extensive study of the clinical efficacy of ginkgo in human trials. In an intent-to-treat analysis conducted by LeBars *et al.* [73] in 1997, gingko was shown to significantly reduce scores for the Alzheimer's Disease Assessment Scale and the Cognitive subscale. Other studies in patients with Alzheimer's have also demonstrated positive effects [74, 75], discussed in a review paper by Kleijnen and Knipschild [76]. Clinical efficacy for dementia has also been demonstrated for the elderly with mild to moderate memory impairment [77, 78]. Adverse effects during ginkgo administration are limited, but include mild gastrointestinal upset, headache, and more significantly spontaneous subdural hematoma [79]. These more significant effects have been reported in patients taking concomitant aspirin, nonsteroid anti-inflamatory drugs (NSAIDS), or anticoagulants [80].

6. VALERIAN FOR INSOMNIA

Valerian or *Valeriana officinalis,* an extract of the valerian root, has been used as a mild tranquilizer and for the treatment of insomnia. Valerian use can result in hypotensive, anticonvulsant, sedative, and hypnotic effects. Animal studies demonstrate biological activity from several of the root components, including valerinic acid, valeranone, valepotriates and gamma-aminobutyric acid, but it remains unclear if these specific compounds are responsible for promoting sleep [81]. Randomized, controlled clinical trials evaluating the use of valerian to treat insomnia are few and have been criticized for the limited number of subjects enrolled. However, one study of eight patients with mild insomnia showed sleep was induced with valerian in an average of 9 minutes compared to 15. 8 minutes for the placebo group [82]. No additional benefit was demonstrated by doubling the dose of valerian from 450 to 900 mg. In a follow-up randomized, controlled study of 128 patients with and without insomnia, Leathwood and Chauffard [83] demonstrated reduced insomnia for those given valerian with the effect being most significant for those with sleep difficulties. The effects of valerian on sleep stages or electroencephalograph spectra have not been studied [84]. A study by Schultz and colleagues [85] showed increased slow-wave sleep and another by Lindahl and Lindwall [86] showed subjective improvement of sleep quality. Valerian root is generally well tolerated; however, some patients have complained of difficulty awakening and some reports suggest a detrimental interaction with alcohol and barbiturates [87].

7. SAW PALMETTO FOR BENIGN PROSTATIC HYPERTROPHY

Saw palmetto, also known as *Serenoa repens,* is a fruit-derived botanical used for the treatment of benign prostatic hypertrophy. The hexane ring isolated from saw palmetto has shown antiandrogenic and estrogenic effects *in vitro* [88].

Two mechanisms have been demonstrated as likely to account for the antihypertrophic effects. First, saw palmetto inhibits dihydrotestosterone and, second, it inhibits 5-α-reductase activity [89]. Two randomized, controlled double-blind studies have been published that showed increased urine flow, decreased residual urine, reduced prostate size, and reduced frequency of urination [90, 91]. In one study, saw palmetto was shown to be more effective in reducing urine residual and improving urine output than a commonly prescribed medication, finasteride [92]. A review of well-controlled studies has been provided by Wilt and colleagues [93]. Saw palmetto is well-tolerated with minimal side effects that are limited to gastrointestinal complaints [94].

8. Feverfew for Migraine Headaches

Feverfew or *Tanacetum parthenium* has received approval by the Canadian Health Protection Branch for use in the treatment of migraine headaches. Both fresh leaf and dried leaf preparations are available and both contain sesquiterpene lactones, which inhibit arterial contraction and induce arterial smooth-muscle contraction. Feverfew, a serotonin antagonist, has been shown to be an inhibitor of prostaglandins [95]. Double-blind, placebo-controlled studies are limited but support an approximate 25% reduction in migraine incidence among migraine patients who take feverfew as a preventive agent [96, 97[.

A summary of the randomized, controlled clinical trial data published in the scientific literature is shown in Table 4.

IV. ADVERSE EFFECTS OF HERBS AND BOTANICALS

A. Incidence

The incidence of adverse effects of herbs and botanicals in the United States is not well documented, but has been reported to be low except when taken in excess of label recommendations [99, 100]. Because the majority of patients do not discuss herbal medicinal use with their physicians, many adverse reactions to these products are thought to go unreported [20]. Physicians use the FDA MedWatch system for reporting adverse drug reactions, but may be less aware of the need to use this same system to report adverse reactions to over-the-counter herbal and botanical supplements. Internationally, studies in Hong Kong [101], Taiwan [102], and the Philippines [103] have documented the extent of adverse reactions seen among users of herbal supplements. A 1995 report from the World Health Organization (WHO), focused on international drug monitoring, indicated that more than 5000 reports of herbal-induced adverse effects have been documented [104]. In contrast, a meta-analysis suggested that pharmaceuticals accounted for more than 100,000 deaths per year in American hospitals [105].

B. Botanicals Associated with Adverse Reactions

Allergic adverse reactions, from dermatitis to anaphylactic shock, are commonly associated with yohimbine [106] and camphor [107]. Toxic reactions have also been documented, including fatal reactions, to pennyroyal [108]. Liver failure has also been reported and is associated with the use of such herbs as germander [109], chaparral [110], comfrey [111], and bajiaolian [112]. An excellent review of adverse reactions associated with herbal medicine use is provided by Ernst [113].

C. Herbal–Medication Interactions

Knowledge of the potential interactions between herbs, botanicals, and prescription medications is critical to their safe application in health care. The review provided focuses on several common botanical–medication interactions. However, for a more in-depth review of the topic, several recently published books are available including one from Brinker [114] and the publishers of *Pharmacy Letters* [115].

Table 5 lists common botanical–medication interactions. The interactions between herbal medicinals and conventional pharmacological agents has been grossly understudied in the scientific literature.

V. REGULATION OF BOTANICAL AND HERBAL MEDICINALS

The regulation of dietary supplements, including botanicals and herbs, changed substantially in 1994 when congress passed the Dietary Supplement Health and Education Act (DSHEA) [116]. This legislation provides an extremely flexible and permissive approach to dietary supplement labeling and excluded dietary supplements from the more stringent approach used in the labeling and marketing of foods. As a result of this legislation, dietary supplement product labels, including herbs and botanicals, can make "structure–function" claims to promote product sales. A structure–function claim would include statements such as "improves prostate health" or "promotes a healthy heart." On the other hand, the regulation requires that no dietary supplement make claims to prevent or treat disease. For example, claims such as "reduces risk for prostate cancer" or "prevents heart disease" are not permissible. For the consumer, this differentiation is not clearly distinct and therefore leads to confusion as to the scientific evidence for efficacy. The label claim must also include the FDA disclaimer, "This statement has not been evaluated by the Food and Drug Administration. This product is not intended to diagnose, treat, mitigate, cure or prevent any disease".

The DHSEA also required that manufacturers provide label information to consumers regarding all of the ingredients contained in the product. The provision of ingredient informa-

TABLE 4 Highlighted Herbs and Evidence of Efficacy

Common name	Species	Indication	Study type[a]	Number of patients	Outcome measures	Benefit
Echinacea	*Echinacea*	Upper respiratory infection (URI) and flu-like illness	DB RCT	180	Flu-like symptoms	Yes
			DB RCT	160	Flu-like symptoms	Yes
			DB RCT	100	URI symptoms	Yes
			DB RCT	120	URI symptoms	Yes
			DB RCT	150	URI symptoms	Yes
			DB RCT	100	URI symptoms	Yes
			DB RCT	100	URI symptoms	Yes
Garlic	*Allium sativum*	Hyperlipidemia	Meta	16 Tr, 952 Pts	Total choles, triglyc	Yes
			Meta	5 Tr, 410 Pts	Total choles, triglyc	Yes
			DB RCT	115	Total choles, triglyc	No
			DB RCT	31	Total choles, triglyc	No
			DB RCT	25	Total choles, triglyc	No
			DB RCT	28	Total choles, triglyc	No
		Hypertension	Meta	Tr, 415 Pts	Blood pressure	Yes
			DB RCT	41	Blood pressure	Yes
Ginger	*Zingiber officinalis*	Motion sickness	SB RCT	36	Nausea, vomiting	Yes
			DB HH RCT	8	Nausea, vomiting	No
			DB RCT	79	Nausea, vomiting	Yes
			DB RCT	8	Nausea, vomiting	No
		Postoperative nausea and vomiting Hyperemesis gravidarum	DB HH RCT	60	Nausea, vomiting	Yes
			DB RCT	120	Nausea, vomiting	Yes
			DB RCT	108	Nausea, vomiting	No
			DB RCT	30	Nausea, vomiting	Yes
Gingko	*Gingko biloba*	Dementia ("cerebral insufficiency")	Review	40 Tr	Various memory and cognition scales	Yes
			DB RCT	27		Yes
			DB RCT	40		Yes
			DB RCT	156		Yes
			DB RCT	202		Yes
St. John's wort	*Hypericum perforatum*	Depression	Meta	23 Tr, 1757 Pts	Various depression scales, especially Hamilton	Yes
			DB HH RCT			Yes
			DB HH RCT			Yes
Valerian	*Valeriana officinalis*	Insomnia	DB RCT	128	Sleep quality	Yes
			DB RCT	8	Sleep latency	Yes
			DB RCT	27	Sleep quality	Yes
			DB RCT	14	Slow-wave sleep	Yes

Source: Reproduced with permission from Barrett, B., Kiefer, D., and Rabago, D. (1999). Assessing the risks and benefits of herbal medicine: An overview of scientific evidence. *Altern. Ther. Health Med.* **5,** 40–49.

[a]DB RCT, double-blind randomized control trial; Meta, meta-analysis; Review, review article. Individual studies are referenced in the original source.

tion provides the FDA with a legal opportunity to challenge product manufacturers who were not reporting impurities, and as a basis for determining the presence of active ingredients. It is the manufacturer's responsibility to provide safe products. It is the responsibility of the FDA to investigate any reported cases of harm, to prove harm was done, and to take the necessary corrective action to ensure public safety.

VI. RECOMMENDATIONS FOR CLINICAL CARE

Are botanical supplements an appropriate therapeutic modality? This is a complex question that warrants careful consideration. Issues of safety, efficacy, ethical behavior, cost effectiveness, and alternative dietary approaches must also

TABLE 5 Herb/Botanical Medication Interactions

Herb/botanical	Pharmacological agent	Adverse effect
Shankhapushpi, ginkgo	Anticonvulsants Phenytoin	Decreased phenytoin levels; loss of seizure control
Licorice	Prednisolone Digitalis	Altered medication pharmacokinetics
Feverfew, garlic, ginkgo, panax, ginseng, red clover, ginger	Anticoagulants—warfarin, aspirin, NSAIDS	Inhibit platelet aggregation, thus enhancing pharmaceutical effects; increased clotting time
Ginkgo	Tricyclic antidepressants	May increase drug activity
Ginseng	Hypoglycemic agents	Lower blood glucose
St. John's wort	Photosensitivity agents piroxicam, tetracycline	Enhance photosensitivity
	MAO inhibitors Indinavir	Concomitant effects on CNS; cytochrome P-450 stimulation
Echinacea	Hepatotoxic medications: anabolic steroids, methotrexate, ketoconazole	Increased risk for hepatic damage
Kava	Alprozolam	Excess sedation
Echinacea, astragalus	Cyclosporine	Reverse desired immunosuppression
Horseradish, kelp	Levothyroxine	Suppress thyroid function, alter medication efficacy
Ginseng, yohimbine	MAO inhibitors	Insomnia, headache, tremors
Evening primrose oil, borage oil	Phenobarbital	Lower seizure threshold
Gossypol	Diuretics Hydrochlorothiazide	Hypokalemia
Siberial ginseng Hawthorne Uzara root	Digitalis	Digoxin toxicity

be considered in the decision to recommend a certain botanical supplement.

A. Legal and Ethical Issues

1. DIETETICS PROFESSIONALS

Professionals who are registered to practice dietetics must adhere to the American Dietetic Association Code of Ethics as the primary source of ethical guidance. State licensure laws also guide ethical decisions for health care professionals. The Code of Ethics for the American Dietetic Association states that dietetics professionals must not "promote or endorse products in a manner that is false or misleading" [117]. Thus, when recommending botanical supplements, it is important that dietetics professionals have a sound knowledge of the subject area and the scientific evidence for efficacy and patient safety. In addition, the American Dietetic Association (ADA) and other professional nutrition science organizations have peer-reviewed position and/or policy statements that each member is expected to uphold. The ADA's position on dietary supplements states: "It is the position of the American Dietetic Association that the best nu-

tritional strategy for promoting optimal health and reducing the risk for chronic disease is to obtain adequate nutrients from a wide variety of foods. Vitamin and mineral supplementation is appropriate when well accepted, peer-reviewed, scientific evidence shows safety and effectiveness" [118]. Standards of professional practice also serve to guide dietetics professionals in the provision of quality nutrition service [119], particularly as dietetics professionals expand their traditional practice roles to include complementary therapeutics including the use of herbs and botanicals [120].

2. MEDICAL PROFESSIONALS

Physicians, unlike dietetics professionals who are guided by the ADA Code of Ethics, have no central governing body that provides such guidance. Many physicians are members of the American Medical Association (AMA) and reference this organization's policies and recommendations. The AMA has an established Code of Ethics that may provide guidance for those who wish to reference it. The AMA has yet to forward a specific policy statement related to herbal and botanical products and the use of these products in clinical practice. The organization has called on the federal government to empower the FDA to place more strict requirements

on the supplement industry with respect to DSHEA. It has also recommended that the AMA itself study DSHEA to determine if it is satisfactory in its present form and to determine whether or not the operations of the regulatory bodies have been appropriate [121].

Physicians, on receiving state licensure, are subject to the state's regulatory authority under police power [122]. This serves to protect a citizen's health and safety by determining who may practice medicine through the establishment of licensing boards. Within this framework, the state will often define the practice of medicine through the use of such language as *diagnosis, treatment* and *cure.* This provides a broad definition of the act of practicing medicine (scope of practice). Scope of practice limitations serve to ensure that providers will only offer services within their level of training and expertise. For physicians, the area of botanical medicine, including the prescribing of herb and botanical supplements, may or may not be an area of formal training and expertise and therefore prescribing botanicals may at times border on licensing limits.

Physicians are not taught botanical medicine in medical school, nor are they routinely educated in these practices during postgraduate training. The proper prescription of herbals and botanicals may be as complicated as knowing the proper pharmaceutical to recommend and comes with experience. Knowledge in this area is often obtained from conferences and/or references rather than through formal educational training. A growing number of medical schools provide some training in complementary and alternative medicine. However, these are usually elective courses [123]. It is therefore necessary for physicians to approach this information with a critical eye. It is also imperative that physicians make every attempt to either educate themselves about this rapidly growing complementary practice, or partner with a practitioner who is well versed in herbal/botanical medicine. Herbal medicine is the fastest growing component of complementary and alternative medicine [13] and an area not without potential problems (medical contraindications, herb–drug interactions). As long as providers either remain uninformed or biased against herbal/botanical medicine, patients will continue to hide their use, thus increasing the possibility of harm. By affording themselves an opportunity to expand their knowledge, physicians will be able provide the quality of care that patients are requesting of them.

B. Cost Effectiveness of Botanical Medicine

Currently, no published reports exist that compare the cost of treating symptoms or chronic disease with botanical versus conventional pharmaceutical-based medicine. The assumption is that botanicals will be more cost effective and have fewer side effects. Clinicians must consider the cost in recommending any botanical supplement. The out-of-pocket cost for botanical therapies may be significantly higher than

that of prescription medications where medical insurance is available. In addition, the use of a botanical or herbal should be considered augmentation of a well-founded dietary (or other) approach to treating the disease or disease manifestations. Without a foundation in dietary intervention, it is unlikely the botanical will be efficacious at the optimal level. Many patients are without adequate dietary advice and may be consuming several botanicals on a daily basis. To ensure efficacy, botanical supplements should be limited to products that have been demonstrated to be effective using scientifically sound methodology. Without evidence for efficacy, expenditures for botanicals cannot be considered cost-effective care.

C. Resources for Medical and Dietetics Professionals

Medical and dietetic professionals must expand their knowledge of botanical use, safety, and therapeutic efficacy and remain informed in this rapidly expanding area of practice. Many professionals may not have been adequately educated in the area of herbal/botanical medicine during their formal training and therefore must rely on self-education to develop this expertise. Developing fundamental knowledge in this area is essential prior to making recommendations to patients. In addition, working collaboratively with physicians, pharmacists, ethnobotanists, and other practitioners trained in the area of botanical medicine is essential to providing optimal care. Table 6 provides a list of reliable, scientifically based resources that can be used to develop expertise in this dynamic area of health care.

VII. SUMMARY

The use of botanical and herbal medicinals to reduce the symptoms of and to treat or prevent chronic disease is on the rise. Medical and dietetic professionals are uniquely positioned to provide patients with reliable, scientifically sound advice on the use of these products in the context of a varied, nutritionally sound diet. Medical and dietetics professionals must be knowledgeable of safety, efficacy, and potential harm for botanical supplements used by their patients. Awareness of ethical and legal considerations when recommending the use or discontinuation of specific botanical supplements is paramount. It is inappropriate for medical and dietetics professionals to recommend any herbal or botanical product to their patients if they stand to achieve financial support for doing so, regardless of the scientific evidence. The use of botanicals and herbal supplements to enhance health is not new to medicine; however, the growing use of these products dictates that dietetics professionals must expand their knowledge and understanding of the growing body of scientific evidence so that optimal nutritional care can be provided to all patients.

TABLE 6   Resources for Botanical Product Use

Organizations/Web sites:

Office of Dietary Supplements
  National Institutes of Health
  Building 31, Room 1B25
  31 Center Drive MSC 2086
  Bethesda, MD 20892
  http://dietary-supplements.info.nih.gov
  301-435-2920

International Bibliographic Information on Dietary Supplements (IBIDS)
  http://odp.od.nih.gov/ods/databases/ibids.html

Council for Responsible Nutrition
  1875 Eye Street NW
  Suite 406
  Washington, DC 20006
  http://www.crnusa.org
  202-872-1488

Food and Drug Administration
  Department of Health and Human Services
  Food and Drug Administration
  Rockville, MD 20857
  http://www.fda.gov

National Center for Complementary & Alternative Medicine
  NCCAM Clearing House
  PO Box 8281
  Silverspring, MD 20907-8218
  http://altmed.od.nih.gov/nccam/resources/cam-ci
  1-888-644-6226

National Council Against Nutrition Fraud, Inc.
  300 E. Pink Hill Road
  Independence, MO 64057
  816-228-4595
  Executive Director: William Jarvis
  909-824-4690

Alternative Medicine Foundation, Inc.
  Bethesda, MD
  HerbalMed: http://www.amfoundation.org/herbmed.htm

Books/Reference Text

- American Dietetic Association. (1999). "Clinician's Guide to Vitamins, Minerals and Other Dietary Supplements." American Dietetic Association, Chicago, IL.
- Gruenwald, J., Brendler, T., and Jaenicke, C. Eds. (1998). "PDR for Herbal Medicines." Medical Economics Company, Montvale, NJ.
- Blumenthal, M., Goldberg, A., Gruenwald, J., Hall, T., Riggins, C. W., and Rister, R. S., Eds. (1998). "The Complete German Commission E Monographs: Therapeutic Guide to Herbal Medicines." American Botanical Councils, Austin, TX.
- Cohen, M. H. (1998). "Complementary and Alternative Medicine: Legal Boundaries and Regulatory Perspectives." John Hopkins University Press, Baltimore, MD.
- Tyler, V. E. (1994). "Herbs of Choice." Haworth Press, Inc., New York.
- Miller, L. G., and Murray, W. J. (1998). "Herbal Medicinals: A Clinician's Guide." Pharmaceutical Products, Press, Binghamton, NY. Available at: http://www.haworthpressinc.com.
- Therapeutic Research Faculty, Pharmacist's Letter (1999). "Natural Medicines Comprehensive Database." Available at http://www.naturaldatabase.com.

References

1. Huxtable, R. J. (1998). Safety of botanicals: Historical perspective [editorial]. *Proc. West. Pharmacol. Soc.* **41,** 1–10.
2. Miller, L. G., and Murray, W. J. (Eds.) (1998). "Herbal Medicinals: A Clinician's Guide." Pharmaceutical Products Press, New York.
3. Duke, J. A. (1997). "The Green Pharmacy." Rodale Press, Emmaus, PA.
4. Tyler, V. E. (1994). "Herbs of Choice: The Therapeutic Use of Phytomedicinals." Pharmaceutical Products Press, New York.
5. Hoffman, F. A., and Leaders, F. E. (1996). Botanical (herbal) medicine in health care: A review from a regulatory perspective. *Pharm. News.* **3,** 23–25.
6. Tyler, V. E. (1993). "The Honest Herbal." Pharmaceutical Products Press, Binghamton, NY.
7. Thomson, C. A., Bloch, A., and Hassler, C. (1999). Position of the American Dietetic Association. *Functional Foods* **99,** 1278–1285.
8. Richman, A., and Witkowski, J. (1997). Herbs by the number. *Whole Foods Magazine* 20–28.
9. Cott, J. (1995). NCDEU update. Natural product formulations available in Europe for psychotropic indications. *Psychopharmacol. Bull.* **31,** 745–751.
10. Aarts, T. (1998). Nutrition industry overview. *Nutr. Bus. J.* **3,** 1–5.
11. Tyler, V. E., and Foster, S. (1996). *In* "Handbook of Nonprescription Drugs," 11th Ed. (T. R. Covington, Ed.), pp. 695–713. American Pharmaceutical Association, Washington, DC.
12. Wright, J. (1997). *In* "Report of the Commission on Dietary Supplement Labels," p. 16. Superintendent of Document, U.S. Government Printing Office #017-00531-2, Washington, DC.
13. Eisenberg, D. M., Davis, R. B., Ettner, S. L., Appel, S., Wilkey, S., Van Rompay, M., and Kessler, R. C. (1998). Trends in alternative medicine use in the United States, 1990–1997: Results of a follow-up national survey. *JAMA* **280**(18), 1569–1575.
14. Johnston, B. A. (1997). One-third of nation's adults use herbal remedies. *Herbalgram* **40,** 49.
15. Brevoort, P. (1997). Overview of the U. S. botanical market. *In* "Third Conference on Botanicals." Drug Information Association, Washington, DC.
16. Eliason, B. C., Kruger, J., Mark, D., and Rasmann, D. N. (1997). Dietary supplement users: Demographics, product use, and medical system interaction. *J. Am. Board Fam. Pract.* **10,** 265–271.
17. Thomson, C. A. (1999). Sorting through the dietary supplement jungle [presentation]. At 82nd Annual Meeting of the American Dietetic Association, Atlanta, GA, October 17.
18. Karch, A. M., and Karch, F. E. (1999). The herb garden. Remember to ask your patients about all preparations. *Am. J. Nurs.* **99,** 12.
19. Eisenberg, D. (1997). Advising patients who seek alternative medicine. *Ann. Intern. Med.* **127,** 61.
20. Barnes, J., Mills, S. Y., Abbot, N. C., Willoughby, M., and Ernst, E. (1998). Different standards for reporting ADRs to herbal remedies and conventional OTC medicines: Face-to-face interviews with 515 users of herbal remedies. *Br. J. Clin. Pharmacol.* **45,** 496–500.

21. American Dietetic Association (2000). "Nutrition and You: Trends 2000" [survey]. American Dietetic Association, Chicago, IL.

22. Groenewegan, W. A., and Heptinstall, S. (1986). Feverfew. *Lancet* **1 (8471)**, 44–45.

23. Liberti, L. E., and DerMarderosian, A. (1978). Evaluation of commercial ginseng products. *J. Pharm. Sci.* **67**, 1487–1489.

24. Alberts, D. S., and Garcia, D. J. (1995). An overview of clinical cancer chemoprevention studies with emphasis on positive phase III studies. *J. Nutr.* **125**, 692S–697S.

25. Lasswell, A., and Thomson, C. (1999). "The American Dietetic Association Physician Nutrition Education Project." American Dietetic Association, Chicago, IL.

26. Wagner, H., and Bladt, S. (1994). Pharmaceutical quality of hypericum extracts. *J. Geriatr. Psychiatry Neurol.* **7**(Suppl. 1), S65–S68.

27. Dimpfel, W., Todorova, A., and Vonderheid-Guth, B. (1999). Pharmacodynamic properties of St. John's wort—A single blind neurophysiological study in healthy subjects comparing two commercial preparations. *Eur. J. Med. Res.* **4**, 303–312.

28. Philipp, M., Kohnen, R., and Hiller, K. O. (1999). Hypericum extract versus imipramine or placebo in patients with moderate depression: Randomised multicentre study of treatment for eight weeks. *Br. Med. J.* **319**, 1534–1539.

29. Vorbach, E. U., Arnoldt, K. H., and Hubner, W. D. (1997). Efficacy and tolerability of St. John's wort extract LI 160 versus imipramine in patients with severe depressive episodes according to ICD–10. *Pharmacopsychiatry* **30**(Suppl. 2), 81–85.

30. Wheatley, D. (1997). LI 160, an extract of St. John's wort, versus amitriptyline in mildly to moderately depressed outpatients—A controlled 6-week clinical trial. *Pharmacopsychiatry.* **30**(Suppl. 2), 77–80.

31. Linde, K., Ramirez, G., Mulrow, C. D., Pauls, A., Weidenhammer, W., and Melchart, D. (1996). St John's wort for depression—An overview and meta-analysis of randomised clinical trials. *Br. Med. J.* **313**, 253–258.

32. Piscitelli, S. C., Burstein, A. H., Chaitt, D., Alfaro, R. M., and Falloon, J. (2000). Indinavir concentrations and St. John's Wort. *Lancet* **355 (9203)**, 547–548

33. Parnham, M. J. (1996). Benefit-risk assessment of the squeezed sap of the purple coneflower (*Echinacea purpurea*) for long-term oral immunostimulation. *Phytomedicine* **3**, 95–102.

34. Bodinet, C., and Beuscher, N. (1991). Antiviral and immunological activity of glycoproteins from *Echinacea purpurea* radix. *Planta Medica* **57**, A33–A34.

35. Wagner, H., Suppner, H., Schafer, W., and Zenk, M. (1988). Immunologically active polysaccharides of *Echinacea purpurea* cell cultures. *Phytochemistry* **27**, 119–126.

36. Melchart, D., Walther, E., Linde, K., Brandmaier, R., and Lersch, C. (1998). Echinacea root extracts for the prevention of upper respiratory tract infections: A double-blind, placebo-controlled randomized trial. *Arch. Fam. Med.* **7**, 541–545.

37. Barnes, J. (1998). Lack of evidence of efficacy of Echinacea in URTI. *Pharm. J.* 260–267.

38. Barrett, B., Vohmann, M., and Calabrese, C. (1999). Echinacea for upper respiratory infection. *J. Fam. Prac.* **48[8]**, 628–35

39. Bräunig, B., and Knick, E. (1993). Therapeutische Erfahrungen mit Echinaceae pallidae bei grippalen Infekten. *Naturheilpraxis* **1**, 72–75.

40. Dorn, M. (1989). Milerung grippaler Effecte durch ein pflanzliches Immunstimulans. *Nuturund Ganzheitsmedizin* 314–319.

41. Hoheisel, O., Sandberg, M., Bertram, S., Bulitta, M., and Schäfer, M. (1997). Echinagard treatment shortens the course of the common cold: A double-blind, placebo-controlled clinical trial. *Eur. J. Clin. Res.* **8**, 261–268.

42. Reitz, H. D. (1990). Immunmodulatoren mit pflanzlichen Wirkstoffen: Eine wissenschaftliche Studie am Beispiel Esberitox N. *Notabene Medici.* **20**, 362–366.

43. Vorberg, G. (1984). Bei Erkältung unspezifische Immunabwehr stimulieran: doppelblindstudie zeigt: das bewährte phytotherapeutikum esberitox verkürzt die symptommatik. *Arztl. Praxis* **36**, 97–98.

44. Vorberg, G., and Schneider, B. (1989). Pflanzliches Immunstimulans verkürzt grippalen Infeckt. Doppelblindstudie belegt die Steigerung der unspezifischen Infektabwehr. *Arztl. Forsch.* **36**, 3–8.

45. Hobbs, C. (1994). Echinacea: a literature review. *Herbalgram* **30**, 33–48.

46. Ernst, E. (1997). Can *Allium* vegetables prevent cancer? *Phytomedicine* **4**, 79–83.

47. Reuter, H. D. (1995). *Allium sativum* and *Allium ursinum,* Part 2: Pharmacology and medicinal applications. *Phytomedicine* **2**, 73–91.

48. Foushee, D. B., Ruffin, J., and Banerjee, U. (1982). Garlic as a natural agent for the treatment of hypertension: a preliminary report. *Cytobios* **34**, 145–152.

49. Malik, Z. A., and Siddiqui, S. (1981). Hypotensive effect of freeze-dried garlic (*Allium sativum*) sap in dog. *J. Pak. Med. Assoc.* **31**, 12–13.

50. Ruffin, J., and Hunter, S. A. (1983). An evaluation of the side effects of garlic as an antihypertensive agent. *Cytobios* **37**, 85–89.

51. Steiner, M., Khan, A. H., Holbert, D., and Lin, R. I. (1996). A double-blind crossover study in moderately hypercholesterolemic men that compared the effect of aged garlic extract and placebo administration on blood lipids. *Am. J. Clin. Nutr.* **64**, 866–870.

52. Silagy, C. A., and Neil, H. A. (1994). A meta-analysis of the effect of garlic on blood pressure. *J. Hypertens.* **12**, 463–468.

53. Lawson, L. D. (1993). *In* "Human Medicinal Agents from Plants" (A. D. Kinghorn and M. F. Barandrin, Eds.), pp. 306–330. American Chemical Society, Washington, DC.

54. Neil, H. A., Silagy, C. A., Lancaster, T., Hodgeman, J., Vos, K., Moore, J. W., Jones, L., Cahill, J., and Fowler, G. H. (1996). Garlic powder in the treatment of moderate hyperlipidaemia: A controlled trial and meta-analysis. *J. R. College Physicians Lond.* **30**, 329–334.

55. Berthold, H. K., Sudhop, T., and von Bergmann, K. (1998). Effect of a garlic oil preparation on serum lipoproteins and cholesterol metabolism: A randomized controlled trial. *JAMA* **279**, 1900–1902.

56. Isaacsohn, J. L., Moser, M., Stein, E. A., Dudley, K., Davey, J. A., Liskov, E., and Black, H. R. (1998). Garlic powder and plasma lipids and lipoproteins: A multicenter, randomized, placebo-controlled trial. *Arch. Intern. Med.* **158**, 1189–1194.

57. Simons, L. A., Balasubramaniam, S., von Konigsmark, M., Parfitt, A., Simons, J., and Peters, W. (1995). On the effect of

garlic on plasma lipids and lipoproteins in mild hypercholes-terolaemia. *Atherosclerosis* **113**, 219–225.

58. Silagy, C., and Neil, A. (1994). Garlic as a lipid lowering agent—a Meta-analysis. *J. R. College Physicians Lond.* **28**, 39–45.

59. Warshafsky, S., Kamer, R. S., and Sivak, S. L. (1993). Effect of garlic on total serum cholesterol. A meta-analysis. *Ann. Intern. Med.* **119**, 599–605.

60. Kleijnen, J., Knipschild, P., and ter Riet, G. (1989). Garlic, onions and cardiovascular risk factors. A review of the evidence from human experiments with emphasis on commercially available preparations. *Br. J. Clin. Pharmacol.* **28**, 535–544.

61. Bleumink, E., Doeglas, H. M., Klokke, A. H., and Nater, J. P. (1972). Allergic contact dermatitis to garlic. *Br. J. Dermatol.* **87**, 6–9.

62. Mowrey, D. B., and Clayson, D. E. (1982). Motion sickness, ginger, and psychophysics. *Lancet* **1 (8273)**, 655–657.

63. Grontved, A., Brask, T., Kambskard, J., and Hentzer, E. (1988). Ginger root against seasickness. A controlled trial on the open sea. *Acta Otolaryngol. (Stockh.)* **105**, 45–49.

64. Wood, C. D., Manno, J. E., Wood, M. J., Manno, B. R., and Mims, M. E. (1988). Comparison of efficacy of ginger with various antimotion sickness drugs. *Clin. Res. Prac. Drug Reg. Aff.* **6**, 129–136.

65. Stewart, J. J., Wood, M. J., Wood, C. D., and Mims, M. E. (1991). Effects of ginger on motion sickness susceptibility and gastric function. *Pharmacology.* **42**, 111–120.

66. Bone, M. E., Wilkinson, D. J., Young, J. R., McNeil, J., and Charlton, S. (1990). Ginger root—A new antiemetic. The effect of ginger root on postoperative nausea and vomiting after major gynaecological surgery. *Anaesthesia* **45**, 669–671.

67. Phillips, S., Ruggier, R., and Hutchinson, S. E. (1993). *Zingiber officinale* (ginger)—An antiemetic for day case surgery. *Anaesthesia* **48**, 715–717.

68. Arfeen, Z., Owen, H., Plummer, J. L., Ilsley, A. H., Sorby-Adams, R. A., and Doecke, C. J. (1995). A double-blind randomized controlled trial of ginger for the prevention of postoperative nausea and vomiting. *Anaesth. Intens. Care* **23**, 449–452.

69. Fischer-Rasmussen, W., Kjaer, S. K., Dahl, C., and Asping, U. (1990). Ginger treatment of hyperemesis gravidarum. *Eur. J. Obstet. Gynecol. Reprod. Biol.* **38**, 19–24.

70. Belew, C. (1999). Herbs and the childbearing woman. Guidelines for midwives. *J. Nurse Midwifery* **44**, 231–252.

71. Backon, J. (1986). Ginger: Inhibition of thromboxane synthetase and stimulation of prostacyclin: Relevance for medicine and psychiatry. *Med. Hypotheses* **20**, 271–278.

72. Wincor, M. Z. (1999). Ginkgo biloba for dementia: A reasonable alternative? *J. Am. Pharm. Assoc. (Wash.)* **39**, 415–416.

73. Le Bars, P. L., Katz, M. M., Berman, N., Itil, T. M., Freedman, A. M., and Schatzberg, A. F. (1997). A placebo-controlled, double-blind, randomized trial of an extract of Ginkgo biloba for dementia. North American EGb Study Group. *JAMA* **278**, 1327–1332.

74. Hofferberth, B. (1994). The efficacy of EGb 761 in patients with senile dementia of the Alzheimer type: A double-blind, placebo-controlled study on different levels of investigation. *Hum. Psychopharmacol.* **9**, 215–222.

75. Kanowski, S., Hermann, W. M., Stephan, K., Wierich, W., and Horr, R. (1997). Proof of efficacy of the Gingko biloba special extract EGb 761 in outpatients suffering from mild to moderate primary dementia of the Alzheimer type or multi-infarct dementia. *Phytomedicine* **4**, 3–13.

76. Kleijnen, J., and Knipschild, P. (1992). Ginkgo biloba for cerebral insufficiency. *Br. J. Clin. Pharmacol.* **34**, 352–358.

77. Rai, G. S., Shovelin, C., and Wesnes, K. A. (1992). A double blind, placebo-controlled study of Ginkgo biloba extract in elderly outpatients with mild to moderate memory impairment. *Curr. Med. Res. Opin.* **12**, 350–355.

78. Vorberg, G. (1985). Ginkgo biloba extract (GBE): A long term study of chronic cerebral insufficiency in geriatric patients. *Clin. Trials J.* **22**, 149–157.

79. Miller, L. G. (1998). Herbal medicinals: Selected clinical considerations focusing on known or potential drug-herb interactions. *Arch. Intern. Med.* **158**, 2200–2211.

80. Rowin, J., and Lewis, S. L. (1996). Spontaneous bilateral subdural hematomas associated with chronic Ginkgo biloba ingestion. *Neurology* **46**, 1775–1776.

81. Houghton, P. J. (1988). The biological activity of valerian and related plants. *J. Ethnopharmacol.* **22**, 121–142.

82. Leathwood, P. D., Chauffard, F., Heck, E., and Munoz-Box, R. (1982). Aqueous extract of valerian root (*Valeriana officinalis* L.) improves sleep quality in man. *Pharmacol. Biochem. Behav.* **17**, 65–71.

83. Leathwood, P. D., and Chauffard, F. (1985). Aqueous extract of valerian reduces latency to fall asleep in man. *Planta Medica* **2**, 144–148.

84. Balderer, G., and Borbely, A. A. (1985). Effect of valerian on human sleep. *Psychopharmacology (Berl.)* **87**, 406–409.

85. Schulz, H., Stolz, C., and Muller, J. (1994). The effect of valerian extract on sleep polygraphy in poor sleepers: A pilot study. *Pharmacopsychiatry* **27**, 147–151.

86. Lindahl, O., and Lindwall, L. (1989). Double blind study of a valerian preparation. *Pharmacol. Biochem. Behav.* **32**, 1065–1066.

87. Hiller, K. O., and Zetler, G. (1996). Neuropharmacological studies on ethanol extracts of *Valeriana officinalis L:* Behavioural and anticonvulsant activities. *Physiother. Res. Int.* **10**, 145–151.

88. Elghamry, M. I., and Hansel, R. (1969). Activity and isolated phytoestrogen of shrub palmetto fruits (*Serenoa repens* Small), a new estrogenic plant. *Experientia* **25**, 828–829.

89. Sultan, C., Terraza, A., Devillier, C., Carilla, E., Briley, M., Loire, C., and Descomps, B. (1984). Inhibition of androgen metabolism and binding by a liposterolic extract of *Serenoa repens* B in human foreskin fibroblasts. *J. Steroid. Biochem.* **20**, 515–519.

90. Champault, G., Patel, J. C., and Bonnard, A. M. (1984). A double-blind trial of an extract of the plant *Serenoa repens* in benign prostatic hyperplasia. *Br. J. Clin. Pharmacol.* **18**, 461–462.

91. Tasca, A., Barulli, M., Cavazzana, A., Zattoni, F., Artibani, W., and Pagano, F. (1985). Trattamento della sintomatologia ostruttiva da adenoma prostatico con estratto di Serenoa repens. Studio clinico in doppio cieco vs placebo. *Minerva Urol. Nefrol.* **37**, 87–91.

92. Bach, D., Schmitt, M., and Ebeling, L. (1997). Phytopharmaceutical and synthetic agents in the treatment of benign prostatic hyperplasia (BPH). *Phytomedicine* **3–4,** 209–213.

93. Wilt, T. J., Ishani, A., Stark, G., MacDonald, R., Lau, J., and Mulrow, C. (1998). Saw palmetto extracts for treatment of benign prostatic hyperplasia: A systematic review. *JAMA* **280,** 1604–1609.

94. Glisson, J., Crawford, R., and Street, S. (1999). The clinical applications of Ginkgo biloba, St. John's wort, saw palmetto, and soy. *Nurse Pract.* **24,** 28.

95. Collier, H. O., Butt, N. M., McDonald-Gibson, W. J., and Saeed, S. A. (1980). Extract of feverfew inhibits prostaglandin biosynthesis. *Lancet* **2 (8200),** 922–923.

96. Johnson, E. S., Kadam, N. P., Hylands, D. M., and Hylands, P. J. (1985). Efficacy of feverfew as prophylactic treatment of migraine. *Br. Med. J. (Clin. Res. Ed.)* **291,** 569–573.

97. Murphy, J. J., Heptinstall, S., and Mitchell, J. R. (1988). Randomised double-blind placebo-controlled trial of feverfew in migraine prevention. *Lancet* **2 (8604),** 189–192.

98. Barrett, B., Kiefer, D., and Rabago, D. (1999). Assessing the risks and benefits of herbal medicine: An overview of scientific evidence. *Altern. Ther. Health Med.* **5,** 40–49.

99. Farnsworth, N. R. (1993). Relative safety of herbal medicines. *Herbalgram* **29,** 36A–36H.

100. Perharic, L., Shaw, D., and Murray, V. (1993) Toxic effects of herbal medicines and food supplements. *Lancet* **342,** 180–181.

101. Chan, T. Y., Chan, A. Y., and Critchley, J. A. (1992). Hospital admissions due to adverse reactions to Chinese herbal medicines. *J. Trop. Med. Hyg.* **95,** 296–298.

102. Lin, S. H., and Lin, M. S. (1993). A survey on drug related hospitalisation in a community teaching hospital. *Int. J. Clin. Pharmacol. Ther. Toxicol.* **31,** 66–69.

103. West, S., Hildesheim, A., and Dosemeci, M. (1993). Nonviral factors for nasopharyngeal carcinoma in the Philippines. *Int. J. Cancer* **55,** 722–727.

104. Edwards, R. (1995). Monitoring the safety of herbal remedies. WHO project is underway. *Br. Med. J.* **311,** 1569–1570.

105. Lazarou, J., Pomeranz, B. H., and Corey, P. N. (1998). Incidence of adverse drug reactions in hospitalized patients: A meta-anaysis of prospective studies. *JAMA* **279**(15), 1200–1205.

106. Sandler, B., and Aronson, P. (1993). Yohimbine-induced cutaneous drug eruption, progressive renal failure, and lupuslike syndrome. *Urology* **41,** 343–345.

107. Marguery, M. C., Rakotondrazafy, J., and El Sayed, F. (1996). Contact allergy to 3-(4'-methylbenzylidene) camphor and contact and photocontact allergy to 4-isopropyl dibenzoylmethane. *Photodermatol. Photoimmunol. Photomed.* **11 (5–6),** 209–212.

108. Anderson, I. B., Mullen, W. H., Meeker, J. E., Khojasteh-Bakht, S. C., Oishi, S., Nelson, S. D., and Blanc, P. D. (1996). Pennyroyal toxicity: Measurement of toxic metabolite levels in two cases and review of the literature. *Ann. Intern. Med.* **124,** 726–734.

109. Larrey, D., Vial, T., Pauwels, A., Castot, A., Biour, M., David, M., and Michel, H. (1992). Hepatitis after germander administration. *Ann. Intern. Med.* **117,** 129–132.

110. Caldwell, S. H., Feeley, J. W., Wieboldt, T. F., Featherston, P. L., and Dickson, R. C. (1994). Acute hepatitis with use of over-the-counter herbal remedies. *VA Med. Q.* **121,** 31–33.

111. Miskelly, F. G., and Goodyer, L. I. (1992). Hepatic and pulmonary complications of herbal medicine. *Postgrad. Med.* **68,** 935–936.

112. Kao, W. F., Hung, D. Z., and Lin, K. P. (1992). Podophyllotoxin intoxication: Toxic effect of Bajiaolian in herbal therapeutics. *Hum. Exp. Toxicol.* **11,** 480–487.

113. Ernst, E. (1998). Harmless herbs? A review of the recent literature. *Am. J. Med.* **104,** 170–178.

114. Brinker, F. J. (1998). "Herb Contraindications and Drug Interactions," 2nd ed. Eclectic Medical Publications, Sandy, OR.

115. Jellin, J. M., Batz, F., and Hitchens, K. (1999). "Pharmacist's Letter/Prescriber's Letter Natural Medicines Comprehensive Database." Therapeutic Research Faculty, Stockton, CA.

116. 103rd Congress, Second Session, Senate (1994). "The Dietary Supplement Health and Education Act of 1994," Report 103–410. Washington, DC.

117. American Dietetic Association (1999). Code of ethics for the profession of dietetics. *J. Am. Diet. Assoc.* **99,** 109–113.

118. American Dietetic Association (2000). "Position of the American Dietetic Association: Vitamin and Mineral Supplementation." Available at http://www. eatright. org/asupple. html.

119. American Dietetic Association (1998). The American Dietetic Association standards of professional practice for dietetics professionals. *J. Am. Diet. Assoc.* **98,** 83–87.

120. Practice and Policy Guidelines Panel, National Institutes of Health Office of Alternative Medicine (1997). "Clinical practice guidelines in complementary and alternative medicine, an analysis of opportunities and obstacles." *Arch. Fam. Med.* **6,** 149–154.

121. American Medical Association, House of Delegates. "Proceedings of the House of Delegates, Resolution 510, I-99." American Medical Association, Chicago.

122. Cohen, M. H. (1998). "Complementary and Alternative Medicine; Legal Boundaries and Regulatory Perspectives." The Johns Hopkins University Press, Baltimore, MD.

123. Wetzel, M. S., Eisenberg, D. M., and Kaptchuk, T. J. (1999). Courses involving complementary and alternative medicine at U.S. medical schools. *JAMA* **280**(9), 784–778.

Disease-Specific Intervention: Prevention and Treatment

A. Cardiovascular Disease

CHAPTER 18

Dietary Macronutrients and Cardiovascular Risk

PENNY KRIS-ETHERTON, KARI HECKER, DENISE SHAFFER TAYLOR, GUIXIANG ZHAO, STACIE COVAL, AND
AMY BINKOSKI
Pennsylvania State University, University Park, Pennsylvania

I. INTRODUCTION

Cardiovascular disease (CVD) is the leading cause of death in the United States accounting for more deaths than all other causes combined. Numerous risk factors for CVD have been identified, many of which are modifiable by diet and lifestyle practices. Major modifiable risk factors include cigarette smoking, elevated total and low-density lipoprotein (LDL) cholesterol levels, overweight and obesity, hypertension, diabetes mellitus, and a sedentary lifestyle. Other important risk factors that are modifiable by diet are a low level of high-density lipoprotein (HDL) cholesterol, elevated levels of triglycerides (TGs), lipoprotein (a), insulin, hypertension, altered hemostatic factors, and small, dense LDL particles.

Diet continues to be an important cornerstone in the prevention and treatment of CVD. Current recommendations are to reduce saturated fat (SFA) and *trans* fatty acids (TFAs) by decreasing total fat and replacing SFA calories with carbohydrate (CHO) resulting in a lower fat, higher CHO diet with protein held constant. An alternative approach is to replace SFA calories with monounsaturated fatty acids (MUFAs), resulting in a diet higher in total fat. Polyunsaturated fatty acids (PUFAs), and omega–3 fatty acids in particular, have been a focus of attention recently because of their striking beneficial effects on CVD risk. The rapid increase in our understanding of fatty acid biology has clearly established the remarkable diversity of the effects of fatty acids on CVD risk factors. These findings underscore the importance of targeting fatty acids to maximally decrease CVD risk. For example, decreasing SFA is an absolute requisite, whereas maintaining or even increasing intake of other fatty acid classes is important for CVD risk reduction.

Historically the emphasis of dietary recommendations has been on modifying the type and amount of fat; however, modifying the type and amount of CHO and protein to lower CVD risk factors has attracted recent attention of scientists. With respect to dietary CHO, researchers are exploring how semi- and nondigestible carbohydrates and the glycemic index of CHO-rich foods affect risk factors for CVD. Likewise, studies are ongoing to unravel the different physio-logical effects that animal and plant proteins appear to elicit on CVD risk. We are transiting an exciting era in which we are gaining a better understanding of how all macronutrients affect CVD risk, and thus, it is not unreasonable to speculate that we will identify more effective dietary approaches for reducing CVD risk.

This chapter will review our present understanding of how changes in the macronutrient profile of the diet affect CVD risk status. We describe various low SFA and cholesterol diets that differ in macronutrient content and present the plasma lipid and lipoprotein responses that have been reported for these diets (Table 1). In addition, there is exciting new information about how diet affects emerging CVD risk factors. Thus, we describe the effect of various low-SFA, low-cholesterol diet options with different macronutrient profiles on newly defined CVD risk factors (Table 2).

II. DIETARY FAT

A. Total Fat

Discussions are ongoing about what the ideal quantity of total fat should be in the diet. Inherent to the discussion about total fat is that SFA and cholesterol should be reduced (i.e., <10% of calories and <300 mg/day, respectively) to most favorably affect risk of CVD and promote weight control. The central question is whether MUFA or CHO should replace SFA calories. A growing body of evidence suggests that replacing SFA with CHO leads to a decrease in HDL cholesterol and an increase in TG [1–3], both of which increase risk of CVD. In contrast, when MUFAs replace SFAs, plasma TGs are decreased and HDL cholesterol is either not decreased or decreased less compared with a high-CHO diet [2–4]. Thus, a high-MUFA, low-SFA diet is thought to result in a more favorable overall CVD risk profile than a low-SFA, high-CHO diet. Advocates of a high-CHO, low-SFA diet, however, argue that this diet will promote weight loss, because fewer calories are consumed and, consequently, elicit a beneficial effect on HDL cholesterol and TGs [5].

TABLE 1   Diets Low in Saturated Fat and Cholesterol with Varying Macronutrient Contents

Dietary Component	High carbohydrate			Higher fat		High protein	
	Step 1 [Ref. 52]	Step 2 [Ref. 52]	Very low fat [Ref. 53]	High MUFA [Ref. 124]	High n-3[a] [Ref. 46]	Animal protein [Ref. 100]	Soy protein [Ref. 110]
Diet composition:							
% CHO	≥55	≥55	≥70	50	50	45–50	45–50
% PRO	15	15	10–15	15	15	20–25	20–25 (25 or more gm of soy)
% FAT	≤30	≤30	≤15	>30 (~35)	>30 (~35)	≤30	≤30
% SFA	8–10	<7	5	<10	<10	8–10	8–10
% MUFA	≤15	≤15	5	≥15	15	≤15	≤15
% PUFA	≤10	≤10	5	<10	7–10	≤10	≤10
% n-6					5.7–8		
% n-3					1.3–2		
n-6:n-3					1–4:1		
Cholesterol (mg)	<300	<200	<100	<300	<300	<300	<300
Fiber (gm)	20–35	20–35	35	20–35	20–35	20–35	20–35
Percent change in blood lipid and lipoproteins[b]:							
Total cholesterol	↓5–15	↓5–20	↓10–20	↓5–15	NC	↓6	↓9
LDL-cholesterol	↓5–20	↓10–25	↓10–20	↓5–20	↑4–11	↓6–9	↓13
HDL-cholesterol	↓0–10	↓0–15	↑ with weight loss ↓ w/o weight loss	NC[c] or slight↓	↑1–3	↑0–12	NC or slight↑
Triglycerides	+5 to −10	+10 to −10	↓ with weight loss ↑ w/o weight loss	NC or slight↓	↓20–33	↓18–23	↓11

[a]9–13 g/day fish oil (1.1–7 g/day n-3 fatty acids).
[b]Compared with an average Western style diet.
[c]NC, no change.

Intertwined in the ongoing discussion is the question of whether a high-MUFA, low-SFA diet (a higher fat diet) leads to an increase in energy consumption, resulting in weight gain and perhaps predisposing one to overweight/obesity. Scientists who favor the position that increasing dietary fat leads to weight gain because of the higher caloric value of fat [6] suggest that we eat a constant volume of food regardless of caloric or macronutrient content. Thus, increasing dietary fat leads to overconsumption of energy [7–11]. In contrast, scientists who oppose this conclusion cite epidemiologic evidence showing little association between total fat intake and the incidence of overweight/obesity [12]. They also argue that fat plays a role in satiety and, thus, helps control calorie intake and body weight [13].

B. Saturated Fatty Acids

The Seven Countries Study [14], a landmark epidemiologic investigation, demonstrated that diet affected serum cholesterol levels and that an elevation in cholesterol increased risk of coronary disease. SFA intake (as a percent of calories) was positively correlated with serum cholesterol levels as well as with 5-year incidence of coronary heart disease

(CHD). Many well-controlled clinical studies followed, resulting in the development of blood cholesterol predictive equations for estimating the changes in total cholesterol in response to changes in type of fat and amount of dietary cholesterol. The original equations developed by Keys *et al.* [15] and Hegsted *et al.* [16] demonstrated that SFA was twice as potent in raising blood cholesterol levels as PUFA was in lowering them. MUFA was shown to have a neutral effect and dietary cholesterol raised the blood cholesterol level but less so than SFA. More recently, predictive equations have been developed for LDL and HDL cholesterol [17–20]. The LDL cholesterol response mimics that for total cholesterol. All fatty acid classes and dietary cholesterol increase HDL cholesterol; SFAs are most potent, PUFAs are least potent, and MUFAs have an intermediate effect.

Recent studies have evaluated the effects of individual fatty acids on plasma lipids and lipoproteins [21]. The effects reported are quite divergent when comparisons are made among the different SFAs. Myristic acid (C14:0) is twice as potent as lauric acid (C12:0) in raising total and LDL cholesterol. However, stearic acid (C18:0) is uniquely different; it has a neutral cholesterol-lowering effect.

TABLE 2   Cardiovascular Risk Factors Modifiable by Diets Low in
Saturated Fat and Cholesterol

Risk factors	Beneficial diet strategies[a]	Potentially adverse diet strategies
Hypercholesterolemia	LF-HC; Hi-MUFA; HP; Soy; Hi-sFib: FOS; Lo-GI	Hi-n-3 (fish oil)
Hypertriglyceridemia	Hi-MUFA; Hi-n-3; HP; Soy; FOS	LF-HC
Low HDL	Hi-MUFA	LF-HC
Small, dense LDL	Hi-MUFA	LF-HC
Insulin resistance	Hi-sFib; Hi-MUFA; Lo-GI; RS; FOS	LF-HC
Platelet aggregation	Hi-n-3; Soy	Unknown
Lipid peroxidation	LF-HC; Soy; Hi-MUFA	Hi-PUFA
Clotting	Hi-n-3; Soy	Unknown
Vascular reactivity	Hi-n-3; Soy	Unknown

[a]*Abbreviations:*
   LF-HC   low-fat, high-carbohydrate
   Hi-MUFA   high monounsaturated fat
   HP   high protein
   Soy   diet high in protein with 25 or more grams of soy protein
   FOS   fructooligosaccharides
   Hi-sFib   high soluble fiber
   Hi-n-3   high omega-3 fatty acid content
   Lo-GI   low-glycemic index
   RS   resistant starch
   Hi-PUFA   high polynsaturated fat

There is some epidemiologic evidence from the Atherosclerosis Risk in Communities Study [22] that a high intake of total fat, SFA, and cholesterol is associated with higher levels of factor VII and fibrinogen, two hemostatic factors that play a role in blood clot formation and are considered risk factors for CVD. Likewise, in the Dietary Effects on Lipoproteins and Thrombogenic Activity Study, a well-controlled multicenter feeding study, a reduction in SFA decreased factor VII [23, 24]. Fibrinogen levels were increased in response to a reduction in total fat [23, 24]. Of note, however, was that the magnitude of the response was modest (i.e., 2–3%).

The evidence is overwhelming that SFA, specifically lauric, myristic, and palmitic acids, have potent total and LDL cholesterol-raising effects. Irrespective of the total amount of fat in the diet, it is imperative that these fatty acids be reduced in the diet to decrease CVD risk.

C. Unsaturated Fatty Acids

1. Monounsaturated Fatty Acids

MUFAs provide great flexibility in diet planning because they can be used to replace SFAs, carbohydrate, or calories from both. Depending on the substitution, there can be a variable change in the total fat content of the diet (i.e., from 15% to 40% of energy), varying from essentially no or little change to an approximate twofold increase. On average, MUFAs provide about 15% of energy to the diet, while a high-MUFA diet typically provides about 20–22% of energy. Currently, there is great interest in MUFAs as a substitute for dietary CHO because of their beneficial effects on CVD risk factors [2, 3]. Diets high in MUFAs (that are low in SFAs and cholesterol) will lower plasma total and LDL cholesterol and TGs and minimize any potential decrease in HDL cholesterol [25]. There is limited evidence indicating that MUFAs may decrease susceptibility of LDL particles to oxidative modification, which is an important initiating event in the development of atherosclerosis, thereby reducing their atherogenic potential [26, 27]. Moreover, a diet higher in total fat has been shown to maintain a higher LDL particle diameter size [28, 29], which is important because small, dense LDLs increase CVD risk [30, 31].

In individuals with type 2 diabetes, a high-MUFA/low-CHO diet decreased both postprandial glucose and plasma insulin by 13.1% (for both) compared with a high-CHO diet [32]. Another study conducted by Garg *et al.* [33], compared a 55% CHO, 30% fat diet with a 40% CHO, 45% fat diet, in which the increase in fat was accomplished with addition of MUFA, on risk of CVD in patients with type 2 diabetes. They reported a significant decrease in a day-long glucose and insulin concentrations with the high-MUFA diet, although there was no change in fasting glucose or insulin in

two diet groups. In addition, in obese patients with type 2 diabetes, substitution of MUFA for CHO in two hypocaloric, weight-loss diets resulted in a greater decrease in both fasting and 24-hour glycemia, although the weight loss was similar in two diet groups [34]. In this same study, postprandial glycemia deteriorated after refeeding subjects with the CHO-enriched but not the MUFA-enriched formula. Collectively, these data suggest that MUFAs may improve the glycemic profile (plasma glucose and insulin levels) in individuals with type 2 diabetes.

2. Trans Fatty Acids

Numerous controlled feeding studies demonstrated that TFAs or hydrogenated fats elicited a blood cholesterol response that was intermediate to that observed for unhydrogenated oils and saturated fats [35]. More recently, studies have been conducted to evaluate the plasma lipid and lipoprotein effects of TFAs. These studies have consistently shown that TFAs increase plasma total and LDL cholesterol relative to unsaturated fatty acids [35]. Compared with SFA, TFAs elicit a similar or perhaps slightly less cholesterol-raising effect [35]. In addition, TFAs lower HDL cholesterol resulting in a worsening of the TC:HDL and LDL:HDL ratios, which, in turn, increase CHD risk [36]. Studies have also reported that TFA intake increases lipoprotein(a) levels [37], which is associated with an increased risk of CVD. Consequently, consumption of products that are low in TFAs and SFAs showed more beneficial effects on serum cholesterol levels [38]. While data from epidemiologic studies related to TFA intake and risk of developing heart disease are inconsistent because of the potential confounding dietary factors, substitution of hydrogenated fat with unhydrogenated fat is recommended in food processing and preparation [39].

D. Polyunsaturated Fatty Acids

1. Omega–6 Fatty Acids

As a result of the early studies by Keys *et al.* [15] and Hegsted *et al.* [16] that demonstrated the hypocholesterolemic effects of PUFAs, clinical trials were conducted to evaluate the effects of a low-SFA diet that was very high in PUFAs ($\sim$16–20.7% of energy) on incidence of CVD. These studies demonstrated a marked cholesterol-lowering effect of a high-PUFA diet (17.6–20.0% reduction in serum cholesterol compared with baseline values) [40, 41]. Importantly, the cholesterol-lowering response was associated with a reduction in the incidence of CVD (16–34%). However, the perception by some that high-PUFA diets may increase risk of certain cancers, despite the lack of strong evidence to support this relationship, diminished support for this diet strategy. This has led to the present recommendation that PUFA calories not exceed 10% of energy.

Recent studies have reported that PUFAs have a slightly greater total and LDL cholesterol-lowering effect versus MUFAs [42]. Thus for practical purposes, MUFAs or PUFAs will elicit effects that are quite similar when incorporated in a diet that meets current recommendations for total fat (30% of energy) and PUFAs (<10% of energy). Some experts advocate, however, that PUFAs not exceed approximately 7% of total energy [43], based on some evidence that PUFAs increase *in vitro* LDL oxidative susceptibility (compared with MUFAs), thereby possibly increasing CVD risk. Thus, a PUFA recommendation of <10% of energy is, at present, prudent.

2. Omega–3 Fatty Acids

The 1970s marked the beginning of extensive scientific evaluation of the role of omega–3 fatty acids in the development of CVD. The seminal studies of Dyerberg *et al.* [44] noted that coronary atherosclerotic disease was rare in Greenland Eskimos and prevalent in a Danish population. These scientists attributed this difference in the incidence of CHD to the high intake of marine oils by the Eskimos and, in particular, eicosapentanoic acid (EPA, C20:5) and docosahexanoic acid (DHA, C22:6). During the past 30 years numerous studies have demonstrated that these fatty acids may confer cardioprotective effects via multiple mechanisms that involve antiarrhythmic actions, sudden death, thrombosis and hemostasis, growth of atherosclerotic plaques, and lipids and lipoproteins.

There is impressive evidence that the omega–3 fatty acid alpha-linolenic acid, reduces coronary morbidity and mortality in patients with heart disease. The Lyon Diet Heart Study [45] reported that any AHA Step 1 Mediterranean dietary pattern (high in alpha-linolenic acid) reduced all cardiac death and nonfatal myocardial infarction by approximately 70% and all coronary events by about 50% despite no improvement in lipids, lipoproteins and adiposity.

Fish oil has a marked hypotriglyceridemic effect in both normotriglyceridemic and hypertriglyceridemic ($\geq$2 mmol/L) individuals. The addition of approximately 9–13 g/day of fish oil (e.g., 1.1–7 g/day of omega-3 fatty acids) resulted in a TG decrease of about 20–25% in normotriglyceridemic individuals and a decrease of about 26–33% in hypertriglyceridemic individuals [46]. However, fish oil elevates LDL cholesterol levels modestly (e.g., 4–5%) in normotriglyceridemic individuals and more so ($\sim$5–11%) in hypertriglyceridemic individuals, and even more so (30%) in some individuals with familial hyperlipidemia (type IV/V) [47]. Thus, fish oil supplements can be an effective treatment for some patients with hypertriglyceridemia, although close monitoring by a physician is essential to ensure that there is no concurrent significant increase in LDL cholesterol.

III. DIETARY CARBOHYDRATE

As discussed in the previous section on dietary fat, there is an ongoing debate about whether it is better to replace saturated fat with calories from MUFAs or CHO to most fa-

vorably impact CVD risk. While both diets lower LDL cholesterol, a low-fat, high-CHO diet, when not accompanied by weight loss, decreases HDL cholesterol and increases TG [48]. This is particularly problematic for people with insulin resistance, whose dyslipidemia often presents as decreased HDL cholesterol and elevated TG [49]. A low-fat, high-CHO diet has also been shown to increase plasma glucose and insulin in individuals with type 2 diabetes [32] and healthy women [50]. On the other hand, it can be argued that a low-fat, high-CHO diet facilitates a reduction in energy intake [51] and effectively reduces and maintains body weight [6], which is a key factor in lowering CVD risk, especially in overweight/obesity.

Among the proponents of high-CHO diets, the National Cholesterol and Education Program (NCEP) [52] recommends that 55% or more energy come from CHO, because total fat is reduced to facilitate a decrease in SFA and help control energy intake. Others advocate a more extreme reduction in fat (10% energy) and thus a much higher CHO (70–80%) diet [53]. This latter approach has been shown to be effective, when combined with other intensive lifestyle changes (e.g., stress management and aerobic exercise), resulting in a reversal of coronary heart disease as measured by percent change in diameter stenosis [54].

While the broader issue is still unresolved as to whether CHO or MUFA should replace SFA calories to lower CVD risk, many scientists are turning their focus to the type of CHO used in a low-fat, high-CHO diet. They argue that low-fat, high-CHO diets have not been adequately evaluated in terms of their effects on the overall CVD risk profile. It has been suggested that in studies comparing high-MUFA to high-CHO diets, part of the explanation for the beneficial effects of MUFA could be due to the specific type of CHO used in the low-fat diets.

When discussing different types of carbohydrate, scientists historically used the terms *complex* versus *simple CHO*. As we gain a better understanding of how CHO affects CVD risk, this terminology is not useful and thus is being phased out. However, there are no well-established categories for CHO as it relates to CVD risk, such as SFA, MUFA, PUFA, and TFA for fat and animal versus plant for protein. This is due in part to the complexity of carbohydrate food sources and their impact on CVD risk. Many foods that are included in a high-CHO diet, such as fruits and vegetables, breads and cereals, and legumes, contain multiple compounds that could favorably affect CVD risk. In this section, we will address a few of the actively researched areas associated with CHO and reduction of CVD risk: the role of glycemic index, dietary fiber, resistant starch, and fructooligosaccharides.

A. Glycemic Index

Carbohydrates differ in terms of their effects on glucose metabolism [55]. Carbohydrates can be classified according to their blood glucose-raising effects using the glycemic index.

Low glycemic index foods, such as mature beans and peas, elicit less of a glycemic response than high glycemic index foods, such as potatoes and ready-to-eat cereals. Low glycemic index diets have been shown to increase insulin sensitivity [56, 57] and decrease total serum cholesterol [56] and LDL cholesterol [57] in people with type 2 diabetes. These findings illustrate the importance of considering not only the macronutrient composition of the diet, but also the type of CHO consumed within the context of a low-fat diet.

In a recent editorial, Grant [58] illustrates the point that in one study, half of the increase in CHO in a low-fat diet was achieved with the addition of sugars [59]. Similar substitutions are evident in another study comparing the effects of high-MUFA and low-fat diets in postmenopausal women. The sample menus reported by the authors show that the low-fat diet contained more sugars or refined foods with a high glycemic index, such as bread, cookies, and potato, than the high-MUFA diet [50].

In general, foods high in soluble fiber have a low glycemic index; however, this is an oversimplification because food preparation and consumption of a specific food in a mixed meal can alter glycemic index. A mixed meal can have a low glycemic index with the selection of certain foods. Because of the complexity of implementing the glycemic index, it likely will be difficult for consumers to adopt at the present time with currently available foods and contemporary lifestyle practices. Furthermore, the concept of glycemic index must also address the role of other nutrients in a way that is consistent with current dietary recommendations. For example, some low glycemic index foods are high in total fat, saturated fat, and sugar and therefore should be limited. Thus, it is apparent that many questions remain about glycemic index. Clearly, additional evidence is needed to refine glycemic index of foods, snacks, meals, and diets and to establish the health effects of glycemic index and how it can be implemented in the population.

B. Dietary Fiber

An abundance of evidence supports a negative association between dietary fiber intake and risk of CVD [60]. Dietary fiber is found naturally in fruits, vegetables, whole-grain cereals, and legumes, and has been supplemented to foods and beverages for several recent studies [61, 62]. Numerous epidemiologic studies support the cardioprotective effect of dietary fiber. For example, data from two large U.S. prospective studies, one including male health professionals [63] and another with female nurses [64], has shown that dietary fiber (most notably cereal fiber) was associated with a reduced risk of fatal and nonfatal myocardial infarction. In addition to epidemiologic evidence, many clinical trials have confirmed the favorable effects of dietary fiber intake on CVD risk factors [65–70].

Soluble fiber, including oat bran, psyllium, guar gum, and pectin, has been shown to reduce CVD risk through its action

on lipids and lipoproteins and glucose metabolism. A recent meta-analysis of 67 controlled human trials [71] determined that various soluble fibers (2–10 g/day) modestly reduced total and LDL cholesterol (2%), and did not affect HDL cholesterol and TGs. In addition, soluble fiber has been shown to lower glucose and insulin levels in healthy individuals [69] and favorably affect insulin sensitivity in individuals with diabetes [68] and moderate hypercholesterolemia [70].

C. Resistant Starch

In recent years, it has become appreciated that the rate of starch hydrolysis can vary from quickly to quite slow. In some instances, the hydrolysis occurs so slowly that some starch may pass into the large intestine undigested. This resistant starch has been defined as "the sum of starch and products of starch hydrolysis not absorbed in the small intestine of healthy individuals" by the European FLAIR Concerted Action on Resistant Starch (euresta) [72].

The beneficial effects of resistant starch on CVD are not well understood. Several animal studies have shown a positive effect on blood lipids and lipoproteins when resistant starch was added to the diet [73, 74]. However, in human studies [75, 76] where free-living normolipidemic subjects were supplemented with two types of resistant starch (retrograded and chemically modified), no effect on serum lipids was observed.

This lack of effect was also observed when examining the effects of resistant starch in hypertriglyceridemic subjects [77]. Although there were no significant effects on serum lipids in the study by Noakes et al. [77], a 17% reduction in postprandial plasma insulin concentrations was observed when high-amylose starch comprised 33% of the carbohydrate content of a test meal. Further research is necessary in various experimental conditions to explore whether resistant starch has a beneficial effect on blood lipids and insulin sensitivity.

D. Fructooligosaccharides

Fructooligosaccharides (FOSs) are indigestible, highly fermentable CHO that occur naturally in foods such as onions, bananas, tomatoes, garlic, and wheat. FOSs can also be produced commercially and have been added to many food products and nutriceuticals [78]. FOSs pass through the intestinal tract undigested and are fermented in the large intestine by bacteria into lactate and short-chain fatty acids [78]. The short-chain fatty acids produced by FOS fermentation ultimately yield 1–2 kcal/g rather than the 4 kcal/g of digestible carbohydrates [79].

A growing body of research has described numerous beneficial effects of FOSs including improvements in plasma lipids and lipoproteins. Evidence from animal studies report that FOSs, as part of a high-CHO, fiber-free, or high-fat diet, reduce total cholesterol and especially TGs [80, 81]. The

TG-lowering action of FOSs occurs as a consequence of a reduction in *de novo* fatty acid synthesis secondary to modification of gene expression of lipogenic enzymes [82, 83]. Additionally, FOS has been found to reduce serum insulin and glucose concentrations in animal models [82].

Studies of the effects of FOSs on lipids and lipoproteins in humans are few in number and have been conflicting. Williams [84] speculates that this inconsistency is due to the significantly lower doses of FOSs administered in human studies compared to the doses used to elicit effects in animals. Most subjects do not tolerate FOS levels greater than 30 g/day due to adverse gastrointestinal symptoms [84]. Some studies have not observed any changes in blood lipids and lipoproteins with FOS intakes ranging between 9 and 20 g/day [85, 86], while others report significant reductions in total and LDL cholesterol or TGs [87, 88]. TGs have been reported to decrease by as much as 27% [87]. It is interesting to note that in hypertriglyceridemic subjects, the TG-lowering action of FOSs may be more pronounced if the diet is high in CHO rather than fat [84]. Furthermore, as observed in animal studies, FOSs have been reported to alter glucose metabolism. Roberfroid [89] and others have demonstrated that the increase of blood glucose and insulin is very low compared to fructose [85, 90, 91].

Future research is needed to assess whether FOSs have a consistent lipid-lowering effect in humans and to assess the dose necessary to achieve beneficial effects. Furthermore, the lipid-lowering mechanisms of FOS remain to be elucidated. However, present data indicate that FOSs reduce total cholesterol and may exert a potentially potent TG-lowering action.

IV. DIETARY PROTEIN

In the attempt to define the optimal ratio of dietary macronutrients for CVD risk reduction, nutrition research has recently turned its attention to the role of protein in cardiovascular health. Available evidence at this time is somewhat limited, but indicates that dietary protein of animal and, particularly, plant (soy) origin may beneficially affect several CVD risk factors.

A. Animal Protein

Early studies reported that hypercholesterolemia and atherosclerosis could be induced in rabbits and other animals by feeding low-fat, cholesterol-free diets containing milk casein as the source of protein [92, 93]. Interestingly, the cholesterol-raising effect of animal protein has not been consistently observed in other animals or in humans [94].

Epidemiologic studies in the 1950s showed strong associations between dietary (animal) protein and mortality from CVD [95]. However, animal protein intake was also significantly correlated with SFA and cholesterol intake—dietary factors known to be hypercholesterolemic and atherogenic

[96]. More recent epidemiologic data, from the Nurses' Health Study, showed that high protein intakes (up to 24% of total energy intake), including animal and plant proteins, significantly reduced the risk of CVD (RR = 0.75; 95% CI: 0.61, 0.92) [97]. In addition, the Cholesterol Lowering Atherosclerosis Study reported a reduction in new coronary artery lesions with increasing dietary protein (low-fat meat and dairy) in place of fat, while persons developing new lesions showed a decrease in mean protein intake [98].

Several controlled feeding studies have found that replacing CHO with low-fat animal protein, such as lean beef, poultry, fish, cottage cheese, and skim milk, can elicit favorable changes in lipid risk factors. In a crossover study conducted by Wolfe *et al.* [99, 100], subjects with moderate hypercholesterolemia were randomly assigned to either a high-protein diet containing 27% protein (79% animal) and 53% CHO or a low-protein diet (11% protein; 65% carbohydrate). Dietary fat (25%), cholesterol (less than 200 mg/ day), and fiber were held constant. Compared to subjects on the low-protein diet, moderately hypercholesterolemic subjects on the high-protein diet experienced a 6% reduction in total and LDL cholesterol, 23% and 28% reductions in TG and very low-density lipoprotein (VLDL), and a 12% increase in HDL cholesterol [99, 100]. Subjects with familial hypercholesterolemia (receiving cholestyramine) experienced similar beneficial changes in plasma lipids with increased dietary protein intake [101]. In another study, normolipidemic subjects consumed either a higher fat (35%), high-protein diet containing 22% protein (70% of animal origin) or a low-protein (12%) diet. Those on the high-protein diet sustained a 6% reduction in total cholesterol, a 9% reduction in LDL cholesterol, an 18% decrease in TG, and a 28% reduction in VLDL compared to subjects who consumed a low-protein diet [102]. In a considerably longer-term study (36 weeks), NCEP Step 1 diets containing primarily lean red meat (beef, veal, pork) or lean white meat (poultry and fish) produced similar reductions in LDL-C and elevations in HDL-C in hypercholesterolemic men and women for the duration of the study [102a].

One recent controlled feeding study, Dietary Approaches to Stop Hypertension (DASH), investigated the effect of dietary patterns, rather than specific compounds on hypertension, a major CVD risk factor. DASH showed that a dietary pattern including animal protein from low-fat dairy products improved blood pressure. Specifically, a diet rich in fruits, vegetables, and low-fat diary products and reduced in saturated fat (18% protein) significantly improved both systolic (decreased by 5.5 mmHg) and diastolic (decreased by 3.0 mmHg) blood pressure beyond that of a lower protein diet (10%) rich in fruits and vegetables [104]. The DASH combination diet is in general accordance with the dietary guidelines established by the American Heart Association and other organizations. It has been reported by Harsha *et al.* [103a] that if the DASH combination diet were strictly adopted by the general American population and resulted in a nationwide blood pressure reduction of the magnitude found in DASH, a 15% decrease in coronary heart disease and about a 27% decrease in stroke incidence would be expected.

Mechanisms in which animal protein may reduce lipid risk factors are uncertain at this time. As opposed to high-CHO diets, high protein diets have been shown to reduce TG and increase HDL cholesterol, and some propose that substituting protein for CHO may increase catabolism or decrease production of VLDL and LDL cholesterol [100]. In rats, a high-protein diet has been reported to significantly decreased hepatic VLDL secretion [104]. Additionally, mild hypercholesterolemia due to increased hepatic HMG-CoA reductase activity was observed in rats fed a low-protein diet (8%) [105].

Though current research suggests that increasing intake of animal protein (20–25% of total energy) as part of a low-fat diet may reduce CVD risk factors, caution may be warranted in recommending a high-protein diet for several reasons. Available evidence supporting the cholesterol-lowering potential of protein is limited and will require more research. Increasing protein intake from animal sources such as meat and dairy can result in increased intakes of saturated fat and cholesterol if lean meats and low-fat dairy products are not chosen. Thus, plasma cholesterol may be adversely affected and override any benefit gained from increasing protein in the diet. Also, high-protein diets may promote the development of renal disease and osteoporosis. Findings in these areas are conflicting and further research to assess the long-term safety of a high-protein diet is needed.

B. Soy (Vegetable) Protein

A multitude of animal studies has reported that blood cholesterol levels are lowered by consumption of soy protein rather than animal protein [106, 107]. In humans, epidemiologic studies report that Asian populations, which consume 30–50 times more soy than Western populations, have a lower prevalence of many chronic diseases, including CVD [108]. A strong correlation between increasing intakes of soy foods and decreasing total cholesterol concentrations in men and women of Asian populations has also been observed [109]. Though many clinical studies reported that substituting soy protein, such as tofu, tempeh, and soy milk, for animal protein reduced plasma cholesterol levels, the results were somewhat inconsistent. However, in 1995, a meta-analysis of 38 controlled clinical trials concluded that soy intakes ranging from 31 to 47 g/day significantly reduced total cholesterol by 9.3%, LDL cholesterol by 12.9%, and TG by 10.5%, with a greater response observed in subjects with higher baseline cholesterol levels [110]. HDL cholesterol was increased modestly (i.e., 2.4%; nonsignificant).

Factors responsible for the antiatherogenic effect of soy remain relatively unknown. Some investigators suggest that soy protein upregulates LDL receptors depressed by hypercholesterolemia [111, 112]. This may explain, in part, why

normolipidemic subjects do not experience significant reductions in total cholesterol subsequent to soy intake [111]. Others hypothesize that the antiatherogenic properties of soy protein are due to its amino acid profile, specifically the low lysine-to-arginine ratio [92, 113]. Arginine is thought to be less hypercholesterolemic than lysine and thus higher concentrations may reduce serum cholesterol levels. Sanchez *et al.* [114] report that the higher amount of arginine in soy protein, roughly twice that of casein, induces a low postprandial insulin-to-glucagon ratio, and decreases serum cholesterol levels by suppressing the lipogenic functions of insulin. In addition to lowering plasma cholesterol levels, the higher concentration of arginine in soy foods is also suggested to improve vascular reactivity. Arginine is the physiological substrate for nitric oxide synthesis, and nitric oxide functions as a potent vasodilator [115].

Various bioactive components in soy, particularly isoflavones, are thought to contribute to its hypocholesterolemic and antiatherogenic properties as well [116]. Several studies have shown that soy protein without isoflavones has little or no effect on serum cholesterol levels [117, 118]. Crouse *et al.* [117] demonstrated a significant dose–response effect where 25 g soy protein with 62 mg isoflavone significantly reduced plasma total and LDL cholesterol compared to soy protein containing 3–27 mg isoflavone. Conversely, other studies have demonstrated that isoflavones alone have very little effect on serum cholesterol levels [119]. Investigators thus propose that synergy between soy protein and its naturally occurring isoflavones is necessary to reduce cholesterol levels [117].

In addition to the effects on plasma cholesterol, soy protein with soy isoflavones is reported to inhibit platelet activation and aggregation [120], LDL oxidative susceptibility [121], and smooth muscle cell migration and proliferation [122]. Soy isoflavones, with and without soy protein, have been shown to improve vascular function [119, 123]. Furthermore, soy isoflavones, also referred to as phytoestrogens, bind to estrogen receptors and may offer cardioprotective effects similar to that of estrogen [116].

The evidence is fairly convincing that consuming 25 g or more of soy protein (with isoflavones) a day beneficially affects other CVD risk factors besides lipids and lipoproteins, particularly in hypercholesterolemic individuals. Whether soy protein or its various bioactive components exert greater cardioprotective action is currently under investigation. However, it is probable that the combination of soy protein and its naturally occurring isoflavones incur the greatest benefit on cardiovascular health.

Research on the effects of protein and CVD risk is promising. Low-fat animal protein (lean meats and low-fat dairy), and especially soy protein, appears to exert many benefits on cardiovascular health. Of specific interest are their effects on TG and HDL cholesterol, as well as hemostasis, platelet function, and vascular reactivity. Therefore, a low-fat, high-protein (20–25% energy from protein) diet may be considered as an alternative to more traditional low-fat, high-CHO diets, particularly in the case of hypertriglyceridemia. Incorporating soy protein (25 g/day) in the diet will improve multiple CVD risk factors.

V. CONCLUSION

Remarkable progress has been made in our knowledge of how diet affects CVD risk. The early studies focused on lipids and lipoprotein risk factors in response to the type of fat in the diet. However, as we have gained a better understanding of how diet affects CVD risk, it has become evident that other risk factors are integral to the progression of CVD. Moreover, it is clear that the other macronutrients, i.e., carbohydrate and protein, affect CVD risk. These observations have led to the development of new diet strategies to target multiple risk factors. At the core of this approach is a reduction of SFA, which unequivocally reduces total and LDL cholesterol levels. Replacing SFA calories with MUFAs has favorable effects on not only total and LDL cholesterol levels, but also HDL cholesterol, TG, insulin levels, and fibrinogen, thereby further reducing CVD risk. Further modifications in CHO (e.g., increasing soluble fiber) and protein (increasing plant protein) also seem to confer additional beneficial effects on CVD risk.

Collectively, we are moving closer to identifying a diet that optimally affects the multitude of CVD risk factors. Identification of this diet will result most likely in the greatest diet-mediated reduction of CVD risk.

References

1. Ginsberg, H. N., Kris-Etherton, P., Dennis, B., Elmer, P. J., Ershow, A., Lefevre, M., Pearson, T., Roheim, P., Ramakrishnan, R., Reed, R., Stewart, K., Stewart, P., Phillips, K., and Anderson, N. (1998). Effects of reducing dietary saturated fatty acids on plasma lipids and lipoproteins in healthy subjects: The DELTA Study, Protocol 1. *Arterioscler. Thromb. Vasc. Biol.* **18,** 441–449.
2. Kris-Etherton, P. M., Pearson, T. A., Wan, Y., Hargrove, R. L., Moriarty, K., Fishell, V., and Etherton, T. D. (1999). High-monounsaturated fatty acid diets lower both plasma cholesterol and triacylglycerol concentrations. *Am. J. Clin. Nutr.* **70,** 1009–1015.
3. Kris-Etherton, P. M., Zhao, G., Pelkman, C. L., Fishell, V. K., and Coval, S. (2000). Beneficial effects of a diet high in monounsaturated fatty acids on risk factors for cardiovascular disease. *Nutr. Clin. Care* **3,** 153–162.
4. Mensink, R. P., and Katan, M. B. (1987). Effect of monounsatured fatty acids versus complex carbohydrates on high-density lipoproteins in healthy men and women. *Lancet* **1,** 122–125.
5. Connor, W. E., and Connor, S. (1997). Should a low-fat, high-carbohydrate diet be recommended for everyone? The case for a low-fat, high-carbohydrate diet. *N. Engl. J. Med.* **337,** 562–563.

6. Bray, G. A., and Popkin, B. M. (1998). Dietary fat intake does affect obesity! *Am. J. Clin. Nutr.* **68**, 1157–1173.

7. Van Stratum, P., Lussenburg, R. N., van Wezel, L. A., Vergoesen, A. J., and Cremer, H. D. (1978). The effect of dietary carbohydrate: Fat ratio on energy intake in adult women. *Am. J. Clin. Nutr.* **31**, 206–212.

8. Lissner, L., Levitsky, D. A., Strupp, B. J., Kalkwarf, H. J., and Roe, D. A. (1987). Dietary fat and the regulation of energy intake in human subjects. *Am. J. Clin. Nutr.* **46**, 886–892.

9. Kendall, A., Levitsky, D. A., Strupp, B. J., and Lissner, L. (1991). Weight loss on a low-fat diet: Consequence of the imprecision of the control of food intake in humans. *Am. J. Clin. Nutr.* **53**, 1124–1129.

10. Stubbs, R. J., Harbron, C. G., Margatroyd, P. R., and Prentice, A. M. (1996). Covert manipulation of dietary fat and energy density; effect on substrate flux and food intake in men eating ad libitum. *Int. J. Obes.* **20**, 651–660.

11. Bell, E. A., Castellanos, V. H., Pelkman, C. L., Thorwart, M. L., and Rolls, B. J. (1998). Energy density of foods affects energy intake in normal-weight women. *Am. J. Clin. Nutr.* **67**, 412–420.

12. Willett, W. C. (1998). Dietary fat and obesity: An uncovering relation. *Am. J. Clin. Nutr.* **98**, 1149–1150.

13. Leibel, R. L., Hirsch, J., Appel, B. E., and Checani, G. C. (1992). Energy intake required to maintain body weight is not affected by wide variation in diet composition. *Am. J. Clin. Nutr.* **55**, 350–355.

14. Keys, A. (1970). "Coronary Heart Disease in Seven Countries," American Heart Association Monograph No. 29, Circulation XLI–XLII, pp. I-1–I-211.

15. Keys, A., Anderson, J. T., and Grande, F. (1965). Serum cholesterol response to changes in the diet. IV. Particular saturated fatty acids in the diet. *Metabolism* **14**, 776–787.

16. Hegsted, D. M., McGandy, R. B., Myers, M. L., and Stare, F. J. (1965). Quantitative effects of dietary fat on serum cholesterol in man. *Am. J. Clin. Nutr.* **17**, 281–295.

17. Mensink, R. P., and Katan, M. B. (1992). Effect of dietary fatty acids on serum lipids and lipoproteins. A meta-analysis of 27 trials. *Arterioscler. Thromb.* **12**, 911–919.

18. Hegsted, D. M., Ausman, L. M., Johnson, J. A., and Dallal, G. E. (1993). Dietary fat and serum lipids: An evaluation of the experimental data. *Am. J. Clin. Nutr.* **57**, 875–883.

19. Yu, S., Derr, J., Etherton, T. D., and Kris-Etherton, P.M. (1995). Plasma cholesterol—Predictive equations demonstrate that stearic acid is neutral and monounsaturated fatty acids are hypocholesterolemic. *Am. J. Clin. Nutr.* **61**, 1129–1139.

20. Clarke, R., Frost, C., Collins, R., Appleby, P., and Peto, R. (1997). Dietary lipids and blood cholesterol: Quantitative meta-analysis of metabolic ward studies. *Br. Med. J.* **314**, 112–117.

21. Kris-Etherton, P. M., and Yu, S. (1997). Individual fatty acid effects on plasma lipids and lipoproteins: Human studies. *Am. J. Clin. Nutr.* **65**(Suppl.), 1628S–1644S.

22. Shahar, E., Folsom, A. R., Wu, K. K., Dennis, B. H., Shimakawa, T., Conlan, M. G., Davis, C. E., and Williams, O. D. (1993). Associations of fish intake and dietary n–3 polyunsaturated fatty acids with a hypocoagulable profile. The Atherosclerosis Risk in Communities (ARIC) Study. *Arterioscler. Thromb.* **13**, 1205–1212.

23. Elmer, P. J. (1995). Effects on lipoproteins and thrombogenic activity: Effects of reducing dietary total and saturated fats on hemostatic factors. *FASEB J.* **9**, A289.

24. Elmer, P. (1996). Effects of a Step I diet and a high monounsaturated fat (MUFA) diet on hemostatic factors in individuals with markers for insulin resistance. *FASEB J.* **10**, A262.

25. Mensink, R. P., and Katan, M. B. (1989). Effect of a diet enriched with monounsaturated or polyunsaturated fatty acids on levels of low-density and high-density lipoprotein cholesterol in healthy women and men. *N. Engl. J. Med.* **321**, 436–441.

26. Gumbiner, B., Low, C. C., and Reaven, P. D. (1998). Effects of a monounsaturated fatty acid-enriched hypocaloric diet on cardiovascular risk factors in obese patients with type 2 diabetes. *Metabolism* **41**, 1373–1378.

27. Reaven, P. D., Parthasarathy, S., Grasse, B. J., Miller, G., Steinberg, D., and Witztum, J. L. (1993). Effects of oleate-enriched and linoleate-enriched diets on the susceptibility of low density lipoprotein to oxidative modification in hypercholesterolemic subjects. *J. Clin. Invest.* **91**, 668–676.

28. Krauss, R. M., and Dreon, D. M. (1995). Low-density lipoprotein subclasses and response to a low-fat diet in healthy men. *Am. J. Clin. Nutr.* **62**, 478S–487S.

29. Reaven, P. D., Grasse, B. J., and Tribble, D. L. (1994). Effects of linoleate-enriched and oleate-enriched diets in combination with alpha-tocopherol on the susceptibility of LDL and LDL subfractions to oxidative modification in humans. *Arterioscler. Thromb.* **14**, 557–566.

30. Austin, M. A. (1994). Small, dense low-density lipoprotein as a risk factor for coronary heart disease. *Int. J. Clin. Lab. Res.* **24**, 187–192.

31. Chait, A., Brazg, R. L., Tribble, D. L., and Krauss, R. M. (1993). Susceptibility of small, dense, low-density lipoproteins to oxidative modification in subjects with the atherogenic lipoprotein phenotype, pattern B. *Am. J. Med.* **94**, 350–356.

32. Parillo, M., Rivellese, A. A., Ciardullo, A. V., Capaldo, B., Giacco, A., Genovese, S., and Riccardi, G. (1992). A high-monounsaturated-fat/low-carbohydrate diet improves peripheral insulin sensitivity in non-insulin-dependent diabetic patients. *Metabolism* **41**, 1373–1378.

33. Garg, A., Bantle, J. P., Henry, R. R., Coulston, A. M., Griver, K. A., Raatz, S. K., Brinkley, L., Chen, Y. D., Grundy, S. M., Huet, B. A., *et al.* (1994). Effects of varying carbohydrate content of diet in patients with non-insulin-dependent diabetes mellitus. *JAMA* **371**, 1421–1428.

34. Low, C. C., Grossman, E. B., and Gumbiner, B. (1996). Potentiation of effects of weight loss by monounsaturated fatty acids in obese NIDDM patients. *Diabetes.* **45**, 569–575.

35. Denke, M. A. (1995). Serum lipid concentrations in humans. *Am. J. Clin. Nutr.* **62**, 693S–700S.

36. Mensink, R. P., and Katan, M. B. (1990). Effect of dietary trans fatty acids on high-density and low-density lipoprotein cholesterol levels in healthy subjects. *N. Engl. J. Med.* **323**, 439–445.

37. Zock, P. L., and Mensink, R. P. (1996). Dietary trans-fatty acids and serum lipoproteins in humans. *Curr. Opin. Lipidol.* **7**, 34–37.

38. Lichtenstein, A. H., Ausman, L. M., Jalbert, S. M., and Schaefer, E. J. (1999). Effects of different forms of dietary hydrogenated fats on serum lipoprotein cholesterol levels. *N. Engl. J. Med.* **340**, 1933–1940.

39. Lichtenstein, A. H. (1997). Trans fatty acids, plasma lipid levels, and risk of developing cardiovascular disease. A statement

for healthcare professionals from the American Heart Association. *Circulation* **95,** 2588–2590.

40. Dayton, S., Pearce, M. L., Hashimoto, S., Dixon, W. J., and Tomiyasu, U. (1969). A controlled clinical trial of a diet high in unsaturated fat in preventing complications of atherosclerosis. *Circulation* **40**(Suppl.), 1–63.

41. Leren, P. (1966). The effects of plasma cholesterol lowering diet in male survivors of myocardial infarction. *Acta Medica Scand.* (Suppl.) **466,** 1–92.

42. Howard, B. V., Hannah, J. S., Heiser, C. C., Jablonski, K. A., Paidi, M. C., Alarif, L., Robbins, D. C., and Howard, W. J. (1995). Polyunsaturated fatty acids result in greater cholesterol lowering and less triacylglycerol elevation than do monounsaturated fatty acids in a dose-response comparison in a multiracial study group. *Am. J. Clin. Nutr.* **62,** 392–402.

43. Grundy, S. M. (1997). What is the desirable ratio of saturated, polyunsaturated, and monounsaturated fatty acids in the diet? *Am. J. Clin. Nutr.* **68,** 142–153.

44. Dyerberg, J., Bang, H. O., and Hjorne, N. (1975). Fatty acid composition of the plasma lipids in Greenland Eskimos. *Am. J. Clin. Nutr.* **28,** 958–966.

45. de Lorgeril, M., Salen, P., Martin, J. L., Monjaud, I., Delaye, J., and Mamelle, N. (1999). Mediterranean diet, traditional risk factors, and the rate of cardiovascular complications after myocardial infarction: Final report of the Lyon Diet Heart Study. *Circulation* **99,** 779–785.

46. Harris, W. S. (1997). n-3 fatty acids and serum lipoproteins: Human studies. *Am. J. Clin. Nutr.* **65**(5 Suppl.), 1645S–1654S.

47. Harris, W. W. (1989). Fish oils and plasma lipid and lipoprotein metabolism in humans: A critical review. *J. Lipid Res.* **30,** 785–807.

48. Yu-Poth, S., Zhao, G., Etherton, T., Naglak, M., Jonnalagadda, S., and Kris-Etherton, P. M. (1999). Effects of the National Cholesterol Education Program's Step I and Step II dietary intervention programs on cardiovascular disease risk factors: A meta-analysis. *Am. J. Clin. Nutr.* **69,** 632–646.

49. DeFronzo, R. A., and Ferrannini, E. (1991). Insulin resistance: A multifaceted syndrome responsible for NIDDM, obesity, hypertension, dyslipidemia, and atherosclerotic cardiovascular disease. *Diabetes Care* **14,** 173–194.

50. Jeppesen, J., Schaaf, P., Jones, C., Zhou, M.-Y., Chen, Y.-D. I., and Reaven, G. M. (1997). Effects of low-fat, high-carbohydrate diets on risk factors for ischemic heart disease in postmenopausal women. *Am. J. Clin. Nutr.* **65,** 1027–1033.

51. Hammer, V. A., and Rolls, B. J. . (1997). Diet composition and the regulation of body weight. *In* "Obesity and Weight Management: The Health Professional's Guide to Understanding and Treatment" (S. Dalton, Ed.), pp. 254–283. Aspen Publishers, Inc., Gaithersburg, MD.

52. Summary of the second report of the National Cholesterol Education Program (NCEP), Expert Panel on Detection, Evaluation, and Treatment of High Blood Cholesterol in Adults (Adult Treatment Panel II). (1993). *JAMA* **269,** 3015–3023.

53. Lichtenstein, A. H., and Van Horn, L. (1998). Very low fat diets. *Circulation* **98,** 935–939.

54. Ornish, D., Scherwitz, L. M., Billings, J. H., Gould, L., Merrit, T. A., Sparler, S., Armstrong, W. T., Ports, T. A., Kirkeeide, R. L., Hogeboom, C., and Brand, R. (1998). Intensive lifestyle changes for reversal of coronary heart disease. *JAMA* **280,** 2001–2007.

55. Wolever, T. M. S. (1999). Dietary recommendations for diabetes: High carbohydrate or high monounsaturated fat. *Nutr. Today* **34,** 73–77.

56. Wolever, T. M. S., Jenkins, D. J. A., Vuksan, V., Jenkins, A. L., Wong, G. S., and Josse, R. G. (1992). Beneficial effects of low-glycemic index diet in overweight NIDDM subjects. *Diabetes Care* **15,** 562–566.

57. Jarvi, A. E., Karlstrom, B. E., Granfeldt, Y. E., Bjorck, I. E., Asp, N. G. L., and Vessby, B. O. H. (1999). Improved glycemic control and lipid profile and normalized fibrinolytic activity on a low-glycemic index diet in type 2 diabetic patients. *Diabetes Care* **22,** 10–18.

58. Grant, W. B. (1999). Low-fat, high-sugar diet and lipoprotein profiles. *Am. J. Clin. Nutr.* **70,** 1111–1113.

59. Dreon, D. M., Fernstrom, H. A., Williams, P. T., and Krauss, R. M. (1999). A very-low-fat diet is not associated with improved lipoprotein profiles in men with a predominance of large, low-density lipoproteins. *Am. J. Clin. Nutr.* **69,** 411–418.

60. Anderson, J. W., and Hanna, T. J. (1999). Impact of nondigestible carbohydrates on serum lipoproteins and risk for cardiovascular disease. *J. Nutr.* **129,** 1457S–1466S.

61. Davidson, M. H., Maki, K. C., Kong, J. C., Dungan, L. D., Torri, S. A., Hall, H. A., Drennan, K. B., Anderson, S. M., Fulgoni, V. L., Saldanha, L. G., and Olson, B. H. (1998). Long-term effects of consuming foods containing psyllium seed husk on serum lipids in subjects with hypercholesterolemia. *Am. J. Clin. Nutr.* **67,** 367–376.

62. Anderson, J. W., Allgood, L. D., Lawrence, A., Altringer, L. A., Jerdack, G. R., Hengehold, D. A., and Morel, J. G. (2000). Cholesterol-lowering effects of psyllium intake adjunctive to diet therapy in men and women with hypercholesterolemia: Meta-analysis of 8 controlled trials. *Am. J. Clin. Nutr.* **71,** 472–479.

63. Rimm, E. B., Ascherio, A., Giovannucci, E., Spiegelman, D., Stampfer, M. J., and Willett, W. C. (1996). Vegetable, fruit, and cereal fiber intake and risk of coronary heart disease among men. *JAMA* **275,** 447–451.

64. Wolk, A., Manson, J. E., Stampfer, M. J., Coldiz, G. A., Hu, F. B., Speizer, F. E., Hennekens, C. H., and Willett, W. C. (1999). Long-term intake of dietary fiber and decreased risk of coronary heart disease among women. *JAMA* **281,** 1998–2004.

65. Olson, B. H., Anderson, S. M., Becker, M. P., Anderson, J. W., Hunninghake, D. B., Jenkins, D. J. A., LaRosa, J. C., Rippe, J. M., Roberts, D. C. K., Stoy, D. B., Summerbell, C. D., Truswell, A. S., Wolever, T. M. S., Morris, D. H., and Fulgoni, V. L., III. (1997). Psyllium-enriched cereals lower blood total cholesterol and LDL cholesterol, but not HDL cholesterol, in hypercholesterolemic adults: Results of a meta-analysis. *J. Nutr.* **127,** 1973–1980.

66. Ripsin, C. M., Keenan, J. M., Jacobs, D. R., Elmer, P. J., Welch, R. R., van Horn, L., Lin, K., Turnbull, W. H., Thye, F. W., Kestin, M., Hegsted, M., Davidson, D. M., Davidson, M. H., Dugan, D., Demark-Wahnefried, W., and Beling, S. (1992). Oat products and lipid lowering. A meta-analysis. *JAMA* **267,** 3317–3325.

67. Anderson, J. W., Deakins, D. A., Floore, T. L., Smith, B. M., and Whitis, S. E. (1990). Dietary fiber and coronary heart disease. *Crit. Rev. Food Sci. Nutr.* **29,** 95–147.

68. Anderson, J. W., Zeigler, J. A., Deakins, D. A., Floore, T. I., Dillon, D. W., Wood, C. L., Oeltgen, O. P. R., and Whitley, R. J. (1991). Metabolic effects of high-carbohydrate, high-fiber diets for insulin-dependent diabetic individuals. *Am. J. Clin. Nutr.* **54,** 936–943.

69. Fukagawa, N. K., Anderson, J. W., Hageman, G., Young, V. R., and Minaker, K. L. (1990). High-carbohydrate, high-fiber diets increase peripheral insulin sensitivity in healthy young and old adults. *Am. J. Clin. Nutr.* **52,** 524–528.

70. Hallfrisch, J., Scholfield, D. J., and Behall, K. M. (1995). Diets containing soluble oat extracts improve glucose and insulin responses of moderately hypercholesterolemic men and women. *Am. J. Clin. Nutr.* **61,** 379–384.

71. Brown, L., Rosner, B., Willett, W., and Sacks, F. (1999). Cholesterol-lowering effects of dietary fiber: A meta-analysis. *Am. J. Clin. Nutr.* **69,** 30–42.

72. Raben, A., Tagliabue, A., Christensen, N. J., Madsen, J., Holst, J. J., and Astrup, A. (1994). Resistant starch: The effect of postprandial glycemia, hormonal response, and satiety. *Am. J. Clin. Nutr.* **60,** 544–551.

73. Cheng, H. H., and Lai, M. H. (2000). Fermentation of resistant rice starch produces propionate reducing serum and hepatic cholesterol in rats. *J. Nutr.* **130,** 1991–1995.

74. Levrat, M. A., Moundras, C., Younes, H., Morand, C., Demigne, C., and Remesy, C. (1996). Effectiveness of resistant starch, compared to guar gum, in depressing plasma cholesterol and enhancing fecal steroid excretion. *Lipids* **31,** 1069–1075.

75. Jenkins, D. J. A, Vuksan, V., Kendall, C. W. C, Wursch, P., Jeffcoat, R., Waring, S., Mehling, C. C., Vidgen, E., Augustin, L. S. A., and Wong, E. (1998). Physiological effects of resistant starches on fecal bulk, short chain fatty acids, blood lipids and glycemic index. *J. Am. College Nutr.* **17,** 609–616.

76. Heijnen, M. L., van Amelsvoort, J. M., Deurenberg, P., and Beynen, A,C. (1996). Neither raw nor retrograded resistant starch lowers fasting serum cholesterol concentrations in healthy normolipidemic subjects. *Am. J. Clin. Nutr.* **75,** 733–747.

77. Noakes, M., Clifton, P. M., Nestel, P. J., Le Leu, R., and McIntosh, G. (1996). Effect of high-amylose starch and oat bran on metabolic variables and bowel function in subjects with hypertriglyceridemia. *Am. J. Clin. Nutr.* **64,** 944–951.

78. Ross Products Division, Abbott Laboratories (1997). "The Benefits of Fructooligosaccharides." Columbus, OH.

79. Molis, C., Flourie, B., Ouarne, F., Gailing, M. F., Lartigue, S., Guibert, A., Bornet, F., and Galmiche, J. P. (1996). Digestion, excretion and energy value of fructooligosaccharides in healthy humans. *Am. J. Clin. Nutr.* **64,** 324–328.

80. Trautwein, E. A., Rieckhoff, D., and Erbersdobler, H. F. (1998). Dietary insulin lowers plasma cholesterol and triacylglycerol and alters bile acid profile in hamsters. *J. Nutr.* **128,** 1937.

81. Delzenne, N., Kok, N., Fiordaliso, M., *et al.* (1993). Dietary fructooligosaccharides modifies lipid metabolism in rats. *Am. J. Clin. Nutr.* **57,** 820S.

82. Delzenne, N. M., and Kok, N. N. (1999). Biochemical basis of oligofructose-induced hypolipidemia in animal models. *J. Nutr.* **129**(Suppl.), 1467S–1470S.

83. Kok, N., Roberfroid, M., and Delzenne, N. (1996). Involvement of lipogenesis in the lower VLDL secretion induced by oligofructose in rats. *Br. J. Nutr.* **76,** 881–890.

84. Williams, C. M. (1999). Effects of insulin on lipid parameters in humans. *J. Nutr.* **129,** 1471S–1473S.

85. Luo, J., Rizkalla, S. W., Alamowitch, C., Boussairi, A., Blayo, A., Barry, J. L., Laffitte, A., Guyon, F., Bornet, F. R., and Slama, G. (1996). Chronic consumption of short-chain fructooligosaccharides by healthy subjects decreased basal hepatic glucose production but had no effect on insulin stimulated glucose metabolism. *Am. J. Clin. Nutr.* **63,** 939–945.

86. Alles, M. S., de Roos, N. M., Bakx, J. C., Van de Lisdonk, E., Zock, P. L., and Hautvast, G. A., Jr., (1999). Consumption of fructooligosaccharides does not favorably affect blood glucose and serum lipid concentrations in patients with type 2 diabetes. *Am. J. Clin. Nutr.* **69,** 64–69.

87. Canzi, E., Brighenti, F., Casiraghi, M. C., Del Puppo, E., and Ferrari, A. (1995). Prolonged consumption of insulin in ready to eat breakfast cereals: Effects on intestinal ecosystem, bowel habits, and lipid metabolism. *In* "Cost 92: Workshop on Dietary Fiber and Fermentation in the Colon."

88. Jackson, K. G., Taylor, G. R. J., Clohessy, A. M., and Williams, C. M. (1999). The effect of the daily intake of insulin on fasting lipid, insulin and glucose concentrations in middle-aged men and women. *Br. J. Nutr.* **82,** 23–30.

89. Roberfroid, M. (1993). Dietary fiber, insulin, and oligofructose: A review comparing their physiological effects. *Crit. Rev. Food Sci. Nutr.* **33,** 102–148.

90. Hidaka, H., Hirayama, M., Tokunaga, T., and Eida, T. (1990). The effects of undigestible fructooligosaccharides on intestinal microflora and various physiological function on human health. *Adv. Exp. Med. Biol.* **270,** 105–117.

91. Yamashita, K., Kawai, K., and Itakura, M. (1984). Effects of fructooligosaccharides on blood glucose and serum lipids in diabetic subjects. *Nutr. Res.* **4,** 961–966.

92. Carroll, K. K. (1992). Dietary protein, cholesterolemia, and atherosclerosis. *Can. Med. Assoc. J.* **147,** 900.

93. Kritchevsky, D., Kolman, R. R., Guttmacher, R. M., and Forbes, M. (1959). Influence of dietary carbohydrate and protein on serum and liver cholesterol in germ-free chickens. *Arch. Biochem. Biophys.* **85,** 444–451.

94. Luhman, C. M., and Beitz, D. C. (1992). Dietary protein and blood cholesterol homeostasis. *In* "Dietary Proteins: How They Alleviate Disease and Promote Better Health" (G. U. Liepa, Ed.), pp. 57–76. American Oil Chemists' Society, Champaign, IL.

95. Terpstra, A. H., Hermus, R. J., and West, C. E. (1983). The role of dietary protein in cholesterol metabolism. *World Rev. Nutr. Diet* **42,** 1–55.

96. Stamler, J. (1979). Population studies. *In* "Nutrition, Lipids, and Coronary Heart Disease" (Levy, Rifkind, Dennis, and Ernst, Eds.), pp. 25–88. Raven Press, New York.

97. Hu, F. B., Stampfer, M. J., Manson, J. E., Rimm, E., Colditz, G. A., Speizer, F. E., Hennekens, C. H., and Willett, W. C. (1999). Dietary protein and risk of ischemic heart disease in women. *Am. J. Clin. Nutr.* **70,** 221–227.

98. Blankenhorn, D. H., Johnson, R. L., Mack, W. J., El Zein, H. A., and Vailas, L. I. (1990). The influence of diet on the appearance of new lesions in human coronary arteries. *JAMA* **263,** 1646–1652.

99. Wolfe, B. M., and Giovannetti, P. M. (1991). Short-term effects of substituting protein for carbohydrate in the diets

of moderately hypercholesterolemic human subjects. *Metabolism* **40**, 338–343.

100. Wolfe, B. M. (1995). Potential role of raising dietary protein intake for reducing risk of atherosclerosis. *Can. J. Cardiol.* **11**(Suppl. G), 127G–131G.

101. Wolfe, B. M., and Giovannetti, P. M. (1992). High protein diet complements resin therapy of familial hypercholesterolemia. *Clin. Invest. Med.* **15**, 349–359.

102. Wolfe, B. M., and Piche, L. A. (1999). Replacement of carbohydrate by protein in a conventional-fat diet reduces cholesterol and triglyceride concentrations in healthy normolipidemic subjects. *Clin. Invest. Med.* **22**, 140–148.

102a. Davidson, M. H., Hunninghake, D., Maki, K. C., Kwiterovich, P. O., Jr., and Kafonek, S. (1999). Comparison of the effects of lean red meat vs. lean white meat on serum lipid levels among free-living persons with hypercholesterolemia: A long-term, randomized clinical trial. *Arch. Intern. Med.* **159**(120), 1331–1338.

103. Svetkey, L. P., Simons-Morton, D., Vollmer, W. M., Appel, L. J., Conlin, P. R., Ryan, D. H., Ard, J., and Kennedy, B. M. (1999). Effects of dietary patterns on blood pressure: Subgroup analysis of the Dietary Approaches to Stop Hypertension (DASH) randomized clinical trial. *Arch. Intern. Med.* **159**, 285–293.

103a. Harsha, D. W., Lin, P-H., Obarzanek, E., Karanja, N. M., Moore, T. J., and Caballero, B. (1999). Dietary approaches to stop hypertension: A summary of study results. *JADA* **99**(Suppl.), S35–S39.

104. Kalopissis, A. D., Griffaton, G., and Fau, D. (1995). Inhibition of hepatic very-low density lipoprotein secretion in obese Zucker rats adapted to a high-protein diet. *Metabolism* **44**, 19–29.

105. Moundra, C., Demigne, C., Morand, C., Levrat, M.-A., and Ramesy, C. (1996). Lipid metabolism and lipoprotein susceptibility to peroxidation are affected by a protein-deficient diet in the rat. *Nutr. Res.* **17**, 125–135.

106. Carroll, K. K., and Kurowska, E. M. (1995). Soy consumption and cholesterol reduction: Review of animal and human studies. *J. Nutr.* **125**, 594S–597S.

107. Kritchevsky, D. (1993). Dietary protein and experimental atherosclerosis. *Ann. N.Y. Acad. Sci.* **676**, 180–187.

108. Coward, L., Barnes, N. C., Setchell, K. D. R., and Barnes, S. (1993). Genistein, daidzein, and their B-glycoside conjugates: Antitumor isoflavones in soybean foods from American and Asian diets. *J. Agr. Food Chem.* **41**, 1961–1967.

109. Nagata, C., Takatsuka, N., Kurisu, Y., and Shimizu, H. (1998). Decreased serum total cholesterol concentration is associated with high intake of soy products in Japanese men and women. *J. Nutr.* **128**, 209–213.

110. Anderson, J. W., Johnstone, B. M., and Cook-Newell, M. E. (1995). Meta-analysis of the effects of soy protein intake on serum lipids. *N. Engl. J. Med.* **333**, 276–282.

111. Sirtori, C. R., Lovati, M. R., Manzoni, C., Monetti, M., Pazzucconi, F., and Gatti, E. (1995). Soy and cholesterol reduction: Clinical experience. *J. Nutr.* **125**, 598S–605S.

112. Meinertz, H., Nilauen, K., and Faergeman, O. (1989). Soy protein and casein in cholesterol-enriched diets: Effects on plasma lipoproteins in normolipidemic subjects. *Am. J. Clin. Nutr.* **50**, 786–793.

113. Kurowska, E. M., and Carroll, K. K. (1990). Essential amino acids in relation to hypercholesterolemia induced in rabbits by dietary casein. *J. Nutr.* **120**, 831–836.

114. Sanchez, A., and Hubbard, R. W. (1991). Plasma amino acids and the insulin/glucagon ratio as an explanation for the dietary protein modulation of atherosclerosis. *Med. Hypotheses* **36**, 27–32.

115. de Lorgeril, M. (1998). Dietary arginine and the prevention of cardiovascular diseases. *Cardiovasc. Res.* **37**, 560–563.

116. Anthony, M. S. (2000). Soy and cardiovascular disease: Cholesterol lowering and beyond. *J. Nutr.* **130**, 662S–663S.

117. Crouse, J. R., Morgan, T., Terry, J. G., Ellis, J., Vitolins, M., and Burke, G. L. (1999). A randomized trial comparing the effect of casein with that of soy protein containing varying amounts of isoflavones on plasma concentrations of lipids and lipoproteins. *Arch. Intern. Med.* **159**, 2070–2076.

118. Sirtori, C. R., Gianazza, E., Manzoni, C., and Lovati, M. R. (1997). Role of isoflavones in the cholesterol reduction by soy proteins in the clinic. *Am. J. Clin. Nutr.* **65**, 166–167.

119. Nestel, P. J., Yamashita, T., Sasahara, T., Pomeroy, S., Dart, A., Komesaroff, P., Owen, A., and Abbey, M. (1997). Soy isoflavones improve systemic arterial compliance but not plasma lipids in menopausal and perimenopausal women. *Arterioscler. Thromb. Vasc. Biol.* **17**, 3392–3398.

120. Williams, J. K., and Clarkson, T. B. (1998). Dietary soy isoflavones inhibit in-vivo constrictor responses of coronary arteries to collagen-induced platelet activation. *Coron. Artery Dis.* **9**, 759–764.

121. Tikkanen, M. J., Wahala, K., Ojala, S., Vihma, V., and Adlercreutz, H. (1998). Effect of soybean phytoestrogen intake on low density lipoprotein oxidation resistance. *Proc. Natl. Acad. Sci. USA* **95**, 3106–3110.

122. Fujio, Y., Fumiko, Y., Takahashi, K., and Shibata, N. (1993). Responses of smooth muscle cells to platelet-derived growth factor are inhibited by herbimycin-A tyrosine kinase inhibitor. *Biochem. Biophys. Res. Commun.* **195**, 79–83.

123. Lieberman, E. H., Gerhard, M. D., Uehata, A., Walsh, B. W., Selwyn, A. P., Ganz, P., Yeung, A. C., and Creager, M. A. (1994). Estrogen improves endothelium-dependent, flow-mediated vasodilation in postmenopausal women. *Arch. Intern. Med.* **121**, 936–941.

124. American Heart Association Nutrition Committee (1999). AHA science advisory: Monounsaturated fatty acids and risk of cardiovascular disease. *Circulation* **100**(11), 1253–1258.

CHAPTER **19**

Other Dietary Components and Cardiovascular Risk

LINDA VAN HORN, SUJATA ARCHER, KIMBERLY THEDFORD, AND AMY BALTES

Northwestern University Medical School, Chicago, Illinois

I. INTRODUCTION

Conclusive data have long established a strong positive association between saturated fat, dietary cholesterol, and elevated levels of total and low-density lipoprotein (LDL) cholesterol [1, 2]. Most national dietary guidelines aimed at reducing cardiovascular risk are based on reductions in saturated fat, dietary cholesterol, and weight loss for those patients who are overweight [3]. The Step 1 and 2 diets recommended by the National Cholesterol Education Program (NCEP) and the American Heart Association (AHA) are based on reduced intakes of total fat, saturated fat, and cholesterol to achieve reductions in population mean blood cholesterol level [1, 4]. These campaigns have been instrumental in achieving the Healthy People 2000 goal mean blood cholesterol level of 200 mg/dL and contributing to the overall reduction in cardiovascular mortality that has occurred in this country during the past three decades [5, 6].

Recent studies have reaffirmed the primary focus on reduced saturated fat and dietary cholesterol intake, but there is also mounting evidence that other dietary factors beyond fat may play a significant supporting role in prevention of heart disease. These include dietary fiber, especially soluble fiber, whole grains, soy, vitamins B_6, B_{12}, and folate, plant stanols and sterols, and a host of phytochemicals. The purpose of this chapter is to summarize current knowledge regarding these dietary factors and their impact on blood lipids and cardiovascular risk. Most of these factors have not merited national dietary guideline status, but as dietary adjuncts they warrant further consideration. The evidence implicating cause and effect surrounding these other factors pales by comparison to that of fatty acid research. This chapter summarizes the quality and quantity of current evidence to place the factors in proper scientific context before considering their potential clinical applications.

II. DIETARY FIBER AND CARDIOVASCULAR RISK

A growing number of prospective studies report a protective benefit of dietary fiber on risk of cardiovascular disease [7–14]. In 1997, the American Dietetic Association published a position statement that "the public should consume adequate amounts of dietary fiber from a variety of plant foods" [15]. General recommendations for intake range between 20–35 g/day or 10–13 g of dietary fiber per 1000 calories [16]. Current population mean intake of dietary fiber is no more than half of the recommended amount [16, 17]. Because nationwide increases in dietary fiber have not accompanied reductions in total and saturated fat intake, other processed fat-modified but non-fiber-rich foods appear to have been substituted instead [16, 18].

The benefits of consuming dietary fiber from carbohydrate foods, including whole grains, cereals, legumes, fruits, and vegetables are many. There is increasing evidence that a dietary pattern rich in these foods not only reduces risk of high blood cholesterol, but also stroke, hypertension, and cancer [14, 19–21]. The AHA, NCEP, and other national health-related organizations emphasize the importance and nutritional benefits of these foods beyond their fiber contributions (1–4). Conversely, diets high in refined carbohydrates and sugars have been linked with adverse effects on high-density lipoprotein (HDL) cholesterol, triglycerides and insulin resistance [18, 22, 23].

A. Definition and Sources of Fiber

Dietary fiber is defined as the storage and cell wall polysaccharide of plants that cannot be hydrolyzed by human digestive enzymes [24, 25]. Dietary fiber includes cellulose, hemicelluloses, pectin, and lignin. Difficulties in perfecting the chemical analysis of fiber had confounded assessment of specific amounts of dietary fiber in previous studies [16]. More reliable methodology for estimating total dietary fiber as well as quantifying soluble fiber content now facilitates research testing specific types of fiber and relationships with lipid metabolism, glucose metabolism, and other biological outcomes [24, 25]. Current nutrient databases document amounts of total dietary fiber as well as soluble and insoluble components making it possible to evaluate biological impacts from different food sources. Table 1 provides data on common sources of dietary fiber [26].

TABLE 1 Sources of Dietary Fiber

Food	Serving size	Soluble g/sv[a]	Insoluble g/sv	Total g/sv
Fruits				
Plums, fresh	1 med	0.3	0.5	0.8
Apricot, dried	4 halves	0.3	0.7	1.0
Apricot, fresh	2 halves	0.4	0.9	1.3
Nectarine, fresh	1 med	0.6	1.0	1.6
Banana	1 med	0.5	1.3	1.8
Prunes, dried	5	1.1	2.0	3.1
Avocado, fresh	1 med	1.2	2.6	3.8
Pear, fresh	1 med	0.7	3.9	4.6
Figs, dried	3	0.5	4.4	4.9
Vegetables/Legumes				
Green beans, fresh cooked	½ cup	0.3	1.3	1.6
Sweet potato, peeled baked	½ cup	0.5	1.4	1.9
Spinach, cooked	½ cup	0.3	2.0	2.3
Brussels sprouts	½ cup	0.4	2.8	3.2
Lima beans	½ cup	0.5	2.9	3.4
Potato, white unpeeled baked	1 med	1.0	3.1	4.1
Kidney beans	½ cup	1.0	3.5	4.5
Baked beans, canned	½ cup	1.7	3.8	5.5
Grains				
Cookie, oatmeal raisin	2 med	0.3	0.6	1.0
Cookie, fig	2 med	0.4	1.0	1.4
Cereal, cream of wheat	¾ cup	0.3	1.1	1.4
Cereal, grapenuts	¼ cup	0.4	1.6	2.0
Cereal, oatmeal	¾ cup	1.2	1.5	2.7
Cereal, Wheat Chex	⅔ cup	0.5	2.3	2.8
Cereal, oat bran (uncooked)	⅓ cup	2.0	3.3	5.3
Cereal, 40% bran flakes	¾ cup	0.6	4.9	5.5

Source: Adapted from Marlett, J. A., and Cheung, T.-F. (1997). Database and quick methods of assessing typical dietary fiber intakes using data for 228 commonly consumed foods. *J. Am. Diet. Assoc.* **97,** 1139–1148.

[a]g/sv = grams per serving.

B. Mechanisms Related to Fiber and Serum Cholesterol Reduction

The exact mechanisms involved in lipid lowering and/or overall risk reduction remain inconclusive. Viscous polysaccharides act in the gastrointestinal tract to reduce blood cholesterol levels by decreasing absorption of cholesterol or fatty acids as well as by decreasing absorption of biliary cholesterol or bioacids [16, 24]. Fiber may also alter serum concentration of hormones and short-chain fatty acids that influence lipid metabolism [25, 27, 28]. β-glucan, the water-soluble fiber prevalent in oats and barley, has been identified in animal models as the active agent influencing cholesterol metabolism reduces LDL cholesterol concentration in human studies [25, 27]. In addition to lipid-lowering benefits, studies on oats and barley have further suggested that α-tocotrienols and other antioxidant components may inhibit HMG-CoA, thereby contributing a weak statin-like influence [25]. The amino acid content of oats or the arginine-to-lysine ratio may also favor the hypocholesterolemic response. Based on more than 40 clinical trials, animal experimental data and meta-analyses, the Food and Drug Administration (FDA), for the first time, adopted a health claim regarding intake of oats as part of a fat-modified diet for reducing risk of coronary heart disease [29]. All prior health claims had been based on specific nutrients or dietary factors, but the oats health claim carried precedent-setting significance for future research on whole foods or food patterns.

C. Psyllium and Lipids

Soon after the oats health claim was established, the FDA approved another health claim for psyllium and cardiovascular disease based on a similar premise [30]. Psyllium, a form of soluble fiber found in a type of grass, can be used as a food supplement. Inherently, psyllium offers no other nutritional benefits compared to foods like oats, barley, beans, or fruits, but studies report LDL cholesterol reductions of 5–15% with 7 or more grams per day [27, 31]. As noted in most other fiber intervention studies, the higher the baseline blood cholesterol level, the greater the LDL cholesterol reduction with psyllium [31, 32]. A meta-analysis of eight studies including psyllium as part of a low-saturated-fat diet reported that consumption of 10.2 g of psyllium per day lowered serum total cholesterol by 4% ($p < 0.0001$) with no effect on serum HDL or triacylglycerol concentrations [32].

D. Summary

Intake of dietary fiber, especially soluble fiber, decreases LDL cholesterol with little or no effect on HDL cholesterol [24, 27, 33–35]. Based on recent epidemiologic evidence, dietary fiber intake is also inversely related to body mass index (BMI) and insulin levels [36]. While impact of soluble fiber on LDL cholesterol lowering is modest, approximately 5% beyond what can be achieved on a fat-modified diet [25], there are other possible health benefits such as increased insulin sensitivity, decreased triglycerides, and improved weight control, that support the dietary recommendations for increased intake of fiber-rich foods [37].

III. HOMOCYSTEINE AND CARDIOVASCULAR DISEASE

Homocysteine is an intermediary amino acid in the pathway of methionine metabolism. Intracellular homocysteine is metabolized by either transsulfuration or remethylation to methionine [38]. Approximately 50% of homocysteine enters the transsulfuration pathway. Condensation of homocysteine with serine is catalyzed by cystathionine-β-synthase, which requires pyridoxal 5'-phosphate, the biologically active form of vitamin B_6 [39, 40]. In the remethylation pathway, methylcobalamin and methyltetrahydrofolate serve as cofactors and cosubstrates for the enzyme 5-methyltetrahydrofolate-homocysteine methyltransferase (methionine synthase) [39]. The second remethylation pathway requires the enzyme betaine-homocysteine methyltransferase [41]. Disruption in the transsulfuration or remethylation pathways results in accumulation of circulating homocysteine, a phenomenon linked with a higher risk for cardiovascular disease [42–44].

Elevated serum homocysteine concentrations are considered an independent risk factor for coronary artery disease (CAD) [39, 42]. The role of homocysteine in vascular disease is postulated to be caused via collagen destabilization, platelet accumulation, or a lowering of serum antithrombin activity [42]. Boushey et al. [45] reported that for women, the odds ratio (OR) for CAD, with a 5 μmol/L increase in total homocysteine was 1.8 (95% CI, 1.3–1.9). The Physicians' Health Study reported that the risk of myocardial infarction even among those who had no history of vascular disease was 3.4-fold greater within 5 years among those with elevated plasma homocysteine concentrations compared to those with lower plasma homocysteine concentrations [46].

Hyperhomocysteinemia is designated as moderate, intermediate and severe corresponding to concentrations of homocysteine between 16–30, 31–100, and greater than 100 nmol/mL, respectively [42]. The normal concentration of homocysteine in plasma is about 10 nmol/mL [42]. Some studies report that elevated plasma homocysteine levels do not pose a risk until levels reach the upper 95th percentile in control subjects [46], whereas others report an increased risk even at lower concentrations [45].

Genetic studies have also identified abnormal thermolabile variants in enzymes such as methlyenetetrahydrofolate reductase, which leads to hyperhomocysteinemia [47]. Only recently has the relationship between circulating vitamins B_{12}, B_6 and folate and plasma homocysteine been addressed.

A. Vitamins and Homocysteine

High levels of plasma homocysteine (>100 nmol/L) can occur due to nutritional deficiencies of vitamins B_{12}, B_6 and folate [42]. Several studies have shown that vitamin B_{12} or folate deficiencies produce elevations in fasting plasma homocysteine levels up to 20 times the upper limits of the normal level (48–50). The influence of vitamin B_6 deficiency with plasma homocysteine is unclear. Some studies have shown tissue depletion of vitamin B_6 with no increase in plasma homocysteine concentrations, whereas others have shown that plasma homocysteine concentrations may be elevated in those who have a vitamin B_6 deficiency (51–53).

In normal metabolism, greater than 50% of homocysteine is recycled into methionine by a transmethylation reaction requiring folate and vitamin B_{12}, whereas vitamin B_6 is a cofactor for the enzyme cystathionine b-synthase in the transsulfuration pathway. Deficiency of this enzyme results in homocystinuria. Several studies have shown an inverse association between blood homocysteine levels with plasma or serum levels of folate, B_6, and B_{12} [54–56].

Selhub et al. [56] reported from the Framingham Study that mean homocysteine levels were significantly higher in the lowest two deciles for folate (15.6 and 13.7 μm/L, respectively) compared with the highest deciles (11.0 μm/L) [57]. It is estimated that there can be a 25% reduction in homocysteine levels with supplementation of 0.5–5.7 mg/day of folate [58]. The Institute of Medicine recommends no more than 1 mg/day of folate supplementation due to the

risk of higher amounts masking signs of a vitamin B_{12} deficiency [58].

In patients with a vitamin B_{12} deficiency who may have intermediate or severe hyperhomocysteinemia, B_{12} can normalize homocysteine levels in 70% of the cases [49]. Vitamin B_{12} intakes of 0.02–0.5 mg/day along with 0.5–5.7 mg/day of folate can lower homocysteine levels up to 7% [58]. Rasmussen *et al.* [59] administered 2 mg of B_{12} along with 10 mg of folate to 126 women and 109 healthy men and reported a decrease of 4.8% in circulating homocysteine levels due to the B_{12} intake. Bronstrup *et al.* [60] provided a supplement with 400 mcg of folate with 6 µg of vitamin B_{12} vs. 400 µg of folate and 400 µg B_{12} and reported a greater reduction in homocysteine levels with the higher B_{12} concentrations vs. the lower dose (−18% vs −11%). Ubbink *et al.* reported a 56.8% prevalence of hyperhomocysteinemia among South African men with suboptimal B_{12} levels [61]. If a patient has a B_{12} deficiency, folate supplementation may be ineffective in reducing homocysteine levels [62].

Supplementation with vitamin B_6 has been shown to enhance the activity of the transsulfuration pathway, which leads to a decrease in elevated circulating homocysteine levels [63]. It is reported that in populations with intakes of less than 1.92 mg/day of B_6 there was a prevalence of high total homocysteine [64]. Some studies report a reduction in homocysteine levels with a supplement of 50 mg B_6 combined with folate and vitamin B_{12}. However not all studies have shown a decrease in plasma homocysteine levels even with high-dose (70–300 mg) supplementation of vitamin B_6 [62]. Vitamin B_6 deficiency is primarily associated with hyperhomocysteinemia after methionine loading. Levels of vitamin B_6 used to treat moderately elevated plasma homocysteine levels range from 25 to 50 mg/day. A concern of vitamin B_6 supplementation relates to sensory neuropathy, which is usually seen in patients treated with dosages greater than 400 mg/day [65].

Long-term supplementation with vitamins to reduce homocysteine levels has not been studied extensively. Ubbink *et al.* [65] studied 22 men who had plasma homocysteine concentrations of >16.3 µmol/L and were given a multivitamin supplementation with 1.0 mg folate, 50 µg B_{12} and 10 mg B_6 for 6 weeks. A decline in circulating homocysteine concentrations was observed from 30.9 to 14.0 µmol/L. Vitamin supplementation was discontinued for 18 weeks and an increase in homocysteine was observed. Treating the patients again with the vitamin formulation for 6 weeks resulted in a decline of homocysteine. Discontinuation of the vitamin therapy and dietary intake aimed at getting foods high in these vitamins resulted in elevated plasma homocysteine concentrations after 18 weeks. The authors concluded that some individuals with hyperhomocysteinemia may be unable to lower plasma homocysteine levels with diet alone [65].

Some other vitamins have been reported to influence plasma homocysteine levels. An intake of 0.6 mg of riboflavin has resulted in a modest decline in plasma homocysteine levels (0.475 mmol/L). Riboflavin functions as a cofactor for methylenetetrahydrofolate reductase [66]. High doses of niacin (3 g/day) have caused an elevation in plasma homocysteine levels [67].

It is unclear if homocysteine should be reduced by diet and/or vitamin therapy [68, 69]. The AHA recommends that intakes of folate, B_{12}, and B_6 be met by intake of vegetables, fruits, legumes, meat, fish, and fortified grains and cereals [68]. The Food and Nutrition Board of the National Academy of Sciences and Institute of Medicine recommends the following RDAs for nonpregnant and nonlactating adults: folate 400 µg, 2.4 µg B_{12}, and 1.7 mg B_6 [58]. Because most of the population does not meet these recommendations, an increase of foods rich in these vitamins is advised. For those who may have malabsorption of some of these vitamins, such as the elderly, foods fortified with these vitamins or a supplement with these vitamins is recommended [59]. An increase in intake of vitamin fortified foods and/or a daily supplement with 0.4 mg folate, 2 mg B_6 and 6 µg B_{12} is recommended when there is a family history of cardiovascular disease, malabsorption, use of certain pharmaceutical agents such as niacin, bile acid-binding resins or L-dopa [70].

B. Summary

In summary, the B vitamins folate, B_{12}, and B_6 play an important role in methionine metabolism and in determining circulating homocysteine levels. However, many questions remain regarding the association of folate, B_{12}, and B_6 with homocysteine levels. Folate supplementation with or without B_{12} and B_6 has been reported to reduce homocysteine levels in hyperhomocysteinemia and in those with normal homocysteine levels. However, data from randomized clinical trials regarding the benefits of folate on cardiovascular disease are lacking [70]. Until such data are available it is recommended that reduction of risks of CAD be achieved via proven methods such as consuming a diet based on the Dietary Guidelines for Americans.

IV. SOY AND CARDIOVASCULAR DISEASE

It has long been recognized that vegetable protein has beneficial health effects compared to animal protein, especially related to serum cholesterol status [1, 2, 71]. Countries with high soy intake have reduced rates of cardiovascular mortality compared with countries consuming primarily animal protein products [3]. During the past 35 years, much research has focused on the relationship between soy intake and reduced risk for cardiovascular and other chronic disease. In a meta-analysis of 38 clinical studies, Anderson *et al.* [72] reported that substitution of soy protein for animal protein was associated with significant decreases in total cholesterol, LDL cholesterol and triglyceride concentration. HDL cholesterol was unchanged in most studies. These data contrib-

uted to the 1999 approval by the FDA of a health claim for reduced cardiovacular risk related to intake of at least 25 g of soy per day [73]. No isoflavone concentration was included in the health claim. Clinical trial data further document that the reductions in LDL cholesterol are greatest among those with the highest baseline levels. This section will briefly review some of these data and the possible mechanisms involved.

A. Is It the Isoflavones?

Soybeans are rich in the isoflavones genistein, daidzein, and to a lesser degree glycitein [74]. These occur primarily as glycoside forms genestin, daidzin, and glycitin [71]. Bacteria in the gut are required to produce the enzymes needed to hydrolyze these glycosides and convert them to the aglycone forms [75]. The isoflavones possess estrogenic activity and binding to estrogen receptors. Levels of these isoflavones vary by the type of product and the degree of processing [76]. Data in animal and human studies report that isoflavones have an independent effect on blood cholesterol [76–80], but dose may dictate response. Cassidy *et al.* [76] reported that 45 mg of isoflavonoids, but not 23 mg of isoflavonoids, resulted in a significant reduction in total and LDL cholesterol concentrations in young females. In an animal study, comparison of soy protein with or without isoflavones lower total cholesterol and LDL cholesterol and higher HDL cholesterol were reported with isoflavones. The prevalence of atherosclerotic lesions was also lower in monkeys fed the soy plus isoflavones [81]. Human data confirming these associations are needed, and national guidelines regarding favorable isoflavone levels have yet to be developed.

B. Possible Mechanisms: Soy Impact on Lipid Lipoproteins

Soy may reduce total cholesterol and LDL cholesterol through various mechanisms. The most commonly accepted hypothesis is that soy may cause possible interruption in hepatobiliary circulation, thereby increasing LDL receptor activity [71]. Another possibility involves hormonal changes in thyroid and insulin-to-glucagan ratio but these remain speculative. Table 2 summarizes possible mechanisms.

C. Increased Apolipoprotein E Receptor Activity

Soy's impact on increased LDL receptor expression in humans [82] may be related to lipid-lowering benefits through an up-regulation of LDL receptors [82–84]. Genetic influences on response may also play a role. Subjects with the apoE2 genotype have less hypercholesterolemia, but the E_2 protein is an inefficient regulator of LDL receptor activity. When the plasma cholesterol responses in individuals with apoE$_2$ versus apoE$_3$ and E$_4$ were compared, the apo E$_2$ carri-

TABLE 2 Soy Protein and Decreased Cardiovascular Risk: Possible Mechanisms

1. ↓ Plasma cholesterol levels, possibly due to:
   a. ↑ bile excretion
   b. ↑ LDL receptor activity
   c. ↑ thyroxine and thyroid-stimulating hormone
   d. ↓ cholesterol absorption
   e. ↑ soy globulins
2. ↓ Susceptibility to LDL oxidation
3. ↑ Arterial compliance
4. Estrogenic activity of soy isoflavones may improve blood lipids

Source: Adapted from Lichtenstein, A. (1998). Soy protein, isoflavones, and cardiovascular disease risk. *J. Nutr.* **128**, 1589–1592.

ers responded weakly to the diet, but not so the E$_3$ and E$_4$ patients. Patients with higher LDL receptor activity seem less likely to show a favorable response to this dietary change as compared to patients whose LDL receptor activity may be relatively suppressed [83].

D. Oxidative Status

As summarized by Lichtenstein [84], the oxidation of LDL increases atherogenicity. Isoflavones appear to inhibit the oxidative modification of LDL by macrophages [85], enhance the resistance of LDL to oxidation [86, 87], and exhibit antioxidant activities in an aqueous phase [88, 89]. Isoflavonoids also appear to scavenge free radicals [90].

V. PHYTOCHEMICALS: PROPOSED ASSOCIATION WITH CARDIOVASCULAR DISEASE

Phytochemicals are biologically active plant compounds found in fruits, vegetables, and whole grains [91]. Interest in phytochemicals has increased due to various epidemiological and clinical studies that report on the benefits of consumption of these compounds for lowering risks for cardiovascular disease and cancer [92–94]. A summary of some of the most frequently reported substances is presented in Table 3. Three classes of phytochemicals—flavonoids, plant sterols, and plant sulfur compounds—have been studied most extensively and will be discussed briefly as they may relate to cardiovascular disease.

A. Flavonoids

Flavonoids are polyphenolic compounds found in fruits, vegetables, nuts, grains, tea, and wine [24, 95]. Flavonols and flavones are subclasses of flavonoids. The presence of polyphenols in plant foods is influenced by genetic factors, environmental conditions, germinations, degree or ripeness, processing, and storage [96]. The average daily intake of

TABLE 3 Phytochemicals with Possible Health Benefits

Active substance	What it may help do	Where it is found
Allylic sulfides	Inhibit cholesterol synthesis	Aged garlic extract, onions, leeks, chives
Alpha-linolenic acid	Reduce inflammation and stimulate the immune system	Flaxseed, soy products, purslane, walnuts
Anthocyanidins	Antioxidant, supports cardiovascular function, may have significant application in the field of ophthalmology	Bilberry, blueberries, grapes
Capsaicin	May support healthy cardiovascular function and digestive function	Cayenne pepper
Carotenoids	Antioxidant properties that may help reduce the accumulation of arterial plaque	Parsley, carrots, winter squash, sweet potatoes, yams, cantaloupe, apricots, spinach, kale, turnip greens, citrus fruit
Catechins	May help the immune system and lower cholesterol	Green tea, berries
Coumarins	Prevents blood clotting	Parsley, carrots, citrus fruit
Curcumins	Antioxidant, modulates prostaglandin	Turmeric, curcumin
Flavonoids	Block receptor sites for certain hormones involved in cancer promotion, antioxidant, supports liver detoxification	Parsley, carrots, citrus fruits, broccoli, cabbage, cucumbers, green tea, squash, yams, tomatoes, eggplant, peppers, soy products, berries, milk thistle, onion, garlic
Gamma-glutamyl allyic cysteines	May have a role in lowering blood pressure and increasing immune system activities	Aged garlic extract
Ginsenoside	Adaptogen, may help to improve the body's ability to adapt to physical or mental stress	Siberian and panax ginseng
Indoles	Induce protective enzymes that deactivate estrogen	Cabbage, brussels sprouts, kale, cauliflower, broccoli
Isoflavones	May inhibit cholesterol production	Soybeans, tofu, soy milk
Isothiocyanates	Powerful inducers of protective enzymes	Mustard, horseradish, radishes, cruciferous vegetables
Lignans	May lower LDL cholesterol, inhibit smooth-muscle proliferation, plaque formation, and activity of thrombin	Soy, whole grains, oats, oat bran, barley, legumes, prunes, apples, carrots, grapefruit, psyllium seed
Limonoids	Powerful inducer of protective enzymes	Citrus fruits
Lycopene	Antioxidant	Tomatoes, red grapefruit, red peppers
Monoterpenes	May inhibit cholesterol production and aid protective enzyme activity	Parsley, carrots, broccoli, cabbage, cucumbers, squash, yams, tomatoes, eggplant, peppers, mint, basil, citrus fruits
Phenolic acids	May inhibit nitrosamine formation	Parsley, carrots, broccoli, cabbage, cucumbers, tomatoes, eggplant, peppers, citrus fruits, whole grains, berries, nuts
Phenylalkylketones	Antioxidant, supports healthy digestive function, modulates prostagladin metabolism	Ginger
Phthalides	Stimulates the production of beneficial enzymes that detoxify carcinogens	Parsley, carrots, celery
Plant sterols	Block estrogen promotion of breast cancer activity; help the absorption of cholesterol	Broccoli, cabbage, cucumbers, squash, yams, tomatoes, eggplant, peppers, soy products, whole grains
Polyacetylenes	Protect against certain carcinogens found in tobacco smoke and help regulate prostagladin production	Parsley, carrots, celery
Proanthocyanidins	Antioxidant, supports healthy capillary integrity, modulates prostaglandin metabolism	Grapes, green tea, wine
Polysaccharides	Supports immune function	Aloe, astragalus
Schisandrins	Adaptogen, may help to improve the body's ability to adapt to physical and mental stressors, supports live function, supports healthy vision	Schisandra
Triterpenoids	May prevent dental decay and act as an antiulcer agent	Citrus fruits, licorice-root extract, soy products

Source: Adapted from Bravo, L. (1998). Polyphenols: Chemistry, dietary sources, metabolism and nutritional significance. *Nutr. Rev.* **56,** 317–333.

dietary flavonoids in the United States is approximately 1.0 g/day, depending on the season [97]. Epidemiological studies have indicated a reduced risk for ischemic heart disease and stroke with the intake of some of the flavonoids [98–100]. However, not all epidemiological and experimental studies have reported an inverse association between flavonoid intake and cardiovascular disease [95, 101]. Different flavonoids exert their influence on reducing CAD risk by varying mechanisms. Soy proteins, rich in isoflavones, have a hypocholesterolemic effect [72]. Quercetin, a flavonol found in broccoli, red grapes, and cereals, is reported to inhibit LDL oxidation [102]. Red wine and grape juice have phenolic flavonoids that act as antioxidants, thereby preventing LDL oxidation [103]. It is also reported that flavones are potent inhibitors of cyclooxygenase activity, thereby inhibiting platelet aggregation [104].

While these potential associations between flavonoids and health are compelling, randomized controlled clinical trials are needed before dietary recommendations and guidelines can be established. The AHA's Scientific Advisory Board recommends that additional research is needed on the classification of flavonoids, their efficacy, and any adverse effects they may have [105]. More specifically, experimental data demonstrating a direct association between flavonoids and platelet aggregation, serum lipoproteins, and blood pressure are needed before cause and effect can be established.

B. Plant Sterols

Plant sterols are another class of phytochemicals that differ from dietary cholesterol due to their side chains. Plant sterols or phytosterols, including sitosterol, stigmasterol, and campesterol, are reported to have serum cholesterol-lowering effects [105]. All vegetable foods have some plant sterol content [106]. The Western diet includes approximately 200–400 mg/day of plant sterols [107].

During the 1950s and 1960s soy sterols were studied extensively and were reported to reduce cholesterol by 10% [108, 109]. The decrease in plasma cholesterol was thought to be via an increase in LDL receptor activity. Animal experimental studies done *in vitro* reported that in isolated rat livers perfused with very low density lipoprotein (VLDL), LDL, and HDL particles obtained from patients with hereditary phytoesterolemia rich in plant sterols showed that only HDL particles provided a vehicle for unesterified cholesterol elimination in bile [110]. Studies with margarines enriched with plant stanol esters reported that an intake of 2–3 g/day reduced total cholesterol by 10% and LDL cholesterol by 15% due to increased cholesterol elimination [111]. Studies on the effects of margarines enriched with different vegetable oil sterols, i.e., margarines with sterol esters from soybean oil (sitosterol, campesterol, and stigmasterol), report them to be as effective as margarines with sitostanol esters

in lowering blood total and LDL cholesterol without influencing HDL cholesterol levels [112].

Plant sterols in products other than margarines may show further benefits. Mice fed a diet supplemented with 2% phytoesterols for 20 weeks increased HDL cholesterol and decreased hepatic lipase activity and plasma fibrinogen concentrations, but clinical studies are needed [113]. Because most studies reporting the benefits of plant sterols on cardiovascular disease have been conducted on hypercholesterolemic patients, data on efficacy and safety long term in normocholesterolemic or mildly hypercholesterolemic people are needed [114]. Also, whether significant decreases in total cholesterol or LDL cholesterol will occur if low doses of these compounds are consumed by individuals is not fully known with no CAD [115].

C. Sulfur-Containing Plant Foods

Sulfur-containing plant foods come from the allium family of vegetables, which includes garlic, onions, and leeks. Garlic and onion have many sulfur-containing active components mainly in the form of cysteine derivatives. These decompose into thiosulfinates and polysulfides by action of allinase on extraction, producing volatile products on decomposition [116]. Onion and garlic have been reported to decrease cholesterol levels, lower risk of thrombosis, and suppress platelet aggregation [117–119].

Garlic is the most widely studied sulfur-containing food. Garlic's putative cardioprotective effects include antithrombotic activity and blood pressure and lipid lowering [120]. It is reported that one-half to one clove of garlic a day reduces hypercholesterolemia by approximately 0.59 mmol/L (23 mg/dL) [116]. However, not all studies report hypocholesterolemic effects of garlic [121, 122]. Some of the concerns about the reported benefits of garlic usage are related to the pharmaceutical dosages required to see results, such as 4–5 g of fresh garlic cloves per day; side effects such as abdominal pain or anemia; differences in garlic manufacturing processes, such as dry powders, oils, freeze-dried preparations and aged extracts; and study designs [120, 121]. Further well-designed clinical studies are required to demonstrate the effect of the sulfur-containing compounds on cardiovascular disease risk factors [94].

D. Summary

Phytochemicals found in fruits and vegetables may play an important cardioprotective role, but well-designed randomized controlled studies are needed to characterize these products and their mode of action. Until such results are available, it is recommended that traditional risk lowering factors such as decreased fat intake, weight loss, and increased physical activity should be addressed. Table 4 summarizes the potential impact of a cumulative beneficial approach.

TABLE 4 Portfolio of Dietary Factors for Cholesterol Reduction

Dietary component	Dietary change	Approximate LDL reduction (%)
Soluble fiber	5–10 g/day	5
Soy protein	25 g/day	5
Plant sterols[a]	1–3 g/day	5
Dietary cholesterol	<200 mg/day	5
Saturated fat[b]	<7% of calories	10
Body weight	Lose 10 lb	5
Total	Full portfolio[c]	35

Source: Adapted from Jenkins, D. J., Kendall, C. W., Axelsen, M., Augustin, L. S., and Vuksan, V. (2000). Viscous and nonviscous fibres, nonabsorbable and low glycaemic index carbohydrates, blood lipid and coronary heart disease. *Curr. Opin. Cardiol.* **11,** 49–56.

[a]Depending on the sterol and stanol.
[b]Reduce *trans* fatty acids as close to zero as possible.
[c]Assuming the effects are additive.

VI. CONCLUSION

There is no question that saturated fat, dietary cholesterol, and obesity are major diet-related risk factors for cardiovascular disease. Building from this base, a host of other nonlipid, dietary factors may also provide important benefits. Dietary fiber, soy, antioxidant vitamins, decreased plasma homocystine levels, phytochemicals, and flavonoids appear to offer advantages that enhance and complement the lipid-modified aspect of the anthiatherogenic diet. Fruits, vegetables, and whole grains are major contributors of these dietary factors and can safely be recommended for other health promoting attributes as well. Future studies will help quantify and validate these associations and also provide evidence of possible long-term benefits.

References

1. The Expert Panel (1993). Summary of the second report of the National Cholesterol Education Program (NCEP) Expert Panel on detection, evaluation and treatment of high blood cholesterol in adults (Adult Treatment Panel II). *JAMA* **269,** 3015–3023.
2. Ginsberg, H. N., Kris-Etherton, P. M., Dennis, B., Elmer, P. J., Ershow, A., Lefevre, M., Pearson, T., Roheim, P., Ramakrishnan, R., Reed, R., Stewart, K., Stewart, P., Phillips, K., and Anderson, N. (1998). Effects of reducing dietary saturated fatty acids on plasma lipids and lipoproteins in healthy subjects. *Arterioscler. Thromb. Vasc. Biol.* **18,** 441–449.
3. National Heart, Lung and Blood Institute (1998). "Clinical Guidelines on the Identification, Evaluation and Treatment of Overweight and Obesity in Adults: The Evidence Report." NIH publication 98–4083. National Institutes for Health, Bethesda, MD.
4. American Heart Association (1996). Dietary guidelines for healthy American adults: A statement for health professionals by the Nutrition Committee. *Circulation* **94,** 1795–1800.
5. U.S. Department of Health and Human Services (2000). "Healthy People 2010: Understanding and Improving Health," conference ed. Government Printing Office, Washington, DC.
6. Life Sciences Research Office, Federation of American Societies for Experimental Biology. U.S. Department of Agriculture (1995). "Third Report on Nutrition Monitoring in the United States," Vol. 2. Prepared for Interagency Board for Nutrition Monitoring and Related Research, U.S. Department of Health and Human Services. Government Printing Office, Washington, DC.
7. Pietinen, P., Rimm, E. B., Korhonen, P., Hartman, A. M., Willett, W. C., Albanes, D., and Virtamo, J. (1996). Intake of dietary fiber and risk of coronary heart disease in a cohort of Finnish men; the alpha-tocopherol, beta-carotene cancer prevention study. *Circulation* **94,** 2720–2727.
8. Morris, J., Marr, J., and Clayton, D. (1977). Diet and heart: A postscript. *Br. Med. J.* **2,** 1307–1314.
9. Kromhout, D., Bosschieter, E., Lezenne, D. C., and Coulander, C. (1982). Dietary fiber and 10-year mortality from coronary heart disease, cancer and all causes: The Zutphen Study. *Lancet* **2,** 518–521.
10. Kushi, L., Lew, R., Stare, F., Ellison, C. R., el Lozy, M., Bourke, G., Daly, L., Graham, I., Hickey, N., Mulcahy, R., and Kevaney, J. (1985). Diet and 20-year mortality from coronary heart disease: The Ireland-Boston Diet Heart Study. *N. Eng. J. Med.* **312,** 811–818.
11. Khaw, K., and Barrett-Connor, E. (1987). Dietary fiber and reduced ischemic heart disease mortality rates in men and women: A 12-year prospective study. *Am. J. Epidemiol.* **126,** 1093–1102.
12. Fehily, A., Yarnell, J., Sweetnam, P., and Elwood, P. (1993). Diet and incident ischemic heart disease: The Carephilly Study. *Br. J. Nutr.* **69,** 303–314.
13. Humble, C., Malarcher, A., and Tyroler, H. (1993). Dietary fiber and coronary heart disease in middle-aged hypercholesterolemic men. *Am. J. Prevent. Med.* **9,** 197–202.
14. Rimm, E. B., Ascherio, A., Giovannucci, E., Spiegellman, D., Stampfer, M. J., and Willett, W. C. (1996). Vegetable, fruit and cereal fiber intake and risk of coronary heart disease among men. *JAMA* **275,** 447–451.
15. Subar, A., Krebs-Smith, S. M., Cook, A., and Kahle, L. L. (1998). Dietary sources of nutrients among U.S. adults, 1989–1991. *J. Am. Diet. Assoc.* **98,** 537–547.
16. Van Horn, L. V. (1997). Fiber, lipids, and coronary heart disease. A statement for healthcare professionals from the Nutrition Committee, American Heart Association. *Circulation* **95,** 2701–2704.
17. Kushi, L., Meyer, K., and Jacobs, Jr., D. (1999). Cereals,legumes and chronic disease risk reduction: Evidence from epidemiologic studies. *Am. J. Clin. Nutr.* **70**(Suppl), 451S–458S.
18. Archer, S., Liu, K., Dyer, A., Ruth, K. J., Jacobs, Jr., D. R., Van Horn, L. V., Hilner, J. E., and Savage, P. J. (1998). Relationship between changes in dietary sucrose and high density lipoprotein cholesterol: The CARDIA study—Coronary Artery Risk Development in Young Adults. *Ann. Epidemiol.* **8,** 433–438.

19. Joshipura, K., Ascherio, A., Manson, J. E., Stampfer, M. J., Rimm, E. B., Speizer, F. E., Hennekens, C. H., Spiegellman, D., and Willett, W. C. (1999). Fruit and vegetable intake in relation to risk of ischemic stroke. *JAMA* **282**, 1233–1239.

20. Liu, S., Manson, J. E., Stampfer, M. J., Hu, F. B., Giovannucci, E., Colditz, G. A., Hennekens, C., and Willett, W. C. (1999). Whole grain intake and risk of coronary heart disease: results from the Nurses Health Study. *Am. J. Clin. Nutr.* **70**, 412–419.

21. Pins, J., and Keenan, J. (1999). Soluble fiber and hypertension. *Prevent. Cardiol.* **2**, 151–158.

22. Turley, M., Skeaff, C., Mann, J., and Cox, B. (1998). The effect of a low-fat, high-carbohydrate diet on serum high density lipoprotein cholesterol and triglyceride. *Eur. J. Clin. Nutr.* **52**, 728–732.

23. Slavin, J., Jacobs, D., and Marquart, L. (1997). Whole grain consumption and chronic disease: Protective mechanisms. *Nutr. Cancer* **27**, 4–21.

24. Anderson, J. W., and Hanna, T. J. (1999). Impact of nondigestible carbohydrates on serum lipoproteins and risk for cardiovascular disease. *J. Nutr.* **129**, 1457S–1466S.

25. Jenkins, D. J., Kendall, C. W., Axelsen, M., Augustin, L. S., and Vuksan, V. (2000). Viscous and nonviscous fibres, nonabsorbable and low glycaemic index carbohydrates, blood lipid and coronary heart disease. *Curr. Opin. Cardiol.* **11**, 49–56.

26. Marlett, J. A., and Cheung, T.-F. (1997). Database and quick methods of assessing typical dietary fiber intakes using data for 228 commonly consumed foods. *J. Am. Diet. Assoc.* **97**, 1139–1148, 1151.

27. Yarnall, S. (1999). The role of soluble fiber in reducing cholesterol levels. *Prevent. Cardiol.* **2**(4), 174–176.

28. Nicolosi, R., Bell, S., Bistrian, B., Greenberg, I., Forse, R., and Blackburn, G. (1999). Plasma lipid changes after supplementation with B-glucan fiber from yeast. *Am. J. Clin. Nutr.* **70**, 208–212.

29. Department of Health and Human Services, Food and Drug Administration. (1996). "Food Labeling: Health Claims; Oats and Coronary Heart Disease. Proposed Rule." *Federal Register* **61**, 296–337.

30. Department of Health and Human Services. (1999). "Food Labeling: Health Claims; Psyllium and Coronary Heart Disease. Proposed Rule." *Federal Register* **63**, 8103–8121.

31. Davidson, M., Maki, K., Kong, J. C., Dugan, L. D., Torri, S. A., Hall, H. A., Drennan, K. B., Anderson, S. M., Fulgoni, V. L., Saldanha, L. G., and Olson, B. H. (1998). Long-term effects of consuming foods containing psyllium seed husk on serum lipids in subjects with hypercholesterolemia. *Am. J. Clin. Nutr.* **67**, 367–376.

32. Anderson, J. W., Allgood, L., Lawrence, A., Altringer, L. A., Jerdack, G. R., Hengehold, D. A., and Morel, J. G. (2000). Cholesterol-lowering effects of psyllium intake adjunctive to diet therapy in men and women with hypercholesterolemia: Meta-analysis of 8 controlled trials. *Am. J. Clin. Nutr.* **71**, 472–479.

33. Ripsin, C., Keenan, J., Jacobs, Jr., D., Elmer, P. J., Welch, R. R., Van Horn, L. V., Liu, K., Turnbull, W. H., Thye, F. W., Kestin, M., Hegsted, M., Davidson, D. M., Davidson, Michael H., Dugan, L. D., Demark-Wahnefried, W., and Beling, S. (1992). Oat products and lipid-lowering: A meta-analysis. *JAMA* **267**, 3317–3325.

34. Hunninghake, D., Miller, V., LaRosa, J., Kinosian, B., Jacobson, T., Brown, V., Howard, W. J., Edelman, D. A., and O'Connor, R. R. (1994). Long-term treatment of hypercholesterolemia with dietary fiber [see comments]. *Am. J. Med.* **97**, 504–558.

35. Hunninghake, D., Miller, V., LaRosa, J., Kinosian, B., Brown, V., Howard, W. J., DiSerio, F. J., and O'Connor, R. R. (1994). Hypocholesterolemic effects of a dietary fiber supplement. *Am. J. Clin. Nutr.* **59**, 1050–1054.

36. Ludwig, D., Pereira, M., Kroenke, C., Hilner, J. E., Van Horn, L. V., Slattery, M. L., and Jacobs, Jr., D. R. (1999). Dietary fiber, weight gain, and cardiovascular disease risk factors in young adults. *JAMA* **282**, 1539–1546.

37. Wolk, A., Manson, J. E., Stampfer, M. J., et al. (1999). Long-term intake of dietary fiber and decreased risk of coronary heart disease among women. *JAMA* **281**, 1998–2004.

38. Finkelstein, J. (1990). Methionine metabolism in mammals. *J. Nutr. Biochem.* **1**, 228–237.

39. Mayer, E., Jacobsen, D., and Robinson, K. (1996). Homocysteine and coronary atherosclerosis. *J. Am. College Nutr.* **27**, 517–527.

40. Ueland, P., Refsum, H., and Brattstrom, L. (1992). Plasma homocysteine and cardiovascular disease. *Atheroscler. Cardiovasc. Dis. Hemostas. Endothel. Func.* 183–236.

41. Ueland, P., and Refsum, H. (1989). Plasma homocysteine, a risk factor for vascular disease: Plasma levels in health, disease and drug therapy. *J. Lab. Clin. Med.* **114**, 473–501.

42. Kang, S. (1996). Treatment of hyperhomcyst(e)inemia: Physiological basis. *J. Nutr.* **126**, 1273S–1275S.

43. Ubbink, J., Becker, P., and Vermaak, W. (1996). Will an increased dietary folate intake reduce the incidence of cardiovascular disease? *Nutr. Rev.* **54**, 213–216.

44. Verhoef, P., Stampfer, M. J., Buring, J., Gaziano, J. M., Allen, R. H., Stabler, S. P., Reynolds, R. D., Kok, F. J., Hennekens, C. H., and Willett, W. C. (1996). Homocysteine metabolism and risk of myocardial infarction: Relation with vitamins B_6, B_{12} and folate. *Am. J. Epidemiol.* **143**, 845–859.

45. Boushey, C., Beresford, S., Omenn, G., and Motulsky, A. (1995). A quantitative assessment of plasma hemocysteine as a risk factor for vascular disease. Probable benefits of increasing folic acid intake. *JAMA* **274**, 1049–1057.

46. Stampfer, M. J., Malinow, M., Willett, W. C., Newcomer, L. M., Upson, B., Ullmann, N. D., Tishler, P. V., and Hennekens, C. H. (1992). A prospective study of plasma homocyst(e)ine and risk of myocardial infarction in U.S. physicians. *JAMA* **324**, 1149–1155.

47. Kang, S., Passen, E., Ruggie, N., Wong, P., and Sora, H. (1993). Thermolabile defect of methylenetetrahydrofolate reductase in coronary artery disease. *Circulation* **88**, 1463–1469.

48. Kang, S., Zhou, J., and Wong, P. (1988). Intermediate homocysteinemia: A thermolabile variant of methylenetetrahydrofolate reductase. *Am. J. Hum. Genet.* **43**, 414–421.

49. Lindenbaum, J., Healton, E., Savage, D., Brust, J. C., Garrett, T. J., Podell, E. R., Marcell, P. D., Stabler, S. P., and Allen, R. H. (1988). Neuropsychiatric disorders caused by cobalamin deficiency in the absence of anemia or macrocytosis. *N. Engl. J. Med.* **318**, 1720–1728.

50. Lindenbaum, J., Savage, D., Stabler, S., and Allen, R. (1990). Diagnosis of cobalamin deficiency: II. Relative sensitivities

of serum cobalamin, methylmalonic acid and total homocysteine concentrations. *Am. J. Hematol.* **34**, 99–107.

51. Shin, H., and Linksweiler, H. (1974). Tryptophan and methionine metabolism of adult females as affected by vitamin B_6 deficiency. *J. Nutr.* **104**, 1248–1255.

52. Park, Y., and Linksweiler, H. (1970). Effect of vitamin B_6 depletion in adult men on the excretion of cystathionine and other methionine metabolism. *J. Nutr.* **100**, 110–116.

53. Ribaya-Mercado, J. (1992). "Vitamin B_6. Nutrition in the Elderly: The Boston Nutritional Status Survey," pp. 127–134. Smith-Gordon and Co. Ltd., London.

54. Kang, S., Wong, P., and Norusis, M. (1987). Homocysteinemia due to folate deficiency. *Metabolism* **36**, 458–462.

55. Robinson, K., Arheart, K., Refsum, H., Crattstrom, L., Boers, G., Ueland, P. M., Rubba, P., Palma-Reis, R., Meleady, R., Daly, L., Witteman, J., and Graham, I. (1998). Low circulating folate and vitamin B_6 concentrations: Risk factors for stroke, peripheral vascular disease, and coronary artery disease: European COMAC Group. *Circulation* **97**, 437–443.

56. Selhub, J., Jacques, P., Wilson, P., Rush, D., and Rosenberg, I. (1993). Vitamin status and intake as primary determinants of homocysteinemia in an elderly population. *JAMA* **270**, 2693–2698.

57. Homocysteine Lowering Trialists' Collaboration. (1998). Lowering blood homocysteine with folic acid based supplements: Meta-analysis of randomised trials. *Br. Med. J.* **316**, 894–898.

58. Food and Nutrition Board, Institute of Medicine (1998). "Dietary Reference Intakes for Thiamin, Riboflavin, Niacin, Vitamin B_6, Folate, Vitamin B_{12}, Panthothenic Acid, Biotin and Choline. National Academy Press, Washington, DC.

59. Rasmussen, K., Moller, J., Lyngbak, A., Hom-Pedersen, M., and Dybkjaer, L. (1996). Age- and gender-specific intervals for total homocysteine and methylmalonic acid in plasma before and after vitamin supplementation. *Clin. Chem.* **42**, 630–636.

60. Bronstrup, A., Hages, M., Prinz-Langenohl, R., and Pietrzik, K. (1998). Effects of folic acid and combinations of folic acid with vitamins B_{12} on plasma homocysteine concentrations in healthy, young women. *Am. J. Clin. Nutr.* **68**, 1104–1110.

61. Ubbink, J. (1997). The role of vitamins in the pathogenesis and treatment of hyperhomocyst(e)inanemia. *J. Inher. Metab. Dis.* **20**, 316–325.

62. Wilcken, D., and Wilcken, B. (1998). B vitamins and homocysteine in cardiovascular disease and aging. *Ann. N.Y. Acad. Sci.* **854**, 361–370.

63. Chasan-Tabar, L., Selhub, J., Rosenberg, I., Malinow, M. R., Terry, P., Tishler, P. V., Willett, W. C., Hennekens, C. H., and Stampfer, M. J. (1996). A prospective study of folate and vitamin B-6 and risk of myocardial infarction in U.S. physicians. *J. Am. College Nutr.* **15**, 136–143.

64. Eikelboom, J., Lonn, E., Genest, J., Graeme, H., and Salim, Y. (1999). Homocyst(e)ine and cardiovascular disease: A critical review of the epidemiological evidence. *Ann. Intern. Med.* **131**, 363–375.

65. Ubbink, J., van der Merwe, A., Vermaak, W., Delport, R., and Potgieter, H. (1993). Hyperhomocysteinemia and the response to vitamin supplementation. *Clin. Invest. Med.* **71**, 993–998.

66. Garg, R., Malinow, M., Pettinger, M., and Hunnighake, D. (1996). Treatment with niacin increases plasma homocyst(e)ine levels [abstract]. *Circulation* **94**(Suppl. I), I-457.

67. Malinow, M., and Stampfer, M. J. (1994). Role of plasma homocyst(e)ine in arterial occlusive diseases. *Clin. Chem.* **40**, 857–858.

68. Malinow, M., Bostom, A., and Krauss, R. (1999). Homocyst(e)ine, diet and cardiovascular disease: A statement for healthcare professionals from the Nutrition Committee, American Heart Association. *Circulation* **99**, 178–182.

69. Stampfer, M. J., and Malinow, M. (1995). Can lowering homocysteine levels reduce cardiovascular risk? *N. Engl. J. Med.* **332**, 328–329.

70. Christen, W., Ajani, U., Glynn, R., and Hennekens, C. (2000). Blood levels of homocysteine and increased risk of cardiovascular disease: Causal or casual? *Arch. Intern. Med.* **160**, 422–434.

71. Potter, S. M. (2000). Soy—New health benefits associated with an ancient food. *Nutr. Today* **35**, 53–60.

72. Anderson, J. W., Johnstone, B. M., and Cook-Newell, M. E. (1995). Meta-analysis of the effects of soy protein intake on serum lipids. *N. Engl. J. Med.* **333**, 276–282.

73. Department of Health and Human Services, Food and Drug Administration (1995). "Food Labeling: Health Claims; Soy Protein and Coronary Heart Disease. *Federal Register* **64**, 57699–57733.

74. Stone, N., Nicolosi, R., Kris-Etherton, P. M., Ernst, N., Krauss, R., and Winston, M. (1996). Summary of the scientific conference on the efficacy of hypocholesterolemic dietary interventions. *Circulation* **94**, 3388–3391.

75. Adlerereutz, H., and Mazur, W. (1997). Phytoestrogens and Western diseases. *Ann. Med.* **29**, 95–120.

76. Cassidy, A., Bingham, S., and Setchell, K. (1995). Biological effects of isoflavonoids in young women: Importance of the chemical composition of soybean products. *Br. J. Nutr.* **74**, 587–601.

77. Anthony, M. S., Clarkson, T., Hughes, C., Morgan, T., and Burke, G. (1996). Soybean isoflavones improve cardiovascular risk factors without affecting the reproductive system of peripubertal rhesus monkeys. *J. Nutr.* **126**, 43–50.

78. Balmir, F., Staack, R., Jeffery, E., Jimerez, M., Wand, L., and Potter, S. M. (1996). An extract of soy flour influences serum cholesterol and thyroid hormones in rats and hamsters. *J. Nutr.* **126**, 3046–3053.

79. Clarkson, T., Anthony, M. S., Williams, J., Honore, E., and Cline, J. (1998). The potential of soybean phytoestrogens for postmenopausal hormone replacement therapy. *Proc. Soc. Exp. Biol. Med.* **217**, 365–368.

80. Pelletier, X., Belbraouet, S., Mirabel, D., Mordret, F., Perrin, J. L., Pages, X., and Debry, G. (1995). A diet moderately enriched in phytosterols lowers plasma cholesterol concentrations in normocholesterolemic humans. *Ann. Nutr. Metabl.* **39**, 291–295.

81. Anthony, M. S., Clarkson, T., Bullock, B., and Wagner, J. (1997). Soy protein versus soy phytoestrogens in prevention of diet-induced coronary artery atherosclerosis of male cynomolgus monkeys. *Arterioscler. Thromb. Vasc. Biol.* **17**, 2524–2531.

82. Lovati, M., Manzoni, C., Canavesi, A., Mordret, F., Perrin, J. L., Pages, X., and Debry, G. (1987). Soybean protein diet increases low density lipoprotein receptor activity in mononuclear cells from hypercholesterolemic patients. *J. Clin. Invest.* **80**, 125–130.

83. Gaddi, A., Ciarocchi, A., Matteuccci, A., Rimondi, S., Ravaglia, G., Descovich, G. C., and Sirtori, C. R. (1991). Dietary treatment for familial hypercholesterolemia—Differential effects of dietary soy protein according to the apolipoprotein E phenotypes. *Am. J. Clin. Nutr.* **53,** 1191–1196.

84. Lichtenstein, A. (1998). Soy protein, isoflavones, and cardiovascular disease risk. *J. Nutr.* **128,** 1589–1592.

85. Kapiotis, S., Hermann, M., Held, I., Seelos, C., Ehringer, H., and Gmeiner, B. (1997). Genistein, the dietary-derived angiogenesis inhibitor, prevents LDL oxidation and protects endothelial cells from damage by atherogenic LDL. *Arterioscler. Thromb. Vasc. Biol.* **17,** 2868–2874.

86. de Whalley, C., Rankin, S., Hoult, J., Jessup, W., and Leake, D. (1990). Flavonoids inhibit the oxidative modification of low density lipoproteins by macrophages. *Biochem. Pharmacol.* **39,** 1743–1750.

87. Kanazawa, T., Osanai, T., Zhang, X., Uemura, T., Yin, X. Z., Onodera, K., Oike, Y., and Ohkubo, K. (1995). Protective effects of soy protein on the peroxidizability of lipoproteins in cerebrovascular disease. *J. Nutr.* **125,** 639S–646S.

88. Ruiz-Larrea, M., Mohan, A., Paganga, G., Miller, N., Bolwell, G., and Rice-Evans, C. A. (1997). Antioxidant activity of phytoestrogenic isoflavones. *Free Rad. Res.* **26,** 63–70.

89. Wei, H., Wei, L., Frenkel, K., Bowen, R., and Barnes, S. (1993). Inhibition of tumor promoter-induced hydrogen peroxide formation in vitro and *in vivo* by genestein. *Nutr. Cancer* **20,** 1–12.

90. Sekizaki, H., Yokosawa, R., Chinen, C., Adachi, H., and Yamane, Y. (1993). Synthesis of isoflavones and their attracting activity to *Aphanomyces euteiches* zoo-spore. *Bio. Pharm. Bull.* **16,** 698–701.

91. Craig, W. (1997). Phytochemicals: Guardians of our health. *J. Am. Diet. Assoc.* **97**(Suppl. 2), S199–S204.

92. Yochum, L., Kushi, L., Meyer, K., and Folsom, A. (1999). Dietary flavonoid intake and risk of cardiovascular disease in postmenopausal women. *Am. J. Epidemiol.* **149,** 943–949.

93. Steinmets, K., and Potter, J. (1991). Vegetables, fruit and cancer. II. Mechanisms. *Cancer Causes Control* **2,** 427–442.

94. Wilcox, J., and Blumenthal, B. (1991). Thrombotic mechanism in atherosclerosis: Potential impact of soy proteins. *J. Nutr.* **125,** 631S–638S.

95. Jannsen, K., Mensink, R., Cox, F., Harryvan, J. L., Hovenier, R., Hollman, P. C. H., and Katan, M. B. (1998). Effects of the flavonoids quercetin and apigenin on hemostasis in healthy volunteers: Results from an in vitro and a dietary supplement study. *Am. J. Clin. Nutr.* **67,** 255–262.

96. Bravo, L. (1998). Polyphenols: Chemistry, dietary sources, metabolism and nutritional significance. *Nutr. Rev.* **56,** 317–333.

97. Kuhnau, J. (1976). The flavonoids: A class of semi-essential food components: Their role in human nutrition. *World Rev. Nutr. Diet.* **24,** 117–191.

98. Hertog, M., Kromhout, D., Aravanis, C., Blackburn, H., Buzina, R., Fidanza, F., Giampaoli, S., Jansen, A., Menotti, A., and Nedeljkovic, S., *et al.* (1995). Flavonoid intake and long-term risk of coronary heart disease and cancer in seven countries. *Arch. Int. Med.* **155,** 381–386.

99. Keli, S., Hertog, M., Feskens, E., and Kromhout, D. (1996). Dietary flavonoids, antioxidant vitamins and incidence of stroke. *Arch. Int. Med.* **156,** 637–642.

100. Knekt, P., Reunanen, R., and Jaatela, J. (1996). Flavonoid intake and coronary mortality in Finland: A cohort study. *Br. Med. J.* **312,** 478–481.

101. Hertog, M., Sweetnam, P., Fehil, A., et al. (1997). Antioxidant flavonols and ischemic heart disease in a Welsh population of men: the Caerphilly Study. *Am. J. Clin. Nutr.* **65,** 1489–1494.

102. Anderson, J. W., Diwadkar, V., and Bridges, S. (1998). Intakes of different antioxidants have different effects on the oxidation of very-low and low-density-lipoproteins from rats. *Proc. Soc. Exp. Biol. Med.* **218,** 376–381.

103. Frankel, E., Kanner, J., German, J., Parks, E., and Kinsella, J. (1993). Inhibition of oxidation of human low-density lipoprotein by phenolic substances in red wine. *Lancet* **341,** 454–457.

104. Landolfi, R., Mower, R., and Steiner, M. (1984). Modification of platelet function and arachidonic acid metabolism by bioflavonoids: Structure-activity relations. *Biochem. Pharmacol.* **33,** 1525–1530.

105. Howard, B., and Kritchevsky, D. (1997). Phytochemicals and cardiovascular disease: A statement for healthcare professionals from the American Heart Association. *Circulation* **95,** 2591–2593.

106. Normen, L., Honsson, M., Anderson, H., can Gameren, Y., and Dutta, P. (1999). Plant sterols in vegetables and fruits commonly consumed in Sweden. *Eur. J. Nutr.* **38,** 84–89.

107. Jones, P. J., MacDougall, D., Ntanios, F., and Vanstone, C. (1997). Dietary phytoesterols as cholesterol-lowering agents in humans. *Can. J. Physiol. Pharm.* **75,** 217–227.

108. Lees, A., Mok, H., Lees, R., McCluskey, M., and Grundy, S. M. (1977). Plant sterols as cholesterol-lowering agents: Clinical trials in patients with hypercholesterolemia and studies of sterol balance. *Atherosclerosis* **28,** 325–338.

109. Vahouny, G., and Kritchevsky, D. (1981). Plant and marine sterols and cholesterol metabolism. *In* "Nutritional Pharmacology" (G. A. Spiller, Ed.), pp. 31–72. Alan R. Liss Inc., New York.

110. Robins, S., and Fasulo, J. (1997). High density lipoproteins, but no other lipoproteins, provide a vehicle for sterol transport to bile. *J. Clin. Invest.* **99,** 380–384.

111. Miettinen, T. A., and Gyllin, H. (1999). Regulation of cholesterol metabolism by dietary plant sterols. *Curr. Opin. Lipidol.* **10,** 9–14.

112. Jones, P. J., and Ntanios, F. (1998). Comparable efficacy of hydrogenated versus nonhydrogenated plant sterol esters on circulating cholesterol levels in humans. *Nutr. Rev.* **56,** 245–248.

113. Moghadasian, M., McManus, B., Godin, D., Rodrigues, B., and Frohlich, J. (1999). Proatherogenic and antiatherogenic effects of probucol and phytoesterols in apolipoprotein E-deficient mice: Possible mechanisms of action. *Circulation* **99,** 1733–1739.

114. Westrate, J., and Meijer, G. (1998). Plant sterol-enriched margarines and reduction of plasma total- and LDL-cholesterol concentrations in normocholesterolaemic and mildly hypercholesterolaemic subjects. *Eur. J. Clin. Nutr.* **52,** 334–343.

115. Denke, M. (1994). Lack of efficacy of low-dose sitostanol therapy as an adjunct to a cholesterol-lowering diet in men with moderate hypercholesterolemia. *Am. J. Clin. Nutr.* **61,** 392–396.

116. Augusti, K. (1996). Therapeutic values of onion (*Allium cepa* L.) and garlic (*Allium sativum* L.). *Ind. J. Exp. Biol.* **34,** 634–640.

117. Warshafsky, S., Kramer, R., and Sivak, S. (1993). Effect of garlic on total serum cholesterol: A meta-analysis. *Ann. Intern. Med.* **119,** 599–605.

118. Ali, M., and Thomson, M. (1995). Consumption of a garlic clove a day could be beneficial in preventing thrombosis. *Prostagland. Leukot. Essent. Fatty Acids* **53,** 211–220.

119. Kendler, B. (1987). Garlic (*Allium sativum*) and onion (*Allium cepa*): A review of their relationship to cardiovascular disease. *Prevent. Med.* **16,** 670–685.

120. Beaglehole, R. (1996). Garlic for flavour, not cardioprotection. *Lancet* **348,** 1186–1187.

121. Berthold, H., Thomas, S., and Bergmann, K. (1998). Effect of garlic oil preparation on serum lipoproteins and cholesterol metabolism: A randomized controlled trial. *JAMA* **279,** 1900–1902.

122. Neil, H., Silagy, C., Lancaster, T., Hodgeman, J., Vos, K., Moore, J. W., Jones, L., Cahill, J., and Fowler, G. H. (1996). Garlic powder in the treatment of moderate hyperlipidaemia: A controlled trial and a meta-analysis. *J. R. College Physicians* **30,** 329–334.

CHAPTER 20

Nutrition, Diet, and Hypertension

MARJI McCULLOUGH[1] AND PAO-HWA LIN[2]

[1]*The American Cancer Society, Atlanta, Georgia*
[2]*Duke University Medical Center, Durham, North Carolina*

I. INTRODUCTION

Approximately 25% of U.S. adults have hypertension,[1] a major risk factor for coronary heart disease, stroke, and premature death [1–3]. Even high normal blood pressure is associated with graded, increased risk of cardiovascular disease [3, 4] (Table 1). In industrialized societies, blood pressure increases with age: by age 60, 50–80% of Americans will be diagnosed with hypertension. It is also more common in people of African-American descent [2]. The cause of hypertension is largely unknown, except that in about 5% of cases it is secondary to underlying pathophysiologic correctable conditions.

Recent reports suggest that more than two-thirds of individuals with hypertension are not well controlled (blood pressure <140 mm Hg systolic/<90 mm Hg diastolic). The full potential of diet modification for treatment of hypertension has likely not yet been realized, because researchers have incompletely identified the dietary causes of hypertension, and because of poor adherence by both the clinicians and the public alike to the established medical and dietary guidelines [5]. Long-standing principal dietary factors thought to be important for blood pressure regulation include salt, alcohol, and body weight, and data to support these are strong. Other nonpharmacologic recommendations include increasing potassium intake and aerobic exercise and smoking cessation [1]. These factors are all recommended as part of the first-line therapy for low-risk individuals, defined as those without diabetes or cardiovascular disease and with systolic blood pressure less than 160 mm Hg and diastolic blood pressure less than 100 mm Hg [1], and as part of the combination therapy program for high-risk individuals. Magnesium, calcium, fiber, fat, protein, and certain carbohydrates have also been hypothesized to affect blood pressure, though information linking these dietary factors to blood pressure reduction is less consistent. Researchers continue to search for additional dietary strategies to prevent and reduce high blood pressure, and to clarify some of the inconsistencies from earlier studies in this area.

In this chapter, we provide an overview of epidemiologic and clinical evidence for established and suspected dietary risk factors for hypertension. Results from the recent Dietary Approaches to Stop Hypertension (DASH) trial [6] and the DASH-Sodium trial [7], both of which demonstrated effective food-based approaches to blood pressure reduction, are also included. We conclude with a summary of qualitative and quantitative recommendations for prevention and control of high blood pressure through dietary means.

A. Methodologic Considerations

Several approaches have been used to study the relationship between diet and blood pressure, and the strengths and limitations of each are worth noting. Cross-sectional observational studies have generated a myriad of hypotheses. However, because these studies cannot determine whether the dietary factor preceded the disease, or whether the diet changed in response to diagnosis or symptoms, they cannot be used to determine causality [8]. Cross-cultural comparisons, another variant of cross-sectional studies, cannot be used to confirm causality because of potentially inadequate control for other confounders of the diet–blood pressure relationship (e.g., body weight, physical activity) that vary among populations [9]. These comparisons are further complicated by possible genetic differences in response to environmental stimuli across populations [10]. Prospective cohort studies provide stronger evidence of cause and effect because the dietary factors of interest are measured at the start of the study, prior to disease diagnosis. The population is then followed over time, and disease risk is estimated according to level of the dietary factor. However, the potential for uncontrolled confounding variables still exists in this type of observational study. Particular methodological issues have the potential to affect the validity of blood pressure studies. For example, because blood pressure varies widely throughout the day, and tends to decrease with repeated measurements, multiple standardized measurements are required, and attention to study design is crucial [11]. Although intervention trials are often of relatively short duration, they offer the most

---

[1]The operational definition of hypertension is a systolic blood pressure of 140 mm Hg or greater, a diastolic blood pressure of 90 mm Hg or greater, or current use of an antihypertensive medication [1]. Finer classifications of high blood pressure, used to guide treatment, are included in Appendix 1.

TABLE 1 Baseline Systolic Blood Pressure and Age-Adjusted 10-Year Mortality from Cardiovascular Disease from the Multiple Risk Factor Intervention Trial

Systolic blood pressure (mm Hg)	n	Deaths	Rate/1,000	Relative risk	Excess deaths	% of all excess deaths
<110	21,379	202	10.5	1.0	0.0	0.0
110–119	66,080	658	11.0	1.0	33.0	1.0
120–129	98,834	1,324	14.3	1.4	375.6	11.5
130–139	79,308	1,576	19.8	1.9	737.6	22.6
						35.1
140–149	44,388	1,310	27.3	2.6	745.7	22.8
150–159	21,477	946	38.1	3.6	592.8	18.2
						41.0
160–169	9,308	488	44.8	4.3	319.3	9.8
170–179	4,013	302	65.5	6.2	220.7	6.8
≥180	3,191	335	85.5	8.1	239.3	7.3
						23.9

Source: Reprinted with permission from Stamler, J. (1991). Blood pressure and high blood pressure: Aspects of risk. *Hypertension* **18**(suppl 1), I95–I107.

Note: Men free of history of myocardial infarction at baseline ($N = 347,978$); Multiple Risk Factor Intervention Trial primary screenees [4].

powerful evaluation of cause and effect because they can address these limitations more fully [12].

Because a comprehensive review of all individual trials in this area is beyond the scope of this chapter, when applicable, we review meta-analyses. These analyses quantitatively pool results from several studies according to specific inclusion criteria and are useful for evaluating consistency in the literature. Some aspects and limitations of this method (especially for pooling observational studies) should be noted [13, 14]: (1) large studies are weighted more heavily, (2) many studies do not control for potential confounders, (3) it is rarely feasible to conduct subanalyses on potentially important modifying factors, and (4) when specific biological markers are not available, accounting for variable dietary adherence among studies is rarely possible.

B. Populations with Low Prevalence of Hypertension

In contrast to the prevalence in the United States, many non-Westernized, remote populations have a low prevalence of hypertension and do not experience an increase in blood pressure with age [10, 15]. Their protection from hypertension is often attributed to a very low salt intake [16–18], though a salt intake similar to U.S. levels has also been documented [19, 20]. Potassium intake tends to be ample or high [18, 20], and these groups tend to be physically active [10]. Low alcohol consumption has been reported in some [18, 21] but not all [22] studies. In most of these societies,

food is obtained primarily from subsistence agriculture, fishing and hunting, and the diet is often high in plant foods and fish.

Migration studies of indigenous populations report increasing prevalence of hypertension with urbanization, providing additional evidence for a role of environmental factors [22, 23]. With urbanization, access to processed food increases, and fresh foods that were previously readily available become less affordable. In addition to other lifestyle changes, increases in body weight, sodium intake, dietary fat, and the ratio of urinary sodium to potassium have been observed during the process of acculturation [21–27]. Assessment of nutrient intake in unacculturated populations may be challenging if there are language barriers and cultural differences in food intake and social norms, and also because nutrient data on commonly consumed local foods may not be available. It is imperative that studies of these groups involve members of the community to facilitate data collection and interpretation [28, 29]. Populations undergoing transition from a traditional to a Westernized lifestyle present a unique opportunity to study the etiology of hypertension. Unfortunately, these opportunities are quickly disappearing.

Vegetarian groups in the United States and abroad have been observed to have lower blood pressure than their non-vegetarian counterparts in many [30, 31] but not all [32] studies. The term *vegetarian* comprises several heterogeneous groups [33], but, in general, the diet tends to be high in whole grains, beans, vegetables, and sometimes fish, dairy products, eggs, and fruit [31]. Aspects of the vegetarian diet

suggested to be protective include a low intake of animal products [31], and a high potassium, magnesium, fiber, and (sometimes) calcium [33, 34] intake. Controlled intervention studies of vegetarian diet patterns report significant reductions in blood pressure in both normotensive [36] and mildly hypertensive [34] groups.

A common dietary pattern among vegetarians and unacculturated groups emerges: plant foods (grains, nuts, seeds, vegetables, and sometimes fruit) provide the bulk of the diet, animal products are limited, and (in some cases) fish consumption is high. Available quantitative nutrient data suggest that these diets are moderate to high in potassium, magnesium and fiber, have a high polyunsaturated-to-saturated fat ratio, and are often—but not always—low in sodium. Clearly, differences in physical activity, stress, alcohol consumption, and other unmeasured factors may also contribute to a lower blood pressure in these groups, but their relative importance is not clear. These observations have nevertheless provided much of the foundation for generating hypotheses for a role of diet in modifying blood pressure.

II. INDIVIDUAL NUTRIENTS AND BLOOD PRESSURE

A. Micronutrients

Micronutrients associated with blood pressure tend to be highly correlated with each other because of their distribution in food sources [37], thus limiting the interpretability of observational studies. For example, foods high in magnesium (e.g., nuts) are also high in fiber and potassium, making it virtually impossible to attribute associations with blood pressure to the effects of a single nutrient. To isolate and test the effect of individual nutrients, intervention studies typically use dietary supplements. In this way, any changes in blood pressure with intervention can be attributed to the nutrient being examined. However, supplements may not be absorbed as well or have similar physiologic effects as when they are consumed in natural form. Varying levels of other components in the diet may also modify the effectiveness of supplements.

1. SODIUM

The potential for sodium reduction to lower blood pressure is supported by a broad range of data, and it is also clear that the association is influenced by genetics [38] and other components in the diet [39, 40]. Whether salt reduction should be broadly recommended to lower blood pressure in individuals without hypertension has been the subject of much controversy [41, 42]. Advocates propose that population-wide sodium reduction of 50–100 mmol/day (1150–2300 mg/day) would substantially lower the incidence of cardiovascular disease in the general population [43, 44]. Some

express concern that sodium reduction may raise vasoconstrictive hormones and lipid levels [45], and increase blood pressure in certain individuals [46, 47], while yet others have concluded that sodium reduction to recommended levels has no adverse effects [48].

Dietary sodium intake is not easily measured by standard dietary assessment methods, because salt added at the table and during cooking is difficult to quantify, and because processed foods vary widely in sodium content. Most often, 24-hour urine collections are used to assess daily sodium intake. Under stable conditions (e.g., adequate health, hydration, no excessive sweating), 90–95% of dietary sodium is excreted in the urine [49]. Wide variations in day-to-day sodium excretion within individuals will weaken the correlation of single 24-hour urinary sodium levels with blood pressure. This weakness may be minimized by collecting multiple samples in individuals or by increasing sample size in group analyses. Several investigators now employ statistical methods to correct for this source of error by using data from repeated collections in a subset of the study population [50, 51]. Improperly collected urine samples and varying geographic conditions (e.g., climate) among populations [10] can introduce additional error.

a. Observational Studies. Observations of a direct relationship between sodium intake and blood pressure across populations support a causal role for sodium in hypertension [52, 53]. The INTERSALT study measured the relationship between 24-hour urinary sodium excretion and blood pressure in 10,079 men and women from 52 centers around the world [54]. A positive relationship between mean urinary sodium excretion by center and blood pressure was noted (Fig. 1a, solid line). When excluding data from the four isolated, traditional populations in whom other unmeasured potentially relevant factors were of particular concern, the association disappeared (dashed line). After adjusting for alcohol and body mass index (Figs. 1b and 1c), a slightly positive relationship was again noted. These investigators also reported a strong positive relationship between sodium intake and the slope of blood pressure increase with age across populations [54], suggesting a role for sodium in age-related blood pressure increase. In a recent reanalysis of the original INTERSALT data, corrected for measurement error due to use of single 24-hour urine collections, results were stronger: a 100 mmol/day (2300 mg sodium) increase in urinary sodium was associated with an increase in systolic blood pressure of 3–6 mm Hg and diastolic blood pressure of 0–3 mm Hg [55]. In a meta-analysis of observational studies, Law *et al.* [56] reported somewhat stronger findings than INTERSALT, especially in the elderly and those with higher baseline blood pressures, but diet and other confounders were not assessed in a standard manner across studies.

Few prospective epidemiologic studies (where sodium intake is measured prior to development of hypertension) have been published. In an analysis of National Health and

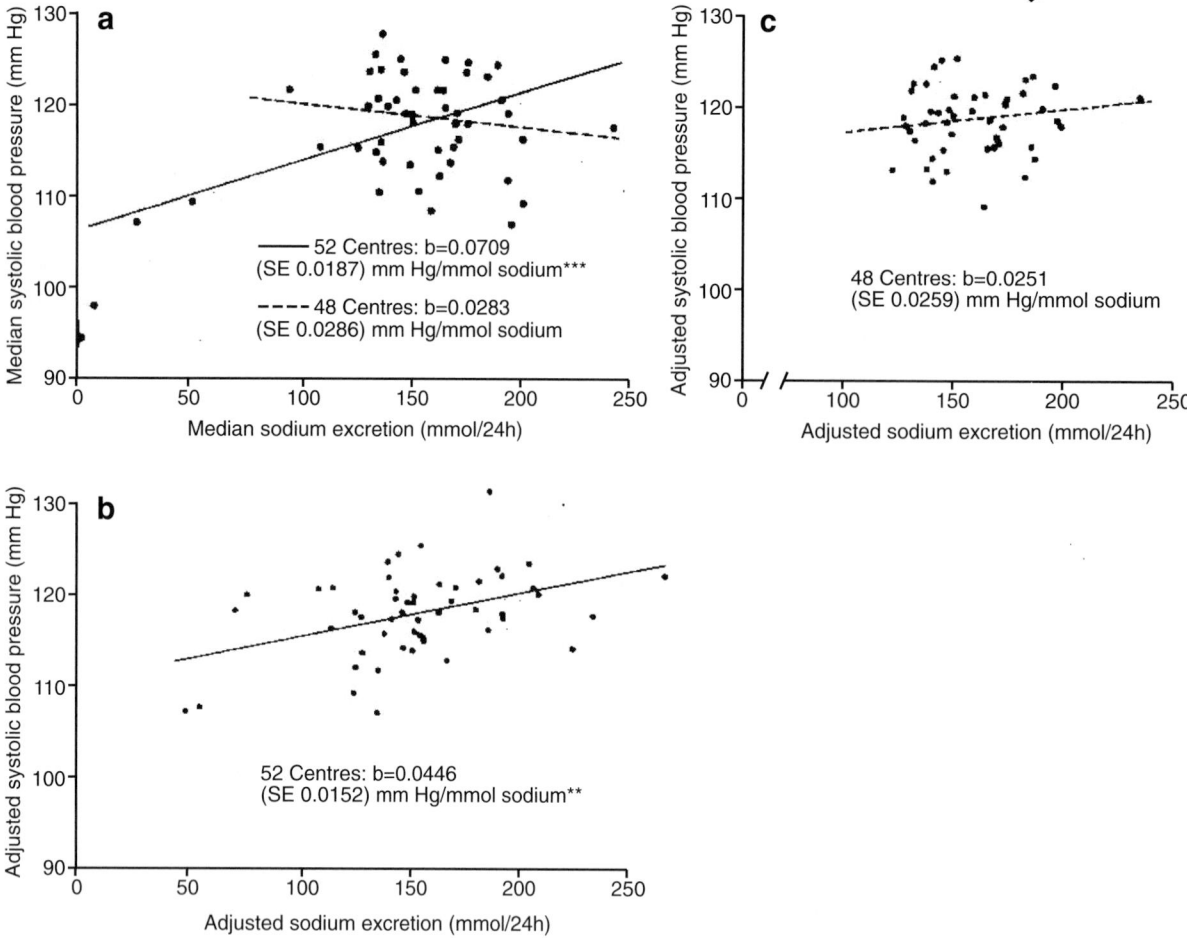

FIGURE 1   Relation between age and sex-adjusted 24-hour urinary sodium excretion and systolic blood pressure in 52 centers from the INTERSALT study. (a) With and without including four remote populations, (b) with additional control for alcohol intake and body mass index in 52 centers, and (c), with control for alcohol intake and body mass index in 48 centers. $*p < 0.05$; $**p < 0.01$; $***p < 0.001$. [Reprinted with permission from Intersalt Cooperative Research Group. (1988). Intersalt: An international study of electrolyte excretion and blood pressure: Results for 24-hour urinary sodium and potassium excretion. *Br. Med. J.* **297,** 319–328.]

Nutrition Examination Survey I (NHANES I) data, a lower sodium intake, unadjusted for energy intake, was associated with higher rates of stroke and all-cause mortality [57]. Similarly paradoxical results were reported in the Scottish Heart Health Study [58]. Limitations in dietary assessment methods, uncontrolled confounding, and a correlation of sodium intake with energy [46, 59] (with higher energy intake often representing higher physical activity) limit the interpretability of these prospective studies. In an analysis of the first NHANES study, He *et al.* [60] found that a 100-mmol increase in dietary sodium was associated with a significant increase in risk of total mortality, a 32% increase in risk of stroke, and an 89% increase in stroke mortality in overweight individuals.

b. Intervention Studies.   The early observation of a large blood pressure reduction in patients with severe hyperten-

sion consuming the Kempner rice diet [61] is often attributed to its low sodium content (7 mmol or 150 mg/day), though the diet was also high in fruit, low in fat and protein, and supplemented with vitamins. The many trials of sodium reduction conducted since then have varied in design, population age, blood pressure status, race and gender composition, amount and form of sodium provided, quantity and control of other nutrients in the diet, trial procedures (inpatient vs. outpatient), and in degree of adherence to the diets. Several meta-analyses of clinical trials of sodium reduction have been published in the last 10 years [43–45, 62]. In a meta-analysis of 28 trials published by Midgely *et al.* [62], a reduction in urinary sodium by 100 mmol/day was associated with a 3.7/0.9 mm Hg lower systolic and diastolic blood pressure, respectively, in individuals with hypertension and 1.0/0.1 mm Hg blood pressure reduction in normotensives. A meta-

analysis by Cutler and others [43] in 1997 of 78 published trials reported stronger results. In people with hypertension, a 100 mmol/day reduction in sodium intake was associated with a 5.8 mm Hg systolic and 2.5 mm Hg diastolic reduction in blood pressure; for normotensives, these reductions were 2.3/1.4 mm Hg in systolic and diastolic blood pressure. Statistical approaches used to quantify the relationship between sodium and blood pressure reduction may partly explain differing conclusions of these investigators.

In the study of Cutler *et al.* [43], the regression line was forced through zero, which assumes that nothing else changed blood pressure during intervention. The regression line was not forced through the origin in the study by Midgley *et al.* [62]; the negative intercept suggested that blood pressure was reduced even without sodium reduction. The recent meta-analysis by Graudal and others [45] included 58 trials in individuals with hypertension and 56 trials in normotensives. Despite greater mean reductions in sodium intake used to estimate the blood pressure-lowering effect (a 118 mmol sodium reduction in individuals with hypertension, and 160 mmol reduction in normotensives), their findings of a 3.9/1.9 mm Hg and 1.2/0.26 mm Hg blood pressure reduction, respectively, were closer to those of Midgley *et al.* [62]. Graudal and colleagues [45] also found that blood pressure regulating hormones, cholesterol and low-density lipoprotein (LDL) cholesterol levels increased on a low-salt diet, more so in studies with extreme sodium reduction.

Graudal *et al.* [45] and Midgely *et al.* [62] included studies of acute sodium reduction (which stimulates blood pressure regulating hormones), while Cutler *et al.* [43] did not. Nevertheless, all meta-analyses reported a direct relationship between sodium and blood pressure, which was consistently significant in hypertensives. The estimate of the magnitude of the reduction varied, at least partly because of statistical methods used, and the choice of studies included in the meta-analyses.

The recently completed DASH-Sodium multicenter trial [7] may help to resolve many issues surrounding the sodium controversy. The study, funded by the National Heart Lung and Blood Institute, compared the effect of three sodium levels (resulting in urinary sodium excretion of 65, 107, and 142 mmol/day) on blood pressure in those with greater than optimal blood pressure or stage 1 hypertension. The sodium intervention was provided in conjunction with a typical U.S. (control) diet or a diet pattern previously shown to lower blood pressure (DASH diet, Appendix 2). The investigators found that the lowest sodium intake (65 mmol/day), superimposed on the already effective DASH diet, provided the most effective blood pressure lowering combination. Compared to the control diet with the highest sodium level, the DASH diet with the lowest sodium level reduced systolic blood pressure by 8.9 mm Hg in participants with hypertension and 7.1 mm Hg in normotensives. The reduction in blood pressure due to sodium was stronger in those consuming the typical American diet than the DASH diet, but was significant in both [7]. Results in the DASH-Sodium trial were seen in hypertensives as well as nonhypertensives, suggesting that a 65 mmol/day general sodium guideline for prevention and treatment of hypertension is warranted [7].

Several long-term, randomized clinical trials have provided evidence that moderate sodium reduction with or without weight loss reduces the incidence of hypertension and cardiovascular events, especially in overweight participants [63]. In the Trial of Nonpharmacologic Interventions in the Elderly (TONE), a 10-pound weight loss and dietary sodium reduction of 40 mmol/day were independently associated with about a 40% reduced risk of hypertension or cardiovascular event after medication withdrawal, compared with those on standard care. In these obese subjects, the combined intervention was associated with a 53% reduced risk of hypertension or CVD event [64]. In the Trials of Hypertension Prevention (TOHP) Phase II, overweight adults who were counseled to reduce sodium achieved a 2.9/1.6 mm Hg blood pressure reduction from sodium reduction alone, and 4.0/2.8 mm Hg when coupled with weight loss, after 6 months. Although effects on average blood pressure declined over time with recidivism, 20% reductions in hypertension incidence were still noted after 48 months of follow-up in each intervention group [65].

c. Salt Sensitivity. Approximately 50% of individuals with hypertension and 25% of normotensives are considered by some to be salt sensitive [66–68], defined arbitrarily as a mean arterial pressure reduction of at least 10 mm Hg or 10% with salt restriction. It is more common in the elderly and in African-Americans [69]. Various protocols have been employed to diagnose salt-sensitivity, including feeding low- and high-sodium diets, and a more rigorous protocol of saline infusion (to expand blood volume), followed by volume contraction with a low-sodium diet and administration of a diuretic [66]. The reasons why certain individuals respond differently to a sodium load are unclear but may be due to differences in the ability of the vascular system to adjust to a change in circulating blood volume, and to blunted sodium excretion [70]. Renal damage will also reduce the ability of the kidney to handle a sodium load. The renin-angiotensin system, activated by many factors, including sodium restriction, stimulates aldosterone secretion, which conserves total body sodium. Physiologic abnormalities, such as low renin hypertension and abnormal modulation ("nonmodulation") of these hormones, predispose to salt sensitivity [71]. Sodium-chloride-induced increases in blood pressure may also be enhanced by a low calcium or potassium intake [40, 72, 73]. Unfortunately, no method is available yet that can be applied clinically to diagnose salt sensitivity. Genetic markers offer promise [74], but much work remains to explain the magnitude of heterogeneity observed. Ideally, future studies will identify markers of susceptibility to aid in targeting interventions.

Sodium is not the only factor that affects blood pressure, and it appears to interact with body weight and levels of other nutrients in the diet. However, sodium reduction is likely to benefit most people, and ultimately the 65 mmol/day recommendation of the DASH-Sodium investigators may prove most effective. Because sodium is ubiquitous in the U.S. food supply, large reductions in intake are not easily attainable. For example, the TOHP Phase I research group reported a mean decrease in sodium excretion of 44 mmol/day after 18 months of intensive dietary counseling in free-living populations [75]. Only 20% of the population met the teaching goal of 60 mmol/day, but 56% were able to reduce sodium to less than 100 mmol/day. Counseling was least effective in men and in African-Americans [75]. Seventy-five percent of sodium intake is derived from processed foods [76], so significant reductions in sodium intake will not be easy to achieve unless sodium is reduced during processing for most foods, including staples such as bread.

2. POTASSIUM

The evidence for a role of potassium in lowering blood pressure is consistent across study types and is biologically plausible. Potassium may lower blood pressure through a direct vasodilatory role, alterations in the renin-angiotensin-aldosterone axis and renal sodium handling, and by natriuretic effects [77].

a. Observational Studies. Epidemiologic observations support a role of dietary potassium in blood pressure control. Both potassium alone (inversely) and the sodium-to-potassium ratio (directly) have been associated with blood pressure in cross-cultural studies [54]. Ophir *et al.* [78] noted that urinary potassium was the strongest discriminating feature related to low blood pressure in vegetarian Seventh Day Adventists in Australia, compared to nonvegetarians; however, their descriptive study also revealed differences in other dietary and lifestyle factors among groups.

b. Intervention Studies. In 1997, Whelton *et al.* [79] published a meta-analysis of randomized clinical trials of potassium and blood pressure. The 33 studies included mostly individuals with hypertension, some of whom were receiving antihypertensive medication. In all studies, potassium was provided as a supplement (median 75 mmol), either superimposed on a controlled research diet or added to participants' usual diets. After excluding one outlier, systolic and diastolic blood pressure were 3.11 and 1.97 mm Hg lower, respectively, with a high potassium intake. Interestingly, greater blood pressure reductions occurred in those with progressively higher urinary sodium excretion during follow-up (measured at the end of the study). This suggests that potassium is more effective at higher levels of sodium intake. In addition, results were significantly stronger in studies that included >80% African-Americans. This meta-analysis reached qualitatively similar conclusions to those of

a 1995 analysis by Cappuccio *et al.* [80], with a roughly 50% overlap in studies included.

In a large intervention trial of U.S. female nurses (Nurses Health Study II), Sacks and colleagues [81] administered supplemental potassium [40 mmol (1560 mg)], calcium [30 mmol (1200 mg)], magnesium [14 mmol (336 mg)], all three minerals, or placebo to women who reported habitually low intakes of these nutrients, for a 6-month period. Potassium, administered alone, was the only intervention that reduced blood pressure [81]. The mild, yet significant reduction occurred even though the women were nonhypertensive (116 ± 8 systolic blood pressure, 73 ± 6 diastolic blood pressure), and were young (mean age 39 years).

Consistent findings in the epidemiologic and clinical literature support a role for potassium in the reduction and prevention of high blood pressure. Considering the markedly lower blood pressure of vegetarians and those living in remote populations compared to industrialized societies, dietary factors other than potassium are also likely to be protective. Other nutrient or non-nutrient factors in a high potassium diet may work additively or interactively with potassium to reduce blood pressure. In the DASH Study [6], the combination dietary pattern lowered blood pressure more than the fruit and vegetable intervention—even though both contained equal levels of potassium and sodium.

3. CALCIUM

Although a modest blood pressure lowering effect of calcium is noted in some observational studies, results from intervention trials have been inconsistent. Studies showing the greatest effect have tended to use dietary sources of calcium (e.g., dairy products), in which several dietary factors change [6]. A blood pressure lowering effect of calcium in certain subgroups (e.g., African-Americans) has been suggested.

a. Observational Studies. The higher calcium and magnesium content of "hard" water, and its inverse relation to cardiovascular mortality [82] initially sparked epidemiologic investigation into the relation of both minerals to blood pressure. Cutler and Brittain [83] reviewed 25 observational studies of calcium and hypertension, 19 of which were cross-sectional, and some of which involved repeated analyses of the same data sets. As a whole, these studies showed only modest associations between calcium and blood pressure. Because most studies used 24-hour recall methods to assess diet, random day-to-day variation may have obscured any relation with blood pressure [83]. It is also worth noting that some low blood pressure populations have minimal calcium intakes [20]—more counter evidence to the link between calcium and blood pressure. Cappuccio and others [84] conducted a meta-analysis of 23 observational studies, and found negligible associations for calcium with both systolic blood pressure and diastolic blood pressure [84], though a reanalysis of this data resulted in a somewhat stronger inverse association [13].

b. Intervention Studies. In 1924, Addison and Clark [85] recorded the blood pressure response to repeated administration and discontinuation of oral calcium supplements in a convenience sample of hospital outpatients and inpatients. They noted that blood pressure decreased after 2 weeks of calcium supplementation and immediately rose with calcium discontinuation. It was not until much later in the century that the calcium hypothesis was tested in a more methodologically rigid fashion in a number of intervention studies.

Several meta-analyses of calcium-intervention trials have been published since 1989 [86–89], all showing only a slight blood pressure reduction, primarily of systolic blood pressure, with calcium supplementation of about 1000 mg. Intervention studies using calcium from food sources have sometimes [90], but not always [91], been more effective, though these studies involve changes in several other nutrients. An interaction between calcium and sodium has been observed [39, 72, 92–94], such that calcium supplementation may prevent a salt-induced rise in blood pressure in susceptible individuals. Inability to either control for sodium intake, or stratify by level of sodium intake in most meta-analyses, may obscure a relationship. Although the interpretation of these studies differs [90], it seems that the modest blood pressure reduction observed with calcium supplementation does not warrant public health recommendations to increase calcium intake specifically for blood pressure control.

4. MAGNESIUM

a. Observational Studies. As with calcium, one of the early suggestions for a role of magnesium in hypertension came from reports that water hardness (increased calcium and magnesium) was associated with lower cardiovascular mortality [82], a finding recently corroborated in Taiwan [95]. Several cross-sectional [96] and prospective observational analyses [97, 98] have found high-magnesium diets to be associated with lower blood pressure. Here again, the major limitation is that high-magnesium diets tend to be high in other beneficial dietary factors as well.

Adequate magnesium is required for the Na/K-ATPase pump, which regulates intracellular calcium—one of the critical determinants of vascular smooth-muscle contraction [99]. Magnesium deficiency is recognized only rarely, being seen usually in the severely malnourished, chronic alcoholics, and in association with malabsorption [99].

b. Intervention Studies. At least 13 randomized intervention trials of magnesium supplementation have been conducted [81, 100–111]. In all but 1 of these studies, volunteers had high blood pressure, and in 5 of these trials, they were receiving antihypertensive medication (primarily diuretics). Magnesium lowered blood pressure in 5 of these studies [100, 101, 107, 108, 110]. Patients were magnesium depleted (due to diuretic treatment) in 2 of the studies [100, 101], and in 1 study an effect was only seen in those with a low baseline intake of dietary magnesium [111]. Kawano *et*

al. [110] found the greatest blood pressure reduction in older men on antihypertensive medications [110]. The majority of studies, however, found no blood pressure lowering effect with magnesium supplementation.

B. Macronutrients

Studies of macronutrients and blood pressure are often subject to various design limitations and thus results can be difficult to interpret. For example, when a study is designed to examine the effect of the amount of fat intake on blood pressure, alteration in fat intake under isocaloric conditions inevitably will change intake of protein and/or carbohydrate and may change the intake of other nutrients as well. As a result, it may be difficult to attribute the effect to only the change in fat intake. In addition, the impact of macronutrients on blood pressure potentially involves the aspect of absolute quantity and the type of macronutrients. Both aspects can affect blood pressure independently, but they are not always distinguishable in research designs.

1. PROTEIN

A high-protein diet has long been suggested to increase kidney load unfavorably and raise blood pressure [112] and may have been the underlying rationale for the Kempner rice diet treatment [61]. However, many epidemiological studies have shown an inverse relationship between dietary protein and blood pressure [113–115]. A detailed review of studies investigating the relationship between dietary protein and blood pressure from 1988 to 1994 has been published [116] and very little new research has been conducted since then.

Overall, high-protein intake, as indicated by urinary nitrogen or dietary protein, was found to be associated with lower diastolic and systolic blood pressures in two large cross-sectional studies in humans [114, 115]. Animal studies also demonstrated that low-protein diets increase blood pressure and stroke, while high-protein diets are protective [117]. However, most intervention trials in humans do not support findings from observational studies. Most human intervention trials use protein supplements and many do not control for other nutrients. Supplements of 7 grams of rice protein to 93 grams of meat protein for 2 weeks to 3 months did not affect blood pressure (118–125). In an 8-week intervention trial, skim milk supplementation reduced blood pressure significantly among 82 normotensive participants [126]. Note that skim milk supplements provided not only additional protein, but also other nutrients, including calcium and magnesium, and both may affect blood pressure. Thus, the blood pressure responses may be caused by multiple factors including protein.

Despite findings from several epidemiological studies demonstrating that blood pressure is associated with only animal protein or only vegetable protein [117, 127, 128],

most intervention trials have not shown such differences [123–125]. The only exception was that vegetable protein did not affect blood pressure in a group of normotensive vegetarians [122], while animal protein raised systolic blood pressure in another group of normotensive vegetarians [121]. The animal protein supplements were given as 250 g of beef (approximately 8 ounces), which contains protein, fat, and other nutrients that may all have contributed to the increases in blood pressure. On the contrary, an epidemiological study demonstrated that animal protein was inversely related to blood pressure [129].

The underlying mechanism by which dietary protein may affect blood pressure is not clear. Specific amino acids, such as arginine, tyrosine, tryptophan, methionine, and glutamate, have been suggested to affect neurotransmitters or humoral factors that affect blood pressure [116]. Soy protein was thus hypothesized to reduce blood pressure because it is rich in arginine, a potential vasodepressor and a precursor for the vasodepressor nitric oxide [130]. In a group of perimenopausal women [131], soy protein supplementation for 6 weeks reduced diastolic blood pressure significantly. However, intakes of other nutrients including calcium, magnesium, and potassium were also increased in the soy protein group. Thus, the blood pressure response may not be attributable to the increase in arginine or soy protein alone. A protein load can increase renal blood flow [132], but the effect of habitual diets on renal blood flow, or the role of renal blood flow in hypertension is not clear [133]. More research is needed to understand the effects of various amino acids in humans, and the mechanisms underlying the relationship between dietary protein and blood pressure if such a relationship exists.

2. DIETARY FAT

Numerous studies have investigated the relationship between dietary fat and blood pressure. However, because of discrepancies in study design, lack of adequate sample size, and other design limitations, the issue is still controversial. Both the absolute total intake of dietary fat and the relative fatty acid composition may be independently related to blood pressure control.

Most observational studies have not found consistent association between total fat intake and blood pressure [134–136]. However, two large European studies [135, 136] but not others [137] show a positive relationship between saturated fatty acids and blood pressure. In clinical intervention trials, lowering total fat intake from 38–40% to 20–25% of energy and/or increasing the polyunsaturated-to-saturated fat ratio from 0.2 to 1.0 reduced blood pressures in several studies [138–141], but not all [142, 143]. As mentioned earlier, any change in total fat intake often introduces changes in other dietary factors as well, so the blood pressure responses may not be attributed solely to the change in fat intake. In addition, it is important to recognize that previous trials

of dietary fat have had small sample sizes, and lacked the sensitivity to detect 3–4 mm Hg effects.

Little is known about the relationship between dietary cholesterol and blood pressure. In the prospective analyses of the Western Electric Study, a significant positive independent relationship was found between dietary cholesterol and systolic blood pressure change during an 8-year period [128, 144]. Stamler et al. [114] also reported that dietary cholesterol was significantly and positively related to blood pressure among the 11,342 participants of the Multiple Risk Factor Intervention Trial. However, in a short-term intervention study, dietary cholesterol at low to moderate levels of intake was found to have no significant effects on blood pressure [145].

Many short-term intervention trials have been undertaken to determine if supplementation of either fish or fish oil lowers blood pressure. Because of variations in research design, participant criteria, dosage and type of supplements, and length of intervention, the results have been inconsistent. Recently, pharmacological dosages of dexapentaenoic acid (DPA) were shown to lower blood pressure, while eicosapentaenoic acid (EPA) was not [146]. It is suggested that the blood pressure lowering effect of fish oil may be strongest in individuals with hypertension and in those with clinical atherosclerotic disease or hypercholesterolemia [147]. In another study, both fish oil and corn oil supplements were shown to reduce blood pressure to similar degrees among elderly hypertensives [148]. Long-term studies are required to confirm if fish oil can lower blood pressure. Until such information is available, it is more advisable to encourage greater fish consumption as part of a healthy diet than taking fish oil supplementation. This is in agreement with the recommendation of the DASH dietary pattern (see later section) to prevent and treat high blood pressure.

A high monounsaturated fatty acid (MUFA) Mediterranean type of diet is also suggested to lower blood pressure mainly based on observational studies. However, little research has been conducted investigating the specific effects of MUFA on blood pressure. A small-scale clinical trial found that a high-MUFA diet (17% of energy) lowered daily antihypertensive medications as compared to a high polyunsaturated fatty acid (PUFA) diet [149]. Another intervention study showed that blood pressure was significantly reduced when 16 persons with diabetes were provided olive oil [150]. Other studies, nevertheless, did not find an effect of a high-MUFA diet on blood pressure [140, 151]. It is important to note that most of these trials of dietary fats and blood pressure have had a small sample size, and lacked sensitivity to detect even 3–4 mm Hg effects in systolic blood pressure. It has been shown that a MUFA-enriched diet produced changes in erythrocyte membrane composition in participants with hypertension [152]. It was hypothesized that the changes in membrane cholesterol modifies the fluidity and the transmembrane fluxes of Na^+ and K^+, which may then indirectly affect blood pressure [153].

It is also possible that fatty acids such as the n-6 and n-3 series may affect blood pressure through the prostaglandin (PG) pathway [154]. Animal studies have shown that n-6 fatty acids increased the tissue and circulating levels of PGs, PGI2, and PGE2, all of which may act as vasodilators [155, 156]. Little research is available in humans examining how fat intake may affect blood pressure through this pathway.

In summary, it is still unclear how fat intake and various fatty acids affect blood pressure and if an interaction exists among these factors. Even though a majority of interventions demonstrate that lowering fat intake reduces blood pressure, the effect may not be attributed to fat alone.

3. CARBOHYDRATES

Very few studies have been designed specifically to investigate the impact of the quantity of carbohydrate intake on blood pressure. Nevertheless, studies of the relationship between fat intake and blood pressure often alter intakes of fat and carbohydrate while keeping protein intake constant. Thus, interpretation of the effect of fat intake on blood pressure is potentially confounded by the effects of carbohydrate intake. An impact of the type of carbohydrate on blood pressure, on the other hand, has been examined in a limited number of studies. In an early study using Wistar rats, Ahrens et al. [157] showed that increasing the proportion of sucrose in the diet to 10–15% of energy for 14 weeks increased blood pressure significantly. These sucrose-fed rats also retained more sodium than the controls, which may have contributed to the blood pressure responses. In addition, the blood pressure of these rats returned to baseline levels when sucrose was replaced with maltose. Other animal studies [158, 159] also showed similar hypertensive effects of sucrose.

Results from human studies have not been consistent. In one study [160], systolic blood pressure rose significantly 1 hour after ingestion of a sucrose solution. However, in an earlier study of patients with coronary artery disease, both systolic and diastolic blood pressures decreased after 4 days of a sucrose load at 4 g/kg/day [161]. In another study that was designed to examine the metabolic effect of sucrose in a group of overweight women, blood pressure levels were not changed after consuming a hypocaloric diet with sucrose as the main source of carbohydrate for 6 weeks [162]. These results are confounded by the concomitant weight reduction diet discussed in the next section.

In the study by Palumbo et al. [161], fructose loading in these patients also reduced blood pressures significantly, but glucose loading had no effect. Similar hypotensive effects of fructose were observed in other studies [163, 164], yet oral glucose loading was found to be either hypertensive [160, 163] or hypotensive [165]. Such inconsistencies in the study of various simple carbohydrates on blood pressure may be due to the differences in study design, study population, inadequate sample size, or length of feeding. More research is needed to clarify the effects of various carbohydrates on

blood pressure using well-controlled designs under long-term situations.

4. FIBER

a. Observational Studies. Both cross-sectional [37, 166, 167] and prospective analyses [97] have demonstrated inverse associations of fiber with blood pressure, but have also noted the high correlation of fiber with other nutrients. In a prospective cohort analysis, Witteman and colleagues [98] found that the protective association with fiber was reduced when magnesium and calcium were used as adjustment factors in the statistical models. Conversely, in the study of Ascherio et al. [97], only dietary fiber remained significantly and inversely related to hypertension when the association was adjusted for other nutrients. Different sources of fiber, including fruit fiber [97] and cereal fiber [166], have been associated with blood pressure reduction in prospective studies.

b. Intervention Studies. Several intervention studies have examined the effect of fiber on blood pressure, with most adding cereal fiber to the diet, and are reviewed by He and Whelton [166]. With an average supplementation of 14 g fiber, systolic and diastolic blood pressure is reduced by about 1.6/2.0 mm Hg [166]. In some studies, fiber has been provided as a combination of soluble and insoluble fibers. Only soluble fiber influences gastrointestinal function and, indirectly, insulin metabolism, a possible mechanism by which fiber may lower blood pressure [166]. The weak effects of fiber in these studies may also be due to small study size, and because many were conducted in young, normotensive individuals, in whom large changes in blood pressure are more difficult to detect. Further studies with adequate power to detect smaller differences in blood pressure are needed to clarify the role of fiber.

III. OTHER DIETARY AND LIFESTYLE MODIFICATIONS

A. Weight Reduction

a. Observational Studies. Observational studies report a positive relationship between several indices of body weight or body fatness and high blood pressure [54, 168–172]. Mechanisms that may be involved in weight loss include suppression of sympathetic nervous system activity, lowered insulin resistance, normalization of blood pressure regulating hormones [173], decreased body sodium stores, decreased blood volume and cardiac output, and higher salt sensitivity in overweight individuals [60, 174, 175].

b. Intervention Studies. Several intervention trials of weight reduction in those with high-normal blood pressure [176–178], often combined with dietary sodium reduction [64, 65], report lower blood pressures with sustained weight

reduction of about 3–7 kg. Of several nonpharmacologic interventions examined in the Trials of Hypertension Prevention Phase I [179], weight loss was found to be the most successful at lowering blood pressure. At the 6-month follow-up visit, men and women in the intervention group had lost 6.5 and 3.7 kg, respectively. This level of weight loss was achieved with a fairly rigorous counseling approach aimed at simultaneously reducing energy intake and increasing exercise [178]. At study termination, blood pressure fell an average of 2.9/2.3 mm Hg overall (after subtracting the blood pressure change in the control group) [178]. In this study, some recidivism occurred, and at 18 months, men had maintained a 4.7-kg reduction, and women, 1.6 kg. After a 7-year follow-up in a subset of study participants, the odds of developing hypertension were reduced by 77% in the weight loss group [180], even though their long-term weight loss was nearly identical to that of the control group (4.9 and 4.5 kg, respectively). This raises the intriguing possibility of long-term effects from previous interventions and deserves further study. Additionally, significant weight loss (5%) is suggested to reduce the need for antihypertensive medication [173].

c. Summary. The high prevalence of overweight and obesity in U.S. adults (54.9%), defined as a body mass index >25 and 30 kg/m^2, respectively [181], is likely to contribute importantly to hypertension, as well as to other chronic diseases and their risk factors. The relative contributions of lower energy intake and exercise [182] in affecting blood pressure change is not completely understood. Weight loss is an effective method to reduce blood pressure but is difficult to implement and maintain [183], particularly among African-Americans, who have a higher prevalence of high blood pressure.

B. Alcohol

a. Observational Studies. Excessive alcohol consumption is associated with higher blood pressure and higher prevalence of hypertension in observational studies [184]. Men who consume ≥3–5 drinks/day [185], and women who consume 2–3 drinks/day [186] may be at particularly higher risk, but levels below this are not associated with increased risk. The relation of alcohol type to risk is inconsistent, and chronic, habitual intake may be more related to blood pressure than recent intake [185]. In one study, men who reduced their alcohol consumption over a 20-year period experienced less age-related increase in blood pressure than those who did not [187].

b. Intervention Studies. The relatively few intervention studies of alcohol and blood pressure have tended to be small and of short duration, and are reviewed by Cushman *et al.* (188). In 9 of 10 studies examined, systolic blood pressure was significantly reduced after a reduction of 1–6 alcoholic beverages per day [188]. The Prevention and Treatment of Hypertension Study (PATHS) was designed to evaluate the long-term blood pressure lowering effect of reducing alcohol consumption in nondependent moderate drinkers (those who consumed >3 alcohol-containing drinks/day) [189]. The goal of intervention in this study was either 2 or fewer drinks daily or a 50% reduction in intake (whichever was less). After 6 months, the intervention group experienced an insignificant (1.2/0.7 mm Hg) reduction in blood pressure compared with the control group, and among individuals with hypertension, this reduction was even more modest. In this study, the intervention group reduced their intake by 2 alcoholic drinks per day, but the control group also lowered their alcohol intake during intervention, so that the difference in intake between the groups was 1.3 drinks/day. Perhaps a greater reduction is necessary to see a stronger effect. However, this level of reduction appears realistic in moderate alcohol drinkers, and is similar to the absolute reduction achieved in an earlier study [190]. In two studies, 6–18 weeks in duration, replacing alcohol with nonalcoholic substitutes resulted in greater reductions [191, 192], suggesting that certain behavioral approaches may promote adherence. In one of these studies, alcohol cessation (from 5 drinks to 0) and energy restriction (mean 9. 6 kg weight loss) combined showed additive effects, and resulted in a reduction in systolic and diastolic blood pressure of 14 and 7 mm Hg, respectively [192].

The exact mechanism for an alcohol–blood pressure association is not clear, but possibilities include a stimulation of the sympathetic nervous system, inhibition of vascular relaxing substances, calcium or magnesium depletion, and increased intracellular calcium in vascular smooth muscle [184, 188]. Variations in study design preclude arriving at a specific cutoff for benefit, but limiting alcohol consumption to two or fewer drinks per day may improve blood pressure control in heavy drinkers. Moderate alcohol consumption also has well-known benefits for overall cardiovascular disease risk [193, 194].

IV. DIETARY PATTERNS

As previously noted, lower blood pressure is often observed among populations who consume a vegetarian-like diet. However, studies on individual nutrients as outlined in previous sections of this chapter, have shown inconsistent results. Explanations for such inconsistencies may include these: (1) The effect of individual nutrients may be too small to be detected, particularly when trials do not contain sufficient sample size and thus statistical power; (2) most intervention studies employed supplements of nutrients, which may function differently from naturally occurring nutrients in foods; (3) other dietary factors naturally occurring in foods that are not hypothesized to affect blood pressure may also have an impact on blood pressure; and (4) nutrients

TABLE 2 Nutrient Targets, Menu Analysis, and Average Daily Servings of Foods, According to Intervention Diet in DASH[a]

Item	Control diet		Fruits-and-vegetables diet		Combination diet	
	Nutrient target	Menu analysis[b]	Nutrient target	Menu analysis[b]	Nutrient target	Menu analysis[b]
Nutrients						
Fat (% of total kcal)	37	35.7	37	35.7	27	25.6
Saturated	16	14.1	16	12.7	6	7.0
Monounsaturated	13	12.4	13	13.9	13	9.9
Polyunsaturated	8	6.2	8	7.3	8	6.8
Carbohydrates (% of total kcal)	48	50.5	48	49.2	55	56.5
Protein (% of total kcal)	15	13.8	15	15.1	18	17.9
Cholesterol (mg/day)	300	233	300	184	150	151
Fiber (g/day)	9	NA	31	NA	31	NA
Potassium (mg/day)	1700	1752	4700	4101	4700	4415
Magnesium (mg/day)	165	176	500	423	500	480
Calcium (mg/day)	450	443	450	534	1240	1265
Sodium (mg/day)	3000	3028	3000	2816	3000	2859
Food groups (no. of servings/day)						
Fruits and juices	1.6		5.2		5.2	
Vegetables	2.0		3.3		4.4	
Grains	8.2		6.9		7.5	
Low-fat dairy	0.1		0.0		2.0	
Regular-fat dairy	0.4		0.3		0.7	
Nuts, seeds, and legumes	0.0		0.6		0.7	
Beef, pork, and ham	1.5		1.8		0.5	
Poultry	0.8		0.4		0.6	
Fish	0.2		0.3		0.5	
Fat, oils, and salad dressing	5.8		5.3		2.5	
Snacks and sweets	4.1		1.4		0.7	

Source: Reprinted with permission from Appel, L. J., Moore, T. J., Obarzanek, E., *et al.* (1997). A clinical trial of the effects of dietary patterns on blood pressure. *N. Engl. J. Med.* **336**, 1117–1124 [6].

[a]Values are for diets designed to provide an energy level of 2100 kcal.

[b]Values are the results of chemical analyses of the menus prepared during the validation phase and during the trial. NA denotes not available.

occurring in foods simultaneously may exert synergistic effects on blood pressure. Thus, the DASH multicenter trial was designed to test the impact of whole dietary patterns on blood pressure while controlling for multiple nutrients and dietary factors simultaneously [195, 196].

A. The Dietary Approaches to Stop Hypertension Trial

Three dietary patterns varying in amounts of fruits, vegetables, and dairy products were developed for the DASH trial [197]. The first dietary pattern was a control diet that mimicked the typical American diet, and contained fewer fruits,

vegetables, and dairy products, and was high in total and saturated fats, cholesterol, and low in dietary fiber, calcium, potassium, and magnesium (Table 2). The "fruits and vegetables" dietary pattern had more fruits and vegetables, and thus higher levels of dietary fiber, potassium, and magnesium as compared to the control diet. The DASH "combination" dietary pattern (also referred to as the DASH diet) emphasizes fruits, vegetables, and low-fat dairy products, includes whole grains, poultry, fish, and nuts, and is reduced in fats, red meat, sweets, and sugar-containing beverages. The DASH diet had reduced amounts of total and saturated fat and cholesterol, and increased amounts of potassium, calcium, magnesium, dietary fiber, and protein. Sodium intake,

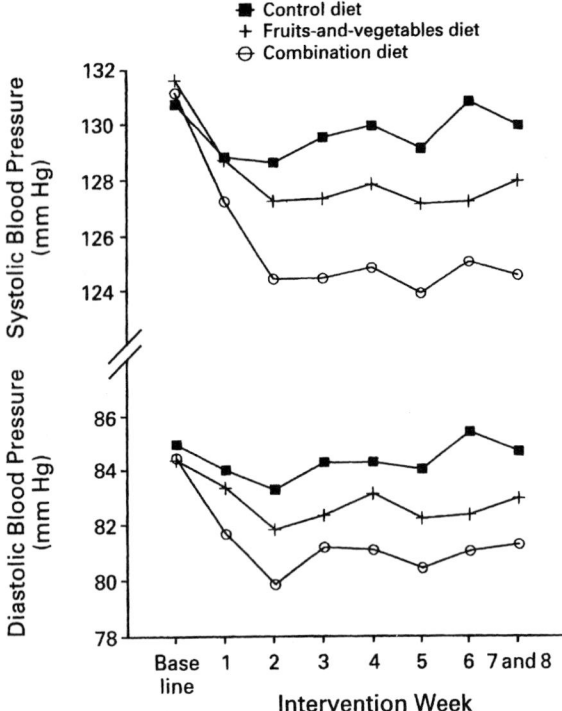

FIGURE 2 Mean systolic and diastolic blood pressures at baseline and during each intervention week, according to diet, for participants in the DASH study. [Reprinted with permission from Ref. [6], Appel, L. J., Moore, T. J., Obarzanek, E., *et al.* (1997). A clinical trial of the effects of dietary patterns on blood pressure. *N. Engl. J. Med.* **336,** 1117–1124.]

body weight, and alcohol consumption were kept constant throughout the intervention.

A total of 459 participants consumed the control diet for the first 3 weeks, and then were randomly assigned to one of the three dietary patterns for an additional 8 weeks. The DASH diet reduced blood pressure by 5.5/3.0 mm Hg (systolic/diastolic) more than the control group (both systolic blood pressure and diastolic blood pressure $p < 0.001$) [6]. The fruits and vegetables diet reduced blood pressures by 2.8/1.1 mm Hg more than the control diet ($p < 0.001$ and $p = 0.07$). The reductions in blood pressures were significant after participants consumed the diets for 2 weeks and were sustained for the following 6 weeks (Fig. 2). In addition, blood pressure lowering was similarly effective in men and women, younger and older persons, and particularly effective among minorities and those who had high blood pressure. These reductions occurred while body weight, sodium intake, alcohol consumption, and exercise patterns remained stable. Among the 133 participants with hypertension (systolic blood pressure ≥ 140 mm Hg; diastolic blood pressure ≥ 90 mm Hg; or both), the combination diet lowered systolic

and diastolic blood pressure by 11.4 and 5.5 mm Hg, respectively. These effects in people with hypertension are similar to reductions seen with single drug therapy.

Even though the DASH trial was not designed to identify specific nutrient(s) responsible for the blood pressure lowering effect, data from the fruits and vegetables group support the hypothesis that increasing potassium, magnesium, and dietary fiber intake reduces blood pressure. In addition, by further lowering total and saturated fat and cholesterol, and increasing low-fat dairy products in the DASH diet, blood pressure reduction was nearly doubled. Because whole-food items rather than single nutrients were manipulated in this trial, other nutrients that were not controlled for in the study, or other beneficial factors as yet unrecognized, may also have contributed to the blood pressure responses. Further research is needed to analyze the specific nutrients or factors responsible for the effect. The nutrient profile of the DASH diet is included in Table 2. Further details on DASH can be found in Appendix 2 and on the following web site: http://dash.bwh.harvard.edu.

V. SUMMARY

The evidence that diet modification can prevent and lower blood pressure is strong, and recommendations are summarized in Table 3. In some cases, the effective intervention strategy and mechanisms involved are still being clarified. Due to various design limitations, inadequate statistical power and measurement issues, studies of single nutrients have generally been inconsistent, except for potassium. However, when multiple nutrients or dietary factors are combined in the same intervention strategy as seen in the DASH study, blood pressure was significantly and effectively reduced. Nutrients may have additive or interactive effects when provided together in the diet. In addition to the DASH pattern, important dietary factors include sodium reduction, weight loss, and avoidance of excessive alcohol. Concurrent adherence to several recommendations is likely to hold the greatest promise for preventing and lowering blood pressure. In addition to addressing unresolved nutritional hypotheses, future research should focus on methods to motivate and maintain dietary changes for blood pressure control. At both the population and individual levels, success in dietary intervention relies on multiple levels of support ranging from clinicians to government agencies to private institutes and industries. In particular, partnering with industry to improve the nutritional value of the food supply, such as reducing the sodium and fat content of processed foods, plays a critical role in implementing dietary changes. Consistent efforts to educate and promote adherence to nutritional guidelines by dietetic and other health care professionals are also instrumental to the prevention and management of hypertension.

TABLE 3 Summary of Evidence Relating Dietary Factors with Blood Pressure

Dietary factors	Strength of relationship with BP[a]	Direction of association	Potential mechanisms	Recommendations	Those most likely to benefit
Sodium	+++	Direct	Changes in blood volume and blood pressure regulating hormones	<65–100 mmol/day	Hypertensives, salt-sensitive individuals, African-Americans, elderly, and those consuming typical American diet
Potassium	+++	Inverse	Vasodilatory; natriuretic	Increase potassium-rich foods	Those on high salt diet
Calcium	+	Inverse	Regulation of parathyroid hormone (PTH) and intracellular calcium; natriuretic	2–3 reduced fat dairy products/day	Possibly salt-sensitive individuals
Magnesium	–	–	Modification of Na-K/ATPase activity	Maintain adequate magnesium intake	Those depleted in magnesium, e.g., from diuretics
Fiber	–	–	Insulin regulation with certain subtypes?	Increase fiber-rich foods for other health benefits	
Fat	++	Direct	Vasodilatory action of prostaglandins (PGE)	Moderate total fat; reduced saturated fat	
Carbohydrates	–	–	Unclear	Consume whole grains	
Protein	+	Inverse	Blood pressure related neurotransmitter by certain amino acids	Consume adequate protein (poultry, fish, nuts, lean meats); limit intake of high fat animal protein	
Alcohol	++	Direct	Unclear	Moderate consumption	Those consuming >2–3 drinks/day
Body weight	+++	Direct	Lowering of blood volume, cardiac output, salt sensitivity, and insulin resistance	Maintain healthy weight; lose weight if overweight	Overweight individuals
Dietary patterns	+++	Depends on factor	Multiple mechanisms, as above	DASH dietary pattern (See Appendix 2)	Those at risk for, or with, hypertension

[a]+++, strong; ++, somewhat consistent and/or likely to benefit certain subgroups; +, data suggestive; –, inconclusive.

APPENDIX 1

Classification of Blood Pressure in Adults Age 18 and Older[a]

Category	Systolic (mm Hg)		Diastolic (mm Hg)
Optimal[b]	<120	and	<80
Normal	<130	and	<85
High–normal	130–139	or	85–89
Hypertension[c]			
Stage 1	140–159	or	90–99
Stage 2	160–179	or	100–109
Stage 3	≥180	or	≥110

Source: The Sixth Report of the Joint National Committee on Prevention, Detection, Evaluation and Treatment of High Blood Pressure, National Institutes of Health, NHLBI, NIH Publication No. 98-4080, November, 1997.

[a]Not taking antihypertensive drugs and not acutely ill. When systolic and diastolic blood pressures fall into different categories, the higher category should be selected to classify the individual's blood pressure status. For example, 160/92 mm Hg should be classified as stage 2 hypertension, and 174/120 mm Hg should be classified as stage 3 hypertension. Isolated systolic hypertension is defined as systolic blood pressure of 140 mm Hg or greater and diastolic blood pressure below 90 mm Hg and staged appropriately (e.g., 170/82 mm Hg is defined as stage 2 isolated systolic hypertension).

[b]Optimal blood pressure with respect to cardiovascular risk is below 120/80 mm Hg. However, unusually low readings should be evaluated for clinical significance.

[c]Based on the average of two or more readings taken at each of two or more visits after an initial screening.

APPENDIX 2

National Institutes of Health

The DASH Diet

This eating plan is from the "Dietary Approaches to Stop Hypertension" (DASH) clinical study. The research was funded by the National Heart, Lung, and Blood Institute (NHLBI), with additional support by the National Center for Research Resources and the Office of Research on Minority Health, all units of the National Institutes of Health. The final results of the DASH study appear in the April 17, 1997, issue of the *New England Journal of Medicine*. The results show that the DASH "combination diet" lowered blood pressure and, so, may help prevent and control high blood pressure.

The "combination diet" is rich in fruits, vegetables, and low-fat dairy foods and low in saturated and total fat. It also is low in cholesterol; high in dietary fiber, potassium, calcium, and magnesium; and moderately high in protein.

The DASH eating plan shown below is based on 2,000 calories a day. Depending on your caloric needs, your number of daily servings in a food group may vary from those listed.

Food Group	Daily Servings	Serving Sizes	Examples and Notes	Significance of Each Food Group to the DASH Diet Pattern
Grains and grain products	7–8	1 slice bread ½ C dry cereal ½ C cooked rice, pasta, or cereal	whole wheat bread, English muffin, pita bread, bagel, cereals, grits, oatmeal	major sources of energy and fiber
Vegetables	4–5	1 C raw leafy vegetable ½ C cooked vegetable 6 oz vegetable juice	tomatoes, potatoes, carrots, peas, squash, broccoli, turnip greens, collards, kale, spinach, artichokes, beans, sweet potatoes	rich sources of potassium, magnesium, and fiber

Fruits	4–5	6 oz fruit juice 1 medium fruit ¼ C dried fruit ¼ C cresh, frozen, or canned fruit	apricots, bananas, dates, grapes, oranges, orange juice, grapefruit, grapefruit juice, mangoes, melons, peaches, pineapples, prunes, raisins, strawberries, tangerines	important sources of potassium, magnesium, and fiber
Low-fat or nonfat dairy foods	2–3	8 oz milk 1 C yogurt 1.5 oz cheese	skim or 1% milk, skim or low-fat buttermilk, nonfat or low-fat yogurt, part-skim mozzarella cheese, nonfat cheese	major sources of calcium and protein
Meats, poultry, and fish	2 or less	3 oz cooked meats, poultry, or fish	select only lean; trim away visible fats; broil, roast, or boil, instead of frying; remove skin from poultry	rich sources of protein and magnesium
Nuts, seeds, and legumes	4–5 per week	1.5 oz or ⅓ C nuts ½ oz or 2 Tbsp seeds ½ C cooked legumes	almonds, filberts, mixed nuts, peanuts, walnuts, sunflower seeds, kidney beans, lentils	rich sources of energy, magnesium, potassium, protein, and fiber

The DASH Diet • Sample Menu • based on 2,000 calories/day

Food	Amount	Servings Provided
Breakfast		
orange juice	6 oz	1 fruit
1% low-fat milk	8 oz (1 C)	1 dairy
corn flakes (with 1 tsp sugar)	1 C	2 grains
banana	1 medium	1 fruit
whole wheat bread (with 1 Tbsp jelly)	1 slice	1 grain
soft margarine	1 tsp	1 fat
Lunch		
chicken salad	¾ C	1 poultry
pita bread	½, large	1 grain
raw vegetable medley:		
carrot and celery sticks	3–4 sticks each	
radishes	2	1 vegetable
loose-leaf lettuce	2 leaves	
part-skim mozzarella cheese	1.5 slice (1.5 oz)	1 dairy
1% low-fat milk	8 oz (1 C)	1 dairy
fruit cocktail in light syrup	½ C	1 fruit
Dinner		
herbed baked cod	3 oz	1 fish
scallion rice	1 C	2 grains
steamed broccoli	½ C	1 vegetable
stewed tomatoes	½ C	1 vegetable
spinach salad:		
raw spinach	½ C	
cherry tomatoes	2	1 vegetable
cucumber	2 slices	
light Italian salad dressing	1 tbsp	½ fat
whole wheat dinner roll	1 small	1 grain
soft margarine	1 tsp	1 fat
melon balls	½ C	1 fruit
Snacks		
dried apricots	1 oz (¼ C)	1 fruit
mini-pretzels	1 oz (¾ C)	1 grain
mixed nuts	1.5 oz (⅓ C)	1 nuts
diet ginger ale	12 oz	0

Total number of servings in 2,000 calories/day menu:

Food Group	Servings
Grains	= 8
Vegetables	= 4
Fruits	= 5
Dairy Foods	= 3
Meats, Poultry, and Fish	= 2
Nuts, Seeds, and Legumes	= 1
Fats and Oils	= 2.5

Tips on Eating the DASH Way

- ❤ Start small. Make gradual changes in your eating habits.

- ❤ Center your meal around carbohydrates, such as pasta, rice, beans, or vegetables

- ❤ Treat meat as one part of the whole meal, instead of the focus.

- ❤ Use fruits or low-fat, low-calorie foods such as sugar-free gelatin for desserts and snacks.

REMEMBER! If you use the DASH diet to help prevent or control high blood pressure, make it a part of a lifestyle that includes choosing foods lower in salt and sodium, keeping a healthy weight, being physically active, and, if you drink alcohol, doing so in moderation.

To learn more about high blood pressure, call 1-800-575-WELL or visit the NHLBI Web site at http://www.nhlbi.nih.gov/nhlbi/nhlbi.htm. DASH is also online at http://dash.bwh.harvard.edu.

Source: The Sixth Report of the Joint National Committee on Prevention, Detection, Evaluation and Treatment of High Blood Pressure, National Institutes of Health, NHLBI, NIH Publication No. 98-4080, November, 1997.

References

1. National Heart Lung and Blood Institute. (1997). "The Sixth Report of the Joint National Committee on Prevention, Detection, Evaluation, and Treatment of High Blood Pressure." National Institutes of Health, Bethesda, MD.

2. Burt, V. L., Whelton, P., Roccella, E. J., Brown, C., Cutler, J. A., Higgins, M., Horan, M. J., and Labarthe, D. (1995). Prevalence of hypertension in the U.S. adult population. Results from the Third National Health and Nutrition Examination Survey, 1988–1991. *Hypertension* **25,** 305–313.

3. Stamler, J. (1991). Blood pressure and high blood pressure. Aspects of risk. *Hypertension* **18,** I-95–I-107.

4. Stamler, J., Neaton, J. D., and Wentworth, D. N. (1989). Blood pressure (systolic and diastolic) and risk of fatal coronary heart disease. *Hypertension* **13,** I-2–I-12.

5. Obarzanek, E., and Moore, T. (1999). Using feeding studies to test the efficacy of dietary interventions: Lessons from the Dietary Approaches to Stop Hypertension trial. *J. Am. Dietet. Assoc.* **99,** S9–S11.

6. Appel, L., Moore, T., Obarzanek, E., Vollmer, W. M., Svetkey, L. P., Sacks, F. M., Bray, G. A., Vogt, T. M., Cutler, J. A., Windhauser, M. M., Lin, P. H., Karanja, N. M., Simons-Morton, D., McCullough, M., Swain, J., Steele, P., Evans, M. A., Miller, E. R., and Harsha, D. W. (1997). A clinical trial of the effects of dietary patterns on blood pressure. *N. Engl. J. Med.* **336,** 1117–1124.

7. Sacks, F. M., Svetkey, L. P., Vollmer, W. M., Appel, L. J., Bray, G. A., Harsha, D., Obarzanek, E., Conlin, P. R., Miller, E. R., Simons-Morton, D. G., Karanja, N M., and Lin, P. H. (2001). Effects on blood pressure of reduced dietary sodium and the Dietary Approaches to Stop Hypertension (DASH) diet. DASH-Sodium Collaborative Research Group. *N. Engl. J. Med.* **344,** 3–10.

8. Denke, M. A., and Obarzanek, E. (1997). The scientific rationale of human feeding studies. *In* "Well-Controlled Diet Studies in Humans" (B. H. Dennis, A. G. Ershow, E. Obarzanek, and B. A. Clevidence, Eds.), pp. 2–9. American Dietetic Association, Chicago, IL.

9. Willett, W. C. (1998). "Nutritional Epidemiology," Second Edition. Oxford University Press, New York.

10. James, G. D., and Baker, P. T. (1990). Human population biology and hypertension. Evolutionary and ecological aspects of blood pressure. *In* "Hypertension: Pathophysiology, Diagnosis and Management" (J. H. Laragh and B. M. Brenner, Eds.), pp. 137–145. Raven Press, Ltd., New York.

11. Knapp, H. R. (1996). Nutritional aspects of hypertension. *In* "Present Knowledge in Nutrition" (E. E. Ziegler and L. J. Filer, Eds.), pp. 438–444. ILSI Press, Washington, DC.

12. Haynes, R. B. (1997). Nature and role of observational studies in public health policy concerning the effects of dietary salt intake on blood pressure. *Am. J. Clin. Nutr.* **65,** 622S–652S.

13. Birkett, N. J. (1998). Comments on a meta-analysis of the relation between dietary calcium intake and blood pressure. *Am. J. Epidemiol.* **148,** 223–228.

14. Stoto, M. A. (1998). Invited commentary on meta-analysis of epidemiologic data: The case of calcium intake and blood pressure. *Am. J. Epidemiol.* **148,** 229–230.

15. Lowenstein, F. W. (1961). Blood-pressure in relation to age and sex in the tropics and subtropics. *Lancet* **1,** 389–392.

16. Page, L. B., Damon, A., and Moellering, R. C. (1974). Antecedents of cardiovascular disease in six Solomon Islands societies. *Circulation* **49,** 1132–1146.

17. Oliver, W. J., Cohen, E. L., and Neel, J. V. (1975). Blood pressure, sodium intake, and sodium related hormones in the Yanomamo Indians, a "no-salt" culture. *Circulation* **52,** 146–151.

18. Carvalho, J. J. M., Baruzzi, R. G., Howard, P. F., Poulter, N., Alpers, M. P., Franco, L., Marcopito, L. F., Spooner, V. J., Dyer, A. R., Elliott, P., Stamler, J., and Stamler, R. (1989). Blood pressure in four remote populations in the INTERSALT study. *Hypertension* **14,** 238–248.

19. Connor, W. E., Cerqueira, M. T., Connor, R. W., Wallace, R. B., Malinow, R., and Casdorph, H. R. (1978). The plasma lipids, lipoproteins, and diet of the Tarahumara Indians of Mexico. *Am. J. Clin. Nutr.* **31,** 1131–1142.

20. Hollenberg, N. K., Martinez, G., McCullough, M., Meinking, T., Passan, D., Preston, M., Rivera, A., Taplin, D., and Vicaria-Clement, M. (1997). Aging, acculturation, salt intake, and hypertension in the Kuna of Panama. *Hypertension* **29,** 171–176.

21. Poulter, N. R., Khaw, K. T., Hopwood, B. E. C., Mugambi, M., Peart, W. S., Rose, G., and Sever, P. S. (1990). The Kenyan Luo migration study: Observations on the initiation of a rise in blood pressure. *Br. Med. J.* **300,** 967–972.

22. He, J., Tell, G. S., Tang, Y.-C., Mo, P.-S., and He, G.-Q. (1991). Effect of migration on blood pressure: The Yi People study. *Epidemiology* **2,** 88–97.

23. Prior, I. A. M. (1974). Cardiovascular epidemiology in New Zealand and the Pacific. *N.Z. Med. J.* **80,** 245–252.

24. Eason, R. J., Pada, J., Wallace, R., Henry, A., and Thornton, R. (1987). Changing patterns of hypertension, diabetes, obesity and diet among Melanesians and Micronesians in the Solomon Islands. *Med. J. Austral.* **146,** 465–473.

25. Zimmet, P., Jackson, L., and Whitehouse, S. (1980). Blood pressure studies in two Pacific populations with varying degrees of modernisation. *N.Z. Med. J.* **91,** 249–252.

26. Hanna, J. M., Pelletier, D. L., and Brown V. J. (1986). The diet and nutrition of contemporary Samoans. *In* "The Changing Samoans: Behavior and Health in Transition" (P. T. Baker, J. M. Hanna, and T. S. Baker, Eds.), pp. 275–296. Oxford University Press, New York.

27. Kaufman, J. S., Owoaje, E. E., James, S. A., Rotimi, C. N., and Cooper, R. S. (1996). Determinants of hypertension in West Africa: Contribution of anthropometric and dietary factors to urban–rural and socioeconomic gradients. *Am. J. Epidemiol.* **143,** 1203–1218.

28. Whiting, S. J., and Mackenzie, M. L. (1998). Assessing the changing diet of indigenous peoples. *Nutr. Rev.* **56,** 248–250.

29. Jerome, N. W. (1997). Culture-specific strategies for capturing local dietary intake patterns. *Am. J. Clin. Nutr.* **65**(Suppl.), 1166S–1167S.

30. Armstrong, B., Van Merwyk, A. J., and Coates, H. (1977). Blood pressure in Seventh-Day Adventist vegetarians. *Am. J. Epidemiol.* **105,** 444–449.

31. Sacks, F. M., Rosner, B., and Kass, E. H. (1974). Blood pressure in vegetarians. *Am. J. Epidemiol.* **100,** 390–398.

32. Burr, M. L., Bates, C. J., Fehily, A. M., and St. Leger, A. S. (1981). Plasma cholesterol and blood pressure in vegetarians. *J. Hum. Nutr.* **35,** 437–441.

33. Beilin, L. J., Rouse, I. L., Armstrong, B. K., Oxon, D., Margetts, B. M., and Vandongen, R. (1988). Vegetarian diet and blood pressure levels: Incidental or causal association? *Am. J. Clin. Nutr.* **48**, 806–810.

34. Margetts, B. M., Beilin, L. J., Vandongen, R., and Armstrong, B. K. (1986). Vegetarian diet in mild hypertension: A randomised controlled trial. *Br. Med. J.* **293**, 1468–1471.

35. Deleted in proof.

36. Rouse, I. L., Beilin, L. J., Armstrong, B. K., and Vandongen, R. (1983). Blood-pressure-lowering effect of a vegetarian diet: Controlled trial in normotensive subjects. *Lancet* **i**, 5–10.

37. Reed, D., McGee, Yano, K., and Hankin, J. (1985). Diet, blood pressure, and multicollinearity. *Hypertension* **7**, 405–410.

38. Luft, F. C., Miller, J. Z., Weinberger, M. H., Christian, J. C., and Skrabal, F. (1988). Genetic influences on the response to dietary salt reduction, acute salt loading, or salt depletion in humans. *J. Cardiovasc. Pharmacol.* **12**, S49–S55.

39. Sowers, J. R., Zemel, M. B., Zemel, P. C., and Standley, P. R. (1991). Calcium metabolism and dietary calcium in salt sensitive hypertension. *Am. J. Hypertens.* **4**, 557–563.

40. Cutler, J. A. (1999). The effects of reducing sodium and increasing potassium intake for control of hypertension and improving health. *Clin. Exp. Hypertens.* **21**, 769–783.

41. McCarron, D. A. (2000). The dietary guideline for sodium: Should we shake it up? Yes! *Am. J. Clin. Nutr.* **71**, 1013–1019.

42. Kaplan, N. M. (2000). The dietary guideline for sodium: Should we shake it up? No. *Am. J. Clin. Nutr.* **71**, 1020–1026.

43. Cutler, J. A., Follmann, D., and Allender, P. S. (1997). Randomized trials of sodium reduction: An overview. *Am. J. Clin. Nutr.* **65**, 643S–651S.

44. Law, M. R., Frost, C. D., and Wald, N. J., III (1991). Analysis of data from trials of salt reduction. *Br. Med. J.* **302**, 819–824.

45. Graudal, N. A., Galloe, A. M., and Garred, P. (1998). Effects of sodium restriction on blood pressure, renin, aldosterone, catecholamines, cholesterols, and triglyceride. A meta-analysis. *JAMA* **279**, 1383–1391.

46. Alderman, M. H., and Lamport, B. (1990). Moderate sodium restriction: Do the benefits justify the hazards? *Am. J. Hypertens.* **3**, 499–504.

47. Luft, F. C. (1988). Sodium: Complexities in a simple relationship. *Hosp. Prac.* 73–80.

48. Kumanyika, S. K., and Cutler, J. A. (1997). Dietary sodium reduction: Is there cause for concern? *J. Am. College Nutr.* **16**, 192–203.

49. Pietinen, P., and Tuomilehto, J. (1980). Estimating sodium intake in epidemiological studies. *In* "Epidemiology of Arterial Blood Pressure" (H. Kestleloot and J. V. Joossens, Eds.), pp. 29–44.

50. Dyer, A. R., Elliott, P., and Shipley, M. (1994). Urinary electrolyte excretion in 24 hours and blood pressure in the INTERSALT study II. Estimates of electrolyte–blood pressure associations corrected for regression dilution bias. *Am. J. Epidemiol.* **139**, 940–951.

51. Frost, C. D., Law, M. R., and Wald, N. J. (1991). Analysis of observational data within populations. *Br. Med. J.* **302**, 815–818.

52. Dahl, L. (1960). Possible role of salt intake in the development of hypertension. *In* "Essential Hypertension: An International Symposium" (P. Cottier and K. D. Bock, Eds.), pp. 53–65. Springer-Verlag, Berling.

53. Elliott, P. (1991). Observational studies of salt and blood pressure. *Hypertension* **17**(Suppl.), I-3–I-8.

54. Intersalt Cooperative Research Group. (1988). Intersalt: An international study of electrolyte excretion and blood pressure: Results for 24-hour urinary sodium and potassium excretion. *Br. Med. J.* **297**, 319–328.

55. Stamler, J. (1997). The INTERSALT study: Background, methods, findings and implications. *Am. J. Clin. Nutr.* **65** (Suppl.), 626S–642s.

56. Law, M. R., Frost, C. D.,and Wald, N. J. (1991). By how much does dietary salt reduction lower blood pressure? I. Analysis of observational data among populations. *Br. Med. J.* **302**, 811–814.

57. Alderman, M. H., Cohen, H., and Madhavan, S. (1998). Dietary sodium intake and mortality: The National Health and Nutrition Examination Survey (NHANES I). *Lancet* **351**, 781–785.

58. Tunstall-Pedoe, H. (1999). Does dietary potassium lower blood pressure and protect against coronary heart disease and death? Findings from the Scottish Heart Health Study. *Semin. Nephrol.* **19**, 500–502.

59. de Wardener, H. E. (1999). Salt reduction and cardiovascular risk: The anatomy of a myth. *J. Hum. Hypertens.* **13**, 1–4.

60. He, J., Ogden, L. G., Vupputuri, S., Bazzano, L. A., Loria, C., and Whelton, P. K. (1999). Dietary sodium intake and subsequent risk of cardiovascular disease in overweight adults. *JAMA* **282**, 2027–2034.

61. Kempner, W. (1948). Treatment of hypertensive vascular disease with rice diet. *Am. J. Med.* **4**, 545–577.

62. Midgley, J. P., Matthew, A. G., Greenwood, C. M. T., and Logan, A. G. (1996). Effect of reduced dietary sodium on blood pressure. *JAMA* **275**, 1590–1597.

63. Chobanian, A. V., and Hill, M. (2000). National Heart, Lung, and Blood Institute workshop on sodium and blood pressure. A critical review of current scientific evidence. *Hypertension* **35**, 858–863.

64. Whelton, P. K., Appel, L. J., Espeland, M. A., Applegate, W. B., Ettingter, W. H., Kostis, J. B., Kumanyika, S., Lacy, C. R., Johnson, K. C., Folmar, S., and Cutler, J. A. (1998). Sodium reduction and weight loss in the treatment of hypertension in older persons: A randomized controlled trial of nonpharmacologic interventions in the elderly (TONE). TONE Collaborative Research Group. *JAMA* **279**, 839–846.

65. The Trials of Hypertension Prevention Collaborative Research Group. (1997). Effects of weight loss and sodium reduction intervention on BP and hypertension incidence in overweight people with high-normal blood pressure: The Trials of Hypertension Prevention, Phase II. *Arch. Intern. Med.* **157**, 657–667.

66. Weinberger, M. H., Miller, J. Z., Luft, F. C., Grim, C. E., and Fineberg, N. S. (1986). Definitions and characteristics of sodium sensitivity and blood pressure resistance. *Hypertension* **8**, II-127–II-134.

67. Kawasaki, T., Delea, C. S., Bartter, F. C., and Smith, H. (1978). The effect of high-sodium and low-sodium intakes on blood pressure and other related variables in human subjects with idiopathic hypertension. *Am. J. Med.* **64**, 193–198.

68. Fujita, T., Henry, W. L., Bartter, F. C., Lake, C. R., and Delea, C. S. (1980). Factors influencing blood pressure in salt-sensitive patients with hypertension. *Am. J. Med.* **69**, 334–344.

69. Luft, F. C., and Weinberger, M. H. (1997). Heterogeneous responses to changes in dietary salt intake: The salt-sensitivity paradigm. *Am. J. Clin. Nutr.* **65**, 612S–617S.

70. Falkner, B. (1988). Sodium sensitivity: A determinant of essential hypertension. *J. Am. College Nutr.* **7**, 35–41.

71. Williams, G. H., and Hollenberg, N. K. (1985). "Sodium-sensitive" essential hypertension. Emerging insights into pathogenesis and therapeutic implications. *In* "Contemporary Nephrology" (S. Klahr and S. G. Massry, Eds.), pp. 303–331. Plenum Publishing Corporation.

72. Zemel, M. B., Kraniak, J., Standley, P. R., and Sowers, J. R. (1988). Erythrocyte cation metabolism in salt-sensitive hypertensive blacks as affected by dietary sodium and calcium. *Am. J. Hypertens.* **1**, 386–392.

73. Kotchen, T. A., and Kotchen, J. M. (1997). Dietary sodium and blood pressure: Interactions with other nutrients. *Am. J. Clin. Nutr.* **65**, 708S–711s.

74. Hunt, S. C., Cook, N. R., Oberman, A., Cutler, J. A., Hennekens, C. H., Allender, P. S., Walker, W. G., Whelton, P. K., and Williams, R. R. (1998). Angiotensinogen genotype, sodium reduction, weight loss, and prevention of hypertension. Trials of Hypertension Prevention, Phase II. *Hypertension* **32**, 393–401.

75. Kumanyika, S. K., Hebert, P. R., Cutler, J. A., Lasser, V. I., Sugars, C. P., Steffen-Batey, L., Brewer, A. A., Cameron, M., Shepek, L. D., Cook, N. R., and Miller, S. T. (1993). Feasibility and efficacy of sodium reduction in the Trials of Hypertension Prevention, Phase I. *Hypertension* **22**, 502–512.

76. National Heart Lung and Blood Institute (1996). "Implementing Recommendations for Dietary Salt Reduction," pp. 1–28. National Institutes of Health, Bethesda, MD.

77. Luft, F. C., Weinberger, M. H., Grim, C. E., and Fineberg, N. S. (1986). Effects of volume expansion and contraction on potassium homeostasis in normal and hypertensive humans. *J. Am. College Nutr.* **5**, 357–369.

78. Ophir, O., Peer, G., Gilad, J., Blum, M., and Aviram, A. (1983). Low blood pressure in vegetarians: The possible role of potassium. *Am. J. Clin. Nutr.* **37**, 755–762.

79. Whelton, P. K., He, J., Cutler, J. A., Brancati, F. L., Appel, L. J., Follmann, D., and Klag, M. J. (1997). Effects of oral potassium on blood pressure. Meta-analysis of randomized controlled clinical trials. *JAMA* **277**, 1624–1632.

80. Cappuccio, F. P., and MacGregor, G. A. (1991). Does potassium supplementation lower blood pressure? A meta-analysis of published trials. *J. Hypertens.* **9**, 465–473.

81. Sacks, F. M., Willett, W. C., Smith, A., Brown, L. E., Rosner, B., and Moore, T. J. (1998). Effect on blood pressure of potassium, calcium, and magnesium in women with low habitual intake. *Hypertension* **31**, 131–138.

82. Crawford, M. D., Gardner, M. J., and Morris, J. N. (1968). Mortality and hardness of local water supplies. *Lancet* **1**, 827–831.

83. Cutler, J. A., and Brittain, E. (1990). Calcium and blood pressure. An epidemiologic perspective. *Am. J. Hypertens.* **3**, 137S–146S.

84. Cappuccio, F. P., Elliott, P., Allender, P. S., Pryer, J., Follman, D. A., and Cutler, J. A. (1995). Epidemiologic association between dietary calcium intake and blood pressure: A meta-analysis of published data. *Am. J. Epidemiol.* **142**, 935–945.

85. Addison, W. L. T., and Clark, H. G. (1924). Calcium and potassium chlorides in the treatment of arterial hypertension. *Can. Med. Assoc. J.* **15**, 913–915.

86. Cappuccio, F. P., Siani, A., and Strazzullo, P. (1989). Oral calcium supplementation and blood pressure: An overview of randomized controlled trials. *J. Hypertens.* **7**, 941–946.

87. Bucher, H. C., Cook, R. J., Guyatt, G. H., Lang, J. D., Cook, D. J., Hatala, R., and Hunt, D. (1986). Effects of dietary calcium supplementation on blood pressure. *JAMA* **275**, 1016–1022.

88. Allender, P. S., Cutler, J. A., Follmann, D., Cappuccio, F. P., Pryer, J., and Elliott, P. (1996). Dietary calcium and blood pressure: A meta-analysis of randomized clinical trials. *Ann. Intern. Med.* **124**, 825–831.

89. Griffith, L. E., Guyatt, G. H., Cook, R. J., Bucher, H. C., and Cook, D. J. (1999). The influence of dietary and nondietary calcium supplementation on blood pressure. An updated meta-analysis of randomized controlled trials. *Am. J. Hypertens.* **12**, 84–92.

90. Cappuccio, F. P. (1999). The "calcium antihypertension theory." *Am. J. Hypertens.* **12**, 93–95.

91. Kynast-Gales, S. A., and Massey, L. K. (1992). Effects of dietary calcium from dairy products on ambulatory blood pressure in hypertensive men. *J. Am. Diet. Assoc.* **92**, 1497–1501.

92. Saito, K., Sano, H., Furuta, Y., and Fukuzaki, H. (1989). Effect of oral calcium on blood pressure response in salt-loaded borderline hypertensive patients. *Hypertension* **13**, 219–226.

93. Rich, G. M., McCullough, M., Olmedo, A., Malarick, C., and Moore, T. J. (1991). Blood pressure and renal blood flow responses to dietary calcium and sodium intake in humans. *Am. J. Hypertens.* **4**, 642S–645S.

94. McCarron, D. A. (1997). Role of adequate dietary calcium intake in the prevention and management of salt-sensitive hypertension. *Am. J. Clin. Nutr.* **65**, 712S–716S.

95. Yang, C. Y., and Chin, H. F. (1999). Calcium and magnesium in drinking water and risk of death from hypertension. *Am. J. Hypertens.* **12**, 894–899.

96. Joffres, M. R., Reed, D. M., and Yano, K. (1987). Relationship of magnesium intake and other dietary factors to blood pressure: The Honolulu heart study. *Am. J. Clin. Nutr.* **45**, 469–475.

97. Ascherio, A., Rimm, E., Giovannucci, E. L., Colditz, G. A., Rosner, B., Willett, W. C., Sacks, F., and Stampfer, M. J. (1992). A prospective study of nutritional factors and hypertension among U.S. men. *Circulation* **86**, 1475–1484.

98. Witteman, J. C. M., Willett, W. C., Stampfer, M. J., Colditz, G. A., Sacks, F. M., Speizer, F. E., Rosner, B., and Hennekens, C. H. (1989). A prospective study of nutritonal factors and hypertension among U.S. women. *Circulation* **80**, 1320–1327.

99. Moore, T. J. (1989). The role of dietary electrolytes in hypertension. *J. Am. College Nutr.* **8**, 1–12.

100. Dyckner, T., and Wester, P. O. (1983). Effect of magnesium on blood pressure. *Br. Med. J.* **286**, 1847–1849.

101. Reyes, A. J., and Leary, W. P., Acosta-Barrios, T. N., and Davis, W. H. (1984). Magnesium supplementation in hypertension treated with hydrochlorothiazide. *Curr. Ther. Res.* **36**, 332–340.

102. Cappuccio, F. P., Markandu, N. D., Beynon, G. W., Shore, A. C., Sampson, B., and MacGregor, G. A. (1985). Lack of

effect of oral magnesium on high blood pressure: A double blind study. *Br. Med. J.* **291,** 235–238.

103. Henderson, D. G., Schierup, J., and Schodt, T. (1986). Effect of magnesium supplementation on blood pressure and electrolyte concentrations in hypertensive patients receiving long term diuretic treatment. *Br. Med. J.* **293,** 664–665.

104. Nowson, C. A., and Morgan, T. O. (1989). Magnesium supplementation in mild hypertensive patients on a moderately low sodium diet. *Clin. Exp. Pharm. Physiol.* **16,** 299–302.

105. Zemel, P. C., Zemel, M. B., Urberg, M., Douglas, F. L., Geiser, R., and Sowers, J. R. (1990). Metabolic and hemodynamic effects of magnesium supplementation in patients with essential hypertension. *Am. J. Clin. Nutr.* **51,** 665–669.

106. Yamamato, M. E., Applegate, W. B., Klag, M. J., Borhani, N. O., Cohen, J. D., Kirchner, K. A., Lakatos, E., Sacks, F. M., Taylor, J. O., and Hennekens, C. H. (1995). Lack of blood pressure effect with calcium and magnesium supplementation in adults with high-normal blood pressure. Results from Phase I of the Trials of Hypertension Prevention (TOHP). *Ann. Epidemiol.* **5,** 96–107.

107. Wirell, M. P., Wester, P. O., and Stegmayr, B. G. (1994). Nutritional dose of magnesium in hypertensive patients on beta blockers lowers systolic blood pressure: A double-blind, cross-over study. *J. Intern. Med.* **236,** 189–195.

108. Witteman, J. C. M., Grobbee, D. E., Derkx, F. H. M., Bouillon, R., de Bruijn, A. M., and Hofman, A. (1994). Reduction of blood pressure with oral magnesium supplementation in women with mild to moderate hypertension. *Am. J. Clin. Nutr.* **60,** 129–135.

109. Sacks, F. M., Brown, L. E., Appel, L., Borhani, N. O., Evans, D., and Whelton, P. (1995). Combinations of potassium, calcium, and magnesium supplements in hypertension. *Hypertension* **26,** 950–956.

110. Kawano, Y., Matsuoka, H., Takishita, S., and Omae, T. (1998). Effects of magnesium supplementation in hypertensive patients. Assessment by office, home, and ambulatory blood pressures. *Hypertension* **32,** 260–265.

111. Lind, L., Lithell, H., Pollare, T., and Ljunghall, S. (1991). Blood pressure response during long-term treatment with magnesium is dependent on magnesium status. A double-blind, placebo-controlled study in essential hypertension and in subjects with high-normal blood pressure. *Am. J. Hypertens.* **4,** 674–679.

112. Meyer, T., Anderson, S., and Brenner, B. (1985). Dietary protein intake and the course of renal disease: The role of capillary hypertension and hyperfusion in the pathogenesis of progressive glomerular sclerosis. *In* "NIH Workshop on Nutrition and Hypertension: Proceedings from a Symposium" (M. Horan, M. Blaustein, J. Dunbar, W. Kachadorian, N. Kaplan, and A. Simopoulos, Eds.). Biomedical Information Corp., New York.

113. Elliott, P., Freeman, J., Pryer, J., Brunner, E., and Marmot, M. (1992). Dietary protein and blood pressure: A report from the Dietary and Nutritonal Survey of British Adults [abstract]. *J. Hypertens.* **10,** S141.

114. Stamler, J., Caggiula, A., and Grandits, G. (1992). Relationships of dietary variables to blood pressure (BP): Findings of the Multiple Risk Factor Intervention Trial (MRFIT) [abstract]. *Circulation* **85,** 867.

115. Stamler, J., Elliott, P., Kesteloot, H., Nichols, R., Claeys, G., Dyer, A. R., and Stamler, R. (1996). Inverse relation of dietary protein markers with blood pressure. Findings for 10,020 men and women in the INTERSALT Study. *Circulation* **94,** 1629–1634.

116. Obarzanek, E., Velletri, P., and Cutler, J. (1996). Dietary protein and blood pressure. **275,** 1598–1603.

117. Yamori, Y., Horie, R., Nara, Y., Ikeda, M., Ooshima, A., and Fukase, M. (1981). Genetics of hypertensive diseases: Experimental studies on pathogenesis, detection of predisposition and prevention. *Adv. Neprhol.* **10,** 51–74.

118. Chapman, C., Gibbons, T., and Henschel, A. (1950). The effect of the rice-fruit diet on the composition of the body. *N. Engl. J. Med.* **243,** 899–905.

119. Hatch, F., Wertheim, A., Eurman, G., Watkin, D., Froeb, H., and Epstein, H. (1954). Effects of diet on essential hypertension, III: Alterations in sodium chloride, protein, and fat intake. *Am. J. Med.* **17,** 499–513.

120. Brussaard, J., van Raakj, J., Strasse-Wolthuis, M., Katan, M., and Hautvast, J. (1981). Blood pressure and diet in normotensive volunteers: Absence of an effect of dietary fiber, protein, or fat. *Am. J. Clin. Nutr.* **34,** 2023–2029.

121. Sacks, F., Donner, A., Castelli, W., Gronemeyer, J., Pletka, P., Margolius, H. S., Landsberg, L., and Kass, E. H. (1981). Effect of ingestion of meat on plasma cholesterol of vegetarians. *JAMA* **246,** 640–644.

122. Sacks, F., Wood, P., and Kass, E. (1984). Stability of blood pressure in vegetarians receiving dietary protein supplements. *Hypertension* **6,** 199–201.

123. Prescott, S., Jenner, D., Beilin, L., Margetts, B., and Vandongen, R. (1987). Controlled study of the effects of dietary protein on blood pressure in normotensive humans. *Clin. Exp. Pharm. Physiol.* **14,** 159–162.

124. Sacks, F., and Kass, E. (1988). Low blood pressure in vegetarians: Effects of specific foods and nutrients. *Am. J. Clin. Nutr.* **48,** 795–800.

125. Kestin, M., Rouse, I., Correll, R., and Nestel, P. J. (1989). Cardiovascular disease risk factors in free-living men: Comparison of two prudent diets, one based on lactoovovegetarianism and the other allowing lean meat. *Am. J. Clin. Nutr.* **50,** 280–287.

126. Buonopane, G., Kilara, A., Smith, J., and McCarthy, R. (1992). Effect of skim milk supplementation on blood cholesterol concentration, blood pressure, and triglycerides in a free-living human population. *J. Am. College Nutr.* **11,** 56–67.

127. Liu, K., Ruth, K., Flack, J., Burke, G., Savage, P., Liang, K-Y., Hardin, M., and Hulley, S. (1992). Ethnic differences in 5-year blood pressure change in young adults: The CARDIA study [abstract]. *Circulation* **85,** 867.

128. Liu, K., Ruth, K., Shekelle, R., and Stamler, J. (1993). Macronutrients and long-term change in systolic blood pressure [abstract]. *Circulation* **87,** 679.

129. Zhou, B., Zhang, X., Zhu, A., Zhao, L., Zhu, S., Ruan, L., Zhu, L., Liang, S. (1994). The relationship of dietary animal protein and electrolytes to blood pressure: A study on three Chinese populations. *Int. J. Epidemiol.* **23,** 716–722.

130. Moncada, S., and Higgs, A. (1993). The L-arginine-nitric oxide pathway. *N. Engl. J. Med.* **329,** 2002–2012.

131. Washburn, S., Burke, G., Morgan, T., and Anthony, M. (1999). Effect of soy protein supplementation on serum lipoproteins, blood pressure, and menopausal symptoms in perimenopausal women. *Menopause* **6,** 7–13.

132. Simon, A. H., Lima, P. R. M., Ribeiro Alves, A. V. F., Bottini, P. V., and Lopes de Faria, J. B. (1998). Renal haemodynamic responses to a chicken or beef meal in normal individuals. *Nephrol. Dial. Transplant* **13,** 2261–2264.

133. Hollenberg, N. K., Rivera, A., Meinking, T., Martinez, G., McCullough, M., Passan, P., Preston, M., Taplin, D., and Vicaria-Clement, M. (1999). Age, renal perfusion and function in island-dwelling indigenous Kuna Amerinds of Panama. *Nephron* **82,** 131–138.

134. Elliott, P., Fehily, A., Sweetnam, P., and Yarnell, J. (1987). Diet, alcohol, body mass, and social factors in relation to blood pressure: The Caerphilly Heart Study. *J. Epidemiol. Commun. Health* **41,** 37–43.

135. Salonen, J., Ruomilehto, J., and Tanskanen, A. (1983). Relation of blood pressure to reported intake of salt, saturated fats, and alcohol in healthy middle-aged population. *J. Epidemiol. Commun. Health* **37,** 7.

136. Salonen, J., Salonen, R., Ihalainen, M., Parviainen, M., Seppanen, R., Kantola, M., Seppanen, K., and Rauramaa, R. (1988). Blood pressure, dietary fats, and antioxidants. *Am. J. Clin. Nutr.* **48,** 1226–1232.

137. Gruchow, H., Sobocinski, K., and Barboriak, J. (1985). Alcohol, nutrient intake and hypertension in U.S. adults. *JAMA* **253,** 1567–1570.

138. Sandstrom, B., Marckmann, P., and Bindslev, N. (1992). An eight-month controlled study of a low-fat high-fiber diet: Effects on blood lipids and blood pressure in healthy young subjects. *Eur. J. Clin. Nutr.* **46,** 95–109.

139. Judd, J., Marshall, M., and Dupont, J. (1989). Relationship of dietary fat to plasma fatty acids, blood pressure, and urinary eicosanoids in adult men. *J. Am. College Nutr.* **8,** 386–399.

140. Mensink, R., Janssen, M., and Katan, M. (1988). Effect on blood pressure of two diets differing in total fat but not in saturated and polyunsaturated fatty acids in healthy volunteers. *Am. J. Clin. Nutr.* **47,** 976–980.

141. Straznicky, N., O'Callaghan, C., Barrington, V., and Louis, W. (1999). Hypotensive effect of low-fat, high carbohydrate diet can be independent of changes in plasma insulin concentrations. *Hypertension* **34**(4, Part 1), 580–585.

142. Aro, A., Peitinen, P., Valsta, L. M., Salminen, I., Turpeinen, A. M., Virtanen, M., Dougherty, R. M., and Iacono, J. M. (1998). Lack of effect on blood pressure by low fat diets with different fatty acids compositions. *J. Hum. Hypertens.* **12,** 383–389.

143. National Diet Heart Study Research Group. (1968). The National Diet Heart Study Final Report. *Circulation* **37,38,** I-228–I-230.

144. Stamler, J., Ruth, K. J., Liu, K., and Shekelle, R. B. (1994). Dietary anti-oxidants and blood pressure change in the Western Electric Study 1958–66 [abstract]. *Circulation* **89,** 932.

145. Sacks, F., Marais, G., Handysides, G., Salazar, J., Miller, L., Foster, J. M., Rosner, B., and Kass, E. H. (1984). Lack of an effect of dietary saturated fat and cholesterol on blood pressure in normotensives. *Hypertension* **6,** 193–198.

146. Mori, T., Bao, D., Burke, V., Puddey, I., and Beilin, L. (1999). Docosahexaenoic acid but not eicosapentaenoic acid lowers ambulatory blood pressure and heart rate in humans. *Hypertension* **34,** 253–260.

147. Morris, M., Sacks, F., and Rosner, B. (1993). Does fish oil lower blood pressure? A meta-analysis of controlled trials. *Circulation* **88,** 523–533.

148. Margolin, G., Huster, G., Glueck, C. J., Speirs, J., Vandegrift, J., Illig, E., Su, J., Streicher, P., and Tracy, T. (1991). Blood pressure lowering in elderly subjects: A double-blind crossover study of w-3 and w-6 fatty acids. *Am. J. Clin. Nutr.* **53,** 562–572.

149. Ferrara, A., Raimondi, A. S., d'Episcopo, L., Guida, L., dello Russo, A., and Marotta, T. (2000). Olive oil and reduced need for antihypertensive medications. *Arch. Intern. Med.* **160,** 837–842.

150. Thomsen, C., Rasmussen, O., Hansen, K., Versterlund, M., and Hermansen, K. (1995). Comparison of the effects on the diurnal blood pressure, glucose, and lipid levels of a diet rich in monounsaturated fatty acids with a diet rich in polyunsaturated fatty acids in type 2 diabetic subjects. *Diabet. Med.* **12,** 600–606.

151. Nielsen, S., Hermansen, K., Rasmussen, O., Thomsen, C., and Mogensen, C. (1995). Urinary albumin excretion rate and 24-h ambulatory blood pressure in NIDDM with microalbuminuria: Effects of a monounsaturated enriched diet. *Diabetologia* **38,** 1069–1075.

152. Ruiz-Gutierrez, V., Muriana, F. J. G., Guerrero, A., Cert, A. M., and Villar, J. (1996). Plasma lipids, erythrocyte membrane lipids and blood pressure of hypertensive women after ingestion of dietary oleic acid from two different sources. *J. Hypertens.* **14,** 1483–1490.

153. Lijnen, P., Fagard, R., Staessen, J., Thijs, L., and Amery, A. (1992). Erythrocyte membrane lipids and cationic transport system in men. *J. Hypertens.* **10,** 1205–1211.

154. Dunn, M., and Grone, H. J. (1985). The relevance of prostaglandins in human hypertension. *Adv. Prostagland. Thrombox. Leukotr. Res.* **13,** 179–187.

155. Adam, O., and Wolfram, G. (1984). Effect of different linoleic acid intakes on prostaglandin biosynthesis and kidney function in man. *Am. J. Clin. Nutr.* **40,** 763–770.

156. Epstein, M., Lifschitz, M., and Rappaport, K. (1982). Augmentation of prostaglandin production by linoleic acid in man. *Clin. Sci.* **63,** 565–571.

157. Ahrens, R. A., Demuth, P., Lee, M. K., and Majkowski, J. W. (1980). Moderate sucrose ingestion and blood pressure in the rat. *J. Nutr.* **110,** 725–731.

158. Preuss, H. G., Knapka, J. J., MacArthy, P., Yousufi, A. K., Sabnis, S. G., and Antonovych, T. T. (1992). High sucrose diets increase blood pressure of both salt-sensitive and salt-resistant rats. *Am. J. Hypertens.* **5,** 585–591.

159. Preuss, H. G., Zein, M., MacArthy, P., Dipette, D., Sabnis, S., and Knapka, J. (1998). Sugar-induced blood pressure elevations over the lifespan of three substrains of Wistar rats. *J. Am. College Nutr.* **17,** 36–47.

160. Hodges, R., and Rebello, T. (1983). Carbohydrates and blood pressure. *Ann. Intern. Med.* **98,** 838–841.

161. Palumbo, P. J., Briones, E. R., Nelson, R. A., and Kottke, B. A. (1977). Sucrose sensitivity of patients with coronary-artery disease. *Am. J. Clin. Nutr.* **30,** 394–401.

162. Surwit, R. S., Feinglos, M. N., McCaskill, C. C., Clay, S. L., Babyak, R. A., Brownlow, B. S., Plaisted, C. S., and Lin, P. H.

(1997). Metabolic and behavioral effects of a high-sucrose diet during weight loss. *Am. J. Clin. Nutr.* **65,** 908–915.

163. Koh, E., and Ard, N. (1988). Effects of fructose feeding on blood parameters and blood pressure in impaired glucose-tolerant subjects. *J. Am. Dietet. Assoc.* **88,** 932–938.

164. Hallfrisch, J., Reiser, S., and Prather, E. S. (1983). Blood lipid distribution of hyperinsulinemic men consuming three levels of fructose. *Am. J. Clin. Nutr.* **37,** 740–748.

165. Jansen, R., Penterman, B., Van Lier, H., and Hoefnagels, W. (1987). Blood pressure reduction after oral glucose loading and its relation to age, blood pressure and insulin. *Am. J. Cardiol.* **60,** 1087–1091.

166. He, J., and Whelton, P. K. (1999). Effect of dietary fiber and protein intake on blood pressure: A review of epidemiologic evidence. *Clin. Exp. Hypertens.* **21,** 785–796.

167. Ascerio, A., Stampfer, M. J., Colditz, G. A., Willett, W. C., and McKinlay, J. (1991). Nutrient intakes and blood pressure in normotensive males. *Int. J. Epidemiol.* **20,** 886–891.

168. Spiegelman, D., Israel, R. G., Bouchard, C., and Willett, W. C. (1992). Absolute fat mass, percent body fat, and body-fat distribution: Which is the real determinant of blood pressure and serum glucose? *Am. J. Clin. Nutr.* **55,** 1033–1044.

169. Stamler, J. (1991). Epidemiologic findings on weight and blood pressure in adults. *Ann. Epidemiol.* **1,** 347–362.

170. Harlan, W. R., Hull, A. L., Schmouder, R. L., Landis, J. R., Thompson, E. E., and Larkin, F. A. (1984). Blood pressure and nutrition in adults. The national health and nutrition examination survey. *Am. J. Epidemiol.* **120,** 17–28.

171. Ford, E. S., and Cooper, R. S. (1991). Risk factors for hypertension in a national cohort study. *Hypertension* **18,** 598–606.

172. Okosun, I. S., Prewitt, T. E., and Cooper, R. S. (1999). Abdominal obesity in the United States: Prevalence and attributable risk of hypertension. *J. Hum. Hypertens.* **13,** 425–430.

173. Dunstan, H. P., and Weinsier, R. L. (1991). Treatment of obesity-associated hypertension. *Ann. Epidemiol.* **1,** 371–379.

174. Rocchini, A. P., Key, J., Bondie, D., Chico, R., Moorehead, C., Katch, V., and Marti. (1989). The effect of weight loss on the sensitivity of blood pressure to sodium in obese adolescents. *N. Engl. J. Med.* **321,** 580–585.

175. McKnight, J. A., and Moore, T. J. (1994). The effects of dietary factors on blood pressure. *Comp. Ther.* **20,** 511–517.

176. Stamler, R., Stamler, J., Gosch, F. C., Civinelli, J., Fishman, J., McKeever, P., McDonald, A., and Dyer, A. R. (1989). Primary prevention of hypertension by nutritional-hygienic means. Final report of a randomized, controlled trial. *JAMA* **262,** 1801–1807.

177. Hypertension Prevention Trial Research Group. (1990). The hypertension prevention trial: Three-year effects of dietary changes on blood pressure. *Arch. Intern. Med.* **150,** 153–162.

178. Stevens, V. J., Corrigan, S. A., Obarzanek, E., Bernauer, E., Cook, N. R., Hebert, P., Mattfeldt-Beman, M., Oberman, A., Sugars, C., Dalcin, A. T., and Whelton, P. K. (1993). Weight loss intervention in Phase I of the trials of hypertension prevention. *Arch. Intern. Med.* **153,** 849–858.

179. The Trials of Hypertension Prevention Collaborative Research Group. (1992). The effects of nonpharmacologic interventions on blood pressure of persons with high normal levels. Results of the Trials of Hypertension, Phase I. *JAMA* **267,** 1213–1220.

180. He, J., Whelton, P. K., Appel, L. J., Charleston, J., and Klag, M. J. (2000). Long-term effects of weight loss and dietary sodium reduction on incidence of hypertension. *Hypertension* **35,** 544–549.

181. Expert Panel on the Identification, Evaluation, and Treatment of Overweight in Adults. (1998). Clinical guidelines on the identification, evaluation, and treatment of overweight and obesity in adults: Executive summary. *Am. J. Clin. Nutr.* **68,** 899–917.

182. Arakawa, K. (1999). Exercise, a measure to lower blood pressure and reduce other risks. *Clin. Exp. Hypertens.* **21,** 797–803.

183. Cutler, J. (1991). Randomized clinical trials of weight reduction in nonhypertensive persons. *Ann. Epidemiol.* **1,** 363–370.

184. MacMahon, S. (1987). Alcohol consumption and hypertension. **9,** 111–121.

185. Klatsky, A. L., Friedman, G. D., and Armstrong, M. A. (1986). The relationships between alcoholic beverage use and other traits to blood pressure: A new Kaiser-Permanente study. *Circulation* **73,** 628–636.

186. Witteman, J. C., Willett, W. C., Stampfer, M. J., Colditz, G. A., Kok, F. J., Sacks, F. M., Speizer, F. E., Rosner, B., and Hennekens, C. H. (1990). Relation of moderate alcohol consumption and risk of systemic hypertension in women. *Am. J. Cardiol.* **65,** 633–637.

187. Gordon, T., and Doyle, J. T. (1986). Alcohol consumption and its relationship to smoking, weight, blood pressure, and blood lipids. *Arch. Intern. Med.* **146,** 262–265.

188. Cushman, W. C., Cutler, J. A., Bingham, S. F., Harford, T., Hanna, E., Dubbert, P., Collins, J. F., Dufour, M., Follman, D., and Allender, P. S. (1994). Prevention and Treatment of Hypertension Study (PATHS). Rationale and design. *Am. J. Hypertens.* **7,** 814–823.

189. Cushman, W. C., Cutler, J. A., Hanna, E., Bingham, S. F., Follmann, D., Harford, T., Dubbert, P., Allender, P. S., Dufour, M., Collins, J. F., Walsh, S. M., Kirk, G. F., Burg, M., Felicetta, J. V., Hamilton, B. P., Katz, L. A., Perry, M., Willenbring, M. L., Lakshman, R., and Hamburger, R. J. (1998). Prevention and Treatment of Hypertension Study (PATHS): Effects of an alcohol treatment program on blood pressure. *Arch. Intern. Med.* **158,** 1197–1207.

190. Wallace, P., Cutler, S., and Haines, A. (1988). Randomised controlled trial of general practitioner intervention in patients with excessive alcohol consumption. *Br. Med. J.* **297,** 663–668.

191. Puddey, I. B., Beilin, L. J., and Vandongen, R. (1987). Regular alcohol use raises blood pressure in treated hypertensive subjects. *Lancet* **1,** 647–651.

192. Puddey, I. B., Parker, M., Beilin, L. J., Vandongen, R., and Masarei, J. R. L. (1992). Effects of alcohol and caloric restrictions on blood pressure and serum lipids in overweight men. *Hypertension* **20,** 533–541.

193. Beilin, L. J. (1995). Alcohol, hypertension and cardiovascular disease. *J. Hypertens.* **13,** 939–942.

194. Rimm, E. B., Giovannucci, E. L., Willett, W. C., Colditz, G. A., Ascerio, A., Rosner, B., and Stampfer, M. J. (1991). A prospective study of alcohol consumption and the risk of coronary disease in men. *Lancet* **338,** 464–468.

195. Sacks, F., Obarzanek, E., Windhauser, M., Svetkey, L. P., Vollmer, W. M., McCullough, M., Karanja, N. M., Lin, P-H.,

Steele, P., Proschan, M. A., Evans, M. A., Appel, L. J., Bray, G. A., Vogt, T. M., and Moore, T. J. (1995). Rationale and design of the Dietary Approaches to Stop Hypertension trial. *Ann. Epidemiol.* **5,** 108–118.

196. Vogt, T., Appel, L., Moore, T., Obarzanek, E., Vollmer, W. M., Svetkey, L. P., Sacks, F. M., Bray, G. A., Cutler, J. A., Windhauser, M. M., Lin, P-H., and Karanja, N. M. (1999). Dietary Approaches to Stop Hypertension: Rationale, design, and methods. *J. Am. Diet. Assoc.* **99**(Suppl.), S12–S18.

197. Karanja, N., Obarzanek, E., Lin, P.-H., McCullough, M. L., Phillips, K. M., Swain, J. F., Champagne, C. M., and Hoben, K. P. (1999). Descriptive characteristics of the dietary patterns used in the Dietary Approaches to Stop Hypertension trial. *J. Am. Diet. Assoc.* **99**(Suppl.), S19–S27.

CHAPTER **21**

Nutrition and Congestive Heart Failure

SUZANNE LUTTON[1] AND NANCY ANZLOVAR
Cleveland Clinic Foundation, Cleveland, Ohio

I. INTRODUCTION

More than 4.8 million Americans are afflicted with congestive heart failure and another 555,000 new cases are diagnosed annually [1]. As the population ages and with improved treatment of other cardiovascular disorders such as myocardial infarction, hypertension, and valvular heart disease, the prevalence of heart failure is anticipated to increase even more. Congestive heart failure (CHF) is actually a constellation of signs and symptoms resulting from impairment of systolic and/or diastolic functioning of the myocardium. Patients with CHF experience difficulties such as shortness of breath, chest discomfort, limitations of exercise capacity, peripheral edema, anorexia, and become fatigued easily.

Many individuals incorrectly interchange the terms *congestive heart failure* and *cardiomyopathy*. Cardiomyopathies are diseases of the myocardium that are associated with cardiac dysfunction and result in the syndrome of congestive heart failure. Cardiomyopathies are divided into several types as defined by the World Health Organization [2] and include the broad categories of dilated, restrictive, hypertrophic, right ventricular, specific, or unclassified. When a patient presents with CHF, it is important to try to identify the underlying cause in order to direct therapy and potentially reverse the disease process. For instance, ventricular dysfunction can be the result of hypertensive cardiomyopathy and aggressive blood pressure lowering can reduce symptoms, diminish left ventricular hypertrophy, and frequently improve the ejection fraction. The symptoms of CHF are often divided into New York Heart Association functional classes (see Table 1). Functional class I is defined as being asymptomatic, even with exertion. Class II patients develop difficulties with moderate exertion such as shortness of breath with walking up hill or climbing stairs. Class III patients have symptoms with mild exertion such as performing the activities of daily living like showering or dressing. Functional Class IV implies symptoms of CHF while at rest.

[1]Current address: Diagnostic Cardiology Associates, Youngstown, Ohio.

II. PATHOPHYSIOLOGY OF HEART FAILURE

The cause of the initial insult to the individual myocyte and myocardium as a whole can vary widely from myocardial infarction to exposure to a toxin such as adriamycin. However, once the injury has occurred, regardless of cause, the heart and cardiovascular system can only respond in a limited number of ways. A decrease in cardiac output from ventricular dysfunction leads to hypoperfusion of vital organs such as the kidneys, with the body inappropriately perceiving a hypovolemic state. This results in activation of the sympathetic nervous, renin-angiotensin-aldosterone, and arginine-vasopressin systems. Consequently, many neurohormones are increased in heart failure, including aldosterone, angiotensin II, atrial natriuretic factor, endothelin, epinephrine, growth hormone, norepinephrine, prostaglandins, renin, tumor necrosis factor-alpha and vasopressin.

Angiotensin II has numerous effects aimed at protecting against hypovolemia and hypotension. Its primary actions are vasoconstriction of the systemic and renal arterioles and stimulation of the production of the potent mineralocorticoid aldosterone by the adrenal glands. Aldosterone and angiotensin II increase sodium reabsorption in the proximal and distal tubules of the kidney. Vasopressin release is also

TABLE 1 New York Heart Association Functional Classes

Functional class	Description
Class I	Asymptomatic; even with heavy exertion
Class II	Slight limitations with exertion; no symptoms at rest
Class III	Marked limitations with exertion; no symptoms at rest
Class IV	Symptoms at rest

triggered by the changes in sodium and water homeostasis, which further exerts antidiuretic and direct, systemic vasoconstrictor effects. The sympathetic nervous system induces systemic vasoconstriction, stimulates additional renin release, and directly and indirectly increases sodium reabsorption in the proximal tubule of the kidney [3].

Although many of these neurohormones are beneficial in acute settings such as cardiogenic shock, in chronic conditions they have detrimental effects on the myocardium and play a significant role in the progressive decline of ventricular function [4, 5]. The chronic actions of all of these neurohormones result in worsening hemodynamics, progressive ventricular dilation and unfavorable remodeling, myocardial fibrosis, and increased morbidity and mortality.

III. STANDARD MEDICAL CARE FOR HEART FAILURE

The main goal in the management and treatment of heart failure is to reduce morbidity and mortality. Heart failure accounts for more than 1 million hospital discharges annually and a 3-month readmission rate of 20–50%. It is essential to try to identify the cause of the cardiomyopathy and any factors that may have contributed to an episode of decompensation. Numerous outstanding articles and guidelines have been previously published that review the standard approach to and medications for the treatment of both acute and chronic heart failure [6–11]. With a better understanding of the pathophysiology of heart failure, including new information from the molecular and cellular levels, the approach to its treatment has evolved dramatically during the last few decades.

Currently, the treatment of CHF involves quadruple therapy, of angiotensin-converting enzyme inhibitors, beta blockers, digoxin, and diuretics as needed. The first aim of therapy for CHF is to relieve the symptoms of vital organ congestion and improve hemodynamics. Diuretics are the mainstay of this therapy. Although diuretics work very well to relieve volume overload and congestion, no studies have demonstrated that diuretics actually improve survival. In fact, there is evidence to suggest that diuretics can be toxic to the myocardium over time through activation of the renin-angiotensin-aldosterone and sympathetic nervous systems. The current recommendations are to use diuretics as needed for symptoms of fluid overload, such as peripheral edema, weight gain, abdominal bloating, increasing cough, or worsening shortness of breath. Once symptomatic improvement occurs and a euvolumic state is achieved, often the diuretic can be decreased or used only on an intermittent basis. Angiotensin-converting enzyme inhibitors are the cornerstone to the long-term treatment of heart failure. They act by preventing the conversion of angiotensin I to angiotensin II and have both hemodynamic and neurohormonal actions.

Large clinical trials such as SOLVD (Studies of Left Ventricular Dysfunction), CONSENSUS (Cooperative North Scandinavian Enalapril Survival Study), SAVE (Survival and Ventricular Enlargement), and V-HeFT-II (Veterans Administration Cooperative Vasodilator Heart Failure Trial II) have provided evidence that angiotensin-converting enzyme inhibitors offer relief from heart failure symptoms and, most importantly, reduce morbidity and mortality [12–15]. Digoxin has been investigated recently in several trials [16–18]. This medication promotes an increase in contractility and also increases baroreceptor sensitivity. It is useful in patients with severe CHF to decrease morbidity, although it does not improve mortality.

One of the newer directions in the treatment of heart failure involves the use of beta-adrenergic receptor blockers to suppress the neurohormonal substances described above in an attempt to improve long-term outcome. Beta-blockers, once contraindicated in heart failure, are now one of the standard medications following their demonstration of safety and improved mortality [19–25]. Aldosterone antagonists, endothelial antagonists, TNF-α antagonists, and several other drug classes are currently being used or are under investigation for the treatment of CHF. In the future, therapy may be directed at altering the cardiovascular system at the genetic and cellular levels before heart failure ever develops.

Another key step in the management of CHF involves modifying any other risk factors for cardiovascular disease. Some of the most important risk factors to control include diabetes, obesity, hypertension, tobacco use, and hyperlipidemia. These risk factors for cardiovascular disease further adversely affect patients already afflicted with CHF. For example, obesity increases systemic vascular resistance, thus increasing the workload of an already failing heart. Weight loss decreases blood pressure, improves lipid and glucose metabolism, and promotes regression of left ventricular hypertrophy [26], all of which improve CHF. These areas are covered in detail in the other chapters on cardiovascular diseases and also under disease-specific interventions in this book. In addition to following standard medical therapy, patients with CHF are encouraged to make lifestyle modifications regarding regular exercise programs and stress management and to follow dietary guidelines. Because of the sodium and water retention present in heart failure, the most important dietary modification is restriction of sodium and water intake.

IV. RESTRICTIONS IN SODIUM

As described above, acute and chronic heart failure results in the activation of the renin-angiotensin-aldosterone, sympathetic nervous, and arginine-vasopressin systems. The kidneys respond to these neurohormones by inappropriately retaining too much sodium and fluid. This leads to further decompensation. Although the measured serum sodium level

TABLE 2   High-Salt Foods[a]

Beverages—soft drinks, tomato juice

Canned foods and soups, bouillon cubes

Cheeses (some)—cottage cheese, American cheese

Condiments and sauces—barbeque sauce, olives, relish,
soy sauce, catsup

Fast foods and many ethnic foods

Frozen main dishes

Pickled vegetables

Shellfish

Smoked, cured, processed meats—hotdogs, ham, bacon, sausage,
corned beef, bologna

Snack foods—salted nuts, potato chips, salted popcorn, pork rinds

[a]Unless product is specifically labeled low sodium or no sodium.

is often normal and sometimes low, the total body store of sodium is markedly elevated. This is a difficult concept for most to understand. A low serum sodium level is an independent predictor of increased mortality. A common response of patients and healthcare providers to a low serum sodium level, unfortunately, is that they may try to increase the level by increasing sodium intake, which only results in further fluid retention. It is essential in CHF to restrict both sodium and water to treat congestion, maintain compensation, and avoid electrolyte derangements.

Most Americans already consume over three times the daily requirement of sodium, sometimes taking in as much as 10 g/day. (One teaspoon is the equivalent of 2.3 g.) In those with mild heart failure, sodium consumption should be limited to 3.0 g a day. Those with moderate to severe heart failure are advised to limit sodium even further to 2.0 g a day. On occasion, patients floridly decompensated may need to temporarily decrease the sodium intake to 0.5–1.0 g/day, although this becomes very difficult to do. The first step in decreasing sodium intake for patients is to completely discontinue use of added salt. To flavor food, a variety of salt substitutes and salt-free seasonings are available on the market. Many of the salt substitutes are high in potassium, which may or may not be desirable for an individual patient. This is usually dependent on the use of other heart failure medications (potassium-wasting vs. potassium-sparing diuretics) and renal function. Patients should consult with their physician regarding use of potassium-containing salt substitutes. Patients should completely avoid high-salt foods (see Table 2). Obvious foods to be avoided are most processed foods, smoked or cured meats, vegetables pickled in brine, tomato sauces, and canned soups, unless they are specifically labeled as containing low or no sodium. The vast majority of fast foods should be eliminated because both the sodium and fat content far exceed recommended intakes.

Label reading is one of the most important means of helping to control sodium intake. The patient and family need to

TABLE 3   Hidden Salts in Foods

Read the ingredient label for		
Disodium phosphate	Sodium bicarbonate	Sodium pectinate
Monosodium glutamate	Sodium caseinate	Sodium propionate
Sodium alginate	Sodium citrate	Sodium sulfite
Sodium benzoate	Sodium hydroxide	

be aware of hidden salts that are used in the preparation, processing, and packaging of foods (see Table 3). Additionally, many medications contain sodium (see Table 4). Generally acceptable foods are those in which the sodium content is less than 0.14 g per serving. Many tables, charts, and books are available to guide patients in food selections.

When patients present with congestion, it is quite common to discover that they have markedly exceeded their sodium intake limits. Routinely obtaining a history of what was consumed in the preceding 24–48 hours can be quite revealing and educational. Often patients think they are following a low-salt diet, yet, unknowingly, their food selections are rather high in salt content. Frequently, patients with mild peripheral edema can be adequately treated with vigilant salt restriction, and thus avoid diuretic therapy.

A common complaint of patients with heart failure is that they are no longer obtaining a brisk response to their diuretic treatment. This may reflect excess sodium intake. Unfortunately, the first response of many practitioners is to simply increase the dosage or change to a different diuretic brand or class. In reality, many cases of apparent "diuretic resistance" are actually due to the fact that the patient has been indiscriminate in sodium consumption. Careful diet control will usually return the urine output to the expected levels.

This apparent resistance can be explained as follows. When a diuretic is first administered and reaches a therapeutic level in the system, naturiesis occurs. However, once the drug level falls out of the effective range, a rebound in sodium resorbed can occur. The amount of sodium reabsorbed by the kidney during this time and until the next dose of diuretic is given can negate the previous losses. Thus, the net sodium loss may be minimal or zero through the entire dosing interval [27]. To maximize the diuretic effects, it is essential that sodium intake be restricted to prevent the kidneys from compensating for the initial losses.

TABLE 4   Sodium in Medications

Alkalizers—sodium citrate

Antacids—sodium bicarbonate

Antibiotics—certain IV forms

Exchange resins—sodium polystyrene sulfonate

Laxatives—sodium phosphate, sodium sulfate

V. RESTRICTIONS IN FLUID INTAKE

The pathophysiology of CHF, as described above, results in chronic fluid and sodium retention. Patients may range from having minimal or no congestion to a tremendous amount of fluid excess. As mentioned earlier, symptoms of fluid overload can include complaints of leg and/or hand swelling, weight gain, abdominal bloating or distention, nausea, early satiety, cough, dyspnea with exertion or at rest, orthopnea, and paroxysmal nocturnal dyspnea. By the time peripheral edema is present and detectable, the patient usually has at least 5 kg of excess fluid. The standard recommendation is to limit total liquid intake to 2 liters (2000 cc) a day or about 64 ounces. Patients who are severely decompensated may require further restrictions to 1000–1500 cc/day. Restricting below this level can be very uncomfortable for patients because of unrelenting thirst, and also increases the risk of kidney failure. Many patients have the incorrect belief that they must consume large quantities of fluid in order to keep the kidneys functioning normally, prevent infections, and help the body "flush out" toxins. Education about not deliberately drinking fluids and providing general guidelines about fluid restriction are some of the first steps in preventing fluid excess and correcting volume overloaded conditions.

Fluid restriction is also of particular importance in the management of hypervolemic hyponatremia. Another common cause for why a patient's diuretic "is not working," besides consuming too much sodium, is that patients will drink as much (or more) volume than they urinate. Total daily input must be less than daily output in order to produce a net diuresis. Excessive fluid consumption can increase the risk for severe electrolyte abnormalities, especially in the setting where a diuretic is being used.

Weight monitoring is very important in the management of congestive heart failure and should be performed after the first morning elimination dressed in a minimal amount of clothing. Patient education focuses on recording body weight and knowledge that a weight increase of more than 2–3 pounds in a day or 5 pounds in a week usually signals fluid retention. Early excess fluid retention frequently can be detected by the scale before edema is physically noted. On these days, patients are encouraged to carefully maintain their prescribed fluid and sodium restriction and even decrease total fluid intake by 1–1.5 cups. Additional diuretics may be necessary in order to reestablish the dry weight if this intervention is unsuccessful. It should be stressed that diuretic therapy alone is insufficient to control and/or prevent excess fluid accumulation.

Patients are encouraged to "visualize" their fluid consumption by using an empty 2-liter bottle. Each time they take a drink, the corresponding amount of fluid is to be placed into the bottle. This enables one to gauge total volume in relation to various household containers. A common misconception is that water is the only fluid that matters. Patients should be reminded that fluid consumption includes foods that become liquid at room temperature, such as ice cream, yogurt, and gelatin desserts. Ice chips or crushed ice are an alternatives to drinking a large glass of water. To accurately assess volume in relation to total fluid allotment, ice chips should be allowed to melt at room temperature. Psychologically, this may have some benefit since a full glass of ice chips is approximately only half the volume of the container once it melts. Placing grapes or strawberries in the freezer or using sugar-free hard candies may also provide relief from excessive thirst and dry mouth. On hot days or where there is excessive perspiration, patients may slightly liberalize their fluid and sodium restrictions. Maintaining a fluid restriction is challenging and there are times that intake exceeds recommendations. If this should occur, the patient should be counseled to be particularly vigilant the following day and decrease intake by at least 1 cup.

VI. RECOMMENDATIONS REGARDING FAT, FIBER, AND CHOLESTEROL

Patients with cardiovascular disease in general should reduce their fat and cholesterol consumption. The current consensus is that total fat intake should be less than 65 g/day and saturated fats should be less than 20 g/day. Overall, fats should be approximately 35% of the total daily energy intake, and cholesterol intake should be less than 0.3 g/day. These general guidelines are reviewed in other chapters of this book. Patients with CHF are generally prescribed the standard cardiovascular prevention guidelines as they apply to their other risk factors such as obesity and hyperlipidemia.

Patients with CHF are typically advised to consume a minimum of 25–35 g of fiber per day and preferably more. The rationale is that patients with heart failure are quite prone to constipation for several reasons, such as from diuretic use and decreased physical activity. Straining can precipitate dysrhythmias and pulmonary edema and must be avoided. An adequate fiber intake can help minimize constipation. High-fiber foods include vegetables, cooked dried peas and beans, whole-grain foods, bran, cereals, pasta, rice, and fresh fruit.

VII. OTHER DIETARY RECOMMENDATIONS

A. Tobacco

All patients with heart failure are advised to quite smoking and discontinue the use of all nicotine products, including snuff and chewing tobacco. Nicotine can increase heart rate and blood pressure by increasing the levels of norepinephrine. Platelets can also be adversely affected, leading to an increased risk of thrombosis, which is particularly problematic in patients with underlying coronary atherosclerosis.

A healthy endothelium in the blood vessels is needed to maintain proper vasodilation and vascular compliance. Endothelial dysfunction is already common in heart failure and it can be further aggravated by smoking, resulting in cell membrane abnormalities, lipid accumulation in the blood vessel walls, increased vascular resistance, and impaired regional blood flow. Finally, cigarette smoking is associated with reduced intake of nutrients such as vitamins E and C [28].

B. Alcohol

Alcoholic cardiomyopathy accounts for about one-third of all the nonischemic, dilated cardiomyopathies [29]. When the cardiovascular system is exposed to ethanol, acute and chronic changes occur in both systolic and diastolic functioning, with the most significant being a depression in contractility. If alcohol consumption continues, 40–50% of patients will die within 3–6 years [30], because continued consumption leads to further myocardial damage and fibrosis. The metabolites of alcohol, acetaldehyde and acetate, can have direct toxic effects on the heart as well. Complete abstinence may stop the progression of heart failure or even allow for recovery in early stages [31–33]. All patients with severe ventricular dysfunction, regardless of cause, should avoid alcohol because of the risk for worsening of their heart failure.

Alcohol can exacerbate many other underlying problems common in patients with CHF. For example, it can have a pressor effect, cause hypertension, and increase left ventricular mass [34]. Those who drink heavily may experience substantial increases in their blood pressure. Alcohol consumption may also lead to deficiencies in magnesium, potassium, phosphorus, and thiamine, which may further exacerbate existing dysfunction. Alcohol can also worsen hyperlipidemia, primarily by elevating the triglyceride levels, although it can also increase both the total cholesterol and low-density lipoprotein concentration [35]. In smaller quantities (less than 1–2 ounces a day), the high-density lipoprotein levels typically increase, thus alcohol may exert a slightly favorable effect. Overall, the risks of continued alcohol consumption outweigh this small benefit of this lipid improvement. The risk of atrial and ventricular dysrhythmias and sudden cardiac death are also increased in this population already prone to these adverse events [36, 37]. Consequently, alcohol consumption should be avoided in all patients with substantial heart failure and in those whose cardiomyopathy is suspected to be primarily from alcohol regardless of severity.

C. Caffeine

There are conflicting studies regarding the effects of caffeine on the cardiovascular system. Caffeine is known to antagonize adenosine receptors and cause phosphodiesterase in-

hibition. The results of acute ingestion are increases in catecholamine and renin levels and an increase in blood pressure. Tolerance quickly develops to caffeine, so it is unclear whether or not there are any long-term harmful effects in patients with CHF. Many are concerned about the potential for arrhythmias; however, studies suggest that moderate amounts of caffeine do not precipitate dysrhythmias [38]. The current recommendations are to limit caffeine to the equivalent of 4–5 cups of coffee in patients with coronary artery disease [39].

VIII. SPECIAL CONSIDERATIONS

A. Nutritional Supplements

Coenzyme Q_{10}, also known as ubiquinone, is a coenzyme for oxidative phosphorylation. It can be found naturally in red meats, fish, soybeans, and vegetable oils. It is present in large quantities in organs that require a fair amount of energy to function adequately, such as the heart, liver, and lung. Coenzyme Q_{10} also has antioxidant properties and acts as a free radial scavenger [40]. The quantity of this coenzyme has been demonstrated to be low in myocardial biopsy specimens of patients with heart failure. Further, the extent of the deficiency correlates with the severity of heart failure [41]. It has been suggested that supplementation with this mitochondrial enzyme might improve energy mechanics, cardiac contractility, and clinical outcomes. Several small studies have suggested possible benefits [42, 43]; however, most of these studies had major design flaws limiting the interpretation and applicability of the results. Two recent, well-conducted studies showed no significant differences in left ventricular ejection fraction, hemodynamics, exercise duration, peak oxygen consumption, cardiac volumes, or quality of life indices after 3–6 months of treatment [44, 45]. It is important to note that coenzyme Q_{10} can adversely interact with warfarin and aspirin and should be avoided when patients are taking these medications [45a–45c].

Taurine is an amino acid found in animal foods such as poultry, beef, pork, fish, and milk. It participates in cell membrane stabilization through modulation of cellular calcium levels, antioxidation [46], and brain and retinal development and it has high concentrations in cardiac tissue. Experimentally, taurine can increase myocardial contractility and potentiate the inotropic response to digoxin presumably by regulating the intracellular calcium concentrations. In laboratory animals with heart failure, taurine has been shown to prevent a reduction in cardiac function, delay the onset of symptoms, and improve survival [47]. Results from very small studies suggest that there may be a beneficial effect in humans [48]. Others suggest that supplementation with this drug, like other oral inotropes studied to date, may actually increase mortality. Investigations with rodents have proposed antiatherosclerotic and hypocholesterolemic effects

TABLE 5 Effect of Food on Common Heart Failure Medications

Absorption delayed	Absorption decreased	Absorption increased
Carvedilol	Aspirin	Chlorothiazide
Enteric coated aspirin	Atenolol	Hydralazine
Digoxin[a]	Catopril[b]	Hydrochlorothiazide
Fosinopril	Quinapril	Labetalol
Furosemide	Sotolol	Metoprolol
Potassium		Propranolol
Quinapril		Spironolactone[c]
Ramapril		
Trandolapril		

[a]Delayed with high bran fiber meals.
[b]Take 1 hour before meals.
[c]Food increases bioavailability, but clinical significance unknown.

[49, 50]. Similar to coenzyme Q_{10}, evidence to suggest a benefit of this supplement is lacking. The current Food and Drug Administration recommended daily intake of taurine is 13 mg/kg/day [51], although supplements as high as 3 g have been suggested for cardiac benefit.

Other nutrients have gained popularity in the field of alternative medications for CHF. Carnitine, L-arginine, and creatine are other supplements that have theoretical benefits in the treatment of CHF. It is known and accepted that carnitine deficiency may result in a dilated or occasionally restrictive cardiomyopathy. Deficiency may also worsen a preexisting cardiomyopathy from other causes. Oral therapy with L-carnitine can be quite effective in this condition [52]. L-Arginine is a precursor or nitric oxide, which induces vasodilation. Heart failure is often associated with endothelial dysfunction, with resultant impairment of nitric oxide-dependent vasodilation. It is postulated that L-arginine, through conversion to nitric oxide, may prevent or correct endothelial dysfunction [53]. However, there have been no proven mortality benefits in large-scale clinical trials of any of these substances. Patients should be reminded that these supplements could be considered in addition to their standard therapy, rather than replacements.

B. Food and Drug Interactions

Many medications commonly used today can be affected by the contents of the gastrointestinal tract. Often the presence of food can delay or decrease the absorption of a medication. The interactions between food and cardiovascular medications are clinically important to understand (see Table 5). Depending on the desired effect, patients need to be instructed when to take their pills in relationship to meals. For instance, food slows down the absorption of carvedilol. If patients take this medication on an empty stomach, they often absorb it too rapidly and, consequently, can experience dizziness and hypotension. In this case, patients are advised to take carvedilol with food to diminish side effects. Finally, some cardiac medications such as amiodarone or furosemide are known to cause nausea or abdominal discomfort and are best taken with a light meal or snack.

C. Cardiac Cachexia

Cardiac cachexia is common in those suffering from chronic, severe CHF. The syndrome is characterized by a drastic reduction in both lean body muscle mass and adipose tissue, with a subsequent decrease in activity level, functional capacity, and strength. Cardiac cachexia is associated with decreased survival. Information gleaned from nutritional surveys obtained on those requiring hospitalization for heart failure have demonstrated that 50–68% of patients are malnourished as determined by total body weight, plasma protein status, and anthropometric measurements [54–56]. The exact mechanism of cachexia is unknown, but most likely many factors contribute to the profound loss (see Table 6).

Many cytokines have been identified that probably play a significant role in the catabolism and weight loss, as reviewed recently by Tisdale [57]. Studies performed in other wasting states, such as malignancies, have shown that increasing nutrient intake alone is unable to reverse this process. Therapies are generally directed toward reversing the possible factors known to impair the ability to eat, such as treating nausea, reducing fluid retention as much as possible, and improving hemodynamics. Small, frequent meals are helpful. At times, some of the restrictions placed on the diet will need to be relaxed so patients can increase their energy intake. An alteration in food composition to be 35% energy from fat, 15% energy from protein and 50% energy from carbohydrate has been suggested to combat the cachexia, although not all agree. Perhaps by decreasing neurohormonal activation, some of the cytokines contributing to the

TABLE 6 Possible Causes of Cardiac Cachexia

Abdominal discomfort, bloating

Altered taste

Anorexia, nausea, and vomiting

Cytokines such as tumor necrosis factor-α, interleukin-1, interferon-γ

Decreased absorption of food

Difficulty eating from shortness of breath

Fluid restriction

Increased caloric expenditure—work of breathing, fever, increased basal metabolic rate

Nutrient losses—renal protein loss, protein-losing enteropathy

Unpalatable diet from restrictions

wasting syndrome will be diminished and patients will stabilize or even increase their muscle mass. Ongoing studies with the use of tumor necrosis factor antagonists and fish oil may reveal interesting outcomes and lead to further therapies directed at this devastating complication of heart failure.

D. Right-Sided Heart Failure

When patients develop CHF, it is sometimes easier to describe their symptoms as either "left sided" or "right sided." Often, both are present simultaneously, although one side typically predominates. The term *right-sided heart failure* implies that the symptoms a patient is experiencing are attributable to dysfunction of the right ventricle. Symptoms can include abdominal discomfort, bloating, leg swelling, early satiety, and nausea. On physical exam, patients can have prominent jugular venous distention, hepatomegaly, splenomegaly, ascites, and pitting edema. The gastrointestinal symptoms occur from both gut edema and organ enlargement. As the liver expands, the capsule around it stretches and becomes quite uncomfortable. It is not uncommon to have right-sided heart failure be confused as an acute abdomen, cholecystitis, appendicitis, or mesenteric ischemia.

Patients with right-sided CHF tend to have difficulties eating an adequate amount. Small, frequent meals are better tolerated than large volumes. Often patients will naturally switch to more liquid meals, which may interfere with fluid and sodium restriction. For example, soups are easier to consume, however, they contribute a high sodium load. Many of the nutritional supplemental drinks on the market can be used, but patients should do so cautiously because some contain large quantities of sodium or are high in sugar and may worsen glucose control in patients with diabetes. Patients again should be encouraged to read labels closely.

Finally, patients with significant edema of the intestinal wall may have decreased absorption of some of their heart failure medications, thus precipitating further decompensation and starting a vicious cycle of deterioration. Hospitalization and conversion of medications to intravenous forms may be necessary until adequate functioning returns.

IX. SUMMARY

Congestive heart failure is the only cardiovascular disorder that is increasing in prevalence. This is mostly due to improved survival from other cardiac conditions such as hypertension and myocardial infarction. Once the initial insult occurs, the renin-angiotensin-aldosterone and sympathetic nervous systems become activated. These neurohormones and other cytokines lead to adverse ventricular remodeling and progressive ventricular dysfunction. Patients are treated routinely now with angiotensin-converting enzyme inhibitors, beta blockers, digoxin, and diuretics. In addition to these medications, diet modification and exercise are also important in controlling the high morbidity and mortality associated with CHF. Sodium restriction to approximately 2 g/day is the most important dietary modification, and this alone will frequently keep patients euvolemic and diminish the need for diuretics.

Excess sodium intake is often the underlying cause for decompensation in a previously stable state. Fluid restriction to 2 L/day is also advisable to decrease fluid retention and assist in net diuresis. This may need to be reduced even further in times of decompensation. Patients with heart failure are also advised to follow the standard guidelines for prevention of cardiovascular disease regarding fat, carbohydrate, and cholesterol intakes. Because patients with CHF are prone to constipation, adequate fiber intake is encouraged.

A number of alternative therapies, such as coenzyme Q_{10} and taurine, have been touted as beneficial in heart failure. These are yet to be scientifically proven to improve morbidity or mortality in large, randomized, placebo-controlled trials. Patients should not use these therapies in place of the standard heart failure medications, which are clearly beneficial. Finally, certain patients with CHF present with further difficulties in obtaining adequate energy and nutrient intakes. As the pathophysiology of the cardiomyopathies becomes better understood and elucidated, medical and nutritional interventions are likely to be even more helpful in the future.

References

1. American Heart Association (2000). "2000 Heart and Stroke Statistical Update." Statistical Supplement. American Heart Association, Dallas, TX.
2. World Health Organization/International Society and Federation of Cardiology Task Force (1996). Definition and classification of cardiomyopathies. *Circulation* **93**, 841–842.
3. Davis, J. O. (1970). The mechanism of salt and water retention in cardiac failure. *Hosp. Prac.* **5**, 63–76.

4. Brunier, M., and Brunner, H. R. (1992). Neurohormonal consequences of diuretics in different cardiovascular syndromes. *Eur. Heart J.* **13**(Suppl. G), 28–33.

5. Kaye, D. M., Lefkovits, J., Jennings, G. L., Bergin, P., Broughton, A., and Esler, M. D. (1995). Adverse consequences of high sympathetic nervous activity in the failing human heart. *J. Am. College Cardiol.* **26**, 1257–1263.

6. ACC/AHA Task Force (1995). Guidelines for the evaluation and management of heart failure. *J. Am. College Cardiol.* **26**, 1376–1398.

7. Dracup, K., Baker, D. W., Dunbar, S. B., Dacey, R. A., Brooks, N. H., Johnson, J. C., Oken, C., and Massie, B. M. (1994). Management of heart failure II: Counseling, education and lifestyle modifications. *JAMA* **272**, 1442–1446.

8. Haas, G. J., and Young, J. B. (1998). Acute heart failure management. *In* "Textbook of Cardiovascular Medicine" (E. J. Topol, Ed.). Lippincott-Raven, Philadelphia, PA.

9. Young, J. B. (1998). Chronic heart failure management. *In* "Textbook of Cardiovascular Medicine" (E. J. Topol, Ed.). Lippincott-Raven, Philadelphia, PA.

10. Konstam, M., Dracup, K., Baker, D., Bottorff, M., Brooks, N., Dacey, R., Dunbar, S., Jackson, A., Jessup, M., Johnson, J., Jones, R., Luchi, R., Massie, B., Pitt, B., Rose, E., Rubin, L., Wright, R., and Hadorn, D. (1994). "Heart Failure: Evaluation and Care of the Patient with Left-Ventricular Systolic Dysfunction. Clinical Practice Guideline," AHCPR Publication No. 94-0612. Agency for Health Care Policy and Research, U.S. Department of Health and Human Services, Rockville, MD.

11. Packer, M., and Cohn, J. (1999). Consensus recommendations for the management of chronic heart failure. *Am. J. Cardiol.* **82**, 2A–38A.

12. The SOLVD Investigators (1992). Effect of enalapril on mortality and on the development of heart failure in asymptomatic patients with reduced left ventricular ejection fractions. *N. Engl. J. Med.* **327**, 685–691.

13. CONSENSUS Trial Study Group. (1987). Effects of enalapril on mortality in severe congestive heart failure: Results of the Cooperative North Scandinavian Enalapril Survival Study (CONSENSUS). *N. Engl. J. Med.* **316**, 1429–1435.

14. Pfeffer, M., Braunwald, E., Moye, L., Basta, L., Brown, E., Cuddy, T., Davis, B., Geltman, E., Goldman, S., Flaker, G., Klein, M., Lamas, G., Packer, M., Rouleau, J., Rouleau, J. L., Rutherford, J., Wertheimer, J., and Hawkins, C. on behalf of the SAVE Investigators (1992). Effect of captopril on mortality and morbidity in patients with ventricular dysfunction after myocardial infarction. Results of the survival and ventricular enlargement trial. *N. Engl. J. Med.* **327**, 669–677.

15. Cohn, J. N., Johnson, G., Ziesche, S., Cobb, F., Francis, G., Tristani, F., Smith, R., Dunkman, W., Loeb, H., Wong, M., Bhat, G., Goldman, S., Fletcher, R., Doherty, J., Hughes, C., Cardon, P., Cintron, G., Shabetai, R., and Haakenson, C. (1991). A comparison of enalapril with hydralazine-isosorbide dinitrate in the treatment of chronic congestive heart failure (VeHEFT-II). *N. Engl. J. Med.* **325**, 303–310.

16. Digitalis Investigation Group (1997). The effect of digoxin on mortality and morbidity in patients with heart failure. *N. Engl. J. Med.* **336**, 525–533.

17. Uretsky, B. F., Young, J. B., Shahidi, F. E., Yellen, L. G., Harrison, M. C., and Jolly, M. K. (1993). Randomized study assessing the effect of digoxin withdrawal in patients with mild to moderate chronic congestive heart failure: Results of the PROVED trial: PROVED Investigative Group. *J. Am. College Cardiol.* **22**, 955–962.

18. Packer, M., Gheorghiade, M., Young, J. B., Costantini, P. J., Adams, K. F., Cody, R. J., Smith, L. K., Van Voorhees, L., Gourley, L. A., and Jolly, M. K. (1993) on behalf of the RADIANCE Study. Withdrawal of digoxin from patients with chronic heart failure treated with angiotensin-converting-enzyme inhibitors. *N. Engl. J. Med.* **329**, 1–7.

19. CIBIS Investigators and Committees (1994). A randomized trial of β-blockade in heart failure: The Cardiac Insufficiency Bisoprolol Study (CIBIS). *Circulation* **90**, 1765–1773.

20. Waagstein, F., Bristow, M. R., Swedberg, K., Camerini, F., Fowler, M. B., Silver, M. A., Gilbert, E. M., Johnson, M. R., Goss, F. G., and Hjalmarson, A. (1993) for the Metoprolol in Dilated Cardiomyopathy (MDC) Trial Study Group. Beneficial effects of metoprolol in idiopathic dilated cardiomyopathy. *Lancet* **342**, 1441–1446.

21. Australia-New Zealand Heart Failure Research Collaborative Group (1997). Randomised, placebo-controlled trial of carvedilol in patients with congestive heart failure due to ischaemic heart disease. *Lancet* **349**, 375–380.

22. Bristow, M. R. (2000). β-adrenergic receptor blockade in chronic heart failure. *Circulation* **101**, 558–569.

23. Packer, M., Bristow, M. R., Cohn, J. N., Colucci, W. S., Fowler, M. B., Gilbert, E. M., and Shusterman, N. H. (1996) for the U.S. Carvedilol Heart Failure Study Group. The effect of carvedilol on morbidity and mortality in patients with chronic heart failure. *N. Engl. J. Med.* **334**, 1349–1355.

24. CIBIS-II Investigators and Committees (1999). The Cardiac Insufficiency Bisoprolol Study II (CIBIS-II): A randomized trial. *Lancet* **353**, 9–13.

25. MERIT-HF Study Group (1999). Effect of metoprolol CR/XL in chronic heart failure: Metoprolol CR/XL Randomised Intervention Trial in Congestive Heart Failure (MERIT-HF). *lancet* **353**, 2001–2007.

26. Albert, M. A., Terry, B. E., Mulekar, M., Cohen, M. V., Massey, C. V., Fan, T. M., Panayiotou, H., and Mukerji, V. (1997). Cardiac morphology and left ventricular function in normotensive morbidly obese patients with and without congestive heart failure, and effect of weight loss. *Am. J. Cardiol.* **80**, 736–740.

27. Wilcox, C. S., Mitch, W. E., Kelly, R. A., Skorechi, K., Meyer, T. W., Friedman, P. A., and Souney, P. F. (1983). Response of the kidney to furosemide. I. Effects of salt intake and renal compensation. *J. Lab. Clin. Med.* **102**, 450–458.

28. Dallongeville, J., Marecaux, N., Fruchart, J. C., and Amouyel, P. (1998). Cigarette smoking is associated with unhealthy patterns of nutrient intake: A meta-analysis. *J. Nutr.* **128**, 1450–1457.

29. Schwarz, F., Mall, G., Zebe, H., Schmitzer, E., Mauthey, J., and Scheusten, H. (1984). Determinants of survival in patients with congestive cardiomyopathy: Quantitative morphologic findings and left ventricular hemodynamics. *Circulation* **70**, 923–928.

30. Kinney, E. L., Wright, R. J., and Caldwell, J. W. (1989). Risk factors in alcoholic cardiomyopathy. *Angiology* **40**, 270–275.

31. Jacob, A. J., McLaren, K. M., and Boon, N. A. (1991). Effects of abstinence on alcoholic heart muscle disease. *Am. J. Cardiol.* **68**, 805–807.

32. Mølgaard, H., Kristensen, B. Ø., and Baandrup, U. (1990). Importance of abstention from alcohol in alcoholic heart disease. *Int. J. Cardiol.* **26**, 373–375.

33. Pavan, D., Nicolosi, G. L., Lestuzzi, C., Burelli, C., Zardo, F., and Zanuttini, D. (1987). Normalization of variables of left ventricular function in patients with alcoholic cardiomyopathy after cessation of excessive alcohol intake: An echocardiographic study. *Eur. Heart J.* **8**, 535–540.

34. Regan, T. J. (1990). Alcohol and the cardiovascular system. *JAMA* **264**, 377–381.

35. Gaziano, J. M., and Manson, J. E. (1996). Diet and heart disease: The role of fat, alcohol and antioxidants. *Cardiol. Clin.* **14**, 69–83.

36. Sharper, A. G., and Wannamethee, G. (1992). Alcohol and sudden cardiac death. *Br. Heart J.* **68**, 443–448.

37. Koskinen, P., and Kupari, M. (1992). Alcohol and cardiac arrhythmias. *Br. Med. J.* **304**, 1394–1395.

38. Myers, M. G. (1991). Caffeine and cardiac arrhythmias. *Ann. Intern. Med.* **114**, 147–150.

39. Lynn, L. A., and Kissinger, J. F. (1992). Coronary precautions. Should caffeine be restricted in patients after myocardial infarction? *Heart Lung* **21**, 365–370.

40. Beyer, R. E., and Emster, L. (1990). The antioxidant role of coenzymes Q. *In* "Highlights in Ubiquinone Research" (G. Lenaz, O. Barnabeli, A. Rabbi, and A. Battino, Eds.), pp. 191–213. Taylor and Francis, London.

41. Folkers, K., Vadhanavikit, S., and Mortensen, S. A. (1985). Biochemical rationale and myocardial tissue data on the effective therapy of cardiomyopathy with coenzyme Q_{10}. *Proc. Natl. Acad. Sci. USA* **82**, 901–904.

42. Langsjoen, P. H., Langsjoen, P. H., and Folkers, K. (1990). Long-term efficacy and safety of coenzyme Q_{10} therapy for idiopathic dilated cardiomyopathy. *Am. J. Cardiol.* **65**, 521–523.

43. Lampertico, M., and Comis, S. (1993). Italian multicentre study on the efficacy and safety of coenzyme Q_{10} as adjuvant therapy in heart failure. *Clin. Invest.* **71**, S129–S133.

44. Watson, P. S., Scalia, G. M., Galbraith, A., Burstow, D. J., Bett, N., and Aroney, C. N. (1999). Lack of effect of coenzyme Q on left ventricular function in patients with congestive heart failure. *J. Am. College Cardiol.* **33**, 1549–1552.

45. Khatta, M., Alexander, B. S., Krichten, C. M., Fisher, M. L., Freudenberger, R., Robinson, S. W., and Gottlieb, S. S. (2000). The effect of coenzyme Q_{10} in patients with congestive heart failure. *Ann. Intern. Med.* **132**, 636–640.

45a. Spigset, O. (1994). Reduced effect of warfarin caused by ubidecarenone. *Lancet* **344**, 1372–1373.

45b. Landbo, C., and Almdal, T. P. (1998). [Interaction between warfarin and coenzyme Q_{10}]. *Ugeskrift for Laeger.* **160**(22), 3226–3227.

45c. Heck, A. M., DeWitt, B. A., and Lukes, A. L. (2000). Potential interactions between alternative therapies and warfarin. *Am. J. Health-System Pharmacy.* **57**, 1221–1230.

46. Cunninham, C., Tipton, K. F., and Dixon, H. B. P. (1998). Conversion of taurine into N-chlorotaurine (taurine chloramine) and sulphoacetaldehyde in response to oxidative stress. *Biochem. J.* **330**, 939–945.

47. Takihara, K., Azuma, J., Awata, N., Ohta, H., Hamaguchi, T., Sawamura, A. Tanaka, Y., Kisimoto, S., and Sperelakis, N. (1986). Beneficial effect of taurine in rabbits with chronic congestive heart failure. *Am. Heart J.* **112**, 1278–1284.

48. Azuma, J., Sawamura, A., and Awata, N. (1992). Usefulness of taurine in chronic congestive heart failure and its prospective application. *Jpn. Circ. J.* **56**, 95–99.

49. Kamata, K., Sugiura, M., Kojima, S., and Kasuya, Y. (1996). Restoration of endothelium-dependent relaxation in both hypercholesterolemia and diabetes by chronic taurine. *Eur. J. Pharmacol.* **303**, 47–53.

50. Yokogoshi, H., Mochizuki, H., Nanami, K., Hida, Y., Miyachi, F., and Oda, H. (1999). Dietary taurine enhances cholesterol degradation and reduces serum and liver cholesterol concentrations in rats fed a high-cholesterol diet. *J. Nutr.* **129**, 1705–1712.

51. National Research Council (1989). "Recommended Dietary Allowances," 10th Ed. National Academy Press, Washington, DC.

52. Tripp, M. E., Katcher, M. L., Peters, H. A., Gilbert, E. F., Arya, S., Hodach, R. J., and Shug, A. L. (1984). Systemic carnitine deficiency presenting as familial endocardial fibroelastosis: A treatable cardiomyopathy. *N. Engl. J. Med.* **310**, 142–148.

53. Hambrecht, R., Hilbrich, L., Erbs, S., Gielen, S., Fiehn, E., Schoene, N., and Schuler, G. (2000). Correction of endothelial dysfunction in chronic heart failure: Additional effects of exercise training and oral l-arginine supplementation. *J. Am. College Cardiol.* **35**, 706–713.

54. Carr, J. G., Stevenson, L. W., Walden, J. A., and Heber, D. (1989). Prevalence and hemodynamic correlates of malnutrition in severe congestive heart failure secondary to ischemic or idiopathic dilated cardiomyopathy. *Am. J. Cardiol.* **63**, 709–713.

55. Mancini, D. M., Walter, G., Reichek, N., Lenkinski, R., McCully, K. K., Mullen, J. L., and Wilson, J. R. (1992). Contribution of skeletal muscle atrophy to exercise intolerance and altered muscle metabolism in heart failure. *Circulation* **85**, 1364–1373.

56. Blackburn, G. L., Gibbons, G. W., Bothe, A., Benotti, P. N., Harken, D. E., and McEnany, T. M. (1977). Nutritional support in cardiac cachexia. *J. Thor. Cardiovasc. Surg.* **73**, 489–495.

57. Tisdale, M. J. (1999). Wasting in cancer. *J. Nutr.* **129**, 243S–246S.

B. Cancer Prevention and Therapy

CHAPTER **22**

Nutrition and Breast Cancer

CHERYL L. ROCK[1] AND WENDY DEMARK-WAHNEFRIED[2]
[1]*University of California at San Diego, La Jolla, California*
[2]*Duke University Medical Center, Durham, North Carolina*

I. INTRODUCTION

Breast cancer is the most common invasive cancer in women in the United States, accounting for approximately 30% of new cancer cases in women. An estimated 192,200 U.S. women will be diagnosed with breast cancer in 2001 [1]. Caucasian women in the United States are more likely to be diagnosed with breast cancer than women of other racial/ethnic groups, but rates of survival for African-American women following diagnosis are lower than for Caucasians [2]. Incidence rates have decreased very slightly during the past several years, following a steady increase since the 1930s. Breast cancer mortality has been declining in recent years, a trend that has been attributed to earlier diagnosis and improvements in initial treatments [3]. As a result, an increasing number of women in the population are breast cancer survivors and are considered at risk for breast cancer recurrence. Recurrence is an important issue in breast cancer management, because the yearly rate of secondary cancer events, even for women who have been diagnosed with very early stage cancers, does not return to the level of similarly aged women who have not been diagnosed with breast cancer [4].

A very large body of scientific evidence on the relationship between nutritional factors and the risk for breast cancer has been accumulated and reported during the past several decades. Notably, research findings in this area are generally characterized by inconsistencies in the evidence for specific dietary factors and divergent views on the interpretation of these data. Much less data on the relationship between factors that may influence risk for recurrence or improve prognosis after the diagnosis of breast cancer (compared with data on primary prevention) have been collected and reported. In addition to dietary and other environmental factors, risk factors that have been linked to risk for breast cancer are gender (women have a 100-fold increased risk compared to men), age (mean age of onset is 66 years), family history (including specific genetic factors), and reproductive history, such as the ages of women at menarche, the birth of the first child, and menopause [1, 5].

A. Mammary Cell Biology and Genetic Factors

Much has been learned about the biology of breast cancer in the past several years. An important and recognized feature of breast cancer is the heterogeneity on a molecular level. As is true of all cancers, mammary carcinogenesis is a multistep process, involving the accumulation of genetic and epigenetic changes that result from the interaction between genetics and the environment [6]. On a cellular level, each case is characterized by a unique disease pathway, with associated genetic changes that may or may not be influenced by different etiological factors or interventions. As discussed by Slattery *et al.* [7], this heterogeneity likely constrains the ability to identify specific links between dietary factors and risk for breast cancer. Variable cellular characteristics also should be anticipated to be among the determinants of response to diet interventions that may reduce risk for breast cancer or cancer recurrence.

In addition to the cellular factors and mitogens that can affect growth regulation and apoptosis and thus influence carcinogenesis in all cell types, an important characteristic of normal cell proliferation and differentiation in the breast is the responsiveness of these cells to ovarian steroids. Estrogens have a direct effect on the mammary gland during various stages of development, such as growth, puberty, pregnancy, and lactation. For example, early full-term pregnancy, a characteristic in the reproductive history that is known to be associated with reduced risk for breast cancer, promotes increased degree of cellular differentiation, a cellular characteristic that is inversely related to the initiation of the neoplastic process [8]. Estrogens also stimulate cell proliferation in breast tissue, which increases the likelihood of random genetic errors and risk for the formation of a malignant phenotype [9]. In laboratory animal experiments, systemic ovarian hormones have been demonstrated to promote breast tumorigenesis [9]. The evidence to support a relationship between serum concentrations of estrogens and risk for breast cancer in human studies is much more inconsistent, which is usually attributed to methodological problems, and laboratory imprecision, and the fact that people are more genetically diverse than laboratory animals. For

example, in premenopausal women, concentrations of hormones in the circulation vary substantially across the menstrual cycle, the timing of which is only crudely assessed in most studies. Breast cancer is considered a hormone-dependent cancer, so nutritional factors that may influence the biosynthesis, metabolism, and inactivation of ovarian hormones, throughout development and adulthood, are suspected to influence risk for breast cancer or recurrence (see Fig. 1). Epidemiological studies have identified some apparent differences in risk factors for breast cancer in premenopausal and postmenopausal women, and menopausal status influences the treatment recommendations on diagnosis, so these subgroups are often (but not always) separated in the analysis of nutrition-related risk factors or response to dietary interventions.

In addition to the ovarian steroids, other growth factors and mitogens that may be modified by nutritional factors and dietary patterns also appear to play an important role in the initiation and promotional phases of breast cancer, based on epidemiological and laboratory studies. Two examples that are currently of intense scientific interest are insulin and insulin-like growth factor 1, and the interactions of these factors with adiposity and weight gain [10, 11], which will be addressed in the sections that follow.

A small proportion of breast cancers can be linked to a specific inherited susceptibility, the most well-known being the highly penetrant, dominant gene mutations, breast cancer gene 1 (*BRCA1*) and *BRCA2* [12]. Both are currently thought to be tumor suppressor genes. The presence of *BRCA1* increases the individual breast cancer risk by approximately 200-fold, but the mutation is rare, accounting for only 5.3% of breast cancer cases in women aged <40 years, 2.2% of cases in women aged 40–49 years, and 1.1% of cases in women aged 50–70 years [12]. The majority of women who are diagnosed with breast cancer do not have this or other specific mutations that have been identified. Inherited variations in other biochemical or metabolic pathways relevant to breast cell biology, such as those involved in estrogen metabolism, are other sources of genetic susceptibility currently under study [13], and their contributions to genetic risk are not yet known.

As discussed in an earlier chapter (see Chapter 13), interactions between genetic and dietary factors also are likely to be among the determinants of risk for breast cancer. Examples of gene–diet interactions currently under study in breast cancer are interactions between polymorphisms of *N*-acetyltransferase and meat consumption [14, 15] and between glutathione *S*-transferase and dietary sources of antioxidants [16].

B. Staging of Breast Cancer and Other Histopathologic and Prognostic Factors

Staging is important in understanding the management of breast cancer because stage at diagnosis determines the choice of recommended treatments and also is a predictive

factor in the overall prognosis. Staging in breast cancer is based on an internationally recognized system [17]. Categorization from stages I through III is based on tumor size and the presence and degree of involvement of axillary lymph nodes and other regional tissues, but no evidence of distant metastases is present in these stages. Stage IV includes the presence of distant metastases. Ductal carcinoma *in situ* and lobular carcinoma *in situ* are not invasive cancers, although these conditions are often treated like invasive breast cancer, because the lesions may progress to invasive breast cancer or be a marker of increased risk for the development of overt carcinoma [18].

The presence (and degree of involvement) of axillary lymph nodes at diagnosis has been found to be the most important predictor of prognosis [19]. However, several other tumor-related factors have been found useful in predicting the prognosis, and these characteristics also may influence the choice of treatments and the response to pharmacological and other interventions. For example, expression of estrogen (and also progesterone) receptors by tumor tissue indicates that normal cellular uptake and response to estrogen has been retained by the cancer cells. In follow-up studies, patients with estrogen receptor-positive tumors have been observed to have better long-term survival than patients with estrogen receptor-negative tumors [19]. Other cellular characteristics that appear to be of prognostic importance include DNA ploidy and S-phase fraction, oncogene amplification, or overexpression of the epidermal growth-factor receptor or *erbB2* (*HER2/neu*), and/or expression of mutant *p53* [18, 19].

II. NUTRITIONAL FACTORS IN THE ETIOLOGY OF BREAST CANCER

A. Primary Cancer Risk

Early interest in the relationship between nutrition and breast cancer was stimulated in large part by data from international comparisons that show a fivefold difference in breast cancer mortality rates across countries that is not explained by different treatment modalities [5]. More importantly, the risk for breast cancer among migrant populations who originate from low-risk countries has been observed to change with relocation (e.g., migration of Japanese women to the United States), subsequently reflecting the rate of the adopted culture and regions with higher breast cancer rates [20–22]. This pattern suggests that environmental factors, such as diet, are likely to play an important etiological role.

1. DIETARY AND NUTRIENT INTAKES AND RISK FOR BREAST CANCER

Clearly, the most well-known hypothesis that has been examined in the investigation of the link between nutrition and risk for breast cancer is that total dietary fat intake may

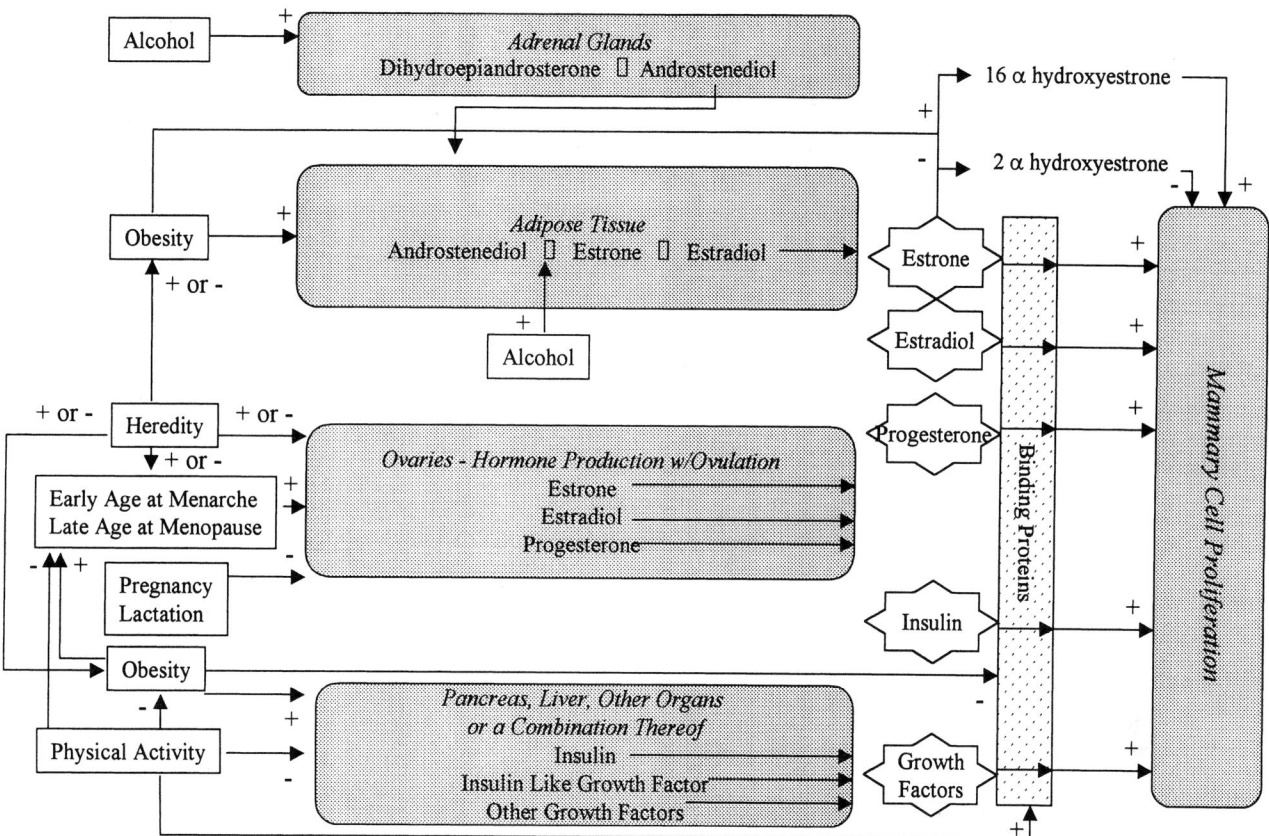

FIGURE 1 Some of the proposed hormonal mechanisms and their associations with mammary cell proliferation.

increase breast cancer risk. More data and resulting reports on this proposed relationship have been collected and published than on any other nutritional or dietary factor and breast cancer. Several eloquent and comprehensive reviews on this topic were published during the 1990s, and the reader is referred to these publications for detailed review and discussion of the evidence collected to date and the challenges in interpreting these data [23–27]. In addition to these comprehensive reviews, several authors have specifically addressed current theories, evidence for the proposed mechanisms, and relevant findings from laboratory animal and cell culture studies [28, 29].

The totality of the evidence suggests great inconsistency, at best, and is not very supportive, particularly when an effort is made to separate the effect of fat intake from the effect of total energy consumption. Although cross-country comparisons from ecological studies demonstrate a striking association between dietary fat intake and incidence of breast cancer [30], data from observational studies conducted within populations generally do not show this relationship, particularly in cohort studies (which exhibit less reporting bias than do simple case-control studies). This can be illustrated by results presented in recent reports. In a pooled analysis involving 4980 cases that arose from 337,819 U.S. women [31], the multivariate pooled relative risk of breast cancer

was 1.05 (95% confidence interval [CI] 0.94–1.16), when comparing women in the highest quintile of energy-adjusted total fat intake compared with women in the lowest quintile. Diet was assessed by means of food frequency questionnaires in all of the studies included in this pooled analysis. Relative risks for intakes of saturated, monounsaturated, and polyunsaturated fat were also were nonsignificant. In a single large cohort study of 88,795 women, of whom 2956 were diagnosed with breast cancer over a follow-up period of 14 years, women consuming 30–35% energy from fat had a relative risk of 1.15 (95% CI 0.73–1.80), compared to women consuming ≤20% energy from fat [32]. In this study by Holmes *et al.* [32], specific types of fat also were not found to be associated with risk of breast cancer, although a small but significant increase in risk was associated with intake of omega-3 fatty acids from fish (relative risk 1.09, 95% CI 1.03–1.16), and *trans* fatty acid intake had a slightly protective effect (relative risk 0.92, 95% CI 0.86–0.98).

Interpretation of these epidemiological data is complicated, of course, by known limitations in dietary assessment methodologies and confounding variables, as discussed in Chapter 4. Measurement error is particularly likely when the evidence relies solely on self-reported dietary data that are collected by instruments with inherent inaccuracy in quantifying nutrient consumption or capturing long-term

dietary intakes [33]. It also has been noted that the range of fat intake among the women in these within-population studies is too limited to enable the identification of a relationship with breast cancer risk, and that the number of women who consume diets that provide ≤20% of energy from fat, even in larger studies, is very small [24].

When testing the relationship between dietary fat and the promotion of breast tumorigenesis in laboratory animal studies, the interpretation of findings also is often difficult, due to the inextricable link between fat intake and energy balance. High-fat diets are energy dense, promoting increased overall growth of the animals and increased adiposity, two factors that independently affect number and size of tumors. However, specific fatty acids do appear to have differential effects on mammary cancer and tumor growth in animal studies. Omega–6 fatty acids have been shown to promote tumor development when fed to laboratory animals, particularly in comparison to omega–3 fatty acid-rich diets [28, 29], theoretically by influencing tumor eicosanoid production and possibly other factors (e.g., protein kinase C, membrane permeability, immune response). The practical significance of these findings from laboratory studies, however, is unclear, because examination of dietary patterns based on food choices does not consistently reveal a protective pattern of specific fatty acids. Also, marked changes in phospholipid and tissue composition of fatty acids may not be readily achieved in humans without fish oil supplements, and fish oil supplements carry some adverse metabolic risk in addition to any possible benefits. In comparison, regular consumption of fish and other food sources of omega-3 fatty acids (e.g., walnuts) could have a more favorable overall risk-to-benefit ratio. This is an area of interest, but consensus does not exist.

A mechanism by which a reduction in dietary fat intake is hypothesized to influence breast cancer risk is that of reducing serum estrogen concentrations. Various feeding and intervention studies have examined the effect of dietary fat reduction on serum estrogen levels. As summarized in a review of these studies by Wu *et al.* [34], estrogen levels generally decreased with fat restriction. Note, however, that significant weight loss occurred in 6 of the 13 studies. Also, intake of dietary fiber was concurrently (and usually substantially) increased in the majority of these studies. Therefore, the interpretation that dietary fat restriction per se promotes a reduction in serum estradiol concentrations can be challenged, because an energy deficit, weight loss, and increased fiber intake could be the true or primary factors that promoted a reduction of hormone levels in these studies.

A relevant theory is that a high-fat (and thus energy-dense) diet during the developmental years may be a determinant of breast cancer risk in adulthood, rather than adult dietary fat intake (for which the evidence has not generally been supportive) [27]. This is a difficult relationship to test and would likely be confounded by the effect of energy density of the diet through childhood and adolescence on anthropometric characteristics (discussed in following sections).

In comparison with dietary fat intake, the evidence is somewhat more consistent for a protective effect of vegetables and fruit intake on risk for breast cancer. Because vegetables and fruits contribute the overwhelming majority of vitamin C and carotenoids in the diet, examination of the relationship between these compounds and breast cancer risk overlaps with investigation of an effect of vegetables and fruit. However, vegetables and fruit provide numerous phytochemicals and also fiber, in addition to the known micronutrients, that may contribute to a protective effect. In a meta-analysis based on 26 studies published from 1982 to 1997, the relationships between risk for breast cancer and intakes of vegetables, fruit, beta-carotene, and vitamin C were examined [35]. High (versus low) consumption of vegetables was found to convey the strongest protective effect (relative risk 0.75, 95% CI 0.66–0.85), with protective effects also evident for beta-carotene and vitamin C intakes as independent variables, but the relationship with fruit consumption was not significant (relative risk 0.94, 95% CI 0.74–1.11) [35].

Recent U.S. case-control and cohort studies provide examples of the degree of risk reduction that has been attributed to these foods. Freudenheim *et al.* [36] examined the association between breast cancer risk and intakes of vegetables, fruit, vitamin C, folate, individual carotenoids, alpha-tocopherol, and dietary fiber in premenopausal women (297 cases and 311 controls) in an analysis that separated the effect of food sources and dietary supplements for the micronutrients. Dietary (but not supplemental) beta-carotene, lutein + zeaxanthin, vitamin C, folate, alpha-tocopherol, and dietary fiber were all found to provide significant protective effects. Most notable was the odds ratio for total vegetable intake, which was 0.46 (95% CI 0.28–0.74), and adjusting only for beta-carotene and lutein + zeaxanthin attenuated this effect. In a large U.S. case-control study that included both premenopausal and postmenopausal women (3543 cases and 9406 controls), eating carrots or spinach more than twice weekly (compared with no intake) was found to be associated with an odds ratio of 0.56 (95% CI 0.34–0.91) [37]. In a U.S. cohort study involving 83,234 women with 2697 incident cases of invasive breast cancer over a 14-year follow-up period [38], strong inverse associations with risk were found for intakes of alpha-carotene, beta-carotene, lutein + zeaxanthin, vitamin C from foods, and total vitamin A. Premenopausal women who consumed ≥5 servings of vegetables and fruit per day had a relative risk of 0.77 (95% CI 0.58–1.02), compared to those consuming <2 servings per day (P = 0.05 for trend), and the effect was stronger among those with a family history or if consumption of ≥15 g alcohol per day was reported. Results of studies in which plasma or adipose tissue concentrations of carotenoids (a marker of vegetable and fruit intake) were quantified have often (but not always) suggested a protective effect in association with higher amounts of these compounds in the tissue [39–41], which would support the observations based on self-reported dietary intakes.

Biologically feasible mechanisms and/or supportive laboratory evidence for several constituents of vegetables and fruits have been reported. In cell cultures, both retinoids and carotenoids have been shown to enhance cellular differentiation and to have marked inhibitory effects on mammary cell growth [42, 43]. Several studies using breast epithelial cells and cell lines have demonstrated that both provitamin A and nonprovitamin A carotenoids, similar to retinoids, promote growth inhibition and apoptosis in transformed cells [43–45]. Vitamin A and carotenoids have a biochemical overlap, because both can be a source of retinoids and exhibit retinoid-like activities. However, the food sources, tissue uptake, regulation, and metabolism of the carotenoids differ from those of preformed vitamin A. Carotenoids can be delivered to peripheral tissue in direct association with intakes across a wide range, with resulting retinoid-like activities in those tissues. In contrast, dietary preformed vitamin A is correlated with biological activity in peripheral tissue only in the lower range of intakes. Another mechanistic theory, which is more limited and not as well supported by current evidence, would group carotenoids with vitamin C and vitamin E, and then assume their mechanistic relationship with breast cancer to be due to an antioxidant effect.

Antioxidants could theoretically reduce the risk for breast cancer by protecting against DNA damage and other free-radical-induced cellular changes that would promote mammary carcinogenesis. However, the relationship between risk for breast cancer and status for vitamin E, which has a well-established function as a biological antioxidant, has been examined in numerous studies, and the results are generally not very supportive [23, 46]. In a large European case-control study among postmenopausal women, adipose tissue concentrations of alpha-tocopherol and beta-carotene and concentration of selenium in toenails were examined in 347 incident cases of breast cancer and 374 controls [47]. Mean levels of these compounds did not differ between the study groups, and analysis did not reveal significant trends suggesting a beneficial effect. U.S. cohort studies also have not generally found an association between vitamin E intake or serum concentrations and risk for breast cancer [48–51].

Another micronutrient of current interest as possibly influencing the risk for breast cancer is folate. Historically, vegetables and fruits have been the major sources of folate in the diet, prior to folic acid fortification. Studies with laboratory animals have demonstrated that folate inadequacy promotes DNA strand breaks and hypomethylation of the *p53* gene [52], indicating a potential biological role in cancer initiation and promotion.

Results from one large prospective study suggest that folate intake, in addition to a possible independent effect, may influence breast cancer risk through an interaction with alcohol [53]. Quite consistently, alcohol intake has been positively associated with risk for breast cancer in epidemiological studies reported during the 1980s and 1990s. The relationship between alcohol intake and breast cancer risk

across the range of alcohol consumption among women in developed countries was examined in a pooled analysis of data from six prospective studies that included a total of 322,647 women [54]. Pooled analysis of data from these cohort studies indicates that alcohol intake exhibits a dose-response relationship with risk for breast cancer, at least up to 60 g/day. The multivariate adjusted relative risk for total alcohol intake of 30–60 g/day (approximately 2–5 drinks/day), compared to nondrinkers, was 1.41 (95% CI 1.18–1.69). Source of alcohol (e.g., wine, beer, spirits) did not influence risk estimates in this pooled analysis. Alcohol has well-known effects on folate status, by interfering with the metabolism of folate and thus increasing the requirement if normal folate-related functions are to be maintained at an optimal level. In a prospective cohort study involving 88,818 women with 3483 incident breast cancer cases over a 16-year follow-up period [53], folate intake $\geq$600 µg/day compared to 150–299 µg/day was associated with a multivariate relative risk of 0.55 (95% CI 0.39–0.76, $P = 0.01$ for trend) among women who consumed $\geq$15 g/day of alcohol. These data would suggest that one mechanism by which alcohol influences risk for breast cancer is through an effect on folate status, because that risk appears to be attenuated by increased folate intake. The prevailing hypothesis has been that alcohol intake promotes increased serum estrogen levels, which could explain the link to breast cancer risk. As reviewed by Ginsburg [55], results from controlled studies suggest that the interaction between alcohol and estrogen is more complicated than has been suggested. In premenopausal women, acute and chronic alcohol consumption appears to increase serum estrogen. In postmenopausal women, acute alcohol consumption increases serum estradiol in users of estrogen replacement therapy, but does not increase circulating estrone or estradiol levels in postmenopausal women who do not use estrogen replacement therapy [55].

As noted above, dietary fiber has been suggested to reduce risk for breast cancer, by perhaps mediating levels of circulating estrogens. This proposed biological mechanism is based on potential interference with enterohepatic estrogen circulation, which is a normal aspect of estrogen metabolism. In this process, about one-third to one-half of the circulating estrogens are secreted in the bile, followed by reabsorption of about 80% of these estrogens [56]. In animal models, dietary fiber has been shown to promote a reduction in circulating estrogen levels as a result of binding in the intestinal lumen, which results in a decreased efficiency of estrogen reabsorption. Among the types of cereal grains and bran that have been tested, those with the highest percentage of lignin, such as wheat bran, exhibit the highest binding affinity for estrogen [57]. However, case-control and cohort studies that have examined the relationship between fiber intake and risk for breast cancer have generally not found a significant protective effect [23, 25]. Limited support for a protective effect of dietary fiber in epidemiological studies, in spite of an evident biological effect in laboratory animal studies, has been attributed to methodological limitations

in diet assessment, which may be greater for fiber than for many other dietary factors, including imprecise food content data and limitations of assessment instruments in categorizing subjects by fiber intake.

In ecological studies, countries that consume greater amounts of soy and soy products, mainly native Japanese and Chinese populations, have historically exhibited the lowest breast cancer mortality rates, when compared with the United States and most European countries [58]. Soy is the richest source of phytoestrogens in the diet, and these soy isoflavones have been shown to exert hormonal effects in cell culture systems and laboratory animal models [59]. Thus, a role in breast cancer prevention for soy and soy isoflavones, as well as other phytoestrogens, has been investigated in numerous laboratory and epidemiological studies. As reviewed by Herman *et al.* [60], both lignans, found in whole grains, fruits, vegetables, and seeds, and the isoflavone phytoestrogens, found in soy and most soy products, have been shown to bind to estrogen receptors and exhibit weak estrogenic activity. Cell culture studies have further shown that genistein, which is the principal isoflavone in soy, has additional biological activities that could be anticarcinogenic in the human biological system, such as an inhibitory effect on tyrosine kinases and related signaling pathways and angiogenesis, and thus could promote differentiation [61]. Because phytoestrogens can act as estrogen agonists as well as antagonists, however, it is possible that phytoestrogens could potentially promote cancer-related changes in mammary cells. This would be most relevant for postmenopausal women, who do not have high levels of endogenous estrogens in the circulation that would compete for estrogen receptor binding sites. Indeed, results from cell culture studies have shown both beneficial and also adverse effects on the growth of mammary epithelial cells, and these observations may be due in part to the concentration of phytoestrogens in the cell culture medium [62].

The reader is referred to Murkies *et al.* [63] for a comprehensive review of the clinical evidence linking phytoestrogens to chronic disease, including breast cancer. Overall, evidence for an effect of soy isoflavones and flaxseed (a source of lignans) on serum hormone concentrations in premenopausal women is inconsistent [59, 64–67]. Clinical evidence for a modest estrogenic effect in response to soy feeding has been observed in studies involving postmenopausal women, as reviewed by Kurzer [59]. Results from case-control studies that have examined the relationship between dietary soy intake and breast cancer risk among Asian and Asian-American populations have been inconclusive [68]. Thus, more clinical studies of the biological effects that might increase or decrease risk for breast cancer are clearly needed before conclusions or consensus opinions on soy or other sources of phystoestrogens can be formulated.

Table 1 lists nutrients and other dietary constituents that have been the focus of research on the link between dietary intakes and risk for breast cancer.

2. ANTHROPOMETRIC CHARACTERISTICS AND RISK FOR BREAST CANCER

a. Associations with Skeletal Markers. Previously thought to be a predictive factor only in populations where energy restriction was significant enough to affect skeletal growth, adult height has emerged as one of the more consistent risk factors for breast cancer in both pre- and postmenopausal women [69–71]. Large cohort and case-control studies conducted among American, European, and Asian women consistently suggest that adult height is a significant risk factor for this disease [71–75]. Among U.S. women ($N = 3430$), Brinton and Swanson [72] found that height greater than 68 inches was associated with breast cancer risks that were 50–80% higher than height ≤ 62 inches. It has been hypothesized that growth factors that drive skeletal development also play a role in stimulating the proliferation of mammary stem cells and thereby increase mammary mass [70]. Although many of these growth factors may be more under the control of heredity rather than diet, recognition of height as a risk factor may be of some benefit by allowing identification of high-risk women who then could be targeted for interventions. Other skeletal indices, such as increased elbow breadth (a marker of frame size), femur length, and bone density also have been associated with increased risk [72, 76]. To date, however, studies have failed to show any association between skeletal markers and disease progression or mortality, in contrast to anthropometric markers of adiposity (discussed in the following section).

b. Associations with Adiposity. Hippocrates was the first to report an association between obesity and breast cancer. The classic studies by Tannenbaum in the 1940s confirmed this premise, and in 1975 deWaard put forth the hypothesis that body nutriture affects risk—an effect mediated by hormonal levels. Despite these observations, it should be noted that a clear discrepancy exists with regard to adiposity and its ability to portend risk for premenopausal versus postmenopausal disease, with relative body leanness serving as a risk factor for disease occurring before menopause and obesity serving as a risk factor for postmenopausal breast cancer [69, 77, 78]. Many have speculated about the reasons for these differences, with some theorizing that body leanness may enhance early detection among younger women, whereas others adhere to the belief that premenopausal breast cancer is distinctly different from postmenopausal disease, being governed more by genetic predisposition and growth factors rather than by long-term exposure to the interacting effects of ovarian steroid hormones and lifestyle factors [70, 79].

In addition to obesity, body fat distribution also appears to play a role in predicting risk for obesity. A majority of studies support central or visceral obesity (primarily assessed via waist:hip ratio) as an additional risk factor [69, 73, 80]. Results from a large cohort study by Sonnenschein *et al.* [81] ($N = 8157$) suggest that waist:hip ratio serves as an independent risk factor for premenopausal breast cancer, in which the increased presence of abdominal fat may be

TABLE 1   Nutrients, Foods, and Other Dietary Factors Suggested to Be Associated with Risk for
Primary Breast Cancer

Strength of current evidence	Nutrient, food, or dietary constituent	Proposed direction of association	Comments
Fairly consistent evidence from epidemiologic analytical research, and biological mechanism(s) are plausible	Vegetable and fruit intake	Decreases risk	Several potential contributing mechanisms, attributable to numerous dietary constituents
	Alcohol intake	Increases risk	Possibly affects risk through hormonal effects, although clinical studies suggest a complicated relationship; possibly linked through effect on folate status
Inconsistent evidence from epidemiologic analytical research, but biological mechanism(s) are plausible and/or demonstrable in laboratory studies	Dietary fiber intake	Decreases risk	Effects on hormonal factors demonstrable in biological systems
	Folate intake	Decreases risk	May contribute to beneficial effects of vegetables and fruits; possibly interacts with alcohol intake
	Carotenoid and vitamin A intake	Decreases risk	May contribute to beneficial effects of vegetables and fruits; strongly supportive evidence from cell culture studies
Evidence from epidemiologic analytical research generally not supportive, but biological mechanism(s) may be plausible or demonstrable	Dietary fat	Decreases risk	Possible effects on hormonal factors, but clinical studies are difficult to interpret due to confounding variables
	Specific fatty acids	Variable effects	Cell culture studies show differential effects of omega-6 and omega-3 fatty acids, but relevance to dietary patterns is not established or evident
	Vitamins E and C and selenium	Decreases risk	Antioxidant effects possible, hypothesized to interact with genetic polymorphisms (e.g., glutathione S-transferase)
Insufficient evidence from epidemiologic analytical research, but biological mechanism(s) may be plausible or demonstrable	Well-done meat	Increases risk	Linked to carcinogens such as heterocyclic amines, hypothesized to interact with genetic polymorphisms (e.g., N-acetyltransferase)
	Soy and soy isoflavones, flaxseed	Variable effects	Although inverse associations suggested by ecologic studies, cell culture studies indicate possibility of adverse effects as well
Evidence from epidemiologic analytical research generally not supportive, and biological mechanism(s) unknown or not demonstrable	Caffeine	—	No association with increased risk found consistently in case-control and cohort studies
	Protein	—	Associated in some case-control but not cohort studies; may be confounded by other characteristics of the diet

linked to increased levels of insulin and related growth factors, whereas among postmenopausal women, waist:hip ratio may serve as another indicator of obesity. Studies by Sellers *et al.* [82] and London *et al.* [83] suggest that risk conferred by either obesity or waist:hip ratio may be further increased by a positive family history.

Given that weight is not a static measure and fluctuates throughout life, it is conceivable that risk may be modified by the presence of obesity or body weight status at differing ages. Although there is a dearth of data, some researchers have speculated that the *in utero* experience, the hormonal milieu of the host mother and her weight gain during pregnancy, may establish a "gonadostat"—a hormonal thermostat that governs the hormonal levels of progeny after birth and thereby influences risk for hormonally linked cancers [78]. Further research is necessary to either support or refute

the presence of hormonal setpoints and the importance of maternal host factors. Indeed, one of the more severe limitations to such research, as well as any studies that assess lifelong exposure, is the reliance on case-control studies and data that for the most part are collected retrospectively.

Studies that have assessed weight prior to or during early adulthood suggest that obesity may actually be protective [84, 85]. This relationship appears logical for premenopausal breast cancer, in which relative obesity is already an acknowledged protective factor. However, given the relationship between increased weight and early menarche, it is difficult to reason why early obesity would be protective for postmenopausal breast cancer. Recent studies, however, indicate that although increased body weight during childhood is predictive of early menarche (among both tall and obese girls), obese girls have significantly fewer ovulatory cycles

and thereby have lower circulating levels of both estrogen and progesterone—hormones that are known to stimulate breast cancer growth [86, 87].

On attainment of adulthood, especially during later adulthood, there appears to be a consistent finding of weight gain and increased body weight being highly associated with increased risk for postmenopausal cancer [69, 71, 77, 88, 89]. The reader is referred to reviews by Ballard-Barbash [69] and Ziegler [71], who provide detailed information and interpretation of body weight and other anthropometric markers in relation to breast cancer risk. In the case of risk associated with adult weight gain, this increased risk has been largely explained by the fact that as women age, their circulating levels of estrogen become more influenced by estrogens produced by adipose tissue rather than those produced by the ovary [79, 89]. Weight gain after age 40 years is also is more likely to be deposited in an android versus gynoid pattern and hence may foretell insulin resistance and the increased production of insulin and insulin-like growth factors that may act synergistically with estrogen to confer risk [69, 77, 88].

Additionally, increased body weight at diagnosis has been recognized as a poor prognostic factor for breast cancer for more than 25 years [90–92]. While obese women are more likely to exhibit advanced stage disease at the time of diagnosis, more than 13 large cohort and case-control studies suggest increased body weight as a risk factor for recurrent disease even after controlling for menopausal status, age, stage, tumor size, and nodal involvement [71, 91–94]. Furthermore, weight gain after diagnosis also increase risk for recurrent disease and mortality (discussed below).

Because body weight is a modifiable risk factor, diet and physical activity may be beneficial for the prevention and management of breast cancer. Few data, however, currently exist regarding weight loss relative to risk. Results are conflicting and confounded by the inability of studies to discern whether reported weight loss was the result of voluntary or involuntary efforts [69].

3. PHYSICAL ACTIVITY AND RISK FOR BREAST CANCER

The first associations between cancer and physical activity were reported by Taylor et al. [95] in 1962. They found that all-cancer mortality rates were significantly increased among sedentary office workers when compared to workers who had more physically demanding positions. During the past 30 years, several investigations have specifically explored the role of physical activity in relation to colon cancer—investigations in which consistent inverse associations have been found [96, 97]. In comparison, far fewer studies that have addressed associations between physical activity and breast cancer have been conducted or reported, and these have been fairly recent. Frisch et al. [98] were the first to report a protective effect of exercise for breast cancer. In a study of 5398 college alumni (2622 of whom were former college athletes and 2766 were nonathletes), they found

that nonathletes had a relative risk of 1.86 (95% CI 1.00–3.47) compared to athletes. The investigators credited risk reduction to the ability of exercise to delay the onset of menarche [98]. Research in this area remained fairly fallow until Bernstein et al. [99] reported findings of a large case-control study (545 breast cancer cases and 545 age, race, parity, and neighborhood-matched controls) that found women who spent 3.8 hours or more per week in physical exercise activities were significantly less likely to develop breast cancer (odds ratio 0.42, 95% CI 0.27–0.64). During the late 1990s, more than two dozen case-control and cohort studies explored associations between physical activity and breast cancer risk. Although findings of these studies have not detected protective effects as strong and consistent as those obtained in studies of colon cancer, a majority of the studies (18 of 26) suggest that increased physical activity is inversely related to breast cancer risk [96, 97, 100, 101]. The reader is referred to comprehensive reviews by Friedenreich and Rohan [100] and Gammon et al. [101]. Because results from animal studies suggest that exercise decreases tumor burden across cancers [102], some speculate that the odds ratios observed in breast cancer studies may be attenuated due to an inability to control for reproductive factors (in many studies, these data were unavailable) or a limitation of instruments to assess physical activity related to housework and childrearing [97]. The protective effects of physical activity are hypothesized to be due to the ability of exercise to mediate levels of endogenous hormones and ovulatory cycles, affect energy balance, and enhance immune response [103]. Studies by Thune et al. [104] and Latikka et al. [105] suggest that exercise may be even more protective among lean women, because they are more likely to become anovulatory with increased physical activity.

B. Nutritional Factors, Prognosis, and Risk for Cancer Recurrence

Factors associated with risk for primary breast cancer are generally assumed to have a high likelihood of association with risk for recurrence following the diagnosis, although actual reported cohort studies addressing this issue are still limited in number (i.e., less than a dozen that examined a role for dietary factors have been published to date). Notably, much of the evidence for biological activity that is cited to support a link between nutritional factors and risk for primary breast cancer is based on studies using cell lines derived from breast cancers or transformed cells (i.e., cells that already have molecular changes leading toward breast cancer). Most of the epidemiological studies that have addressed whether nutritional factors might be associated with improved prognosis or longer breast cancer-free survival time have relied on data that were collected at the time of diagnosis. This approach assumes that spontaneous, substantial changes in food choices or other factors would be unlikely or difficult for individuals following the diagnosis, which may or may not be true. Risk for recurrence and/or

overall survival (i.e., risk of death) are the dependent variables in these investigations, and associations with nutritional factors are typically similar for these two outcomes because they are highly correlated. Another important characteristic that affects interpretation of results from the studies that attempt to link diet with survival is the adjustment for factors that are known to influence survival, such as stage at diagnosis. If not considered in the analysis, these characteristics could confound the associations and may even influence factors such as body weight and food choices at diagnosis.

As noted above, the most consistent association with survival, among the various nutritional factors, is the link between degree of overweight at diagnosis and risk for recurrence. For example, in 557 women diagnosed with negative-node-negative breast cancer, those with body weight greater than 25% of desirable weight for height at diagnosis had significantly reduced rates of disease-free survival compared with nonobese women (hazard ratio 1.93, 95% CI 1.29–2.88) [106]. Among 735 women with lymph node-positive breast cancer who received adjuvant chemotherapy, the adjusted proportional-hazards regression model indicates that risk for disease recurrence over a 10-year period for patients more than 20% over desirable weight for height was 1.33 times that of patients not more than 20% overweight (95% CI 1.05–1.68) [107]. In the Iowa Women's Health Study, women in the highest tertile of body mass index at diagnosis of breast cancer had an age-adjusted 1.9-fold higher risk (95% CI 1.0–3.7) of dying during a median follow-up time of 2.9 years after diagnosis, when adjusted for other prognostic variables [108].

Several studies have associated decreased survival with dietary fat intake at diagnosis, adjusted [109–111] or unadjusted [108, 112, 113] for energy, whereas others [114–116] did not detect this association. The issue of energy adjustment is illustrated in the findings from a study by Saxe et al. [117], in which both energy (hazard ratio 1.58, 95% CI 1.05 –2.38) and total fat (hazard ratio 1.46, 95% CI 1.05–2.01) intakes were directly associated with risk for recurrence, but the significance of the association with fat intake disappeared when energy-adjusted. In a study that used a food-based approach to describing dietary intake, risk for recurrence was associated with intakes of butter, margarine, and lard (servings/day) with a risk ratio of 1.67 (95% CI 1.17–2.39) among premenopausal women, adjusted for disease stage and age [118]. In a prospective study by Holmes et al. [119] involving 1982 women diagnosed with breast cancer, in which dietary data (from food frequency questionnaires) were collected preceding and following the diagnosis, and numerous adjustments were performed to separate the influence of dietary factors, no apparent association between fat intake and mortality was observed. However, protein intake, mainly linked to poultry, fish, and dairy food sources, was found to exert a protective effect (relative risk 0.65, 95% CI 0.47–0.88).

Protective effects for vegetables and fruits and the associated micronutrients, vitamin C and the carotenoids, also have been observed in several of these follow-up cohort studies [109, 111, 119, 120], with more consistency than has been observed for dietary fat. Rohan et al. [111] found that women consuming ≥8058 mg beta-carotene per day at diagnosis, compared to women consuming ≤3051 mg/day, had a 32% reduction in risk of death over a mean of 5.5 years follow-up, although this difference was only marginally significant ($P = 0.075$ for trend) when adjusted for energy and other risk factors. Ingram [120] found total fruit and vegetable ($P = 0.04$), beta-carotene ($P = 0.001$), and vitamin C ($P = 0.03$ for trend) intakes at diagnosis to be associated with increased likelihood of survival in a cohort of 103 women diagnosed with breast cancer and followed for 6 years, although this analysis was not adjusted for stage at diagnosis. Similar findings were reported from a cohort of 678 women diagnosed with breast cancer followed for nearly 8 years [109]. The hazard ratio for dying of breast cancer in this study was 0.48 (95% CI 0.23–0.99) for the highest compared to the lowest quartile of beta-carotene intake, and was 0.43 (95% CI 0.21–0.86) for vitamin C intake, adjusted for stage, tumor characteristics, age, and menopausal status. In the largest cohort of this type reported to date (described above), increased vegetable and fruit intake (≥4.2 versus ≤2.1 servings/day) was associated with decreased mortality in the women without metastatic disease at diagnosis [119]. This association was generally supported by data on the relevant individual nutrients provided by these foods. For example, the multivariate relative risk of death for lutein + zeaxanthin intake was 0.87 (95% CI 0.62–1.21, $P = 0.04$ for trend), comparing the highest to the lowest quintile.

Although alcohol intake has been identified as a risk factor for primary breast cancer, as discussed above, follow-up studies in which this variable has been examined have rather consistently not found a relationship between alcohol intake and overall survival [110, 111, 117, 119]. Earlier cohort studies of women diagnosed with breast cancer also did not find an association between dietary fiber intake and likelihood of survival [109–111, 120], although data from more recent reports are not in agreement. Energy-adjusted bread and cereal consumption was found to be protective against recurrence, although quantified dietary fiber intake per se was not significantly associated, in a recent cohort study of 149 women followed for >5 years following diagnosis [117]. In the largest of this type of cohort followed to date, relative risk of death was significantly linked to dietary fiber intake (relative risk 0.69, 95% CI 0.50–0.97), comparing the highest to the lowest quintile [119].

III. NUTRITIONAL ISSUES FOLLOWING THE DIAGNOSIS OF BREAST CANCER

During the 1980s and 1990s, the development and use of effective screening technologies have resulted in an increased ability to detect cancers at earlier stages when treatments are most effective. With increased breast cancer

awareness and the use of screening mammography, a majority of all breast cancers are now diagnosed at a localized stage, with 96% 5-year relative survival rates [121]. These successes have resulted in a paradigm shift, because breast cancer is now managed largely as a chronic disease, rather than treated as an acute fatality [122]. Therefore, although the next section will address nutritional concerns that may emerge in the months that immediately follow diagnosis, nutrition interventions for patients with breast cancer have become largely focused on promoting long-term health via healthful eating, a physically active lifestyle, and the avoidance of obesity [123–125]. However, little is known about what constitutes an optimal diet during the initial treatment for breast cancer, no diets or dietary supplements have yet to be proven to be helpful, and little is currently known about nutrient-treatment modality interactions [126]. Indeed, further research is sorely needed in this area.

A. Issues and Interventions in the Initial Treatment of Breast Cancer

1. SURGERY-RELATED NUTRITIONAL ISSUES

Almost all patients with breast cancer, except those with inflammatory breast cancer, receive surgery (i.e., either mastectomy or lumpectomy) as a primary treatment for their disease. Some receive axillary node dissection or sentinel node biopsy to provide additional information that can be used to help guide decision making for adjuvant forms of treatment. In some cases, such as when tumors are excessively large, diffuse, or difficult to excise, neoadjuvant therapy is given prior to surgery with the expectation that this will reduce the tumor and thus make it easier to remove. In most cases, however, surgery is usually the first, and sometimes the only, treatment received [127].

In contrast to other cancers, such as head and neck, in which patients often are malnourished on diagnosis, or in some gastrointestinal cancers in which prolonged postsurgical recovery may impinge upon nutritional status, patients with breast cancer are unlikely to have nutritional deficiencies and are also unlikely to manifest them either at diagnosis or during the postsurgical period [128]. This includes any additional surgeries that might be pursued for reconstructive purposes. Therefore, there is seldom a need to promote any particular diet other than one that is healthful. Exceptions to the rule, however, do occur and standard procedures to assess nutritional status and to intervene, if necessary, are still warranted (discussed below).

Given the important role of obesity in influencing risk for breast cancer among postmenopausal women, and the role it plays as an unfavorable prognostic factor in both pre- and postmenopausal disease, patients with breast cancer should be encouraged to achieve a desirable weight [69, 77, 129]. Interventions that promote the avoidance of weight gain are prudent during surgical recovery, and also during the completion of any adjuvant chemotherapy and/or radiation ther-

apy [129]. Active efforts toward weight loss, however, are most often delayed until wound healing and adjuvant treatment are complete, given concern that energy restriction may adversely affect immune function and healing [130].

2. ADJUVANT CHEMOTHERAPY

Chemotherapy is usually offered to breast cancer patients who are either at increased risk for systemic disease or among those in whom metastases have been identified. Side effects of chemotherapy include hair loss, neutropenia, mucositis, dysphagia, dysgeusia, nausea, vomiting, and, surprisingly, weight gain [91, 92].

In recent years, the development and use of antiemetic agents have greatly relieved the side effects of nausea and vomiting. However, a substantial number of patients with breast cancer still report these effects. Small and frequent feedings that are low in fat and comprised primarily of carbohydrates are often effective in relieving symptoms. Altered sense of taste also is frequently reported, with many patients complaining that foods do not taste as they used to, "sweet foods taste too sweet, " and "meats taste metallic." In responding to these taste alterations, some patients may gravitate toward bland foods, such as rice, potatoes, and gelatin, whereas others seek out salty, spicy, or tart foods [131].

A smaller number of patients develop mucositis, which generally appears in mid- to late therapy [127]. Mouth sores may be exacerbated by foods with high acidity, such as salad dressings and fruit juices, as well as flinty foods such as tortilla chips. Difficulty swallowing is even more rare, and appropriate intake usually can be achieved with cool soothing foods such as gelatins and yogurts, as well as the use of sauces or gravies on solid food items. Fortunately, these symptoms are often short lived, usually lasting for a portion of the week following chemotherapy administration.

Seemingly in direct contrast to these side effects is the side effect of weight gain. Previous studies suggest that weight gain is especially pronounced among premenopausal women, and among those who have nodal involvement and who receive multiagent regimens [91, 92]. Gains in weight commonly range from 2.5 to 6.2 kg; however, greater gains are not unusual. Boyd reports that one out of four premenopausal patients with breast cancer gains more than 11 kg during the course of adjuvant chemotherapy [132].

This weight gain is undesirable for several reasons. First, it may negatively affect quality of life. Previous studies indicate that a majority of patients with breast cancer find weight gain distressing and report it as a major concern [133–136]. Second, this weight gain may predispose women to other diseases and weight-related problems, such as hypertension, cardiovascular disease, gallbladder disease, orthopedic disturbances, and diabetes mellitus [122, 137]. Such disease can cause significant morbidity and mortality, which continues once management of breast cancer is achieved. Finally, although not conclusive, there is evidence to sug-

gest that weight gain adversely affects disease-free survival. Camoriano et al. [133] followed 646 patients with breast cancer for a median of 6.6 years and found that premenopausal patients who gained more than the median amount of weight (5.9 kg) were 1.5 times more likely to relapse and 1.6 times more likely to die of their breast cancer. Results from studies conducted by Chlebowski et al. [138] and Goodwin et al. [139] parallel these findings and suggest a need for interventions that prevent the prevalent problem of weight gain in this population.

To date, only a handful of interventions to prevent gains in weight that specifically occur during adjuvant chemotherapy have been tested, and these have been met with mixed results. In a randomized trial of 104 early stage breast cancer patients, Loprinzi et al. [140] found that patients who received intensive diet counseling on energy-restricted diets failed to gain significantly less weight than those assigned to the control arm. In contrast, a phase II study by Goodwin et al. [141], who tested a structured program of diet (an energy-restricted, low-fat, and high-fiber diet) and exercise on 61 newly diagnosed, loco-regional breast cancer patients, found this multifaceted intervention to be successful. Follow-up analyses revealed that the strongest predictor of this program's success was increased physical activity, not diet. A cross-sectional study by Rock et al. [142] also points to the role of physical activity as an important factor governing weight gain in women following the diagnosis of breast cancer.

Although much more research is needed, results of these studies provide support for interventions to include, if not center on, physical activity. This premise is further supported by findings of Aslani et al. [143], Cheney et al. [144], Demark-Wahnefried et al. [145, 146], and Kutynec et al. [147], who by differing methods (i.e., dual energy X-ray absorptiometry, computer-assisted tomography, in vivo neutron capture analysis) found that the weight gain experienced by patients with breast cancer occurs either in the absence of any gains in lean tissue or in the presence of lean tissue loss. This distinctive weight gain pattern, increased gains in adipose tissue with concurrent with losses of muscle mass, is a condition usually associated with the chronic use of corticosteroids, hypopituitarism, neuromuscular diseases, hypogonadism, prolonged inactivity or bed rest, and menopause, and one in which resistance training and aerobic activity represent the cornerstones of treatment. Because most physical activity interventions directed toward this population have either been inadequately controlled or focused on other endpoints (i.e., improvement in quality of life, reduction of nausea), much more research is necessary to determine optimal interventions for this population with regard to both content and delivery [148]. Given that most well-controlled studies do not support increased energy intake as a cause of weight gain in this population, it is doubtful that energy restriction should play a major role in these interventions. Also, an overemphasis on dieting or energy restriction may exacerbate eating pathology and psychological distress in these patients [149]. However, these patients may benefit from programs that promote plant-based diets that are high in calcium and low in fat [92, 131, 146, 147, 150]. Furthermore, there may be a need to develop discrete interventions that respond to the specific needs of both premenopausal and postmenopausal patients.

3. NUTRITIONAL ISSUES ASSOCIATED WITH RADIATION THERAPY

Radiation therapy is often used to establish local control of breast cancer. Because radiation fields rarely include the alimentary tract, there are usually no direct nutrition-related effects. Indeed, side effects appear to be limited to mild erythema and fatigue [151]. As with chemotherapy, patients actually may feel energized if they pursue routine physical activity during the period that they receive these treatments (usually a time period of 6 weeks). Several physical activity interventions have been pursued within this population as a means to improve quality of life and increased functional capacity; however, for the most part, these efforts have been uncontrolled and small in size [148].

4. NUTRITIONAL ISSUES ASSOCIATED WITH HORMONAL THERAPY

Megestrol acetate is a long-standing hormonal agent used in the treatment of breast cancer [91]. Today, the use of megestrol acetate is usually confined to women who have later stage disease. One of the more noteworthy side effects of this agent is weight gain, an effect so reliable that megestrol acetate is marketed as an anticachexic agent for other cancers. Although one might assume that the issue of weight gain would be less of a concern among women with later stage disease, a study by Kornblith et al. [152] suggests that most patients still find this side effect distressing. To date, no interventions aimed at weight control have been reported in this select patient population.

Tamoxifen and next-generation selective estrogen receptor modulators represent hormonal agents that have been offered to women with earlier stage disease. In the past, these were only offered to women with estrogen receptor-positive tumors; however, recently their use has become more widespread, as agents for cancer control and as agents for cancer prevention [153]. Reports of weight gain with tamoxifen have been mixed, with some studies reporting gains [154] and some not [153]. A body composition study by Ali et al. [155], however, suggests that irrespective of weight gain, tamoxifen is associated with increases in body fatness. Thus, women prescribed tamoxifen and/or next-generation estrogen receptor modulators also may benefit from interventions that include increased physical activity; however, no such studies have been reported to date.

An additional concern with these hormonal agents is their potential interaction with foods or supplements that are rich in phytoestrogens, such as soy foods and soy supplements.

Speculation exists that specific phytoestrogenic compounds may interfere with the action of hormonal agents and reduce their effect, or perhaps stimulate the growth of initiated breast cancers by themselves [156]. Further research is necessary to determine potential interactions or direct effects, but until then, the risks and/or benefits of supplemental genistein, daidzein, or other related compounds are unknown and they cannot be recommended. Likewise, the use of soy foods above moderate levels also cannot be supported without further research.

5. ADDITIONAL CONCERNS

In 1993, Monnin *et al.* [136] reported the results of a descriptive study of 143 early stage breast cancer patients who were participating in a community-based Reach to Recovery Program. Respondent interest was high for diets aimed at cancer prevention (60%), reduced fat (56%), and weight reduction (48%). Although somewhat dated, this study suggests that patients with breast cancer are interested in nutrition-related programs, findings that were supported in a study by Demark-Wahnefried *et al.* [157], who found high levels of interest in both diet (57% were ''very'' to ''extremely'' interested) and exercise (56% were ''very'' to ''extremely'' interested) programs among 531 breast cancer survivors. Fifty-two percent of these respondents indicated a preference for interventions to be offered within 3 months of diagnosis. These findings suggest that interventions are likely to be greeted with good reception and high levels of interest; however, again more research is necessary to truly discern the unique barriers, the specific content, and the methods of delivery in order to promote optimal efficacy.

Previous studies also suggest that the majority of patients with breast cancer use either vitamin or mineral or herbal supplements [136, 157, 158]. While general concerns relating to herbal supplements (see Chapter 17) and vitamin and mineral supplements [159] have been previously addressed, there is a paucity of well-controlled research studies that have either supported or refuted the use of supplements among women who have already been diagnosed with breast cancer. Concern exists, however, with regard to supplement use during treatment, because of speculation that high-dose supplemental nutrients may stimulate cell repair of neoplastic cells, which are the intended targets of both chemotherapy and radiation therapy, while others argue that supplements may render cancer cells more chemosensitive by enhancing cell cycling [160]. Again, further research is necessary to determine the potential benefits and/or risks of nutritional and herbal supplements with respect to their use during treatment.

B. The Long-Term Perspective: Issues and Interventions under Study

Nutrition and breast cancer is currently an active area of research, with several studies testing the relationship between dietary intake and cancer incidence. In addition to studies aimed at primary prevention, two large ongoing multicenter studies are examining whether diet modification can influence the risk for recurrence and the overall survival following the diagnosis of breast cancer.

In the Women's Health Initiative, postmenopausal women aged 50–79 years are enrolled at 40 clinical centers nationwide into a clinical trial ($N = 64,000$) or an observational study ($N = 100,000$) [161]. One arm of the randomized clinical trial is testing whether a low-fat eating pattern ($\leq20\%$ of energy from fat, ≥5 servings/day vegetables and fruits, ≥6 servings/day grain products) may help to prevent breast cancer, with colorectal cancer and cardiovascular disease as additional study outcomes under evaluation in that arm. The Canadian Diet and Breast Cancer Prevention Trial, a multicenter randomized controlled study, is testing whether a low-fat (15% of energy), high-carbohydrate diet intervention can reduce the incidence of breast cancer over a 10-year period among women aged 30–65 years who have increased mammographic density [162]. Studies suggest that mammographic density is a marker of histopathologic changes in breast tissue associated with increased risk for cancer [163], and preliminary studies indicate that a reduction in dietary fat intake may promote a reduction of mammographic density in the breast [164, 165]. Other studies are targeting women with a family history of breast cancer, testing whether a low-fat diet ($<15\%$ of energy) and/or nine daily servings of vegetables and fruits is feasible in this group and is associated with changes in oxidative DNA levels [166, 167].

Table 2 summarizes the key features of two ongoing multicenter randomized clinical trials that are testing whether diet intervention can reduce risk for recurrence in women who are breast cancer survivors. In the Women's Intervention Nutrition Study, the primary dietary goal is a reduction in dietary fat intake ($\leq15\%$ energy from fat) [168]. Preliminary data indicate good adherence, with an average reduction from 33% to 20% energy from fat at 6 months into the study [168]. In the Women's Healthy Eating and Living Study, the primary emphasis is on increased vegetable and fruit intake, with daily dietary goals of five vegetable servings, 16 ounces of vegetable juice, three fruit servings, 15–20% energy from fat, and 30 g dietary fiber. Feasibility study reports and preliminary trial data from this study also indicate excellent adherence [169–171]. Key outcomes of interest in both of these studies are recurrence-free survival and overall survival, and study participants are followed for an average of 6 years.

Until more definitive evidence becomes available, published dietary guidelines, such as those from the American Cancer Society [172, 173] and the American Institute for Cancer Research [174], form the basis of current recommendations. Among the published dietary guidelines, those that appear to be most relevant to the prevention and control of breast cancer, based on current knowledge, emphasize plant-based diets with increased intake of vegetables and fruit, the

TABLE 2 Key Features of Two Large Ongoing Multicenter Randomized Clinical Trials Testing Whether Diet Intervention Can Reduce Risk for Recurrence of Breast Cancer in Women Diagnosed with Early Stage Disease

Study characteristics	Women's Intervention Nutrition Study	Women's Healthy Eating and Living Study
Subjects	$N = 2500$; recruited from clinical sites nationwide	$N = 3000$; recruited from clinical sites in California, Arizona, Texas, and Oregon
Anticipated study end	2005	2004
Key eligibility criteria	Aged 48–78 years at time of diagnosis Diagnosed with primary operable invasive breast carcinoma categorized as stage I, stage II, or stage IIIA Randomized within 12 months of primary surgery Excluded if <20% energy from fat in baseline diet	Aged 18–70 years at time of diagnosis Diagnosed with primary operable invasive breast carcinoma categorized as stage I (≥1 cm), stage II, or stage IIIA within the previous 4 years Randomized after completion of initial therapies (e.g., radiation therapy, adjuvant chemotherapy) Pre-enrollment diet not considered in inclusion or exclusion criteria
Dietary goals for the intervention group	Reduced dietary fat (<15% of energy)	Daily dietary goals are five vegetable servings, 16 ounces vegetable juice, three fruit servings, 30 g fiber, and 15–20% energy from fat
Primary intervention method	Individualized counseling provided by a nutritionist at the clinical sites, plus quarterly group sessions	Centralized telephone counseling protocol, plus monthly cooking classes at the clinical sites

promotion of increased physical activity to promote healthy weight management, and limited consumption of alcohol (for primary prevention).

The risk for morbidity and mortality from causes other than breast cancer should be considered in dietary recommendations for breast cancer survivors, especially those diagnosed with early stage cancers [124]. Due to heightened health concerns, patients with breast cancer often are highly motivated to adhere to dietary recommendations that may improve overall health. For example, even though the current evidence to support a link between fat intake and risk for breast cancer (or the prognosis following diagnosis) is not strongly supportive, limiting saturated fat intake is a well-established strategy to promote a plasma lipoprotein and lipid profile that is associated with reduced risk for cardiovascular disease (see Chapter 18). Similarly, eating a diet with adequate dietary fiber has been associated with decreased risk of coronary heart disease in women [175] and may contribute to overall health, irrespective of a possible link between fiber and breast cancer.

A long-term effect of chemotherapy that can occur in women who are premenopausal at diagnosis is ovarian dysfunction. In women at risk for breast cancer recurrence, whatever their age, estrogen replacement therapy may not be an option, so dietary factors and lifestyle behaviors that may reduce risk for osteoporosis can be important in long-term care. Although tamoxifen and other selective estrogen receptor modulators have been observed to promote maintenance of bone density in postmenopausal women [176], many women are not prescribed these drugs because they are not considered good candidates for this type of pharmacologic treatment and, when prescribed, the treatment duration is

typically ≤5 years. Sufficient dietary calcium, adequate vitamin D intake, and increased physical activity are particularly appropriate recommendations to maintain bone health in this population.

IV. SUMMARY AND CONCLUSIONS

Breast cancer is the most common cancer among women in the United States and is a disease associated with multiple genetic, hormonal, environmental, and lifestyle factors. Diet is presumed to play a significant role in both the risk of breast cancer and the progression of disease. To date, however, given the dearth of findings from randomized, controlled clinical trials, which represent the ultimate test of the effects of nutritional factors on disease, there is little that can be definitively stated. Fortunately, within the next decade, results from large diet intervention trials should be able to provide solid information that can be used to develop evidence-based interventions and guidelines for both the prevention and treatment of breast cancer. Until then, findings from epidemiologic and laboratory studies provide some insight. Currently, good support exists for women to choose diets that are plant based (i.e., rich in vegetables and fruits) and limited in alcohol, which may reduce risk for primary breast cancer. While support for fat restriction in the prevention of breast cancer is conflicting, it must be borne in mind that although breast cancer is a major health concern for U.S. women, cardiovascular disease remains the largest cause of mortality. Limiting intake of fat, especially saturated fat, may help to reduce cardiovascular disease risk for all women, including breast cancer survivors. Physical activity

also can play a significant role in weight regulation and therefore is encouraged.

Although other factors hypothesized to influence risk may hold promise, to date, studies on these factors have had sufficient limitations in design and/or execution, or have been too small in size, to produce definitive findings. Therefore, nutrition and breast cancer remains a dynamic area in which much more research is needed.

References

1. Greenlee, R. T., Hill-Harmon, M. B., Murray, T., and Thun, M. (2001). Cancer statistics, 2001. *CA Cancer J. Clin.* **51,** 15–36.
2. Dignam, J. J. (2000). Differences in breast cancer prognosis among African-American and Caucasian women. *CA Cancer J. Clin.* **50,** 50–64.
3. Chu, K., Tarone, R., Kessler, L. G., Ries, L. A. G., Hankey, B. F., Miller, B. A., and Edwards, B. K. (1996). Recent trends in U.S. breast cancer incidence, survival, and mortality rates. *J. Natl. Cancer Inst.* **88,** 1571–1579.
4. Hayes, D. F., and Kaplan, W. (1996). Evaluation of patients after primary therapy. *In* "Diseases of the Breast" (J. R. Harris, M. E. Lippman, M. Morrow, and S. Hellman, Eds.). Lippincott-Raven, Philadelphia, PA.
5. Harris, J. R., Lippman, M. E., Veronesi, U., and Willett, W. (1992). Breast cancer (first of three parts). *N. Engl. J. Med.* **320,** 319–328.
6. Harris, C. C. (1991). Chemical and physical carcinogenesis: Advances and perspectives for the 1990s. *Cancer Res.* **51** (Suppl.), 5023S–5044S.
7. Slattery, M. L., O'Brian, E., and Mori, M. (1995). Disease heterogeneity: Does it impact our ability to detect dietary associations with breast cancer? *Nutr. Cancer* **24,** 213–220.
8. Russo, J., and Russo, I. H. (1994). Toward a physiological approach to breast cancer prevention. *Cancer Epidemiol. Biomarkers Prev.* **3,** 353–364.
9. Snekeker, S. M., and Diaugustine, R. P. (1996). Hormonal and environmental factors affecting cell proliferation and neoplasia in the mammary gland. *In* "Cellular and Molecular Mechanisms of Hormonal Carcinogenesis: Environmental Influences" (J. Huff, J. Boyd, and J. C. Barrett, Eds.). Wiley-Liss, Inc., New York.
10. Pollak, M. N. (1998). Endocrine effects of IGF-I on normal and transformed breast epithelial cells: Potential relevance to strategies for breast cancer treatment and prevention. *Breast Cancer Res. Treat.* **47,** 209–217.
11. Del Giudice, M. E., Fantus, I. G., Ezzat, S., McKeown-Eyssen, G., Page, D., and Goodwin, P. J. (1998). Insulin and related factors in premenopausal breast cancer risk. *Breast Cancer Res. Treat.* **47,** 111–120.
12. Ford, D., Easton, D. F., and Peto, J. (1995). Estimates of the gene frequency of BRCA1 and its contribution to breast and ovarian cancer incidence. *Am. J. Hum. Genet.* **57,** 1457–1462.
13. Sellers, T. A. (1997). Genetic factors in the pathogenesis of breast cancer: Their role and relative importance. *J. Nutr.* **127,** 929S–932S.
14. Ambrosone, C. B., Freudenheim, J. L., Sinha, R., Graham, S., Marshall, J. R., Vena, J. E., Laughlin, R., Nemoto, T., and Shields, P. G. (1998). Breast cancer risk, meat consumption and *N*-acetyltransferase (*NAT2*) genetic polymorphisms. *Int. J. Cancer* **74,** 825–830.
15. Zheng, W., Deitz, A. C., Campbell, D. R., Wen, W. Q., Cerhan, J. R., Sellers, T. A., Folsom, A. R., and Hein, D. W. (1999). *N*-acetyltransferase 1 genetic polymorphism, cigarette smoking, well-done meat intake, and breast cancer risk. *Cancer Epidemiol. Biomarkers Prev.* **8,** 233–239.
16. Ambrosone, C. B., Coles, B. F., Freudenheim, J. L., and Shields, P. G. (1999). Glutathione-*S*-transferase (GSTM1) genetic polymorphisms do not affect human breast cancer risk, regardless of dietary antioxidants. *J. Nutr.* **129,** 565S–568S.
17. Fleming, I. D., Cooper, J. S., Henson, D. E., Hutter, R. V. P., Kennedy, B. J., Murphy, G. P., O'Sullivan, B., Sabin, L. H., and Yarbro, J. W., Eds. (1997). "American Joint Committee on Cancer Staging Manual," 5th ed. J. B. Lippincott, Philadelphia, PA.
18. Harris, J. R., Lippman, M. E., Veronesi, U., and Willett, W. (1992). Breast cancer (second of three parts). *N. Engl. J. Med.* **327,** 390–398.
19. Donegan, W. L. (1997). Tumor-related prognostic factors for breast cancer. *CA Cancer J. Clin.* **47,** 28–51.
20. Kelsey, J. L., and Horn-Ross, P. L. (1993). Breast cancer: Magnitude of the problem and descriptive epidemiology. *Epidemiol. Rev.* **15,** 7–16.
21. McMichael, A. J., and Giles, G. G. (1988). Cancer in migrants in Australia: Extending descriptive epidemiological data. *Cancer Res.* **48,** 751–756.
22. Ziegler, R. G., Hoover, R. N., Pike, M. C., Hildesheim, A., Nomura, A. M., West, D. W., Wu-Williams, A. H., Kolonel, L. N., Horn-Ross, P. L., Rosenthal, J. F., and Myer, M. B. (1993). Migration patterns and breast cancer risk in Asian-American women. *J. Natl. Cancer Inst.* **85,** 1819–1827.
23. Hunter, D. J., and Willett, W. C. (1996). Nutrition and breast cancer. *Cancer Causes Control* **7,** 56–68.
24. Wynder, E. L., Cohen, L. A., Muscat, J. E., Winters, B., Dwyer, J. T., and Blackburn, T. (1997). Breast cancer: Weighing the evidence for a promoting role of dietary fat. *J. Natl. Cancer Inst.* **89,** 766–775.
25. Clavel-Chapelon, F., Niravong, M., and Joseph, R. R. (1997). Diet and breast cancer: Review of the epidemiologic literature. *Cancer Detect. Prev.* **21,** 426–440.
26. Greenwald, P. (1999). Role of dietary fat in the causation of breast cancer: Point. *Cancer Prev. Biomarkers Control* **8,** 3–7.
27. Hunter, D. J. (1999). Role of dietary fat in the causation of breast cancer: Counterpoint. *Cancer Prev. Biomarkers Control* **8,** 9–13.
28. Rose, D. P. (1997). Dietary fatty acids and cancer. *Am. J. Clin. Nutr.* **66**(Suppl.), 998S–1003S.
29. Guthrie, N., and Carroll, K. K. (1999). Specific versus nonspecific effects of dietary fat on carcinogenesis. *Prog. Lipid Res.* **38,** 261–271.
30. Armstrong, B., and Doll, R. (1975). Environmental factors and cancer incidence and mortality in different countries with special reference to dietary practices. *Int. J. Cancer* **15,** 617–631.
31. Hunter, D. J., Spielgelman, D., Adami, H. O., Beeson, L., Van Den Brandt, P. A., Folson, A. R., Fraxer, G. E., Goldbohm, R. A., Graham, S., Howe, G. R., Kushi, L. H., Marshall, J. R., McDermott, A., Miller, A. B., Speizer, F. E., Wolk, A., Yaun, S. S., and Willett, W. (1996). Cohort studies of fat intake and

the risk of breast cancer—a pooled analysis. *N. Engl. J. Med.* **334,** 356–361.

32. Holmes, M. D., Hunter, D. J., Colditz, G. A., Stampfer, M. J., Hankinson, S. E., Speizer, F. E., Rosner, B., and Willett, W. C. (1999). Association of dietary intake of fat and fatty acids with risk of breast cancer. *JAMA* **281,** 914–920.

33. Prentice, R. L. (1996). Measurement error and results from analytic epidemiology: Dietary fat and breast cancer. *J. Natl. Cancer Inst.* **88,** 1738–1747.

34. Wu, A. H., Pike, M. C., and Stram, D. O. (1999). Meta-analysis: Dietary fat intake, serum estrogen levels, and the risk of breast cancer. *J. Natl. Cancer Inst.* **91,** 529–534.

35. Gandini, S., Merzenich, H., Robertson, C., and Boyle, P. (2000). Meta-analysis of studies on breast cancer risk and diet: The role of fruit and vegetable consumption and the intake of associated micronutrients. *Eur. J. Cancer* **36,** 636–646.

36. Freudenheim, J. L., Marshall, J. R., Vena, J. E., Laughlin, R., Brasure, J. R., Swanson, M. K., Nemoto, T., and Graham, S. (1996). Premenopausal breast cancer risk and intake of vegetables, fruits, and related nutrients. *J. Natl. Cancer Inst.* **88,** 340–348.

37. Longnecker, M. P., Newcomb, P. A., Mittendorf, R., Greenberg, E. R., and Willett, W. C. (1997). Intake of carrots, spinach, and supplements containing vitamin A in relation to risk of breast cancer. *Cancer Epidemiol. Biomarkers Prev.* **6,** 887–892.

38. Zhang, S., Hunter, D. J., Forman, M. R., Rosner, B. A., Speitzer, F. E., Colditz, G. A., Manson, J. E., Hankinson, S. E., and Willett, W. C. (1999). Dietary carotenoids and vitamins A, C, and E and risk of breast cancer. *J. Natl. Cancer Inst.* **91,** 547–556.

39. Potischman, N., McCulloch, C. E., Byers, T., Nemoto, T., Subbe, N., Milch, R., Parker, R., Rasmussen, K. M., Root, M., Graham, S., and Campbell, T. C. (1990). Breast cancer and dietary and plasma concentrations of carotenoids and vitamin A. *Am. J. Clin. Nutr.* **52,** 909–915.

40. Zhang, S., Tang, G., Russell, R. M., Mayzel, K. A., Stampfer, M. J., Willett, W. C., and Hunter, D. J. (1997). Measurement of retinoids and carotenoids in breast adipose tissue and a comparison of concentrations in breast cancer cases and control subjects. *Am. J. Clin. Nutr.* **66,** 626–632.

41. Yeum, K. J., Ahn, S. H., Rupp de Paiva, S. A., Lee-Kim, Y., Krinsky, N. I., and Russell, R. M. (1998). Correlation between carotenoid concentrations in serum and normal breast adipose tissue of women with benign breast tumor or breast cancer. *J. Nutr.* **128,** 1920–1926.

42. Rock, C. L., Kusluski, R. A., Galvez, M. M., and Ethier, S. P. (1995). Carotenoids induce morphological changes in human mammary epithelial cell cultures. *Nutr. Cancer* **23,** 319–333.

43. Prakash, P., Krinsky, N. I., and Russell, R. M. (2000). Retinoids, carotenoids, and human breast cell cultures: A review of differential effects. *Nutr. Rev.* **58,** 170–176.

44. Dawson, M. I., Chao, W., Pine, P., Jong, L., Hobbs, P. D., Rudd, C. K., Quick, T. C., Niles, R. M., Zhang, X., Lombardo, A., Ely, K. R., Shroot, B., and Fontana, J. A. (1995). Correlation of retinoid binding affinity to retinoic acid receptor alpha with retinoid inhibition of estrogen receptor-positive MCF-7 mammary carcinoma cells. *Cancer Res.* **55,** 4446–4451.

45. Sumantran, V. N., Zhang, R., Lee, D. S., and Wicha, M. S. (2000). Differential regulation of apoptosis in normal versus transformed mammary epithelium by lutein and retinoic acid. *Cancer Epidemiol. Biomarkers Prev.* **9,** 257–263.

46. Stoll, B. A. (1998). Breast cancer and the Western diet: Role of fatty acids and antioxidant vitamins. *Eur. J. Cancer* **34,** 1852–1856.

47. Van't Veer, P., Strain, J. J., Fernandez-Crehuet, J., Martin, B. C., Thamm, M., Kardinaal, A. F., Kohlmeier, L., Huttunen, J. K., Martin-Moreno, J. M., and Kok, F. J. (1996). Tissue antioxidants and postmenopausal breast cancer: The European Community Multicentre Study on Antioxidants, Myrocardial Infarction, and Cancer of the Breast. *Cancer Epidemiol. Biomarkers Prev.* **5,** 441–447.

48. Graham, S., Zielezny, M., Marshall, J., Priore, R., Freudenheim, J., Brasure, J., Haughey, B., Nasca, P., and Zdeb, M. (1992). Diet in the epidemiology of postmenopausal breast cancer in the New York State Cohort. *Am. J. Epidemiol.* **136,** 1327–1337.

49. Hunter, D. J., Manson, J. E., Colditz, G. A., Stampfer, M. J., Rosner, B., Hennekens, C. H., Speizer, F. E., and Willett, W. C. (1993). A prospective study of the intake of vitamins C, E, and A and the risk of breast cancer. *N. Engl. J. Med.* **329,** 234–240.

50. Kushi, L. H., Fee, R. M., Sellers, T. A., Zheng, W., and Folsom, A. R. (1996). Intake of vitamins A, C, and E and postmenopausal breast cancer. The Iowa Women's Health Study. *Am. J. Epidemiol.* **144,** 165–174.

51. Dorgan, J. F., Sowell, A., Swanson Potischman, N., Miller, R., Schussler, N., and Stephenseon, H. E. (1998). Relationships of serum carotenoids, retinol, alpha-tocopherol, and selenium with breast cancer risk: Results from a prospective study in Columbia, Missouri (United States). *Cancer Causes Control* **9,** 89–97.

52. Kim, Y. I., Pogribny, I. P., Basnakian, A. G., Miller, J. W., Selhub, J., James, S. J., and Mason, J. B. (1997). Folate deficiency in rats induces DNA strand breaks and hypomethylation within the p53 tumor suppressor gene. *Am. J. Clin. Nutr.* **65,** 46–52.

53. Zhaang, S., Hunter, D. J., Hankinson, S. E., Giovannucci, E. L., Rosner, B. A., Colditz, G. A., Speizer, F. E., and Willett, W. C. (1999). A prospective study of folate intake and the risk of breast cancer. *JAMA* **281,** 1632–1637.

54. Smith-Warner, S. A., Spiegelman, D., Yaun, S. S., Van Brandt, P. A., Folson, A. R., Goldbohm, A., Graham, S., Holmberg, L., Howe, G. R., Marshall, J. R., Miller, A. B., Potter, J. D., Speizer, F. E., Willett, W. C., Wolk, A., and Hunter, D. J. (1998). Alcohol and breast cancer in women. A pooled analysis of cohort studies. *JAMA* **279,** 535–540.

55. Ginsburg, E. S. (1999). Estrogen, alcohol and breast cancer risk. *J. Steroid. Biochem. Molec. Biol.* **69,** 299–306.

56. Aldercreutz, H. (1974). Hepatic metabolism of estrogen in health and disease. *N. Engl. J. Med.* **xxx,** 1081–1083.

57. Arts, C. J. M., Govers, C., Van Den Berg, H., Wolters, M. G. E., Van Leeuwen, P., and Thussen, J. H. H. (1991). In vitro binding of estrogens by dietary fiber and the in vivo apparent digestibility tested in pigs. *J. Steroid. Biochem. Molec. Biol.* **38,** 621–628.

58. Henderson, B. E., and Bernstein, L. (1991). The international variation in breast cancer rates: An epidemiological assessment. *Breast Cancer Res. Treat.* **18**(Suppl.), S11–S17.

59. Kurzer, M. S. (2000). Hormonal effects of soy isoflavones: Studies in premenopausal and postmenopausal women. *J. Nutr.* **130**(Suppl.), 660S–661S.

60. Herman, C., Adlercreutz, T., Goldin, B. R., Gorbach, S. L., Hockerstedt, K. A. V., Watanabe, S., Hamalainen, E. K., Hase, T. A., and Fotsis, T. (1995). Soybean phytoestrogen intake and cancer risk. *J. Nutr.* **125**(Suppl.), 757S–770S.

61. Barnes, S. (1995). Effect of genistein on in vitro and in vivo models of cancer. *J. Nutr.* **125**(Suppl.), 777S–783S.

62. Wang, C., and Kurzer, M. S. (1997). Phytoestrogen concentration determines effects on DNA synthesis in human breast cancer cells. *Nutr. Cancer* **28**, 236–247.

63. Murkies, A. L., Wilcos, G., and Davis, S. R. (1998). Phytoestrogens. *J. Clin. Endocrin. Metab.* **83**, 297–303.

64. Adlercreutz, H., Hockerstedt, K., Bannwart, C., Bloigu, S., Hamalainen, E., Fotsis, T., and Ollus, A. (1987). Effect of dietary components, including lignans and phytoestrogens, on enterohepatic circulation and liver metabolism of estrogens, and on sex hormones binding globulin (SHBG). *J. Steroid. Biochem.* **27**, 1135–1144.

65. Cassidy, A., Bingham, S., and Setchell, K. D. (1994). Biological effects of a diet of soy protein rich in isoflavones on the menstrual cycle of premenopausal women. *Am. J. Clin. Nutr.* **60**, 333–340.

66. Lu, L. J. W., Anderson, K. E., Grady, J. J., and Nagamani, M. (1996). Effects of soya consumption for one month on steroid hormones in premenopausal women: Implications for breast cancer risk reduction. *Cancer Epidemiol. Biomarkers Prev.* **5**, 63–70.

67. Phipps, W. R., Martini, M. C., and Lampe, J. W. (1993). Effect of flaxseed ingestion on the menstrual cycle. *J. Clin. Endocrin. Metab.* **77**, 1215–1219.

68. Wu, A. H., Ziegler, R. G., Nomura, A. M. Y., West, D. W., Kolonel, L. N., Horn-Ross, P. L., Hoover, R. N., and Pike, M. C. (1998). Soy intake and risk of breast cancer in Asians and Asian Americans. *Am. J. Clin. Nutr.* **68**(Suppl.), 1437S–1443S.

69. Ballard-Barbash, R. (1994). Anthropometry and breast cancer. Body size—a moving target. *Cancer* **74**(Suppl.), 1090–1100.

70. Clinton, S. K. (1997). Diet, anthropometry and breast cancer: Integration of experimental and epidemiologic approaches. *J. Nutr.* **127**(Suppl.), 916S–920S.

71. Ziegler, R. G. (1997). Anthropometry and breast cancer. *J. Nutr.* **127**(Suppl.), 924S–928S.

72. Brinton, L. A., and Swanson, C. A. (1992). Height and weight at various ages and risk of breast cancer. *Ann. Epidemiol.* **2**, 597–609.

73. Ng, E. H., Gao, F., Ji, C. Y., Ho, G. H., and Soo, K. C. (1997). Risk factors for breast carcinoma in Singaporean Chinese women: The role of central obesity. *Cancer* **80**, 725–731.

74. Swanson, C. A., Jones, D. Y., Schatzkin, A., Brinton, L. A., and Ziegler, R. G. (1988). Breast cancer risk assessed by anthropometry in the NHANES I epidemiological follow-up study. *Cancer Res.* **48**, 5363–5367.

75. DeWaard, F. (1975). Breast cancer incidence and nutritional status with particular reference to body weight and height. *Cancer Res.* **35**, 3351–3356.

76. Modina, R., Borsellino, G., Poma, S., Baroni, M., DiNubila, B., and Sacchi, P. (1992). Breast carcinoma and skeletal formation. *Eur. J. Cancer* **28A**, 1068–1070.

77. Carroll, K. K. (1998). Obesity as a risk factor for certain types of cancer. *Lipids* **33**, 1055–1059.

78. Cleary, M. P., and Maihle, N. J. (1997). The role of body mass index in the relative risk of developing premenopausal versus postmenopausal breast cancer. *Proc. Soc. Exp. Biol. Med.* **216**, 28–43.

79. Vinko, R., and Apter, D. (1989). Endogenous steroids in the pathophysiology of breast cancer. *Crit. Rev. Oncol. Hematol.* **9**, 1–16.

80. Schapira, D. V., Clark, R. A., Wolff, P. A., Jarrett, A. R., Kumar, N. B., and Aziz, N. M. (1994). Visceral obesity and breast cancer risk. *Cancer* **74**, 632–639.

81. Sonnenschein, E., Toniolo, P., Terry, M. B., Bruning, P. F., Kato, I., Koenig, K. L., and Shore, R. E. (1999). Body fat distribution and obesity in pre- and postmenopausal breast cancer. *Int. J. Epidemiol.* **28**, 1026–1031.

82. Sellers, T. A., Drinkard, C., Rich, S. S., Potter, J. B., Jeffery, R. W., Hong, C. P., and Folsom, A. R. (1994). Familial aggregation and heritability of waist-to-hip ratio in adult women: The Iowa Women's Health Study. *Int. J. Obes. Relat. Metab. Disord.* **18**, 607–613.

83. London, S. J., Colditz, G. A., Stampfer, M. J., Willett, W. C., Rosner, B. R., and Spetzer, F. E. (1989). Prospective study of relative weight, height and risk of breast cancer. *JAMA* **262**, 2853–2858.

84. LeMarchand, L., Kolonel, L. N., Earle, M. E., and Mi, M. P. (1988). Body size at different periods of life and breast cancer risk. *Am. J. Epidemiol.* **128**, 137–152.

85. Radimer, K., Siskind, V., Bain, C., and Schofield, F. (1993). Relation between anthropometric indicators and risk of breast cancer among Australian women. *Am. J. Epidemiol.* **138**, 77–89.

86. Apter, D. (1996). Hormonal events during female puberty in relation to breast cancer risk. *Eur. J. Cancer Prev.* **5**, 476–482.

87. Stoll, B. A. (1997). Impaired ovulation and breast cancer risk. *Eur. J. Cancer* **33**, 1532–1535.

88. Stoll, B. A. (1999). Western nutrition and the insulin resistance syndrome: A link to breast cancer. *Am. J. Clin. Nutr.* **53**, 83–87.

89. Kumar, N. B., Lyman, G. H., Allen, K., Cox, C. E., and Schapira, D. V. (1995). Timing of weight gain and breast cancer risk. *Cancer* **76**, 243–249.

90. Abe, R., Kumago, N., Kimura, M., Hirosaki, A., and Nakamura, T. (1976). Biological characteristics of breast cancer in obesity. *Tokyo J. Exp. Med.* **120**, 351–359.

91. Demark-Wahnefried, W., Winer, E. P., and Rimer, B. K. (1993). Why women gain weight with adjuvant chemotherapy for breast cancer. *J. Clin. Oncol.* **11**, 1418–1429.

92. Demark-Wahnefried, W., Rimer, B. K., and Winer, E. P. (1997). Weight gain in women diagnosed with breast cancer. *J. Am. Diet. Assoc.* **97**, 519–529.

93. Wee, C. C., McCarthy, E. P., Davis, R. B., and Phillips, R. S. (2000). Screening for cervical and breast cancer: Is obesity an unrecognized barrier to preventive care? *Ann. Intern. Med.* **132**, 697–704.

94. Tretli, S., Haldorsen, T., and Ottestad, L. (1990). The effect of pre-morbid height and weight on the survival of breast cancer patients. *Br. J. Cancer* **62**, 299–303.

95. Taylor, H. L., Klepetar, E., Keys, A., Parlin, W., Blackburn, H., and Puchner, T. (1962). Death rates among physically

active and sedentary employees of the railroad industry. *Am. J. Public Health* **52,** 1697–1707.

96. Lee, I.-M. (1995). Exercise and physical health: Cancer and immune function. *Res. Q. Exerc. Sport* **66,** 286–292.

97. McTiernan, A., Ulrich, C., Slate, S., and Potter, J. (1998). Physical activity and cancer etiology: Associations and mechanisms. *Cancer Causes Control* **9,** 487–509.

98. Frisch, R. E., Wyshak, G., Albright, N. I., Albright, T. F., Schiff, I., and Witischi, J. (1985). Lower prevalence of breast cancer and cancers of the reproductive system among former college athletes compared to non-athletes. *Br. J. Cancer* **52,** 885–891.

99. Bernstein, L., Henderson, B. E., Hanisch, R., Sullivan-Hally, J., and Ross, R. K. (1994). Physical exercise and reduced risk of breast cancer in young women. *J. Natl. Cancer Inst.* **86,** 1403–1408.

100. Friedenreich, C. M., and Rohan, T. E. (1995). A review of physical activity and breast cancer. *Epidemiology* **6,** 311–317.

101. Gammon, M. D., John, E. M., and Britton, J. A. (1998). Recreational and occupational physical activities and risk of breast cancer. *J. Natl. Cancer Inst.* **90,** 100–117.

102. Daneryd, P. L., Hafstrom, L. R., and Karlberg, I. H. (1990). Effects of spontaneous physical exercise on experimental cancer anorexia and cachexia. *Eur. J. Cancer* **26,** 1083–1088.

103. Hoffman-Goetz, L., Apter, D., Demark-Wahnefried, W., Goran, M. I., McTiernan, A., and Reichman, M. E. (1998). Possible mechanisms mediating an association between physical activity and breast cancer. *Cancer* **83,** 621–628.

104. Thune, I., Brenn, T., Lund, E., and Gaard, M. (1997). Physical activity and the risk of breast cancer. *N. Engl. J. Med.* **336,** 1269–1275.

105. Latikka, P., Pukkala, E., and Vihko, V. (1998). Relationship between the risk of breast cancer and physical activity. An epidemiological perspective. *Sports Med.* **26,** 133–143.

106. Senie, R. T., Rosen, P. P., Rhodes, P., Lesser, M. L., and Kinne, D. W. (1992). Obesity at diagnosis of breast carcinoma influences duration of disease-free survival. *Ann. Intern. Med.* **116,** 26–32.

107. Bastarrachea, J., Hortobagyi, G. N., Smith, T. L., Kau, S. C., and Buzdar, A. U. (1993). Obesity as an adverse prognostic factor for patients receiving adjuvant chemotherapy for breast cancer. *Ann. Intern. Med.* **119,** 18–25.

108. Zhang, S., Folsom, A. R., Sellers, I. A., Kushi, L. H., and Potter, J. D. (1995). Better breast cancer survival for postmenopausal women who are less overweight and eat less fat. The Iowa Women's Health Study. *Cancer* **76,** 275–283.

109. Jain, M., Miller, A. B., and To, T. (1994). Premorbid diet and the prognosis of women with breast cancer. *J. Natl. Cancer Inst.* **86,** 1390–1397.

110. Holm, L. E., Nordevang, E., Hjalmar, M. L., Lindbrink, E., Callmer, E., and Nilsson, B. (1993). Treatment failure and dietary habits in women with breast cancer. *J. Natl. Cancer Inst.* **85,** 32–36.

111. Rohan, T. E., Hiller, J. E., and McMichael, A. J. (1993). Dietary factors and survival from breast cancer. *Nutr. Cancer* **20,** 167–177.

112. Nomura, A. M. Y., Le Marchand, L., Kolonel, L. N., and Hankin, J. H. (1991). The effect of dietary fat on breast cancer survival among Caucasian and Japanese women in Hawaii. *Breast Cancer Res. Treat.* **18**(Suppl.), 135–141.

113. Gregorio, D. I., Emrich, L. J., Graham, S., Marshall, J. R., and Nemoto, T. (1985). Dietary fat consumption and survival among women with breast cancer. *J. Natl. Cancer Inst.* **75,** 37–41.

114. Kyogoku, S., Hirohata, T., Nomura, Y., Shigematsu, T., Takeshita, S., and Hirohata, I. (1992). Diet and prognosis of breast cancer. *Nutr. Cancer* **17,** 271–277.

115. Erwertz, M., Gillanders, S., Meyer, L., and Zedeler, K. (1991). Survival of breast cancer patients in relation to factors which affect the risk of developing breast cancer. *Int. J. Cancer* **49,** 526–530.

116. Newman, S. C., Miller, A. B., and Howe, G. R. (1986). A study of the effect of weight and dietary fat on breast cancer survival time. *Am. J. Epidemiol.* **123,** 767–774.

117. Saxe, G. A., Rock, C. L., Wicha, M. S., and Schottenfeld, D. (1999). Diet and risk for breast cancer recurrence and survival. *Breast Cancer Res. Treat.* **53,** 241–253.

118. Hebert, J. R., Hurley, T. G., and Ma, F. (1998). The effect of dietary exposures on recurrence and mortality in early stage breast cancer. *Breast Cancer Res. Treat.* **51,** 17–28.

119. Holmes, M. D., Stampfer, M. J., Colditz, G. A., Rosner, B., Hunter, D. J., and Willett, W. C. (1999). Dietary factors and the survival of women with breast carcinoma. *Cancer* **86,** 826–835.

120. Ingram, D. (1994). Diet and subsequent survival in women with breast cancer. *Br. J. Cancer* **69,** 592–595.

121. American Cancer Society (2000). "Cancer Facts and Figures 2000." American Cancer Society, Atlanta, GA.

122. Li, F. P., and Stovall, E. (1998). Long-term survivors of cancer. *Cancer Epidemiol. Biomarkers Prev.* **7,** 269–270.

123. Meadows, A. T., Varricchio, C., Crosson, K., Harlan, L., McCormick, P., Nealon, E., Smith, M., and Ungerleider, R. (1998). Research issues in cancer survivorship. *Cancer Epidemiol. Biomarkers Prev.* **7,** 1145–1151.

124. Holmes, M. D., and Willett, W. C. (1995). Can breast cancer be prevented by dietary and lifestyle changes? *Ann. Med.* **27,** 429–430.

125. Byers, T., Rock, C. L., and Hamilton, K. K. (1997). Dietary changes after breast cancer. What should we recommend? *Cancer Prac.* **5,** 317–320.

126. Jatoi, A., and Loprinzi, C. L. (1999). Nutritional determinants of survival among patients with breast cancer. *Surg. Clin. North Am.* **79,** 1145–1156.

127. NIH web site (2000). Available at *http://cancernet.nci.nih. gov/cancer_types/breast_cancer.shtml.*

128. Rose, M. A. (1989). Health promotion and risk prevention: Applications for cancer survivors. *Oncol. Nurs. Forum* **16,** 335–340.

129. Goodwin, P. J., and Boyd, N. F. (1990). Body size and breast cancer prognosis: A critical review of the evidence. *Breast Cancer Res. Treat.* **16,** 205–214.

130. Greenhalgh, D. G., and Gamelli, R. L. (1987). Is impaired wound healing caused by infection or nutritional depletion? *Surgery* **102,** 306–312.

131. Grindel, C. G., Cahill, C. A., and Walker, M. (1989). Food intake of women with breast cancer during their first six months of chemotherapy. *Oncol. Nurs. Forum* **16,** 401–407.

132. Boyd, N. F. (1993). Nutrition and breast cancer. *J. Natl. Cancer Inst.* **85,** 6–7.

133. Camoriano, J. K., Loprinzi, C. L., Ingle, J. N., Therneau, T., Krook, J., and Veeder, M. (1990). Weight change in women treated with adjuvant therapy or observed following mastectomy for node-positive breast cancer. *J. Clin. Oncol.* **8,** 1327–1334.

134. Ganz, P. A., Schag, C. C., and Polinsky, M. L. (1987). Rehabilitation needs and breast cancer: The first month after primary therapy. *Breast Cancer Res. Treat.* **10,** 243–253.

135. Goodwin, P. J., Ennis, M., Pritchard, K. I., McCready, D., Koo, J., Sidlofsky, S., Trudeau, M., Hood, N., and Redwood, S. (1999). Adjuvant treatment and onset of menopause predict weight gain after breast cancer diagnosis. *J. Clin. Oncol.* **17,** 120–129.

136. Monnin, S., Schiller, M. R., Sachs, L., and Smith, A. M. (1993). Nutritional concerns of women with breast cancer. *J. Cancer Educ.* **8,** 63–89.

137. Brown, B. W., Brauner, C., and Minnotte, M. C. (1993). Non-cancer deaths in white adult cancer patients. *J. Natl. Cancer Inst.* **85,** 979–997.

138. Chlebowski, R. T., Weiner, J. M., Reynolds, R., Luce, J., Bulcavage, L., and Bateman, L. (1986). Long-term survival following relapse after 5-FU but not CMF adjuvant breast cancer therapy. *Breast Cancer Res. Treat.* **7,** 23–29.

139. Goodwin, P. A., Panzarella, T., and Boyd, N. F. (1988). Weight gain in women with localized breast cancer—A descriptive study. *Breast Cancer Res. Treat.* **11,** 59–66.

140. Loprinzi, C. L., Athmann, L. M., Kardinal, C. G., O'Fallon, J. R., See, J. A., Bruce, B. K., Dose, A. M., Miser, A. W., Kern, P. S. Tschetter, L. K., and Rayson, S. (1996). Randomized trial of dietitian counseling to try to prevent weight gain associated with breast cancer adjuvant chemotherapy. *Oncology* **53,** 228–232.

141. Goodwin, P., Esplen, M. J., Butler, K., Winocur, J., Pritchard, K., Brazel, S., Gao, J., and Miller, A. (1998). Multidisciplinary weight management in locoregional breast cancer: Results of a phase II study. *Breast Cancer Res. Treat.* **48,** 53–64.

142. Rock, C. L., Flatt, S. W., Newman, V., Caan, B. J., Haan, M. N., Stefanick, M. L., Faerber, S., and Pierce, J. P. (1999). Factors associated with weight gain in women after diagnosis of breast cancer. *J. Am. Diet. Assoc.* **99,** 1212–1221.

143. Aslani, A., Smith, R. C., Allen, B. J., Pavalis, N., and Levi, J. A. (1999). Changes in body composition during breast cancer chemotherapy with the CMF-regimen. *Breast Cancer Res. Treat.* **57,** 285–290.

144. Cheney, C. L., Mahloch, J., and Freeny, P. (1997). Computerized tomography assessment of women with weight changes associated with adjuvant treatment for breast cancer. *Am. J. Clin. Nutr.* **66,** 141–146.

145. Demark-Wahnefried, W., Hars, V., Conaway, M. R., Havlin, K., Rimer, B., McElveen, G., and Winer, E. P. (1997). Reduced rates of metabolism and decreased physical activity in breast cancer patients receiving adjuvant chemotherapy. *Am. J. Clin. Nutr.* **65,** 1495–1501.

146. Demark-Wahnefried, W., Peterson, B. L., Winer, E. P., Marcom, P. K., Marks, L., Hardenbergh, P., Aziz, N., and Rimer, B. R. (in press). Changes in weight, body composition and factors influencing energy balance among premenopausal breast cancer patients receiving adjuvant chemotherapy—A case for sarcopenic obesity. *J. Clin. Oncol.* (in press).

147. Kutynec, C. L., McCargar, L., Barr, S. I., and Hislop, T. G. (1999). Energy balance in women with breast cancer during adjuvant chemotherapy. *J. Am. Diet. Assoc.* **99,** 1222–1227.

148. Friedenreich, C. M., and Courneya, K. S. (1996). Exercise as rehabilitation for cancer patients. *J. Sports Med.* **6,** 237–242.

149. Rock, C. L., McEligot, A. J., Flatt, S. W., Sobo, E. J., Wilfley, D. E., Jones, V. E., Hollenbach, K. A., and Marx, R. D. (2000). Eating pathology and obesity in women at risk for breast cancer recurrence. *Int. J. Eating Dis.* **27,** 172–179.

150. Foltz, A. (1985). Weight gain among stage II breast cancer patients: A study of five factors. *Oncol. Nurs. Forum* **12,** 21–26.

151. Mock, V., Dow, K. H., Meares, C. J., Grimm, P. M., Dienemann, J. A., Haisfield-Wolfe, M. E., Quitasol, W., Mitchell, S., Chakravarthy, A., and Gage, I. (1997). Effects of exercise on fatigue, physical functioning and emotional distress during radiation therapy for breast cancer. *Oncol. Nurs. Forum* **24,** 991–1000.

152. Kornblith, A. B., Hollis, D. R., and Zuckerman, E. (1993). Effect of megestrol acetate on quality of life in a dose-response trial in women with advanced breast cancer. *J. Clin. Oncol.* **11,** 2081–2089.

153. Day, R., Ganz, P. A., Costantino, J. P., Cronin, W. M., Wickerham, D. L., and Fisher, B. (1999). Health-related quality of life and tamoxifen in breast cancer prevention: A report from the National Surgical Adjuvant Breast and Bowel Project P-1 Study. *J. Clin. Oncol.* **17,** 2659–2669.

154. Hoskin, P. J., Ashley, S., and Yarnold, J. R. (1992). Weight gain after primary surgery for breast cancer—effect of tamoxifen. *Breast Cancer Res. Treat.* **22,** 129–132.

155. Ali, P. A., al-Ghorabie, F. H., Evans, C. J., el-Sharkawi, A. M., and Hancock, D. A. (1998). Body composition measurements using DXA and other techniques in tamoxifen-treated patients. *Appl. Radia. Isot.* **49,** 643–645.

156. Boyle, F. M. (1997). Adverse interaction of herbal medicine with breast cancer treatment. *Med. J. Austral.* **167,** 286.

157. Demark-Wahnefried, W., Peterson, B., McBride, C., Lipkus, I., and Clipp, E. (2000). Current health behaviors and readiness to pursue lifestyle change among men and women diagnosed with early stage prostate and breast cancers. *Cancer* **88,** 674–684.

158. Newman, V., Rock, C. L., Faerber, S., Flatt, S. W., Wright, F. A., and Pierce, J. P. (1998). Dietary supplement use by women at risk for breast cancer recurrence. *J. Am. Diet. Assoc.* **98,** 285–292.

159. American Dietetic Association (2001). Position of the American Dietetic Association: Food fortification and dietary supplements. *J. Am. Diet. Assoc.* **101,** 115–125.

160. Clifford, C., and Kramer, B. (1993). Diet as risk and therapy for cancer. *Med. Clin. N. Am.* **77,** 725–744.

161. The Women's Health Initiative Study Group. (1998). Design of the Women's Health Initiative Clinical Trial and Observational Study. *Control. Clin. Trials* **19,** 61–109.

162. Boyd, N. F., Fishell, E., Jong, R., MacDonald, J. C., Sparrow, R. K., Simor, I. S., Kriukov, V., Lockwood, G., and Tritchler, D. (1995). Mammographic densities as a criterion for entry to a clinical trial of breast cancer prevention. *Br. J. Cancer* **72,** 476–479.

163. Boyd, N. F., Lockwood, G. A., Byng, J. W., Tritchler, D. L., and Yaffe, M. J. (1998). Mammographic densities and breast cancer risk. *Cancer Epidemiol. Biomarkers Prev.* **7**, 1133–1144.

164. Boyd, N. F., Greenberg, C., Lockwood, G., Little, L., Martin, L., Byng, J., Yaffe, M., and Tritchler, D. (1997). Effects at two years of a low-fat, high-carbohydrate diet on radiologic features of the breast: Results from a randomized trial. *J. Natl. Cancer Inst.* **89**, 488–496.

165. Knight, J. A., Martin, L. J., Greenberg, C. V., Lockwood, G. A., Byng, J. W., Yaffe, M. J., Tritchler, D. L., and Boyd, N. F. (1999). Macronutrient intake and change in mammographic density at menopause: Results from a randomized trial. *Cancer Epidemiol. Biomarkers Prev.* **8**, 123–128.

166. Simon, M. S., Heilbrun, L. K., Boomer, A., Kresge, C., Depper, J., Kim, P. N., Valeriote, F., and Martino, S. (1997). A randomized trial of a low-fat dietary intervention in women at high risk for breast cancer. *Nutr. Cancer* **27**, 136–142.

167. Djuric, Z., Depper, J. B., Uhley, V., Smith, D., Lababidi, S., Martino, S., and Heilbrun, L. K. (1998). Oxidative DNA damage levels in blood from women at high risk for breast cancer are associated with dietary intakes of meats, vegetables, and fruits. *J. Am. Diet. Assoc.* **98**, 524–528.

168. Chlebowski, R. T., Blackburn, G. L., Buzzard, I. M., Rose, D. P., Martino, S., Khandekar, J. D., York, R. M., Jeffery, R. W., Elashoff, R. M., and Wynder, E. L. (1993). Adherence to a dietary fat intake reduction program in postmenopausal women receiving therapy for early breast cancer. *J. Clin. Oncol.* **11**, 2072–2080.

169. Pierce, J. P., Faerber, S., Wright, F. A., Newman, V., Flatt, S. W., Kealey, S., Rock, C. L., Hryniuk, W., and Greenberg, E. R. (1997). Feasibility of a randomized trial of a high-vegetable diet to prevent breast cancer recurrence. *Nutr. Cancer* **28**, 282–288.

170. Rock, C. L., Flatt, S. W., Wright, F. A., Faerber, S., Newman, V., Kealey, S., and Pierce, J. P. (1997). Responsiveness of serum carotenoids to a high-vegetable diet intervention designed to prevent breast cancer recurrence. *Cancer Epidemiol. Biomarkers Prev.* **6**, 617–623.

171. Rock, C. L., Thomson, C., Caan, B. J., Flatt, S. W., Newman, V., Ritenbaugh, C., Marshall, J. R., Hollenbach, K. A., Stefanick, M. L., and Pierce, J. P. (2001). Reduction in fat intake is not associated with weight loss in most women after breast cancer diagnosis. *Cancer,* **91**, 25–34.

172. The American Cancer Society 1996 Advisory Committee on Diet, Nutrition and Cancer Prevention (1996). Guidelines on diet, nutrition, and cancer prevention: Reducing the risk of cancer with healthy food choices and physical activity. *CA Cancer J. Clin.* **46**, 325–342.

173. American Cancer Society Workgroup on Nutrition and Physical Activity for Cancer Survivors (2000). "Nutrition after Cancer: A Guide for Informed Choices." American Cancer Society, Atlanta, GA.

174. World Cancer Research Fund/American Institute for Cancer Research (1997). "Food, Nutrition and the Prevention of Cancer: A Global Perspective." American Institute for Cancer Research, Washington, DC.

175. Wolk, A., Manson, J. E., Stampfer, M. J., Colditz, G. A., Hu, F. B., Speizer, F. E., Hennekens, C. H., and Willett, W. C. (1999). Long-term intake of dietary fiber and decreased risk of coronary heart disease among women. *JAMA* **281**, 1998–2004.

176. Chlebowski, R. T. (2000). Reducing the risk of breast cancer. *N. Engl. J. Med.* **343**, 191–198.

CHAPTER 23

Nutrition and Colon Cancer

MARTHA L. SLATTERY[1] AND BETTE J. CAAN[2]
[1]University of Utah, Salt Lake City, Utah
[2]Kaiser Foundation Research Institute, Oakland, California

I. INTRODUCTION

In the United States, approximately 130,000 new cases and 55,000 deaths are attributed to colorectal cancer yearly, making it one of the most common cancers for both men and women [1]. Worldwide, an estimated 875,000 cases of colorectal cancer occurred in 1996, accounting for 8.5% of all incident cancers [2]. A 20-fold variation in reported incidence of colorectal cancer has been noted around the world, with developed countries having high incidence rates and developing countries having much lower incidence rates. Furthermore, migrant populations who move from countries of low to high incidence adopt the rates of the host country [3]. These facts suggests that changes in diet and lifestyle that correlate with changes in populations as they become more developed are associated with colorectal cancer. Much research attention has been focused on diet—with the expectation that identification of specific dietary factors that contribute to the observed variation and to changing incidence rates will provide avenues for prevention of colorectal cancer.

One way to explore dietary links to colorectal cancer is through ecological studies, which correlate differences in colorectal cancer mortality with differences in population intakes of nutrients such as fat, fiber, and calcium [4–6]. Although far from definitive, these studies suggest that populations with diets low in fat and high in fiber or calcium have lower mortality from colorectal cancer. Another approach is analytic epidemiological studies, which have produced inconsistent findings regarding the relationship between many dietary factors and colorectal cancer.

Case-control studies comparing recalled dietary differences in those with and without cancer, and cohort studies linking reported diet to disease development have also singled out many suspect dietary components. More than 75 case-control and cohort studies have been conducted, often with inconsistent findings. Conflicting results can stem from many sources, including study design, methods used to collect and analyze data, age and sex of the population being studied, range of dietary exposures captured from the questionnaire, the referent period for which the dietary data were collected, and possibly the tumor site itself. In the case-control study, participants are asked to recall past dietary intake; it is possible that recalled dietary intake might be influenced by changes in diet as a result of disease. Cohort studies frequently have limited ranges of dietary exposure, because they are often based on a more select population than population-based case-control studies. If dietary factors are only linked at high levels of intake, associations might be missed in cohort studies because of a truncated range of dietary intake. Data are usually obtained from self-administered questionnaires in cohort studies, therefore less detailed information on diet and other possible exposures is obtained than with the interviewer-administered questionnaires usually used in case-control studies. These differences can lead to misclassification of levels of dietary intake. For more information on strengths and weaknesses of epidemiological research see Chapter 4.

Results from controlled clinical trials of diet and colonic polyps are providing credence to associations for some dietary factors. Although polyps are precursor lesions to colon tumors, not all polyps progress to tumors. Thus some differences in dietary associations could be expected for studies that focus on adenomas versus adenocarcinomas.

Several major hypotheses for mechanisms have emerged in research on nutrition and adenocarcinoma of the colon (Table 1). These hypotheses are overlapping and complementary. They stress the complexity of colon cancer and the difficulty of identifying individual mechanisms, and also elucidate the diverse approaches being used to examine the links between nutrition and colon cancer.

In this chapter we discuss five different models describing mechanisms by which diet may either promote or prevent colon cancer and review the supporting epidemiologic data (Table 2) for each.

II. MODEL 1: BILE ACIDS, FAT/FIBER, AND MEATS/VEGETABLES

Perhaps the oldest theory that has guided epidemiologic studies on diet and colon cancer has focused on bile acids [7]. This model and closely related ones focus on a variety of nutrients and form the bulk of the epidemiologic literature.

357

TABLE 1 Summary of Some of the Hypothesized Mechanisms Related to a Diet and Colon Cancer Relationship

Model	Hypotheses
Bile acid/volatile fatty acid	Bile acid metabolism is central to colon cancer. A high-fat diet increases levels of bile acids, and bile acids damage cells in the colon and induce proliferation.
Fat and fiber	International correlation studies suggest that dietary fat increases risk of colon cancer; fat is associated with bile acid metabolism. Colon cancer was rare among Africans who ate a diet high in whole grains; early case-control studies supported this.
Meats and vegetables	A variation of the fat and fiber hypothesis. Data suggest variability in cancer risk that correlates with the spectrum of meat and vegetables in the diet [31].
Cooked foods	Meat prepared at high temperatures increases heterocyclic amines and polycyclic aromatic hydrocarbons. These carcinogens increase risk of colon cancer.
Insulin resistance	Insulin resistance hypothesis links many of the previously identified risk factors for colon cancer. Increased insulin levels influence cell proliferation and stimulate growth of colon tumors.
DNA methylation	Dietary factors such as folate, vitamin B_6, vitamin B_{12}, methionine, and alcohol are involved in DNA methylation pathways. Levels of intake of these nutrients that lead to availability of low levels of methyl groups cause hypomethylation of DNA. DNA damage leads to colon cancer.
Growth medium	Dietary factors act as initiators and promoters of the transition from normal to malignant cell. Dietary factors are involved in apoptosis and cell growth and regulation.

TABLE 2 Summary of Epidemiological Studies of Diet and Colon Cancer Associations

Dietary factor	Risk estimates	Supporting evidence	Comments
Model 1: Bile acids, fat/fiber, meats/vegetables (plant foods)			
Fat	0.8–3.0	Older case/control studies and those that did not adjust for total energy more likely to report associations.	Specific types of fat may be important. Association with fat may be confounded by total energy.
Fiber	0.6–1.0	Most case-control and cohort studies report reduced risk at high levels of fiber intake.	Association may be dependent on level of fiber intake.
Meats	0.7–2.5	Many cohort and case-control studies observed no increased risk.	Associations may depend on amount of meat eaten at a given time, method of preparation, age of the population, or other factors that could modify these effects.
Vegetables	0.8–0.5	Most studies observed reduced risk.	Some vegetables may be more important than others. Studies examining cruciferous vegetables are inconclusive in their findings.
Fruits	0.8–1.2	No consistent association	Specific types of fruits may be important, such as apples and apricots.
Whole grains	0.6–1.0	Many studies support inverse association.	Different definitions of whole grains are used. Some studies have not adjusted for dietary fiber.
Beta-carotene	~ 1.0	Inconsistent associations	Some studies show an increased risk with higher levels of intake among smokers.
Lutein	0.6–0.8	Report from one study	Associations appear to be stronger for younger people and those with proximal tumors. Lutein is a good marker for green vegetable intake.
Lycopene	0.8–1.0	Report from one study	Although protective effect not observed, high intake of tomatoes has been reported as protective in three studies that examined the association.
Vitamin E	0.6–1.0	Inconclusive	Strong protective effect reported from cohort study of older women; other studies have not identified similar protective effect.
Vitamin C	0.6–1.0	Inconclusive	Although plausible mechanisms exist, studies have generally not detected associations.

(continues)

TABLE 2 (*continued*)

Dietary factor	Risk estimates	Supporting evidence	Comments
Model 2: Cooked foods			
Fried foods	Null–6.0	Inconclusive	Many studies show no association; three show strong associations for highly browned or processed food.
Model 3: Insulin resistance			
Energy intake	RR: 0.8–1.8	Case-control studies report increased risk, with associations that are generally not observed in cohort studies.	Possible recall bias in case-control studies; cohort studies have narrower range of exposures. Some studies suggest that risk associated with energy intake is related to level of energy expenditure.
Sucrose	1.0–2.0	Inconsistent	Many studies have examined sugar-containing foods rather than sucrose. Sucrose-to-dietary fiber ratio better indicator of risk than sucrose alone in one study.
Refined grains	1.1–2.0	Most studies suggest an increase in risk.	Different definitions of refined grains are used.
Glycemic index	1.5	Limited data available	Results mainly from one study.
Model 4: DNA methylation			
Folate	0.7–1.1	Inconsistent	Some data support a protective effect in conjunction with other related factors; however, few studies show significant reduction in risk for dietary folate. Folate supplements have been associated with reduced risk if taken for 15 or more years.
Vitamin B_6	0.6–0.9	Suggestive of protective effect	Few studies have evaluated intake of this vitamin; however, it appears that it may reduce risk of colon cancer.
Methionine	0.7–1.1	Inconsistent	May be associated with risk in conjunction with other related dietary factors, although not all studies that examined the combined effect of these DNA-related factors observed an association.
Alcohol	0.7–7.0	Inconsistent	Some studies suggest stronger associations for distal and rectal tumors. Association may be confounded by cigarette smoking.
Model 5: Cell growth regulators			
Calcium	0.5–1.6	Inconsistent	Studies with a wide range of calcium intake generally show a protective effect. Clinical trials of polyps support the association. Most studies show reduced risk, although sometimes the reduced risk is not statistically significant.
Vitamin D	0.5–1.0	Inconsistent	Few studies have evaluated vitamin D, although most show a reduction in risk. Some studies have shown that supplement vitamin D reduces risk. May be an important factor.

Note: Nutrients fit into multiple models. They are listed with the model with which they have been most aligned.

This hypothesis suggests that high-fat consumption stimulates bile acid output and higher concentrations of conjugated bile acid in the colonic contents. In the colon, bile acids are deconjugated and dehydroxylated to form secondary bile acids that, in turn, damage cells and induce proliferation. In more recent years, this model has incorporated both fat and fiber. Fat stimulates bile acids and fiber binds bile acids. Dietary fiber also reduces transit time, increases stool bulk, and helps ferment volatile fatty acids—all of which may help reduce the conversion of primary to secondary bile

acids in the colon [8]. The products of fermentable volatile fatty acids include butyrate, which, in addition to being a major colonic epithelial cell fuel, may play a role in apoptosis and cell replication [9]. Pectin, a water-soluble fiber, reduces the rate of glucose absorption and decreases the rate of absorption and/or availability of lipids.

Meat and vegetable intake is also relevant to this hypothesis [7]. Meat contains high levels of fat and protein that may be harmful to the colon, while vegetables are rich sources of vitamins, minerals, fiber, and phytochemicals

(plant substances) that may protect against the development of colon cancer.

A. Dietary Fat

Ecological studies have reported that fat in diets varies directly with rates of colon cancer deaths [6]. While many early case-control and cohort studies detected an increased risk of colon cancer with increasing intake of dietary fat [4], more recent cohort, large case-control, and a pooled analysis of 13 case-control studies [10–12] have failed to find an association between dietary fat and colon cancer. The Nurse's Health Study is one of the few cohort studies that has detected an association between dietary fat and colon cancer [13]. In that study, a twofold increased risk of colon cancer was associated with high fat intake. In contrast, a cohort study of colorectal cancer in Hawaiian-Japanese men reported an inverse association, higher intakes of total fat associated with lower colon cancer risk. [11].

Studies examining specific types of fat in the diet as potential risk factors for colon cancer have similarly been inconclusive. The Nurse's Health Study and Male Professional Study found an increased risk of colon cancer associated with high intakes of animal fat [12–13]. On the other hand, the Netherlands cohort identified no increased risk associated with types of dietary fat [14], as have other studies attempting to look at specific fatty acids in the diet [15–17].

Although the data only weakly support an association between dietary fat and colon cancer, there are plausible biological explanations in addition to its role in bile acid production that support an association between specific types of fat and colon cancer. Specific fatty acids such as butyric acid have been shown to influence apoptosis [9], eicosanoids derived from 20-carbon polyunsaturated fatty acids have been shown to regulate cell proliferation and immune response [18], and linoleic acid has been shown to be involved in prostaglandin synthesis as well as acting synergistically with other growth factors [19, 20]. Early studies linking dietary fats to colon cancer could have been confounded by the effect of total energy, because fats are major contributors to variability in total energy in the diet, and statistical methods to sort these factors were often not employed [21–23]. Studies that have tried to separate the effects have generally not shown an association for dietary fat [24]. It is possible that fat is only important at high levels of intake and, because fat consumption is decreasing, important associations are no longer detected. It is also possible that other factors that modify the harmful effects of dietary fat are changing in the population.

B. Meat

Given the inconsistent associations between dietary fat and colon cancer, it is possible that red meat, a major source of animal fat, may actually be the agent responsible for the increased risk attributed to dietary fat. However, associations between red meat and colon cancer are also inconsistent for both case-control and cohort studies. While two cohort studies found increased risk with higher consumption of red meat, processed meat, or other types of meat [12, 13], 10 other cohort studies did not find an association [25]. Only with a Norwegian cohort was there an increased risk associated with sausage intake as a main meal in women, but not in men [26]. Case-control studies are likewise inconsistent [4, 27, 28]. Some studies detected associations [29], while others did not [30]. Manousos et al. [31] has shown an eightfold variation in colon cancer rates based on the combined intake of meat and vegetables. In a study of Seventh Day Adventists, meat was associated with colon cancer only among those who did not eat legumes [32].

C. Dietary Fiber

Fiber has been associated with reduced risk of colon cancer in numerous studies [4, 33–37]. Types of fiber may be important, although a recent study with the power to examine specific types of dietary fiber did not observe differences in risk from soluble and insoluble fiber [38]. In that study it was observed that the strongest associations were for older people and those with proximal tumors, possibly explaining the lack of association observed in some cohorts of younger people [39]. Level of fiber intake may also be an important determinate of risk. Some research based on a wide range of intake shows protection only at high levels of fiber intake [38]; other studies may fail to identify the association because of truncated levels of fiber intake [39].

Despite the relatively consistent association between dietary fiber and colon cancer in both case-control and cohort studies, two randomized intervention studies have failed to detect reduced polyp recurrence between groups that consumed high intakes of fiber and those that did not. In the Polyp Prevention Trial [39a], a randomized study of 2079 men and women with recently detected colorectal adenomas, an increase in dietary fiber intake (from approximately 10–17 g/1000 kcal) combined with reduction in dietary fat (from 35% to 24% of energy) and increased consumption of fruits and vegetables did not reduce the likelihood of having recurrent adenomatous polyps during the 4-year follow-up. Similarly, Alberts and colleagues [39b] did not observe an effect on risk for recurrence of polyps at 3-year follow-up with dietary supplementation of 13.5 g wheat bran fiber/day in a randomized study of 1303 men and women. These studies point out the limitations of clinical trials. Nutrition intervention studies generally use polyps as the endpoint instead of cancer. While polyps are generally considered precursors to cancer, the majority of polyps do not advance to cancer. In intervention trials, such as these, many of the initial polyps were small. The critical time for inervention is possibly earlier than after the development of polyps. Participants in clinical trials often change other behaviors, some of which

may directly influence the effect of the dietary intervention itself. Thus, the interpretation of these nutrition intervention studies is not always clear and straightforward.

D. Plant Foods: Vegetables, Fruits, Legumes, and Grains

Plant foods, in addition to fiber, are the custodians of numerous dietary constituents, including vitamins, minerals, and other potentially anticarcinogenic factors. Vegetables, specific types of vegetables, fruits, legumes, whole grains, and refined grains have all been examined in relationship to colon cancer. Of these plant foods, vegetables are perhaps one of the most consistently identified factors associated with a reduced risk of colon cancer [4]. Most studies report a 30–40% reduction in risk in those with the highest level of vegetable intake relative to those with the lowest level of intake [33, 38, 40–42]. According to the World Cancer Research Fund report, "Evidence that diets rich in vegetables protect against cancer of the colon and rectum is convincing" [42].

Cruciferous vegetables are the most widely studied type of vegetable, with inconsistent results associated with high levels of intake [4]. Other specific types of vegetables reported to reduce risk of colon cancer are dark yellow vegetables [odds ratio (OR) 0.7; 95% confidence interval (CI) 0.6–1.0] and tomatoes (OR 0.6; 95% CI 0.4–0.8) [38]. La Vecchia [43], for example, reported a significant 20–60% reduction in colon and rectal cancer risk for high consumption of tomatoes. Levi *et al.* [29] noted a significant inverse association between garlic consumption and colorectal cancer (OR 0.3; 95% CI 0.2–0.6).

Associations between fruits and colon cancer are much less consistent than those found for vegetables. While some studies report inverse associations [40], others report null associations, or even a slight increase in risk for canned fruits and juices (OR 1.2; 95% CI 0.9–1.5) [38]. Levi and colleagues [29] observed a halving of risk of colorectal cancer associated with high levels of citrus fruit intake (OR 0.5; 95% CI 0.3–0.8).

Wholegrain and refined grain products have also been evaluated, with some studies showing that wholegrain products reduce risk of colon cancer while more refined grains are associated with an increased risk (34, 35, 38, 44). Levi *et al.* [29] observed an 80% increased risk (95% CI 1.1–52.9) of colorectal cancer associated with refined grains, whereas a halving of risk was observed for high levels of wholegrain intake (OR 0.5; 95% CI 0.3–0.9). A study conducted in France similarly found a twofold increase in colorectal cancer associated with high intake of refined grains [30].

Studies that have tried to ferret out the association between the different compounds present in plant foods and colon cancer have shown that, even when controlling for dietary fiber, trace minerals, antioxidants, and other nutrients found in plant foods, vegetables still remain significantly inversely associated with colon cancer [38]. This implies that other unmeasured compounds contained in vegetables are protective. However, these bioactive compounds are unavailable in standard nutrient databases, leaving assessment of foods that contain these compounds as a surrogate for their intake.

E. Dietary Antioxidants

Vitamins with antioxidant properties, including beta-carotene, vitamin E, and vitamin C, are associated with decreased colon cancer risk in some but not all studies [4, 41, 45–47]. Enger and colleagues [48] observed that beta-carotene intake was inversely associated with polyp development. However, several clinical trials [45, 49–51] have found that high-dose beta-carotene supplementation increases risk of colorectal cancer and adenomas among smokers. In addition, the Australian Polyp Study [45] associated higher levels of beta-carotene with greater risk of recurrence of large polyps. On the other hand, a study in the Netherlands [14] linked a high vitamin C intake with a marked decrease in colon cancer risk (OR 0.5; 95% CI 0.3–0.9).

Few investigators have examined the relationship between colon cancer risk and individual carotenoids other than beta-carotene [52]. Carotenoids, long recognized for their antioxidant properties, are of increasing interest in relation to cancer because of their effect on regulation of cell growth and modulation of gene expression, as well as their possible effect on immune response [53]. Data from a large case-control study revealed an inverse relationship between lutein intake and colon cancer (40% to 10% lower risk depending on subgroup). The association was strongest for proximal tumors and in those diagnosed when younger. Lycopene-rich tomatoes have also been associated with reduced risk of colon cancer [38, 54], while another study examining lycopene failed to show an association [52].

Vitamin E has also been inversely associated with colon cancer in some but not all studies [4, 41, 55, 56]. This vitamin represents a group of tocol and tocotrienol derivatives that may have specific biological mechanisms of action [57]. Alpha-tocopherol is the most biologically active tocopherol and has been the major tocopherol considered in dietary calculations of vitamin E intake. Despite the lower biological activity of other tocopherols, such as beta-, gamma-, and delta-tocopherol, their presence in the diet in amounts two to four times that of alpha-tocopherol makes them potentially important chemopreventive agents [57].

The association between colorectal cancer and vitamin E, mainly in the form of alpha-tocopherol, is mixed among analytic epidemiologic studies [55, 56, 58, 59] and clinical trials [60, 61]. The work of Bostick and colleagues [58] provides the strongest evidence of an association between vitamin E and colon cancer. In that cohort of women living in Iowa, a strong protective effect was seen in women categorized in the upper quintile of vitamin E, after adjusting for other confounding factors. Women younger than 59 years

old were the most protected by vitamin E; and supplemental vitamin E appeared to be more protective than vitamin E from dietary sources. On the other hand, clinical trials have not supported the observation that vitamin E supplements decrease risk of colorectal polyps, a precursor to colon cancer [60, 61], nor have data from a large case-control study of colon cancer, after adjusting for related dietary and lifestyle factors [62]. In work by Longnecker and colleagues [59], the association between serum vitamin E and cancers of the colon and rectum was not statistically significant after adjusting for serum cholesterol. Examination of various forms of Vitamin E in conjunction with colon cancer risk also failed to show an inverse association [62].

III. MODEL 2: COOKED FOODS

More recently it has been suggested that the methods used to cook meat and other foods are more important than the foods themselves[63–65]. Diets high in fat and protein—high-meat diets, for example—contain greater amounts of heterocyclic amines when cooked at high temperatures. Greater exposure to these carcinogens increases cancer risk. Cooked sucrose may also be harmful in that it has been shown to promote aberrant crypt foci in rodents [66].

Using data from a case-control study, Gerhardsson de Verdier *et al.* [67] reported an increased risk of colon cancer (OR 2.7; 95% CI 1.4–5.9), comparing most frequent consumers of fried meat with a heavily browned surface to those who did not use these cooking methods; associations in this study were higher for rectal cancer than for colon cancer (OR 6.0; 95% CI 2.9–12.6). Schiffman and Felton [68] reported more than a threefold increase in risk associated with consuming well-done meat. Other studies failed to detect these associations or reported much weaker associations (OR 1.3; 95% CI 1.0–1.7), using an index based on frequency of meat consumption and temperature of cooking [28].

IV. MODEL 3: INSULIN RESISTANCE

An emerging and potentially important hypothesis relates nutrition to colon cancer through dietary contributions to insulin resistance. McKeown-Eyssen [69] first proposed this theory and Giovannucci [70] provided additional support in a literature review. The insulin resistance hypothesis pulls together many risk factors into a central biological mechanism. Physical activity, being protective for colon cancer [71], is inversely associated with blood glucose levels [72]; body size is directly associated with glucose levels as well as with colon cancer [73, 74]; and diets high in fiber and low in sucrose are inversely associated with both glucose levels and colon cancer [75, 76]. Moreover, increased levels of blood glucose and/or triglycerides can result in increased insulin levels that may in turn influence cell proliferation and stimulate growth of colon tumors.

A. Energy and Energy Balance

Energy intake, energy expenditure, and body size are factors that have been repeatedly studied in relation to colon cancer. Briefly, high levels of energy intake are associated with increased risk of colon cancer in many case-control studies, although cohort studies generally have not observed the association [4, 42]. In contrast, high levels of physical activity are consistently associated with reduced risk of colon cancer (this association has not been detected in studies of rectal cancer) [4]. Having a large body mass has also been associated with a greater risk of colon cancer, especially in men [74].

Given the connection of these factors to each other, the importance of energy balance has also been examined in relation to colon cancer [77]. High energy intake and high body mass both become highly significantly associated with colon cancer when levels of physical activity are low. Similarly, being physically active is most critical when energy intake is high. Thus, the underlying activity level of the population studied may be important to detect associations between colon cancer and energy intake.

B. Sugar and Glycemic Index

Levels of simple sugar consumption also vary from country to country and may typify a Western-style diet. High consumption of simple sugars may result in increased triglyceride and plasma glucose levels, especially among those who are insulin resistant [78].

In addition to examining dietary sugar, many studies have focused on high sucrose-containing foods [79–83]. Bostick and colleagues [79], for example, in a cohort of older women, observed that sucrose-containing foods showed stronger associations with colon cancer than did sucrose itself, with the strongest associations being observed when dairy foods that were high in sugar, such as ice cream, were excluded. Others have demonstrated links to specific foods [81, 82], although the high sugar content by itself may not be driving the association [81, 83]. Desserts or dairy products with a high-sugar content, for instance, have other components, such as fat or calcium, that may account for the observed associations with colon cancer. Findings reported by Slattery and colleagues [84] and Bostick and colleagues [79] suggest that the strongest associations are among older women. Findings regarding sucrose itself have been mixed [84–90]. Of the studies reported, only two found a significant association between sucrose and colon or colorectal cancer [8, 85]. Some of these discrepancies could be accounted for by age of study participants.

Although most studies in this area have focused on sugars themselves and foods high in sugars and starches, few attempts have been made to estimate a metabolic response based on consumption of foods. The variation in reported risk estimates between studies for high-sugar foods and/or sugar may be the result of different metabolic responses to specific foods. The glycemic index was proposed to provide

an indication of plasma glucose response to diet [91, 92]. One study noted a 40–60% increase in colon cancer risk among those with the highest dietary glycemic index [84]. Glycemic index, however, does not correlate with simple sugar intake.

V. MODEL 4: DNA METHYLATION

Methylation of DNA is one step in the regulation of gene activity [93–96]. Disturbances in DNA methylation are thought to result in abnormal expression of oncogenes and tumor suppressor genes [96–98]. In the case of colorectal tumors, for example, both generalized genomic hypomethylation and hypermethylation of usually unmethylated sites occur frequently [97–99]. Several dietary components, including folate, methionine, vitamin B_{12}, and vitamin B_6, are involved either directly or indirectly in DNA methylation [99, 100]. Alcohol may also alter DNA methylation patterns indirectly by affecting the intestinal absorption, hepatobiliary metabolism, and renal excretion of folate [101, 102]. Dietary involvement in the DNA methylation process has become a focus of research into the nutrition and colon cancer relationship

A. Folate, Vitamin B_6, and Methionine

Freudenheim and colleagues [103] originally observed that high intakes of dietary folate in women, but not men, were inversely associated with colon cancer, with stronger associations observed as the tumor site became more distal. In that study, the energy-adjusted risk estimate for the highest quartile of intake relative to the lowest quartile of intake (relative risk, RR) for women was 0.69 (95% CI 0.36–1.30), and for men was 1.03 (95% CI 0.56–1.89). In a large case-control study, folate intake was associated with a slight decrease in risk, with risk estimates for upper quintile of intake for women ranging from 0.7 to 0.9 and ORs for men ranging from 0.8 to 1.1, depending on age and site-specific subgroup [100]. Adjustment for dietary fiber attenuated the association in that study, although Freudenheim and colleagues [103] did not observe an alteration in risk after adjustment for fiber from vegetables. Giovannucci et al. [104] observed that men in the highest quintile of dietary folate intake were not at reduced risk (RR 0.85; 95% CI 0.54–1.39).

Inclusion of vitamin supplement data had little effect in findings reported either by Giovannucci et al. [104] or Slattery et al. [100]. One study noted that people taking folate supplements for 15 or more years were at reduced risk of colon cancer, but there was no effect from folate supplements taken for less than 15 years [105]. It is not clear if this finding is one of chance, if it points to a time when folate supplementation may have had important protective influences, or if it points to other characteristics that may be linked to reduced colon cancer risk in a small subset of the population.

Other nutrients involved in this pathway have been examined less extensively than dietary folate. Methionine was not associated with risk of colon cancer in a large case-control study [10], although Giovannucci and colleagues [104] observed that those with the highest intake were at reduced risk (RR 0.65; 95% CI 0.42–1.02) in their cohort study. Vitamin B_6 intake has also been shown by some investigators to reduce risk of colon cancer [101].

B. Alcohol

The association of alcohol with colon cancer has been inconsistent, with approximately half of all studies showing an increase in risk [4, 106] and the rest showing no association [107–109]. Evidence linking alcohol and colorectal cancer has usually been more consistent and stronger for more distal or rectal tumors, and some investigators have pointed to cigarette smoking as a confounding variable [109].

It is possible that interaction between nutrients is needed to create a situation that can lead to disturbances in DNA methylation. For instance, in the study by Freudenheim and colleagues [103], men at highest risk for rectal cancer were those who consumed large amounts of alcohol and had low intakes of dietary folate; similar results were not reported for colon cancer. Giovannucci et al. [104] found the greatest increase in risk of colon cancer when a combination of factors was present: high alcohol and low folate or low methionine. However, the study by Slattery and colleagues [100], in which a large sample size provided the most power to detect an association, found no significant increase in risk of colon cancer with a dietary profile that could be considered "high risk" with respect to alcohol and folate intakes [100]. Because several genetic variants have been identified that may impact this pathway, these potential interactions are being investigated and will be discussed later in this chapter.

VI. MODEL 5: CELL GROWTH REGULATORS

Given that dietary factors act as initiators and promoters of tumors that advance along the continuum from polyp, the common precursor lesion, to colon cancer, this model of cell growth regulation encompasses several dietary factors because the proliferative activity of colon mucosa is modified by different nutrients [110, 111]. Newmark and colleagues [112] have suggested that calcium may induce saponification of free fatty acids and bile acids, thereby diminishing the proliferative stimulus of these compounds on the colon mucosa. Calcium might also directly influence proliferation by inducing cell differentiation [113]. Few data are available for vitamin D, but animal and human experimental studies suggest inhibition of cell proliferation by vitamin D, either directly or by way of its effect on calcium absorption [112–114].

A. Calcium

As concluded in a meta-analysis conducted in 1996 [115] and in a recent review [116], epidemiological data on calcium and colon cancer are not conclusive. However, results published subsequently add support to the hypothesis that calcium has a protective role. A cohort study in Finland, for example, found a significant reduction in risk at high levels of calcium intake [15], as did a large multicenter case-control study from the United States [117] and a case-control study conducted in Wisconsin [118]

Although several studies support reduced risk of colon cancer with calcium, with risk estimates for high levels of intake being 0.5 [117–121], other studies do not confirm these results [115, 116]. A prospective study among Iowa women, including 241 colon cancer cases after 10 years of follow-up, suggested an inverse association between calcium and colon cancer only among those without a family history of colorectal cancer among first-degree relatives [122]. Support for an association between calcium and colon cancer also comes from controlled studies which show that epithelial proliferation of the colon mucosa, a presumed intermediate marker of colorectal carcinogenesis, is diminished by calcium supplementation in humans [123]. Additionally, a double-blind, placebo-controlled clinical trial of calcium in sporadic adenoma patients showed that, although the overall proliferation rate was unchanged, the distribution of proliferating cells was favorably altered [124]. And recently, a large controlled clinical trial demonstrated that polyp recurrence was reduced by 15–20% with calcium supplementation [125].

Inconsistent findings in epidemiologic studies examining the relationship between calcium and colon cancer may be explained by methodological issues related to an observational epidemiologic study design. For instance, the variation in calcium intake in some studies may have been insufficient to detect differences in risk across categories. In studies that observed a weak inverse association, the differences in median dietary calcium values between the lowest and the highest category of intake ranged between 500 and 700 mg/day, whereas in a larger multicenter study of colon cancer [117], in which an inverse association was detected, the median dietary calcium values between the lowest and highest quintile of intake were 1601 mg for men and 1236 mg for women. That study noted that the protective effect was essentially limited to the highest quintile of intake and that looking only at the fourth quintile of intake one might consider the results as null or only weakly protective.

B. Vitamin D

As reviewed by Martinez and Willett [116], epidemiological data on vitamin D and colorectal cancer are sparse and suggest protective effects of vitamin D on colon cancer risk. In large studies—both case control and cohort—the inverse association between dietary vitamin D and colorectal cancer ranges between 0.5 and 0.9, although not always reaching statistical significance after multivariate adjustment [117–121, 126–128]. An inverse association was detected in the Iowa Women's Health Study among those with a negative family history of colorectal cancer but not among those with a positive family history [122]. Supplemental vitamin D has been significantly inversely related to colon cancer [118]. Most studies where an inverse association with vitamin D intake was found are prospective cohort studies in which exposure is assessed many years before diagnosis. Vitamin D may have a protective effect on early stages of tumor development that is not captured in case-control studies.

VII. FOOD INTAKE RELATIONSHIPS

A. Dietary Patterns

Diet is complex. Patterns of consumption are not focused on a single food or nutrient, despite the fact that our assessment of risk generally takes a one nutrient or specific food approach. It is possible that the overall pattern of intake is more important than any single food. To assess this possibility, several groups have identified dietary patterns and evaluated their association with risk of developing colon cancer. For example, when a large case-control study identified eating patterns using factor analyses [129], two major dietary patterns emerged.

Although the descriptive labels were arbitrarily given, foods clustering together represent what could be described as the "Western diet" and the "prudent diet." The Western diet represented an eating pattern characterized by high intakes of red meat, fast foods, high-fat dairy foods, refined grains, and foods with a high sugar content. The prudent diet, on the other hand, was typified by high intakes of fruits, vegetables, whole grains, and fish and poultry. Subsequent to the initial study, these same dietary patterns were identified and validated using data from a large cohort study [130].

Assessment of these dietary patterns revealed that the Western dietary pattern was associated with increased risk of colon cancer, while the prudent dietary pattern was inversely associated with colon cancer. While the link with individual food items is not consistent between studies, the data are unified on the more broadly focused eating patterns. The dietary pattern can also modify the risk associated with a family history of colorectal cancer [131].

B. Dietary and Genetic Interactions

Genetic susceptibility can take two forms: inheritance of high-penetrance genes, such as the adenomatous polyposis coli (*APC*) gene [132], or mismatch repair genes leading to hereditary nonpolyposis colon cancer (*HPNCC*) [133], or low-penetrance genes, such as the ones discussed below.

TABLE 3   Interrelationship between Diet and Genetic Factors

Disease pathways	Genetic factors[a]	Dietary factors
Meat/fat/cooking	NAT2/NAT1/CYP1A1 GST	Meat, protein, fat, cruciferous vegetables, coffee
DNA methylation	MTHFR	Folate, vitamin B_{12}, vitamin B_6
	Metehionine synthase	Methionine
	Alcohol dehydrogenases	Alcohol
Insulin	IGF	Sugar, fat, energy balance
Cell growth regulation	TGFβ	
	VDR	Calcium, vitamin D
	ApoE	Fat, sugar

[a]NAT2 = N-acetyltransferase 2
NAT1 = N-acetyltransferase 1
CYP1A1 = cytochrome P450 1A1
GST = glutathione-S-transferase
MTHFR = methylenetetrahydrofolate reductase
IGF = Insulin-like growth factor
TGFβ = Transforming growth factor beta
VDR = Vitamin D receptor
ApoE = Apolipoprotein E

Susceptibility associated with inheritance of low-penetrance genes, while carrying a much lower independent risk than high-penetrance genes, is relatively common. Thus, low-penetrance genes may be associated with a much higher population attributable risk than high-penetrance genes [133], especially when coupled with dietary factors that may serve as modulators. (See Chapter 13.) Table 3 summarizes some of the suspected relationships between diet and genetic factors.

Carcinogens in meat prepared at high temperatures contain heterocyclic amines and polycyclic aromatic hydrocarbons that are metabolized by enzymes such as N-acetyltransferase and glutathione S-transferase (GST) [134]. The internal dose and actual DNA exposure to heterocyclic amines, polycyclic aromatic hydrocarbons, and *N*-nitrosocompounds seems to be particularly important for those who are rapid metabolizers of these compounds. Refined grains and fats also contain polycyclic aromatic hydrocarbons and heterocyclic amines and may also interact with variants of these low-penetrance genes [135, 136]. Increased risk of colon cancer among rapid acetylators who consume high levels of meat has been observed in some populations [137–139] or population subsets, i.e., only older men [139], but not in other studies [28].

Several constituents of cruciferous vegetables, including isothiocyanates and indoles, have been hypothesized to reduce risk of cancer through activation of GST [140, 141]. Sulforaphane, an isothiocyanate compound found predominately in broccoli, is one of the most potent inducers of GST [142–144]. Differences in observed associations between cruciferous vegetables and colon cancer could be the result of genetic variants that alter susceptibility from exposure to these vegetables. One study has examined the interaction between colon cancer and cruciferous vegetable consumption and *GST*μ-*1* genotype [145]. In that study those most influenced by the combination of cruciferous vegetable consumption and *GST*μ-*1* genotype were younger individuals who smoked cigarettes. A study linking colonic adenomas with cruciferous vegetables found that those with the *GST*μ-*1* null genotype received more protection from ingestion of large amounts of broccoli than did those with *GST*μ-*1* positive genotype [146].

Kahweol palmitate and cafestol palmitate are two other potent inducers of GST found in green coffee beans and roasted coffee beans [144]. Mice fed green coffee beans have a six- to sevenfold increased level of GST activity [147], and similar effects have been observed for roasted coffee beans. Epidemiologic studies have generally reported an inverse association between high consumption of coffee and risk of colon cancer [148], although the mechanism is not well known.

Methylenetetrahydrofolate reductase (*MTHFR*) is a key enzyme in the conversion to 5-methyltetrahydrofolate, the major circulating form of folate in the body and the primary methyl donor for the methylation of homocysteine to methionine. This enzyme is also key in the methylation process of DNA. A polymorphism of the human *MTHFR* gene that leads to reduced *MTHFR* activity resulting in elevated plasma homocysteine levels has been described [149].

Investigators have evaluated the interaction between folate, vitamin B_{12}, vitamin B_6, alcohol and the presence of *MTHFR* polymorphisms. One large case-control study did not observe significant interaction between these dietary factors and *MTHFR* genotype [150]. Others have shown more

variation in risk estimates [151, 152] by *MTHFR* genotype, although estimates of association have generally been imprecise because of small sample sizes [153]. Other genes involved in methylation processes, such as methionine synthase [154] and alcohol dehydrogenase, may also be influenced by dietary factors. However, one study evaluating methionine synthase did not find variation in risk by genotype in conjunction with either alcohol or folate intake [155].

Another way in which dietary factors may influence colon cancer risk is by interacting with genetic variants that influence insulin levels, apoptosis, and cell growth. For example, variants of genes for the insulin-like growth factor *(IGF)* [156, 157], vitamin D receptor *(VDR)* [158], apolipoprotein E *(apoE)* [159], and the transforming growth factor *(TGFβ)* [160] may be associated with colon cancer.

Potentially important diet and genetic interactions may occur for each hypothesized model of the relationship between diet and colon cancer [161]. Because we are only beginning to explore and understand various disease pathways, our knowledge of such interactions is in its infancy. As we gain a better grasp of the genes involved in disease pathways, possible dietary interactions with those genes will undoubtedly become clearer.

C. Diet and Specific Mutations in Tumors

A spectrum of mutations occurs in colon cancer tumors, implying that multiple pathways to disease exist. The primary genetic mutations observed in colon tumors are mutations in the *APC* gene, *Ki-ras* gene, *p53,* and microsatellite instability [162]. Studies have reported approximately 85–90% of colon tumors with an *APC* mutation. Most population-based studies estimate that 30–40% of colon tumors have *Ki-ras* mutations [163, 164], while microsatellite instability has been found to occur in between 14 and 18% of cases [165]. The prevalence of *p53* mutations, the most commonly mutated gene in most cancers including colon cancer, varies by the method used to detect the abnormality [166, 167]. While immunohistochemistry studies estimate the prevalence of *p53* overexpression at 50–75% of colon tumors, studies attempting to identify mutations provide much lower estimates of closer to 40% of tumors [167, 168].

Few studies have examined the association between diet and these distinct tumor mutations. *Ki-ras* mutations have been evaluated in two studies of cancer and one of colonic polyps. The first study found that calcium intake reduced risk of *Ki-ras* mutations, while monounsaturated fat intake increased risk of these mutations [169]. The second study, being much larger, detected mutation-specific associations [163]. Whereas dietary fat intake increased risk of G → T mutations, low levels of dietary factors associated with DNA methylation actually reduced the risk of having a G → A mutation. This information is inconsistent with that presented by Martinez and colleagues [164] in their study of adenomas. They observed that supplemental folate reduced

the risk of having a *Ki-ras* mutation, while dietary intake of folate was unrelated to *Ki-ras* mutations.

Dietary associations with *p53* mutations have been reported for two studies. In one study [168], fat intake was associated with a greater likelihood of a *p53* mutation, especially transversions. In another study, beef intake was more strongly associated with *p53* negative cases than *p53* positive cases [170]. Associations between dietary factors and microsatellite instability have not been reported.

VIII. PREVENTION OF COLON CANCER

The link between diet and colon cancer is undoubtedly complex. Given that the effects of individual nutrients and overall dietary composition will vary depending on genetic predisposition and other environmental influences, it is somewhat understandable that attempts to identify consistent associations between dietary factors and colon cancer are difficult. However, there is now adequate evidence to put forth several important public health recommendations that may aid in the prevention of colorectal cancer and will promote lifestyle patterns consistent with healthy living.

The World Cancer Research Fund, in their report *Food, Nutrition and the Prevention of Cancer: A Global Perspective* [42] concludes the following:

> The most effective ways of preventing colorectal cancer are consumption of diets high in vegetables and regular physical activity and low consumption of red and processed meat. Possible further means of preventing this cancer, are maintenance of body weight within recommended levels throughout life, and consumption of diets high in non-starch polysaccharides, starch and carotenoids and low in sugar, fat and eggs.

These are applicable and recommended for prevention of colon cancer based on current knowledge.

As future research continues to focus on the interactions between diet and genetics, we should be able, within subsets of the population with specified susceptibilities, to identify stronger and more consistent associations as well as develop targeted interventions with specific dietary recommendations.

References

1. American Cancer Society. (1997). "Cancer Facts and Figures." American Cancer Society, Atlanta, GA.
2. World Health Organization. (1997). "The World Health Report." World Health Organization, Geneva, Switzerland.
3. Haenszel, W., and Kurihara, M. (1968). Studies of Japanese migrants. I. Mortality from cancer and other diseases among Japanese in the United States. *J. Natl. Cncer Inst.* **40,** 43–68.
4. Potter, J. D,, Slattery, M. L., Bostick, R. M., and Gapstur, S. M. (1993). Colon cancer: A review of the epidemiology. *Epidemio. Rev.* **15,** 499–545.

5. Sorenson, A. W., Slattery, M. L., and Ford, M. H. (1988). Calcium and colon cancer: A review. *Nutr. Cancer* **11**(3), 135–145.

6. Adlercreutz, H. (1990). Western diet and Western diseases: Some hormonal and biochemical mechanisms and associations. *Scand. J. Clin. Lab. Invest.* **50**, 3–23.

7. Potter, J. D. (1992). Reconciling and epidemiology, physiology, and molecular biology of colon cancer. *J. A. M. A.* **268**, 1573–1578.

8. Hill, M. J. (1998). Cereals, cereal fibre and colorectal cancer risk: A review of the epidemiological literature. *Euro.J. Cancer Prev.* **7**, S5–S10.

9. Hague, A., Elder, D. J. E., Hicks, D. J., and Prasleva, C. (1995). Apoptosis in colorectal tumour cells: Induction by the short chain fatty acids butyrate, proprionate and acetate and by the bile salt deoxycholate. *Int. J. Cancer* **60**, 400–406.

10. Howe, G. R., Aronson, K. J., Benito, E., Castelleto, R., Cornee, J., Esteve, J., Gallagher, R. P., Iscovich, J. M., Deng-ao, J., Kaaks, R., Kune, G. A., Kune, S., Lee, H. P., Lee, M., Miller, A. B., Peters, R. K., Potter, J. D., Riboli, E., Slattery, M. L., Trichopoulos, D., Tuyns, A., Tzonou, A., Whittemore, A. S., Wu-Williams, A. H., and Shu, Z. (1997). The relationship between dietary fat intake and risk of colorectal cancer: Evidence from the combined analysis of 13 case-control studies. *Cancer Causes Control* **8**, 215–228.

11. Le Marchand, L., Wilkens, L. R., Hankin, J. H., Kolonel, L. N., and Lyu, L. C. (1997). A case-control study of diet and colorectal cancer in a multiethnic population in Hawaii (United States): Lipids and foods of animal origin. *Cancer Causes Control* **8**, 637–648.

12. Giovannucci, E., Rimm, E. B., Stampher, M. J., Colditz, G. A., Ascher, A., Willett, W. C. (1994). Intake of fat, meat, and fiber in relation to risk of colon cancer in men. *Cancer Res.* **54**, 2390–2397.

13. Willett, W. C., Stampher, M. J., Colditz, G. A., Rosner, B. A., Speizer, F. E. (1990). Relation of meat fat and fiber intake to the risk of colon cancer in a prospective study among women. *N. Engl. J. Med.* **323**, 1664–1672.

14. van den Brandt, P. A., Goldbohm, R.A., Van't Veer, P., Volovics, A., Hermus, R. J. J., and Sturmans, F. (1990). A large-scale prospective cohort study on diet and cancer in The Netherlands. *J. Clin. Epidemiol.* **43**, 285–295.

15. Pietinen, P., Malila, N., Virtanen, M., Hartman, T. J., Tangrea, J. A., Albanes, D., and Virtamo, J. (1999). Diet and risk of colorectal cancer in a cohort of Finnish men. *Cancer Causes* **10**, 389–396.

16. Slattery, M. L., Potter, J. D., Duncan, D., and Berry, T. D. (1997). Dietary fats and colon cancer: Assessment of risk associated with specific fatty acids. *Int. J. Cancer* **73**, 670–677.

17. Franceschi, S., LaVecchia, C., Russo, A., Favero, A., Negri, E., Conti, E., Montella, M., Filiberti, R., Amadori, D., and Decarli, A. (1999). Macronutrient intake and risk of colorectal cancer in Italy. *Int. J. Cancer* **75**, 321–324.

18. Sears, B. (1993). Essential fatty acids, eicosanoids, and cancer. *In* "Adjuvant Nutrition in Cancer Treatment" (P. Quillin and E. M. Williams, Eds.), pp. 267–282. Cancer Treatment and Research Foundation, Arlington Heights, IL.

19. Hsiao, W. L. W., Pai, H. L. H., Matsui, M. S., and Weinstein, I. B. (1994). Effects of specific fatty acids on cell transformation induced by an activated c-H-*ras* oncogene. *Oncogene,* **5**, 417–421.

20. Rose, D. P., and Connolly, J. M. (1990). Effects of fatty acids and inhibitors in eicosanoid synthesis on the growth of a human breast cancer cell line in culture. *Cancer Res.* **50**, 139–144.

21. Willett, W,, Stampfer, M. J. (1986). Total energy intake: Implications for epidemiologic analyses. *Am. J. Epidemiol.* **124,** 17–27.

22. Brown, C. C,, Kipnis, V,, Freedman, L. S., Hartman, A. M,, Schatzkin, A., and Wacholder, S. (1994). Energy adjustment methods for nutritional epidemiology: The effect of categorization. *Am. J. Epidemiol.* **139,** 323–338.

23. Wacholder, S., Schatzkin, A., Freedman, L. S., Kipnis, V., Hartman, A., and Brown, C. C. (1994). Can energy adjustment separate the effects of energy from those of specific macronutrients? *Am. J. Epidemiol.* **140,** 848–855.

24. Slattery, M. L., Caan, B. J., Potter, J. D., Berry, T. D., Coates, A., Duncan, D., and Edwards, S. L. (1997). Dietary energy sources and colon cancer risk. *Am. J. Epidemiol.* **145**(3), 199–210.

25. Hill, M. J. (1999). Meat or wheat for the next millennium? A debate pro meat. Meat and colorectal cancer. *Pro. Nutr. Soc.* **58,** 261–264.

26. Gaard, M., Tretli, S., and Loken, E. B. (1996). Dietary factors and risk of colon cancer: A prospective study of 50,535 young Norwegian men and women. *Eur. J. Cancer Prev.* **5,** 445–454.

27. Kampman, E., Verhoeven, D., Sloots, L, and van't Veer, P. (1995). Vegetable and animal products as determinants of colon cancer risk in Dutch men and women. *Cancer Causes Control* **6,** 225–234.

28. Kampman, E., Slattery, M. L., Bigler, J., Leppert, M., Samowitz, W., Caan, B. J., and Potter, J. D. (1999). Meat consumption, genetic susceptibility, and colon cancer risk: A U.S. multicenter case-control study. *Cancer Epidemiol. Biomarkers Prev.* **8,** 15–24.

29. Levi, F., Pasche, C., La Vecchia, C., Lucchini, F., and Franceschi, S. (1998). Food groups and colorectal cancer risk. *Brit. J. Cancer* **79,** 1283–1287.

30. Boutron-Ruault, M. C., Senesse, P., Faivre, J., Chatelain, N., Belghiti, C., and Meance, S. (1999). Foods as risk factors for colorectal cancer: A case-control study in Burgundy (France). *Eur. J. Cancer Prev.* **8,** 229–235.

31. Manousos, O., Day, N. E., Trichopoulos D., Gerovassilis, G., and Tzonou, A. (1983). Diet and colorectal cancer: A case-control study in Greece. *Int. J. Cancer* **32,** 1–5.

32. Singh, P. N., and Fraser, G. E. (1997) Dietary risk factors for colon cancer in a low-risk population. *Am. J. Epidemiol.* **148,** 761–774.

33. Howe, G., Benito, E., Castelleto, R., Cornee, J., Esteve, J., Gallagher, R. P., Iscovich, J. M., Deng-ao, J., Kaaks, R., Kune, G. A., Miller, A., Peters, R., Potter, J., Riboli, E., Slattery, M., Trichopoulos, D., Tuyns, A., Tzonou, A., Whittemore, A. S., Wu-Williams, A. H., and Shu, Z. (1992). Dietary intake of fibre and decreased risk of cancers of the colon and rectum: Evidence from the combined analysis of 13 case-control studies. *J. Natl. Cancer Inst.* **84**(24), 1887–1896.

34. Trock, B., Lanza, E., and Greenwald, P. (1990). Dietary fiber, vegetables, and colon cancer: Critical review and meta-analyses of the epidemiologic evidence. *J. Natl. Cancer Inst.* **82,** 650–661.

35. Lipkin, M., Reddy, B., Newmark, H., and Lamprecht, S. A. (1999). Dietary factors in human colorectal cancer. *Annu. Rev. Nutr.* **19,** 545–586.

36. Negri, E., Franceschi, S., Parpinel, M., and La Vecchia, C. (1998). Fiber intake and risk of colorectal cancer. *Cancer Epidemiol. Biomarkers, Prev.* **7,** 667–671.

37. Jensen, M. C. J. F., Bueno-de-Mesquita, H. B., Buzina, R., Fidanza, F., Menotti, A., Blackburn, H., Nissinen, A. M., Kok, F. J., and Kromhout, D., for the Seven Countries Study Research Group. (1998). Dietary fiber and plant foods in relation to colorectal cancer mortality: The Seven Countries Study. *Int. J. Cancer* **81,** 174–179.

38. Slattery, M. L., Potter, J. D., Coates, A, Ma, K., Duncan, D. M., Berry, T. D., and Caan, B. J. (1997). Plant foods and colon cancer: An assessment of specific foods and their related nutrients. *Cancer Causes Control* **8,** 575–590.

39. Fuchs, C. S., Giovannucci, E. L., Colditz, G. A., Hunter D. J., Stampfer, M. J., Rosner, B., Speizer, F. E., Pilch, S. M. and Willett, W. C. (1999). Dietary fiber and the risk of colorectal cancer and adenoma in women. *N. Engl. J. Med.* **340,** 169–176.

39a. Schatzkin, A., Lanza, E., Corle, D., Lance, P., Iber, F., Caan, B., Shike, M., Weissfeld, J., Burt, R., Cooper, M. R., Kikendall, J. W., Cahill, J. and the Polyp Prevention Trial Study Group. (2000). Lack of effect of a low-fat diet on the recurrence on colorectal adenomas. *N. Engl. J. Med.* **342,** 1149–1155.

39b. Alberts, D. D., Martinez, M. E., Roe, D. J., Gullen-Rodriguez, J. M., Marshall, J. R., Van Leeuwen, J. B., Reid, M. E., Ritengaugh, C., Vargus, P. A., Bhattacharyva, A. B., Earnest, D. L., Sampliner, R. E., and the Phoenix Colon Cancer Prevention Physician's Network. (2000). Lack of effect of a high-fiber cereal supplement on the recurrence of colorectal adenomas. *N. Engl. J. Med.* **342,** 1156–1162.

40. Shannon, J., White, E., Shattuck, A. L., and Potter J. D. (1995). Relationship of food groups and water intake to colon cancer risk. *Cancer Epidemiol. Biomarkers Prev.* **5,** 495–502.

41. Steinmetz, K. A., and Potter, J. D. (1991). Vegetables, fruit, and cancer. I. Epidemiology. *Cancer Causes Control* **2,** 325–357.

42. World Cancer Research Fund. (1997). "Food, nutrition and the Prevention of Cancer: A Global Perspective." American Institute for Cancer Research, Washington, DC.

43. La Vecchia, C. (1998). Mediterranean epidemiological evidence on tomatoes and the prevention of digestive-tract cancers. *Proc. Soc. Exp. Biol. Med.* **218,** 125–128.

44. Jacobs, D. R., Slavin, J., and Marquart, L. (1995). Whole grain intake and cancer: A review of the literature. *Nutr. Cancer* **24,** 221–229.

45. MacLennan, R., Macrae, F., Bain, C., Banistutta, D., Chapuis, P., Gratten, H., Lambert, J., Newland,R. C., Ngu, M., Russell, A., Ward, M., Wahlquist, M. L. (1995). The Australian Polyp Prevention Project. Randomized trial of intake of fat, fiber, and beta carotene to prevent colorectal adenoma. *J. Nat. Cancer Inst.* **87,** 1760–1766.

46. Dorgan, J. F., and Schatzkin, A. (1991). Antioxidant micronutrients in cancer prevention. *Hematol. Oncol. Clin. N. Am.* **5,** 43–68.

47. Hennekens, C. H. (1994). Antioxidant vitamins and cancer. *Am. J. Med.* **97,** 2S–4S, 22S–28S.

48. Enger, S. M., Longnecker, M. P., Chen, M. J., Harper, J. M., Lee, E. R., Frankl, H. D., and Haile, R. W. (1996). Dietary intake of specific carotenoids and vitamins A, C, and E and prevalence of colorectal adenomas. *Cancer Epidemiol. Biomarkers Prev.* 5, 147–153.

49. Omenn, G. S., Goodman, G. E., Thornquist, M. D., Balmes, J., Cullen, M. R., Glass, A., Koegh, J. P., Meyskens, F. L., Volanis, B., Williams, J. H., Barnhart, S., Cherniack, M. G., Brodkin, C. A., and Hammul, S. (1996). Risk factors for lung cancer and for intervention effects in CARET, the Beta-carotene and Retinol Efficacy Trial. *J. Natl. Cancer Inst.* **88,** 1550–1559.

50. Alpha-Tocopherol, Beta Carotene Cancer Prevention Study Group. (1994). The effect of vitamin E and beta carotene on the incidence of lung cancer and other cancers in male smokers. *N. Eng. J. Med.* **330,** 1029–1035.

51. Hennekens, C. H., Buring, J. E., Manson, J. E., Stampfer, M., Rosner, B., Cook, N., Belanger, C., LaMotte, F., Gaziano, J. M., Ridker, P., Willett, W., and Peto, R. (1996). Lack of effect of long-term supplementation with β-carotene on the incidence of malignant neoplasma and cardiovascular disease. *N. Eng. J. Med.* **334,** 1145–1149.

52. Slattery, M. L., Benson, J., Curtin, K., Ma, K, N., Schaeffer, D., and Potter, J. D. (2000). Carotenoids and colon cancer. *Am. J. Clin. Nutr.* **71,** 575–582.

53. Rock, C. L. (1997). Carotenoids: Biology and treatment. *Pharmacol. Ther.* **75,** 185–197.

54. Le Marchand, L., Franke, A. A., Custer, L., Wilkens, L. R., and Cooney, R. V. (1997). Lifestyle and nutritional correlates of cytochrome CYP1A2 activity: Inverse associations with plasma lutein and alpha-tocopherol. *Pharmacogenetics* 7, 11–19.

55. Flagg, E. W., Coates, R. J., and Greenberg, R. S. (1995). Epidemiologic studies of antioxidants and cancer in humans. *J. Am. College Nutr.* **14,** 419–427.

56. Byers T., and Guerrero, N. {1995). Epidemiologic evidence for vitamin C and vitamin E in cancer prevention. *Am. J. Clin. Nutr.* **62,** 1385S–1392S.

57. Stone, W. L., and Papas, A. M. (1997). Tocopherols and the etiology of colon cancer. *J. Natl. Cancer Inst.* **89,** 1006–1014.

58. Bostick, R. M., Potter, J. D., McKenzie, D. R., Sellers, T. A., Kushi, L. H., Steinmetz, K. A., and Folsom, A. R. (1993). Reduced risk of colon cancer with high intake of vitamin E: The Iowa Women's Health Study. *Cancer Res.* **53,** 4230–4237.

59. Longnecker, M. P., Martin-Moreno, J. M., Knekt, P., Nourma, A. M. Y., Schober, S. E., Stahelin, H. B., Wald, N. J., Grey, K. F., and Willett, W. C. (1992). Serum a-tocopherol concentration in relation to subsequent colorectal cancer: Pooled data from five cohorts. *J. Natl. Cancer Inst.* **84,** 430–435.

60. McKeown-Eyssenm, G., Holloway, C., Jazmaji, V., Bright-See, E., Dion, P., and Bruce, W. R. (1988). A randomized trial of vitamins C and E in the prevention of recurrence of colorectal polyps. *Cancer Res,* **48,** 4701–4705.

61. Greenberg, E. R., Baron, J. A., Tosteson, T. D., Freeman, D. H., Beck, G. J., Bond, J. H., Colacchio, T. A., Coller, J. A., Frankl, H. D., Haile, R. W., Mandel, J. S., Nierenberg, D., Rothstein, R., Snover, D., Stevens, M., Summers, R., and van Stolk, R. (1998). A clinical trial of antioxidant vitamins to prevent colorectal adenoma. *N. Eng. J. Med.* **331,** 141–147.

62. Slattery, M. L., Edwards, S. L., Anderson, K. E., and Caan, B. J. (1998). Vitamin E and colon cancer: Is there an association? *Nutr. Cancer* **30**(3), 201–206.

63. Sinha, R., Rothman, N., Brown, E. D., Levander, O. A., Davies, D. S., Lang, N. P., Kadluber, F. F., and Hoover, R. N. (1995), High concentrations of the carcinogen 2-amino-1-methyl-6-phenylimidazo-[4, 5B] pyridine (PhIP) occur in chicken and are dependent on the cooking method. *Cancer Res.* **55**, 4516–4519.

64. Hayatsu, H., Hayatsu, T., Wataya, W., and Mowel, H. F. (1985). Fecal mutagenicity arising from ingestion of fried ground beef in the human. *Mutat. Res.* **143**, 207–211.

65. Skog, K., Steineck, G., Augustsson, K., and Jagerstad, M. (1995). Effect of cooking temperature on the formation of heterocyclic amines in fried meat products and pan residues. *Carcinogenesis (Lond.)* **16**, 861–867.

66. Corpet, D., Stamp, D., Medline, A., Minkin, S., Archer, M. C., and Bruce, W. R. (1990).Promotion of colonic microadenoma growth in mice and rats fed cooked sugar or cooked casein and fat. *Cancer Res.* **50**, 6955–6958.

67. Gerhardsson de Verdier, M., Hagman, U., Peters, R. K., Steineck, G., and Overvik, E. (1991). Meat, cooking methods and colorectal cancer: A case-referent study in Stockholm. *Int. J. Cancer* **49**, 520–525.

68. Schiffman, M. H., and Felton, J. S. (1990). Re: Fried foods and risk of colon cancer. *Am. J. Epidemiol.* **131**, 378–378.

69. McKeown-Eyssen, G. (1994). Epidemiology of colorectal cancer revisited: are serum triglycerides and/or plasma glucose associated with risk? *Cancer Epidemiol. Biomarkers Prev.* **3**, 687–695.

70. Giovannucci, E. (1995). Insulin and colon cancer. *Cancer Causes Control* **6**, 164–179.

71. Slattery, M. L., Edwards, S. L., Ma, K. N., Friedman, G. F., and Potter, J. D. (1997). Physical activity and colon cancer: A public health perspective. *Ann. Epidemiol.* **7**, 137–145.

72. Huttunen, J. K., Lansimies, E., Voutilainen, E., Ehnholm, E., Hietanen, E., Pentilla, I., Siltonen, B., and Rauramaa, R. (1979). Effect of moderate physical exercise on serum lipoproteins: A controlled clinical trial with special reference to serum high-density lipoproteins. *Circulation* **60**, 1220–1229.

73. Krotkiewski, M., Bjorntorp, P., Sjostrom, L., and Smith, U. (1983). Impact of obesity on metabolism in men and women. Importance of regional adipose tissue distribution. *J. Clin. Invest.* **72**, 1150–1162.

74. Caan, B. J., Coates, A. O., Slattery, M. L., Potter, J. D., Quesenberry, C. P., Jr,, and Edwards, S. (1998). Body size and colon cancer in a large case-control study. *Int. J. Obes. Relat. Metab. Dis.* **22**, 178–184.

75. Coulston, A., Lui, C. G., and Reaven, C. G. (1983). Plasma glucose, insulin, and lipid responses to high-carbohydrate low-fat diets in normal humans. *Metabolism* **32**, 52–56.

76. Tuyns, A. J., Haelterman, M., Kaaks, R. (1987). Colorectal cancer and intake of nutreints: Oligosaccharides are a risk factor, fats are not. A case-control study in Belgium. *Nutr. Cancer* **10**, 181–186.

77. Slattery, M. L., Potter, J. D., Caan, B. J., Edwards, S. L., Coates, A., Berry, D. T., and Mori, M. (1997). Energy balance and colon cancer—beyond physical activity. *Cancer Res.* **57**, 75–80.

78. Kim, Y. I. (1998). Diet, lifestyle, and colorectal cancer: Is hyperinsulinemia the missing link? *Nutr. Rev.* **56**, 275–279.

79. Bostick, R. M., Potter, J. D., Kushi, L. H., Sellers, T. A., Steinmetz, K. A., McKenzie, D. R., Gapstur, S. M., and Folsom A. R. (1994). Sugar, meat, and fat intake, and non-dietary risk factors for colon cancer incidence in Iowa women (United States). *Cancer Causes Control* **5**, 38–52.

80. Philips, R. (1975). Role of life-style and dietary habits in risk of cancer among Seventh-Day Adventists. *Cancer Res.* **35**, 3513–3522.

81. Miller, A. B., Howe, G. R., Jain, M., Craib, D. J. P., and Harrison, L. (1983). Food items and food groups as risk factors in a case-control study of diet and colorectal cancer. *Int. J. Cancer* **32**, 155–161.

82. Tuyns, A. J., Kaaks, R., and Haelterman, M. (1988). Colorectal cancer and the consumption of foods: A case-control study in Belgium. *Nutr. Cancer* **11**, 189–204.

83. Pickle, L. W., Greene, M. H., Ziegler, R. G., Toledo, A., Hoover, R., and Lynch, H. T. (1984). Colorectal cancer in rural Nebraska. *Cancer Res.* **44**, 363–369.

84. Slattery, M. L., Benson, J., Berry, T. D., Duncan, D., Edwards, S. L., Caan, B. J., and Potter, J. D. (1997). Dietary sugar and colon cancer. *Cancer Epidemiol. Biomarkers Pre.* **6**, 677–685.

85. Bristol, J. B., Emmett, P. M., Heaton, K. W., and Williamson R. C. N. (1985). Sugar, fat, and the risk of colorectal cancer. *Br. Med. J.* **291**, 1467–1470.

86. Macquart-Moulin, G., Riboli, E., Cornee, J., Charnay, B., Berthezene, P., and Day, N. (1986). Case-control study on colorectal cancer and diet in Marseilles. *Int. J. Cancer* **38**, 183–191.

87. LaVecchia, C., Negri, E., Decarli, A., D'Avanzo, B., Gallotti, L., Gentile, A., and Franceschi, S. (1988). A case-control study of diet and colorectal cancer in northern Italy. *Int. J. Cancer* **41**, 492–498.

88. Bidoli, E., Franceschi, S., Talamini, R., Barra, S., and LaVecchia, C. (1992). Food consumption and cancer of the colon and rectum in north-eastern Italy. *Int. J. Cancer* **50**, 223–229.

89. Benito, E., Obrador, A., Stiggelbout, A., Bosch, F. X., Mulet, M., Munoz, N., and Kaldor, J. (1990). A populaiton-based case-control study of colorectal cancer in Majorca. I. Dietary factors. *Int. J. Cancer* **45**, 69–76.

90. Peters, R. K., Pike, M. C., Garabrant, D., and Mack, T. M. (1992). Diet and colon cancer in Los Angeles County, California. *Cancer Causes Control* **3**, 456–473.

91. Crapo, P. A., Reaven, G., and Olefsky, J. (1977). Postpradial plasma-glucose and -insulin responses to different complex carbohydrates. *Diabetes* **26**, 1178–183.

92. Vaaler, S., Hanssen, K. F., and Aagenaes, O. (1980). Plasma glucose and insulin responses to orally administered carbohydrate-rich foodstuffs *Nutr. Metab.* **24**, 168–175.

93. Laird, P. W., and Jaenisch, R. (1994). DNA methylation and cancer. *Hum. Mole. Genet.* **3**, 1487–1495.

94. Cedar, H. (1988). DNA methylation and gene activity. *Cell* **53**, 3–4.

95. Issa, J. P., Vertino, P. M., Wui, J., Sazawal, S., Celano, P., Neikin, B. D., Hamilton, S. R., Baylin, S. B. (1993). Increased cytosine DNA-methyltransferase activity during colon cancer progression. *J. Natl. Cancer Inst.* **85**, 1235–1240.

96. Goelz, S. E,, Vogelstein, B., Hamilton, S. R., and Feinberg, A. P. (1985). Hypomethylation of DNA from benign and malignant human colon neoplasms. *Science* **228**, 187–200.

97. Makos, M., Nelkin, B. D., Lerman, M. I., Latif, F., Abar, B., and Baylin, S. B. (1992). Distinct hypermethylation patterns occur at altered chromosome loci in human lung and colon cancer. *Proc. Natl. Acad. Sci. USA* **89**, 1929–1933.

98. Baylin, S. B., Makos, M., We, J., Chiu Yen, R. W., de Bustros, A., Vertino, P., and Nelkin, B. D. (1991). Abnormal patterns of DNA methylation in human neoplasia: Potential consequences for tumor progression. *Cancer Cells* **3**, 382–390.

99. Giovannucci, E., Stampfer, M. J., Colditz, G. A., Rimm, E. B., Trichopoulos, D., Rosner, B. A., Speizer, F. E., and Willett, W. C. Folate, methionine, and alcohol intake and risk of colorectal adenoma. *J. Natl. Cancer Institute.* **85**, 875–884.

100. Slattery, M. L., Schaeffer, D., Edwards, S. L., Ma, K. N., and Potter, D. J. (1997). Are dietary factors involved in DNA methylation associated with colon cancer? *Nutr. and Cancer* **28**, 52–62.

101. Shaw, S., Jayatilleke, E., Herbert, V., and Colman, N. (1899). Cleavage of folates during ethanol metabolism. Role of acetaldehyde/xanthine oxidase-generated superoxide. *Biochem. J.* **257**, 277–280.

102. Seitz, H. K., and Simanowski, U. A. (1988). Alcohol and carcinogenesis. *Ann. Rev. Nutr.* **8**, 99–119.

103. Freudenheim, J. L., Graham, S., Marshall, J. R., Haughey, B. P., Cholewinski, S., and Wilkinson, G. (1991). Folate intake and carcinogenesis of the colon and rectum. *Int. J. Epidemiol.* **20**, 368–374.

104. Giovannucci, E., Stampfer, M. J., Colditz, G. A., Rimm, E. B., Trichopoulos, D., Rosner, B. A., Spezer, F. E., Willett, W. C. (1993). Folate, methionine, and alcohol intake and risk of colorectal adenoma. *J. Natl. Cancer Institute* **85**, 875–884.

105. Giovannucci, E., Stampfer, M. J., Colditz, G. A., Hunter, D. J., Fuchs, C., Rosner, B. A., Speizer, F. E., and Willett, W. C. (1998). Multivitamin use, folate, and colon cancer in women in the Nurses' Health Study. *Ann. Intern. Med.* **129**, 517–524.

106. Munoz, S. E., Navarro, A., Lantieri, M. J., Fabro, M. E., Peyrano, M. G., Ferraroni, M., Decarli, A., La Vecchia, C., and Eynard, A. R. (1998). Alcohol, methylxanthine-containing beverages, and colorectal cancer in Cordoba, Argentina. *Eur. J. Cancer Prev.* **7**, 207–213.

107. Kune, G. A., and Vitetta, L. (1992). Alcohol consumption and the etiology of colorectal cancer: A review of the scientific evidence from 1957 to 1991. *Nutr. Cancer* **18**, 97–111,

108. Hsing, A. W., McLaughlin, J. K., Chow, W. H., Schuman, L. M., Chen, H. T. C., Gridley, G., Bielke, E., Wacholder, S., and Blot, W. J. (1998). Risk factors for colorectal cancer in a prospective study among U. S. white men. *Int. J. Cancer* **77**, 549–553.

109. Slattery, M. L., West, D. W., Robison, L. M., French, T. K,, Ford, M., and Sorenson, A. W.. (1990) Tobacco, alcohol, coffee, and caffeine as risk factors for colon cancer in a low-risk population. *Epidemiology* **1**(2), 141–145.

110. Risio, M., Lipkin, M., Newmark, H., Yang, K., Rossini, F. P., Steele, N. E., Boone, C. W., and Keloff, G. J. Apoptosis, cell replication, and Western-style diet-induced tumorigenesis in mouse colon. *Cancer Res.* **56**, 4910–4916.

111. Stamp, D., Zhang, S. M., Medline, A., Bruce, W. R., and Archer, M. C. (1993). Sucrose enhancement of the early steps of colon carcinogenesis in mice. *Carcinogenesis* **14**, 777–779.

112. Newmark, H. L., Wargovich, M. J., and Bruce, W. R. (1984). Colon cancer and dietary fat, phosphate, and calcium: A hypothesis *J. Natl. Cancer Inst.* **72**, 1323–1325.

113. Buset, M., Lipkin, M., Winawer, S., Swaroop, S., and Friedman, E. (1986). Inhibition of human colonic epithelial cell proliferation in vivo and in vitro by calcium. *Cancer Res.* **46**, 5426–5430.

114. Shabahang, M., Buras, R. R., Davoodi, F., Schumaker, L. M., Naua, R. J., Uskokovic, M. R., Brenner, R. V., Evans, S. R. (1994). Growth inhibition of HT–29 human colon cancer cells by analogues of 1, 25-dihydroxyvitamin D3. *Cancer Res.* **54**, 4057–4064.

115. Bergsma-Kadijk, J. A., van't Veer, P., Kampman E., and Burema, J. (1996). Calcium does not protect against colorectal neoplasia. *Epidemiology* **7**, 590–597.

116. Martinez, M. E., and Willett, W. C. (1998). Calcium, vitamin D, and colorectal cancer: A review of the epidemiologic evidence. *Cancer Epidemiol. Biomarkers Prev.* **37**, 163–168.

117. Kampman, E., Slattery, M. L., Caan, B. J., amd Potter, J. D. (2000). Calcium, vitamin D, sunshine exposure, dairy products, and colon cancer risk. *Cancer Causes Control* **11**, 459–466.

118. Marcus, P. M., and Newcomb, P. A. The association of calcium and vitamin D, and colon and rectal cancer in Wisconsin women. *Int. J. Epidemiol.* **27**, 788–793.

119. Pritchard, R. S., Baron, J. A., and Gerhardsson de Verdier, M. (1996). Dietary calcium, vitamin D, and risk of colorectal cancer in Stockholm, Sweden. *Cancer Epidemiol. Biomarkers Prev.* **5**, 897–900

120. Kearney, J., Giovannucci, E., Rimm, E. B., Ascherio, A., Stampfer M. J., Colditz, G. A., Wing, A., Kampman, E., and Willett, W. C. (1996). Calcium, vitamin D, and dairy foods and the occurrence of colon cancer in men. *Am. J. Epidemiol.* **143**, 907–917.

121. Zheng, W., Anderson, K. E., Kushi, L. H., Sellers, T. A., Greenstein, J., Hong, C. P., Cerhan, J. R., Bostick, R. M., and Folsom, A. R. (1998). A prospective cohort study of intake of calcium, vitamin D, and other micronutrients in relation to incidence of rectal cancer among postmenopausal women. *Cancer Epidemiol. Biomarkers Prev.* **7**, 221–225.

122. Sellers, T. A., Bazyk, A. E., Bostick, R. M., Kush, L. H., Olson, J. E., Anderson, K. E., Lazovich, D., and Folsom, A. R. (1998). Diet and risk of colon cancer in a large prospective study of older women: An analysis stratified on family history (Iowa, United States). *Cancer Causes Control* **9**, 357–367.

123. Bostick, R. M. (1997). Human studies of calcium supplementation and colorectal epithelial cell proliferation. *Cancer Epidemiol. Biomarkers Prev.* **6**, 971–980.

124. Bostick, R. M., Fosdick, L., Wood, J. R., Grambsch, P., Grandits, G. A., Lillemore, T. J., Louis, T. A., and Potter, J. D. (1995). Calcium and colorectal epithelial cell proliferation in sporadic adenoma patients: A randomized, double-blind, placebo-controlled clinical trial. *J. Natl. Cancer Inst.* **87**, 1307–1315.

125. Baron, J. A., Beach, M., Mandel, J. S., van Stolk, R. U., Haile, R. W., Sandler, R. S., Rothstein, R., Summers, R. W., Snover, D. C., Beck, G. J., Bond, J. H., and Greenberg, E. R. (1999). Calcium supplements for the prevention of colorectal adenomas. *N. Engl. J. Med.* **340**, 101–107.

126. Martinez, M. E., Giovannucci, E. L., Colditz, G. A., Stampfer, M. J., Hunter, D. J., Speizer, F. E., Wing, A., and Willett,

W. C. (1996). Calcium, vitamin D, and the occurrence of colorectal cancer among women. *J. Natl. Cancer Inst.* **88,** 1375–1382.

127. Bostick, R. M., Potter, J. D., Sellers, T. A., McKenszie, D. R., Kushi, H., and Folsom, A. R. (1993). Relation of calcium, vitamin D, and dairy food intake to incidence of colon cancer in older women. *Am. J. Epidemiol.* **137,** 1302–1317.

128. Kampman, E., Goldbohm, R. A., Van den Brandt, P. A., and Van't Veer, P. Fermented dairy products, calcium, and colorectal cancer in the Netherlands Cohort Study. *Cancer Res.* **54,** 3186–3190.

129. Slattery, M. L., Boucher, K. M., Caan, B. J., Potter, J. D., and Ma, K. N. (1998). Eating patterns and colon cancer. *Am. J. Epidemiol.* **148,** 4–16.

130. Hu, F. B., Rimm, E., Smith-Warner, S. A., Feskanich, D., Stampfer, M. J., Ascherio, A., Sampson, L., and Willett, W. C. (1999). Reproducibility and validity of dietary patterns assessed with a food-frequency questionnaire. *Am. J. Clin. Nutr.* **69**(2), 243–249.

131. Le Marchand, L., Wilkens, L. R., Hankin, J. H., Kolonel, L. N., and Lyu, L. C. (1999). Independent and joint effects of family history and lifestyle on colorectal cancer risk: Implications for prevention. *Cancer Epidemiol. Biomarkers Prev.* **8,** 45–52.

132. Groden, J., Thliveris, A., Samowitz, W., Carlson, M., Gelbert, L., Albertsen, H., Josyln, G., Steves, J., Spirol, L., and Robertson, M. (1991). Identification and characterization of the familial adenomatous polyposis coli gene. *Cell* **66,** 589–600.

133. Toniolo, P., Boffetta, P., Shuker, D. E. G., Rothman, N., Hulka, B., and Pearce, N. (1997). "Application of Biomarkers in Cancer Epidemiology," IARC Scientific Publication. No. 142. Oxfold, UK.

134. Dennis, M. J., Massey, R. C., Cripps, G., Venn, I., Howarth, N., and Lee, G. (1991). Factors affecting the polycyclic aromatic hydrocarbon content of cereals, fats and other products. *Food Additives Contamin.* **8,** 517–530.

135. Takeuchi, M., Hara, M., Inoue, T., and Kada, T. (1988). Adsorption of mutagens by refined corn bran. *Muta. Res.* **204,** 263–267.

136. Vineis, P., and McMichael, A. (1996). Interplay between heterocyclic amines in cooked meat and metabolic phenotype in the etiology of colon cancer. *Cancer Causes Control* **7,** 479–486.

137. Welfare, M. R., Cooper, J., Bassendine, M. F., and Daly, A. K. (1997). Relationship between acetylator status, smoking, diet and colorectal cancer risk in the northeast of England. *Carcinogenesis* **18,** 1351–1354.

138. Roberts-Thomson, I. C., Ryan, P., Khoo, K. K., Hart, W. J., McMichael, A. J., and Butler, R. N. (1996). Diet, acetylator phenotype, and risk of colorectal neoplasia. *Lancet* **347,** 1372–1374.

139. Chen, J., Stampfer, M. J., Hough, H. L., Garcia-Closas, M., Willett, W. C., Hennekens, C. H., Kelsey, K. T., and Hunter, D. J. (1998). A prospective study of N-acetyltransferase genotype, red meat intake, and risk of colorectal cancer. *Cancer Res.* **8,** 3307–3311.

140. Wattenberg, L. W. (1990). Inhibition of carcinogenesis by minor nutrient constituents of the diet. *Proc. Nutr. Soc.* **49,** 173–183.

141. Zhang, Y., and Talalay, P. (1994). Anticarcinogenic activities of organic isothiocyanates: Chemistry and mechanisms. *Cancer Res.* **54,** 1976S–1981S

142. Gerhauser, C., You, M., Liu, J., Moriarty, R. M., Hawthorne, M., Mehta, R. G., Moon, R. C., and Pezzuto, J. M. (1997). Cancer chemopreventive potential of sulforamate, a novel analogue of sulforaphane that induces phase 2 drug-metabolizing enzymes. *Cancer Res.* **57,** 272–278.

143. Fahey, J. W., Zhang, Y., and Talalay, P. (1997). Broccoli sprouts: An exceptionally rich source of inducers of enzymes that protect against chemical carcinogens. *Proc. Natl. Acad. Sci. USA* **94,** 10367–10372.

144. Sreerama, L., Hedge, M. W., and Sladek, N. E. (1995). Identification of a class 3 aldehyde dehydrogenase in human saliva and increased levels of this enzyme, glutathione S-transferases and DT-diaphorase in the saliva of subjects who continually ingest large quantities of coffee or broccoli. *Clin. Cancer Res.* **1,** 1153–1163.

145. Slattery M. L., Kampman, E., Samowitz, W., Caan, B. J., and Potter, J. D. (2000). Interplay between dietary inducers of GST and the *GSTM*-1 genotype in colon cancer. *Int. J. Cancer* **87,** 728–733.

146. Lin, H. J., Probst-Hensch, N. M., Louie, A. D., Kau, I. H., Witte, J. S., Ingles, S. A., Frankl, H. D., Lee, E. R., and Haile, R. W. (1998). Glutathione transferase null genotype, broccoli, and lower prevalence of colorectal adenomas. *Cancer Epidemiol. Biomarkers Prev.* **7,** 647–652.

147. Lam, L. K. T., Sparnins, V. L., and Wattenberg, L. W. (1982). Isolation and identification of kahweol palmitate and cafestol palmitate as active constituents in green coffee beans that enhance glutathion S-transferase activity in the mouse. *Cancer Res.* **42,** 1193–1198.

148. Giovannucci, E. (1998). Meta-analysis of coffee consumption and risk of colorectal cancer. *Am. J. Epidemiol.* **147,**(11), 1043–1052.

149. Frosst, P., Blom, H. J., Milos, R., Goyette, P., Sheppard, C. A., Matthews, R. G., Boers, G. J. H., den Heijer, M., Kluijtmans, L. A. J., van den Heuvel, and L., Rozen, R. (1995). A candidate genetic risk factor for vascular disease: A common mutation in methylenetetrahydrofolate reductase. *Nat. Gen.* **10,** 111–113.

150. Slattery, M. L., Potter, J. D., Samowitz, Schaffer, D., Caan, B., and Leppert, M. (1999). Methylenetetrahydrofolate reductase, diet, and risk of colon cancer. *Cancer Epidemiol. Biomarkers Prev.* **8,** 513–518.

151. Chen, J., Giovannucci, E., Kelsey, K., Rimm, E. B., Stampfer, M. J., Colditz, G. A., Spiegelman, D., Willett, W. C., and Hunter, D. J. (1996). A methylenetetrahydrofolate reductase polymorphism and the risk of colorectal cancer. *Cancer Res.* **56,** 4862–4864.

152. Ma, J., Stampher, M. J., Giovannucci, E., Artigas, C., Hunter, D. J., Fuchs, C., Willett, W. C., Selhub, J., Hennekens, C. H., and Rozen, R. (1997). Methylenetetrahydrofolate reductase polymorphism, dietary interactions and risk of colorectal cancer. *Cancer Res.* **57,** 1098–1102.

153. Chen, J., Giovannucci, E. L., Hunter, D. J. (1999). MTHFR polymorphism, methyl-replete diets and the risk of colorectal carcinoma and adenoma among U. S. men and women: An example of gene-environment interactions in colorectal tumorigenesis. *J. Nutr.* **129**(2S Suppl.), 560S–564S.

154. Chen, L. H., Liu, M-L, Hwang, H-Y, Chen, L-S, Korenberg, J., and Shane, B. (1997). Human methionine synthase. CDNA cloning, gene localization and expression. *J. Biolog. Chem.* **272,** 3628–3634.

155. Ma, J., Stampfer, M. J., Christensen, B., Giovannucci, E., Hunter, D. J., Chen, J., Willett, C., Selhub, J., Hennekens, C. H., Gravel, R, and Rozen, R. (1999). A polymorphism of the methionine synthase gene: Association with plasma folate, vitamin B12, homocyst(e)ine, and colorectal cancer risk. *Cancer Epidemiol. Biomarkers Prev.* **8**(9), 825–929.

156. Guo, Y., Narayan, S., Yallampalli, C., Singh, P. (1992). Characterization of insulinlike growth factor I receptors in human colon cancer. *Gastroenterology* **102,**1101–1108.

157. Giovannucci, E. (1999). Insulin-like growth factor-I and binding protein–3 and risk of cancer. *Horm. Res.* **51,** (Suppl. S3), 34–41.

158. Cross, H. S., Bajna, E., Bises, G., Genser, D., Kallay, E., Potzi, R., Wenzl, E., Wrba, F., Roka, R., and Peterlik, M. (1996). Vitamin D receptor and cytokeratin expression may be progression indicators in human colon cancer. *Anticancer Res.* **16,** 2333–2337.

159. Davidson, N. (1996). Apolipoprotein E polymorphism: Another player in the genetics of colon cancer susceptibility? *Gastroenterology* **110,** 2006–2009.

160. Pasche, B., Kolachana, P., Nafa, K., Satagopan, J., Chen, Y. C., Lo, R. S., Brener, D., Yang, D., Kirstein, L., Oddoux, C., Ostrer, H., Vineis, P., Varesco, L., Jhanwar, S., Luzzatto, L., Massague, J., and Offit, K. (1999). TGFbR–1 (6A) is a candidate tumor susceptibility allele. *Cancer Res.* **59,** 5678–5682.

161. Gertig, D. M., and Hunter, D. J. (1998). Genes and environment in the etiology of colorectal cancer. *Cancer Biol.* **8,** 285–298.

162. Vogelstein, B., Fearon, E. R., Hamilton, S. R., Kern, S. E., Presinger, B. A., Leppert, M., Nakamura, Y., White, R., Smits, A. M. M., and Boss J. L. (1988). Genetic alterations during colorectal-tumor development. *New Eng. J. Med.* **319,** 525–532.

163. Slattery, M. L., Curtin, K., Ma, K., Anderson, K., Edwards, S., Leppert, M., Potter, J., Schaffer, D., and Samowitz, W. (2000). Associations between dietary intake and Ki-ras mutations in colon tumors:A population-based study. *Cancer Res.* **60,** 3935–6941.

164. Martinez, M. E., Maltzman, T., Marshall, J. R,, Einspahr, J., Reid, M. E., Sampliner, R, Ahnen, D. J., Hamilton, S. R., and Alberts, D. S. (1999). Risk factors for Ki-ras protooncogene mutation in sporadic colorectal adenomas. *Cancer Res.* **59,** 5181–5185.

165. Thibideau, S. N., Bren, G., and Schald, D. (1993). Microsatellite instability in cancer of the proximal colon. *Science* **260,** 816–819.

166. Baker, S. J., Fearon, E. R., Nigro, J. H., Hamilton, S. R., Preisinger, A. C., Jessup, J. M., Vantuinen, P., Ledbetter, D. H., Barker, D. F., Nakamura, Y., White, R., and Vegelstein, B. (1989). Chromosome 17 deletions and p53 mutations in colorectal carcinomas. *Science* **244,** 217–222.

167. Fearon, E. R. (1994). Molecular genetic studies of the adenoma-carcinoma sequence. *Adv. Intern. Med.* **39,** 123–146.

168. Voskuil, D. W., Kampman, E., van Kraats, A. A., Balder, H. F., van Muijen, G. N. P., Goldbohm A. R., and van't Veer, P. (1999). *p53* over-expression and *p53* mutations in colon arcinomas: Relation to dietary risk factors. *Int. J. Cancer* **81,** 675–681.

169. Bautista, D., Obrador, A., Moreno, V., Cabeza, E., Canet, R., Benito, E., Bosch, Costa, J. (1997). Ki-ras mutation modifies the protective effect of dietary monounsaturated fat and calcium on sporadic colorectal cancer. *Cancer Epidemiol. Biomarkers Prev.* **6,** 57–61.

170. Freedman, A. N., Michalek, A. M., Marshall, J. R., Mettlin, C. J., Petrelli, N. J., Black, J. D., Zhang, Z. F., Satchidanand, S., and Asirwatham, J. E. (1996). Familial and nutritional risk factors for p53 overexpression in colorectal cancer. *Cancer Epidemiol. Biomarkers Prev.* **5,** 285–291.

CHAPTER 24

Nutrition and Prostate Cancer

LAURENCE N. KOLONEL
University of Hawaii, Honolulu, Hawaii

I. INTRODUCTION

This chapter discusses the epidemiologic evidence for associations of dietary factors with prostate cancer risk, and the potential for diet to play a role in prostate cancer prevention. Some findings from animal and *in vitro* studies, as well as possible mechanisms for the carcinogenic effects, are presented in support of the epidemiologic findings.

A. Normal Prostate Anatomy and Function

The normal adult prostate gland is a walnut-sized organ that surrounds the urethra and the neck of the bladder. The gland is composed of three distinct zones: peripheral, central, and transition. The peripheral zone is comprised of left and right lobes that can be palpated during digital rectal examination. The transition zone is the region that enlarges in benign prostatic hyperplasia, which is common in older men [1]. The prostate gland is a male secondary sex organ that secretes one fluid component of semen. Prostatic fluid is essential for male fertility.

Normal growth and activity of the prostate gland is under the control of androgenic hormones. Circulating testosterone, primarily produced in the testes, diffuses into the prostate where it is irreversibly converted by the enzyme steroid 5α-reductase type II to dihydrotestosterone (DHT), a metabolically more active form of the hormone. Dihydrotestosterone binds to the androgen receptor, and this complex then translocates to the cell nucleus where it activates selected genes [2].

B. Pathology and Diagnosis of Prostate Cancer

Almost all prostate tumors are classified as adenocarcinomas (i.e., they arise from the glandular epithelial cells), and occur most commonly in the peripheral zone of the gland. Accordingly, they can often be felt by the physician during digital rectal examination. A unique feature of human prostate cancer is the high frequency of small, latent tumors in older men. A clear relationship between these occult tumors and those which become clinically apparent has not been established, although it is commonly assumed that the latter

evolve from the former as a consequence of additional genetic mutations.

Generally, prostate cancer in its early stages is asymptomatic. Enlargement of the prostate gland, (benign prostatic hyperplasia or BPH) commonly begins after the age of 45, ultimately leading to urinary tract symptoms (difficult and frequent urination). Many cases of prostate cancer are diagnosed as a result of digital rectal examination performed when a man visits his physician for relief of these symptoms. (Suspicious lesions on examination may be confirmed by transrectal ultrasound, followed by a biopsy of the gland.) In recent years, the prostate-specific antigen (PSA) test has come into widespread use. This test is not specific for prostate cancer, however, and gives an abnormal result if there is any increased tissue growth in the gland, such as occurs in BPH. Because of its sensitivity, the PSA test can lead to the diagnosis of very early, microscopic tumors. Although such lesions might never progress to clinical disease, surgical removal carries a risk of major complications (notably incontinence and/or impotence), leading to controversy regarding the proper use of PSA as a screening test for early prostate cancer [3].

II. DESCRIPTIVE EPIDEMIOLOGY OF PROSTATE CANCER

A. Incidence and Mortality Trends

Prostate cancer is a common cancer among men in many Western countries, and is the leading male incident cancer in the United States, where 180,400 new cases are projected for the year 2000 [4, 5]. Incidence trends in the United States show a rather slow increase over most of the last 50 years, with a rather striking increase between 1989 and 1992, attributable in large measure to the widespread adoption of the PSA screening test, which first became available in the early 1980s [6]. Since 1992, the incidence has declined, reflecting an end to the surge in cases due to the introduction of this new screening procedure [7], as well as, perhaps, to the more judicious application of PSA screening. Moreover, mortality from prostate cancer is low relative to its incidence. This is because prostate cancer is generally well controlled by

TABLE 1   Proposed Risk Factors for Prostate Cancer

Category	Characteristic or Exposure
Demographic	Age, ethnicity, geography
Genetic	Family history (father, brothers); major predisposing genes
Occupational	Cadmium products, rubber industry, agricultural chemicals
Hormonal	Androgens (testosterone, dihydrotestosterone)
Lifestyle	Sexually transmitted agent, smoking, alcohol, vasectomy, physical activity, diet

treatment (surgery, radiation, and androgen ablation) and occurs at relatively late ages, so that even men who are not cured of the disease often die from other causes. Interestingly, a parallel increase in prostate cancer mortality did not occur during the period 1989–1992, presumably because most of the additional cases diagnosed would not otherwise have led to fatal outcomes.

B. Risk Factors for Prostate Cancer

Few risk factors for prostate cancer have been established. Proposed factors are listed in Table 1. Age is the strongest risk factor. Prostate cancer incidence increases more sharply with age than does any other cancer; more than 50% of cases in the United States are diagnosed in men above the age of 70 [4, 8].

Race/ethnicity is a second risk factor for prostate cancer. In the United States, the lowest incidence rates are seen among Korean and Vietnamese men, both relatively recent immigrant groups from Asia; the rates are somewhat higher among Chinese, American Indian, Alaska Native, and Native Hawaiian men. Caucasian men have very high rates, but by far, the highest incidence of this cancer is among African-American men [9].

The incidence of prostate cancer varies more than 60-fold in populations around the world (Fig. 1). Indeed, of all common cancers, this site shows the widest variation between low- and high-risk countries or populations. High rates are seen in developed, especially Western, countries, including the United States, Canada, parts of Europe, and Australasia. Low rates tend to occur in Asia, particularly China [4, 10]. The highest reported rates in the world are among African-Americans, whereas the lowest reported rates are among Chinese men in Shanghai. Interestingly, Chinese men in more developed areas of Asia (Singapore and Hong Kong) and Chinese men in the United States have much higher incidence rates than men in mainland China (see cross-hatched populations in Fig. 1). Furthermore, immigrants from Japan to Brazil and the United States have higher rates than do men in Japan [8]. Although the incidence of prostate cancer in Japan increased about threefold between 1970 and

1990, which was similar to the rate of increase in the United States during the same period, the actual incidence in Japan remains very low.

Men with a first-degree male relative who has had prostate cancer are at a two- to threefold increased risk; whether this reflects an inherited predisposition for the disease or a shared environmental exposure has not been confirmed [11, 12]. The search for major predisposing genes for prostate cancer has identified some candidates, though none has yet been confirmed (discussed below).

Apart from these few established risk factors, the etiology of prostate cancer is unknown. Among the several potential causal agents, apart from diet, that have been proposed are (1) occupational exposures (rubber industry; manufacture of products containing cadmium, such as paints and batteries; use of agriculture chemicals); (2) sexually transmitted agents (e.g., cytomegalovirus); (3) smoking; (4) alcohol use; (5) vasectomy; and (6) physical activity [11, 13–15]. However, the evidence is not yet convincing for any of these exposures.

Although it is suspected that most exogenous factors affecting prostate cancer risk exert their influence by altering endogenous androgen levels [16], epidemiologic studies have not yet clearly established the role of androgens in prostate cancer. Studies of prediagnostic circulating levels of individual androgens generally showed no clear association with prostate cancer [11, 17–19]. However, two studies showed weak positive relationships between the ratio of testosterone to dihydrotestosterone and prostate cancer [20, 21]. A third study showed a strong positive association of plasma testosterone with prostate cancer only after adjustment for the sex hormone binding globulin level [22]. The latter finding suggests that the level of free (unbound) testosterone may be most relevant.

The most promising area of research on the etiology of prostate cancer pertains to diet.

III. STUDIES OF DIET IN RELATION TO PROSTATE CANCER

A. Origin of the Diet–Prostate Cancer Hypothesis

The descriptive patterns of prostate cancer, especially data showing very different rates of the disease in the same ethnic/racial group living in different geographic settings, as well as changing rates in migrants and their offspring [8], prompted investigators to seek environmental risk factors for this cancer. Diet became an important focus of this research because (1) geographic variations in food and nutrient intakes are known to be large [10]; and (2) components of the diet can influence the levels of circulating androgens [23, 24], which, as noted above, are thought to play a role in prostate cancer risk. Many different dietary factors, including both foods

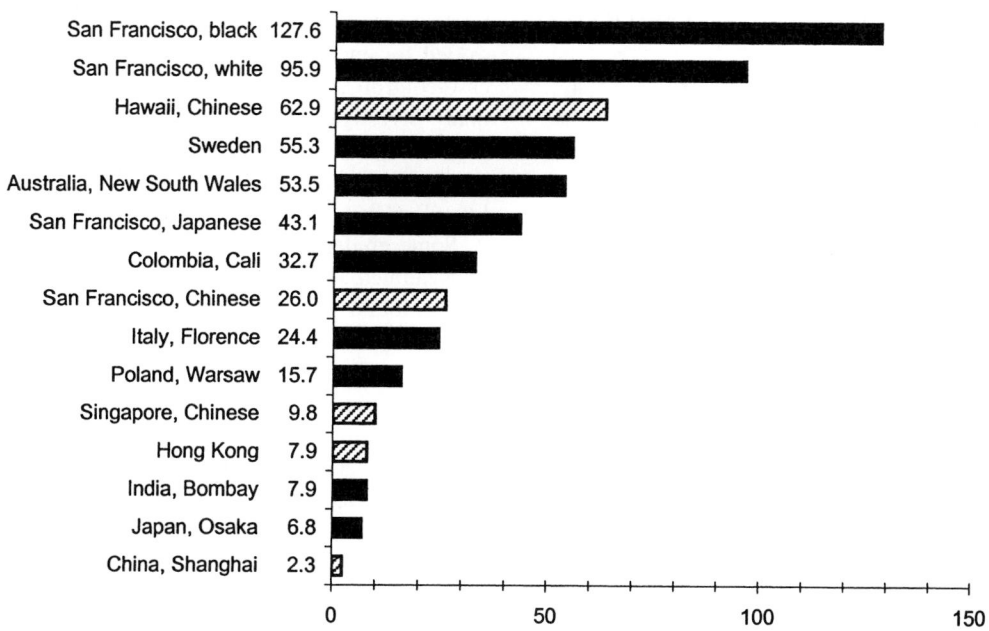

FIGURE 1   Prostate cancer incidence in selected populations, 1988–1992 (rates age adjusted to the world standard population).

and particular constituents of foods, have been proposed and studied. Some of these appear to increase risk, while others are possibly protective. These factors are listed in Table 2, and the supporting evidence is discussed in the following sections of this chapter.

B. Dietary Factors That Increase Risk

1. FOODS AND BEVERAGES

a. Red Meat.   Many epidemiologic investigations of different designs, including ecologic [25–27], case-control [28–33], and cohort [34–37] studies, have reported positive associations between the consumption of meat, especially red meat, and prostate cancer. However, not all studies reproduced this finding [38–43].

Explaining the association with meat is not straightforward. Initially, the finding was thought to reflect a high exposure to dietary fat, especially saturated fat, because meat and dairy products are the major contributors to fat intake in the Western diet. However, because the findings on dietary fat per se and prostate cancer are equivocal (discussed below), other explanations for the association should be considered. There are several possibilities: (1) In the American diet, red meat is a major source of zinc, which is essential for testosterone synthesis and may have other effects in the prostate (discussed below). (2) Diets high in meat and other animal products may be relatively deficient in certain anticarcinogenic constituents found primarily in plant foods. (3) Most intriguingly, many meats are cooked at high temperatures, such as by pan-frying, grilling, or barbecuing. Cooking meats at high temperatures can result in the forma-

tion of heterocyclic amines, which are potent carcinogens in animals, including the rat prostate [44]. Furthermore, when meats are cooked on charcoal grills, rendered fat is pyrolized by the coals, leading to the deposition of polycyclic aromatic hydrocarbons, which are also carcinogenic in animals, on the outer surface of the meat [45]. Few epidemiologic studies have been able to examine the relationship of such exposures to prostate cancer risk, because their levels in the diets of individuals cannot be easily and precisely assessed. An epidemiologic study which estimated heterocyclic amine intake

TABLE 2   Proposed Dietary Risk Factors for Prostate Cancer

Increasing Risk	Decreasing Risk
Foods & Beverages	
Red meat	Vegetables
Dairy products	Fruits
Alcohol	Legumes
	Tea
Food Components	
Total energy	Vitamin D
Fat	Vitamin E
Calcium	Carotenoids
Zinc	Fructose
Cadmium	Selenium
	Isoflavonoids
Diet-Associated Factors	
Obesity	Physical activity

from cooked meat and risk of prostate cancer did not lead to a clear result [46].

b. Dairy Products. Several case-control [28, 31, 32, 47, 48] and cohort [34, 37, 49] studies found positive associations between the consumption of milk and other dairy products and the risk of prostate cancer. Nevertheless, other studies did not find this association [33, 38, 41, 43, 50]. One explanation for the positive association could be an adverse effect on the prostate of the high fat, especially saturated fat, content of dairy products. Another prominent constituent of these foods is calcium, which has also been proposed as a risk factor for prostate cancer (discussed below).

c. Alcoholic Beverages. Most case-control studies showed no association of prostate cancer with either total alcohol intake or with the intake of specific types of alcoholic beverages [30, 38, 39, 51–53], although a study among U.S. black and white males found a positive association for total alcohol intake in both groups [54]. Although some cohort studies also found no association [34, 37, 55], a few did see an effect, including a cohort study in Japan [56] that found an increased risk for alcohol drinkers in general, a U.S. cohort [43] that found an elevated risk for drinkers of beer, and a European cohort that found some evidence of an elevated risk for drinkers of white (but not red) wine [57]. Some general mechanisms by which alcohol might enhance carcinogenesis have been proposed, including the activation of environmental nitrosamines, production of carcinogenic metabolites (acetaldehyde), immune suppression, and secondary nutritional deficiencies [54, 57].

2. NUTRIENTS AND OTHER FOOD CONSTITUENTS

a. Energy. Total energy intake was not reported in early epidemiologic studies of diet and prostate cancer, because the dietary assessment methods used at the time were incomplete. However, several studies in recent years have examined this variable, particularly in relation to the effects of dietary fat intake. The findings have been very inconsistent. Some studies reported a positive association for energy intake and no independent association with dietary fat [58, 59]. Others reported an effect of dietary fat, but no independent effect of energy [32, 50, 60, 61]. One study reported a positive association with both total energy and total fat [33], and two studies found no association with either total energy or fat [39, 62]. An experimental study in rodents (rats and mice) found that energy restriction reduced prostate tumor growth, possibly by inhibiting tumor angiogenesis [63].

b. Fat. Dietary fat has been the most studied nutrient with regard to effects on prostate cancer risk. This topic was recently reviewed in detail [64]. Total fat intake has been associated with the risk of prostate cancer in several case-control studies [30, 51, 65–67], although most found the association to be strongest for saturated or animal fat [29, 60, 65–68]. In two cohort studies that examined total and saturated fat, one [62] found no evidence of an effect on prostate cancer, and the other [36] found an elevated risk for

total, but not saturated, fat. When limited to studies that controlled for energy intake, however, the findings from both case-control and cohort studies are more equivocal, with many investigations showing no independent effect of fat [39, 58, 59, 61, 62]. In some studies, the association with total and saturated fat was stronger for the advanced cases [36, 60, 67].

Some epidemiologic studies examined intakes of monounsaturated and polyunsaturated fat as well. Most of these studies found no association of either of these classes of fat with prostate cancer [62, 64], although a few case-control studies reported positive associations [41, 50, 67].

A few studies in recent years also examined specific fatty acids (including several omega-3 and omega-6 polyunsaturated fatty acids, as well as monounsaturated fatty acids), based either on dietary intake data or biochemical measurements in blood or adipose tissue [62, 64]. Most studies found no significant associations, although the data are not consistent, and no conclusions as to the role of specific fatty acids on the risk of prostate cancer can be reached on the basis of current data.

Some animal experiments have tested the fat–prostate cancer hypothesis. For example, a high-fat diet increased prostate cancer incidence and shortened the latency period in Lobund Wistar rats treated with exogenous testosterone to induce the tumors [69]. Conversely, prostate tumor growth rate was reduced by a fat-free diet in Dunning rats [70] or by lowering dietary fat intake in athymic nude mice injected with LNCaP cells (a human prostate cancer cell line) [71]. With regard to specific types of fat, fish oils containing high levels of omega-3 fatty acids, such as eicosapentaenoic and docosahexaenoic acids, generally suppressed prostate tumor growth in rodents, whereas omega-6 polyunsaturated fatty acids, such as linoleic and linolenic acids, promoted tumor growth [72, 73]. However, because most animal studies have been conducted in rodents, whose prostate glands differ anatomically from that of the human, extrapolation of these findings to humans is particularly tenuous.

A number of plausible mechanisms by which dietary fat could increase cancer risk have been proposed. These include the formation of lipid radicals and hydroperoxides that can produce DNA damage, increased circulating androgen levels, decreased gap-junctional communication between cells, altered activity of signal transduction molecules, effects on eicosanoid metabolism, and decreased immune responsiveness [64].

c. Calcium. As noted above, a number of studies that have examined the relationship of dairy product consumption to prostate cancer risk found a positive association. Dairy products could be a marker of exposure to calcium as well as saturated or animal fat, because this food group is a major source of both nutrients in the Western diet. Data on calcium specifically are more limited, but one case-control study [48] and a cohort study [74] both reported statistically significant positive associations, especially with advanced or

metastatic cancer. However, a case-control study among U.S. whites and blacks did not show an effect of calcium on prostate cancer risk [32].

A mechanism for an adverse effect of calcium on prostate carcinogenesis has been proposed, based on the observation that a high intake of calcium decreases the circulating levels of $1,25(OH)_2$ vitamin D, which may inhibit cell proliferation and promote differentiation in prostatic tissue [75]. The role of vitamin D in prostatic carcinogenesis is discussed below.

d. Zinc and Cadmium. The trace elements zinc and cadmium are considered together because they act as antagonists in biological systems. Few epidemiologic studies have examined dietary zinc in relationship to prostatic cancer. Most of the studies found no effect of zinc, especially after energy adjustment [39, 50, 58, 67], although a positive association was suggested in two reports [66, 76]. The frequent association of prostate cancer risk with high intake of red meat (discussed above) could also be explained by a higher intake of zinc, rather than animal fat, because meat, especially red meat, is an important source of zinc in the American diet (other sources are shellfish, whole-grain cereals, nuts, and legumes) [77]. Reports based on zinc levels in serum or prostatic tissue of patients with cancer and controls have not been consistent [78, 79], but such studies are unreliable, because the levels of zinc measured after diagnosis in the cases may reflect physiologic changes in the prostate as a result of the cancer.

As a major constituent of prostatic fluid [80, 81], zinc is essential for normal prostate function. Zinc is also essential for normal testicular function, and high levels of zinc have been proposed to increase the production of testosterone, leading to enhanced tissue growth in the prostate. Plasma levels of zinc have been positively correlated with testosterone and dihydrotestosterone levels in men [82, 83]. Furthermore, in the rat prostate, zinc has been shown to increase 5α-reductase activity [84] and to potentiate androgen receptor binding [85]. Thus, one might speculate that higher intake of zinc could partially offset the normal decline in testosterone levels with age [86–88], thereby contributing to prostate cancer risk.

Epidemiologic evidence for cadmium as a risk factor for prostate cancer is also limited. Only two studies attempted to assess dietary exposure [89, 90], and neither found very convincing evidence for an effect of diet alone, although both studies found some evidence for a positive association when combined cadmium exposure from multiple sources (diet, cigarette smoking, occupation) was considered. Most studies of cadmium and prostate cancer have been among exposed workers in industries that utilize cadmium, and the findings of those investigations are only weakly suggestive of an adverse effect [11]. Cadmium is a competitive inhibitor of zinc in enzyme systems and accumulates in the body throughout life, because no mechanism exists for excreting it. Thus, the hypothesis that cadmium may be carcinogenic

for the prostate has biologic plausibility. This hypothesis is further supported by studies showing that cadmium is carcinogenic in animals, and that the effect can be blocked by simultaneous injection of zinc [91, 92].

3. DIET-ASSOCIATED RISK FACTORS
a. Obesity. Prostate cancer is sometimes considered a male counterpart to breast cancer in women, for which there is clear evidence of a positive association with obesity, especially in postmenopausal cases. However, evidence for a similar association of adult obesity with prostate cancer is limited. Although a few epidemiological studies reported a significant positive association [28, 49, 93], most studies found no clear relationship of measures of obesity to prostate cancer risk [35, 37, 51, 59, 60, 65–67, 94–96]. Even when limited to prospective cohort investigations, the findings have been inconsistent, and some studies even showed inverse associations [e.g., 97–100]. The influence of obesity at younger ages is also unclear. One study suggested that childhood obesity may be protective against adult prostate cancer [99], but another study found that obesity at age 20 years was associated with an increased risk [97].

The basis for an association between obesity and prostate cancer could involve endocrine factors, because adult obesity in men has been associated with decreased circulating levels of testosterone and increased levels of estrogen [101]. This mechanism would suggest an inverse rather than a direct association between obesity and this cancer.

C. Dietary Factors That Decrease Risk

1. FOODS AND BEVERAGES
a. Vegetables. Intake of vegetables has been inversely associated with cancer risk at many sites. This has led to strong recommendations to consume significant quantities of these foods as part of a healthful diet. However, the evidence for a beneficial effect of vegetables on prostate cancer risk is not overwhelming. Although some case-control studies showed inverse associations with selected vegetables or vegetable groupings, including green and yellow vegetables, cruciferous vegetables, and carrots [30, 33, 102–105], others showed no significant associations [28, 31, 32, 40, 41, 106, 107]. The findings from prospective cohort studies have been mostly null [35, 43, 49, 108–110]. The findings for legumes, a vegetable subgroup, are considered separately (discussed below), and the findings for tomatoes are included in the later discussion of carotenoids.

Because vegetables contain numerous compounds that can act through a variety of mechanisms to inhibit carcinogenesis [111], an inverse association between vegetables and prostate cancer is plausible. Some of these mechanisms are discussed with respect to specific food constituents below.

b. Fruits. The epidemiologic data on fruits and prostate cancer are also inconsistent, but interestingly, several studies, both case-control [40, 66, 102, 103] and cohort [34,

110], showed a direct (positive) association. Other case-control [31–33, 41, 50, 104, 105] and cohort [35, 43, 49, 108, 109] studies showed either no association or a statistically nonsignificant inverse relationship to prostate cancer risk. In one cohort study [74], a statistically significant inverse association was found for fruit intake and advanced prostate cancer; this finding did not persist after adjustment for total fructose intake.

Why intake of fruits might have an adverse effect on the prostate is not clear. Fruits contain many of the same compounds with anticarcinogenic properties that are found in vegetables, such as various carotenoids and vitamin C [111]. Although this finding is not yet established firmly, it does appear that fruit intake has no particular benefit with regard to the risk of prostate cancer.

c. Legumes, Including Soy Products. Legumes, and particularly soy products, have recently become a focus of research on prostate cancer. Prostate cancer rates have traditionally been low in populations, such as those of Japan and China, where the intake of soy products is relatively high. A few case-control [39, 40, 103, 104] and cohort [34, 35, 110, 112] studies have reported inverse associations between intake of legumes and prostate cancer, including soyfoods specifically [34, 40, 104, 112]. At present, the data are suggestive of a beneficial effect of legumes, but not soy products uniquely. Additional research may clarify this issue.

In the past, legumes were of interest in nutritional epidemiology primarily because of their important contribution to fiber intake. However, these foods also contain phytoestrogens, plant constituents that have mild estrogenic properties. Because estrogens are associated with lower risk of prostate cancer and are used in prostate cancer therapy, there is a good rationale for the hypothesis that phytoestrogen intake can protect against prostate cancer. Soybeans and many products made from soy, such as tofu, are rich in a class of phytoestrogens known as isoflavones (other classes of phytoestrogens include the coumestans and lignans). The main isoflavones found in soy include genistein, daidzein, and glycetein [113, 114]. Although the mechanism for a protective effect of soy products on prostate carcinogenesis could entail the estrogenic effects of isoflavones, other actions of these compounds, such as inhibition of protein tyrosine phosphorylation, induction of apoptosis, and suppression of angiogenesis, have also been proposed [115]. Laboratory data based on human tissue as well as animal models offer support for the hypothesis that soy products may protect against prostate cancer [115]. For example, in a xenograft model for prostate cancer in mice, a low-fat diet combined with soy protein and isoflavones produced lower tumor growth rates and reduced final tumor weights compared with mice on a high-fat diet (with or without the soy/isoflavone supplement), or a low-fat diet without the soy/isoflavone supplement, suggesting that both low-fat and high-soy diets may be important in reducing the risk of prostate cancer [116].

Although soy products and isoflavones are of particular interest, legumes contain other bioactive microconstituents, including saponins, protease inhibitors, inositol hexaphosphate, γ-tocopherol, and phytosterols; mechanisms by which each of these compounds can inhibit carcinogenesis have been proposed [111, 115, 117–119].

d. Tea. Only a few studies have examined the relationship between tea consumption and prostate cancer risk, and the findings have been inconsistent. One cohort study in Hawaii showed an inverse relationship between daily tea consumption and prostate cancer risk [120], but other cohort [34, 121] and case-control [39, 40] studies did not reproduce this finding.

Tea contains polyphenols that are potentially anticarcinogenic because of their antioxidant properties, effects on signal transduction pathways, inhibition of cell proliferation, and other actions in the body [122].

2. NUTRIENTS AND OTHER FOOD CONSTITUENTS

a. Vitamin D. Evidence for a protective effect of vitamin D against prostate cancer is limited. In one cohort study [74] and two case-control studies [33, 48], estimates of dietary vitamin D intake, whether from foods or supplements, were not associated with risk. Four cohort studies that examined the relationship of prediagnostic 1,25-dihydroxyvitamin D ($1,25(OH)_2D$), the biologically active form of the vitamin, in serum to subsequent development of prostate cancer produced discrepant results. One study found a clear inverse association [123], but the other three studies did not reproduce this finding [124–126].

Vitamin D reduces cell proliferation in the prostate (and other tissues) and enhances cell differentiation, both of which would be expected to lower the risk of cancer [75]. In a mouse model, a $1,25(OH)_2D$ analog inhibited the growth of prostate tumors [127].

b. Vitamin E. The intake of vitamin E is not adequately assessed with dietary histories, because much of the vitamin is obtained from fats and oils added during food preparation; estimating the amounts of added fats and oils is especially difficult. Nevertheless, a few epidemiologic studies attempted to determine vitamin E intake, with variable results. Two case-control studies [58, 59] found no association with prostate cancer risk. Another case-control study [41] found an inverse association with risk. Use of vitamin E supplements was not associated with prostate cancer risk overall in a cohort of U.S. men [128], although a reduced risk for advanced cancers was seen among current smokers and recent ex-smokers. Some cohort studies reported on findings for vitamin E and prostate cancer based on prediagnostic serum levels. In one report, an inverse association was seen [129], whereas in three others, no association was found [130–132]. In an intervention trial among male heavy smokers in Finland, an incidental finding was a reduced risk of prostate cancer associated with intake of vitamin E supplements [133, 134]. Because the study was not specifically designed

to test hypotheses related to prostate cancer, these results need confirmation. Furthermore, neither dietary nor serum vitamin E level at baseline was associated with subsequent development of prostate cancer in the non-vitamin E supplementation group [135].

Vitamin E inhibits the growth of human prostate tumors in nude mice [136]. As a powerful antioxidant, one mechanism for a protective effect of vitamin E against carcinogenesis in the prostate could be inhibition of lipid peroxidation [137].

c. Carotenoids (β-Carotene and Lycopene).

The epidemiologic evidence related to carotenoids and prostate cancer is inconsistent. The results of case-control studies on β-carotene intake are mixed. Although some studies reported an inverse association [47, 51, 67, 102], most offered no support for a protective effect of this nutrient [33, 39, 50, 58, 59, 61, 66, 105, 107]. Furthermore, the findings often differed between younger and older men. Cohort studies have reported that dietary intake of β-carotene decreased risk [43] or had no effect on risk [108, 109], but, like the case-control studies, the findings sometimes differed between younger and older men [43]. One of these studies also showed no effect of α-carotene, β-cryptoxanthin, or lutein on the risk of prostate cancer [109]. Studies based on prediagnostic serum have reported both an increased risk [138] and no association [130, 139] with elevated β-carotene levels. (A recent study showed that circulating levels of β-carotene are significantly correlated with the levels in prostatic tissue [140].) Finally, in an intervention trial in Finland, β-carotene supplementation was associated with a decreased risk of prostate cancer among nondrinkers of alcohol, but an increased risk among drinkers [133].

A carotenoid of current interest with regard to prostate cancer is lycopene, found primarily in tomatoes and tomato products (other food sources include watermelon, grapefruit, and guava). Although a few case-control studies showed an inverse association between tomato consumption, particularly cooked tomatoes [32, 41, 103], most studies have found no association [39, 40, 104–107]. Of the studies that estimated actual lycopene intake, none showed a clear inverse relationship to prostate cancer risk [33, 39, 103, 107]. One study [32] found a weak inverse association with raw tomatoes but not cooked tomatoes (which is surprising, because the lycopene should be more bioavailable in the cooked tomatoes due to enhanced absorption as a result of heat processing and the presence of lipids [141]). The findings from cohort studies are also inconsistent: Two found a significant inverse association [35, 109], while a third found no association [110]. The results of studies based on prediagnostic circulating levels of lycopene are also inconsistent, two showing an inverse relationship [139, 142], and one, no association [130].

β-Carotene, lycopene, and other carotenoids are widely distributed in human tissues, including the prostate [140, 143], where, as potent antioxidants, they help protect cell membranes, DNA, and other macromolecules from damage by reactive oxygen species. Other biological activities of carotenoids, such as the upregulation of gap-junctional communication [144] may also contribute to their anticarcinogenic effects. In three human prostate cancer cell lines (PC-3, DU 145, and LNCaP), β-carotene significantly inhibited in vitro growth rates [145].

d. Fructose.

Intake of fructose was inversely associated with the risk of prostate cancer in one cohort study [74], which found a similar relationship for the intake of fruit, a major source of fructose in the diet. Although other epidemiologic studies have not assessed fructose intake per se, several, as noted earlier, examined the relationship of fruit intake to prostate cancer and most did not find an inverse association. However, the metabolism of calcium, phosphorus, fructose, and vitamin D are interrelated, and unless all components are considered simultaneously in an analysis, their individual effects could be missed [74].

The hypothesis for the protective effect of fructose is that it reduces plasma phosphate levels, resulting in increased levels of circulating $1,25(OH)_2$ vitamin D, which in turn may reduce the risk of prostate cancer [74, 146] (discussed above).

e. Selenium.

Only a few epidemiologic studies have examined selenium and prostate cancer. Two case-control studies [67, 103] found no association between estimated selenium intake and prostate cancer risk, and baseline selenium intake was not associated with subsequent development of prostate cancer in a Finnish intervention trial [135]. In addition, prediagnostic serum selenium was not related to prostate cancer in a prospective cohort in Finland [147]. In contrast, prediagnostic selenium levels in toenails were inversely associated with advanced prostate cancer [148] and, in a selenium intervention trial to prevent skin cancer, an incidental finding was a reduced incidence of prostate cancer [149]. Because prostate cancer was not the primary endpoint of the trial, this finding needs to be confirmed.

Selenium is a component of glutathione peroxidase, an important enzyme in certain antioxidative pathways. In an in vitro experiment, selenium was shown to inhibit the growth of human (DU-145) prostate carcinoma cells [150]. Selenium may exert its anticancer effects through any of several proposed mechanisms, such as antioxidation, enhanced immune function, inhibition of cell proliferation, and induction of apoptosis [151].

f. Isoflavonoids.

The potential role of isoflavonoids in prostate carcinogenesis was discussed above in the section on legumes.

3. DIET-ASSOCIATED PROTECTIVE FACTORS

a. Physical Activity.

The role of physical activity in human prostate caricinogensis is at present quite unclear. Several epidemiologic studies have examined this relationship, but the findings have been inconsistent. Although some studies showed an inverse association, others showed no association or a positive association with prostate cancer risk [13,

152, 153]. These discrepancies may be resolved if future studies distinguish better between different types of physical activity, and can establish the time of life (e.g., young adulthood versus older ages) that may be most relevant.

Because exercise influences androgen levels in the body, an effect of physical activity on prostate cancer risk is biologically plausible. Exercise lowers testosterone in the blood, and also raises the level of sex hormone binding globulin, which reduces the circulating free testosterone levels; both effects would be expected to lower prostate cancer risk [13, 154].

IV. GENETICS AND GENE–ENVIRONMENT INTERACTIONS

As noted above, prostate cancer shows a familial association (i.e., men whose fathers or brothers have had prostate cancer are at a two- to threefold risk of getting the disease as men without such a family history). The search for one or more highly penetrant genes that predispose to prostate cancer and that may explain at least part of this familial association has not yet been successful. Several candidate genes have been identified thus far, including a promising locus at q24-25 on chromosome 1 [155–157].

However, genetic predisposition may have a more indirect relationship to prostate cancer. Cell growth and differentiation in the prostate are regulated by androgens and various growth factors. It has been shown that several genes related to these cellular constituents are polymorphic (i.e., exist in variant forms) [158]. Some of these variants may have functional effects, leading to altered activity of the gene product. For example, a variant form, A49T, of the gene *SRD5A2* (steroid 5α-reductase type II) that encodes the enzyme responsible for converting testosterone to dihydrotestosterone in the prostate, was recently found to have lower activity in an *in vitro* assay [159]. Such functional consequences of genetic polymorphisms in constitutional DNA could lead to differing susceptibilities to prostate cancer. Indeed, men with the less active variant form (A49T) of the *SRD5A2* gene were found to be at a greater risk for prostate cancer [159]. Variant forms of the androgen receptor gene (*AR*), the vitamin D receptor gene (*VDR*), and the insulin-like growth factor 1 gene *(IGF-1)* have also been examined in relation to prostate cancer risk [160–164]. Such polymorphisms may not only affect the risk for prostate cancer, but also the pathological characteristics of the tumors and hence prognosis [165].

Because diet (and other behaviors, such as physical activity [166]) can influence androgen, vitamin D, and IGF-1 levels in the body, interactions may occur between dietary exposures and inherited susceptibilities in determining actual risk for prostate cancer. Thus, men who consume an unhealthful diet and who also carry the high-risk variant of one or more of the genes mentioned above may be at especially high risk for prostate cancer. Such gene–environment interactions offer considerable potential for elucidating the etiology of prostate cancer and will no doubt be explored in future research.

V. DIETARY INTERVENTION TRIALS

A randomized intervention trial is the closest method to an experimental design that can be implemented in human subjects. Such a trial should be conducted only when there is considerable evidence for a beneficial effect, without apparent harm, based on observational studies and supported by animal and *in vitro* studies. As the preceding review indicates, the data in support of most dietary factors are either limited or inconsistent, and would not justify the expense and risks of an intervention trial specifically for prostate cancer. However, two recent randomized intervention trials that were conducted for other purposes have shown unexpected reductions in prostate cancer incidence in the intervention groups. One of these studies [149, 167] was designed to test the potential of a daily selenium supplement (200 μg) to reduce the occurrence of basal and squamous cell skin cancers in men with a prior history of such lesions. The second trial [133, 134] tested the effects of daily β-carotene (20 mg) and/or vitamin E (50 mg *dl*-α-tocopherol acetate) on the risk of lung cancer in a group of male smokers. In both trials, the incidence of prostate cancer was significantly lower in the men who received the intervention compared with the placebo groups. In the lung cancer trial, the reduced incidence was in the men who received vitamin E rather than β-carotene. However, because protection against prostate cancer was not a prespecified hypothesis in either trial, the results cannot be taken as definitive. Based on these findings, and the supportive evidence from other epidemiologic and laboratory research, a double-blind randomized trial to test the potential benefit of supplemental selenium (200 μg/day) and vitamin E (400 mg/day), alone and in combination, is about to begin in the United States [168]. However, the results will not be available for several years.

VI. CONCLUSIONS AND IMPLICATIONS FOR PREVENTION AND TREATMENT

Considering the combined evidence from descriptive epidemiologic studies (especially the remarkable changes in migrant populations), analytic epidemiologic studies in widely varying populations, experimental studies in animals, and *in vitro* studies, the likelihood that certain dietary components or general patterns of eating influence the risk of prostate cancer remains high. However, at the present time, no specific relationships have been established conclusively. Continued research on this topic should be a high priority because diet is a modifiable risk factor and because prostate cancer incidence is extremely high in many populations. In

addition, further research on genetic polymorphisms that affect susceptibility to prostate cancer should contribute to better identification of high-risk groups of men who can be targeted for future preventive dietary interventions.

Currently, the primary treatment modalities for prostate cancer consist of surgery, radiation, and hormonal therapy. The fact that the findings for many dietary factors were stronger in advanced or metastatic cases of prostate cancer (e.g., saturated fat, calcium) indicates that dietary effects can occur very late in the disease process. This suggests that dietary interventions have the potential not only to reduce the incidence, but also to improve the survival rates of the disease, providing another possible form of therapy. Indeed, a recent study showed significantly worse survival for prostate cancer patients in the upper tertile of saturated fat intake (>13.2% of calories) compared with men in the lower tertile (<10.8% of calories) [169]. A possible mechanism to explain this result is reduced circulating androgen levels in the men with lower fat intake [23, 24], since prostate tumors are androgen sensitive, at least early in their clinical course.

Based on current knowledge, it is not prudent to make very specific dietary recommendations to prevent or treat prostate cancer. However, taken as a whole, the evidence offers reasonably strong support for a diet that emphasizes vegetables, including legumes, and is moderate or low in the consumption of meat, especially red meat, and dairy products.

References

1. Bostwick, D. G., Amin, M. B. (1996). Prostate and seminal vesicles. In "Anderson's Pathology, " 10th ed. (I. Damjanov and J. Linder, Eds.), Vol. 2, pp. 2197–2230. Mosby, St. Louis, MO.

2. Partin, A. W., and Coffey, D. S. (1998). The molecular biology, endocrinology and physiology of the prostate and seminal vesicles. In "Campbell's Urology," 7th ed. (P. C. Walsh, A. B. Retik, E. D. Vaughan, Jr., and A. J. Wein, Eds.), Vol. 2, pp. 1381–1428. W. B. Saunders, Philadelphia, PA.

3. Barry, M. J. (1998). PSA screening for prostate cancer: The current controversy—A viewpoint. Patient Outcomes Research Team for Prostatic Diseases. Ann. Oncol. 9, 1279–1282.

4. Parkin, D. M., Whelan, S. L., Ferlay, J., Raymond, L., and Young, J., Eds. (1997). "Cancer Incidence in Five Continents," Vol. VII. IARC Sci. Pub. No. 143, IARC, Lyon, France.

5. American Cancer Society (2000). "Cancer Facts and Figures 2000." American Cancer Society, Atlanta, GA.

6. Hankey, B. F., Feuer, E. J., Clegg, L. X., Hayes, R. B., Legler, J. M., Prorok, P. C., Ries, L. A., Merrill, R. M., and Kaplan, R. S. (1999). Cancer surveillance series: Interpreting trends in prostate cancer—Part I: Evidence of the effects of screening in recent prostate cancer incidence, mortality, and survival rates. J. Natl. Cancer Inst. 91, 1017–1024.

7. Legler, J. M., Feuer, E. J., Potosky, A. L., Merrill, R. M., and Kramer, B.S. (1998). The role of prostate-specific antigen (PSA) testing patterns in the recent prostate cancer incidence decline in the United States. Cancer Causes Control 9, 519–527.

8. Kolonel, L. N. (1997). Racial and geographic variations in prostate cancer and the effect of migration. In "Accomplishments in Cancer Research 1996" (J. G. Fortner and P. A. Sharp, Eds.), pp. 221–230. Lippincot-Raven, Philadelphia, PA.

9. Miller, B. A., Kolonel, L. N., Bernstein, L., Young, J. L., Jr., Swanson, G. M., West, D., Key, C. R., Liff, J. M., Glover, C. S., and Alexander, G. A., Eds. (1996). "Racial/Ethnic Patterns of Cancer in the United States 1998–1992." NIH Pub. No. 96-4104. National Cancer Institute, Bethesda, MD.

10. World Cancer Research Fund/American Institute for Cancer Research. (1997). "Food, Nutrition and the Prevention of Cancer: A Global Perspective," Chap. 1, pp. 20–52. American Institute for Cancer Research, Washington, DC.

11. Nomura, A. M. Y., and Kolonel, L. N. (1991). Prostate cancer: A current perspective. Am. J. Epidemiol. 13, 200–227.

12. Whittemore, A. S., Wu, A. H., Kolonel, L. N., John, E. M., Gallagher, R. P., Howe, G. R., West, D. W., Teh, C.-Z., and Stamey, T. (1995). Family history and prostate cancer risk in black, white, and Asian men in the United States and Canada. Am. J. Epidemiol. 141, 732–740.

13. McTiernan, A., Ulrich, C., Slate, S., and Potter, J. (1998). Physical activity and cancer etiology: Associations and mechanisms. Cancer Causes Control 9, 487–509.

14. Parker, A. S., Cerhan, J. R., Putnam, S. D., Cantor, K. P., and Lynch, C. F. (1999). A cohort study of farming and risk of prostate cancer in Iowa. Epidemiology 10, 452–455.

15. John, E. M., Whittemore, A. S., Wu, A. H., Kolonel, L. N., Hislop, T. G., Howe, G. R., West, D. W., Hankin, J., Dreon, D. M., Teh, C.-Z., Burch, J. D., and Paffenbarger, R. S., Jr. (1995). Vasectomy and prostate cancer: Results from a multiethnic case-control study. J. Natl. Cancer Inst. 87, 662–669.

16. Wilding, E. (1995). Endocrine control of prostate cancer. Cancer Surveys 23, 43–62.

17. Nomura, A. M. Y., Stemmermann, G. N., Chyou, P.-H., Henderson, B. E., and Stanczyk, F. Z. (1996). Serum androgens and prostate cancer. Cancer Epidemiol. Biomarkers Prev. 5, 621–625.

18. Guess, H. A., Friedman, G. D., Sadler, M. C., Stanczyk, F. Z., Vogelman, J. H., Imperato-McGinley, J., Lobo, R. A., and Orentreich, N. (1997). 5α-Reductase activity and prostate cancer: A case-control study using stored sera. Cancer Epidemiol. Biomarkers Prev. 6, 21–24.

19. Vatten, L. J., Ursin, G., Ross, R. K., Stanczyk, F. Z., Lobo, R. A., Harvei, S., and Jellum, E. (1997). Androgens in serum and the risk of prostate cancer: A nested case-control study from the Janus Serum Bank in Norway. Cancer Epidemiol. Biomarkers Prev. 6, 967–969.

20. Nomura, A., Heilbrun, L. K., Stemmermann, G. N., and Judd, H. L. (1988). Prediagnostic serum hormones and the risk of prostate cancer. Cancer Res. 48, 3515–3517.

21. Hsing, A. W., and Comstock, G. W. (1993). Serological precursors of cancer: Serum hormones and risk of subsequent prostate cancer. Cancer Epidemiol. Biomarkers Prev. 2, 27–32.

22. Gann, P. H., Hennekens, C. H., Ma, J., Longcope, C., and Stampfer, M. J. (1996). Prospective study of sex hormone levels and risk of prostate cancer. J. Natl. Cancer Inst. 88, 1118–1126.

23. Hamalainen E, Adlercreutz H, Puska P, and Pietinen P. (1984). Diet and serum sex hormones in healthy men. J. Steroid. Biochem. 20, 459–464.

24. Hill, P., Wynder, E. L., Garbaczewski, L., Garnes, H., and Walker, A. R. (1979). Diet and urinary steroids in black and white North American men and black South African men. *Cancer Res.* **39**, 5101–5105.

25. Howell, M. A. (1974). Factor analysis of international cancer mortality data and per capita food consumption. *Br. J. Cancer* **29**, 328–336.

26. Armstrong, B., and Doll, R. (1975). Environmental factors and cancer incidence and mortality in different countries, with special reference to dietary practices. *Int. J. Cancer* **15**, 617–631.

27. Koo, L. C., Mang, O. W., and Ho, J. H. (1997). An ecological study of trends in cancer incidence and dietary changes in Hong Kong. *Nutr. Cancer* **28**, 289–301.

28. Talamini, R., La Vecchia, C., Decarli, A., Negri, E., and Franceschi, S. (1986). Nutrition, social factors and prostatic cancer in a Northern Italian population. *Br. J. Cancer* **53**, 817–821.

29. Bravo, M. P., Castellanos, E., and del Rey Calero, J. (1991). Dietary factors and prostatic cancer. *Urol. Int.* **46**, 163–166.

30. Walker, A. R. P., Walker, B. F., Tsotetsi, N. G., Sebitso, C., Siwedi, D., and Walker, A. J. (1992). Case-control study of prostate cancer in black patients in Soweto, South Africa. *Br. J. Cancer* **65**, 438–441.

31. Talamini, R., Franceschi, S., La Vecchia, C., Serraino, D., Barra, S., and Negri, E. (1992). Diet and prostatic cancer: A case-control study in Northern Italy. *Nutr. Cancer* **118**, 277–286.

32. Hayes, R. B., Ziegler, R. G., Gridley, G., Swanson, C., Greenberg, R. S., Swanson, G. M., Schoenberg, J. B., Silverman, D. T., Brown, L. M., Pottern, L. M., Liff, J., Schwartz, A. G., Fraumeni, J. F., Jr., and Hoover, R. N. (1999). Dietary factors and risks for prostate cancer among blacks and whites in the United States. *Cancer Epidemiol. Biomarkers Prev.* **8**, 25–34.

33. Deneo-Pellegrini, H., De Stefani, E., Ronco, A., and Mendilaharsu, M. (1999). Foods, nutrients and prostate cancer: A case-control study in Uruguay. *Br. J. Cancer* **80**, 591–597.

34. Severson, R. K., Nomura, A. M. Y., Grove, J. S., and Stemmermann, G. N. (1989). A prospective study of demographics, diet and prostate cancer among men of Japanese ancestry in Hawaii. *Cancer Res.* **49**, 1857–1860.

35. Mills, P. K., Beeson, W. L., Phillips, R. L., and Fraser, G. E. (1989). Cohort study of diet, lifestyle and prostate cancer in Adventist men. *Cancer* **64**, 598–604.

36. Giovannucci, E., Rimm, E. B., Colditz, G. A., Stampfer, M. J., Ascherio, A., Chute, C. C., and Willett, W. C. (1993). A prospective study of dietary fat and risk of prostate cancer. *J. Natl. Cancer Inst.* **85**, 1571–1579.

37. Le Marchand, L., Kolonel, L. N., Wilkens, L. R., Myers, B. C., and Hirohata, T. (1994). Animal fat consumption and prostate cancer: A prospective study in Hawaii. *Epidemiology* **5**, 276–282.

38. Gronberg, H., Damber, L., and Damber, J. E. (1996). Total food consumption and body mass index in relation to prostate cancer risk: A case-control study in Sweden with prospectively collected exposure data. *J. Urol.* **155**, 969–974.

39. Key, T. J., Silcocks, P. B., Davey, G. K., Appleby, P. N., and Bishop, D. T. (1997). A case-control study of diet and prostate cancer. *Br. J. Cancer* **76**, 678–687.

40. Villeneuve, P. J., Johnson, K. C., Kreiger, N., and Mao, Y., for the Canadian Cancer Registries Epidemiology Research Group. (1999). Risk factors for prostate cancer: Results from the Canadian National Enhanced Cancer Surveillance System. *Cancer Causes Control* **10**, 355–367.

41. Tzonou, A., Signorello, L. B., Lagiou, P., Wuu, J., Trichopoulos, D., and Trichopoulou, A. (1999). Diet and cancer of the prostate: A case-control study in Greece. *Int. J. Cancer* **80**, 704–708.

42. Hirayama, T. (1979). "Epidemiology of Prostate Cancer with Special Reference to the Role of Diet," pp. 149–155. National Cancer Institute Monograph No. 53. U.S. Government Printing Office, Washington, DC.

43. Hsing, A. W., McLaughlin, J. K., Schuman, L. M., Bjelke, E., Gridley, G., Wacholder, S., Chien, H. T., and Blot, W. J. (1990). Diet, tobacco use, and fatal prostate cancer: Results from the Lutheran brotherhood cohort study. *Cancer Res.* **50**, 6836–6840.

44. Shirai, T., Sano, M., Tamano, S., Takahashi, S., Hirose, M., Futakuchi, M., Hasegawa, R., Imaida, K., Matsumoto, K., Wakabayashi, K., Sugimura, T., and Ito, N. (1997). The prostate: A target for carcinogenicity of 2-amino-1 methyl-6-phenylimidazo[4,5-b]pyridine (PhIP) derived from cooked foods. *Cancer Res.* **57**, 195–198.

45. Lijinsky, W., and Shubik, P. (1964). Benzo(a)pyrene and other polynuclear hydrocarbons in charcoal-broiled meat. *Science* **145**, 53–55.

46. Norrish, A. E., Ferguson, L. R., Knize, M. G., Felton, J. S., Sharpe, S. J., and Jackson, R. T. (1999). Heterocyclic amine content of cooked meat and risk of prostate cancer. *J. Natl. Cancer Inst.* **91**, 2038–2044.

47. Mettlin, C., Selenskas, S., Natarajan, N., and Huben, R. (1989). Beta-carotene and animal fats and their relationship to prostate cancer risk. A case-control study. *Cancer* **64**, 605–612.

48. Chan, J. M., Giovannucci, E., Andersson, S.-O., Yuen, J., Adami, H.-O., and Wolk, A. (1998). Dairy products, calcium, phosphorous, vitamin D, and risk of prostate cancer (Sweden). *Cancer Causes Control* **9**, 559–566.

49. Snowdon, A. A., Phillips, R. L., and Choi, W. (1984). Diet, obesity, and risk of fatal prostate cancer. *Am. J. Epidemiol.* **120**, 244–250.

50. Lee, M. M., Wang, R.-T., Hsing, A. W., Gu, F.-L., Wang, T., and Spitz, M. (1998). Case-control study of diet and prostate cancer in China. *Cancer Causes Control* **9**, 545–552.

51. Ross, R. K., Shimizu, H., Paganini-Hill, A., Honda, G., and Henderson, B. E. (1987). Case-control studies of prostate cancer in blacks and whites in Southern California. *J. Natl. Cancer Inst.* **78**, 869–874.

52. Yu, H., Harris, R. E., and Wynder, E. L. (1988). Case-control study of prostate cancer and socioeconomic factors. *Prostate* **13**, 317–325.

53. Tavani, A., Negri, E., Franceschi, S., Talamini, R., and La Vecchia, C. (1994). Alcohol consumption and risk of prostate cancer. *Nutr. Cancer* **21**, 25–31.

54. Hayes, R. B., Brown, L. M., Schoenberg, J. B., Greenberg, R. S., Silverman, D. T., Schwartz, A. G., Swanson, G. M., Benichou, J., Liff, J. M., Hoover, R. N., and Pottern, L. M. (1996). Alcohol use and prostate cancer risk in U.S. blacks and whites. *Am. J. Epidemiol.* **143**, 692–697.

55. Hiatt, R. A., Armstrong, M. A., Klatsky, A. L., and Sidney, S. (1994). Alcohol consumption, smoking, and other risk factors

and prostate cancer in a large health plan cohort in California (United States). *Cancer Causes Control* **5**, 66–72.

56. Hirayama, T. (1992). "Life-Style and Cancer: From Epidemiological Evidence to Public Behavior Change to Mortality Reduction of Target Cancers," pp. 65–74. National Cancer Institute Monograph No. 12. U.S. Govt. Printing Office, Washington, DC.

57. Schuurman, A. G., Goldbohm, R. A., and van den Brandt, P. A. (1999). A prospective cohort study on consumption of alcoholic beverages in relation to prostate cancer incidence (The Netherlands). *Cancer Causes Control* **10**, 597–605.

58. Andersson, S. O., Wolk, A., Bergstrom, R., Giovannucci, E., Lindgren, C., and Baron, J. (1996). Energy, nutrient intake and prostate cancer risk: A population-based case-control study in Sweden. *Int. J. Cancer* **68**, 716–722.

59. Rohan, T. E., Howe, G. R., Burch, J. D., and Jain, M. (1995). Dietary factors and risk of prostate cancer: A case-control study in Ontario, Canada. *Cancer Causes Control* **6**, 145–154.

60. Whittemore, A. S., Kolonel, L. N., Wu, A. H., John, E. M., Gallagher, R. P., Howe, G. W., Burch, J. D., Hankin, J. H., Dreon, D. M., West, D. W., Teh, C.-Z., and Paffenbarger, R. S., Jr. (1995). Prostate cancer in relation to diet, physical activity and body size in blacks, whites and Asians in the U.S. and Canada. *J. Natl. Cancer Inst.* **87**, 652–661.

61. Ghadirian, P., Lacroix, A., Maisonneuve, P., Perret, C., Drouin, G., Perrault, J. P., Beland, G., Rohan, T. E., and Howe, G. R. (1996). Nutritional factors and prostate cancer: A case-control study of French Canadians in Montreal, Canada. *Cancer Causes Control* **7**, 428–436.

62. Schuurman, A. G., van den Brandt, P. A., Dorant, E., Brants, H. A. M., and Goldbohm, R. A. (1999). Association of energy and fat intake with prostate carcinoma risk. *Cancer* **86**, 1019–1027.

63. Mukherjee, P., Sotnikov, A. V., Mangian, H. J., Zhou, J.-R., Visek, W. J., and Clinton, S. K. (1999). Energy intake and prostate tumor growth, angiogenesis, and vascular endothelial growth factor expression. *J. Natl. Cancer Inst.* **91**, 512–523.

64. Kolonel, L. N., Nomura, A. M. Y., and Cooney, B. (1999). Dietary fat and prostate cancer: Current status. *J. Natl. Cancer Inst.* **91**, 414–428.

65. Graham, S., Haughey, B., Marshall, J., Priore, R., Byers, T., Rzepka, T., Mettlin, C., and Pontes, J. E. (1983). Diet in the epidemiology of carcinoma of the prostate gland. *J. Natl. Cancer Inst.* **70**, 687–692.

66. Kolonel, L. N., Yoshizawa, C. N., and Hankin, J. H. (1988). Diet and prostate cancer: A case-control study in Hawaii. *Am. J. Epidemiol.* **127**, 999–1012.

67. West, D. W., Slattery, M., Robison, L. M., French, T. K., and Mahoney, A. W. (1991). Adult dietary intake and prostate cancer risk in Utah: A case-control study with special reference to aggressive tumors. *Cancer Causes Control* **2**, 85–94.

68. Harvei, S., Bjerve, K. S., Tretli, S., Jellum, E., Robsahm, T. E., and Vatten, L. (1997). Prediagnostic level of fatty acids in serum phospholipids: ω-3 and ω-6 fatty acids and the risk of prostate cancer. *Int. J. Cancer* **71**, 545–551.

69. Pollard, M., and Luckert, P. H. (1986). Promotional effects of testosterone and high fat diet on the development of autochthonous prostate cancer in rats. *Cancer Lett.* **32**, 223–237.

70. Clinton, S. K., Palmer, S. S., Spriggs, C. E., and Visek, W. J.. (1988). Growth of Dunning transplantable prostate adenocarcinoma in rats fed diets with various fat contents. *J. Nutr.* **118**, 908–914.

71. Wang, Y., Corr, J. G., Thaler, H. T., Tao, Y., Fair, W. R., and Heston, W. D. (1995). Decreased growth of established human prostate LNCaP tumors in nude mice fed a low-fat diet. *J. Natl. Cancer Inst.* **87**, 1456–1462.

72. Pandalai, P. K., Pilat, M. J., Yamazaki, K., Naik, H., and Pienta, K. J. (1996). The effects of omega-3 and omega-6 fatty acids on *in vitro* prostate cancer growth. *Anticancer Res.* **16**, 815–820.

73. Karmali, R. A., Reichel, P., Cohen, L. A., Terano, T., Hirai, A., Tamura, Y., and Yoshida, S. (1987). The effects of dietary omega-3 fatty acids on the DU-145 transplantable human prostatic tumor. *Anticancer Res.* **7**, 1173–1179.

74. Giovannucci, E., Rimm, E. B., Wolk, A., Ascherio, A., Stampfer, M. J., Colditz, G. A., and Willett, W. C. (1998). Calcium and fructose intake in relation to risk of prostate cancer. *Cancer Res.* **58**, 442–447.

75. Feldman, D., Zhao, X. Y., and Krishnan, A. V. (2000). Vitamin D and prostate cancer. *Endocrinology* **141**, 5–9.

76. Schrauzer, G. N., White, D. A., and Schneider, C. J. (1977). Cancer mortality studies—III: Statistical associations with dietary selenium intakes. *Bioinorgan. Chem.* **7**, 23–34.

77. Shils, M. E., Olson, J. A., and Shike, M., Eds. (1994). "Modern Nutrition in Health and Disease," 8th ed. Lea & Febiger, Philadelphia, PA.

78. Feustel, A., and Wennrich, R. (1986). Zinc and cadmium plasma and erythrocyte levels in prostatic carcinoma, BPH, urological malignancies, and inflammations. *Prostate* **8**, 75–79.

79. Whelan, P., Walker, B. E., and Kelleher, J. (1983). Zinc, vitamin A and prostatic cancer. *Br. J. Urol.* **55**, 525–528.

80. Tisell, L.-E., Fjelkegard, B., and Leissner, K.-H. (1982). Zinc concentration and content of the dorsal, lateral and medial prostatic lobes and of periurethral adenomas in man. *J. Urol.* **128**, 403–405.

81. Feustel, A., and Wennrich, R. (1984). Determination of the distribution of zinc and cadmium in cellular fractions of BPH, normal prostate and prostatic cancers of different histologies by atomic and laser absorption spectrometry in tissue slices. *Urol. Res.* **12**, 253–256.

82. Habib, F., Mason, M., Smith, P., and Stitch, S. (1979). Cancer of the prostate: Early diagnosis by zinc and hormone analysis. *Br. J. Cancer* **39**, 700–704.

83. Hartoma, T., Nahoul, K., and Netter, A. (1977). Zinc, plasma androgens and male sterility. *Lancet* **2**, 1125–1126.

84. Om, A.-S., and Chung, K.-W. (1996). Dietary zinc deficiency alters 5 alpha reduction and aromatization of testosterone and androgen and estrogen receptors in rat liver. *J. Nutr.* **126**, 842–848.

85. Colvard, D. S., and Wilson, E. M. (1984). Zinc potentiation of androgen receptor binding to nuclei in vitro. *Biochemistry* **23**, 3471–3478.

86. Vermeulen, A., Kaufman, J. M., and Giagulli, V. A. (1996). Influence of some biological indexes on sex hormone-binding globulin and androgen levels in aging or obese males. *J. Clin. Endocrin. Metab.* **8l**, 1821–1826.

87. Wu, A. H., Whittemore, A. S., Kolonel, L. N., John, E. M., Gallagher, R. P., West, D. W., Hankin, J., Teh, C. Z., Dreon, D. M., and Paffenbarger, R. S., Jr. (1995). Serum androgens

and sex hormone-binding globulins in relation to lifestyle factors in older African-American, white, and Asian men in the United States and Canada. *Cancer Epidemiol. Biomarkers Prev.* **4,** 735–741.

88. Gray, A., Feldman, H., McKinlay, J., and Longcope, C. (1991). Age, disease and changing sex hormone levels in middle-aged men: Results of the Massachusetts male aging study. *J. Clin. Endocrin. Metab.* **73,** 1016–1025.

89. Kolonel, L. N, and Winkelstein, W., Jr. (1977). Cadmium and prostatic carcinoma. *Lancet* **2,** 566–567.

90. Abd Elghany, N., Schumacher, M. C., Slattery, M. L., West, D. W., and Lee, J. S. (1990). Occupation, cadmium exposure, and prostate cancer. *Epidemiology* **1,** 107–115.

91. Haddow, A., Roe, F. J. C., Dukes, C. E., and Mitchley, B. C. (1964). Cadmium neoplasia: Sarcomata at the site of injection of cadmium sulphate in rats and mice. *Br. J. Cancer* **18,** 667–673.

92. Gunn, S. A., Gould, T. C., and Anderson, W. A. D. (1964). Effects of zinc on cancerogenesis by cadmium. *Proc. Soc. Exp. Biol. Med.* **115,** 653–657.

93. Lew, E. A., and Garfinkel, L. (1979). Variations in mortality by weight among 750,000 men and women. *J. Chron. Dis.* **32,** 563–576.

94. Nomura, A., Heilbrun, L. K., and Stemmermann, G. N. (1985). Body mass index as a predictor of cancer in men. *J. Natl. Cancer Inst.* **74,** 319–323.

95. Thompson, M. M., Garland, C., Barrett-Connor, E., Khaw, K. T., Friedlander, N. J., and Wingard, D. L. (1989). Heart disease risk factors, diabetes and prostatic cancer in an adult community. *Am. J. Epidemiol.* **129,** 511–517.

96. Nilsen, T. I. L., and Vatten, L. J. (1999). Anthropometry and prostate cancer risk: A prospective study of 22,248 Norwegian men. *Cancer Causes Control* **10,** 269–275.

97. Schuurman, A. G., Goldbohm, R. A., Dorant, E., and van den Brandt, P. A. (2000). Anthropometry in relation to prostate cancer risk in the Netherlands Cohort Study. *Am. J. Epidemiol.* **151,** 541–549.

98. Cerhan, J. R., Torner, J. C., Lynch, C. F., Rubenstein, L. M., Lemke, J. H., Cohen, M. B., Lubaroff, D. M., and Wallace, R. B. (1997). Association of smoking, body mass, and physical activity with risk of prostate cancer in the Iowa 65+ Rural Health Study (United States). *Cancer Causes Control* **8,** 229–238.

99. Giovannucci, E., Rimm, E. B., Stampfer, M. J., Colditz, G. A., and Willett, W. C. (1997). Height, body weight, and risk of prostate cancer. *Cancer Epidemiol. Biomarkers Prev.* **6,** 557–563.

100. Andersson, S.-O., Wolk, A., Bergstrom, R., Adami, H.-O., Engholm, G., Englund, A., and Nyren, O. (1997). Body size and prostate cancer: A 20-year follow-up study among 135,006 Swedish construction workers. *J. Natl. Cancer Inst.* **89,** 385–389.

101. Pasquali, R., Casimirri, F., Cantobelli, S., Melchionda, N., Morselli Labate, A. M., Fabbri, R., Capelli, M., and Bortoluzzi, L. (1991). Effect of obesity and body fat distribution on sex hormones and insulin in men. *Metabolism* **40,** 101–104.

102. Ohno, Y., Yoshida, O., Oishi, K., Okada, K., Yamabe, H., and Schroeder, F. H. (1988). Dietary beta-carotene and cancer of the prostate: A case-control study in Kyoto, Japan. *Cancer Res.*. **48,** 1331–1336.

103. Jain, M. G., Hislop, G. T., Howe, G. R., and Ghadirian, P. (1999). Plant foods, antioxidants, and prostate cancer risk: Findings from case-control studies in Canada. *Nutr. Cancer* **34,** 173–184.

104. Kolonel, L. N., Hankin, J. H., Whittemore, A. S., Wu, A. H., Gallagher, R. P., Wilkens, L. R., John, E. M., Howe, G. R., Dreon, D. M., West, D. W., and Paffenbarger, R. S., Jr. (2000). Vegetables, fruits, legumes and prostate cancer: A multiethnic case-control study. *Cancer Epidemiol. Biomarkers Prev.* **9,** 795–804.

105. Cohen, J. H., Kristal, A. R., and Stanford, J. L. (2000). Fruit and vegetable intakes and prostate cancer risk. *J. Natl. Cancer Inst.* **92,** 61–68.

106. Le Marchand, L., Hankin, J. H., Kolonel, L. N., and Wilkens, L. R. (1991). Vegetable and fruit consumption in relation to prostate cancer risk in Hawaii: A re-evaluation of the effect of dietary beta-carotene. *Am. J. Epidemiol.* **133,** 215–219.

107. Norrish, A. E., Jackson, R. T., Sharpe, S. J., and Skeaff, C. M. (2000). Prostate cancer and dietary carotenoids. *Am. J. Epidemiol.* **151,** 119–123.

108. Shibata, A., Paganini-Hill, A., Ross, R. K., and Henderson, B. E. (1992). Intake of vegetables, fruits, beta-carotene, vitamin C and vitamin supplements and cancer incidence among the elderly: A prospective study. *Br. J. Cancer* **66,** 673–679.

109. Giovannucci, E., Ascherio, A., Rimm, E. B., Stampfer, M. J., Colditz, G. A., and Willett, W. C. (1995). Intake of carotenoids and retinol in relation to risk of prostate cancer. *J. Natl. Cancer Inst.* **87,** 1767–1776.

110. Schuurman, A. G., Goldbohm, R. A., Dorant, E., and van den Brandt, P. A. (1998). Vegetable and fruit consumption and prostate cancer risk: A cohort study in the Netherlands. *Cancer Epidemiol. Biomarkers Prev.* **7,** 673–680.

111. Steinmetz, K. A., and Potter, J. D. (1991). Vegetables, fruit, and cancer. II. Mechanisms. *Cancer Causes Control* **2,** 427–442.

112. Jacobsen, B. K., Knutsen, S. F., and Fraser, G. E. (1998). Does high soy milk reduce prostate cancer incidence? The Adventist Health Study (United States). *Cancer Causes Control* **9,** 553–557.

113. Wang, H., and Murphy, P. A. (1994). Isoflavone content in commercial soybean foods. *J. Agri. Food Chem.* **42,** 1666–1673.

114. Franke, A. A., Custer, L. J., Wang, W., and Shi, S. J. (1998). HPLC analysis of isoflavonoids and other phenolic agents from foods and from human fluids. *Proc. Soc. Exp. Biol. Med.* **211,** 163–173.

115. Fournier, D. B., Erdman, J. W., Jr., and Gordon, G. B. (1998). Soy, its components and cancer prevention: A review of the in vitro, animal, and human data. *Cancer Epidemiol. Biomarkers Prev.* **7,** 1055–1065.

116. Aronson, W. J., Tymchuk, C. N., Elashoff, R. M., McBride, W. H., McLean, C., Wang, H., and Heber, D. (1999). Decreased growth of human prostate LNCaP tumors in SCID mice fed a low-fat, soy protein diet with isoflavones. *Nutr. Cancer* **35,** 130–136.

117. Rao, A. V., and Sung, M. K. (1995). Saponins as anticarcinogens. *J. Nutr.* **125**(3 Suppl.), 717S–724S.

118. Kennedy, A. R. (1998). The Bowman-Birk inhibitor from soybeans as an anticarcinogenic agent. *Am. J. Clin. Nutr.* **68**(Suppl.), 1406S–1412S.

119. Wyatt, C. J., Carballido, S. P., and Mendez, R. O. (1998). α- and γ-tocopherol content of selected foods in the Mexi-

can diet: Effect of cooking losses. *J. Agri. Food Chem.* **46**, 4657–4661.

120. Heilbrun, L. K., Nomura, A., and Stemmermann, G. N. (1986). Black tea consumption and cancer risk: A prospective study. *Br. J. Cancer* **54**, 677–683.

121. Kinlen, L. J., Willows, A. N., Goldblatt, P., and Yudkin, J. (1988). Tea consumption and cancer. *Br. J. Cancer* **58**, 397–401.

122. Yang, C. S., Chung, J. Y., Yang, G., Chhabra, S. K., and Lee, M. J. (2000). Tea and tea polyphenols in cancer prevention. *J. Nutr.* **130**(2S Suppl.), 472S–478S.

123. Corder, E. H., Guess, H. A., Hulka, B. S., Friedman, G. D., Sadler, M., Vollmer, R. T., Lobaugh, B., Drezner, M. K., Vogelman, J. H., and Orentreich, N. (1993). Vitamin D and prostate cancer: A prediagnostic study with stored sera. *Cancer Epidemiol. Biomarkers Prev.* **2**, 467–472.

124. Gann, P. H., Ma, J., Hennekens, C. H., Hollis, B. W., Haddad, J. G., and Stampfer, M. J. (1996). Circulating vitamin D metabolites in relation to subsequent development of prostate cancer. *Cancer Epidemiol. Biomarkers Prev.* **5**, 121–126.

125. Braun, M. M., Helzlsouer, K. J., Hollis, B. W., and Comstock, G. W. (1995). Prostate cancer and prediagnostic levels of serum vitamin D metabolites. *Cancer Causes Control* **6**, 235–239.

126. Nomura, A. M., Stemmermann, G. N., Lee, J., Kolonel, L. N., Chen, T. C., Turner, A., and Holick, M. F. (1998). Serum vitamin D metabolite levels and the subsequent development of prostate cancer. *Cancer Causes Control* **9**, 425–432.

127. Schwartz, G. G., Hill, C. C., Oeler, T. A., Becich, M. J., and Bahnson, R. R. (1995). 1,25-dihydroxy-16-ene-23-yne-vitamin D₃ and prostate cancer cell proliferation in vivo. *Urology* **46**, 365–369.

128. Chan, J. M., Stampfer, M. J., Ma, J., Rimm, E. B., Willett, W. C., and Giovannucci, E. L. (1999). Supplemental vitamin E intake and prostate cancer risk in a large cohort of men in the United States. *Cancer Epidemiol. Biomarkers Prev.* **8**, 893–899.

129. Eichholzer, M., Stahelin, H. B., Gey, F. K., Ludin, E., and Brnasconi, F. (1996). Prediction of male cancer mortality by plasma level of interacting vitamins: 17-year follow-up of the Basel study. *Int. J. Cancer* **55**, 145–150.

130. Nomura, A. M. Y., Stemmermann, G. N., Lee, J., and Craft, N. E. (1997). Serum micronutrients and prostate cancer in Japanese Americans in Hawaii. *Cancer Epidemiol. Biomarkers Prev.* **6**, 487–492.

131. Comstock, G. W., Bush, T. L., and Helzlsouer, K. (1992). Serum retinol, beta-carotene, vitamin E and selenium as related to subsequent cancer of specific sites. *Am. J. Epidemiol.* **135**, 115–121.

132. Knekt, P., Aromaa, A., Maatela, J., Aaran, R., Nikkari, T., Hakama, M., Hakulinen, T., Peto, R., Saxen, E., and Teppo, L. (1988). Serum vitamin E and risk of cancer among Finnish men during a 10-year follow-up. *Am. J. Epidemiol.* **127**, 28–41.

133. Heinonen, O. P., Albanes, D., Virtamo, J., Taylor, P. R., Huttunen, J. K., Hartman, A. M., Haapakoski, J., Malila, N., Rautalahti, M., Ripatti, S., Maenpaa, H., Teerenhovi, L., Koss, L., Virolainen, M., and Edwards, B. K. (1998). Prostate cancer and supplementation with α-tocopherol and β-carotene: Incidence and mortality in a controlled trial. *J. Natl. Cancer Inst.* **90**, 440–446.

134. The Alpha-tocopherol, Beta Carotene Cancer Prevention Study Group. (1994). The effect of vitamin E and beta carotene on the incidence of lung cancer and other cancers in male smokers. *N. Engl. J. Med.* **330**, 1029–1035.

135. Hartman, T. J., Albanes, D., Pietinen, P., Hartman, A. M., Rautalahti, M., Tangrea, J. A., and Taylor, P. R. (1998). The association between baseline vitamin E, selenium, and prostate cancer in the Alpha-Tocopherol, Beta-Carotene Cancer Prevention Study. *Cancer Epidemiol. Biomarkers Prev.* **7**, 335–340.

136. Fleshner, N., Fir, W. R., Huryk, R., and Heston, W. D. (1999). Vitamin E inhibits the high-fat diet promoted growth of established human prostate LNCaP tumors in nude mice. *J. Urol.* **161**, 1651–1654.

137. Burton, G. W., and Ingold, K. U. (1981). Autooxidation of biological molecules. 1. The antioxidant activity of vitamin E and related chain-breaking phenolic antioxidants *in vivo*. *J. Am. Chem. Soc.* **103**, 6472–6477.

138. Knekt, P., Aromaa, A., Maatela, J., Aaran, R. K., Nikkari, T., Hakama, M., Hakulein, T., Peto, R., and Teppo, L. (1990). Serum vitamin A and subsequent risk of cancer: Cancer incidence follow-up of the Finnish Mobile Clinic Health Examination Survey. *Am. J. Epidemiol.* **132**, 857–870.

139. Hsing, A. W., Comstock, G. W., Abbey, H., and Polk, B. F. (1990). Serologic precursors of cancer. Retinol, carotenoids, and tocopherol and risk of prostate cancer. *J. Natl. Cancer Inst.* **82**, 941–946.

140. Freeman, V. L., Meydani, M., Yong, S., Pyle, J., Wan, Y., Arvizu-Durazo, R., and Liao, Y. (2000). Prostatic levels of tocopherols, carotenoids, and retinol in relation to plasma levels and self-reported usual dietary intake. *Am. J. Epidemiol.* **151**, 109–118.

141. Sies, H., and Stahl, W. (1998). Lycopene: Antioxidant and biological effects and its bioavailability in the human. *Proc. Soc. Exp. Biol. Med.* **218**, 121–124.

142. Gann, P. H., Ma, J., Giovannucci, E., Willett, W., Sacks, F., Hennekens, C. H., and Stampfer, M. J. (1999). Lower prostate cancer risk in men with elevated plasma lycopene levels: Results of a prospective analysis. *Cancer Res.* **59**, 1225–1230.

143. Clinton, S. K., Emenhiser, C., Schwartz, S. J., Bostwick, D. G., Williams, A. W., Moore, B. J., and Erdman, W. J., Jr. (1996). Cis-trans lycopene isomers, carotenoids, and retinol in the human prostate. *Cancer Epidemiol. Biomarkers Prev.* **5**, 823–833.

144. Bertram, J. S. (1999). Carotenoids and gene regulation. *Nutr. Rev.* **57**, 182–191.

145. Williams, A. W., Boileau, T. W., Zhou, J. R., Clinton, S. K., and Erdman, J. W., Jr. (2000). Beta-carotene modulates human prostate cancer cell growth and may undergo intracellular metabolism to retinol. *J. Nutr.* **130**, 728–732.

146. Giovannucci, E. (1998). Dietary influences of 1,25(OH)₂ vitamin D in relation to prostate cancer: A hypothesis. *Cancer Causes Control* **9**, 567–582.

147. Knekt, P., Aromaa, A., Maatela, J., Alfthan, G., Aaran, R., Hakama, M., Hakulinen, T., Peto, R. P., and Teppo, L. (1990). Serum selenium and subsequent risk of cancer among Finnish men and women. *J. Natl. Cancer Inst.* **32**, 864–868.

148. Yoshizawa, K., Willett, W. C., Morris, S. J., Stampfer, M. J., Speigelman, D., Rimm, E. B., and Giovannucci, E. (1998). Study of prediagnostic selenium levels in toenails and the

risk of advanced prostate cancer. *J. Natl. Cancer Inst.* **90**, 1219–1224.

149. Clark, L. C., Combs, G. F., Turnbull, B. W., Slate, E. H., Chalker, D. K., Chow, J., Davis, L. S., Glover, R. A., Graham, G. F., Gross, E. G., Krongrad, A., Lesher, J. L., Park, H. K., Sanders, B. B., Smith, C. L., and Taylor, J. R. (1996). Effects of selenium supplementation for cancer prevention in patients with carcinoma of the skin. A randomized controlled trial. *JAMA* **276**, 1957–1963.

150. Webber, M. M., Perez-Ripoll, E. A., and James, G. T. (1985). Inhibitory effects of selenium on the growth of DU–145 human prostate carcinoma cells in vitro. *Biochem. Biophys. Res. Commun.* **130**, 603–609.

151. Medina, D. (1986). Mechanisms of selenium inhibition of tumorigenesis. *Adv. Exp. Med. Biol.* **206**, 465–472.

152. Liu, S., Lee, I.-M., Linson, P., Ajani, U., Buring, J. E., and Hennekens, C. H. (2000). A prospective study of physical activity and risk of prostate cancer in U.S. physicians. *Int. J. Epidemiol.* **29**, 29–35.

153. Giovannucci, E., Leitzmann, M., Spiegelman, D., Rimm, E. B., Colditz, G. A., Stampfer, M. J., and Willett, W. C. (1998). A prospective study of physical activity and prostate cancer in male health professionals. *Cancer Res.* **58**, 5117–5122.

154. Hackney, A. C., Fahrner, C. L., and Gulledge, T. P. (1998). Basal reproductive hormonal profiles are altered in endurance trained men. *J. Sports Med. Phys. Fitness* **38**, 138–141.

155. Goode, E. L., Stanford, J. L., Chakrabarti, L., Gibbs, M., Kolb, S., McIndoe, R. A., Buckley, V. A., Schuster, E. F., Neal, C. L., Miller, E. L., Brandzel, S., Hood, L., Ostrander, E. A., and Jarvik, G. P. (2000). Linkage analysis of 150 high-risk prostate cancer families at 1q24–25. *Genet. Epidemiol.* **18**, 251–275.

156. Xu, J. (2000). Combined analysis of hereditary prostate cancer linkage to 1q24–25: Results from 772 hereditary prostate cancer families from the International Consortium for Prostate Cancer Genetics. *Am. J. Hum. Genet.* **66**, 945–957.

157. Xu, J., Meyers, D., Freije, D., Isaacs, S., Wiley, K., Nusskern, D., Ewing, C., Wilkens, E., Bujnovszky, P., Bova, G. S., Walsh, P., Isaacs, W., Schleutker, J., Matikainen, M., Tammela, T., Visakorpi, T., Kallioniemi, O. P., Berry, R., Schaid, D., French, A., McDonnell, S., Schroeder, J., Blute, M., Thibodeau, S., Grönberg, H., Emanuelsson, M., Damber, J.-E., Bergh, A., Jonsson, B.-A., Smith, J., Bailey-Wilson, J., Carpten, J., Stephan, D., Gillanders, E., Amundson, I., Kainu, T., Freas-Lutz, D., Baffoe-Bonnie, A., Van Aucken, A., Sood, R., Collins, F., Brownstein, M., and Trent, J. (1998). Evidence for a prostate cancer susceptibility locus on the X chromosome. *Nat. Genet.* **20**, 175–179.

158. Ross, R. K., Pike, M. C., Coetzee, G. A., Reichardt, J. K. V., Yu, M. C., Feigelson, H., Stanczyk, F. Z., Kolonel, L. N., and Henderson, B. E. (1998). Androgen metabolism and prostate cancer: Establishing a model of genetic susceptibility. *Cancer Res.* **58**, 4497–4504.

159. Makridakis, N. M., Ross, R. K., Pike, M. C., Crocitto, L. E., Kolonel, L. N., Pearce, C. L., Henderson, B. E., and Reichardt, J. K. V. (1999). Association of mis-sense substitution in SRD5A2 gene with prostate cancer in African-American and Hispanic men in Los Angeles, U.S.A. *Lancet* **354**, 975–978.

160. Platz, E. A., Giovannucci, E., Dahl, D. M., Krithivas, K., Hennekens, C. H., Brown, M., Stampfer, M. J., and Kantoff, P. W. (1998). The androgen receptor gene GGN microsatellite and prostate cancer risk. *Cancer Epidemiol. Biomarkers Prev.* **7**, 379–384.

161. Stanford, J. L., Just, J. J., Gibs, M., Wicklund, K. G., Neal, C. L., Blumenstein, B. A., and Ostrander, E. A. (1997). Polymorphic repeats in the androgen receptor gene: Molecular markers of prostate cancer risk. *Cancer Res.* **57**, 1194–1198.

162. Habuchi, T., Suzuki, T., Sasaki, R., Wang, L., Sato, K., Satoh, S., Akao, T., Tsuchiya, N., Shimoda, N., Wada, Y., Koizumi, A., Chihara, J., Ogawa, O., and Kato, T. (2000). Association of vitamin D receptor gene polymorphism with prostate cancer and benign prostatic hyperplasia in a Japanese population. *Cancer Res.* **60**, 305–308.

163. Ingles, S. A., Ross, R. K., Yu, M. C., Irvine, R. A., La Pera, G., Haile, R. W., and Coetzee, G. A. (1997). Association of prostate cancer risk with genetic polymorphisms in vitamin D receptor and androgen receptor. *J. Natl. Cancer Inst.* **89**, 166–170.

164. Takacs, I., Koller, D. L., Peacock, M., Christian, J. C., Hui, S. L., Conneally, P. M., Johnston, C. C., Jr., Foroud, T., and Econs, M. J. (1999). Sibling pair linkage and association studies between bone mineral density and the insulin-like growth factor I gene locus. *J. Clin. Endocrin. Metab.* **84**, 4467–4471.

165. Jaffe, J. M., Malkowicz, B., Walker, A. H., MacBride, S., Peschel, R., Tomaszewski, J., Van Arsdalen, K., Wein, A. J., and Rebbeck, T. R. (2000). Association of SRD5A2 genotype and pathological characteristics of prostate tumors. *Cancer Res.* **60**, 1626–1630.

166. Tymchuk, C. N., Tessler, S. B., Aronson, W. J., and Barnard, R. J. (1998). Effects of diet and exercise on insulin, sex hormone-binding globulin, and prostate-specific antigen. *Nutr. Cancer* **31**, 127–131.

167. Clark, L. C., Dalkin, B., Krongrad, A., Combs, G. F., Jr., Turnbull, B. W., Slate, E. H., Witherington, R., Herlong, J. H., Janosko, E., Carpenter, D., Borosso, C., Falk, S., and Rounder, J. (1998). Decreased incidence of prostate cancer with selenium supplementation: Results of a double-blind cancer prevention trial. *Br. J. Urol.* **81**, 730–734.

168. Klein, E. A., Thompson, I. M., Lippman, S. M., Goodman, P. J., Albanes, D., Taylor, P. R., and Coltman, C. (2000). SELECT: The selenium and vitamin E cancer prevention trial–rationale and design. *Prostate Cancer Prostat. Dis.* **3**, 145–151.

169. Meyer, F., Bairati, I., Shadmani, R., Fradet, Y., and Moore, L. (1999). Dietary fat and prostate cancer survival. *Cancer Causes Control* **10**, 245–251.

CHAPTER **25**

Nutrition and Lung Cancer

SUSAN T. MAYNE
Yale University School of Medicine, New Haven, Connecticut

I. INTRODUCTION

Lung cancer is the most common cause of cancer death in both men and women in the United States. An estimated 171,600 persons were diagnosed with lung cancer in the United States in 1999 (94,000 men and 77,600 women), and 158,900 persons died of lung cancer during the same time [1]. Cigarette smoking is established as the dominant risk factor for lung cancer. With progress in tobacco cessation in American men, mortality from lung cancer has declined significantly in this group (-1.6% per year from 1991 to 1995 [1]). The gains made with regard to declining rates in men are encouraging, but must be considered against the rates for women, which continue to increase, although the rate of increase has begun to slow [1]. Also, tobacco use in youth is increasing, indicating that tobacco prevention and cessation continue to be public health priorities as the primary strategies for reducing lung cancer morbidity and mortality.

Another possible approach for reducing lung cancer deaths is detection of lung cancer when the disease is still localized. Early detection of lung cancer has great potential; the 5-year relative survival rate for lung cancer diagnosed when the disease is still localized is 50% [1]. In contrast, the 5-year relative survival rate for all stages of lung cancer combined is only 14%. A variety of approaches for early detection are being investigated; one newer approach that has been suggested to have potential is low-dose computed tomography screening [2].

While tobacco is clearly the predominant risk factor for lung cancer, other risk factors have also been identified, including exposure to certain industrial and organic chemicals; radon and asbestos exposure; radiation exposure; air pollution; personal history of tuberculosis and other prior lung diseases; family history of lung cancer; and exposure to environmental tobacco smoke for nonsmokers [1, 3]. Also, as detailed below, dietary factors have been associated with lung cancer risk. Many of these risk factors are potentially modifiable, particularly certain occupational and environmental exposures and diet, offering opportunities to further reduce risk of lung cancer. However, it cannot be overly emphasized that tobacco prevention and cessation remain the foundation of public health efforts for lung cancer prevention; all other approaches should be viewed as adjunct approaches to tobacco control.

II. DIETARY CONSTITUENTS AND PRIMARY PREVENTION OF LUNG CANCER

There are some excellent, comprehensive reviews on the topic of nutrition in the etiology of lung cancer [4, 5]. This chapter will attempt to summarize and interpret the current literature on the topic of nutrition and lung cancer, drawing primarily from observational epidemiology studies and human intervention trials.

A. Fruit and Vegetable Consumption

Lung cancer is a highly prevalent disease in many countries of the world, therefore, it is not surprising that numerous observational studies, both case-control and cohort, have examined the association between consumption of various foods and food groups and lung cancer risk. In reviewing this literature, the most consistent observation seen is that increased consumption of fruits and/or vegetables is associated with a lower risk of lung cancer. This inverse association has been noted for decades, has been observed in studies from many different countries, has been seen in both smokers as well as nonsmokers, is observed in both men and women, and has been observed for all histologic types of lung cancer [4]. The World Cancer Research Fund, in association with the American Institute for Cancer Research, recently concluded that "seven cohort and 17 case-control studies are almost entirely consistent with a protective effect of vegetables and fruits against lung cancer. The evidence that diets high in vegetables and fruits decrease the risk of lung cancer is convincing" [5]. In some studies, the magnitude of the inverse association for fruits exceeds that of vegetables, while in others, the converse appears to hold. An inverse association has been seen with many different types of fruits and vegetables; the evidence is the most abundant for green vegetables and carrots [5]. The majority of studies that examined the association between consumption

of cruciferous vegetables and lung cancer risk also find strong or moderate decreases in risk at the highest consumption levels [5].

These results from observational studies are reasonably consistent; however, observational studies cannot prove that there is a causal relationship between low fruit and vegetable intake and lung cancer risk. That is, observational studies are susceptible to confounding, and thus can only demonstrate associations (see Chapter 4). Confounding occurs if some other factor is associated with both low fruit and vegetable consumption and lung cancer risk. One such possible confounder is tobacco use itself, in that it is clearly associated with lung cancer risk, and studies also demonstrate that cigarette smokers report consuming significantly less vitamin C and beta-carotene (markers of fruit and vegetable consumption [6]) as compared to nonsmokers [7]. In most of the epidemiologic studies of fruit and vegetable consumption and lung cancer risk, investigators have appropriately controlled or adjusted their estimates for tobacco use. However, residual confounding, due to imperfect measurement of tobacco, remains a concern.

One approach for minimizing the potential for confounding by smoking in studies of diet and lung cancer risk is to examine the association between diet and lung cancer risk in nonsmokers. Several case-control studies of lung cancer in nonsmokers and some cohort studies with nonsmoking lung cancer cases are available. For example, Kalandidi et al. [8] examined passive smoking and diet as risk factors for lung cancer among Greek women, the majority of whom were lifelong nonsmokers. In this study, high consumption of fruits was associated with a significantly lower lung cancer risk. The associations of lung cancer risk with passive smoking and reduced fruit intake were independent and did not confound each other. Inverse associations between fruit intake and lung cancer risk were also noted in a study of Chinese women in Hong Kong who never smoked [9]. Candelora et al. [10] also examined the association between diet and lung cancer risk in women who never smoked; increased consumption of vegetables was associated with a significantly lower lung cancer risk. Mayne et al. [11] studied both men and women nonsmokers with lung cancer, and reported inverse associations of lung cancer risk with increased consumption of fruits and vegetables; the association was strongest for raw fruit and vegetables. The previous studies in nonsmokers were all case-control studies, but the results are supported by cohort data as well. For example, Knekt et al. [12] reported that nonsmokers who consumed the lowest tertile of fruits and berries had a relative risk for lung cancer sevenfold greater than nonsmokers who consumed the highest tertile of fruits and berries ($p = 0.001$ for trend). Thus, these studies of lung cancer risk in nonsmokers appear to indicate that protective associations observed for fruits and/or vegetables do not appear to be due to confounding by tobacco, although confounding by other lifestyle factors still remains a possibility.

While most of the studies of diet and lung cancer have emphasized the role of diet in the etiology of lung cancer, some literature suggests that diet could be important in lung cancer prognosis. For example, Goodman et al. [13] used dietary data collected as part of two case-control studies on lung cancer to examine a possible association between diet 1 year prior to diagnosis and lung cancer survival. The results suggested that increased consumption of all vegetables combined was associated with a significant reduction in the risk of death in women but not men. Fruit intake was also associated with increased survival among women. The authors concluded that certain components of fruits and vegetables may prolong survival in some lung cancer patients.

Fruits and vegetables are complex mixtures of many different compounds, several of which might have cancer-preventive properties [14]. Much research has been targeted toward identifying the components of fruits and vegetables that might have cancer-preventive activity. Although several components, such as carotenoids and vitamin C, have received considerable study as discussed below, it is presently unknown which components/combinations of components in fruits and vegetables are thought to influence human lung carcinogenesis.

B. Vitamins and Minerals

1. CAROTENOIDS AND RETINOL

Carotenoids are plant pigments that are found primarily in a variety of fruits and vegetables. The most commonly ingested carotenoids in human populations include beta-carotene, alpha-carotene, lycopene, lutein and zeaxanthin, and beta-cryptoxanthin. Intake of carotenoids is highly correlated with intake of fruits and vegetables; carotenoids as measured in blood or other tissues are considered one of the best biomarkers for fruit and vegetable intake [15, 16]. Given this, it is not surprising that epidemiologic studies generally find inverse associations between consumption of carotenoids or blood levels of carotenoids and lung cancer risk, as reviewed elsewhere [4, 17].

Numerous studies have examined the association between the carotenoid beta-carotene, in diet or in serum/plasma, and lung cancer risk. A recent review of this literature by the International Agency for Research on Cancer [17] concluded that the association of lower serum or plasma beta-carotene with lung cancer risk was remarkably consistent. For example, three of three cohort studies, six of seven nested case-control studies, and five of five case-control studies reported an inverse association between plasma or serum beta-carotene concentrations and lung cancer risk. There was evidence of a dose–response in 12 of the 15 total studies reviewed. Considering estimated intake of carotenoids in diet, in nearly all studies reviewed, risk for lung cancer was lower among people with a high dietary intake of beta-carotene or carotenoids [17]. Some studies have used recently available food composition databases for carotenoids

to estimate consumption of the major dietary carotenoids. In these studies, no particular carotenoid has consistently emerged as being associated with reduced risk of lung cancer. Some studies have suggested that higher intake of alpha-carotene, in particular, seems to be more strongly associated with lower lung cancer risk [18, 19]. Other studies have reported comparable inverse associations for alpha-carotene, beta-carotene, and lutein [20]. However, other studies have observed no association with alpha-carotene but inverse associations with beta-cryptoxanthin and lutein + zeaxanthin [21], or with lycopene [22]. The majority of studies, however, found stronger inverse trends with vegetable and fruit intake than with estimated carotenoid intake [17]. Le Marchand *et al.* [20], for example, concluded that their data supported greater protection afforded by consuming a variety of vegetables compared to only foods rich in a particular carotenoid.

Certain carotenoids, known as provitamin A carotenoids, can be metabolically converted into retinol. Provitamin A carotenoids include beta-carotene, alpha-carotene, and beta-cryptoxanthin. Many of the early epidemiologic studies of diet and lung cancer examined the association of total vitamin A in the diet with lung cancer risk [4]. In 1975, for example, Bjelke [23] noted an association between dietary vitamin A and human lung cancer risk. As investigators began to examine associations separately for carotenoids versus retinol (preformed vitamin A), it became apparent that inverse associations with vitamin A were largely being driven by provitamin A carotenoids [4]. That is, the evidence from observational studies linking retinol with reduced lung cancer risk is inconsistent and weak at present.

Given the consistency of the results of epidemiologic studies on beta-carotene, coupled with chemopreventive efficacy of beta-carotene in animal models of skin carcinogenesis and buccal pouch carcinogenesis [17], several intervention trials of beta-carotene for the prevention of lung and other cancers were implemented in the 1980s and early 1990s. The first lung cancer prevention trial involving beta-carotene to be completed was the Alpha-Tocopherol Beta-Carotene (ATBC) Study [24], which involved 29,133 Finnish males ages 50–69 who were heavy cigarette smokers at entry (average one pack/day for 36 years). The study design was a 2×2 factorial with participants randomized to receive either supplemental beta-carotene (20 mg/day), alpha-tocopherol (50 mg/day), the combination, or placebo for 5–8 years. Unexpectedly, participants receiving beta-carotene (alone or in combination with alpha-tocopherol) had a statistically significant 18% increase in lung cancer incidence and 8% increase in total mortality relative to participants receiving placebo. Supplemental beta-carotene did not appear to affect the incidence of other major cancers occurring in this population.

The Carotene and Retinol Efficacy Trial (CARET) was a multicenter lung cancer prevention trial of supplemental beta-carotene (30 mg/day) plus retinyl palmitate (25,000 IU/day) versus placebo in asbestos workers and smokers [25]. CARET was terminated nearly 2 years early in January 1996, because interim analyses of the data indicated that, should the trial have continued for its planned duration, it is highly unlikely that the intervention would have been found to be beneficial. Furthermore, the interim results indicated that the supplemented group was developing more lung cancer, not less, consistent with the results of the ATBC trial. Overall, lung cancer incidence and total mortality were significantly increased by 28% and 17%, respectively, in the supplemented subjects. The increase in lung cancer following supplementation with beta-carotene and retinyl palmitate was observed for current, but not former, smokers.

In contrast to these findings are the results of the Physicians' Health Study (PHS) of supplemental beta-carotene versus placebo in 22,071 U.S. male physicians [26]. There was no effect—positive or negative—after 12 years of supplementation with beta-carotene (50 mg every other day) on total cancer, lung cancer, or cardiovascular disease. The relative risk for lung cancer was reduced by a nonsignificant 10% in current smokers randomized to beta-carotene and a nonsignificant 22% in nonsmokers randomized to beta-carotene as compared to placebo. The apparent lack of an effect of long-term supplementation of beta-carotene on lung cancer incidence, even in baseline smokers who were administered the supplements for up to 12 years, is noteworthy. A similar lack of effect of supplemental beta-carotene on overall cancer incidence was seen in the Women's Health Study [27], although the duration of intervention was short (median 2.1 years).

A clear mechanism to explain the apparent enhancement of lung carcinogenesis by supplemental beta-carotene, alone or in combination with retinol, in smokers has yet to emerge. As detailed elsewhere [28], it should be noted that the two trials that observed this enhancing effect [24, 25] had higher median plasma beta-carotene concentrations in their intervention groups relative to trials that did not observe an enhancing effect on lung cancer [26, 29]. Thus, it is possible that high tissue concentrations of beta-carotene in the presence of strongly oxidative tobacco smoke cause an interaction that promotes carcinogenesis. A recent animal study has suggested that this effect might be mediated by altered retinoid signaling [30].

The surprising results of the intervention trials involving beta-carotene and lung cancer prevention emphasize the value of results from randomized intervention trials prior to establishing public policy on the basis of observational data. Many have interpreted the observational data as being contradictory with the intervention trial results, but they really are not contradictory when it is recognized that the observational data that are derived from fruits and vegetables reflect relatively low doses of carotenoids in a complex matrix involving many other compounds, and generally reflect dietary patterns that may have been in existence for decades. The trials, in contrast, reflect one specific carotenoid given in a highly bioavailable preparation for a relatively short time period, and administered relatively late in the carcinogenic

process to a high-risk group of subjects. The intervention trial data involving high-dose supplemental beta-carotene should not be interpreted as evidence against possible benefits of fruits and vegetables; there are currently no data to suggest that fruits and vegetables might have adverse effects with regard to lung cancer.

2. VITAMIN C

Most of the early studies on dietary factors and lung cancer were designed to examine the association of carotenoids or vitamin A with lung cancer risk. Consequently, many of these studies did not use food frequency questionnaires designed to estimate intake of vitamin C, omitting foods such as potatoes that are important sources of vitamin C but are not important sources of carotenoids or retinol. Also, relatively few studies on diet and lung cancer performed plasma vitamin C measurements, because samples were not specifically preserved at the time of sample collection, which is necessary for vitamin C measurements. Given this, the literature on vitamin C and lung cancer risk is not as extensive as that on carotenoids and lung cancer; however, several studies are available.

The available literature on vitamin C and lung cancer risk has been reviewed elsewhere [4, 5, 31]. In general, most studies indicate that persons who consume more vitamin C in the diet are at reduced risk of lung cancer, although some studies find no association between vitamin C and lung cancer risk. According to the most recent review [5], "most of six cohort and eleven case-control studies have found some degree of decreased risk of lung cancer with higher vitamin C intake, although these associations were in many cases only weak or moderate; no studies found a strong increase in risk." Some of the studies examined associations of both vitamin C and fruit/vegetable intake in relation to lung cancer risk; the majority found more consistent and/or stronger inverse associations with fruit and/or vegetable consumption [4]. Thus, it seems probable that the observed decrease in risk is really attributable to some other component of vitamin C-containing foods (vegetables and fruits), and not to vitamin C itself [5].

Randomized trials of supplemental vitamin C for lung cancer prevention have not been initiated, although large trials are ongoing that include supplemental vitamin C as one of several factors being studied for chronic disease prevention. One such trial is the Women's Antioxidant Cardiovascular Study (WACS), which is randomizing 8000 female health professionals with a prior cardiovascular event or with three or more coronary risk factors to antioxidant nutrients [32]. The nutrients included are beta-carotene (50 mg), alpha-tocopherol (600 IU), or vitamin C (500 mg; all given every other day) in a $2 \times 2 \times 2$ factorial design. Another such trial is Physicians' Health Study II (PHS II), an extension of the original Physicians' Health Study of aspirin and beta-carotene. PHS II is a randomized trial enrolling 15,000 eligible male physicians aged 55 years and older to a 2×2 $\times 2 \times 2$ factorial design of antioxidant vitamins in the prevention of total and prostate cancer, cardiovascular disease, and cataract and macular degeneration [33]. The antioxidant nutrients being studied in this trial are vitamin E (400 IU every other day), beta-carotene (50 mg every other day), vitamin C (500 mg every day), and a multivitamin (Centrum Silver daily). While neither of these trials is specifically designed nor powered to evaluate an effect of vitamin C on lung cancer, they are some of the largest trials yet under way to investigate the effects of vitamin C as a single agent on chronic disease outcomes.

3. VITAMIN E

Some epidemiologic studies have attempted to quantitate intake of vitamin E from foods, but the intake estimates are generally considered to be somewhat unreliable [34]. Vitamin E is concentrated in many vegetable oils and fats and the amount of fats and oils added during food preparation is difficult to assess. Also, different oils have different concentrations of tocopherols, and food labels often do not provide the specific fat or oil in the product, and manufacturers may substitute fat sources depending on availability and cost. Given this situation, epidemiologic studies of vitamin E and cancer generally rely on biochemical markers of exposure, such as plasma concentrations of alpha-tocopherol. In studies that rely on biochemical markers, greatest weight should be given to cohort studies, where bloods are obtained prior to lung cancer diagnosis, rather than case-control studies, where bloods are obtained postdiagnosis.

A recent review of this literature [35] indicates that results are somewhat mixed, with some studies suggesting an inverse association with plasma vitamin E but other studies failing to observe such an association. For example, a Finnish study of male smokers participating in the ATBC trial (discussed above) examined the association between prediagnostic serum vitamin E and lung cancer risk [36]. Those in the highest quintile of serum alpha-tocopherol had 19% lower lung cancer incidence compared to those in the lowest quintile [relative risk (RR) = 0.81, 95% confidence interval (CI) = 0.67 − 0.97]. This suggestion of a protective effect was especially strong among men younger than 60 years and men with less cumulative tobacco exposure. Results from a cohort of Chinese tin miners [37] also suggested an inverse association between serum alpha-tocopherol and lung cancer risk among men less than 60 years of age ($p = 0.002$ for trend). Although an early analysis of members of the Washington County, Maryland, cohort revealed significantly lower serum vitamin E levels among cases compared to controls [38], this result was not replicated in a subsequent analysis [39]. Several other prospective studies suggested nonsignificant inverse associations in a variety of different populations; however, inverse associations were not observed in other studies, as reviewed elsewhere [35].

Results from a large intervention trial of vitamin E for lung cancer prevention are available. That is, the ATBC Trial

discussed previously investigated both beta-carotene and alpha-tocopherol in the primary prevention of lung cancer [24]. The trial was conducted in Finnish male smokers. The RR of lung cancer in men randomized to receive vitamin E (50 mg/day) for 5–8 years was 0.98 [95% CI, 0.86–1.12]. The dose of vitamin E is relatively modest; trials with higher doses of vitamin E are under way [32, 33]. However, lung cancer is not the primary endpoint for ongoing trials involving vitamin E, thus their statistical power with regard to lung cancer endpoints is likely to be limited.

4. SELENIUM

Selenium is widely present in the food supply, although the selenium content of food varies, depending on the selenium content of the soil where the plant was grown or where the animal (which ingests local forage crops) was raised. The amount of selenium in soil can vary substantially, and the same food items may have more than a 10-fold difference in selenium content [34]. For these reasons, estimation of selenium exposure through dietary assessment is generally considered unreliable, with most epidemiologic studies relying on biomarkers for assessing selenium status, such as blood-based measures or toenail clippings.

As reviewed elsewhere [35], several observational studies have examined the association between selenium status and lung cancer risk with mixed results. Van den Brandt and colleagues [40] detected a strong inverse relationship between toenail selenium and lung cancer risk in a large Dutch cohort followed for 3.3 years ($p = 0.006$ for trend). An inverse association of serum selenium and lung cancer risk was also observed in a large cohort of Finnish subjects [41, 42]. However, at least five other studies have not observed an inverse association between selenium status and lung cancer risk (reviewed in [35]).

Results of one clinical trial involving selenium are pertinent to the issue of selenium and lung cancer prevention. The Nutritional Prevention of Cancer Trial was a placebo-controlled, randomized clinical trial, designed to test the ability of high-selenium yeast supplements (200 μg/day) to reduce second skin cancer in 1312 men and women who had a recent history of nonmelanoma skin cancer [43]. Participants were selected from dermatology clinics located in regions of the United States with high rates of nonmelanoma skin cancer and with low levels of soil selenium. While selenium supplementation was of no benefit in terms of preventing new skin cancers, persons randomized to selenium supplementation as compared to the placebo group had statistically significant decreases in risk of total cancer ($p = 0.002$) and cancers of the lung ($p = 0.04$), colorectum ($p = 0.03$), and prostate ($p = 0.002$). A total of 17 lung cancers occurred in the selenium group as compared to 31 in the placebo group (RR = 0.54, 95% CI = 0.30–0.98). The possibility that supplemental selenium might help reduce the risk of lung cancer is provocative, but it should be noted that the findings with regard to lung and other cancers were un-

expected, based on small numbers, and require confirmation in subsequent trials. Also, participants in the selenium trial were selected from low-selenium regions of the United States, so the results may not be generalizable. Finally, selenium is a trace mineral with a relatively narrow range of safety. That is, the tolerable upper limit for selenium as set by the National Academy of Sciences is 400 μg/day [34]. Usual selenium intake from foods averages around 100 μg/day in the United States [34]. Supplementation can thus readily elevate total selenium intake to levels approaching or exceeding the upper limit, increasing the probability of encountering adverse effects of selenosis (most notably hair and nail brittleness).

5. FOLATE

Folate has recently been of considerable interest with regard to a possible role in cancer prevention. Folate is crucial to the synthesis of nucleic acids and thus to normal cell replication. Also, folate is involved in methyl transfer reactions; abnormalities in DNA methylation are known to occur during carcinogenesis. Folate is also concentrated in fruits and vegetables, particularly green leafy vegetables, leading to the suggestion that folate might account for some of the lower risks observed with regard to green vegetables, for example.

Only a few epidemiologic studies have specifically reported on associations between dietary folate and lung cancer risk. In the Netherlands Cohort Study on Diet and Cancer [21], the association between dietary folate and risk of lung cancer was evaluated. After 6.3 years of follow-up in the cohort, a total of 939 male lung cancer cases were identified. Using a case-cohort analysis, the authors reported that higher dietary folate was associated with a lower risk of lung cancer overall (adjusted RR = 0.70, 95% CI = 0.51–0.95 comparing fifth quintile to first quintile of intake). Inverse trends were noted in both former and current smokers, with a statistically significant trend in the latter ($p = 0.0001$ for trend). The authors also stratified by histologic subtype; higher dietary folate was inversely associated with risk of small cell carcinomas, squamous cell carcinomas, and adenocarcinomas. As expected, dietary folate was correlated with intake of many other micronutrients ($r = 0.66$ for vitamin C, $r = 0.62$ for beta-carotene). The authors concluded that folate and vitamin C had stronger protective associations with lung cancer risk than the carotenoids, but noted that the inverse associations might reflect a generalized fruit and vegetable effect rather than effects of specific nutrients. Another cohort study also noted a highly significant inverse association between dietary folate and lung cancer risk [44]. In this analysis, the protective effect of folate was stronger for heavy smokers, and was limited to cases with squamous cell carcinomas. In contrast, no association between total folate consumption (diet and supplements) was noted in the Nurses' Health Study cohort [45].

No trials using folate for the primary prevention of cancer have been completed; however, one randomized and blinded

trial of folate investigated effects on an intermediate end-point for lung cancer. In this trial, smoking men with squamous metaplasia of the lung were randomized to either high-dose supplements of folate (10 mg/day) and vitamin B_{12} (500 μg/day) or placebo for 4 months [46]. The authors noted a significantly greater reduction in atypical cells in sputum in the intervention group as compared to the placebo group ($p = 0.02$). However, the authors cautioned overinterpretation of their findings given the small study population ($n = 73$ total), the supraphysiological doses used, and the substantial spontaneous variation in sputum cytologies.

C. Macronutrients and Related Substances

1. ENERGY BALANCE/ADIPOSITY

Obesity has been shown to increase the risk for many cancers, such as postmenopausal breast cancer, endometrial cancer, and colon adenomas and adenocarcinomas, as discussed elsewhere [47]. Suggestive positive associations have also been noted for prostate cancer. However, lung cancer (along with premenopausal breast cancer) stands out in that most of the current literature suggests that obesity, as measured by the body mass index, is associated with a lower risk [47]. The interpretation of an inverse association between obesity and lung cancer risk, however, is complicated in that this relationship has been observed in smoking populations, where the well-known impact of smoking on both body fatness and on lung cancer risk may obscure true relationships (i.e., confounding). Most investigators adjust their estimates for the effects of smoking, but it is not clear that statistical adjustment can fully compensate for the effects of smoking.

Studies of the relationship of obesity to lung cancer risk in nonsmokers thus afford another approach for examining this relationship while minimizing potential confounding by tobacco. One large, population-based case-control study is now available on the association between obesity and lung cancer risk in nonsmokers [47]. This analysis of 412 case-control pairs indicated a positive relationship between body mass index [weight (kg)/height (m²)] and lung cancer risk for those who had never smoked and those who formerly smoked. The risk was particularly noted at high levels of adiposity; a body mass index > 30.84 kg/m² (highest octile) was associated with a threefold greater risk of lung cancer as compared to a body mass ≤ 21.26 kg/m² (lowest octile). These results require replication in other large population-based case-control studies of nonsmokers or pooled cohort studies of nonsmokers, but if replicated, they suggest that lung cancer may well be added to the lengthy list of chronic diseases in which risk increases with obesity.

2. DIETARY FAT, SATURATED FAT, AND CHOLESTEROL

Possible associations between total fat, saturated fat, cholesterol, and lung cancer risk have been reviewed comprehensively elsewhere [4, 5]. Approximately six cohort and six case-control studies have examined some aspects of dietary fat or cholesterol in relation to lung cancer risk. Overall, the evidence regarding total fat and lung cancer risk is somewhat inconsistent, with some studies indicating higher risk with higher intake levels, but other studies failing to observe any association. Associations with dietary fat might reflect residual confounding by smoking; again, studies of nonsmokers can be informative in this regard. One of the strongest associations noted for dietary fat and lung cancer risk comes from a study of nonsmoking women in Missouri [48]. Risk of lung cancer increased with increasing levels of total fat; the effects seemed to be particularly attributable to saturated fat. The adjusted risk estimate for saturated fat was 6-fold greater for the highest quintile of fat intake and was even more pronounced among women with adenocarcinoma, reaching 11-fold for this histologic type. However, following this initial publication, the authors reported that the odds ratios for saturated fat were highly sensitive to the method used for energy adjustment, due to the high correlation between saturated fat and total energy [49]. Adjustment using the nutrient residual method reduced the magnitude of the odds ratios to 1.78 for the highest quintile of saturated fat as compared to the lowest quintile. The same investigators did another case-control study of lung cancer in Missouri women, most of who were smokers [50]. In this analysis, an association between dietary fats, frequency of meat consumption, and lung cancer risk was observed. However, after adjusting for potential confounders and removing data from proxy respondents, dietary fat and consumption of red meat were no longer associated with lung cancer risk. These studies illustrate the difficulties in analyzing and interpreting effects of dietary fats on risk of lung and other cancers.

A tangential link between fats and lung cancer risk comes from some interesting studies on cooking practices and lung cancer risk in Chinese women. Chinese cooking often involves frying ingredients in oil at high temperatures, which produces fumes to which the cook is exposed. In Taiwanese women nonsmokers, lung cancer risk increased with the number of meals cooked per day [51]. The risk was also greater if women usually waited until fumes were emitted from the cooking oil before they began cooking. Shields *et al.* [52] examined the production of potentially mutagenic substances emitted from a variety of cooking oils heated to the temperatures typically encountered in wok cooking. Their results suggested that unrefined Chinese rapeseed oil, in particular, produced significant quantities of mutagenic compounds. Lowering the cooking temperature or adding an antioxidant to the oil reduced volatile emissions.

3. HETEROCYCLIC AMINES

As described above, some epidemiologic studies suggest that increased consumption of fat, saturated fat, and cholesterol increases the risk of lung cancer. Meat is a rich dietary source of these nutrients, and meats cooked at high temperatures are known to contain various pyrolysis products, such

as heterocyclic amines. Heterocyclic amines are known to be highly mutagenic, and their production in meats is a function of cooking method. Pan-frying and grilling/barbecuing, in particular, promote heterocyclic amine formation. Given this, some recent epidemiologic studies have investigated a possible association of meat intake and meat cooking practices as determinants of lung cancer risk. In a case-control study of women with lung cancer, Sinha *et al.* [53] reported that lung cancer risk was increased with higher consumption of total meat, red meat, well-done meat, and fried meat. Not all types of red meat were associated with an increased risk; for example, higher consumption of red meat cooked by microwave was associated with a significantly lower risk of lung cancer. The authors suggest that variable effects of meat-cooking practices on lung cancer risk may explain some of the inconsistent results in prior epidemiologic studies of meat consumption and lung cancer risk [53], and suggest a need for future studies to collect detailed information on meat cooking practices.

III. DIETARY CONSTITUENTS AND PREVENTION OF SECOND LUNG CANCER

Early stage lung cancers can be surgically resected, but patients remain at risk for second lung cancers. Thus, interest has been shown in interventions, nutritional or other, aimed at reducing the risk of second lung cancers. Two adjuvant chemoprevention trials involving retinyl palmitate have now been completed. In the first trial, patients with stage I non-small-cell lung cancer ($n = 307$) who had been treated surgically were assigned randomly to treatment with retinyl palmitate (300,000 IU) for 1 year or observation [54]. At a median follow-up of 46 months, survival trends favored retinyl palmitate over no therapy in estimated 5-year disease-free survival (64% vs. 51%, $p = 0.054$) and overall survival (62% vs. 54%, $p = 0.44$). Eighteen patients in the retinyl palmitate arm developed a second primary tumor compared with 29 patients developing 33 second primaries in the control group. Retinyl palmitate toxicity was frequent, occurring in the majority of treated patients.

These promising results, however, were not replicated in a much larger trial, known as Euroscan [55], a multicenter trial employing a 2 × 2 factorial design to test 2 years of intervention with retinyl palmitate and *N*-acetylcysteine in preventing second primary tumors in 2592 patients. Patients in the Euroscan trial had completed definitive therapy for non-small-cell lung cancer (40% of those randomized) or for early stage head and neck cancer (60% of those randomized). The dose of retinyl palmitate in this trial was 300,000 IU daily for the first year followed by 150,000 IU daily for a second year. After a median follow-up of 49 months, there was no benefit for either retinyl palmitate or *N*-acetylcysteine with regard to survival, event-free survival, or second primary tumors. Second primary tumors developed in 54 patients in

the combined intervention group, 61 patients in the retinyl palmitate only group, 61 patients in the *N*-acetylcysteine only group, and 32 in the no intervention group (not significant). Thus, current evidence does not support a role for high-dose vitamin A in second primary lung cancer prevention.

IV. CONCLUSIONS AND RECOMMENDATIONS

The available literature on diet and lung cancer can be readily summarized into the following general statement: Dietary patterns characterized by higher consumption of fruits and vegetables and the nutrients concentrated in these foods (carotenoids, vitamin C, folate) are associated with a lower risk of lung cancer, and diets characterized by higher consumption of meats, total fat, and saturated fat are associated with greater lung cancer risk. Nutrient supplements have not been shown to be of value in the primary or secondary prevention of lung cancer. As noted by others [56], the evidence of a protective effect of fruits and vegetables is more consistently observed in case-control studies compared to cohort studies. Moreover, the magnitude of a possible protective effect of fruits and vegetables in the cohort studies is generally less than what one would have expected based on ecologic evidence and case-control studies [56]. Koo [57] has noted that much of the available literature is based on studies of white male smokers in North America and Europe; these populations are known to be low consumers of fruit and vegetables (relative to nonsmokers) and are less likely to pursue perceived healthier lifestyles. Koo thus suggests that some of the epidemiologic findings on diet and lung cancer are artifacts due to inadequate adjustment for behavioral correlates of smoking. While this may be true in part, it must be noted that fruits and/or vegetables have been observed to be protective in other racial and ethnic populations [58]. Also, several studies of diet and lung cancer risk in nonsmokers, including those who have never smoked, suggest protective effects of fruits and vegetables. It remains possible that protective effects are due to behavioral correlates of increased fruit and vegetable consumption (i.e., confounding), but this can only be evaluated by randomized trials. To date, no trials of fruit and vegetable intake for lung cancer prevention have been initiated, but ongoing dietary intervention trials such as the Women's Health Initiative [59] and the Women's Healthy Eating and Living Study [60] can certainly examine lung cancer incidence by treatment arm, although with uncertain statistical power.

Given the enormous costs and difficulties of conducting large-scale intervention trials, observational studies remain the primary approach for elucidating diet and chronic disease relationships. With a disease as frequent as lung cancer, cohort studies are clearly viable and will continue to be used in etiologic research. A new emphasis, however, on more diverse cohorts is clearly needed. As discussed by Riboli and

Kaaks [56], multicenter cohorts offer one possible approach in that they allow for the selection of populations with varying dietary habits within the same cohort. One such cohort is the multiethnic cohort in Hawaii and Los Angeles, which includes subcohorts from different ethnic groups in these areas [61]. Another large, multicenter cohort is the European Prospective Investigation into Cancer and Nutrition [62]. Utilization of large, diverse cohorts such as these, along with biochemical markers of nutrient status, where appropriate, may increase confidence in diet and disease relationships observed.

In the meantime, however, the optimal approach for lung cancer prevention should emphasize the proven benefits of tobacco cessation and prevention, in addition to what can be considered "prudent" recommendations to increase consumption of fruits and vegetables of all types, and to reduce intake of meat, total fat, and saturated fat. This dietary pattern is associated not only with a lower risk of lung cancer, but also with lower risk of many other chronic diseases, as described elsewhere in this volume.

References

1. American Cancer Society (1999). "Cancer Facts and Figures—1999." American Cancer Society, Atlanta, GA.

2. Henschke, C. I., McCauley, D. I., Yankelevitz, D. F., Naidich, D. P., McGuinness, G., Miettinen, O. S., Libby, D. M., Pasmantier, M. W., Koizumi, J., Altorki, N. K., and Smith, J. P. (1999). Early Lung Cancer Action Project: Overall design and findings from baseline screening. *Lancet* **354**, 99–105.

3. Blot, W. J., and Fraumeni, J. F., Jr. (1996). Cancers of the lung and pleura. *In* "Cancer Epidemiology and Prevention" (D. Schottenfeld and J. F. Fraumeni, Jr., Eds.), 2nd ed., pp. 637–665. Oxford University Press, New York.

4. Ziegler, R. G., Mayne, S. T., and Swanson, C. A. (1996). Nutrition and lung cancer. *Cancer Causes Control* **7**, 157–177.

5. World Cancer Research Fund (1997). "Food, Nutrition and the Prevention of Cancer: A Global Perspective." American Institute for Cancer Research, Washington, DC.

6. Drewnowski, A., Rock, C. L., Henderson, S. A., Shore, A. B., Fischler, C., Galan, P., Preziosi, P., and Hercberg, S. (1997). Serum beta-carotene and vitamin C as biomarkers of vegetable and fruit intakes in a community-based sample of French adults. *Am. J. Clin. Nutr.* **65**, 1796–1802.

7. Dallongeville, J., Marecaux, N., Fruchart, J.-C., and Amouyel, P. (1998). Cigarette smoking is associated with unhealthy patterns of nutrient intake: A meta-analysis. *J. Nutr.* **128**, 1450–1457.

8. Kalandidi, A., Katsouyanni, K., Voropoulou, N., Bastas, G., Saracci, R., and Trichopoulos, D. (1990). Passive smoking and diet in the etiology of lung cancer among non-smokers. *Cancer Causes Control* **1**, 15–21.

9. Koo, L. C. (1988). Dietary habits and lung cancer risk among Chinese females in Hong Kong who never smoked. *Nutr. Cancer* **11**, 155–172.

10. Candelora, E. C., Stockwell, H. G., Armstrong, A. W., and Pinkham, P. A. (1992). Dietary intake and risk of lung cancer in women who never smoked. *Nutr. Cancer* **17**, 263–270.

11. Mayne, S. T., Janerich, D. T., Greenwald, P., Chorost, S., Tucci, C., Zaman, M. B., Melamed, M. R., Kiely, M., and McKneally, M. F. (1994). Dietary beta carotene and lung cancer risk in U.S. nonsmokers. *J. Natl. Cancer Inst.* **86**, 33–38.

12. Knekt, P., Jarvinen, R., Seppanen, R., Rissanen, A., Aromaa, A., Heinonen, O. P., Albanes, D., Heinonen, M., Pukkala, E., and Teppo, L. (1991). Dietary antioxidants and the risk of lung cancer. *Am. J. Epidemiol.* **134**, 471–479.

13. Goodman, M. T., Kolonel, L. N., Wilkens, L. R., Yoshizawa, C. N., Le Marchand, L., and Hankin, J. H. (1992). Dietary factors in lung cancer prognosis. *Eur. J. Cancer* **28**, 495–501.

14. Dragsted, L. O., Strube, M., and Larsen, J. C. (1993). Cancer protective factors in fruits and vegetables: Biochemical and biological background. *Pharmacol. Toxicol.* **72**(Suppl.), S116–S135.

15. McEligot, A. J., Rock, C. L., Flatt, S. W., Newman, V., Faerber, S., and Pierce, J. P. (1999). Plasma carotenoids are biomarkers of long-term high-vegetable intake in women with breast cancer. *J. Nutr.* **129**, 2258–2263.

16. Campbell, D. R., Gross, M. D., Martini, M. C., Grandits, G. A., Slavin, J. L., and Potter, J. D. (1994). Plasma carotenoids as biomarkers of vegetable and fruit intake. *Cancer Epidemiol. Biomarkers Prev.* **3**, 493–500.

17. International Agency for Research on Cancer (IARC) (1998). "IARC Handbooks of Cancer Prevention. Carotenoids," Vol. 2. Oxford University Press, Carey, North Carolina.

18. Ziegler, R. G., Colavito, E. A., Hartge, P., McAdams, M. J., Schoenberg, J. B., Mason, T. J., and Fraumeni, J. F., Jr. (1996). Importance of α-carotene, β-carotene, and other phytochemicals in the etiology of lung cancer. *J. Natl. Cancer Inst.* **88**, 612–615.

19. Knekt, P., Jarvinen, R., Teppo, L., Aromaa, A., and Seppanen, R. (1999). Role of various carotenoids in lung cancer prevention. *J. Natl. Cancer Inst.* **91**, 182–184.

20. Le Marchand, L., Hankin, J. H., Kolonel, L. N., Beecher, G. R., Wilkens, L. R., and Zhao, L. P. (1993). Intake of specific carotenoids and lung cancer risk. *Cancer Epidemiol. Biomarkers Prev.* **2**, 183–187.

21. Voorrips, L. E., Goldbohm, R. A., Brants, H. A. M., van Poppel, G. A. F. C., Sturmans, F., Hermus, J. J., and van den Brandt, P. A. (2000). A prospective cohort study on antioxidants and folate intake and male lung cancer risk. *Cancer Epidemiol. Biomarkers Prev.* **9**, 357–365.

22. Garcia-Closas, R., Agudo, A., Gonzalez, C. A., and Riboli, E. (1998). Intake of specific carotenoids and flavonoids and the risk of lung cancer in women in Barcelona. *Nutr. Cancer* **32**, 154–158.

23. Bjelke, E. (1975). Dietary vitamin A and human lung cancer. *Int. J. Cancer* **15**, 561–565.

24. The Alpha-Tocopherol, Beta Carotene Cancer Prevention Study Group (1994). The effect of vitamin E and beta carotene on the incidence of lung cancer and other cancers in male smokers. *N. Engl. J. Med.* **330**, 1029–1035.

25. Omenn, G. S., Goodman, G. E., Thornquist, M. D., Balmes, J., Cullen, M. R., Glass, A., Keogh, J. P., Meyskens, F. L., Jr., Valanis, B., Williams, J. H., Barnhart, S., and Hammar, S. (1996). Effects of a combination of beta carotene and vitamin A on lung cancer and cardiovascular disease. *N. Engl. J. Med.* **334**, 1150–1155.

26. Hennekens, C. H., Buring, J. E., Manson, J. E., Stampfer, M., Rosner, B., Cook, N. R., Belanger, C., LaMotte, F., Gaziano,

J. M., Ridker, P., Willett, W., and Peto, R. (1996). Lack of effect of long-term supplementation with beta carotene on the incidence of malignant neoplasms and cardiovascular disease. *N. Engl. J. Med.* **334,** 1145–1149.

27. Lee, I. M., Cook, N. R., Manson, J. E., Buring, J. E., and Hennekens, C. H. (1999). Beta-carotene supplementation and incidence of cancer and cardiovascular disease: The Women's Health Study. *J. Natl. Cancer Inst.* **91,** 2102–2106.

28. Mayne, S. T. (1998). Beta-carotene, carotenoids, and cancer prevention. *In* "Principles and Practice of Oncology (PPO) Updates" (V. T. DeVita, Jr., S. Hellman, and S. A. Rosenberg, Eds.), Vol. 12, pp. 1–15. Lippincott Raven Healthcare, Cedar Knolls, NJ.

29. Blot, W. J., Li, J.-Y., Taylor, P. R., Guo, W., Dawsey, S., Wang, G.-Q., Yang, C. S., Zheng, S.-F., Gail, M., Li, G.-Y., Yu, Y., Liu, B.-Q., Tangrea, J., Sun, Y.-H., Liu, F., Fraumeni, J. F., Jr., Zhang, Y.-H., and Li, B. (1993). Nutrition intervention trials in Linxian, China: Supplementation with specific vitamin/mineral combinations, cancer incidence, and disease-specific mortality in the general population. *J. Natl. Cancer Inst.* **85,** 1483–1492.

30. Wang, X-D., Liu, C., Bronson, R. T., Smith, D. E., Krinsky, N. I., and Russell, R. M. (1999). Retinoid signaling and activator protein-1 expression in ferrets given beta-carotene supplements and exposed to tobacco smoke. *J. Natl. Cancer Inst.* **91,** 60–66.

31. Block, G. (1991). Vitamin C and cancer prevention: The epidemiologic evidence. *Am. J. Clin. Nutr.* **53,** 270S–282S.

32. Manson, J. E., Gaziano, J. M., Spelsberg, A., Ridker, P. M., Cook, N. R., Buring, J. E., Willett, W. C., and Hennekens, C. H. (1995). A secondary prevention trial of antioxidant vitamins and cardiovascular disease in women: Rationale, design and methods. *Ann. Epidemiol.* **5,** 261–269.

33. Christen, W. G., Gaziano, J. M., and Hennekens, C. H. (2000). Design of Physicians' Health Study II—a randomized trial of beta-carotene, vitamins E and C, and multivitamins, in prevention of cancer, cardiovascular disease, and eye disease, and review of results of completed trials. *Ann. Epidemiol.* **10,** 125–134.

34. Institute of Medicine, National Academy of Sciences, Food and Nutrition Board, Panel on Dietary Antioxidants and Related Compounds (2000). "Dietary Reference Intakes for Vitamin C, Vitamin E, Selenium, and Carotenoids." National Academy Press, Washington, DC.

35. Mayne, S. T., and Vogt, T. M. (2000). Antioxidant nutrients in cancer prevention. *In* "Principles and Practice of Oncology (PPO) Updates" (V. T. DeVita, Jr., S. Hellman, and S. A. Rosenberg, Eds.), Vol. 14, pp. 1–12. Lippincott Williams & Wilkins Healthcare, New York.

36. Woodson, K., Tangrea, J. A., Barrett, M. J., Virtamo, J., Taylor, P. R., and Albanes, D. (1999). Serum alpha-tocopherol and subsequent risk of lung cancer among male smokers. *J. Natl. Cancer Inst.* **91,** 1738–1743.

37. Ratnasinghe, D., Tangrea, J. A., Forman, M. R., Hartman, T., Gunter, E. W., Qiao, Y. L., Yao, S. X., Barett, M. J., Giffen, C. A., Erozan, Y., Tockman, M. S., and Taylor, P. R. (2000). Serum tocopherols, selenium and lung cancer risk among tin miners in China. *Cancer Causes Control* **11,** 129–135.

38. Menkes, M. S., Comstock, G. W., Vuilleumier, J. P., Helsing, K. J., Rider, A. A., and Brookmeyer, R. (1986). Serum beta-carotene, vitamins A and E, selenium, and the risk of lung cancer. *N. Engl. J. Med.* **315,** 1250–1254.

39. Comstock, G. W., Alberg, A. J., Huang, H.-Y., Wu, K., Burke, A. E., Hoffman, S. C., Norkus, E. P., Gross, M., Cutler, R. G., Morris, J. S., Spate, V. L., and Helzlsouer, K. J. (1997). The risk of developing lung cancer associated with antioxidants in the blood: Ascorbic acid, carotenoids, alpha-tocopherol, selenium, and total peroxyl radical absorbing capacity. *Cancer Epidemiol. Biomarkers Prev.* **6,** 907–916.

40. van den Brandt, P. A., Goldbohm, A., van't Veer, P., Bode, P., Dorant, E., Hermus, R. J., and Sturmans, F. (1993). A prospective cohort study on selenium status and the risk of lung cancer. *Cancer Res.* **53,** 4860–4865.

41. Knekt, P., Aromaa, A., Maatela, J., Alfthan, G., Aaran, R. K., Hakama, M., Hakulinen, T., Peto, R., and Teppo, L. (1990). Serum selenium and subsequent risk of cancer among Finnish men and women. *J. Natl. Cancer Inst.* **82,** 864–868.

42. Knekt, P., Marniemi, J., Teppo, L., Heliovaara, M., and Aromaa, A. (1998). Is low selenium status a risk factor for lung cancer? *Am. J. Epidemiol.* **148,** 975–982.

43. Clark, L. C., Combs, G. F., Turnbull, B. W., Slate, E. H., Chalker, D. K., Chow, J., Davis, L. S., Glover, R. A., Graham, G. F., Gross, E. G., Krongrad, A., Lesher, J. L., Jr., Park, H. K., Sanders, B. B., Jr., Smith, C. L., and Taylor, J. R. (1996). Effects of selenium supplementation for cancer prevention in patients with carcinoma of the skin. *JAMA* **276,** 1957–1963.

44. Bandera, E. V., Freudenheim, J. L., Marshall, J. R., Zielezny, M., Priore, R. L., Brasure, J., Baptiste, M., and Graham, S. (1997). Diet and alcohol consumption and lung cancer risk in the New York State cohort (United States). *Cancer Causes Control* **8,** 828–840.

45. Speizer, F. E., Colditz, G. A., Hunter, D. J., Rosner, B., and Hennekens, C. (1999). Prospective study of smoking, antioxidant intake, and lung cancer in middle-aged women (USA). *Cancer Causes Control* **10,** 475–482.

46. Heimburger, D. C., Alexander, C. B., Birch, R., Butterworth, C. E., Bailey, W. C., and Krumdieck, C. L. (1988). Improvement in bronchial squamous metaplasia in smokers treated with folate and vitamin B_{12}: Report of a preliminary randomized, double-blind intervention trial. *JAMA* **259,** 1525–1530.

47. Rauscher, G. H., Mayne, S. T., and Janerich, D. T. (2000). Relation between body mass index and lung cancer risk in men and women never and former smokers. *Am. J. Epidemiol.* **152,** 506–513.

48. Alavanja, M. C. R., Brown, C. C., Swanson, C., and Brownson, R. C. (1993). Saturated fat intake and lung cancer risk among nonsmoking women in Missouri. *J. Natl. Cancer Inst.* **85,** 1906–1916.

49. Swanson, C. A., Brown, C. C., Brownson, R. C., and Alavanja, M. C. R. (1997). Re: Saturated fat intake and lung cancer risk among nonsmoking women in Missouri. *J. Natl. Cancer Inst.* **89,** 1724–1725.

50. Swanson, C. A., Brown, C. C., Sinha, R., Kulldorff, M., Brownson, R. C., and Alavanja, M. C. (1997). Dietary fats and lung cancer risk among women: The Missouri Women's Health Study (United States). *Cancer Causes Control* **8,** 883–893.

51. Ko, Y.-C., Cheng, L. S.-C., Lee, C.-H., Huang, J.-J., Huang, M.-S., Kao, E.-L., Wang, H.-Z., and Lin, H.-J. (2000). Chinese

food cooking and lung cancer in women nonsmokers. *Am. J. Epidemiol.* **151,** 140–147.

52. Shields, P. G., Xu, G. X., Blot, W. J., Fraumeni, J. F., Jr., Trivers, G. E., Pellizzari, E. D., Qu, Y. H., Gao, Y. T., and Harris, C. C. (1995). Mutagens from heated Chinese and U.S. cooking oils. *J. Natl. Cancer. Inst.* **87,** 836–841.

53. Sinha, R., Kulldorff, M., Curtin, J., Brown, C. C., Alavanja, M. C. R., and Swanson, C. A. (1998). Fried, well-done red meat and risk of lung cancer in women (United States). *Cancer Causes Control* **9,** 621–630.

54. Pastorino, U., Infante, M., Maioli, M., Chiesa, G., Buyse, M., Firket, P., Rosmentz, N., Clerici, M., Soresi, E., Valente, M., Belloni, P. A., and Ravasi, G. (1993). Adjuvant treatment of stage I lung cancer with high-dose vitamin A. *J. Clin. Oncol.* **11,** 1216–1222.

55. van Zandwijk, N., Dalesio, O., Pastorino, U., de Vries, N., and van Tinteren, H., for the European Organization for Research and Treatment of Cancer, Head and Neck and Lung Cancer Cooperative Groups (2000). EUROSCAN, a randomized trial of vitamin A and *N*-acetylcysteine in patients with head and neck cancer or lung cancer. *J. Natl. Cancer Inst.* **92,** 977–986.

56. Riboli, E., and Kaaks, R. (2000). Invited commentary: The challenge of multi-center cohort studies in the search for diet and cancer links. *Am. J. Epidemiol.* **151,** 371–374.

57. Koo, L. C. (1997). Diet and lung cancer 20+ years later: More questions than answers? *Int. J. Cancer* **10**(Suppl.), 22–29.

58. Pillow, P. C., Hursting, S. D., Duphorne, C. M., Jiang, H., Honn, S. E., Chang, S., and Spitz, M. R. (1997). Case-control assessment of diet and lung cancer risk in African Americans and Mexican Americans. *Nutr. Cancer* **29,** 169–173.

59. The Women's Health Initiative Study Group (1998). Design of the Women's Health Initiative clinical trial and observational study. *Controll. Clin. Trials* **19,** 61–109.

60. Rock, C. L., Newman, V., Flatt, S. W., Faerber, S., Wright, F. A., and Pierce, J. P. (1997). Nutrient intakes from foods and dietary supplements in women at risk for breast cancer recurrence. The Women's Healthy Eating and Living Study Group. *Nutr. Cancer* **29,** 133–139.

61. Kolonel, L. N., Henderson, B. E., and Hankin, J. H. (2000). A multiethnic cohort in Hawaii and Los Angeles: Baseline characteristics. *Am. J. Epidemiol.* **151,** 346–357.

62. Riboli, E., and Kaaks, R. (1997). The EPIC project: Rationale and study design. *Int. J. Epidemiol.* **26,** S6–S14.

CHAPTER **26**

Nutrition and the Patient with Cancer

BARBARA ELDRIDGE,[1] CHERYL L. ROCK,[2] AND PAULA DAVIS McCALLUM[3]

[1]*University of Colorado Health Sciences Center, Denver, Colorado*
[2]*University of California at San Diego, La Jolla, California*
[3]*Advantage Nutrition, Ltd., Chagrin Falls, Ohio*

I. INTRODUCTION

Nutrition is an important component of the management of individuals diagnosed with cancer. Whether undergoing active therapy, recovering from cancer treatment, or in remission and aiming to avoid recurrence, the potential importance of optimal energy and nutrient intake has been examined in numerous studies, with general agreement that there is a role for nutrition intervention specific to the situation and needs of the patient [1, 2]. The primary goals for nutrition intervention in cancer are to prevent or reverse nutrient deficiencies, to preserve lean body mass, to minimize nutrition-related side effects, and to maximize the quality of life. Consistent screening practices to identify patients at risk for malnutrition are essential. Nutrition therapy is an integral part of cancer care from diagnosis through treatment and recovery. Moreover, patients view diet and nutrition as a way to participate in their care. Providing sound, individualized nutritional guidance can be challenging due to the vast and often contradictory amount of information that is currently available. This chapter discusses nutrition issues that are pertinent for patients with cancer throughout the continuum of care and also presents practical nutrition management strategies for dealing with treatment-related side effects.

II. RATIONALE AND IMPORTANCE OF OPTIMAL NUTRITION

From an historical perspective, providing nutritional care to the patient with cancer has not always been believed to be wise or useful to incorporate in overall management. A few decades ago, fear that nutritional repletion would stimulate tumor growth, based on early studies with animal models, was a barrier to pursuing nutrition interventions in the patient with cancer [3]. In cell culture and animal studies, starvation has indeed been observed to slow tumor growth and proliferation of cancer cells [4, 5]. However, the health status of the host is concurrently adversely affected by nutritional depletion, and the malnutrition that results when nutrition intervention is not provided to the patient with cancer was historically a major cause of cancer-related mortality [6].

More recent laboratory studies have shown that when cancer is being treated, providing adequate energy and essential nutrients may possibly improve the efficacy and reduce the toxicity of chemotherapy and other cancer treatments [7], suggesting a potential beneficial role for maintaining adequate intake given the current improved approaches to cancer management. A number of clinical research studies have examined whether improving nutritional status can improve tolerance to oncologic therapies and reduce surgical complications in patients with cancer, and important factors determining benefit include the degree of risk for malnutrition that is present and the aggressiveness (with associated risk) of the nutrition intervention (discussed below).

The presence of cancer and cancer therapy can alter nutritional status significantly. Substantial weight loss and poor nutritional status have been documented in more than 50% of patients at the time of cancer diagnosis in clinical series reports [8, 9], although the prevalence of weight loss and malnutrition varies widely across cancer types. This point can be illustrated by results from a classic study of the prevalence and prognostic effect of weight loss prior to chemotherapy [10], in which data from 3,047 patients enrolled in 12 chemotherapy protocols of the Eastern Cooperative Oncology Group were examined and grouped according to weight loss as a percent of pre-illness weight. Patients with non-Hodgkin's lymphoma subtypes with favorable tumor tissue characteristics, breast cancer, acute nonlymphocytic leukemia, and sarcomas had the lowest prevalence of weight loss, with 60–69% of patients with those cancer types having no weight loss. Intermediate prevalence of weight loss, which was defined as a frequency of 48–61%, was observed in those with unfavorable non-Hodgkin's lymphoma subtypes, colon cancer, prostatic cancer, and lung cancer. The highest frequency of weight loss (83–87%) was observed in patients with pancreatic or gastric cancer, with approximately one-third of these patients reporting a loss of >10% of prediagnosis body weight. Also, these investigators found that when grouped by cancer type, tumor extent, and activity level, median survival time was shorter in those who had experienced weight loss compared with those who had not experienced weight loss [10].

Weight loss and poor nutritional status also have been suggested to be associated with lower scores on quality-of-life

measures in patients with cancer. For example, in a case series of 119 patients with gastrointestinal cancer [11], weight-stable patients (compared to weight-losing patients) had significantly higher scores in response to queries addressing physical, cognitive, and social functioning, although a causal relationship cannot be assumed in this cross-sectional study. However, depression and the loss of independence that result from nutritional depletion and debilitation are well-known clinical sequelae of malnutrition in patients with cancer [12], and the response of family and friends to cancer-related weight loss can add additional stress and anxiety to the patient's situation [4].

III. CANCER CACHEXIA

The predominant nutritional problem in patients diagnosed with cancer is a variant of protein energy malnutrition, which is commonly noted as a secondary diagnosis. Termed *cancer cachexia,* the syndrome is characterized by weight loss, anorexia, muscle wasting, increased basal metabolic rate, immunosuppression, and abnormalities in fluid status and energy metabolism. It differs from simple starvation-related protein energy malnutrition primarily because the compensatory mechanisms that would promote the preservation of muscle mass and adaptation to alternate fuels are apparently not operating.

The etiology of cancer cachexia is not entirely understood, and it can manifest in patients with metastatic cancer, as well as in patients with localized disease. Energy imbalance in these patients can be due to reduced intake and/or increased expenditure, with metabolic alterations contributing to the depletion of lean muscle mass.

A. Anorexia and Inadequate Dietary Intake

Inadequate dietary intake may be caused by anorexia or altered taste perceptions, or may be the result of systemic effects of the neoplastic process or tumor-related symptoms (especially if gastrointestinal tract malignancies are present) [13, 14]. Psychological problems such as anxiety, depression, and the emotional stress of diagnosis and treatment can also alter eating patterns and cause reduced intake. Anorexia is basically defined as loss of appetite or loss of the desire to eat [15]. Alterations in taste acuity and taste preferences also are often reported by patients diagnosed with cancer and may contribute to reduced dietary intake [16]. However, observations of taste perception abnormalities in patients with cancer must be interpreted cautiously if not adjusted for age or other factors known to influence this characteristic [17], and malnutrition itself is associated with changes in taste perception and preferences. An additional causal factor that can reduce the spontaneous intake of many patients with cancer is chemotherapy-induced changes in taste perceptions.

If the tumor involves the gastrointestinal tract, obstructions or tumor-related gastrointestinal symptoms, such as pain

or altered sensations when swallowing, can cause intake to be markedly reduced [18]. Ovarian cancer and metastatic melanoma tumors can cause external impingement on the gastrointestinal tract, so that eating is uncomfortable [14]. Treatments for cancer, including surgery, radiation therapy, and chemotherapy (discussed below), have associated side effects that can influence appetite and ability to eat comfortably.

Current evidence suggests that anorexia in patients with cancer also is likely caused in large part by systemic appetite-suppressing factors, such as cytokines, that are produced by the tumor cells and the immune cells [4]. These are the same factors that promote the metabolic alterations observed in cancer cachexia that result in the depletion of lean muscle mass (discussed below). Additionally, these factors also increase resting energy expenditure, so many patients experience weight loss despite normal or even above-normal dietary intake. The primary mechanism believed to be responsible for both anorexia and the metabolic characteristics of cancer cachexia is the interaction between the growing tumor and the immune system, which results in the production of cytokines (tumor necrosis factor, interleukin 1, interleukin 6, and alpha and gamma interferon), in addition to the secretion of hormonal factors that promote wasting [8, 9, 13].

B. Metabolic Abnormalities in Cancer Cachexia

The reader is referred to several comprehensive reviews of the metabolic alterations characteristic of cancer cachexia and the evidence linking the syndrome to the various circulating factors currently believed to be the primary causal agents [4, 8, 14, 19]. The overall features of cancer cachexia are similar to an acute metabolic stress response, in that the usual energy-conserving and protein-sparing metabolic adjustments to starvation are paradoxically absent in cancer cachexia.

Increased basal metabolic expenditure is often, but not always, observed in association with cancer cachexia [4]. Inconsistency in the findings in this area are likely due to patients being studied at various stages of illness and with differing nutritional status, as well as the methodological limitations in getting accurate measures in acutely ill and often hospitalized patients. In one clinical study involving patients with small cell lung cancer, a reduced or normalized level of basal energy expenditure was observed to occur in those who responded to chemotherapy, whereas patients who were nonresponders did not exhibit changes in basal energy expenditure [20], which supports the hypothesized causal role of tumor–host interactions. However, patients with cancer who are symptomatic or involved in treatments typically have lower amounts of physical activity, so their total energy expenditure may be similar to healthy subjects, despite increased levels of basal energy expenditure.

In contrast, increased protein turnover is quite consistently observed in patients with cancer cachexia, with skeletal muscle wasting resulting from increased glycolysis and decreased muscle protein synthesis [21]. Also typically present are increased lipolysis and decreased fat synthesis, due

to decreased lipoprotein lipase activity, which can result in elevated serum lipids [8]. Abnormalities of carbohydrate metabolism include decreased glucose tolerance, increased glucose uptake, and increased lactate production. The fundamental problem is cytokine-induced gluconeogenesis and the increasing utilization of protein stores for fuel, which also has been hypothesized to be linked to increased tumor uptake of glucose as a preferential substrate [22]. However, it has been well established in animal models that this metabolic problem is caused by the presence of the tumor and the associated circulating factors [4, 8, 19], so limiting the intake of carbohydrate (either sources or amounts), which has been suggested among various cancer-fighting strategies in popular literature aimed toward patients with cancer, would be unlikely to alter the prognosis or progression. With or without exogenous glucose and regardless of carbohydrate sources in the diet, endogenous glucose production (from protein stores) would continue to be stimulated by the cytokines and other tumor factors until the tumor is resected or the cancer is in remission.

In summary, the anorexia-cachexia syndrome is multifactorial. In addition to metabolic aberrations, patients with cancer may experience a gamut of nutrition-related symptoms that affect their ability to eat. It is important to note that many of these symptoms are interrelated and may be relieved by a combination of nutritional counseling or support and pharmaceutical management.

C. Pharmaceutical Management of Cancer Cachexia

Some patients suffer quite specifically from a lack of appetite as a primary factor leading to poor intake and weight loss. Those patients may benefit from appetite stimulants, which are ideally administered in combination with nutritional counseling and, in some cases, an anabolic agent. Published reviews on this topic include one on clinical studies of appetite-stimulating medications by Ottery *et al.* [23] and reviews on the rationale and research on pharmaceutical approaches to the management of cancer cachexia by Barber *et al.* [19] and Chlebowski [24].

Table 1 provides a list of common nutrition-related symptoms and the supportive drugs therapies that are used to manage them. Many of these medications can be administered concomitantly and are ideally accompanied by nutritional counseling.

IV. BASIC NUTRITION CONCEPTS FOR MANAGING PATIENTS WITH CANCER

Whatever the phase of treatment or recovery, individuals with cancer should strive to consume a nutritionally adequate diet. Eating well means including a variety of foods daily and consuming a diet that contains recommended amounts of the essential nutrients, including protein, carbo-

hydrate, fat, vitamins, minerals, and water, necessary to maintain health (see Chapter 48). During times of illness and recovery from cancer treatments, nutritional requirements are often increased and individuals may benefit from encouragement to consume nutrient-dense foods to ensure adequate nutrition and weight maintenance. As noted above, individuals that maintain body weight and nutrient stores may be able to better tolerate treatment-related side effects and recover from therapy more quickly. Improved nutrition status helps to maintain strength and energy, enhance quality of life, and repair and rebuild tissues that have been affected by cancer therapy [11, 25].

The American Cancer Society's Guidelines on Diet, Nutrition and Cancer Prevention (shown in Table 2 [26]) also provides sound advice regarding healthy eating for cancer prevention for all individuals, including cancer survivors [11]. An additional resource from the American Cancer Society summarizes current knowledge on nutrition for cancer survivors [27].

A. Intakes of Energy and Protein and Body Weight

Nutrition intervention for patients with cancer is basically supportive therapy, regardless of whether the current goal of care is curative or palliative. Patients often need encouragement to consume sufficient energy and protein to maintain their stores. Achievement and maintenance of an appropriate weight for their height can be another important issue. During the course of therapy and recovery, some individuals may need to increase their energy consumption for weight maintenance or desired weight gain, while others may need to decrease their energy intake for desired weight loss. However, weight lost during initial cancer therapy is more likely due to the loss of muscle (lean body mass) than fat stores. The loss of lean body mass can contribute to fatigue, adversely impact the immune system, and delay and lengthen recovery. Thus, even if patients are overweight, the maintenance of lean tissue and body cell mass should be encouraged during treatment and recovery. The reader is referred to a review of approaches to estimating energy requirements in Chapter 2.

Currently, the most widely used tool to estimate desirable body weight for height is the body mass index (see Chapter 31). Body mass index adjusts for height and has been shown to be highly correlated with actual adiposity. Based on available evidence, a body mass index range for best health is currently defined as 20–25 kg/m². Because more precise measures of body composition are generally not available for use in usual patient care settings, due to their high cost and limited accessibility, bioelectric impedance analysis is often used in this setting to estimate body composition, although there are some known limitations to this methodology. Even skinfold measurements and waist and hip circumferences can provide some insight about body composition in the patient with cancer.

TABLE 1   Common Supportive Drug Therapies for Nutrition-Related Symptoms

Nutrition-related symptom	Drug category	Drug(s)
Anemia	Hematopoietic agents	Epoetin alpha
Anorexia	Appetite stimulants	Dronabinol; megestrol acetate; corticosteroids
Constipation	Laxatives	Lactulose; bisacodyl; magnesium–citrate, hydroxide, sulfate; senna; cascara; casanthranol
	Stool softeners	Docusate sodium
Diarrhea	Antidiarrheals	Bismuth subsalicylate; loperimide; tincture of opium; diphenoxylate with aptropine; sandostatin
	Bulk-forming agents	Dietary fiber—psyllium, methycellulose
Early satiety	Prokinetic agents	Metoclopromide
Flatulence/bloating	Antacids	Aluminum hydroxide; magnesium hydroxide
	Antiflatulents	Simethicone
Malabsorption	Pancreatic enzymes	Pancrelipase; lactase; pancreatin
Mucositis	Topical anesthetics	Viscous xylocaine
	General mouth care	Sodium bicarbonate or saline mouth rinse; glutamine
Nausea	Antiemetics	Ondansetron hydrochloride; prochlorperazine; dronabinol; scopolamine
	Prokinetics	Metoclopromide
Neutropenia	Hematopoietic agents	Filgastim
Odynophagia	Topical anesthetics	Viscous xylocaine
	Analgesics	Nonopioids
	Narcotics	Opioids
Oral candidiasis	Antifungal agents	Fluconazole; ketoconazole; nystatin; clotrimazole lozenges
Pain	Analgesics	Nonopioids; acetaminophen; nonsteroidal antiinflammatories
	Narcotics	Opioids; morphine; hydromorphone
Taste changes	General mouth care	Sodium bicarbonate or saline mouth rinse
Thrombocytopenia	Hematopoietic agents	Sargramostim
Vomiting	Antiemetics	Ondansetron hydrochloride; prochlorperazine; dronabinol; scopolamine
	Cough suppressants and expectorants (for vomiting due to cough)	Guaifenesin; dextromethorphan hydrobromide
Weight loss	Anabolic agents	Oxandrolone; growth hormone
Xerostomia	General mouth care	Sodium bicarbonate or saline mouth rinse
	Mouth moisturizers	Saliva substitutes; lemon glycerine swabs
	Saliva stimulants	Pilocarpine hydrochloride

Source: Data drawn from [13, 71–73].

Protein needs are also increased in times of illness, therapy, and recovery. Extra protein is needed by the body to repair and to rebuild tissues affected by treatment and to maintain a healthy immune system. However, nitrogen and energy balance are inextricably linked, and if adequate energy is not consumed during times of stress, the body will use its protein reserves (lean body mass) as a fuel substrate.

B. Micronutrients

Some patients with cancer take large amounts of vitamin and mineral supplements because they are led to believe that these products can help to combat cancer or enhance their immune systems. Although essential micronutrients are necessary for optimal health, controlled clinical trials have not shown that vitamin and mineral supplements, even at high dosages, are useful in promoting cancer remission or improving cancer-related symptoms [27–29]. In fact, large doses of some vitamins can cause adverse side effects such as gastrointestinal discomfort [30], which can exacerbate eating problems in patients with cancer. Another current issue relates specifically to the antioxidant micronutrients, which are promoted for their ability to protect cells from free radical damage or oxidation. Radiation therapy and alkylating chemotherapy agents kill cancer cells by oxidative damage, so some researchers have expressed concern that large

TABLE 2 American Cancer Society Guidelines on Diet, Nutrition, and Cancer Prevention

1. Choose most of the foods you eat from plant sources.
   - Eat five or more servings of fruits and vegetables each day.
   - Eat other foods from plant sources, such as breads, cereals, grain products, rice, pasta, or beans several times each day.
2. Limit your intake of high-fat foods, particularly from animal sources.
   - Choose foods low in fat.
   - Limit consumption of meats, especially high-fat meats.
3. Be physically active—achieve and maintain a healthy weight.
   - Be at least moderately active for 30 minutes or more on most days of the week.
   - Stay within your healthy weight range.
4. Limit alcoholic beverages, if you drink at all.

Source: From American Cancer Society (1996). Advisory Committee on Diet, Nutrition, and Cancer Prevention (1996). Guidelines on diet, nutrition, and cancer prevention: Reducing the risk of cancer with healthy food choices and physical activity. *CA Cancer J. Clin.* **46,** 325–342.

doses of antioxidants, especially single nutrients, just before and during therapy may actually interfere with the action of prescribed anticancer therapeutic regimens [31]. Results from other studies using cell cultures, however, have suggested that antioxidants may enhance the effects of standard radiation and chemotherapy [32]. Thus, this is a controversial issue that is not fully resolved at this time.

When patients are able to consume a reasonably nutritious diet with adequate energy and protein, supplementation with vitamins and minerals is usually not necessary [27, 33]. Because non-nutrient constituents of foods may provide many health benefits, supplements should never replace the intake of regular foods and the goal of eating a healthy diet. However, if patients are experiencing difficulty eating and treatment-related side effects, the use of a multivitamin and mineral supplement that provides no more than 100% of the U.S. Recommended Dietary Allowances, is generally considered to be safe [34–37]. Patients should also be encouraged to communicate with their health care providers regarding their use of vitamin and mineral supplements. Developing and maintaining a good rapport and avoiding a judgmental attitude and demeanor can help to promote good communications and reduce the likelihood of harm from self-treatment with high-dose micronutrient supplements.

C. Importance of Regular Physical Activity

Although information is limited regarding the role of physical activity in the management of cancer patients and survival [27], regular physical activity is known to be associated with numerous health benefits. Increased physical activity has been shown to increase energy, improve of quality of life, and reduce fatigue and anxiety in patients with cancer [38]. Other benefits include improved maintenance of lean body mass, maintenance of mobility, and stress reduction. However, before participating in any type of physical activity or exercise program, patients with cancer should be advised to obtain an evaluation by qualified professionals for an individualized physical assessment and plan specific to their capabilities and needs.

D. Complementary and Alternative Medicine

Survey studies suggest that more than half of all patients with cancer use some form of complementary or alternative therapies [39]. Patients seek complementary and alternative medicine for a variety of reasons: to promote health and prevent cancer; to replace conventional therapies that have been exhausted, shown to be ineffective, or are associated with side effects and significant risk; or to gain control over their own care [40]. The American Cancer Society defines complementary therapies as supportive methods that are used to complement evidence-based treatment, to help control symptoms, and to improve well-being and quality of life [41]. Alternative therapies refer to treatments that are promoted as cancer cures and are unproven or scientifically disproved methods. Categories of nutrition-related complementary and alternative therapies include vitamin and mineral supplementation, single- or multinutrient preparations; herbals (leaves of a plant) and botanicals (seeds, stem, roots); and nutrition (diet) and metabolic therapies. Examples of complementary and alternative medicines commonly used by patients with cancer are listed in Table 3.

Currently, the U.S. Food and Drug Administration does not regulate herbal and botanical products, and patients need to be aware that just because products may be "natural" they may not be safe (see Chapter 17). General guidelines for selecting herbals and botanicals include using only standardized extracts or products that list plant components and their quantities; buying products manufactured by reputable companies that are prepared, standardized, and manufactured with quality control; and using low, conservative doses. Patients should also be advised that many of the alternative nutrition and diet therapies advocated require substantial changes in regular eating habits and may be nutritionally inadequate. As noted above, patients need to be encouraged to discuss their use of complementary and alternative therapies with their health care professionals.

V. NUTRITION ISSUES THROUGHOUT THE CONTINUUM OF CARE

Cancer and cancer therapy can increase nutritional needs significantly, as well as affect normal digestion, absorption, and metabolism. Many individuals experience treatment-related side effects such as fatigue, loss of appetite, taste alterations, nausea, vomiting, and changes in bowel function that can further impair their ability to consume adequate

TABLE 3 Common Complementary and Alternative Medicines for Patients with Cancer

Herbals and botanicals	Proposed uses and cautions
Echinacea (purple cone flower)	*Proposed use:* Colds, flu, fever; respiratory and lower urinary tract infections. *Caution:* Contraindicated for individuals with autoimmune diseases and allergies to daisies; numbing of the tongue; not for long-term use.
Zingiber officinale (ginger)	*Proposed use:* Antiemetic; calming odor and aroma. *Caution:* While effective in motion-related nausea, may not be effective in chemotherapy-induced nausea.
Caulophyllum thalictroides (black cohosh)	*Proposed use:* Management of menopausal symptoms (hot flashes and dysmenorrhea) *Caution:* Large doses may cause dizziness, nausea, headaches, hypotension.
Serenoa repens (saw palmetto)	*Proposed use:* Relief of urinary symptoms in benign prostate hyperplasia; no scientific evidence that it is an effective treatment for prostate cancer. *Caution:* Rare headaches, mild abdominal pain, nausea and dizziness; antiestrogen.
PC-SPECS (combination of seven Chinese herbs and saw palmetto)	*Proposed use:* Has estrogenic activity and can cause decreases in blood testosterone levels; not a proven treatment for prostate cancer, although clinical trials are underway. *Caution:* Potential side effects include elevation of blood pressure, increased levels of estrogen, and formation of blood clots in legs and lungs.
Silybum marianum (milk thistle)	*Proposed use:* Antioxidant; limited evidence to support that use will prevent liver damage during and following chemotherapy. *Caution:* May delay the clearance of chemotherapeutic agents by the liver.
Flaxseed (containing omega-3, -6, and -9 fatty acids) and fish oils (containing omega-3 fatty acids)	*Proposed use:* In animal studies have been shown to have a possible anticancer effect; fish oils linked with cardiovascular disease prevention and an anti-inflammatory agent. *Caution:* Flaxseed contains compounds that may be estrogenic; gastrointestinal upset with ingestion of large amounts; fish oils may worsen glucose tolerance and can increase bleeding time.
Soy and soy foods	*Proposed use:* Inconsistent scientific evidence in the use of soy foods in primary and secondary cancer prevention. *Caution:* May not be appropriate for women with hormone-responsive cancers.
Teas	*Proposed use:* Antioxidant; enhances immune system. *Caution:* Due to the caffeine content may cause insomnia, nervousness, and irregular heart rate; available in decaffeinated forms; antiplatelet effect.

Nutrition (diet) therapies	Overview and reason for caution
Macrobiotic diet	*Overview:* Emphasis on whole foods (grains, cereals, vegetables, sea vegetables, beans, fermented soy, fruits, nuts, seeds, and soups); individualized diet based on whether cancer is "yin," "yang," or "neutral." *Caution:* May be inadequate in energy and micronutrients; restrictive; considerable meal planning and preparation.
Gerson therapy	*Overview:* Cleansing and detoxifying program, raw fruit and vegetable regimen that includes juice therapy (13 glasses/day) and fresh calf's liver solution daily. *Caution:* Restrictive; difficult to follow.
Kelley regime	*Overview:* Includes the consumption of 25 nutritional supplements and digestive enzymes, detoxifying treatments such as coffee enemas, moderate exercise, fasting, and purging. *Caution:* Restrictive; difficult to follow.
Juice therapies	*Overview:* Uses fresh fruit and vegetable juice regimen to cleanse and detoxify the body. *Caution:* Inadequate in energy and macro/micronutrients; may eliminate fiber found in whole fruits and vegetables, depending on the juicer used.

Source: Data from [74–81].

energy and essential nutrients. Side effects of therapy are usually temporary, although some individuals may experience lasting changes that affect their ability to eat and maintain optimal nutritional status.

A. Nutritional Screening and Assessment of the Patient with Cancer

Screening and nutritional assessment should be interdisciplinary; the health care team (e.g., physicians, nurses, registered dietitians, social workers) should all be involved in the nutritional management of patients throughout the continuum of care. Basic concepts and components of nutritional assessment are described in Part 1 of this text and are reviewed in detail elsewhere [42]. In the clinical setting, indices that incorporate several aspects of nutritional assessment are often useful. An example of one of these nutritional screening and assessment tools is the Scored Patient-Generated Subjective Global Assessment. This global assessment tool is adapted from the original Subjective Global Assessment, developed by Detsky, to include the patient responses and more cancer-specific symptoms [43, 44]. The scored version is a further adaptation by Ottery and colleagues that also includes guidelines for the triage of nutritional therapy [45].

The Scored Patient-Generated Subjective Global Assessment is an easy-to-use, inexpensive approach that can be used in multiple clinical settings and is ideal for interdisciplinary use. Patients and/or caregivers complete sections on weight history, food intake, symptoms, and functioning. A health care team member evaluates weight loss, disease, and metabolic stress and performs a nutrition-related physical examination. A score is generated from the information collected. The need for nutrition intervention is determined according to the score.

B. Routes of Providing Nutritional Support and Care

Ideally, all patients with cancer should be screened and assessed for nutritional risk at the time of diagnosis and reevaluated throughout the course of their treatment and recovery. In general, care of the patient with cancer involves individualized guidance on the appropriate routes of intake and on how best manage treatment-related side effects. Prompt determination and early intervention of nutrition-related problems are vital for improving outcomes.

Because of the well-established adverse effect of poor nutritional status on morbidity and mortality, and the high prevalence of malnutrition in this population, numerous clinical trials of the effect of nutrition intervention on various outcome measures in patients with cancer have been conducted and reported during the 1980s and 1990s. However, the overwhelming majority of these intervention trials have involved total parenteral nutrition, which carries risk for infection and other complications. In contrast, few research

efforts have tested the efficacy of lower risk nutrition interventions, such as nutritional counseling and dietary manipulations, and more research on these interventions in this patient population is sorely needed.

1. ORAL INTAKE

If at all possible, oral nutrition is the preferred route for feeding. Specifically, several strategies have been proposed for modifying the diet according to patients' specific needs as dictated by their disease processes and treatment-related side effects (see Table 4). Also, the use of liquid nutritional supplements may be necessary for patients unable to consume sufficient energy and protein to maintain their weight and optimum nutritional status (see Chapters 15 and 16).

A telephone-based follow-up study of nutrition counseling was reported by Schiller et al. [46], with a study population consisting of 400 patients who had been referred for nutrition counseling, of whom 4% of the sample were patients with cancer. Overall, the counseling interaction was found to be well received by the patients, with 85% reporting at follow-up that they knew what to eat after talking with the dietitian, and 62% reporting that they had changed their diets following the counseling while 44% reported health-related changes. In a study of diet modification specifically relevant to patients with cancer, Menashian et al. [47] tested the effect of a modified diet to help control nausea and vomiting in 19 patients receiving cisplatin chemotherapy. Patients in the study group who were advised to consume the modified diet, which consisted of foods observed clinically to be better tolerated during chemotherapy, experienced fewer episodes of emesis when compared to the control subjects and 57% less volume of emesis on the first day of treatment.

2. ENTERAL NUTRITION

When patients are unable to meet their nutritional needs orally, other routes of nutrition support need to be considered. Enteral nutrition is indicated when patients cannot eat due to mechanical obstruction or prolonged anorexia, or if they cannot consume adequate oral intake due to treatment-related toxicities (i.e., odynophagia, mucositis, esophagitis) [48]. Feeding enterally, rather than parenterally, helps to reduce infectious complications such as bacterial translocation, by preserving gut barrier and immune function. Enteral nutritional formulas may be administered via nasoenteric tube for short-term use. A nasoenteric tube may be advanced through the stomach to the proximal duodenum to reduce the risk for aspiration. More permanent feedings may be administered via gastrostomy or jejunostomy directly into stomach or small intestine, respectively (see Chapter 16 for a more detailed discussion). This approach has been demonstrated to be an efficient method of providing long-term enteral nutrition support and is generally more acceptable to patients than using a nasoenteric tube [48].

Based on nutritional status at presentation, existing comorbidity, and prescribed cancer treatments, many patients

TABLE 4   Nutrition Management Strategies for Patients with Cancer

Nutrition-related side effect	Nutrition management strategies
Anorexia (loss of appetite)	Eat smaller, more frequent meals and snacks. Include energy-dense, high-protein foods and snacks throughout the day. Keep easy-to-prepare and easy-to-eat foods on hand. Create pleasant meal settings. Experiment with new foods. Light exercise. Pharmaceutical approach—Appetite stimulants may be indicated.
Constipation	Use of a fiber-rich diet, including the consumption of fresh fruits and vegetables, dried fruits, nuts, seeds, whole grains, and cereals. Drink lots of fluids to help keep stools soft. Light exercise. Avoidance of gas-forming foods and beverages (e.g., dried beans and peas, cruciferous vegetables, melons, carbonated beverages). Pharmaceutical approach—Use of stool softeners and laxatives may be indicated.
Diarrhea	Use of a low-residue or fiber-restricted diet. Eat smaller, more frequent meals and snacks. If lactose intolerance is present, avoidance of lactose-containing foods and beverages. If fat intolerance is present, avoidance of high-fat, greasy foods. Drink lots of fluids for minimizing the occurrence of dehydration. Avoidance of gas-forming foods and beverages (e.g., dried beans and peas, cruciferous vegetables, melons, carbonated beverages). Avoidance of coffee and other caffeinated beverages. Pharmaceutical approach—Use of antidiarrheals, bulk-forming agents, or pancreatic enzymes may be indicated.
Early satiety (feeling of fullness)	Eat smaller, more frequent meals and snacks. Include energy-dense, high-protein foods and snacks throughout the day. Avoidance of gas-forming foods and beverages (e.g., dried beans and peas, cruciferous vegetables, melons, carbonated beverages) may be beneficial. Avoidance of high-fat or greasy foods that are more slowly digested and absorbed. Avoid drinking large amounts of fluids at one time.
Fatigue	Eat smaller, more frequent meals and snacks. Include energy-dense, high-protein foods and snacks throughout the day. Keep easy-to-prepare and easy-to-eat foods on hand. Light activity may be beneficial. Accept help from friends and family members for help with food procurement and meal preparation.
Flatulence/bloating/gas	Eat smaller, more frequent meals and snacks. Avoidance of gas-forming foods and beverages (e.g., dried beans and peas, cruciferous vegetables, melons, carbonated beverages). Avoidance of high-fat or greasy foods that are more slowly digested and absorbed. Light activity. Pharmaceutical approach—Use of antiflatulents and antacids may be indicated.
Hyperglycemia	Limit the amounts of total carbohydrate consumed, if excessive. Regularly scheduled meals and snacks each day—do not skip meals. Consumption of a balanced diet at each meal eaten—including a source of fat and protein at each meal. Attention to portion size. If thirsty, quench thirst with water or other noncaloric beverages. Weight maintenance. Light activity. Pharmaceutical approach—Use of antihyperglycemics may be indicated.
Mucositis and stomatitis	Avoidance of tart, acidic, or spicy foods and beverages. Avoidance of rough-textured foods. Cool foods and beverages may be more soothing. Use of a semisolid or soft food diet. Keep mouth clean—good oral care is essential (i.e., regular brushing and rinsing). Pharmaceutical approach—Use of topical anesthetics may be indicated.

(continues)

TABLE 4 *(continued)*

Nutrition-related side effect	Nutrition management strategies
Nausea and vomiting	Eat smaller, more frequent meals and snacks. Eat slowly. Use bland, easy-to-digest foods and beverages. Drink lots of fluids throughout the day for minimizing the occurrence of dehydration. Avoidance of strong cooking odors. Avoidance of gas-forming foods and beverages (e.g., dried beans and peas, cruciferous vegetables, melons, carbonated beverages). Avoidance of high-fat or greasy foods that are more slowly digested and absorbed. Light activity. Pharmaceutical approach—Use of antiemetics may be indicated.
Neutropenia (low blood counts)	Cook all foods thoroughly; avoid raw eggs, fish, meat, and poultry. Wash hands frequently. Keep hot foods hot and cold foods cold. Avoidance of spoiled, moldy, or damaged foods—cheeses, fruits, and vegetables. Do not buy or use canned or packaged foods and beverages that are swollen, dented, or damaged. Check expiration dates on all canned or packaged foods and beverages. Avoid salad bars, food buffets, and large groups of people when dining out. Avoid untested well water. Avoid unpasteurized beverages. Pharmaceutical approach—Use of hematopoietic agents may be indicated.
Odynophagia and dysphagia	Avoidance of rough-textured foods. Cool foods and beverages may be more soothing. Use of a semisolid or soft food diet. Pharmaceutical approach—Use of topical anesthetics and pain medications may be indicated.
Pain	Take pain medications with food. Eat smaller, more frequent meals and snacks. Include energy-dense, high-protein foods and snacks throughout the day. If present, management of constipation. Pharmaceutical approach—Use of opioids and other medications for pain may be indicated.
Taste and odor changes	Serve foods cold, because hot foods produce stronger flavors and smells. Experiment with new foods, seasonings, marinades, and flavors. Use mints, lemon drops, or gum throughout the day to leave a more pleasing taste in the mouth. Keep mouth clean—good oral care is essential (regular brushing and rinsing). If a metallic taste is present, the use of plastic and glass utensils and cookware may be beneficial.
Weight gain	Regularly scheduled meals and snacks each day—do not skip meals. Consumption of a balanced diet at each meal eaten. Attention to portion size. Regular light activity and exercise. Limit obviously energy-dense and high-fat foods. Drink plenty of water and other noncaloric beverages throughout the day. Weight maintenance while on active cancer therapy.
Weight loss	Eat smaller, more frequent meals and snacks. Include energy-dense, high-protein foods and snacks throughout the day. Keep easy-to-prepare and easy-to-eat foods on hand. Use of liquid nutrition supplements and homemade drinks/shakes. To gain lean body mass, a combination of regular light activity and an additional 500–1000 kcal/day above the normal requirement is needed. Pharmaceutical approach—Appetite stimulants or anabolics may be indicated.
Xerostomia	Drink plenty of fluids throughout the day. Use of a semisolid or soft food diet. Use sugarless mints, lemon drops, or gum throughout the day to leave a more pleasing taste in the mouth. Keep mouth clean—good oral care is essential (regular brushing and rinsing). Add moisture (broth, sauces, gravies, butter, or margarine) to foods and meals consumed. Avoid commercial mouthwashes containing alcohol. Use of a humidifier to moisten room air especially at night. Pharmaceutical approach—Use of saliva stimulants or substitutes may be indicated.

may benefit from prophylactic placement of percutaneous endoscopic gastrostomy feeding tubes to deliver enteral nutrition support [49]. Feeding tubes usually need to remain in place through recovery to ensure normalization of oral intake and weight. One instance in which enteral (tube) feeding may be superior to oral feeding is when elemental diets are used. These diets may help to maintain energy and nutrient intakes in some circumstances, for example, during pelvic radiation therapy, when absorptive capabilities are limited.

3. PARENTERAL NUTRITION

The reader is referred to several recent [4, 8, 14, 19, 48] and early [24, 50, 51] reviews of the numerous clinical trials of total parenteral nutrition in the care of patients before and during treatments for cancer. This approach, when applied without specific inclusion criteria, has not been shown to improve nutritional measures in the average patient with cancer and is actually associated with increased risk of complications such as infections. In 1989, the American College of Physicians published a position paper concluding that parenteral nutrition support was associated with net harm in patients with cancer [52].

However, parenteral nutrition support may be appropriate for some patients with cancer for whom oral intake or enteral nutrition is not an option. The main concern is with the indiscriminate use in patients who are undergoing routine cytotoxic treatments and who do not have preexisting malnutrition. For example, in the classic Veterans Affairs Total Parenteral Nutrition Cooperative Study [53], 395 patients who required laparotomy or noncardiac thoracotomy, with the majority having a diagnosis of cancer, were randomly assigned to receive either total parenteral nutrition for 7–15 days prior to surgery and 3 days afterward or no perioperative parenteral nutrition support. Overall, there were more infectious complications in the parenteral nutrition group than in the controls. However, among those who were severely malnourished based on global assessment score, patients who received total parenteral nutrition had fewer noninfectious complications than controls (relative risk 0.12, 95% confidence interval 0.02–0.91) with no increase in infectious complications [52]. Another situation in which total parenteral nutrition is currently believed to be beneficial in the management of patients with cancer is in bone marrow transplantation (discussed below) [14]. As summarized by Mercadante [48], the use of parenteral nutrition support should be considered adjuvant treatment and support during therapy for malnourished patients or in those with severely impaired gastrointestinal function who are otherwise expected to survive.

In the care of patients who are managed with parenteral nutrition, complications include potential for fluid overload in patients receiving blood products, chemotherapy and medications via peripheral or central access; hyperglycemia secondary to the high concentration of dextrose present in parenteral mixtures and insulin resistance associated with

severe illness; electrolyte imbalance; and increased triglycerides in patients receiving lipid emulsions. Intense monitoring of parenteral nutrition is required to minimize possible complications and to ensure that nutritional needs are being met appropriately.

C. Nutritional Effects of Cancer Therapies

Conventional methods of cancer treatment include surgery, radiation therapy, and chemotherapy. In many instances, patients receive multimodality therapy to most effectively treat their cancers. Prompt nutritional screening and assessment followed by appropriate pharmaceutical intervention and nutritional counseling to manage treatment-related side effects may help improve tolerance to therapy and enable patients to recover more quickly. Patients receiving aggressive cancer therapy (e.g., bone marrow transplantation) typically need aggressive nutrition support. The following sections review common treatment-related side effects and possible nutrition implications.

1. SURGERY

After surgery, sufficient energy and protein are required for wound healing and recovery. Many patients experience pain, fatigue, and loss of appetite, and are unable to consume their regular diet because of surgery-related side effects. The surgical removal or resection of any part of the alimentary tract can impair digestion (including mastication) and absorption substantially. Most side effects are temporary and dissipate within a few days of the surgical procedure. Some surgical interventions, however, may have long-lasting nutritional implications. Medications, adherence to postsurgery discharge instructions, and changes in diet can help reduce the side effects experienced. Most patients benefit from some type of a diet progression (i.e., clear liquids, then easy-to-digest foods, then regular diet) in the first few days postoperatively. Table 5 lists common side effects of cancer surgery.

2. CHEMOTHERAPY

Chemotherapy involves the use of chemical agents and medications to treat cancer and is a systemic therapy that affects the whole body [14]. The action of chemotherapeutic agents can be cytotoxic to normal cells as well as malignant cells, in particular cells with a rapid turnover such as bone marrow, hair follicles, and mucosa of the alimentary tract. Common side effects with nutritional implications include loss of appetite, fatigue, nausea, vomiting, mucositis, taste alterations, xerostomia, dysphagia, and changes in bowel function. These agents can also adversely impact renal and hepatic function, as well as cause damage to the gastrointestinal tract, which can result in the impairment of digestion and absorption, further compromising nutritional status. Chemotherapy can also cause immunosuppression, resulting in neutropenia, thrombocytopenia, and anemia. The severity

TABLE 5 Common Side Effects of Cancer Surgery

Surgery site	Commonly experienced side effects
Tongue	Difficulty with chewing and swallowing Sore mouth Dysgeusia Xerostomia Loss of appetite Fatigue
Mandible	Difficulty with chewing Taste changes Xerostomia Sore mouth Loss of appetite Fatigue
Esophagus	Acid reflux Indigestion Difficulty with swallowing Loss of appetite Fatigue
Stomach	Early satiety Gastric reflux Dumping syndrome Dehydration Loss of appetite Fatigue
Small intestine	Malabsorption Fat intolerance Lactose intolerance Diarrhea Dehydration Loss of appetite Fatigue
Colon—resection	Increased transit time Diarrhea Dehydration Bloating, cramping, and/or gas Loss of appetite Fatigue
Rectum—resection	Increased rectal pressure Changes in usual bowel habits Loss of appetite Fatigue
Pancreas	Loss of appetite Alterations in carbohydrate metabolism (hyperglycemia) Bloating, cramping, and/or gas Changes in usual bowel habits Fat intolerance Fatigue
Lung	Shortness of breath Loss of appetite Early satiety Fatigue
Breast	Fatigue Loss of appetite Weight gain

(continues)

TABLE 5 *(continued)*

Surgery site	Commonly experienced side effects
Prostate	Changes in urination habits Loss of appetite Fatigue
Brain	If on corticosteroids, changes in sleep and appetite and possible elevation in blood glucose levels Nausea Fatigue
Gynecological	Bloating or gas Fatigue Early satiety Loss of appetite

of the side effects experienced is related to the prescribed treatment regimen: single or combination agent therapy, dose administration, planned number of cycles, individual response, and current health status. The timely and appropriate use of supportive therapies and medications are important to the effective management of treatment-related side effects.

3. RADIATION THERAPY

Radiation therapy can be delivered from an outside source into the body (external beam therapy) or by placing a radioactive source inside the body (brachytherapy or internal therapy). Whereas chemotherapy is a systemic treatment, radiation therapy and surgery only affect the tumor and the area surrounding it. Some chemotherapy agents may be given in combination with radiation therapy due to their radiation-enhancing effects. Patients receiving multimodality therapy may manifest side effects sooner and with greater toxicity. Side effects are most commonly site specific (i.e., limited to the area being treated). Patients generally begin to notice the effects of external beam radiation therapy after 8–10 days of treatment, and side effects usually resolve within 2–4 weeks after treatment is complete. Regardless of the site of radiation therapy, patients usually experience some degree of fatigue, loss of appetite, and skin changes and hair loss in the treated area. Use of supportive therapies and medications are important in the management of treatment-related side effects. Table 6 lists common side effects of radiation therapy.

D. Nutrition Concerns during and after Recovery from Cancer Therapy

After treatment ends, optimal nutrient intake and physical activity are vital to the recovery process. Lingering effects of treatment may require continued attention and appropriate nutrition intervention. Patients should be encouraged to strive for weight stabilization or increased energy and

TABLE 6 Common Side Effects of Radiation Therapy

Site of radiation therapy	Commonly experienced side effects
Brain	Nausea; vomiting; elevated blood glucose due to steroid administration; fatigue; loss of appetite
Head and neck	Xerostomia; sore mouth; dysphagia; odynophagia; taste alterations; mucositis; fatigue; loss of appetite
Lung, esophagus, and breast	Dysphagia; heartburn; fatigue; loss of appetite
Abdomen	Nausea; vomiting; fatigue; loss of appetite
Pelvis	Changes in bowel function—diarrhea, gas, bloating, cramping; milk intolerance; fatigue; loss of appetite
Bone	Fatigue; loss of appetite; constipation due to pain medication

TABLE 7 Late-Occurring Side Effects with Nutritional Implications

Osteoradionecrosis of the mandible and increased incidence of dental caries in patients following head and neck irradiation— Difficulty with chewing and swallowing.

Fibrosis of the esophagus after head and neck irradiation— Dilation of the esophagus may be necessary and/or a speech pathology consultation for swallowing evaluation and management is indicated.

Pneumenitis after lung irradiation—Difficulty with breathing and increased fatigue.

Chemotherapy-induced neuropathies of the fingers and toes— Patients may experience decreased sensation, causing difficulty with food procurement and food preparation.

Radiation enteritis after pelvic irradiation—Alterations in digestion and absorption; patients may need to restrict (or limit) lactose, fiber, and/or fat.

Bowel obstruction following pelvic irradiation for gynecological cancer—Often requires the use of enteral nutrition to bypass the obstructed area, or parenteral nutrition may be indicated.

protein intake to achieve and maintain normal body weight. The ideal is to return to normal eating and to achieve a weight that is appropriate for height. For many patients, their precancer diagnosis diets may have been poor, and due to increased health concerns, they may be interested in improving their eating habits.

Whereas the acute toxicities of surgery, chemotherapy, and radiation therapy may become apparent during the course of treatment, some side effects may not manifest until several weeks, months, or even years after the treatment has been completed. Examples of treatment-related late-occurring side effects with nutrition implications are listed in Table 7. Patients living with chronic treatment-related side effects face challenges with eating. Patients need to be reassessed during follow-up for late effects of treatment and receive appropriate nutrition intervention.

E. Nutritional Care for Advanced Cancer and Palliative Care

Management of nutrition-related symptoms continues in the care of patients living with advanced cancer. Emphasis should be placed on enhancing quality of life. Assisting patients in symptom management eases feelings of anxiety and fear, and helps them to maintain their sense of independence. The reader is referred to previous reviews on the ethical and feeding issues in advanced disease [54, 55].

VI. SPECIAL SITUATIONS

A. Bone Marrow Transplantation

Bone marrow and stem cell transplant procedures can impact nutrition status significantly, and nutrition is an important part of the management of patients who are recipients of bone marrow transplantation. To eradicate malignant cells, cytotoxic conditioning regimens are given with or without total body irradiation, followed by an intravenous infusion of bone marrow or stem cells. Effects of therapy include immunosuppression lasting 2–4 weeks post-transplant, anorexia, xerostomia, dysgeusia, stomatitis, oral and esophageal mucositis, and diarrhea. Immunosuppressive medications also have significant nutrition implications that can result in multiple problems with eating. Using isotopic dilution technology to assess body composition, Cheney et al. [56] documented decreased body cell mass and negative nitrogen balance in patients receiving bone marrow transplantation for acute lymphocytic leukemia. Thiamin deficiency, a reduction in the plasma pool of vitamin E, and electrolyte and trace element deficiencies also have been observed in patients receiving bone marrow transplantation [57–59]. A majority of these patients currently receive much of their care outside of the hospital, so nutritional assessment and monitoring is critically important in their care.

Awareness of the actions and the nutrition implications of cytotoxic and immunosuppressive agents can help health care professionals be proactive in patient care in this circumstance. Because the majority of patients undergoing bone marrow transplantation are unable to eat sufficient quantities of food to achieve the estimated energy requirement (or maintain the level of intake reported at admission), alternative routes to nutrition support are usually considered and have become a standardized component of care at most transplant centers.

Historically, parenteral nutrition has been considered the method of choice for ensuring nutritional adequacy in bone marrow transplantation, mainly due to the likelihood that

gastrointestinal symptoms of considerable severity may be present. Because of the high level of risk for nutritional problems in these patients, parenteral nutrition support may even be initiated and utilized as prophylaxis, and is usually not discontinued until the patient demonstrates the ability to consume a sufficient amount of the oral diet to achieve a predetermined goal level of nutritional requirements (ranging from 50% to 70%). The usefulness of tube feeding is often limited by the presence of mucosal and esophageal ulceration, nausea and vomiting, and local infection of the mouth and esophagus, even when gut function appears normal. In clinical trials, total parenteral nutrition has been shown to result in significantly higher energy and protein intake when compared with allowing patients to consume an oral diet *ad libitum* [60]. However, parenteral nutrition has not been consistently associated with favorable effects on duration of hospitalization, episodes of bacteremia, or total number of complications in these patients, and it has been suggested that intestinal mucosal integrity is better maintained by using enteral rather than parenteral nutrition support [57, 61]. In practice, aggressive parenteral nutrition support is also more likely to result in fluid overload, hyperglycemia, and catheter-related complications in these patients [62]. The goal is always to promote the progression toward achieving regular oral intake as a component of normal functioning and recovery, which may be impeded or delayed when patients are discharged on parenteral nutrition. In a controlled trial in which outpatient parenteral nutrition was compared with intravenous hydration, parenteral nutrition was associated with delayed resumption of oral intake after transplantation, while failing to provide any substantial improvement in patient outcome [63].

In another prospective randomized study [64], total parenteral nutrition was compared with an individualized enteral feeding program that involved close monitoring, snacks, and/or tube feeding. Approximately one-quarter of the patients assigned to the enteral nutrition group ultimately had to receive parenteral nutrition due to intolerance of the tube feeding, but parenteral nutrition did not shorten the duration of marrow aplasia and was associated with more complications related to feeding route (i.e., fluid overload requiring diuretics). Also worth noting is that the cost of the enteral nutrition intervention (which included individualized attention and snacks) for the 28-day feeding period was less than half that of the parenteral nutrition approach. Results from other studies of enteral nutrition support suggest that, when tolerated, this approach is effective, probably underutilized, and may even impart some special protective effects [57, 61].

Modifications in the parenteral nutrition solutions used in the nutrition support of bone marrow transplant patients, such as the addition of certain amino acids (i.e., glutamine, arginine) or omega–3 fatty acids, are also currently under study. The addition of glutamine, which is not considered an essential amino acid, is based on the rationale that it may improve intestinal mucosal integrity, reduce the incidence of

bacterial translocation, and improve nitrogen balance. In a small clinical trial, Ziegler *et al.* [65] demonstrated that glutamine-supplemented parenteral nutrition after bone marrow transplantation was associated with improved nitrogen balance, reduced incidence of clinical infection, lower rates of microbial colonization, and reduced hospital stay compared with patients receiving standard parenteral nutrition support. However, no differences in the incidence of fever or time of recovery from myelosuppression were observed. This is currently an area of great interest.

A major complication of allogenic transplant (related or unrelated donor) is graft-versus-host disease, in which donor cells react against the tissues of the host. Graft-versus-host disease can manifest in up to two-thirds of bone marrow transplant recipients and may occur as early as 7–10 days after the bone marrow infusion [66]. Although rare, graft-versus-host disease has also been documented in patients receiving autologus (patient's own bone marrow) and stem cell transplants. Major organs affected by graft-versus-host disease are the intestinal tract, skin, and liver. Side effects of graft-versus-host disease include skin rash, nausea, vomiting, abdominal cramping and/or pain, secretory diarrhea, malabsorption, and liver dysfunction. Patients with acute gut involvement require nutritional management that consists of bowel rest and parenteral nutrition followed by a diet progression for reintroducing foods.

Following transplantation, patients become immunocompromised, so supportive therapy to prevent infection is essential. In general, patients need to be instructed on food safety practices including avoidance of eating foods that contain unsafe levels of bacteria (raw meats, spoiled or moldy foods, and unpasteurized beverages); importance of thorough hand washing; special handling of raw meats, fish, poultry, eggs, utensils, cutting boards and countertops; and storage of foods at appropriate temperatures (below 40°F and above 140°F).

A low-microbial or low-bacteria diet, which is based primarily on empiric knowledge of the distribution of microorganisms in the food supply, is often prescribed for these patients. These diets consist mainly of cooked foods, because the major limitation imposed is on fresh or uncooked food items. In a few previous studies, the microbial content of several food items has been actually evaluated [67, 68]. Only a few previous studies have evaluated the acceptability and efficacy of low-microbial diets in patients receiving bone marrow transplantation. The large variability in how these diets are actually defined across institutions contributes to the difficulty in examining the clinical impact. In an early review of studies on immunosuppressed patients with cancer who were treated with sterile, low-microbial, or regular diets, it was concluded that the question of whether infection, morbidity, mortality, and response to therapy are affected by this strategy cannot be adequately addressed, due in part to variability across patients, interventions, and other influencing factors [69]. Because many food restrictions are imposed

with this strategy if strictly followed, the nutrient adequacy of actual intake of patients who are prescribed the low-microbial diet should be monitored.

B. Nutritional Care for Pediatric Patients with Cancer

Working with pediatric cancer patients can be challenging, due to their fears of cancer treatment and their apprehension regarding unfamiliar routines and caregivers. In addition, parents and family members may feel overwhelmed by the demands of their child's therapy, as well as the treatment-related side effects that their child may experience. The overall goals for nutritional care of the child with cancer include the management of nutrition-related symptoms and side effects, and the provision of adequate energy and nutrients for proper growth and development. The reader is referred to Andrassy and Chwals [70] for a review of the issues and scientific basis of nutritional support of the pediatric patient with cancer.

VII. SUMMARY AND CONCLUSIONS

Nutrition plays an important role in the management of the patient with cancer. Metabolic alterations caused by the presence of cancer and numerous adverse effects of treatments for cancer increase the risk for malnutrition in this patient population. Appropriate nutritional care may improve the patient's tolerance of treatments and also the quality of life during treatment and recovery. Patients with cancer have increased likelihood of using complementary and alternative approaches to care, some of which involve nutritional supplements and dietary manipulations. Although a variety of techniques and strategies may be useful in the nutritional care of these patients, more clinical studies are needed to demonstrate the specific usefulness of these approaches and the overall efficacy of nutrition intervention.

References

1. Rivlin, R. S., Shils, M. E., and Sherlock, P. (1983). Nutrition and cancer. *Am. J. Med.* **75**, 843–854.
2. McCallum, P., and Polisana, C. (2000). "The Clinical Guide to Oncology Nutrition." American Dietetic Association, Chicago, IL.
3. Copeland, E. M. (1998). Historical perspective on nutritional support of cancer patients. *CA Cancer J. Clin.* **48**, 67–68.
4. Brody, J. J. (1999). The syndrome of anorexia-cachexia. *Curr. Opin. Oncol.* **11**, 255–260.
5. Torosian, M. H., and Donoway, R. B. (1991). Total parenteral nutrition and tumor metastasis. *Surgery* **109**, 597–601.
6. Warren, S. (1932). The immediate cause of death in cancer. *Am. J. Med. Sci.* **184**, 610.
7. Branda, R. F., Nigels, E., Lafayette, A. R., and Hacker, M. (1998). Nutritional folate status influences the efficacy and toxicity of chemotherapy in rats. *Blood* **92**, 2471–2476.
8. Langstein, H., and Norton, J. (1991). Mechanisms of cancer cachexia. *Hematol. Oncol. Clin. North Am.* **5**, 103–123.
9. McMahon, K., Decker, G., and Ottery, F. (1998). Integrating proactive nutritional assessment in clinical practices to prevent complications and cost. *Semin. Oncol.* **25**, 20–27.
10. DeWys, W. D., Begg, C., Lavin, P. T., Band, P. R., Bennett, J. M., Bertino, J. R., Cohen, M. H., Douglass, H. O., Engstrom, P. F., Ezdinli, E. Z., Horton, J., Johnson, G. J., Moertel, C. G., Oken, M. M., Perlia, C., Rosenbaum, C., Silverstein, M. N., Skeel, R. T., Sponzo, R. W., and Tormey, D. C. (1980). Prognostic effect of weight loss prior to chemotherapy in cancer patients. Eastern Cooperative Oncology Group. *Am. J. Med.* **69**, 491–497.
11. O'Gorman, P., McMillan, D. C., and McArdle, C. S. (1998). Impact of weight loss, appetite, and the inflammatory response on quality of life in gastrointestinal cancer patients. *Nutr. Cancer* **32**, 76–80.
12. Wilkes, G. (2000). Nutrition: The forgotten ingredient in cancer care. *Am. J. Nurs.* **100**, 46–51.
13. Nelson, K., Walsh, D., and Sheehan, F. (1994). The anorexia-cachexia syndrome. *J. Clin. Oncol.* **12**, 213–225.
14. Rivadeneira, D. E., Evoy, D., Fahey, T. J., Lieberman, M. D., and Daly, J. M. (1998). Nutritional support of the cancer patient. *CA Cancer J. Clin.* **48**, 69–80.
15. Cangiano, C., Laviano, A., Muscaritoli, M., Meguid, M. M., Cascino, A., and Fanfelli, F. R. (1996). Cancer anorexia: New pathogenic and therapeutic insights. *Nutr.* **12**(Suppl.), S41–S51.
16. Trant, A. S., Serin, J., and Douglass, H. O. (1982). Is taste related to anorexia in cancer patients? *Am. J. Clin. Nutr.* **36**, 45–58.
17. Drewnowski, A. (1997). Taste preferences and food intake. *Ann. Rev. Nutr.* **17**, 237–253.
18. Machin, J., and Shaw, C. (1998). A multidisciplinary approach to head and neck cancer. *Eur. J. Cancer Care* **7**, 93–96.
19. Barber, M. D., Ross, J. A., and Fearon, K. C. H. (2000). Disordered metabolic response with cancer and its management. *World J. Surg.* **24**, 681–689.
20. Jebb, S. A., Osborne, R. J., Dixon, A. K., Bleehen, N. M., and Elia, M. (1994). Measurements of resting energy expenditure and body composition before and after treatment of small cell lung cancer. *Ann. Oncol.* **5**, 915–919.
21. Shaw, J. H., Humberstone, D. M., Douglas, R. G., and Korea, J. (1991). Leucine kinetics in patients with benign disease, non-weight-losing cancer, and cancer cachexia: Studies at the whole-body and tissue level and the response to nutritional support. *Surgery* **109**, 37–50.
22. Kallinowski, F., Schlenger, K. H., Runkel, S., Kloes, M., Stoherrer, M., Okunieff, P., and Vaupel, P. (1989). Blood flow, metabolism, cellular microenvironment and growth rate of human xenografts. *Cancer Res.* **49**, 3759–3764.
23. Ottery, F. D., Walsh, D., and Strawford, A. (1998). Pharmacologic management of anorexia/cachexia. *Semin. Oncol.* **25** (Suppl.), 35–44.
24. Chlebowski, R. T. (1991). Nutritional support of the medical oncology patients. *Hematol. Oncol. Clin. N. Am.* **5**, 147–160.
25. Levy, M., Ottery, F., and Hermann, J. (1992). Supportive care in oncology. *Curr. Prob. Cancer* **16**, 329–418.

26. The American Cancer Society 1996 Advisory Committee on Diet, Nutrition, and Cancer Prevention (1996). Guidelines on diet, nutrition, and cancer prevention: Reducing the risk of cancer with healthy food choices and physical activity. *CA Cancer J. Clin.* **46,** 325–342.

27. American Cancer Society Workgroup on Nutrition and Physical Activity for Cancer Survivors (2001). Nutrition after cancer: A guide for informed choices. *CA Cancer J. Clin.* **51** (in press).

28. Creagan, E. T., Moertel, C. G., O'Fallon, J. R., Schutt, A. J., O'Connell, M. J., Rubin, J., and Frytak, S. (1979). Failure of high-dose vitamin C (ascorbic acid) therapy to benefit patients with advanced cancer. A controlled trial. *N. Engl. J. Med.* **301,** 687–690.

29. Moertel, C. G., Fleming, T. R., Creagan, E. T., Rubin, J., O'Connell, M. J., and Ames, M. M. (1985). High-dose vitamin C versus placebo in the treatment of patients with advanced cancer who have had no prior chemotherapy. A randomized double-blind comparison. *N. Engl. J. Med.* **312,** 137–141.

30. Miller, D. R., and Hayes, K. C. (1982). High dose vitamin C versus placebo in the treatment of patients with advanced cancer who have had no prior chemotherapy. *N. Engl. J. Med.* **312,** 137–141.

31. Bruemmer, B. (1997). Nutrition dialogue. *Marrow Transpl. Nutr. Network* **4,** 3.

32. Prasad, K., Kumar, A., Kochupillai, V., and Cole, W. (1999). High doses of multiple antioxidant vitamins: Essential ingredients in improving the effectiveness of standard cancer therapy. *J. Am. College Nutr.* **18,** 13–25.

33. American Dietetic Association (1996). Position of the American Dietetic Association: Vitamin and mineral supplementation. *J. Am. Diet. Assoc.* **96,** 73–77.

34. Monsen, E. R. (2000). Dietary reference intakes for the antioxidant nutrients: Vitamin C, vitamin E, selenium, and carotenoids. *J. Am. Diet. Assoc.* **100,** 637–640.

35. Food and Nutrition Board, Institute of Medicine (2000). "Dietary Reference Intakes for Vitamin C, Vitamin E, Selenium, and Carotenoids." National Academy Press, Washington, DC.

36. Food and Nutrition Board, Institute of Medicine (1998). "Dietary Reference Intakes for Calcium, Phosphorus, Magnesium, Vitamin D, and Fluoride." National Academy Press, Washington, DC.

37. Food and Nutrition Board, Institute of Medicine (1998). "Dietary References Intakes for Thiamin, Riboflavin, Niacin, Vitamin B6, Folate, Vitamin B12, Pantothenic Acid, Biotin, and Choline." National Academy Press, Washington, DC.

38. Courneya, K., and Friedenreich, C. (1999). Physical exercise and quality of life following cancer diagnosis: A literature review. *Ann. Behav. Med.* **21,** 1–9.

39. Brigden, M. (1993). Unproven (questionable) cancer therapies. *West. J. Med.* **163,** 463–469.

40. Eisenberg, D. (1997). Advising patients who seek alternative medical therapies. *Ann. Intern. Med.* **127,** 61–69.

41. American Cancer Society (1999). "American Cancer Society Operation Statement on Complementary and Alternative Methods of Cancer Management." American Cancer Society, Atlanta, GA.

42. Simko, M. D., Cowell, C., and Gilbride, J. A. (1995). "Nutrition Assessment." Aspen, Gaithersburg, MD.

43. Detsky, A., McLaughlin, J., Baker, J., Johnston, N., Whittaker, S., Mendelson, R. A., and Jeejeebhoy, K. N. (1987). What is subjective global assessment of nutritional status? *J. Parenteral Enteral Nutr.* **11,** 8–13.

44. Ottery, F. (1996). Definition of standardized nutritional assessment and interventional pathways in oncology. *Nutrition* **12**(Suppl.), S15–S19.

45. McCallum, P. (2000). Patient-generated subjective global assessment. *In* "Clinical Guide to Oncology Nutrition" (P. D. McCallum and C. G. Polisena, Eds.), pp. 11–23. The American Dietetic Association, Chicago, IL.

46. Schiller, M. R., Miller, F., Moore, C., Davis, E., Dunn, A., Mulligan, K., and Zeller, P. (1998). Patients report positive nutrition counseling outcomes. *J. Am. Diet. Assoc.* **98,** 977–982.

47. Menashian, L., Flam, M., Douglas-Paxton, D., and Raymond, J. Improved food intake and reduced nausea and vomiting in patients given a restricted diet while receiving cisplatin chemotherapy. *J. Am. Diet. Assoc.* **92,** 58–61.

48. Mercadante, S. (1998). Parenteral versus enteral nutrition in cancer patients: Indications and practice. *Support Care Cancer* **6,** 85–93.

49. Eldridge, B. (1992). Effectiveness of percutaneous endoscopic feeding tubes placed in head and neck radiation therapy patients. *J. Parenteral Enteral Nutr.* **16**(Suppl.).

50. Lipman, T. O. (1991). Clinical trials of nutritional support in cancer. *Hematol. Oncol. Clin. North Am.* **5,** 91–102.

51. Chen, M. K., Souba, W. W., and Copeland, E. M. (1991). Nutritional support of the surgical oncology patient. *Hematol. Oncol. Clin. North Am.* **5,** 125–145.

52. American College of Physicians (1989). Parenteral nutrition in patients receiving cancer chemotherapy. *Ann. Intern. Med.* **110,** 734–736.

53. The Veterans Affairs Total Parenteral Nutrition Cooperative Study Group (1991). Perioperative total parenteral nutrition in surgical patients. *N. Engl. J. Med.* **325,** 525–532.

54. American Dietetic Association (1992). Position of the American Dietetic Association: Issues in feeding the terminally ill adults. *J. Am. Diet. Assoc.* **92,** 996–1002.

55. Burck, R. (1996). Feeding, withdrawing, and withholding: Ethical perspectives. *Nutr. Clin. Prac.* **11,** 2143–2153.

56. Cheney, C. L., Abson, K. G., Aker, S. N., Lenssen, P., Cunningham, B. A., Buergel, N. S., and Thomas, E. D. (1987). Body composition changes in marrow transplant recipients receiving total parenteral nutrition. *Cancer* **59,** 1515–1519.

57. Hermann, V. M., and Petruska, P. J. (1993). Nutrition support in bone marrow transplant recipients. *Nutr. Clin. Prac.* **8,** 19–17.

58. Rovelli, A., Bonomi, M., Murano, A., Locasciulli, A., and Uderzo, C. (1990). Severe lactic acidosis due to thiamine deficiency after bone marrow transplantation in a child with acute monocytic leukemia. *Haematologica* **75,** 579–581.

59. Clemens, M. R., Ladner, C., Ehninger, G., Einsele, H., Renn, W., Buhler, E., Waller, H. D., and Gey, K. F. (1990). Plasma vitamin E and β-carotene concentrations during radiochemotherapy preceding bone marrow transplantation. *Am. J. Clin. Nutr.* **51,** 216–219.

60. Weisdorf, S. A., Lysne, J., Wind, D., Haake, R. J., Sharp, H. L., Goldman, A., Schissel, K., McGlave, P. B., Ramsay, N. K., and Kersey, J. H. (1987). Positive effect of prophylactic total parenteral nutrition on long-term outcome of bone mineral transplantation. *Transplantation* **43,** 833–838.

61. Papadopoulou, A., MacDonald, A., Williams, M. D., Darbyshire, P. J., and Booth, I. W. (1997). Enteral nutrition after bone marrow transplantation. *Arch. Dis. Child.* **77,** 131–136.

62. Taveroff, A., McArdle, A. H., and Rybka, W. B. (1991). Reducing parenteral energy and protein intake improves metabolic homeostasis after bone marrow transplantation. *Am. J. Clin. Nutr.* **54,** 1087–1092.

63. Charuhus, P. M., Fosberg, K. L., Bruemmer, B., Aker, S. N., Leisenring, W., Seidel, K., and Sullivan, K. M. (1997). A double-blind randomized trial comparing outpatient parenteral nutrition with intravenous hydration: Effect on resumption of oral intake after marrow transplantation. *J. Parenteral Enteral Nutr.* **21,** 157–161.

64. Szeluga, P. J., Stuart, R. K., Brookmeyer, R., Utermohlen, V., and Santos, G. (1987). Nutritional support of bone marrow transplant recipients: A prospective, randomized clinical trial comparing total parenteral nutrition to an enteral feeding program. *Cancer Res.* **47,** 3309–3316.

65. Ziegler, T. R., Young, L. S., Benfell, K., Scheltinga, M., Hortos, K., Bye, R., Morrow, F. D., Jacobs, D. O., Smith, R. J., Antin, J. H., and Wilmore, D. W. (1992). Clinical and metabolic efficacy of glutamine-supplemented parenteral nutrition after bone marrow transplantation. *Ann. Intern. Med.* **116,** 821–828.

66. Charuhas, P. (1993). Dietary management during antitumor therapy of cancer patients. *Topics Clin. Nutr.* **9,** 42–53.

67. Pizzo, P. A., Purvis, D. S., and Water, C. (1982). Microbiological evaluation of food items. *J. Am. Diet. Assoc.* **82,** 272–279.

68. Moe, G. (1991). Enteral feeding and infection in the immunocompromised patient. *Nutr. Clin. Prac.* **6,** 55–64.

69. Aker, S. N., and Cheney, C. L. (1983). The use of sterile and low microbial diets in ultraisolation environments. *J. Parenteral Enteral Nutr.* **7,** 390–397.

70. Andrassy, R. J., and Chwals, W. J. (1998). Nutritional support of the pediatric oncology patient. *Nutrition* **14,** 124–129.

71. Murphy, S., and Von Roenn, J. (2000). Pharmacological management of anorexia and cachexia. *In* "Clinical Guide to Oncology Nutrition" (P. D. McCallum and C. G. Polisena, Eds.), pp. 127–133. The American Dietetic Association, Chicago, IL.

72. Eldridge, B. (2000). Chemotherapeutic and nutrition implications. *In* "Clinical Guide to Oncology Nutrition" (P. D. McCallum and C. G. Polisena, Eds.), pp. 61–69. The American Dietetic Association, Chicago, IL.

73. Levy, M. (1991). Constipation and diarrhea in cancer patients. *Cancer Bull.* **43,** 412–422.

74. Blumenthal, M., Busse, W. R., Goldberg, A., Hall, T., Riggins, C. W., and Rister, R. S., eds.; Klein, S., and Rister, R. S., translators (1998). "The Complete German E Monographs: The Therapeutic Guide to Herbal Medicines." American Botanical Council, Austin, TX.

75. Cassielith, B. (1998). "The Alternative Medicine Handbook." W.W. Norton, New York.

76. Montbriand, M. (1994). An overview of alternative therapies chosen by patients with cancer. *Oncol. Nurs. Forum* **21,** 1547–1554.

77. Spaulding-Albright, N. (1997). A review of some herbal and related products commonly used in cancer patients. *J. Am. Diet. Assoc.* **97**(Suppl.), S208–S215.

78. Tyler, V., and Foster, S. (1999). "The Honest Herbal," 4th Edition. Haworth Press, Binghamton, NY.

79. Tyler, V. (1994). "Herbs of Choice." Haworth Press, Binghamton, NY.

80. (1998). "Physician's Desk Reference on Herbal Medicine." Medical Economics, Montvale, NJ.

81. Molseed, L. (2000). Alternative therapies in oncology. *In* "Clinical Guide to Oncology Nutrition" (P. D. McCallum and C. G. Polisena, Eds.), pp. 150–159. The American Dietetic Association, Chicago, IL.

C. Diabetes Mellitus

CHAPTER **27**

Obesity and the Risk for Diabetes

REJEANNE GOUGEON
McGill University, Montreal, Quebec, Canada

I. INTRODUCTION

It has long been recognized that one of the medical consequences of obesity is development of type 2 diabetes mellitus. Epidemiological studies, both cross sectional [1–12] and prospective [8, 13–22], show a positive relationship between degree of obesity, notably that of central adiposity [7, 11, 15, 16], and the risk for diabetes. Two large prospective studies have examined the impact of obesity on the incidence of diabetes in women [23] and in men [22] and calculated that 77% of new cases in women and 64% in men could be prevented if body mass index [BMI, weight (kg)/height (m²)] were maintained below 25 kg/m². An increase in the prevalence of obesity in certain countries may well explain the concurrent increase in diabetes prevalence [24, 25]. Furthermore, body fat mass has also been shown to be associated with an increase in the risk of prediabetic conditions such as glucose intolerance and insulin resistance [6].

Despite these strong associations with diabetes, obesity does not appear to be an essential condition for type 2 diabetes to express itself in a genetically predisposed person. Indeed, 20–25% of persons with type 2 diabetes are not obese [23, 26, 27], and 80% of individuals with elevated BMI and indicators of high intra-abdominal adiposity do not develop diabetes [23]. Still, the improvement in diabetes control observed with weight loss [27–30] indicates that obesity has an impact on diabetes and its prevention and management. This chapter will examine some of the mechanisms that relate increased adiposity to diabetes, and the independent contribution of risk factors for obesity such as low physical activity level and unhealthy diets to the development of diabetes. This chapter (1) provides the current definitions and diagnostic criteria of obesity and diabetes, (2) reexamines some of the evidence that suggests a major role for excess adiposity in the etiology of diabetes and its complications, and (3) describes the contributions of weight loss and energy restriction in the management of the obese persons with diabetes.

II. DEFINITIONS AND CLASSIFICATIONS OF OBESITY AND DIABETES

A. Obesity

Obesity has been explained as the result of an imbalance between the intake of energy substrates and energy utiliza-

tion [31]. This imbalance promotes the shunting of substrates into anabolic pathways for synthesis and storage of fat [31]. Obesity is referred to as a condition when fat accumulation is excessive to an extent that it increases risk of ill health [32], especially if it is stored in the abdominal region [33]. Obesity may well represent a heterogeneous group of conditions. Because obesity has been poorly defined, it has been difficult to establish what role it plays in the etiology of diabetes. A World Health Organization (WHO) expert committee has proposed cutoff points for the classification of overweight and obesity [34] such that it would be possible to identify individuals or groups at risk and to compare weight status across populations. A classification can also provide a basis for the evaluation of interventions. Body mass index values (using BMI calculated as the weight in kilograms divided by the square of height in meters) have been used to classify obesity in populations because they correlate with percentage of body fat and with mortality and morbidity. Furthermore, the values are the same for both sexes because the relationship between BMI and mortality is similar in men and women. Because women have a higher percentage body fat for a comparable weight than men, this indicates that women can carry fat better than men. It has been suggested that they do so because their excess fat is mainly subcutaneous and peripherally distributed (thighs, buttocks, breasts) compared with men in whom fat is stored in the abdominal region [35].

The classification proposed by WHO [Table 1 [34]) is based on the relationship between BMI and mortality. BMIs between 18.5 and 24.9 kg/m² are defined as normal, between 30 and 39 as obese, and >40 as severely obese [35]. A BMI >30 does not always correspond to excess adiposity. A muscle builder may have a BMI of 30 that is associated with a large muscle mass. Ethnic groups with deviating body proportions, such as being very tall and thin, have healthy BMIs ranging from 17 to 22 kg/m² and have excessive fat mass at a BMI of 25 [36].

Cutoff points have also been defined for waist circumference, which is another simple measure for predicting excess visceral adipose tissue [37]. It also predicts risk of cardiovascular disease and relates to both BMI and the waist: hip ratio.

Waist circumference ≥94 cm in men [37 inches] and ≥80cm [32 inches] in women indicates a need for concern [38]and ≥102 cm [40 inches] in men and ≥88 cm [35 inches]

TABLE 1 Cutoff Points for Body Mass Index

BMI (kg/m²)	WHO classification of obesity
<18.5	underweight
18.5–24.9	normal range
25.0–29.9	grade 1 overweight
30.0–39.9	grade 2 overweight
≥40.0	grade 3 overweight

Source: World Health Organization (1997). Obesity: Preventing and managing the global epidemic. Report of a WHO Consultation presented at the World Health Organization, June 3–5, 1997. Publication WHO/NUT/NCD/98.1. World Health Organization, Geneva, Switzerland.

in women are critical levels of intra-abdominal fat [37] that indicate a need for action and intervention (Table 2).

A decrease in waist circumference in response to intervention is an indication of a decrease in risk for chronic disease [39]. The waist circumference measured at the narrowest part of the torso, at midpoint between the lower border of the rib cage and the iliac crest, alone, is considered a useful tool for initial screening and follow-up assessment of change.

Visceral fat prediction can be obtained by more complex methods such as computed tomography scans [40]. These can measure sagittal diameters from which abdominal subcutaneous fat measured by ultrasound can be subtracted for more precision [41].

B. Diabetes Mellitus

Diabetes mellitus is a heterogeneous group of metabolic diseases characterized by elevated blood glucose concentration and disturbances of carbohydrate, fat, and protein metabolism secondary to absolute or relative deficiency in insulin action and/or secretion [42, 43].

An untreated person with diabetes will present the following symptoms: excessive thirst, polyuria, pruritus, blurred vision, and unexplained weight loss. Asymptomatic diabetes, particularly type 2 diabetes mellitus, may be diagnosed when abnormal blood or urine glucose levels are found during routine testing. Exposure to chronic hyperglycemia is associated with pathologic and functional changes in organs such as the eyes, blood vessels, heart, kidneys, and nerves [43].

The classification of diabetes mellitus is based primarily on its clinical description and comprises four major types: type 1, type 2, other specific types, and gestational diabetes mellitus. All differ in their etiology. For example, type 1 diabetes, which is prone to ketoacidosis, is due to autoimmune or idiopathic destruction of the β cells of the pancreas, destruction that results in a deficiency in insulin secretion. Type 2 diabetes is due to metabolic abnormalities leading to a diminished response to the action of insulin, along with a defect in insulin secretion. Other types relate to genetic defects, pancreatopathy or are first diagnosed during pregnancy

TABLE 2 Cutoff Points for Waist Circumferences

Waist circumference	Men	Women
Need for concern	≥94cm	≥80cm
Critical level	≥102cm	≥88cm

Source: National Heart, Lung, and Blood Institute, Obesity Education Initiative Expert Panel (1998). Clinical guidelines on the identification, evaluation, and treatment of overweight and obesity in adults: The evidence report. *Obes. Res.* **6** (Suppl. 2), 51S–209S.

(such as gestational diabetes), and may or may not subsequently develop into diabetes after parturition [44].

The classification also includes impaired glucose tolerance and impaired fasting glucose because of their association with increased risk of developing diabetes and cardiovascular disease [45].

In a previous classification [42], subgroups were identified to distinguish obese and non obese persons within the type 2 diabetes and impaired glucose tolerance categories; insulin resistance was reported to be accentuated in subjects who have central obesity and are physically inactive, implicating body weight and fat distribution as risk factors for glucose intolerance.

1. WHO HAS DIABETES?

Although diabetes is characterized by alterations of fat [46] and of protein metabolism [47, 48], glucose impairment remains the hallmark of diabetes diagnosis and control.

The diagnosis of diabetes mellitus is made using one of three methods recommended by the American Diabetes Association:

1. A person shows symptoms of diabetes (polyuria, polydipsia, unexplained weight loss) and has a plasma glucose concentration, measured at any time of day, regardless of time of meal, greater than 11.1 mmol/L (≥200 mg/dL).
2. A person has a fasting plasma glucose concentration ≥7.0 mmol/L (≥126 mg/dL), with fasting meaning at least 8 hours after food consumption.
3. A person has a plasma glucose concentration ≥11.1 mmol/L (≥200 mg/dL) two hours after an oral intake of 75 g anhydrous glucose dissolved in water; this procedure is called an oral glucose tolerance test (OGTT). The 11.1 mmol/L cutoff point for the 2-hour postload glucose of the OGTT has been chosen because in large population studies, it is approximately at that point that the prevalence of complications specific to diabetes, such as retinopathy and nephropathy, increases significantly and dramatically [43]. Studies in Pima Indians, in Egyptians, and in the National Health and Nutrition Examination Survey (NHANES) III (reported in [43]) show strong associations between retinopathy and both fasting plasma glucose and 2-hour postload glucose concentrations. Furthermore, the prevalence of arterial

disease strongly relates with fasting plasma glucose and 2-hour postload glucose concentrations [49], and their thresholds for increased risk of macrovascular disease correspond with the values recommended for the diagnosis of diabetes.

Fasting plasma glucose values have been established to define normality: fasting plasma glucose < 6.1 mmol/L (<110 mg/dL) and to define an intermediate category that is too high to be considered normal but too low for a diagnosis of diabetes. That category is called impaired fasting glucose and corresponds to glucose values between 6.1 and 7.0 mmol/L (110 and 126 mg/dL).

The results of an OGTT are classified within one of three categories:

1. One of normal glucose tolerance when the 2-hour postload glucose is <7.8 mmol/L (<140 mg/dL).
2. One of impaired glucose tolerance when the 2-hour postload glucose is ≥7.8 mmol/L (≥140 mg/dL) but <11.1 mmol/L (<200 mg/dL).
3. One of a provisional diagnosis of diabetes that needs to be confirmed on a subsequent day, when the 2-hour postload glucose is ≥11.1 mmol/L (≥200 mg/dL)

Criteria have been established [43] to determine when testing for diabetes should be done in order to optimize the prevention of the disease and its complications. These criteria recommend that testing be done in all individuals over 45 and, when results are normal, be repeated every 3 years thereafter. However, testing should be done at a younger age and more frequently in individuals who are obese or have a BMI >27 kg/m². This indicates that obese individuals are considered more at risk of having undiagnosed diabetes and experiencing chronic hyperglycemia, a factor known to contribute to microvascular and macrovascular diseases. The early detection and treatment of this disease could decrease mortality and minimize complications, especially those related to renal disease, peripheral vascular disease, and cardiovascular disease [42]. Thus testing individuals at high risk becomes highly cost effective and has implications in the prevention of diabetes [42]. Obese individuals are such individuals at high risk [43].

III. WHY ARE THE OBESE AT RISK?

A. Epidemiological Evidence

Obesity has been implicated as a risk factor for diabetes in cross-sectional [50–52] and longitudinal studies [53–61]. Population-based studies have shown strong associations between central adiposity, assessed by measurements of skinfolds on the trunk, and type 2 diabetes [59, 62, 63]. Ratios of waist-to-hip circumferences have been reported to be highly predictive of not only abnormal blood lipids and lipoproteins, but of glucose intolerance as well [1–21, 64–69]. Prospective studies have provided evidence that, as overall adiposity and upper-body adiposity increased, so did the risk of developing diabetes [69, 70]. Elevated glucose concentrations were likewise associated with a greater risk for diabetes [70, 71]. One prospective study of Mexican-Americans, a population at high risk for this disorder [72], reported that the subjects who developed diabetes after a follow-up of 8 years had initially higher BMIs and central adiposities and were characterized by higher fasting glucose and insulin concentrations [17]. However, although BMI and ratio of subscapular-to-triceps skinfolds related to onset of diabetes in an univariate analysis, they no longer were significant predictors of diabetes in a multivariate analysis that included glucose and insulin concentrations. Such results indicated that obesity per se was not essential for the development of diabetes, but that diabetes most likely resulted from alterations in insulin metabolism.

The hyperinsulinemia, an indirect indicator of insulin resistance, mediated the development of diabetes in subjects characterized by an unfavorable body fat distribution [72]. However, in other population studies carried out in whites [56], Nauruans [73], and Japanese [74], obesity remained an independent predictive factor after adjusting for glucose and insulin, indicating that it may act through other pathways than insulin action and secretion. Even if insulin and glucose concentrations are better predictors of diabetes and their screening identifies the subjects who could benefit from intervention, it remains true that more obese than lean persons are at risk of being resistant to insulin and are candidates who can benefit from weight loss and improved physical fitness. Oral glucose tolerance tests were used to assess type 2 diabetes mellitus and IGT in a large multiethnic population in Mauritius. In that population, age, family history, overall body mass, abdominal fat, and low physical activity scores were independent risk factors for diabetes [5]. However, there were ethnic differences in the relative importance of some factors. For example, physical inactivity had a lower impact in the Chinese of both sexes and so did the waist-to-hip ratio, than in Muslim women. In other ethnic groups, the waist-to-hip ratio was a stronger predictor for glucose intolerance than BMI in women compared to men, for whom it was the reverse.

The data analyzed from a large cohort of 51, 529 U.S. male health professionals, 40–75 years of age, and followed during 5 years, show that as BMI increased beyond 24 kg/m², the risk for diabetes increased. It was 77 times greater in men whose BMI was >35 kg/m² than in lean men. This study provides strong evidence that weight gain during adult life increases the risk of developing diabetes. In men who had gained more than 11 kg, their relative risk was amplified according to their BMI at age 21 years by 6.3 with a BMI <22, by 9.1 with a BMI of 22–23 and by 21.1 with a BMI >24 kg/m² [22].

The data also suggested that waist circumference was a better predictor of diabetes than waist:hip ratio [22]. The reliability of waist and hip measurements is limited by their difficulty and the fact that they are taken at different sites of the body in various studies. Nevertheless, population data report strong associations between waist-to-hip ratio and

glucose intolerance [8], accounting for the associations with body mass index. A high prevalence of diabetes has been found in populations that have a tendency for central adiposity and have been exposed to the Westernization of their lifestyle and its consequence, weight gain [75].

B. Fetal Origins of Type 2 Diabetes and Obesity

Some individuals may be more prone to insulin resistance and diabetes with weight gain if they have been malnourished *in utero*. Malnutrition during pregnancy forces the fetus to adapt during its development to an extent that permanent changes occur in the structure and the physiology of its body [76]. These changes seen in low-birth-weight infants have been identified as contributing factors in adult life to chronic diseases like type 2 diabetes mellitus, coronary heart disease, stroke and hypertension [76–78]. It was first reported in England at the beginning of the 1990s that middle-aged adults who had low weights at birth and during infancy were at greater risk of type 2 diabetes and insulin resistance [78]. This association was confirmed in later studies in Europe and the United States [79–81] suggesting that endocrine and metabolic adaptations induced by malnutrition could explain insulin resistance in skeletal muscle.

These associations only applied to infants born of mothers without gestational diabetes. The infants of the latter, by contrast, tended to be of high birth weight (macrosomia), but also at risk for developing type 2 diabetes as adults [81].

Prenatal exposure to the Dutch famine in 1944 was associated with lower glucose tolerance and insulin resistance in the offsprings once adults, even if the famine had little effect on their birth weights [82]. These associations support a role for prenatal nutrition in type 2 diabetes.

In the Nurses' Health Study [81], the inverse association between birth weights and diabetes remained significant even after adjustment for adult adiposity. The higher relative risk was seen among lean, moderate, and obese women, indicating that *in utero* growth had independent effects from adult body weight on the risk for developing type 2 diabetes. The greatest risk remained, however, in women of low birth weight who developed obesity as adults [81].

Data obtained from rat studies confirm human observations. Pregnant rats fed isoenergetic protein restricted diets gave birth to offsprings with low birth weights, reduced pancreatic β-cell mass and islet vascularization, and an impaired insulin response [83, 84], conditions that were not restored by normal nutrition after birth [84]. These offspring experienced diabetic pregnancies, exposing their fetus to hyperglycemia, and increasing their risk of becoming diabetic adults. These observations indicated that *in utero* environment affects endocrine function and when deficient, contributes to insulin resistance and β-cell dysfunction that may lead to type 2 diabetes, especially in the presence of obesity [75].

Most prospective studies of prediabetic individuals demonstrate that they are hyperinsulinemic [85], or have impaired

insulin secretion, subtle abnormalities of β-cell function that may be present before overt diabetes develops. Absence of rapid oscillations of insulin has been reported in first degree relatives of patients with type 2 diabetes [86]. Other abnormalities include a greater proportion of proinsulin in plasma of patients with type 2 diabetes [87].

C. Visceral Obesity and Insulin Resistance: Major Predictors of Diabetes

Type 2 diabetes is a syndrome of diseases with different causes. For a minority of patients, these include mutations in some genes, such as the insulin receptor gene, that appear to cause insulin resistance, or in other genes that impair β-cell functions, compromise the glucose-sensing mechanism in the β cell and appear to be a mild form of the autoimmune disease [88, 89]. Not all individuals with identified mutations express the diabetic phenotype [90]. It is conceivable that other gene mutations not yet identified and environmental factors, including nutrition and physical activity modulate its expression [90]. But for the majority of patients, the best predictor of the future onset of type 2 diabetes is insulin resistance. Insulin resistance is closely related to abdominal adiposity, contributing to glucose intolerance also in the aged [91]. Insulin resistance is common in obesity [91–94] and is characterized by hyperinsulinemia. Thus, visceral adiposity is considered a risk factor for diabetes because of its associated insulin resistance. A prospective study [95] that followed second- and third- generation Japanese-Americans for up to 10 years confirms that the amount of intraabdominal fat plays an important role in the development of diabetes. In this study, visceral adiposity, measured by computed tomography, was predictive of diabetes incidence, regardless of age, sex, family history of diabetes, fasting insulin, insulin secretion, glycemia, and total and regional adiposity. Incremental insulin response to an oral glucose challenge, an assessment of insulin secretion, was depressed in the older generation, suggesting that a failure in β-cell function preceded the onset of diabetes [96]. Impaired insulin secretion may reflect a genetic susceptibility to impaired glucose tolerance and type 2 diabetes [97, 98]. By increasing the demand for insulin, insulin resistance becomes a risk factor for diabetes, causing glucose intolerance in subjects who have impaired insulin secretory capacity and a reduction in the glucose potentiation of insulin secretion [99]. Insulin resistance was also associated with an impaired suppression of glucagon secretion by glucose in impaired glucose tolerance, suggesting that β-cell dysfunction and local insulinopenia may exaggerate glucagon secretion because the α cell becomes less sensitive to glucose [99].

D. Parallel in the Increasing Prevalences of Obesity and Diabetes

Obesity is considered a risk factor for diabetes also because its reported increasing prevalence parallels that of type 2

diabetes [100]. Two massive cross-sectional surveys carried out from 1984 to 1986 and from 1995 to 1997 revealed that mean BMI increased substantially from 27.2 to 29 kg/m2 in diabetic and from 25.1 to 26.3 kg/m² in nondiabetic subjects, and that the proportion with BMI >30.0 kg/m² went from 8 to 14% of nondiabetic men and from 13 to 18% of nondiabetic women, in all ages combined [100]. It was in the younger age group (20–39 years) that the increase in obesity was the greatest, paralleled by the greatest increase in known diabetes. Although mean physical activity did not change between surveys, the data indicated that the most overweight persons reported the least amount of leisure time spent on physical activity [100]. The authors concluded that this rapid increase in obesity in the younger population may worsen the predicted increase in the prevalence of diabetes as that cohort of the population ages, and reaches an age when diabetes becomes more prevalent. This distressful prediction is highly probable unless strategies are implicated to radically change lifestyles and body weight.

E. Insulin Insensitivity in Nonobese with Visceral Adiposity

The effects of nutrition and physical inactivity on body composition and metabolic fitness are becoming the burden of those who are not obese as well. Normal weight individuals also display a cluster of characteristics that predispose them to type 2 diabetes. Thirteen young women were identified in a cohort of 71 healthy nonobese women as being insulin insensitive to glucose [101]. The same women had a higher percentage of body fat and higher subcutaneous and visceral adiposity compared to the insulin-sensitive group. The energy expended in physical activity, measured by doubly labeled water methodology and indirect calorimetry, was less (2.7 ± 0.9 vs. 4.4 ± 1.5 MJ/day, $p = 0.01$) than in the insulin-sensitive group. This study indicates that body fat and inactivity override body weight in determining glucose metabolism. Furthermore, there is evidence that there is a high prevalence of these individuals in the general population [102]. Although assessed from self-reported questionnaires, physical activity has been shown to be inversely related to the incidence of type 2 diabetes [103].

F. Metabolic Alterations in Obesity That Predispose to Type 2 Diabetes Mellitus

Total fatness and a body fat distribution that favors visceral fat cell hypertrophy [65, 66] alter the metabolism of glucose (see Fig. 1 and Table 3). Both are associated with more insulin resistance than observed in individuals who are obese with lower body adiposity [104, 105], greater breakdown of the stored triacylglycerol in adipose cells [106], and elevated plasma nonesterified free fatty acid concentrations, which can lead to impaired glucose tolerance [107–110].

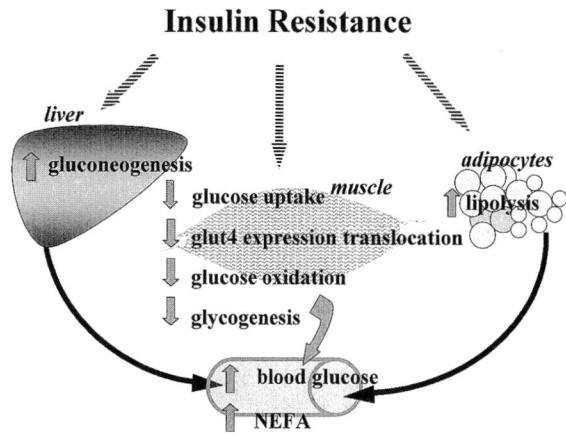

FIGURE 1 As fat mass and abdominal obesity increase, insulin sensitivity in skeletal muscle falls, leading to a decrease in glucose uptake, glucose oxidation (especially postprandially), and glycogen stores. In the liver, insulin clearance contributes to hyperinsulinemia, and gluconeogenesis increases as does glucose output. Enlarged visceral adipose tissue is associated with less response to the antilipolytic action of insulin, and more response to the lipolytic action of catecholamines is associated with increased nonesterified fatty acids (NEFA) in circulation.

1. VISCERAL FAT ALTERATIONS IN OBESITY

The extent of fat storage as triacylglycerol in adipocytes will depend on the balance between its formation and its mobilization. Both processes are under hormonal and nervous system regulations. Insulin plays a major role in suppressing the breakdown of triglycerides or lipolysis, by lowering cyclic AMP concentrations [111], which causes a disphosphorylation of hormone-sensitive lipase and, especially after food intake, by activating the enzyme lipoprotein

TABLE 3   Metabolic Alterations in Obesity Related to Diabetes

α_2 adrenoceptor activity in abdominal tissue of men that favors greater visceral adiposity

β_3-adrenoceptor sensitivity in visceral fat that increases the lipolity response to catecholamine

Strong relationship between insulin resistance and visceral adiposity

Overproduction of tumour-necrosis factor α by specific adipocytes, altering insulin action

Reduction of hepatic insulin clearance in upper-body obesity leading to hyperinsulinemia

Defects in intracellular glucose transporters (GLUT 4)

Less suppression of fat mobilization by insulin in visceral fat

Hypercortisolism in upper body obesity that favors lipolysis

Metabolic inflexibility of oxidation fuel selection in skeletal muscle

Endothelial dysfunction

lipase. Lipoprotein lipase releases fatty acids from chylomicrons and very low density lipoproteins (VLDL) in the circulation. Half of those are taken up for storage [112]. Catecholamines can suppress lipolysis [113] via their action on α_2 adrenoceptors, but they mostly have the opposite effect of insulin and by acting on β adrenoreceptors, they increase cyclic AMP and the phosphorylation of hormone-sensitive lipase, stimulating lipolysis and the release of fatty acids in the circulation [113].

Body fat distribution may be influenced by differences in lipoprotein lipase activity. In premenopausal women, lipoprotein lipase activity is higher in femoral and gluteal compared with abdominal regions, where fat cells are larger. These differences are not seen in men nor in postmenopausal women [114]. Furthermore it has been suggested that a greater α_2 activity in the abdominal tissue of men may explain greater adiposity in that location [115].

Body fat distribution also affects the lipolytic response to the catecholamine norepinephrine. It has been reported that in men and women, the response is greater in abdominal compared with gluteal and femoral adipose tissues, abdominal adipocytes having greater β_3-adrenoceptor sensitivity. Receptor numbers are reported to be increased in obese subjects [116]. Lipolysis being relatively more elevated in visceral fat cells, subjects with upper-body obesity would be exposed to a greater release of free fatty acids into the portal system.

2. INSULIN SENSITIVITY IN OBESITY

Studies measuring insulin sensitivity showed a positive correlation between the degree of upper body adiposity and the steady-state plasma glucose, an index of the capacity a subject has to dispose of a glucose challenge under insulin stimulus [65]. The correlation between abdominal fat and insulin resistance has been shown to be independent of total body fatness [65, 117, 118]. Overall glucose disposal by skeletal muscle in premenopausal women was lower with greater upper body fatness [119]. Insulin resistance of glucose in skeletal muscle is seen in both obesity and type 2 diabetes mellitus. The decreased efficiency in glucose disposal has been related to the reduction in insulin-stimulated activity of the glucose-6-phosphate independent form of glycogen synthase. Other factors that may explain why insulin resistance worsens in some obese individuals and not in others as their fat mass increases are the overproduction by specific adipocytes of proinflammatory cytokines such as tumor necrosis factor α(TNF-α). These cytokines block the effect of insulin on glucose transport in skeletal muscle by producing nitric oxide in excess via the induction of the expression of inducible nitric oxide synthase [120, 121]. TNF-α mRNA expression in adipose tissue and skeletal muscle correlates with BMI and plasma insulin levels. It inhibits the tyrosine kinase activity of the insulin receptor, altering its action and possibly leading to insulin resistance [122].

Fractional hepatic clearance of insulin, postabsorptive and during stimulation by intravenous glucose or an oral glucose load, is reduced in upper body obesity compared with lower body obesity, despite indications that the portal plasma insulin levels do not differ [123].

Less hepatic insulin extraction leads to greater peripheral insulin concentrations and hyperinsulinemia. This effect may be a consequence of elevated levels of free testosterone and decreased sex hormone-binding globulin [124] that characterize upper-body obesity [67].

The transport of glucose into the adipose cell was reduced in obesity and more so in type 2 diabetes because of a depletion of intracellular glucose transporters and of carriers for their recruitment to the plasma membrane of the cell [125]. Although the content in intracellular glucose transporters did not differ in the skeletal muscle of subjects who were obese compared with controls, the defect associated with impaired responsiveness to insulin was a loss in the functional activity of the transporters or a decrease in their translocation to the cell surface. The latter may be a consequence of long-term exposure to hyperglycemia in type 2 diabetes [126].

Visceral adipose tissue shows a greater response to lipolytic stimuli but is less sensitive to suppression of fat mobilization by insulin than subcutaneous adipose tissue. The elevated concentrations in insulin in upper body obesity will have a greater inhibitory effect on lipolysis in subcutaneous adipose fat and proportionally a greater amount on nonesterified fatty acids will be mobilized from visceral fat [127]. It is conceivable that more portal nonesterified fatty acids be conducive to greater hepatic and skeletal muscle insulin resistance [128].

Upper-body obesity is associated with hypercortisolism, characterized by increased degradation and clearance rates of cortisol that are compensated by increased production rates. Cortisol favors lipolysis by inhibiting the action of insulin and permitting that of catecholamines [129]. Because visceral fat shows a higher density of glucocorticoid receptors compared to subcutaneous fat, hypercortisolism in obesity may contribute to more portal nonesterified fatty acids and hepatic and skeletal muscle insulin resistance.

Circulating nonesterified fatty acids concentrations increase as fat mass increases [128]. Furthermore, as insulin action diminishes with obesity, suppression of nonesterified fatty acids is decreased and their concentrations in plasma increased [130]. The larger supply of fatty acids to the liver, particularly if they are not totally suppressed after meals, is associated with accumulation of acetyl CoA and inhibition of pyruvate carboxylase altering glucose utilization and stimulating gluconeogenesis and inappropriate hepatic glucose production. In muscle, maintaining or increasing plasma nonesterified fatty acids concentrations decreased insulin-stimulated glucose uptake.

Using the euglycemic-hyperinsulinemic clamp and indirect calorimetry, lipid infusions produced a decrease in insulin-stimulated glucose oxidation and a greater decrease in

glycogen synthesis [131]. These results suggested that in insulin-resistant states with increased lipid availability and oxidation, glucose oxidation was reduced. However, by contrast, in fasting conditions, hyperglycemia in type 2 diabetes was shown to override the effect of increased lipid availability and be associated with increased glucose oxidation in leg muscle. Normalization of the leg muscle hyperglycemia with a low dose of insulin increased fat oxidation [132]. There is evidence (reviewed in [133]) to suggest that, postabsorptively, skeletal muscle fat oxidation in insulin-resistant states is decreased. This decrease is explained by the presence in muscle of carbohydrate-derived malonyl CoA, which inhibits carnitine palmitoyl transferase blocking the entry of free fatty acids into the mitochondria [134]. Carnitine palmitoyl transferase activity has been shown to be reduced in the vastus lateralis muscle of insulin-resistant individuals who are obese [135]. The excess free fatty acids may increase long-chain acyl CoA concentrations and diacylglycerol, leading to the accumulation of lipids in muscle, an effect conducive to alterations of insulin signaling and insulin action.

Human studies suggest that muscle lipid content in obesity could be a determinant of insulin insensitivity [136, 137], independently of visceral fat [136]. Lipid accumulation in muscle is observed in trained athletes who are insulin sensitive but who have a great metabolic capacity for lipid utilization, which is not the case in muscles of sedentary individuals who are obese. Obese subjects appear to display metabolic inflexibility of oxidative fuel selection [133]. Compared with insulin-sensitive lean individuals, obese subjects have shown lower fat oxidation after an overnight fast, as indicated by higher leg respiratory quotient (RQ), and less capacity to switch to glucose in insulin-stimulated conditions, as indicated by an absence of increase in leg RQ. Furthermore, high levels of fatty acids may suppress insulin secretion and their effect may be toxic to the β cells of the pancreas, becoming an important contributor to the pathogenesis of obesity-dependent type 2 diabetes [45]. Excess nonesterified fatty acids reduces hepatic insulin extraction, further increasing its serum concentration [128].

The prevalence of visceral fat measured by computer tomography correlated with endothelial dysfunction, independently of BMI in otherwise healthy women who are obese [138]. Endothelial dysfunction was also closely associated with a marker of insulin sensitivity. The authors attributed these early alterations involved in the atherosclerotic process to high nonesterified fatty acids levels.

Forty percent of the insulin secreted by the pancreas is removed by the liver. Defects in hepatic insulin clearance can contribute to hyperinsulinemia, a downregulation of insulin receptors and aggravation of insulin resistance [130]. As long as the pancreas maintains sufficient insulin secretion to compensate for insulin resistance, glycemia remains within the normal range. Once the β cells fail to compensate, insulin response is decreased and glucose uptake by muscle diminished. Then, the liver oxidizes preferentially fatty acids and gluconeogenesis is stimulated. The consequences are a conversion from normal to impaired glucose tolerance and, in genetically susceptible individuals, to diabetes [139].

G. Psychological Stress, Diabetes, and Visceral Adiposity Associations

Björntorp [140] has formulated a theory that links stress and diabetes because of the endocrine abnormalities that result from psychological stress-induced activation of the hypothalamo-pituitary-adrenal axis. Stress can be associated with high cortisol and low sex steroid concentrations. These antagonize insulin action and cause visceral adiposity, which may contribute to insulin resistance and the onset of type 2 diabetes mellitus. Psychological stress is known to aggrevate glycemia in diabetes [141]. The effect of major stressful life events over 5 years on the prevalence of type 2 diabetes was assessed in a Caucasian population aged 50–74 years. The results support Björntorp's theory by showing a greater prevalence of previously undetected diabetes with more stressful events reported [142]; the age- and sex-adjusted association between major life changes and diabetes was independent of family history of diabetes, physical activity, heavy alcohol use, or low level of education. There was no association between work-related stressful events and type 2 diabetes in this cross-sectional study. A weak positive association was found with waist-to-hip ratio, but visceral fat was not the main mediating factor between stress and diabetes. It has been suggested that the link between stress and diabetes may be through other factors such as the chronic stimulation of the autonomic nervous system and its resulting hyperglycemia [142, 143]. Whether central obesity is a response to psychological stress, and both in turn increased the risk of glucose intolerance over time, remains to be evaluated in longitudinal studies [142].

Although it is not an obligatory factor, obesity may increase the risk of developing diabetes in susceptible individuals. The majority of persons with type 2 diabetes are obese [42]. Data from a prospective study in men aged 40–59 years at screening and followed for a period of 12 years showed that the risk increased progressively with increasing BMI. Weight gain of >10% over time increased the risk even in overweight individuals with initial BMI of 25.0–27.9 kg/m². Both the magnitude of BMI and the duration of obesity increased the risk of diabetes. The risk in men who had a BMI >30 kg/m² for more than 5 years was eight times that of men who were not overweight. Weight fluctuation did not affect the risk of diabetes but there was a trend for weight loss to be associated with a decrease in risk [144].

H. Improvement in Insulin Sensitivity with Weight Loss and Energy Intake Restriction

In obesity characterized by diminished insulin action, any treatment associated with weight loss improves insulin sensitivity

and fasting plasma glucose; these improvements are related to losses of abdominal fat [145, 146]. Fujioka *et al.* [145] measured the changes in body fat distribution and those in metabolic disorders after an 8-week energy intake restricted diet (800 kcal/day) in 40 women aged 38 ± 9 (mean + SD) years with uncomplicated obesity. Body fat was determined by the CT scan method and 14 women were characterized as having visceral fat obesity rather than subcutaneous fat obesity with a visceral/subcutaneous measurement of >0.4. They found that at week 8 of diet, the decrease in visceral fat volume was more sharply correlated with the changes in plasma glucose and in lipid metabolism than the decrease in body weight, total fat or subcutaneous fat volume, and that these correlations were independent of total fat loss. The reduction in visceral fat was more pronounced compared with subcutaneous fat.

Another study [146] reported that the improvements in fasting plasma glucose and insulin sensitivity with weight loss were related to losses of abdominal fat. That study was designed to distinguish the effects of energy intake restriction before substantial weight loss from those of a weight loss of 6.3 ± 0.4 kg on glycemia, hepatic glucose production, and insulin action and secretion in 20 overweight subjects with or without type 2 diabetes. At day 4 of reducing energy intake by 50%, a significant decrease was observed in basal hepatic glucose output with a greater insulin suppression of endogenous glucose production in all subjects, measured during a hyperinsulinemic euglycemic clamp. Although the decrease in glucose output was counteracted by a decrease in metabolic clearance rate of glucose, it resulted in a fall in fasting plasma glucose. This fall related to the decrease in carbohydrate intake and possibly an associated reduction in hepatic glycogen content. At day 4 of energy intake restriction, fat oxidation was increased as were the nonesterified fatty acids levels. With substantial weight loss (at day 28 of the energy intake restricted diet), plasma glucose was further decreased in the diabetic subjects only, a decrease associated with increased metabolic clearance rates. Fasting insulin concentrations were reduced compared with those preceding weight loss and insulin sensitivity was improved in both groups. These improvements were associated with a reduction in the abdominal fat depot. These data support a role for central adiposity in the alterations of glucose metabolism observed in obesity. Pascale *et al.* [147] also reported a significant decrease in the waist-to-hip ratio of 69 overweight type 2 diabetic subjects after a loss of more than 13 kg at 6 months of a behavioral weight-loss program. Waist-to-hip ratio had decreased by 2.6 and 2.0% in men and women, respectively. These subjects were characterized by upper-body obesity. Waist circumferences also decreased from 121 ± 17 to 106 ± 11 cm in women and from 120 ± 10 to 108 ± 16 cm in men. Changes in waist circumferences related significantly with weight loss ($p \geq 0.01$) Baseline waist-to-hip ratio correlated significantly with change in waist-to-hip ratio at 6 months. Although the improvements

in glycemic control indicated by decreases in hemoglobin A_{1c}, plasma glucose, and insulin concentrations correlated with weight loss, they did not with changes in waist-to-hip ratio.

The improvement in glycemia observed with weight loss underlines the impact of obesity in the development of type 2 diabetes. Pories *et al.* [148] reported that 90% of the glucose intolerant or diabetic obese subjects who had lost 50 kg, 12 months after gastric bypass surgery, achieved normoglycemia and maintained it for up to 14 years.

I. Obesity and Treatment of Diabetes

The conclusions of the UK Prospective Diabetes Study [149] are that optimal diabetic control aiming at a hemoglobin A_{1c} level of $<7.0\%$ must be achieved if morbidity is to be prevented significantly. To do so, intensive therapy using insulin alone or combined with oral hypoglycemic agents may be required. Results from the Finnish Multicenter Insulin Therapy Study, in which 100 insulin-treated type 2 diabetic patients were followed for 12 months, showed that good glycemic control started to deteriorate after 3 months, and more so in the obese subjects, the latter being attributed to the greater insulin resistance in these subjects. Control was best achieved in the nonobese subjects whether with insulin alone or in combination with other therapeutic agents. However, the combination therapy was associated with less weight gain [150].

Obesity in persons with type 1 diabetes can affect their insulin requirements by aggravating their insulin resistance. The consequences of increasing the insulin dosages can be further weight gain associated with the lipogenic effects of insulin and the additional eating in reaction to the hypoglycemic events often seen with intensive therapy [151]. Weight gain with insulin therapy is often associated with a higher waist-to-hip ratio [149]. Given the associations between obesity and dyslipidemia, atherosclerosis, and hypertension, intensive therapy of diabetes should aim at not producing weight gain [149].

IV. CONCLUSION

Family history of diabetes and age are recognized risk factors for diabetes [18], but they cannot be controlled. Recommendations for prevention of diabetes address factors that can be controlled. Because the hallmark of diabetes control is glycemia, the goals of the treatment of type 2 diabetes have been primarily to normalize blood glucose. Tight control of glycemia is necessary to prevent microvascular complications [149]. However, the increased cardiovascular risk associated with the disease commands that therapeutic strategies be devised to correct the factors related to that risk. These include elevated blood pressure, smoking, abnormal lipid profile, low physical activity and obesity. Current data

support that to reduce the incidence of diabetes it is advisable to achieve a healthy weight when young and maintain it throughout life [22]. Prevention of overall obesity should be the result of a lifestyle that includes healthy eating habits and levels of physical activity associated with the maintenance of optimal fitness for age [122]. Innovative ways are especially needed to promote and achieve proficient physical activity and exercise habit in those who are obese and have diabetes [152].

References

1. Haffner, S. M., Stern, M. P., Hazuda, H. P., Pugh, J., and Patterson, J. K. (1987). Do upper-body and centralized adiposity measure different aspects of regional body-fat distribution? Relationship to non-insulin-dependent diabetes mellitus, lipids, and lipoproteins. *Diabetes* **36,** 43–51.
2. van Noord, P. A., Seidell, J. C., den Tonkelaar, I., Baanders-van Halewijn, E. A., and Ouwehand, I. J. (1990). The relationship between fat distribution and some chronic diseases in 11,825 women participating in the DOM-project. *Int. J. Epidemiol.* **19**[3], 546–570.
3. Skarfors, E. T., Selinus, K. I., and Lithell, H. O. (1991). Risk factors for developing non-insulin dependent diabetes: A 10 year follow-up of men in Uppsala. *Br. Med. J..* **303,** 755–760.
4. Shelgikar, K. M., Hockaday, T. D., and Yajnik, C. S. (1991). Central rather than generalized obesity is related to hyperglycemia in Asian Indian subjects. *Diab. Med.* **8,** 712–717.
5. Dowse, G. K., Zimmet, P. Z., Gareeboo, H., George, K., Alberti, M. M., Tuomilehto, J., Finch, C. F., Chitson, P., and Tulsidas, H. (1991). Abdominal obesity and physical inactivity as risk factors for NIDDM and impaired glucose tolerance in Indian, Creole, and Chinese Mauritians. *Diabetes Care* **14,** 271–282.
6. Tai, T. Y., and Chuang, L. M., Wu, H. P., and Chen, C. J. (1992). Association of body build with non-insulin dependent diabetes mellitus and hypertension among Chinese adults: A 4-year follow-up study. *Int. J. Epidemiol.* **21,** 511–517.
7. Schmidt, M., Duncan, B. B., Canani, L. H., Karohl, C., and Chambless, L. (1992). Associations of waist-hip ratio with diabetes mellitus. Strength and possible modifiers. *Diabetes Care* **15,** 912–914.
8. McKeigue, P. M., Pierpoint, T., Ferrie, J. E., and Marmot, M. G. (1992). Relationship of glucose intolerance and hyperglycemia to body fat pattern in South Asians and Europeans. *Diabetologia* **35,** 785–791.
9. Shaten, B. J., Smith, G. D., Kuller, L. H., and Neaton, J. D. (1993). Risk factors for the development of type II diabetes among men enrolled in the usual care group of the Multiple Risk Factor Intervention Trial. *Diabetes Care* **16,** 1331–1339.
10. Marshall, J. A., Hamman, R. F., Baxter, J., Mayer, E. J., Fulton, D. L., Orleans, M., Rewers, M., and Jones, R. H. (1993). Ethnic differences in risk factors associated with the prevalence of non-insulin-dependent diabetes mellitus. The San Luis Valley Diabetes Study. *Am. J. Epidemiol.* **137,** 706–718.
11. Collins, V. R., Dowse, G. K., Toelupe, P. M., Imo, T. T., Aloaina, F. L., Spark, R. A., and Zimmet, P. Z. (1994). Increasing prevalence of NIDDM in the Pacific island popula-

tion of Western Samoa over a 13-year period. *Diabetes Care* **17,** 288–296.
12. Chou, P., Liao, M. J., and Tsai, S. T. (1994). Associated risk factors of diabetes in Kin-Hu, Kinmen. *Diabet. Res. Clin. Prac.* **26,** 229–235.
13. Ohlson, L. O., Larsson, B., Svardsudd, K., Welin, L., Eriksson, H., Wilhelmsen, L., Bjorntorp, P., and Tibblin, G. (1985). Influence of body fat distribution on the incidence of diabetes mellitus. 13. 5 years of follow-up of the participants in the study of men born in 1913. *Diabetes* **34,** 1055–1058.
14. Modan, M., Karasik, A., Halkin, H., Fuchs, Z., Lusky, A., Shitrit, A., and Modan, B. (1986). Effect of past and concurrent body mass index on prevalence of glucose intolerance and type 2 (non-insulin-dependent) diabetes and on insulin response. *Diabetologia* **29,** 82–89.
15. Lundgren, H., Bengtsson, C., Blohme, G., Lapidus, L., Sjostrom, L. (1989). Adiposity and adipose tissue distribution in relation to incidence of diabetes in women: Results from a prospective population study in Gothenburg, Sweden. *Int. J. Obes.* **13**(4), 413–423.
16. Lemieux, S., Prud'homme, D., Nadeau, A., Tremblay, A., Bouchard, C., Despres, J. P. (1996). 7-year changes in body-fat and visceral adipose-tissue in women—associations with indexes of plasma glucose-insulin homeostasis. *Diabetes Care* **19,** 983–991.
17. Haffner, S. M., Stern, M. P., Mitchell, B. D., Hazuda, H. P., and Patterson, J. K. (1990). Incidence of type II diabetes in Mexican Americans predicted by fasting insulin and glucose levels, obesity, and body-fat distribution. *Diabetes* **39,** 283–288.
18. Colditz, G. A., Willett, W. C., Stampfer, M. J., Manson, J. E., Hennekens, C. H., Arky, R. A., and Speizer, F. E. (1990). Weight as a risk factor for clinical diabetes in women. *Am. J. Epidemiol.* **132,** 501–513.
19. Knowler, W. C., Pettitt, D. J., Saad, M. F., Charles, M. A., Nelson, R. G., Howard, B. V., Bogardus, C., and Bennett, P. H. (1991). Obesity in the Pima Indians: Its magnitude and relationship with diabetes. *Am. J. Clin. Nutr.* **53**(6 Suppl.), 1543S–1551S.
20. Charles, M. A., Fontbonne, A., Thibult, N., Warnet, J. M., Rosselin, G. E., and Eschwege, E. (1991). Risk factors for NIDDM in white population. Paris prospective study. *Diabetes* **40,** 796–799.
21. Cassano, P. A., Rosner, B., Vokonas, P. S., and Weiss, S. T. (1992). Obesity and body fat distribution in relation to the incidence of non-insulin-dependent diabetes mellitus. A prospective cohort study of men in the normative aging study. *Am. J. Epidemiol.* **136,** 1474–1486.
22. Chan, J. M., Rimm, E. B., Colditz, G. A., Stampfer, M. J., and Willett, W. C. (1994). Obesity, fat distribution, and weight gain as risk factors for clinical diabetes in men. *Diabetes Care* **17** 961–969.
23. Colditz, G. A., Willett, W. C., Rotnitzky, A., and Manson, J. E. (1995) Weight gain as a risk factor for clinical diabetes mellitus in women. *Ann. Intern. Med.* **122,** 481–486.
24. Ruwaard, D., Gijsen, R., Bartelds, A. I., Hirasing, R. A., Verkleij, H., and Kromhout, D. (1996). Is the incidence of diabetes increasing in all age-groups in the Netherlands? *Diabetes Care* **19,** 214–218.
25. Midthjell, K., Kruger, O., Holmen, J., Tverdal, A., Claudi, T., Bjorndal, A., and Magnus, P. (1999). Rapid changes in the

prevalence of obesity and known diabetes in an adult Norwegian population. *Diabetes Care* **22,** 1813–1820.

26. Hadden, D. R., Montgomery, D. A., Skelly, R. J., Trimble, E. R., Weaver, J. A., Wilson, E. A., and Buchanan K. D. (1975). Maturity onset diabetes mellitus: Response to intensive dietary management. *Br. Med. J.* **3,** 276–278.

27. Lean, M. E. J., Powrie, J. K., Anderson, A. S., and Garthwaite, P. H. (1990). Obesity, weight loss and prognosis in type 2 diabetes. *Diab. Med.* **7,** 228–233.

28. U.K. Prospective Diabetes Study Group (1990). UK Prospective Diabetes Study 7. Response of fasting plasma glucose to diet therapy in newly presenting type II diabetic patients. *Metabolism* **39,** 909–912.

29. Vessby, B., Boberg, M., Karlstrom, B., Lithell, H., and Werner, I. (1984). Improved metabolic control in overweight diabetic patients. *Acta Med. Scand.* **216,** 67–74.

30. Williamson, D. F., Pamuk, E., Thun, M., Flanders, D., Byers, T., and Heath, C. (1995). Prospective study of intentional weight loss and mortality in never smoking U.S. white women. *Am. J. Epidemiol.* **141:**1128–1141.

31. Rosenbaum, M., Leibel, R. L., and Hirsch, J., (1997). Obesity. *N. Engl. J. Med.* **337**(6), 396–407.

32. Garrow, J. S. (1988). Health implications of obesity. In: "Obesity and Related Diseases," pp. 1–16. Churchill Livingstone, London.

33. Vague, J. (1956). The degree of masculine differentiation of obesities—a factor determining predisposition to diabetes, atherosclerosis, gout and uric calculous disease. *Am. J. Clin. Nutr.* **4,** 20–34.

34. WHO Expert Committee (1995). "Physical Status: The Use and Interpretation of Anthropometry," WHO Technical Report No. 854. World Health Organization, Geneva, Switzerland.

35. Seidell, J. C., and Flegal, K. M. (1997). Assessing obesity: Classification and epidemiology. *British Medical Bulletin* **53,** 238–253.

36. Norgan, N. G., and Jones, P. R. M. (1995). The effect of standardising the body mass index for relative sitting height. *Int. J. Obes.* **19,** 206–208.

37. Lemieux, S., Prud'homme, D., Bouchard, C., Tremblay, A., and Despres, J. P. (1996). A single threshold value of waist girth identifies normal-weight and overweight subjects with excess visceral adipose tissue. *Am. J. Clin. Nutr.* **64,** 685–693.

38. Lean, M. E. J., Han, T. S., and Morrison, C. E. (1995). Waist circumference indicates the need for weight measurement., *Br. Med. J.* **311,** 158–161.

39. Lean, M. E., Han, T. S., and Morrison, C. E. (1995). Waist circumference action levels in the identification of cardiovascular risk factors: Prevalence study in a random sample. *Br. Med. J.* **311,** 1401–1405.

40. Sjostrom, L., Kvist, H., and Tylen, U. (1985). Methodological aspects of measurements of adipose tissue distribution. *In* "Metabolic Complications of Human Obesities" (J. Vague, P. Björntorp, B. Guy Grand, M. Rebuffe-Scrive, and P. Vague, Eds.), pp. 13–19. Excerpta Medica, Amsterdam.

41. Armellini, F., Zamboni, M., Harris, T., Micciolo, R., and Bosello, O. (1997). Sagittal diameter minus subcutaneous thickness. An easy-to-obtain parameter that improves visceral fat prediction. *Obes. Res.* **5,** 315–320.

42. WHO Study Group (1994). "Prevention of Diabetes Mellitus," WHO Technical Report No. 844. World Health Organization, Geneva, Switzerland.

43. "Report of the Expert Committee on the Diagnosis and Classification of Diabetes Mellitus" (2000). *Diabetes Care* **23** (Suppl. 1), S4–S19.

44. Stern, M. P. (1988). Type II diabetes mellitus. Interface between clinical and epidemiological investigation. *Diabetes Care* **11,** 119–126.

45. Fuller, J. H., Shipley, M. J., Rose G., Jarret R. J., and Keen, H. (1980). Coronary heart disease risk and impaired glucose tolerance: The Whitehall Study. *Lancet* **1,** 1373–1376.

46. Unger, R. H. (1995). Lipotoxicity in the pathogenesis of obesity-dependent NIDDM. Genetic and clinical implications. *Diabetes* **44,** 863–870.

47. Nair, K. S., Garrow, J. S., Ford, C., Mahler, R. F., and Halliday, D. (1983). Effect of poor diabetic control and obesity on whole body protein metabolism in man. *Diabetologia* **25,** 400–403.

48. Gougeon, R., Styhler, K., Morais, J. A., Jones, P. J. H., and Marliss, E. B. (2000). Effects of oral hypoglycemic agents and diet on protein metabolism in Type 2 diabetes. *Diabetes Care* **23,** 1–8.

49. Beks, P. J., Mackay, A. J. C., de Neeling, J. N. D., de Vries, H., Bouter, L. M., and Heine, R. J. (1995). Peripheral arterial disease in relation to glycaemia level in elderly Caucasian population: The Hoorn Study. *Diabetologia* **38,** 86–96.

50. King, H., Zimmet, P., Raper, L. R., and Balkau, B. (1984). Risk factors for diabetes in three Pacific populations. *Am. J. Epidemiol.* **119,** 396–409.

51. King, H., Taylor, R., Koteka, G., Nemaia, H., Zimmet, P. Z., Bennett, P. H., Raper, andL. R. (1986). Glucose tolerance in Polynesia: Population-based surveys in Rarotonga and Niue. *Med. J. Austral.* **145,** 505–510.

52. McLarty, D. G., Swai, A. B. M., Kitange, H. M., Masuki, G., Mtinangi, G. L., Kilima, P. M., Makene, W. J., Chuwa, L. M., and Alberti, K. G. M. M. (1989). Prevalence of diabetes and impaired glucose tolerance in rural Tanzania. *Lancet* **1,** 871–875.

53. Medalie, J. H., Papier, C. M., Goldbourt, U., and Herman, J. B. (1975). Major factors in the development of diabetes mellitus in 10,000 men. *Arch. Intern. Med.* **135,** 811–817.

54. Stanhope, J. M., and Prior, I. A. M. (1980). The Tokelau island migrant study: Prevalence and incidence of diabetes mellitus. *N.Z. Med. J.* **92,** 417–421.

55. Knowler, W. C., Pettitt, D. J., Bennett, P. H., and Savage, P. J. (1981). Diabetes incidence in Pima Indians: Contributions of obesity and parental diabetes. *Am. J. Epidemiol.* **113,** 144–156.

56. Keen, H., Jarrett, R. J., and McCartney, P. (1982). The tenyear follow-up of the Bedford survey (1962–1972): Glucose tolerance and diabetes. *Diabetologia* **22,** 73–78.

57. Butler, W. J., Ostrander, L. D., Carman, W. J., and Lamphiear, D. E. (1982). Diabetes mellitus in Tecumseh, Michigan: Prevalence, incidence and associated conditions. *Am. J. Epidemiol.* **116,** 971–980.

58. Balkau, B., King, H., Zimmet, P., and Raper, L. R. (1985). Factors associated with the development of diabetes in the Micronesian population of Nauru. *Am. J. Epidemiol.* **122,** 594–605.

59. Haffner, S. M., Stern, M. P., Hazuda, H. P., Rosenthal, M., Knapp, J. A., and Malina, R. M. (1986). Role of obesity and fat distribution in non-insulin-dependent diabetes mellitus in Mexican Americans and Non-Hispanic whites. *Diabetes Care* **9**, 153–161.

60. Ohlson, L. O., Larsson, B., Bjorntorp, P., Eriksson, H., Svardsudd, K., Welin, L., Tibblin, G., and Wilhelmsen, L. (1988). Risk factors for type 2 (non-insulin-dependent) diabetes mellitus: Thirteen and one-half years of follow-up of the participants in a study of Swedish men born in 1913. *Diabetologia* **31**, 798–805.

61. Schranz, A. G. (1989). Abnormal glucose tolerance in the Maltese: A population-based longitudinal study of the natural history of NIDDM and IGT in Malta. *Diab. Res. Clin. Prac.* **7**, 7–16.

62. Feldman, R., Sender, A. J., and Seigelbaum, A. B. (1969). Difference in diabetic and non-diabetic fat distribution patterns by skinfold measures. *Diabetes* **18**, 478–486.

63. Joos, S. K., Mueller, W. H., Hanis, C. L., and Schull, W. J. (1984). Diabetes alert study. Weight history and upper body obesity in diabetic and non-diabetic Mexican American adults. *Ann. Hum. Biol.* **11**, 167–171.

64. Kissebah, A. H., Vydelingum, N., Murray, R., Evans, D. J., Hartz, A. M., Kalfhuff, R. K, and Adams, P. W. (1982). Relationship of body fat distribution to metabolic complications of obesity. *J. Clin. Endocrinol. Metab.* **54**, 254–260.

65. Krotkiewski, M., Björntorp, P., Sjöström, C., and Smith, U. (1983). Impact of obesity on metabolism in men and women: Importance of regional adipose distribution. *J. Clin. Invest.* **72**, 1150–1162.

66. Evans, D. J., Hoffman, R. G., Kalkhoff, R. K., and Kissebah, A. H. (1983). Relationship of androgenic activity to body fat topography, fat cell morphology, and metabolic aberrations in premenopausal women. *J. Clin. Endocrinol. Metab.* **57**, 304–310.

67. Hartz, A. J., Rupley, D. C., and Rimm, A. H. (1984). The association of girth measurements with disease in 32, 856 women. *Am. J. Epidemiol.* **119**, 71–80.

68. Evans, D. J., Hoffman, R. G., Kalkhoff, R. K., and Kissebah, A. H. (1984). Relationship of body fat topography to insulin sensitivity and metabolic profiles in premenopausal women. *Metabolism.* **33**, 68–75.

69. Ohlson, L. O., Larsson, B., Svärdsudd, K., Eriksson, H., Wilhelmsen. L., Björntorp, P., and Tibblin, G. (1985). The influence of body fat distribution on the incidence of diabetes mellitus: 13.5 year follow-up of the participants in the study of men born in 1913. *Diabetes* **34**, 1055–1058.

70. Keen, H., Jarrett R. J., and McCarthey, P. (1982). The ten-year follow-up of the Bedford Survey (1962–72): Glucose intolerance and diabetes. *Diabetologia* **22**, 73–78.

71. Saad, M. F., Knowler, W. C., Pettitt, D. J., Nelson, R., Mott, D. M., and Bennett, P. H. (1988). The natural history of impaired glucose tolerance in Pima Indians. *N. Engl. J. Med.* **319**, 1500–1506.

72. Diehl, A. K., and Stern, M. P. (1989). Special health problems of Mexican Americans: Obesity, gallbladder disease, diabetes mellitus and cardiovascular disease. *Adv. Intern. Med.* **34**, 79–96.

73. Sicree, R. A., Zimmet, P. Z., King, H. O. M, and Coventry, J. S. (1987). Plasma insulin response among Nauruans: Pre-diction of deterioration in glucose tolerance over 6 yr. *Diabetes.* **36**, 179–186.

74. Kadowaki, T., Miyake, Y., Hagura, R., Akanuma, Y., Kajinuma, H., Kuzuya, N., Takafu, F., and Kosaka K. (1984). Risk factors for worsening to diabetes in subjects with impaired glucose tolerance. *Diabetologia* **26**, 44–49.

75. Wilding, J., and Williams, G. (1998). Diabetes and obesity. *In* "Clinical Obesity" (P. G. Kopelman and M. J. Stock, Eds.), pp. 309–349. Blackwell Science, Cambridge.

76. Barker, D. J. P. (1998). Mothers, Babies and Health in Later Life. 2nd ed. Churchill Livingston, Edinburgh.

77. Barker, D. J. (1995). Fetal origins of coronary heart disease. *Br. Med. J.* **311**, 171–174.

78. Hales, C. N., Barker, D. J., Clark, P. M., Cox, L. J., Fall, C., Osmond, C., and Winter, P. D. (1991). Fetal and infant growth and impaired glucose tolerance at age 64. *Br. Med. J.* **303**, 1019–1022.

79. Lethell, H. O., McKeigue, P. M., Berglund, L., Mohsen, R., Lithell, U. B., and Leon, D. A. (1996). Relation of size at birth to non-insulin dependant diabetes and insulin concentrations in men aged 50–60 years. *Br. Med. J.* **312**, 406–410.

80. McCance, D. R., Pettitt, D. J., Hanson, R. L., Jacobsson, L. T., Knowler, W. C., and Bennett, P. H. (1994). Birth weight and non-insulin dependent diabetes: thrifty genotype, thrifty phenotype or surviving small baby genotype? *Br. Med. J.* **308**, 942–945.

81. Rich-Edwards, J. W., Colditz, G. A., Stampfer, M., Willett, W. C., Gillman, M. W., Hennekens, C. H., Speizer, F. E., and Manson, J. E. (1999). Birth weight and the risk for Type 2 diabetes mellitus in adult women. *Ann. Intern. Med.* **130**, 278–284.

82. Ravelli, A. C., van der Meulen, J. H., Michels, R. P., Osmond, C., Barker, D. J., and Hales, C. N. (1998). Glucose tolerance in adults after prenatal exposure to famine. *Lancet* **351**, 173–177.

83. Snoeck, A., Remacle, C., Reusens, B., and Hoet, J. J. (1990). Effect of a low protein diet during pregnancy on the fetal rat endocrine pancreas. *Biol. Neonate* **57**, 107–118.

84. Dahri, S., Snoeck, A., Reusens-Billen, B., Remacle, C., and Hoet, J. J. (1991). Islet function in offspring of mothers on low-protein diet during gestation. *Diabetes* **40**(Suppl. 2), 115–120.

85. Martin, B. C., Warram, J. H., Krolewski, A. S., Bergman, R. N., Soeldner, J. S., and Kahn, C. R. (1992). Role of glucose and insulin resistance in development of type 2 diabetes mellitus: Results of a 25-year follow-up study. *Lancet* **340**, 925–929.

86. O'Rahilly, S., Turner, R. C., and Matthews, D. R. (1988). Impaired pulsatile secretion of insulin in relatives of patients with non-insulin-dependent diabetes. *N. Engl. J. Med.* **318**, 1225–1230.

87. Porte, D. J., and Kahn, S. E. (1989). Hyperproinsulinemia and amyloid in NIDDM. Clues to etiology of Islet beta-cell dysfunction? *Diabetes* **38**, 1333–1336.

88. Steiner, D. F., Tager, H. S., Chan, S. J., Nanjo, K., Sanke, T., and Rubenstein, A. H. (1990). Lessons learned from molecular biology of insulin-gene mutations. *Diabetes Care* **13**, 600–609.

89. Froguel, P., Zouali, H., Vionnet, N., Velho, G., Vaxillaire, M., Sun, F., Lesage, S., Butel, M. O., Stoffel, M., Takeda, J.,

Robert, J. J., Paisa, P., Permutt, M. A., Beckmann, J. S., Bell, G. I., and Cohen, D. (1993). Familial hyperglycemia due to mutations in glucokinase: Definition of a new subtype of non-insulin-dependent (type 2) diabetes mellitus. *N. Engl. J. Med.* **328,** 697–702.

90. Taylor, S. I., Accili, D., and Imai, Y. (1994). Insulin resistance or insulin deficiency. Which is the primary cause of NIDDM. *Diabetes* **43,** 735–740.

91. Kohrt, W. M., Kirwan, J. P., Staten, M. A., Bourey, R. E., King, D. S, and Holloszy, J. O. (1993). Insulin resistance in aging related to abdominal obesity. *Diabetes* **42,** 273–281.

92. DeFronzo, R. A., and Ferranini, E. (1991). Insulin resistance: A multifaceted syndrome responsible for NIDDM, obesity, hypertension, dyslipidemia and atherosclerotic cardiovascular disease. *Diabetes Care* **14,** 175–194.

93. Beard, J. C., Ward, W. K, Halter, J. B., Wallum, B. J., and Porte, D., Jr. (1987). Relationship of islet function to insulin action in human obesity. *J. Clin. Endocrin. Metab.* **65,** 59–64.

94. Prager, R., Wallace P., and Olefsky, J. M. (1986). In vivo kinetics of insulin action, peripheral glucose disposal and hepatic glucose output in normal and obese subjects. *J. Clin. Invest.* **78,** 472–481.

95. Boyko, E. J., Fujïmoto, W. Y., Leonetti, D. L., and Newell-Morris, L. (2000). Visceral adiposity and risk of type 2 diabetes. *Diabetes Care* **23,** 465–471.

96. Samaras, K., and Campbell, L. V. (2000). Increasing incidence of type 2 diabetes in the third millennium. Is abdominal fat the central issue? *Diabetes Care* **23,** 441–442.

97. Gerich, J. (1998). The genetic basis of type 2 diabetes mellitus: impaired insulin secretion versus impaired insulin sensitivity. *Endocrin. Rev.* **19,** 491–503.

98. Vauhkonen, I., Niskanen, L., Vanninen, E., Kainulainen, S., Uusitupa, M., and Laakso, M. (1997). Defects in insulin secretion and action in non-insulin-dependent diabetes are inherited: metabolic studies on offspring of diabetes probonds. *J. Clin. Invest.* **100,** 86–89.

99. Larsson, H., and Ahrin, B. (2000). Islet dysfunction in insulin resistance involves impaired insulin secretion and increased glucagon secretion in postmenopausal women with impaired glucose tolerance. *Diabetes Care* **23**, 650–657.

100. Midthjell, K., Krüger, O., Holmer, J., Tverdal, A., Claudi, T., Bjorndal, A., and Magnus, P. (1999). Rapid changes in the prevalence of obesity and known diabetes in an adult Norwegian population. *Diabetes Care* **22,** 1813–1820.

101. Dvorak, R. V., De Nino, W. F., Ades, P. A., and Poehlman, E. T. (1999). Phenotypic characteristics associated with insulin resistance in metabolically obese but normal-weight young women. *Diabetes* **48,** 2210–2214.

102. Ruderman, N., Chisholm, D., Pi-Sunyer, X., and Schneider, S. (1998). The metabolically obese, normal-weight individual revisited. *Diabetes* **47,** 699–713.

103. Helmovich, S. P., Ragland, D. R., Leung, R. W., and Paffenbarger, R. S., Jr. (1991). Physical activity and reduced occurrence of non-insulin-dependent diabetes mellitus. *N. Engl. J. Med.* **325,** 147–152.

104. Salans, L. B., Knittle, J. L., and Hirsch, J. (1968). The role of adipose cell size and adipose tissue insulin sensitivity in the carbohydrate intolerance of human obesity. *J. Clin. Invest.* **47,** 153–165.

105. Olefsky, J. M. (1976). The insulin receptor: Its role in the insulin resistance of obesity and diabetes. *Diabetes* **25,** 1154–1162.

106. Goldrick, R. B., and McLoughlin, G. M. (1970). Lipolysis and lipogenesis from glucose in human fat cells of different sizes: Effects of insulin, epinephrine and theophyeline. *J. Clin. Invest.* **40,** 1213–1223.

107. Björntorp, P., Bengtsson, C., Blohmé, G., Jonsson, A., Sjöström, L., Tibblin, E., Tibblin G., and Wilhelmsen, L. (1971). Adipose tissue fat cell size and number in relation to metabolism in randomly selected middle-aged men and women. *Metab. Clin. Exp.* **20,** 927–935.

108. Björntorp, P. (1984). Hazards in subgroups of human obesity. *Eur. J. Clin. invest.* **14,** 239–241.

109. Randle, P. J., Garland, P. B., Hales, C. N., and Newholme, E. A. (1963). The glucose–fatty acid cycle. Its role in insulin sensitivity and the metabolic abnormalities of obesity. *Lancet* **1,** 785–789.

110. Stern, M. P., Olefsky, J. Farquhar, J., and Reaven, G. (1973). Relationship between fasting plasma lipid levels and adipose tissue morphology. *Metabolism* **22,** 1311–1317.

111. Smith, C. J., Vasta, V., Degerman, E., Belfrage, P., and Manganiello, V. C. (1991). Hormone-sensitive cyclic GMP-inhibited cyclic AMP phosphodiesterase in rat adipocytes. Regulation of insulin and c. AMP-dependent activation by phosphorylation. *J. Biol. Chem.* **266**(133), 85–90.

112. Eaton, R. P., Berman, M., and Steinberg, D. (1969). Kinetic studies of plasma free fatty acid and triglyceride metabolism in man. *J. Clin. Invest.* **48,** 1576–1579.

113. Lafontan, M., and Berlan, M. (1993). Fat cell adrenergic receptors and the control of white and brown fat cell function. *J. Lipid Res.* **34,** 1057–1091.

114. Rebuffe-Scrive, M., and Björntorp, P. (1985). Regional adipose tissue metabolism in man. *In* "Metabolic Complications of Human Obesities" (J. Vague, P. Björntorp, and B. Guy-Grand, Eds.), pp. 149–159. Excerpta Medica, Amsterdam.

115. Lafontan, M., Dang-Tran, L., and Berlan, M. (1975). Alpha-adrenergic antipolytic effect of adrenaline in human fat cells of the thigh: Comparison with adrenal responsiveness of different fat deposits. *Eur. J. Clin. Invest.* **9,** 261–266.

116. Lonnqvist, F., Thorne, A., Nilsell, K, Hoffstedt, J., and Arner, P. (1995). A pathogenic role of visceral fat B$_3$ adrenoceptors in obesity. *J. Clin. Invest.* **95,** 1109–1116.

117. Carey D. G., Jenkins, A. B., Campbell, L. V., Freund, J., and Chisholm, D. J. (1996). Abdominal fat and insulin resistance in normal and overweight women. *Diabetes* **45,** 633–638.

118. Després, J. P. (1993). Abdominal obesity as important component of insulin resistance syndrome. *Nutrition* **9,** 452–459.

119. Evans, D. J., Murray, R., and Kissebah, A. H. (1984). Relationship between skeletal muscle insulin resistance, insulin-mediated glucose disposal and insulin binding effects of obesity and body fat topography. *J. Clin. Invest.* **74,** 1515–1525.

120. Bédard, S., Marcotte, B., and Marette, A. (1997). Cytokines modulate glucose transport in skeletal muscle by inducing the expression of inducible nitric oxide synthase. *Biochem. J.* **325,** 487–493.

121. Kapur, S., Bédard, S., Marcotte, B., Côté, C., and Marette, A. (1997). Expression of nitric oxide synthase in skeletal muscle: A novel role for nitric oxide as a modulator of insulin action. *Diabetes* **46,** 1691–1700.

122. Hotamisligil, G. S., and Spiegelman, B. M. (1994). Tumor-necrosis-factor-alpha: A key component of the obesity-diabetes link. *Diabetes* **43**, 1271–1278.

123. Peiris, A. N., Mueller, R. A., and Smith, G. A. (1986). Splanchnic insulin metabolism in obesity: Influence of body fat distribution. *J. Clin. Invest.* **78**, 1648–1657.

124. Kissebah A. H., Evans D. J., Peiris A., and Wilson, C. R. (1985). Endocrine characteristics in regional obesities: role of sex steroids. *In* "Metabolic Complications of Human Obesities" (J. Vague, P. Björntorp, B. Guy-Grand, M. Rebuffé-Scrive, and P. Vague, Eds.), pp. 115–130. Elsevier, Amsterdam.

125. Garvey, W. T., Maianu, L., Huecksteadt, T. P., Birnbaum, M. J., Molina, J. M., and Ciaraldi, T. P. (1991). Pretranslational suppression of a glucose transporter protein causes cellular insulin resistance in non-insulin dependent diabetes and obesity. *J. Clin. Invest.* **87**, 1072–1081.

126. Garvey, W. T., Olefsky, J. M., Matthaei, S., and Marshall, S. (1987). Glucose and insulin coregulate the glucose transport system in primary cultured adipocytes. *J. Biol. Chem.* **262**, 189–197.

127. Rebuffe-Scrive, M., Andersson, B., Olbe, L., and Björntorp, P. (1989). Metabolism of adipose tissue in intraabdominal depots of non-obese men and women. *Metabolism* **38**, 453–461.

128. Boden, G. (1997). Role of fatty acids in the pathogenesis of insulin resistance and NIDDM. *Diabetes* **46**, 3–10.

129. Cigolini, M., and Smith, U. (1979). Human adipose tissue in culture. VIII. Studies on the insulin-antagonistic effect of glucocorticoids. *Metabolism* **28**, 502–510.

130. Campbell, P. J., Carlson, M. G., and Nurjhan, N. (1994). Fat metabolism in human obesity. *Am. J. Physiol.* **266**, E600–E605.

131. Kelley, D. E., Mokan, M., Simoneau, J.-A., and Mandarino, L. J. (1993). Interaction between glucose and free fatty acid metabolism in human skeletal muscle. *J. Clin. Invest.* **92**, 93–98.

132. Kelley, D. E., and Mandarino, L. J. (1990). Hyperglycemia normalizes insulin-stimulated skeletal muscle glucose oxidation and storage in noninsulin-dependent diabetes mellitus. *J. Clin. Invest.* **86**, 1999–2007.

133. Kelley, D. E., and Mandarino, L. J. (2000). Fuel selection in human skeletal muscle in insulin resistance. A reexamination. *Diabetes* **49**, 677–683.

134. Winder, W. W., Arogyasami, J., Elayan, I. M., and Dartmill, D. (1990). Time course of exercise-induced decline in malinoyl-CoA in different muscle types. *Am. J. Physiol.* **259**, E266–E271.

135. Simoneau, J.-A., Veerkamp, J. H., Turcotte, L. P., and Kelley, D. E. (1999). Markers of capacity to utilize fatty acids in human skeletal muscle: Relation to insulin resistance and obesity and effects of weight loss. *FASEB J.,* **13**, 2051–2060.

136. Pan, D. A., Lillioja, S., Kriketos, A. D., Milner, M. R., Baur, L. A. Bogardus, C., Jenkins, A. B., and Storlein, L. H. (1997). Skeletal muscle triglycerides levels are inversely related to insulin action. *Diabetes* **46**, 983–988.

137. Goodpaster, B. H., Thaete, F. L., Simoneau, J.-A., and Kelley, D. E. (1997). Subcutaneous abdominal fat and thigh muscle composition predict insulin sensitivity independently of visceral fat. *Diabetes* **46**, 1579–1585.

138. Arcaro, G., Zamboni, M., Rossi, L., Turcato, E., Covi, G., Armellini, F., Bosello, O., and Lechi, A. (1999). Body fat distribution predicts the degree of endothelial dysfunction in uncomplicated obesity. *Int. J. Obes.* **23**, 936–942.

139. Reaven, G. M. (1995). The fourth musketeer—from Alexander Dumas to Claude Bernard. *Diabetologia* **38**, 3–13.

140. Björntorp, P. (1997). Body fat distribution, insulin resistance, and metabolic diseases. *Nutrition.* **13**, 795–803.

141. Surwit, R. S., Schneider, M. S., and Fernglos, M. N. (1992). Stress and diabetes mellitus. *Diabetes Care* **15**, 1413–1422.

142. Mooy, J. M., de Vries, H., Grootenhuis, P. A., Bonter, L. M., and Heine, R. J. (2000). Major stressful life events in relation to prevalence of undetected Type 2 diabetes. *Diabetes Care* **23**, 197–201.

143. Surwit, R. S., and Funglos, M. N. (1988). Stress and autonomic nervous system in Type 2 diabetes: A hypothesis. *Diabetes Care* **11**, 83-85.

144. Wannamethee, S. G., and Shaper, A. G. (1999). Weight change and duration of overweight and obesity in the incidence of type 2 diabetes. *Diabetes Care* **22**, 1266–1272.

145. Fujioka, S., Matsuzawa, Y., Tokunaga, K., Kawamoto, T., Kobatake, T., Keno, Y., Kotani, K., Yoshida, S., and Tarui, S. (1990). Improvement of glucose and lipid metabolism associated with selective reduction of intra-abdominal visceral fat in premenopausal women with visceral fat obesity. *Int. J. Obes.* **15**, 853–859.

146. Markovic, T. P., Jenkins, A. B., Campbell, L. V. Furler, S. M., Kraegen, E. W., and Chisholm, D. J. (1998). The determinants of glycemic responses to diet restriction and weight loss in obesity and NIDDM. *Diabetes Care* **21**, 687–694.

147. Pascale, R. W., Wing, R. R., Blair, E. H., Harvey, J. R., and Guare, J. C. (1996). The effect of weight loss on change in waist-to-hip ratio in patients with type II diabetes. *Int. J. Obes.* **16**, 59–65.

148. Pories, W. J., Swanson, M. S., Macdonald, K. G., Long, S. B., Morris, P. G., Brown, B. M., Barakat, H. A., deRamon, R. A., Israel, G., and Dolezal, J. M. (1995). Who would have thought it? An operation proves to be the most effective therapy for adult-onset diabetes-mellitus. *Ann. Surg.* **222**, 339–352.

149. UK Prospective Diabetes Study (UKPDS) Group (1998). Intensive blood-glucose control with sulfonylureas or insulin compared with conventional treatment and risk of complications in patients with type 2 diabetes (UKPDS 33). *Lancet* **353**, 837–853.

150. Yki-Järvinen, H., Ryysy, L., Kauppila, M., Kujansuu, E., Lahti, J., Marjanen, T., Niskanen, L., Rajala, S., Salo, S., Seppala, P., Tulokas, T., Viikari, J., and Taskinen, M. R. (1997). Effect of obesity on the response to insulin therapy in noninsulin-dependent diabetes mellitus. *J. Clin. Endocrin. Metab.* **82**, 4037–4043.

151. Diabetes Control and Complications Trial Research Group (1993). The effect of intensive treatment of diabetes on the development and progression of long-term complications in insulin dependent diabetes mellitus. *N. Engl. J. Med.* **329**, 977–986.

152. Pronk, N. P., and Wing, R. R. (1994). Physical activity and long term maintenance of weight loss. *Obes. Res.* **2**, 587–599.

CHAPTER 28

Nutrition Management for Type 1 Diabetes

ANN ALBRIGHT

Sacramento, California

I. INTRODUCTION

Diabetes is one of the most common diseases that nutrition and other health professionals encounter. Both health professionals and people with diabetes have identified medical nutrition therapy as an extremely challenging aspect of diabetes care [1]. While nutrition has long been viewed as a cornerstone in the treatment of diabetes, the information on which many of the nutrition recommendations are based is evolving. During the last decade, landmark research has been conducted that has significantly changed how diabetes is treated. The patient is the key decision maker in diabetes care. The meal plan must be individualized and based on the patient's usual eating habits and preferences. The insulin regimen is then integrated into the patient's lifestyle. This is a significant shift from previous diet plans that were based primarily on energy intake and structured to meet the insulin regimen.

The role of the nutrition professional is to work with the patient and other members of the health care team to set and help patients achieve their nutrition goals. Once the goals have been established, the nutrition professional works with patients to select tools for making nutrition decisions based on the most current information and guides them in their decision making. To provide the most accurate information to patients, it is imperative that health professionals have the most current information available on medical nutrition therapy for diabetes care. In addition, nutrition professionals must also understand and use self-monitoring of blood glucose results and have a thorough understanding of medications and of physical activity. Optimal management of type 1 diabetes requires the health care provider to integrate all of this information into patient care.

II. DEFINITION AND BURDEN OF TYPE 1 DIABETES

Type 1 diabetes accounts for approximately 10% of the diabetic cases and is characterized by an inability to produce insulin, resulting in hyperglycemia [2]. Insulin, a hormone produced by the beta cells of the pancreas, is needed by muscle, adipose tissue, and the liver to utilize glucose. The hyperglycemia of diabetes places individuals with this disease at risk for developing microvascular complications, including retinopathy (eye disease) and nephropathy (kidney disease), macrovascular disease (including heart disease and stroke), and various neuropathies (both autonomic and peripheral).

The two subgroups within type 1 diabetes are immune-mediated and idiopathic diabetes. Type 1 immune-mediated diabetes was formerly known as juvenile-onset or insulin-dependent diabetes. This form of the disease usually occurs before the age of 30 with most cases occurring in childhood or adolescence. However, it is now estimated that 10–20% of Caucasians developing diabetes in adulthood may have immune-mediated beta cell destruction [3]. The immune destruction of the beta cells may occur over several months to years. In young people, the onset of symptoms is usually abrupt and rapid treatment is necessary to correct ketoacidosis and prevent death. The beta cell destruction in adults that develop type 1 diabetes may be much more gradual and an absolute requirement for insulin may not be necessary for many years [2].

Type 1 immune-mediated diabetes is considered an autoimmune disease in which the immune system attacks the body's own tissues. It is currently unclear what triggers the immune process leading to type 1 diabetes, but the process is identified by the presence of islet-cell antibodies, insulin autoantibodies, and autoantibodies to glutamic acid decarboxylase. Type 1 diabetes does not develop in all patients with these antibodies, but at least one of these antibodies is present in 85–90% of patients at the time of diagnosis [4]. The predisposition to type 1 immune-mediated diabetes is inherited as a multigenic trait with low penetrance. Genetic markers have been identified which indicate the potential vulnerability to this subgroup of type 1 diabetes [5]. At least one human leukocyte antigen (HLA) class II DR3 or DR4 antigen is found in 95% of type 1 patients. Also linked to type 1 diabetes are DR1, DR16, and DR8, while DR15 and DR11 are considered to confer protection. Class II DQ genes are also linked to type 1 diabetes and, although these HLA

429

types are necessary, they are not sufficient for developing type 1 diabetes.

Type 1 idiopathic diabetes is a new subgroup and represents only a small number of people with beta-cell destruction. These patients have variable insulin deficiency and only intermittently require insulin treatment. This form of diabetes is strongly inherited, but does not have HLA association or evidence of autoimmunity. When seen, it is more often found in those of African and Asian background [4].

III. DIABETES MEDICAL NUTRITION THERAPY

Four steps have been identified that are necessary for accomplishing diabetes medical nutrition therapy: (1) a comprehensive nutrition assessment that addresses metabolic, nutrition, and lifestyle factors; (2) setting practical, achievable goals with the patient that have been mutually agreed on by the patient and the dietitian; (3) identifying nutrition interventions that the patient can understand and is most likely to use; and (4) evaluating progress toward meeting the goals and identifying areas in need of future attention [6]. These steps have been identified in and are supported for diabetes by the Diabetes Control and Complications Trial (DCCT) [7], the American Diabetes Association nutrition recommendations [1], and the nutrition practice guidelines for type 1 diabetes developed and tested by the Diabetes Care and Education Practice Group of the American Dietetic Association [8].

The DCCT was designed to compare intensive with conventional diabetes treatment on the development and progression of early vascular and neurologic complications of type 1 diabetes [7]. This multicenter clinical trial randomized 1441 patients between the ages of 13 and 39 with type 1 diabetes into two treatment groups, conventional or intensive. Within each of the treatment groups, there were patients with no sign of diabetic retinopathy at baseline (primary prevention) and patients with mild diabetic retinopathy at baseline (secondary prevention). Intensive therapy consisted of three or more insulin injections per day or insulin pump therapy and self-monitoring of blood glucose at least four times per day. Insulin dose adjustments were made according the results of self-monitoring of blood glucose, food intake, and anticipated exercise. These patients also had frequent contact with members of the health care team. Conventional therapy consisted of one or two daily insulin injections, daily self-monitoring of blood glucose or urine testing for glucose, and education about diet and exercise. Daily adjustments in insulin were not usually made and the goal of therapy was the absence of symptoms of hyperglycemia, normal growth and development, and no severe or frequent hypoglycemia. These patients had standard follow-up with health care professionals. The DCCT conclusively demonstrated that intensive blood glucose management can significantly reduce

TABLE 1 Diabetes Control and Complications Trial Results

Intensive management/blood glucose control made a difference
76% reduction in retinopathy
60% reduction in neuropathy
54% reduction in albuminuria
39% reduction in microalbuminuria
Implication: Improved blood glucose control also applies to persons with type 2 diabetes.

Source: Reprinted with permission from Diabetes Control and Complications Trial Research Group (1993). The effect of intensive treatment of diabetes on the development and progression of long-term complications in insulin-dependent diabetes mellitus. *N. Engl. J. Med.* **329,** 977–986.

the risk for microvascular complications of type 1 diabetes (Table 1).

The DCCT showed that medical nutrition therapy is essential in achieving optimal glucose control [9, 10]. The nutrition interventions used in the DCCT were tailored to fit the patient's lifestyle, motivation, and learning level. Insulin adjustments were made to fit the selected nutrition plan. The dietitians implemented a variety of nutrition strategies to assist patients in the intensive therapy groups attain near euglycemia. The nutrition approaches ranged from the general recommendations of the Healthy Food Choices to the more detailed approach of total available glucose (discussed below). Recognizing the need for flexibility in the nutrition plan for patients with type 1 diabetes, and working with the patient to select the approach used, contributed to the reduction in hemoglobin A_{1c} in the DCCT.

Historically, nutrition recommendations for those with diabetes have spanned everything from starvation diets to high-fat diets. In 1994 the American Diabetes Association developed nutrition guidelines that presented a major change in the philosophy of nutrition care for those with diabetes [1]. An individually developed dietary plan based on metabolic, nutrition, and lifestyle requirements replaced the defined caloric prescription. These nutrition recommendations acknowledged that a single diet does not appropriately treat all types of diabetes. The goals of medical nutrition therapy in diabetes care are (1) maintenance of near-normal blood glucose levels by balancing food intake with insulin (exogenous or endogenous) and physical activity, (2) achievement of optimal lipid levels, (3) provision of adequate energy for maintaining or attaining reasonable weight and normal growth, (4) prevention and treatment of acute and chronic complications of diabetes, and (5) improvement of overall health through optimal nutrition.

The recommendations for protein, fat, and carbohydrate are designed to achieve the goals of medical nutrition therapy. They emphasize the need to individually assess the patient and make macronutrient selections based on patient outcome goals and not just generic percentages.

A. Protein

Variations in dietary protein intake can influence blood glucose levels in diabetes by modifying the availability of gluconeogenic substrates, as well as insulin and counterregulatroy hormone secretion. There are limited scientific data on which to establish firm recommendations for protein intake in diabetes. Because evidence does not support that protein requirements for type 1 patients are higher or lower than the general population, the recommended protein intake for those with diabetes is 10–20% of total energy. In a study of 12 patients with type 1 diabetes, glucose response and insulin requirements were measured by a glucose controlled insulin infusion system for 5 hours after ingestion of three different meals: 450 kilocalories standard meal, the standard meal with 200 kilocalories (equivalent to 7 ounces of lean meat) of added protein, and the standard meal with 200 kilocalories of added fat [11]. The glucose response to the protein meal was greater ($p = 0.005$) than the response to either the standard or fat-added meals due to an increase in the late (last 150 minutes) glucose response. The late insulin response was also greater ($p < 0.005$) for the protein-added meal. This effect was seen with 7 ounces of protein. Whether people with diabetes who eat 1–2 ounces of protein with a snack to prevent subsequent hypoglycemia (especially hypoglycemia during the night) will have the same results remains unknown. If protein does affect blood glucose levels, it is likely due to stimulation of glucagon by protein [12]. The increase in glucagon exerts a transient increase in hepatic glucose release so it is not likely to provide protection against subsequent hypoglycemia.

Excessive protein intake has been implicated in the pathogenesis of diabetic nephropathy since high protein intake increases glomerular filtration rate (GFR) [13]. Some studies conducted in people with diabetes suggest that the use of low-protein diets may modify the underlying glomerular injury of diabetes and delay the progression of nephropathy [14, 15]. There is evidence that the protein source may influence the progression of renal disease. Amino acids from meat proteins may adversely affect GFR and the progression of renal disease compared to vegetable, egg white, cheese, or cooked soybean proteins [16–18]. Most data support some restriction of protein intake to prevent or delay diabetic nephropathy, but more data are necessary to determine the optimal protein content and the stage of renal disease that responds to protein restriction. Currently, a protein intake similar to the adult Recommended Dietary Allowances (0.8 g/kg), approximately 10% of the daily energy, is considered sufficiently restrictive for individuals with evidence of diabetic nephropathy [1].

B. Fat/Carbohydrate

The remaining 80–90% of energy must be distributed between fat and carbohydrate [1]. The decisions about amount of fat and carbohydrate are guided by the patient's metabolic goals, eating habits, weight issues (if any), and the elevated risk for cardiovascular disease (CVD) in those with diabetes. Modification of CVD risk factors is especially important because diabetes is a strong independent risk factor for CVD [19]. It is recommended that saturated fat intake be less than 10% of energy, polyunsaturated fat intake be up to 10% of energy, and cholesterol be limited to 300 mg or less daily. The remaining 60–70% of energy comes from monounsaturated fats and carbohydrate.

People with type 1 diabetes who are taking adequate amounts of insulin usually have plasma cholesterol, very low density lipoprotein (VLDL) cholesterol, low-density lipoprotein (LDL) cholesterol, and triglyceride concentrations similar to those without diabetes of the same age and gender, but have higher than average high-density lipoprotein (HDL) cholesterol levels [20, 21]. Uncontrolled type 1 diabetes is associated with elevated lipid levels, but adequate insulin usually normalizes them. Many studies, but not all, suggest that blood glucose control directly influences the levels of several plasma lipid concentrations [22]. Abnormalities in size and density of lipoprotein composition can exist in these patients even when the plasma lipid measurements are normal.

If elevated LDL cholesterol is the primary problem, the National Cholesterol Education Program (NCEP) Step 2 guidelines (7% of total energy from saturated fat and 200 mg dietary cholesterol) should be implemented. If elevated triglycerides and VLDL cholesterol are primary concerns, a moderate increase in monounsaturated fat and a moderate intake of carbohydrate may be implemented [6]. Some studies have shown that an increase in monounsaturated fat lowered triglycerides and blood glucose more than a high-carbohydrate intake in some individuals [23, 24].

The percentage of carbohydrates is individualized based on eating habits, glucose and lipid goals, and the presence of other medical conditions. Relative differences in plasma glucose responses to various carbohydrates have been reported and published in a tool called the glycemic index. The clinical utility of this information has raised many questions, however. If a patient is encouraged to only eat low glycemic index foods, food choices will be severely limited. Priority should first be given to the total amount of carbohydrate consumed rather than the source of the carbohydrate. The form of carbohydrate (liquid or solid) is also an important consideration since liquids are absorbed more quickly.

The most widely held belief about the dietary treatment of diabetes is that simple sugars must be avoided and replaced with complex carbohydrates. This belief is based on the assumption that sugars are more rapidly digested and absorbed than starch and, hence, aggravate hyperglycemia. There is no scientific evidence to support this assumption. When examined as a single nutrient, sucrose produces a glycemic response lower than that of bread, rice, and potatoes [25]. Fruits and milk are reported to have lower glycemic

TABLE 2   Studies Comparing Glycemic Effects of Isocaloric Amounts of Sucrose and Starch in Diabetic Subjects[a]

Study	Number of diabetic subjects	Duration	Percent calories from sucrose	Sucrose found to have adverse effects on glycemia?
[40]	22	Single meal	25	No
[41]	18	Single meal	14	No
[42]	21	Single meal	15	No
[43]	6	Single meal	15	No
[44]	18	Single meal	14	No
[45]	24	8 days	23	No
[46]	16	5 days	7	No
[47]	10	2 days	10	No
[48]	18	4 weeks	38	No
[49]	12	4 weeks	19	No

Source: Reprinted with permission from Franz, M. J., Horton, E. S., Bantle, J. P., Beebe, C. A., Brunzell, J. D., Coulston, A. M., Henry, R. R., Hoogwerf, B. J., and Stacpoole, P. W. (1994). Nutrition principles for the management of diabetes and related complications. *Diabetes Care* **17,** 490–518.

[a]Meals were provided to subjects by the investigators.

responses than many starches [1]. At least 10 studies have been conducted that show isocaloric amounts of sucrose and starch produce similar blood glucose responses (Table 2). In particular, a crossover design study in children with type 1 diabetes compared the glycemic effect of isocaloric diets containing 2% total calories as sucrose and 10% total calories from sucrose [26]. Both diets provided 50% energy from carbohydrate, 30% from fat, and 20% from protein in three meals and three snacks. Glucose, fructose, and dietary fiber

content of the diets were identical. Sucrose isocalorically replaced part of the complex carbohydrate at each meal and for the afternoon snack. Insulin doses remained constant. The blood glucose responses are depicted in Fig 1.

When making decisions about sucrose-containing foods in the meal plan, it is important to remember that one of the goals of the nutrition recommendations is improvement of health through optimal nutrition. Sucrose can be substituted for other carbohydrates, gram for gram in the context of a

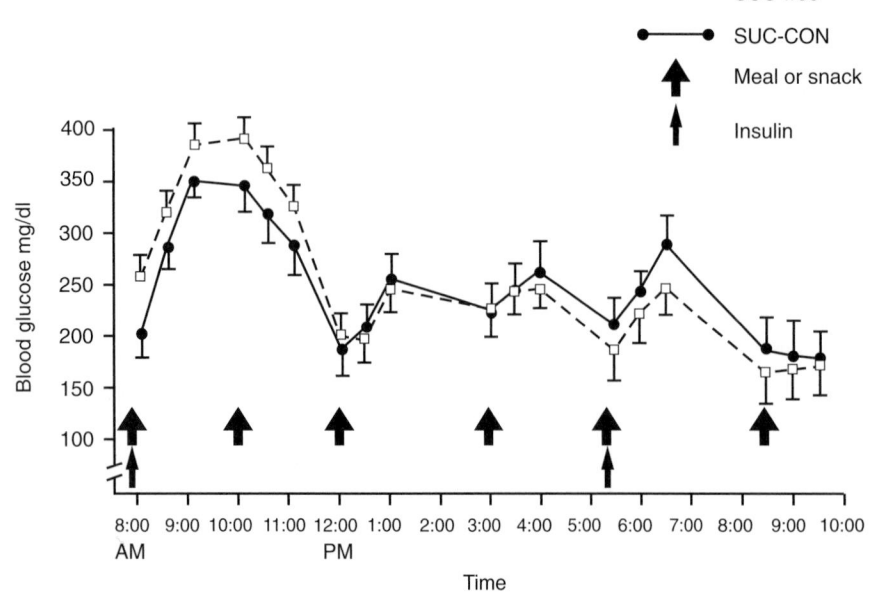

FIGURE 1   Blood glucose concentrations (mean ± SEM) from 8 A.M. to 9:30 P.M. for sucrose-free and sucrose-containing diet periods (2 days per diet period; 10 children). [From Loghmani, E., Richard, K., Washburne, L., Vandagriff, H., Fineberg, N., and Golden, M. (1991). Glycemic response to sucrose-containing mixed meals in diets of children with insulin-dependent diabetes mellitus. *J. Pediatr.* **119,** 531–537. Reprinted with permission from Mosby, Inc.]

healthy diet. Foods containing sucrose are usually high in fat and contain minor amounts of vitamins and minerals. It is also important to clearly articulate to the patient that sucrose and sucrose-containing foods must be substituted for other carbohydrates, not just added to the meal plan, and these choices should be made with attention to a healthy diet.

C. Nutrition Practice Guidelines

The Nutrition Practice Guidelines for Type 1 Diabetes (practice guidelines) were developed by the Diabetes Care and Education Practice Group of the American Dietetic Association [8]. The practice guidelines are intended to serve as a guide for provision of consistent, quality care to those with type 1 diabetes. The objectives of establishing the practice guidelines were to define responsibilities of dietetics professionals who work with patients who have type 1 diabetes, guide practice decisions, promote self-management training, and define state-of-the-art medical nutrition therapy. Four principles were used to guide the development and testing of the practice guidelines and are summarized as follows: The practice guidelines (1) guide practitioners about appropriate health care decisions for specific circumstances; (2) are based on the best available research and professional judgment; (3) are comprehensive, specific, and manageable; and (4) are thoroughly researched and validated through field testing by a reasonable pool of practitioners.

The practice guidelines are summarized in Fig. 2. A referral by the patient's primary care provider initiates the process. At this point, the dietitian must make a decision about the appropriateness of the referral. For example, the patient may require an intervention such as psychological counseling before referral to the dietitian can be productive. At a minimum, data that include the reason for referral, current medical condition, pertinent laboratory data, and diabetes management goals should accompany the referral. Follow-up with the referring provider should summarize the assessment findings, recommendations, intervention provided, and treatment plan.

The second area of the practice guidelines is a thorough assessment of the patient. Table 3 provides sample questions that guide the dietitian through this assessment. In addition to the topics identified in Table 3, it is important to assess the patient's beliefs and attitudes about chronic disease and his or her readiness to change. Once an assessment is completed, it is followed by setting realistic goals. Short- and long-term, clinical, and behavioral goals can be set. The goals must be set mutually by the clinician and the patient. The patient should not feel overwhelmed by the goals and, if necessary, goals should be adjusted to help the patient experience success. Once realistic goals have been established, the level of nutrition care needed is identified, a nutrition prescription developed, and a meal plan approach (discussed below) selected.

The dietitian must also determine which educational strategies (e.g., visual learner) are most effective for the patient (see discussion in Chapter 8). These educational strategies should be used to help the patient most effectively apply the interventions. Finally, evaluation of the patient's progress must occur regularly. This will allow adjustments to be made as necessary and assist the patient in achieving goals. A schedule for follow-up with the patient must also be developed. The frequency for follow-up can range from daily when initiating or intensifying therapy to quarterly for patients who are in the maintenance phase. Throughout the entire implementation of medical nutrition therapy it is important to document and communicate information about the assessment, the goals, the selected interventions, the nutrition prescription, and the follow-up plan to all members of health care team.

The practice guidelines were field tested in a variety of practice settings to determine the impact on patients' glycemic levels and perceptions about quality of care [27]. The results showed that dietitians in the practice guidelines group spent 63% more time with patients and were more likely to do an assessment and discuss the results with patients than dietitians in the usual care group. The patients who were receiving care according to the practice guidelines achieved greater reductions in hemoglobin A_{1C} that were statistically and clinically significant.

IV. INSULIN REGIMENS

Insulin is required for the treatment of type 1 diabetes. Several researchers contributed to the discovery of insulin, but credit is given to Banting and Best for first isolating insulin in 1921. At the time, insulin was considered a cure for diabetes because, without it, certain death was in store for those with type 1 diabetes. Soon after its discovery, processes were developed for isolation and commercial production of insulin from beef and pork pancrease. Over time, a number of modifications in the production of insulin have occurred, resulting in improved purity, varying action profiles (rapid-acting, short-acting, intermediate-acting, and long-acting), and structure identical to native human insulin [28]. In the intervening years since its discovery, we have clearly learned that insulin is a lifesaving medication, but it is not a cure for diabetes.

In an effort to duplicate the normal physiologic functions of insulin, it is important to understand the onset, peak, and duration of the various insulins. Table 4 summarizes this information for the insulins currently available.

Other factors that must be considered in the use of insulin include pharmacokinetics of insulin absorption, injection site, and timing of premeal insulin injections. An important determinant of insulin availability is its absorption from subcutaneous tissue. There is intra-individual variation in insulin absorption of approximately 25% from day to day and interindividual variation of up to 50% [28]. Although this percentage variation is the same for all insulins, in absolute terms (minutes or hours) there will be much less variation in

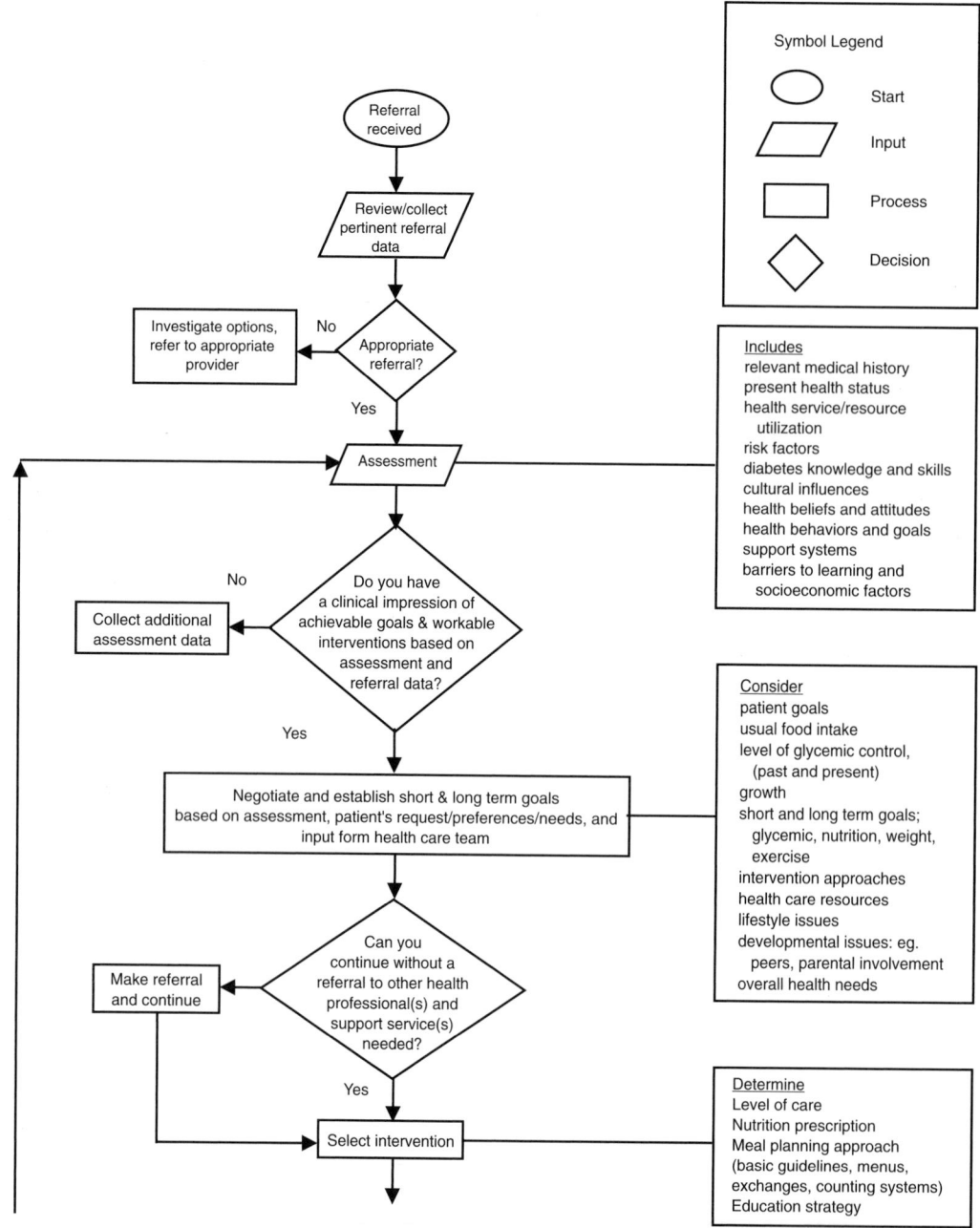

FIGURE 2   Flowchart for Nutrition Practice Guidelines for Type 1 Diabetes Mellitus. [From Kulkarni, K., Castle, G., Gregory, R., Holmes, A., Leontos, C., Powers, M., Snetselaar, L., Splett, P., and Wylie-Rosett, J. (1997). Nutrition practice guidelines for Type 1 diabetes: An overview of the content and application. *Diabetes Spectrum* **10**(4), 248–256. Reprinted with permission from the American Diabetes Association, Inc.]

the absorption of rapid-acting insulins and greater variation in absorption of longer-acting preparations.

The injection site also affects absorption. Absorption is usually fastest from the abdomen, followed by the arms, buttocks, and thighs. The difference in absorption rates among these sites is likely due to blood flow [28]. The variability is great enough that random rotation of injection sites should be avoided. It is better to rotate inject sites within a region rather than between regions. For example, any particular in-

jection (e.g., prebreakfast) should be rotated within a site such as the abdomen rather than rotating it among the abdomen, arm, and thigh.

Blood flow, skin thickness, ambient temperature, smoking, and massage of injection site also influence insulin absorption rate [28]. Because physical activity increases blood flow to an exercising part of the body, it can accelerate the absorption of insulin and contribute to hypoglycemia. The greater the time interval between the injection and the exer-

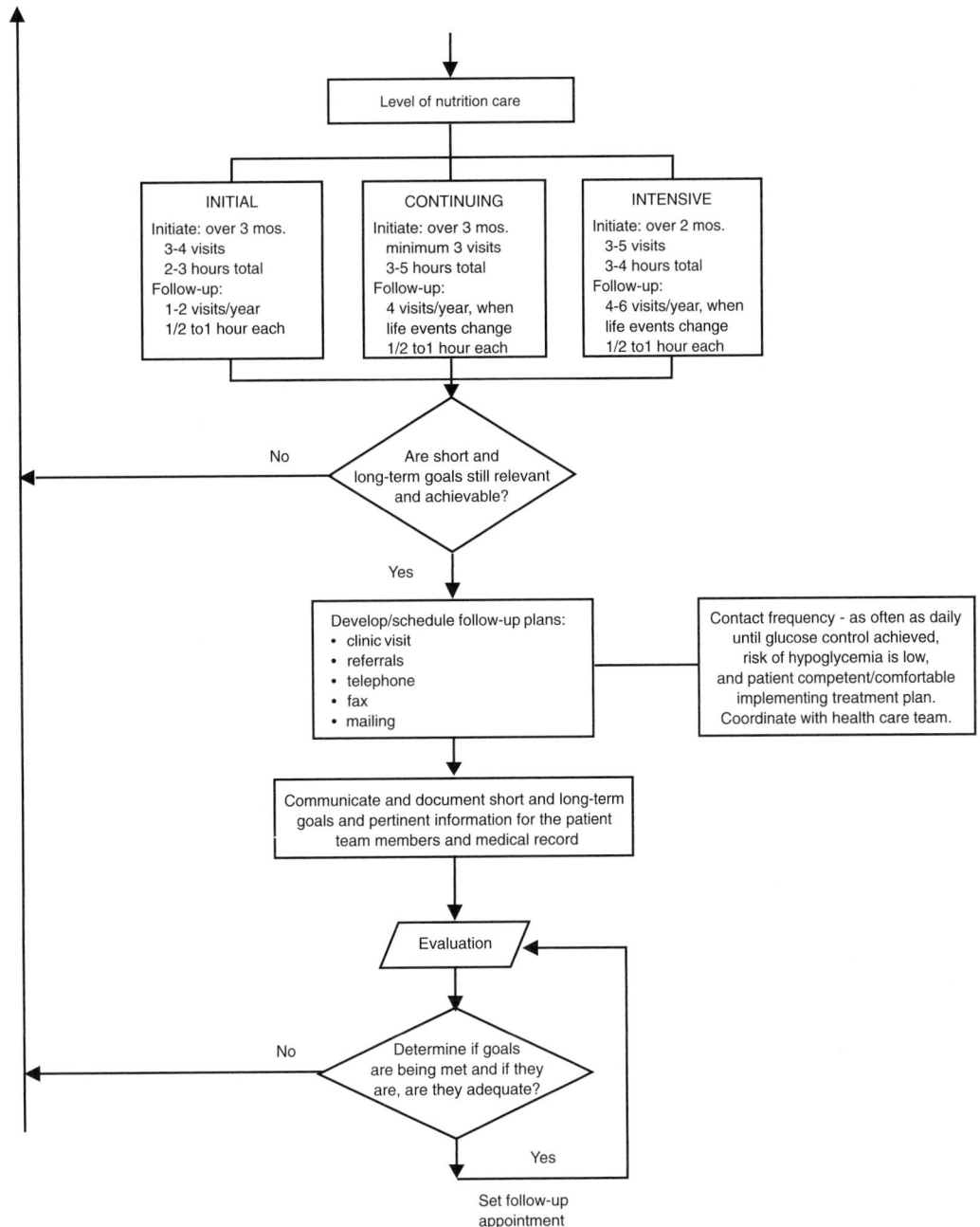

FIGURE 2 *(continued)*

cise (>60–90 minutes), the less effect injection site has on absorption rate [29]. The timing of an insulin injection relative to exercise must be evaluated to decrease the likelihood of hypoglycemia.

As seen from the information in Table 4, there is variability in the onset and peak of insulin action. In an effort to match blood glucose and insulin levels following a meal, it is important to consider the timing of premeal insulin injections. For example, regular insulin should optimally be administered 30–60 minutes before eating, allowing the insulin level in the blood to better match the glucose level. The purpose of insulin is to keep the blood glucose from getting too high postprandially. This means that insulin should be appropriately used to prevent an abnormal rise in blood glucose and not be used to chase high blood glucose levels. It is important to remember that the current insulin preparations and regimens do not guarantee perfect blood glucose control. Support and instruction need to be provided to the patient to help them most effectively use insulin and not feel defeated when the blood glucose results are not always consistently normal.

Patients with type 1 diabetes may be using conventional or intensive insulin therapy. In conventional therapy, insulin administration usually consists of twice daily injections of

TABLE 3 Minimum Assessment Data for Type 1 Diabetes

Content area	Sample questions for minimum assessment
Medical history/present health status	Tell me about any health problems you have. What are you taking? Include over-the-counter medications.
Risk assessment	Determine risk for acute and chronic complications—hypoglycemic unawareness (long-standing diabetes, lack of symptoms), microproteinuria, and so on.
Diabetes knowledge and skills	What have you been told about diabetes? Tell me what you do differently now that you have diabetes. Tell me about how you make food choices now that you have diabetes. Are you using a specific meal planning method (i.e., exchanges, carbohydrate counting, menus, etc.)? Are you presently doing self-monitoring of blood glucose? If yes, tell me what you do with the results.
Lifestyle/cultural influences	Tell me about your day. When do you get up, eat, and so on? How do some days vary from this day? Who lives with you? How do they affect your daily schedule?
Health beliefs and attitudes	Do you think your diabetes can get better?

Health behaviors and goals	Goals
	  Tell me about your goals related to diabetes care.
	  Do you have target blood glucose goals? If yes, what are they?
	  What are your specific nutrition-related goals?
	Usual eating habits
	  Tell me how you decide what you are going to eat.
	  What are two typical days of food intake? Are weekends different from weekdays? How often do you eat out?
	Exercise
	  Are you willing to continue or expand activity?
	Other
	  Do you have any problems chewing your food?

Barriers to learning	Tell me about any difficulties you have had when trying to make changes in your life. Why is it difficult?

Source: Kulkarni, K., Castle, G., Gregory, R., Holmes, A., Leontos, C., Powers, M., Snetselaar, L., Splett, P., Wylie-Rosett, J. (1997). Nutrition practice guidelines for Type I diabetes: An overview of the content and application. *Diabetes Spectrum* **10**(4), 248–256.

TABLE 4 Time Course of Action of Insulin Preparations[a]

Insulin preparation	Onset of action (hour)	Peak action (hour)	Duration of action (hour)
Rapid onset Regular (crystalline; soluble)	½–1	2–4	4–6
Rapid onset Lispro (analogue)	¼–½	1–2	3–5
Intermediate acting NPH (isophane)	1–4	8–10	12–20
Intermediate acting Lente (insulin zinc suspension)	2–4	8–12	12–20
Long acting Ultralente (extended insulin zinc suspension)	3–5	10–16	18–24
Combinations 70/30–70% NPH, 30% regular	½–1	Dual	12–20
Combinations 50/50–50% NPH, 50% regular	½–1	Dual	12–20

Source: Reprinted with permission from Skyler, J. S. (1998). *In* "Insulin Therapy in Type I Diabetes Mellitus," Vol. I, pp. 36–49. Mosby-Year Book, St. Louis, MO.
[a]Based on doses of 0.1–0.2 U/kg, in the abdomen, for human insulin.

short-acting and intermediate-acting insulin before breakfast and dinner. This method of therapy provides less flexibility for the patient and it requires that the patient be more consistent with timing of insulin administration and food intake. In intensive therapy, insulin administration is by multiple daily injections or by continuous subcutaneous insulin infusion, also called insulin pump therapy. Use of intensive insulin therapy provides more flexibility for the patient, but does require more injections and blood glucose monitoring. Intensive therapy increases the likelihood of hypoglycemia and can result in weight gain. It is essential that before patients are started on intensive therapy they have detailed information about food, physical activity, and insulins. They must also be willing to test blood glucose levels four to six times a day to make treatment plan adjustments and be able to gauge the success of these adjustments [8].

The DCCT has shown that better blood glucose control is achieved with intensive therapy, but there may some patients for whom intensive therapy is too risky and they will be better managed by conventional therapy. Patients for whom intensive therapy may be inappropriate include those with hypoglycemia unawareness and/or history of severe hypoglycemia, advanced complications, or psychological limitations [30]. Other nutrition-related risks include eating disorders or fear of weight gain [8].

Insulin can be administered by syringe or insulin pen, jet injector, or continuous subcutaneous insulin infusion. Appropriate instruction is required to teach patients how to fill the syringe and inject properly. An insulin pen makes dosage accuracy much easier since the dose is made by turning a knob. The jet injector forces insulin into the skin through pressure and not a needle. The continuous subcutaneous insulin infusion or insulin pump is a device about the size of a pager that is connected to a cannula inserted under the skin; it delivers rapid-acting insulin (Regular or Lispro) continually. The amount of insulin needed by the patient in the fasted state, known as the basal rate, must be determined first. This information is programmed into the insulin pump and the patient will receive these microliter amounts continuously. The pump can be reprogrammed to change the basal rate(s) if necessary. Prior to eating, the patient must determine how much rapid-acting or short-acting insulin will be required to cover the meal. This insulin dose (called a bolus) is delivered by pushing a button on the pump. The pump does not make insulin dosage decisions for the patient, but it does allow flexibility in eating and exercise.

A. Self-Monitoring of Blood Glucose

Self-monitoring of blood glucose is also an important part of managing diabetes. A variety of blood glucose monitoring devices is now available that allows those with diabetes to test their own blood glucose. These devices became widely available in the 1980s and have improved in accuracy and sophistication in the intervening years. All people with diabetes should test their blood glucose regardless of whether or not they use insulin, although those who use insulin are likely to have to test more frequently. There is no standard frequency for self-monitoring, but it should be done frequently enough to help the patient meet treatment goals. Increased frequency of testing is often required when initiating an exercise program to assess blood glucose response to exercise and allow safe exercise participation. Patients must be given instruction on how to operate, clean, and calibrate the device, and—most importantly—guidance on how to use the information to make food, exercise, and medication adjustments.

Health professionals must use patient blood glucose monitoring results to help the patient assess and make adjustments in their meal plan. It is not possible to appropriately assist patients with diabetes in developing and adjusting their meal plan without using blood glucose records. All nutrition and other health professionals who work with diabetic patients must develop the necessary skills to interpret and use blood glucose monitoring information. Reviewing these records with the patient reinforces the need to keep records. The reecord allows the patient and the health care professional to identify blood glucose patterns to make adjustments in therapy.

B. Meal Planning Approaches

Several meal planning approaches are used in diabetes care and they vary in complexity and the ability to make insulin adjustments. When practicing intensive therapy, the meal planning approach used must provide enough information to allow for accurate adjustments in insulin. None of the meal planning approaches has been scientifically validated. The plan selected should be one that the individual with diabetes can understand and which helps them select appropriate foods and achieve their glycemic goals.

Carbohydrate counting is not a new meal planning approach, but has recently gained renewed interest. This technique is based on the premise that the carbohydrate found in foods is the major factor influencing postprandial blood glucose excursions [31]. The focus is on total carbohydrate eaten, not the source of carbohydrate. Many consider carbohydrate counting to be a simpler method because it focuses on one macronutrient. When using this approach, patients must still learn about protein and fat intake, even though they have minimal direct effect on blood glucose when consumed in usual amounts. They do contribute to energy intake and weight gain may become an issue when dietary protein and fat are ignored. In addition, large amounts of fat can delay the postprandial peak in blood glucose and this can have an impact on glucose control [11].

Three levels of carbohydrate counting have been developed that progress from basic (level 1) to intermediate (level 2) to advanced (level 3) [32–34]. Level 1 introduces the concept of carbohydrate counting, identifies foods that contain

carbohydrate, sources of carbohydrate information (e.g., label reading), how to count grams of carbohydrate in food, and consistent carbohydrate intake. When introducing this phase, the patient records their usual carbohydrate intake and, with the dietitian, target carbohydrate goals are determined.

Level 2 focuses on pattern management, which is used to identify blood glucose patterns that are affected by food, physical activity, and insulin. These patterns are important to identify since they allow more logical adjustments to be made in insulin, carbohydrate, or physical activity. In the intermediate level of carbohydrate counting, the emphasis is on identifying blood glucose patterns, interpreting the data, and determining the possible actions necessary to alter blood glucose levels. In addition, information is given about subtracting the carbohydrate contribution from fiber if the food contains more than 5 g per serving amount and helping the patient avoid hypoglycemia and weight gain.

Level 3 is for those patients on intensive therapy who use carbohydrate-to-insulin ratios to make insulin dosage decisions and choose to use more detailed information. In the advanced level of carbohydrate counting, the concept of carbohydrate-to-insulin ratio, the amount of carbohydrate that is covered by 1 unit of fast-acting or rapid-acting insulin, is introduced. For example, a patient who eats 75 g of carbohydrate and requires 5 units of insulin has a ratio of 15 g of carbohydrate to 1 unit of insulin. The dietitian assists the patient in calculating the ratio for each meal and snack using food, insulin, and blood glucose records.

All levels of carbohydrate counting require that the person with diabetes practice estimating portion sizes and develop a reasonable skill level. This technique helps those with diabetes understand the relationships among food, insulin, physical activity, and blood glucose level. Armed with this information, patients are often better able to make appropriate adjustments in their management plan [35].

Total available glucose is another meal planning approach that some have found useful [9]. This system is based on the premise that 100% of carbohydrate content, 58% of the protein content, and 10% of the fat content of foods become glucose. In this system a total available glucose-to-insulin ratio is established that requires counting the glucose contribution of all macronutrients. More recent data have shown, however, that although 50–60% of protein has the potential to be used for gluconeogenesis, it has little effect on postmeal blood glucose [11, 36]. It is speculated that this system probably works because both protein and fat require insulin for metabolism although they have minimal effect on postmeal glucose level [11].

For many years, the most widely used method in diabetic meal planning was the exchange system [37]. This system was developed in 1950 and represented the first organized meal approach that was agreed to by the organizations involved in diabetes and nutrition care. Because of the historical contribution of this technique, it has been taught as the standard meal planning tool for people with diabetes. It is a useful technique, but it is not necessarily the best tool for all patients.

Foods are organized into three main groups: carbohydrate, meat and meat substitutes, and fat. Foods are further divided into specific exchange lists that contain a listing of weighed or measured foods of approximately the same nutritional value. Because of this arrangement, foods on each list can be substituted or "exchanged" with other foods on the same list. The meal plan for a patient is devised in terms of the number of exchanges they should consume at a meal or snack.

There are also more simplified meal planning approaches such as the food guide pyramid or Healthy Food Choices [39]. These options provide basic information about healthy eating and are very visual, but they do not provide enough detail for most patients with type 1 diabetes to make premeal insulin adjustments.

V. CONCLUSION

The management of type 1 diabetes is challenging for both the patient and health care professional. Over the years it has become much clearer that the management of this complex disease is more successfully accomplished when the patient is at the center of the team and when the various health care professionals necessary to treat diabetes work as a team. The question in diabetes care is no longer whether blood glucose control is important for decreasing the risk for complications of diabetes, but it is now a question of how best to achieve appropriate blood glucose control. Several meal planning approaches can be utilized depending on patient needs and preferences. Patients with type 1 diabetes must be given adequate information, coaching, and support so they can make their own decisions about food choices. In addition to using current information about medical nutrition therapy, nutrition and other health professionals must be knowledgeable about and make use of blood glucose records and information on insulin to more appropriately assist the patient with nutrition and exercise decisions in their diabetes management.

References

1. Franz, M., Horton, E., Bantle, J., Beebe, C., Brunzell, J., Coulston, A., Henry, R., Hoogwerf, B., and Stacpoole, P. (1994). Nutrition principles for the management of diabetes and related complications. *Diabetes Care* **17,** 490–518.
2. Expert Committee on the Diagnosis and Classification of Diabetes Mellitus (1997). Report of the expert committee on the diagnosis and classification of diabetes mellitus. *Diabetes Care* **30,** page numbers to come.
3. Zimmet, P. Z., Tuomi, T., Mackay, R., Rowley, M. J., Knowles, W., Cohen, M., and Lang, D. A. (1994). Latent autoimmune diabetes mellitus in adults (LADA): The role of antibodies to glutamic acid decarboxylase in diagnosis and prediction of insulin dependency. *Diabet. Med.* **11,** 299–303.

4. Branson, R., Davis, J., and Remington, P. (1998). *In* "Chronic Disease Epidemiology and Control," Vol. II, pp. 421–464. United Book Press, Frederick, Maryland.

5. Atkinson, M. A., and Maclaren, N. K. (1994). The pathogenesis of insulin dependent diabetes. *N. Engl. J. Med.* **331**, 1428–1436.

6. Holler, H., and Pastors, J. (1997). *In* "Management of Diabetes: Medical Nutrition Therapy," Vol. I, pp. 15–28. American Dietetic Association, Chicago, IL.

7. Diabetes Control and Complications Trial Research Group (1993). The effect of intensive treatment of diabetes on the development and progression of long-term complications in insulin-dependent diabetes mellitus. *N. Engl. J. Med.* **329**, 977–986.

8. Diabetes Care and Education, a practice of group of The American Dietetic Association, Kulkarni, K. D., Castle, G., Gregory, R., Holmes, A., Leontos, C., Powers, M. A., Snetselaar, L., Splett, P. L., and Wylie-Rosett, J. (1997). Nutrition practice guidelines for Type I diabetes: An overview of the content and application. *Diabetes Spectrum* **10**, 248–256.

9. DCCT Research Group. (1993). Nutrition interventions for intensive therapy in the Diabetes Control and Complications Trial. *J. Am. Diet. Assoc.* **93**, 768–772.

10. Delahanty, L., and Halford, B. (1993). The role of diet behaviors in achieving improved glycemic control in intensively treated patients in the Diabetes Control and Complications Trial. *Diabetes Care* **16**, 1453–1458.

11. Peters, A. L., and Davidson, M. B. (1993). Protein and fat effects on glucose responses and insulin requirements in subjects with insulin-dependent diabetes mellitus. *Am. J. Clin. Nutr.* **58**, 555–560.

12. Ahmed, M., Nuttall, F. Q., Gannon, M. C., and Lamusga, R. F. (1980). Plasma glucagon and alpha-amino acid nitrogen response to various diets in normal humans. *Am. J. Clin. Nutr.* **33**, 1917–1924.

13. Brenner, B. M., Meyer, T. W., and Hostetter, T. H. (1982). Dietary protein intake and the progressive nature of kidney disease: The role of hemodynamically mediated glomerular injury in the pathogenesis of progressive glomerular sclerosis in aging, renal ablation and intrinsic renal disease. *N. Engl. J. Med.* **307**, 652–659.

14. Zeller, K. R. (1991). Low-protein diets in renal disease. *Diabetes Care* **14**, 856–866.

15. Friedman, E. A. (1982). Diabetic nephropathy: Strategies in prevention and management. *Kidney Int.* **21**, 780–791.

16. Kontessis, P., Jones, S., Dodds, R., Trevisan, R., Nosadini, R., Fioretto, P., Brosato, M., Sacerdoti, D., and Viberti, G. C. (1990). Renal metabolic and hormonal responses to ingestion of animal and vegetable proteins. *Kidney Int.* **38**, 136–144.

17. Jibani, M. M., Bloodworth, L. L., Foden, E., Griffiths, K. D., and Galpin, O. P. (1991). Predominantly vegetarian diet in patients with incipient and early clinical diabetic nephropathy: Effects on albumin excretion rate and nutritional status. *Diab. Med.* **8**, 949–953.

18. Nakamura, H., Ito, S., Ebe, N., and Shibata, A. (1993). Renal effects of different types of protein in healthy volunteer subjects and diabetic patients. *Diabetes Care* **16**, 1071–1075.

19. Stamler, J., Vaccaro, O., Neaton, J. D., and Wentworth, D., for the Multiple Risk Factor Intervention Trial Research Group (1993). Diabetes, other risk factors, and 12-yr cardiovascular mortality for men screened in the Multiple Risk Factor Intervention Trial. *Diabetes Care* **16**, 434–444.

20. Nikkila, E. A., and Hormila, P. (1978). Serum lipids and lipoprotein in insulin-treated diabetes: demonstration of increased high density lipoprotein concentrations. *Diabetes* **27**, 1078–1086.

21. Kern, P. (1987). Lipid disorders in diabetes mellitus. *Mt. Sinai J. Med.* **54**, 245–252.

22. Dunn, F. L. (1992). Plasma lipid and lipoprotein disorders in IDDM. *Diabetes* **41**, 102–106.

23. Garg, A., Bonanome, A., Grundy, S. M., Zhang, A. J., and Unger, R. H. (1988). Comparison of a high-carbohydrate diet with high-monounsaturated-fat diet in patients with non-insulin-dependent diabetes mellitus. *N. Engl. J. Med.* **391**, 829–834.

24. Parillo, M., Rivellese, A. A., Ciardullo, A. V., Capaldo, B., Giacco, A., Genovese, S., and Ricardi, G. (1992). A high-monounsaturated-fat/low-carbohydrate diet improves peripheral insulin sensitivity in non-insulin-dependent diabetic patients. *Metabolism* **41**, 1371–1378.

25. Jenkins, D. J. A., Woever, T. M. S., Jenkins, A. L., Josse, R. G., and Wong, G. S. (1984). The glycaemic response to carbohydrate foods. *Lancet* **2**, 388–391.

26. Loghmani, E., Richard, K., Washburne, L., Vandagriff, J., Fineberg, N., and Golden, M. (1991). Glycemic response to sucrose-containing mixed meals in diets of children with insulin-dependent diabetes mellitus. *J. Pediatr.* **119**, 531–537.

27. Kulkarni, K., Castle, G., Gregroy, R., Holmes, A., Leontos, C., Powers, M., Snetselaar, L., Splett, P., and Wylie-Rosett, J., for the Diabetes Care and Education Dietetic Practice Group (1998). Nutrition practice guidelines for type 1 diabetes mellitus positively affect dietitian practices and patient outcomes. *J. Am. Diet. Assoc.* **98**, 62–70.

28. Skyler, J. S. (1998). *In* "Insulin therapy in Type I Diabetes Mellitus," Vol. I, pp. 36–49. Mosby Year Book, St. Louis, MI.

29. Berger, M. (1995). *In* "Adjustment of Insulin Therapy," Vol. I., pp. 117–132. American Diabetes Association, Inc., Alexandria, VA.

30. Diabetes Control and Complications Trial Research Group (1995). Implementation of treatment protocols in the Diabetes Control and Complications Trial. *Diabetes Care* **18**, 361–376.

31. Nuttall, F. Q. (1993). Carbohydrate and dietary management of clients with insulin- requiring diabetes. *Diabetes Care* **16**, 1039–1042.

32. American Diabetes Association and American Dietetic Association (1995). "Carbohydrate Counting: Getting Started." American Diabetes Association, Alexandria, VA, and American Dietetic Association, Chicago, IL.

33. American Diabetes Association and American Dietetic Association (1995). "Carbohydrate Counting: Moving On." American Diabetes Association, Alexandria, VA, and American Dietetic Association, Chicago, IL.

34. American Diabetes Association and American Dietetic Association (1995). "Carbohydrate Counting: Carbohydrate/Insulin Ratios." American Diabetes Association, Alexandria, VA, and American Dietetic Association, Chicago, IL.

35. Gillespi, S., Kulkarni, K., and Daly, A. (1998). Using carbohydrate counting in diabetes clinical practice. *J. Am. Diet. Assoc.* **98**, 897–899.

36. Franz, M. J. (1997). Protein: Metabolism and effect on blood glucose levels. *Diabetes Ed.* **23,** 651–663.

37. American Diabetes Association and American Dietetic Association (1995). "Exchange Lists for Meal Planning." American Diabetes Association, Alexandria, VA, and American Dietetic Association, Chicago, IL.

38. American Diabetes Association and The American Dietetic Association (1995). "The First Step in Diabetes Meal Planning." American Diabetes Association, Alexandria, VA, and American Dietetic Association, Chicago, IL.

39. American Diabetes Association and The American Dietetic Association (1986). "Healthy Food Choices." American Diabetes Association, Alexandria, VA, and The American Dietetic Assocaition, Chicago, IL.

40. Bantle, J. P., Laine, D. C., Castle, G. W., Thomas, J. W., Hoogwerf, B. J., and Goetz, F. C. (1983). Postprandial glucose and insulin responses to meals containing different carbohydrates in normal and diabetic subjects. *N. Engl. J. Med.* **309,** 7–12.

41. Slama, G., Haardt, M. J., Jean-Joseph, P., Costagliola, D., Goicolea, I., Bornet, F., Elgrably, F., and Tchobroutsky, G. (1984). Sucrose taken during mixed meal has no additional hyperglycemic action over isocaloric amounts of starch in well-controlled diabetics. *Lancet* **2,** 122–125.

42. Bornet, F., Haardt, M. J., Costagliola, D., Blayo, A., and Slama, G. (1985). Sucrose or honey at breakfast have no additional acute hyperglycemic effect over an isoglucidic amount of bread in type ii diabetic patients. *Diabetologia* **28,** 213–217.

43. Forlani, G., Galuppi, V., Santacroce, G., Braione, A. F., Giangiulio, S., Ciavarella, A., and Vannini, P. (1989). Hyperglycemic effect of sucrose ingestion in IDDM patients controlled by artificial pancreas. *Diabetes Care* **12,** 296–298.

44. Peters, A. L., Davidson, M. B., and Eisenberg, K. (1990). Effect of isocaloric substitution of chocolate cake for potato in type I diabetic patients. *Diabetes Care* **13** 888–892.

45. Bantle, J. P., Laine, C. W., and Thomas, J. W. (1986). Metabolic effects of dietary fructose and sucrose in types I and II diabetic subjects. *JAMA* **256,** 3241–3246.

46. Wise, J. E., Keim, K. S., Huisinga, J. L., and Willmann, P. A. (1989). Effect of sucrose-containing snacks on blood glucose control. *Diabetes Care* **12,** 423–426.

47. Loghmani, E., Richard, K., Washburne, L., Vandagriff, H., Fineberg, N., and Golden, M. (1991). Glycemic response to sucrose-containing mixed meals in diets of children with insulin-dependent diabetes mellitus. *J. Pediatr.* **119,** 531–537.

48. Abraira, C., and Derler, J. (1988). Large variations of sucrose in constant carbohydrate diets in type II diabetes. *Am. J. Med.* **84,** 193–200.

49. Bantle, J. P., Swanson, J. E., Thomas, W., and Laine, D. C. (1993). Metabolic effects of dietary sucrose in type II diabetic subjects. *Diabetes Care* **16,** 1301–1305.

CHAPTER 29

Nutritional Management for Type 2 Diabetes

ANN M. COULSTON
Woodside, California

I. INTRODUCTION

Diabetes mellitus is a group of metabolic disorders characterized by hyperglycemia resulting from defects in insulin secretion, insulin action, or both. The hyperglycemia of diabetes increases the risk of a variety of complications including cardiovascular disease, stroke, visual impairment and blindness, nephropathy leading to renal failure, and neuropathy. Diabetes imposes a major public health burden in the United States and is associated with more than 300,000 deaths and about $100 billion in total costs annually [1].

Broadly, diabetes is classified into two major forms. Type 1 diabetes is characterized by a complete inability of the beta cells of the pancreas to produce insulin. It most commonly occurs during childhood and young adulthood and accounts for about 10% of all persons diagnosed with diabetes. Type 2 diabetes is a combination of a defect in insulin secretion and insulin resistance at the site of insulin action in the muscle, liver, and adipose tissue [2]. It is the most common form of the disease, affecting 90% of individuals with diabetes [3]. Most people with type 2 diabetes are obese, and obesity itself causes some degree of insulin resistance. Insulin secretion improves with weight loss but hyperglycemia seldom returns to normal. Type 2 diabetes has a gradual onset usually beginning with an impairment of glucose tolerance that frequently goes undiagnosed. It is estimated that, at diagnosis, most adults with type 2 diabetes have had the disease for an average of 7 years [4].

Only recently have individuals with type 2 diabetes been treated aggressively. This is partially accounted for by the fact that we are witnessing a trend toward an increase in younger individuals developing type 2 diabetes in association with an increase in childhood obesity. Also, because of the gradual disease onset, many patients, at diagnosis, have had the disease for several years and the ravages of chronic hyperglycemia may already be damaging vital body tissues [5]. Results of the United Kingdom Prospective Diabetes Study (UKPDS) [6] demonstrated that the hyperglycemia in type 2 diabetes is no less deadly than that in type 1 diabetes [7].

The management of type 2 diabetes is complex. Patients require a combination of medications and lifestyle changes to achieve blood glucose control [8]. They are frequently older and may have associated disease states that also require medical management, such as hypertension. Many are obese or overweight and this problem must also be addressed. Larger amounts of fat in the abdominal area are most closely associated with insulin resistance and type 2 diabetes [9]. Duration and degree of obesity can affect insulin secretion rates. Once diabetes is diagnosed, time continues to be a factor as beta-cell exhaustion progresses and eventually necessitates the use of insulin secretagogues or exogenous insulin therapy. Early detection followed by early intervention might slow this progress and reduce complications [4]. Reduced energy intake and moderate weight loss improve insulin sensitivity and lower blood glucose levels in type 2 patients [10]. Glycemic improvement, as a result of energy restriction, is due to the combined effects of reduced calories and carbohydrate intake.

Nutrition therapy is an important part of the overall management of diabetes. Current nutrition recommendations to achieve and maintain glucose, lipid, and blood pressure goals are simple to state, but difficult to initiate and even more difficult to maintain. Nutrition therapy can be summarized as follows: Lose weight if overweight (more than 30 kg/m²), restrict saturated fat intake, and divide total nutrient intake throughout the day [11, 12]. These nutrition recommendations are necessarily vague due to the heterogeneous nature of type 2 patients, which makes it impossible to recommend one dietary pattern. Available research data to substantiate more precise guidelines are lacking. As with all treatment regimens for chronic diseases, behavior modification and lifestyle change are essential.

In addition to providing guidelines to correct blood glucose and blood lipid levels, patients with type 2 diabetes need to receive information about basic nutrition needs [12a]. The traditional approach to medical management of type 2 diabetes, consisting of monotherapy, a weight-loss or "no sugar" diet, and advice to "get some exercise," will not yield desired medical outcomes. Current recommendations are for patients to have targeted blood glucose levels, whereby patients know and attempt to achieve their blood glucose goals. This kind of therapy is made possible by

feedback from daily self-monitoring of blood glucose and routine laboratory evaluations. Ongoing training programs for educators of patients with diabetes are essential [12b]. Table 1 defines glycemic control goals for type 2 diabetes.

This chapter will address the nutritional management of adults with type 2 diabetes. Nutrition issues for people with type 1 diabetes and with gestational diabetes are discussed in other chapters in this volume (Chapters 28 and 30).

II. ENERGY INTAKE AND BODY WEIGHT MANAGEMENT

Approximately 80–90% of people with type 2 diabetes are overweight [4]. Exercise and restriction of energy intake can improve glucose tolerance, diminish insulin resistance, and improve coronary risk factors in many patients with established type 2 diabetes, especially those who are hyperinsulinemic and insulin resistant. On the other hand, the therapeutic efficacy of diet and exercise in such patients has been limited because most individuals with this disorder are more than 40 years old at the time of diagnosis and many tend to be resistant to lifestyle changes [13].

Obesity, upper-body obesity in particular [9], aging, and a sedentary lifestyle are independent environmental factors that contribute to insulin resistance [14]. Weight loss improves blood glucose control by decreasing insulin resistance, which improves glucose uptake and reduces hepatic glucose output [15]. Studies have evaluated blood glucose control during weight loss and demonstrate that metabolic changes occur with as little as a 10 kg weight loss [10, 16]. Blood glucose levels and insulin sensitivity continue to improve as weight loss progresses on an energy-restricted constant diet [16]. Patients with hyperinsulinemia respond most dramatically to weight loss, thus early intervention before beta-cell exhaustion occurs provides the best possibility for improving blood glucose control with weight loss. Because we know that 30–40% of patients diagnosed with type 2 diabetes already have clinically significant ischemic heart disease, microvascular disease, and neuropathy at the time of diagnosis [5], diet and exercise may be more beneficial if instituted earlier in life, before the onset of hyperglycemia [17]. Glycemic control begins to improve within 24 hours of initiating a hypocaloric diet, even before any weight is lost [10]. In fact, within 10 days of a controlled hypocaloric diet 87% of the eventual drop in blood glucose occurs. These metabolic changes are temporary and require continuation of an energy intake that maintains a decreased body weight.

Many suggestions have been proposed for the most effective macronutrient composition to achieve weight loss in patients with diabetes. Traditionally, weight-loss diets are high in carbohydrate and low in fat. However, because of the carbohydrate intolerance of patients with diabetes, scientists have questioned the wisdom of this approach. At the same time there is concern that higher fat diets might promote obesity. Two reports in the literature have shown equal amounts of weight loss on hypocaloric, low-fat or higher fat diets [18, 19]. When metabolic parameters were examined during weight loss, investigators found that energy restriction and weight loss improved glycemic control, lipid profiles, and blood pressure independent of diet composition. In another report, the cardiovascular risk profile was improved when monounsaturated fatty acids or carbohydrate replaced saturated fatty acids on weight loss diets [20]. Very-low-calorie diet therapy consisting of 400–800 kcal/day has been shown to be safe in obese individuals with diabetes [21]. However this is a weight reduction method that can only be used for 3–4 months and then weight maintenance or moderately restricted diets must be initiated. To determine how this technique might work for the long-term, Wing and colleagues [21, 22] studied short periods of energy restriction, ranging from 1 day/week to 1 week/month to enhance weight loss efforts. One characteristic that all current weight loss methods have in common is that actual long-term weight loss is difficult and results are not dramatically different between weight loss regimens. Unfortunately, weight loss is very difficult to achieve and maintain in obese patients in general, and even more so in patients with type 2 diabetes, especially those on oral medications [23]. The metabolic explanation for increased difficulty with weight loss in diabetics is yet to be fully explained. The complexity of weight management has led clinicians to adopt the philosophy that absence of weight gain is itself a reputable goal.

III. MACRONUTRIENT INTAKE

A. Protein

Historically, the protein content, both type and amount, of the diet in patients with type 2 diabetes has played a secondary role to carbohydrate and fat content. General concerns for dietary protein adequacy have been to maintain lean body mass and nitrogen balance whether people have diabetes or not.

Body proteins are continuously being synthesized and degraded. The estimated turnover is about 280 g/day [24]. The amino acids resulting from protein degradation can be recycled, but this process is incomplete. Current data indicate that the efficiency with which amino acids are recycled may be regulated by the amount of protein in the diet [24]. The lower the protein content of the diet, the more efficiently amino acids are utilized. The current recommended amount, 0.8 g/kg body weight, represents an intake of about 11% of energy from protein. The estimated amount of protein ingested by the general population in the United States represents 15–20% of energy intake or 1.1–1.4 g/kg body weight based on 2000 kcal/day. This is considerably more than the minimum protein necessary even in people with diabetes. Campbell and associates [25] evaluated the protein requirements for older adults (56–80 years of age) and found that 1.0–1.25 g/kg is necessary to maintain lean body mass [25].

TABLE 1 Glycemic Control for Type 2 Diabetes

Biochemical index	Normal	Goal	Additional action suggested
Fasting/preprandial glucose	<110 mg/dL	80–120 mg/dL	<80 or >140 mg/dL
Bedtime glucose	<120 mg/dL	100–140 mg/dL	<100 or >160 mg/dL
Glycosylated hemoglobin	<6%	<7%	>8%

Source: Adapted from Zimmerman, B. R. (Ed.). (1998). "Medical Management of Type 2 Diabetes," 4th ed., p. 35. American Diabetes Association, Alexandria, VA.

Specific dietary protein recommendations for people with diabetes have not been established. An increased loss of body protein with severe insulin deficiency has been known for years [26, 27]. This is especially striking in patients with type 1 diabetes in whom withdrawal of insulin results in a marked increase in protein loss [28]. When insulin is replaced in the management of type 1 diabetes, the protein requirement is considered to be similar to that for nondiabetic individuals. More recent studies indicating increased leucine turnover suggest that the minimum protein requirement is likely to be increased in most people with type 1 diabetes [29]. If so, the reason protein malnutrition is uncommon is probably that the amount of dietary protein ingested by the average adult regularly exceeds the required amount.

In people with established renal insufficiency, with or without diabetes, a restriction in dietary protein has been considered desirable to modify the progression of the disease. This is controversial and there is concern that frank protein deficiency may result [30, 31]. At the present time, there is no evidence that restricting protein in the diet of people with diabetes will prevent or delay the onset of renal insufficiency.

From reports in the literature, we know that the minimum amount of protein necessary to replace body stores is relatively small, and the amount of protein that can be tolerated without toxic effects is high [32]. Data to support beneficial effects of protein in the diet lower or higher than the typical Western diet, which contains approximately 15–20% of calories from protein, are lacking. The position of the American Diabetes Association recommends 10–20% of calories from protein, with the lower amount being recommended for patients with overt nephropathy [11].

From anecdotal information, diets composed mainly of lean meat in quantities to meet energy requirements are not readily acceptable. Even isocaloric diets containing 40–45% of energy from protein are not acceptable. This was confirmed by Nuttall and colleagues [33] feeding normal young volunteers diets of 41% energy from protein. Although these diets were isocaloric, subjects commented that this amount of food was more than they were comfortable eating. They also complained of malaise and lethargy after ingesting the high-protein diet. Keep in mind that the so-called "high-protein diets" being promoted in the popular weight loss diet literature recommend 30% of energy from protein in the context of a hypocaloric, not isocaloric, energy level. Thus, the actual recommended amount of protein in grams in such diets is not likely to be more than "high normal" for an isocaloric diet.

In the liver, amino acids that are not required to replace body proteins, particularly nonessential amino acids, are deaminated [34]. The amino group is condensed with carbon dioxide to form urea, which is then carried to the kidneys and excreted in the urine. The amount of urea excreted per day is an index of the amount of protein metabolized, although about 14% of newly synthesized urea is utilized by bacteria in the colon [35]. Small amounts of amino acids are also metabolized (deaminated) in the kidney [36]. The carbon skeletons remaining after deamination can be converted to glucose. The resulting glucose may contribute to plasma glucose concentration. Despite the conversion of amino acids to glucose, controlled feeding studies of known amounts of protein do not result in the predicted (calculated) increase in peripheral glucose concentration in normal or type 2 subjects [37, 38]. Further studies designed to elucidate these findings are described below.

It is known that the carbon skeleton of all amino acids derived from protein digestion, with the exception of leucine, can be used to synthesize glucose. Theoretically, ingestion of 100 g protein can yield 50–80 g glucose depending on the amino acid composition of the protein. Using isotope dilution techniques combined with determination of urea formation rates, it was calculated that ingestion of 50 g of cottage cheese protein would result in 34 g being deaminated over the 8-hour period of the study in normal subjects. However, the amount of glucose entering the circulation was only 9.7 g [39]. Thus, the amount of glucose produced was considerably less than the amount theorized by about 25 g. A similar technique, applied to patients with type 2 diabetes following the ingestion of beef protein, found that of the 50 g protein ingested only ~2 g could be accounted for by the appearance of glucose in the circulation over an 8-hour period [40]. Thus, in patients with diabetes, the amount of glucose appearing in the circulation was even less than in normal subjects. From the beef protein load, 28 g glucose was predicted. The fate of the remaining carbon skeletons is unknown.

In healthy people, protein is a weak insulin stimulator compared with glucose; however, in patients with type 2 diabetes, protein and glucose are equipotent in stimulating insulin secretion. After the ingestion of protein, the circulating insulin concentration is increased in both healthy subjects and patients with type 2 diabetes [41, 42]. When protein is

ingested with glucose, healthy subjects have an additive insulin response [43], whereas obese subjects with type 2 diabetes exhibit a synergistic insulin response [44].

Protein-containing foods are generally classified as plant or animal based. Studies comparing animal to plant proteins are confounded by the fact that ingestion of plant protein diets is accompanied by additional dietary fiber, while diets based on animal protein are associated with an increased ingestion of dietary fat. Animal studies have demonstrated an atherogenecity of animal protein diets as compared to plant- or soy protein-based diets [45]. However, it is not possible with the data currently available to draw conclusions as to the benefits or hazards of either plant or animal proteins in the diets of people with type 2 diabetes.

B. Carbohydrate

Fasting blood glucose is determined by the overproduction of glucose from the liver and the body's ability to remove glucose from the blood stream. The amount of glucose absorbed from a meal largely determines the blood glucose response in the postprandial state. Patients with type 2 diabetes require from 3 to 4 hours for blood glucose to return to fasting or premeal levels after eating. However, gastric emptying rate, intestinal motility, and factors that affect glucose removal from the circulation, such as insulin response or insulin resistance, modify the absolute plasma glucose response. Thus, plasma glucose concentration at any given time is the result of the action of medication, glucose absorption from meals, and endogenous production of glucose mainly from the liver.

Prior to the availability of insulin and other pharmaceutical agents, both glucose overproduction and the impaired ability to metabolize absorbed glucose were shown to be treatable by dietary manipulations. In the early 1900s semi-starvation or low-calorie diets controlled overproduction of glucose. The amount of carbohydrate in the diet depended on the severity of diabetes and was tailored to the individual utilization rate [46]. Dietary patterns were low in carbohydrate and very high in fat as an energy fuel. Adhering to these diets was difficult, and semi-starvation could only be followed for a limited time.

Following the availability of insulin and oral agents for the treatment of diabetes, food energy restriction and the carbohydrate content of the diet have been greatly relaxed. In fact, there has been a universal trend toward advocating a higher and higher carbohydrate content in the diet, not only for people with diabetes, but also for the general population [47, 48]. An increase in carbohydrate intake allows a decrease in fat intake to meet overall energy needs. The protein content of the diet remains relatively constant. This high-carbohydrate dietary recommendation was driven by the concern that dietary fat, especially saturated fat, in the diet was responsible for the increasing incidence of cardiovascular disease.

Because cardiovascular disease is more common in people with diabetes and accounts for the majority of deaths in patients with diabetes [49–51] early dietary recommendations followed the American Heart Association and recommended a high-carbohydrate, low-fat diet [47]. However, the American Heart Association guidelines were aimed primarily at people with hypercholesterolemia. The most frequent lipid abnormalities in patients with type 2 diabetes are hypertriglyceridemia, increased very low density lipoprotein (VLDL) cholesterol, and reduced HDL cholesterol [52]. Plasma concentrations of total and low-density lipoprotein (LDL) cholesterol are similar to those in the general population. However, about 40% of patients with type 2 diabetes have an elevated LDL cholesterol [53]. The hypertriglyceridemia of type 2 diabetes is believed to be due in part to increased hepatic production of triglyceride-rich VLDL particles induced by increased dietary carbohydrate intake. An increase in small, dense LDL particles along with decreased HDL cholesterol and hypertriglyceridemia appear to be sequelae of insulin resistance, although a complete understanding of the mechanism remains to be elucidated [52, 54]. The insulin resistance of type 2 diabetes results in hyperinsulinemia in the face of hyperglycemia. Epidemiological studies have demonstrated that, in addition to the dyslipidemia of type 2 diabetes, hyperglycemia and hyperinsulinemia contribute to an increased risk for cardiovascular disease in people with diabetes [55, 56].

Dietary intervention studies of high-carbohydrate, low-fat diets as compared to moderate-carbohydrate, higher fat diets have indicated that the risk factors for cardiovascular disease in people with type 2 diabetes are exacerbated with high-carbohydrate, low-fat diets [57, 58]. Diets with relatively high fat (40–45% of energy from fat) in which monounsaturated and polyunsaturated fatty acids predominate demonstrate an improved lipid profile, and the increase in dietary fat does not hinder glucose disposal [59]. As a result of studies that demonstrate that higher intakes of carbohydrate accentuate plasma glucose, insulin, and triglyceride response, general nutrition recommendations currently are to individualize the amount of carbohydrate in the diet to optimize patient blood glucose and lipid goals [12].

Unresolved questions about the best type of dietary carbohydrate for people with type 2 diabetes remain. For many years, it was felt that refined sucrose (i.e., table sugar) should be eliminated from the diets of people with diabetes despite the lack of convincing scientific data. More recent evidence indicates that the amount of sucrose typically found in the American diet does not have an adverse effect on blood glucose control [60, 61]. Consequently, current dietary recommendations from the American Diabetes Association do not prohibit sucrose or any type of dietary carbohydrate [11]. Rather the focus is on the amount of all dietary carbohydrate at each meal and for the total day because the amount of carbohydrate at meals and throughout the day has a major impact on daylong blood glucose control.

In recent years, interest in dietary fiber has increased. The American Diabetes Association has suggested 20–35 g dietary fiber/day for people with diabetes [12]. This amount

represents an increase from the recent reports of dietary fiber intake of 17 g/day for the general population and 16 g/day for people with diabetes [62]. Increasing consumption of soluble fiber has been shown to reduce serum cholesterol and improve colonic function [63]. Whether or not patients with type 2 diabetes can achieve improved glycemic control by consuming diets high in dietary fiber, and especially soluble fiber, has been debated. Studies have shown that mixing viscous, nonstarch polysaccharides with carbohydrate-rich foods reduces the postprandial plasma glucose response, presumably by slowing the intestinal absorption of glucose [64, 65]. However, the amounts required to achieve these one-meal test results are too high to be acceptable in a routine diet. Nevertheless, high-fiber diets had been encouraged for people with diabetes with the rationale that dietary fiber would delay or reduce the absorption of glucose from the intestine.

In early studies of mixed diets, which varied in total dietary fiber from a variety of food sources, fed to patients with type 2 diabetes, no improvement in plasma glucose response was noted [66]. In this same study, higher fiber diets did not show any benefit to plasma cholesterol levels beyond that which can be achieved with a reduction in saturated fatty acid intake [66, 67]. A more recent report led to different conclusions. Diets for patients with type 2 diabetes that contained 50 g total dietary fiber, of which 25 g were from soluble fiber and all fiber from nonfortified foods, found significant improvement in both plasma glucose control and decreased fasting plasma lipid concentrations [68]. This report is very convincing; however, the lifestyle change to consume 50 g dietary fiber/day may be difficult for a population with reported usually intake of 16 g/per day as reported by the National Health and Nutrition Examination Survey (NHANES III) [62].

Finally, dietary fiber has been encouraged for all to prevent colon cancer. However, two recent intervention trials in normal glycemic individuals found no association between dietary fibers from fruits, vegetables, and whole grains on the recurrence of adenomatous polyps, thought to be the early signs of developing colon cancer [69, 70]. Whether the subjects were able to consume the level of fiber-rich foods recommended is not substantiated in the research report. In addition, many scientists believe that dietary fiber is only one risk factor in the development of colon cancer. It would be naïve, however, to suggest that dietary fiber has no role in colorectal cancer from these reports.

During the past century, investigators have reported differences in the plasma glucose response to the ingestion of different carbohydrate-containing foods despite the foods being matched for total carbohydrate content [71, 72]. Dietary carbohydrate foods are composed of a variety of mono-, di-, and polysaccharide structures. These sugars and starches are hydrolyzed into constituent glucose molecules by a combination of pancreatic amylase and intestinal mucosal glucosidase and maltase enzymes. These enzymes are present in excess so the rate-limiting process is not related to hydrolysis but rather the physical state of the starch. Uncooked starch in general is poorly digested and, thus, not well absorbed. Another hydrolysis factor is how readily the starch granules, which differ in size and structure depending on the plant source, undergo gelatinization. As a result, starch in many foods is not completely hydrolyzed or digestible.

Sugars, on the other hand, are readily digested and absorbed in the intestine. However, the monosaccharide fructose does not cause an elevation in blood glucose in normal glycemic or in patients treated for diabetes. Recently Gannon and colleagues [73] verified this concept by comparing the daylong plasma glucose and insulin response to identical carbohydrate content meals in patients with type 2 diabetes. One day the meals were high in starch foods and the other day in sugars from fruit, vegetables, and dairy products. On the day of the higher sugars diet, plasma glucose and insulin were significantly lower following each meal. Although these findings are interesting and help explain the glycemic impact of foods, dietary patterns are a combination of starches and sugars. Consequently, when individual carbohydrate-containing foods are tested for their glycemic response, foods differ.

Jenkins and colleagues [74, 75] tested a large number of foods and compared them to the plasma glucose response for pure glucose or white bread and developed a "glycemic index." Of concern for the nutritional management of patients with diabetes is to determine whether or not these differences in glycemic response have clinical relevance. Recent reports from the Health Professionals Follow-up Study cohort and the Nurses' Health Study cohort indicate that over time, diets high in glycemic load and low in cereal fiber significantly increase the risk of type 2 diabetes [76, 77]. These observational studies need to be addressed in research settings with careful controls on potential confounding factors and in settings where the mechanisms of disease can be studied. Controlled intervention studies have failed to show clinically significant differences between so-called high and low glycemic index foods in the context of a total day's meal [78, 79]. As additional studies have appeared in the literature, generally conducted with intervention techniques relying on dietary advice and lists of foods to choose and avoid, the use of the glycemic index has been criticized and its utility in nutritional management of people with diabetes questioned [80, 81].

C. Fat

Because diabetes is associated with a marked increase in coronary artery disease, there is a strong focus on dietary fatty acid intake [51]. Several studies have shown that increased cardiovascular risk factors, including hypertension, precede the onset of type 2 diabetes [82]. In most studies the excess risk of cardiovascular disease is relatively greater in women with diabetes than men [51].

People with type 2 diabetes have a dyslipidemia, as mentioned earlier, consisting of increased triglyceride concentrations and decreased HDL cholesterol levels, and small dense

LDL cholesterol particles that do not normalize with improved glycemic control [54, 83]. This dyslipidemia is strongly associated with increased central (visceral) obesity, insulin resistance, and cardiovascular disease [54, 84–86]. Much has been written about the association of hyperinsulinemia and/or insulin resistance with cardiovascular disease [87]. The study by Despres and colleagues [88] provides the strongest evidence that hyperinsulinemia is associated prospectively with the development of cardiovascular disease. LDL cholesterol is usually not different in people with or without diabetes, but a number of metabolic and compositional changes in LDL particles have been described. A preponderance of smaller denser LDL particles (subclass pattern B) has been identified as a risk for cardiovascular disease [86]. Although this has not been studied extensively in people with type 2 diabetes, small, dense LDL particles are associated with increased triglyceride and decreased HDL cholesterol levels, male sex, hyperinsulinemia, and insulin resistance [54]. People with type 2 diabetes and hypertriglyceridemia usually have both overproduction and impaired catabolism of VLDL triglyceride. Lipoprotein lipase (LPL) activity can be reduced in patients with poor glucose control and profound hypertriglyceridemia [89]. Decreased HDL cholesterol levels may be due to increased catabolism, or to decreased production of HDL due to impaired catabolism of VLDL and decreased LPL activity [90]. For additional information, Ginsberg [91] has reviewed the pathophysiology of dyslipemia in diabetes and Haffner [92] has recently reviewed the effectiveness of medical therapy for the dyslipidemia of adults with type 2 diabetes.

Before 1971, most advice on nutritional therapy for diabetes was to restrict dietary carbohydrate and increase dietary fat to meet daily caloric needs [93]. However, epidemiological studies in the 1960s showed a cardiovascular disease risk associated with increased intake of total and saturated fat [94]. As it became apparent that cardiovascular disease was a leading cause of death in people with diabetes [50], nutrition recommendations for people with diabetes called for reduction in total fat and saturated fats to <30% and <10% of calories, respectively [95]. Controversy has arisen over recommending a low-fat, high-carbohydrate diet to these patients because of concern that this may worsen triglyceride and HDL abnormalities and ultimately increase cardiovascular risk [96]. Another concern is whether overweight and obese people with type 2 diabetes will be able to lose weight on a higher fat diet.

Current American Diabetes Association and American Dietetic Association dietary guidelines permit either a high-carbohydrate, low-fat diet, or a moderate carbohydrate, higher fat diet enriched with polyunsaturated or monounsaturated fat. The issue of whether a high-monounsaturated-fat diet is preferable to a high-carbohydrate diet remains controversial [97]. In short term studies, a high-carbohydrate diet has been associated with higher triglyceride levels and lower HDL levels than a higher fat diet [98, 99]. The nutrition practice guidelines of the American Dietetic Association

suggest a 4- to 6-month trial of nutrition intervention before lipid-lowering pharmacological treatment is initiated [100]. However if the patient has preexisting cardiovascular disease or already has made all of the lifestyle changes he or she is willing or able to make, pharmacological intervention may be initiated sooner.

It has been demonstrated in numerous studies that glycemic control and insulin action are improved—or at least not made worse—when the diet is restricted in saturated fatty acids [101–103]. The debate, therefore, is not whether saturated fat should be limited to 10% or less of total caloric intake, as is currently recommended by the National Cholesterol Education Program (NCEP) for the prevention of cardiovascular risk, but what is the best alternative energy source for the patient with diabetes. Dietary protein is generally ~10–20% of total daily energy intake. This leaves roughly 70–80% of energy intake to be derived from a combination of polyunsaturated fats, monounsaturated fats, and carbohydrates.

Several short-term studies have been conducted that have explored diets of greater than 30% energy from fat with the extra fat coming from monounsaturated fatty acids [58, 98, 99]. In these isocaloric studies, saturated fatty acids were maintained at 10% of energy. At the end of each diet phase, fasting glucose and insulin concentrations, and total cholesterol and LDL cholesterol concentrations, did not differ between the two diets. However, fasting triglyceride levels, VLDL cholesterol, and postprandial excursions of glucose, insulin, and triglycerides were higher while fasting HDL cholesterol levels decreased during the high-carbohydrate diet period. The authors emphasize that the lower total glucose load keeps postprandial glucose and insulin concentrations reduced, low dietary saturated fat keeps LDL cholesterol in check, and the higher monounsaturated and polyunsaturated content of the diet prevents HDL cholesterol decrease and triglyceride concentration increase. With attention to food choices, it is possible to keep the saturated fat content of the diet low without decreasing the total dietary fat intake. The addition of unsaturated fatty acids to the diet to maintain energy needs appears to be the optimal approach to nutrition management, especially for patients with the typical dyslipidemia of type 2 diabetes and with insulin resistance.

IV. TRACE MINERAL REQUIREMENTS

A. Magnesium

Magnesium levels remain remarkably constant in people without diabetes, due to regulatory mechanisms. However, those with diabetes appear to be prone to low serum magnesium levels [104, 105]. The clinical significance of this finding remains undefined, because only about 0.3% of total body magnesium is in the blood. Low serum levels may be related to increased urinary magnesium losses secondary to glycosuria-induced renal wasting [106], although short-term

improvement in glycemic control has not been shown to restore serum magnesium levels [107].

Magnesium is intimately involved in a number of important biochemical reactions, particularly processes that involve the formation and use of high-energy phosphate bonds. As a cofactor in more than 300 enzyme reactions, it modulates glucose transport through membranes and is a cofactor in several enzymatic systems involving glucose oxidation [108]. Some believe that magnesium deficiency may increase or cause insulin resistance [109].

Low levels of magnesium have been associated with hypertension, cardiac arrhythmia, congestive heart failure, retinopathy, and insulin resistance [110–112]. Magnesium depletion in a few studies has been shown to result in insulin resistance as well as impaired insulin secretion and thereby may worsen control of diabetes [112]. Nadler and colleagues [113] conducted a magnesium depletion study. Men were fed 12 mg magnesium daily for 3 weeks. Intravenous glucose tolerance tests performed at the beginning and end of the 3-week period revealed a significant increase in insulin sensitivity. These findings raise the possibility that insulin resistance and abnormal glucose tolerance might be due to inadequate magnesium. In fact, Paolisso and colleagues [114] have shown magnesium supplementation to improve glucose tolerance in nondiabetic elderly, and improve insulin response in elderly, type 2 patients with diabetes. It is possible that decreased magnesium levels may represent a marker rather than a cause of the disease. In a recent report on the role of magnesium deficiency in the pathogenesis of type 2 diabetes from the large (12,218 adults) Atherosclerosis Risk in Communities (ARIC) Study, the authors demonstrated in white, but not black, adults a strong relationship between type 2 diabetes and serum magnesium levels [115]. Findings in this study suggest that modification of magnesium intake by dietary means alone is insufficient to achieve an effect to prevent type 2 diabetes. Whether pharmacological doses of magnesium coupled with other risk factors for diabetes can reduce long-term risk remains to be studied.

Until magnesium depletion studies conducted in normal individuals can relate specific dietary intake levels with abnormal glucose tolerance testing or other indicators of glucose metabolism, it is premature to consider the prevalence of diabetes mellitus as a functional indicator of adequacy for magnesium [116]. The revised Recommended Dietary Allowance (RDA) value for magnesium for women over 50 years of age is 320 mg/day and 420 mg/day for men in the same age group [116]. A review of the literature by the Standing Committee resulted in a gradual increase in the RDA for magnesium with age. Thus, it makes sense, at the least, to assess the dietary intake of older patients with type 2 diabetes for magnesium adequacy. The American Diabetes Association consensus statement on magnesium supplementation for patients with diabetes concluded that until accurate indexes of magnesium deficiency are available, routine evaluation of magnesium status in otherwise healthy individuals with diabetes is not recommended [107].

B. Chromium

In laboratory animals chromium deficiency is associated with an increase in blood glucose, cholesterol, and triglyceride concentrations. This observation has led to the investigation of chromium status in humans. The biologically active elemental chromium product is called glucose tolerance factor [117]. Glucose tolerance factor is composed of nicotinic acid, elemental chromium, and the amino acids glutamic acid, glycine, and cysteine. It acts as a cofactor for insulin and may facilitate insulin-membrane receptor interaction. However, glucose tolerance factor lowers plasma glucose only in the presence of insulin (postprandial state) and not in overnight fasted animals [118].

Most chromium supplements are poorly absorbed, but when combined with picolinate, absorption is improved. Because no method exists to determine chromium deficiency, the prevalence of a deficiency is unknown. Rabinowitz and colleagues [119] studied chromium in hair, serum, urine, and red blood cells and could not identify a deficiency of chromium in people with or without diabetes. In three double-blind crossover studies in patients with diabetes, chromium supplementation failed to improve glucose and lipid levels [120–122].

Recent evidence from China suggests a role for chromium supplementation in people with type 2 diabetes. Individuals with type 2 diabetes were randomly divided into three groups and supplemented with 1000 μg/day or 2000 μg/day chromium or placebo. In all three groups, fasting, 2-hour glucose concentrations and glycosylated hemoglobin values decreased but the decreases in the subjects receiving supplemental chromium were much larger. Fasting and 2-hour insulin concentrations were also lowered in the two supplemented groups. Total plasma cholesterol concentration decreased in the group receiving supplements, but there was no impact of supplementation on HDL cholesterol, triglyceride concentration, or body weight [123].

However, before chromium supplementation can be recommended, double-blind crossover studies of the effect of chromium supplementation in people with diabetes with known dietary intake of chromium need to be conducted. Until proven otherwise, it is assumed that chromium functions as a nutrient, not as a therapeutic agent, and that it benefits only individuals with marginal glucose intolerance whose signs and symptoms are due to marginal or overt chromium deficiency [124].

V. CONCLUSION

We are witnessing a surge in public and media attention on type 2 diabetes mellitus. This is due in part to the increasing worldwide incidence of type 2 diabetes and to the reports of disease management studies that continue to show marked improvement in disease outcome with improved glycemic control. Nutrition intervention remains a key component of type 2 diabetes management.

In this chapter, nutrient components of the diet are discussed in relation to the impact they have on diabetes treatment. The entire disease management process has been enhanced due to the advances in oral medications for glucose and lipid control. In addition, with an increased focus on near-normal glycemic control in this population, all health care team members are more closely involved in assisting the patients with disease management.

The use of herbal products (commonly viewed as a component of nutrition therapy) in disease prevention and treatment is gaining in popularity [125]. Despite the tremendous recent growth in popularity, carefully controlled studies are few. For these reasons, no discussion of this topic has been included here. However, with the development of guidelines for clinical investigation, this is an area that will expand in the future [126].

The public health burden of type 2 diabetes causes us to take notice not only for treatment following diagnosis, but more importantly, disease prevention for those genetically susceptible and attention to the current epidemic of obesity in adults and children. The role for nutrition is expanding as our knowledge and treatment options increase.

References

1. Brancati, F. L., Kao, W. H. L., Folsom, A. R., Watson, R. L., and Szklo, M. (2000). Incident type 2 diabetes mellitus in African American and white adults. *JAMA* **283**, 2253–2259.

2. DeFronzo, R. (1988). Lilly lecture 1987. The triumvirate: Beta-cell, muscle, liver. *Diabetes* **37**, 667–687.

3. Kenny, S. J., Aubert, R. E., and Geiss, L. S. (1995). Prevalence and incidence of non-insulin-dependent diabetes. *In* "Diabetes in America" (National Diabetes Data Group, Ed.), pp. 47–68. U.S. Dept. of Health and Human Services, Public Health Service, National Institutes of Health, Bethesda, MD.

4. American Diabetes Association (2000). Report of the expert committee on the diagnosis and classification of diabetes mellitus [committee report]. *Diabetes Care* **23**(Suppl. 1), S4–S19.

5. Harris, MI. (1995). Undiagnosed NIDDM: Clinical and public health issues. *Diabetes Care* **18**, 258–268.

6. U.K. Prospective Diabetes Study Group (1998). Intensive blood glucose control with sulfonylureas or insulin compared with conventional treatment and risk of complications in patients with type 2 diabetes (UKPDS 33). *Lancet* **352**, 837–853.

7. Diabetes Control and Complications Trial Research Group (1993). The effect of intensive treatment of diabetes on the development and progression of long-term complications of insulin-dependent diabetes mellitus. *N. Engl. J. Med.* **329**, 977–986.

8. Turner, R. C., Cull, C. A., Frighi, V., and Holman, R. R., for the U.K. Prospective Diabetes Study (UKPDS) Group (1999). Glycemic control with diet, sulfonylurea, metformin, or insulin in patients with type 2 diabetes mellitus. *JAMA* **281**, 2005–2012.

9. Kissebah, A. H., Vydelingum, N., Murray, R., Evans, D. F., Hartz, A. J., Kalkhoff, R. K., and Adams, P. W. (1982). Relationship of body fat distribution to metabolic complications of obesity. *J. Clin. Endocrinol. Metab.* **54**, 254–260.

10. Henry, R. R., Schaefer, L., and Olefsky, J. M. (1985). Glycemic effects of intensive caloric restriction and isocaloric refeeding in noninsulin dependent diabetes mellitus. *J. Clin. Endocrinol. Metab.* **61**, 917–925.

11. American Diabetes Association (2000). Nutrition recommendations and principles for people with diabetes mellitus [position statement]. *Diabetes Care* **23**(Suppl. 1), S43–S46.

12. Franz, M. J., Horton, E. S., Bantle, J. P., Beebe, C. A., Brunzell, J. D., Coulston, A. M., Henry, R. R., Hoogwerf, B. J., and Stackpoole, P. W. (1994). Nutrition principles for the management of diabetes and related complications [technical review]. *Diabetes Care* **17**, 490–518.

12a. Lipkin, E. (1999). New strategies for the treatment of type 2 diabetes. *J. Am. Diet. Assoc.* **99**, 329–334.

12b. Lorenz, R. A., Gregory, R. P., Davis, D. L., Schlundt, D. G., and Wermager, J. (2000). Diabetes training for dietitians: Needs assessment, program description and effects on knowledge and problem solving. *J. Am. Diet. Assoc.* **100**, 225–228.

13. Skarfors, E. T., Wegener, T. A., Lithell, H., and Selinus, I. (1987). Physical training as treatment for type 2 diabetes in elderly men: A feasibility study over 2 years. *Diabetologia* **30**, 930–933.

14. Eriksson, K. F., and Lindgarde, F. (1996). Poor physical fitness and impaired early insulin response but late hyperinsulinemia, as predictors of NIDDM in middle-aged Swedish men. *Diabetologia* **39**, 573–579.

15. Ruderman, N., Chisholm, D., Pi-Sunyer, X., and Schneider, S. (1998). The metabolically obese, normal-weight individual revisited. *Diabetes* **47**, 699–713.

16. Wing, R. R., Koeske, R., Epstein, L. H., Nowarlk, M. P., Gooding, W., and Becker, D. (1987). Long-term effects of modest weight loss in type 2 diabetic patients. *Arch Intern Med* **147**, 1749–1753.

17. Ruderman, N. B., Schneider, S. H., and Berchtold, P. (1981). The "metabolically-obese," normal-weight individual. *Am. J. Clin. Nutr.* **34**, 1617–1621.

18. Low, C. C., Grossman, E. B., and Gumbiner, B. (1995) Potentiation of effects of weight loss by monounsaturated fatty acids in obese NIDDM patients. *Diabetes* **45**, 569–571.

19. Golay, A., Allaz, A. F., Morel, Y., de Tonnac, N., Tankova, S., and Reaven, G. (1996) Similar weight loss with low or high carbohydrate diets. *Am. J. Clin. Nutr.* **63**, 174–178.

20. Heilbronn, L. K., Noakes, M., and Clifton, P. M. (1999). Effect of energy restriction, weight loss and diet composition on plasma lipids and glucose in patients with type 2 diabetes. *Diabetes Care* **22**, 889–895.

21. Wing, R. R., Blair, E., and Marcus, M. (1994). Year-long weight loss treatment for obese patients with type 2 diabetes: Does inclusion of an intermittent very low calorie diet improve control? *Am. J. Med.* **97**, 354–362.

22. Williams, K., Mullen, M., Kelly, D., and Wing, R. (1998). The effect of short periods of caloric restriction on weight loss and glycemic control in type 2 diabetes. *Diabetes Care* **21**, 2–8.

23. Kelley, D. E., Wing, R., Buonocore, C., Sturis, J., Polonsky, K., and Fitzsimmons, M. (1993). Relative effects of caloric restriction and weight loss in non-insulin-dependent diabetes mellitus. *J. Clin. Endocrinol. Metab.* **77**, 1287–1293.

24. Newby, F. D., and Price, S. R. (1998). Determinants of protein turn-over in health and disease. *Mineral Electrolyte Metab.* **24,** 6–12.

25. Campbell, W. W., Crim, M. C., Dallal, G. E., Young, V. R., and Evans, W. J. (1994). Increased protein requirements in elderly people: New data and retrospective reassessments. *Am. J. Clin. Nutr.* **60,** 501–509.

26. Reed, J. A. (1954). Aretaeus, the Cappadocian. *Diabetes* **3,** 419–421.

27. Frank, L. L. (1957). Diabetes mellitus in the text book of old Hindu medicine. *Am. J. Gastroenterol.* **27,** 76–95.

28. Nair, K. S., Garrow, J. S., Ford, C., Mahler, R. F., and Halliday, D. (1983). Effect of poor diabetic control and obesity on the whole body protein metabolism in man. *Diabetologia* **25,** 400–403.

29. Hoffer, L. J. (1993). Are dietary protein requirements altered in diabetes mellitus? *Can. J. Physiol. Parmacol.* **71,** 633–638.

30. Henry, R. R. (1994). Protein content of the diabetic diet. *Diabetes Care* **17,** 1502–1513.

31. Maroni, B. J., and Mitch, W. E. (1997). Role of nutrition in prevention of the progression of renal disease. *Annu. Rev. Nutr.* **17,** 435–455.

32. Gannon, M. C., and Nuttall, F. Q. (1999). Protein and diabetes. *In* "American Diabetes Association Guide to Medical Nutrition Therapy for Diabetes" (M. J. Franz and J. P. Bantle, Eds.), pp. 107–125. American Diabetes Association, Alexandria, VA.

33. Nuttall, F. Q., Gannon, M. C., Wald, J. L., and Ahmed, M. (1985). Plasma glucose and insulin profiles in normal subjects ingesting diets of varying carbohydrate, fat, and protein content. *J. Am. College Nutr.* **4,** 437–450.

34. Wahren, J., Felig, P., and Hagenfeldt, L. (1976). Effect of protein ingestion on splanchnic and leg metabolism in normal men and in patients with diabetes mellitus. *J. Clin. Invest.* **57,** 987–999.

35. Vilstrup, H. (1980). Synthesis of urea after stimulation with amino acids: Relation to liver function. *Gut* **21,** 990–995.

36. Ganong, W. F. (1979). "Review of Medical Physiology." Lange Medical Publications, Los Altos, CA.

37. Nuttal, F. Q., and Gannon, M. C. (1991). Plasma glucose and insulin response to macronutrients in nondiabetic and NIDDM subjects. *Diabetes Care* **14,** 824–838.

38. Gannon, M. C., Nuttal, F. Z., Lane, J. T., and Burmeister, L. A. (1992). Metabolic response to cottage cheese or egg white protein, with or without glucose in type 2 diabetic subjects. *Metabolism* **41,** 1137–1145.

39. Kahn, M. A., Gannon, M. C., and Nuttall, F. Q. (1992). Glucose appearance rate following protein ingestion in normal subjects. *J. Am. College Nutr.* **11,** 701–706.

40. Gannon, M. C., and Nuttall, F. Q. (1997). The metabolic response to dietary protein in subjects with type 2 diabetes (abstract). *J. Am. College Nutr.* **16,** 478.

41. Floyd, J. C., Fajans, S. S., Conn, J. W., Knopf, R. F., and Rull, J. (1996). Insulin secretion in response to protein ingestion. *J. Clin. Invest.* **45,** 1479–1486.

42. Rabinowitz, D., Merimee, T. J., Maffezzoli, R., and Burggess, J. A. (1966). Patterns of hormonal release after glucose, protein, and glucose plus protein. *Lancet* **2,** 454–457.

43. Krezowski, P. A., Nuttall, F. Q., Gannon, M. C., and Bartosh, N. H. (1986). The effect of protein ingestion on the metabolic

response to oral glucose in normal individuals. *Am. J. Clin. Nutr.* **44,** 847–856.

44. Gannon, M. C., Nuttall, F. Q., Neil, B. J., and Westphal, S. A. (1988). The insulin and glucose responses to meals of glucose plus various proteins in type 2 diabetic subjects. *Metabolism* **37,** 1081–1088.

45. Carroll, K. K., and Kurowska, E. M. (1995). Soy consumption and cholesterol reduction: Review of animal and human studies. *J. Nutr.* **125,** 594S–597S.

46. Nuttall, F. Q., and Gannon, M. C. (1999). Carbohydrate and diabetes. *In* "American Diabetes Association Guide to Medical Nutrition Therapy for Diabetes" (M. J. Franz, and J. P. Bantle, Eds.) pp. 85–106. American Diabetes Association, Alexandria, VA.

47. American Heart Association (1988). Dietary guidelines for healthy American adults: A statement for physicians and health professionals by the Nutrition Committee, American Heart Association. *Circulation* **77,** 721A.

48. Expert Panel on Detection, Evaluation, and Treatment of High Blood Cholesterol in Adults (1993). Summary of the Second Report of the National Cholesterol Education Program (NCEP) Expert Panel on Detection, Evaluation, and Treatment of High Blood Cholesterol in Adults (Adult Treatment Panel II). *JAMA* **269,** 3015–3023.

49. Klienman, J. C., Donahue, P. R., Harris, M. I., Finucane, F. F., Madans, J. H., and Dwight, B. B. (1988). Mortality among diabetics in a national sample. *Am. J. Epidemiol.* **128,** 389–401.

50. Stamler, J., Vaccaro, O., Neaton, J. D., and Wentworth, D., for the Multiple Risk Factor Intervention Trial Research Group (1993). Diabetes, other risk factors, and 12-yr cardiovascular mortality for men screened in the Multiple Risk Factor Intervention Trial. *Diabetes Care* **16,** 434–444.

51. Wingard, D. L., and Barrett-Connor, E. (1995). Heart disease and diabetes. *In* "Diabetes in America," 2nd ed. (M. I. Harris, Ed.), pp. 429–448. U.S. Govt. Printing Office, Washington, DC.

52. Reaven, G. M. (1992). The role of insulin resistance and hyperinsulinemia in coronary heart disease. *Metabolism* **41,** 16–19.

53. Stern, M. P., Patterson, J. K., Haffner, S. M., Hazuda, H. P., and Mitchell, B. D. (1989). Lack of awareness and treatment of hyperlipidemia in type 2 diabetes in a community survey. *JAMA* **262,** 360–364.

54. Reaven, G. M, Chen, Y. D., Jeppesen, J., Maheux, P., and Krause, R. (1993). Insulin resistance and hyperinsulinemia in individuals with small, dense, low density lopoprotein particles. *J. Clin. Invest.* **92,** 141–146.

55. Fontbonne, A., Eschwege, E., Cambien, F., Richard, J. L., Ducimetiere, P., Thibult, N., Warnet, J. M., Claude, J. R., and Rosselin, G. E. (1989). Hypertriglyceridemia as a risk factor of coronary heart disease mortality in subjects with impaired glucose tolerance or diabetes. Results from the 11-year follow-up of the Paris Prospective Study. *Diabetes Care* **3,** 300–304.

56. Fontbonne, A. M., and Eschwege, E. M. (1991). Insulin and cardiovascular disease: Paris Prospective Study. *Diabetes Care* **14,** 461–469.

57. Coulston, A. M., Hollenbeck, C. B., Swislocki, A. L. M., Chen, Y.-D. I., and Reaven, G. M. (1987). Deleterious metabolic effects of high-carbohydrate, sucrose-containing diets

in patients with non-insulin-dependent diabetes mellitus. *Am. J. Med.* **82,** 213–220.

58. Garg, A., Bantle, J. P., Henry, R. R., Coulston, A. M., Griver, K. A., Raatz, S. K., Brinkley, L., Chen, Y.-D. I., Grundy, S. M., Huet, B. A., and Reaven, G. M. (1994). Effects of varying carbohydrate content of the diet in patients with non-insulin-dependent diabetes mellitus. *JAMA* **271,** 1421–1428.

59. Reaven, G. M. (1997). Do high carbohydrate diets prevent the development or attenuate the manifestations (or both) of syndrome X? A viewpoint strongly against. *Curr. Opin. Lipidol.* **8,** 23–27.

60. Coulston, A. M., Hollenbeck, C. B., Donner, C. C., Williams, R., Chiou, Y.-A. M., and Reaven, G. M. (1985). Metabolic effects of added dietary sucrose in individuals with non-insulin-dependent diabetes mellitus (NIDDM). *Metabolism* **34,** 962–966.

61. Bantle, J. P., Swanson, J. E., Thomas, W., and Laine, D. C. (1993). Metabolic effects of dietary sucrose in type 2 diabetic subjects. *Diabetes Care* **16,** 1301–1305.

62. "National Health and Nutrition Examination Survey III, 1988–94." (April 1998). NCHS CD-ROM series 11, No 2A (ASCII version). National Center for Health Statistics, Hyattsville, MD.

63. Bruce, B., Spiller, G. A., Klevay, L. M., and Gallagher, S. K. (2000). A diet high in whole and unrefined foods favorably alters lipids, antioxidant defenses, and colonic function. *J. Am. College Nutr.* **19,** 61–67.

64. Nuttall, F. Q. (1997). Dietary fiber in the management of diabetes. *Diabetes* **42,** 503–508.

65. Wursch, P., and Pi-Sunyer, F. X. (1997). The role of viscous soluble fiber in the metabolic control of diabetes: A review with special emphasis on cereals rich in beta-glucan. *Diabetes Care* **20,** 1774–1780.

66. Hollenbeck, C. B., Coulston, A. M., and Reaven, G. M. (1986). To what extent does increased dietary fiber improve glucose and lipid metabolism in patients with non-insulin-dependent diabetes mellitus (NIDDM)? *Am. J. Clin. Nutr.* **43,** 16–24.

67. Usitupa, M., Sutonen, O., Savolainen, K., Silvasti, M., Penttila, I., and Parvianinen, M. (1989). Metabolic and nutritional effects of long-term use of guar gum in the treatment of non-insulin-dependent diabetes of poor metabolic control. *Am. J. Clin. Nutr.* **49,** 345–351.

68. Chandalia, M., Garg, A., Lutjohann, D., von Bergmann, K., Grundy, S. M., and Brinkley, L. J. (2000). Beneficial effects of high dietary fiber intake in patients with type 2 diabetes mellitus. *N. Engl. J. Med.* **342,** 1392–1398.

69. Schatzkin, A., Lanza, E., Corle, D., Lance, P., Iber, F., Caan, B., Shike, M., Weissfeld, J., Burt, R., Cooper, M. R., Kikendall, W., and Cahill, J., and the Polyp Prevention Trial Study Group (2000). Lack of effect of a low-fat, high-fiber diet on the recurrence of colorectal adenomas. *N. Engl. J. Med.* **342,** 1149–1155.

70. Alberts, D. S., Martinez, M. E., Roe, D. J., Guillen-Rodriguez, J. M., Marshall, J. R., van Leeuwen, B., Reid, M. E., Rittenbaugh, C., Vargas, P. A., Bhattacharyya, A. B., Earnest, D. L., and Sampliner, R. E., and the Phoenix Colon Cancer Prevention Physicians' Network (2000). Lack of effect of a high-fiber cereal supplement on the recurrence of colorectal adenomas. *N. Engl. J. Med.* **342,** 1156–1162.

71. Labbe, M. (1907). Tolerame comparee des divers hydrates de carbone part l'organisme des diabetiques. *Bull. Mem. Soc. Med. Hosp.* **24,** 221–234.

72. Otto, H., Bleyer, G., and Pehhartz, M. (1983). Kehlenhydrataustausch nac biologischen Aquivalenten. *In* "Diatetik bei Diabetes Mellitus," pp 41–51. Verlag Has Huber, Bern, Switzerland.

73. Gannon, M. C., Nuttall, F. Q., Westphal, S. A., Fang, S., and Ercan-Fang, N. (1998). Acute metabolic response to high-carbohydrate, high-starch meals compared with moderate-carbohydrate, low-starch meals in subjects with type 2 diabetes. *Diabetes Care* **21,** 1619–1626.

74. Jenkins, D. J. A., Wolever, T. M. S., and Taylor, R. H. (1981). Glycemic index of foods: A physiological basis for carbohydrate exchange. *Am. J. Clin. Nutr.* **34,** 362–366.

75. Wolever, T. M. S., Katzman-Relle, L., Jenkins, A. L., Vuksan, V., Josse, R. G., and Jenkins, D. J. A. (1994). Glycemic index of 102 complex carbohydrate foods in patients with diabetes. *Nutr. Res.* **14,** 651–669.

76. Salmeron, J., Mason, J. E., Stampfer, M. J., Colditz, G. A., Wing, A. L., and Willett, W. C. (1997). Dietary fiber, glycemic load, and risk of non-insulin-dependent diabetes mellitus in women. *JAMA* **277,** 472–477.

77. Salmeron, J., Ascherio, A., Rimm, E. B., Colditz, G. A., Spiegelman, D., Jenkins, D. J., Stamfer, M. J., Wing, A. L., and Willett, W. C. (1997). Dietary fiber, glycemic load, and risk of NIDDM in men. *Diabetes Care* **20,** 545–550.

78. Laine, D. C., Thomas, W., Levitt, M. D., and Bantle, J. P. (1987). Comparison of predictive capabilities of diabetic exchange lists and glycemic index of foods. *Diabetes Care* **10,** 387–394.

79. Coulston, A. M., Hollenbeck, C. B., Swislocki, A. L. M., and Reaven, G. M. (1987). Effect of source of dietary carbohydrate on plasma glucose and insulin responses to mixed meals in subjects with NIDDM. *Diabetes Care* **10,** 395–400.

80. Calle-Pascual, A. L., Gomez, V., Leon, F., and Bordiu, E. (1988). Foods with a low glycemic index do not improve glycemic control of both type 1 and type 2 diabetic patients after one month of therapy. *Diabetes Metab.* **14,** 629–633.

81. Coulston, A. M., and Reaven, G. M. (1997). Much ado about (almost) nothing. *Diabetes Care* **20,** 241–243.

82. Haffner, S. M., Stern, M. P., Hazuda, H. P., Mitchell, B. D., and Patterson, J. K. (1990). Cardiovascular risk factors in confirmed prediabetic individuals: Does the clock for coronary heart disease start ticking before the onset of clinical diabetes? *JAMA* **263,** 2893–2898.

83. Stewart, M. W., Laker, M. F., Dyer, R. G., Game, F., Mitcheson, J., Winocour, P. H., and Alberti, K. G. M. M. (1993). Lipoprotein compositional abnormalities and insulin resistance in type 2 diabetic patients with mild hyperlipidemia. *Arterioscler. Thromb.* **13,** 1046–1052.

84. Kissebah, A. H., and Krakower, G. R. (1994). Regional adiposity and morbidity. *Physiol. Rev.* **74,** 761–811.

85. Gardner, C. D., Fortmann, S. P., and Krauss, R. M. (1996). Association of small low-density lipoprotein particles with the incidence of coronary artery disease in men and women. *JAMA* **276,** 875–881.

86. Stampfer, M. J., Krauss, R. M., Ma, J., Blanche, P. H., Holl, L. G., Sacks, F. M., and Hennekens, C. H. (1996). A prospec-

tive study of triglyceride level, low-density lipoprotein particle diameter, and risk of myocardial infarction. *JAMA* **276,** 882–888.

87. Reaven, G. M. (1988). 1988 Banting Lecture: Role of insulin resistance in human disease. *Diabetes* **37,** 1595–1607.

88. Despres, J. P., Lamarch, B., Mauriege, P., Cantin, B., Dagenais, G. R., Moorjani, S., and Lupien, P. J. (1996). Hyperinsulinemia as an independent risk factor for ischemic heart disease. *N. Engl. J. Med.* **334,** 952–957.

89. Taskinen, M.-R., Beltz, W. F., Harper, I., Fields, R. M., Schonfeld, G., Grundy, S. M., and Howard, B. V. (1986). Effects of NIDDM on very-low-density lipoprotein triglyceride and apolipoprotein B metabolism: Studies before and after sulfonylurea therapy. *Diabetes* **35,** 1268–1277.

90. Golay, A., Zech, L., Shi, M. Z., Chiou, Y. A., Reaven, G. M., and Chen, Y. D. (1987). High-density lipoprotein (HDL) metabolism in non-insulin dependent diabetes mellitus: Measurement of HDL turnover using tritiated HDL. *J. Clin. Endocrinol. Metab.* **65,** 512–518.

91. Ginsberg, H. (1991). Lipoprotein physiology in non-diabetic and diabetic states: Relationship to atherogenesis. *Diabetes Care* **14,** 839–855.

92. Haffner, S. M. (1998). Management of dyslipidemia in adults with diabetes (a technical review). *Diabetes Care* **21,** 160–178.

93. Bierman, E. L., Albrink, M. J., Arky, R. A., Conner, W. E., Dayton, S., Spritz, N., and Steinberg, D. (1971). Principles of nutritional and dietary recommendations for patients with diabetes mellitus. *Diabetes* **20,** 633–634.

94. Keys, A. (1970). Coronary heart disease in seven countries. *Circulation* **41** (Suppl. 1), 1–211.

95. American Diabetes Association (1987). Nutritional recommendations and principles for individuals with diabetes mellitus. *Diabetes Care* **10,** 126–132.

96. Garg, A. (1994). High-monounsaturated fat diet for diabetic patients: Is it time to change the current dietary recommendations? *Diabetes Care* **17,** 242–246.

97. Berry, E. M. (1997). Dietary fatty acids in the management of diabetes mellitus. *Am. J. Clin. Nutr.* **66,** 991S–997S.

98. Garg, A., Bonanome, A., Grundy, S. M., Zhang, A. J., and Unger, R. H. (1988). Comparison of high-carbohydrate diet with high monounsaturated-fat diet in patients with non-insulin-dependent diabetes mellitus. *N. Engl. J. Med.* **391,** 829–834.

99. Coulston, A. M., Hollenbeck, C. B., Swislocki, A. L. M., and Reaven, G. M. (1989). Persistence of hypertriglyceridemic effect of low-fat high-carbohydrate diets in NIDDM patients. *Diabetes Care* **12,** 94–101.

100. Monk, A., Barry, B., McClain, K., Weaver, T., Cooper, N., and Franz, M. J. (1995). Practice guidelines for medical nutrition therapy provided by dietitians for persons with non-insulin dependent diabetes mellitus. *J. Am. Diet. Assoc.* **95,** 999–1006.

101. Stone, D. B., and Conner, W. E. (1963). The prolonged effects of a low cholesterol, high carbohydrate diet upon the serum lipids in diabetic patients. *Diabetes* **12,** 127–132.

102. Anderson, J. W., and Ward, K. (1979). High-carbohydrate, high fiber diets for insulin-treated men with diabetes mellitus. *Am. J. Clin. Nutr.* **32,** 2312–2321.

103. Kolterman, O. G., Greenfiled, M., Reaven, G. M., Saekow, M., and Olefsky, J. M. (1979). Effect of a high carbohydrate diet on insulin binding to adipocytes and on insulin action in vivo in man. *Diabetes* **28,** 731–736.

104. Nadler, J. L., Malayan, S., Luong, H., Shaw, S., Natarajan, R. D., and Rude, R. K. (1992). Intracellular free magnesium deficiency plays a key role in increased platelet reactivity in type II diabetes mellitus. *Diabetes Care* **15,** 835–841.

105. Lima, J. D. L., Cruz, T., Pousada, J. C., Rodrigues, L. E., Barbosa, K., and Cangucu, V. (1990). The effect of magnesium supplementation in increasing doses on the control of type 2 diabetes. *Diabetes Care* **21,** 682–686.

106. Rude, R. K. (1993). Magnesium metabolism and deficiency. *Endocrinol. Metab. Clin. North Am.* **22,** 377–395.

107. American Diabetes Association (1992). Magnesium supplementation in the treatment of diabetes (consensus statement). *Diabetes Care* **15,** 1065–1067.

108. Mooradian, A. D., Faila, M., Hoogwerf, B., Isaac, R., Maryniuk, M., and Wylie-Rosett, J. (1994). Selected vitamins and minerals in diabetes mellitus [technical review]. *Diabetes Care* **17,** 464–479.

109. Alzaid, A., Dinneen, S., Moyer, T., and Rizza, R. (1995). Effects of insulin on plasma magnesium in non-insulin dependent diabetes mellitus: Evidence for insulin resistance. *J. Clin. Endocrinol. Metab.* **80,** 1376–1381.

110. Whelton, P. K., and Klag, M. J. (1989). Magnesium and blood pressure: Review of the epidemiologic and clinical trial experience. *Am. J. Cardiol.* **63,** 26G–30G.

111. Shattock, M. J., Hearse, D. J., and Fry, C. H. (1987). The ionic basis of anti-ischemic and anti-arrhythmic properties of magnesium in the heart. *J. Am. College Nutr.* **6,** 27–33.

112. Paolisso, G., Scheen, A., D'Onofrio, E., and Lefebvre, P. (1990). Magnesium and glucose homeostasis. *Diabetologia* **33,** 511–514.

113. Nadler, J. L., Buchanan, T., Natarajan, R., Antonipillai, I., Bergman, R., and Rude, R. K. (1993). Magnesium deficiency produces insulin resistance and increased thromboxane synthesis. *Hypertension* **21,** 1024–1029.

114. Paolisso, G., Sgambato, S., Gambardella, A., Pizza, G., Tesauro, P., Varricchio, M., and D'Onofrio, F. (1992). Daily magnesium supplements improve glucose handling in elderly subjects. *Am. J. Clin. Nutr.* **55,** 1161–1167.

115. Kao, W. H. L., Folsom, A. R., Nieto, F. J., Mo, J.-P., Watson, R. S., and Brancati, F. L. (1999). Serum and dietary magnesium and the risk for type 2 diabetes mellitus: The Atherosclerosis Risk in Communities Study. *Arch. Intern. Med.* **159,** 2151–2159.

116. Food and Nutrition Board, Institute of Medicine, National Academy of Sciences (1997). "Dietary Reference Intakes for Calcium, Phosphorus, Magnesium, Vitamin D, and Fluoride." National Academy Press, Washington, DC.

117. Schwarz, K., and Mertz, W. (1957). A glucose tolerance factor and its differentiation from factor 3. *Arch. Biochem. Biophys.* **72,** 515–518.

118. Truman, R. W., and Doisy, R. J. (1977). Metabolic effects of the glucose tolerance factor (GTF) in normal and genetically diabetic mice. *Diabetes* **26,** 820–826.

119. Rabinowitz, M. B., Levin, S. R., and Gonick, J. E. (1980). Comparisons of chromium status in diabetic and normal men. *Metabolism* **29,** 355–364.

120. Rabinowitz, M. B., Gonick, H. C., Levin, S. R., Davidson, M. B. (1983). Effect of chromium and yeast supplements on carbohydrate and lipid metabolism. *Diabetes Care* **6,** 319–327.

121. Sherman, L., Glennon, J. A., Brech, W. J., Klomberg, G. H., and Gordon, E. S. (1968). Failure of trivalent chromium to improve hyperglycemia in diabetes mellitus. *Metabolism* **17,** 439–442.

122. Usitupa, M. I. J., Kumpulainen, J. T., and Voutilainen, E. (1983). Effect of inorganic chromium supplementation on glucose intolerance, insulin response and serum lipids in non-insulin-dependent diabetics. *Am. J. Clin. Nutr.* **38,** 404–410.

123. Anderson, R. A., Cheng, N., Bryden, N. A., Polansky, M. M., Cheng, N., Chi, J., and Feng, J. (1997). Elevated intakes of supplemental chromium improve glucose and insulin variables in individuals with type 2 diabetes. *Diabetes* **46,** 1786–1791.

124. Liu, V. J. K., and Morris, J. S. (1978). Relative chromium response as an indicator of chromium status. *Am. J. Clin. Nutr.* **31,** 972–976.

125. Eisenberg, D. M., Davis, R. B., Ettner, S. L., Appel, S., Wilkey, S., Van Rompay, M., and Kessler, R. C. (1998). Trends in alternative medicine use in the United States, 1990–1997: Results of a follow-up national survey. *JAMA* **280,** 1569–1575.

126. Margolin, A., Avants, S. K., and Kleber, H. (1998). Investigating alternative medicine therapies in randomized controlled trials. *JAMA* **280,** 1626–1628.

CHAPTER 30

Nutritional Management for Gestational Diabetes

LYNNE LYONS[1] AND DIANE READER[2]
[1]Burlingame, California
[2]International Diabetes Center, Minneapolis, Minnesota

I. INTRODUCTION

Gestational diabetes mellitus (GDM), carbohydrate intolerance of variable severity with onset or first recognition during pregnancy [1], occurs on average in 4% of all pregnancies in the United States. The incidence of GDM varies throughout the United States, due to the diversity of ethnic groups and maternal ages. The risk of GDM increases with age, obesity, and genetic predisposition or family history of diabetes. It is interesting to note that the incidence of diabetes in certain ethnic groups may be different in the country of origin compared to the same ethnic group in their country of immigration. Ethnic groups with high rates of type 2 diabetes have a high rate of GDM. Because GDM is more likely to occur in overweight women who lead a sedentary life and are older, immigrants with these characteristics and who have adopted such a lifestyle will, in turn, develop GDM at the same rate as the adopted country [2].

II. SCREENING AND DIAGNOSIS

In 1952, Jackson [3] observed a perinatal (fetal and newborn) mortality rate of 8% in pregnant women who later developed diabetes in midlife compared to a perinatal mortality rate of 2% in the control group. These observations led to the development of the 50 g oral glucose screening test. At Boston City Hospital and Lying-In-Hospital in 1954, the first major prospective study of abnormal carbohydrate metabolism in pregnancy began. [4] The 50 g glucose load was taken without regard to the previous meal or time of day. A subsequent 1-hour blood glucose sample was obtained. From this work, it was determined that an upper limit blood glucose value of 140 mg/dL would fail to detect approximately 10% of GDM cases. In contrast, lowering the value to 130 mg/dL would increase by 15–25% the number of women requiring a 100-g oral glucose tolerance test (OGTT). However, if the 50 g glucose load is taken in the fasting state, the 140 mg/dL upper limit detects approximately the same number of elevations as the 130 mg/dL upper limit. When the

result of the 50 g glucose is elevated, the next step is the 100-g, 3-hour OGTT.

In 1964, O'Sullivan and Mahan [5] introduced the first set of diagnostic criteria to predict future diabetes. As part of this series of studies, they found an increased rate of fetal macrosomia and stillbirth in pregnant women with elevated blood glucose values. A controlled trial in which 50% of the pregnant women were treated with insulin therapy demonstrated a lower rate of these complications [5]. These values were retrospectively applied to 1013 women who were tested in pregnancy and followed for 5–10 years to monitor the development of diabetes. These data were based on the predictive value of the pregnant woman developing diabetes later in life rather than a focus on the effect to the fetus [6].

The method of venous whole-blood glucose analysis employed during the time of O'Sullivan and Mahan was the Somogyi-Nelson technique [6]. This method of blood glucose analysis has been replaced by the glucose oxidase method, which utilizes venous plasma instead of whole blood. In 1979, the National Diabetes Data Group suggested that the O'Sullivan criteria should be adjusted downward by 15% to approximate the values in plasma to account for the higher glucose concentration [7]. In 1982, Coustan and Carpenter [6] proposed a new set of criteria developed using the glucose oxidase method of plasma glucose analysis.

Controversy continues over which diagnostic criteria are most clinically appropriate. As recently as the 1997 Fourth International Workshop–Conference on Gestational Diabetes Mellitus, consensus on glucose testing criteria had not been reached. However, the American Diabetes Association recommends use of the Coustan–Carpenter modified criteria. Most countries outside the United States use the World Health Organization criteria for the diagnosis of GDM, a 75-g 2-hour OGTT [6]. However, this test is not as well validated as the 100-g OGTT [8] and controversy remains [9]. Many clinical scientists believe that the establishment of a definition and method of detection for GDM will not be agreed on worldwide until a worldwide, multicenter trial is conducted.

The American Diabetes Association Clinical Practice Recommendations 2000 suggests that for high-risk women,

a 100-g OGTT alone should be utilized to diagnose GDM [8]. Risk factors include marked obesity, GDM in a prior pregnancy, glucosuria, or a strong family history of diabetes. This "one-step approach" to diagnosing GDM is more cost effective in high-risk patients or populations. The one-step approach deletes the 50-g glucose screen and moves directly to the 100-g OGTT. The "two-step approach" is employed for women at average risk for GDM. The first step is the 50-g glucose screening test. If this test is elevated, the 100-g OGTT, the second step, is used to diagnose the presence of GDM (Table 1).

III. RISKS AND COMPLICATIONS

The risk of fetal complications parallels the rise in maternal blood glucose levels. If maternal blood glucose is maintained at normal levels, the risk of complications decreases. The most common complication associated with GDM is fetal macrosomia, weight of ≥ 4500 g (2 standard deviations above the normal for the reference population). Maintenance of maternal blood glucose levels close to the upper end of normal are necessary to prevent the overstimulation of fetal insulin, which can, in turn, cause deposition of fetal adipose tissue, most importantly in the trunk and shoulders. Macrosomia is associated with increased birth trauma (shoulder dystocia, clavicular fracture, brachial palsy) and higher rates of Cesarean section.

If maternal blood glucose is elevated during the latter stages of pregnancy, the newborn is at higher risk for hypoglycemia. With maternal hyperglycemia, the fetal beta cells are stimulated to produce excess insulin. If maternal glucose levels have been elevated, high fetal insulin is present at delivery. This is one of the causes of newborn hypoglycemia. Newborns of GDM mothers have their blood glucose tested a short time after delivery, and if the blood glucose is low, oral dextrose is administered. In some cases, the newborn is unable to maintain normal blood glucose and must receive dextrose intravenously. If blood glucose levels remain low, coma and brain damage can occur. Persson and Hanson [10] suggest that sustained hyperglycemia and hyperinsulinemia may also cause fetal acidemia and hypoxia *in utero*.

Another possible consequence of fetal hyperinsulinemia is cardiac hypertrophy with impaired circulatory function and pulmonary maturation; this may cause respiratory distress. Respiratory distress syndrome is one of the leading causes of admission into the neonatal intensive care unit for babies of GDM mothers. Polyhydramnios (excess amniotic fluid), hyperbilirubinemia, polycythemia, and hypocalcemia are also related to GDM.

Additionally, congenital anomalies are generally associated with poor glucose control during organogenesis, which occurs in the first trimester of pregnancy. GDM develops in midpregnancy; therefore, blood glucose levels have been normal during organogenesis. Fetal anomalies are usually associated with pregnancy in women with type 1 or 2 diabetes.

IV. TREATMENT AND MONITORING

Nutrition therapy is the primary treatment for GDM. If the blood glucose levels cannot be normalized with nutrition therapy, insulin therapy is added to the treatment regime. Self-monitoring of blood glucose provides information to determine the success of the therapies and predict risks to the fetus.

A. Blood Glucose Monitoring

Self-monitoring of blood glucose allows women to apply self-management skills to control hyperglycemia and prevent hypoglycemia [11]. Time points most commonly tested are fasting and postprandial. Patients receive immediate feedback on the impact of food intake, exercise, or insulin on blood glucose levels, and health professionals are better able to individualize the treatment plan. Frequent (2–5 times daily) blood glucose monitoring provides adequate information to direct the treatment plan. Levels and frequency of elevated blood glucose values indicate fetal risk. Postprandial peak blood glucose values correlate better to fetal risk than preprandial glucose values, and also indicate the need for insulin therapy or insulin dose adjustment. In one study, a group of women in the postprandial monitoring group had lower rates of neonatal hypoglycemia, had less large-for-gestational-age infants, and lower rates of Cesarean section than the women in the preprandial testing group [12].

Several reliable blood glucose meters are available. One feature that should be considered when selecting a blood glucose meter for pregnancy is the hemoglobin range. Pregnant women have lower hematocrit values, and some meters are not accurate with a hematocrit of $\leq 30\%$. Additional features to consider are a memory with time and date and data downloading capabilities. These features are helpful if the patient's record keeping is inconsistent, inaccurate, or disorganized. A percentage of patients chooses to falsify their data in an attempt to avoid insulin therapy, hide dietary indiscretions, please clinicians, or simply hide the fact that they did not test their blood glucose levels. A comparison of patient hand-written blood glucose records to values in the meter memory revealed that 25% of the values were omitted from the record and 28% of the values were added to the record [13]. The majority of clinical management decisions are based on the information provided by blood glucose testing; therefore, it is imperative that the information be reliable.

B. Nutrition Therapy

It is important to determine the desired clinical outcome before appropriate nutrition therapy can be prescribed. Clinical

TABLE 1 Screening and Diagnosis of GDM

Low risk for GDM—No screening necessary
  Age < 25 years; weight normal before pregnancy; member of an ethnic group with a low
  prevalence of GDM; no known diabetes in first-degree relatives; no history of abnormal
  glucose tolerance; no history of poor obstetric outcome

Average risk for GDM—Screening between 24 and 28 weeks' gestation

High risk for GDM—Screening at first obstetrical visit; subsequent screening between 24
and 28 weeks' gestation
  Marked obesity; personal history of GDM; glucosuria; strong family history of diabetes

50-g oral glucose screen—Abnormal values require oral glucose tolerance OGTT as soon as
  possible; for values > 195 mg/dL (mmol/L), skip the OGTT and refer directly for treatment
  of GDM

100-g OGTT—Two abnormal values diagnose GDM; one abnormal value requires retesting
in 2–4 weeks
  Fasting blood glucose ≥95 mg/dL (5.3 mmol/L)
  One-hour blood glucose ≥180 mg/dL (10.0 mmol/L)
  Two-hour blood glucose ≥155 mg/dL (8.6 mmol/L)
  Three-hour blood glucose ≥140 mg/dL (7.8 mmol/L)

Postpartum (6 weeks after delivery) 75-g OGTT

	Normal	Impaired glucose tolerance	DM[a]
Fasting blood glucose	<110 mg/dL	≥110 and <126 mg/dL	≥126 mg/dL
Two-hour blood glucose	<140 mg/dL	≥140 and <200 mg/dL	≥200 mg/dL
Retest at a minimum of 3 years		Retest at more frequent intervals	

Source: Adapted from American Diabetes Association (2000). Gestational diabetes mellitus. *Diabetes Care* **23**(Suppl. 1), S77–S79.
  [a]DM if, symptoms of DM and random plasma glucose concentration ≥200 mg/dL.

outcomes will guide the nutrition prescription for each specific patient, such as changes in nutrition therapy at follow-up appointments and the initiation of insulin therapy.

Three clinical outcomes are generally agreed on: blood glucose values within target range before and after eating, adequate nutrient intake for pregnancy, and appropriate weight gain based on body mass index (BMI). An additional clinical outcome used by some practitioners is negative fasting urinary ketone levels. The first clinical outcome is specific to GDM and seeks to produce the blood glucose levels of a pregnant woman without GDM. The second and third outcomes are common to all pregnant women. The reason they are highlighted is that weight gain or energy and nutrient intake can be adversely affected in an effort to achieve normal blood glucose levels. If all three clinical outcomes cannot be achieved with nutrition therapy alone, then insulin is indicated (Table 2).

C. Self-Management or Behavioral Outcomes

Management of any type of diabetes, including GDM, requires the patient to learn self-management techniques. The two self-management tools that help the provider guide de-

cision making are the blood glucose monitoring record and the food intake record.

The health care provider or dietitian needs to ensure that the patient can test her blood glucose level with a self-

TABLE 2 Clinical Outcomes for Gestational Diabetes

Blood glucose within target range	Fasting 60–90 mg/dL	
	Postmeal <120–140 mg/dL at 1 hour	
	Postmeal <120 mg/dL at 2 hours	
Appropriate weight gain based on BMI	*Pounds*	*Gain per week*
<19.8	28–40	Slightly more than 1 lb/week
19.8–26.0	25–35	Approx. 1 lb/week
>26.0–29	15–25	Slightly less than 1 lb/week
>29.0	15	Individualize
Adequate nutrient intake	Dairy foods: 3–4 servings per day	
	Protein: 0.8 g/kg per day	
	Vegetables: 2–3 servings per day	
	Fruit: 2–3 servings per day	
	Grains/starches: 6–8 servings per day	

monitoring meter. This tool provides valuable information on the impact of specific foods and meals on blood glucose values. Blood glucose values are tested before breakfast (fasting) and after each meal. The after-meal test can be done at 1 or 2 hours postprandial. The blood glucose standard is different for each time point (Table 2). Patients should test according to a consistent time schedule.

Another self-monitoring tool that is essential to the management of GDM is the daily food record. The food record provides information to determine the energy intake; carbohydrate, protein, and fat intake; the frequency and timing of meals and snacks; and the nutritional adequacy for vitamins, minerals, and protein. Although a daily food record often provides an incomplete picture of a woman's actual intake, it is the only tool that allows the diet counselor to make specific nutrition recommendations.

As a group, pregnant women are usually motivated to do what is necessary to deliver a healthy baby and readily comply with nutrition and testing recommendations. A sample daily food record is shown in Table 3.

D. Referral

For most women, the initial treatment for GDM is nutrition therapy. Therefore, a consultation with a dietitian is essential as soon as possible following the diagnosis. Unlike other types of diabetes, GDM is a short-lived condition lasting only until the baby is born. With this in mind, it is important to implement nutrition therapy quickly and make the nutrition prescription easy to follow.

E. Achieving Clinical Outcomes with Nutrition Therapy

Dietary carbohydrates are the main nutrient affecting blood glucose levels. Therefore, nutrition therapy is primarily a carbohydrate-controlled food plan. The goal of carbohydrate control is to achieve specific blood glucose values after eating. The problem to overcome is insulin resistance or a relative insulin deficiency. In the nonpregnant state, a woman is able to make adequate amounts of insulin to keep blood glucose in a normal range. As the pregnancy progresses, hormone levels associated with pregnancy increase, which increases insulin resistance and, thus, a need for additional insulin. Most pregnant women can compensate and maintain normal glucose levels. About 4% of pregnant women cannot compensate for this state of relative insulin inadequacy and develop gestational diabetes. By controlling the carbohydrate content of the diet, the insulin requirements are controlled and minimized. Carbohydrate control is achieved in the many ways (Table 4).

1. TOTAL CARBOHYDRATE

The ideal amount of carbohydrate is unknown, but generally comprises about 40–45% of total daily calories, which is usually a reduction from the prepregnancy diet. Major and colleagues [14] determined that GDM women, following a diet less than 42% of energy from carbohydrate, had lower postprandial blood glucose values, reduced incidence of insulin treatment, and better perinatal outcomes as compared to GDM women following a diet 45–50% energy from carbohydrate. Typically for the pregnant woman, this reduction in carbohydrate is stated in per-meal terms rather than in per-day terms, such as limit dinner to 60 g carbohydrate, rather than limit carbohydrate to 42% of total energy.

Why not eliminate all carbohydrate foods entirely due to their blood glucose elevating effect? The human body prefers carbohydrate for energy needs. If the carbohydrate content of the diet dips too low, the body uses fat for energy and ketone production results. High levels of the ketone, beta-hydroxybutyrate, in the maternal blood have been correlated to lower scores on Stanford-Binet intelligence tests in children [15]. Carbohydrate-rich foods also provide essential nutrients, such as calcium from milk and milk products and vitamin C from fruit. Blood glucose control is not the only goal; adequate nutrition for the growing fetus is also a high priority.

2. DISTRIBUTION OF CARBOHYDRATE

In the meal plan, carbohydrate is distributed throughout the day, into 3 meals and 2–4 snacks. Smaller, more frequent feedings help decrease postprandial hyperglycemia and maintain the necessary energy intake. Some women find that the frequent meals and snacks help in the prevention of hunger, ketone production, heartburn, and nausea. Blood glucose testing guides the distribution of carbohydrate. For example, a high blood glucose level after lunch may indicate the need to decrease the planned lunch carbohydrate and compensate for the decrease in energy by adding a protein-rich food.

3. MORNING CARBOHYDRATE

Carbohydrate is not as well tolerated at breakfast compared to other meals. During pregnancy, increased nocturnal levels of cortisol and growth hormone appear to contribute to morning glucose intolerance. Excess carbohydrate at breakfast may aggravate this situation and contribute to even higher blood glucose values. Some clinicians have suggested that the carbohydrate consumption at the breakfast meal be limited to 15–30 g [16, 17]. The food record and blood glucose record are used to evaluate postprandial control. If the woman desires more carbohydrate-rich foods and postprandial glucose goals can be maintained, more carbohydrate can be added to the diet. Continued blood glucose monitoring and vigilance with dietary recommendations are needed throughout pregnancy, because placental lactogen levels increase insulin resistance. Tolerance to carbohydrate can change as the pregnancy progresses. Protein-rich foods should be added to the breakfast meal in place of carbohydrate to satisfy hunger. Protein-rich foods also stimulate

TABLE 3 Sample Daily Food Record

Normal fasting blood glucose concentration is 60–99 mg/dL

One hour after meal blood glucose concentration is 100–129 mg/dL

Please record the time you finish eating and everything you eat and drink in portion sizes. Example: 8 oz. 2% milk, 2 slices bread, 3 oz. turkey, 1 tsp mayonnaise

Please bring your records and blood glucose meter to each appointment

Day, date, and time	Breakfast	Snack	Lunch	Snack	Dinner	Snack
Monday, 2/4	2 slices of wheat bread with peanut butter, herb tea 30 g carbohydrate Time: 8:20	One small peach, 6 crackers, & string cheese 30 g carbohydrate Time: 10:30	1½ cups pasta, 1 slice French bread, tomato & sausage sauce, grated cheese on top, water 60 g carbohydrate Time: 12:25	8 oz. no sugar added fruit yogurt & ½ banana 30 g carbohydrate Time: 3:30	1 cup rice, chicken breast, 1 cup of broccoli, diet soda 45 g carbohydrate Time: 8:25	8 oz. 2% milk, 6 saltine crackers, 1–2 oz. ham 30 g carbohydrate Time: 10:30
Fasting blood glucose: 83 Time: 8:09	1 hour after meal blood glucose: 118 Time: 9:23		1 hour after meal blood glucose: 137, 15 g too much carbohydrate Time: 1:29		1 hour after meal blood glucose: 122 Time: 9:20	
Activity, stress, comments	15-Minute walk after breakfast		Cafeteria at work		Home	Prenatal vitamin supplement
Tuesday, 2/5	One wheat English muffin, 2 eggs, 2 tsp margarine, herb tea 30 g carbohydrate Time: 8:45	1 cup watermelon, 8 oz. 2% milk 30 g carbohydrate Time: 11:05	Tuna sandwich on wheat bread, small apple, water 45 g carbohydrate Time: 12:45	1¼ cup strawberries, ½ cup no sugar added chocolate ice cream 30 g carbohydrate Time: 4:10	1 cup mashed potato, ½ cup corn, BBQ ribs, green salad, lemonade with Equal 45 g carbohydrate Time: 8:15	8 oz. 2% milk, 6 crackers & cheese 30 g carbohydrate Time: 10:45
Fasting blood glucose: 79 Time: 8:13	1 hour after meal blood glucose: 134 Time: 9:50		1 hour after meal blood glucose: 117 Time: 1:43		1 hour after meal blood glucose: 122 Time: 9:20	
Activity, stress, comments	Didn't go for a walk, feeling tired		Brought from home		Dinner with friends, went for a 20-minute walk after dinner	Prenatal vitamin supplement

TABLE 4 Dietary Carbohydrate Guidelines

Total carbohydrate intake	40–45% of energy
Distribution of carbohydrate	3 meals and 2–4 snacks
Morning carbohydrate	Restrict to about 30 g
Type of carbohydrate	Use blood glucose monitoring to identify
Sugars	Eliminate and/or evaluate foods such as juice, desserts, or cereal with blood glucose monitoring
Consistency of carbohydrate intake	Balance with insulin therapy and prevent carbohydrate undereating or overeating

insulin secretion from the pancreas and, thus, do not contribute significantly to postprandial glucose elevations.

Continued blood glucose monitoring is needed throughout pregnancy. Determination of the best distribution and type of carbohydrate-containing foods tolerated at the various times of day is achieved with the information provided by the food intake record and blood glucose monitoring. This information will also help prevent unnecessary food restrictions.

4. TYPE OF CARBOHYDRATE

Many clinicians find that certain foods give a higher glycemic response, causing a higher elevation in postprandial blood glucose. Many studies in nonpregnant populations of people with diabetes have shown that the type and amount of carbohydrate in the diet influences blood glucose levels [18, 19]. Women with gestational diabetes often observe great variation in postprandial blood glucose values, even though the carbohydrate amount is consistent.

Clinical observation in women with GDM indicates that ready-to-eat cereal, fruit juices, and other highly refined products tend to result in a higher postprandial blood glucose level [20]. Some health care providers or dietitians recommend that their patients consume unrefined, whole-grain breads, old-fashioned oatmeal, nuts, legumes, and lentils because of their lower glycemic response. Clapp and colleagues [21] compared two isocaloric, high-carbohydrate diets on the whole-blood glucose and insulin response to mixed energy intake and exercise in healthy nonpregnant and pregnant women. They reported a difference following exercise and postprandial blood glucose response between low-glycemic and high-glycemic index diets. Thus, instead of decreasing the amount of carbohydrate, the type or form of the carbohydrate could be altered to improve postprandial glycemia. Instead of labeling foods as acceptable or unacceptable for GDM, the clinician and the patient with GDM can evaluate her glycemic response to particular foods.

a. Simple Carbohydrate. Eliminating foods high in sucrose and other simple carbohydrates helps attain blood glucose goals. Elimination of these foods usually results in an

overall reduction of carbohydrate intake. Sweet foods, such as soft drinks, lemonade, juices, candy, and desserts, are usually eliminated in the nutritional management of women with GDM to allow intake of carbohydrate-rich foods with essential nutrients.

Many research studies in nonpregnant patients with type 1 and type 2 diabetes report that refined carbohydrates can be included in the diet without compromising glucose control [21a–21c]. In the GDM population these foods are eliminated because they provide no nutrient value, the glucose control is more stringent, a usual portion provides too much carbohydrate, and the food restriction is for a short period of time [22]. Many women with GDM will have a very difficult time completely avoiding all "sweets." In some situations, small portions containing about 15 g of carbohydrate per serving may be consumed as long as glucose control is not compromised.

5. CONSISTENCY OF CARBOHYDRATE

Carbohydrate consistency is encouraged, specifically to prevent undereating and to assist with postprandial blood glucose evaluation. If insulin therapy is added to nutrition therapy, it becomes essential to maintain carbohydrate consistency at meals and snacks to facilitate making insulin dose adjustments.

Recommendations are usually made for a specific carbohydrate amount at meals and snacks, with emphasis on consistency. An example might be 30 g carbohydrate at breakfast and 45 g carbohydrate at lunch and dinner, with remaining carbohydrate, approximately 30 g each, at snacks. Some women are taught to adjust short or rapid-acting insulin based on their preprandial blood glucose level and the amount of carbohydrate they plan to eat at that meal [11].

6. PROTEIN

Protein inclusion in meals and snacks does not significantly affect blood glucose excursions and, thus, can provide additional energy in place of carbohydrate. Blood glucose monitoring will determine if protein is helpful in controlling blood glucose for a particular individual. Generally, paring of carbohydrate and protein at meals and bedtime provides a better postprandial blood glucose due to the delayed absorption of the carbohydrate caused by the protein and fat. The Recommended Dietary Allowance (RDA) for protein in pregnancy is 60 g/day [23]. The RDA for protein is easily met in meal plans for GDM, because protein generally comprises 20–25% of energy.

7. FAT

In the treatment of GDM, the percentage of energy from fat may be higher than generally recommended. The increase in fat is due to a decrease in carbohydrate intake and increased animal protein intake, which inherently adds fat. Fat usually ranges from 30% to 40% of total energy in GDM management. Because GDM is a short-term condition, the total amount of fat is not designed to be a long-term recom-

mendation. Large amounts of fat beyond total energy needs should, however, be avoided to prevent excessive weight gain, which, in turn, can result in further insulin resistance.

Because GDM is a condition of insulin resistance, some scientists suggest that reducing fat intake may decrease insulin resistance and improve blood glucose levels. Preliminary research indicates that a higher polyunsaturated-to-saturated fat (P:S) ratio may protect against the development of GDM [24]. In one study, women with a higher saturated fat intake developed GDM independent of their weight status [24]. This has implications for women that are at high risk of developing GDM as well as women who have GDM. Further research is needed to evaluate this theory. Low-fat diets would need to be closely evaluated for use in GDM. Adequate fat intake is needed during pregnancy to provide essential fatty acids needed for fetal brain development [25].

8. Energy Intake and Weight Gain

Energy intake should be sufficient to promote appropriate weight gain while preventing hyperglycemia and ketonuria or ketonemia. Energy recommendations are monitored by weight gain patterns, ketone testing, appetite assessment, and review of food records.

No agreement has been reached on a minimum energy requirement for women with GDM [26]. Total energy expenditure and basal metabolic rate do not differ between GDM and control pregnant women [27]. Individual needs for energy intake vary according to body size and physical activity. A minimum of approximately 1700–1800 kcal/day of carefully chosen food choices has been shown to prevent ketosis [28]. Intakes below this level are generally not advised and often result in inadequate weight gain, weight loss, and/or ketosis [15].

The specific level of energy intake should be individualized, based on assessment of prepregnancy weight, physical activity level, and pregnancy weight gain to date.

Most clinicians prefer to base energy intake recommendations on a woman's actual intake rather than energy prediction formulas. However, if someone is not adept in assessing energy intake, lacks the time to make that assessment, or prefers to start with a standard calculation, the Harris-Benedict formula is recommended. Some clinicians use an adjusted, prepregnancy body weight for obese women (adjusted body weight = [(actual body weight − desirable body weight) × 0.25] + desirable body weight). Add 300 kcal for the second and third trimester of pregnancy [29].

The use of energy restriction or hypocaloric diets has been proposed as a method to improve blood glucose control in obese women. While some studies report a reduction in macrosomia, concerns with this treatment are for the safety of the fetus. Restrictive energy intake can lead to ketone production, which may harm the fetus and is to be avoided for all pregnant women [15]. Maggee and colleagues [30] showed that a 50% energy reduction (1200 kcal/day) resulted in ketone production; however, a follow-up study, reducing energy by 33%, did not produce ketonuria [31].

9. Artificial Sweeteners

Non-nutritive sweeteners available in the United States have been deemed safe for consumption during pregnancy [32]. Moderation is encouraged and defined on an individual basis. A maximum of 3 servings of non-nutritive sweetener per day is often considered reasonable. The primary concern is that high consumption of artificially sweetened foods replaces more nutritious choices.

Aspartame, made of the amino acids aspartic acid and phenylalanine, has shown to pose no risk to the fetus when ingested in amounts at least three times the accepted daily intake. Women with phenylketonuria must monitor their intake of all sources of phenylalanine. Phenylalanine does cross the placenta; however, foods sweetened with aspartame contain less phenylalanine than protein foods in a meal [33]. Similarly, acesulfame potassium also has been shown to pose no risk. Multigenerational studies show no effect on fertility, number of offspring, birth weight, or mortality [34].

There is no current evidence that saccharin is harmful to the fetus, but, because it crosses the placenta, the use of saccharin during pregnancy is not recommended [32].

F. Assessing Clinical Outcomes

The individual who provides nutrition therapy is often the person who recognizes when the limits of nutrition therapy have been met and insulin therapy is needed. Follow-up appointments are needed in order to determine if the patient is achieving clinical outcomes and using self-management techniques correctly. It is generally considered appropriate to schedule a follow-up appointment 1 week after the initial consult and plan to have at least a second follow-up appointment in 2 or 3 weeks [29].

A variety of factors interfere with achieving clinical outcomes. Some factors relate to patient behaviors and knowledge level and others relate to hormonal and metabolic factors beyond patient control. At each follow-up visit, the following should be assessed: records of food intake, ketone and blood glucose monitoring; body weight change; patient's ability to understand and follow regimen; and patient questions and concerns. Changes to the nutrition plan or further education to improve implementation may be recommended. Some women will not be able to achieve blood glucose targets despite their best efforts. At this point, insulin therapy is needed to supplement nutrition therapy (see Table 5).

G. Insulin Therapy

If postprandial blood glucose levels are higher than the clinical goal at the same meal on two or more occasions during the week, insulin therapy is recommended to control the blood glucose at that particular meal. This decision is made regardless of the cause of the elevations. Despite the patient's best effort to follow the nutrition therapy, some women demonstrate an extreme sensitivity to excess or simple carbohydrate intake. Insulin is the drug of choice. Oral

TABLE 5 Assessment of Clinical Outcomes and Solutions

Test and results	Possible causes	Possible solutions
Elevated postprandial blood glucose	Excessive food intake/large portions	Evaluate meal plan and redistribute carbohydrate intake
	Not following food plan	Determine reasons why patient is not following meal plan
	Eating foods with large amounts of carbohydrate, such as dessert-type foods or sweetened beverages	Evaluate meal plan; decrease carbohydrate intake and keep isocaloric by increasing protein and/or fat intake
	A particular food raises blood glucose	Evaluate form of carbohydrate consumed
	Meals and/or snacks eaten too close together	Space meals and snacks evenly throughout the day so feedings are about 2.5–3 hours apart
	Timing of exogenous insulin injection and meals not coordinated	Coordinate time of meal and insulin to match action times of injected insulin
	Decreased physical activity	Increase physical activity after meals
	Increased stress	
	Brief illness/infection/pain	
	Needs insulin/inadequate dose of insulin	Initiate insulin or increase current dosage
	Bed rest	
	Tocolytic drugs or steroids	
Weight loss	Undereating to control blood glucose/avoid insulin	Discuss importance of adequate energy intake
		Initiate insulin therapy
	Insufficient energy intake prescribed	Increase energy intake of food plan prescribed
	Nausea, vomiting, heartburn, or illness that is inhibiting adequate intake	Diet modifications for nausea, vomiting, heartburn, illness
	Errors in portioning foods—portion sizes too small	Initial adjustment to meal plan
	Skipping meals or snacks	Verify with patient the ability to consume prescribed meals and snacks
	Increased physical activity	
	Undereating to avoid weight gain	
	Pica	Refer to appropriate provider for pica counseling
Excessive weight gain	Food intake above needs	Decrease energy intake by adjusting meal plan
	Decreased physical activity	Increase physical activity
	Excessive insulin dosage, which may be promoting excessive food intake	Measure food portions
	Cultural beliefs that promote weight gain	Cultural sensitivity and lifestyle counseling
	Fluid retention/edema	Evaluate insulin dosage

Source: Adapted from American Dietetic Association (2001). Nutrition practice guidelines for gestational diabetes. www.eatright.org.

hypoglycemic medications used in the treatment of type 2 diabetes have not been tested in pregnancy and are not recommended during pregnancy.

Postprandial blood glucose is best controlled with premeal rapid or short-acting insulin. The ratio of rapid or short-acting insulin to grams of carbohydrate intake will vary depending on the level of insulin resistance. Generally, more insulin is required at breakfast to cover carbohydrate intake than at lunch and dinner. For example, the rapid or short-acting insulin-to-carbohydrate ratio at breakfast may be 1 unit to 8 g carbohydrate, compared to 1 unit to 10 g carbohydrate at lunch and dinner. To avoid three to four injections daily, the prebreakfast injection may be a combination of rapid or short-acting and intermediate-acting insulins. This regime

would eliminate a prelunch injection because the lunchtime carbohydrate would be controlled by the intermediate-acting insulin given in the morning [35]. The lunch meal carbohydrate may need to be limited to 45 or 60 g because a higher dose of prebreakfast intermediate-acting insulin may cause midmorning hypoglycemia. An estimate of total daily insulin dose can be calculated as follows: present body weight (kg) × 0.8 to 1.0 units (during the second and third trimester) = total daily insulin units (units/kg body weight). These units are then divided between prebreakfast and predinner treatments. Two-thirds of the total daily insulin units are administered before breakfast, with a further division of two-thirds administered as intermediate-acting insulin and one-third as rapid or short-acting insulin. The predinner dose is

one-third of the total daily insulin dose, with further division between one-half as intermediate-acting insulin and one-half as rapid or short-acting insulin [36].

When fasting blood glucose levels are elevated predinner or bedtime, intermediate-acting insulin is needed. Diet and exercise have little effect on fasting glucose levels. There is general consensus that one should not delay insulin initiation, because glucose intolerance and insulin resistance only worsen as the pregnancy continues.

Women who require insulin therapy vary according to ethnicity, clinical goals, and testing regimens. A 1990 survey of obstetricians and maternal–fetal medicine physicians, showed the following treatment pattern: forty percent treated ≤ 10% with insulin, 31% treated 20%, 23% treated 20–30%, 5% treated ≥ 50%, and 2% treated 100% of their patients with insulin [35]. In contrast, 20 years of national and international research effort have resulted in reports of 30–60% of GDM treated with insulin [35].

V. POSTPARTUM RECOMMENDATIONS AND CONSIDERATIONS

Women with a history of GDM have a 17–63% risk of developing type 2 diabetes 5–16 years after the first pregnancy with GDM. The risk of diabetes is particularly high in women who have marked hyperglycemia during or soon after pregnancy, women who are obese, and women whose gestational diabetes was diagnosed before 24 weeks of gestation [37]. These risk factors are markers that correspond to insulin resistance, diminished beta-cell function, and increased endogenous glucose production. Maternal postpartum testing with a 75-g OGTT should be administered at 6 weeks' postpartum in order to assess glycemic status. Repeat 75-g OGTT tests should be conducted at 3-year intervals. Impaired glucose tolerance or impaired fasting glucose are intermediate stages between normal glucose metabolism and diabetes. Women that appear to have impaired glucose tolerance or impaired fasting glucose should receive testing at more frequent intervals [8]. Efforts to prevent diabetes should be directed at maintenance of a normal body weight, regular physical exercise, and avoidance of drugs that increase insulin resistance, such as steroids and high-dose combination or progestin-only oral contraceptives.

In utero exposure to hyperglycemia may have far-reaching consequences. The offspring of women with GDM have a higher risk of obesity and abnormal glucose metabolism when they are children and young adults. Large-for-gestational-age offspring of GDM mothers have a higher BMI at 4–7 years when compared to average for gestational age offspring of GDM mothers [38]. A high maternal prepregnant BMI is a significant indicator for large-for-gestational-age infants [38]. Even though obesity usually resolves during the first year of life, it reappears by 14–17 years of age with a mean BMI of 24.6 kg/m². Excess fetal insulin production is a predictor for both obesity and impaired glucose tolerance

in adolescence. Aberrant maternal metabolism as measured by hemoglobin A_1c, fasting plasma glucose levels, and blood ketone or beta-hydroxybutyrate concentration is associated with poorer intellectual and psychomotor development in offspring [39]. The female offspring of GDM mothers have a higher risk of GDM during their pregnancies. Once again, measures to reduce insulin resistance and obesity will benefit the offspring as well as the parents in prevention of type 2 diabetes.

The method of infant feeding also seems to have an influence on later development of diabetes. The best source of these retrospective correlation studies comes from populations with high incidences of diabetes. The Pima Indians have a 50% rate of GDM. The offspring of GDM mothers had a lower incidence of type 2 diabetes if they were breast fed for at least 2 months and their birth weight was between 2500 and 3500 g. Birth weights of <2000 g or >4000 g are associated with higher incidence of diabetes as the offspring age (25–35 years old) [40].

VI. CONCLUSION

In summary, gestational diabetes mellitus is a type of diabetes first diagnosed during pregnancy. The primary treatment for GDM is nutrition therapy. Generally, the diet plan is carbohydrate controlled, with 40–45% of total energy from carbohydrate. Nutrition therapy provides all of the nutrient requirements for pregnancy as well as adequate energy to meet the weight gain goal based on prepregnant weight status. If blood glucose levels cannot be maintained at acceptable values, insulin therapy is implemented to supplement nutrition therapy. Insulin therapy is individualized based on the hyperglycemia patterns revealed with blood glucose monitoring.

Generally, GDM resolves immediately postpartum. However, a postpartum 75-g OGTT should be performed at 6–8 weeks' postpartum to determine the resolution of GDM. Women who develop GDM are at a high risk of developing type 2 diabetes due their genetic predisposition. GDM is a window into the woman's metabolic future. To reduce the risk or delay the onset of type 2 diabetes, women should be advised to maintain a normal weight, exercise regularly, and eat a diet low in saturated fats.

References

1. Metzger, B. E. (1990). ADA Workshop-Conference Organizing Committee: Summary and recommendations of the Third International Workshop-Conference on Gestational Diabetes Mellitus. *Diabetes* **40**(Suppl. 2), 197–201.
2. King, H. (1998). Epidemiology of glucose intolerance and gestational diabetes in women of childbearing age. *Diabetes Care* **21**(Suppl. 2), B9–B13.
3. Jackson, W. P. U. (1952). Studies in pre-diabetes. *Br. Med. J.* **3**, 690–696.
4. Wilkerson, H. L. C., and Remein, Q. R. (1957). Studies of abnormal carbohydrate metabolism in pregnancy. *Diabetes* **6**, 324–329.

5. O'Sullivan, J. B., and Mahan, C. B. (1964). Criteria for the oral glucose tolerance in pregnancy. *Diabetes* **13,** 278–285.

6. Coustan, D. R., and Carpenter, M. W. (1998). The diagnosis of gestational diabetes. *Diabetes Care* **21**(Suppl. 2), B5–B8.

7. Ramus, R. M., and Kitzmiller, J. L. (1994). Diagnosis and management of gestational diabetes. *Diabet. Mellit. Rev.* **2**(1), 43–52.

8. American Diabetes Association (2000). Gestational diabetes mellitus. *Diabetes Care* **23**(Suppl. 1), S77–S79.

9. Gabbe, S. G. (1998). The gestational diabetes mellitus conferences. *Diabetes Care* **21**(Suppl. 2), B1–B4.

10. Persson, B., and Hanson, U. (1998). Neonatal morbidities in gestational diabetes mellitus. *Diabetes Care* **21**(Suppl. 2), B79–B84.

11. Kitzmiller, J. L. (1993). Sweet success with diabetes. The development of insulin therapy and glycemic control for pregnancy. *Diabetes Care* **16**(Suppl. 3), 107–121.

12. DeVeciana, M., Major, C., Morgan, M., Asrat, T., Toohey, J., Lien, J., and Evans, A. (1995). Postprandial versus preprandial blood glucose monitoring in women with gestational diabetes mellitus requiring insulin therapy. *N. Engl. J. Med.* **333**(19), 1237–1283.

13. Langer, O., and Mazze, R. (1986). Diabetes in pregnancy: Evaluating self-monitoring performance and glycemic control with memory-based reflectance meters. *Am. J. Obstet. Gynecol.* **155,** 635–637.

14. Major, C., Henry, J., DeVeciana, M., and Morgan, M. (1998). The effects of carbohydrate restriction in patients with diet-controlled gestational diabetes. *Obstet. Gynecol.* **91,** 600–604.

15. Rizzo, T., Metzger, B., Burns, W., and Burns, K. (1991). Correlations between antepartum maternal metabolism and intelligence of offsprings. *N. Engl. J. Med.* **316,** 911–916.

16. Fagen, C., King, J., and Erick, M. (1995). Nutrition management in women with gestational diabetes mellitus: A review by ADA's Diabetes Care and Education dietetic practice group. *J. Am. Diet. Assoc.* **95,** 460–467.

17. Lerner, R. A. (1976). Studies of gylcemia and glucosuria in diabetics after breakfast meals of different composition. *Am. J. Clin. Nutr.* **29,** 716–725.

18. Ahern, J. A., Gatcomb, P. M., Held, N. A., Pettit, W. A., and Tamborlane, W. V. (1993). Exaggerated hyperglycemia after a pizza meal in well-controlled diabetes. *Diabetes Care* **16,** 578–580.

19. Collier, G. R., Wolever, T. M. S., Wong, G. S., and Josse, R. G. (1988). Prediction of glycemic response to mixed meals in non-insulin dependent diabetic subjects. *Am. J. Clin. Nutr.* **3,** 85–88.

20. Lock, D. R., Bar-eyal, A., Voet, H., and Madar, Z. (1988). Glycemic indices of various foods given to pregnant diabetic subjects. *Obstet. Gynecol.* **71,** 180–183.

21. Clapp, J. F. (1998). Effect of dietary carbohydrate on the glucose and insulin response to mixed caloric intake and exercise in both caloric intake and exercise in both nonpregnant and pregnant women. *Diabetes Care,* **21**(Suppl. 2), B107–B112.

21a. Peterson, D. B., Lambert, J., Gerring, S., Darling, P., Carter, R. D., Jelfs, R., and Mann, J. I. (1986). Sucrose in the diet of diabetic patients—just another carbohydrate? *Diabetologia* **29,** 216–220.

21b. Bantle, J. P., Laine, D. C., Castle, G. W., Thomas, J. W., Hoogwerf, B. J., and Goetz, F. C. (1983). Postprandial glucose and insulin response to meals containing different carbohydrates in normal and diabetic subjects. *N. Engl. J. Med.* **309,** 7–12.

21c. Bantle, J. P., Swanson, J. E., Thomas, W., and Laine, D. C. (1993). Metabolic effects of sucrose in type 2 diabetic subjects. *Diabetes Care* **16,** 1301–1305.

22. Lyons, L., and Flanagan, G. (1994). Do the new nutrition guidelines apply to pregnancy? Perinatal Nutrition Report.

23. Food and Nutrition Board. (1989). "Recommended Dietary Allowances," 10th ed., pp. 33–34. National Academy of Sciences, Washington, DC.

24. Wang, Y., Storlien, L., Jenkins, A., Tapsell, L., Jin, Y., Pan, J., Shao, Y., Calvert, G., Moses, R., Shi, H., and Zhu, X. (2000). Dietary variables and glucose tolerance in pregnancy. *Diabetes Care* **23**(4), 460–464.

25. Conner, W. E. (2000). Importance of M-3 fatty acids in health and disease. *Am. J. Clin. Nutr.* **71**(Suppl.), 171S–175S.

26. Metzger, B., and Coustan, D. C., and the Organizing Committee (1998). Summary and recommendations of the Fourth International Workshop-Conference on Gestational Diabetes Mellitus. *Diabetes Care* **21**(Suppl. 2), xxx–xxx.

27. Butte, N. (2000). Carbohydrate and lipid metabolism in pregnancy: Normal compared with gestational diabetes mellitus. *Am. J. Clin. Nutr.* **71**(Suppl.), 1256S–1261S.

28. Jovanovic-Peterson, L., and Peterson, C. M. (1992). Nutritional management of the obese gestational diabetic pregnant woman (editorial). *J. Am. College Nutr.* **11**(3), 246–250.

29. American Dietetic Association (2001). Nutrition practice guidelines for gestational diabetes. www.eatright.org.

30. Maggee, M. S., Knopp, R. H., and Benedetti, T. J. (1990). Metabolic effects of 1200 kcal diet in obese pregnant women with gestational diabetes. *Diabetes* **39,** 234–240.

31. Knopp, R. H., Magee, M. S., Raisys, V., et al. (1991). Hypocaloric diets and ketogenesis in the management of obese gestational diabetic women. *J. Am. College Nutr.* **10,** 649–667.

32. American Dietetic Association (1993). Position of the American Dietetic Association: Use of nutritive and non-nutritive sweeteners. *J. Am. Diet. Assoc.* **93**(17), 816–821.

33. Pitkin, R. M. (1984). Aspartame ingestion during pregnancy. *In* "Aspartame" (L. D. Steginck and J. F. Filer, Eds.), pp. 555–563. Marcel Dekker, New York.

34. World Health Organization Expert Committee on Food Additives (1981, 1983). "Toxicological Evaluation of Certain Food Additives and Food Contaminants." No. 16, pp. 11–27, and No. 18, pp. 12–14. World Health Organization, Geneva.

35. Langer, O. (2000). Management of gestational diabetes. *In* "Clinical Obstetrics and Gynecology" (R. M. Pitkin and J. R. Scott, Eds.), Vol. 43, pp. 106–115.

36. (1998). "Sweet Success Guidelines for Care." California Diabetes and Pregnancy Program.

37. Kjos, S. L., and Buchanan, T. A. (1999). Gestational diabetes mellitus. *N. Engl. J. Med.* **341**(23), 1749–1756.

38. Vohr, B. R., McGarvey, S. T., and Tucker, R. (1999). Effects of maternal gestational diabetes on offspring adiposity at 4–7 years of age. *Diabetes Care* **22**(8), 1284–1291.

39. Silverman, B. L., Rizzo, T. A., Cho, N. H., and Metzger, B. E. (1998). Long term effects of the intrauterine environment. *Diabetes Care* **21**(Suppl. 2), B142–B149.

40. Pettitt, D. J., and Knowler, W. C. (1998). Long term effects of the intrauterine environment, birth weight, and breast-feeding in Pima Indians. *Diabetes Care* **21**(Suppl. 2), B138–B141.

D. Obesity

CHAPTER 31

Obesity: Overview of Treatments and Interventions

HELEN M. SEAGLE, HOLLY WYATT, AND JAMES O. HILL

University of Colorado Health Sciences Center, Denver, Colorado

I. INTRODUCTION

Obesity is a pervasive disease in our world: Currently an estimated 1.2 billion of the global population are overweight [1]. In the United States, more than half of the population is either overweight or obese, and this disease affects all age, sex, and race-ethnic groups [2]. The prevalence of overweight and obesity made a dramatic leap upward toward the end of the twentieth century; in 1960 only about one-third of the U.S. population was overweight [2]. Because excess weight is associated with a higher incidence of diseases such as diabetes, cardiovascular diseases, osteoarthritis, and some cancers [3], the burden of obesity is high. In the United States alone, the total economic cost of this disease is estimated to be about $117.73 billion per year (2000 dollars) with more than half of that cost being derived from direct medical care expenses [4, economic costs updated from 1995 costs reported in source]. Health care providers and policymakers alike are faced with the dilemma of managing this obesity epidemic and preventing this situation from worsening.

Obesity is a complex disease of multifactorial origins. However, there is simplicity in the underlying model of body weight change. The energy balance equation dictates that in order for body weight to change, there must be an energy imbalance. Either a change in energy intake or a change in energy output must occur so that body stores of energy are altered, causing a change in total body weight [5]. Therefore, treatments of obesity must either focus on diminishing energy intake (e.g., diet, medications, surgery) or increasing energy output (e.g., physical activity) or a combination of both (e.g., behavior modification addressing changes in dietary intake and physical activity). However, it is imperative that any intervention for overweight and obesity address both weight gain prevention and weight maintenance as well as body weight reduction [6].

The primary care physician is often the first person to assess an individual's need for obesity treatment. Ideally, the physician would then refer the client to a comprehensive weight management program or obesity specialist, or recommend a commercial weight loss program and provide follow-up care to monitor progress. If the primary care physician decides to treat the client, referrals should be made for additional services, e.g., psychologist, exercise physiologist, or registered dietitian [7]. Determining the appropriate treatment approach for an individual requires a careful assessment of an individual's needs [6]. An obese person with two or three comorbidities clearly requires a more aggressive approach than an overweight individual suffering no medical impact from excess body fat. The use of a tailored approach to obesity treatment will ensure that more people become successful in their weight management efforts. Obesity treatment is one arena where a one-size-fits-all approach does not ensure success.

II. ASSESSMENT OF OVERWEIGHT AND OBESITY

Obesity is characterized by the accumulation of excess body fat. Although accurate methods to measure body fat do exist, they are expensive and impractical for general use. Body weight has traditionally been used as a surrogate measure of excess body fat. In the past, an obese or overweight body weight was based on ideal body weight tables established by The Metropolitan Life Insurance Company [8]. These insurance tables estimated an "ideal" weight for a given height, frame size, and gender based on collected mortality data. Overweight and obesity were then defined as some percentage above the estimated ideal body weight. Although widely used, these tables were criticized for being derived from populations with body fat contents that did not reflect those of the general public, for using frame size (an arbitrary assessment), and for being based on mortality outcomes alone without evaluating morbidity data [6].

A. Clinical Assessments of Body Fat

1. BODY MASS INDEX

In recent years, the use of a body mass index (BMI) has replaced the insurance tables and has become the recommended method to estimate body fat and to define both overweight and obesity in a clinical setting [1, 6]. BMI is determined by weight in kilograms divided by height

ft/in lbs.	4'10"	4'11"	5'0"	5'1"	5'2"	5'3"	5'4"	5'5"	5'6"	5'7"	5'8"	5'9"	5'10"	5'11"	6'0"	6'1"	6'2"	6'3"	6'4"
120	25	24	23	23	22	21	21	20	19	19	18	18	17	17	16	16	15	15	15
125	26	25	24	24	23	22	22	21	20	20	19	18	18	17	17	17	16	16	15
130	27	26	25	25	24	23	22	22	21	20	20	19	19	18	18	17	17	16	16
135	28	27	26	26	25	24	23	23	22	21	21	20	19	19	18	18	17	17	16
140	29	28	27	27	26	25	24	23	23	22	21	21	20	20	19	19	18	18	17
145	30	29	28	27	27	26	25	24	23	23	22	21	21	20	20	19	19	18	18
150	31	30	29	28	27	27	26	25	24	24	23	22	22	21	20	20	19	19	18
155	32	31	30	29	28	28	27	26	25	24	24	23	22	22	21	20	20	19	19
160	34	32	31	30	29	28	28	27	26	25	24	24	23	22	22	21	21	20	19
165	35	33	32	31	30	29	28	28	27	26	25	24	24	23	22	22	21	21	20
170	36	34	33	32	31	30	29	28	27	27	26	25	24	24	23	22	22	21	21
175	37	35	34	33	32	31	30	29	28	27	27	26	25	24	24	23	23	22	21
180	38	36	35	34	33	32	31	30	29	28	27	27	26	25	24	24	23	22	22
185	39	37	36	35	34	33	32	31	30	29	28	27	27	26	25	24	24	23	22
190	40	38	37	36	35	34	33	32	31	30	29	28	27	27	26	25	24	24	23
195	41	39	38	37	36	35	34	33	32	31	30	29	28	27	27	26	25	24	24
200	42	40	39	38	37	36	34	33	32	31	30	30	29	28	27	26	26	25	24
205	43	41	40	39	38	36	35	34	33	32	31	30	29	29	28	27	26	26	25
210	44	43	41	40	38	37	36	35	34	33	32	31	30	29	29	28	27	26	26
215	45	44	42	41	39	38	37	36	35	34	33	32	31	30	29	28	28	27	26
220	46	45	43	42	40	39	38	37	36	35	34	33	32	31	30	29	28	27	27
225	47	46	44	43	41	40	39	38	36	35	34	33	32	31	31	30	29	28	27
230	48	47	45	44	42	41	40	38	37	36	35	34	33	32	31	30	30	29	28
235	49	48	46	44	43	42	40	39	38	37	36	35	34	33	32	31	30	29	29
240	50	49	47	45	44	43	41	40	39	38	37	36	35	34	33	32	31	30	29
245	51	50	48	46	45	43	42	41	40	38	37	36	35	34	33	32	32	31	30
250	52	51	49	47	46	44	43	42	40	39	38	37	36	35	34	33	32	31	30
255	53	52	50	48	47	45	44	43	41	40	39	38	37	36	35	34	33	32	31
260	54	53	51	49	48	46	45	43	42	41	40	38	37	36	35	34	33	33	32

FIGURE 1   Body mass index using height in feet and inches and weight in pounds.

in meters squared ($BMI = kg/m^2$). The formula: weight (pounds)/height (inches)^2 × 704.5 can be used to convert height in inches and weight in pounds directly into BMI units [9]. Figure 1 converts measures of height and weight into BMI units.

BMI is a better estimate of body fat than body weight [6, 10] and has advantages over the ideal body weight estimation that preceded it. Unlike the ideal body weight tables that were based on mortality data alone, BMI correlates with morbidity. The relationship between a given BMI and the risk of both mortality and morbidity has been assessed in several large epidemiological studies [11–13]. BMI does not require a subjective assessment for frame size and the same formula is used for both men and women (unlike the insurance tables, which were specific for gender). However, there are limitations to the usefulness of the BMI. BMI may overestimate total body fat in persons who are very muscular (such as elite athletes) and may underestimate body fat in persons who have lost muscle mass (such as the elderly). Additionally, BMI will inaccurately reflect body fat in edematous states or in individuals who are less than 5 feet tall. Clinical judgment must always be used in the interpretation of BMI on an individual case basis.

Despite the above limitations, the correlation between BMI and excess body fat in the general population is good [14]. Both the National Institutes of Health and the World Health Organization have defined overweight as a BMI of $25.0–29.9 kg/m^2$, and obesity as a BMI of $30 kg/m^2$ or greater [1, 6]. These BMI cutoffs were determined using studies evaluating the relationship between BMI and mortality and morbidity risk [11, 12]. In general, morbidity and mortality risk increases as BMI rises, but this relationship is curvilinear. Increases in BMI between 20 and $25 kg/m^2$ alter the morbidity and mortality risk less than increases in BMI above $25 kg/m^2$. For example, in the Nurses' Health Trial, relative to a woman with a $BMI < 21 kg/m^2$, heart disease risk was 1.8 times greater in women with a BMI between 25 and $29 kg/m^2$ but 3.3 times greater for women with a BMI greater than $29 kg/m^2$ [11, 15]. Gender does not alter this relationship; therefore, the same cutoff points are used to

TABLE 1 Risk Factors That Increase the Need for Weight Reduction

Very high risk	High risk	Other risk factors
Coronary heart disease	Three or more of the following cardiovascular risk factors:	Physical inactivity
Presence of atherosclerotic diseases	Cigarette smoking	High serum triglycerides
Type 2 diabetes mellitus	Hypertension	
Sleep apnea	Elevated low-density lipoprotein cholesterol	
	Impaired fasting glucose	
	Family history of premature coronary heart disease	
	Age $\geq$45 years for men or age $\geq$55 years for women	

define obesity (BMI $\geq$ 30 kg/m^2) and overweight (BMI 25–29.9 kg/m^2) in both men and women [16].

2. WAIST CIRCUMFERENCE

The waist circumference is an assessment tool that can complement the BMI measurement for assessment of disease risk. Excess fat located in the upper abdominal region (visceral fat) is associated with a greater risk than fat located in other areas [17]. Abdominal fatness is an independent risk factor (even when BMI is not increased) and is predictive of comorbidities and mortality [17, 18]. Sex-specific cutoffs for waist circumference can be used for adults with a BMI less than 35 kg/m^2. In individuals with a BMI above 35 kg/m^2, a waist circumference does not confer additional disease risk and therefore it is not necessary to measure waist circumference in patients with BMI > 35 kg/m^2.

High risk is defined by a waist circumference > 40 inches (102 cm) for men and > 35 inches (88 cm) for women [6]. The power of waist circumference to predict disease risk may vary by ethnicity and age [14]. For example, waist circumference is a better indicator of disease risk than BMI in Asian-Americans and in older individuals. For this reason, waist circumference cutoffs may need to be adjusted, in the future, based on age and ethnicity.

B. Assessment of Risk Factors

Patients should be assessed for the presence of concomitant cardiovascular risk factors or comorbidities. Some obesity-associated diseases and cardiovascular risk factors will place the patient in a very high risk category for morbidity and mortality and, therefore, the aggressiveness of the obesity intervention or treatment should be increased.

If a patient has three or more cardiovascular risk factors, they can be classified as being at a *high risk* for obesity-related disorders. Cardiovascular risk factors include cigarette smoking, hypertension, a low-density lipoprotein cholesterol $\geq$160 mg/dL (4.1 mmol/L), a high-density lipoprotein cholesterol <35 mg/dL (0.9 mmol/L), an impaired fasting glucose (fasting glucose of 110–125 mg/dL, or 6.1–6.9 mmol/L), a family history of premature heart disease, and age $\geq$ 45 years for men and age $\geq$ 55 years or postmenopausal for women. The presence of these risk factors heightens the need for

obesity treatment and concomitant lipid lowering therapy and blood pressure management when appropriate. Patients are considered to be at *very high risk* if they have existing coronary heart disease, atherosclerotic diseases, type 2 diabetes mellitus, or sleep apnea. This would include patients that have had a myocardial infarction, angina pectoris, a history of heart surgery, or angioplasty. Table 1 summarizes additional risk factors that increase the need for weight reduction and place the individual in a very high risk or high-risk category [6].

C. Assessment of Readiness

After assessing the patient's need for weight reduction, the health care provider must assess the patient's readiness to participate in treatment. Even when a patient is seriously overweight, he or she may not be ready to make a commitment to weight reduction [7]. Providers need to determine if the patient recognizes the need for weight loss and is willing (and able) to sustain a weight loss effort. A series of questions developed by Brownell can be used to help assess a patient's readiness to accept and participate in a long-term treatment plan [19, 20].

D. Selecting Treatment Options

Many options are available for treating overweight and obese individuals. For each patient, the risks of each treatment option must be weighed against the benefit of the potential weight loss produced by that treatment. This risk/benefit assessment must take into account a patient's BMI, waist circumference, and the presence of comorbidities and cardiovascular risk factors. Patients at a higher BMI or with existing obesity-related diseases are at more risk from their excess weight and, therefore, more aggressive treatments such as pharmacotherapy and surgery become appropriate options. For each patient, there is a level of obesity where the risk of the treatment is outweighed by the benefit the patient would receive from a long-term reduction in weight. Each treatment plan must be tailored to meet the BMI and risk/benefit assessment for each patient. Table 2 shows recommended treatment options based on BMI and the presence or absence of a serious health complication [21].

TABLE 2   Selecting Treatment Options Based on BMI and Comorbidities

Body mass index	Comorbidities[a] present	Diet	Exercise	Behavioral therapy	Pharmacotherapy	Surgery
25–26.9	No	_[b]	_[b]	_[b]	–	–
	Yes	+	+	+	–	–
27–29.9	No	_[b]	_[b]	_[b]	–	–
	Yes	+	+	+	+	–
30–34.9	No	+	+	+	+	–
	Yes	+	+	+	+	–
35–39.9	No	+	+	+	+	–
	Yes	+	+	+	+	+
≥40	No	+	+	+	+	+
	Yes	+	+	+	+	+

Source: Based on "NIH Clinical Guidelines on the Identification, Evaluation, and Treatment of Overweight and Obesity in Adults: The Evidence Report" (1998). National Institutes of Health, Bethesda, MD.
    + indicates appropriate treatment option; – indicates inappropriate treatment option.
    [a]Comorbidities include hypertension, sleep apnea, dyslipidemia, coronary heart disease, and type 2 diabetes.
    [b]Prevention of weight gain with diet, exercise, and behavioral therapy is indicated.

E. Appropriate Goal Setting

The evidence-based NIH clinical guidelines for obesity treatment set the following general goals for weight loss and management: (1) to prevent further weight gain, (2) to reduce body weight, and (3) to maintain a lower body weight long term [6]. Traditionally, the goal of obesity treatment was to achieve an ideal body weight, and for many people this meant losing extremely large amounts of weight. However, a reduction to ideal body weight is not necessary for health improvement and risk reduction. Clinical studies indicate that moderate weight reduction (i.e., 5–10% of the initial body weight) can correct or ameliorate many of the metabolic abnormalities associated with obesity and that small weight losses are associated with improvements in hypertension, dyslipidemia, and type 2 diabetes mellitus [22–24]. Prescribing a weight loss goal of 5–10% sets a reasonable and achievable goal that may be more easily maintained. Unfortunately, many patients are not satisfied with weight reduction in this range and the provider must work closely with the patient to help set realistic expectations and provide guidance in this area.

III. LIFESTYLE MODIFICATION

Lifestyle modification, in particular, the modification of a person's diet and physical activity, is the cornerstone of most obesity treatment programs. For most people this treatment incurs no side effects, has minimal cost, and, if the lifestyle changes can be maintained, has great potential for long term effectiveness [25]. In addition to creating changes in diet and physical activity patterns, the lifestyle modification component of obesity interventions usually also includes some form of behavioral treatment to enhance the long-term effectiveness of the program.

A. Dietary Modification

At any one time, about 70% of U.S. adults are trying to lose or maintain their weight [26] and almost all report modifying their diet in some way to achieve their goals [26, 27]. Because the prevalence of overweight and obesity is also at an all-time high, this interest in dieting and attempts to modify diet appear to be contradictory. This contradiction underscores the difficulty people face in making seemingly simple changes to their dietary intake in an environment that encourages easy overconsumption of energy.

1. CREATING AN ENERGY DEFICIT

The universal component of dietary interventions for weight loss is a creation of an energy deficit [1, 6]. Most recommendations encourage a slow rate of weight loss through an energy deficit (energy output minus energy intake) of 500–1000 kcal/day [1, 6]. This recommendation is based on the energy cost of burning 1 pound of excess body weight per week. Typically, the composition of the weight loss is about 25% fat-free mass and 75% fat mass. Metabolically, the more obese person can handle a greater energy deficit, as demonstrated by a lower protein oxidation rate during fasting, than a lean person [28]. It is important to monitor the rate of weight loss during the active weight loss phase. Initially, particularly at the greater energy deficits, diuresis may occur and weight will be dropped quickly. However, after this initial drop in weight, the rate of weight loss will slow and should not be greater than 1% body weight per week [29]. An energy deficit of 500–1000 kcal/day should produce about a 10% body weight reduction over 6 months [6].

Many healthcare providers prescribe a standard weight loss diet of a preset calorie level, e.g., 1200 or 1500 kcal/day. This approach has the advantage of allowing the health care provider to give out preprinted diet plans already designed to achieve the calculated energy level. The disadvantages of this approach include inappropriately low energy intakes (i.e., >1000 kcal/day deficits) in very large individuals with high energy requirements, and diet plans that are not tailored to an individual's lifestyle. To avoid inappropriate energy deficits, it makes more sense to estimate a person's energy expenditure and subtract 500–1000 kcal/day (the greater energy deficit should be reserved for the heavier individuals). Estimating a person's energy expenditure based on sex, body weight, and age [30] is preferable to using self-reported food intakes, which are notoriously unreliable, particularly among obese subjects [31, 32]. Alternatively, as a general rule, an appropriate energy level can be determined by assigning 12 kilocalories per pound of current body weight and then subtracting 500–1000 calories to create an energy deficit. The NIH Clinical Guidelines recommend 1000–1200 kcal/day for women and 1200–1500 kcal/day for men [6]. However, they emphasize the need for dietary education and tailoring the diet plan to accommodate individual food preferences.

Decreasing one's food consumption without ensuring an intake of a variety of foods may compromise a person's nutrient intake, particularly of calcium, iron, and vitamin E. At energy intakes below 1200 kcal/day, it is difficult to consume an adequate intake of essential vitamins and minerals. Multivitamin and mineral supplements are recommended for intakes below 1200 kcal/day and for individuals whose food choices limit their ability to consume a satisfactory nutrient intake.

2. VERY LOW CALORIE/ENERGY DIETS

Some dietary regimens, such as very low calorie diets (VLCDs), establish a greater than 1000 kcal/day energy deficit. A VLCD is typically a liquid formulation that contains up to 800 kcal/day (3350 kJ/day) [33]. VLCDs are enriched in protein of high biologic value (0.8–1.5 g/kg of ideal body weight per day), and are supplemented with essential vitamins, minerals, electrolytes, and fatty acids. A typical VLCD program lasts for 12–16 weeks and the liquid formula completely replaces all usual foods. A structured period of refeeding usually occurs after a VLCD, with solid foods slowly being reintroduced into the patient's diet.

VLCDs are effective in producing a weight loss quickly. The mean weight loss for a 12- to 16-week program (including the long-term weight loss of dropouts) is about 20 kg [34]. Weight losses on VLCDs are greater for men than women [34], and heavier people lose more than lighter people [35]. It has been hypothesized that, beyond the greater than usual energy deficit, the form of these diets is an important factor in the effectiveness of a VLCD to produce a weight loss [34, 35]. That is, the structured feeding regimen of a VLCD encourages excellent adherence to the low-calorie

plan; a patient does not have to make food choices and refrains from making impulsive high-calorie selections.

Although effective at producing a quick weight loss, VLCDs have not proven to be effective for long-term weight loss maintenance. Now, many programs combine VLCD with behavior modification and this combination has slightly improved the long-term weight maintenance outcomes [36]. Other disadvantages of VLCDs include the expense of the programs and the side effects of the quick weight loss. The most serious side effects include hyperuricemia, gout, gallstones, and cardiac complications. These serious side effects underscore the need for (1) appropriate medical assessment for patients entering a program; (2) use of VLCDs in only obese patients (i.e., BMI > 30), especially those individuals with co-morbid conditions that would be responsive to weight loss, e.g., diabetes, sleep apnea, or presurgery; and (3) ongoing medical supervision during the course of the program [1, 33]. VLCDs are not recommended for use in obesity treatment by the NIH Clinical Guidelines [6].

3. MEAL REPLACEMENTS

Meal replacement drinks are sometimes used in weight loss programs. These differ from VLCDs in that they are designed to replace only one or 2 of the day's meals rather than the whole day's intake, and they are sold over the counter. The advantage of a meal replacement drink is that it can replace a person's most problematic meal of the day with a drink of a known energy and macronutrient content, thus helping to achieve a targeted energy intake goal. Few studies have specifically evaluated the efficacy of meal replacement drinks for weight loss [37]. A recent 27-month study [38] showed a significantly greater weight loss in people following a low-calorie plan utilizing two meal replacement drinks per day versus people following a conventional low-calorie plan (11.3 ± 6.8% vs. 5.9 ± 5.0% of initial body weight, $p < 0.0001$). Additionally, meal replacement drinks may be useful for weight maintenance or weight gain prevention. A study conducted in rural Wisconsin evaluated the efficacy of meal replacement drink treatment against the backdrop of weight gain experienced by matched controls over a 5-year period [39]. A total of 134 men and women participated in a self-management meal replacement drink program that included a 3-month active weight loss phase (two meal replacement drinks per day with weekly weigh-ins) and a maintenance phase (self-monitoring of weight and use of a meal replacement drink if weight gain occurred). During the same 5-year period, 86% of the meal replacement drink participants were *at least* weight stable (≤0.8 kg weight gain), while only 25% of the matched controls had prevented weight gain [39]. However, further research is required to verify the efficacy of this weight loss treatment.

4. MACRONUTRIENT COMPOSITION

A negative energy balance is the most important factor affecting the amount, rate, and composition of weight loss. The macronutrient composition of the diet has no significant

additive effect on these weight loss parameters during the course of a usual obesity treatment program [40]. However, it is apparent that the macronutrient composition of a weight loss diet may have an important effect on behavioral compliance with a dietary regimen.

In feeding experiments, it has been shown that people typically eat a constant daily weight of food regardless of the type of diet consumed [41]. Because fat contains more kilocalories per gram than either protein or carbohydrate (9 vs. 4 kcal/g), more energy is likely to be consumed when high-fat versus low-fat foods are eaten [41]. Additionally, fat has been proposed to have a weak effect on both satiation (process controlling meal size) and satiety (process controlling subsequent hunger and eating) [42] (see Chapter 35). "Passive overconsumption" is a term used to describe the likelihood of increased energy intake that occurs during high-fat feeding due to the combination of these two factors: high energy value of fat and its weak effect on both satiation and satiety [42]. For these reasons a low-fat diet (less than 30% energy from fat) is currently the typical recommended macronutrient guideline for weight loss [1, 6, 43]. Because diabetes and cardiovascular disease are frequent comorbidities of obesity, it is also recommended to modify the fat content of the diet to be low in saturated and *trans* fatty acids, and higher in monounsaturated fats [43].

Manufacturers have responded to consumer demand for lower fat versions of foods, and the number of fat-modified foods has increased dramatically in the marketplace [44]. Some fat-modified foods are still high in calories or may be consumed in larger than usual portions and therefore may not promote an energy deficit in an individual trying to lose weight. Mistakenly, people have assumed that a low-fat, high-carbohydrate diet can promote weight loss regardless of energy intake. Although weight loss has occurred in studies that have evaluated the use of a low-fat diet with *ad libitum* feeding [45], it is possible for a positive energy balance to occur. High-carbohydrate diets consumed in excess of energy requirements will promote fat storage despite higher carbohydrate oxidation rates [46].

Replacing some of the fat in the diet with protein may be an effective way to promote adherence to a weight loss plan. Acute appetite studies indicate that, calorie for calorie, protein exerts a more powerful effect on satiety than either fat or carbohydrate and may increase adherence to a reduced-energy, low-fat diet [42]. In a recent study, increasing the protein content to 25% of total energy intake of an *ad libitum* fat-reduced diet significantly improved weight loss over an *ad libitum* fat-reduced diet with a protein content of 12% [47]. Studies like this must be repeated in other populations and under different experimental conditions before specific recommendations can be made for protein content of a weight loss diet.

More recently, energy density (energy/food weight) of foods and diets has been evaluated as a potential dietary attribute that could be manipulated to influence energy in-

take [48]. However, the role that energy density plays in weight regulation is unclear, and currently there are no recommendations regarding the appropriate energy density of a weight loss diet.

5. NOVEL DIETS

Many people become frustrated with their perceived inability to change their body weight in a timely manner and are enticed by quick and painless weight loss promised by popular diet programs and books. These diets tend to be very limiting in food choices (e.g., grapefruit diet), restrictive of at least one macronutrient (e.g., Atkins diet), or rely on novel food combinations (e.g., the zone diet). If a person is able to adhere to one of these diets (which are typically hypocaloric), then weight loss usually occurs, and in that respect these diets do work. However, despite the anecdotal evidence provided by these programs and books, there are currently no carefully controlled trials evaluating the efficacy of any of these diets for weight loss or for weight loss maintenance. The initial dramatic weight loss that occurs on many of these diets is often due to the diuresis that occurs as glycogen stores are depleted in response to a low carbohydrate intake. This weight loss is temporary and if carbohydrate intake is increased, the glycogen stores are repleted and body weight increases accordingly. On very low carbohydrate diets, the body goes through a period of ketogenesis to provide fuel that can be utilized by the brain cells. Ketones are potent appetite depressants and lack of appetite may be one reason why individuals, at least temporarily, follow such restrictive diets.

The major criticism of these restrictive diets is that they promote rapid weight loss but do not address long-term weight maintenance. Because these diets tend to be very restrictive, many people may not be able to adhere to the regimen long term. Typically there is no education component on how to make appropriate healthful food choices after returning to a normal diet to promote long-term weight maintenance. In addition, these diets may be associated with the overconsumption of foods rich in saturated fat, a risk factor for the development of coronary artery disease.

6. THE NONDIET APPROACH

Recently, there has been a movement toward replacing restrictive diet approaches and unrealistic weight goals with promotion of healthful food choices and size acceptance. Proponents cite two rationales for adopting this approach: (1) there is no long-term effective strategy for treating obesity and (2) pressure to be thin impairs the psychological and social well-being of both people who are overweight and those who are not [49]. The focus of the nondiet approach is to encourage people to improve their self-acceptance (self-image) regardless of their current weight and to adopt healthy practices to promote physical well-being, e.g., promoting fitness and healthful food choices. Very few studies have carefully evaluated the result of the nondiet approaches

on weight loss or the reduction of comorbidities associated with obesity [50]. Repeated weight loss (also termed weight cycling) does not appear to be associated with psychopathology or changes in weight- and eating-related constructs [51]. However, it is apparent that more research is needed to conclusively determine the psychological effect of repeated episodes of dieting and weight loss.

B. Physical Activity Modification

In general, physical activity has been used as a key component of obesity treatment. However, studies looking at physical activity per se for weight loss have found only modest reductions in body weight using this strategy [52]. Weight losses in the range of 0.09–0.1 kg/week have been reported when exercise is used alone compared to a no-treatment control group [52, 53]. Exceptions to this trend have been reported with extreme levels of exercise as is seen in military-type training. Combining exercise with dietary restriction produces only a slight increase in weight loss over dietary restriction alone [52]. In general, groups using diet restriction plus exercise lost more weight than the diet-alone condition, but the magnitude of the difference was not significant in most studies.

A possible explanation for the relatively modest effect of physical activity on weight loss is that the energy cost of exercise is minimal compared to potential changes in energy intake. Subjects who exercise for 30 minutes 5 days a week may only burn 1000 kcal more per week depending on their size, fitness level, and intensity of exercise. In comparison, subjects may consume an extra 1000 kcal in one or two unplanned snacks and easily negate the energy expended in exercise for the entire week.

Although its impact on weight loss may be minimal, physical activity appears to have a crucial role in the long-term maintenance of a weight loss (i.e., the prevention of weight regain). Many correlation studies show a strong association between self-reported exercise at follow-up and maintenance of a weight loss [52]. Studies using doubly labeled water suggest physical activity in the range of 11–12 kcal/kg/day may be necessary to prevent weight regain following a weight loss [54].

Data from the National Weight Control Registry (NWCR) also support the concept that high levels of physical activity are crucial in preventing weight regain following a weight loss. The NWCR is a registry of more than 2000 individuals who have maintained a minimum of a 30-pound weight loss for at least 1 year. These individuals report using a variety of methods to lose weight initially, but more than 90% report exercise as a key element in maintaining the loss long term. They report expending, on average, 2682 kcal/week in physical activity [25]. This is approximately the equivalent of walking 4 miles 7 days a week, and many report much higher levels. This suggests that while physical activity may not have been essential for weight loss in these subjects, they

believe it to be essential in prevention of weight regain. A complete review of the role of physical activity in obesity intervention appears in Chapter 32.

C. Behavior Modification

Group behavioral programs, conducted on a weekly basis in university or hospital clinics, have been reported to produce average reductions of 8–10% of initial body weight over 16–26 weeks [7]. The key behavioral modification components utilized in obesity treatment include self-monitoring, stimulus control, and relapse prevention strategies [55]. Self-monitoring commonly includes the systematic recording of food intake, exercise activities, and/or weight change. The available scientific literature on obesity suggests that consistent self-monitoring, particularly of food intake, is associated with improved treatment outcome [56, 57], even during high-risk periods such as holidays [58].

Use of stimulus control involves the identification and modification of environmental cues associated with overeating and sedentary activity and is widely accepted as clinically effective [59].

Relapse prevention strategies involve training patients to prepare for lapses in the weight loss process and to utilize coping strategies to prevent complete relapse of behavior change efforts [60].

Finally, group-based behavior modification training is used in a variety of obesity treatment formats, including university-based programs, commercial weight management programs (e.g., Weight Watchers, Jenny Craig), and self-help programs (e.g., Take Off Pounds Sensibly, Overeaters Anonymous). Although preliminary research indicates that group-based interventions may be equally as effective as individual interventions for a variety of problem behaviors, there has been no systematic assessment to date on the group process specifically for obesity intervention [61]. As such, a variety of important questions including optimal number of group participants, frequency and length of meetings, critical group leader skills, and strategies to identify the optimal candidates for group-based interventions remain unanswered [61]. Most behavioral modification techniques utilized in a group setting can be effectively incorporated into weight loss counseling provided to an individual [7, 62].

IV. PHARMACEUTICAL INTERVENTION

A. Background

While diet, physical activity and behavior modification remain the cornerstone of obesity management, pharmaceutical intervention has become a legitimate therapeutic option for obesity treatment in the last 10 years. The increasing interest in pharmaceutical interventions has primarily been fueled by the realization that obesity in the United States has

reached epidemic proportions with no sign of slowing down. Additionally, the old perception that obesity is caused by a lack of willpower or gluttony has been replaced with a better scientific understanding of the genetics and biology that predispose certain individuals to gain weight in our current environment [63].

The discovery of leptin in the mid-1990s established the existence of a genetically controlled complex biological system for food intake and weight regulation. The view of obesity has shifted away from that of a behavioral problem occurring in people lacking in self-control and discipline to that of a chronic disease model with genetic, biological, and behavioral roots. This critical shift in thinking also changed the view of drug therapy for obesity from that of a short-term quick fix for a social problem to a long-term treatment for a chronic disease. It is now acknowledged that obesity, like other chronic diseases such as hypertension or diabetes, will require long-term treatment.

Weight loss medications were previously viewed as unsuccessful because weight was always regained following the withdrawal of the drug. Now it is recognized that medications need to be given long term to be effective in obesity treatment [64]. A landmark long-term weight loss trial using the combination of phentermine and fenfluramine was published by Weintraub and coworkers in 1992 [65]. This trial showed these medications' efficacy in maintenance of a weight loss over 4 years. This long-term pharmaceutical treatment data, along with the view of obesity as a chronic disease, marked the acceptance of pharmacotherapy as legitimate intervention in obesity treatment.

In the mid-1990s, dexfenfluramine alone and fenfluramine in combination with phentermine were used for long-term treatment of obesity. In September 1997, reported concerns about serious unacceptable side effects, such as valvular heart lesions, led to the withdrawal of dexfenfluramine and fenfluramine from the market. This left no long-term FDA-approved medications for obesity treatment. Since that time, the FDA has approved two new medications for long-term use in the treatment of obesity. Neither of these drugs (to date) has been associated with heart valve lesions. All other weight loss medications approved by the FDA for weight loss are approved only for short-term use (Table 3). Because obesity is a chronic disease and must be managed for long periods of time, if not a lifetime, only medications approved for long-term use are of real interest in obesity treatment.

B. Medications Approved for Short-Term Use in Weight Loss

The FDA has approved several medications for short-term use (less than 3 months). These drugs include mazindol, phentermine, and diethylpropion. These are noradrenergic or sympathomimetic drugs that either stimulate release or block reuptake of norepinephrine. In general, these medications have produced more weight loss than placebo in most short-term clinical trials, but the magnitude of the weight loss was variable [66, 67]. Large clinical trials evaluating these drugs for efficacy and safety in long-term obesity treatment are scarce and the FDA has not approved their use for longer than 3 months.

Phenylpropanolamine (PPA), available over the counter, is classified by the FDA as "possibly effective" in weight loss treatment and has provisional approval for weight loss [66, 67]. PPA produces more weight loss than placebo in short-term studies [68, 69]. In the one controlled trial of PPA that lasted 20 weeks, at 6 weeks the PPA-treated group had lost 2.4 kg compared with a 1.1 kg loss in the placebo group. In the optional 14-week extension to the study the PPA group lost 5.1 kg (6.5%) and the placebo group lost 0.4 kg (0.5%) of initial body weight [67]. Safety is an issue, because PPA is an over-the-counter medication and may be associated with slight elevations in blood pressure. Maximum dosage for PPA should not exceed 75 mg/day [64, 70].

C. Medications with No Approval for Use to Promote Weight Loss

Fluoxetine and ephedrine/caffeine have been evaluated in several weight loss trials [23, 71, 72], but do not have FDA approval for weight loss. Patients taking fluoxetine in doses greater than 60 mg/day have shown more weight loss than placebo in clinical trials. However, the long-term efficacy of fluoxetine is questionable, because weight regain, while *continuing* the medication, was also demonstrated [23, 72].

The ephedrine/caffeine combination has also been evaluated as a potential weight loss medication. The effects of ephedrine are amplified by caffeine and this combination is more efficacious than either compound alone in safe doses. Patients receiving the ephedrine/caffeine combination (caffeine 600 mg/day and ephedrine 60 mg/day) showed significantly more weight loss than patients receiving placebo (16.6 vs. 13.2 kg at 24 weeks, $p < 0.01$) [71]. Side effects of this combination include tremor and insomnia.

Ephedrine is derived from a natural ephedra herb (also known as *ma huang*), and many herbal preparations exploit the ephedrine/caffeine combination. More than 800 reports of side effects, including arrhythmias, increases in blood pressure, and death, have been reported to the Food and Drug Administration (FDA) by consumers taking herbal weight loss medications containing the ephedra herb. It is unclear what dosages, combinations, and circumstances may have lead to or caused the reported side effects since the herbal or so-called "natural" preparations are not governed by the FDA. Studies are under way to determine whether *ma huang* and other herbal products are safe and effective for weight loss, but currently there is no evidence to support their safety or use. The NHLBI Guidelines do not recommend the use of herbal preparations for weight loss at this time [6].

TABLE 3 Pharmaceutical Interventions Used in Obesity Treatment

Drug	Mechanism of action	Administration	Daily dose range (mg)	FDA approval for use
Benzphetamine	Stimulates NE release	Start with 25 mg qd; max dose 25–50 mg po tid	25–150	Short term
Phendimetrazine	Stimulates NE release	35 mg po tid before meals or 105 mg SR qd	35–105	Short term
Diethylproprion	Stimulates NE release	25 mg po tid or 75 mg SR qd	25–75	Short term
Mazindol	Blocks NE reuptake	Start with 1 mg po qd; max dose 1 mg po tid with meals	1–3	Short term
Phentermine	Stimulates NE release	15, 30, or 37.5 mg po qd in the AM	15–37.5	Short term
Phenylpropalamine	Alpha-1 agonist	25 mg po tid or 75 mg SR qd	25–75	Provisional (over the counter)
Fluoxetine	Serotonin reuptake inhibitor	60 mg po qd	60	None
Ephedrine/caffeine	Stimulates NE release	Ephedrine 20 mg po tid Caffeine 200 mg po tid	Ephedrine 20–60 Caffeine 200–600	None
Sibutramine	Serotonin and NE reuptake inhibitor	Start with 10 mg po qd; may increase or decrease to 5–15 mg po qd	5–15	Long term
Orlistat	Lipase inhibitor	120 mg taken with each meal po tid	120–360	Long term

Key: po = by mouth; qd = once a day; tid = three times a day; SR = slow release capsule; NE = norepinephrine.

D. Medications Approved for Long-Term Use

1. SIBUTRAMINE

Sibutramine was approved in 1997 for long-term treatment of obesity. Sibutramine is a combination serotonin and norepinephrine reuptake inhibitor. Unlike the fenfluramine–phentermine combination, sibutramine does not stimulate the release of either of these neurotransmitters and this may be why valvular heart lesions have not been associated with the use of this drug [73]. Sibutramine's main mechanism of action is a reduction in food and energy intake. In laboratory animals, sibutramine also increases total metabolic rate by an increase in thermogenesis but this effect remains in question in humans and is small in magnitude if present [74–76].

The long-term efficacy of sibutramine has been evaluated in several 6- and 12-month double-blind randomized studies [77–79]. Sibutramine-treated patients lose significantly more weight, on average, than placebo-treated patients in these studies. For example, a greater than 10% weight loss was achieved by 30–39% of the sibutramine-treated patients (on 10 and 15 mg/day, respectively) versus only 8% of the placebo group achieving this level of weight loss in a 12-month study [77].

Side effects for sibutramine include headache, dry mouth, constipation, and insomnia. Increases in heart rate and blood pressure have been reported and, therefore, blood pressure should be monitored before and regularly after starting the medication. A few patients (<5%) may have a significant increase in blood pressure and, therefore, uncontrolled hypertension, a history of heart disease, heart failure, stroke, and arrhythmia are contraindications to the use of this drug.

Sibutramine is also contraindicated with monoamine oxidase inhibitors and other serotonin uptake inhibitors, which include medications for depression and migraines. Sibutramine is available in 5-, 10-, and 15-mg tablets and is taken once a day. Weight loss is dose related with the 10- and 15-mg dose. Most patients should be started on the 10-mg dose and adjustments made as necessary.

2. ORLISTAT

The FDA approved the use of orlistat for the long-term treatment of obesity in 1999. Orlistat is a minimally absorbable agent (<1%) that works in the gastrointestinal tract by blocking gastrointestinal lipases and reducing the subsequent absorption of ingested fat by approximately 30% [80]. Orlistat has been studied in 1- and 2-year clinical trials [81–83]. In general, the orlistat-treated groups lost more weight and had a higher percentage of subjects able to achieve a 10% weight loss than subjects in the placebo-treated group [84]. In a large study evaluating over 600 patients, 38.8% of the patients in the orlistat group achieved a 10% or greater weight loss compared to only 17.7% in the placebo group [85]. Orlistat's use for weight loss maintenance has been evaluated in 2-year studies. In these studies, a hypocaloric diet in combination with orlistat was used for weight loss in the first year, and then a eucaloric diet with orlistat or placebo was used in the second year to evaluate weight loss maintenance. In a large study by Davidson and coworkers [82], almost twice as many patients (34.1%) in the orlistat group were able to maintain a ≥10% weight loss for the 2-year period compared to the placebo group (17%) [82]. Sim-

ilar results indicate that mean body weight regain is less with orlistat treatment than placebo (32.4 versus 56.0%; orlistat and placebo respectively) [81]. In these clinical trials, orlistat was used in combination with either a low-fat hypocaloric diet for weight loss or a eucaloric diet for weight maintenance, and a portion of the benefit seen in these trials must be attributable to that diet.

The optimal dosing of orlistat is 120-mg po tid with meals that contain fat. Higher doses do not have any additional efficacy in weight loss and may result in more adverse events [86]. Orlistat is minimally absorbed; therefore, any systemic adverse events would be expected to be negligible. Orlistat should be used with a diet that is less than 30% energy from fat to prevent adverse side effects that include oily stools, oily spotting, flatus with discharge, fecal urgency, and fecal incontinence [86]. These events are due to the drug inhibiting fat absorption rather than a direct effect of the drug itself. Patients should be advised to maintain a low-fat diet while using the medication, because these side effects increase with diets over 30% energy from fat. In general, these events tend to decrease over time.

Mean plasma levels of vitamins A, D, E, and β-carotene were monitored during the trials. In general, plasma levels of these vitamins decreased but remained in the reference range [85, 86]; however, in the United States a multivitamin supplement is recommended for patients prescribed orlistat and should be taken 2 hours before or after the dose of orlistat.

E. Risk/Benefit Ratio

1. SELECTING PATIENTS FOR PHARMACOTHERAPY

After the degree of obesity has been assessed and the presence of comorbidities determined, the potential risks and benefits of a particular pharmacotherapy should be determined for each patient. The risk of the potential side effects of the medication must be carefully weighed against the benefits of the weight loss as a result of the treatment. The risk of not losing weight or even gaining weight must also be considered in the decision-making process. Additionally, many clinicians require that patients attempt weight loss in a structured program of diet, exercise, and behavioral modification before being considered for pharmacotherapy [7]. Severe obesity (BMI > 35 kg/m²) carries a high risk of morbidity and mortality [87], and intensive therapeutic approaches are indicated for most individuals. The lower BMI threshold for pharmaceutical intervention is not as easily defined, and other factors such as a high waist circumference, recent weight gain, family history and the presence of comorbidities become important considerations in the decision to treat with weight loss medications. Cosmetic weight loss attempts for patients who want to lose a few pounds are not appropriate. The risk of the medication in this case is not outweighed by the benefit since a reduction in weight at a lean weight (BMI ≤ 25 kg/m²) is not associated with

significant improvements in health risks. Currently, the evidence and the NHLBI guidelines justify the use of a weight loss medication in patients with BMIs ≥ 30 kg/m² or ≥ 27 kg/m² if comorbidities such as hypertension or diabetes are present [6].

2. PREDICTORS OF EFFICACY

Not every patient responds to drug therapy. Therefore, it is important to monitor patients on weight loss medications, not only for potential side effects, but also for the efficacy of the medication itself. Clinical trials have shown that initial responders tend to continue to lose weight, whereas initial nonresponders continue to be nonresponders. The initial rate of weight loss has been frequently noted to predict subsequent weight loss. If the patient does not lose weight or maintain a previous weight loss with the medication, the medication should be discontinued. In this case, the risk of the medication is not outweighed by the weight loss, because there has not been a reduction in weight. As a general guideline, patients who do not lose 1% of body weight during their first month of treatment should discontinue treatment [74].

F. Medications Combined with Lifestyle Modification

It is important to emphasize that weight loss medications should be prescribed in combination with a diet, exercise, and behavioral modification program. Medications are not a substitute for, but an adjunct to, lifestyle intervention, providing additional benefit by helping patients adhere to the necessary diet and exercise changes. For some individuals, diet and exercise alone may be enough to produce a 10% weight loss and long-term maintenance. For others, medications may provide a necessary additional intervention to allow weight loss success.

V. SURGICAL TREATMENT

In general, surgical intervention is considered the most effective treatment for weight loss and long-term weight maintenance. Surgery, with its inherent permanence, clearly has an advantage in long-term success [88]. It is reserved for patients with severe disease that have failed less invasive interventions and are at a very high risk for obesity-related morbidity and mortality. In the past, practitioners have used a rough guide of an excess weight of 100 pounds (45.5 kg) as an indication to consider a surgical intervention. In 1991, The National Institute of Health Consensus Development Conference on gastrointestinal surgery for severe obesity set the patient selection criterion for surgery as a BMI exceeding 40 kg/m² [89]. In certain instances, an obese patient with a BMI between 35 and 40 kg/m² may be considered for a surgical procedure if a severe comorbidity is present [89].

These life-threatening comorbidities commonly include sleep apnea, hypertension, diabetes, heart failure, and vertebral disc herniation [90]. There is no recommendation at this time for children or adolescents. As the procedures for obesity surgery improve, it is expected that the BMI criteria for surgical candidates will be reduced.

Similar to pharmacotherapy, the use of a surgical intervention in obesity requires a risk/benefit analysis for each case. Those patients that have a low probability of success with nonsurgical interventions and who meet BMI criteria may be considered for surgery. Patients who have been determined to have acceptable operative risks should be well informed and motivated. They must understand how their lives may change after the operation and be able to participate in treatment and long-term follow-up. A surgeon experienced with the procedure (and working in a clinical setting with adequate support) should carry out the procedure.

A. Surgical Procedures

Two principal types of procedures, vertical banded gastroplasty and a Roux-en-Y gastric bypass, have become the current standard in weight loss surgery [88]. The vertical banded gastroplasty is a gastric resection procedure that consists of constructing a small pouch with a restricted outlet along the lesser curvature of the stomach. A Roux-en-Y gastric bypass procedure involves constructing a small gastric pouch whose outlet is a Y-shaped limb of small bowel. The procedure results in ingested food bypassing the majority of the stomach and varying lengths of the small intestine.

1. Amount of Weight Loss

Of the two major types of surgical procedures, the vertical banded gastroplasty and the gastric bypass, the gastric bypass produces a slightly greater weight loss. This increase in weight loss has to be balanced against a higher risk of nutritional deficiencies associated with the Roux-en-Y gastric bypass procedure. On average, weight losses produced by these procedures result in a 20–35% reduction in initial weight or 40–50% of excess weight [88, 90, 91]. Inadequate weight loss is between 20% and 25% with gastric restriction procedures and 5% with a gastric bypass [88]. In both procedures weight loss occurs over a period of 18–24 months and weight loss is typically well maintained for as long as 14 years [91].

2. Reduction in Obesity-Related Comorbid Conditions

Most patients experience substantial improvements in obesity-related comorbidities such as sleep apnea, glycemic control, and hypertension [91]. Studies looking at quality of life also report improvements following the surgical procedure and weight loss [92, 93]. The Swedish Obesity Study, a large prospective randomized study, has provided encouraging interim data that weight reduction following surgery reduced the 2-year incidence of diabetes, hypertension, and other health risks by 3- to 32-fold [94].

3. Complications and Side Effects

For centers that specialize in obesity surgery, the immediate operative mortality for both the vertical banded gastroplasty and Roux-en-Y gastric bypass procedures are relatively low and usually in the range of 0.5–1% [88, 90]. Morbidity in the early postoperative period may be as high as 10–20% [88]. These postoperative complications include wound infections, wound dehiscence, leaks from the staple line breakdown, stomal stenosis, marginal ulcers, pulmonary problems, and deep venous thrombosis. Other problems may arise in the later postoperative period. These include pouch and distal esophageal dilation, incisional hernias, strictures, persistent vomiting, cholecystitis, and diarrhea.

In the long-term, micronutrient deficiencies of vitamin B_{12}, folate, and iron are common and must be treated. Nutritional deficiencies are more likely in the bypass versus the gastric restriction procedures. Patients must be willing to take supplements postoperatively and must be monitored closely. Nutritional deficiencies are of particular concern in women of childbearing years because nutrient deficiencies carry a high risk of fetal damage.

"Dumping syndrome," a side effect of a gastric bypass procedure, is characterized by tachycardia, palpitations, diaphoresis, and nausea. Ingestion of energy-dense high-carbohydrate food, which is rapidly emptied into the small intestine, causes the release of vasoactive gastrointestinal polypeptides that may lead to the syndrome. Up to 70% of patients undergoing a gastric bypass procedure will experience some degree of a "dumping syndrome."

Vomiting and intolerance to solid food are the most common side effect of a gastric restrictive procedure. Most vomiting following a restrictive procedure is behavioral, but stricture and stenosis must be ruled out.

VI. SPECIAL ISSUES IN THE TREATMENT OF PEDIATRIC OBESITY

Data from national surveys indicate a significant increase in the prevalence of overweight and obesity in children and adolescents [95]. Obesity now affects one in five children and is considered to be the most prevalent pediatric nutrition disease in the United States [96]. Because obese children tend to become obese adults and face an increased risk of chronic diseases, e.g., diabetes and cardiovascular diseases, pediatric obesity is considered a major public health problem. However, even during childhood and adolescence, disorders such as hyperlipidemia, hypertension, and abnormal glucose tolerance occur with increased frequency in overweight and obese children [96]. In addition to the metabolic sequelae, significant negative psychosocial consequences of obesity are observed in this population [96].

Treatment goals for pediatric obesity are different than those for adult obesity. Because children are still growing with increases in lean body mass, treatment focuses on preventing weight gain rather than the weight loss focus of adult treatment [1]. Additionally, any treatment aimed at regulating body weight and body fat must also provide adequate nutrition for the growth and development of the child. It is also important that the health care provider evaluate the physiological and psychological impact of an obesity treatment for children and adolescents. Pharmacological and surgical obesity treatments have not been well evaluated in the pediatric population and are currently not recommended interventions [1, 6]. Therefore, the only recommended treatments involve changes in dietary intake, increases in physical activity and the utilization of behavior modification techniques. For a more complete review of all pediatric obesity treatments the reader is referred to Epstein *et al.* [97]. A summary of the special issues of pediatric obesity interventions is presented below.

Any dietary intervention to regulate a child's body weight must provide sufficient energy for growth and development. In particular, micronutrients such as iron and calcium must be adequately provided by the diet. Dietary advice and modification are most likely to be effective if there is parental involvement because parental attitudes, purchase, and presentation of food as well as modeling of eating behavior can impact a child's intake [1]. Some child-feeding practices can have negative (and unintended) effects on a child's food preferences and ability to control food intake [98]. For example, stringent parental control can increase a child's preference for high-energy-dense foods and limit a child's acceptance of a wide variety of foods [98]. Parental support involves being a positive role model for healthful feeding behavior as well as providing a wide array of healthful food choices in a supportive eating context [99]. Finally, because the potential for emergence of eating disorders is high in both children and adolescents, dietary modifications must occur in the context of the promotion of realistic body weight goals, positive self-esteem, and body image satisfaction.

It has been stated that our current environment facilitates underactivity through increased opportunity for sedentary activities [100]. This statement is just as true for children as it is for adults with sedentary activities (e.g., television viewing, video game playing) frequently taking prominence in children's lives. Physical activity interventions in the treatment of pediatric obesity often include decreasing these sedentary behaviors [101, 102]. Studies have shown this approach to be effective both in increasing physical activity and producing relative changes in BMI [101, 102]. In addition, because children are more likely to continue being active if they are able to choose their own activity, providing a choice of activities appears to be superior to providing a specific exercise prescription [101].

The fact that children routinely attend school, an environment that has continuous and intensive contact with children, creates a unique opportunity for pediatric obesity intervention. Schools have the necessary resources to promote physical activity (e.g., gym equipment, playing fields), they provide at least one meal a day where children can be exposed to healthful food choices, and many schools have access to school nurses or health clinics, which could potentially provide services to overweight children [103]. Obese children in treatment groups in school-based interventions have shown greater reductions in percentage overweight than untreated obese controls [1]. The effectiveness of school-based programs for the treatment of obesity has been modest but the results are encouraging and are worthy of more research.

VII. ACUTE WEIGHT LOSS VERSUS MAINTAINING LONG-TERM WEIGHT LOSS

Until recently, obesity was viewed as an acute disorder and so typical treatment was a single short-term intervention. However, weight loss can rarely be maintained for long periods, e.g., longer than 1 year, with only one short-term intervention. Therefore the real challenge of the obesity epidemic lies in the *prevention* of weight regain, not in the accomplishment of weight loss itself.

To address the chronic nature of the disease, a treatment plan for obesity must be long term and focused on both achieving and maintaining a weight loss. It may be useful to view weight loss separately from weight loss maintenance, and to consider different strategies for each. Weight loss requires creating a negative energy balance (intake < expenditure) for a relatively short period of time while weight loss maintenance requires a patient to be in energy balance (intake = expenditure) for a very long period of time. In the weight maintenance period the patient can maintain a weight loss at any level of intake, but must match expenditure to that level for long-term success. Treatments that produce the largest deficit in intake will produce the most weight loss but these treatments may not be easy to maintain chronically. Similarly, the treatments that most effectively maintain a weight loss may not be very effective in producing weight loss.

For example, VLCDs are a well-established method for safely achieving a substantial weight loss but individuals treated with VLCDs frequently regain the majority of their weight loss. They are very successful at producing a weight loss but do not easily nor safely continue for very long periods of time. Regular physical activity, on the other hand, does not produce large amounts of weight loss as an acute intervention by itself, but it has proven to be a critical strategy in long-term weight loss maintenance [25, 54]. The best overall treatment for an obese individual may incorporate treatments for acute weight loss paired with a different treatment in the weight maintenance phase. Potentially, weight loss medications may have their greatest role in helping obese individuals maintain a weight loss achieved by differ-

ent interventions (such as diet and exercise) that may be very difficult to maintain at the necessary level for long periods of time.

VIII. THE FUTURE OF WEIGHT MANAGEMENT

Prevention of obesity is the true future of weight management. Preventing excess weight gain from ever occurring should be an easier task than treating obesity once it is present. However, there has been surprisingly little research into obesity prevention and, to date, prevention efforts have met with modest success at best. While obesity prevention can be targeted as a high priority, there is much to learn about how to do it effectively.

The prevention of obesity should not focus exclusively on the behavior of an individual. Prevention should address the larger environmental and societal factors that ultimately influence an individual's behavior. The current environment in the United States promotes weight gain and obesity by encouraging excessive food consumption and discouraging physical activity. We live in an environment that has an abundance of cheap, good-tasting, energy-dense foods but requires little physical exertion for day-to-day living. It is difficult for individuals in this environment to consistently maintain behaviors that would support a healthy body weight.

There is a need for a concerted, integrated effort from all sectors of society to create an environment that is less obesity conducive. Despite the daunting nature of this task, the rapidity of the increase in obesity underscores the urgency in addressing the issue.

References

1. World Health Organization (1997). Obesity: Preventing and managing the global epidemic. Report of a WHO Consultation presented at the World Health Organization, June 3–5, 1997. Publication WHO/NUT/NCD/98.1. World Health Organization, Geneva, Switzerland.
2. Flegal, K. M., Carroll, M. D., Kuczmarski, R. J., and Johnson, C. L. (1998). Overweight and obesity in the United States: Prevalence and trends, 1960–1994. *Int. J. Obes. Rel. Med. Dis.* **22**(1), 39–47.
3. Must, A., Spadano, J., Coakley, E. H., Field, A. E., Colditz, G., and Dietz, W. H. (1999). The disease burden associated with overweight and obesity. *JAMA* **282**, 1523–1529.
4. Wolf, A. M., and Colditz, G. A. (1998). Current estimates of the economic cost of obesity in the United States. *Obes. Res.* **6**(2), 97–106.
5. Hill, J. O. (1997). Energy metabolism and obesity. *In* "Clinical Research in Diabetes and Obesity, Vol. II: Diabetes and Obesity" (B. Drazin and R. Rizza, Eds.), pp. 3–12. Humana Press, Inc., Totowa, NJ.
6. National Heart, Lung, and Blood Institute, Obesity Education Initiative Expert Panel (1998). Clinical guidelines on the identification, evaluation, and treatment of overweight and obesity in adults: The evidence report. *Obes. Res.* **6**(Suppl. 2), 51S–209S. http://www.nhlbi.nih.gov/guidelines/obesity/ob_home.htm.
7. Anderson, D., and Wadden, T. (1999). Treating the obese patient: Suggestions for primary care practice. *Arch. Fam. Med.* **8**, 156–167.
8. Metropolitan Life Insurance Company (1983). Metropolitan height and weight tables. *Stat. Bull. Met. Life Ins. Co.* **64**, 2.
9. Stensland, S., and Margolis, S. (1990). Simplifying the calculation of body mass index for quick reference. *J. Am. Diet. Assoc.* **90**, 856.
10. Heymsfield, S. B., Allison, D. B., Heshka, S., and Pierson, R. N. (1995). "Handbook of Assessment Methods for Eating Behavior and Weight Related Problems: Measures, Theory, and Research," pp. 515–560. Sage Publications, Thousand Oaks, CA.
11. Manson, J. E., Willett, W. C., Stampfer, M. J., Colditz, G. A., Hunter, D. J., Hankinson, S. E., Hennekens, C. H., and Speizer, F. E. (1995). Body weight and mortality among women. *N. Engl. J. Med.* **333**, 677–685.
12. Lew, E. A., and Garfinkel, L. (1979). Variations in mortality by weight among 750,000 men and women. *J. Chronic Dis.* **32**, 563–576.
13. Gordon, T., and Doyle, J. T. (1988). Weight and mortality in men: The Albany Study. *Int. J. Epidemiol.* **17**, 77–81.
14. Gallagher, D., Visser, M., Sepulveda, D., Pierson, R. N., Harris, T., and Heymsfield, S. B. (1996). How useful is body mass index for comparison of body fatness across age, sex, and ethnic groups? *Am. J. Epidemiol.* **143**, 228–239.
15. Bray, G. A. (1996). Health hazards of obesity. *Endocrin. Metab. Clin. No. Am.* **4**, 907–919.
16. Seidel, J. (1998). Epidemiology: Definition and classification of obesity. *In* "Clinical Obesity" (P. G. Kopleman and M. J. Stock, Eds.), pp. 1–17. Blackwell Science, Malden, MA.
17. Despres, J. P., Moorjani, S., Lupien, P. J., Tremblay, A., Nadeau, A., and Bouchard, C. (1990). Regional distribution of body fat, plasma lipoproteins, and cardiovascular disease. *Arteriosclerosis* **10**, 497–511.
18. Lemieux, S., Prud'homme, D., Bouchard, C., Tremblay, A., and Despres, J. P. (1996). A single threshold value of waist girth identifies normal-weight and overweight subjects with excess visceral adipose tissue. *Am. J. Clin. Nutr.* **64**, 685–693.
19. Brownell, K. D. (1990). Dieting readiness. *Weight Control Digest* **1**, 1–9.
20. Bray, G. A. (1998). The dieting readiness test. *In* "Contemporary Diagnosis and Management of Obesity," pp. A1–A7. Handbooks in Health Care, Newtown, PA.
21. North American Association for the Study of Obesity. (1998). "The Practical Guide to the Identification, Evaluation, and Treatment of Overweight and Obese Adults. National Institutes of Health, National Heart, Lung, and Blood Institute, Bethesda, MD.
22. Wing, R., Koeske, R., Epstein, Z. L., Norwalk, M. P., Gooding, W., and Becker, D. (1987). Long-term effects of modest weight loss in type II diabetic patients. *Arch. Intern. Med.* **147**, 1749–1753.
23. Goldstein, D. J., Rampey, A. H., Roback, P. J., Wilson, M. G., Hamilton, S. H., Sayler, M. E., and Tollefson, G. D. (1995). Efficacy and safety of long-term fluoxetine

treatment of obesity—maximizing success. *Obes. Res.* **3** (Suppl. 4), 481S–490S.

24. Dattilo, A. M., and Kris-Etherton, P. M. (1992). Effects of weight reduction on blood lipids and lipoproteins: A meta-analysis. *Am. J. Clin. Nutr.* **56**, 320–328.

25. Klem, M. L., Wing, R. R., McGuire, M. T., Seagle, H. M., and Hill, J. O. (1997). A descriptive study of individuals successful at long-term maintenance of substantial weight loss. *Am. J. Clin. Nutr.* **66**, 239–246.

26. Serdula, M. K., Mokdad, A. H., Williamson, D. F., Galuska, D. A., Mendlein, J. M., and Heath, G. W. (1999). Prevalence of attempting weight loss and strategies for controlling weight. *JAMA* **282**, 1353–1358.

27. French, S. A., Jeffrey, R. W., and Murray, D. (1999). Is dieting good for you?: Prevalence, duration and associated weight and behavior changes for specific weight loss strategies over four years in U.S. adults. *Int. J. Obes.* **23**, 320–327.

28. Elia, M., Stubbs, R. J., and Henry, C. J. K. (1999). Differences in fat, carbohydrate, and protein metabolism between lean and obese subjects undergoing total starvation. *Obes. Res.* **7**, 597–604.

29. VanItallie, T. B. (1999). Treatment of obesity: Can it become a science? *Obes. Res.* **7**, 605–606.

30. Food and Agricultural Organization/World Health Organization/United Nations University. (1985). "Report of a Joint Expert Consultation: Energy and Protein Requirement of Adults." Technical Report No. 724. World Health Organization, Geneva.

31. Schoeller, D. A., Bandini, L. G., and Dietz, W. H. (1989). Inaccuracies in self-reported intake identified by comparison with the doubly labeled water method. *Can. J. Physiol. Pharmacol.* **68**, 941–949.

32. Lichtman, S. W., Pisarska, K., Berman, E. R., Pestone, M., Dowling, H., Offenbacher, E., Weisel, H., Heshka, S., Matthews, D. E., and Heymsfield, S. B. (1992). Discrepancy between self-reported and actual caloric intake and exercise in obese subjects. *N. Engl. J. Med.* **327**, 1893–1898.

33. National Task Force on the Prevention and Treatment of Obesity (1993). Very low-calorie diets. *JAMA* **270**, 967–974.

34. Wadden, T. A. (1993). Treatment of obesity by moderate and severe caloric restriction. Results of clinical research trials. *Ann. Intern. Med.* **119**, 688–693.

35. Wing, R. R. (1992). Don't throw out the baby with the bathwater. A commentary on very-low-calorie diets. *Diabetes Care* **15**, 293–296.

36. Wadden, T. A., Sternberg, J. A., Letizia, K. A., Stunkard, A. J., and Foster, G. D. (1989). Treatment of obesity by very low calorie diet, behavior therapy, and their combination: A five-year perspective. *Int. J. Obes.* **13**(Suppl. 2), 39–46.

37. Heber, D., Ashley, J. M., Wang, H. J., and Elashoff, R. M. (1994). Clinical evaluation of a minimal intervention meal replacement regimen for weight reduction. *J. Am. College. Nutr.* **13**, 608–614.

38. Ditschuneit, H. H., Flechtner-Mors, M., Johnson, T. D., and Adler, G. (1999). Metabolic and weight-loss effects of a long-term dietary intervention in obese patients. *Am. J. Clin. Nutr.* **69**, 198–204.

39. Quinn Rothacker, D. (2000). Five-year self-management of weight using meal replacements: Comparison with matched controls in rural Wisconsin. *Nutrition* **16**, 344–348.

40. Hill, J. O., Drougas, H., and Peters, J. C. (1993). Obesity treatment: Can diet composition play a role? *Ann. Intern. Med.* **119**, 694–697.

41. Lissner, L., Levitsky, D. A., Strupp, B. J., Kalkwarf, H. J., and Roe, D. A. (1987). Dietary fat and the regulation of energy intake in human subjects. *Am. J. Clin. Nutr.* **46**, 886–892.

42. Blundell, J. E., and Stubbs, R. J. (1999). High and low carbohydrate and fat intakes: Limits imposed by appetite and palatability and their implications for energy balance. *Eur. J. Clin. Nutr.* **53**, S148–S165.

43. Krauss, R. M., Deckelbaum, R. J., Ernst, N., Fisher, E., Howard, B. V., Knopp, R. H., Kotchen, T., Lichtenstein, A. H., McGill, H. C., Pearson, T. A., Prewitt, T. E., Stone, N. J., Horn, L. V., and Weinberg, R. (1996). Dietary guidelines for healthy American adults. A statement for health professionals from the nutrition committee, American Heart Association. *Circulation* **94**, 1795–1800.

44. Calorie Control Council (2000). "Fat Replacers: Food Ingredients for Health Eating." Available at: http://www.caloriecontrol.org/fatrepl.html.

45. Astrup, A., Ryan, L., Grunwald, G. K., Storgaard, M., Saris, W., Melanson, E., and Hill, J. O. (2000). The role of dietary fat in body fatness: Evidence from a preliminary meta-analysis of ad libitum low-fat diet intervention studies. *Br. J. Nutr.* **83**, S25–S32.

46. Horton, T. J., Drougas, H., Brachey, A., Reed, G. W., Peters, J. C., and Hill, J. O. (1995). Fat and carbohydrate overfeeding in humans: Different effects on energy storage. *Am. J. Clin. Nutr.* **62**, 19–29.

47. Skov, A. R., Toubro, S., Ronn, B., Holm, L., and Astrup, A. (1999). Randomized trial on protein vs carbohydrate in ad libitum fat reduced diet for the treatment of obesity. *Int. J. Obes.* **23**, 528–536.

48. Bell, E. A., Castellanos, V. A., Pelkman, C. L., Thorwart, M. L., and Rolls, B. J. (1998). Energy density of foods affects energy intake in normal-weight women. *Am. J. Clin. Nutr.* **67**, 412–420.

49. Ikeda, J. P., Hayes, D., Satter, E., Parham, E. S., Kratina, K., Woolsey, M., Lowey, M., and Tribole, E. (1999). A commentary on the new obesity guidelines from NIH. *J. Am. Diet. Assoc.* **99**, 918–919.

50. Higgins, L., and Gray, W. (1999). What do anti-dieting programs achieve? A review of research. *Austral. J. Nutr. Diet.* **56**, 128–136.

51. Foster, G. D., Sarwer, D. B., and Wadden, T. A. (1997). Psychological effects of weight cycling in obese persons: A review and research agenda. *Obes. Res.* **5**, 474–488.

52. Wing, R. R. (1999). Physical activity in the treatment of the adulthood overweight and obesity: Current evidence and research issues. *Med. Sci. Sports Exerc.* **30**(11), S547–S552.

53. Zachwieja, J. J. (1996). Exercise as treatment for obesity. *Endocrinol. Metab. Clin. N. Am.* **25**(4), 965–988.

54. Schoeller, D. A., Shay, K., and Kushner, R. F. (1997). How much physical activity is needed to minimize weight gain in previously obese women? *Am. J. Clin. Nutr.* **66**, 551–556.

55. Foreyt, J. P., and Poston, W. S., II (1998). What is the role of cognitive-behavior therapy in patient management? *Obes. Res.* **6**, 18S–22S.

56. Boutelle, K. N., and Kirshenbaum, D. S. (1998). Further support for consistent self-monitoring as a vital component of successful weight control. *Obes. Res.* **6**, 219–224.

57. Streit, K. J., Stevens, N. H., Stevens, V. J., and Rossner, J. (1991). Food records: A predictor and modifier of weight change in a long-term weight loss program. *J. Am. Diet. Assoc.* **91,** 213–216.

58. Boutelle, K. N., Kirshenbaum, D. S., Baker, R. C., and Mitchell, M. E. (1999). How can obese weight controllers minimize weight gain during high risk holiday season? By self-monitoring very consistently. *Health Pysch.* **18,** 364–368.

59. Foreyt, J. P., and Goodrick, G. K. (1993). Evidence for success of behavior modification in weight loss and control. *Ann. Intern. Med.* **119,** 698–701.

60. Foreyt, J. P., and Poston, W. S., II (1998). The role of the behavioral counselor in obesity treatment. *J. Am. Diet. Assoc.* **98,** S27–S30.

61. Hayaki, J., and Brownell, K. D. (1996). Behaviour change in practice: Group approaches. *Int. J. Obes.* **20,** S27–S30.

62. Frank, A. (1998). A multidisciplinary approach to obesity management: The physician's role and team care alternatives. *J. Am. Diet. Assoc.* **98,** S44–S48.

63. Comuzzie, A. G., and Allison, D. B. (1998). The search for human obesity genes. *Science* **280,** 1374–1377.

64. Bray, G. A. (1998). Drug treatment of overweight. *In* "Contemporary Diagnosis and Management of Obesity," pp. 246–273. Handbooks in Health Care, Newtown, PA.

65. Weintraub, M., Sundaresan, P. R., and Cox, C. (1992). Long-term weight control study VI. *Clin. Pharmacol. Ther.* **51,** 619–633.

66. Ryan, D. H. (1996). Medicating the obese patient. *Endocrinol. Metab. Clin. N. Am.* **25,** 989–1004.

67. Bray, G. A., and Greenway, F. L. (1999). Current and potential drugs for treatment of obesity. *Endocrinol. Rev.* **20**(6), 805–875.

68. Weintraub, M. (1985). Phenylpropanolamine as an anorexic agent in weight control: A review of published and unpublished studies. *Clin. Pharmacol. Ther.* **5,** 53–79.

69. Greenway, F. (1992). Clinical studies with phenylpropanolamine: A meta-anlaysis. *Am. J. Clin. Nutr.* **55,** 203S–205S.

70. Morgan, J. P., and Funderburk, F. R. (1992). Phenylpropanolamine and blood pressure: A review of prospective studies. *Am. J. Clin. Nutr.* **55,** 206S–210S.

71. Astrup, A., Breum, L., Tiubro, S., Hein, P., and Quaade, F. (1992). The effect and safety of an ephedrine/caffeine compound compared to ephedrine, caffeine and placebo in obese subjects on an energy restricted diet: A double blinded trial. *Int. J. Obes.* **16,** 269–277.

72. Darga, L. L., Carroll-Michals, L., Botsford, S. J., and Lucas, C. P. (1991). Fluoxetine's effects on weight loss in obese subjects. *Am. J. Clin. Nutr.* **54,** 321–325.

73. Heal, D. J., Aspley, S., Prow, M. R., Jackson, H. C., Martin, K. F., and Cheetham, S. C. (1998). Sibutramine: A novel anti-obesity drug. A review of the pharmacological evidence to differentiate it from amphetamine and d-fenfluramine. *Int. J. Obes.* **22**(Suppl. 1), S18–S28.

74. Astrup, A., Hansen, H. L., Lundsgaard, C., and Toubro, S. (1998). Sibutramine and energy balance. *Int. J. Obes.* **22** (Suppl. 1), S30–S35.

75. Seagle, H. M., Bessesen, D. H., and Hill, J. O. (1998). Effects of sibutramine on resting metabolic rate and weight loss in overweight women. *Obes. Res.* **6,** 115–121.

76. Hansen, D. L., Toubro, S., Macdonald, I., Stock, M. J., and Astrup, A. (1997). Thermogenic properties of sibutramine in humans. *Int. J. Obes.* **22**(Suppl. 2), 102A.

77. Jones, S. P., Smith, I. G., Kelly, F., and Gray, J. A. (1995). Long-term weight loss with sibutramine. *Int. J. Obes.* **19** (Suppl. 2), 41.

78. Apfelbaum, M., Vague, P., Ziegler, O., Hanotin, C., Thomas, F., and Leutenegger, E. (1999). Long-term maintenance of weight loss after a very-low calorie diet: A randomized blinded trial of the efficacy and tolerability of sibutramine. *Am. J. Med.* **106,** 179–184.

79. Bray, G. A. (1996). Health hazards of obesity. *Endocrinol. Metab. Clin. N. Am.* **25,** 907–919.

80. Zhi, J., Melia, A. T., Funk, C., Viger-Chougnet, A., Hopfartner, G., Lausecker, B., Wang, K., Fulton, J. S., Gabriel, L., and Mulligan, T. E. (1996). Metabolic profiles of minimally absorbed orlistat in obese/overweight volunteers. *J. Clin. Pharmacol.* **36,** 1006–1011.

81. Hill, J. O., Hauptman, J., Anderson, J. W., Fujioka, K., O'Neil, P. M., Smith, D. K., Zavoral, J. H., and Aronne, L. J. (1999). Orlistat, a lipase inhibitor, for weight maintenance after conventional dieting: A 1-y study. *Am. J. Clin. Nutr.* **69,** 1108–1116.

82. Davidson, M. H., Hauptman, J., Di Girolamo, M., Foreyt, J. P., Halsted, C. H., Heber, D., Heimburger, D. C., Lucas, C. P., Robbins, D. C., Chung, J., and Heymsfield, S. B. (1999). Weight control and risk factor reduction in obese subjects treated with orlistat: A randomized, controlled trial. *JAMA* **281,** 235–242.

83. James, W. P. T., Avenell, A., Broom, J., and Whitehead, J. (1997). A one-year trial to assess the value of orlistat in the management of obesity. *Int. J. Obes. Metab. Disord.* **21** (Suppl.), 24–30.

84. Hill, J. O., and Wyatt, H. R. (1999). The efficacy of orlistat (xenical) in promoting weight loss and preventing weight regain. *Curr. Prac. Med.* **2**(11), 228–231.

85. Sjostrom, L. M., Rissanen, A., Andersen, T., Boldrin, M., Golay, A., Koppeschaar, H. P., and Krempf, M., for the European Multi-Center Orlistat Study Group (1998). Randomised placebo-controlled trial of orlistat for weight loss and prevention of weight regain in obese patients. *Lancet* **352,** 167–172.

86. Van Gaal, L. F., Broom, J. I., Enzi, G., and Toplak, H., for the Orlistat Dose-Ranging Group. (1998). Efficacy and tolerability of orlistat in the treatment of obesity: A 6-month dose ranging study. *Eur. J. Clin. Pharmacol.* **54,** 125–132.

87. Sjostrom, L. V. (1992). Mortality of severely obese subjects. *Am. J. Clin. Nutr.* **55,** 516S–523S.

88. Greenway, F. L. (1996). Surgery for obesity. *Endocrinol. Metab. Clin. N. Am.* **25**(4), 1005–1027.

89. National Institutes of Health, Consensus Development Conference (1992). Gastrointestinal surgery for severe obesity. *Am. J. Clin. Nutr.* **55,** 487S–619S.

90. Kral, J. (1998). Surgical treatment of obesity. *In* "Handbook of Obesity" (G. A. Bray, C. Bouchard, and W. P. James, Eds.), pp. 977–993. Marcel Dekker, New York.

91. Poiries, W. J., Swanson, M. S., MacDonald, K. G., Long, S. B., Morris, P. G., Brown, B. M., Barakat, H. A., de Ramon, R. A., Israel, G., Dolezal, J. M., and Dohm, L. (1995). Who would have thought it? An operation proves to be the most effective therapy for adult onset diabetes mellitus. *Ann. Surg.* **222,** 339–352.

92. Castelnuovo-Tedesco, P. (1986). Psychiatric complications of surgery for superobesity: A review and reappraisal. *Clin. Nutr.* **5**(Suppl.), 163–166.

93. Rand, S. W., and Macgregor, M. C. (1991). Successful weight loss following obesity surgery and the perceived liability of morbid obesity. *Int. J. Obes.* **15,** 577–579.

94. Sjostrom, L. (1998). What does SOS teach us in 1998? *Int. J. Obes.* **22**(Suppl. 3), S93.

95. Troiano, R. P., and Flegal, K. M. (1998). Overweight children and adolescents: Description, epidemiology, and demographics. *Pediatrics* **101,** 497–504.

96. Dietz, W. H. (1998). Health consequences of obesity in youth: Childhood predictors of adult disease. *Pediatrics* **101,** 518–525.

97. Epstein, L. H., Myers, M. D., Raynor, H. A., and Saelens, B. E. (1998). Treatment of obesity. *Pediatrics* **101,** 554–570.

98. Birch, L. L., and Fisher, J. O. (1998). Development of eating behaviors among children and adolescents. *Pediatrics* **101,** 539–549.

99. Satter, E. M. (1996). Internal regulation and the evolution of normal growth as the basis for prevention of obesity in children. *J. Am. Diet. Assoc.* **96,** 860–864.

100. Hill, J. O., and Peters, J. C. (1998). Environmental contributions to the obesity epidemic. *Science* **280,** 1371–1374.

101. Epstein, L. H., Paluch, R. A., Gordy, C. C., and Dorn, J. (2000). Decreasing sedentary behaviors in treating pediatric obesity. *Arch. Pediatr. Adolesc. Med.* **154,** 220–226.

102. Robinson, T. N. (1999). Reducing children's television viewing to prevent obesity. *JAMA* **282,** 1561–1567.

103. Story, M. (1999). School-based approaches for preventing and treating obesity. *Int. J. Obes.* **22,** S43–S51.

CHAPTER **32**

Obesity: Role of Physical Activity

MARCIA L. STEFANICK
Stanford University, Palo Alto, California

I. INTRODUCTION

The prevalence of obesity, defined as having a body mass index (BMI) greater than or equal to 30 kg/m² [1], increased markedly in the United States between the second (1976–1980) and third (1988–1994) National Health and Nutrition Examination Surveys (NHANES II and III). Specifically, the percent of the U.S. population aged 20 years or older that is obese increased from 14.5% to 22.5% between surveys, while the prevalence of overweight (i.e., BMI of 25–29.9 kg/m² [1]), persisted at 32.0% across surveys, to total 54.5% of U.S. adults who are overweight or obese [2]. This information prompted the NHLBI Obesity Education Initiative (OEI) Expert Panel to develop evidence-based "Clinical Guidelines on the Identification, Evaluation, and Treatment of Overweight and Obesity in Adults," which specifies three general goals of weight loss and management: to prevent further weight gain, to reduce body weight, and to maintain a lower body weight over the long term [3].

The guidelines include the recommendation that physical activity be "part of a comprehensive weight loss therapy and weight control program, because it: modestly contributes to weight loss in overweight and obese adults, may decrease abdominal fat, increases cardiorespiratory fitness, and may help with maintenance of weight loss" [3]. The exercise prescription is the same as that recommended by the Centers for Disease Control and Prevention and the American College of Sports Medicine (ACSM) in 1995 [4], then endorsed by the NIH Consensus Development Panel on Physical Activity and Cardiovascular Health [5] and incorporated into the Report of the Surgeon General [6]. The prescription is that moderate levels of physical activity for 30–45 minutes, 3–5 days a week should be encouraged initially, with a long-term goal of accumulating at least 30 minutes or more of moderate-intensity physical activity on most, and preferably all, days of the week [3].

Subsequent to the release of the OEI guidelines, an ACSM roundtable was convened to review more carefully the literature pertaining to the role of physical activity in the prevention and treatment of obesity and its comorbidities, using a similar evidence-based approach [7]. Drawing from the wealth of information assembled for the development of the ACSM consensus statement [8], and other sources, the

role of physical activity in adult obesity, as a population level characteristic and at the level of the individual, will be reviewed here. Although it is recognized that the prevalence of obesity in U.S. children and adolescents is increasing, the complex issues underlying the relationship of physical activity and body composition changes in children and prepubertal and postpubertal adolescents are beyond the scope of this review; therefore, the reader is referred to a recent review by Epstein and Goldfield on physical activity and childhood obesity [9]. Note that *obesity* refers to excess body fatness, which is not always present with a high BMI, such as in bodybuilders; however, the percent of the population that is lean at a high BMI is relatively small and has only a small impact on population data.

II. RELATIONSHIP OF PHYSICAL ACTIVITY TO THE PREVALENCE OF OBESITY IN POPULATIONS

Despite methodological issues that preclude accurate assessment of the relationship of physical activity to body weight and adiposity, an inverse association between physical activity or exercise and body weight has been reported in many cross-sectional epidemiologic studies [10]. In the 1996 U.S. Behavioral Risk Factor Surveillance System (BRFSS), the prevalence of inactivity was high in both normal weight (defined as BMI < 25 kg/m²) and overweight men (26.8% and 25.6%, respectively) and women (27.8% and 31.7%, respectively), but was considerably higher in obese men (32.7%) and women (40.9%), while participation in recommended physical activity was low in both normal weight and overweight men (29.3% and 29.2%, respectively) and women (30.7% and 26.0%, respectively), but was substantially lower among obese men (23.5%) and women (18.9%) [11].

The observation has often been made that the level of physical activity is a better predictor of weight gain than estimates of energy or fat intake [8]. A decrease in physical activity has been inferred in several studies that have reported secular decreases in energy intake concurrent with increases in weight and/or fatness; and in one study that had both energy intake and physical activity data, an analysis of secular trends in obesity were accompanied by changes in

transport to work, work-related activity, and/or changes in leisure-time activity [12]. Several large-scale observational studies have also justified a relationship between higher physical activity at baseline or improvements in physical activity and either attenuated weight gain or a lower odds of significant weight gain [13]. An inverse relationship between physical activity and weight change was reported in a 4- to 7-year (median 5.7-year) study involving more than 12,500 Finnish adults, aged 25–64 years [14] and across 4 years in about 10,000 U.S. male health professionals aged 45–64 years [15], as well as over a 2-year period in approximately 3500 men and women in Minnesota, of a mean age of 38 years [16], and in nearly 2000 Chinese women, aged 20–45 [17]. In addition, prospective data from the Aerobics Center Longitudinal Study (ACLS) [18] and the biracial CARDIA cohort [19] showed that improved cardiorespiratory fitness over 7.5 and 7 years, respectively, relates inversely to weight change.

The longitudinal evidence suggests that habitual physical activity plays a greater role in attenuating age-related weight gain, rather than in promoting weight loss [13]. Recent data from a cross-sectional analysis from the National Runner's Health Study suggest that substantial increases in activity level are necessary to maintain body weight with age [20], findings that have been corroborated by the Male Health Professional Follow-up [15] and ACLS [18] cohort data. Results from more than 9000 adults responding to the NHANES I Epidemiologic Follow-up Study (1971–1975 to 1982–1984) suggest that even relative to people who stay very active over time, sedentary people who increase activity can minimize the risk of major weight gain compared to people who decrease their activity, thus supporting the notion that increasing physical activity over time reduces the risk of becoming overweight [21].

III. PHYSICAL ACTIVITY AND DETERMINANTS AND ETIOLOGY OF OBESITY

It is generally accepted that the development of obesity in any given individual requires that energy intake exceed energy expenditure over a period of time. To prevent weight gain, one must balance energy intake and energy expenditure long term. To lose weight, one must expend more energy than is consumed. Energy expenditure is composed of the resting metabolic rate (RMR), a measurement of the energy expended to maintain normal body functions and homeostasis at rest, in the postabsorptive state; the thermic effect of food (TEF), which includes the energy costs of food absorption, metabolism, and storage of substrates; and physical activity, which includes the energy expended above RMR and TEF, for both voluntary exercise and involuntary activity such as shivering, fidgeting, and postural control. In general, RMR accounts for about 60–75% of daily energy expenditure, TEF for 5–10%, and physical activity for 15% in sed-

entary individuals and up to 30% or more in highly active individuals [22].

The amount of fat-free mass (FFM) in the body is the primary determinant of RMR, which is also influenced by age, gender, and genetics [22]. There is no indication that RMR has declined during the past few decades [23], so it is unlikely that RMR is a major factor in the increased prevalence of obesity in the population; however, small perturbations in RMR can substantially impact the regulation of body weight in a given individual. RMR decreases as adults age, about 2–3% per decade, primarily due to loss of FFM [22]; thereby, slowly shifting the energy balance in favor of fat weight gain if energy intake and physical activity are held constant. In older individuals, aerobic exercise does not appear to increase FFM; however, it may provide an adequate stimulus to maintain FFM with age [24]. In contrast, resistance exercise increased FFM (1.1–2.1 kg) in 15 out of 29 studies in older adults [24], while also reducing fat mass similar to changes induced by aerobic exercise (resistance exercise: -1.7 ± 0.4; aerobic exercise: -1.9 ± 0.8 kg).

A modest suppression of RMR is also generally seen in response to energy restriction (i.e., dieting), ranging between 5% and 25%, with an average maximum change of about 15% [25], largely due to a decrease in FFM, which often accompanies diet-induced weight loss. Several studies have reported that aerobic exercise and strength training may help preserve metabolically active, lean body mass during dieting, and prevent diet-induced reductions in RMR [6, 25, 26].

Controversy persists over whether the thermic effect of food ingestion increases if physical activity follows a meal and whether physical activity before a meal reduces appetite [6, 27]. The evidence suggests that physical activity programs do not necessarily produce a compensatory increase in food intake in obese individuals [6] and, overall, the literature points to a rather weak coupling between energy intake and physical activity-induced energy expenditure, suggesting that increasing energy expenditure through physical activity (or maintaining an active lifestyle) can cause weight loss or prevent weight gain [27].

Physical activity includes activities of daily living, work-related physical activity, and leisure-time physical activity. The first two have declined considerably during the past several decades and may be primary factors contributing to the increased prevalence of obesity [23]. In contrast, leisure-time physical activity has not decreased appreciably, but is very low, as the 1996 BRFSS data verify [11]. Adopting the exercise prescription presented in the OEI guidelines [3] would result in an energy expenditure of approximately 1000 kcal (4184 kJ) per week; however, the amount of physical activity that protects against obesity has not been established and it is unclear whether this prescription is adequate.

Fat weight loss and preservation of lean body mass should be the goals of a weight loss program. Fat weight loss may be slow, relative to weight loss strategies aimed at total weight, in which loss of water and stored carbohydrate may occur quickly. Fat, the most abundant energy reserve, is a

very efficient fuel source. It has been estimated that 1 kg of body fat supplies enough energy to support about 100 km of walking or jogging, or comparable activities. Nonetheless, as little as a 2.5-km walk or jog (a 20- to 30-minute effort) five times a week, which conforms to the exercise prescription recommended in the OEI guidelines, would bring about a loss of 6.5 kg of fat over the course of a year, assuming one does not consume excess energy or expend less energy in the remaining 23.5 hours of the day. If fat loss were to be achieved solely through the direct energy cost associated with increased physical exercise, a person must be committed to expending the energy over a reasonable period of time, with respect to his or her weight loss goal.

Considerable research has been conducted during the past several decades on adaptations of muscle and fat tissue to exercise training; body composition changes associated with exercise-induced weight loss; differences between lipolytic responses of subcutaneous and intra-abdominal (visceral) fat in response to norepinephrine, which may influence differential mobilization of fat stores during exercise; and interactions between exercise and diet (both energy intake and relative contributions from fat, carbohydrate, and protein) during weight loss [26]. A clear physiological rationale supports the notion that exercise could bring about loss of excess body fat and/or serve to maintain weight loss and/or prevent accumulation of excess adipose tissue over time. Metabolic rate during exercise can increase up to 20 times above resting levels; therefore, it seems obvious that if a person were to engage in exercise regularly without increasing energy intake appreciably, weight loss should occur.

It is well known, of course, that within any given environment, there is considerable variation in body fatness among people who are in energy balance, due to genetic factors, which have been estimated to contribute anywhere from 25% to 70% of the variability in adiposity [28–31]; however, because the U.S. genotype has not changed substantially enough during the past few decades to explain the increased prevalence of obesity, it seems that a focus on increasing physical activity remains appropriate. A recent study of nearly 1000 female twins showed that current physical activity was a stronger predictor of total-body and central adiposity of healthy middle-aged women than dietary intake or smoking; furthermore, participants with a predisposition to adiposity did not show a lesser effect of physical activity on body mass [32].

IV. ROLE OF PHYSICAL ACTIVITY IN TREATMENT (WEIGHT LOSS) OF OVERWEIGHT AND OBESITY: EVIDENCE FROM RANDOMIZED CONTROLLED TRIALS

Both the OEI Panel [3] and the consensus committee assembled for the ACSM Roundtable [7, 8] considered data arising from a substantial number of randomized controlled trials,

involving a substantial number of participants, as providing the highest quality evidence. After reviewing the literature, four sets of tables were developed for this review, each of which presents the basic study design (randomized intervention groups); the number of subjects (N) completing the trial versus, in parentheses, the number randomized; key subject recruitment criteria; length of training period; initial obesity status; and weight changes. Studies were included if they were of at least 3 months' duration, had at least 20 participants completing the trial, and enabled assessment of the role of the intervention on body weight.

The first two tables present randomized controlled trials of aerobic exercise versus control and trials of aerobic exercise plus diet versus diet only. Although an attempt was made to identify as many studies that met the basic criteria as possible, it is likely that many small studies that would meet these criteria were not identified; however, the reader should take others that they identify into account in relationship to those that appear here. In these tables, the studies are separated by BMI categories for normal weight, overweight, and obese, using initial mean BMI. Earlier trials often reported baseline weight, without height, and did not report BMI, thereby making it difficult to determine the initial obesity status of the participants, especially when data are not separated by gender. For the purpose of categorizing these studies, an average height of 178 cm was assumed for men and 166 cm for women. It is important to note that many studies reported significant weight changes within groups, that is, baseline versus post-treatment weights, without specifying whether there were significant differences between groups, thereby making poor use of the control group. Furthermore, in studies with more than two treatment groups, pairwise comparisons are often made without an initial analysis of variance for all randomized participants; therefore, the significance of differences between the aerobic exercise only group versus control is not always clear.

Details regarding the exercise prescriptions for the majority of the trials presented in these tables were provided in a recent review that appeared in the American Heart Association monograph on "Obesity: Impact on Cardiovascular Disease" [33]. For the most part, these prescriptions conform to the OEI guidelines [3]; however, adherence to the prescriptions is generally not reported, so it is not clear what percent of participants randomized to the aerobic exercise or resistance training programs were achieving the recommended levels of activity. Although it is assumed that most of the randomized controlled trials published "intention-to-treat" analyses on all who completed the trial, this is often not clarified.

A. Randomized Controlled Trials of Aerobic Exercise Only

Table 1 presents the randomized controlled trials that included an aerobic exercise only and a control group. Noting the caveats discussed above, regarding some uncertainties in

TABLE 1   Randomized Trials with Aerobic Exercise Only versus Control Groups

Study	Interventions: treatment groups	N post (randomized)[a] sex; basic (key) inclusion criteria	Training period duration	Initial BMI [or weight in kg]	Weight (kg) [or BMI] change	Differences between groups (weight changes)
A. Trials in normal weight individuals, i.e., mean BMI < 25.0 kg/m^2						
Huttunen (1979)[34]	1: Aerobic exericse 2: Control	90 (100) men; middle-aged	4 months	1: [78.4] 2: [79.9]	1: −0.9 2: −0.6	NS[b]
Wood (1983)[35]	1: Aerobic exercise 2: Control	78 (81) men; sedentary	9–12 months	1: [76.4] 2: [78.0]	1: −1.9 2: +0.6	$p = 0.002$
Duncan (1991)[43]	1: Aerobic walking (8.0 km/hr) 2: Brisk walking (6.4 km/hr) 3: Strolling (4.8 km/hr) 4: Control	59 (102) women, premenopausal; sedentary	24 weeks	1: [60.3] 2: [64.2] 3: [62.0] 4: [66.5]	1: +1.1 2: +0.1 3: +0.8 4: +3.7	2 vs 4, $p < 0.05$ No other differences
B. Trials in overweight individuals, i.e., mean BMI 25.0–29.9 kg/m^2						
King (1991)[38]	1: Aerobic exercise—higher intensity, group-based 2: Aerobic exercise—higher intensity, home-based 3: Aerobic exercise—lower intensity, home-based 4: Control	167 (197) men; sedentary 160 (131), women postmenopausal but not on hormone replacement therapy; sedentary	9–12 months	1: 27.4 2: 28.0 3: 27.1 4: 27.0 1: 26.3 2: 27.1 3: 25.7 4: 27.1	1: [−0.2] 2: [−0.2] 3: [−0.9] 4: [+0.1] 1: [+0.4] 2: [+0.1] 3: [−0.6] 4: [0.0]	No group differences in either sex
Hellenius (1993)[36]	1: Aerobic exercise 2: Low-fat diet 3: Aerobic exercise + low-fat diet 4: Control	157 (158) men; mildly elevated total cholesterol	6 months	1: 26.1 2: 25.3 3: 25.2 4: 24.5	1: [−0.3] 2: [−0.3] 3: [−0.6] 4: [+0.3]	1 & 2 vs. 4, $p < 0.01$ 3 vs. 4, $p < 0.001$
Anderssen (1995)[39]	1: Aerobic exercise 2: Energy-restricted (low-fat) diet 3: Aerobic exercise + energy-restricted diet 4: Control	209 (198+21) men + women, BMI = 24 kg/m^2, elevated diastolic blood pressure	1 year	All (mean) 28.8	1: [−0.3] 2: [−1.2] 3: [−1.8] 4: [+0.3]	1 vs. 4 NS 2 vs. 3 NS 2 & 3 vs. 4, $p < 0.05$
Pritchard (1997)[37]	1: Aerobic exercise (weight loss) 2: Energy-restricted, low-fat diet 3: Control (weight maintenance)	58 (66) men; overweight	12 months	1: 29.2 2: 29.0 3: 28.6	1: −2.6 2: −6.3 3: +0.9	1 & 2 vs. 3, $p < 0.05$ Pre vs. post: 1: $p < 0.05$ 2: $p < 0.001$
Stefanick (1998)[40]	1: Aerobic exercise 2: Low-fat diet 3: Aerobic exercise + low-fat diet 4: Control	190 (197) men, 177 (180) women, postmenopausal; low HDL cholesterol plus elevated LDL cholesterol	9–12 months	All: Men: 27.0 [84.2] Women: 26.3 [69.6]	1: −0.6 2: −2.8 3: −4.2 4: +0.5 1: −0.4 2: −2.7 3: −3.1 4: +0.8	1 vs. 4, NS 1 vs. 2, $p < 0.05$ 1 vs. 3, $p < 0.001$ 2 & 3 vs. 4, $p < 0.001$ 1 vs. 4 NS 1 vs. 2 $p < 0.05$ 1 vs. 3, $p < 0.01$ 2 & 3 vs. 4, $p < 0.001$
C. Trials in obese individuals, i.e., mean BMI ≥30.0 kg/m^2						
Ronnemaa (1986)[45]	1: Aerobic exercise 2: Control	25 (30) men (33%) + women with type 2 diabetes	4 months	1: [85.2] 2: [82.8]	1: −2.0 2: +0.5	Not reported Pre vs post: 1: $p < 0.05$
Wood (1988)[41]	1: Aerobic exercise (weight loss) 2: Energy-restricted diet (weight loss) 3: Control (weight maintenance)	131 (155) men; 120–160% ideal wt, sedentary	9–12 months	1: [94.1] 2: [93.0] 3: [95.4]	1: −4.0 2: −7.2 3: +0.6	1 & 2 vs. 3, $p < 0.001$ 1 vs. 2, $p < 0.01$

(continues)

TABLE 1 *(continued)*

Study	Interventions: treatment groups	N post (randomized)[a] sex; basic (key) inclusion criteria	Training period duration	Initial BMI [or weight in kg]	Weight (kg) [or BMI] change	Differences between groups (weight changes)
Raz (1994)[46]	1: Aerobic exercise 2: Control	26 men + 14 women; 50–70 yrs old, with type 2 diabetes	12 weeks	1: 31.8 2: 30.2	1: [−0.3] 2: [+0.4]	NS
Katzel (1995)[42]	1: Aerobic exercise with no weight change (low-fat diet) 2: Energy-restricted, low-fat diet 3: Control	111 (170) men; 120–160% ideal wt, sedentary	9 months	1: 30.4 2: 30.8 3: 29.5	1: −0.5 2: −9.5 3: +0.2	None reported Pre vs. post: 2: $p < 0.05$
Ready (1995)[44]	1: Aerobic exercise (walking) 2: Control	25 (40) women, postmenopausal; high total cholesterol, sedentary	6 months	1: 29.4 2: 32.1	1: −1.9 2: −0.6	$p < 0.05$

[a]N post = number of subjects completing the trial; in parentheses, number of randomized subjects.
[b]NS = not significant.

assuming significant differences between groups, one [34] of two [34, 35] trials of normal weight men, two [36, 37] of five [36-40] trials of overweight men, and one [41] of two [41, 42] trials of obese men reported significant, albeit modest, weight reduction with aerobic exercise versus control. It is worth noting that the study design of the second trial of obese men [42] required that exercisers not lose weight, as discussed below. The one trial that included aerobic exercise only in premenopausal women [43] was in normal weight women who were assigned to control or one of three exercise programs, only one of which was reported to reduce weight versus control. This trial is discussed below. Neither of the large trials of overweight, postmenopausal women [38, 40] reported weight loss by exercise only, despite significant increases in VO_{2max}; however, a small trial of borderline obese postmenopausal women reported a modest weight reduction in women assigned to walking versus control [44]. Two similarly sized studies that mixed obese men and women with type 2 diabetes found no effect of exercise on weight [45, 46].

The two trials of normal weight men [34, 35] differed primarily in their length. The Stanford Exercise Study [34] involved a 9- to 12-month intervention, compared to only 4 months for the Finnish study [35], but also, the Finnish men were assigned to individualized training programs, albeit under the supervision of an exercise physiologist at least once a month. The Stanford study provided supervised exercise sessions, with choices as to exercise volume and intensity, three times a week. Another difference was that the Stanford men were provided no dietary instruction, whereas the both exercisers and controls in the Finnish study were instructed to reduce dietary saturated fat intake, simple carbohydrate-rich foods, and alcohol, but not encouraged to lose weight; a small, but significant reduction in mean body weight occurred within each group, with no differences seen between

groups. In the Stanford study, secondary analyses [34], which separated exercisers into four "treatment-dose" groups (based on weekly jogging/walking distance: 0–6.2, 6.3–12.6, 12.7–20.6, and 20.8+ km), showed that distance correlated significantly with body fat changes ($r = -0.49$; $p = 0.002$).

In one of the trials of overweight men who lost weight with aerobic exercise versus control [36], the exercisers were advised to increase exercise gradually until they could do regular aerobic type exercise (e.g., walking, jogging) 2–3 times a week at an intensity of 60–80% of maximal heart rate and lasting 30–45 minutes. In the second, smaller trial of overweight men who lost weight with exercise versus control [37], exercisers selected their own aerobic exercise regimen, with a minimum participation set at three sessions of 30 minutes per week at 65–75% of maximum heart rate. Of the 21 exercisers, 11 walked, 4 jogged (2 alternated jogging with swimming), 3 attended a gymnasium (45 minutes of aerobic workout, 15 minutes resistance, anaerobic) and 3 rode an exercise bike. Dual-energy X-ray absorptiometry (DXA) scans revealed that more than 80% of weight loss by exercisers was fat; whereas 40% of weight lost in a third, diet only group, was lean tissue.

In one of the three trials of overweight men that reported no significant weight loss with exercise [38], participants were assigned to control or one of three different exercise programs: group-based, higher intensity (73–88% peak heart rate); home-based, higher intensity; home-based, lower intensity (60–73%). Those assigned to group-based, higher intensity were encouraged to attend an exercise program consisting primarily of walking and jogging 3 times a week during which they were expected to have at least 40 minutes of higher intensity exercise. Participants assigned to home-based exercise were expected to do either higher intensity exercise 3 times per week or lower intensity exercise 5 times

per week, depending on assignment, with the goal of achieving an equal volume of exercise in all groups. All three exercise conditions improved VO_{2max} ($p < 0.03$), by approximately a 5% increase, compared to controls.

The Oslo Diet and Exercise Study (ODES) investigated exercise and diet effects on blood pressure in normotensives and mild hypertensives [39], and BMI changes were reported by diastolic blood pressure tertiles (<84, $84–91$, >91 mm Hg) for each treatment group, rather than by treatment assignment, requiring some manipulation of the data to estimate an overall mean BMI change for each treatment group. Statistical comparisons were inferred from those reported for each treatment group within blood pressure tertiles. Participants were offered a supervised program of 1 hour 3 times per week, with a focus on endurance-type exercise at an intensity of 60–80% of peak heart rate, such as aerobics, circuit training, and fast walking/jogging.

The Diet and Exercise for Elevated Risk (DEER) trial [40] involved randomization to an aerobic exercise consisting of 45 minutes of walking, jogging, or comparable activity, at 60–80% of maximum heart rate, at least 3 times per week, which resulted in a significant increase in aerobic capacity of 2.7 mL/kg/min. Closer scrutiny of the energy intake data, determined through five unannounced 24-hour dietary recall telephone interviews, revealed increases in the exercise only men (on the order of about 100 kcal per day) compared to other groups, and although these were not significant, this would certainly counteract the 700–900 kcal/week energy expenditure achieved by most exercisers. Lean mass loss, assessed by hydrostatic weighing, was significantly greater in DEER men assigned to a low-fat diet, with or without the addition of exercise (1.3 kg for both), compared to exercise only men.

Specific exercise-related weight goals were integral to the study design in the two major trials of borderline obese men in Table 1. The exercise prescription for the first Stanford Weight Control Project, SWCP-I [41], consisted of approximately 45 minutes of supervised walking or jogging 3 times per week and was integrated into a goal of reducing body fat, rather than total weight, by one-third over the 9- to 12-month intervention period. Energy intake, assessed by 7-day food records, did not differ between exercisers and controls at either 7 months or 1 year. The greater initial adiposity of the exercisers in the SWCP-I trial may partially explain the greater weight loss seen in this group compared to the studies of overweight men; however, of greater interest is the fact that exercise-induced weight loss was successfully achieved. It is worth noting that the OEI Panel [3] unknowingly included two additional publications from this trial among its set of randomized controlled trials that reported successful weight loss by aerobic exercise only [33], thereby inappropriately strengthening the data in support of the role of aerobic exercise in producing weight loss. Meta-analyses reviewed by the panel may have made similar errors.

In the Katzel *et al.* [42] study, exercisers were instructed for 3 months prior to baseline tests on an isoenergetic reduced-fat diet, which they were encouraged to continue, without losing weight, throughout the trial. Their exercise consisted of 45 minutes of treadmill and cycle ergometer workouts, 3 times per week. Of those who completed the trial, exercisers increased VO_{2max} 17% above baseline ($p < 0.001$), but did not change average weight; however, percent body fat was decreased 0.8% ($p < 0.005$), compared to controls ($p < 0.001$).

An earlier metabolic study by Sopko *et al.* [47], designed to tease apart the relationships of diet- and exercise-induced weight loss on lipid changes, involved 40 initially sedentary men, aged 19–44, who were slightly overweight (110% of standard weight). Men were randomly assigned for 12 weeks to control, weight loss by energy restriction, weight loss by exercise, and exercise with weight maintenance. Meals were prepared in a metabolic kitchen for all groups and were fixed at 40% energy from fat. Energy intake was adjusted to maintain weight every 3 days, according to group assignment. Exercisers engaged in supervised treadmill walking with an energy expenditure of 700 kcal per session, 5 times a week, to total 3500 kcal per week, at a pace of 5.6–6.4 km/hr for most subjects. Significant weight was lost by men assigned to weight loss by exercise (-6.2 kg), but not to control (-0.5 kg) or exercise with weight maintenance (-0.5 kg). Together with the SWCP-I [41] and Katzel *et al.* [42] trials, these data highlight the role of energy intake in determining the effectiveness of exercise on weight loss in overweight and obese men.

The trial of exercise in normal weight premenopausal women [43] required assignment to control or three different exercise intensities: aerobic walking (8.0 km/hr), brisk walking (6.4 km/hr) or strolling (4.8 km/hr), with each group walking a distance of 2.4 km, 5 days per week initially, and increasing this to 4.8 km by the seventh week, which was maintained through the remainder of the 24-week trial. Weight loss was reported for women who were doing brisk walking versus control, but not by those doing an equal amount of exercise as aerobic walking (8.0 km/hr), which resulted in the greatest increase in VO_{2max}, or strolling (4.8 km/hr), and it is unclear that the ANOVA was significant across the four groups.

In the small trial of borderline obese women, those assigned to walking attended supervised sessions twice a week for the first 2 weeks and once a week thereafter. Average walking speed increased from 5.5 to 6.0 km/hr. The estimated weekly energy expenditure was 6367 kJ. The 6-month program resulted in an increase in VO_{2max} of 11% in walkers ($p < 0.01$ versus controls). Analysis of 3-day food records indicated that there were no significant changes in energy intake or diet composition throughout the program. Walkers lost a small but significant amount of fat mass (-1.7 kg) compared with controls ($p < 0.05$).

In summary, the randomized controlled trials reviewed here, which involved randomization of about 1000 men and 300 women to exercise only or control, generally show only modest (or no) weight loss with aerobic exercise pro-

grams that meet the recommended exercise prescription, even though these result in improved cardiorespiratory fitness. Due to an absence of trials, the evidence that exercise without dietary change will reduce body weight in overweight or obese women is extremely weak, particularly in premenopausal women. Men seem more likely to lose weight with exercise than postmenopausal women, but this is clearly dependent on attention to energy intake. It is important to point out, however, that these studies do not exceed 1 year, and as pointed out earlier, considerable time is necessary to achieve fat loss with exercise; furthermore, if lean mass is increased, total weight will not reflect the improved body composition achieved.

Of considerable interest is a review by Toth *et al.* [24] of aerobic exercise and resistance exercise in older adults, which included data from hydrostatic (underwater) weighing or DXA and revealed that aerobic exercise was effective in reducing body fat stores in 20 of 22 studies and that the changes in fat were related to the total number of exercise sessions. The initial obesity status of the participants in these trials was not included in the review; however, this report suggests that older adults may benefit more from aerobic exercise than those studied in the trials reviewed here.

B. Trials of Aerobic Exercise Plus Diet versus Diet Only for Weight Loss

The Expert Panel stated that a combination of a reduced-energy diet and increased physical activity produces greater weight loss than diet alone or exercise alone, based on results from 12 studies [36, 39, 40, 48–56] which are listed in Table 2, with seven additional trials that seem to meet the criteria of the Expert Panel [57–63]. These studies include fairly equal numbers of overweight men and women, but nearly twice as many obese women as men, including women who are considerably more obese than those who are included in studies listed in Table 1. None of the five trials of overweight individuals, which included more than 100 premenopausal women, 300 postmenopausal women, and about 550 men, reported greater weight loss in men or women assigned to aerobic exercise plus diet versus to diet only [36, 39, 40, 48, 49]; however, both treatments resulted in significant weight loss compared to controls in all five trials. Only one [48] of the nine trials [48, 50–52, 57–62] of obese class 1 (BMI = 30.0–34.9 kg/m^2) individuals, which included more than 300 women, mostly premenopausal, and approximately 300 men, reported greater weight loss in the exercise plus diet group versus the diet only group. The one trial that showed greater weight loss with the addition of exercise to diet versus diet only, the second Stanford Weight Control Project (SWCP-II), found this outcome in men, but not in the women, whose BMI fell within the overweight group [48]. Only one [53] of five trials [53–56, 63] in obese class 2 (BMI = 35–39.9 kg/m^2) individuals, which also included more than 300 women but only about 25 men, reported

greater weight loss in the exercise plus diet group versus the diet only group, and this was a small study that mixed 9 men and 21 women and did not have a control (no weight loss treatment) group [53].

In summary, only 2 of 19 studies involving about 2000 overweight or obese women and men showed a significant benefit of the addition of aerobic exercise to a weight-reducing diet for weight loss. These data provide little support for the contention that the addition of exercise to an energy-restricted diet will result in significant additional weight loss in a majority of overweight or obese individuals; however, the majority of these studies included fewer than 20 participants per treatment assignment, whereas the SWCP-II trial [48] included more than twice that number.

One additional trial, not shown on the table, compared a dietary intervention with and without the addition of exercise in individuals with mean BMI < 25.0 kg/m^2 from a South Asian population. The Diet and Moderate Exercise Trial [64] randomly assigned 419 men and 44 women, who had one or more coronary heart disease (CHD) risk factors, to one of two groups for 24 weeks:

Group A: American Heart Association (AHA) Step I (reduced-fat) diet + fruits and vegetables + exercise, consisting of brisk walking, 3–4 km/day, or spot running, 10–15 min/day ($N = 231$)
Group B: AHA Step I diet only ($N = 232$).

At 24 weeks, after 20 weeks of exercise in addition to the dietary regimen, group A had lost 6.5 kg (9.8% reduction from baseline), while group B had lost only 0.3 kg ($p < 0.01$ versus A). Whether this difference should be attributed primarily to the exercise or to the addition of fruits and vegetables to the diet may be worthy of further investigation in overweight or obese individuals.

C. Role of Resistance Exercise in Weight Control

Considerably less information is available on the potential role of resistance exercise or strength training, which presumably favors retention of lean body mass, in managing weight control than has accumulated for aerobic exercise. The most recent ACSM recommendations for the quantity and quality of exercise to be achieved by adults includes a progressive resistance training component that provides a stimulus to all major muscle groups, with the plan to complete 10–15 repetitions of a set of 8–10 exercises, 2–3 days/week [65]. Although these guidelines do not address obesity management, researchers have begun to assess the possible role of such activity in bringing about weight loss. Two of the trials of obese class 1 women, Sweeny *et al.* [59] and Marks *et al.* [52], and three of the trials of obese class 2 women, Donnelly *et al.* [63], Andersen *et al.* [54], and Wadden *et al.* [56], that appear on Table 2, compare aerobic exercise with resistance exercise or strength training. None

TABLE 2 Randomized Trials with Aerobic Exercise Plus Diet versus Diet Only Groups

Study	Interventions: treatment groups	N post (randomized)[a] sex; basic (key) inclusion criteria	Training period duration	Initial BMI [or weight in kg]	Weight (kg) [or BMI] change	Differences between groups (weight changes)
A. Trials in overweight individuals, i.e., mean BMI 25.0–29.9 kg/m²						
Wood (1991)[48]	1: Aerobic exercise + energy-restricted low-fat diet 2: Energy-restricted, low-fat diet 3: Control	112 (132) women, premenopausal; BMI = 24–30, sedentary	1 year	Women: 27.9 [75.0]	1: −5.1 2: −4.1 3: +1.3	1 vs. 2, NS[b] 1 & 2 vs. 3 $p < 0.001$
Svendsen (1993)[49]	1: Aerobic + anaerobic exercise + energy-restricted (formula) diet 2: Energy-restricted (formula) diet 3: Control	118 (121) women, postmenopausal; BMI = 25 kg/m²	12 weeks	1: [78.1] 2: [78.1] 3: [76.6]	1: −10.3 2: −9.5 3: +0.5	1 vs. 2, NS 1 & 2 vs. 3, $p < 0.001$
Hellenius (1993)[36]	1: Aerobic exercise + low-fat diet 2: Low-fat diet 3: Aerobic exercise 4: Control	157 (158) men; mildly elevated total cholesterol	6 months	1: 25.2 2: 25.3 3: 26.1 4: 24.5	1: [−0.6] 2: [−0.3] 3: [−0.3] 4: [+0.3]	1 vs. 2, NS 1 vs. 3, NS 1 vs. 4, $p < 0.001$
Anderssen (1995)[39]	1: Aerobic exercise + energy-restricted diet 2: Energy-restricted, low-fat diet 3: Aerobic exercise 4: Control	209 (198 + 21) men + women, BMI = 24 kg/m²; elevated diastolic blood pressure	1 year	All (mean) 28.8	1: [−1.8] 2: [−1.2] 3: [−0.3] 4: [+0.3]	1 vs. 2, NS 1 & 2 vs. 4, $p < 0.05$ 3 vs. 4, NS
Stefanick (1998)[40]	1: Aerobic exercise + low-fat diet 2: Low-fat diet 3: Aerobic exercise 4: Control	190 (197) men, 177 (180) women, postmenopausal; with low HDL cholesterol plus elevated LDL cholesterol	9–12 months	All: Men: 27.0 [84.2]	1: −4.2 2: −2.8 3: −0.6 4: +0.5	1 vs. 2, NS 1 vs. 3, $p < 0.001$ 2 vs. 3, $p < 0.05$ 1 & 2 vs. 4, $p < 0.001$
				Women: 26.3 [69.6]	1: −3.1 2: −2.7 3: −0.4 4: +0.8	1 vs. 2, NS 1 vs. 3, $p < 0.01$ 2 vs. 3, $p < 0.05$ 1 & 2 vs. 4, $p < 0.001$
B. Trials in obese (Class I) individuals, i.e., mean BMI 30.0–34.9 kg/m²						
Hammer (1989)[50]	1: Aerobic exercise + energy-restricted diet 2: Energy-restricted diet 3: Aerobic exercise + control diet 4: Control-low-fat, *ad libitum* diet	26 (36) women, premenopausal	16 weeks	1: 32.2 2: 32.2 3: 30.6 4: 37.0	1: −12.9 2: −9.5 3: −6.7 4: −5.8	1 vs. 2, not reported 1, 2, & 3 vs. 4, $p < 0.05$
Hill (1989)[57]	1: Aerobic exercise + constant 1200 kcal/day diet 2: Constant 1200 kcal/day diet 3: Aerobic exercise + alternating (600, 900, 1200, 1500 kcal/day) diet 4: Alternating diet	32 (40) women; 130–160% ideal body wt	12 weeks	1: 30 2: 31 3: 31 4: 31	1 + 3: −8.6 2 + 4: −6.5 1 + 2: −7.9 3 + 4: −7.7	1 + 3 vs. 2 + 4, $p < 0.05$ 1 + 2 vs. 3 + 4, NS
Bertram (1990)[58]	Energy-restricted (5000 kJ) diet + 1: Aerobic exercise + stretch/strengthen 2: Diet lectures 3: Control	36 (45) women; obese	1 year	1: 34.6 2: 34.3 3: 34.8	1: −7.0 2: −9.3 3: −8.1	No differences Pre vs. post: $p < 0.01$ for all
Wood (1991)[48]	1: Aerobic exercise + energy-restricted, low-fat diet 2: Energy-restricted, low-fat diet 3: Control	119 (132) men; BMI = 28–34, sedentary	1 year	All: 30.7 [98.4]	1: −8.7 2: −5.1 3: +1.7	1 vs. 2, $p < 0.01$ 1 & 2 vs. 3, $p < 0.001$
Sweeney (1993)[59]	Energy-restricted diet—severe (40%) + moderate (70%) (combined) 1: Aerobic exercise (walking) 2: No exercise 3: Aerobic exercise + circuit weight training	30 (47) women, premenopausal; 135–185% ideal body wt	6 months	1: 34.9 2: 33.4 3: 37.1	1: −15 2: −13 3: −11 based on graph	No group differences

TABLE 2 (continued)

Study	Interventions: treatment groups	N post (randomized)[a] sex; basic (key) inclusion criteria	Training period duration	Initial BMI [or weight in kg]	Weight (kg) [or BMI] change	Differences between groups (weight changes)
Dengel (1994)[60]	1: Aerobic exercise + energy-restricted low-fat diet 2: Energy-restricted, low-fat diet 3: Control	66 (148) men; 120–160% wt, sedentary, > 45 yrs old	10 months	1: 30.3 2: 30.1 3: 29.5	1: −8.1 2: −9.3 3: +0.4	1 vs. 2, NS 1 & 2 vs. 3, $p < 0.05$
Blonk (1994)[51]	1: Aerobic exercise + behavior + diet 2: Energy-restricted diet	53 (20 + 40) men + women; BMI > 27, with type 2 diabetes	24 months	1: 31.3 2: 32.8	1: −3.5 2: −2.1	NS
Marks (1995)[52]	1: Aerobic exercise (cycling) + diet 2: Energy-restricted, low-fat diet 3: Resistance training + diet 4: Aerobic exercise + resistance training + diet 5: Control	80 women, premenopausal 120–150% ideal body wt	20 weeks	1: 28.7 2: 30.1 3: 30.4 4: 31.3 5: 29.4	1: −4.5 2: −3.7 3: −3.5 4: −5.4 5: +1.5	1 or 3 vs. 2, NS 1, 2, 3, & 4 vs. 5, $p < 0.005$ No other group differences
Fox (1996)[61]	1: Aerobic + resistance exercise (200 kcal/day expenditure) + energy-restricted (−500 kcal/day) diet 2: Energy-restricted diet (−500 kcal/day) 3: Energy-restricted diet (−700 kcal/day)	40 (46) women, postmenopausal; 120–140% ideal wt, 60 yrs old	24 weeks	1: 30.6 2: 29.8 3: 30.4	1: −7.1 2: −6.6 3: −5.8	No group differences
Evans (1999)[62]	1: Aerobic exercise + energy-restricted diet 2: Energy-restricted diet 3: Control-low-fat, ad libitum diet	26 (36) women, premenopausal; BMI > 27, sedentary	16 weeks	1: 29.6 2: 31.9 3: 31.9	1: −3.9 2: −7.2 3: +1.2	1 vs. 2, NS 1 & 2 vs. 3, $p < 0.05$

C. Trials in obese (Class II) individuals, i.e., mean BMI 35.0–39.9 kg/m^2

Study	Interventions: treatment groups	N post (randomized)[a] sex; basic (key) inclusion criteria	Training period duration	Initial BMI [or weight in kg]	Weight (kg) [or BMI] change	Differences between groups (weight changes)
Wing (1988)[53]	1: Aerobic exercise + energy-restricted diet 2: Energy-restricted diet	9 men + 21 women; > 20% ideal wt, 30–65 yrs old, with type 2 diabetes	10 weeks + 1 year follow-up	1: 37.5 2: 37.9	1: −9.3 2: −5.6	1 vs. 2, $p < 0.01$
Donnelly (1991)[63]	Energy-restricted (liquid) diet 1: Aerobic (endurance) exercise 2: No exercise 3: Weight training 4: Endurance exercise + weight training	69 women [women could self-select group]	90 days	1: 37.5 2: 38.2 3: 38.2 4: 38.3	1: −21.4 2: −20.4 3: −20.9 4: −22.9	No group differences
Andersen (1995)[54]	Energy-restricted (liquid) diet + 1: Aerobic exercise 2: Strength training 3: Aerobic exercise + strength training 4: No exercise	53 (66) women; obese	48 weeks	All (mean) 36.2	1: −13.4 2: −17.9 3: −15.3 4: −12.9	No group differences
Gordon (1997)[55]	1: Aerobic exercise + low-fat diet 2: Low-fat diet 3: Aerobic exercise	48 (17 + 38) men + women; 21–65 yrs old, with systolic blood pressure = 130–179 and/or diastolic blood pressure = 85–109	12 weeks	1: [92.7] 2: [100.5] 3: [101.9]	1: −7.1 2: −5.8 3: −1.0	1 vs. 2, NS 1 & 2 vs. 3, $p < 0.001$
Wadden (1997)[56]	Very low energy diet + 1: Aerobic exercise 2: Strength training 3: Aerobic exercise + strength training 4: No exercise	120 (128) women; obese	48 weeks	1: 37.3 2: 36.5 3: 35.3 4: 36.4	1: −13.7 2: −17.2 3: −15.2 4: −14.4	No group differences

[a]N post = number of subjects completing the trial; in parentheses, number of randomized subjects.
[b]NS = not significant.

of these show a difference in weight loss between these forms of exercise when combined with the diets; however, the greater interest would be in the maintenance of lean body mass. In a trial that included measurement of adipose tissue by magnetic resonance imaging[66], 24 women with BMI over 27 kg/m^2 and waist-to-hip ratio greater than 0.85 were randomly assigned to aerobic exercise or resistance exercise for 16 weeks, with both groups instructed on an energy-restricted diet. The aerobic exercise group, which started at a mean BMI of 34.4 kg/m^2, lost 10.9 kg, while the resistance exercise group started at mean BMI of 31.8 kg/m^2 and lost 10.1 kg. These differences were not significant among groups, and both groups reduced their volume ratio of visceral to subcutaneous fat, with no differences between groups [66].

In a 12-week strength training study of 22 obese women (mean BMI of 31.4 kg/m^2 for the resistance exercise group and 32.8 kg/m^2 for the controls), total weight was increased 1.4 kg in resistance exercise and 0.4 kg in controls, but there were no significant differences between groups [67]. The fact that weight was increased, rather than decreased, emphasizes the need to separate possible lean body mass gain and fat weight loss in such studies. As reported above, resistance exercise increased fat-free mass in 15 out of 28 studies of older adults, and also reduced fat mass and total mass in a majority of these studies [24], suggesting that resistance training may have a role to play in weight control.

D. Role of Physical Activity in the Maintenance of Weight Loss

It is generally believed that exercise is important for preventing weight regain; however, there are few randomized controlled trials that include long-term follow-up. A meta-analysis [68] noted that 1-year follow-up patients in the diet only group maintained a weight loss of 6.6 kg, whereas those in the diet plus exercise group maintained a weight loss of 8.6 kg; however, neither the overall weight loss nor the percent of weight loss retained differed significantly between conditions. Table 3 presents several long-term follow-up studies from randomized controlled trials of exercise plus diet versus diet only.

Wing *et al.* [53] published two small trials and their follow-up studies in one report. The 2-year weight change data for the study with aerobic exercise plus diet (−7.9 kg) versus diet only (−3.8 kg) were similar to the data for the study of aerobic exercise plus diet (−7.8 kg) versus a low-intensity, flexibility ("placebo") exercise plus diet group (−4.0 kg); however, the differences among groups reached significance in the first study, but not the second.

Pavlou *et al.* [69] conducted a complicated study involving randomization of 160 men to four different diets and to exercise or no exercise (eight groups). To present the weight loss phase data by exercise status, tabulated data for the four diet groups were combined by exercise treatment arm to determine the mean initial weight and first-year weight loss; however, the follow-up data were provided only as a graph for all eight groups, requiring some gross estimation of weight change. However, it was fairly clear that the four groups assigned to exercise maintained weight loss quite successfully compared to the non-exercising groups.

Svendsen *et al.* [70] published a 6-month follow-up to the 12-week study, shown on Table 2. Both the exercise plus diet and diet only women gained about 2 kg during this period, and although weight loss was still significant versus control, it remained not significant between the combined and diet only women.

Skender *et al.* [71] published a one-year follow-up to a trial in which obese men and women had been randomly assigned to a Help Your Heart Eating Plan (HYHEP) or to aerobic exercise, primarily walking, for 3–5 45-minute periods per week, at an intensity that subjectively was perceived as "vigorous" but not "strenuous," without changing diet; or to exercise plus the eating plan. At 1 year, the exercise only group (−2.9 kg) had lost less weight than the diet only (−6.8 kg) or exercise plus diet group (−8.9 kg), ANOVA $p < 0.09$; however, both the diet only and exercise plus diet groups regained weight during the second year, while the exercise only group maintained its weight loss. Weight change from baseline to year 2 for 86 (of an original 127) women who returned was diet only (+0.9), exercise only (−2.7 kg), and diet plus exercise (−2.2 kg).

Wadden *et al.* [72] reported 1-year follow-up data for the study shown on Table 2. All groups, regardless of assignment to aerobic exercise, strength training, a combination, or no exercise gained back a substantial portion of the weight they had lost in the initial year and there were no differences among groups.

These few studies provide only minimal support for the notion that the addition of exercise to diet is effective for maintenance of weight loss over time; however, the data are clearly very limited. The Skender *et al.* study [71] is particularly intriguing because it suggests that exercise only may be a better approach for long-term benefits, despite the modest weight loss that is observed initially. Long-term follow-up studies are needed to evaluate the real value of any given weight loss strategy, particularly aerobic exercise, before drawing any conclusions.

Although the randomized controlled trial data do not provide strong evidence, there is considerable anecdotal support for the belief that exercise is important in weight maintenance after losses of substantial weight. In a study involving interviews of 44 obese women who regained weight after successful weight reduction (relapsers), 30 formerly obese, average-weight women who maintained weight loss (maintainers), and 34 women who had always remained at the same average, nonobese weight ($n = 34$), 90% of maintainers and 82% of controls reported exercising regularly, compared to only 34% of relapsers [73]. The National Weight Control Registry, a large study of successful long-term maintainers of weight loss, includes 629 women and 155 men who lost an average of 30 kg and maintained a required

TABLE 3 Follow-up Studies of Trials with Aerobic Exercise Plus Diet versus Diet Only

Study	Interventions: treatment groups	N post (randomized)[a] sex; basic (key) inclusion criteria	Training period duration	Initial BMI [or weight in kg]	Weight (kg) change in Year 1	Weight (kg) change by Year 2
Wing (1988)[53]	Energy-restricted diet + 1: Aerobic exercise 2: Control	28 (30) men + women; >20% ideal wt, 30–65 yrs old, with type 2 diabetes	10 weeks + 1 year follow-up	1: 37.5 2: 37.9	1: −9.3 2: −5.6	1: −7.9 2: −3.8 1 vs. 2, $p < 0.01$
Wing (1988)[53]	Energy-restricted diet + 1: Aerobic exercise (walking) 2: Low intensity, flexibility exercise	19 (25) men + women; >20% ideal wt, 30–65 yrs old, with type 2 diabetes	10 weeks + 1-year follow-up	1: 38.1 2: 37.5	1: −8.5 2: −7.3	1: −7.8 2: −4.0 1 vs. 2, NS[a]
Pavlou (1989)[69]	8 groups: one of 4 diets (balanced energy deficit; protein-sparing modified fast; 420 kcal; 800 kcal) 1: Aerobic exercise 2: No exercise	160 men; averaged 122% ideal wt, 26–52 yrs old	8 weeks + 18 months follow-up	Mean by EX across 4 diets 1: [100.4] 2: [103.0]	1: −12 2: −10 NS	1: −10 2: −2 $p < 0.01$
Svendsen (1994)[70]	1: Aerobic + anaerobic exercise + energy-restricted (formula) diet 2: Energy-restricted (formula) diet 3: Control	110 (118) women, postmenopausal; BMI = 25 kg/m²	12 weeks	1: [78.1] 2: [78.1] 3: [76.6]	1: −10.3 2: −9.5 3: +0.5 1 vs. 2, NS	1: −8.5 2: −7.5 3: +0.5 1 vs. 2, NS
Skender (1996)[71]	1: Aerobic exercise + HYHEP diet 2: Diet (HYHEP) 3: Aerobic exercise	86 (127) men + women; 25–45 yrs old, 14 kg overweight, sedentary Year 2: 88 (61)	Year 1: weight loss intervention Year 2: follow-up	1: [100.1] 2: [98.5] 3: [93.7]	1: −8.9 2: −6.8 3: −2.9 ANOVA $p < 0.09$	1: −2.2 2: +0.9 3: −2.7
Wadden (1998)[72]	Energy-restricted diet + 1: Aerobic exercise 2: Strength-training 3: Aerobic exercise + strength training 4: No exercise	77 (99) women; obese	Year 1: weight loss intervention Year 2: follow-up	All: 36.5 [95.8]	1: −13.5 2: −17.3 3: −17.3 4: −15.3	1: −8.5 2: −10.1 3: −8.6 4: −6.9 No group differences

[a]N post = number of subjects completing the trial; in parentheses, number of randomized subjects.

[b]NS = not significant.

minimum weight loss of 13.6 kg for 5 years [74]. These men and women report using both diet and exercise to maintain weight loss, and report a very high activity level of approximately 11,830 kJ being expended through physical activity per week. This exceeds the ACSM recommendation of 2000 kcal/week (8368 kJ/week) energy expenditure as optimal physical activity, a goal that was achieved by 52% of the registry sample (50% of women, 62% of men) [74].

E. Weight Loss in Trials Designed to Study Adherence to Different Exercise Programs

Table 4 presents a set of behaviorally based exercise studies, in order of increasing obesity level of the participants, which were designed to determine better adherence strategies, in-

cluding determination of optimal exercise dose and volume (i.e., frequency, duration, intensity) and whether breaking up daily exercise into multiple short bouts, rather than employing single long bouts, will improve adherence and thus outcomes. It is unclear whether the Duncan et al. study [43] demonstrated that a brisk walking pace is more likely to bring about weight loss than strolling or going at a race-walking speed, due to possible errors in the analytic approach, but this is an intriguing question. The King et al. [38] study, which focused on adherence issues surrounding group- versus home-based exercise as well as optimal intensity of exercise, did not identify a better approach to weight loss during the initial year; however, although groups did not differ in weight changes during a second year, the higher intensity, group-based men and women increased BMI

TABLE 4 Randomized Trials of Different Exercise Programs

Study	Interventions: treatment groups	N post (randomized)[a] sex; basic (key) inclusion criteria	Training period duration	Initial BMI [or weight in kg]	Weight (kg) [or BMI] change	Differences between groups (weight changes)
Duncan (1991)[43]	1: Aerobic walking (8.0 km/hr) 2: Brisk walking (6.4 km/hr) 3: Strolling (4.8 km/hr) 4: Control	59 (102) women, premenopausal; sedentary	24 weeks	1: [60.3] 2: [64.2] 3: [62.0] 4: [66.5]	1: +1.1 2: +0.1 3: +0.8 4: +3.7	2 vs. 4, $p < 0.05$ No other differences
King (1991)[38]	1: Aerobic exercise—higher intensity, group-based 2: Aerobic exercise—higher intensity, home-based 3: Aerobic exercise—lower intensity, home-based 4: Control	167 (197) men; 131 (160) women, postmenopausal; not on HRT; sedentary	9–12 months	1: 27.4 2: 28.0 3: 27.1 4: 27.0 1: 26.3 2: 27.1 3: 25.7 4: 27.1	1: [−0.2] 2: [−0.2] 3: [−0.9] 4: [+0.1] 1: [+0.4] 2: [+0.1] 3: [−0.6] 4: [0.0]	No group differences in either sex
Dunn (1999)[76]	1: Structured aerobic exercise (3–5 group sessions/week) 2: Lifestyle physical activity (accumulate 30 min moderate-intensity exercise most days)	190 (235) men + women (50%); 35–60 yrs old, sedentary	24 months	1: 28.0 2: 28.4	1: +0.7 2: −0.1	NS[b]
Andersen (1999)[77]	Behavioral (+ diet) weight loss + 1: Structured aerobic exercise 2: Lifestyle physical activity	38 (40) women; 15 kg ideal wt	16 weeks	1: 31.4 2: 32.4	1: −8.3 2: −7.9	NS
Jakicic (1999)[79]	Energy-restricted, low-fat diet + 1: Long-bout aerobic exercise 2: Short-bout aerobic exercise 3: Short-bout aerobic exercise + exercise equipment	115 (148) women; 25–45 yrs old, 120–175% ideal wt, sedentary	(6, 12) 18 months	1: 32.9 2: 33.2 3: 32.1	1: −5.3 2: −3.4 3: −7.0	1 vs. 2, NS 1 vs. 3, NS 2 vs. 3, $p < 0.01$
Jakicic (1995)[78]	Energy-restricted, low-fat diet + 1: Long-bout aerobic exercise 2: Short-bout aerobic exercise	52 (56), women; 120–175% ideal wt, sedentary	20 weeks	1: 33.8 2: 34.1	1: −6.5 2: −8.9	NS
Perri (1997)[80]	Behavioral (diet) weight loss + 1: Group-based exercise 2: Home-based exercise	41 (49) women; BMI = 27–45, 40–60 yrs old	15 months	1: 34.0 2: 33.1	1: −7.0 2: −11.7	$p < 0.05$
Wing (1988)[53]	1: Aerobic exercise (moderate intensity, walking) + energy-restricted diet 2: Low-intensity, flexibility exercise + energy-restricted diet	21 women + 4 men; > 20% ideal wt, 30–65 yrs old, with type 2 diabetes	10 weeks	1: 38.1 2: 37.5	1: −8.5 2: −7.3	1 vs. 2, NS Pre vs. post: 1 & 2, $p < 0.001$

[a]N post = number of subjects completing the trial; in parentheses, number of randomized subjects.

[b]NS = not significant.

slightly (0.1 and 0.2 kg/m² respectively) from baseline to 24 months, whereas, the higher intensity, home-based men and women decreased BMI slightly (−0.1 kg/m² each), as did the lower intensity, home-based men and women (−0.2 and −0.4 kg/m², respectively), which is generally not what happens to older adults over a 2-year period [75].

The effect of accumulating activity over the course of the day through "lifestyle activity" versus structured aerobic

exercise has received interest from exercise researchers in recent years. Dunn et al. [76] demonstrated that a lifestyle physical activity intervention was as effective as a structured exercise program in improving physical activity, cardiorespiratory fitness, and blood pressure in a moderately overweight cohort of men and women; however, neither group changed their weight, which is not surprising considering the modest effect on weight loss associated with structured aer-

obic exercise. Andersen *et al.* [77] combined these exercise options with a low-fat energy-restricted diet in a 16-week randomized trial of obese women. Weight loss was similar between groups, with no difference between them; however, the aerobic group lost less fat-free mass. During a 1-year follow-up, the aerobic group regained 1.6 kg, while the lifestyle group regained 0.08 kg, suggesting that lifestyle intervention may be better for weight maintenance.

Jakicic *et al.* [78, 79] have published two studies of effects of doing exercise in multiple short bouts. In the first [78], obese women, aged 25–50 years, were randomly assigned to a behavioral weight loss program consisting of an energy-restricted diet combined with 5 days per week of either single aerobic exercise bouts per day, starting as 20-minute bouts (weeks 1–4), increasing to 30-minute bouts (weeks 5–8) and to 40-minute bouts (weeks 9–20); or multiple 10-minute bouts per day, starting as 2 bouts per day, increasing to 3, then 4, respectively [23]. Both groups reduced energy intake and percent energy from fat significantly. Women performing multiple short bouts lost 8.9 kg in the 20-week period, while those exercising in single long bouts lost 6.4 kg (n.s., not significant) Because the dietary changes (energy restriction) probably contributed the most to weight loss, it was not possible to determine the independent contribution of the exercise components; however, exercising in multiple short bouts was shown to improve adherence to exercise and to result in significantly greater improvement in aerobic capacity, as well as a trend for greater weight loss. In the second trial [79], obese women were assigned to one of three treatment groups, all of which included an energy-restricted diet: long-bout exercise, multiple short-bout exercise, or multiple short-bout exercise with home exercise equipment using a treadmill. Total and fat weight loss was significantly greater in the short-bout exercise with home exercise equipment group compared to multiple short-bout exercise, but did not differ between long-bout exercise and either multiple short-bout exercise or short-bout exercise with home exercise equipment.

Another study that compared a 15-month group-based exercise behavioral weight loss program to a home-based program, involving moderate intensity walking (30 min/day, 5 days/week) revealed that obese women in the home-based program lost significantly more weight than those in the group program, presumably due to greater adherence to exercise [80].

V. ROLE OF PHYSICAL ACTIVITY IN PREVENTING AND TREATING OBESITY-RELATED COMORBIDITIES

The evidence for a relationship of overweight and obesity and central or upper body fat distribution with type 2 diabetes, hypertension, dyslipoproteinemias, in particular low high-density lipoprotein (HDL) cholesterol and elevated

plasma triglyceride concentrations, and CHD is reasonably strong [81]. In addition, obesity is related to gallbladder disease, respiratory disease, certain cancers (in particular, colorectal and prostate, endometrial, cervical, and breast), and osteoarthritis [81]. The role of physical activity in treating these obesity-related disorders is therefore of great interest.

A. Type 2 Diabetes Mellitus

The evidence is reasonably strong that physical activity has favorable effects on reducing insulin resistance in obesity and among patients with type 2 diabetes mellitus [82]. Improvement in glucose tolerance is less consistently observed and is related to exercise intensity, changes in adiposity, the interval between exercise and glucose tolerance testing, and severity of glucose intolerance before initiating an exercise training program [82].

B. Hypertension

Epidemiological studies show an inverse relationship between the incidence of high blood pressure and physical activity or fitness, which is either more pronounced in the overweight or independent of body size [83]. Based on a review of 68 study groups with normotensive and hypertensive subjects of both sexes, the weighted net reduction of blood pressure in response to dynamic physical training was determined to average 3.4/2.4 mm Hg ($p < 0.001$), unrelated to initial BMI [83]. Exercise seems to be less effective than diet in lowering blood pressure ($p < 0.02$) and adding exercise to diet yields no further benefit [83].

C. Dyslipoproteinemia

Evidence to support a role of physical activity in raising HDL cholesterol or lowering plasma triglyceride concentrations independent of weight loss is weak, particularly at the recommended levels of moderate intensity exercise [42]; however, if sufficient weight is lost by an energy-restricted diet or exercise without dietary change, without concomitant reductions in dietary fat, HDL cholesterol is likely to be increased and triglyceride levels decreased, particularly in overweight or obese men [35, 41, 42, 84]. The addition of exercise is also effective in preventing the diet-induced reduction in HDL cholesterol that accompanies a reduction in dietary fat, in both men and women [48, 84]. Finally, the addition of exercise to a low-fat, low-cholesterol diet enhances the low density lipoprotein lowering effect of the diet in men and postmenopasual women with unfavorable lipoprotein profiles [40, 84]

D. Coronary Heart Disease

The report of the surgeon general [6] provided strong evidence for a role of physical activity in reducing the risk of

CHD, which is an obesity-related comorbidity. A prospective study of walking compared to vigorous exercise revealed that even moderate levels of activity are associated with significant reduction in CHD risk for both nonobese and obese women; furthermore, women who were physically active were leaner and had a lower prevalence of hypertension, diabetes, and hypercholesterolemia [85].

E. Cancers

The evidence to support a role for physical activity in preventing colon cancer is reasonably convincing [86]. Though not as strong, there is also considerable evidence of a protective role of physical activity on hormone-dependent cancers, particularly endometrial, and gallstones [86]. Unfortunately, the data are not clear on whether physical activity in overweight and obese adults is associated with benefits compared to sedentary overweight adults.

F. Central Adiposity

There is insufficient evidence to support the belief that physical activity will bring about preferential reduction in visceral fat and central adiposity, due to a paucity of studies that have adequately assessed this issue. Exercise intervention trials have not shown a reduction in waist circumference in the absence of weight loss; however, a modest reduction (about 3 cm) has been reported in response to exercise-induced weight loss of approximately 3 kg [87]

VI. CONCLUSIONS

Epidemiological studies suggest that physical inactivity is related to obesity and that active adults are less likely to be obese or to gain weight as they age; however, it is unclear whether a sedentary lifestyle actually causes obesity or that physical activity prevents weight gain or promotes normal weight. There is ample biological rationale to support the contention that being more physically active and maintaining lean body mass, through resistance exercise and possibly aerobic exercise, will facilitate weight control. The value of exercise may be best seen in older adults, for whom preserving lean body mass may be as important as reducing body fat.

Unfortunately, the evidence from clinical trials to support a strong role for adopting a more active lifestyle to bring about weight loss in overweight or obese adults is weak, particularly in women. However, it should be recognized that changes in body composition derived solely from aerobic exercise, without dietary change, will occur slowly, because fat is a very efficient fuel. The addition of resistance exercise might increase lean body mass, which would result in even slower changes in total body weight. In general, neither aerobic exercise nor resistance exercise seem to be powerful enough to cause major weight loss, without the addition of restriction of energy intake, nor do the available studies provide strong evidence that exercise will bring about long-term maintenance of weight loss. Unfortunately, the studies to date have been small and have not provided enough information on adherence to the exercise protocols to enable one to assess the true value of aerobic or resistance exercise. Because diet-induced weight loss is not associated with long-term success, it is important to work toward improving adherence to exericise programs and to recognize that patience may be required to accept the slow weight loss achieved through exercise.

In the meantime, the evidence that exercise improves other disease risk factors associated with obesity continues to accumulate. It is becoming increasingly clear that engaging in exercise at the recommended 30 minutes per day dose may provide the overweight and obese individual many benefits, even if it facilitates only modest weight loss and/or maintenance.

References

1. World Health Organization (1998). "Obesity: Preventing and Managing the Global Epidemic." World Health Organization, Geneva.
2. Flegal, K. M., Carroll, M. D., Kuczmarski, R. J., and Johnson, C. L. (1998). Overweight and obesity in the United States: Prevalence and trends, 1960–1994. *Int. J. Obes.* **22**, 39–47.
3. Expert Panel on the Identification, Evaluation, and Treatment of Overweight in Adults (1998). Clinical guidelines on the identification, evaluation, and treatment of overweight and obesity in adults—The evidence report. *Obes. Res.* **6**(Suppl. 2), 51S–209S.
4. Pate, R. R., Pratt, M., Blair, S. N., Haskell, W. L., Macera, C. A., Bouchard, C., Buchner, D., Ettinger, W., Heath, G. W., King, A. C., Kriska, A., Leon, A. S., Marcus, B. H., Morris, J., Paffenbarger, R. S., Jr., Patrick, K., Pollock, M. L., Rippe, J. M., Sallis, J., and Wilmore, J. H. (1995). Physical activity and public health: A recommendation from the Centers for Disease Control and Prevention and the American College of Sports Medicine. *JAMA* **273**, 402–407.
5. NIH Consensus Development Panel on Physical Activity and Cardiovascular Health (1996). Physical activity and cardiovascular health. *JAMA* **276**, 241–246.
6. U.S. Department of Health and Human Services (1996). "Physical Activity and Health: A Report of the Surgeon General." U.S. Department of Health and Human Services, Centers for Disease Control and Prevention, National Center for Chronic Disease Prevention and Health Promotion, Atlanta, GA.
7. Bouchard, C., and Blair, S. N. (1999). Introductory comments for the consensus on physical activity and obesity. *Med. Sci. Sports Exerc.* **31**, S498–S501.
8. Grundy, S. M., Blackburn, G., Higgins, M., Lauer, R., Perri, M. B., and Ryan, D. (1999). Physical activity in the prevention and treatment of obesity and its comorbities: Evidence report of independent panel to assess the role of physical activity in the treatment of obesity and its comorbidities. *Med. Sci. Sports Exerc.* **31**, 1493–1500.

9. Epstein, L. H., and Goldfield, G. S. (1999). Physical activity in the treatment of childhood overweight and obesity: Current evidence and research issues. *Med. Sci. Sports Exerc.* **31**, S553–S559.

10. DiPietro, L. (1995). Physical activity, body weight, and adiposity: An epidemiologic perspective. *Exerc. Sports Sci. Rev.* **23**, 275–303.

11. Pratt, M., Macera, D. A., and Blanton, C. (1999). Levels of physical activity and inactivity in children and adults in the United States: Current evidence and research issues. *Med. Sci. Sports Exerc.* **31**, S526–S533.

12. Jebb, S. A., and Moore, M. S. (1999). Contribution of a sedentary lifestyle and inactivity to the etiology of overweight and obesity: Current evidence and research issues. *Med. Sci. Sports Exerc.* **31**, S534–S541.

13. DiPietro, L. (1999). Physical activity in the prevention of obesity: Current evidence and research issues. *Med. Sci. Sports Exerc.* **31**, S542–S546.

14. Rissanen, A. M., Heliovaara, M., Knekt, P., Reunanen, A., and Aroma, A. (1991). Determinants of weight gain and overweight in adult Finns. *Eur. J. Clin. Nutr.* **45**, 419–430.

15. Coakley, E. H., Rimm, E. B., Colditz, G., Kawachi, I., and Willett, W. (1998). Predictors of weight change in men: Results from the Health Professionals Follow-Up Study. *Int. J. Obes.* **22**, 89–96.

16. French, S. A., Jeffery, R. W., Forster, J. L., McGovern, P. G., Kelder, S. H., and Baxter, J. E. (1994). Predictors of weight change over two years among a population of working adults: The Healthy Worker Project. *Int. J. Obes.* **18**, 145–154.

17. Paeratukul, S., Popkin, B. M., Keyou, G., Adair, L. S., and Stevens, J. (1998). Changes in diet and physical activity affect the body mass index of Chinese adults. *Int. J. Obes.* **22**, 424–431.

18. DiPietro, L., Kohl, H. W., III, Barlow, C. W., and Blair, S. N. (1998). Improvements in cardiorespiratory fitness attenuate age-related weight gain in healthy men and women: The Aerobics Center Longitudinal Study. *Int. J. Obes.* **22**, 55–62.

19. Lewis, C. E., Smith, B. E., Wallace, O. D., Williams, O. D., Bild, D. E., and Jacobs, D. R. (1997). Seven year trends in body weight and associations of weight change with lifestyle and behavioral characteristics in black and white young adults: The CARDIA Study. *Am. J. Public Health* **87**, 635–642.

20. Williams, P. T. (1997). Evidence for the incompatibility of age-neutral overweight and age-neutral physical activity standards from runners. *Am. J. Clin. Nutr.* **65**, 1391–1396.

21. Williamson, D. R., Kahn, H. S., Remington, P. L., and Anda, R. F. (1990). The 10-year incidence of overweight and major weight gain in U.S. adults. *Arch. Intern. Med.* **150**, 665–672.

22. Poehlman, E. T., Melby, C., and Goran, M. I. (1991). The impact of exercise and diet restriction on daily energy expenditure. *Sports Med.* **11**, 78–101.

23. Hill, J. O., and Melanson, E. L. (1999). Overview of the determinants of overweight and obesity: Current evidence and research issues. *Med. Sci. Sports Exerc.* **31**, S515–S521.

24. Toth, M. J., Beckett, T., and Poehlman, E. T. (1999). Physical activity and the progressive change in body composition with aging: Current evidence and research issues. *Med. Sci. Sports Exerc.* **31**, S590–S596.

25. Prentice, A. M., Goldberg, F. R., Jebb, S. A., Black, A. E., Murgatroyd, P. R., and Diaz, E. O. (1991). Physiological responses to slimming. *Proc. Nutr. Soc.* **50**, 441–458.

26. Stefanick, M. L. (1993). Exercise and weight control. *Exerc. Sports Sci. Rev.* **21**, 363–396.

27. Blundell, J. E., and King, N. A. (1999). Physical activity and regulation of food intake: Current evidence. *Med. Sci. Sports Exerc.* **31**, S573–S583.

28. Stunkard, A. J., Foch, T. T., and Hrubec, Z. (1986). A twin study of human obesity. *JAMA* **256**, 51–54.

29. Stunkard, A. J., Sorenson, T. I., and Hanis, C. (1986). An adoption study of human obesity. (1986). *N. Engl. J. Med.* **314**, 193–198.

30. Bouchard, C., and Tremblay, A. (1990). Genetic effects in human energy expenditure components. *Int. J. Obes.* **14**, 49–55.

31. Cardon, L. R., Carmelli, R. D., Fabsitz, R. R., and Reed, T. (1994). Genetic and environmental correlations between obesity and body fat distribution in adult male twins. *Hum. Biol.* **66**, 465–479.

32. Samaras, K., Kelly, P. J., Chiano, M. N., Spector, T. D., and Campbell, L. V. (1999). Genetic and environmental influences on total-body and central abdominal fat: The effect of physcial activity in female twins. *Ann. Intern. Med.* **130**, 873–882.

33. Stefanick, M. L. (1999). Physical activity in the management of obesity: Issues and implementation. *In* Obesity: Impact on Cardiovascular Disease (G. F. Flecther, S. M. Grundy, and L. L. Hayman, Eds.), pp. 261–293. Futura Publishing Co., Inc., Armonk, NY.

34. Huttunen, J. H., Lansimies, E., Voutilainen, E., Ehnholm, C., Hietanen, E., Pentila, I., Siitonen, O., and Rauramaa, R. (1979). Effect of moderate physical exercise on serum lipoproteins: A controlled clinical trial with special reference to serum high-density lipoproteins. *Circulation* **60**, 1220–1229.

35. Wood, P. D., Haskell, W. L., Blair, S. N., Williams, P. T., Krauss, R. M., Lindgren, F. T., Albers, J. J., Ho, P. H., and Farquhar, J. W. (1983). Increased exercise level and plasma lipoprotein concentrations: A one-year, randomized, controlled study in sedentary, middle-aged men. *Metabolism* **32**, 31–39.

36. Hellenius, M. L., de Faire, U. H., Berglund, B. H., Hamsten, A., and Krakau, I. (1993). Diet and exercise are equally effective in reducing risk for cardiovascular disease. Results of a randomized controlled study in men with slightly to moderately raised cardiovascular risk factors. *Atherosclerosis* **103**, 81–91.

37. Pritchard, J. E., Nowson, C. A., and Wark, J. D. (1997). A worksite program for overweight middle-aged men achieves lesser weight loss with exercise than with dietary change. *J. Am. Diet. Assoc.* **97**, 37–42.

38. King, A. C., Haskell, W. L., Taylor, C. B., Kraemer, H. C., and DeBusk, R. F. (1991). Group- vs home-based exercise training in healthy older men and women: A community-based clinical trial. *JAMA* **266**, 1535–1542.

39. Anderssen. S., Holme, I., Urdal, P., and Hjermann, I. (1995). Diet and exercise intervention have favourable effects on blood pressure in mild hypertensives: The Oslo Diet and Exercise Study (ODES). *Blood Press* **4**, 343–349.

40. Stefanick, M. L., Mackey, S., Sheehan, M., Ellsworth, N., Haskell, W. L., and Wood, P. D. (1998). Effects of diet and exercise in men and postmenopausal women with low levels of HDL cholesterol and high levels of LDL cholesterol. *N. Engl. J. Med.* **339**, 12–20.

41. Wood, P. D., Stefanick, M. L., Dreon, D. M., Frey-Hewit, B., Garay, S. C., Williams, P. T., Superko, H. R., Fortmann, S. P., Albers, J. J., Vranizan, K. M., Ellsworth, N. M., Terry, R. B., and Haskell, W. L. (1988). Changes in plasma lipids and lipoproteins in overweight men during weight loss through dieting as compared with exercise. *N. Engl. J. Med.* **319**, 1173–1179.

42. Katzel, L. I., Bleecker, E. T., Colman, E. G., Rogus, E. M., Sorking J. D., and Goldberg, A. P. (1995). Effects of weight loss vs aerobic exercise training on risk factors for coronary disease in healthy, obese, middle-aged and older men: A randomized controlled trial. *JAMA* **274**, 1915–1921

43. Duncan, J. J., Gordon, N. F., and Scott, C. B. (1991). Women walking for health and fitness: How much is enough? *JAMA* **266**, 3295–3299.

44. Ready, A. E., Drinkwater, D. T., Ducas, J., Fitzpatrick, D. W., Brereton, D. G., and Oades, S. C. (1995). Walking program reduces elevated cholesterol in women postmenopause. *Can. J. Cardiol.* **11**, 905–912.

45. Ronnemaa, T., Mattila, K., Lehtonen, A., and Kallio, V. (1986). A controlled randomized study on the effect of long-term physical exercise on the metabolic control in type 2 diabetic patients. *Acta Med. Scand.* **220**, 219–224.

46. Raz, I., Hauser, E., and Bursztyn, M. (1994). Moderate exercise improves glucose metabolism in uncontrolled elderly patients with non-insulin-dependent diabetes mellitus. *Isr. J. Med. Sci.* **30**, 766–770.

47. Sopko, G., Leon, A. S., Jacobs, D. R., Foster, N., Moy, J., Kuba, K., Anderson, J. T., Casal, D., McNally, C., and Frantz, I. (1985). The effects of exercise and weight loss on plasma lipids in young obese men. *Metabolism* **34**, 227–236.

48. Wood, P. D., Stefanick, M. L., Williams, P. T., and Haskell, W. L. (1991). The effects on plasma lipoproteins of a prudent weight-reducing diet, with or without exercise, in overweight men and women. *N. Engl. J. Med.* **325**, 461–466.

49. Svendsen, O. L., Hassager, C., and Christiansen, C. (1993). Effect of an energy-restrictive diet with or without exercise on lean tissue, resting metabolic rate, cardiovascular risk factors, and bone in overweight postmenopausal women. *Am. J. Med.* **95**, 131–140.

50. Hammer, R. L., Barrier, C. A., Roundy, E. S., Bradford, J. M., and Fisher, A. G. (1989). Calorie-restricted low-fat diet and exercise in obese women. *Am. J. Clin. Nutr.* **49**, 77–85.

51. Blonk, M. C., Jacobs, M. A. J. M., Biesheuvel, E. H. E., Weeda-Mannak, W. L., and Heine, R. J. (1994). Influences on weight loss in type 2 diabetic patients: Little long-term benefit from group behaviour therapy and exercise training. *Diab. Med.* **11**, 449–457.

52. Marks, B. L., Ward, A., Morris, D. H., Castellani, J., and Rippe, J. M. (1995). Fat-free mass is maintained in women following a moderate diet and exercise program. *Med. Sci. Sports Exerc.* **27**, 1243–1251.

53. Wing, R. R., Epstein, L. H., Paternostro-Bayles, M., Nowalk, M. P., and Gooding, W. (1988). Exercise in a behavioural weight control programme for obese patients with Type 2 (non-insulin-dependent) diabetes. *Diabetologia* **31**, 902–909.

54. Andersen, R. E., Wadden, T. A., Bartlett, S. J., Vogt, R. A., and Weinstock, R. S. (1995). Relation of weight loss to changes in serum lipids and lipoproteins in obese women. *Am. J. Clin. Nutr.* **62**, 350–357.

55. Gordon, N. F., Scott, C. B., and Levine, B. D. (1997). Comparison of single versus multiple lifestyle interventions: Are the antihypertensive effects of exercise training and diet-induced weight loss additive? *Am. J. Cardiol.* **79**, 763–767.

56. Wadden, T. A., Vogt, R. A., Andersen, R. E., Bartlett, S. J., and Foster, G. D. (1997). Exercise in the treatment of obesity: Effects of four interventions on body composition, resting energy expenditure, appetite, and mood. *J. Consult. Clin. Pschyol.* **65**, 269–277.

57. Hill, J. O., Schlundt, D. G., Sbrocco, T., Sharp, T., Pope-Cordle, J., Stetson, B., Kaler, M., and Heim, C. (1989). Evaluation of an alternating-calorie diet with and without exercise in the treatment of obesity. *Am. J. Clin. Nutr.* **50**, 248–254.

58. Bertram, S. R., Venter, I., and Stewart, R. I. (1990). Weight loss in obese women—exercise v. dietary education. *S. Afr. Med. J.* **78**, 15–18.

59. Sweeney, M. E., Hill, J. O., Heller, P. A. Baney, R., and Di-Girolamo, M. (1993). Severe vs moderate energy restriction with and without exercise in the treatment of obesity: Efficiency of weight loss. *Am. J. Clin. Nutr.* **57**, 127–134.

60. Dengel, D. R., Hagberg, J. M., Coon, P. J., Drinkwater, D. T., and Goldberg, A. P. (1994). Effects of weight loss by diet alone or combined with aerobic exercise on body composition in older obese men. *Metabolism* **43**, 867–871.

61. Fox, A. A., Thompson, J. L., Butterfield, G. E., Gylfadottir, U., Moynihan, S., and Spiller, G. (1996). Effects of diet and exercise on common cardiovascular disease risk factors in moderately obese older women. *Am. J. Clin. Nutr.* **63**, 225–233.

62. Evans, E. M., Saunders, M. J., Spano, M. A., Arngrimsson, S. A., Lewis, R. D., and Cureton, K. J. (1999). Effects of diet and exercise on the density and composition of the fat-free mass in obese women. *Med. Sci. Sports Exerc.* **31**, 1778–1787.

63. Donnelly, J. E., Pronk, N. P., Jacobsen, D. J., Pronk, S. J., and Jakicic, J. M. (1991). Effects of a very-low-calorie diet and physical-training regimens on body composition and resting metabolic rate in obese females. *Am. J. Clin. Nutr.* **54**, 56–61.

64. Singh, R. B., Rastogi, S. S., Ghosh, S., Niaz, M. A., and Singh, N. K. (1993). The Diet and Moderate Exercise Trial (DAMET): Results after 24 weeks. *Acta Cardiol.* **48**, 543–557.

65. American College of Sports Medicine (1998). The recommended quantity and quality of exercise for developing and maintaining cardiorespiratory and muscular fitness, and flexibility in healthy adults. *Med. Sci. Sports Exerc.* **30**, 975–991.

66. Ross, R., and Rissanen, J. (1994). Mobilization of visceral and subcutaneous adipose tissue in response to energy restriction and exercise. *Am. J. Clin. Nutr.* **60**, 695–703.

67. Manning, J. M., Dooly-Manning, C. R., White, K., Kampa, I., Silas, S., Kesselhaut, M., and Ruoff, M. (1991). Effects of a resistive training program on lipoprotein-lipid levels in obese women. *Med. Sci. Sports Exerc.* **23**, 1222–1226.

68. Miller, W. C., Koceja, D. M., and Hamilton, E. J. (1997). A meta-analysis of the past 25 years of weight loss research using diet, exercise or diet plus exercise intervention. *Int. J. Obes.* **21**, 941–947.

69. Pavlou, K. N., Krey, S., and Steffee, W. P. (1989). Exercise as an adjunct to weight loss and maintenance in moderately obese subjects. *Am. J. Clin. Nutr.* **49**, 1115–1123.

70. Svendsen, O. L., Hassager, C., and Christiansen, C. (1994). Six months' follow-up on exercise added to a short-term diet in

overweight postmenopausal women—Effects on body composition, resting metabolic rate, cardiovascular risk factors and bone. *Int. J. Obes.* **18,** 692–698.

71. Skender, M. L., Goodrick, G. K., Del Junco, D. J., Reeves, R. S., Darnell, L., Gotto, A. M., and Foreyt, J. P. (1996). Comparison of 2-year weight loss trends in behavioral treatments of obesity, diet, exercise, and combination interventions. *J. Am. Diet. Assoc.* **96,** 342–346.

72. Wadden, T. A., Vogt, R. A., Foster, G. D., and Anderson, D. A. (1998). Exercise and the maintenance of weight loss: 1-year follow-up of a controlled clinical trial. *J. Consult. Clin. Pschyol.* **66,** 429–433.

73. Kayman, S., Bruvol, W., and Stern, J. S. (1990). Maintenance and relapse after weight loss in women: Behavioral aspects. *Am. J. Clin. Nutr.* **52,** 800–807.

74. Klem, M. L., Wing, R. R., McGuire, M. T., Seagle, H. M., and Hill, J. O. (1997). A descriptive study of individuals successful at long-term maintenance of substantial weight loss. *Am. J. Clin. Nutr.* **66,** 239–246.

75. King, A. C., Haskell, W. L., Young, D. R., Oka, R. K., and Stefanick, M. L. (1995). Long-term effects of varying intensities and formats of physical activity on participation rates, fitness, and lipoproteins in men and women aged 50–65 years. *Circulation* **91,** 2596–2604.

76. Dunn, A. L., Marcus, B. H., Kampert, J. B., Garcia, M. E., Kohl, H. W., III, and Blair, S. N. (1999). Comparison of lifestyle and structured interventions to increase physical activity and cardiorespiratory fitness: A randomized trial. *JAMA* **281,** 327–334.

77. Andersen, R. E., Wadden, T. A., Bartlett, S. J., Zemel, B., Verde, T. J., and Franckowiak, S. C. (1999). Effects of lifestyle activity vs structured aerobic exercise in obese women: A randomized trial. *JAMA* **281,** 335–340.

78. Jakicic, J. M., Wing, R. R., Butler, B. A., and Robertson, R. J. (1995). Prescribing exercise in multiple short bouts versus one continuous bout: Effects on adherence, cardiorespiratory fitness, and weight loss in overweight women. *Int. J. Obes.* **19,** 893–901.

79. Jakicic, J. M., Winters, C., Lang, W., and Wing, R. R. (1999). Effects of intermittent exercise and use of home exercise equipment on adherence, weight loss, and fitness in overweight women: A randomized trial. *JAMA* **282,** 1554–1560.

80. Perri, M. G., Marin, A. D., Leermakers, E. A., Sears, S. F., and Notelovitz, M. (1997). Effects of group- versus home-based exercise in the treatment of obesity. *J. Consult. Clin. Psychol.* **65,** 278–285.

81. Pi-Sunyer, F. X. (1999). Comorbities of overweight and obesity: Current evidence and research issues. *Med. Sci. Sports Exerc.* **31,** S602–S608.

82. Kelley, D. E., Goodpaster, B. H. (1999) Effects of physical activity on insulin action and glucose tolerance in obesity. *Med. Sci. Sports Exerc.* **31,** S619–S623.

83. Fagard, R. H. (1999). Physical activity in the prevention and treatment of hypertension in the obese. *Med. Sci. Sports Exerc.* **31,** S624–S630.

84. Stefanick, M. L. (1999). Physical activity for preventing and treating obesity-related dyslipoproteinemias. *Med. Sci. Sports Exerc.* **31,** S609–S618.

85. Manson, J. E., Hu, F. B., Rich-Edwards, J. W., Colditz, G. A., Stamper, M. J., Willett, W. C., Speizer, F. E., and Hennekens, C.H. (1999). A prospective study of walking as compared with vigorous exercise in the prevention of coronary heart disease in women. *N. Engl. J. Med.* **341,** 650–658.

86. Rissanen, A., and Fogelholm, M. (1999). Physical activity in the prevention and treatment of other morbid conditions and impairments associated with obesity: Current evidence and research issues. *Med. Sci. Sports Exerc.* **31,** S635–S645.

87. Ross, R., and Janssen, I. (1999). Is abdominal fat preferentially reduced in response to exercise-induced weight loss? *Med. Sci. Sports Exerc.* **31,** S568–S572.

CHAPTER 33

Macronutrient Intake and the Control of Body Weight

DAVID A. LEVITSKY
Cornell University, Ithaca, New York

I. INTRODUCTION

Scholars of the control of food intake and the regulation of body weight have given little attention to the role played by macronutrients until fairly recently. Most researchers in this field were convinced by the dictum issued by the famous physiologist, Adolph [1], who declared that "Within limits, rats eat for calories," a conclusion readily transferred to humans as well. Although Mayer [2] and Mellinkoff *et al.* [3] tried to argue particular roles for their pet nutrients (glucose and amino acids, respectively), the domination of the field by the set-point theories of body weight [4–17] shifted the focus of research from dietary variables to physiology in the search for those mechanisms that controlled body weight through the control of food intake.

Meanwhile, the public was being fed (sold) great dreams of easy weight reduction and magical cures by eating certain macronutrients and avoiding others. In 1972, Robert Atkins was one of the first of a series of diet gurus to pontificate the virtues of eating a high-protein, low-carbohydrate, high-fat diet as a means of losing weight and curing obesity. He was followed by a rash of other "non-nutritionist" experts who pushed their own versions of the single macronutrient theory (carbohydrate is the culprit) and made lots of money and converts of the public on the way to their bank.

Fortunately, in the last 20 years the medical/nutritional establishment has begun to listen to the public's questions and have generated a considerable amount of research on the role macronutrients play in the control of food intake and body weight. In some areas, there is almost complete agreement. In others, the answers are split almost down the middle. The purpose of this chapter is to review this literature and reveal what we do and do not know about the role played by macronutrients in determining energy intake and, ultimately, body weight.

II. FAT CHANCE

The macronutrient that has received the most attention in the scientific appetite and body weight literature is dietary fat.

The relationship between dietary fat and body weight has been examined almost at every level of analysis from molecular to epidemiological. The epidemiological literature on the relationship between fat intake and body weight was critically reviewed by Lissner and Heitmann [18]. Although the data are not entirely consistent, they concluded that the greater the amount of dietary fat humans consume, the greater their body weight. Although the preponderance of the data indicate a direct relationship between fat consumption and body weight, they probably *underestimated* the effect for two reasons. First, poor measures of food consumption lead to an underestimation of the magnitude of the effect, and most measures of food consumption in the home environment are quite poor. Even more serious, though, is the problem that the underestimation of fat intake and energy is directly related to body weight. The larger the person, the greater they underestimate their energy intake [19–24]. Expressing fat intake as a percent of energy ingested reduces this problem somewhat, but not entirely. Despite these limitations, the literature supports the conclusions reached by Lissner and Heitmann [18]. As depicted in Fig. 1, the preponderance of studies that have addressed this issue have found that a positive and significant relationship exists between dietary fat and body weight and/or fat composition. The greater the amount of fat consumed, the greater the amount of body fat.

III. ESTABLISHING CAUSAL LINKS

However, because the epidemiological data reported above are correlational, they do not prove that eating a diet rich in fat causes an increase in body weight. It is possible that having a body composed of a high percent of fat causes an increased preference for dietary fat. Establishing a causal link between dietary fat and body weight requires an experimental design where the amount of fat that people consume must be experimentally manipulated and its effects on food intake or body weight (fat) measured. Two kinds of studies

Number of studies demonstrating a positive relationship between dietary fat and BMI or fat composition

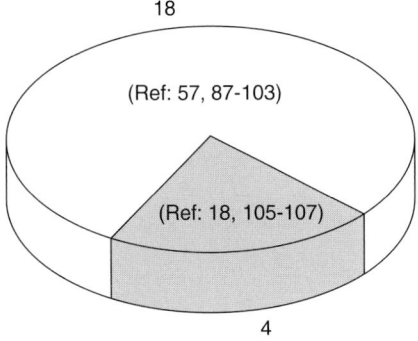

Number of studies failing to demonstrate a positive relationship between dietary fat and BMI or fat composition

FIGURE 1 Distribution of ecological studies relating body composition to dietary fat.

Number of studies demonstrating a positive relationship between dietary fat and food intake

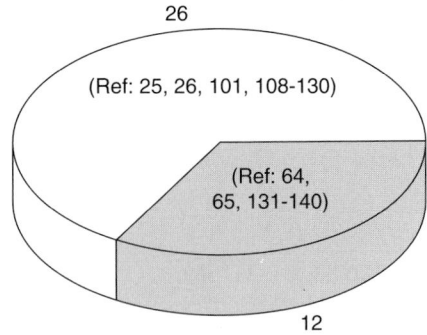

Number of studies failing to demonstrate a positive relationship between dietary fat and food intake

FIGURE 2 Distribution of experimental studies on the effects of dietary fat on food intake.

have been used to examine the causal links between macronutrient intake and body weight: laboratory studies and clinical studies.

A. Laboratory Studies

Unfortunately, studies of the effects of macronutrients in the laboratory rarely are of long enough duration to observe changes in body weight or fat composition. The dependent measure in most of these studies is the amount of food consumed. In many ways, this is a far more accurate measure of energy balance than body weight or even body composition measures, particularly if the design utilizes each subject as his or her own control. Any inaccuracy in estimating the energy or nutrient content of the food is nullified because each subject is tested under all conditions.

Figure 2 illustrates the results of studies on the effects of alterations of dietary fat on energy consumption. Although the weight of the evidence appears to support the epidemiological studies (people consume fewer calories when the diet contains less fat) important and interesting methodological differences exist that are cause for concern.

Most of the studies that failed to find that humans change the amount of food they consume (compensate) for changes in dietary fat had altered the fat content of all the foods that were accessible to the subjects. For most of these studies, all foods offered to the subjects were approximately of the same relative fat content. Therefore, when the fat content was reduced, the fat content of all foods was decreased. Consequently, the only way subjects could avoid reducing their daily energy intake when faced with a low-fat diet was to increase the amount of lower fat foods that they consumed.

Most of those studies that did find that subjects do compensate for alterations in dietary fat manipulated the fat content only of a single meal such as lunch or changed the fat

content of only particular foods in the diet. Poppitt and Swann [25] provided a direct comparison of the two methodologies within a single study. Their results are replotted in Fig. 3. Under conditions where the fat content of only the lunch was manipulated (left panel), subjects appear to energetically compensate by changing the amount of food they consumed. However, as the right panel indicates, when the fat content of all the food is altered, humans do not compensate for the reduced energy content and, therefore, energy intake is diminished.

This dependence of finding energetic compensation on specific methodology is quite important, but not understood. More importantly, if energy compensation for low-fat foods does exist when subjects have free access to foods of different fat composition, as suggested by these studies, then eating low-fat foods in the "real world" will never succeed as a strategy to chronically suppress in body weight, unless one ate only low-fat foods. The examination of clinical studies, however, indicates that people do lose weight when they use some low-fat foods, suggesting that the laboratory conditions or procedures may produce an artifact making it difficult to extrapolate the results to the "real world." It is also possible that if conditions are sufficiently well controlled in the laboratory, people will demonstrate physiological regulation, but that the external variables associated with eating behavior in humans are so powerful as to easily obscure its demonstration.

B. Clinical Studies

Clinical studies are more realistic than laboratory studies. However, it is usually quite difficult to obtain weighed food intake measures from subjects in a clinical study as a measure of energy intake. Therefore, such studies require subjects to prepare their own meals and record what they eat.

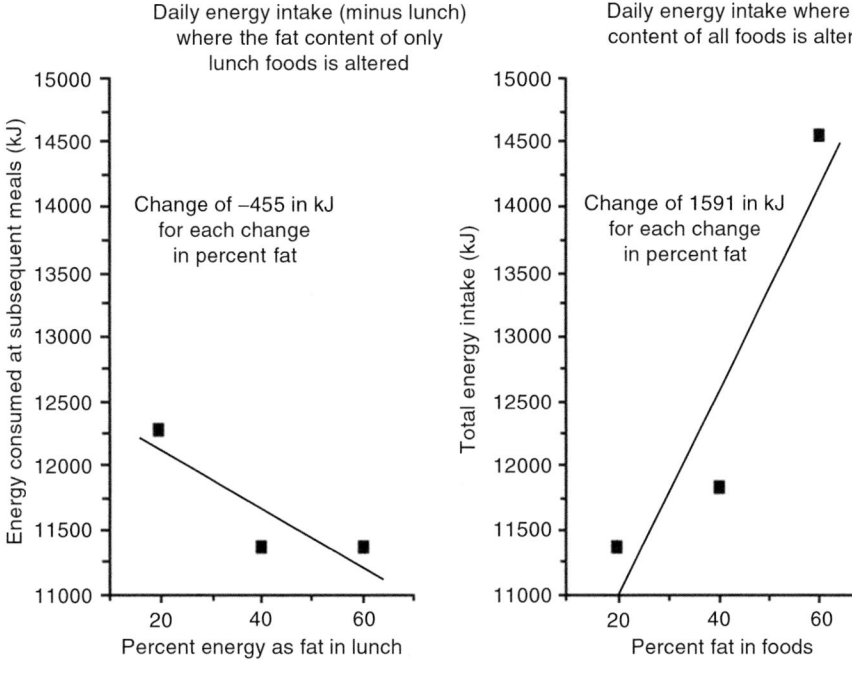

FIGURE 3   Energy intake as a function of level of dietary fat. (Left) Only the fat content of the lunch was varied. (Right) Fat content of all foods were varied. [Adapted from Poppitt, S. D., and Swann, D. L. (1998). Dietary manipulation and energy compensation. *Int. J. Obes. Relat. Metab. Disord.* **22,** 1024–1031.]

Such records, unfortunately, involve large measurement errors. As a consequence, clinical studies rely on physiological measures to corroborate their energy intake measures such as body weight or blood lipid concentrations.

Figure 4 shows the results of 21 published clinical studies in which the fat content of the diet was changed and body weights of subjects in the community were measured at the beginning and the end of the study. This figure clearly illustrates that changes in dietary fat in the "real world" are not totally compensated for by an accurate adjustment of energy intake. A reduction of 1% in the fat composition of the diet results in a average weight loss of 0.25 kg. It is important to note that the study by Kendall *et al.* [26] is the only study in which food intake was actually dispensed and measured throughout the study. In this study the amount of fat consumed was also measured. The amount of weight loss observed falls exactly on the regression line generated by the other studies, indicating that the change in fat intake and body weight of the other studies must have been fairly accurate.

These data confirm the majority of laboratory studies and the epidemiological studies that have indicated that humans do not accurately compensate for changes in the fat content of the diet and either gain or lose weight depending on the amount of fat in the diet.

IV. IS IT FAT OR ENERGY DENSITY?

The fact that high-fat diets cause an increase in energy intake and obesity in animals has been evident for a long time in the animal feeding literature (see West and York [27] for a thorough review). Whereas this effect was thought to occur because of some unique property relating to the chemical structure of fat, Ramirez and Friedman [28] performed a series of interesting studies demonstrating that the excessive energy intake was due to an increase in the energy density of the diet rather than because of the fat content per se.

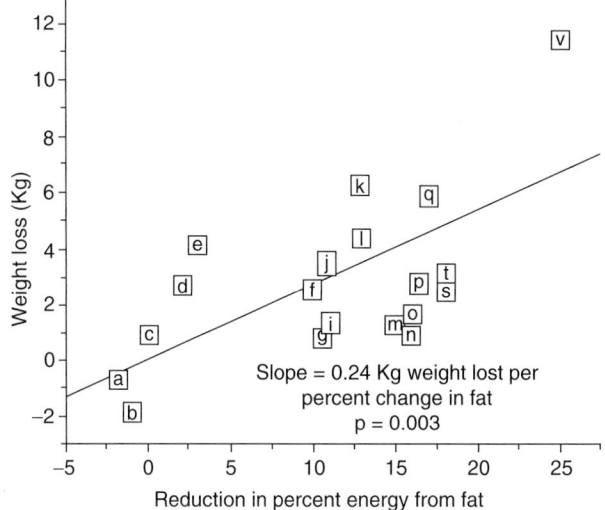

FIGURE 4   Maximum weight loss as a function of percent calories from fat. a. Marckmann* (190); b. Simon *et al.* (191); c. Bloomberg *et al.* (192); d. Stefanick *et al.* (193); e. Singh *et al.* (194); f. Kendall *et al.* (26); g. Lee-Han *et al.* (195); i. Raben *et al.* (196), Jeffrey *et al.* (197); j. Siggaard *et al.* (198); k. Pritchard *et al.* (199); l. Shah *et al.* (200); m. Hunninghake *et al.* (201); n. Boyd *et al.* (202); o. Insull *et al.* (203); p. Buzzard *et al.* (204); q. Toubro & Astrup (205); s. Kasim *et al.* (206), Schlundt *et al.* (207); t. Sheppard *et al.* (208); u. Ornish *et al.* (209). Data adapted from Hill *et al.* (210). *Data point derived from Marckmann (190).

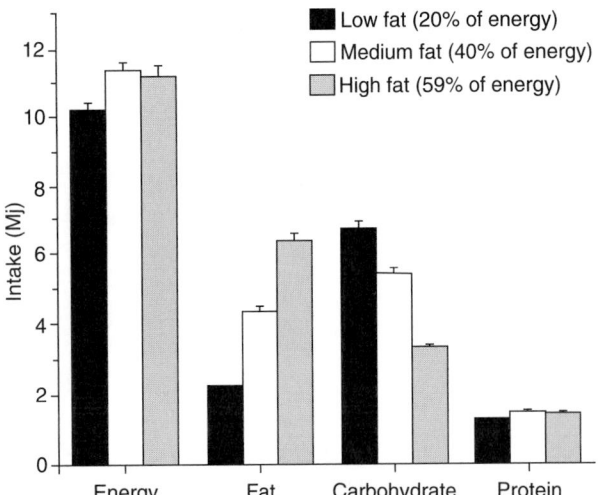

FIGURE 5 Intake of energy and macronutrients as a function of dietary fat when the energy density of the diet is held constant. [Adapted from Stubbs, R. J., Harbron, C. G., and Prentice, A. M. (1996). Covert manipulation of the dietary fat to carbohydrate ratio of isoenergetically dense diets. *Int. J. Obes. Relat. Metab. Disord.* **20,** 651–660.]

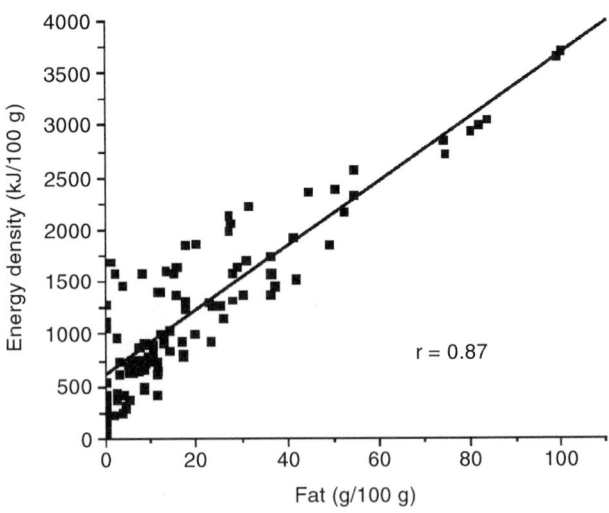

FIGURE 6 Relationship between energy density and fat concentration of 125 randomly selected foods. [Data from USDA (1996). "Continuing Survey of Food Intakes by Individuals (CSFII): Diet and Health Knowledge Survey, 1994. Department of Agriculture, Beltsville Human Nutrition Research Center/ARS.]

In one of the few human studies that failed to observe an increase in energy intake with increasing dietary fat, van Stratum *et al.* [29] examined the effects of introducing liquid diets that varied in the amount of fat and carbohydrate they contained, but were of equal energy density. They failed to find a difference in total energy intake between the two liquid diets either in the amount of liquid diet consumed or the amount of solid food eaten during the rest of the day. Stubbs *et al.* [30] reported similar results using a more elegant experimental design in which the amount of dietary fat was varied (20, 40, and 59%), but where the energy density of the three diets was maintained constant. A 3-day menu rotation was used for 14 days and was repeated three times; each time all the foods contained one of the three amounts of dietary fat. Subjects were free to eat as much or as little as they desired. The results of this extraordinary study are shown in Fig. 5 and are very consistent with the work of Ramirez and Friedman [28] in animals and with van Stratum *et al.* [29] in humans. Total energy intake did not differ between any condition despite the large differences between fat and carbohydrate. The study quite clearly demonstrates that the reason humans (and animals) overeat on a high-fat diet is because of the high energy density of fat and not because of any unique metabolic or physical property of high dietary fat.

This idea that energy density is the cause of overeating on a high-fat diet has been firmly confirmed by more recent studies [30–36]. These studies make it increasingly clear that humans not only fail to adjust the volume of food they consume to compensate for varying levels of fat in their food, but are equally as imprecise in adjusting the volume of

food they consume when the energy density of the diet is altered with carbohydrates, water, or fiber. Daily energy intake is a direct function of the energy density (calories per weight) of the diet [33–38].

Although this finding is of major theoretical and applied significance, in reality, the major determinant of energy density is the amount of fat in food. Figure 6 shows the relationship between the fat content and energy density for 125 randomly selected foods. The foods were consumed by subjects in the 1994 Continuing Survey of Food Intakes of Individuals conducted by the U. S. Department of Agriculture (USDA) [39]. A similar function was observed by Poppitt [37]. Thus, the easiest and most practical way to reduce energy density is to choose to eat foods low in fat content. Unless there is a reduction in energy expenditure, such a strategy must result in a chronic reduction in body weight.

V. ARE CARBOHYDRATES THE CULPRIT RESPONSIBLE FOR OVERWEIGHT?

Although Fig. 4 clearly indicates that energy density is determined primarily by dietary fat, there is a popular notion that carbohydrates are mainly responsible for overweight and obesity. Carbohydrates have been blamed as the culprit for obesity in such best selling books as "Dine Out and Lose Weight: The French Way to Culinary 'Savoir Vivre'" by Michel Montignac [40], "Sugar Busters! Cutting Sugar to Trim Fat" by H. Leighton Steward *et al.* [41], "Dr. Atkins' New Diet Revolution" by Robert C. Atkins [42] (actually an evolution from his previous book, "Dr. Atkins' Diet Revolution: The High Calorie Way to Stay Thin Forever" [43]),

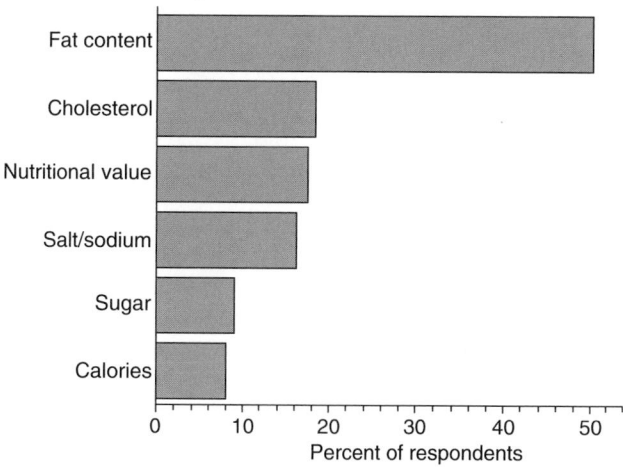

FIGURE 7 Nutritional concerns of supermarket consumers. [Adapted from Food Marketing Institute (1999). "Trends in the United States—Consumer Attitudes and the Supermarket." Food Marketing Institute, Washington, DC.

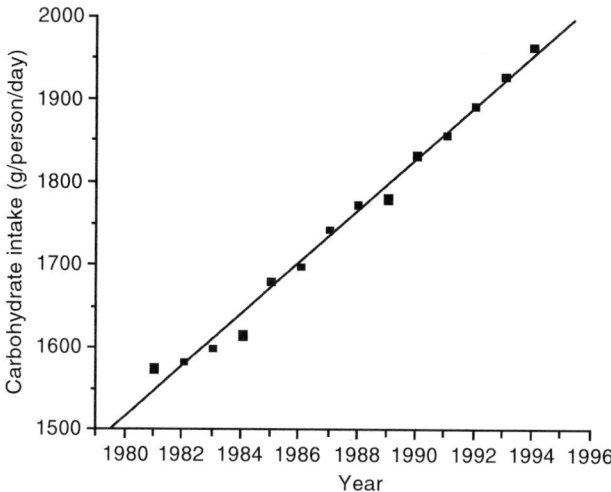

FIGURE 8 U.S. per-capita intake of carbohydrate, 1988–1995. [Data from USDA (1996). "Continuing Survey of Food Intakes by Individuals (CSFII): Diet and Health Knowledge Survey, 1994. Department of Agriculture, Beltsville Human Nutrition Research Center/ARS.] Beltsville, Maryland.

"The Zone" by Barry Sears and Bill Lawren [44]; "The Carbohydrate Addict's Diet: The Lifelong Solution to Yo-Yo Dieting" by Rachael and Richard Heller [45], and "Protein Power: The High-Protein/Low-Carbohydrate Way to Lose Weight, Feel Fit, and Boost Your Health—in Just Weeks" by Rachael and Michael Eades [46].

The basic premise behind all of these money-making books is that despite the fact that Americans are more concerned about fat than any other aspect of food, as is depicted in Fig. 7, and have been reducing their consumption of fat [47], Americans are still getting fatter [48]. Therefore, these nutrition gurus would argue that it is not dietary fat that is causing the overweight and obesity; it is the carbohydrate content that is the culprit.

There is little doubt that daily carbohydrate intake has been increasing during the past 20 years. The data displayed in Fig. 8 are taken from USDA disappearance data [39] and show this trend quite well. However what is the evidence that carbohydrates actually cause overweight and obesity?

Figure 9 shows the number of studies that have examined the relationship between carbohydrate intake and body weight and/or fat composition. The overwhelming majority of these studies find an *inverse* relationship between carbohydrate intake and body weight, not a direct one. Larger people are associated with eating less carbohydrate, not more. Only two studies failed to find a relationship. No study has found a positive relationship.

But what about sugar? Doesn't the consumption of sugar lead to increased body weight? Apparently not. Figure 10 shows the number of studies that have examined the relationship between sugar consumption and body weight. The data are quite similar to the study relating total carbohydrate to body weight—the more sugar consumed, the smaller the body weight. These studies shed considerable doubt on the

major premise promulgated by the popular diet books: Body size is not related to the consumption of carbohydrate, but rather to dietary fat or the concentration of energy.

VI. ENERGY COMPENSATION FOR FAT AND SUGAR SUBSTITUTES

If we can generalize from the majority of studies cited above that humans appear to demonstrate very little energy compensation for reductions in either dietary fat or carbohydrate, then using palatable, low-calorie fat or sugar substitutes should be an effective way to reduce daily energy intake.

Number of studies demonstrating a negative correlation between carbohydrate intake and BMI or fat composition

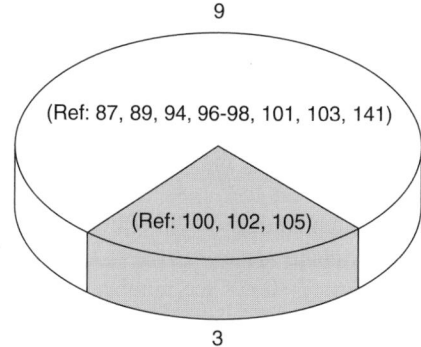

Number of studies failing to demonstrate a negative correlation between carbohydrate intake and BMI or fat composition

FIGURE 9 Correlational studies on the relationship between carbohydrate consumption and BMI or fat composition.

Number of studies demonstrating a negative correlation
between sugar intake and BMI or fat composition

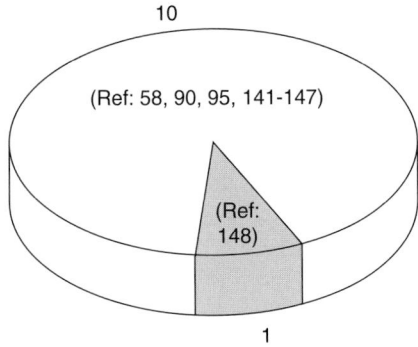

Number of studies failing to demonstrate a negative correlation
between sugar intake and BMI or fat composition

FIGURE 10   Distribution of ecological studies on the relationship between sugar consumption and body weight.

Number of studies demonstrating little or no
energetic compensation for the ingestion of fat substitutes

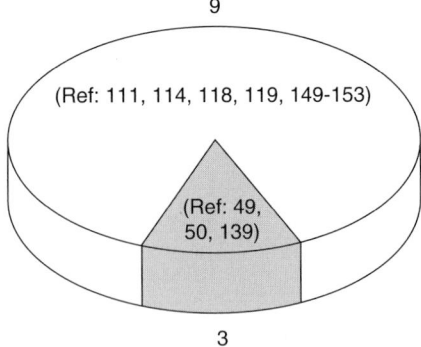

Number of studies demonstrating energetic
compensation for the ingestion of fat substitutes

FIGURE 11   Distribution of studies of energy compensation in response to the consumption of fat substitutes.

Indeed, in many respects, the use of fat substitutes is a better test of the role of dietary fat on energy balance than merely reducing the amount of fat, because it replaces the food with a product of similar properties. The results of studies that have examined the relationship between fat and sugar substitutes and energy intake are presented in Figs. 11 and 12. Similar to the studies on the effect of decreasing fat intake, the majority of published studies demonstrate that humans do not accurately compensate for the reduced energy when the fat in the diet is replaced by a fat substitute, as can be seen in Fig. 11. The study by Cotton *et al.* [49] is particularly important because although they found about 72% energy compensation, the level of dietary fat was reduced to about 20% of energy from 34%. This high degree of fat restriction is substantially more than what was observed in other studies. The study by Kelly *et al.* [50] failed to show a difference in energy intake between a group receiving sucrose polyester in place of dietary fat for a 3-month trial. However, it was very possible that the measure of energy intake (dietary records) was too variable to allow accurate assessment. This interpretation is supported by the fact that the dietary change was sufficient to cause a statistically significant reduction in blood lipid and in body weight of the group receiving the fat substitute. A reduction in energy may have occurred in this group as a function of eating the fat substitutes, but the intake measure could have been too insensitive to detect it.

The experimental studies on the effects of sugar substitutes on energy intake are even clearer than those for fat substitutes. Figure 12 shows the number of studies where sugar substitutes are used in place of sugars and its effects on intake are measured. As is evident from this figure, the vast majority of studies fail to find energy compensation for the energy lost when the sugar in foods is replaced by noncaloric sweeteners regardless of the particular food in which the sweetener was added, for example, water, soft drinks,

yogurt, and cheese. With such a preponderance of studies showing lack of energy compensation when noncaloric sweeteners are substituted for sugar in the diet, one would expect it to be easy to demonstrate that the use of these sweeteners should facilitate weight loss. Unfortunately, the data are not clear and are riddled with controversy.

Two papers that fueled the controversy appeared in 1986 and caused a stir in the popular press and in the scientific community. In a fascinating, but brief, letter to *The Lancet*, Blundell and Hill [51] reported that the ingestion of aspartame caused an increase in hunger ratings in human subjects, and in another paper, Stellman and Garfinkel [52] reported that women who consumed the sweetener saccharine were more likely to gain body weight than nonusers of saccharine. Rogers and Blundell [53] extended their finding by demonstrating that following the ingestion of saccharine, not only

Number of studies demonstrating little or no
energetic compensation for the ingestion of sugar substitutes

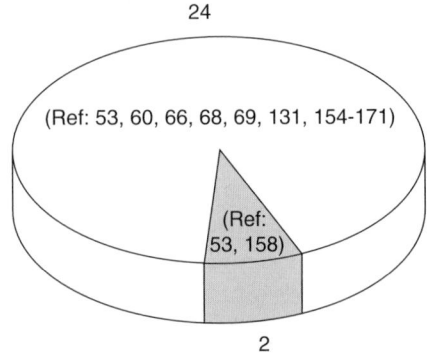

Number of studies demonstrating energetic
compensation for the ingestion of fat substitutes

FIGURE 12   Distribution of studies of energy compensation in response to the consumption of sugar substitutes.

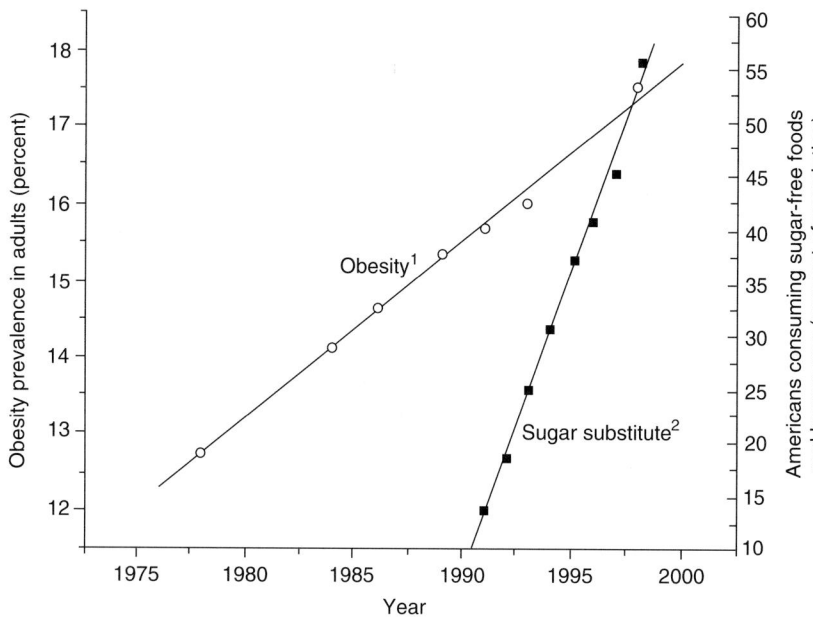

FIGURE 13 Prevalence of obesity and consumption of low-calorie sweeteners, 1978–1998. [Adapted from [1]Mokdad, A. H., Serdula, M. K., Dietz, W. H., Bowman, B. A., Marks, J. S., and Koplan, J. P. (1999). the spread of the obesity epidemic in the United States, 1991–1998. *JAMA* **282**, 1519–1522; and [2]Calorie Control Council (2000). Most popular low calorie, sugar free products: Trends and statistics, Calorie Control Council national consumer survey. Available at http://www.caloriecontrol.org/.]

are subjects hungrier, but they increased their food intake. Thus, rather than being an aid to weight reduction, these studies were suggesting that artificial sweeteners may actually cause a gain in body weight.

Conflicts in science usually resolve themselves with replication and increased scrutiny. As evidence in Figure 12 indicates, the effect observed by Rogers and Blundell [53] was never replicated by any other investigator and may be attributed to a type 2 statistical error. Most researchers fail to find energy compensation for sweetener consumption. In a thorough critic of the Stellman and Garfinkel [52] paper, Renwick [54] pointed out major weaknesses of this study that shed considerable doubt as to its conclusion: (1) The data were based on the subject's memory of their body weight, not measured body weight and (2) anyone who actively tried to lose body weight was eliminated from the analysis. Either of these conditions would have led to the *false* conclusion that weight gain is *related* to sweetener use.

Other published papers in the literature also shed doubt that low-calorie sweeteners could be a significant aid to weight control. No difference in body weight was observed between low-calorie sweetener users and nonusers [55, 56]. Colditz *et al.* [57] reported a *positive* relationship between the use of the sweetener saccharine and a gain in body weight. These results would suggest that sweeteners are not effective in reducing body weight. However, it might be argued that those subjects with the largest body weight had the greatest need for sweeteners to reduce their caloric intake, but apparently, this is not the case. Richardson [58] found no difference in sweetener use between people who restrict their sugar intake compared to those who do not. Consequently, the "need" to use sweeteners for weight reduction explanation cannot explain these results.

These studies clearly raise serious doubts as to whether humans use low-calorie sweeteners as substitutes for sugar as originally intended. Even more disturbing from an energetic perspective is that if consumers did substitute low-calorie sweeteners for sugar, then the proportion of their total energy intake derived from fat would increase [59–61]. As is evident from the data presented above, increasing the percentage of energy from fat may result in an increase in body weight, not a decrease.

One of the few studies that examined the issue of how consumers were using sugar substitutes was provided by Chen and Parham [62]. They found that consumers, college students, were not using the sugar substitutes to substitute for carbohydrates, but rather they were consuming foods containing the sweeteners in addition to the sugars consumed in their diet. This pattern of behavior was not seen when low-calorie sweeteners were substituted covertly for sugar in the diet [60]. It seems that the knowledge of the contents of foods drastically changes the decision to consume it or not, an effect well documented in the laboratory [63–65], although not universally [66]. Miller *et al.* [67] found that information about the caloric content of potato chips significantly affected restrained eaters, but had no effect on unrestrained eaters.

Nevertheless, the relationship between the effectiveness of artificial sweeteners as a weight reduction aid is tenuous at best, particularly in light of the data presented in Fig. 13. This figure shows that the per-capita consumption of low-calorie sweeteners has been increasing, yet so has the incidence of obesity. Despite the fact that a reduction in body weight is the ultimate test of the effectiveness of sweeteners, remarkably few studies have examined this question. An early study by Porikos *et al.* [68] suggested that lean and

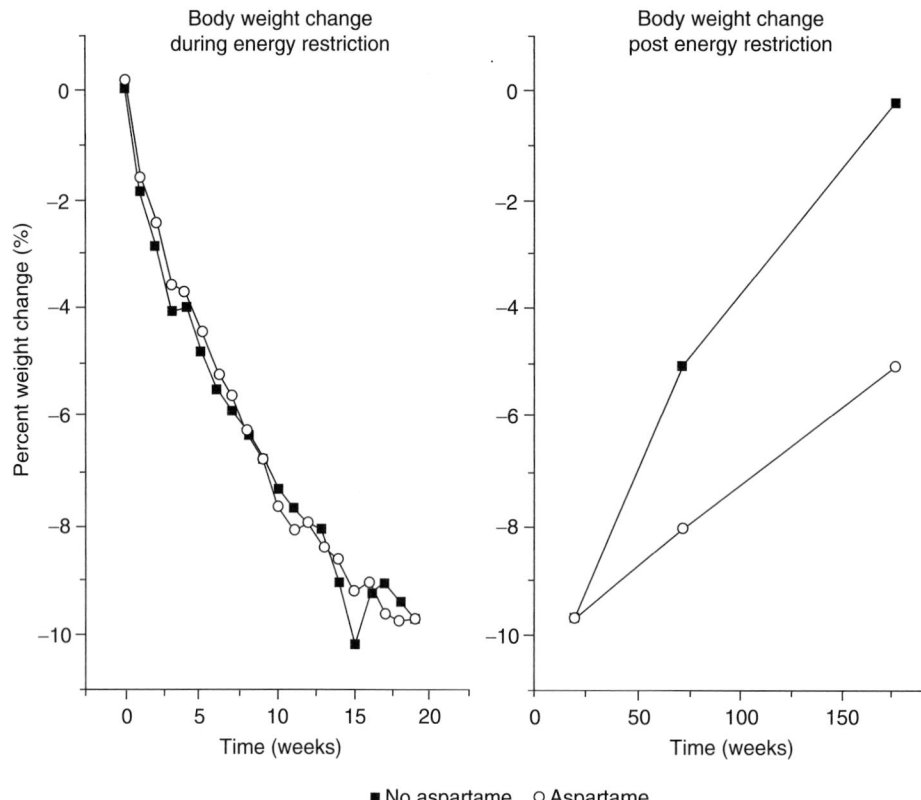

FIGURE 14   Effect of asparatame on the change in body weight during weight reduction and recovery. [Adapted from Blackburn, G. L., Kanders, B. S., Lavin, P. T., Keller, S. D., and Whatley, J. (1997). The effect of aspartame as part of a multidisciplinary weight-control program on short- and long-term control of body weight. *Am. J. Clin. Nutr.* **65,** 409–418.]

obese subjects lose weight when low-calorie sweeteners are substituted for sugar and gain weight when the substitutes are replaced by sugar, but several methodological problems leave this conclusion guarded.

Tordoff and Alleva [69] showed that drinking sodas only sweetened with aspartame for 3 weeks produced a significant loss in weight at the end of a 3-week period. However, the magnitude of the weight changes were less than 1 kg in 3 weeks. Perhaps the best evidence that the use of low-calorie sweeteners can produce weight loss was published by Blackburn and his associates [70] who performed one of the only long-term studies of the effectiveness of sugar substitutes in a weight reduction program. Their results can be seen in Fig. 14. All subjects in this study were prescribed a 4180-kJ diet for 16 weeks, then observed for 2 years. The left panel illustrates that the weight loss in the group who used aspartame was not different from the group that did not use aspartame. However, the right panel shows the typical weight recovery that follows diet-induced weight loss programs. The group that had used aspartame during the dieting phase continued to use it during the follow-up phase and showed less rapid relapse than the group that did not use asparatme. Unfortunately, linear regression analysis of the weight loss

at 77 weeks indicated that the sustained weight loss was unrelated to aspartame use. Most probably, the subject's measures of aspartame use were too inaccurate to observe such a relationship. Nevertheless, at present no clear demonstration exists in the literature that sustained use of low-calorie sweeteners produces a significant weight loss.

VII. PROTEIN PARADOX

Although all the popular books cited above blame carbohydrates in our diet as being the major culprit responsible for our expanding waistlines, the solution they propose is a diet that is not only low in carbohydrate, but high in protein (30% of energy or greater). Figure 15 shows the relationship between the protein and fat content of 500 randomly selected foods from the USDA food consumption survey [39]. This figure shows clearly that a diet high in protein is very likely to be high in dietary fat.

The problem is that the scientific evidence cited above indicates that a high-fat diet would not only be ineffective as a weight reduction tool, but should actually cause a weight gain. Do the gurus of the lay nutrition press know something

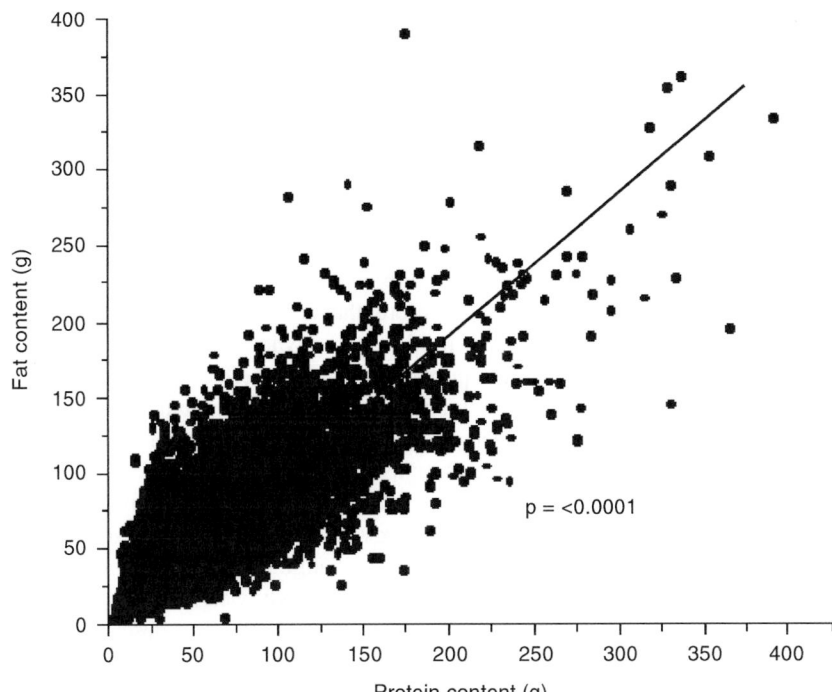

FIGURE 15 Relationship between protein content and fat content of 500 randomly selected foods. [Data from USDA (1996). "Continuing Survey of Food Intakes by Individuals (CSFII): Diet and Health Knowledge Survey, 1994." Department of Agriculture, Beltsville Human Nutrition Research Center/ARS.] Beltsville, Maryland.

about macronutrients and body weight that the scientific community does not?

One possible resolution to this paradox is that protein may cause a better suppression of appetite and food intake than carbohydrate and therefore adhering to a high-protein, high-fat, low-carbohydrate diet is easier than reducing the consumption of high-fat foods. There is reason for suspecting this to be true. It has been known for almost a century that feeding high-protein diets to animals produces a very significant reduction in spontaneous food intake [71–79]. Because of the robustness of this phenomenon, many attempts have been made to identify the critical aspects of the protein metabolism that may be responsible for the dramatic suppression in food intake caused by high protein diets [3, 76, 80, 81].

Unfortunately, the literature on the possible appetite-suppressing effects of protein in humans is not clear. Figure 16 indicates that regardless of whether one measures appetite ratings or grams of food consumed, slightly more studies indicate that protein has a greater satiety effect than carbohydrate, but the number of studies is evenly split on this issue when energy intake is measured.

Several classic, but long forgotten, nutritional studies of chronic feeding of a high-protein diet may shed some light on this protein paradox. McClellan and DuBois [82] fed two (and monitored a third) "normal" men who consumed solely a meat diet for a period of 1 year. All three subjects lost body weight. Yudkin and Carey [83] challenged the conclusion of an earlier and provocative paper by Kekwick and Pawan [84] who argued, as do their modern-day counterparts, that diets

composed primarily of protein and fat have a particular "metabolic effect" that facilitates weight loss. Their subjects maintained exhaustive, weighed dietary records of everything they ate during a 2-week control period, then again during the next 2 weeks, during which time they were instructed to minimize their consumption of carbohydrate and eat as much protein and fat as they desired. The results for all six of their study subjects are shown in Fig. 17. There are several remarkable features about this work that should give us insight as to why the population is buying into the high-protein, high-fat diets, the most important of which is that all the subjects lost weight. The reason for the weight loss is shown in the top left panel of this figure. Restricting the carbohydrate in the diet reduced the total calories consumed. All six subjects did what they were told by reducing the amount of carbohydrate they ate as seen in the top right panel, but their consumption of protein and fat (lower two panels) was unaffected by their restriction of carbohydrate. The average reduction in energy intake was quite large, approximately 37%. In a subsequent replication, Stock and Yudkin [85] examined 11 more subjects in a very similar experimental paradigm. They observed a 33% decrease in energy intake and, again, no change was observed in the amount of protein or fat consumed, only a reduction in carbohydrate intake.

These two older studies may be criticized because they had subjects record their own data and did not use a crossover design. However, similar observations were made by Skov et al. [86], who also observed a reduction in energy intake on a low-carbohydrate, high-protein diet using a more

Number of studies demonstrating a greater
"satiety effect" of protein than carbohydrate

9

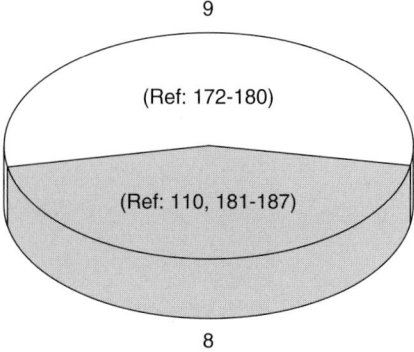

(Ref: 172-180)

(Ref: 110, 181-187)

8

Number of studies failing to demonstrate a greater
"satiety effect" of protein than carbohydrate

Number of studies demonstrating a greater
suppression of energy intake after ingestion of protein
relative to carbohydrate

7

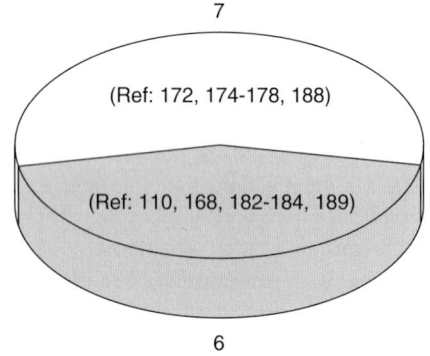

(Ref: 172, 174-178, 188)

(Ref: 110, 168, 182-184, 189)

6

Number of studies failing to demonstrate a greater
suppression of energy intake after ingestion of protein
relative to carbohydrate

FIGURE 16 Distribution of studies of the relative "satiety effect" of protein in relation to carbohydrate on appetite (top) and energy intake (bottom).

experimentally sophisticated design, more subjects, and measured over a longer period of time (26 weeks). They observed an approximately 18% reduction in energy intake in a group of overweight and obese subjects who ate *ad libitum* from a menu composed of high-protein (22%), low-carbohydrate (46%) foods prepared by their staff compared to a matched group of subjects who consumed a high-carbohydrate (59%), low-protein (12%) diet.

One reason why the Skov *et al.* study [86] observed a smaller difference in energy intake than the Yudkin [85] group may be due to the greater degree of experimental control. Skov *et al.* controlled the composition of the diet consumed by their subjects. The reduction in energy derived from dietary carbohydrate was offset by an increase in the amount of energy derived from protein. In the Yudkin studies, the subjects determined the composition of the diet and did not increase the amount of protein in response to the decrease in carbohydrate. This control allowed Skov and his associates to rule out palatability and energy density as factors contributing to their results. What we don't know is what changes the public makes when they try to follow these high-protein, low-carbohydrate diets.

It appears, therefore, that at least two processes are operating to make the low-carbohydrate, high-protein diet appealing to the public as an easy and effective means of losing weight. Protein appears to have a slight, but significant, satiating property compared to carbohydrate or fat when it is eaten in large amounts consistently. Even more intriguing is the possibility that a large reduction in carbohydrate foods does not result in energy compensation in a free-living population. Thus, without a change in energy expenditure, energy intake will be low, and body weight will be lost. For how long, we don't know. Clearly, this area deserves serious research by the scientific community.

VIII. SUMMARY AND IMPLICATIONS OF THE RESEARCH ON MACRONUTRIENTS AND INTAKE

In viewing the long list of studies in macronutrients and food intake, it becomes apparent that humans do not eat for energy. In fact, it appears that humans possess very poor mechanisms to adjust the volume of food they consume in response to alterations in energy density of the foods they consume. If these observations are true, then the use of "artificial" sweeteners and fats should successfully cause a sustained reduction in the body weight in our population. Why sweeteners and fat substitutes do not cause a greater weight loss than they do requires more research as to how consumers use these products. If energy concentration is the major determinant of human energy intake, as suggested by this research, then the major thrust of any programs aimed at weight reduction or obesity prevention should concentrate on the consumption of energy-dilute foods such as soups, salads, and casseroles.

From a more theoretical perspective, the plasticity of body weight, rather than the constancy of body weight, that occurs when macronutrients are manipulated should evoke a reevaluation of the theory that energy intake in humans is well controlled and that body weight is well regulated. It is quite possible that humans maintain a vestigial process that "controls" our behavior of eating, but that this system is easily dominated by more powerful environmental determinants. If this is the case, then it is not too optimistic to believe that by understanding more about these environmental determinants, such as macronutrient composition, it may be possible to not only understand why we are getting fatter, but

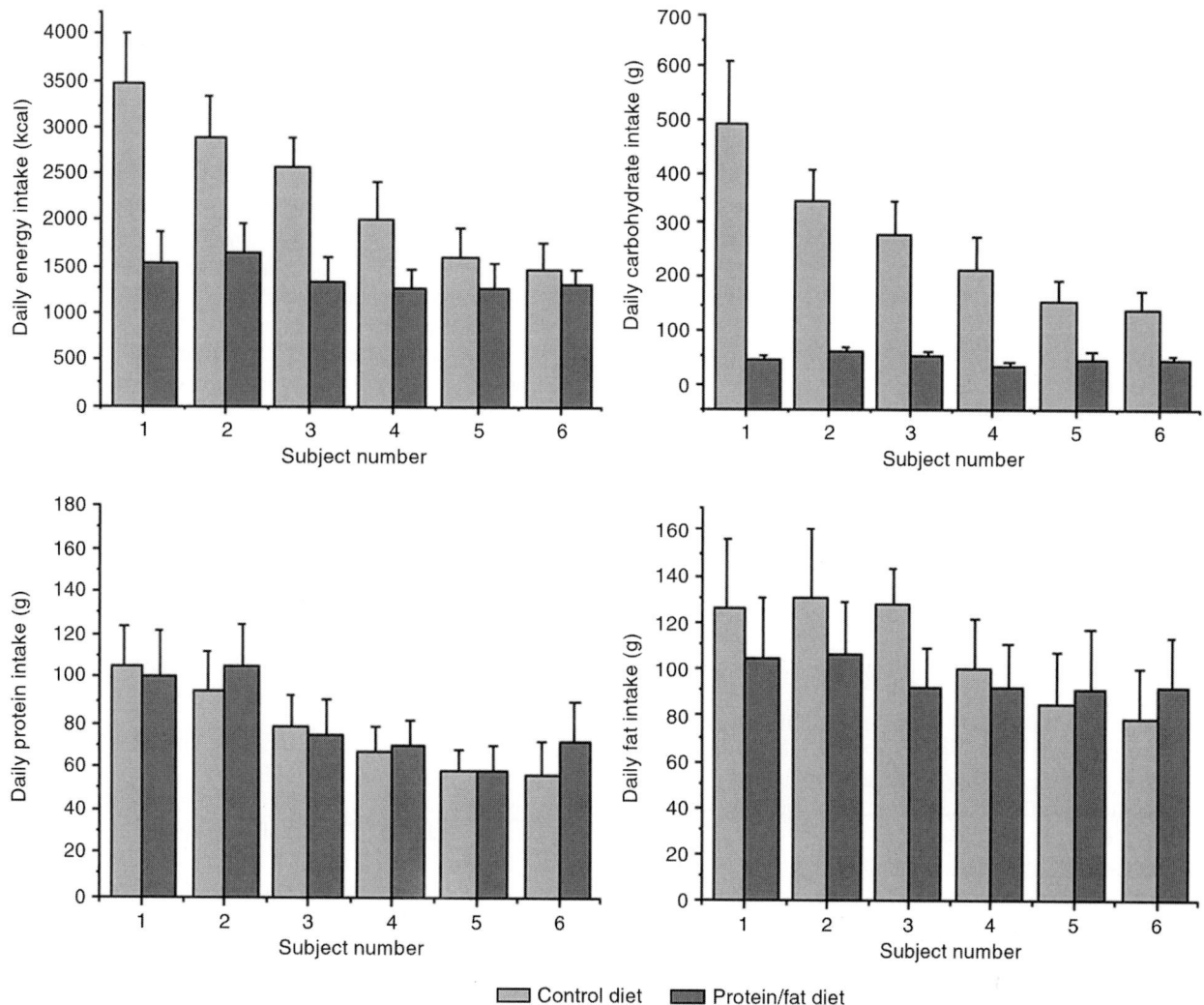

FIGURE 17 Daily caloric and macronutrient intake of six subjects consuming a high-protein, low-carbohydrate diet. [Adapted from Yudkin, J., and Carey, M. (1960). The treatment of obesity by the "high-fat" diet: The inevitability of calories. *Lancet* **2,** 939–941.]

also and, most importantly, be able to reduce and even prevent some of the overweight obesity from occurring.

References

1. Adolph, E. F. (1947). Urges to eat and drink in rats. *Am. J. Physiol.* **151,** 110–125.
2. Mayer, J. (1955). Regulation of energy intake and the body weight: The glucostatic theory and the lipostatic hypothesis. *Ann. NY Acad. Sci.* **63,** 15–43.
3. Mellinkoff, S. M., Franklin, M., Boyle, D., and Geipell, M. (1956). Relationship between serum amino acid concentration and fluctuation in appetite. *J. Appl. Physiol.* **8,** 535–538.
4. Michel, C., and Cabanac, M. (1999). Effects of dexamethasone on the body weight set point of rats. *Physiol. Behav.* **68,** 145–150.
5. Cabanac, M., and Morrissette, J. (1992). Acute, but not chronic, exercise lowers the body weight set-point in male rats. *Physiol. Behav.* **52,** 1173–1177.
6. Garn, S. M. (1992). Role of set-point theory in regulation of body weight [letter; comment]. *FASEB J.* **6,** 794.
7. Cabanac, M. (1991). Role of set-point theory in body weight [letter; comment]. *FASEB J.* **5,** 2105–2106.
8. Bernardis, L. L., McEwen, G., and Kodis, M. (1986). Body weight set point studies in weanling rats with dorsomedial hypothalamic lesions (DMNL rats). *Brain Res. Bull.* **17,** 451–460.
9. Fantino, M., Faion, F., and Rolland, Y. (1986). Effect of dex-fenfluramine on body weight set-point: Study in the rat with hoarding behaviour. *Appetite* **7**(Suppl), 115–126.
10. Fantino, M., and Brinnel, H. (1986). Body weight set-point changes during the ovarian cycle: Experimental study of rats using hoarding behavior. *Physiol. Behav.* **36,** 991–996.

11. Harris, R. B., and Martin, R. J. (1984). Recovery of body weight from below "set point" in mature female rats. *J. Nutr.* **114,** 1143–1150.

12. Keesey, R. E., and Corbett, S. W. (1984). Metabolic defense of the body weight set-point. *Res. Publ. Assoc. Res. Nerv. Ment. Dis.* **62,** 87–96.

13. Stunkard, A. J. (1982). Anorectic agents lower a body weight set point. *Life Sci.* **30,** 2043–2055.

14. De Castro, J. M., Paullin, S. K., and DeLugas, G. M. (1978), Insulin and glucagon as determinants of body weight set point and microregulation in rats. *J. Comp. Physiol. Psychol.* **92,** 571–579.

15. Garrow, J. S., and Stalley, S. (1975). Is there a "set point" for human body-weight? *Proc. Nutr. Soc.* **34,** 84A–85A.

16. Barnes, D. S., Mrosovsky, N. (1974). Body weight regulation in ground squirrels and hypothalamically lesioned rats: Slow and sudden set-point changes. *Physiol. Behav.* **12,** 251–258.

17. Myers, R. D., and Martin, G. E. (1973). 6-OHDA lesions of the hypothalamus: Interaction of aphagia, food palatability, set-point for weight regulation, and recovery of feeding. *Pharmacol. Biochem. Behav.* **1,** 329–345.

18. Lissner, L., and Heitmann, B. L. (1995). Dietary fat and obesity: Evidence from epidemiology. *Eur. J. Clin. Nutr.* **49,** 79A–90A.

19. Black, A. E., Goldberg, G. R., Jebb, S. A., Livingstone, M. B., Cole, T. J., and Prentice, A. M. (1991). Critical evaluation of energy intake data using fundamental principles of energy physiology: 2. Evaluating the results of published surveys. *Eur. J. Clin. Nutr.* **45,** 583–599.

20. Heitmann, B. L. (1993). The influence of fatness, weight change, slimming history and other lifestyle variables on diet reporting in Danish men and women aged 35–65 years. *Int. J. Obes. Relat. Metab. Disord.* **17,** 329–336.

21. Heitmann, B. L., and Lissner, L. (1995). Dietary underreporting by obese individuals—is it specific or non-specific? *Br. Med. J.* **311,** 986–989.

22. Heitmann, B. L., Lissner, L, Sorensen, T. I., and Bengtsson, C. (1995). Dietary fat intake and weight gain in women genetically predisposed for obesity. *Am. J. Clin. Nutr.* **61,** 1213–1217.

23. Heitmann, B. L., Lissner, L., and Osler, M. (2000). Do we eat less fat, or just report so? *Int. J. Obes. Relat. Metab. Disord.* **24**(4), 435–442.

24. Prentice, A. M., Black, A. E., Coward, W. A., Davies, H. L., Golderg, G. R., Murgatroyd, P. R., Ashford, J., Sawyer, M., and Whitehead, R. G. (1986). High levels of energy expenditure in obese women. *Br. Med. J. Clin. Res. Ed.* **292,** 983–987.

25. Poppitt, S. D., and Swann, D. L. (1998). Dietary manipulation and energy compensation: Does the intermittent use of low-fat items in the diet reduce total energy intake in free-feeding lean men? *Int. J. Obes. Relat. Metab. Disord.* **22,** 1024–1031.

26. Kendall, A., Levitsky, D. A., Strupp, B. J., and Lissner, L. (1991). Weight loss on a low-fat diet: Consequence of the imprecision of the control of food intake in humans. *Am. J. Clin. Nutr.* **53,** 1124–1129.

27. West, D. B., and York, B. (1998). Dietary fat, genetic predisposition, and obesity: Lessons from animal models. *Am. J. Clin. Nutr.* **67,** 505S–512S.

28. Ramirez, I., and Friedman, M. I. (1990). Dietary hyperphagia in rats: Role of fat, carbohydrate, and energy content. *Physiol. Behav.* **47,** 1155–1163.

29. van Stratum, P., Lussenburg, R. N., van Wezel, L. A., Vergroesen, A. J., and Cremer, H. D. (1978). The effect of dietary carbohydrate to fat ratio on energy intake by adult women. *Am. J. Clin. Nutr.* **31,** 206–212.

30. Stubbs, R. J., Harbron, C. G., and Prentice, A. M. (1996). Covert manipulation of the dietary fat to carbohydrate ratio of isoenergetically dense diets: Effect on food intake in feeding men ad libitum. *Int. J. Obes. Relat. Metab. Disord.* **20,** 651–660.

31. Stubbs, R. J., Johnstone, A. M., O'Reilly, L. M., Barton, K., and Reid, C. (1998). The effect of covertly manipulating the energy density of mixed diets on ad libitum food intake in "pseudo free-living" humans. *Int. J Obes. Relat. Metab. Disord.* **22,** 980–987.

32. Saltzman, E., Dallal, G. E., and Roberts, S. B. (1997). Effect of high-fat and low-fat diets on voluntary energy intake and substrate oxidation: Studies in identical twins consuming diets matched for energy density, fiber, and palatability. *Am. J. Clin. Nutr.* **66,** 1332–1339.

33. Bell, E. A., Castellanos, V. H., Pelkman, C. L., Thorwart, M. L., and Rolls, B. J. (1998). Energy density of foods affects energy intake in normal-weight women. *Am. J. Clin. Nutr.* **67,** 412–420.

34. Rolls, B. J., and Bell, E. A. (1999). Intake of fat and carbohydrate: Role of energy density. *Eur. J. Clin. Nutr.* **53**(Suppl 1), S166–S173.

35. Rolls, B. J., Bell, E. A., and Thorwart, M. L. (1999). Water incorporated into a food but not served with a food decreases energy intake in lean women. *Am. J. Clin. Nutr.* **70,** 448–455.

36. Rolls, B. J., Bell, E. A., Castellanos, V. H., Chow, M., Pelkman, C. L., and Thorwart, M. L. (1999). Energy density but not fat content of foods affected energy intake in lean and obese women. *Am. J. Clin. Nutr.* **69,** 863–871.

37. Poppitt, S. D. (1995). Energy density of diets and obesity. *Int. J. Obes.* **19,** S20–S26.

38. Poppitt, S. D., and Prentice, A. M. (1996). Energy density and its role in the control of food intake: Evidence from metabolic and community studies. *Appetite* **26,** 153–174.

39. USDA (1996). Continuing Survey of Food Intakes by Individuals (CSFII): Diet and Health Knowledge Survey, 1994. Department of Agriculture, Beltsville Human Nutrition Research Center/ARS, Maryland.

40. Montignac, M. (1989). "Dine Out and Lose Weight: The French Way to Culinary 'Savoir Vivre.'" Montignac: USA, Inc.

41. Steward, H. L., Bethea, M. C., Andrews, S. S., Brennan, R. O., and Balart, L. A. (1998). "Sugar Busters! Cut Sugar to Trim Fat." Ballantine Books, New York.

42. Atkins, R. C. (1998). "Dr. Atkins' New Diet Revolution." Avon Books, New York.

43. Atkins, R. C. (1972). "Dr. Atkins' Diet Revolution: The High Calorie Way to Stay Thin Forever." David MacKay Co. Inc., New York.

44. Sears, B., and Lawren, B. (1995). "The Zone: A Dietary Road Map to Lose Weight Permanently, Reset Your Genetic Code, Prevent Disease, and Achieve Maximum Physical Performance." Harper Collins, New York.

45. Heller, R. F. and Heller, R. F. (1993). "The Carbohydrate Addict's Diet: The Lifelong Solution to Yo-Yo Dieting." Signet, New York.

46. Eades, M. R., and Eades, M. D. (1997). "Protein Power: The High-Protein/Low-Carbohydrate Way to Lose Weight, Feel Fit, and Boost Your Health—in Just Weeks!" Bantam Books, New York.

47. Stephen, A., and Wald, N. J. (1990). Trends in individual consumption of dietary fat in the United States, 1920–1984. *Am. J. Clin. Nutr.* **52,** 457–469.

48. Heini, A. F., and Weinsier, R. L. (1997). Divergent trends in obesity and fat intake patterns: The American paradox. *Am. J. Med.* **102,** 259–264.

49. Cotton, J. R., Weststrate, J. A., and Blundell, J. E. (1996). Replacement of dietary fat with sucrose polyester: Effects on energy intake and appetite control in nonobese males. *Am. J. Clin. Nutr.* **63,** 891B–896B.

50. Kelly, D.E., Wing, R., Buonocore, C., Sturis, J., Polonsky, K., and Fitzsimmons, M. (1993). Relative effects of calorie restriction and weight loss in noninsulin-dependent diabetes mellitus. *J. Clin. Endocr. Metab.* **77,** 1287–1293.

51. Blundell, J. E., and Hill, A. J. (1986). Paradoxical effects of an intense sweetener (aspartame) on appetite [letter]. *Lancet* **1,** 1092–1093.

52. Stellman, S. D,, and Garfinkel, L. (1986). Artificial sweetener use and one-year weight change among women. *Prevent. Med* **15,** 195–202.

53. Rogers, P. J., and Blundell, J. E. (1989). Separating the actions of sweetness and calories: Effects of saccharin and carbohydrates on hunger and food intake in human subjects. *Physiol. Behav.* **45,** 1093–1099.

54. Renwick, A. G. (1994). Intense sweeteners, food intake, and the weight of a body of evidence. *Physiol. Behav.* **55,** 139–143.

55. McCann, M. B., Brulson, M. F., and Stulb, S. C. (1956). Noncaloric sweeteners and weight reduction. *J. Am. Diet. Assoc.* **32,** 327–330.

56. Parham, E. S., and Parham, A. R. J. (1980). Saccharin use and sugar intake by college students. *J. Am. Diet. Assoc.* **76,** 560–563.

57. Colditz, G. A., Willett, W. C., Stampfer, M. J., London, S. J., Segal, M. R., and Speizer, F. E. (1990). Patterns of weight change and their relation to diet in a cohort of healthy women. *Am. J. Clin. Nutr.* **51,** 1100–1105.

58. Richardson, J. F. (1972). The sugar intake of businessmen and its inverse relationship with relative weight. *Br. J. Nutr.* **27,** 449–460.

59. Beaton, G. H., Tarasuk, V., and Anderson, G. H. (1992). Estimation of possible impact of noncaloric fat and carbohydrate substitutes on macronutrient intake in the human. *Appetite* **19,** 87–103.

60. Naismith, D. J., and Rhodes, C. (1995). Adjustment in energy intake following the covert removal of sugar from the diet. *J. Hum. Nutr. Diet.* **8,** 167–175.

61. Mela, D. J. (1997). Fat and sugar substitutes: Implications for dietary intakes and energy balance. *Proc. Nutr. Soc.* **56,** 827–840.

62. Chen, L. N., and Parham, E. S. (1991). College students' use of high-intensity sweeteners is not consistently associated with sugar consumption. *J. Am. Diet. Assoc.* **91,** 686–690.

63. Wooley, S. C. (1972). Physiologic versus cognitive factors in short term food regulation in the obese and nonobese. *Psychosom. Med.* **34,** 62–68.

64. Caputi, F. A., and Mattes, R. D. (1993). Human dietary responses to perceived manipulation of fat content in a midday meal. *Int. J. Obes. Relat. Metab. Disord.* **17,** 237–240.

65. Shide, D. J., and Rolls, B. J. (1995). Information about the fat content of preloads influences energy intake in healthy women. *J. Am. Diet. Assoc.* **95,** 993–998.

66. Rolls, B. J., Laster, L. J., and Summerfelt, A. (1989). Hunger and food intake following consumption of low-calorie foods. *Appetite* **13,** 115–127.

67. Miller, D. L., Castellanos, V. H., Shide, D. J., Peters, J. C., and Rolls, B. J. (1998). Effect of fat-free potato chips with and without nutrition labels on fat and energy intakes. *Am. J. Clin. Nutr.* **68,** 282–290.

68. Porikos, K. P., Hesser, M. F., and Van Itallie, T. B. (1982). Caloric regulation in normal-weight men maintained on a palatable diet of conventional foods. *Physiol. Behav.* **29,** 293–300.

69. Tordoff, M. G., and Alleva, A. M. (1990). Effect of drinking soda sweetened with aspartame or high-fructose corn syrup on food intake and body weight. *Am. J. Clin. Nutr.* **51,** 963–969.

70. Blackburn, G. L., Kanders, B. S., Lavin, P. T., Keller, S. D., and Whatley, J. (1997). The effect of aspartame as part of a multidisciplinary weight-control program on short- and long-term control of body weight. *Am. J. Clin. Nutr.* **65,** 409–418.

71. Osborn, T. P., and Mendel, L. B. (1921). Growth on diets containing more than ninety percent of protein. *In* "Scientific Proceedings Abstracts of Communications, 114th Meeting," pp. 167–168. Cambridge University Press, Cambridge.

72. Reader, V. B., and Drumond, J. C. (1925). Further observations on nutrition with diets rich in protein. *J. Physiol.* 59, 472–478.

73. Krauss, R. M., and Mayer, J. (1965). Influence of protein and amino acids on food intake in the rat. *Am. J. Physiol.* **209,** 479–483.

74. Peng, Y. S., Meliza, L. L., Vavich, M. G., and Kemmerer, A. R. (1974). Changes in food intake and nitrogen metabolism of rats while adapting to a low or high protein diet. *J. Nutr.* **104,** 1008–1017.

75. Semon, B. A., Leung, P. M., Rogers, Q. R., and Gietzen, D. W. (1987). Effect of type of protein on food intake of rats fed high protein diets. *Physiol. Behav.* **41,** 451–458.

76. Semon, B. A., Leung, P. M., Rogers, Q. R., and Gietzen, D. W. (1988). Increase in plasma ammonia and amino acids when rats are fed a 44% casein diet. *Physiol. Behav.* **43,** 631–636.

77. Harper, A. E. (1976). Protein and amino acids in the regulation of food intake. *In* "Hunger: Basic Mechanisms and Clinical Implications" (D. Novin, W. Wyrwicka, and G. A. Bray, Eds.) pp. 103–113. Raven Press, New York.

78. Hannah, J. S., Dubey, A. K., and Hansen, B. C. (1990). Post-ingestional effects of a high-protein diet on the regulation of food intake in monkeys. *Am. J. Clin. Nutr.* **52,** 320–325.

79. McArthur, L. H., Kelly, W. F., Gietzen, D. W., and Rogers, Q. R. (1993). The role of palatability in the food intake response of rats fed high-protein diets. *Appetite* **20,** 181–196.

80. Anderson, G. H., and Li, E. T. S. (1987). Protein and amino acids in the regulation of quantitative and qualitative aspects of food intake. *Int. J. Obes.* **11,** 97–108.

81. Peters, J. C., and Harper, A. E. (1987). Acute effects of dietary protein on food intake, tissue amino acids, and brain serotonin. *Am. J. Physiol.* **252,** R902–R914.

82. McClellan, W. S., and DuBois, E. F. (1930). Prolonged meat diets with a study of kidney function and ketosis. *J. Biol. Chem.* **37,** 651–668.

83. Yudkin, J., and Carey, M. (1960). The treatment of obesity by the "high-fat" diet: The inevitability of calories. *Lancet* **2,** 939–941.

84. Kekwick, A., and Pawan, G. L. S. (1956). Calorie intake in relation to body weight changes in the obese. *Lancet* **2,** 155–161.

85. Stock, A. L., and Yudkin, J. (1970). Nutrient intake of subjects on low carbohydrate diet used in treatment of obesity. *Am. J. Clin. Nutr.* **23,** 948–952.

86. Skov, A. R., Toubro, S., Ronn, B., Holm, L., and Astrup, A. (1999). Randomized trial on protein vs carbohydrate in ad libitum fat reduced diet for the treatment of obesity. *Int. J. Obes. Relat. Metab. Disord.* **23,** 528–536.

87. Dreon, D. M., Frey-Hewitt, B., Ellsworth, N., Williams, P. T., Terry, R. B., and Wood, P. D. (1988). Dietary fat to carbohydrate ratio and obesity in middle-aged men. *Am. J. Clin. Nutr.* **47,** 995–1000.

88. Gazzaniga, J. M., and Burns, T. L. (1993). Relationship between diet composition and body fatness, with adjustment for resting energy expenditure and physical activity, in preadolescent children. *Am. J. Clin. Nutr.* **58,** 21–28.

89. George, V., Tremblay, A., Despres, J. P., Leblanc, C., and Bouchard, C. (1990). Effect of dietary fat content on total and regional adiposity in men and women. *Int. J. Obes.* **14,** 1085–1094.

90. Gibson, S. A. (1993). Consumption and sources of sugars in the diets of British schoolchildren—are high sugar diets nutritionally inferior? *J. Hum. Nutr. Diet.* **6,** 355–371.

91. Klesges, R. C., Klesges, L. M., Haddock, C. K., and Eck, L. H. (1992). A longitudinal analysis of the impact of dietary intake and physical activity on weight change in adults. *Am. J. Clin. Nutr.* **55,** 818–822.

92. Kulesza, W. (1982). Dietary intake in obese women. *Appetite* **3,** 61–68.

93. Lissner, L. (1987). Dietary correlates of human obesity: The role of dietary fat. Cornell University, Ithaca, NY.

94. Maffeis, C., Provera, S., Filippi, L., Sidoti, G., Schena, S., Pinelli, L., and Tato, L. (2000). Distribution of food intake as a risk factor for childhood obesity. *Int. J. Obes.* **24,** 75–80.

95. Macdiarmid, J. I., Vail, A., Cade, J. E., and Blundell, J. E. (1998). The sugar–fat relationship revisited: Differences in consumption between men and women of varying BMI. *Int. J. Obes. Relat. Metab. Disord.* **22,** 1053–1061.

96. Miller, W. C., Lindeman, A. K., Wallace, J, and Niederpruem, M. (1990). Diet composition, energy intake, and exercise in relation to body fat in men and women. *Am. J. Clin. Nutr.* **52,** 426–430.

97. Nelson, L. H., and Tucker, L. A. (1996). Diet composition related to body fat in a multivariate study of 203 men. *J. Am. Diet. Assoc.* **96,** 771–777.

98. Ortega, R. M., Requejo, A. M., Andres, P., Lopez Sobaler, A. M., Redondo, R., and Gonzalez Fernandez, M. (1995). Relationship between diet composition and body mass index in a group of Spanish adolescents. *Br. J. Nutr.* **74,** 765–773.

99. Pudel, V., and Westenhoefer, J. (1992). Dietary and behavioural principles in the treatment of obesity. *In* "International Monitor on Eating Patterns and Weight Control," Vol. 1, pp. 2–7. Medicon/Servier. Cited in Lissner and Hutman (18).

100. Romieu, I., Willett, W. C., Stampfer, M. J., Colditz, G. A., Sampson, L., Rosner, B., Hennekens, C. H., and Speizer, F. E. (1988). Energy intake and other determinants of relative weight. *Am. J. Clin. Nutr.* **47,** 406–412.

101. Tremblay, A., Plourde, G., Despres, J. P., and Bouchard, C. (1989). Impact of dietary fat content and fat oxidation on energy intake in humans. *Am. J. Clin. Nutr.* **49,** 799–805.

102. Tucker, L. A., and Kano, M. J. (1992). Dietary fat and body fat: A multivariate study of 205 adult females. *Am. J. Clin. Nutr.* **56,** 616–622.

103. Tucker, L. A., Seljaas, G. T., and Hager, R. L. (1997). Body fat percentage of children varies according to their diet composition. *J. Am. Diet. Assoc.* **97,** 981–986.

104. Keys, A. (1970). Coronary heart disease in seven countries. *Circulation* **1,** 1–191.

105. Lissner, L., and Lindroos, A. K. (1994). Is dietary underreporting macronutrient-specific? *Eur. J. Clin. Nutr.* **48,** 453–454.

106. Robertson, S. M., Cullen, K. W., Baranowski, J., Baranowski, T., Hu, S. H., and de Moor, C. (1999). Factors related to adiposity among children aged 3 to 7 years. *J. Am. Diet. Assoc.* **99,** 938–943.

107. Slattery, M. L., McDonald, A., Bild, D. E., Caan, B. J., Hilner, J. E., Jacobs, D. R. J. and Liu, K. (1992). Associations of body fat and its distribution with dietary intake, physical activity, alcohol, and smoking in blacks and whites. *Am. J. Clin. Nutr.* **55,** 943–949.

108. Blundell, J. E., Burley, V. J., Cotton, J. R., and Lawton, C. L. (1993). Dietary fat and the control of energy intake: Evaluating the effects of fat on meal size and postmeal satiety. *Am. J. Clin. Nutr.* **57,** 772S–777S.

109. Cotton, J. R., Burley, V. J., Weststrate, J. A., and Blundell, J. E. (1994). Dietary fat and appetite: Similarities and differences in the satiating effect of meals supplemented with either fat or carbohydrate. *J. Hum. Nutr. Diet.* **7,** 11–24.

110. de Graaf, C., Hulshof, T., Weststrate, J. A., and Jas, P. (1992). Short-term effects of different amounts of protein, fats, and carbohydrates on satiety. *Am. J. Clin. Nutr.* **55,** 33–38.

111. de Graaf, C., Drijvers, J. J. M. M., Zimmermanns, N. J. H., Hof, K. H. V., Westrate, J. A., van den Berg, H., Velthuis-te, W., Westerterp, K. R., Verboeket-van de Venne, W. P. H., and Westerterp-Plantenga, M. S. (1997). Energy and fat compensation during long term consumption of reduced fat products. *Appetite* **29,** 305–323.

112. Duncan, K. H., Bacon, J. A., and Weinsier, R. L. (1983). The effects of high and low energy density diets on satiety, energy intake, and eating time of obese and nonobese subjects. *Am. J. Clin. Nutr.* **37,** 763–767.

113. Durrant, M. L., Royston, J. P., Wloch, R. T., and Garrow, J. S. (1982). The effect of covert changes in energy density of preloads on subsequent ad libitum energy intake in lean and obese human subjects. *Hum. Nutr. Clin Nutr.* **36,** 297–306.

114. Glueck, C. J., Hastings, M. M., Allen, C., Hogg, E., Baehler, L., Gartside, P. S., Phillips, D., Jones, M., Hollenback, E. J., Braun, B., and Anastasia, J. V. (1982). Sucrose polyester and covert caloric dilution. *Am. J. Clin. Nutr.* **35,** 1352–1359.

115. Green, S. M., Burely, V. J., and Blundell, J. E. (1994). Effect of fat- and sucrose-containing foods on the size of eating episodes and energy intake in lean males: Potential for causing overconsumption. *Eur. J. Clin. Nutr.* **48,** 547–555.

116. Green, S. M., and Blundell, J. E. (1996). Subjective and objective indices of the satiating effect of foods. Can people predict how filling a food will be? *Eur. J. Clin. Nutr.* **50,** 798–806.

117. Hill, A. J., Leathwood, P. D., and Blundell, J. E. (1987). Some evidence for short-term caloric compensation in normal weight human subjects: The effects of high- and low-energy meals on hunger, food preference and food intake. *Hum. Nutr. Appl. Nutr.* **41,** 244–257.

118. Hulshof, T., de Graaf, C., and Weststrate, J. A. (1993). The effects of preloads varying in physical state and fat content on satiety and energy intake. *Appetite* **21,** 273–286.

119. Hulshof, T., de Graaf, C., and Weststrate, J. A. (1995). Short-term effects of high-fat and low-fat/high-SPE croissants on appetite and energy intake at three deprivation periods. *Physiol. Behav.* **57,** 377–383.

120. Lawton, C. L., Burley, V. J., Wales, J. K., and Blundell, J. E. (1993). Dietary fat and appetite control in obese subjects: Weak effects on satiation and satiety. *Int. J. Obes. Relat. Metab. Disord.* **17,** 409–416.

121. Lawton, C. L., Delargy, H. J., Smith, F. C., Hamilton, V., and Blundell, J. E. (1998). A medium-term intervention study on the impact of high- and low-fat snacks varying in sweetness and fat content: Large shifts in daily fat intake but good compensation for daily energy intake. *Br. J. Nutr.* **80,** 149–161.

122. Lissner, L., Levitsky, D. A., Strupp, B. J., Kalkwarf, H. J., and Roe, D. A. (1987). Dietary fat and the regulation of energy intake in human subjects. *Am. J. Clin. Nutr.* **46,** 886–892.

123. Murgatroyd, P. R., Goldberg, G. R., Leahy, F. E., Gilsenan, M. B., and Prentice, A. M. (1999). Effects of inactivity and diet composition on human energy balance. *Int. J. Obes. Relat. Metab. Disord.* **23,** 1269–1275.

124. Rolls, B. J., Kim-Harris, S., Fischman, M. W., Foltin, R. W., Moran, T. H., and Stoner, S. A. (1994). Satiety after preloads with different amounts of fat and carbohydrate: Implications for obesity [see comments]. *Am. J. Clin. Nutr.* **60,** 476–487.

125. Spiegel, T. A. (1973). Caloric regulation of food intake in man. *J. Comp. Physiol. Psychol.* **84,** 24–37.

126. Stubbs, R. J., Ritz, P., Coward, W. A., and Prentice, A. M. (1995). Covert manipulation of the ratio of dietary fat to carbohydrate and energy density: Effect on food intake and energy balance in free-living men eating ad libitum. *Am. J. Clin. Nutr.* **62,** 330A–337A.

127. Stubbs, R. J., Harbron, C. G., Murgatroyd, P. R., and Prentice, A. M. (1995). Covert manipulation of dietary fat and energy density: Effect on substrate flux and food intake in men eating ad libitum. *Am. J. Clin. Nutr.* **62,** 316B–329B.

128. Stubbs, R. J., O'Reilly, L. M., Johnstone, A. M., Harrison, C. L., Clark, H., Franklin, M. F., Reid, C. A., and Mazlan, N. (1999). Description and evaluation of an experimental model to examine changes in selection between high-protein, high-carbohydrate and high-fat foods in humans. *Eur. J. Clin. Nutr.* **53,** 13–21 [erratum **53**(3), 247].

129. Thomas, C. D., Peters, J. C., Reed, G. W., Abumrad, N. N., Sun, M., and Hill, J. O. (1992). Nutrient balance and energy expenditure during ad libitum feeding of high-fat and high-carbohydrate diets in humans. *Am. J. Clin. Nutr.* **55,** 934–942.

130. Tremblay, A., Lavallee, N., Almeras, N., Allard, L., Despres, J. P., and Bouchard, C. (1991). Nutritional determinants of the increase in energy intake associated with a high-fat diet. *Am. J. Clin. Nutr.* **53,** 1134–1137.

131. Foltin, R. W., Fischman, M. W., Emurian, C. S., and Rachlinski, J. J. (1988). Compensation for caloric dilution in humans given unrestricted access to food in a residential laboratory. *Appetite* **10,** 13–24.

132. Foltin, R. W., Fischman, M. W., Moran, T. H., Rolls, B. J., and Kelly, T. H. (1990). Caloric compensation for lunches varying in fat and carbohydrate content by humans in a residential laboratory. *Am. J. Clin. Nutr.* **52,** 969–980.

133. Foltin, R. W., Rolls, B. J., Moran, T. H., Kelly, T. H., McNelis, A. L., and Fischman, M. W. (1992). Caloric, but not macronutrient, compensation by humans for required-eating occasions with meals and snack varying in fat and carbohydrate. *Am. J. Clin. Nutr.* **55,** 331–342 [erratum **56**(5), 954].

134. Gatenby, S. J., Aaron, J. I., Morton, G. M., and Mela, D. J. (1995). Nutritional implications of reduced-fat food use by free-living consumers. *Appetite* **25,** 241–252.

135. Gatenby, S. J., Aaron, J. I., Jack, V. A., and Mela, D. J. (1997). Extended use of foods modified in fat and sugar content: Nutritional implications in a free-living female population. *Am. J. Clin. Nutr.* **65,** 1867–1873.

136. Goldberg, G. R., Murgatroyd, P. R., McKenna, A. P., Heavey, P. M., and Prentice, A. M. (1998). Dietary compensation in response to covert imposition of negative energy balance by removal of fat or carbohydrate [see comments]. *Br. J. Nutr.* **80,** 141–147.

137. Mattes, R., Pierce, C. B., and Friedman, M. I. (1988). Daily caloric intake of normal-weight adults: Response to changes in dietary energy density of a luncheon meal. *Am. J. Clin. Nutr.* **48,** 214–219.

138. Rolls, B. J., Kim, S., McNelis, A. L., Fischman, M. W., Foltin, R. W., and Moran, T. H. (1991). Time course of effects of preloads high in fat or carbohydrate on food intake and hunger ratings in humans. *Am. J. Physiol.* **260,** R756–R763.

139. Rolls, B. J., Pirraglia, P. A., Jones, M. B., and Peters, J. C. (1992). Effects of olestra, a noncaloric fat substitute, on daily energy and fat intakes in lean men. *Am. J. Clin. Nutr.* **56,** 84–92.

140. van het Hof, K. H., Weststrate, J. A., van den Berg, H., Velthuis-te, W. E., de Graaf, C., Zimmermanns, N. J., Westerterp, K. R., Westerterp-Plantenga, M. S., and Verboerket-van, D. V. (1997). A long-term study on the effect of spontaneous consumption of reduced fat products as part of a normal diet on indicators of health. *Int. J. Food Sci. Nutr.* **48,** 19–29.

141. Keen, H., Thomas, B. J., Jarrett, R. J., and Fuller, J. H. (1979). Nutrient intake, adiposity, and diabetes. *Br. Med. J.* **1,** 655–658.

142. Bolton-Smith, C., and Woodward, M. (1994). Dietary composition and fat to sugar ratios in relation to obesity. *Int. J. Obes. Relat. Metab. Disord.* **18,** 820–828.

143. Gibson, S. A. (1996). Are diets high in non-milk extrinsic sugars conducive to obesity? An analysis from the dietary and nutritional survey of British adults. *J. Hum. Nutr. Diet.* **9,** 283A–292A.

144. Gibson, S. A. (1996). Are high-fat, high-sugar foods and diets conducive to obesity? *Int. J. Food Sci. Nutr.* **47.** 405B–415B.

145. Kaufmann, N. A., Poznanski, R., and Guggenheim, K. (1975). Eating habits and opinions of teenagers on nutrition and obesity. *J. Am. Diet. Assoc.* **66,** 264–268.

146. Lewis, C. J., Park, Y. K., Dexter, P. B., and Yetley, E. A. (1992). Nutrient intakes and body weights of persons consuming high and moderate levels of added sugars. *J. Am. Diet. Assoc.* **92,** 708–713.

147. Stam-Moraga, M. C., Kolanowski, J., Dramaix, M., De Backer, G., and Kornitzer, M. D. (1999). Sociodemographic and nutritional determinants of obesity in Belgium. *Int. J. Obes.* **23,** 1–9.

148. Morgan, K. J., Johnson, S. R., and Stampley, G. L. (1983). Children's frequency of eating, total sugar intake and weight/ height stature. *Nutr. Res.* **3,** 635–652.

149. Cotton, J. R., Burley, V. J., Weststrate, J. A., and Blundell, J. E. (1996). Fat substitution and food intake: Effect of replacing fat with sucrose polyester at lunch or evening meals. *Br. J. Nutr.* **75,** 545A–556A.

150. de Graaf, C., and Hulshof, T. (1995). The effect of nonabsorbable fat on energy and fat intake. *Eur. J. Med. Res.* **1,** 72–77.

151. de Graaf, C., Hulshof, T., Weststrate, J. A., and Hautvast, J. G. (1996). Nonabsorbable fat (sucrose polyester) and the regulation of energy intake and body weight. *Am. J. Physiol.* **270,** R1386–R1393.

152. Hill, J. O., Seagle, H. M., Johnson, S. L., Smith, S., Reed, G. W., Tran, Z. V., Cooper, D., Stone, M., and Peters, J. C. (1998). Effects of 14 d of covert substitution of olestra for conventional fat on spontaneous food intake. *Am. J. Clin. Nutr.* **67,** 1178–1185.

153. Westerterp-Plantenga, M. S., Wijckmans-Duijsens, N. E., ten Hoor, F., and Weststrate, J. A. (1997). Effect of replacement of fat by nonabsorbable fat (sucrose polyester) in meals or snacks as a function of dietary restraint. *Physiol. Behav.* **61,** 939–947.

154. Anderson, G. H., Savavis, S., Schacher, R., Zlotkin, S., and Leiter, L. A. (1989). Aspartame: Effect on lunch-time food intake, appetite and hedonic response in children. *Appetite* **13,** 93–103.

155. Beridot-Therond, M. E., Arts, I., Fantino, M., and De, L. G. (1998). Short-term effects of the flavour of drinks on ingestive behaviours in man. *Appetite* **31,** 67–81.

156. Black, R. M., Tanaka, P., Leitter, L. A., and Anderson, G. H. (1991). Soft drinks with aspartame: Effect on subjective hunger, food selection, and food intake of young adult males. *Physiol. Behav.* **49,** 803–810.

157. Black, R. M., Leiter, L. A., and Anderson, G. H. (1993). Consuming aspartame with and without taste: Differential effects on appetite and food intake of young adult males. *Physiol. Behav.* **53,** 459–466.

158. Birch, L. L., McPhee, L., and Sullivan, S. (1989). Children's food intake following drinks sweetened with sucrose or aspartame: Time course effects. *Physiol. Behav.* **45,** 387–395.

159. Canty, D. J., and Chan, M. M. (1991). Effects of consumption of caloric vs noncaloric sweet drinks on indices of hunger and food consumption in normal adults. *Am. J. Clin. Nutr.* **53,** 1159–1164.

160. Drewnowski, A., Massien, C., Louis-Sylvestre, J., Fricker, J., Chapelot, D., and Apfelbaum, M. (1994). The effects of aspartame versus sucrose on motivational ratings, taste prefer- ences, and energy intakes in obese and lean women. *Int. J. Obes. Relat. Metab. Disord.* **18,** 570A–578A.

161. Drewnowski, A., Massien, C., Louis-Sylvestre, J., Fricker, J., Chapelot, D., and Apfelbaum, M. (1994). Comparing the effects of aspartame and sucrose on motivational ratings, taste preferences, and energy intakes in humans. *Am. J. Clin. Nutr.* **59,** 338B–345B.

162. Lavin, P. T., Sanders, P. G., Mackey, M. A., and Kotsonis, F. N. (1994). Intense sweeteners use and weight change among women: A critique of the Stellman and Garfinkel study. *J. Am. Coll. Nutr.* **13,** 102–105.

163. Mattes, R. (1990). Effects of aspartame and sucrose on hunger and energy intake in humans. *Physiol. Behav.* **47,** 1037–1044.

164. Rodin, J. (1990). Comparative effects of fructose, aspartame, glucose, and water preloads on calorie and macronutrient intake. *Am. J. Clin. Nutr.* **51,** 428–435.

165. Rogers, P. J., Carlyle, J. A., Hill, A. J., and Blundell, J. E. (1988). Uncoupling sweet taste and calories: Comparison of the effects of glucose and three intense sweeteners on hunger and food intake. *Physiol. Behav.* **43,** 547–552.

166. Rogers, P. J., Pleming, H. C., and Blundell, J. E. (1990). Aspartame ingested without tasting inhibits hunger and food intake. *Physiol. Behav.* **47,** 1239–1243.

167. Rogers, P. J., Keedwell, P., and Blundell, J. E. (1991). Further analysis of the short-term inhibition of food intake in humans by the dipeptide L-aspartyl-L-phenylalanine methyl ester (aspartame). *Physiol. Behav.* **49,** 739–743.

168. Rolls, B. J., Hetherington, M., and Laster, L. J. (1988). Comparison of the effects of aspartame and sucrose on appetite and food intake. *Appetite* **11**(Suppl. 1), B62–B67.

169. Rolls, B. J., Kim, S., and Fedoroff, I. C. (1990). Effects of drinks sweetened with sucrose or aspartame on hunger, thirst and food intake in men. *Physiol. Behav.* **48,** 19–26.

170. Ryan-Harshman, M., Leiter, L. A., and Anderson, G. H. (1987). Phenylalanine and aspartame fail to alter feeding behavior, mood and arousal in men [see comments]. *Physiol. Behav.* **39,** 247–253.

171. Van Itallie, T. B., Yang, M. U., and Porikos, K. P. (1988). Use of aspartame to test the "body weight set point" hypothesis. *Appetite* **11(Suppl. 1),** 68–72.

172. Barkeling, B., Rossner, S., and Bjorvell, H. (1990). Effects of a high-protein meal (meat) and a high-carbohydrate meal (vegetarian) on satiety measured by automated computerized monitoring of subsequent food intake, motivation to eat and food preferences. *Int. J. Obes.* **14,** 743–751.

173. Booth, D. A, Chase, A., and Campbell, A. T. (1970). Relative effectiveness of protein in the late stages of appetite suppression in man. *Physiol. Behav.* **5,** 1299–1302.

174. Hill, A. J., and Blundell, J. E. (1990). Sensitivity of the appetite control system in obese subjects to nutritional and serotoninergic challenges. *Int. J. Obes.* **14,** 219–233.

175. Johnson, J., and Vickers, Z. (1993). Effects of flavor and macronutrient composition of food servings on liking, hunger and subsequent intake. *Appetite* **21,** 25–39.

176. Johnstone, A. M., Stubbs, R. J., and Harbron, C. G. (1996). Effect of overfeeding macronutrients on day-to-day food intake in man. *Eur. J. Clin. Nutr.* **50,** 418–430.

177. Latner, J. D., and Schwartz, M. (1999). The effects of a high-carbohydrate, high-protein or balanced lunch upon later food intake and hunger ratings. *Appetite* **33,** 119–128.

178. Poppitt, S. D., McCormack, D., and Buffenstein, R. (1998). Short-term effects of macronutrient preloads on appetite and energy intake in lean women. *Physiol. Behav.* **64,** 279–285.

179. Stubbs, R. J., van Wyk, M. C., Johnstone, A. M., and Harbron, C. G. (1996). Breakfasts high in protein, fat or carbohydrate: Effect on within-day appetite and energy balance. *Eur. J. Clin. Nutr.* **50,** 409B–417B.

180. Wadden, T. A., Stunkard, A. J., Day, S. C., Gould, R. A., and Rubin, C. J. (1987). Less food, less hunger: Reports of appetite and symptoms in a controlled study of a protein-sparing modified fast. *Int. J. Obes.* **11,** 239–249.

181. Geliebter, A. A. (1979). Effects of equicaloric loads of protein, fat, and carbohydrate on food intake in the rat and man. *Physiol. Behav.* **22,** 267–273.

182. Johnstone, A. M., Shannon, E., Whybrow, S., Reid, C. A., and Stubbs, R. J. (2000). Altering the temporal distribution of energy intake with isoenergetically dense foods given as snacks does not affect total daily energy intake in normal-weight men. *Br. J. Nutr.* **83,** 7–14.

183. Lang, V., Bellisle, F., Oppert, J. M., Craplet, C., Bornet, F. R., Slama, G., and Guy-Grand, B. (1999). Satiating effect of proteins in healthy subjects: A comparison of egg albumin, casein, gelatin, soy protein, pea protein, and wheat gluten. *Am. J. Clin. Nutr.* **67,** 1197–1204.

184. Lang, V., Bellisle, F., Alamowitch, C., Craplet, C., Bornet, F. R., Slama, G., and Guy-Grand, B. (1999). Varying the protein source in mixed meal modifies glucose, insulin and glucagon kinetics in healthy men, has weak effects on subjective satiety and fails to affect food intake. *Eur. J. Clin. Nutr.* **53,** 959–965.

185. Rolls, B. J., Hetherington, M., and Burley, V. J. (1988). The specificity of satiety: The influence of foods of different macronutrient content on the development of satiety. *Physiol. Behav.* **43,** 145A–A153.

186. Sunkin, S., and Garrow, J. S. (1982). The satiety value of protein. *Hum. Nutr. Appl. Nutr.* **36,** 197–201.

187. Stockley, L., Jones, F. A., and Broadhurst, A. J. (1984). The effects of moderate protein or energy supplements on subsequent nutrient intake in man. *Appetite* **5,** 209–219.

188. Araya, H., Hills, J., Alvina, M., and Vera, G. (2000). Short-term satiety in preschool children: A comparison between a high protein meal and a high complex carbohydrate meal. *Int. J. Food Sci. Nutr.* **51,** 119–124.

189. Marmonier, C., Chapelot, D., and Louis-Sylvestre, J. (2000). Effects of macronutrient content and energy density of snacks consumed in a satiety state on the onset of the next meal. *Appetite* **34,** 161–168.

190. Marckmann, P. (1994). Fat from fish oil? *Int. J. Obes.* **18,** 185.

191. Simon, M. S., Heilbrun, L. K., Boomer, A., Kresge, C., Depper, J., Kim, P. N., Valeriote, F., and Martino, S. (1997). A randomized trial of a low-fat dietary intervention in women at high risk for breast cancer. *Nutr. Cancer* **27,** 136–142.

192. Bloomberg, B. P., Kromhout, D., Goddijn, H. E., Jansen, A., and Obermann-de Boer, G. L. (1991). The impact of the Guidelines for a Healthy Diet of The Netherlands Nutrition Council on total and high density lipoprotein cholesterol in hypercholesterolemic free-living men. *Am. J. Epidemiol.* **134,** 39–48.

193. Stefanick, M. L., Mackey, S., Sheehan, M., Ellsworth, N., Haskell, W. L., and Wood, P. D. (1998). Effects of diet and exercise in men and postmenopausal women with low levels of HDL cholesterol and high levels of LDL cholesterol. *N. Eng. J. Med.* **339,** 12–20.

194. Singh, R. B., Rastogi, S. S., Verma, R., Laxmi, B., Singh, R., Ghosh, S., and Niaz, M. A. (1992). Randomised controlled trial of cardioprotective diet in patients with recent acute myocardial infarction: results of one year follow up [see comments]. *Br. Med. J.* **304,** 1015–1019.

195. Lee-Han, H., Cousins, M., Beaton, M., McGuire, V., Kriukov, V., Chipman, M., and Boyd, N. (1988). Compliance in a randomized clinical trial of dietary fat reduction in patients with breast dysplasia. *Am. J. Clin. Nutr.* **48,** 575–586.

196. Raben, A., Jensen, N. D., Marckmann, P., Sandstrom, B., and Astrup, A. (1995). Spontaneous weight loss during 11 weeks' ad libitum intake of a low fat/high fiber diet in young, normal weight subjects. *Int. J. Obes. Relat. Metab. Disord.* **19,** 916–923.

197. Jeffrey, R. W., Hellerstedt, W. L., French, S. A., and Baxter, J. E. (1995). A randomized trial of counseling for fat restriction versus calorie restriction in the treatment of obesity. *Int. J. Obes. Relat. Metab. Disord.* **19,** 132–137.

198. Siggaard, R., Raben, A., and Astrup, A. (1996). Weight loss during 12 weeks' ad libitum carbohydrate-rich diet in overweight and normal-weight subjects at a Danish work site. *Obes. Res.* **4,** 347–356.

199. Pritchard, J. E., Nowson, C. A., and Wark, J. D. (1996). Bone loss accompanying diet-induced or exercise-induced weight loss: A randomised controlled study. *Int. J. Obes. Relat. Metab. Disord.* **20,** 513–520.

200. Shah, M., McGovern, P., French, S., and Baxter, J. (1994). Comparison of a low-fat, ad libitum complex-carbohydrate diet with a low-energy diet in moderately obese women. *Am. J. Clin. Nutr.* **59,** 980–984.

201. Hunninghake, D. B., Stein, E. A., Dujovne, C. A., Harris, W. S., Feldman, E. B., Miller, V. T., Tobert, J. A., Laskarzewski, P. M., Quiter, E., and Held, J. (1993). The efficacy of intensive dietary therapy alone or combined with lovastatin in outpatients with hypercholesterolemia [see comments]. *N. Engl. J. Med.* **328,** 1213–1219.

202. Boyd, N. F., Cousins, M., Beaton, M., Fishell, E., Wright, B., Fish, E., Kruikov, V., Lockwood, G., Tritchler, D., and Hanna, W. (1988). Clinical trial of low-fat, high-carbohydrate diet in subjects with mammographic dysplasia: Report of early outcomes. *J. Natl. Cancer Inst.* **80,** 1244–1248.

203. Insull, W. J., Henderson, M. M., Prentice, R. L, Thompson, D. J., Clifford, C., Goldman, S., Gorbach, S., Moskowitz, M., Thompson, R., and Woods, M. (1990). Results of a randomized feasibility study of a low-fat diet. *Arch. Intern. Med.* **150,** 421–427.

204. Buzzard, I. M., Asp, E. H., Chlebowski, R. T., Boyar, A. P., Jeffrey, R. W., Nixon, D. W., Blackburn, G. L., Jochimsen, P. R., Scanlon, E. F., and Insull, W. J. (1990). Diet intervention methods to reduce fat intake: Nutrient and food group composition of self-selected low-fat diets. *J. Am. Diet. Assoc.* **90,** 42–50, 53.

205. Toubro, S, and Astrup, A. (997). Randomised comparison of diets for maintaining obese subjects' weight after major weight loss: Ad lib, low fat, high carbohydrate diet v fixed energy intake. *Br. Med. J.* **314,** 29–34.

206. Kasim, S. E., Martino, S., Kim, P. N., Khilnani, S., Boomer, A., Depper, J., Reading, B. A., and Heilbrun, L. K. (1993). Dietary and anthropometric determinants of plasma lipopro-

teins during a long-term low-fat diet in healthy women. *Am. J. Clin. Nutr.* **57,** 146–153.

207. Schlundt, D. G., Hill, J. O., Pope-Cordle, J., Arnold, D., Virts, K. L., and Katahn, M. (1993). Randomized evaluation of a low fat ad libitum carbohydrate diet for weight reduction. *Int. J. Obes. Relat. Metab. Disord.* **17,** 623–629.

208. Sheppard, L., Kristal, A. R., and Kushi, L. H. (1991). Weight loss in women participating in a randomized trial of low-fat diets. Am. J. Clin. Nutr. **54,** 821–828.

209. Ornish, D., Brown, S. E., Scherwitz, L. W., Billings, J. H., Armstrong, W. T., Ports, T. A., McLanahan, S. M., Kirkeeide, R. L., Brand, R. J., and Gould, K. L. (1990). Can lifestyle changes reverse coronary heart disease? The Lifestyle Heart Trial [see comments]. *Lancet* **336,** 129–133.

210. Hill, J. O., Melanson, E. L., and Wyatt, H. T. (2000). Dietary fat intake and regulation of energy balance: Implications for obesity. *J. Nutr.* **130,** 284S–288S.

211. Food Marketing Institute (1999). "Trends in the United States—Consumer Attitudes and the Supermarket." Food Marketing Institute, Washington, DC.

212. Mokdad, A. H., Serdula, M. K., Dietz, W. H., Bowman, B. A., Marks, J. S., and Koplan, J. P. (1999). The spread of the obesity epidemic in the United States, 1991–1998. *JAMA* **282,** 1519–1522.

213. Calorie Control Council (2000). Most popular low calorie, sugar free products: Trends and statistics, Calorie Control Council national consumer survey. Available at http://www.caloriecontrol.org/.

CHAPTER **34**

Behavioral Risk Factors for Obesity: Diet and Physical Activity

NANCY E. SHERWOOD, MARY STORY, AND DIANNE NEUMARK-SZTAINER
University of Minnesota, Minneapolis, Minnesota

I. INTRODUCTION

Obesity is a significant problem that affects children, adolescents, and adults across gender, race, and socioeconomic strata. Dramatic increases in the prevalence of obesity in recent years have focused attention on this important public health problem. Comprehensive data of trends in the prevalence of obesity provided by national surveys (NHES I, 1960–1962; NHANES I, 1971–1974; NHANES II, 1976–1980; NHANES III, 1988–1994) show that the percentage of obese adults has increased over time, particularly during the past two decades (Fig. 1) [1]. The percentage of adults classified as obese, that is, those with a body mass index (BMI) $\geq$ 30 kg/m^2, increased from 14% in NHANES II to 23% in NHANES III. An additional 32% of adults in NHANES III were classified as overweight according to the BMI $\geq$ 25 kg/m^2 standard. According to these national data, an estimated 97 million adults (or 55% of the adult population) are classified as overweight. Prevalence rates of obesity and overweight among children and adolescents have also

increased dramatically since the mid-1960s and appear to be on the rise. NHANES data indicate that the prevalence of overweight (BMI $\geq$ 95th percentile) among youth doubled from 1976–1980 to 1988–1994, increasing from 8% to 14% for 6–11 year olds and from 6% to 12% for 12–17 year olds [2]. Currently about 11% of U.S. children and adolescents are overweight, and an additional 14% have a BMI between the 85th and 95th percentiles, indicating risk of overweight (Fig. 2). The higher prevalence of obesity among children is of particular concern given that childhood-onset obesity often tracks with adult obesity [3].

The alarming increase in the prevalence of obesity during the last few decades has raised concerns about associated health risks for children, adolescents, and adults. Persistence of this trend could lead to substantial increases in the number of people affected by obesity-related health conditions and premature mortality. The health risks associated with obesity are numerous and include hypertension, type 2 diabetes mellitus, dyslipidemia, stroke, gallbladder disease, osteoarthritis, sleep apnea, respiratory problems, and certain cancers (e.g.,

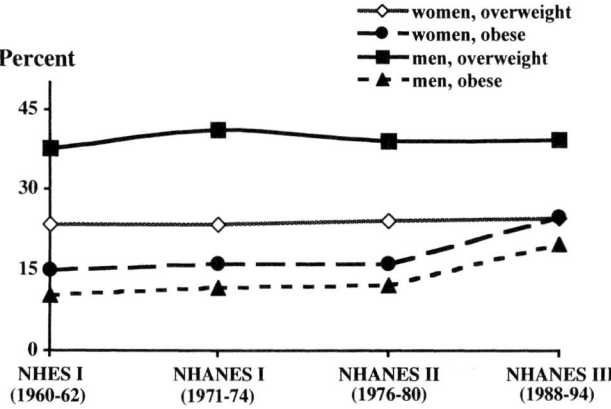

FIGURE 1 Proportion of overweight (BMI 26–29.9 kg/m^2) and obese (BMI $\geq$ 30 kg/m^2) adult men and women (by gender for selected years, United States 1960–1994). [Adapted from National Institutes of Health, National Heart, Lung and Blood Institute (1999). "Clinical Guidelines on the Identification, Evaluation, and Treatment of Overweight and Obesity in Adults." NHLBI, National Institutes of Health, Bethesda, MD.]

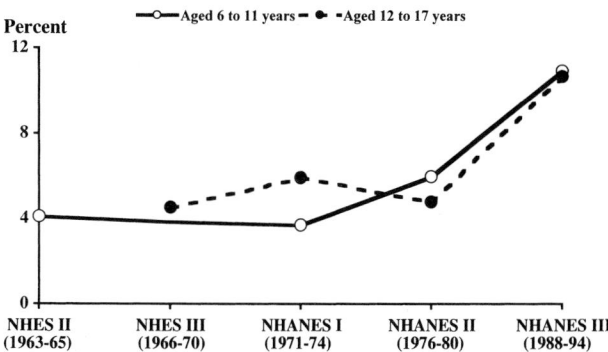

FIGURE 2 Proportion of overweight children and adolescents (by age for selected years, United States, 1963–1994). Overweight is defined as at or above the gender- and age-specific 95th percentile of BMI based on a preliminary analysis of data from the year 2000 growth charts. [Adapted from Troiano, R. P., and Flegal, K. M. (1998). Data reported in: Overweight children and adolescents: Description, epidemiology, and demographics. *Pediatrics* **101**(Suppl. 1), 497–504. Reproduced with permission from *Pediatrics*, Vol. 101, Pages S497–S504, Table 4, copyright 1998.]

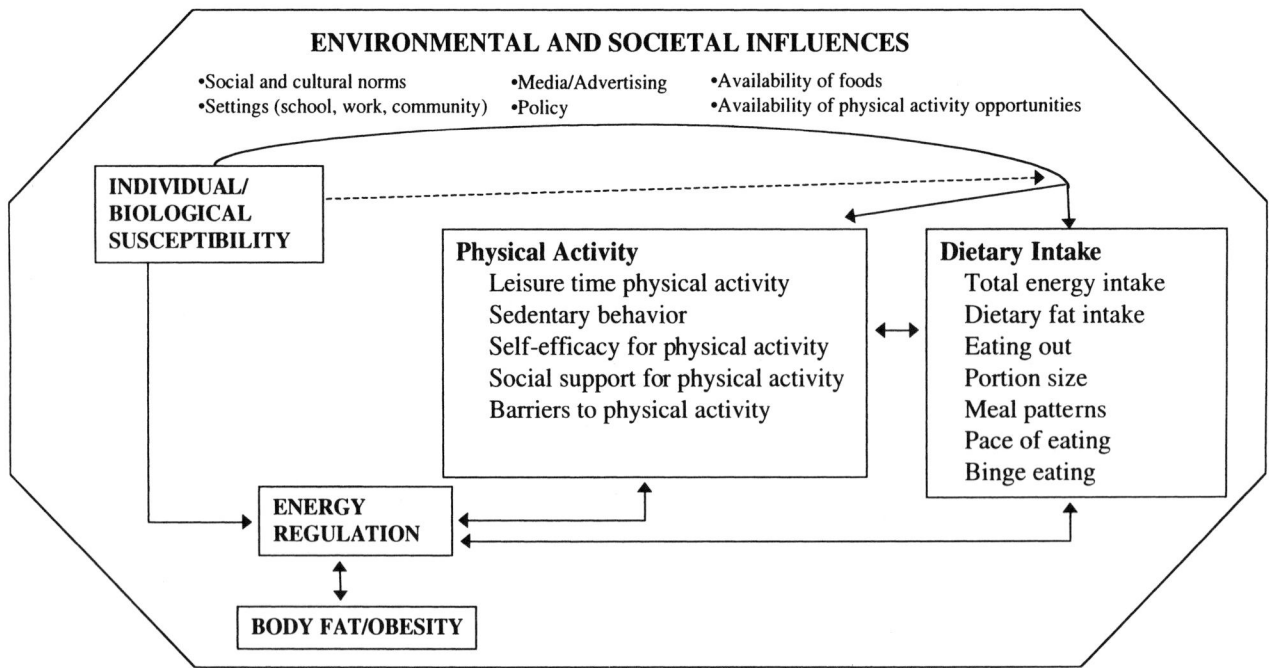

FIGURE 3   Influences on energy balance and obesity. This model shows the direct and indirect influence of biological susceptibility on energy regulation and obesity. This model also shows that both biological susceptibility and environmental factors influence dietary intake and physical activity, which, in turn, directly affect energy regulation and obesity. [Adapted with permission from World Health Organization (1997). "Obesity: Preventing and Managing the Global Epidemic," Report of a WHO Consultation on Obesity, Geneva, June 3–5, 1997. World Health Organization, Geneva.]

endometrial, breast, prostate, and colon) [3, 4]. Obesity is also associated with psychosocial problems such as binge eating disorders and depression for some individuals [5]. Individuals who are obese are also adversely impacted by social bias and discrimination [6–8]. The economic burden of obesity is sizable because of its impact on individual health, costs to society due to lost productivity, and premature mortality and treatment costs [9–11]. Estimates of the economic burden of obesity are as high as $100 billion per year [4].

Obesity and overweight are multidetermined chronic problems resulting from complex interactions between genes and an environment characterized by energy imbalance due to sedentary lifestyles and ready access to an abundance of food [3]. Research suggests that obesity runs in families and that some individuals are more vulnerable than others to weight gain and developing obesity [12]. Various mechanisms through which genetic susceptibility to weight gain have been proposed include low resting metabolic rate, low level of lipid oxidation rate, low fat-free mass, and poor appetite control [3]. Genetic research holds considerable promise for understanding the development of obesity and identifying those at risk for obesity. However, the rapid increase in rates of obesity has occurred over too brief a time period for there to have been significant genetic changes in the population. Although body weight is primarily regulated by a series of physiological processes, it is also influenced by behavioral and environmental factors [3]. Recent epide-

miological trends in obesity have been linked to behavioral and environmental changes that have occurred in recent years. The higher proportion of fat and the higher energy density of the diet in combination with reductions in physical activity levels and increases in sedentary behavior have been implicated as significant contributors to the obesity epidemic [3, 4]. Importantly, these dietary and activity behavioral risk factors are modifiable and can be targets for change in obesity prevention and treatment efforts.

Understanding the determinants of obesity and developing appropriate prevention and treatment strategies requires an in-depth examination of behavioral risk factors for obesity. The goal of this chapter is to review available data regarding behavioral and environmental determinants of dietary intake and physical activity and to discuss implications for future public health research and intervention. The review will focus on behavioral risk factors for obesity in both children and adults. Figure 3 presents a conceptual model for understanding how behavior risk factors influence weight regulation and obesity.

II. PHYSICAL ACTIVITY

This section examines the role of physical activity in the development of obesity. Multiple factors that influence physical activity levels will be discussed, including sedentary be-

havior, psychological variables such as self-efficacy, social support, and environmental and societal influences.

Prominent among the health benefits associated with a physically active lifestyle is the protective effect of physical activity on obesity. An abundance of cross-sectional research shows that lighter individuals are more active than heavier individuals and prospective research indicates that changes in physical activity level are associated with changes in body weight in the direction predicted by the energy balance equation [13–22]. The majority of studies conducted in children also find that physical activity levels and body weight are negatively associated [23]. Exercise has also been shown to improve short- and long-term weight loss in experimental studies in both children and adults [19, 23].

A. Prevalence of Leisure-Time Physical Activity in Adults

Despite the benefits of physical activity for body weight regulation and health, we are in the midst of a sedentary behavior epidemic. Only 15% of U.S. adults engage regularly in vigorous physical activity during leisure time, defined as 3 times a week for a minimum of 20 minutes [24]. Only 22% of adults report engaging in regular physical activity, defined as a minimum of 30 minutes of moderate to vigorous activity on most days of the week [24]. Twenty-five percent of adults report that they never engage in physical activity during leisure time [24]. Demographic differences in physical activity levels have also been observed, with men more likely to be physically active than women [25]. Approximately 60% of American women do not participate in any form of regular physical activity [26, 27]. Physical activity also declines with age, with women experiencing a greater decline in older age groups than men [27]. African-American and Hispanic adults are less physically active than Caucasians [24, 26]. Education and income are also both positively associated with physical activity level [25, 28–30].

B. Prevalence of Leisure-Time Physical Activity in Youth

Although estimates of physical activity levels among youth are slightly higher than self-reports by adults, the prevalence of regular physical activity is still surprisingly low. According to data from the Youth Risk Behavior Survey (YRBS) and the National Health Interview Survey–YRBS, about half of young people in the United States (age 12–21) regularly participate in vigorous physical activity, with one-fourth reporting no vigorous physical activity and 14% reporting no vigorous or light to moderate physical activity [24]. Data from the National Children and Youth Fitness studies [31, 32] indicate that about 60% of children in elementary through the high school years reported engaging in moderate to higher intensity physical activities throughout the year. Similar to activity patterns with adults, girls tend to be less active than boys and declines with age are more striking for girls compared to boys [24]. African-American girls, in particular, appear to be at greater risk for inactivity [24]. Representative survey data on the physical activity patterns of young children are not available, in part because of methodological difficulties in collecting such data from children. Young children are limited in their ability to accurately recall their activity patterns and the unplanned, unstructured nature of children's physical activity patterns does not lend itself well to the self-report format employed in large-scale surveys.

C. Sedentary Behavior

Although low levels of leisure-time physical activity likely contribute to the epidemic of obesity, it is noteworthy that among adults, leisure-time activity has remained stable or increased since the mid-1980s, the time period during which the prevalence of obesity increased [24]. The past century, however, has produced dramatic changes in physical activity patterns in the United States. Machines with motors have replaced human labor in virtually every aspect of life, so that the energy expenditure now required for daily life is a fraction of what it was a generation or two ago. The consequences of this dramatic change are far reaching and only now are beginning to be carefully studied. It is likely that increases in sedentary activities such as television watching and computer use and decreases in lifestyle, household, and occupational activity that have been less carefully measured have contributed to reductions in overall energy expenditure at the population level. Television viewing is a major source of inactivity and has received considerable attention as a risk factor for obesity [33–35]. In addition to potentially contributing to lower energy expenditure by displacing time potentially spent in more active pursuits, television viewing has been hypothesized to contribute to excess energy intake. Television watching can serve as a cue for eating given the numerous references to food and commercials for food, often high-fat, high-calorie foods, on television [35, 36].

According to data provided by A.C. Nielsen Company, the average household television set was turned on for more than 7 hours per day in 1998 [37]. Survey data estimating the frequency of television watching are necessary, however, because television viewing is not necessarily the primary activity when the television set is turned on. Data from the Americans' Use of Time study show that free time spent watching television increased from about 10.4 hours per week in 1965 to about 15.1 hours in 1985 [38]. Survey data from adults also indicate that time spent watching television averages about 2–3 hours a day [39–41]. Dietz and Gortmaker [35] report that children in the United States spend, on average, as much time watching television each year as they do attending school. Data from the 1990 YRBS showed that more than 70% of students in grades 9 through 12 reported watching at least 1 hour of television each school day

and more than 35% reported watching television 3 or more hours per day [42]. Other national data show that the average amount of television viewing is about 5 hours per day among 10- to 15-year-old children [33]. About one-third of these children watched more than 5 hours per day and only 1% watched 0–2 hours per day.

Cross-sectional research has shown that there is generally a positive relationship between television watching and obesity in children [33, 35, 43–55] and adults [39, 40, 56, 57]. Prospective relationships between television watching and weight are unclear with some studies showing that frequency of television watching is weakly or moderately associated with future weight gain [35, 58, 59], and other studies not detecting an association [39]. Although it has been hypothesized that television watching influences obesity by replacing time that could otherwise be spent engaging in more active pursuits, only some studies have shown that children and adults who watch more television are less physically active [43, 48, 52, 56, 57]. Crawford et al. [39] caution that the link between obesity and television watching appears to be complex and that targeting television viewing alone would not be an adequate public health strategy for addressing the obesity epidemic. They also suggest that better ways of conceptualizing and measuring sedentary behavior are necessary to fully understand its impact on the development of obesity.

Despite the fact that relationships between sedentary behavior and obesity are somewhat unclear, intervention research with children and adolescents that has focused on reducing television watching shows promise as an obesity prevention and treatment strategy. The work of Epstein et al. [36, 60–62] has figured prominently in the literature on decreasing sedentary activity as a strategy for promoting higher levels of physical activity. According to Epstein, the principles of behavioral economics or behavioral choice theory can be applied to sedentary individuals who, given the opportunity to choose between sedentary and physically active alternatives, will consistently choose the sedentary alternative. Choice of a given alternative, in this case, sedentary behavior, depends on the behavioral "cost" of that choice. Epstein argues and has demonstrated empirically in the laboratory that reducing the accessibility of sedentary behaviors or increasing the cost of being sedentary are both methods for reducing sedentary behavior. Epstein and colleagues [60] have also demonstrated that obese children participating in family-based weight control programs show the best changes when they are reinforced for being less sedentary as opposed to being reinforced for being more active.

School-based research targeting change in sedentary behaviors also shows promise. Robinson [63] conducted a small randomized trial in which one elementary school received an 18-lesson, 6-month classroom curriculum to reduce television, videotape, and video game use, and one school served as the control group. At follow-up, children in

the intervention school had lower BMIs, tricep skinfold thicknesses, waist circumferences, and waist-to-hip ratios relative to children in the control school. Significant differences were also observed in children's reported television viewing and meals eaten in front of the television although no signficant differences were observed for moderate-to-vigorous physical activity levels, cardiorespiratory fitness, or high-fat food intake. The Planet Health Program, another school-based obesity prevention trial, found that the decreasing television component of their multicomponent program appeared to contribute most to the decrease in prevalence of obesity observed among girls [64]. The effectiveness of reducing sedentary behaviors in preventing and treating obesity clearly deserves further exploration. One reason for the success of such strategies may be the simplicity or clarity of the intervention message.

D. Self-Efficacy for Physical Activity

Exercise self-efficacy is one of the strongest and most consistent predictors of exercise behavior. Self-efficacy predicts both exercise intention and several forms of exercise behavior [18, 65–75]. Self-efficacy is an individual's beliefs in his or her ability to successfully engage in a given behavior. It is theorized to influence the activities that individuals choose to approach, the effort expended on such activities, and the degree of persistence demonstrated in the face of failure or aversive stimuli [76]. Exercise self-efficacy is the degree of confidence an individual has in his or her ability to be physically active under a number of specific/different circumstances or, in other words, efficacy to overcome barriers to exercise [67]. Among adults, self-efficacy is thought to be particularly important in the early stages of exercise [71]. In the early stage of an exercise program, exercise frequency is related to one's general beliefs regarding physical abilities and one's confidence that continuing to exercise in the face of barriers will pay off. Self-efficacy has also been shown to be highly related to physical activity in youth. Children with higher perceived self-efficacy for physical activity and for overcoming barriers to physical activity were more active [77–80]. Gender differences in self-efficacy have also been observed, with boys reporting higher self-efficacy than girls [80].

Given that self-efficacy for exercise is such a strong predictor of exercise behavior, enhancing self-efficacy should figure prominently in physical activity intervention programs [81]. Strategies for enhancing self-efficacy could include teaching individuals how to overcome barriers to exercise, creating opportunities for positive experiences with physical activity, and providing positive feedback regarding exercise performance [72, 81, 82]. Self-monitoring can be also be used as a tool for those who exercise on their own to monitor performance and provide evidence regarding physical activity accomplishments [81, 83]. Emphasis should

also be placed on increasing girls' self-efficacy for exercise, given observed gender differences in exercise self-efficacy and physical activity levels.

E. Exercise History

Prior history of physical activity should positively influence future physical activity behavior by promoting and shaping self-efficacy for exercise and by developing physical activity skills. The observed relationship between exercise history and exercise behavior varies, however, depending on how exercise history is defined and the time period over which physical activity behavior is "tracked." Physical activity has been shown to track in early childhood [84]. Recent exercise history is generally predictive of future exercise behavior [85]. Childhood exercise history, however, is inconsistently related to physical activity in adulthood [68, 86]. Childhood physical activity experiences are also only modestly predictive of adult self-efficacy and exercise behavior [86]. The perception of the exercise experience as a child may be as important as amount of childhood exercise. One recent study found that recalling being forced to exercise as a child was associated with lower levels of physical activity in adulthood [87]. A child's enjoyment of physical activity [78, 80] and enjoyment of physical education experiences [88] are significant predictors of physical activity levels. Creating positive environments for physical activity for youth is likely a key factor in promoting higher levels of physical activity as a lifestyle habit.

F. Social Support for Physical Activity

Social support is another strong correlate of physical activity for both youth and adults. Adults who engage in regular exercise report more support for activity from people in their home and work environments [18, 68, 89, 90]. Adults who are initiating exercise programs are more likely to perceive their families as being supportive of their desire to maintain good health [91]. Additionally, individuals who joined a fitness program with their spouse had higher rates of adherence at 12 months compared to those who joined without a spouse [92]. Carron et al. [93] examined six major sources of social influence on physical activity, including important others such as physicians or work colleagues, family member, exercise instructors or other in-class professionals, co-exercisers, and members of exercise groups in a comprehensive review. The authors concluded that social influence generally has a small to moderate effect on exercise to behavior. Moderate to large effect sizes were found for family support and attitudes about exercise, important others and attitudes about exercise, and family support and compliance behavior.

Family support for physical activity is a robust correlate of physical activity for both boys and girls [77–79, 88]. Parental prompts for children to play outdoors instead of watching television or playing video games have been shown to positively influence children's activity levels [94]. Parental prompts to be active have also been shown to be related to young children's activity levels in some [95–97], but not all studies [98, 99]. Taylor et al. [100] argue that age of the child needs to be taken into account when understanding the impact of parental behavior on children's activity levels. Specifically, as children make the transition to school and spend more time in broader social contexts, other social influences may become more prominent. Not surprisingly, social support for physical activity from peers is also positively correlated with physical activity levels [31, 79]. Taylor et al. [100] also suggest that attention should be paid to children's perception of parents' social influence and potential adverse forms of social influence such as nagging, discouragement, or excessive pressure to be physically active.

G. Barriers to Physical Activity

1. TIME

Among adults, time constraints are the most frequent barriers to exercise and are reported by both sedentary and active individuals [89, 101]. Even among regular exercisers, scheduling efficacy remains an important and significant predictor of adherence [67]. Therefore, to maintain exercise adherence, regular exercisers have to become adept at dealing with time as a barrier. The time barrier may be a particular problem for certain population subgroups. For example, Schmitz et al. [102] reported that becoming a parent is associated with reductions in physical activity for mothers. Time spent caring for children may make it difficult for parents to maintain a regular physical activity program.

Several physical activity intervention approaches geared toward addressing the time barrier have been developed in recent years. Although group exercise programs can provide support and structure for participants, these advantages may be outweighed by the long-term costs involved in traveling to exercise sites at specific times for physical activity involvement [103]. Home-based physical activity programs appear to be a positive option for many adults [89, 104–108]. In the context of a weight loss program, Perri and colleagues [105] compared the effects of two exercise regimens, a group-based program versus a home-based program, on exercise participation, adherence, and fitness. Their results indicated that participants in the home-based program demonstrated better adherence and exercise performance data, particularly at 12-month follow-up. Two recent studies, which compared structured exercise program to a lifestyle approach, reported that the lifestyle program was as effective as the structured exercise program in improving physical activity and health outcomes including body weight and cardiorespiratory fitness [107, 108]. The recent focus on the health benefits of short bouts versus long bouts of activity given the public health recommendation to accumulate 30

minutes of physical activity on most days of the week also has implications for addressing the problem of time as a barrier to activity [109–113]. Short bouts of activity may be easier for people to incorporate into their schedules and may be particularly suitable for those initiating physical activity. Research suggests that multiple short bouts of exercise have been effective at promoting adherence to exercise programs [107, 108, 112, 113]. Interestingly, Epstein and colleagues [62, 114] have also reported that a lifestyle approach to exercise is associated with better adherence and greater weight loss in children.

2. Access

Another barrier that has received some attention in the determinants literature is access to exercise facilities. Distance between individuals' homes and exercise facilities has been shown to be negatively correlated with exercise behavior in adults [115]. Depending on an individual's activity preference, access to exercise facilities may or may not be related to exercise levels. For those individuals who prefer exercises such as walking or running, which can be done anywhere, access to facilities may be less relevant. Additionally, for those who exercise with home equipment, which could include stationary bikes, treadmills, and even exercise videos, access to facilities may also not affect exercise adherence. Regardless, the extent to which environments are conducive to physical activity (i.e., walking/biking paths, safe streets) likely has a strong impact on population activity levels. One recent study examining the association between neighborhood safety and sedentary behavior in a population-based sample found that there was a higher prevalence of physical inactivity among persons who perceived their neighborhoods as unsafe [116]. Better measurement of environmental resources for physical activity and strategies for improving access to physical activity facilities are needed.

3. Environmental Factors

Physical activity among youth appears to be particularly strongly influenced by environmental factors. First of all, the amount of time children spend playing outside has been shown to be a strong correlate of physical activity levels [98, 117]. Clearly, children who live in neighborhoods where play spaces are not adequate are going to have more difficulty achieving recommended levels of physical activity. Use of after-school time for sports and physical activity [88], access to community sports activities [80], and frequency of parents transporting children to activity locations have all been shown to be correlates of physical activity in boys and girls [99, 118]. The extent to which families have time and resources to support their children in physical activity pursuits will also have a strong impact on children's activity levels. Anecdotal reports suggest that children spend less time in unstructured physical activities (e.g., neighborhood pick-up games, hide and seek, tag) than in previous years. In contrast, there appears to have been an increase in community-

organized sports (e.g., traveling soccer and basketball teams) that require increased parental time, involvement, and financial resources. These factors may potentially contribute to decreases in physical activity and increased socioeconomic differences in physical activity and obesity risk among youth and is an area worthy of further exploration.

4. Overweight and/or Discomfort with Physical Activity

Clearly, body weight and physical activity are inextricably linked. Although it is clear that increasing physical activity is an important factor in regulating body weight, weight status may serve as a barrier to physical activity. Sedentary individuals may be heavier than those who initiate exercise programs [91]. This is due in part to physical activity being less pleasurable (i.e., it is uncomfortable for people to exercise when they are heavier), and in part because of embarrassment (i.e., individuals report feeling embarrassed about being seen in public in exercise clothes, at gyms, etc., due to weight status). However, weight status can also be a motivator for initiating exercise. One of the most common reasons adults give for exercising is weight control. Also, dieting to control weight is positively associated with frequency of participation in both high and moderate intensity physical activity [16]. Physical activity promotion programs, however, need to be modified to address the needs of overweight youth and adults.

Another important aspect of physical activity promotion for weight control is how much exercise to recommend. Data from studies of successful weight loss maintainers suggest that the optimal exercise recommendations for weight control likely exceed current public health recommendations. Optimal exercise levels for weight maintenance may be close to 1 hour of moderate to vigorous activity on most days of the week [119, 120]. This higher level of activity may be perceived as intimidating and difficult to achieve for those who have a history of sedentary behavior and are overweight. Strategies and support for helping individuals gradually increase their physical activity level while remaining injury free are needed.

III. DIETARY FACTORS

This section examines the role of dietary factors in the development of overweight and obesity. Multiple factors that influence food intake will be discussed, including the macronutrient composition of the diet, environmental and societal influences, and specific eating patterns.

A. Macronutrient Composition

1. Energy Intake

The relationship between trends in obesity and in greater fat or energy intake has not been clearly established. Labo-

ratory experiments in animals and human clinical studies have repeatedly shown that the level of fat and energy intake in the diet is strongly and positively related to excess body weight. In contrast, population-based surveys of diet and obesity have reported inconsistent results [3].

In adults, data from two national surveys suggest that energy intakes have increased slightly [121, 122], while in one national survey energy intake declined [123]. Findings from the USDA 1977–1978 Nationwide Food Consumption Survey (NFCS) and the USDA 1994–1996 Continuing Survey of Food Intakes of Individuals (CSFII) indicate that reported daily energy intakes increased from 2239 to 2455 calories in men and from 1534 to 1646 in women [122, 124]. Findings from NHANES I (1971–1974) and NHANES II (1976–1980) found that daily mean energy intakes were approximately 100–300 calories higher in NHANES III (1988–1994) compared to NHANES II [121]. Dietary data from the 1987 and 1992 National Health Interview Surveys suggest that energy intake declined slightly between 1997 and 1992 (on average about 100 calories/day) for adults [123].

Secular trends in energy intakes of youth aged 2–19 have also been examined. Data from NHANES found that mean energy intake changed little from the 1970s to 1988–1994, except for an increase among adolescent girls [125]. Between NHANES II and NHANES III, mean energy intake increased 1–4% among most age groups under age 20; mean intakes declined 3% for ages 6–11 years and increased 16% in females ages 16–19 years [126]. Among adolescent girls, energy intake increased by 225 calories. The increase between surveys for black females aged 12–19 was even larger at 249 calories. Mean energy intakes from the USDA's national food consumption surveys showed little change for young children and slightly lower mean intakes for adolescents in 1989–1991 compared to 1977–1978 [124].

The inconsistencies in secular-trend surveys have been attributed to a number of factors, including weaknesses in the study design, methodological flaws, confounders, and random or systematic measurement error in the dietary data [3]. For example, the procedural changes between NHANES II and III in dietary survey methodologies, and survey food coding and nutrient composition databases make comparisons between the two surveys difficult [121]. Some evidence suggests that people participating in nutrition surveys underreport the food they eat, either by completely omitting food items or by inaccurately estimating the amount eaten [122]. Underreporting of food intake is discussed below.

The mixed dietary results of national surveys and the paradoxical findings that energy and fat intakes have decreased or stayed about the same, despite an increase in overweight prevalence, has led some researchers to conclude that the observed trend in obesity is not related to a shift in energy and fat intake but rather a decline in physical activity. Secular trends in energy intake suggest that increased intake over time is not the major contributor to the increased prevalence of overweight among Americans and that decreased physical activity may play a more important role in overweight population prevalence [125]. However, given the problems inherent in measuring dietary intakes, and methodological survey issues, it should be noted that under more controlled laboratory conditions consistent findings show a strong association between dietary factors and obesity [3] (see Chapter 2, Energy Requirement Methodology).

In understanding the development of obesity, an important question is whether obese individuals eat more than leaner individuals. In most studies with both adults and children, energy intake has not been found to correlate with the degree of obesity [24]. However, this may be due, in part, to underreporting of food intake by the obese.

2. UNDERREPORTING OF FOOD INTAKE

In contrast to measures of body weight, dietary intake is difficult to measure accurately. Underreporting must be considered when interpreting dietary survey data. Studies have documented that food consumption is underreported by about 20–25% by people participating in dietary studies and occurs more often in women, overweight persons, and weight-conscious persons [121, 127, 128]. Discrepancies between reported energy intakes and measured energy expenditures (with the doubly labeled water method) of 20–50% have been described in overweight individuals [127, 129]. The systematic bias of underreporting in both overweight and nonoverweight individuals may be due to socially desirable responses, poor memory for foods consumed, lack of awareness of food consumed, difficulty with portion size estimation, or undereating (consuming less food than usual because of the requirement to record food intake). A recent study of underreporting of habitual food intake in obese men found that about 70% of the total underreporting was due to a diminished intake of food over the reporting period; that is, subjects changed their food patterns during the recording period [129]. Selective underreporting of fat intake was also found. The magnitude of underestimations observed in various studies indicates the considerable error in dietary intake data and highlights the need for improved techniques of data collection [130] (see discussion in Chapter 2).

3. FAT INTAKE

Dietary fat has a higher energy density than either protein or carbohydrates. Controversy remains about whether the percentage of dietary fat plays an important role in development of obesity and in its treatment once it has developed [131, 132]. There is evidence that consumption of high-fat diets increases total energy intake and that excess dietary fat is stored with a greater efficiency than similar excesses of dietary carbohydrate or protein [131, 133]. On the other hand, it has been argued that in short-term studies only a modest reduction in body weight is typically seen in individuals assigned to diets with a lower percentage of dietary fat,

which suggests that dietary fat does not play a role in the development of obesity [132]. Results of studies in laboratory animals and metabolic studies clearly and strongly show that a high percentage of fat in the diet relative to other macronutrients contributes to the development of obesity. These kinds of research, however, do not prove causality in humans [131, 133, 134]. It has also been pointed out that the focus on dietary fat may have been overemphasized at the expense of total energy intake. Total energy balance is what matters most and the focus on dietary fat intake must be viewed through its effects on total energy intake [133]. Reduction of dietary fat is one of the most practical ways to reduce energy density of the diet.

National data show that Americans have dramatically lowered the percent of energy intake from total fat during the last three decades. The reduction is from about 45% of energy in 1965 to about 34% in 1995 [135]. Levels, though, continue to be higher than the 30% recommended. Interestingly, the percent of calories from fat continued to decrease from 1990 to 1995 even as the daily grams of fat intake remained steady or increased. The explanation for this paradox is that although daily fat consumption was increasing or remained unchanged, the total caloric intake was increasing at a faster pace. A higher number of calories consumed will reduce the percentage of calories from fat even when there is no decrease in total fat consumption. Therefore, the decrease in percent of calories from fat observed recently may be a result of increased total caloric intake and not necessarily due to decreased fat consumption [135].

4. Sugar Intake

Americans are consuming record high amounts of caloric sweeteners, mainly sucrose and corn sweeteners. Per-capita consumption increased 45 pounds or 41% between 1950–1959 and 1997 [136]. In 1997, Americans consumed on average 154 pounds of caloric sweeteners and when adjusted for losses this is 33 teaspoons of added sugar per person per day [137]. Regular (nondiet) soft drinks are the major contributor of added sweeteners in the American diet and account for one-third of the intake of added sweeteners [138]. There has been a 47% increase in annual per-capita consumption of regular carbonated soft drinks, from 28 gallons per person in 1986 to 41 gallons in 1997.

Guthrie and Morton [138] found increased intake of regular soft drinks to be one of the major changes in children's diets between 1989–1991 and 1994–1995. High soft drink consumption may lead to excessive energy intake (a 12-ounce soft drink contains approximately 150 kcal), which theoretically may contribute to obesity. Harnack and colleagues [139] found that energy intake was positively associated with consumption of regular soft drinks. Energy intake was higher for those in the highest soft drink consumption category. In this study the association of obesity and soft drink consumption was not assessed. However, using NHANES III data, Troiano *et al.* [125] reported that soft drink energy contribution was higher among overweight children and adolescents.

There is no consensus regarding the role of sugar intake on body weight regulation. A preference for sweet-fat foods has been observed in obese individuals, which may be a factor in promoting excess energy consumption [3]. However, the notion that a sensory "sweet tooth," that is, a heightened preference for sweet taste, is a direct cause of obesity is not well supported [140].

B. Environmental Influences

1. U.S. Food Supply

Data of dietary levels of individuals provide key information on energy and nutrient intakes. However, food supply data can also provide a measure of changes in food consumption over time and estimated nutrient content of the food supply. Food supply data, also known as food disappearance data, reflect the amount of food commodities entering the market, regardless of final use. USDA's Economic Research Service (ERS) has developed methods to adjust the food supply for spoilage, plate waste, and other losses. USDA's Center for Nutrition Policy and Promotion provides food supply nutrient estimates derived from the ERS data [137]. These data are used as a proxy to estimate human consumption. Adjusted food supply data suggest that average daily calorie intake increased 14.7%, or about 340 calories, between 1984 and 1994.

USDA food supply data indicate that Americans are consuming record amounts of some high-fat dairy products (e.g., cheese) and caloric sweeteners and near record amounts of added fats, including salad and cooking oils and baking fats. The hefty increase in grain consumption reflects higher consumption of mostly refined rather than high-fiber, whole-grain products [136]. On the positive side, fruit and vegetable consumption continues to rise. Americans consumed about a fifth (22%) more fruit and vegetables in 1997 than in the 1970s [137]. Supermarket produce departments carry more than 400 produce items today, up from 250 in the late 1980s and 150 in the mid-1970s. Also, the number of ethnic and natural foodstores that offer fresh produce continue to increase [137].

The food industry has responded to consumer demand for lower fat products. For example, 2076 new food products introduced in 1996 claimed to be reduced in fat or fat free—nearly 16% of all new food products introduced that year, and more than twice the number just 3 years earlier. The number dropped in 1997 and it is unclear whether that represents a backlash to health concerns [141]. The Calorie Control Council reports a notable rise in the percentage of the U.S. population consuming low-calorie products: 19% of the population in 1978, 29% in 1984, and 76% in 1991 [142]. Still, the use of these products has not prevented the progression of obesity in the population. It should be pointed out that many commercially available low-fat or fat-free

foods are not lower in energy density than their full-fat counterparts [143].

2. EATING OUT

During the past 20 years, one of the most noticeable changes in eating patterns of Americans has been the increased popularity of eating out [144]. The proportion of meals and snacks eaten away from home increased by more than two-thirds between 1977–1978 and 1995, rising from 16% of all meals and snacks in 1977–1978 to 27% in 1995 [145]. Almost half of all adults (46%) were restaurant patrons on a typical day during 1998 [146]. Currently, almost half (47%) of a family's food budget is spent on away-from-home food [147]. In 1970, the family food expenditure on away-from-home eating was only 26% of total food spending [145]. The restaurant industry projects that in the 2000s, 53% of the food dollar will be spent away from home [146]. Food away from home includes foods obtained at restaurants, fast-food places, school cafeterias, and vending machines. A number of factors account for the increasing trend in eating out, including a growing number of working women (75% of women 25–50 years old are in the workforce), more two-earner households, higher incomes, a desire for convenience foods because of busy lifestyles and little time for preparing meals, more fast-food outlets offering affordable food, smaller families, and increased advertising and promotion by large food service chains and fast-food outlets [144].

The trend in eating out may be related to the observed increase in caloric intake among Americans, because food away from home is generally higher in calories and fat than food consumed at home [137, 145]. Many table-service restaurants provide 1000–2000 calories per meal, amounts equivalent to 35–100% of a full day's energy requirement for most adults [148]. Data from USDA's food intake surveys conducted during the past 20 years have been analyzed to compare the nutritional qualities of at-home and away-from-home foods and changes over time. In 1995, the average total fat and saturated fat content of away-from-home foods, expressed as a percentage of calories, was 38% and 13%, respectively, compared with 32% and 11% for at-home foods [145]. Foods eaten away from home provided 34% of total food energy consumption in 1995, up from 19% in 1977–1978. The 1995 data also suggest that, when eating out, people tend to eat larger amounts, eat higher calorie foods, or both [137]. Lin and colleagues [144] at the USDA calculated that if away-from-home food had the same average nutrient densities as food at home in 1995, Americans would have consumed 197 fewer calories per day, and reduced their fat intake to 31.5% of calories from fat (instead of 33.6%).

Consumers may view food differently when eating out than when eating at home. Consumers may view eating away from home as an exception to their usual dietary patterns, regardless of how frequently it occurs, and an opportunity to

"splurge" [149]. Consumers also may not be aware of the fat or calorie content of prepared foods because nutrition information is generally not provided in restaurants and other eating places. Restaurants generally do not provide detailed nutritional profiles of foods served, although some fast-food restaurants have this information available on request. New restaurant regulations mandate that menu items labeled as low-fat must comply with defined standards. However, consumers by and large must rely on their own knowledge to identify healthful menu options [149]. Because the trend of eating out is expected to increase even more in the next decade, nutrition interventions to improve the nutritional quality of food choices made away from home are needed. Such interventions should include both environmental changes (e.g., nutrition information on foods) and efforts to change consumer attitudes toward eating out and increase motivation to make healthier choices [145, 149].

3. FAST FOODS

Fast food has become a significant part of the American diet. In the United States, more than 200 people are served a hamburger every second of the day [3]. The number of fast-food outlets in the United States has risen steadily during the past 25 years, increasing from roughly 75,000 outlets in 1972 to almost 200,000 in 1997 [150]. Fast-food sales in the United States rose 56% to $102,387 million between 1988 and 1998 [151]. Many fast foods are high in fat. The fat density of fast foods is about 40% of total calories. Recently, several fast-food restaurants have introduced large-size burgers that are exceptionally high in fat and calories. For example, McDonald's Big Xtra with Cheese burger has 810 calories and 46 grams of fat; Burger King's Double Whopper with Cheese burger has 960 calories and 63 grams of fat; and Hardee's Monster Burger has 970 calories with 67 grams of fat. In addition, large soft drinks containing substantial amounts of sugar are often consumed as part of the fast-food meal and are high in calories [3, 145].

Several fast-food chains have tried to introduce reduced-fat entrees, but later withdrew them because of slow sales. For example, in 1991, McDonald's introduced the McLean Deluxe, which used a 91% fat-free beef patty, but due to slow sales and poor public acceptance it was taken off the market after a few years. Taco Bell introduced a line of low-fat menu items in 1994, called Border Lights, but these were also largely removed because of sluggish sales [150]. Many fast-food chains offer other low-fat items, such as grilled chicken sandwiches, wraps, and salads.

One notable trend in fast-food outlets is toward larger portion sizes or super sizes that give the impression of "better value" for money and encourage overeating. Increasing the portion size on beverages and french fries, two of the most profitable fast-food items, and offering a "trade-up" is a common menu option. For example, what used to be a large portion on the standard combo menu at one fast-food restaurant, that is, a 21-ounce beverage and 5 ounces of fries,

has been renamed medium. Customers can pay 40 cents to trade up to a 32-ounce beverage and 6-ounce fries, and another 40 cents to go up to the new top tier of 42-ounce soft drink and 7-ounce fries [152]. A 42-ounce soft drink has 410 calories and 7 ounces of fries has 610 calories.

Despite these food service trends, direct evidence that increased fast-food consumption leads to obesity is lacking. One recent study examined the relationship between fast-food eating and body mass index in 1059 adult men and women over 1 year. The researchers found that the number of meals eaten at fast-food restaurants per week was positively associated with energy intake and body mass index in women but not in men. The strongest relationship was observed among low-income women [58]. Another recent study assessed energy intake and the frequency of consuming food from seven fast-food and table-service restaurants in 73 adults [153]. The researchers found that the frequency of consuming restaurant food was positively associated with body fatness, and total daily energy intake and fat intake. More such studies are warranted to assess whether frequency of fast-food consumption and eating out is related to the secular trends in obesity prevalence in the United States and globally.

Fast-food outlets are receiving increasing competition from supermarkets and other establishments offering fully or partially prepared entrees or multicourse meals for eat-in or carry-out. On an average day in 1998, 21% of U.S. households used some form of takeout or delivery [146]. Home meal replacements, as they are called, are intended to be easily reheated in the oven or microwave and are designed to eliminate the need to cook at home by providing a wide variety of higher quality foods that are as convenient and affordable as fast food [150]. The widespread adoption of microwave ovens by U.S. households (now in nearly 90% of homes) contributes to the convenience of home meal replacements for takeout [150]. Driven by consumer demand for convenience due to hectic schedules, the market for home meal replacements will continue to rise. It is speculated that miniaturized outlets offering hot fast-food meals might one day be as common in public buildings as soft drink machines are today [150]. This speaks to the need for consumer education and nutrition labeling of these products.

4. CHANGING PORTION SIZES

It has been suggested that food portion sizes in food service establishments have become larger and thereby have increased energy intake, which may lead to obesity. However, empirical data to support this association are lacking. It is noticeable, though, that many restaurants, especially fast-food restaurants, in recent years are offering large and extra-large portion sizes of products and meals at low cost. A comparison of food service portion sizes during the past 30 years is remarkable. Putnam [137] reports that the typical fast-food outlet's hamburger in 1957 contained a little more than 1 ounce of cooked meat, compared with up to 6 ounces

in 1997. Soda pop was 8 ounces in 1957, compared with 32 ounces to 64 ounces in 1997. A theater serving of popcorn was 3 cups in 1957, compared with 16 cups (medium size popcorn) in 1997. A muffin was less than 1.5 ounces in 1957, compared with 5–8 ounces in 1997.

5. FOOD ADVERTISING

Advertising and promotion are central to the marketing of the American food supply. Although the food industry is certainly not to be blamed for the epidemic of obesity, because the food market is so competitive, advertising encourages Americans to eat and buy more palatable food. The U.S. food marketing system is the second largest advertiser in the economy (after the automobile industry), and a leading supporter of network, spot, and cable television, newspapers, magazines, billboards, and radio. The food industry spends about $11 billion annually on advertising; of this, about $7 billion was spent by food manufacturer's and $3 billion by food establishments, mainly fast-food restaurants [154]. Most of the advertising focuses on highly packaged and processed foods. Advertising expenditures on fruits and vegetables are negligible. In 1997–1998, advertising expenditures for candy and gum were $765 million, soft drinks $549 million, and McDonald's spent just over $1 billion [148, 154]. In contrast, the USDA spent $333.3 million on nutrition education, evaluation, and demonstrations. The food industry advertising expenditures also dwarf the National Cancer Institute's annual budget of $1 million for the educational component of the 5-a-Day campaign to promote fruit and vegetable consumption [148].

Television is the favorite medium used by the food industry [154]. Children are exposed to much television advertising. One study examined food advertising during children's Saturday morning television programming and found that over half (56%) of all advertisements were for food. The foods promoted were predominantly high in fat or sugar, and many were low in nutritional value. As such, the diet presented on Saturday morning television is the antithesis of what is recommended for healthful eating for children [155].

There is also a growing trend toward food commercialism and marketing in schools. Corporations are interested in the youth market to build brand loyalty and because they represent a large and growing market. A study by the Consumers Union Education Services [156] found that direct advertising in schools has mushroomed. Examples include school bus advertising for soft drinks and fast-food restaurants; "free" textbook covers advertising candy, chips, and soft drinks; ads for high-sugar, high-fat products on wall boards and in hallways, in student publications such as newsletters and yearbooks, and on sports scoreboards; and product giveaways in coupons. In addition, Channel One, the daily news program that is broadcast to millions of students in grades 6–12 in thousands of schools, has 2 minutes out of each daily 12-minute program devoted to paid commercials for products that include candy bars, snack chips, and soft drinks

[156]. A worrisome trend in schools is exclusive marketing agreements for soft drinks in vending machines. Some school districts have signed exclusive contracts and expect to generate as much as $11 million over a 10-year contract [157].

There is no evidence that food advertising is linked to the epidemic of obesity. It is unlikely that food advertising would have a direct influence on obesity. However, advertising does affect food choices. In halting the epidemic of obesity, the food industry needs to be involved with other sectors of society in developing public health strategies to prevent obesity and creating an environment that supports healthy eating. Policies to create more healthful environments for children are discussed later.

C. Eating and Dietary Practices

The majority of research examining the potential role of diet in the etiology of obesity has focused on associations between obesity and dietary intake (e.g., intake of energy, macronutrients, and food groups). As previously discussed, findings from this large body of research leave many questions unanswered. Fewer studies have examined associations between obesity and eating practices such as the pace of eating, meal patterns, dieting, and binge eating. In this section, we highlight some of the research that examines associations between specific eating practices and obesity, identifies questions that remain unanswered, and makes some recommendations based on this body of research for future studies and for interventions aimed at obesity prevention/treatment.

1. PACE OF EATING

Eating practices aimed at eating at a slower pace are often encouraged in obesity treatment programs. Efforts to slow down the pace of eating may assist certain individuals to consume smaller amounts of food. However, research findings comparing the pace of eating among overweight and nonoverweight individuals have not been consistent. Some studies have shown that overweight individuals do have a rapid eating pace [158–160]. However, other studies have not found a characteristic eating style among overweight individuals [161, 162]. Based on findings from their work and the work of others, Terri and Beck [162] have concluded that differences in eating behaviors between overweight and nonoverweight individuals are "extremely variable and cannot be presumed." Therefore, they suggest that individual assessment is required before embarking on a treatment program that attempts to modify eating behaviors in overweight individuals [162]. For overweight individuals who tend to eat large amounts of food at a quick pace, behavioral strategies aimed at slowing the pace of eating may be helpful, whereas for others these strategies may not be suitable.

2. MEAL PATTERNS

Concerns about skipping meals exist in that meals are important for ensuring an adequate nutrient intake, socializing (if done with family and/or friends), and for avoiding hunger, which may then lead to binge-eating episodes. Meal skipping has been found to be higher among overweight adolescents than among their nonoverweight peers. In a cross-sectional study of more than 8000 adolescents, usual breakfast consumption was reported by 53% of nonoverweight youth, 48% of moderately overweight youth (85th–95th percentile), and 43% of very overweight youth (BMI > 95th percentile) [163]. Due to the cross-sectional nature of these findings, it is not clear whether breakfast skipping leads to obesity (i.e., in that it may be associated with higher energy intake at later times in the day) or rather that breakfast-skipping was a consequence of obesity (i.e., meals are being skipped for weight control purposes).

Meal skipping is frequently used as a weight control method. Among adolescents and adults trying to control their weight, Neumark-Sztainer et al. [164] found that skipping meals was commonly reported; 18.6% of adult males and females, 22.8% of adolescent females, and 14.1% of adolescent males trying to control their weight reported skipping meals. An important question relates to the impact of skipping meals on overall energy and nutrient intake. In a study of women participating in a weight gain prevention study, skipping meals for weight control purposes was not associated with overall energy intake [165]. However, meal skippers reported higher percentages of total energy intake from fat and from sweets, lower percentages of total energy intake from carbohydrates, and lower fiber intakes than women who did not report meal skipping [165].

In summary, existing research suggests that meal skipping is associated with a poorer nutrient intake and with obesity status [163, 165, 166]. However, it is not clear whether meal skipping plays an etiological role in the onset of obesity or rather is a consequence of obesity. Prospective studies are needed to assess causality. However, in light of the inverse associations between meal skipping and nutrient intake, and the potential for leading to uncontrolled eating due to hunger, meal skipping should not be recommended as a weight control strategy. Rather, careful planning of meals with nutrient-dense foods that are low in fat and calories should be encouraged.

3. DIETING BEHAVIORS AND DIETARY RESTRAINT

Research findings clearly indicate that overweight individuals are more likely to report engaging in dieting and other weight control behaviors than nonoverweight individuals. For example, in a large cross-sectional study of adolescents, dieting behaviors were reported by 17.5% of underweight girls (BMI ≤ 15th percentile), 37.9% of average weight girls (BMI: 15th–85th percentile), 49.3% of moderately overweight girls (BMI: 85th–95th percentile), and 52.1% of very overweight girls (BMI ≥ 95th percentile)

[167]. Due to the cross-sectional nature of this study, it is not clear whether dieting led to higher BMI values or rather that overweight status led to increased dieting behaviors. The latter assumption is usually taken to be the more probable one in that social norms emphasize the importance of thinness, and overweight girls may be trying to modify their body weight to better fit these norms.

In a prospective study on adolescent girls by Stice and his colleagues [168], baseline dieting behaviors and dietary restraint were found to be associated with obesity onset 4 years later. After controlling for baseline BMI values, the hazard for obesity onset over the 4-year study period was 324% greater for baseline dieters than for baseline non-dieters. For each unit increase on the restraint scale, there was a corresponding 192% increase in the hazard for obesity onset [168]. These findings suggest that for some individuals self-reported dieting may be associated with a higher energy intake, and not a lower energy intake as intended. One explanation for this is that self-reported "dieting" may represent a temporary change in eating behaviors, which may be alternated with longer term eating behaviors that are not conducive to weight control. Another explanation is that self-reported dieting and dietary restraint may be associated with increased binge-eating episodes resulting from excessive restraint, control, and hunger. Indeed, Stice and his colleagues did report positive, albeit modest, associations between binge eating and both dieting behaviors ($r = 0.20$) and dietary restraint ($r = 0.20$). Other researchers have also suggested that dietary restraint may lead to binge-eating behaviors [169, 170], thereby placing individuals at risk for weight gain, rather than the intended weight loss or maintenance.

It is noteworthy that retrospective studies of adults who have been successful in losing weight and in maintaining their weight loss over extended periods of time suggest that modifications in eating and physical behaviors are helpful strategies. The National Weight Control Registry is a large study of individuals who have been successful at long-term maintenance of weight loss [119]. The most common dietary strategy used by these successful weight loss maintainers was limiting intake of certain types or classes of foods. Other commonly used dietary strategies included limiting quantities of food eaten, limiting the percentage of daily energy from fat, and counting calories. Meal patterns tended to be regular; on average, subjects reported eating nearly 5 times per day and only a small proportion ate less than 2 times per day. Also, most members of the registry reported increasing physical activity levels as part of their weight loss effort [119].

4. BINGE EATING

Overweight individuals are more likely to engage in binge-eating behaviors than their nonoverweight counterparts [5]. In a nonclinical sample of adult women enrolled in a weight gain prevention program, binge eating was reported by 9% of nonoverweight women and 21% of overweight women [171]. Furthermore, binge eating tends to be more prevalent among overweight individuals seeking treatment for weight loss. Based on a review of the literature, Devlin *et al.* [172] have estimated that between 25% and 50% of overweight people seeking treatment for weight loss engage in binge eating. Factors contributing to the higher rates of binge eating among overweight individuals, as compared to nonoverweight individuals, may include the following: greater appetites brought on by higher physiological needs of a larger body size, greater emotional disturbances (e.g., depressive symptoms) or different responses to stressful situations, greater exposure to stressful situations (e.g., related to weight stigmatization), increased weight preoccupation and dieting behaviors, and stronger dietary restraint.

In working with overweight individuals within health care and other settings, it is essential to be sensitive to the daily struggles they may face within thin-oriented societies. Overweight clients may be reluctant to share their binge-eating experiences; therefore a nonjudgmental attitude on the part of the health care provider is critical. For some individuals, hunger resulting from dieting or meal skipping may be a major cause of binge eating while for others binge eating may be a response to stress. Some individuals may be experiencing cyclical patterns; for example, emotional stress leads to binge eating, which leads to further emotional stress, which leads to further binge eating. Strategies for avoiding binge eating should be linked to factors that appear to be leading to binge eating for each individual.

5. FAMILY INFLUENCES ON DIETARY INTAKE AND EATING PRACTICES

Research has demonstrated that familial factors contribute to the etiology of obesity via genetic and shared environmental factors [173, 174]. A considerable amount of research has been devoted to the role of the family in the etiology, prevention, and treatment of obesity [175–177]. With regard to dietary intake and eating practices, questions arise as to how the family environment influences individual family members' eating behaviors and what the family can do to improve eating behaviors of its members. The aim is clearly to provide for an environment in which healthful food is available, eaten in an enjoyable manner, and consumed in appropriate amounts. Most of the research in this area has focused on the influence of parents on their children's eating behaviors.

Parents/caretakers may influence their children's dietary intake and eating practices via numerous channels. Some of the key channels include food availability within the home setting (including food purchasing, food preparation, and food accessibility), family meal patterns, infant and child feeding practices, role modeling of eating behaviors and body image attitudes, and verbal encouragement of specific eating practices.

In focus group discussions, adolescents reported that their parents influence their food choices in different ways: parental eating and cooking behaviors, parental food purchasing

patterns, parental concern about foods their children eat, family meal patterns, overall parent–child relations, and family cultural/religious practices [167]. Adolescents also perceived that they were more likely to eat healthier foods when eating meals with their families, than when eating in other situations [178, 179].

Research in the arena of adolescent health indicates that general family context variables are strongly associated with the emotional well-being of adolescents and with eating and other health-related behaviors [180]. For example, Neumark-Sztainer and her colleagues [181, 182] found that low family connectedness (i.e., perceived level of caring and communication within the family) placed adolescents at increased risk for inadequate intake of fruit, vegetables, and dairy foods. Furthermore, among overweight youth, Mellin and her colleagues [183] found that high family connectedness was associated with more regular breakfast eating, increased fruit and vegetable consumption, and lower rates of unhealthy dieting behaviors. These findings indicate the importance of a positive familial environment for adolescents and, in particular, for overweight youth who may be experiencing social stigmatization and need additional support.

An important question relates to how involved parents should be in their children's eating practices; that is, what is an appropriate parental role? Birch and her colleagues [184, 185] have examined associations between child-feeding practices and children's ability to regulate their energy intake. Birch and Fisher [184] have suggested that individual differences in self-regulation of energy intake are associated with differences in child-feeding practices and with children's adiposity. They state that "initial evidence indicates that imposition of stringent parental controls can potentiate preferences for high-fat, energy-dense foods, limit children's acceptance of a variety of foods, and disrupt children's regulation of energy intake by altering children's responsiveness to internal cues of hunger and satiety." In a study of 77 three- to five-year-old children, Johnson and Birch [185] found that children with greater body fat stores were less able to regulate energy intake accurately. The strongest predictor of children's ability to regulate energy intake was parental control in the feeding situation; mothers who were more controlling of their children's food intake had children who showed less ability to self-regulate energy intake ($r = -0.67$). They concluded from this study that "the optimal environment for children's development of self-control of energy intakes is that in which parents provide healthy food choices but allow children to assume control of how much they consume."

Parents of overweight children and adolescents are often in a difficult situation in that they want to be supportive of their children, yet also want to help them to modify behavioral patterns that may increase their risk of obesity. Furthermore, they may feel as though they are being blamed for their child's obesity. Existing research suggests that parental involvement and support is important [177, 183], but efforts to control a child's intake may be counterproductive [184,

185], Further studies are needed to explore how parents can best help their overweight children develop a positive self-image and healthy eating and physical activity behaviors.

IV. SUMMARY AND PUBLIC HEALTH RECOMMENDATIONS

We have reviewed the literature on key physical activity and diet-related risk factors for obesity in children and adults. Highlights of the review from the physical activity domain include (1) the importance of addressing the influence of both leisure-time physical activity and sedentary behavior to total energy expenditure, (2) the importance of fostering both self-efficacy and social support for physical activity to promote higher levels of physical activity, and (3) the influence of environmental factors on physical activity levels. Highlights related to dietary intake include (1) recognizing the contribution of both dietary fat intake and total energy intake to energy regulation; (2) the importance of accurately assessing portion size; (3) the influence of eating practices such as eating out, meal skipping, restrained eating and binge eating on obesity; and (4) social and environmental factors that promote excess energy intake.

To effectively combat the public health problem of obesity, interventions that target change in dietary intake and physical activity are necessary. Intervention efforts must take into account that dietary intake and physical activity are complex, multidetermined behaviors influenced by individual, social, and environmental factors. Although obesity intervention approaches have traditionally focused primarily on an individual's change, both individual- and population-level approaches are essential. Community-based interventions including school-based programs, after-school programs and work-site programs as well as clinic-based programs focused on diet, physical activity and weight management all have the potential to effectively address the problem of obesity. Environmental and policy interventions to prevent obesity have also begun to receive greater attention [103, 148, 186].

A. School and Community-Based Youth Programs

The increasing prevalence of obesity in adults and children, coupled with difficulty in successfully treating adult obesity, highlight the urgent need for prevention approaches geared toward children. Table 1 provides an overview of essential components for obesity prevention programs in schools. School-based programs must encompass both educational and environmental strategies to promote health eating and activity levels among students. A number of school-based programs targeting physical activity and eating behaviors have shown that is possible to modify school environments and show improvements in diet and physical activity levels [64, 187–190].

TABLE 1   Strategies for School Programs to Promote Healthy Eating and Physical Activity

Healthy eating	Physical activity
• Supply health education regarding nutrition and healthy weight management as part of required curriculum for health education.	• Require and fund daily physical education and sports programs in primary and secondary schools.
• Train staff involved in nutrition education and offer work-site health promotion opportunities for staff.	• Provide adequate training for physical education teachers to promote higher levels of physical activity during classes.
• Educate children on the influence of food advertising on eating habits.	• Ensure the provision of adequate space and necessary athletic/sports equipment.
• Ban required watching of commercials for foods high in calories, fat, or sugar on school television programs.	• Provide a positive environment regarding physical activity to promote the development of self-efficacy and enjoyment of physical activity for all students.
• Conduct school-wide media campaigns to promote healthy eating (e.g., the "5 a day message").	• Provide after-school physical education/sports opportunities for students.
• Modify cafeteria staff food preparation practices (e.g., low-fat food preparation methods).	• Incorporate traditional and "nontraditional" (e.g., dance) types of activities in physical education classes.
• Increase availability of fresh fruits, vegetables, and low-fat milk and low-fat choices in cafeterias.	• Incorporate strategies to promote decreases in sedentary behavior.
• Reduce the availability of vending machines with soft drinks, high-fat, high-sugar snack foods.	• Involve families and communities in supporting and reinforcing higher levels of physical activity.
• Involve families and communities in supporting and reinforcing healthy eating patterns.	• Provide links to community programs and resources for physical activity.

Although the majority of health promotion programs for children are provided in school settings [191], community-based programs have considerable potential for helping children acquire positive health behaviors. The school environment confers many advantages including the reduction of barriers of cost and transportation and the provision of access to a large, already-assembled population. Community-based, after-school programs have the potential to complement health promotion and education efforts made by schools for several reasons. Although children spend a large proportion of time in school each day, after-school hours constitute a substantial amount of time each week. Often children do not have opportunities to spend this time constructively, particularly in at-risk communities. According to the National Education Longitudinal Survey, the average eighth grader spends between 2 and 3 hours a day at home alone after school [192]. These hours have been shown to be those when many youth engage in high-risk behaviors due to lack of supervision. When young people are provided with safe and healthy activities in which to participate during critical gap periods (e.g., after school, on weekends), they are less likely to have time to participate in the high-risk, unhealthy activities that can delay or derail positive development [193–195].

Community-based, after-school programs provide multiple opportunities for teaching and reinforcing healthy patterns of physical activity and eating. Through their involvement in such programs, children can be educated about healthful eating habits and active lifestyles, but also have ample opportunity to practice these new habits and skills. Classroom-based eating habit programs that emphasize the behavioral skills needed for planning, preparing, and selecting healthy foods can be easily adapted for this setting. Children may have the opportunity to practice new skills in such pro-grams by engaging in activities such as planning and preparing healthy snacks. According to Sallis and McKenzie [196], physical activity programs for children should include (1) activities and skills that have the potential for carryover into adult life, (2) moderate intensity activities, and (3) a focus on maximizing the participation of all children. Community based, after-school programs are ideal for achieving such goals.

B. Policy Recommendations

Table 2 provides a thorough overview of policy recommendations for obesity prevention across a number of domains. These policy recommendations acknowledge the multiple levels at which change must occur from city, state, and federal tax programs to fund campaigns to promote healthy eating and physical activity and curb unhealthy patterns to developing better walking/biking paths for the purposes of both recreation and transportation to work [148]. Recommendations for work-site programs are also made including environmental changes in work setting such as promoting healthy eating by increasing the availability of healthy food choices in cafeterias, instituting work-site campaigns to promote physical activity and healthy eating, and providing tax incentives to employers for providing weight management programs.

V. CONCLUSION

The recently released goals of Healthy People 2010 are to reduce the prevalence of obesity among adults from 23% to 15% and to reduce the prevalence of obesity among children and adolescents from 11% to 5% [197, 198]. The etiology of

TABLE 2 Reducing the Prevalence of Obesity: Policy Recommendations

Education
- Provide federal funding to state public health department for mass media health promotion campaigns that emphasize healthful eating and physical activity patterns.
- Require instruction in nutrition and weight management as part of the school curriculum for future health education teachers.
- Make a plant-based diet the focus of dietary guidance.
- Ban required watching of commercials for foods high in calories, fat, or sugar on school television programs (for example, Channel One).
- Declare and organize an annual National "No-TV" Week.
- Require and fund daily physical education and sports programs in primary and secondary schools, extending the school day if necessary.
- Develop culturally relevant obesity prevention campaigns for high-risk and low-income Americans.
- Promote healthy eating in government cafeterias, Veterans Administration medical centers, military installations, prisons, and other venues.
- Institute campaigns to promote healthy eating and activity patterns among federal and state employees in all departments.

Food labeling and advertising
- Require chain restaurants to provide information about calorie content on menus or menu boards and nutrition labeling on wrappers.
- Require that containers for soft drinks and snacks sold in movie theaters, convenience stores, and other venues bear information about calories, fat, or sugar content.
- Require nutrition labeling on fresh meat and poultry products.
- Restrict advertising of high-calorie, low-nutrient foods on television shows commonly watched by children or require broadcasters to provide equal time for messages promoting healthy eating and physical activity.
- Require print advertisements to disclose the caloric content of the foods being marketed.

Food assistance programs
- Protect school food programs by eliminating the sale of soft drinks, candy bars, and foods high in calories, fat, or sugar in school buildings.
- Require that any foods that compete with school meals be consistent with federal recommendations for fat, saturated fat, cholesterol, sugar, and sodium content.
- Develop an incentive system to encourage food stamp recipients to purchase fruits, vegetables, whole grains, and other healthful foods, such as by earmarking increases in food stamp benefits for the purchase of those foods.

Health care and training
- Require medical, nursing, and other health professions curricula to teach the principles and benefits of healthful diets and exercise patterns.
- Require health care providers to learn about behavioral risks for obesity and how to counsel patients about health-promoting behavior change.
- Develop and fund a research agenda focused on behavioral as well as metabolic determinants of weight gain and maintenance, and on the most cost-effective methods for promoting healthful diet and activity patterns.
- Revise Medicaid and Medicare regulations to provide incentives to health care providers for nutrition and obesity counseling and other interventions that meet specified standards of cost and effectiveness.

Transportation and urban development
- Provide funding and other incentives for bicycle paths, recreation centers, swimming pools, parks, and sidewalks.
- Develop and provide guides for cities, zoning authorities, and urban planners on ways to modify residential neighborhoods, workplaces, and shopping centers to promote physical activity.

Taxes
- Levy city, state, or federal taxes on soft drinks and other foods high in calories, fat, or sugar to fund campaigns to promote good nutrition and physical activity.
- Subsidize the costs of low-calorie nutritious foods, perhaps by raising the costs of selected high-calorie, low-nutrient foods.
- Remove sales taxes on, or provide other incentives for, purchase of exercise equipment.
- Provide tax incentives to encourage employers to provide weight management programs.

Policy development
- Use the National Nutrition Summit to develop a national campaign to prevent obesity.
- Produce a *Surgeon General's Report on Obesity Prevention*.
- Expand the scope of the President's Council on Physical Fitness and Sports to include nutrition and to emphasize obesity prevention.
- Develop a coordinated federal implementation plan for the Healthy People 2010 nutrition and physical activity objectives.

Source: Nestle, M., and Jacobson, M. F. (2000). Halting the obesity epidemic: A public health policy approach. *Public Health Rep.* **115,** 12–24.

obesity is complex and encompasses a wide variety of social, behavioral, cultural, environmental, physiological, and genetic factors. To achieve these ambitious goals, considerable effort must be focused on helping individuals at the population level modify their diets and increase their physical activity levels, key behaviors involved in the regulation of body weight. Educational and environmental interventions that support diet and exercise patterns associated with healthy body weight must be developed and evaluated. Prevention of obesity should begin early in life and involve the development and maintenance of healthy eating and physical activity patterns. These patterns need to be reinforced at home, in schools, and throughout the community. Public health agencies, communities, government, health organizations,

the media, and the food and health industry must form alliances if we are to combat obesity.

References

1. Flegal, K. M., Carroll, M. D., Kuczmarski, R. J., Johnson, C. L. (1998). Overweight and obesity in the United States: Prevalence and trends, 1960–1994. *Int. J. Obes. Relat. Metab. Disord.* **22,** 39–47.

2. Troiano, R. P., Flegal, K. M. (1998). Overweight children and adolescents: Description, epidemiology, and demographics. *Pediatrics* **101**(Suppl. 1), 497–504.

3. World Health Organization (1997). "Obesity: Preventing and Managing the Global Epidemic," Report of a WHO Consultation on Obesity, Geneva, June 3–5, 1997. World Health Organization, Geneva.

4. National Institutes of Health, National Heart, Lung, and Blood Institute (1999). "Clinical Guidelines on the Identification, Evaluation, and Treatment of Overweight and Obesity in Adults." National Institutes of Health, National Heart, Lung, and Blood Institute, Bethesda, MD.

5. Marcus, M. (1993). Binge eating in obesity. *In* "Binge Eating: Nature, Assessment, and Treatment" (C. G. Fairburn and G. T. Wilson, Eds.), pp. 77–96. Guilford Press, New York.

6. Falkner, N. H., French, S. A., Jeffery, R. W., Neumark-Sztainer, D., Sherwood, N. E., and Morton, N. (1999). Mistreatment due to weight: Prevalence and sources of perceived mistreatment in women and men. *Obes. Res.* **7,** 572–576.

7. Wadden, T. A., and Stunkard, A. J. (1985). Social and psychological consequences of obesity. *Ann. Intern. Med.* **103,** 1062–1067.

8. Gortmaker, S. L., Must, A., Perrin, J. M., Sobol, A. M., and Dietz, W. H. (1993). Social and economic consequences of overweight in adolescence and young adulthood [see comments]. *N. Engl. J. Med.* **329,** 1008–1012.

9. Oster, G., Thompson, D., Edelsberg, J., Bird, A. P., and Colditz, G. A. (1999). Lifetime health and economic benefits of weight loss among obese persons. *Am. J. Public Health* **89,** 1536–1542.

10. Thompson, D., Edelsberg, J., Kinsey, K. L., and Oster, G. (1998). Estimated economic costs of obesity to U.S. business. *Am. J. Health Promot.* **13,** 120–127.

11. Wolf, A. M., and Colditz, G. A. (1996). Social and economic effects of body weight in the United States. *Am. J. Clin. Nutr.* **63,** 466S–469S.

12. Bouchard, C., and Perusse, L. (1988). Heredity and body fat. *Annu. Rev. Nutr.* **8,** 259–277.

13. Dannenberg, A. L., Keller, J. B., Wilson, P. W., and Castelli, W. P. (1989). Leisure time physical activity in the Framingham Offspring Study. Description, seasonal variation, and risk factor correlates. *Am. J. Epidemiol.* **129,** 76–88.

14. DiPietro, L., Williamson, D. F., Caspersen, C. J., Eaker, E. (1993). The descriptive epidemiology of selected physical activities and body weight among adults trying to lose weight: The Behavioral Risk Factor Surveillance System Survey, 1989. *Int. J. Obes. Relat. Metab. Disord.* **17,** 69–76.

15. Folsom, A. R., Caspersen, C. J., Taylor, H. L., Jacobs, D. R., Jr., Luepker, R. V., Gomez-Marin, O., Gillum, R. F., and Blackburn, H. (1985). Leisure time physical activity and its relationship to coronary risk factors in a population-based sample. The Minnesota Heart Survey. *Am. J. Epidemiol.* **121,** 570–579.

16. French, S. A., Jeffery, R. W., Forster, J. L., McGovern, P. G., Kelder, S. H., and Baxter, J. E. (1994). Predictors of weight change over two years among a population of working adults: The Healthy Worker Project. *Int. J. Obes. Relat. Metab. Disord.* **18,** 145–154.

17. Gibbons, L. W., Blair, S. N., Cooper, K. H., and Smith, M. (1983). Association between coronary heart disease risk factors and physical fitness in healthy adult women. *Circulation* **67,** 977–983.

18. Hovell, M., Sallis, J., Hofstetter, R., Barrington, E., Hackley, M., Elder, J., Castro, F., and Kilbourne, K. (1991). Identification of correlates of physical activity among Latino adults. *J. Community Health* **16,** 23–36.

19. King, A. C., and Tribble, D. L. (1991). The role of exercise in weight regulation in nonathletes. *Sports Med.* **11,** 331–349.

20. Slattery, M. L., McDonald, A., Bild, D. E., Caan, B. J., Hilner, J. E., Jacobs, D. R., Jr., and Liu, K. (1992). Associations of body fat and its distribution with dietary intake, physical activity, alcohol, and smoking in blacks and whites. *Am. J. Clin. Nutr.* **55,** 943–949.

21. Voorrips, L. E., Lemmink, K. A., van Heuvelen, M. J., Bult, P., and van Staveren, W. A. (1993). The physical condition of elderly women differing in habitual physical activity. *Med. Sci. Sports Exerc.* **25,** 1152–1157.

22. Voorrips, L. E., van Staveren, W. A., Hautvast, J. G. (1991). Are physically active elderly women in a better nutritional condition than their sedentary peers? *Eur. J. Clin. Nutr.* **45,** 545–552.

23. Epstein, L. H. (1995). Exercise in the treatment of childhood obesity. *Int. J. Obes. Relat. Metab. Disord.* **19**(Suppl. 4), S117–121.

24. U.S. Department of Health and Human Services (1988). "Surgeon General's Report on Nutrition and Health." U.S. Department of Health and Human Services, Public Health Service, Washington, DC.

25. Caspersen, C. J., and Merritt, R. K. (1992). Trends in physical activity patterns among older adults: The Behavioral Risk Factor Surveillance System, 1986–1990. *Med. Sci. Sports Exerc.* **24,** 526.

26. Caspersen, C. J.,and Merritt, R. K. (1995). Physical activity trends among 26 states, 1986–1990. *Med. Sci. Sports Exerc.* **27,** 713–720.

27. Caspersen, C. J., Merritt, R. K., Health, G. W., and Yeager, K. K. (1990). Physical activity patterns of adults aged 60 years and older. *Med. Sci. Sports Exerc.* **22,** S79.

28. Bauman, A., Owen, N., and Rushworth, R. L. (1990). Recent trends and socio-demographic determinants of exercise participation in Australia. *Community Health Studies* **14,** 19–26.

29. Folsom, A. R., Cook, T. C., Sprafka, J. M., Burke, G. L., Norsted, S. W., and Jacobs, D. R., Jr. (1991). Differences in leisure-time physical activity levels between blacks and whites in population-based samples: The Minnesota Heart Survey. *J. Behav. Med.* **14,** 1–9.

30. King, A. C., Blair, S. N., Bild, D. E., Dishman, R. K., Dubbert, P. M., Marcus, B. H., Oldridge, N. B., Paffenbarger, R. S. J., Powell, K. E., and Yeager, K. K. (1992). Determinants

of physical activity and interventions in adults. *Med. Sci. Sports Exerc.* **24,** S221–S236.

31. Ross, J. G., and Gilbert, G. G. (1985). The National Children and Youth Fitness Study. A summary of findings. *J. Phys. Educ. Recreat. Dance* **56,** 45–50.

32. Ross, J. G., and Pate, R. R. (1987). The National Children and Youth Fitness Study. *J. Phys. Educ. Recreat. Dance* **58,** 51–56.

33. Gortmaker, S. L., Must, A., Sobol, A. M., Peterson, K., Colditz, G. A., and Dietz, W. H. (1996). Television viewing as a cause of increasing obesity among children in the United States, 1986–1990. *Arch. Pediatr. Adolesc. Med.* **150,** 356–362.

34. Dietz, W. H., and Strasburger, V. C. (1991). Children, adolescents, and television. *Curr. Probl. Pediatr.* **21,** 8–31; discussion 32.

35. Dietz, W. H., Jr., and Gortmaker, S. L. (1985). Do we fatten our children at the television set? Obesity and television viewing in children and adolescents. *Pediatrics* **75,** 807–812.

36. Epstein, L. H. (1992). Exercise and obesity in children. *J. Appl. Sport Psychol.* **4,** 120–133.

37. AC Nielsen Company. (2000). "2000 Report on Television. The First 50 Years." Nielsen Media Research, New York.

38. Robinson, J., and Godbey, G. (1997). "Time for Life." Pennsylvania State University Press, University Park.

39. Crawford, D. A., Jeffery, R. W., and French, S. A. (1999). Television viewing, physical inactivity and obesity. *Int. J. Obes. Relat. Metab. Disord.* **23,** 437–440.

40. Sidney, S., Sternfeld, B., Haskell, W. L., Jacobs, D. R., Jr., Chesney, M. A., and Hulley, S. B. (1996). Television viewing and cardiovascular risk factors in young adults: The CARDIA study. *Ann. Epidemiol.* **6,** 154–159.

41. Coakley, E. H., Rimm, E. B., Colditz, G., Kawachi, I., and Willett, W. (1998). Predictors of weight change in men: Results from the Health Professionals Follow-up Study. *Int. J. Obes. Relat. Metab. Disord.* **22,** 89–96.

42. Heath, G. W., Pratt, M., Warren, C. W., and Kann, L. (1994). Physical activity patterns in American high school students. Results from the 1990 Youth Risk Behavior Survey. *Arch. Pediatr. Adolesc. Med.* **148,** 1131–1136.

43. Pate, R. R., and Ross, J. G. (1987). The national children and youth fitness study II: Factors associated with health-related fitness. *J. Phys. Educ. Recreat. Dance* **58,** 93–95.

44. Obarzanek, E., Schreiber, G. B., Crawford, P. B., Goldman, S. R., Barrier, P. M., Frederick, M. M., and Lakatos, E. (1994). Energy intake and physical activity in relation to indexes of body fat: The National Heart, Lung, and Blood Institute Growth and Health Study. *Am. J. Clin. Nutr.* **60,** 15–22.

45. Shannon, B., Peacock, J., and Brown, M. J. (1991). Body fatness, television viewing and calorie-intake of a sample of Pennsylvania sixth grade children. *J. Nutr. Educ.* **23,** 262–268.

46. Locard, E., Mamelle, N., Billette, A., Miginiac, M., Munoz, F., and Rey, S. (1992). Risk factors of obesity in a five year old population. Parental versus environmental factors. *Int. J. Obes. Relat. Metab. Disord.* **16,** 721–729.

47. Andersen, R. E., Crespo, C. J., Bartlett, S. J., Cheskin, L. J., and Pratt, M. (1998). Relationship of physical activity and television watching with body weight and level of fatness among children: Results from the Third National Health and Nutrition Examination Survey [see comments]. *JAMA* **279,** 938–942.

48. Robinson, T. N., Hammer, L. D., Killen, J. D., Kraemer, H. C., Wilson, D. M., Hayward, C., and Taylor, C. B. (1993). Does television viewing increase obesity and reduce physical activity? Cross-sectional and longitudinal analyses among adolescent girls [see comments]. *Pediatrics* **91,** 273–280.

49. Robinson, T. N., and Killen, J. D. (1995). Ethnic and gender differences in the relationships between television viewing and obesity, physical activity and dietary fat intake. *J. Health Educ.* **26,** S91–S98.

50. Tucker, L. A. (1986). The relationship of television viewing to physical fitness and obesity. *Adolescence* **21,** 797–806.

51. Wolf, A. M., Gortmaker, S. L., Cheung, L., Gray, H. M., Herzog, D. B., and Colditz, G. A. (1993). Activity, inactivity, and obesity: Racial, ethnic, and age differences among schoolgirls. *Am. J. Public Health* **83,** 1625–1627.

52. DuRant, R. H., Baranowski, T., Johnson, M., and Thompson, W. O. (1994). The relationship among television watching, physical activity, and body composition of young children. *Pediatrics* **94,** 449–455.

53. DuRant, R. H., Thompson, W. O., Johnson, M., and Baranowski, T. (1996). The relationship among television watching, physical activity, and body composition of 5- or 6-year-old children. *Pediatr. Exerc. Sci.* **8,** 15–26.

54. Dwyer, J. T., Stone, E. J., Yang, M., Feldman, H., Webber, L. S., Must, A., Perry, C. L., Nader, P. R., and Parcel, G. S. (1998). Predictors of overweight and overfatness in a multiethnic pediatric population. Child and Adolescent Trial for Cardiovascular Health Collaborative Research Group. *Am. J. Clin. Nutr.* **67,** 602–610.

55. Armstrong, C. A., Sallis, J. F., Alcaraz, J. E., Kolody, B., McKenzie, T. L., and Hovell, M. F. (1998). Children's television viewing, body fat, and physical fitness. *Am. J. Health Promot.* **12,** 363–368.

56. Tucker, L. A., and Friedman, G. M. (1989). Television viewing and obesity in adult males. *Am. J. Public Health* **79,** 516–518.

57. Tucker, L. A., and Bagwell, M. (1991). Television viewing and obesity in adult females. *Am. J. Public Health* **81,** 908–911.

58. Jeffery, R. W., and French, S. A. (1998). Epidemic obesity in the United States: Are fast foods and television viewing contributing? *Am. J. Public Health* **88,** 277–280.

59. Ching, P. L., Willett, W. C., Rimm, E. B., Colditz, G. A., Gortmaker, S. L., and Stampfer, M. J. (1996). Activity level and risk of overweight in male health professionals. *Am. J. Public Health* **86,** 25–30.

60. Epstein, L. H., Valoski, A. M., Vara, L. S., McCurley, J., Wisniewski, L., Kalarchian, M. A., Klein, K. R., and Shrager, L. R. (1995). Effects of decreasing sedentary behavior and increasing activity on weight change in obese children. *Health Psychol.* **14,** 109–115.

61. Epstein, L. H., Saelens, B. E., Myers, M. D., and Vito, D. (1997). Effects of decreasing sedentary behaviors on activity choice in obese children. *Health Psychol.* **16,** 107–113.

62. Epstein, L. H. (1998). Integrating theoretical approaches to promote physical activity. *Am. J. Prevent. Med.* **15,** 257–265.

63. Robinson, T. N. (1999). Reducing children's television viewing to prevent obesity: A randomized controlled trial. *JAMA* **282,** 1561–1567.

64. Gortmaker, S. L., Peterson, K., Wiecha, J., Sobol, A. M., Dixit, S., Fox, M. K., and Laird, N. (1999). Reducing obesity

via a school-based interdisciplinary intervention among youth: Planet Health. *Arch. Pediatr. Adolesc. Med.* **153,** 409–418.

65. Brawley, L. R., and Rodgers, W. M. (1993). Social psychological aspects of fitness promotion. *In* "Exercise Psychology" (P. Seraganian, Ed.), pp. 254–298. Wiley, New York.

66. Courneya, K. S., and McAuley, E. (1993). Can short-range intentions predict physical activity participation? *Percept. Mot. Skills* **77,** 115–122.

67. DuCharme, K. A., and Brawley, L. R. (1995). Predicting the intentions and behavior of exercise initiates using two forms of self-efficacy. *J. Behav. Med.* **18,** 479–497.

68. Hovell, M. F., Sallis, J. F., Hofstetter, C. R., Spry, V. M., Faucher, P., and Caspersen, C. J. (1989). Identifying correlates of walking for exercise: An epidemiologic prerequisite for physical activity promotion. *Prevent. Med.* **18,** 856–866.

69. Marcus, B. H., Pinto, B. M., Simkin, L. R., Audrain, J. E., and Taylor, E. R. (1994). Application of theoretical models to exercise behavior among employed women. *Am. J. Health Promot.* **9,** 49–55.

70. Marcus, B. H., Selby, V. C., Niaura, R. S., and Rossi, J. S. (1992). Self-efficacy and the stages of exercise behavior change. *Res. Q. Exerc. Sport.* **63,** 60–66.

71. McAuley, E. (1992). The role of efficacy cognitions in the prediction of exercise behavior in middle-aged adults. *J. Behav. Med.* **15,** 65–88.

72. McAuley, E., and Jacobson, L. (1991). Self-efficacy and exercise participation in sedentary adult females. *Am. J. Health Promot.* **5,** 185–191.

73. Poag, K., and McAuley, E. (1992). Goal setting, self-efficacy, and exercise bahavior. *J. Sport Exerc. Psychol.* **14,** 352–360.

74. Poag-DuCharme, K. A., and Brawley, L. R. (1993). Self-efficacy theory: Use in the prediction of exercise behavior in the community setting. *J. Appl. Sport Pscyhol.* **5,** 178–194.

75. Rodgers, W. M., and Brawley, L. R. (1993). Using both self-efficacy theory and the theory of planned behavior to discriminate adherers and dropouts from stuctured programs. *J. Appl. Sport Psychol.* **5,** 195–206.

76. Bandura, A. (1986). "Social Foundations of Thought and Action: A Social Cognitive Theory." Prentice Hall, Englewood Cliffs.

77. O'Loughlin, J., Paradis, G., Kishchuk, N., Barnett, T., and Renaud, L. (1999). Prevalence and correlates of physical activity behaviors among elementary schoolchildren in multiethnic, low income, inner-city neighborhoods in Montreal, Canada. *Ann. Epidemiol.* **9,** 397–407.

78. DiLorenzo, T. M., Stucky-Ropp, R. C., Vander Wal, J. S., and Gotham, H. J. (1998). Determinants of exercise among children. II. A longitudinal analysis. *Prevent. Med.* **27,** 470–477.

79. Simons-Morton, B. G., McKenzie, T. J., Stone, E., Mitchell, P., Osganian, V., Strikmiller, P. K., Ehlinger, S., Cribb, P., and Nader, P. R. (1997). Physical activity in a multiethnic population of third graders in four states. *Am. J. Public Health* **87,** 45–50.

80. Trost, S. G., Pate, R. R., Saunders, R., Ward, D. S., Dowda, M., and Felton, G. (1997). A prospective study of the determinants of physical activity in rural fifth-grade children. *Prevent. Med.* **26,** 257–263.

81. McAuley, E., Lox, C., and Duncan, T. E. (1993). Long-term maintenance of exercise, self-efficacy, and physiological change in older adults. *J. Gerontol.* **48,** 218–224.

82. McAuley, E., Courneya, K. S., and Lettunich, J. (1991). Effects of acute and long-term exercise on self-efficacy responses in sedentary, middle-aged males and females. *Gerontologist* **31,** 534–542.

83. Williams, P., and Lord, S. R. (1995). Predictors of adherence to a structured exercise program for older women. *Psychol. Aging* **10,** 617–624.

84. Pate, R. R., Baranowski, T., Dowda, M., and Trost, S. G. (1996). Tracking of physical activity in young children. *Med. Sci. Sports Exerc.* **28,** 92–96.

85. Dishman, R. K., and Sallis, J. F. (1994). Determinants and interventions for physical activity and exercise. *In* "Physical Activity, Fitness, and Health: International Proceedings and Consensus Statement" (C. Bouchard, R. J. Shephard, and T. Stephens, Eds.), pp. 214–238. Hum. Kinet, Champaign.

86. Hoftstetter, C. R., Hovell, M. F., and Sallis, J. F. (1990). Social learning correlates of exercise self-efficacy: Early experiences with physical activity. *Soc. Sci. Med.* **31,** 1169–1176.

87. Taylor, W. C., Blair, S. N., Cummings, S. S., Wun, C. C., and Malina, R. M. (1999). Childhood and adolescent physical activity patterns and adult physical activity. *Med. Sci. Sports Exerc.* **31,** 118–123.

88. Sallis, J. F., Prochaska, J. J., Taylor, W. C., Hill, J. O., and Geraci, J. C. (1999). Correlates of physical activity in a national sample of girls and boys in grades 4 through 12. *Health Psychol.* **18,** 410–415.

89. King, A. C., Taylor, C. B., Haskell, W. L., and DeBusk, R. F. (1990). Identifying strategies for increasing employee physical activity levels: Findings from the Stanford/Lockheed Exercise Survey. *Health Educ. Q.* **17,** 269–285.

90. Treiber, F. A., Baranowski, T., Braden, D. S., Strong, W. B., Levy, M., and Knox, W. (1991). Social support for exercise: Relationship to physical activity in young adults. *Prevent. Med.* **20,** 737–750 [erratum **21**(3), 392].

91. Hooper, J. M., and Veneziano, L. (1995). Distinguishing starters from nonstarters in an employee physical activity incentive program. *Health Educ. Q.* **22,** 49–60.

92. Wallace, J. P., Raglin, J. S., and Jastremski, C. A. (1995). Twelve month adherence of adults who joined a fitness program with a spouse vs without a spouse. *J. Sports Med. Phys. Fitness* **35,** 206–213.

93. Carron, A. V., Hausenblaus, H. A., and Mack, D. (1996). Social influence and exercise: A meta-analysis. *J. Sports Exerc. Psychol.* **18,** 1–16.

94. Epstein, L. H., Smith, J. A., Vara, L. S., and Rodefer, J. S. (1991). Behavioral economic analysis of activity choice in obese children. *Health Psychol.* **10,** 311–316.

95. Klesges, R. C., Costes, T. J., Moldenhauer-Klesges, L. M., Holzer, B., Gustavson, J., and Barnes, J. (1984). The FATS: An observational system for assessing physical activity in children and associated parent behavior. *Behav. Assess.* **6,** 333–345.

96. Klesges, R. C., Malott, J. M., Buschee, P. F., and Weber, J. M. (1986). The effects of parental influences on children's food intake, physical activity and relative weight. *Int. J. Eat. Disord.* **5,** 335–346.

97. McKenzie, T. L., Sallis, J. F., Nader, P. R., Patterson, T. L., Elder, J. P., Berry, C. C., Rupp, J. W., Atkins, C. J., Buono, M. J., and Nelson, J. A. (1991). BEACHES: An observational system for assessing children's eating and physical activity

behaviors and associated events. *J. Appl. Behav. Anal.* **24,** 141–151.

98. Klesges, R. C., Eck, L. H., Hanson, C. L., Haddock, C. K., and Klesges, L. M. (1990). Effects of obesity, social interactions, and physical environment on physical activity in preschoolers. *Health Psychol.* **9,** 435–449.

99. Sallis, J. F., Alcaraz, J. E., McKenzie, T. L., Hovell, M. F., Kolody, B., and Nader, P. R. (1992). Parental behavior in relation to physical activity and fitness in 9-year-old children. *Am. J. Dis. Child.* **146,** 1383–1388.

100. Taylor, W. C., Baranowski, T., and Sallis, J. F. (1994). Family determinants of childhood physical activity. *In* "Advances in Exercise Adherence" (R. Dishman, Ed.). Human Kinetics, Champaign, IL.

101. Dishman, R. K., Sallis, J. F., and Orenstein, D. R. (1985). The determinants of physical activity and exercise. *Public Health Rep.* **100,** 158–171.

102. Schmitz, M. K. H., Jacobs, D. R., French, S., Lewis, C. E., Caspersen, C. J., and Sternfeld, B. (1999). The impact of becoming a parent on physical activity: The CARDIA Study. *Circulation* **99,** 1108.

103. King, A. C. (1994). Community and public health approaches to the promotion of physical activity. *Med. Sci. Sports Exerc.* **26,** 1405–1412.

104. Sherwood, N. E., Morton, N., Jeffery, R. W., French, S. A., Neumark-Sztainer, D., and Falkner, N. H. (1998). Consumer preferences in format and type of community-based weight control programs. *Am. J. Health Promot.* **13,** 12–18.

105. Perri, M. G., Martin, A. D., Leermakers, E. A., Sears, S. F., and Notelovitz, M. (1997). Effects of group- versus home-based exercise in the treatment of obesity. *J. Consult. Clin. Psychol.* **65,** 278–285.

106. Craighead, L. W., and Blum, M. D. (1989). Supervised exercise in behavioral treatment for moderate obesity. *J. Behav. Med.* **20,** 49–60.

107. Andersen, R. E., Wadden, T. A., Bartlett, S. J., Zemel, B., Verde, T. J., and Franckowiak, S. C. (1999). Effects of lifestyle activity vs structured aerobic exercise in obese women: A randomized trial. *JAMA* **281,** 335–340.

108. Dunn, A. L., Marcus, B. H., Kampert, J. B., Garcia, M. E., Kohl, H. W., III, and Blair, S. N. (1999). Comparison of lifestyle and structured interventions to increase physical activity and cardiorespiratory fitness: A randomized trial. *JAMA* **281,** 327–334.

109. Murphy, M. H., and Hardman, A. E. (1998). Training effects of short and long bouts of brisk walking in sedentary women. *Med. Sci. Sports Exerc.* **30,** 152–157.

110. DeBusk, R. F., Stenestrand, U., Sheehan, M., and Haskell, W. L. (1990). Training effects of long versus short bouts of exercise in healthy subjects. *Am. J. Cardiol.* **65,** 1010–1013.

111. Ebisu, T. (1985). Splitting the distances of endurance training: On cardiovascular endurance and blood lipids. *Jpn. J. Phys. Educ.* **32,** 37–43.

112. Jakicic, J. M., Wing, R. R., Butler, B. A., and Robertson, R. J. (1995). Prescribing exercise in multiple short bouts versus one continuous bout: Effects on adherence, cardiorespiratory fitness, and weight loss in overweight women. *Int. J. Obes. Relat. Metab. Disord.* 893–901.

113. Jakicic, J. M., Winters, C., Lang, W., and Wing, R. R. (1999). Effects of intermittent exercise and use of home exercise equipment on adherence, weight loss, and fitness in overweight women: A randomized trial. *JAMA* **282,** 1554–1560.

114. Epstein, L. H., Valoski, A., Wing, R. R., and McCurley, J. (1994). Ten-year outcomes of behavioral family-based treatment for childhood obesity [see comments]. *Health Psychol.* **13,** 373–383.

115. Sallis, J. F., Hovell, M. F., Hofstetter, C. R., Elder, J. P., Hackley, M., Caspersen, C. J., and Powell, K. E. (1990). Distance between homes and exercise facilities related to frequency of exercise among San Diego residents. *Public Health Rep.* **105,** 179–185.

116. (1999). Neighborhood safety and the prevalence of physical inactivity—Selected states, 1996. *MMWR Morbid. Mortal. Wkly. Rep.* **48,** 143–146.

117. Baranowski, T., Thompson, W. O., DuRant, R. H., Baranowski, J., and Puhl, J. (1993). Observations on physical activity in physical locations: Age, gender, ethnicity, and month effects. *Res. Q. Exerc. Sport.* **64,** 127–133.

118. Sallis, J. F., Alcaraz, J. E., McKenzie, T. L., and Hovell, M. F. (1999). Predictors of change in children's physical activity over 20 months. Variations by gender and level of adiposity. *Am. J. Prevent. Med.* **16,** 222–229.

119. Klem, M. L., Wing, R. R., McGuire, M. T., Seagle, H. M., and Hill, J. O. (1997). A descriptive study of individuals successful at long-term maintenance of substantial weight loss. *Am. J. Clin. Nutr.* **66,** 239–246.

120. McGuire, M. T., Wing, R. R., Klem, M. L., and Hill, J. O. (1999). Behavioral strategies of individuals who have maintained long-term weight losses. *Obes. Res.* **7,** 334–341.

121. McDowell, M. A., Briefel, R. R., Alaimo, K., Bischof, A. M., Caughman, C. R., Carroll, M. D., Loria, C. M., and Johnson, C. L. (1994). Energy and macronutrient intakes of persons ages 2 months and over in the United States: Third National Health and Nutrition Examination Survey, Phase 1, 1988–91. *Adv. Data* **255,** 1–24.

122. Tippett, K. S., and Cleveland, L. E. (1999). How current diets stack up: Comparison with dietary guidelines. *In* "America's Eating Habits: Changes and Consequences" (E. Frazao, Ed.), pp. 51–70. USDA, Washington, DC.

123. Norris, J., Harnack, L., Carmichael, S., Pouane, T., Wakimoto, P., and Block, G. (1997). U.S. trends in nutrient intake: The 1987 and 1992 National Health Interview Surveys. *Am. J. Public Health* **87,** 740–746.

124. Federation of Associated Societies for Experimental Biology (1995). "Third Report on Nutrition Monitoring in the United States." U.S. Government Printing Office, Washington, DC.

125. Troiano, R. P., Briefel, R. R., Carroll, M. D., and Bialostosky, K. (2000). Energy and fat intake of children and adolescents in the United States. Data from the National Health and Nutrition Examination Surveys. *Am. J. Clin. Nutr.* **72,** 1343S–1354S.

126. Briefel, R. R., McDowell, M. A., Alaimo, K., Caughman, C. R., Bischof, A. L., Carroll, M. D., and Johnson, C. L. (1995). Total energy intake of the U.S. population: The third National Health and Nutrition Examination Survey, 1988–1991. *Am. J. Clin. Nutr.* **62,** 1072S–1080S.

127. Schoeller, D. A. (1990). How accurate is self-reported dietary intake? *Nutr. Rev.* **48,** 373–379.

128. Bingham, S. A. (1987). The dietary assessment of individuals; Methods, accuracy, new techniques and recommendations. *Nutr. Abstr. Rev.* **57,** 705–742.

129. Goris, A. H., Westerterp-Plantenga, M. S., and Westerterp, K. R. (2000). Undereating and underrecording of habitual food intake in obese men: Selective underreporting of fat intake. *Am. J. Clin. Nutr.* **71,** 130–134.

130. Jonnalagadda, S. S., Mitchell, D. C., Smiciklas-Wright, H., Meaker, K. B., Heel, N. V., Karmally, W., Ershow, A. G., and Kris-Etherton, P. M. (2000). Accuracy of energy intake data estimated by a multiple-pass, 24-hour dietary recall technique. *J. Am. Diet. Assoc.* **100,** 303–308; quiz 309–311.

131. Bray, G. A., and Popkin, B. M. (1998). Dietary fat intake does affect obesity! *Am. J. Clin. Nutr.* **68,** 1157–1173.

132. Willett, W. C. (1998). Is dietary fat a major determinant of body fat? *Am. J. Clin. Nutr.* **67,** 556S–562S.

133. Hill, J. O., Melanson, E. L., and Wyatt, H. T. (2000). Dietary fat intake and regulation of energy balance: Implications for obesity. *J. Nutr.* **130,** 284–288S.

134. West, D. B., and York, B. (1998). Dietary fat, genetic predisposition, and obesity: Lessons from animal models. *Am. J. Clin. Nutr.* **67,** 505S–512S.

135. Anand, R. S., and Basiotis, P. P. (1998). Is total fat consumption really decreasing? *Family Econom. Nutr. Rev.* **11,** 58–60.

136. Putnam, J., and Gerrior, S. (1999). Trends in the U.S. food supply, 1970–1997. *In* "America's Eating Habits: Changes and Consequences" (E. Frazao, Ed.), pp. 133–160. USDA, Washington, DC.

137. Putnam, J. (1999). U.S. food supply providing more food and calories. *FoodReview* **22,** 2–12.

138. Guthrie, J. F., and Morton, J. F. (2000). Food sources of added sweeteners in the diets of Americans. *J. Am. Diet. Assoc.* **100,** 43–51, quiz 49–50.

139. Harnack, L., Stang, J., and Story, M. (1999). Soft drink consumption among U.S. children and adolescents: Nutritional consequences. *J. Am. Diet. Assoc.* **99,** 436–441.

140. Drewnowski, A. (1997). Taste preferences and food intake. *Annu. Rev. Nutr.* **17,** 237–253.

141. Weimer, J. (1999). Accelerating the trend toward healthy eating. *In* "America's Eating Habits: Changes and Consequences" (E. Frazao, Ed.), pp. 385–401. USDA, Washington, DC.

142. Heini, A. F., and Weinsier, R. L. (1997). Divergent trends in obesity and fat intake patterns: The American paradox. *Am. J. Med.* **102,** 259–264.

143. Bell, E. A., Castellanos, V. H., Pelkman, C. L., Thorwart, M. L., and Rolls, B. J. (1998). Energy density of foods affects energy intake in normal-weight women. *Am. J. Clin. Nutr.* **67,** 412–420.

144. Lin, B. H., Guthrie, J., and Frazao, E. (1999). Nutrient contribution of food away from home. *In* "America's Eating Habits: Changes and Consequences" (E. Frazao, Ed.), pp. 213–242. USDA, Washington, DC.

145. Lin, B. H., Guthrie, J., and Frazao, E. (1998). Popularity of dining out presents barrier to dietary improvements. *FoodReview* **21,** 2–10.

146. National Restaurant Association (2000). "Restaurant Industry Pocket Factbook." National Restaurant Association, Washington, DC.

147. Clauson, A. (1999). Share of food spending for eating out reaches 47%. *FoodReview* **22,** 20–33.

148. Nestle, M., and Jacobson, M. F. (2000). Halting the obesity epidemic: A public health policy approach. *Public Health Rep.* **115,** 12–24.

149. Guthrie, J. F., Derby, B. M., and Levy, A. S. (1999). What people know and do not know about nutrition. *In* "America's Eating Habits: Changes and Consequences" (E. Frazao, Ed.), pp. 243–280. USDA, Washington, DC.

150. Jekanowski, M. D. (1999). Causes and consequences of fast food sales growth. *FoodReview* **22,** 11–16.

151. Anonymous (1999). Food away from home sales at a glance 1988–98. *FoodReview* **22,** 26.

152. Howard, T. (1999). McD's rejiggers menu for trade-ups. *Brandweek* **40,** 8.

153. McCrory, M. A., Fuss, P. J., Hays, N. P., Vinken, A. G., Greenberg, A. S., and Roberts, S. B. (1999). Overeating in America: Association between restaurant food consumption and body fatness in healthy adult men and women ages 19 to 80. *Obes. Res.* **7,** 564–571.

154. Gallo, A. E. (1999). Food advertising in the United States. *In* "America's Eating Habits: Changes and Consequences" (E. Frazao, Ed.), pp. 173–180. USDA, Washington, DC.

155. Kotz, K., and Story, M. (1994). Food advertisements during children's Saturday morning television programming: Are they consistent with dietary recommendations? *J. Am. Diet. Assoc.* **94,** 1296–1300.

156. Consumers Union Education Services (1995). "Captive Kids: Commercial Pressures on Kids at School." Consumers Union of United States, Yonkers, NY.

157. Jacobson, M. F. (1998). "Liquid Candy. How Soft Drinks are Harming Americans' Health." Center for Science in the Public Interest, Washington, DC.

158. Keane, T. M., Geller, S. E., and Scheirer, C. J. (1981). A parametric investigation of eating styles in obese and nonobese children. *Behav. Ther.* **12,** 280–286.

159. LeBow, M. D., Goldberg, P. S., and Collins, A. (1977). Eating behavior of overweight and nonoverweight persons in the natural environment. *J. Consult. Clin. Psychol.* **45,** 1204–1205.

160. Barkeling, B., Ekman, S., and Rossner, S. (1992). Eating behaviour in obese and normal weight 11-year-old children. *Int. J. Obes. Relat. Metab. Disord.* **16,** 355–360.

161. Adams, N., Ferguson, J., Stunkard, A. J., and Agras, S. (1978). The eating behavior of obese and nonobese women. *Behav. Res. Ther.* **16,** 225–232.

162. Terry, K., Beck, S. (1985). Eating style and food storage habits in the home. Assessment of obese and nonobese families. *Behav. Modif.* **9,** 242–261.

163. Boutelle, K., Neumark-Sztainer, D., Story, M., Resnick, M. (submitted). Weight control behaviors among overweight adolescents.

164. Neumark-Sztainer, D., Rock, C., Thornquist, M., Cheskin, L., Neuhouser, M., and Barnett, M. (2000). Weight control behaviors among adults and adolescents. *Prevent. Med.* **30,** 381–391.

165. Neumark-Sztainer, D., French, S. A., and Jeffery, R. W. (1996). Dieting for weight loss: Associations with nutrient intake among women. *J. Am. Diet. Assoc.* **96,** 1172–1175.

166. Nicklas, T. A., Bao, W., Webber, L. S., and Berenson, G. S. (1993). Breakfast consumption affects adequacy of total daily intake in children. *J. Am. Diet. Assoc.* **93,** 886–891.

167. Neumark-Sztainer, D., Story, M., Falkner, N. H., Behuring, T., and Resnick, M. D. (1999). Sociodemographic and personal characteristics of adolescents engaged in weight loss

and weight/muscle gain behaviors: Who is doing what? *Prevent. Med.* **28,** 4–5.

168. Stice, E., Cameron, R. P., Killen, J. D., Hayward, C., and Taylor, C. B. (1999). Naturalistic weight-reduction efforts prospectively predict growth in relative weight and onset of obesity among female adolescents. *J. Consult. Clin. Psychol.* **67,** 967–974.

169. Wardle, J., and Beinart, H. (1981). Binge eating: A theoretical review. *Br. J. Clin. Psychol.* **20,** 97–109.

170. Polivy, J., and Herman, C. P. (1985). Dieting and binging. A causal analysis. *Am. Psychol.* **40,** 193–201.

171. French, S. A., Jeffery, R. W., Sherwood, N. E., and Neumark-Sztainer, D. (1999). Prevalence and correlates of binge eating in a nonclinical sample of women enrolled in a weight gain prevention program. *Int. J. Obes. Relat. Metab. Disord.* **23,** 576–585.

172. Devlin, M. J., Walsh, B. T., Spitzer, R. L., and Hasin, D. (1992). Is there another binge eating disorder? A review of the literature on overeating in the absence of bulimia nervosa. *Int. J. Eating Disord.* **11,** 333–340.

173. Teasdale, T. W., Sorensen, T. I., and Stunkard, A. J. (1990). Genetic and early environmental components in sociodemographic influences on adult body fatness. *Br. Med. J.* **300,** 1615–1618.

174. Bouchard, C. (1989). Genetic factors in obesity. *Med. Clin. N. Am.* **73,** 67–81.

175. Nader, P. R. (1993). The role of the family in obesity prevention and treatment. *Ann. NY Acad. Sci.* **699,** 147–153.

176. Golan, M., Fainaru, M., and Weizman, A. (1998). Role of behaviour modification in the treatment of childhood obesity with the parents as the exclusive agents of change. *Int. J. Obes. Relat. Metab. Disord.* **22,** 1217–1224.

177. Epstein, L. H. (1985). Family-based treatment for preadolescent obesity. *Adv. Devel. Behav. Pediatr.* **6,** 1–39.

178. Neumark-Sztainer, D., Story, M., Ackard, D., Moe, J., and Perry, C. (2000). The "family meal": Views of adolescents. *J. Nutr. Educ.* **32,** 329–354.

179. Neumark-Sztainer, D., Story, M., Ackard, D., Moe, J., and Perry, C. (2000). Family meals among adolescents: Findings from a pilot study. *J. Nutr. Educ.* **32,** 335–340.

180. Resnick, M. D., Bearman, P. S., Blum, R. W., Bauman, K. E., Harris, K. M., Jones, J., Tabor, J., Beuhring, T., Sieving, R. E., Shew, M., Ireland, M., Bearinger, L. H., and Udry, J. R. (1997). Protecting adolescents from harm. Findings from the National Longitudinal Study on Adolescent Health. *JAMA* **278,** 823–832.

181. Neumark-Sztainer, D., Story, M., Resnick, M. D., and Blum, R. W. (1996). Correlates of inadequate fruit and vegetable consumption among adolescents. *Prevent. Med.* **25,** 497–505.

182. Neumark-Sztainer, D., Story, M., Dixon, L. B., Resnick, M., and Blum, R. (1997). Correlates of inadequate consumption of dairy products among adolescents. *J. Nutr. Educ.* **29,** 12–20.

183. Mellin, A., Neumark-Sztainer, D., Story, M., Ireland, M., and Resnick, M. (submitted). Unhealthy behaviors and psychosocial difficulties among overweight youth: The potential impact of familial factors.

184. Birch, L. L., and Fisher, J. O. (1998). Development of eating behaviors among children and adolescents. *Pediatrics* **101,** 539–549.

185. Johnson, S. L., and Birch, L. L. (1994). Parents' and children's adiposity and eating style. *Pediatrics* **94,** 653–661.

186. Sallis, J. F., Bauman, A., and Pratt, M. (1998). Environmental and policy interventions to promote physical activity. *Am. J. Prevent. Med.* **15,** 379–397.

187. Nader, P. R., Stone, E. J., Lytle, L. A., Perry, C. L., Osganian, S. K., Kelder, S., Webber, L. S., Elder, J. P., Montgomery, D., Feldman, H. A., Wu, M., Johnson, C., Parcel, G. S., and Luepker, R. V. (1999). Three-year maintenance of improved diet and physical activity: The CATCH cohort. Child and Adolescent Trial for Cardiovascular Health. *Arch. Pediatr. Adolesc. Med.* **153,** 695–704.

188. Lytle, L. A., Stone, E. J., Nichaman, M. Z., Perry, C. L., Montgomery, D. H., Nicklas, T. A., Zive, M. M., Mitchell, P., Dwyer, J. T., Ebzery, M. K., Evans, M. A., and Galati, T. P. (1996). Changes in nutrient intakes of elementary school children following a school-based intervention: Results from the CATCH Study. *Prevent. Med.* **25,** 465–477.

189. McKenzie, T. L., Nader, P. R., Strikmiller, P. K., Yang, M., Stone, E. J., Perry, C. L., Taylor, W. C., Epping, J. N., Feldman, H. A., Luepker, R. V., and Kelder, S. H. (1996). School physical education: Effect of the Child and Adolescent Trial for Cardiovascular Health. *Prevent. Med.* **25,** 423–431.

190. Sallis, J. F., McKenzie, T. L., Alcaraz, J. E., Kolody, B., Faucette, N., and Hovell, M. F. (1997). The effects of a 2-year physical education program (SPARK) on physical activity and fitness in elementary school students. Sports, Play and Active Recreation for Kids. *Am. J. Public Health* **87,** 1328–1334.

191. Contento, I., Blach, G., Bronner, Y., Lytle, L., Maloney, S., Olson, C., and Swadener, S. (1995). The effectiveness of nutrition education and implications for nutrition education policy, programs and research: A review of research. *J. Nutr. Educ.* **27,** 284–418.

192. U.S. Department of Education, Office of Education Research and Improvement NCFES (1990). "A Profile of the American Eighth Grader: NEL: 88 Description Summary." U.S. Government Printing Office, Washington, DC.

193. Carnegie Council on Adolescent Development (1992). "Matter of Time: Risk and Opportunity in the Nonschool Hours." Carnegie Council on Adolescent Development, Waldorf, MD.

194. Carnegie Council of Adolescent Development (1995). "Great Transitions: Preparing Adolescents for a New Century." Carnegie Corporation, New York.

195. Mulhall, P. F., Stone, D., and Stone, B. (1996). Home alone: Is it a risk factor for middle school youth and drug use? *J. Drug Educ.* **26,** 39–48.

196. Sallis, J. F., and McKenzie, T. L. (1991). Physical education's role in public health. *Res. Q. Exerc. Sport.* **62,** 124–137.

197. U.S. Department of Health and Human Services (2000). "Healthy People 2010: Conference Edition, Vol I." U.S. Department of Health and Human Services, Washington, DC.

198. U.S. Department of Health and Human Services (2000). "Healthy People 2010: Conference Edition, Vol II." U.S. Department of Health and Human Services, Washington, DC.

CHAPTER **35**

Role of Taste and Appetite in Body Weight Regulation

ADAM DREWNOWSKI AND VICTORIA WARREN-MEARS
University of Washington, Seattle, Washington

I. INTRODUCTION

More than 50% of all adults in the United States are classified as being either overweight or obese [1]. The prevalence of obesity has increased dramatically in the last two decades, especially among ethnic minorities and the poor [1–3]. Given that human physiology and genetics have changed little during that time, the explanation must lie in reduced physical activity or altered eating habits. Although the mainstream of obesity research continues to focus on genetic, metabolic, and physiological factors in weight gain [1], the obesity epidemic is most likely caused by a profound change in dietary behaviors. Changes in the global food supply may also play a part [4, 5]. Dietary Guidelines for Americans 2000 now suggest that rising obesity rates are tied to the wide availability of cheap and palatable foods [6].

Taste and palatability are among the key influences on food choice [7–9]. According to consumer studies [9], adults' food choices are determined by food taste, cost, and convenience, rather than by concerns with nutrition or health. The best tasting and most palatable foods are often those that provide the maximum amount of energy per unit weight [9]. Many such foods contain fat, sugar, or both. Inaccessible to most people on a daily basis until the last century, corn sugars and vegetable oils are now among the cheapest food commodities available [10–11]. The question is whether sensory mechanisms that have evolved to maintain energy supply when food was scarce can effectively adapt to dietary excess. Examining taste responses and appetite for sweet and high-fat foods in relation to body weight is the main focus of this chapter.

II. GENETICS AND BODY WEIGHT

Obesity is said to be a heritable trait [12, 13]. The fact that obese parents tend to have obese children [14–15] was taken as evidence that obesity had a familial origin. Studies of Danish adoptees showed that obesity, or more correctly body mass, was an inherited variable [16]. Another line of evidence was provided by studies of monozygotic and dizygotic twins [17]. Identical twins had the same patterns of weight gain in response to overfeeding and a similar distribution of body fat [17]. Twin studies now suggest that genes may account for as much as 75–80% of the variance in percent body fat among children aged 3–17 years [18].

Some people may be more vulnerable than others to excess weight gain. According to the "thrifty gene" hypothesis [10], evolutionary selection may have favored those people who were best able to store body fat when food became available. Because gene expression is modulated by nutrients, the heritable trait may not be obesity per se, but rather a vulnerability or predisposition to excessive weight gain [19, 20]. The expression of obesity among susceptible individuals must involve some aspect of dietary behavior, not to mention exposure to an obesity-promoting diet. The continuing search for an obese phenotype has focused on those "obese" behaviors, including taste-related ones, that might show a genetic component.

Body metabolism, physical activity, and dietary choices are each influenced by genetic traits [12]. Studies explored whether infants born to obese mothers had lower metabolic rates [21], distinct eating behaviors, or showed an elevated sensory response to sweet [22]. Most of those studies were inconclusive. Sweet taste responses of obese adults have also been investigated [23–25]. For the most part, studies failed to show a consistent "obese" pattern of sweet taste responses, eating behaviors, or eating styles. While there was a great deal of individual variation in taste responsiveness, few systematic differences by body-weight category were observed. Moreover, there was no evidence that any of the taste-related behaviors had a genetic component.

The fact that obesity rates have increased so sharply during the past two decades suggests that changing dietary choices and increasingly sedentary lifestyles—rather than genetics—are the key factors in the obesity epidemic. If obesity is multiply determined, then the search for a single obese genotype is likely to be fruitless. Contrary to the notion that obesity is a random "genetic lottery," the distribution of obesity in the United States varies in a predictable manner with age, race/ethnicity, education, and income. With obesity rates reaching 90% in some populations [26–28], it

would appear that most people are vulnerable in some degree to excess weight gain. Instead of actively promoting obesity, genetic factors may provide an inadequate protection against an energy-rich dietary environment. Instead of being a rare and abnormal state, obesity may represent a normal adaptive response to the prevailing environmental and dietary conditions.

III. TASTE FACTORS AND FOOD CHOICES

The chief role of the taste system is to promote and maintain eating behavior. The pleasure response to sweet taste is present at birth. A newborn's reaction to sweet has been assessed using facial expressions captured during the first few hours of life [29]. In 3-day-old infants, the taste response to sucrose causes relaxation, a slight smile, and licking of the upper lip. Three-day-old infants prefer sucrose solutions to water, prefer sweeter over less sweet sugars, and selectively consume the most concentrated sugar solutions [29]. This sensory reflex serves to orient and maintain the feeding response, assuring a constant supply of dietary energy. The key sensory characteristic of mother's milk is its sweet taste. Sugar is a major source of energy. Studies on the development of food preferences in young children suggest that novel flavors are accepted most readily when they are paired with a concentrated source of energy, most often sugar or fat [30]. Taste behaviors, orienting the newborn toward sugar and fat, most likely evolved because they were crucial to survival [31, 32].

Foods that are described as good tasting are often concentrated sources of energy and contain fat, sugar, or both [7–9]. The concept of food palatability includes taste, aroma, and texture. Sweetness is a basic taste, perceived through receptors located in taste buds, distributed through the oral cavity, and concentrated on the dorsal area of the tongue. The sensation of fatness is mediated through the perception of texture and mouthfeel. Such texture attributes as smoothness, creaminess, crunchiness, or tenderness are all associated with the fat content of foods. In addition, many of the volatile flavor molecules are fat soluble such that the characteristic aroma of many foods is linked to their fat content. Studies in humans and rats suggest that sensory preferences for fat are either innate or acquired very early in life.

There is no question that the enjoyment of sweetness and fat has a physiological basis [31]. Placing a sweet substance on the tongue of a crying newborn has a remarkable calming effect. This persists for several minutes and can be used to calm the infant during blood draws and other painful procedures. Studies have linked taste responses to sweetness to the endogenous opiate peptide system. Further evidence that taste responses to sweetness and fat are mediated by endorphins is provided by clinical studies in adult women. Infusions of the opiate agonist naloxone suppressed sensory

preferences for sweetened dairy products and selectively reduced the consumption of sweet high-fat foods such as cookies or chocolate. This effect was strongest among women diagnosed with the binge-eating disorder [33], suggesting that some food cravings may be mediated by endorphins. Although naloxone is not an effective agent for weight loss, opiate blockade may prevent palatability-induced overeating [34].

The pleasure response to foods is thought to serve the physiological needs of the organism [31]. According to some theories, sweet taste preferences are linked to both short- and long-term energy needs (see [23] for review). In laboratory studies, taste response to sweetness declined after a meal, or following the ingestion of sweet glucose solutions [31]. There was some question whether this satiety response was linked to energy content, because a similar suppression in sweet taste preference was also obtained with noncaloric aspartame solutions [23]. Other studies attempted to link sweet taste preferences with the physiological set point of body weight. In that view, a drop in body weight below set point would lead to increased sweet preferences. Conversely, an increase in body weight above set point should lead to an observable decrease in sweet preferences. However, given that the set point was a theoretical construct as opposed to a measurable variable, that hypothesis could never be tested appropriately [23]. While preferences for sweet solutions vary across individuals, they have not been linked to any particular body weight.

As shown in Fig. 1, obese male patients showed a diversity of responses to milk and cream sweetened with different amounts of sucrose, up to 16% sucrose wt/wt. Each panel represents data for a different patient ($n = 9$). Hedonic ratings measured along a five-point category scale either rose (top five panels) or declined with increasing sucrose concentrations (bottom four panels), consistent with previous results. Individual patterns of response to sucrose were much the same before and after weight loss. Even a very substantial loss in body weight in excess of 40 kg failed to alter the type of taste response to sweetness.

Studies on obesity and sensory response to fat were more convincing, showing that obese women patients gave the highest hedonic ratings to energy-rich mixtures of cream and sugar. In some studies, taste preferences were associated with food preferences and selective consumption of sweet and high-fat foods. There was also evidence that the diets of obese men and women tended to be higher in fat than those of lean controls. However, such diets were probably more energy dense, providing more energy per unit weight or volume.

Sensory preferences for dietary fats have been linked to body mass index and body fatness in children, adolescents, and adults [35, 36]. In clinical studies using sweetened dairy foods, obese women selected taste stimuli that were high in fat over those that were intensely sweet [25]. In contrast,

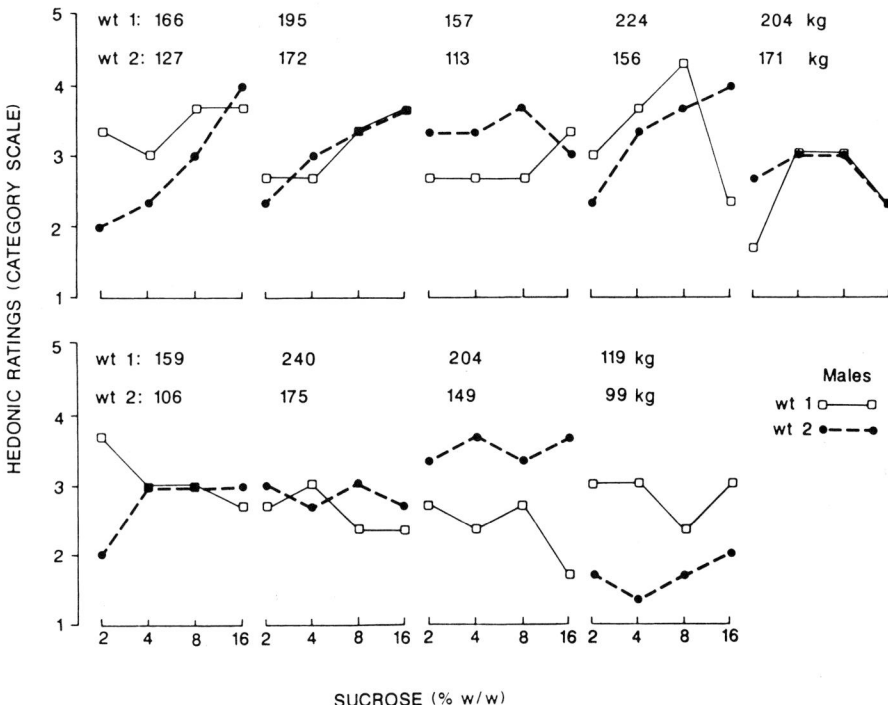

FIGURE 1 Hedonic ratings for milk and cream sweetened with different amount of sucrose. Data are presented separately for nine obese males before and after weight loss. Initial (wt 1) and final (wt 2) weights (kg) are indicated.

emaciated females with anorexia nervosa liked sweet taste but showed an aversion to dairy fat. These studies were later confirmed by the observation that fatter persons tended to select higher-fat foods [35]. In a laboratory study, preferences for fat in foods were linked with the respondents' own body fatness [35]. A related study conducted with 3- to 5-year-old children showed that the children's fat preferences were influenced by the body mass of the parents, suggesting that fat preferences may be a heritable trait [36]. It is as yet unclear whether the preferences were for fat per se, or for those fat-rich stimuli that provided maximal energy per unit weight or volume. Because fats provide a concentrated source of dietary energy, they have an impact on hunger, appetite, and satiety [37–40].

IV. HUNGER, APPETITE, AND SATIETY

People eat food several times per day. These eating occasions can be divided into larger meals and smaller snacks. People begin to eat when they are hungry and stop when they are satiated. While *hunger* is defined as a generalized state of energy depletion, the term *appetite* often denotes a desire to eat a given food [8, 9]. In studies with rats, the onset of eating was preceded by a transient drop in plasma glucose.

Several theories have been developed to account for the seeming day-to-day control of food intake [41–43]. The glucostatic theory held that food consumption was triggered by a drop in the availability of glucose to cells and tissues. The lipostatic theory held that a drop in body fat stores would provoke feeding behavior, while the aminostatic theory suggested that feeding occurred to maintain amino acid homeostasis. What these early theories shared was the common premise that hunger and appetite triggered food consumption, primarily in response to energy needs. In contrast, the current focus is on mechanisms that may halt food consumption in response to energy surplus. Instead of hunger and appetite, the current research emphasis is on the physiological mechanisms of satiety [44, 45].

Satiety refers to reduced hunger and faster termination of eating [8, 9]. Foods that deliver fewer kilocalories per meal are, by definition, more satiating [7–9]. In contrast, foods that tend to be overeaten have, by definition, less of an effect on satiety. There has been some argument whether fat-rich foods are overeaten because of their high energy density or because of their fat content [45]. If satiety is macronutrient driven, fat may be overeaten because it affects satiety less than a corresponding amount (in kcalories) of carbohydrate or protein [46].

Some researchers separate the concepts of satiation, measured by meal size, and the state of postmeal satiety, as

measured by the time delay until the next meal [38–40]. The distinction was meant to account for the puzzling phenomenon that though energy-dense fat ought to promote satiety, high-fat foods were often eaten to excess. The favored explanation was that fats had a weak effect on satiation but a much stronger effect on satiety [38–40]. Satiety is typically associated with delayed gastric emptying, elevated plasma glucose and insulin levels, and a postmeal elevation in plasma lipids.

Both hunger and satiety are thought to be under neural regulatory control [41]. In animal studies, the initiation and termination of feeding can be achieved by manipulating central neurotransmitters and peptides [41, 42]. Studies of such mechanisms have led to the development of pharmacological agents for obesity treatment. Again, the focus has shifted from reducing appetite to promoting satiety. Whereas amphetamine-like substances that reduce hunger and appetite are no longer in common use, selective serotonin reuptake inhibitors that promote satiety are the current drugs of choice [43]. However, centrally acting pharmacological agents are only sporadically effective, have potential for causing side effects, and lead to only minor weight loss. Research has also addressed the role of gut peptides such as bombesin and cholecystokinin in promoting satiety; however, they do not appear to be effective in most human studies. Similarly, leptin, a hormone secreted by the adipose tissue, is largely ineffective in promoting satiety, reducing food intakes, or causing weight loss in humans.

Some researchers have argued that taste factors override normal satiety signals, leading to overeating and overweight [46, 47]. Sweet taste has been singled out for special blame. The addition of sugars to foods was reported to stimulate appetite and increase food consumption [48, 49]. Identical claims were made for noncaloric sweeteners, suggesting that sweet taste, and not the presence of sugar, was the key factor. Curiously, similar claims regarding fat were based not on taste but on its energy density. Energy density of fats, the argument went, suppressed satiety signals and led to "passive overeating" [46] of fat-rich foods. Of course, energy-dense foods tend to be palatable and vice versa.

In principle, consumption of more satiating foods ought to lead to lower energy intakes and therefore weight loss. However, palatability and satiety are mirror-image terms that are linked, moreover, to the energy density of foods. Palatability, sometimes measured in terms of hedonic response or predisposition toward a given food, is said to heighten appetite and so increase the amount of food consumed. In contrast, satiety, often measured in terms of fullness or reduced liking for a given food, is said to reduce the amount of food consumed [7–9, 43–46]. Given that palatability and satiety are measured in terms of actual consumption, their relationship is by definition, reciprocal. Palatable foods that are overeaten are thereby, by definition, the least satiating [8]. Conversely, the highly satiating foods are, also by definition,

the least palatable. The creation of palatable and yet satiating foods, the avowed goal of the weight loss industry, is a contradiction in terms.

V. ENERGY DENSITY OF FOODS

Energy density is said to be the key factor in the regulation of food intake [50–52]. Under *ad libitum* conditions in the laboratory, young people tend to consume a constant weight of food rather than a constant amount of energy [53]. Foods with high energy density, that is, more kilocalories per unit weight, deliver more kilocalories per eating occasion than do energy-dilute foods [53, 54]. In contrast, lower energy density is associated with lower energy intakes per meal.

Energy-dilute foods are more bulky and so provide fewer kilocalories per eating occasion. By definition then, energy-dilute foods are more satiating than are energy-dense foods [51–53]. Chocolate cake, hamburgers, and French fries provide from 3 to 5 kcal/g. Chocolate candy and peanut butter provide 5 to 6 kcal/g. In contrast, most raw vegetables and salad greens are energy-dilute foods, providing between 0.1 and 0.5 kcal/g.

Because energy-dense foods deliver more energy per eating occasion, they are—by definition—less satiating. A study of 38 common foods [55] measured satiety ratings every 15 minutes for 2 hours following the consumption of equicaloric (240 kcal) amounts of food. That amount of energy can be provided by less than 50 g of chocolate or by more than 1000 g of boiled spinach. The satiety index was calculated by dividing the area under the satiety response curve for the test foods by the mean satiety curve for white bread and multiplying by 100%. Satiety indices correlated most highly with the weight of foods consumed that ranged from a low of 38 g for peanuts to a high of 625 g for oranges [60].

Analyses of satiety ratings showed that cake, cookies, and chocolate were less satiating than were porridge, potatoes, and boiled fish [55]. However, porridge and boiled fish were rated as significantly less palatable than cookies and chocolate [55]. It would appear that energy-dense foods are palatable but not satiating, whereas energy dilute foods are satiating but not palatable [7–9]. Although studies [51, 52, 56] have sometimes contrived to separate energy density, nutrient composition, and palatability, these factors are rarely separable in real life. Generally, higher fat diets are more enjoyable and varied and tend to provide more energy per unit weight than do the more bulky low-fat or fat-free diets. Factors that influence food choices in real life, such as cost, accessibility, and convenience [57], are generally ignored in laboratory studies where a variety of foods is provided to the respondent at no cost.

The energy-density approach to dieting has been the topic of many articles and popular books. If people consume a

constant weight of food each day, then choosing energy-dense foods will lead to higher energy intakes. Conversely, selecting foods with low energy density should lead—in principle—to lower energy intakes and eventual weight loss [53]. The idea that fat and protein had different effects on satiety has already been exploited by the weight loss industry. Most liquid formula diets are simply mixtures of protein, fiber, and water, together with small amounts of carbohydrate. Alhough they represent a major commercial success, their availability has not reduced the growing rates of overweight and obesity. [58]

Two main problems are associated with the energy-density approach to weight loss. First, energy density of foods is almost completely determined by their water and fat content [8, 9]. Generally, energy-dense foods are dry, high in fat, and sometimes high in sugar (e.g., chocolate). In contrast, energy-dilute foods are high in water, fiber, and sometimes protein (e.g., spinach). Multiple regression analyses of some 100 common foods in the U.S. diet showed that water content alone accounted for 85% of the variance, while water and fat accounted for 99% of the variance. Sugar, fiber, and protein content played a decidedly lesser role [9].

Second, the more energy-dense foods are usually more palatable. Classic studies on U.S. Army food preferences [59] showed that steak, milkshakes, and cake were preferred over broccoli and yogurt. A study of food preferences of obese men and women likewise showed that cakes and desserts were preferred over fresh vegetables and fruit. Whereas obese men listed steak and meat dishes among their favorite foods, obese women selected foods that were both sweet and rich in fat. Such foods included chocolate, ice cream, doughnuts, cookies, and cake [25]. Only women with anorexia nervosa have been observed to consistently list energy-dilute vegetables and salads among their favorite foods [60].

VI. APPETITE FOR ENERGY

Obesity is the long-term outcome of excess energy intake relative to energy expenditure [61]. Studies using doubly labeled water techniques have established that obese patients expend, and also consume, more energy than do lean controls [62]. Though energy imbalance is the chief—and maybe the only—reason for body weight gain, studies have sought to link obesity rates with excess consumption of a single nutrient or a given food. In some studies, obesity was linked with excess consumption of simple sugars, including sweets, snacks, desserts, and carbonated soft drinks [63–65]. Obesity has also been linked with excess fat consumption, including frequent consumption of fast foods [66, 67]. Studies have even linked obesity with greater dietary variety [68] and with higher frequency of food consumption away from home [69].

The once-popular externality hypothesis held that obese persons were more attuned to external variables, such as the taste of food, as opposed to the internal signals of hunger and satiety [8]. Subsequent research showed the obese were no more sensitive to sweet taste, did not necessarily prefer sweet solutions, and showed the same satiety response to sweetness as did normal-weight controls [8].

At this time, there is no convincing evidence to link obesity with specific macronutrient appetites. Although obesity has been blamed on excessive consumption of fast foods or carbonated soft drinks, no study has shown that obese persons have a selective appetite for either sugar or fat. It may be that obesity is associated with an appetite for energy-dense foods, whatever their nutrient content may be. For the most part, given the nature of the food supply, such foods will contain either sugar or fat.

The role of dietary fat in promoting weight gain has proven to be controversial [67, 70–72]. Noting that obesity rates in the United States have risen, while the proportion of fat energy in the diet has dropped, some scientists [71] have questioned the connection between fat consumption and obesity. However, the proportion of fat in the diet is not as important as the total amount of energy consumed. As shown by National Health and Nutrition Examination Survey III data, both energy intakes and fat consumption in grams per day actually increased between 1976–1980 and 1988–1994, this for both women and men [73]. Total energy intakes, and not percentage of fat in the diet, are likely to be more predictive of weight gain.

Why the energy imbalance is not redressed by the physiological mechanisms of hunger, appetite, or satiety is a good question. From the evolutionary standpoint, sensory mechanisms regulating food intake were meant to protect the organism against starvation and respond primarily to energy needs. A plentiful food supply is a very recent phenomenon [10, 74]. The question is whether taste mechanisms, geared toward the acceptance of sugar and fat, can also protect us from the potential ill effects of dietary excess now that sugar and fat are the most common foodstuffs available [10]. It is possible that they cannot. Far from being an abnormality or a disease, obesity may represent an adaptive response to the current environmental conditions

References

1. National Heart, Lung, and Blood Institute, Obesity Initiative Task Force (1998). Clinical guidelines on the identification, evaluation, and treatment of overweight and obesity in adults—The evidence report. *Obes. Res.* **6** (Suppl. 2), 1S–210S.
2. Flegal, K. M., Carroll, M. D., Kuczmarski, R. J., and Johnson, C. L. (1998). Overweight and obesity in the United States: Prevalence and trends, 1960 to 1994. *Int. J. Obes.* **22,** 39–47.
3. Mokdad, A. H., Serdula, M. K., Dietz, W. H., Bowman, B. A., Marks, J. S., and Koplan, J. P. (1999). The spread of the obesity epidemic in the United States 1991–1998. *JAMA* **282,** 1519–1522.

4. Harnack, L. J., Jeffery, R. W., and Boutelle, K. N. (2000). Temporal trends in energy intake in the United States: An ecologic perspective. *Am. J. Clin. Nutr.* **71**(6), 1478–1484.

5. Cavadini, C., Siega-Riz, A. M., and Popkins, B. M. (2000). U.S. adolescent food intake trends from 1965 to 1996. *Arch. Dis. Child.* **83**(1), 18–24.

6. USDA (2000). "Dietary Guidelines for Americans." Available at http://www.ars.usda.gov.

7. Drewnowski, A. (1997). Taste preferences and food intake. *Annu. Rev. Nutr.* **17,** 237–250.

8. Drewnowski, A. (1998). Palatability and satiety: Models and measures. *Ann. Nestle* **56,** 32–42.

9. Drewnowski, A. (1998). Energy density, palatability, and satiety: Implications for weight control. *Nutr. Rev.* **56,** 347–353.

10. Groop, L. C., and Tuomi, T. (1997). Non-insulin-dependent diabetes mellitus—A collision between thrifty genes and an affluent society. *Ann. Med.* **29,** 37–53.

11. Drewnowski, A., and Popkin, B. M. (1997). The nutrition transition: New trends in the global diet. *Nutr. Rev.* **55,** 31–43.

12. Weinsier, R. L., Hunter, G. R., Heini, A. F., Goran, M. I., and Sell, S. M. (1998). The etiology of obesity: Relative contribution of metabolic factors, diet and physical activity. *Am. J. Med.* **105**(2), 145–150.

13. Perusse, L., and Bouchard, C. (1999). Genotype–environment interaction in human obesity. *Nutr. Rev.* **57**(5), (II)S31–S38.

14. Garn, S. M., Sullivan, T. V., and Hawthorne, V. M. (1989). Fatness and obesity of the parents of obese individuals. *Am. J. Clin. Nutr.* **50**(6), 1308–1313.

15. Stunkard, A. J., Berkowitz, R. I., Stallings, V. A., and Cater, J. R. (1999). Weights of parents and infants: Is there a relationship? *Int. J. Obes. Relat. Metab. Disord.* **23**(2), 159–162.

16. Stunkard, A. J., Sorensen, T. I., Hanis, C., Teasdale, T. W., Chakraborty, R., Schull, W. J., and Schulsinger, F. (1986). An adoption study of human obesity. *N. Engl. J. Med.* **314,** 193–198.

17. Bouchard, C., Tremblay, A., Despres, J. P., Nadeau, A., Lupien, P. J., Theriault, G., Dussault, J., Moorjani, S., Pinault, S., and Fournier, G. (1990). The response to long-term overfeeding in identical twins. *N. Engl. J. Med.* **322,** 1477–1482.

18. Faith, M. S., Pietrobelli, A., Nunez, C., Heo, M., Heymsfield, S. B., Allison, D. B. (1999). Evidence for independent genetic influences on fat mass and body mass index in a pediatric twin sample. *Pediatrics* **104,** 61–67.

19. Stunkard, A. J. (1996). Current views on obesity. *Am. J. Med.* **100,** 230–236.

20. Grundy, S. M. (1998). Multifactorial causation of obesity: Implications for prevention. *Am. J. Clin. Nutr.* **67**(Suppl.), 536S–572S.

21. Roberts, S. B., Savage, J., Coward, W. A., Chew, B., and Lucas, A. (1988). Energy expenditure and intake in infants born to lean and overweight mothers. *N. Engl. J. Med.* **318,** 461–466.

22. Nisbett, R. E., and Gurwitz, S. B. (1970). Weight, sex, and eating behavior of human newborns. *J. Comp. Physiol. Psychol.* **73,** 245–253.

23. Drewnowski, A. (1987). Sweetness and obesity. *In* "Sweetness" (J. Dobbing, Ed.), pp. 177–190. Springer-Verlag, London.

24. Drewnowski, A., Brunzell, J. D., Sande, K., Iverius, P. H., and Greenwood, M. R. C. (1985). Sweet tooth reconsidered: Taste responsiveness in human obesity.

25. Drewnowski, A., Kurth, C., Holden-Wiltse, J., and Saari, J. (1992). Food preferencees in human obesity: Carbohydrates versus fats. *Appetite* **18,** 207–221.

26. Seidell, J. C. (1997). Time trends in obesity: An epidemiological perspective. *Horm. Metab. Res.* **29**(4), 155–158.

27. Martorell, R., Khan, L. K., Hughes, M. L., and Grummer-Strawn, L. M. (2000). Obesity in women from developing countries. *Eur. J. Clin. Nutr.* **54**(3), 247–252.

28. Centers for Disease Control and Prevention, Centers for Health Statistics (2000). Obesity rates. Available at http://www.cdc.gov.

29. Mennella, J. A., Beauchamp, G. K. (1998). Early flavor experiences: research update. *Nutr. Rev.* **56,** 205–211.

30. Birch, L. L. (1999). Development of food preferences. *Annu. Rev. Nutr.* **19,** 41–62.

31. Cabanac, M. (1971). Physiological role of pleasure. *Science* **173,** 1103–1107.

32. De Graaf, C., and Zandstra, E. H. (1999). Sweetness intensity and pleasantness in children, adolescents, and adults. *Physiol. Behav.* **67**(4), 513–520.

33. Drewnowski, A., Krahn, D. D., Demitrack, M. A., Nairn, K., and Gosnell, B. A. (1995). Naloxone, an opiate blocker, reduces the consumption of sweet high-fat foods in obese and lean female binge eaters. *Am. J. Clin. Nutr.* **61**(6), 1206–1212.

34. Mercer, M. E., and Holder, M. D. (1997). Food cravings, endogenous opioid peptides, and food intake: A review. *Appetite* **29**(3), 325–352.

35. Mela, D. J., and Sacchetti, D. A. (1991). Sensory preferences for fats: Relationships with diet and body composition. *Am. J. Clin. Nutr.* **53,** 908–915.

36. Fisher, J. O., and Birch, L. L. (1995). Fat preferences and fat consumption of 3- to 5-year-old children are related to parental adiposity. *J. Am. Diet. Assoc.* **95,** 759–764.

37. Drewnowski, A. (1987). Fats and food texture: Sensory and hedonic evaluations. *In* "Food Texture" (H. R. Moskowitz, Ed.), pp. 217–250. Marcel Dekker, New York.

38. Blundell, J. E., and Macdiarmid, J. I. (1997). Fat as a risk factor for overconsumption: Satiation, satiety and patterns of eating. *J. Am. Diet. Assoc.* **97**(Suppl.), S63–S69.

39. Blundell, J. E., Burley, V. J., Cotton, J. R., and Lawton, C. L. (1993). Dietary fat and the control of energy intake: Evaluating the effects of fat on meal size and post-meal satiety. *Am. J. Clin. Nutr.* **57,** 772S–778S.

40. Green, S. M., Burley, V. J., and Blundell, J. E. (1994). Effect of fat- and sucrose-containing foods on the size of eating episodes and energy intake in lean males: Potential of causing overconsumption. *Eur. J. Clin. Nutr.* **48,** 547–555.

41. Woods, S. C., Seeley, R. J., Porte, D., and Schwartz, M. W. (1998). Signals that regulate food intake and energy homeostasis. *Science* **280**(5368), 1378–1383.

42. Seeley, R. J., and Berthoud, H. R. (2000). Neural and metabolic control of macronutrient selection: Consensus and controversy. *In* "Neural and Metabolic Control of Macronutrient Intake" (H.-R. Berthoud and R. J. Seeley, Eds.), pp. 489–496. CRC Press, New York.

43. Halford, J. C., and Blundell, J. E. (2000). Pharmacology of appetite suppression. *Prog. Drug. Res.* **54,** 25–58.

44. Rolls, B. J., Hetherington, M., and Burley, V. J. (1988). The specificity of satiety: The influence of foods of different macronutrient content on the development of satiety. *Physiol. Behav.* **43,** 145–153.

45. Rolls, B. J., Fedoroff, I. C., Guthrie, J. F., and Laster, L. J. (1990). Foods with different satiating effects in humans. *Appetite* **15,** 115–126.
46. Blundell, J. E., Lawton, C. L., Cotton, J. R., and Macdiarmid, J. I. (1996). Control of human appetite: Implications for the intake of dietary fat. *Annu. Rev. Nutr.* **16,** 285–319.
47. Gibson, S. A. (1996). Are high-fat, high-sugar foods and diets conducive to obesity? *Int. J. Food Nutr. Sci.* **47,** 405–415.
48. Rogers, P. J., Carlyle, J., Hill, A. J., and Blundell, J. E. (1988). Uncoupling sweet taste and calories: Comparison of the effects of glucose and three intense sweeteners on hunger and food intake. *Physiol. Behav.* **43,** 547–552.
49. Rogers, P. J., and Blundell, J. E. (1989). Separating the actions of sweetness and calories: Effects of saccharin and carbohydrates on hunger and food intake in human subjects. *Physiol. Behav.* **45,** 1093–1099.
50. Poppitt, S. D. (1995). Energy density of diets and obesity. *Int. J. Obes.* **19**(Suppl.), S20–S26.
51. Stubbs, R. J., Harbron, C. G., and Prentice, A. M. (1996). Covert manipulation of the dietary fat to carbohydrate ratio of isoenergetically dense diets: Effects on food intake in feeding men ad libitum. *Int. J. Obes.* **20,** 651–660.
52. Prentice, A. M., and Poppit, S. D. (1996). Importance of energy density and macronutrients in the regulation of food intake. *Int. J. Obes.* **20**(Suppl.), S18–S23.
53. Rolls, B. J., and Bell, E. A. (1999). Intake of fat and carbohydrate: Role in energy density. *Eur. J. Clin. Nutr.* **53,** S166–S173.
54. Seagle, H. M., Davy, B. M., Grunwald, G., and Hill, J. O. (1997). Energy density of self-reported food intake: Variation and relationship to other food components. *Obes. Res.* **5** (Suppl.), S87.
55. Holt, S. H. A., Brand Miller, J. C., Petocz, P., and Farmakalidis, E. (1995). A satiety index of common foods. *Eur. J. Clin. Nutr.* **49,** 675–690.
56. Rolls, B. J., Kim-Harris, S., Fischman, M. W., Foltin, R. W., Moran, T. H., and Stoner, S. H. (1994). Satiety after preloads with different amounts of fat and carbohydrate: Implications for obesity. *Am. J. Clin. Nutr.* **60,** 476–487.
57. Glanz, K., Basil, M., Maibach, E., Goldberg, J., and Snyder, D. (1998). Why Americans eat what they do: Taste, nutrition, cost, convenience and weight control concerns as influences on food consumption. *J. Am. Diet. Assoc.* **98,** 1118–1126.
58. Drewnowski, A. (1993). Low-calorie foods and the prevalence of obesity. *In* "Low-Calorie Foods Handbook" (A. M. Altschul, Ed.), pp. 513–534. Marcel Dekker, New York.
59. Meiselman, H. L., Waterman, D., and Symington, L. E. (1974). "Armed Forces Food Preferences." U.S. Army Natick Development Center Technical Report TR-75-63-FSL.
60. Drewnowski, A., Pierce, B., and Halmi, K. A. (1988). Fat aversion in eating disorders. *Appetite* **10,** 119–131.
61. Goran, M. I. (2000). Energy metabolism and obesity. *Med. Clin. N. Am.* **84**(2), 347–362.
62. Schoeller, D. A. (1999). Recent advances from application of doubly labeled water to measurement of human energy expenditure. *J. Nutr.* **129**(10), 1765–1768.
63. Wildey, M. B., Pampalone, S. Z., Pelletier, R. L., Zive, M. M., Elder, J. P., and Sallis, J. F. (2000). Fat and sugar levels are high in snacks purchased from student stores in middle schools. *J. Am. Diet. Assoc.* **100,** 319–322.
64. Farris, R. P., Nicklas, T. A., Myers, L., and Berenson, G. S. (1998). Nutrient intake and food group consumption of 10-year-olds by sugar intake level: The Bogalusa Heart Study. *J. Am. College Nutr.* **17,** 579–585.
65. Harnack, L., Stang, J., and Story, M. (1999). Soft drink consumption among U.S. children and adolescents: Nutritional consequences. *J. Am. Diet. Assoc.* **99,** 436–411.
66. Jeffery, R. W., French, S. A. (1998). Epidemic obesity in the United States: Are fast foods and television viewing contributing? *Am. J. Public Health* **88,** 277–280.
67. Bray, G., and Popkin, B. M. (1998). Dietary fat intake does effect obesity. *Am. J. Clin. Nutr.* **68,** 1157–1173.
68. McCrory, M. A., Fuss, P. J., McCallum, J. E., Yao, M., Vinken, A. G., Hays, N. P., and Roberts, S. B. (1999). Dietary variety within food groups: Association with energy intake and body fatness in men and women. *Am. J. Clin. Nutr.* **69**(3), 440–447.
69. McCrory, M. A., Fuss, P. J., Hays, N. P., Vinken, A. G., Greenberg, A. S., and Roberts, S. B. (1999). Overeating in America: Association between restaurant food consumption and body fatness in healthy adult men and women ages 19 to 80. *Obes. Res.* **7**(6), 564–571.
70. Hill, J. O., Melanson, E. L., and Wyatt, H. T. (2000). Dietary fat intake and regulation of energy balance: Implications for obesity. *J. Nutr.* **130**(Suppl. 2), 284S–288S.
71. Willett, W. C. (1998). Dietary fat and obesity: An unconvincing relation. *Am. J. Clin. Nutr.* **68,** 1149–1150.
72. Willett, W. C. (1998). Is dietary fat a major determinant of body fat? *Am. J. Clin. Nutr.* **67**(Suppl. 3), 556S–562S.
73. McDowell, M. A., Briefel, R. R., Alaimo, K., Bischof, A. M., Caughman, C. R., Carroll, M. D., Loria, C. M., and Johnson, C. L. (1994). Energy and macronutrient intakes of persons ages 2 months and over in the United States: Third National Health and Nutrition Examination Survey, Phase 1, 1988–91. *Vital Health Statis. NCHS* **255,** 1–24.
74. Trichopoulou, A., and Lagiou, P. (1997). Worldwide patterns of dietary lipids intake and health implications. *Am. J. Clin. Nutr.* **66**(Suppl.), 961S–964S.

E. Gastrointestinal Diseases

CHAPTER 36

Nutrition in the Prevention and Treatment of Common Gastrointestinal Symptoms

LAWRENCE J. CHESKIN[1] AND DEBRA L. MILLER[2]

[1]*Johns Hopkins Bayview Medical Center, Baltimore, Maryland*
[2]*Central Soya Co., Inc., Fort Wayne, Indiana*

I. INTRODUCTION

The prevalence of episodic gastrointestinal complaints in the general population is quite high and can take many forms. In a recent national survey in which respondents were asked about digestive symptoms (pain, bloating, loose stools), 40.5% reported having one or more digestive complaints in the month prior to the interview [1]. Gastrointestinal complaints include acute symptoms such as abdominal pain, bloating, excessive gas or burping, diarrhea, heartburn, constipation, and nausea. These symptoms may occur for varying amounts of time and with varying degrees of severity. Other gastrointestinal problems are syndromes or diseases and are thus more chronic in nature; the most common include irritable bowel syndrome and gastroesophageal reflux disease. Others are less common but important causes of morbidity, for example, inflammatory bowel diseases (ulcerative colitis and Crohn's disease) and celiac disease.

Some of these conditions are attributed directly to the ingestion of certain foods or are potentially aggravated by specific foods. Another recent survey, which assessed the prevalence of various gastrointestinal complaints (cramps, nausea, excessive burping and gas, bloating, constipation, diarrhea, heartburn), found that individuals who reported having these complaints frequently attribute them to foods and beverages consumed. Table 1 shows the percentages of attribution of gastrointestinal complaints to foods and beverages in general and to specific foods [2]. While it is noteworthy that a large fraction of people surveyed attribute gastrointestinal symptoms to diet, in many cases this is anecdotal information and there are no scientific data to support a causative link [3].

It is thought that this predilection toward gastrointestinal distress from foods is a rather recent phenomenon in human history. In prehistoric time, our ancestors rarely experienced such ailments as constipation, heartburn, gas, or irritable bowel syndrome [4]. This seems surprising given that early humans consumed nearly everything in their environment

including most of the plants, roots, animals, and insects. Because early humans consumed all components of foodstuffs including husks, skins, pit, and seeds, the digestive tract needed to be an efficient processor of food and, indeed, this is what it evolved to be. However, since the 19th century, milling and processing of food (outside of the gastrointestinal tract) have become commonplace. Through milling procedures, raw foods are processed into flour, sugar, and oils. Much dietary fiber and other nutrients are lost in this process. Nutrition scientists have recently begun to recognize the importance of fiber and other natural components of foods in gastrointestinal health. Some foods, however, are indeed more likely to cause negative digestive consequences than others. The goals of this chapter are to focus on the common acute gastrointestinal complaints/symptoms: excessive gas, heartburn, diarrhea, constipation, and nausea/vomiting; to discuss specific foods that are associated with such symptoms; and, finally, to identify nutritional and other practices that may be therapeutic for such ailments.

II. EXCESSIVE GAS

A. Prevalence and Causes

Having intestinal gas is normal; however, having excess gas can be uncomfortable or even embarrassing. Gas in the intestines comes from three sources: swallowed air, intralumenal production resulting from the normal breakdown of certain undigested foods by the harmless bacteria that are naturally present in the large intestine, and from diffusion from the blood [5]. While the self-reported frequency of excessive intestinal gas varies, humans have a relatively consistent amount of gas (~200 mL) in their small and large bowel in both the fasting state and after a meal [6]. However, the rate of excretion of gas varies greatly between individuals, ranging from 476 to 1491 mL/day (mean 705 mL/day) [7]. In one British study, participants who ingested their usual diet

TABLE 1   Attribution of Gastrointestinal Symptoms (in Past Month) to Foods or Beverages
by American Adults (947 Interviews)

	Excessive gas	Bloating	Heartburn	Diarrhea	Constipation	Nausea
Number of gastrointestinal events reported by respondents[a]	151	92	220	172	119	94
Percentage of respondents attributing gastrointestinal symptoms to foods and/or beverages	78.2	62.0	79.1	54.1	43.7	25.5
Percentages for specific foods to which symptoms were attributed[b]						
Spicy foods	38.1	36.8	66.5	23.7	7.7	45.0
Beans	44.9	21.2	10.3	10.8	9.6	0
Vegetables	25.4	12.3	3.5	16.1	7.7	0
Fruit	8.5	10.5	4.6	16.1	13.5	4.2
Fried/greasy foods	22.9	35.1	36.8	34.4	23.1	41.7
Milk, cheese, lactose	25.4	26.3	8.1	16.1	40.4	16.7
Sugar substitutes	0	1.8	0.6	2.2	1.9	4.2
Fat substitutes	0.9	1.8	0.6	2.2	5.8	4.2
Bran/high-fiber foods	10.2	12.3	1.7	12.9	1.9	0
Alcohol	2.5	5.3	12.6	9.7	0	12.5
Coffee	5.9	5.3	15.5	7.5	3.9	12.5
Other	14.4	17.5	13.2	23.7	30.8	16.7

[a]Respondents could report multiple events.
[b]Respondents could attribute symptoms to multiple foods and/or beverages.

passed gas per rectum an average of 8 times/day [7], whereas a study of healthy American participants (aged 20–60) passed gas on an average frequency of 10 times per day with an upper limit of normal (mean ± 2 SD) of 20 times per day [8].

B. Production and Composition of Intestinal Gas

Three gases—CO_2, H_2, and CH_4—are produced in appreciable quantity in the bowel lumen. Carbon dioxide (CO_2) is thought to account for 50–60% of flatus volume, and such levels are usually associated with high concentrations of H_2. Because the only bowel source of H_2 is bacterial metabolism, flatus CO_2 similarly appears to be derived from fermentation reactions. Intestinal bacteria liberate H_2 during fermentation of either carbohydrate or protein; however, H_2 production from amino acids is appreciably less than that from sugars.

Comprehensive tests of why some individuals have increased rectal gas have not been done; however, it has been determined that neither age nor sex correlated with the frequency of the passage of flatus [8]. Increased gas is often attributed to dietary factors. In individuals with intestinal disorders, carbohydrates and proteins, which are completely absorbed by the normally functioning intestine, may be malabsorbed and provide a substrate for colonic H_2 production.

Like H_2, the sole source of CH_4 (methane) in humans is the metabolism of the colonic bacteria. A person's tendency to produce methane is usually a fairly consistent trait over a period of several years. This tendency appears to be related more to genetic factors than to diet or other environmental factors. People who consistently produce large quantities of CH_4 have stools that float in water due to a decreased fat-to-gas ratio in the density of the stool [9]. Although there has been some speculation that persons who produced larger amounts of CH_4 may be at higher risk of colon cancer, this has not been substantiated by recent studies [10].

Interestingly, the three main gases in flatus or intestinal gas are not those that produce noxious or unpleasant odors. Rather, odor is attributed to trace amounts of sulfur-containing compounds such as methanethiol, dimethylsulfide, and hydrogen sulfide [11]. The majority of ingested sulfur is from the amino acids: methionine, cystine, and cysteine. Specific foods that contain these compounds are high-protein foods like meats and eggs. Sulfur is also a component of the vitamins thiamin and biotin.

C. Excess Gas and Specific Foods

Foods particularly associated with the production and excretion of excess gas include fruits and vegetables (particularly

TABLE 2 Foods Associated with Excessive Intestinal Gas

Category	Foods
Carbonated beverages	Sodas
	Some juices
	Beer
	Some wine coolers
Legumes/beans	Kidney
	Black
	Black-eyed peas
	Northern
	Pinto
	Garbanzo
	Lentils
	Navy
Cruciferous vegetables	Broccoli
	Cauliflower
	Brussels sprouts
	Cabbage
Fruit	Apples
	Pears
Starches	Potatoes
	Wheat
	Oats
	Corn
	Noodles
Dairy products (for those who are lactose intolerant)	Milk
	Ice cream
	Cheese

legumes [12]), which contain high concentrations of oligosaccharides that cannot be digested by the enzymes of the normal small bowel. Instead, the oligosaccharides are fermented by the colonic bacteria, resulting in the production of gas. Of the numerous oligosaccharide-containing foods alleged to increase the excretion of rectal gas, baked beans, which contain a large amount of the complex sugar raffinose, are the only natural food that has been carefully studied. In one study, a diet containing 51% of its calories as baked beans increased flatus elimination from a basal level of 15 to 176 mL/hour [12a]. Table 2 includes a list of foods associated with intestinal gas [5].

Other foods and food components that have been shown to increase H_2 production in healthy participants after ingestion include flours made with wheat, oats, potatoes, and corn (see Table 2), because these foods are rich in polysaccharides (not oligosaccharides). Complex carbohydrates other than oligosaccharides may not be completely absorbed [13].

Excess gas production is not limited to complex carbohydrates; some commonly used sweeteners and fibers have been associated with increased H_2 excretion. Fructose, present in exceptionally large quantities in sodas, juices, and other soft drinks, is malabsorbed by a sizable proportion of the healthy population [14]. Also, sorbitol, widely used as a low-calorie sugar substitute, is also poorly absorbed, and is readily fermented by colonic bacteria, causing gas production. Studies of the gas-producing effects of various fiber sources have shown that only pectin (found in apples and other fruits and vegetables) and hemicelluloses (the main structural fiber in cereals) appreciably increase H_2 excretion [15].

Lactose intolerance is caused by a deficiency in the intestinal enzyme, lactase, which is necessary for the digestion of the disaccharide, lactose, a sugar found almost exclusively in dairy products. Lactase deficiency is the most common enzyme deficiency in humans. This common condition is thought to contribute to gastrointestinal complaints of gas and bloating, among other symptoms (see Chapter 37 on lactose intolerance). Lactose intolerance contributes to excessive gas production when unabsorbed lactose provides a substrate for H_2 production by colonic bacteria.

Abdominal distention and bloating, thought to be caused by "too much gas," are two of the most frequently encountered gastrointestinal complaints. However, there is no evidence that excessive bowel gas is the primary cause of bloating and distention. The frequent complaint that certain foods "give me gas" or "make me bloated" may actually be more related to a hypersensitivity to bowel distention. Specific foods may actually stimulate abnormal motility rather than cause increased production of gas.

D. Therapy for Excess Gas

In trying to eliminate foods from the diet that may cause excess gas [e.g., cauliflower, brussels sprouts, dried beans (legumes), broccoli, cabbage and bran], foods that are high in fiber and food for the overall health of your digestive system may also be eliminated. Because of this, these foods may best be consumed in moderation rather than completely eliminated from the diet. For individuals who experience excess gas production as a result of eating foods containing wheat or corn flours, experimenting with rice flour as an alternative may be of benefit. Rice flour is the only complex carbohydrate that has been shown to be almost completely absorbed [13].

Digestive aids such as Beano® reduce gas by facilitating the digestion of raffinose, the sugar in beans and many gas-producing vegetables. Simethicone-containing products, such as Mylicon® and Gas X®, reduce bloating by reducing surface tension and coalescing bubbles of gas. Table 3 contains a list of medications for gas. Other foods that are thought to produce gas that may be eliminated from the diet include sorbitol-containing chewing gum and hard candy (such foods may also cause excess air swallowing because of constant chewing) and carbonated beverages. Exercise can also aid in stimulating the passage of gas through the digestive tract.

For individuals with lactase deficiency, restriction of lactose-containing foods (milk and milk products), ingestion of oral lactase enzyme preparations (Lactaid®), or the substitution of yogurt for milk has been thought to be of benefit to

TABLE 3 Medications for Symptomatic Relief of GI Symptoms

GI symptom	Drug category	Brand name example(s)	Comments
Gas	Enzymes	Beano® Lactaid®	Should be taken before food is eaten.
	Simethicone	Mylicon® Gas X®	
Heartburn	Antacids	Tums® Rolaids®	Should not be taken every day.
	H₂ receptor antagonists	Pepcid AC® Zantac® Tagamet®	May take up to 30 minutes to provide relief; may be taken before eating if irritating food is to be eaten.
Diarrhea	Bismuth subsalicylate	Pepto Bismol®	Decreases the secretions of the intestines; turns stool black.
	Loperamide diphenoxylate	Imodium AD® or Lomotil®	Slows down the movement of the intestines and its secretion but may worsen or prolong the illness by retarding the evacuation of infectious agents.
	Non-absorbable mixtures of kaolin and pectin	Kaopectate®	Makes stools more bulky.
Constipation	Osmotic laxatives	Correctol®	May increase intestinal water content enough to cause diarrhea.
	Bulk laxatives	Metamucil®	Does not provide immediate relief for constipation symptoms.
Nausea/vomiting	Dimenhydrinate	Dramamine®	For motion sickness; also causes drowsiness.
	Prochlorperazine/promethazine	Compazine® Phenergan®	Suppositories.

lactose maldigesters with gas problems. However, a controlled, blinded study of participants with self-diagnosed, severe lactose intolerance showed that symptoms following ingestion of 1 cup of regular milk and 1 cup of lactose-free milk were not different [16] (see Chapter 37).

III. HEARTBURN AND GASTROESOPHAGEAL REFLUX DISEASE

A. Prevalence and Causes

Heartburn is the most common specific gastrointestinal complaint in the Western Hemisphere. Nearly every middle-aged American adult has had one or more episodes of heartburn. Surveys have found that about 40% of U.S. adults experience heartburn at least once a month [17, 18], while roughly 10% suffer with heartburn daily [19]. Heartburn is also common during pregnancy, particularly in the third trimester, with 90% of pregnant women experiencing some type of reflux symptoms [20].

Gastroesophageal reflux disease (GERD) occurs when the muscle connecting the esophagus with the stomach does not function properly, allowing stomach acids and contents to enter the esophagus. Heartburn begins as a burning pain that starts behind the breastbone and radiates upward toward the back of throat. The description of "burning" or "hot"

or "acidic" sensations is typically used. Often there is a sensation of food coming back into the mouth, accompanied by an acid or bitter taste. Heartburn can become intense enough to cause pain that radiates throughout the chest region upward toward the neck and throat and occasionally to the back and arms.

Heartburn, the classic manifestation of GERD, is a commonly used but frequently misunderstood term. It has many synonyms, including "indigestion," "acid regurgitation," "sour stomach," and the more general "chest pain." The precise physiologic mechanisms that produce heartburn are, surprisingly, poorly understood. Although the reflux of gastric acid is most commonly associated with heartburn, the same symptoms may be elicited by other gastrointestinal events (esophageal distention, reflux of bile salts, and acid-induced motility disorders).

The pain associated with heartburn seems best explained by the stimulation of chemoreceptors due to the sensitivity of the esophagus to the presence of acid, as demonstrated during perfusion studies or by monitoring the esophageal pH of people with GERD. These receptors, however, are not superficial and their specific location is not known [21]. Correlations between discrete episodes of acid reflux and actual pain are poor; therefore, painful symptoms seem to require more than just the presence of acid in the esophagus [22]. One contributing factor may be the disruption of the mucous membrane in the esophagus, although most symptomatic

patients do not show such a disruption. Another possibility is hydrogen ion concentrations in the esophagus that alter its pH. One study found that 25 participants with reflux disease experienced heartburn-like symptoms when infused with solutions of pH 1.0 and 1.5, but only one-half had such symptoms with solutions of pH 2.5–6.0 [23]. Other factors may include inflammation with increased polymorphonuclear leukocytes, acid clearance mechanisms, salivary bicarbonate concentration, volumes of refluxed acid, and the interaction of pepsin with acid [5].

B. Heartburn and Food

Heartburn is predictably aggravated by many factors, food in particular. Symptoms usually present within an hour of eating, particularly after consuming the largest meal of the day. Foods high in fat, chocolate, onions, or carminatives (peppermint and spearmint) may aggravate heartburn by decreasing lower esophageal sphincter pressure [24, 25]. While the lower esophageal sphincter is not an actual sphincter, but rather a muscular structure that acts as a sphincter, it normally remains contracted, closing the entrance to the stomach and preventing reflux of the stomach contents into the lower esophagus [5]. When lower esophageal sphincter pressure is lowered, stomach contents and acid may flow upward into the esophagus. Diminished lower esophageal sphincter pressure may result from hormonal (gastrin, secretin, cholecystokinin, and glucagon) action, muscle abnormalities, or impaired nerve innervation [5].

Intake of foods such as peppermint, spearmint, chocolate, alcohol, and fats (especially fat in whole milk) may alter the hormonal milieu of the esophagus and reduce lower esophageal sphincter pressure [26]. In contrast, coffee contains the methylxanthines caffeine and theophylline, which may increase lower esophageal sphincter pressure by inhibiting phosphodiesterase, in turn, increasing intracellular concentrations of cyclic adensosine monophosphate in the lower esophageal sphincter [26]. Other studies, however, have found that theophylline decreases lower esophageal sphincter pressure and that caffeine had no effect [26]. Another study found that both caffeinated and decaffeinated coffee decreased lower esophageal sphincter pressure [26], indicating that there may an unknown substance in coffee other than caffeine that affects lower esophageal sphincter pressure. How peppermint and spearmint increase lower esophageal sphincter pressure is unknown.

Other foods commonly associated with heartburn include highly acidic foods such as citrus products and tomato-based foods, and spicy foods. These foods do not affect lower esophageal sphincter pressure. Rather, they directly irritate the inflamed esophageal mucosa by increasing the presence of acid, lowering pH, or increasing osmolarity [5]. Many beverages, including citrus juices, soft drinks, coffee, and alcohol, also cause heartburn by more than one mechanism. Wine drinkers may have heartburn after hearty red wines, but not after delicate white wines. The exact reason for this is not known.

In addition, generalized chest pain, characterized as a squeezing or burning substernal sensation, radiating to the back, neck, jaw, or arms (sometimes indistinguishable from angina), is associated with the ingestion of very hot or very cold liquids. The mechanism for this is not well understood. One possible cause may be esophageal distention resulting from the activation of stretch receptors in response to a cold substance [24]. Such distention and pain are also experienced with acute food impaction, the drinking of carbonated beverages (in some individuals), and dysfunction in the belch reflex.

Other factors that may aggravate heartburn include running; however, riding a stationary bicycle or using other exercise machines does not seem to have this effect and, thus, may be good exercise for those with GERD. Cigarette smoking exacerbates heartburn because nicotine lowers lower esophageal sphincter pressure. Air swallowing, which often accompanies inhalation of smoke, also tends to relax the lower esophageal sphincter. A number of medications may also cause or exacerbate heartburn by decreasing lower esophageal sphincter pressure. Aspirin may directly irritate the inflamed esophagus. Finally, emotions such as fear, anxiety, and worry may aggravate heartburn symptoms, probably through the amplification of symptoms rather than by increasing the amount of acid reflux.

C. Therapy

GERD can be lessened by following a few guidelines. In addition to limiting the foods known to precipitate heartburn symptoms, decreasing the amount eaten at meals, and not eating 2–3 hours prior to lying down or going to bed may also help reduce symptoms. Foods to avoid due to heartburn include high-fat foods, peppermint/spearmint, caffeinated foods and beverages (coffee, tea, chocolate, colas), alcohol, citrus fruits and juices, tomatoes and tomato products, and pepper. However, citrus fruits and tomatoes are good sources of vitamin C.

Because heartburn is such a common gastrointestinal complaint, many of those who suffer its effects do not consult a physician and seek relief from over-the-counter preparations such as antacids and H_2 receptor antagonists (e.g., Pepcid AC®, Zantac®, Tagamet®) (Table 3). In a recent study of patients who use antacids daily, more than half had evidence of erosive esophagitis. Individuals with frequent or daily heartburn and pregnant women are advised to consult their physician for evaluation and individualized therapies.

IV. DIARRHEA

A. Prevalence and Causes

Diarrhea is best defined as an increased liquidity or decreased consistency of stools [5]. There are four mechanisms of diarrhea. The first is osmotic diarrhea, which is caused by

the presence of unusually large amounts of poorly absorbed, osmotically active solutes—such as dietary carbohydrate or laxative—in the gut lumen. In osmotic diarrhea, the ingested solute or solutes exert an osmotic force across the intestinal mucosa causing an increase in water in the large intestine. Hallmarks of osmotic diarrhea include the following:

1. Fecal water output is directly related to the fecal output of the solute or solutes exerting osmostic pressure across the intestinal mucosa.
2. Diarrhea stops with fasting or the termination of ingesting the poorly absorbed solute (carbohydrate or laxatives)
3. Stool analysis reveals an osmotic gap that is much more than the normal osmolarity of fecal fluid that exits the rectum (290 mOsm/kg).

The second mechanism is secretory diarrhea, which refers to the diarrhea that is caused by abnormal ion transport in intestinal epithelial cells. This condition is not marked by an osmotic gap, but may occur in tandem with osmotic diarrhea. Infectious diseases of the gastrointestinal tract often result in secretory diarrhea.

The third mechanism of diarrhea is altered gut motility. Gut motility is the process and pace by which food is physically transported through the gastrointestinal tract. Enhanced motility may result in diarrhea by propelling boluses of fluid quickly through the gut, thereby decreasing the contact time with the absorptive epithelial-sometimes called "intestinal hurry" [5]. Conversely, abnormally slow motility may allow bacteria to "overgrow" in the small intestine and cause diarrhea or steatorrhea (an excess amount of fat in the feces).

The final mechanism of diarrhea is exudation. Exudation, as it relates to diarrhea, is usually the result of inflammation or ulceration and causes the escape of mucus, fluid, serum proteins, and blood from the intestinal mucosa [5]. These components are deposited in the gut lumen and expelled in the feces. This type of diarrhea is associated with dysentery and ulcerative colitis [5].

Because secretory, altered motility and exudation mechanisms for diarrhea are associated with infectious diseases of the gastrointestinal tract or more chronic types of diarrhea, this discussion will focus on osmotic diarrhea, the mechanism most associated with acute bouts of diarrhea related to the ingestion of food.

B. Diarrhea and Food

As noted, malabsorbed carbohydrates, such as starches, lactose, and fructose, can contribute to osmotic diarrhea. When carbohydrates are not absorbed in the small intestine, they remain in the lumen and are a potential source of osmotically active particles. Two main factors determine the severity of diarrhea that results from carbohydrate malabsorption in sensitive individuals: (1) the type and amount of carbohydrate ingested and (2) the rate at which carbohydrate reaches the colon. If relatively large amounts of malabsorbed carbohy-

drate are present in the gut (e.g., lactose intolerance), diarrhea is likely to result. Smaller amounts of malabsorbed carbohydrate, such as after ingestion of a sorbitol-containing food, may result only in bloating, distention. and excessive flatus (see Section II on excessive gas).

Malabsorbed dietary fat, which can be normal with high-fat diets, can also contribute to diarrhea. When dietary fatty acids not properly absorbed by the small intestine reach the colon, a portion of them is hydroxylized by bacterial enzymes [5]. Under experimental conditions, fatty acids and hydroxy-fatty acids have been shown to inhibit fluid absorption from both the small intestine and colon [27–29]. This is the proposed mechanism by which steatorrhea causes excessive fecal fluid losses [5]. Controversy has arisen over whether the nonabsorbable, lipid-based fat replacer, olestra, causes diarrhea. In a placebo-controlled trial, consumption of olestra-containing potato chips did not result in increased reports of diarrhea or other gastrointestinal complaints compared to triglyceride-containing potato chips [3]. Unpublished data from the olestra postmarketing surveillance study also indicate no dose–response relationship between diarrhea and olestra intake [2].

Diarrhea is also a common complaint in individuals who consume large amounts of alcohol (acutely or chronically). Ethanol (the alcohol found in alcoholic beverages) has numerous effects on the gastrointestinal tract that contribute to diarrhea. Ethanol ingestion alters gut motility, causing rapid transit and heightened propulsive movements, resulting in food malabsorption [30, 31]. Alcohol also decreases the activity of enzymes that break down disaccharides, decreases bile secretion (when liver disease is present), and can cause malabsorption of fat, thiamin, vitamin B^{12}, folate, glucose, amino acids, water, and sodium [5]. Many binge drinkers are also at higher risk of steatorrhea due to decreased pancreatic exocrine function from chronic pancreatitis [5]

Another common food-related cause of diarrhea is so-called, "traveler's diarrhea," which refers to the gastrointestinal infections often acquired when an individual travels from industrialized to developing areas of the world. The condition is usually defined, in the setting of recent travel, as the passage of three or more unformed stools in a 24-hour period in association with one or more of the following: nausea, vomiting, cramps, fever, fecal urgency, and bloody stools [32]. Traveler's diarrhea is acquired when fecally contaminated foods or water are ingested. Infectious agents present in fecal matter such as bacteria, viruses, and parasites are the primary cause of the disorder [32]. Table 4 provides a list of high- and low-risk foods to avoid when traveling to high-risk areas and what areas of the world represent the greatest risk for travelers.

Diarrhea is one of the most common side effects of drugs. Antibiotics are especially associated with diarrhea. A major mechanism of this effect is through antibiotic interference with the ecology of gut bacteria, suppressing growth of natural bacteria and favoring the growth of other bacteria

TABLE 4 High- and Low-Risk Foods and Risk Areas of the World
for Traveler's Diarrhea

High-risk foods	Low-risk foods
Raw/undercooked meats, seafood	Water when:
Uncooked vegetables	bottled
Tap water	treated by filtration, reverse osmosis, or
Ice	chemical disinfection
Unpasteurized milk and dairy products	boiled
	Bottled sodas, juices
	Bottled beers, wines

High-risk areas	Intermediate-risk areas	Low-risk areas
Latin America	Russia	Canada
Middle East	China	United States
Africa	Some Caribbean Islands	Northern Europe
Much of Asia		Japan
		New Zealand
		Australia
		Some Caribbean Islands

(such as *Clostridium difficile*). This causes inflammation and injury of the gut lining and stimulates the secretion of fluid [4].

Laxative abuse is a self-induced cause of diarrhea that is seen in young women with eating disorders in an attempt to control body weight by decreasing food absorption; however, even large doses of Correctol® have been shown to decrease energy absorption by only about 5%. Weight loss from this practice is primarily fluid loss [33]. Finally, diarrhea may also occur in runners, "runners trots," especially those beginning a running training program [34]. Causes for this are speculative, but may include osmotic activity due to excess intake of fiber or carbohydrate, or increased motility from the physical impact of running [35, 36].

C. Therapy

Because a multitude of foods may contribute to diarrhea in different people, individuals must try to eliminate "suspected" food and experiment with others. During an episode of diarrhea, it may be helpful to briefly limit food intake to cooked food (no raw foods) and, depending on the severity, consume clear broths, teas, gelatin, bottled non-carbonated water, and drinks that replenish electrolytes such as sports drinks. Low-fat high-protein foods are also usually tolerated (i.e., skinless chicken or fish, egg whites) and should be added to improve protein content of the diet. Dairy products may be added as symptoms and time pass. Raw fruits and salads should be added last. Extended dietary restrictions to manage diarrhea (e.g., beyond a few days) can delay the healing process due to impaired nutritional status. Table 3 provides a list of medications for symptomatic relief of diarrhea.

If lactose intolerance is suspected, intake of dairy products should be greatly reduced. If this results in the disappearance of diarrhea, lactose intolerance is likely and treatment with restriction or avoidance of dairy products, supplemental lactase tablets (such as Lactaid), or lactose-reduced dairy products is helpful.

For traveler's diarrhea, the best treatment for mild symptoms without fever includes rehydration from a safe source (bottled water, soda, juice, or canned soup) coupled with a source of sodium such as salted crackers, and avoiding other solid foods until symptoms dissipate [32]. Subsalicylates or loperamide can provide symptom relief. With moderate to severe symptoms plus fever or dysentery, antibacterial agents may be necessary, in which case, travelers must seek medical treatment [32].

When diarrhea results from running, moderating dietary fiber, waiting several hours after eating before running, and attempting to have a bowel movement before running may be helpful. The diarrhea produced by laxative abuse should improve once such abuse ceases; however, edema may develop following more severe or prolonged abuse. This edema, however, usually spontaneously resolves (see Chapter 43 on eating disorders). Finally, if diarrhea is caused by antibiotic use, the general recommendations listed above are appropriate, in addition to consulting the prescribing physician and considering stopping the possible offending agent or changing to another, less problematic antibiotic if further treatment is needed. Because antibiotic use and other infections can deplete the gut of bacteria necessary for digestion, consuming yogurt with live or active cultures (lactobacillus) may help replenish these bacteria.

It is also noteworthy that, even when there is an underlying, non-food-related cause for diarrhea (such as chronic

pancreatitis), avoidance of large amounts of certain foods (such as fatty foods in chronic pancreatitis) is useful nutritional therapy for reducing diarrhea.

V. CONSTIPATION

A. Prevalence and Causes

The concept of constipation differs greatly between individuals, and between the medical and lay definitions. Difficult defecation with straining and hard or infrequent stools are symptoms most often associated with constipation by the lay public. Other symptoms sometimes associated with constipation include no urge to have bowel movements, a sense of incomplete evacuation, anal or perineal pain, soiling of clothes, and discomfort (pain/bloating). Abdominal pain relieved by defecation, a hard stool, straining at defecation, incomplete evacuation and abdominal discomfort are each reported by 5–30% of individuals in surveyed populations in developed nations [5]. Bowel frequency of less than three stools per week, the requirement for meeting the medical definition of constipation, is reported by about 4% of respondents, and fewer than two stools per week by 1–2% of respondents.

Individual characteristics associated with constipation include increased age and nonwhite ethnicity (living in Western society). Also, constipation is more prevalent in women than men [37]. Specific symptoms associated with constipation are more common [38] and infrequent stools (1–2/week) tend to be reported almost entirely by women [39]. In one study of 220 healthy participants consuming their normal diet, 17% of women, but only 1% of men, passed less than 50 g of stool per day [40]. Also, many women (about 40%) experience some type of constipation during pregnancy [41]. The reason for this sex difference is unknown and does not seem to be related to circulating levels of sex hormones or other hormones [42]. Elderly persons report more straining during defecation rather than decreased bowel frequency [5]. In the United States, constipation is 30% more common among nonwhites than whites, with similar increases in prevalence with age [37, 43]. In native populations of Africa and India, however, constipation appears to be quite rare, likely because differences in the diet between native and Americanized populations [40].

This discussion will focus primarily on diet-related causes of constipation; however, there are other factors that may cause or exacerbate constipation. Any factor that increases water absorption from the colon and leads to smaller, harder stools could theoretically cause constipation. Just as reduced contact time between gut contents and the colonic mucosa favors decreased water absorption and diarrhea, increased contact time increases water absorption and can cause constipation. Individuals with wide and/or long colons are likely to have slower transit rates and increased likelihood of constipation [44]. Also, in some individuals the frequency and

duration of peristaltic colonic waves are reduced or nonexistent. This condition causes very slow transit time and the passage of one or fewer bowel movements per week [5]. Other physiological factors that may contribute to constipation are failure of relaxation of the anal sphincter, diminished rectal sensation, and diseases such as hypothyroidism, diabetes mellitus, Parkinson's disease, multiple sclerosis, and spinal cord injuries or lesions [5].

Interestingly, some psychological factors also seem related to constipation. In one study of 21 healthy males, stool weight and bowel frequency were significantly correlated with personality traits such as being socially outgoing, energetic, and optimistic [45]. Patients with the diagnoses of anorexia or bulimia nervosa often complain of constipation, and prolonged whole-gut transit time has been shown in patients with both conditions [46].

B. Constipation and Food

In contrast to previously discussed gastrointestinal complaints such as diarrhea, constipation is not commonly aggravated by the ingestion of specific foods. Rather, constipation is most commonly associated with the omission of fiber in the diet. Fiber is often defined as a plant food component that cannot be digested. Many forms of fiber are polysaccharides made of sugar units joined in unique linkages that render the molecule resistant to degradation by digestive enzymes. Thus, fiber is, by and large, undigestable carbohydrate.

Increased intake of fiber helps to prevent the development of constipation in two ways: (1) fiber increases stool volume and weight and (2) fiber decreases colonic transit time. Fiber adds to stool weight both directly and indirectly. Because fiber is not degradable, this nondigested bulk contributes directly to stool weight. In addition, some types of fiber can hold water within their cellular structure, adding further bulk to the stool as well. Fiber ingestion contributes indirectly to stool bulk by increasing the proliferation of intestinal bacteria, which, in turn, increases stool weight.

Ingested dietary fiber has been clearly shown to decrease colonic transit time (i.e., increase the speed at which undigested material moves through the colon). A meta-analysis of 20 studies (including normal control participants, those with irritable bowel syndrome, and those with constipation) revealed that the addition of fiber to the diet consistently resulted in decreased transit time [47]. The mechanism by which this occurs is not fully understood, but it is thought that the increased bulk created by ingested fiber in the colonic lumen stimulates propulsive motor activity [5]. However, other factors may be involved. In a study comparing coarse and fine bran given twice daily, the coarse bran reduced colonic transit time while the fine bran had no effect [48]. Another study found that inert plastic particles of the same size as coarse bran increased fecal output and decreased transit time similar to coarse bran [49]. Thus, it is

possible that colonic stimulation is dependent on the size and/or nature of the particulate fiber.

C. Therapy

When an individual with normal colonic function adds fiber to the diet, stool weight increases in proportion to its baseline weight [5]. When an individual with frequent constipation (those who pass small stools) increases fiber intake, the resulting stool weight may still be below normal. In a study of 10 constipated women given a 20 g/day supplement of wheat bran, stool weight increased from an initial 30 to 60 g/day and bowel movement frequency increased from a mean two to three times weekly [50]. However, this output is still only about half as large as the average stool weight of those with normal function. Thus, increased fiber intake as the treatment for frequent constipation is often disappointing. However, increased fiber intake is the simplest, least expensive, and most natural treatment for constipation. Thus, most constipated individuals are advised to increase dietary fiber intake by about 30 g of nonstarch polysaccharide per day [5]. Increased intake of fiber has also been shown helpful in decreasing risk of colorectal cancer, diverticular disease, irritable bowel syndrome, and hemorrhoids.

Methods to increase fiber intake include:

- Adding more fruits and vegetables to the diet (especially carrots, apples, oranges, celery)
- Substituting whole-grain foods for refined products (e.g., whole wheat bread instead of white bread, brown rice for white rice)
- Add wheat or oat bran to muffin or baked good recipes
- Add legumes (beans and nuts) in side dishes or in casseroles

It is best to introduce additional fiber to the diet gradually, so that the gastrointestinal tract can adapt to fiber-related changes in bacterial proliferation, gas production, and transit time. For some, especially women, added fiber may aggravate abdominal distention and discomfort [51]. Symptoms usually subside within 1–2 weeks. Bran fiber treatment may not be appropriate for young people with congenital megacolon (Hirschprung's disease), and, in some elderly individuals, if it exacerbates incontinence [5].

Fluid intake is another important component of therapy for constipation. The combination of added water and fiber increases stool bulk, while dehydration or salt depletion is likely to lead to increased salt and water absorption by the large intestine, resulting in small, hard stools. Drinking eight, 8-ounce glasses of liquids per day is recommended. While any liquid is better than no liquid, some are better than others. Water is best, followed by vegetable juice, fruit juice (but these are often high in energy), milk, broth (although often high in sodium), and beverages such as coffee, tea (iced or hot), and soft drinks.

For more chronic forms of constipation, a bulk laxative may be helpful (see Table 3). Bulk laxatives are a concentrated form of nonstarch polysaccharides useful for patients who cannot consume dietary fiber in adequate quantities. These products are based on wheat, plant seed mucilage, plant gums, or synthetic methylcellulose derivatives [5]. Bulk laxatives are appropriate as treatment for constipation over the long-term and should not be expected to provide immediate relief of constipation. Bulking agents may be quite useful in constipation experienced during pregnancy.

For more severe forms of constipation or impaction, a stepped care approach is usually employed. This approach would first address lifestyle factors such as low dietary fiber and fluid intake and then add progressively more potent laxatives. A physician should be consulted to determine the proper sequence and choice of treatment options.

VI. NAUSEA AND VOMITING

A. Causes and Prevalence

1. COMPONENTS OF VOMITING

There are three components of vomiting: nausea, retching (dry heaves), and emesis (vomiting) [5].

1. *Nausea* is an extremely unpleasant, uneasy sensation that is difficult to describe and may or may not precede vomiting. A variety of stimuli may contribute to nausea (labyrinthine stimulation, visceral pain, negative psychological issues) [5]. The neural pathways mediating nausea are not known, but are thought to be the same as those for vomiting. It is possible that mild stimulation of this pathway results in nausea, while more intense activation results in vomiting [5].
2. *Retching* is the sensation of "dry heaves." It consists of spasms and abortive respiratory movements with the glottis (visible part of the larynx in the rear of the throat) closed. During an episode of retching, muscular mechanisms of breathing become opposed. The chest wall and diaphragm are coordinated in an inhalation muscular contraction (motions of breathing in) while abdominal muscles are in expiratory contractions (motions associated with breathing out). During retching, the distal portion of the stomach (antrum) contracts, whereas the upper portions (the fundus and cardiac) relax. The mouth is closed. Retching may or may not be followed by vomiting.
3. *Vomiting* occurs when the gastric contents are forced up and out of the mouth, "throwing up." This occurs by forceful and sustained contraction of the abdominal muscles and diaphragm at a time when the cardia of the stomach is raised and open and the pylorus is contracted [5]. This elevation of the cardia eliminates the intra-abdominal portion of the esophagus, which, if present, would tend to prevent the high intragastric pressure from

forcing gastric contents into the esophagus [5]. The mechanism by which the cardia opens during vomiting is not clear.

2. MECHANISMS OF NAUSEA AND VOMITING

The neurophysiology of nausea and vomiting has been extensively studied in cats by Borison and colleagues [52, 53]. Vomiting involves a complex set of neurologic activities that suggests some central "vomiting center" in the dorsal part of the medulla [52, 53]. Electrical stimulation of this area in cats has induced vomiting [52, 53]. Other studies have suggested that there is a certain portion of the medulla that is associated with vomiting, but does not respond to electrical stimulation. Rather, this area responds to chemical stimulation and has been called the *chemoreceptor trigger zone* [52–56]. However, because most of this work has been done in cats, caution must be exercised when extrapolating these results to human causes and controls of vomiting.

3. OTHER PHENOMENA ASSOCIATED WITH NAUSEA AND VOMITING

1. *Hypersalivation* is an increase in saliva production, is often experienced prior to vomiting, and is thought to result from the proximity of the proposed vomiting center in the medulla to the medullary control center for salivation.
2. *Tachycardia* (increased heart rate) usually accompanies nausea, and retching is accompanied by *bradycardia* (decreased heart rate). Retching and vomiting have been associated with the onset of an arrhythmia (atrial fibrillation) and termination of other arrhythmias (e.g., ventricular tachycardia) [57, 58].
3. *Defecation,* the passing of stool, may also occur with vomiting. Similar to the association with salivation, the central control of defecation is also thought to be mediated in the medulla. Increased stimulation of the medulla, thus, may also cause these associated physiologic responses [52].

B. Conditions Causing Nausea and Vomiting

1. INFECTIONS OF THE GASTROINTESTINAL TRACT

Infection of the gastrointestinal tract may result in sudden outbreaks of vomiting, usually early in the morning. The urge to vomit may be so intense that individuals may vomit in bed and also experience headaches, muscle aches, giddiness, diarrhea, sweating, and fever. Many viruses and other infectious agents may cause such symptoms; however, for most gastrointestinal infections, recovery is generally fast.

2. MEDICATIONS

Taking medications, especially new medications, is also associated with nausea and vomiting. It is thought that many medications act on the chemoreceptor trigger zone to induce nausea and vomiting [5]. Major offenders include dopamine agonists, opiate analgesics, antibiotics, and cancer chemotherapy agents, though virtually all medications are sometimes associated with this side effect. Sensitivity to the effects of medications on nausea and vomiting may be predicted if an individual has a history of motion sickness [59].

3. MOTION SICKNESS

Sweating, dizziness, headache, and nausea that may or may not lead to vomiting while in motion in cars, trains, and airplanes is referred to as motion sickness. It is thought to be caused by conflicting sensory activation of the vestibular system (which regulates balance) in the inner ear and visual sensory input. In other words, the eyes do not detect motion to the same degree as the balance mechanism in the inner ear, leading to a stress-producing phenomenon that activates the nausea and/vomiting center of the brain.

4. MORNING SICKNESS

Nausea and vomiting during early pregnancy are common and often occur soon after waking. Nausea occurs in 50–90% of pregnancies and vomiting in 24–55% [60, 61] and is more common in first pregnancies, younger women, nonsmokers, obese women, those with <12 years of education, and women whose corpus luteum is primarily on the right side of the uterus. The onset of these symptoms is generally at 4–5 weeks of pregnancy [20] and may reach a peak of severity and frequency around 12 weeks [20]. The exact cause of morning sickness is not known. The two main theories are that women who are prone to morning sickness may have (1) abnormal hormone levels (human chorionic gonadotropin, progesterone, and andogrens) and/or (2) unstable gastric electrical activities and a reduced response to the ingestion of food. A severe form of morning sickness, hyperemesis gravidarum, occurs in 3.5 per 1000 pregnancies [5]. This condition is marked by severe vomiting, which results in nutritional and/or electrolyte disturbances in early pregnancy. Causes of this condition are not known.

5. PSYCHOGENIC VOMITING

Psychological factors are also associated with nausea and vomiting.

1. *Food aversions.* It is also possible that the mere smell, taste, or even sight of a specific food can produce a psychologically associated nausea. When individuals eat foods prior to an episode of gastrointestinal infection or other nausea/vomiting causing condition, such foods may become associated with nausea or vomiting. This may lead to the development of a food aversion. Although such associations were important evolutionary survival aids, teaching that eating certain foods may

result in illness, modern humans can inappropriately develop these aversions, even with long delays between foods and symptoms, or even when the individual is certain that the food did not cause the illness [62].

2. *Self-induced vomiting.* This behavior is most often seen in young women with eating disorders such as anorexia or bulimia nervosa who regurgitate ingested food and beverages in an attempt to lose or control body weight. These individuals may become very skilled at concealing their vomiting.

3. *Erotic vomiting.* Some women with underlying psychological aberrations induce vomiting to obtain sexual gratification.

Other conditions associated with nausea and vomiting may be of a more chronic nature. Causes for chronic symptoms may include mechanical obstruction of the gastrointestinal tract, brain tumors, or metabolic or endocrine disorders.

C. Vomiting and Food

The timing of nausea and vomiting following a meal may partially indicate its cause. Nausea or vomiting occurring within 1 hour of a meal may indicate a peptic ulcer or a psychological disorder [5]. Nausea or vomiting occurring 1–8 hours after a meal may indicate food poisoning [5].

The main food-related problem that may cause nausea and vomiting is food-borne illness or "food poisoning." Most cases of food poisoning result from the ingestion of food containing bacteria such as salmonella, *Campylobacter jejuni, Escherichia coli,* or many others. These different bacteria and even different strains of similar bacteria can cause a variety of symptoms that range in severity from traveler's diarrhea (in developing countries) to death (as witnessed in 1993 in children who ate bacteria-infested ground beef from a fast-food chain).

Major nutritional and metabolic consequences of acute and chronic vomiting may occur. Acute vomiting can result in metabolic derangements such as these:

- *Potassium deficiency.* This deficiency may lead to overall muscle weakness, poor intestinal tone with gastrointestinal bleeding, heart rhythm and conduction abnormalities, and weakness of respiratory muscles.
- *Sodium depletion.* When the serum and body stores of sodium are depleted rapidly, as can occur with intense vomiting episodes, extreme lethargy can result. An individual may also become irritable, confused, weak, and sometimes hostile. Sodium depletion can also lead to alkalosis [a condition in which the blood has an excess of base-forming elements (pH>7.4)] and further nausea and vomiting if not repleted.

Chronic vomiting may lead to other nutritional concerns such as reduced energy intake, malnutrition, and deficiency states for various nutrients.

TABLE 5 Guidelines for Conducting a Thorough Medical Work-Up for Nausea or Vomiting

Contact a physician or seek medical attention if:

For adults and children:
- Vomitus contains blood or "coffee grounds"
- Stools contain blood or are black or tarry
- Nausea lasts for more than 1 week (in women, pregnancy may be a possibility)
- Severe headache
- Lethargy
- Confusion
- Decreased alertness
- Severe abdominal pain

For children 6 years and younger:
- Vomiting lasts more than a few hours
- Diarrhea is also present
- There are signs of dehydration (dry mouth, eyes, skin, and/or sunken eyes and confusion)
- Accompanied by a fever >100°F

For children older than 6:
- Vomiting lasts for more than 1 day
- There are signs of dehydration (see above)
- Accompanied by a fever of >102°F

D. Therapy

Most vomiting episodes subside within 6–24 hours of onset and can be treated at home [5]. A number of pharmaceutical products (Table 3) are available for the treatment of the nausea and vomiting associated with motion sickness, medication usage and gastrointestinal infections. See Table 5 for guidelines suggesting when a comprehensive examination and work-up should be conducted for vomiting. Avoidance of nausea and vomiting associated with stomach-irritating medications can sometimes be improved by taking the medication with food.

A number of dietary practices have been suggested traditionally to ease nausea. These include drinking cold beverages slowly, eating salty foods, eating slowly, and eating smaller, more frequent meals. Eating light meals of low-fat, starchy foods and avoiding strong-smelling or tasting foods has been shown to lessen the nausea associated with motion sickness. Avoiding certain foods such as fried, greasy, or very sweet foods may also help prevent nausea. Strong smelling or strong tasting foods are often those associated with food aversions and nausea.

If an individual feels nauseated, vomiting may be prevented by drinking small amounts of clear, sweetened liquids such as carbonated beverages or fruit juices. Resting is also advised, because activity may worsen nausea. Mechanisms for why these therapies prevent or ease nausea have not been extensively studied.

One food that has been studied in regard to its effects on nausea is ginger root. Ginger root and ginger-containing

foods have long been regarded as digestive aids in Chinese medicine [63]. A number of studies have investigated ginger as an antiemetic [64, 65] and an antinausea treatment [66–68]. In one study, participants given 1 g of powdered ginger prior to surgery had significantly fewer incidents of nausea than the group receiving a placebo dosage [65]. Other studies have found similar results under different experimental conditions (postoperative dosage [64], prior to sea voyage [69], and prior to administration of certain nausea-causing medications [67]. Thus, ginger powder may be of aid in nausea.

To avoid vomiting and other gastrointestinal symptoms that are caused by food poisoning or contamination, standard food preparation and storage precautions should be used. The reader is referred to current guidelines and summaries on this topic [70, 71].

If persistent vomiting results in potassium or sodium loss, it is best to replace these nutrients through dietary sources to minimize the possibility of excess intake. Good sources of dietary potassium include spinach, bananas, mushrooms, broccoli, and milk. Salty crackers, broths, or other low-fat, salt-containing foods can help replace sodium. Drinking plenty of water is important to prevent or treat dehydration.

VII. CONCLUSION

Given the preceding discussion, it is evident that diet plays a large role in managing common gastrointestinal complaints. Both the inclusion and exclusion of specific foods and food categories can contribute to gastrointestinal symptoms. Although there may not be one "diet" per se to prevent all gastrointestinal ills, there are common characteristics of a diet appropriate for general health that may be applicable. Tenets of such a healthy diet to prevent gastrointestinal symptoms include:

1. Consume an adequate, but not excess, amount of energy. Maintaining normal body weight is important.
2. Reduce dietary fat intake, especially saturated fat. High-fat foods, such as fried foods, are often linked to gastrointestinal complaints of heartburn, gas, diarrhea, and constipation, as well as gallstones and exacerbation of symptoms such as bloating in chronic pancreatitis and other causes of malabsorption. Excessive fat intakes can also contribute to bloating due to steatorrhea.
3. Increase fiber intake. Daily intake of 30–40 g of fiber can improve gastrointestinal health by increasing gut motility and adding to stool weight. This can be accomplished by increasing the number of daily servings of fruit and vegetables and choosing natural and not processed grains. Fiber sources should be added to the diet incrementally to avoid producing excess gas. If certain healthy foods are problematic, they may be able to be consumed in moderation or in small amounts.
4. Eat slowly and chew food thoroughly. When food is consumed slowly the mechanisms that regulate hunger and satiety are able to communicate appropriate messages for terminating a meal. Eating slowly also allows for improved gastric emptying and lessens the sensation of bloating and risk of developing heartburn.
5. Consume alcohol and caffeine in moderation (<2 alcohol- or caffeine-containing drinks per day. Excess alcohol intake causes general irritation of the upper gastrointestinal tract especially.
6. Exercise regularly. Running or jogging may not be advisable for those who are sensitive to diarrhea, but other more stationary forms of aerobic exercise are advisable for both gastrointestinal and cardiovascular health.
7. Do not assume that a specific food is problematic in causing gastrointestinal complaints. If a specific food is suspected to be not tolerated, the use of commercially available supplemental enzymes (such as lactase for lactose intolerance) may allow individuals to consume foods that provide important nutrients.

Following such guidelines may bring modern food intake and behavior into better balance with a gastrointestinal tract that evolved to suit the diet of Paleolithic ancestors. In addition, being aware of potential hazards to gastrointestinal health such as traveling in developing countries and proper food safety procedures can also help prevent troubling gastrointestinal symptoms.

References

1. Sandler, R. S., Stewart, W. F., Liberman, J. N., Ricci, J. A., and Zorich, N. L. (2000). Abdominal pain, bloating and diarrhea in the United States: Prevalence and impact. *Dig. Dis. Sci.* **45,** 166–171.
2. Miller, D. L., and Cheskin, L. J. GI symptoms associated with specific ingestion of specific foods. Unpublished data from the Olestra Post-Marketing Surveillance Study.
3. Cheskin, L. J., Midday, R., Zorich, N., and Filloon, T. (1998). Gastrointestinal symptoms following consumption of olestra or regular triglyceride potato chips. *JAMA* **279,** 150–152.
4. Janowitz, H. D. (1997). "Good Food for Bad Stomachs." Oxford University Press, New York.
5. Feldman, M., Scharschmidt, B. F., and Sleissinger, M. H. (1998). "Gastrointestinal and Liver Disease: Pathophysiology, Diagnosis and Management. W. B. Saunders, Philadelphia, PA.
6. Lasser, R. B., Bond, J. H., and Levitt, M. D. (1975). The role of intestinal gas in functional abdominal pain. *N. Engl. J. Med.* **293,** 524–526.
7. Tomlin, J., Lowis, C. and Read, N. W. (1991). Investigation of normal flatus production in healthy volunteers. *Gut* **32,** 665–669.
8. Olsson, S., Furne, L., and Levitt, M. D. (1995). Relationship of gaseous symptoms to intestinal gas producton: Symptoms do not equal increased production. *Gastroenterology* **108**(Suppl.), A28.
9. Levitt, M. D. and Duane, W. C. (1972). Floating stools—flatus versus fat. *N. Engl. J. Med.* **286,** 973–975.

10. Karlin, D. A., Jones, R. D., Stroeleim, J. R., Mastromarino, A. J., and Potter, G. D. (1982). Breath methane excretion in patients with unresected colorectal cancer. *J. Natl. Cancer Inst.* **69,** 573–576.

11. Moore, J. G., Jessop, L. D. and Osborne, D. N. (1987). A gas chromatographic and mass spectrometric analysis of the odor of human feces. *Gastroenterology* **93,** 1321–1329.

12. Steggerda, F. R. (1968). Gastrointestinal gas following food consumption. *Ann. N.Y. Acad. Sci.* **150,** 57–66.

12a. Steggerda, F. R. (1968). Gastrointestinal gas following food consumption. *Ann. N.Y. Acad. Sci.* **150,** 57–69.

13. Levin, M. D., Hirsch, P., Fetzer, C. A., Sheehan, M., and Levine, A. S. (1987). H2 excretion after ingestion of complex carbohydrates. *Gastroenterology* **92,** 383–389.

14. Ravich, W. J., Bayless, T. M., and Thomas, M. (1983). Fructose: Incomplete intestinal absorption in humans. *Gastroenterology* **84,** 26–29.

15. Tadesse, K., and Eastwood, M. A. (1978). Metabolism of dietary fiber components in man assessed by breath hydrogen and methane. *Br. J. Nutr.* **40,** 393–396.

16. Suarez, F., Savaiano, D. A., and Levitt, M. D. (1995). A comparison of symptoms with milk or loacrose-hydrolyzed milk in people with self-reported severe lactose intolerance. *N. Engl. J. Med.* **333,** 1–4.

17. Gallup Organization (1988). "Survey on Heartburn across America." Gallup Organization, Pinceton, NJ.

18. Nebel, O. T., Fornes, M. F., and Castell, D. O. (1976). Symptomatic gastroesophageal reflux: Incidence and precipitating factors. *Dig. Dis. Sci.* **21,** 953–956.

19. Thompson, W. A., and Heaton, K. W. (1982). Heartburn and globus in apparently healthy people. *Can. Med. Assoc. J.* **126,** 46–48.

20. Johnson, R. V. (1994). "The Mayo Clinic Complete Book of Pregnancy and Baby's First Year." William Morrow & Company, Inc., New York.

21. Hookman, P., Siegel, C. I., and Hendrix, T. R. (1966). Failure of oxethazaine to alter acid induced espohageal pain. *Am J. Dig. Dis.* **11,** 811–813.

22. Johnson, D. A., Winters, C., Spurling, T. J., Chobanian, S. J., and Cattau, E. L. (1989). Esophageal acid sensitivity in Barrett's esophagus. *J. Clin. Gastroenterol.* **9,** 23–26.

23. Smith, J. L., Opekum, A. R., Larkai, E., and Graham, D. Y. (1989). Sensitivity of the esophageal mucosa to pH in gastroesophageal reflux disease. *Gastroenterology* **96,** 683–689.

24. Tradifilipoulos, G. (1989). Nonobstructive dysphagia in reflux esophagitis. *Am. J. Gastroenterol.* **84,** 614–618.

25. Feldman, M., and Barnett, C. (1995). Relationship between acidity and osmolarity of popular beverages and reported postprandial heartburn. *Gastroenterology* **108,** 125–131.

26. Zeman, F. J. (1991). "Clinical Nutrition and Dietetics," pp. 197. Macmillan Publishing Company, New York.

27. Bright-Asare, P., and Binder, H. J. (1973). Stimulation of colonic secretion of water and electrolytes by hydroxy fatty acids. *Gastroenterology* **64,** 81–88.

28. Ammon, H. V., and Phillips, S. F. (1973). Inhibition of colonic water and electrolyte absorption by fatty acids in man. *Gastroenterology* **65,** 744–749.

29. Ammon, H. V., and Phillips, S. F. (1974). Inhibition of ileal water absorption by intraluminal fatty acids. Influence of chain length, hydroxylation and conjugation of fatty acids. *J. Clin. Invest.* **53,** 205–210.

30. Martin, J. L., Justus, P. G., and Mathias, J. A. (1980). Altered motility of the small intestine in response to ethanol (ETOH): An explanation for the diarrhea associated with the consumption of alcohol. *Gastroenterology* **78,** 1218.

31. Wegener, M., Schaffstein, J., Dilger. U., Coenen, C., Wedmann, B., and Schmidt, G. (1991). Gastrointestinal transit of solid–liquid meal in chronic alcoholics. *Dig Dis Sci.* **36,** 917–923.

32. De Las Casas, C., Adachi, J., and Dupont, H. (1999). Travelers' diarrhea [review]. *Aliment. Pharmacol. Ther.* **13,** 1373–1378.

33. Bo-Linn, G. W., Santa Ana, C. A., Morawski, S. G., and Fordtran, J. S. (1983). Purging and calorie absorption in bulimic patients and normal women. *Ann. Intern. Med* **99,** 14–17.

34. Sullivan, S. N. (1981). The gastrointestinal symptoms of running [letter]. *N. Engl. J. Med.* **304,** 915.

35. Sullivan, S. N. (1987). Exercise-associated symptoms in triathletes. *Phys. Sports Med.* **15,** *105–108.*

36. Cheskin, L. J., Crowell, M. D., Kamal, N., Rosen, B., Schuster, M. M., and Whitehead, W. E. (1990). The effects of acute exercise on gastrointestinal motility. *J. Gastrointest. Motil.* **4,** 173–177.

37. Johanson, J. F., Sonnenberg, A., and Koch, T. R. . (1989). Clinical epidemiology of chronic constipation. *J. Clin. Gastroenterol.* **11,** 525–536.

38. Talley, N. J., Weaver, A. L., Zinmeister, A. R., and Melton, L. J. (1993). Functional constipation and outlet delay: A population-based study. *Gastroenterology* **105,** 781–790.

39. Heaton, K. W., Radvan, J., Cripps, H., Mountford, R. A., Braddon, F. E., and Hughes, A. O. (1992). Defecation frequency and timing, and stool form in the general population. *Gut* **33,** 818–824.

40. Cummings, J. H., Bingham, S. A., Heaton, K. W., and Eastwood, M. A. (1992). Fecal weight, colon cancer risk and dietary intake of nonstarch polysaccharides (dietary fiber). *Gastroenterology* **103,** 1783–1789.

41. Andersen, A. S. (1986). Dietary factors in the aetiology and treatment of constipation during pregnancy. *Br. J. Obstet. Gynaecol.* **93,** 245–249.

42. Kamm, M. A., Farthing, M. J. G., Lennard-Jones, J. E., Perry, L. A., and Chard, T. (1991). Steroid hormone abnormalities in women with severe idiopathic constipation. *Gut* **32,** 80–84.

43. Talley, N. J., O'Keefe, E. S., Zinmeister, A. R. (1992). Prevalence of gastrointestinal symptoms in the elderly: A population-based study. *Gastroenterology* **102,** 895–901.

44. Preston, D. M., Lennard-Jones, J. E., and Thomas, B. M. (1985). Towards a radiologic definition of idiopathic megacolon. *Gastrointest. Radiol.* **10,** 167–169.

45. Tucker, D. M., Sandstead, H. H., Logan, G. M., Kelvay, L. M., Mahalko, J., Johnson, L. K., Inman, L., and Inglett, G. E. (1981). Dietary fiber and personality factors as determinants of stool output. *Gastroenterology* **81,** 879–883.

46. Kamal, N., Chami, T., Andersen, A., Rosell, F. A., Schuster, M. M., and Whitehead, W. E. (1991). Delayed gastrointestinal transit times in anorexia nervosa and bulimia nervosa. *Gastroenterology* **101,** 1320–1324.

47. Muller-Lissner, S. A. (1988). Effect of wheat bran on weight of stool and gastrointestinal transit time: A meta-analysis. *Br. Med. J.* **296,** 615–617.

48. Kirwas, W. O., Smith, A. N., McConnell, A. A., Mitchell, W. D., and Eastwood, M. A. (1974). Action of different bran preparations on colonic function. *Br. Med. J.* **4,** 187–189.

49. Tomlin, J., and Read, N. W. (1988). Laxative properties of indigestible plastic particles. *Br. Med. J.* **297,** 1175–1176.
50. Graham, D. Y., Moser, S. E., and Estes, M. K. (1982). The effect of bran on bowel function in constipation. *Am. J. Gastroenterol.* **77,** 599–603.
51. Preston, D. M., and Lennard-Jones, J. E. (1986). Severe chronic constipation of young women: "Idiopathic slow transit constipation." *Gut* **27,** 41–48.
52. Borison, H. L., Borison, R., and McCarthy, L. S. (1984). Role of the area postrema in vomiting and related functions. *Fed. Proc.* **43,** 2955–2958.
53. Borison, H. L., and Wang, S. C. (1953). Physiology and pharmacology of vomiting. *Pharmacol. Rev.* **5,** 193.
54. Baker, P. C. H., and Bernat, J. L. (1985). The neuroanatomy of vomiting in man: Tegmentum of the pons and middle cerebellar peduncle. *J. Neurol. Neurosurg. Psychiat.* **48,** 1165–1168.
55. Miller, A. D. (1993). Neuroanatomy and physiology. *In* "The Handbook of Nausea and Vomiting" (M. H. Sleisenger, Ed.), pp. 1–9. Parthenon, New York.
56. Carpentar, D. O. (1990). Neural mechanisms of emesis. *Can. J. Physiol. Pharmacol.* **68,** 230–236.
57. Wilson, C. L., and Davis, S. J. (1978). Recurrent atrial fibrillation with nausea and vomiting. *Aviat. Space. Environ. Med.* **49,** 624–625.
58. Lyon, L. J., and Nevins, M. A. (1978). Retching and termination of ventricular tachycardia. *Chest* **74,** 110–113.
59. Morrow, G. R. (1985). The effect of susceptibility to motion sickness on the side effects of cancer chemotherapy. *Cancer* **55,** 2766–2770.
60. Baron, T., Ramirez, B., and Richter, J. E. (1993). Gastrointestinal motility disorders during pregnancy. *Ann. Intern. Med.* **118,** 366–375.
61. Deuchar, N. (1995). Nausea and vomiting in pregnancy: A review of the problem with particular regard to psychological and social aspects. *Br. J. Obstet Gynaecol.* **102,** 6–8.
62. Logue, A. W. (1986). "The Psychology of Eating: An Introduction," 2nd ed., p. 108. W. H. Freeman and Company, New York.
63. Bone, F. (1997). Ginger. *Br. J. Physiother.* **4,** 110–120.
64. Bone, M. E., Wilkinson, D. J., Young, J. R., McNeil, J., and Charlton, S. (1990). Ginger-root, a new anti-emetic: The effect of ginger root on postoperative nausea and vomiting after major gynaecological surgery. *Anaesthesia.* **45,** 669–671.
65. Phillips, S. R., Ruggier, S. E., and Hutchison, S. E. (1993). *Zingiber officinale* (ginger)—An anti-emetic for day case surgery. *Anaesthesia* **48,** 715–717.
66. Afreen, A. (1995). A double-blind randomized controlled trial of ginger for the prevention of postoperative nausea and vomiting. *Anaesth. Intens. Care* **23,** 449–452.
67. Meyer, K., Schwarz, J., Crater, D., and Keyes, B. (1995). *Zingiber officinale* (ginger) used to prevent 8-MOP associated nausea. *Dermatol. Nurs.* **7,** 242–244.
68. Pace, J. C. (1987). Oral ingestion of encapsulated ginger and reprted self-care actions for the relief of chemotherapy-associated nausea and vomiting. *Dis. Abstr. Int. (Sci.)* **47,** 3297.
69. Grontved, A., Brask, T., Kambskard, J., and Hentzer, E. (1988). Ginger root against seasickness: A controlled trial on the open sea. *Acta Otolaryngol.* **105,** 45–49.
70. www.mywebmd.com/content/article/1739.50624.
71. www.foodsafety.gov.

CHAPTER **37**

Nutrient Considerations in Lactose Intolerance

DENNIS SAVAIANO,[1] STEVE HERTZLER,[2] KARRY A. JACKSON,[1] AND FABRIZIS L. SUAREZ[3]

[1]Purdue University, West Lafayette, Indiana
[2]Ohio State University, Columbus, Ohio
[3]Minneapolis Veteran's Administration Medical Center, Minneapolis, Minnesota

I. INTRODUCTION

Ingestion of a large, single dose of lactose (e.g., 50 g, the quantity in a quart of milk) by lactose maldigesters commonly results in diarrhea, bloating, and flatulence [1]. The wide dissemination of this information has led some of the lay population and a fraction of the medical community to attribute common gastrointestinal symptoms to lactose intolerance, independent of the dose of lactose ingested. As a result, a segment of the population avoids dairy products due to the belief that even trivial doses of lactose will induce diarrhea or gas. However, multiple factors affect the ability of lactose to induce perceptible symptoms. These factors include residual lactase activity [2], gastrointestinal transit time [3], lactose consumed with other foods [4], lactose load [5], and colonic fermentation [6]. In the United States, approximately 72 million individuals are lactose maldigesters, many of whom are Asian-Americans, African-Americans, and Hispanics (Table 1). These minority groups are rapidly growing segments of the population. Thus, the overall number of lactose maldigesters will grow in the United States in coming years.

This chapter will (1) review the pathophysiology of lactose maldigestion, (2) attempt to correct common misconceptions concerning the frequency and severity of lactose intolerance symptoms, and (3) provide dietary strategies to minimize symptoms of intolerance.

II. LACTOSE IN THE DIET

Lactose is the primary disaccharide in virtually all mammalian milks. It is unique among the major dietary sugars because of the (β-1 $\rightarrow$ 4 linkage between its component monosaccharides, galactose and glucose. Lactose production in nature is limited to the mammalian breast, which contains the enzyme system (lactose synthase) necessary to create this linkage [7]. Human milk contains approximately 7% lactose by weight, which is among the highest lactose concentrations of all mammalian milks [5]. Cow's milk contains 4–5% lactose. Lactose, being water soluble, is associated with the whey portion of dairy foods. Thus, hard cheeses (with the whey removed from the curds) contain very little lactose compared to fluid milk.

TABLE 1 Projections of Lactose Maldigestion in the United States

	Percentage lactose maldigesters (LM)	Population 1990 (millions)	LM 1990 (millions)	Population 2000 (millions)	LM 2000 (millions)	Population 2025 (millions)	LM 2025 (millions)
African-Americans	75	30	23	34	25.5	44	33
Asian-Americans	100	7	7	11	11	20.5	20.5
Caucasian	20	188	37.6	197	39.4	209	41.8
Hispanic (all races)	60	22	13	31	18.6	60	36
Native Americans	100	2	2	2	2	2.5	2.5
Total	29	249	82.6	275	96.5	336	133.8
Percentage lactose maldigesters			33		35		40

Source: Estimates based on U.S. Department of Commerce, 1990 Census.

In addition to food sources of lactose, small amounts of lactose are found in a wide variety of medications due to the excellent tablet-forming properties of lactose [5]. However, lactose is usually present in milligram, rather than gram, quantities in most medications and the amount is biologically insignificant.

III. DIGESTION OF LACTOSE

The small intestine is normally impermeable to lactose. Lactose must first be hydrolyzed to glucose and galactose, which are subsequently absorbed. Inability to digest lactose is referred to as *lactose maldigestion.* Lactose digestion is dependent on the enzyme lactase-phlorizin hydrolase (LPH), a microvillar protein that has at least three enzyme activities: galactosidase, phlorizin hydrolase, and glycosylceramidase [8, 9]. Synthesis of LPH occurs in enterocytes, with the highest and most uniform synthesis being in the jejunum in humans [10]. The LPH gene is located on chromosome 2 and directs the synthesis of a pre-proLPH that is processed intracellularly (and possibly by pancreatic proteases) into the mature form that is anchored in the cell membrane at the brush border [11, 12]. Lactase activity develops late in gestation compared to other disaccharidases. Lactase activity in a fetus at 34 weeks is only 30% that of a full-term infant, rising to 70% of the full-term activity by 35–38 weeks [13].

IV. LOSS OF LACTASE ACTIVITY

Full-term infants possess high lactase activity, except for *congenital lactase deficiency,* in which lactase is completely absent at birth. Holzel *et al.* [14] first described congenital lactase deficiency in 1959. A very rare condition even in Finland (where it is most common), only 42 cases were diagnosed from 1966 to 1998 [11]. Lactase activity in jejunal biopsy specimens from infants with congenital lactase deficiency is reduced to 0–10 IU/g protein, and severe diarrhea results from unabsorbed lactose [11]. Treatment with a lactose-free formula eliminates symptoms and promotes normal growth and development [15].

Primary acquired hypolactasia, in which there is up to a 90–95% reduction in lactase activity, is much more common than congenital lactase deficiency (alactasia) [16]. The preferred term for this type of hypolactasia is *lactase nonpersistence* (LNP). It is estimated that approximately 75% of the world's population are LNP (see Table 2), with the exception of Northern Europeans and a few pastoral tribes in Africa and the Middle East that maintain infantile levels of lactase throughout life [17]. Thus, LNP is not a "lactase deficiency" disease, but is the normal pattern in human physiology, similar to the physiology of other mammalian species. This permanent loss of lactase occurs sometime after 3–5 years of age [9, 18]. It is hypothesized that *lactase persistence* is the result of a genetic mutation 3000–5000 years ago in populations where dairy foods had become an important component of the adult diet [19]. A gene mutation may have conferred a selective evolutionary advantage in these populations [20]. Lactase persistence is inherited as an autosomal dominant characteristic [17].

The genetic regulation of LPH has been studied extensively. Most evidence supports reduced levels of lactase mRNA in lactose maldigesters, suggesting that regulation is primarily at the level of transcription [21–24]. However, hypolactasia is sometimes present even when lactase mRNA is abundant, suggesting that post-transcriptional factors play a role [10, 25, 26]. One potential reason for conflicting results is the intestinal segment examined (duodenum versus jejunum). Lactase expression is higher and more uniform in the jejunum compared to the duodenum [27, 28]. Another potential discrepancy is the age of the subjects studied. A poor correlation between lactase mRNA and lactase activity was reported in intestinal biopsies from children, although the biopsy specimens in this study were duodenal [26]. Lactase activity in the jejunal enterocytes is found in a "mosaic"-type pattern [29]. In hypolactasic individuals, some jejunal enterocytes produce high amounts of lactase while others, even those sharing the same villus, do not produce lactase [10]. Thus, rather than a uniform reduction in lactase production among all enterocytes, a hypolactasic individual may have a "patchy" distribution of lactose-producing enterocytes that are low in number relative to the non-lactase-producing enterocytes. In lactase persistent individuals, all villus enterocytes may produce lactase. Current evidence suggests that the regulation of lactase is accomplished primarily at the level of transcription, although post-transcriptional factors (e.g., degradation of mRNA and post-translational processing of the LPH protein) could be important in some individuals.

Secondary hypolactasia occurs as the result of damage to the enterocytes via disease, medications, surgery, or radiation to the gastrointestinal tract (see Table 3) [5, 30, 31]. For example, the prevalence of microsporidiosis, which is associated with hypolactasia, can be as high as 50% in HIV-infected patients [32]. Seventy percent of HIV-infected patients showed evidence of lactose maldigestion compared to only 34% of controls [33]. In addition, the severity of lactose maldigestion increases in the more advanced stages of the disease. In general, secondary hypolactasia is reversible once the underlying cause is treated, but this reversal may require 6 months or more of diet therapy [5].

V. DIAGNOSIS OF LACTOSE MALDIGESTION

A. Direct Assessment Methods

Lactose digestion can be assessed directly or indirectly. The direct method involves obtaining a biopsy specimen of intes-

TABLE 2 Projections of Lactose Maldigestion around the World

	Percentage lactose maldigesters (LM)	Population 1995 (millions)	LM 1995 (millions)	Population 2000 (millions)	LM 2000 (millions)	Population 2025 (millions)	LM 2025 (millions)
Africa	75	753	565	877	658	1642	1231
Asia	100	3299	3299	3543	3543	4466	4466
Europe	20	809	162	827	165	893	893
Latin America	70	501	351	550	385	786	786
North America	25	286	72	297	74	347	347
Oceania	25	28	7	30	8	39	39
Total		5676	4456	6127	4833	8177	6523
Percentage lactose maldigesters			**78%**		**79%**		**80%**

Source: Population estimates from the United Nations.

tinal tissue and assaying for lactose activity or by intestinal perfusion studies [34]. While these tests can accurately measure lactase activity, they are invasive and seldom used clinically.

B. Indirect Assessment Methods

Several indirect methods for assessing lactose digestion are available, including blood, urine, stool, and breath tests. Blood tests involve feeding a standard 50-g lactose dose and measurement of plasma glucose every 15–30 minutes over a period of 30 minutes to 2 hours. A rise in blood glucose of at least 25–30 mg/dL (1.5–1.7 mmol/L) is indicative of normal lactose digestion [34]. Unfortunately, blood glucose lev-

els are subject to a variety of hormonal influences, reducing the reliability of this test. A blood test for galactose has been developed to correct this problem. The lactose dose is administered with a 500 mg/kg dose of ethanol (to prevent conversion of galactose to glucose in the liver) [34]. The galactose test is more reliable than the glucose test, but the ethanol exposure and invasive blood sampling are disadvantages.

A commonly used urine test involves the measurement of galactose in the urine, rather than the blood, during the lactose tolerance test with ethanol. Another urine test is conducted by simultaneously administering lactose and lactulose (a nonabsorbable disaccharide) [34]. Small amounts of lactose (up to 1% of the ingested dose) and lactulose diffuse unmediated across the intestinal mucosa and are

TABLE 3 Potential Causes of Secondary Hypolactasia

Diseases		
Small bowel	**Multisystem**	**Iatrogenic**
HIV enteropathy	Carcinoid syndrome	Chemotherapy
Regional enteritis (e.g., Crohn's disease)	Cystic fibrosis	Radiation enteritis
Sprue (celiac and tropical)	Diabetic gastropathy	Surgical resection of intestine
Whipple's disease (intestinal lipodystrophy)	Protein energy malnutrition	Medications
Ascaris lumbricoides infection	Zollinger-Ellison syndrome	Colchicine (antigout)
Blind loop syndrome	Alcoholism	Neomycin (antibiotic)
Giardiasis	Iron deficiency	Kanamycin (antibiotic)
Infectious diarrhea		Aminosalicylic acid (antibiotic)
Short gut		

Sources: Adapted with permission from:

Srinivasan, R., and Minocha, A. (1998). When to suspect lactose intolerance: Symptomatic, ethnic, and laboratory issues. *Postgrad. Med.* **104**(3), 109–123;

Scrimshaw, N. S., and Murray, E. B. (1998). The acceptability of milk and milk products in populations with a high prevalence of lactose intolerance. *Am. J. Clin. Nutr.* **48**, 1083–1159; and

Savaiano, D. A., and Levitt, M. D. (1987). Milk intolerance and microbe-containing dairy foods. *J. Dairy Sci.* **70**, 397–406.

excreted in the urine. The ratio of lactose to lactulose in the urine (collected over 10 hours) is determined by the hydrolysis of lactose. A value of less than 0.3 indicates normal lactose digestion and a ratio approaching 1.0 is observed in hypolactasia [34].

The measurement of stool pH and reducing substances in the stools has been used to assess lactose digestion in children. The analyses are easy to perform and convenient for the patient. However, stool pH has been shown to be unreliable in the diagnosis of hypolactasia in children and adults [34]. Furthermore, changes in gut motility and water excretion can alter the level of reducing substances in the stool. Thus, diagnosis of hypolactasia should not be based on stool tests alone [34].

Breath tests are most widely used to diagnose maldigestion. The principle behind breath tests is that lactose, which escapes digestion in the small intestine, is fermented by bacteria in the colon, producing short-chain fatty acids and hydrogen, carbon dioxide, and methane (in some individuals) gases. One breath test measures the amount of $^{13}CO_2$ excreted in the breath following administration of ^{13}C-lactose [34]. This stable isotope test has the advantage over older tests employing radioactive ^{14}C-lactose, but the high cost of the equipment prohibits widespread use of this method.

The current "gold standard" for diagnosis of carbohydrate maldigestion is the breath hydrogen test. Bacterial fermentation is the only source of molecular hydrogen in the body. A portion of the hydrogen produced in the colon diffuses into the blood, with ultimate pulmonary excretion [35]. The hydrogen breath test is widely used because it is noninvasive and easy to perform. Typically, a subject is given an oral dose of lactose following an overnight (≥ 12 hours) fast. Breath samples are collected at regular intervals for a period of 3–8 hours. In early studies, 50 g of lactose was used as a challenge dose. Almost all lactose maldigesters will experience intolerance symptoms following a dose of lactose this large [30], and yet many will be able to tolerate smaller, more physiologic doses of lactose. Doses of lactose that are in the range of 1–2 cups (240–480 ml) of milk (12–24 g lactose) have recently been more frequently used [36]. The dose of lactose used in the breath hydrogen test influences the diagnostic criterion for lactose maldigestion. Early studies with 50 g lactose showed perfect separation of lactose digesters from maldigesters using a rise in breath hydrogen of greater than 20 parts per million (ppm) above the fasting level [37]. More recently, Strocchi *et al.* [38] evaluated different criteria for diagnosis of carbohydrate maldigestion, using small doses of carbohydrate (10 g lactulose). Using a cutpoint of ≥ 10 ppm rise in breath hydrogen above fasting over an 8-hour period resulted in improved sensitivity (93% vs. 76%) and only a slight decrease in specificity (95% vs. 100%) compared to the 20-ppm cutoff. Further, it was shown that using a sum of hydrogens from hours 5, 6, and 7 and a ≥ 15-ppm above fasting cutpoint resulted in 100% sensitivity and specificity.

Despite the advantages of breath hydrogen testing, care must be taken to ensure an accurate test. First, it is important to establish a low baseline breath hydrogen value, to which subsequent values are compared. This is accomplished by fasting before and after consumption of the lactose dose. In addition, it has been shown that a meal low in nondigestible carbohydrate (e.g., white rice and ground meat) the evening before the test results in lower baseline hydrogen [39]. Second, it is possible that some individuals may have a colonic microflora that is incapable of producing hydrogen. However, these individuals are rare and the possibility of a non-hydrogen-producing flora can be ruled out by the administration of lactulose [38]. Third, approximately 40% of adults harbor significant numbers of methane-producing bacteria in the colon [40]. Because methanogenic bacteria consume four parts of hydrogen to produce one part methane [40], some authors have suggested that simultaneous measurement of methane will improve the accuracy of breath hydrogen testing in methane-producing subjects [41]. The availability of gas chromatographs that can analyze both hydrogen and methane in breath samples eliminates this potential problem. Finally, a number of factors (sleep, antibiotics, smoking, bacterial overgrowth of the small intestine, and exercise) may complicate the interpretation of breath hydrogen tests [34]. Therefore, standardization of the breath test protocol and appropriate controls are important.

VI. LACTOSE MALDIGESTION AND INTOLERANCE SYMPTOMS

A positive breath hydrogen test is indicative of lactose maldigestion. However, reduced lactase levels do not necessarily lead to intolerance symptoms. Symptoms of intolerance occur when the amount of lactose consumed exceeds the ability of both the small intestine and colon to effectively metabolize the dose. Unhydrolyzed lactose passes from the small intestine to the large intestine where it is fermented by enteric bacteria, producing the gases that are partially responsible for causing intolerance symptoms. The intensity of symptoms varies with the amount of lactose consumed [31, 42–44], the degree of colonic adaptation [45, 46] and the physical form of the lactose-containing food [47].

The correlation between lactose maldigestion and reported intolerance symptoms is unclear. Most maldigesters can tolerate the amount of lactose in up to 1–2 cups of milk without experiencing severe symptoms. However, some lactose maldigesters believe that small amounts of lactose, such as the amount used with coffee or cereal, cause gastrointestinal distress [48]. Individual differences observed in symptom reporting may reflect learned behaviors, cultural attitudes, or other social issues.

Lactose maldigesters, unselected for their degree of lactose intolerance, tolerated a cup of milk without experiencing appreciable symptoms [49–51]. However, the results of these studies did not gain general acceptance, in part because of failure to utilize subjects with "severe" lactose intolerance. In 1995, Suarez *et al.* [48] conducted a study in 30

self-described "severely lactose intolerant individuals." Initial breath hydrogen test measurements indicated that approximately 30% (9 of 30) of the subjects claiming severe lactose intolerance were digesters and, thus, had no physiological basis for intolerance symptoms. These findings further demonstrate how strongly behavioral and psychological factors influence symptom reporting. Additional research is necessary to evaluate the psychological component of symptom reporting in lactose maldigesters.

VII. LACTOSE DIGESTION, CALCIUM, AND OSTEOPOROSIS

Individuals who are lactose intolerant can tolerate moderate amounts of lactose with minimal to no gastrointestinal discomfort [48, 52], however, some lactose maldigesting individuals may unnecessarily restrict their intake of lactose-containing, calcium-rich dairy foods, thus compromising calcium intake. Milk and milk products contribute 73% of the calcium to the U.S. food supply [53]. Lactose maldigestion is associated with lower calcium intakes and is more frequent in osteoporotic patients than in controls [54–57]. For example, Newcomer et al. [54] found that 8 of 30 women with osteoporosis were lactose maldigesters compared to only 1 of 30 controls. In addition, calcium intakes of LNP postmenopausal women in this study (530 mg/day) were significantly lower than in the lactase persistent women (811 mg/day). Interestingly, in this report, and another by Horowitz et al. [55], few of the LNP subjects reported a history of milk intolerance and yet they still restricted milk intake. The lower milk intakes in these subjects may have been due to factors other than lactose intolerance. However, it is also possible that these subjects restricted their milk intakes due to lactose intolerance in childhood, forgot that they had done so, and simply maintained that pattern of milk intake throughout life.

Another potential explanation for the increased prevalence of osteoporosis among lactose maldigesters is that maldigestion of lactose decreases absorption of calcium. Human and animal studies suggest that lactose stimulates the intestinal absorption of calcium [53]. However, there is considerable disagreement regarding the influence of lactose and lactose maldigestion on calcium absorption in adults. This disagreement results from a number of factors including the dose of lactose given, the choice of method for assessing calcium absorption (single isotope, double isotope, balance methods), prior calcium intake of the subjects, and the form in which the calcium is given (milk vs. water).

Kocian et al. [58], using a single-isotope (^{47}Ca) method, demonstrated improved absorption of a 972-mg calcium dose from lactose-hydrolyzed milk as compared to milk containing lactose in lactose maldigesters. Conversely, the regular milk resulted in increased calcium absorption versus the lactose-hydrolyzed milk in lactose digesters. Another study, using dual-isotope methods, a 50-g lactose load, and 500 mg

of calcium chloride in water found similar results [59]. Total fractional calcium absorption was decreased in maldigesters and increased in digesters with lactose feeding. However, the doses of lactose given in these studies (39–50 g or the equivalent of 3–4 cups of milk) were unphysiologic and may have resulted in more rapid intestinal transit than would be observed with more physiologic amounts of lactose.

Several studies have been conducted with physiologic doses of lactose. Griessen et al. [60], using dual-isotope methods, found that lactose maldigesters ($n = 7$) had a slightly, but not statistically significantly, greater total fractional calcium absorption from 500 mL of milk compared to 500 mL of lactose-free milk. They also observed a nonsignificant decline in fractional calcium absorption in normal subjects ($n = 8$) when comparing lactose-free milk with regular milk. In another dual-isotope study, lactose maldigesters absorbed more calcium from a 240-mL dose of milk than did digesters (about 35% vs. 25%), which was thought to be due to lower calcium intakes in the lactose maldigesting group [61]. Most importantly, however, no difference was observed in fractional calcium absorption between lactose-hydrolyzed and regular milk in either group of subjects. Finally, calcium absorption from milk and yogurt, each containing 270 mg of calcium, was studied in our laboratory using a single-isotope method [62]. No significant differences were observed in calcium absorption between milk and yogurt in either the lactose maldigesting or digesting subjects. Interestingly, yogurt resulted in slightly, but significantly ($p < 0.05$), greater calcium absorption in lactose maldigesters when compared to lactose digesters.

Differences in study methodology (milk vs. water, dose of lactose, and the choice of method for determining calcium absorption) may explain contrasting results. Physiologic doses of lactose (e.g., amounts provided by up to 2 cups of milk) are not likely to have a significant impact on calcium absorption. The increased prevalence of osteoporosis in lactose maldigesters is most likely related to inadequate calcium intake rather than impaired intestinal calcium absorption.

VIII. DIETARY MANAGEMENT FOR LACTOSE MALDIGESTION

It is difficult for lactose maldigesters to consume adequate amounts of calcium if dairy products are eliminated from the diet. Fortunately, lactose intolerance is easily managed. Dietary management approaches that effectively reduce or eliminate intolerance symptoms are discussed below and shown in Table 4.

A. Dose Response to Lactose

There is a clear-cut relationship between the dose of lactose consumed and the symptomatic response. Small doses (up to

TABLE 4   Dietary Strategies for Lactose Intolerance

Factors affecting lactose digestion	Dietary strategy	References
Dose of lactose	Consume a cup of milk or less at a time, containing up to 12 g lactose.	Suarez *et al.* (1995)[48] Hertzler *et al.* (1996)[6] Suarez *et al.* (1997)[52]
Intestinal transit	Consume milk with other foods, rather than alone, to slow the intestinal transit of lactose.	Solomons *et al.* (1985)[69] Martini and Savaiano (1988)[4] Dehkordi *et al.* (1995)[70]
Yogurts	Consume yogurts containing active bacteria cultures. A serving, or even two, should be well tolerated. Lactose in yogurts is better digested than the lactose in milks.	Kolars *et al.* (1984)[77] Gilliland and Kim (1984)[83] Savaiano *et al.* (1984)[47] Shermak *et al.* (1995)[82]
	Pasteurized yogurts do not improve lactose digestion; however, these products, when consumed, produce little to no symptoms.	Savaiano *et al.* (1984)[47] Kolars *et al.* (1984)[83] Gilliland and Kim (1984)[77]
Digestive aids	Over-the-counter lactase supplements (pills, capsules, and drops) may be used when large doses of lactose (>12 g) are consumed at once.	Moskovitz *et al.* (1987)[97] Lin *et al.* (1993)[94] Ramirez *et al.* (1994)[98]
	Lactose-hydrolyzed milks also are well tolerated	Nielsen *et al.* (1984)[104] Biller *et al.* (1987)[109] Rosado *et al.* (1989)[106] Brand and Holt (1991)[102]
Colon adaptation	Consume lactose-containing foods daily to increase the colon bacteria's ability to metabolize undigested lactose.	Perman *et al.* (1981)[116] Florent *et al.* (1985)[46] Hertzler *et al.* (1996)[6]

12 g of lactose) yield no symptoms [1, 48, 50–52], whereas high doses (>20–50 g of lactose) produce appreciable symptoms in most individuals [1, 63–65]. In a well-controlled trial, Newcomer *et al.* [1] demonstrated that >85% of lactose maldigesters developed intolerance symptoms after consuming 50 g of lactose (the approximate amount of lactose in 1 quart of milk) as a single dose. The frequency of reported symptoms may be attributed to the nonphysiologic nature of the lactose dose and the physical form of lactose load administered. A physiologic dose containing 15–25 g of lactose is adequate to produce appreciable symptoms in some subjects [30, 66]. The incidence of symptom reporting generally remains above 50% with intermediate doses. However, the frequency varies from less than 40% to greater than 90% [30]. In a double-blind protocol, Suarez *et al.* [48] demonstrated that feeding 12 g of lactose with a meal resulted in minimal to no symptoms in maldigesters. Interestingly, in unblinded studies [66, 67], lactose maldigesters more frequently reported intolerance symptoms after consuming lactose loads similar to that given by Suarez *et al.* Recently, Suarez *et al.* [52] provided further evidence that individuals who are lactose intolerant can consume lactose-containing foods without experiencing appreciable symptoms by feeding lactose maldigesters 2 cups of milk daily. One cup of milk was given with breakfast, and the second was given

with the evening meal. The symptoms reported by maldigesters after consumption of 2 cups of milk were trivial.

Symptoms from excessive lactose in the intestine may increase out of proportion to dosage, which raises the possibility that the absorption efficiency decreases with increased loads. Fractional lactose absorption is most likely influenced by dosage, with more effective absorption of small loads and less effective utilization of larger doses. Hertzler *et al.* [43], using breath hydrogen as an indicator, suggested that 2 g of lactose is almost completely absorbed, whereas there was some degree of maldigestion when a 6-g load was ingested. The only study directly measuring the lactose absorption efficiency in lactose maldigesting subjects is that of Bond and Levitt [68], who intubated the terminal ileum and then fed the subjects ^{14}C lactose mixed with polyethylene glycol, a nonabsorbable volumetric marker. Analysis of the ratio of ^{14}C lactose to polyethylene glycol passing through the terminal ileum allowed researchers to calculate the percentage of lactose absorbed. On average, maldigesters absorbed about 40% of a 12.5-g lactose load, whereas the other 60% passed to the terminal ileum. However, sizable differences were seen in absorption efficiency among lactose maldigesters. These differences could represent differences in residual lactase efficiency and/or gastric emptying and intestinal transit time.

B. Factors Affecting Gastrointestinal Transit of Lactose

Consuming milk with other foods, rather than alone, can minimize symptoms from lactose maldigestion [4, 69, 70]. A probable explanation for these findings is that the presence of additional foods slows the intestinal transit of lactose. Slowed transit allows more contact between ingested lactose and residual lactase in the small intestine, thus improving lactose digestion. It is also possible that additional foods may simply slow the rate at which lactose arrives in the colon, because a delay in peak breath hydrogen production, rather than a significant decrease in total hydrogen production has been reported [4]. The slower fermentation of lactose might allow for more efficient disposal of fermentation gases, reducing the potential for symptoms.

The energy content, fat content, and added components such as chocolate may influence gastrointestinal transit of lactose and subsequent lactose digestion. Leichter [71] showed that 50 g of lactose from whole milk (1050 mL) resulted in fewer symptoms (abdominal discomfort, bloating, and flatulence) compared to 50 g of lactose from either skim milk (1050 mL) or an aqueous solution (330 mL). However, only blood glucose was measured to determine lactose digestion and no statistical evaluation of symptoms was done in this study. Recent studies have demonstrated that higher fat milk may slightly decrease breath hydrogen relative to skim milk [70], but not improve intolerance [70, 72, 73]. Further, increasing the energy content or viscosity of milk has not been effective in improving lactose digestion or tolerance [74, 75].

Chocolate milk has been recommended for individuals who are lactose intolerant. Apparently, chocolate milk empties from the stomach more slowly than unflavored milk, possibly due to its higher osmolality or energy content [3]. Two reports have demonstrated improved lactose digestion (i.e., reduced breath hydrogen) from chocolate milk [70, 76], with fewer symptoms reported in one of these studies [76].

Clearly, consumption of milk with other foods results in improved tolerance compared to milk alone. Therefore, consuming small amounts of milk routinely with meals is a recommended approach for individuals who are lactose intolerant to obtain sufficient calcium from dairy products. These individuals might also try chocolate milk to improve tolerance.

C. Yogurts

The lactose in yogurt with live cultures is digested better than lactose in milk and is well tolerated by those who are lactose intolerant [77]. Prior to fermentation, most commercially produced yogurt is nearly 6% lactose due to the addition of milk solids to milk during yogurt production. However, as the lactic acid bacteria (*Lactobacillus delbrueckii* subsp. *bulgaricus* and *Streptococcus salivarius*

subsp. *thermophilus*) multiply to nearly 100 million organisms per milliliter, 20–30% of the lactose is utilized, decreasing the lactose content of yogurt to approximately 4% [78]. During fermentation, the activity of the β-galactosidase enzyme substantially increases. Casein, calcium phosphate, and lactate in yogurt act as buffers in the acidic environment of the stomach, thus protecting a portion of the microbial lactase from degradation and allowing the delivery of intact cells to the small intestine [79, 80]. In the duodenum, once the intact bacterial cells interact with bile acids, they are disrupted allowing substrate access to enzyme activity.

Yogurt consumption results in enhanced digestion of lactose and improved tolerance [47, 77, 81–83]. In 1984, Kolars *et al.* [77] and Gilliland and Kim [83] reported enhanced lactose digestion from yogurt in lactose maldigesters. In both studies, breath hydrogen excretion was significantly reduced with the consumption of live culture yogurt. Furthermore, Kolars *et al.* [77] found that an 18-g load of lactose in yogurt resulted in significantly fewer intolerance symptoms reported by subjects as compared to the other forms of lactose given. Also in 1984, Savaiano *et al.* [47] demonstrated that yogurt feeding resulted in one-third to one-fifth less hydrogen excretion as compared to other lactose-containing dairy foods with no symptoms. Shermak *et al.* [82] reported that a 12-g load of lactose in yogurt resulted in lower peak hydrogen in children with a delay in the time for breath hydrogen to rise when compared to a similar lactose load given in milk. Moreover, the children experienced significantly fewer intolerance symptoms with yogurt consumption.

Yogurt pasteurization following fermentation has been somewhat controversial [83]. One advantage of pasteurizing yogurt is a longer shelf life. However, removing the active cultures that are partly responsible for improved lactose digestion may increase lactose maldigestion and intolerance symptoms and cause lactose maldigesters to avoid yogurt products. Pasteurizing yogurt increases the maldigestion of lactose [47, 82, 83]. However, pasteurized yogurt is moderately well tolerated, producing minimal symptoms [47, 81, 82]. Because pasteurized yogurt is relatively well tolerated, other factors such as the physical form, or gelling, and the energy density of yogurt may play a role in tolerance. The level of the β-galactosidase enzyme in yogurt may not be the limiting factor for improving lactose digestion because not all yogurts have the same level of lactase activity [84]. Martini *et al.* [84] fed yogurts with varying levels of microbial β-galactosidase. The remaining characteristics of the test yogurts (pH, cell counts, and lactose concentrations) were similar. Despite the different levels of β-galactosidase activity, all yogurts equally improved lactose digestion and minimized intolerance symptoms.

D. Unfermented Acidophilus Milk

Individuals who are lactose maldigesters [85–87] may consume unfermented milk containing cultures of *Lactobacillus*

acidophilus in an effort to consume adequate amounts of calcium and avoid intolerance symptoms. Various strains of *L. acidophilus* exist, however strain NCFM has been most extensively studied and used in commercial products. Unfermented acidophilus milk tastes identical to unaltered milk because the NCFM strain does not multiply in the product, provided that the storage temperature is below 40°F (5°C) [85, 86, 88]. *Lactobacillus acidophilus* strain NCFM is derived from human fecal samples [79] and contains β-galactosidase (lactase). The effectiveness of acidophilus milk on improving lactose digestion and intolerance symptoms has been evaluated. Most evidence suggests that unfermented acidophilus milk does not enhance lactose digestion or reduce intolerance symptoms [47, 88–90] primarily due to the low concentration of the species in the milk. Improved lactose digestion has been observed by some [91]; however, the test milk in this study contained a much higher concentration of *L. acidophilus* than is normally used to produce commercial acidophilus milks.

Further, the microbial lactase from *L. acidophilus* may not be available to hydrolyze the lactose *in vivo* [84, 86, 90]. *Lactobacillus acidophilus* is not a bile-sensitive organism [79, 88]. Therefore, once the intact bacterial cells reach the small intestine, bile acids may not disrupt the cell membrane to allow the release of the microbial lactase. However, sonicated acidophilus milk improved lactose digestion by reducing breath hydrogen [92]. Thus, if less bile-resistant strains were developed and used in adequate amounts, these strains may allow the β-galactosidase to be released, possibly yielding an effective approach to the dietary management of lactose maldigestion.

E. Lactase Supplements and Lactose-Reduced Milks

The use of lactase supplements and lactose-reduced dairy products is steadily growing in the United States. The leading brand in this industry, "Lactaid," reported $126 million in sales for fiscal 1997. The number of new dairy product introductions categorized as low- or no-lactose rose 50% from 1992 to 1997 [93].

Lactase pills, capsules, and drops contain lactase derived from yeast (*Kluyveromyces lactis*) or fungal (*Aspergillus niger, A. oryzae*) sources. Dosages of lactase per pill or caplet vary from 3000 to 9000 FCC units [94, 95]. Since 1984, these over-the-counter preparations have been generally recognized as safe by the U.S. Food and Drug Administration [96]. Additionally, milk that has been treated with lactase, resulting in a 70–100% reduction in lactose, is commercially available [95].

A number of studies have evaluated the effectiveness of these products. Doses of 3000–6000 Food Chemicals Codex (FCC) units of lactase administered just prior to milk consumption decrease both breath hydrogen and symptom responses to lactose loads ranging from 17 to 20 g [94, 97, 98].

The decrease in breath hydrogen and symptoms is generally dose dependent. Doses up to 9900 FCC units may be needed for digestion of a large lactose load, such as 50 g of lactose [94, 99, 100].

Lactose-hydrolyzed milks also improve lactose tolerance in both children and adults [64, 65, 101–111]. A by-product of lactose-hydrolyzed milk is increased sweetness, due to the presence of free glucose [48]. This increased sweetness may increase its acceptability in children [104].

F. Colonic Fermentation and Colonic Bacterial Adaptation of Lactose

The colonic bacteria ferment undigested lactose and produce short-chain fatty acids (SCFA) and gases. Historically, this fermentation process was viewed as a cause of lactose intolerance symptoms. However, it is now recognized that the fermentation of lactose, as well as other nonabsorbed carbohydrates, plays an important role in the health of the colon and impacts the nutritional status of the individual.

The loss of intestinal lactase activity in lactose maldigesters is permanent. Studies from Israel, India, and Thailand have reported that feeding 50 g of lactose or more per day for periods of 1–14 months has no impact on jejunal lactase activity [17, 112, 113]. Despite this fact, milk has been used successfully in the treatment of malnourished children in areas of the world where lactose maldigestion is common. In Ethiopia, for example, 100 schoolchildren, aged 6–10 years, were fed 250 mL of milk per day for a period of 4 weeks [114]. While the children initially experienced some degree of gastrointestinal symptoms, the symptoms rapidly abated and returned to pretrial levels within 4 weeks. Similar results were observed with schoolchildren in India [112]. Finally, a study of African-Americans, who were lactose maldigesting and lactose intolerant aged 13–39 years, showed that 77% of the subjects could ultimately tolerate ≥12 g of lactose if lactose was increased gradually and fed daily over a period of 6–12 weeks [115]. Approximately 80% of the subjects (18 of 22) had rises in breath hydrogen of at least 10 ppm above baseline at the maximum dose of lactose tolerated, suggesting that improved digestion of lactose in the small intestine was not responsible for the increased tolerance. Therefore, the authors proposed that colonic bacterial adaptation was a likely explanation for these findings.

Evidence for colonic bacterial adaptation to disaccharides (lactulose, lactose) is substantial. Perman *et al.* [116] fed adults 0.3 g/kg lactulose per day for 7 days and observed a decrease in fecal pH from 7.1 ± 0.3 to 5.8 ± 0.6. The breath hydrogen response to a challenge dose of lactose (0.3 g/kg) fell significantly after lactulose adaptation. Employing the same experimental design and doses of lactulose, Florent *et al.* [46] measured fecal β-galactosidase, colonic pH, breath hydrogen, fecal carbohydrates, SCFA, and ¹⁴C-lactulose catabolism in subjects before and after the 7-day lactulose maintenance period. Fecal β-galactosidase was six times

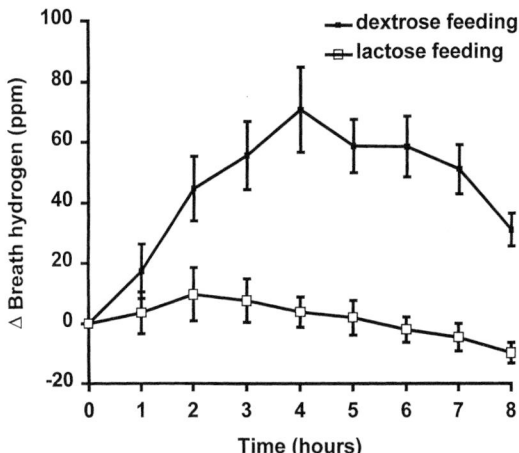

FIGURE 1 Breath hydrogen response to a lactose challenge after lactose (□) or dextrose (■) feeding periods. Data are the means ± SEM, n = 20. [Reprinted with permission from Hertzler, S. R., and Savaiano, D. A. (1996). Colonic adaptation to daily lactose feeding in lactose maldigesters reduces lactose intolerance. *Am. J. Clin. Nutr.* **64,** 232–236.]

greater after lactulose feeding and breath hydrogen fell significantly. Breath $^{14}CO_2$ (indicating catabolism of ^{14}C-lactulose) increased and fecal outputs of lactulose and total hexose units were low after the lactulose feeding. Symptoms were not measured; however, a follow-up study showed that adaptation to lactulose (40 g/day for 8 days) reduced symptoms of diarrhea induced by a large dose (60 g) of lactulose [117]. Breath hydrogen decreased significantly and fecal β-galactosidase activity increased as in the previous study.

Finally, two feeding trials adapting lactose maldigesters to lactose have been reported. The first was a blinded, crossover study from our laboratory at the University of Minnesota [45]. Feeding increasing doses of lactose (from 0.3 up to 1.0 g/kg/day) for 16 days resulted in a threefold increase in fecal β-galactosidase activity, which returned to baseline levels within 48 hours after substitution of dextrose for lactose. Further, 10 days of lactose feeding (from 0.6 up to 1.0 g/kg/day), compared to dextrose feeding, dramatically decreased the breath hydrogen response to a lactose challenge dose (0.35 g/kg) (see Fig. 1). In fact, after lactose adaptation, the subjects no longer appeared to be lactose maldigesters, based on a 20-ppm rise in breath hydrogen above fasting. The large doses of lactose fed during the adaptation period (averaging 42–70 g/day) resulted in only minor symptoms. Additionally, the severity and frequency of flatus symptoms in response to the lactose challenge dose were reduced by 50%.

The second study was a double-blind, placebo-controlled trial conducted in France with a group of 46 subjects who were lactose intolerant [118]. Following a baseline lactose challenge with 50 g of lactose, subjects were randomly assigned to either a lactose-fed group (n = 24) or a sucrose-fed control group (n = 22). Subjects were fed 34 g of either lactose or sucrose per day for 15 days. Fecal β-galactosidase increased and breath hydrogen decreased as the result of lactose feeding. Clinical symptoms (except diarrhea) were 50% less severe after lactose feeding. However, the sucrose-fed control group also experienced a comparable decrease in symptoms, despite no evidence of metabolic adaptation. Thus, these authors concluded that the improvements in symptoms resulted from familiarization with the test protocol rather than from metabolic adaptation.

Colonic bacteria develop an increased ability to ferment lactose (indicated by increased fecal β-galactosidase) following prolonged lactose feeding. Because hydrogen gas is an endproduct of fermentation, one might expect that the increased ability to ferment lactose would result in an increase, rather than the observed decrease, in breath hydrogen. However, breath hydrogen excretion represents the net of bacterial hydrogen production and consumption in the colon [40]. A decrease in net production of hydrogen could result from either decreased bacterial production or increased consumption. To examine the mechanism for decreased breath hydrogen after lactose adaptation, we employed metabolic inhibitors of bacterial hydrogen consumption (methanogenesis, sulfate reduction, and acetogenesis) to obtain measures of absolute hydrogen production [119]. Subjects were fed increasing amounts of lactose or dextrose in a manner similar to previous studies. Fecal samples were assayed *in vitro* for absolute hydrogen production and hydrogen consumption. Absolute hydrogen production after 3 hours of incubation with lactose was threefold lower after lactose adaptation (242 ± 54 μL) compared to the dextrose feeding period (680 ± 79 μL, $p = 0.006$). Fecal hydrogen consumption was unaffected by either feeding period. These findings tend to support the hypothesis that prolonged lactose feeding favors the growth or metabolic activity of bacteria (e.g., bifidobacteria, lactic acid bacteria) that can ferment lactose without the production of hydrogen. Feeding lactose, lactulose, and nonabsorbable oligosaccharides stimulates the proliferation of lactic acid bacteria in the colon [120–122]. Additionally, high populations of bifidobacteria inhibit the growth of known hydrogen-producing organisms, such as clostridia or *Escherichia coli* [123].

Colonic bacterial adaptation to lactose does occur. Although the role of colonic adaptation in improving symptoms is not firmly established, it is clear that many individuals who are lactose intolerant can develop a tolerance to milk if they consume it regularly. This may represent a simpler and less expensive solution than the use of lactose digestive aids.

IX. GENE THERAPY FOR LACTOSE INTOLERANCE

Although conventional dietary therapies for lactose intolerance exist, the possibility of gene therapy for lactase nonpersistence was examined by During *et al.* [124]. An

adeno-associated virus vector was orally administered to hypolactasic rats to increase lactase mRNA. The adeno-associated virus vector is a defective, helper-dependent virus and the wild type is nonpathogenic in humans and other species. Following a single administration of a recombinant adeno-associated virus vector expressing β-galactosidase, all rats treated with this vector ($n = 4$) were positive for *lacZ* mRNA in the proximal intestine within 3 days. There was no lactase mRNA in the rats treated with the control vector. On day 7, following vector administration, the rats were challenged with a lactose solution. The treated rats had a rise in blood glucose from 114 ± 4 to 130 ± 3 mg/dL after 30 minutes, while the control rats had a flat blood glucose curve. Further, the treated rats still displayed similar lactase activity when challenged with lactose 6 months later. Thus, the potential of gene therapy for lactose intolerance exists.

X. SUMMARY

A majority of the world's population and approximately 25% of the U.S. population are lactose maldigesters. Milk and milk products not only contain lactose, but are also important sources of calcium, riboflavin, and high-quality protein. Some maldigesters may avoid dairy products due to the perception that intolerance symptoms will inevitably follow dairy food consumption. Avoiding dairy products may limit calcium intake and bone density, thus increasing the risk for osteoporosis. Avoidance of milk and milk products is unnecessary since moderate lactose consumption does not produce a symptomatic response in maldigesters. Additionally, various dietary strategies effectively manage lactose intolerance by reducing or eliminating gastrointestinal symptoms. Dairy food consumption is possible for individuals who are lactose intolerant if simple dietary management strategies are incorporated into daily living.

References

1. Newcomer, A. D., McGill, D. B., Thomas, P. J., and Hofmann, A. F. (1978). Tolerance to lactose among lactase deficient American Indians. *Gastroenterology* **74,** 44–46.
2. Ravich, W. J., and Bayless, T. M. (1983). Carbohydrate absorption and malabsorption. *Clin. Gastroenterol.* **12,** 335–356.
3. Welsh, J. D., and Hall, W. H. (1977). Gastric emptying of lactose and milk in subjects with lactose malabsorption. *Am. J. Dig. Dis.* **22,** 1060–1063.
4. Martini, M. C., and Savaiano, D. A. (1988). Reduced intolerance symptoms from lactose consumed with a meal. *Am. J. Clin. Nutr.* **47,** 57–60.
5. Scrimshaw, N. S., and Murray, E. B. (1988). The acceptability of milk and milk products in populations with a high prevalence of lactose intolerance. *Am. J. Clin. Nutr.* **48,** 1083–1159.
6. Hertzler, S. R., Levitt, M. D., and Savaiano, D. A. (1996). Colonic adaptation to the daily lactose feeding in lactose maldigesters reduces lactose tolerance. *Am. J. Clin. Nutr.* **64,** 1232–1236.
7. Kretchmer, N., and Sunshine, P. (1967). Intestinal disaccharidase deficiency in the sea lion. *Gastroenterology* **53,** 123–129.
8. Zeccha, L., Mesonero, J. E., Stutz, A., Poiree, J-C., Giudicelli, J., Cursio, R., Gloor, S. M., and Semenza, G. (1998). Intestinal lactase-phlorizin hydrolase (LPH): The two catalytic sites; the role of the pancreas in pro-LPH maturation. *FEBS Lett.* **435,** 225–228.
9. Montgomery, R. K., Buller, H., Rings, E. H. H. M., and Grand, R. J. (1991). Lactose intolerance and the genetic regulation of intestinal lactase phlorizin hydrolase. *FASEB J.* **5,** 2824–2832.
10. Rossi, M., Maiuri, L., Fusco, M. I., Salvati, V. M., Fuccio, A., Aurrichio, S., Mantei, N., Zecca, L., Gloor, S. M., and Semenza, G. (1997). Lactase persistence versus decline in human adults: Multifactorial events are involved in downregulation after weaning. *Gastroenterology* **112,** 1506–1514.
11. Järvelä, I., Enattah, N. S., Kokkonen, J., Varilo, T., Sahvilahti, E., and Peltonen, L. (1998). Assignment of the locus for congenital lactase deficiency to 2q21, in the vicinity of but separate from the lactase-phlorizin hydrolase gene. *Am. J. Hum. Genet.* **63,** 1078–1085.
12. Sterchi, E. E., Mills, P. R., Fransen, J. A. M., Hauri, H.-P., Lentze, M. J., Naim, H. Y., Ginsel, L., and Bond, J. (1990). Biogenesis of intestinal lactase-phlorizin hydrolase in adults with lactose intolerance: Evidence for reduced biosynthesis and slowed-down maturation in enterocytes. *J. Clin. Invest.* **86,** 1329–1337.
13. Kien, C. L., Heitlinger, L. A., Li, U., and Murray, R. D. (1989). Digestion, absorption, and fermentation of carbohydrates. *Semin. Perinatol.* **13,** 78–87.
14. Holzel, A., Schwarz, V., and Sutcliffe, K. W. (1959). Defective lactose absorption causing malnutrition in infancy. *Lancet* **1,** 1126–1128.
15. Sahvilahti, E., Launiala, K., and Kuitunen, P. (1983). Congenital lactase deficiency. *Arch. Dis. Child.* **58,** 246–252.
16. Newcomer, A. D., and McGill, D. B. (1984). Clinical consequences of lactase deficiency. *Clin. Nutr.* **3,** 53–58.
17. Sahi, T. (1994). Genetics and epidemiology of adult-type hypolactasia. *Scand. J. Gastroenterol.* **29,** 7–20.
18. Gilat, T., Russo, S., Gelman-Malachi, E., and Aldor, T. A. M. (1972). Lactase in man: A nonadaptable enzyme. *Gastroenterology* **62,** 1125–1127.
19. Simoons, F. J. (1978). The geographic hypothesis and lactose malabsorption—A weighing of the evidence. *Am. J. Dig. Dis.* **23,** 963–980.
20. McCracken, R. D. (1970). Adult lactose tolerance [letter]. *J. Am. Med. Assoc.* **213,** 2257–2260.
21. Lee, M.-F., and Krasinski, S. D. (1998). Human adult-onset lactase decline: An update. *Nutr. Rev.* **56,** 1–8.
22. Lloyd, M., Mevissen, G., Fischer, M., Olsen, W., Goodspeed, D., Genini, M., Boll, W., Semenza, G., and Mantei, N. (1992). Regulation of intestinal lactase in adult hypolactasia. *J. Clin. Invest.* **89,** 524–529.
23. Fajardo, O., Naim, H. Y., and Lacey, S. W. (1994). The polymorphic expression of lactase in adults is regulated at the messenger RNA level. *Gastroenterology* **106,** 1233–1241.
24. Eschler, J. C., de Koning, N., van Engen, C. G. J., Arora, S., Buller, H. A., Montgomery, R. K., and Grand, R. J. (1992).

Molecular basis of lactase levels in adult humans. *J. Clin. Invest.* **89**, 480–483.

25. Sebastio, G., Villa, M., Sartorio, R., Guzetta, V., Poggi, V., Aurrichio, S., Boll, W., Mantei, N., and Semenza, G. (1989). Control of lactase in human adult-type hypolactasia and in weaning rabbits and rats. *Am. J. Hum. Genet.* **45**, 489–497.

26. Olsen, W. A., Li, B. U., Lloyd, M., and Korsmo, H. (1996). Heterogeneity of intestinal lactase activity in children: Relationship to lactase-phlorizin hydrolase messenger RNA abundance. *Pediatr. Res.* **39**, 877–881.

27. Newcomer, A. D., and McGill, D. B. (1966). Distribution of disaccharidase activity in the small bowel of normal and lactase-deficient subjects. *Gastroenterology* **51**, 481–488.

28. Triadou, N., Bataille, J., and Schmitz, J. (1983). Longitudinal study of the human intestinal brush border membrane proteins. *Gastroenterology* **85**, 1326–1332.

29. Maiuri, L., Rossi, M., Raia, V., Garipoli, V., Hughes, L. A., Swallow, D., Noren, O., Sjostrom, H., and Aurrichio, S. (1994). Mosaic regulation of lactase in human adult-type hypolactasia. *Gastroenterology* **107**, 54–60.

30. Savaiano, D. A., and Levitt, M. D. (1987). Milk intolerance and microbe-containing dairy foods. *J. Dairy Sci.* **70**, 397–406.

31. Srinivasan, R., and Minocha, A. (1998). When to suspect lactose intolerance: Symptomatic, ethnic, and laboratory clues. *Postgrad. Med.* **104**, 109–123.

32. Schmidt, W., Schneider, T., Heise, W., Schulze, J.-D., Weinke, T., Ignatius, R., Owen, R. L., Zeitz, M., Riecken, E.-O., and Ulrich, R. (1997). Mucosal abnormalities in microsporidiosis. *AIDS* **11**, 1589–1594.

33. Corazza, G. R., Ginaldi, L., Furia, N., Marani-Toro, G., Di Giammartino, D., and Quaglino, D. (1997). The impact of HIV infection on lactose absorptive capacity. *J. Infect.* **35**, 31–35.

34. Arola, H. (1994). Diagnosis of hypolactasia and lactose malabsorption. *Scand. J. Gastroenterol.* **29**, 26–35.

35. Levitt, M. D., and Donaldson, R. M. (1970). Use of respiratory hydrogen (H2) excretion to detect carbohydrate malabsorption. *J. Lab. Clin. Med.* **75**, 937–945.

36. Solomons, N. W. (1984). Evaluation of carbohydrate absorption: The hydrogen breath test in clinical practice. *Clin. Nutr.* **3**, 71–78.

37. Metz, G., Jenkins, D. J., Peters, J. J., Newman, A., and Blendis, L. M. (1975). Breath hydrogen as a diagnostic method for hypolactasia. *Lancet* **1**, 1155–1157.

38. Strocchi, A., Corazza, G., Ellis, C. J., Gasbarrini, G., and Levitt, M. D. (1993). Detection of malabsorption of low doses of carbohydrate: Accuracy of various breath hydrogen criteria. *Gastroenterology* **105**, 1404–1410.

39. Anderson, I. H., Levine, A. S., and Levitt, M. D. (1981). Incomplete absorption of the carbohydrate in all-purpose wheat flour. *N. Engl. J. Med.* **304**, 891–892.

40. Levitt, M. D., Gibson, G. R., and Christl, S. U. (1995). Gas metabolism in the large intestine. In "Human Colonic Bacteria: Role in Nutrition, Physiology, and Disease" (G. R. Gibson and G. T. Macfarlane, Eds.), pp. 131–154. CRC Press, Boca Raton, FL.

41. Bjorneklett, A., and Jenssen, E. (1982). Relationships between hydrogen (H₂) and methane (CH₄) production in man. *Scand. J. Gastroenterol.* **17**, 985–992.

42. Gudmand Høyer, E. (1994). The clinical significance of disaccharide maldigestion. *Am. J. Clin. Nutr.* **59**, 735S–741S.

43. Hertzler, S. R., Huynh, B., and Savaiano, D. A. (1996). How much lactose is "low lactose"? *J. Am. Diet. Assoc.* **96**, 243–246.

44. Vesa, T. H., Korpela, R. A., and Sahi, T. (1996). Tolerance to small amounts of lactose in lactose maldigesters. *Am. J. Clin. Nutr.* **64**, 197–201.

45. Hertzler, S. R., and Savaiano, D. A. (1996). Colonic adaptation to daily lactose feeding in lactose maldigesters reduces lactose intolerance. *Am. J. Clin. Nutr.* **64**, 232–236.

46. Florent, C., Flourie, B., Leblond, A., Rautureau, M., Bernier, J.-J., and Rambaud, J.-C. (1985). Influence of chronic lactulose ingestion on the colonic metabolism of lactulose in man (an in vivo study). *J. Clin. Invest.* **75**, 608–613.

47. Savaiano, D. A., AbouElAnouar, A., Smith, D. E., and Levitt, M. D. (1984). Lactose malabsorption from yogurt, pasteurized yogurt, sweet acidophilus milk, and cultured milk in lactase-deficient individuals. *Am. J. Clin. Nutr.* **40**, 1219–1223.

48. Suarez, F. L., Savaiano, D. A., and Levitt, M. D. (1995). A comparison of symptoms after the consumption of milk or lactose-hydrolyzed milk by people with self-reported severe lactose intolerance. *N. Engl. J. Med.* **333**, 1–4.

49. Rorick, M. H., and Scrimshaw, N. S. (1979). Comparative tolerance of elderly from differing ethnic background to lactose-containing and lactose-free daily drinks: A double-blind study. *J. Gerontol.* **34**, 191–196.

50. Haverberg, L., Kwon, P. H., and Scrimshaw, N. S. (1980). Comparative tolerance of adolescents of differing ethnic backgrounds to lactose-containing and lactose-free dairy drinks. I. Initial experience with a double-blind procedure. *Am. J. Clin. Nutr.* **33**, 17–21.

51. Unger, M., and Scrimshaw, N. S. (1981). Comparative tolerance of adults of differing ethnic backgrounds to lactose-free and lactose-containing dairy drinks. *Nutr. Res.* **1**, 1227–1233.

52. Suarez, F. L., Savaiano, D. A., Arbisi. P., and Levitt, M. D. (1997). Tolerance to the daily ingestion of two cups of milk by individuals claiming lactose intolerance. *Am. J. Clin. Nutr.* **65**, 1502–1506.

53. Miller, G. D., Jarvis, J. K., and McBean, L. D. (2000)."Handbook of Dairy Foods and Nutrition," 2nd ed., pp. 311–54. CRC Press, Boca Raton, FL.

54. Newcomer, A. D., Hodgson, S. F., McGill, D. B., and Thomas, P. J. (1978). Lactase deficiency: Prevalence in osteoporosis. *Ann. Intern. Med.* **89**, 218–220.

55. Horowitz, M., Wishart, J., Mundy, L., and Nordin, B. E. C. (1987). Lactose and calcium absorption in postmenopausal osteoporosis. *Arch. Intern. Med.* **147**, 534–536.

56. Finkenstedt, G., Skrabal, F., Gasser, R. W., and Braunsteiner, H. (1986). Lactose absorption, milk consumption, and fasting blood glucose concentrations in women with idiopathic osteoporosis. *Br. Med. J.* **292**, 161–162.

57. Corazza, G. R., Benati, G., DiSario, A., Tarozzi, C., Strocchi, A., Passeri, M., and Gasbarrini, G. (1995). Lactose intolerance and bone mass in postmenopausal Italian women. *Br. J. Nutr.* **73**, 479–487.

58. Kocian, J., Skala, I., and Bakos, K. (1973). Calcium absorption from milk and lactose-free milk in healthy subjects and patients with lactose intolerance. *Digestion* **9**, 317–324.

59. Cochet, B., Jung, A., Griessen, M., Bartholdi, P., Schaller, P., and Donath, A. (1983). Effects of lactose on intestinal calcium absorption in normal and lactase-deficient subjects. *Gasterenterology* **84,** 935–940.

60. Griessen, M., Cochet, B., Infante, F., Jung, A., Bartholdi, P., Donath, A., Loizeau, E., and Courvoisier, B. (1989). Calcium absorption from milk in lactase-deficient subjects. *Am. J. Clin. Nutr.* **49,** 377–384.

61. Tremaine, W. J., Newcomer, A. D., Riggs, L., and McGill, D. B. (1986). Calcium absorption from milk in lactase-deficient and lactase-sufficient adults. *Dig. Dis. Sci.* **31,** 376–378.

62. Smith, T. M., Kolars, J. C., Savaiano, D. A., and Levitt, M. D. (1985). Absorption of calcium from milk and yogurt. *Am. J. Clin. Nutr.* **42,** 1197–1200.

63. Johnson, A. O., Semenya, J. G., Buchowski, M. S., Enwonwu, C. O., and Scrimshaw, N. S. (1993). Correlation of lactose maldigestion, lactose intolerance, and milk intolerance. *Am. J. Clin. Nutr.* **57,** 399–401.

64. Reasoner, J., Maculan, T. P., Rand, A. G., and Thayer, W. R., Jr. (1981). Clinical studies with low-lactose milk. *Am. J. Clin. Nutr.* **34,** 54–60.

65. Pedersen, E. R., Jensen, B. H., Jensen, H. J., Keldsbo, I. L., Moller, E. H., and Rasmussen, S. N. (1982). Lactose malabsorption and tolerance of lactose-hydrolyzed milk: A double-blind controlled crossover trial. *Scand. J. Gastroenterol.* **17,** 861–864.

66. Bayless, T. M., Rothfeld, B., Masser, C., Wise, L., Paige, D., and Bedine, M. S. (1975). Lactose and milk intolerance: Clinical implications. *N. Engl. J. Med.* **292,** 1156–1159.

67. Rosado, J. L., Gonzales, C., Valencia, M. E., Lopez, B., Mejia, L., and Del Carmen Baez, M. (1994). Lactose maldigestion and milk intolerance: A study in rural and urban Mexico using physiological doses of milk. *J. Nutr.* **124,** 1052–1059.

68. Bond, J. H., and Levitt, M. D. (1976). Quantitative measurement of lactose absorption. *Gastroenterology* **70,** 1058–1062.

69. Solomons, N. W., Guerrero, A.-M., and Torun, B. (1985). Dietary manipulation of postprandial colonic lactose fermentation: I. Effect of solid foods in a meal. *Am. J. Clin. Nutr.* **41,** 199–208.

70. Dehkordi, N., Rao, D. R., Warren, A. P., and Chawan, C. B. (1995). Lactose malabsorption as influenced by chocolate milk, skim milk, sucrose, whole milk, and lactic cultures. *J. Am. Diet. Assoc.* **95,** 484–486.

71. Leichter, J. L. (1973). Comparison of whole milk and skim milk with aqueous lactose solution in lactose tolerance testing. *Am. J. Clin. Nutr.* **26,** 393–396.

72. Vesa, T. H., Lember, M., and Korpela, R. (1997). Milk fat does not affect the symptoms of lactose intolerance. *Eur. J. Clin. Nutr.* **51,** 633–636.

73. Cavalli-Sforza, L. T., and Strata, A. (1986). Double-blind study on the tolerance of four types of milk in lactose malabsorbers and absorbers. *Hum. Nutr. Clin. Nutr.* **40C,** 19–30.

74. Vesa, T. H., Marteau, P. R., Briet, F. B., Boutron-Ruault, M.-C., and Rambaud, J.-C. (1997). Raising milk energy content retards gastric emptying of lactose in lactose-intolerant humans with little effect on lactose digestion. *J. Nutr.* **127,** 2316–2320.

75. Vesa, T. H., Marteau, P. R., Briet, F. B., Flourie, B., Briend, A., and Rambaud, J.-C. (1997). Effects of milk viscosity on gastric emptying and lactose intolerance in lactose maldigesters. *Am. J. Clin. Nutr.* **66,** 123–126.

76. Lee, C. M., and Hardy, C. M. (1989). Cocoa feeding and human lactose intolerance. *Am. J. Clin. Nutr.* **49,** 840–844.

77. Kolars, J. C., Levitt, M. D., Aouji, M., and Savaiano, D. A. (1984). Yogurt—An autodigesting source of lactose. *N. Engl. J. Med.* **310,** 1–3.

78. Răsic, J., and Kurmans, J. A. (1978). The nutritional-physiological value of yoghurt. In "Yogurt; Scientific Grounds, Technology, Manufacture and Preparations," pp. 99–137. Tech. Dairy Pub. House, Copenhagen, Denmark.

79. Savaiano, D. A., and Kotz, C. (1988). Recent advances in the management of lactose intolerance. *Contemp. Nutr.* **13,** no. 9, 10.

80. Pochart, P., Dewit, O., Desjeux, J.-H., and Bourlioux, P. (1989). Viable starter culture, β-galactosidase activity, and lactose in doudenum after yogurt ingestion in lactase-deficient humans. *Am. J. Clin. Nutr.* **49,** 828–831.

81. Lerebours, E., N'Djitoyap Ndam, C., Lavoine, A., Hellot, M. F., Antoine J. M., and Colin, R. (1989). Yogurt and fermented-then-pasteurized milk: Effects of short-term and long-term ingestion on lactose absorption and mucosal lactase activity in lactase-deficient subjects. *Am. J. Clin. Nutr.* **49,** 823–827.

82. Shermak, M. A., Saavedra, J. M., Jackson, T. L., Huang, S. S., Bayless, T. M., and Perman, J. A. (1995). Effect of yogurt on symptoms and kinetics of hydrogen production in lactose-malabsorbing children. *Am. J. Clin. Nutr.* **62,** 1003–1006.

83. Gilliland, S. E., and Kim, H. S. (1984). Effect of viable starter culture bacteria in yogurt on lactose utilization in humans. *J. Dairy Sci.* **67,** 1–6.

84. Martini, M. C., Lerebours, E. C., Lin, W.-J., Harlander, S. K., Berrada, N. M., Antoine, J. M., and Savaiano, D. A. (1991). Strains and species of lactic acid bacteria in fermented milks (yogurts): Effect on *in vivo* lactose digestion. *Am. J. Clin. Nutr.* **54,** 1041–1046.

85. Lin, M.-Y., Savaiano, D., and Harlander, S. (1991). Influence of nonfermented dairy products containing bacterial starter cultures on lactose maldigestion in humans. *J. Dairy Sci.* **74,** 87–95.

86. Hove, H., Nørgaard, H., and Mortensen, P. B. (1999). Lactic acid bacteria and the human gastrointestinal tract. *Eur. J. Clin. Nutr.* **53,** 339–350.

87. Gilliland, S. E. (1989). Acidophilus milk products: A review of potential benefits to consumers. *J. Dairy Sci.* **72,** 2483–2494.

88. Newcomer, A. D., Park, H. S., O'Brein, P. C., and McGill, D. B. (1983). Response of patients with irritable bowel syndrome and lactase deficiency using unfermented acidophilus milk. *Am. J. Clin. Nutr.* **38,** 257–263.

89. Payne, D. L., Welsh, J. D., Manion, C. V., Tsegaye, A., and Herd, L. D. (1981). Effectiveness of milk products in dietary management of lactose malabsorption. *Am. J. Clin. Nutr.* **34,** 2711–2715.

90. Onwulata, C. I., Rao, D. R., and Vankineni, P. (1989). Relative efficiency of yogurt, sweet acidophilus milk, hydrolyzed-lactose milk, and a commercial lactase tablet in alleviating lactose maldigestion. *Am. J. Clin. Nutr.* **49,** 1233–1237.

91. Kim, H. S., and Gilliland S. E. (1984). *Lactobacillus acidophilus* as a dietary adjunct for milk to aid lactose digestion in humans. *J. Dairy Sci.* **66,** 959–966.

92. Mcdonough, F. E., Hitchins, A. D., Wong, N. P., Wells, P., and Bodwell, C. E. (1987). Modification of sweet acidophilus

milk to improve utilization by lactose-intolerant persons. *Am. J. Clin. Nutr.* **45,** 570–574.

93. Lower lactose can create higher profits: Perceived intolerance to dairy products creates new niche. (1998). Dairy Field 181, 20.

94. Lin, M.-Y., DiPalma, J. A., Martini, M. C., Gross, C. J., Harlander, S. K., and Savaiano, D. A. (1993). Comparative effects of exogenous lactase (β-galactosidase) preparations on in vivo lactose digestion. *Dig. Dis. Sci.* **38,** 2022–2027.

95. McNeil, P. P. C. (2000). "About Lactaid and Lactaid Ultra." Available at http://www.lactaid.com.

96. Lactase preparation from *K. lactis* affirmed as GRAS. (1984). *Food Chem. News* December 10, p. 30.

97. Moskovitz, M., Curtis, C., and Gavaler, J. (1987). Does oral enzyme replacement therapy reverse intestinal lactose malabsorption? *Am. J. Gastroenterol.* **82,** 632–635.

98. Ramirez, F. C., Lee, K., and Graham, D. Y. (1994). All lactase preparations are not the same: Results of a prospective, randomized, placebo-controlled trial. *Am. J. Gastroenterol.* **89,** 566–570.

99. DiPalma, J. A., and Collins, M. S. (1989). Enzyme replacement for lactose malabsorption using a beta-D-galactosidase. *J. Clin. Gastroenterol.* **11,** 290–293.

100. Sanders, S. W., Tolman, K. G., and Reitberg, D. P. (1992). Effect of a single dose of lactase on symptoms and expired hydrogen after lactose challenge in lactose-intolerant adults. *Clin. Pharm.* **11,** 533–538.

101. Cheng, A. H., Brunser, O., Espinoza, J., Fones, H. L., Monckeberg, F., Chichester, C. O., Rand, G., and Hourigan, A. G. (1979). Long-term acceptance of low-lactose milk. *Am. J. Clin. Nutr.* **32,** 1989–1993.

102. Brand, J. C., and Holt, S. (1991). Relative effectiveness of milks with reduced amounts of lactose in alleviating milk intolerance. *Am. J. Clin. Nutr.* **54,** 148–151.

103. Turner, S. J., Daly, T., Hourigan, J. A., Rand, A. J., and Thayer, W. R., Jr. (1976). Utilization of a low-lactose milk. *Am. J. Clin. Nutr.* **29,** 739–744.

104. Nielsen, O. H., Schiotz, P. O., Rasmussen, S. N., and Krasilnikoff, P. A. (1984). Calcium absorption and acceptance of low-lactose milk among children with lactase deficiency. *J. Pediatr. Gastroenterol.* **3,** 219–223.

105. Paige, D. M., Bayless, T. M., Mellits, E. D., Davis, L., Dellinger, W. S., Jr., and Kreitner, M. (1979). Effects of age and lactose tolerance on blood glucose rise with whole cow and lactose-hydrolyzed milk. *J. Agric. Food Chem.* **27,** 677–680.

106. Rosado, J. L., Morales, M., and Pasquetti, A. (1989). Lactose digestion and clinical tolerance to milk, lactose-prehydrolyzed milk, and enzyme-added milk: A study in undernourished continuously enteral-fed patients. *J. Parenteral Enteral Nutr.* **13,** 157–161.

107. Nagy, L., Mozsik, G., Garamszegi, M., Sasreti, E., Ruzsa, C., and Javor, T. (1983). Lactose-poor milk in adult lactose intolerance. *Acta Med. Hung.* **40,** 239–245.

108. Payne, D. L., Welsh, J. D., Manion, C. V., Tsegaye, A., and Herd, L. D. (1981). Effectiveness of milk products in dietary management of lactose malabsorption. *Am. J. Clin. Nutr.* **34,** 2711–2715.

109. Biller, J. A., King, S., Rosenthal, A., and Grand, R. J. (1987). Efficacy of lactase-treated milk for lactose-intolerant pediatric patients. *J. Pediatr.* **111,** 91–94.

110. Rosado, J. L., Morales, M., Pasquetti, A., Nobara, R., and Hernandez, L. (1988). Nutritional evaluation of a lactose-hydrolyzed milk-based enteral formula diet: I. A comparative study of carbohydrate digestion and clinical tolerance. *Rev. Invest. Clin.* **40,** 141–147.

111. Payne-Bose, D., Welsh, J. D., Gearhart, H. L., and Morrison, R. D. (1977). Milk and lactose-hydrolyzed milk. *Am. J. Clin. Nutr.* **30,** 695–697.

112. Reddy, V., and Pershad, J. (1972). Lactase deficiency in Indians. *Am. J. Clin. Nutr.* **25,** 114–119.

113. Keusch, G. T., Troncale, F. J., Thavaramara, B., Prinyanot, P., Anderson, P. R., and Bhamarapravthi, N. (1969). Lactase deficiency in Thailand: Effect of prolonged lactose feeding. *Am. J. Clin. Nutr.* **22,** 638–641.

114. Habte, D., Sterky, G., and Hjalmarsson, B. (1973). Lactose malabsorption in Ethiopian children. *Acta Pediatr. Scand.* **62,** 649–654.

115. Johnson, A. O., Semenya, J. G., Buchowski, M. S., Enwonwu, C. O., and Scrimshaw, N. S. (1993). Adaptation of lactose maldigesters to continued milk intakes. *Am. J. Clin. Nutr.* **58,** 879–881.

116. Perman, J. A., Modler, S., and Olson, A. C. (1981). Role of pH in production of hydrogen from carbohydrates by colonic bacterial flora: Studies in vivo and in vitro. *J. Clin. Invest.* **67,** 643–650.

117. Flourie, B., Briet, F., Florent, C., Pellier, P., Maurel, M., and Rambaud, J.-C. (1993). Can diarrhea induced by lactulose be reduced by prolonged ingestion of lactulose? *Am. J. Clin. Nutr.* **58,** 369–375.

118. Briet, F., Pochart, P., Marteau, P., Flourie, B., Arrigoni, E., and Rambaud, J. C. (1997). Improved clinical tolerance to chronic lactose ingestion in subjects with lactose intolerance: A placebo effect? *Gut* **41,** 632–635.

119. Hertzler, S. R., Savaiano, D. A., and Levitt, M. D. (1997). Fecal hydrogen production and consumption measurements: Response to daily lactose ingestion by lactose maldigesters. *Dig. Dis. Sci.* **42,** 348–353.

120. Terada, A., Hara, H., Kataoka, M., and Mitsuoka, T. (1992). Effect of lactulose on the composition and metabolic activity of the human fecal flora. *Microb. Ecol. Health Dis.* **5,** 43–50.

121. Gibson, G. R., Beatty, E. R., Wang, X., and Cummings, J. H. (1995). Selective stimulation of bifidobacteria in the human colon by oligofructose and insulin. *Gastroenterology* **108,** 975–982.

122. Ito, M., and Kimura, M. (1993). Influence of lactose on faecal microflora in lactose maldigesters. *Microb. Ecol. Health Dis.* **6,** 73–76.

123. Gibson, G. R., and Wang, X. (1994). Regulatory effects of bifidobacteria on the growth of other colonic bacteria. *J. Appl. Bacteriol.* **77,** 412–420.

124. During, M. J., Xu, R., Young, D., Kaplitt, M. G., Sherwin, R. S., and Leone, P. (1998). Peroral gene therapy of lactose intolerance using an adeno-associated virus vector. *Nat. Med.* **4,** 1131–1135.

CHAPTER 38

Nutrient Considerations in Inflammatory Bowel Disease and Short Bowel Syndrome

PETER L. BEYER

University of Kansas Medical Center, Kansas City, Kansas

I. INTRODUCTION

The two primary forms of idiopathic inflammatory bowel disease, Crohn's disease and ulcerative colitis, are characterized as chronic, inflammatory diseases of varying severity. The cause is unknown but the disease appears to involve significant interaction of the intestinal wall with intestinal microbes, ingested foods and beverages, gastrointestinal secretions, local and systemic immune components, and genetic factors. The disease may result in malabsorption of nutrients, obstruction of the gastrointestinal tract, decreased oral intake, increased nutrient requirements, and adverse response to ingested foods. Malnutrition is common. Medications and other therapies employed in treating inflammatory bowel disease can further compromise nutritional status.

Specific dietary factors may enhance or attenuate the underlying inflammatory processes involved in the disease, and certain dietary habits can worsen or reduce the severity of symptoms of inflammatory bowel disease. Surgery is common in the life of patients with inflammatory bowel disease and, in some cases, may significantly affect the ability of the patient to maintain adequate nutritional status without specialized nutrition care. Consequently, dietary interventions have a significant role in the management of inflammatory bowel disease, its symptoms, and its consequences. In the first section of this chapter, characteristics of inflammatory bowel disease, the nature of the inflammatory process, and the potential role for nutrition interactions are reviewed. In the second section, nutrition and short bowel syndrome, one of the potential complications of Crohn's disease and other gastrointestinal maladies, are discussed.

II. INFLAMMATORY BOWEL DISEASE

Inflammatory bowel disease refers to any type of inflammatory disorder involving the small and/or large intestine including those caused by infectious, immunologic, or toxic agents. Crohn's disease and ulcerative colitis are the two most common forms of idiopathic inflammatory bowel disease and will be the only forms considered here. Although Crohn's disease and ulcerative colitis share many clinical, genetic, and pathologic features, they also exhibit distinguishing characteristics.

A. Characteristics of Inflammatory Bowel Disease

In both Crohn's disease and ulcerative colitis, risk of weight loss, growth failure, anemia, diarrhea, fever, arthritic and dermatologic manifestations, nutrient deficiencies, and colon cancer are increased. Although malnutrition can occur in both disorders, it is more likely to occur in Crohn's disease primarily due to the involvement of the small bowel and as a result of small intestinal resections. See Table 1 for common disease characteristics.

In Crohn's disease, malabsorption, abdominal pain, mucosal thickening, strictures, obstruction, abscesses and fistula formation and nephrolithiasis are more common. (See Figs. 1 and 2 for representation of normal small intestine and colon, Fig. 3 for Crohn's disease, and Fig. 4 for ulcerative colitis; for Figs. 3 and 4, see color plate at the back of the book.) Crohn's disease may appear anywhere along the gastrointestinal tract although it most commonly occurs in the ileum and colon together (in about 40–55% of the cases), in the colon alone (15–30% of cases), or in the small intestine alone (about 30%). Diseased bowel may be adjacent to "skipped" areas that appear normal. In contrast to ulcerative colitis, the disease is transmural rather than mucosal. Over the course of the disease, about 70% of persons with Crohn's disease will eventually have at least one surgery. Surgery does not guarantee a cure and it is not uncommon to encounter persons with Crohn's disease who have had numerous surgical procedures.

In ulcerative colitis, only the colon is involved. In about 30% of patients, the disease remains confined to the rectum.

TABLE 1   Characteristics of Crohn's Disease and Ulcerative Colitis

Features common to both Crohn's disease and ulcerative colitis
Chronic episodes of relapse and remission with varying degrees of duration and severity
Diarrhea
Extraintestinal manifestations to varying degrees
Fever
Increased risk of colorectal cancer
Characteristics more common in Crohn's disease
Any area of the gastrointestinal tract but more commonly involves the distal small bowel and colon, with a smaller percentage involving just the small bowel or just the colon
Skipped areas
Transmural, thickening of the intestinal wall
70% have surgery in their lifetime; surgery does not guarantee a cure
Abscesses, sinus tract, fistulas
Strictures
Hyperoxaluria, oxalate stones
Characteristics more common in ulcerative colitis
Mucosal layer only
Confined to the colon
Surgical resection of the colon eliminates the disease
Normally originates in the distal colon and migrates proximally
Gastrointestinal bleeding

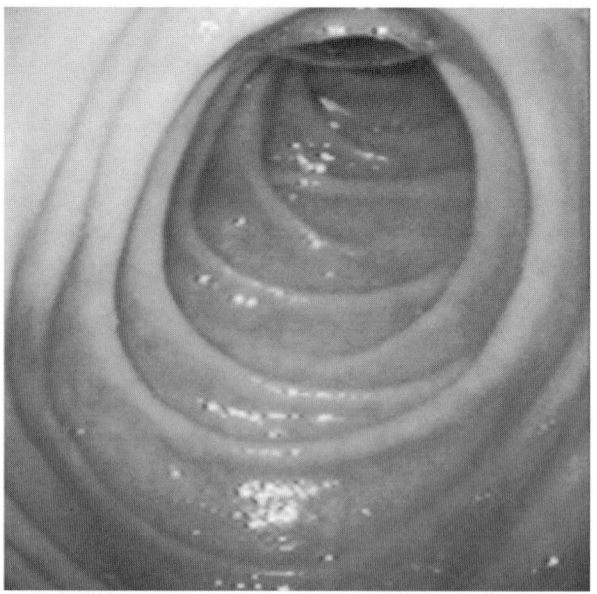

FIGURE 1   Normal small intestine. Photo courtesy of Dr. Gottumukkala Raju, Kansas University Medical Center, Division of Gastroenterology.

Worldwide, the incidence of Crohn's disease ranges from less than 1 new case per 100,000 annually to 12 per 100,000 annually. The broad range perhaps reflects the genetic influence and, to varying degrees, the sophistication of the systems in place for identifying and reporting the disease throughout the world. In the United States, the incidence of new cases of Crohn's disease is about 5–7 per 100,000 and

In about 25–50% of those who present with proctitis, the disease progresses eventually to more extensive colonic involvement. The disease begins distally in the rectum and moves proximally when it progresses. Diarrhea is the most common symptom but crampy abdominal pain and rectal bleeding are also common presentations. One-third or fewer of persons with ulcerative colitis eventually require colectomy during their lifetime. After colectomy, however, the disease does not recur anywhere else in the intestinal tract [1–4].

B. Incidence, Prevalence, and Course

Inflammatory bowel disease may occur at any age, but the onset most frequently occurs between the ages of 15–30 years; a smaller rise in occurrence is seen after the sixth decade [2, 4]. Neither Crohn's disease nor ulcerative colitis is common but because of the frequency of clinic and hospital visits associated with the diseases, health care professionals tend to have a distorted sense of the prevalence.

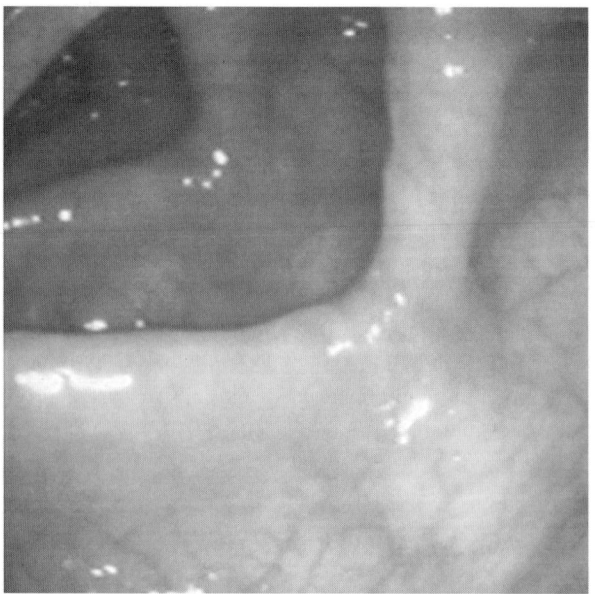

FIGURE 2   Normal colon (cecum). Photo courtesy of Dr. Gottumukkala Raju, Kansas University Medical Center, Division of Gastroenterology.

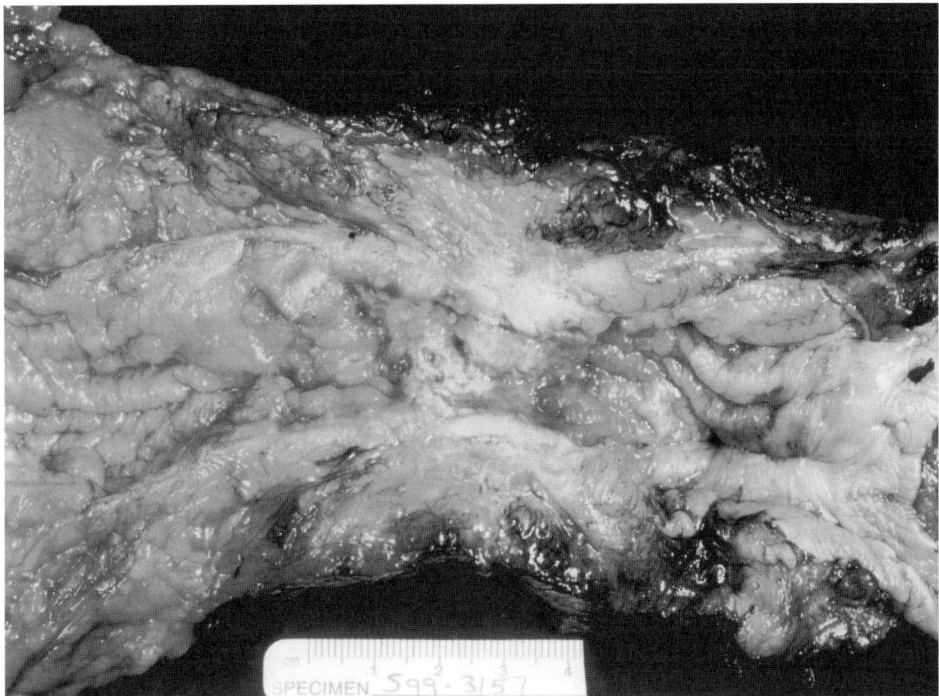

FIGURE 3 Crohn's disease. Photo courtesy of Ossama Tawfik, MD, PhD, Director, Surgical Pathology, University of Kansas Medical Center.

for ulcerative colitis is about 10–12 per 100,000. According to the Crohn's Colitis Society [5], the prevalence of inflammatory bowel disease is approximately 150 cases per 100,000 persons and the risk of developing Crohn's disease in an individual who had a relative with Crohn's disease is increased 10-fold. If siblings or both parents have Crohn's

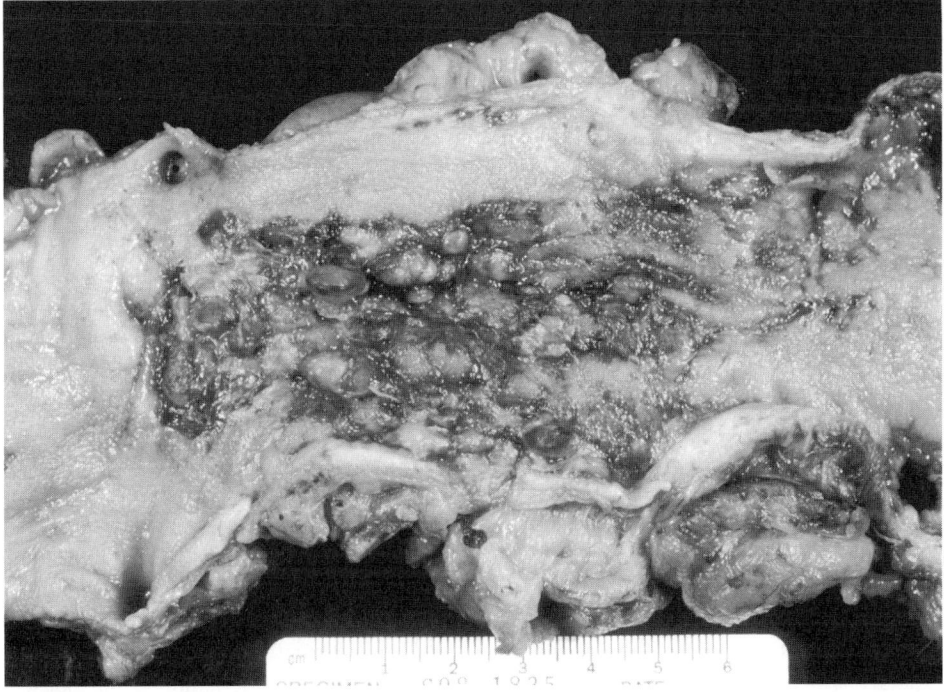

FIGURE 4 Ulcerative colitis. Photo courtesy of Ossama Tawfik, MD, PhD, Director, Surgical Pathology, University of Kansas Medical Center.

disease, the risk increases to 30 times normal. Because of the variance in the prevalence, severity, and course of the disease, several genes are suspected to be involved. Initial research appears to be consistent with the concept that Crohn's disease and ulcerative colitis are polygenic in nature [4, 6, 7].

The course of inflammatory bowel disease can vary from tranquil to severe and intermittent to unrelenting. In persons with more severe and active forms of disease, symptoms, health care requirements, dietary changes, and anxiety (regarding procedures, symptoms, normal aberrations in bowel habit, concern about surgery, social embarrassment) can significantly affect the quality of life [3, 4, 8, 9]. The factors involved in the onset, course, and outcomes of the disease are multifactorial and include the interactions of genetic susceptibility, environmental influence and therapeutic interventions. These factors taken together affect the overall course, severity, and outcomes of the disease [4, 6]. Nutrition appears to play a role in the clinical profile, treatment, and perhaps onset of the disease, but the impact of nutrition is not as well understood in some aspects of the disease as in others.

C. Inflammatory Events in Crohn's Disease and Ulcerative Colitis

In any discussion of nutritional aspects of an inflammatory disease, a review of the pathologic events in the inflammatory process is appropriate. Several dietary factors may be involved in the exacerbation, modulation, or resolution of the inflammatory state.

The inflammatory process is typically initiated by microbial invasion, physical trauma, exposure to toxic agents, or autoimmune reactions and subsequently a cascade of events occurs [10–12]. Events include recruitment and proliferation of leukocytes; release of eicosanoids, proinflammatory and regulatory cytokines; release of proteases and generation of oxygen radicals; activation of clotting mechanisms; and production of fibrous tissue. The normal inflammatory response is directed toward containment of the injury, destruction of invading microbes, inactivation of toxins, and repair of the injured tissue. Overzealous inflammatory response, which may result from extreme or chronic injury, however, can result in serious damage to tissues and organs.

The term *inflammatory bowel* is an appropriate descriptor for Crohn's disease and ulcerative colitis because the classic events of acute and chronic inflammation are exhibited with each disease. In inflammatory bowel disease, sufficient evidence exists that the factors that drive the inflammatory response and/or the inappropriate reaction to the initiating agent are responsible for the symptoms and the physical and pathological changes seen in the disorders. Dietary lipids, antioxidants, and dietary antigens have the potential to influence the inflammatory response and, consequently, the inflammatory response affects nutrient intake, nutrient pro-

TABLE 2 Inflammatory Events Identified in Patients with Active Inflammatory Bowel Disease

Entry and proliferation of macrophages, neutrophils, and lymphocytes into the area of active disease

Release of inflammatory metabolites of arachidonic acid (e.g., leukotriene B_4)

Release of proinflammatory cytokines (e.g., TNF, IL-1, 6, 8, and 12) and anti-inflammatory cytokines (e.g., 4, 10, 11)

Involvement and hypersensitivity of mucosal T cells

Increased peroxidation, generation of oxygen radicals, and release of proteolytic enzymes

Increased permeability (gut edema, pro loss and entry)

Increased fibrin/collagen formation; increased thickness of the gut wall

Damage/dysfunction in secretion, digestion, absorption, and the barrier against microbes/proteins

Increased synthesis of acute phase proteins and activation of the clotting cascade

Fatigue, anorexia, malaise, and arthritic and other systemic complications

cessing, and requirements. A brief overview, therefore, of the inflammatory process in inflammatory bowel disease and the potential role of nutrients is appropriate.

Several features of active immune and inflammatory processes have been demonstrated in both Crohn's disease and in ulcerative colitis (see Table 2). Most of the inflammatory events are localized to the bowel, but at least in active states, signs of systemic activity are also apparent. Infiltration and proliferation of macrophages, neutrophils, lymphocytes, and/or fibroblasts are seen in the intestinal crypts, wall, lamina propria, and mesentery [3, 6, 13]. Evidence also exists that eosinophils are involved in the active disease [14]. Proinflammatory eicosanoids (e.g., leukotriene B_4) are released from cell walls of leukocytes and somatic cells. Eicosanoids may be viewed as metabolic endproducts of arachidonic acid, which is produced endogenously from dietary n-6 fatty acids and incorporated into membrane phospholipids [15]. Proinflammatory cytokines, for example, tumore necrosis factor (TNF), interleukin-1 (IL-1), IL-6, and IL-8, are released in increased amounts and appear to reflect, at least to some degree, the severity of the disease [15–19]. Regulatory or anti-inflammatory cytokines (e.g., IL-10, and IL-11) are also increased but at levels insufficient to effectively counteract the overall proinflammatory state. Levels of peroxidation and generation of oxygen radicals are increased [20], and circulating levels of antioxidants may be decreased [21]. Consistent with the inflammatory process, platelets, prothrombin, fibrinogen, and collagen formation are increased, resulting in increased risk of systemic thromboembolic episodes, local fibrosis, and thickening of the bowel wall (most notably in Crohn's disease) [22].

TABLE 3 Possible Causes of Inflammatory Bowel Disease

Virus or bacterium

Defective mucosal barrier functions

Increased permeability to microbes, toxins, and antigens

Abnormal response to pathogens/antigens

Abnormal response to normal flora

Imbalance of proinflammatory/anti-inflammatory cytokine homeostasis

Autoimmune component

Dietary (e.g., sugar/refined diet, lipids, dietary antigens)

As a result of the release of histamine, cytokines, and eicosanoids, increased gut permeability, local edema, ulceration, and damage to the intestinal architecture may occur. Gastrointestinal secretion, digestion, absorption, and motility may be abnormal, especially in active stages, and the normal barrier to microbial fragments, toxins and large peptides may be compromised. As in any significant inflammatory response, acute phase proteins are found in increased levels and may serve, along with specific cytokine and leukotriene levels, as markers of the disease. Fatigue, malaise, anorexia, and disturbances in sleep patterns and mood can be seen in active disease [23].

D. Etiology of Inflammatory Bowel Disease

The cause of Crohn's disease and ulcerative colitis is unknown, but several possibilities have been evaluated (see Table 3). Under normal circumstance the gastrointestinal tract is continuously exposed to potential antigens and toxins in the form of microbes, dietary components, and medications. Normally, physical and immunologic barriers prevent undue host interaction with the luminal environment. The combination of some form of exogenous luminal stimuli and dysregulated endogenous response appears to bring on and allow the disease process to takes its course. One of the most popular hypotheses is an abnormal immune response to normal gastrointestinal flora or hyperreactivity to common pathogens [24].

In the pathology of inflammatory bowel disease, bacteria and viruses have long been etiologic candidates because of (1) associations between the incidence of inflammatory bowel and community exposure to microbial infections, (2) antibodies in tissues to specific microbial fragments, or (3) gastrointestinal damage provoked by infectious agents. Measles virus, strains of *Eschericia coli* and *Mycobacterium paratuberculosis* have all been implicated, but not proven as causal factors [1, 3, 6]. Other hypotheses include a defective mucosal barrier, which allows increased interaction with luminal contents of the gut [25]; an imbalance of proinflammatory to anti-inflammatory cytokines [26]; downregulation

of glucocorticoid receptors [27]; hyperresponsiveness of mucosal T cells [28]; increased nitric oxide production [29]; and increased production of oxidative compounds or decreased protection by antioxidants [20, 21].

Several forms of genetic susceptibility appear to play a role in the endogenous response to whatever environmental stimuli may be involved [6, 7], but the disease process and the associated inflammatory response combine to confound the ability to identify clear-cut relationships. Identifying the initial trigger for disease onset is difficult. A number of years may elapse between the first symptoms of the disease and its diagnosis, and the initiation of the disease may occur long before symptoms become apparent. The disease process and the inflammatory response result in pathologic changes (e.g., increased gut permeability and antigen exposure), which creates the problem of identifying whether the disease or the antigen came first.

1. Do Dietary Factors Cause or Promote Inflammatory Bowel Disease?

Although certain foods or food types have been associated with changes in the incidence of inflammatory bowel disease, no specific foods have been proven to *cause* inflammatory bowel disease. Also, no single food has consistently and objectively been identified in the onset of an acute inflammatory episode or, when withdrawn, consistently has shown to induce remission. This is not to say that patients with inflammatory bowel disease might not have food allergies, that foods might not serve to heighten the immunologic activity, or that certain food types might not aggravate symptoms [29a].

Russel and colleagues [30] attempted to associate the rising incidence of inflammatory bowel disease with changes in dietary consumption patterns. The authors showed a positive risk for inflammatory bowel disease with increases in consumption of cola beverages, chocolate, and chewing gum, but negative risk for consumption of citrus fruits. As noted by these investigators, these nutritional items could be true risk factors or they could be coincidental dietary patterns adopted during the same time period. Joachim [31] reported subjective responses to foods of 60 patients with inflammatory bowel disease. Patients were asked to report whether specific foods made them feel better or worse. Patients reported an increased number of problems with chocolate, dairy products, fats, and artificial sweeteners. Unfortunately, only 122 foods were included on the questionnaire and the author did not report the number of problem foods in matched healthy controls or patients with other forms of gastrointestinal illness.

Several investigations have been centered on the lipid content of the diet [32, 33]. High-fat diets and an increased ratio of n-6 to n-3 fatty acids have been associated with the increased occurrence of inflammatory bowel disease and perhaps the duration of remission. Consumption of predominantly n-6 lipid increases the potential to produce leukotrienes

and prostaglandins from arachidonic acid released from cell membrane phospholipids during inflammation. The eicosanoids produced from n-6 fatty acids are more inflammatory and aggregatory than those from n-3 fatty acids. Leukotriene B_4, for example, induces recruitment and activation of neutrophils, monocytes, and eosinophils. It also stimulates the production of a number of proinflammatory cytokines and chemical mediators [34, 35]. Reducing consumption of dietary n-6 fatty acids relative to n-3 fatty acid intake may attenuate synthesis of proinflammatory cytokines secreted by leukocytes, such as TNF-α and IL-1 mediators.

Geerling and associates [33] examined the fatty acid intake and the fatty acid composition of plasma phospholipids and adipose tissue in 20 newly diagnosed patients with Crohn's disease, 32 patients with long-standing Crohn's disease in remission, and matched controls. Fatty acid intake was not different between cases and controls but a lower percentage of the sum of n-3 fatty acids and other changes in the lipid profile were seen in the patients. Kuroki and colleagues [36] measured serum fatty acid levels in 20 patients with Crohn's disease without major resections and 18 healthy controls. Unexpectedly, they found adequate amounts of both essential n-6 and n-3 fatty acids. Increasing levels of n-3 fatty acids, however, were associated with a decreased Crohn's disease activity index. Other dietary lipids, such as gamma linolenic acid, may play anti-inflammatory roles by modifying ratios of chemical mediators [37]. As is the case of other dietary factors examined thus far, lipids appear to be an associated rather than an independent etiologic factor.

2. Do Food Allergies Bring On or Cause the Disease?

The lumen of the gastrointestinal tract is normally filled with antigens that have the potential to initiate at least part of the local immune and inflammatory processes. However, the role of food allergies as a major player in the cause of inflammatory bowel disease has not been established. For example, Bichoff and associates [38] studied 375 adults with gastrointestinal disorders, including inflammatory bowel disease, for objective evidence of intestinal allergic reactions. Thirty-two percent of the individuals complained of adverse reactions to foods as a cause of their abdominal symptoms, 14% had indirect evidence of allergic manifestations, but only 3% of the cases could be confirmed by allergen provocation, elimination, and rechallenge testing. The authors concluded that food antigens could be a factor in a subgroup of persons with inflammatory and functional disease. The incidence of allergies in the gastrointestinal patients (3.2%) was only slightly greater than the approximately 1.5% occurrence seen in the overall adult population [39].

In several earlier reports, milk allergy was suggested as a cause or trigger in the relapse of ulcerative colitis. Increased antibodies to milk protein have been reported [1], but their presence did not correlate with other markers of allergy or severity of symptoms. Withdrawal of milk or any other specific food does not consistently result in remission of active disease. After studying the sera of patients with Crohn's disease, Huber and colleagues [40] detected no food-specific IgE. Local allergic response to foods in the gastrointestinal tract does not appear to be a primary component of the pathology of inflammatory bowel disease [41]. However, if mucosal permeability is compromised, food antigens may contribute to the disease process. Additional work is needed to clarify the role of allergies to specific foods in the overall disease process.

In earlier reports, consumption of sucrose, refined cereals, fast foods, and fat have been positively associated with either the incidence of inflammatory bowel disease or with its onset. Intake of dietary fiber, fruits and vegetables, and specific nutrients, on the other hand, were negatively associated with the onset of inflammatory bowel disease [42, 43]. In more recent reviews, however, no consistent relationship of such foods with either the onset or management of inflammatory bowel disease could be demonstrated [44, 45]. The association between intake of foods and inflammatory bowel disease may simply reflect food intake patterns when the initial onset or relapse of the disease occurs. Establishing that specific foods may trigger the onset of a disease flare is difficult, partly because of the fact that the delay between specific dietary behaviors and notable symptoms may be lengthy. The heightened inflammatory state associated with the disease process and the resulting increased intestinal permeability may simply allow entry and reaction to certain foods that may otherwise be well tolerated. Tolerance of dietary components may be compromised simply as a result of changes in secretion, motility, digestion, absorption, or intestinal flora. Intolerance to some foods in patients with inflammatory bowel disease may also be easily predicted by their effects in normal individuals, such as consumption of excess amounts of lactose, caffeine, dietary fiber, or legumes.

E. Nutrition-Related Problems in Inflammatory Bowel Disease

Patients often share concerns regarding their symptoms and potential outcomes, as outlined in Table 4. Patients with Crohn's disease may have experienced prolonged episodes of bloating, cramping, nausea, and vomiting as a result of intestinal obstruction. Patients with either Crohn's or ulcerative colitis disease may have experienced prolonged periods of diarrhea, with 15 or more stools daily. Healthy persons normally endure various types of minor abdominal pains and changes in bowel habit with little thought. Patients with inflammatory bowel disease, however, associate gastrointestinal signals with symptoms that previously preceded exacerbation of disease, surgery, diagnostic procedures, or prolonged hospitalizations. Patients with Crohn's disease

TABLE 4 Concerns Expressed by Patients with Inflammatory Bowel Disease in Surveys, Internet Newsgroups, and Support Groups

Need for procedures, surgery/ostomy/hospitalization

Sources/significance of pain and other symptoms

Diarrhea, incontinence

Occurrence of obstruction/fistulae

Possibility that symptoms will lead to initial or repeat surgery

Symptoms or appliances interfering with daily activity, quality of life, interactions with others

Concern whether nutrient intake and digestion/absorption are adequate

Side effects of medications

Incomplete understanding of symptoms; no definite etiology for the disease

Inconsistent advice/answers from health care professional and others

TABLE 5 Nutrition-Related Problems in Inflammatory Bowel Disease

Diarrhea

Anemias (from blood loss, decreased intake, or malabsorption of iron, vitamin B_{12}, or folate)

Anorexia

Weight loss

Hypoalbuminemia

Growth failure in children

Malnutrition (macro- and micronutrients)

Incomplete and/or limited diet

Malabsorption

Vitamin and mineral depletion

Bone demineralization (due to poor intake and malabsorption of vitamin D, calcium)

Food intolerances, food aversions, fear of eating

---

who have already had significant small bowel resections may worry about their ability to absorb sufficient food and liquid, and persons with more severe forms of both Crohn's disease and ulcerative colitis may worry about ostomy surgery and its sequelae. Because neither the cause nor the triggers for the onset of the disease are clear, frustration is common among patients attempting to resolve or temper their disease activity [4, 8, 9]. Moreover, anxiety itself may worsen the manifestations of the disease.

Diarrhea, with or without malabsorption, and weight loss are the most common nutritional problems seen in inflammatory bowel disease [1–3]. In flares of inflammatory bowel disease and after small bowel resections in Crohn's disease, diarrhea may be severe enough to cause dehydration and electrolyte disturbances. Incontinence, increased stool frequency, and the occurrence of anal burning may make the diarrhea even more unpleasant.

Several forms of anemia may occur as a result of inadequate intake, malabsorption, increased requirements, and drug–nutrient interactions. Microcytic anemia in ulcerative colitis is more commonly related to blood loss than poor iron intake or malabsorption. Macrocytic anemia due to vitamin B_{12} deficiency is more likely to be seen in Crohn's patients who have had resections of the terminal ileum, the site of active absorption of vitamin B_{12} [46]. Anemia related to folate deficiency can occur as a result of poor intake, poor absorption, or drug–nutrient interactions [47, 48]. See Table 5 for a list of nutrition-related problems.

Numerous reports of micronutrient deficiencies in persons with inflammatory bowel disease have been published during the last two or three decades [46–50], especially when literature from around the world is reviewed. However, today, the likelihood of micronutrient deficiency is less likely. Widespread use of enteral nutrition formulas, vitamin and mineral supplements, and fortified foods reduces the risk of deficiencies.

Despite the availability of micronutrients, some vitamin and mineral deficiencies do occur. Vitamin B_{12}, folate, zinc, calcium, iron, magnesium, selenium, copper, and vitamin A, D, and E inadequacies have all been reported in patients with inflammatory bowel disease [46–52]. Fear of eating, food aversions, self-imposed or iatrogenic diet restrictions, surgical resections, and drug–nutrient interactions are likely to increase the risk of micronutrient deficiencies. Because the cells lining the gastrointestinal tract are especially metabolically active, macro- and micronutrient deficiencies have the potential to contribute to the pathology of the disease and compromise its resolution.

Anorexia may be related to the patient's symptoms of abdominal pain, bloating, nausea, or diarrhea. Increased levels of several cytokines may also contribute to anorexia [23, 53]. Patients may be afraid to eat specific foods or food types either because they have heard that specific foods may worsen symptoms or they have had adverse experiences with specific foods. Food aversions and questionable associations of foods with subsequent symptoms are not uncommon. The pattern is not unlike that seen in cancer patients who undergo aggressive chemotherapy, become ill as a result of the side effects of therapy, and associate the illness with ingestion, taste, or smell of foods.

Patients may associate adverse symptoms with consumption of specific foods or food types and may be on restricted diets imposed by health professionals, by themselves, or on the advice of "self-proclaimed" nutrition experts. The reason for food restrictions may be to prevent symptoms, maintain remission, or treat the disease.

Weight loss, growth failure, and delayed maturation are some of the most common problems in inflammatory bowel disease. Although the inflamed gastrointestinal tract may not

TABLE 6   Primary Treatment Options
for Inflammatory Bowel Disease

Medications—Anti-inflammatory agents, immune modulators, antibiotics

Surgery—Repair strictures, resections of small and large bowel

Psychosocial—Counseling, education, support

Nutrition—Restore deficiencies, reduce symptoms, prevent relapse (induce remission?)

TABLE 7   Medical Management of Inflammatory
Bowel Disease—Common Agents

Anti-inflammatory drugs—Corticosteroids, sulfasalazine, 5-aminosalicylic acid (5-ASA or Mesalamine)

Immune modulators or suppressants—Methotrexate, azathioprine, 6-mercaptopurine, cyclosporine, monoclonal antibody to TNF-α (Infliximab)

Antibiotics—Metronidazole, ciprofloxacin

be as efficient at absorbing macronutrients, compared to the healthy gastrointestinal tract, most investigators and experienced clinicians attribute the nutritional inadequacy to lack of sufficient food intake [54–56]. In severe stages of either Crohn's disease or ulcerative colitis, varying degrees of malabsorption may occur, but the primary cause of malabsorption is major intestinal resection in Crohn's disease and, to a lesser extent, the disease process itself. Decreased levels of transport proteins such as albumin, transferrin, or prealbumin may be related to the shift in priority in protein synthesis in the liver that occurs with physiologic stressors. Also, increased intestinal loss of nitrogen with disease relapse, or prolonged or acute periods of decreased protein and total energy intake, may worsen the level of transport proteins.

F. Treatment of Inflammatory Bowel Disease

Treatment of inflammatory bowel disease usually involves several strategies, including medications, surgery, nutrition, and psychosocial support (see Table 6). The goals of treatment are essentially to promote remission (or at least resolve symptoms), treat and prevent complications, restore and maintain nutrition status, and improve quality of life. Because the etiology of inflammatory bowel disease is unknown and no single therapy is completely effective in accomplishing the overall goals, therapies are used in combination and are based on individual needs.

1. MEDICAL MANAGEMENT

Over the course of a lifetime, patients with inflammatory bowel disease are likely to be treated with several medications. Drugs may be used for inducing remission, maintaining remission, and treating specific symptoms of the disease. Medications may be used in different combinations depending on the severity and presentation of the disease. General categories of medications commonly used to treat the primary events of inflammatory bowel disease include anti-inflammatory agents, immunomodulator/suppressive drugs, and antibiotics. Several other medications, however, may also be used specifically to treat symptoms at various stages of the disease such as antidiarrhea or antiemetic medications [1–3, 57–60].

Although most of the agents are used for both Crohn's disease and ulcerative colitis, some differences in application

and effectiveness do occur. Drugs may be required for prolonged periods of time and at high doses to cause remission. Sometimes even combinations of approaches may fail. No single medication is consistently effective at quenching active disease or maintaining continuous remission. Use of medications brings additional costs, potential short-term and long-term side effects, and drug–drug and drug–nutrient interactions. They invariably alter daily life patterns. See Table 7 for a listing of commonly used medications.

To treat moderate to severe disease in both Crohn's disease and ulcerative colitis, several classes of drugs may be used singly or in combination, but corticosteroids remain the principal drug of choice. Because of the metabolic, cosmetic, and psychogenic complications associated with use of corticosteroids, however, large doses and prolonged treatment are avoided when possible. Corticosteroids are not considered a valuable alternative in maintaining remission in either form of inflammatory bowel disease. Cyclosporine has been used in severe cases and as an alternative to surgery when the disease is resistant to steroid therapies [60]. Infliximab, a monoclonal antibody to TNF-α, has recently been approved for treatment of chronic active Crohn's disease and for the treatment of fistulas [59]. Its use has not been extended to the management of ulcerative colitis. Infliximab has been shown to have some benefit in the treatment of pouchitis [61], a complication in some patients who have had ileorectal pouches created as fecal reservoirs after colectomy.

Agents used as primary treatment of mild to moderate active disease include topical corticosteroids, sulfasalazine, 5-aminosalicylic acid, azathioprine, 6-mercaptopurine, methotrexate, and the antibiotics ciprofloxacin and metronidazole. The medications can be used in combination with steroids. To maintain remission, sulfasalazine, 5-aminosalicylic acid, metronidazole, azathioprine, or 6-mercaptopurine are normally used. All of the medications may be justified in the management of various stages of inflammatory bowel disease, but mild to significant adverse side effects occur in approximately 5–60% of percent of patients [2, 59, 60].

A number of new agents are being evaluated for treatment of inflammatory bowel disease, including anti-inflammatory cytokines, such as IL-10 and IL-11 [62]; growth hormone [62a]; neutralizing antibodies of specific proinflammatory cytokines [63]; inhibitors of, and antibodies to, inflammatory leukotrienes or their precursors [64]; nicotine (for patients

with ulcerative colitis) [57]; bismuth compounds [65]; intravenous heparin [66], and a protease inhibitor from soy [67]. Other approaches also include use of other forms of antibiotics, adrenocorticotropic hormone (ACTH) [68], and leukocytapheresis [69].

2. SURGICAL TREATMENT

Indications for surgery typically include severe, unrelenting disease, strictures, obstruction, hemorrhage, increased risk of cancer, repair of fistulas, and failure of medical therapy [70, 71]. In ulcerative colitis, colectomy "cures" the disease in that the disease does not subsequently occur elsewhere in the gastrointestinal tract. Approximately half of patients with ulcerative colitis have surgery in the first 10 years after diagnosis [70]. The most common form of surgery is colectomy with the creation of an ileoanal pouch (commonly called a J-pouch or W-pouch), using folds of ileum pulled into the rectal canal and anastomosed to the rectum. The pouch develops a flora and serves, to some degree, as a colonic/rectal reservoir. Another form is the continent ileostomy or Kock pouch in which folds of ileum are used to create an internal reservoir, which is drained with a catheter several times per day [1, 2]. No appliance is worn. The traditional colectomy involves the creation of an ileostomy and the use of an external stool collection appliance. Patient problems or concerns associated with the ileostomy may include stomal irritation, irritation of the skin surrounding the ostomy, leakage or dislodgment of the ostomy bag, odors, and social stigmata associated with the use of an external appliance. Most patients appear to do well with the ostomy and feel, in general, that being disease-free outweighs the inconvenience of an ostomy [72].

With Crohn's disease, surgical resection of severely involved segments of small or large bowel does not, unfortunately, bring resolution of the disease. Endoscopic evidence of disease recurrence is seen in half or more of patients within a year after surgery. Duration of clinical remission varies greatly. In some patients, relapse may occur in month, and in other patients, apparent remission may last for years. Seventy to 90% of patients with Crohn's disease eventually have at least one surgery during their lifetime. Strictureplasty has been used in relatively uncomplicated cases of Crohn's disease to relieve narrowed segments of bowel [70]. In some cases, patients with prolonged severe courses of Crohn's disease have multiple resections resulting in short bowel syndrome and the attendant nutritional and medical consequences.

3. NUTRITIONAL TREATMENT

Nutrition and dietary patterns may play several roles in the management of inflammatory bowel disease. Nutritional rehabilitation may be required after acute or prolonged reduction in the quantity or quality of dietary intake. Dietary modifications may be required to increase the tolerance of foods during exacerbation of the active disease. Changes in nutritional practices may be needed to be able to provide

TABLE 8 Potential Roles of Nutrition in Inflammatory Bowel Disease

Restore nutrition status after prolonged or acute illness; prevent malnutrition lifelong

Provide nutrients and fuels for enterocytes, colonocytes

Provide fuel for and alter gastrointestinal flora

Reduce gastrointestinal symptoms during acute stages or prevent complications

Modify the immune and inflammatory response

Induce and maintain remission

Help patient understand roles of diet/foods and digestive and absorptive functions; sort out food associations and intolerances

adequate nourishment with complications such as short bowel syndrome, strictures, or fistulas. Refeeding protocols may be appropriate after severe malnutrition, after severe bouts of the disease, or after surgical procedures. Nutrition may also have some role in the regulation of the inflammatory response and inducing or maintaining remission. Restoration of nutrition status may include a carefully selected oral diet, vitamin and mineral supplements, or special enteral and/or parenteral nutrition. See Table 8 for a summary of factors impacting nutrition.

As a result of extensive resections and severe stages of the disease, malabsorption of macro- and micronutrients could occur. Medications may also limit appetite, produce gastrointestinal-related symptoms, and result in decreased intake, decreased absorption, and/or increased requirement for nutrients.

G. Nutrition Assessment in Inflammatory Bowel Disease

A comprehensive assessment is required when evaluating nutrition risk and considering nutritional interventions in inflammatory bowel disease. Nutrition assessment for the person with inflammatory bowel disease would likely include (1) consideration of several elements of the patient's medical and surgical history (e.g., duration and severity of the disease, presence of strictures, fistulas, resections, ostomies); (2) presence of nutrition-related symptoms, such as diarrhea (e.g., stool volume, frequency) or malabsorption (increased fecal fat, abdominal cramping, bloating, or distension); (3) physical measures such as growth rate for age, body mass index, weight changes; (4) a diet history that includes habitual food intake, quantity and quality of the diet, intolerance and aversions to various foods, perceived and documented food allergies; (5) use of herbal and nutritional supplements, alternative therapies, prescription and over-the-counter medications; and (6) pertinent laboratory data that reflect protein energy and micronutrient status. The nutrition assessment should also include an evaluation of the patient's

understanding of his or her nutrition status, needs, problems, and therapeutic options.

Energy requirements of persons with inflammatory bowel disease are not usually increased except with sepsis and fever, but protein requirements are increased. Energy requirements may be increased to restore weight, to return to normal growth curves, or to compensate for malabsorption. The presence of active disease by itself, however, does not appear to raise energy requirements appreciably [54, 55]. Protein needs may be increased more significantly due to gastrointestinal nitrogen losses, the inflammatory response, and the need for new tissue for weight gain and growth.

H. Modification of Specific Dietary Factors in Management

Patients may be taught to help themselves manage nutrition-related symptoms such as abdominal bloating, gas and diarrhea, strictures, malabsorption, and nutritional deficiencies. Current evidence suggests that dietary practices might also alter the severity of the disease, increase the effectiveness medications, or prolong remission.

1. LIPIDS

The amount and nature of the fatty acids consumed in the diets may play a role in the management of several inflammatory diseases, including inflammatory bowel. The ratio of n-6 polyunsaturated fatty acids consumed to n-3 unsaturated fatty acid in the Western diet greatly favors n-6 fatty acids. Estimates of the ratio of n-6 to n-3 fatty acids consumed in various parts of the world range from approximately 9:1 [73] to 30:1 [74]. Consumption of oils such as corn, cottonseed, safflower, and sunflower were originally encouraged for their cholesterol-lowering effect and as a source of linoleic acid, an n-6 essential fatty acid. Most vegetable oils are rich in n-6 fatty acid and low in n-3. In the last two or three decades, consumption of polyunsaturated n-6 fatty acids largely replaced a significant portion of saturated fats that had been habitually consumed. Consumption of marine and terrestrial sources of preformed and precursor n-3 fatty acids is now receiving more attention because of their potential to impact several forms of inflammatory and chronic disease. Recently the ratio of fatty acid consumption has begun to shift slightly more toward n-3 fatty acids primarily as a result of increased consumption of soy and canola oils [73]. When dietary lipids are ingested, the fatty acids serve not only as a fuel but also become components of the phospholipids in virtually every cell membrane in the body. The nature of the fatty acids in the cell membranes affects the physical, chemical, and functional properties of the cell and cell wall. Lipids also serve as precursors for potent mediators in many physiologic reactions, including the immune and inflammatory response.

Consumption of a diet that contains predominantly n-6 fatty acids, for example, results in adipose lipid and cell membrane phospholipids that are high in n-6 fatty acyl groups. When macrophages, neutrophils, lymphocytes, and other cells are activated, they release membrane lipids that are precursors of potent regulators of the inflammatory response. Their release and synthesis can affect recruitment and proliferation of other leukocytes and fibroblasts, alter the permeability of tissues, increase adherence of leukocytes and platelets, increase the generation of harmful oxygen metabolites, and increase the synthesis of proinflammatory eicosanoids. Eicosanoids produced from the metabolism of polyunsaturated fatty acids of the n-6 family (linoleic acid) tend to be proinflammatory and aggregatory, whereas those from n-3 fatty acids in general tend to be anti-inflammatory and decrease cellular adherence. In animal and human studies, supplemental feeding of n-3 fatty acids in the form of linolenic acid and preformed eicosapentaenoic and docosahexaenoic acids has been shown to reduce the synthesis and levels of proinflammatory cytokines, such as TNF-α and IL-1, and reduce the generation of potent leukotrienes and prostaglandins, which enhance leukocyte chemotaxis and membrane permeability [74–76]. In clinical trials the value of n-3 fatty acids in the management of inflammatory bowel disease has been considered promising but more as a complementary approach rather than single independent treatment [77].

In general, n-3 fatty acid content of the diet may be especially low in some patients with inflammatory bowel disease. The n-3 fatty acids appear to be reasonably safe in the amounts required to alter membrane eicosanoids and may have value in either sparing other therapies or independently tempering the inflammatory process and its consequences.

Gamma-linolenic acid (C18-3 n-6) and dihomo-gamma-linolenic acid, the elongase catalyzed product of gamma-linolenic acid, have also been shown to alter membrane lipids in inflammatory cells [78, 79]. These n-6 fatty acids have been evaluated in animals and in humans in the attenuation of inflammatory and proliferative disorders, but not to the same extent as n-3 fatty acids. Initial reports have shown reduced levels of proinflammatory cytokines, and later leukotriene synthesis and modulated autoimmune activity. Sources of the fatty acids include borage oil and evening primrose oil. Conjugated linoleic acids are a group of isomers of linoleic acid found in bovine lipids and in other ruminant animals that have been shown to have antiproliferative properties against several cancer cell lines [80]. The lipids also tend to reduce cell adhesion, decrease platelet aggregation, and alter several chemical mediators in the immune and inflammatory processes [81]. Their role in inflammatory bowel disease, however, has not been evaluated.

Medium-chain triglycerides may have little to do with the inflammatory process, but they may be valuable as an energy source in patients with lipid malabsorption. Absorption of long-chain fatty acids may be compromised during prolonged intestinal disease because of bile salt malabsorption that accompanies ileal resection. Medium-chain triglycerides are known to enter the portal route without the more exten-

sive processing that long-chain fats undergo, but preliminary studies suggest that medium-chain triglycerides may also serve as an energy substrate for colonocytes in the same manner as short-chain fatty acids [82].

2. DIETARY FIBER, RESISTANT STARCHES, AND SHORT-CHAIN FATTY ACIDS

Consumption of dietary fiber and carbohydrates that are incompletely digested or absorbed have the potential to alter colonic flora and affect several gastrointestinal functions. The malabsorbed polysaccharides and sugars serve as substrates for microbes in the colon and the endproducts of microbial fermentation can, in turn, serve as a primary fuel for cells lining the colon and modify their metabolic activity. Inulin, fructose oligosaccharides, pectin, banana, oat and soy fiber, and several resistant carbohydrates contain indigestible carbohydrates that have been shown to alter microbial populations in the colon [83–85]. Several have been shown to increase, at least transiently, bifidobacteria and lactobacillus members that are viewed as healthful microbes. Various saccharides have also been shown to reduce the growth of potentially pathogenic microbial populations such as *Clostridium difficile* [83–87].

The endproducts of fiber and carbohydrate fermentation in the colon are short-chain fatty acids and gases. Short-chain fatty acids and, in particular, butyrate serve as a primary and preferred fuel for colonocytes and appear to be semi-essential for their normal function. In several animal and human studies, addition of various fermentable saccharides or short-chain fatty acids has been reported to increase colonic blood flow, maintain normal mucosal barrier function, enhance fluid and electrolyte absorption (at least at physiologic doses), prevent antibiotic-associated diarrhea, provide protection from toxins, reduce the potential for inflammatory activity, and maintain normal proliferation and differentiation of colonocytes [83–87]. In several trials, addition of dietary fiber sources or topical administration of short-chain fatty acids has been shown to have some value in treating mild forms of ulcerative colitis or in maintaining remission—either as single agents or when used in combination with more traditional therapies. The effect is modest, but further work with the sources of fermentable saccharides and combinations of short-chain fatty acids may bring more effective therapies [88, 89]. Most of the work with dietary fiber has appropriately been focused toward ulcerative colitis, but use of fiber sources has been considered in the management of Crohn's disease.

Dietary fiber intake is relatively low in the U.S. diet, and patients with inflammatory bowel disease may consume even less. Fear of obstruction, increased gas, or concern about coarseness of fibrous foods may result in very low intakes, making the patient more susceptible to the reported effects of insufficient colonic substrate. Use of dietary fiber sources, even if in powdered or blenderized form, may be helpful in the diets of persons with inflammatory bowel dis-

ease and especially in ulcerative colitis. Because some fibrous foods are not greatly changed until they reach the colon, caution is advised in patients with strictures. Boluses of powdered sources have been shown to cause obstruction in the upper gastrointestinal tract. Thus the best approach is to use whole foods as the fiber source. Fruits, vegetables, and whole grains are excellent sources of fiber, vitamins, minerals, trace elements, and numerous potentially protective phytochemicals that may favorably affect the health of the gastrointestinal tract and the individual.

3. DIETARY SUGARS

High sugar intake and consumption of refined foods, at least in some countries, has been linked to the preillness diet or rise in the incidence of inflammatory bowel disease [42–44]. No causal association, however, has been demonstrated [3, 45]. On the other hand, consumption of large amounts of sugars could displace foods that provide other nutrients. Certain sugars (e.g., lactose, fructose, alcohol sugars) are not as well absorbed as other carbohydrates and may contribute to symptoms such as bloating, gas, and diarrhea. Malabsorption and fermentation of relatively modest amounts of small molecular weight sugars can result in osmotic diarrhea [90–92].

4. VITAMINS, MINERALS, AND ANTIOXIDANT NUTRIENTS

Micronutrient and antioxidant status may be compromised in patients with inflammatory bowel disease, by a combination of an incomplete diet, malabsorption, and the inflammatory process. When in remission, persons with inflammatory bowel disease can consume a good diet as a source of essential micronutrients, antioxidants, and protective phytochemicals not found in nutrient supplements. If, however, the patient is unable or unwilling to consume a complete diet, then certainly vitamin-mineral supplements and/or liquid nutrition supplements may be appropriate. Numerous oral supplements are available with different lipid mixtures, protein sources, fiber, and other additives to meet patient needs. Some patients will have selective nutritional problems, such as vitamin B_{12} malabsorption due to ileal resection or calcium and vitamin D inadequacy due to avoidance of lactose. (Refer to Chapter 16 on enteral and parenteral nutrition.)

I. Parenteral and Enteral Nutrition Support

Although the cause of inflammatory bowel disease is unknown, current information suggests that inflammatory bowel disease occurs when genetic aberrations and environmental triggers interact. The primary environmental factors to which the gastrointestinal tract is exposed are foods and microbes. Both dietary factors and elements of the gastrointestinal flora have been scrutinized, but no specific etiologic agent(s) have been identified as yet. Regular diets, however, are a potential source of antigens, contain elements that may

serve as inflammatory or suppressive agents, and provide a major source of fuels for both cells lining the gastrointestinal tract and microbes residing in the gastrointestinal tract.

1. DOES NUTRITION SUPPORT INDUCE REMISSION?

The extent to which nutritional measures can induce and maintain remission remains an interesting and unresolved issue. Parenteral nutrition was initially considered an appropriate approach because one could restore the individual's nutritional status and provide sufficient energy for growth and weight gain. Use of parenteral nutrition and withdrawal of oral nutrition was seen as "bowel rest" and provided an opportunity to reduce both the antigenic load from food and reduce microbial populations. Use of parenteral nutrition has not, however, been as successful as hoped as a primary therapy in treating Crohn's disease and has been even less effective in treating ulcerative colitis [2, 94]. Although a small percentage of patients may benefit with a reasonable length of remission, short-term remission is the more common outcome. Withholding enteral nutrition may also be considered undesirable because it may compromise gut integrity.

Although not entirely nutritionally complete, parenteral nutrition has served as a valuable tool for providing nutritional support for patients with gastrointestinal obstruction, perforation, and toxic megacolon, and it can provide a primary source of nutrition in patients with malabsorption after major small bowel resection. Parenteral nutrition does not obviously contain the phytonutrients and wide range of lipids and microelements found in a normal diet. Additional study with other supportive additives such as specific amino acids, lipids, and selected micronutrients may in the future provide more effective parenteral solutions.

The effectiveness of various forms of enteral feedings as a primary treatment for inflammatory bowel disease has been evaluated in several reviews and meta-analyses [94–103]. In almost all the reviews, Crohn's disease appeared to be more amenable to enteral feeding treatment than ulcerative colitis, although in a few individual studies, such interventions were reported to have some value in managing ulcerative colitis. In ulcerative colitis, therapeutic trials with fermentable fibers, short-chain and medium-chain fatty acids, and n-3 fatty acids may ultimately achieve success more than the use of standard parenteral and enteral formulas [88, 89]. With few exceptions, enteral nutrition appears to be more effective than parenteral nutrition, but whether enteral nutrition as a sole therapy is as effective as or better than medications is less clear.

In many of the reports, corticosteroids and other medical treatments were considered clear-cut choices and enteral nutrition seen as supportive care. In other reports, enteral diets were said to be the preferred route and were considered to be at least as effective as medications. For example, Messori et al. [95] performed a meta-analysis of the effectiveness of chemically defined diets versus corticosteroids from seven randomized clinical trials. The authors concluded that steroids were significantly more effective than diet in inducing

remission in active Crohn's disease. The authors also separated patients who failed to complete the enteral trial because they did not tolerate the formula and concluded that steroids were still superior.

In another meta-analysis, Schwab al al. [96] reviewed 18 studies, which included 295 patients treated with elemental diets, 214 with oligopeptide diets, and 62 with polymeric diets. When the data were adjusted for patients who completed the course of enteral diet treatment, 73, 70, and 67%, respectively, of the patients achieved remission with the three types of diets. The authors considered the rates of remission with diet to be comparable to rates achieved with corticosteroids. Heuschkel and Walker-Smith [97] reviewed several enteral diet studies and their own experiences with use of enteral nutrition in children. These authors concluded that the studies reviewed suggested that enteral nutrition may promote healing of the intestinal mucosa better than corticosteroids, but admitted that 40–60% of children will still become symptomatic within a year of treatment.

Examination of similarities and differences in the design of the dozens of individual studies in which enteral diet or medications were considered more efficacious does not entirely clarify the situation. Numerous criteria were used to describe the severity of the patient's disease both when the therapy started and when remission was achieved. Initial disease activity ranged from mild to severe. Severity of disease and/or resolution of disease have been measured using clinical measures such as diarrhea, weight change, and ratings of well-being. In other studies, more objective indicators, such as endoscopic and histologic evidence, levels of inflammatory mediators, or measures of gastrointestinal structure/permeability, were used. Duration of the patient's disease prior to initiating enteral nutrition nutrition or medical therapy may or may not have been reported. In some of the study designs, diet therapy may have been evaluated with and without various medications to determine whether diet improved the overall management, and dose and route of administration of medications varied greatly. Duration of treatment with enteral therapy ranged from 2 to 8 weeks or longer and the diet may have been fed orally, by tube, or by combinations of routes. Indeed, one of the problems identified by even the proponents of nutritional therapy was that some of the diets were unpalatable or it was difficult for some patients to take the majority of their diet in the form of an enteral formula. Improved nutritional status was considered one of the measures of success in many of the studies but nutritional status may not have been well described or was described in a variety of ways. Severity of disease, degree of control required, and type of health care system employed in the various countries may have influenced the need for and duration of hospitalization.

In earlier studies, "elemental" or chemically defined type diets were preferred because they tended to be low in fat and the nitrogen was in the form of amino acids and small peptides. More recently, use of "polymeric" and whole-protein nitrogen sources and even regular foods have claimed to be

as effective as elemental diets in allowing remission of Crohn's disease. In addition to differences in the approaches to comparisons with diet and medications, it should be noted that the natural course of inflammatory bowel disease includes unexplained exacerbations and remission. In the history of therapeutic interventions with medications, 30–60% of patients may improve with placebo alone [3, 94].

2. How Might Diets Work as Therapy?

Selected enteral feedings could play several roles in the management of the disease. Patients with inflammatory bowel disease are often malnourished and have inadequate intake of protein, energy, and micronutrients. This malnutrition may create changes in gastrointestinal barrier functions and digestive functions and alter immune mechanisms. Individual dietary components may act as antioxidants, serve as precursors to inflammatory mediators, and alter the relative types of microbes existing in the gastrointestinal tract. Dietary excesses may also bring about undue symptoms even though they may have nothing to do with the pathology of the disease. Many of the formulations used in past studies did not include many of the newer individual nutrient additives or modifications, yet many appeared to achieve some level of success in treatment of inflammatory bowel disease or at least tolerance. Continued trials, for example, with lipids, amino acids, short-chain fatty acids and fiber sources, antioxidant nutrients, and phytochemicals, may make enteral diets more effective in managing inflammatory bowel disease.

Whether or not nutrition support is effective as a primary therapy, both parenteral and enteral feedings are valuable in restoring nutritional reserves and allowing growth and maturation in children. Enteral nutrition would appear to be an appropriate first choice of nutrition therapy. Appropriate selection and use of enteral nutrition has the potential to provide enterocytes and colonocytes with a direct source of preferred fuels, and allow normal proliferation and differentiation of those cells, increase gut barrier functions, and suppress the proliferation of unhealthy microbes. If diet does serve as a source of antigens, inflammatory stimulants, or toxins, enteral formulas may be designed specifically to reduce the offending agents yet provide reasonable nutrition support. Sufficient success with nutrition as a sole therapy alone and in combination with other treatments warrants additional study in inducing and maintaining remission in both Crohn's disease and ulcerative colitis.

III. SHORT BOWEL SYNDROME

A. Definition

Short bowel syndrome refers to the set of symptoms and complications that occurs after significant small bowel resection. Resection of the colon or stomach does not constitute or result in short bowel syndrome, but loss of either can compromise the patient who has had a small intestinal resection. The syndrome and its consequences are primarily related to the inability to absorb digested foods and to reabsorb endogenous secretions. Malabsorption of macronutrients, micronutrients, fluids, and electrolytes occurs but the severity varies considerably. Weight loss, growth retardation, diarrhea, dehydration, electrolyte disturbances, bone loss, renal oxalate stones, gallstones, lactic acidosis, and bacterial overgrowth may occur depending on the extent and nature of the resection [104, 105]. The syndrome may be permanent, as is the case with severe shortening of the gastrointestinal tract, or temporary with less drastic resections. The symptoms will appear immediately after the resection and continue unless sufficient adaptation occurs and/or medical, nutritional, or surgical interventions are successful. Typically, maximal adaptation of the remaining intestine takes months or years to occur.

B. Causes

In adults, Crohn's disease is the principal cause of short bowel syndrome, accounting for about 60–70% of the cases. Mesenteric infarct, radiation enteritis, and volvulus are less common etiologies. In infants and children, atresia, volvulus, gastroschisis, and necrotizing enterocolitis are more common reasons for significant resections leading to short bowel syndrome [104]. The incidence and prevalence are not known but the number of persons supported on total or supplemental parenteral nutrition number in the tens of thousands.

C. Predictors of the Severity and Duration of the Syndrome

The severity and duration of symptoms, the patient's need for nutrition support, and the survival of the patient all depend on the length and function of the remaining gastrointestinal tract and the health of the host. Patients who survive without parenteral nutrition tend to adapt more completely, have fewer adverse symptoms, and are at decreased nutritional risk. They tend to be patients who are very young, have remaining distal ileum and ileocecal valve, have retained colon, and are otherwise healthy and well nourished. Alternatively, predictors of poor survival include dependence on parenteral nutrition support, increased nutrition risk, more complications, and compromised quality of life. These patients tend to have loss of terminal ileum and ileocecal valve, advanced age at resection, loss of the colon in addition to small bowel, and presence of residual gastrointestinal disease [104–109].

D. Variants of Short Bowel Syndrome

Requirements for nutritional, medical, and surgical care of the patient after bowel resections can be predicted somewhat by the normal physiologic role and capacity of segments

TABLE 9   Predictors of Severity of
Nutrition Risk in
Short Bowel Syndrome

Loss of distal ileum
Loss of ileocecal valve
Loss of colon in addition to small bowel
Advanced age
Residual disease
Mesenteric infarct as cause for bowel resection

removed and remaining. See Table 9 for predictors of severity of short bowel syndrome and nutrition risk. Figure 5 illustrates normal events in gastrointestinal secretion, digestion, absorption, and fermentation processes for comparison with changes following bowel resections.

1. JEJUNAL RESECTIONS

Despite the fact that most gastrointestinal fluids are secreted into the proximal small intestine and the jejunum is normally the site of intense digestive activity, loss of the entire jejunum in infants or adults typically results in only transient and relatively mild malabsorption as long as the patient and the remaining gastrointestinal tract are healthy (see Fig. 6 for depiction of jejunal resection). Initially, the patient will require parenteral nutrition support but will be able to begin consuming small, frequent, simple meals as soon as bowel motility returns. Adaptation of the remaining intestine will likely to occur during the next several months. The patient will likely be able to consume regular foods with only limited restrictions and minimal compromise in digestive and absorptive capacity. The remaining gastrointestinal tract has sufficient reserve to compensate for the decreased surface area. Because lactase enzyme is produced primarily in the cells of the proximal small intestine, jejunal resection typically results in lactose malabsorption. The patient may also have slightly more rapid overall transit through the gastrointestinal tract and may not tolerate consumption of large quantities of hyperosmolar or highly concentrated foods and beverages. Net protein and energy intake, and fluid and electrolyte utilization, are not seriously threatened. The efficiency of absorption of certain nutrients such as iron, calcium, magnesium, and some lipid-soluble nutrients may be slightly compromised.

2. ILEAL RESECTIONS

Major resections of the ileum create several problems in maintaining nutrition [104, 110–113] (see Fig. 7 for depiction of ileal resection). A summary of the consequences of ileal resection can be found in Table 10. Normally, adults consume about 2 liters of fluid per day and the proximal gastrointestinal tract secretes approximately 7–9 liters of fluid per day into the intestinal tract. A significant amount of

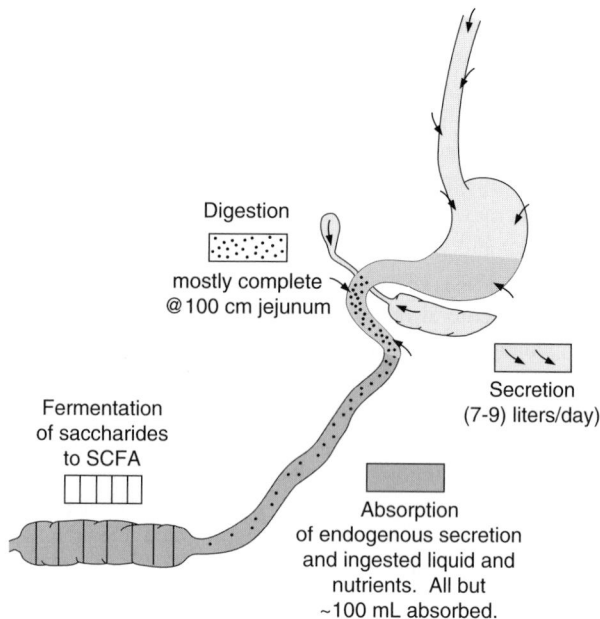

FIGURE 5   Normal gastrointestinal tract.

fluid is normally absorbed in the distal small intestine and normally only 1–1.5 liters of liquid chyme per day enters the colon. Only about 100 mL of water is lost in the feces daily. When ileal resections occur, the remaining small and large intestine must absorb the residual fluid. If colon is resected

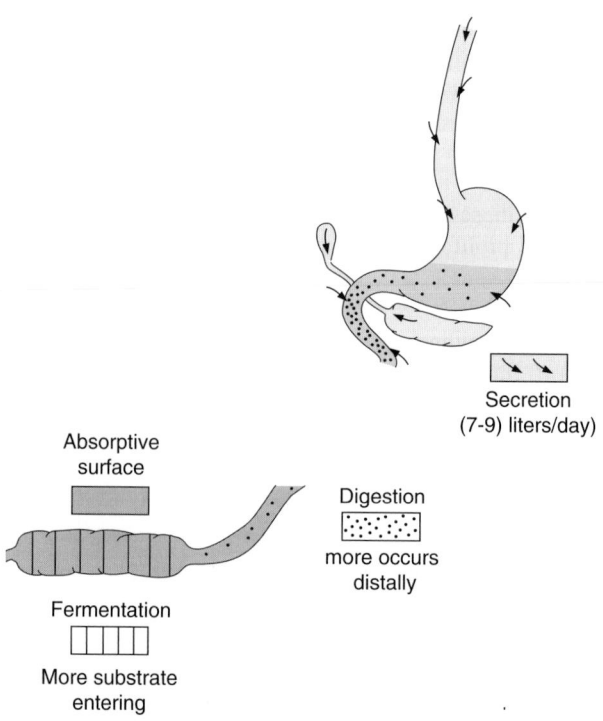

FIGURE 6   Jejunal resection.

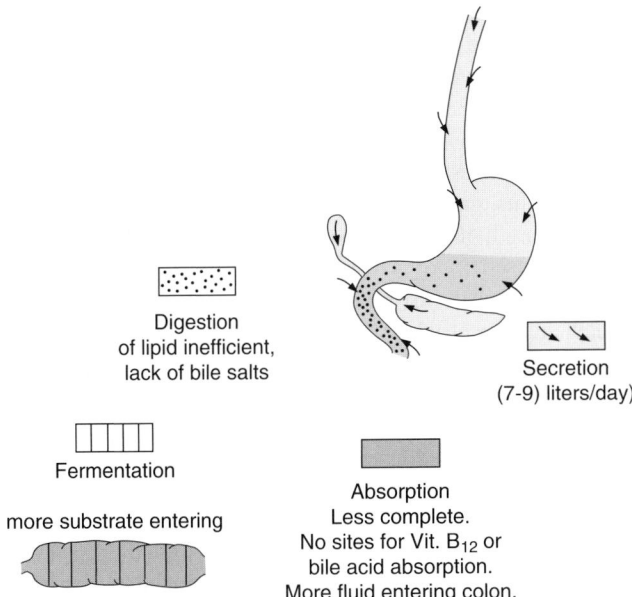

FIGURE 7 Ileal resection.

TABLE 10 Consequences of Ileal Resection, Especially with Loss of Ileocecal Valve

Increased fluid loss

Shorter transit

Bile acid malabsorption; insufficient *de novo* bile salt synthesis

Fat, fatty acid malabsorption

Malabsorption of fat-soluble nutrients

Decreased calcium, zinc, magnesium absorption

If colon remains:
—Increased colonic oxalate absorption
—Increased secretion from malabsorbed bile acids and fatty acids
—Increased risk of small bowel overgrowth

in addition to the ileum, maintaining adequate hydration and electrolyte status is difficult.

The last meter of ileum is also the primary site for the absorption of vitamin B_{12} intrinsic factor complex and is the only site for reabsorption of bile acids entering the intestine from the biliary tract. Healthy adults usually have sufficient stores of vitamin B_{12} to last for 3 years or so and after ileal resection receive periodic injections of vitamin B_{12}. More importantly, loss of the distal ileal segment, where 90% or more of bile salts are reabsorbed, results in a significant malabsorption cascade. The role of bile salts is to provide surfactant action to help reduce the particle size of lipid droplets and to participate in the formation of micelles. Micelles are the polar particles in which free fatty acids, monoglycerides, and fat-soluble vitamins are absorbed into cells of the small intestine. When bile salts are no longer "recycled" in the distal ileum, *de novo* synthesis in the liver from the sterol pool cannot supply sufficient bile salts for adequate absorption of lipids and lipid-soluble nutrients. In addition, unabsorbed bile acids entering the colon are considered "irritants" and serve as secretagogues at a time when colon is already burdened with the task of absorbing extraordinary amounts of fluid. Increased amounts of unabsorbed fatty acids in the lumen of the bowel can result in the formation of fatty acid soaps with calcium, magnesium, and zinc, which interfere with the absorption of these minerals. The malabsorbed fatty acids may also serve as secretagogues in the colon.

Dietary oxalate normally binds with calcium and other divalent cations to form insoluble complexes, but free oxalate becomes more available for absorption in the colon. In both ileal resections and long-term Crohn's disease involv-

ing the ileum, hyperoxaluria and renal stone formation are not uncommon. In an attempt to bind bile acids, improve colonic fluid and electrolyte absorption, and reduce absorption of oxalate colestyramine, supplemental calcium, and modest dietary oxalate restriction are often prescribed [104, 110].

Another potential complication of distal ileal resections, especially involving loss of the ileocecal valve, is bacterial overgrowth in the small intestine. The small intestine is normally relatively sterile, but with loss of the one-way barrier provided by the ileocecal valve, microbes from the colon may more readily mix with small bowel contents. Bacterial overgrowth is usually treated with antibiotics but more recently use of small bowel irrigation, probiotics, and prebiotic foods have been tried with some success [114].

3. LOSS OF ILEUM AND COLON

If both the ileum and colon are resected (see Fig. 8), maintenance of adequate hydration and energy balance becomes more difficult. Although only 1–1.5 liters of fluid normally enters the colon, a healthy colon is capable of

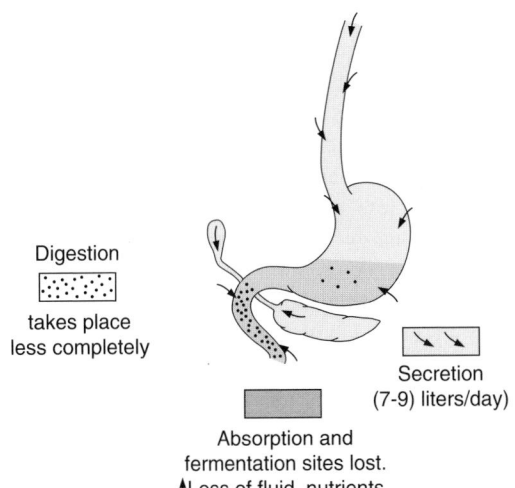

FIGURE 8 Resection of both ileum and colon.

absorbing 3–4 liters. With only a jejunum, patients have difficulty absorbing ingested fluid and endogenous gastrointestinal secretions. Fecal outputs from jejunostomies may exceed 3–5 liters daily and patients may lose 100–200 mEq sodium in the effluent. In addition to increased risk of hypovolemia, patients are also more at risk for hypokalemia and hypomagnesemia and other forms of nutrient depletion [104, 110, 112].

The presence of foodstuffs or partially digested foods in the distal intestine normally stimulates the release of neuroendocrine secretions, including glucagon-like peptide-1 (GLP-1) [115], peptide tyrosine tyrosine (peptide YY), or neuropeptide-Y [116], which may downregulate the secretory and motor activity of the stomach and proximal small intestine. Short-chain fatty acids produced in the colon from fermentation of carbohydrate and fiber may also slow gastric emptying [117]. The net effect of the ileal or ileocolonic "brake" in the normal, intact gastrointestinal tract is to retard gastric emptying, reduce secretions from the proximal gastrointestinal tract, and decrease motility. The mechanism is not completely understood and current hypotheses are likely oversimplified. However, the colonic brake mechanisms are reasonable explanations for the normal regulation of the volume of food released and propagated through the gastrointestinal tract and for the observed clinical maladjustment in short bowel syndrome. Regardless of the exact mechanism, the loss of distal ileum and colon appears to result in the loss of the ileocolonic brake phenomenon that slows entry of food and secretions into the intestine.

The colon also serves to salvage energy from malabsorbed substrates. In humans, the role of the colon in extracting energy from foodstuffs is normally relatively minor. In short bowel syndrome, however, more carbohydrate, lipids, and nitrogenous compounds enter the colon than usual. The amount of energy the colon can extract after small bowel resections from malabsorbed substrates varies with the length of small intestine remaining. In normal individuals consuming a typical diet, only about 5–10% of energy is salvaged by colonic fermentation and absorption [110]. Nordgaard and colleagues [118] demonstrated using bomb calorimetry the fecal energy losses that occur with and without the colon. Patients who had 150–200 cm of small intestine without a colon excreted only 0.8 MJ/day (110 kcal) more than those with an intact colon. But when patients had only 100 cm or less small bowel remaining, preservation of the colon for energy salvage from malabsorbed substrates became much more important. Colectomy resulted in an extra loss of 4.9 MJ/day (about 1150 kcal).

Colonocytes cannot absorb long-chain fatty acids to any significant degree, but short-chain fatty acids produced from microbial fermentation of fiber, carbohydrate, and, to a lesser extent, amino acids can be used by the colonocytes and the host. Recently, investigators have shown that medium-chain fatty acids can also be used by colonocytes and absorbed systemically [119, 120]. Loss of the colon and ileum not only results in loss of the energy salvage mechanism, but also decreased fluid and electrolyte absorption, more rapid transit, and overall decreased efficiency of absorption of foodstuffs.

4. MAJOR INTESTINAL RESECTIONS

Volvulus, gastroschisis, or atresias often result in a small bowel length of only a 100 cm or less. The same risk factors for increased morbidity apply in infants including loss of ileum, ileocecal valve, and colon, except infants appear to adapt significantly better after resections than adults. In normal healthy infants and children, intestinal growth occurs from preterm until early adulthood. Weaver and associates [121] studied 1010 necropsy specimens from preterm fetuses and subjects up to 20 years of age. Small bowel length more than doubled from 20 to 40 weeks' gestation and almost doubled again from term (275 cm) to age 10 years (500 cm). From 10 to 20 years intestinal length increased only an additional 75 cm. The extent to which lengthening and other forms of adaptation occur after resection (beyond normal growth) is not clear, but infants appear to function reasonably well with very short intestinal remnants. In infants, survival without parenteral nutrition has been reported with as little as approximately 20–60 cm of small bowel if the children have retained ileocecal valve and as little as 30–100 cm without the ileocecal valve [105–109]. If the ileocecal valve is lost, retained colon becomes more important for maintenance of electrolyte balance and adequate hydration, and to salvage malabsorbed substrates [109, 110, 118]. Adults typically require at least 100–200 cm of small intestine to avoid at least partial dependence on parenteral nutrition and adaptation may be more prolonged and less complete [104, 112–113, 122]. For children with extremely short small bowel lengths who cannot adapt, several options remain. They can remain on parenteral nutrition, undergo small bowel lengthening procedures, or undergo small bowel transplantation. Parenteral nutrition imposes on the quality of life for the patient and caretakers and carries increased risk of infection, hepatic failure, gallstone formation, and nutrient deficiencies [123, 124].

The ability to tolerate major bowel resections in adults is considerably less than in children. If the patient has residual disease and has had other changes in gastrointestinal pathology due to radiation enteritis, atherosclerosis, diabetes, or inflammatory bowel disease, then bowel resections pose greater risk. In patients with radiation enteritis, even relatively small resections of the ileum, especially if the resection includes the ileocecal valve, can create short bowel syndrome.

Patients who suffer mesenteric infarct may lose almost the entire small intestine and most of the colon. Because mesenteric infarct typically occurs in older patients as a result of arteriosclerotic vascular disease, adaptation of the remaining segment may not be sufficient. The patient may require lifelong support with at least supplemental parenteral

nutrition. Persons with massive resections and their caretakers will need to be patient and cautious with oral and enteral feedings. Maximal adaptation may require up to 2 years. Reintroduction and advancement of foods should be gradual. Unfortunately, some patients may never be able to absorb sufficient amounts of nutrients by way of the gastrointestinal tract. Overeating or overfeeding, especially with hypertonic and large volumes of foods, may result in net loss of endogenous fluid and electrolyte [110, 125].

E. Principles of Nutrition Care and Feeding in Short Bowel Syndrome

One of the primary principles of managing patients with short bowel syndrome is to start using the gut as soon as possible. Foods and the gastrointestinal secretions are trophic to the small bowel and malnutrition compromises the adaptive process [126–128]. In laboratory animal studies, the gastrointestinal tract has been shown to atrophy markedly during starvation and parenteral nutrition. In humans, the degree of gut atrophy during parenteral nutrition may not be as striking as in animal models, but it appears to occur. Biasco et al. [129] described the gastrointestinal response in a patient fed by parenteral and oral nutrition after a subtotal resection for mesenteric obstruction. The patient had 30 cm of proximal jejunum anastomosed to his descending colon. The patient was fed exclusively by parenteral nutrition for 30 days, and then oral nutrition was gradually introduced during the next 30 days. Jejunal biopsies were taken during parenteral and oral periods and examined for cell kinetic studies. Hypoplasia was demonstrated soon after parenteral nutrition was initiated and remained until oral nutrition was started. Hyperplasia occurred soon after oral feeding, and after 14 days crypt depth and villous height had increased by approximately 50%.

A significant portion of the energy supplied to the small intestine comes from sugars, keto acids, and amino acids (notably glutamine) from the lumen of the gastrointestinal tract. An even greater percent of the energy for colonocytes come from substrates in the lumen, in this case primarily short-chain fatty acids produced in fermentation of saccharides. Enteral nutrition then provides fuels for both the intestine and the host.

In short bowel syndrome, the desired and observed response to feeding after major bowel resection is vigorous hyperplasia, hypertrophy, and increased length and diameter of the remaining small bowel. If oral or enteral feeding is not provided, atrophy occurs. Even small amounts of foodstuffs provide sufficient stimulus for intestinal growth. Initial feedings after bowel resections may include small frequent meals, sips of liquid supplements, or dilute enteral feedings to gradually restore gastrointestinal function and stimulate adaptation.

Adaptation in the gastrointestinal tract is not as complete as that seen in other organ systems, and when adaptation is maximal, the patient may still have inadequate absorptive function. The extent to which adaptation takes place depends on the age of the individual, the health and vascular patency of the remaining intestine, and nutritional factors. Relatively few studies have been reported in which changes in intestinal length and diameter of the bowel following intestinal resection have been measured. Shin et al. [130] studied the adaptive response in dogs with massive resections after receiving nutrition support in the sequence normally recommended for human patients. Seven mongrel dogs had surgical resections, leaving 20 cm of proximal jejunum anastomosed to the mid-transverse colon. The dogs were initially fed by parenteral nutrition and, after 4 days, oral food and water were reintroduced. Parenteral nutrition was continued in addition to the oral diet for 30 days and was then stopped. Parenteral nutrition proved to be essential initially because oral feeding induced massive stool outputs. Six weeks after the resection, the five dogs that survived were reexplored and the remaining small bowel was examined. The length and circumference of the jejunum increased by 30%, and the crypt depth, number of villi and the width of the villi, had each increased by approximately 20%. Stool volume and frequency gradually decreased but were still abnormal.

Solhaug [131] studied five female patients who had undergone jejuno-ileal bypass procedures for treatment of obesity. Patients had end-to-end anastomosis of their proximal jejunum to their distal ileum and had undergone a second operation because of complications or unsuccessful weight loss. The remaining segments of small intestine increased during a 1- to 2-year period from a mean of 52 to 82 cm while the subjects consumed an ad libitum diet. The bypassed segments essentially remained unchanged. Mucosal thickness was approximately 20–40% greater than the bypassed segment, villous height was 25–50% greater and small intestinal circumference was double that of the bypassed segment.

When starting feedings in patients with short bowel, the diet is normally provided in very small meals or in sips of dilute formula diets [110, 113, 132]. During the advancement of feeding, the patient is normally supported at least in part by parenteral feeding so that oral feeding proceeds gradually to allow the gut to adapt and to prevent diarrhea and malabsorption. If the patient is unable or unwilling to eat consistently in a controlled or scheduled manner, enteral feedings can be provided in frequent mini meals or delivered by tube feeding. Tube feedings can be scheduled at night or between meals as needed, then decreased as the patient is able to take more foods and beverages orally. Many patients are anorectic initially and may later become hyperphagic [125]. Overfeeding foods and beverages, especially at the beginning of refeeding, can easily result in loss of more fluid than was originally consumed. Patients sometimes express extreme hunger and weakness. They may subsequently consume large volumes of food and beverages only to experience malabsorption of foodstuffs and large fluid

effluent. Typically, dietary modifications are included to assure adequate nutriture without overwhelming digestive and absorptive capacity.

Principles of managing nutritional aspects of short bowel syndrome are based on the sites and capacities of digestion and absorption [110, 126, 128, 132, 133]. The mainstays of the diet are starches and lean animal products with modest amounts of fat. Patients with retained colon may do better with relatively higher amounts of starches and lower amounts of fat (20–20% of energy from fat) than those without. Sources of both n-6 and n-3 fatty acids should be provided. Medium-chain triglyceride-containing products can be helpful in providing a source of energy, especially in patients without the distal ileum. Poorly absorbed sugars (e.g., fructose, alcohol sugars) and consumption of large volumes of all hyperosmolar sugar sources should be limited. The lactase enzyme may be lacking in some patients but reasonable amounts of lactose can be tolerated especially when supplied in foods such as cheeses, yogurts, or mixed foods rather than milk as a beverage [134]. Commercially available lactase enzyme can also be used to improve the tolerance to foods high in lactose.

Some foods are discouraged simply because they provide little or no nutrient value and may displace better sources of nutrients in the diet. Caffeinated and alcoholic beverages tend to increase gastrointestinal secretions, alter motility, or increase permeability and contribute little to nutritional value. The diet need not be devoid of fiber; in fact, modest amounts of dietary fiber may help to regulate gastric emptying. If the patient has a residual colon, fiber may be fermented to short-chain fatty acids to enhance gastrointestinal function and increase absorption of fluid and electrolytes. In patients with strictures, dietary fiber may need to be in the form of small particulate matter and added to juices or other foods.

A typical diet in the patient with short bowel may include small but frequent portions of foods such as eggs, meats, poultry, fishes, breads and cereals, rice, potatoes, pastas, vegetables, and vegetable juices. Specially tailored oral electrolyte replacement fluids [135] may be used, as needed, but low-calorie, caffeine-free beverages or flavored waters can also be used, preferably taken frequently in small quantities. Use of vitamin and mineral supplements should be tailored to the patient's dietary habits, tolerances, and absorptive capacity. Because transit through the remaining gastrointestinal tract may be rapid, tablets may not disintegrate in time for maximal absorption, so supplements may need to be crushed or provided in liquid form.

F. Nutrients, Growth Factors, and Medical and Surgical Therapies

Several specific nutrients and neuroendocrine agents are being evaluated to hasten or enhance the adaptive process including supplemental glutamine, growth hormone, epider-

mal growth factor, insulin-like growth factor 1, n-3 fatty acids, nucleotides, fermentable fibers, or short-chain fatty acids [128, 132, 136–139].

Wilmore [132] has described the use of a combination of growth hormone, supplemental dietary glutamine, and a low-fat diet high in complex carbohydrate in managing more than 300 patients who were dependent on parenteral nutritional support or considered to be at significant risk for nutritional inadequacies. Wilmore and his group report that the combined therapy has been successful in increasing body weight and lean mass, reducing dependence on parenteral nutrition, and improving overall well-being of patients with short bowel syndrome. Other investigators [140, 141] have not been as enthusiastic about this approach. Scolapio [140], for example, in a randomized, placebo-controlled, double-blind crossover trial, studied growth hormone and supplemented glutamine in eight patients who had been dependent on parenteral nutrition for 3–19 years. While receiving the treatment, patients gained fluid weight and lean mass but only as long as the therapy was continued and the patients did not demonstrate increased fluid and macronutrient absorption during the 21-day trial. Based on their study with animal models, Vanderhoof et al. [141] concluded that any adaptive response was more likely to be the result of enteral nutrition rather than the combined glutamine-growth hormone treatment.

Dietary fiber or short-chain fatty acids have been studied in the regulation of normal gastrointestinal function as a therapeutic agent in the management of gastrointestinal disease and as a regulatory agent in short bowel syndrome. Dietary fiber may help regulate gastric emptying by increasing the viscosity of gastric contents or as a result of a feedback mechanism when dietary fiber and resistant starch are fermented to short-chain fatty acids in the colon [120, 139, 142]. Short-chain fatty acids and certain dietary fibers may also regulate colonic cellular differentiation and serve to prevent the overgrowth of potentially pathogenic organisms [142].

Patients with short bowel syndrome may be also treated with several medications to improve symptoms, decrease gastrointestinal secretions, delay gastric emptying, slow intestinal transit, or bind bile acids. Histamine-2 receptor blockers or proton pump inhibitors may be used in the initial stages of gastric acid hypersecretion; loperamide, atropine, opiates, and octeotide may be used for management of diarrhea; and cholestyramine can be used to bind bile acids [104, 112]. Other agents are being studied in the management and prevention of complications of short bowel symptoms.

Several surgical procedures have been considered in the management of extreme short bowel and intestinal failure, including intestinal tapering and lengthening procedures, intestinal loops, reversal of intestinal segments, insertion of colonic segments (which normally exhibit slower transit), insertion of reversed segments colon, creation of intestinal loops and valve-type passages, and, most recently, intestinal

transplant [143–148]. Small bowel transplant may include small intestinal segments alone, small intestine with colon, and intestine with liver transplant. Transplant may be the only alternative when prolonged treatment of gut failure with total parenteral nutrition leads to liver failure. The treatments that appear to be considered the best for improving existing short bowel are small intestinal lengthening [145, 146] and, for gut failure, total parenteral nutrition and intestinal transplant [147, 148]. Transplant procedures and immunosuppresive therapy are improving and with time may provide an option for more patients in the future.

IV. CONCLUSION

Both inflammatory bowel disease and short bowel syndrome are gastrointestinal disorders that may lead to serious nutrition-related consequences, including diarrhea and malabsorption, weight loss, growth retardation, dehydration, micronutrient deficiencies, electrolyte disturbances, and bone loss. Each disorder requires thorough evaluation of the patient's nutrition status and each requires that nutrition intervention be tailored to the individual. Nutrition interventions typically take the form of dietary modifications, enteral and parenteral nutrition support, nutrition supplements, and education of the patient and his or her caregivers. Newer medical, surgical, and nutritional approaches to prevention and treatment continue to improve the survival and quality of life in patients with inflammatory bowel disease and short bowel syndrome. However, despite the numerous investigations already performed related to nutrition in inflammatory bowel disease and short bowel, the knowledge and science base for practice of nutrition in the treatment of these disorders is still in its infancy.

References

1. Jewel, D. P. (1998). Ulcerative colitis. *In* "Gastrointestinal and Liver Disease" (M. Feldman, H. H. Sleisenger, and B. F. Scharschmidt, Eds.), 6th ed., pp. 1735–1760. W. B. Saunders, Philadelphia, PA.
2. Brown, M. O. (1999). Inflammatory bowel disease. *Primary Care* **26**, 141–170.
3. Kornbluth, A., Sachar, D. B., and Salomon, P. (1998). Crohn's disease. *In* "Gastrointestinal and Liver Disease" (M. Feldman, H. H. Sleisenger, and B. F. Scharschmidt, Eds.), 6th ed., pp. 1708–1734. W. B. Saunders, Philadelphia, PA.
4. Andres, P., and Friedman, L. (1999). Epidemiology and the natural course of inflammatory bowel disease. *Gastroenterol. Clin. N. Am.* **28**, 225–281.
5. Facts about the epidemiology of inflammatory bowel disease. (1999). Crohn's Colitis Foundation of America Library. New York. Available at http://www.ccfa.org.
6. Papadakis, K. A. (1999). Current theories on the causes of inflammatory bowel disease. *Gastroenterol. Clin. N. Am.* **28**, 283–296.
7. Pena, A. S. (1999). Genetics of inflammatory bowel disease. The candidate gene approach: Susceptibility versus disease heterogeneity. Dig Dis. **16**, 356–363.
8. Moody, G., Eaden, J. E., and Mayberry, J. F. (1999). Social implications of childhood Crohn's disease. *J. Pediatr. Gastroenterol. Nutr.* **28**, S43–S45.
9. Akobeng, A. K., Suresh-Babu, M. V., Firth, D., Miller, V., Mir, P., and Thomas, A. G. (1999). Quality of life in children with Crohn's disease: A pilot study. *J. Pediatr. Gastroenterol. Nutr.* **28**, S37–S39.
10. Ward, P., and Lentsch, A. (1999). The acute inflammatory response and its regulation. *Arch. Surg.* **134**, 666–669.
11. Azimakopoulos, G. (1999). Mechanisms of the systemic immune response. *Perfusion* **114**, 269–277.
12. Boyle, E., Jr., Pohlman, T., Johnson, M., and Verrier, E. (1997). Endothelial cell injury in cardiovascular surgery: The systemic inflammatory response. *Ann. Thorac. Surg.* **63**, 277–284.
13. Azakura, H., Suzuki, A., Ohtsuka, K., Hasegawa, K., and Sugimura K. (1999). Gut associated lymphoid tissues in ulcerative colitis. *J. Parenteral Enteral Nutr.* **23**, 25S–28S.
14. Troncone, R., Caputo, N., Esposito., V., Campanozzi, A., Campanozzi, F., Auricchio, R., Greco, L., and Cucchiara, S. (1999). Increased concentration of eosinophilic cationic protein in whole gut lavage fluid from children with inflammatory bowel disease. *J. Pediatr. Gastroenterol. Nutr.* **28**, 164–168.
15. Van Dullemen, H., Meenan, J., Stronkhorst, G. N. J., and Van Deventer, S. J. H. (1997). Mediators of mucosal inflammation: Implications for therapy. *Scand. J. Gastroenterol.* **223**(Suppl.), 92–98.
16. Rogler, G., and Andus, T. (1998). Cytokines in inflammatory bowel disease. *World J. Surg.* **22**, 382–389.
17. Guimbaud, R., Bertrand, V., Chauvelot-Moachon, L., Quartier, G., Vidon, N., Giroud, J., Couturier, D., and Chaussade, S. (1998). Network of inflammatory cytokines and correlation with disease activity in ulcerative colitis. *Am. J. Gastroentrol.* **93**, 2397–2404.
18. Niederau, C., Backmerhoff, F., Schumacher, B., and Niederau, C. (1997). Inflammatory mediators and acute phase proteins in patients with Crohn's disease and ulcerative colitis. *Hepatogastroenterology* **44**, 90–107.
19. Ishiguro, Y. (1999). Cytokine production correlates with endoscopic acitvity of ulcerative colitis. *J. Gastroenterol.* **34**, 66–74.
20. Thompson, A., Hemphill, D., and Jeejeebhooy, K. N. (1998). Oxidative stress and antioxidants in intestinal disease. *Dig. Dis.* **16**, 152–158.
21. Ramakrishna, B., Varghese, R., Jayakumar, S., Mathan, M., and Balasubramanian, K. (1997). Circulating antioxidants in ulcerative colitis and their relationship to disease severity and activity. *J. Gastroenterol. Hepatol.* **12**, 490–494.
22. Kjeldsen, J., Lassen, J., Brandslund, I., and Schaffalitzky de Muckadell, O. (1998). Markers of coagulation and fibrinolysis as measures of dietary activity in inflammatory bowel disease. *Scand. J. Gastroenterol.* **33**, 637–643.
23. Murch, S. (1998). Local and systemic effects of macrophage cytokines in intestinal inflammation. *Nutrition* **14**, 780–783.
24. Nielsen, O. H., and Rask-Madsen, J. (1996). Mediators of inflammation in chronic inflammatory bowel disease. *Scand. J. Gastroenterol.* **216**(Suppl.), 149–159.

25. Russell, A. L. (1999). Glycoaminoglycan (GAG) deficiency in protective barrier as an underlying, primary cause of ulcerative colitis, Crohn's disease interstitial cystitis and possibly Reiter's syndrome. *Med. Hypotheses* **52,** 297–301.

26. Nogauchi, M., Hiwatachi, N., Liu, Z., and Toyota, T. (1998). Secretion imbalance between tumor necrosis factor and its inhibitor in inflammatory bowel disease. *Gut* **43,** 203–209.

27. Franchimont, D., Louis, E., Dupont, P., Vrindts-Gevaert, Y., Chrousos, G., Geenen, V., and Belaiche, J. (1999). Decreased corticosensitivity in quiescent Crohn's disease: An ex vivo study using whole blood cell cultures. *Dig. Dis. Sci.* **44,** 1208–1215.

28. Kugathasan, S., Willis, J., Dahms, B., O'Riordan, M., Hupertz, V., Binion, D., Boyle, J., and Fiocchi, C. (1998). Intrinsic hyperreactivity of mucosal T cells to interleukin–2 in pediatric Crohn's disease. *J. Pediatr.* **133,** 675–681.

29. Iwashita, E. (1998). Greatly increased mucosal nitric oxide in ulcerative colitis determined in situ by a novel nitric oxide-selective microelectrode. *J. Gastroenterol. Hepatol.* **13,** 391–394.

29a. Santos, J., Bayarri, C., Saperas, E., Nogeiras, C., Antolin, M., Cadahia, A., and Malagelada, J. R. (1999). Characterisation of immune mediator release during the immediate response to segmental mucosal challenge in the jejunum of patients with food allergy. *Gut* **45,** 553–558.

30. Russel, M. G., Engels, L. G., Muris, J. W., Limonard, C. B., Volovics, A., Brummer, R. J., and Stockbrugger, R. W. (1998). Modern life in the epidemiology of inflammatory bowel disease: A case control study with special emphasis on nutritional factors. *Eur. J. Gastroenterol. Hepatol.* **10,** 243–249.

31. Joachim, G. (1999). The relationship between habits of food consumption and reported reactions to food in people with inflammatory bowel disease—testing the limits. *Nutr. Health* **13,** 69–83.

32. Shoda, R., Matsueda, K., Yamato, S., and Umeda, N. (1996). Epidemiologic analysis of Crohn disease in Japan: Increased dietery intake of n–6 polyunsaturated fatty acids and animal protein relates to the increased incidence in Japan. *Am. J. Clin. Nutr.* **63,** 741–745.

33. Geerling, B. J., v-Houwelingen, A. C., Badart-Smook, A., Stockbrugger, R. W., and Burmmer, R. J. (1999). Fat intake and fatty acid profile in plasma phospholipids and adipose tissue in patients with Crohn's disease. *Am. J. Gastroenterol.* **94,** 410–417.

34. Heller, A., Koch, T., Schmeck, J., and van-Ackern, K. (1998). Lipid mediators I: Inflammatory disorders. *Drugs* **55,** 487–496.

35. Crooks, S. W., and Stockley, R. A. (1998). Leukotriene B4. *Int. J. Biochem. Cell. Biol.* **30,** 173–178.

36. Kuroki, F., Iida, M., Matsumoto, T., Aoyagi, K., Kanamoto, K., and Fujishima, M. (1997). Serum n3 polyunsaturated fatty acids are depleted in Crohn's disease. *Dig. Dis. Sci.* **42,** 1137–1141.

37. Purasiri, P., Mckechnie, A., Heys, S. D., and Eremin, O. (1997). Modulation in vitro of human natural cytotoxicity, lymphocyte proliferative response mitogens and cytokine production by essential fatty acids. *Immunology* **92,** 166–172.

38. Bichoff, S. C., Herrmann, A., and Manns, M. P. (1996). Prevalence of adverse reactions to food in patients with gastrointestinal disease. *Allergy* **51,** 811–818.

39. Sampson, H. A. (1997). Food allergy. *JAMA* **278,** 1888–1894.

40. Huber, A., Genser, D., Spitzauer, S., Scheiner, O., and Jensen-Jarolim, E. (1998). IgE/anti-IgE immune complexes in sera from patients with Crohn's disease do not contain food specific IgE. *Int. Arch. Allergy Immunol.* **115,** 67–72.

41. Mowat, A. M., and Viney, J. L. (1997). The anatomical basis of intestinal immunity. *Immunol. Rev.* **156,** 145–166.

42. Persson, P. G., Ahlbom, A., and Hellers, G. (1992). Diet and inflammatory bowel disease: A case-control study. *Epidemiology* **3,** 47–52.

43. Reif, S., Klein, I., Farbstein, M., Hallak, A., and Gilat, T. (1997). Pre-illness dietary factors in inflammatory bowel disease. *Gut* **40,** 754–760.

44. Hunter, J. O. (1998). Nutritional factors in inflammatory bowel disease [comment]. *Eur. J. Gastroenterol. Hepatol.* **10,** 235–237.

45. Riordan, A. M., Ruxton, C. H., and Hunter, J. O. (1998). A review of associations between Crohn's disease and consumption of sugars. *Eur. J. Clin. Nutr.* **52,** 229–238.

46. Solomons, N. W. (1983). Micronutrient deficiencies in inflammatory bowel disease. *Clin. Nutr.* **2,** 19–25.

47. Steger, G. G., Mader, R. M., Vogelsang, H., Schofl, R., Lochs, H., and Ferenci, P. (1994). Folate absorption in Crohn's disease. *Digestion* **55,** 234–238.

48. Imes, S., Pinchbeck, B. R., Dinwoodie, A., Walker, K., and Thompson, A. B. (1987). Iron, folate, vitamin B–12, zinc and copper status in outpatients with Crohn's disease. *J. Am. Diet. Assoc.* **87,** 928–930.

49. (1988). Sulfasalazine inhibits folate absorption. *Nutr. Rev.* **49,** 320–323.

50. Rath, H. C., Caesar, I., Roth, M., and Scholmerich, J. (1998). Nutritional deficiencies and complications in chronic inflammatory bowel disease. *Med. Klin.* **93,** 6–10.

51. Spiegel, J. E., and Willenbucher, R. F. (1999). Copper deficiency in a patient with Crohn's disease receiving parenteral nutrition. *J. Parenteral Enteral. Nutr.* **23,** 169–172.

52. Rannem, T., Ladefoged, K., Hylander, E., Hegnhoj, J., and Staun, M. (1998). Selenium depletion in patients with gastrointestinal diseases: Are there any predictive factors? *Scand. J. Gastroenterol.* **33,** 1057–1061.

53. Plata-Salaman, C. R. (1998). Cytokine-induced anorexia. Behavorial, cellular, and molecular mechanisms. *Ann. N.Y. Acad. Sci.* **856,** 160–170.

54. Rigaud, D., Angel, L. A., Cerf, M., Carduner, M. J., Melchior, J.-C., Sautier, C., Rene, E., Apfelbaum, M., and Mignon, M. (1994). Mechanisms of decreased food intake during weight loss in adult Crohn's disease patients without obvious malabsorption. *Am. J. Clin. Nutr.* **60,** 775–781.

55. Schneeweiss, B., Lochs, H., Zauner, C., Fischer, M., Wyatt, J., Maier-Dobersberger, T., and Schneider, B. (1999). Energy and substrate metabolism in patients with active Crohn's disease. *J. Nutr.* **129,** 844–848.

56. O'Keefe, S. J. (1996). Nutrition and gastrointestinal disease. *Scand. J. Gastroenterol.* **220**(Suppl.), 52–59.

57. Stein, R. B. (1999). Medical therapy for inflammatory bowel disease. *Gastroenterol. Clin. N. Am.* **28,** 297–321.

58. Michetti, P., and Peppercorn, M. A. (1999). Medical therapy of specific clinical presentations. *Gastroenterol. Clin. N. Am.* **28,** 353–370.

59. Present, D. H., Rutgeerts, P., Targan, S., Hanauer, S. B., Mayer, L., van Hogezand, R. A., Podolsky, D. K., Sands,

B. E., Braakman, T., DeWoody, K. L., Schaible, T. F., and vanDeventer, S. J. (1999). Infliximab for the treatment of fistulas in patients with Crohn's disease. *N. Engl. J. Med.* **340,** 1398–1405.

60. Stack, W. A., Long, R. G., and Hawkey, C. J. (1998). Short- and long-term outcome of patients treated with cyclosporine for severe acute ulcerative colitis. *Aliment. Pharmacol. Ther.* **12,** 973–978.

61. Ricart, E., Panaccione, R., Loftus, E. V., Tremaine, W. J., and Sandborn, W. J. (1999). Successful management of Crohn's disease of ileoanal pouch with infliximab. *Gastroenterology* **117,** 429–432.

62. Robinson, M. (1998). Medical therapy of inflammatory bowel disease for the 21st century. *Eur. J. Surg.* **582**(Suppl.), 90S–98S.

62a. Slonim, A. E., Bulone, L., Damore, M. B., Goldgerg, T., Wingertzahn, M. A., and McKinley, M. J. (2000). A preliminary study of growth hormone therapy for Crohn's disease. *N. Engl. J. Med.* **342,** 1633–1637.

63. Schrieber, S. (1998). Experimental immunomodulatory therapy of inflammatory bowel disease. *Neth. J. Med.* **53,** S24–S31.

64. Muller-Peddinghaus, R. (1997). Leukotriene synthesis inhibitor effects of 5-lipoxygenase inhibition—Exemplified by the leukotriene synthesis inhibitor BAY X 1005. *J. Physiolol. Pharmacol.* **48,** 529–536.

65. Suarez, F. L., Furne, J. K., Springfield, J., and Levitt, M. D. (1998). Bismuth subsalicylate markedly decreases hydrogen sulfite release in the human colon. *Gastroenterology* **114,** 923–929.

66. Folwaczny, C., Wiebecke, B., and Loeschke, K. (1999). Unfractioned heparin in the therapy of patients with highly active inflammatory bowel disease. *Am. J. Gastroenterol.* **94,** 1551–1555.

67. Ware, J. H., Wan, X. S., Newberne, P., and Kennedy, A. R. (1999). Birman-Birk inhibitor concentrate reduces colon inflammation in mice with dextran sulfate sodium-induced ulcerative colitis. *Dig. Dis. Sci.* **44,** 986–990.

68. Chun, A., Chadi, R. M., Korelitz, B. I., Colonna, T., Felder, J. B., Jackson, M. H., Morgenstern, E. H., Rubin, S. D., Sacknoff, A. G., and Gliem, G. M. (1998). Intravenous corticotrophin vs hydrocortisone in the treatment of hospitalized patients with Crohn's disease: A randomized double-blind study and follow-up. *Inflamm. Bowel Dis.* **4,** 171–181.

69. Kosaka, T., Sawada, K., Ohnishi, K., Egashira, A., Yamamura, M., Tanida, N., Satomi, M., and Shimoyama, T. (1999). Effect of leukocytapheresis therapy using a leukocyte removal filter in Crohn's disease. *Intern. Med.* **38,** 102–111.

70. Becker, J. M. (1999). Surgical therapy for ulcerative colitis and Crohn's disease. *Gastroenterol. Clin. N. Am.* **28,** 371–390.

71. Patel, H. I., Leichtner, A. M., Colodny, A. H., and Shamberger, R. C. (1997). Surgery for Crohn's disease in infants and children. *J. Pediatr. Surg.* **32,** 1063–1067.

72. Cohen, R. D., Broadski, A. L., and Hanauer, S. B. (1999). A comparison of quality of life in patients with severe ulcerative colitis after total colectomy versus medical treatment with intravenous cyclosporine. *Inflamm. Bowel Dis.* **5,** 1–10.

73. Kris-Etherton, P. M., Taylor D. S., Yu-Poth, S., Huth, P., Moriarty, K., Fishell, V., Harbrove, R. L., Zhao, G., and Etherton, T. D. (2000). Polyunsaturated fatty acids in the food chain in the United States. *Am. J. Clin. Nutr.* **71**(Suppl.), 179S–188S.

74. Simopoulos, A. P. (1999). Essential fatty acids in health and chronic disease. *Am. J. Clin. Nutr.* **70**(Suppl.), 560S–569S.

75. Kinsella, J. E. (1991). Alpha-linolenic acid: Functions and effects on linoleic acid metabolism and eicosanoid-mediated reactions. *Adv. Food Nutr. Res.* **35,** 1–184.

76. Miura, S., Tsuzuki, Y., Hokari, R., and Ishii, H. (1998). Modulation of intestinal immune system. *J. Gastroenterol. Hepatol.* **13,** 1183–1190.

77. Buzzi, A., Boschi, S., Brignola, C., Munarini, A., Carinani, G., and Miglio, F. (2000). Polyunsaturated fatty acids and inflammatory bowel disease. *Am. J. Clin. Nutr.* **71**(Suppl.), 339S–342S.

78. Johnson, M. M., Swan, D. D., Surette, M. E., Stegner, J., Chilton, T., Fonteh, A. N., and Chilton, F. H. (1997). Dietary supplementation with gamma-linolenic acid alters fatty acid content and eicosanoid production. *J. Nutr.* **127,** 1435–1444.

79. Mancuso, P., Whelan, J., DeMichele, S. J., Snider, C. C., Guszcza, J. A., and Karlstad, M. D. (1997). Dietary fish oil and fish and borage oil suppress intrapulmonary proinflammatory eicosanoid biosynthesis and attenuate pulmonary neutrophil accumulation in endotoxic rats. *Crit. Care. Med.* **25,** 1198–1206.

80. Parodi, P. W. (1997). Cows' milk fat components as potential anticarcinogenic agents. *J. Nutr.* **127,** 1055–1060.

81. Sugano, M., Tsujita, A., Yamasaki, M., Noguchi, M., and Yamada, K. (1998). Conjugated linoleic acid modulates tissue levels of chemical mediators and immunoglobulins in rats. *Lipids* **33,** 521–527.

82. Jeppeson, P. B., and Mortensen, P. B. (1999). Colonic digestion and absorption of energy from carbohydrates and medium-chain triglycerides in small bowel failure. *J. Parenteral Enteral Nutr.* **23**(Suppl.), S101–S105.

83. Bengmark, S., and Jeppsson, B. (1995). Gastrointestinal surface protection and reconditioning. *J. Parenteral Enteral Nutr.* **19,** 410–415.

84. Gibson, G. R. (1998). Dietary modulation of the human gut mircroflora using prebiotics. *Br. J. Nutr.* **80,** S209–S212.

85. Emery, E. A., Ahmad, S., Koethe, J. D., Skipper, A., Peerlmutter, S., and Paskin, D. L. (1997). Banana flakes control diarrhea in enterally fed patients. *Nutr. Clin. Prac.* **12,** 72–75.

86. Oli, M. W., Petschow, B. W., and Buddington, R. K. (1998). Evaluation of fructooligosaccharide supplementation of oral electrolyte solutions for treatment of diarrhea: Recovery of the intestinal bacteria. *Dig. Dis. Sci.* **43,** 138–147.

87. Andoh, A., Bamba, T., and Sasaki, M. (1999). Physiologic roles of dietary fiber and butyrate in intestinal functions. *J. Parenteral Enteral Nutr.* **23,** S70–S73.

88. Fernandez-Banares, F., Hinojosa, J., Sanchez-Lombrana, J. L., Navarro, E., Martinez-Salmeron, J. F., Garcia-Puges, A., Gonzales-Huix, F., Riera, J., Gonzolez-Lara, V., Dominguez Abascal, F., Gine, J. J., Moles, J., Gomollon, F., and Gassull, M. A. (1999). Randomized cllinical trial of plantago ovata seeds (dietary fiber) as compared to mesalamine in maintaining remission in ulcerative colitis. Spanish Group for the Study of Crohn's Disease and Ulcerative Colitis. *Am. J. Gastroenterol.* **94,** 427–433.

89. Breuer, R. I., Soergel, K. H., Lashner, B. A., Christ, M. L., Hanauer, S. B., Vanagunas, A., Harig, J. M., Keshavarzian, A., Robinson, M., Sellen, J. M., Weinberg, D., Vidican, D. E., Flemal, K. L., and Rademaker, A. W. (1997). Short chain fatty

acid rectal irrigation for left-sided ulcerative colitis: A randomized, placebo controlled trial. *Gut* **40,** 485–491.

90. Clausen, M. R., Jorgensen, J., and Mortensen, P. B. (1998). Comparison of diarrhea induced by ingestion of fructo-oligosaccharide Idolax and disaccharide lactulose: Role of osmolarity versus fermentation of malabsorbed carbohydrate. *Dig. Dis. Sci.* **43,** 2696–2707.

91. Hyams, J. (1983). Sorbitol intolerance: An unappreciated cause of functional gastrointestinal complaints. *Gastroenterology* **84,** 30–33.

92. Smith, M. M., and Lifshitz, F. (1994). Excess fruit juice consumption as a contributing factor in nonorganic failure to thrive. *Pediatrics* **93,** 438–443.

93. United States Department of Agriculture (1999). "Food and Nutrient Intake by Individuals in the United States by Sex and Age, 1994–1996," NSF Report No. 96-2, NTIS Accession No. PB99-117251. National Technical Information Service, Springfield, VA.

94. Sitrin, M. D. (1992). Nutrition support in inflammatory bowel disease. *Nutr. Clin. Prac.* **7,** 53–60.

95. Messori, A., Trallori, G., D'Albasio, G., Milla, M., and Pacini, F. (1996). Defined-formula diets versus steroids in the treatment of active Crohn's disease: A meta-analysis. *Scand. J. Gastroenterol.* **31,** 267–272.

96. Schwab, D., Raithel, M., and Hahn, E. G. (1998). Enteral nutrition in acute Crohn's disease. *Z. Gastroenterol.* **36,** 983–995.

97. Heuschkel, R. B., and Walker-Smith, J. A. (1999). Enteral nutrition in inflammatory bowel disease of childhood. *J. Parenteral Enteral Nutr.* **23,** S29–S32.

99. Polk, D. B., Hattner, J. T., and Kerner, J. A. (1992). Improved growth and disease activity after intermittent administration of a defined formula diet in children with Crohn's disease. *J. Parenteral Enteral Nutr.* **16,** 499–504.

100. Han, P. D., Burke, A., Baldassano, R. N., Rombeau, J. L., and Lichtenstein, G. R. (1999). Nutrition and inflammatory bowel disease. *Gastroenterol. Clin. N. Am.* **28,** 423–443.

101. Lewis, J. D., and Fisher, R. L. (1994). Nutrition support in inflammatory bowel disease. *Med. Clin. N. Am.* **78,** 1443–1456.

102. Lindor, K., Fleming, R., Burnes, J., Nelson, J., and Ilstrup, D. (1992). A randomized prospective trial comparing a defined formula diet, corticosteroids, and a defined formula diet plus corticosteroids in active Crohn's disease. *Mayo Clin. Proc.* **67,** 328–333.

103. Fukada, Y., Kosaka, T., Okui, M., Hirakawa, H., and Shimoyama, T. (1995). Efficacy of nutritional therapy for Crohn's disease. *J. Gastroenterol.* **8**(Suppl.), 83–87.

104. Westergaard, H. (1998). Short bowel syndrome. *In* "Gastrointestinal and Liver Disease" (M. Feldman and M. H. Sleisenger, Eds.), 6th ed., pp. 1548–1560. W. B. Saunders, Philadelphia, PA.

105. Vanderhoof, J. A., and Langnas, A. N. (1997). Short-bowel syndrome in children and adults. *J. Gastroenterol.* **115,** 1767–1778.

106. Mayer, J. M., Schober, P. H., Weissensteiner, U., and Hollwarth, M. E. (1999). Morbidity and mortality of the short-bowel syndrome. *Eur. J. Pediatr. Surg.* **9,** 121–125.

107. Vanderhoof, J. A., and Matya, S. M. (1999). Enteral and parenteral nutrition in patients with short-bowel syndrome. *Eur. J. Pediatr. Surg.* **9,** 214–219.

108. Goulet, O. (1998). Short bowel syndrome in pediatric patients. *Nutrition* **14,** 784–787.

109. Carbonnel, F., Cosnes, J., Chevret, S., Beaugerie, L., Ngo, Y., Malafosse, M., Rolland, P., Quintrec, Y., and Gendre, J. P. (1996). The role of anatomic factors in nutritional autonomy after extensive small bowel resection. *J. Parenteral Enteral Nutr.* **20,** 275–279.

110. Beyer, P. L. (1998). Short-bowel syndrome. *In* "Dietitian's Handbook of Enteral and Parenteral Nutrition" (A. Skipper, Ed.), 2nd ed., pp. 418–436. Aspen Publishers, Gaithersburg, MD.

111. Purdum, P. P., III, and Kirby, D. F. (1991). Short-bowel syndrome: A review of the role of nutrition support. *J. Parenteral Enteral Nutr.* **15,** 93–101.

112. Nightingale, J. M. (1999). Management of patients with a short bowel. *Nutrition* **15,** 633–637.

113. Vanderhoof, J. A., and Langnas, A. N. (1997). Short-bowel syndrome in children and adults. *Gastroenterology* **113,** 1767–1778.

114. Vanderhoof, J. A., Young, R. J., Murray, N., and Kaufman, S. S. (1998). Treatment strategies for small bowel bacterial overgrowth in short bowel syndrome. *J. Pediatr. Gastroenterol. Nutr.* **27,** 155–160.

115. Wojdemann, M., Wettergren, A., Sternby, B., Holst, J. J., Lawsen, S., Rehfeld, J. F., and Olsen, O. (1998). Inhibition of human gastric lipase secretion by glucagon-like peptide-1. *Dig. Dis. Sci.* **43,** 700–805.

116. Chen, C. H., Stephens, R. L., Jr., and Rogers, R. C. (1997). PYY and NPY: Control of gastric motility via action on R1 and Y2 receptors in the DVC. *Neurogastroenterol. Motil.* **9,** 109–116.

117. Cuche, G., and Malbert, C. H. (1999). Ileal short chain fatty acids inhibit transpyloric flow in pigs. *Scand. J. Gastroenterol.* **34,** 149–155.

118. Nordgaard, I., Hansen, B. S., and Mortensen, P. B. (1996). Importance of colonic support for energy absorption as small-bowel failure proceeds. *Am. J. Clin. Nutr.* **64,** 222–231.

119. Jeppesen, P. B., and Mortensen, P. B. (1998). The influence of a preserved colon on the absorption of medium chain fat in patients with small bowel resection. *Gut* **43,** 478–483.

120. Jorgensen, J. R., Clausen, M. R., and Mortensen, P. B. (1997). Oxidation of short and medium chain C2-C8 fatty acids in Sprague-Dawley rat colonocytes. *Gut* **40,** 400–405.

121. Weaver, L. T., Austin, S., and Cole, T. J. (1991). Small intestinal length: A factor essential for gut adaptation. *Gut* **32,** 1321–1323.

122. Messing, B., Crenn, P., Beau, P., Boutron-Rualt, M. C., Rambaud, J. C., and Matchuansky, C. (1999). Long-term survival and parenteral nutrition dependence in adult patients with the short bowel syndrome. *Gastroenterology* **117,** 1043–1050.

123. Suita, S., Masumoto, K., Yamanouchi, T., Nagano, M., and Nakamura, M. (1999). Complications in neonates with short bowel syndrome and long term parenteral nutrition. *J. Parenteral Enteral Nutr.* **23**(Suppl.), S106–S109.

124. Jeppesen, P. B., Langholz, E., and Mortensen, P. B. (1999). Quality of life in patients receiving home parenteral nutrition. *Gut* **44,** 844–852.

125. Cosnes, J., Lamy, P. H., Beaugerie, L., LeQuintrec, M., Gendre, J. P., and LeQuintrec, Y. (1990). Adaptive hyperphagia

in patients with postsurgical malabsorption. *Gastroenterology* **99**, 1814–1819.

126. Bragg, L. E., Thompson, J. S., and Rikkers, L. F. (1991). Influence of nutrient delivery on gut structure and function. *Nutrition* **7**, 237–243.

127. Firmansyah, A., Penn, D., and Lebenthal, E. (1989). Isolated coloncyte metabolism of glucose, glutamine, n-butyrate and beta-hydroxybutyrate in malnutrition. *Gastroenterology* **97**, 622–629.

128. Ziegler, T. R., Estvariz, C. F., Jonas, C. R., Gu, L. H., Jones, D. P., and Leader, L. M. (1999). Interactions between nutrients and peptide growth factors in intestinal growth, repair and function. *J. Parenteral Enteral Nutr.* **23**, S174–S182.

129. Biasco, G., Callegari, C., Lami, F., Minarini, A., Miglioli, M., and Barbara, L. (1984). Intestinal morphological changes during oral refeeding in a patient previously treated with total parenteral nutrition for small bowel resection. *Am. J. Gastroenterol.* **79**, 585–588.

130. Shin, C. S., Chaudhry, A. G., Khaddam, M. H., Penha, P. D., and Dooner, R. (1980). Early morphologic changes in the intestine following massive resection of the small intestine and parenteral nutrition therapy. *Surg. Gynecol. Obstet.* **151**, 246–250.

131. Solhaug, H. (1976). Morphometric studies of the small intestine following jejunoileal shunt operation. *Scand. J. Gastroent.* **11**, 155–160.

132. Wilmore, D. W. (1999). Growth factors and nutrients in the short bowel syndrome. *J. Parenteral Enteral Nutr.* **23**, S117–S120.

133. Lykins, T. C., and Stockwell, J. (1998). Comprehensive modified diet simplifies nutrition management of adults with short-bowel syndrome. *J. Am. Diet. Assoc.* **98**, 309–315.

134. Arrigoni, E., Marteau, P., Briet, F., Pochart, P., Rambaud, J. C., and Messing, B. (1994). Tolerance and absorption of lactose from milk and yogurt during short-bowel syndrome in humans. *Am. J. Clin. Nutr.* **60**, 926–929.

135. Beaugerie, L., Cosnes, J., Verwaerde, F., Dupas, H., Lamy, P., Gendre, J. P., and LeQuintrec, Y. (1991). Isotonic high-sodium oral rehydration solution for increasing sodium absorption in patients with short-bowel syndrome. *Am. J. Clin. Nutr.* **53**, 769–772.

136. Thompson, J. S. (1999). Epidermal growth factor and the short bowel syndrome. *J. Parenteral Enteral Nutr.* **23**, S113–S116.

137. Iijima, S., Tsujinaka, T., Kido, Y., Hayashida, Y., Ishida, H., Homma, T., Yokoyama, H., and Mori, T. (1993). Intravenous administration of nucleosides and a nucleotide mixture diminishes intestinal mucosal atrophy induced by total parenteral nutrition. *J. Parenteral Enteral Nutr.* **17**, 265–270.

138. Murphy, M. S. (1998). Growth factors and the gastrointestinal tract. *Nutrition* **14**, 771–774.

139. Bengmark, S. (2000). Colonic food: Pre- and probiotics. *Am. J. Gastroenterol.* **95**(Suppl.), S5–S7.

140. Scolapio, J. S. (1999). Effect of growth hormone, glutamine, and diet on body composition in short bowel syndrome: A randomized, controlled study. *J. Parenteral Enteral Nutr.* **23**, 309–313.

141. Vanderhoof, J. A., Kollman, K. A., Griffin, S., and Adrian, T. E. (1997). Growth hormone and glutamine do not stimulate intestinal adaptation following massive small bowel resection in the rat. *J. Pediatr. Gastroenterol. Nutr.* **25**, 327–331.

142. Scheppach, W. (1994). Effects of short chain fatty acids on gut morphology and function. *Gut* **35**(Suppl.), S35–S38.

143. Thompson J. S., and Langnas, A. N. (1999). Surgical approaches to improving intestinal function in the short-bowel syndrome. *Arch. Surg.* **134**, 706–709.

144. Goulet, O., Jan, D., Lacaille, F., Colomb, V., Michel, J. L., Damotte, D., Jouvet, P., Brousse, N., Faure, C., Cezard, J. P., Sarnacki, S., Peuchmaur, M., Hubert, P., Ricour, C., and Revillon, Y. (1999). Intestinal transplantation in children: Preliminary experience in Paris. *J. Parenteral Enteral Nutr.* **23**(Suppl.), S121–S125.

145. Bianchi, A. (1997). Longitudinal intestinal lengthening and tailoring: Results in 20 children. *J. R. Soc. Med.* **90**, 429–432.

146. Figueroa, C. R., Harris, P. R., Birdsong, E., Franklin, F. A., and Georgeson, K. E. (1996). Impact of intestinal lengthening on the nutritional outcome for children with short bowel syndrome. *J. Pediatr. Surg.* **31**, 912–916.

147. Amii, L. A., and Moss, R. L. (1999). Nutritional support of the pediatric surgical patient. *Curr. Opin. Pediatr.* **11**, 237–240.

148. Thompson, J. S. (1999). Intestinal transplantation. Experience in the United States. *Eur. J. Pediatr. Surg.* **9**, 271–273.

CHAPTER **39**

Nutrition and Liver Disease

SARAH H. RIGBY AND KATHLEEN B. SCHWARZ
Johns Hopkins Children's Center, Baltimore, Maryland

I. INTRODUCTION

The liver plays a central role in the metabolism of carbohydrates, proteins, lipids, vitamins, and minerals. As a result, diseases of the liver can disrupt this metabolism and adversely affect nutritional status. Acute and chronic liver diseases occur in both children and adults, and malnutrition often accompanies the disease. Many known and suspected factors contribute to malnutrition, and they will be discussed in the following sections. Liver transplantation is a viable option for many children and adults with end-stage liver disease, and good nutritional status is of utmost importance for these patients. The nutritional management of liver disease is an exciting field in which much research still needs to be done to address the many questions surrounding adequate and appropriate nutrition intervention for each disease and for the different stages of liver disease.

II. PATHOGENESIS OF MALNUTRITION

A. Mechanisms of Malnutrition

1. ACUTE LIVER DISEASE

Acute liver disease can result in weight loss due to nausea, vomiting, anorexia, and diarrhea. Increases in energy expenditure could also affect weight loss; however, it is unclear whether or not energy expenditure is altered in acute liver disease [1, 2]. Malnutrition is not normally a sequela of acute disease if premorbid nutritional status was normal. Acute liver disease may resolve or advance to chronic liver disease.

Fulminant hepatic failure is an acute condition that results in hepatic encephalopathy and coagulopathy. Hepatic encephalopathy must occur for the diagnosis of fulminant hepatic failure. With the development of hepatic encephalopathy, there are elevated levels of ammonia, a decrease in the plasma concentrations of the branched-chain amino acids, and an increase in the concentrations of the aromatic amino acids [3, 4]. Malnutrition can occur as a result of disordered metabolism of carbohydrates, proteins, and fats in addition to possible iatrogenic restrictions on nutrient intake.

2. CHRONIC LIVER DISEASE

Chronic liver disease can progress through stages of fibrosis to the end-stage disease, cirrhosis. Cirrhosis is irreversible and is defined by fibrosis, damage and regeneration of hepatocytes, altered hepatic architecture, and decreased hepatic function. Patients with chronic liver disease may present with cholestasis or with anicteric cirrhotic liver disease.

Many patients with chronic liver disease are predisposed to malnutrition as a result of many factors, including inadequate intake and malabsorption [5, 6]. Decreased appetite, nausea, vomiting, and restrictive diets can result in inadequate nutrient intake. Ascites itself can also affect intake, because the ascites may result in increased intra-abdominal pressure, which leads to early satiety. Cholestasis, cirrhosis, portal hypertension, and pancreatic insufficiency can all contribute to malabsorption [7]. Elevated energy expenditure and altered protein metabolism may also contribute to the development of malnutrition [1, 5, 8].

B. Specific Nutritional Issues and Inadequacies

1. CARBOHYDRATES

The metabolism of carbohydrates in the liver includes glycogenesis, glycogenolysis, and gluconeogenesis. Glycogenesis is the process of storing excess glucose for use by the body at a later time. Glycogenolysis occurs when the body, which prefers glucose as an energy source, needs energy. The glycogen previously stored by the liver is broken down to glucose and dispersed throughout the body. When glycogen stores are depleted and glucose is required by the body, the liver initiates the production of glucose from amino acids, lactate, and glycerol in a process called gluconeogenesis.

Most studies of energy metabolism in liver disease have focused on adults with cirrhosis. Results of such studies indicate that glucose intolerance and insulin resistance are common findings in this population; however, for most patients, these findings do not appear to be clinically significant [9, 10]. The production of glucose may be subnormal and the liver's capacity to store glycogen may be decreased as a result of the fibrosis that occurs with cirrhosis [11].

2. PROTEIN

The synthesis of certain proteins, including albumin, protease inhibitors, acute-phase reactants, storage and iron-binding proteins, and coagulation factors, occurs predominantly in the liver. Protein synthesis may not be adversely affected until the liver disease is late stage or in fulminant hepatic failure [12]. On the other hand, protein degradation is possibly increased even in earlier stages of disease [5, 13]. As a result, the provision of adequate protein to ensure positive nitrogen balance is imperative, because this will allow for regeneration of hepatocytes.

Increased plasma concentrations of aromatic amino acids and decreased plasma concentrations of branched-chain amino acids are seen in many patients with chronic liver disease [3, 4, 14]. The utilization of branched-chain amino acids to correct these abnormalities appears to be indicated only in fulminant hepatic failure and patients with chronic protein-induced encephalopathy [9, 15]. In patients with liver disease, standard amino acids in amounts sufficient to prevent negative nitrogen balance are recommended except in those patients who are truly protein intolerant [9].

3. FAT

Lipids are also synthesized and catabolized in the liver. The synthesis of lipids, lipogenesis, occurs with an influx of excess carbohydrate. The catabolism of fatty acids produces ketone bodies, which can be used by the brain and heart as a source of energy when glucose is not available or in short supply.

Patients with cirrhosis derive a greater than normal percentage of their energy from the catabolism of fat, which may be attributed to lower stores of glycogen [11, 16]. This utilization of fat as an energy source resembles a body's reaction in a state of starvation [2, 11]. Steatorrhea, the malabsorption of dietary fat, can occur in liver disease when bile acid flow to the intestines is insufficient. Biliary insufficiency can result in inadequate absorption of fat and other nutrients and decreased energy intake, which may lead to malnutrition.

4. FAT-SOLUBLE VITAMINS

Fat-soluble vitamins are absorbed after undergoing micellar solubilization, a bile salt-dependent process, and are metabolized and/or stored in the liver. Deficiencies occur with steatorrhea, because malabsorption of fat results in concomitant malabsorption of fat-soluble vitamins. Vitamin A deficiency can result in growth failure, anorexia, decreased resistance to infections, keratinization of epithelium, and night blindness. Vitamin D deficiency can result in rickets in children and osteomalacia in adults. Vitamin E deficiency can result in neurological disorders including peripheral neuropathy and myopathy. Vitamin K deficiency can impair clotting factor synthesis, which may result in a propensity for bleeding, bruising, and hemorrhage. The impaired syn-

thesis of clotting factors may also result from hepatic failure. Supplementation with water-miscible fat-soluble vitamins may help correct these deficiencies; however, patients must be closely monitored for toxicity.

5. WATER-SOLUBLE VITAMINS

Children with chronic liver disease may be at risk for water-soluble vitamin deficiencies due to decreased intake and malabsorption; however, the incidence of these deficiencies has not been widely studied. Adults with alcoholic liver disease, and some with nonalcoholic liver disease, have been observed to exhibit deficiencies of folate, thiamin, niacin, and vitamin B_{12}.

6. TRACE ELEMENTS

Adults and children with liver disease may be at risk for metabolic derangements in zinc, selenium, chromium, and copper. Zinc deficiency may occur in liver disease as a result of poor dietary intake, increased urinary losses, decreased absorption, and altered metabolism [17, 18]. This deficiency may present as impaired night vision, macular degeneration, anorexia, changes in taste, skin lesions, depressed immune function, decreased protein synthesis, and slow wound healing [19]. Supplementation has been recommended and appears to be effective in correcting the deficiency [19].

Selenium deficiency may exist in patients with liver disease [20, 21]; however, methods that have been used to assess deficiency are questionable [19]. If a true selenium deficiency is identified, supplementation should be administered because selenium deficiency may result in cardiomyopathy.

Copper deficiency is unlikely in liver disease because the liver excretes copper in bile. Patients with cholestasis could potentially have copper toxicity as a result of decreased excretion. Wilson's disease, which causes liver disease due to increased copper levels, is discussed below.

7. IRON AND CALCIUM

The potential causes of malnutrition in adults and children with liver disease, as discussed above, may predispose to iron and calcium deficiencies. In addition, those patients with recurrent esophageal variceal bleeding are prone to be iron deficient. Calcium deficiency may occur with apparent vitamin D deficiency as a result of disordered metabolism rather than impaired calcium absorption [22, 23]. Supplementation with 25 (OH) vitamin D may be beneficial.

III. MAJOR LIVER DISEASES

Diseases of the hepatobiliary system may be subdivided according to the location of the initial insult—either in the liver (hepatocellular) or in the biliary system. However, as the

disease process advances, both hepatocellular and biliary tract disease may result, regardless of the site of initial insult.

A. Hepatocellular

1. ALCOHOLIC LIVER DISEASE

The intake and metabolism of alcohol play a major role in the development of alcoholic liver disease and associated malnutrition. Intake of alcohol may replace other foods in the diet and thus decrease the total intake of nutrients from other sources, thereby predisposing a person to inadequate nutrient intake. Alcohol oxidation takes precedent over lipid oxidation in the liver; as a result, lipids accumulate in the liver causing fatty liver. It has been suggested that acetaldehyde, a product of alcohol oxidation, may exert a hepatotoxic effect at high levels [24].

Alcoholic liver disease is a progressive disease that is defined by three stages: hepatic steatosis (fatty liver), alcoholic hepatitis, and cirrhosis. Hepatic steatosis symptoms include fatigue, anorexia, nausea, vomiting, and hepatomegaly. Some patients in this stage may present with portal hypertension, bleeding esophageal varices, and low serum albumin [25, 26]. Abstinence from alcohol with adequate nutrient intake may reverse hepatic steatosis.

Alcoholic hepatitis is an inflammation of the liver secondary to the toxic effect of alcohol. Hepatitis occurs in many, but not all, patients who initially present with hepatic steatosis. The incidence of excessive alcohol intake often precipitates hepatitis. Symptoms are similar to those for hepatic steatosis with the addition of fever and possibly acute weight loss. Low serum albumin and prolonged prothrombin time may also be present. The acute symptoms of alcoholic hepatitis can resolve with abstinence and adequate nutrition; alternately, it may progress to liver failure, hepatic encephalopathy, or cirrhosis.

Cirrhosis develops in only 10–20% of chronic alcoholics. Symptoms include fatigue, anorexia, nausea, and sometimes hepatic encephalopathy and bleeding esophageal varices. Malnutrition is common in patients with alcoholic hepatitis and cirrhosis, because anorexia, nausea, and vomiting lead to decreased intake. The substitution of alcohol for food results in decreased intake of nutrients [5, 27–29]. Malabsorption and reduced vitamin intake also adversely affect nutritional status. Ascites can cause premature satiety, thereby decreasing intake. Increased energy expenditure may also play a role in the development of malnutrition [1, 30]. Malnutrition has been associated with increased mortality in alcohol-related liver disease [31]; therefore, recognition of the disease and initiation of appropriate nutritional therapy is imperative.

Specific vitamin and mineral deficiencies occur in alcoholic liver disease. Thiamin deficiency (i.e., beriberi, Wernicke-Korsakoff syndrome) occurs as a result of decreased intake and the interference of alcohol with thiamin metabolism. Supplementation is not effective unless there is abstinence from alcohol. Beriberi is characterized by either peripheral neuropathy (dry beriberi) or edema and heart failure (wet beriberi). Severe thiamin deficiency, Wernicke's encephalopathy, is characterized by mental confusion, ataxia, and coma. Wernicke-Korsakoff syndrome, a progressive degenerative disease affecting memory, can be a sequela to Wernicke's encephalopathy. Patients with niacin deficiency, pellegra, present with psychosis, dermatitis, and diarrhea. Alcohol also interferes with the metabolism of vitamin B_6 and folate, which can result in neurological abnormalities and anemia, respectively.

Nutritional therapy involves abstinence from alcohol and provision of adequate nutrients. Intake may be affected by symptoms mentioned previously, as well as by the palatability of the diet provided in a hospital setting [9]. Restrictions on protein and sodium may be initiated; however, protein restriction is not recommended unless a patient has chronic protein-induced encephalopathy [9]. For those patients unable to take adequate nutrition, the initiation of supplemental feedings is recommended.

2. VIRAL HEPATITIS

Viral hepatitis is an inflammation of the liver secondary to direct or indirect damage due to viral infection, including but not limited to hepatitis A, B, C, D, and E; Epstein-Barr virus; and cytomegalovirus. Viral hepatitis can result in acute and chronic disease states. Chronic hepatitis is defined by hepatic inflammation that persists for greater than 6 months in combination with abnormally elevated liver enzymes. The severity of chronic hepatitis ranges from elevated liver enzymes without other symptoms to hepatic failure.

Hepatitis A virus is usually transmitted via a fecal–oral pathway from contaminated water or food. Nausea, vomiting, anorexia, and abdominal pain may occur, thereby placing the patient at risk for inadequate nutritional intake. Hepatitis A causes acute hepatitis without subsequent chronic disease or carrier state.

Hepatitis B virus is transmitted through the exchange of blood or other body fluids. This virus can cause acute or chronic hepatitis, cirrhosis, hepatic failure, or a carrier state. Hepatitis D virus occurs only in the presence of hepatitis B and is therefore thought to be transmitted via similar routes. Hepatitis D can present as a coinfection with hepatitis B or as a superimposed infection in a patient who is a viral hepatitis B carrier. Patients may become carriers of D virus, have acute and chronic disease, or present with fulminant hepatic failure.

Hepatitis C virus is transmitted via blood and blood products. Hepatitis C virus can also cause acute or chronic hepatitis, cirrhosis, or a carrier state. Hepatitis E virus may be transmitted via a fecal–oral pathway from contaminated water and may only cause acute infection. Non-A, non-B hepatitis is transmitted via contaminated water and transfusions. It can cause acute and chronic hepatitis, fulminant hepatic failure, or a carrier state.

Epstein-Barr virus causes infectious mononucleosis, and hepatitis is often a symptom of this disease. The hepatitis usually resolves without progression. Cytomegalovirus is usually asymptomatic in adults but children often are affected by complications. Transmission can occur during delivery from mother to infant or later to the infant via breast milk. Transfusions have also been indicated in transmission of this virus. It can cause jaundice and hepatitis in the newborn; however, progression to cirrhosis is uncommon.

Medically, the treatment goal is to reduce hepatic inflammation using steroids or antiviral drugs if needed. Patients with end-stage liver disease due to hepatitis B virus or hepatitis C virus may be candidates for liver transplant; however, reccurence of the virus is common [32]. Nutritionally, provision of adequate intake for all stages is the primary goal because symptoms may predispose patients to decreasing intake. Patients with chronic hepatitis are more at risk for developing malnutrition due to long-term inadequate intake and hepatic dysfunction. Cirrhosis may develop and cause cholestasis, which occurs when bile flow is obstructed and bile salts accumulate in the liver. As previously discussed, malabsorption occurs with the potential for the development of malnutrition. Chronic hepatitis may also lead to portal hypertension and ascites. Ascites can cause early satiety in patients, thereby decreasing nutritional intake. Sodium-restricted diets are often initiated for patients with ascites in an effort to decrease fluid retention, and sodium restriction may decrease the palability of the diet, further reducing intake [9].

Fulminant hepatic failure and occasionally chronic hepatitis result in hepatic encephalopathy. This is a state in which plasma ammonia levels are elevated, plasma branched-chain amino acids are decreased, and plasma aromatic amino acids are elevated. Nutritional goals in hepatic encephalopathy include provision of adequate energy to prevent catabolism and provision of sufficient protein for positive nitrogen balance. Patients with hepatic encephalopathy as a result of fulminant hepatic failure may better tolerate branched-chain amino acids as a source of protein; however, the majority of cirrhotic patients with hepatic encephalopathy can tolerate normal levels of standard protein [9].

3. AUTOIMMUNE HEPATITIS

Autoimmune hepatitis is an inflammation of the liver with unknown etiology. It is defined by the presence of periportal hepatitis, elevated gammaglobulin levels, and autoantibodies, and on the exclusion of viral hepatitis and other hepatic disorders [33]. Autoimmune hepatitis typically presents in young women and its etiology is unknown. Symptoms may include nausea, vomiting, jaundice, fatigue, and hepatomegaly. Weight loss is not a common finding. Treatment involves the use of prednisone and azathioprine. Long-term side effects of prednisone in children include stunting, and in adults, osteopenia. Supplementation with calcium and vitamin D is recommended. Liver transplantation is considered

for patients who have failed medical therapy; however, the disease may recur after transplant [34, 35].

4. NONALCOHOLIC STEATOHEPATITIS

Nonalcoholic steatohepatitis is a disease that presents with similar features of alcoholic liver disease in patients who are not alcoholics. Patients are commonly obese females who have hyperlipidemia and hyperglycemia [36, 37]. Symptoms may include fatigue, abdominal pain, and hepatomegaly. Nutritional therapy focuses on weight loss and control of hyperlipidemia and hyperglycemia. Unfortunately, improvement of nutritional status may not affect progression of the disease.

5. PREGNANCY-RELATED HEPATIC DISORDERS

Intrahepatic cholestasis of pregnancy usually presents later in pregnancy with pruritis and increased levels of bile acid [38]. Steatorrhea as a result of cholestasis may, as previously discussed, lead to malabsorption. Maternal long-term health is not affected by intrahepatic cholestasis of pregnancy and the disease usually resolves after delivery. Conversely, intrahepatic cholestasis of pregnancy appears to cause increased risk of prematurity, fetal distress, and stillbirths [38, 39]. Nutritional goals are aimed at providing sufficient energy to promote growth and development of the fetus and at preventing fat-soluble vitamin deficiencies.

Liver disease often occurs as a complication of preeclampsia, which is diagnosed by the presence of hypertension and proteinuria. A related entity is the HELLP syndrome, characterized by hemolysis, elevated liver enzymes, and low platelets. Symptoms include nausea, vomiting, and fatigue. Management includes close monitoring of the mother and fetus and provision of adequate nutrition; however, preeclampsia may prevent fetal growth secondary to hypertension-induced placental damage [40, 41]. This syndrome can progress to a fatal outcome as a result of a spontaneous rupture of the liver.

Acute fatty liver of pregnancy occurs during the third trimester and patients may present with nausea, vomiting, ascites, hypoglycemia, preeclampsia, coagulopathy, and encephalopathy. Hepatic failure can lead to maternal and fetal death, therefore early diagnosis and subsequent delivery are imperative. Complete recovery is expected after delivery [42].

6. NEONATAL HEPATITIS

Neonatal hepatitis is a cholestatic disease for which all other known causes of cholestasis, including infectious, metabolic, genetic, and toxic, have been ruled out. Patients present with hyperbilirubinemia and many present with hepatosplenomegaly and failure to thrive. Cholestasis is a result of decreased bile flow and the accumulation of substances normally excreted in bile. The decreased availability of bile in the intestines can lead to growth failure because bile is needed for the formation of micelles, which aid in the

absorption of long-chain triglycerides. Treatment for growth failure includes administration of medium-chain triglycerides, which are absorbed directly into the portal vein without the aid of bile. Medium-chain triglyceride oil does not contain linoleic acid nor does it carry fat-soluble vitamins, so a source of essential fatty acids must be supplemented. Two to 4% of total energy intake from a source of essential fatty acids is recommended to prevent a deficiency [43].

7. GENETIC DEFECTS IN BILE ACID METABOLISM

Cholestasis and chronic degeneration of the liver can occur in patients with genetic defects in bile acid metabolism. Enzyme deficiencies result in an inability to produce primary bile acids, which leads to the accumulation of toxic intermediaries in the pathway producing bile acids. Medical treatment includes attempted inhibition of bile production and stimulation of bile secretion to decrease toxin accumulation. Nutritional therapy includes use of medium-chain triglyceride oil and supplementation of essential fatty acids, if needed.

8. METABOLIC LIVER DISEASE

a. Glycogen Storage Diseases.
Glycogen is the primary storage form of glucose, and patients with glycogen storage diseases have deficiencies of various enzymes involved in the metabolism of glycogen. There are at least 12 different types of glycogen storage disease but only three predominantly involve the liver.

Glycogen storage disease I (von Gierke's disease) is the most common and is due to inadequate glucose-6-phosphatase activity. This enzyme hydrolyzes glucose-6-phosphate to produce free glucose. Infants present with hypoglycemia, hepatomegaly, and growth failure. Hypoglycemia occurs in the fasting state because glycogen cannot be converted to glucose. Hyperlipidemia, lactic acidemia, and metabolic acidosis occur in many patients as well.

Nutritionally, the goal is to provide an almost continuous supply of glucose to prevent hypoglycemia. Infants and young children with glycogen storage disease I require frequent (every 2–3 hours) daytime feedings and continuous feeds overnight. The provision of a fructose- or galactose-free formula for infants may be beneficial because these sugars are converted to glucose-6-phosphate [44]. Older children and adults can include cornstarch with meals to avoid frequent feedings. Cornstarch, highly branched chains of glucose, is slowly broken down into glucose and provides a steady supply of glucose to the body during fasting periods. Glycogen storage disease I does not normally result in hepatic failure or cirrhosis; however, hepatic adenomas develop in many patients. Glycogen storage disease I is an indication for liver transplant and does not appear to recur in patients with transplants [45–48].

Glycogen storage disease III (Forbes' disease) is a deficiency of amylo-1,6-glucosidase glycogen debranching enzyme, which leads to glycogen accumulation and decreased glucose release. Patients present with hypoglycemia, hepatomegaly, and growth failure and may have muscle weakness and myopathy. This disease is less severe than glycogen storage disease I in that gluconeogenesis can occur via other pathways; however, glycogen storage disease III may eventually progress to fibrosis and cirrhosis. Some patients may need cornstarch therapy for better glycemic control, but in general, a high-protein, low-carbohydrate diet is recommended [49, 50]. This will provide usable substrates for gluconeogenesis and will decrease the storage of glycogen. The presence of cirrhosis may indicate a need for liver transplantation, which corrects the metabolic disorder [51, 52].

Glycogen storage disease IV (Andersen's disease) is a deficiency of the branching enzyme 1,4-glucan-6-glycosyltransferase (amylopectinosis) in which glycogen and amylopectin accumulate in the liver and other organs. Hypoglycemia is not common, but symptoms include hepatomegaly, growth failure, and hypotonia. Glycogen storage disease IV commonly progresses to cirrhosis. Appropriate dietary therapy is unclear, and both high-carbohydrate and high-protein diets have been suggested [50]. Liver transplantation has been performed successfully in patients with glycogen storage disease IV [45].

b. Tyrosinemia.
Tyrosinemia is caused by a deficiency of fumarylacetoacetate hydrolase, an enzyme in the tyrosine degradation pathway. Metabolic intermediaries that accumulate in this disease are toxic. Infants may present with vomiting, cirrhosis, ascites, hypophosphatemic rickets, and coagulopathy. Older patients may experience renal and neurological involvement.

Nutritional therapy consists mainly of restriction of tyrosine and phenylalanine to prevent accumulation of toxic intermediaries. Sufficient energy is required to prevent catabolism and promote growth. A high-carbohydrate, low-protein diet is recommended; however, appropriate dietary management does not slow the progression of liver disease [53, 54]. Liver transplantation corrects the enzyme deficiency and can reverse any renal or neurological damage [48, 53–58].

c. Urea Cycle Defects.
Urea cycle defects are a result of absolute or relative deficiencies in enzymes required for protein degradation. These defects can result in hyperammonemia with intake of protein, which may be exacerbated by metabolic stress. Infants present with vomiting, respiratory distress, lethargy, and coma secondary to hyperammonemia. Permanent damage to the nervous system occurs if hyperammonemia persists.

Treatment includes reducing ammonia levels with drugs and alteration of diet. In the acute stage when ammonia levels are high, the goal is to reduce those levels. Tube feedings with minimal protein, high energy, and additional arginine are recommended. If unable to feed enterally, parenteral nutrition without amino acids should be initiated. Amino acids or protein can be reintroduced slowly after ammonia levels have decreased.

Chronically, therapy is aimed at maintaining levels of ammonia less than 50 μmol and to provide sufficient protein for growth and development. A low-protein diet, in addition to sodium benzoate, which increases excretion of nitrogen, are standard therapies. Supplementation with arginine, a conditionally essential amino acid, is necessary except in patients with arginase deficiency because it also increases excretion of nitrogen [59–61]. Liver transplantation has been successfully performed in patients with urea cycle disorders [62].

d. Byler's Syndrome. Byler's syndrome, also known as progressive familial intrahepatic cholestasis, is a disease in which there is apparently a defect in the canicular secretion of bile acids. These children have normal synthesis of bile acids but a decreased bile acid secretion in bile [63]. The accumulation in the liver of the bile acids is hepatotoxic. Cholestasis, pruritis, and failure to thrive in the first few months of life are typical presentations of this disease. Rickets may develop as a result of steatorrhea secondary to decreased bile acids. Fibrosis, cirrhosis, and hepatic failure develop in most patients. If cirrhosis has not developed, surgical therapy may be considered. A partial biliary diversion allows bile to drain into a stoma and can improve symptoms [64, 65]; however, liver transplant is needed if cirrhosis develops. Recurrence of Byler's disease post-transplant has not been reported [66, 67].

e. Cystic Fibrosis. Cystic fibrosis is a multisystem disease caused by altered sodium chloride transport through certain endothelial-lined organ systems, including the lungs, pancreas, and hepatobiliary system. Dysfunction of the hepatobiliary system can occur when thickened secretions cause obstructions. Many patients with cystic fibrosis can present with hepatobiliary complications including fatty liver, cirrhosis, cholelithiasis, common bile duct stenosis, portal hypertension, and hepatic failure [68, 69]. Decreased bile acids in the intestines will compound the malabsorption that is frequently associated with pancreatic deficiencies. Pancreatic enzymes are given as standard therapy for patients with cystic fibrosis and pancreatic dysfunction; however, the enzymes may not be as effective for patients with decreased bile flow. In the event of liver failure, transplantation is an option for patients with stable pulmonary function [70–73]. Cystic fibrosis is discussed in more detail in Chapter 45.

f. Wilson's Disease. In Wilson's disease, copper metabolism is disrupted, resulting in accumulation of copper in the liver, brain, and kidneys. The mechanism of accumulation is unknown, but it is suggested that it is a result of a decrease in the amount of copper excreted in bile. Wilson's disease usually presents after the first few years of life as acute or chronic hepatitis. Cholestasis, cirrhosis, or liver failure may also occur along with neurological and psychiatric symptoms.

A copper chelating drug, D-penicillamine, is the major therapy for this disease; however, a low-copper diet is also recommended. Foods with high copper levels such as shellfish, legumes, nuts, mushrooms, chocolate, and liver should be avoided.

If the disease progresses to liver failure, transplantation is recommended. Liver transplant has been performed successfully with post-transplant improvement in metabolic and neurological symptoms [67, 74–78].

g. Galactosemia. Galactosemia is an inherited disorder of galactose metabolism in which there is a deficiency of galactose-1-phosphate uridyltransferase. Galactose-1-phosphate accumulates in the liver and other organs and can cause end-stage liver disease and death if not treated. Newborns present with vomiting, diarrhea, growth failure, cataracts, and cholestasis when fed formulas containing galactose or lactose. Lactose, the predominant carbohydrate in mammalian milk, is a disaccharide formed from glucose and galactose. Treatment includes eliminating galactose from the diet. If galactose is excluded early enough, acute symptoms may resolve and long-term complications may be avoided.

h. Hereditary Fructose Intolerance. Hereditary fructose intolerance is the result of a deficiency of the enzyme fructose-1-phosphate aldolase, which causes fructose-1-phosphate to accumulate in the liver. Fructose-1-phosphate is a competitive inhibitor of phosphorylase, an enzyme that regulates the conversion of glycogen to glucose. With high levels of fructose-1-phosphate, the conversion of glycogen to glucose is decreased, resulting in lactic acidosis and hypoglycemia, which may precipitate seizures. Infants with hereditary fructose intolerance present with vomiting, diarrhea, cholestasis, and hepatomegaly. Excluding fructose and sucrose (the disaccharide of glucose and fructose) from the diet is standard treatment. Early treatment results in resolution of symptoms with a normal life expectancy.

i. Alagille Syndrome. Alagille syndrome is defined in part by the decreased number of interlobular (intrahepatic) bile ducts found in the liver. Patients typically present with congenital heart disease, bone defects, opthalmologic defect, distinct facial features, chronic cholestasis, pruritis, hypercholesterolemia, and xanthomas. Fat and fat-soluble vitamin malabsorption often occurs, which can lead to growth failure. The use of formulas containing medium-chain triglyceride oil may be required in addition to vitamin supplementation. The severity of fat malabsorption may necessitate supplemental tube feedings for infants or older children to provide sufficient energy to meet nutritional needs. Liver transplantation is an option for children who progress to end-stage liver disease [56, 79].

B. Biliary Tract

1. BILIARY ATRESIA

Biliary atresia results from a progressive degeneration of the biliary tract. The destruction results in obstructed bile flow, which leads to cholestasis, fibrosis, and cirrhosis. Sur-

gical therapy consists of a Kasai procedure (hepatic portoenterostomy), in which there is a direct anastamosis of the liver with the small intestines in the hopes of creating an alternative path for bile drainage. This should be done soon after diagnosis, around 6–8 weeks of age, prior to development of advanced fibrosis. Biliary atresia is the leading cause of liver transplant in children [56, 80]. Transplant is standard therapy for patients in which the Kasai procedure has failed [80, 81].

Biliary atresia results in decreased intraluminal bile acids, which leads to fat and fat-soluble malabsorption. Nutritional therapy includes infant formulas containing medium-chain triglyceride oils to optimize fatty acid absorption and, if needed, supplemental feeds to provide sufficient energy for growth. Maintenance of nutritional status is of utmost importance for patients awaiting liver transplantation [82, 83].

2. CHOLEDOCHAL CYSTS

Choledochal cysts are formed by dilatation of the common bile duct and if untreated may result in biliary obstruction and cirrhosis. Infants can present with jaundice, vomiting, and acholic stools. Older patients may present with jaundice, abdominal pain, and abdominal mass. Definitive therapy is surgical, and complete excision of the cyst is recommended, both to prevent biliary cirrhosis and because the cyst is premalignant.

3. PRIMARY SCLEROSING CHOLANGITIS

Primary sclerosing cholangitis is characterized by inflammation and progressive destruction of the biliary tract. Patients may present with abdominal pain, jaundice, pruritis, steatorrhea, and hepatomegaly. The majority of patients with primary sclerosing cholangitis also have inflammatory bowel disease [84, 85]. Primary sclerosing cholangitis progresses despite medical therapy and liver transplantation is usually indicated [81, 86]; however, primary sclerosing cholangitis may recur after transplant [35].

4. CHOLEDOCHOLITHIASIS

Choledocholithiasis occurs when gallstones obstruct the common bile duct. Obstruction of the flow of bile results in malabsorption of fat and fat-soluble vitamins and can result in cholecystitis and secondary biliary cirrhosis if untreated.

5. PRIMARY BILIARY CIRRHOSIS

Primary biliary cirrhosis is a chronic degenerative liver disease found predominantly in middle-aged women. The etiology of primary biliary cirrhosis is unknown, but it has been suggested that it may be secondary to an autoimmune process [87]. Thus, an inflammatory process causes gradual destruction of bile ducts, which leads to fibrosis and then cirrhosis. With progressive destruction of the bile ducts, there is a decrease in the secretion of bile into the intestinal lumen. This decrease, as mentioned previously, can result in fat and fat-soluble vitamin malabsorption. Other symptoms

TABLE 1   Evaluation of Nutritional Assessment Parameters in Childhood Liver Disease

	Valuable	Misleading
Body weight		X
Height	X	
Upper extremity anthropometrics	X	
Lower extremity anthropometrics		X
Plasma proteins		X
Nitrogen balance studies		X
Creatinine–height index		X
Immune status		X
Subjective assessment	X	
24-hour dietary recall	X	

Source: Reprinted from Novy, M. A., and Schwarz, K. B. (1997). Nutritional considerations and management of the child with liver disease. *Nutrition* **13(3)** 177–184, with permission from Elsevier Science.

of primary biliary cirrhosis include fatigue, osteopenia, pruritis, hypercholesterolemia, and hyperlipidemia. Patients may be asymptomatic for years; however, most patients experience a slow progression of the disease with gradual development of symptoms [88, 89]. There is some evidence that resting metabolic rate increases as the disease progresses [90]. The use of medium-chain triglyceride oil can improve nutritional status when fat malabsorption is present [91]. Fat-soluble vitamin supplementation may be required to prevent deficiencies. Liver transplantation is an option for patients with advanced primary biliary cirrhosis; however, primary biliary cirrhosis may recur after transplant [35, 92–95].

IV. NUTRITIONAL MANAGEMENT OF LIVER DISEASES

A. Assessment of Nutritional Status

Consistent and careful monitoring of nutritional status is necessary to identify and treat malnutrition. However, this monitoring can be challenging, because many parameters routinely used for assessment are affected by the liver disease itself (Table 1). Body weight may be elevated due to the fluid retention of ascites, edema, and hepatosplenomegaly, whether or not these symptoms are appreciable [96, 97]. True body weight decreases, therefore, may not be evident [98]. A better parameter for assessment in children may be height, because a reduced height for age can be indicative of chronic malnutrition [99]. However, use of height may be misleading because liver disease can affect skeletal development resulting in baseline short stature [96, 100].

Some of the more accurate parameters for assessment may be triceps skinfold and arm muscle and fat measurements, despite the possible existence of unappreciable edema

[96]. The upper extremities are less prone to fluid accumulation, and measurements may be more accurate if done regularly by the same person.

Visceral proteins, including albumin, transferrin, prealbumin, and retinol-binding protein, are typically used to assess nutritional status because they are synthesized in the liver. Alterations in serum levels can occur with liver disease as a result of malnutrition or as a result of decreased hepatic function [101, 102]. Albumin synthesis may be preserved until end-stage liver disease [12], but synthesis will be affected by inadequate protein intake [7].

Nitrogen balance, measured using 24-hour urine collection and diet recall, can be inaccurate due to inability of the liver to detoxify ammonia, which results in decreased production of urea secondary to hepatic dysfunction. A creatinine–height index may be useful in assessing muscle mass if renal function is normal [103].

Cell-mediated immunity as a marker for nutritional status is assessed using the total lymphocyte count and delayed cutaneous hypersensitivity [104, 105]. However, total lymphocyte count can be decreased and hypersensitivity tests can be abnormal in patients with liver disease [106].

Subjective global assessment, if combined with diet history, calorie intake records, physical examination with assessment for vitamin deficiencies, and arm anthropometric measurements may be the most useful method of determining malnutrition in patients with liver disease [106, 107].

B. Acute Liver Failure

Nutritional management of acute liver disease, assuming normal nutritional status prior to the injury, is primarily supportive. Malnutrition does not normally develop; therefore, maintenance of current nutritional status is the focus. Provision of the Recommended Dietary Allowances (RDA) for energy and protein should be adequate in most cases. Fulminant hepatic failure is an exception, because hepatic encephalopathy with hyperammonemia makes nutritional management more challenging. The provision of adequate protein to prevent catabolism is the goal, and recommended protein amounts for infants and adults are 1.0–1.5 g/kg/day [7, 108]. Protein recommendations for children and teenagers are 0.5–1.0 g/kg/day [7]. If standard protein intake worsens the encephalopathy, it may be necessary, in addition to medical therapy, to utilize branched-chain amino acid administration to provide sufficient protein. Vegetable protein is another alternative that is sometimes better tolerated; however, intake of adequate protein is difficult due to the volume of foods that must be consumed to meet needs. Energy recommendations for adults range from 25 to 35 kcal/kg/day with all stages of encephalopathy [108]. For children, at least the RDA level for energy should be provided, with higher amounts given as needed to prevent hypoglycemia and protein catabolism [7]. Ideal body weight or dry weight should be used in determining energy and protein needs when fluid overload is evident or suspected. Maintenance of nutritional status and prevention of deterioration are important aspects of the supportive care given to patients with fulminant hepatic failure as transplantation may be the only option for many patients.

C. Chronic Liver Diseases

1. CHOLESTATIC LIVER DISEASE

Nutritional goals of chronic liver disease are to provide adequate energy and protein to prevent energy deficit and protein catabolism and to promote regeneration of hepatic cells [109]. Infants and children with cholestatic liver disease require at least 125–150% of the RDA for adequate energy intake, and adults with cholestatic liver disease may also have increased energy requirements [43, 90, 96, 110, 111]. Infants need at least 3 g/kg/day of protein [43], while the minimum protein intake for children and adults should be the RDA level for age. For both children and adults, energy from fat is often provided in the form of medium-chain triglyceride oil to optimize absorption [91, 112, 113]. As previously mentioned, medium-chain triglyceride oil does not contain linoleic acid or transport fat-soluble vitamins, so a source of essential fatty acids must be supplemented. Two to 4% of total energy intake from a source of essential fatty acids is generally needed to prevent deficiency [43].

Supplementation of water-miscible fat-soluble vitamins is standard therapy for patients with cholestatic disease; however, close monitoring of serum levels is needed to prevent toxicity. Doses for correcting deficiencies will vary, but, in general, children should receive 5000–25,000 IU vitamin A/day, 3–5 µg 25-hydroxyvitamin D/kg/day, 15–25 IU vitamin E/day given as alpha tocopherol polyethylene glycol-succinate, and 2–5 mg vitamin K twice a week [114]. Supplements of calcium and phosphorus may also be indicated using 25–100 mg/kg/day of elemental calcium and 25–50 mg/kg/day of phosphorus [114]. Copper and manganese are excreted by the liver in bile; therefore, supplementation should be avoided in cholestatic patients.

For adults with cholestatic liver disease and deficiencies, supplementation with 5000–25,000 IU vitamin A/day and 5–10 mg/day of oral vitamin K are recommended [114a]. An intake of 1000–1500 mg calcium/day, and, in patients with deficiencies, 400 IU of vitamin D/day is recommended to help prevent osteoporosis [115]. Zinc, selenium, and iron should be supplemented if deficiencies are found [116].

Sodium and fluid restrictions may be necessary if ascites and edema are problematic, and this often decreases the palability and therefore the intake of the diet. If patients are unable to consume adequate energy and protein by mouth, supplemental enteral feedings are beneficial [117–120]. Providing enteral feedings at night and allowing patients to eat during the day is one option that can help meet estimated nutritional needs. If patients are unable to eat or are eating poorly, bolus feeds can be given at meal times or after at-

tempts to eat. Patients with ascites or severe glycemic changes may benefit from continuous feedings to decrease the sensation of fullness and better maintain blood glucose levels.

2. ANICTERIC CIRRHOTIC LIVER DISEASE

Patients with noncholestatic liver disease should not be supplemented with vitamins or minerals unless a deficiency has been documented. Sodium and fluid restrictions may be necessary, with the potential for a resultant decrease in dietary intake, as mentioned above.

D. End-Stage Liver Disease

Cirrhosis is the end stage of liver disease, and almost all liver diseases may potentially progress to this stage. Cirrhosis can be stable or unstable, with varying presentations. Energy and protein recommendations for adults with uncomplicated cirrhosis are 25–30 kcal/kg/day and 0.8 g protein/kg/day [9, 108]. Adults with complicated cirrhosis require 25–35 kcal/kg/day and 1.0–1.2 g protein/kg/day [9, 108]. Infants and children with end-stage liver disease need an estimated 150% of the RDA for energy and at least 3 g protein/kg/day [43, 111, 121].

Fat-soluble vitamin deficiencies should be identified prior to supplementation in patients with noncholestatic liver disease [9]. Water-soluble vitamin deficiencies are common in patients with alcoholic liver disease and may be present in patients with other liver diseases as a result of malabsorption or hepatic dysfunction. Supplementation of these vitamins is recommended to correct the deficiency.

Hepatic encephalopathy may occur in patients with end-stage liver disease and some patients may benefit from supplementation with branched-chain amino acids [122, 123]. Formulas with branched-chain amino acids may be more beneficial than partially hydrolyzed protein in improving nutritional status of children with end-stage liver disease [116]. However, for both children and adults, standard protein formulations are appropriate unless a patient is protein intolerant [9, 121].

V. PREPARATION FOR LIVER TRANSPLANT

Indications for liver transplant include fulminant hepatic failure, progressive hepatic degenerative diseases, metabolic diseases, and end-stage liver disease. Several surgical options are available for transplant candidates. Orthotopic whole-organ liver transplant is possible when the donor organ is size compatible with the recipient. Split-liver transplants allow for two patients to receive reduced-sized grafts. Living-related transplants involve transplanting the donor's left lateral segment, often to a small child [56, 67, 80, 124, 125].

Patients awaiting liver transplantation are often malnourished as a result of the many disease conditions previously discussed. Improving nutritional status prior to transplant is imperative because malnutrition affects morbidity and mortality post-transplant [124, 126–129]. Identification of degree of malnutrition is useful in determining aggressiveness of nutritional support [99]; however, as previously discussed, parameters of assessing nutritional status are affected by the liver disease itself and limitations must be recognized [97]. Optimal nutritional support may not completely reverse malnutrition prior to transplant [130], but can improve nutritional status [131]. Improvement of nutritional status may improve immune system response and decrease the possibility of pre- and post-transplant infections and complications [98].

Post-transplant nutritional support may also be necessary to reverse malnutrition or continue pre-transplant improvement of nutritional status [121, 132]. Studies have shown that children do exhibit catch-up growth post-transplantation, yet linear growth resumes at a slower rate [130, 132–135]. In addition to increased survival, post-transplant quality of life improves in comparison to life pre-transplant [136, 137].

VI. SUMMARY AND CONCLUSIONS

The liver is an important organ in the metabolism and utilization of all macro- and micronutrients. The presence of liver diseases can have a profound effect on nutritional status. Nutrition interventions play a key role in the overall management of liver diseases.

References

1. Shanbhogue, R. L., Bistrian, B. R., Jenkins, R. L., Jones, C., Benotti, P., and Blackburn, G. L. (1987). Resting energy expenditure in patients with end-stage liver disease and in normal population [see comments]. *J. Parenteral Enteral Nutr.* **11**, 305–308.
2. Schneeweiss, B., Graninger, W., Ferenci, P., Eichinger, S., Grimm, G., Schneider, B., Laggner, A. N., Lenz, K., and Kleinberger, G. (1990). Energy metabolism in patients with acute and chronic liver disease. *Hepatology* **11**, 387–393.
3. Morgan, M. Y., Milsom, J. P., and Sherlock, S. (1978). Plasma ratio of valine, leucine and isoleucine to phenylalanine and tyrosine in liver disease. *Gut* **19**, 1068–1073.
4. Weisdorf, S. A., Freese, D. K., Fath, J. J., Tsai, M. Y., and Cerra, F. B. (1987). Amino acid abnormalities in infants with extrahepatic biliary atresia and cirrhosis. *J. Pediatr. Gastroenterol. Nutr.* **6**, 860–864.
5. McCullough, A. J., and Tavill, A. S. (1991). Disordered energy and protein metabolism in liver disease. *Semin. Liver Dis.* **11**, 265–277.
6. Mendenhall, C. L., Moritz, T. E., Roselle, G. A., Morgan, T. R., Nemchausky, B. A., Tamburro, C. H., Schiff, E. R., McClain, C. J., Marsano, L. S., and Allen, J. I. (1995). Protein energy malnutrition in severe alcoholic hepatitis: Diagnosis

and response to treatment. The VA Cooperative Study Group #275. *J. Parenteral Enteral Nutr.* **19,** 258–265.

7. Novy, M. A., and Schwarz, K. B. (1997). Nutritional considerations and management of the child with liver disease. *Nutrition* **13,** 177–184.

8. Swart, G. R., van den Berg, J. W., Wattimena, J. L., Rietveld, T., van Vuure, J. K., and Frenkel, M. (1988). Elevated protein requirements in cirrhosis of the liver investigated by whole body protein turnover studies. *Clin. Sci.* **75,** 101–107.

9. McCullough, A. J., Teran, J. C., and Bugianesi, E. (1998). Guidelines for nutritional therapy in liver disease. *In* "The A.S.P.E.N. Nutrition Support Practice Manual" (R. Merritt, Ed.), pp. 12-1–12-12. American Society for Parenteral and Enteral Nutrition, Silver Spring, MD.

10. Muller, M. J., Pirlich, M., Balks, H. J., and Selberg, O. (1994). Glucose intolerance in liver cirrhosis: Role of hepatic and non-hepatic influences. *Eur. J. Clin. Chem. Clin. Biochem.* **32,** 749–758.

11. Owen, O. E., Reichle, F. A., Mozzoli, M. A., Kreulen, T., Patel, M. S., Elfenbein, I. B., Golsorkhi, M., Chang, K. H., Rao, N. S., Sue, H. S., and Boden, G. (1981). Hepatic, gut, and renal substrate flux rates in patients with hepatic cirrhosis. *J. Clin. Invest.* **68,** 240–252.

12. O'Keefe, S. J., Ogden, J., and Rund, J. (1989). The use of 14C labeled phenylalanine to trace deranged aromatic amino acid metabolism in liver failure: A functional indicator with prognostic potential [abstract]. *Gastroenterology* **96,** A641.

13. Pierro, A., Koletzko, B., Carnielli, V., Superina, R. A., Roberts, E. A., Filler, R. M., Smith, J., and Heim, T. (1989). Resting energy expenditure is increased in infants and children with extrahepatic biliary atresia. *J. Pediatr. Surg.* **24,** 534–538.

14. Blonde-Cynober, F., Aussel, C., and Cynober, L. (1999). Abnormalities in branched-chain amino acid metabolism in cirrhosis: Influence of hormonal and nutritional factors and directions for future research. *Clin. Nutr.* **18,** 5–13.

15. Morgan, T. R., Moritz, T. E., Mendenhall, C. L., and Haas, R. (1995). Protein consumption and hepatic encephalopathy in alcoholic hepatitis. VA Cooperative Study Group #275. *J. Am. College Nutr.* **14,** 152–158.

16. Owen, O. E., Trapp, V. E., Reichard, G. A., Jr., Mozzoli, M. A., Moctezuma, J., Paul, P., Skutches, C. L., and Boden, G. (1983). Nature and quantity of fuels consumed in patients with alcoholic cirrhosis. *J. Clin. Invest.* **72,** 1821–1832.

17. Kahn, A. M., Helwig, H. L., Redeker, A. G., and Reynolds, T. B. (1965). Urine and serum zinc abnormalities in disease of the liver. *Am. J. Clin. Pathol.* **44,** 426–435.

18. Hambidge, K. M., Krebs, N. F., Lilly, J. R., and Zerbe, G. O. (1987). Plasma and urine zinc in infants and children with extrahepatic biliary atresia. *J. Pediatr. Gastroenterol. Nutr.* **6,** 872–877.

19. McClain, C. J., Marsano, L., Burk, R. F., and Bacon, B. (1991). Trace metals in liver disease. *Semin. Liver Dis.* **11,** 321–339.

20. Aaseth, J., Thomassen, Y., Alexander, J., and Norheim, G. (1980). Decreased serum selenium in alcoholic cirrhosis [letter]. *N. Engl. J. Med.* **303,** 944–945.

21. Thuluvath, P. J., and Triger, D. R. (1992). Selenium in chronic liver disease. *J. Hepatol.* **14,** 176–182.

22. Bucuvalas, J. C., Heubi, J. E., Specker, B. L., Gregg, D. J., Yergey, A. L., and Vieira, N. E. (1990). Calcium absorption in bone disease associated with chronic cholestasis during childhood. *Hepatology* **12,** 1200–1205.

23. Wills, M. R., and Savory, J. (1984). Vitamin D metabolism and chronic liver disease. *Ann. Clin. Lab Sci.* **14,** 189–197.

24. Lieber, C. S. (1993). Herman Award Lecture, 1993: A personal perspective on alcohol, nutrition, and the liver. *Am. J. Clin. Nutr.* **58,** 430–442.

25. Leevy, C. M. (1962). Fatty liver: A study of 270 patients with biopsy proven fatty liver and a review of the literature. *Medicine* **41,** 249–278.

26. Mezey, E. (1993). Treatment of alcoholic liver disease. *Semin. Liver Dis.* **13,** 210–216.

27. Mezey, E. (1991). Interaction between alcohol and nutrition in the pathogenesis of alcoholic liver disease. *Semin. Liver Dis.* **11,** 340–348.

28. Lieber, C. S. (1988). The influence of alcohol on nutritional status. *Nutr. Rev.* **46,** 241–254.

29. Mendenhall, C., Bongiovanni, G., Goldberg, S., Miller, B., Moore, J., Rouster, S., Schneider, D., Tamburro, C., Tosch, T., and Weesner, R. (1985). VA Cooperative Study on Alcoholic Hepatitis. III: Changes in protein-calorie malnutrition associated with 30 days of hospitalization with and without enteral nutritional therapy. *J. Parenteral Enteral Nutr.* **9,** 590–596.

30. Jhangiani, S. S., Agarwal, N., Holmes, R., Cayten, C. G., and Pitchumoni, C. S. (1986). Energy expenditure in chronic alcoholics with and without liver disease. *Am. J. Clin. Nutr.* **44,** 323–329.

31. Mendenhall, C. L., Tosch, T., Weesner, R. E., Garcia-Pont, P., Goldberg, S. J., Kiernan, T., Seeff, L. B., Sorell, M., Tamburro, C., and Zetterman, R. (1986). VA Cooperative Study on Alcoholic Hepatitis. II: Prognostic significance of protein-calorie malnutrition. *Am. J. Clin. Nutr.* **43,** 213–218.

32. Dodson, S. F., Issa, S., and Bonham, A. (1999). Liver transplantation for chronic viral hepatitis. *Surg. Clin. N. Am.* **79,** 131–145.

33. Johnson, P. J., and McFarlane, I. G. (1993). Meeting report: International Autoimmune Hepatitis Group. *Hepatology* **18,** 998–1005.

34. Neuberger, J., Portmann, B., Calne, R., and Williams, R. (1984). Recurrence of autoimmune chronic active hepatitis following orthotopic liver grafting. *Transplantation* **37,** 363–365.

35. Balan, V., Abu-Elmagd, K., and Demetris, A. J. (1999). Autoimmune liver diseases. Recurrence after liver transplantation. *Surg. Clin. N. Am.* **79,** 147–152.

36. Powell, E. E., Cooksley, W. G., Hanson, R., Searle, J., Halliday, J. W., and Powell, L. W. (1990). The natural history of nonalcoholic steatohepatitis: A follow-up study of forty-two patients for up to 21 years. *Hepatology* **11,** 74–80.

37. Ludwig, J., Viggiano, T. R., McGill, D. B., and Oh, B. J. (1980). Nonalcoholic steatohepatitis: Mayo Clinic experiences with a hitherto unnamed disease. *Mayo Clin. Proc.* **55,** 434–438.

38. Reyes, H., and Simon, F. R. (1993). Intrahepatic cholestasis of pregnancy: An estrogen-related disease. *Semin. Liver Dis.* **13,** 289–301.

39. Davidson, K. M. (1998). Intrahepatic cholestasis of pregnancy. *Semin. Perinatol.* **22,** 104–111.
40. Shipp, T. D., and Wilkins-Haug, L. (1997). The association of early-onset fetal growth restriction, elevated maternal serum alpha-fetoprotein, and the development of severe preeclampsia. *Prenat. Diagn.* **17,** 305–309.
41. Odendaal, H. J., Pattinson, R. C., and Toit, R. D. (1987). Fetal and neonatal outcome in patients with severe pre-eclampsia before 34 weeks. *S. Afr. Med. J.* **71,** 555–558.
42. Bacq, Y. (1998). Acute fatty liver of pregnancy. *Semin. Perinatol.* **22,** 134–140.
43. Kaufman, S. S., Murray, N. D., Wood, R. P., Shaw, B. W., Jr., and Vanderhoof, J. A. (1987). Nutritional support for the infant with extrahepatic biliary atresia. *J. Pediatr.* **110,** 679–686.
44. Wiechmann, D. A., and Balistreri, W. F. (1998). Inherited metabolic disorders of the liver. *In* "Sleisenger and Fordtran's Gastrointestinal and Liver Disease" (M. Feldman *et al.,* Eds.), 6th ed., Vol. 2, pp. 1083–1097. W. B. Saunders Co., Philadelphia, PA.
45. Selby, R., Starzl, T. E., Yunis, E., Todo, S., Tzakis, A. G., Brown, B. I., and Kendall, R. S. (1993). Liver transplantation for type I and type IV glycogen storage disease. *Eur. J. Pediatr.* **152**(Suppl. 1), S71–S76.
46. Malatack, J. J., Finegold, D. N., Iwatsuki, S., Shaw, B. W., Jr., Gartner, J. C., Zitelli, B. J., Roe, T., and Starzl, T. E. (1983). Liver transplantation for type I glycogen storage disease. *Lancet* **1,** 1073–1075.
47. Sokal, E. M., Lopez-Silvarrey, A., Buts, J. P., and Otte, J. B. (1993). Orthotopic liver transplantation for type I glycogenosis unresponsive to medical therapy. *J. Pediatr. Gastroenterol. Nutr.* **16,** 465–467.
48. Martinez, I., V, Margarit, C., Tormo, R., Infante, D., Iglesias, J., Allende, H., Lloret, J., Jimenez, A., and Boix-Ochoa, J. (1987). Liver transplantation in metabolic diseases. Report of five pediatric cases. *Transplant. Proc.* **19,** 3803–3804.
49. Gremse, D. A., Bucuvalas, J. C., and Balistreri, W. F. (1990). Efficacy of cornstarch therapy in type III glycogen-storage disease. *Am. J. Clin. Nutr.* **52,** 671–674.
50. Goldberg, T., and Slonim, A. E. (1993). Nutrition therapy for hepatic glycogen storage diseases. *J. Am. Diet. Assoc.* **93,** 1423–1430.
51. Matern, D., Starzl, T. E., Arnaout, W., Barnard, J., Bynon, J. S., Dhawan, A., Emond, J., Haagsma, E. B., Hug, G., Lachaux, A., Smit, G. P., and Chen, Y. T. (1999). Liver transplantation for glycogen storage disease types I, III, and IV. *Eur. J. Pediatr.* **158**(Suppl. 2), S43–S48.
52. Haagsma, E. B., Smit, G. P., Niezen-Koning, K. E., Gouw, A. S., Meerman, L., and Slooff, M. J. (1997). Type IIIb glycogen storage disease associated with end-stage cirrhosis and hepatocellular carcinoma. The Liver Transplant Group. *Hepatology* **25,** 537–540.
53. Freese, D. K., Tuchman, M., Schwarzenberg, S. J., Sharp, H. L., Rank, J. M., Bloomer, J. R., Ascher, N. L., and Payne, W. D. (1991). Early liver transplantation is indicated for tyrosinemia type I. *J. Pediatr. Gastroenterol. Nutr.* **13,** 10–15.
54. Mieles, L. A., Esquivel, C. O., Van Thiel, D. H., Koneru, B., Makowka, L., Tzakis, A. G., and Starzl, T. E. (1990). Liver transplantation for tyrosinemia. A review of 10 cases from the University of Pittsburgh. *Dig. Dis. Sci.* **35,** 153–157.
55. Paradis, K., Weber, A., Seidman, E. G., Larochelle, J., Garel, L., Lenaerts, C., and Roy, C. C. (1990). Liver transplantation for hereditary tyrosinemia: The Quebec experience. *Am. J. Hum. Genet.* **47,** 338–342.
56. Rosenthal, P., Podesta, L., Sher, L., and Makowka, L. (1994). Liver transplantation in children. *Am. J. Gastroenterol.* **89,** 480–492.
57. Shoemaker, L. R., Strife, C. F., Balistreri, W. F., and Ryckman, F. C. (1992). Rapid improvement in the renal tubular dysfunction associated with tyrosinemia following hepatic replacement. *Pediatrics* **89,** 251–255.
58. Mohan, N., McKiernan, P., Preece, M. A., Green, A., Buckels, J., Mayer, A. D., and Kelly, D. A. (1999). Indications and outcome of liver transplantation in tyrosinaemia type 1. *Eur. J. Pediatr.* **158**(Suppl. 2), S49–S54.
59. Brusilow, S. W. (1984). Arginine, an indispensable amino acid for patients with inborn errors of urea synthesis. *J. Clin. Invest.* **74,** 2144–2148.
60. Brusilow, S. W., and Batshaw, M. L. (1979). Arginine therapy of argininosuccinase deficiency. *Lancet* **1,** 124–127.
61. Batshaw, M. L. (1984). Hyperammonemia. *Curr. Prob. Pediatr.* **14,** 1–69.
62. Saudubray, J. M., Touati, G., Delonlay, P., Jouvet, P., Narcy, C., Laurent, J., Rabier, D., Kamoun, P., Jan, D., and Revillon, Y. (1999). Liver transplantation in urea cycle disorders. *Eur. J. Pediatr.* **158**(Suppl. 2), S55–S59.
63. Jacquemin, E., Dumont, M., Bernard, O., Erlinger, S., and Hadchouel, M. (1994). Evidence for defective primary bile acid secretion in children with progressive familial intrahepatic cholestasis (Byler disease). *Eur. J. Pediatr.* **153,** 424–428.
64. Emond, J. C., and Whitington, P. F. (1995). Selective surgical management of progressive familial intrahepatic cholestasis (Byler's disease). *J. Pediatr. Surg.* **30,** 1635–1641.
65. Whitington, P. F., Freese, D. K., Alonso, E. M., Schwarzenberg, S. J., and Sharp, H. L. (1994). Clinical and biochemical findings in progressive familial intrahepatic cholestasis. *J. Pediatr. Gastroenterol. Nutr.* **18,** 134–141.
66. Soubrane, O., Gauthier, F., DeVictor, D., Bernard, O., Valayer, J., Houssin, D., and Chapuis, Y. (1990). Orthotopic liver transplantation for Byler disease. *Transplantation* **50,** 804–806.
67. Haberal, M., Buyukpamukcu, N., Bilgin, N., Telatar, H., Besim, A., Simsek, H., Arslan, G., Ekici, E., Velidedeoglu, E., and Cuhadaroglu, S. (1994). Segmental living related liver transplantation in pediatric patients. *Transplant. Proc.* **26,** 183–184.
68. Gaskin, K. J., Waters, D. L., Howman-Giles, R., de Silva, M., Earl, J. W., Martin, H. C., Kan, A. E., Brown, J. M., and Dorney, S. F. (1988). Liver disease and common-bile-duct stenosis in cystic fibrosis. *N. Engl. J. Med.* **318,** 340–346.
69. Weber, A. M., Roy, C. C., Morin, C. L., and Lasalle, R. (1973). Malabsorption of bile acids in children with cystic fibrosis. *N. Engl. J. Med.,* **289,** 1001–1005.
70. Couetil, J. P., Soubrane, O., Houssin, D. P., Dousset, B. E., Chevalier, P. G., Guinvarch, A., Loulmet, D., Achkar, A., and Carpentier, A. F. (1997). Combined heart-lung-liver, double lung-liver, and isolated liver transplantation for cystic fibrosis in children. *Transpl. Int.* **10,** 33–39.
71. Noble-Jamieson, G., Valente, J., Barnes, N. D., Friend, P. J., Jamieson, N. V., Rasmussen, A., and Calne, R. Y. (1994).

Liver transplantation for hepatic cirrhosis in cystic fibrosis. *Arch. Dis. Child.* **71,** 349–352.

72. Sharp, H. L. (1995). Cystic fibrosis liver disease and transplantation [editorial]. *J. Pediatr.* **127,** 944–946.

73. Mack, D. R., Traystman, M. D., Colombo, J. L., Sammut, P. H., Kaufman, S. S., Vanderhoof, J. A., Antonson, D. L., Markin, R. S., Shaw, B. W., Jr., and Langnas, A. N. (1995). Clinical denouement and mutation analysis of patients with cystic fibrosis undergoing liver transplantation for biliary cirrhosis. *J. Pediatr.* **127,** 881–887.

74. Bellary, S., Hassanein, T., and Van Thiel, D. H. (1995). Liver transplantation for Wilson's disease. *J. Hepatol.* **23,** 373–381.

75. Chen, C. L., Chen, Y. S., Lui, C. C., and Hsu, S. P. (1997). Neurological improvement of Wilson's disease after liver transplantation. *Transplant. Proc.* **29,** 497–498.

76. Diaz, J., Acosta, F., Canizares, F., Bueno, F. S., Tornel, P. L., Tovar, I., Contreras, R. F., Marquez, M., Martinez, P., and Parrilla, P. (1995). Does orthotopic liver transplantation normalize copper metabolism in patients with Wilson's disease? *Transplant. Proc.* **27,** 2306.

77. Khanna, A., Jain, A., Eghtesad, B., and Rakela, J. (1999). Liver transplantation for metabolic liver diseases. *Surg. Clin. N. Am.* **79,** 153–162.

78. Lui, C. C., Chen, C. L., Cheng, Y. F., and Lee, T. Y. (1998). Recovery of neurological deficits in a case of Wilson's disease after liver transplantation. *Transplant. Proc.* **30,** 3324–3325.

79. Marino, I. R., ChapChap, P., Esquivel, C. O., Zetti, G., Carone, E., Borland, L., Tzakis, A. G., Todo, S., Rowe, M. I., and Starzl, T. E. (1992). Liver transplantation for arteriohepatic dysplasia (Alagille's syndrome). *Transpl. Int.* **5,** 61–64.

80. Reyes, J., and Mazariegos, G. V. (1999). Pediatric transplantation. *Surg. Clin. N. Am.* **79,** 163–189.

81. Alagille, D. (1987). Liver transplantation in children—Indications in cholestatic states. *Transplant. Proc.* **19,** 3242–3248.

82. Cywes, C., and Millar, A. J. (1990). Assessment of the nutritional status of infants and children with biliary atresia. *S. Afr. Med. J.* **77,** 131–135.

83. Shiga, C., Ohi, R., Chiba, T., Nio, M., Endo, N., Mito, S., and Hino, M. (1997). Assessment of nutritional status of postoperative patients with biliary atresia. *Tohoku J. Exp. Med.* **181,** 217–223.

84. LaRusso, N. F., Wiesner, R. H., Ludwig, J., and MacCarty, R. L. (1984). Current concepts. Primary sclerosing cholangitis. *N. Engl. J. Med.* **310,** 899–903.

85. Lefkowitch, J. H. (1982). Primary sclerosing cholangitis. *Arch. Intern. Med.* **142,** 1157–1160.

86. Gordon, R. D., Shaw, B. W., Jr., Iwatsuki, S., Esquivel, C. O., and Starzl, T. E. (1986). Indications for liver transplantation in the cyclosporine era. *Surg. Clin. N. Am.* **66,** 541–556.

87. Heathcote, J. (1997). The clinical expression of primary biliary cirrhosis. *Semin. Liver Dis.* **17,** 23–33.

88. Metcalf, J. V., James, O. F., Palmer, J. M., Bassendine, M. F., Jones, D. E., and Mitchinson, H. C. (1996). True positive AMA and normal alkaline phosphatase: Is this primary biliary cirrhosis (PBC)—10 years on, the answer is yes [abstract]. *Gut* **38,** A634.

89. Mahl, T. C., Shockcor, W., and Boyer, J. L. (1994). Primary biliary cirrhosis: Survival of a large cohort of symptomatic and asymptomatic patients followed for 24 years. *J. Hepatol.* **20,** 707–713.

90. Green, J. H., Bramley, P. N., and Losowsky, M. S. (1991). Are patients with primary biliary cirrhosis hypermetabolic? A comparison between patients before and after liver transplantation and controls. *Hepatology* **14,** 464–472.

91. Ros, E., Garcia-Puges, A., Reixach, M., Cuso, E., and Rodes, J. (1984). Fat digestion and exocrine pancreatic function in primary biliary cirrhosis. *Gastroenterology* **87,** 180–187.

92. Haagsma, E. B. (1999). Clinical relevance of recurrence of primary biliary cirrhosis after liver transplantation. *Eur. J. Gastroenterol. Hepatol.* **11,** 639–642.

93. Portmann, B. C. (1999). Recurrence of primary biliary cirrhosis after transplantation. The pathologist's view. *Eur. J. Gastroenterol. Hepatol.* **11,** 633–637.

94. Neuberger, J., Portmann, B., Macdougall, B. R., Calne, R. Y., and Williams, R. (1982). Recurrence of primary biliary cirrhosis after liver transplantation. *N. Engl. J. Med.* **306,** 1–4.

95. Samuel, D., Gugenheim, J., Mentha, G., Castaing, D., Degos, F., Benhamou, J. P., and Bismuth, H. (1990). Liver transplantation for primary biliary cirrhosis. *Transplant. Proc.* **22,** 1497–1498.

96. Sokol, R. J., and Stall, C. (1990). Anthropometric evaluation of children with chronic liver disease. *Am. J. Clin. Nutr.* **52,** 203–208.

97. Hehir, D. J., Jenkins, R. L., Bistrian, B. R., and Blackburn, G. L. (1985). Nutrition in patients undergoing orthotopic liver transplant. *J. Parenteral Enteral Nutr.* **9,** 695–700.

98. Porayko, M. K., DiCecco, S., and O'Keefe, S. J. (1991). Impact of malnutrition and its therapy on liver transplantation. *Semin. Liver Dis.* **11,** 305–314.

99. Goulet, O. J., de Ville, D. G., Otte, J. B., and Ricour, C. (1987). Preoperative nutritional evaluation and support for liver transplantation in children. *Transplant. Proc.* **19,** 3249–3255.

100. Roggero, P., Cataliotti, E., Ulla, L., Stuflesser, S., Nebbia, G., Bracaloni, D., Lucianetti, A., and Gridelli, B. (1997). Factors influencing malnutrition in children waiting for liver transplants. *Am. J. Clin. Nutr.* **65,** 1852–1857.

101. Crawford, D. H., Cuneo, R. C., and Shepherd, R. W. (1993). Pathogenesis and assessment of malnutrition in liver disease. *J. Gastroenterol. Hepatol.* **8,** 89–94.

102. Carpentier, Y. A., Barthel, J., and Bruyns, J. (1982). Plasma protein concentration in nutritional assessment. *Proc. Nutr. Soc.* **41,** 405–417.

103. Pirlich, M., Selberg, O., Boker, K., Schwarze, M., and Muller, M. J. (1996). The creatinine approach to estimate skeletal muscle mass in patients with cirrhosis. *Hepatology* **24,** 1422–1427.

104. Dominioni, L., and Dionigi, R. (1987). Immunological function and nutritional assessment. *J. Parenteral Enteral Nutr.* **11,** 70S–72S.

105. O'Keefe, S. J., El Zayadi, A. R., Carraher, T. E., Davis, M., and Williams, R. (1980). Malnutrition and immuno-incompetence in patients with liver disease. *Lancet* **2,** 615–617.

106. Munoz, S. J. (1991). Nutritional therapies in liver disease. *Semin. Liver Dis.* **11,** 278–291.

107. Detsky, A. S., Baker, J. P., O'Rourke, K., Johnston, N., Whitwell, J., Mendelson, R. A., and Jeejeebhoy, K. N. (1987). Predicting nutrition-associated complications for patients undergoing gastrointestinal surgery. *J. Parenteral Enteral Nutr.* **11,** 440–446.

108. Plauth M., Merli, M., Kondrup, J., Weimann, A., Ferenci, P., and Muller, M. J. (1997). ESPEN guidelines for nutrition in liver disease and transplantation. *Clin. Nutr.* **16,** 43–55.

109. Diehl, A. M. (1991). Nutrition, hormones, metabolism, and liver regeneration. *Semin. Liver Dis.* **11,** 315–320.

110. Kondrup, J., and Muller, M. J. (1997). Energy and protein requirements of patients with chronic liver disease. *J. Hepatol.* **27,** 239–247.

111. Shetty, A. K., Schmidt-Sommerfeld, E., and Udall, J. N., Jr. (1999). Nutritional aspects of liver disease in children. *Nutrition* **15,** 727–729.

112. Beath, S., Johnson, T., Willis, I., Hooley, G., Brown, G., Booth, I. W., and Kelly, D. (1993). Superior absorption of medium-chain triacylglycerols compared with conventional dietary long-chain fats in children with chronic liver disease. *Proc. Nutr. Soc.* **52,** 253A.

113. Cohen, M. I., and Gartner, L. M. (1971). The use of medium-chain triglycerides in the management of biliary atresia. *J. Pediatr.* **79,** 379–384.

114. Sokol, R. J. (1987). Medical management of the infant or child with chronic liver disease. *Semin. Liver Dis.* **7,** 155–167.

114a. Wolfe, M. M. (2000). Primary sclerosing cholangitis. *In* "Therapy of Digestive Disorders: A Companion to Sleisenger and Fordtran's Gastrointestinal and Liver Disease (S. Cohen, G. L. Davis, R. A. Giannella, S. B. Hanauer, W. Silen, and P. P. Toskes, Eds.), 1st ed., pp. 219–226. W. B. Saunders Co., Philadelphia, PA.

115. Vleggaar, F. P., van Buuren, H. R., Wolfhagen, F. H., Schalm, S. W., and Pols, H. A. (1999). Prevention and treatment of osteoporosis in primary biliary cirrhosis. *Eur. J. Gastroenterol. Hepatol.* **11,** 617–621.

116. Chin, S. E., Shepherd, R. W., Thomas, B. J., Cleghorn, G. J., Patrick, M. K., Wilcox, J. A., Ong, T. H., Lynch, S. V., and Strong, R. (1992). The nature of malnutrition in children with end-stage liver disease awaiting orthotopic liver transplantation. *Am. J. Clin. Nutr.* **56,** 164–168.

117. Duche, M., Habes, D., Lababidi, A., Chardot, C., Wenz, J., and Bernard, O. (1999). Percutaneous endoscopic gastrostomy for continuous feeding in children with chronic cholestasis. *J. Pediatr. Gastroenterol. Nutr.* **29,** 42–45.

118. Holt, R. I., Miell, J. P., Jones, J. S., Mieli-Vergani, G., and Baker, A. J. (2000). Nasogastric feeding enhances nutritional status in paediatric liver disease but does not alter circulating levels of IGF-I and IGF binding proteins. *Clin. Endocrinol. (Oxf.)* **52,** 217–224.

119. Charlton, C. P., Buchanan, E., Holden, C. E., Preece, M. A., Green, A., Booth, I. W., and Tarlow, M. J. (1992). Intensive enteral feeding in advanced cirrhosis: Reversal of malnutrition without precipitation of hepatic encephalopathy. *Arch. Dis. Child.* **67,** 603–607.

120. Kearns, P. J., Young, H., Garcia, G., Blaschke, T., O'Hanlon, G., Rinki, M., Sucher, K., and Gregory, P. (1992). Nutritional therapy for alcoholic hepatitis: Are we there yet [abstract]? *Hepatology* **16,** 846.

121. Protheroe, S. M. (1998). Feeding the child with chronic liver disease. *Nutrition* **14,** 796–800.

122. O'Keefe, S. J., Ogden, J., and Dicker, J. (1987). Enteral and parenteral branched chain amino acid-supplemented nutritional support in patients with encephalopathy due to alcoholic liver disease. *J. Parenteral Enteral Nutr.* **11,** 447–453.

123. Marchesini, G., Dioguardi, F. S., Bianchi, G. P., Zoli, M., Bellati, G., Roffi, L., Martines, D., and Abbiati, R. (1990). Long-term oral branched-chain amino acid treatment in chronic hepatic encephalopathy. A randomized double-blind casein-controlled trial. The Italian Multicenter Study Group. *J. Hepatol.* **11,** 92–101.

124. Kelly, D. A. (1998). Current results and evolving indications for liver transplantation in children. *J. Pediatr. Gastroenterol. Nutr.* **27,** 214–221.

125. Alonso, M. H., and Ryckman, F. C. (1998). Current concepts in pediatric liver transplant. *Semin. Liver Dis.* **18,** 295–307.

126. Beath, S., Brook, G., Kelly, D., McMaster, P., Mayer, D., and Buckels, J. (1994). Improving outcome of liver transplantation in babies less than 1 year. *Transplant. Proc.* **26,** 180–182.

127. Halliday, A. W., Benjamin, I. S., and Blumgart, L. H. (1988). Nutritional risk factors in major hepatobiliary surgery. *J. Parenteral Enteral Nutr.* **12,** 43–48.

128. Shepherd, R. W., Chin, S. E., Cleghorn, G. J., Patrick, M., Ong, T. H., Lynch, S. V., Balderson, G., and Strong, R. (1991). Malnutrition in children with chronic liver disease accepted for liver transplantation: Clinical profile and effect on outcome. *J. Paediatr. Child Health* **27,** 295–299.

129. Moukarzel, A. A., Najm, I., Vargas, J., McDiarmid, S. V., Busuttil, R. W., and Ament, M. E. (1990). Effect of nutritional status on outcome of orthotopic liver transplantation in pediatric patients. *Transplant. Proc.* **22,** 1560–1563.

130. van Mourik, I. D., Beath, S. V., Brook, G. A., Cash, A. J., Mayer, A. D., Buckels, J. A., and Kelly, D. A. (2000). Long-term nutritional and neurodevelopmental outcome of liver transplantation in infants aged less than 12 months. *J. Pediatr. Gastroenterol. Nutr.* **30,** 269–275.

131. Chin, S. E., Shepherd, R. W., Cleghorn, G. J., Patrick, M., Ong, T. H., Wilcox, J., Lynch, S., and Strong, R. (1990). Preoperative nutritional support in children with end-stage liver disease accepted for liver transplantation: An approach to management. *J. Gastroenterol. Hepatol.* **,** **5,** 566–572.

132. Shepherd, R. W. (1996). Pre- and postoperative nutritional care in liver transplantation in children. *J. Gastroenterol. Hepatol.* **11,** S7–S10.

133. Rodeck, B., Melter, M., Hoyer, P. F., Ringe, B., and Brodehl, J. (1994). Growth in long-term survivors after orthotopic liver transplantation in childhood. *Transplant. Proc.* **26,** 165–166.

134. Sarna, S., Sipila, I., Jalanko, H., Laine, J., and Holmberg, C. (1994). Factors affecting growth after pediatric liver transplantation. *Transplant. Proc.* **26,** 161–164.

135. Holt, R. I., Broide, E., Buchanan, C. R., Miell, J. P., Baker, A. J., Mowat, A. P., and Mieli-Vergani, G. (1997). Orthotopic liver transplantation reverses the adverse nutritional changes of end-stage liver disease in children. *Am. J. Clin. Nutr.* **65,** 534–542.

136. Burdelski, M., Nolkemper, D., Ganschow, R., Sturm, E., Malago, M., Rogiers, X., and Brolsch, C. E. (1999). Liver transplantation in children: Long-term outcome and quality of life. *Eur. J. Pediatr.* **158**(Suppl. 2), S34–S42.

137. Zitelli, B. J., Gartner, J. C., Malatack, J. J., Urbach, A. H., Miller, J. W., Williams, L., Kirkpatrick, B., Breinig, M. K., and Ho, M. (1987). Pediatric liver transplantation: Patient evaluation and selection, infectious complications, and lifestyle after transplantation. *Transplant. Proc.* **19,** 3309–3316.

F. Other Major Diseases

CHAPTER **40**

Nutrition and Renal Disease

D. JORDI GOLDSTEIN[1] AND BETH McQUISTON[2]
[1]IVonyx, Inc., Reno, Nevada
[2]Park Ridge, Illinois

I. INTRODUCTION

Historically, nutrition science research in renal disease has been mainly directed toward determining if nutrients modulate progressive renal disease, influence metabolic abnormalities associated with established disease, and serve as a therapy for the nutritional consequences associated with chronic renal failure. While initially descriptive in nature, current studies are mechanistic in scope, providing insight as to how nutrients interact with cellular functions. These data allow a sophistication in understanding the interaction between nutrients and how they might modulate mechanisms of renal disease. Clinical research completed in the past decade has established a relationship between nutritional status and outcome (i.e., morbidity and mortality) in patients who require dialysis therapy. These data impact the clinical arena through increased attention to nutrition assessment, monitoring, and intervention as components of medical care.

It is the intent of this chapter to summarize the past and present nutrition science base underlying current nutrition recommendations and treatment for the patient with chronic renal insufficiency, the patient requiring renal replacement therapy, and care during post-transplantation.

II. CHRONIC RENAL FAILURE

As of 1997, there were 304,083 patients in the United States receiving treatment for end-stage renal disease (ESRD) [1]. The approximate rate of new growth for the period of 1992–1997 was 6% per year [2]. The financial burden for ESRD in 1997 by all payers was estimated at $15.64 billion, an increase from $14.55 billion in 1996 [2]. Chronic renal failure is a disease syndrome where progressive, irreversible losses of the excretory, endocrine, and metabolic capacities of the kidney occur due to kidney damage. The mechanisms as to how and why kidney disease progresses to end stage, even following treatment of the initial insult, continue to be studied. Examples of primary diseases leading to chronic renal failure include diabetes, hypertension, glomerulonephritis and cystic disease. The nature of the disease and the portion of the nephron that becomes damaged determines the symptoms, diagnosis, and treatment [3]. Chronic renal failure

(CRF) progresses slowly over time [4]. Once the disease progresses to end stage, continuance of life requires the initiation of renal replacement therapy or kidney transplantation.

Consideration of the role that certain nutrients might have in causing or contributing to progressive renal disease has been an active area of research for more than 20 years. In the study of a relationship between nutrients and progressive disease, dietary protein [5–9] has been the most extensively studied, and more recently fatty acids [10–12].

It has long been recognized in rats with experimental CRF that high-protein diets lead to increased proteinuria, mortality, and renal damage, whereas restriction of dietary protein results in improvement [4]. In humans, low-protein diets initiated early in chronic renal failure have been shown to ameliorate clinical uremic symptoms by decreasing the formation of nitrogenous compounds [13–15]. However, the beneficial effect of dietary protein restriction with or without ketoacid analogues or essential amino acid supplementation on human renal disease progression [13–20] has not been consistently reproducible [4, 8].

During the 1970s, implementation of dietary protein restriction as low as 0.3 grams of dietary protein per kilogram body weight per day (g/kg/day) with supplementation of ketoacid analogue or essential amino acid for the patient with chronic renal insufficiency was not uncommon [13–20]. The rationale for the use of these preparations was the observation that ammonium nitrogen derived from urea hydrolysis in the gut was capable of aminating the ketoacid analogue into essential amino acid that could then be used as protein by the body [13, 14, 16–19]. This not only exploits a valuable source of nitrogen [18], but permits daily essential amino acid requirements to be met despite the adherence to an almost nitrogen-free diet [19]. The advantage was to avoid the side effects of malnutrition, which were often observed in patients trying to adhere to a low-protein diet alone [13–15, 17]. However, these diets were difficult to adhere to and patients often became malnourished. The benefits of these diets had not been demonstrated, and there was no information related to how dietary protein restriction might be a beneficial intervention for the failing kidney.

In 1982, Brenner and colleagues [21] reported that ingestion of protein-rich meals in animals, and infusion of high amino acid nutrient solutions in humans, led to renal

hemodynamic changes indicative of increased renal workload. They observed elevated total renal blood flow, glomerular pressures, and glomerular filtration rate. This led to the hypothesis that high-protein diets increase renal workload and might be detrimental for the patient with chronic renal failure. The role of the renin-angiotensin system in modulating renal hemodynamics is now well established. There is increasing evidence that protein intake may alter the activity of the renin-angiotensin system and the renal production and urinary excretion of eicosanoids [5, 22]. Ongoing studies have determined that an increase in protein intake stimulates the secretion of several hormones including glucagon, vasopressin, eicosanoids, dopamine, and renin.

It has been postulated that renal progression may result from increased glomerular perfusion and elevated intraglomerular capillary pressures once a critical reduction in renal mass has occurred. In this hypothesis, global sclerosis causes diseased glomeruli to stop functioning. Remaining glomeruli undergo compensatory hyperperfusion, which results in intraglomerular hypertension leading to injury, progressive sclerosis, and total loss of glomeruli. How intraglomerular hypertension develops and modifies glomerular cell functions is not clear. In rats with subtotal nephrectomy, protein restriction has been found to suppress the early hemodynamic changes and minimize later glomerular changes. In rats with a remnant kidney, a low-protein diet reduces glomerular hypertension and glomerulosclerosis. The reverse is observed with high-protein diets. In addition, the class of eicosanoids secreted with high-protein feeding promotes renal vasoconstriction [4, 5, 21, 22].

Due to the inconsistent nature of results of clinical studies, the utility of dietary protein restriction for the treatment of progressive renal disease remains controversial. In 1990, a multicenter trial, the Modification of Diet in Renal Disease (MDRD) study [21, 22] was implemented to clarify the effectiveness of protein-restricted diets. Two groups of patients were studied. Group A patients had glomerular filtration rates (GFRs) in the range of 25–55 mL/min/1.73 m^2 and were randomized to a diet of ≥ 1 g protein/kg/day or 0.6 g protein/kg/day. Mean blood pressures were maintained at 105 or 92 mm Hg. Group B patients had GFRs in the range of 13–24 mL/min/1.73 m^2 and assigned diets that were 0.6 g/kg/day or 0.3 g/kg/day protein plus a ketoacid supplement. Blood pressure goals were the same. Renal function was monitored for 2.2 years by measuring ^{125}I-iothalamate renal clearance.

Study results demonstrated that neither the low-protein diet or blood pressure control decreased the loss of GFR. Therefore, prescription of a low-protein diet alone is not sufficient to slow progression. Trends that were observed included a beneficial affect of low-protein diet for patients with proteinuria that exceeded 1 g/day. Also, patients with polycystic kidney disease did not demonstrate any response to therapy [4]. A recent study [23] reports that a very low protein diet, providing 0.3 g protein, 35 kcal, 5–7 mg inorganic phosphorus/kg/day, supplemented with ketoacid ana-

logues or essential amino acid, calcium carbonate, iron, and multivitamins, preserved nutritional status, corrected uremic symptoms, and deferred initiation of dialysis in 239 patients followed for 13 years. There was no correlation found between patient outcome and treatment with the low-protein, supplemented diet. To date, dietary protein restriction has not been demonstrated to stop the progression of chronic renal failure. However, the majority of studies suggest that at the least, protein restriction offers clinical benefits for the metabolic consequences of uremia.

Research interest has also been directed toward dietary fatty acids, in response to a growing body of evidence implicating eicosanoid metabolism in the pathophysiology of progressive renal disease [24]. It has been demonstrated that altering the availability of essential fatty acids can influence the natural course of several important diseases in the mammalian organism [25]. For example, epidemiological studies of the Dutch, Japanese, and native Greenland Eskimo populations attribute their low incidence of heart disease to a fish diet high in omega-3 fatty acids [25]. Several investigations exploring the effects of polyunsaturated fatty acid supplemented diets in experimental immune and nonimmune models of renal disease have been reported. Beneficial observations have included an improved lipid profile [26, 27], prolonged survival [28, 29], improved renal function [29], improved proteinuria [27, 30], and delay in progression [31].

Dietary essential fatty acids are the direct precursors to the biologically diverse and potent class of compounds, the eicosanoids. Several chronic inflammatory and renal diseases are characterized in part by an overproduction of eicosanoids [24]. These facts suggest that manipulation of dietary fatty acids might contribute a therapeutic influence by altering gene expression and proinflammatory and other activated pathways in disease processes [32–34]. Fatty acid manipulation has been reported to modify macrophage function, production of vasoactive substances, and membrane signal transduction. Alteration of phospholipid fatty acid composition in cell membranes achieved by manipulation of cell medium fatty acid content has been reported to affect many cellular properties. Examples include cell membrane fluidity, receptor binding, cell-mediated transport, ion channels, eicosanoid formation, and intracellular calcium concentration [24, 33, 35, 36].

Despite the encouraging experimental results that have been reported, human trials have had inconsistent results [37–44]. The exception is in patients with IgA nephropathy. Renal disease progression was reduced when patients were administered a fish oil supplement enriched with eicosapentaenoic acid and docosahexaenoic acid [10, 11]. A recent report indicates that docosahexaenoic acid, not eicosapentaenoic acid, inhibits mesangial cell proliferation and may offer a clinical benefit during acute phases or relapses of glomerulopathies [12].

There are not enough data at present to justify any specific dietary recommendations regarding fatty acid modification for patients with chronic renal insufficiency. However, due

to the controversial and suggestive nature of the literature on dietary protein, current recommendations include dietary protein restriction (see Table 1).

III. NUTRITION FOR THE PATIENT REQUIRING RENAL REPLACEMENT THERAPY

A. Renal Dialysis

Since the introduction of dialysis in the 1960s, significant advances have dramatically changed the way ESRD patients are managed and treated [45, 46]. The pioneering efforts by Scribner, Boen, Tenckhoff, and Popovich in the late 1950s to the mid-1960s led to what we know today as dialysis therapy. Scribner, the forefather of hemodialysis, established an acute dialysis program at the University of Washington in Seattle in the late 1950s. He later developed the Scribner shunt, and with Babb, succeeded in building the first home hemodialysis machine. Similarly, the efforts by Boen, Tenckhoff, and Popovich developed peritoneal dialysis access and paved the way for this treatment modality [46].

Dialysis can be defined as a process whereby the solute composition of a solution is altered by exposure to another solution through a semipermeable membrane [46, 47]. Small to mid-molecular weight solutes and water molecules can pass through the membrane, whereas larger molecular solutes cannot [47]. Utilization of hemodialysis or peritoneal dialysis is based on clinical condition, lifestyle, and psychosocial considerations. Psychosocial considerations include quality-of-life factors, depression [48–50], and compliance with dietary, fluid, and treatment modalities [51].

Of paramount importance is the viability of a patent dialysis access. Access to the bloodstream is both the lifeline and the "Achilles heel" of dialysis. A well-functioning access is crucial to provide adequate dialysis and optimal medical care of the ESRD patient regardless of treatment modality. If hemodialysis is selected, blood is removed from the arterial side of the patient's access, via an arteriovenous fistula, arteriovenous graft, or catheter. It is processed through a dialyzer and then returned through the venous side of the access. This process occurs repeatedly over the course of several hours. Whenever possible, the order of preference for placement of different blood vessel access is fistula, graft, and, as a temporizing measure or if the aforementioned accesses are not viable options, a cuffed tunneled central venous catheter [52]. A fistula, the anastomosis of an artery to a vein, is the preferred and best form of hemodialysis access due to longevity and low incidence of complications. If creating a fistula is not a viable option, synthetic tubing, such as polytetrafluoroethylene, can be used to create an arteriovenous graft in the arm or the thigh [46].

In peritoneal dialysis, the body's own peritoneal membrane serves as the semipermeable membrane across which solutes and water pass. Generally, 1–3 liters of a dextrose salt solution is infused into the peritoneal cavity. The rate of solute transport, the type of number of peritoneal dialysis exchanges, and solution dwell times vary among patients. A method to determine membrane function and the optimal peritoneal dialysis method for each patient is the peritoneal equilibration test [53]. Rate of solute transport ranges from low to high and can be measured via this test. Peritoneal solute and solvent movement rates vary among patients and, over time, may vary even within the same patient [54]. A variety of types of peritoneal dialysis exist with the two main types being continuous ambulatory peritoneal dialysis and continuous cycling peritoneal dialysis. Similar to the decision to choose hemodialysis or peritoneal dialysis, which type of peritoneal dialysis is performed is dependent on lifestyle and clinical considerations.

Whether a patient receives hemodialysis or peritoneal dialysis, adequacy of dialysis is of paramount importance to optimize patient nutritional status and, ultimately, morbidity and mortality. The landmark National Cooperative Dialysis Study provided a longitudinal evaluation of hemodialysis patients dialysis regimen over 1 year's time. Participants were divided into four treatment groups in order to assess the minimum dialysis time that would provide adequate outcome [55]. Ultimately, inadequate protein intake was associated with inadequate dialysis (as defined by an elevated blood urea nitrogen level) and increased mortality [56]. These results have since been confirmed and expanded [57–63]. Similar results were obtained in a larger, retrospective study conducted by Owen et al. [64]. The records of 13,473 patients were evaluated to determine the effects of blood urea nitrogen reduction during dialysis and nutritional adequacy on mortality. The odds ratio for death increased dramatically with poor nutritional status (as assessed by a low serum albumin) and inadequate dialysis (as assessed by urea reduction ratio). Specifically, patients with a serum albumin of 3.5–3.9 and 3.0–3.4 had odds ratios for death of 1.48 and 3.13, respectively. Patients with a urea reduction ration less than 60% also had a higher odds ratio for death compared with a urea reduction ratio of 65–69%. Hakim et al. [65] conducted a prospective study on 130 hemodialysis patients over 3 years. Differences in delivered dose of dialysis were evaluated with a 25% increase in delivered dialysis dose being correlated with a decrease in annual mortality rate. In addition, increased protein intake, as measured by protein catabolic rate, was demonstrated with increased dose of dialysis.

The methods and recommendations with how dialysis is performed as well as dietary recommendations for ESRD patients have been transformed by these results. Historically, dialysis prescriptions were empirically prescribed (Table 2). Currently, however, dialysis prescriptions are individualized and closely monitored. Although in the past, blood urea nitrogen levels or urea reduction ratios have been used to assess adequacy of dialysis, with the advent of computerized programs, urea kinetic modeling techniques should be used to assess, measure, and individualize the adequacy and

TABLE 1   Nutrition Recommendations for Patients with Chronic Renal Failure
Not Undergoing Dialysis[a,b,c]

Protein	
Low-protein diet (g/kg/day)	0.55–0.60 including ≥0.35 of high-biologic-value protein
Energy (kcal/kg/day)	≥35 unless the patient's relative body weight is greater than 120% of ideal or the patient gains or is afraid of gaining unwanted weight
Fat (percentage of total energy intake)[d,e]	30
Polyunsaturated to saturated fatty acid ratio[e]	1.0:1.0
Carbohydrate[e,f]	Rest of nonprotein calories
Total fiber intake (g/day)[e]	20–25
Minerals (range of intake)	
Sodium (mg/day)	1000–3000[g]
Potassium (mEq/day)	40–70
Phosphorus (mg/kg/day)	5–10[h]
Calcium (mg/day)	1400–1600[i]
Magnesium (mg/day)	200–300
Iron (mg/day)	≥10–18[j]
Zinc (mg/day)	15
Water (mL/day)	Up to 3000 as tolerated[g]
Vitamins	
Thiamin (mg/day)	1.5
Riboflavin (mg/day)	1.8
Pantothenic acid (mg/day)	5
Niacin (mg/day)	20
Pyridoxine HCl (mg/day)	5
Vitamin B_{12} (μg/day)	3
Vitamin C (mg/day)	60
Folic acid (mg/day)	1
Vitamin A	No addition
Vitamin D	Individualized
Vitamin E (IU/day)	15
Vitamin K	None[k]

Source: Reprinted with permission from Kopple, J. (1997). Nutrition management of nondialyzed patients with chronic renal failure. *In* "Nutritional Management of Renal Disease" (J. D. Kopple and S. G. Massey, Eds.), p. 495.

[a]GFR above 4–5 mL/min/1.73 m² and less than 25 mL/min/1.73 m².

[b]The protein intake is increased by 1.0 g/day of high-biologic-value protein for each gram per day of urinary protein loss.

[c]When recommended intake is expressed per kilogram body weight, this refers to the patient's normal weight, as determined from the NHANES data, or adjusted body weight.

[d]Refers to percentage of total energy intake (diet plus dialysate). If triglyceride levels are very high, the percentage of fat in the diet may be increased to about 40% of total calories; otherwise, 30% of total calories is preferable.

[e]These dietary recommendations are considered less crucial than the others. They are only emphasized if the patient has a specific disorder that may benefit from this modification or has expressed interest in this dietary prescription and is complying well to more important aspects of the dietary treatment.

[f]Should be primarily complex carbohydrates.

[g]Can be higher in patients who have greater urinary losses.

[h]Phosphate binders (aluminum carbonate or hydroxide, or calcium carbonate, acetate, or citrate) often are needed to maintain normal serum phosphorus levels.

[i]Dietary intake usually must be supplemented to provide these levels. Higher daily calcium intakes are commonly ingested because of the use of calcium binders of phosphate.

[j]≥10 mg/day for males and nonmenstruating females; ≥18 mg/day for menstruating females.

[k]Vitamin K supplements may be needed for patients who are not eating and who receive antibiotics.

TABLE 2   History of Diet Changes for Hemodialysis Patients

Nutrient	1960s	1970s	1980s	1990s
Protein	20–40 g/day	0.75–1.0 g/kg/day	1.0–1.1 g/kg/day	1.1–1.4 g/kg/day
Phosphorus	Not restricted	700 mg/day	1000–1200 mg/day	10–17 mg/kg/day
Potassium	2500 mg/day	1800–2300 mg/day	2000–3000 mg/day	40 mg/kg/day
Sodium	0.5 g/day	1.0–2.5 g/day	2–3 g/day	2–3 g/day
Fluid	500–800 mL/day	500 mL/day	1000 mL/day	500–750 mL/day

Source: Adapted from Jacobs, L., Rubens-Kenler, S., and Dwyer, J. (1996). *Topics Clin. Nutr.* **12**, 6–17.

quality of dialysis [66, 67]. *Kt/V* is a measure of the dose of dialysis given in a single treatment where *K* is the dialyzer urea clearance, *t* is the total treatment time, and *V* is the total volume within the body that urea is distributed [68]. *Kt/V* and creatinine clearance are two methods to determine adequacy of dialysis and should be calculated using formal urea kinetic modeling. Hemodialysis patients should receive a single pool *Kt/V* of at least 1.2 per treatment [66]. Continuous ambulatory peritoneal dialysis, nightly intermittent dialysis, and continuous cycling peritoneal dialysis patients need to obtain a weekly *Kt/V*$_{urea}$ of 2.0, 2.2, and 2.3 with a weekly creatinine clearance of 60, 66, and 64 L/1.73 m², respectively [67]. One notable exception is for continuous ambulatory peritoneal dialysis patients that are low transporters. For this subgroup of patients, creatinine clearance should be at least 50 L/week/1.73 m² with a weekly creatinine clearance of 2.0 or greater [69]. Because nutritional status and morbidity and mortality are closely linked with adequacy of dialysis, these guidelines should be rigorously followed.

B. Comorbid Conditions Associated with ESRD

ESRD patients have a higher mortality compared with age-matched controls in the general population [70]. Moreover, most ESRD patients have comorbid conditions that further increase their relative risk of death such as cardiovascular disease, bone disease, secondary hyperparathyroidism, anemia, and malnutrition.

1. Cardiovascular Disease

Cardiovascular disorders have a high prevalence in the ESRD patients and account for approximately 50% of deaths for this patient population [70–71]. Common cardiovascular abnormalities in these patients include heart disease, congestive heart failure, left ventricular hypertrophy, hypertension, and peripheral vascular disease [70]. Malnutrition, oxidative stress, and genetic components may play a synergistic effect on rapid development of atherosclerosis [72]. While a variety of comorbid conditions contribute to cardiovascular disease (CVD) in this population, renal failure also adds independent cardiovascular risk factors such as derange-

ments in lipoprotein metabolism and elevated homocysteine levels [70, 73].

2. Abnormalities in Lipoprotein Metabolism

Hypertriglyceridemia with decreased high-density lipoprotein (HDL) cholesterol occurs in 50–70% of ESRD patients [74]. Due to the high prevalence of CVD in ESRD, these patients need to be screened for hyperlipidemia and treated [75]. Even in patients having normal HDL cholesterol, low-density lipoprotein (LDL) cholesterol, and triglyceride levels, very low density lipoprotein (VLDL) cholesterol levels may be elevated due to impaired catabolism. Moreover, ESRD patients tend to have increased lipoprotein(a) levels and increased small dense LDL particles [74, 76, 77]. Furthermore, these lipoprotein particles are subject to increased oxidation due to the effect of uremic toxins and may cause vascular injury [78]. Thus, even in the appearance of normal lipoprotein levels, significant lipoprotein derangements may increase the risk of CVD. In addition to pharmacological interventions, dietary modification to lower lipid levels may be attempted; however, dietary restriction of fat/cholesterol has not been definitely shown to improve CVD risk in this patient population, and ensuring adequate energy and protein intake may take precedence.

3. Hyperhomocysteinemia

Homocysteine may directly damage vascular endothelium [47], and hyperhomocysteinemia has been found to increase the odds ratio for vascular events [79] and has been linked with an increased mortality rate in ESRD patients. The landmark study by Wilcken *et al.* [80] and confirmed by others [81–84], demonstrated higher plasma homocysteine levels in ESRD patients compared with the general population. With kidney failure, there is decreased metabolism of homocysteine by the renal parenchyma. In addition, increased losses of the necessary cofactors for homocysteine metabolism, such as folate, vitamin B$_6$, and vitamin B$_{12}$, may occur due to the dialysis process itself. Moreover, decreased intake of these vital nutrients may occur due to the dietary restrictions.

Vascular damage occurs due to generation of hydrogen peroxide and free radicals when homocysteine is oxidized to

its disulfide form [85–87]. Other proposed mechanisms for vascular damage include impairment of endothelial-derived relaxing factor on nitric oxide production, damage to the endothelium by the inhibition of prostacyclin production (a prostaglandin antagonist of platelet aggregation), and the oxidative effects on LDL by homocysteine-induced hydrogen peroxide production [88–92]. Optimizing intake of folate, vitamin B_{12}, and vitamin B_6 intake has been demonstrated to decrease serum homocysteine levels by 30–50% [93] and may have cardioprotective effects [80, 83, 84, 91–93]. Supplementation of folate, vitamin B_6, and B_{12} should be considered [80, 91, 92].

In addition to diabetes and blood pressure control, management of hyperlipidemia and homocystemia may help decrease CVD risk [70–72, 91, 93–95].

4. BONE DISEASE

Bone disease diagnoses in ESRD include osteitis fibrosa, osteomalacia, osteosclerosis, and osteoporosis [96] and are associated with increased mortality. Contributors to renal osteodystrophy include decreased conversion of vitamin D to the active form, 1,25-dihydroxycholecalciferol, by the kidney, resulting in low serum calcium and elevated parathyroid hormone levels. In addition, serum phosphorus levels are typically elevated due to decreased renal excretion. Alterations in vitamin D metabolism and increased phosphorus levels result in the development of secondary hyperparathyroidism and contribute to increased mortality [97–100].

A landmark study by Block *et al.* [98] clearly delineated the adverse consequences of elevated parathyroid hormone, phosphorus, and the product of the serum calcium level multiplied by the serum phosphorus level (Ca × P). Retrospective analysis of data from more than 6400 hemodialysis patients demonstrated that elevated serum phosphorus, Ca × P, and parathyroid hormone levels were independently associated with increased morbidity and mortality. After adjustment for comorbid conditions, patients with a phosphorus level > 6.5 mg/dL had a 27% higher death risk than patients with a serum phosphorus between 2.4 and 6.5. Of note, 39% of these patients had a serum phosphorus > 6.5, thus placing them at increased risk of mortality. Similarly, elevated Ca × P was associated with increased mortality, reaching statistical significance with Ca × P >72. Specifically, patients with a Ca × P >72 had a 34% higher risk of death relative to those with a Ca × P between 42 and 52. Parathyroid hormone levels > 975 pg/mL also were associated with an increased mortality rate. Studies conducted by Lowrie and Lew [57] found that patients with a serum phosphorus between 7 and 11 mg/dL had a twofold higher relative risk of death than patients with phosphorus levels between 5 and 7 mg/dL.

Thus, reduction of serum phosphorus, Ca × P, and parathyroid hormone levels is imperative to prevent or improve many pathological consequences, such as left ventricular hypertrophy, anemia, immune suppression, hypertriglyceride-mia, vascular complications, and renal osteodystrophy [71, 97, 98].

Historically, the emphasis has been placed on preventing high bone turnover in this patient population; however, a recent study by Atsumi *et al.* [101] illustrates negative consequences of low bone turnover. Male patients with parathyroid hormone levels in the lowest tertile (mean parathyroid hormone 32.9 pg/mL) had a 31% prevalence of vertebral fractures compared with only a 13% and 17% incidence in those patients in the middle (mean parathyroid hormone 116 pg/mL) and highest (mean parathyroid hormone 502 pg/mL) tertile, respectively. Thus, both high and low bone turnover are associated with adverse outcomes.

Most ESRD patients will require management of secondary hyperparathyroidism with dietary phosphorus restriction, phosphate binder use, and oral or intravenous supplementation of vitamin D or vitamin D analogues. Serum parathyroid hormone, calcium, and phosphorus levels should be closely monitored for ESRD patients, especially those who are administered vitamin D therapy.

A variety of oral and intravenous vitamin D or vitamin D analogs are available. The dose must be titrated based on individual patient need to prevent over- or undersuppression of parathyroid hormone. Phosphate binders, such as calcium acetate, calcium carbonate, or sevelamar hydrochloride, should be individualized and prescribed with meals in order to be effective in controlling serum phosphorus levels.

5. ANEMIA

The majority of ESRD patients have decreased hematocrit (Hct) and hemoglobin (Hgb) levels because they are unable to synthesize adequate amounts of erthyropoietin, a hormone produced by renal tubular cells [102, 103]. They also have increased blood loss from dialysis procedures. The resulting anemia is treated with recombinant human erythropoietin (rHuEPO) and iron [104]. Prior to 1989, the main therapeutic treatment option for treating anemia in this patient population repeated blood transfusions. This was not ideal and contributed to iron overload [105]. With the advent of rHuEPO, renal anemia can be effectively treated and alleviated in the majority of ESRD patients [106–108]. If left untreated, a wide variety of adverse events occur, such as cardiac enlargement, ventricular hypertrophy, angina, congestive heart failure, malnutrition, and impaired immunological response [109–118]. Uncorrected, anemia is associated with increased mortality [119, 120]. Thus, the development of rHuEPO dramatically and significantly improved the health and well-being of ESRD patients.

Recommended hematocrit and hemoglobin target levels for the ESRD population are 33–36% and 11–12 g/dL, respectively [121]. Some studies suggest higher levels may be desirable in certain patients [105, 122–125]. Subcutaneous administration is preferred over intravenous for pre-ESRD and ESRD patients because lower doses of rHuEPO can be used to maintain hematocrit levels > 33% [106, 121, 126–

129]. Generally, for adult patients, 80–120 units rHuEPO/kg/week in two to three doses is recommended for subcutaneous administration. If administered intravenously, generally 120–180 units/kg/week rHuEPO should be given over three dialysis sessions [121]. However, the absolute dose depends on the individual patient response.

Most patients on dialysis will receive recombinant human erythropoietin to promote synthesis of red blood cells and will require iron supplementation [104, 130–132]. Although many factors may contribute to rHuEPO hyporesponsiveness, such as infections, chronic inflammation, secondary hyperparathyroidism, and occult blood loss, among others [108], the most frequent contributor is iron deficiency [108, 133, 134]. Current recommendations to assess iron stores and appropriate iron therapy are used to determine if serum transferrin saturation levels are greater than 20% and if serum ferritin levels are greater than 100 units [121]. Although various oral iron preparations are available, intestinal iron absorption may be impaired in dialysis patients [135, 136]. A trial of oral iron may be tried, particularly in peritoneal dialysis patients [137–140]; however, for most hemodialysis and many peritoneal dialysis patients, intravenous iron supplementation is more effective in treating iron deficiency anemia [121, 130, 132, 141–143]. If oral iron is to be used, 200 mg of elemental iron should be provided per day in two to three divided doses, preferably between meals and not with phosphate binders [121, 131]. If intravenous iron is to be used, a maintenance dose of 25–100 mg per week is recommended [121, 131]. Prior to maintenance, a typical course of intravenous iron therapy is 1 g over 10 dialysis treatments (i.e., 100 mg per treatment). A variety of intravenous iron preparations are available in the United States and include iron dextran, iron gluconate, and—soon to be available—iron sucrose, also known as iron saccharate [144].

6. MALNUTRITION

Malnutrition is an important and modifiable risk for mortality in the ESRD population [57, 64, 145–151]. Causes of inadequate nutritional status in this population include anorexia, catabolic state, loss of amino acids during the dialysis process, and complement activation due to exposure to various dialyzer membranes [152].

The landmark National Cooperative Dialysis Study found the number of hospitalizations per year was highest in patients with the lowest protein intake as determined by protein catabolic rate [153]. Similarly, work conducted by Lowrie and Lew [57] on more than 14,000 hemodialysis patients found a strong association between low serum albumin and mortality. Of note, nearly 70% of patients had serum albumin levels of less than 4.0 g/dL, and 15% had serum albumins less than 3.5 g/dL. Patients with a serum albumin <2.5 g/dL had a 20 times higher risk of death than patients with an albumin >4.0 g/dL. Somewhat surprisingly, patients with albumin levels of 3.5–4.0 g/dL still had a two times higher

risk of death than patients with albumin levels >4.0 g/dL. The importance of nutritional status was not universally accepted and recognized until these outcome studies were reported. Both individualized dialysis prescription and dietary guidelines are essential to optimize nutritional status of ESRD patients.

Nutritional assessment, monitoring, and interventions are critical to prescribe appropriate clinical nutrition therapies and, ultimately, to improve patient outcomes. Improvements in quality of life may be demonstrated with improved nutritional status [49, 154]. Similarly, poor nutritional status may be associated with decreased quality-of-life scores [50].

C. Nutrition Assessment

Because malnutrition is so strongly correlated with mortality, nutrition assessment and monitoring are vital. Registered dietitians are especially skilled in this area and should be consulted [155]. A complete nutrition assessment will include a number of parameters including clinical findings, body composition, weight, dietary assessment, and biochemical indices (Table 3).

1. SUBJECTIVE GLOBAL ASSESSMENT

Subjective global assessment is a method of history taking and physical examination that can be quickly and effectively performed to assess and monitor the nutritional status of patients [152, 156–160]. The subjective global assessment was originally developed for use in surgical patients, but has since been validated for use in ESRD patients. Patients are assigned to a risk category based on subjective global assessment ratings. A low or downward trend in an subjective global assessment rating would suggest compromised nutritional status and require intervention.

2. ANTHROPOMETRICS

Common anthropometric measurements obtained in this population include height, weight, triceps skinfold, subscapular skinfold, arm circumference, abdominal circumference, calf circumference, knee height, and elbow breadth [161, 162]. Obtained measurements are compared to standardized percentiles; however, no current standards are available that are specific to the ESRD population.

Anthropometric measurements can also be combined in the evaluation of nutritional status. For example, weight for height has been demonstrated to be a strong predictor of 12-month mortality in hemodialysis patients [163]. Mortality rate appears to decrease as a patient's weight for height increases. Similarly, patients with a higher body mass index (BMI) may have a lower mortality rate than those with a lower BMI [164]. Use of correct body weight is essential for patient assessment and for determination of dietary needs. A variety of definitions of weight have been used for nutritional assessment such as usual body weight, standard body

TABLE 3   Data Categories and Constituents Inherent to Nutritional Assessment

1. Clinical	2. Food and diet intake	3. Biochemical	4. Body weight	5. Body composition
Physical examination	Diet history	Visceral protein stores	History	Adipose stores
Nutrient physical examination	Appetite assessment	Static protein reserves	Actual	Lean body mass (skeletal muscle)
Medical history	Quantitative food intake	Other estimates of protein nutriture	Compared to standards	—
Psychosocial history	Qualitative food intake	Immune competence	Body mass index	—
Demographics	Food habits and patterns	Vitamins, minerals, and trace elements	Weight change over time	—
Physical activity level	Fluid intake/balance	Fluid, electrolyte, and acid–base balance	Goal weight	—
Current medical/ surgical issues	—	Lipid status	—	—

Source: Reprinted with permission from Goldstein, D. J. (1998). Assessment of nutritional status in renal disease. *In* "Handbook of Nutrition and the Kidney" (W. E. Mitch and S. Klahr, Eds.), pp. 45–86. Lippincott Williams & Wilkins, Philadelphia, PA.

weight, and ideal body weight. The current recommendation of the Nutrition Dialysis Outcomes Quality Initiative committee suggests use of the edema-free body weight (also known as dry weight) when the patient is between 90% and 115% median standard weight as determined by the National Health and Nutrition Examination Survey (NHANES) II weight tables (Table 4). If the patient's body weight is outside this range, adjusted edema-free body weight should be used (Fig. 1).

3. DIETARY ASSESSMENT

Controversy exists on the best method for dietary assessment of this population. Some studies suggest that 7-day diet records are necessary [165], whereas others suggest that a 24-hour recall is just as accurate and may increase the likelihood of successful data collection in this group [166]. Assessment of the patient's typical food intake can identify areas of educational need as well as provide valuable information for individualizing dietary counseling. Nutrition screening is a first step in identifying nutrition-related issues in renal patients. Figure 2 provides an example of an excellent nutrition screening tool.

4. BIOCHEMICAL INDICES

The results of a variety of biochemical indices and calculations need to be integrated in order to evaluate nutritional status in ESRD patients. Table 5 categorizes a number of these parameters. The most widely used parameters are highlighted below.

a. Serum Albumin. A low serum albumin is strongly correlated with increased morbidity and mortality and may be related to poor nutritional intake [57, 59, 61, 70]. Ideally, serum albumin levels should be maintained greater than 4.0 g/dL. Of note, hospital admissions have been demon-

strated to be shorter with higher serum albumin levels [61]. Although serum albumin may provide information regarding the patient's nutritional status, it is adversely influenced by the coexistence of chronic inflammatory states, liver disease, pancreatic disease, and nephrotic syndrome, among others, and must be interpreted accordingly [70, 96].

b. Serum Prealbumin. Serum prealbumin has a half-life of only 2 days, making it a potentially more sensitive marker of protein status than albumin, and is another predictor of morbidity and mortality in patients with ESRD. More specifically, a prealbumin <30 mg/dL may indicate malnutrition [149]. Patients with ESRD initiating dialysis with a prealbumin >30 mg/dL were found to have a higher observed and expected survival than those who did not [167].

Of note, serum prealbumin levels are related to the level of renal function and may increase with declining renal function (due to decreased catabolism), regardless of nutritional status [168]. Evaluation of prealbumin levels may be most helpful once a patient's kidney function is in a steady state [169, 170]. Similar to albumin, prealbumin is also adversely influenced by infection, inflammation, and comorbid conditions.

c. Serum Cholesterol. Low serum cholesterol levels may indicate protein energy malnutrition or be a reflection of other comorbid conditions. A low serum cholesterol, <150 mg/dL, may be a higher risk factor for mortality than an elevated serum cholesterol level in this patient population [59, 171, 172]. A desirable serum cholesterol level is between 150 and 200 mg/dL. Importantly, cholesterol levels may be affected by acute infection, malnutrition, and nephrotic syndrome, or elevated by use of glucocorticoids [96]. If serum cholesterol levels are substantially elevated, patients with ESRD may benefit from a fibric acid analogue or statin therapy [71, 173]. However, the long-term safety of

TABLE 4 Average Weights for Men and Women, by Age and Height in the United States

		Age (years)					
		18–24	25–34	35–44	45–54	55–64	65–74
	Height (in)	Weight (pounds)					
Men	62	140	139	150	142	145	161
	64	139	147	154	150	158	154
	65	160	161	166	164	163	159
	68	157	165	170	174	172	164
	70	165	180	179	183	173	174
	72	169	188	183	183	177	188
	74	185	182	204	203	216	
Women	58	121	121	117	117	136	140
	60	122	124	138	137	148	142
	62	128	133	143	143	159	154
	64	126	140	147	155	156	158
	66	142	139	148	157	145	154
	68	131	150	160	189	158	200
	Height (cm)	Weight (kg)					
Men	157	63.64	63.18	68.18	64.55	65.91	73.18
	163	63.18	66.82	70.00	72.27	71.82	70.00
	168	72.73	73.18	75.45	74.55	74.09	72.27
	173	71.36	75.00	77.27	79.09	78.18	74.55
	178	75.00	81.82	81.36	83.18	78.64	79.09
	183	76.82	85.45	83.18	83.18	80.45	85.45
	188	84.09	82.73	92.73	92.27	98.18	
Women	147	55.00	55.00	53.18	53.18	61.82	63.64
	152	55.45	56.36	62.73	62.27	67.27	64.55
	157	58.18	60.45	65.00	65.00	72.27	70.00
	163	57.27	63.64	66.82	70.45	70.91	71.82
	168	64.55	63.18	67.27	71.38	65.91	70.00
	173	59.56	68.15	72.73	76.82	71.82	90.91

Source: "Clinical Practice Guidelines for Nutrition" (1999). NFK-DOQL. National Kidney Foundation, New York.

lipid-lowering agents in this population has not been established [71].

d. Serum Creatinine and Creatinine Index. Serum creatinine and creatinine index measures can be useful in evaluation of patients with ESRD who have negligible renal function. Creatinine is formed at a relatively constant rate from muscle tissue and thus may be used in a patient with a stable GFR to assess muscle mass. The creatinine index is defined as the creatinine synthesis rate [152] and is directly related to skeletal muscle mass.

A low serum creatinine or creatinine index may be indicative of decreased muscle mass and/or low dietary protein intake [174] and is correlated with increased mortality [59, 171, 175]. Specifically, assuming minimal residual renal function, mortality risk increases with serum creatinine levels of <9–11 mg/dL [59, 169, 171, 176] and/or a creatinine index that is low or declining [177]. In patients with significant residual renal function, serum creatinine may not be as

$$aBW_{ef} = BW_{ef} + [(SBW - BW_{ef}) \times 0.25]$$

where BW_{ef} = edema free body weight and SBW = standardized body weight as determined by NHANES II data.

FIGURE 1 Calculation of adjusted body weight. [Reprinted with permission from K/DOQN nutrition in chronic renal failure: Adult guidelines (2000). *Am. J. Kidney Dis.* **35**(6), S17–S104.]

Use this Checklist to determine whether your patient may have a nutrition related problem. Do not overlook the warning signs of poor nutrition.

Read the statements below to your patient. Place a check mark in the yes column if the statement applies to the patient. Place a check mark in the no column if it does not apply to the patient. If your patient has a nutrition related problem, you can use the Renal DETERMINE Nutrition Screening Reference Sheets to determine what the appropriate interventions are to help the patient resolve their problem.

	Yes	No
In addition to your kidney disease, do you have one or more of these problems: high blood pressure, high blood cholesterol, diabetes, heart disease, or stomach problems? (Circle those that apply to the patient)		
Do you have mouth, chewing, or swallowing problems that make it hard for you to eat?		
Do you have problems with your medications?		
Do you forget to take your medications more than two times a week?		
Without wanting to, have you lost 10 pounds in the last 6 months?		
Are you following a special diet?		
Do you have questions or problems with your special diet?		
Do you have a poor appetite?		
Does food not taste good to you?		
Do you eat fewer than 2 meals per day?		
Are you ever too tired to cook or eat?		
Do you have trouble paying for the food, medications, or medical care that you need?		
Do you eat alone most of the time?		

Additional questions for dialysis patients:

	Yes	No
Is your appetite poor on dialysis days?		
Is your appetite poor on non-dialysis days?		
Is your appetite poor all the time?		
Do you miss meals on dialysis days?		
Do you have a lot of stomach aches or gas that affects how much and what you eat?		

Additional questions for transplant patients:

	Yes	No
Have you developed an infection since your trnasplant that affects how much and what you eat?		
Have you had rejection problems since your transplant that affects how much and what you eat?		
Have you had reactions to drugs since your transplant that affects how much and what you eat?		

FIGURE 2 DETERMINE checklist. [Reprinted with permission from Leung, J., and Dwyer, J. (1998). Renal DETERMINE nutrition awareness checklist for health care professionals. *J. Renal Nutr.* **2,** 95–103.]

TABLE 5 Biochemical Parameters for Assessing the Nutritional Status of the Patient with Renal Disease

A. *Visceral protein stores*
  Albumin
  Prealbumin (thyroxin binding prealbumin)
  Retinol-binding protein
  Transferrin (siderophilin)
  Somatomedin c (insulin-like growth factor 1)
  Acute-phase proteins (ceruloplasmin, complement components, c-reactive protein, fibrinogen)
  Fibronectin
  Pseudocholinesterase
  Ribonuclease
  Total protein
  Albumin/globulin ratio
B. *Static (somatic) protein reserves*
  Urinary and serum creatinine
  Creatinine height index
  3-Methylhistidine
C. *Other estimates of protein reserves*
  Plasma amino acid profiles
  Protein turnover studies
  Biochemical analysis of skeletal muscle
  Nitrogen balance
D. *Immune competence*
  Total lymphocyte counts
  Delayed cutaneous hypersensitivity responses: *Candida,* mumps, *Trichophyton,* streptokinase-streptodornase (sksd), and purified protein derivative (ppd)
  Specific immunoglobulin levels
  Complement proteins
E. *Vitamins, mineral, trace element nutriture*
  Serum levels of water-soluble vitamins, fat-soluble vitamins, and specific minerals and trace elements
  Nutrition physical examination
F. *Fluid, electrolyte, and acid–base status*
  Serum chemistries: sodium, potassium, calcium, phosphorus, bicarbonate, chloride, glucose
G. *Indirect indices of renal function and dialysis adequacy*
  Serum creatinine
  Blood urea nitrogen
H. *Anemia*
  Hemoglobin
  Hematocrit
  Mean cell corpuscular volume
  Total iron-binding capacity
  Serum iron
  Percent transferrin saturation
  Ferritin
  Red blood cell count
  Reticulocyte count
  White blood cell count
I. *Hyperlipidemia*
  Serum: cholesterol, triglycerides
J. *Renal osteodystrophy*
  Serum: calcium, vitamin D, alkaline phosphatase

Source: Reprinted with permission from Goldstein, D. J. (1998). Assessment of nutritional status in renal disease. *In* "Handbook of Nutrition and the Kidney" (W. E. Mitch and S. Klahr, Eds.), pp. 45–86. Lippincott Williams & Wilkins, Philadelphia, PA.

useful in evaluating nutritional status. In this case, serum creatinine will be lower because the kidney will be excreting higher levels of creatinine into the urine.

Another technique to assess protein status in patients with ESRD is protein catabolic rate. Protein catabolic rate measures net protein degradation and protein intake in stable hemodialysis and peritoneal dialysis patients and is a derivative of urea kinetic modeling. It reflects the amount of protein that a patient is catabolizing per day and is useful in reviewing patient food intake. In a patient that is nutritionally stable and not catabolic, the protein catabolic rate equals the dietary protein intake [178, 179]. Low values may be reflective of poor nutritional intake and are strongly correlated with increased morbidity and mortality [145, 153, 180]. Of note, protein catabolic rate can be falsely elevated if a patient is catabolic and falsely low if a patient is anabolic [152].

D. Nutrition Recommendations

1. PROTEIN AND ENERGY

In general, the dietary needs of patients on chronic hemodialysis are high in energy and protein, and restricted in phosphorus, sodium, potassium, and fluid. Nitrogen balance studies on hemodialysis patients have demonstrated a 30% higher nitrogen appearance rate during dialysis versus the interdialytic period [181, 182], indicating that the dialysis process itself increased net protein catabolism. The dialysis process causes loss of amino acids and stimulates the inflammatory process, thus increasing protein breakdown [96]. Based on studies providing protein and energy supplementation to hemodialysis patients, 1.2 g protein/kg body weight and 35 kcal/kg body weight are general recommendations [183]. Peritoneal dialysis patients generally have a more liberalized diet, higher in protein, sodium, potassium, and fluid, due to increased losses during the dialysis process, but are restricted in phosphorus. Based on current literature and research, Table 6 lists nutrition recommendations; however, more research is necessary to verify the efficacy of these guidelines. Frequently, actual energy and protein intake for hemodialysis and peritoneal dialysis patients are below these parameters [184]. When estimating a peritoneal dialysis patient's energy intake, the energy available from the dialysate should also be considered.

2. VITAMIN AND MINERAL SUPPLEMENTATION

Some patients may require supplementation of water-soluble vitamins due to increased losses during the dialysis process coupled with anorexia and poor food intake [92, 96]. Vitamins specially designed for this patient population are available and should be used if vitamin supplementation is prescribed [91, 92]. In general, a vitamin designed for the ESRD population contains B vitamins, folic acid, and vitamin C (Table 7). Fat-soluble vitamins and minerals are intentionally omitted. The majority of patients will require

TABLE 6 Daily Nutrient Recommendations for ESRD Based on Treatment Modality

Nutrient	Hemodialysis	Peritoneal dialysis
Protein (g/kg)[a]	1.2–1.3; at least 50% high biological value	1.2–1.3; at least 50% high biological value
Energy (kcal/kg or [kJ/kg])[a] If patient <90% or >115% of median standard weight, use aBW$_{ef}$	30–35 [125–145] if 60 years of age or older; 35 [145] if less than 60 years of age	30–35 [125–145] if 60 years of age or older; 35 [145] if less than 60 years of age
Phosphorus	800–1200 mg/day or <17 mg/kg[a]	1200 mg/day or <17 mg/kg[a]
Sodium	2000–3000 mg/day (88–130 mmol/day)	Individualize based on blood pressure and weight; CAPD and APD, 3000–4000 mg/day (130–175 mmol/day)
Potassium	40 mg/kg[a] or approximately 2000–3000 mg/day (50–80 mmol/day)	Generally unrestricted with CAPD and APD (approximately 3000–4000 mg/day (80–106 mmol/day) unless serum level is increased or decreased
Fluid	500–1000 ml/day plus daily urine output	CAPD and APD approximately 2000–3000 mL/day based on daily weight fluctuations, urine output, ultrafiltration, and blood pressure; unrestricted if weight and blood pressure are controlled and residual renal function = 2–3 L/day
Calcium	Approximately 1000–1800 mg/day; supplement as needed to maintain normal serum level	Same as for hemodialysis

Source: Modified with permission from "Manual of Clinical Dietetics," 6th ed. © 2000 American Dietetic Association, Chicago, IL, and Canadian Dietetic Association.

[a]To come.

[b]For continuous ambulatory peritoneal dialysis (CAPD) and automated or "cycler" peritoneal dialysis (APD), include dialysate calories.

specific and titrated supplementation of iron and vitamin D or vitamin D analogue.

IV. NUTRITIONAL REQUIREMENTS OF THE POST-TRANSPLANT PATIENT

The overall goal of the post-transplant diet is to normalize electrolyte imbalances, promote blood pressure control, prevent weight gain, maximize bone density, control blood glucose, and promote overall good nutritional status [185–187]. Although renal transplantation restores near-normal renal function, other abnormalities may arise primarily as a consequence of antirejection medications [188]. Specifically, more than 60% of renal transplant patients demonstrate hyperlipidemia. This is primarily due to necessary corticosteroids, and antirejection medications, such as cyclosporin A, as well as antihypertensive medications. Post-transplant patients are also at increased risk of CVD [189–195]. Approximately 60% of renal transplant patients have elevated serum cholesterol levels with about 40% of deaths post-transplant attributable to CVD [196]. To control body weight, serum triglyceride and serum cholesterol levels, a low-fat diet and an exercise plan are generally recommended [187,

197–199]. Many patients will also require lipid-lowering medication. Moreover, glucose intolerance is a frequent occurrence post-transplant, primarily due to corticosteroids and other antirejection medications such as cyclosporin A [200, 201]. Importantly, in addition to the hyperglycemic effects

TABLE 7 Vitamin Recommendations for ESRD Patients Undergoing Chronic Dialysis

Nutrient	ESRD
Vitamin C	60 mg/day
Vitamin B$_1$	1.5 mg/day
Vitamin B$_2$	1.7 mg/day
Niacinamide	20 mg/day
Vitamin B$_6$	5–10 mg/day
Vitamin B$_{12}$	0.006 mg/day
Pantothenic acid	10 mg/day
Folic acid	0.8–1.0 mg/day
Biotin	0.3 mg/day

Source: Adapted from "Comparison of Vitamin Formulations Prescribed for Renal Patients" (2000). R&D Laboratories, Marina Del Rey, CA.

TABLE 8 Nutrition Guidelines for Adult Kidney Transplant Recipients

Nutrient	Prescription	Purpose
First 6–8 weeks following transplant and during treatment for acute rejection:		
Protein	1.3–1.5 g/kg	Counteract protein catabolism; promote wound healing
Calories	30–35 kcal (125–145 kJ)/kg	Meet postsurgery energy demands and allow protein to be used for anabolism
After 6–8 weeks:		
Protein	1.0 g/kg	Minimize muscle protein wasting
Calories	Sufficient to achieve optimal weight for height	Achieve/maintain optimal weight
At all times:		
Carbohydrates	Consistent carbohydrate intake; increase fiber content	Meet energy demands; promote bowel regularity
Fats	No more than 30% of calories; cholesterol <300 mg/day	Reduce post-transplant hyperlipidemia; help prevent progression of atherosclerosis
Potassium	Variable; restrict or supplement as necessary based on serum level	Maintain acceptable potassium level
Sodium	2–4 g (87–175 mmol) may be necessary	Maintain blood pressure control in salt-sensitive individuals; minimize edema
Calcium	1000–1500 mg	Minimize further bone demineralization; correct calcium/phosphorus imbalance
Phosphorus	1200–1500 mg; some patients may require supplements	Minimize further bone demineralization; correct calcium/phosphorus imbalance
Fluids	Ad lib	Maintain adequate hydration

Source: Modified with permission from "Manual of Clinical Dietetics," 6th ed. © 2000 American Dietetic Association, Chicago, IL, and Canadian Dietetic Association.

on CVD, post-transplant patients with glucose intolerance have a higher risk for infection and decreased survival rates [202, 203]. Thus, appropriate control of blood glucose is warranted.

Excessive weight gain is a frequent problem that can exacerbate hyperlipidemia and glucose intolerance. Weight control may be problematic in this patient population because many of the antirejection medications may stimulate appetite. Excess weight gain may have adverse effects on heart disease, lipids, blood pressure, diabetes [199], and, although controversial, possibly increase graft rejection [204, 205].

In addition to increased CVD, glucose intolerance, and increased weight gain, bone disease and altered bone mineral metabolism is a significant problem post-kidney transplant. Hypophosphatemia occurs in as many as 50% of post-transplant patients [206]. In addition, studies show a 10% decrease in bone density by 5 months post-transplant [207].

In the post-transplant state, during adaptation to the kidney and medication regimen, the patient may present with electrolyte imbalances. Due to the effects of immunosuppressive medications on bone mineral metabolism, post-transplant patients will need to increase their phosphorus and calcium intake and/or may need supplementation to prevent bone demineralization. Serum electrolytes should be closely monitored with appropriate interventions taken as warranted.

Of note, protein and energy needs are increased during the first 4–8 weeks post-transplantation. In general, post-kidney transplant patients will require a high-protein, low-fat diet [187]. Nutrition guidelines for post-transplant patients are summarized in Table 8.

V. CONCLUSION

Nutritional factors play an important role in the etiology and management of chronic renal disease. During the past several years, important research questions in this area have been addressed in large-scale clinical studies, which have involved the assessment of nutritional factors as predictors of outcome and randomized controlled diet intervention trials. However, much remains to be learned, and important clinical questions are not yet fully resolved. Nutritional recommendations for the clinical management of patients with chronic renal failure are likely to evolve with increased efforts to expand the knowledge base in this area.

References

1. U.S. Renal Data System (1999). Annual Data Report. II. Incidence and prevalence of ESRD. *Am. J. Kidney Dis.* **34,** S40–S50.

2. U.S. Renal Data System (1999). Annual Data Report. Executive Summary. *Am. J. Kidney Dis.* **34,** S9–S19.

3. Burton, B., and Hirschman, G. (1983). Current concepts of nutritional therapy in chronic renal failure: An update. *J. Am. Diet. Assoc.* **82,** 359–63.

4. Mitch, W. E. (1997). Influences of diet on the progression of chronic renal insufficiency. *In* "Nutritional Management of Renal Disease" (J. D. Kopple and S. G. Massry, Eds.), pp. 317–340. Williams & Wilkins, Baltimore, MD.

5. Klahr, S. (1989). Effects of protein intake on the progression of renal disease. *Annu. Rev. Nutr.* **9,** 87–108.

6. Rosman, J. B., Meijer, S., Sluiter, W. J., Ter Wee, P. M., Piers-Becht, T. P., and Donker, A. J. M. (1984). Prospective randomised trial of early dietary protein restriction in chronic renal failure. *Lancet* **2,** 1291–1295.

7. Fouque, D., Laville, M., Boissel, J. P., Chifflet, R., Labeeuw, M., and Zech, P. Y. (1992). Controlled low protein diets in chronic renal insufficiency: Meta-analysis. *Br. Med. J.* **304,** 216–220.

8. Klahr, S., Levey, A. S., Beck, G. J., Caggiula, A. W., Hunsicker, L., Kusek, J. W., and Striker, G. (1994). The effects of dietary protein restriction and blood pressure control on the progression of chronic renal failure. Modification of Diet in Renal Disease Study Group. *N. Engl. J. Med.* **330,** 878–884.

9. Levey, A. S., Adler, S., Caggiula, A. W., England, B. K., Greene, T., Hunsicker, L. G., Kusek, J. W., Rogers, N. L., and Teschan, P. E. (1996). Effects of dietary protein restriction on the progression of advanced renal disease in the Modification of Diet in Renal Disease Study. *Am. J. Kidney Dis.* **27,** 652–663.

10. Donadio, J. V., Bergstralh, E. J., Offord, K. P., Spencer, D. C., and Holley, K. E. (1994). A controlled trial of fish oil in IgA nephropathy. *N. Engl. J. Med.* **331,** 1194–1199.

11. Donadio, J. V., Dart, R. A., Grande, J. P., Bergstralh, E. J., and Spencer, D. C. (1999). The long-term outcome of patients with IgA nephropathy treated with fish oil in a controlled trial. *J. Am. Soc. Nephrol.* **10,** 1772–1777.

12. Grande, J. P., Walker, J. J., Holub, B. J., Warner, G. M., Keller, D. M., Haugen, J. D., Donadio, J. V., and Dousa, T. P. (2000). Suppressive effects of fish oil on mesangial cell proliferation in vitro and in vivo.

13. Ell, S., Fynn, M., Richards, P., and Halliday, D. (1978). Metabolic studies with keto acid diets. *Am. J. Clin. Nutr.* **31,** 1776–1783.

14. Heidland, A., Kult, J., Rockel, A., and Heidbreder, E. (1978). Evaluation of essential amino acids and keto acids in uremic patients on low-protein diet. *Am. J. Clin. Nutr.* **31,** 1784–1792.

15. Bauerdick, H., Spellerberg, P., and Lamberts, B. (1978). Therapy with essential amino acids and their nitrogen-free analogues in severe renal failure. *Am. J. Clin. Nutr.* **31,** 1793–1796.

16. Burns, J., Cresswell, E., Eill, S., Fynn, M., Jackson, M. A., Lee, H. A., Richards, P., Rowlands, A., and Talbot, S. (1978). Comparison of the effects of keto acid analogues and essential amino acids on nitrogen homeostasis in uremic patients on moderately protein-restricted diets. *Am. J. Clin. Nutr.* **31,** 1767–1775.

17. Furst, P., Ahlberg, M., Alvestrand, A., and Bergstrom, J. (1978). Principles of essential amino acid therapy in uremia. *Am. J. Clin. Nutr.* **31,** 1744–1755.

18. Walser, M. (1978). Principles of keto acid therapy in uremia. *Am. J. Clin. Nutr.* **31,** 1756–1760.

19. Walser, M. (1975). Nutritional effects of nitrogen-free analogues of essential amino acids. *Life Sci.* **17,** 1011–1020.

20. Bergstrom, J., Ahlberg, M., Alvestrand, A., and Furst, P. (1978). Metabolic studies with keto acids in uremia. *Am. J. Clin. Nutr.* **31,** 1761–1766.

21. Brenner, B. M., Meyer, T. W., and Hostetter, T. H. (1982). Dietary protein intake and the progressive nature of kidney disease: The role of hemodynamically mediated glomerular injury in the pathogenesis of progressive glomerular sclerosis in aging, renal ablation, and intrinsic renal disease. *N. Engl. J. Med.* **307,** 652–659.

22. Klahr, S. (1996). Low-protein diets and angiotensin-converting enzyme inhibition in progressive renal failure. *In* "Renal Disease Progression and Management" (M. M. Avram and S. Klaher, Eds.), pp. 36–41. W. B. Saunders, Philadelphia, PA.

23. Aparicio, M., Chauveau, P., De Precigout, V., Bouchet, J.-L., Lasseur, C., and Combe, C. (2000). Nutrition and outcome on renal replacement therapy of patients with chronic renal failure treated by a supplemented very low protein diet. *J. Am. Soc. Nephrol.* **11,** 708–716.

24. Keane, W., O'Donnel, M., Kasiske, B., and Schmitz, P. (1990). Lipids and the progresion of renal disease. *J. Am. Soc. Nephrol.* **1,** S69–S74.

25. Weber, P. (1988). Membrane phospholipid modification by dietary n-3 fatty acids: Effects on eicosanoid formation and cell function. *Prog. Clin. Biol. Res.* **282,** 263–274.

26. Ito, Y., Barcelli, U., Yamashita, W., Weiss, M., Glas-Greenwalt, P., and Pollak, V. (1988). Fish oil has beneficial effects on lipids and renal disease of nephrotic rats. *Metabolism* **37,** 352–357.

27. Goldstein, D. J., Wheeler, D., Dandstrom, D. J., Kawachi, H., and Salant, D. J. (1995). Fish oil ameliorates renal injury and hyperlipidemia in the Milan normotensive rat model of focal glomerulosclerosis. *J. Am. Soc. Nephrol.* **6,** 1468–1475.

28. Prickett, J., Robinson, D., and Steinberg, A. (1981). Dietary enrichment with the polyunsaturated fatty acid eicosapentaenoic acid prevents proteinuria and prolongs survival in NZB x NZW F1 mice. *J. Clin. Invest.* **68,** 556–559.

29. Weiss, M., Hitzemann, R., and Pollak, V. (1986). Beneficial effects of polyunsaturated fatty acids in partially nephrectomized rats. *Prostaglandins* **32,** 211–219.

30. Weise, W. J., Natori, Y., Levine, J. S., O'Meara, Y. M., Minto, A., Manning, E. C., Goldstein, J. J., Abrahamson, D. R., and Salant, D. J. (1993). Fish oil has preventive and therapeutic effects on proteinuria in passive Heymann nephritis. *Kidney Int.* **43,** 359–368.

31. Robinson, D., Prickett, J., Makoul, G., Steinberg, A., and Colvin, R. (1986). Dietary fish oil reduces progression of established renal disease in (NZB x NZW)F1 mice and delays renal disease in BXSB and MRL/1 strains. *Arthritis Rheum.* **29,** 539–546.

32. Worgall, T. S., and Deckelbaum, R. J. (1999). Fatty acids: Links between genes involved in fatty acid and cholesterol metabolism. *Curr. Opin. Clin. Nutr. Metab. Care* **2,** 127–133.

33. Simopoulos, A. P. (1999). Essential fatty acids in health and chronic disease. *Am. J. Clin. Nutr.* **70**(3 Suppl.), 560S–569S.

34. Jump, D. B., and Clarke, S. D. (1999). Regulation of gene expression by dietary fat. *Annu. Rev. Nutr.* **19,** 63–90.

35. Goldstein, D. J., Wheeler, D. C., and Salant, D. J. (1996). Effects of omega-3 fatty acids on complement-mediated glomerular epithelial cell injury. *Kidney Int.* **50**, 1863–1871.

36. Hwang, D., and Rhee, S. H. (1999). Receptor-mediated signaling pathways: Potential targets of modulation by dietary fatty acids. *Am. J. Clin. Nutr.* **70**(4), 545–556.

37. Hamazaki, T., Tateno, S., and Shishido, H. (1984). Eicosapentaenoic acid and IgA nephropathy. *Lancet* **1**, 1017–1018.

38. Schaap, G., Bilo, H., Popp-Snijders, C., Mulder, C., and Donker, A. (1987). Effects of protein intake variation and omega-3 polyunsaturated fatty acids on renal function in chronic renal disease. *Life Sci.* **41**, 2759–2765.

39. Bennett, W., Walker, R., and Kincaid-Smith, P. (1989). Treatment of IgA nephropathy with eicosapentaenoic acid (EPA): A two-year prospective trial. *Clin. Nephrol.* **31**, 128–131.

40. Clark, W., Parbtani, A., Huff, M., Reid, B., Holub, B., and Falardeau, P. (1989). Omega-3 fatty acid dietary supplementation in systemic lupus erythematosus. *Kidney Int.* **36**, 653–660.

41. Cheng, I., Chan, P., and Chan, M. (1990). The effects of fish-oil diet supplement on the progression of mesangial IgA glomerulonephritis. *Nephrol. Dial. Transplant.* **5**, 241–246.

42. Westburg, G., and Tarkowski, A. (1990). Effect of MaxEPA in patients with SLE. A double-blind crossover study. *Scand. J. Rheumatol.* **19**, 137–143.

43. D'Amico, G., Remuzzi, G., Maschio, G., Gentile, M., Gotti, E., Oldrizzi, L., Manna, G., Mecca, G., Rugiu, C., and Gellin, G. (1991). Effect of dietary proteins and lipids in patients with membranous nephropathy and nephrotic syndrome. *Clin. Nephrol.* **35**, 237–242.

44. Clark, W. P., Parbtani, A., Naylor, D., Levinton, C., Muirhead, N., Spanner, E., Huff, M., Philbrick, D., and Holub, B. (1993). Fish oil in lupus nephritis: Clinical findings and methodological implications. *Kidney Int.* **44**, 75–86.

45. St. Joer, S. T. (1996). Renal nutrition therapy in historical perspective. *Top. Clin. Nutr.* **12**, 1–5.

46. Ahmad, S. (1999). "Manual of Clinical Dietetics," 1st ed. Scientific Press, London.

47. Zawada, E. T. (1994). Indications for dialysis. *In* "Handbook of Dialysis" (J. T. Daugirdas and I. S. Ing, Eds.), 2nd ed., pp. 3–12. Little Brown and Co., Boston.

48. Kimmel, P. L., Phillips, T. M., Simmens, S. J., Peterson, R. A., Weihs, K. L., Alleyne, S., Cruz, I., Yanovsju, H. A., and Veis, J. H. (1998). Psychosocial factors, behavioral compliance and survival in urban hemodialysis patients. *Kidney Int.* **54**, 245–254.

49. Heacock, P., Nabel, J., Norton, P., Heile, S., and Royse, D. (1996). An exploration of the relationship between nutritional status and quality of life in chronic hemodialysis patients. *J. Renal Nutr.* **6**, 152–157.

50. Ohri-Vachaspati, P., and Sehgal, A. R. (1999). Quality of life implications of inadequate protein nutrition among hemodialysis patients. *J. Renal Nutr.* **9**, 9–13.

51. Sensky, T., Leger, C., and Gilmour, S. (1996). Psychosocial and cognitive factors associated with adherence to dietary and fluid restriction regimens by people on chronic haemodialysis. *Psychother. Psychosomat.* **65**, 36–42.

52. National Kidney Foundation "Clinical Practice Guidelines for Vascular Access" (1997). NKF-DOQI. National Kidney Foundation, New York.

53. Twardowski Z. J. (1987). Peritoneal equilibration test. *Perit. Dial. Bull.* **7**, 138–140.

54. Sorkin, M. I., and Diaz-Buxo, J. A. (1994). Physiology of Peritoneal Dialysis. *In* "Handbook of Dialysis" (J. T. Daugirdas and T. S. Ing, Eds.), 2nd ed., pp. 245–262. Little Brown and Co., Boston.

55. Wineman R. J. (1983). Rationale of the National Cooperative Dialysis Study. *Kidney Int.* **23**, 8–11.

56. Schoenfeld, P. Y., Henry, R., Laird, N. M., and Roxe, D. M. (1983). Assessment of nutritional status of the National Cooperative Dialysis Study population. *Kidney Int.* **23**, S80–S88.

57. Lowrie, E. G., and Lew, N. L. (1990). Death risk in hemodialysis patients: The predictive value of commonly measured variables and an evaluation of death rate between facilities. *Am. J. Kidney Dis.* **15**, 458–482.

58. Collins, A. J., Ma, J. Z., Umen, A., and Keshaviah, P. (1994). Urea index and other predictors of hemodialysis patient survival. *Am. J. Kidney Dis.* **23**, 272–282.

59. Lowrie, E. G., Huang, W. H., and Lew, N. L. (1995). Death risk predictors among peritoneal dialysis and hemodialysis patients: A preliminary comparison. *Am. J. Kidney Dis.* **26**, 220–228.

60. Churchill, D. H., Taylor, D. W., and Keshaviah, P. R. (1996). Adequacy of dialysis and nutrition in continuous peritoneal dialysis: Association with clinical outcomes. *J. Am. Soc. Nephrol.* **7**, 198–207.

61. Fung, L., Pollock, C. A., Caterson, R. J., Mahony, F. J., Waugh, D. A., Macadam, C., and Ibels, L. S. (1996). Dialysis adequacy and nutrition determine prognosis in continuous ambulatory peritoneal dialysis patients. *J. Am. Soc. Nephrol.* **7**, 737–744.

62. Bargman, J. M., Bick, J., Cartier, P., Dasgupta, M. K., Fine A., Lavoie, S. D., Spanner, E., and Taylor, P. A. (1999). Guidelines for adequacy and nutrition in peritoneal dialysis. Canadian Society of Nephrology. *J. Am. Soc. Nephrol.* **10**, S311–S321; Held, P. J., Port, F. K., Wolfe, R. A., Stannard, D. C., Carroll, C. E., Daugirdas, J. T., Greer, J. W., and Hakim, R. M. (1996). The dose of hemodialysis and patient mortality. *Kidney Int.* **50**, 550–556.

63. Chatoth, D. K., Golper, T. A., and Gokal, R. (1999). Morbidity and mortality in redefining adequacy of peritoneal dialysis: A step beyond the National Kidney Foundation Dialysis Outcomes Quality Initiative. *Am. J. Kidney Dis.* **33**, 617–632.

64. Owen, W. F., Lew, N. L., Liu, Y., Lowrie, E. G., and Lazarus, J. M. (1993). The urea reduction ratio and serum albumin concentration as predictors of mortality in patients undergoing hemodialysis. *N. Engl. J. Med.* **329**, 1001–1006.

65. Hakim, R. M., Breyer, J., Ismail, N., and Schulman, G. (1994). Effects of dose of dialysis on morbidity and mortality. *Am. J. Kidney Dis.* **23**, 661–669.

66. National Kidney Foundation "Clinical Practice Guidelines for Hemodialysis Adequacy" (1997). NKF-DOQI. National Kidney Foundation, New York.

67. National Kidney Foundation "Clinical Practice Guidelines for Peritoneal Dialysis Adequacy" (1997). NKF-DOQI. National Kidney Foundation, New York.

68. Depner, T. A. (1994). Assessing adequacy of hemodialysis: Urea modeling. *Kidney Int.* **45**, 1522–1535.

69. Churchill, D. H., Thorpe, K. E., Nolph, K. D., Keshaviah P. R., Oreopoulus, D. G., and Page, D. (1998). Increased

peritoneal membrane transport is associated with decreased patient and technique survival for peritoneal dialysis patients. The Canada-USA (CANUSA) Peritoneal Dialysis Study Group. *J. Am. Soc. Nephrol.* **9,** 1285–1292.

70. Prichard, S. S. (2000). Comorbidities and their impact on outcome in patients with end stage renal disease. *Kidney Int.* **57,** S100–S104.

71. Wheeler, D. C. (1997). Cardiovascular risk factors in patients with chronic renal failure. *J. Renal Nutr.* **7,** 182–186.

72. Steinvinkel, P., Hemburger, O., Paultine, F., Diczfalvisy, O., Wang, T., Berglund, L., and Jogestrand, T. (1999). Strong association between malnutrition, inflammation, and atherosclerosis in chronic renal failure. *Kidney Int.* **55,** 1899–1911.

73. Prichard, S. (1999). Major and minor risk factors for cardiovascular disease in continuous ambulatory peritoneal dialysis patients. *Perit Dial Int.*

74. Attman, P. O., Samuelsson, O., and Alavpovic, P. (1993). Lipoprotein metabolism and renal failure. *Am. J. Kidney Dis.* **21,** 573–592.

75. Kasiske, B. L. (1998). Hyperlipidemia in patients with chronic renal disease. *Am. J. Kidney Dis.* **32,** S142–S156.

76. Kronenberg, F., Utermann, G., and Dieplinger, H. (1996). Lipoprotein(a) in renal disease. *Am. J. Kidney Dis.* **27,** 1–25.

77. O'Neal, D., Lee, P., Murphy, B., and Best, J. (1996). Low density lipoprotein particle size distribution in end stage renal disease treated with hemodialysis or peritoneal dialysis. *Am. J. Kidney Dis.* **27,** 84–91.

78. Daschner, M., Lenhartz, H., Botticher, D., Schaefer, F., Wollschlager, M., Mehls, O., and Leichsenring, M. (1996). Influence of dialysis on plasma lipid peroxidation products and antioxidant levels. *Kidney Int.* **50,** 1268–1272.

79. Dennis, V. W., and Robinson, K. (1996). Homocysteinemia and vascular disease in end stage renal disease. *Kidney Int.* **57,** S11–S17.

80. Wilcken, D. E., Dudman, N. P. B., Tyrrell, P. A., Robertson, M. R. (1988). Folic acid lowers elevated plasma homocysteine in chronic renal insufficiency: Possible implications for prevention of vascular disease. *Metabolism* **37,** 697–701.

81. Chauveau, P., Chadefaux, B., Coude, M., Aupetit, J., Hannedouche, T., Kamoon, P., and Jungers, P. (1993). Hyperhomocysteinemia: A risk factor for atherosclerosis in chronic uremic patients. *Kidney Int.* **43,** S72–S77.

82. Bostom, A. G., Shemin, D., Lapane, K. L., Miller, J. W., Sutherland, P., Nadeau, M., Seyoum, E., Hartman, W., Prior, R., Wilson, P. W. (1995). Hyperhomocysteinemia and traditional cardiovascular disease risk factors in end stage renal disease patients on dialysis: A case control study. *Atherosclerosis* **93,** 114.

83. Bostom, A. G., Shemin, D., Lapane, K. L., Nadeau, M. R., Sutherlans, P. C., Rozen, R., Yoburn, D., Jacques, P. F., Selhub J., and Rosenberg, I. H. (1996). Folate status is the major determinant of fasting total plasma homocysteine levels in maintenance dialysis patients. *Atherosclerosis* **123,** 193–202.

84. Bostom, A. F., Shemin, D., Verhoef, P., Nadau, M. R., Jacques, P. F., Aelhub, J., Dworkin, L., and Rosenberg, I. H. (1997). Elevated fasting total plasma homocysteine levels and cardiovascular disease outcomes in maintenance dialysis patients. A prospective study. **17,** 2554–2558.

85. Sacks, T., Moldow, C. F., Craddoxk, P. R., Bowers, T. K., and Jacob, H. S. (1978). Oxygen radical mediated endothelial

cell damage by complement stimulated granuloycytes. An in vitro model of immune vascular damage. *J. Clin. Invest.* **6,** 1161–1167.

86. Wall, R. T., Harlan, J. M., Harker, L. A., and Striker, G. E. (1980). Homocysteine induced endothelial cell injury in vitro: A model for the study of vascular injury. *Thromb. Res.* **18,** 113–121.

87. Martin, W. J. (1984). Neutrophils kill pulmonary endothelial cells by a hydrogen peroxide dependent pathway: An in vitro model of neutrophil mediated lung injury. *Am. Rev. Resp. Dis.* **130,** 209–213.

88. Bunting, S., Gyrglewski, R., Mondaca, S., and Vane, J. R. (1976). Arterial walls generate from prostaglandin endoperoxides a substance (prostaglandin X) which relaxes strips of mesenteric and coeliac arteries and inhibits platelet aggregation. *Prostaglandins* **12,** 897–913.

89. Partasarthys, ?? (1987). Oxidation of low density lipoprotein by thiol compounds leads to its recognition by the acetyl LDL receptor. *Biochem. Biophys. Acta* **917,** 337–340.

90. Stamler, J. S., Osborne, J. A., Jaraki, O., Rabbani, L. E., Mullins, M., Singel, D., and Loscalzo, J. (1993). Adverse vascular effects of homocysteine are modulated by endothelial derived relaxing factor and related oxides of nitrogen. *J. Clin. Invest.* **91,** 308–318.

91. Makoff, R., Dwyer, J., and Rocco, M. V. (1996). Folic acid, pyridoxine, cobalamin, and homocysteine and their relationship to cardiovascular disease in end-stage renal disease. *J. Renal Nutr.* **6,** 2–11.

92. Rocco, M. V., and Makoff, R. (1997). Appropriate vitamin therapy for dialysis patients. *Semin. Dial.* **10,** 272–277.

93. Dierkes, J., Domrose, U., Ambrosch, A., Bosselman, H. P., Neumann, K. H., and Luley, C. (1999). Response of hyperhomocysteinemia to folic acid supplementation in patients with end stage renal disease. *Clin. Nephrol.* **51,** 108–115.

94. Parfrey, P. S., Foley, R. N., Harnett, J. D., Kent, G. M., Murray, D. C., Barr,e P. E. (1996). Outcome and risk factors for left ventricular disorders in chronic uraemia. *Nephrol. Dial. Transplant.* **11,** 1277–1285.

95. Zagler, P. G., Nikolic, J., Brown, R. H., Campbell, M. A., Hunt, W. C., Peterson, D., Van Stone, J., Levey, A., Meyer, K. B., Klag, M. J., Johnson, H. K., Clark, E., Sadler, J. H., Teredesai, P. (1998). U curve association of blood pressure and mortality in hemodialysis patients. *Kidney Int.* **54,** 561–569.

96. Goldstein, D. J. (1998). Assessment of nutritional status in renal disease. *In* "Handbook of Nutrition and the Kidney" (W. E. Mitch and S. Klahr, Eds.), pp. 45–86. Lippincott-Raven, Philadelphia.

97. Bro, S., Olgaard, K. (1997). Effects of excess parathyroid hormone on nonclassical target organs. *Am. J. Kidney Dis.* **30,** 606–620.

98. Block, G. A., Hulbert-Shearon, T. E., Levin, N. W., Port, F. K. (1998). Association of serum phosphorus and calcium X phosphate product with mortality risk in chronic hemodialysis patients: A national study. *Am. J. Kidney Dis.* **31,** 607–617.

99. Levin, N. W., Hulbert-Shearon, T. E., Strawderman, R., Port, F. (1998). Which causes of death are related to hyperphosphatemia in hemodialysis (HD) patients? *J. Am. Soc. Nephrol.* **9,** 217A.

100. Slatopolsky, E., Dusso, A., and Brown, A. J. (1999). The role of phosphorus in the development of secondary hyperpara-

thyroidism and parathyroid cell proliferation in chronic renal failure. *Am. J. Med. Sci.* **317,** 370–376.

101. Atsumi, K., Kushida, K., Yamazaki, K., Shimizu, S., Ohmura A., and Inoue, T. (1999). Risk factors for vertebral fractures in renal osteodystophy. *Am. J. Kidney Dis.* **33,** 287–293.

102. McGonigle, R. S. R., Wallin, J. D., Shadduck, R. K., and Fisher, J. W. (1984). Erythropoietin deficiency and erythropoiesis in renal insufficiency. *Kidney Int.* **25,** 437–444.

103. Nissenson, A. R., and Strobos, J. (1999). Iron deficiency in patients with renal failure. *Kidney Int.* **55,** S18–S21.

104. Frankenfield, D., Johnson, C. A., Wish, J. B., Rocco, M. V., Madore, F., and Owen, W. F. (2000). Anemia management of adult hemodialysis patients in the U.S.: Results from the 1997 ESRD Core Indicators project. *Kidney Int.* **57,** 578–589.

105. Nissenson, A. R., Pickett, J. L., Theberge, D. C., Brown, W. S., and Schweitzer, S. V. (1996). Brain function is better in hemodialysis patients when hematocrit is normalized with erythropoietin. *J. Am. Soc. Nephrol.* **7,** 1459.

106. Eschbach, J. W., Kelly, M. R., Haley, N. R., Abels, R. I., and Adamson J. W. (1989). Treatment of the anemia of progressive renal failure with recombinant human erythropoietin. *N. Engl. J. Med.* **321,** 158–163.

107. Schaefer, R. M., Horl, H., and Massry, S. G. (1989). Treatment of renal anemia with recombinant human erythropoietin. *Am. J. Nephrol.* **9,** 353–362.

108. Tarng, D., Huang, T., Chen, T. W., and Yang, W. (1999). Erythropoietin hyporesponsiveness: From iron deficiency to iron overload. *Kidney Int.* **55,** S107–S118.

109. Canaud, B., Bouloux, C., Rivory, J. P., Taib, J., Garrad, L. J., Florence, P., and Mion, C. (1990). Erythropoietin-induced changes in protein nutrition: Quantitative assessment by urea kinetic modeling analysis. *Blood Purif.* **8,** 301–308.

110. MacDougall, I. C., Lewis, N. P., Saunders, M. J., Cochlin, D. L., Davies, M. E., Hutton, R. D., Fox, K. A. A., Coles, G. A., and Williams, J. D. (1990). Long-term cardiorespiratory effects of amelioration of renal anaemia by erythropoietin. *Lancet* **335,** 489–493.

111. Barany, P., Pettersson, E., Ahlberg, M., Hultman, E., and Bergstrom, J. (1991). Nutritional assessment in anemic hemodialysis patients treated with recombinant human erythropoietin. *Clin. Nephrol.* **35,** 270–279.

112. Pascual, J., Teruel, J. L., Moya, J. L., Liano, F., Jimenez-Mena, M., and Ortuno, J. (1991). Regression of left ventricular hypertrophy after partial correction of anemia with erythropoietin in patients on hemodialysis. A prospective study. *Clin. Nephrol.* **35,** 280–287.

113. Wizemann, V., Kaufmann, J., and Kramer, W. (1992). Effect of erythropoietin on ischemic tolerance in anemic hemodialysis patients with confirmed coronary artery disease. *Nephron* **62,** 161–165.

114. Vanholder, R., Van Biesen, W., and Ringoir, S. (1993). Contributing factors to the inhibition of phagocytosis in hemodialyzed patients. *Kidney Int.* **44,** 208–214.

115. Wizemann, V., Schafer, R., and Kramer, W. (1993). Follow up of cardiac changes induced by anemia compensation in normotensive hemodialysis patients with left ventricular hypertrophy. *Nephron* **64,** 202–206.

116. Gafter, U., Kalechman, Y., Orlin, J. B., Levi, J., and Sredni, B. (1994). Anemia of uremia is associated with reduced in vitro cytokine secretion: Immunopotentiating activity of red blood cells. *Kidney Int.* **45,** 224–231.

117. Harnett, J. D., Foley, R. N., Kent, G. M., Barre, P. E., Murray, D., and Parfrey, P. S. (1995). Congestive heart failure in dialysis patients: Prevalence, incidence, prognosis and risk factors. *Kidney Int.* **47,** 884–890.

118. Tarng, D. C., Huang, T. P., and Doong, T. I. (1998). Improvement of nutritional status in patients receiving maintenance hemodialysis after correction of renal anemia with recombinant human erythropoietin. *Nephron* **78,** 253–259.

119. Madore, F., Bridges, K., Lew, N., Lowrie, E., Lazarus, J. M., and Owen, W. F. (1997). Anemia in hemodialysis patients: Variables impacting this outcome predictor. *J. Am. Soc. Nephrol.* **8,** 1921–1929.

120. Ma, J., Ebben, J., Hong, X., and Collins, A. (1999). Hematocrit level and associated mortality in hemodialysis patients. *J. Am. Soc. Nephrol.* **10,** 610–619.

121. National Kidney Foundation "Clinical Practice Guidelines for the Treatment of Anemia of Chronic Renal Failure" (1997). NKF-DOQI. National Kidney Foundation, New York.

122. Benz, R. L., Pressman, M. R., Hovick, E. T., and Peterson, D. D. (1996). Relationship between anemia of chronic renal failure and sleep, sleep disorders and daytime alertness: Benefits of normalizing hematocrit. *J. Am. Soc. Nephrol.* **7,** 1473.

123. Sangkabutra, T., McKenna, M. J., Mason, K., Crankshaw, D. P., and McMahon, L. P. (1997). Effects of K, pH and different haemoglobin levels on maximal exercise performance in haemodialysis patients. *Nephrology* **3,** S304.

124. Besarb, A., Bolton, K., Browne, J., Egrie, J., Nissenson, A., Okamoto, D., Schwab, S., and Goodkin, D. (1998). The effects of normal as compared with low hematocrit values in patients with cardiac disease who are receiving hemodialysis and Epoetin. *N. Engl. J. Med.* **339,** 584–590.

125. Moreno, F., Sanz-Guajardo, D., Lopez-Gomez, J. M., Jofre, R., and Valderrabano, F. (2000). Increasing the hematocrit has a beneficial effect on quality of life and is safe in selected hemodialysis patients. *J. Am. Soc. Nephrol.* **11,** 335–342.

126. Schaller, R., Sperschneider, H., Thieler, H., Dutz, W., Hans, S., Voigt, D., Marx, M., Engelmann, J., Schoter, K. H., Scigalla, P., and Stein, G. (1994). Differences in intravenous and subcutaneous application of recombinant human erythropoietin: A multicenter trial. *Artific. Organs* **18,** 552–558.

127. Albitar, S., Meulders, Q., Hammond, H., Soutif, C., Bouvier, P., and Pollini, J. (1995). Subcutaneous versus intravenous administration of erythropoietin improves its efficiency for the treatment of anaemia in haemodialysis patients. *Nephrol. Dial. Transplant.* **10,** 40–43.

128. Paganini, E. P., Eschbach, J. W., Lazarus, J. M., Van Stone, J. C., Gimenez, L. F., Graber, S. E., Egrie, J. C., Okamoto, D. M., and Goodkin, D. A. (1995). Intravenous versus subcutaneous dosing of epoetin alfa in hemodialysis patients. *Am. J. Kidney Dis.* **26,** 331–340.

129. Jensen, J. D., Madsen, J. K., and Jensen, L. W. (1996). Comparison of dose requirement, serum erythropoietin and blood pressure following intravenous and subcutaneous erythropoietin treatment of dialysis patients. *Eur. J. Clin. Pharmacol.* **50,** 171–177.

130. Cohen, D., and Bloom, R. (1996). Erythropoietin requirements are inversely related to iron saturation levels in chronic stable hemodialysis patients. *J. Am. Soc. Nephrol.* **7,** 1442.

131. Fishbane, S., Mittal, S. K., Maesaka, J. K. (1999). Beneficial effects of iron therapy in renal failure patients on hemodialysis. *Kidney Int.* **55,** S67–S70.

132. Vychytil, A., and Haag-Weber, M. (1999). Iron status and iron supplementation in peritoneal dialysis patients. *Kidney Int.* **55,** [69], S71–S78.

133. MacDougall, I. C., Cavill, I., Hulme, B., Bain, B., McGregor, E., McKay, P., Sauders, E., Coles, G. A., and Williams, J. D. (1992). Detection of functional iron deficiency during erythropoietin treatment. A new approach. *Br. Med. J.* **304,** 225–226.

134. Tarng, D. C., Chen, T. W., Huang, T. P. (1995). Iron metabolism indices for early detection of the response and resistance to erythropoietin therapy in maintenance hemodialysis patients. *Am. J. Nephrol.* **15,** 230–237.

135. Donnelly, S. M., Posen, G. A., All, M. A. (1991). Oral absorption in hemodialysis patients treated with erythropoietin. *Clin. Invest. Med.* **14,** 271–276.

136. Kooistra, M. P., Van Es, A., Struyvenburg, A., and Marx, J. J. M. (1995). Low iron absorption in erythropoietin hemodialysis patients. *J. Am. Soc. Nephrol.* **6,** 543.

137. Schaefer, R. M., and Schaefer, L. (1992). Management of iron substitution during rHuEPO therapy in chronic renal failure patients. *Erythropoiesis* **3,** 71–75.

138. Horl, W. H., Cavill, I., MacDougall, I. C., Schaeffer R. M., and Sunder-Plassmann, G. (1996). How to diagnose and correct iron deficiency during rHuEPO therapy: A consensus report. *Nephrol. Dial. Transplant.* **11,** 246–250.

139. Drueke, T. B., Barany, P., Cazzola, M., Eshbach, J. W., Grutz-macher, P., Kaltwasser, J. P., Koch, K. M., Macdougall, I. C., Pippard, M. J., Shaldon, S., and Van Wyck, D. B. (1997). Management of iron deficiency in renal anemia: Guidelines for the optimal therapeutic approach in erythropoietin treated patients. *Clin. Nephrol.* **48,** 1–8.

140. Fishbane, S., and Maesaka, J. K. (1997). Iron management in renal disease. *Am. J. Kidney Dis.* **29,** 319–333.

141. Nyvad, O., Danielsen, H., and Madsen, S. (1994). Intravenous iron-sucrose complex to reduce epoetin demand in dialysis patients. *Lancet* **344,** 1305–1306.

142. Fishbane, S., Frei, G. L., and Maesaka, J. (1995). Reduction of recombinant human erythropoietin doses by use of chronic intravenous iron supplementation. *Am. J. Kidney Dis.* **26,** 41–46.

143. Sunder-Plassmann, G., and Hurl, W. H. (1997). Erythropoietin and iron. *Clin. Nephrol.* **47,** 141–157.

144. Baile, G. R., Johnson, C. A., and Mason, N. A. (2000). Parenteral iron use in the management of anemia in end-stage renal disease patients. *Am. J. Kidney Dis.* **35,** 1–12.

145. Harter, H. R. (1983). Review of significant findings from the National Cooperative Dialysis Study and recommendations. *Kidney Int.* **13,** S107.

146. Parker, T. F. I., Laird, N. M., and Lowrie, E. G. (1983). Comparison of the study groups in the national cooperative dialysis study and a description of morbidity, mortality, and patient withdrawal. *Kidney Int.* **23**(13), S42–S49.

147. Collins, A. J., Hanson, G., Umen, A., Kiellstrand, C., and Keshaviah, P. (1990). Changing risk factor demographics in end-stage renal disease patients entering hemodialysis and the impact on long term mortality. *Am. J. Kidney Dis.* **15,** 422–432.

148. Kopple, J. D. (1994). Effect of nutrition on morbidity and mortality in maintenance dialysis patients. *Am. J. Kidney Dis.* **24,** 1002–1009.

149. Ikizler, T. A., and Hakim, R. M. (1996). Nutrition in end stage renal disease. *Kidney Int.* **50,** 343–357.

150. Ikizler, T. A., Wingard, R. L., Harvell, J., Shyr, Y., and Hakim, R. (1999). Association of morbidity with markers of nutrition and inflammation in chronic hemodialysis patients: A prospective study. *Kidney Int.* **55,** 1945–1951.

151. Herselman, M., Moosa, M. R., Kotze, T. J., Kritzinger, M., Wuister, S., Mostert, D. (2000). Protein-energy malnutrition as a risk factor for increased morbidity in long term hemodialysis patients. *J. Renal Nutr.* **10,** 7–15.

152. National Kidney Foundation "Clinical Practice Guidelines for Nutrition" (In press). NKF-DOQI. National Kidney Foundation, New York.

153. Acchiardo, S. R., Moore, L. W., snf Latour, P. A. (1983). Malnutrition as the main factor in morbidity and mortality of hemodialysis patients. *Kidney Int.* **16,** S199.

154. Stewart, J., Schvaneveldt, N. B., and Christensen, N. K. (1993). The effect of computerized dietary analysis nutrition education on nutrition knowledge, nutrition status, dietary compliance and quality of life of hemodialysis patients. *J. Renal Nutr.* **3,** 177–185.

155. National Institutes of Health Consensus Statement (1993). "Morbidity and Mortality of Dialysis." U.S. Department of Health and Human Services, Bethesda, MD.

156. Young, G. A., Kopple, J. D., Lindholm, B., Vonesh, E. F., De, V. A., Scalamogna, A., Castelnova, C., Oreopoulos, D. G., Anderson, G. H., Bergstrom, J., et al. (1991). Nutritional assessment of continuous ambulatory peritoneal dialysis patients: An international study. *Am. J. Kidney Dis.* **17,** 462–471.

157. Enia, G., Sicuso, C., Alati, G., and Zoccali, C. (1993). Subjective global assessment of nutrition in dialysis patients. *Nephrol. Dial. Transplant.* **8,** 1094–1098.

158. Canada-USA (CANUSA) Peritoneal Dialysis Study Group (1996). Adequacy of dialysis and nutrition in continuous peritoneal dialysis: Association with clinical outcomes. *J. Am. Soc. Nephrol.* **7,** 198–207.

159. Jones C. H., Newstead C. G., Will E. J., Smye S. W., and Davison A. M. (1997). Assessment of nutritional status in continuous ambulatory peritoneal dialysis patients: Serum albumin is not a useful measure. *Nephrol. Dial. Transplant.* **12,** 1406–1413.

160. Kuhlmann, M. K., Winkelspecht, B., Hammers, A., and Kohler, H. (1997). [Malnutrition in hemodialysis patients. Self assessment, medical evaluation and verifiable parameters] [German]. *Medizinische Klinik* **92,** 13–17.

161. Chumlea, W. C. (1997). Anthropometric assessment of nutritional status in renal disease. *J. Renal Nutr.* **7,** 176–181.

162. Yates, L. A. (1996). Anthropometric worksheet for use with hemodialysis patients. *J. Renal Nutr.* **6,** 162–164.

163. Kopple, J. D., Zhu, X. F., Lew, N. L., and Lowrie E. G. (1999). Body weight-for-height relationships predict mortality in maintenance hemodialysis patients. *Kidney Int.* **56,** 1136–1148.

164. Fleischmann, E., Teal, N., Dudley, J., May, W., Bower, J. D., and Salahudeen, A. K. (1999). Influence of excess weight on mortality and hospital stay in 1346 hemodialysis patients. *Kidney Int.* **55,** 1560–1567.

165. Kloppenburg, W. D., Stegeman, C. A., Hooyschuur M., van der Ven, J., de Jong, P. E., and Huisman, R. M. (1999). Assessing dialysis adequacy and dietary intake in the individual hemodialysis patient. *Kidney Int.* **55**, 1961–1969.

166. Griffiths, A., Russell, L., Breslin, M., Russell, G., and Davies, S. (1999). A comparison of two methods of dietary assessment in peritoneal dialysis patients. *J. Renal Nutr.* **9**, 26–31.

167. Sreedhara, R., Avram, M. M., Blanco, M., Batish, R., Avram, M. M., and Mittman, N. (1996). Prealbumin is the best nutritional predictor of survival in hemodialysis and peritoneal dialysis. *Am. J. Kidney Dis.* **28**, 937–942.

168. Adoncecchi, L., Marrocco, W., Sucraci C., Pecora, P., Gallinella, B., Porra, R., and Cavina, G. (1984). Effect of renal and liver failure on blood levels of vitamin A, its precursor and its carrier proteins, prealbumin and retinol binding protein. *Bollettino-Societa Italiana Biolgia Sperimentale* **60**, 881–886.

169. Avram, M. M., Goldwasser, P., Erroa, M., and Fein, P. A. (1994). Predictors of survival in continuous ambulatory peritoneal dialysis patients: The importance of prealbumin and other nutritional and metabolic markers. *Am. J. Kidney Dis.* **23**, 91–98.

170. Goldwasser, P., Michel, M. A., Collier, J., Mittman, N., Fein, P., Gusik, S., and Avram, M. M. (1993). Prealbumin and lipoprotein(a) in hemodialysis: Relationships with patient and vascular access survival. *Am. J. Kidney Dis.* **22**, 215–225.

171. Avram, M. M., Mittman, N., Bonomini, L., Chattopadhyay, J., and Fein, P. (1995). Markers for survival in dialysis: A seven year prospective study. *Am. J. Kidney Dis.* **26**, 209–219.

172. Iseki, K., Miyasato, F., Tokuyama, K., Nishime, K., Uehara, H., Shiohira, Y., Sunagawa, H., Yoshihara, K., Yoshi, S., Toma, S., Kowatari, T., Wake, T., Oura, T., Fukiyama, K. (1997). Low diastolic blood pressure, hypoalbuminemia and risk of death in a cohort of chronic hemodialysis patients. *Kidney Int.* **51**, 1212–1217.

173. Massy, Z. A., MA, J. Z., Louis, T. A., Kasiske, B. (1995). Lipid lowering therapy in patients with renal disease. *Kidney Int.* **48**, 188–198.

174. Blumenkrantz, M. J., Kopple, J. D., Gutman, R. A., Chan, Y. K., Barbour, G. L., Roberts, C., Shen, F. H., Gandhi, V. C., Tucker C. T., Curtis, F. K., and Coburn, J. W. (1980). Methods for assessing nutritional status of patients with renal failure. *Am. J. Clin. Nutr.* **33**, 1567–1585.

175. Avram, M. M., Fein, P. A., Bonomini, L., Mittman, N., Loutoby, R., Avram D., K., and Chattopadhyay, J. (1996). Predictors of survival in continuous ambulatory peritoneal dialysis patients: A five year prospective study. *Periton. Dial. Int.* **16**, S190–S194.

176. DeLima, J., Sesso, R., Abensur, H., Lopes, H. F., Giorgi, M. C., Krieger, E. M., and Pileggi, F. (1995). Predictors of mortality in long term haemodialysis patients with a low prevalence of comorbid conditions. *Nephrol. Dial. Transplant.* **10**, 1708–1713.

177. Canaud, B., Garred, L. J., Argiles, A., Flavier, J. L., Bouloux, C., and Mion, C. (1995). Creatinine kinetic modelling: A simple and reliable tool for the assessment of protein nutritional status in haemodialysis patients. *Nephrol. Dial. Transplant.* **10**, 1405–1410.

178. Goldstein, D. J., and Frederico, C. B. (1987). The effect of urea kinetic modeling on the nutrition management of hemodialysis patients. *J. Am. Diet. Assoc.* **4**, 474–479.

179. Gotch, F. A. (1995). Kinetic modeling in hemodialysis, *In* "Clinical Dialysis" (A. R. Nissenson, R. N. Fine, and D. E. Gentile, Eds.), 3rd ed., pp. 156–188. Appleton and Lange, Norwalk, CT.

180. Gotch, F. A., and Sargent, J. A. (1985). A mechanistic analysis of the National Cooperative Dialysis Study. *Kidney Int.* **28**, 526–534.

181. Ward, R. A., et al. (1978). Protein catabolism during hemodialysis. *Am. J. Clin. Nutr.* **32**, 243.

182. Farrell, P. C., and Hone, P. W. (1980). Dialysis induced catabolism. *Am. J. Clin. Nutr.* **33**, 1417.

183. Kluthe, R., Luttgen, F. M., Capetianu, T., Heinze, V., Katz, N., and Sudhoff, A. (1998). Protein requirements in maintenance hemodialysis. *Am. J. Clin. Nutr.* **31**, 1812.

184. Kopple, J. D. (1998). Dietary protein and energy requirements in ESRD patients. *Am. J. Kidney Dis.* **32**, S97–S104.

185. Perez, R. (1993). Managing nutrition problems in transplant patients. *Nutr. Clin. Prac.* **8**, 28–32.

186. Weil, S. E. (1996). Nutrition in the kidney transplant recipient. *In* "Handbook of Kidney Transplantation" (G. M. Danovitch, Ed.), 2nd ed., pp. 321–335. Little Brown and Co., Boston.

187. Hines, L. (2000). Can low-fat/cholesterol nutrition counseling improve food intake habits and hyperlipidemia of renal transplant patients? *J. Renal Nutr.* **10**(1), 30–35.

188. Jaggers, H. J., Allman, M. A., and Chan, M. (1996). Changes in clinical profile and dietary considerations after renal transplantation. *J. Renal Nutr.* **6**, 12–20.

189. Ibels, L. S., Alfrey, A., Weil, R. (1978). Hyperlipidemia in adult, pediatric and diabetic renal transplant recipients. *Am. J. Med.* **64**, 634–643.

190. Ponticelli, C., Barbi, G. L., Cantaluppi, A., Donati, C., Annoni, G., and Brancaccio, D. (1978). Lipid disorders in renal transplant recipients. *Nephron* **20**, 189–195.

191. Chan, M. K., Varghese, Z., Persaud, J. W., Fernando, O. N., and Moorhead, J. F. (1981). The role of multiple pharmacotherapy in the pathogenesis of hyperlipidemia after renal transplantation. *Clin. Nephrol.* **15**, 309–313.

192. Jackson, J. M., and Lee, H. A. (1982). The role of propanolol therapy and proteinuria in the etiology of post renal transplantation hyperlipidemia. *Clin. Nephrol.* **18**, 95–100.

193. Shen, S. Y., Lukens, C. W., Alongi, S. V., Sfeir, R. E., Dagner, F. J., and Sadler, J. H. (1983). Patient profile and effect of dietary therapy on post transplant hyperlipidemia. *Kidney Int.* **24**, S147–S152.

194. Kasiske, B. L., and Umen, A. J. (1987). Persistent hyperlipidemia in renal transplant patients. *Medicine* **66**, 309–316.

195. Raine, A. E., Carter, R., Mann, J. I., and Morris, P. J. (1988). Adverse effects of cyclosporine on plasma cholesterol in renal transplant recipients. *Nephrol. Dial. Transplant.* **3**, 458–463.

196. Wolfe, R. A., et al. (1998). Causes of death, U.S. Renal Data System. *Am. J. Kidney Dis.* **32**, S85–S86.

197. Devine, W. (1994). Review of nutritional status on diet in dialysis and transplant patients. *Dial. Transplant.* **23**, 38–41, 47–48.

198. Sullivan, S. S., Anderson, E. J., Best, S., et al. (1996). The effect of diet on hypercholesterolemia in renal transplant recipients. *J. Renal Nutr.* **6**, 141–151.

199. Patel, M. D. (1998). The effect of dietary intervention on weight gain after renal transplantation. *J. Renal Nutr.* **8**, 137–141.

200. Nakai, I., Omoni, Y., Aikawa, I., Yasumura, T., Suzuki, S., Yoshimura, N., Arakawa, K., Matsui, S., and Oka, T. (1988). Effect of cyclosporine on glucose metabolism in kidney transplant recipients. *Transplant Proc.* **20,** 969–978.

201. Roth, D., Milgrom, N., Esquenazi, V., Fuller, L., Burke, G., and Miller, J. (1989). Post transplant hyperglycemia: Increased incidence in cyclosporine treated allograft recipients. *Transplantation* **47,** 278–281.

202. Friedman, E. A., Shyh, T., Beyer, M. M., Maris, T., and Butt, K. M. (1985). Post transplant diabetes in kidney transplant recipients. *Am. J. Nephrol.* **5,** 196–202.

203. Bordreaux, J. P., McHugh, L., Canfax, D. M., Ascher, N., Sutherland, D. E., Payne, W., Simmons, R. L., Najarian, J. S., and Fryd, D. S. (1987). The impact of cyclosporine and combination immunosuppression on the incidence of posttransplant diabetes in renal allograft recipients. *Transplantation* **44,** 371–381.

204. Pirsch, J. D., Armbrust, M. D., Knechtle, S. J., D'Allessandro, A. M., Sollinger, H. W., Heisey, D. M., and Belzer, F. O. (1995). Obesity as a risk factor following renal transplantation. *Transplantation* **59,** 631–663.

205. Dimeny, E., and Fellstrom, B. (1997). Metabolic abnormalities in renal transplant recipients. Risk factors and predictors of chronic graft dysfunction. *Nephrol. Dial. Transplant.* **12,** 21–24.

206. Massari, P. U. (1997). Disorders of bone and mineral metabolism after renal transplantation. *Kidney Int.* **52,** 1412–1421.

207. Horber, F., Casez, J., Steiger, U., Czerniak, A., Montando, A., and Jaeger, P. (1994). Changes in bone mass early after kidney transplantation. *J. Bone Mineral Res.* **9,** 1–9.

CHAPTER 41

Nutritional Management of Parkinson's Disease and Other Conditions Like Alzheimer's Disease

CHRISTY TANGNEY

Rush Presbyterian St. Luke's Medical Center, Chicago, Illinois

I. INTRODUCTION

Neurodegenerative disorders commonly increase in incidence with advancing age. These disorders broadly can be classified into two categories: (1) cognitive decline, such as Alzheimer's disease, vascular dementia, and Parkinson's disease; and (2) physical decline, which may also include these disorders. Alzheimer's disease is the most common form of dementia observed after 60 years of age. From 6% to 8% of those older than 65 have Alzheimer's disease with the prevalence doubling every 5 years after age 60 [1]. Parkinson's disease is the second most common neurodegenerative disorder after Alzheimer's disease, with a prevalence of 2% among persons over the age of 65 years [2]. Parkinson's disease has an unknown etiology, affects more than 1 million people in North America, and has serious health consequences. Mortality is 2–5 times as high among affected persons as among age-matched controls [3–5]. The average age at diagnosis is 57 years, and the disease is rarely seen in those under 30, becoming more common after age 55 years.

Cognitive performance and nutritional status are important indications of general health and functional status in elderly persons. Nutrition and cognition are interrelated. Nutrition surveys of the elderly often indicate increased risk of malnutrition, most often subclinical deficiencies (i.e., folate, vitamin B_{12}), which can impair cognition and mood. Impaired cognition and depression, in turn, decrease appetite.

This chapter will address the interrelationship of nutrition and cognition. In the broadest sense, the primary objective is to review the evidence for nutritional components as potential risk factors for cognitive decline, Alzheimer's disease, and Parkinson's disease. The literature to be reviewed includes animal studies, pathological comparisons, retrospective case-control studies, cross-sectional studies, and longitudinal studies. Evidence from clinical trials for use of specific nutritional therapies for Alzheimer's disease and Parkinson's disease will be described. Finally, nutritional management issues specific for Alzheimer's disease and Parkinson's disease will be examined.

II. NUTRITIONAL FACTORS IN RELATION TO COGNITIVE FUNCTION

A. Laboratory Animal Studies

To define a relationship between a dietary component and cognitive performance, it is important to demonstrate that varying dietary consumption can be reflected in changes in brain tissue, which affect changes in cognitive function. Laboratory animal studies provide a means to illustrate this cause-and-effect relationship. A number of animal studies have examined the influence of specific dietary nutrients at inadequate, adequate, and supranormal levels on tissue concentrations and, specifically, critical regions of the brain, such as the hippocampus, cortex, and striatum. For example, there is ample evidence that tissue levels of alpha-tocopherol are increased with dietary supplementation, but longer feeding periods are required to elevate vitamin E concentration in cerebrum, especially in older animals [6–10]. Serum, adipose tissues, and other organs exhibit increases more rapidly than brain, suggesting that serum levels may not be a good indicator of brain tissue content. Moreover, even with vitamin E-adequate diets, older animals were more likely to manifest lipofuscin, an indicator of lipid peroxidative damaged proteins, than younger animals [10]. In humans, studies suggest that age may exert an effect on serum vitamin E concentrations independent of intake of vitamin E [11].

Because animal brain tissue levels of vitamin E can be elevated with dietary and supplemental vitamin E, what is the evidence that such changes alter cognitive performance? In aged laboratory animals, chronic supranormal feeding of antioxidants may improve cognitive skills. For example, Socci and colleagues [12] found that 24-month-old rats administered intraperitoneal injections of alpha-tocopherol (200 mg/kg/day body weight) and of a spin trapping compound at 32 mg/kg body weight, and vitamin C in their drinking water (600 mg/week) for 2 months had a greater rate of acquisition and greater memory retention than vehicle-treated animals. Motor activity was not changed [12]. Other groups have also

found that vitamin E supplementation in older animals not only elevates brain vitamin E content, but also is associated with improved cognitive performance and less oxidative damage [13–16]. Martin and colleagues [14] fed 6-month-old rats diets enriched in vitamin E (500 mg all rac-alpha-tocopherol acetate/kg diet), spinach, or strawberry extracts for 8 months and observed a marked enhancement in striatal dopamine release in those fed diets enriched in fruits and vegetables but low in vitamin E or those enriched in vitamin E content as compared to controls. Cortex, hippocampus, cerebellum, and striatum vitamin E concentrations were significantly increased in response to supplementation. The risk of neurologic degeneration was reduced with alpha-tocopherol treatment of transgenic mice expressing human variants of amyloid precursor protein, a protein generally considered to reflect brain damage seen in Alzheimer's disease [17].

B. Case-Control, Cross-Sectional, and Prospective Studies of Dietary Components in Relation to Cognitive Function

A number of cross-sectional and longitudinal studies provide both dietary and biochemical evidence (largely serum, plasma, or erythrocyte concentrations) of possible relationships between nutritional factors and cognitive changes. Diet is a particularly difficult exposure to measure because of its complexity. As outlined in Table 1 [18–35], the majority of studies in the literature represent cross-sectional comparisons. For example, when cognitive scores using the Mattis dementia rating in relatively healthy older adults, aged 50–75 years, were dichotomized according to age and education, plasma alpha-tocopherol concentrations were found to be highly correlated with cognitive function [29]. Although a number of antioxidant compounds such as carotenoids and vitamin C were quantified in this large sample, many other dietary components were not examined. In one of the largest cross-sectional studies of the relationship between cognitive performance (memory) and serum antioxidant micronutrient concentrations (vitamin E, vitamin C, beta-carotene, vitamin A, and selenium), low vitamin E/cholesterol ratios were highly predictive of poor memory performance after adjustment for age, education, income, vascular risk factors, and other trace elements (Table 2) [32]. Years of education was a predictor of memory performance [odds ratio (OR) 3.3, $p < 0.0001$]. As found in the entire sample, a strong direct relationship between blood vitamin E/cholesterol levels and memory was also observed in Mexican-Americans and non-Hispanic Caucasians [OR = 4.1, 95% confidence intervals (CI), 1.4–11.99, $p < 0.02$ and OR 2.32, CI 1.0–5.4, $p < 0.05$]. A trend was also observed among non-Hispanic African-Americans, but this association was nonsignificant. Only 7% of the entire sample presented with poor memory overall, 5.9% among individuals who had ever smoked versus 8.4% who had never smoked, and in 14% with a history of prior strokes and 6.6% with no previous stroke.

It has been suggested that estimating the influence of single nutrients rather than dietary patterns is too restrictive. Certainly people eat foods, not nutrients, and the combination of nutrients usually ingested is what may afford protection against cognitive decline. In a cross-sectional study derived from five older male cohorts (aged 70–91 years) from the Seven Countries Study, Huijbregts and colleagues [36] looked at overall dietary quality (obtained through diet histories and evaluated using the Healthy Diet Indicator) and found that this indicator was associated with better cognitive function using the Mini Mental Status Examination.

Relatively few studies examined dietary components in relation to future cognitive performance. These longitudinal studies afford greater confidence in possible relationships between biochemical indices or dietary intakes and functioning. In the cross-sectional analyses of elderly Swiss individuals, for example, blood concentrations of vitamin C and beta-carotene, but not those of vitamin E, were found to be correlated with cognitive function in 442 subjects [28]. Again, concurrent status may not necessarily reflect what is available for specific brain regions. Cross-sectional analyses are particularly prone to selection biases and do not account for the latency period between exposures and cognitive decline. In the longitudinal analyses by the same group, however, both beta-carotene and vitamin C status remained significant predictors of cognition.

In another study of 137 elderly individuals from the New Mexico Aging Project [27], both past (6 years) and concurrent nutrition status (assessed by dietary records and blood indicators) were also related to cognitive performance. These investigators performed an extensive nutrition evaluation that included vitamin C, vitamin E, many B vitamins (i.e., folate, vitamin B_{12}), and several minerals. In many cases, both dietary and biochemical indices indicated potential protective effects against cognitive decline. Surprisingly, no biochemical determinations of vitamin E were reported in this study. Several longitudinal studies in which food frequency questionnaires or queries regarding supplement use appear to confirm the possible role afforded by vitamin E [21, 28, 34, 35] and/or vitamin C [21, 30, 34, 35]. Finally, fish intake appears to have a protective effect on stroke and dementia [25]. Estimating fish intake on the basis of response to four fish items on the Chicago Health and Aging Project food frequency questionnaire, and cognitive performance data measured at baseline, and at both 6-month and 3-year follow-up revealed less decline in cognitive function among persons with higher fish intake (p for trend = 0.04 for fish consumption ranging from several times per month to more than 2 times per week). Whether the reduction in cognitive decline is attributable to fish consumption patterns, specific fatty acids (i.e., omega 3 fatty acids), or some unidentified covariates requires further study.

The inconsistencies between these findings are notable. There are many possible reasons for these differences, which may include the study sample, the type of cognitive tests

TABLE 1 Biochemical and Dietary Studies of Dietary Components in Relation to Cognitive Performance

Investigators	Population	Design	Nutrient measures	Beta-carotene	Vitamin E	Vitamin C	Vitamin B$_{12}$	Vitamin B$_6$	Thiamin	Vitamin B$_2$	Folate	Zinc
			Dietary components (↓ signifies a protective association found; 0, no association; ↑, a negative association or enhanced risk with increased amounts)									
Goodwin et al. [18]	260 men and women aged 60 years and older	Cross-sectional	Plasma concentrations			↓	↓			↓	↓	
			3-day weighed food records			↓					↓	
Spindler and Renvall [19]	73 clinical patients	Cross-sectional	Erythrocyte enzyme activities								↓	
			3 day food records			0						
Haines et al. [20]	75 London residents	Case-control	Plasma concentrations			0						0
Masaki et al. [21]	3735 Japanese-American men	Cross-sectional	Supplement use		↓	↓						
		4-Year prospective			↓	↓						
		20-Year prospective			↓	↓						
Gale et al. [22]	921 British residents aged 65 years and older	Cross-sectional	Plasma concentrations		↓	↓						
			7-day weighed food records		↓	↓						
Jama et al. [23]	5182 Rotterdam residents	Cross-sectional	Food frequency questionnaire	↓	0	0						
Seneca investigators [24]	880 persons from 11 European countries	Cross-sectional	Plasma concentrations	↓	↓		↓				↓	
Kalmijn et al. [25]	1176 Zutphen men	Cross-sectional	Diet history	0	0	0						
		3-Year prospective		0	0	0						
Ortega et al. [26]	260 Spanish seniors aged 65 years and older	Cross-sectional	7-day weighed food record	↓		↓	0		↓	0	↓	↓
La Rue et al. [27]	137 New Mexico seniors aged 66 years and older	Cross-sectional	3-day food records		↓	↓	0		↓	↓	↓	
		6-Year prospective			↓	0	↓		0	0	↓	
		Cross-sectional	Erythrocyte enzyme activities			↓		↓	↓	↓		
		6-Year prospective	Plasma and erythrocyte concentrations				0				0↓	
Perrig et al. [28]	442 Swiss senior residents	Cross-sectional	Plasma concentrations	↓	0	↓						
		22-Year prospective		↓	0	↓						
Schmidt et al. [29]	1769 Austrian subjects aged 50–75 years	Cross-sectional	Plasma concentrations	0	↓	0						
Paleologos et al. [30]	117 Australians	4-Year prospective	Supplement use			↓						
			Food frequency questionnaire			↓						
Berr et al. [31]	1389 French adults	Cross-sectional	Plasma and erythrocyte concentrations	?								
Perkins et al. [32]	4809 NHANES III sample, aged 60 years and older	Cross-sectional	Serum concentrations	0	↓	0		—				
Lindeman et al. [33]	251 New Mexican adults	Cross-sectional	Serum concentrations			0	0				↓	
Morris et al. [35]	2878 Chicago elderly	3-Year prospective	Food frequency questionnaire		↓	↓						

TABLE 2 Proportion and Odds of Having Poor Memory for Selected
Demographic Attributes and Biochemical Measures of Antioxidants in 4809
U.S. Elderly from NHANES III, 1988–1994

Attributes or intake of blood antioxidant concentration	Percentage with poor memory	Odds ratio 95% confidence interval	Level of significance (*p* values)
Sex			
Male	8.4	1.95 (1.30–2.94)	
Female	6.0	1.00[a]	0.002
Alcohol consumption			
Lifetime abstention	13.7	1.98 (1.42–2.77)	
No abstention	5.4	1.00[a]	<0.0001
Education (yr)			
0–8	17.1	3.29 (2.04–5.31)	
9–11	7.0	1.96 (1.10–3.48)	
12	3.7	1.47 (0.85–2.54)	
13	2.6	1.00[a]	<0.0001
Annual income			
<$20,000	11.2	1.74 (1.24–2.44)	
≥$20,000	3.0	1.00[a]	0.002
Vitamin E/cholesterol concentrations			
<4.8	11.3	2.09 (1.02–4.26)	
4.8–5.8	6.9	1.42 (0.79–2.55)	
5.8–7.2	5.0	1.03 (0.62–1.71)	
>7.2	4.1	1.00[a]	0.025
Selenium (mg/dL)			
<113.4	9.8	1.15 (0.72–1.82)	
113.4–121.4	6.2	1.04 (0.64–1.69)	
124.1–135.4	6.0	1.08 (0.59–1.98)	
>135.4	5.3	1.00[a]	0.505
Vitamin C (mg/dL)			
<0.53	10.4	1.07 (0.69–1.06)	
0.53–0.86	7.0	0.89 (0.59–1.32)	
0.87–1.15	4.2	0.79 (0.51–1.22)	
>1.15	5.2	1.00[a]	0.650
Beta-carotene/cholesterol concentrations			
<0.06	6.6	0.79 (0.45–1.38)	
0.06–0.09	6.6	0.99 (0.60–1.63)	
0.09–0.15	6.7	0.91 (0.62–1.33)	
>0.15	7.4	1.00[a]	0.552

Source: Adapted from Perkins, A. J., Hendrie, H. C., Callahan, C. M., Gao, S., Unverzagt, F. W., Xu, Y., Hall, K. S., and Hui, S. L. (1999). Association of antioxidants with memory in a multiethnic elderly sample using the Third National Health and Nutrition Survey. *Am. J. Epidemiol.* **150,** 37–44 [32].

[a]Reference category.

used, and the ability of such tests to detect specific cognitive deficits. Results are also influenced by the type of food or nutrient exposure and the period of time this index reflects (dietary tool, static biochemical indicator in plasma or erythrocyte, or a functional index such as enzyme activity). Serum vitamin E concentration, when expressed per unit of serum cholesterol, was associated with memory performance of participants in National Health and Nutrition Examination

Survey (NHANES) III [32]. Only one other group corrected for cholesterol concentration [28], which provides greater accuracy in assessment.

Several vitamins, including folate, vitamin B_6, and vitamin B_{12}, are involved in methylation reactions in brain tissue and, indirectly, in the prevention of homocysteinemia, which has been associated with increased risk of vascular occlusive disease, stroke, and thrombosis [37]. Many have proposed that a loss of cognitive function may be related to inadequate status for these vitamins via reduced production of S-adenosylmethionine [38], which serves as one of the universal methyl donors in a variety of reactions including the biosynthesis of neurotransmitters [39]. As briefly summarized in Table 1 and more extensively addressed in an excellent review [40], mostly positive or null associations between status for these vitamins and cognitive function have been reported.

III. NUTRITIONAL FACTORS IN RELATION TO ALZHEIMER'S DISEASE AND PARKINSON'S DISEASE

A. Pathological Studies in Alzheimer's Disease and Parkinson's Disease

When postmortem brain tissues of neurological normal controls and groups of patients with neurodegenerative disorders such as Alzheimer's disease and Parkinson's disease were compared to specific micronutrients, such as vitamin E, the results are far from definitive. Some data suggest higher levels in brains of patients with Alzheimer's disease and Parkinson's disease; others do not [41–43]. Vitamin C and beta-carotene concentrations in brain tissue were not quantified in these studies.

In pathological comparisons of Alzheimer's disease cases and controls, comparisons of postmortem brains of controls and Parkinson's disease cases suggest that basal lipid peroxidation is exaggerated in nigral tissue of Parkinson's disease on the basis of higher levels of malondialdehyde (an intermediate product of lipid peroxidation) concentrations and lower concentrations of polyunsaturated fatty acids in Parkinson's disease cases [43, 44]. Postmortem findings are far from conclusive because tissues are susceptible to complications and artifacts with sample processing. Cerebrospinal fluids may afford the ideal biological matrix because these can be obtained in living patients and controls. Here again, some controversy concerning the site of fluid sampling clouds the picture. An important concentration gradient may exist for vitamin E from ventricular to lumbar fluids. Stepped increases in vitamin E supplements (400–4000 IU/day) did not appear to elevate *ventricular* cerebrospinal fluid of patients with Parkinson's disease with Ommaya shunts [45], but *lumbar* cerebrospinal fluids of patients with Parkinson's disease did reflect vitamin E supplementation (2000 IU/day),

with increases being directly related to the duration of supplementation [46]. Lumbar cerebrospinal fluid concentration of alpha-tocopherol were also markedly reduced in patients with Alzheimer's disease when compared to those of controls [47]. Ikeda and coworkers [48] showed lower vitamin B_{12} concentrations in cerebrospinal fluid, but not plasma of patients with Alzheimer's disease as compared to those of patients with other dementias. Further work in this area may clarify the reasons for these seemingly disparate results.

B. Observational Studies of Nutritional Factors in Relation to Alzheimer's Disease

With chronic diseases such as Alzheimer's disease and Parkinson's disease, disease onset is usually a long period of time prior to actual diagnosis. Case-control studies are cost-effective designs for uncommon disease, but as a result are more prone to biased estimates of exposure than are longitudinal studies. A number of case-control studies exist for Alzheimer's disease [49–53] with no consistent outcomes that identify nutritional components. Folate and antioxidant nutrient inadequacies such as vitamin E are most often cited as possible risk factors. In a longitudinal study of aging and Alzheimer's disease in a community of nuns, the severity of atrophy of the cortex (via postmortem magnetic resonance imaging) was examined in relation to serum folate levels. The age-adjusted correlation between cortical atrophy and serum folate levels for all 30 deceased participants was -0.40, $p = 0.03$; no other nutrients examined (including vitamin B_{12}, vitamin B_6, thiamin, vitamin E, and carotenoids) showed any linear relationship to cortical atrophy [54]. In many studies, serum alpha-tocopherol levels were found to be lower in persons with Alzheimer's disease [50, 55–58], but not all studies found this relationship [20].

Longitudinal studies of subjects before the onset of overt symptoms of Alzheimer's disease provide greater confidence in the relationships between nutrient exposures and disease. In a random sample acquired from a prospective study of elderly residents of Boston, the relationship between incident Alzheimer's disease and use of vitamin C and vitamin E supplements was examined [34]. After 4.3 years of follow-up, 91 of the 642 sample participants with vitamin information met the accepted criteria for diagnosis of Alzheimer's disease. None of the 27 vitamin E supplement users had Alzheimer's disease, compared to 3.9 predicted, based on the crude observed incidence among nonusers ($p = 0.04$). Alzheimer's disease incidence for supplement users when adjusted for sex, age, years of education, and length of follow-up was not significant ($p = 0.1$). In contrast, the adjusted number of Alzheimer's disease cases among vitamin C users were significantly less than among nonusers ($p = 0.04$). No relationship was detected for incident Alzheimer's disease with multivitamin use. The relationship for other nutritional supplements could not be examined because too few persons in the cohort reported use of these supplements. A major

TABLE 3 Annual Change in Global Cognitive Score over 3 Years by Quintile of Intake of Vitamins E and C among 2878 Participants Based on Random Effects Models Adjusted for Age, Sex, Race, Education, and Total Energy Intake

Variable	Quintile of intake				
	1	2	3	4	5
Vitamin E median intake (IU/day)	6.8	8.6	10.6	29.1	386.1
Change in score per year	−0.7	−0.05	−0.06	−0.07	−0.05[a]
	(referent)	(−0.07, −0.04)	(−0.07, −0.04)	(−0.08, −0.06)	(−0.06, −0.03)
Vitamin C median intake (mg/day)	63.2	110.8	156.2	221.2	683.2
Change in score per year	−0.07	−0.06	−0.05	−0.07	−0.05[b]
	(referent)	(−0.07, −0.04)	(−0.07, −0.06)	(−0.09, −0.06)	(−0.06, −0.03)

Source: Adapted from [35].
[a] $p = 0.01$.
[b] $p = 0.07$.

strength of this study was that the information regarding vitamin supplement use obtained through direct observation of all medications from the entire cohort. Hence, biased estimates of vitamin use are unlikely. The small number of persons taking vitamin supplements raises the possibility that the findings may be due to chance. Results may also be biased due to the selected participant and nonparticipant bias (i.e., 20% refused to participate, 13% died). The absence of an association among multivitamin users may be the result of low statistical power; thus, investigators were unable to detect a small effect of lower doses of these vitamins or other vitamins in multivitamin mixtures. Large-scale randomized trials will likely resolve some of these issues. Equally important is the addition of more longitudinal studies that examine diet and the incidence of Alzheimer's disease that may confirm or refute these findings.

In preliminary analyses of biracial community participants in the Chicago Health and Aging Project, a significant inverse relationship between total intake (diet and supplements combined) of vitamin E and change in global cognitive score over 3 years (using the average of Z-transformed scores for four cognitive tests) was found [35]. Compared with an average decline of 0.07 standard deviation (SD)/year for a person with an intake in the lowest quintile, the average decline in the global Z-score in the highest quintile was 0.05 SD/year (Table 3). There was also a marginally significant reduction in cognitive decline in those with the highest intake of vitamin C. Because there was a significant reduction in cognitive decline in the highest quintile of vitamin E intake (median 386 IU/day), these data suggest that supplement use probably contributes to this relationship. When intakes of these vitamins from food sources were examined separately, decline in global score was reduced by 0.03 SD/year per log (IU) increase in vitamin E intake ($p = 0.0005$). Intake from dietary vitamin C was not associated with change in cognitive decline [35]. Dietary intake data were based on a food frequency questionnaire, and a preliminary

data provide support for the accuracy of this instrument with respect to vitamin supplement reporting behaviors [59]. If food intake is more stable over time than supplement use, the observed inverse relationship suggests that vitamin E intake from foods may be sufficient to protect against cognitive decline.

In another community study of 3777 elderly subjects aged >65 years living in southwestern France, mean alcohol consumption through use of a structured questionnaire was recorded with the main objective of identifying new Alzheimer's disease cases after 1 and 3 years [60]. After 3 years, the incidence of Alzheimer's disease was lower in those who drank a moderate amount of wine (3–4 glasses/day) compared to nondrinkers (adjusted OR = 0.28, $p < 0.05$) and for mild drinkers (<1–2 glasses per day), the adjusted OR for Alzheimer's disease was 0.55, $p < 0.05$. Further information is needed to provide confirmation of this finding. The antioxidant contribution of wine is consistent with findings for vitamin C and vitamin E, mentioned above.

C. Observational Studies of Nutritional Factors in Relation to Parkinson's Disease

Parkinson's disease is less common than Alzheimer's disease, and there are a greater number of case-control studies addressing potential dietary risk factors and Parkinson's disease (Table 4) [61–73]. There are several reasons to examine diet as a possible exposure that may explain Parkinson's disease. First, the rare disease, amyotrophic lateral sclerosis-parkinsonism-dementia, observed in the islands of Guam and Rota, is thought to be caused by a dietary toxin from the cycad plant [74]. Second, a number of neuropathological studies implicate oxidative stress in the pathogenesis of Parkinson's disease [43, 44]. Also, it was discovered that a synthetic heroin analogue, 1-methyl-4-phenyl-1,2,3,6-tetrahydropyridine (MPTP) was selectively toxic to dopaminergic neurons in the substantia nigra. The toxicity attributable

TABLE 4 Biochemical and Dietary Studies of Parkinson's Disease

Investigators	Study sample	Design	Nutrient exposure measurement	Relationships noted
Golbe et al. [61]	81 Cases; 81 controls (New Jersey)	Case-control	Food preference lists, early adulthood	Peanuts, salad oil/dressing, and plums consumption less likely in cases than controls.
Tanner et al. [62]	35 Cases; 70 controls (Chicago)	Case-control	Vitamin supplement use during early childhood and adult years	Vitamin E supplements and use of cod liver oil is protective against Parkinson's disease.
Fernandez-Calle et al. [63]	42 Cases; 42 spouse controls (Spain)	Case-control	Serum concentration	No association.
Tangney et al. [64]	100 Cases; 200 controls (China)	Case-control	Food frequency questionnaire; under 30 and 30–50 years old	No association for vitamins C, E, or beta-carotene intakes.
Cerhan et al. [65]	41,836 Women	Prospective longitudinal; 6 year	Food frequency questionnaire	Protective effect for vitamin C and manganese intakes; vitamin A intake associated with increased risk of disease.
Hellenbrand et al. [66]	342 Cases; 342 controls (Germany)	Case-control	Food frequency questionnaire	Lower consumption of carbohydrates (OR = 2.7, 1.3–6.1), higher consumption of vitamin C (OR = 0.60, 0.33–1.09) and niacin (OR = 0.15, 0.07–0.33) are associated with risk of Parkinson's disease. No association with vitamin E intake.
Logroscino et al. [67]	104 Cases; 352 controls (Italy)	Case-control	Food frequency questionnaire	Consumption of animal fats was associated with 9-fold increase in risk of Parkinson's disease with low transferrin saturation, indicative of low iron stores. No direct association between dietary iron and risk of Parkinson's disease.
Morens et al. [3]	84 Cases; 336 controls (Honolulu)	Nested case-control	Food frequency questionnaire and 24 hour dietary recall	No association for dietary or supplemental vitamin E, but prior consumption of legumes was highly related to Parkinson's disease (OR = 0.27, 0.09–0.78).
Ross et al. [68]	8004 Japanese-American men 45–68 years old (Honolulu Heart Program)	Prospective longitudinal	Food frequency questionnaire	Incident Parkinson's disease declines consistently with increased coffee intake from 10.4 per 10,000 person years in no coffee drinkers to 1.9 in men who drank more than 28 oz/day.
Anderson et al. [69]	103 Cases; 156 controls (Washington)	Case-control	Food frequency questionnaire	Consumption of animal fats (OR = 3.3, 1.4–7.6) associated with Parkinson's disease. No other relationships.
De Rijk et al. [70]	5342 Adults, 55–95 years old	Cross-sectional	Food frequency questionnaire	Vitamin E intakes (OR = 0.5, 0.2–0.9) in a dose-dependent manner protective against Parkinson's disease. Others examined: beta-carotene, vitamin C, and flavonoids, with marginal odds ratios.
Foy et al. [72]	51 Cases; 41 controls	Case-control	Plasma concentration	Lower vitamins A, C, beta-carotene, and E in Alzheimer's disease; lower vitamin C and lycopene in Parkinson's disease. No differences between cases and controls.
Fall et al. [73]	113 Cases; 263 controls (Sweden)	Case-control	Frequency of intake of 29 food items	Higher consumption of meats, smoked ham, eggs, French bread, tomatoes, coffee, tea, and alcohol among cases.

to MPTP involves oxidation and the formation of a reactive intermediate that impairs mitochondrial function and results in cell death in the substantia nigra pars compacta and promotes oxidative stress [75]. The appealing attribute of the oxidative stress hypothesis is that cumulative oxidative damage over time could account for the late life onset and the progressive nature of this disorder.

Two retrospective case-control studies suggest an inverse association between vitamin E and Parkinson's disease which initiated considerable interest in antioxidant protection and Parkinson's disease [61, 76]. Dietary intake was not quantified directly, but patients with Parkinson's disease rate their food consumption of specific foods different than that of their spouses. Consumption of foods rich in vitamin E and possibly other antioxidant-rich foods (e.g., salad dressing, peanuts, plums) were inversely associated with risk of Parkinson's disease. Tanner and colleagues [62] found that early life use of multivitamins, vitamin E supplements, and cod liver oil was greater among 70 controls as compared to 35 Parkinson's disease subjects. In a secondary analyses of these data, acquired by interviewer-administered food frequency questionnaires using a well-recognized nutrient database (University of Minnesota Nutrient Data System, version 2.4), yielded a null finding, except when females, ages 31–50 years, were examined separately, $OR = 0.89$, $p = 0.01$ [64]. Another two case-control studies found no inverse relationship for any antioxidant nutrients examined, although the designs were fraught with problems [66, 67]. Finally, in a nestled case-control study of Hawaiian men of Japanese ancestry, an inverse association was shown between Parkinson's disease and consumption of foods containing vitamin E (in particular, legumes) [3]. Intriguingly, three of these case-control studies suggest that consumption of animal fats or meats is associated with increased risk for Parkinson's disease [67, 69, 73]. Thus far, the most compelling data are those from a recent large community-based study in which vitamin E intakes assessed from an interviewer-administered food frequency questionnaire were significantly lower ($p = 0.03$) in those with Parkinson's disease ($n = 31$) than those without Parkinson's disease ($n = 5311$) [70]. Those with higher vitamin E intakes had Parkinson's disease significantly less often than those with lower vitamin E intakes ($OR = 0.5$, 95% CI, 0.2–0.9). Even excluding those with late stage Parkinson's disease and supplement users, the associations did not change. When vitamin E, beta-carotene, vitamin C, and flavonoid intakes were categorized into tertiles, a dose-dependent trend for vitamin E intakes and risk for Parkinson's disease was observed. These findings need to be confirmed in prospective studies in which dietary habits have been measured before the onset of Parkinson's disease. The Rotterdam study may provide such data shortly [70–71]. In addition, further investigation of the role of animal fats and meats should be explored in longitudinal studies in which clinical diagnoses of Parkinson's disease can be ascertained.

At present there are two large prospective studies reporting relationships between diet and Parkinson's disease incidence. As is characteristic of longitudinal studies, subjects were disease free when reporting their usual dietary intakes via dietary history questionnaire or food frequency questionnaire. In the first of these studies, 41,836 women from Iowa Women's Health Study were followed up for an average of 6 years. A significant protective effect was noted for vitamin C and manganese intakes while increased risk was observed for vitamin A intake [65]. Unfortunately, these results are only available as a preliminary report and more information is needed. The Honolulu Heart Program followed Hawaiian men of Japanese and Okinawan ancestry in a nested case-control design [3]. Once again, consumption of foods containing vitamin E 25 years earlier appear to protect against Parkinson's disease. In the longitudinal analyses [68], incident Parkinson's disease and coffee intake were compared in a 30-year follow-up of the 8004 men in the study. Age-adjusted incidence of Parkinson's disease declined consistently with increased coffee intake from 10.4 per 10,000 person years in no coffee drinkers to 1.9 in men who drank more than 28 oz/day. Similar relationships were observed for total caffeine intake and appeared independent of smoking. Further studies are warranted to confirm or refute these findings.

IV. SPECIFIC NUTRITIONAL TRIALS IN COGNITIVE, ALZHEIMER'S, AND PARKINSON'S DISEASES

While reports of several trials aimed at treating cognitive impairment or dementia are available [77, 78], few can truly be classified as rigorous double-blind, clinical trials with random assignment of treatments. On the other hand, rigorously controlled clinical trials have limitations when studying these diseases. First, if the chronic disease has a long latency period, is it appropriate to test whether short-term nutrient exposure affords protection in individuals with advanced disease? The second important issue is to examine extant observational studies and neuropathological studies in order to test the hypothesis of nutrient exposure and disease risk. More of a nutrient is not always better.

With respect to alternative therapies with free radical scavenging properties, Gingko biloba extract Egb 761 (containing terpenoids and several organic acids) has been shown to inhibit toxicity of beta amyloid peptide (a marker of Alzheimer's disease on hippocampal neuronal cultures [79]. Egb 761 has been studied extensively in Germany and the United States and approved in the former for the treatment of dementia [80, 81]. In the former trial, in which 200 demented patients received either 40 mg Egb 761, three times/day, or placebo for 1 year, modest improvements were observed in cognitive performance and social functioning, but these changes were large enough to be discerned by a caregivers' scale. A small but significant improvement on cog-

nitive function has also been noted following a review of more than 30 studies of Egb 761 [82]. A major clinical trial is currently under way to test the efficacy of a daily supplement (240 mg) in 1500 subjects against 1500 subjects assigned placebo over 5 years of treatment.

A. Alzheimer's Disease Trials

At this point in time, we are aware of only one completed double-blind clinical trial, the Alzheimer's Disease Cooperative Study of 324 subjects with moderate disease. The main objective of this placebo-controlled, parallel group, factorial design, multicenter trial was to determine whether vitamin E (2000 IU/day or 1342 alpha-tocopherol equivalents/day) or selegiline (10 mg/day) or both could slow functional decline in Alzheimer's disease patients [83]. Selegiline is a monoamine oxidase B inhibitor with antioxidant properties [84]. Time to functional decline was operationalized as the time to reach any one of the following endpoints: institutionalization, loss of basic activities of daily living as measured [85], severe dementia as defined by a clinical rating of 3 [86], or death. Risk of reaching this outcome was significantly reduced by vitamin E ($p < 0.001$), selegiline ($p < 0.01$), and combined treatments ($p < 0.05$). There was no evidence of additional improvement with both treatments over each treatment alone, however. Although significant benefits of vitamin E supplementation alone as compared to placebo were found for functional assessments, none was shown for cognitive tests. A large proportion of subjects were unable to complete the cognitive testing at the end of 2 years. The lack of cognitive benefit has also been ascribed to the relatively advanced nature of the disease of subjects at study entry. Therefore, Grundman and others [87] have proposed a primary prevention trial with 2000 IU/day vitamin E or placebo in those at risk for Alzheimer's disease who have minor cognitive deficits that are insufficient to meet clinical criteria for Alzheimer's disease.

B. Parkinson's Disease Trials

A double-blind clinical trial of the monoamine oxidase B inhibitor, selegiline, and alpha-tocopherol, known as the deprenyl and tocopherol antioxidant therapy of Parkinson's disease or DATATOP, was designed to test whether either treatment or both might retard the progression of Parkinson's disease. Initial analyses at the end of the trial showed that vitamin E at 2000 IU/day was without effect [88] but selegiline markedly delayed the onset of disability. Follow-up studies showed that the effects were not sustained [89, 90]. One concern with DATATOP and the Alzheimer's Disease Cooperative Study is that the latency period for development of the disease with that afforded by the nutrient exposure is missed. A 2- or 4-year follow-up may be too brief to discern any treatment effect in patients with established disease.

Identification of subjects at high risk of either disease rather than patients with clearly defined diagnosis and long-term nutrient (or food) exposure may be necessary to truly illustrate neuroprotection. Again, the vitamin E dose selected for aforementioned trials is thought to elevate brain levels by as much as 50%, which is consistent with animal studies suggesting increases in vitamin E levels in brain by 30–60% of the elevation seen in plasma [8, 10, 91], as well as lumbar cerebrospinal fluid levels observed in DATATOP participants [8]. On the other hand, data from both ventricular cerebrospinal fluid levels of patients with Parkinson's disease on stepped doses from 400 to 4000 IU/day of vitamin E [45] and prospective data [23, 70, 71] suggest that even lower doses may be effective.

Another randomized clinical trial is currently recruiting young and older patients with Parkinson's disease and age-matched controls in order to determine whether glucose aides memory in healthy elderly and young people, and second, whether glucose facilitates working memory in people with Parkinson's disease. The premise for the use of glucose relies on its role as a precursor of acetylcholine synthesis as well as the fact that many drugs used for cognition enhancement produce their effect through enhanced glucose utilization [92]. Moreover, glucose may enhance retention and or retrieval from long-term verbal memory [93]. In a series of experiments, older men were shown to be more susceptible to cognitive impairment during hypoglycemia than were young men [94]. Additionally, a recent review by Benton and Parker [95] shows that breakfast consumption influences cognition, primarily memory, through a variety of mechanisms, one of which is through an elevation of blood and brain glucose levels.

V. NUTRITIONAL MANAGEMENT ISSUES IN NEUROCOGNITIVE DISORDERS

One important component of nutritional management of patients with any neurodegenerative disorder is rigorous scrutiny of weight change patterns of patients, because weight loss is so common, particularly in advanced stages. Because cognitive deficiencies lead to orientation disturbances, loss of independence, and altered eating behaviors, the nutritional care of patients with these diseases becomes critical.

A. Weight Loss in Patients with Alzheimer's Disease

The National Institute of Neurological and Communicative Disorders and Strokes Task Force included weight loss as a clinical sign of Alzheimer's disease [96]. Alzheimer's disease was a risk factor for weight loss in 467 subjects ages 65 years and older followed for 5 annual exams in the Chicago Health and Aging Project, but weight loss was not associated with disease severity [97]. Conversely, changes in stage of Alzheimer's disease were significantly related to weight

change, and losses greater than 5% were highly predictive of mortality [98]. Equally important to evaluate is the perceived burden of the caregivers [99], which has been shown to be highly predictive of weight loss in Alzheimer's disease [100].

It is unclear why weight loss occurs in Alzheimer's disease. Contrary to earlier studies in which only resting energy expenditure was measured [101, 102], increased total energy expenditures cannot explain observed weight losses, even those with severe cachexia (weight loss >2 kg over the 12-month period). In fact, both lower physical activity and lower resting energy expenditures were observed in Alzheimer's disease [103]. Because both weight gain as well as weight loss are observed in patients with Alzheimer's disease, some aberration in weight regulation may be present. Grundman and colleagues [104] showed that atrophy of the mesial temporal cortex in Alzheimer's disease patients is associated with lower body mass index and lower cognitive function. Because the mesial temporal cortex plays an important role in eating behavior, memory, and emotions, this relationship should be explored further.

Documentation of food intakes of patients with Alzheimer's disease are sparse in the literature. Refusal of food is a commonly reported problem and may be related to abnormalities in the neuroendocrine system. Neurotransmitters such as neuropeptide Y and norepinephrine are reduced in patients with Alzheimer's disease type dementia [105]. Little research has explored these possibilities, however [106]. One group examined the use of dronabinol in 15 patients with Alzheimer's disease who were refusing food in whom weight gain, but no change in energy intake, was observed. Some of the behaviors associated with food refusal may be due to dysphagia or failure to recognize edible items as food (agnosia) [107]. Refusal to eat may even be a symptom of depression; antidepressant therapy has been shown to improve intakes even in severely demented patients [108].

B. Weight Loss in Parkinson's Disease

In patients with Parkinson's disease, impaired cognition and motor disturbances (i.e., dysphagia) may result in marked anorexia. The prevalence of weight loss (as well as a reduction in muscle mass) in Parkinson's disease will vary with the degree of gastrointestinal dysfunction. Dysphagia and constipation are not a sequelae of the disease but often the result of the medications used to treat Parkinson's disease. Weight loss estimates vary from 20 to 50% of patients with Parkinson's disease [109, 110]. In one study, patients with Parkinson's disease were four times more likely than age-matched controls to lose more than 10 pounds [111]. In a doubly labeled water studies of patients with Parkinson's disease and healthy controls, Toth and coworkers [112] have shown that although resting energy expenditures are greater among patients with Parkinson's disease (1655 ± 283 versus 1561 ± 219 kcal/day), physical activity expenditure is considerably less. Again, as observed for patients with Alz-

heimer's disease, daily total energy expenditures are nearly 15% lower (2214 ± 460 kcal/day versus 2590 ± 497 kcal/day) in patients with Parkinson's disease, when compared to controls.

Tanner and colleagues [62] have summarized three general gastrointestinal disorders in Parkinson's disease: motility disorders (including dysphagia and constipation), sialorrhea, and appetite disorders. Aspiration and malnutrition are common outcomes of these disorders. Because swallowing abnormalities and excessive drooling are often related, it is important that swallowing studies be performed to define the nature of the dysphagia and presence or absence of silent aspiration. Soft diets can help most types of dysphagia by making it easier to move foods through the mouth and esophagus. These foods can also minimize aspiration by reducing the need for separate fluid intake [113]. The use of feeding gastrostomies or jejunostomies should be the last alternative.

In the case of patients with Parkinson's disease, constipation management is important. This consists of dietary changes, exercise, and pharmacotherapy. High-fiber foods should be encouraged along with increased fluids (in particular, water) [114, 115], and exercise should be as vigorous as possible. Use of stool softeners can be added if given with meals. Patients with Parkinson's disease are also at risk for osteoporosis [116, 117]. Patients following any protein redistribution or restriction plan (discussed below) are often prone to inadequate calcium intakes [118, 119].

C. Protein Modified Diets in Parkinson's Disease

Advanced Parkinson's disease and prolonged levodopa treatment can cause patients to become more resistant to levodopa therapy [120]. Approximately 50% of patients with Parkinson's disease prescribed levodopa for 3 or more years experience motor-response fluctuations [121], an unpredictable "on" and "off" of motor function. Periods of drug unresponsiveness in Parkinson's disease may be due to the competition between the large neutral amino acids and levodopa across the blood brain barrier [120, 122–125]. This competition decreases the availability of levodopa for the brain, thereby resulting in reduced ability to control motor functions. Although there is no specific definition, low-protein diets typically limit total daily protein intakes to 0.8 g/kg body weight, which is lower than the average American intake of 1.6 g/kg [124, 126–128]. A protein-restricted or redistributed diet is one in which daytime protein intake is usually below 10 g with unrestricted evening intake. The rationale for this approach is that levodopa will be better absorbed and effective during the restrictive protein period when mobility is most desired. Other factors may also play a role in the effectiveness of levodopa treatment, such as time between levodopa administration and the meal, frequency of meals, usual dietary intake of energy, carbohy-

TABLE 5 Nutrient Content of Milkshakes Provided in a Crossover Study

	High-protein shake[a]	Low-protein shake[a]
Protein (g)	5.4	0.8
Carbohydrates (g)	12.3	14.9
Fat (g)	7.3	8.4
Carbohydrate to protein ratio	2.3:1	18.6:1
Fiber (g)	0	0
Energy (kcal)	136.1	138.1

Source: Adapted from Tsui, J. K., Ross, S., Poulin, K., Douglas, J., Postnikoff, D., Calne, S., Woodward, W., and Calne, D. B. (1989). The effect of dietary protein on the efficacy of L-dopa: A double blind study. *Neurology* **39,** 549–552 [124].

[a]Values are per 100-mL milkshake.

drates, fat, or fiber. Unfortunately, little systematic study of factors other than protein intake has been addressed by investigators.

Low-protein and protein redistribution studies have been associated with positive effects for some patients suffering from "on–off" fluctuations. In a double-blind crossover study, Tsui and coworkers [124] compared the motor performance and blood levels of levodopa in 10 fluctuating patients with Parkinson's disease on high- (80 or 70 g protein/day for men and women, respectively) and low-protein milkshakes (50 or 40 g protein/day for men and women, respectively). For 5 days, subjects were given either a high- or low-protein milkshake for breakfast and lunch and ate a regular diet in the evening. After a 2-day rest period, the subjects were given the alternate milkshake for another 5 days. Although plate waste studies were done, no record was made of fat, carbohydrate, or fiber content of the participants' diets other than the amount found in the milkshakes (Table 5). Seven out of 10 patients reported a statistically significant improvement ($p < 0.05$) in performance while on a low-protein diet, but blood levodopa levels did not differ. Because the intervention was so short and intake data are incomplete, no firm conclusions can be drawn concerning the efficacy of this dietary manipulation for patients with Parkinson's disease suffering from motor oscillation.

Carter and coworkers [127] also looked at the effectiveness of protein restriction and redistribution in five elderly patients. Subjects were prescribed a high-protein diet (1.6 g/kg/day) for 1 day and then changed to either a protein-restricted diet (0.8 g/kg body weight/day consumed throughout the day) or a protein-redistributed diet (0.8 gm/kg body weight/day in which 90% of the protein is consumed at night) for 3 consecutive days. Patients experienced significantly better motor performance and reduced levels of plasma large neutral amino acid concentrations ($p < 0.001$) on the protein-restricted diet and protein-redistributed diet

than on a high-protein diets. During the day, the patients on the protein-redistributed diet had the most "on" time as compared the protein-restricted diet and the high-protein diet (77%, 67%, and 51%, respectively). Although these investigators reported dietary intakes of energy, protein, carbohydrate, and fat, no information regarding fiber intakes or background dietary patterns was provided. Again, these findings suggest that such strategies may provide some additional motor control, but further research that carefully defines the dietary patterns of patients prior to the test diet and careful dietary monitoring with long-term follow-up is warranted.

The relative amounts of carbohydrate and protein in foods consumed together may also influence how much levodopa enters the brain and, thereby, may modify unpredictable fluctuations [128]. Nine men suffering from unpredictable motor oscillations (mean age of 60) were fed three diets in which the carbohydrate-to-protein ratio was varied: 21:1, 5:1, and 0.3:1; a crossover design was used [128]. Plasma levels of large neutral amino acids were 24% higher and 18% lower on the 0.3:1 and the 21:1 diets, respectively ($p<0.001$) as compared to those when on the 5:1 plan. Consumption of the 0.3:1 diet caused increased Parkinsonian symptoms while with the 21:1 diet, patients became dyskinetic. A decrease in motor performance, assessed by decreased ability to place pegs in a peg board and a decrease in accuracy in writing, was also observed in patients on the 0.3:1 and the 21:1 diets. The patients on a 5:1 diet maintained stable plasma large neutral amino acids ($<3\%$ change), while motor performance on the pegboard and their writing improved. Based on these outcomes, the researchers concluded that the 5:1 diet was associated with improved clinical performance and recommended further study with manipulations. Further work by Feldman [129] and O'Brien [118] confirm that in the short-term, milkshakes with a 5:1 or 7:1 provide enhanced motor function. However, no evidence is available concerning the likelihood of long-term compliance with such dietary plans or whether the observed motor improvements can be sustained. Pare and coworkers [119] examined the impact of protein-restricted diets in patients with Parkinson's disease who were prescribed these dietary plans (maximum of 10 g protein before evening) on nutritional adequacy based on food records completed by the study participants. Calcium, iron, phosphorus, and niacin intakes were marginal (Table 6). We have also found that, in designing a strict 7:1 dietary plan, a multivitamin multimineral supplement is indicated [130].

Finally, data are very limited regarding the value of fiber-rich diets and an improvement in motor skills of patients with Parkinson's disease with unpredictable fluctuations. Nineteen fluctuating patients with Parkinson's disease (13 women and 6 men) suffering from constipation consumed a 28 g fiber/day diet [131]. A supplement of 18 g dietary fiber (made of wheat, pectin, and dimethylpolyoxylhexane) was mixed with water and administered to all the subjects in addition to 10 g fiber consumed in their diet. Disability

TABLE 6 Mean Energy and Nutrient Intakes in Patients with Parkinson's Disease during Usual Diet and Protein-Restricted Diet Periods

Dietary component	Regular diet[a]	Protein-restricted diet
Energy (kcal/day)		
Females ($n = 6$)	1975 ± 196	1759 ± 290
Males ($n = 6$)	2351 ± 413	2460 ± 611
Protein (g/day)		
Females	71 ± 11	54 ± 13
Males	83 ± 11	63 ± 13
Calcium (mg/day)		
Females	716 ± 110	463 ± 159
Males	857 ± 238	633 ± 229
Iron (mg/day)		
Females	15 ± 2	12 ± 2
Males	17 ± 3	15 ± 3
Riboflavin (mg/day)		
Females	1.6 ± 0.2	1.2 ± 0.3
Males	1.7 ± 0.3	1.5 ± 0.3
Niacin (mg/day)		
Females	31 ± 6	24 ± 5
Males	38 ± 5	30 ± 6
Phosphorus (mg/day)		
Females	1200 ± 139	870 ± 243
Males	1487 ± 247	1136 ± 194

Source: Adapted from Pare, S., Barr, S. I., and Ross, S. E. (1992). Effect of daytime protein restriction on nutrient intakes of free-living Parkinson's disease patients. *Am. J. Clin. Nutr.* **55,** 701–707 [119].

[a]Values represent mean $\pm$ standard deviation.

scores were measured using the United Parkinson's Disease Rating Scale motor exam before the study began, at 2 weeks into the study, and at the end of 2 months. With significant improvement ($p<0.0001$) in frequency of bowel movements came borderline significant improvement in gait ($p = 0.05$) and reduction in 3-*O*-methyl dopamine ($p = 0.034$). The compound 3-*O*-methyl dopamine reflects the amount of dopamine metabolized in the periphery. The investigators suggest that levodopa absorption was accelerated by increased gastric motility and shortened gastric emptying, which may improve clinical response [131]. Unfortunately, dietary intakes prior to the intervention as well as those during the intervention were not recorded, so again, this study cannot provide support for a unique role of such diets in motor performance.

VI. SUMMARY

There is definitely a need to explore the possible protective and negative associations between specific exposures of both food and nutrients as well as overall usual dietary patterns (quantified by tools such as the Healthy Diet Indicator [36], the Healthy Eating Index [132] or the Dietary Quality Index–Revised [133]) and cognitive performance. Because further information is needed to estimate intake levels associated with change in cognitive performance, several ongoing longitudinal studies provide a unique opportunity to examine these factors in their study populations. We await future reports from many of these studies, including the Rotterdam, Iowa Women's Health, SENECA, and CHAP studies. Equally important is the need to define better small-scale clinical studies to address the efficacy of modified protein, and fiber-enriched dietary patterns on the motor function of patients with Parkinson's disease. Finally, it is paramount that evaluation of depression and cognitive impairment be a routine component of every nutritional assessment.

References

1. Small, G. W., Rabins, P. V., Barry, P. P., Buckholtz, N. S., DeKosky, S. T., Ferris, S. H., Finkel, S. I., Gwyther, L. P., Khachaturian, Z. S., Lebowitz, B. D., McRae, T. D., Morris, J. C., Oakley, F., Schneider, L. S., Streim, J. E., Sunderland, T., Teri, L. A., and Tunek, L. E. (1997). Diagnosis and treatment of Alzheimer's disease and related disorders. Consensus statement of the American Association for Geriatric Psychiatry, the Alzheimer's Association and the American Geriatrics Society. *JAMA* **278,** 1363–1371.

2. Martin, J. A. (1999). Mechanisms of disease: Molecular basis of the neurodegenerative disorders. *N. Engl. J. Med.* **340,** 1970–1980.

3. Morens, D. M., Grandinetti, A., Waslien, C. I., Park, C. B., Ross, G. W., and White, L. R. (1996). Case-control study of idiopathic Parkinson's disease and dietary vitamin E intake. *Neurology* **46,** 1270–1274.

4. Louis, E. D., Marder, K., Cote, L., Tang, M., and Mayeux, R. (1997). Mortality from Parkinson's disease. *Arch. Neurol.* **54,** 260–264.

5. Bennett, D. A., Beckett, L. A., Murray, A. M., Shannon, K. M., Goetz, C. G., Pilgrim, D. M., and Evans, D. A. (1996). Prevalence of parkinsonian signs and associated mortality in the community residents of older people. *N. Engl. J. Med.* **334,** 71–76.

6. Zhang, J.-R., Andrus, P. K., and Hall, E. D. (1993). Age-related changes in hydroxyl radical stress and antioxidants in gerbil brain. *J. Neurochem.* **61,** 1640–1647.

7. Vatassery, G. T. (1979). Alpha tocopherol levels in various regions of the central nervous systems of the rat and guinea pig. *Lipids* **13,** 828–833.

8. Vatassery, G. T., Brin, M. F., Fahn, S., Kayden, H. J., Traber, M. G. (1988). Effect of high doses of vitamin E on the concentrations of vitamin E in several brain regions, plasma liver, and adipose tissue of rats. *J. Neurochem.* **51,** 621–623.

9. Bourre, J.-M., and Clement, M. (1991). Kinetics of rat peripheral nerve, forebrain, and cerebellum alpha tocopherol depletion: Comparison with different organs. *J. Nutr.* **121,** 1204–1207.

10. Monji, A., Morimoto, N., Okuyama, I., Yamashita, N., and Tashiro, N. (1994). Effect of dietary vitamin E on lipofuscin

accumulation with age in the rat brain. *Brain Res.* **634,** 62–168.

11. Ford, E. S., and Sowell, A. (1999). Serum alpha-tocopherol status in the United States population: Findings from the Third National Health and Nutrition Examination Survey. *Am. J. Epidemiol.* **150,** 290–300.

12. Socci, D. J., Crandall, B. M., and Arendash, G. W. (1995). Chronic antioxidant treatment improves cognitive performance of aged rats. *Brain Res.* **693,** 88–94.

13. Pillai, S. R., Traber, M. G., Steiss, J. E., Kayden, H. J., and Cox, N. R. (1993). Alpha tocopherol concentrations of the nervous system and selected tissues of adult dogs fed three levels of vitamin E. *Lipids* **28,** 1101–1105.

14. Martin, A., Prior, R., Shukitt-Hale, B., Cao, G., and Joseph, J. A. (2000). Effects of fruits and vegetables or vitamin E-rich diet on vitamins E and C distribution in peripheral and brain tissues: Implications for brain function. *J. Gerontol.* **55A,** B144–B151.

15. Joseph, J. A., Shukitt-Hale, B., Denisova, N. A., Prior, R. L., Cao, G., Martin, A., Taglialatela, G., and Bickford, P. C. (1998). Long-term dietary strawberry, spinach or vitamin E supplementation retards the onset of age-related neuronal signal-transduction and cognition-behavioral deficits. *J. Neurosci.* **18,** 8047–8055.

16. Hara, H., Kato, H., and Kogure, K. (1990). Protective effect of alpha-tocopherol on ischemic neuronal damage in gerbil hippocampus. *Brain Res.* **510,** 335–338.

17. Hsiao, K. K., Borchelt, D. R., Olson, K., Johannsdottir, R., Kitt, C., Yunis, W., Xu, S., Eckman, C., Younkin, S., and Price, D. (1995). Age-related CNS disorder and early death in transgenic FVB/N mice overexpressing Alzheimer amyloid precursor proteins. *Neuron* **15,** 1203–1218.

18. Goodwin, J. S., Goodwin, J. M., and Garry, P. J. (1983). Association between nutritional status and cognitive functioning in a healthy elderly population. *JAMA* **249,** 2917–2921.

19. Spindler, A. A., and Renvall, M. A. (1989). Nutritional status and psychometric test scores in cognitively impaired elders. *Ann. N.Y. Acad. Sci.* **301,** 167–177.

20. Haines, A., Iliffe, S., Morgan, P., Dormandy, T., and Wood, B. (1991). Serum aluminum and zinc and other variables in patients with and without cognitive impairment in the community. *Clin. Chim. Acta* **198,** 261–266.

21. Masaki, K. H., Losonczy, K. G., Izmirlian, G., Foley, D. J., Ross, G. W., Petrovitch, H., Havlik, R., and White, L. R. (2000). Association of vitamin E and C supplement use with cognitive function and dementia in elderly men. *Neurology* **54**(6), 1265–1272.

22. Gale, C. R., Martyn, C. N., and Cooper, C. (1996). Cognitive impairment and mortality in a cohort of elderly people. *Br. Med. J.* **312,** 608–611.

23. Jama, J. W., Launer, L. J., Witteman, J. C. M., den Breeijen, J. H., Breteler, M. M., Grobbee, D. E., and Hofman, A. (1996). Dietary antioxidants and cognitive function in a population-based sample of older persons: The Rotterdam study. *Am. J. Epidemiol.* **144,** 275–280.

24. Seneca Investigators: De Groot, C. P., van Stavaren, W. A., Dirren, H., and Hautvast, J. G. (1996). Summary and conclusions of the report on the second data collection period and longitudinal analyses of the SENECA study. *Eur. J. Clin. Nutr.* **50**(Suppl. 2), S123–S124.

25. Kalmijn, S., Feskens, E. J. M., Laner, L. J., and Kromhout, D. (1997). Polyunsaturated fatty acids, antioxidants, and cognitive function in very old men. *Am. J. Epidemiol.* **145,** 33–41.

26. Ortega, R. M., Requejo, A. M., Andres, P., Lopez-Sobaler, A. M., Quintas, M. E., Redondo, M. R., Navia, B., and Rivas, T. (1997). Dietary intake and cognitive function in a group of elderly people. *Am. J. Clin. Nutr.* **66,** 803–809.

27. LaRue, A., Koehler, K. M., Wayne, S. J., Chiulli, S. J., Haaland, K. Y., and Garry, P. J. (1997). Nutritional status and cognitive functioning in a normally aging sample: A 6-y reassessment. *Am. J. Clin. Nutr.* **65,** 20–29.

28. Perrig, W. J., Perrig, P., and Stahelin, B. (1997). The relation between antioxidants and memory performance in the old and very old. *J. Am. Geriatr. Soc.* **45,** 718–724.

29. Schmidt, R., Hayn, M., Reinhart, B., Roob, G., Schmidt, H., Schumacher, M., Watzinger, N., and Launer, L. J. (1998). Plasma antioxidants and cognitive performance in middle-aged and older adults: Results of the Austrian Stroke Prevention Study. *J. Am. Geriatr. Soc.* **46,** 1407–1410.

30. Berr, C., Richard, M. J., Roussel, A. M., and Bonithon-Kopp, C. (1998). Systemic oxidative stress and cognitive performance in the population-based EVA study. *Free Radical Biol. Med.* **24,** 1202–1208.

31. Paleologos, M., Cumming, R. G., and Lazarus, R. (1998). Cohort study of vitamin C intake and cognitive impairment. *Am. J. Epidemiol.* **148,** 45–50.

32. Perkins, A. J., Hendrie, H. C., Callahan, C. M., Gao, S., Unverzagt, F. W., Xu, Y., Hall, K. S., and Hui, S. L. (1999). Association of antioxidants with memory in a multiethnic elderly sample using the Third National Health and Nutrition Survey. *Am. J. Epidemiol.* **150,** 37–44.

33. Lindeman, R. D., Romero, L. J., Koehler, K. M., Liang, H. C., LaRue, A., Baumgartner, R. N., and Garry, P. J. (2000). Serum vitamin B_{12}, C and folate concentrations in the New Mexico Elder Health Survey: Correlations with cognitive and affective function. *J. Am. College Nutr.* **19,** 68–76.

34. Morris, M. C., Beckett, L. A., Scherr, P. A., Hebert, L. E., Bennett, D. A., and Field, T. S. (1998). Vitamin E and vitamin C supplement use and risk of incident Alzheimer disease. *Alzheimer Dis. Assoc. Disord.* **12,** 121–126.

35. Morris, M. C., Evans, D. A., Bienias, J. L., Wilson, R. S., and Tangney, C. C. (2000). Dietary intake of vitamin E and vitamin C and cognitive decline in a biracial community population. *Neurobiol. Aging* **21**(Suppl 1), S202.

36. Huijbregts, P. P. C. W., Feskens, E. J. M., Rasanen, L., Fidanza, F., Nissinen, A., Menotti, A., and Kromhout, D. (1998). Dietary patterns and cognitive function in elderly men in Finland, Italy, and Netherlands. *Eur. J. Clin. Nutr.* **52,** 826–831.

37. Boushey, C. J., Beresford, S. A. A., Omenn, G. S., and Motulsky, A. G. (1995). A quantitative assessment of plasma homocysteine as a risk factor for vascular disease. *JAMA* **274,** 1049–1057.

38. Rosenberg, I. H., and Miller, J. W. (1992). Nutritional factors in physical and cognitive functions of elderly people. *Am. J. Clin. Nutr.* **55,** 1237S–1243S.

39. Bressa, G. M. (1994). S-adenosyl-1-methionine (SAMe) as antidepressant: meta-analysis of clinical studies. *Acta Neurol. Scand.* **154**(Suppl.), 7–14.

40. Selhub, J., Bagley, L. C., Miller, J., and Rosenberg, I. H. (2000). B vitamins, homocysteine, and neurocognitive function in the elderly. *Am. J. Clin. Nutr.* **71**, 514S–520S.

41. Adams, J. D. Jr., Klaidman, L. K., Odunze, I. N., Shen, H. C., and Miller, C. A. (1991). Alzheimer's and Parkinson's disease. Brain levels of glutathione, glutathione disulfide, and vitamin E. *Mol. Chem. Neuropathol.* **14**, 213–226.

42. Metcalfe, T., Bowen, D. M., and Muller, D. P. (1989). Vitamin E concentrations in human brain of patients with Alzheimer's disease, fetuses with Down's syndrome, centenarians, and controls. *Neurochem. Res.* **13**, 1209–1212.

43. Dexter, D. T., Carter, C. J., Wells, F. R., Javoy-Agid, F., Agid, Y., Lees, A., Jenner, P., and Marsden, C. D. (1989). Basal lipid peroxidation in substantia nigra is increased in Parkinson's disease. *J. Neurochem.* **52**, 381–389.

44. Dexter, D. T., Holley, A. E., Flitter, W. D., Slater, T. F., Wells, F. R., Daniel, S. E., Lees, A. J., Jenner, P., and Marsden, C. D. (1994). Increased levels of lipid hydroperoxides in parkinsonian substantia nigra: An HPLC and ESR study. *Movement Disord.* **9**, 92–97.

45. Pappert, E. J., Tangney, C., Goetz, C. G., Ling, Z. D., Lipton, J. W., Stebbins, G. T., and Carvey, P. M. (1996). Alpha tocopherol in ventricular cerebrospinal fluid of Parkinson's disease patients: Dose-response study and correlations with plasma levels. *Neurology* **47**, 1037–1042.

46. Vatassery, G. T., Fahn, S., Kuskowski, M. A., and the Parkinson Study Group (1998). Alpha tocopherol in CSF of subjects taking high-dose vitamin E in the DATATOP study. *Neurology* **50**, 1900–1902.

47. Tohgi, H., Abe, T., Nakanishi, M., Hamato, F., Sasaki, K., and Takahashi, S. (1995). Concentrations of alpha-tocopherol and its quinone derivative in cerebrospinal fluid from patients with vascular dementia of the Binswanger type and Alzheimer type dementia. *Neurosci. Lett.* **174**, 73–76.

48. Ikeda, T., Furukawa, Y., Mashimoto, S., Takahashi, K., and Yamada, M. (1990). Vitamin B$_{12}$ levels in serum and cerebrospinal fluid of people with Alzheimer's disease. *Acta Psychiatr. Scand.* **82**, 327–329.

49. Joosten, E., Lesaffre, E., Riezler, R., Ghekiere, V., Dereymaeker, L., Pelemans, W., and Dejaeger, E. (1997). Is metabolic evidence for vitamin B12 and folate deficiency more frequent in elderly patients with Alzheimer's disease? *J. Gerontol. A: Biol. Sci. Med. Sci.* **52**, M76–M79.

50. Agbayema, M., Bruce, V., and Siemens, V. (1992). Pyridoxine, ascorbic acid and thiamine in Alzheimer and comparison subjects. *Canad. J. Psych.* **37**, 661–662.

51. Renvall, M. J., Spindler, A. A., Ramsdell, J. W., and Paskvan, M. (1989). Nutritional status of free-living Alzheimer's patients. *Am. J. Med. Sci.* **298**, 20–27.

52. Levitt, A. J., and Karlinsky, H. (1992). Folate, vitamin B12 and cognitive impairment in patients with Alzheimer's disease. *Acta Psychiatr. Scand.* **86**, 301–305.

53. Kristensen, M. O., Gulmann, N. C., Christensen, J. E. J., Ostergaard, K., and Rasmussen, K. (1993). Serum cobalamin and methylmalonic acid in Alzheimer dementia. *Acta Neurol. Scand.* **87**, 475–481.

54. Snowdon, D. A. (2000). Serum folate and the severity of atrophy of the neocortex in Alzheimer disease: Findings from the Nun Study. *Am. J. Clin. Nutr.* **71**, 993–998.

55. Jackson, C. V. E., Holland, A. J., Williams, C. A., and Dickerson, J. W. T. (1988). Vitamin E and Alzheimer's disease in subjects with Down's syndrome. *J. Ment. Def. Res.* **32**, 479–484.

56. Nes, M., Sem, S., Rousseau, B., Bjorneboe, G. E., Engedal, K., Trygg, K., and Pedersen, J. I. (1988). Dietary intakes and nutritional status of old people with dementia living at home in Oslo. *Eur. J. Clin. Nutr.* **42**, 581–593.

57. Jeandel, C., Nicholas, M., Dubois, F., Nabet-Belleville, F., Penin, F., and Cuny, G. (1989). Lipid peroxidation and free radical scavengers in Alzheimer's disease. *Gerontology* **35**, 275–282.

58. Zaman, Z., Roche, S., Fielden, P., Frost, P. G., Niriella, D. C., and Cayley, A. C. (1992). Plasma concentrations of vitamins A and E and carotenoids in Alzheimer's disease. *Age Aging* **21**, 91–94.

59. Tangney, C. C., Evans, D. A., Morris, M. C. (2000). Validity of a food frequency questionnaire in the reporting of vitamin and mineral supplement use in an older biracial community population. Presented at "Fourth International Conference on Dietary Assessment Methods."

60. Orgogozo, J. M., Dartigues, J. F., LaFont, S., Letenneur, L., Commenges, D., Salamon, R., Renaud, S., and Breteler, M. B. (1997). Wine consumption and dementia in the elderly: A prospective community study in the Bordeaux area. *Rev. Neurol.* **153**, 185–192.

61. Golbe, L. I., Farrell, T. M., and Davis, P. H. (1988). Case-control study of early life dietary factors in Parkinson's disease. *Arch. Neurol.* **45**, 1350–1353.

62. Tanner, C. M., Cohen, J. A., Sommerville, B. C., and Goetz, C. G. (1988). Vitamin use and Parkinson's disease. *Ann. Neurol.* **23**, 182–185.

63. Fernandez-Calle, P., Molina, J. A., Jimenez-Jimenez, F. J., Vazquez, A., Pondal, M., Garcia-Ruiz, P. J., Urra, D. G., Domingo, J., and Codoceo, R. (1992). Serum levels of alpha-tocopherol (vitamin E) in Parkinson's disease. *Neurology* **42**, 1064–1066.

64. Tangney, C. C., Chao, C., and Tanner, C. M. (1993). Dietary antioxidant intakes of Parkinson's disease patients and controls: Secondary analyses using the Minnesota Dietary Analysis System. *J. Am College Nutr.* **13**, 126A.

65. Cerhan, J. R., Wallace, R. B., and Folsom, A. R. (1994). Antioxidant intake and risk of Parkinson's disease (PD) in older women. *Am. J. Epidemiol.* **139**, S65.

66. Hellenbrand, W., Boeing, H., Robra, B. P., Seidler, A., Vieregge, P., Nischan, P., Joerg, J., Oertel, W. H., Schneider, E., and Ulm, G. (1996). Diet and Parkinson's disease II: A possible role for the past intake of specific nutrient-results from a self-administered food frequency questionnaire in a case-control study. *Neurology* **47**, 644–650.

67. Logroscino, G., Marder, K., Cote, L., Tang, M. X., Shea, S., and Mayeux, R. (1996). Dietary lipids and antioxidants in Parkinson's disease: A population-based, case-control study. *Ann. Neurol.* **39**, 89–94.

68. Ross, G. W., Abbott, R. D., Petrovitch, H., Morens, D. M., Grandinetti, A., Tung, K. H., Tanner, C. M., Masaki, K. H., Blanchette, P. L., Curb, J. D., Popper, J. S., and White, L. R. (2000). Association of coffee and caffeine intake with the risk of Parkinson disease. *JAMA* **282**, 2674–2679.

69. Anderson, C., Checkoway, H., Franklin, G. M., Beresford, S., Smith-Weller, T., and Swanson, P. D. (1999). Dietary factors in Parkinson's disease: The role of food groups and specific foods. *Movement Disord.* **14,** 21–27.

70. De Rijk, M. C., Breteler, M. M., den Breeijen, J. H., Launer, L. J., Grobbee, D. E., van der Meche, F. G., and Hofman, A. (1997). Dietary antioxidants and Parkinson disease. The Rotterdam Study. *Arch. Neurol.* **54**(6), 762–765.

71. DeRijk, M. C., Launer, L. J., Berger, K., Breteler, M. M, Dartigues, J. F., Baldereschi, M., Fratiglioni, L., Lobo, A., Martinez-Lage, J., Trenkwalder, C., and Hofman, A. (1997). Prevalence of parkinsonism and Parkinson's disease in Europe: the EUROPARKINSON Collaborative Study. *J. Neurol. Neurosurg. Psychiatry* **62,** 10–15.

72. Foy, C. J., Passmore, A. P., Vahidassr, M. D., Young, I. S., and Lawson, J. S. (1999). Plasma chain breaking antioxidants in Alzheimer's disease, vascular dementia, and Parkinson's disease. *Q. J. Med.* **92,** 39–45.

73. Fall, P. A., Fredrikson, M., Axelson, A., and Ogranerus, A. K. (1999). Nutritional and occupational factors influencing the risk of Parkinson's disease: A case-control study in southeastern Sweden. *Movement Disord.* **14,** 28–37.

74. Spencer, P. (1993). Guam ALS/parkinsonism-dementia: A long-latency neurotoxic disorder caused by a "slow toxin(s)" in food? *Can. J. Neurol.* **43,** 1173–1180.

75. Singer, T. P., Castagnoli, N., Jr., Ramsay, R. R., and Trevor, A. J. (1987). Biochemical events in the development of parkinsonism induced by 1-methyl-4-phenyl-1,2,3,6-tetrahydropyridine. *J. Neurochem.* **49,** 1–8.

76. Golbe, L. I., Farrell, T. M., and Davis, P. H. (1990). Followup study of early life protective and risk factors in Parkinson's disease. *Movement Disord.* **5,** 66–70.

77. Eastley, R., Wilcox, G. K., and Bucks, R. S. (2000). Vitamin B_{12} deficiency in dementia and cognitive impairment: The effects of treatment on neuropsychological function. *Int. J. Geriatr. Psych.* **15,** 226–233.

78. Baker, H., DeAngelis, B., Naker, E. R., Frank, O., and Jaslowdagger, S. P. (1999). Lack of effect of 1 year intake of a high-dose vitamin and mineral supplement on cognitive function in elderly women. *Gerontology* **45,** 195–199.

79. Bastianetto, S., Ramassamy, C., Christen, Y., Poirier, J., and Quirion, E. (2000). Ginkgo biloba extract (EGb 761) protects in vitro rat hippocampal cells against toxicity induced by β-amyloid peptides. *Eur. J. Neurosci.* **12,** 1882–1890.

80. LeBars, P. L., Katz, M. M., Berman, N., Itil, T., Freedman, A. M., and Schalzberg, A. F. (1997). A placebo-controlled, double-blind, randomized trial of an extract of Ginkgo biloba for dementia. *JAMA* **278,** 1327–1332.

81. Kanowski, S., Herrmann, W. M., Stephan, K., Wierich, W., and Hörr, R. (1996). Proofs of efficacy of the Ginkgo biloba special extract EGb 761 in outpatients suffering from mild to moderate primary degenerative dementia of the Alzheimer type or multi-infarct dementia. *Pharmacopsychiatry* **29,** 47–56.

82. Oken, B. S., Storzbach, D. M., and Kaye, J. A. (1998). The efficacy of Ginkgo biloba on cognitive function in Alzheimer disease. *Arch. Neurol.* **55,** 1409–1415.

83. Sano, M., Ernesto, C., Thomas, R. G., Klauber, M. R., Schafer, K., Grundman, M., Woodbury, P., Growdon, J, Cotman, C. W., Pfeiffer, E., Schneider, L. S., and Thal, L. J.

84. Jenner, P., and Olanow, C. W. (1996). Oxidative stress and the pathogenesis of Parkinson's disease. *Neurology* **47,** S161–S170.

85. Blessed, G., Tomlinson, B. E., and Roth, M. (1968). The association between quantitative measures of dementia and senile changes in the grey matter of elderly subjects. *Br. J. Psychiatr.* **114,** 797–811.

86. Morris, J. C. (1993). The Clinical Dementia Rating (CDR): Current version and scoring rules. *Neurology* **43,** 2412–2414.

87. Grundman, M. (2000). Vitamin E and Alzheimer disease: The basis for additional clinical trials. *Am. J. Clin. Nutr.* **71,** 630S–636S.

88. Parkinson Study Group (1993). Effects of tocopherol and deprenyl on the progression of disability in early Parkinson's disease. *N. Engl. J. Med.* **328,** 176–183.

89. Parkinson Study Group. (1996). Effects of deprenyl and tocopherol treatment on Parkinson's disease in DATATOP subjects requiring levodopa. *Ann. Neurol.* **39,** 37–45.

90. Parkinson Study Group. (1996). Effects of deprenyl and tocopherol treatment on Parkinson's disease in DATATOP subjects not requiring levodopa. *Ann. Neurol.* **39,** 29–36.

91. Meydani, M., Macauley, J. B., and Blumberg, J. B. (1986). Influence of dietary vitamin E, selenium, and age on regional distribution of alpha tocopherol in the rat brain. *Lipids* **21,** 786–791.

92. Wenk, G. L. (1989). An hypothesis on the role of glucose in the mechanism of action of cognition enhancers. *Psychopharmacology* **99,** 431–438.

93. Foster, J. K., Lidder, P. G., and Sunram, S. I. (1998). Glucose and memory: Fractionation of enhancement effects? *Psychopharmacology* **137,** 259–270.

94. Matyka, K., Evans, M., Lomas, J., Cranston, I., Macdonald, I., and Amiel, S. A. (1997). Altered hierarchy of protective responses against severe hypoglycemia in normal aging in healthy men. *Diabetes Care* **20,** 135–141.

95. Benton, D., and Parker, P. Y. (1998). Breakfast, blood glucose, and cognition. *Am. J. Clin. Nutr.* **67,** 772S–778S.

96. McKhann, G., Drachman, D., Folstein, M., Katzman, R., Price, D., and Stadlan, E. M. (1984). Clinical diagnosis of Alzheimer's disease: Report of the NINCDS-ADRDA Work Group under the auspices of Department of Health and Human Services Task Force on Alzheimer's Disease. *Neurology* **34,** 939–944.

97. Cronin-Stubbs, D., Beckett, L. A., Scherr, P. A., Field, T. S., Chown, M. J., Pilgrim, D. M., Bennett, D. A., and Evans, D. A. (1997). Weight loss in people with Alzheimer's disease: A prospective population-based analysis. *Br. Med. J.* **314,** 178–179.

98. White, H., Pieper, C., and Schmader, K. (1998). The association of weight change in Alzheimer's disease with severity of disease and mortality: A longitudinal analysis. *J. Am. Geriatr. Soc.* **46,** 1223–1227.

99. Zarit, S. H., Todd, P. A., and Zarit, J. M. (1982). Families under stress: Interventions of caregivers of senile dementia patients. *Psychotherapy* **19,** 461–471.

100. Guyonnet, S., Nourhashemi, F., Andrieu, S., Reyes-Ortega, G., de Glisezinski, L., Adoue, D., Riviere, D., Vellas, B., and

Albarede, J. L. (1998). A prospective study of changes in nutritional status in Alzheimer's patients. *Arch. Gerontol. Geriatr.* **12S** (Suppl), 255–262.

101. Wolfe-Klein, G. P., Silverstone, F. A., Lansey, S. C., Tesi, D., Ciampaglia, C., O'Donnell, M., Galkowski, J., Jaeger, A., Wallenstein, S., and Leleiko, N. S. (1995). Energy requirements in Alzheimer's disease patients. *Nutrition* **11**, 264–268.

102. Reyes-Ortega, G., Guyonnet, S., Ousset, P. J., Nourhashemi, F., Vellas, B., Albarede, J. L., De Glizezinski, I., Riviere, D., and Fitten, L. J. (1997). Weight loss in Alzheimer's disease and resting energy expenditure (REE), a preliminary report. *J. Am. Geriatrics. Soc.* **45**, 1414–1415.

103. Poehlman, E. T., Toth, M. J., Goran, M. I., Carpenter, W. H., Newhouse, P., and Rosen, C. J. (1997). Daily energy expenditure in free-living non-institutionalized Alzheimer's patients: A doubly labeled water study. *Neurology* **48**, 997–1002.

104. Grundman, M., Corey-Bloom, J., Jernigan, T., Archibald, S., and Thal, L. J. (1996). Body weight in Alzheimer's disease is associated with mesial temporal cortex atrophy. *Neurology* **46**, 1585–1591.

105. Morley, J. E., Mooradian, A. D., Silver, A. J., Heber, D., and Alfin-Slater, R. B. (1988). Nutrition in the elderly. *Ann. Intern. Med.* **109**, 890–904.

106. Ferry, M., Alix, E., Brocker, P., Haller, J., and Weggemans, R. M. (1996). Nutrition et demence de type Alzheimer. *In* "Nutrition de la personne agee. Aspects Fundamentaux, Cliniques et Psychosociaux," (S. Berger-Levrault, Ed.), pp. 87–96. Berger-Levrault, Paris.

107. Volicer, L., Seltzer, B., Rheaume, Y., Karner, J., Glennon, M., Riley, M. E., and Crino, P. (1989). Eating difficulties in patients with probable dementia of the Alzheimer type. *J. Geriatr. Psych. Neurol.* **2**, 188–195.

108. Volicer, L., Rheaume, Y., and Cyr, D. (1994). Treatment of depression in advanced Alzheimer's disease. *J. Geriatr. Psych. Neurol.* **7**, 227–229.

109. Abbott, R. A., Cox, H., Marcus, H., and Tomkins, A. (1992). Diet, body size and micronutrient status in Parkinson's disease. *Eur. J. Clin. Nutr.* **46**, 879–884.

110. Morris, M. C. Bennett, D. A., Cronin-Stubbs, D., Beckett, L. A., and Tangney, C. C. (1996). Parkinsonian signs and weight loss in a community-based sample of older persons in East Boston. *Am. J. Epidemiol. Res.* **143**, S65.

111. Beyer, P. L., Palarino, M. Y., Michalek, D., Busenbark, K., and Koller, W. C. (1995). Weight change and body composition in patients with Parkinson's disease. *J. Am. Diet. Assoc.* **95**, 979–983.

112. Toth, M. J., Fishman, P. S., and Poehlman, E. T. (1997). Free-living daily energy expenditure in patients with Parkinson's disease. *Neurol.* **48**(1), 88–91.

113. Jost, W. H. (1997). Gastrointestinal motility problems in patients with Parkinson's disease. Effects of antiparkinsonian treatment and guidelines for management. *Drugs Aging* **10**, 249–258.

114. Weingart, J., Tangney, C. C., Murtaugh, M., and Domas, A. J. "Estimating Usual Dietary Intakes of Men and Women with Moderate Parkinson's Disease on Levodopa." Master's thesis, 1997. Rush University, Chicago, IL.

115. Holden, K. (1998). "Eat Well, Stay Well with Parkinson's Disease," pp. 13–27. Five Star Living, Fort Collins, CO.

116. Yamada, T., Kachi, T., and Ando, K. (1995). Osteoporosis and fractures in Parkinson's disease. *Jpn J. Geriatrics.* **32**, 637–640.

117. Taggart, H., and Crawford, V. (1995). Reduced bone density of the hip in elderly patients with Parkinson's disease. *Age Aging* **24**, 326–328.

118. O'Brien, C. E., Tangney, C. C., and Ho-Dong, R. (1993). *In* "Quality of Life through Balanced Nutrition" (C. E. O'Brien, C. C. Tangney, and R. Ho-Dong, Eds.). Patient handbook. Pp. 1–90. Elan Nutra Pharma, Jacksonville, FL.

119. Pare, S., Barr, S. I., and Ross, S. E. (1992). Effect of daytime protein restriction on nutrient intakes of free-living Parkinson's disease patients. *Am. J. Clin. Nutr.* **55**, 701–707.

120. Juncos, J. L., Fabbrini, G., Mouradian, M. M., Serrati, C., and Chase, T. N. (1987). Dietary influences on the antiparkinson response to levodopa. *Arch. Neurol.* **44**, 1003–1005.

121. Marsden, C. D., and Parkes, J. D. (1977). Success and problems of long-term levodopa therapy in Parkinson's disease. *Lancet* **1**, 345–349.

122. Nutt, J. G., Woodward, W. R., Hammerstad, J. P., Carter, J. H., and Anderson, J. L. (1984). The "on-off" phenomenon in Parkinson's disease: Relation to levodopa absorption and transport. *N. Engl. J. Med.* **310**, 483–488.

123. Gimenez-Rolden, S., and Mateo, D. (1991). Predicting beneficial responses to a protein-redistribution diet in fluctuating Parkinson's disease. *Acta Neurol. Belg.* **91**, 189–200.

124. Tsui, J. K., Ross, S., Poulin, K., Douglas, J., Postnikoff, D., Calne, S., Woodward, W., and Calne, D. B. (1989). The effect of dietary protein on the efficacy of L-dopa: A double blind study. *Neurology* **39**, 549–552.

125. Karstaedt, P. J., and Pincus, J. H. (1992). Protein redistribution diet remains effective in patients with fluctuating Parkinsonism. *Arch. Neurol.* **49**, 149–151.

126. Food and Nutrition Board. (1989). "Recommended Dietary Allowances." National Academy of Sciences, Washington, DC, National Academy Press.

127. Carter, J. H., Nutt, J. G., Woodward, W. F., Hatcher, L. F., and Trotman, T. L. (1989). Amounts and distribution of dietary protein affect clinical response to levodopa in Parkinson's disease. *Neurology* **39**, 552–556.

128. Berry, E. M., Growden, J. H., Wurtman, J. J., Caballero, B., and Wurtman, R. J. (1991). A balanced carbohydrate:protein diet in the management of Parkinson's disease. *Neurology* **41**, 1295–1297.

129. Feldman, R. G. (1994). A pilot study of EL-422. *Drug Nutrients Neurol.* 36–42.

130. Tangney, C. C. (1994). A review of low-protein and high-carbohydrate diets in Parkinson's disease. *Drugs Nurtrients Neurol.* 24–33.

131. Astarloa, R., Mena, M. A., Sanchez, V., dela Vega, L., and deYebenes, J. G. (1992). Clinical and pharmocokinetic effects of a diet rich in insoluble fiber on Parkinson's disease. *Clin. Neuropharmacol.* **15**, 375–380.

132. U.S. Department of Agriculture, Center for Nutrition Policy and Promotion (1998). "The Healthy Eating Index 1994–1996," CNPP-5. U.S. Department of Agriculture, Washington, D.C.

133. Haines, P. S., Siega-Riz, A. M., and Popkin, B. M. (1999). The diet quality index revised: A measurement instrument for populations. *J. Am. Dietet. Assoc.* **99**, 697–704.

CHAPTER **42**

Osteoporosis

ROBERT HEANEY
Creighton University, Omaha, Nebraska

I. INTRODUCTION

In 1990 osteoporosis was redefined, for the first time in nearly a century, as a condition of skeletal fragility due to decreased bone mass and to microarchitectural deterioration of bone tissue, with consequent increased risk of fracture [1]. This definition was conceptually important because it both acknowledged and encouraged a shift in thinking about osteoporosis from an anatomic to a dynamic condition. Low bone mass became a risk factor for fracture, rather than, as formerly, the defining characteristic of the disease. This redefinition accompanied a growing recognition that osteoporosis is not a single disorder, but a group of more or less discrete fracture syndromes, multifactorial both in etiology and in pathogenesis.

The recognition not only of a multiplicity of pathogenetic factors, but of *disease* heterogeneity adds another dimension of complexity that must be considered when describing and assessing the role of any single factor, whether hormones, exercise, or nutrition (as in this case). Thus, not only is nutrition just one of several interacting factors in any given fracture syndrome, but it may play quite different roles, or none at all, in certain of those syndromes, while being of greater importance in others. This was first suggested in the 1979 report by Matkovic and his colleagues [2] from Croatia, which showed that high calcium intake was associated with strikingly reduced hip fracture risk, but not with altered risk of distal forearm fracture in the same population.

II. NUTRITION IN THE OSTEOPOROTIC FRACTURE CONTEXT

Nutrition affects bone health in two qualitatively distinct ways. Bone tissue deposition, maintenance, and repair are the result of cellular processes, and the cells of bone responsible for these functions are as dependent on nutrition as are the cells of any other tissue. The production of bone matrix, for example, requires the synthesis and post-translational modification of collagen and an array of other proteins. Nutrients involved in such synthesis include protein, the vitamins C, D, and K, and the minerals copper, manganese, and

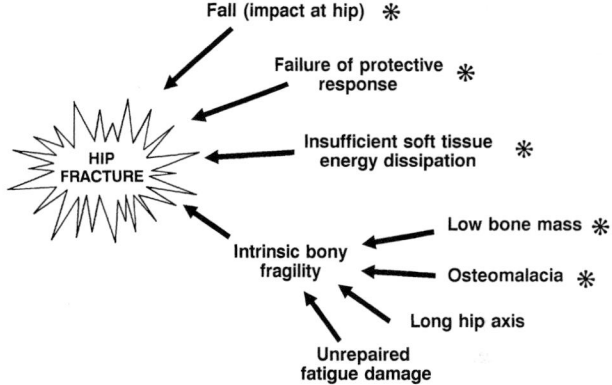

FIGURE 1 Schematic representation of the interplay of principal factors thought to be important in hip fracture. Asterisks denote factors with a recognized nutritional determinant. (Copyright Robert P. Heaney, 1995. Reproduced with permission.)

zinc. Phosphorus also is indirectly involved in these cellular activities. Additionally, the skeleton serves as a very large nutrient reserve for two minerals, calcium and phosphorus, and the size of that reserve (i.e., the massiveness of the skeletal structures) will be dependent in part on the daily balance between absorbed intake and excretory loss of these two minerals. Bone mass is also dependent on a variety of nonnutritional factors, such as genetics, mechanical loading, hormonal status, and others. These dependencies complicate the interpretation of low bone mass values because, while low bone mass always means a reduced calcium reserve, simple reduction in bone mass does not necessarily mean that it had a nutritional cause.

Factors involved in osteoporotic fractures can be organized hierarchically to include the injury itself, the strength of the bone, the mass and density of the bone, and the adequacy of nutrition as it affects bone mass. Hip fracture is perhaps the most serious of the fragility fractures, inasmuch as it carries an excess mortality, is expensive, and causes significant deterioration in quality of life for most of its survivors. It is, as well, a good example of the many interacting factors that constitute this fracture domain, and I will use it as such in this preliminary overview. Figure 1 illustrates, schematically, how the various contributing factors interact for hip

fracture. It also highlights probable sites in this schema at which nutrition plays a role.

A. Frailty and Injury

Almost all fractures, even those we term *low trauma,* occur as a result of some injury—the application of more force to the bone than it is able to sustain.Usually this is a result of a fall or the application of bad body mechanics (e.g., bending forward to lift a heavy object). Although fracture incidence patterns differ somewhat from site to site, the risk of virtually all fractures rises with age, and all fractures contribute to the burden of illness, disability, and expense that the elderly (and society) bear.

The first factor to consider is the fall itself. Normally postural reflexes operate to get the arms into position to break the force of the fall or to swing the body so that it lands on the buttocks (or both). These reflexes are almost always effective in younger individuals, but they commonly fail in the elderly. As a result, young people rarely strike the lateral portion of the trochanteric region of the hip when they fall, whereas the fragile elderly more commonly do so. The force of the impact, when falling from standing height, may well be sufficient to break even a healthy femur if that force is concentrated in a small enough impact area [3]. Additionally, hip fracture is a particularly serious problem in undernourished elderly individuals who have less muscle and fat mass around the hip, and therefore less soft tissue through which the force of the impact can be distributed to a larger area of the lateral surface of the trochanter.

Nutrition enters into this region of the fracture domain both through its effect on propensity to fall [4] and on maintenance of the soft tissue mass. This latter factor, particularly, is the rationale for the development and successful deployment of hip pads as protection against hip fracture in the elderly [5]. In some cases, nutrition may also influence central nervous system processing time or contribute to the general feebleness that predisposes to falling. The implication here is that we should attempt to improve general nutrition in the elderly or, failing that, we should certainly attend to coexisting nutritional problems at the time of fracture repair.

B. Intrinsic Bony Strength and Fragility

Strength in bone, as in most engineering structures, is dependent on its mass density, on the three-dimensional arrangement of its material in space, and upon the intrinsic strength of its component material (particularly, in bone, as that strength is influenced over long periods of use by the accumulation of unrepaired fatigue damage). All three factors play some role in most low-trauma fractures, and it is not possible to say which may be the most important in any given case. Nevertheless, most of the investigative effort in this regard in the past 30 years has been devoted to the measurement of bone mass and density, and hence much of what we know about bone strength in living individuals comes

from our observation of this facet of the bone strength triad. There is, in fact, a general consensus that decreased bone mass produces a decrease in bone strength.

But, clearly, other fragility factors exist as well, although there is less of a consensus as to how large a role they play [6]. The data of Ross *et al.* [7] show that prior spine fracture signifies the presence of fragility independent of, and at least as, important as the fragility due to low bone density. Similarly Hui *et al.* [8] showed that the fracture risk gradient for age, holding density constant, was greater than the risk gradient for density itself. These effects, independent of bone mass, may be partly explained by structural and qualitative defects in bone.

For example, individuals with compression fractures of the vertebrae have been found to have excessive loss of horizontal, cross-bracing trabeculae in their cancellous bone [9, 10], whereas other individuals with the same overall degree of bone loss, but with the bracing trabeculae maintained intact, are less apt to fracture. This may be the basis for the predictive value of prior spine fracture [7]. It appears that women, in particular, are more prone to loss of horizontal trabeculae than are men, and this fact is probably also the explanation for the 6:1 to 8:1 female:male sex differential in vertebral osteoporosis. The data of Eventov *et al.* [11] indicate the probable importance of repair of fatigue damage. Faulkner *et al.* [12] and Glüer *et al.* [13] have called attention to a probable role of geometric factors at the hip, specifically to hip axis length, and Gilsanz *et al.* [14] to the importance of vertebral body size.[1] In summary, evidence from several quarters makes it clear that bony fragility has bases other than reduced bone density.

Nevertheless, fracture risk rises by a factor in the range of 1.5–2.5 times for every drop in bone mass/density of one standard deviation. And whatever may be the role of nonmass factors, it is an inescapable fact that most elderly individuals have bone mass values that are more than two standard deviations below the young adult mean; hence, they all can be said to be at considerably increased risk for fragility fracture. Why some older persons do fracture and others do not appears to be explainable by a combination of random chance, differences in falling patterns, and the structural differences just described.

Nutrition enters into this portion of the fracture domain predominantly through its influence on bone mass (or density). Because nonmass factors also influence bone strength, nutritional inadequacies can never explain more than a part of the problem, and nutritional interventions can never completely eliminate fragility fractures. It may also be that trace nutrients such as certain of the vitamins (e.g., C, D, K) or minerals such as manganese, copper, and zinc (see below) directly influence the remodeling process and/or the character of the remodeled bone, and hence affect bone strength

---

[1]Other things being equal, a long hip axis increases hip fracture risk, and a small cross-sectional area for vertebral bodies increases spine fracture risk.

through their impact on the repair of inevitable fatigue damage. However, little is known about these possibilities in the adult skeleton. Hence, in most of what follows, the emphasis will be on the nutritional factors that influence bone *mass*.

C. Bone Mass and Density

Bone mass and density are themselves influenced by many factors. Holding body weight constant, the three most important—or at least the three most commonly found to be limiting in industrialized nations—are physical activity, gonadal hormones, and nutrition. In adults of industrialized nations the nutrients most critical for bone health are calcium and vitamin D. Calcium intake, specifically, may be inadequate for the straightforward reason that it is low; however, even when statistically "normal," it may still be inadequate because of subnormal absorption [16] or greater than normal excretory loss [17, 18]. Other nutrients are also essential for building a healthy skeleton, but, except for calcium, their effects are usually seen most clearly during growth. Once built, the skeleton tends to be relatively insulated from many subsequent nutritional deficiencies. In addition, a number of other factors also influence bone mass, such as smoking, alcohol abuse, and various drugs used to treat a variety of medical illnesses, as well as those illnesses themselves.

The effects of each of these factors are largely independent. In other words, altering any one of them will not substitute for, or compensate for, adverse effects of the others. Thus, a high calcium intake will not prevent the loss of bone that occurs immediately following menopause in women or castration in men. Similarly, physical activity will not compensate for an inadequate calcium intake. Neither will a high calcium intake offset the effects of alcohol abuse or smoking. Much of the apparent confusion in the bone field during the past 25 years could have been avoided if we had better understood that these factors, while interactive, are substantially independent.

Finally, although much of the following discussion will focus on calcium, it is necessary to stress what should perhaps go without saying, that calcium is a nutrient, not a drug, and hence its beneficial effects will be confined to individuals whose intake of calcium is insufficient. Also, calcium is not an isolated nutrient; it occurs in foods along with other nutrients, and it has been shown that diets low in calcium tend also to be inadequate in other respects as well [19, 20]. Thus, while it is necessary to deal with nutrients one at a time in an analysis such as this, the disorders in our patients are likely to be more complex.

III. PROBLEMS IN THE INVESTIGATION OF NUTRITIONAL EFFECTS ON BONE

Significant problems arise for both observational and experimental approaches to the elucidation of nutrient effects on the skeleton, and failure to recognize or overcome them has led both to seemingly contradictory results among various studies and to substantial confusion about the role of nutrition in bone health. Some of these problems are nutrition specific; others are inherent in bone biology.

A. Nutrition-Specific Problems

1. ESTIMATION OF NUTRIENT INTAKE

Two nutrients with clearly established effects on bone are vitamin D and calcium. For both, there are substantial difficulties in estimating intake [21, 22]. Vitamin D is found naturally in very few foods (mostly fish oils and, to a limited extent, egg yolks).[2] For primitive humans, solar exposure would have been the principal source of vitamin D, as is still the case in rural cultures and in the young of even many urbanized societies. Vitamin D is added as a fortificant to fluid and dry milk in the United States and Canada (but not to most other dairy foods).[3] Serum 25(OH vitamin D levels have long been recognized as the best available indicator of vitamin D status. Even so, their significance is not fully clear [26]. Furthermore, such levels are affected by season, so no single value in any given individual adequately captures his or her year-round average. Such measurements are also sufficiently costly and invasive so as to be precluded in most epidemiological studies involving large numbers of subjects. Finally, while vitamins D_2 and D_3 have heretofor been considered equivalent in potency (and both measured and used as a fortificant interchangeably), Vieth [27] has shown that D_2 exhibits only 60% the potency of D_3 in humans.

Calcium also presents serious difficulties to the investigator who would attempt to estimate its intake. Food calcium content often varies widely from published food table values—sometimes by a factor of 2–3—reflecting variations in soil mineral content and plant tissue hydration (among other factors). Even commercial milk exhibits 10–20% variability from dairy to dairy or state to state. Charles

---

[2]One could argue that vitamin D ought not be considered a nutrient at all, because it is not a constituent of most foods and is naturally synthesized in abundance in our skin, given adequate solar exposure. But it was lumped accidentally with the other vitamins (nutrients in the strict sense) in the early days of development of nutritional science, and that is where we treat it and think about it today. That is not just an historical curiosity. Nutritionists in the past have often held that one can get all the nutrients one needs from a balanced, varied diet, and have been slow to embrace the notions of engineered foods and food fortification. That clearly is a misguided approach to an accidental nutrient such as vitamin D. As the species moved out of equatorial regions, humans did not hesitate to develop warm clothing and shelter as protection from a cold environment. For vitamin D, at least, the same approach would seem to be indicated, now that the biochemistry involved is understood. The industrialized nations of the high latitudes have done that for infants and children for the past 60+ years, and rickets is rare today in those countries, but vitamin D insufficiency is still common among adults—particularly among the elderly (see section below on vitamin D).

[3]Unfortunately quality control has been poor in the past [23–25], i.e., the level of fortification can be highly variable (ranging from near-toxic levels to absent altogether in many skim milk samples—despite what may appear on the label). For both reasons, it has been extremely difficult to assess effective vitamin D intake by any sort of questionnaire.

[28] found, in a chemical analysis of foods consumed in a series of metabolic balance studies, that less than 70% of the actual variability in intake among a group of subjects was reflected in the *calculated* intakes derived from food table values for the foods consumed, despite the fact that the precise quantities of every food eaten were known with high accuracy. Outside of the metabolic ward environment, and particularly in epidemiological studies, there is the added uncertainty of portion size estimation and food item recall. Another problem is presented by large differences in bioavailability. The calcium of kale or collard greens is highly available [29], while that of spinach is nearly totally unavailable [30]. Thus *actual* intake and *effective* intake can differ substantially. Finally, broad daily and seasonal variations are seen in intake patterns. In this regard, Heaney *et al.* [31] showed, in a large series of 7-day consecutive diet records, that any random day elected out of the total record captured only 12.6% of the interday variance, and that the error of the estimate of the 7-day average from one of its days was ± 178 mg (which means that the 95% confidence interval covers a range of more than 700 mg!).

The difficulty of estimating effective calcium intake is compounded by two further problems. First is the use of calcium salts as excipients or "inert" ingredients in many medications or as non-nutritive additives to various bulk foods. In both cases their calcium content goes unrecognized and often unacknowledged on the product label. Second is the increased use of explicit calcium supplements since 1982. This should not, of itself, create a problem for estimating calcium intake. However, many tablets in the past exhibited highly variable pharmaceutical formulations [32, 33], and, hence, unpredictable absorbability. Excipient calcium will not often produce major errors in intake estimates unless food source intakes are low (in which case undocumented medication calcium can easily account for half the actual calcium intake); nevertheless Heaney *et al.* [31] reported several cases in which such unrecognized calcium contributed more than 1000 mg/day to the intake.

In any event, both causes can lead to serious misclassification of individual intakes in observational or epidemiological studies, therefore biasing toward the null any investigation dependent on intake estimates. An illustration of the effect of this bias is found in a meta-analysis by Heaney [34] of 28 studies in late postmenopausal women published between 1988 and 1992. Twenty-three of these 28 studies reported a positive effect of calcium intake on bone mass, bone loss, or fracture. However, when they were subdivided according to whether the investigators controlled the calcium intake directly or relied on estimates of intake derived from questionnaires and food records, it turned out that all of the 12 studies in which investigators controlled the intake had demonstrated a significant calcium benefit, while all of the inconclusive studies had been those in which intake had been merely estimated. The difference is explainable by errors in intake estimates in the questionnaire-based studies.

2. MAGNITUDE OF NUTRIENT–NUTRIENT INTERACTIONS

It is a commonplace of nutritional science that nutrients interact, thereby altering one another's requirements.[4] It is to be expected, therefore, that the nutrients important for bone health would also exhibit this sort of interaction. What may not have been expected is the very considerable magnitude of those interactions with regard to critical bone nutrients. Co-ingested nutrients alter both obligatory renal loss and intestinal absorption of calcium and phosphorus. While effects on absorption are comparatively modest, effects on obligatory loss can alter the minimum daily requirement for calcium very substantially. (These effects are covered in more detail later in this chapter.)

For our purposes here, it is sufficient only to note that other nutrients, ingested within the normal range of human intakes, so alter ability to maintain calcium equilibrium as to produce a fourfold difference between the lowest and the highest values for the minimum requirement. This is a quite extraordinary range and is virtually without parallel among other nutrients. It is for this reason that it is usually misleading to make comparisons among populations that may differ not only in calcium intake, but in intakes of protein and sodium particularly, as well as in the proportion of animal and vegetable food sources in the customary diet. It is likely that much of the seeming differences in the relationship of calcium to bone status across populations [35] can be attributed to differences in minimum requirement related to nutrient–nutrient interactions, and much of the apparent confusion surrounding this topic attributed to failure to give adequate consideration to the influence of these interactions.

B. Bone-Specific Problems

1. THE BONE REMODELING TRANSIENT

The bone remodeling transient is dealt with in greater depth elsewhere [36, 37]. It is important to mention it briefly in this context because, whenever bone remodeling is altered by an intervention (nutritional in this context), the changes in calcium balance or bone mass that follow will, for a period of 6–12 months, reflect not the effects (if any) of the intervention on *steady-state* bone balance, but shrinkage or expansion of the bone remodeling space caused by asynchrony of the changes produced in bone formation and resorption.

This is a particular problem for calcium, because calcium alters endogenous parathyroid hormone production, and parathyroid hormone is the principal determinant of the amount of global skeletal remodeling. But any other nutrient (such as vitamin D or phosphorus), that also alters parathyroid hormone production (whether directly or indirectly) may produce qualitatively similar effects.

---

[4]Recommended dietary allowances (RDAs) are designed, in theory, to be generous enough to accommodate this food-related variability in requirement.

Thus, the classical stratagem of measuring nutrient balance in individuals on differing intake levels for periods of up to a few weeks, then giving them a short rest period, then trying yet another intake for a few more weeks (and so forth), will not work for bone or its measurable surrogates. Unfortunately, there are no easy alternatives. Balance for nutrients that are bulk bone constituents can be assessed only under steady-state conditions, and for calcium, that means either studying persons on their habitual intakes, or deferring study for 6–12 months after altering intake of a given nutrient. Both options severely limit what the investigator can do to test various hypotheses involving nutrition and bone status.

2. ISOLATION OF BULK BONE FROM CURRENT NUTRITIONAL INFLUENCES

Bone is very much a living tissue, with its cells responding both to systemic influences and to strain patterns within the bony structure. Nevertheless, the mechanical properties of bone reside exclusively in the intercellular, nonliving, two-phase composite of fibrous protein and mineral. With the exception of use-related, accumulating fatigue damage, the inherent mechanical properties of this material are largely (though not entirely) determined at the time a unit of bone is formed. The entire skeleton is turned over at a rate of only 8–10% per year (and some regions much more slowly). Because only currently forming bone will be affected by current conditions, nutritional stresses have predictably small effects on current bone strength. The bulk of bone is, in effect, isolated from the systemic and environmental influences that can rapidly produce outspoken effects in soft tissues. This is not to say that there are *no* effects on bone. It is possible that bone cells, damaged by current nutritional problems, may die or otherwise fail in one or another of their monitoring functions. But the effects of that failure may become evident only years in the future, and they are, accordingly, extremely difficult to study.

3. SLOW RESPONSE TIME OF BONE

A corollary of the slow turnover of bone tissue is that bone mass changes relatively slowly in response to nutritional influences, either positive or negative. A gain or loss of bone amounting to at most 1–2% per year is typically all that many interventions can produce in adults. Continued over many years, such a rate of change can have profound effects on skeletal strength, but it is a change that is hard to detect by absorptiometric methods in short-term investigations, and essentially impossible to detect reliably in individuals. Although the gain or loss associated with a nutritional intervention may be real enough, its presence is dwarfed by the relatively huge mass of preexisting bone, and its detection tends to be swamped by the inevitable noise of measurement. Balance studies can sensitively detect much smaller changes (since the background bone mass is not reflected in the balance value), but they are subject to the problem of the remodeling transient discussed earlier, and sufficient time

must be allowed for the system to come into equilibrium if they are to be useful. Serum and urine biomarkers can sensitively signal qualitative changes in bone remodeling processes, but they are not sufficiently quantitative to tell us the size of any change in bone balance that may have been produced by an intervention.

4. LIFE PHASE SPECIFICITY OF BONY RESPONSE

As will be developed in more detail below, the skeleton is the body's reserve of the nutrient, calcium. It is the largest reserve of all the nutrients, and one that has acquired an unrelated function in its own right—the mechanical support of our bodies. While bone strength is clearly an inverse function of bone density, and any decrease in bone density must have mechanical consequences, nevertheless reserves, by their very nature, are designed to be called on, and it should not be surprising to find that there may be physiological circumstances in which the reserve will reduce some of its store of mineral, not always because the diet is insufficient to offset excretory and dermal losses, but precisely because the physiological situation demands it or because the body senses that some of the reserve is no longer needed. Lactation may be one such situation and menopause another. In any event, nutritional interventions should be expected to produce qualitatively different effects when they are deployed under such differing physiological circumstances.

5. COMMENT

This discussion of investigative problems is, of necessity, brief. My purpose has been to highlight the inherent difficulty involved in investigating problems at the interface of nutrition and bone status. Failure of bone biologists to recognize nutritional measurement problems and failure of nutritionists to reckon adequately with the complexities of bone biology will lead (and has led) to badly designed, inconclusive, or misleading investigations. This is a problem not only for investigators, but for those who attempt to make sense of what they report. It is not that easy alternatives are being overlooked. Rather, there are no easy alternatives. But, while the problems are difficult, they are not intractable.

IV. THE NOTION OF A NUTRIENT REQUIREMENT

Nutritional science was born about a century ago with the then-revolutionary recognition that the absence of something could produce disease.[5] Once nutritional deficiency was accepted as the cause of disease the notion of a requirement centered on the intake needed to avoid the recognizable deficiency disease concerned. While the science of nutrition

---

[5]The prevailing notion at the time was that all disease was caused by infections or intoxications—i.e., by some noxious influence from outside the organism.

has advanced notably since its beginnings, particularly in understanding precisely what various nutrients do in the body, our definitions of a requirement are still often pegged to early 20th-century ability to recognize and characterize disease. There is growing dissatisfaction with this disease-centered approach, and increasingly one reads that the field ought to redefine a requirement as the intake needed to produce optimal health. But the main problem with the traditional approach to a requirement is not that it is negative (i.e., disease centered) but that its definition of disease is primitive. It is centered on disorders that develop rapidly and have distinct clinical expression recognizable with the tools of 70 years ago. However, a deficiency that takes 10 years to develop or to make its presence evident is no less a deficiency than one that develops in 10 days.[6]

Vitamin K deficiency, for example, produces a bleeding disorder, and this is the defining disease associated with the nutrient. Does absence of bleeding mean that vitamin K nutriture is adequate? We now recognize that vitamin K is necessary for gamma-carboxylation of a large number of proteins in addition to the clotting factors, three of them involved in bone matrix (see section below on vitamin K). We also recognize that gamma-carboxylation of these proteins can be very incomplete even when the clotting factors are normally carboxylated, and that physiological vitamin K supplementation completely repairs this deficit. It is not known whether this undercarboxylation expresses itself as disease, but our ignorance in that regard does not guarantee that the absence of clotting disturbance means vitamin K sufficiency.

In this chapter I define a requirement as the intake that ensures full expression of known functions of the nutrient concerned, and I will presume that any substantial deviation from full physiological expression is harmful until proved safe.

V. THE NATURAL INTAKE OF CALCIUM AND VITAMIN D

It has only recently been recognized that both calcium and vitamin D were present in superabundance in the environment in which the human species evolved. It seems likely that, over the millennia of evolution, human physiology developed mechanisms to protect the organism from getting too much of these important nutrients. By contrast, contemporary adult humans, living in industrialized nations at higher latitudes, have intakes of these nutrients that are often only a small fraction of what their primitive ancestors experienced, and our physiologies are, therefore, maladapted to what our environment currently provides.

---

[6]The first clearly identified deficiency disease, beriberi, typically develops in 30–90 days after onset of thiamin deprivation, and it responds to treatment with roughly equal speed. One can speculate whether nutritional science would have developed at all if its disease states had typically had long latency periods.

Vitamin D is produced normally in the skin by a photochemical reaction in which ultraviolet light from the sun changes 7-dehydrocholesterol into previtamin D. As the human species evolved in equatorial East Africa, with ample sunlight year-round, two mechanisms coevolved that prevented the accumulation of an excess of vitamin D. One was skin pigmentation, which slowed the photochemical reaction, and the other was the fact that continued solar radiation degrades previtamin D to inert products before it is taken up into the circulating blood. As a result, vitamin D accumulation in the skin plateaus after a few minutes of sun exposure, with the time varying with skin pigmentation. Circulating levels of 25(OH) vitamin D under early conditions can be estimated from values observed in dark-skinned, outdoor laborers at tropical latitudes, which have been reported to be in the range of 150 nmol/L [27] or ~4–6 times what is typically measured in city dwellers at midlatitudes.

As humans moved farther and farther north (away from the equator), and needed all the ultraviolet they could get, skin pigmentation became lighter and lighter. Still, in latitudes such as that of Boston and farther north, the sun is so low in the sky in winter that effectively none of the responsible ultraviolet rays gets through the atmosphere, even on a sunny day [38]. As a result, vitamin D tends to be a scarce nutrient at high latitudes, and without careful attention to maintaining adequacy, varying degrees of vitamin D insufficiency will be common. Just 75 years ago, more than 80% of the children in England showed evidences of rickets [39]. Thanks to nearly universal vitamin D prophylaxis in children, rickets is now a relatively rare disorder.

Calcium, too, was present in abundance in the environment in which the human species evolved. The plant foods eaten by hunter-gatherers provided a calcium intake that, adjusted for differences in body size, would have been in the range of 2000–4000 mg/day for 60–70 kg adults [40, 41]. (Contrast that figure with the median value for women 20 and over in the United States in the NHANES III study: in the range of 600 mg/day [42].) Sources available to our ancestors included a very large number of greens, tubers, roots, nuts, and berries, many of them with very high calcium nutrient densities [41]. Moreover, invertebrate and reptilian sources of animal protein typically have calcium-to-calorie ratios that are six-fold higher than fish or mammalian meats [43]. By contrast, cultivated cereal plants, legumes, and fruits—the plant foods modern humans mainly consume—exhibit augmented levels of carbohydrate and/or fat without a proportionate increase in minerals and vitamins; thus, they almost always have lower calcium densities than do their wild cousins.

The agricultural/pastoral revolution, which occurred from roughly 3000 to 10,000 years ago in various parts of the world, made it possible to feed vastly more people than the hunter-gatherer mode permitted. This was partly because of the increased energy content of polyploid cereal mutants (which occur spontaneously, but which, because of their greater seed weight, need human intervention for their effi-

cient propagation). At the same time the agricultural revolution produced striking changes in micronutrient intake, generally for the worse. We see this reflected in modern times in the nutritional deficiencies that result when hunter-gatherers such as the !Kung San people are forced by restriction of their range to take up farming [44].

The effect on the calcium density of the diet is depicted in Figure 2. Diets of hunter-gatherers would have been in the range of 70–90 mg calcium/100 kcal (somewhat higher if invertebrate protein sources featured prominently in the diet). Those who then domesticated animals and lived mainly off their milk (as do the Masai, the Ariaal, and, indeed, all pastoralist societies today) would have had a shift in diet to somewhere in the neighborhood of 200 mg calcium/100 kcal.[7] By contrast, those who settled on the land and subsisted mainly on cereal crops and legumes would, at least from these food sources alone, have had diets with calcium densities under 20 mg/100 kcal. While vegetable greens would have helped when available, calcium intakes based solely on cereals and legumes would probably not have been sufficient to sustain bone health. However, there are numerous, well-attested examples of peoples living in stable equilibrium with their environments who have developed nonfood ways of augmenting the meager calcium intake provided by a diet based on seed foods. The addition of lime to corn meal by indigenous peoples in Central America is one well-known example. Less well known is the practice of pregnant Southeast Asian women of drinking a liquid produced by soaking bones in vinegar [45]. Andean Indians have been reported to add both a particular plant ash and a heat-treated rock powder to their cereal gruel [46]. All of these practices represent a kind of conscious addition of a substance that, *de facto,* augmented the calcium intake of a cereal-based diet.

It seems likely that *unconscious* additions of the same sort were nearly universal among neolithic farming communities. The archaeological record has preserved numerous examples of stone mortars used for dehulling cereal grains and stone querns for grinding the seeds into flour [47]. In the fertile crescent at least, limestone would have been the most readily available and the most workable stone, and the hours of hand grinding of dehulled cereal grains would inevitably have added substantial calcium (as calcium carbonate) to the resulting flour.[8] As technology advanced, and millstones were made of harder and harder rock (usually silicon- and aluminum-based rather than calcium-based minerals), aggregate calcium intakes would have declined toward the lower line depicted in Figure 2. Thus, the low calcium intakes

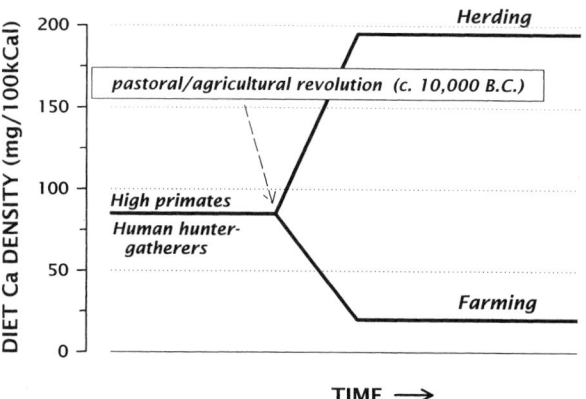

FIGURE 2 Changes in calcium concentration of the diet associated with the agricultural/pastoral revolution. (Copyright Robert P. Heaney, 1995. Reproduced with permission.)

that we take for granted today are relatively quite late arrivals on the human diet scene.

Because hominid and early human diets were very rich in calcium, the human intestine either failed to develop effective absorptive transport mechanisms or actually developed an absorptive barrier to protect against too much calcium. Nor did mechanisms to conserve absorbed calcium develop. (Presumably, there would be little need to conserve in the face of environmental surfeit.) Humans typically absorb only about 25–35% of the calcium in contemporary diets [48] and put about 150 mg/day back into the gut in the digestive secretions [49]. Thus, net absorption of a dietary calcium increment is usually in the range of 10–15% even during growth when skeletal need is greatest [50]. Additionally, dermal losses are completely unregulated and renal conservation is limited as well. These are precisely the physiological patterns one would expect with an environmentally abundant nutrient.[9]

This is the background to why, despite a high standard of living and the potential to nourish ourselves at a level never previously achieved in the history of the race, civilized diets tend to be deficient in precisely these two critical nutrients, calcium and vitamin D.

VI. CALCIUM

A. The Skeleton as a Nutrient Reserve

Throughout the course of vertebrate evolution, bone developed several times and has served many functions, such as dermal armor and internal stiffening [51]. Evidence from a variety of lines suggests that the most primitive function of the skeleton is actually to buffer the internal milieu for

---

[7]The Masai typically have calcium intakes in the range of 6000–7000 mg calcium/day, essentially all from milk.

[8]The addition of calcium carbonate to bread flour in the United Kingdom during and after World War II and in Japan in the postwar years, as well as the recent fortification of certain breads in the United States with calcium sulfate, are but modern, conscious instances of what must have been an unwitting ancient practice.

[9]It is instructive to compare the body's handling of calcium with that of sodium, which was an environmentally scarce nutrient during hominid evolution. By contrast with calcium, essentially 100% of dietary sodium is absorbed, and dermal and renal sodium losses can be reduced to near zero.

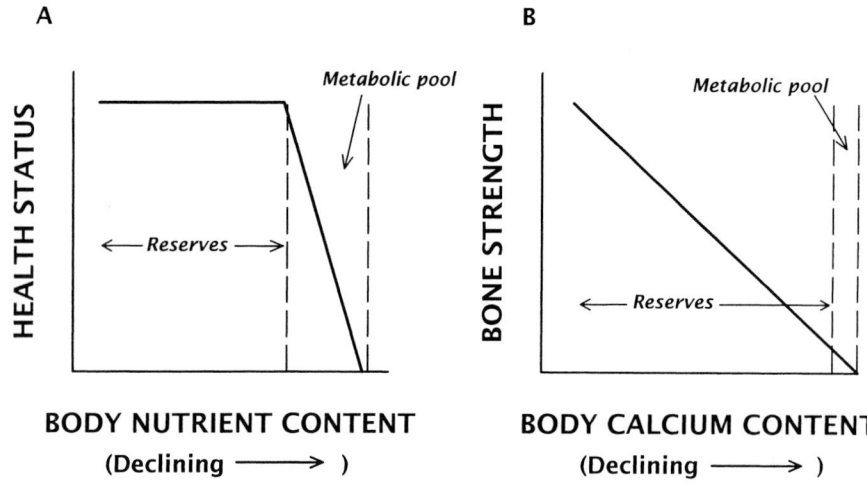

FIGURE 3 Schematic illustration of the relationship between health status and body depletion of a nutrient. (A) Depletion of body stores of a typical nutrient after placing the organism on a deficient intake. (B) In the pattern exhibited by calcium, the reserve is very large relative to the metabolic pool, but health, as reflected in skeletal strength, declines steadily as the reserve itself is depleted. (Copyright Robert P. Heaney, 1995. Reproduced with permission.)

several essential minerals, notably calcium and phosphorus [52]. In some species, phosphorus would have been the critical element; in others, calcium. For both nutrients, the skeleton serves both as a source and as a sink, that is, as a reserve to offset shortages and, to a limited extent, as a place for safely storing surpluses.

We see this reserve feature of skeletal function expressed in diverse ways. For example, there is the long-established fact that laboratory animals such as cats, rats, and dogs will reduce bone mass as needed to maintain near constancy of calcium levels in the extracellular fluid [53–55]. This activity is mediated by parathyroid hormone and involves actual bone destruction, not leaching of calcium from bone. When calcium-deprived animals are parathyroidectomized, bone is spared, but severe hypocalcemia develops [56]. More physiologically, perhaps, deer temporarily increase bone resorption each year to meet the calcium and phosphorus demands of annual antler formation (which exceed the nutrient supply of late winter and spring foliage) [57]. Finally, we see the opposite side of the same function expressed in the now well-established fact that augmented calcium intake will slow or reduce age-related bone loss in humans (see below).[10]

While retaining this primitive, reserve function, bone in the higher, terrestrial vertebrates acquired a second role, namely, internal stiffening and rigidity—what is today the most apparent feature of the skeleton. As such, calcium (or phosphorus) is the only nutrient with a reserve that possesses such a secondary function (with the possible exception of the thermal insulation provided by energy reserves). Figure 3 presents this situation schematically and contrasts calcium with the bulk of other nutrients, depicting what happens for

each when intake is curtailed. For typical nutrients, the reserve is first depleted, without detectable impact on the health or functioning of the organism. Then, after the reserve is exhausted and the metabolic pool begins to be depleted, clinical disease expresses itself. For some nutrients (e.g., vitamin A—energy), the reserve can be quite large, and the latent period may last many months. But for others (e.g., thiamin, the reserve may be very small, and detectable dysfunction develops soon after intake drops.

With calcium, the reserve is vast relative to the cellular and extracellular metabolic pools of calcium. As a result, dietary insufficiency virtually never impairs biochemical functions that are dependent on calcium, at least in ways we can now recognize. However, because bone strength is a function of bone mass, it follows inexorably that any decrease whatsoever in the size of the calcium reserve—any decrease in bone mass—will produce a corresponding decrease in bone strength. We literally walk about on our calcium reserve. It is this unique relationship that is both the basis for the linkage of calcium nutriture with bone status and the explanation why reduction in the size of the reserve is the sole defining characteristic of the major human calcium deficiency syndrome.

B. Defining the Requirement for Calcium

Unlike other nutrients, the requirement for calcium relates solely to this secondary function, i.e., to the size of the calcium reserve, in other words, to total skeletal and regional bone mass. However, unlike energy, which can be stored as fat without practical limit, the size of the calcium reserve is limited, even in the face of dietary surfeit, by genetic and mechanical factors (see below). As a result, calcium functions as a threshold nutrient, much as does iron. This means that, below some critical value, the effect (bone mass for calcium, or hemoglobin mass for iron) will be limited by available supplies, while above that value, i.e., the *threshold*,

---

[10]That this reduction in bone loss is not simply a pharmacologic effect of calcium, as suggested by Kanis and Passmore [58], is indicated by two facts: (1) The effects are greater in those with low baseline calcium intakes and (2) even the augmented intakes employed in these studies are usually well below what primitive humans would have ingested, i.e., they are in the *nutritional* range, not the *pharmacological* range, of calcium intakes.

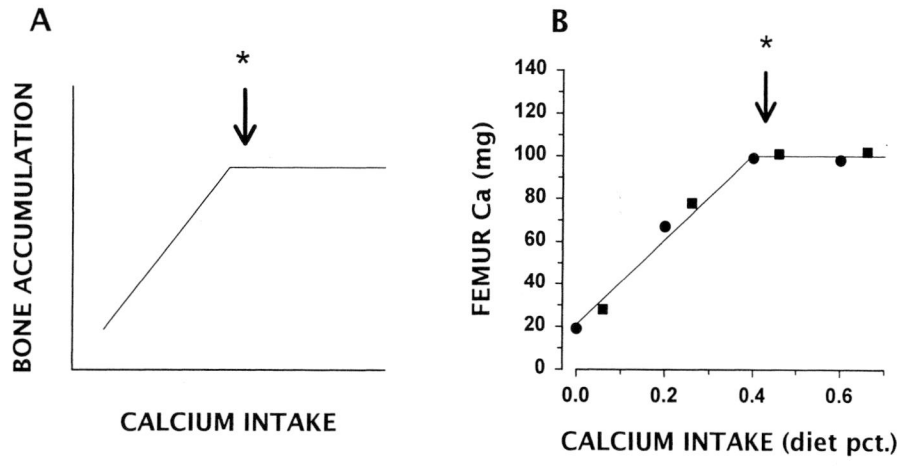

*** Minimum requirement**

FIGURE 4 Threshold behavior of calcium intake. (A) Theoretical relationship of bone accumulation to intake. Below a certain value—the threshold—bone accumulation is a linear function of intake (the ascending line); in other words, the amount of bone that can be accumulated is limited by the amount of calcium ingested. Above the threshold (the horizontal line), bone accumulation is limited by other factors and is no longer related to changes in calcium intake. (B) Actual data from two experiments in growing rats, showing how bone accumulation does, in fact, exhibit a threshold pattern. (Redrawn from data in Forbes *et al.* [59]. Copyright Robert P. Heaney, 1992. Reproduced with permission.)

no further benefit will accrue from additional intake. This biphasic relationship is depicted schematically in Figure 4, in which the intake-effect relationship is depicted schematically in Figure 4A, and then exemplified in Figure 4B by data derived from a growing animal model. In Figure 4B, the effect of the nutrient is expressed directly as the amount of bone calcium an animal is able to accumulate from any given intake.

However, if *effect* is broadened to mean "any change whatsoever," then the diagram fits all life stages, even when bone may be undergoing some degree of involution. This generalized form of the threshold diagram is set forth in Figure 5, which shows schematically what the intake/retention curves look like during growth, maturity, and involution. In brief, the plateau occurs at a positive value during growth, at zero retention in the mature individual, and sometimes at

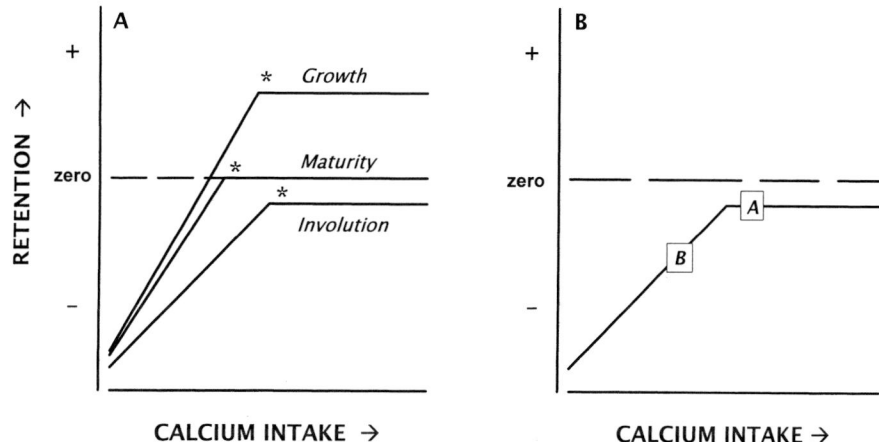

FIGURE 5 (A) Schematic calcium intake and retention curves for three life stages. Retention is greater than zero during growth, zero at maturity, and may be negative during involution. Asterisks represent minimum daily requirement. (B) The involution curve only. Point B designates an intake below the maximal calcium retention threshold, whereas point A designates an intake above the threshold. (Copyright Robert P. Heaney, 1998. Reproduced with permission.)

TABLE 1   Various Estimates of the Calcium Requirement in Women

Age (years)	1989 RDA[a]	NIH[b]	1998 DRI[c]	Balance[d]
1–5	800	800	—	1100
6–10	800	800–1200	960	1100
11–24	1200	1200–1500	1560	1600
Pregnancy/lactation	1200	1200–1500	1200–1560	—
24–50/65	800	1000	1200	800–1000
65–	800	1500	1440	1500–1700

[a]From Ref. 73.

[b]Recommendations for women as proposed by the Consensus Development Conference on Optimal Calcium Intake [61].

[c]The so-called "adequate intakes" of the new DRI values, multiplied by a factor of 1.2 to convert them into RDA format [60].

[d]Estimates derived from published balance studies [50].

a negative value in the elderly. (Available evidence suggests that there are probably several involutional curves, with the plateau during involution at a negative value in the first 3–5 years after menopause, at zero for approximately the next 10 years, and then at increasingly negative values with advancing age.)

In Figure 5B, which shows only a composite involutional curve, two points are identified: one below (B) and one above (A) the threshold. At A, calcium retention is negative for reasons intrinsic to the skeleton, whereas at B, involutional effects are compounded by inadequate intake, which makes the balance more negative than it needs to be. Point B (or below) is probably where most older adults in the industrialized nations would be situated today. The goal of calcium nutrition in this life stage is to move them to point A, thereby making certain that insufficient calcium intake is not aggravating any underlying bone loss.

The functional indicator of nutritional adequacy for such a threshold nutrient is termed *maximal retention* and can be located in Figures 4A and 5A at the asterisks above the curves. The intake corresponding to this point represents the minimum daily requirement. Calcium retention in this sense is "maximal" only in that further intake of calcium will produce no further retention. (This is in contrast to treatment with hormones or drugs, which can sometimes produce further calcium retention.) This approach was used by the Food and Nutrition Board of the National Academy of Sciences for the first time in its development of recommended intakes for calcium in 1997 [60].

Much uncertainty and confusion have arisen in recent years about what the threshold intake may be for various ages and physiological states. With the 1994 Consensus Development Conference on Optimal Calcium Intake [61] and the report of the Panel on Calcium and Related Nutrients [60], the bulk of that confusion has been resolved. The evidence for the intakes recommended by the consensus panel is summarized both in the conference and panel reports and

in recent reviews of the relationship of nutrition and osteoporosis [34, 62], and will be summarized only briefly in ensuing sections of this chapter.

It is worth noting, however, that the recommendations of the consensus conference, while expressed in quantitative terms, were basically qualitative: Contemporary calcium intakes in North America and Northern Europe, by both men and women, are too low for optimal bone health in Caucasian individuals. The most persuasive of the evidence leading to this conclusion came in the form of several randomized controlled trials showing both reduction in age-related bone loss and reduction in fractures following augmentation of prevailing calcium intakes [63–72]. But randomized controlled trials, at least as performed to date, are not well suited to dose ranging (largely because of the problem of the remodeling transient; see above). Hence, while the panel was convinced that prevailing intakes were too low, their recommended levels in several cases involved ranges, and were clearly prudential judgments, centered of necessity on intakes employed in the trials concerned.

It is instructive, therefore, to review all the recent recommendations, in concert with the evidence from balance studies (to be discussed further below). Table 1 sets forth these various recommendations. As can be seen, while the 1994 NIH recommendations are, for most ages, substantially higher than the 1989 RDAs [73], they are actually quite close both to values derivable from available balance studies and to the 1997 recommendations of the Food and Nutrition Board.

C. The Requirement at Various Life Stages

In excess of 140 studies have been published relating calcium intake to bone status as summarized and reviewed elsewhere [62]. In more than 40% of this total, the investigators controlled calcium intake, and essentially all of these studies showed that calcium intakes above the then-prevailing RDAs

conferred a bone benefit. Even among the observational studies, in which calcium intake was not investigator controlled and could only be estimated, about 80% were positive. There is, thus, an overwhelming mass of evidence establishing the importance both of calcium for bone and of ensuring intakes higher than prevailing levels or former recommendations. What cannot easily be determined from controlled trials (as has already been noted) is the precise location of the intake threshold, i.e., the point where bony retention is maximal and further intake confers no further bony benefit. The following sections focus on estimating this intake level by age and physiological state.

1. Growth

The human skeleton at birth contains approximately 25 g calcium and, in adult women, 1000–1200 g. All of this difference must come in by way of the diet. Further, unlike other structural nutrients such as protein, the amount of calcium retained is always substantially less than the amount ingested. This is because, as already noted, absorption efficiency is relatively low even during growth, and because calcium is lost daily through shed skin, nails, hair, and sweat, as well as in urine and nonreabsorbed digestive secretions. The gap between calcium intake and calcium retention is larger than is generally appreciated. In the adult with a modest but repairable skeletal deficiency, only about 4–8% of ingested calcium is retained. While retention efficiency is generally higher during growth, even when bone accumulation is most rapid, less than half of the intake is actually retained—ranging from a high of 40% in term infants to 20% in young adults [50]. Even premature infants, with a permeable gut membrane and a relatively huge mineralization demand, exhibit net absorption of less than 60% [74], and dermal and urinary losses mean that they retain even less than that figure. This inefficient retention is not so much because ability to build bone is limited but because, as noted elsewhere, human physiology is optimized to prevent calcium intoxication, not to cope with chronic shortage.

Aside from the obvious fact that one cannot store what one does not ingest, how does suboptimal calcium intake limit bone mass accumulation? Except in unusual circumstances, it is not through limiting bone deposition. In most animal experiments as well as human observations, low calcium intake probably does not limit the growth in bone length or breadth. This is because bone-forming sites do not "see" the diet. They are exposed only to circulating levels of calcium, phosphorus, and the calciotrophic hormones, and even in the face of frank dietary calcium restriction, blood calcium levels change very little. An inadequate calcium intake does, however, result in a bone with a thinner cortex and fewer, thinner trabeculae. This comes about through modulation of the balance between the normal, ongoing processes of bone formation and bone resorption.

To understand how dietary intake interacts with the modeling process, it is necessary to recall that bone reshapes itself continuously during growth. In growing long bones, new bone is deposited at the periosteal surface of the midshaft, at the endosteal surface of the submetaphyseal shaft, and at the growth plate. At the same time, bone is resorbed at the endosteal-trabecular surface and on the outer surface of the metaphyseal funnel. This produces concentric expansion of both external shaft diameter and medullary cavity diameter. This dual process reshapes bones so that they conform to growth in body size. The difference between the amount deposited and the amount resorbed is equal to the net bone gain (or loss).

When ingested calcium is less than optimal, the endosteal-trabecular resorptive process increases, and the balance between formation and resorption, normally positive during growth, falls toward zero. This occurs because parathyroid hormone augments bone resorption at the endosteal-trabecular surface in order to sustain the level of ionized calcium in the extracellular fluid. When the demands of mineralization at the periosteum and growth plates exceed the amount of calcium absorbed from the diet and released from growth-related bone modeling, more parathyroid hormone is secreted and resorption increases still further, until balance becomes zero or even negative. If calcium is the only limiting nutrient, it is usually considered that growth in size continues normally, but that a limited quantity of mineral now has to be redistributed over an ever larger volume.

Usually children's diets in Western nations are not so calcium deprived as to preclude entirely any increase in bone mass, but occasional instances of severe restriction have been reported. Then, high levels of parathyroid hormone drive phosphorus levels in the extracellular fluid so low that mineralization is inhibited and a rachitic type of lesion develops [75, 76], even though vitamin D status may be normal. In such circumstances, bone growth does slow.[11] Short of such extreme situations, the principal perceptible effect of inadequate calcium intake during growth in developed countries is a skeleton of low mass—normally shaped and sized, but containing a smaller than normal amount of bone tissue.

Having said that, it must be noted that at least two studies suggest that augmented calcium intake may influence bone size as well as bone mass [77, 78]. The first [77] is difficult to interpret because the supplementation included extra protein, phosphorus, and other key nutrients as well as calcium. But the second [78], with better matching of other nutrient intakes, also showed a small effect of extra calcium on both bone mass and stature.

Most of the periosteal expansion and growth in length and much of the endosteal expansion during growth are genetically and mechanically determined. Studies in twins have shown that a large fraction of the variability in peak

---

[11]This issue is complicated by the fact that diets so severely deficient in calcium are commonly inadequate on other grounds as well, e. g., protein and energy. Consequently, the growth-stunting undoubtedly has multiple causes.

bone mass is accounted for by the genetic program [79]. However, as already noted, endosteal expansion can be increased in the face of insufficient calcium intake beyond what would be dictated by the genetic program. Thus, while an abundant diet will not produce more bone than the genetic program calls for, a deficient diet must restrict what a person is able to accumulate. Optimal peak bone mass for any given individual can be defined as a skeleton in which the balance between the concentric expansions of growth is solely determined by the individual's genetic program and is not reduced by an exogenous shortage of calcium. Correspondingly, optimal calcium intake can be operationally defined as the intake that permits this full expression of the genetic program.

As just noted, net bone accumulation will be greater as calcium intake increases, but only to the point where endosteal-trabecular resorption is due solely to the genetic program governing growth, and is not being driven by body needs for calcium. Above that level, as seen in Figures 4 and 5, further increases in calcium intake will produce no further bony accumulation. The intake required to achieve the full genetic program, and thus to ensure peak bone mass, is the intake that corresponds to the beginning of the plateau region in Figs. 4 and 5. This value will be different for different stages of growth, in part because growth rates are not constant and also because, as body size increases, obligatory calcium losses through skin and excreta increase as well.

The best approach to determine this value in humans lies, as with the laboratory animal, in testing various intakes for their influence on calcium retention, i.e., finding the plateau and locating its threshold. (In healthy individuals, calcium retention amounts to the same thing as bone tissue accumulation, because calcium is normally stored in the body only in the form of bone.) Over the past 75 years, many such studies have been performed. When these reports are combined, it is possible to make out the pattern of plateau behavior found in laboratory animals and, from the aggregated data, to estimate the intake values that correspond to the threshold [50]. Figure 6 represents one example of the relationship between intake and retention, combining the results of many published studies of calcium balance. It is derived from a subset of the adolescents whose balances were assembled by Matkovic [80]. More recently, Jackman *et al.* [81] studied a series of adolescent girls (each at two intakes, varying from subject to subject), and reported an intake threshold at very nearly the same level as that found by Matkovic and Heaney in their meta-analysis [50]. Both approaches clearly show the plateau type of behavior that both animal studies and theoretical considerations predict. They also confirm that, at intakes less than the plateau threshold, daily storage is less than optimal, i.e., accumulation of bone is being limited by intake. Any such limiting intake must be considered inadequate.

Table 2 and Figure 7 summarize some of the relevant calculations flowing from the type of analysis of aggregated balance data exemplified in Fig. 6 for various stages of

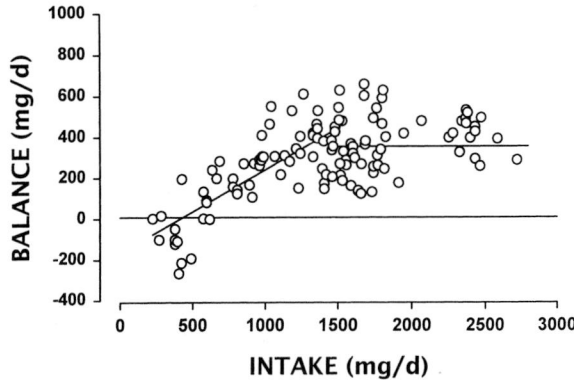

FIGURE 6   The relationship of calcium intake, on the horizontal axis, to calcium retention (balance), on the vertical axis, for a subset of the adolescents described by Matkovic and Heaney [50]. Note that, despite the "noisiness" that is inevitable in measurements of balance in humans, there is clear evidence of an intake plateau, as observed in the animal experiments of Fig. 4. Note also that, for this age, the threshold of the plateau occurs at about 1500 mg calcium/day. (Copyright Robert P. Heaney, 1992. Reproduced with permission.)

growth [50]. First are the threshold intake values, as judged from the assembled balance studies. In some instances these values are slightly higher than both the NIH consensus conference figures and current Recommended Dietary Intakes (RDIs) (Table 1), but, in general, the various recent estimates are quite close to one another. Aside from the usefulness of these threshold values themselves, one especially notable feature of the data in Table 2 is that even after linear growth has ceased (i.e., in young adults), calcium retention still occurs if the intake is high enough to support it. In other words, bony consolidation can continue after growth in stature has ceased. For this reason, calcium intake in young adults needs to be sufficient not only to maintain skeletal equilibrium but to support this continuing augmentation of bone mass.

Figure 7 shows, for the four age groups delineated in Table 2, the best-fit regression lines for the intake regions

TABLE 2   Critical Values for Calcium Intake and Retention Efficiency by Age[a]

Intake threshold		Subthreshold retention efficiency[b]	X-axis intercept (mg/day)
Age (years)	(mg/day)		
0–1	1090	+0.407	13
2–8	1390	+0.238	183
9–17	1480	+0.356	320
18–30	957	+0.200	732

[a]Derived from analyses of published balance studies during growth [50].

[b]Slope of the relationship of retention on intake.

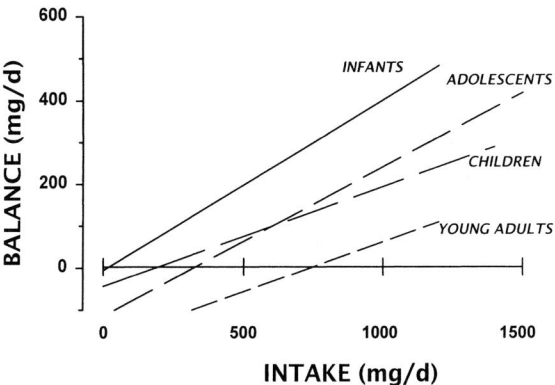

FIGURE 7 Regression lines for the subthreshold regions of the intake-balance relationships in infants, children, adolescents, and young adults, from the data of Matkovic and Heaney [50]. (Copyright Robert P. Heaney, 1992. Reproduced with permission.)

below the age-specific thresholds. This analysis of the data reveals a number of interesting features. First, although the slopes are qualitatively similar, there are nevertheless some important quantitative differences among the age groups. The ability to make use of an increment in calcium intake is greater in infancy and adolescence (i.e., the slope is larger) when skeletal growth is most rapid, and lower in childhood and the young adult years, when growth is slower, as would be expected. Perhaps of even greater interest is the rightward displacement of the regression lines in Figure 6 with advancing age. This phenomenon, reflected in the values in Table 2 for the X-axis intercept, reflects the effect of age on obligatory loss. While zero balance is obviously not healthy for a *growing* organism, these zero-balance intake values are useful in that they reflect how much calcium an individual must ingest just to stay even (i.e., not to *lose* bone) at the ages concerned. As Figure 7 shows, infants can reduce calcium loss to nearly zero on zero calcium intake. For older children and young adults, larger and larger calcium intakes are required to sustain even zero balance. Most of this effect is accounted for by a rise in urine calcium with age. It is probably body size that is forcing the higher obligatory requirement since, in a multiple regression model of these data, body size continues to have an effect even after controlling for age [50].

At least 10 randomized controlled trials of calcium supplementation in children and adolescents have been published [66, 67, 78, 81–83], together with several longitudinal observational studies in young adults [84]. All of the controlled trials were positive, as were three-fourths of the observational studies. As mentioned above, the bone remodeling transient contributes to the measured difference in these controlled trials. The relative size of its contribution remains uncertain; nevertheless, simulation of the remodeling transient indicates that the gain reported in these studies is greater than can be explained by that mechanism alone. In all studies, supplemental calcium elevated the children's in-

takes above the 1989 RDAs. The finding of greater bone gain in the supplemented children than in the control group underscores the inadequacy of the earlier RDA values. In other words, they indicate that the RDAs for 1989 and earlier lie on the ascending portion of the threshold curves of Figures 4 and 5, rather than on the plateau. Hence, these studies reinforce the higher requirement values set forth in Table 2.

In a third trial [80], one group of pubescent girls received approximately the 1989 RDA while the other group was held to a calcium intake of 450 mg/day (far less than the RDA but unfortunately not uncommon for girls of that age). As predicted, growth in stature was the same in both groups, but bone mass failed to increase in the low intake group, while it did in the high intake group. Matkovic *et al.* [85] had previously shown that intakes as low as 450 mg per day in adolescent girls did not support positive calcium balance, mainly because, despite intense skeletal demand at that life stage, urinary conservation of calcium remained inefficient. While this third study does not specifically address the issue of what the intake requirement ought to be during adolescence, it does clearly document the deleterious effects of intakes well below the RDA.

All of these intervention studies, as already noted, produce a remodeling transient. None was designed to evaluate steady-state changes, and hence their positive findings cannot be translated directly into a specific intake recommendation. However, the 4-year longitudinal study of young adults by Recker and his colleagues [84] involved no alteration of calcium intake and hence avoided the problem of the transient. This study showed prospectively that bone augmentation continues well into the third decade. Bone mass gains in their subjects ranged from 0.5% per year for the forearm to 1.25% per year for total body bone mineral. The single most important correlate of the rate of bone accumulation in this Caucasian group of women was calcium intake. The rate of accumulation was inversely proportional to age, with the best estimate of the age at which the rate reached zero being approximately 29–30 years. This suggests that the window of opportunity to achieve the full genetic program appears to remain at least partly open until about age 30. It is not certain that the gains observed in this study were as great as might have been possible, since subjects were studied on their habitual calcium intakes, which were below the threshold values of Table 2. Nevertheless, these observations of Recker *et al.* [84] provide qualitative confirmation of the analyses for this age group derived from the balance studies (Table 2), which showed that young adults were able to retain calcium if intakes were at or above the threshold. They also illustrate well how the data from observational studies can complement the data from controlled trials.

The importance of ensuring full realization of the genetic potential for skeletal development lies in the fact that bone mass seems to track throughout life. Newton-John and Morgan [86] first noted this phenomenon more than 30 years ago

in cross-sectional data, and Matkovic *et al.* [87] showed very clearly in their study of two Croatian populations that those who had higher mass at age 30 remained higher than the others out to age 75, even though both groups were apparently losing bone with age. The same phenomenon has been seen in shorter term, longitudinal studies [88–90], both across puberty and in the postmenopausal years. Dertina *et al.* [88] have gone so far as to suggest that those most at risk for late life osteoporosis can be detected before puberty.

2. MATURITY

Once peak bone mass has been achieved, the principal force acting on the skeleton is no longer the impetus of growth, but the mechanical loads imposed in ordinary, everyday usage. Skeletal structures, like all engineering structures, deform slightly under load. The skeleton senses that degree of deformation, and attempts to adjust its mass (by controlling the balance between bone resorption and bone formation) so that this deformation remains on the order of 0.1–0.15% in any given dimension. If a bone is loaded so heavily that it consistently bends more than that amount, then the balance between local formation and resorption is adjusted to favor formation, thus making that region stiffer. Conversely, if a bony segment is little used, and its bending is less than that critical amount, the skeleton senses that it has an excess of bone in the region concerned, and adjusts remodeling balance to remove some of the apparent surplus.

This reference level of bending is one of the fascinating physiological constants of nature. Across the vertebrates, for all species and all bones studied to date, bone mass is regulated such that any given bone deforms by about that critical 0.1–0.15% in ordinary use. This reference level of bending is termed a *setpoint,* and the bone remodeling apparatus operates to minimize local deviations from this critical value. The cellular basis for the setpoint and the precise nature of the apparatus that detects departures from it remain unknown[12]; however, there is suggestive evidence that localizes this sensing apparatus to the network of osteocytes embedded in bone. For several years, it has seemed likely that one of the principal determinants of the setpoint of this mass-regulating system is the level of gonadal hormones. Circumstantial evidence in support of this connection includes the facts that estrogen receptors in bone are concentrated in osteocytes [91], and that true bone density rises sharply at puberty [92] and declines by about the same amount at menopause (whether natural or artificial) [93]. These life-phase changes are what one would expect if estrogen influences the setpoint.[13]

---

[12]Bone is not unique in this regard: The molecular basis for the setpoint in most biological feedback systems is not known.

[13]The same level of bending sensed as tolerable in an estrogen-deprived state lies above the reference level when estrogen is present (and the setpoint is lower). The bone remodeling apparatus responds by adding bone to reduce the size of the difference from the reference level of bending.

While adjustments in mass around the setpoint presume an adequate calcium intake, it turns out that prevailing intakes tend to be closer to adequate during the ages 25–50 in women, since estrogen improves the efficiency of intestinal calcium absorption [48, 93] and of renal calcium conservation [94, 95]. Thus estrogen not only increases the reference level of bone density, but it helps the body access and retain the mineral necessary to augment bone to that higher level. For this reason, except for the special circumstances of pregnancy and lactation (discussed below), the years from 25 to 50 are a time in life when a woman's skeletal calcium need is at its lowest. She is no longer storing calcium, and her absorption and retention are operating at their adult peak efficiency.

Welten *et al.* [96] in a meta-analysis of 33 studies performed in adults between 18 and 50 years of age, found a positive association between calcium intake and bone mass in this age group, and noted that it seemed prudent to maintain an intake of 1500 mg/day during this life period. This is a higher figure than either the NIH consensus conference recommendations or the 1997 DRIs of Table 1. Heaney *et al.* [94], using balance methods in estrogen-replete women ingesting their habitual calcium intakes, found a mean intake for zero balance of slightly under 1000 mg/day, and Nordin *et al.* [97], also using balance methods, arrived at a figure slightly above 800 mg/day. Recker *et al.* [98], in a small prospective study of bone mass in premenopausal women found no detectable bone loss over a 2-year period on an estimated mean calcium intake of 651 mg. Baran *et al.* [99], studying women in their fifth decade, found bone loss in a control group receiving 892 mg calcium/day. Loss occurred only from year 2 to year 3, and not during the first 2 years of observation, and it is not clear from that paper whether the apparent loss in year 3 was related to the loss of sampling units that occurred between years 2 and 3, or whether there was actual loss in those who remained in the study.

Requirement estimates based on balance studies make no provision for sweat loss of calcium since, by design, balance methods usually eliminate vigorous exercise. The importance of sweat loss has been highlighted by a study in male college athletes showing sweat calcium losses of over 200 mg in a single vigorous workout session [100]. Moreover, there was a perceptible loss of bone mineral density across a playing season that was preventable by adding calcium supplements to the athletes' already good diets. It is likely that the lost bone would have been regained after the playing season was over (as long as the diet was adequate); that is, that the skeleton was acting in its capacity as a calcium reserve during the playing season. Nevertheless, the study makes clear how large and important sweat losses can be. Undoubtedly such losses contribute to the low bone mass described in women athletes who often have less than generous calcium intakes.

In conclusion, the bulk of the available evidence suggests that it is important to maintain an intake of 1000–1500 mg/

day during the mature years. Moreover, there are other health reasons for maintaining a high calcium intake during this period [101], even if bone health can be supported adequately by an intake in the range of 800–1000 mg/day.

3. PREGNANCY AND LACTATION

Pregnancy and lactation are circumstances in which the mother must provide for maintenance of her own skeleton as well as for construction of her child's. Specifically, during the 9 months of pregnancy, she provides the fetus with 25–30 g calcium, and in her milk during the ensuing nine months of lactation, another 50–75 g. This aggregate is in the range of 7–10% of her own total body calcium and would, presumably, produce a corresponding decrease in bone mass if she were not able to obtain some or all of the required quantities from ingested calcium. It has always seemed intuitively attractive, therefore, to recommend an increased calcium intake during these physiologically demanding life-stages [73] (see also Table 1). Moreover, given the relatively low calcium intakes of modern industrialized societies, one might have expected that a history of multiparity and extended lactation would be associated with lower bone mass and increased risk of osteoporosis. In general, however, epidemiological studies have found, if anything, the contrary. Most studies report a positive association between parity and bone mass density [102–107], although occasional reports of negative associations can be found [108]. Much of the positive association turns out to be due to increased ponderosity, and after correcting for weight, the positive correlations tend to become statistically nonsignificant. Nevertheless, most are still on the positive side, and there is little or no hint in the available evidence that the calcium drain of pregnancy and lactation adversely affects the maternal skeleton.

Bone remodeling accelerates in pregnancy [109–114], and maternal intestinal calcium absorption efficiency increases to the highest level since early infancy. Both changes begin well before significant fetal skeletal accumulation of calcium [109, 115]. Both humans and rats show anticipatory storage of skeletal minerals prior to onset of fetal skeletal mineralization [107, 109], and Heaney and Skillman [109] estimated, from balance studies in pregnant women studied on their habitual calcium intakes, that cumulative calcium balance at term exceeded fetal needs, and that the mother, therefore, went into lactation with a skeletal surplus. Brommage and Baxter [110] reported data consistent with a skeletal surplus in rats at delivery, and ultrasound methods suggest that the same occurs in pregnant mares [111]. However, this will not be possible if calcium intake is very low. Barger-Lux et al. [116] reported bone loss across pregnancy in young women with dietary calcium to protein ratios averaging 6.6 mg/g.

During lactation, the majority of reports indicate that some degree of bone loss regularly occurs [101, 102, 105–108, 112, 113, 117–120], particularly in presumably reactive bony sites such as the centers of the vertebral bodies and the ultradistal radius [117, 118]. On the other hand, this loss appears to reverse after weaning and may, therefore, represent to some extent a negative remodeling transient like what occurs in deer at the time of antler formation [57]. Immediately following delivery, absorption efficiency falls to or toward nonpregnant, nonlactating levels and remains at this relatively low level throughout lactation, despite the continuing drain of lactational calcium loss [109, 113, 121]; however, urinary calcium falls at the same time and remains low throughout lactation and for several months post-weaning [112], while bone remodeling remains elevated [112, 113]. This is a physiological situation conducive to replacement of lost bone.[14]

Lactating rats lose nearly one-third of their skeleton during milk production [119]. This loss doubles if the animals are fed low- calcium diets, but it does not diminish when the normally high calcium diet of a rat is increased as much as threefold [119]. It is likely that this bone loss represents an anticipatory phenomenon; that is, rather than the calcium being drawn out of bone by the drain of lactation, the bone pumps calcium into the circulation for milk production. This is suggested by the reduced parathyroid hormone levels during lactation [122], by the usually reported failure of increased calcium intake to reduce the loss, and by the high serum phosphorus levels during lactation.[15] How this outpouring of skeletal mineral for the benefit of lactation occurs is less clear, although it is certainly plausible that the hypoestrin state of lactation would, like menopause or athletic amenorrhea, shift the bone setpoint, and result in some downward reduction in bone density (thereby, effectively, releasing stored calcium and phosphorus).

While Kalkwarf et al. [123] found no effect of calcium supplementation, a few reports suggest that even the modest reductions in bone mass normally found during human lactation can be reduced or eliminated by extra calcium [117, 118]. The relatively slow growth of human infants (in comparison, for example, with rats) imposes a lower lactational burden on a human mother, and some of the differences between species may be attributable to quite significant differences in lactational demands for mineral.

Given the concordance of the balance data and the epidemiological evidence, it seems likely either that adaptive mechanisms are usually sufficient to accommodate the calcium demands of pregnancy and lactation or that postweaning adjustments compensate for whatever bone may have been lost. As it turns out, there is physiological evidence to indicate that both occur.

---

[14]The importance of urinary loss for balance is discussed in the section on nutritional factors that influence the requirement.

[15]In this latter respect, phosphate is as necessary for milk production as is calcium, and high serum phosphorus levels serve that important purpose. The contrary causal flow, that is, lactation pulling calcium out of bone, would work against the lactational need for phosphorus, since parathyroid hormone, mediating the response to all calcium needs, lowers serum phosphorus.

Compensatory physiological adjustments surrounding pregnancy and lactation are more vigorous than at other lifestages, and the current consensus is that a high calcium intake makes less long-term difference to a woman's skeleton at this lifestage than at most other times in her life. In summarizing the available literature, the panel responsible for the 1997 DRIs noted that there was no evidence on which to base a recommendation for a higher calcium intake during pregnancy and lactation than that considered optimal for other women of the same age. They did add, however, that the situation with adolescent pregnancy was problematic and inadequately studied, and that perhaps some increment above the adolescent recommendation in such individuals might be prudent.

4. MENOPAUSE

It has been noted already that estrogen seems to adjust the bending setpoint of bone. Accordingly, whenever women lose ovarian hormones, either naturally at menopause or earlier as a result of anorexia nervosa or athletic amenorrhea, the skeleton seems to sense that it has more bone than it needs, and hence allows resorption to carry away more bone than formation replaces. (Precisely the same change occurs when men lose testosterone for any reason.) This is equivalent to raising the bone bending setpoint, as described above. While varying somewhat from site to site across the skeleton, the downward adjustment in bone mass due to lack of gonadal hormone amounts to approximately 10–15% of the bone a woman had in the lumbar spine and 6 percent at the total hip prior to menopause [93].

The importance of this phenomenon in a discussion of nutrient effects is to help distinguish menopausal bone loss from nutrient deficiency loss and to stress that menopausal loss, which is due to absence of gonadal hormones, not to nutrient deficiency, cannot be substantially influenced by diet. Almost all of the published studies of calcium supplementation within 5 years following menopause failed to prevent bone loss [63, 124, 125]. Even Elders *et al.*, [125] who employed a calcium intake in excess of 3000 mg/day, succeeded only in slowing menopausal loss, not in preventing it. However, Dutch women tend to be calcium replete, because of high national dairy product consumption, and other studies have shown effects of calcium supplementation in the early menopausal years that are intermediate between placebo and estrogen [72, 124, 125]. It is likely that, in any group of early menopausal women, there are some whose calcium intake is so inadequate that they are losing bone for two reasons (estrogen lack plus calcium insufficiency).

As important as menopausal bone loss is, it is only a one-time, downward adjustment, and, if nutrition is adequate, the loss continues for only a few years, after which the skeleton comes into a new steady state (although at a 5–15% lower bone mass). It is in this context that the importance of a high peak skeletal mass becomes apparent. One standard deviation for lumbar spine bone mineral content in normal women

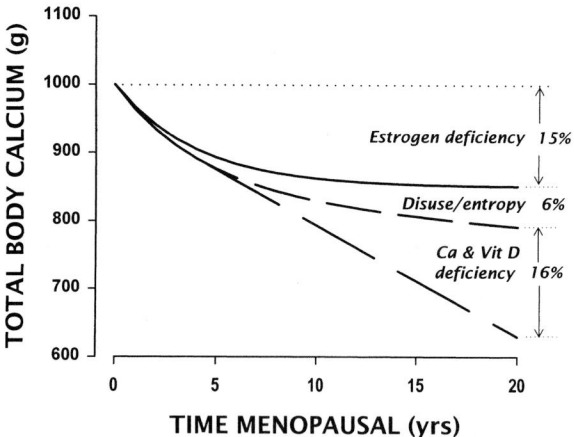

FIGURE 8   Partition of age-related bone loss in a typical postmenopausal woman with an inadequate calcium intake. Based on a model described in detail elsewhere [93]. (Copyright Robert P. Heaney, 1990. Reproduced with permission.)

is about 10–15% of the young adult mean, and for total body bone mineral, about 12%. Hence a woman at or above one standard deviation above the mean can sustain the 15% menopausal loss and still end up with as much bone as the average woman has before menopause. By contrast, a woman at or under one standard deviation below the young adult mean premenopausally drops to two standard deviations below the mean as she crosses menopause and is, therefore, by the WHO criteria [127], already osteopenic and verging on frankly osteoporotic.

As noted, the menopausal bone mass adjustment amounts to a loss at the spine of 10–15%, and at the hip, ~6% [128]. Hip bone change, both immediately before and after this menopausal downward adjustment, averages about −5% per year, while, except for the menopausal loss, the spine curve is flat. But this is so only as long as calcium intake is adequate. In this regard, it is important to recall the nonskeletal effects of estrogen described above; improvement of intestinal absorption and renal conservation [48, 94, 95]. Because of these effects, an estrogen-deficient woman has a higher calcium requirement, and unless she raises her calcium intake after menopause, she will continue to lose bone after the estrogen-dependent quantum has been lost, even if the same diet would have been adequate to maintain her skeleton before menopause. In other words, early in the menopausal period, her bone loss is mainly (or entirely) because of estrogen withdrawal, while later it is because of inadequate calcium intake.

Figure 8 assembles, schematically, the set of factors contributing to bone loss in the postmenopausal period. The figure shows both the self-limiting character of the loss due to estrogen deficiency and the usually slower, but continuing, loss due to nutritional deficiency, when present. Unlike the estrogen-related loss, which mostly plays itself out in 3–6 years, an ongoing calcium deficiency loss will continue

to deplete the skeleton indefinitely for the remainder of a woman's life, that is, unless calcium intake is raised to a level sufficient to stop it. Furthermore, since both absorption efficiency [48] and calcium intake [42] decline with age, the degree of calcium shortfall typically worsens with age.

Thus it is important for a woman to increase her calcium intake after menopause, even though, for the first few years, doing so will not prevent estrogen-withdrawal bone loss. Both the 1984 NIH consensus conference on osteoporosis [129], and the 1994 Consensus Conference on Optimal Calcium Intake [61] recommended intakes of 1500 mg/day for estrogen-deprived postmenopausal women. It may be that the optimal intake is somewhat higher still (see below), but median intake in the United States for women of this age is in the range of 500–600 mg/day [42], and if the bulk of the diets could be raised even to 1500 mg/day, the impact on skeletal health would be considerable.

5. SENESCENCE

There is general agreement that bone is lost with aging. Early cross-sectional data suggested that spine loss began as early as age 30–35, but, except for the hip, longitudinal studies have not borne that out for most skeletal regions (e.g., spine, forearm) [98]. Significant loss probably does not begin until sometime in the sixth or seventh decade.[16] This age-related bone loss occurs in both sexes, regardless of gonadal hormone levels. However, it is obscured at the commonly measured spine site in the years immediately following menopause in women by the substantially larger effect of estrogen withdrawal (see Figure 8). It probably occurs, however, even in estrogen-treated women, at about the same rate as in men. This rate varies by skeletal region and is generally reported to be on the order of 0.5–1.0% per year by the seventh decade, and accelerates with advancing age. Age-related loss involves both cortical and trabecular bone and can be due to several causes. These include disuse atrophy consequent upon reduced physical activity, an entropic kind of loss due to accumulation of random remodeling errors which, of their nature tend to be irreversible[17]; reduction in androgenic steroid levels, and finally nutritional deficiency loss. These types of bone loss are summarized in Figure 8.

While nutrient deficiency is clearly only a part of the problem, nevertheless it is common. Intestinal calcium absorption efficiency declines with age [48], at the same time as nutrient intake itself generally declines [42]; the result is that the diet of aging individuals becomes doubly inadequate. This inadequacy is clearly expressed, for example, in

the rate of bone loss reported by Chapuy et al. [64] in the untreated control group of their large randomized trial of calcium and vitamin D supplementation. These women, with an average age of 84 and with calcium intakes that averaged 514 mg/day, were losing bone from the femur at rates of slightly more than 35% per year. That there was a causal connection between intake and bone loss is demonstrated by the fact that the loss was completely obliterated with calcium (and vitamin D) supplementation.

It is in this age group that the most dramatic and persuasive evidence for the importance of a high calcium intake has been produced in recent years. This is primarily because most fragility fractures rise in frequency with age and, hence, the opportunity to see a fracture benefit (if one exists) is greater then.[18] Chapuy et al. [64] showed a reduction in hip fracture risk of 43% by 18 months after starting supplementation with calcium and vitamin D, and a 32% reduction in other extremity fractures. Chevalley et al. [68], in another study in elderly women, resolved the question left unanswered in the study of Chapuy et al. (whether the calcium or the vitamin D was responsible for the effect) by giving vitamin D to both controls and treated subjects, but calcium only to the treated group. They, too, found a reduction in femoral bone loss and in fracture incidence (vertebral in this case) in the calcium-supplemented women. Recker et al. [69] in a 4-year, randomized controlled trial in elderly women (mean age 73), showed that a calcium supplement reduced both age-related bone loss and incident vertebral fractures. Their subjects had all received a multivitamin supplement containing 400 IU of vitamin D; hence, most or all of the effect in the calcium-supplemented group can be attributed to the calcium alone.

The studies of Chevalley et al. [68] and Recker et al. [69] should not be interpreted to mean that vitamin D is unimportant in this age group. It is likely that intakes of both calcium and vitamin D are commonly inadequate in the elderly (see below), and the high prevalence of combined deficiency has complicated study of the actual requirements of either nutrient in this age group. The importance of these studies lies in the fact that, even after ensuring vitamin D repletion, there was still a calcium benefit and, hence, presumptively a calcium deficiency in this age group. Heikinheimo et al. [132] had earlier shown the converse in an elderly Finnish population. Vitamin D supplementation in this population (which tends to be calcium replete) significantly reduced all fractures, both in institutionalized and in free-living individuals.

The calcium intake achieved in the Chapuy et al. [64] study was about 1700 mg/day, in the Chevalley et al. [68] study, 1400 mg/day, and in the Recker et al. [69] study, about 1600 mg/day. These values are in the range of the intake

---

[16]For certain bony regions, *density* may begin to decline earlier [130], but in most such instances a countervailing periosteal expansion occurs such that total regional bone mass remains constant and bone strength is, if anything, greater.

[17]Examples include overlarge Haversian cavities, fenestrated trabecular plates, and severed trabecular spicules that, once disconnected, become unloaded and hence are subject to rapid resorption [131].

---

[18]Reduction in bone loss is only presumptively beneficial. Until it can be shown that fracture incidence is reduced, bone mass effects are less persuasive, and despite the abundant theoretical underpinnings of why bone mass should be important, only fracture reduction is ultimately convincing.

found by Heaney *et al.* [94, 133] to be the mean requirement for healthy estrogen-deprived older women (1500–1700 mg/day). All of these studies are, therefore, fully consistent with the more recent recommendations in the range of 1500 mg/day (Table 1).

An important feature of these controlled trials in already elderly individuals was that bone mass was low in both treated and control groups at the start of the study, and while a significant difference in fracture rate was produced by calcium supplementation, even the supplemented groups would have to be considered as having an unacceptably high fracture rate. What these studies do not establish is how much lower the fracture rate might have been if a high calcium intake had been provided for the preceding 20–30 years of these women's lives. The studies of Matkovic *et al.* [4] and Holbrook *et al.* [134], although not randomized trials, strongly suggest that the effect may be larger than has been found with treatment started in the eighth and ninth decades of life. Both of these observational studies reported a hip fracture rate that was roughly 60% lower in elderly whose habitual calcium intakes had been high. While findings from observational studies such as these had not been considered persuasive in the absence of proof from controlled trials, the trials with fracture endpoints have now met that need.

Additional reinforcement comes from recent work of McKane *et al.* [135], who studied the effect of a large calcium supplement on parathyroid hormone secretory dynamics in elderly women. In brief, a mean calcium intake of 2413 mg/day lowered parathyroid hormone levels 40% to the young normal range, and normalized the abnormal parathyroid hormone secretory dynamics typical of the elderly female. They concluded that the combination of declining oral calcium intake, deteriorating vitamin D status, reduced calcium absorption, and impaired renal conservation of calcium in the elderly lead to parathyroid gland hyperactivity and increased bone resorption.

Together the aggregate of available studies underscores the importance of achieving at least the 1400–1500 mg/day target figure of the new recommendations for the elderly. At the same time it must be stressed, once again, that osteoporosis is a multifactorial condition, and that removing one of these factors (i.e., ensuring an adequate calcium intake) cannot be expected to eradicate all osteoporotic fractures.

D. Nutritional Factors That Influence the Requirement

Several nutritional factors influence or have been proposed to influence the calcium requirement (Table 3). The principal interacting nutrients are sodium, protein, caffeine, and fiber. Fiber and caffeine influence calcium absorption [136–138] and typically exert relatively minor effects, while sodium and protein influence urinary excretion of calcium [136, 137], and can be of much greater significance for the calcium economy. Phosphorus and fat are sometimes mentioned in

TABLE 3 Food Factors and the Calcium Requirement

	Negative effects	Positive effects
Absorption	Fiber	Fiber
	Phytate	Food
	Oxalate	Lactose
	Caffeine	Carbohydrates
	Fat	Lysine
	Phosphorus	Fat
Excretion	Protein	Phosphorus
	Sodium	Alkaline ash
	Chloride	
	Acid ash	
	[Aluminum hydroxide]	

connection with calcium absorption, but their effect in humans seems minor to nonexistent.

The basis for the importance of nutrients acting on absorption and excretion is illustrated in Fig. 9, which partitions the variance in calcium balance observed in 560 balances in healthy middle-aged women studied in the author's laboratory. As Fig. 9 shows, only 11% of the variance in balance among these women is explained by differences in their calcium intakes, and absorption efficiency explains only another 15%. By contrast, urinary losses explain slightly more than 50%.[19] The dominance in Fig. 9 of renal excretion would be trivial in primary bone-losing syndromes, but it is particularly noteworthy that it appears to be operative in conditions of health, because it means that obligatory losses through the kidney pull calcium out of the skeleton. This is a concept for which we are particularly indebted to the work of Nordin and his associates [139, 140].

[19]I have already remarked on the importance of urinary calcium loss in the context of the declining retention efficiency with age in growing children, and have noted that the drop in urine calcium during lactation and postweaning helps to compensate for lactational demands.

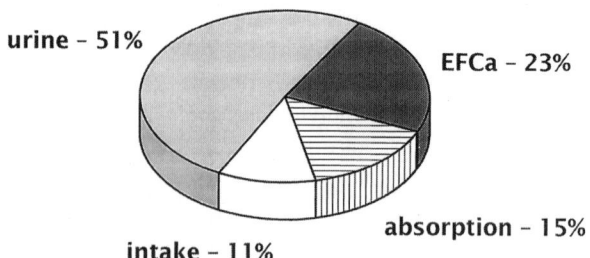

FIGURE 9 Partition of variance in calcium balance in normal women among the input–output processes involved in calculation of balance. (Copyright Robert P. Heaney, 1994. Reproduced with permission.)

1. INFLUENCES ON INTESTINAL ABSORPTION OF CALCIUM

a. Fiber. The effect of fiber is variable, and generally small. In acute, single-meal absorption tests, many kinds of fiber have no influence at all on absorption, such as the fiber in green, leafy vegetables [30, 34]. Moreover, fibers of the class termed nondigestible oligosaccharides, rather than interfering with absorption, have been shown in rats to increase both mucosal mass and calcium absorption [141], and there are reports in humans suggesting a similar effect, at least on absorption [142, 143] (which is why fiber is listed in both columns of Table 3). The current theory is that volatile fatty acids produced in fermentation of the nondigestible oligosaccharides by colonic flora evoke gut hormone responses that regulate mucosal mass (thereby serving to match the metabolic cost of replacing the mucosa every 5 days to the level of food intake). The fiber in wheat bran, by contrast, reduces absorption of co-ingested calcium in single-meal tests, although except for extremes of fiber intake [144], the antiabsorptive effect is generally relatively small.

Often lumped together with fiber are associated food constituents such as phytate and oxalate, both of which can reduce the availability of any calcium contained in the same food. For example, for equal ingested loads, the calcium of beans is only about half as available as the calcium of milk [145], while the calcium of spinach and rhubarb is nearly totally unavailable [30, 146]. For spinach and rhubarb, the inhibition is mostly due to oxalate. For common beans, phytate is responsible for about half the interference, and oxalate, the other half. The effects of phytate and oxalate are highly variable. There is a sufficient quantity of both antiabsorbers in beans to complex all the calcium also present, and yet their combined absorptive interference is only half what might have been predicted. With the exception of bran, these interferences generally operate only on calcium contained in the same food. This is because the antiabsorber is usually already fully complexed with calcium in the ingested food. Thus, spinach does not typically interfere with absorption of co-ingested milk calcium.

b. Caffeine. Often considered to have a deleterious effect on the calcium economy, caffeine actually has the smallest effect of the known interacting nutrients. A single cup of brewed coffee causes deterioration in calcium balance of 3 mg [137, 138, 147], mainly by reducing absorption of calcium [137]. The effect is probably on active transport, although this is not known for certain. This effect is so small as to be more than adequately offset by a tablespoon or two of milk [137, 147]; and café au lait or caffe latte produce a substantial net calcium gain, despite their caffeine content.

c. Fat. Fat also has sometimes been presumed to reduce calcium absorption by a similar mechanism, that is formation of calcium soaps with unesterified fatty acids released in the chyme by intestinal lipases. However, in healthy adult humans, no appreciable effect of fat intake on calcium absorption has been found. This is at least partly explained, as with

phosphorus (see below), by the fact that the normal small intestine absorbs fat much more avidly than it does calcium. At intakes in the range of recommended levels, the feces contain a considerable stoichiometric excess of calcium relative to fatty acids.

2. INFLUENCES ON RENAL CONSERVATION OF CALCIUM

a. Protein and Sodium. As noted, the effects of protein and of sodium are substantial [17, 18, 138, 148]. Both nutrients increase urinary calcium loss across the full range of their own intakes, from very low to very high—so it is not a question of harmful effects of an excess of these nutrients. Sodium and calcium share the same transport system in the proximal tubule, and every 2300 mg sodium excreted by the kidney pulls 20–60 mg of calcium out with it. And every gram of protein metabolized in adults causes an increment in urine calcium loss of about 1 mg.[20] This latter effect is probably due to excretion of the sulfate load produced in the metabolism of sulfur-containing amino acids (and is thus a kind of endogenous analog of the acid rain problem). At low sodium and protein intakes, the minimum calcium requirement for skeletal maintenance for an adult female may be as little as 450 mg/day [139], whereas if her intake of both nutrients is high, she may require as much as 2000 mg/day to maintain calcium balance. A forceful illustration of the importance of sodium intake is provided by the report of Matkovic *et al.* [85] that urine calcium remains high in adolescent girls on calcium intakes too low to permit bone gain. The principal determinant of urinary calcium in such young women is sodium intake [149], not calcium intake.

Differences in protein and sodium intake from one national group to another are part of the explanation of why studies in different countries have shown sometimes strikingly different calcium requirements [35]. At the same time, one usually finds a positive correlation between calcium intake and bone mass within the national range of intakes [150]. Hence, while sodium (and protein) intake differences across cultures may obscure the calcium effect, they do not obliterate it.

The acid/alkaline ash characteristic of the diet is also important, although the quantitative relationship of this diet feature to the calcium requirement is less completely developed. Nevertheless, it has clearly been shown that substitution of metabolizable anions (e.g., bicarbonate or acetate) for fixed anions (e.g., chloride) in various test diets will lower obligatory urinary calcium loss substantially [151, 152]. This suggests that primarily vegetarian diets create a lower calcium requirement, and provides a further explanation for the seemingly lower requirement in many nonindustrialized

---

[20]This protein effect would be predicted to be less during growth, and particularly when growth is rapid, as in infancy. Then, much of the ingested protein is incorporated into tissue, while in adults, with no net tissue gain, protein catabolism matches protein intake.

populations. However, it is not yet clear whether, within a population, vegetarians have higher bone mass values than omnivores [153], and such limited data as are available suggest, in fact, the contrary [154–156].

b. Phosphorus. Phosphorus is commonly believed to reduce calcium absorption, but the evidence for that effect is scant to nonexistent, and there is much contrary evidence. Spencer *et al.* [157] showed no effect of even large increments in phosphate intake on overall calcium balance at low, normal, and high intakes of calcium. In adults, calcium to phosphorus ratios ranging from 0.2 to above 2.0 are without effect on calcium balance when studied under metabolic ward conditions and adjustments are made for calcium intake [138]. Still phosphorus intake is not without effect on the calcium economy. It depresses urinary calcium loss and elevates digestive juice secretion of calcium by approximately equal amounts (which is why there is no net effect on balance [49, 148]). While it is true that stoichiometric excesses of phosphate will tend to form complexes with calcium in the chyme, various calcium phosphate salts have been shown to exhibit absorbability similar to other calcium salts [158], and phosphate is, of course, a principal anion of the major food source of calcium (dairy products). In any case, phosphate itself is more readily absorbed than calcium (by a factor of at least 2–3 times), and at intakes of both nutrients in the range of their respective DRIs, absorption will leave a stoichiometric excess of calcium in the ileum, not the other way around. This explains the seeming paradox that high calcium intakes can block phosphate absorption (as in management of end-stage renal disease), while achievably high phosphate intakes have little or no effect on calcium absorption.

c. Aluminum. Although not in any sense a nutrient, aluminum, in the form of aluminum-containing antacids, also exerts significant effects on obligatory calcium loss in the urine [159]. By binding phosphate in the gut, these substances reduce phosphate absorption, lower integrated 24-hour serum phosphate levels, and thereby elevate urinary calcium loss. This is the opposite of the more familiar hypocalciuric effect of oral phosphate supplements. Therapeutic doses of Aluminum-containing antacids can elevate urine calcium by 50 mg/day or more.

3. Enhancers of Calcium Absorption

Relatively little work has been done on enhancers of calcium absorption. Lactose is said to improve absorption, but the effect may be confined to the rat. Human studies using various carbohydrates have generally shown some enhancement [160], but the effect may be confined to intestines damaged by disease or surgery, because it has been hard to find in healthy subjects [161]. Also, the effect of various carbohydrates may be nonspecific, due instead to alteration of the gastric emptying pattern associated with co-ingestion of other food constituents—what we have elsewhere characterized as the "meal effect" [162]. (That is the meaning of the entry "food" in Table 3.)

Nevertheless, given the generally low absorbability of calcium, the prospect of finding substances that might improve calcium bioavailability has enticed many food processors. Various food fractions, such as casein phosphopeptide, derived from milk, have been found to improve calcium absorbability in certain experimental systems [163], although its effect in humans is probably small [164]. Likewise, certain amino acids, notably lysine, have been thought to enhance calcium absorption [165], but human evidence in their regard is sparse and inconsistent. Even fat might theoretically be viewed as an enhancer, since it is known to slow gastric emptying. However, we have been unable to find, using multiple regression methods, any effect of even large variations in fat intake on absorption fraction in our observational study of middle-aged women.

4. Intake vs Interference

For diets high in calcium, as would have been the case for our hunter-gatherer ancestors, high protein and possibly high sodium intakes could have been handled by the body without adverse effects. These nutrients create problems for the calcium economy of contemporary adult humans mainly because we typically have calcium intakes that are low relative to those of preagricultural humans. This is because at prevailing low intakes, compensatory adjustment mechanisms are already operating, and for many individuals, capacity for further adaptation (e.g., increased absorption efficiency) is very limited. An increased demand for only 40 mg calcium/day would require a nearly 40% increase in intestinal absorption at intakes at the bottom quartile for North American and European women today, while the same demand can be met by an increase of only 1–2% in absorption efficiency at intakes such as those that prevailed during hominid evolution. The former is not possible, while the latter is easily accomplished. Thus, while there is some emphasis today among nutritionists on regulating intake of interfering nutrients, the real problem is not so much that the intakes of these other nutrients are high, as that calcium intake is too low to allow us to adjust to the inevitable nutrient–nutrient interactions that occur with any diet.

VII. VITAMIN D

It has long been recognized that vitamin D is important for absorption of calcium from the diet. Its role in that regard lies in facilitating active transport, probably by inducing the formation of a calcium-binding transport protein in intestinal mucosal cells. This function is particularly important for adaptation to low intakes. There is also, apparently, a second vitamin D-related absorption mechanism, transcaltachia [166], which is nongenomic in expression but nevertheless requires occupancy of the classical vitamin D receptor. Finally, absorption also occurs passively, probably mainly by way of paracellular diffusion. This route is not dependent on

vitamin D and is not as well studied. The proportion of absorption by the three mechanisms varies with intake and is not well characterized in humans; at high calcium intakes (above 2000 mg/day) the absorption fraction approaches that observed in anephric individuals (~10–15% of intake). Under these circumstances it is likely that active transport contributes relatively little to the total absorbed load. Nevertheless, it is clear, at prevailing calcium intakes, that vitamin D status influences absorptive performance and that it thereby influences the minimum calcium requirement.

A simple calculation suffices to establish the magnitude of this influence. Assume an intake of 1000 mg calcium/day. To that is added about 150 mg in the form of digestive secretions and sloughed off mucosa. If passive absorption is at a level of 12.5% of intake, net absorption would amount to 144 mg, leaving the individual in *negative* balance across the gut of ~6 mg/day (and, of course, producing no calcium gain for the body to offset renal and dermal losses). If, however, vitamin D-mediated, active transport is operating, so that, for example, total absorption was 27.5%, net absorption becomes +109 mg. The relationship of active transport to net absorption is shown graphically, for various intakes, in Fig. 10, which makes clear that meeting physiological demands for calcium would require very high calcium intakes in the absence of vitamin D. (That situation is depicted by the bottom line in the figure, which is the net absorption contour for zero active absorption, as well as by the other lines depicting lower levels of active transport, reflecting, in turn, varying degrees of vitamin D insufficiency.)

A principal storage form of the vitamin is 25-hydroxyvitamin D (25OHD), and its plasma level is generally regarded as the best clinical indicator of vitamin D status. Although usually considered to be about three orders of magnitude less potent than calcitriol in promoting active transport in animal receptor assays, there is growing evidence that it may possess physiological functions in its own right [167–172], and in the only human dose–response studies performed to date, 25OHD was found to have a molar potency in the range of 1/125 to 1/400 that of 1,25(OH)$_2$D$_3$ [171–173], not the 1/2000 figure usually considered to reflect relative 25OHD activity.

Vitamin D status commonly deteriorates in the elderly, whose plasma 25OHD levels are generally lower than in young adults [174, 175]. These elderly persons, without histological or biochemical evidence of osteomalacia, nevertheless exhibit high parathyroid hormone levels, high serum alkaline phosphatase levels, and low absorptive performance, all of which move to or toward normal with physiological amounts of supplemental vitamin D [174–177]. The rate of age-related loss of bone has been found to be inversely correlated to dietary vitamin D [178]. Low dosage vitamin D supplementation of ostensibly healthy postmenopausal women significantly slows wintertime bone loss and reduces the annual parathyroid-mediated activation of the bone remodeling system that occurs in winter through late spring [175]. These changes all suggest relative vitamin D insufficiency.

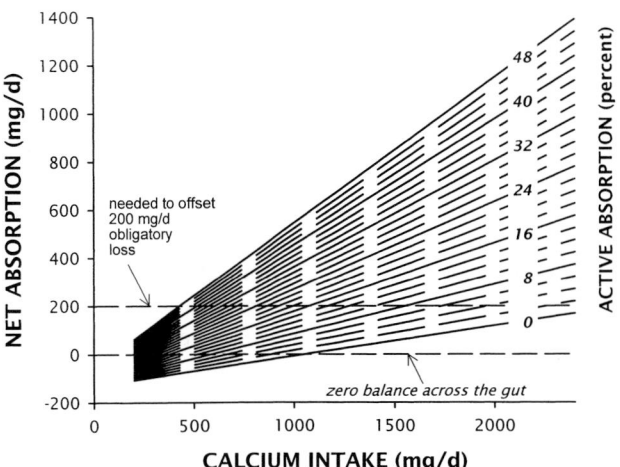

FIGURE 10   Relationship of vitamin D-mediated, active calcium absorption, calcium intake, and net calcium gain across the gut. Each of the contours represents a different level of active absorption above a baseline passive absorption of 12.5%. (The values along each contour represent the sum total of passive and variable active absorption.) The horizontal, dashed lines indicate zero and 200 mg/day net absorption, respectively. The former is the value at which the gut switches from a net excretory to a net absorptive mode, and the latter is the value needed to offset typical urinary and dermal losses in mature adults. (Copyright Robert P. Heaney, 1999. Reproduced with permission.)

Low 25OHD levels in the elderly are partly due to decreased solar exposure, partly to decreased efficiency of skin vitamin D synthesis, and partly to decreased intake of milk, the principal dietary source of the vitamin in North America. Moreover, the elderly exhibit other abnormalities of the vitamin D endocrine system, which may further impair their ability to adapt to reduced calcium intake. These include decreased responsiveness of the renal 1-α-hydroxylase to parathyroid hormone [179] and possibly, also, decreased mucosal responsiveness to calcitriol [180] (although available data do not permit distinguishing a decrease in mucosal responsiveness from a simple decrease in mucosal mass).

For all of these reasons, there is a growing body of opinion that the requirement for vitamin D rises with age [27, 176, 181–184], and a body of data that strongly suggests that relative vitamin D deficiency plays a role in several components of the osteoporosis syndrome. Perhaps most persuasive of all is the finding by Heikinheimo *et al.* [132], in a randomized, controlled trial, of substantial reduction in all fractures in an elderly Finnish population given a single injection of 150,000–300,000 IU vitamin D each fall.[21] Lips *et al.* [185], on the other hand, found no benefit from an additional 400 IU of vitamin D in a Dutch population.

The foregoing studies (as well as others) lead inexorably to the conclusion that vitamin D insufficiency is prevalent in

---

[21]This dose amounts to a daily average exposure of 410–820 IU and can thus be considered a physiological intake.

the middle-aged and elderly of Northern Europe and North America. Moreover, in virtually none of the studies showing a benefit of supplemental vitamin D was frank osteomalacia a significant feature of the problem. Hence, as discussed above, this criterion for true vitamin D deficiency may well be much too strict to be nutritionally useful today. How the vitamin D requirement ought to be defined is another matter. Holick [184] has presented data showing that it takes an intake of at least 600 IU/day, from all sources, to sustain serum 25(OH)D levels, and the doses of vitamin D used in the studies summarized above also suggest that an intake in the range of 500–800 IU/day is required for full expression of the known effects of vitamin D in adults. Vieth [27] presents evidence that the requirement may be higher still.

What is not clear from the above is how much of the effect of vitamin D in studies such as the fracture prevention trial of Heikinheimo *et al.* [132] is due to facilitating gut adaptation to marginal calcium intakes, and how much may represent an extraintestinal effect of the vitamin in its own right, for example, on muscle tone or coordination. Calcitriol receptors are widely distributed in many tissues, and calcitriol enhances parathyroid hormone-mediated bone resorption and exhibits autocrine action in cell differentiation and in the immune response. Furthermore, calcitriol elicits a prompt and sizable increase in osteoblast synthesis of osteocalcin [186]. Additionally, elevating serum 25OHD levels in the elderly improves the often incomplete gamma carboxylation of osteocalcin (see next section). Nevertheless, patients with vitamin D-dependent rickets type II, who lack functional calcitriol receptors, show essentially complete remission of most of their skeletal pathophysiology with intravenous calcium infusions alone [187]. Furthermore, while subtle impairment of immune function can be demonstrated in nutritional vitamin D deficiency, the defects appear to be sufficiently mild to be of little or no clinical consequence in most individuals. Hence the issue of the extraintestinal importance of vitamin D remains unclear.

VIII. VITAMIN K

The chemistry and physiology of vitamin K have been extensively reviewed elsewhere [186, 188–191]. In brief, vitamin K is necessary for the gamma-carboxylation of glutamic acid residues in a large number of proteins. Most familiar are those related to coagulation, in which seven vitamin K-dependent proteins are involved in one way or another. The gamma-carboxyglutamic acid residues in the peptide chain bind calcium, either free or on the surface layers of crystals, and have been thought to function in varying ways including catalysis of the coagulation cascade, inhibiting mineralization (as in urine) [192], and serving as osteoclast chemotactic signals [193]. Vitamin K deficiency classically produces bleeding disorders, but the liver, where the clotting factors are produced, is highly efficient in extracting vita-

min K from the circulation, and gamma-carboxylation declines substantially in other tissues before the deficiency is severe enough to result in bleeding disorders. It may thus be that the bleeding tendencies that have been the hallmark of vitamin K deficiency are, in fact, the *last* manifestation of deficiency. If so, what the other clinical expressions of deficiency may be remain uncertain.

Three vitamin K-dependent proteins are found in bone matrix: osteocalcin (bone gla protein), matrix gla-protein, and protein S. Only osteocalcin is unique to bone. There is also a kidney gla protein (nephrocalcin) [194], that may be involved in renal conservation of calcium. Osteocalcin binds avidly to hydroxyapatite (but not to amorphous calcium phosphate) and is chemotactic for bone-resorbing cells. Originally thought to be synthesized and gamma-carboxylated by osteoblasts as they deposit bone matrix, it now seems that osteocalcin is synthesized by osteocytes [195], particularly those newly embedded in forming bone matrix. Roughly 30% of the synthesized osteocalcin is not incorporated into matrix, but is released instead into the circulation, where, like alkaline phosphatase, it can be measured and used as an indicator of new bone formation.

In vitamin K deficiency, such as would occur with coumarin anticoagulants, serum osteocalcin levels decline, and the degree of carboxylation of the circulating osteocalcin falls dramatically. Further, binding to hydroxyapatite of the osteocalcin produced under these conditions falls precipitously soon after starting anticoagulant therapy. It would seem, therefore, that vitamin K deficiency would have detectable skeletal effects. The problem is that they have been very hard to find. Rats reared and sustained to adult life under near total suppression of osteocalcin gamma-carboxylation show only minor skeletal defects, mostly related to abnormalities in the growth apparatus [186]. Warfarin anticoagulation therapy in humans has generally not been found to be associated with decreased bone mineral density or increased fractures [196, 197]. However, an osteocalcin knockout mouse exhibits a skeleton significantly more dense than normal [198], a finding compatible with osteocalcin's playing a role in facilitating resorption. In aging humans, the problem of detecting skeletal abnormalities is compounded by the relative isolation of bone from current nutritional stresses, discussed briefly above.

Various vitamin K-related abnormalities have been described in association with osteoporosis, but their pathogenetic significance remains unclear. Circulating vitamin K and menaquinone levels are low in hip fracture patients [199], but since these levels reflect only recent dietary intake [200, 201], it is uncertain to what extent they reflect prefracture vitamin K status. Osteocalcin is undercarboxylated in osteoporotics, and this defect responds to physiological doses of vitamin K [202]. Finally, urine calcium has been reported to be high in some patients with osteoporosis and to fall in response to physiological doses of vitamin K [203, 204]. In the same subjects, urine hydroxyproline was also

found to be high and to fall on vitamin K treatment. The effect was confined to subjects with pretreatment hypercalciuria, and could plausibly be explained as a defect first in a calcium transport protein, with a consequent renal leak of calcium, and a corresponding parathyroid hormone-mediated increase in bone resorption (reflected in the increased hydroxyproline excretion). In a prospective study Feskanich *et al.* [205] found lower hip fracture rates in those with the highest vitamin K intakes, but the cohort was relatively young (mean age: 61) and the relevance of this finding to more typical hip fracture patients is uncertain.

Whether or not vitamin K is important for bone health, serum vitamin K levels are indicators of general nutritional status, and it may simply be that the observation of low vitamin K levels in osteoporotics, especially in those with hip fracture, is a reflection mainly of the often poor nutrition of these individuals [206–208]. Manifestly, much about vitamin K and bone health remains unclear and more work must be done. Until such questions are resolved, it would seem prudent to ensure in the elderly a sufficient vitamin K intake to achieve full expression of the gamma-carboxylation of all vitamin-K dependent proteins.

IX. OTHER ESSENTIAL NUTRIENTS

A. Magnesium

Magnesium is an essential intracellular cation, a cofactor of many basic cellular processes, particularly those involving energy metabolism. In the face of true magnesium deficiency, there is widespread cellular dysfunction, including the cells and tissues that control the calcium economy and bone remodeling, among others. While slightly more than half the body magnesium is contained in the mineral of bone, it is less certain whether it plays any role there or is, like zinc (see below), present simply accidentally, insofar as it was present in the extracellular fluid bathing the mineralizing site. On the other hand, magnesium alters the surface properties of calcium phosphate crystals, and its concentration in bone is sufficiently high to exert such an effect there. However, the physical-chemical equilibrium between bone crystals and the dissolved minerals in the extracellular fluid is itself poorly understood; hence, any role of magnesium therein is correspondingly uncertain.

Magnesium deficiency clearly occurs in humans of all ages, most often resulting from severe alcoholism or intestinal magnesium leaks, as from sprue or from ileostomy losses. One well-studied manifestation is hypocalcemia, now recognized to be due to refractoriness of the parathyroid glands to the hypocalcemic stimulus itself, coupled with refractoriness of the bone resorption apparatus to parathyroid hormone.

Low bone mass is also a common feature in these situations. But individuals with magnesium deficiency commonly have calcium deficiency as well, and for the same reasons— a varying combination of low intake, renal wastage, and intestinal leakage. One would therefore expect osteoporosis to be very common in such individuals, as is the case. How much of this bony deficit is due to the magnesium deficiency and how much to the calcium deficiency is unclear. (In a clinical sense the question is moot: both deficiencies need repair.) Treating the underlying condition and replacing lost calcium increases bone density in these patients, but Rude and Olerich [209] have shown that even when the underlying condition is controlled and serum magnesium seemingly normal, additional magnesium supplementation will produce a further increase in bone mineral density.

This latter observation highlights one of the difficulties besetting this field—the assessment of magnesium status. Serum magnesium is recognized not to be a reliable indicator of tissue magnesium repletion. Many investigators favor the magnesium tolerance test [210], that is, measuring percent retention of an intravenous infusion of magnesium. This is, of course, not practical in clinical practice. Nevertheless the observations of Rude and Olerich [209] highlight the fact that serum magnesium values within the "normal" reference range may mask a capacity to respond to further magnesium supplementation.

This is precisely the point at which magnesium intersects the arena of the pathogenesis and treatment of common postmenopausal osteoporosis. Unfortunately no segment of the osteoporosis field is probably more beset with poorly designed, poorly executed, and inadequately powered studies than this one. For example, two small trials, one not randomized, the other with high loss of subjects during the trial, reported bone gain in postmenopausal women given a supplement containing magnesium [211, 212]. Neither study constitutes persuasive evidence of a magnesium effect. The upshot of these and many other even weaker studies is that it is simply not possible to say with any certainty what, if any, role magnesium plays in pathogenesis or treatment of osteoporosis.

One fact seems certain: in any unselected group of individuals with low bone mass, calcium and/or vitamin D supplementation results in clear skeletal benefits (see above), *without using extra magnesium*. And despite the fact that magnesium may be necessary for the functioning of such cells as those responsible for synthesizing $1,25(OH)_2D$ [213], there is clear proof that supplemental magnesium does not enhance calcium absorption in ostensibly healthy older adults. Spencer *et al.* [214] more than doubled daily magnesium intake in a group of volunteers and could find no effect on calcium absorption, whether from low or normal calcium intakes. Similarly, the many randomized controlled trials demonstrating efficacy of calcium supplementation in reducing age-related bone loss and fractures all achieved their effect without supplementing with magnesium.

But absence of proof is not the same as absence of effect. One cannot say, in the routine management of osteoporosis,

that the results would not have been even better had extra magnesium been provided as well. Because sprue syndromes can be silent [215], subtle magnesium deficiency could well exist in some individuals with otherwise typical osteoporosis (to mention only one potential cause of magnesium deficiency). Hence, lacking the ability easily to identify individuals with unrecognized magnesium deficiency, it is hard to argue against prudent attention to magnesium supplementation in individuals who have osteoporosis or are at high risk for fragility fractures.

B. Trace Minerals

Several trace minerals, notably zinc, manganese, and copper, are essential metallic cofactors for enzymes involved in synthesis of various bone matrix constituents. Vitamin C (along with zinc) is needed for collagen cross-links. In growing animals, diets deficient in these nutrients produce definite skeletal abnormalities [216, 217]. Additionally, zinc deficiency is well known to produce growth retardation and other abnormalities in humans. But it is not known with certainty whether significant deficiencies of these elements develop in previously healthy adults, or at least, if they do, whether such deficiencies contribute detectably to the osteoporosis problem.

1. Copper

Copper is of particular interest. The principal sources of copper in the diet are shellfish, nuts, legumes, whole-grain cereals, and organ meats. True dietary copper deficiency is considered to be rare and to be confined to special circumstances, such as with total parenteral nutrition or infants recovering from malnutrition. Recognized manifestations in humans have usually centered on disorders of hemopoiesis, mainly as an iron-refractory, hypochromic anemia and leukopenia. Osteoporosis or fragility fractures have not been generally considered to be a part of the syndrome. However, copper-deficient premature infants have underdeveloped, weak bones that fracture easily and respond to copper supplementation [218], and in one human with copper deficiency due to a copper transport defect, the patient's morbidity included osteoporosis [219].

Copper is a necessary cofactor for lysyl oxidase, one of the principal enzymes involved in collagen cross-linking. These cross-links are important for connective tissue strength, both in tension and in compression, because they prevent the fibrils from sliding along one another's length. Bone formed under conditions of lysyl oxidase inhibition is mechanically weak, independent of mass. Copper deficiency is reported to be associated with osteoporotic lesions in sheep, cattle, and rats [216, 220]. Copper has not been much studied in connection with human osteoporosis, but in one study in which serum copper was measured, levels were negatively correlated with lumbar spine bone mineral density, even after ad-

justing for body weight and dietary calcium intake [221]. In another [222] postmortem specimens of bone from osteoporotic individuals were reported to contain fewer cross-links than bone from age-matched controls.

2. Zinc

Zinc is a known constituent of about 300 enzymes, including alkaline phosphatase, and it plays a role with other proteins, such as the estrogen receptor molecule. Its principal sources in the human diet are red meat, whole-grain cereals, shellfish, and legumes. A 70-kg adult body contains 2–3 g zinc, about half in bone. Most of this bony zinc is located on the surfaces of the calcium phosphate crystals and probably has no metabolic significance. (Many cations present in the mineralizing environment adsorb to the oxygen-rich phosphate groups on crystal surfaces and get stuck there as free water is displaced by new mineral deposition.) A fortuitous consequence of this situation is that urine zinc reflects bone resorption. Thus, Herzberg et al. [223] have shown that urine zinc rises with age, is higher in patients with osteoporosis, and is reduced when postmenopausal women are given estrogen [224]. While some etiologic connection between zinc and osteoporosis cannot be ruled out, these observations are most easily explained as reflections of the enhanced bone resorption found in many patients with osteoporosis, the elevated resorption of the estrogen-deprived, postmenopausal state, and the well-known antiresorptive effect of estrogen. Urinary zinc excretion probably functions as a marker for bone resorption, rather than as a reflection of the underlying disease mechanisms.

On the other hand, of known nutrients, zinc is the one most strongly related to serum IGF-1 [225], a growth factor known to be osteotrophic even in adults. In this connection, Schürch et al. [226] have shown the importance of IGF-1 in recovery from hip fracture. In an observational study from Sweden, fracture risk was higher in individuals with low zinc intakes [227], and, after adjusting for other nutrients, the risk gradient showed the expected dose–response relationship. New et al. [228], in a dietary survey of nearly 1000 British premenopausal women, found high zinc intakes to be associated with higher bone density values at both spine and hip.

Suggestive paleolithic evidence connecting zinc intake with bone status is provided by ancient skeletons discovered in Canary Island cave burials (where contamination by, or leeching of minerals into, groundwater is considered not to have occurred). Bones with normal zinc content per unit ash, concentrated in one region of the islands, tended to be robust, while those with low zinc contents, on another island, were found to be osteoporotic [229]. Zinc content of bone, as suggested above, is determined by the circulating zinc levels when bone is mineralizing, and thus low bone zinc probably reflects low zinc intake throughout life. Whether this exposure played an etiologic role in the low bone mass of these skeletal remains is conjectural.

3. MANGANESE

Although manganese is also recognized as an essential nutrient, its precise role in nutrition is much less well characterized than that of copper and zinc. Although manganese deficiency is well recognized in both laboratory and farm animals, there is no generally recognized manganese deficiency syndrome in humans. Manganese is widely distributed in foods and is especially rich in tea.

Bone manganese content is, like that of copper and zinc, a reflection mainly of serum levels prevailing at the time bone is formed, and thus a reflection of dietary manganese. Bone manganese probably has no other metabolic significance per se. Manganese is capable of activating many enzymes, but for most the effect is nonspecific. Manganese is, however, believed to be the preferred metal ion for certain glycosylation reactions involved in mucopolysaccharide synthesis. In this connection, manganese deficiency could interfere with both cartilage and bone matrix formation.

Animals reared on manganese-deficient diets exhibit general growth retardation, but careful measurements indicate that long bone growth is disproportionately affected [230], possibly reflecting a specific problem with endochondral bone formation. There is also indication of delayed skeletal maturation, suggesting a role of manganese in chondrogenesis. Strause et al. [231] showed this quite nicely in a rat model in which demineralized bone powder is implanted subcutaneously. In control animals cartilage forms around the powder implant, then osteogenesis occurs. In manganese-deficient animals neither development took place. In further work, Strause et al. [232] showed that manganese-deficient rats had both disordered regulation of calcium homeostasis and decreased bone mineral density. Because histology was not performed, it is not possible to say whether this represented impaired mineralization or osteoporosis. Finally, Reginster et al. [233] found low serum manganese in a group of 10 women with osteoporosis. What significance any of these findings may have for the bulk of human osteoporosis is uncertain.

In one four-way, randomized intervention trial, a trace mineral cocktail including copper, zinc, and manganese slowed bone mineral loss in postmenopausal women, when given either with or without supplemental calcium [234]. There appeared to be a small additional benefit from the extra trace minerals; however, the only statistically significant effect in this study was associated with the calcium supplement. This could mean that trace mineral deficiency plays no role in osteoporosis, but it could also mean that not all of the women treated suffered from such deficiency. In fact, because both osteoporotic and age-related bone loss are multifactorial, one would presume that only some of the subjects in such a study would be deficient, since there is no known way to select subjects for inclusion on the basis of presumed trace mineral need. Thus, the suggestive findings of this study have to be considered grounds for further exploration of this issue.

X. CONCLUSION

Many nutrients and lifestyle interact to determine bone density and risk for osteoporosis. Knowledge of bone acquisition during childhood and adolescents has assumed a key role in predicting age-related bone loss in later years. There are also unique issues of bone metabolism that occur with pregnancy and lactation that help determine nutrient intake recommendations for women during those years. Although dietary adequacy of calcium is primarily associated with bone density, many other vitamins and minerals play important roles in the development and maintenance of normal bone. Vitamin D adequacy and its metabolites play a key role, especially with advancing age. In addition, newer information on vitamin K and its role in bone acquisition has expanded our understanding of the role of nutrition in bone health. As the older adult population increases in the United States, the public health consequences of bone health become an important factor in morbidity, mortality, and quality of life.

References

1. Consensus Development Conference. (1991). Prophylaxis and treatment of osteoporosis. *Am. J. Med.* **90,** 107–110.
2. Matkovic, V., Kostial, K., Simonovic, I., Buzina, R., Brodarec, A., and Nordin, B. E. C. (1979). Bone status and fracture rates in two regions of Yugoslavia. *Am. J. Clin. Nutr.* **32,** 540–549.
3. Robinovitch, S. N., Hayes, W. C., and McMahon, T. A. (1991). Prediction of femoral impact forces in falls on the hip. *J. Biomechan. Eng.* **113,** 366–374.
4. Vellas, B., Baumgartner, R. N., Wayne, S. J., Concelcao, J., Lafont, C., Albarede, J.-L., and Garry, P. J. (1992). Relationship between malnutrition and falls in the elderly. *Nutrition* **8,** 105–108.
5. Lauritzen, J. B., Petersen, M. M., and Lund, B. (1993). Effect of external hip protectors on hip fracture. *Lancet* **341,** 11–13.
6. Heaney, R. P. (1993). Is there a role for bone quality in fragility fractures? *Calcif. Tissue Int.* **53,** S3–S5.
7. Ross, P. D., Davis, J. W., Epstein, R. S. and Wasnich, R. D. (1991). Pre-existing fractures and bone mass predict vertebral fracture incidence in women. *Ann. Intern. Med.* **114,** 919–923.
8. Hui, S. L. Slemenda, C. W., and Johnston, C. C., Jr. (1988). Age and bone mass as predictors of fracture in a prospective study. *J. Clin. Invest.* **81,** 1804–1809.
9. Kleerekoper, M. Feldkamp, L. A., Goldstein, S. A., Flynn, M. J., and Parfitt, A, M. (1987). Cancellous bone architecture and bone strength. *In* "Osteoporosis 1987" (C. Christiansen, J. S. Johansen, and B. J. Riis, Eds.), pp. 294–300. Norhaven A/S, Viborg, Denmark.
10. Aaron, J. E., Makins, N. B., and Sagreiya, K. (1987). The microanatomy of trabecular bone loss in normal aging men and women. *Clin. Orthop. Rel. Res.* **215,** 260–271.
11. Eventov, I., Frisch, B., Cohen, Z., and Hammel, I. (1991). Osteopenia, hematopoiesis and osseous remodeling in iliac

crest and femoral neck biopsies: A propecive study of 102 cases of femoral neck fractures. *Bone* **12,** 1–6.

12. Faulkner, K. G., Cummings, S., Black, D., Palermo, L., Glüer, C. C., and Genant, H. K. (1993). Simple measurement of femoral geometry predicts hip fracture: The study of osteoporotic fractures. *J. Bone Miner. Res.* **8,** 1211–1217.

13. Glüer, C.-C., Cummings, S. R., Pressman, A., Li, J., Glüer, K., Gaulkner, K. G., Grampp, S., and Genant, H. K. (1994). Prediction of hip fractures from pelvic radiographs: The study of osteoporotic fractures. *J. Bone Miner. Res.* **9,** 671–677.

14. Gilsanz, V., Loro, L. M., Roe, T. F., Sayre, J., Gilsanz, R., and Schulz, E. E. (1995). Vertebral size in elderly women with osteoporosis. *J. Clin. Invest.* **95,** 2332–2337.

15. Heaney, R. P. (1989). Osteoporotic fracture space: An hypothesis. *Bone Miner.* **6,** 1–13.

16. Heaney, R. P., and Recker, R. R. (1986). Distribution of calcium absorption in middle-aged women. *Am. J. Clin. Nutr.* **43,** 299–305.

17. Nordin, B. E. C., Polley, K. J., Need, A. G., Morris, H. A., and Marshall, D. (1987). The problem of calcium requirement. *Am. J. Clin. Nutr.* **45,** 1295–1304.

18. Nordin, B. E. C., Need, A. G., Morris, H. A., and Horowitz, M. (1991). Sodium, calcium and osteoporosis. *In* "Nutritional Aspects of Osteoporosis" (P. Burckhardt and R. P. Heaney, Eds.) pp. 279–295. Raven Press, New York.

19. Barger-Lux, M. J., Heaney, R. P., Packard, P. T., Lappe, J. M., and Recker, R. R. (1992). Nutritional correlates of low calcium intake. *Clin. Appl. Nutr.* **2,** 39–44.

20. Devine, A., Prince, R. L., and Bell, R. (1996). Nutritional effect of calcium supplementation by skim milk powder or calcium tablets on total nutrient intake in postmenopausal women. *Am. J. Clin. Nutr.* **64,** 731–737.

21. Barrett-Connor, E. (1991). Diet assessment and analysis for epidemiologic studies of osteoporosis. *In* "Nutritional Aspects of Osteoporosis" (P. Burckhardt and R. P. Heaney. Eds.) pp. 91–98. Raven Press, New York.

22. Heaney, R. P. (1991). Assessment and consistency of calcium intake. *In* "Nutritional Aspects of Osteoporosis" (P. Burckhardt and R. P. Heaney, Eds.), pp. 99–104. Raven Press, New York.

23. Jacobus, C. H., Holick, M. F., Shao, Q., Chen, T. C., Holm, I. A., Kolodny, J. M., Fuleihan, G. E.-H., and Seely, E. W. (1992). Hypervitaminosis D associated with drinking milk. *N. Engl. J. Med.* **326,** 1173–1177.

24. Holick, M. F., Shao, Q., Liu, W. W., and Chen, T. C. (1992). The vitamin D content of fortified milk and infant formula. *N. Engl. J. Med.* **326,** 1178–1181.

25. Chen, T. C., Heath, H. H., III, and Holick, M. F. (1993). An update on the vitamin D content of fortified milk from the United States and Canada. *N. Engl. J. Med.* **329,** 1507.

26. Barger-Lux, M. J., Heaney, R. P., Lanspa, S. J., Healy, J. C., and DeLuca, H. F. (1995). An investigation of sources of variation in calcium absorption efficiency. *J. Clin. Endocrinol. Metab.* **80,** 406–411.

27. Vieth, R. (1999). Vitamin D supplementation, 25-hydroxyvitamin D concentrations, and safety. *Am. J. Clin. Nutr.* **69,** 842–856.

28. Charles, P. (1989). Metabolic bone disease evaluated by a combined calcium balance and tracer kinetic study. *Dan. Med. Bull.* **36,** 463–479.

29. Heaney, R. P., Weaver, C. M., Hinders, S. M., Martin, B., and Packard, P. (1993). Absorbability of calcium from Brassica vegetables. *J. Food Sci.* **58,** 1378–1380.

30. Heaney, R. P., Weaver, C. M., and Recker, R. R. (1988). Calcium absorbability from spinach. *Am. J. Clin. Nutr.* **47,** 707–709.

31. Heaney, R. P., Davies, K. M., Recker, R. R., and Packard, P. T. (1990). Long-term consistency of nutrient intakes. *J. Nutr.* **120,** 869–875.

32. Carr, C. J., and Shangraw, R. F. (1987). Nutritional and pharmaceutical aspects of calcium supplementation. *Am. Pharm.* NS27: **4950,** 54–57.

33. Shangraw, R. F. (1989). Factors to consider in the selection of a calcium supplement. *In* "Proceedings of the 1987 Special Topic Conference on Osteoporosis." Public Health Reports S104, pp. 46–50. USDHHS, Washington, DC, Public Health Service.

34. Heaney, R. P. (1993). Nutritional factors in osteoporosis. *Ann. Rev. Nutr.* **13,** 287–316.

35. Hegsted, D. M. (1986). Calcium and osteoporosis, *J. Nutr.* **116,** 2316–2319.

36. Parfitt, A. M. (1980). Morphologic basis of bone mineral measurements: Transient and steady state effects of treatment in osteoporosis. *Miner. Electrolyte Metab.* **4,** 273–287.

37. Heaney, R. P. (1994). The bone remodeling transient: Implications for the interpretation of clinical studies of bone mass change. *J. Bone Miner. Res.* **9,** 1515–1523.

38. Webb, A. R., Kline, L. W., and Holick, M. F. (1988). Influence of season and latitude on the cutaneous synthesis of vitamin D_3: Exposure to winter sunlight in Boston and Edmonton will not promote vitamin D_3 synthesis in human skin. *J. Clin. Endocrinol. Metab.* **67,** 373–378.

39. Harris, L. J. (1956). Vitamin D and bone. *In* "The Biochemistry and Physiology of Bone" (G. H. Bourne, Ed.), pp. 581–622. Academic Press, New York.

40. Eaton, S. B., and Konner, M. (1985). Paleolithic nutrition. A consideration of its nature and current implications. *N. Engl. J. Med.* **312,** 283–289.

41. Eaton, S. B., and Nelson, D. A. (1991). Calcium in evolutionary perspective. *Am. J. Clin. Nutr.* **54,** 281S–287S.

42. Alaimo, K., McDowell, M. A., Briefel, R. R., Bischof, A. M., Caughman, C. R., Loria, C. M., and Johnson, C. L. (1994). "Dietary Intake of Vitamins, Minerals, and Fiber of Persons Ages 2 Months and Over in the United States: Third National Health and Nutrition Examination Survey, Phase 1, 1988–1991," advance data from Vital and Health Statistics, No. 258. National Center for Health Statistics, Hyattsville, MD.

43. Brand Miller, J., James, K. W., and Maggiore, P. M. A. (1997). "Tables of Composition of Australian Aboriginal Foods." Aboriginal Studies Press, Canberra.

44. Fernandes-Costa, F. J., Marshall, J., Ritchie, C., van Tonder, S. V., Dunn, D. S., Jenkins, T., and Metz, J. (1984). Transition from a hunter–gatherer to a settled lifestyle in the ¡Kung San: Effect on iron, folate and vitamin B12 nutrition. *Am. J. Clin. Nutr.* **40,** 1295–1303.

45. Rosanoff, A., and Calloway, D. H. (1982). Calcium source in Indochinese immigrants. *N. Engl. J. Med.* **306,** 239–240.

46. Baker, P. T., and Mazess, R. B. (1963). Calcium: Unusual sources in the highland Peruvian diet. *Science* **142,** 1466–1467.

47. Molleson, T. (1994). The eloquent bones of Abu Hureyra. *Sci. Am.* **271**(2), 70–75.

48. Heaney, R. P., Recker, R. R., Stegman, M. R., and Moy, A. J. (1989). Calcium absorption in women: Relationships to calcium intake, estrogen status, and age. *J. Bone Miner. Res.* **4,** 469–475.

49. Heaney, R. P., and Recker, R. R. (1994). Determinants of endogenous fecal calcium in healthy women. *J. Bone Miner. Res.* **9,** 1621–1627.

50. Matkovic, V., and Heaney, R. P. (1992). Calcium balance during human growth. Evidence for threshold behavior. *Am. J. Clin. Nutr.* **55,** 992–996.

51. Urist, M. R. (1964). The origin of bone. *Discovery* **25,** 13–19.

52. Urist, M. R. (1962). The bone–body fluid continuum. *Perspect. Biol. Med.* **6,** 75–115.

53. Bauer, W., Aub, J. C., and Albright, F. (1929). Studies of calcium and phosphorus metabolism. *J. Exp. Med.* **49.** 145.

54. Gershon-Cohen, J., and Jowsey, J. (1964). The relationship of dietary calcium to osteoporosis. *Metabolism* **13,** 221.

55. Bodansky, M., and Duff, V. B. (1939). Regulation of the level of calcium in the serum during pregnancy. *JAMA* **112,** 223–229.

56. Jowsey, J., and Raisz, L. G. (1968). Experimental osteoporosis and parathyroid activity. *Endocrinology* **82,** 384–396.

57. Banks, W. J., Jr., Epling, G. P. Kainer, R. A., and Davis, R. W. (1968). Antler growth and osteoporosis. *Anat. Rec.* **162,** 387–398.

58. Kanis, J. A., and Passmore, R. (1989). Calcium supplementation of the diet—I and II. *Br. Med.J.* **298,** 137–140, 205–208.

59. Forbes, R. M., Weingartner, K. E., Parker, H. M., Bell, R. R., and Erdman, J. W., Jr. (1979). Bioavailability to rats of zinc, magnesium and calcium in cassein-, egg- and soy protein-containing diets. *J. Nutr.* **109,** 1652–1660.

60. Food and Nutrition Board, Institute of Medicine (1997). "Dietary Reference Intakes for Calcium, Magnesium, Phosphorus, Vitamin D, and Fluoride." National Academy Press, Washington, DC.

61. NIH Consensus Development Conference (1994). Optimal calcium intake. *JAMA* **272,** 1942–1948.

62. Heaney R. P. (2000). Calcium, dairy products, and osteoporosis. *J. Am. College Nutr.* **19,** 83S–99S.

63. Dawson-Hughes, B., Dallal, G. E., Krall, E. A., Sadowski, L., Sahyoun, N., and Tannenbaum, S. (1990). A controlled trial of the effect of calcium supplementation on bone density in postmenopausal women. *N. Engl. J. Med.* **323,** 878–883.

64. Chapuy, M. C., Arlot, M. E., Duboeuf, F., Brun, J., Crouzet, B., Arnaud, S., Delmas, P. D., and Meunier, P. J. (1992). Vitamin D₃ and calcium to prevent hip fractures in elderly women. *N. Engl. J. Med.* **327,** 1637–1642.

65. Reid, I. R., Ames, R. W., Evans, M. C., Gamble, G. D., and Sharpe, S. J. (1993). Effect of calcium supplementation on bone loss in postmenopausal women. *N. Engl. J. Med.* **328,** 460–464.

66. Johnston, C. C., Jr., Miller, J. Z., Slemenda, C. W., Reister, T. K., Hui, S., Christian, J. C., and Peacock, M. (1992). Calcium supplementation and increases in bone mineral density in children. *N. Engl. J. Med.* **327,** 82–87.

67. Lloyd, T., Andon, M. B., Rollings, N., Martel, J. K., Landis, J. R., Demers, L. M., Eggli, D. F., Kieselhorst, K., and Kulin, H. E. (1993). Calcium supplementation and bone mineral density in adolescent girls. *JAMA* **270,** 841–844.

68. Chevalley, T., Rizzoli, R., Nydegger, V., Slosman, D., Rapin, C.-H., Michel, J.-P., Vasey, H., and Bonjour, J. P. (1994). Effects of calcium supplements on femoral bone mineral density and vertebral fracture rate in vitamin D-replete elderly patients. *Osteoporos. Int.* **4,** 256–252.

69. Recker, R. R., Hinders, S., Davies, K. M., Heaney, R. P., Stegman, M. R., Kimmel, D. B., and Lappe, J. M. (1996). Correcting calcium nutritional deficiency prevents spine fractures in elderly women. *J. Bone Miner. Res.* **11,** 1961–1966.

70. Dawson-Hughes, B., Harris, S. S., Krall, E. A., and Dallal, G. E. (1997). Effect of calcium and vitamin D supplementation on bone density in men and women 65 years of age or older. *N. Engl. J. Med.* **337,** 670–676.

71. Reid, I. R., Ames, R. W., Evans, M. C., Sharpe, S. J., and Gamble, G. D. (1994). Determinants of the rate of bone loss in normal postmenopausal women. *J. Clin. Endocrinol. Metab.* **79,** 950–954.

72. Aloia, J. F., Vaswani, A., Yeh, J. K., Ross, P. L., Flaster, E., and Dilmanian, F. A. (1994). Calcium supplementation with and without hormone replacement therapy to prevent postmenopausal bone loss. *Ann. Intern. Med.* **120,** 97–103.

73. Food and Nutrition Board, Commission on Life Sciences, National Research Council (1989). "Recommended Dietary Allowances," 10th ed. National Academy Press, Washington, DC.

74. Bronner, F., Salle, B. L., Putet, G., Rigo, J., and Senterre, J. (1992). Net calcium absorption in premature infants: Results of 103 metabolic balance studies. *Am. J. Clin. Nutr.* **56,** 1037–1044.

75. Pettifor, J. M., Ross, P., Wang, J., Moodley, G., and Couper-Smith, J. (1978). Rickets in children of rural origin in South Africa—a comparison between rural and urban communities. *J. Pediatr.* **92,** 320–324.

76. Oginni, L. M., Sharp, C. A., Worsfold, M., Badru, O. S., and Davie, M. W. J. (1999). Healing of rickets after calcium supplementation. *Lancet* **353,** 296–297.

77. Leighton, G., and McKinley, P. L. (1930). "Milk Consumption and the Growth of School Children." Dept. of Health for Scotland, H.M.S.O.

78. Bonjour, J.-P., Carrie, A.-L., Ferrari, S., Clavien, H., Slosman, D., Theintz, G., and Rizzoli, R. (1997). Calcium-enriched foods and bone mass growth in prepubertal girls: A randomized, double-blind placebo-controlled trial. *J. Clin. Invest.* **99,** 1287–1294.

79. Christian, J. C., Yu, P. L., Slemenda, C. W., and Johnson, C. C., Jr. (1989). Heritability of bone mass: A longitudinal study in aging male twins. *Am. J. Hum. Genet.* **44,** 429–433.

80. Matkovic, V. (1991). Calcium metabolism and calcium requirements during skeletal modeling and consolidation of bone mass. *Am. J. Clin. Nutr.* **54,** 245S–260S.

81. Jackman, L. A., Millane, S. S., Martin, B. R., Wood, O. B., McCabe, G. P., Peacock, M., and Weaver, C. M. (1997). Calcium retention in relation to calcium intake and postmenarcheal age in adolescent females. *Am. J. Clin. Nutr.* **66,** 327–333.

82. Chan, G. M., Hoffman, K., and McMurray, M. (1995). Effects of dietary products on bone and body composition in pubertal girls. *J. Pediatr.* **126,** 551–556.

83. Cadogan, J., Eastell, R., Jones, N. and Barker, M. E. (1997). Milk intake and bone mineral acquisition in adolescent girls: Randomised, controlled intervention trial. *Br. Med. J.* **315**, 1255–1260.

84. Recker, R. R., Davies, K. M., Hinders, S. M., Heaney, R. P., Stegman, M. R., and Kimmel, D. B. (1992) Bone gain in young adult women. *JAMA* **268**, 2403–2408.

85. Matkovic, V., Fontana, D., Tominac, C., Goel, P., Chesnut, C.H., III. (1990). Factors that influence peak bone mass formation: A study of calcium balance and the inheritance of bone mass in adolescent females. *Am. J. Clin. Nutr.* **52**, 878–888.

86. Newton-John, H. F., and Morgan, B. D. (1970). The loss of bone with age: Osteoporosis and fractures. *Clin. Orthrop.* **71**, 229–232.

87. Matkovic, V., Kostial, K., Simonovic, I., Buzina, R., Brodarec, A., and Nordin, B. E. C. (1979). Bone status and fracture rates in two regions of Yugoslavia. *Am. J. Clin. Nutr.* **32**, 540–549.

88. Dertina, D., Loro, M. L., Sayre, J., Kaufman, F., and Gilsanz, V. (1998). Childhood bone measurements predict values at young adulthood. *Bone* **23**, S288.

89. Ferrari, S., Rizzoli, R., Slosman, D., and Bonjour, J.-P. (1998). Familial resemblance for bone mineral mass is expressed before puberty. *J. Clin. Endocrinol. Metab.* **83**, 358–361.

90. Slemenda, C. W., Hui, S. L., Longcope, C., Wellman, H., and Johnston, C. C., Jr. (1990). Predictors of bone mass in perimenopausal women. *Ann. Intern. Med.* **112**, 96–101.

91. Braidman, I. P., Davenport, L. K., Carter, D. H., Selby, P. L., Mawer, E. B., and Freemont, A. J. (1995). Preliminary in situ identification of estrogen target cells in bone. *J. Bone Miner. Res.* **10**, 74–80.

92. Gilsanz, V., Gibbens, D. T., Roe, T. F., Carlson, M., Senac, M. O., Boechat, M. I., Huang, H. K., Schulz, E. E., Libanati, C. R., and Cann, C. C. (1988) Vertebral bone density in children: Effect of puberty. *Radiology* **166**, 847–850.

93. Heaney, R. P. (1990). Estrogen–calcium interactions in the postmenopause: A quantitative description. *Bone Miner.* **11**, 67–84.

94. Heaney, R. P., Recker, R. R., and Daville, P. D. (1978). Menopausal changes in calcium balance performance. *J. Lab. Clin. Med.* **92**, 953–963.

95. Nordin, E. C., Need, A. G., Morris, H. A., Horowitz, M. and Robertson, W. G. (1991). Evidence for a renal calcium leak in postmenopausal women. *J. Clin. Endocrinol. Metab.* **72**, 401–407.

96. Welten, D. C., Kemper, H. C. G., Post, G. B., and van Staveren, W. A. (1995). A meta-analysis of the effect of calcium intake on bone mass in females and males. *J. Nutr.* **125**, 2802–2813.

97. Nordin, B. E. C. (1997). Calcium and osteoporosis. *Nutrition* **13**, 664–686.

98. Recker, R. R., Lappe, J. M., Davies, K. M., and Kimmel, D. B. (1992). Change in bone mass immediately before menopause. *J. Bone Miner. Res.* **7**, 857–862.

99. Baran, D., Sorensen, A., Grimes, J., Lew, R., Karellas, A., Johnson, B., and Roche, J. (1989). Dietary modification with dairy products for preventing vertebral bone loss in premenopausal women: A three-year prospective study. *J. Clin. Endocrinol. Metab.* **70**, 264–270.

100. Klesges, R. C., Ward, K. D., Shelton, M. L., Applegate, W. B., Cantler, E. D., Palmieri, G. M., Harmon, K., and Davis, J. (1996). Changes in bone mineral content in male athletes. *JAMA* **276**, 226–230.

101. Heaney, R. P. (2001). Calcium intake and the prevention of chronic disease. *In* "Frontiers in Nutrition" (T. Wilson and N. Temple, Eds.), pp. 31–50. Humana Press, Totowa, NJ.

102. Koetting, C. A., and Wardlaw, G. M. (1988). Wrist, spine, and hip bone density in women with variable histories of lactation. *Am. J. Clin. Nutr.* **48**, 1479–1481.

103. Byrne, J., Thomas, M. R. and Chan, G. M. (1987). Calcium intake and bone density of lactating women in their late childbearing years. *J. Am. Diet. Assoc.* **87**, 883–887.

104. Hansen, M. A., Overgaard, K., Riis, B. J., and Christiansen, C. (1991). Potential risk factors for development of postmenopausal osteoporosis, examined over a 12-year period. *Osteoporos. Int.* **1**, 95–102.

105. Laitinen, K., Valimaki, M., and Keto, P. (1991). Bone mineral density measured by dual-energy X-ray absorptiometry in healthy Finnish women. *Calcif. Tissue Int.* **48**, 224–231.

106. Walker, A. R. P., and Walker, F. (1972). The influence of numerous pregnancies and lactations on bone dimensions in South African Bantu and Caucasian mothers. *Clin. Sci.* **42**, 189–196.

107. Kritz-Silverstein, D., Barrett-Connor, E., and Hollenbach, K. A. (1992). Pregnancy and lactation as determinants of bone mineral density in psotmenopausal women. *Am. J. Epidemiol.* **136**, 1052–1059.

108. Lissner, L., Bengtsson, C., and Hansson, T. (1991). Bone mineral content in relation to lactation history in pre- and postmenopausal women. *Calcif. Tissue Int.* **48**, 319–325.

109. Heaney, R. P., and Skillman, T. G. (1971). Calcium metabolism in normal human pregnancy. *J. Clin. Endocrinol. Metab.* **33**, 661–670.

110. Brommage, R., and Baxter, D. C. (1988). Elevated calcium, phosphorus, and magnesium retention in pregnant rats prior to the onset of fetal skeletal mineralization. *J. Bone Miner. Res.* **3**, 667–672.

111. McGlade, M. J. (1993). Effects of gestation, lactation, and maternal calcium intake on mechanical strength of equine bone. *J. Am. College Nutr.* **12**, 372–377.

112. Miller, M. A., Omura, T. H., and Miller, S. C. (1989). Increased cancellous bone remodeling during lactation in beagles. *Bone* **10**, 279–285.

113. Kent, G. N., Price, R. I., Gutteridge, D. H., Smith, M., Allen, J. R., Bhagat, C. I., Barnes, M. P., Hickling, C. J., Retallack, R. W., and Wilson, S. G. (1990). Human lactation: Forearm trabecular bone loss, increased bone turnover, and renal conservation of calcium and inorganic phosphate with recovery of bone mass following weaning. *J. Bone Miner. Res.* **5**, 361–369.

114. Cross, N. A., Hillman, L. S., Allen, S. H., Krause, G. F., and Vieira, N. E. (1995). Calcium homeostasis and bone metabolism during pregnancy, lactation and postweaning: A longitudinal study. *Am. J. Clin. Nutr.* **61**, 514–523.

115. Kent, G. N., Price, R. I., Gutteridge, D. H., Rosman, K. J., Smith, M., Allen, J. R., Hickling, C. J., and Blakeman, S. L. (1991). The efficiency of intestinal calcium absorption is increased in late pregnancy but not in established lactation. *Calcif. Tissue Int.* **48**, 293–295.

116. Barger-Lux, M. J., Heaney, R. P., Davies, K. M., Chin, B. K. (1999). Bone mass before and after full-term pregnancy in young women with histories of dietary calcium deficiency. *J. Bone Miner. Res.* **14,** S393.

117. Chan, G. M., McMurry, M., Westover, K., Engelbert-Fenton, K., and Thomas, M. R. (1987). Effects of increased dietary calcium intake upon the calcium and bone mineral status of lactating adolescent and adult women. *Am. J. Clin. Nutr.* **46,** 319–323.

118. Morales, A., Tud-Tud Hans, L., Herber, M., Taylor, A. K., and Baylink, D. J. (1993). Lactation is associated with an increase in spinal bone density. *J. Bone Miner. Res.* **8,** S156.

119. Brommage, R., and DeLuca, H. F. (1985). Regulation of bone mineral loss during lactation. *Am. J. Physiol. Endocrinol. Metab.* **11,** E182–E187.

120. Sowers, M. F., Corton, G., Shapiro, B., Jannausch, M. L., Crutchfield, M., Smith, M. L., Randolph, J. F., and Hollis, B. (1993). Changes in bone density with lactation. *JAMA* **269,** 3130–3135.

121. Specker, B. L., Vieira, N. E., O'Brien, K. O., Ho, M. L., Heubi, J. E., Abrams, S. A., and Yergey, A. L. (1994). Calcium kinetics in lactating women with low and high calcium intakes. *Am. J. Clin. Nutr.* **59,** 593–599.

122. Kalkwarf, H. J., Specker, B. L., and Ho, M. (1999). Effects of calcium supplementation on calcium homeostatis and bone turnover in lactating women. *J. Clin. Endocrinol. Metab.* **84,** 464–470.

123. Kalkwarf, H. J., Specker, B. L., Bianchi, D. C., Ranz, J., and Ho, M. (1997). The effect of calcium supplementation on bone density during lactation and after weaning. *N. Engl. J. Med.* **337,** 523–528.

124. Riis, B., Thomsen, K., and Christiansen, C. (1987). Does calcium supplementation prevent postmenopausal bone loss? *N. Engl. J. Med.* **316,** 173–177.

125. Elders, P. J. M., Netelenbos, J. C., Lips, P., van Ginkel, F. C., Khoe, E., Leeuwenkamp, O. R., Hackeng, W. H. L., and van der Stelt, P. F. (1991). Calcium supplementation reduces vertebral bone loss in perimenopausal women: A controlled trial in 248 women between 46 and 55 years of age. *J. Clin. Endocrinol. Metab.* **73,** 533–540.

126. Recker, R. R., Saville, P. D., and Heaney, R. P. (1977). The effect of estrogens and calcium carbonate on bone loss in postmenopausal women. *Ann. Intern. Med.* **87,** 649–655.

127. Kanis, J. A., Melton, L. J., III, Christiansen, C., Johnston, C. C., and Khaltaev, N. (1994). The diagnosis of osteoporosis. *J. Bone Miner. Res.* **9,** 1137–1141.

128. Recker, R. R., Lappe, J. M., Davies, K. M., and Heaney, R. P. (2000). Characterization of perimenopausal bone loss: A prospective study. *J. Bone Miner. Res.* **15,** 1965–1973.

129. NIH Consensus Conference on Osteoporosis, (1984). *JAMA* **252,** 799–802.

130. Matkovic, V., Jelic, T., Wardlaw, G. M., Ilich, J. A., Goel, P. K., Wright, J. K., Andon, M. D., Smith, K. T., and Heaney, R. P. (1994). Timing of peak bone mass in Caucasian females and its implication for the prevention of osteoporosis. *J. Clin. Invest.* **93,** 799–808.

131. Lis, M. (1990). Consequences of the remodeling process for vertebral trabecular bone structure: A scanning electron microscopy study (uncoupling of unloaded structures.) *Bone Miner.* **10,** 13–35.

132. Heikinheimo, R. J., Inkovaara, J. A., Harju, E. J., Haavisto, M. V., Kaarela, R. H., Kataja, J. M., Kokko, A. M. L., Kolho, L. A., and Rajala, S. A. (1992). Annual injection of vitamin D and fractures of aged bones. *Calcif. Tissue Int.* **51,** 105–110.

133. Heaney, R. P. (1989). The calcium controversy: A middle ground between the extremes. In "Proceedings of the 1987 Special Topic Conference on Osteoporosis," Public Health Reports S104, pp. 36–46. USDHHS, Washington, DC, Public Health Service.

134. Holbrook, T. L., Barrett-Connor, E., and Wingard, D. L. (1988). Dietary calcium and risk of hip fracture: 14-year prospective population study. *Lancet* **2,** 1046–1049.

135. McKane, W. R., Khosla, S., Egan, K. S., Robins, S. P., Burritt, M. F., and Riggs, B. L. (1996). Role of calcium intake in modulating age-related increases in parathyroid function and bone resorption. *J. Clin. Endocrinol. Metab.* **81,** 1699–1703.

136. Pilch, S. M., (Ed.). (1987). "Physiological Effects and Health Consequences of Dietary Fiber," prepared for the Center for Food Safety and Applied Nutrition, Food and Drug Administration by the Life Sciences Research Office, Federation of American Societies for Experimental Biology. FASEB Special Publications Office, Bethesda, MD.

137. Barger-Lux, M. J., and Heaney, R. P. (1995). Caffeine and calcium economy revisited. *Osteoporos. Int.* **5,** 97–102.

138. Heaney, R. P., and Recker, R. R. (1982). Effects of nitrogen, phosphorus, and caffeine on calcium balance in women. *J. Lab. Clin. Med.* **99,** 46–55.

139. Nordin, B. E. C., Need, A. G., Morris, H. A., and Horowitz, M. (1993). The nature and significance of the relationship between urinary sodium and urinary calcium in women. *J. Nutr.* **123,** 1615–1622.

140. Nordin, B. E. C., Need, A. G., Morris, H. A., Horowitz, M., Chatterton, B. E., and Sedgwick, A. W. (1995). Bad habits and bad bones. In "Nutritional Aspects of Osteoporosis '94" P. Burckhardt and R. P. Heaney, Eds., Challenges of Modern Medicine, Vol. 7, pp. 1–25. Ares-Serono Symposia Publications, Rome, Italy.

141. Demigne, C., Levrat, M. A., and Remesy, C. (1989). Effects of feeding fermentable carbohydrates on the cecal concentations of minerals and their fluxes between the cecum and blood plasma in the rat. *J. Nutr.* **119,** 1625–1630.

142. Coudray, C., Bellanger, J., Castiglia-Delavaud, C., Rémésy, C., Vermorel, M., and Rayssignuier, Y. (1997). Effect of soluble or partly soluble dietary fibres supplementation on absorption and balance of calcium, magnesium, iron and zinc in healthy young men. *Eur. J. Clin. Nutr.* **51,** 375–380.

143. van den Heuvel, E. G. H. M., Muys, T., van Dokkum, W., and Schaafsma, G. (1999). Oligofructose stimulates calcium absorption in adolescents. *Am. J. Clin. Nutr.* **69,** 544–548.

144. Weaver, C. M., Heaney, R. P., Martin, B. R., and Fitzsimmons, M. L. (1991). Human calcium absorpion from whole wheat products. *J. Nutr.* **121,** 1769–1775.

145. Weaver, C. M., Heaney, R. P., Proulx, W. R., Hinders, S. M., and Packard, P. T. (1993). Absorbability of calcium from common beans. *J. Food Sci.* **58,** 1401–1403.

146. Weaver, C. M., Heaney, R. P., Nickel, K. P., and Packard, P. T. (1997). Calcium bioavailability from high oxalate vegetables: Chinese vegetables, sweet potatoes, and rhubarb. *J. Food Sci.* **62,** 524–525.

147. Barrett-Connor, E., Chang, J. C., and Edelstein, S. L. (1994). Coffee-associated osteoporosis offset by daily milk consumption. *JAMA* **271**, 280–283.

148. Heaney, R. P. (1993). Protein intake and the calcium economy. *J. Am. Diet. Assoc.* **93**, 1261–1262.

149. Matkovic, V., Ilich, J. Z., Andon, M. B., Hsieh, L. C., Tzagournis, M. A., Lagger, B. J., and Goel, P. K. (1995). Urinary calcium,, sodium, and bone mass of young females. *Am. J. Clin. Nutr.* **62**, 417–425.

150. Lau, E. M. C., Cooper, C., and Woo, J. (1991). Calcium deficiency—A major cause of osteoporosis in Hong Kong Chinese. *In* "Nutritional Aspects of Osteoporosis" (P. Burckhardt and R. P. Heaney, Eds.), pp. 175–180. Raven Press, New York.

151. Berkelhammer, C. H., Wood, R. J., and Sitrin, M. D. (1988). Acetate and hypercalciuria during total parenteral nutrition. *Am. J. Clin. Nutr.* **48**, 1482–1489.

152. Sebastian, A., Harris, S. T., Ottaway, J. H., Todd, K. M., and Morris, Jr., R. C. (1994). Improved mineral balance and skeletal metabolism in postmenopausal women treated with potassium bicarbonate. *N. Engl. J. Med.* **330**, 1776–1781.

153. Reed, J. A., Anderson, J. J. B., Tylasky, F. A., and Gallagher, P. N., Jr. (1994). Comparative changes in radial-bone density in elderly female lacto-ovo-vegetarians and omnivores. *Am. J. Clin. Nutr.* **59**, 1197S–1202S.

154. Barr, S. I., Prior, J. C., Janelle, K. C., and Lentle, B. C. (1998). Spinal bone mineral density in premenopausal vegetarian and nonvegetarian women: Cross-sectional and prospective comparisons. *J. Am. Diet. Assoc.* **98**, 760–765.

155. Chiu, J.-F., Lan, S.-J., Yang, C.-Y., Wang, P.-W., Yao, W.-J., Su, I.-H., and Hsieh, C.-C. (1997). Long-term vegetarian diet and bone mineral density in postmenopausal Taiwanese women. *Calcif. Tissue Int.* **60**, 245–249.

156. Lau, E. M. C., Kwok, T., Woo, J., and Ho, S. C. (1998). Bone mineral density in Chinese elderly female vegetarians, vegans, lacto-vegetarians and omnivores. *Eur. J. Clin. Nutr.* **52**, 60–64.

157. Spencer, H., Kramer, L., Osis, D., and Norris, C. (1978). Effect of phosphorus on the absorption of calcium and on the calcium balance in man. *J. Nutr.* **108**, 447–457.

158. Heaney, R. P., Recker, R. R., and Weaver, C. M. (1990). Absorbability of calcium sources: The limited role of solubility. *Calcif. Tissue Int.* **46**, 300–304.

159. Spencer, H., Kramer, L., Norris, C., and Osis, D. (1982). Effect of small doses of aluminum-containing antacids on calcium and phosphorus metabolism. *Am. J. Clin. Nutr.* **36**, 32–40.

160. Kelly, S. E., Chawla-Singh, K., Sellin, J. H., Yasillo, N. J., and Rosenberg, I. H. (1984). Effect of meal composition on calcium absorption: Enhancing effect of carbohydrate polymers. *Gastroenterology* **87**, 596–600.

161. Sheikh, M. S., Santa Ana, C. A., Nicar, J. J., Schiller, L. R., and Fordtran, J. S. (1988). Calcium absorption: Effect of meal and glucose polymer. *Am. J. Clin. Nutr.* **48**, 312–315.

162. Heaney, R. P., Smith, K. T., Recker, R. R., and Hinders, S. M. (1989). Meal effects on calcium absorption. *Am. J. Clin. Nutr.* **49**, 372–376.

163. Mykkanen, H. M., and Wasserman, R. H. (1980). Enhanced absorption of calcium by casein phosphopeptides in rachitic and normal chicks. *J. Nutr.* **110**, 2141–2148.

164. Heaney, R. P., Saito, Y., and Orimo, H. (1994). Effect of caseinphosphopeptide on absorbability of co-ingested calcium in normal postmenopausal women. *J. Bone Miner. Metab.* **12**, 77–81.

165. Agnusdei, D., Civitelli, R., Camporeale, A., Hardi, P., and Gennari, C. (1995). Dietary L-lysine and calcium metabolism in humans. *In* "Nutritional Aspects of Osteoporosis '94" (P. Burckhardt and R. P. Heaney, Eds.), Challenges of Modern Medicine, Vol. 7, pp. 263–271. Ares-Serono Symposia Publications, Rome, Italy.

166. Norman, A. W. (1990). Intestinal calcium absorption: A vitamin-D hormone-mediated adaptive response. *Am. J. Clin. Nutr.* **51**, 290–300.

167. Bell, N. H., Epstein, S., Shary, J., Greene, V., Oexmann, M. J., and Shaw, S. (1988). Evidence of a probable role for 25-hydroxyvitamin D in the regulation of calcium metabolism. *J. Bone Miner. Res.* **3**, 489–495.

168. Barger-Lux, M. J., Heaney, R. P., Lanspa, S. J., Healy, J. C., and DeLuca, H. F. (1995). An investigation of sources of variation in calcium absorption physiolgy. *J. Clin. Endocrinol. Metab.* **80**, 406–411.

169. Francis, R. M., Peacock, M., Storer, J. H., Davies, A. E. J., Brown, W. B., and Nordin, B. E. C. (1983). Calcium malabsorption in the elderly: The effect of treatment with oral 25-hydroxyvitamin D$_3$. *Eur. J. Clin. Invest.* **13**, 391–396.

170. Reasner, C. A., Dunn, J. F., Fetchick, D., Liel, Y., Hollis, B. W., Epstein, S., Shary, J., Mundy, G. R., and Bell, N. H. (1990). Alteration of vitamin D metabolism in Mexican-Americans [letter]. *J. Bone Miner. Res.* **5**, 793–794.

171. Colodro, I. H., Brickman, A. S., Coburn, J. W., Osborn, T. W., and Norman, A. W. (1978). Effect of 25-hydroxy-vitamin D$_3$ on intestinal absorption of calcium in normal man and patients with renal failure. *Metabolism* **27**, 745–753.

172. Devine, A., Dick, I. M., Wilson, S., and Prince, R. L. (1999). Vitamin D status is unrelated to bone density or turnover in elderly postmenopausal women: A cross-sectional and longitudinal vitamin D intervention study. *J. Bone Miner. Res.* **14**, S382.

173. Heaney, R. P., Barger-Lux, M. J., Dowell, M. S., Chen, T. C., and Holick, M. F. (1997). Calcium absorptive effects of vitamin D and its major metabolites. *J. Clin. Endocrinol. Metab.* **82**. 4111–4116.

174. McKenna, J. M., Freaney, R., Meade, A., and Muldowney, F. P. (1985). Hypovitaminosis D and elevated serum alkaline phosphatase in elderly Irish people. *Am. J. Clin. Nutr.* **41**, 101–109.

175. Dawson-Hughes, B., Dallal, G. E., Krall, E. A., Harris, S., Sokoll, L. J., and Galconer, G. (1991). Effect of vitamin D supplementation on wintertime and overall bone loss in healthy postmenopausal women. *Ann. Intern. Med.* **115**, 505–512.

176. Heaney, R. P. (1986). Calcium, bone health, and osteoporosis. *In* "Bone and Mineral Research," Annual IV (W. A. Peck, Ed.), pp. 225–301. Elsevier Science Publishers, Amsterdam.

177. Krall, E. A., Sahyoun, N., Tannenbaum, S., Dallal, G. E., and Dawson-Hughes, B. (1989). Effect of vitamin D intake on seasonal variations in parathyroid hormone secretion in postmenopausal women. *N. Engl. J. Med.* **321**, 1777–1783.

178. Lukert, B., Higgins, J., and Stoskopf, M. (1992). Menopausal bone loss is partially regulated by dietary intake of vitamin D. *Calcif. Tissue Int.* **51**, 173–179.

179. Slovik, D. M., Adams, J. S., Neer, R. M., Holick, M. F., and Potts, J. T., Jr. (1981). Deficient production of 1,25-dihydroxyvitamin D in elderly osteoporotic patients. *N. Engl. J. Med.* **305,** 372–374.

180. Francis, R. M., Peacock, M., Taylor, G. A., Storer, J. H., and Nordin, B. E. C. (1984). Calcium malabsorption in elderly women with verteral fractures: Evidence for resistance to the action of vitamin D metabolites on the bowel. *Clin. Sci.* **66,** 103–107.

181. Gloth, F. M., III, Tobin, J. D., Sherman, S. S., and Hollis, B. W. (1991). Is the recommended daily allowance for vitamin D too low for the homebound elderly? *J. Am. Geritr. Soc.* **39,** 137–141.

182. Parfitt, A. M., Gallagher, J. C., Heaney, R. P., Johnson, C. C., Jr., Neer, R., and Whedon, G. D. (1982). Vitamin D and bone health in the elderly. *Am. J. Clin. Nutr.* **36,** 1014–1031.

183. Suter, P. M., and Russell, R. M. (1987). Vitamin requirements of the elderly. *Am. J. Clin. Nutr.* **45,** 501–512.

184. Holick, M. F. (1995). Sources of vitamin D: Diet and sunlight. *In* "Nutritional Aspects of Osteoporosis" (P. Burckhardt and R. P. Heaney, Eds.), Challenges in Modern Medicine, Vol. 7, pp. 289–309. Ares-Serono Symposia Publications, Rome, Italy.

185. Lips, P., Graafmans, W. C., Ooms, M. E., Bezemer, P. D., and Bouter, L. M. (1996). Vitamin D supplementation and fracture incidence in elderly persons. *Ann. Intern. Med.* **124,** 400–406.

186. Price, P. A. (1988). Role of vitamin-K dependent proteins in bone metabolism. *Ann. Rev. Nutr.* **8,** 565–583.

187. Bliziotes, M., Yergey, A. L., Nanes, M. S., Muenzer, J., Begley, M. G., Vieira, N. E., Kher, K. K., Brandi, M. L., and Marx, S. J. Absent intestinal response to calciferols in hereditary resistance to 1,25-dihydroxyvitamin D: Documentation and effective therapy with high dose intravenous infusions. *J. Clin. Endocrinol. Metab.* **66,** 294–300.

188. Olson, R. E. (1984). The function and metabolism of vitamin K. *Ann. Rev. Nutr.* **4,** 281–337.

189. Szulc, P., and Delmas, P. D. (1995). Is there a role for vitamin K deficiency in osteoporosis? *In* "Nutritional Aspects of Osteoporosis" (P. Burckhardt and R. P. Heaney, Eds.), Challenges in Modern Medicine, Vol. 7, pp. 357–366. Ares-Serono Publications, Rome, Italy.

190. Vermeer, C., Knapen, M. H. J., and Jie, K.-S. G. (1995). Increased vitamin K-intake may retard postmenopausal loss of bone mass. *In* "Nutritional Aspects of Osteoporosis" (P. Burckhardt and R. P. Heaney, Eds.). Challenges in Modern Medicine, Vol. 7, pp. 367–379. Ares-Serono Publications, Rome, Italy.

191. Binkley, N. C., Suttie, J. W. (1995). Vitamin K nutrition and osteoporosis. *J. Nutr.* **125,** 1812–1821.

192. Nakagawa, Y., Ahmed, M. A., Hall, S. L., Deganello, S., and Coe, F. L. (1987). Isolation from human calcium oxalate renal stones of nephrocalcin, a glycoprotein inhibitor of calcium oxalate crystal growth. *J. Clin. Invest.* **79,** 1782–1787.

193. Hauschka, P. V., Lian, J. B., Cole, D. E. C., and Gundberg, C. M. (1989). Osteocalcin and matrix gla protein: Vitamin K-dependent proteins in bone. *Physiol. Rev.* **69,** 990–1047.

194. Nakagawa, Y., Abram, V., Kezdy, F. J., Kaiser, E. T., and Coe, F. L. (1983). Purification and characterization of the principal inhibitor of calcium monohydrate crystal growth in human urines. *J. Biolog. Chem.* **258,** 12594–12600.

195. Kasai, R., Bianco, P., Robey, P. G., and Kahn, A. J. (1994). Production and characterization of an antibody against the human bone GLA protein (BGP/osteocalcin) propeptide and its use in immunocytochemistry of bone cells. *Bone Miner.* **25,** 167–182.

196. Jamal, S. A., Browner, W. S., Bauer, D. C., and Cummings, S. R. (1998). Warfarin use and risk for osteoporosis in elderly women. *Ann. Intern. Med.* **128,** 829–832.

197. Caraballo, P. J., Gabriel, S. E., Castro, M. R., Atkinson, E. J., and Melton, L. J., III. (1999). Changes in bone density after exposure to oral anticoagulants: A meta-analysis: *Osteoporos. Int.* **9,** 441–448.

198. Ducy, P., Desbois, C., Boyce, B., Pinero, G., Story, B., Dunstan, C., Smith, E., Bonadio, J., Goldstein, S., Gundberg, C., Bradley, A., and Karsenty, G. (1996). Increased bone formation in osteocalcin-deficient mice. *Nature* **382,** 448–452.

199. Hodges, S. J., Pilkington, M. J., Stamp, T. C. B., Catterall, A., Shearer, M. J., Bitensky, L., and Chayen, J. (1991). Depressed levels of circulating menaquinones in patients with osteoporotic fractures of the spine and femoral neck. *Bone* **12,** 387–389.

200. Gerland, G., Sadowski, J. A., and O'Brien, M. D. (1993). Dietary induced subclinical vitamin K deficiency in normal human subjects. *J. Clin. Invest.* **91,** 1761–1768.

201. Roberts, N. B., Holding, J. D., Walsh, H. P. J., Klenerman, L., Helliwell, T., King, D., and Shearer, M. (1996). Serial changes in serum vitamin K$_1$, triglyceride, cholesterol, osteocalcin and 25-hydroxyvitamin D3 in patients after hip replacement for fractured neck of femur or osteoarthritis. *Eur. J. Clin. Invest.* **26,** 24–29.

202. Plantalech, L. C., Chapuy, M. C., Guillaumont, M., Chapuy, P., Leclerq, M., and Delmas, P. D. (1990). Impaired carboxylation of serum osteocalcin in elderly women: Effect of vitamin K$_1$. *In* "Osteoporosis 1990," (C. Christiansen and K. Overgaard, Eds.), pp. 345–347. Osteopress Ap, Copenhagen.

203. Knapen, M. H. J., Hamulyak, K., and Vermeer, C. (1989). The effect of vitamin K supplementation on circulating osteocalcin (bone gla protein) and urinary calcium excretion. *Ann. Intern. Med.* **111,** 1001–1005.

204. Vermeer, C., and Hamulyak, K. (1991). Pathophysiology of vitamin K-deficiency and oral anticoagulants. *Thromb. Haemostas.* **66,** 153–159.

205. Feskanich, D., Weber, P., Willett, W. C., Rockett, H., Booth, S. L., and Colditz, G. A. (1999). Vitamin K intake and hip fractures in women: A prospective study. *Am. J. Clin. Nutr.* **69,** 74–79.

206. Geinoz, G., Rapin, C. H., Rizzoli, R., Kraemer, R., Buchs, B., Slosman, D., Michel, J. P., and Bonjour, J. P. (1993). Relationship between bone mineral density and dietary intakes in elderly. *Osteoporos. Int.* **3,** 242–248.

207. Rico, H., Refilla, M., Villa, L. F., Hernandez, E. R., and Fernandez, J. P. (1992). Crush fracture syndrome in senile osteoporosis: A nutritional consequence. *J. Bone Miner. Res.* **7,** 317–319.

208. Delmi, M., Rapin, C.-H., Bengoa, J.-M., Delmas, P. D., Vasey, H., and Bonjour, J.-P. (1990). Dietary supplementation in elderly patients with fractured neck of the femur. *Lancet* **335,** 1013–1016.

209. Rude, R. K., and Olerich, M. (1996). Magnesium deficiency: Possible role in osteoporosis associated with gluten-sensitive enteropathy. *Osteoporos. Int.* **6,** 453–461.

210. Ryzen, E., Elbaum, N., Singer, F. R., and Rude, R. K. (1985). Parenteral magnesium tolerance testing in the evaluation of magnesium deficiency. *Magnesium* **4,** 137–147.
211. Abraham, G. E. (1991). The importance of magnesium in the management of primary postmenopausal osteoporosis. *J. Nutr. Med.* **2,** 165–178.
212. Stendig-Lindberg, G., Tepper, R., and Leichter, I. (1994). Trabecular bone density in a two-year controlled trial of peroral magnesium in osteoporosis. *Magnesium Res.* **6,** 155–163.
213. Rude, R. K., Adams, J. S., Ryzen, E., Endres, D. B., Niimi, H., Horst, R., Haddad Jr., J. G., and Singer, F. R. (1985). Low serum concentrations of 1,25-dihydroxyvitamin D in human magnesium deficiency. *J. Clin. Endocrinol. Metab.* **61,** 933–940.
214. Spencer, H., Fuller, H., Norris, C., and Williams, D. (1994). Effect of magnesium on the intestinal absorption of calcium in man. *J. Am. College Nutr.* **13,** 485–492.
215. Ott, S., Tucci, J. R., Heaney, R. P., and Marx, S. J. (1997). Hypocalciuria and abnormalities in mineral and skeletal homeostatis in patients with celiac sprue without intestinal symptoms. *Endocrinol. Metab.* **4,** 201–206.
216. Davis, G. K., and Mertz, W. (1987). Copper. *In* "Trace Elements in Human and Animal Nutrition," 5th ed. (W. Mertz, Ed.), Vol. I, pp. 301–364. Academic Press, Inc., San Diego, CA.
217. Mertz, W. (Ed.) (1987). "Trace Elements in Human and Animal Nutrition," 5th ed. Academic Press, San Diego, CA.
218. Schmidt, H., Herwig, J., and Greinacher, I. (1991). The skeletal changes in premature infants with copper deficiency. Rofo. *Fortschritte aud dem Gebiete der Rontgenstrahlen und der Neuen Bildgebenden Verfahren* **155,** 38–42.
219. Buchman, A. L., Keen, C. L., Vinters, H. V. Harris, E., Chugani, H. T., Bateman, B., Rodgerson, D., Vargas, J., Verity, A., and Ament, M. (1994) Copper deficiency secondary to a copper transport defect: A new copper metabolic disturbance. *Metabolism* **43,** 1462–1469.
220. Strain, J. J. (1988). A reassessment of diet and osteoporosis—Possible role for copper. *Med. Hypotheses* **27,** 333–338.
221. Howard, G., Andon, M., Bracker, M., Saltman, P., and Strause, L. (1992). Low serum copper, a risk factor additional to low dietary calcium in postmenopausal bone loss. *J. Trace Elements Exp. Med.* **5,** 23–31.
222. Oxlund, H., Mosekilde, L., and Ortoft, G. (1996). Reduced concentration of collagen reducible cross-links in human trabecular bone with respect to age and osteoporosis. *Bone* **19,** 479–484.

223. Herzberg, M., Foldes, J., Steinberg, R., and Menczel, J. (1990). Zinc excretion in osteoporotic women. *J. Bone Miner. Res.* **5,** 251–257.
224. Herzberg, M., Lusky, A., Blonder, J., and Frenkel, Y. (1996). The effect of estrogen replacement on zinc in serum and urine. *Obstet. Gynecol.* **87,** 1035–1040.
225. Devine, A., Rosen, C., Mohan, S., Baylink, D. J., and Prince, R. L. (1998). Effects of zinc and other nutritional factors on IGF-1 and IGF binding proteins in postmenopausal women. *Am. J. Clin. Nutr.* **68,** 200–206.
226. Schürch, M. A., Rizzoli, R., Slosman, D., and Bonjour, J.-Ph. (1996). Protein supplements increase serum IGF-1 and decrease proximal femur bone loss in patients with a recent hip fracture. *In* "Osteoporosis 1996," (S. E. Papapoulos, P. Lips, H. A. P. Pols, C. C. Johnston, and P. D. Delmas, Eds.), pp. 327–329. Elsevier Science B. V., Amsterdam.
227. Elmstahl, S., Gullberg, B., Janzon, L., Johnell, O., and Elmstahl, B. (1998). Increased incidence of fractures in middle-aged and elderly men with low intakes of phosphorus and zinc. *Osteoporos. Int.* **8,** 333–340.
228. New, S. A., Bolton-Smith, C., Grubb, D. A., and Reid, D. M. (1997). Nutritional influences on bone mineral density: A cross-sectional study in premenopausal women. *Am. J. Clin. Nutr.* **65,** 1831–1839.
229. González-Reimers, E., and Arnay-de-la-Rosa, M. (1992). Ancient skeletal remains of the Canary Islands: Bone histology and chemical analysis. *Anthrop. Anz.* **50,** 201–215.
230. Asling, C. W., and Hurley, L. S. (1963). The influence of trace elements on the skeleton. *Clin. Orthop.* **27,** 213–264.
231. Strause, L., Saltman, P., and Glowacki, J. (1987). The effect of deficiencies of manganese and copper on osteoinduction and on resorption of bone particles in rats. *Calcif. Tissue Int.* **41,** 145–150.
232. Strause, L. G., Hegenauer, J., Saltman, P., Cone, R., and Resnick, D. (1986). Effects of long-term dietary manganese and copper deficiency on rat skeleton. *J. Nutr.* **116,** 135–141.
233. Reginster, J. Y., Strause, L. G., Saltman, P., and Franchimont, P. (1988). Trace elements and postmenopausal osteoporosis: A preminary study of decreased serum manganese. *Med. Sci. Res.* **16,** 337–338.
234. Strause, L., Saltman, P., Smith, K. T., Bracker, M., and Andon, M. B. (1994) Spinal bone loss in postmenopausal women supplemented with calcium and trace minerals. *J. Nutr.* **124,** 1060–1064.

CHAPTER **43**

Eating Disorders: Anorexia Nervosa, Bulimia Nervosa, and Binge Eating Disorder

CHERYL L. ROCK[1] AND WALTER H. KAYE[2]

[1]*University of California at San Diego, La Jolla, California*
[2]*University of Pittsburgh Medical Center, Pittsburgh, Pennsylvania*

I. INTRODUCTION

As a general theme, the eating disorders are characterized by abnormal eating patterns and cognitive distortions related to food and weight, which, in turn, result in adverse effects on nutritional status, medical complications, and impaired health status and function. Diagnostic criteria for the eating disorders and the approaches to management have evolved through various stages during the past several decades, and research efforts continue to increase knowledge of the biological and behavioral aspects of eating pathology.

II. DEFINITIONS AND DIAGNOSTIC CRITERIA

A. Diagnostic Criteria and Distinguishing Characteristics

Clinical diagnosis of these disorders is based on the psychological, behavioral, and physiological characteristics described by the *Diagnostic and Statistical Manual of Mental Disorders,* fourth edition (DSM-IV), criteria [1]. Current DSM-IV criteria for anorexia nervosa, bulimia nervosa, eating disorder not otherwise specified, and binge eating disorder are listed in Table 1. For anorexia nervosa, the diagnostic criteria specify body weight <85% of that expected based on age and height (with the latter cutpoint typically interpreted as being a body mass index ≤ 17.5 kg/m^2 in adults), intense fear of gaining weight, disturbance in the way in which body size or weight is perceived, and amenorrhea if the patient is a postmenarchal female. With the most recent DSM criteria, subgroups of anorexia nervosa are further defined as restricting type and binge eating/purging type. Criteria for the diagnosis of bulimia nervosa are recurrent binge eating, recurrent purging behavior or excessive exercise or fasting, excessive concern about body weight or shape, and absence of anorexia nervosa. Patients with bulimia nervosa are also categorized on the basis of the nature

of the behavior utilized to prevent weight gain despite recurrent binge eating episodes. A clinically relevant concept that results from these criteria is that a patient cannot be diagnosed with both anorexia nervosa and bulimia nervosa at any given point in time.

A third major diagnostic category, eating disorder not otherwise specified, is used to describe patients who meet most but not all of the criteria for the better defined disorders, patients who practice other types of behavior to prevent weight gain (such as chewing and spitting out food), and diagnoses for which more research is believed necessary to better define the condition. Binge eating disorder is currently considered as the latter type and is classified within this grouping, although provisional criteria have been developed for binge eating disorder and are being used until further refinements are established. The provisional criteria for binge eating disorder include recurrent episodes of binge eating, associated with at least three behavioral and attitudinal characteristics, such as eating large amounts when not physically hungry or feeling disgusted or guilty after overeating. In binge eating disorder, the absence of compensatory behaviors despite recurrent episodes of overeating typically results in obesity, although the diagnostic criteria for this condition do not specifically define or address body weight.

Over a lifetime, some patients may meet diagnostic criteria for more than one of these conditions, suggesting a continuum of eating disorders [2], and there is substantial overlap in attitudes and behaviors relating to food and weight. However, distinctive patterns of comorbidity and risk factors have been identified for each of these disorders, and the nutritional and medical consequences differ a great deal. The different types of eating disorders and their subtypes are associated with different nutritional problems and management issues, despite attitudinal and behavioral similarities.

B. Prevalence

Current prevalence of the clinical eating disorders in the general population has been estimated to be 0.5–1% for anorexia

Nutrition in the Prevention and Treatment of Disease

685

TABLE 1   Current Diagnostic Criteria for Various Eating Disorders

Diagnostic citeria for anorexia nervosa

A. Refusal to maintain body weight at or above a minimally normal weight for age and height (e.g., weight loss leading to maintenance of body weight <85% of that expected; or failure to make expected weight gain during period of growth, leading to body weight <85% of that expected).

B. Intense fear of gaining weight or becoming fat, even though underweight.

C. Disturbance in the way in which one's body weight or shape is experienced, undue influence of body weight or shape on self-evaluation, or denial of the seriousness of the current low body weight.

D. In postmenarchal females, amenorrhea, i.e., the absence of at least three consecutive menstrual cycles. (A woman is considered to have amenorrhea if her periods occur only following hormone, e.g., estrogen, administration.)

Specify type:

Restricting type: during the current episode of anorexia nervosa, the person has not regularly engaged in binge eating or purging behavior (i.e., self-induced vomiting or the misuse of laxatives, diuretics, or enemas).

Binge eating/purging type: during the current episode of anorexia nervosa, the person has regularly engaged in binge eating or purging behavior (i.e., self-induced vomiting or the misuse of laxatives, diuretics, or enemas).

Diagnostic criteria for bulimia nervosa

A. Recurrent episodes of binge eating. An episode of binge eating is characterized by both of the following:
(1) eating, in a discrete period of time (e.g., within any 2-hour period), an amount of food that is definitely larger than most people would eat during a similar period of time and under similar circumstances;
(2) a sense of lack of control over eating during the episode (e.g., a feeling that one cannot stop eating or control what or how much one is eating).

B. Recurrent inappropriate compensatory behavior in order to prevent weight gain, such as self-induced vomiting; misuse of laxatives, diuretics, enemas, or other medications; fasting; or excessive exercise.

C. The binge eating and inappropriate compensatory behaviors both occur, on average, at least twice a week for 3 months.

D. Self-evaluation is unduly influenced by body shape and weight.

E. The disturbance does not occur exclusively during episodes of anorexia nervosa.

Specify type:

Purging type: during the current episode of bulimia nervosa, the person has regularly engaged in self-induced vomiting or the misuse of laxatives.

Non-purging type: during the current episode of bulimia nervosa, the person has used other inappropriate compensatory

behaviors, such as fasting or excessive exercise, but has not regularly engaged in self-induced vomiting or the misuse of laxatives, diuretics, or enemas.

Diagnostic criteria for eating disorder not otherwise specified

This category is for disorders of eating that do not meet the criteria for any specific eating disorder. Examples include:

A. All of the criteria for anorexia nervosa are met except the individual has regular menses.

B. All of the criteria for anorexia nervosa are met except that, despite substantial weight loss, the individual's current weight is in the normal range.

C. All of the criteria for bulimia nervosa are met except binges occur at a frequency of less than twice a week or for a duration of less than 3 months.

D. An individual of normal body weight who regularly engages in inappropriate compensatory behavior after eating small amounts of food (e.g., self-induced vomiting after the consumption of two cookies).

E. An individual who repeatedly chews and spits out, but does not swallow, large amounts of food.

F. Binge eating disorder; recurrent episodes of binge eating in the absence of the regular use of inappropriate compensatory behaviors characteristic of bulimia nervosa.

Provisional criteria for binge eating disorder

A. Recurrent episodes of binge eating. An episode of binge eating is characterized by both of the following:
(1) eating, in a discrete period of time (e.g., within any 2-hour period), an amount of food that is definitely larger than most people would eat in a similar period of time under similar circumstances;
(2) a sense of lack of control over eating during the episode (e.g., a feeling that one cannot stop eating or control what or how much one is eating).

B. The binge eating episodes are associated with three (or more) of the following:
(1) eating much more rapidly than normal;
(2) eating until feeling uncomfortably full;
(3) eating large amounts of food when not feeling physically hungry;
(4) eating alone because of being embarrassed by how much one is eating;
(5) feeling disgusted with oneself, depressed, or very guilty after overeating.

C. Marked distress regarding binge eating is present.

D. The binge eating occurs, on average, at least 2 days a week for 6 months.

E. The binge eating is not associated with the regular use of inappropriate compensatory behaviors (e.g., purging, fasting, excessive exercise) and does not occur exclusively during the course of anorexia nervosa.

Source: Reprinted with permission from *Diagnostic and Statistical Manual of Mental Disorders,* Fourth Edition. Copyright 1994 Psychiatric Association, Washington, DC.

nervosa, 2% for bulimia nervosa, and 2% for binge eating disorder [2]. Overall, the overwhelming majority (>95%) of patients diagnosed with clinical eating disorders are female. An epidemic of eating disorders among high school students

and on college campuses has been suggested in some reports, based on variable criteria and approaches to estimate prevalence of the problem, but the figures cited do not necessarily reflect the actual prevalence of clinically diagnosable eating

TABLE 2 Various Factors Associated with Increased Risk for Eating Disorders

Female gender

Family history of eating disorders

Affective disorders

Substance abuse

Certain character traits (i.e., perfectionism, excessive compliance)

Low self-esteem

Family dysfunction

Profession or pursuit that stresses maintaining a certain body weight (i.e., dance, modeling, acting, athletics)

Diseases for which management involves emphasis on diet and diet regulations (i.e., type 1 diabetes mellitus, cystic fibrosis)

disorders [3–7]. Epidemiological studies often report numbers of subjects with mild eating disturbances or bulimic behavior, typically based on self-report survey data, rather than using the DSM criteria [3, 6]. Many young women engage in pathological dieting behaviors without meeting the current diagnostic criteria for anorexia or bulimia nervosa and may be regarded as having subclinical eating disorders. For example, 40–60% of high school girls in the United States are reported to be dieting to lose weight, and about 13% induce vomiting or use diet pills, laxatives, or diuretics [7]. In one university survey study, 32% of women reported binge eating at least twice per month, but only 2.7% reported that they feared loss of control over eating during binges, and even fewer (1.2%) met additional criteria for bulimia nervosa [8]. Other studies of college student populations have found that at least 30% of women of reproductive age are practicing some pathological weight control activities, with 15% regularly engaging in bulimic behaviors, including both binge eating and purging [4, 5].

Current evidence suggests that the clinical eating disorders are only the most extreme form of pathological eating attitudes and behaviors that are present in many young women. As described by Fairburn and Beglin [3], a broad spectrum of eating psychopathology likely exists in the general population, as a continuum of dieting behavior and weight concerns, especially among women. Knowledge of risk factors, demographic characteristics, and comorbidities of the eating disorders are likely distorted by the nature of the subgroup that seeks treatment, because many individuals with eating disorders do not seek treatment.

III. ETIOLOGY

Eating disorders have many causes, and it is likely that several factors contribute to the development of the disorder in any given case. Table 2 lists various factors associated with increased risk for eating disorders. Sociocultural influences may explain why eating disorders are mainly observed in economically advantaged communities and countries, and a cultural obsession with weight and thinness in women has been linked with increasing incidence during the past two decades [6]. Interpersonal factors and family interactions have also been suggested to contribute to risk, based on interviews and observations of patients and their families [9].

A. Nutritional and Dietary Risk Factors

Nutritional factors and dieting behavior may contribute to the development and course of eating disorders. In the pathogenesis of anorexia nervosa, dieting or other purposeful changes in food choices contribute enormously to the course of the disease because the physiological and psychological consequences of starvation serve as perpetuating factors. In bulimia nervosa, dieting precedes the development of the pattern of binge eating compensatory behaviors for the majority of patients with this disorder, although a minority (approximately 15%) report that they started binge eating prior to dieting [10]. The onset of bulimia nervosa usually follows a period of dieting to lose weight [10, 11], and a causative link between dietary restraint and bulimia is strengthened by similar behavior among obese patients who binge eat following diet restriction and among normal subjects following a period of food deprivation [12, 13]. Abnormal eating patterns, as well as their physiological consequences, serve to perpetuate the disorder and contribute to its often intractable nature. Higher prevalence rates among specific groups, such as athletes and patients with type 1 diabetes mellitus, support the concept that increased risk occurs with conditions in which dietary restraint and body weight assume great importance. However, only a small proportion of individuals who diet or restrict intake develop an eating disorder.

B. Genetic and Biologic Factors

Results from recent family and twin studies suggest that eating disorders are highly heritable conditions [14, 15]. This raises the possibility that biological factors may be crucial determinants of vulnerability, with certain individuals more susceptible to developing an eating disorder in response to the environmental factors that increase risk. For example, recent evidence suggests that both anorexia nervosa and bulimia nervosa are familial and that clustering of the disorders in families may arise partly from genetic transmission of risk [16, 17]. Moreover, a more broadly defined eating disorder phenotype that differs from anorexia nervosa or bulimia nervosa in degree of severity occurs far more often in relatives of both anorexia and bulimia nervosa probands compared to relatives of normal controls. Likewise, analysis of data from a large epidemiological sample of twins obtained via the Virginia Twin Registry [18, 19] adds to evidence of a strong association between anorexia nervosa and bulimia nervosa. In short, evidence suggests at least some sharing of

familial risk and liability factors between anorexia nervosa and bulimia nervosa. Paralleling these accounts are several reports of greater pairwise concordance rates of eating disorders in monozygotic compared to dyzygotic twin pairs, with several large-scale, community-based studies suggesting that as much as 50–80% of the variance in the development of eating disorders is due to genetic factors [15].

Various general psychiatric symptoms are found commonly in patients with anorexia nervosa or bulimia nervosa. In many cases, they develop secondary to malnutrition and other disabling psychological effects of aberrant eating psychological disability, as noted above; yet, in some, they clearly antedate disordered eating, or arise following recovery from low body weight or binge eating. Whether or not particular psychiatric disorders increase liability to eating disorders or are expressions of a shared underlying diathesis is a question of heuristic and clinical importance. For example, anorexia nervosa and bulimia nervosa often co-occur with major mood disorders, but the two conditions do not seem to express a single, shared transmitted liability [20]. Similarly, despite the high prevalence of substance abuse in bulimia nervosa, these appear to be independently transmitted disorders [21–23]. On the other hand, preliminary data suggest a common familial transmission of anorexia nervosa and obsessive compulsive personality disorder [16], thus suggesting the existence of a broad, genetically influenced phenotype with core features of rigid perfectionism and propensity for extreme behavioral constraint.

Determining whether behavioral symptoms are a consequence or a potential cause of pathological feeding behavior or malnutrition is a major methodological issue in the study of eating disorders. It is impractical to study eating disorders prospectively due to the young age of onset and difficulty in premorbid identification of people who will develop an eating disorder. However, subjects can be studied after long-term recovery from an eating disorder. The assumed absence of confounding nutritional influences in recovered women raises a possibility that persistent psychobiological abnormalities might be trait related and potentially contribute to the pathogenesis of this disorder. Investigators [24–27] have found that women who are long-term recovered from anorexia nervosa have a persistence of obsessional behaviors as well as inflexible thinking, restraint in emotional expression, and a high degree of self- and impulse-control. In addition, they have social introversion, overly compliant behavior, and limited social spontaneity as well as greater risk avoidance and harm avoidance. Moreover, long-term recovered anorexics have been found to have continued core eating disorder symptoms, such as ineffectiveness, a drive for thinness, and significant psychopathology related to eating habits. Similarly, people who have recovered from bulimia nervosa continue to be over concerned with body shape and weight, abnormal eating behaviors, and dysphoric mood [28–32]. Individuals recovered from anorexia nervosa or bulimia nervosa have increased perfectionism, and their most common

obsessional target symptoms are the need for symmetry and ordering/arranging. Considered together, these residual behaviors can be characterized as over concerns with body image and thinness, obsession with symmetry, exactness, and perfectionism, and dysphoric/negative affect. In general, pathologic eating behavior and malnutrition appear to exaggerate the magnitude of these concerns. Thus, the intensity of these symptoms is reduced after recovery but the content of these concerns remains unchanged. The persistence of these symptoms after recovery raises the question of whether a disturbance of such behaviors indicates morbid traits contributing to the pathogenesis of anorexia nervosa and bulimia nervosa.

There has been considerable interest in the role that serotonin may play in anorexia nervosa and bulimia nervosa. That is because brain serotonin pathways have been implicated in behaviors typically found in people with eating disorders, such as disturbance of feeding, mood, impulse regulation, and obsessionality. A substantial number of studies have shown alterations in serotonergic activity in the ill state [33, 34]. While less well studied, serotonergic disturbances appear to persist after recovery in both anorexia nervosa and bulimia nervosa. For example, both recovered anorexics and bulimic women have been found to have elevated levels of cerebrospinal fluid concentrations of 5-hydroxyindoleacetic acid (5-HIAA), the major metabolite of serotonin [31, 35]. *Low* levels of cerebrospinal fluid 5-HIAA are associated with impulsive and nonpremeditated aggressive behaviors, which cut across traditional diagnostic boundaries [36]. Behaviors noted after recovery from anorexia nervosa or bulimia nervosa, such as obsessions with symmetry, exactness, and perfectionism, and negative affect tend to be opposite in character to behaviors displayed by people with low 5-HIAA levels. These data support the hypothesis that increased cerebrospinal fluid 5-HIAA concentrations may be associated with exaggerated anticipatory overconcern with negative consequences (i.e., harm avoidance), while the lack of such concerns may explain impulsive, aggressive acts that are associated with low cerebrospinal fluid 5-HIAA levels.

IV. ANOREXIA NERVOSA

A. Diagnosis and Nutritional Assessment

Anorexia nervosa occurs much more often in girls and women (compared with males), in adolescence and early adulthood (rather than later in life), and in higher (versus lower) income groups. However, it does occur in males and can be diagnosed at any age and in any socioeconomic or cultural subgroup. By definition, patients with anorexia nervosa present with a very low weight for height, with marked reductions in both adipose tissue stores and lean body mass. In contrast with the patient who is underweight due to a condition such as infection or malabsorption, low

body weight in the patient with anorexia nervosa is the result of a purposeful effort to lose weight and maintain low weight by limiting energy intake and/or increasing energy expenditure, typically over a period of months.

1. PHYSICAL EXAMINATION AND CLINICAL DIAGNOSIS

In patients with eating disorders, a full physical examination should be performed by a physician familiar with common findings, with particular attention to vital signs; physical and sexual growth and development (including height and weight); the cardiovascular system; and evidence of dehydration, acrocyanosis, lanugo, salivary gland enlargement, and scarring on the dorsum of the hands (Russell's sign). A dental examination should also be performed. It is generally useful to assess growth, sexual development, and general physical development in younger patients. The use of a pediatric growth chart may permit identification of patients who have failed to gain weight and who have growth retardation. A discussion of pertinent laboratory evaluations and physical findings is provided in detail in the *Practice Guidelines for the Treatment of Patients with Eating Disorders* [37].

2. ENERGY REQUIREMENTS

Some investigators and clinicians have hypothesized that patients with anorexia nervosa may have increased energy requirements due to psychological stress or other metabolic abnormalities, which would theoretically facilitate weight loss. However, current evidence suggests that resting energy expenditure in anorexia nervosa patients who are maintaining a low body weight does not differ from control subjects when expressed as a function of lean body mass [38]. In ambulatory anorexia nervosa patients maintaining low body weights, Casper *et al.* [39] demonstrated that substantially increased levels of physical activity (rather than hypermetabolism per se) explain higher-than-expected total energy expenditure in low-weight patients. During the refeeding process, resting energy expenditure increases dramatically compared to prediction equations derived from observations of normal subjects who are not eating high-energy diets [40], presumably as a result of metabolic effects of the refeeding regimen. In clinical practice, this means that higher-than-expected levels of intake may be necessary to enable progressive weight restoration. Some differences in energy expenditure have been observed across subgroups of patients, with the restricting subtype observed to require more energy to promote weight gain than the binge eating/purging type during the refeeding and immediate postweight restoration phases [41].

3. CLINICAL LABORATORY FINDINGS AND VITAMIN AND MINERAL STATUS

Table 3 lists clinical and laboratory abnormalities that are common in anorexia nervosa patients. The endocrine abnormalities are a consequence of low body weight and malnu-

TABLE 3 Clinical and Laboratory Abnormalities That Are Commonly Observed in Patients with Anorexia Nervosa

Clinical abnormalities
Hypothermia
Dehydration
Hypotension, bradycardia, prolonged QT interval, arrhythmia
Decreased heart size
Dry skin
Acrocyanosis
Lanugo hair growth
Delayed gastric emptying
Severe constipation, bowel obstruction
Swollen salivary glands, dental caries, and erosion of enamel (if self-induced vomiting present)
Osteopenia
Laboratory abnormalities
Leukopenia, neutropenia, anemia, thrombocytopenia
Abnormal liver enzyme concentrations
Hypoglycemia
Hypercortisolemia, elevated urinary free cortisol
Hypercholesterolemia
Hypercarotenemia
Low T3 levels, sick euthyroid syndrome
Electolyte disturbances (hypokalemia, hyponatremia, hypomagnesemia, hyperphosphatemia)
Low serum estradiol (testosterone, if male) concentration
Increased growth hormone

trition and are reversible with weight restoration. Electrolyte disturbances are more likely to occur in the binge eating/purging type than in the restricting type. Circulating concentrations of secretory proteins that are often used as laboratory markers of overall nutritional status, such as serum albumin, are sometimes (but not always) reduced, depending in part on the state of hydration of the patient when the blood sample was collected and the severity of the weight loss.

Notably, clinical laboratory data must be interpreted within the context of the neuroendocrine and other physiological abnormalities that are present in starvation [42–44]. For example, hypercholesterolemia, if present, is a consequence of thyroid abnormalities in response to dietary restriction. Hypercarotenemia is often present in these patients due to the consumption of high-carotenoid foods (i.e., deeply pigmented vegetables and fruits) by a low-weight individual [45] and is innocuous. Carotenoid absorption is inefficient but unregulated, so peripheral tissue concentrations are largely determined by intake versus relative body mass and tissue capacity (e.g., an individual with a smaller body mass has a higher tissue concentration than an individual with greater body mass, at a given dose of carotenoid intake). The conversion of

provitamin A carotenoids to vitamin A is very well regulated, so hypercarotenemia does not cause hypervitaminosis A.

Results from clinical studies and case series reports suggest that vitamin deficiencies occur in up to one-third of anorexia nervosa patients [46–49]. Overall, inadequate dietary intake and poor overall nutritional status are major causative factors. Recent evidence suggests that thyroid hormone abnormalities that result from severe dietary restriction may adversely affect riboflavin status by causing an impaired metabolism of the vitamin to the active coenzyme forms [50]. The latter finding is of clinical importance because this suggests that an improvement in energy balance and, thus, overall nutritional status (rather than simply providing the vitamin) may be necessary to correct the problem.

Osteopenia is a serious and possibly irreversible medical complication of anorexia nervosa, with 50% of patients having bone density measurements greater than two standard deviations below age- and gender-matched controls [51]. Results from several studies indicate that some recovery of trabecular bone may be possible with weight restoration and recovery, but compromised bone density and deficits in bone mineral are evident after 11 years of follow-up after weight restoration and recovery [52–54]. Several causative factors have been identified, including hypoestrogenemia, elevated cortisol levels, decreased calcium intake, deficiency of insulin-like growth factor-1 (a nonspecific result of compromised nutritional status), and excessive physical activity [51, 55]. Unlike other conditions in which low circulating estrogen concentrations are associated with bone loss (i. e., the perimenopause), providing exogenous estrogen has not been shown to preserve or restore bone mass in the majority of patients with anorexia nervosa [56]. Calcium supplementation alone, even at a level of 1500 mg/day, has also not been found to promote increased bone density in these patients [51, 56]. Factors most consistently observed to be associated with lower bone mineral density in these patients at diagnosis and follow-up are longer duration of illness, which is often reflected in years of amenorrhea, and lower current and/or lowest relative body weight [51–54, 57, 58].

B. Medical and Nutritional Management of Anorexia Nervosa

Weight restoration is the most critical component of the treatment of anorexia nervosa [37, 59, 60]. However, weight restoration alone clearly does not indicate recovery, and forcing weight gain without psychological support and counseling is ill advised. The treatment of the patient with anorexia nervosa involves a concerted and rigorous effort to improve nutritional status and restore body weight, concurrent with intensive psychotherapeutic counseling that often involves family therapy if the patient is young or resides at home.

1. Nutritional Management

Weight restoration is best achieved by ensuring sufficient energy intake to promote weight gain, facilitated by nutri-

tional counseling to provide guidance, reassurance, and assistance with specific food choices. Hospitalization is indicated for refeeding if the patient is severely nutritionally compromised (e.g., <75% of recommended weight for height) [37]. Weight restoration can also be achieved through outpatient medical care and counseling, although a slower rate of weight gain should be expected with that approach. The usual strategy is to set a target weight goal and aim for a weight gain of 2–3 pounds/week for inpatients and 1–2 pounds/week for outpatients during weight restoration.

Most patients with anorexia nervosa are initially very conflicted about their involvement in treatment programs, because maintaining a low body weight and other aspects of the eating disorder are serving as coping mechanisms, and the eating disorder may also be the sole source of identity. Rather than perceiving the patient as being manipulative and treatment resistant, the informed view is to recognize that the behaviors are simply being tenaciously held until belief in the ability to develop another way of life and self-identify, as well as new thinking patterns, can enable the patient to relinquish the eating disorder thinking patterns and behavior. Several treatment team members are involved in the long-term care, and frequent contact and good communications among the members of the treatment team are essential.

The nutritional counseling process consists of establishing and monitoring dietary and behavioral goals in a stepwise manner, with the application of counseling strategies to help the patient expand his or her diet [60]. Typically, the patient is terrified of weight gain and may be struggling with hunger and urges to binge eat, yet the food choices allowed (by the patient) are too limited to enable sufficient energy intake. Thus, individualized guidance and a meal plan that provides a framework for meals and food choices can be enormously helpful. Specific strategies for effective nutrition intervention and counseling techniques have been described [60, 61]. Cognitive restructuring, which involves challenging deeply held beliefs and thought patterns with more accurate and healthy perceptions and interpretations, also includes nutrition education and the provision of factual information regarding dieting, nutrition, and the relationship between starvation and physical symptoms. Nutrition counseling begins with assessment and the development of short-term and long-term goals, as rapport and a trusting relationship develop, and extends over some time with counseling sessions scheduled at a frequency that is individualized for the patient and his or her needs.

In most inpatient treatment programs, certain dietary rules about food choices and goals for energy intake must be agreed on and followed in order for patients to normalize meals and eating patterns. Typically, patients are permitted to select a limited number of foods (i.e., three to five) that they may refuse to eat, and some personal preferences can be accommodated. For example, a lactovegetarian diet can be nutritionally adequate and sufficiently dense in energy to enable weight restoration, while more extreme diets (i.e., one that excludes all animal products) present more problems

because of difficulty in achieving adequate energy and nutrient intakes.

Water retention during refeeding should be anticipated, due to shifts in the secretion of aldosterone in response to changes in dietary intake and other hormonal changes. Also, guidance with food choices to promote normal bowel function can be helpful, such as increased intake of grain products that are high in insoluble fiber. Delayed gastric emptying and related gastrointestinal complaints (i.e., bloating) resolve with continued refeeding and weight restoration. Fluid intake and output, electrolytes (especially phosphate and potassium), body weight, and vital signs should be monitored during refeeding.

Results from several clinical studies provide some insight about changes in body composition that may be anticipated to occur in the anorexia nervosa patient during weight restoration. In a recent study of 26 low-weight female anorexia nervosa patients in which dual-energy X-ray absorptiometry and skinfold measurements were used to monitor body composition and fat distribution, increased energy intake to promote weight restoration was associated with significant increases in all major body compartments (e.g., body fat, lean body mass, bone mineral content) [62]. Although fat comprised the largest amount of the weight gained in this study by Orphanidou et al. [62], results from the skinfold measurements did not suggest preferential fat deposition in any area. As observed in previous reports [63], even though a greater net gain of body fat typically results from weight restoration in these patients, their body fat usually remains considerably lower than healthy control subjects. A critical concept is that change in weight or body mass index does not necessarily predict change in lean tissue or fat mass, and a meaningful change in fat mass or fat-free mass may occur without a change in body mass index or weight [64]. This is a clinically relevant issue because weight gain has historically been used as evidence of adherence to target eating patterns and, thus, is often an inaccurate basis for expanded privileges and rewards in behavioral therapy-based programs.

In very rare instances, enteral or parenteral feeding may be necessary. However, risks associated with aggressive nutrition support in these patients are hypophosphatemia, refeeding edema, cardiac failure, seizures, aspiration of enteral formula, and death [37, 65]. Thus, in the rare cases in which enteral or parenteral nutrition support may be necessary, careful and knowledgeable medical monitoring is of paramount importance. Notably, reliance on foods (rather than enteral or parenteral nutrition support) as the primary method of weight restoration contributes a great deal to the long-term recovery. The overall goal is to help the patient normalize eating patterns, and learning that behavior must involve planning and practicing with real food.

In the initial treatment phases, physical activity almost always must be limited, due to risk for injury and to create an energy balance that permits weight gain. The counseling effort should communicate that in the healthy state, exercise is an activity that should be undertaken for enjoyment and fitness (rather than a strategy to simply expend energy and promote weight loss), and that excessive exercise is often a common component of the eating disorder itself. Supervised, low-weight strength training is less likely to impede weight gain than other forms of activity and can be psychologically helpful for patients.

Weight restoration is the only specific factor or intervention that has been consistently observed to promote recovery of bone mass [51, 52]. However, ensuring adequate vitamin D (400 IU/day) and calcium (1000–1500 mg/day) intakes is an additional consideration in management [37, 43, 51, 66], because these dietary factors enable bone mineralization with improved endocrine and nutritional status.

2. PHARMACOLOGIC MANAGEMENT AND PSYCHOLOGIC THERAPIES

Patients with anorexia nervosa often do not respond effectively to treatment [67]. Extended hospitalizations can be lifesaving because such treatment can restore weight to emaciated people, which, in turn, reverses medical complications. However, such hospitalizations can be lengthy and expensive, and relapse after hospitalization has been reported to be high [68]. Limited efficacy of pharmacologic and psychologic treatment in anorexia nervosa may be due, in part, to the fact that past treatments have focused mainly on attempts to increase the rate of weight gain of emaciated patients in a hospital setting. Inpatient treatment, consisting of nursing care, behavior modification and supportive psychotherapy, succeeds in restoring the weight of most emaciated anorectics. Thus, the evaluation of the efficacy of medications in augmenting weight gain in anorexia nervosa has been limited, because most trials have been conducted on outpatients or inpatients already participating in behavioral and nutritional eating disorders treatment programs, which are themselves effective in the short run. In these settings, controlled trials have not provided consistent evidence for the efficacy of antidepressant medications in the treatment of anorexia nervosa [69–71].

A more recent series of randomized controlled studies have examined the efficacy of various types of psychological therapies in promoting weight gain in acutely ill patients [68, 72]. Overall, the results indicate that substantial improvement in body mass and general psychosocial adjustment can be achieved in some subjects with anorexia nervosa using cognitive-behavioral, psychoeducational, and family therapy techniques (in some studies, coupled with dietary counseling), although treatment gains are not as robust in patients with more chronic, long-standing disability. A few recent studies have focused on preventing relapse in anorexia nervosa and appear to show more promise [68, 72]; for example, some psychotherapies specifically developed to treat anorexia nervosa appear to show reduced relapse at 1–2 years follow-up.

Recent studies suggest that fluoxetine may be useful in the prevention of relapse in anorexia nervosa. In separate open and double-blind placebo-controlled studies, fluoxetine

was shown to improve outcome and reduce relapse when administered *after* weight restoration [73, 74], associated with a significant reduction in core eating disorder symptoms, depression, anxiety, and obsessions and compulsions. In a recent double-blind, placebo-controlled study, 10 of 16 (63%) subjects on fluoxetine remained well during 1 year of outpatient follow-up, whereas only 3 of 19 (16%) remained well on placebo ($P = 0.006$) [74]. Fluoxetine administration was associated with a significant weight gain and a significant reduction in obsessions and compulsions and, thus, appears to improve outcome in patients with anorexia nervosa by reducing symptoms and helping to maintain a healthy body weight in continuing outpatient treatment.

Interestingly, two studies [75, 76] have found that selective serotonin reuptake inhibitors are specifically not useful when patients with anorexia nervosa are malnourished and underweight. As noted by Tollefson [77], these medications are dependent on neuronal release of serotonin for their action. If the release of serotonin from presynaptic neuronal storage sites is substantially compromised, and net synaptic serotonin concentration is negligible, a clinically meaningful response to a selective serotonin reuptake inhibitor might not occur. In fact, malnourished individuals with anorexia nervosa have reduced cerebrospinal fluid 5-HIAA, the major serotonin metabolite in the brain [78], suggesting that there are reduced levels of synaptic serotonin. This could be due to reduced availability of tryptophan, the essential amino acid precursor to serotonin [79]. This link between dietary intake and efficacy of selective serotonin reuptake inhibitors is supported by data that have consistently shown that dieting in healthy normal-weight and obese women reduces tryptophan availability, thereby limiting potential serotonergic production [80]. Moreover, studies in animals show that food restriction decreases serotonin and its synthesis rate in the brain [81]. In addition, depletion of tryptophan, the precursor of serotonin, reverses the effects of selective serotonin reuptake inhibitors in depressed patients [82] and plasma tryptophan was observed to be inversely related to depression scores. In anorexia nervosa, weight restoration promotes normalized nutritional status, and cerebrospinal fluid 5-HIAA concentrations then become elevated [35]. These changes in nutritional status and serotonergic activity might explain why individuals with anorexia nervosa may become responsive to fluoxetine after weight restoration.

V. BULIMIA NERVOSA

A. Diagnosis and Nutritional Assessment

Patients with bulimia nervosa are usually within the normal range of weight for height. The diagnostic criteria focus on the binge eating (and purging) behaviors, but another key characteristic aspect of the dietary pattern in bulimia nervosa is dietary restriction. In fact, the patient's efforts to restrict his or her diet according to rules such as good or bad and safe or forbidden (rather than simply calories per se), may actually set the stage for binge eating when the forbidden foods are consumed or the allowed level of intake is exceeded [83, 84]. A small subgroup of patients with bulimia nervosa reports that binge eating preceded dieting, and these patients appear to more closely resemble individuals with binge eating disorder (discussed below), with consistently higher body weights [10]. The majority of patients with bulimia nervosa use purging behaviors to prevent weight gain, and self-induced vomiting is the most common strategy utilized [2, 11, 37]. Purging behaviors do not completely prevent the utilization of energy from episodic binge eating, and an average retention of approximately 1200 kcal from binges of various sizes and energy contents was observed in one study [85].

Laxative abuse is also very common among patients with bulimia nervosa (as well as among patients with binge eating/purging type anorexia nervosa). Patients often use laxatives to reduce anxiety and feelings of fullness or bloating [86], although laxatives, even at the high doses used by patients with eating disorders, have been shown to have a minimal effect on absorption of energy-producing macronutrients [87].

1. PHYSICAL EXAMINATION AND CLINICAL DIAGNOSIS

By definition, patients with bulimia nervosa do not present with low body weight, as is characteristic of anorexia nervosa. Clinical evidence of purging behavior, such as dental changes, dehydration, salivary gland enlargement, and scarring on the dorsum of the hands (Russell's sign), are likely to be present. Gastrointestinal complaints, such as bloating, flatulence, and constipation, are common in bulimia nervosa, and the severity of these complaints has been found to correlate with severity of depression [88]. Ipecac, an over-the-counter emetic, is used by some patients with bulimia nervosa (and also by some patients with binge eating/purging type anorexia nervosa). Chronic ipecac use can result in skeletal myopathy, electrocardiographic changes, and cardiomyopathy resulting in congestive heart failure and arrhythmia [89]. Dental complications caused by self-induced vomiting can be serious and permanent, and the typical appearance of the characteristic dental erosion that results from this behavior allows it to be distinguished from other causes [90].

2. CLINICAL LABORATORY FINDINGS

Clinical and laboratory abnormalities observed in the patient with bulimia nervosa are very similar to those observed in anorexia nervosa (see Table 3), with the degree of nutritional compromise and starvation being the most important determinant of risk for these abnormalities. Depending on the nonbinge diet, various degrees of energy imbalance occur in bulimia nervosa, so abnormalities that result from a severe energy deficit (i.e., low serum estradiol, hypercholes-

terolemia, osteopenia) are often, but not always, observed in these patients. Dehydration and electrolyte abnormalities caused by purging, such as hypokalemia and hypochloremic alkalosis, are common [37].

B. Medical and Nutritional Management of Bulimia Nervosa

The majority of patients with bulimia nervosa are managed as outpatients, in private practice settings, or in day treatment programs. Hospitalization is considered necessary only when life-threatening medical problems or risk for suicide is present [37]. Monitoring of electrolytes, vital signs, and body weight are the major components of medical management. Cognitive-behavioral therapy, interpersonal psychotherapy, and pharmacologic treatments have all been shown to be effective in the treatment of bulimia nervosa.

1. NUTRITIONAL MANAGEMENT

The primary goal of nutritional management is to normalize the patient's eating pattern, which is typically very chaotic and characterized by an overall pattern of food rules, restrictions, or dieting, regularly interspersed with episodes of binge eating and purging. Although many patients with bulimia nervosa desire weight loss (whether or not they are truly overweight), it is important to communicate that the sole and primary goal of intervention is to normalize the eating patterns and discontinue purging behavior.

Cognitive-behavioral therapy, which is the most well-established, effective treatment of bulimia nervosa, includes dietary guidance and nutrition education as core components of the therapy [37, 91]. The primary nutritional aspects of cognitive-behavioral therapy include meal planning, encouraging a pattern of regular eating, and discouraging dieting. Didactic nutrition education includes teaching about body weight regulation, energy balance, the psychological and physiological effects of starvation, misconceptions about dieting and weight control, and physical consequences of bulimic behavior. Patients are encouraged to eat three planned meals (plus two to three planned snacks) each day, with a minimum of 1500 kcal/day to prevent hunger, because hunger has been shown to greatly increase susceptibility to binge eating. Helping the patient expand her diet to begin to include forbidden foods (initially, under controlled circumstances) is usually necessary and helpful. Severe and self-imposed dietary restraint regarding specific food types and choices also promotes perpetuation of the binge eating pattern. Other strategies that are helpful include keeping food records, weighing no more than once per week, and stimulus control (i.e., not shopping while hungry). Nutritional counseling includes developing a food plan and individualized guidance with specific dietary goals that are established and monitored as the diet is expanded, and a regular eating pattern is established. Additional counseling strategies have been summarized [60].

Discontinuing purging behaviors is an important aspect of intervention for most patients with bulimia nervosa, and this usually results in rebound fluid retention that is very disturbing to the patient due to overconcern with weight. Discussing the nature of this temporary weight gain is helpful, and encouraging a focus on fitness and lean body tissue (rather than body weight per se) can be reassuring. Regular eating, activity, and sleeping patterns, plus consistent daily intakes of carbohydrate, sodium, and energy, will eventually result in normal sodium (and fluid) balance. Severe dietary sodium restriction may actually aggravate the problem of fluid retention in these patients, because counterregulatory mechanisms, such as increased aldosterone secretion, are highly responsive due to periods of dehydration and electrolyte depletion. Education and guidance with the effects of withdrawal from stimulant laxatives is also often necessary, and specific clinical protocols for normalizing bowel function have been reported [37, 86]. Useful dietary strategies include increased intakes of whole grains, wheat bran, and bulk-forming agents, concurrent with adequate fluids to reduce risk for bowel obstruction.

Although the goal is to eliminate self-induced vomiting behavior, strategies to minimize loss of dental enamel until that point is reached have been suggested. For example, toothbrushing after vomiting should be discouraged, because the enamel is particularly susceptible to abrasion at that time, but rinses with bicarbonate and fluoride solutions after vomiting, in addition to regular topical fluoride applications, may help to minimize enamel loss [90].

2. PHARMACOLOGIC MANAGEMENT AND PSYCHOLOGICAL THERAPIES

It is fair to say that progress to date in establishing the efficacy of specific psychological and pharmacological therapies for eating disorders has been more dramatic for bulimia nervosa than for anorexia nervosa [67, 91, 92]. With regard to psychotherapy, although the number of controlled clinical trials is still small, most indicate that cognitive-behavioral therapy is an effective treatment for upwards of 60–70% of individuals with bulimia nervosa, with remission of binge eating and purging achieved in 30–50% of cases. Direct comparisons of cognitive-behavioral therapy with other psychological treatments suggest that this modality is more effective than psychodynamically oriented supportive expressive psychotherapy in reducing core symptoms of bulimia nervosa, and is more effective than a strictly behavioral treatment in preventing early relapse into dietary restriction, binge eating, and purging. Evidence further suggests that cognitive-behavioral therapy results in improvements in certain core features of the illness, such as body dissatisfaction, pursuit of thinness, and perfectionism.

Evidence for the efficacy of antidepressant pharmacotherapy in bulimia nervosa is impressive; however, the benefits may diminish over time in a significant proportion of individuals with bulimia nervosa who respond initially, and

only a minority have complete suppression of their symptoms with antidepressant monotherapy [69–71]. The results of most double-blind, placebo-controlled randomized trials reported to date indicate that antidepressants show at least some superiority over placebo in reducing the frequency of binge eating episodes. In addition, some studies show a reduction in intensity of some other symptoms commonly seen in bulimia nervosa, such as preoccupation with food and depression. These findings have been demonstrated with a variety of antidepressive medications, including tricyclic agents, monoamine oxidase inhibitors, and selective serotonin reuptake inhibitors. Patients participating in these trials typically reported from 8–10 episodes of binge eating per week at baseline. The average decrease in binge frequency for patients receiving the antidepressant medication has been observed to be about 55%, with wide variation across studies. Placebo responses were similarly variable, but generally the decrease of binge frequency was less than half of the magnitude of the response for the active treatment. However, only a minority of the patients actually achieved full abstinence from binge eating and purging behaviors. Most trials have shown no correlation between improvement in mood and reduction in symptoms of bulimia nervosa. Additionally, antidepressants suppress symptoms of bulimia nervosa also in nondepressed bulimic patients, suggesting a mode of action other than through their antidepressant effects. In some studies, the patients receiving the antidepressive medication demonstrated a reduction in the tendency for stressors to trigger binge eating.

A few studies [93–98] have assessed the relative efficacy of combining psychotherapy (in most trials, of the cognitive-behavioral therapy type) and antidepressants for the management of bulimia nervosa, compared with the isolated treatments themselves. Although differing in many respects, these studies suggest that the improvement in symptoms of bulimia nervosa with cognitive-behavioral therapy alone was greater than with the medication alone. Adding medication to the psychotherapy generally did not significantly improve the outcome over psychotherapy alone in terms of eating behaviors, nor did it increase the speed of the therapeutic response. However, one prolonged follow-up evaluation found that combined treatment was more effective for a number of eating variables than cognitive-behavioral therapy alone. Another study showed the superiority of combined therapy in reducing the rates of anxiety and depression.

VI. EATING DISORDER NOT OTHERWISE SPECIFIED

A. Overview of Eating Disorder Not Otherwise Specified

Eating disorder not otherwise specified is a large and heterogeneous diagnostic category that is applicable for individuals who have clinically significant eating disorders but who fail to meet all of the diagnostic criteria for the main eating disorders, anorexia nervosa or bulimia nervosa [99]. Binge eating disorder is included in this category at this time, as evidence accumulates to sufficiently support the specific diagnostic criteria for this disorder [1].

Patients with this diagnosis can have serious eating problems that adversely affect health status, and the nutritional and medical management issues in these patients are similar to those in the patient with anorexia nervosa or bulimia nervosa. For example, some women can menstruate at a very low body weight, possibly due to a biological adaptation to the low weight, although they are otherwise comparable to the patient who meets the full diagnostic criteria for anorexia nervosa (which includes amenorrhea for at least three consecutive menstrual cycles). Another example is an obese individual who has lost a substantial amount of weight due to extreme and unhealthy eating patterns and cognitive distortions related to food and weight, but whose current weight is in the normal range. The eating problems and attitudes of the latter type of patient are characterized by an intense fear of regaining weight. Individuals with unusual food rules or eating patterns to promote weight loss or maintenance of low body weight, although not below a weight that meets the criteria for anorexia nervosa, and associated with psychological distress and abnormal attitudes about food, would also be assigned to this diagnostic category.

Because this is a heterogeneous group, the medical and nutritional management of a patient with a diagnosis of eating disorder not otherwise specified is determined by the specific eating behaviors and attitudes and clinical problems that are present. In general, the same issues, principles and treatment strategies relevant to the other eating disorders are applicable to these patients.

B. Binge Eating Disorder

1. DIAGNOSIS AND NUTRITIONAL ASSESSMENT OF BINGE EATING DISORDER

The diagnostic criteria for binge eating disorder are considered provisional rather than definite at this time, because less evidence has been accumulated to define the disorder and to differentiate it from other eating disorders as a distinct condition [1]. Also, fewer studies that might support the efficacy of various treatments and interventions have been conducted and reported, compared to research in anorexia nervosa and bulimia nervosa [100–102].

Patients with binge eating disorder do not use purging behaviors on a regular basis, yet they binge eat regularly, so they are typically obese [12]. Patients with binge eating disorder are usually identified when they seek treatment for their obesity, rather than presenting for treatment of an eating disorder. In fact, >20% of individuals seeking weight loss treatment from university or commercial programs report binge eating problems and related psychological distress

[12]. The characteristics and behaviors of patients with binge eating disorder have been compared with those of non-binge-eating obese patients in several studies. A consistent finding in these studies is that patients with binge eating disorder are typically more obese than non-binge-eating obese patients [103]. Another consistent finding is that patients with binge eating disorder, compared to non-binge-eating obese patients, have an increased frequency of psychiatric symptoms and diagnoses, independent of degree of obesity [101–104]. Major depression accounts for the greatest difference between these two groups.

While anorexia nervosa and bulimia nervosa occur predominantly in women, males comprise a comparatively higher percentage of patients with binge eating disorder (suggested to be 40% of patients with this disorder), and similar prevalence rates have been observed in men and women in community and college samples [105, 106]. Another demographic feature that distinguishes binge eating disorder from the other eating disorders is that it appears to occur at similar rates across different racial and ethnic groups [106–108].

Although the majority of patients with binge eating disorder report frequent dieting and concern with body weight, a pattern of dieting behavior preceding binge eating is not characteristic of patients with binge eating disorder, in contrast with the temporal sequence that occurs in the majority of patients with bulimia nervosa [102]. Approximately 50% of patients with binge eating disorder report that they started binge eating before they started dieting or trying to lose weight [109, 110]. Because of the concern that dietary restriction increases the susceptibility to binge eating in bulimia nervosa, normalized eating patterns and guidance away from energy restriction is stressed in bulimia nervosa treatment programs. However, this concern may not be as relevant in the treatment of binge eating disorder, in which patients appear to have a more generalized and consistent lack of control over their eating patterns and food choices, even when they are not binge eating.

2. Psychological, Medical, and Nutritional Management of Binge Eating Disorder

Similar to bulimia nervosa, cognitive-behavioral therapy, interpersonal psychotherapy, and pharmacologic treatments have all been shown to have utility in the treatment of binge eating disorder [102]. Psychotherapy has been shown to be effective in reducing the frequency of binge eating in patients with binge eating disorder, but cognitive behavior therapy (adapted from protocols used in the treatment of bulimia nervosa) and interpersonal therapy are the approaches most often utilized [12, 101, 102].

a. Nutritional Management. In the adaptation of cognitive-behavioral therapy to the treatment of binge eating disorder, the goal is reduced frequency of binge eating and also a pattern of overall moderation of food intake. Although a framework or meal plan for regular meals may be useful for many patients, strict food rules and rigid diet plans are discouraged. The goal is to promote a healthy overall pattern of eating and exercise, and achieving that goal is accomplished by planning and by identifying and modifying maladaptive thoughts and beliefs that lead to overeating and binge eating. Nutritional guidance emphasizes three planned meals and two to three planned snacks each day, no more than a 3-hour interval between meals or snacks, a varied and balanced diet, and food servings that are of average portion size. Many patients with binge eating disorder benefit from basic nutrition education on the components of a healthy diet and discussion to dispel common myths about diet and nutrition.

An important issue in the nutritional management of patients with binge eating disorder is whether weight loss should be a goal of the intervention, in addition to normalized eating patterns. For the vast majority of these patients, obesity is the major health risk resulting from the disorder. Efforts that are focused solely on eliminating binge eating have not been shown to result in weight loss in the majority of patients with binge eating disorder [110–114]. Also, studies suggest that guidance toward energy restriction through the application of behavioral weight control strategies does not appear to exacerbate binge eating in these patients [101, 102, 111]. However, the long-term effects on weight management that may be achieved in these patients by behavioral intervention programs that incorporate energy restriction are unknown. Decades of research and long-term follow-up of participants in behavioral treatment programs aimed toward weight reduction suggest that few patients are likely to sustain the energy deficit necessary for continued weight loss and maintenance without considerable motivation and lifestyle modification (see Chapter 34). Thus, the cognitive-behavioral treatment programs for binge eating currently place the greatest emphasis on the goal of normalized eating patterns, clarifying with patients that simply eliminating the binge eating is unlikely to cause substantial weight loss.

b. Pharmacologic Management. The use of antidepressants, such as the tricyclic antidepressants, in binge eating disorder has been suggested to have a possible role in the treatment of binge eating disorder, based on results from some studies [101]. However, a role for pharmacotherapy has not been firmly established at this point, and more studies are needed.

VII. OUTCOME

As recently reviewed by Pike [115], most studies of long-term outcome of patients with anorexia nervosa suggest that 50–75% of patients achieve a good to intermediate outcome and 15–25% are chronically symptomatic, although the length of time of follow-up contributes to large variability in these figures. Estimates of overall mortality associated with anorexia nervosa range up to 20%, mainly due to starvation-related medical problems and suicide. In a 10- to 15-year

follow-up study conducted by Strober and colleagues [116], nearly 76% of 95 adolescent patients with anorexia nervosa experienced full recovery, defined as being free of all criterion symptoms of anorexia nervosa or bulimia nervosa for not less than 8 consecutive weeks. Nearly 14% failed to achieve even partial recovery at any time during the follow-up period, although no deaths occurred in this case series. Time to recovery ranged from 57 to 79 months, but once recovered, subsyndromal relapse was rare (observed in only 7% of patients who achieved full recovery, and most of these patients returned to full recovery).

In another long-term follow-up study of 84 female patients with anorexia nervosa reported by Zipfel and colleagues [117], 51% of the patients had achieved full recovery, 10% still met full diagnostic criteria for anorexia nervosa, and 16% had died from causes related to anorexia nervosa, after an average of 21 years following the initial inpatient treatment. Significant predictors of poorer outcome were longer duration of illness before first admission, low body mass index, inadequate weight gain during the first hospitalization, and severe psychological or social problems.

Similar to long-term follow-up studies of anorexia nervosa, outcome data on bulimia nervosa vary considerably across studies, with recovery rates ranging from 13% to 71% [118]. Factors reported to be predictive of poorer outcome in bulimia nervosa were severity of eating pathology, frequency of vomiting at baseline, extreme weight fluctuations, comorbid disorders, impulsivity, low self-esteem, and suicidal behavior. In a follow-up study of patients with bulimia nervosa who were followed for an average of 11.5 years [119], full or partial remission occurred in nearly 70% of the 173 patients. Of the remainder, 11% still met full criteria for bulimia nervosa, 18.5% met criteria for eating disorder not otherwise specified, and 1 patient died.

Although long-term follow-up data on binge eating disorder are scant, good outcome of 68 patients with binge eating disorder over a 6-year course has been reported [120], with the majority having no eating disorder at follow-up. Nearly 6% still met criteria for binge eating disorder, 7.4% met criteria for bulimia nervosa, 7.4% met criteria for eating disorder not otherwise specified, and 1 patient died.

VIII. PREVENTION OF EATING DISORDERS

Few would argue that prevention or early detection and treatment are the best approaches to reducing the morbidity and mortality associated with the eating disorders. Although current evidence suggests that genetic factors play a crucial role in determining the individual susceptibility to eating disorders, familial, sociocultural, and nutritional factors (i.e., dieting behavior) create the environment in which the susceptibility is more likely to result in a full-blown eating disorder. Chaotic eating patterns and malnutrition adversely affect cognitive function and response to psychotherapy, so early intervention and restoration of good nutritional status can be important in determining the course of the disorder.

Although there is general agreement that prevention is a good strategy, the best focus of these efforts is still unclear [121]. Organized prevention efforts, which are typically provided and evaluated in school and university settings [122–124], usually emphasize the value of individuality, promoting increased self-confidence and self-esteem, and encouraging the development of skills to resist social pressure [125, 126]. Attitudes and beliefs that promote dieting are driven by powerful sociocultural attitudes that may be resistant to change. However, health care providers can be sensitive to the attitudes about food, nutrition, and body weight that are communicated to individual patients and community groups, recognizing the potential impact of these communications on dieting behavior and weight concerns in those at risk.

IX. SUMMARY AND CONCLUSIONS

Nutrition is an important aspect of the prevention and treatment of the eating disorders, which appear to develop as a consequence of both genetic and environmental factors in susceptible individuals. Although the specific nutritional issues and intervention strategies differ across these conditions, a unifying concept is the goal of achieving a normal eating pattern and healthy body weight, which involves cognitive restructuring, behavioral skills training, and nutrition education. Overall, the long-term outcome for the majority of patients with eating disorders is good, despite the severity of the disturbance in eating behaviors and attitudes that characterizes these disorders at diagnosis.

References

1. American Psychiatric Association (1994). "Diagnostic and Statistical Manual of Mental Disorders," 4th ed. American Psychiatric Association, Washington, DC.
2. Schweiger, U., and Fichter, M. (1997). Eating disorders: Clinical presentation, classification and aetiological models. *Bailliere's Clin. Psych.* **3,** 199–216.
3. Fairburn, C. G., and Beglin, S. J. (1990). Studies of the epidemiology of bulimia nervosa. *Am. J. Psychiatry* **147,** 401–408.
4. Drewnowski, A., Hopkins, S. A., and Kessler, R. C. (1988). The prevalence of bulimia nervosa in the U.S. college population. *Am. J. Public Health* **78,** 1322–1325.
5. Drewnowski, A., Yee, D. K., Kurth, C. L., and Krahn, D. D. (1994). Eating pathology and DSM-III-R bulimia nervosa: A continuum of behavior. *Am. J. Psychiatry* **151,** 1217–1219.
6. Hsu, L. K. G. (1996). Epidemiology of the eating disorders. *Psych. Clin. N. Am.* **19,** 681–700.
7. Steiner, H., and Lock, J. (1998). Anorexia nervosa and bulimia nervosa in children and adolescents: A review of the past 10 years. *J. Am. Acad. Child Adolesc. Psychiatry* **37,** 352–359.

8. Schotte, D. E., and Stunkard, A. J. (1987). Bulimia vs bulimic behaviors on a college campus. *J.A.M.A.* **258,** 1213–1215.

9. Bruch, H. (1973). "Eating Disorders: Obesity, Anorexia Nervosa, and the Person Within." Basic Books, New York.

10. Haiman, C., and Devlin, M. J. (1999). Binge eating before the onset of dieting: A distinct subgroup of bulimia nervosa. *Int. J. Eating Disord.* **25,** 151–157.

11. Kirkley, B. G. (1986). Bulimia: Clinical characteristics, development, and etiology. *J. Am. Diet. Assoc.* **86,** 486–472.

12. Marcus, M. D. (1993). Binge eating in obesity. *In* "Binge Eating" (C. G. Fairburn and G. T. Wilson, Eds.), pp. 77–96. Guilford Press, New York.

13. Keys, A., Brozek, J., Henschel, A., Mickelson, O., and Taylor, H. L. (1950). "The Biology of Human Starvation," University of Minnesota Press, Minneapolis.

14. Lilenfeld, L. R., Kaye, W. H., and Strober, M. (1997). Genetics and family studies of anorexia nervosa and bulimia nervosa. *Bailliere's Clin. Psych.* **3,** 177–197.

15. Bulik, C., Sullivan, P., and Kendler, K. (1998). Heritability of binge eating and bulimia nervosa. *Biolog. Psychiatry* **44,** 1210–1218.

16. Lilenfeld, L. R., Kaye, W. H., Greeno, C. G., Merikangas, K., Plotnicov, K. H., Pollice, C. P., Rao, R., Strober, M., Bulik, C. M., and Nagy, L. (1998). A controlled family study of anorexia and bulimia nervosa: Psychiatric and effects of proband comorbidity. *Arch. Gen. Psychiatry* **55,** 603–610.

17. Strober, M., Freeman, R., Lampert, C., Diamond, J., and Kaye, W. H. (2000). Controlled family study of anorexia nervosa and bulimia nervosa: Evidence of shared liability and transmission of partial syndromes. *Am. J. Psychiatry* **157,** 393–401.

18. Kendler, S. K., MacLean, C., Neale, M., Kessler, R., Heath, A., and Eaves, L. (1991). The genetic epidemiology of bulimia nervosa. *Am. J. Psychiatry* **148,** 1627–1637.

19. Walters, E. E., and Kendler, K. S. (1995). Anorexia nervosa and anorexic-like syndromes in a population-based twin sample. *Am. J. Psychiatry* **152,** 64–71.

20. Strober, M. (1991). Family-genetic studies of eating disorders. *J. Clin. Psychiatry* **52,** 9–12.

21. Kaye, W. H., Lilenfeld, L. R., Plotnicov, K., Merikangas, K. R., Nagy, L., Strober, M., Bulik, C. M., Moss, H., and Greeno, C. G. (1996). Bulimia nervosa and substance dependence: Association and family transmission. *Alcohol Clin. Exp. Res.* **20,** 878–881.

22. Schuckit, M. A., Tipp, J. E., Anthenelli, R. M., Bucholz, K. K., Hesselbrock, V. M., and Nurnberger, J. l. (1996). Anorexia nervosa and bulimia nervosa in alcohol-dependent men and women and their relatives. *Am. J. Psychiatry* **153,** 74–82.

23. Kendler, K. S., Walters, E. E., Neale, M. C., Kessler, R. C., Heath, A. C., and Eaves, L. J. (1995). The structure of the genetic and environmental risk factors for six major psychiatric disorders in women. *Arch. Gen. Psychiatry* **52,** 374–383.

24. Casper, R. C. (1990). Personality features of women with good outcome from restricting anorexia nervosa. *Psychosom. Med.* **52,** 156–170.

25. O' Dwyer, A. M., Lucey, J. V., and Russell, G. F. (1996). Serotonin activity in anorexia nervosa after long-term weight restoration: Response to D-fenfluramine challenge. *Psycholog. Med.* **26,** 353–359.

26. Srinivasagam, N. M., Kaye, W. H., Plotnicov, K. H., Greeno, C., Weltzin, T. E., and Rao, R. (1995). Persistent perfectionism, symmetry, and exactness after long-term recovery from anorexia nervosa. *Am. J. Psychiatry* **152,** 1630–1634.

27. Strober, M. (1980). Personality and symptomatological features in young, nonchronic anorexia nervosa patients. *J. Psychosom. Res.* **24,** 353–359.

28. Collings, S., and King, M. (1994). Ten-year follow-up of 50 patients with bulimia nervosa. *Br. J. Psychiatry* **164,** 80–87.

29. Fallon, B. A., Walsh, B. T., Sadik, C., Saoud, J. B., and Lukasik, V. (1991). Outcome and clinical course in inpatient bulimic women: A 2- to 9-year follow-up study. *J. Clin. Psychiatry* **52,** 272–278.

30. Johnson-Sabine, E., Reiss, D., and Dayson, D. (1992). Bulimia nervosa: A 5-year follow-up study. *Psychological Med.* **22,** 951–959.

31. Kaye, W. H., Greeno, C. G., Moss H., Fernstrom, J., Fernstrom, M., Lilenfeld, L. R., Weltzin, T. E., and Mann, J. J. (1998). Alterations in serotonin activity and psychiatric symptoms after recovery from bulimia nervosa. *Arch. Gen. Psychiatry* **55,** 927–935.

32. Norring, C. E., and Sohlberg, S. S. (1993). Outcome, recovery, relapse and mortality across six years in patients with clinical eating disorders. *Acta Psychiatrica Scand.* **87,** 437–444.

33. Brewerton, T. D. (1995) Toward a unified theory of serotonin dysregulation in eating and related disorders. *Psychoneuroendocrinology* **20,** 561–590.

34. Jimerson, D. C., Lesem, M. D., Kaye, W. H., Hegg, A. P., and Brewerton, T. D. (1990) Eating disorders and depression: Is there a serotonin connection? *Biolog. Psychiatry* **28,** 443–454.

35. Kaye, W. H., Gwirtsman, H. E., George, D. T., and Ebert, M. H. (1991). Altered serotonin activity in anorexia nervosa after long-term weight restoration. *Arch. Gen. Psychiatry* **48,** 556–562.

36. Stein, D. J., Hollander, E., and Liebowitz, M. R. (1993). Neurobiology of impulsivity and impulse control disorders. *J. Neuropsychiatry Clin. Neurosci.* **5,** 9–17.

37. American Psychiatric Association (2000). Practice guidelines for the treatment of patients with eating disorders. *Am. J. Psychiatry* **157**(Suppl.), 1–39.

38. Obarzanek, E., Lesem, M. D., and Jimerson, D. C. (1994). Resting metabolic rate of anorexia nervosa patients during weight gain. *Am. J. Clin. Nutr.* **60,** 666–675.

39. Casper, R. C., Schoeller, D. A., Kushner, R., Hnilicka, J., and Gold, S. T. (1991). Total daily energy expenditure and activity level in anorexia nervosa. *Am. J. Clin. Nutr.* **53,** 1143–1150.

40. Krahn, D. D., Rock, C. L., Dechert, R. E., Nairn, K. K., and Hasse, S. A. (1993). Changes in resting energy expenditure in anorexia nervosa patients during refeeding. *J. Am. Diet. Assoc.* **93,** 434–438.

41. Neuberger, S. K., Rao, R., Welstzin, T. E., Greeno, C., and Kaye, W. H. (1995). Differences in weight gain between restrictor and bulimic anorectics. *Int. J. Eating Disord.* **17,** 331–335.

42. Rock, C. L., and Curran-Celentano, J. (1996). Nutritional management of eating disorders. *Psych. Clin. N. Am.* **19,** 701–713.

43. Becker, A. E., Grinspoon, S. K., Kubanski, A., and Herzog, D. B. (1999). Eating disorders. *N. Engl. J. Med.* **340,** 1092–1098.

44. Gold, P. W., Gwirtsman, H., Avgerinos, P. C., Neiman, L. K., Gallucci, W. T., Kaye, W., Jimerson, D., Ebert, M., Rittmaster, R., Loriaux, L., and Chrousos, G. P. (1986). Abnormal hypothalamic–pituitary–adrenal function in anorexia nervosa. *N. Engl. J. Med.* **314,** 1335–1342.

45. Rock, C. L., and Swendseid, M. E. (1993). Plasma carotenoid levels in anorexia nervosa and in obese patients. *Methods. Enzymol.* **214,** 116–123.

46. Van Binsbergen, C. J. M., Okink, J., Van Den Berg, H., Koppeschaar, H., and Bennink, H. J. T. C. (1988). Nutritional status in anorexia nervosa: Clinical chemistry, vitamins, iron and zinc. *Eur. J. Clin. Nutr.* **42,** 929–937.

47. Langan, S. M., and Farrell, P. M. (1985). Vitamin E, vitamin A and essential fatty acid status of patients hospitalized for anorexia nervosa. *Am. J. Clin. Nutr.* **41,** 1054–1060.

48. Phillipp, E., Pirke, K. M., Seidl, M., Tuschl, R. J., Fichter, M. M., Eckert, M., and Wolfram, G. (1988). Vitamin status in patients with anorexia nervosa and bulimia nervosa. *Int. J. Eating Disord.* **8,** 209–218.

49. Rock, C. L., and Vasantharajan, S. (1995). Vitamin status of eating disorder patients: Relationship to clinical indices and effect of treatment. *Int. J. Eating Disord.* **18,** 257–262.

50. Capo-chichi, C. D., Gueant, J. L., Lefebvre, E., Bennani, N., Lorentz, E., Vidailhet, C., and Vidailhet, M. (1999). Riboflavin and riboflavin-derived cofactors in adolescent girls with anorexia nervosa. *Am. J. Clin. Nutr.* **69,** 672–678.

51. Grinspoon, S., Herzog, D., and Klibanski, A. (1997). Mechanisms and treatment options for bone loss in anorexia nervosa. *Psychopharmacol. Bull.* **33,** 399–404.

52. Bachrach, L. K., Katzman, D. K., Litt, I. F., Guido, D., and Marcus, R. (1991). Recovery from osteopenia in adolescent girls with anorexia nervosa. *J. Clin. Endocrin. Metab.* **72,** 602–606.

53. Herzog, W., Minne, H., Deter, C., Leidig, G., Schellberg, D., Wuster, C., Gronwald, R., Sarembe, E., Kroger, F., Bergmann, G., Petzold, E., Hahn, P., Schepank, H., and Ziegler, R. (1993). Outcome of bone mineral density in anorexia nervosa patients 11. 7 years after first admission. *J. Bone Miner. Res.* **8,** 597–605.

54. Ward, A., Brown, N., and Treasure, J. (1997). Persistent osteopenia after recovery from anorexia nervosa. *Int. J. Eating Disord.* **22,** 71–75.

55. Carmichael, K. A., and Carmichael, D. H. (1995). Bone metabolism and osteopenia in eating disorders. *Medicine* **74,** 254–267.

56. Klibanski, A., Biller, B. M. K., Schoenfeld, D. A., Herzog, D. B., and Saxe, V. C. (1995). The effects of estrogen administration on trabecular bone loss in young women with anorexia nervosa. *J. Clin. Endocrinol. Metab.* **89,** 898–904.

57. Goebel, G., Schweiger, U., Kruger, R., and Fichter, M. M. (1999). Predictors of bone mineral density in patients with eating disorders. *Int. J. Eating Disord.* **25,** 143–150.

58. Hay, P. J., Delahunt, J. W., Hall. A., Mitchell, A. X., Harger, G., and Salmond, C. (1992). Predictors of osteopenia in premenopausal women with anorexia nervosa. *Calcif. Tissue Int.* **50,** 498–501.

59. Beumont, P. J. V., Russell, J. D., and Touyz, S. W. (1993). Treatment of anorexia nervosa. *Lancet* **341,** 1635–1640.

60. Rock, C. L. (1997). Nutritional management of anorexia and bulimia nervosa. *Balliere's Clin. Psychiatry* **3,** 259–273.

61. Rock, C. L., and Yager, J. (1987). Nutrition and eating disorders: a primer for clinicians. *Int. J. Eating Disord.* **6,** 267–280.

62. Orphanidou, C. I., McCargar, L. J., Birmingham, C. L., and Belzberg, A. S. (1997). Changes in body composition and fat distribution after short-term weight gain in patients with anorexia nervosa. *Am. J. Clin. Nutr.* **65,** 1034–1041.

63. Russell, J. D., Mira, M., Allen, B. J., Stewart, P. M., Vizzard, J., Arthur, B., and Beaumont, P. J. V. (1994). Protein repletion and treatment in anorexia nervosa. *Am. J. Clin. Nutr.* **59,** 98–102.

64. Trocki, O., and Shepherd, R. W. (2000). Change in body mass index does not predict change in body composition in adolescent girls with anorexia nervosa. *J. Am. Diet. Assoc.* **100,** 457–459.

65. Birmingham, C. L., Alothman, A. F., and Goldner, E. M. (1996). Anorexia nervosa: Refeeding and hypophosphatemia. *Int. J. Eating Disord.* **20,** 211–213.

66. Food and Nutrition Board (1997). "Dietary Reference Intakes for Calcium, Phosphorus, Magnesium, Vitamin D, and Fluoride." National Academy Press, Washington, DC.

67. Herzog, D. B., Keller, M. B., Strober, M., Yeh, C. J., and Pai, S. Y. (1992). The current status of treatment for anorexia nervosa and bulimia nervosa. *Int. J. Eating Disord.* **12,** 215–220.

68. Russell, G. F., Szmukler, G. I., Dare, C., and Eisler, I. (1987). An evaluation of family therapy in anorexia nervosa and bulimia nervosa. *Arch. Gen. Psychiatry* **44,** 1047–1056.

69. Jimerson, D. C., Wolfe, B. E., Brotman, A. W., and Metzger, E. D. (1996). Medications in the treatment of eating disorders. *Psych. Clin. N. Am.* **19,** 739–754.

70. Mitchell, J. E., Raymond, N., and Specker, S. (1993). A review of controlled trials of pharmacotherapy and psychotherapy in the treatment of bulimia nervosa. *Int. J. Eating Disord.* **14,** 229–247.

71. Walsh, B. T. (1991). Psychopharmacological treatment of bulimia nervosa. *J. Clin. Psychiatry* **52,** 34–38

72. Treasure, J., Todd, G., Brolly, M., Tiller, J., Nehmed, A., and Denman, F. (1995). A pilot study of a randomized trial of cognitive analytical therapy vs educational behavioral therapy for adult anorexia nervosa. *Behav. Res. Ther.* **33,** 363–367.

73. Kaye, W. H., Weltzin, T. E., Hsu, L. K. G., and Bulik, C. M. (1991). An open trial of fluoxetine in patients with anorexia nervosa. *J. Clin. Psychiatry* **52,** 464–471.

74. Kaye, W. H., Nagata, T., Hsu, L. K. G., Sokol, M. S., McConaha, C., Plotnicov, K. H., Weise, J., and Deep, D. (In press). Double-blind placebo-controlled administration of fluoxetine in restricting-type anorexia nervosa. *Am. J. Psychiatry.*

75. Attia, E., Haiman, C., Walsh, B. T., and Flater, S. R. (1998). Does fluoxetine augment the inpatient treatment of anorexia nervosa? *Am. J. Psychiatry* **155,** 548–551.

76. Ferguson, C. P., La Via, M. C., Crossan, P. J., and Kaye, W. H. (1999). Are SSRI's effective in underweight anorexia nervosa? *Int. J. Eating Disord.* **25,** 11–17.

77. Tollefson, G. D. (1995). Selective serotonin reuptake inhibitors. *In* Textbook of Psychopharmacology'' (A. F. Schatzberg and C. B. Nemeroff, Eds.), pp. 161–182. American Psychiatric Press, Washington, DC.

78. Kaye, W. H., Ebert, M. H., Raleigh, M., and Lake, R. (1984). Abnormalities in CNS monoamine metabolism in anorexia nervosa. *Arch. Gen. Psychiatry* **41,** 350–355.

79. Schweiger, U., Warnhoff, M., Pahl, J., and Pirke, K. M. (1986). Effects of carbohydrate and protein meals on plasma large neutral amino acids, glucose, and insulin levels of anorexic patients. *Metabolism* **35,** 938–943.

80. Anderson, I. M., Parry-Billings, M., Newsholme, E. A., Fairburn, C. G., and Cowen, P. J. (1990). Dieting reduces plasma tryptophan and alters brain 5-HT function in women. *Psycholog. Med.* **20,** 785–791.

81. Haleem, D. J., and Haider, S. (1996). Food restriction decreases serotonin and its synthesis rate in the hypothalamus. *Neuro. Report* **7,** 1153–1155.

82. Delgado, P. L., Price, L. H., Aghajanian, G. K., Landis, H., and Heninger, G. R. (1990). Serotonin function and the mechanism of antidepressant action. Reversal of antidepressant-induced remission by rapid depletion of plasma tryptophan. *Arch. Gen. Psychiatry* **47,** 411–418.

83. Kales, E. F. (1990). Macronutrient analysis of binge eating in bulimia. *Physiol. Behav.* **43,** 837–840.

84. Heatherington, M. M., Altemus, M., and Nelson, M. L. (1994). Eating behavior in bulimia nervosa: Multiple meal analyses. *Am. J. Clin. Nutr.* **60,** 864–873.

85. Kaye, W. H., Weltzin, T. E., Hsu, L. K., McConaha, C. W., and Bolton, B. (1993). Amount of calories retained after binge eating and vomiting. *Am. J. Psychiatry* **150,** 969–971.

86. Colton, P., Woodside, D. B., and Kaplan, A. S. (1999). Laxative withdrawal in eating disorders: treatment protocol and 3- to 20-month follow-up. *Int. J. Eating Disord.* **25,** 311–317.

87. Bo-Linn, G. W., Santa Ana, C. A., Morawski, S. G., and Fordtran, J. S. (1983). Purging and calorie absorption in bulimic patients and normal women. *Ann. Intern. Med.* **99,** 14–17.

88. Chami, T. N., Anderson, A. E., Crowell, M. D., Schuster, M. M., and Whitehead, W. E. (1995). Gastrointestinal symptoms in bulimia nervosa: Effects of treatment. *Am. J. Gastroenterol.* **90,** 88–92.

89. Palmer, E. P., and Guay, A. T. (1985). Reversible myopathy secondary to abuse of ipecac in patients with major eating disorders. *N. Engl. J. Med.* **313,** 1457–1459.

90. Bouquot, J. E., and Seime, R. J. (1997). Bulimia nervosa: Dental perspectives. *Prac. Periodont. Aesth. Dentistry* **9,** 655–663.

91. Fairburn, C. G., Marcus, M. D., and Wilson, G. T. (1993). Cognitive-behavioral therapy for binge eating and bulimia nervosa. *In* "Binge Eating, " (C. B. Fairburn and G. T. Wilson, Eds.), pp. 361–404. Guilford Press, New York.

92. Arnow, B. (1997). Psychotherapy of anorexia and bulimia. *Balliere's Clin. Psych.* **3,** 235–257.

93. Agras, W. S., Rossiter, E. M., Arnow, B., Schneider, J. A., Telch, C. F., Raeburn, S. D., Bruc, B., Perl, M., and Koran, L. M. (1992). Pharmacologic and cognitive-behavioral treatment for bulimia nervosa: A controlled comparison. *Am. J. Psychiatry* **149,** 82–87.

94. Fichter, M. M., Leibl, K., Rief, W., Brunner, E., Schmidt-Auberger, S., and Engel, R. R. (1991). Fluoxetine versus placebo: a double-blind study with bulimic inpatients undergoing intensive psychotherapy. *Pharmacopsychiatry* **24,** 1–7.

95. Goldbloom, D. S., Olmsted, M., Davis, R., Clewes, J., Heinmaa, M., Rockert, W., and Shaw, B. (1997). A randomized controlled trial of fluoxetine and cognitive behavioral therapy for bulimia nervosa: Short-term outcome. *Behav. Res. Ther.* **35,** 803–811.

96. Leitenberg, J., Rosen, J. C., Wolf, J., Vara, L. S., Detzer, M. J., and Srebnik, D. (1994). Comparison of cognitive-behavior therapy and desipramine in the treatment of bulimia nervosa. *Behav. Res. Ther.* **32,** 37–45.

97. Mitchell, J. E., Pyle, R. L., Eckert, E. D., Hatsukami, D., Pomeroy, C., and Zimmerman, R. (1990). A comparison study of antidepressants and structured intensive group psychotherapy in the treatment of bulimia nervosa. *Arch. Gen. Psychiatry* **47,** 149–157.

98. Walsh, B. T., Wilson, G. O., Leob, K. L., Devlin, M. J., Pike, K. M., Roose, S. P., Fleiss, J., and Waternaux, C. (1997). Medication and psychotherapy in the treatment of bulimia nervosa. *Am. J. Psychiatry* **154,** 523–531.

99. Walsh, B. T., and Garner, D. M. (1997). Diagnostic issues. *In* "Handbook of Treatment for Eating Disorders," 2nd ed. (D. M. Garner, and P. E. Garfinkel, Eds.), pp. 25–33. Guilford Press, New York.

100. Baker, C. W., and Brownell, K. D. (1999). Binge eating disorder: Identification and management. *Nutr. Clin. Care* **2,** 344–353.

101. Devlin, M. J. (1996). Assessment and treatment of binge-eating disorder. *Psych. Clin. N. Am.* **19,** 761–772.

102. Marcus, M. D. (1997). Adapting treatment for patients with binge-eating disorder. *In* "Handbook of Treatment for Eating Disorders," 2nd ed. (D. M. Garner and P. E. Garfinkel, Eds.), pp. 484–493. Guilford Press, New York.

103. Telch, C. F., Agras, W. S., and Rossiter, E. M. (1988). Binge eating increases with increasing adiposity. *Int. J. Eating Disord.* **7,** 115–119.

104. Marcus, M. D., Wing, R. R., Ewing, L., Kern, E., Gooding, W., and McDermott, M. (1996). Psychiatric disorders among obese binge eaters. *Int. J. Eating Disord.* **19,** 45–52.

105. Yanovski, S. Z., Nelson, J. E., Dubbert, B. K., and Spitzer, R. L. (1993). Association of binge eating disorder and psychiatric comorbidity in obese subjects. *Am. J. Psychiatry* **150,** 1472–1479.

106. Spitzer, R. L., Yanovski, S. Z., Wadden, T., Wing, R., Marcus, M. D., Stunkard, A., Devlin, M., Mitchell, J., Hasin, D., and Horne, R. L. (1993). Binge eating disorder: Its further validation in a multisite study. *Int. J. Eating Disord.* **13,** 137–153.

107. Smith, D. E., Marcus, M. D., Lewis, C., Fitzgibbon, M., and Schreiner, P. (1998). Prevalence of binge eating disorder, obesity, and depression in a biracial cohort of young adults. *Ann. Behav. Med.* **20,** 277–232.

108. Smith, D. E. (1995). Binge eating in racial minority groups. *Addict. Behav.* **20,** 695–703.

109. Wilson, G. T., Nonas, C. A., and Rosenblum, G. D. (1993). Assessment of binge-eating in obese patients. *Int. J. Eating Disord.* **13,** 25–33.

110. Mussell, M. P., Mitchell, J. E., Weller, C. L., Raymond, N. C., Crow, S. F., and Crosby, R. D. (1995). Onset of binge eating, dieting, obesity, and mood disorders among subjects seeking treatment for binge eating disorder. *Int. J. Eating Disord.* **17,** 395–410.

111. Marcus, M. D., Wing, R. R., and Fairburn, C. G. (1995). Cognitive treatment of binge eating versus behavioral weight control in the treatment of binge eating disorder. *Ann. Behav. Med.* **17,** S090.

112. Wilfley, D. E., Agras, W. S., Telch, C. F., Rossiter, E. M., Schneider, J. A., Cole, A. G., Sifford, L. A., and Raeburn, S. D. (1993). Group cognitive-behavioral therapy and group interpresonal therapy for the nonpurging bulimic individual: A controlled comparison. *J. Consult. Clin. Psychol.* **61,** 296–305.

113. Carter, J. C., and Fairburn, C. G. (1998). Cognitive-behavioral self-help for binge eating disorder: A controlled effectiveness study. *J. Consult. Clin. Psychol.* **66,** 616–623.

114. Tech, C. F., Agras, W. S., Rossiter, E. M., Wilfley, D., and Kenardy, J. (1990). Group cognitive-behavioral treatment for the nonpurging bulimic: An initial evaluation. *J. Consult. Clin. Psych.* **58,** 629–635.

115. Pike, K. M. (1998). Long-term course of anorexia nervosa: Response, relapse, remission, and recovery. *Clin. Psychol. Rev.* **18,** 447–475.

116. Strober, M., Freeman, R., and Morrell, W. (1997). The long-term course of severe anorexia nervosa in adolescents: Survival analysis of recovery, relapse, and outcome predictors over 10–15 years in a prospective study. *Int. J. Eating Disord.* **22,** 339–360.

117. Zipfel, S., Lowe, B., Reas, D. L., Deter, H. C., and Herzog, W. (2000). Long-term prognosis in anorexia nervosa: lessons from a 21-year follow-up study. *Lancet* **355,** 721–722.

118. Herzog, D. B., Nussbaum, K. M., and Marmor, A. K. (1996). Comorbidity and outcome in eating disorders. *Psych. Clin. N. Am.* **19,** 843–859.

119. Keel, P. K., Mitchell, J. E., Miller, K. B., Davis, T. L., and Crow, S. J. (1999). Long-term outcome of bulimia nervosa. *Arch. Gen. Psychiatry* **56,** 63–69.

120. Fichter, M. M., Quadflieg, N., and Gnutzmann, A. (1998). Binge eating disorder: Treatment outcome over a 6-year course. *J. Psychosom. Res.* **44,** 385–405.

121. Huon, G. F., Braganza, C., Brown, L. B., Richie J. E., and Roncolato, W. G. (1998). Reflections on prevention in dieting-induced disorders. *Int. J. Eating Disord.* **23,** 455–458.

122. Rosen, D. S., and Neumark-Sztainer, D. (1998). Review of options for primary prevention of eating disturbances among adolescents. *J Adolesc. Health* **23,** 354–363.

123. Schwitzer, A. M., Bergholz, K., Dore, T., and Salimi, L. (1998). Eating disorders among college women: Prevention, education, and treatment responses. *J. Am. College Health* **46,** 199–207.

124. Neumark-Sztainer, D. (1996). School-based programs for preventing eating disturbances. *J. School Health* **66,** 64–71.

125. Killen, J. D., Taylor, B. C., Hammer, L. D., Litt, I., Wilson, D. M., Rich, T., Hayward, C., Simmonds, B., Krawmer, H., and Varady, A. (1993). An attempt to modify unhealthful eating attitudes and weight regulation practices of young adolescent girls. *Int. J. Eating Disord.* **13,** 369–384.

126. Huon, G. F. (1994). Towards the prevention of dieting-induced disorders: Modifying negative food- and body-related attitudes. *Int. J. Eating Disord.* **16,** 395–399.

CHAPTER **44**

Nutrition and Food Allergy

ABBA I. TERR
San Francisco, California

I. INTRODUCTION

Food is the primary source of nutrients required for maintaining the structure and continued functioning of the body. It is also a potential source of disease. Excessive, insufficient, or improper balance of foods in the diet may cause pathologic conditions such as obesity or malnutrition. Foods and their natural or artificial additives and contaminants can be the source of infection, toxic diseases, or allergy.

Food allergy has been recognized since antiquity. It is based on the fact that foods are chemically foreign to the body. An allergic reaction can range in severity from an annoyance to death. Thus, diagnosing food allergy and identifying the specific food that caused it are essential, so that future reactions can be avoided.

Food allergy is a confusing and often misunderstood subject. It is frequently misdiagnosed. This chapter will focus on the mechanisms of disease and the methods of diagnosis and treatment that are based on current scientific evidence.

II. DEFINITIONS

Confusion about what constitutes food allergy occurs among medical professionals as well as the public. This can often be traced to a lack of precise terminology and clear understanding of physiologic mechanisms of food-induced disease.

Adverse reactions are any conditions—whether pathologic or only subjective—that occur when a particular food is eaten. *Food allergy* is one of main adverse reactions and refers to disease in which a component of food, most often a protein, is an antigen that induces an immune response in the patient. The antigen responsible for allergy is called an *aller-gen*. Not all immune responses to food antigens result in allergy.

Allergy refers to immune responses to environmental allergens that result in inflammation detrimental to the patient. In contrast, *immunity* refers to immune responses that protect from infectious microorganisms or toxic chemicals.

There are a number of allergic diseases, reflecting the complexity of the immune response. They are classified by the Gell and Coombs system, which is based on the particular immune pathway involved in the disease (Table 1). This classification system is fully discussed later in the chapter.

Food intolerance is the term used by allergists for adverse reactions that are not allergic. Certain foods contain chemicals that have *pharmacologic* effects, such as caffeine in coffee causing stimulation, or histamine-like compounds in wines causing flushing and headache (Table 2). Some persons are susceptible to these effects, while others are not. Those who are may misinterpret their symptoms as an allergy. *Toxicity* is likewise a direct effect of either a naturally occurring chemical in the food, such as mushroom poisoning, or a toxin from a bacterial contaminant, such as the *Staphyloccocus* or *Escherichia coli*.

III. THE IMMUNE RESPONSE AND ALLERGY

The immune response is a complicated process by which the immune system generates both antibodies and sensitized lymphocytes that recognize a specific antigen. Antibodies are referred to chemically as *immunoglobulins*. The five different classes of immunoglobulin molecules are IgG, IgA, IgM, IgD, and IgE. Antibodies of the IgG class are the most

TABLE 1 Gell and Coombs Classification of Allergic Diseases

Type	Immune reactant	Class	Mediator	Reaction
I	Antibody	IgE	Mast cell	Imflammation
II	Antibody	IgG/IgM	Complement	Cytolysis
III	Antibody	IgG/IgM	Complement	Inflammation
IV	Sensitized cell	T lymphocyte	Cytokines	Inflammation

TABLE 2   Some Foods with Naturally Occurring Chemicals That May
Simulate the Effects of Allergy

Chemical	Food	Effect
Histamine	Parmesan, Roquefort cheeses Spinach Eggplant Red wines Some Chinese food	Increased vascular permeability, vasodilatation, pruritus
Caffeine	Coffee Cola	Central nervous system stimulation
Tyramine	Cheese	Headache
Phenylethylamine	Cheese Red wine Chocolate	Central nervous system stimulation
Serotonin	Banana Avocado Tomato	Central nervous system stimulation
Theobromine	Chocolate	Central nervous system stimulation

abundant in the serum and are responsible for long-lasting immunity. IgM antibodies are the ones that are produced first during the immune response. IgE antibodies are responsible for the most common forms of allergic diseases. Because immune responses are normal processes, small amounts of antibodies to foods are normal and do not cause disease or interfere with health.

Specificity and cross-reactivity are important concepts in allergic disease. *Specificity* refers to the ability of the immune system to recognize very small differences between "foreign" proteins (i.e., those from the environment) and proteins that exist in the person's own body. Each individual's immune responses are determined by his or her genetic makeup. This fact is especially evident when immunologic rejection of a tissue or organ graft occurs.

Cross-reactivity arises when two or more different proteins have the same or closely similar chemical structure so that they are recognized by the same antibody. There are numerous examples, especially among food allergens and among allergens in foods and other environmental substances, such as pollens and natural rubber latex (Table 3).

Any food protein is a potential allergen. Nevertheless, the majority of people tolerate all of the food proteins they eat, even though these protein products are rapidly and efficiently absorbed from the gastrointestinal mucosa and reach the systemic circulation, from where they have access to the immune system. The immune system does, in fact, recognize many food protein products as antigenic and does make specific IgG, IgA, and IgM antibodies and T-cell immune responses to them. However, these are normal and do not cause disease. They may be present in higher amounts in infants who are weaned early.

The gastrointestinal tract has a unique immune system of its own, called the gastrointestinal associated lymphoid tis-

sue, which is a part of the larger mucosal associated lymphoid tissue of the gastrointestinal tract, respiratory mucosa, and the ductal tissue of the mammary gland during lactation. Gastrointestinal associated lymphoid tissue consists of lymphoid tissue that includes the Peyer's patches of the intestinal mucosa, the lymphoid follicles in the appendix, lymphocytes and plasma cells in the intestinal lamina propria, the intraepithelial lymphocytes, and the mesenteric lymph nodes.

A unique feature of gastrointestinal associated lymphoid tissue is the production of secretory IgA antibodies (sIgA). These antiodies form molecular complexes with their corresponding food antigens (Ag). The Ag–sIgA complexes are retained in the glycocalyx, slowing absorption of food antigens and promoting digestion by proteolytic enzymes.

Immunological tolerance refers to the failure of the immune system to respond to an antigen. An individual's own protein molecules (and other potential allergens) are normally in a state of immunologic self-tolerance. There are certain "autoimmune" diseases, such as systemic lupus erythematosus, in which self-tolerance to some of the body's natural chemicals is lost, so that the immune system produces autoantibodies and autoimmune disease. *Oral tolerance* can be produced experimentally in animals by the oral administration of antigen. This causes a decreased or absent systemic immune response. It requires a high dose of antigen, and the effect is specific for that antigen only and is not a general immune depression. The significance of oral tolerance as a normal process is not certain. However, eating food exposes the immune system to large oral quantities of potential food antigens, so it is possible that oral immunologic tolerance to foods may be necessary for normal health.

It has been postulated that a decrease in oral tolerance to foods may enhance production of IgE antibodies and lead to food allergy. Several studies show that exclusive breast feed-

TABLE 3 Cross-Reactivity of Foods and Other Allergens

Other allergens	Foods
Pollens	
Ragweed	Melons
	Banana
Birch	Apple
	Pear
	Potato
	Hazelnut
	Carrot
	Celery
	Kiwi
Mugwort	Celery
Natural rubber latex	Banana
	Chestnut
	Avocado
	Kiwi

ing increases oral tolerance and helps prevent food allergy. Although this is theoretical, allergists and pediatricians encourage breast feeding, hoping to prevent or delay the development of allergy in infants.

A. The Allergic Response

Allergy is a two-step process. The first step is *sensitization.* The immune system recognizes a foreign protein (e.g., in a food) as an antigen when it enters the body. It generates an immune response consisting of specific antibodies or specifically sensitized T lymphocytes. The antibodies or lymphocytes are "specific" because they carry the information needed to recognize the corresponding antigen. If the antibody is an IgE antibody, it will respond to the presence of the allergen by generating an inflammatory reaction, called *allergy.* Thus, allergy refers to disease and not simply to the existence of antibodies.

The distinction between sensitization (sensitivity) and allergy is important. An allergy test is not a test of allergic disease. It shows sensitization, i.e., that a person has the specific antibodies or T cells being tested. Sensitization is necessary but not alone sufficient to have an allergic disease. Many people have specific antibodies to one or more food allergens, yet they have no reaction when eating the food. Treatment, including elimination diets, must not be recommended on the basis of a positive allergy test only.

B. Types of Allergic Diseases

The classification of allergic diseases is based on the mechanisms of immunopathology and, therefore, the clinical manifestations (Table 1). A description of these mechanisms and their resulting diseases follows.

Type I reactions are mediated by IgE antibodies that react with the allergen on tissue mast cells or circulating basophils. Once the interaction between the allergen and the IgE antibody occurs, these cells rapidly generate and release certain chemical mediators, such as histamine, which results in pathologic effects locally or systemically. These mediators have effects on blood vessels causing vasodilatation, which causes erythema and, if extensive, could lead to hypotension and shock. Cutaneous effects almost invariably result in pruritus and flushing, usually accompanied by urticaria and/or angioedema because of increased vascular permeability. Airborne allergens cause conjunctival and eyelid itching, rhinitis, and bronchospasm. Orally ingested allergens cause itching and swelling of the lips, tongue, and palate; laryngeal edema; and gastrointestinal smooth muscle spasm resulting in vomiting, diarrhea, and pain. Obviously, not all of these effects necessarily occur with each allergen exposure. If the exposure is by injection or oral ingestion, multiple organs may be involved, and this is referred to as systemic anaphylaxis.

Type II reactions are mediated by IgG or IgM antibodies, which have the property of activating the complement system when combined with antigen to form immune complexes. If the antigen is on a cell, such as a virus or a transfused red blood cell, complement activation causes lysis (destruction) of the cell. This is useful in responding to a viral infection, but undesirable in the case of a mismatched blood transfusion. Type II allergic reactions are caused by drugs that bind to the patient's blood cells, and they have been postulated to occur in very rare instances of milk-induced thrombocytopenia.

Type III reactions also involve IgG or IgM antibodies and complement, but in this case the result is tissue or organ inflammation. This mechanism may be important in celiac disease and dermatitis herpetiformis. It has also been attributed to a form of food allergy in some cases of arthritis, pulmonary hemosiderosis, and intestinal blood loss, but so far without scientifically supportive evidence.

Type IV reactions are cell-mediated forms of hypersensitivity that do not involve antibodies. This is the mechanism of allergic contact dermatitis, but the same mechanism has been postulated as contributing to celiac disease, dermatitis herpetiformis, enterocolitis, and even some cases of malabsorption.

Atopy is the most common manifestation of type I allergy, affecting about 20% of the population who produce IgE antibodies to certain proteins from organic sources in the everyday environment. The allergens include organic airborne particles: pollens of trees, grasses, and weeds; mold spores; the house dust mite; and emanations from animals, such as cats, dogs, and horses. They also include—but to a lesser extent—some of the natural proteins in foods. The atopic diseases are allergic rhinitis, bronchial asthma, and atopic dermatitis. One or more may coexist in the same patient. A number of genes predispose to atopy, so the condition is often familial. In the 80% of the population without the genetic predisposition to atopy, no amount of natural exposure to allergens in pollens, molds, dust, or foods will induce the

formation of specific IgE antibodies and atopic disease. Atopic persons frequently have IgE antibodies to food allergens that sensitize without causing clinical allergic disease.

Anaphylaxis, a less common form of type I allergy, is a systemic disease caused by IgE antibodies that is a medical emergency with a rapid appearance of urticaria, angioedema, bronchospasm, shock, and effects on other organs. It may be fatal. The allergens that are most often responsible for anaphylaxis are proteins and nonprotein organic chemicals, especially drugs, foods, and venom from *Hymenoptera* stinging insects. Exposure is therefore by injection or ingestion. Rarely, in a highly sensitive patient, inhalation or contact of the allergen on a mucous membrane or on the skin may trigger anaphylaxis. *Urticaria/angioedema* is a limited form of anaphylaxis involving the skin only, and it is caused by similar allergens. Anaphylaxis and urticaria/angioedema may affect either atopic or nonatopic persons.

Serum sickness is a disease characterized by skin rash, joint inflammation, and fever. It is an allergic reaction to drugs but has never been clearly associated with foods. It is caused by IgG or IgM antibodies, which activate the complement system, generating systemic inflammation. It resolves when the patient discontinues using the drug that caused the disease.

Allergic contact dermatitis is an acute inflammatory disease of the skin causing redness, swelling, papules, vesicles, and scaling that appears directly on the area of skin in contact with the allergen. It does not involve antibodies, but is caused by a particular immune cell, the effector T lymphocyte, that specifically recognizes the contact allergen. The most common contact allergen is urushiol, a chemical in poison ivy, poison oak, and poison sumac. Allergic contact dermatitis is also frequently caused by allergens in jewelry, perfumes, cosmetics, rubber products, some topical medications, and other items that may contact the skin. Allergic contact dermatitis can also be caused by food allergy, in which a skin eruption appears where the food has contacted the skin, primarily around the mouth in infants and on the hands as an occupational disease of food handlers. Unlike diseases caused by IgE antibodies, which begin within minutes after exposure to the allergen, allergic contact dermatitis caused by T lymphocytes requires many hours, typically 1 to several days, after skin contact with the food before the reaction begins. It is thus called *delayed hypersensitivity,* and the delayed latency period makes diagnosing the condition more challenging. IgE-mediated allergic diseases, both atopy and anaphylaxis, are often referred to an *immediate hypersensitivity.*

IV. PREVALENCE OF FOOD ALLERGY

Food allergy is much less common than is perceived by the general public. A number of surveys indicate that about 20% of the population consider themselves to be allergic to foods [1, 2]. However, subjective self-diagnosis cannot be con-

firmed scientifically in a vast majority of these cases. Research by allergy specialists who base a definitive diagnosis on an expert history and examination, proper testing, and confirmation by double-blind placebo-controlled food challenge—the "gold standard" for diagnosis—reveals a more accurate estimate that only 1–2% of adults have bona fide food allergy [3]. Furthermore, the prevalence of food allergy differs among different population groups. It depends on age (most common prior to age 2), atopy (more common, especially in patients with atopic dermatitis), diet (availability of particular foods, depending on geography and culture), breast feeding practices and the presence of other diseases. Anaphylaxis, the most serious form of food allergy, occurs in 0.004% of the U.S. population (1 in 250,000).

Allergy to food additives is difficult to estimate because different criteria have been used for diagnosis, but most studies report that it affects between 0.01% and 0.20% in the general population [4], although one report from Denmark documented a 1–2% prevalence in schoolchildren [5]. These figures may be much higher than the true prevalence as determined by blinded placebo-controlled food challenge.

There is also a strong public perception that food additives frequently cause allergy [6]. Estimates of prevalence vary at least 100-fold and are related to the type of data with subjective reports being the least reliable. Double-blind challenges are the only reliable methods for accurate diagnosis. Based on challenge data, prevalence in atopic children is 1–2%, in atopic adults <0.15% but possibly as low as 0.03%. This includes all adverse reported events, many of which are not allergic, such as subjective headache and behavioral/mood changes [6].

V. FOOD ALLERGENS

Any food is potentially allergenic, but certain foods cause allergic reactions more commonly than others. In almost all cases the allergen is a protein, usually about 10,000–60,000 (10–60 kDa) in molecular weight. Each foodstuff typically contains a number of different proteins, but not all are allergens. The protein allergens in foods, like those in airborne particles such as pollens, often contain a small amount of carbohydrate and are therefore called glycoproteins, but the allergen is in the protein and not the carbohydrate portion of the molecule. The common allergens are called major and those found infrequently are considered minor.

Many common food allergen molecules have been isolated from food and purified. The purified allergens are named using an abbreviated form of the scientific name of their biologic source (Table 4).

Cow's milk contains numerous proteins, many of which have been identified as allergens [7]. They are present in both the casein and whey fractions. Pasteurization—flash heating to destroy pathogenic microbes—does not significantly denature the proteins, so the allergens survive this

TABLE 4 Nomenclature of Selected Food Allergens

Food	Allergen	Nomenclature
Cow (*Bos domesticus*) milk	Alpha-lactalbumin	Bos d 4
	Beta-lactoglobulin	Bos d 5
	Serum albumin	Bos d 6
Soy (*Glycine max*)	Hydrophobic seed protein	Gly m 1
	Profilin	Gly m 3
Chicken (*Gallus domesticus*) egg	Ovomucoid	Gal d 1
	Ovalbumin	Gal d 2
	Lysozyme	Gal d 4
Shrimp (*Metapeneus ensis*)	Tropomysin	Met e 1
Peanut (*Arachis hypogaea*)	Vicilin	Ara h 1
	Conglutin	Ara h 2
Lobster (*Panulirus stimpsoni*)	Tropomysin	Pan s 1
Cod (*Gadus callarias*)	Parvalbumin-beta	Gad c 1

process. Most patients with cow's milk allergy tolerate beef without reactions, even though they may have a positive skin test to beef. On the other hand, a high degree of cross-reactivity is seen with goat and sheep milk, so these may not be suitable substitutes in cases of cow's milk allergy.

Chicken egg allergy is almost always an allergy to the egg white and not the yolk. Egg white contains 23 different glycoproteins, and 4 of these are major allergens, of which ovomucoid is the most frequent [8]. Although most patients who are allergic to chicken egg can tolerate the chicken meat (muscle, skin), a few with exquisite anaphylactic sensitivity may react to the meat also. Cross-reactions with egg allergens from other birds, such as ducks, turkeys, and geese, are common [9].

Legumes are the most common foods causing food allergy in the United States. *Peanut* allergy is a particularly prominent cause of food-induced anaphylaxis and therefore the subject of considerable research interest. Sixteen allergenic proteins have been identified to date, and 3 of them are major peanut allergens. The allergenicity is not found in peanut oil, but it remains in processing of virtually all peanut products, such as flour. *Soybean* allergy occurs especially in children and infants, and this is a problem that must be considered in those infants fed on a soy-based formula because of their allergy or intolerance to cow's milk. Soy is extensively used in many food preparations because of its high protein content and low cost. Several allergenic soy proteins have been identified. These are not found in pure soybean oil, but some allergens are present in commercial sources of the oil, in lecithin preparations, and in margarines. There is extensive potential allergic cross-reaction among legumes when tested in the laboratory, but other legumes such as beans, peas, and licorice are far less likely to cause clinical allergic reactions. Most peanut-sensitive patients can tolerate other legumes [10].

Tree nuts cause allergy especially in adults. These include brazil nuts, cashews, filberts (hazelnut), hickory nuts, pecans, pine nuts, pistachios, and walnuts. Cross-reactions among these are common but not always present. There is no known allergenic cross-reactivity between any of these tree nuts and any legumes, including peanut.

Fish is very likely the most common type of food causing allergy in adults [11]. There are hundreds of edible species of fish, and cross-reactivity is extensive.

Crustaceans and mollusks are also important, although the majority of allergy-like reactions, especially urticaria and angioedema, are not immunologic. Allergenic cross-reactivity occurs among different crustaceans and among different mollusks, but not between them.

Cereal grains are a more important cause of allergy in children than in adults. They include wheat, barley, rye, oats, rice, corn, sorghum, and millet, accounting for 70% of the world protein consumption. The allergens vary by disease, e.g., globulin and glutenin in IgE oral allergy, and albumin in baker's asthma. Gliadin is the protein that causes celiac disease. Allergenic cross-reactivity among grains is common. Occupational food allergy is usually manifested as asthma, rhinitis, and/or dermatitis and is cased by inhalation of airborne flour dust. In baker's asthma, skin tests to cereal grains are positive in 54% of cases, whereas clinical disease occurs in only 20% [12]. Most patients wih baker's asthma have no reaction to the ingestion of the same food causing the asthma.

VI. CLINICAL MANIFESTATIONS OF FOOD ALLERGY

Allergic diseases from foods are best classified and understood on the basis of their immunologic mechanism (Table 1).

A. Type I—IgE-Mediated Allergic Diseases

IgE antibodies cause the large majority of well-documented food allergies. They are recognized by (1) the rapid onset of the clinical symptoms and signs following ingestion of the food, (2) objective evidence of allergic inflammation, and (3) evidence that the patient has the specific IgE antibody to the food that initiated the reaction. In some cases, the fact that the disease is caused by IgE antibody is supported by pathologic evidence of eosinophils in the affected tissue or organ and positive therapeutic response to appropriate medications. IgE-mediated reactions to foods, including anaphylaxis and urticaria, can be mimicked by certain chemicals present in some foods that are capable of causing nonallergic reactions.

Anaphylaxis is the most serious form of allergy because of the potential for a rapid fatal outcome. Food allergy is a frequent cause of anaphylaxis [13]. About 100 fatalities occur per year in the United States from food-induced anaphylaxis [14], and an estimated 1000 cases are severe but not fatal [10]. As a general rule, the more quickly the reaction begins after the food is eaten, the more severe the reaction will become. The amount of allergen causing anaphylaxis can be exceedingly small. The likelihood of a fatal outcome is increased in patients with asthma, even if the asthma is not active at the time of the reaction. Although atopic diseases (allergic rhinitis, asthma, atopic dermatitis) and anaphylaxis are both cased by IgE antibodies, atopy is not a prerequisite for anaphylaxis. Nevertheless, most patients with anaphylaxis to a food are in fact atopic. Anaphylaxis to a food affects females twice as often as males. In some infants, the reaction occurs on the first feeding of the food, in which case it is likely that sensitization occured from exposure to the allergen through breast feeding. In most cases, however, the patient reports a history of prior ingestion of the food without a reaction.

In nonfatal reactions, anaphylaxis can be mild to severe. The reaction may consist of pruritus, urticaria, angioedema, contact urticaria, erythema, laryngeal edema, rhinitis, conjunctivitis, bronchospasm, hypotension or shock, nausea, vomiting, abdominal cramps, diarrhea, and uterine or bladder cramps. Not all of these findings occur in every case, but at least two organ systems are involved. Immediate treatment is essential in order for the reaction to subside without permanent organ damage.

The allergist evaluating a patient for food anaphylaxis generally does so after the incident has passed and therefore relies on the patient's history. Review of an emergency room record, if available, will provide the necessary information to confirm the presence and severity of the reaction. The most common foods reported to cause anaphylaxis are wheat, shellfish, fruit, milk, celery, and fish. Although peanut and egg white are reported less frequently, they are especially important because minute amounts may be present in some food preparations in a form in which they are likely to be unknowingly ingested by a patient with a known allergy to that food. The allergen is particularly hidden when it is contained in a pastry, salad, sandwich, hors d'ouvres, or candy. Testing to confirm the specific food sensitivity is done by either the skin test method or by the radioallergosorbent test, which detects the specific IgE antibody in the patient's serum. Either test is usually highly reliable to confirm the specific sensitivity, and double-blind, placebo-controlled challenge is almost never used because of the potentially severe nature of this disease.

By definition, anaphylaxis is a systemic disease. However, the term *gastrointestinal anaphylaxis* may be used for a reaction that begins within minutes and less than 2 hours after ingestion of a food and results in symptoms of nausea, abdominal pain, cramps, vomiting, and sometimes diarrhea, but without any other symptoms or signs of systemic anaphylaxis. In some children with a mild form of this condition who eat the food frequently, it may cause poor appetite and abdominal pain.

Food-dependent, exercise-induced anaphylaxis is an IgE-mediated food reaction that occurs in a patient who exercises 2–3 hours or less either after or before eating a meal containing the food allergen [15–17]. In some cases, urticaria or anaphylaxis without other systemic effects may occur. Foods that are especially likely to be implicated in this rare disease are celery, shrimp, oyster, chicken, peach, and wheat. The patient can eat the food without a reaction if there is no physical exercise within 2 hours of ingestion. Exercise in the absence of eating the food during this time interval also does not cause anaphylaxis.

An *anaphylactoid reaction* is identical to anaphylaxis, but the patient is not allergic to the agent that causes the reaction. Certain chemicals are capable of directly activating mast cells or basophils without the need for IgE antibodies. This causes the cells to release the same mediators that cause allergic anaphylaxis. Chemicals capable of doing this are present in some foods, especially shellfish or berries, although the precise chemicals that are responsible are unknown. Unlike allergic anaphylaxis, it does not occur each time the food is eaten, and the risk is higher if a large quanity is eaten or if the food is not fresh and possibly contaminated with bacteria or other microorganisms. The distinction between anaphylactic and anaphylactoid reactions should be made in each case by an allergic evaluation and proper testing, because the food causing anaphylaxis must be avoided, whereas avoidance might not be necessary if there is no allergy to the food.

Cutaneous reactions are common. Immediate reactions caused by IgE antibodies produce acute urticaria, angioedema, or both. These occur especially after ingestion of fish, shellfish, tree nuts, and peanuts in adults, and eggs, milk, peanuts, and tree nuts in children. The reaction subsides promptly and does not recur unless the food is eaten again. Contact urticaria results from direct skin contact with raw meats, fish, fruits, and occasionally other foods. The

urticarial lesions appear only on the areas of contact with the food. Chronic urticaria/angioedema is a condition of frequently recurring hives or swelling that persists for weeks or months and is rarely if ever caused by foods. In fact, it is almost always idiopathic, because a search for any causative allergen or condition is usually negative.

Urticaria or angioedema may result from eating a food in the absence of an IgE allergy to the food. This is analogous to an anaphylactoid reaction as discussed above, and the same foods (shellfish and berries) are the usual causes.

Atopic dermatitis is one of the three manifestation of atopy. Patients with this disease may also have asthma and/or allergic rhinitis in addition to the skin disease. Allergy testing will frequently, but not always, show evidence of IgE sensitivities to inhalant allergens, especially the house dust mite, and foods. Nevertheless, the role of food allergy in causing or exacerbating the skin eruption is controversial and frequently disputed.

It is unusual for a patient with atopic dermatitis to report a history of a flare of the dermatitis following ingestion of certain foods and improvement on elimination diets. However, when 400 children with atopic dermatitis were challenged with a double-blind, placebo-controlled food challenge in a research setting, one-third demonstrated an immediate allergic reaction [3]. These children had severe atopic dermatitis, high total serum IgE levels, and most of them had respiratory allergy as well. Reactions occurred in minutes and almost always within 2 hours. Seventy-five percent of the food reactions involved the skin, and 30% involved the skin only. The reactions were pruritus, erythema, and morbilliform eruptions, especially at sites of existing eczema. In individual cases, the allergy was limited to only a few foods. Elimination of the food from the diet then resulted in improvement or clearing of the rash in some of the cases, and later challenge with the same food caused urticaria in those whose eczema had cleared. These children usually have positive skin tests or radioallergosorbent tests to some foods. Only 50% of the foods with a positive skin test produced a positive challenge, and foods that gave a negative skin test almost always resulted in a negative challenge. Gastrointestinal symptoms occurred in 51% of the challenges, although there was no history of these symptoms occurring prior to the challenge testing. Upper respiratory symptoms occurred in 45%, with wheezing in 15%. A positive challenge was associated with a significant rise in plasma histamine, consistent with an immediate-phase IgE allergic response. Many of the reactions included a pruritic rash that appeared 4–8 hours after the food challenge, accompanied by blood and tissue biopsy evidence consistent with a late-phase IgE allergic response. Long-term elimination diets achieved significant clinical improvement, including elimination of subclinical gastrointestinal malabsorption. Ninety percent of these food reactions to double-blind, placebo-controlled food challenges were to egg, milk, peanut, soy, and wheat. After 1–2 years of elimination of the allergenic food from the diet,

food hypersensitivity was permanently lost in a third of the patients, especially to soy, but only rarely to peanut. The positive skin test reactions persisted. Based on these and other findings, it is likely that only about one-third of children—and very few adults—with atopic dermatitis have demonstrable food allergy.

The *oral allergy syndrome* is a localized "contact" allergic reaction of the oropharynx. The symptoms are pruritus and angioedema of the lips, tongue, palate, and throat, beginning about 5 minutes after the food is eaten and resolving promptly thereafter. It results especially from eating uncooked fruits and vegetables, and it occurs in patients with allergy to those food allergens that cross-react with certain plant pollens (Table 3). These patients usually also have symptomatic allergic rhinoconjunctivitis to the cross-reacting pollen [18].

Allergic eosinophilic gastroenteritis is an uncommon condition in some atopic patients who are allergic to both inhalant and food allergens. In adults with this disease, the ingestion of the food allergen causes postprandial nausea and vomiting, abdominal pain, diarrhea, and occasionally steatorrhea and weight loss [19]. Complications include hypoalbuminemia and iron deficiency anemia. In infants it causes failure to thrive, and in some cases a protein-losing enteropathy may result [20]. The food allergen can be identified by skin test or radioallergosorbent test, and when it is eliminated from the diet the disease resolves, although this may take up to 12 weeks of avoidance of the food. Laboratory studies confirm the allergic nature of the disease. Peripheral blood eosinophilia may be as high as 50%, and eosinophils are present in intestinal secretions and in ascites fluid. There is eosinophilic inflammation of the esophagus, stomach, or intestine, involving the mucosa, muscular, or serosal layers, and Charcot-Leyden crystals can be found in stool samples. Compared to normals, there is an increase in the total amount of IgE normally found in duodenal secretions and serum.

Some children and adolescents with this disease do not have specific IgE antibody to the food that causes the disease to flare. A very low protein diet for these patients may cause resolution in 6–8 weeks. The condition also responds favorably to systemic corticosteroid therapy if the specific causative food is not identified and eliminated.

Respiratory food hypersensitivity is rare. Patients with asthma sometimes suspect that their attacks are caused by certain foods, but double-blind, placebo-controlled food challenge—the only reliable way to prove food-induced asthma—rarely provokes an asthma attack. In cases where this does happen, it is almost always in an atopic child, and the reaction is accompanied by a skin rash or a gastrointestinal response as well. Interestingly, however, ingestion of food allergens may increase a state of nonspecific bronchial hyperreactivity, as shown by methacholine challenge testing. The clinical significance of this is unknown.

Some patients with exquisite sensitivity to a food may experience an allergic reaction by simply inhaling fumes of the food. This may cause symptoms of allergic rhinitis,

conjunctivitis, laryngeal edema, bronchospasm, vomiting, and even on rare occasions anaphylactic shock [21]. The foods most commonly responsible are fish, mollusks, crustaceans, eggs, and peanut.

B. Type II—IgG- or IgM-Mediated Cytotoxic Allergic Diseases

Allergic reactions to drugs that adhere to blood cells in which the cell is destroyed because of antibody to the drug have been recognized for many years. There have been rare reports of thrombocytopenia apparently caused by milk [22], possibly by this mechanism.

C. Type III—IgG- or IgM-Mediated Inflammatory Allergic Diseases

Rare instances of inflammatory gastrointestinal and respiratory conditions that are caused by a particular food and ameliorated when the food is eliminated from the diet have been suspected to be allergic diseases mediated by IgG antibodies. As discussed earlier, small amounts of IgG antibodies are normal and harmless, but in these cases, an IgG antibody to the food is present in unusually large amounts, and the inflammation is thought to be a consequence of immune complexes that activate complement. The diagnosis of a specific food causing the disease should be made by clinical evidence of improvement when the food is eliminated and exacerbation when the food is reintroduced before an elimination diet is prescribed for treatment.

Heiner's syndrome is a rare disease of infants who have produced high concentrations of IgG antibodies to milk because of frequent aspiration [23]. As a consequence, ingestion of milk triggers a type III immune complex allergic reaction in the lung, causing pulmonary infiltrates. Recurrent attacks may result in anemia and in some cases pulmonary hemosiderosis. The diagnosis can be confirmed by measuring precipitating antibodies to milk in the serum.

D. Type IV—T-Cell-Mediated Allergic Diseases

There are two types of contact dermatitis: allergic and irritant. The latter is an irritation where the food contacts the skin, because of a chemical or physical property of the food. It does not involve the immune system [24]. The allergen in *allergic contact dermatitis* to a food is usually an organic chemical contained naturally within the food or an additive, rather than a food protein. It is first suspected by the history and skin examination and then confirmed by a 48-hour skin patch test.

The condition is an inflammatory dermatitis, which is pruritic and may be similar in appearance to atopic eczema, but with a tendency to include vesicles and blisters. Numerous foods have been shown to cause the disease. Garlic and onion are the most common, especially among people who

handle food often [25]. Citrus fruits, many green vegetables, and some spices should also be suspected.

Some potent contact allergens, especially metals such as nickel, cobalt, and chrome, may occur naturally in certain foods. Patients sensitized by contact from jewelry or from an occupational exposure can experience a flare of the dermatitis after ingesting food that contains the metal allergen [26]. A special diet free of that particular metallic ion may then be necessary. There is also a problem of cross-reactivity between an allergen in a plant and an unrelated food. Urushiol, the allergen in the poison ivy leaf, is antigenically similar to a chemical in the oil of cashew nut and in mango. A person with severe poison ivy sensitivity may experience a rash from contact with those foods or exacerbation of the poison ivy rash from eating the food.

VII. NONALLERGIC IMMUNOLOGIC DISEASES

There are a group of conditions that are caused by nonallergic intolerance to certain foods in which the immune system nevertheless plays a role. A common one is gluten-sensitive enteropathy, also known as *celiac disease,* in which the intestinal mucosa becomes inflamed and atrophic from ingestion of gliadin, a component of gluten in wheat and other grains [27]. Ingestion of gliadin causes diarrhea, steatorrhea, weight loss, malabsorption, and other clinical manifestations. Immunologic involvement includes IgA antibodies to gliadin [28], lymphocyte inflammation of the intestinal mucosa, and some evidence of cell-mediated (T-cell) immunity to gliadin. It is unclear whether these specific immune responses are the cause or the effect of the disease, and there is some feeling that the cause is a toxic effect of gluten [29]. Nevertheless, a lifelong gluten-free diet keeps the condition under control.

Dermatitis herpetiformis is a skin disease that is associated with gluten-sensitive enteropathy [30, 31]. The skin eruption consists of a pruritic symmetric rash that is papulovesicular. Like celiac disease, there is a genetic predisposition in persons with certain HLA haplotypes. The gastrointestinal pathology is similar to celiac disease, and IgA is deposited in the skin. It responds to a gluten-free diet.

Enterocolitis syndrome is a disease of infants 1 week to 3 months of age, who have protracted vomiting and diarrhea resulting in dehydration, acidosis, and methemoglobinemia [32]. Cow's milk and soy are the predominant foods eaten at that age, but occasionally other foods may cause a similar disease in older children, and rarely seafoods may do so in adults. The stools contain blood, eosinophils, and neutrophils. Jejunal biopsy reveals flattened villi, edema, lymphocytes, eosinophils, and mast cells. Deliberate diagnostic challenge with the suspected food causes diarrhea and vomiting in 1–3 hours. Skin testing is negative to the food that is responsible for the disease. It is not an IgE-mediated allergic

disease, and the immunopathogenesis is uncertain at this time. Symptoms resolve in 72 hours when the food is eliminated from the diet.

Eosinophilic colitis occurs during the first few months of life in infants who are fed cow's milk and/or soy, but it may also occur in breast-fed infants [33]. There is no apparent gastrointestinal discomfort in the infant, but there is gross or occult blood in the stools. Microscopic pathology includes eosinophilia in the epithelium and lamina propria and edema and neutrophils in the distal colon. Elimination of the responsible food results in clearing in 72 hours.

Enteropathy is also a disease of early infancy. There is diarrhea with or without vomiting, failure to thrive, and malabsorption. Cow's milk is the usual cause, but soy, egg, wheat, rice, chicken, or fish may also be responsible [34]. Biopsy of the intestinal tract shows patchy villous atrophy, milk lymphocytic infiltration, and edema.

VIII. NONIMMUNOLOGIC REACTIONS TO FOODS

Gustatory rhinorrhea refers to a condition of excessive and annoying nasal secretions that some persons experience after eating. It may occur after eating certain foods, especially spicy ones, or after any meal. The mechanism of rhinorrhea is probably a simple stimulation of muscarinic parasympathetic nerves.

Lactose intolerance results from deficient intestinal lactase so that dietary lactose ferments in the bowel, with excessive production of gas. Primary lactase deficiency varies in prevalence among different ethnic and geographic populations. Secondary lactase deficiency is transient and may last for 2 weeks or more after an acute gastrointestinal infection. More persistent secondary deficiency complicates chronic gastrointestinal diseases. (See Chapter 37 on lactose intolerance).

Scombroid fish poisoning results from contamination by *Klebsiella* of spoiled tuna, mackerel, bonito, mahi, and bluefish. The bacterial decarboxylate histidine [35] generates histamine and simulates an allergic reaction. Symptoms are a sharp peppery taste, burning of the mouth, vomiting, diarrhea, nausea, facial flushing, and headache.

IX. CONDITIONS WITH NO PROVEN RELATIONSHIP TO FOODS

So many medical and nonmedical conditions have been incorrectly attributed to "food allergy" that only a few will be reviewed here.

Infantile colic affects 15–20% of infants [36], causing uncontrollable crying and abdominal distension. It starts before age 6 weeks and lasts for 3–6 months. Despite numerous theories, the cause remains unknown. Although food allergy is claimed to contribute in up to 10–15% of cases [37], there is no scientific proof that colic is an allergic condition, and it occurs regardless of the diet, even with exclusive breastfeeding.

Behavioral changes in children and even in adults have often been attributed to the ingestion of certain foods and food additives. Sugar, dietary salicylates, aspartame and certain other chemicals, food preservatives, and food coloring agents have achieved popular notoriety as the cause of attention deficit hyperactivity disorder, but properly controlled food challenge and elimination protocols fail to substantiate these claims [38].

The *Chinese restaurant syndrome* encompasses a variety of symptoms such as headache, sweating, thirst, facial flushing, facial burning, abdominal pain, tearing of eyes, and a crawling sensation of the skin. It begins 15–20 minutes after eating and subsides several hours later without treatment. Although widely attributed to monosodium glutamate, controlled deliberate challenge studies frequently fail to reproduce the symptoms [39]. There is no evidence that it is caused by allergy to monosodium glutamate or to Chinese food.

Food allergy has also been claimed to cause sudden infant death syndrome, allergic tension-fatigue syndrome, enuresis, and headache in children, and rheumatoid arthritis, chronic fatigue syndrome, migraine, epilepsy, and inflammatory bowel disease (Crohn's disease or chronic ulcerative colitis) in adults and children. There is no scientific proof for any of these conditions being caused by food allergy.

X. DIAGNOSIS OF FOOD ALLERGY

The diagnostic process begins with a thorough history and complete physical examination to establish the nature, extent, and duration of symptoms and their association with the ingestion of a suspected food. Important information includes the timing of the reaction after the food is eaten, the quantity of food required, and consistency of the reaction to the food over time. The history is generally more reliable for acute reactions than for chronic diseases. A hidden ingredient must also be considered. A personal and family history of atopy or other diseases may be important. A complete physical examination is critical to detect objective signs of allergic inflammation and to rule out other possible diseases. In some cases the diagnosis may be obvious, as in a child with recurrent anaphylactic reactions to peanut. In most cases, however, a differential diagnosis and appropriate testing are necessary.

Diet-symptom diaries have the advantage that they provide a prospective "history" of reactions and a more accurate documentation than is possible by recall. They are especially useful for disproving a false assumption that a particular food caused reactions. Diaries are especially helpful for patients with intermittent urticaria/angioedema.

TABLE 5   Tests of Specific Immune Responses for Each Type of Allergic
Reaction, Based on the Gell and Coombs Classification

Class	Skin test	*In vitro* test
I	Immediate wheal/erythema prick test	Radioallergosorbent test Enzyme-linked immunosorbent assay
II	Not applicable	Not applicable
III	Intradermal arthus test	Serum precipitin test
IV	Patch test (for allergic contact dermatitis) Intradermal 48-hour delayed hypersensitivity test	*In vitro* lymphocyte transformation test

Diagnostic elimination diets, accompanied by a written diary, have long been used by allergists. They are generally based on the results of skin testing and/or from the history. To be accurate, the diary must include the timing of every item of food eaten, all symptoms or reactions, and any other items or events that may explain the patient's symptoms, such as medications. The purpose of the diet is to eliminate symptoms and/or objective physical or laboratory findings. When this occurs, an open challenge is performed with one of the suspect foods. The other foods are then challenged one at a time while the diary record is maintained. If a particular food causes a reaction consistent with the previous symptoms, it is again eliminated and rechallenged. In general, three successive positive provocative unblinded tests to a food can be considered probably significant, although the mechanism must then be determined. A reaction to the challenge suggests the cause but not the mechanism. For example, provoking a food reaction in an open challenge could result from allergy, toxicity, an enzyme deficiency, or even a psychological response. If ongoing chronic symptoms fail to improve in 2 weeks, the diet should be abandoned.

Tests for a specific immune response must be appropriate to the suspected allergic reaction (Table 5). In most cases, the suspected disease is caused by IgE antibodies, and both the immediate wheal/erythema skin test and the *in vitro* serum assay for specific IgE antibodies to foods are reliable. The skin test is more sensitive, but reading and interpreting the result is subjective and requires training and experience. Immediate skin testing to food allergens is done by the prick testing method [40]. A false negative result can occur from an inactive extract, because some food allergens are labile. Skin testing is most useful for suspected food allergy causing anaphylaxis.

The standard *in vitro* test is the radioallergosorbent test, which measures the quantity of specific IgE antibodies in a sample of the patient's serum. Most commercial medical laboratories offer a limited panel of foods. A negative test to a food by either skin testing or radioallergosorbent test virtually ensures that the patient does not have an IgE-mediated allergic reaction to that food. On the other hand, a positive test in a child indicates only a 50% chance of clinical allergy, while in adults it is only about 3%.

Patch testing to foods is used for suspected allergic contact dermatitis. It is accurate because it simulates the disease "in miniature." The food extract is applied to a small area of skin for 48 hours. A positive test consists of a localized skin inflammation at the patch test site [40].

Endoscopy of the stomach or small bowel during oral challenge with a food allergen to observe for objective changes, with or without biopsy, may be required in some patients with suspected food-induced gastroenteropathy.

The *double-blind, placebo-controlled food challenge* is the gold standard for proof of a specific food-induced disease [41], but a positive result does not mean that the disease is necessarily allergic. It is usually appropriate to perform oral food challenge unblinded or single-blind first. If these are negative, there is no need to proceed further. The double-blind, placebo-controlled food challenge is an essential method for many clinical research studies in food allergy, and it has been especially valuable for analyzing food-related complaints without objective evidence of a physical reaction.

The procedure for double-blind, placebo-controlled food challenge is demanding [42, 43]. The suspect food is eliminated from the diet for 7–13 days, or longer if necessary, until the patient is asymptomatic. The challenges are administered while the patient is fasting and free of antihistamines or any other drug that might prevent or mask the reaction. The first challenge is performed with a dose selected as unlikely to cause a reaction. Subsequent challenges are doubled in dose and administered every 15–60 minutes until a reaction occurs or until 10 g of the test food is tolerated, at which time the test is considered negative. Food extracts and an equal number of placebo controls are given in random order. The food challenges are administered as lyophilized extracts packed into capsules or dissolved in liquid. Because rare false-negative reactions (2–5%) have occurred, a negative result should be repeated with an open challenge. Following the session, the patient should be observed for up to 2 hours

if an IgE reaction is suspected, up to 4–8 hours for milk enterocolitis, and up to 24–48 hours for other gastrointestinal reactions. Wherever appropriate and possible, an objective measure consistent with the disease should be included, such as pulmonary function testing, nasal smear for eosinophils, or histamine or tryptase content of plasma or urine.

XI. DIFFERENTIAL DIAGNOSIS

The diagnosis of food allergy rests on the identification of the disease as an allergy, objective evidence of sensitization to a food, and reasonable assurance that the food is responsible for the disease. This requires a suspicion that the patient has food allergy and elimination of other possible diseases and other potential adverse effects from foods. Gastrointestinal anatomic abnormalities, infection, peptic ulcer disease, and gall bladder disease are some conditions that can be misdiagnosed as gastrointestinal food allergy. Nonallergic reactions from foods include poisoning, intolerance because of intestinal enzyme deficiency, and a response to foods from psychosocial factors.

XII. TREATMENT

The only sure treatment of food allergy is elimination of the food from the diet. In most cases, allergy is limited to one food, one class of food, or a small number of different foods. Therefore, avoidance therapy is not likely to cause nutritional deficiency. Some infants and a few adults, however, have multiple specific food allergies, requiring diet supplements to maintain good nutritional status.

In some cases, incomplete elimination accompanied by appropriate drug therapy is possible. Drugs that may offer such protection in IgE-mediated disease include antihistamines, mast cell stabilizers (cromolyn, ketotifen), and corticosteroids. The efficacy of leukotriene inhibitors alone or in combination with other drugs has yet to be studied.

The acute anaphylactic reaction is treated with epinephrine, intravenous fluid replacement for shock, bronchodilator drugs, antihistamines, and maintenance of the circulation and airways.

Immunotherapy (desensitization) for IgE-mediated food allergy could theoretically eliminate or reduce allergic sensitivity to foods. It has long been established as effective and safe for patients with allergic rhinitis caused by inhalant allergens and for those with anaphylaxis to venom from the stings of *Hymenoptera* insects. Currently, uncertainty remains about its effectiveness in allergic asthma from inhalant allergens. Clinical trials using extracts of foods in patients with food-induced anaphylaxis to date have been frustrated by excessive numbers of serious and even fatal systemic reactions. Clinical studies of food immunotherapy are continuing, however, and may eventually prove to be useful. If

so, it is likely to require some type of modification of the allergen to avoid reactions from the treatment itself.

A small number of atopic infants and small children have severe allergic reactions to multiple food proteins with gastrointestinal and skin involvement. They are unable to tolerate enough variety of foods to permit adequate intake of nutrients. The disease usually begins when foods are first introduced into the diet. These are believed to be true IgE-mediated allergic sensitivities. Various "elemental" amino acid-based formula diets have been devised to satisfy all of the infant's nutritional needs for protein to sustain growth.

XIII. PROGNOSIS OF FOOD ALLERGY

There is very little reliable information about the prognosis of food allergy. In infants and children, allergy to foods frequently remits after several years [44], with the notable exception of anaphylaxis, especially to nuts and peanut. Children with documented food allergy should be monitored by serial skin testing on an annual basis. They should scrupulously avoid the allergenic food as long as the skin test remains positive. Only when the test reverts to negative should careful administration of a small test dose of the food be given. This is best done in a medical facility where appropriate treatment is available for immediate use.

Most adult-onset food allergy reactions are also transient, although they may persist for years before remitting. Celiac disease, which is an immunologically mediated disease but not an allergic one, is a permanent condition.

Multiple food allergies encompassing almost all ingested proteins in infants persist for 1 to several years with gradual loss of food sensitivities over a period of a number of years, permitting slow and gradual introduction of natural foods into the diet.

XIV. PREVENTION OF FOOD ALLERGY

Allergists have long been interested in preventing the development of allergic diseases and specific allergies, including foods. Expectant parents who are allergic frequently request strategies to prevent, diminish, or at least delay the onset of allergy in their offspring. A number of dietary measures have been tried empirically, and limited clinical research has been done on this important issue. At this time, there are no firm recommendations for primary prevention (i.e., before the onset of the disease).

In 12 studies published to date [45], various "highly allergenic" foods such as egg, cow milk, peanut, fish, soy, and others were eliminated for varying periods of time from the diet of the mother (during pregnancy, after delivery, or both) and/or from the infant. Follow-up evaluations were typically done after 18 months, but they ranged from 12 months to 15 years. Ten studies reported some reduction in severity of the

infant's atopic disease, especially dermatitis, but no effect was observed in the other two studies. There were significant differences in the protocols, and even the best results suggest that a highly restrictive diet that is difficult to follow for either the pregnant woman or the infant cannot be recommended as a reliable prevention strategy for infants of allergic parents-to-be. Nevertheless, most allergists do recommend breast feeding to delay the introduction of cow's milk for the infant, delayed introduction of solid foods until about 6 months, and elimination of milk, egg, nuts, and fish until 12 months [45]. These particular foods are selected empirically, because there is obviously no way to know what foods should be avoided in a diet for primary prevention before allergies are present.

XV. FOOD ADDITIVES

Approximately 3000 different substances are intentionally added to the food supply to provide color, flavor, appearance, nutritional value, disease prevention, (e.g., antimicrobials, vitamins, minerals), texture, preservative properties, or enhanced cooking properties. They may or may not be listed as ingredients in the final product. Additives may be foodstuffs (e.g., sugar, cornstarch), minerals, synthetic organic compounds, or natural organic compounds [4, 46–47].

Unintentional additives may also appear in the final food product during processing of the food by inadvertent mixture or by contamination with microorganisms.

It is possible that any one of these food additives can cause an adverse reaction, including allergy, and many people believe they do so frequently. The additives most often claimed to cause allergic or allergic-like reactions are synthetic colorants, sulfites, monosodium glutamate, aspartame, and benzoates. Controlled challenge studies to date indicate that adverse reactions to food additives are actually very rare.

Sulfites in foods cause an allergy-like reaction in some asthmatic patients. The bronchial mucosa in asthma is unusually sensitive to certain irritants and chemicals, including sulfur-containing compounds such as sulfites [48]. Inhalation of sulfur fumes or sulfur dioxide gas results in an acute asthmatic attack and may be fatal. Because sulfites are widely added to certain foods to prevent oxidation, eating such foods may cause acute bronchospasm [49]. This occurs only in persons with asthma. The reaction probably results from inhaling sulfur dioxide fumes generated from the sulfites while the food is being chewed. The reaction is not an allergic one, and no immunologic mechanism is involved. Some asthmatic patients are especially sensitive, because they are deficient in the enzyme sulfite oxidase. Those who have experienced exacerbation of their disease from eating sulfite-containing foods should always avoid such foods, and some allergists recommend avoidance for all persons with asthma. The foods most likely to contain sulfites are listed in Table 6.

TABLE 6 Some Foods Containing Sulfites Likely to Exacerbate Asthma

High content	Medium content
Wine	Wine vinegar
Most dried fruits	Dried potatoes
Some fruit juices	Some commercial gravies
Molasses	Some commercial sauces
Sauerkraut juice	Fruit toppings
	Maraschino cherries
	Pectin
	Sauerkraut
	Fresh shrimp
	Pickled foods
	Cocktail onions
	Relishes

Source: Adapted from Simon, R. A. (1996). Adverse reactions to food and drug additives. *Immunol. Allergy Clin. N. Am.* **16,** 137.

Some allergists believe that chronic urticaria/angioedema in certain patients is caused by food additives, especially tartrazine (yellow dye #5). However, the reaction cannot be confirmed in patients who report hives from tartrazine when they are challenged in a double-blind protocol [50].

Vegetable gums are natural products that are added to many foods as thickeners and to increase the bulk of the product. They have long been suspected to cause IgE-mediated allergic reactions and are frequently included in the standard skin testing panel used by allergists. Although some atopic patients do react to these skin tests and there is an occasional case report [51], no data are available on the actual prevalence, if any, of clinical reactions to vegetable gums. Their presence in a particular food is not always indicated on the product label.

Antioxidants, especially butylated hydroxyanisol, butylated hydroxytoluene, nitrates, nitrites, citric acid, and benzoates, have all been suspected to cause allergy, especially chronic urticaria. In fact, there is no documentation that any of these cause allergic disease. They may have other adverse health effects in some patients, but these are pharmacologic or toxic, not allergic.

XVI. GENETICALLY ENGINEERED FOODS

The science and methods of biotechnology are being increasingly applied to agriculture for selectively producing crops with desirable characteristics, such as enhanced nutritional properties or resistance to herbicides. This is done by inserting DNA with the genetic code for a desired trait into the chromosome of the plant cells in the laboratory, then culturing the cells to produce plantlets that are eventually trans-

ferred to soil and propagated. The resulting bioengineered foods in theory could have been produced by the traditional breeding methods that have been used for more than a century, but bioengineering is much more specific and predictable.

Although there is concern about the safety of genetically engineered foods, includng the possible emergence of new food allergens, this has yet to occur. In fact, it is theoretically possible to produce crops, such as peanuts, that lack the known major allergens, and attempts along these lines are currently in progress.

References

1. Young, E., Stoneham, M. D., Petruckevitch, A., Barton, J., and Rona, R. (1994). A population study of food intolerance. *Lancet* **93,** 446–456

2. Altman, D. R., and Cerement, L. T. (1996). Public perceptions of food allergy. *J. Allergy Clin. Immunol.* **97,** 1247–1251.

3. Sampson, H., and Metcalfe, D. D. (1991). Immediate reactions to foods. *In* "Food Allergy: Adverse Reactions to Foods and Food Additives" (D. D. Metcalfe, H. Sampson, and R. A. Simon, Eds.), pp. 100–112. Blackwell Scientific Publications, Boston.

4. Bush, R. K., and Taylor, S. L. (1989). Adverse reactions to food and drug additives. *In* "Allergy: Principles and Practice," 5th ed. (E. Middleton, Jr., C. E. Reed, E. F. Ellis, N. F. Atkinson, Jr., J. W. Yunginger, and W. W. Busse, Eds.), Chap. 83, pp. 1183–1198. Mosby, St. Louis.

5. Fuglsang, G., Madsen, C., and Saval, P. (1993). Prevalence of intolerance to food additives among Danish schoolchildren. *Pediatr. Allergy Immunol.* **4,** 123–129.

6. Madsen, C. (1994). Prevalence of food additive intolerance. *Hum. Exp. Toxicol.* **13,** 393–399.

7. Bleumink, E., and Young, E. (1968). Identification of the atopic allergens in cow's milk. *Int. Arch. Allergy Appl. Immunol.* **34,** 521–543.

8. Hoffman, D. R. (1983). Immunochemical identification of the allergens in egg white. *J. Allergy Clin. Immunol.* **71,** 481–486.

9. Langland, T. (1983). A clinical and immunological study of hen's egg white. VI. Occurrence of proteins cross-reacting with allergens in hen's egg white as studied in egg white from turkey, duck, goose, seagull, and in hen's egg yolk, and hen and chicken sera and flesh. *Allergy* **38,** 399–412.

10. Bock, S. A., and Atkins, F. M. (1989). The natural history of peanut allergy. *J. Allergy Clin. Immunol.* **83,** 900–904.

11. Aas, K. (1966). Studies of hypersensitivity to fish: A clinical study. *Int. Arch. Allergy Appl. Immunol.* **29,** 346–363.

12. Thiel, H., and Ulmer, W. (1980). Baker's asthma: Development and possibility for treatment. *Chest* **78,** 400–405.

13. Kemp, S. F., Lockey, R. F., Wolf, B. L., and Lieberman, P. (1995). Anaphylaxis: A review of 266 cases. *Arch. Intern. Med.* **155,** 1749–1754.

14. Yunginger, J. W., Sweeney, K. G., Sturner, W. Q., Giannandrea, L. A., Teigland, J. D., Bray, M., Benson, P. A., York, J. A., Biedrzycki, L., and Squillace, D. L. (1988). Fatal food-induced anaphylaxis. *JAMA* **260,** 1450–1452.

15. Kidd, J. M., III, Cohen, S. H., Sosman, A. J., and Fink, J. N. (1983). Food-dependent exercise-induced anaphylaxis. *J. Allergy Clin. Immunol.* **71,** 407–411.

16. Dohi, M., Suko, M., Sugiyami, H., Yamashita, N., Tadokoro, K., Juji, F., Okudaira, H., Sano, Y., Ito, K., and Miyamoto, T. (1991). Food-dependent, exercise-induced anaphylaxis: A study of 11 Japanese cases. *J. Allergy Clin. Immunol.* **87,** 34–40.

17. Horan, R., and Sheffer, A. (1991). Food-dependent, exercise-induced anaphylaxis. *Immunol. Allergy Clin. N. Am.* **11,** 757–766.

18. Anderson, L. B., Dreyfuss, E. M., Logan, J., Johnstone, D. E., and Glaser, J. (1970). Melon and banana sensitivity coincident with ragweed pollinosis. *J. Allergy* **45,** 310–319.

19. Min, K., and Metcalfe, D. (1991). Eosinophilic gastroenteritis. *Immunol. Allergy Clin. N. Am.* **11,** 799–813.

20. Moon, A., and Kleinman, R. (1995). Allergic gastroenteropathy in children. *Ann. Allergy Asthma Immunol.* **74,** 5–12.

21. Crespo, J. F., Pascual, C., Dominguez, C., Ojeda, I., Munoz, F. M., and Esteban, M. M. (1995). Allergic reactions associated with airborne fish particles in IgE-mediated fish hypersensitive patients. *Allergy* **50,** 257–261.

22. Caffrey, E. A., Sladen, G. E., Isaacs, P. E. T., and Clark, K. G. A. (1981). Thrombocytopenia caused by cow's milk. *Lancet* **2,** 226–240.

23. Heiner, D. C., and Sears, J. W. (1960). Chronic respiratory disease associated with multiple circulating precipitins to cow's milk. *Am. J. Dis. Child.* **100,** 500–502.

24. Beltrani, V. S., and Beltrani, V. P. (1997). Contact dermatitis: A review. *Ann. Allergy* **78,** 160–195.

25. Burks, J. W. (1954). Classic aspects of onion and garlic dermatitis in housewives. *Ann. Allergy* **12,** 592–595.

26. Rietschel, R. L., and Fowler, J. F., Jr. Eds. (1996). "Fisher's Contact Dermatitis," 4th ed., p. 813–814. Williams & Wilkins, Baltimore, MD.

27. Trier, J. S. (1991). Celiac sprue. (1991). *N. Engl. J. Med.* **325,** 1709–1719.

28. Scott, H., Fausa, O., Ek, J., and Brandtzaeg, P. (1984). Immune response patter in coeliac disease: Serum antibodies to dietary antigens measured by an enzyme-linked immunosorbent assay. *Clin. Exp. Immunol.* **57,** 25–32.

29. Cornell, H. J. (1988). Amino acid composition of peptides remaining after in vitro digestion of gliadin sub-fraction with duodenal mucosa from patients with coeliac disease. *Clin. Chim. Acta* **176,** 279–289.

30. Hall, R. P. (1987). The pathogenesis of dermatitis herpetiformis: Recent advances. *J. Am. Acad. Dermatol.* **16,** 1129–1144.

31. Katz, A. I., Hall, R. P., Lawley, T. J., and Strober, W. (1980). Dermatitis herpetiformis: The skin and the gut. *Ann. Intern. Med.* **93,** 857–874.

32. Powell, G. K. (1978). Milk- and soy-induced enterocolitis of infancy. *J. Pediatr.* **93,** 553–560.

33. Machida, H. M., Catto Smith, A. G., Gall, D. G., Trevenen, C., and Scott, R. B. (1994). Allergic colitis of infancy: Clinical and pathologic aspects. *J. Pediatr. Gastroenterol.* **19,** 22–26.

34. Kuitunen, P., Visakorpi, J. K., Savilahti, E., and Pelkonen, P. (1975). Malabsorption syndrome with cow's milk intolerance: Clinical findings and course in 54 cases. *Arch. Dis. Child.* **50,** 351–356.

35. Hughes, J. M., and Merson, M. H. (1976). Fish and shellfish poisoning. *N. Engl. J. Med.* **2295,** 1117–1120.

36. Hide, D. W., and Guyer, B. M. (1982). Prevalence of infantile colic. *Arch. Dis. Child.* **57,** 559–560.

37. Taubman, B. (1988). Parental counseling compared with elimination of cow's milk or soy milk protein for the treatment of infant colic syndrome: A randomized trial. *Pediatrics* **81,** 756–761.

38. Consensus Conference. (1982). Defined diets and childhood hyperactivity. *JAMA* **248,** 290–292.

39. Filer, L. J., and Stegink, L. D. (1994). A report of the proceedings of an MSG workshop held August 1991. *CRC Crit. Rev. Food. Sci. Nutr.* **34,** 159–174.

40. Terr, A. I. (1997). Mechanisms of hypersensitivity. *In* "Human Immunology," 9th ed. (D. P. Stites, A. I. Terr, and T. G. Parslow, Eds.), Chap. 26, pp. 376–388. Appleton & Lange, Stamford, CT.

41. Sampson, H. A., and Metcalfe, D. D. (1992). Food allergies. *JAMA* **268,** 2840–2844.

42. Bock, S. A., Sampson, H. A., Atkins, F. M., Zeiger, R. S., Lehrer, S., Sachs, M., Bush, R. K., and Metcalfe, D. D. (1988). Double-blind, placebo-controlled food challenge (DBPCFC) as an office procedure: A manual. *J. Allergy Clin. Immunol.* **82,** 986–997.

43. Metcalfe, D., and Sampson, H. (1990). Workshop on experimental methodology for clinical studies of adverse reactions to foods and food additives. *J. Allergy Clin. Immunol.* **86,** 421–442.

44. Bock, S. A. (1982). The natural history of food sensitivity. *J. Allergy Clin. Immunol.* **69,** 173–177.

45. Hill, D. J., and Hosking, C. S. (1999). The management and prevention of food allergy. *In* "Food Hypersensitivity and Adverse Reactions: A Practical Guide for Diagnosis and Management" (M. Frieri and B. Kettelhut, Eds.), Chap. 21, pp. 423–448. Marcel Dekker, New York.

46. Simon, R. A. (1996). Adverse reactions to food and drug additives. *Immunol. Allergy Clin. North Am.* **16,** 137–176.

47. Finegold, I. (1999). Adverse reactions to food additives. *In* "Food Hypersensitivity and Adverse Reactions: A Practical Guide for Diagnosis and Management" (M. Frieri and B. Kettelhut, Eds.), Chap. 6, p. 117. Marcel Dekker, New York.

48. Stevenson, D. D., and Simon, R. A. (1981). Sensitivity to ingested metabisulfites in asthmatic subjects. *J. Allergy Clin. Immunol.* **68,** 26–32.

49. Delohery, J., Simmul, R., Castle, W. D., and Allen, D. H. (1984). The relationship of inhaled sulfur dioxide reactivity to ingested metabisulfite sensitivity in patients with asthma. *Am. Rev. Resp. Dis.* **130,** 1027–1032.

50. Stevenson, D. D., Simon, R. A., Lumry, W. R., and Mathison, D. A. (1986). Adverse reactions to tartrazine. *J. Allergy Clin. Immunol.* **78,** 182–191.

52. Danoff, D., Lincoln, L., Thomson, D. M., and Gold, P. (1978). "Big Mac attack." *N. Engl. J. Med.* **298,** 1095–1096.

CHAPTER **45**

Nutrition and Cystic Fibrosis

PHILIP M. FARRELL AND HUI-CHUAN LAI
University of Wisconsin—Madison, Madison, Wisconsin

I. INTRODUCTION

Cystic fibrosis (CF) is the most common, life-threatening autosomal recessive disorder with estimated incidences of 1 in 2900 white live births, 1 in 17,000 black live births, and 1 in 90,000 Asian live births [1, 2]. CF was recognized as a distinct clinical entity in 1938. It is a generalized disease of the exocrine glands characterized by abnormal sodium and chloride transport, leading to elevated electrolyte levels in the sweat glands [3]. Dysfunction of the other exocrine glands occurs, producing viscid secretions of low water content. This results in pancreatic insufficiency, which leads to malabsorption and failure to gain weight, as well as airway obstructions, which leads to increased susceptibility to recurrent bronchial infection, progressive lung damage, and eventual respiratory failure.

A. Clinical Presentation

The three categories of major clinical abnormalities in CF are (1) gastrointestinal tract involvement, characterized by pancreatic insufficiency leading to malabsorption and malnutrition; (2) respiratory tract involvement, characterized by chronic obstructive pulmonary disease with recurrent infections; and (3) salt loss in sweat that can lead to severe hyponatremic dehydration. The pancreatic disturbance begins prenatally and can cause intestinal obstruction in newborns with CF (a problem referred to as meconium ileus). It has been estimated that 85–90% of CF patients have functional pancreatic insufficiency [4], and 15–20% have meconium ileus [5]. Unlike pancreatic insufficiency, pulmonary status of patients with CF often appears normal at birth, however, it inevitably shows obstruction and infection. The onset and rate of progression of CF lung disease are not well understood but appear to vary widely among individuals [6, 7]. Other complications may occur as the disease progresses. For example, glucose intolerance and diabetes mellitus are prevalent [8] and about 15% of adults with CF develop diabetes requiring insulin therapy [9]; up to 5% of CF patients develop overt liver disease in adolescence or adulthood [10]; and infertility in males with CF is virtually universal [11].

B. Pathogenesis

On the basis of molecular genetics research [12, 13], CF fundamentally can be attributed to mutations occurring in the long arm of chromosome 7. With cloning of the CF gene, it has been demonstrated that the most common mutation is a 3-base-pair deletion, which results in the loss of a phenylalanine residue at amino acid position 508 of the predicted gene product, namely, the cystic fibrosis transmembrane regulator *(CFTR)* [13, 14]. The 3-base-pair deletion mutant (commonly referred to as the $\Delta F508$ mutation) occurs in about 70% of the CF chromosomes [14, 15] and more than 85% of CF patients in the United States have at least one $\Delta F508$ allele [16]. However, more than 800 other DNA mutations in the CF gene have been identified.

The abnormal CFTR protein is the underlying pathogenic factor in the disease process due to its role in regulating ion transport across the apical membrane of epithelial cells, particularly chloride conductance, which is invariably defective in CF [2, 17]. The most recent research suggests that the CFTR protein is a structural component of the chloride channel and may itself account for the channel core [13].

C. Diagnosis and Treatment

The diagnosis of CF is customarily made because of (1) a positive family history, (2) the occurrence of meconium ileus, or (3) symptoms of intestinal malabsorption or pulmonary disease with infection, which occur at variable ages [18, 19]. Once the characteristic signs and symptoms become evident, the diagnosis of CF can be readily established by performing a sweat test using pilocarpine iontophoresis [20]. Although these traditional methods are generally effective in diagnosing CF, there are often delays in diagnosis and referral to a CF center. Accordingly, there has been considerable interest in establishing neonatal screening methods for detection of presymptomatic cases for the purpose of instituting early treatment and preventing ameliorating symptoms. In 1979, Crossley *et al.* [21] first described the use of dry-blood specimen obtained from the newborns to measure immunoreactive trypsinogen level, which was shown to be highly elevated in patients with CF [21, 22]. The discovery of the

Copyright © 2001 by Academic Press.
All rights of reproduction in any form reserved.

CFTR gene in 1989 [12] has promoted the development of new screening methods where the immunoreactive trypsinogen test is coupled with detection of the most common mutant allele *(ΔF508)* or with *CFTR* mutation analysis [23]. The potential benefits and risks associated with CF neonatal screening programs have been under investigation in various regions of the world [24–27] In several recent reports [27–32], clear evidence of nutritional benefits attributable to early diagnosis was demonstrated by anthropometric indexes. The most convincing evidence was obtained from a randomized clinical trial in Wisconsin after 10 years of investigation [28, 29]. Although some other states and all of Australia have implemented routine neonatal screening for CF, more evidence of pulmonary benefits and information on cost effectiveness are needed before other regions proceed to implement this method of early diagnosis.

Clinical management of CF involves treatment programs with three principal objectives: (1) improve nutritional status, (2) promote clearance of respiratory secretions, and (3) control bronchopulmonary infections. Care programs for CF patients in North America and many European countries are organized in specialized regional centers. These centers have placed particular emphasis on enhancing nutritional status and using aggressive strategies to prevent progressive pulmonary disease [33]. Although CF lung disease cannot be cured, treatment programs have been generally effective, as evidenced by the increasing longevity of CF patients in the United States from less than 20 years to approximately 30 years during the past two decades [9, 34]. The primary causes of deaths in patients with CF are cardiorespiratory complications, accounting for 85% of the deaths from CF that occurred in 1997 [9]. For this reason, most CF Centers in the United States place a great deal of emphasis on respiratory management for patients with CF.

II. OVERVIEW OF NUTRITIONAL PROBLEMS IN CYSTIC FIBROSIS

CF is associated with an increased risk of protein energy malnutrition, as well as deficiencies in fat-soluble vitamins and other micronutrients. At the mild end of the malnutrition spectrum, CF patients may have depleted stores or low circulating concentrations of a given nutrient, but no associated signs or symptoms. More pronounced nutritional deficiencies lead to metabolic abnormalities, structural changes, functional disturbances, growth failure, developmental delay, and a variety of other characteristics of malnutrition. Malnutrition is most likely to occur during periods of rapid growth when nutritional requirements are high, during pulmonary exacerbations, and with increased severity of lung disease.

Historically, malnutrition in patients with CF was thought to represent either an inherent consequence of disease process or a physiologic adaptation to advanced pulmonary dis-

TABLE 1 Factors Contributing to Malnutrition in Cystic Fibrosis

Disease factors
Presence of pancreatic insufficiency
Severity of pancreatic insufficiency (the degree of steatorrhea and azotorrhea)
Partial intestinal resection secondary to bowel obstruction (caused by meconium ileus)
Severity of respiratory disease
Loss of bile salts associated with steatorrhea
Cholestatic liver disease
Diabetes mellitus
Nutritional factors
Growth velocity (of particular concern in young children and adolescents with CF)
Macronutrient intakes (e.g., the quantity and quality of food consumed)
Micronutrient deficiencies (e.g., vitamin E)
Energy expenditure
Eating behaviors

ease. However, it is now recognized that the causes of malnutrition in CF are multiple and can be attributed to three primary mechanisms [35–37]: increased energy and nutrient losses, increased energy expenditure; and decreased energy and nutrient intakes. Table 1 lists the major risk factors for malnutrition associated with CF.

A. Causes of Malnutrition

1. INCREASED LOSSES
Maldigestion or malabsorption resultant from pancreatic insufficiency is the primary factor contributing to energy and nutrient losses in patients with CF. Approximately 85% of CF patients have pancreatic insufficiency at the time of diagnosis. However, the severity of maldigestion and/or malabsorption depends on the residual pancreatic function and varies greatly among individual CF patients. In addition to pancreatic insufficiency, losses of bile salts and bile acids are commonly associated with steatorrhea and can exacerbate maldigestion and malabsorption. Patients presenting with meconium ileus, in particular those who have undergone intestinal resection, have further reduction in intestinal absorptive capabilities. Other factors may also contribute to energy and nutrient losses. For example, diabetes mellitus may increase energy losses due to glycosuria if not adequately controlled.

2. INCREASED REQUIREMENT
Energy requirements in patients with CF are highly variable. Several studies have reported that patients with CF have increased energy expenditure compared with non-CF

patients [38–41]. A variety of explanations have been proposed to explain the increased energy expenditure observed in CF patients. These include chronic lung infection, increase in work of breathing, genetic and cellular defects, and changes in body composition.

Chronic lung infections, particularly with *Pseudomonas aeruginosa,* have been shown to be associated with 25–80% increase in metabolic rate and energy requirements [42]. The link between CF genotype and energy requirement was reported in a study by Tomezsko *et al.* [41], who demonstrated that energy expenditure was increased by 23% in CF patients with homozygous $\Delta F508$ mutation as compared with non-CF controls [41]. The hypothesis that a basic cellular defect may increase energy requirement was supported by *in vitro* studies showing that mitochondria from cultured fibroblasts obtained from CF patients had higher rates of oxygen consumption compared with control tissues [43, 44]. Last, the observation that CF patients often have a lower percentage of body stores of metabolic substrates relative to their muscle mass compared with non-CF individuals [41] may contribute to increased energy expenditure in CF.

3. DECREASED CONSUMPTION

The appetite or energy intake of CF patients may be limited due to a variety of disease complications. Acute respiratory exacerbations are a common cause of anorexia, and chest infections often give rise to nausea and vomitting, which may further reduce intake [35]. The biochemical causes of anorexia associated with acute infection are unclear, but elevated circulating levels of tumor necrosis factor may play a role [45]. In addition to pulmonary complications, a variety of gastrointestinal complications also contribute to anorexia and inadequate caloric intake [35]. Increased occurrence of gastroesophageal reflux and esophagitis are observed in patients with CF. Distal intestinal obstruction syndrome, a form of subacute or chronic partial bowel obstruction, usually occurs in older patients with pancreatic insufficiency. Large fecal masses, palpable in the abdomen, give rise to intermittent abdominal distention and cramping accompanied with reduced appetite. Constipation in the absence of distal intestinal obstruction syndrome is another cause of anorexia and abdominal discomfort in older patients with CF.

B. Common Nutritional Deficiencies

1. ENERGY AND MACRONUTRIENTS

As discussed earlier, patients with CF are at high risk of energy inadequacy due to their increased requirement and decreased consumption. Fat is the highest density source of energy and is needed to provide sufficient essential fatty acids. However, prior to 1980, restriction of fat intake was often recommended in an effort to lessen the symptoms of steatorrhea and malabsorption.

Protein poses less of a nutritional problem than does fat in the CF population. The major risk of protein deficiency in CF patients occurs during the first year of life, when the average requirement is at least three times as great as that in adulthood. Human milk, which is relatively low in protein (7% of energy), and soy-based formula have been particularly associated with hypoproteinemic edema and growth retardation before instituting pancreatic enzyme therapy. It is recommended that protein should provide at least 15% of total daily energy intake for CF patients with pancreatic insufficiency.

2. FAT-SOLUBLE VITAMINS

Deficiencies of fat-soluble vitamins in the CF population have been demonstrated in many studies [46–53]. Vitamin A and E are of the greatest concern, particularly in patients with severe malabsorption or liver disease. Deficiencies in Vitamin D or vitamin K are less common, and most likely occur in association with advanced cholestatic liver disease.

Vitamin A deficiency was the first micronutrient deficit demonstrated in patients with CF. Clinical symptoms of vitamin A deficiency reported in CF patients include keratinizing metaplasia of the bronchial epithelium, xerophthalmia, and night blindness. Several mechanisms for vitamin A deficiency in CF have been proposed, ranging from a defect in the mobilizing hepatic storage of vitamin A due to liver disease to low levels of retinol binding protein, which is responsible for transporting vitamin A in the circulation [48, 49].

Vitamin E deficiency in CF is most commonly evidenced by low plasma levels of α-tocopherol, which has been shown to be prevalent in infants with CF identified from neonatal screening programs [48, 54]. Vitamin K deficiency has not been routinely demonstrated in patients with CF. However, vitamin K deficiency is likely to develop in patients with CF who also have severe cholestatic liver disease, short-bowel syndrome, and lung disease requiring frequent antibiotic use [53].

3. MINERALS

Macrominerals of concern in CF include sodium, calcium, and phosphorus. Sodium is of concern in CF patients because of its abnormally high content in the sweat. In hot climates, salt depletion can be catastrophic, leading to severe hyponatremic dehydration and shock. Therefore, sodium requirement may be considerably higher for CF patients than that of normal individuals. Nevertheless, routine sodium supplements appear to be unnecessary because the average American diet contains an overabundance of sodium. Sodium supplements are needed only in conditions that may cause prolonged sweat loss.

There is no clear evidence of deficiency in trace minerals in patients with CF. However, low plasma levels of zinc, calcium, magnesium, and iron in patients with CF have all been reported [55, 56]. In particular, iron-deficiency anemia

with low serum ferritin has been shown to be quite frequent in CF patients with advanced pulmonary disease [56, 57].

4. ESSENTIAL FATTY ACIDS

Essential fatty acid (EFA) deficiency has been known to occur in patients with CF [54, 58–60]. In infancy, particularly before diagnosis, EFA deficiency can occur with desquamating skin lesions, increased susceptibility to infection, poor wound healing, thrombocytopenia, and growth retardation. In older patients who are adequately treated, clinical evidence of EFA deficiency is rare, although biochemical abnormalities of EFA status remain common [61–63]. The major abnormalities in fatty acid profile found in patients with CF is a low level of linoleic acid and elevated levels of palmitoleic, oleic, and eicosatrienoic acid.

Multiple hypotheses have been proposed to explain the underlying mechanisms of abnormal EFA status associated with CF. Fat malabsorption secondary to pancreatic insufficiency is the most common explanation for EFA. However, some investigators have postulated a primary metabolic defect in fatty acid metabolism [61–63]. In addition, van Egmond and colleagues [64] found that the growth rates of infants with CF were closely correlated with linoleic acid status.

III. PREVALENCE OF MALNUTRITION

Malnutrition associated with CF is characterized by its early onset, and is often present at the time of CF diagnosis. Growth impairment, abnormalities in the biochemical markers of nutritional status, and clinical symptoms of malnutrition all have been reported in patients with CF. Because CF is associated with many risk factors of malnutrition, and growth impairment is very common in children with CF, there have been doubts whether normal growth can occur in children with CF [65]. The recent results from the Wisconsin CF neonatal screening study [28, 29] demonstrated unequivocally that young children with CF who are diagnosed early can grow normally with energy intakes averaging 110% of RDA. The prevalence of growth impairment, biochemical abnormalities, and suboptimal intakes is discussed further below.

A. Growth Impairment

Weight retardation and linear growth failure are the most common observations documented in the CF clinics [66, 67], although its severity and prevalence vary greatly. Accurate estimates on the prevalence of malnutrition in the North American CF populations have been difficult to obtain in the past, due to lack of sufficient data. In recent years, national databases compiled by the U.S. and Canadian Cystic Fibrosis Foundations, known as the CF Foundation Patient Registries, have become available, making it possible to determine population estimates on the prevalence of malnutrition associated with CF. In a comprehensive study by Lai *et al.* [68], the nutritional status of more than 13,000 pediatric patients with CF seen in 144 CF centers in the United States during 1993 was examined using anthropometric criteria. Physical growth of children with CF was found to be substantially below normal at all ages, when plotted against growth curves developed by the National Center for Health Statistics for U.S. children [69], as shown in Fig. 1. The prevalence of stunting, defined as height below the 5th percentile, and underweight, defined as weight below the 5th percentile, was at approximately 25%. In addition, malnutrition was found to be particularly prevalent in infants (47%) and adolescents (34%) as compared with children at other ages (22%), and in patients with newly diagnosed, untreated CF (44%). In another study by Lai *et al.* [70], underweight was also found to be prevalent in adults with CF. Approximately 35% of the 7200 adults with CF documented in the 1992–1994 U.S. and Canadian CF Foundation Patient Registries were below the 5th percentile for weight when evaluated based on adult weight standards published from the second National Health and Nutrition Examination Survey [71].

B. Biochemical Abnormalities

In addition to growth impairment, abnormalities in the biochemical indexes of nutritional status also exist in patients with CF. Serum markers of protein status (e.g., albumin, prealbumin, retinol binding protein), fat (e.g., cholesterol, EFA profile), and fat-soluble vitamins (e.g., retinol, α-tocopherol) are typically found to be low in patients with CF. Abnormalities in biochemical indices are particularly prevalent in newly diagnosed infants with CF. Sokol *et al.* [72] reported that, of the 36 infants identified via CF newborn screening, 36% were hypoalbuminemic, 21% had low serum retinol, 35% had low serum 25-hydoxyvitamin D, and 38% had low serum α-tocopherol. Similarly, Lai *et al.* [54] reported that, of the 50 infants diagnosed before 3 months of age via neonatal screening, 46% had low serum albumin levels, 40% had low serum retinol levels, 72% had low α-tocopherol levels, and 50% had low plasma linoleic acid levels. Normalization of the biochemical nutritional indices can occur following comprehensive nutrition therapy. As observed by Marcus *et al.* [73], the prevalence of low serum albumin and retinol reduced substantially after 6 months of treatment. However, plasma α-tocopherol and linoleic acid remained low in 20–30% of patients despite ongoing nutrition therapy. In another recent cross-sectional study by Benabdeslam *et al.* [74], who examined 56 patients with CF aged 4–26 years, the prevalence of low plasma levels of albumin, cholesterol, and retinol binding protein remained high at 42, 25, and 12%, respectively, despite regular treatment. Serum concentrations of retinol and α-tocopherol were also significantly lower in CF patients compared to those of non-CF controls.

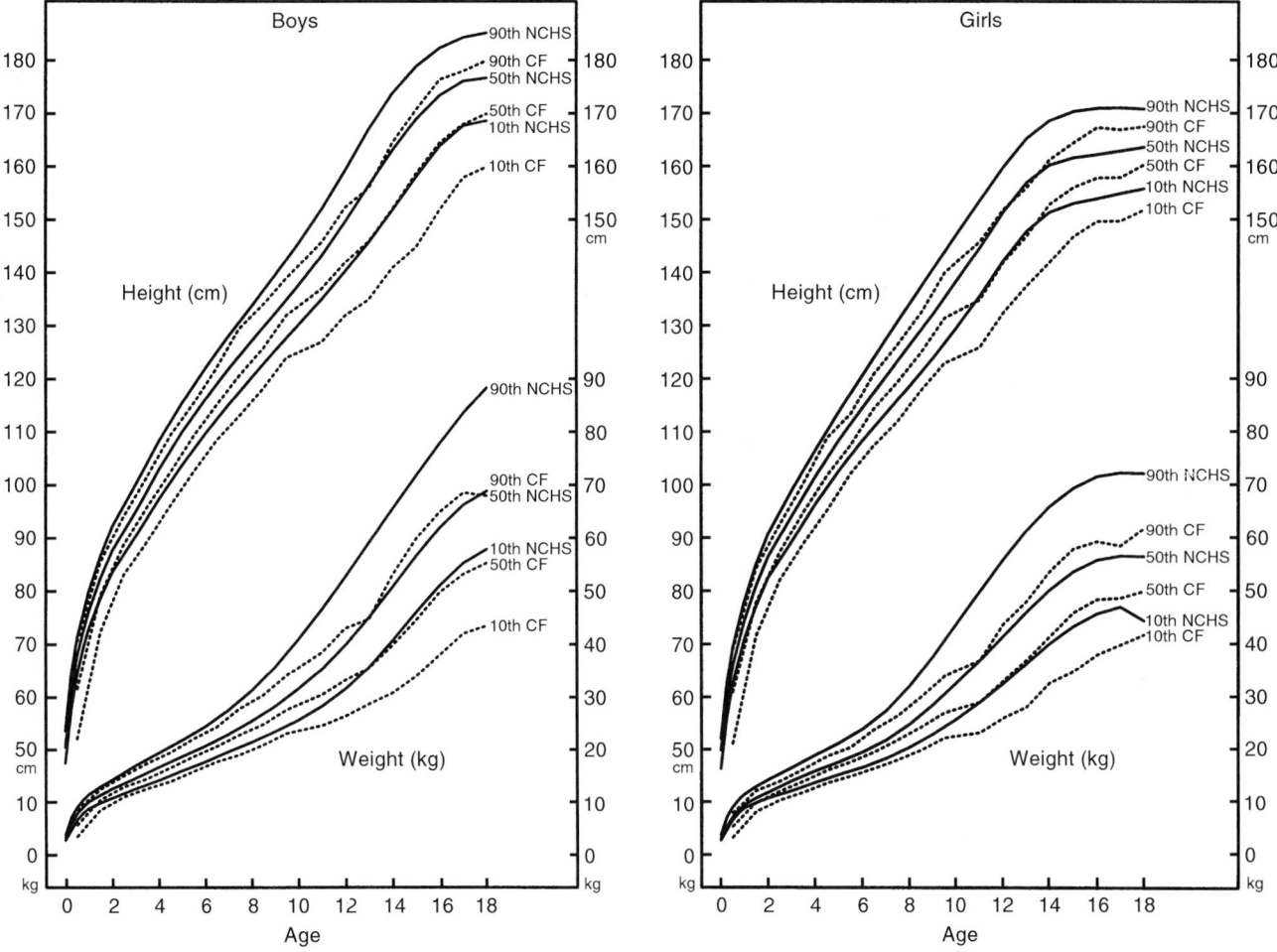

FIGURE 1   Height and weight percentile curves of children with CF (dotted curves) compared with those of the National Center for Health Statistics reference population (solid curves). [Modified from Lai, H. C., Kosorok, M. R., Sondel, S. A., Chen, S. T., FitzSimmons, S. C., Green, C., Shen, G., Walker, S., and Farrell, P. M. (1998). Growth status in children with cystic fibrosis based on National Cystic Fibrosis Patient Registry data: Evaluation of various criteria to identify malnutrition. *J. Pediatr.* **132,** 478–485.]

C. Suboptimal Dietary Intakes

The literature often describes infants and young children with CF as having voracious appetites. However, a number of dietary surveys particularly during the 1970s and early 1980s, when patients with CF were commonly prescribed with fat-resricted diets on the assumption that a reduction in dietary fat intake might improve bowel symptoms, indicate that patients with CF often eat less than normal. [75]. The observation of better growth and survival in patients with CF who received an unrestricted-fat, high-energy diet in combination with pancreatic enzyme supplementation compared with those who received low-fat diet in the early 1980s has changed dietary practices in most CF centers [76]. Energy intakes of 120% or greater than the Recommended Dietary Allowances (RDA), with 40% of energy from fat are now recommended for patients with CF [77]. However, patients

with CF often fail to consume such high amounts of energy and/or fat because of their disease manifestation. In several cross-sectional or short-term studies [78–82] and a small prospective 3-year study of 25 patients [83], energy and fat intakes of patients with CF were reported to be much lower than these recommendations. More recently, a longitudinal study [84] evaluating dietary intake patterns in children with CF from the time of diagnosis to age 10 years revealed that mean energy intake was at ~110% of RDA with fat consisting of ~37% of energy.

IV. NUTRITIONAL ASSESSMENT AND INTERVENTION

Frequent monitoring of the nutritional status for patients with CF is ential to ensure early detection of any deterioration and

TABLE 2 Guidelines for Assessment of Nutritional Status in Patients with Cystic Fibrosis

Index	Minimum frequency	Indication
1990 Guidelines		
Anthropometric assessment		
Length (0–2 years) and height (2–20 years)	Every 3 months	At diagnosis, routine care
Weight and percentage of ideal weight-for-height	Every 3 months	At diagnosis, routine care
Head circumference (0–2 years)	Every 3 months	At diagnosis, routine care
Midarm circumference and triceps skinfold thickness	Yearly	At diagnosis, routine care
Biochemical assessment		
Complete blood count[a]	Yearly	At diagnosis, routine care
Serum/plasma retinol and α-tocopheral	Yearly	At diagnosis, routine care
Albumin	As indicated	At diagnosis, weight loss, growth failure, clinical deterioration
Electrolyte and acid–base balance	As indicated	At diagnosis, infancy, breast feeding, prolonged fever, summer heat
Dietary assessment		
Dietary intakes[b]	Yearly	At diagnosis, routine care
3-Day fat balance[c]	As indicated	At diagnosis, weight loss, growth failure, clinical deterioration
Proposed additional guidelines (2001)		
Length/height adjusting for parental stature	Every 3 months	At diagnosis, routine care
Body mass index	Every 3 months	At diagnosis, routine care
Head circumference (3–6 years)	Yearly	At diagnosis, routine care
Assessment of puberty (9–20 years)	Yearly	At diagnosis, routine care
Plasma fatty acid status	Yearly	At diagnosis, routine care

Source: 1990 Guidelines: Adapted from Ramsey, B. W., Farrell, P. M., and Pencharz, P., for the Consensus Committee (1992). Nutritional assessment and management in cystic fibrosis: A consensus report. *Am. J. Clin. Nutr.* **55,** 108–116. Proposed Additional Guidelines (2001): Cystic Fibrosis Foundation Consensus Committee on Nutrition, March 2001.

[a]If there is any evidence of iron deficiency, iron status should be measured (i.e., serum iron, iron-binding capacity, and serum ferritin).

[b]Usually consists of a 24-hour dietary recall with assessment of dietary patterns; should be performed by a dietitian.

[c]Include both dietary records to determine energy and fat intakes as well as a determination of stool fat excretion concurrent with evaluation of dietary fat intake to permit calculation of absorption coefficient and assessment of the degree of malabsorption.

prompt initiation of nutrition intervention. Patients with CF are most vulnerable to developing nutrition deficiencies during times of rapid growth, e.g., during infancy and adolescence, and during periods of pulmonary declines. During these periods, close monitoring and intervention are critical to prevent nutritional failure. Guidelines for nutritional assessment and intervention for patients with CF were developed in the early 1990s and reported by the US Cystic Fibrosis Foundation [85, 86]. The following section describes these guidelines. In addition, the Consensus Committee on Nutrition from the Cystic Fibrosis Foundation is in the process of updating the 1990 guidelines.

A. Guidelines for Nutritional Assessment

Assessment of nutritional status for patients with CF must include anthropometric, biochemical, and dietary assessments. The frequency at which the different indices of nutritional status monitoring should be measured is given in Table 2.

1. ANTHROPOMETRIC ASSESSMENT

Anthropometric assessment, with an emphasis on physical growth, is an important component of nutritional assessment in children with CF. Measurements of height (or length in children aged 0–2 years), weight, and head circumference (in children aged 0–2 years) should be obtained at each clinic visit. To evaluate if deviation from normal growth occurs, sequential measurements of height and weight should be plotted on standard growth charts and converted to sex- and age-specific percentiles. The growth charts developed by the National Center for Health Statistics can be used for this purpose [69, 87]. The infant growth charts should be used for children aged 0–3 years, and the 2- to 18-year charts should be used for older children. For adolescents with CF, it is recommended to supplement National Center for Health Statistics growth charts with the Tanner charts to monitor growth and pubertal development [88].

In addition to height/length and weight, it is important to evaluate whether the patient's weight is ideal for his or her height. For this purpose, the Cystic Fibrosis Foundation recommends the use of a weight-for-height index [89], which is referred as the percentage of ideal weight-for-height and can be calculated by the following steps:

Step 1. Plot the patient's height/length on the growth chart and determine the height percentile.
Step 2. Determine the patient's "ideal weight," which is the weight at the same percentile as that for his or her height. For example, for a 6-year-old girl with a height on the 25th percentile, her ideal weight is the weight that corresponds to the 25th percentile weight at age 6 year.
Step 3. Express actual weight as a percentage of ideal weight, that is,
Percentage of ideal weight = (actual weight/ideal weight) × 100.
Step 4. Classify nutritional status using the following criteria:
Normal—90–100%
Underweight—85–89%
Mild malnutrition—80–84%
Moderate malnutrition—75–79%
Severe malnutrition—<75%.

Special attention should be given to patients with poor growth. Using various height and weight indices, the following criteria are recommended to identify patients with nutritional failure:

For patients <5 years of age—a weight-for-height index <85% of ideal weight, weight loss for >2 months, or a plateau in weight gain for 2–3 months
For patients 5–18 years of age—weight-for-height index <85% of ideal weight, weight loss for >2 months, or a plateau in weight gain for 6 months

For patients >18 years of age—a weight-for-height index <85% of ideal weight, or weight loss >5% for >2 months.

In addition to the above, body mass index, midarm circumference, and skinfold thickness should be used to further assess the patient's lean body mass and body fatness.

2. BIOCHEMICAL ASSESSMENT

Routine measurements of the following biochemical indices of nutritional status should be obtained: electrolytes and acid–base status, complete blood count (CBC), serum albumin, retinol, and α-tocopherol. In addition to these routine measurements, when the results of CBC show evidence of iron deficiency, iron status should be assessed (i.e., serum iron, iron-binding capacity, and serum ferritin).

Routine assessments of vitamin D (25-hydroxycholecalciferol), vitamin K status, and EFA status are not presently regarded as necessary. However, annual assessments of these nutrients are likely to be recommended in the update guidelines because recent findings indicate increased prevalence of abnormal status of these nutrients among patients with CF [52–54, 62].

3. DIETARY ASSESSMENT

Assessments of energy requirement and dietary intakes are important ways of determining whether the patient is in negative energy balance. Energy requirements vary greatly among individual CF patients due to their wide range of the degree of malabsorption and hypermetabolism. Therefore, energy requirements for patients with CF are best determined by estimating the basal metabolic rate, the degree of malabsorption, and the severity of pulmonary disease. For patients who are growing normally and whose steatorrhea is under good control, the estimated energy requirement is consistent with that recommended by the RDA for their gender and age [90]. For patients with increased energy requirement due to malabsorption and/or pulmonary disease, energy requirement can be estimated by the following method:

Step 1. Estimate basal metabolic rate by using the equations provided by the World Health Organization [91].
Step 2. Estimate daily energy expenditure using the following equation:
Daily energy expenditure = basal metabolic rate × (activity coefficient + disease coefficient)
where the activity coefficient is 1.3 (confine to bed), 1.5 (sedentary) or 1.7 (active), and the disease coefficient is 0 (normal lung function, i.e., forced expiratory volume in one second (FEV_1) >80% predicted), 0.2 (moderate lung disease, i.e., FEV_1 40–79% predicted), or 0.3 (severe lung disease, i.e., FEV_1 <40%).
Step 3. Estimate daily energy requirement, taking into account the degree of fat malabsorption, which can be

estimated by the coefficient of fat absorption based on 3-day fat balance studies:

a. Pancreatic-sufficient patients (including patients on enzyme with coefficient of fat absorption ≥93%), daily energy requirement = daily energy expenditure.

b. For pancreatic-insufficient patients with a coefficient of fat absorption <93%, daily energy requirement = daily energy expenditure × (0.93/coefficient of fat absorption).

c. For pancreatic-insufficient patients whose coefficient of fat absorption has not been determined, an approximate value of 0.85 may be used to estimate daily energy requirement, i.e., daily energy requirement = daily energy expenditure × (0.93/0.85).

Evaluation of dietary intake is best performed by nutritionists specializing in the care of patients with CF. For patients with good nutritional status, a dietitian may assess dietary habits and the quality of dietary intake using a 24-hour dietary recall. However, for patients with suboptimal nutritional status, a 3-day prospective food record is the best way to obtain quantitative estimates of energy and nutrient intakes. This assessment can then be used as the basis for initiating appropriate nutrition intervention.

B. Guidelines for Nutrition Management

Nutrition management for patients with CF varies and depends on the patient's age and disease severity. Nutrition intervention begins at the time of CF diagnosis, which corresponds to the first 2 years of life in the majority of patients with CF. After the diagnosis of CF, nutrition management is based on the clinical status of patients with CF and can be categorized into five response categories: routine management, anticipatory guidance, supportive intervention, rehabilitative care, and resuscitative and palliative care. The goals of the nutritional management for each response category are summarized in Table 3.

1. AT DIAGNOSIS

The time of diagnosis is a crucial period for beginning nutritional education, dietary counseling, and therapeutic interventions. All nutritional indices should be measured at the time of CF diagnosis. These include anthropometry (height, weight, and/or head circumference), biochemical nutritional markers (serum or plasma albumin, vitamin A, vitamin E, and EFA), and dietary intake. In addition, assessment of pancreatic function status is essential, and is best determined based on a 3-day fat balance study. If maldigestion and malabsorption are identified, pancreatic enzyme replacement therapy should be initiated. Nutritional interventions can then be individualized to each patient's needs. Extensive discussion of nutritional management with patients and/or parents is another important aspect of care during this period of time. By concentrating on nutrition during the family's first few

visits to the CF center, care-givers will be able to stress the importance of establishing and maintaining good nutrition.

2. ROUTINE MANAGEMENT

The primary goal of routine nutrition management is to optimize pancreatic enzyme replacement, as well as nutritional and vitamin supplements. Management should be based on the patient's clinical status and energy requirement. Nutritional status should be assessed at each clinic visit. Presently, the Cystic Fibrosis Foundation recommends that patients with CF be seen on a routine follow-up basis every 3–4 months. Thus, at a minimum, growth and nutritional status should be monitored at these intervals. Because nutritional requirements are influenced by age, routine management from infancy to adulthood is further discussed below.

a. Infancy to 2 Years. The first 2 years represent the phase of life with the highest growth rate and energy requirement. Infants diagnosed with CF vary widely with regard to their presenting symptoms. Infants diagnosed as a result of gastrointestinal and/or pulmonary symptoms often present with growth failure at the time of CF diagnosis. These infants should be evaluated weekly or every other week until normal weight gain has been established.

Infants born with meconium ileus, in particular, those who have bowel resection resultant from intestinal surgery, represent another special group with high risk of nutritional failure. To promote optimal growth, these infants may require enteral or parenteral nutrition support in addition to predigested formula and pancreatic enzyme therapy. Intensive monitoring on growth, biochemical nutritional indices, and dietary intake are critical in maintaining proper growth rate in CF patients with meconium ileus.

Unlike infants with more severe CF as described above, infants identified through a positive family history or through neonatal screening within the first 3 months of life are often asymptomatic and show relatively good growth at the time of CF diagnosis. The goals of nutrition management for this group of infants are to maintain normal growth and to prevent the occurrence of malnutrition.

Milk products serve as the predominant source of nutrients for infants with CF during the first year of life. Breast feeding is encouraged in infants who show appropriate growth. However, breast-fed infants should be closely monitored with regard to their growth velocity, protein status, and electrolyte status. Supplementation with formula should be initiated if growth faltering is observed. If an infant with CF is growing at a normal rate, a change to whole cow's milk may be recommended beginning at 12 months of age, although formula feeding may be continued up to 24 months of age. Introduction of solid food should be made according to the guidelines of the American Academy of Pediatrics, namely, between 4 and 6 months of age or earlier if necessary.

b. Toddlers to Preschool (Ages 2–6 years). Children in this age group have developed self-feeding behaviors and express individual food preferences. Dietary intake and de-

TABLE 3 Guidelines for Nutritional Management in Patients with Cystic Fibrosis

Category	Target group	Goals
At diagnosis and routine management	All patients	Nutritional education and dietary counseling; pancreatic enzyme replacement and vitamin supplementation for patients with pancreatic insufficiency
Anticipatory guidance	Patients at risk of developing energy imbalance (i.e., severe pancreatic insufficiency, frequent pulmonary infections, periods of rapid growth) but maintaining a weight-for-height index of ≥90% of ideal weight	Further education to prepare patients for increased energy needs; increased monitoring of dietary intakes; increased caloric density in diet as needed; behavioral assessment and counseling
Supportive intervention	Patients with decreased weight velocity and/or a weight-for-height index of 85–90% of ideal weight	All of the above plus oral supplements as needed
Rehabilitative care	Patients with a weight-for-height index consistently ≤85% of ideal weight	All of the above plus enteral supplementation via nasogastric tube or enterostomy as indicated
Resuscitative and palliative care	Patients with a weight-for-height index consistently ≤75% of ideal weight or with progressive nutritional failure	All of the above plus continuous enteral feeds or total parenteral nutrition

Source: Adapted from Ramsey, B. W., Farrell, P. M., and Pencharz, P., for the Consensus Committee (1992). Nutritional assessment and management in cystic fibrosis: A consensus report. *Am. J. Clin. Nutr.* **55,** 108–116.

gree of physical activity vary from day to day. For these reasons, close monitoring of dietary habits, energy intake, and growth velocity are important.

c. School Age (Ages 6–12 years). Children in this age group are exposed to significant degrees of peer pressure and are challenged to self-manage their disease. Compliance with prescribed medications such as pancreatic enzymes and fat-soluble vitamins can become a major problem during this period. In addition, acceptance and understanding by teachers and fellow students may be lacking, further stressing a child with CF.

d. Adolescence and Puberty (Ages 12–18 years). This developmental stage represents another vulnerable period of developing malnutrition because of increased nutritional requirement associated with accelerated growth, endocrine development, and high levels of physical activity. In addition, pulmonary disease often becomes more severe in this period, increasing energy requirement. Pubertal delay and growth failure are common and come at a time of extreme psychosocial stresses.

Frequent monitoring of dietary intake, growth velocity, and nutritional status are important; every 3 months is optimal. Nutritional counseling must be directed toward the patient rather than the parents.

e. Adulthood. Patients with CF who reach adulthood are usually responsible for the entire management of their disease, as well as for the financial burden of a chronic illness. While in college or working, adults with CF are constantly adapting to new schedules and stresses. The goal of nutrition management is to maintain ideal weight-for-height and to prevent weight loss. Nutritional counseling must be practical and pragmatic to help adults adjust to these changes.

f. Pregnancy and Lactation. Widespread experience in recent years has demonstrated that pregnancy and lactation can be accomplished successfully by some women with CF. Pregnant women with CF should follow the RDA guidelines for nutrient intakes. In addition, special attention should be given to appropriate weight gain, particularly during the last trimester of pregnancy. In addition to the usual multivitamin supplementation for CF, one prenatal vitamin should be consumed daily. During lactation, marked increase in energy intake is necessary to meet the high energy requirement during this period.

g. Vitamin Supplementation. In CF patients with pancreatic insufficiency, vitamin supplementation is necessary to prevent the occurrence of deficiencies. For infants and children younger than 2 years of age, liquid multivitamin supplementation at a dose equivalent to 1 mL of polyvisol (Mead Johnson Nutritionals, Evansville, IN), has been shown to provide sufficient vitamins A and D. Children aged 2–8 years need a standard multivitamin containing 400 IU vitamin D and 5000 IU vitamin A in a dose of 1 tablet/day. Older children, adolescents and adults need a standard adult multivitamin preparation, 1–2 tablets/day.

In addition to standard multivitamin supplementation, additional supplementation with vitamin E with the following doses are recommended: ages 0–6 months, 25 IU/day; 6–12 months, 50 IU/day; ages 1–4 years, 100 IU/day; 4-10 years, 100-200 IU/day; and >10 years, 200–400 IU/day. For the first 2 years of life, vitamin E is given as Aquasol E (Rover

Pharmaceuticals, Fort Washington, PA) or liquid-E (Twin Labs, Ronkonkoma, NY). More research is needed to define the optimal supplementation regimen for vitamin K in patients with CF. Until further information is available, recommendations are to prescribe vitamin K supplementation as follows: age 0–12 months, 2.5 mg/week, or 2.5 mg twice weekly if on antibiotics; ages >1 year, 5.0 mg twice weekly when on antibiotics or if cholestatic liver disease is present.

3. GUIDELINES FOR NUTRITIONAL SUPPORT

For CF patients who are at risk of developing, and those who are experiencing, nutritional failure, nutritional support beyond the level of routine maintenance care is required. Nutritional support is delivered at various levels, beginning with dietary modification, to oral supplementation, to enteral and parenteral supplementation. Guidelines for nutritional support of these patients are divided into four categories based on the severity of malnutrition (Table 3).

a. Anticipatory Guidance. Patients with CF in this category maintain relatively normal nutritional status (i.e., weight-for-height index >90%), but are at high risk of developing energy deficiencies. These include patients who are growing rapidly, e.g., infants and adolescents, and patients who have more severe clinical symptoms, e.g., pancreatic insufficiency, meconium ileus, and frequent pulmonary infections. Nutrition counseling is directed to dietary and behavioral modifications for the purpose of increasing energy intake and minimizing the risk of nutritional decline by introducing the concept of boosted oral intake. This concept considers the patient's usual food preferences and habits and then increases the nutrient density of the diet without dramatically increasing the amount of food consumed. For example, margarine or butter may be added to many foods, and light cream can be used in place of skim milk or water when preparing canned soup. Instead of snacks like fruit juice, nutrient-dense foods such as nuts, cheese and crackers, cold cuts, whole milk, peanut butter sandwiches, and pizza may be provided to patients requiring additional nutrients.

In addition to the quality of the diets, psychosocial and behavioral problems can have significant impact on the nutritional status of patients with CF. An in-depth assessment of eating behavior, feeding patterns, and family interactions at mealtimes should be performed when a patient shows signs of decline in nutritional status.

b. Supportive Intervention. This level of nutritional support is initiated when patients with CF show signs of mild malnutrition, as indicated by a weight-for-height index between 85% and 90%. Initial management follows the same guidelines as outlined in "anticipatory guidance." However, additional oral supplements in the form of homemade or proprietary products are strongly encouraged to maximize caloric and nutrient intakes. Homemade supplements are often more palatable and less expensive than commercial products, although the latter may be more convenient. If these treatments are not successful within 3 months or if the patient's weight falls below 85% of ideal, more aggressive nutritional management should be considered, as described below.

c. Rehabilitative Care. This level of nutritional support is initiated for CF patients who are experiencing nutritional failure (as indicated by a weight below 85% of ideal) and who are unable to improve weight gain with the use of oral supplementation and behavioral modification. In this case, further nutrition intervention with nocturnal enteral feedings can be helpful. Several studies have shown that this intervention improves body composition, increases strength and sense of well-being, increases sense of mastery over body weight, improves body image, encourages normal pubertal development, and reduces weight loss during pulmonary exacerbations.

Enteral feeding can be delivered via nasogastric tubes, gastrostomy tubes, and jejunostomy tubes. The choice of an enterostomy tube and technique for its placement should be based on local factors and the expertise of the CF center involved. Nasogastric tubes are appropriate for short-term nutritional support in highly motivated patients. Patients can learn to pass soft Silastic feeding tubes to receive overnight feeding. High-calorie formula can be infused, allowing patients to receive up to 50% of their energy requirement while asleep.

Gastrostomy tubes can be used for patients who need chronic enteral nutritional support. Gastrostomy tubes or buttons can be placed by the percutaneous endoscopic route or surgically. Gastroesophageal reflux may occur with gastrostomy tube feeding. This problem can often be alleviated by adjusting the feeding rate, the patient's positioning during sleep, and administration of prokinetic agents (e.g., domperidone). Jejunostomy feedings potentially increase the problem of nutrient malabsorption, but have been used very successfully in some CF centers. Use of predigested or elemental formula may be needed with jejunostomy feeding.

d. Resuscitative and Palliative Care. This level of nutritional support is targeted to CF patients who are severely malnourished, with a weight below 75% of the ideal. Aggressive nutritional rehabilitation in terminally ill patients is usually not medically indicated (unless the patients are awaiting organ transplantation). Nevertheless, parenteral nutrition may be used for short-term support when enteral feedings are contraindicated, for example, for patients with short-gut syndrome, pancreatitis, and severe gastroenteritis, and during postoperative period after intestinal surgery.

V. CONCLUSIONS

The clear associations between nutritional status and clinical outcomes in CF mandate careful nutritional assessment, management, and monitoring of all patients with CF. In recent years, there has been a shift away from the idea that malnutrition is inevitable for most patients with CF toward the more optimistic view that normal nutrition and growth

are possible if early diagnosis and aggressive nutritional monitoring and therapy are made to each individual patient, based on high-quality scientific studies. This task is best accomplished by involving a multidisciplinary team that includes a dietitian in the care and management of CF patients. In this way, the goals of normal growth and prevention of malnutrition can be attained, which will improve the prognosis and quality of life for patients with CF.

References

1. Kosorok, M. R., Wei, W. H., and Farrell, P.M. (1996). The incidence of cystic fibrosis. Stat Med 1996 **15,** 449–462.

2. Boat, T. F., Welsh, M. J., and Beaudet, A. L. (1989). Cystic Fibrosis. *In* "The Metabolic Basis of Inherited Disease" (C. R. Scriver, Al L. Beaudet, W. S. Sly, and D. Valle Eds.), pp. 2649–2680. McGraw-Hill, New York.

3. di Sant'Agnese, P. A., and Davis, P. B. (1976). Research in cystic fibrosis. *N. Engl. J. Med.* **295,** 481–485.

4. Waters, D. L., Dorney, S. F. A., Gaskin, K. J., Gruca, M. A., O'Halloran, M., and Wilcken, B. (1990). Pancreatic function in infants identified as having cystic fibrosis in a neonatal screening program. *N. Engl. J. Med.* **322,** 303–308.

5. Kerem, E., Corey, M., Kerem, B., Durie, P., Tsui, L. C., and Levison, H. (1989). Clinical and genetic comparisons of patients with cystic fibrosis, with or without meconium ileus. *J. Pediatr.* **114,** 767–773.

6. Corey, M. L. (1980). Longitudinal studies in cystic fibrosis. *In* "Perspectives in Cystic Fibrosis," pp. 246–261. Canadian Cystic Fibrosis Foundation, Toronto.

7. Katz, J. N., Horwitz, R. I., Dolan, T. F., and Shapiro, E. D. (1986). Clinical features as predictors of functional status in children with cystic fibrosis. *Pediatrics* **108,** 352–358.

8. Hardin, D. S., and Moran, A. (1999). Diabetes mellitus in cystic fibrosis. *Endocrinol. Metab. Clin. of N. Am.* **28,** 787–800.

9. Cystic Fibrosis Foundation. (1998). "National Cystic Fibrosis Patient Registry Annual Data Report, 1997." Cystic Fibrosis Foundation, Bethesda. MD.

10. Scott-Jupp, R., Lana, M., and Tanner, M. S. (1991). Prevalence of liver disease in cystic fibrosis. *Arch. Dis. Child.* **66,** 698–701.

11. Kaplan, E., Shwachman, H., Perlmutter, A. D., Rule, A., Khaw, K. T., and Holsclaw, D. S. (1968). Reproductive failure in males with cystic fibrosis. *N. Engl. J. Med.* **279,** 65–69.

12. Kerem, B. S., Rommens, J. M., Buchanan, J. A., Markiewicz, D., Cox, T. K., Chakravarti, A., Buchwald, M., and Tsui, L. C. (1989). Identification of the cystic fibrosis gene: Genetic analysis. *Science* **245,** 1073–1080.

13. Collins, F. S. (1992). Cystic fibrosis: Molecular biology and therapeutic implications. *Science* **256,** 29–33.

14. Tsui, L. C., and Buchwald, M. (1991). Biochemical and molecular genetics of cystic fibrosis. *In* "Advances in Human Genetics" (H. Harris and K. Hirschhorn, Eds.), pp. 153–266. Plenum Press, New York.

15. Gregg, R. G., Simantel, A., Farrell, P. M., Koscik, R., Kosorok, M. R., Laxova, A., Laessig, R., Hoffman, G., Hassemer, D., Mischler, E. H., and Splaingard, M. (1997). Newborn screening for cystic fibrosis in Wisconsin: Comparison of biochemical and molecular methods. *Pediatrics* **99,** 819–824.

16. The Cystic Fibrosis Genotype–Phenotype Consortium. (1993). Correlation between genotype and phenotype in patients with cystic fibrosis. *N. Engl. J. Med.* **329,** 1308–1313.

17. Anderson, M. P., Rich, D. P., Gregory, R. J., Smith, A. E., and Welsh, M. J. (1991). Generation of cAMP-activated chloride currents by expression of CFTR. *Science* **251,** 679–682.

18. Blythe, S. A., and Farrell, P. M. (1984). Advances in the diagnosis and management of cystic fibrosis. *Clin. Biochem.* **17,** 277–283.

19. Rosenstein, B. J., Langbaum, T. S., and Metz, S. J. (1982). Cystic fibrosis: Diagnostic considerations. *Johns Hopkins Med. J.* **150,** 113–120.

20. di Sant'Agnese, P. A., and Farrell, P. M. (1976). Neonatal and general aspects of cystic fibrosis. *In* "Current Topics in Clinical Chemistry—Clinical Biochemistry of the Neonate" (D. S. Young and J. M. Hicks, Eds.), pp. 199–217. Wiley, New York.

21. Crossley, J. R., Elliot, R. B., and Smith, R. A. (1979). Dried blood spot screening for cystic fibrosis in the newborn. *Lancet* **1,** 472–474.

22. Heely, A. F., Heely, M. E., King, D. N., Kuzemko, J. A., and Walsh, M. P. (1982). Screening for cystic fibrosis by dried blood spot trypsin assay. *Arch. Dis. Child.* **57,** 18–21.

23. Farrell, P. M., Mischler, E. H., Fost, N. C., Wilfond, B. S., Tluczek, A., Gregg, R. G., Bruns, W. T., Hassemer, D. J., and Laessig, R. H. (1991). Current issues in neonatal screening for cystic fibrosis and implications of the CF gene discovery. *Pediatr. Pulmonol.* **57,** 11–18.

24. Farrell, P. M., and Mischler, E. H. (1992). Newborn screening for cystic fibrosis. *Adv. Pediatr.* **39,** 31–64.

25. Mastella, G., Barlocco, E. G., Antonacci, B., Borgo, G., Braggion, C., Cazzola, G., Conforti, M., Doro, R., Faraguna, D., Giglio, L., Miano, A., Parmelli, C., and Riggio, S. (1988). Is neonatal screening for cystic fibrosis advantageous? The answer of a wide 15 years follow-up study. *In* "Mucoviscidose: Depistage Neonatal et Prise en Charge Precoce Caen," pp. 127–143. CHRU de Caen.

26. Wilcken, B. (1993). Newborn screening for cystic fibrosis: Its evolution and a review of the current situation. *Screening* **2,** 43–62.

27. Dankert-Roelse, J. E., te Meerman, G. J., Martin, A., ten Kate, L. P., and Knol, K. (1989). Survival and clinical outcome in patients with cystic fibrosis, with or without neonatal screening. *J. Pediatr.* **114,** 362–367.

28. Farrell, P. M., Kosorok, M. R., Laxova, A., Shen, G., Koscik, R. E., Bruns, W. T., Splaingard, M., and Mischler, E. H. (1997). Nutritional benefits of neonatal screening for cystic fibrosis. *N. Engl. J. Med.* **337,** 963–969.

29. Farrell, P. M., Kosorok, M. R., Rock, M. J., Laxova, A., Zeng, L., Lai, H. C., Hoffman, G., Laessig, R. H., Splaingard, M. L., and the Wisconsin Cystic Fibrosis Neonatal Screening Study Group (2001). Early diagnosis of cystic fibrosis through neonatal screening prevents severe malnutrition and improves long-term growth. *Pediatrics* **107,** 1–13.

30. Bronstein, M. N., Sokol, R. J., Abman, S. H., Chatfield, B. A., Hammond, K. B., Hambidge, K. M., Stall, C. D., and Accurso, F. J. (1992). Pancreatic insufficiency, growth, and nutrition in infants identified by newborn screening as having cystic fibrosis. *J. Pediatr.* **120,** 533–540.

31. Waters, D. L., Wilcken, B., Irwing, L., van Asperen, P., Mellis, C., Simpson, J. M., Brown, J., and Gaskin, K. J. (1999).

Clinical outcomes of newborn screening for cystic fibrosis. *Arch. Dis. Child.* **80,** F1–F7.

32. Ghosal, S., Taylor, C. J., Pickering, M., and McGaw, J. (1996). Head growth in cystic fibrosis following early diagnosis by neonatal screening. *Arch. Dis. Child.* **75,** 191–193.

33. Cystic Fibrosis Foundation (1997). "Clinical Practice Guidelines for Cystic Fibrosis." Cystic Fibrosis Foundation, Bethesda, MD.

34. FitzSimmons, S. C. (1993). The changing epidemiology of cystic fibrosis. *J. Pediatr.* **122,** 1–9.

35. Durie, P. R., and Pencharz, P. B. (1992). Nutrition in cystic fibrosis. *Br. Med. Bull.* **48,** 823–847.

36. Pencharz, P. B., and Durie, P. R. (1993). Nutritional management of cystic fibrosis. *Annu. Rev. Nutr.* **13,** 111–136.

37. Stallings, V. A. (1994). Nutritional deficiencies in cystic fibrosis:Causes and consequences. *New Insights Cyst. Fibros.* **2,** 1–5.

38. Vaisman, N., Pencharz, P. B., Corey, M., Canny, G. J., and Hahn, E. (1987). Energy expenditure of patients with cystic fibrosis. *J. Pediatr.* **111,** 496–500.

39. Buchdahl, R. M., Cox, M., Fulleylove, C., Marchant, J. L., Tomkins, A. M., Brueton, M. J., and Warner, J. O. (1988). Increased resting energy expenditure in cystic fibrosis. *J. Appl. Physiol.* **64,** 1810–1816.

40. Anthony, H., Bines, J., Phelan, P., and Paxton, S. (1998). Relation between dietary intake and nutritional status in cystic fibrosis. *Arch. Dis. Child.* **78,** 443–447.

41. Tomezsko, J. L., Stallings, V. A., Kawchak, D. A., Goin, J. E., Diamond, G., and Scanlin, T. F. (1994). Energy expenditure and genotype of children with cystic fibrosis. *Pediatr. Res.* **35**(4, Pt. 1), 451–460.

42. Pencharz, P., Hill, R., Archibald, E., Levy, L., and Newth, C. (1984). Energy needs and nutritional rehabilitation in undernourished adolescents and young adult patients with cystic fibrosis. *J. Pediatr. Gastroenterol. Nutr.* **3,** S147–S153.

43. Feigal, R. J., and Shapiro, B. L. (1979). Mitochondrial calcium uptake and oxygen consumption in cystic fibrosis. *Nature (Lond.)* **278,** 276–277.

44. Stutts, M. J., Knowles, M. R., Gatzy, J. T., and Boucher, R. C. (1986). Oxygen consumption and ouabain binding sites in cystic fibrosis nasal epithelium. *Pediatr. Res.* **20,** 1316–1320.

45. Norman, D., Elborn, J. S., Cordon, S. M., Rayner, R. J., Wiseman, M. S., Hiller, E. J., and Shale, D. J. (1991). Plasma tumour necrosis factor alpha in cystic fibrosis. *Thorax* **46,** 91–95.

46. Farrell, P. M. (1991). Nutrition in malabsorptive disorders. *In* "Rudolph's Pediatrics," 19th ed. (A. M. Rudolph, Ed.), Chap. 9.14.3, pp. 249–252. Appleton and Lange, San Mateo, CA.

47. Congden, P. J., Bruce, G., Rothburn, M. M., Clarke, P. C., Littlewood, J. M., Kelleher, J., and Losowsky, M. S. (1981). Vitamin status in treated patients with cystic fibrosis. *Arch. Dis. Child.* **81,** 708–714.

48. Feranchak, A. P., Sontag, M. K., Wagener, J. S., Hammond, K. B., Accurso, F. J., and Sokol, R. J. (1999). Prospective, long-term study of fat-soluble vitamin status in children with cystic fibrosis identified by newborn screen. *J. Pediatr.* **135,** 601–610.

49. Ahmed, F., Ellis, J., Murphy, J., Wootton, S., and Jackson, A. A. (1990). Excessive faecal losses of vitamin A (retinol) in cystic fibrosis. *Arch. Dis. Child.* **65,** 589–593.

50. Wilfond, B. S., Farrell, P. M., Laxova, A., and Mischler, E. (1994). Severe hemolytic anemia associated with vitamin E deficiency in infants with cystic fibrosis. Implications for neonatal screening. *Clin. Pediatr.* **33,** 2–7.

51. Lancellotti, L., D'Orazio, C., Mastella, G., Mazzi, G., and Lippi, U. (1996). Deficiency of vitamins E and A in cystic fibrosis is independent of pancreatic function and current enzyme and vitamin supplementation. *Eur. J. Pediatr.* **155,** 281–285.

52. Henderson, R. C., and Lester, G. (1997). Vitamin D levels in children with cystic fibrosis. *Southern Med. J.* **90,** 378–383.

53. Durie, P. R. (1994). Vitamin K and the management of patients with cystic fibrosis. *Can. Med. Assoc. J.* **15,** 933–936.

54. Lai, H. C., Kosorok, M. R., Laxova, A., Davis, L. A., FitzSimmons, S., and Farrell, P. M. (2000). Nutritional status of patients with cystic fibrosis with meconium ileus: A comparison with patients without meconium ileus and diagnosed early through neonatal screening. *Pediatrics* **105,** 53–61.

55. Vormann, J., Gunther, T., Magdorf, K., and Wahn, U. (1992). Mineral metabolism in erythrocytes from patients with cystic fibrosis. *Eur. J. Clin. Chem. Clin. Biochem.* **30,** 193–196.

56. Pond, M. N., Morton, A. M., and Conway, S. P. (1996). Functional iron deficiency in adults with cystic fibrosis. *Resp. Med.* **90,** 409–413.

57. Ater, J. L., Herbst, J. J., Landaw, S. A., and O'Brien, R. T. (1983). Relative anemia and iron deficiency in cystic fibrosis. *Pediatrics* **71,** 810–814.

58. Farrell, P. M., Mischler, E. H., Engle, M. J., Brown, D. J., and Lau, S. (1985). Fatty acid abnormalities in cystic fibrosis. *Pediatr. Res.* **19,** 104–109.

59. Christophe, A., and Robberecht, E. (1996). Current knowledge on fatty acids in cystic fibrosis. *Prostagland. Leukotr. Essent. Fatty Acids* **55**(3), 129–138.

60. Roulet, M., Frascarolo, P., Rappaz, I., and Pilet, M. (1997). Essential fatty acid deficiency in well nourished young cystic fibrosis patients. *Eur. J. Pediatr.* **156,** 952–956.

61. Ozsoylu, S. (1998). Clinical importance of essential fatty acid deficiency. *Eur. J. Pediatr.* **157,** 779.

62. Lloyd-Still, J. D., Bibus, D. M., Powers, C. A., Johnson, S. B., and Holman, R. T. (1996). Essential fatty acid deficiency and predisposition to lung disease in cystic fibrosis. *Acta Paediatr.* **85,** 1426–1432.

63. Hubbard, V. S., Dunn, D. G., and di Sant Agnese, P. A. (1977). Abnormal fatty acid composition of plasma lipids in cystic fibrosis: A primary or secondary effect? *Lancet* **2,** 1302–1304.

64. van Egmond, A. W., Kosorok, M. R., Koscik, R., Laxova, R., and Farrell, P. M. (1996). Effect of linoleic acid intake on growth of infants with cystic fibrosis. *Am. J. Clin. Nutr.* **63,** 746–752.

65. Davis, P. B., and Kercsmar, C. M. (2000). Growth in children with chronic lung disease. *N. Engl. J. Med.* **342,** 887–888.

66. Kraemer, R., Rudeberg, A., Hadorn, B., and Rossi, E. (1978). Relative underweight in cystic fibrosis and its prognostic value. *Acta Paediatr. Scand.* **67,** 33–37.

67. Soutter, V. L., Kristidis, P., Gruca, M. A., and Gaskin, K. J. (1986). Chronic undernutrition/growth retardation in cystic fibrosis. *Clin. Gastroenterol.* **15,** 137–154.

68. Lai, H. C., Kosorok, M. R., Sondel, S. A., Chen, S. T., FitzSimmons, S. C., Green, C., Shen, G., Walker, S., and Farrell,

P. M. (1998). Growth status in children with cystic fibrosis based on National Cystic Fibrosis Patient Registry data: Evaluation of various criteria to identify malnutrition. *J. Pediatr.* **132,** 478–485.

69. Hamill, P. V. V., Drizd, T. A., Johnson, C. L., Reed, R. B., Roche, A. F., and Moore, W. M. (1979). Physical growth: National Center for Health Statistics percentiles. *Am. J. Clin. Nutr.* **55,** 108–116.

70. Lai, H. C., Corey, M., FitzSimmons, S. C., Kosorok, M. R., and Farrell, P. M. (1999). Comparison of growth status in patients with cystic fibrosis in the United States and Canada. *Am. J. Clin. Nutr.* **69,** 531–538.

71. U.S. Department of Health and Human Services (1987). "Anthropometric Reference Data and Prevalence of Overweight, United States, 1976–1980," data from the National Health Survey Series 11, No. 238, DHHS Publication No. (PHS) 87-1688. NCHS, Hyattsville, MD.

72. Sokol, R. J., Reardon, M. C., Accurso, F. J., Stall, C., Narkewicz, M., Abman, S. H., and Hammond, K. B. (1989). Fat-soluble vitamin status during the first year of life in infants with cystic fibrosis identified by screening of newborns. *Am. J. Clin. Nutr.* **50,** 1064–1071.

73. Marcus, M. S., Sondel, S. A., Farrell, P. M., Laxova, A., Carey, P. M., Langhough, R., and Mischler, E. H. (1991). Nutritional status of infants with cystic fibrosis associated with early diagnosis and intervention. *Am. J. Clin. Nutr.* **54,** 578–585.

74. Benabdeslam, H., Garcia, I., Bellon, G., Gilly, R., and Revol, A. (1998). Biochemical assessment of the nutritional status of cystic fibrosis patients treated with pancreatic enzyme extracts. *Am. J. Clin. Nutr.* **67,** 912–918.

75. Dodge, J. A., and Yassa, J. G. (1980). Food intake and supplemental feeding programs. *In* "Perspectives in Cystic Fibrosis" (J. M. Sturgess, Ed.), pp. 125–136. Canadian Cystic Fibrosis Foundation, Toronto.

76. Corey, M., McLaughlin, F. J., Williams, M., and Levison, H. (1988). A comparison of survival, growth, and pulmonary function in patients with cystic fibrosis in Boston and Toronto. *J. Clin. Epidemiol.* **41,** 583–591.

77. Pencharz, P. B. (1983). Energy intakes and low-fat diets in children with cystic fibrosis. *J. Pediatr. Gastroenterol. Nutr.* **2,** 400–402.

78. Bell, D., Durie, P., and Forstner, G. G. (1984). What do children with cystic fibrosis eat? *J. Pediatr. Gastroenterol. Nutr.* **3**(Suppl. 1), S137–S146.

79. Buchdahl, R. M., Fulleylov, C., Matchant, J. L., Warner, J. O., and Brueton, M. J. (1989). Energy and nutrient intakes in cystic fibrosis. *Arch. Dis. Child.* **64,** 373–378.

80. Hodges, P., Sauriol, D., Man, S. F., Reichert, A., Grace, M., Talbot, T. W., Brown, N., and Thomson, A. B. (1984). Nutrient intake of patients with cystic fibrosis. *J. Am. Diet. Assoc.* **84,** 664–669.

81. Lloyd-Still, J. D., Smith, A. E., and Wessel, H. U. (1989). Fat intake is low in cystic fibrosis despite unrestricted dietary practices. *J. Parenteral Enteral Nutr.* **13,** 296–298.

82. Tomezsko, J. L., Stallings, V. A., and Scanlin, T. F. (1992). Dietary intake of healthy children with cystic fibrosis compared with normal control children. *Pediatrics* **90,** 547–553.

83. Kawchak, D. A., Zhao, H., Scanlin, T. F., Tomezsko, J. L., Cnaan, A., and Stallings, V. A. (1996). Longitudinal, prospective analysis of dietary intake in children with cystic fibrosis. *J. Pediatr.* **129,** 119–129.

84. Lai, H. C., Kosorok, M. R., Laxova, A., Davis, L. A., and Farrell, P. M. (1999). Long-term dietary intakes in children with cystic fibrosis: Evaluation from diagnosis to age 10 years. *Pediatr. Pulmonol.* (Suppl.), 297.

85. Ramsey, B. W., Farrell, P. M., and Pencharz, P., for the Consensus Committee (1992). Nutritional assessment and management in cystic fibrosis: A consensus report. *Am. J. Clin. Nutr.* **55,** 108–116.

86. Cystic Fibrosis Foundation (1997). "Clinical Practice Guidelines for Cystic Fibrosis." Cystic Fibrosis Foundation, Bethesda, MD.

87. Kuczmarski, R. J., Ogden, C. L., Grummer-Strawn, L. M., Flegal, K. M., Guo, S. S., Wei, R., Mei, Z., Curtin, L. R., Roche, A. F., and Johnson, C. L. (2000). "CDC Growth Charts: United States," advanced data from Vital and Health Statistics, No. 314. National Center for Health Statistics, Hyattsville, MD.

88. Tanner, J. M., and Whitehouse, R. H. (1976). Clinical longitudinal standards for height, weight, height velocity, weight velocity, and stages of puberty. *Arch. Dis. Child.* **51,** 170–179.

89. Moore, D. J., Durie, P. R., Forstner, G. G., and Pencharz, P. B. (1985). The assessment of nutritional status in children. *Nutr. Res.* **5,** 797–799.

90. National Research Council (1989). "Recommended Dietary Allowances," 10th ed. National Academy Press, Washington, DC.

91. World Health Organization (1985). "Energy and Protein Requirements." WHO Tech. Report Series No. 724. World Health Organization, Geneva.

CHAPTER **46**

Osteomalacia

ROBERT MARCUS

Stanford University, Palo Alto, California

I. INTRODUCTION

Mature human bone is a proteinaceous matrix that embeds a highly organized crystalline mineral, hydroxyapatite. The mineral phase of adult bone normally approximates about 40% of the total bone mass. In osteoporotic patients, despite the occasional presence of subtle abnormalities of bone mineralization, the customary ratio of mineral to matrix is not seriously altered. *Osteomalacia* is the name given a condition in which the total amount of bone may be low, normal, or high, but in which the matrix is notably undermineralized (Fig. 1). The mechanical consequences of undermineralization may be severe. Osteomalacic bone behaves poorly in standardized tests of bone strength, and long bones may deform in response to routine mechanical loads.

The term *osteomalacia* describes a disorder of adult bone. In children, circumstances leading to osteomalacia also produce the specific disorder of growth plates known as rickets. The bones of children with rickets also undermineralize, and are therefore osteomalacic. If untreated, affected children may experience potentially serious consequences of osteomalacia, including reduced pulmonary function due to poor chest expansion and inability to undergo normal childbearing due to pelvic deformity.

This chapter reviews adult osteomalacia with a primary focus on its antecedents. It describes the clinical settings in which osteomalacia likely occurs and briefly summarizes elements of diagnosis and management of this condition. To begin, it briefly summarizes normal bone mineralization and the disruptions in this process that lead to osteomalacia.

II. MINERALIZATION

The concentrations of calcium and phosphate found normally in extracellular fluid substantially exceed their solubility product in aqueous solution. The normal extracellular fluid ionized Ca^{2+} activity in most species approximates 2.5 mEq/L (1.25 mM), whereas concentrations of inorganic phosphate, which fluctuate considerably with dietary intake, are generally about 1 mM in fasting adult humans. Thus, the degree of body fluid saturation can be expressed as a simple ion product $(Ca^{2+} \times P_i^{-3}) = \sim1.3$ mM^2, which approaches

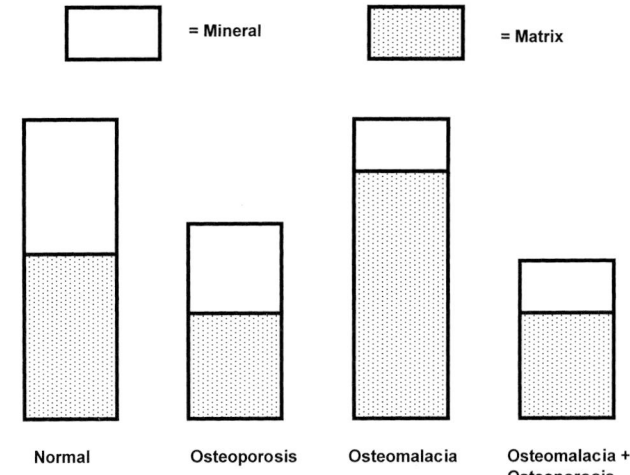

FIGURE 1 Relative proportion of bone mineral and matrix in normal, osteoporotic, and osteomalacic bone.

the effective solubility of aqueous calcium-phosphate. In the absence of a catalyzing nucleus on which orderly crystal growth can proceed, crystal precipitation will not occur in stable supersaturated solutions with $(Ca^{2+} \times PO_4^{-3})$ ion products even as high as 6 mM^2 because of a thermodynamic barrier related to mineral complexity.

In bone, a number of organic molecules influence the nucleation process and thereby serve to initiate crystal deposition. Matrix components with clustered phosphate groups bind calcium and promote mineralization. Once nucleation occurs, crystal growth proceeds rapidly in proportion to the concentrations of the mineral constituents. One model for this process involves the osteoblast enzyme, alkaline phosphatase, which is thought to initiate nucleation by hydrolyzing organic phosphates, thereby raising the local concentration of inorganic phosphate above supersaturation [1]. The specific phosphate-containing substrates for this process have not been identified, but likely include matrix phosphoproteins and phospholipids.

Given the fact that extracellular fluids are supersaturated with mineral, why, as with Lot's wife, does mineralization not occur everywhere all the time? To a major degree, the *metastable* condition of bone reflects the existence of small

729

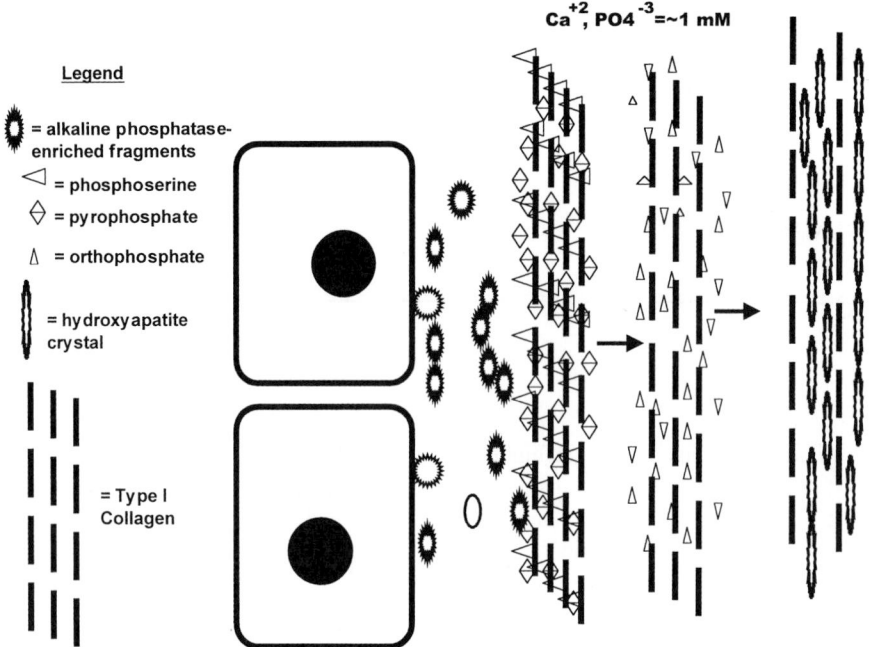

FIGURE 2 General scheme for bone mineralization.

inorganic, as well as proteinaceous, compounds that act as mineralization inhibitors. The first of these to be identified was pyrophosphate [2]. This ubiquitous by-product of ATP hydrolysis circulates in extracellular fluids at millimolar concentration, which suffices to inhibit mineral deposition. In aqueous solutions of inorganic calcium and phosphorus, pyrophosphate constrains both mineral growth and dissolution in super- and undersaturated conditions, respectively.

After osteoblasts have laid down new bone matrix, cleavage of pyrophosphate and possibly other phosphorylated molecules, such as phosphoserine residues in type I collagen, must occur before mineral can be deposited. Pyrophosphate cleavage is accomplished by the skeletal enzyme alkaline phosphatase, which is incorporated into the osteoblast plasma membrane. As osteoblasts move away from their newly secreted osteoid, membrane fragments are torn from the cells, permitting alkaline phosphatase to establish contact with and hydrolyze pyrophosphate and other phosphorus-containing mineralization inhibitors, so that mineral precipitation ensues (Fig. 2). Other mineralization inhibitors are also found in bone, including citrate, magnesium, and the large molecular weight glycosaminoglycans, but their relative importance to normal mineral deposition and crystal growth is not certain.

Collagen fibers in bone are highly ordered and thus direct the nucleation of mineral from metastable solutions. This is termed *heterogeneous nucleation,* as opposed to the spontaneous precipitation of mineral from supersaturated solutions. Deposition of mineral into collagen is not a random event. Indeed, the structural periodicity of pores and spaces in and around the collagen fibers creates specific sites at which a nidus of mineralization occurs. The initial crystals are

formed within the hole zones that result from the quarter-stagger of collagen molecules (Fig. 3) [3, 4]. Thus, mineralization does not occur as a wave throughout collagen fibers, but rather by nucleation at multiple, independent sites in the hole zones. It is likely that other matrix components, especially phosphoproteins, also facilitate nucleation at these sites [5–8]. With time, the entire collagenous structure becomes encased in mineral so that the final product, mature calcified bone, is analogous to a freeway tower in which the original interconnected steel poles and girders are encased in cement.

To succeed, mineral deposition must satisfy multiple conditions, including adequate local concentrations of calcium and phosphorus, normally active alkaline phosphatase, ability of collagen to undergo crystal nidation and foster mineral accumulation, and, finally, absence of nondegradable mineralization inhibitors. Failure to satisfy any of these conditions can jeopardize final mineralization and give rise to osteomalacia (Fig. 4).

III. OSTEOMALACIC BONE

Abnormalities encountered on routine skeletal radiographs of osteomalacic bone reflect the decrease in the amount of mineralized bone along with an increased prevalence of undermineralized bone surfaces (Fig. 5). These include an overall washed out appearance of the skeleton, coarsened trabecular patterns with poorly defined edges, and, in severe cases, bony deformation and pseudofractures. The latter, known also as Looser's zones, represent incomplete fragility

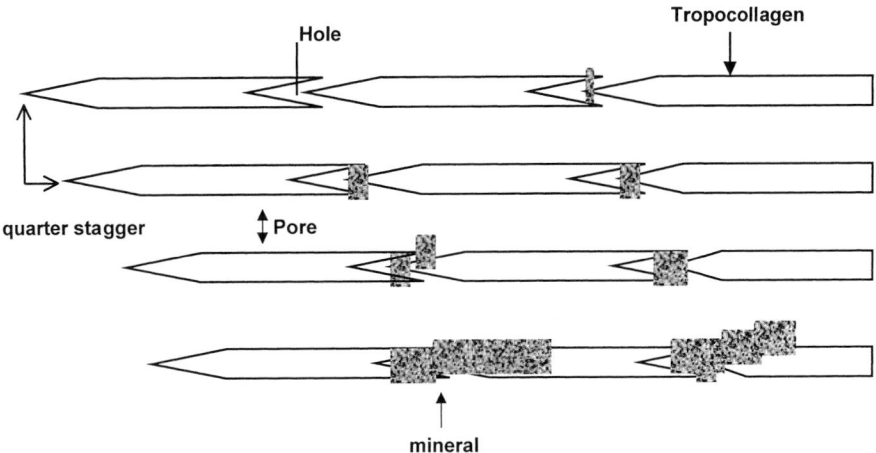

FIGURE 3 Mineral deposition on collagen.

fractures that show focal accumulation of osteoid. They tend to be oriented perpendicularly to the long axis of the cortical surface and are frequently bilateral, occurring commonly in the scapulae, pubic rami, proximal femurs, ribs, and long bones [9].

One hallmark of osteomalacic bone is its histologic appearance. Bone remodeling normally occurs on about 10% of bony surfaces, the remainder being quiescent. Sites that have been subjected to recent bone resorption contain surfaces that are actively replacing lost bone with fresh bone matrix. Although this new bone is destined ultimately to be fully calcified, a number of bone surfaces that have not yet mineralized will persist until the process has gone to comple-

tion. These partially mineralized surfaces reveal a thin covering of unmineralized matrix, or *osteoid*. Under normal circumstances the total prevalence of osteoid-lined surfaces is low, and the osteoid layers themselves do not exceed 15 micrometers in average thickness (Fig. 6, top; see color plate at the back of the book). By contrast, osteomalacic bone is characterized by the diffuse accumulation of thick osteoid clumps over the majority of, or even the entire, trabecular surface (Fig. 6, bottom) [10].

It may be difficult at times to distinguish true osteomalacia from a state in which an increased prevalence of osteoid-covered surfaces reflects increased whole-body bone remodeling activity (so-called "high-turnover" states), as happens

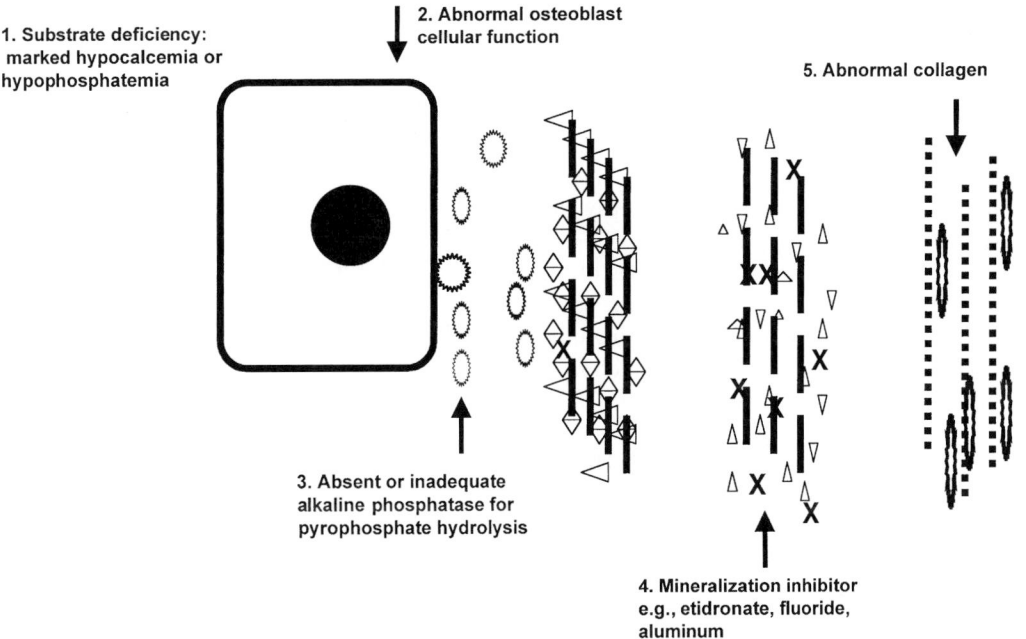

FIGURE 4 Disruptors of mineralization.

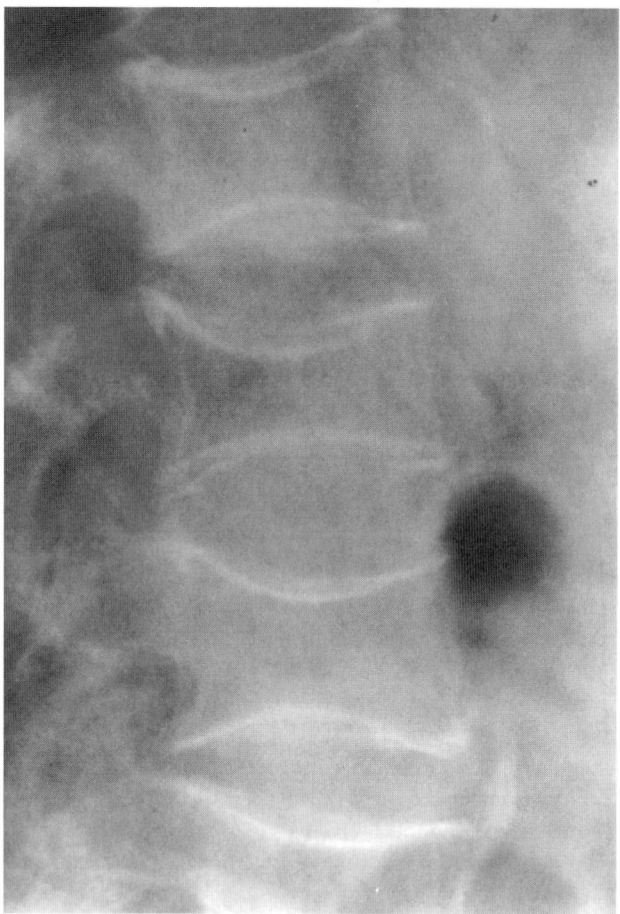

FIGURE 5 Radiographic appearance of osteomalacic bone. [Reprinted with permission from Steiner, E. J., Jergas, M., and Genant, H. K. (1995). Radiology of osteoporosis. *In* "Osteoporosis" (R. Marcus, D. Feldman, and J. Kelsey, Eds.), pp. 1019–1954. Academic Press, San Diego.]

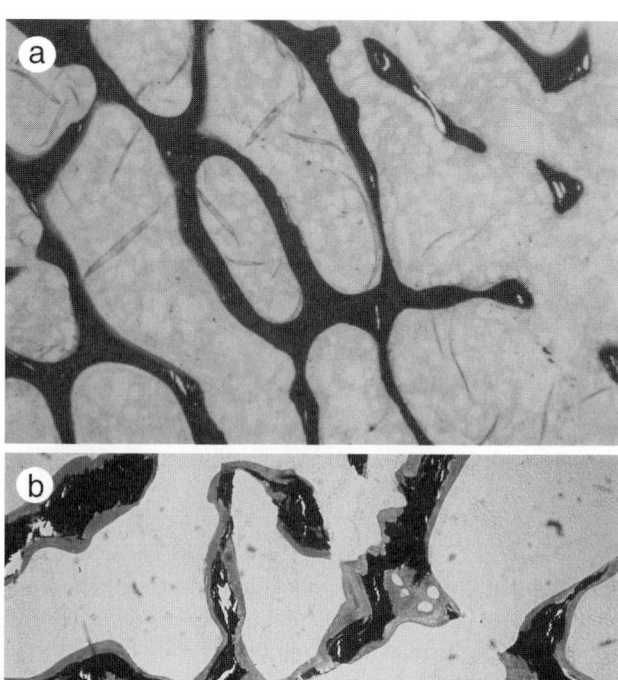

FIGURE 6 Histologic appearance of normal (top) and osteomalacic (bottom) bone. [Reprinted with permission from Compston, J. (1997). Bone histomorphometry. *In* "Vitamin D" (D. G. Feldman, F. H. Glorieux, and J. W. Pike, Eds.), pp. 573–586. Academic Press, San Diego.]

frequently in hyperthyroidism, hyperparathyroidism, and hypervitaminosis A or D. To distinguish these two conditions requires that an iliac crest bone biopsy be obtained in which bone is labeled *in vivo* prior to taking the biopsy (so-called "dynamic histomorphometry"). A typical method to accomplish this is to administer two separate doses of the antibiotic, tetracycline, approximately 10 days apart. Tetracycline binds avidly to bone matrix at sites of ongoing mineral deposition. When examined under ultraviolet light, areas of tetracycline uptake are denoted as bands of yellow fluorescence. When the patient is doubly labeled, two bands appear, and the average distance between them, divided by the number of days between dose administration, gives a value called the mineral apposition rate representing the amount of new bone mineralized per day (Fig. 7; see color plate at the back of the book) [9]. The mineral apposition rate is normally about 70 μm per day. In states of high bone turnover, surface prevalence of tetracycline uptake is high and the mineral apposition rate is normal or high. By contrast, osteomalacia shows both a reduction in the number of bone surfaces taking up tetracycline and a very low mineral apposition rate.

This discussion gains particular relevance in light of the nutritional focus of this volume. Several nutritionally based clinical situations lead to increased osteoid prevalence on bone surfaces. These multiple states are associated with increased secretion of parathyroid hormone, such as in response to low calcium intake, or as a toxic manifestation of high-dose vitamins A or D. In these instances, normal mineral apposition rates on tetracycline-labeled biopsies indicate a generalized increase in bone turnover rate but are not compatible with a diagnosis of osteomalacia.

IV. CAUSES OF OSTEOMALACIA

A. Vitamin D Deficiency

1. VITAMIN D PHYSIOLOGY

Vitamin D, whether obtained through the action of ultraviolet light on 7-dehydrocholesterol in the skin or through

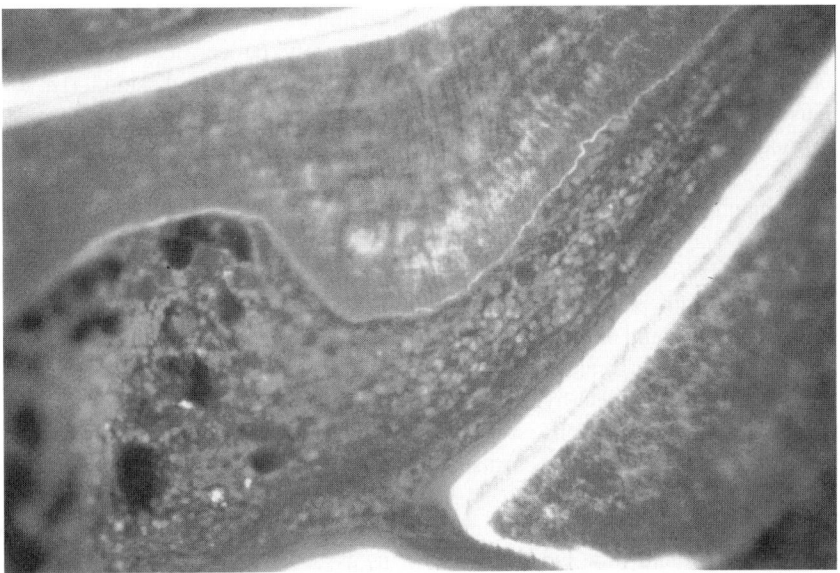

FIGURE 7 Dynamic histomorphometry of trabecular bone shown by tetracycline double labeling. [Reprinted with permission from Compston, J. (1997). Bone histomorphometry. *In* "Vitamin D" (D. G. Feldman, F. H. Glorieux, and J. W. Pike, Eds.), pp. 573–586. Academic Press, San Diego.]

dietary ingestion, is biologically inert until it is converted to its polar active metabolites by hydroxylation (Fig. 8). The first step in this pathway involves a hepatic cytochrome *P*-450 enzyme that hydroxylates the parent vitamin in the 25 position. The resulting compound, 25-hydroxyvitamin D (25OHD) constitutes the most abundant circulating form of vitamin D. In the circulation, 25OHD binds highly to a specific vitamin D binding globulin. The metabolic fate of 25OHD is determined by the relative activities of two enzymes located in the renal tubules. The first, the 1-α hydroxylase, converts 25OHD into its most active form, 1,25-dihydroxyvitamin D, or *calcitriol*. The alternative step involves a 24-hydroxylase that converts 25OHD into the practically inert product, 24, 25-dihydroxyvitamin D [11].

The major regulators of calcitriol synthesis are parathyroid hormone, hypophosphatemia, and hypocalcemia. In the face of dietary calcium deficiency, small reductions in plasma ionized calcium activity lead to compensatory hypersecretion of parathyroid hormone, which in turn stimulates the 1-α hydroxylase to promote calcitriol production. Parathyroid hormone also indirectly stimulates this enzyme by causing the kidney tubule to reabsorb less phosphate, thereby creating a state of renal phosphate depletion. Phosphate depletion exerts a powerful stimulatory effect on 1-α hydroxylase. Because serum calcium concentrations actually increase (and those of parathyroid hormone decrease) in the presence of hypophosphatemia, the increased hydroxylase activity must be a direct response to low phosphorus content rather than to parathyroid hormone [12]. Increased calcitriol production results in higher circulating concentrations of this metabolite and, therefore, increased vitamin D action on the

intestine to enhance calcium absorption efficiency. Thus, the primary physiological role for vitamin D is to increase intestinal calcium absorption efficiency [13].

Although considered a "prehormone" insofar as it is a substrate for calcitriol synthesis, 25OHD itself possesses

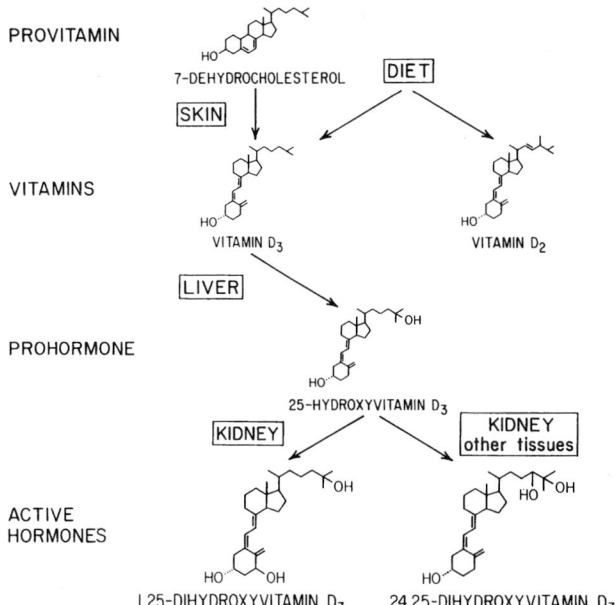

FIGURE 8 Vitamin D pathway. [Reprinted with permission from Henry, H. (1997). The 25-hydroxyvitamin D1 alpha-hydroxylase. *In* "Vitamin D" (D. G. Feldman, F. H. Glorieux, and J. W. Pike, Eds.), pp. 41–68. Academic Press, San Diego.]

intrinsic bioactivity. Indeed, 25OHD has an affinity for the vitamin D receptor that is only 1:1000 that of calcitriol, but as it circulates at 1000-fold molar excess relative to calcitriol (~30 ng/mL versus 30 pg/mL), 25OHD actually accounts for an important fraction of total vitamin D activity *in vivo*.

An additional feature of vitamin D physiology warranting comment is the suggestion that vitamin D metabolites normally are excreted into the bile, only to be reabsorbed further down the intestine (so-called "enterohepatic circulation"). If such a process does truly occur, it would explain the vitamin D deficiency states associated with surgical diversion of biliary contents, as occurs with jejunal or ileal bypass surgery, or use of bile acid sequestering medications, such as cholestyramine. Evidence for an enterohepatic mechanism includes the recovery of radioactivity in the bile following injection of isotopic 25OHD [14]. In a recent review of this topic, however, Mawer *et al.* [15] found little evidence to support the biological significance of those metabolites that are excreted into the bile, and concluded it is "unlikely that any enterohepatic circulation of vitamin D metabolites that does occur is . . . of physiologic significance."

As stated, the primary action of vitamin D is to increase the efficiency of intestinal calcium absorption. Calcium is normally absorbed by two distinct processes. The first, which is sensitive to vitamin D, involves an active transport process confined largely to the duodenum. The second, which is independent of vitamin D, involves facilitated diffusion throughout the small intestine (transcaltachia). Although multiple and diverse effects of vitamin D metabolites have been demonstrated in bone and kidney, the increase in intestinal calcium absorption has by far the greatest importance for skeletal homeostasis.

2. VITAMIN D ADEQUACY, INADEQUACY, AND DEFICIENCY

The definition of vitamin D adequacy remains a controversial topic (see review by Chapuy and Meunier [16]). Clinical laboratories generally publish a "normal" range for 25OHD spanning 10–50 ng/mL. Consensus exists that values below this range, particularly below 6 ng/mL, are highly associated with clinical, biochemical, and histological evidence of osteomalacia. However, evidence suggests that values above 10 ng/mL are not necessarily adequate for optimal bone balance. A highly significant inverse relationship exists between circulating concentrations of 25OHD and parathyroid hormone. Thus, in the presence of low circulating 25OHD, parathyroid hormone secretion increases, leading to higher rates of bone turnover and loss. However, at circulating 25OHD concentrations in excess of ~30 ng/mL, the negative association with parathyroid hormone loses significance, suggesting that a vitamin D replete state exists. Although extremely low 25OHD concentrations are, at most, uncommon in the general population of Western countries, values associated with increased parathyroid hormone se-

cretion (<~20 ng/mL), which are very common, might legitimately be considered to reflect a degree of vitamin "inadequacy." At substantial risk for vitamin D inadequacy are people living in the Northern tier of the United States, in Canada, or in Northern or Central Europe, particularly during winter months. Vitamin D inadequacy is also frequently encountered, even in more temperate climates, among shut-ins and others who avoid sunlight exposure, as well as institutionalized patients who do not receive full-spectrum ultraviolet light. Many studies indicate that low vitamin D concentrations are very common in elderly men and women. There is marked seasonal variation in circulating 25OHD, so that the prevalence of vitamin D insufficiency during the winter ranges, depending on country, from 8% to 60% [17–19].

Full discussion of vitamin D adequacy exceeds the scope of this chapter, but this issue bears directly on the consideration of osteomalacia. Earlier descriptions of "osteomalacia" in association with various medications and pathological states frequently offered no histological corroboration of the diagnosis, and even when that was done, did not apply contemporary diagnostic criteria for osteomalacia. Examination of this literature, particularly with respect to so-called "anticonvulsant osteomalacia," indicates that many reports more likely represented examples of secondary hyperparathyroidism and "high-turnover" osteoporosis due to modest or moderate vitamin D inadequacy [20].

3. VITAMIN D DEFICIENCY BASED ON POOR VITAMIN INTAKE OR SUNLIGHT EXPOSURE

Florid vitamin D deficiency characterized life in Northern Europe during the 18th and 19th centuries, but overt vitamin D deficiency is rare today in industrialized societies. That being said, it is true that certain ethnic groups may undertake dietary and clothing habits that place them at higher risk for deficiency. The primary dietary sources of vitamin D include fish oils and supplemented dairy products. In the United States, milk is supplemented to a nominal concentration of 400 units vitamin D per quart, albeit with great variability in quality control. Milk supplementation is not frequent in other countries. Some [21, 22] albeit not all [23] studies indicate that the cutaneous production of vitamin D in response to ultraviolet irradiation declines with age. Older men and women who may not achieve adequate solar exposure, and who drink little milk, are at particular risk for marked vitamin D inadequacy, if not of true deficiency.

Inadequate solar exposure has been identified as a cause of florid osteomalacia, particularly in women, when traditional dress and indoor lifestyles keep people from receiving even a modicum of sunlight. Osteomalacia on this basis has been reported even from areas of the world, such as Turkey and the Arabian peninsula, that are drenched in sunlight most of the year [24]. In addition, use of sun block creams reduces the rise in vitamin D concentration following a standard dose of solar exposure, leading to lower circulating 25OHD concentrations [25, 26].

4. Vitamin D Deficiency Based on Gastrointestinal Pathology

In Western society, true vitamin D deficiency commonly occurs when intestinal function has been disrupted. Affected individuals include those who have undergone gastroduodenal (Billroth I) or gastrojejunal (Billroth II) anastomoses or jejuno- or ileal-bypass surgery, individuals with bowel infarction, or patients with malabsorption syndromes such as those associated with coeliac or inflammatory bowel disease and extensive diverticulosis. Patients with primary biliary disorders or those taking medications, such as bile acid sequestrants (Cholestyramine, Questran®) or products aimed at inducing fat malabsorption (Orlistat, Xenical®) may also be at added risk for vitamin D deficiency.

Patients who have undergone gastrojejunal bypass surgery suffer a very high prevalence of osteoporosis and, to a lesser extent, osteomalacia, although when osteomalacia is assessed using iliac crest biopsy criteria, the prevalence may exceed 20% [15, 27]. Abnormalities in mineral metabolism in these patients reflect multiple deficits in intestinal function. Vitamin D-sensitive active calcium absorption occurs relatively high in the duodenum, so that bypassing this portion of the gut severely jeopardizes the adaption to low calcium intake. Patients with intestinal bypass surgery experience deficits in both vitamin D and calcium homeostasis resulting in a state of secondary hyperparathyroidism to maintain plasma calcium normalcy. High circulating concentrations of parathyroid hormone in turn promote urinary phosphate excretion and hypophosphatemia, all of which contribute to osteomalacia. As discussed above, the possibility that vitamin D metabolites in bile undergo enteric recirculation has been considered a convenient explanation for the depletion of 25OHD in patients undergoing intestinal bypass surgery. However, the importance of this mechanism has been placed into serious question [15]. Alternatively, it has been shown that hyperparathyroid states are associated with increased clearance of 25OHD, and that clearance normalizes when parathyroid hormone concentrations are reduced by calcium supplementation [28]. Thus, the 25OHD depletion characteristic of intestinal bypass patients may be due to compensatory parathyroid hormone hypersecretion.

Unfortunately, many patients who have undergone disruptive intestinal operations fail to receive adequate medical follow-up once the acute postoperative period has passed. Because of the insidious onset of bone disease, skeletal complaints develop very slowly, generally coming to medical attention only decades later, at which time the patients frequently neglect to mention (or their physicians neglect to ask about or even recognize the significance of) the previous surgical history.

Osteomalacia and osteoporosis, occasionally severe, are recognized to occur in the setting of chronic liver disease. Early studies indicating a high prevalence of osteomalacia were based on relatively nonrigorous histological analyses. Recent studies indicate that true osteomalacia is actually very uncommon in liver disease, although it occurs occasionally in association with severe vitamin D deficiency [29, 30].

5. Inherited Forms of Vitamin D Deficiency or Resistance

Mutations in the 1-α hydroxylase enzyme (vitamin D-dependent rickets) lead to a condition of extreme vitamin D resistance and are associated with very low blood concentrations of calcitriol [31, 32]. Affected children respond exuberantly to small doses of exogenous calcitriol and, if treated in a timely fashion, experience cure of rickets and do not subsequently develop osteomalacia. By contrast, children with mutations in the vitamin D receptor have profound hypocalcemia, rickets and osteomalacia, and total body alopecia. They show normal to high circulating concentrations of vitamin D and its metabolites, but fail completely to respond to the exogenous administration of these agents [33]. Clinical and biochemical remissions have been observed in these children with long-term administration of calcium infusions. These children tend to undergo a substantial degree of remission when they enter puberty, and adult osteomalacia has not been a major problem.

X-linked hypophosphatemic rickets (or vitamin D-resistant rickets) is an inherited disorder of renal tubular function resulting in wasting of inorganic phosphorus and hypophosphatemia and leading clinically to rickets and osteomalacia. Clinical expression of this disorder is highly variable, ranging from very mild to severe rickets and/or osteomalacia. In adults with X-linked hypophosphatemic rickets, serum concentrations of 250HD are normal, and those of calcitriol are either normal or only mildly depressed [34]. However, given the degree of hypophosphatemia that occurs in this disorder, much higher concentrations of calcitriol would be predicted. Thus, regulation of the renal 1α-hydroxylase appears to be abnormal [35]. Recent discovery of the *PHEX* gene and its gene product, a membrane-bound endopeptidase, has clarified the genetic, if not the physiologic, basis of this disorder. It is speculated that inactivating mutations of *PHEX* produce X-linked hypophosphatemic rickets because affected people fail to break down phosphatonin, a (still hypothetical) hormone that is predicted to promote hypophosphatemia by impairing renal tubular reabsorption of phosphorus [36]. In addition to X-linked hypophosphatemic rickets, other forms of hereditary rickets/osteomalacia have been described [35].

B. Phytate Ingestion

About 30 years ago, attention was called to a substantial prevalence of rickets and osteomalacia in Pakistani and Indian immigrants to Great Britain [37, 38]. Multiple reasons can be invoked to explain such an occurrence, including changes imposed on these people in diet, dress, and sunlight access. However, one additional aspect of this condition, shared also with Bedouins living in the Middle East, is exposure to unleavened bread made from a high phytate flour

(the traditional chapati bread) [39]. Phytate is a 6-carbon cyclic compound in which each carbon atom is linked covalently to a phosphate moiety. These multiple phosphate groups effectively chelate calcium ions, thereby preventing their absorption.

C. Inadequate Calcium Intake

Because ionized calcium is critical for proper function of nerves, heart and other muscles, and other vital physiological processes, maintaining its circulating concentration within fairly narrow limits is a matter of high priority. Humans, mammals, and indeed birds, reptiles, and amphibia, possess an elaborate parathyroid-vitamin D axis that compensates for inadequate intake or intestinal absorption of calcium by drawing on skeletal reserves to support the plasma calcium concentration. Hence, although isolated calcium inadequacy, if extremely severe, could theoretically cause osteomalacia, this must be a very rare occurrence. It is likely that a calcium deficiency state of sufficient magnitude and duration to overwhelm the parathyroid compensatory mechanism might actually prove lethal to neurological and cardiac function before clinical osteomalacia could emerge.

Despite the fact that tropical countries have abundant sunlight, nutritional rickets remains prevalent in such countries. The possibility has been raised that dietary calcium deficiency may be the underlying factor in such cases. In a Nigerian study [40], 123 children with rickets were observed to have very low calcium intakes averaging 200 mg/day. Children were treated with vitamin D (600,000 U intramuscularly at enrollment and at 12 weeks), calcium (1000 mg daily), or a combination of both. Treatment produced a smaller increase in the average serum calcium concentration in the vitamin D intervention group ($\sim$0.5 mg/dL at 24 weeks) than in either the calcium ($\sim$1.5 mg/dL, $P < 0.001$) or combination-therapy groups ($\sim$1.4 mg/dL, $P < 0.001$). A greater proportion of children in the calcium and combination-therapy groups than in the vitamin D group reached desired clinical outcomes, i.e., suppression of serum alkaline phosphatase activity and radiographic healing of rickets [39]. Thus, the results suggest a contribution of inadequate dietary calcium to the pathogenesis of rickets in these children. A similar suggestion has been made for a cohort of Bangladeshi children with rickets [41].

An occasional patient with chronic anorexia nervosa has been found to have osteomalacia. However, given the global nature of nutritional deficits in this disorder, it is not possible to assign sole culpability to calcium deficiency in these cases [42].

D. Phosphorus Depletion

Sustained decreases in the plasma phosphorus concentration reliably induce osteomalacia in experimental animals and emerge as a common basis for osteomalacia in humans. Hypophosphatemia (inorganic phosphate concentrations below 1 mM, or $\sim$3.0 mg/dL) is encountered in diverse clinical situations. Intestinal causes include impaired phosphorus absorption due to vitamin D deficiency or resistance, and excessive ingestion of phosphorus-binding aluminum-containing antacids or laxatives. Compelling evidence was presented several decades ago that sustained use of phosphate-binding antacids (primarily aluminum hydroxide) produced hypophosphatemia and muscle weakness typical of patients with osteomalacia [43]. During the past decade, these compounds have been virtually abandoned for antacid use and have been replaced by calcium carbonate for the control of serum phosphorus concentrations in renal failure patients. Osteomalacia rarely has been described in patients subjected to chronic laxative abuse.

E. Tumor-Induced Osteomalacia

Beginning more than 50 years ago, a series of case reports brought attention to an association of hypophosphatemic osteomalacia with the presence of unusual tumors [44, 45]. Patients complained typically of progressive weakness, primarily involving large muscle groups of the legs, with marked limitation in the ability to rise from a chair or climb stairs. Hypophosphatemia was severe, with serum phosphate concentrations frequently below 2.0 mg/dL. Generalized bone pain was also frequent. Symptoms and metabolic abnormalities were characteristically present for years before a tumor was discovered. Some tumors were extremely small, being found as tiny skin nodules or lumps in the webs of toes. In some cases, tumor resection led rapidly to dramatic resolution of biochemical features and symptoms. In many cases, however, tumors were inoperable or surgery was only partly successful. Histologically, these tumors have been highly unusual in their appearance. They have been variably called hemangiopericytomas and ossifying or nonossifying fibromas, among other names.

Some progress has been made in understanding the underlying mechanism of tumor-induced osteomalacia. The syndrome is characterized by paraneoplastic defects in vitamin D metabolism, abnormal proximal renal tubular function, and grossly diminished renal phosphate reabsorption. Serum calcitriol concentrations are vanishingly low, which, in the face of profound hypophosphatemia, constitutes *prima facie* evidence for defective synthesis or accelerated removal of this hormone. Most investigators consider it likely that these tumors produce humoral factor(s) that alter renal proximal tubular function [35]. Evidence from a single instructive case suggests that the tumor produces a phosphaturic protein or proteins, which could explain the defective phosphorus reabsorption, although it does not suggest a basis for the low calcitriol values [46]. For patients in whom a tumor is discovered, surgical excision may be curative. When the

causative tumor cannot be found or completely resected, palliative treatment with calcium, vitamin D, and phosphate replacement is helpful [47].

Osteomalacia has also been noted to occur in patients with a variety of other tumor types, including typical carcinomas, myelomas, and lymphomas. Whether osteomalacia in such patients reflects a mechanism similar to that of tumor-induced osteomalacia, described above, is uncertain because it generally has not been possible to resect the tumors. Alternatively, the bone disorder could be a reflection of severe cachexia associated with systemic malignancy. Osteomalacia also has been reported in association with neurofibromatosis, but nothing definitive can be stated about its cause [35].

F. Renal Tubular Defects

The Fanconi syndrome is a generalized disorder of proximal renal tubular transport. Its features include wasting of phosphate, glucose, bicarbonate, uric acid, and one or more amino acids [48]. In addition to several hereditary forms, Fanconi syndrome can also be produced by renal tubular toxins, including heavy metals [49, 50], drugs (outdated tetracyclines) and precipitated immunoglobulins or their subunits, as in myeloma, amyloidosis, and paraprotein states [51]. Osteomalacia occurs in Fanconi syndrome as a consequence of profound phosphorus wasting.

Some patients who have undergone ureterosigmoidostomy have developed osteomalacia. The underlying pathophysiology is not entirely clear, but appears to reflect the degree of metabolic acidosis that develops in these patients [52].

G. Deficits in Osteoblast Function

As described above, normal initiation of mineralization requires the initial action of skeletal alkaline phosphatase on pyrophosphate. Hypophosphatasia is a genetic disorder characterized by severe deficiency or complete absence of multiple isoforms of alkaline phosphatase [53] and which on iliac crest biopsy shows osteomalacia. Although profound deficits in phosphatase activity have been demonstrated in diverse tissues, it is the absence of this enzyme in bone that underlies the clinically important manifestations of the disease. Severely affected individuals experience bone pain, fractures, and deformity. Rarely, homozygous individuals may die in infancy, the cause of death perhaps related to increased intracranial pressure due to premature craniosynostosis (closure of cranial sutures). Less severely affected children may show rickets, dental hypoplasia, craniosynostosis, ectopic soft-tissue calcifications and growth retardation. Biochemical features include increased plasma concentrations of pyridoxal 5'-phosphate and an increased urinary excretion of phosphatidyl ethanolamine [54]. At present, there is no specific or effective therapy for patients with hypophosphatasia. In this disorder, high doses of vitamin D and phosphate are probably ineffective at best, and potentially dangerous.

H. Presence of Mineralization Inhibitors

Fluoride is the most common naturally occurring inhibitor of mineralization. Indeed, although pitting of dental enamel is the hallmark of mild fluoride toxicity, severe endemic fluorosis leads to profound osteomalacia and bony sclerosis. This condition occurs primarily in areas of the world in which groundwater fluoride content is naturally high. Such areas include portions of Southern Italy, Central Europe, and arid regions of India. Skeletal fluorosis is commonly observed in deer and other animals that graze in those areas [55]. In the United States, groundwater in sections of Colorado and the arid Southwest have very high natural fluoride content, and endemic fluorosis in grazing animals is frequent. Human skeletal fluorosis does not occur in the United States because federal statutes require communities having excessive water fluoride content to adjust the ambient fluoride concentration or to provide all children a supply of freshwater within tolerable fluoride limits. Industrial fluoride exposure may sometimes reach toxic levels in aluminum smelter workers, and there are occasional reports of patients experiencing acute fluoride toxicity in response to a breakdown in hemodialysis quality control.

Human osteomalacia related to fluoride exposure has been a frequent concern with respect to therapeutic fluoride treatment of osteoporosis. The risk of osteomalacia is particularly high when adequate vitamin D and supplemental calcium are not also prescribed. In addition, the bisphosphonate etidronate (Didronel®) has been known to cause osteomalacia since its early use at high dose (15–20 mg/kg/day) for management of Paget's disease of bone. Even at lower doses (5 mg/kg/day), continuous use of this agent has been associated with focal osteomalacia. This attribute of etidronate limits its use in the treatment of osteoporosis, because it is necessary to prescribe it on a cyclical basis if osteomalacia is to be avoided. For example, in one standard treatment regimen, etidronate is generally given for 14 days every 3 months with adequate provision of calcium and vitamin D for the remaining 76 days [55a]. Second- and third-generation potent bisphosphonates, such as alendronate (Fosamax®), pamidronate (Aredia®), or risedronate (Actonel®) do not impair mineralization, and therefore do not cause osteomalacia at clinically relevant doses.

Aluminum constitutes a special case of mineralization inhibitor. Its role in preventing intestinal phosphorus absorption has been described above. In addition, it has been implicated as the cause of a severe form of osteomalacia in patients with chronic renal failure who have received aluminum-containing antacids for control of plasma phosphorus concentration. Bone biopsy specimens in such patients

reveal extensive accumulation of aluminum at mineralizing surfaces and are reported as indicative of a very low turnover (adynamic) state. Treatment of aluminum-related osteomalacia requires its removal with desferroxamine, a chelating agent [56]. Although this therapy is often dramatically successful, the frequency of serious infections in treated individuals has raised concern about the strategy of treating all patients who have been exposed to aluminum. At present, it is recommended that treatment be reserved for patients with symptomatic aluminum-related toxicity. Despite the fact that aluminum antacids have been replaced by calcium salts as the mainstay for managing hyperphosphatemia, adynamic osteomalacia unrelated to aluminum exposure persists and has actually increased in prevalence as an important clinical problem for patients with chronic renal failure. The basis remains obscure.

V. TREATMENT OF OSTEOMALACIA

Successful therapy of osteomalacia requires elimination of its underlying factors in individual cases. For patients who suffer nutritional vitamin D deficiency, restoration of normal circulating concentrations of 25OHD is the desired endpoint. Multiple treatment schedules have been described. Therapy can be initiated with high doses of vitamin D, such as 25,000 units/day, for 6 months, at which time the dose can be reduced toward maintenance amounts (400–800 units/day). Adequate supplemental calcium, perhaps 1500 mg/day, should also be provided. For patients with short-bowel syndromes, intestinal bypass, or other disruptions of normal bowel architecture, vitamin D should be administered by a parenteral route. Intramuscular injection of 50,000–100,000 units/month is sufficient. The rare child who is completely refractory to the actions of calcitriol generally requires long-term administration of intravenous calcium infusions, at least until the time of puberty.

For patients with renal phosphorus wasting, restoration of tissue phosphorus content is the primary aim. This generally involves the oral administration of various phosphate salts in amounts sufficient to provide 1–2 g/day of elemental phosphorus. Preparations that are currently available include sodium/hydrogen salts (e.g., Fleet's PhosphoSoda®), or mixtures of sodium and potassium phosphate (e.g., K-Phos®). The latter may be preferable for patients who cannot tolerate large sodium loads. Tolerability of phosphate salts may be limited by diarrhea. Some patients develop hypocalcemia and secondary hyperparathyroidism in response to phosphorus supplementation. When that occurs, additional vitamin D and calcium may be required.

In patients with primary abnormalities in osteoblastic function, such as those with hypophosphatasia, administration of excess vitamin D and calcium may be counterproductive and actually toxic. These patients should be treated only to be certain that vitamin D deficiency does not confound the underlying disorder. For patients with tumor-related osteomalacia, all attempts should be made to locate and extirpate the tumor.

Finally, where osteomalacia is based on excessive exposure to fluoride, etidronate, or nonabsorbable antacids, the offending exposure must be terminated. Unfortunately, the skeletal half-life of fluoride and bisphosphonate is long, and resolution of osteomalacia may require years of follow-up. Such patients do respond, at least partially, to vitamin D and calcium therapy. Aluminum excess is successfully treated by infusions of desferroxamine [56].

References

1. Robison, R. (1923). The possible significance of hexosephosphonic esters in ossification. *Biochem. J.* **17,** 286–293.
2. Fleisch, H., and Neuman, W. F. (1961). Mechanisms of calcification: Role of collagen, polyphosphates and phosphatase. *Am. J. Physiol.* **200,** 1296–1300.
3. Fleisch, H., Russell, R. G. G., and Francis, M. D. (1969). Diphosphonates inhibit hydroxyapatite dissolution *in vitro* and bone resorption in tissue culture and in vivo. *Science* **165,** 1262–1264.
4. Glimcher, M. J., Hodge, A. J., and Schmitt, F. O. (1957). Macromolecular aggregation states in relation to mineralization: The collagen–hydroxyapatite system as studied in vitro. *Proc. Natl. Acad. Sci. USA* **43,** 860–867.
5. Koutsoukos, P. G., and Nancollas, G. H. (1987). The mineralization of collagen in vitro. *Colloids Surf.* **28,** 95–105.
6. Cohen-Solal, L., Cohen-Solal, M., and Glimcher, M. J. (1979). The identification of gamma glutamyl phosphate in the alpha 2 chain of chicken bone collagen. *Proc. Natl. Acad. Sci. USA* **76,** 4327–4330.
7. Maier, G. D., Lechner, J. H., and Veis, A. (1983). The dynamics of formation of a collagen-phosphophoryn conjugate in relation to the passage of the mineralization front in rat incisor dentin. *J. Biol. Chem.* **258,** 1450–1455.
8. Glimcher, M. J. (1989). Mechanisms of calcification: Role of collagen fibrils and collagen-phosphoprotein complexes *in vitro* and *in vivo*. *Anat. Rec.* **224,** 139–153.
9. Steiner, E., Jergas, M., and Genant, H. K. (1995). Radiology of Osteoporosis. *In* "Osteoporosis" (R. Marcus, D. Feldman, and J. Kelsey, Eds.), pp. 1019–1054. Academic Press, San Diego.
10. Compston, J. (1997). Bone Histomorphometry. *In* "Vitamin D" (D. G. Feldman, F. H. Glorieux, and J. W. Pike, Eds.), pp. 573–586. Academic Press, San Diego.
11. Henry, H. L. (1997). The 25-hydroxyvitamin D1 alpha-hydroxylase. *In* "Vitamin D" (D. G. Feldman, F. H. Glorieux, and J. W. Pike, Eds.), pp. 41–68. Academic Press, San Diego.
12. Horst, R. L., and Reinhardt, T. A. (1997). Vitamin D metabolism. *In* "Vitamin D" (D. G. Feldman, F. H. Glorieux, and J. W. Pike, Eds.), pp. 13–31. Academic Press, San Diego.
13. Wasserman, R. H. (1997). Vitamin D and the intestinal absorption of calcium and phosphorus. *In* "Vitamin D" (D. G. Feldman, F. H. Glorieux, and J. W. Pike, Eds.), pp. 259–274. Academic Press, San Diego.
14. Arnaud, S. B., Goldsmith, R. S., Lambert, P. W., and Go, V. L. W. (1975). 25-hydroxyvitamin D3: Evidence of an enterohepatic circulation in man. *Proc. Soc. Exp. Biol.* **149,** 570–572.

15. Mawer, E. B., and Davies, M. (1997). Bone disorders associated with gastrointestinal and hepatobiliary disease. *In* "Vitamin D" (D. G. Feldman, F. H. Glorieux, and J. W. Pike, Eds.), pp. 831–847. Academic Press, San Diego.

16. Chapuy, M.-C., and Meunier, P. J. (1997). Vitamin D insufficiency in adults and the elderly. *In* "Vitamin D" (D. G. Feldman, F. H. Glorieux, and J. W. Pike, Eds.), pp. 679–693. Academic Press, San Diego.

17. Stamp, T. C. B., and Round, J. M. (1974). Seasonal changes in human plasma levels of 25-hydroxyvitamin D. *Nature (Lond.),* **247,** 563–565.

18. Lund, B., and Sorenson, O. H. (1979). Measurement of 25-hydroxyvitamin D in serum and its relation to sunshine, age, and vitamin D. *Scand. J. Clin. Lab. Invest.* **39,** 23–30.

19. Gloth, F. M., and Tobin, J. D. (1995). Vitamin D deficiency in older people. *J. Am. Geriatr. Soc.* **43,** 822–828.

20. Weinstein, R. S., Bryce, G. F., Sappington, L. J., King, D. W., and Gallagher, B. B. (1984). Decreased serum ionized calcium and normal vitamin D metabolite levels with anticonvulsant drug treatment. *J. Clin. Endocrinol. Metab.* **58,** 1003–1009.

21. MacLaughlin, J., and Holick, M. F. (1985). Aging decreases the capacity of human skin to produce vitamin D3. *J. Clin. Invest.* **76,** 1536–1538.

22. Holick, M. F., Matsuoka, L. Y., and Wortsman, J. (1989). Age, vitamin D and solar ultraviolet. *Lancet* **2,** 1104–1105.

23. Davie, M., and Lawson, D. E. M. (1980). Assessment of plasma 25-hydroxyvitamin D response to ultraviolet irradiation over a controlled area in young and elderly subjects. *Clin. Sci.* **58,** 235–242.

24. Gullu, S., Erodgan, M. F., Uysal, A. R., Baskal, N., Kamel, A. N., and Erdogan, G. (1998). A potential risk for osteomalacia due to sociocultural lifestyle in Turkish women. *Endocrine J.* **45,** 675–678.

25. Matsuoka, L. Y., Ide, L., Wortsman, J., MacLaughlin, J. A., and Holick, M. F. (1987). Sunscreens suppress cutaneous vitamin D3 synthesis. *J. Clin. Endocrinol. Metab.* **64,** 1165–1168.

26. Matsuoka, L. Y., Wortsman, J., Hanifan, N., and Holick, M. F. (1988). Chronic sunscreen use decreases circulating concentrations of 25-hydroxyvitamin D: A preliminary study. *Arch. Dermatol.* **124,** 1802–1804.

27. Eddy, R. L. (1971). Metabolic bone disease after gastrectomy. *Am. J. Med.* **50,** 442–449.

28. Davies, M., Heys, S. E., Selby, P. S., Berry, J. L., and Mawer, E. B. (1997). Increased catabolism of 25-hydroxyvitamin D in patients with partial gastrectomy and elevated 1,25-dihydroxyvitamin D levels. Implications for metabolic bone disease. *J. Clin. Endocrinol. Metab.* **82,** 209–212.

29. Compston, J. E., Crowe, J. P., Wells, I. P., Horton, L. W. L., Hirst, D., Merrett, A. L., Woodhead, J. S., and Williams, R. (1980). Vitamin D prophylaxis and osteomalacia in chronic cholestatic liver disease. *Dig. Dis. Sci.* **25,** 28–32.

30. Parfitt, A. M. (1990). Osteomalacia and related disorders. *In* "Metabolic Bone Disease and Clinically Related Disorders" (S. M. Avioli, Ed.), pp. 329–396. W. B. Saunders, Philadelphia, PA.

31. Scriver, C. R. (1970). Vitamin D dependency. *Pediatrics* **45,** 361–363.

32. Fraser, D., Kooh, S. W., Kind, H. P., Hollick, M. F., Tanaka, Y., and DeLuca, H. F. (1973). Pathogenesis of hereditary vitamin D dependent rickets. An inborn error of vitamin D metabolism involving defective conversion of 25-hydroxyvitamin D to 1-alpha, 25-dihydroxyvitamin D. *N. Engl. J. Med.* **289,** 817–822.

33. Malloy, P. J., Pike, J. W., and Feldman, D. (1997). Hereditary 1,25-dihydroxyvitamin D resistant rickets. *In* "Vitamin D" (D. G. Feldman, F. H. Glorieux, and J. W. Pike, Eds.), pp. 765–788. Academic Press, San Diego.

34. Lyles, K. W., Clark, A. G., and Drezner, M. K. (1982). Serum 1,25-dihydroxyvitamin D levels in subjects with X-linked hypophosphatemic rickets and osteomalacia. *Calcif. Tiss. Intl.* **34,** 125–130.

35. Drezner, M. K. (1997). Clinical disorders of phosphate homeostasis. *In* "Vitamin D" (F. H. Feldman, and J. W. Pike, Eds.), pp. 733–753. Academic Press, San Diego.

36. Drezner, M. K. (2000). PHEX gene and hypophosphatemia. *Kidney Int.* **57,** 9–18.

37. Hodgkin, P., Hine, P. M., Kay, G. H., Lumb, G. A., and Stanbury, S. W. (1973). Vitamin D-deficiency in Asians at home and in Britain. *Lancet* **2,** 167–171.

38. Holmes, A. M., Enoch, B. A., Taylor, J., and Jones, M. E. (1973). Occult rickets and osteomalacia amongst the Asian immigrant population. *Quart. J. Med.* **42,** 125–149.

39. Berlyne, G. M., Ben-Ari, J., and Norde, E. (1973). Bedouin osteomalacia due to calcium deprivation caused by high phytic acid content of unleavened bread. *Am. J. Clin. Nutr.* **26,** 910–911.

40. Thacher, T. D., Fischer, P. R., Pettifor, J. M., Lawson, J. O., Isichei, C. O., Reading, J. C., and Chan, G. M. (1999). A comparison of calcium, vitamin D, or both for nutritional rickets in Nigerian children. *N. Engl. J. Med.* **341,** 602–604.

41. Fischer, R., Rahman, A., Cimma, J., Kyaw-Myint, T. O., Kabir, A. R., Talukder, K., Hassan, N., Manaster, B. J., Staab, D. B., Duxbury, J. M., Welch, R. M., Meisner, C. A., Haque, S., and Combs, G. F., Jr. (1999). Nutritional rickets without vitamin D deficiency in Bangladesh. *J. Trop. Pediatr.* **45,** 291–293.

42. Oliveri, B., Gomez Acotto, C., and Mautalen, C. (1999). Osteomalacia in a patient with severe anorexia nervosa. *Rev. Rhum. (Engl. ed.)* **66,** 505–508.

43. Lotz, M., Zisman, E., and Bartter, F. C. (1968). Evidence for a phosphorus-depletion syndrome in man. *N. Engl. J. Med.* **278,** 409–415.

44. Salassa, R. M., Jowsey, J., and Arnaud, C. D. (1970). Hypophosphatemic osteomalacia associated with "nonendocrine" tumors. *N. Engl. J. Med.* **283,** 65–70.

45. Evans, D. J., and Azzopardi, J. G. (1972). Distinctive tumours of bone and soft tissue causing acquired vitamin-D resistant osteomalacia. *Lancet* **1,** 353–354.

46. Cai, Q., Hodgson, S. F., Kao, P. C., Lennon, V. A., Klee, G. G., Zinsmiester, A. R., and Kumar, R. (1994). Brief report: Inhibition of renal phosphate transport by a tumor product in a patient with oncogenic osteomalacia. *N. Engl. J. Med.* **330,** 1645–1649.

47. Yeung, S. J., McCutcheon, I. E., Schultz, P., Gagel, R. F. (2000). Use of long-term intravenous phosphate infusion in the palliative treatment of tumor-induced osteomalacia. *J. Clin. Endocrinol. Metab.* **85,** 549–555.

48. Lee, D. B., Drinkard, J. P., Rosen, V. J., and Gonick, H. (1972). The adult Fanconi syndrome: Observations on etiology, morphology, renal function and mineral metabolism in three patients. *Medicine* **51,** 107–138.

49. Adams, R. G., Harrison, J. F., and Scott, P. (1969). The development of cadmium-induced proteinuria, impaired renal function, and osteomalacia in alkaline battery workers. *Quart. J. Med.* **38,** 425–443.

50. Emmerson, B. T. (1970). "Ouch-ouch" disease: The osteomalacia of cadmium nephropathy. *Ann. Intern. Med.* **73,** 854–855.

51. Bate, K. L., Clouston, D., Packham, D., Ratnaike, S., and Ebeling, P. R. (1998). Lambda light chain induced nephropathy: A rare cause of the Fanconi syndrome and severe osteomalacia. *Am. J. Kidney. Dis.* **32,** E3.

52. Donohoe, J. F., Freaney, R., and Muldowney, F. P. (1969). Osteomalacia in ureterosigmoidostomy. *Irish J. Med. Sci.* **8,** 523–530.

53. Henthorn, P. S., Raducha, M., Fedde, K. N., Lafferty, M. A., and Whyte, M. P. (1992). Different missense mutations at the tissue-nonspecific alkaline phosphatase gene locus in autosomal recessively inherited forms of mild and severe hypophosphatasia. *Proc. Natl. Acad. Sci. USA* **89,** 9924–9928.

54. Whyte, M. P. (1989). Hypophosphatasia. *In* "The Metabolic Basis of Inherited Disease," 6th ed. (C. B. Scriver, W. S. Sly, and D. Valle, Eds.), pp. 2843–2856. McGraw-Hill, New York.

55. Schultz, M., Kierdorf, U., Sedlacek, F., and Kierdorf, H. (1998). Pathological bone changes in the mandibles of wild red deer. (*Cervas elaphus L.*) exposed to high environmental levels of fluoride. *J. Anat.* **193,** 431–432.

55a. Watts, N. B., Harris, S. T., Genant, H. K., Wasnich, R. D., Miller, P. D., Jackson, R. D., Licata, A. A., Ross, P., Woodson, G. C., III, Yanover, M. J., Mysiw, J., Kohse, L., Rao, M. B., Steiger, P., Richmond, B., and Chesnut, C. H., III (1990). Intermittent cyclical etidronate treatment of postmenopausal osteoporosis. *N. Engl. J. Med.* **323,** 73–79.

56. Malluche, H. H., Smith, A. J., Abreo, K., and Faugere, M. C. (1984). The use of desferoxamine in the management of aluminum accumulation in bone in patients with renal failure. *N. Engl. J. Med,* **311,** 140–144.

CHAPTER 47

Nutrition and Immunodeficiency Syndromes

JUL GERRIOR AND CHRISTINE WANKE
Tufts University School of Medicine, Boston, Massachusetts

I. INTRODUCTION

As we enter the third decade of the acquired immunodeficiency syndrome (AIDS) epidemic, nutrition and metabolic concerns continue to challenge health professionals, medical scientists, and individuals infected with the human immunodeficiency virus (HIV). In the developed world, the rate of death caused by HIV and AIDS has declined largely due to the advent of highly active antiretroviral therapy. However, even in the setting of advanced HIV treatment, complications of infection continue. In countries where there is limited access to medicine, the mortality and infection rate has grown substantially, contributing to abbreviated life expectancy. Weight loss and other nutritional factors have been and continue to be problems for HIV-infected patients. Malnutrition is a common complication of HIV infection and is an independent predictor of morbidity and mortality [1]. Compromised nutritional status continues to exist as well as a newly described metabolic syndrome called lipodystrophy or fat redistribution syndrome.

This chapter summarizes the available data on nutrition and AIDS including the wasting syndrome, HIV-related weight loss, and the lipodystrophy syndrome. A significant portion of this chapter will be devoted to addressing the clinical importance of assessment as well as relevant data on intervention strategies for HIV-related weight loss. Because the metabolic abnormalities and associated body shape changes are often clinically disturbing to the patient and also the providers, we will discuss the role of assessment and possible intervention strategies for this syndrome.

II. HIV-ASSOCIATED WEIGHT LOSS

The wasting syndrome is defined as progressive involuntary weight loss of >10% of baseline body weight in the setting of a chronic infection and/or chronic diarrhea, and it has distinct features. It is classically associated with advanced and possibly untreated HIV disease [2]. HIV-associated weight and muscle loss was noted early in the AIDS epidemic. In fact, HIV infection or AIDS is known in Africa as "slim disease" [3]. In Africa and other developing countries, wasting is due both to HIV infection opportunistic infections, such as gastrointestinal infections, and tuberculosis. Before the antiretroviral therapy era, opportunistic infections also had a clinical impact on weight loss, because fever, anorexia, and malabsorption accelerated the rate of weight loss in the developed world as well. Even in the active antiretroviral therapy era, the etiology of continued weight loss is not so clear, in spite of maximal viral suppression.

In the past, wasting syndrome, determined by physical examination, presented as loss of body weight and lean body mass. Today, there are validated techniques to measure more accurately body composition of HIV-infected patients. Although the wasting syndrome may appear obvious upon physical examination, further definition of the overall complexity and nature of HIV-associated weight loss is possible.

The Center for Disease Control (CDC) definition of wasting syndrome as an AIDS-defining illness is: "Involuntary weight loss of >10% of baseline body weight plus either chronic diarrhea defined as at least one stool per day for >30 days. Or chronic weakness and fever for >30 days in the absence of a condition other than HIV infection that could explain the findings (e.g., tuberculosis, cancer, or microsporidiosis)" [2].

Nahlen and colleagues [4] studied the prevalence of wasting syndrome between 1987 and 1991 for the CDC. They reported a 17.8% wasting syndrome in the 16,773 females and 130,852 males studied [4]. This study examined the prevalence data in a cohort of cases reported to the CDC. Despite issues raised of ethnic or racial bias of case reporting, the highest percentage of wasting syndrome was seen in Hispanics, followed by African Americans, Caucasians, and Asians/others. A report [5] on a longitudinal study in Puerto Rico, during a similar time period, demonstrated that HIV wasting syndrome accounted for 9.7% of 1520 cases between May 1992 to December 1996. This is comparable to the percentage of Caucasians with AIDS-defining wasting syndrome from the CDC report.

Among other analyses from the CDC data set include gender differences in AIDS-defining wasting syndrome. These data reported a higher incidence of AIDS wasting in

females (10.2%) compared to males (6.7%) [4]. Thus, the conclusion of this report stated AIDS wasting to be significant in both genders, but more common in women.

To further assess the incidence of wasting syndrome prior to the highly active antiretroviral therapy era, a study was conducted in a cohort of homosexual males. The multicenter AIDS cohort study [6], established to assess the progression of HIV infection to AIDS, also led to an accumulation of data available to determine the incidence of weight loss in this cohort. A longitudinal, prospective study that drew from populations in the Baltimore, Washington (DC), Chicago, Pittsburgh, and Los Angeles areas was included. Weight loss occurred during 6 months before recognized seroconversion and up to 18 months prior to the onset of AIDS. The data analysis determined that weight loss was an early predictor of progression to AIDS in this cohort [6].

Weight loss associated with HIV infection is multifactorial and not completely understood. It is recognized that wasting, particularly of lean muscle mass, is an independent predictor of death [1]. In addition to the devastation of morbidity and mortality due to wasting syndrome, many have described other related consequences of weight loss including increased progression of disease, decline in function and strength, and loss of muscle protein [7–11]. Despite the potency of antiretroviral therapy today and a noted decline in secondary infections, HIV-related weight loss continues to occur across all categories [12].

Wanke and colleagues [12] assessed the prevalence of wasting in a large cohort of HIV-positive subjects treated with active antiretroviral therapy and found that 33.6% of all participants met the study definition of wasting. They defined the wasting syndrome as loss of >10% body weight since diagnosis, loss of >5% of body weight in the past 6 months, and sustained body mass index of <20 kg/m² since the previous 6-month visit. These data suggest that wasting in the era of active antiretroviral therapy remains a problem and cannot be ignored even when patients are on potent therapy.

Criticism of the CDC definition for wasting includes a lack of specification of "baseline body weight," a time frame for weight loss, and lack of criteria for body composition. Defining wasting as a sustained body weight loss of 5% over 6 months serves to represent nutritional risk better than 10% body weight loss from baseline or preinfection body weight.

III. HIV-ASSOCIATED LIPODYSTROPHY SYNDROME

A newly identified nutritional-related complication has been observed in HIV-infected patients. It is referred to by many pseudonyms such as "lipodystrophy syndrome," "fat redistribution syndrome," "peripheral lipodystrophy syndrome," "crix-belly," and "protease paunch." The etiology of this complication (similar to wasting) is unclear and does not have a generally accepted definition. This syndrome will be referred to as *lipodystrophy* in the context of this chapter.

Lipodystrophy is associated with body shape changes and metabolic abnormalities, but should not to be equated with classic lipodystrophy. The most common change in body shape is enlarged truncal girth resulting from a deposit of adipose tissue in the visceral area. In some cases, patients develop a dorsocervical fat pad or "buffalo hump" on the posterior neck. Alternatively, this syndrome may be limited to or include peripheral fat atrophy of the extremities, buttocks, and face. It is common to observe increasing venous markings in the periphery due to the frank loss of fatty tissue. Initially, these changes in body shape were thought to be associated with protease inhibitor therapy. More careful observation noted that these changes occur with or without protease inhibitor therapy [13–18].

Metabolic complications have also been documented in the lipodystrophy syndrome. These include, but are not limited to hyperlipidemia, insulin resistance, and, rarely, hyperglycemia [15, 19]. The lipodystrophy syndrome will be discussed in more detail as part of the assessment and intervention strategies of this chapter.

IV. CAUSES OF WEIGHT LOSS IN HIV/AIDS

As suggested above, weight loss due to HIV infection is complex, multifaceted, and not completely understood. The associated causes of weight loss include inadequate intake induced by loss of appetite, malabsorption caused by intestinal dysfunction or diarrheal illness, metabolic abnormalities related to cytokines or the HIV infection itself, or hormonal imbalances. Each of these components may be present independent of one another or in combination.

Malnutrition in HIV infection may be classified as starvation or cachexia. Starvation is simply a lack of food, such as is seen in developing countries or in poverty-stricken areas of developed countries. It may occur either voluntarily or involuntarily and be reversed by providing sufficient energy, electrolytes, and water. Long-term starvation often leads to a physiological response noted by a decrease in energy expenditure, preservation of glucose and protein metabolism, and an increase in lipid oxidation. In comparison, cachexia is defined as a depletion or breakdown of lean body mass. This is commonly associated with an acute illness or an infection, because the body expends protein and glucose substrate in response to an acute insult. This metabolic alteration is significant and life sustaining in the short term, but in the long term will result in nitrogen and protein depletion. Starvation can be corrected by refeeding, but for the cachectic patient, alterations in carbohydrate and protein metabolism have to be closely monitored.

A. Anorexia and Oral Intake

Anorexia is a common manifestation in HIV infection and AIDS. Two studies have documented that negative energy balance is the primary determinant of HIV-associated weight loss [20, 21]. The causes of inadequate intake include a variety of metabolic, gastrointestinal, and neurologic symptoms. HIV-induced proinflammatory cytokines may contribute to anorexia as does HIV infection itself. The majority of antiviral medications for HIV have anorexigenic effects. Many patients are taking up to 30 or more pills daily in an attempt to control the virus and related infections. Side effects from these agents commonly cause nausea, vomiting, or diarrhea. Other barriers to adequate intake may be due to taste changes, difficulty swallowing, malignancies (Kaposi's sarcoma), opportunistic infections, such as oral thrush, cytomegalovirus, herpes, and apthous ulcers. Dental infections may also contribute to inadequate intake and subsequent weight loss.

Psychological issues as well as mood-altering medications may cause changes in appetite and often contribute to a disinterest in food. "Battle fatigue" is a common term associated with HIV-infected individuals who have been fighting this disease for many years. They often complain of overall exhaustion for a variety of reasons. Some may be preparing to give up the fight. This in itself can be both a physical and a psychological reason for appetite loss. Economic, social, and cultural factors may limit adequate nutritional intake in some patients.

B. Diarrhea and Malabsorption in HIV and AIDS

Chronic diarrhea and malabsorption of nutrients is common in these patients. In the United States, 60% of all HIV-infected patients experience diarrhea at some point in the course of their disease. The incidence of diarrhea is 100% of HIV-infected patients in developing countries [22]. A population survey reported chronic diarrhea in 3–24% of patients and correlated with reduced quality of life. In the same survey, when patients were further questioned, the prevalence of diarrhea reported increased to 38% [23]. These data suggest that the prevalence of diarrhea is likely to be higher than expected due to interpretation of questionnaires and definitions of diarrhea. Weight loss due to malabsorption of nutrients is more common in patients who experience small bowel diarrhea, where most nutrient absorption occurs, than large bowel diarrhea. Symptoms of small bowel diarrhea include frequent, high-volume stools often accompanied by discomfort in the abdomen, dehydration, and weight loss. Large bowel diarrhea is commonly associated with urgency or tenesmus. Dehydration is common with both types of diarrhea and leads to skin breakdown.

Pathogens most likely found in HIV-infected patients include the bacteria *Salmonella, Campylobacter, Shigella, My-* *cobacterium avium,* and *Clostridium difficile*; the protozoa *Cryptosporidia, Isospora belli,* and *microsporidium*; and cytomegalovirus, adenovirus, and herpes simplex virus. Enteroaggregative *Escherichia coli* has been described in HIV infection and may be the cause of chronic diarrhea [24].

After a complete workup of potential causes for diarrhea in HIV-infected patients, 10–20% of cases have no identifiable pathogen. In the setting of idiopathic diarrhea, other probable causes may include chronic inflammation of the small intestinal mucosa, atrophy of the villi, or pancreatic insufficiency. Primary HIV infection of the enterocytes adhering to the small intestine or invading the gut-associated lymphoid tissue has been postulated to be causal but this remains unclear. Other possible explanations for persistent diarrhea and malabsorption include the presence of unidentified pathogens, motility issues, autonomic dysfunction, colonic inflammation, bacterial overgrowth, medications, dietary habits, and oral nutrition supplements [25, 26].

C. Metabolic Abnormalities

Weight loss due to metabolic abnormalities or alterations has been described in HIV/AIDS patients. It has been documented that total energy expenditure and resting energy expenditure increase in HIV infection; however, data do not agree whether weight loss is due to increased energy expenditure or associated with decreased energy intake [20, 21]. Macallan and colleagues [20] assessed resting energy expenditure, total energy expenditure, and energy intake in 27 men with HIV infection. The results indicated no difference in total energy expenditure as compared to HIV-negative controls. However, there was a positive association between the rate of weight loss and decreased total energy expenditure in all subjects. These changes were correlated with a reduction in physical activity and energy intake. Conclusions from this study indicate that total energy expenditure is reduced during episodes of weight loss and the primary determinant is due to a deficit in energy intake and reduced activity level.

Grunfeld and colleagues [21] reported an increase in resting energy expenditure in HIV-positive subjects at varying stages of disease. Resting energy expenditure was increased in 11% of HIV-positive subjects, in 25% with CDC-defined AIDS, and in 29% of AIDS subjects with secondary infections. Kotler and colleagues [27] reported a reduction in resting energy expenditure, predicted by the Harris-Benedict equation, in clinically stable, HIV-infected men compared to controls. It is clear from these studies that energy expenditure appears to be altered by HIV disease and therefore energy requirements need to be carefully determined for medical nutrition therapy.

An alteration in intermediary metabolism has been described in HIV/AIDS patients, but the mechanism remains unclear. An increase in plasma triglyceride concentration and acceleration of protein turnover has been documented in AIDS wasting patients with weight loss [28, 29]. Furthermore,

carbohydrate oxidation is suppressed and insulin resistance is increased resulting in an increase in fat storage rather than lean tissue [30]. Another explanation derived to understand HIV-related weight loss is the role that cytokine production may play. The production of tumor necrosis factor (TNF), interferon α (IFN-α), interleukin 1 (IL-1), interleukin 6 (IL-6), and possibly other cytokines may be partly responsible for anorexia and wasting as part of an inflammatory response to infection [31]. Elevated plasma triglyceride and cholesterol concentration, insulin resistance, and, in some cases, the development of diabetes have been associated with HIV infection, specifically in the extended life span associated with the active antiretroviral therapy era. These metabolic abnormalities are often associated with the lipodystrophy syndrome. Similar to the derangement in metabolism described in HIV-related weight loss, the phenomenon described in HIV-associated lipodystrophy is poorly understood. Intervention strategies for this myriad of syndromes will be examined later in this chapter.

V. HORMONAL IMBALANCES

The most common endocrine abnormality in men with HIV infection is testosterone deficiency, which results in hypogonadism [32]. Symptoms include low sex drive, weight loss, and fatigue. Testosterone, a major anabolic hormone in men, occurs in low levels in women. In men, chronically low testosterone levels may lead to reduced anabolism and poor lean tissue preservation. Low testosterone may be seen in patients who experience an acute insult or acute infection followed by weight loss. Other reported endocrine manifestations associated with HIV infection include the thyroid, pituitary, and adrenal glands. Adrenal insufficiency, growth hormone abnormalities, and low thyroid function have been associated with HIV infection [33]. Because wasting syndrome is poorly understood, so are the endocrine abnormalities.

VI. NUTRITIONAL ASSESSMENT

An assessment of nutritional status in HIV/AIDS is similar to that in other disease states. The information gathered in a nutritional assessment should provide appropriate and relevant data toward the development of intervention and monitoring strategies of individual patients. The goal of this section is to suggest assessment parameters that are critical in the evaluation of nutritional status in HIV infection in both general terms and specific concerns for those experiencing lipodystrophy syndrome. In addition, the American Dietetic Association has prepared a useful clinical guide and a position statement for professionals working in HIV [34, 35]. The guidelines state the minimum nutrition services that should be provided to children, women, and men infected with HIV.

A standard nutritional evaluation of HIV-infected adults should include the following parameters: body weight, ideal and usual body weight, body mass index, and biochemical indices. Clinical research studies are evaluating the use of bioelectrical impedance analysis as a supplement to anthropometry for body composition analysis. Appetite status, dietary intake, and gastrointestinal symptoms are also included. Other relevant clinical data may include duration of HIV infection, age, sex, medication and medication history, medical history, socioeconomic status (including access to food), and psychosocial history.

For patients with the lipodystrophy syndrome, body shape changes result in an evaluation that differs from a standard nutrition assessment of HIV-infected adults. Assessment for patients with lypodystrophy includes waist and hip circumference, waist:hip ratio, midarm circumference, midthigh circumference, and skinfold thickness over the triceps, suprailiac, subscapular, and thigh. If applicable, photographic evaluation of body habitus, including the dorsocervical fat pad and facial wasting if present, may be used to monitor body shape changes over time and impact of clinical interventions. In research settings, visceral adipose tissue evaluation may be achieved through the use of computed tomography imaging or dual-energy x-ray absorptiometry calibrated for body composition, not bone density. Other assessment parameters to evaluate lipodystrophy may include plasma lipid and glucose concentrations, oral glucose tolerance test, insulin sensitivity studies, and careful clinical examination of arms, legs, and face to identify venous markings due to fat atrophy.

A. Body Weight Assessment

Although body weight is documented in most routine assessments, in patients with HIV/AIDS, body composition is a better predictor of nutritional and health status than body weight. Although body weight can serve as a convenient and simple predictor of general nutritional status, it is often subject to errors in interpretation due to fluid retention associated with cardiac, renal, and hepatic diseases, or dehydration from diarrhea or chronic illness. Nonetheless, body weight is useful to document so trends can be examined over time. Obtain a weight history prior to HIV infection, during HIV infection, and recently. These questions may be a useful way to characterize the complete weight history of an individual. From the information provided, the clinician can establish baseline data and determine therapeutic goals.

1. IDEAL AND USUAL BODY WEIGHT FOR HEIGHT
Estimating usual and ideal body weight is another key component in the nutrition assessment. This allows determination of percent weight change from actual weight to usual body weight. Estimation of ideal body weight can be

done by consulting the weight–height reference chart established from Metropolitan Life Insurance Company actuarial data [36]. The Metropolitan height–weight tables do not offer ideal body weights of individuals from ethnic and low socioeconomic background because the data are derived from healthy men and women who were offered life insurance in the late 1950s. However, this does present a point of reference for an estimated ideal body weight for individuals so is often used in clinical settings. A practical approach to estimate ideal body weight for height involves selecting the midpoint of the medium frame and determine an ideal body weight with a range of ± 5%.

Once this information is established, develop an understanding of the patient's perception of his or her own ideal body weight. Discrepancy between the provider and the patient may occur if there is not a clear understanding of patient needs.

2. Body Mass Index

Body mass index (BMI) is a ratio of weight to height used to assess degree of fatness or adiposity of an individual [37]. The measurement is obtained from the calculation of weight in kilograms divided by height in meters squared. BMI is an assessment tool used to estimate degree of overweight or obesity. In the general population, a BMI of 30 kg/m^2 or above indicates obesity. A BMI below 19 kg/m^2 indicates a risk of malnutrition. However, BMI is only one component of nutrition assessment and, like body weight, it should not be the only data used to assess nutritional status especially in diseases like AIDS, which can greatly alter body composition.

B. Body Composition Assessment

Body composition provides information on amounts of various body tissues beyond total weight. In this section, we will discuss the techniques that are useful in the clinical assessment of body composition in HIV/AIDS and review the relevance of the specific body compartments.

1. Bioelectrial Impedance Analysis

Bioelectrical impedance analysis is a method used to estimate body compartments through a mechanism of resistance and reactance. The compartments measured include body cell mass, fat mass, extracellular tissue, and fat-free mass. The fact that the analyzer is portable and the measurement quick and without discomfort makes bioelectrical impedance analysis popular in the clinical setting. The analyzer detects resistance and reactance and, at high frequencies, total body water is the conducting medium. At low frequencies, the membrane lipid content of the body cell mass compartment acts as a capacitor, which limits the flow to intracellular space only. The calculations estimate different body compartments [38]. Accuracy of the measurements depends on adequate hydration. Estimates of lean body mass

are improved when age, sex, and body weight are included in the calculation. In addition to these compartments, estimates of total body water along with extracellular and intracellular water are obtained.

The importance of body composition analysis in HIV/AIDS is to estimate the amount and percentage of body cell mass present in these patients. As we described earlier, the prevalence of wasting (loss of body cell mass) persists despite improved treatment regimens. Thus, early detection and monitoring of body cell mass is critical, because it is the compartment of body tissue that is most representative of functional status. This compartment accounts for intracellular water, red blood cells, and organ and skeletal tissue, and is the site of all metabolic activity [39]. Ideal body cell mass in men is estimated as 40–45% of ideal body weight for height. For women, the ideal body cell mass is estimated at 30–35% of ideal body weight for height.

Other compartments of clinical significance include fat mass, extracellular tissue, and fat-free mass. Fat mass is the compartment of tissue responsible for stored energy or fuel and insulation for temperature regulation of organs. Depletion of fat stores is commonly seen during starvation or insufficient energy intake. During starvation, the body becomes efficient at sparing proteins and lean tissue; however, in the setting of HIV infection, the opposite occurs. Fat stores remain as depletion of body cell mass occurs in HIV infection. Ideal fat mass for men is estimated to be between 10–20% of actual body weight. Ideally, 16–19% is a more suitable fat mass for HIV/AIDS infection. Ideal fat mass for women is estimated at 20–30% of actual body weight.

Extracellular tissue is the transport and structure compartment that includes bone, collagen, cartilage, and other tissues. Assessment of extracellular tissue can provide information pertaining to hydration status. Low extracellular tissue indicates that dehydration may be present. Normal or euhydration status will return extracellular tissue to normal. Edema will often cause extracellular tissue to appear abnormally high. This fluid shift occurs to provide more transport fluid to the "stressed" area. When extracellular tissue continues to increase, this indicates poor response to nutritional repletion. This may also identify a candidate for anabolic therapy in the setting of advanced weight loss. Ideal extracellular tissue should be the same as estimated body cell mass requirements, 40–45% of ideal body weight for height should contain extracellular tissue in men, and the estimated extracellular tissue for women is 30–35% of ideal body weight for height.

Fat-free mass is total body weight minus fat mass. This compartment contains extracellular tissue and body cell mass and therefore does not represent ideal functional tissue. Anthropometric assessment using skinfold thickness measurements will yield a two-compartment model containing fat-free mass and fat mass. In a research setting, common skinfold thickness sites measured include fat tissue over the

triceps, subscapular, suprailiac, and thigh, performed in triplicate. These measurements are use in calculations of fat-free mass and fat mass percentages [40].

C. Nutrition Assessment in Lipodystrophy Syndrome

The lipodystrophy syndrome, as described earlier, is associated with metabolic abnormalities including elevated plasma lipid levels, glucose intolerance, insulin resistance, and changes in body shape. Because clinical focus has shifted from the wasting syndrome to the lipodystrophy syndrome, it is as important to obtain data relevant to body shape and body image as it is to obtain body weight. Nutritional assessment of lipodystrophy requires additional information, compared to the standard nutritional assessment for HIV/AIDS, but how to characterize these changes is not yet defined.

Fat accumulation and fat atrophy are the two body shape changes seen with lipodystrophy syndrome. Although it is important to define usual and ideal body weight in lipodystrophy syndrome, it is especially useful to examine body deposition of fat and/or areas of fat atrophy. The waist-to-hip measurement ratio provides an important indicator of central obesity. The standard waist measurement should be performed directly under the lowest rib or usually at the narrowest point around the waist. The standard hip measurement is directed at the maximum extension point around the buttocks. Normality is defined in men as waist circumference <88.2 cm and waist-to-hip ratio ≤0.95, and in women, a waist circumference <75.3 cm and waist-to-hip ratio ≤0.9 for decreased risk of cardiovascular disease [41]. Note that although there are standard methods to measure waist and hip, the distribution of body fat seen in these patients might affect the interpretation of these values.

Measuring body composition in lipodystrophy syndrome is complicated by the abnormal distribution of body fat. In research settings, magnetic resonance imaging and computed tomography scan can also be used to define the extent of visceral abdominal fat. Dual-energy x-ray absorptiometry (DXA) can be calibrated to determine regional body fat as well. Their high cost and limited accessibility makes these approaches less likely to be used in routine clinical care. Total body magnetic resonance imaging may be the most ideal and accurate method to quantify fat distribution in lipodystrophy. Increased visceral fat on magnetic resonance imaging has been correlated to waist circumference in lipodystrophy; therefore, measuring waist and hip circumferences seems a reliable, valid, and practical method of assessment, although some HIV-infected individuals may also have increased subcutaneous fat [42].

Fat accumulation may be associated with insulin resistance, lipid abnormalities, and increased cardiac risk in patients with this syndrome [43]. Computed tomography imaging is a common research method of evaluating this area of prominent fat accumulation seen in this syndrome. Serial

measurements of DXA, magnetic resonance imaging, or computed tomography scans will allow for comparison of longitudinal data over time.

D. Biochemical Indices of Nutrition Assessment

Routine biochemical parameters in HIV/AIDS nutrition assessment include the serum albumin concentrations, fasting cholesterol concentrations, fasting triglyceride concentrations, electrolyte concentrations, and complete blood count. Symptoms of fatigue, weight loss, and low sexual drive may be suggestive of hypogonadism. As discussed earlier, the role of testosterone status in HIV-associated weight loss suggests that the evaluation of testosterone levels may be important in HIV/AIDS and should include total and free testosterone, specifically in the presence of the described symptoms.

Chronic diarrhea or loose stools is another common complication in HIV/AIDS and suggests an evaluation of malabsorption and micronutrient levels when diarrhea persists in the absence of negative stool cultures or other potential gastrointestinal illnesses. The following tests may be recommended: serum zinc and magnesium concentrations, vitamin B_{12} concentrations, D-xylose, 24–72 hour fecal fat test, and folate concentrations. Evaluation of gastrointestinal symptoms is essential and should be addressed with a gastrointestinal specialist. Recommendations of gastrointestinal assessment parameters include stool number and consistency; severity of abdominal bloating, cramping, and pain; routine stool examination for opportunistic pathogens; and upper and lower endoscopy and biopsy (if necessary).

For the lipodystrophy syndrome, evaluation of biochemical metabolic parameters may include fasting blood glucose concentration, lipoprotein profile, oral glucose tolerance test, and serum insulin concentrations.

HIV monitoring should involve a specialist in infectious diseases or a clinician with experience in the treatment of HIV infection. Common immune or HIV-related parameters are absolute CD4 count and percentage, absolute CD8 count and percentage, and viral load or the amount of virus present in blood.

E. Appetite Status and Assessment of Oral Intake

Of primary importance in the nutritional management of HIV/AIDS is the assessment of appetite status and nutrient intake. Earlier in this chapter many potential causes of anorexia in HIV/AIDS were described. Medications, opportunistic infections, and depression are among a few of the possible causes of anorexia in HIV infection. The consequences of anorexia often result in low energy intake and subsequent weight loss. In the clinical setting, the three most common methods to evaluate estimated oral intake include 24-hour recall, food frequency questionnaire, and 3-day food

diary [44]. Each method has its advantages and limitations. Chapter 1 of this text discusses these methods in detail.

VII. NUTRITIONAL RECOMMENDATIONS

Many pharmacological agents are available to enhance or optimize the nutritional health of individuals infected with HIV infection. These include appetite stimulants, anabolic analogues, and anticytokine therapies. A majority of the evidence suggests that these therapies may play a role in the improvement of nutritional status, but a detailed review is beyond the scope of this chapter. The goal of this section is to address the specific nutritional needs of HIV/AIDS individuals and provide recommendations for intervention.

A. Recommended Energy Needs

Studies of resting energy expenditure in patients with HIV infection were described above and these data suggest that resting energy expenditure increases 10–25% due to the progression of disease or, specifically, an acquired opportunistic infection. [20–23]. Therefore, it is reasonable to recommend an increase is estimated energy requirement by 10–15%. If an HIV-infected individual is weight stable without weight loss, a 10% increase from the estimated basal energy expenditure needs is recommended. However, if weight loss is evident, estimated energy needs should be adjusted to 15% above the basal energy expenditure requirements. The estimated energy calculation is based on the Harris-Benedict equation for energy needs plus an additional 10–15% for HIV infection and an activity factor.

A simple guideline to assist patients with achieving energy needs is to encourage the intake of six small meals or three adequate meals and two snacks daily. If appropriate, an energy-dense, high-protein oral liquid supplement may be needed.

B. Recommended Protein Needs

Much attention has been given to protein status and the maintenance of the immune system [45]. Low serum albumin is an indicator of worsening nutritional status and is seen with disease progression. The Recommended Dietary Allowance (RDA) for protein is 0.8–1.0 g/kg body weight for a healthy person [46]. However, based on data in HIV/AIDS, protein requirements are estimated to be 1.2–2.0 g/kg body weight [47, 48]. For example, in the 70-kg male, the estimated protein needs would be 84–140 g/day. A general daily approximation of estimated protein needs is 100–150 g/day for men and 80–100 g/day for women. To maintain the optimal protein intake, protein supplementation may be considered.

C. Vitamin and Mineral Recommendations

Altered nutritional status may influence the course of HIV disease progression and survival [49, 50]. Micronutrient deficiencies, widespread among various HIV-infected cohorts, cause disruption in immune function, disease progression, viral expression, and related morbidity [51, 52]. Decreased plasma concentrations of zinc, selenium, and vitamins B_6, B_{12}, A, and E are evident and appear to be functionally relevant in maintaining the integrity of immune responses. Baum and colleagues [53] reported a low concentration of vitamins A and E in the plasma of homosexual males with HIV infection. In the same study, 40–50% of HIV-infected men and women who abuse drugs also had severely decreased plasma concentrations of vitamins A and E. In a cohort of pediatric patients, perinatally exposed, aged 15–18 months, a high proportion had zinc and selenium deficiency [54].

Selenium deficiency has been demonstrated to be a significant predictor of HIV-related mortality, independent of CD4 counts over time or antiretroviral therapy. Others have demonstrated selenium deficiency to be predictive of HIV-related prognosis, immune dysfunction, and decreased survival [55, 56]. This antioxidant at the cellular level is an integral part of the enzyme glutathione peroxidase system, which increases the oxygen consumption of cells and protects membranes against oxidative stress. Selenium status may have an important role in slowing the progression of HIV disease and oxidative stress in HIV disease may be an important mechanistic factor [57]. Recent investigations indicate that supplementation of selenium at doses of 200 mcg/day may help to increase the enzymatic defense systems in patients with HIV infection [58].

Recent studies have also suggested that vitamin E, another antioxidant nutrient, may be able to increase the CD4-to-CD8 cell ratio and increase lymphocyte counts while reducing levels of suppressor cells [59]. A study evaluating vitamin E status in HIV-infected patients showed that those patients who had the highest plasma concentrations of vitamin E had a 34% decrease in risk progression to AIDS compared to the lowest quartile [60]. In a review of the immune effects of vitamin E, Allard and colleagues [61] examined the effects of vitamin E supplementation (800 IU) in HIV-infected patients. They showed an increase in plasma alpha-tocopherol concentration ($p < 0.0005$), a reduction in lipid peroxidation ($p < 0.025$), and also a reduction in plasma HIV viral load ($p < 0.1$) compared to placebo.

Based on these observations of micronutrient status and possible physiological role in HIV/AIDS, supplementation with vitamins C, E, beta-carotene, and selenium may be warranted.

D. Glutamine and Cysteine Status

Glutamine has been noted to have an effect on enhancing lean body mass in HIV infected patients as well as supporting

the integrity of the gut mucosa [62–68]. It has been shown that HIV-infected individuals may have abnormal levels of the amino acids cysteine and glutathione, complicating the body's ability to maintain lean body mass [63]. Supplementation with N-acetyl-cysteine has been postulated as a modality to enhance glutathione levels in these patients [64]. Glutathione plays an important role in the maintenance of cellular function and immunological reactivity [62]. Recognizing the importance of maintaining cellular and skeletal lean body mass, supplementation with cysteine and glutamine may be recommended.

E. Nutritional Recommendations for the Lipodystrophy Syndrome

Because there is no clear definition of the lipodystrophy syndrome, there are also no specific dietary considerations established. For HIV-infected patients with the lipodystrophy syndrome, weight gain is not an issue, rather the distribution of body weight and body fat is the concern. Weight loss is typically not the goal for patients in this situation. A recommendation to promote normal blood lipid levels is a standard clinical approach. Because these patients have insulin resistance, a dyslipidemia develops when low-fat, high-carbohydrate diets are followed. Like patients with type 2 diabetes (see Chapter 29), plasma lipid normalization results from diets containing moderate amounts of unsaturated fatty acids and moderate in total carbohydrate.

VIII. NUTRITIONAL COUNSELING

Data are limited on the effectiveness of nutrition counseling and outcome of enhanced oral intake and body weight. A recent study compared nutritional counseling alone versus nutritional counseling and enteral supplements for 6 weeks in malnourished patients with HIV infection. Half of the patients in each treatment group achieved at least 80% of their target energy intake and the supplement group had larger increases in fat-free mass and grip strength [69]. An earlier study, conducted before the availability of active antiretroviral therapy, concluded that malnourished HIV-infected patients who received oral supplementation and nutritional counseling for 6 weeks achieved a mean weight gain of 1.1 kg [70]. These data are useful and demonstrate that nutrition counseling may assist patients with increasing energy and protein intakes; however, more outcome data are needed.

To standardize care for HIV/AIDS patients and foster outcome data collection, a nutrition therapy guideline has been developed [34]. The protocol, designed for HIV-infected adults, children, and adolescents, provides details for screening and nutrition therapy delivered with expected outcomes. Major goals are to optimize nutrition status, prevent the development of nutrient deficiencies, prevent loss of weight and lean body mass, maximize the effectiveness of medical and pharmacological treatments, and minimize health care costs [34].

IX. SUMMARY

Nutrition complications in HIV/AIDS include HIV-associated weight loss, the wasting syndrome, and the lipodystrophy syndrome. Metabolic abnormalities may include dyslipidemia, insulin resistance, and in some cases type 2 diabetes mellitus. The lipodystrophy syndrome may cause body shape changes including increased truncal fat, a dorsocervical fat pad, thinning of the extremities, and loss of facial fat. Adequate energy and protein intake is necessary to maintain adipose reserve and lean body cell mass. Specific micronutrients of particular importance for HIV/AIDS patients are antioxidant nutrients because requirements may be increased due to oxidative stress. Nutritional therapy is an important component of the overall health care of patients who live with HIV/AIDS.

References

1. Kotler, D. P., Tierney, A. R., Wang, J., and Pierson, R. N., Jr. (1989). The magnitude of body cell mass depletion determines the timing of death from wasting in AIDS. *Am. J. Clin. Nutr.* **50,** 444–447.
2. Centers for Disease Control (1987). Revision of the CDC surveillance case definition for acquired immunodeficiency syndrome. *Mortal. Morbid. Wkly. Rept.* **36,** 3–15.
3. Serwadda, D., Mugerwa, R., and Sewankambo, N. (1985). Slim disease: A new disease in Uganda and its association with HTLV-III infection. *Lancet* **2,** 849–852.
4. Nahlen, B. L., Chu, S. V., Nwanyanwu, O. C., Berkelman, R. L., Martinez, S. A., and Rullan, J. V. (1993). HIV wasting syndrome in the United States. *AIDS* **7,** 183–188.
5. Gomez, M. A., Valezquez, M., and Hunter, R. F. (1997). Outline of the human retrovirus registry: Profile of Puerto Rican HIV infected population. *Boetin Asociacion Medica de Puerto Rico* **89,** 111–116.
6. Graham, N. M. H., Munoz, A., Bacellar, H., Kingsley, L. A., Visscher, B. R., and Phair, J. P. (1993). Clinical factors associated with weight loss related to infection with human immunodeficiency virus type 1 in the Multicenter AIDS cohort study. *Epidemiology* **137,** 439–446.
7. Chlebowski, R., Grosvenor, M., Bernhard, N. H., Morales, L. S., and Bulcavage, L. M. (1989). Nutritional status, gastrointestinal dysfunction, and survival in patients with AIDS. *Am. J. Gastroenterol.* **84,** 1288–1293.
8. Guenter, P., Muurahainen, N., Kosok, A., Cohan, G. R., Rudenstein, R., and Turner, J. (1993). Relationships among nutritional status, disease progression, and survival in HIV infection. *J. AIDS* **6,** 1130–1138.
9. Suttman, U., Ockenga, J., Selberg, O., Hoogestraat, L., Deicher, H., and Muller, M. (1995). Incidence and prognostic value of malnutrition and wasting in human immunodeficiency virus-infected outpatients. *J. AIDS* **8,** 239–246.

10. Yarasheski, K., Zachwieja, J., Gischler, J., Crowley, J., Horgan, M., and Powderly, W. G. (1998). Increased plasma Gln and Leu R (a) and inappropriately low muscle protein synthesis rate in AIDS wasting. *Am. J. Physiol.* **275,** E577–E583.

11. Wheeler, D., Gibert, C., Launer, C., Muurahainen, N. Elion, R., Abrams, D., and Bartsch, G. (1998). Weight loss as a predictor of survival and disease progression in HIV infection. *J. AIDS* **18,** 80–85.

12. Wanke, C., Silva, M., Knox, T., Forrester, J., Speigelman, D., and Gorbach, S. (2000). Weight loss and wasting remain common complications in individuals infected with HIV in the era of highly active antiretroviral therapy. *Clin. Infect. Dis.* **31,** 803–805.

13. Carr, A., Samaras, K., Burton, S., Law, M., Freund, J., Chisolm, D. J., and Cooper, D. A. (1998). A syndrome of peripheral lipodystrophy, hyperlipidemia, and insulin resistance due to HIV protease inhibitors. *AIDS* **12,** F51–F58.

14. Miller, K. D., Jones, E., Yanovski, J. A., Shankar, R., Feuerstein, I., and Falloon, J. (1998). Visceral abdominal-fat accumulation associated with use of indinavir. *Lancet* **351,** 87–85.

15. Rosenburg, H. E., Mulder, J., Septowitz, K. A., and Giordano, M. F. (1998). "Protease-paunch" in HIV+ persons receiving protease inhibitor therapy: Incidence, risks, and endocrinologic evaluation. *In* "5th Conference on Retrovirus and Opportunistic Infections."

16. Herry, I., Bernard, L., de Truchis, P., and Perronne, C. (1997). Hypertrophy of the breasts in a patient treated with indinavir. *Clin. Infect. Dis.* **25,** 937–938.

17. Roth, V. R., Kravcik, S., and Angel, J. B. (1998). Development of cervical pads following therapy with human immunodeficiency virus type 1 protease inhibitors. *Clin. Infect. Dis.* **27,** 68–72.

18. Lo, J. C., Mulligan, K., Tai, V. W., Algren, H., and Schambelan, M. (1998). "Buffalo hump" in HIV infected patients on antiretroviral therapy. *Lancet* **351,** 867–870.

19. Vigouroux, C., Gharakhanian, S., Salhi, Y., Nguyen, T. H., Chevenne, D., Capeau, J., and Rozenbaum, W. (1999). Diabetes, insulin resistance and dyslipidemia in lipodystrophic HIV-infected patients on highly active antiretroviral therapy (HAART). *Diabet. Metab.* **25**(3), 225–232.

20. Macallan, D. C., Noble, C., Baldwin, C., Foskett, M., McManus, T., and Griffin, G. (1995). Energy expenditure and wasting in human immunodeficiency virus infection. *N. Eng. J. Med.* **333,** 83–88.

21. Grunfeld, C., Pang, M., Shimizu, L., Shigenaga, J., Jensen, P., and Feingold, K. (1992). Resting energy expenditure, caloric intake and short-term weight change in human immunodeficiency infection and the acquired immunodeficiency syndrome. *Am. J. Clin. Nutr.* **588,** 317–318.

22. Kotler, D. P., Francisco, A., Clayton, F., Scoles, J. V., and Orenstein, J. M. (1990). Small intestinal injury and parasitic diseases in AIDS. *Ann. Intern. Med.* **113,** 444–449.

23. Watson, A., Samore, M. H., and Wanke, C. A. (1996). Diarrhea and quality of life in ambulatory HIV-infected patients. *Dig. Dis. Sci.* **41,** 1794–1800.

24. Mayer, H. B., and Wanke, C. A. (1995). Enteroaggregative *Esherichia coli* as a possible cause of diarrhea in an HIV infected patient. *N. Eng. J. Med.* **332,** 273–274.

25. Gillin, J. S., Shike, M., Alcock, N., Urmacher, C., Krown, S., Kurtz, R., Lightdale, E., and Winawer, S. J. (1985). Malabsorption and mucosal abnormalities of the small intestine in the acquired immunodeficiency syndrome. *Ann. Intern. Med.* **102,** 619–622.

26. Lambl, B. B., Federman, M., Pleskow, D., and Wanke, C. (1996). Malabsorption and wasting in AIDS patients with microsporidia and pathogen-negative diarrhea. *AIDS* **10,** 1–5.

27. Kotler, D. P., Tierney, A. R., Brenner, S. K., Couture, S., Wang, J., and Pierson, R. N. (1990). Preservation of short-term energy balance in clinically stable patients with AIDS. *Am. J. Clin. Nutr.* **51,** 7–13.

28. Grunfeld, C., and Feingold, K. R. (1992). Metabolic disturbances and wasting in the acquired immunodeficiency syndrome. *N. Eng. J. Med,* **327,** 329–337.

29. Grunfeld, C., Kotler, D. P., Hamadeh, R., Tierney, A., Wang, J., and Pierson, R. N. (1989). Hypertriglyceridemia in the acquired immunodeficiency syndrome. *Am. J. Med.* **86,** 27–31.

30. Hommes, M. T., Romijn, J. A., Endert, E., Eeftinck Schattenkerk, J. K., and Sauerwein, H. P. (1991). Insulin sensitivity and insulin clearance in human immunodeficiency virus-infected men. *Metabolism* **40,** 651–656.

31. Suttmann, U., Selberg, O., Gallati, H., Ockenga, J., Deicher, M., and Muller, M. (1994). Tumor necrosis factor receptor levels are linked to the acute phase response and malnutrition in human immunodeficiency virus-infected patients. *Clin. Sci.* **86,** 461–467.

32. Coodley, G. O., Loveless, M. O., Nelson, H. D., and Coodley, M. K. (1994). Endocrine function in the HIV wasting syndrome. *J. AIDS* **7,** 46–51.

33. Masharani, U., and Schambelan, M. (1993). The endocrine complications of acquired immunodeficiency syndrome. *Adv. Intern. Med.* **38,** 323–336.

34. Los Angeles County Commission on HIV Health Services. (1999). "Guidelines for Implementing HIV/AIDS Medical Nutrition Therapy Protocols" Los Angeles, CA.

35. American Dietetic Association (2000). Position of the American Dietetic Association and Dietitians of Canada: Nutrition intervention in the care of persons with human immunodeficiency virus infection. *J. Am. Diet. Assoc.* **100,** 708–717.

36. Metropolitan Life Insurance Co. (1959; revision 1983). "Statistical Bulletin: Build and Blood Pressure Study."

37. Heimburger, D., and Weinsier, R. (1997). Obesity. *In* "Handbook of Clinical Nutrition," 3rd ed. Mosby-Year Book, St. Louis, MO.

38. Lukaski, H. C. (1987). Methods for the assessment of human body composition: Traditional and new. *Nutrition* **46,** 537–556.

39. Moore, F. D., and Boyden, C. M. (1963). Body cell mass and limits of hydration: Their relation to estimated skeletal weight. *Ann. N.Y. Acad. Sci.* **110,** 62–71.

40. Durnin, J. V. G. A., and Wormersley, J. (1974). Body fat assessed from total body density and its estimation from skinfold thickness: Measurement of 481 men and women aged 16–72 years. *Bri. J. Nutr.* **32,** 77–96.

41. Molarius, A., and Seidell, J. C. (1998). Selection of anthropometric indicators for classification of abdominal fatness—A critical review. *Int. J. Obes. Relat. Metab. Disord.* **22,** 719–727.

42. Engleson, E. S., Kotler, D. P., Agin, D., Wang, J., Pierson, R. N., and Heymsfield, S. (1999). Fat distribution in HIV-infected patients reporting truncal enlargement quantified by whole-body magnetic resonance imaging. *Am. J. Clin. Nutr.* **69,** 1162–1169.

43. Kosminski, L., Kuritzkes, D., Lichtenstein, K., Greenberg, K., Ehrlich, J., and Eckel, R. H. (1999). An increase in abdominal girth on protease inhibitor therapy is associated with visceral obesity and metabolic disturbances that closely resemble syndrome X. *Antivir. Ther.* **4,** 54.

44. American Dietetic Association (1991). "Handbook of Clinical Dietetics," Vol. 1, pp. 24–26. Yale University Press, New Haven, CT.

45. Gray, R. H. (1983). Similarities between AIDS and PCM. *Am. J. Public Health* **73,** 1332.

46. National Academy of Sciences (1989). "Recommended Dietary Allowances," 10th ed. National Academy Press, Washington, DC.

47. Sharkey, S. J., Sharkey, K. A., Sutherland, L. R., Church, D. L., and the GI/HIV Study Group. Nutritional status and food intake in human immunodeficiency virus infection. (1992). *J. AIDS* **5,** 1091–1098.

48. Chandra, R. K. (1992). Protein energy malnutrition and immunological responses. *J. Nutr.* **122** (Supplement); 597–600.

49. Baum, M. K., Shor-Posner, G., Lu, Y., Rosner, B., Sauberlick, H. E., Fletcher, M. A., Szapocznik, J., Eisdorfer, C., Burning, J. E., and Hennekens, C. H. (1995). Micronutrients and HIV progression. *AIDS* **9,** 1051–1056.

50. Semba, R. D., Graham, N., Caiaffa, W. T., Clement, L., Iviahov, D., and Margolick, J. B. (1993). Increased mortality associated with vitamin A deficiency during human immunodeficiency virus-type infection. *Arch. Intern. Med.* **153,** 2149–2154.

51. Shor-Posner, G., and Baum, M. K. (1996). Nutritional alterations in HIV–1 seropositive and seronegative drug users. *Nutrition* **12,** 555–556.

52. Beach, R. S., Mantero-Atienza, E., Shor-Posner, G., Javier, J. J., Szapocznik, J., Morgan, R., Sauberlick, H., Cornwell, P. E., Eisdorfer, C., and Baum, M. K. (1992). Specific nutrient abnormalities in asymptomatic HIV infection. *AIDS* **6,** 701–708.

53. Baum, M. K., Shor-Posner, G., and Lai, H. (1997). High risk of mortality in HIV infection is associated with selenium deficiency. *J. AIDS* **15,** 370–374.

54. Campa, A., Shor-Posner, G., and Zhang, G. (1997). Nutritional status of HIV-infected children: Survivors versus progressors. Conference on nutrition and immunology. Atlanta, GA, May 5–7.

55. Constans, J., Pellegrin, J. L., Sergeant, C., Simonoff, M., Fleury, H., Ling, B., and Conri, C. (1995). Serum selenium predicts outcome in HIV infection [letter]. *J. AIDS* **10,** 392.

56. Bologna, R., Indacochea, F., and Shor-Posner, G. (1994). Selenium and immunity in HIV-infected pediatric patients. *J. Nutr. Immun.* **3,** 41–49.

57. Malvy, D., Richard, M., Arnaud, J., Favier, A., and Amedee-Menesme, C. (1994). Relationship of plasma malondialdehyde, vitamin E, and antioxidant mircronutrients to human immunodeficiency virus–1 seropositivity. *Clin. Chim. Acta,* **224,** 89–94.

58. Delmas-Beauvieux, M. C., Peuchant, E., and Coucouron, A. (1996). The enzymatic antioxidant system in blood and glutathione status in human immunodeficiency virus (HIV)-infected patients: Effect of supplementation with selenium or beta carotene. *Am. J. Clin. Nutr,* **64,** 101–107.

59. Pacht, E. R., Diaz, P., Clanton, T., Hart, J., and Gadek, J. E. (1997). Serum vitamin E decreases in HIV-seropositive patients over time. *J. Lab. Clin. Med,* **130,** 293–296.

60. Tang, A. M., Graham, N., Semba, R. D., and Saah, A. J. (1997). Association between serum vitamin A and E levels and HIV-1 disease progression. *AIDS* **11,** 613–620.

61. Allard, J. P., Aghclassi, E., Chau, J., Tam, C., Kovacs, C., Salit, I., and Walmsley, S. (1998). Effects of vitamin E and C supplementation on oxidative stress and viral load in HIV-infected subjects. *AIDS* **12,** 1653–1659.

62. Beutler, E. (1989). Nutritional and metabolic aspects of glutathione. *Annu. Rev. Nutr.* **9,** 287–302.

63. Droge, W., Eck, H. P., Haher, H., Pekar, U., and Daniel, V. (1988). Abnormal amino acid concentrations in the blood of patients with acquired immunodefiency syndrome (AIDS) may contribute to the immunological defect. *Biol. Chem. Hoppe-Seyler* **369,** 143–148.

64. Droge, W., and Breitkreutz, R. (1999). N-Acetyl-cysteine in the therapy of HIV-positive patients. *Curr. Opin. Clin. Nutr. Metabol. Care* **2,** 493–498.

65. Shabert, J. K., and Wilmore, D. W. (1996). Glutamine deficiency as a cause of human immunodeficiency virus wasting. *Med. Hypoth.* **46,** 252–256.

66. Shabert, J., Winslow, C., Lacey, J. and Wilmore, D. (1999). Glutamine-antioxident supplementation increases body cell mass in AIDS patients with weight loss: A randomized double-blind controlled trial. *Nutrition* **15,** 860–864.

67. Clark, R. H., Feleke, G., Din, M., Yasmin, T., Singh, G., Khan, F., and Rathmacher, J. (2000). Nutritional treatment for acquired immunodeficiency virus-associated wasting using β-hydroxy, β-methylbutyrate, glutamine, and arginine: A randomized, double-blind, placebo-controlled study. *J. Parenteral Enteral Nutr.* **24,** 133–139.

68. Souba, W. W., Klimberg, V. S., Plumley, D. A., Salloum, R., Flynn, T., Bland, K., and Copeland, E. (1990). The role of glutamine in maintaining a healthy gut and supporting the metabolic response to injury and infection. *J. Surg. Res.* **48,** 383–391.

69. Rabeneck, L., Palmer, A., Knowles, J. B., Seidehamel, R. J., Harris, C. L., Merkel, K. L., Risser, J., and Akrabawi, S. (1998). A randomized controlled trial evaluating nutrition counseling with or without oral supplementation in malnourished HIV-infected patients. *J. Amer. Diet. Assoc.* **98,** 434–438.

70. Stack, J. A., Bell, S. J., Burke, P. A., and Forse, R. A. (1996). Use of supplements in patients with human immunodeficiency virus infection. *J. Amer. Diet. Assoc.* **96,** 337–341.

G. Overall Disease Prevention

CHAPTER **48**

Nutrition Guidelines to Maintain Health

SUZANNE P. MURPHY

University of Hawaii, Honolulu, Hawaii

I. INTRODUCTION

Nutrition guidelines for Americans fall into two broad categories: those that focus primarily on nutrient intakes and those that are primarily oriented to food choices. In addition, clinicians and researchers have come to realize that healthy food and nutrient intakes are inevitably linked to healthy activity levels, so that physical activity guidance is often included with dietary guidance.

The Food and Nutrition Board of the National Academy of Sciences has periodically released recommendations for nutrient intakes by Americans. The last complete set of recommendations was published in 1989 [1], but these Recommended Dietary Allowances are now being replaced by Dietary Reference Intakes (DRIs), most recently in 2000 [2–4]. DRI is an umbrella term for four types of nutrient recommendations:

- Estimated average requirement
- Recommended Dietary Allowance
- Adequate intake
- Tolerable upper intake level.

To date, DRIs have been set for 17 nutrients. Until the DRI process is complete, health professionals and the public will need to use a combination of the new DRIs and the 1989 RDAs when deciding what nutrient intakes are appropriate (Tables 1–3).

Three types of guidance have been developed by federal government agencies to help consumers make healthy food and nutrient choices. The Dietary Guidelines for Americans have been jointly issued by USDA and USDHHS every 5 years since 1980. The most recent were released in 2000 [5, 6]. The number of guidelines has been increased from 7 to 10 (Table 4). Two of the three new guidelines result from dividing previous guidelines: recommendations regarding fruit and vegetable intakes have been separated from those regarding grain intake; and the former guideline suggesting balancing food intake with physical activity now is divided into a guideline on healthy weight and a guideline on physical activity. An entirely new guideline on food safety reflects the increasing importance of food safety when selecting and preparing foods.

The Food Guide Pyramid is a tool that is widely used in nutrition education efforts, and has proved to be particularly useful in helping the public make healthy food choices [7]. The Food Guide Pyramid translates the guidance offered by both the RDAs and the dietary guidelines into a graphic format that illustrates the recommended number of servings from each of six food groups (Figs. 1 and 2). Nutrition facts labels [8] and supplement facts labels [9] are now required by law, and provide consumers with useful information at the point of purchase.

Physical activity guidance has been offered by several organizations, but the most widely disseminated recent recommendation is that from the Centers for Disease Control and Prevention and the American College of Sports Medicine: "Exercise moderately for 30 minutes almost every day of the week" [10]. The new dietary guideline on physical activity states "Be physically active every day." Physical activity guidance now frequently accompanies dietary guidance because health professionals recognize that maintenance of a healthy body size and sustained cardiopulmonary fitness can only be achieved through an active lifestyle coupled with healthy dietary choices.

II. GUIDELINES FOR NUTRIENT ADEQUACY AND SAFETY

A. Dietary Reference Intakes for Nutrient Adequacy

The DRIs offer guidance on the level of nutrient intake that will promote health and reduce the risk of chronic disease. The process for setting the new DRIs was developed by the Food and Nutrition Board after substantial feedback from the nutrition professionals [11]. Several new concepts were incorporated:

- An increased focus on reduction of chronic disease risk as well as the prevention of nutritional deficiencies.
- Determination of an estimated average requirement (EAR), which would be the intake that would be adequate for approximately 50% of a healthy population.
- Calculation of a Recommended Dietary Allowance (RDA) from the EAR, by adding two standard deviations of the requirement distribution. The RDA is thus the level of intake that would be adequate for 97.5% of the population.

TABLE 1 Dietary Reference Intakes: Recommended Intakes for Individuals; Food and Nutrition Board, Institute of Medicine, National Academies

Life stage group	Calcium (mg/d)	Phosphorus (mg/d)	Magnesium (mg/d)	Vitamin D (μg/d)[a,b]	Fluoride (mg/d)	Thiamin (mg/d)	Riboflavin (mg/d)	Niacin (mg/d)[c]	Vitamin B$_6$ (mg/d)	Folate (μg/d)[d]	Vitamin B$_{12}$ (μg/d)	Pantothenic Acid (mg/d)	Biotin (μg/d)	Choline[e] (mg/d)	Vitamin C (mg/d)	Vitamin E (mg/d)[f]	Selenium (μg/d)
Infants																	
0–6 mo	210*	100*	30*	5*	0.01*	0.2*	0.3*	2*	0.1*	65*	0.4*	1.7*	5*	125*	40*	4*	15*
7–12 mo	270*	275*	75*	5*	0.5*	0.3*	0.4*	4*	0.3*	80*	0.5*	1.8*	6*	150*	50*	6*	20*
Children																	
1–3 y	500*	460	80	5*	0.7*	0.5	0.5	6	0.5	150	0.9	2*	8*	200*	15	6	20
4–8 y	800*	500	130	5*	1*	0.6	0.6	8	0.6	200	1.2	3*	12*	250*	25	7	30
Males																	
9–13 y	1,300*	1,250	240	5*	2*	0.9	0.9	12	1.0	300	1.8	4*	20*	375*	45	11	40
14–18 y	1,300*	1,250	410	5*	3*	1.2	1.3	16	1.3	400	2.4	5*	25*	550*	75	15	55
19–30 y	1,000*	700	400	5*	4*	1.2	1.3	16	1.3	400	2.4	5*	30*	550*	90	15	55
31–50 y	1,000*	700	420	5*	4*	1.2	1.3	16	1.3	400	2.4	5*	30*	550*	90	15	55
51–70 y	1,200*	700	420	10*	4*	1.2	1.3	16	1.7	400	2.4[g]	5*	30*	550*	90	15	55
>70 y	1,200*	700	420	15*	4*	1.2	1.3	16	1.7	400	2.4[g]	5*	30*	550*	90	15	55
Females																	
9–13 y	1,300*	1,250	240	5*	2*	0.9	0.9	12	1.0	300	1.8	4*	20*	375*	45	11	40
14–18 y	1,300*	1,250	360	5*	3*	1.0	1.0	14	1.2	400[h]	2.4	5*	25*	400*	65	15	55
19–30 y	1,000*	700	310	5*	3*	1.1	1.1	14	1.3	400[h]	2.4	5*	30*	425*	75	15	55
31–50 y	1,000*	700	320	5*	3*	1.1	1.1	14	1.3	400[h]	2.4	5*	30*	425*	75	15	55
51–70 y	1,200*	700	320	10*	3*	1.1	1.1	14	1.5	400	2.4[g]	5*	30*	425*	75	15	55
>70 y	1,200*	700	320	15*	3*	1.1	1.1	14	1.5	400	2.4[g]	5*	30*	425*	75	15	55
Pregnancy																	
≤18 y	1,300*	1,250	400	5*	3*	1.4	1.4	18	1.9	600[i]	2.6	6*	30*	450*	80	15	60
19–30 y	1,000*	700	350	5*	3*	1.4	1.4	18	1.9	600[i]	2.6	6*	30*	450*	85	15	60
31–50 y	1,000*	700	360	5*	3*	1.4	1.4	18	1.9	600[i]	2.6	6*	30*	450*	85	15	60
Lactation																	
≤18 y	1,300*	1,250	360	5*	3*	1.4	1.6	17	2.0	500	2.8	7*	35*	550*	115	19	70
19–30 y	1,000*	700	310	5*	3*	1.4	1.6	17	2.0	500	2.8	7*	35*	550*	120	19	70
31–50 y	1,000*	700	320	5*	3*	1.4	1.6	17	2.0	500	2.8	7*	35*	550*	120	19	70

Note: This table presents Recommended Dietary Allowances (RDAs) in bold type and Adequate Intakes (AIs) in ordinary type followed by an asterisk (*). RDAs and AIs may both be used as goals for individual intake. RDAs are set to meet the needs of almost all (97 to 98 percent) individuals in a group. For healthy breastfed infants, the AI is the mean intake. The AI for other life-stage and gender groups is believed to cover needs of all individuals in the group, but lack of data or uncertainty in the data prevent being able to specify with confidence the percentage of individuals covered by this intake.

Source: Reprinted with permission from "Dietary Reference Intakes." Copyright 2000 by the National Academy of Sciences. Courtesy of the National Academy Press, Washington, DC.

[a] As cholecalciferol. 1 μg cholecalciferol = 40 IU vitamin D.

[b] In the absence of adequate exposure to sunlight.

[c] As niacin equivalents (NE). 1 mg of niacin = 60 mg of tryptophan; 0–6 months = preformed niacin (not NE).

[d] As dietary folate equivalents (DFE). 1 DFE = 1 μg food folate = 0.6 μg of folic acid from fortified food or as a supplement consumed with food = 0.5 μg of a supplement taken on an empty stomach.

[e] Although AIs have been set for choline, there are few data to assess whether a dietary supply of choline is needed at all stages of the life cycle, and it may be that the choline requirement can be met by endogenous synthesis at some of these stages.

[f] As α-tocopherol. α-Tocopherol includes *RRR*-α-tocopherol, the only form of α-tocopherol that occurs naturally in foods, and the 2*R*-stereoisomeric forms of α-tocopherol (*RRR*-, *RSR*-, *RRS*-, and *RSS*-α-tocopherol) that occur in fortified foods and supplements. It does not include the 2*S*-stereoisomeric forms of α-tocopherol (*SRR*-, *SSR*-, *SRS*-, and *SSS*-α-tocopherol), also found in fortified foods and supplements.

[g] Because 10 to 30 percent of older people may malabsorb food-bound B$_{12}$, it is advisable for those older than 50 years to meet their RDA mainly by consuming foods fortified with B$_{12}$ or a supplement containing B$_{12}$.

[h] In view of evidence linking folate intake with neural tube defects in the fetus, it is recommended that all women capable of becoming pregnant consume 400 μg from supplements or fortified foods in addition to intake of food folate from a varied diet.

[i] It is assumed that women will continue consuming 400 μg from supplements or fortified food until their pregnancy is confirmed and they enter prenatal care, which ordinarily occurs after the end of the periconceptual period—the critical time for formation of the neural tube.

TABLE 2 Recommended Dietary Allowances[a], Revised 1989 (Abridged), Designed for the Maintenance of Good Nutrition of Practically All Healthy People in the United States, Food and Nutrition Board, National Academy of Sciences, National Research Council

Category	Age (years) or condition	Weight[b] (kg)	Weight[b] (lb)	Height[b] (cm)	Height[b] (in)	Protein (g)	Vitamin A (µg RE)[c]	Vitamin K (µg)	Iron (mg)	Zinc (mg)	Iodine (µg)
Infants	0.0–0.5	6	13	60	24	13	375	5	6	5	40
	0.5–1.0	9	20	71	28	14	375	10	10	5	50
Children	1–3	13	29	90	35	16	400	15	10	10	70
	4–6	20	44	112	44	24	500	20	10	10	90
	7–10	28	62	132	52	28	700	30	10	10	120
Males	11–14	45	99	157	62	45	1,000	45	12	15	150
	15–18	66	145	176	69	59	1,000	65	12	15	150
	19–24	72	160	177	70	58	1,000	70	10	15	150
	25–50	79	174	176	70	63	1,000	80	10	15	150
	51+	77	170	173	68	63	1,000	80	10	15	150
Females	11–14	46	101	157	62	46	800	45	15	12	150
	15–18	55	120	163	64	44	800	55	15	12	150
	19–24	58	128	164	65	46	800	60	15	12	150
	25–50	63	138	163	64	50	800	65	15	12	150
	51+	65	143	160	63	50	800	65	10	12	150
Pregnant						60	800	65	30	15	175
Lactating	1st 6 months					65	1,300	65	15	19	200
	2nd 6 months					62	1,200	65	15	16	200

Source: Reprinted with permission from "Recommended Dietary Allowances," 10th ed. Copyright 1989 by the National Academy of Sciences. Courtesy of the National Academy Press, Washington, DC.

Note: This table does not include nutrients for which Dietary Reference Intakes have recently been established (see "Dietary Reference Intakes for Calcium, Phosphorus, Magnesium, Vitamin D, and Fluoride" [1997], "Dietary Reference Intakes for Thiamin, Riboflavin, Niacin, Vitamin B_6, Folate, Vitamin B_{12}, Pantothenic Acid, Biotin, and Choline" [1998], and "Dietary Reference Intakes for Vitamin E, Vitamin C, Selenium, and Carotenoids" [2000]).

[a]The allowances, expressed as average daily intakes over time, are intended to provide for individual variations among most normal persons as they live in the United States under usual environmental stresses. Diets should be based on a variety of common foods in order to provide other nutrients for which human requirements have been less well defined.

[b]Weights and heights of Reference Adults are actual medians for the U.S. population of the designated age, as reported by NHANES II. The median weights and heights of those under 19 years of age were taken from Hamill et al. (1979). The use of these figures does not imply that the height-to-weight ratios are ideal.

[c]Retinol equivalents. 1 retinol equivalent = 1 µg retinol or 6 µg β-carotene.

- Use of an adequate intake (AI) when the scientific database is not sufficient to set an EAR (and its associated RDA).
- Determination of a tolerable upper intake level (UL), which represents the upper level of intake that poses a low risk of adverse effects. Usual intakes above this level are not recommended.

To date, DRIs have been set for the bone-related nutrients (calcium, phosphorus, magnesium, vitamin D, and fluoride) [2], for the B vitamins (thiamin, riboflavin, niacin, vitamin B_6, vitamin B_{12}, folate, and choline) [3], and for the antioxidant nutrients (vitamin C, vitamin E, and selenium) [4]. Reports are expected by the time of publication on micronutrients (vitamins A and K, iron, zinc, copper, molybdenum, boron,

etc.) and on macronutrients (energy, protein, fat, carbohydrates, and dietary fiber). As mentioned earlier, until DRIs have been set for all nutrients, health professionals will need to use a combination of the new DRIs and the former RDAs, as shown in Tables 1 through 3.

Because there are many new uses of the DRIs, a Subcommittee on Uses and Interpretation of the DRIs was convened, and will publish two reports: one on assessing intakes [12] and the other on planning intakes (expected in mid-2001).

When offering guidance to consumers on healthy nutrient intakes, health professionals should suggest the RDA (or the AI if an RDA is not available) as the appropriate target. Because an individual's actual requirement is almost never known, the goal is to reduce to a very low level the risk that an intake is inadequate. By definition, usual intake at the

TABLE 3 Dietary Reference Intakes: Tolerable Upper Intake Levels (UL[a]); Food and Nutrition Board, Institute of Medicine, National Academies

Life stage group	Calcium (g/day)	Phosphorus (g/day)	Magnesium (mg/day)[b]	Vitamin D (μg/day)	Fluoride (mg/day)	Niacin (mg/day)[c]	Vitamin B6 (mg/day)	Folate (μg/day)[c]	Choline (g/day)	Vitamin C (mg/day)	Vitamin E (mg/day)[d]	Selenium (μg/day)
Infants												
0–6 months	ND[e]	ND	ND	25	0.7	ND	ND	ND	ND	ND	ND	45
7–12 months	ND	ND	ND	25	0.9	ND	ND	ND	ND	ND	ND	60
Children												
1–3 years	2.5	3	65	50	1.3	10	30	300	1.0	400	200	90
4–8 years	2.5	3	110	50	2.2	15	40	400	1.0	650	300	150
Males, females												
9–13 years	2.5	4	350	50	10	20	60	600	2.0	1,200	600	280
14–18 years	2.5	4	350	50	10	30	80	800	3.0	1,800	800	400
19–70 years	2.5	4	350	50	10	35	100	1,000	3.5	2,000	1,000	400
>70 years	2.5	3	350	50	10	35	100	1,000	3.5	2,000	1,000	400
Pregnancy												
≤18 years	2.5	3.5	350	50	10	30	80	800	3.0	1,800	800	400
19–50 years	2.5	3.5	350	50	10	35	100	1,000	3.5	2,000	1,000	400
Lactation												
≤18 years	2.5	4	350	50	10	30	80	800	3.0	1,800	800	400
19–50 years	2.5	4	350	50	10	35	100	1,000	3.5	2,000	1,000	400

Source: Reprinted with permission from "Dietary Reference Intakes." Copyright 2000 by the National Academy of Sciences. Courtesy of the National Academy Press, Washington, DC.

[a]UL = The maximum level of daily nutrient intake that is likely to pose no risk of adverse effects. Unless otherwise specified, the UL represents total intake from food, water, and supplements. Due to lack of suitable data, ULs could not be established for thiamin, riboflavin, vitamin B$_{12}$, pantothenic acid, or biotin. In the absence of ULs, extra caution may be warranted in consuming levels above recommended intakes.

[b]The ULs for magnesium represent intake from a pharmacological agent only and do not include intake from food and water.

[c]The ULs for niacin and folate apply to synthetic forms obtained from supplements, fortified foods, or a combination of the two.

[d]As α-tocopherol; applies to any form of supplemental α-tocopherol.

[e]ND = Not determinable due to lack of data of adverse effects in this age group and concern with regard to lack of ability to handle excess amounts. Source of intake should be from food only to prevent high levels of intake.

level of the RDA or AI has a low risk of inadequacy (2–3% for the RDA). For example, the appropriate target for magnesium intake for a woman 31–50 years of age is the RDA of 320 mg/day (Table 1). Her target for calcium intake should be the AI of 1000 mg/day.

To reflect newer information on bioavailability, the RDAs for two nutrients are in different forms than were used in the past: folate is in micrograms of dietary folate equivalents rather than total micrograms, while vitamin E is in milligrams of α-tocopherol, rather than in milligrams of α-tocopherol equivalents. For folate, the new dietary folate equivalent unit reflects an increased availability of fortification and supplemental forms of folate, and thus will tend to increase estimated intakes of this nutrient.

The situation is reversed for vitamin E. Forms of tocopherol other than α-tocopherol (such as λ-tocopherol and β-tocopherol) are not considered active forms of the vitamin due to poor transport from the liver. Furthermore, the activity of the all rac-α-tocopherol form that is commonly used for fortification and in dietary supplements has a lower activity because only the 2R stereoisomers of α-tocopherol (which constitute 50% of all rac-α-tocopherol) are maintained in human plasma and thus serve as vitamin E in tissues. However, the current unit for measuring vitamin E intake is α-tocopherol equivalents, which includes all forms of tocopherol (although the activity is less for forms other than α) and all the stereoisomers of α-tocopherol. Therefore, intakes measured in α-tocopherol equivalents will overestimate intakes of the 2R stereoisomers of α-tocopherol.

B. The Tolerable Upper Intake Level: A New DRI to Reduce the Risk of Adverse Effects

For the first time, the nutrient intake recommendations from the Food and Nutrition Board also include a level of intake that should not be exceeded. The tolerable upper intake level may be used by health professionals and consumers to ensure that nutrient intakes are not too high. Table 3 shows the ULs that have been set for the first three sets of nutrients. For example, the UL for calcium is 2500 mg/day for children and adults. It is unlikely that this level of intake could be achieved from unfortified foods alone. However, through the use of heavily fortified foods, calcium supplements and/or antacids, intake exceeding 2500 mg/day is possible. Intakes above the UL for calcium carry an increased risk of milk-alkalai syndrome, a potentially serious metabolic disorder.

The UL for magnesium for adults is 350 mg/day from pharmacologic forms. Because magnesium salts can cause osmotic diarrhea, intakes above 350 mg/day are not recommended. Food sources of magnesium do not cause diarrhea, and thus are not included in this UL. Indeed, the UL for magnesium is below the RDA for magnesium for adult men (420 mg/day), reflecting the different forms of the nutrient in each of these DRIs. Several other nutrient DRIs also use different forms for the RDA and the UL: niacin and folate

TABLE 4 Dietary Guidelines for Americans

Aim for Fitness	Aim for a healthy weight.
	Be physically active each day.
Build a Healthy Base	Let the Pyramid guide your food choices.
	Choose a variety of grains daily, especially whole grains.
	Choose a variety of fruits and vegetables daily.
	Keep food safe to eat.
Choose Sensibly	Choose a diet that is low in saturated fat and cholesterol and moderate in total fat.
	Choose beverages and foods to moderate your intake of sugars.
	Choose and prepare foods with less salt.
	If you drink alcoholic beverages, do so in moderation.

Source: U.S. Department of Agriculture and U.S. Department of Health and Human Services (2000). "Dietary Guidelines for Americans," 5th ed., Home and Garden Bulletin No. 232. U.S. Government Printing Office, Washington, DC.

(for which the UL is from fortification or supplemental forms only), and vitamin E (where the UL is for all forms of α-tocopherol, whereas the RDA is only for the 2R stereoisomers of α-tocopherol).

ULs are not available for all nutrients, not because intake at any level in considered safe, but because scientific data were not sufficient to set an upper level. ULs should never be considered a target intake; the RDA and AI are the appropriate targets. In some instances, controlled trials, feeding studies, or theraputic prescriptions may utilize nutrient levels above the UL. In these cases, when medical supervision is provided, intakes above the UL may be appropriate.

C. How Do Current Nutrient Intakes Compare to the RDAs and DRIs?

Evaluating nutrient intakes of either individuals or of groups presents many challenges, as noted by a number of authors [12–17]. National nutrition surveys are conducted periodically by both the U.S. Department of Agriculture (the Continuing Survey of Food Intakes by Individuals, CSFII) and the U.S. Department of Health and Human Services (the National Health and Nutrition Examination Survey, NHANES). Table 5 gives some examples of possible ways to evaluate the intake data from these surveys, illustrated using intake data for men and women 31–50 years of age.

Because a complete evaluation of nutrient intakes at this time requires using a combination of the 2000 DRIs and the 1989 RDAs, the recommended intakes shown in Table 5 are DRI–RDAs for vitamin C, vitamin E, magnesium, vitamin B_6, and folate, DRI–AI for calcium, and 1989 RDAs for iron, zinc, and vitamin A.

Food Guide Pyramid
A Guide to Daily Food Choices

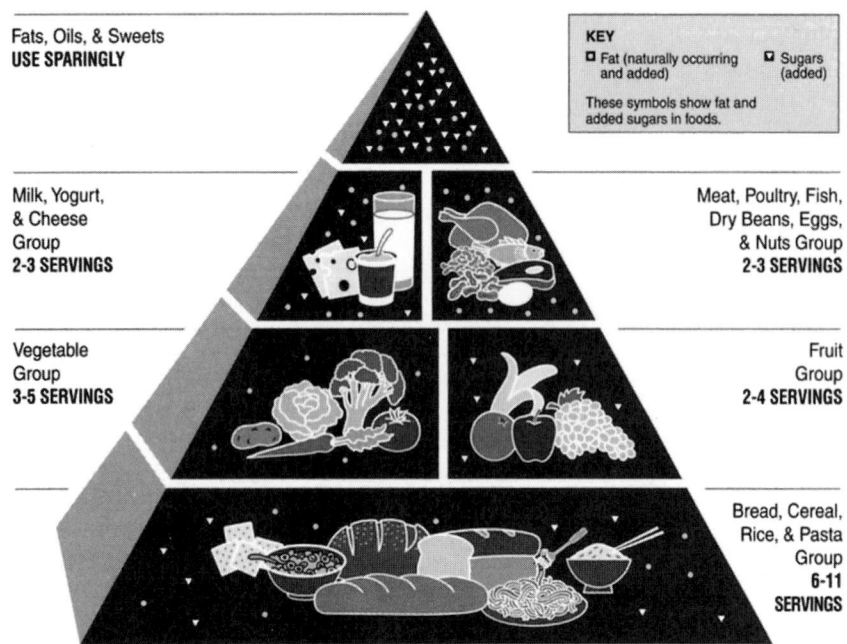

KEY
□ Fat (naturally occurring and added) ▣ Sugars (added)
These symbols show fat and added sugars in foods.

Fats, Oils, & Sweets
USE SPARINGLY

Milk, Yogurt, & Cheese Group
2-3 SERVINGS

Meat, Poultry, Fish, Dry Beans, Eggs, & Nuts Group
2-3 SERVINGS

Vegetable Group
3-5 SERVINGS

Fruit Group
2-4 SERVINGS

Bread, Cereal, Rice, & Pasta Group
6-11 SERVINGS

Source: U.S. Department of Agriculture/U.S. Department of Health and Human Services

FIGURE 1 The Food Guide Pyramid, a guide to daily food choices. [From U.S. Department of Agriculture and U.S. Department of Health and Human Services (2000). "Dietary Guidelines for Americans," 5th ed., Home and Garden Bulletin No. 232. U.S. Government Printing Office, Washington, DC.]

HOW MANY SERVINGS DO YOU NEED EACH DAY?

Food group	Children ages 2 to 6 years, women, some older adults (about 1,600 calories)	Older children, teen girls, active women, most men (about 2,200 calories)	Teen boys, active men (about 2,800 calories)
Bread, Cereal, Rice, and Pasta Group (Grains Group)–especially whole grain	6	9	11
Vegetable Group	3	4	5
Fruit Group	2	3	4
Milk, Yogurt, and Cheese Group (Milk Group)–preferably fat free or low fat	2 or 3*	2 or 3*	2 or 3*
Meat, Poultry, Fish, Dry Beans, Eggs, and Nuts Group (Meat and Bean Group)–preferably lean or low fat	2, for a total of 5 ounces	2, for a total of 6 ounces	3, for a total of 7 ounces

Adapted from U.S. Department of Agriculture, Center for Nutrition Policy and Promotion. The Food Guide Pyramid, Home and Garden Bulletin Number 252, 1996.

*The number of servings depends on your age. Older children and teenagers (ages 9 to 18 years) and adults over the age of 50 need 3 servings daily. Others need 2 servings daily. During pregnancy and lactation, the recommended number of milk group servings is the same as for nonpregnant women.

FIGURE 2 How many servings do you need each day? [From U.S. Department of Agriculture and U.S. Department of Health and Human Services (2000). "Dietary Guidelines for Americans," 5th ed., Home and Garden Bulletin No. 232. U.S. Government Printing Office, Washington, DC.]

TABLE 5 How Well Are American Adults Meeting the RDAs?
Selected Nutrients for Men and Women 31 to 50 Years Old

Nutrient	Gender	Recommended intake[a]	Reported mean intake	EAR[a]	Percent below the EAR[b]
Vitamin C (mg/day)	Men	90	187[c]	75	~25%
	Women	75	165[c]	50	~5%
Vitamin E (mg α-tocopherol/day)	Men	15	17[c,d]	12	>50% (αte)
	Women	15	30[c,d]	12	>50% (αte)
Calcium (mg/day)	Men	1000	913[e]	None	N/A
	Women	1000	637[e]	None	N/A
Magnesium (mg/day)	Men	420	341[e]	350	~50%
	Women	320	236[e]	265	~70%
Vitamin B$_6$ (mg/day)	Men	1.3	6.9[c]	1.1	~5%
	Women	1.3	4.9[c]	1.1	~10%
Folate (μg DFE/day)	Men	400	708[c,f]	320	~8%
	Women	400	718[c,f]	320	~15%
Iron (mg/day)	Men	10	18.7[g]	None	N/A
	Women	15	12.4[g]	None	N/A
Zinc (mg/day)	Men	15	14.9[g]	None	N/A
	Women	12	9.5[g]	None	N/A
Vitamin A (RE/day)	Men	1000	1238[g]	None	N/A
	Women	800	869[g]	None	N/A

[a]From Ref. [4] for vitamin C and vitamin E; Ref. [2] for calcium and magnesium; Ref. [3] for vitamin B$_6$ and folate; and Ref. [1] for iron, zinc, and vitamin A.

[b]The percent below the EAR approximates the percent of the population with inadequate nutrient intakes. N/A indicates that the percent below the EAR cannot be determined because an EAR is not available; no EAR was set for nutrients in 1989, and an AI, rather than an EAR and RDA, was set for calcium. All intake data are adjusted for day-to-day variation in intakes before examining the proportion below the EAR.

[c]Intake of food and supplements as reported in NHANES III 1988–1994. From Ref. [4] for vitamin C and vitamin E; Ref. [3] for vitamin B$_6$; and Ref. [18] for folate. Due to the large variance in intakes, mean nutrient intakes at the RDA do not ensure that there is a low prevalence of dietary inadequacy for a population.

[d]Intake data for vitamin E are in milligrams of α-tocopherol equivalents, while the recommendations are in milligrams of α-tocopherol. Thus actual intake data in milligrams of α-tocopherol would be lower because forms other than α (such as γ and β) are not included, and the availability of fortification and supplemental all rac-α-tocopherol is reduced.

[e]Intake from food only as reported in CSFII 1994–1996. From Ref. [3]. Due to the large variance in intakes, mean nutrient intakes at the RDA do not ensure that there is a low prevalence of dietary inadequacy for a population. Mean intakes would increase if supplements were included.

[f]Folate intake data are in micrograms of dietary folate equivalents, and assumes current levels of fortification of cereal grains with folate. They reflect intake from food plus supplements for men 45–69 years of age and women 20–49 years of age in NHANES III (no data were given for men 20–49 years of age). From Ref. [18].

[g]Intake from food only as reported in NHANES III 1988–1991. Average for ages 30–39 and 40–49. From Ref. [20]. Due to the large variance in intakes, mean nutrient intakes at the RDA do not ensure that there is a low prevalence of dietary inadequacy for a population. Mean intakes would increase if supplements were included.

Food composition tables, and thus intakes estimated from the national surveys, usually are not in dietary folate equivalents. Thus, folate intakes will be underestimated. Furthermore, at the time the surveys were conducted, folate fortification of grain products was not required. Since 1998, however, folate intake will have risen as a result of folate fortification of grains. A recent analysis of the NHANES III data has been published showing folate intakes adjusted for the new dietary folate equivalents and for grain fortification [18]. To illustrate the importance of these intake adjustments,

the adjusted total folate intake (from food and supplements) shown in Table 5 can be compared to the unadjusted total intakes that have been published [3]. For example, for men 45–69 years of age, mean intake of folate after adjustment was 709 μg dietary folate equivalents/day, compared to 429 μg/day (for men aged 51–70 years) without the adjustment. For women, the differences are also large: 710 μg dietary folate equivalents/day if adjusted (women 20–49 years of age) versus 407 μg/day unadjusted (women 31–50 years of age). Although the age groups do not match exactly, it is still possible to conclude that estimated intakes would be much higher if the recommended adjustments are made. The adjustments also have a large impact on the percent of the population below the EAR (an estimate of the prevalence of inadequacy): For men in the above age groups, the prevalence is only 8% with adjusted data, but more than 50% with unadjusted data. For women, the comparable figures are 15% versus more than 50%.

For vitamin E, the intakes shown in Table 5 are probably underestimates because the intake data are in α-tocopherol equivalents. An additional consideration is the difficulty of accurately measuring vitamin E intakes, because this vitamin is most concentrated in oils, and these foods are frequently underreported in surveys [19]. Underreporting of fats could lead to underreporting of vitamin E and, in turn, to overestimates of the prevalence of inadequacy. It is difficult to know how the combination of these two effects would change the evaluation of vitamin E intake.

An important issue to consider when evaluating intakes is whether all sources of a nutrient are measured and included in total intake. In particular, many Americans take dietary supplements, and the contribution of supplements to intakes should be considered before evaluating the adequacy of an individual diet or the prevalence of inadequacy for a group of individuals. NHANES III, conducted in 1988 to 1994, collected and quantified nutrient intakes from supplements, but the 1994–1996 CSFII did not. Table 5 shows total intakes for vitamins C and E, and for vitamin B_6 and folate. However, total intake data for calcium, magnesium, iron, zinc, and vitamin A have not been published, so the values in Table 5 are for food sources only. Therefore, the mean intakes for these nutrients are lower than they would have been with supplements included, and the percent below the EAR is probably an overestimate of the true prevalence of dietary inadequacy.

When evaluating intakes from the national surveys, it is desirable to know the percent of the population below the EAR, because that percentage is an accurate estimate of the prevalence of inadequate intakes for most nutrients (this approach cannot be used if requirements are skewed, however, such as with iron requirements for menstruating women). Of the nutrients shown in Table 5, only five currently have an EAR, so the prevalence of dietary inadequacy can only be estimated for these five nutrients. The findings for vitamin E illustrate the importance of examining the distribution of in-

takes, not just the means. More than 50% of the population was below the EAR, although mean vitamin E intake was well above the RDA of 15 mg/day. The intake data are obviously skewed by supplement users, whose high intakes raise the mean, but have little effect on the percent of the population below the EAR.

Thus, nutrient intakes appear to be low for several nutrients for adults aged 31–50 years. Although comparable analyses have not been summarized here for other age and gender groups, others have reported low intakes of several nutrients for most age groups [2–4, 20, 21]

III. GUIDELINES FOR HEALTHY FOOD CHOICES

A. Dietary Guidelines for Americans

By law, the secretaries of Agriculture and of Health and Human Services are required to jointly issue dietary guidelines for Americans every five years. The recently released Dietary Guidelines for Americans [5, 6] fulfill that requirement for the year 2000. Changes in both the number and content strengthen the guidelines [22]. Because the number of guidelines increased to 10, the committee advising the federal agencies recommended an overarching theme that would help consumers remember the purpose of the guidelines. Thus, the guidelines were put into three categories with an ABC theme: **A**im for Fitness, **B**uild a Healthy Base, **C**hoose Sensibly. As shown in Table 4, the 10 guidelines fall under one of these three themes.

1. AIM FOR FITNESS

Two guidelines are included under the Aim for Fitness category: the healthy weight guideline ("Aim for a healthy weight") and the physical activity guideline ("Be physically active every day"). In the past, there was a single guideline promoting a healthy weight through appropriate dietary choices as well as sufficient physical activity. However, the remarkable increases in the rates of obesity among Americans have added urgency to the need to find better ways to help individuals avoid accumulating body fat [23, 24]. Using the newer range for healthy weight as a body mass index between 19.0 and 25.0, only 41% of all individuals 20 years of age and older were classified as having a healthy weight (39% of men and 44% of women) [25]. Furthermore, the low rates of physical activity among both youth and adults are a cause for concern not only as a contributing factor to the percent of the population that is overweight and obese, but also to a declining level of muscular and cardiopulmonary fitness that is likely to be associated with cardiovascular disease, diabetes, and osteoporosis, especially among older adults [26]. Physical activity is discussed in more detail later (Section IV.A).

2. BUILD A HEALTHY BASE

For the first time since the initiation of the dietary guidelines, there is not a guideline focusing on dietary variety ("Eat a variety of foods" was included with the guidelines from 1980 through 1995). Instead, the 2000 guideline reads "Let the Pyramid guide your food choices." Several advantages are seen for this new wording. First, the primary purposes of the guideline are to communicate the importance of consuming a nutritionally adequate diet and to provide specific information on how to achieve this goal. Although eating a variety of foods indeed helps to promote better nutrient intakes within a population [27], there is no guarantee that variety alone will allow individuals to ensure that their diets meet the nutrient recommendations (such as the RDAs and AIs discussed in the previous section). The Food Guide Pyramid was specifically developed to provide guidance on the type of dietary pattern that can promote nutritional adequacy (see Fig. 1). It has been a very successful nutrition education tool and is widely incorporated into educational messages and programs. The Food Guide Pyramid was the central focus of the previous variety guideline, so it follows that incorporating a reference to the pyramid directly into the guideline text more clearly communicates the essence of a guideline to achieve nutritional adequacy. Secondly, there was some concern that a broad guideline to increase variety might inadvertently promote overconsumption of energy. There is some evidence that a variety of carbohydrate foods, for example, is associated with a higher body fatness [28]. Finally, it was clear that consumers did not always realize that a variety of *healthy* foods was being suggested—not a variety of snack foods and desserts. More information on the Food Guide Pyramid is given in the next section.

The concept of variety is still a valid one, however, as long as consumers understand that a variety of nutrient-dense foods are being promoted. Thus, both the grain guideline ("Eat a variety of grains daily, especially whole grains") and the fruit and vegetable guideline ("Eat a variety of fruits and vegetables daily") specifically mention the desirability of selecting a variety of these foods. The separation of the former fruit/vegetable/grain guideline into two guidelines emphasizes the importance these foods play in a healthy diet. They are the base of the Food Guide Pyramid, and form the foundation of a diet that is nutritionally adequate. In addition, high consumption of these foods has been shown to reduce the risk of a variety of chronic diseases, including cardiovascular disease and cancer [29–31]. Indeed, the association between fruit, vegetable, and whole-grain intakes and reduced risk of disease is often stronger than the association between intakes of their nutrient components (such as fiber, vitamins and minerals, or carotenoids) and risk. The reasons why this occurs are not well understood, but might include unmeasured food components, interactions among the components within a food, and inaccurate composition data for the components. Furthermore, fruits, vegetables, and whole grains tend to be low in both fat and energy, and thus can be consumed in greater volume than more energy-dense foods without exceeding energy needs. There is evidence that a diet that is based on foods with a low energy density can both promote weight loss and prevent weight gain [32, 33].

A food safety guideline ("Keep food safe to eat") was included for the first time in response to increasing concerns about foodborne illness. The U.S. Government Accounting Office has estimated a range of 6.5 to 33 million cases of foodborne illness a year [34]. More recently, the Centers for Disease Control and Prevention estimated that foodborne diseases cause approximately 76 million illnesses, 325,000 hospitalizations, and 5000 deaths in the United States each year [35]. The estimates are difficult to derive because the majority of cases are not reported to health care providers. Even the lower end of the range raises substantial concern about the burden of illness (and the cost of lost productivity) attributable to these illnesses. Although consumers cannot control all sources of food contamination, there is reason to believe that high-risk behaviors by consumers contribute to a substantial portion of foodborne illness [36]. Therefore, an important objective of this guideline is to improve food handling practices. The advice to consumers follows the same four topics that are promoted by the FightBAC! campaign by the Partnership for Food Safety Education [37]:

- Clean (wash hand and surfaces often)
- Separate (separate raw, cooked, and ready-to-eat foods while shopping, preparing, or storing)
- Cook (cook foods to a safe temperature)
- Chill (refrigerate perishable foods promptly).

3. CHOOSE SENSIBLY

The first two of the "Choose Sensibly" guidelines focus on fat and sugar intakes. The fat guideline ("Choose a diet that is low in saturated fat and cholesterol and moderate in total fat") represents recent research on the role of fat intake on overall health. First, the evidence is strong that intakes of both saturated fat and cholesterol are positively associated with cardiovascular disease [38, 39] (see Chapter 18). Thus, the guideline continues to promote a maximum of 10% of energy from saturated fat, and a maximum of 300 mg/day of dietary cholesterol. Table 6 shows that more than 70% of Americans are meeting the cholesterol goal, but only 36% meet the saturated fat goal. The guideline also continues to recommend that less than 30% of energy intake come from fat, as has been suggested by a variety of public and private health organizations. However, the guideline committee recognized that very low fat diets (those well below 30% of energy from fat) may not be ideal for all individuals and, indeed, that diets that are high in carbohydrates may actually contribute to cardiovascular disease for some people [40, 41]. Therefore, the guideline was worded to suggest a "moderate" consumption of total fat, to avoid the implication that all individuals should aim for fat intakes below 30% of

TABLE 6 How Well Are Americans Following the Food Guide
Pyramid and the Dietary Guidelines for Fat Intake?

	Recommended intake[a]	Average intake[b]	Percent meeting recommendation[c]
Grain group	6–11 servings/day	6.8 servings/day	38
Vegetable group	3–5 servings/day	3.4 servings/day	42
Fruit group	2–4 servings/day	1.5 servings/day	22
Dairy group	2–3 servings/day	1.5 servings/day	23[d]
Meat group	5–7 ounces	4.5 ounces	30
Discretionary fat	Use sparingly	24.9% of energy	Not quantified
Added sugars	Use sparingly	16.1% of energy	Not quantified
Total fat	<30% of energy	32.7% of energy	34
Saturated fat	<10% of energy	11.2% of energy	36
Cholesterol	<300 mg/day	247 mg/day	72

[a]From Refs. [5] and [7].

[b]All individuals aged 2 years and older. From Refs. [21] and [50]. Reflects 2-day averages based on data reported in the 1996 CSFII, except for fat, saturated fat, and cholesterol, where only the first day of data is used in calculating the averages. Excludes breast-fed children.

[c]Based on servings recommended for a specific caloric intake (for example, 6 servings/day of grains if 2200 kcal/day or less; 9 servings/day if 2200 to 2800 kcal/day; and 11 servings/day if greater than 2800 kcal/day) [7]. Two-day averages are used when determining the percent below the recommendations.

[d]Uses 3 servings/day as the recommendation for women who were pregnant or lactating, and for individuals aged 11–24 years (USDA FGP booklet). This percentage would be likely to decrease if the newer guideline was used: 3 servings/day for all individuals over age 50 and for those aged 9–18 years, based on the increased calcium recommendations for these age categories; 2 servings/day for younger children, and for persons aged 19–50 years; no increased dairy intake is necessary during pregnancy and lactation [5].

energy. As explained in an earlier chapter of this book (Chapter 18), advice regarding the distribution of macronutrients in a diet should be tailored, whenever possible, to an individual's specific risk factors (such as low-density lipoprotein and high-density lipoprotein cholesterol levels).

The sugar guideline ("Choose beverages and foods to moderate your intake of sugars") reflects concerns that Americans are overconsuming energy in the form of sugar. Although sugars are chemically identical whether they are added to foods or occur naturally, the intent of the guideline was to suggest a reduction in intake of foods that are high in sugar and low in vitamins and minerals, particularly for individuals with low energy intakes or those wishing to reduce their energy intakes. For example, many fruits, vegetables, and dairy products are high in sugars such as fructose and lactose, but these foods are also important sources of many vitamins and minerals. In contrast, foods such as nondiet carbonated beverages or fruit-flavored punches usually supply very few nutrients other than energy. Thus, the guideline urges Americans to avoid foods that are high in added sugars (and the text lists examples of these foods: soft drinks, cakes, cookies, pies, fruitades and fruit punch, ice cream, and candy). Furthermore, dairy product consumption among

children and adolescents is decreasing at the same time that soft drink consumption is increasing [42]. Thus, there is concern that high intakes of carbonated beverages may be replacing milk intake among adolescents, for whom bone mineral accretion is especially important if osteoporosis later in life is to be avoided [43]. High intakes of sugars are also associated with an increased incidence of dental caries, providing yet another reason to moderate intake of sugar [44].

The remaining two guidelines in this section on choosing sensibly address salt intake ("Choose and prepare foods with less salt") and alcohol intake ("If you drink alcoholic beverages, do so in moderation). Although the wording has changed somewhat since the 1995 guidelines, the intent of these two guidelines remains essentially unchanged. The salt guideline refers to the 2400-mg daily value for sodium that is listed on the nutrition facts label on food products, but does not specifically state this should be the upper limit of intake (see Section III.D for more details on daily values). Moderate intake of alcohol is defined as no more than one drink per day for women and two drinks per day for men, where 12 ounces of beer, 5 ounces of wine, or 1.5 ounces of distilled spirits count as a serving. The alcohol guideline also lists individuals who should not drink:

- Children and adolescents
- Individuals of any age who cannot restrict their drinking to moderate levels
- Women who are pregnant or may become pregnant
- Individuals who plan to drive, operate machinery, or take part in other activities that require attention, skill, or coordination
- Individuals taking prescription or over-the-counter medications that can interact with alcohol.

B. The Food Guide Pyramid

The Food Guide Pyramid was released by the USDA in 1992 [7], and has been widely distributed to both health professionals and consumers. Its appeal is twofold: It is a simple and actionable graphic, and it is based on detailed analyses that demonstrate its scientific accuracy. Both the form and the content of the Food Guide Pyramid underwent extensive testing. Numerous focus groups were conducted to ensure that consumers understood the messages being conveyed, and that the pyramid was a meaningful graphic for offering dietary guidance [45]. In addition, extensive analyses were conducted to determine what guidance would ensure adequacy (provision of recommended levels of nutrients) and moderation (low-fat, low-energy choices from each of the groups) [45]. Finally, typical dietary patterns in the United States were considered, which led to the selection of the food groups, and the number of servings of each, that would provide the recommended levels of nutrients at three daily energy levels (1600, 2200, and 2800 kcal/day) as shown in Fig. 2. Because the food groups are broadly defined, they can be adapted to meet specific cultural and personal preferences. Thus, the Food Guide Pyramid combines the dietary guidelines and the RDAs/DRIs into a single tool that is both scientifically based and consumer friendly.

Serving sizes for the foods in each Food Guide Pyramid food group, except the tip, are specified [7] as shown in Fig. 3. Serving sizes are smaller than many typical portions. For example, a slice of bread or one-half cup of pasta is a serving of the grains group, although typical portions are substantially larger than these. (Adults typically consume about two slices of bread per eating occasion, and about one cup of pasta [46].)

Many variations of the Food Guide Pyramid have been proposed, but most are specific interpretations of the pyramid's more general guidance. For example, a children's pyramid was released by the USDA in 1999 that offers a graphic that includes foods frequently consumed by children [47] (see Fig. 4). It is also a departure from the original (adult) Food Guide Pyramid, in that the importance of physical activity is emphasized with pictures of children engaged in several types of physical activity shown around the pyramid graphic. Although pyramids for various cultural or ethnic groups have been proposed, there is seldom the same level of analytic research for these variations as was conducted for the original, more general, Food Guide Pyramid. Health professionals should be cautious about recommending food guides that have not undergone the rigorous testing of the Food Guide Pyramid.

The Food Guide Pyramid is based on the 1989 RDAs and on the 1990 dietary guidelines. As explained in Section II of this chapter, the 1989 RDAs are being substantially revised as part of the process of setting the new DRIs. In addition, the dietary guidelines have been modified and expanded twice (in 1995 and 2000) since the pyramid was developed. To date, the only change in either type of guidance that is likely to significantly affect the Food Guide Pyramid is the increased recommendation for calcium. As reflected in the Food Guide Pyramid that is included in the 2000 dietary guidelines [5], three (rather than two) servings of dairy products would be required for adults over the age of 50 in order to meet the new AI for calcium of 1200 mg/day. Three servings would also be recommended for children and young adults 9–18 years of age (rather than those 13–24 years of age). It is anticipated that the Food Guide Pyramid will be reevaluated when the process of setting the DRIs is complete.

C. Food Exchanges to Design Meal Plans

Food exchanges were originally developed by the American Dietetic Association and the American Diabetes Association as a consumer-friendly tool that health professionals could use in meal planning for diabetic patients [48]. Starting in 1989, the exchange lists were adapted for use in weight management as well. These exchanges have been widely used by dietitians to provide simple guidelines for their clients who wished to control macronutrient intake. Although the food exchanges were developed many years before the Food Guide Pyramid was published in 1992, the format of the exchanges is remarkably similar to the food groups used in the pyramid. These are the exchange list food groups:

- Starch/bread
- Meat: lean, medium-fat, and high-fat
- Vegetable
- Fruit
- Milk: skim, low-fat, whole
- Fat.

Each of the exchanges is assigned an approximate value for energy and for grams of carbohydrate, protein, and fat. A dietitian or diabetes educator can then plan a diet for a patient to include a specified number of exchanges from each group. Once the number of exchanges is determined, the grams of the macronutrients and the energy content of the diet can be easily estimated.

The patient then uses the booklet to decide what food selections fit within each exchange. For example, if a patient's

WHAT COUNTS AS A SERVING?

Bread, Cereal, Rice, and Pasta Group (Grains Group)–whole grain and refined

- 1 slice of bread
- About 1 cup of ready-to-eat cereal
- 1/2 cup of cooked cereal, rice, or pasta

Vegetable Group

- 1 cup of raw leafy vegetables
- 1/2 cup of other vegetables–cooked or raw
- 3/4 cup of vegetable juice

Fruit Group

- 1 medium apple, banana, orange, pear
- 1/2 cup of chopped, cooked, or canned fruit
- 3/4 cup of fruit juice

Milk, Yogurt, and Cheese Group (Milk Group)*

- 1 cup of milk** or yogurt**
- 1 1/2 ounces of natural cheese** (such as Cheddar)
- 2 ounces of processed cheese** (such as American)

Meat, Poultry, Fish, Dry Beans, Eggs, and Nuts Group (Meat and Beans Group)

- 2–3 ounces of cooked lean meat, poultry, or fish
- 1/2 cup of cooked dry beans# or 1/2 cup of tofu counts as 1 ounce of lean meat
- 2 1/2-ounce soyburger or 1 egg counts as 1 ounce of lean meat
- 2 tablespoons of peanut butter or 1/3 cup of nuts counts as 1 ounce of meat

NOTE: Many of the serving sizes given above are smaller than those on the Nutrition Facts Label. For example, 1 serving of cooked cereal, rice, or pasta is 1 cup for the label but only 1/2 cup for the Pyramid.

* This includes lactose-free and lactose-reduced milk products. One cup of soy-based beverage with added calcium is an option for those who prefer a non-dairy source of calcium.

** Choose fat-free or reduced-fat dairy products most often.

Dry beans, peas, and lentils can be counted as servings in either the meat and beans group or the vegetable group. As a vegetable, 1/2 cup of cooked, dry beans counts as 1 serving. As a meat substitute, 1 cup of cooked, dry beans counts as 1 serving (2 ounces of meat).

FIGURE 3   What counts as a serving? [From U.S. Department of Agriculture and U.S. Department of Health and Human Services (2000). "Dietary Guidelines for Americans," 5th ed., Home and Garden Bulletin No. 232. U.S. Government Printing Office, Washington, DC.]

plan includes six starch/bread exchanges, he or she may choose among a variety of cereals, grains, pasta, beans, starchy vegetables such as corn or potatoes, bread, and crackers. High-fat starchy foods like muffins or french fried potatoes count as a starch exchange *and* a fat exchange. Portion sizes for one exchange of each food are specified, such as one (1-ounce) slice of bread or one-half cup of mashed potatoes.

When using exchanges, health professionals should be aware that while the exchange food groups and the Food Guide Pyramid food groups are similar, there are some important differences that may lead to confusion if a patient is also familiar with the Food Guide Pyramid. For example, as mentioned above, potatoes count as a starch exchange, not as a vegetable. Dried beans and peas, and corn, are also considered starches. High-fat foods like nuts and seeds, avocados, and bacon count as fat exchanges only. Many vegetables are considered "free" foods, rather than vegetables, because they contain very few calories per serving (e.g., lettuce, cabbage, cucumber, celery, and zucchini). Furthermore, there are several differences in the portion sizes for foods in the exchange groups compared to these same foods in the Food Guide Pyramid servings (e.g., meat exchanges are measured in ounces, not in 2- to 3-ounce servings like the pyramid).

A primary appeal of the exchange lists continues to be the flexibility offered to the health professional in planning macronutrient-controlled diets for patients. If combined with the minimum recommended number of servings from the Food Guide Pyramid, the exchange lists provide an attractive alternative for a health professional who wishes to work with a client to design a meal plan that is nutritionally adequate as well as individually tailored for the client's specific macronutrient goals.

D. The Role of Food and Supplement Labels in Helping Consumers Follow the Dietary Guidelines

The nutrition facts on food labels provide information that can help consumers follow the dietary guidelines (see Fig. 5). The Nutrition Labeling and Education Act (NLEA) of 1990 requires a nutrition facts panel on most packaged food products [8]. Consumers can use this information to monitor their consumption of energy, fat, saturated fat, sugar, and sodium, as recommended in the body weight, fat, sugar, and sodium guidelines. Persons who wish to increase their intakes, for example of vitamins, minerals, and dietary fiber, also will find the nutrition facts useful. For example, tofu may be a good source of calcium if it is precipitated with a

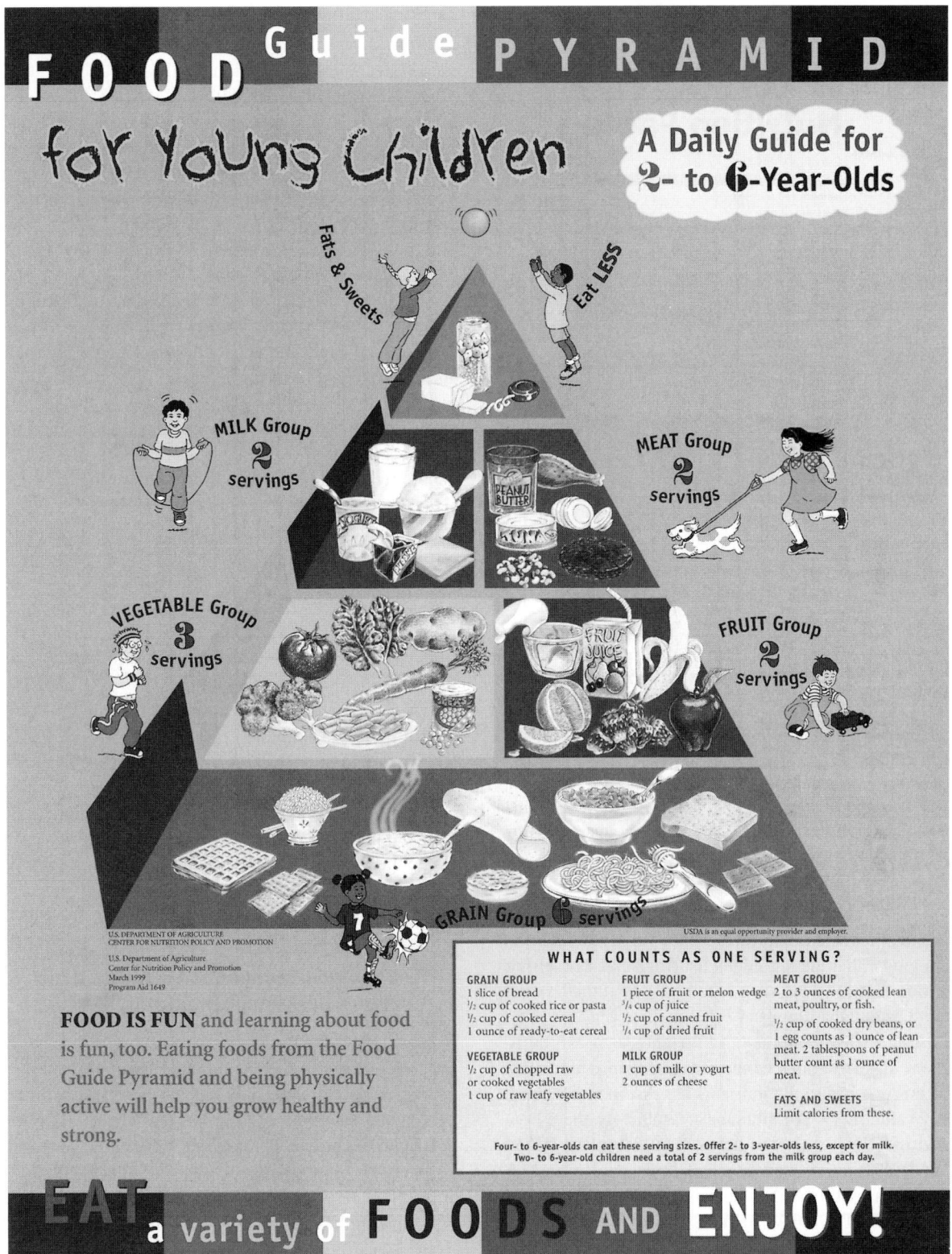

FIGURE 4   Food Guide Pyramid for young children; a daily guide for 2- to 6-year-olds. [From U.S. Department of Agriculture (1999). "Tips for Using the Food Guide Pyramid for Young Children 2 to 6 Years Old," Program Aid 1647. U.S. Department of Agriculture, Center for Nutrition Policy and Promotion, Washington, DC.]

HOW TO READ A NUTRITION FACTS LABEL

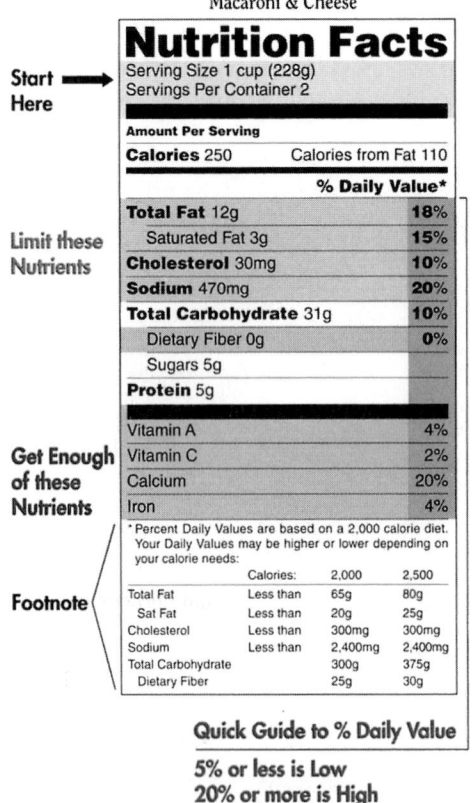

FIGURE 5 How to read a nutrition facts label. [From U.S. Department of Agriculture and U.S. Department of Health and Human Services (2000). "Dietary Guidelines for Americans," 5th ed., Home and Garden Bulletin No. 232. U.S. Government Printing Office, Washington, DC.]

calcium salt, but some tofu products have very little calcium. By examining either the ingredient list (for a calcium salt) or the nutrition facts, it is possible to tell quickly if the product provides substantial amounts of calcium.

For most nutrients, amounts in weights such as grams, milligrams, or micrograms would not be meaningful to most consumers. As a result, the nutrients are shown as a percent of a daily value (DV). For vitamins and minerals, these DVs are based on RDIs, which in turn are based on the RDAs from 1968 [49]. For macronutrients, cholesterol, fiber, sodium, and potassium, the DVs are based on Daily Reference Values (DRVs). The DRVs parallel the recommendations from the dietary guidelines regarding fat (less than 30% of energy intake) and saturated fat (less than 10% of energy intake) consumption. The DV for dietary fiber intake is 11.5 g/1000 kcal, for cholesterol is 300 mg/day, for sodium is 2400 mg/day, and for potassium is 3500 mg/day. For example, for a 2000-calorie diet, the DV for fat is 65 g/day, the DV for saturated fat is 20 g/day, and the DV for dietary fiber

is 25 g. The DVs for two calorie intake levels (2000 and 2500 kcal/day) are specified on the label for total fat, saturated fat, cholesterol, sodium, total carbohydrate, and dietary fiber. The percent of the 2000 kcal/day DV that is contained in the specific product is also given in larger type in the center of the panel. For calories, calories from fat, total fat, saturated fat, cholesterol, and sodium, the actual amount per serving is also given. For example, the macaroni and cheese nutrition facts shown in Fig. 5 indicate that one serving of this product (1 cup) contains 18% of the DV for total fat (12 g) and 15% of the DV for saturated fat (3 g). Consumers can readily scan the %DVs to see if this food item is a high or low source of specific nutrients. Nutrition information on unpackaged fruits and vegetables must be posted in the produce department of grocery stores.

Because they serve different purposes, the serving sizes used for the food label do not always correspond to those used for the Food Guide Pyramid. The servings on the food label are specified by the NLEA and are intended to reflect usual portion sizes that a consumer might typically select. In contrast, the Food Guide Pyramid servings were not necessarily usual portion sizes, but rather were portions that allowed flexibility in providing dietary guidance. In most cases, the pyramid serving size is smaller than the corresponding food label serving size. For example, as noted above, a Food Guide Pyramid serving of pasta is one-half-cup, although a typical portion is closer to 1 cup. Thus, the serving size of pasta on the food label is 1 cup to correspond to this typical portion.

Starting in March 1999, a supplement facts label was required for most dietary supplements [9]. The format of this label is similar to that for the nutrition facts label on foods, but also allows for more flexibility in reporting nonnutrient components. For example, a ginseng supplement would indicate the number of micrograms in the supplement, but no daily value is given.

E. How Do Current Food Group Intakes Compare to Recommendations?

Table 6 shows the recommended servings from the five major food groups of the Food Guide Pyramid, and the actual intakes reported by a national sample of Americans [50]. Although mean intakes of grains and vegetables exceed the minimum recommended number of servings (six and three, respectively), approximately 60% of the population is not meeting the recommendations. The minimum number of servings applies to persons who are consuming a diet of 1600 kcal (or less), so those with higher energy intakes should also have a higher number of servings from each of the pyramid food groups (up to the maximum number of servings shown in Fig. 2, for a 2800-kcal diet). Intakes of fruit, dairy, and meats or meat substitutes are even lower, with only 22–30% of Americans reporting diets that meet these recommendations.

As can also be seen in Table 6, Americans consume a substantial portion of their energy intake as discretionary fat and added sugar; together these items contribute 41% of the calories in a typical American diet. For the average sedentary woman, low-fat choices from the Food Guide Pyramid would total about 1220 kcal for a 1600-kcal diet, or about 75% of caloric intake [43]. For a sedentary man, appropriate Food Guide Pyramid choices would total about 1650 kcal for a 2200-kcal diet, which is also about 75% of caloric intake. Clearly, individuals who are consuming 41% of their energy from discretionary fat and added sugars are either substituting these items for foods that are more nutrient dense, or are adding these items to their diets at the risk of overconsumption of energy. Although the contribution of fat and sugar to obesity has been difficult to quantify (probably in large part due to underreporting of these foods by survey subjects [19]), if energy consumption exceeds energy expenditure (and, for children and adolescents, the energy requirements for growth), fat storage will occur. Until the role of these foods as a factor in obesity can be better understood, it remains appropriate to encourage a reduction in the use of foods with a low nutrient-to-calorie ratio.

About one-third of the population reported diets that met the guidelines for total fat (less than 30% of energy intake) or for saturated fat (less than 10% of energy intake). However, the cholesterol goal (less than 300 mg/day) was being met by more than 70% of the sample.

Overall, Americans are not choosing diets that follow either the dietary guidelines or the Food Guide Pyramid. The only recommendation that is being met by at least half the population is the one for cholesterol. The Healthy Eating Index provides a tool for evaluating overall conformance with the dietary guidelines [51, 52]. An individual is scored on 10 dietary parameters, most of which are shown in Table 6 (consumption of the correct number of food group servings, and meeting the guidelines for fat and cholesterol; in addition, a diet is scored for the level of sodium intake, and also for a measure of dietary variety based on the number of different food commodities that were consumed). Out of a possible score of 100, the average was 64 in 1994–1996 [52]. By this measure as well, there is room for substantial improvement in the pattern of the American diet.

IV. BEYOND FOOD AND NUTRIENT GUIDELINES: PHYSICAL ACTIVITY GUIDELINES

A. A New Dietary Guideline on Physical Activity

Increasing concerns about both the fitness level and the obesity rates among Americans have led to a dietary guideline that focuses specifically on physical activity: "Be physically active every day." The text following the guidelines gives specific advice on a minimum level of physical activity: 30 minutes of moderate physical activity most days of the week, preferably daily, for adults, and 60 minutes for children.

Chapter 32 examined the role of inactivity in the etiology of obesity. Inactivity not only predisposes an individual to weight gain, but also can reduce the efficacy of weight loss attempts [26]. Obesity in turn is a risk factor for a variety of chronic diseases. Furthermore, an inactive lifestyle is a direct risk factor for several chronic diseases, beyond the indirect role of inactivity in promoting obesity [26]. The roles of both obesity and inactivity as risk factors for chronic disease are discussed elsewhere in this book: osteoporosis (Chapter 42), colon cancer (Chapter 23), cardiovascular disease (Chapters 18 through 21), and diabetes (Chapter 27).

In addition, an active lifestyle can promote a healthy diet by increasing energy requirements. With a larger energy "budget," individuals can spare calories for optional foods containing added sugars and discretionary fats, without displacing foods from the healthy foundation of their diets. The ability to choose a larger variety of foods, without gaining weight, also increases the enjoyment of eating, and decreases the guilt associated with occasional choices of foods of low nutrient density.

The text in the dietary guidelines booklet lists the following benefits of regular physical activity:

- Increases physical fitness.
- Helps build and maintain healthy bones, muscles, and joints.
- Builds endurance and muscular strength.
- Helps manage weight.
- Lowers risk factors for cardiovascular disease, colon cancer, and type 2 diabetes.
- Helps control blood pressure.
- Promotes psychological well-being and self-esteem.
- Reduces feelings of depression and anxiety.

B. Other Recommendations

The physical activity dietary guideline is a simplified version of the guidance offered in 1995 by the Centers for Disease Control and Prevention and the American College of Sports Medicine: "Every U.S. adult should accumulate 30 minutes or more of moderate-intensity physical activity on most, preferably all, days of the week" [10, p. 402]. This message has been widely disseminated, and provides an achievable goal for most Americans. One of the appealing concepts for the public has been the ability to count short periods of exercise toward the daily goal of 30 minutes. Thus, walking up stairs, or walking an extra few blocks to work, can accumulate toward the total, as long as the activity is carried out at a moderate pace. Moderate activity is defined as an activity that requires three to six metabolic equivalents, where a metabolic equivalent is the ratio of the metabolic rate while

TABLE 7   How Well Are Americans Following the Physical Activity Guidelines? Changes in Physical Activity Rates and Year 2000 Targets

Healthy People 2000 objective	Age group	Percent at baseline (year)	Percent at most recent measure (year)	Increase or decrease	Target for 2000
Light to moderate activity, at least 5 times per week	18–74 years	22% (1985)	23% (1995)	Slight increase	30%
Light to moderate activity, at least 7 times per week	18–74 years	16% (1985)	16% (1995)	No change	30%
Vigorous activity, at least 3 times per week	10–17 years	59% (1984)	N/A[a]	N/A[a]	75%
	Grades 9–12	N/A[a]	64% (1997)	N/A[a]	75%
	18 years and older	12% (1985)	16% (1995)	Increase	20%
Sedentary lifestyle	18 years and older	24% (1985)	23% (1995)	Slight decrease	15%
Daily school physical education	Grades 1–12	36% (1984–1986)	N/A[a]	N/A[a]	50%
	Grades 9–12	42% (1991)	27% (1997)	Decrease	50%
Active physical education class time, at least 30 minutes, at least once a week	Grades 9–12	24% (1991)	21% (1997)	Decrease	50%

Source: Adapted from U.S. Department of Health and Human Services (1999). "Healthy People 2000 Review, 1998–99," Publication No. (PS) 99-1256. U.S. Department of Health and Human Services, Centers for Disease Control and Prevention, National Center for Health Statistics, Hyattsville, MD.

[a]N/A = not available.

performing the activity to the resting metabolic rate (measured in kcal/min.). Examples of moderate activity include walking briskly (3–4 mph), cycling for pleasure or transportation, and swimming [10]. Numerous activities that can contribute to the 30 minutes of daily exercise are given in the dietary guidelines book [5].

The guidance for children's physical activity is based primarily on recommendations from the Centers for Disease Control and Prevention [53] suggesting that 60 minutes of moderate activity per day is appropriate. In addition, evidence linking television watching and body weight and level of fatness suggest that television viewing should be limited for children [54].

C. How Do Current Activity Levels Compare to These Guidelines?

Data on activity levels for Americans are given in the 1998–1999 Healthy People 2000 Review [55] and are summarized in Table 7. Few American adults (only 16%) engage in even light to moderate activity daily, and only 23% engage in this level of activity at least five times per week. Furthermore, improvements between 1985 and 1995 are almost nonexistent. Clearly, it would take a substantial change in lifestyle to

expand daily light to moderate activities to most American adults. A similar number of adults (about 16%) engage in vigorous activity at least three times per week, although this number has increased (from 12%) since 1985. Furthermore, the number of adults with a sedentary lifestyle is essentially unchanged, at almost one-fourth of the population. Data from the 1994 Behavioral Risk Factor Surveillance System indicate that 33% of overweight men and 41% of overweight women 18 years of age and older reported no leisure time physical activity during the previous month [56].

For adolescents in grades 9–12, physical activity in the schools is declining (Table 7). The percent engaging in daily physical education declined from 42% to only 27% between 1991 and 1997, and those engaging in active physical education time at least 30 minutes per week declined from 24% to 21% over this same time period. No recent data have been compiled for younger children, but in 1984–1986, only 36% of children in grades 1–12 participated in daily school physical education.

However, there is some evidence of an increase in the percent of adolescents who engage in vigorous activity at least three times per week: Although the groups are not exactly comparable, 59% of children 10–17 years of age exercised vigorously at least three times per week in 1984, while

the comparable figure was 64% for those in grades 9–12 in 1997, 13 years later. Because physical activity in schools appears to be declining, these increases in vigorous activity may be attributable to after-school sports or similar non-school activities.

Thus, a public health priority is to identify ways to provide safe and enjoyable opportunities to engage in physical activity for both adults and children. Physical education in schools provides an obvious opportunity to increase the activity level of younger children. For older children, team sports may offer more appeal. Community-based activities may be the best way to reach the large majority of sedentary adults. It will take a concerted effort by health professionals if activity levels in America are to increase substantially.

V. SUMMARY

Currently a variety of consumer-friendly tools are available to promote the consumption of healthful diets and the need for daily physical activity. In general, these interact smoothly to provide incentives for the selection of nutritious foods and at least moderately strenuous activity levels.

However, despite these educational tools, consumers do not appear to be motivated to make the dietary changes recommended by these nutrient and food guidelines, or to select more frequent or more strenuous physical activities. As can be seen from the survey summaries in Tables 5, 6, and 7, many improvements could be made to American food and activity choices. The burden falls on nutrition educators and behavioral scientists to provide approaches that will inspire the public to change their food practices and activity levels in a positive direction. The rewards are many, both at the individual level (in reduced rates of chronic disease) and the societal level (in reduced medical care costs and lost productivity). A recent estimate suggests that 14% of all deaths in the United States in 1990 (300,000 deaths) were due to poor diet and activity patterns [57]. The challenge for health professionals is to provide the motivation and the environment that will facilitate more healthful diet and activity patterns by the American public. Successful and practical intervention programs are greatly needed.

References

1. National Research Council, Food and Nutrition Board (1989). "Recommended Dietary Allowances." National Academy Press, Washington, DC.
2. Institute of Medicine (1997). "Dietary Reference Intakes for Calcium, Phosphorus, Magnesium, Vitamin D, and Fluoride." National Academy Press, Washington, DC.
3. Institute of Medicine (1998). "Dietary Reference Intakes for Thiamin, Riboflavin, Niacin, Vitamin B6, Folate, Vitamin B12, Pantothenic Acid, Biotin, and Choline." National Academy Press, Washington, DC.
4. Institute of Medicine (2000). "Dietary Reference Intakes for Vitamin C, Vitamin E, Selenium, and Carotenoids." National Academy Press, Washington, DC.
5. U.S. Department of Agriculture and U.S. Department of Health and Human Services (2000). "Dietary Guidelines for Americans," 5th ed., Home and Garden Bulletin No. 232. U.S. Government Printing Office, Washington, DC.
6. U.S. Department of Agriculture (2000). "Report of the Dietary Guidelines Advisory Committee on the Dietary Guidelines for Americans, 2000." U.S. Government Printing Office, Washington, DC.
7. U.S. Department of Agriculture (1992). "The Food Guide Pyramid," Home and Garden Bulletin No. 252. U.S. Government Printing Office, Washington, DC.
8. Kurtzweil, P. (1993). Nutrition facts to help consumers eat smart. *FDA Consumer* **27**(4), 22–27.
9. Kurtzweil, P. (1998). An FDA guide to dietary supplements. *FDA Consumer* **32**(5), 28–35.
10. Pate, R. R., Pratt, M., Blair, S. N., Haskell, W. L., Macera, C. A., Bouchard, C., Buchner, D., Ettinger, W., Heath, G. W., King, A. C., Kriska, A., Leon, A.S., Marcus, B. H., Morris, J., Paffenbarger, R. S., Patrick, K., Pollack, M. L., Rippe, J. M., Sallis, J., and Wilmore, J. H. (1995). Physical activity and public health—A recommendation from the Centers for Disease Control and Prevention and the American College of Sports Medicine. *JAMA* **273**, 402–407.
11. Institute of Medicine (1994). "How Should the Recommended Dietary Allowances Be Revised?" National Academy Press, Washington, DC.
12. Institute of Medicine (2000). "Dietary Reference Intakes: Applications in Dietary Assessment." National Academy Press, Washington, DC.
13. National Research Council, Food and Nutrition Board (1986). "Nutrient Adequacy: Assessment Using Food Consumption Surveys." National Academy Press, Washington, DC.
14. Life Sciences Research Office, Federation of American Societies for Experimental Biology (1986). "Guidelines for Use of Dietary Intake Data." Life Sciences Research Office, Bethesda, MD.
15. Thompson, F. E., and Beyers, T. (1994). Dietary assessment resource manual. *J. Nutr.* **124**, 2245S–2317S.
16. Buzzard, I. M., and Willett, W. C., Eds. 1994. Dietary assessment methods. *Am. J. Clin. Nutr.* **59**, 143S–306S.
17. Willett, W. C., and Sampson, L., Eds. (1997). Dietary assessment methods. *Am. J. Clin. Nutr.* **65**, 1097S–1368S.
18. Lewis, C. J., Crane, N. T., Wilson, D. B., and Yetley, E. A. (1999). Estimated folate intakes: Data updated to reflect food fortification, increased bioavailability, and dietary supplement use. *Am. J. Clin. Nutr.* **70**, 198–207.
19. Briefel, R. R., Sempos, C. T., McDowell, M. A., Chien, S., and Alaimo, K. (1997). Dietary methods research in the Third National Health and Nutrition Examination Survey: Underreporting of energy intake. *Am. J. Clin. Nutr.* **65**, 1203S–1209S.
20. Alaimo, K., McDowell, M. A., Briefel, R. R., Bischof, A. M., Caughman, C. R., Loria, C. M., and Johnson, C. L. (1994). "Dietary Intake of Vitamins, Minerals, and Fiber of Persons Ages 2 Months and Over in the United States: Third National Health and Nutrition Examination Survey, Phase 1, 1988–91," Advance Data No. 258. National Center for Health Statistics, Hyattsville, MD.

21. U.S. Department of Agriculture, Food Surveys Research Group (1997). "Data Tables: Results from USDA's 1996 Continuing Survey of Food Intakes by Individuals and 1996 Diet and Health Knowledge Survey." U.S. Department of Agriculture, Riverdale, MD.

22. Johnson, R. K., and Kennedy, E. (2000). The 2000 Dietary Guidelines for Americans: What are the changes and why were they made? *J. Am. Diet. Assoc.* **100,** 769–774.

23. Kuczmrski, R. J., Flegal, K. M., Campbell, S. M., and Johnson, C. L. (1994). Increasing prevalence of overweight among U.S. adults. *JAMA* **272,** 205–211.

24. National Center for Health Statistics, Centers for Disease Control and Prevention (1997). Update: Prevalence of overweight among children, adolescents, and adults—United States 1988–1994. *Morbid. Mortal. Wkly Rept* **46,** 199–202.

25. U.S. Department of Health and Human Services, Office of Public Health and Science (1998). "Healthy People 2010 Objectives: Draft for Public Comment." U.S. Department of Health and Human Services, Washington, DC.

26. U.S. Department of Health and Human Services (1996). "Physical Activity and Health: A Report of the Surgeon General." U.S. Department of Health and Human Services, Centers for Disease Control and Prevention, National Center for Chronic Disease Prevention and Health Promotion, Atlanta, GA.

27. Krebs-Smith, S. M., Smiciklas-Wright, H., Guthrie, H. A., and Krebs-Smith, J. (1987). The effects of variety in food choices on dietary quality. *J. Am. Diet. Assoc.* **87,** 897–903.

28. McCrory, M. A., Fuss, P. J., McCallum, J. E., Yao, M., Vinken, A. G., Hays, N. P., and Roberts, S. B. (1999). Dietary variety within foodgroups: Association with energy intake and body fatness in men and women. *Am. J. Clin. Nutr.* **69,** 440–447.

29. Steinmetz, K. A., and Potter, J. D. (1996). Vegetables, fruit, and cancer prevention: A review. *J. Am. Diet. Assoc.* **96,** 1027–1039.

30. Ness, A. R., and Powles, J. W. (1997). Fruit and vegetables, and cardio-vascular disease: A review. *Int. J. Epidemiol.* **26,** 1–13.

31. Jacobs, D. R., Jr., Meyer, K. A., Kushi, L. H., and Folsom, A. R. (1998). Whole grain intake may reduce the risk of ischemic heart disease death in postmenopausal women: The Iowa Women's Health Study. *Am. J. Clin. Nutr.* **68,** 248–257.

32. Rolls, B. J., Bell, E. A., Castellanos, V. H., Chow, M., Pelkman, C. L., and Thorwart, M. L. (1999). Energy density but not fat content of foods affected energy intake in lean and obese women. *Am. J. Clin. Nutr.* **69**(5), 863–871.

33. Rolls, B. J., Castellanos, V. H., Halford, J. C., Kilara, A., Panyam, D., Pelkman, C. L., Smith, G. P., and Thorwart, M. L. (1998). Volume of food consumed affects satiety in men. *Am. J. Clin. Nutr.* **67,** 1170–1177.

34. U.S. General Accounting Office (1996). "Food Safety: Information on Foodborne Illnesses: Report to Congressional Committees," GAO/RCED-96-96. U.S. General Accounting Office, Washington, DC.

35. Mead, P. S., Slutsker, L., Dietz, V., McCaig, L. F., Bresee, J. S., Shapiro, C., Griffin, P. M., and Tauxe, R. V. (1999). Food-related illness and death in the United States. *Emerg. Infect. Dis.* **5,** 607–625.

36. Yang, S., Leff, M. G., McTague, D., Horvath, K. A., Jackson-Thompson, J., Murayi, T., Boeselager, G. K., Melnik, T. A., Gildemaster, M. C., Ridings, D. L., Altekruse, S. F., and Angulo, F. J. (1998). Multistate surveillance for food-handling, preparation, and consumption behaviors associated with food-borne diseases: 1995 and 1996 BRFSS food-safety questions. *Morbid. Mortal. Wkly Rept* **47,** 33–57.

37. Kurtzweil, P. (1998). A year of food safety accomplishments. *FDA Consumer* **32**(5), 8–9.

38. Gordon, D. J. (1995). Cholesterol and mortality: What can meta-analyses tell us? *In* "Cardiovascular Disease" (L. L. Gallo, Ed.), pp. 333–340. Plenum Press, New York.

39. Gordon, D. J. (1995). Cholesterol lowering and total mortality. *In* "Lowering Cholesterol in High Risk Individuals and Populations" (B. M. Rifkind, Ed.), pp. 33–48. Marcel Dekker, New York.

40. Grundy, S. M. (1998). Overview: Second International Conference on Fats and Oil Consumption in Health and Disease: How we can optimize dietary composition to combat metabolic complications and decrease obesity. *Am. J. Clin. Nutr.* **67**(3), 497S–499S.

41. Krauss, R. M. (1998). Triglycerides and atherogenic lipoproteins: Rationale for lipid management. *Am. J. Med.* **105**(1A), 58S–62S.

42. Morton, J. F., and Guthrie, J. F. (1998). Changes in children's total fat intakes and their food group sources of fat, 1989–91 versus 1994–95: Implications for diet quality. *Fam. Econ. Nutr. Rev.* **11,** 44–57.

43. Harnack, L., Stang, J., and Story, M. (1999). Soft drink consumption among U.S. children and adolescents: Nutritional consequences. *J. Am. Diet. Assoc.* **99,** 436–441.

44. Depaola, D. P., Faine, M. P., and Palmer, C. A. (1999). Nutrition in relation to dental medicine. *In* "Modern Nutrition in Health and Disease," 9th ed. (M. E. Shils, J. A. Olson, M. Shike, and A. C. Ross, Eds.), pp. 1099–1124. Williams and Wilkins, Baltimore, MD.

45. U.S. Department of Agriculture, Human Nutrition Information Service (1993). "USDA's Food Guide: Background and Development," Misc. Pub. No. 1514. U.S. Department of Agriculture, Hyattsville, MD.

46. Krebs-Smith, S. M., Guenther, P. M., Cook, A., Thompson, F. E., Cucinelli, J., and Ulder, J. (1997). "Foods Commonly Consumed Per Eating Occasion and in a Day, 1989–91," NFS Report No. 91-3. U.S. Government Printing Office, Washington, DC.

47. U.S. Department of Agriculture (1999). "Tips for Using the Food Guide Pyramid for Young Children 2 to 6 Years Old," Program Aid 1647. U.S. Department of Agriculture, Center for Nutrition Policy and Promotion, Washington, DC.

48. American Dietetic Association and American Diabetes Association (1995). "Exchange Lists for Meal Planning." American Dietetic Association, Chicago, IL.

49. Kurtzweil, P. (1993). Daily values encourage healthy diet. *FDA Consumer* **27**(4), 28–32.

50. U.S. Department of Agriculture, Food Surveys Research Group (1997). "Pyramid Servings Data: Results from USDA's 1995 and 1996 Continuing Survey of Food Intakes by Individuals." U.S. Department of Agriculture, Riverdale, MD.

51. U.S. Department of Agriculture, Center for Nutrition Policy and Promotion (1995). "The Healthy Eating Index," CNPP-1. U.S. Department of Agriculture, Center for Nutrition Policy and Promotion, Washington, DC.

52. Bowman, S. A., Lino, M., Gerrior, S. A., and Basiotis, P. P. (1998). "The Healthy Eating Index 1994–96." CNPP-5. U.S.

Department of Agriculture, Center for Nutrition Policy and Promotion, Washington, DC.

53. Centers for Disease Control and Prevention (1997). Guidelines for school and community health programs to promote lifelong physical activity among young people. *Morbid. Mortal. Wkly Rept* **46**(RR-6), 1–34.

54. Andersen, R. E., Crespo, C. J., Bartlett, S. J., Cheskin, L. J., and Pratt, M. (1998). Relationship of physical activity and television watching with body weight and level of fatness among children: Results from the Third National Health and Nutrition Examination Survey. *JAMA* **279**, 938–942.

55. U.S. Department of Health and Human Services (1999). "Healthy People 2000 Review, 1998–99," Publication No. (PS) 99-1256. U.S. Department of Health and Human Services, Centers for Disease Control and Prevention, National Center for Health Statistics, Hyattsville, MD.

56. Centers for Disease Control and Prevention (1996). Prevalence of physical inactivity during leisure time among overweight persons—Behavioral Risk Factor Surveillance System, 1994. *Morbid. Mortal. Wkly Rept* **45**, 185–188.

57. McGinnis, J. M., and Foege, W. H. (1993). Actual causes of death in the United States. *JAMA* **270**, 2207–2212.

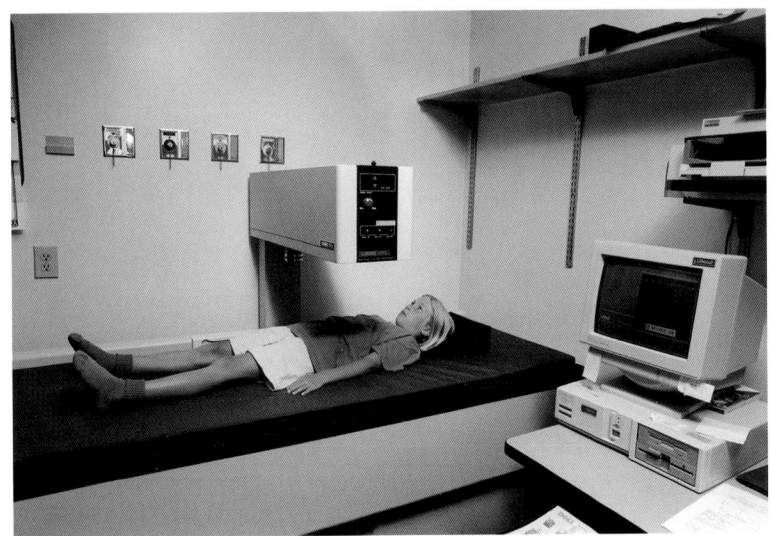

Chapter 2, Figure 2 Dual-energy x-ray absorptiometry is a scanning technique that accurately estimates bone mineral, fat, and fat-free soft tissue.

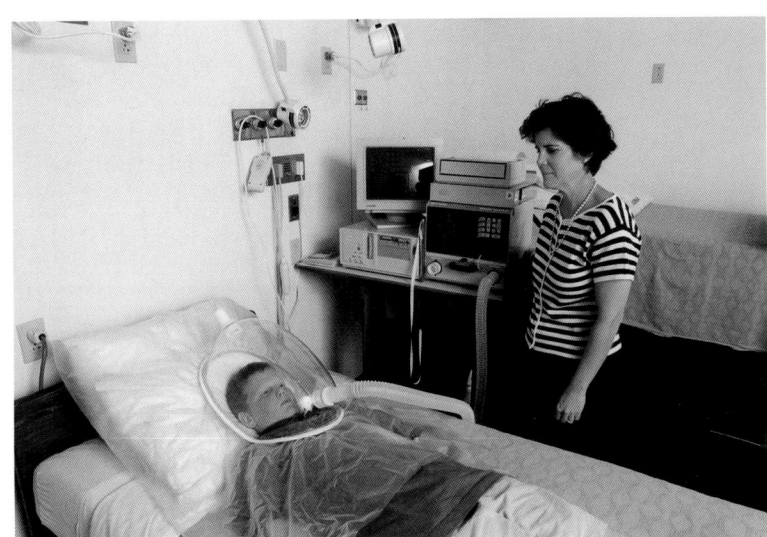

Chapter 2, Figure 3 Measurement of resting metabolic rate using indirect calorimetry.

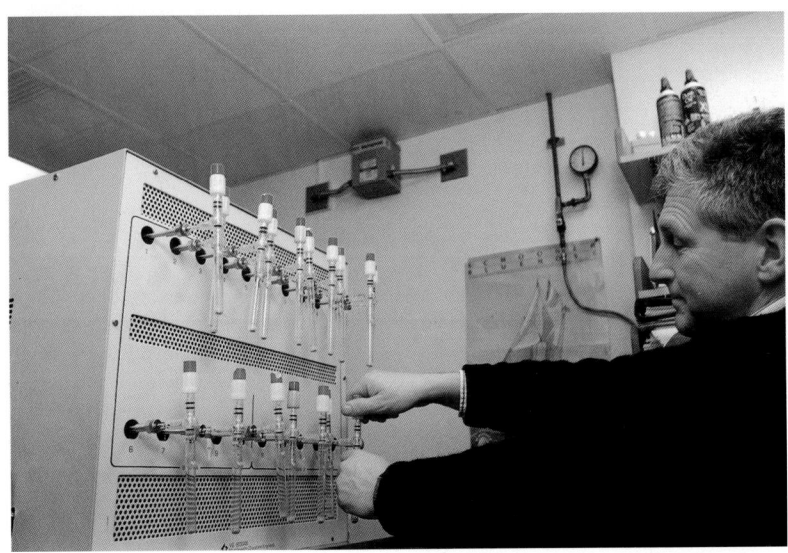

Chapter 2, Figure 4 Mass spectrometer used for the analysis of isotope enrichments in the DLW method.

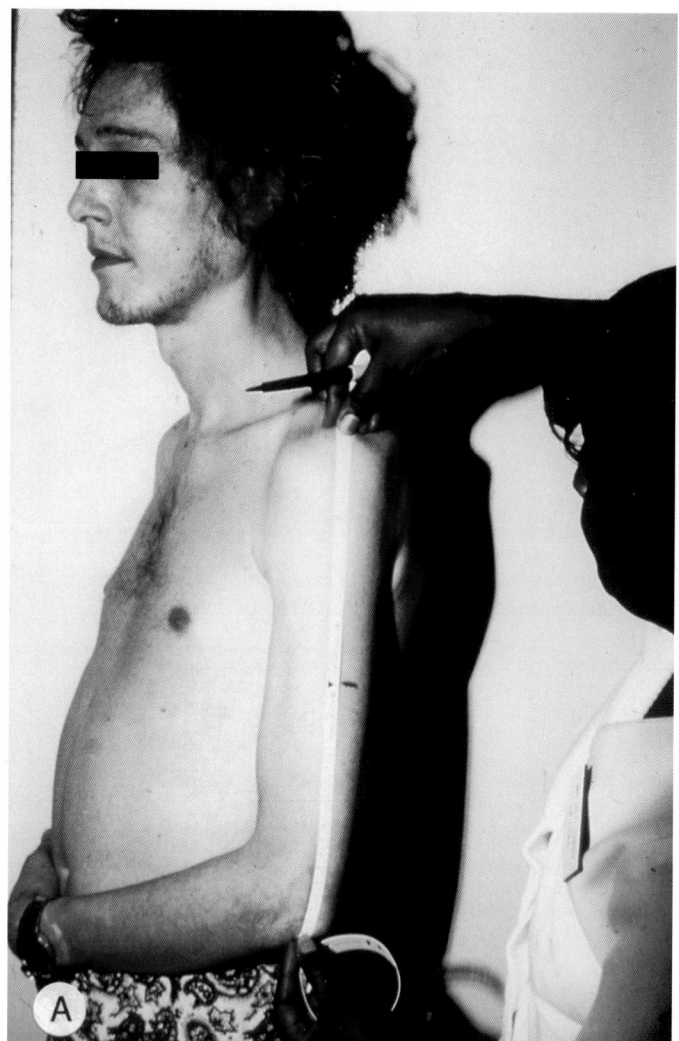

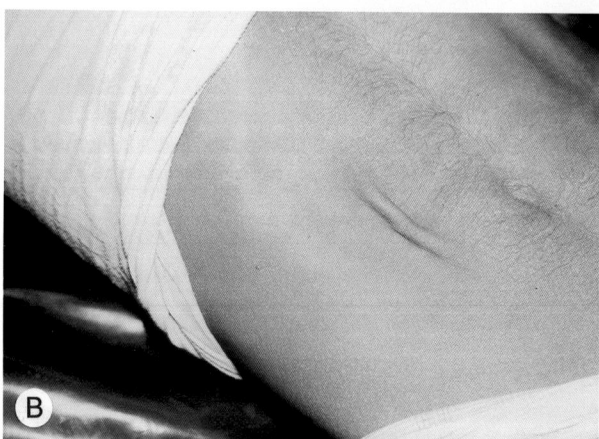

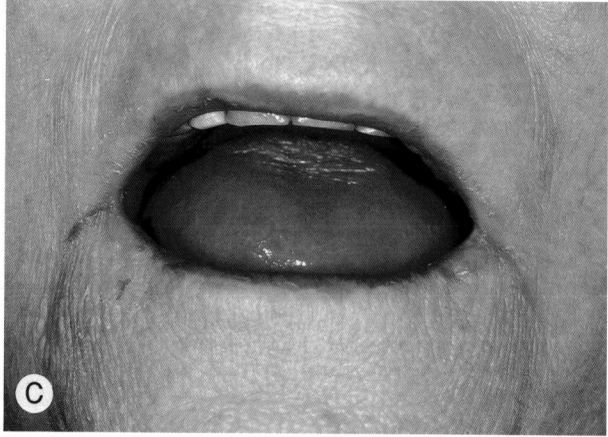

Chapter 3, Figure 4 Physical signs associated with nutrient deficiencies. (A) Muscle wasting in severe protein energy malnutrition. (B) Tenting of skin in dehydration; the skin retains the tented shape after being pinched. (C) Glossitis and angular stomatitis associated with multiple B vitamin deficiencies. (D) Dermatitis associated with zinc deficiency. (E) Cheilosis, or vertical fissuring of the lips, associated with multiple B vitamin deficiencies. (F) Bitot's spot accompanying vitamin A deficiency. (Photos courtesy of Dr. Robert Russell and Dr. Joel Mason.)

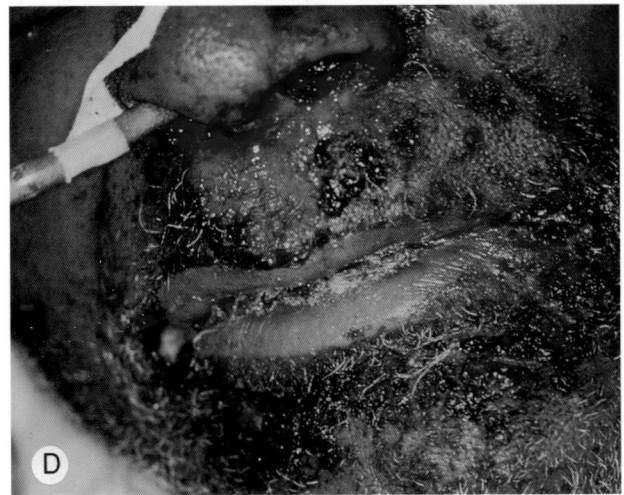

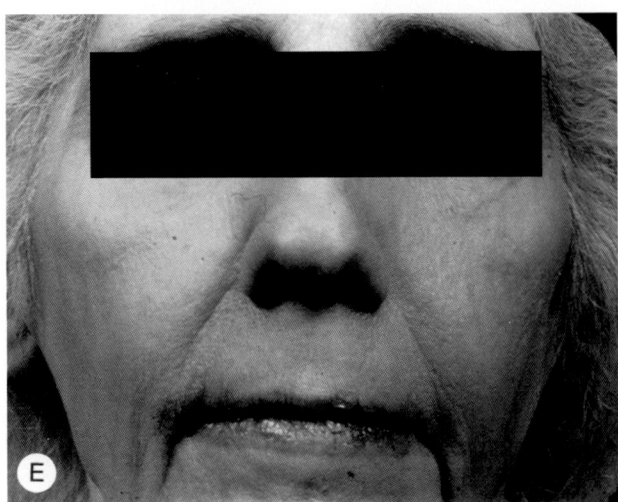

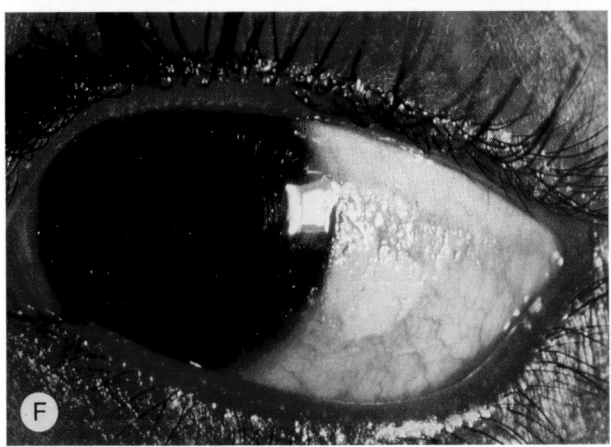

Chapter 3, Figure 4 *continued*

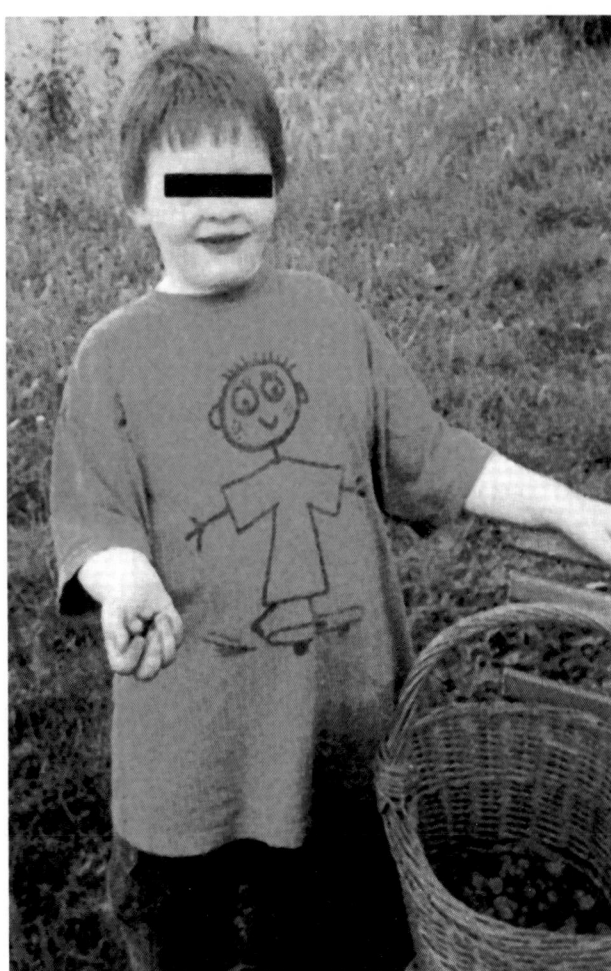

Chapter 12, Figure 2 Photo of 5-year-old boy with early-onset obesity, adrenal insufficiency, and red hair caused by mutation of the *POMC* gene. This patient had early hypoglycemia and hyponatriaemia due to ACTH deficiency. Birth weight was normal but, due to hyperphagia, obesity was apparent by 5 months of age. [Reprinted with permission from Krude, H., Biebermann, H., Luck, W., Horn, R., Brabant, G., and Grüters, A. (1998). Severe early-onset obesity, adrenal insufficiency, and red hair pigmentation caused by *POMC* mutations in humans. *Nature Genet.* **19**, 155–157.]

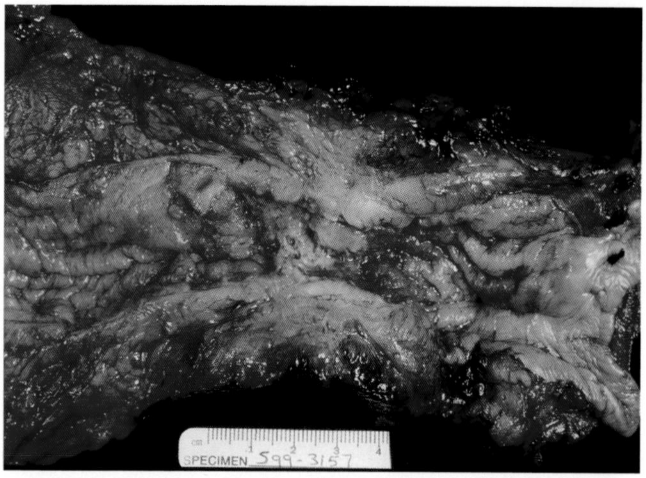

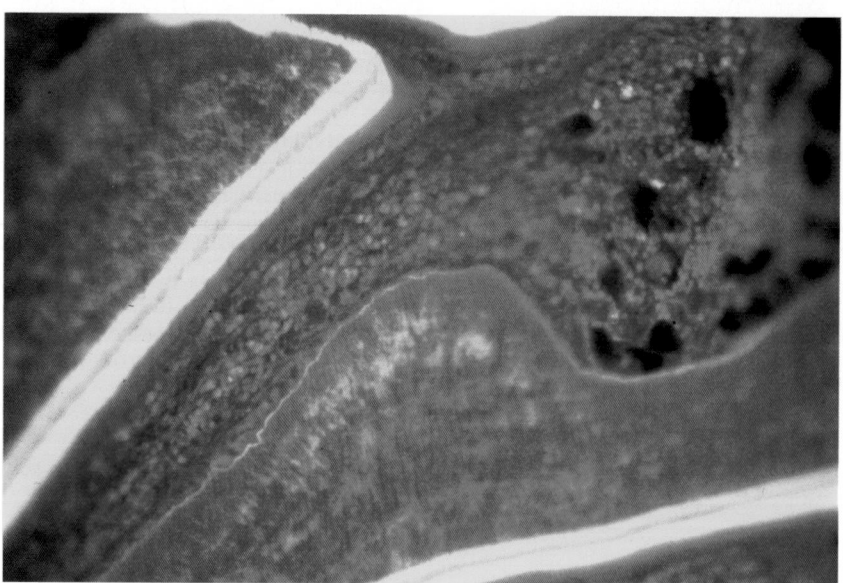

Chapter 38, Figure 3

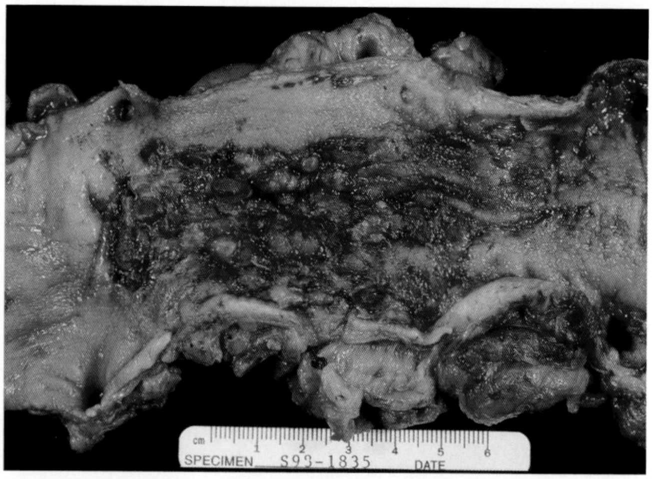

Chapter 38, Figure 4

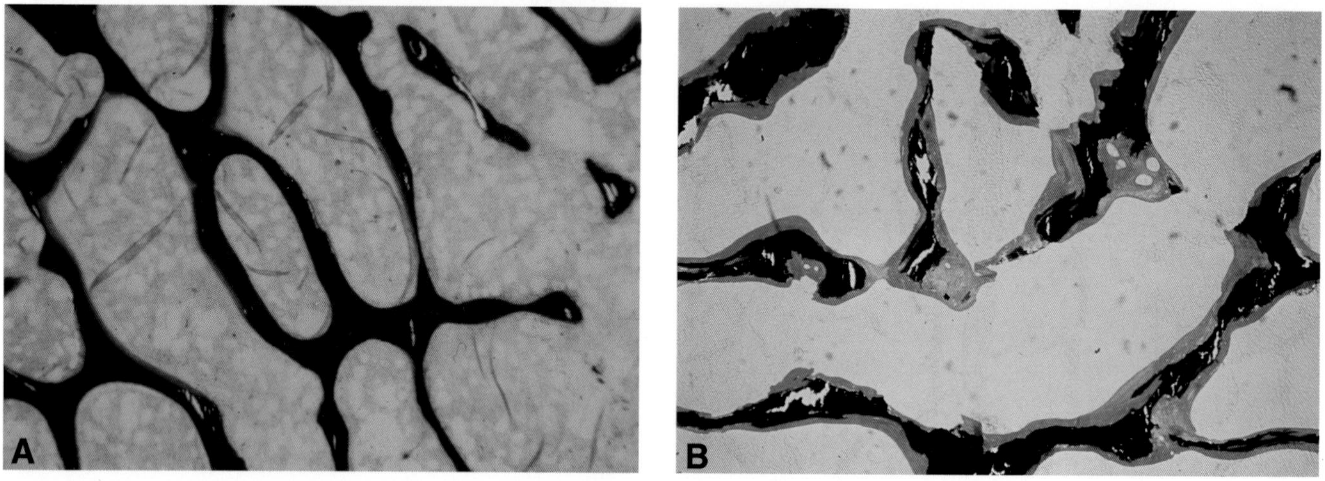

Chapter 46, Figure 6 Histologic appearance of normal (A) and osteomalacic (B) bone. [Reprinted with permission from Compston, J. (1997). Bone histomorphometry. *In* "Vitamin D" (F. H. Glorieux, D. G. Feldman, and J. W. Pike, Eds.), pp. 573–586. Academic Press, San Diego.]

Chapter 46, Figure 7 Dynamic histomorphometry of trabecular bone shown by tetracycline double labeling. [Reprinted with permission from Compston, J. (1997). Bone histomorphometry. *In* "Vitamin D" (F. H. Glorieux, D. G. Feldman, and J. W. Pike, Eds.), pp. 573–586. Academic Press, San Diego.]

Epilogue

JANET KING

USDA, Western Human Nutrition Research Center, University of California at Davis, Davis, California

This book, *Nutrition in the Prevention and Treatment of Disease,* emphasizes the past and current scientific evidence of the role played by nutrition in the prevention and treatment of chronic disease. New emerging areas of study are discussed with an emphasis on the *evolutionary* process in science and its application. Thus, the book prepares the clinical nutrition investigator or practitioner for a lifelong commitment to learning and change.

As we start the 21st century, we have entered a new era of nutrition in the prevention and treatment of disease. The definition of clinical nutrition has changed. Today, clinical nutrition involves the integration of diet, genetics, environment, and behavior to promote health and well-being throughout life. This definition requires the capacity to deal with complexity and to utilize multidisciplinary approaches. Now, more than ever before, nutritionists need broad training in a variety of disciplines while being expert in one well-defined aspect.

The complexity of the relationship between diet, genetics, environment, and behavior is demonstrated by the unfolding story of diet and atherosclerotic heart disease. Early investigators discovered the links between dietary cholesterol, saturated fats, and atherosclerosis. Later, relationships with polyunsaturated fats were explored. This led to studies of monounsaturates, fish oils, and *trans* fatty acids. More recently, body iron and ferritin levels have been linked to coronary heart disease, as have intakes of antioxidants and folic acid. Also, evidence is emerging that immune function may play a role. The picture becomes much less clear as conflicting data on the role of specific fats, other nutrients, food components, and dietary patterns evolve. This is only part of the picture, however. Epidemiological studies show that gender, perhaps racial and ethnic background, and personal behaviors, such as physical activity, also influence progression of the disorder.

When one adds the effect of the interindividual variations in genes on risk factors for heart disease, the situation becomes overwhelming. Studies in the United States show that 50% of the variance in plasma cholesterol concentration is genetically determined, and the response of plasma cholesterol to dietary interventions is heterogeneous. For example, on a low-fat/high-cholesterol diet, individuals with apoE4/4

phenotype respond with an increase in serum cholesterol whereas those with apoE2/2, 3/2, and 3/4 do not [1]. Genetics and diet also influence low-density lipoprotein peak particle size. Low-fat diets induce an atherogenic lipoprotein phenotype characterized by a predominance of small, dense low-density lipoprotein particles (subclass pattern B) in healthy subjects who originally had large low-density lipoprotein particles (subclass pattern A) [2]. Also, feeding a very low-fat (10% of energy) diet to children of parents with pattern B induces the atherogenic small dense low-density lipoproteins; this did not occur in children of parents with pattern A [3]. Thus, the influence of genetics on response to a dietary intervention is evident in childhood. These data imply that it is not prudent to recommend a low-fat diet for all children and adults until the complex interaction between diet, genetics, and environment is better defined.

During the last 25 years, the impact of diet and environment on disease was uncovered; during the next two decades, the impact of genetics will be added into the equation. This integration will not be easy. First, changes in the diet induce many regulatory responses that attenuate the effect of these changes on the organism's metabolism, making the response of individual genes subtle. Also, many genes are involved in the metabolic pathways so that any differences observed are due to groups of genes rather than individual genes. Furthermore, although the human genome has been identified, functions of the genes have only been described for a small portion of the DNA sequences. As we await data on gene function, new information about the phenotypic responses to dietary interventions, such as increases in serum cholesterol and lipoprotein concentrations, will be helpful in deriving appropriate dietary interventions. Data on phenotypic responses to diets can be used to match a dietary intervention to an individual's specific genetic pattern.

Epidemiological studies help describe the link between diet and phenotypic responses. Nutritional epidemiology, or the study of diet and the occurrence of disease in human populations, also emerged within the past 25 years. During the next 25 years, nutritional and molecular epidemiology will merge. This will enable large-scale, population studies of the associations between dietary patterns and phenotypes for chronic disease. To date, most of the studies have linked

dietary patterns with the *occurrence* of disease, i.e., *trans* fatty acid intake and cardiovascular disease, β-carotene intake and breast or lung cancer, and dietary fiber and colorectal cancer. Knowledge of the associations between diet and early biomarkers of disease is much more useful. That information will emerge as phenotypes associated with high risk for chronic disease are identified.

In sum, the tool chest of the clinical nutritionist 25–30 years ago included a diet manual, a good dietary history and food composition data table, a tape measure, and a pair of skinfold calipers. Using empirical data generated from those tools, simple dietary prescriptions were derived. Today, in the 21st century, the clinical nutritionist must have a broad understanding of the scientific basis for disease and the influence of diet, genetics, and the environment on the progress of the disorder. The capacity to deal with complex interactions across multiple disciplines is essential. At the same time, the clinical nutritionist or investigator in human nutrition needs a thorough, in-depth understanding of cultural and socioeconomic influences on food behaviors and the competency to integrate that knowledge with phenotypic or functional markers of the disease. Comprehensive textbooks, such as this one, that integrate basic principles and concepts across disciplines while showing how to apply this knowledge in new, creative ways are an essential part of the tool chest needed in this new era of practice.

References

1. Miettinen, T. A., Gylling, H., and Sanhanen, H. (1988). Serum cholesterol response to dietary cholesterol and apolipoprotein E phenotype. *Lancet* **2,** 1261.
2. Dreon, D. M., Fernstrom, H. A., Miller, B., and Krauss, R. M. (1995). Apolipoprotein E isoform phenotype and LDL subclass response to a reduced-fat diet. *Arterioscler. Thromb. Vasc. Biol.* **15,** 105–111.
3. Dreon, D. M., Fernstrom, H. A., Williams, P. T., and Krauss, R. M. (2000). Reduced LDL particle size in children consuming a very-low-fat diet is related to parental LDL-subclass patterns. *Am. J. Clin. Nutr.* **71,** 1611–1616.

Index

Dear Student,

Thank you for purchasing this textbook. We hope you find it a useful tool as you examine the topic of taxation.

A Study Guide is available through your bookstore. The purpose of the Study Guide is to assist you in studying and reviewing the text material and provide you with a means of self-testing. The Study Guide provides a chapter review, study exercises, true-false and multiple- choice questions.

If the Study Guide is not in stock in your bookstore, ask the bookstore manager to order a copy for you. In addition, the Study Guide may be purchased at **academic.cengage.com/taxation**. Simply select your course type, and then choose your text from the titles listed. At the shopping resources page, select "Book Supplements" and click on the link for "Study Guide."

Best wishes for a great year!

Cordially,
James W. Pratt and William N. Kulsrud

TAXATION SERIES

Federal Taxation

2010 EDITION

JAMES W. PRATT
WILLIAM N. KULSRUD

CONTRIBUTING AUTHORS

GREGORY A. CARNES, PH.D., C.P.A. | The University of North Alabama
MARGUERITE R. HUTTON, PH.D., C.P.A. | Western Washington University
ROBERT W. JAMISON, PH.D., C.P.A. | Indiana University
WILLIAM N. KULSRUD, PH.D., C.P.A. | Indiana University
NATHAN OESTREICH, PH.D., C.P.A. | San Diego State University
JAMES W. PRATT, D.B.A., C.P.A. | University of Houston
EDWARD J. SCHNEE, PH.D., C.P.A. | University of Alabama
STEVEN C. THOMPSON, PH.D., C.P.A. | Texas State University
JOHN C. TRIPP, PH.D., C.P.A. | University of Denver
MICHAEL J. TUCKER, J.D., PH.D., C.P.A. | Quinnipiac College
JAMES L. WITTENBACH, D.B.A., C.P.A. | University of Notre Dame

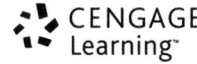
CENGAGE
Learning

Australia　Brazil　Canada　Mexico　Singapore　Spain　United Kingdom　United States

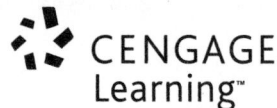

Federal Taxation
2010 Edition

James W. Pratt
William N. Kulsrud

Executive Editors:
Maureen Staudt
Michael Stranz

Senior Project Development Manager:
Linda DeStefano

Marketing Specialists:
Sara Mercurio
Lindsay Shapiro

Senior Production/Manufacturing Manager:
Donna M. Brown

PreMedia Supervisor:
Joel Brennecke

Permissions Specialists:
Kalina Hintz
Todd Osborne

Product Development Manager:
Greg Albert

Developmental Editor:
Sarah Blasco

Custom Production Editor:
Jennifer Flinchpaugh

Senior Project Coordinator:
Robin Richie

Cover and Preface Designer:
Candice Swanson

Compositor:
Pre-Press PMG

Cover and Chapter Opener Images:
© 2009 Jupiterimages Corporation

For product information and technology assistance, contact us at
Cengage Learning Customer & Sales Support, 1-800-354-9706

For permission to use material from this text or product,
submit all requests online at **cengage.com/permissions**
Further permissions questions can be emailed to
permissionrequest@cengage.com

Library of Congress Control Number: 2009924613

ISBN-13: 978-1-4240-6375-8 | PKG ISBN-13: 978-1-4240-6986-6

ISBN-10: 1-4240-6375-2 | PKG ISBN-10: 1-4240-6986-6

Cengage Learning
5191 Natorp Blvd.
Mason, OH 45040
USA

Cengage Learning is a leading provider of customized learning solutions with office locations around the globe, including Singapore, the United Kingdom, Australia, Mexico, Brazil, and Japan. Locate your local office at: **international.cengage.com/region**

Cengage Learning products are represented in Canada by Nelson Education, Ltd.

For your lifelong learning solutions, visit **cengage.com/custom**

Visit our corporate website at **cengage.com**

Printed in the United States of America

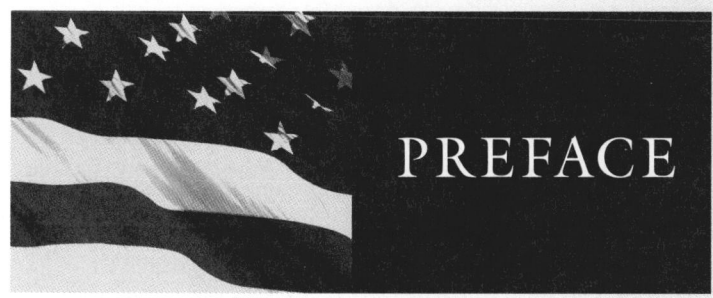

WELCOME TO THE
PRATT & KULSRUD TAXATION SERIES

For more than 20 years, the Pratt & Kulsrud Taxation Series has provided educators, students and professionals an engaging and clear presentation of tax law. In 1984 the series began with *Federal Taxation*, a first-of-its-kind textbook exploring issues relating to the taxation of individuals and businesses. The success of that text and the demand for additional topics led to the creation of two separate texts: *Corporate, Partnership, Estate and Gift Taxation* and *Individual Taxation*.

Through each edition, the series has consistently held to the principle that the key to learning taxation is to understand the underlying purpose behind every rule. For this reason, the authors and editors have made a concerted effort to provide the conceptual background and historical foundation they believe are essential for comprehension. This approach is bolstered by more than 1,000 examples and review questions that address the most important aspects of the law. This edition continues the tradition of excellence with timely updates reflecting the latest in tax laws, the integration of H&R Block TaxCut® Home & Business software, and rich online resources for instructors.

THE 2010 EDITION

The 2010 edition has been revised to reflect changes in the tax law and significant judicial and administrative developments during the past year. Since the 2009 edition went to press, Congress enacted several major changes to the tax law, including the *American Recovery and Reinvestment Act of 2009*, the *Emergency Economic Stabilization Act of 2008*, the *Energy Improvement and Extension Act of 2008*, and the *Heartland, Habitat, Harvest, and Horticulture Act of 2008*. As these became law, online supplements were provided that keyed the changes to the relevant chapters and pages of the text. The changes brought about by the new legislation are now incorporated in the 2010 text. As we go to press with this edition, there are various tax proposals being considered in Congress that may lead to significant and immediate changes in the tax law. Should any of these proposals be enacted, we will continue our long-standing policy of posting these changes online for current users of the text at **custom.cengage.com/pktax**.

FEATURES FOR LEARNERS

- **H&R Block TaxCut® Home & Business Software:** Every new copy of this text automatically comes packaged with H&R Block TaxCut Home & Business software to provide students an additional tax-preparation tool. Practical and remarkably easy to use, the software contains features for both basic and complex problems. H&R Block TaxCut Home & Business allows students to prepare returns for individuals, C and S corporations, partnerships, estates and trusts. The TaxCut website (**taxcut.com**) offers useful tips, calculators and other up-to-the-minute, relevant, tax information. We do not anticipate any problems loading the software; however, Cengage Learning Technical Support (1-800-423-0563) is available for help if necessary.

- **Learning Objectives:** A summary of key points can be found at the beginning of each chapter. The summary outlines what students should understand after reading the chapter.

- **Problem Materials:** Available at the end of each chapter, a variety of assessment tools are offered to gauge comprehension. These tools include discussion questions and computational problems, as well as tax-return problems that highlight topics discussed in the chapter.

- **You Make the Call:** Students are challenged by hypothetical situations that require reasoning and judgment to resolve practical tax examples.

- **Check Your Knowledge:** Throughout the text, objective and short-answer review questions are provided that address key concepts. These review questions ensure that students grasp the critical aspects of each topic.

In addition, an accompanying Study Guide (ISBN 1-4240-7090-2) to this text is available. The Study Guide provides chapter reviews, study exercises, true-false and multiple-choice questions. These may be used in both your initial study of the chapter material and in your review. The Study Guide may be purchased through your bookstore or at **academic.cengage.com/taxation**. Simply select your course type, and then choose your text from the titles listed. At the shopping resources page, select "Book Supplements" and click on the link for "Study Guide."

ENHANCED SUPPORT FOR INSTRUCTORS

Support Web Site
custom.cengage.com/pktax
This support site is your one stop for test banks, the latest tax updates, inflation adjustments posted on a regular basis, and PowerPoint® slides. Designed for classroom use, there are slides for each chapter, as well as slides containing solutions for many problems.

Go to the support site for the following resources:

Solutions Manual: This manual contains solutions to the discussion questions and computational problems at the end of each chapter. These solutions reference specific pages and examples from the text, and supporting statutory or administrative authorities, where appropriate.

Instructor's Resource Guide and Test Bank: This guide includes solutions to comprehensive and tax research problems, tax-return problems, and a test bank containing more than 750 objective questions (true-false and multiple choice), with answers that reference specific pages and examples in the text.

Instructor's Resource CD with ExamView®: Key instructor ancillaries listed below are provided on CD-ROM — giving instructors the ultimate tool for preparing and customizing lectures and presentations.

- Instructor's resource guide and test bank
- Solutions to tax-research and tax-return problems
- Additional test items and solutions
- The test bank files on the CD are provided in ExamView® format and in Word file format.

ExamView® is an easy-to-use test creation software compatible with Microsoft Windows®.

CENGAGE LEARNING CUSTOM SOLUTIONS

Cengage Learning Custom Solutions can work with you to develop a specialized publication that will make the educational experience unique and personal for all learners. Through our Custom publishing service, authors can publish original learning materials as a standalone book or as a supplement to another text; your materials can then be bundled with other Cengage Learning products. Our Custom services give you nearly limitless options for developing materials tailored to suit individual needs.

- Derivative solutions let you build a book or a collection of course material using content from previously published Cengage textbooks. Include your own content to customize your materials even more.

- TextChoice, our database publishing program, uses our online database of content to develop your custom learning materials. Select readings, chapters or excerpts from more than 40 subject areas. Visit **textchoice.com**.

- Our recently expanded Cover Gallery allows you to select a professional cover design to complement your customized book, or create a unique, course-specific design. Visit our online gallery at **custom.cengage.com/covers**.

- Custom Solutions can publish your original learning materials with the help of our Custom publishing editors and our original works program. Textbooks, supplements, study guides... the possibilities are endless!

- Technology Services can provide you with tailored learning materials in a variety of delivery methods.

For more information on Cengage Learning Custom Solutions' services, visit custom.cengage.com.

ADDITIONAL OFFERINGS FROM THE
PRATT & KULSRUD TAXATION SERIES

The series includes new editions of:

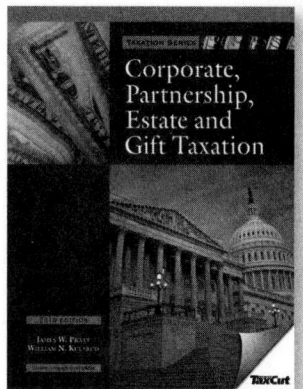

Corporate, Partnership, Estate and Gift Taxation
2010 Edition
ISBN 1-4240-6988-2

Areas of taxation essential to the education of individuals pursuing careers in taxation or tax-related fields are emphasized. The first eight chapters are devoted to the tax problems of regular corporations and their shareholders. Two chapters consider the taxation of partnerships and partners, while one chapter examines S corporations. These chapters are followed by a separate chapter examining the special problems of international taxation, an area of growing importance. Another chapter discusses Federal estate and gift taxation. And two additional chapters contain related topics for the income taxation of estates, trusts and beneficiaries, and the major aspects of family tax planning. The text also includes a chapter on state and local taxation. The scope of this text is intentionally broad to accommodate a variety of uses and to provide flexibility for instructors designing advanced tax courses. Includes H&R Block TaxCut®.

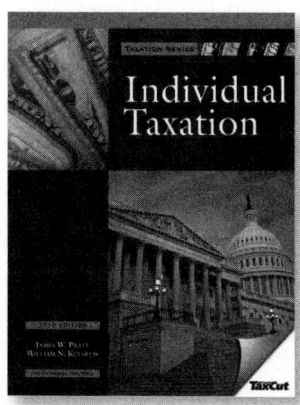

Individual Taxation
2010 Edition
ISBN 1-4240-6987-4

Numerous examples and computational illustrations explain the more complex rules concerning the Federal income taxation of individuals, making this text ideal for a first course in Federal taxation, undergraduate or graduate accounting, business or law students. Includes H&R Block TaxCut®.

ACKNOWLEDGEMENTS

The editor and author team would like to thank particularly Linda Curry of Indiana University, Karen Davis of Quinnipiac University and Leonard Goodman of Rutgers University for their comments and suggestions. In addition, the editors and authors would like to acknowledge the tireless efforts of Cengage Learning Custom Solutions' Developmental Editor Sarah Blasco and Custom Production Editor Jennifer Flinchpaugh. Their work on this edition has led to a strong revision that will benefit both student and instructor. Thanks also to our Executive Editor Maureen Staudt and Marketing Specialist Sara Mercurio. Finally, we appreciate the efforts of the Custom Solutions editors and South-Western sales representatives who put this book into your hands for adoption consideration.

ABOUT THE EDITORS

James W. Pratt

James W. (Jim) Pratt is the PriceWaterhouse Coopers Professor of Accountancy & Taxation at the University of Houston's C.T. Bauer College of Business. Jim joined the faculty in 1972 after receiving his doctorate degree from the University of Southern California. He has published articles in leading professional journals, such as the *Journal of Accountancy*, *Journal of Taxation*, *Journal of Corporate Taxation*, *Journal of Partnership Taxation*, and *The Tax Adviser*. In addition to his contributions as an author and editor, Jim has received several awards for outstanding teaching. He has also taught in continuing professional education programs for more than 30 years and has served as a tax training consultant for several national and local accounting firms.

William N. Kulsrud

William N. (Bill) Kulsrud is an Associate Professor of Accounting at the Kelley School of Business of Indiana University, Indianapolis/Bloomington, and serves as Chair of the Master of Science in Accounting and Master of Science in Taxation programs. Bill joined the faculty in 1979 after receiving his Ph.D. from the University of Texas. He has published numerous articles, which have appeared in leading professional journals such as the *Journal of Taxation*, *Journal of Corporate Taxation*, *The Tax Adviser*, *Taxation for Accountants*, and *Taxes — The Tax Magazine*. He has also served as an editorial adviser to *The Tax Adviser*, *Journal of Accountancy* and *Journal of the American Taxation Association*. In addition to his contributions as an author and editor, Bill has received many awards for outstanding teaching. In 1990 he was named Accounting Educator of the Year by the Indiana C.P.A. Society. He has also taught hundreds of professional education programs for national and local accounting firms and has developed materials used in their continuing education programs. Bill is currently the co-coordinator of the National Tax Education Program sponsored by the AICPA.

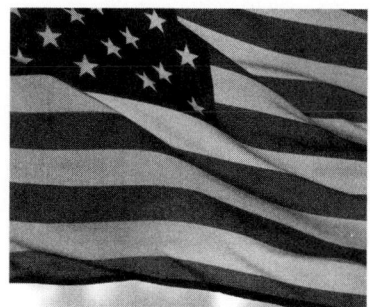

★ CONTENTS IN BRIEF ★

ix

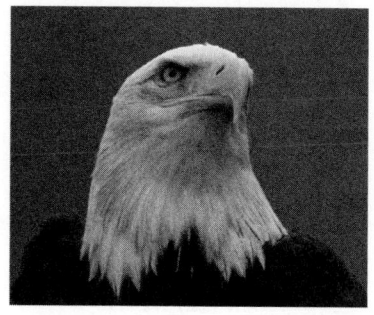

★ CONTENTS ★

PART I
INTRODUCTION TO THE FEDERAL TAX SYSTEM

Chapter 1   AN OVERVIEW OF FEDERAL TAXATION

Chapter 2   TAX PRACTICE AND RESEARCH

Chapter 3   TAXABLE ENTITIES, TAX FORMULA, INTRODUCTION TO PROPERTY TRANSACTIONS

Chapter 4   PERSONAL AND DEPENDENCY EXEMPTIONS; FILING STATUS; DETERMINATION OF TAX FOR AN INDIVIDUAL; FILING REQUIREMENTS

PART II
GROSS INCOME

Chapter 5   GROSS INCOME

Chapter 6   GROSS INCOME: INCLUSIONS AND EXCLUSIONS

PART III
DEDUCTIONS AND LOSSES

Chapter 7   OVERVIEW OF DEDUCTIONS AND LOSSES

Chapter 8   EMPLOYEE BUSINESS EXPENSES

Chapter 9 CAPITAL RECOVERY: DEPRECIATION, AMORTIZATION, AND DEPLETION

Chapter 10 CERTAIN BUSINESS DEDUCTIONS AND LOSSES

Chapter 11 ITEMIZED DEDUCTIONS

Chapter 12 DEDUCTIONS FOR CERTAIN INVESTMENT
            EXPENSES AND LOSSES

PART IV
ALTERNATIVE MINIMUM TAX AND TAX CREDITS

Chapter 13 THE ALTERNATIVE MINIMUM TAX AND TAX CREDITS

PART V
PROPERTY TRANSACTIONS

Chapter 14   PROPERTY TRANSACTIONS: BASIS DETERMINATION AND RECOGNITION OF GAIN OR LOSS

Chapter 15   NONTAXABLE EXCHANGES

Chapter 16 PROPERTY TRANSACTIONS: CAPITAL GAINS AND LOSSES

Chapter 17   PROPERTY TRANSACTIONS: DISPOSITIONS OF TRADE OR BUSINESS PROPERTY

PART VI
EMPLOYEE COMPENSATION AND RETIREMENT PLANS

Chapter 18   EMPLOYEE COMPENSATION AND RETIREMENT PLANS

PART VII
CORPORATE TAXATION

Chapter 19 CORPORATIONS: FORMATION AND OPERATION

Chapter 20   CORPORATE DISTRIBUTIONS, REDEMPTIONS AND LIQUIDATIONS

Chapter 21   TAXATION OF CORPORATE ACCUMULATIONS

PART VIII
FLOW-THROUGH ENTITIES

Chapter 22   TAXATION OF PARTNERSHIPS AND PARTNERS

Chapter 23   S CORPORATIONS

PART IX
FAMILY TAX PLANNING

Chapter 24   THE FEDERAL TRANSFER TAXES

Chapter 25   INCOME TAXATION OF ESTATES AND TRUSTS

Chapter 26   FAMILY TAX PLANNING

APPENDICES AND INDEX

INTRODUCTION TO THE FEDERAL TAX SYSTEM

★ ★ ★ ★ CONTENTS ★ ★ ★ ★

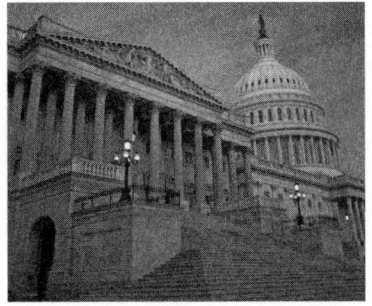

★ CHAPTER ONE ★

AN OVERVIEW OF FEDERAL TAXATION

LEARNING OBJECTIVES

Upon completion of this chapter you will be able to:

▸ Trace the historical development of our Federal income tax system

▸ Explain the key terms used to describe most taxes

▸ Identify the different types of Federal taxes found in the United States, including

  ▸ Income taxes

  ▸ Wealth transfer taxes

  ▸ Employment taxes

  ▸ Excise taxes

▸ Understand the relationship between estate and gift taxes

▸ Explain the differences in the employment taxes levied on employees versus those levied on self-employed individuals

▸ Identify some of the more common social and economic goals of our Federal tax system

---

CHAPTER OUTLINE

INTRODUCTION

The United States has developed what is perhaps the most sophisticated and complex national tax programs in the world today. This system of taxation has an impact on almost every business and investment decision as well as many personal decisions. Decisions a business enterprise must make, such as the form it will take (i.e., sole proprietorship, partnership, limited liability company, or corporation), the length and nature of its operations, and the manner in which it will be terminated cannot be made without consideration of the tax consequences. An individual's decisions regarding employment contracts and alternative forms of compensation, as well as place and duration of employment, will be affected by the Federal tax structure. Even such personal choices as housing, family size, marital relationships, and termination of these relationships by divorce or death involve some of the most complex rules of the Federal tax law. This complexity places a *premium* on knowledge of the various types of Federal taxes imposed on those who by chance or choice must operate within the system's boundaries.

The purpose of this book is to introduce the reader to the major elements of Federal taxation. A corollary objective of the authors is to aid the reader in the development of his or her *tax awareness* (i.e., ability to recognize tax problems, pitfalls, and planning opportunities). Such an awareness is not only an important attribute of accountants and lawyers—it is *essential* for everyone who chooses a career in business.

THE NATURE OF A TAX

The Supreme Court of the United States has defined a *tax* as "an exaction for the support of the Government."[1] Thus, what a tax does is to provide a means through which the government derives a majority of the revenues necessary to keep it in operation. A tax is not merely a source of revenue, however. As discussed in a later section of this chapter, taxes have become a powerful instrument that policymakers use to attain social as well as economic goals.

A tax normally has one or more of the following characteristics:

1. There is no *direct relationship* between the exaction of revenue and any benefit to be received by the taxpayer. Thus, a taxpayer cannot trace his or her tax payment to an Army jeep, an unemployment payment, a weather satellite, or any of the myriad expenditures that the Federal government authorizes.

2. Taxes are levied on the basis of *predetermined criteria*. In other words, taxes can be objectively determined, calculated, and even planned around.

3. Taxes are levied on a *recurring* or *predictable* basis. Most taxes are levied on an annual basis, although some, like the estate tax, are levied only once.

4. Taxes *may be distinguished* from regulations or penalties. A regulation or penalty is a measure specifically designed to control or stop a particular activity. For instance, at one time Congress imposed a charge on the products of child labor. This charge was specifically aimed at stopping the use of children in manufacturing and thus was a regulation rather than a tax, even though it was called a "tax." Also, taxes can be distinguished from licenses and fees, which are payments made for some special privilege granted or services rendered (e.g., marriage license or automobile registration fee).

---

[1] *U.S. v. Butler*, 36-1 USTC ¶9039, 16 AFTR 1289, 297 U.S. 1, 70 (USSC, 1936). An explanation of case citations such as this is presented in Chapter 2.

The major types of taxes imposed by taxing authorities within the United States (e.g., income, employment, and wealth transfer taxes) are discussed later in this chapter. As will be noted, one or more of the above characteristics can be found in each of these various taxes.

DEVELOPMENT OF U.S. TAXATION

The entire history of the United States, from its beginnings as a colony of England to the present day, is entwined with the development of Federal taxation. From its infancy until well into the current century, the United States Federal tax system closely paralleled the tax laws of its mother country, England.[2]

EXCISE AND CUSTOMS DUTIES

Shortly after the colonies won independence and became the United States of America, tariffs became the Federal government's principal revenue-raising source.[3] At the time of its adoption in 1789, the U.S. Constitution gave Congress the power to levy and collect taxes. Promptly exercising this authority, Congress passed as its first act the Tariff Act of 1789, which imposed a system of duties (called excise taxes) on imports.

FEDERAL INCOME TAX

As time passed and the Federal government enlarged the scope of its activities, it became more and more apparent to political leaders that they would have to identify additional sources of revenue to supplement the tariff system. A tax on income was a likely alternative, but Congress was concerned about the constitutionality of an income tax. Under the original Constitution, any *direct* tax imposed by Congress was required to be *apportioned* among the states on the basis of relative populations. Under such a system the Federal tax rates that apply to citizens of one state may be different from those that apply to another state because the sizes of the states' populations differed. If such a system had been tried, it would have been politically and practically unworkable.

Example 1. Assume that Congress imposed a $50,000 tax on income. Assume further that the United States was composed of only three states with populations as follows: Vermont—2,000; Texas—3,000; and New York—5,000. Under the original Constitution, if the income tax were a direct tax, it would be allocated among the states according to population, and each state's tax burden would be as follows: Vermont, $10,000 (20% of total population × $50,000 tax); Texas, $15,000 (30% of $50,000); and New York, $25,000 (50% of $50,000).

Example 2. Assume the sum of the residents' income in each state above was as follows: Vermont—$100,000; Texas—$300,000; and New York—$1,000,000. In such a case, the average rate of tax on income in each state would be as follows: Vermont, 10% ($10,000 tax ÷ $100,000 income); Texas, 5% ($15,000 ÷ $300,000); and New York, 2.5% ($25,000 ÷ $1,000,000). Since incomes are not distributed among the states in the same proportion as residents, the Federal government would be required to

---

[2] The states in turn have developed their own systems of taxation which often parallel—but sometimes diverge from—the Federal tax system.

[3] A tariff is a duty imposed on an importer. Since it is a cost of the product being imported, it usually is passed on to the consumer as part of the product's price. Thus, the higher the tariff imposed on a product, the higher must be its price if importation is to be profitable.

assess taxes on citizens of different states at *different rates*—a resident of Vermont might pay taxes at a rate of 10% while a resident of New York paid only 2.5%.

Despite the apportionment requirement, Congress enacted the first Federal income tax in 1861 to finance the vastly increased expenditures brought on by the Civil War. The tax was applied uniformly to all residents—the apportionment requirement being ignored, apparently on the belief that the income tax was not a direct tax. In *Springer v. U.S.*,[4] however, a taxpayer challenged the Civil War income tax, asserting that the tax was unconstitutional because it was direct, and that any direct tax required apportionment.

The distinction between *direct* taxes and indirect taxes has never been completely clarified. According to some, a direct tax is one that cannot be avoided or at least shifted to another with ease. Two taxes generally considered direct taxes are head taxes and property taxes; neither of these can be escaped without difficulty. Customs duties and other excise taxes are normally considered indirect taxes, since they can be avoided by not purchasing the particular good. Beyond these examples, however, the issue is unresolved. In *Springer*, the Supreme Court specifically addressed the question of whether an income tax was a direct tax and, therefore, whether apportionment was required. The Court held that only head taxes and real estate taxes were direct taxes and all other taxes, including the income tax, were indirect. Thus Congress had not violated the Constitution in ignoring the apportionment clause when it imposed the income tax. Although this case dealt squarely with the issue, the decision did not end the controversy.

The income tax was allowed to expire shortly after the Civil War, in 1872, but was reenacted in almost identical form in 1894. Upon reinstatement, it again was attacked as a direct tax requiring apportionment. In *Pollock v. Farmers' Loan and Trust Co.*,[5] the Supreme Court focused specifically on the income tax as it applied to income from real estate. The Court believed this case to be different from *Springer* and held that a tax on income from real estate was the equivalent of a tax on the real estate itself. Accordingly, the Court held that the tax was unconstitutional because it was a direct tax imposed without apportionment. After this decision, the constitutionality of an income tax was again suspect.

Undaunted by the *Pollock* decision, proponents of a Federal income tax continued their efforts and in 1909 were successful in bringing about a corporate income tax. This tax was upheld by the Supreme Court in *Flint v. Stone Tracy Co.*[6] when the Court held that it was an excise tax measured by corporate income, rather than a direct tax.

Concurrent with its passage of the 1909 corporate income tax, Congress proposed an amendment to the Constitution that would allow it to levy a tax on *all* incomes *without* apportionment among the states based on population. This effort culminated in the passage of the Sixteenth Amendment on February 25, 1913, which provided that,

> The Congress shall have the power to lay and collect taxes on incomes from whatever source derived, without apportionment among the several States, and without regard to any census or enumeration.

Without hesitation, Congress enacted the Revenue Act of 1913 on October 3, 1913 and made it retroactive to March 1, 1913.

Because of special exemptions and the progressive tax rates of the 1913 income tax law, it too was challenged as a denial of due process of law as guaranteed by the Fifth Amendment to the Constitution. In 1916 the Supreme Court upheld the validity of

---

[4]   102 U.S. 586 (USSC, 1880).

[5]   3 AFTR 2602, 157 U.S. 429 (USSC, 1895).

[6]   3 AFTR 2834, 220 U.S. 107 (USSC, 1911).

the new income tax law in *Brushaber v. Union Pacific Railroad Co.*[7] Although many changes have taken place, the United States has not been without a Federal income tax since 1913.

As historical conditions changed and the Federal government's need for additional revenues increased, Congress exercised its income taxing authority by the passage of many separate pieces of legislation that resulted in greater complexity in the Federal income tax law. Each new revenue act was a reenactment of a previous revenue act with added amendments. This process created great confusion for those working with the law, since it could be necessary to research more than 100 separate sources to determine exactly what law was currently in effect. In addition, the reenactment of a statute sometimes suggested that any intervening interpretation of that statute (law) by the courts or the Treasury was approved by Congress, although no such Congressional approval was expressly stated. Congress resolved the confusion in 1939 with its systematic arrangement of all tax laws into the Internal Revenue Code of 1939, a permanent codification that required no reenactment.

The 1939 Code was revised in 1954 and again in 1986. Thus, today's governing Federal tax law is the *Internal Revenue Code of 1986*. The 1986 Code has been amended by significant tax changes made since 1986, and it will continue to be amended to incorporate changes in the tax law as those changes are enacted.

FEDERAL WEALTH TRANSFER TAXES

In 1916, the very same year the Supreme Court upheld the constitutionality of the Federal income tax, Congress enacted the first Federal law to impose a tax on the transfer of property triggered by the death of an individual. The value of the transfer was measured by the fair market value of the various assets included in the decedent's estate, and consequently the tax imposed on the transfer is referred to as the estate tax. The Federal estate tax imposed a progressive tax on the value on the decedent's taxable estate.

Because an individual could avoid the imposition of the Federal estate tax simply by giving away his or her property before death, Congress enacted the first Federal gift tax in 1924[8] to prevent full scale avoidance of the estate tax.

Like the Federal income tax, these Federal wealth transfer taxes have undergone significant changes since first enacted, adding to their complexity. These taxes are discussed later in this chapter.

FEDERAL TAXES AS A SOURCE OF REVENUE

Among sources of revenue, only the Federal income tax can claim a dominant role in providing the funds with which the U.S. government operates. The chart in Exhibit 1-1 illustrates the role of the Federal income tax in providing funding for President Bush's proposed 2009 budget. Note the limited role of excise taxes. Federal transfer taxes are even less significant and are included in the "other" category as a revenue source.

KEY TAX TERMS

Before examining the various types of Federal taxes in more detail, the reader must first become familiar with basic tax terminology. Some of the more common terms are briefly presented below.

---

[7]   240 U.S. 1 (USSC, 1916).

[8]   Although repealed in 1926, the Federal gift tax was reinstated in 1932.

Tax Base. A tax base is that amount upon which a tax is levied. For instance, in the case of Federal income taxation, the tax base is *taxable income.* Taxable income is the taxpayer's total income less exclusions, deductions, and exemptions that might be available to a particular taxpayer. In the case of the Federal wealth transfer taxes, the tax base is the fair market value of the property transferred by gift or at death *reduced* by certain exclusions, exemptions, or deductions allowed by Congress.

EXHIBIT 1-1
2009 Proposed Budget

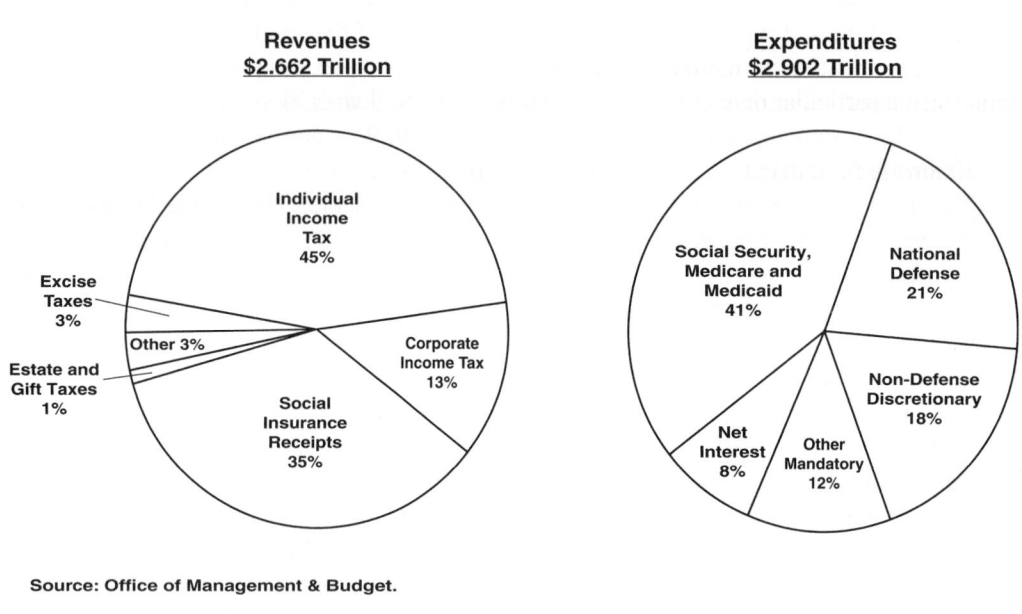

Source: Office of Management & Budget.

Income. Any *permanent* increment to wealth generally is defined as income. Temporary increments such as loans are not considered to be income. Sometimes income is subject to Federal taxation and other times it is not. The taxability of these increments to wealth generally depends upon whether Congress has *exempted* a particular form of income from taxation. Increments to wealth take many forms. Such increments may take the form of cash, property other than cash, or even services that are rendered to the taxpayer. As a general rule, Congress—and the various Federal courts assigned to interpret its laws—consider *any* increment to wealth to be taxable income *unless* it is *excluded* by definition (e.g., loans that must be repaid), by specific statutory authority in the Internal Revenue Code of 1986, or by the Constitution. Each of these possibilities is examined in detail in Chapters 5 and 6, which deal with gross income.

Exclusion. Certain increments to wealth that are *not included* in a particular Federal tax base are referred to as exclusions. Since the Constitution grants Congress the authority to tax income *from whatever source derived,* exclusions are the creations of Congress. For various social, political, or economic reasons, Congress has chosen to exclude many sources of income and wealth transfers from their usual Federal tax base. The more common Congressional objectives of exclusions are discussed in a later section of this chapter.

Example 3. N receives a $13,000 graduation gift from her aunt. N does not have to include this amount in determining taxable income because Congress has specifically excluded gifts from income. If N had received the $13,000 in exchange for rendering services to her aunt, or if N had received the $13,000 for appearing on a television game show, then in both cases she would have to include (report) the amount in income subject to taxation.

Example 4. Refer to *Example 3* above. If N's aunt transfers $13,000 to N in the current year as a graduation gift, and this is the only gift made by the aunt to N in the current year, this transfer will not be subjected to the Federal gift tax. Congress has provided an annual exclusion from gift taxation of $13,000 per donee in 2009.

Deduction. A deduction is a reduction in the gross (total) amount that must be included in the taxable base. For instance, when an individual taxpayer incurs expenses such as medical expenses, interest on a home mortgage, or property taxes, he or she generally will be allowed to deduct these expenses to arrive at taxable income for Federal tax purposes. Similarly, corporations are allowed to deduct most of their costs of doing business to determine corporate taxable income. It is *extremely important* to note, however, that deductions are a matter of legislative grace—unless Congress has specifically authorized a particular deduction, the expense will not be deductible.

Example 5. Individual T purchased his family residence in 2002 for $90,000. T sells his home in 2009 for $80,000. T may not take a deduction for the $10,000 loss (a permanent reduction in wealth) in determining his taxable income *because* Congress has not authorized a deduction for this particular type of loss.

Most deductions available to individual taxpayers and to other taxable entities (i.e., corporations, estates, and trusts) are discussed in detail in Chapters 7 through 12 of this text.

Tax Rates. A tax rate is some percentage applied to the tax base to determine a taxpayer's liability. Tax rate structures usually are either proportional or progressive. A *proportional* tax rate is one that remains at a constant percentage regardless of the size of the tax base. A *progressive* tax rate structure is one in which an increasing percentage rate is applied to increasing increments of the tax base. A *regressive* tax rate structure is one in which a decreasing percentage rate is applied to increasing increments of the tax base.

Example 6. B has a tax base of $5,000 and pays a tax of $500, or 10% of the tax base. C's tax base is $10,000 and the tax on this amount is $1,000, or 10%. If the same constant rate of 10% is applied to any amount of tax base, the tax is proportional.

Example 7. R has a tax base of $10,000 and pays a tax of $500 on the first $5,000, and a tax of $1,000 on the next $5,000. The total tax of $1,500 was calculated by applying a 10% rate to the first $5,000 increment of the tax base and then applying a 20% rate to the excess tax base over $5,000. Since a higher percentage rate is applied as the tax base increases, this is a progressive rate structure.

Most excise taxes (e.g., sales taxes) employ a proportional tax rate. However, both the Federal income and transfer tax rates, as well as most state income tax rates, are progressive. The 2009 Federal income tax rate schedules for individual taxpayers appear on the inside front cover of this text for ready reference. The income tax rates for corporations, estates, and trusts are presented on the inside back cover of the text. The Federal gift and estate tax rates are reproduced in Appendix A-3 at the back of the text. A glance at either of these sources will indicate the progressive nature of the Federal tax system.

Marginal, Average, and Effective Tax Rates. It is not surprising that tax rates receive a great deal of attention. Since taxes have such a significant impact on taxpayer's lives, everyone has an interest in—as well as an opinion about—tax rates. Are tax rates too high or too low? Are they too progressive or too flat? In any dialogue regarding tax rates, it is important to understand the terminology and distinguish between three different tax rate concepts: the marginal rate, the average rate and the effective tax rate.

Marginal Tax Rates. The marginal tax rate of any tax rate structure is that percentage at which the next unit of the tax base will be taxed. For example, in the case of the income tax, if a taxpayer earns an additional dollar of income, the marginal rate would be the rate that applied to that dollar. The marginal tax rates of the Federal income tax rate structure for single and married taxpayers for 2009 and the amounts of income to which they apply are shown below:

Tax Rate	Single Taxpayers Taxable Income	Married Taxpayers Taxable Income
10%	$ 0 – $ 8,350	$ 0 – $ 16,700
15	8,350 – 33,950	16,700 – 67,900
25	33,950 – 82,250	67,900 – 137,050
28	82,250 – 171,550	137,050 – 208,850
33	171,550 – 372,950	208,850 – 372,950
35	Over 372,950	Over 372,950

Note the progressive nature of the rate structure. There are currently six marginal tax rates for individuals, starting at 10% and climbing to a high of 35%. Each of these rates applies to a range of income known as a tax bracket. It is not uncommon to hear people say they are in a particular tax bracket. If a single person says he is in the "25% bracket," it simply means that his taxable income is at a level ($33,950 – $82,250 in 2009) such that the next dollar of income is taxed at 25%. While the tax rates for married taxpayers are the same as those for singles, they generally apply to different brackets of income. For the 10% and 15% rates, the married brackets are exactly twice the size of those for single taxpayers but vary thereafter until the top rate is reached. The potential for implicit tax "penalties" for being married or single, depending on a couple's income, who earns it and other factors, is discussed in Chapter 4.

Over the years, the tax rates and ranges of income to which they apply have varied dramatically. The first income tax that applied in 1913 had seven rates, ranging from 1% to 7%. In contrast, in 1962 there were 23 brackets, beginning at a rate of 22% and ending at 91%! No doubt rates and brackets will continue to change as Congress deems it necessary to balance the budget, raise revenues or to provide a tax cut. A typical tax computation using the current tax rate schedule is illustrated below.

Example 8. H, an unmarried taxpayer, has taxable income of $35,000 for 2009. Referring to tax rate Schedule X on the inside front cover of this text, an unmarried taxpayer with taxable income of $35,000 has a tax of $4,937.50 as computed below. H's marginal tax rate is 25%.

2009 tax on $33,950	$4,675.00
Plus: Tax on income above $33,950 [($35,000 – $33,950 = $1,050) × 25%]	262.50
Tax liability	$4,937.50

A taxpayer's knowledge of his or her marginal tax rate is essential in any tax-planning effort to minimize taxes. Without such knowledge, the tax impact of an additional dollar of the tax base or an additional dollar deduction cannot be determined.

Example 9. Refer to *Example 8*. If unmarried taxpayer H, age 40, is considering depositing $5,000 in an Individual Retirement Account (the maximum amount allowed in 2009 as a deduction for Federal income tax purposes), he could determine his immediate tax savings to be $1,250 (the 25% marginal tax rate × the $5,000 income not taxed). Similarly, if H had a 33% marginal tax rate and wanted to know the after-tax amount of a proposed $10,000 increase in salary, he would simply multiply $10,000 by 67% (100% − 33%). In such case, the after-tax value of the $10,000 salary increase would be $6,700.

Many individuals, including those who are highly educated, do not understand the marginal tax rate concept. All too often one hears the expression, "I can't afford to earn more because it will throw me into a higher tax bracket and I will keep less than I do now after taxes." This theoretically cannot occur unless the marginal tax rate exceeds 100 percent.

While the rates above normally are used to compute an individual's tax liability, a lower rate can apply. An individual's gains from the sale of so-called capital assets (e.g., corporate stocks) held for more than a year receive preferential treatment. Such gains, referred to as long-term capital gains, usually are taxed at 15 percent but could be taxed as high as 28 percent. However, for 2008 and 2009 any long-term capital gains of taxpayers in either the 10 or 15 percent income tax bracket will be tax-free. Gains from sales of capital assets that are held for a year or less, short-term capital gains, are tax at an individual's ordinary rates.

Corporate tax rates, like individual rates, are progressive (see inside back cover). The rates run from 15% to 35%. Corporations with taxable incomes less than $75,000 may take advantage of the lower rates. When taxable income exceeds the $75,000 threshold, corporations generally face marginal rates of 34% up to $10,000,000 of taxable income and 35% for taxable incomes exceeding the $10,000,000 mark. The long-term capital gains of a corporation receive no preferential treatment and are taxed at regular rates.

Average Tax Rates. The average rate is computed by dividing the taxpayer's tax liability by the tax base. For the income tax, the average tax rate is simply the tax divided by taxable income (tax ÷ taxable income).

Example 10. K, an unmarried taxpayer, has 2009 taxable income of $82,250 and pays a tax of $16,750. Although her marginal tax rate is 25%, K's average tax rate is only 20.36% ($16,750 ÷ $82,250).

Average tax rates are a bit misleading in that they seem to suggest that all units of the tax base (e.g., all dollars of income) are treated equally. But as seen above, in a progressive tax rate system where marginal rates increase as income increases, some dollars of income are taxed higher than others. The average tax rate is just that, an average. While providing some insight about the overall rate structure, average rates say little about the true impact of a tax on the taxpayer. For this information, effective tax rates are the preferred statistic.

Effective Tax Rates. The effective tax rate is computed by dividing the tax by some broader measure other than the tax base, often some quantity reflecting taxpayer's ability to pay. For example, for the income tax, the effective tax rate is normally determined by dividing the tax by total economic income (tax ÷ total economic income).

Example 11. Assume the same facts as in *Example 10* except that K's total economic income is $100,000 the $17,750 difference between total income and taxable income being attributable to exclusions and deductions (e.g., interest on tax-exempt bonds and the personal exemption). In such case, K would pay taxes at an effective rate of 16.75% [$16,750 ÷ $100,000].

Marginal rates are often confused with average rates and effective rates. For example, in decrying the harshness of the income tax, people often point to their marginal rate and declare that they are paying that percent (e.g., 25%) of their income to the government. A comparison of Examples 10 and 11 above reveals that this clearly is not the case. Although the taxpayer has a marginal tax rate of 25%, the average rate is 20.36% and the effective rate is only 16.75%.

While effective tax rates provide meaningful information about a taxpayer's tax burden, it is not without problems, the most difficult of which is that there is no uniform definition of total economic income or the amount that will serve as the denominator in the formula. Any use of effective tax rates must recognize this potential weakness. In practice, however, the denominator for any particular purpose such as financial reporting or economic studies is usually well-defined from the outset. As a result, effective tax rates (ETRs) usually provide a relatively straightforward measure of the percentage of income siphoned away by taxes. For this reason, ETRs are of great interest not only to individual taxpayers but also businesses, governments (U.S. and foreign), investors, analysts, academics, public interest groups and others.

One of the most common uses of the ETR concept can be found in financial reporting. Since taxes have a significant impact on a company's earnings, management, investors, creditors and other users of financial statements are particularly interested in the company's ETR. Due to the importance of taxes on a company's net income, generally accepted accounting principles—specifically FAS 109 and its interpretations—require public companies to provide additional disclosures, a detailed footnote, regarding the impact of income taxes on financial statement income (book income).[9] This information includes the company's ETR. In this context, ETR generally is the percentage of taxes paid on pre-tax book income (tax ÷ pre-tax book income). Although a corporation's statutory U.S. tax rate is normally a flat 35 percent, the ETR usually differs. For example, the footnotes to the financial statements of Microsoft reported an ETR of 31% in 2006 and 26.3% in 2005. Such differences occur because book income may be higher or lower than taxable income. For example, interest income from municipal bonds is included in book income but is excluded from taxable income. Similarly dividend income is fully included in book income but corporations normally pay taxes on only 30 percent of their dividends. On the expense side, book income includes fines and penalties and life insurance premiums on key executives but taxable income does not allow deductions for such costs. In addition, book income includes income from foreign subsidiaries but is not included in a corporation's consolidated taxable income (until is repatriated or paid back to the U.S. usually through dividend payments).

The ETR is a useful tool since it provides a snapshot of whether a business is or is not paying taxes and if so, how much. In addition, the ETR provides a criterion for determining how well a business is managing its tax liability relative to other firms in the same industry or businesses as a whole.

Tax Credits. A tax credit is a dollar-for-dollar offset against a tax liability. A credit is quite different from a deduction, since it directly reduces the tax liability itself, whereas a deduction simply reduces the base amount subject to the tax.

---

[9] See *Accounting for Income Taxes*, Statement of Financial Accounting Standards No. 109, Financial Accounting Standards Board, 1992. For financial statement purposes, FAS 109 requires income tax expense to be based on financial statement income rather than actual taxable income. Thus actual taxes paid may differ significantly from the reported amount. The ETR provides a picture of the taxes actually paid relative to book income rather than taxable income.

Example 12. T is a single taxpayer with a 28% marginal tax rate. An additional $100 tax deduction would reduce T's tax by $28 (28% × $100). If the $100 qualified as a tax credit, however, T would have a $100 tax reduction—the equivalent of a $357 tax deduction at a marginal tax rate of 28% ($357 × 28% = $100).

Tax credits are discussed in detail in Chapter 13 of this text.

MAJOR TYPES OF TAXES

Taxing authorities within the United States have a wide array of taxes with which they raise revenues or attempt to effect social, political, or economic change. The average individual will feel the impact of quite a number of taxes during his or her lifetime. Any attempt to accumulate wealth requires diligent tax planning, and to ignore the impact of Federal, state, and local taxes will serve no useful purpose toward this end. Although the principal thrust of this text is aimed at the Federal income and wealth transfer taxes, some of the other types of taxes merit a brief introduction.

INCOME TAXES

An income tax is an extraction of some of the taxpayer's economic gain, usually on a periodic basis. In addition to the Federal government, many states and some local governments impose a tax on income. For example, New York City residents could pay not only a federal income tax of 35 percent but also a state income tax of 7.7 percent and a city income tax of 4.45 percent. As noted earlier in Exhibit 1-1, the individual income tax was expected to provide 45 percent of the Federal government's fiscal 2009 revenues. Of all the sources providing revenues to the Federal government, the individual income tax is the largest. In contrast, the corporate income tax was expected to provide only 11 percent of the Federal government's projected revenues in fiscal 2009.[10]

The Federal government imposes an income tax on individuals, corporations, estates, and trusts. Usually, a final tax reckoning (reporting and paying taxes due) is made at the end of each year. In order to ensure tax collections, however, Congress has created a pay-as-you-go requirement. Basically, this process requires employers to withhold and remit to the Federal government income taxes on wages paid to employees. Individuals with income from sources other than wages, and most other taxable entities, are required to make estimated tax prepayments during the year.[11]

Application of the Federal income tax to individuals is discussed in Chapters 3 and 4. Computation of a corporation's Federal income tax is explained in Chapter 19. The Federal income taxation of partnerships, estates, and trusts is examined in Chapters 22 and 25. For now, the procedures for determining the Federal income tax liability of corporate and individual taxpayers are reduced to computational formulas presented in Exhibits 1-2 and 1-3 as follows. The components of these formulas are introduced and discussed in greater detail in Chapter 3.

---

[10] Such heavy reliance on the income tax as a source of government revenues is peculiar to the United States. Most Western European nations have turned to a Value-Added Tax (VAT). A VAT is a system of taxing the increment in value of goods as they move through the production and manufacturing process to the market place. The VAT operates very much like a national sales tax and has occasionally been proposed, though unsuccessfully, for the United States.

[11] This procedure was developed by Congress during World War II to accelerate annual tax payments needed to finance the war effort. The process served so well to increase compliance with, and facilitate administration of, the Federal income tax law that Congress chose not to abandon it at the close of the war.

EXHIBIT 1-2

Tax Formula For Corporate Taxpayers

Income (from whatever source)	$xxx,xxx
Less: Exclusions from gross income	−xx,xxx
Gross income	$xxx,xxx
Less: Deductions	−xx,xxx
Taxable income	$xxx,xxx
Applicable tax rates	xx%
Gross tax	$ xx,xxx
Less: Tax credits and prepayments	−x,xxx
Tax due (or refund)	$ xx,xxx

EXHIBIT 1-3

Tax Formula for Individual Taxpayers

Income (from whatever source)		$xxx,xxx
Less: Exclusions from gross income		−xx,xxx
Gross income		$xxx,xxx
Less: Deductions for adjusted gross income		−xx,xxx
Adjusted gross income		$xxx,xxx
Less: 1. The larger of:		
a. Standard deduction	$x,xxx	
or	*or*	−x,xxx
b. Total itemized deductions	$x,xxx	
2. Personal and dependency exemptions ×		
exemption amount		−x,xxx
Taxable income		$xxx,xxx
Applicable tax rates (from Tables or Schedules X, Y, or Z)		xx%
Gross tax		$ xx,xxx
Less: Tax credits and prepayments		−x,xxx
Tax due (or refund)		$ xx,xxx

Most states in the United States impose an income tax of some sort.[12] Generally, state income taxes are designed to operate much like the Federal income tax. Almost all the states have a tax-withholding procedure and most use the income determination for Federal income tax purposes as the tax base. Some states allow a deduction for Federal income taxes, while others exclude income that is subject to Federal income taxation. Interest income from Federal government obligations is not subject to state income taxation, and interest income from state and local government obligations generally is not

---

[12] States *not* currently imposing an income tax on individuals are Alaska, Florida, Nevada, South Dakota, Texas, Washington, and Wyoming. Tennessee and New Hampshire impose an income tax on an individual's dividend and interest income. Every state imposes either a corporate income tax or a tax on the privilege of conducting business within the state's boundaries. See subsequent discussion of franchise taxes.

subject to either Federal or state income taxation. Most states have developed their own set of rates, exemptions, and credits; however, the filing date for the state income tax return generally coincides with the due date of the taxpayer's Federal income tax return.[13]

One particular problem that has developed in the area of state taxation is the so-called unitary tax. Several states[14] tax businesses on the basis of their global activities, not just their local operations. This asserted right to tax income that has not been earned within the state's boundaries has been subjected to many challenges in the courts; but, as of this date, the unitary tax has not been struck down as unconstitutional.[15] Foreign corporations object to this worldwide combined reporting for many reasons, the most obvious being that it may result in the imposition of state taxation even when no taxable income has been generated by intrastate operations.

WEALTH TRANSFER TAXES

Unlike Federal and state income taxes, wealth transfer taxes are not significant revenue producers. For example, Federal transfer tax revenues for fiscal year 2009 represent less than 1 percent of Federal government revenues.[16] Historically, the primary function of wealth transfer taxes has been to *hinder* the accumulation of wealth by family units. Thus, the goal of wealth redistribution generally underlies the design of estate and gift tax systems.

The estate tax and its partner, the gift tax, are both excise taxes on the transfers of property. The estate tax is imposed on the amount of a decedent's *net* wealth (fair market value of total assets less debts and expenses) that passes to his or her heirs at death. Absent any other rule, the estate tax easily could be avoided by giving away property before death. For this reason, Congress enacted a tax on gifts. The gift tax is imposed on the value of property transferred during an individual's life. As explained below, only a relatively small percentage of taxpayers are affected by the gift or estate tax since they apply only when the transfer of wealth is substantial, (e.g., more than $1,000,000 during life or $3,500,000 at death). But for those to whom the taxes do apply, the cost can be significant.

Prior to 1977, the gift tax and estate tax were two separate taxes. Taxable gifts made during life generally did not impact the estate tax calculation. However, in 1976, the gift tax and estate tax were combined into what is conceptually a unified transfer tax. The taxes are unified in the way that the taxes are calculated. As an individual makes taxable gifts during life, the gift tax is computed on a cumulative basis. To calculate the tax on current year gifts, the donor must add all taxable gifts made in prior years (since 1976) to the current gifts, calculate the gross tax on the sum of the lifetime transfers, and then subtract gift taxes assessed on the prior years' gifts. The remainder is the current year gift tax. When the individual dies, the estate tax is computed in a similar manner by adding all prior taxable gifts to the taxable estate, applying the appropriate rate and subtracting any prior gift taxes assessed. It is sometimes useful to think of the transfer at death as the final gift. Note that in both cases, the addition of prior taxable gifts does not result in the gifts being taxed twice but only raises the marginal rate at which the current transfers are taxed. Like the Federal income tax rate structure, the gift tax and the estate tax rates are progressive.

As a practical matter, the estate and gift tax do not apply to most taxpayers. For starters, to eliminate the vast administrative problems that would result if the gift tax were

---

[13]   For individuals and partnerships, the due date of the Federal income tax return is the fifteenth day of the fourth month following the close of the tax year. For corporate taxpayers, the due date of the Federal return is the fifteenth day of the *third* month following the close of the tax year.

[14]   Among those states that tax businesses on the basis of worldwide income are Alaska, California, Colorado, Florida, Idaho, Illinois, Indiana, Massachusetts, Montana, New Hampshire, New York (oil companies only), North Dakota, Oregon, and Utah.

[15]   The U.S. Supreme Court upheld California's system of taxing global profits of U.S.-based multinational businesses in *Container Corporation of America v. Franchise Tax Board*, 103 S.Ct. 2933 (USSC, 1983).

[16]   Office of Management and Budget, 2009 *Fiscal Year Budget*.

imposed on all gifts (e.g., birthday presents), the tax is imposed only on those transfers that exceed a certain threshold. In 2009, this amount is $13,000. Technically, individuals are entitled to an exclusion of $13,000 per donee per year. The exclusion enables an individual to make an unlimited number of gifts as long as they do not exceed $13,000 per donee in one year. For married couples, these rules permit a husband and wife to give $26,000 a year to a particular donee (e.g., a child) tax free. In addition, to the annual exclusion, gifts to a spouse, charity or transfers for educational or medical purposes normally are not taxable.

Provisions also exist to ensure that only transfers of substantial wealth are subject to tax. For gift tax purposes, gifts in excess of amounts excluded are not subject to tax until the cumulative amount of all gifts exceeds $1,000,000. Similarly, at death, in 2009, there is no estate tax unless total transfers during life and at death exceed $3,500,000. It should be noted that once transfers exceed these levels, the tax is quite high. When total gifts exceed the $1,000,000 mark, the marginal rate begins at 41 percent and rises to 45 percent. When the estate (including lifetime gifts) exceeds the $3,500,000 amount, the marginal rate is 45 percent for 2009. A more detailed discussion of these taxes is provided below.

The Federal Estate Tax. Discussed in detail in Chapter 24, the procedure for computing the Federal estate tax liability is illustrated in Exhibit 1-4.

EXHIBIT 1-4
Computation of Federal Estate Tax Liability

Gross estate		$x,xxx,xxx
Less the sum of:		
Expenses, indebtedness, and taxes	$ xx,xxx	
State death taxes	x,xxx	
Losses	x,xxx	
Charitable bequests	xx,xxx	
Marital deduction	xxx,xxx	−xxx,xxx
Taxable estate		$ xxx,xxx
Plus: Taxable gifts made after December 31, 1976		+xx,xxx
Total taxable transfers		$ xxx,xxx
Tentative tax on total transfer		$ xxx,xxx
Less the sum of:		
Gift taxes paid on post-1976 taxable gifts	$ x,xxx	
Estate tax credit	xx,xxx	
Other tax credits	x,xxx	−xx,xxx
Estate tax liability		$ xx,xxx

A decedent's gross estate includes the value of *all* property owned at date of death, wherever located. This includes the proceeds of an insurance policy on the life of the decedent if the decedent's estate is the beneficiary, or if the decedent had any ownership rights[17] in the policy at time of death. Property is generally included in the gross estate at its *fair market value* as of the date of death.[18]

---

[17] Ownership rights in a life insurance policy include the power to change the policy's beneficiary, the right to cancel or assign the policy, and the right to borrow against the policy.

[18] An executor of a taxable estate may elect an alternative valuation date of six months after death. See Chapter 24 for more details.

The taxable estate is the gross estate reduced by deductions allowed for funeral and administrative expenses, debts of the decedent, certain taxes and losses, state dealth taxes and charitable gifts made from the decedent's estate. It is important to note that there is no limit imposed on the charitable deduction. If an individual is willing to leave his or her entire estate for public, charitable, or religious use, there will be no taxable estate. Finally, an *unlimited* marital deduction is allowed for the value of property passing to a surviving spouse. Thus, if a married taxpayer leaves all of his or her property to the surviving spouse, no Federal estate tax will be imposed on the estate. On the death of the surviving spouse, the couple's wealth may be subject to taxation.[19]

Under current Federal estate tax laws, taxable gifts made after 1976 are added to the taxable estate to arrive at total taxable transfers. A tentative estate tax is then computed on the base amount. All gift taxes paid on post-1976 gifts, as well as certain tax credits, are subtracted from this tentative tax in arriving at the Federal estate tax due, if any. Most estate tax credits have a single underlying purpose—to reduce or eliminate the effect of multiple taxation of a single estate. Estate taxes paid to the various states or foreign countries on property owned by the decedent and located within their boundaries are examples of estate tax credits. However, the major credit available to reduce the Federal estate tax has been the *unified credit*.

The unified credit was a lifetime credit available for all taxable transfers, including taxable gifts made after 1976 through 2003. It had to be used when available; a taxpayer could not decide to postpone use of the credit if he or she made a taxable transfer in any given year. Over the years, the relief provided by the unified credit slowly eroded away with inflation. As a result, more and more taxpayers feared that they would be required to pay estate taxes. With the *Taxpayer Relief Act of 1997*, Congress responded to this fear by increasing the amount of the unified credit to an equivalent exemption of $1,000,000. This amount was further increased by the *Economic Growth and Tax Relief Reconciliation Act of 2001*. Under the 2001 legislation, the unified credit became two separate credits—one for estate tax and another one for gift tax. The estate tax credit was scheduled to grow over the eight years beginning in 2001, eventually reaching an equivalent exclusion amount of $3,500,000. However, the gift tax credit was set at a maximum of $345,800 (an exemption equivalent of $1,000,000). The credit increase for estate taxes occurs ratably as follows:

	Credit		Exemption Equivalent	
Year	Estate Tax	Gift Tax	Estate Tax	Gift Tax
2002–03	$ 345,800	$345,800	$1,000,000	$1,000,000
2004–05	555,800	345,800	1,500,000	1,000,000
2006–08	780,800	345,800	2,000,000	1,000,000
2009	1,455,800	345,800	3,500,000	1,000,000
2010	Repealed	345,800	Repealed	1,000,000

In 2010, the estate tax, but *not* the gift tax, is scheduled for repeal. The repeal is currently legislated for one year only, however. In 2011, the estate tax returns, with the exemption equivalent amount reverting back to $1 million. The gift tax exemption equivalent amount is increased to $1 million in 2001 and stays there unless and until it is further changed in subsequent legislation.

In 2009, the estate tax credit is $1,455,800. This amount of credit completely offsets the tax on $3,500,000 of taxable transfers (see Appendix A for the Estate and Gift Transfer Tax Rate Schedules currently in effect). Thus, an individual may make substantial transfers of wealth *before* any tax liability is incurred.

---

[19] Planning for maximizing the benefit of the unlimited marital deduction is discussed in Chapter 26 .

Example 13. In 2009, D died owning Google stock worth $3,500,000. D had never made a taxable gift. D was not married and had no deductions. In such case, the taxable estate and total taxable transfers would be $3,500,000, and there would be no estate tax computed as follows:

Taxable estate and total taxable transfers	$3,500,000
Gross estate tax (see Appendix A-3).	$1,455,800
Estate tax credit.	(1,455,800)
Tax due.	$ 0

Note how the estate tax credit operates to exempt $3,500,000 of total taxable transfers from tax. For this reason, it is commonly said that taxpayers have an estate tax exemption equal to $3,500,000.

The Federal Gift Tax. The purpose of the federal gift tax is to prevent a taxpayer's avoidance of the federal estate tax simply by giving away his or her property prior to death. The procedure for computing the federal gift tax liability is presented as a formula in Exhibit 1-5. To arrive at taxable gifts for the year, the taxpayer's total gifts may be reduced by the annual exclusion and by the deductions allowed for property transferred to a spouse or charity. In computing taxable gifts for the current year, note that a donor is allowed an annual exclusion of $13,000 per donee in 2009. The annual exclusion is allowed *each year* even if the donor has made gifts in the prior years to the same donee.

EXHIBIT 1-5
Computation of Federal Gift Tax Liability

Fair market value of all gifts made in the current year		$xxx,xxx
Less the sum of:		
Annual exclusions ($13,000 per donee in 2009)	$ xx,xxx	
Marital deduction	xx,xxx	
Charitable deduction	x,xxx	−xx,xxx
Taxable gifts for current year		$xxx,xxx
Plus: Taxable gifts made in prior years		+xx,xxx
Taxable transfers to date		$xxx,xxx
Tentative tax on total transfers to date		$ xx,xxx
Less the sum of:		
Gift taxes computed at current rates on prior years' taxable gifts	$ x,xxx	
Gift tax credit	x,xxx	−x,xxx
Gift tax due on current gifts.		$ xx,xxx

Example 14. T, a widower, wanted his son, daughter-in-law, and their five children to share his wealth. On December 25, 2009 he gave $13,000 to each family member. He repeats these gifts in 2010. Although T has transferred $182,000 [$13,000 × 7 (number of donees) × 2], he has not made taxable gifts in either 2009 or 2010.

The marital and charitable deductions for Federal gift tax purposes are the same as for the Federal estate tax—*unlimited*. Thus, if a taxpayer gives his or her spouse a $2,000,000 anniversary present or transfers $100,000 to his or her church, a taxable gift has not been made.

If taxable gifts have been made for the current year, the cumulative computational procedure of the gift transfer tax must be applied.

Example 15. In 2000, X made his first taxable gift of $100,000 (after the exclusion). The tax (before credits) on this amount was $23,800. X made a second taxable gift of $85,000 in 2009. The tax (before credits) on the second gift is $26,200, computed as follows:

2000 taxable gift	$100,000
2009 taxable gift	+85,000
Cumulative gifts.	$185,000
Tax on cumulative taxable gifts of $185,000.	$ 50,000
2000 taxable gift.	−23,800*
Tax on 2009 gift.	$ 26,200

* See the estate and gift transfer tax rate schedules in Appendix A. Note that the current year's tax rate is used to compute the tax reduction for the 2000 gift.

Note that the cumulative system of wealth transfer taxation *and* the progressive rate schedule cause a higher tax on the 2009 gift, even though the 2009 gift was $15,000 *less* than the 2000 gift.

The tentative tax liability in the above example is reduced by the unified credit available for the gift tax, $345,800. The gift tax credit is the only credit available to offset the federal gift tax liability.

The unified credit for the gift tax is $345,800 and is equivalent to an exemption of $1,000,000. In applying the credit, it is important to understand that whatever amount is used in one year reduces the amount of the credit available in future years or at death. In other words, if a taxpayer makes no taxable gifts during his or her lifetime, the entire unified credit of $1,455,800 in 2009 is available to reduce any estate taxes that otherwise may be due at the taxpayer's death (see Example above). In contrast, if the taxpayer uses all $345,800 of the unified credit to reduce gift taxes, such amount is not available at death.

Example 16. Prior to 2009, T had never made a taxable gift. In 2009, T made her first *taxable* gift of $1,000,000. Using the rate schedule, the gift tax on the $1,000,000 taxable transfer prior to application of the unified credit would be $345,800. However, the credit of $345,800 would completely eliminate the tax. The calculation is shown below:

Current taxable gift	$1,000,000
Prior taxable gifts.	—
Total taxable gifts	$1,000,000
Tax	$ 345,800
Unified credit	(345,800)
Gift tax due.	$ 0

Example 17. In 2000, Y made her first taxable gift of $350,000. Assume the tax calculated on this gift is $104,800. Y is required to use any available gift tax credit. Consequently, she used $104,800 of her available gift tax credit so that the actual gift tax due is reduced to zero. In 2009, Y makes her second taxable gift of $2,000,000. The tax on this gift is computed as follows:

Taxable gift for 2009		$ 2,000,000
Plus: 2000 taxable gift		+350,000
Taxable transfers to date		$ 2,350,000
Tentative tax on total transfers		
to date (see Appendix A for tax rates)		$ 938,300
Less: Gift taxes calculated on 2000 gift		−104,800
Tentative tax on 2009 gift		$ 833,500
Less: Remaining gift tax credit:		
Total gift credit available for 2009	$ 345,800	
Less: Gift tax credit		
used in 2000.	− 104,800	− 241,000
Gift tax due on 2009 gift		$ 592,500

Another unique feature of the Federal gift tax involves the *gift-splitting* election available to a married donor. If a donor makes the election on his or her current gift tax return, one half of all gifts made during the year will be considered to have been made by the donor's spouse. The election is valid *only if* both spouses *consent* to gift-splitting.

Example 18. In 2009 husband H makes two gifts of $100,000 each to his son and daughter. His wife W makes a gift of $5,000 to the daughter only. H and W elect gift-splitting on their 2009 gift tax returns. As a result, H will report a gift to the son of $50,000 and a gift to the daughter of $52,500 [$1/2$ of ($100,000 + $5,000)], and will claim two $13,000 gift tax exclusions. W will report exactly the same gifts and claim two annual exclusions. Without gift-splitting, H would still be entitled to $26,000 of exclusions, but W could only claim an exclusion of $5,000 for her gift to the daughter. Thus, by electing to split gifts, a married donor can, in effect, make use of any annual exclusions not needed by his or her spouse. More importantly, if taxable gifts are made under a gift-splitting arrangement, H can use his unified credit and W can use her lifetime credit to reduce the tax liability.

State and Local Transfer Taxes. Many states and some local jurisdictions impose an inheritance tax on the *right to receive* property at death. Unlike an estate tax, which is imposed on the estate according to value of property transferred by the decedent at death, an inheritance tax is imposed on the recipient of property from an estate.[20] The amount of an inheritance tax payable usually is directly affected by the degree of kinship between the recipient and the decedent. The inheritance tax typically provides an exemption from the tax, which increases as the relationship between the recipient (e.g., surviving spouse, children, grandchildren, parents, etc.) and the decedent becomes closer. In addition, as the relationship becomes closer, the transfer tax rates decrease. Thus, the more closely related one is, the smaller the inheritance tax will be. Generally, little if any inheritance tax exemption is available for transfers to unrelated recipients, and the highest rate is imposed.

---

[20] It is not uncommon for the decedent's will to provide that his or her estate pay any inheritance tax imposed on the recipient of property from the estate.

Example 19. The Indiana inheritance tax is similar to most inheritance taxes. For example, transfers to a surviving spouse and charities are totally exempt. In contrast, the exemption for transfers to children and grandchildren is $100,000, and the rates on the excess run from 1 to 10 percent. As the relationship between the decedent and the beneficiary grows more distant, the exemption shrinks and the rates grow. The exemption for transfers to brothers and sisters and their descendants (e.g., nieces and nephews) is only $500, and the rates range from 7 to 15 percent. Finally, transfers to nonrelatives (e.g., friends) are subject to an even lower exemption, $100, and the rates extend from 10 to 20 percent.

In addition to state and local inheritance taxes on beneficiaries, many states also impose estate taxes on the decedent's estate. The rates imposed on the taxable estate are considerably lower than those of the federal estate tax rates.[21] Beginning in 2005, any inheritance or estate taxes imposed by a state are deductible in computing the Federal taxable estate. While most states impose some type of death tax, only a few states have a gift tax. In those states where there is no gift tax, wholesale avoidance of any state death tax is prohibited by certain special rules. For example, a state law may require that transfers made within one year of death to be included in the death tax base.

EMPLOYMENT TAXES

The Federal government and most states impose some form of employment tax on either self-employed individuals, employees,[22] or employers. The most common form of state employment tax is levied on wages, with the proceeds used to finance the state's unemployment benefits program. State unemployment taxes are imposed on employers who have employees working within the state's boundaries, but only if the employees would be eligible for unemployment benefits from the state. Most states' unemployment taxes are based on the same taxable wage base as that used for the Federal unemployment tax (see discussion below), and employers are allowed to take state unemployment taxes paid as a credit against the Federal unemployment tax liability.

The Federal government imposes two types of taxes on employment—a social security tax and an unemployment tax. The Federal Insurance Contribution Act (FICA) imposes a tax on self-employed individuals, employees, and employers. The FICA tax is paid by both an employee and his or her employer if the employee is eligible for social security and Medicare health insurance benefits. Although subject to a different tax rate, self-employed individuals are required to pay FICA taxes on net earnings from self-employment. The Federal Unemployment Tax Act (FUTA) imposes a tax *only* on the employer. Self-employed individuals are not eligible for unemployment benefits and thus are not subject to the FUTA tax. The tax base and rate structure of both these Federal employment taxes are presented below.

FICA Taxes. FICA taxes, often referred to as Social Security and Medicare taxes, have a long history. Both taxes help pay for a variety of federal programs that together assist individuals in times of need such as old-age, disability, death and illness. Social Security was enacted in 1935 to pay a guaranteed source of income to retired workers normally when they reach age 65. Since 1935 the Act has been modified many, many

---

[21] States that impose both an estate and inheritance tax generally allow a credit against the state estate tax for any inheritance tax imposed on the heirs.

[22] The term "employee" is used to identify persons whose work effort, tools, place of work, and work time periods are subject to the supervision and control of another (the employer). A person who provides his or her own tools and who has the *right* to exercise control over when, where, and for whom services are rendered (i.e., an independent contractor) generally is classified as self-employed rather than as an employee. See Chapter 8 for a discussion of the importance this classification has in the deductions allowed to individuals for Federal income tax purposes.

times, providing more and more benefits. For example, major additions occurred in 1956 and 1960 when the Act was amended to extend benefits for most disabled workers and their families. The programs established by these amendments are now collectively known as the Old Age, Survivors and Disability Insurance (OASDI) programs. In addition to these programs, Congress addressed problems of health care for the aged with the creation of Medicare Health Insurance (MHI) in 1965. Medicare helps pay hospital and medical expenses for persons who have reached age 65. In 2006, Medicare was amended to help pay for prescription drugs.

The Social Security and Medicare programs are paid for primarily through taxes on wages and self-employment income. Taxes to pay for Social Security benefits were first collected in January 1937 at a rate of 1 percent on the first $3,000 of wages or a maximum of only $30! In 1966, tax collections began for Medicare at a rate of .35 percent on the same wage base as for Social Security. At that point, 1966, the total tax for the two components of FICA, Social Security and Medicare, was 4.2 percent (3.85 + .35) on wages of $6,600 or a maximum of $2,772. Since those early days both the tax rates as well as the base have swelled. The rates stopped climbing–at least temporarily–in 1990 when they reached what they are currently: 6.2 percent for Social Security and 1.45 percent for Medicare. The wage base for Social Security changes every year and in 2009 is $106,800. Until 1992, the wage base for Medicare was the same as for Social Security but starting in 1993 the base for Medicare became unlimited and remains unlimited today.

Employees and Employers. FICA taxes are imposed at the combined rate of 7.65 percent (6.2% social security + 1.45% MHI) on each dollar of an employee's wages up to $106,800 plus 1.45 percent on each additional dollar of wages in 2009. As explained above, there is no maximum amount on the MHI component of the FICA tax because the 1.45 percent MHI tax is applicable to *all* compensation. The employer is required to pay a matching amount of FICA taxes for each employee (i.e., the same tax rates on each employee's wage base up to the same limits).[23]

> **Example 20.** During 2009 employee E earns wages of $70,000. As a result, E will pay $5,355 (7.65% × $70,000) FICA taxes, and her employer must pay the same amount as an employment tax.

> **Example 21.** During 2009 employee F earns wages of $240,000. As a result F will pay $10,102 FICA taxes, and her employer must pay the same amount as an employment tax. It is important to note that the 1.45% MHI tax has no ceiling amount. The calculation is as follows:

Social security portion = 6.2% × $106,800 limit	$ 6,622
Plus: MHI portion = 1.45% × $240,000	+3,480
Total FICA taxes	$10,102

An employer is required to withhold both Federal income taxes and FICA taxes from each employee's wages paid during the year. The employer is then required to remit these withheld amounts plus the employer's matching FICA taxes for each employee to the IRS on a regular basis, usually weekly or monthly.[24] Employers also are required to file Form 941, Employer's Quarterly Federal Tax Return, by the end of the first month following each quarter of the calendar year (e.g., by April 30, 2009 for the quarter ended

---

[23] Employers are allowed a tax deduction for all payroll taxes. See Chapter 7 for a discussion of business deductions.

[24] The frequency of these payments depends on the total amount of Federal income taxes withheld and the FICA taxes due on the employer's periodic payroll. The amount of Federal income and FICA taxes to be withheld from each employee's wages, and the reporting and payment requirements are specified in Circular E, *Employer's Tax Guide*, a free publication of the Internal Revenue Service.

March 31, 2009), and pay any remaining amount of employment taxes due for the previous quarter.[25]

In some instances, an employee who has had more than one employer during the year may have paid *excess* FICA taxes for the year and will be entitled to a Federal income tax credit or refund for the excess.

> **Example 22.** During 2009 E earned $100,000 from his regular job and $50,000 from a part-time job. E's full time employer withheld $7,650 ($100,000 × 7.65%) and E's part time employer withheld $3,825 ($50,000 × 7.65%). Each employer made matching contributions and paid the withheld amount and the employer's match to the IRS. Since E has paid a total of $11,475 ($7,650 + $3,825) FICA taxes and the maximum amount due for 2009 is $8,797 [($106,800 × 6.2% = $6,622) + ($150,000 × 1.45% = $2,175)], E will be entitled to a tax credit or refund of the $2,678, the difference between the $11,475 he paid and the $8,797 that is due. Note that this simply represents the FICA taxes withheld on E's wages in excess of the $102,000 maximum amount subject to the 6.2% Social Security rate in 2009 ($150,000 − $106,800 = $43,200 × 6.2% = $2,678).

Self-Employed Taxpayers. Like employees, self-employed individuals are normally required to pay FICA taxes on their self-employment income (commonly known as self-employment tax or the SE tax). The social security portion of self-employment tax rate is 12.4 percent and the MHI portion is 2.9 percent. These rates are *twice* the FICA tax rates imposed on an employee's wages. In 2009, the ceiling amount for the social security portion of the SE tax is $106,800, the same as for employees. As a result, taxpayers with self-employment income not exceeding this amount will pay an SE tax of 15.3 percent on their self-employment income. This tax is computed as part of Form 1040 on Schedule SE. (See Appendix B for this form.) Note that a taxpayer is not required to pay self-employment taxes unless he or she has self-employment income of $400 or more.[26]

Self-Employment Income. Self-employed persons do not receive wages. Employees receive wages. The equivalent of wages for a self-employed person is self-employment income. Self-employment income is generally the trade or business income earned by an individual as an independent contractor, a sole proprietor or a general partner in a partnership. Self-employment income does not include income passive in nature or investment income such as interest, dividends or rents. Nor does it include gains from the sale of property (other than sales of inventory or property customarily held for sale to customers). Note that self-employment income is a "net" concept so expenses related to producing the income may be subtracted in reaching the base.

The most common type of self-employment income is that received by for providing services *other than in an employee capacity.* For example, it includes income earned by accountants, tax preparers, doctors, dentists, veterinarians, engineers, lawyers and consultants as long as they are independent contractors, sole proprietors or general partners. But self-employment income is not limited to income earned by professionals. It also includes income earned by such persons as farmers, fisherman, contractors, subcontractors, massage therapists, graphic designers, hair stylists, salesmen and freelance writers. Income from odd jobs also counts as self-employment income such as income from babysitting and child care, mowing lawns, driving a taxi, painting, tutoring, selling

---

[25] Because of significant penalties for underpayment of these Federal employment taxes, most employers exercise great care to make payments on a timely basis. See Circular E for a discussion of these penalties and due dates.

[26] Technically, self-employment income is defined as "net earnings from self-employment." Because the amount of net earnings from self-employment is 92.35% of self-employment income, there is no self-employment tax unless the taxpayer's self-employment income is $433 ($400/92.35%) or more. See §§ 1401 and 1402(b).

handicrafts, operating a bed and breakfast or serving on a board of directors. In all cases, the services must have been performed as an independent contractor, sole proprietor or partner to be considered self-employment income.

Whether an individual is an independent contractor or an employee depends on the facts in each case. An individual is normally considered an independent contractor if the payer has the right to control or direct only the result of the work and not how it will be done. Unfortunately, this is a dreadfully controversial area. As might be expected, payers, wanting to avoid payment of a 7.65 percent employment tax, are inclined to call a worker an independent contractor. Conversely, the government, hoping to ensure the collection of employment and income taxes, wants to classify the worker as an employee. To dissuade employers from misclassification, the government imposes severe penalties if the employer intentionally classifies a worker as an independent contractor when it is clear he or she is an employee.

In most cases, an independent contractor's self-employment income is reported to the taxpayer on Form 1099. Just like an employer that must provide an employee with a Form W-2 reporting wages earned, businesses must give a Form 1099 to any "independent contractor" who provides $600 or more of services to the business during the year. Generally a payer is not required to provide a Form 1099 to a corporation but there are a number of exceptions. For example, businesses must always give attorneys a Form 1099 regardless of the form of business in which the attorneys perform their services. Note that while the reporting threshold for a payer is $600, an individual is not required to pay self-employment tax unless his or her total self-employment income is $400 or more.

Calculation of Self-Employment Tax. As a general rule, the self-employment tax is 15.3 percent of self-employment income. However, in computing the amount of a taxpayer's self-employment income subject to tax, a special adjustment is required as explained in the following example.

> **Example 23.** S is a sole proprietor who prepares tax returns. This year his income from operations net of all expenses *except* the self-employment tax related to such income is $10,000. To arrive at the correct measure of *net* income for the sole proprietorship, the taxpayer must reduce the $10,000 by the portion of the self-employment tax that represents a cost of doing business. This is analogous to an employer whose labor expenses include the 7.65 percent FICA tax on an employee's wages (i.e., the employer's matching share of FICA). A self-employed person incurs a similar cost and that cost is one-half of the individual's self-employment tax. Consequently, to determine the self-employment tax base, the tax preparer's income of $10,000 is reduced by one-half of the hypothetical self-employment tax on the $10,000 or $765 [$10,000 × 7.65% (15.3% × $^1/_2$)]. This results in self-employment income subject to tax of $9,235 ($10,000 − $765). The actual self-employment tax is $1,412.96 (15.3% × $9,235).

Following the approach above, in computing the amount subject to tax for each of the self-employment tax bases (both the 12.4 percent and the 2.9 percent), the taxpayer always reduces net earnings from self-employment by an amount equal to one-half the combined 15.3 percent tax rate times net earnings from self-employment (i.e., 7.65% × net earnings from self-employment).[27] Note that this adjustment applies only in the computation of the amount of the self-employment tax bases. However, consistent with the theory above, a self-employed individual is entitled to an actual deduction for one-half of the self-employment tax as a business expense in computing adjusted gross income. Using the facts of the example, the actual deduction would be $706.48 (1/2 × actual self-employment tax of $1,412.96). Observe that the actual deduction in computing adjusted

---

[27] § 1402(a)(12).

gross income is $706.48 and not the $765 used to compute the self-employment tax bases. Examples of these calculations are given below.

Each component of the self-employment tax required to be paid is computed as follows:

1. Multiply net earnings from self-employment by one-half of the self-employment tax rate, 7.65% (1/2 × 15.3%) and subtract that amount to reach a tentative tax base of 92.35% of the original amount.[28]

2. Compare the result in step 1 with the maximum base amount for the social security portion of the self-employment tax ($106,800 for 2009) and select the smaller amount.

3. Multiply the amount in step 1 by the Medicare rate of 2.9% and the amount in step 2 by the Social Security rate of 12.4%.

4. Add the amounts of the separate components from step 3. This is the amount of self-employment tax required to be paid.

Example 24. Individuals C and D have net earnings from self-employment for 2009 of $50,000 and $150,000, respectively. Self-employment taxes for C and D are determined as follows:

Self-employment tax computation	C		D	
Social Security (12.4% portion)				
Net earnings from self-employment..........	$50,000		$150,000	
− (1/2 × 15.3% = 7.65%) of net earnings	(3,825)		(11,475)	
SE tax base (92.35% net earnings)*	$46,175		$138,525	
Smaller of SE tax base above or				
maximum wage base ($106,800 for 2009) ..	$46,175		$106,800	
× _____ 12.4%	× 12.4%		× 12.4%	
Social Security tax		$5,726		$13,243
MHI (2.9% portion)				
Net earnings from self-employment..........	$50,000		$150,000	
− (1/2 × 15.3% = 7.65%) of net earnings	(3,825)		(11,475)	
SE tax base (92.35% net earnings)**	$46,175		$138,525	
× _____ 2.9%	× 2.9%		× 2.9%	
MHI tax		1,339		4,017
Total self-employment tax		$7,065		$17,260
Deduct 1/2 SE tax for A.G.I..................		$3,533		$ 8,630

 * Not to exceed wage base − wages received
**No reduction for wages

C will be allowed to deduct $3,533 (one-half of $7,065 self-employment tax paid) for income tax purposes, and D will be allowed to deduct $8,630 (one-half of $17,260).

---

[28] Note that the steps can be combined simply by multiplying the individual's net earnings from self-employment by 100% − one-half the current combined self-employment tax rate (i.e., 100% − 7.65% = 92.35%).

Although both will receive a benefit from the income tax deduction, note that only C has received any benefit from the so-called second deduction in arriving at his self-employment tax base for the social security component. Because D's reduced net earnings for self-employment are still greater than the maximum tax base for the social security component, she is required to pay the maximum amount of this component of the self-employment tax for 2009 (i.e., $106,800 × 12.4% = $13,243$).

In some instances, a self-employed individual may also earn wages subject to FICA withholding while working as a full or part-time employee. In such a case, the maximum earnings base subject to the social security component of the self-employment tax is reduced by the wages earned as an employee.

Example 25. During 2009 T received wages of $88,000 and had self-employment income of $50,000. In computing T's self-employment tax, the maximum taxable base for the social security tax is reduced by the wages paid because T's employer has already withheld the appropriate FICA amount on these wages.

	Social Security
Maximum tax base	$106,800
Less: Wages subject to FICA tax	(88,000)
Reduced maximum tax base	$ 18,800
Net earnings from self-employment	$ 50,000
Subtract: 7.65% of net earnings from self-employment	(3,825)
	$ 46,175
Smaller of reduced maximum tax base or amount determined above	$ 18,800
Times: Social security tax rate	× 12.4%
Tax on social security component	$ 2,331
Social security tax	$ 2,331
Plus: MHI tax ($46,175 × 2.9%)	1,339
Equals: T's self-employment tax	$ 3,670

T will also have an income tax deduction of $1,835 (one-half of the $3,670 self-employment taxes paid).

FUTA Taxes. A Federal unemployment tax is imposed on employers who pay wages of $1,500 or more during any calendar quarter in the calendar year, or who employ at least one individual on each of some 20 days during the calendar year or previous year.[29] Certain exceptions are made for persons employing agricultural or domestic workers.

FUTA tax revenues are used by the Federal government to augment unemployment benefit programs of the various states. The current FUTA tax rate is 6.2 percent of the first $7,000 of wages paid during the year to each covered employee. This translates into a *maximum* FUTA tax of $434 (6.2% × $7,000) *per employee* per year. Since most states also impose an unemployment tax on employers, a credit is allowed against an employer's FUTA tax liability for any similar tax paid to a state. Currently, the maximum FUTA tax credit allowed for this purpose is 5.4 percent of the covered wages

---

[29] § 3306(a)(1).

(i.e., maximum of $378 per employee). Thus, the maximum FUTA tax paid is normally $56 ($434 − $378, or 0.8% × $7,000) per employee.

All employers subject to FUTA taxes must file Form 940, Employer's Annual Federal Unemployment Tax Return, on or before January 31 of the following year. If the employer's tax liability exceeds certain limits, estimated tax payments must be made during the year.[30] Most states require an employer to file unemployment tax returns and make tax payments quarterly.

EXCISE TAXES

The purpose of an excise tax is to tax certain privileges as well as the manufacture, sale, or consumption of specified commodities. Federal excise taxes are imposed on the sale of specified articles, various transactions, occupations, and the use of certain items. This type of tax is not imposed on the profits of a business or profession, however. The major types of excise taxes are as follows:

1. Occupational taxes;
2. Facilities and services taxes;
3. Manufacturers' taxes; and
4. Retail sales of products and commodities taxes.

Occupational Taxes. Some businesses must pay a fee before engaging in their business. These types of businesses include, but are not limited to, liquor dealers, dealers in medicines and dealers in firearms.

Facilities and Services Taxes. The person who pays for services and facilities must pay the tax on these items. The institution or person who furnishes the facilities or services must collect the tax, file returns, and turn over the taxes to the taxing authorities. A few of the common services subject to the facilities and services excise tax include air travel, hotel or motel lodging, and telephone service.

Manufacturers' Taxes. As a rule, certain manufactured goods are taxed at the manufacturing level to make collection easier. Most of these items are of a semi-luxurious or specialized nature, such as sporting goods or firearms. This excise tax applies to the sale or use by the manufacturer, producer, or importer of specified articles. The taxes may be determined by quantity of production (e.g., pounds or gallons) or by a percentage of the sales price. When sales price is used as an index, the tax is based on the sales price of the manufacturer, producer, or importer.

Retail Sales of Products and Commodities Taxes. This excise tax applies to the retail sale or use of diesel fuel, special motor fuels, and fuel used in noncommercial aviation. The tax is collected from the person buying the product by the seller, and the seller must file and pay the tax unless the buyer purchased it tax-free.

State Excise Taxes. Many states and local governments also have excise taxes. They vary in range of coverage and impact, but most parallel the Federal excise taxes. For instance, most states have an excise tax on gasoline, liquor, and cigarettes, as does the Federal government.

---

[30] See instructions in Circular E, *Supra*, Footnote 25.

ADDITIONAL TYPES OF TAXES

Many other types of taxes are used to augment state, local, and Federal income, employment, excise, and wealth transfer taxes. The three levels of government have never been reluctant to exercise their imagination in creating and developing new ways of supplementing governmental revenues. A few of the other more common types of taxes are briefly explained below.

Franchise Tax. A franchise tax is a tax on the privilege of doing business in a state or local jurisdiction. The measure of the tax generally is the net income of the business or the value of the capital used within the taxing authority's jurisdiction.

Sales Tax. A sales tax is imposed on the gross receipts from the retail sale of tangible personal property (e.g., clothing, automobiles, and equipment) and certain services. Each state or local government determines the tax rate and the services and articles to be taxed. The seller will collect the tax from the consumer at the time of the sale, and then periodically remit the taxes to the appropriate taxing authority. Often a state or local government allows the seller to retain a nominal percentage of the collected taxes to compensate for the additional costs incurred by the seller in complying with the tax requirements.

Use Tax. A use tax is a tax imposed on the use within a state or local jurisdiction of tangible property on which a sales tax was not paid. The tax rate normally equals that of the taxing authority's sales tax.

Doing-Business Penalty. This penalty tax is imposed on a business that has not obtained authorization from the state or local government to operate within its border. Usually, a business must pay a fee for a state charter or some other kind of license as permission to enter business within the state.

Real Property Tax. A real property tax is a tax on the value of realty (land, buildings, homes, etc.) owned by nonexempt individuals or organizations within a jurisdiction. Rates vary with location. This type of tax normally supports local services, such as the public school system or the fire department, and is levied on a recurring annual basis.

Tangible Personal Property Tax. This tax is levied on the value of tangible personalty located within a jurisdiction. Tangible personalty is property not classified as realty and includes such items as office furniture, machinery and equipment, inventories, and supplies. The tax normally must be paid annually, with each local jurisdiction determining its own tax rate and the items to tax.

Intangible Personal Property Tax. This tax is imposed on the value of intangible personalty (i.e., stocks, bonds, and accounts and notes receivable) located within a jurisdiction. The tax generally is paid annually, with each local jurisdiction setting its own tax rate and items to be taxed.

GOALS OF TAXATION

In subsequent chapters, the specific provisions that must be followed to compute the Federal income tax will be discussed in detail. Some may view this discussion as a hopeless attempt to explain what seems like an endless barrage of boring rules—rules that, despite their apparent lack of "rhyme or reason," must be considered if the final tax liability is to be determined. The frustration that students of taxation often feel when

studying the rules of Federal tax law is not completely unfounded. Indeed, a famous tax scholar, Boris Bittker, once commented on the increasing intricacy of the tax law, saying, "Can one hope to find a way through a statutory thicket so bristling with detail?"[31] As this statement suggests, many provisions of the law are, in fact, obscure and often appear to be without purpose. However, each provision of the tax law originated with some goal, even if no more than to grant a benefit to some Congressperson's constituency. A knowledge of the goals underlying a particular provision is an important first step toward a comprehension of the provision. An understanding of the purpose of the law is an invaluable tool in attacking the "statutory thicket." In studying taxation, it becomes apparent that many provisions have been enacted with similar objectives. The following discussion reviews some of the goals of taxation that often serve as the reasons behind the rule.

ECONOMIC OBJECTIVES

At first glance, it seems clear that the primary goal of taxation is to provide the resources necessary to fund governmental expenditures. At the Federal level, however, this is not entirely true. As many economists have pointed out, any taxing authority that has the power to control the money supply—as does our Federal government—can satisfy its revenue needs by merely creating money. Nevertheless, complete reliance on the Treasury's printing press to provide the needed resources is not a viable alternative. If the government's expenditures were financed predominantly with funds that it created rather than those obtained through taxation, excess demand would result, which in turn would cause prices to rise, or inflation. Thus, taxation in serving a revenue function also operates along with other instruments of policy to attain a stable price level.

Although Congress can create its own resources, revenue objectives often can explain a particular feature of the law. Consider the personal and dependency exemption deductions, the purpose of which is to free from tax the income needed to maintain a minimum standard of living. Although the cost of living has risen substantially over the years, Congress has been reluctant to increase the amount of these exemptions. The exemption deduction was set at $600 from 1948 to 1969. It slowly crept to $1,000 in 1979 where it essentially stayed until Congress started requiring inflation adjustments in 1985. In effect, the deduction has changed very little over the years, despite significant increases in the price level during this time. The reluctance to alter the exemption amount derives primarily from the potential impact on revenues. A slight increase in the exemption without a corresponding increase in revenues from other sources would result in a tremendous revenue loss because of the number of exemptions taxpayers claim—approximately 259 million in 2002. For similar reasons, Congress has refrained, until recently, from adjusting the tax rate schedules to compensate for inflation, since to do so would significantly reduce its inflow of resources. In 1985, however, both the personal and dependency exemption amount, the standard deduction *and* the individual tax rate schedules were adjusted (indexed) for the increase in the Consumer Price Index that occurred during the previous year.

Revenue considerations also can explain why tax accounting methods sometimes differ from those used for financial accounting. Prior to 1954, an accrual basis taxpayer could neither defer taxation of prepaid income nor deduct estimates of certain expenses, such as the expected costs of servicing warranty contracts. In 1954, the treatment of such items was changed to conform with financial accounting principles that permit deferral of income and accrual of expenses in most situations. The expected revenue loss attributed to this change was $50 million. Within a year after the change, however, the Treasury requested that Congress repeal the new provisions retroactively because estimates of the

---

[31] Boris I. Bittker and Lawrence M. Stone, *Federal Income Taxation*, 5th Ed. (Boston: Little, Brown & Co., 1980) 1iii.

revenue loss were in excess of several billion dollars. In short, Congress responded and, as a result, the treatment of prepaid income and certain accruals for tax and financial accounting purposes differs—a difference attributable to revenue considerations.

The role of Federal taxation in carrying out economic policy extends beyond the realm of revenue raising and price stability. Taxation is a major tool used by the government to attain satisfactory economic growth with full employment. The title of the 1981 tax bill is illustrative: *The Economic Recovery Tax Act of 1981* (ERTA). As the title suggests, a major purpose of this legislation was directed toward revitalizing the health of the economy. ERTA significantly lowered tax rates to spur the economy out of a recession. Its objective was to place more *after-tax* income in the hands of taxpayers for their disposal. By so doing, it was hoped that taxpayers would consume more and thus increase aggregate demand, resulting in economic growth.

Congress also has used the tax structure to directly attack the problem of unemployment. In 1977, employers were encouraged to increase employment by the introduction of a general jobs tax credit, which effectively reduced the cost of labor. In 1978, Congress eliminated the general jobs credit and substituted a targeted jobs credit. This credit could be obtained only if employers hired certain targeted groups of individuals who were considered disadvantaged or handicapped. This credit was expanded in 1983 to stimulate the hiring of economically disadvantaged youth during the summer. The credit was further refined and is now referred to as the work opportunity credit. As the credit for jobs suggests, Congress believes that major economic problems can be solved using the tax system.

A subject closely related to economic growth and full employment is investment. To stimulate investment spending, Congress has enacted numerous provisions. For example, accelerated depreciation methods—the modified accelerated cost recovery system (MACRS)—may be used to compute the deduction for depreciation, thus enabling rapid recovery of the taxpayer's investment.

Congress encourages certain industries by granting them favorable tax treatment. For example, the credit for research and experimental expenditures cited above clearly benefits those engaged in technology businesses. Other tax provisions are particularly advantageous for other groups such as builders, farmers, and producers of natural resources. Special incentives also are available for manufacturers. As will become clear in later chapters, the income tax law is replete with rules designed to encourage, stimulate, and assist various enterprises as Congress has deemed necessary over the years.

SOCIAL OBJECTIVES

The tax system is used to achieve not only economic goals but social objectives as well. Some examples are listed below:

1. The deduction for charitable contributions helps to finance the cost of important activities that otherwise would be funded by the government.

2. The deduction for interest on home mortgages subsidizes the cost of a home and thus encourages home ownership.

3. The work opportunity credit noted above exists to fight unemployment problems of certain disadvantaged groups of citizens.

4. Larger standard deductions are granted to taxpayers who are 65 or over, or who are blind, to relieve their tax burden.

5. Deductions for contributions to retirement savings accounts encourage individuals to provide for their future needs.

These examples are representative of the many provisions where social considerations provide the underlying rationale.

The above discussion is but a brief glimpse of how social and economic considerations have shaped our tax law. Interestingly, most of the provisions mentioned have been enacted in the past 25 years. During this time, Congress has relied increasingly on the tax system as a means to strike at the nation's ills. Whether the tax law can be used successfully in this manner is unclear. Many believe that attacking such problems should be done directly through government expenditure programs—not through so-called *tax expenditures*. A *tax expenditure* is the estimated amount of revenue lost for failing to tax a particular item (e.g., scholarships), for granting a certain deduction (e.g., charitable contributions), or for allowing a credit (e.g., work opportunity credit). The concept of tax expenditures was developed by noted tax authority Stanley S. Surrey. While Assistant Secretary of the Treasury for Tax Policy during 1961–1969, Surrey and his supporters urged that certain activities should not be encouraged by subsidizing them through reduced tax liabilities. They argued that paying for government-financed activities in such a roundabout fashion makes their costs difficult if not impossible to determine. In addition, they asserted that such expenditures are concealed from the public eye as well as from the standard budgetary review process.[32] Others, however, argued that the tax system could be used effectively for this purpose. Whether either view is correct, Congress currently shows no apparent signs of discontinuing use of the tax system to influence taxpayers' behavior.

OTHER OBJECTIVES

Although social and economic goals provide the rationale for much of our tax law, many provisions can be explained in terms of certain well-established principles of taxation. These principles are simply the characteristics that "good" taxes exhibit. Most tax experts agree that a tax is good if it satisfies the following conditions:[33]

1. The tax is *equitable* or fair;

2. The tax is *economically efficient* (i.e., it advances a goal where appropriate and otherwise is as neutral as possible);

3. The tax is *certain* and not arbitrary;

4. The tax can be administered by the government and complied with by the taxpayer at a *low cost* (i.e., it is *economical* to operate); and

5. The tax is *convenient* (i.e., administration and compliance can be carried out with the utmost simplicity).

These five qualities represent important principles of taxation that must be conformed with in pursuing social and economic goals. As discussed below, these criteria have greatly influenced our tax law.

Equity. A tax system is considered equitable if it treats all persons who are in the same economic situation in the same fashion. This aspect of equity is referred to as *horizontal equity*. In contrast, *vertical equity* implies that taxpayers who are not in the same situation will be treated differently—the difference in treatment being fair and just.

---

[32] The annual U.S. budget now contains a projection of annual tax expenditures.

[33] These qualities were first identified by Adam Smith. See The *Wealth of Nations*, Book V, Chapter II, Part II (New York: Dutton, 1910).

There are two major obstacles in implementing the equity concept as explained. First, there must be some method to determine when taxpayers are in the same economic situation. Second, there must be agreement on reasonable distinctions between those who are in different situations. The manner in which these obstacles are addressed explains two significant features of our tax system.

As indicated above, the first major difficulty in implementing the equity concept is identification of some technique to determine when taxpayers are similarly situated. For tax purposes, it is well settled that similarity is measured in terms of a taxpayer's *ability to pay*. Hence, taxpayers with equal abilities to pay should pay equal taxes. To the dismay of some tax policymakers, however, there is no simple, unambiguous index of an individual's ability. A taxpayer's ability to pay is the composite of numerous factors including his or her wealth, income, family situation, health, and attitude. Clearly, no one measure captures all of these factors. This being so, tax specialists generally have agreed that the best objective measure of ability to pay is income. This agreement, that income is a reasonable surrogate for ability to pay and thus serves the equity principle, explains in part why the primary tax used by the Federal government is an *income* tax.

The second obstacle in implementing the equity concept concerns the treatment of taxpayers who are differently situated. In terms of income, the problem may best be explained by reference to two taxpayers, A and B. If A's income (e.g., $100,000) exceeds B's (e.g., $20,000), it is assumed that A has more ability to pay and thus should pay more tax. The dilemma posed is not whether A and B should pay differing amounts of tax, but rather, what additional amount may be fairly charged to A. If a proportional tax of five percent is levied against A and B, A pays $5,000 (5% of $100,000) and B pays $1,000 (5% of $20,000). While application of this tax rate structure results in A paying $4,000 more than B absolutely, A pays the same amount in relative terms; that is, they both pay the *same* 5 percent. Those charged with the responsibility of developing Federal tax policy have concluded that paying more tax in absolute terms does not adequately serve the equity goal. For this reason, a progressive tax rate structure is used, requiring relatively more tax to be paid by those having more income. With respect to A and B above, this structure would require that A pay a greater percentage of his income than B.

The equity principle explains (at least partially) not only the basic structure of our predominant tax device—an income tax and its progressive tax rate structure—but also explains many other provisions in our law. In fact, some of the factors mentioned earlier that affect a taxpayer's ability to pay are recognized explicitly by separate provisions in the Code. For example, a taxpayer may deduct medical expenses and casualty losses—items over which the taxpayer has little or no power—if such items exceed a certain level. Similarly, a taxpayer's family situation is considered by allowing exemption deductions for dependents whose support is the taxpayer's responsibility.

There are many other specific situations where the equity principle controls the tax consequences. For example, fairness dictates that taxes should not be paid when the taxpayer does not have the *wherewithal to pay* (i.e., the money to pay the tax). This is true even though the transaction results in income to the taxpayer.

> **Example 26.** Upon the theft of valuable machinery, LJM Corporation received a $20,000 insurance reimbursement. Assuming the machinery had a cost (adjusted for depreciation) of $5,000, LJM has realized a $15,000 gain ($20,000 − $5,000). Although the corporation has realized a gain, it also has lost the productive capacity of the machinery. If LJM reinvests the entire $20,000 proceeds in similar assets within two years of the theft, the gain is not taxed but rather deferred. This rule derives from Congressional belief that equity would not be served if taxes were levied when the taxpayer did not have the wherewithal to pay. In addition, the taxpayer's total economic situation has not been so materially altered as to require recognition of the gain.

Administrative Concerns. The final three qualities of a good tax—certainty, economy, and simplicity—might be aptly characterized as administrative in nature. Numerous provisions exist to meet administrative goals. Some of these are so obvious as to be easily overlooked. For example, the certainty requirement underlies the provision that a tax return generally is due each April 15, while economy of collection is the purpose, at least in part, for withholding. Similarly, provisions requiring the taxpayer to compute the tax using tables provided by the IRS are motivated by concerns for simplicity.

Perhaps the most important aspect of the administrative principles is that they often conflict with other principles of taxation. Consequently, one principle must often be adhered to at the expense of another. For example, our tax system could no doubt be more equitable if each individual's ability to pay was personally assessed, much like welfare agents assess the needs of their clients. However, this improvement could be obtained only at a substantial administrative cost. The administrative principle is first in importance in this case, as well as in many others.

A PRELUDE TO TAX PLANNING

Although taxes affect numerous aspects of our lives, their impact is not uncontrollable. Given an understanding of the rules, taxes can be managed with considerable success. Successful management, however, is predicated on good tax planning.

Tax planning is simply the process of arranging one's actions in light of their potential tax consequences. It should be emphasized that the tax consequences sometimes turn on how a particular transaction is structured—that is, *form* often controls taxation.

Example 27. Z is obligated to make monthly payments of interest and principal on a note secured by his home. During the year, he was short of cash so his mother, B, who lives with Z, made the payments for him. Even though B made the payments directly, she may not deduct the interest expense because interest is deductible only if it relates to a debt for which the taxpayer is personally liable. Moreover, her son cannot deduct the expense since he did not make payment. Note that the deduction could have been obtained had the payment been structured properly. If Z had received a gift of cash from his mother and then made payment, he could have claimed the interest deduction. Alternatively, if B had been jointly liable on the note, she could have deducted the interest payments she made.

In the example above, note that regardless of how the transaction is structured, the result is the same *except for* the tax ramifications. By merely planning and changing the form of the transaction, tax benefits are obtained. Before jumping to the conclusion that form always governs taxation, a caveat is warranted. Courts often are obliged to disregard form and let substance prevail. Notwithstanding the form versus substance difficulty, the point to be gained is that the pattern of a transaction often determines the tax outcome.

The obvious goal of most tax planning is the minimization of the amount that a person or other entity must transfer to the government. The legal minimization of taxes is usually referred to as *tax avoidance*. Although the phrase "tax avoidance" may have a criminal connotation, there is no injustice in legally reducing one's taxes. The most profound statement regarding the propriety of tax avoidance is found in a dissenting opinion authored by Judge Learned Hand in the case of *Commissioner v. Newman*. Judge Hand wrote:[34]

---

[34] 159 F.2d 848 (CA-2. 1947).

Over and over again courts have said that there is nothing sinister in so arranging one's affairs so as to keep taxes as low as possible. Everybody does so, rich or poor, and all do right, for nobody owes any public duty to pay more than the law demands: taxes are enforced exactions, not voluntary contributions. To demand more in the name of morals is pure cant.

This statement is routinely cited as authority for taking those steps necessary to reduce one's taxes. It should be emphasized that tax planning and tax avoidance involve only those actions that are legal. *Tax evasion* is the label given to illegal activities that are designed to reduce the tax liability.

The planning effort for Federal income taxation (the principal area covered in this text) requires an understanding of the answer to *four* basic questions regarding the flow of cash and cash equivalents into and out of various tax entities. These questions regard the amount, character, and timing of income, deductions and credits, and recognition (reporting) of these items. The answers depend upon the tax entity that receives or transfers the cash or cash equivalents, its tax accounting period and methods, and whether the entity is considered a taxpayer separate from its owners or simply a conduit through which items of income, gain, loss, deduction, or credit flow to its owners. The tax entities recognized for Federal tax purposes, and the tax planning questions, are presented in Exhibit 1-6.

Tax planning efforts often involve deferring the recognition of income or shifting the incidence of its tax to a lower tax bracket entity (e.g., from parents to children), or accelerating, deferring, or shifting deductions and credits to tax periods or among tax entities with higher or lower tax rates. Keeping this overall scheme of tax minimization in mind, many of the subsequent chapters of this text conclude with a discussion of tax planning considerations.

EXHIBIT 1-6
Tax Planning Perspective

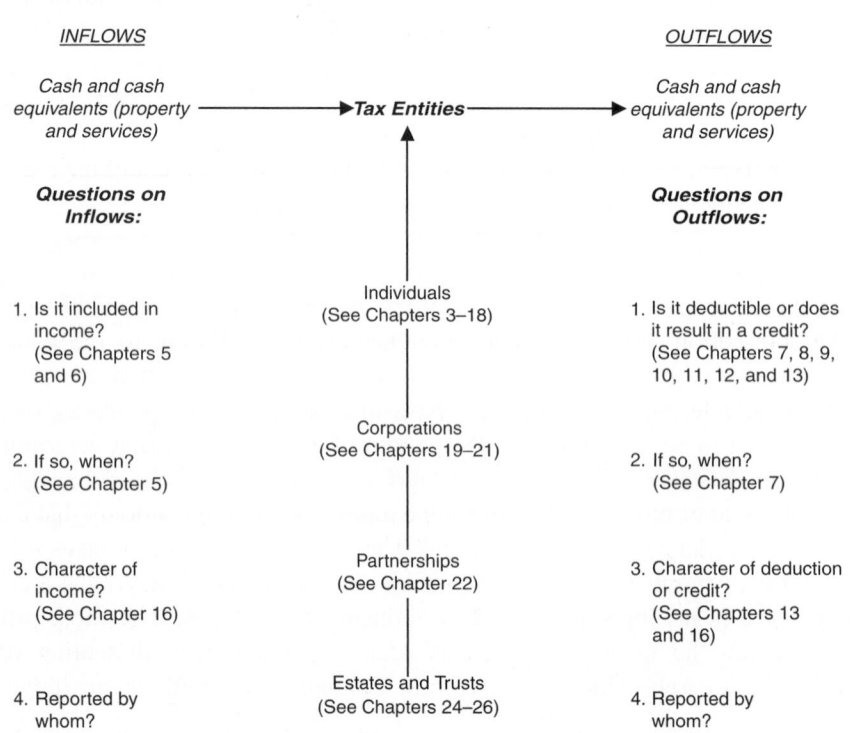

PROBLEM MATERIALS

DISCUSSION QUESTIONS

1-1   *Tax Bases.* Describe the tax bases for the Federal income tax and for each of the Federal wealth transfer taxes.

1-2   *Tax Rates.* Distinguish between a proportional tax rate structure and a progressive tax rate structure. What is the significance of the marginal tax rate under either a proportional or a progressive rate structure?

1-3   *Progressive, Proportional, and Regressive Taxes.* The media often refer to sales taxes as regressive. Similar comments are made when discussing social security taxes (FICA). Are the media correct? Include in your comments an explanation of the different types of tax rate structures.

1-4   *Deduction versus Credit.* Distinguish between a deduction and a credit. If a credit is allowed for 20 percent of an expenditure in lieu of a deduction for the total expenditure, under what circumstances should you prefer the credit? The deduction?

1-5   *Individual versus Corporate Taxable Income.* Based on the tax formulas contained in Exhibits 1-2 and 1-3, what are the significant differences in computing a corporation's taxable income as opposed to computing an individual's taxable income?

1-6   *Withholding Taxes at Source.* What do you believe is the principal reason that Congress continues the pay-as-you-go requirements of employers withholding Federal income taxes from the wages paid their employees?

1-7   *Marital Deduction.* Describe the marital deduction allowed for Federal estate and gift taxes. How might an individual use this deduction to avoid all Federal wealth transfer taxes?

1-8   *Estate Tax Credit.* How is the estate transfer tax credit applied in determining taxable wealth transfers?

1-9   *Annual Gift Tax Exclusion.* What is the amount of the annual Federal gift tax exclusion? If a widow were interested in making gifts to her daughter and seven grandchildren, how much could she transfer to them in any given year before incurring a taxable gift?

1-10   *Gift-Splitting Election.* What is the gift-splitting election allowed for Federal gift tax purposes? How might the marital deduction be used to explain why Congress allows this election?

1-11   *Estate versus Inheritance Taxes.* Distinguish between an estate and an inheritance transfer tax.

1-12   *Federal Employment Taxes.* Distinguish between FICA and FUTA taxes. Between an employee and his or her employer, who bears the greater burden of these taxes?

1-13   *Unemployment Taxes.* For 2009 what is the maximum FUTA tax an employer can expect to pay if he or she has three employees during the year and the minimum salary paid is $10,000? If the employer also is subject to state unemployment taxes, what is the maximum amount of credit he or she will be allowed against the FUTA tax liability?

1-14 *Sales versus Use Tax.* Distinguish between a sales and a use tax. Assume you live in state A but near the border of state B and that state A imposes a much higher sales tax than does state B. If you were planning to purchase a new automobile, what might you be tempted to do? How might state A discourage your plan?

1-15 *Tax Expenditures.* It is often suggested that many of our social problems can be cured through use of tax incentives.
    a. Discuss the concept of tax expenditures.
    b. Expand on the text's discussion of the pros and cons of tax expenditures vis-a-vis direct governmental expenditures.

1-16 *Goals of Taxation.* In a recent discussion concerning what a fair tax is, the following comments were made: (1) the fairest tax is one that someone else has to pay; (2) people should be taxed in accordance with the benefits they obtain (i.e., taxes are the price paid for the benefit); (3) a head tax would be the fairest; and (4) why tax at all?—just use the printing press. Discuss the first three of these comments in terms of equity and explain whether the fourth represents a viable alternative.

PROBLEMS

1-17 *Marginal Tax Rates.* T, a single taxpayer, has taxable income of $40,000 for 2009. If T anticipates a marginal tax rate of 15 percent for 2010, what income tax savings could she expect by accelerating $1,000 of deductible expenditures planned for 2010 into the 2009 tax year?

1-18 *Tax Rate Schedules and Rate Concepts.* An examination of the tax rate schedules for single taxpayers (see the inside cover of the text) indicates that the tax is a "given dollar amount" plus a percentage of taxable income exceeding a particular level.
    a. Explain how the "given dollar amounts" are determined.
    b. Assuming the taxpayer has a taxable income of $50,000 and is single, what is his tax liability for 2009?
    c. Same facts as (b). What is the taxpayer's marginal tax rate?
    d. Same facts as (b). What is the taxpayer's average tax rate?
    e. Assuming the taxpayer has tax-exempt interest income from municipal bonds of $30,000, what is the taxpayer's effective tax rate?

1-19 *Tax Equity.* Taxpayer R has income of $20,000. Similarly, S has income of $20,000. Each taxpayer pays a tax of $1,000 on his income.
    a. Discuss whether the tax imposed is equitable. Include in your discussion comments concerning horizontal and vertical equity.
    b. Assume S has a taxable income of $40,000 and pays a tax of $2,000 on his income. Discuss whether the tax imposed is equitable in light of this new information.

1-20 *Tax Fairness.* R and S both own homes in Houston. Both have an appraised value of $200,000 and, consequently, both R and S pay $5,000 in real property taxes. Explain why such a tax may be considered fair by some and unfair by others.

1-21 *Understanding Tax Rate Concepts.* Indicate whether the following statements are true or false and, if false, explain why.
    a. Tax-exempt income would cause the taxpayer's average tax rate to increase.
    b. Tax-exempt income would cause the taxpayer's marginal tax rate to decrease.
    c. Tax-exempt income would cause the taxpayer's effective tax rate to decrease.

1-22   *Understanding Tax Rate Concepts.* Indicate whether the following statements are true or false and, if false, explain why.
   a.   From a technical point of view, sales taxes are progressive.
   b.   From a popular point of view, sales taxes are regressive.
   c.   From a popular point of view, sales taxes are proportional.
   d.   From a technical point of view, there are no regressive taxes in the United States.

1-23   *Think Tax.* From a tax perspective, a transaction that may make sense for one taxpayer may be complete nonsense for another. Consider two married taxpayers, H and W who earn $500,000 per year and L and M who earn $20,000 per year. Both plan on buying interest-paying bonds with a face value of $1,000, either State of Indiana bonds paying 6% tax-exempt interest or AT&T bonds paying eight percent taxable interest. Assume the bonds are in all other respects equivalent (e.g., price, risk, etc.). Show (with calculations) why it would make perfect sense for H and W to buy the Indiana bonds but it would be foolish for L and M to buy the Indiana bonds.

1-24   *Identifying Tax Expenditures.* Indicate whether the following would be considered a tax expenditure.
   a.   Tax deduction allowed for payment of gasoline purchased by a taxicab driver who owns and operates his own taxicab business.
   b.   Deduction for charitable contributions made by individual taxpayers.
   c.   Postponement of taxation of income earned on an individual's savings in an Individual Retirement Account until such income is distributed.
   d.   Straight-line depreciation of an office building used in a trade or business.
   e.   Tax credit for purchase of electric automobile.
   f.   Deduction for interest paid on a home mortgage.

1-25   *Advantages and Disadvantages of Tax Expenditures.* Indicate whether the following would be considered an advantage or disadvantage of a tax expenditure.
   a.   Administrative costs less than other forms of government financial assistance
   b.   Beneficiaries easily identified
   c.   Only those entitled to financial assistance receive it
   d.   Costs and budgetary effects readily assessed
   e.   Benefits (e.g., from deductions) rise and fall without direct approval from the government
   f.   Less palatable to beneficiaries
   g.   Effect on tax system

1-26   *Taxable Gifts.* M made the following cash gifts during 2009:

To her son	$50,000
To her daughter	50,000
To her niece	10,000

   a.   If M is unmarried, what is the amount of taxable gifts she has made in 2009?
   b.   If M is married and her husband agrees to split gifts with her, what is the total amount of taxable gifts made by M and her husband for 2009?

1-27   *Taxable Estate.* R dies in 2009. R made taxable gifts during his lifetime in 1988, 1989, 1991, 1995, and 1997 but paid no Federal transfer taxes due to the unified transfer tax credit in effect in those years. What effect will these taxable gifts have on determining the following:
   a.   R's Federal taxable estate?
   b.   The rates imposed on the Federal taxable estate?

1-28 *Estate Tax Computation.* T died on January 4, 2009. He owned the following property on his date of death:

Cash	$10,000,000
Stocks and bonds	700,000
Residence	800,000
Interest in partnership	350,000
Miscellaneous personal property	25,000

Upon T's death, he owed $80,000 on the mortgage on his residence. T also owned a life insurance policy. The policy was term life insurance which paid $200,000 to his mother upon his death. Its value immediately before his death was $0. T had all of the incidents of ownership with regard to the policy.

During his life, T had made only one gift. He gave a diamond ring worth $30,000 (it was an old family heirloom) to his daughter in 1995. No gift taxes were paid on the gift due to the annual exclusion (gift-splitting was elected) and the unified transfer tax credit in effect for that year. The ring was worth $50 000 on his date of death.

T's will contained the following provisions:

a. To my wife I leave all of the stocks and bonds.

b. To my alma mater, State University, I leave $50,000 to establish a chair for a tax professor in the Department of Accounting in the School of Business.

c. The residue of my estate is to go to my daughter.

Compute T's estate tax before any credits other than the Federal estate tax credit.

1-29 *Inheritance Taxes.* This year Bob died, leaving $500,000 to his heirs. His state of residence imposes an inheritance tax. Indicate whether the following statements are true or false and, if false, explain why. Consider using the Internet to find information on how the inheritance tax laws of your state operate.

a. The amount of the inheritance tax is $0 since Bob's estate does not exceed the 2009 taxable threshold of $2 million.

b. Assume Bob is single. The amount of inheritance tax due from Bob's estate, like the Federal estate tax, is the same regardless of whom he names as the beneficiaries.

c. Assume Bob is married. The amount of inheritance tax due from Bob's estate—like the Federal estate tax—is zero if he leaves the entire amount to his surviving spouse or children.

d. Any inheritance tax paid by Bob's estate may be used to reduce any Federal estate tax his estate owes.

1-30 *Excess FICA Taxes.* During 2009 E earned $70,000 of wages from employer X and $50,000 of wages from employer Y. Both employers withheld and paid the appropriate amount of FICA taxes on E's wages.

a. What is the amount of excess taxes paid by E for 2009?

b. Would it make any difference in the amount of E's refund or credit of the excess of FICA taxes if he was a full-time employee of each employer for different periods of the year, as opposed to a full-time employee of X and a part-time employee of Y for the entire year?

1-31 *Self-Employment Tax.* During 2009 H had earnings from self-employment of $50,000 and wages of $78,000 from employer X. Employer X withheld and paid the appropriate amount of FICA taxes on H's wages. Compute H's self-employment tax liability for 2009. What is the amount of H's income tax deduction for the self-employment taxes paid?

1-32 *Tax Awareness.* Assume that you are currently employed by Corporation X in state A. Without your solicitation, Corporation Y offers you a 20 percent higher salary if you will relocate to state B and become its employee. What tax factors should you consider in making a decision as to the offer?

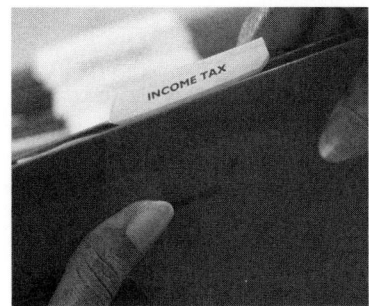

★ CHAPTER TWO ★

TAX PRACTICE AND RESEARCH

LEARNING OBJECTIVES

Upon completion of this chapter you will be able to:

- Describe the basic features of tax practice: compliance, planning, litigation, and research

- Identify typical career paths in taxation

- Understand the rules of conduct that must be followed by those who perform tax services

- Appreciate the role of ethics in tax practice and the responsibilities of tax practitioners

- Explain the key penalties that influence positions taken on tax returns

- Describe the process in which Federal tax law is enacted and subsequently modified or evaluated by the judiciary

- Interpret citations to various statutory, administrative, and judicial sources of the tax law

- Identify the source of various administrative and judicial tax authorities

- Locate most statutory, administrative, and judicial authorities

- Evaluate the relative strength of various tax authorities

- Understand the importance of communicating the results of tax research

CHAPTER OUTLINE

INTRODUCTION

Before jumping into the rules and regulations that must be applied to determine the taxpayer's tax liability, one should have at least an appreciation of the basic nature of tax practice and how to go about finding answers to tax questions. This chapter lays the necessary foundation by first exploring exactly what it is that tax professionals do and the rules of conduct that they must observe while doing it. The chapter concludes by identifying the various sources of tax law and how they may be accessed and used to solve a particular tax question.

TAX PRACTICE IN GENERAL

There are essentially four aspects of tax practice: compliance, planning, litigation, and research. Although these may be thought of as discrete areas, as a practical matter, tax professionals are normally involved in all four.

Tax Compliance. The area of tax compliance generally encompasses all of the activities necessary to meet the statutory requirements of the tax law. This largely involves the preparation of the millions of tax returns that must be filed by individuals and other organizations each year. Interestingly, the reliance of individuals on professional return preparation is rather a recent phenomenon. There was a time when most individuals prepared their own returns and H&R Block was unheard of. However, the ever-increasing complexity of the tax law has made professional assistance almost a necessity and in fact created a tax preparation industry. In 2006, 59.2 percent of all the individual tax returns filed were completed by a paid preparer.[1] Tax preparation services are typically

---

[1]   See "Tax Stats at a Glance," IRS Statistics of Income (preliminary data, revised June 4, 2008) http://www.irs.gov/taxstats

performed by Certified Public Accountants (CPAs), attorneys, enrolled agents (individuals who have passed a two-day examination given by the IRS), and commercial tax return preparation services. But there are no special requirements that must be met to become a tax return preparer. Consequently, anyone willing to try his or her hand at mastering the tax law—as well as any shysters who think there is a buck to be made—can hang out a shingle. In fact, the advent of personal computers and sophisticated yet user-friendly software have made tax preparation easier for everyone, including those who want to get into the tax preparation business. Note, however, that only CPAs, attorneys, and enrolled agents are authorized to practice before the IRS and are therefore able to represent taxpayers beyond the initial audit (e.g., at the Appellate level).

As might be imagined, the day-to-day tasks of those working in the tax compliance area typically surround preparation of a tax return. They collect the appropriate information from the taxpayer and then analyze and evaluate such data for use in preparing the required tax return or other tax filing. But tax compliance goes far beyond merely placing numbers in boxes. In many cases, completion of the return requires tax research to determine the appropriate treatment of a particular item. Preparation of a return may also uncover tax planning opportunities that can be shared with the client to obtain future savings. In addition, tax compliance involves representation of the taxpayer before the IRS during audits and appeals.

Tax Planning. Perhaps the most rewarding part of tax practice is tax planning and the sense of satisfaction one gets from helping clients minimize their tax liability. As explained in the previous chapter, tax planning is simply the process of arranging one's financial affairs in light of their potential tax consequences. Unlike the weather, taxpayers often have some degree of control over their tax liability, and it is the job of the tax adviser to help the taxpayer whenever possible. A great deal of tax planning is simply an outgrowth of the tax compliance process. Well-trained tax professionals often recognize a situation where a little planning could have brought a more favorable result. In these so-called *closed fact* situations, it is typically too late to do anything until the opportunity once again presents itself, typically the next year. On the other hand, taxpayers about to embark on a transaction—an *open fact* situation—may engage a tax adviser to determine the tax consequences and how to structure the transaction to obtain the most beneficial outcome.

Tax Litigation. As might be expected, taxpayers and the IRS do not always agree on the tax treatment of a particular item. Many disputes and controversies are settled during an appeals process within the IRS itself. Others, however, are ultimately resolved in a court of law. Tax litigation is a very specialized but often lucrative area of tax practice. In most cases, tax litigation is conducted only by licensed attorneys. However, accountants and others, including the taxpayer himself, can represent the taxpayer in certain situations. In addition, accountants often assist legal counsel and provide litigation support.

Tax Research. Most practitioners believe that tax research is the most interesting part of tax practice. Tax research is simply the process of obtaining information and synthesizing it to answer a particular tax question. Regardless of the area of tax practice—compliance, planning, or litigation—tax research plays an important part.

Tax research generally involves identifying tax issues, finding relevant information on the issues, and assessing the pertinent authority to arrive at a conclusion. Unfortunately, the law is not so straightforward that the answer to any tax question is readily available. Consequently, being able to do the research is an important skill for anyone involved in tax. For example, a decorator that works out of her home may want to know whether the cost of maintaining a home office can be deducted in computing taxable income. It may seem that a common problem like this could be easily resolved, but it is

often much more difficult than might be imagined. To answer this question, the tax adviser may be required to sift through mounds of information—rules, regulations, IRS pronouncements, and court cases—in order to determine the proper treatment. Even if an answer seems apparent, the dynamic nature of the tax law often requires the practitioner to constantly update his or her research to ensure that it is current and has not been changed by some recent development.

TAXATION AS A PROFESSIONAL CAREER

The need for tax advisory services has grown almost exponentially in recent years. The growth is not surprising given the growth in the tax law. Over the past 35 years, there have been tax law changes virtually every year. During this time Congress has turned to the tax system again and again to attack not only the country's economic ills but its social problems as well. The end result is a tax law, both Federal and state, that is forever changing and quite complex. Consequently, individuals and organizations have increasingly needed to call upon tax specialists to help them cope with the law. These demands on the tax profession have created tremendous opportunities for those interested in careers in taxation.

The tax specialists of today wear a number of hats. They act as tax consultants as well as business advisers. They help individuals and business owners with tax compliance, keep them informed of changes in the tax law, and assist them in personal financial planning. Tax advisers not only consult on Federal and state income tax matters; they also prepare sales, payroll, and franchise tax returns. Industry and government also employ tax specialists who are involved in planning and compliance. Here are some examples of activities in which the tax specialist might be involved:

▶ A husband and wife want to transfer their business to their children. Should they sell the business to the kids or would they be better off just giving it to them? A tax specialist can compare the income tax consequences of a sale to that of a gift or bequest and help design the best plan in light of the couple's wishes.

▶ A taxpayer wants to sell her corporation. Should she sell the stock or cause the corporation to sell its assets? A tax specialist can explain the tax and nontax factors affecting the decision.

▶ An individual and his son are forming a new business. Should it be operated as a corporation, an S corporation, a partnership, or a limited liability company? A tax specialist can help with the analysis.

▶ A corporation is planning on opening operations in a foreign country. A tax specialist can help reorganize the company to help minimize U.S. and foreign taxes.

▶ A corporation is considering the establishment of a retirement plan. A tax adviser who specializes in employee benefits can provide information regarding the tax considerations.

▶ A taxpayer is seeking a divorce. A tax specialist can explain the tax consequences.

▶ A corporation and its subsidiaries are thinking about filing a consolidated tax return. The tax specialist can assist the taxpayer in filing such a return, preparing estimated tax payments, or reviewing a corporation's tax returns.

▶ The IRS wants to deny the taxpayer a deduction for meals and entertainment. The tax specialist might represent an individual during the IRS examination or present oral and written arguments before an IRS appeals conference and (if qualified) before the U.S. Tax Court.

In these and similar matters, the tax specialist is often an important member of the client's professional advisory team and works with other high-caliber individuals to minimize client costs. For example, if a business owner is seeking estate planning advice, the team typically includes the individual's attorney, accountant, life insurance agent, and tax adviser.

Thousands of men and women enjoy successful careers in taxation. They are highly respected as professionals and are well compensated for their work. Those in tax rarely find their jobs boring or dull. Tax work, particularly once one has paid one's dues and built a firm foundation, is interesting and challenging. Moreover, working in a tax department along with other professionals with like interests can be a vastly rewarding personal experience. Tax professionals also serve the public good by raising the standard of tax practice and administration and by working with other groups to improve the tax system.

SOURCES AND APPLICATIONS OF TAX LAW

As stated at the outset of this chapter, before delving into the rules and regulations of taxation, it is important at a minimum to have an appreciation of not only the nature of tax practice but also the sources of the tax law and how they can be used for solving questions. The second half of this chapter identifies the various components of the tax law, explains how they can be accessed, and reviews the basic methods of tax research.

AUTHORITATIVE SOURCES OF TAX LAW

Sources of tax law can be classified into two broad categories: (1) the law, and (2) official interpretations of the law. The law consists primarily of the Constitution, the Acts of Congress, and tax treaties. In general, these sources are referred to as the *statutory* law. Most statutory law is written in general terms for a typical situation. Since general rules, no matter how carefully drafted, cannot be written to cover variations on the normal scheme, interpretation is usually required. The task of interpreting the statute is one of the principal duties of the Internal Revenue Service (IRS) as representative of the Secretary of the Treasury. The IRS annually produces thousands of releases that explain and clarify the law. To no one's surprise, however, taxpayers and the government do not always agree on how a particular law should be interpreted. In situations where the taxpayer or the government decides to litigate the question, the courts, as final arbiters, are given the opportunity to interpret the law. These judicial interpretations, administrative interpretations, and the statutory law are considered in detail below.

STATUTORY LAW

The Constitution of the United States provides the Federal government with the power to tax. Disputes concerning the constitutionality of an income tax levied on taxpayers without apportionment among the states were resolved in 1913 with passage of the Sixteenth Amendment. Between 1913 and 1939, Congress enacted revenue acts that amounted to a complete rewrite of all tax law to date, including the desired changes. In 1939, due primarily to the increasing complexity of the earlier process, Congress codified all Federal tax laws into Title 26 of the *United States Code*, which was then called the *Internal Revenue Code of 1939*. Significant changes in the Federal tax laws were made during World War II and the postwar period of the late 1940s. Each change resulted in amendments to the 1939 Code. By 1954, the codification process had to be repeated in order to organize all additions to the law and to eliminate obsolete

provisions. The product of this effort was the *Internal Revenue Code of 1954*. After 1954, Congress took great care to ensure that each new amendment to the 1954 Code was incorporated within its organizational structure with appropriate cross-references to any prior provisions affected by a new law. In 1986, Congress again made substantial revision in the tax law. Consistent with this massive redesign of the 1954 Code, Congress changed the title to the *Internal Revenue Code of 1986*. Like the 1954 Code, the 1986 Code is subject to revisions introduced by a new law. Recent changes incorporated into the 1986 Code include the Economic Stimulus Act of 2008, the Emergency Economic Stabilization Act of 2008, the Heroes Earnings Assistance and Relief Act of 2008, and the American Recovery and Reinvestment Tax Act of 2009, just to name a few of the many during the last year.

The legislative provisions contained in the Code are by far the most important component of tax law. Although procedure necessary to enact a law is generally well known, it is necessary to review this process with a special emphasis on taxation. From a tax perspective, the *intention* of Congress in producing the legislation is extremely important since the primary purpose of tax research is to interpret the legislative intent of Congress.

THE MAKING OF A TAX LAW

Article I, Section 7, Clause 1 of the Constitution provides that the House of Representatives of the U.S. Congress has the basic responsibility for initiating revenue bills.[2] The Ways and Means Committee of the House of Representatives must consider any tax bill before it is presented for vote by the full House of Representatives. On bills of major public interest, the Ways and Means Committee holds public hearings where interested organizations may send representatives to express their views about the bill. The first witness at such hearings is usually the Secretary of the Treasury, representing the President of the United States. In many cases, proposals for new tax legislation or changes in existing legislation come from the President as a part of his political or economic programs.

After the public hearings have been held, the Ways and Means Committee usually goes into closed session, where the Committee prepares the tax bill for consideration by the entire House. The members of the Committee receive invaluable assistance from their highly skilled staff, which includes economists, accountants, and lawyers. The product of this session is a proposed bill that is submitted to the entire House for debate and vote.

After a bill has been approved by the entire House, it is sent to the Senate and assigned to the Senate Finance Committee. The Senate Finance Committee may also hold hearings on the bill before its consideration by the full Senate. The Senate's bill generally differs from the House's bill. In these situations, both versions are sent to the Joint Conference Committee on Taxation, which is composed of members selected from the House Ways and Means Committee and from the Senate Finance Committee. The objective of this Joint Committee is to produce a compromise bill acceptable to both sides. On occasion, when compromise cannot be achieved by the Joint Committee or the compromise bill is unacceptable to the House or the Senate, the bill "dies." If, however, compromise is reached and the Senate and House approve the compromise bill, it is then referred to the President for his or her approval or veto. If the President vetoes the bill, the legislation is "killed" unless two-thirds of both the House and the Senate vote to override the veto. If the veto is overridden, the legislation becomes law.

When a bill is signed into law by the President it is sent to the Office of the Federal Register to be assigned a "public law number." For example, the Tax Reform Act of 1986 is designated P.L. 99-514 and is explained in the following diagram.

---

[2] Tax bills do not originate in the Senate, except when they are attached to other bills.

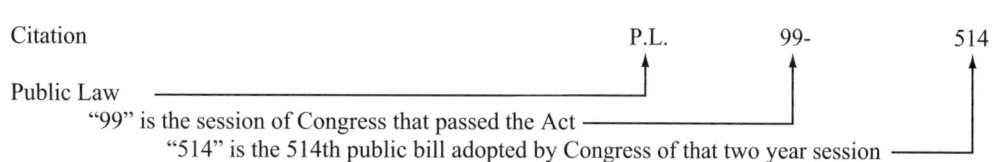

Citation   P.L.   99-   514

Public Law
    "99" is the session of Congress that passed the Act
        "514" is the 514th public bill adopted by Congress of that two year session

References to the various laws are often made using their public law numbers. Unfortunately, the public law number does not indicate the year in which the bill was enacted. However, the legislative session in which a public law was enacted can be determined using the following formula:

$$\text{(Session number} \times 2) - 112 = \text{Second year of session}$$

Using this formula, P.L. 99-514 was enacted during the 1985–1986 legislative session ($99 \times 2 = 198 - 112 = 86$). The Tax Relief and Health Care Act of 2006 was P.L. 109-432. Using the formula reveals that this Act was enacted during the 2005–2006 legislative session ($109 \times 2 = 218 - 112 = 106$)

COMMITTEE REPORTS

It should be noted that at each stage of the legislative process, information is produced that may be useful in assessing the intent of Congress. One of the better sources of Congressional intent is a report issued by the House Ways and Means Committee. This report contains the bill as well as a general explanation. This explanation usually provides the historical background of the proposed legislation along with the reasons for enactment. The Senate Finance Committee also issues a report similar to that of the House. Because the Senate often makes changes in the House version of the bill, the Senate's report is also an important source. Additionally, the Joint Conference Committee on Taxation issues its own report, which is sometimes helpful. Two other sources of intent are the records of the debates on the bill and publications of the initial hearings.

Committee reports and debates appear in several publications. Committee reports are officially published in pamphlet form by the U.S. Government Printing Office as the bill proceeds through Congress. The enacted bill is published in the *Internal Revenue Bulletin* and the *Internal Revenue Cumulative Bulletin*. The debates are published in the *Congressional Record*. In addition to these official government publications, several commercial publishers make this information available to subscribers.

The diagram below illustrates the normal flow of a bill through the legislative process and the documents that are generated in this process.

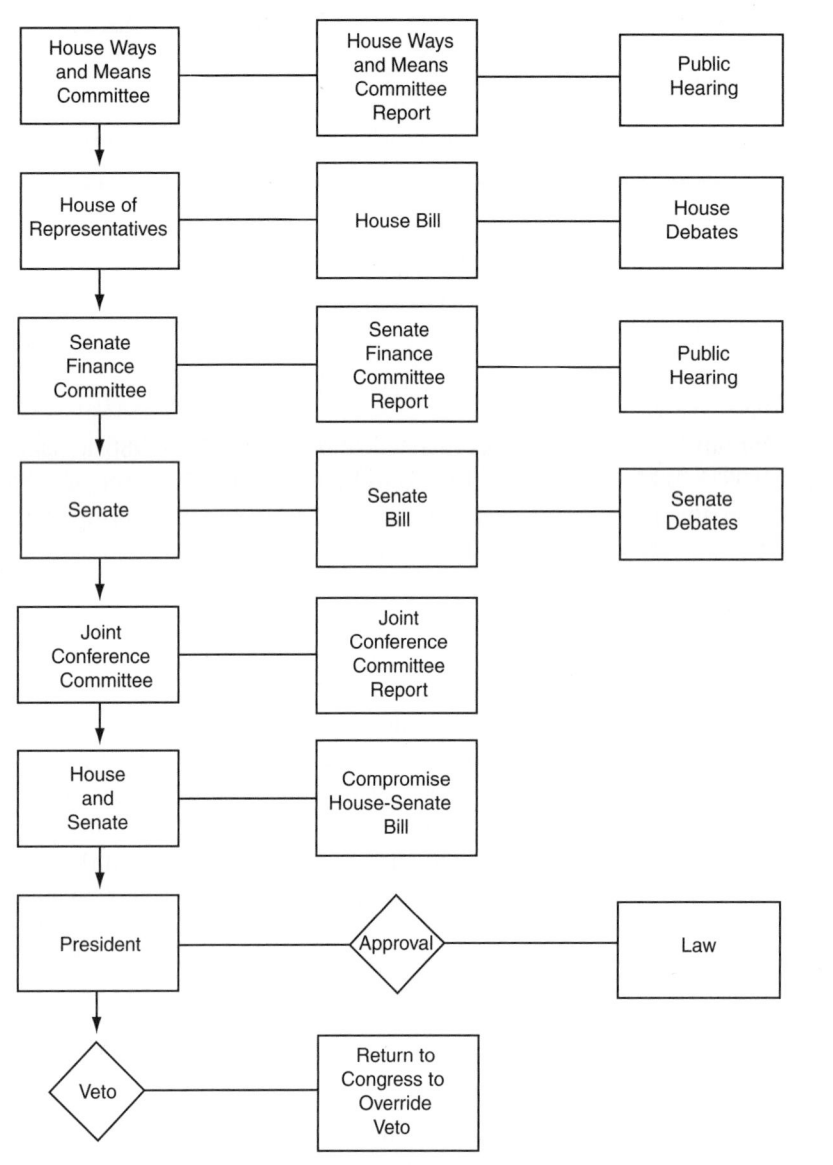

ORGANIZATION OF THE INTERNAL REVENUE CODE

Once a tax bill becomes tax law, it is incorporated into the existing structure of the U.S. federal laws known as the *United States Code*. As mentioned above, the *U.S. Code* is the collection of all laws enacted by Congress. Laws concerning the same subject matter (e.g., taxation) are consolidated in a single "title." As shown in Exhibit 2-1, there are 50 titles. Tax laws are incorporated directly into Title 26 entitled *Internal Revenue Code*.[3]

---

[3]   All future use of the term Code or Internal Revenue Code refers to the *Internal Revenue Code of 1986*, as amended.

EXHIBIT 2-1
United States Code

TITLE NUMBER	TITLE NAME	TITLE NUMBER	TITLE NAME
Title 1	General Provisions	**Title 26**	**Internal Revenue Code**
Title 2	The Congress	Title 27	Intoxicating Liquors
Title 3	The President	Title 28	Judiciary and Judicial Procedure
Title 4	Flag and Seal, Seat Of Government, ...	Title 29	Labor
Title 5	Government Organization and Employees	Title 30	Mineral Lands and Mining
Title 6	Domestic Security	Title 31	Money and Finance
Title 7	Agriculture	Title 32	National Guard
Title 8	Aliens and Nationality	Title 33	Navigation and Navigable Waters
Title 9	Arbitration	Title 34	Navy (repealed)
Title 10	Armed Forces	Title 35	Patents
Title 11	Bankruptcy	Title 36	Patriotic Societies and Observances
Title 12	Banks and Banking	Title 37	Pay and Allowances Of the Uniformed Services
Title 13	Census	Title 38	Veterans' Benefits
Title 14	Coast Guard	Title 39	Postal Service
Title 15	Commerce and Trade	Title 40	Public Buildings, Property, and Works
Title 16	Conservation	Title 41	Public Contracts
Title 17	Copyrights	Title 42	The Public Health and Welfare
Title 18	Crimes and Criminal Procedure	Title 43	Public Lands
Title 19	Customs Duties	Title 44	Public Printing and Documents
Title 20	Education	Title 45	Railroads
Title 21	Food and Drugs	Title 46	Shipping
Title 22	Foreign Relations and Intercourse	Title 47	Telegraphs, Telephones, and Radiotelegraphs
Title 23	Highways	Title 48	Territories and Insular Possessions
Title 24	Hospitals and Asylums	Title 49	Transportation
Title 25	Indians	Title 50	War and National Defense

Title 26 (the Internal Revenue Code) is further divided as follows:

> **Title 26** of the United States Code (referred to as the Internal Revenue Code)
> **Subtitle A**—Income Taxes
> **Chapter 1**—Normal Taxes and Surtaxes
> **Subchapter A**—Determination of Tax Liability
> **Part I**—Tax on Individuals
> **Sections**—1 through 5

Exhibit 2-2 reveals the contents of the various subdivisions. As a practical matter, virtually all of a tax practitioner's work is done in Subtitle A, Chapter 1, which deals with income taxes. Note that subtitles are further divided into chapters, subchapters, parts, subparts and finally the most important element: sections.

EXHIBIT 2-2

Internal Revenue Code: Subtitles, Chapters, Subchapters

Subtitle	Subject	First Code Section
Subtitle A	Income Taxes	§ 1
Subtitle B	Estate and Gift Taxes	§ 2001
Subtitle C	Employment Taxes	§ 3101
Subtitle D	Miscellaneous Excise Taxes	§ 4001
Subtitle E	Alcohol, Tobacco, and Certain Other Excise Taxes	§ 5001
Subtitle F	Procedure and Administration	§ 6001
Subtitle G	The Joint Committee on Taxation	§ 8001
Subtitle H	Financing of Presidential Election Campaigns	§ 9001
Subtitle I	Trust Fund Code	§ 9501

Chapters in Subtitle A	Name	First Code Section
1	Income Taxes	§ 1
2	Tax on Self-Employment Income	§ 1401
3	Withholding of Tax on Nonresident Aliens and Foreign Corporations	§ 1441
4	[Repealed]	
5	[Repealed]	§ 1491
6	Consolidated Returns	§ 1501

Selected Subchapters of Chapter 1	Name	Code Sections
A	Determination of Tax Liability	§§ 1-59B
B	Computation of Taxable Income	§§ 61-291
C	Corporate Distributions and Adjustments	§§ 301-385
D	Deferred Compensation, etc.	§§ 401-436
E	Accounting Periods and Methods of Accounting	§§ 441-483
F	Exempt Organizations	§§ 501-530
G	Corporations Used to Avoid Income Tax on Shareholders	§§ 531-565
H	Banking Institutions	§§ 581-597
I	Natural Resources	§§ 611-638
J	Estates, Trusts, Beneficiaries, and Decedents	§§ 641-692
K	Partners and Partnerships	§§ 701-777
L	Insurance Companies	§§ 801-848
M	Regulated Investment Companies and Real Estate Investment Trusts	§§ 851-860L
N	Tax Based on Income From Sources Within or Without the United States	§§ 861-999
O	Gain or Loss on Disposition of Property	§§ 1001-1111
P	Capital Gains and Losses	§§ 1201-1298
S	Tax Treatment of S Corporations and Their Shareholders	§§ 1361-1379

The most critical portions of the Internal Revenue Code are its "sections." The sections contain the laws—often referred to as provisions or rules—that a taxpayer must follow to determine taxable income and ultimately the final tax liability. For example, the starting point in determining taxable income is gross income and Code Section 61 provides the definition of gross income as follows: income. Section 61 appears below.

Section 61: Gross Income Defined

(a)   *General definition. Except as otherwise provided in this subtitle (A), gross income means all income from whatever source derived, including (but not limited to) the following items:*

    (1)   *Compensation for services, including fees, commissions, fringe benefits, and similar items;*

    (2)   *Gross income derived from business;*

    (3)   *Gains derived from dealings in property*

    (4)   *Interest*

    (5)   *Rents*

       .

       .

       .

    (14)   *Income in respect of a decedent and*

    (15)   *Income from an interest in an estate or trust.*

The ability to use the Internal Revenue Code is essential for all individuals who have any involvement with the tax laws.

When working with the tax law, it is often necessary to make reference to, or *cite*, a particular source with respect to the Code. The *section* of the Code is the source normally cited. A complete citation for a section of the Code would be too cumbersome. For instance, a formal citation for Section 1 of the Code would be "Subtitle A, Chapter 1, Subchapter A, Part I, Section 1." In most cases, citation of the section alone is sufficient. Sections are numbered consecutively throughout the Code so that each section number is used only once. Currently the numbers run from Section 1 through Section 9833. Not all section numbers are used, so that additional ones may be added by Congress in the future without the need for renumbering.[4]

Citation of a particular Code section in tax literature ordinarily does not require the prefix "Internal Revenue Code" because it is generally understood that, unless otherwise stated, references to section numbers concern the Internal Revenue Code of 1986 as amended. However, since most Code sections are divided into subparts, reference to a specific subpart requires more than just its section number. Section 170(a)(2)(B) serves as an example.

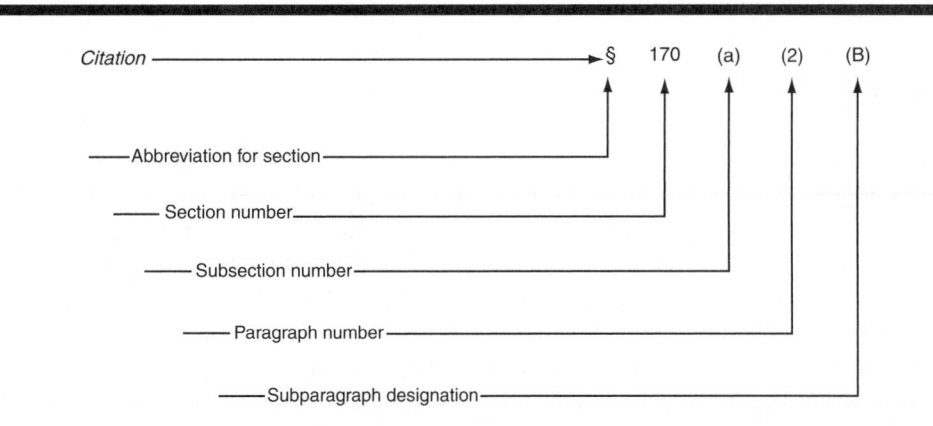

---

4   It is interesting to note that when it adopted the 1954 Code, Congress deliberately left section numbers unassigned to provide room for future additions. Recently, however, Congress has been forced to identify new sections by alphabetical letters following a particular section number. See, for example, Sections 280, 280A, 280B, and 280C of the 1986 Code.

All footnote references used throughout this text are made in the form given above. In most cases, the "§" or "§§" symbols are used in place of the terms "section" or "sections," respectively.

Single-volume or double-volume editions of the Internal Revenue Code are published after every major change in the law. Private publishing companies such as Commerce Clearing House, Inc. (CCH) and the Research Institute of America (RIA) publish these editions as well as a wealth of other tax information. All of this tax information is included in so-called tax services–massive tax libraries–compiled and published by these companies and others. The major tax services, all available electronically, are discussed in a later section of this chapter.

TAX TREATIES

The laws contained in tax treaties represent the third and final component of the statutory law. Tax treaties (also referred to as tax conventions) are agreements between the United States and other countries that provide rules governing the taxation of residents of one country by another. For example, the tax treaty between the United States and France indicates how the French government taxes U.S. citizens residing in France and vice versa. Tax treaties, as law, have the same authority as those laws contained in the Code.[5] Treaty provisions may override provisions of the Internal Revenue Code if the treaty was signed after August 16, 1954.[6] For this reason, persons involved with an international tax question must be aware of tax treaties and recognize that the Code may be superseded by a tax treaty.

ADMINISTRATIVE INTERPRETATIONS

After Congress has enacted a tax law, the Executive branch of the Federal government has the responsibility for enforcing it. In the process of enforcing the law, the Treasury interprets, clarifies, defines, and analyzes the Code in order to apply Congressional intention of the law to the specific facts of a taxpayer's situation. This process results in numerous administrative releases including the following:

1. Regulations

2. Revenue rulings and letter rulings

3. Revenue procedures

4. Technical advice memoranda

REGULATIONS

Regulations are the Treasury's official interpretation of the Internal Revenue Code. To illustrate, consider the problem of a couple who discovered $4,467 of old currency in a piano seven years after they purchased it at an auction for $15.[7] Is this taxable income? Note that the definition of gross income contained in § 61 above provides little guidance, indicating only that "income is income from whatever source derived." However, one of the regulations explaining what constitutes gross income, Reg. § 1.61-14, indicates that buried treasure is to be included in income. Other regulations concerning gross income discuss in detail the treatment of such items as dividends, interest and rents. The major

---

[5]   See Code § 7852(d)(1).

[6]   § 7852(d)(2).

[7]   *Ermenegildo Cesarini v. U.S.*, 69-1 USTC ¶9270, 23 AFTR 2d 69-997, 296 F Supp 3 (DC-OH, 1969).

purpose of the regulations is to interpret, explain, clarify and elaborate on the various provisions of the Internal Revenue Code.

Code § 7805(a) authorizes the Secretary of the Treasury to "prescribe all needful rules and regulations for the enforcement of this title, including all rules and regulations as may be necessary of any alteration of law in relation to internal revenue." Section 7805(b) provides authority to the Secretary to prescribe the extent, if any, to which any ruling or regulation relating to the internal revenue laws will be applied without retroactive effect. In most cases the Secretary delegates the power to write the regulations to the Commissioner of the Internal Revenue Service. In practice, this means that the regulations are written by the technical staff of the IRS or by the office of the Chief Counsel of the IRS, an official who is also an assistant General Counsel of the Treasury Department.

Regulations are issued in the form of *Treasury Decisions* (often referred to as TDs), which are published in the *Federal Register* and sometimes later in the *Internal Revenue Bulletin*. The *Federal Register* is the official publication for regulations and legal notices issued by the executive branch of the Federal government. The *Federal Register* is published every business day. Before a TD is published in final form, it must be issued in proposed form, a *proposed regulation*, for a period of at least 30 days before it is scheduled to become final.

Upon publication, interested parties have at least 30 days to comment on proposed regulations. In addition, public hearings are often scheduled. In theory, at the end of this comment period, the Treasury responds in any one of three ways; it may withdraw the proposed regulation, amend it, or leave it unchanged. In the latter two cases, the Treasury normally issues the regulation in its final form as a TD, published in the *Federal Register*. The final version of any given regulation is quite frequently significantly different from the proposed version.

Afterwards, the new regulation is included in Title 26 of the *Code of Federal Regulations*. In fact, however, proposed regulations sometimes remain in proposed form for many years. Proposed regulations do not have the force of law and are not the Treasury's official position on a particular issue.

Temporary Regulations. The National Office of the Treasury issues temporary regulations as the need arises. Often such regulations are issued in response to substantive changes in the tax law when tax practitioners, in particular, need immediate guidance in applying a new or revised statute. Such regulations usually deal with immediate filing requirements or details regarding a mandated accounting method change. Temporary regulations are effective immediately without the comment period. This is true even though temporary regulations normally are also issued as proposed regulations which are subject to the comment period. Temporary regulations expire three years after issuance and are given the same respect and precedential value as final regulations.

The primary purpose of the regulations is to explain and interpret particular Code sections. Although regulations have not been issued for all Code sections, they have been issued for the great majority. In those cases where regulations exist, they are an important authoritative source on which one can usually rely. Regulations can be classified into three groups: (1) legislative; (2) interpretive; and (3) procedural.

Legislative Regulations. Occasionally, Congress will give specific authorization to the Secretary of the Treasury to issue regulations on a particular Code section. For example, under § 1502, the Secretary is charged with prescribing the regulations for the filing of a consolidated return by an affiliated group of corporations. There are virtually no Code sections governing consolidated returns, and the regulations in effect serve in lieu of the Code. In this case and others where it occurs, the regulation has the force and effect of a law,

with the result that a court reviewing the regulation usually will not substitute its judgment for that of the Treasury Department unless the Treasury has clearly abused its discretion.[8]

Interpretative Regulations. Interpretative regulations explain the meaning of a Code section and commit the Treasury and the Internal Revenue Service to a particular position relative to the Code section in question. This type of regulation is binding on the IRS but not on the courts, although it is "a body of experience and informed judgment to which courts and litigants may properly resort for guidance."[9] Interpretive regulations have considerable authority and normally are invalidated only if they are inconsistent with the Code or are unreasonable.

Procedural Regulations. Procedural regulations cover such areas as the information a taxpayer must supply to the IRS and the internal management and conduct of the IRS in certain matters. Those regulations affecting vital interests of the taxpayers are generally binding on the IRS, and those regulations stating the taxpayer's obligation to file particular forms or other types of information are given the effect of law.

Citation for Regulations. Regulations are arranged in the same sequence as the Code sections they interpret. Thus, a regulation begins with a number that designates the type of tax or administrative, definitional, or procedural matter and is followed by the applicable Code section number. For example, Treasury Regulation Section 1.614-3(f)(5) serves as an illustration of how regulations are cited throughout this text.

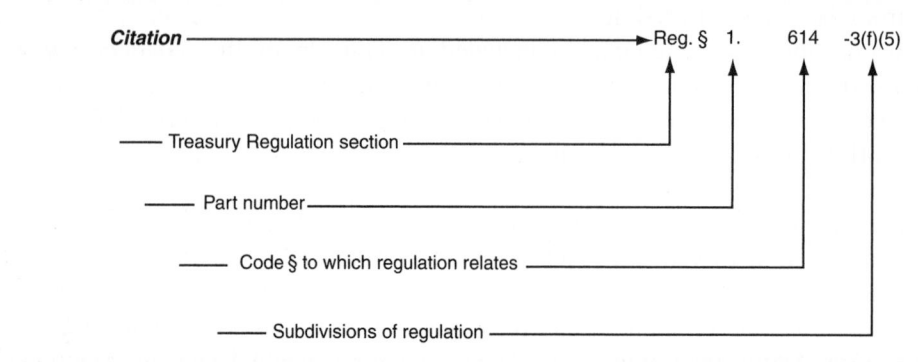

The part number of a Treasury regulation is used to identify the general area covered by the regulation as follows:

Part Number	Law Subject
1	Income Tax
20	Estate Tax
25	Gift Tax
31	Employment Tax
48–49	Excise Tax
301	Procedural Matters

The various subdivisions of a regulation are not necessarily related to a specific subdivision of the Code.

---

[8] *Anderson, Clayton & Co. v. U.S.*, 77-2 USTC ¶9727, 40 AFTR2d 77-6102, 562 F.2d 972 (CA-5, 1977), Cert. den. at 436 U.S. 944 (USSC, 1978).

[9] *Skidmore v. Swift and Co.*, 323 U.S. 134 (USSC, 1944).

Sometimes the Treasury issues temporary regulations when it is necessary to meet a compelling need. For example, temporary regulations are often issued shortly after enactment of a major change in the tax law. These temporary regulations have the same binding effect as final regulations until they are withdrawn or replaced. Such regulations are cited as Temp. Reg. §.

Temporary regulations should not be confused with proposed regulations. The latter have no force or effect.[10] Nevertheless, proposed regulations provide insight into how the IRS currently interprets a particular Code section. For this reason, they should not be ignored.

REVENUE RULINGS

Revenue rulings also are official interpretations of the Federal tax laws and are issued by the National Office of the IRS. Revenue rulings do not have quite the authority of regulations, however. Regulations are a direct extension of the law-making powers of Congress, whereas revenue rulings are an application of the administrative powers of the Internal Revenue Service. In contrast to rulings, regulations are usually issued only after public hearings and must be approved by the Secretary of the Treasury.

Unlike regulations, revenue rulings are limited to a given set of facts. For example, in Rev. Rul. 97-9, the IRS addressed whether the provision that concerns medical expenses, § 213, allowed a deduction for the costs of controlled substances such as marijuana when used for medical care. The ruling evaluated § 213 as it applied to this specific set of facts and held that because such purchases were in violation of Federal law they were not deductible.

Taxpayers may rely on revenue rulings in determining the tax consequences of their transactions; however, taxpayers must determine for themselves if the facts of their cases are substantially the same as those set forth in the revenue ruling.

Revenue rulings are published in the weekly issues of the *Internal Revenue Bulletin*. The information contained in the *Internal Revenue Bulletins* (including, among other things, revenue rulings) is accumulated and usually published semiannually in the *Cumulative Bulletin*. The *Cumulative Bulletin* reorganizes the material according to Code section. Citations for the *Internal Revenue Bulletin* and the *Cumulative Bulletin* are illustrated below.

REVENUE PROCEDURES

Revenue procedures are statements reflecting the internal management practices of the IRS that affect the rights and duties of taxpayers. Occasionally they are also used to announce procedures to guide individuals in dealing with the IRS or to make public something the IRS believes should be brought to the attention of taxpayers. For example, each year the IRS announces the rate at which business mileage can be deducted (e.g., Rev. Proc. 2008-72 provides that the rate for 2009 is 55 cents per mile).

Revenue procedures are published in the weekly *Internal Revenue Bulletins* and bound in the *Cumulative Bulletin* along with revenue rulings issued in the same year. The citation system for revenue procedures is the same as for revenue rulings except that the prefix "Rev. Proc." is substituted for "Rev. Rul."

---

[10]   Federal law (i.e., the Administrative Procedure Act) requires any federal agency, including the Internal Revenue Service, that wishes to adopt a substantive rule to publish the rule in proposed form in order to give interested persons an opportunity to comment. Proposed regulations are issued in compliance with this directive.

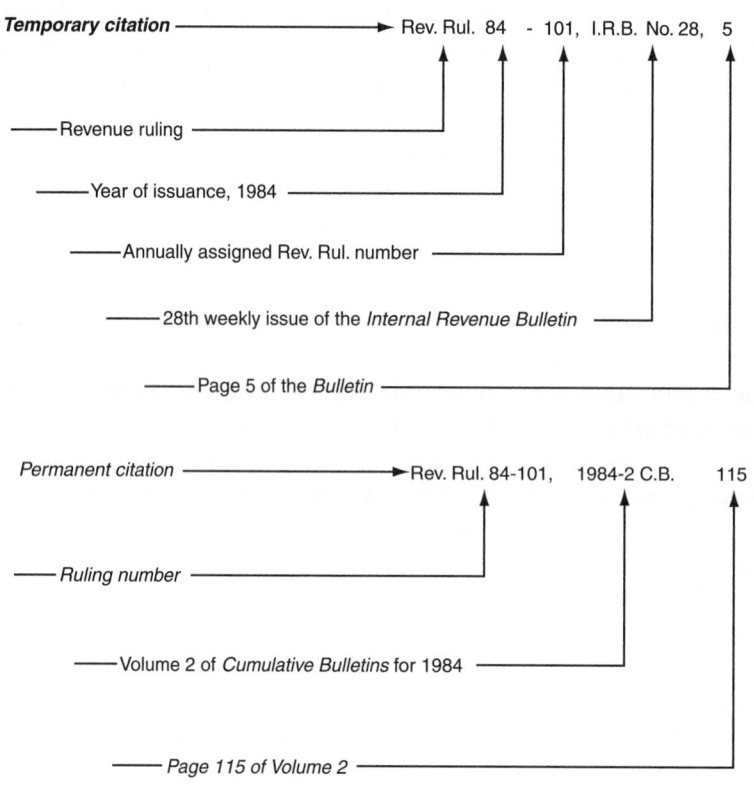

LETTER RULINGS

The term *letter ruling* actually encompasses three different types of rulings: private letter rulings, determination letters, and technical advice memoranda. These items are not published in an official government publication but are available from commercial sources.

Private Letter Ruling. Taxpayers who are in doubt about the tax consequences of a contemplated transaction can ask the National Office of the IRS for a ruling. Generally, the IRS has discretion about whether to rule or not, and it has issued guidelines describing the circumstances under which it will rule.[11]

Unlike revenue rulings, private letter rulings apply only to the particular taxpayer asking for the ruling and are thus not applicable to taxpayers in general. Section 6110(j)(3) specifically states that "unless the Secretary otherwise establishes by regulations, a written determination may not be used or cited as a precedent." Recently, however, the IRS has expanded the list of authorities constituting "substantial" authority for Section 6662 purposes to include private letter rulings. As discussed in the previous section, § 6662 imposes an accuracy-related penalty equal to 20 percent of the underpayment unless the taxpayer can cite "substantial authority" for his or her position.

For those requesting a ruling, the IRS's response might provide insurance against surprises. As a practical matter, a favorable ruling should preclude any controversies with the IRS on an audit of that transaction, at least with respect to the matters addressed in the private letter ruling. During the process of obtaining a private letter

---

[11]   See Rev. Proc. 2009-3, 2009-1 I.R.B. 107 for a description of the areas in which the IRS has refused to issue advanced rulings. Note, also, that the IRS is required to charge taxpayers a fee for letter rulings, opinion letters, determination letters, and similar requests. A sense of the various fees charged can be found in Rev. Proc. 2009-1, 2009-1 IRB 1 248, (Appendix A). See § 6591.

ruling, the IRS often recommends changes in a proposed transaction to assist the taxpayer in achieving the tax result he or she wishes. Since 1976, the IRS has made individual private letter rulings publicly available after deleting names and other information that would tend to identify the taxpayer. Private letter rulings are published by both CCH and RIA.

Determination Letter. A determination letter is similar to a private letter ruling, except that it is issued by the office of the local IRS district director, rather than by the National Office. Unlike private letter rulings, determination letters usually relate to completed transactions. Like private letter rulings, they are not published in any official government publication but are available commercially. In most instances, determination letters deal with issues and transactions that are not overtly controversial. Obtaining a determination letter in order to ensure that a pension plan is qualified is a typical use of a determination letter.

Technical Advice Memorandum. A technical advice memorandum ("tech advice") is typically requested by an IRS agent during an audit. The request is normally made to the National Office when the agent has a question that cannot be answered by sources in his or her local office. The technical advice memorandum only applies to the taxpayer for whose audit the technical advice was requested and cannot be relied upon by other taxpayers. Technical advice memoranda are available from private publishers but are not published by the government.

Citations for letter rulings and technical advice follow a multi-digit file number system. IRS Letter Ruling 200434039 serves as an example.

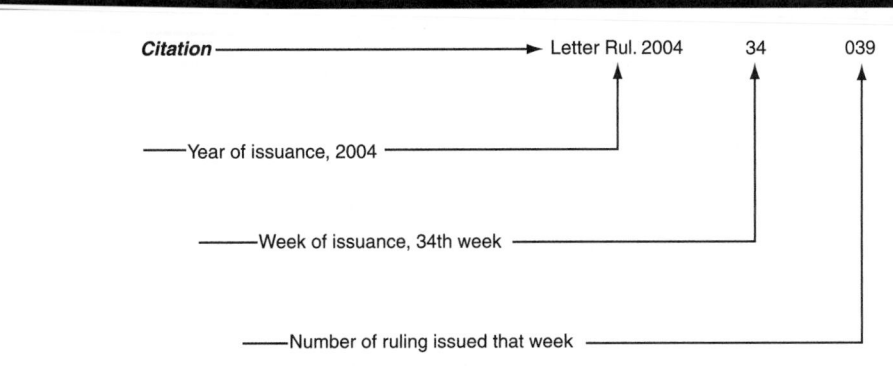

JUDICIAL INTERPRETATIONS

The Congress passes the tax law and the Executive branch of the Federal government enforces and interprets it, but under the American system of checks and balances, it is the Judiciary branch that ultimately determines whether the Executive branch's interpretation is correct. This provides yet another source of tax law—court decisions. It is therefore absolutely essential for the student of tax as well as the tax practitioner to have a grasp of the judicial system of the United States and how tax cases move through this system.

Before litigating a case in court, the taxpayer must have exhausted the administrative remedies available to him or her within the Internal Revenue Service. If the taxpayer has not exhausted his or her administrative remedies, a court will deny a hearing because the claim filed in the court is premature.

All litigation begins in what are referred to as *courts of original jurisdiction*, or *trial courts*, which "try" the case. There are three trial courts: (1) the Tax Court;

(2) the U.S. District Court; and (3) the U.S. Court of Federal Claims. Note that the taxpayer may select any one (and only one) of these three courts to hear the case. If the taxpayer or government disagrees with the decision by the trial court, it has the right to appeal to either the U.S. Court of Appeals or the U.S. Court of Appeals for the Federal Circuit, whichever is appropriate in the particular case. If a litigating party is dissatisfied with the decision by the appellate court, it may ask for review by the Supreme Court, but this is rarely granted. The judicial system is illustrated and discussed on the following page.

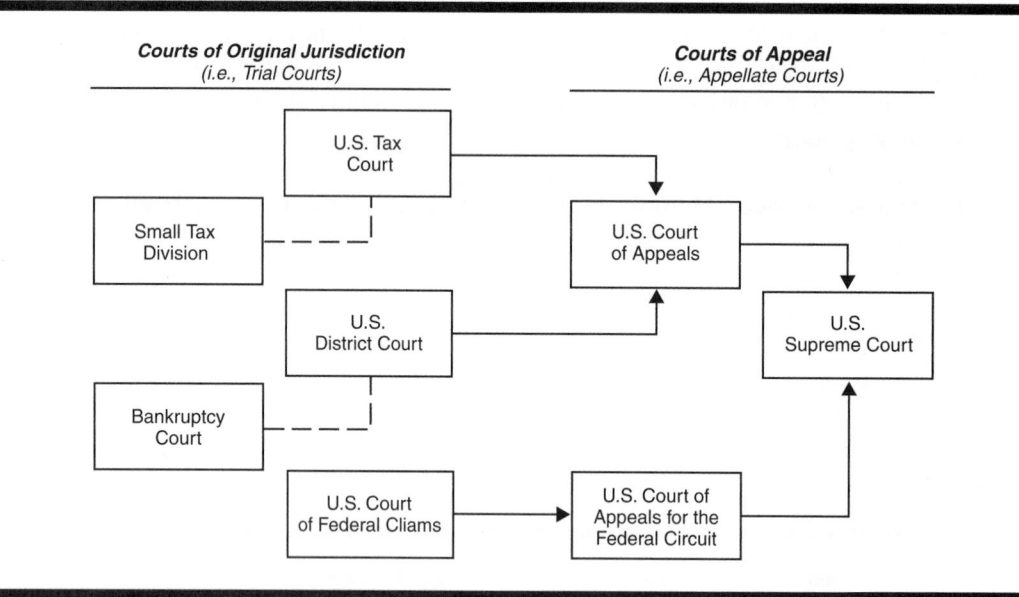

TRIAL COURTS

U.S. Tax Court. The Tax Court, as its name suggests, specializes in tax matters and hears no other types of cases. The judges on the court are especially skilled in taxation. Usually, prior to being selected as a judge by the President, the individual was a practitioner or IRS official who was noted for his or her expertise. This Court is composed of 19 judges who "ride circuit" throughout the United States (i.e., they travel and hear cases in various parts of the country as can be seen in the map contained in Exhibit 2-3). Occasionally, the full Tax Court hears a case, but most cases are heard by a single judge who submits his or her opinion to the chief judge, who then decides whether the full court should review the decision.

Besides its expertise in tax matters, two other characteristics of the Tax Court should be noted. Perhaps the most important feature of the Tax Court is that the taxpayer does not pay the alleged tax deficiency before bringing his or her action before the court. The second facet of the Tax Court that bears mentioning is that a trial by jury is not available.

U.S. District Courts. For purposes of the Federal judicial system, the United States is divided into 11 geographic areas called circuits, which are subdivided into districts. For example, the second circuit, which is composed of Vermont, Connecticut, and New York, contains the District Court for the Southern District of New York, which covers parts of New York City. Other districts may include very large areas, such as the District Court for the State of Arizona, which covers the entire state. A taxpayer may take a case into the District Court for the district in which he or she resides, but only after the disputed tax deficiency has been paid. The taxpayer then sues the IRS for a refund of the disputed amount. The District Court is a court of general jurisdiction and hears many

types of cases in addition to tax cases. This is the only court in which the taxpayer may obtain a jury trial. The jury decides matters of fact but not matters of law. However, even in issues of fact, the judge may, and occasionally does, disregard the jury's decision.

U.S. Court of Federal Claims. The United States Court of Federal Claims hears cases involving certain claims against the Federal government, including tax refunds. The Court is made up of 16 judges and usually meets in Washington, D.C. A taxpayer must pay the disputed tax deficiency before bringing an action in this court, and may not obtain a jury trial. Appeals from the U.S. Court of Federal Claims are taken to the U.S. Court of Appeals for the Federal Circuit.

The chart below illustrates the position of the taxpayer in bringing an action in these courts.

Small Claims Cases. When the amount of tax and penalties or a claim for refund are $50,000 per year or less, the taxpayer may elect to submit the case to the division of the Tax Court hearing small claims cases, called the Small Tax Division of the Tax Court. This procedure allows a taxpayer to obtain a decision with a minimum of formality, delay, and expense. However, the taxpayer loses the right to appeal the decision. The Small Tax Division is administered by the chief judge of the Tax Court, who is authorized to assign small claims cases to special trial judges. These cases receive priority on the trial calendars, and relatively informal rules are followed whenever possible. The special trial judges' opinions are published on these cases, but the decisions are not reviewed by any other court or treated as precedents in any other case.

Bankruptcy Court. Under limited circumstances, it is possible for the bankruptcy court to have jurisdiction over tax matters. The filing of a bankruptcy petition prevents creditors, including the IRS, from taking action against a taxpayer, including the filing of a proceeding before the Tax Court if a notice of deficiency is sent after the filing of a petition in bankruptcy. In such cases, a tax claim may be determined by the bankruptcy court.

	U.S. Tax Court	U.S. District Court	U.S. Court of Federal Claims
Jurisdiction	Nationwide	Specific district in which court is sitting	Nationwide
Subject Matter	Tax cases only	Many different types of cases, both criminal and civil	Claims against the Federal government, including tax refunds
Payment of Contested Amount	Taxpayer does not pay deficiency, but files suit against IRS Commissioner to stop collection of tax	Taxpayer pays alleged deficiency and then files suit against the U.S. government for refund	Taxpayer pays alleged deficiency and then files suit against the U.S. government for refund
Availability of Jury Trial	No	Yes	No
Appeal Taken to	U.S. Court of Appeals	U.S. Court of Appeals	U.S. Court of Appeals for the Federal Circuit
Number of Courts	1	95	1
Number of Judges per Court	19	1	16

APPELLATE COURTS

U.S. Courts of Appeals. Which appellate court is appropriate depends on which trial court hears the case. Taxpayer or government appeals from the District Courts and the Tax Court are taken to the U.S. Court of Appeals that has jurisdiction over the court in which the taxpayer lives. Appeals from the U.S. Court of Federal Claims are taken to the U.S. Court of Appeals for the Federal Circuit, which has the same powers and jurisdictions as any of the other Courts of Appeals except that it only hears specialized appeals. Courts of Appeals are national courts of appellate jurisdiction. With the exceptions of the Court of Appeals for the Federal Circuit and the Court of Appeals for the District of Columbia, these appellate courts are assigned various geographic areas of jurisdiction as shown in the map in Exhibit 2-3 and in the table below.

Court of Appeals for the Federal Circuit (CA-FC)	District of Columbia Circuit (CA-DC)	First Circuit (CA-1)		
U.S. Court of Federal Claims	District of Columbia	Maine Massachusetts New Hampshire Puerto Rico Rhode Island		

Second Circuit (CA-2)	Third Circuit (CA-3)	Fourth Circuit (CA-4)	Fifth Circuit (CA-5)	Sixth Circuit (CA-6)
Connecticut New York Vermont	Delaware New Jersey Pennsylvania Virgin Islands	Maryland N. Carolina S. Carolina Virginia W. Virginia	Louisiana Mississippi Texas	Kentucky Michigan Ohio Tennessee

Seventh Circuit (CA-7)	Eighth Circuit (CA-8)	Ninth Circuit (CA-9)	Tenth Circuit (CA-10)	Eleventh Circuit (CA-11)
Illinois Indiana Wisconsin	Arkansas Iowa Minnesota Missouri Nebraska N. Dakota S. Dakota	Alaska Arizona California Guam Hawaii Idaho Montana Nevada Oregon Washington	Colorado New Mexico Kansas Oklahoma Utah Wyoming	Alabama Florida Georgia

EXHIBIT 2-3

United State Tax Court: Places of Trial and U.S. Courts of Appeals

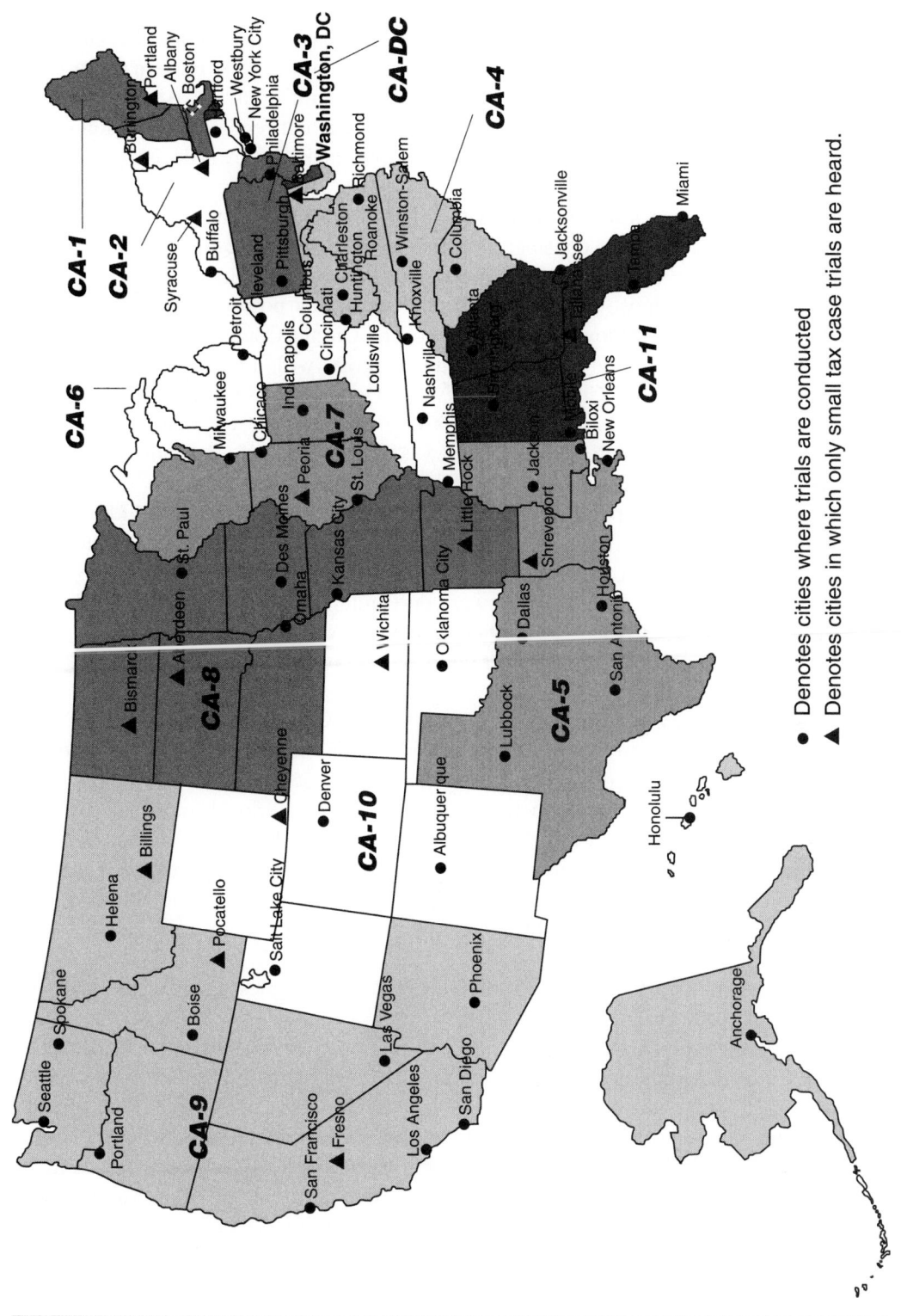

• Denotes cities where trials are conducted

▲ Denotes cities in which only small tax case trials are heard.

Taxpayers may appeal to the Courts of Appeal as a matter of right, and the Courts must hear their cases. Very often, however, the expense of such an appeal deters many from proceeding with an appeal. Appellate courts review the record of the trial court to determine whether the lower court completed its responsibility of fact finding and applied the proper law in arriving at its decision.

District Courts must follow the decision of the Appeals Court for the circuit in which they are located. For instance, the District Court in the Eastern District of Missouri must follow the decision of the Eighth Circuit Court of Appeals because Missouri is in the Eighth Circuit. If the Eighth Circuit has not rendered a decision on the particular issue involved, then the District Court may make its own decision or follow the decision in another Circuit.

The Tax Court is a national court with jurisdiction throughout the entire country. Prior to 1970, the Tax Court considered itself independent and indicated that it would not be bound by the decisions of the Circuit Court to which its decision would be appealed. In *Golsen*,[12] however, the Tax Court reversed its position. Under the *Golsen rule*, the Tax Court now follows the decisions of the Circuit Court to which a particular case would be appealed. Even if the Tax Court disagrees with a Circuit Court's view, it will decide based upon the Circuit Court's view. On the other hand, if a similar case arises in the jurisdiction of another Circuit Court that has not yet ruled on the same issue, the Tax Court will follow its own view, despite its earlier decision following a contrary Circuit Court decision.

The U.S. Courts of Appeals generally sit in panels of three judges, although the entire court may sit in particularly important cases. They may reach a decision that affirms the lower court or that reverses the lower court. Additionally, the Appellate Court could send the case back to the lower court (remand the case) for another trial or for rehearing on another point not previously covered. It is possible for the Appellate Court to affirm the decision of the lower court on one particular issue and reverse it on another.

Generally, only one judge writes a decision for the Appeals Court, although in some cases no decision is written and an order is simply made. Such an order might hold that the lower court is sustained, or that the lower court's decision is reversed as being inconsistent with one of the Appellate Court's decisions. Sometimes other judges (besides the one assigned to write the opinion) will write additional opinions agreeing with (concurring opinion) or disagreeing with (dissenting opinion) the majority opinion. These opinions often contain valuable insights into the law controlling the case, and often set the ground for a change in the court's opinion at a later date.

U.S. Supreme Court. The U.S. Supreme Court is the highest court of the land. No one has a *right* to be heard by this Court. It only accepts cases it wishes to hear, and generally those involve issues that the Court feels are of national importance. The Supreme Court generally hears very few tax cases. Consequently, taxpayers desiring a review of their trial court decision find it solely at the Court of Appeals. Technically, cases are submitted to the Supreme Court through a request process known as the "Writ of Certiorari." If the Supreme Court decides to hear the case, it grants the Writ of Certiorari; if it decides not to hear the case, it denies the Writ of Certiorari. It is important to note that there is another path to review by the U.S. Supreme Court—*by appeal*—as opposed to by Writ of Certiorari. This "review by appeal" may be available when a U.S. Court of Appeals has held that a state statute is in conflict with the laws or treaties of the United States. The "review by appeal" may also be available when the highest court in a state has decided a case on grounds that a Federal statute or treaty is invalid, or when the state court has held a state statute valid despite the claim of the

---

[12] *Jack E. Golsen.* 54 T.C. 742 (1970).

losing party that the statute is in conflict with the U.S. Constitution or a Federal law. Review by the U.S. Supreme Court is still discretionary, but a Writ of Certiorari is not involved.

The Supreme Court, like the Courts of Appeals, does not conduct another trial. Its responsibility is to review the record and determine whether or not the trial court correctly applied the law in deciding the case. The Supreme Court also reviews the decision of the Court of Appeals to determine if the court used the correct reasoning.

In general, the Supreme Court hears cases only when one or more of the following conditions apply:

1. When the Court of Appeals has not used accepted or usual methods of judicial procedure or has sanctioned an unusual method by the trial court;

2. When a Court of Appeals has settled an important question of Federal law and the Supreme Court feels such an important question should have one more review by the most prestigious court of the nation;

3. When a decision of a Court of Appeals is in apparent conflict with a decision of the Supreme Court;

4. When two or more Courts of Appeals are in conflict on an issue; or

5. When the Supreme Court has already decided an issue but feels that the issue should be looked at again, possibly to reverse its previous decision.

CASE CITATION

Tax Court Decisions. Prior to 1943, the Tax Court was called the Board of Tax Appeals. The decisions of the Board of Tax Appeals were published as the *United States Board of Tax Appeals Reports* (BTA). Board of Tax Appeals cases are cited as follows:

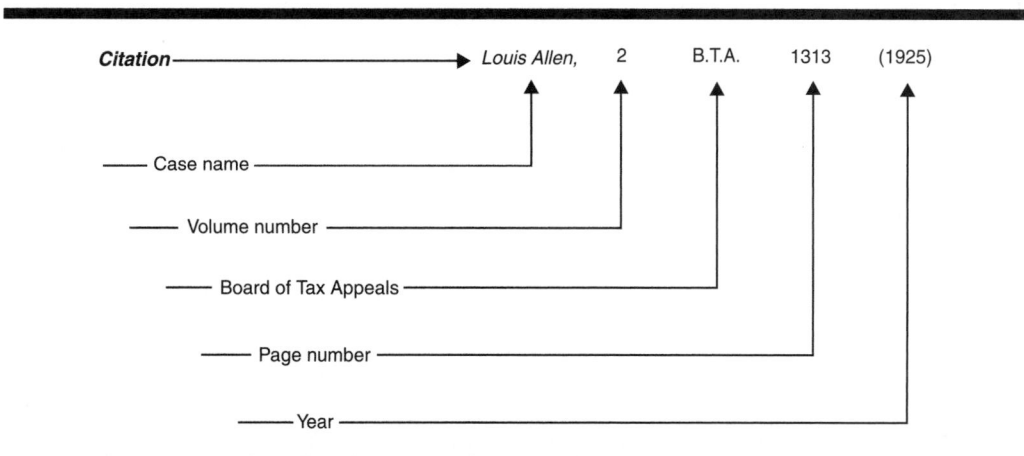

The Tax Court renders two different types of decisions with two different citation systems: Regular decisions and Memorandum decisions.

Tax Court *Regular* decisions deal with new issues that the court has not yet resolved. In contrast, decisions that deal only with the application of already established principles of law are called *Memorandum* decisions. The United States government publishes Regular decisions in *United States Tax Court Reports* (T.C.). Tax Court Regular decisions are cited as follows:

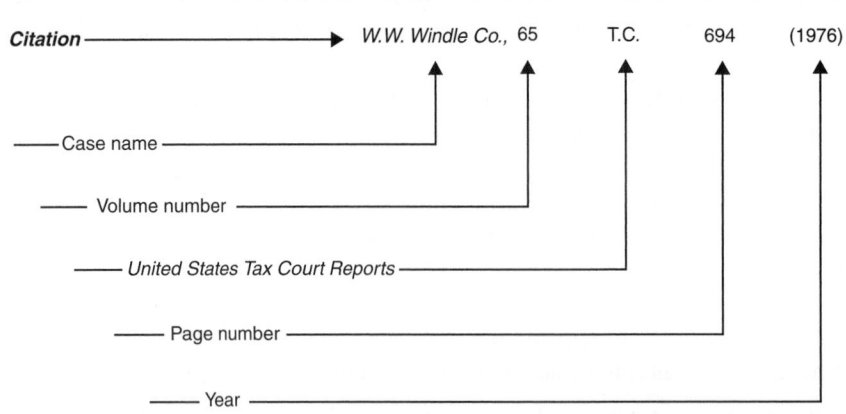

Citation ⟶ *W.W. Windle Co.,* 65 T.C. 694 (1976)

——— Case name ———

——— Volume number ———

——— *United States Tax Court Reports* ———

——— Page number ———

——— Year ———

Like revenue rulings and the *Cumulative Bulletins*, there is a time lag between the date a Tax Court Regular decision is issued and the date it is bound in a *U.S. Tax Court Report* volume. In this case, the citation appears as follows:

Temporary Citation:

W.W. Windle Co., 65 T.C. ————— , No. 79(1976).

Here the page is left out, but the citation tells the reader that this is the 79th Regular decision issued by the Tax Court since Volume 64 ended. When the new volume (65th) of the Tax Court Report is issued, then the permanent citation may be substituted for the old one. Both CCH and RIA have tax services that allow the researcher to find these temporary citations.

The IRS has adopted the practice of announcing whether it agrees or disagrees with a decision issued by a court by announcing its acquiescence or nonacquiescence. Until 1991, this practice was limited to certain Regular decisions of the Tax Court. At that time, however, the IRS began to acquiesce or nonacquiesce to other cases where it thought it would be useful.[13] The IRS may withdraw its acquiescence or nonacquiescence at any time and may do so even retroactively. Acquiescences and nonacquiescences are published in the weekly *Internal Revenue Bulletins* and the *Cumulative Bulletins*.

The U.S. government publishes the Tax Court's Regular decisions, and also posts the decisions to its website (http://www.ustaxcourt.gov). The website currently has both Regular and Memorandum decisions since September 25, 1995. The Tax Court does not publish memorandum decisions. However, both CCH and RIA publish them. CCH publishes the memorandum decisions under the title *Tax Court Memorandum Decisions* (TCM), while RIA publishes these decisions as *Tax Court Reporter and Memorandum Decisions* (T.C. Memo). In citing Tax Court memorandum decisions, some authors prefer to use both the RIA and the CCH citations for their cases.

Decisions of the Small Claims division of the Tax Court were first published on the U.S. Tax Court Web site as U.S. Tax Court Summary Opinions in 2001. All of these decisions appear with the caveat that such cases may not be treated as precedent for any other case.

In an effort to provide the reader the greatest latitude of research sources, this dual citation policy has been adopted for this text. The case of *Alan K. Minor* serves as an example of the dual citation of Tax Court memorandum decisions.

---

[13] The IRS's acquiescence is symbolized by "A" or "Acq." and its nonacquiescence by "NA" or "Nonacq."

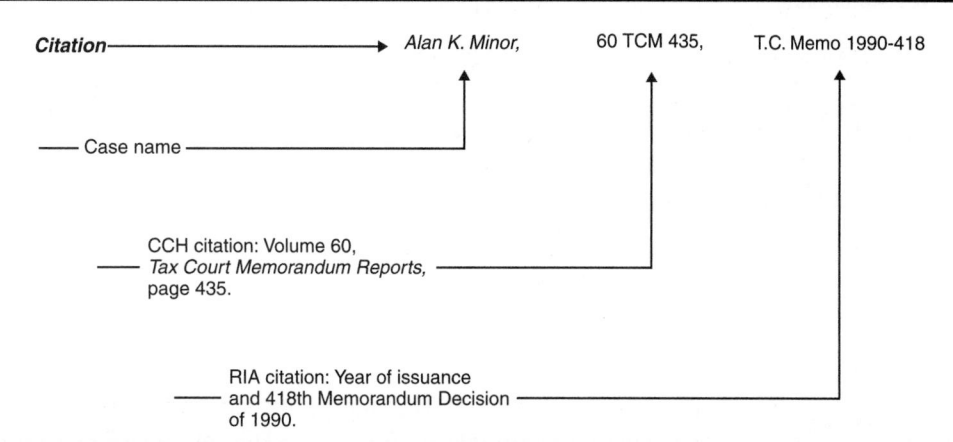

As noted above, Tax Court Summary Opinions can be found at the website of the Tax Court or through RIA and CCH. All use the same form of citation. For example, the decision in Richard Bradley on January 21, 2006 would be cited as follows:

   Richard Bradley, T.C. Summary Opinion, 2006–61

Citations for U.S. District Court, Court of Appeals, and Claims Court. Commerce Clearing House, Research Institute of America, and West Publishing Company all publish decisions of the District Courts, Courts of Appeals, and the Court of Federal Claims. When available, all three citations of a case are provided in this text.[14] CCH publishes the decisions of these courts in its *U.S. Tax Cases* (USTC—not to be confused with the *U.S. Tax Court Reports*) volumes, and RIA offers these decisions in its *American Federal Tax Reports* (AFTR) series.[15] West Publishing Company reports these decisions in either its *Federal Supplement Series* (F. Supp.—District Court decisions), or its *Federal Second Series or Federal Third Series* (F.2d or F.3d—Court of Federal Claims and Courts of Appeals decisions).

The citation of the U.S. District Court decision of *Cam F. Dowell, Jr. v. U.S.* is illustrated for each of the three publishing companies as follows:

CCH Citation:

   Cam F. Dowell, Jr. v. U.S., 74-1 USTC ¶9243, (D.Ct. Tx., 1974).

Interpretation: This case is reported in the first volume of the *U.S. Tax Cases*, published by CCH for calendar year 1974 (74-1), located at paragraph (¶) 9243, and is a decision rendered in 1974 by a U.S. District Court located in Texas (Tx.).

RIA Citation:

   Cam F. Dowell, Jr. v. U.S., 33 AFTR2d 74-739, (D.Ct. Tx., 1974).

Interpretation: Reported in the 33rd volume of the second series of the *American Federal Tax Reports* (AFTR2d), published by RIA for 1974, and located at page 739.

---

14   When all three publishers have not printed the case, only the citations to the cases published are provided.

15   Until the acquisition of Prentice Hall by RIA, Prentice Hall published cases under its own name. Accordingly, researchers needing cases from before 1993 will often encounter Prentice Hall as publisher of these reporters now carried under RIA's name.

West Citation:

> *Cam F. Dowell, Jr. v. U.S.*, 370 F.Supp. 69 (D.Ct. Tx., 1974).

Interpretation: Located in the 370th volume of the *Federal Supplement Series* (F.Supp), published by West Publishing Company, and located at page 69.

The multiple citation of the U.S. District Court case illustrated above appears as follows:

> *Cam F. Dowell, Jr. v. U.S.*, 74-1 USTC ¶9243, 33 AFTR2d 74-739, 370 F.Supp. 69 (D.Ct. Tx., 1974).

Decisions of the Court of Federal Claims (Ct. Cls.), the Courts of Appeals (e.g., CA-1, CA-2, etc.), and the Supreme Court (USSC) are published by CCH and RIA in the same reporting source as District Court decisions (i.e., USTCs and AFTRs). Court of Federal Claims and Court of Appeals decisions are reported by West Publishing Company in its *Federal Second Series* (F.2d) or *Federal Third Series* (F.3d). West also publishes the *Federal Appendix* (Fed. Appx.) which includes opinions not selected by the Courts of Appeals for publication in the Federal reporters. Supreme Court decisions are published by West Publishing Company in its *Supreme Court Reports* (S.Ct.), and the U.S. Government Printing Office publishes Supreme Court decisions in its *Supreme Court Reports* (U.S.).

An example of the multiple citation of a Court of Appeals decision follows:

Citation:

> *Millar v. Comm.*, 78-2 USTC ¶9514, 42 AFTR2d 78-5246, 577 F.2d 212 (CA-3, 1978).

A multiple citation of a Supreme Court decision would appear as follows:

Citation:

> *Fausner v. Comm.*, 73-2 USTC ¶9515, 32 AFTR2d 73-5202, 413 U.S. 838 (USSC, 1973).

Note that in each of the citations above, the designation "Commissioner of the Internal Revenue Service" is simply abbreviated to "Comm." In some instances, the IRS or U.S. is substituted for Comm., and older cases used the Commissioner's name. For example, in *Gregory v. Helvering*, 293 U.S. 465 (USSC, 1935), Mr. Helvering was the Commissioner of the Internal Revenue Service at the time the case was brought to the Court. Also note that the citation contains a reference to the Appellate Court rendering the decision (i.e., CA-3, or USSC) and the year of issuance.

Exhibits 2-4 and 2-5 summarize the sources of case citations from various reporter services.

EXHIBIT 2-4
Reporters of Tax Court Decisions

Reporter	Abbr.	Type	Publisher
Tax Court Reports	TC	Regular	Government Printing Office
Tax Court Memorandum Decisions	TCM	Memorandum	Commerce Clearing House
Tax Court Memorandum Decisions	TC Memo	Memorandum	Research Institute of America

EXHIBIT 2-5
Reporters of Decisions Other Than Tax Court

Reporter	Abbr.	Courts Reported	Publisher
Supreme Court Reports	U.S.	Supreme Court	Government Printing Office
Supreme Court Reporter	S.Ct	Supreme Court	West Publishing
Federal Supplement	F.Supp	District Courts	West Publishing
Federal Reporter	F. F.2d F.3d	Cts. of Appeals and Ct. of Fed. Cls.	West Publishing
Federal Appendix	Fed. Appx.	Cts. of Appeals Unreported cases	West Publishing
American Federal Tax Reports	AFTR2d	Ct. of Fed. Cls. Cts. of Appeals, and Supreme Ct.	Research Institute of America
United States Tax Cases	USTC	Same as AFTR and AFTR2d	Commerce Clearing House

SECONDARY SOURCES

The importance of understanding the sources discussed thus far stems from their role in the taxation process. As mentioned earlier, the statutory law and its official interpretations constitute the legal authorities that set forth the tax consequences for a particular set of facts. These legal authorities, sometimes referred to as *primary authorities*, must be distinguished from so-called *secondary sources* or *secondary authorities*. The secondary sources of tax information consist mainly of books, periodicals, articles, newsletters, and editorial judgments in tax services. When working with the tax law, it must be recognized that secondary sources are unofficial interpretations—mere opinions—that have no legal authority.

Although secondary sources should not be used as the supporting authority for a particular tax treatment (except as a supplement to primary authority or in cases where primary authority is absent), they are an indispensable aid when seeking an understanding of the tax law. Several of these secondary materials are discussed briefly below.

TAX SERVICES

"Tax service" is the name given to a set of organized materials that contains a vast quantity of tax-related information organized so as to make it useful and accessible to tax practitioners. In general, a tax service is a paper or electronic compilation of some or all of the following: the Code, regulations, court decisions, IRS releases, and explanations of these primary authorities by the editors. As the listing of contents suggests, a tax service is invaluable since it contains, all in one place, a wealth of tax information, including both primary and secondary sources. Most tax services are available on CD-ROM or the Internet, or both. Moreover, these materials are updated constantly to reflect current developments—an extremely important feature given the dynamic nature of tax law. The major tax services are:

Publisher	Name of Publications
Commerce Clearing House	*Standard Federal Tax Reporter—Income Taxes*
Research Institute of America	*United States Tax Reporter and Federal Tax Coordinator—2nd Series*
The Bureau of National Affairs, Inc.	*Tax Management Portfolios—U.S. Income*

The widespread use of computers has found applications in tax research. For example, *LEXIS* is a computerized data base that a user can access through his or her personal computer. The *LEXIS* data base contains almost all information available in an extensive tax library. Suppliers of tax services currently make computer-based tax liabraries available to their customers. Undoubtedly computers are basic to tax research.

Commerce Clearing House, Research Institute of America, and other publishers issue weekly summaries of important cases and other tax developments that many practitioners and scholars find helpful in keeping current with developments in the tax field. The Bureau of National Affairs publishes the *Daily Tax Bulletin*, a comprehensive daily journal of late-breaking tax news that often reprints entire cases or regulations of particular importance. *Tax Notes*, published by Tax Analysts, is a weekly publication addressing legislative and judicial developments in the tax field. *Tax Notes* is particularly helpful in following the progress of tax legislation through the legislative process.

TAX PERIODICALS

In addition to these services, there are a number of quality publications (usually published monthly) that contain articles on a variety of important tax topics. These publications are very helpful when new tax acts are passed, because they often contain clear, concise summaries of the new law in a readable format. In addition, they serve to convey new planning opportunities and relay the latest IRS and judicial developments in many important sub-specialities of the tax profession. Some of the leading periodicals include the following:

ATA Journal of Legal Tax Research	*Taxes—The Tax Magazine*
Estate Planning	*The International Tax Journal*
Journal of Corporate Taxation	*The Review of Taxation of Individuals*
Journal of Partnership Taxation	*The Tax Advisor*
Journal of Real Estate Taxation	*The Tax Executive*
Journal of Taxation	*The Tax Lawyer*
Tax Law Journal	*Trusts and Estates*
Tax Law Review	

In addition to these publications, many law journals contain excellent articles on tax subjects.

Several indexes exist that may be used to locate a journal article. Through the use of a subject index, author index, and in some instances a Code section index, articles dealing with a particular topic may be found. Three of these indexes are:

Title	Publisher
Index to Federal Tax Articles	Warren, Gorham and Lamont
Federal Tax Articles	Commerce Clearing House
The Accountant's Index	American Institute of Certified Public Accountants

In addition, the *United States Tax Reporter*, published by RIA, contains a section entitled "Index to Tax Articles."

TAX RESEARCH

Having introduced the sources of tax law, the remainder of this chapter is devoted to working with the law—or more specifically, the art of tax research. Tax research may be defined as the process used to ascertain the optimal answer to a question with tax implications. Although there is no perfect technique for researching a question, the following approach normally is used:

1. Obtain all of the facts

2. Diagnose the problem from the facts

3. Locate the authorities

4. Evaluate the authorities

5. Derive the solution and possible alternative solutions

6. Communicate the answer

Each of these steps is discussed below.

OBTAINING THE FACTS

Before discussing the importance of obtaining all the facts, the distinction between closed fact research and open- or controlled-fact research should be noted. If the research relates to a problem with transactions that are complete, it is referred to as closed-fact research and normally falls within the realm of tax practice known as tax compliance. On the other hand, if the research relates to contemplated transactions, it is called controlled- or open-fact research and is an integral part of tax planning.

In researching a closed-fact problem, the first step is gathering all of the facts. Unfortunately, it is difficult to obtain all relevant facts upon first inquiry. This is true because it is essentially impossible to understand the law so thoroughly that all of the proper questions can be asked before the research task begins. After the general area of the problem is identified and research has begun, it usually becomes apparent that more facts must be obtained before an answer can be derived. Consequently, additional inquiries must be made until all facts necessary for a solution are acquired.

DIAGNOSING THE ISSUE

Once the initial set of facts is gathered, the tax issue or question must be identified. Most tax problems involve very basic questions such as these:

1. Does the taxpayer have gross income that must be recognized?

2. Is the taxpayer entitled to a deduction?

3. Is the taxpayer entitled to a credit?

4. In what period is the gross income, deduction, or credit reported?

5. What amount of gross income, deduction, or credit must be reported?

As research progresses, however, such fundamental questions can be answered only after more specific issues have been resolved.

Example 1. R's employer owns a home in which R lives. The basic question that must be asked is whether use of the home constitutes income to R. After consulting the

various tax sources, it can be determined that § 61 requires virtually all benefits to be included in income unless another provision specifically grants an exclusion. In this case, § 119 allows a taxpayer to exclude the value employer-provided of housing if the housing is on the employer's premises, the lodging is furnished for the convenience of the employer, and the employee is required by the employer to accept the housing. Due to the additional research, three more specific questions must be asked:

1. Is the home on the employer's premises?

2. Is the home provided for the employer's convenience?

3. Is R required to live in the home?

As the above example suggests, diagnosing the problem requires a continuing refinement of the questions until the critical issue is identified. The refinement that occurs results from the awareness that is gained through reading and rereading the primary and secondary authorities.

> **Example 2.** Assume the same facts as in *Example 1*. After determining that one of the issues concerns whether R's home is on the business premises, a second inquiry is made of R concerning the location of his residence. (Note that as the research progresses, additional facts must be gathered.) According to R, the house is located in a suburb, 25 miles from his employer's downtown office. However, the house is owned by the employer, and hence R suggests that he lives on the employer's premises. He also explains that he often brings work home and frequently entertains clients in his home. Having uncovered this information, the primary authorities are reexamined. Upon review, it is determined that in *Charles N. Anderson*,[16] the court indicated that an employee would be considered on the business premises if the employee performed a significant portion of his duties at the place of lodging. Again the question must be refined to ask: Do R's work and entertainment activities in the home constitute a significant portion of his duties?

LOCATING THE AUTHORITIES

Identification of the critical issue presented by any tax question begins by first locating, then reading and studying the appropriate authority. Locating the authority is ordinarily done using a tax service. With the issue stated in general terms, the subject is found in the index volume and the location is determined. At this point, the appropriate Code sections, regulations, and editorial commentary may be perused to determine their applicability to the question.

> **Example 3.** In the case of R above, the problem stated in general terms concerns income. Using an index, the key word, *income*, could be located and a reference to information concerning the income aspects of lodging would be given.

Once information relating to the issue is identified, the authoritative materials must be read. That is, the appropriate Code sections, regulations, rulings, and cases must be examined and studied to determine how they relate to the question. As suggested above, this process normally results in refinement of the question, which in turn may require acquisition of additional facts.

---

[16]   67-1 USTC ¶9136, 19 AFTR2d 318, 371 F.2d 59 (CA-6, 1966).

EVALUATING THE AUTHORITY

After the various authorities have been identified and it has been *verified* that they are applicable, their value must be appraised. This evaluation process, as will become clear below, primarily involves appraisal of court decisions and revenue rulings.

The Code. The Internal Revenue Code is the final authority on most tax issues since it is the Federal tax law as passed by Congress. Only the courts can offset this authority by declaring part of the law unconstitutional, and this happens rarely. Most of the time, however, the Code itself is only of partial help. It is written in a style that is not always easy to understand, and it contains no examples of its application. Accordingly, to the extent the Code can be understood as clearly applicable, no stronger authority exists, except possibly a treaty. But in most cases, the Code cannot be used without further support.

Treasury Regulations. As previously discussed, the regulations are used to expand and explain the Code. Because Congress has given its authority to make laws to the Executive branch's administrative agency—the Treasury—the regulations that are produced are a very strong source of authority, second only to the Code itself. Normally, the major issue when a regulation is under scrutiny by a Court is whether the regulation is consistent with the Code. If the regulations are inconsistent, the Court will not hesitate to invalidate them.

Judicial Authority. The value of a court decision depends on numerous factors. On appraising a decision, the most crucial determination concerns whether the outcome is consistent with other decisions on the same issue. In other words, consideration must be given to how other decisions have evaluated the one in question. An invaluable tool in determining the validity of a case is a *citator*. A tax citator provides an alphabetical listing by last name of virtually all tax cases and other administrative pronouncements (e.g. rulings). After the name of each case, there is a record of other decisions that have cited (in the text of their facts and opinions) the first case. The list of cases is organized by type of court and then by year. Exhibit 2-4 provides sample entries from the citators published by RIA and CCH for the Supreme Court's decision in *Indianapolis Power and Light Co.*

Example 4. Refer to Exhibit 2-6 and the sample entries from the RIA and CCH citators. Observe that the Supreme Court's decision in *Indianapolis Power and Light Co. (IPL)* was cited (mentioned) in a number of cases at various levels as well in several rulings. For instance, the *IPL* decision was cited by the Supreme Court in *Banks II*, by the Ninth Circuit in *Westpac-Pacific Foods* and by the Tax Court in *Tampa Bay Devil Rays, Ltd.* Similarly, *IPL* was cited in Rev. Proc. 91-31 and Rev. Rul. 2003-39.

It is important to note that tax citators often use abbreviations for subsequent case history. For example, the abbreviations *aff'g* and *aff'd* mean "affirming" and "affirmed" and indicate that an appeals court has upheld the decision in question. Similarly, *rev'g* and *rev'd* mean "reversing" and "reversed" and indicate that a trial court's decision was overturned. Finally, *rem'g* and *rem'd* mean "remanding" and "remanded" and indicate that the case has been sent back to a lower court for reconsideration.

The validity of a particular decision may be assessed by examining how the subsequent cases viewed the cited decision. For example, subsequent cases may have agreed or disagreed with the decision in question, or distinguished the facts of the cited case from those examined in a later case. In this regard, note how the RIA citator provides a notation, indicating the relationship between the cited and citing cases. For example, the Banks II decision is shown as having "cited favorably" the IPL decision. The CCH citator does not provide this information.

EXHIBIT 2-6
Tax Citators: RIA and CCH

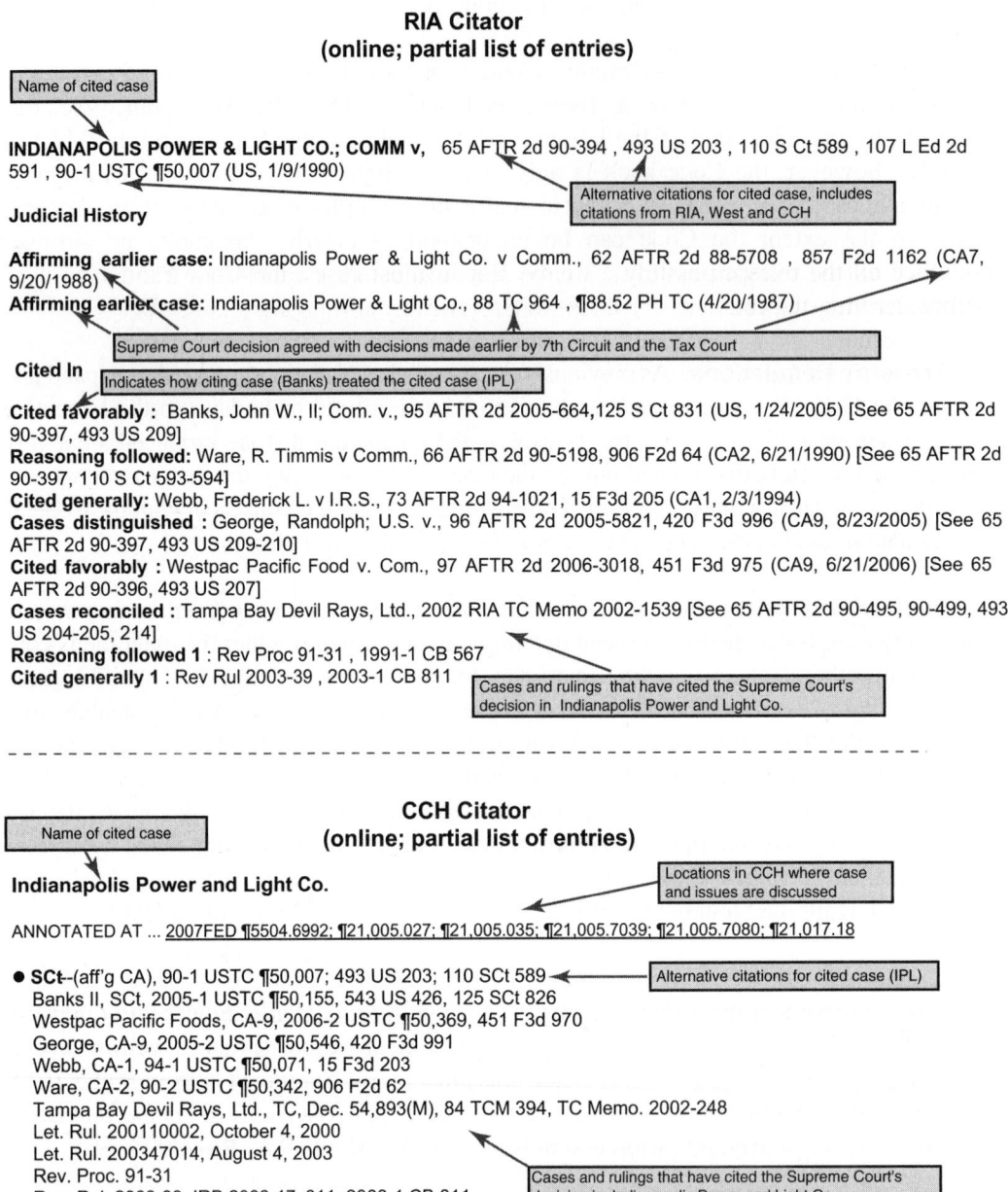

Another important factor that must be considered in evaluating a court decision is the level of the court that issued it. Decisions issued by trial courts have less value than those issued by appellate courts. And, of course, decisions of the Supreme Court are the ultimate authority.

A court decision's value rises appreciably if the IRS agrees with its result. As discussed earlier, the IRS usually indicates whether it acquiesces or does not acquiesce to Regular Tax Court decisions. The position of the Service may also be published in a revenue ruling.

Rulings. The significance of revenue rulings lies in the fact that they reflect current IRS policy. Since agents of the IRS are usually reluctant to vary from that policy, revenue rulings carry considerable weight.

Revenue rulings are often evaluated in court decisions. Thus, a tax service should be used to determine whether relevant rulings have been considered in any decisions. By examining the Court's view of the ruling, possible flaws may be discovered.

The IRS must adhere to private letter rulings issued to the taxpayer as long as the transaction is carried out in the manner initially approved. Variation from the facts on which the ruling was based permits the Service to revise its position. As mentioned earlier, a private letter ruling applies only to the particular taxpayer to whom it was issued. It does not apply to other taxpayers. However, such a ruling should prove helpful to any other taxpayer faced with a substantially identical fact pattern.

DERIVING THE SOLUTION

Once all the relevant authorities have been evaluated, a conclusion must be drawn. Before deriving the final answer or answers, however, an important caveat is warranted: the researcher must ensure that the research reflects all current developments. The new matters section of a tax service can aid in this regard. The new matters section updates the textual discussion with any late-breaking developments. For instance, the section will contain any new cases, regulations, or pronouncements of the Internal Revenue Service that may bear on the discussion of the topic covered in the main text.

COMMUNICATING THE FINDINGS

The final product of the research effort is a memorandum recording the research and a letter to the interested parties. Although many formats are suitable for the memorandum, one technique typically used is structured as follows:

1. Description of the facts

2. Statement of the issues or questions researched

3. Report of the conclusions (brief answers to the research questions)

4. Discussion of the rationale and authorities that support the conclusions

5. Summary of the authorities consulted in the research

A good tax memorandum is essential. If the research findings are not communicated intelligently and effectively, the entire research effort is wasted.

RULES OF TAX PRACTICE: RESPONSIBILITIES AND ETHICS

Over the past several years there has been a great deal of attention focused on ethics in business. The world of taxation has not escaped this attention. Unethical behavior of taxpayers and tax preparers has always been a serious concern of the tax system, primarily because of its reliance on voluntary compliance.

Anyone who has ever filed an income tax return recognizes the potential for bilking the system. It is as easy as underreporting income or overstating deductions. What is perhaps more important is that it can be done with so little risk. The current audit rate is so low—approximately 1 percent—that many dishonest taxpayers think they can exploit the system with little chance that they will ever get caught. That the tax system is such an easy mark was underscored recently in testimony given before the House Ways and Means Oversight Subcommittee by two practitioners convicted of tax fraud for illegal refund schemes. In his testimony, Barry Becht, a 36-year-old former tax return preparer, explained that, before he was convicted and sent to Federal prison, he had "helped" his clients reduce their tax liabilities by over $750,000 simply by overstating their

deductions. Surprisingly, Becht did not share in his client's windfalls. Allegedly his only purpose was to build up his practice! The other convicted felon, Frazier Todd, reported that he had gained more than $500,000 in only two years using electronic filing schemes. Shortly after college and with the help of a few courses on computers, accounting, and business, Todd had set up a tax-preparation service near public housing in Atlanta. There he was able to strike deals with low-income taxpayers who allowed him to use their names and social security numbers to falsify wage statements (W-2 forms). He then proceeded to file returns electronically, which enabled him to obtain a refund before the IRS discovered that the returns were phony. Unfortunately, the stories of Becht and Todd are just two illustrations of how easy it is to abuse the system. Near the close of 1993, the IRS estimated that the "tax gap," the amount of unpaid taxes (income, payroll, and excise) due to cheating and fraud, was over $150 billion annually. By 2001, the gap had increased to as much as $353 billion.[17]

The problems of tax fraud do not go unnoticed, however. To safeguard the system, encourage compliance, and promote ethical behavior, the government has adopted a number of mechanisms. Among these is an intricate set of penalties that can be applied to both taxpayers and tax return preparers. These penalties cover a variety of violations, such as failure to file and pay taxes on a timely basis, negligence in preparing the tax return, and outright fraud. While the penalties are usually monetary in nature, criminal penalties—such as the jail sentences given to Mr. Becht and Mr. Todd—may result if the taxpayer goes beyond these civil offenses and purposefully attempts to evade tax. The failure-to-file and failure-to-pay penalties—penalties that typically result not because taxpayers are trying to deceive the government but simply because they are late in filing and paying their taxes—are discussed in Chapter 4. The focus in this chapter is on the responsibilities of taxpayers and tax return preparers in filing returns and the major penalties that may be imposed with respect to positions taken on returns.

TAXPAYER PENALTIES

In a 1985 IRS survey, one out of every five people reported that they cheated on their tax return. In the same survey, 41 percent said they believed that their fellow taxpayers also cheated. Similarly, Professor Peggy Hite found in a 1993 survey of Indiana residents that 40 percent of the individuals asked indicated that they definitely would not voluntarily report prize income, such as money won in a lottery or similar contests and sweepstakes.[18] Another 30 percent were somewhat wishy-washy in their answers, suggesting that, depending on the circumstances, they also would not report the income. But anyone thinking about cheating should recognize that it can be quite expensive. The IRS has over 140 penalties in its arsenal that it could apply. In their simplest form, these penalties provide that as long as taxpayers do not cheat and make a good faith effort to determine their tax liability, they have no reason to worry. But in reality the ethical problems created by the tax system for taxpayers and tax preparers can be difficult to resolve. Unfortunately, the law rarely provides clear-cut answers, leaving taxpayers wondering what they should do.

As an illustration, consider two taxpayers, both with bad backs, who bought $5,000 hot tubs on the hope that they might have some therapeutic value. Can the taxpayers deduct their costs as a medical expense? Even if they researched the question every day of the week for a month, the answer may not be clear. Should the fact that the answer is not clear preclude them from deducting their expenses? Some taxpayers might be inclined to simply abandon the issue, pay the tax and never worry about it again. But others might believe that there is some support for their position and want to take the deduction. So

---

[17]   IR News Release 2005-38 (Mar. 29, 2005).

[18]   "Nearly 1 in 3 Would Cheat on Taxes," *The Indianapolis Star*, April 7, 1994, B1.

assume in this case taxpayer A deducts the expense and taxpayer B deducts not only the cost of the tub but, banking on the audit lottery, also deducts the entire cost of the house on the grounds that it serves as a rehabilitation facility. What happens if both returns are audited and the agent rejects the deductions of both taxpayers? Obviously the system of punishment should fit the crime. And this is what Congress has attempted to do by creating a penalty system that fairly treats taxpayers who in good faith believe that their position has validity but at the same time discourages taxpayers from taking frivolous positions, hoping that the audit lottery will never pick their number.

As the penalty discussion below will reveal, the tax law has its own way of dealing with taxpayers who stray too far from the correct position. While the system is complex, it is somewhat analogous to the way a mother treats her teenage son who is apt to stay out beyond his 12 o'clock curfew. If the son is a few minutes late, there will probably be no penalty if he has a reasonable explanation. On the other hand, if he gets home two hours late, the penalty will probably be severe unless he called to say he would be late. But if he never called, punishment is a virtual certainty unless his story is truly believable and backed by witnesses. And, of course, if her son lies, he will be grounded forever. Although the rules for breaking curfew are not completely analogous to those for taxpayers that take erroneous positions on returns, the comparison may be useful. If a taxpayer takes an incorrect position with respect to a *small* amount, there will be no penalty as long as there is a *reasonable basis* for the position. On the other hand, if the tax dollars involved are *substantial*, a penalty is normally imposed unless the taxpayer has *substantial authority* for the position or, alternatively, has disclosed the position and has a reasonable basis for it. Of course, if the taxpayer commits blatant fraud, the penalties could be quite harsh. These ethical standards for taxpayers are embedded in two types of penalties: accuracy-related penalties and penalties for fraud.

ACCURACY-RELATED PENALTIES

What happens if a waiter simply fails to report all of his tips? What if a 70-year-old grandmother fails to file her return believing that senior citizens do not have to pay tax? And what if the taxpayer deducts the cost of his daughter's wedding as business entertainment? As might be expected, the IRS does not treat such transgressions lightly. If the taxpayer's behavior can be characterized as negligent, a penalty in addition to the regular tax may be imposed. In 1989, Congress consolidated several existing penalties relating to negligence into a so-called accuracy-related penalty. The accuracy-related penalty is generally 20 percent of the portion of the tax underpayment. The principal accuracy-related penalties include:[19]

- ▸ Negligence or disregard of rules and regulations
- ▸ Substantial understatement of income tax
- ▸ Substantial valuation misstatement.

Note that these penalties do not stack on top of each other. The IRS must pick which one it wants to assess.

Negligence Penalty (Insubstantial). The negligence penalty, as an accuracy-related penalty, is 20 percent of the portion of the tax underpayment that is attributable to negligence or disregard of the rules and regulations.[20] For example, assume a taxpayer forgets to report $1,000 that he received for consulting during the year. If the taxpayer is in the 28 percent tax bracket, the underpayment is $280 and the penalty would be $56 (20% ×

---

[19] § 6662.

[20] § 6662(c).

$280). Note that when the day of reckoning comes, the taxpayer will be required to pay the underpayment, interest on the underpayment from the original due date, and the penalty, if any. The taxpayer may also owe interest on the penalty. Interest on the penalty generally starts to run when the taxpayer has been notified of the penalty, usually sometime after the audit. Under § 6601(e)(2)(B) interest must be paid on the failure-to-file penalty, accuracy-related penalties, and the fraud penalty.

Negligence is generally defined as any failure to do what a reasonable and ordinarily prudent person would do under the circumstances. To avoid the negligence penalty, the taxpayer must make a reasonable attempt to comply with the law. The negligence penalty is usually imposed when the taxpayer fails to report income or claims large amounts of unsubstantiated expenses. For example, a waitress who fails to report her cash tips would probably get hit with the penalty, as would the businessperson who claims thousands of dollars of business entertainment expenses with little or no substantiation—a specific requirement for travel and entertainment expenses. A taxpayer is automatically considered negligent and liable for the 20 percent penalty if he or she fails to report any type of income for which there is an information return filed by the party paying the income (e.g., Form 1099). In other situations, determination of whether the penalty should be imposed is in the hands of the auditor. It is important to note, however, that taxpayers who intentionally attempt to deceive the government are normally not subject to the negligence penalty but rather the more severe fraud penalty discussed below.

For most taxpayers, the most important aspect of the negligence penalty concerns its relationship to positions taken on returns.

> **Example 5.** This year D graduated with a marketing degree from the University of Arkansas and immediately took a job with a publishing company as a sales representative. The company did not provide her with an office, so she worked out of her home. After talking with her boss at work, she found out that he deducted his home office expenses as business expenses on his return. Knowing little about tax, she followed her boss's lead and deducted $3,000 of expenses related to her home office. Two years later D's return was audited and the agent informed her that he planned to deny her deduction for the home office expenses. Assuming the agent is correct, another issue is raised: should the negligence penalty apply since D has taken an incorrect position on the return?

Prior to 1994, the taxpayer could avoid the negligence penalty as long as the position was not frivolous and it was disclosed on the return. But that approach inspired taxpayers to play the audit lottery. For example, aggressive taxpayers might take a questionable deduction, disclose it, then hope that they would never be audited. Even if they got caught, there was little risk of punishment since disclosure protected them against a negligence penalty in every situation except where the position was frivolous or patently improper. In other words, as long as the position was nonfrivolous—that is, the taxpayer had some basis on which to argue the disclosed position (e.g., a merely arguable or merely colorable claim)—the negligence penalty could be avoided.[21] Believing that the ethical standard set by this rule was far too low, the Revenue Reconciliation Act of 1993 changed the rules. Under the current approach, taxpayers are forced to be more cautious about the positions they take on their returns.

A negligence penalty can be assessed unless the taxpayer has a *reasonable basis* for the position taken on the return regardless of whether it is disclosed on the return.[22] What

---

[21]   Reg. §§ 1.6662-3(b)(3) and 1.6694-2(c)(2).

[22]   See Predmore, "New Reasonable Basis Standard for Return Disclosure Likely to Be Troublesome," *Journal of Taxation* (January, 1994), p. 25, which indicates that, until the regulations are modified, "disclosure of a not frivolous position should suffice to avoid the negligence penalty." Discussions with other practitioners suggest that nonfrivolous positions probably can no longer be protected through disclosure.

the current approach means to taxpayers is that in situations where the potential tax understatement is insubstantial they can ethically take a position that is contrary to the rules and regulations without fear of the negligence penalty as long as there is a reasonable basis for believing that if the matter were litigated, the taxpayer would prevail against the IRS. Of course, the critical issue here is what constitutes a reasonable basis.

Although any definition of a "reasonable basis" would be subject to debate, the regulations do provide some guidance. According to the regulations, the reasonable basis standard is met if the return position is "arguable, but fairly unlikely to prevail in court."[23] Practitioners generally interpret this to mean that a position has a reasonable basis if it has at least a 20 percent chance of succeeding (without regard to the possibility that it might not be discovered at all). Apparently, this represents a slight increase in the level of support required by the nonfrivolous standard for disclosed positions under prior law. In the final analysis, however, the standard leaves a great deal to be desired. The regulations do provide one additional insight that may be useful: the "too good to be true" rule. This rule indicates that the reasonable basis standard is not met if the taxpayer fails to make a reasonable attempt to determine the correctness of a position that seems too good to be true.

Substantial Understatement Penalty. The substantial understatement penalty, like its sibling, the negligence penalty, is an accuracy-related penalty that is 20 percent of the portion of the underpayment of tax due to any substantial understatement of income tax.[24] The understatement is considered substantial if it exceeds the larger of (1) 10 percent of the correct tax or (2) $5,000.

The major difference between the substantial understatement penalty and the negligence penalty concerns the level of authority required to avoid penalty for an erroneous *undisclosed* position. In effect, Congress is telling taxpayers that if the risky position they are taking involves a substantial amount of tax and they are *unwilling to disclose* the position, the degree of support they must have is greater than simply a reasonable basis. The substantial understatement penalty applies to undisclosed positions unless the taxpayer has *substantial authority* for the position. It is unclear what the substantial authority requirement calls for, but it seems clear that it is somewhat more stringent than the 1 in 3 test of the realistic possibility of success standard discussed below but less demanding than the more-likely-than-not requirement, a more than 50 percent chance, related to certain positions taken with respect to certain tax shelter investments. For purposes of the substantial authority analysis, only materials published by Congress, the IRS, and the courts are relevant. Conclusions suggested by tax professionals in treatises, legal periodicals (which provide the basis of many arguments), or the like are not to be considered.[25]

The degree of support necessary to avoid the substantial understatement penalty drops down a notch if the taxpayer is willing to disclose the position. The substantial understatement penalty can be avoided if the taxpayer makes *adequate disclosure* and has a *reasonable* basis for his position. What constitutes adequate disclosure is clearer than what constitutes a reasonable basis. Disclosure is considered adequate if the position is explained on a special form intended just for this purpose. Form 8275 or 8275-R, or on the return in accordance with rules issued by the IRS each year.[26] In effect, when the tax dollars involved are material, taxpayers must meet a much higher standard— substantial authority—than is normally applied unless they are willing to disclose the position.

---

[23] § 6662(d).

[24] § 6662(d)(2)(B). A corporate taxpayer has a substantial understatement if the amount of the understatement exceeds the lesser of (1) 10% of the tax required to be shown on the return for the tax year (or, if greater, $10,000), or (2) $10 million.

[25] Reg. § 1.6692-4(d)(3)(iii).

[26] Reg. § 1.6694-2(c)(3).

Substantial Valuation Misstatement. The tax law often requires taxpayers and tax return preparers to provide valuations for certain items. For example, taxpayers are generally entitled to a deduction for the fair market value of property given to qualified charitable organizations. What happens if a taxpayer in the 30 percent bracket gives a work of art that he says is worth $6,000 when its value is really closer to $2,000? The answer is that he has saved $1,200 ($4,000 × 30%) if he wins the audit lottery. But if the IRS does catch him, the taxpayer may face an accuracy-related penalty for substantial valuation misstatement. A 20 percent penalty is imposed on the underpayment of tax attributable to the misstatement.[27] The taxpayer avoids the penalty, however, if the misstatement does not exceed 150 percent of the correct value or if the amount of tax underpayment attributable to the misstatement is less than $5,000 ($10,000 for corporations). Thus the taxpayer above, who overstated the correct value by 300 percent, would still escape the valuation penalty since the amount of tax attributable to the misstatement, $1,200, is less than the $5,000 threshold. However, the taxpayer could still be subject to the negligence or the substantial understatement penalties.

Summary of Penalties for Inaccurate Returns. There is a great deal of confusion over penalties concerning erroneous positions on tax returns and what one can do to avoid them. Nevertheless, Exhibit 2-7 summarizes the three accuracy-related penalties discussed above and what defenses are available to the taxpayer. After a great deal of studying, it may become clear that the likelihood of a penalty depends on three factors: the amount of the potential understatement, whether the taxpayer has disclosed the position adequately, and the level of support that there is for the position. As a rule, if the tax dollars are not significant, a reasonable basis protects the taxpayer from penalty. On the other hand, if the tax dollars are substantial, the taxpayer is protected only if

EXHIBIT 2-7
The 20 Percent Penalty for Inaccurate Returns and Defenses: § 6662

1. Negligence (insubstantial)
   ▶ Defined: Reasonable attempt to comply with the tax laws
   ▶ Defenses:
     ◦ Reasonable basis (disclosure is unnecessary)
     ◦ Exercise of reasonable care in preparing tax return
     ◦ Reasonable cause and good faith

2. Substantial understatement
   ▶ Defined: Understatement greater than 10% of tax or $5,000, whichever is larger
   ▶ Defenses:
     ◦ Understatement does not exceed threshold
     ◦ Disclosure with reasonable basis
     ◦ No disclosure with substantial authority
     ◦ Reasonable cause and good faith

3. Substantial valuation misstatement
   ▶ Defined: Misstatement more than 150% of correct valuation
   ▶ Defenses:
     ◦ Misstatement does not exceed threshold
     ◦ Amount of underpayment of tax is less than $5,000
     ◦ Reasonable cause and good faith

---

[27] § 6662(e). The penalty is 40 percent if the claimed value is 200 percent or more of the correct value.

EXHIBIT 2-8

Standards of Compliance Required to Avoid Penalties

1. Frivolous position
   - Defined: Patently improper
     - No protection for frivolous positions

2. Not frivolous position
   - Defined: Not patently improper, merely arguable
     - Pre-1994: Protection against negligence with disclosure
     - Post-1993: Apparently no protection

3. Reasonable basis
   - Defined: Arguable but fairly unlikely to prevail in court
     - Protects against insubstantial negligence
     - Protects against substantial understatement if position disclosed

4. Realistic possibility of success
   - Defined: More than one in three chances for success
     - Protects against insubstantial negligence without disclosure
     - Protects against substantial negligence with disclosure

5. Substantial authority
   - Defined: Supporting authorities are substantial (Congress, IRS, or court cases)
     - Protects against insubstantial and substantial negligence without disclosure (except tax shelter items)

6. More-likely-than-not
   - Defined: Greater than 50 percent chance of prevailing against the IRS if the matter were litigated
     - Protects against insubstantial and substantial negligence without disclosure related to certain positions taken with respect to certain tax shelter investments

7. Reasonable cause and good faith
   - Defined: Facts and circumstances determination
     - Protects normally against all penalties

---

there is substantial authority or if there is disclosure with reasonable basis. Exhibit 2-8 summarizes the various standards of compliance and ranks them according to their level of certainty. Note that in all cases the taxpayer can avoid the penalties by showing that there was *reasonable cause* for the position taken or that he or she acted in *good faith*. Obviously, these are both purely subjective determinations based on the individual facts and circumstances.

FRAUD

When the taxpayer attempts to defraud the government, the tax law imposes a minimum penalty equal to 75 percent of the amount of underpayment attributable to the fraud.[28] *In addition*, the taxpayer may also be subject to the criminal penalties for fraud. Criminal penalties can be as high as $100,000 ($500,000 for corporate taxpayers) and imprisonment for up to five years. Despite these penalties, taxpayers by the thousands are willing to play the audit lottery, including some rich and famous tax felons:[29]

---

[28] § 6663.

[29] See in part "Famous Faces from IRS Hall of Shame," *Sacramento Bee*, March 29, 1994. Metro Final Scene, D3.

- Leona Helmsley, New York hotel magnate, who will forever be remembered for her offhand comment to her housekeeper, "we don't pay taxes; only the little people pay taxes." Helmsley, convicted in 1992 for deducting millions of dollars of personal expenses, including renovations to her personal residence, was fined more than $7 million and sentenced to four years in prison (served 18 months).

- Pete Rose, baseball player and all-time leader in hits (4,256). Rose failed to report income from memorabilia shows and gambling and served five months in prison.

- Spiro Agnew, vice-president during the Nixon era. Agnew, who failed to report income from bribes, was fined $10,000 and had a three-year suspended sentence.

- Chuck Berry, famous rock and roll star of Johnny B. Goode fame. Berry underreported his income by $110,000 in 1979 and served four months in prison.

- Aldo Gucci, famous designer. Gucci pleaded guilty to $7 million of tax fraud in 1989 and was sentenced to one year in jail and fined $30,000.

- Al Capone, racketeer and mobster. Capone, convicted of tax evasion in 1931, was fined $50,000 and served eight years of a ten-year sentence, then retired to his Miami estate.

- Willie Nelson, country and western singing star. Nelson ran up his tax bill to over $32 million. He served no time in prison, but part of the bill was paid from part of his ranch, which was seized by the IRS.

- Richard Hatch, winner in the debut season of reality show "Survivor." Hatch failed to report $1,000,000 and pay taxes on the winnings. He reportedly asked an accountant to prepare two tax returns, one with the winnings and the other without, and chose to file the latter. Hatch was found guilty of tax evasion and was sentenced in 2006 to serve 51 months in prison.

Civil fraud has not been clearly defined, but it requires more than simply negligent acts or omissions by the taxpayer. There is a fine line between fraud and negligence (to which a lesser penalty applies, as explained above). Fraud does not occur by accident. It is a willful and deliberate attempt to evade tax. For example, consider a taxpayer who is entitled to a deduction of $19,000. What penalty applies if he transposed the digits and claimed a deduction of $91,000? Fraud occurs only if it can be shown that the taxpayer knew that the amounts reported on the return were false. In this regard, the IRS must prove this to be true by a "preponderance of evidence." Thus for the transposition error above, the fraud penalty can be upheld if the IRS can carry its burden of proof and show that the taxpayer intentionally transposed the numbers. Lacking this, the negligence or substantial understatement penalty would probably be assessed. Note that before the *criminal* fraud penalty can be imposed, the IRS must show that the taxpayer intentionally tried to evade tax "beyond a shadow of any reasonable doubt." All of those in the "hall of shame" above found that this is not an impossible task. As a practical matter, the penalty imposed—negligence, civil, or criminal fraud—depends on the severity of the offense and the ability of the IRS to carry the burden of proof.

> **Example 6.** Dr. Bradford Calloway paid his children, all of whom were under 12 years of age, $11,000 for performing various tasks relating to his business. The kids did such chores as mail sorting, trash collecting, and answering the telephone. Although expenses incurred in carrying on a business such as these are normally deductible, the IRS did not believe that children that age could perform work worth that much money for any business. The Tax Court agreed with the IRS, and the judge added a fraud penalty, explaining that "We find it inherently incredible that Calloway, an intelligent and educated professional man, would pay a total of

$11,138.56 for such services, performed by small children on a part-time basis, or that he could seriously believe that such payments represented reasonable and deductible compensation for services rendered in his medical practice . . . particularly in the face of his accountant's contrary advice."[30]

TAX PREPARER PENALTIES

Understanding the penalty structure becomes doubly hard when a tax preparer is involved. What are the responsibilities of tax preparers when the client is unscrupulous or simply wants to take an aggressive position? As a practical matter, it is not the totally dishonest taxpayer that presents difficulties for tax return preparers. Most practitioners can easily walk away from such engagements. The more perplexing and more common problems concern situations where the client wants the preparer to take an aggressive position on issues for which the answer is unclear. Similarly, taxpayers may want to pursue a particular position because they view the law as arbitrary or capricious or they are not receptive to the preparer's response. These situations often present an ethical dilemma for the preparer. What side should the practitioner take? Should the preparer sign the return if he or she disagrees with the taxpayer? First, it needs to be emphasized that the tax practitioner is being paid to be an advocate for the client, not an independent third party hired to provide an unbiased or neutral opinion. It is the job of the tax expert to explain the relevant considerations and possible consequences, including positions that may be contrary to the law but which may be defensible. That done, it is not the right of the practitioner to impose his or her own set of moral values on the client. The final decision is to be made by the client after reviewing the alternatives provided. If the practitioner believes that the client's actions violate his or her personal code of ethics, the practitioner should withdraw from the engagement.

Beyond the basic preparer-client relationship, there are a number of other forces at work that affect whether the preparer signs the return containing a risky position. First, even if an answer to a particular question does exist, the costs of uncovering it probably cannot be recovered from the client. Second, given the small percentage of tax returns that are audited, there is only a slight chance that either the taxpayer or preparer will ever come face to face with the IRS. Third, preparers, like most people, want to please their customers and find it hard to just say no. When these dynamics are present, they make it relatively easy for practitioners to resolve an issue in favor of the client, notwithstanding the lack of reasonable support for the position. This is particularly true when the practitioner knows that the unprincipled competitor down the street will do whatever the client wants and at a cheaper price. On the other hand, the practitioner's sense of public duty, concern about his or her personal and professional reputation, and possible legal liability may cause him or her to be something less than an advocate for the client. As might be expected, the practitioner's proper role in these situations is not clearly defined. There are, however, in addition to the preparer's own personal code of ethics, some guidelines that a preparer generally must follow in carrying on a tax practice.

Individuals who prepare tax returns are subject to a variety of rules regulating their professional conduct. The rules governing tax practice are contained in Treasury Circular 230 and various provisions of the Internal Revenue Code. In addition, CPAs and attorneys engaged in tax practice must also follow the rules of conduct imposed by their professional organizations: the American Institute of Certified Public Accountants (AICPA) and the American Bar Association (ABA). The general rules of conduct prescribed by the AICPA for all CPAs concern a variety of matters such as independence,

---

[30] A. J. Cook, *A. J.'s Tax Court* (St. Luke's Press, 1987), p. 96.

integrity, objectivity, advertising, contingent fees, and responsibilities of the accountant when undertaking an engagement—but none of these are directly related to tax practice. Acknowledging that individuals engaged in tax practice have ethical concerns beyond those covered in the general rules of conduct, the AICPA has developed Statements on Standards for Tax Services (SSTSs). These statements, currently eight in number, provide additional guidelines for professional conduct of CPAs in tax practice. Similarly, the ABA Standing Committee on Ethics and Professional Responsibility has also issued certain opinions regarding an attorney's conduct when practicing before the IRS.

Tax Return Positions. As might be imagined, the rules and applicable penalties concerning practitioner conduct as set forth by Circular 230, the Internal Revenue Code, the AICPA, and the ABA deserve a chapter devoted solely to these topics. In essence, however, the most important penalty for those preparing returns is that contained in § 6694(a) as recently revised in 2008. Section 6694(a) provides that a penalty of $1,000 (or if greater, 50% of the income from preparing the return) is imposed on the preparer of a tax return if any part of an understatement of the liability on a return is due to an unreasonable position taken on the tax return and the return preparer knew (or reasonably should have known) of the position.[31] If the position is properly disclosed on the return, the penalty does not apply if there was a reasonable basis for the position.[32] If the position is not disclosed, the penalty applies unless there is substantial authority for the position. As noted earlier, substantial authority includes the Internal Revenue Code, Regulations (final, temporary and proposed), court cases, tax treaties, and administrative pronouncements (Revenue Rulings, Revenue Procedures, Private Letter Rulings, Technical Advice Memoranda, Notices and similar documents). If the position is with respect to a tax shelter investment, the threshold for authority is raised, and the penalty is imposed unless it was reasonable to believe that the position would "more likely than not" be sustained on its merits if the position were litigated. The preparer penalty is not imposed in any case if it is shown that there is reasonable cause for the understatement and the preparer acted in good faith. Note that the penalty applies to any paid preparer regardless of whether the person is a CPA, enrolled agent, friend, or relative. If the preparer is compensated, the penalty could apply.[33]

> **Example 7.** T purchased a computer this year that he uses in his job as a financial planner. His friends at the office say that he can deduct it. His accountant, P, explained that it might be deductible but only if T can demonstrate that the computer's use is for his employer's convenience and not his own. If the position is disclosed, neither P nor T will be subject to penalty if there is a reasonable basis for the position. If the position is not disclosed, then normally substantial authority must exist to avoid penalty.

At first glance, it would appear that the size of penalty imposed by the IRS, $1,000, is so small that it would do little to dissuade preparers from taking whatever position

---

[31] The penalty increases to the greater of $5,000 or 50% of the income derived from preparation of the return if it is attributable to willful or reckless conduct. See § 6694(b).

[32] Disclosure must be made on Form 8275 or, when the position is contrary to a Regulation, Form 8275-R. See Reg. § 1.6694-2(c)(3)(i).

[33] See § 7701(a)(36) for a definition of preparer.

a client wishes. What may not be apparent, however, is the significance of this standard *and* its violation should a disgruntled client end up suing the preparer for malpractice. In a civil action against a preparer, the courts, both judges and juries, typically rely on expert testimony to assess whether the preparer should be held liable. In such case, it is not too hard to imagine a judge or jury believing that the preparer was negligent once an expert has explained that the preparer has already been penalized under § 6694(a). Even if the preparer is ultimately exonerated, the costs to defend such action could be substantial. Moreover, failing to observe such a standard could ultimately cost the practitioner the loss of his or her professional license to practice as a CPA or attorney. In short, it is not the size of the penalty that the practitioner fears but the other consequences that the penalty may trigger.

> **Example 8.** T, a CPA, has prepared the tax return for D&G Home Products for the past 15 years. It is normally a week-long job and worth well over $10,000 to T's practice. He also does the monthly preparation of financial statements worth another $20,000 per year. This year G spent more than $100,000 on a Super Bowl excursion for its customers. In preparing the return, D&G insists that it should be able to deduct all of the expenses, but T has some reservations. T understands there have been some recent changes in the law in this area but does not have time to adequately research the issue, and, even if he did, he doubts whether he could charge for the time spent. He also knows that this is a lucrative engagement and he wants to continue the relationship with the client. Finally, T recognizes that it is highly unlikely that the return will ever be audited. Consequently, T decides to sign the return and worry about it only if a problem arises. But what happens if the return is audited, the position is overturned, and a preparer penalty is assessed on the grounds that the return contained an undisclosed position that did not have substantial authority supporting it. While the penalty would be monetarily small, the real concern is the effect of the reversal on the client. D&G may have a short memory once it is forced to pay the tax, interest, and perhaps a substantial understatement penalty and interest on the penalty. It may not remember conversations with T and his admonitions. In the end, the corporation may feel that it was misled and sue T for malpractice and thousands of dollars. In such a proceeding, D&G may have the upper hand since it has been determined by a court of law that the position was unrealistic under that standards of § 6694(a) and T has therefore failed to meet his ethical responsibilities.

The decision that all practitioners ultimately face with every return they prepare is whether they can in good faith sign the tax return as preparer. Under the current rules, preparers normally will be reluctant to sign if the return contains an undisclosed position that does not have substantial authority.[34]

In addition to the $1,000 penalty, the tax law provides a number of other penalties to encourage ethical conduct by preparers. For example, a penalty of $1,000 per return is imposed where the preparer willfully attempts to understate the liability of the taxpayer or where the preparer understates the taxpayer's liability by reckless or intentional disregard of the rules or regulations.[35] The law also contains a number of

---

[34] Prop. Reg. § 10.34.

[35] § 6694(b).

criminal penalties for preparers with fines of up to $10,000 and imprisonment for up to three years.[36]

Other Guidelines for CPAs. As suggested above, the Statements on Standards for Tax Services provide a number of other guidelines for members of the AICPA who are tax practitioners. There are currently eight statements. *SSTS No. 1*, regarding tax positions, was mentioned above. The remaining statements generally fall into one of two categories: (1) return preparation issues (SSTS Numbers 2, 3, and 4) and (2) issues that arise after a return is filed (SSTS Numbers 5, 6, and 7). Some of these statements are summarized below.

▸ *SSTS No. 2: Answers to Questions on the Return.* When there are questions on a return that have not been answered, the CPA should make a reasonable effort to obtain appropriate answers from the taxpayer and provide the answers to the questions on the return. The significance of the question in terms of the information's effect on taxable income or loss and tax liability may be considered in determining whether the answer to a question may be omitted. However, omission of an answer is not justified simply because the answer may prove to be disadvantageous to the taxpayer.

▸ *SSTS No. 3: Certain Procedural Aspects of Preparing Returns.* In preparing or signing a return, a CPA may, without verification, rely in good faith on information furnished by the taxpayer or a third party. However, the CPA cannot ignore the implications of information furnished, and should make reasonable inquiries if the information appears to be incorrect, incomplete, or inconsistent either by itself or on the basis of other facts known to the CPA. When preparing the current return, the CPA should make use of returns from prior years wherever feasible. If the tax law or regulations impose conditions with respect to the tax treatment of an item (e.g., substantiating documentation), the CPA should make appropriate inquiries to determine if the conditions are met. In addition, when preparing a return, the CPA should consider relevant information known to the CPA from the tax return of another taxpayer, but should also consider any legal limitations relating to confidentiality.

▸ *SSTS No. 4: Use of Estimates.* Unless it is prohibited by the Internal Revenue Code or other tax rule, a CPA may prepare returns involving the use of the taxpayer's estimates, if under the circumstances, exact data cannot be obtained in a practical manner. When estimates are used, they should be presented in such a manner as to avoid the implication of greater accuracy than that which exists. The CPA should be satisfied that estimated amounts are reasonable under the circumstances.

▸ *SSTS No. 6: Knowledge of Error (Return Preparation).* A CPA should advise the taxpayer promptly upon learning of an error in a previously filed return, or upon learning of a taxpayer's failure to file a required return. The advice of the CPA may be oral, and should include a recommendation of the measures to be taken. The CPA is not obliged to inform the IRS and may not do so without the permission of the taxpayer, except where required by law. If the CPA is requested to prepare the current year's return and the taxpayer has not taken appropriate steps

---

[36]   See §§ 7206, 7207, and 7216.

to correct an error on a prior year's return, the CPA should consider whether to withdraw from preparing the return and whether to continue a professional or employment relationship with the taxpayer.

▸ *SSTS No. 7: Knowledge of Error (Administrative Proceeding).* When the CPA represents a taxpayer in an administrative proceeding regarding a return with an error known to the CPA that has resulted or may result in more than an insignificant effect on the taxpayer's tax liability, the CPA should notify the taxpayer and recommend corrective measures to be taken. The recommendations may be given orally. The CPA is not obligated to inform the IRS or other taxing authority, and may not do so without the taxpayer's permission, except where required by law. However, the CPA should request permission from the taxpayer to disclose the error to the IRS. Absent such permission, the CPA should consider withdrawing from the engagement.

Circular 230 Changes. In 2005, Circular 230 was changed to require those who practice before the IRS to disclose to their clients when the advice they give to them cannot be relied on for purposes of mitigating penalties that might be imposed on them. In practice, this means that lawyers, CPAs and other tax practitioners affix a disclaimer somewhat like that which follows to all written communications with clients that do not constitute a full legal option. The disclaimer must be placed on faxes, e-mails, blackberries and regular written correspondence.

> DISCLAIMER: Any federal tax advice contained in this communication (including attachments) was not intended or written to be used, and it cannot be used, by you for the purpose of (1) avoiding any penalty that may be imposed by the Internal Revenue Service or (2) promoting, marketing or recommending to another party any transaction or matter addressed herein.

The above discussion is just a brief introduction to the penalties and rules of practice that serve to define the proper conduct for taxpayers and preparers. In reality, there are a number of other penalties and rules that may apply in certain situations.[37] Nevertheless, this introduction may provide a sense of what are the most common ethical problems facing tax practitioners. Moreover, it underscores the importance of being able to find authoritative answers for questions, the subject of the next section.

✓ CHECK YOUR KNOWLEDGE

Review Question 1. The system of penalties provides an escape for taxpayers if the positions taken on their returns meet certain standards. In effect, meeting a certain standard enables the taxpayer to avoid a penalty. Practitioners generally associate a probability of success rate for each standard. What probabilities would you assign?

Frivolous	_____
Substantial authority	_____
Nonfrivolous	_____
More-likely-than-not	_____
Reasonable basis	_____
Realistic possibility of success	_____

None of these probabilities other than *realistic possibility of success* have been quantified by the law. However, practitioners would typically rank the standards in the following

---

[37] For a more complete discussion, see the related text, *Corporate Partnership, Estate and Gift Taxation, 2010 Edition*, Chapter 18.

order with the associated probabilities of success. Although the probabilities might vary from firm to firm and practitioner to practitioner, the order would remain the same.

1.	More-likely-than-not	> 50%
2.	Substantial authority	≥ 40
3.	Realistic possibility of success	≥ 33
4.	Reasonable basis	≥ 20
5.	Nonfrivolous	≥ 5
6.	Frivolous	< 5

Review Question 2. Pete Hartman operates an accounting practice in northern Virginia just outside of Washington. One of his long-time clients is Jim Anderson. Last year the IRS audited Jim's 2007 tax return, and he ultimately had to pay additional taxes as well as interest on that amount. Jim now wants to deduct a portion of this interest as a business expense. He reasons that because business expenses are deductible and the interest was directly attributable to back taxes on business income, the deduction should be allowed. There has also been another development this year. Jim's daughter has been diagnosed to have dyslexia. The problem is not severe but it was enough to cause Jim to enroll his daughter in a private school that is better equipped to provide the additional help she needs. The tuition for the school is $20,000, and Jim wants to deduct the cost as a medical expense. After some research, Pete believes that both positions are somewhat risky. Jim has asked Pete about the downside risk of taking this position on his return. Pete estimates that taking the deduction for the interest will reduce Jim's tax liability of $30,000 about $1,000. If he were to claim only the medical expense deduction by itself, it would reduce his tax liability by about $6,000. Try to answer the following questions.

a. What is the maximum penalty that Jim might pay if he deducts only the interest and it is considered erroneous but not fraudulent?

Jim would be subject to an accuracy-related penalty (negligence), which is 20 percent of the amount of the underpayment due to the overstatement of deductions. In this case, the penalty would be $200 (20% × $ 1,000). In addition, Jim would owe the additional $1,000 in tax plus interest on the underpayment *and* interest on the penalty.

b. True-False. Jim will not be subject to penalty with respect to the interest deduction as long as his position has a reasonable basis even if he does not specifically disclose the position on the return since the amount of tax at stake is not substantial.

True. The negligence penalty will not be assessed as long as the taxpayer has a reasonable basis for the position regardless of whether the position is disclosed on the tax return.

c. True-False. Jim will not be subject to penalty with respect to the tuition deduction as long as his position has a reasonable basis even if he does not specifically disclose the position on the return.

False. In this situation, Jim's $6,000 understatement would be considered substantial since it exceeds the larger of $5,000 or 10 percent of the correct tax, $3,000 (10% × $30,000). When the understatement in question is substantial, the substantial understatement penalty applies. This penalty can be avoided only if the taxpayer has substantial authority for his position *or* he discloses the position and such position has reasonable basis. Here Jim will not have disclosed the position, so a reasonable basis for the position will not suffice.

d. Jim has indicated that he does not want to flag either position. Pete would not be subject to a preparer penalty with respect to the tuition deduction if the position is *not* disclosed as long as the position:
  (1) has a reasonable basis
  (2) is nonfrivolous
  (3) has a realistic possibility of success
  (4) has a more-likely-than-not chance of prevailing
  (5) all of the above

(4). To avoid the $1,000 preparer penalty of § 6694(a), an undisclosed position must be supported with substantial authority. However, if the position is disclosed, the preparer penalty will not apply as long as it there is a reasonable basis for the position.

e. Pete understands that the SSTS indicate that he is not supposed to sign the return where there is an undisclosed position unless the position has a realistic possibility of success. However, he has no real idea whether the chances are 20 percent, 30 percent, 40 percent, or whatever based on what he has found. Can Pete sign a return containing a position for which there is no reasonable basis without violating the AICPA statements if he discloses the position?

Yes. The SSTS provide that a practitioner can sign any return as long as the position is disclosed and it is not frivolous.

PROBLEM MATERIALS

DISCUSSION QUESTIONS

2-1 *Taxpayer Penalties.* In reviewing his last year's return, T noticed that he had inadvertently deducted the entire cost of a new air-conditioning system. Such cost should have been capitalized and depreciated.
  a. T wants to know what penalties, if any, might be assessed if his return is audited and the IRS uncovers his mistake.
  b. What should T do?

2-2 *Tax Positions.* R operates a small accounting practice in Columbus, Ohio. While preparing the return for his long-time client C, he found out that C wants to deduct the cost of lawn care for her home. C is a landscape architect who recently started using a room at her home as an office. She feels that this is clearly a business expense. During the interview she seemed to have a point. "What if my clients came to my house and the yard was less than picture perfect? It would kill my business," she explained. R has reviewed the proposed regulations on the home office deduction, and they specifically state that lawn care is not deductible. Nevertheless, he understands C's point. R just cannot say no, and he is thinking about preparing the return and deducting a portion of lawn care allocable to C's home office.
  a. Assume the position is erroneous and is not disclosed. Will C be subject to any penalty? Explain.
  b. Assume the position is erroneous and is disclosed. Will C be subject to any penalty? Explain.

2-3 *Avoiding Preparer Penalties.* H recently quit a national public accounting firm and purchased the practice of a local accountant. Her first busy season with this new set of clients has been eye-opening. Some of the taxpayers have been taking very questionable positions on certain recurring items. Somewhat paranoid, H is now quite concerned about incurring penalties. What can she do to guard against possible preparer penalties?

2-4 *Knowledge of Error.* Last March, P put the finishing touches on the tax return of one of his most prized clients, Great Buy Corporation. When preparing the monthly financial statement for June, P noticed that $30,000 of sales somehow got left off of the return. What should P do?

2-5 *Knowledge of Error.* This year P got a new client from the firm down the street, Dewey, Cheatham and Howe. After reviewing the client's prior year return, he found, as he had expected, an error in the way Dewey had computed depreciation. What should P do?

2-6 *Making a New Tax Law.* Describe the Congressional process of making a tax bill into final law.

2-7 *Legislative versus Interpretative Regulations.* Explain the difference between a legislative Treasury Regulation and an interpretative Regulation.

2-8 *Proposed versus Final Regulations.* Distinguish between proposed and final Regulations. How would either type of Regulation involving Code § 704 be cited?

2-9 *Revenue Rulings and Revenue Procedures.* Distinguish between a Revenue Ruling and a Revenue Procedure. Where can either be found in printed form?

2-10 *Private versus Published Rulings.* Distinguish between a private letter ruling and a Revenue Ruling. Under what circumstances would a taxpayer prefer to rely on either of these sources?

2-11 *Technical Advice Memoranda.* What are Technical Advice Memoranda? Under what circumstances are they issued?

2-12 *Trial Courts.* Describe the trial courts that hear tax cases. What are the advantages or disadvantages of litigating a tax issue in each of these courts?

2-13 *The Appeals Process.* A taxpayer living in Indiana has exhausted her appeals within the IRS. If she chooses to litigate her case, trace the appeals process assuming she begins her effort in each of the following trial courts:
a. The U.S. Court of Federal Claims
b. The U.S. District Court
c. The U.S. Tax Court
d. The Small Tax Division of the U.S. Tax Court

2-14 *Tax Court Decisions.* Distinguish between a Regular Tax Court decision and a Memorandum decision.

2-15 *Authority of Tax Law Sources.* Assuming that you have discovered favorable support for your position taken in a controversy with an IRS agent in each of the sources listed below, indicate how you would use these authoritative sources in your discussion with the agent.
a. A decision of the U.S. District Court having jurisdiction over your case if litigated
b. Treasury Regulation
c. The Internal Revenue Code

    d. A decision of the Supreme Court

    e. A decision by the Court of Appeals

    f. A decision of the Small Claims Court

    g. A decision of the U.S. Tax Court

    h. A private letter ruling issued to another taxpayer

    i. A Revenue Ruling

    j. A tax article in a leading periodical

2-16 *Tax Services.* What materials are generally found in leading tax services? Which does your library have?

❓ YOU MAKE THE CALL

2-17 T is the owner of a small CPA firm that has developed a very good auditing and tax practice over the years. Recently, while visiting the home of S, his best client (revenues of about $50,000 annually for audit and tax services), T learned some very disturbing information about S's business practices. During a tour of her home, S accidentally revealed that some very expensive personal entertainment equipment acquired in 2009 had been charged to her corporation (cost of approximately $100,000). S stated that everyone she knew charged personal assets to their business accounts and that it appeared to be generally accepted practice. She said she hoped T would not mind.

    When T returned to his office, he immediately checked S's 2009 corporate income tax return and found that depreciation had been taken on the $100,000 cost of assets listed simply as "Equipment." Of course, T never suspected the assets were for personal use in S's home.

    What should T do? This client is too good to lose, but T is worried about the consequences of allowing this type of behavior to continue.

PROBLEMS

2-18 *Interpreting Citations.* Interpret each of the following citations:

    a. Reg. § 1.721-1(a).

    b. Rev. Rul. 60-314, 1960-2 C.B. 48.

    c. Rev. Proc. 86-46, 1986-2 C.B. 739.

    d. Rev. Rul. 98-36, I.R.B. No. 31, 6.

    e. § 351.

2-19 *Citation Abbreviations.* Explain each of the abbreviations below.

    a. B.T.A.

    b. Acq.

    c. D. Ct.

    d. CA-9

    e. F.Supp.

    f. NA.

    g. Ct. Cls.

    h. USTC

    i. AFTR

    j. *Cert. Den.*

    k. *aff'g* and *aff'd*

    l. *rev'g* and *rev'd*

    m. *rem'g* and *rem'd*

2-20   *Interpreting Citations.* Identify the publisher and interpret each of the following citations:
  a.   41 TCM 289.
  b.   93 S. Ct. 2820 (USSC, 1973).
  c.   71-1 USTC ¶9241 (CA-2, 1971).
  d.   236 F.Supp. 761 (D. Ct. Va., 1974).
  e.   T.C. Memo 1977-20.
  f.   48 T.C. 430 (1967).
  g.   6 AFTR2d 5095 (CA-2, 1960).
  h.   589 F.2d 446 (CA-9, 1979).
  i.   277 U.S. 508 (USSC, 1928).

2-21   *Citation Form.* Record the following information in its proper citation form.
  a.   Part 7, subdivision (a)(2) of the income tax Regulation under Code § 165
  b.   The 34th Revenue Ruling issued March 2, 1987, and printed on pages 101 and 102 of the appropriate document
  c.   The 113th letter ruling issued the last week of 1986

2-22   *Citation Form.* Record the following information in its proper citation form.
  a.   A 1982 U.S. Tax Court case in which Roger A. Schubel sued the IRS Commissioner for a refund, published in volume 77 on pages 701 through 715 as a Regular decision
  b.   A 1974 U.S. Tax Court case in which H. N. Schilling, Jr. sued the IRS Commissioner for a refund, published by (1) Commerce Clearing House in volume 33 on pages 1097 through 1110 and (2) Prentice Hall as its 246th decision that year
  c.   A 1966 Court of Appeals case in which Boris Nodiak sued the IRS Commissioner in the second Circuit for a refund, published by (1) Commerce Clearing House in volume 1 of that year at paragraph 9262, (2) Prentice Hall in volume 17 on pages 396 through 402, and (3) West Publishing Company in volume 356 on pages 911 through 919.

RESEARCH PROBLEMS

2-23   *Using a Citator.* Use either the Commerce Clearing House or Research Institute of America Citator in your library and locate *Richard L. Kroll, Exec. v. U.S.*
  a.   Which Court of Appeals Circuit heard this case?
  b.   Was this case heard by the Supreme Court?
  c.   James B. and Doris E. Wallach are included in the listing below the citation for Kroll. In what court was the Wallach case heard?

2-24   *Using a Citator.* Using any available citator, locate the case of *Corn Products v. Comm.*, 350 U.S. 46. What effect did the decision in *Arkansas Best v. Comm.* (58 AFTR2d 86-5748, 800 F.2d 219) have on the precedential value of the *Corn Products* case?

2-25   *Locating Court Cases.* Locate the case of *Robert Autrey, Jr. v. United States*, 89-2 USTC ¶9659, and answer the following questions.
  a.   What court decided the case on appeal?
  b.   What court originally tried the case?
  c.   Was the trial court's decision upheld or reversed?

2-26   *Locating Court Cases.* Locate the case of *Fabry v. Commissioner*, 111 T.C. 305, and answer the following questions.
  a.   What court tried the case?
  b.   Identify the various types of precedential authority the judge used in framing his opinion.

2-27 *Locating Court Cases.* Locate the cited court cases and answer the questions below.

    a. *Stanley A. and Lorriee M. Golanty*, 72 T.C. 411 (1979). Did the taxpayers win their case?

    b. *Hamilton D. Hill*, 41 TCM 700, T.C. Memo ¶71,127 (1971). Who was the presiding judge?

    c. *Patterson (Jefferson) v. Comm.*, 72-1 USTC ¶9420, 29 AFTR2d 1181 (Ct. Cls., 1972). What was the issue being questioned in this case?

2-28 *Completing Citations.* To the extent the materials are available to you, complete the following citations:

    a. Rev. Rul. 98-60, _____C.B. _____.

    b. *Lawrence W. McCoy*, _____T.C. _____(1962).

    c. *Reginald Turner* _____ TCM _____ T.C. Memo 1954-38.

    d. *RCA Corp. v. U.S.*, _____ USTC _____ (CA-2, 1981).

    e. *RCA Corp. v. U.S.*, _____ AFTR2d _____ (CA-2, 1981).

    f. *RCA Corp. v. U.S.*, _____ F.2d _____ (CA-2, 1981).

    g. *Comm. v. Wilcox*, _____ S. Ct. _____ (USSC, 1946).

    h. _____, 79-1 USTC ¶9139 (USSC, 1979).

    i. _____, 34 T.C. 842 (1960).

    j. *Brian E. Knutson*, 60 TCM 540, T.C. Memo _____.

    k. *Samuel B. Levin v. Comm.*, 43 AFTR2d 79-1057 (_____).

2-29 *Examination of Tax Sources.* For each of the tax sources listed below, identify at least one of the tax issues involved. In addition, if the source has a temporary citation, provide its permanent citation (if available).

    a. *Battelstein Investment Co. v. U.S.*, 71-1 USTC ¶9227, 27 AFTR2d 71-713, 442 F.2d 87 (CA-5, 1971).

    b. *Joel Kerns*, 47 TCM, _____T.C. Memo 1984-22.

    c. *Patterson v. U.S.*, 84-1 USTC ¶9315 (CA-6, 1984).

    d. *Webster Lair*, 95 T.C. 484 (1990).

    e. *Thompson Engineering Co., Inc.*, 80 T.C. 672 (1983).

    f. *Towne Square, Inc.*, 45 TCM 478, T.C. Memo 1983-10.

    g. Rev. Rul. 85-13, I.R.B. No. 7, 28.

    h. Rev. Proc. 85-49, I.R.B. No. 40, 26.

    i. *William E Sutton, et al. v. Comm.*, 84 T.C. _____No. 17.

    j. Rev. Rul. 86-103, I.R.B. No. 36, 13.

    k. *Hughes Properties, Inc.*, 86-1 USTC ¶9440, 58 AFTR2d 86-5062, _____U. S. _____(USSC, 1986).

    l. Rev. Rul. 98-27, I.R.B. No. 22, 4.

2-30 *Office in the Home.* T comes to you for advice regarding the deductibility of expenses for maintaining an office in his home. T is currently employed as an executive vice president for Zandy Corporation. He has found it impossible to complete his job responsibilities during the normal forty-hour weekly period. Although the office building in which he works is open nights and weekends, the heating and air-conditioning systems are shut down at night (from 6 p.m.) and during the entire weekend. As a result, T has begun taking work home with him on a regular basis. The work is generally done in the den of T's home. Although T's employer does not require him to work at home, T is convinced that he would be fired if his work assignments were not completed on a timely basis. Given these facts, what would you advise T about taking a home-office deduction?

    Partial list of research aids:

        § 280A

        Proposed Reg. § 1.280A

        M.G. Hill, 43 TCM 832, T.C. Memo 1982-143

2-31   *Journal Articles.* Refer to *Problem 2-30.* Consult an index to periodicals (e.g., AICPA's *Accountants Index*; Warren, Gorham, and Lamont's *Index to Federal Tax Articles*; or CCH's *Federal Tax Articles*) and locate a journal article on the topic of tax deductions for an office in the home. Copy the article. Record the citation for the article (i.e., author's name, article title, journal name, publication date, and first and last pages of the article) at the top of your paper. Prepare a two-page summary of the article, including all relevant issues, research sources, and conclusions. Staple your two-page summary to the article. The grade for this exercise will be based on the relevance of your article to the topic, the accuracy and quality of your summary, and the quality of your written communication skills.

2-32   *Deductible Medical Expenses.* B suffers from a severe form of degenerative arthritis. Her doctor strongly recommended that she swim for at least one hour per day in order to stretch and exercise her leg and arm muscles. There are no swimming pools nearby, so B spent $15,000 to have a swimming pool installed in her back yard. This expenditure increased the fair market value of her house by $5,000. B consults you about whether she can deduct the cost of the swimming pool on her individual tax return. What do you recommend?

   Hint: You should approach this problem by using the tax service volumes of either Commerce Clearing House or Research Institute of America. Both tax services are organized according to Code Sections, so you should start with Code § 213. You will find the Code Sections on the back binding of the volumes. Research Institute of America has a very extensive index, so look under the term "medical expenses."

2-33   *Deductible Educational Expenses.* T is a CPA with a large accounting firm in Houston, Texas. He has been assigned to the international taxation group of his firm's tax department. As a result of this assignment, T enrolls in an international tax law course at the University of Houston Law School. The authorities of the University require T to enroll as a regular law student; and, theoretically, if he continues to attend courses, T will graduate with a law degree. Will T be able to deduct his tuition for the international tax law course as a business expense?

   Hint: Go to either the RIA or CCH tax service and use it to find the analysis of Code § 162. When you have found the discussion of § 162, find that part of the subsection dealing with educational deductions. Read the appropriate Regulations and then note the authorities listed after the Regulations. Read over the summaries provided and then choose those you think have the most relevance to the question asked above. Read these cases and other listed authorities, and formulate a written response to the question asked in light of these cases and other authorities Finally, for the authorities you choose, go to the RIA or CCH Citator and use it to ensure that your authorities are current.

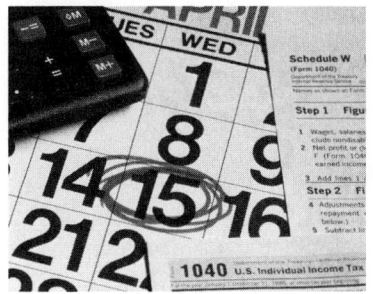

CHAPTER THREE

TAXABLE ENTITIES, TAX FORMULA, INTRODUCTION TO PROPERTY TRANSACTIONS

LEARNING OBJECTIVES

Upon completion of this chapter you will be able to:

▸ Identify the entities that are subject to the Federal income tax

▸ Explain the basic tax treatment of individuals, corporations, partnerships, S corporations, and fiduciary taxpayers (trusts and estates)

▸ Understand the basic tax formulas to be followed in computing the tax liability for individuals and corporations

▸ Define many of the basic terms used in the tax formula such as gross income, adjusted gross income, taxable income, exclusion, deduction, and credit

▸ Calculate the gain or loss on the disposition of property and explain the tax consequences, including the special treatment of capital gains and losses

---

CHAPTER OUTLINE

INTRODUCTION

The amount of income tax ultimately paid by any taxpayer is determined by applying the many rules comprising our income tax system. This chapter examines some of the fundamental features of this system. They are

- *Taxable Entities*—those entities that are subject to taxation and those that are merely conduits
- *Tax Formulas*—the mathematical relationships used to compute the tax for the various taxable entities
- *Property Transactions*—the tax treatment of sales, exchanges, and other dispositions of property

This chapter, in covering the essentials, provides a bird's-eye view of the entire income tax system. For many, this may be sufficient. This one chapter may contain enough tax law and have more than enough detail for some. Nevertheless, it is just part of the picture. Many of the details as well as the conceptual basis for some of these provisions are left to later chapters. This can be frustrating to those who want more or know that more exists, but the major purpose of this chapter is to establish the basic framework in which the implications of any particular transaction on taxable income can be assessed. To this end, the chapter gives not only a brief description of what is taxable and what is deductible but also a glimpse of such complex topics as the passive loss rules and the alternative minimum tax. Remember, the goal is not necessarily to provide a detailed discussion of all the rules but to provide a foundation so that problems, pitfalls, and opportunities can be recognized.

THE TAXABLE ENTITY

The income tax is imposed on the income of some type of entity. Unfortunately, there is no uniform agreement on what is the theoretically correct unit of taxation. There are a variety of legal, economic, social, and natural entities that Congress could select: individuals (natural persons), family units, households (those living together), sole proprietorships, partnerships, corporations, trusts, estates, governments, religious groups, nonprofit organizations, and other voluntary or cooperative associations. Despite the disagreement over which of these or other entities are the proper choices, Congress has provided that only certain entities are responsible for actually paying the tax. According to the Code, individuals, most corporations, and fiduciaries (estates and trusts) are taxable entities. Other entities, such as sole proprietorships, partnerships, and so-called "S" corporations, are not required to pay tax on any taxable income they might have. Instead, the taxable income of these entities is passed through or allocated to their owners, who bear the responsibility for paying any tax that may be due. For this reason, these entities are often referred to as flow-through entities or conduits. Exhibit 3-1 summarizes the various types of entities.

EXHIBIT 3-1
Types of Entities

Taxpaying Entities	Flow-Through Entities or Conduits
Individuals	Sole proprietorships
C Corporations (regular corporations)	Partnerships and limited liability companies
Trusts	S corporations
Estates	

Example 1. R and S are equal partners in a partnership that had taxable income of $50,000 in the current year. The partnership does not pay tax on the $50,000. Rather, the income is allocated equally between R and S. Thus, both R and S will report $25,000 of partnership income on their individual returns and pay the required tax regardless of whether they received distributions from the partnership.

In the following sections, the general tax treatment of the taxable entities—individuals, corporations, and fiduciaries—is explained along with the treatment of flow-through entities, sole proprietorships, partnerships and "S" corporations. The specific tax treatment of entities other than individuals is discussed separately in later chapters. However, it should be emphasized that many of the tax rules applying to one entity also apply to other entities. These similarities are pointed out as the various rules are discussed.

TAXABLE ENTITIES

INDIVIDUAL TAXPAYERS

The primary target for the income tax is the *individual* taxpayer. For 2007, 138.4 million individual returns were filed (Forms 1040, 1040A and 1040 EZ), and these were responsible for 51 percent of the total tax revenue collected by the federal government. This amount easily exceeded the second and third place finishers, employment taxes (31.6 percent) and corporate income taxes (14.7 percent). These statistics leave little doubt about the importance of the individual income tax in the United States.

Citizens and Residents of the United States. Section 1 of the Internal Revenue Code provides that a tax is imposed on the taxable income of all individuals. As might be expected, the term *individual* generally applies to U.S. citizens. However, it also includes persons who are *not* U.S. citizens but who are considered residents, so-called *resident aliens*. Thus, if Prince Harry decides to move to New York to escape the tabloids of London, he could be subject to U.S. taxes even though he is not a U.S. citizen. The same could be said for a Japanese citizen working for Honda in Marysville, Ohio or a Canadian citizen who lives and works in Detroit. Whether these people are residents requires application of a complicated test.[1] The key point to remember is that foreign citizens who are not merely visiting but stay for an extended period must worry about the need for filing.[2] As discussed below, the tax would be levied on both their U.S. income and any foreign income.

Foreign Taxpayers. Individuals who are not U.S. citizens and who do not qualify as residents may be subject to U.S. tax. These persons, referred to as *nonresident aliens*, are taxed on certain types of income that are received from U.S. sources.[3] If the income is derived from a trade or business carried on in the United States, that income is taxed in the same way as it is for a citizen or resident. Most other income earned in the United States is taxed at a flat rate of 30 percent. However, there are a number of special rules that must be observed.

Age. It should be noted that the age of an individual is not a factor in determining if he or she is a taxpaying entity. Whether the individual is eight years old or eighty years

---

[1]   See § 7701(b) for a definition of the "substantial presence test" that is used to determine if an individual is a resident alien and subject to U.S. tax.

[2]   Reg. § 1.871-2(b).

[3]   § 871.

old, he or she is still subject to tax on any taxable income received. Contrary to the belief of some people, a child's income is taxed to the child and not the parent. As explained later, age may have an impact on *both* the method of computing the tax and the amount of tax owed; it does not, however, impact the individual's status as a taxpayer.

Worldwide Income. The Federal income tax on individuals applies not only to domestic (U.S.) source income, but also to income from foreign sources. In other words, a U.S. citizen is subject to U.S. taxation on his or her worldwide income regardless of where he or she lives (e.g., Rhode Island or Rome) or the source of the income (e.g., Connecticut or Copenhagen). It is therefore possible to have foreign source income taxed by more than one country (e.g., the foreign country and the United States). Several provisions exist to prevent or minimize double taxation, however. For example, U.S. citizens and residents living abroad may claim either the foreign tax credit (a direct reduction in the tax)[4] or deduct such taxes.[5]

In lieu of claiming a credit or deduction for foreign taxes, a U.S. citizen who works and lives in a foreign country may exclude from his or her U.S. income certain amounts of income earned abroad.[6] The foreign earned income exclusion is adjusted annually for inflation and for 2009 is $91,400. An individual qualifies for the exclusion if he or she maintains his tax home in a foreign country (i.e., his principal place of business is in the foreign country) and he or she is either a bona fide resident of a foreign country or is physically present in a foreign country for 330 days in any 12 consecutive months.

Example 2. Z, a U.S. citizen, is an aircraft mechanic who was temporarily assigned to a lucrative job in Seoul, South Korea. Z lived in Seoul all of 2009 except for two weeks when he came back to the United States to visit relatives. From his Korean job, he earned $101,400 in 2009. Because Z's tax home is in a foreign country and he was present in the foreign country for at least 330 days during 12 consecutive months, he meets the physical presence test and may exclude $91,400 of his $101,400 salary. The remaining $10,000 plus any other income, such as dividends and interest, are subject to tax.

In addition to the relief measures mentioned above, taxpayers may exclude, subject to certain limitations, allowances (in-kind or cash) for foreign housing. Also, tax treaties often exist that deal with the problem of double taxation by the United States and foreign countries.

State Income Taxes. While virtually the entire focus of this text is on the federal income tax, state income taxes cannot be ignored. All but seven states have a state income tax imposed on individuals. The seven that do not have an income tax are: Alaska, Florida, Nevada, South Dakota, Texas, Washington and Wyoming. However, the income taxes of New Hampshire and Tennessee extend only to interest and dividends. Thus the vast majority of all individuals must pay not only federal income taxes but also state and local income taxes.

As might be expected, states that impose an income tax do not necessarily follow the federal rules. Each has its own unique method to compute taxable income. Of the 41 states with an income tax, 25 begin their calculation with federal adjusted gross income, 8 use federal taxable income as the starting point and 3 use the federal income tax liability as the basis for their tax. To make matters more challenging, some states conform with the

---

[4] § 901.

[5] § 164(a).

[6] § 911(a).

methods allowed for federal tax purposes (e.g., depreciation) while others do not. As might be imagined, the world of state and local taxes can become quite complex.

The important concept to grasp here is not how the various state laws work but whether they apply to the taxpayer at all. Those working in tax must not overlook the possibility that a taxpayer may be responsible not only for federal taxes but for state or local taxes as well. For example, consider a professional football player, say Peyton Manning of the Indianapolis Colts who lives in Indianapolis and files an Indiana income tax return. If he plays a game in Philadelphia, must he file a state income tax return for Pennsylvania and perhaps another return for the city of Philadelphia? Similarly, if a staff accountant working for a national accounting firm in Chicago is assigned temporarily to an audit in Denver, must he pay income taxes in Colorado? If a son is a professor at Michigan State but is a shareholder in his father's S corporation that operates a farm in Iowa, must the son pay Iowa taxes? At this juncture, the answer is not as important as asking the question!

CORPORATE TAXPAYERS

Section 11 of the Internal Revenue Code imposes a tax on all corporations. The corporate income tax applies to both domestic corporations and foreign corporations with trades or businesses operated in the United States.[7] However, the federal tax treatment of a corporation differs depending on whether it is a "C" corporation (a regular corporation) or an "S" corporation. For tax purposes, a corporation is treated as a C corporations unless it is eligible and elects to be treated as an S corporation. C corporations, like individuals, are treated as separate taxable entities. On the other hand, S corporations normally are not separate taxable entities but are treated as conduits, passing their income and losses through to their shareholders (as discussed below). It should be emphasized that this difference–C or S–is made only for tax purposes. For all other purposes (e.g., liability), the applicable state laws make no distinction.

The overall income tax treatment of corporations is quite similar to that of individuals. In fact, all of the basic rules governing income, exclusions, deductions, and credits apply to individuals as well as C corporations and, for that matter, fiduciaries. For example, the general rule concerning what is deductible, found in § 162, allows *all* taxpayers a deduction for trade or business expenses. Similarly, § 103 provides that *all* taxpayers are allowed to exclude interest income from state and local bonds. Although many of the general rules are the same for both individuals and corporations, there are several key differences.

The most obvious difference can be seen by comparing the corporate and individual formulas for determining taxable income as found in Exhibits 3-2 and 3-3. The concepts of adjusted gross income and itemized deductions found in the individual tax formula are conspicuously absent from the corporate formula. Other major differences in determining taxable income involve the treatment of particular items, such as dividend income and charitable contributions. These and other differences are discussed in detail in Chapter 19. It should be emphasized once again, however, that most of the basic rules apply whether the taxpayer is a corporation or an individual.

One difference in the taxation of individuals and corporations that is not apparent from the basic formula, but which should be noted, concerns the tax rates that each uses in computing the tax liability (see the inside back cover of the text). A comparison of the individual and corporate tax rates shows a somewhat similar progression: 10 to 35 percent for individuals and 15 to 39 percent for corporations. But note that the rates apply at quite different levels of income.

---

[7]   § 882(a). See Chapter 19 for more details.

EXHIBIT 3-2

Tax Formula for Corporate Taxpayers

Total Income (from whatever source)	$xxx,xxx
Less: Exclusions from gross income	− xx,xxx
Gross income	$xxx,xxx
Less: Deductions	− xx,xxx
Taxable income	$xxx,xxx
Applicable tax rates	xx%
Gross tax	$ xx,xxx
Less: Tax credits and prepayments	− x,xxx
Tax due (or refund)	$ xx,xxx

EXHIBIT 3-3

Tax Formula for Individual Taxpayers

Total income (from whatever source)			$xxx,xxx
Less:	Exclusions from gross income		− xx,xxx
Gross income			$xxx,xxx
Less:	Deductions *for* adjusted gross income		− xx,xxx
Adjusted gross income			$xxx,xxx
Less:	1. The larger of:		
	a. Standard deduction	$x,xxx	
	or	or	− x,xxx
	b. Total itemized deductions	$x,xxx	
	2. Number of personal and dependency exemptions ×		
	exemption amount		− x,xxx
Taxable income			$xxx,xxx
Applicable tax rates (from Tables or Schedules X, Y, or Z)			xx%
Gross income tax			$ xx,xxx
Plus:	Additional taxes (e.g., self-employment tax, alternative		
	minimum tax, recapture of tax credits)		+ x,xxx
Less:	Tax credits and prepayments		− x,xxx
Tax due (or refund)			$ xx,xxx

Perhaps the most critical aspect of corporate taxation that is generally not shared with any other taxable entity concerns the potential for double taxation. When a corporation receives income and subsequently distributes that income as a dividend to its shareholders, the effect is to tax the income twice: once at the corporate level and again at the shareholder level. Double taxation can occur because the corporation is not allowed to deduct any dividend payments to its shareholders. As one might suspect, many have questioned the equity of this treatment, arguing that it penalizes those who elect to do business in the corporate form. Note, however, that this treatment is consistent with the fact that the corporation is considered a separate legal entity. Moreover,

it is often argued that the corporation and its owners in reality do not bear the burden of the corporate tax. According to the argument, corporations are able to shift the tax burden either to consumers by charging higher prices or to employees by paying lower wages. In addition, those who reject the double tax theory often note that closely held corporations, whose owners may also be employees of the business, are able to avoid double taxation to the extent they can characterize any corporate distributions as deductible salary payments rather than nondeductible dividends. Whether in fact double taxation does or does not occur, it appears that this feature, which has been part of the U.S. tax system since its inception, is unlikely to change in the immediate future.

Example 3. J owns all of the stock of ZZ Inc., a C corporation. This year ZZ reported taxable income of $1,000,000 before considering any distributions to J. Assume that ZZ is in the 34 percent marginal tax bracket while J is in 35 percent bracket. J plans on withdrawing $600,000 from the corporation. Ignoring payroll taxes, is J better off if he causes the corporation to distribute $600,000 as a qualifying dividend or $600,000 as a salary?

Distribution Treated as a Dividend	ZZ Inc.	J	Total
Taxable income before distributions to J	$1,000,000		
Distributions to J			
Nondeductible dividend	—	$600,000	
Taxable income	$1,000,000	$600,000	
Tax rate	x 34%	x 15%	
Total tax	$340,000	90,000	$430,000
Distribution Treated as a Salary			
Taxable income before distributions to J	$1,000,000		
Distributions to J			
Deductible salary	(600,000)	$600,000	
Taxable income	$400,000	$600,000	
Tax rate	x 34%	x 35%	
Total tax	$136,000	$210,000	$346,000
Savings			$ 84,000

As calculated above, J saves $84,000 by withdrawing the $600,000 as a salary rather than as a dividend. The savings result because $600,000 of the total income is taxed twice when it is distributed as a dividend (once at the corporate level and again at the individual level) but only once when the distribution is treated as a salary because the corporation is allowed to deduct the salary payment as a business expense. Note that currently the qualifying dividend is taxed at a maximum rate of 15 percent (2009 and 2010). In 2011 dividends are scheduled to be treated as ordinary income potentially taxed at the highest marginal rate as they were prior to 2003.

Special rules apply to the formation of a corporation, corporate dividend distributions, and distributions made to shareholders in exchange for their stock. Penalty taxes also may be assessed against corporations that try to shelter income from high personal tax rates by accumulating it in the corporation, rather than making dividend distributions. These topics and others related to the income taxation of corporations and their owners are discussed in Chapters 19, 20, and 21.

FIDUCIARY TAXPAYERS

A *fiduciary* is a person who is entrusted with property for the benefit of another, the *beneficiary*. The individual or entity that acts as a fiduciary is responsible for managing and administering the entrusted property, at all times faithfully performing the required duties with the utmost care and prudence.

Two types of fiduciary relationships are the trust and the estate. The trust is a legal entity created when the title of property is transferred by a person (the *grantor*) to the fiduciary (the *trustee*). The trustee is required to implement the instructions of the grantor as specified in the trust agreement. Typically, the property is held in trust for a minor or some other person until he or she reaches a certain age or until some specified event occurs.

An estate is also recognized as a legal entity, established by law when a person dies. Upon the person's death, his or her property generally passes to the estate, where it is administered by the fiduciary until it is distributed to the beneficiaries. Both trusts and estates are treated as taxpaying entities.

The Code specifically provides for a tax on the taxable income of estates and trusts.[8] Determining the tax for such entities is very similar to determining the tax for individuals, with one major exception.[9] When distributions are made to beneficiaries, the distributed income is generally taxed to the beneficiary rather than to the estate or trust.[10] In essence, the trust or estate is permitted to reduce its taxable income by the amount of the distribution—acting as a *conduit*, since the distributed income flows through to the beneficiaries.

> **Example 4.** T is the trustee of a trust established for the benefit of A and B. The trust generated $4,000 of income subject to tax for the current year and no distributions were made to either A or B during the year. The trustee files an annual fiduciary tax return for the year and pays the tax based on the $4,000 taxable amount.

> **Example 5.** Assume that for the next year the trust in *Example 4* had $10,000 of income subject to tax and that distributions of $2,000 each were made to A and B. The trustee files an annual trust return for the year and pays a tax based on $6,000 ($10,000 taxable income − $4,000 distributions). A and B each include $2,000 in their income tax returns for the year.

Distributions made by a trust or estate from its corpus (also called the trust property or principal), including undistributed profits from prior years, generally are not taxable to the beneficiary.[11] This is because these distributions are part of a gift or inheritance or have been taxed previously. Similarly, the trust or estate is not entitled to deductions for these nontaxable distributions.[12]

FLOW-THROUGH ENTITIES

SOLE PROPRIETORSHIPS

The first of the nontaxpaying, flow-through entities is the sole proprietorship. A sole proprietorship is commonly defined as an unincorporated business owned by one

---

[8]   §§ 1(e) and 641(a).

[9]   § 641(b).

[10]   §§ 651 and 661.

[11]   § 662.

[12]   § 661. These and other provisions related to the Federal taxation of estates, trusts, and beneficiaries are discussed in Chapter 25.

individual. The definition includes essentially all individuals who are in business for themselves. Indeed, while they may not think of themselves as proprietors, individuals who are self-employed (e.g., doctors, lawyers, accountants, consultants, plumbers, carpenters) as well as independent contractors are taxed as sole proprietorships. In addition, for tax purposes, a single member limited liability company (SMLLC) that does not elect to be treated as a corporation is disregarded as an entity separate from its owner and is treated as a sole proprietorship.

The tax treatment of sole proprietorships differs somewhat from that of financial accounting. For financial accounting purposes, the business activities of the proprietor are treated as distinct from other activities of the owner. The sole proprietorship is considered a totally independent accounting entity for which separate records and reports are maintained. For tax purposes, a similar approach applies except the sole proprietorship is not a separate taxable entity. For this reason, it does not file its own tax return. Instead, the income and deductions from operating a proprietorship are summarized and reported on Schedule C of the owner's personal income tax return along with other tax items (See Appendix B for Form 1040 and Schedule C).

Although some might not consider a sole proprietorship as a "flow-through" entity in the same sense that partnerships and S corporations are, they clearly function in much the same way. In essence, a sole proprietorship serves as a conduit through which its net income or loss flows through to the individual. Any item of income or deduction of the proprietorship that might receive some type of special treatment had the owner received or paid it directly—rather than running it through the business—is not included on the Schedule C but is reported separately on the owner's personal return (e.g., interest income, capital gains, charitable contributions). Distributions or withdrawals that an owner receives from a proprietorship are not considered salary or other income since all of the proprietorship income is included on the individual's return regardless of whether it is distributed. Therefore, a proprietor's "draw" is ignored.

> **Example 6.** K is employed as a law professor at State University, where she earns a salary of $102,000. K also operates a part-time consulting practice as a sole proprietorship. She maintains a separate checking account for the business. The business earned net income of $30,000 this year before considering $50 of interest earned on the money in the business' checking account, a $100 charitable contribution drawn on the business account to the United Way and a withdrawal of $18,000. How are the activities reported?
>
> The sole proprietorship does not file a separate return and pay tax. Instead, K reports the sole proprietorship's income of $30,000 on her Schedule C. This amount is subsequently combined with her salary of $102,000 and other income and deductions on her return to compute her taxable income. She then pays both the income and self-employment taxes required. The $50 of interest income is not considered part of the proprietorship income but is aggregated with other interest income that K might have and is reported separately (Schedule B). The same approach is used for the charitable contribution. The contribution is treated as if K had made it personally and would be deducted as an itemized deduction on Schedule A if K itemizes. The $18,000 withdrawal is ignored since it represents either part of her original investment in the business or income that is currently or previously reported on Schedule C.

It is easy to dismiss sole proprietorships in a world dominated by multinational corporations and partnerships. Indeed IRS statistics bare this out, indicating that in 2005, proprietorships accounted for only 9.7 percent of the net income reported by businesses. Nevertheless, based on returns filed for that year, proprietorships cannot be ignored. The number of proprietorships

far exceeded the number of corporations and partnerships: 21.4 million proprietorships (71.8%) versus 5.7 million corporations (19%) and 2.7 million partnerships (9.2%).[13]

PARTNERSHIPS

A partnership is a conduit for Federal income tax purposes. This means that the partnership itself is not subject to Federal income tax and that all items of partnership income, expense, gain, loss, or credit pass through to the partners and are given their tax effect at the partner level.[14] The partnership is required to file an information return (Form 1065) reporting the results of the partnership's transactions and how those results are divided among the partners. Each partner's share of the various items are reported to the partner on Schedule K-1. Using this information, the partners each report their respective shares of the items on their own tax returns.[15] Because partners pay taxes on their shares of the partnership income regardless of whether it is distributed, distributions made by the partnership generally are not taxable to the partners.[16]

> **Example 7.** For its current calendar year, EG Partnership had taxable income of $18,000. During the year, each of its two equal partners received cash distributions of $4,000. The partnership is not subject to tax, and each partner must include $9,000 in his annual income tax return, despite the fact that each partner actually received less than this amount in cash. The distributions normally are not taxable since they represent previously taxed income. The partnership must file an annual information return reporting the results of its operations and the effect of these operations on each partner.

A characteristic of a partnership (as well as an S corporation or sole proprietorship) that deserves special emphasis is the treatment of losses. If a business is typical, it will take several years of operation before it can be declared a profitable venture. Until that time, expenses normally exceed revenues and the result is a net loss. In the case of a conduit entity such as a partnership, that net loss flows through to the owners, who are generally allowed to offset it against any other income they may have. In contrast, if a regular C corporation sustains a loss, referred to as a net operating loss, or NOL, the shareholders do not benefit from that loss directly. A C corporation is allowed, like individuals, to use the loss to offset taxable income of prior or subsequent years. Generally, losses are carried back two years and forward 20 years. For example, the taxpayer would first carry back the loss to the second prior year and offset it against any taxable income. In such case, the taxpayer would file a claim for a tax refund. Any remaining loss is carried to the first prior year. Any remaining loss is carried forward for 20 years. The key point to remember is that the losses of a partnership flow through and thus may provide immediate benefit, whereas those of a C corporation do not flow through and can be used only if the corporation has income in other tax years.

In some respects, the partnership is treated as a separate entity for tax purposes. For example, many tax elections are made by the partnership,[17] and a partnership interest

---

[13]   *The 2009 Statistical Abstract (Table 722. Number of Tax Returns, Receipts, and Net Income by Type of Business: 1990 to 2005)*, U.S. Census Bureau.

[14]   § 701.

[15]   § 702(a).

[16]   § 731(a).

[17]   § 703(b).

generally is treated as a single asset when sold.[18] On the other hand, transactions between the partners and partnership are sometimes treated as if the partner was an independent third party and sometimes special rules apply.[19] For example, an individual partner who performs services for the partnership in his or her role as a partner is generally not considered an employee for tax purposes. Such payments are not considered salaries or wages. Consequently, the payments are not subject to withholding or employment taxes and are not reported to the partner at the end of the year on form W-2. Instead, these so-called "guaranteed payments" are reported to the partner on a Schedule K-1 and are subject to self-employment taxes. Consistent with this approach, a partner does not qualify for the favorable tax treatment of certain employee fringe benefits (see Chapter 6). In addition, a partner's share of any trade or business income of the partnership is generally subject to self-employment taxes. These and other controlling provisions related to the Federal income tax treatment of partnerships are covered in detail in Chapter 22.

ELECTING SMALL BUSINESS CORPORATIONS: "S" CORPORATIONS

The Internal Revenue Code allows certain closely held corporations to elect to be treated as conduits (like partnerships) for Federal income tax purposes. The election is made pursuant to the rules contained in Subchapter S of the Code.[20] For this reason, such corporations are referred to as *S corporations*. Not all corporations are eligible to elect S status. The only corporations that qualify are those that have 100 or fewer shareholders and meet certain other tests.

If a corporation elects S corporation status, it is taxed in virtually the same fashion as a partnership. Like a partnership, the S corporation's items of income, expense, gain, or loss pass through to the shareholders to be given their tax effect at the shareholder level. Salaries and wages of shareholders who work for the corporation and other employees are reported on a Form W-2 and are subject to withholding of income taxes and FICA (that is matched by the employer corporation). Although employees generally qualify for favorable treatment of fringe benefits, shareholder-employees owning 2 percent or more of the corporation's stock do not. As a result, the value of any fringe benefits, such as medical insurance coverage, is taxable as compensation to the employee-shareholder (who is allowed to deduct it). Distributions from an S corporation, like those from partnerships, normally are nontaxable since they usually represent previously taxed income.

The S corporation files an information return (Form 1120S) similar to that of a partnership, reporting the results of the corporation's transactions and how those results are allocated among the shareholders. The individual shareholders report their respective shares of the various items on their own tax returns. Chapter 23 contains a detailed discussion of the taxation of S corporations and their shareholders.

LIMITED LIABILITY COMPANIES

All 50 states and the District of Columbia have passed legislation creating a relatively new form of business entity: the limited liability company (LLC). What is this new creature and how is it taxed? Perhaps the best characterization of an LLC is that it is a cross between a partnership and a corporation. LLCs are created under state law by filing articles of organization. The owners of an LLC are called members and can be individuals, partnerships, regular corporations, S corporations, trusts, or other LLCs. Although some states allow single-member LLCs, two or more members usually form the entity.

---

[18] § 741 states that the sale or exchange of an interest in a partnership shall generally be treated as the sale of a capital asset.

[19] § 707(a).

[20] §§ 1361 through 1379.

Like a corporation, an LLC can act on its own behalf and sue and be sued. Also like a corporation, members generally possess limited liability except that they may be liable for their own acts of malpractice in those states that allow professionals to form LLCs.

The tax law does not specifically address the tax treatment of an LLC. Initially, this omission caused some uncertainty as to whether an LLC should be taxed as a corporation or a partnership. To eliminate this confusion, the Treasury issued the so-called check-the-box regulations.[21] Under these rules, an LLC with two or more owners is treated as a partnership for tax purposes unless it elects to be treated as a corporation (i.e., the LLC is a partnership unless it checks the box on Form 8832 to be treated as a regular C corporation). An LLC with only one member is disregarded and treated as a sole proprietorship, unless it elects to be treated as a corporation.

The treatment of LLCs for self-employment tax purposes has also produced some confusion. As noted above, in the case of a partnership, a partner's share of partnership income is generally self-employment income subject to self-employment taxes. However, this rule is true only for general partners. Historically, limited partners have been treated differently on the theory that their role is similar to that of an investor rather than someone who is actively involved in the business. Consequently, a limited partner's share of partnership income has been viewed more similar to investment income (e.g., dividends and interest) than business income. Section 1402 (a)(13) reflects this line of reasoning, providing that a limited partner's share of partnership income is not subject to self-employment tax. However, based on this approach, it was not clear whether a member of an LLC was to be treated like a limited partner, in which case the LLC's income would escape employment taxes. Hoping to eliminate this potential loophole, proposed regulations created new rules to test limited partners as well as LLC members. Under the proposed regulations, a limited partner or LLC member must treat his or her share of income as self-employment income if any of the following tests are met:[22]

1. The individual has personal liability for the debts of or claims against the business by reason of being a partner. This rule should rarely apply to a member of an LLC.

2. The individual has authority to contract on behalf of the entity.

3. The individual participates in the entity's trade or business for more than 500 hours during the year.

4. Substantially all of the activities of the entity involve the performance of services in the fields of health, law, engineering, architecture, accounting, actuarial science, or consulting.

Although these proposals provide needed guidance, they were heavily criticized. As a result, Congress intervened in 1997, passing legislation that postponed their implementation.[23] Since that time there has been no further action and the treatment of LLCs for purposes of self-employment taxes is still unresolved.

TAX-EXEMPT ORGANIZATIONS

Since inception, U.S. tax laws have exempted from federal income taxation charitable and religious organizations as well as a variety of nonprofit associations. The vast majority of tax-exempt organizations obtain their tax exempt status from § 501(c)(3).

---

[21] Reg. § 301.7701-3.

[22] Prop. Reg. § 1.1402(a)-2(h).

[23] See § 935 of the Tax Reform Act of 1997.

Under this provision, corporations that are organized and operated exclusively for religious, charitable, scientific, literary, or educational purposes are exempt, assuming certain requirements are met. It is often said that these organization are twice blessed since not only are they exempt from tax but contributions they receive are deductible.

Although tax-exempt entities usually do not pay tax, there are exceptions. If a nonprofit organization conducts a business unrelated to the purpose for which its exemption was granted, any taxable income resulting from that business would be subject to tax. The tax is referred to as the unrelated business income tax (UBIT). The UBIT rules are designed to prevent unfair competition that would otherwise arise between taxable and nontaxable entities that carry on the same business. If the tax-exempt entity is organized as a corporation, its tax on unrelated business taxable income is computed in the same manner as a regular corporation. Also note that if unrelated business income comprises a substantial portion of the organization's income, it could lose its tax-exempt status.

> **Example 8.** HHH Corporation is a nonprofit organization that operates a health agency. It collects dues from all of its members that number over 50,000. The dues income is nontaxable. Each month it e-mails a monthly newsletter to its members. Recently, several companies expressed interest in advertising in its newsletter. Would the advertising income be considered unrelated business income?
>
> Yes. Even though the corporation is a nonprofit organization, the advertising income would be taxable since the sale of ads is sufficiently commercial in nature to constitute a business activity that is carried on regularly (e.g., monthly). Moreover, if the advertising income comprised a substantial portion of the organization's income, it could lose its tax-exempt status.

> **Example 9.** The Mudville Little League Baseball Organization is a tax-exempt organization. Every spring it holds a car wash to raise money for its operation. Is the income subject to tax?
>
> No. The income from the car wash is exempt because the activity is not regularly carried on as a business.

As the examples might suggest, whether an otherwise tax-exempt organization has unrelated taxable income is often unclear. The point to grasp at this level is that even those organizations that might seem exempt—churches, universities, foundations and the like—may produce taxable income and, if the amount is substantial, they may lose their tax-exemption.

✔ CHECK YOUR KNOWLEDGE

Review Question 1. Section 1 of the Internal Revenue Code imposes a tax on all individuals. If taken literally, this would mean that the United States taxes not only Oprah Winfrey but also Fidel Castro and Elton John. Are these foreign citizens subject to U.S. tax?

The U.S. income tax generally applies to the worldwide income of U.S. citizens and resident aliens. As a result, it would not apply to Mr. Castro and Mr. John since they are not citizens and do not live in the United States. The key question for an alien is whether the individual could be considered a resident. Whether a foreign citizen is considered a resident is normally based on the period of time he or she is present in the United States. For this purpose, an alien who is a mere transient (e.g., a foreigner who vacations in the United States) is not a resident.

Although foreign citizens such as Castro and John usually are not subject to U.S. tax, they can be. Nonresident aliens are taxed on their income from U.S. sources. Based on this rule, income earned from a job or a business in the United States is subject to U.S. tax. In

addition, nonresident aliens who receive investment income from U.S. sources, such as dividends on U.S. stocks, normally must pay U.S. taxes on such income.

Review Question 2. Child actors and actresses have made millions of dollars from their movie appearances (e.g., Hannah Montana, Macaulay Culkin).

a. Must these children file their own returns and report the income, or do their parents simply include it on their return?

Although there are some special rules that can apply, parents normally do not report the income of their children on their return. A child is treated as a taxable entity, separate and distinct from his or her parents. Consequently, if a child's income exceeds the filing requirement threshold, he or she must usually file a return.

b. Do you think there could be any advantage derived from the fact that a child is a separate taxpayer?

Besides all of the other things that children are—both good and bad—they can also be mini-tax shelters. Since they are separate taxpayers, they have their own set of tax rates and other tax characteristics. Therefore, to the extent that parents are able to shift income from the parents' high bracket to the child's low bracket (and still control the use of the income), taxes can be saved. These opportunities and some limitations that restrict such schemes are discussed more fully in Chapter 4 and Chapter 5.

Review Question 3. After all these years, Bob decided to start his own business: Bob's Bar and Grill. He has even convinced his wife, Jane, to help. Bob has everything ready but still must decide what form the business should take. Originally, he did not even think about it. Bob simply thought he would operate the business as a sole proprietorship.

a. If Bob does pursue this course, will he need to file a separate return for the business?

A sole proprietorship is not considered a separate taxable entity. Instead, all of the information related to the proprietorship is included on the individual's personal tax return. The results of operation are summarized on Schedule C. The net profit or loss is transferred from Schedule C to page 1 of Form 1040. In addition, since such income is also subject to self-employment tax, the net profit is also transferred to Schedule SE, where the special computation is made. It is important to note that either Bob or Jane can be the proprietor—but not both. If Jane is to be the proprietor, she must own the business. If Jane wishes to compensate Bob, she can pay him a salary or wages. However, if Bob and Jane both wish to be owners, they must use another form of business.

b. After Bob and Jane talked to their attorney, it was clear that they did not want to be a general partnership (where each and every partner is liable for partnership obligations) or a sole proprietorship. Why?

Typically, individuals want to protect their personal assets from the liabilities of risky ventures. While insurance may provide some protection, most individuals want the added safety of limited liability that only the corporate or LLC form offers. A *limited* partnership allows some partners protection, but this business form requires that there must be at least one *general* partner (who would have unlimited liability).

c.   At first Bob and Jane thought they would be a corporation. But according to their accountant, this new thing called an LLC allows business owners to achieve what he believes is tax nirvana. What is all the fuss about LLCs? Can you not get the same thing with S corporations? What do you think? How are LLCs taxed? What form of business organization seems best for Bob and Jane's business?

The beauty of an LLC is that all of the owners have limited liability yet the entity is usually taxed like a partnership. As a result, all of the income, as well as any loss, flows through to the partners. The significance of this treatment is twofold. First, if any loss occurs, it can be used to offset any other income Bob and Jane may have. If a C corporation is chosen, early losses do not provide any benefit until the business starts to make money. The NOL carryback feature for corporations is useless, because the business is brand new. Moreover, if it is like most businesses, Bob and Jane's operation will experience losses—at least until the clientele develop a love for Bob's cooking. The second attraction of an LLC is the fact that its income avoids the double tax that can occur with C corporations. But why opt for an LLC? Is not this same treatment available with an S corporation? In this regard, the LLC is virtually identical to an S corporation, but there are many differences that some argue make the LLC more attractive. The only difference that can be gleaned from the discussion above is that an S corporation is limited to 100 shareholders while a partnership or LLC can have an unlimited number of owners. This may be irrelevant for Bob and Jane but could be extremely important for some businesses (e.g., a large public accounting firm). Another difference concerns the type of owner allowed. For example, an S corporation can generally have only individuals (and no nonresident aliens) as shareholders, but there are no restrictions on the type of partner or member that a partnership or an LLC can have. This too may be unimportant for Bob and Jane but there are still other considerations too technical to touch on here.

As a practical matter, prior to the advent of the LLC, most advisers would have suggested that Bob and Jane choose to be an S corporation. Since 1986 S corporations have generally been the most popular form of conducting business—at least when there were no more than the maximum shareholders allowed—because they were the only form of business that offered limited liability to all of its owners and a single level of tax. But the advent of the LLC changes all of this. As time passes, it will be interesting to see if LLCs become more popular than S corporations. In any event, they provide yet one more option for the business owner to select.

TAX FORMULA

Computing an income tax liability is normally uncomplicated, requiring only a few simple mathematical calculations.[24] These steps, referred to as the tax formula, are shown in Exhibits 3-2 and 3-3. The tax formula is presented here in two forms: the simpler general formula that establishes the basic concepts as applicable to corporate taxpayers (Exhibit 3-2) and the more complex formula for individual taxpayers (Exhibit 3-3). The formulas in Exhibits 3-2 and 3-3 are useful references while studying the various aspects of Federal income tax law in the subsequent chapters. To make such reference easier, both formulas are reproduced on the inside back cover of the text.

[24]   §§ 1 and 63.

The tax formula for each type of entity is incorporated into the Federal income tax forms. Exhibit 3-2 may be compared with Form 1120 (the annual income tax return for corporations) and Exhibit 3-3 with Form 1040 (the return for individuals). These forms are included in Appendix B at the back of the text.

Examination of the two formulas reveals the importance of tax terms such as *gross income, deductions, and exemptions.* Each of these terms and countless others used in the tax law have very specific meanings. Indeed, as later chapters will show, taxpayers often have been involved in litigation solely to determine the definition of a particular term. For this reason, close attention must be given to the terminology used in taxation.

ANALYZING THE TAX FORMULA

Income. The tax computation begins with a determination of the taxpayer's total income, both taxable and nontaxable. As the formula in Exhibit 3-3 suggests, income is defined very broadly to include income from any source.[25] The list of typical income items in Exhibit 3-4 illustrates its comprehensive nature. A specific definition of income is developed in Chapter 5.

EXHIBIT 3-4
Partial List of Items Included in Gross Income

Alimony and separate maintenance payments	Income from rental operations
Annuities	Income in respect of a decedent
Awards	Interest
Bonuses	Pensions and other retirement benefits
Commissions	Prizes and gambling or lottery winnings
Debts forgiven to debtor by a creditor	Pro rata share of income of a partnership
Dividends from corporations	Pro rata share of income of an S corporation
Employee expense reimbursements	Punitive damages
Fees and other compensation for personal services	Rewards
	Royalties
Gains from illegal transactions	Salaries and wages
Gains from transactions in property	Social Security benefits (zero or a portion)
Gross profit from sales	Tips and gratuities
Hobby income	Trade or business income
Income from an interest in an estate or trust	Unemployment compensation

Exclusions. Although the starting point in calculating the tax is determining total income, not all of the income identified is taxable. Over the years, Congress has specifically exempted certain types of income from taxation, often in an attempt to accomplish some specific goal.[26] In tax terminology, income exempt from taxation and thus not included in a taxpayer's gross income is referred to as an "exclusion." Exhibit 3-5 shows a sample of the numerous items that can be excluded when determining gross income. Exclusions are discussed in detail in Chapter 6.

Gross Income. The amount of income remaining after the excludable items have been removed is termed *gross income.* When completing a tax return, gross income is usually the only income disclosed, because excluded income normally is not reported.

---

[25] § 61(a).

[26] See Chapter 6 for a discussion of the social and economic reasons for excluding certain items of income from taxation.

EXHIBIT 3-5
Partial List of Exclusions from Gross Income

Amounts received from employer-financed health and accident insurance to the extent of expenses	Interest on most state and local government debt
	Meals and lodging furnished for the convenience of one's employer
Amounts received from health, accident, and disability insurance financed by the taxpayer	Personal damage awards (physical injury or sickness)
Amounts received under qualified educational assistance plans	Premiums paid by employer on group-term life insurance (for coverage up to $50,000)
	Proceeds of life insurance paid on death
Certain specified employee fringe benefits	Proceeds of borrowing
Child support payments received	Qualified transportation plan benefits
Contributions by employer to employer-financed accident and health insurance coverage	Scholarship and fellowship grants (but only for tuition, fees, books, and supplies)
Dependent care assistance provided by employer	Social Security benefits (within limits)
Gifts and inheritances	Veteran's benefits
Improvements by lessee to lessor's property	Welfare payments

Example 10. E is divorced and has custody of her only child. E's income for the current year is from the following sources:

Salary	$34,000
Alimony from former spouse	12,000
Child support for child	6,000
Interest from First Savings & Loan	1,200
Interest on U.S. Government Treasury Bonds	1,600
Interest on State of Texas Bonds	2,000
Total	$56,800

Even though E's total income is $56,800, her gross income for tax purposes is only $48,800 because the child support and the interest income from the State of Texas are excluded. All the other items are included in gross income. Note that the interest from the Federal government is taxable, even though interest from state and local governments is generally excluded from gross income.

Deductions. *Deductions* are those items that are subtracted from gross income to arrive at taxable income. The deductions normally allowed may be classified into two major groups:

1. *Business and Production-of-Income Expenses*—deductions for expenses related to carrying on a trade or business or some other income-producing activity, such as an investment.[27]

2. *Certain Personal Expenses*—deductions for a few expenses of an individual taxpayer that are primarily personal in nature, such as charitable contributions and medical expenses.[28]

Observe that the Code allows a deduction only for business or investment expenses. Personal expenses—other than a handful of special items—are not deductible. As someone once said, the Code's treatment of deductions is relatively simple: the costs of earning a

[27] §§ 162 and 212.
[28] §§ 170 and 213.

living are deductible but the costs of living are not. The problem is determining into which category the expense falls.

A trade or business is an activity that is entered into for profit and involves significant taxpayer participation, either personally or through agents. It typically involves providing goods or services to customers, clients, or patients. If the activity qualifies as a trade or business, all the costs normally associated with operating the business are generally deductible. In most cases, it is easy to determine whether a taxpayer is engaged in a trade or business, but not always. For example, consider a taxpayer who travels around the world looking for antiques and incurs $10,000 of travel expenses but ultimately sells one item for a $100 profit. In this situation, the taxpayer might argue that he has a $9,900 loss from the activity that he should be able to offset against other income. On the other hand, it could easily be argued that the taxpayer was not really trying to make a profit. In such case, the IRS may deny the taxpayer's deduction. In these and similar situations, the determination of whether the taxpayer is truly in a trade or business must be based on all the facts and circumstances.

It should also be noted that the law takes the view that an individual who is employed is in the business of providing services. This is an extremely important assumption since it enables employees to deduct their business expenses (e.g., professional dues, subscriptions, and similar costs).[29]

Although business expenses are deductible, the line between a deductible business expense and a nondeductible personal expense is not always clear. For this reason, the Code often contains additional rules or requires certain conditions to be met to ensure that the expense is truly for business. For example, the Code addresses the personal element of business meals and entertainment that are not reimbursed by limiting the deduction to only 50 percent of their cost. Similarly, expenses related to education, travel, transportation, moving or a home office are not deductible unless they meet a laundry list of requirements. Most of these special rules are discussed in detail in Chapter 8.

The rental of real estate is generally not considered to be a trade or business, unless the tenants are transient (i.e., stay for short periods of time, as in a hotel or motel) or there are extraordinary services provided to tenants (e.g., a nursing home). Nevertheless, the expenses are normally deductible as expenses related to an income-producing activity and are classified as deductions for adjusted gross income.

As one might suspect at this point, Congress is quite cautious in granting deductions. There are rules, rules, and more rules that try to ensure that only true business expenses are deductible. The tax law is particularly concerned about deduction of losses (i.e., the excess of deductions over revenues) from activities in which the taxpayer has an interest. The problem became particularly acute in the 1970s and 1980s, when certain activities were designed primarily to generate tax losses (tax shelter limited partnerships and rental real estate were the biggest culprits). In an attempt to eliminate widespread abuse, Congress enacted the so-called *passive loss* rules in 1986. These highly complex rules generally limit the deduction of losses from activities, including rental real estate, in which the taxpayer is a mere investor and does not materially participate. The passive loss rules are covered in detail in Chapter 12.

Classifying Deductions. A comparison of the general tax formulas used by corporations and by individuals reveals some differences in the treatment of deductions. For a corporate taxpayer, all deductions are subtracted directly from gross income to arrive at taxable income. In contrast, the individual formula divides deductions into two groups:[30] one group of deductions is allowed to reduce gross income, resulting in what is referred to as *adjusted gross income* (A.G.I.), while a second group is subtracted from A.G.I. As

---

[29]   See Reg. § 1.162-6 and *David J. Primuth*, 54 T.C. 374 (1970).

[30]   § 62.

explained more fully below, the first group of deductions is generally composed of certain business expenses and other special items. The deductions in this group are referred to as deductions *for* adjusted gross income. The second group of expenses consists of two categories of allowable deductions: (1) deductions *from* adjusted gross income, and (2) deductions for personal and dependency exemptions. Deductions from adjusted gross income, normally referred to as *itemized deductions*, may be deducted only if they exceed a stipulated amount known as the *standard deduction* (e.g., in 2009 $5,700 for single taxpayers and $11,400 for married taxpayers filing jointly). The deduction for any personal and dependency exemptions claimed (e.g., $3,650 per exemption in 2009) is deductible regardless of the amount of other deductions.

Dividing deductions into two groups is done primarily for administrative convenience. Congress substantially reduced the number of individuals who claim itemized deductions because such deductions need to be reported only if they exceed the taxpayer's standard deduction. This reduction in the number of tax returns with itemized deductions significantly reduced the IRS audit procedures involving individual taxpayers. In recent years, only about 35 percent of taxpayers have itemized their deductions. Since corporate taxpayers have only business deductions, no special grouping was needed and thus the term *adjusted gross income* does not exist in the corporate formula.

Adjusted Gross Income. The amount of an individual taxpayer's adjusted gross income (A.G.I.) serves two primary purposes. First, it is simply a point of reference used for classifying deductions: deductions are classified as either for or from A.G.I. Second, the calculation of many deductions, credits and other tax items is made with reference to A.G.I. For example, medical expenses are deductible only if they exceed 7.5 percent of A.G.I., while personal casualty losses may be deducted only if they exceed 10 percent of A.G.I. In addition, recent changes in the tax law make A.G.I. even more important for some taxpayers. As explained below, most itemized deductions and the deduction for exemptions are reduced if adjusted gross income exceeds certain levels.

Example 11. This year proved to be very difficult for T; his divorce became final, and shortly thereafter he became very sick. For the year, he earned $45,000 and paid $5,000 in alimony to his ex-wife and $10,000 for medical expenses that were not reimbursed by insurance. T's A.G.I. is $40,000 ($45,000 − $5,000) because alimony is a deduction for A.G.I. As computed below, T's medical expense deduction is limited to $7,000 because he is allowed to deduct only the amount that exceeds 7.5% of his A.G.I.

Medical expenses (unreimbursed)		$10,000
Adjusted gross income	$40,000	
Times:	× 7.5%	
Threshold	$ 3,000	(3,000)
Deductible medical expenses		$ 7,000

Deductions for Adjusted Gross Income. Code § 62 specifically lists the deductions that are subtracted from gross income to determine A.G.I. This listing is a potpourri of items, as illustrated in Exhibit 3-6. Over the years, this group of deductions has gone by various names. For example, practitioners often refer to this category of deductions as being "above the line"—the line being A.G.I. Some commentators and authors label these as deductions from gross income. For years, the Form 1040 listed these deductions as "adjustments" to income, although this label is no longer used (see Form 1040 in Appendix B). This text will use the "deduction for" terminology. Classification of a deduction as one for A.G.I. is significant for numerous reasons, as explained fully in

Chapter 7. The most important of these reasons, however, is that unlike itemized deductions, deductions for A.G.I. need not exceed a minimum level before they are subtracted when computing taxable income.

EXHIBIT 3-6
List of Deductions for Adjusted Gross Income

Alimony and separate maintenance payments paid

Attorney fees and court costs related to unlawful discrimination cases

Certain deductions of life tenants and income beneficiaries of property

Certain portion of lump-sum distributions from pension plans subject to the special averaging convention

Certain required repayments of supplemental unemployment compensation benefits

Contributions to health savings accounts

Contributions to pension, profit sharing, and other qualified retirement plans on behalf of a self-employed individual

Contributions to the retirement plan of an electing Subchapter S corporation on behalf of an employee/shareholder

Deduction for domestic production activities

Deductions attributable to property held for the production of rents and royalties (reported on Schedule E)

Educator expenses

Individual retirement account contributions (within limits)

Losses from the sale or exchange of property

Moving expenses

One-half of any self-employment tax

Penalties for premature withdrawal of deposits from time savings accounts

Reforestation expenses

Reimbursed trade or business expenses of employees (only if the employee adequately accounts to the employer under an accountable plan in which case neither the reimbursement nor the expense is reported (see Chapter 8; see also expenses of statutory employees)

State and local official's deductible expenses

Statutory employee's deductions (life insurance salespersons, traveling salespersons and certain others report income and deductions on Schedule C; see Chapters 7 and 8)

Student loan interest

Trade or business deductions of self-employed individuals (including deductions claimed on Schedule C and unreimbursed expenses of qualified performing artists)

Tuition payments up to $4,000 for some students

Itemized Deductions and the Standard Deduction. Itemized deductions are all deductions other than the deductions for A.G.I. and the deduction for personal and dependency exemptions.[31] While deductions for A.G.I. are deductible without limitation, itemized deductions are deducted only if their total exceeds the taxpayer's *standard deduction.* For example, if in 2009 T has total itemized deductions of $3,900 and his standard deduction amount is $5,700, he normally would claim the standard deduction in lieu of itemizing deductions. In contrast, if T's itemized deductions were $7,000, he would no doubt elect to itemize in order to maximize his deductions.

The standard deduction was introduced along with the concept of adjusted gross income and deductions *for* and *from* A.G.I. as part of the overall plan to eliminate the need for every taxpayer to list or itemize certain deductions on his or her return. As suggested above, by allowing the taxpayer to claim some standard amount of deductions in lieu of itemizing each one, the administrative problem of verifying the millions of deductions that otherwise would have been claimed has been eliminated. The standard deduction also simplifies return preparation since most individuals no longer have to determine the amount of most of

---

[31] § 63.

the deductions to which they are entitled. For this reason, the amount of the standard deduction is theoretically set at a level that equals or exceeds the average person's expenditures for those items qualifying as deductions from A.G.I. Consequently, the great majority of taxpayers claim the standard deduction in lieu of itemizing deductions.

After changes in 2008, the standard deduction is the sum of four components:

1. Basic standard deduction

2. Increase for individuals who are age 65 or over and/or blind

3. Increase for real property taxes paid

4. Increase for disaster losses in federally declared disaster areas

5. Increase for qualified motor vehicle taxes

Basic Standard Deduction. The basic amount of each taxpayer's standard deduction differs depending on his or her filing status.[32] The amounts for each filing status are adjusted annually for inflation. For 2008 and 2009, the amounts are shown below:

Filing Status	Standard Deduction Amount	
	2008	2009
Single	$ 5,450	$ 5,700
Unmarried head of household	8,000	8,350
Married persons filing a joint return (and surviving spouse)	10,900	11,400
Married persons filing a separate return	5,450	5,700

Additional Standard Deduction for Elderly or Blind Taxpayers. Congress has long extended some type of tax relief to the elderly and blind to take into account their special situations. Currently, an unmarried taxpayer who is either blind or age 65 at the close of the taxable year is allowed to increase his or her basic standard deduction by an additional $1,400 (2009).[33] If an unmarried taxpayer is *both* blind and 65 or older, he or she is allowed to increase the standard deduction by $2,800. If a taxpayer is married, he or she is allowed only $1,100 (2009) for each status for a maximum increase on a joint return of $4,400 [($1,100 × 2 for the husband = $2,200) + ($1,100 × 2 for the wife = $2,200)].

> **Example 12.** In 2009, S, single, celebrated her sixty-fifth birthday. Instead of using the $5,700 standard deduction amount allowed for single taxpayers for 2009, S will be allowed a standard deduction of $7,100 ($5,700 basic standard deduction + $1,400 additional standard deduction).
>
> If S were married filing a joint return for 2009, the standard deduction amount allowed would be $12,500 ($11,400 + $1,100). If both S and her husband were 65 or older, the standard deduction would be $13,600 [$11,400 standard deduction + (2 × $1,100 additional standard deduction)].

Both age and blindness are determined at the close of the taxable year. Guidelines are provided for determining whether an individual is legally blind, and specific filing

---

[32] § 63(c) contains the standard deduction amounts for 1988. The amounts for subsequent years are adjusted for inflation and announced by the IRS annually. Filing status is discussed in Chapter 4.

[33] § 63(f).

[34] §§ 151(d) and 151(d)(3). A taxpayer is legally blind if he or she cannot see better than 20/200 in the better eye with corrective lenses, or the taxpayer's field of vision is not more than 20 degrees. A statement prepared by a physician or optometrist must be attached to the return when a taxpayer is less than totally blind. Reg. § 1.151-1(d)(2).

requirements must be met.[34] An individual is considered to have attained age 65 on the day *preceding* his or her sixty-fifth birthday.[35] Thus, if a taxpayer's sixty-fifth birthday is January 1, 2010, he or she is considered to be 65 on December 31, 2009.

Additional Standard Deduction for Real Property Taxes. The Housing Assistance Act of 2008 added a new twist to the standard deduction. As a general rule, taxpayers are allowed an itemized deduction for real property taxes (e.g., the property taxes paid with respect to a personal residence). However, many homeowners who pay property taxes are not able to itemize and claim the deduction because their itemized deductions do not exceed the standard deduction. This is particularly true for retired homeowners. Retirees often have paid off the mortgages on their homes and do not itemize because they no longer have deductible mortgage interest. Yet they still have property taxes. To help these homeowners, the Housing Act modified the standard deduction. In addition to the increases to the normal standard deduction for being elderly and blind, taxpayers may increase the standard deduction for a limited amount of state and local real property taxes paid, $500, or in the case of joint filers, $1,000.[36] The increase is not restricted to real property taxes on a principal residence. For example, property taxes on a vacation home or land held for investment would qualify. Any real property taxes that are claimed as deductions for A.G.I. are not taken into account in determining the increase. Note that at the time of this writing, the increase is for 2008 and 2009 only.

> **Example 13.** H and W are married and file a joint return. They are both age 62. In 2008, they pay $1,400 in state and local real property taxes. However, their other itemized deductions (e.g., charitable contributions, mortgage interest, and state income taxes) are not sufficient to itemize. Consequently, they claim the standard deduction. What is the couple's standard deduction?
>
> The couple's standard deduction is $12,400 ($11,400 basic standard deduction for joint filers plus the $1,000 increase for real property taxes allowed to joint filers). The balance of the real property taxes, $400, is not deductible. Note if either H or W had been age 65 or older or blind, they could increase their standard deduction by those allowances as well.

Additional Standard Deduction for Disaster Losses. The final component of the standard deduction is the increase for certain casualty losses. This component was added in 2008 to provide relief to those taxpayers who suffered casualty losses and who did not itemize their deductions. An increase is allowed for the amount of personal casualty losses attributable to a federally declared disaster occurring in a disaster area as determined by the President.[37] Note that only the personal casualty losses in excess of personal casualty gains are taken into account. The increase applies only for 2008 and 2009.

> **Example 14.** H, age 40, is single and lives in Kansas. This year a tornado struck his car resulting in a casualty loss after insurance reimbursement of $10,000. The tornado was a federally declared disaster and his home was in the disaster area. He had other itemized deductions of $1,000. What is the H's standard deduction?
>
> H's standard deduction is $15,700 ($5,700 basic standard deduction for single filers plus the $10,000 increase for disaster loss). Note that H will not itemize in this case since his itemized deductions would have been $11,000 which is less than the increased standard deduction of $15,700.

---

[35]   Reg. § 1.151-1(c)(2).

[36]   § 63(c)(1)(C).

[37]   § 63(c)(1)(D). The 10 percent floor for net personal casualty losses does not apply for purposes of this provision (see Chapter 10).

Additional Standard Deduction for Qualified Motor Vehicle Taxes. The American Reinvestment and Recovery Act of 2009 added still another element to the standard deduction. For 2009 only, taxpayers may deduct qualified motor vehicle taxes as either a part of the standard deduction or as an itemized deduction.

Qualified motor vehicle taxes generally include sales and excise taxes on a purchase of a passenger automobile or light duty truck (gross vehicle weight of not more than 8,500 pounds), a motorcycle or a motor home. The deduction is available only for purchases of new vehicles (i.e., the original use begins with the taxpayer) and is limited to the amount of taxes attributable to the first $49,500 of the purchase price. The deduction is phased out ratably for a taxpayer with modified adjusted gross income between $125,000 and $135,000 ($250,000 and $260,000 on a joint return).

Limitations on Use of Standard Deductions. Not all individuals are entitled to the full benefit of the standard deduction.[38] For example, a married person filing a separate return is not allowed a standard deduction if his or her spouse itemizes. This prevents a married couple from increasing their total deductions by having one spouse claim all of the itemized deductions and the other spouse claiming the standard deduction. Nonresident aliens are also denied use of the standard deduction. In addition, the standard deduction is limited for an individual who is claimed as a dependent on another taxpayer's return. This limitation is discussed in Chapter 4.

Itemized Deductions. As explained above, itemized deductions simply are those deductions that are not deductible for A.G.I. The majority of itemized deductions are for selected personal, family and living expenses that Congress believed should be allowed for various policy reasons. These include medical expenses, state and local property, income and sales taxes, home mortgage interest, charitable contributions and casualty and theft losses. A partial list of itemized deductions is provided in Exhibit 3-7. In addition to these, a special subset of itemized deductions, so-called "miscellaneous itemized deductions" are allowed as discussed below.

Miscellaneous Itemized Deductions. Itemized deductions are also allowed for a group of other expenses referred to as *miscellaneous itemized deductions.* Miscellaneous itemized deductions include the deductions for unreimbursed employee business expenses (e.g., dues to professional organizations, subscriptions to professional journals, travel and others that are not reimbursed under an accountable plan), tax return preparation fees and related costs, and certain investment expenses (e.g. safety deposit boxes, investment advice).[39] The classification of an expense as a miscellaneous itemized deduction is extremely important because a limitation is imposed on their deduction. Only the portion of miscellaneous itemized deductions exceeding 2 percent of adjusted gross income is deductible. Congress imposed this limitation in hopes of simplifying the law. The 2 percent floor is intended to relieve taxpayers of the burden of recordkeeping (unless they expect to incur substantial expenditures) and relieve the IRS of the burden of auditing these expenditures.

Example 15. R, single, is employed as an architect for the firm of J&B Associates where he earned $50,000. His itemized deductions for the year were interest on his home mortgage, $5,000; charitable contributions, $900; tax return preparation fee,

---

[38]   See § 63(c)(6) for this exception and others.

[39]   An employee's business expenses are treated as reimbursed under §62 only if the employee adequately accounts for the expense to his or her employer (e.g., submits documentation) under the accountable plan rules. In such case the employee reports neither income nor expense and the expense is essentially the employer's. Otherwise the employee reports the income and claims the expense as a miscellaneous itemized deduction. See Reg. §1.62-2 and Chapter 8.

EXHIBIT 3-7
Partial List of Itemized Deductions

Not Subject to 1 Percent Cutback Rule

Medical expenses (amount in excess of 7.5 percent of A.G.I.):
    Prescription drugs and insulin
    Medical insurance premiums
    Fees of doctors, dentists, nurses, hospitals, etc.
    Medical transportation
    Hearing aids, dentures, eyeglasses, etc.
Investment interest (to extent of investment income)
Casualty and theft losses (amount in excess of 10 percent of A.G.I.)
Wagering losses (to the extent of wagering income)

Subject to 1 Percent Cutback Rule

Certain state, local, and foreign taxes:
    State, local, and foreign income taxes
    State, local, and foreign real property taxes
    State and local personal property taxes
    State and local sales taxes
Mortgage interest on personal residences (limited)
Mortgage insurance on personal residences
Charitable contributions (not to exceed 50 percent of A.G.I.)
Miscellaneous itemized deductions (amount in excess of 2 percent of A.G.I.):
    Costs of preparation of tax returns
    Fees and expenses related to tax planning and advice
    Investment counseling and investment expenses
    Certain unreimbursed employee business expenses (including travel and transportation, professional
        dues, subscriptions, continuing education, union dues, and special work clothing)

$300; and unreimbursed professional dues, $800. R's total itemized deductions are computed as follows:

Miscellaneous itemized deductions:	
Tax return preparation fee	$ 300
Professional dues	800
Total miscellaneous itemized deductions	$ 1,100
A.G.I. limitation (2% × $50,000)	(1,000)
Total deductible miscellaneous itemized deductions	$ 100
Other itemized deductions:	
Interest on home mortgage	5,000
Charitable contributions	900
Total itemized deductions	$ 6,000

Because R's itemized deductions of $6,000 exceed the standard deduction for single persons, $5,700 (2009), he will deduct the entire $6,000. Note that only $100 of R's miscellaneous itemized deductions is deductible, whereas all of his other itemized deductions are deductible.

Deduction Cutback Rule. In search of more revenue, Congress imposed a limitation on the amount of itemized deductions that high-income taxpayers may deduct. Since 1990 taxpayers must reduce total itemized deductions otherwise allowable (*other than* medical

expenses, casualty and theft losses, investment interest and certain gambling losses) by 1 percent (2 percent for 2006 and 2007, 3 percent for prior years) of their A.G.I. in excess of $166,800 ($83,400 for married individuals filing separately).[40] However, this reduction cannot exceed 26.67 percent of the deductions (53.33% in 2006 and 2007, 80% for prior years). This 26.67 percent limit ensures that taxpayers subject to the cutback rule can deduct at least 73.33 percent of their so-called 1 percent deductions. As a result, a taxpayer's itemized deductions are never completely phased out.

> **Example 16.** J and K are married and file a joint return for 2009. Their combined adjusted gross income is $189,600 and they are entitled to itemized deductions of $16,500 and exemption deductions of $7,300 (2 × $3,650). Due to the cutback rule, their deductible itemized deductions must be reduced (i.e., cut back) by $228 [($189,600 − $166,800 = $22,800) × 1%], leaving $16,272 ($16,500 − $228). J and K have taxable income calculated as follows:

Adjusted gross income	$189,600
Minus: Deductible itemized deductions after cutback	− 16,272
Minus: Exemption deductions ($3,650 × 2)	− 7,300
Equals: Taxable Income	$166,028

The 1 percent cutback rule on itemized deductions should not be confused with the 2 percent limitation on miscellaneous itemized deductions discussed above. Miscellaneous itemized deductions that exceed the 2 percent of A.G.I. threshold are still subject to the 1 percent cutback rule. The deduction cutback rule, which is scheduled to expire in 2010, is discussed in detail in Chapter 11.

Exemptions. Congress has always recognized the need to insulate from tax a certain amount of income required by the taxpayer to support himself and others. For this reason, every individual taxpayer is entitled to a basic deduction for himself and his dependents. This deduction is called an *exemption*. For 2009, an individual taxpayer is entitled to a deduction of $3,650 for each *personal* and *dependency* exemption.[41] *Personal exemptions* are those allowed for the taxpayer. Generally, every taxpayer is entitled to claim a personal exemption for himself or herself. However, taxpayers *cannot* claim a personal exemption on their own return if they can be claimed as a dependent on another taxpayer's return.[42] If husband and wife file a joint return, they are treated as two taxpayers and are therefore entitled to claim two personal exemptions. *Dependency exemptions* may be claimed for qualifying individuals who are supported by the taxpayer.[43] In addition to the 1 percent cutback in itemized deductions, high-income taxpayers are required to reduce the amount of their total deduction for personal and dependency exemptions. All the special rules governing deductions for exemptions are discussed in detail in Chapter 4.

Taxable Income and Tax Rates. After all deductions have been identified, they are subtracted from gross income to arrive at taxable income. Taxable income is the tax base to which the tax rates are applied to determine the taxpayer's gross tax liability (i.e., the tax liability before any credits or prepayments).

---

[40] Technically, § 68 provides a 3% cutback limited to 80% of the deductions. However, for 2006–2007, the cutback was 2/3 of this amount or 2% (53.34% maximum) and for 2008–2009 it is only 1/3 or 1% (26.67% maximum). For this reason, throughout the text this provision is referred to as the 1% cutback rule. Practitioners also refer to this rule as the phase-out or phase-down rule. The cutback rule is scheduled to expire after 2009.

[41] § 151(d)(1). For 1989 the exemption was $2,000. For years *after* 1989, the amount has been indexed for inflation.

[42] § 151(d)(2).

[43] § 152.

The tax rate schedule to be used in computing the tax varies, depending on the nature of the taxable entity. For example, one set of tax rates applies to all regular corporations (see inside back cover of text). In contrast, individuals use one of four tax rate schedules (see inside front cover) depending on their filing status, of which there are four. These are:

1. Unmarried individuals (i.e., single) who are not surviving spouses or heads of household

2. Heads of household

3. Married individuals filing jointly and surviving spouses

4. Married individuals filing separately

These tax rate structures are all graduated with the rates of 10, 15, 25, 28, 33, and 35 percent. Although the rates in each schedule are identical, the degree of progressivity differs. For example, in 2009 the 28 percent marginal rate applies to single taxpayers when income exceeds $82,250, but this rate does not apply to married individuals filing jointly until income exceeds $137,050. The various filing statuses and rate schedules are discussed in Chapter 4.

> **Example 17.** H and W are married and file a joint return for 2009. They have adjusted gross income of $151,000, two dependents, and itemized deductions of $31,400. Their taxable income is $105,000, computed as follows:

Adjusted gross income		$151,000
Minus: Itemized deductions	$31,400	
Personal exemptions ($3,650 × 4)	+ 14,600	− 46,000
Equals: Taxable income		$ 105,000

> The tax for a married couple filing jointly on this amount computed using the rate schedules is $18,625 as shown below.

Tax on $67,900	$ 9,350.00
Plus: Tax on excess at 25% [($105,000 − $67,900 = $37,100) × .25]	9,275.00
Equals: Total tax	$18,625.00

Credits. Unlike a deduction, which reduces income in arriving at taxable income, a credit is a direct reduction in tax liability. Normally, when the credit exceeds a person's total tax, the excess is not refunded—hence, these credits are referred to as *nonrefundable* credits. In some instances, however, the taxpayer is entitled to receive a payment for any excess credit. This type of credit is known as a *refundable* credit.

Credits have frequently been preferred by Congress and theoreticians because they affect all taxpayers equally. In contrast, the value of a deduction varies with the taxpayer's marginal tax rate. However, credits often have complicated rules and limitations. A partial list of tax credits is included in Exhibit 3-8.

EXHIBIT 3-8
Partial List of Tax Credits

Foreign tax credit	Credit for the elderly
Child tax credit	Credit for producing fuel from a nonconventional source
Earned income credit	Credit for increasing research activities
Child and dependent care credit	Welfare to work credit
Credit for adoption expenses	Work opportunity credit
Hope scholarship credit	Low income housing credit
Lifetime learning credit	Credit for rehabilitating certain buildings

Prepayments. Attempting to accelerate the collection of revenues for the war effort in 1943, Congress installed a "pay-as-you-go" system for certain taxes. Under this system, income taxes are paid in installments as the income is earned.

Prepayment, or advance payment, of the tax liability can be made in several ways. For individual taxpayers, the two most common forms of prepayment are Federal income taxes withheld from an employee's salaries and wages and quarterly estimated tax payments made by the taxpayer. Certain corporate taxpayers must make quarterly estimated tax payments as well. Quarterly estimated tax payments are required for taxpayers who have not prepaid a specified level of their anticipated Federal income tax in any other way, and there are penalties for failure to make adequate estimated prepayments.

These prepayments serve two valuable purposes. As suggested above, prepayments allow the government to have earlier use of the tax proceeds. Secondly, prepayments reduce the uncertainty of collecting taxes since the government, by withholding at the source, gets the money before the taxpayer has a chance to put it to a different use. In effect, the government collects the tax while the taxpayer has the wherewithal (ability) to pay the tax.

Other Taxes. There are several types of other taxes that must be reported and paid with the regular Federal income tax. A partial list of these taxes is included in Exhibit 3-9. Two deserve special mention.

EXHIBIT 3-9
Partial List of Other Taxes

Alternative minimum tax
Self-employment tax
Social security tax on tip income not reported to employer
Tax on premature withdrawal from an Individual Retirement Account
Tax from recapture of investment credit
Uncollected employee F.I.C.A. and R.R.T.A. tax on tips

Self-Employment Tax. As explained in Chapter 1, self-employed individuals as well as general partners in partnerships are, like employees, required to pay FICA taxes (commonly known as self-employment taxes). Since the tax is paid on income from sole proprietorship and partnership businesses carried on by individual partners, it is convenient for the IRS to collect this tax along with the income tax on Form 1040. The individual calculates the tax on Schedule SE and claims the income tax deduction for one-half of the self-employment tax paid on page 1 of Form 1040.

Alternative Minimum Tax. In 1969 there was an outcry by the media and others that the rich did not pay their fair share of taxes. Indeed, the House Ways and Means Committee Report indicated that in 1964 over 1,100 returns with adjusted gross incomes over $200,000 paid an average tax of 22 percent. Moreover, it reported that there were a significant number of cases where taxpayers with economic income of $1 million or more paid an effective tax amounting to less than 5 percent of their income. As might be expected, faced with such facts Congress decided to take action. However, instead of risking the wrath of their constituents by simply repealing the various loopholes that enabled these taxpayers to avoid taxes, Congress elected to take a politically cautious approach: a direct tax on the loopholes. In effect, the taxpayer simply added up all of the loopholes and paid a flat tax on them. As a result, the minimum tax was born. The whole thrust of this new tax was to ensure that all individuals paid a minimum tax on their income. It currently applies to all taxpayers, individuals, corporations, and fiduciaries.

Over the years, the minimum tax evolved into a monster and was adorned with its current name, the alternative minimum tax (AMT). Despite the changes and increased

complexity, it remains basically the same. The mathematical steps for computing the AMT are relatively simple:

	Regular taxable income	
±	Adjustments and preferences	
	Alternative minimum taxable income	
−	Exemption (subject to phase-out)	
	Tax base	
×	Rate	
	Tentative alternative minimum tax	
−	Regular tax	
	Alternative minimum tax	

As the formula above illustrates, the taxpayer starts with taxable income and then adds certain income that is excluded for regular tax purposes and adds back certain deductions that are normally allowed. These modifications to regular taxable income are referred to as *preference items* and *adjustments*. In this regard, it is important to recognize that the AMT effectively functions as an entirely separate system with its own rules. For example, while most interest from state and local bonds is not taxable, such interest is taxable for AMT purposes if the bonds are used to fund some private activity such as a downtown mall. Similarly, deductions that are usually allowed for regular tax purposes, such as exemptions, miscellaneous itemized deductions, and state and local taxes, are not allowed in computing the AMT. In effect, there are two rules for some items: one rule for regular tax purposes and another for AMT purposes. After taking into account all of the special adjustments required under this alternative system, the new result is called alternative minimum taxable income. This amount is then reduced by an allowable exemption to arrive at the tax base. For 2009 the exemption amounts are $70,950 for joint filers ($35,475 for those filing separately) and $46,700 for single and head-of-household taxpayers. The exemption is reduced by 25% for each dollar by which AMTI exceeds certain levels (e.g. $150,000 for joint filers, $112,500 for singles). A two-tier rate structure is then applied to the tax base (26 percent on the first $175,000 and 28 percent on the excess). The product is referred to as the tentative AMT. This amount is compared to the regular tax, and the taxpayer pays the higher. Technically, the excess of the tentative AMT over the regular tax is the AMT, but the bottom line is that the taxpayer pays the higher amount.

Example 18. H and W are married with four children. For 2009, they filed a joint return, reporting gross income of $400,000 and regular taxable income of $180,000. Various adjustments required under the AMT were $40,550. Using the 2009 exemption and 2009 regular tax rates, the couple must pay an AMT of $4,818, computed as follows:

	Regular taxable income	$180,000
±	Adjustments	40,550
	Alternative minimum taxable income	$220,550
−	Exemption [$70,950 − $17,637 (25% × ($220,550 − $150,000 = 70,550))]	(53,313)
	Tax base	$167,237
×	Rate	× 26%
	Tentative alternative minimum tax	$ 43,482
−	Regular tax (2009 rates)	(38,664)
	Alternative minimum tax	$ 4,818

Note that the AMT is only $4,818, but the taxpayer must pay a total of $43,482 (regular tax of $38,664 + AMT of $4,818).

There is no good rule of thumb as to when the AMT is triggered. For the vast majority of taxpayers it is simply not an issue. These individuals are not subject to the tax since they have low to moderate taxable incomes with few adjustments, causing them to fall below the exemption amounts. It is typically high-income taxpayers who have substantial adjustments, and other taxpayers who are successful in avoiding the regular tax, that fall prey to the AMT. Obviously the key lies in the nature of the adjustments. For now it is sufficient to say that beyond the few preferences and adjustments mentioned above there are several more such as those relating to depreciation, depletion, and stock options. Full coverage of the AMT is deferred until Chapter 13. Nevertheless, even at this early juncture it is important to recognize that the AMT exists and often alters what appears to be very favorable tax treatment for some items. More importantly, the net of the AMT has started catching far more taxpayers than Congress ever intended.

✔️ CHECK YOUR KNOWLEDGE

Review Question 1. It's time for "Tax Jeopardy." Here are the answers; supply the questions.

   a.   The type of expenses all taxpayers can deduct.

What are business expenses? Around tax time, there is a single question that can be heard reverberating across the land: What can I deduct? The answer is business expenses. All taxpayers are allowed to deduct the ordinary and necessary expenses incurred in carrying on a trade or business. The vast majority of all deductions fall into this category. Note also that this rule allows the deduction of employee business expenses. In addition, taxpayers are entitled to deduct expenses related to investment activities (e.g., investment advice or repairs and maintenance on rental property).

   b.   The type of expenses taxpayers normally cannot deduct.

What are personal expenses? Although business expenses are deductible, personal expenses normally are not deductible. For example, the costs of food, shelter, clothing, and personal hygiene cannot be deducted. However, there are some exceptions.

   c.   Five notable exceptions to the rule that personal expenses are not deductible. (Hint: they are all reported on Schedule A of Form 1040, found in Appendix B of this book.) What are the following?

      1.   Medical expenses (but only if they exceed 7.5 percent of A.G.I.)

      2.   Taxes

            ▸ State and local income or sales taxes but not both
            ▸ Real estate taxes
            ▸ Personal property taxes

      3.   Interest

            ▸ Home mortgage interest
            ▸ Student loan interest (maximum of $2,500)
            ▸ Investment interest (but only to the extent of investment income)

      4.   Charitable contributions

      5.   Casualty and theft losses

d. The type of business expenses that are deductible as itemized deductions.

What are unreimbursed employee business expenses? For example, if an employee pays for a business meal and his or her employer reimburses the cost of the meal, the expense is deductible in arriving at A.G.I. if the employer includes the reimbursement in the employee's gross income. Technically, if the employee adequately accounts to the employer under the accountable plan rules, the employee has no income for the reimbursement nor any deduction for the expense (see Chapter 8). However, when the expense is not reimbursed, it is allowable only as a miscellaneous itemized deduction subject to the 2 percent floor. Other common examples of employee business expenses that are frequently deductible as miscellaneous itemized deductions are unreimbursed professional expenses (e.g., subscriptions, dues, license fees), union dues, and special clothing (when deductible).

e. The only type of tax-exempt income reported on the return. (Hint: see page 1 of Form 1040.)

What is tax-exempt interest income (reported on line 8b of page 1 of Form 1040)?

f. Something the individual tax formula has that the corporate tax formula does not have.

What is adjusted gross income? What is the standard deduction? What are exemptions?

g. A benefit received by the elderly and blind.

What is the increased standard deduction for taxpayers who are age 65 or over or who are blind?

h. Deductions that are deductible for individuals even if the taxpayer does not itemize deductions.

What are deductions for A.G.I.? In addition, deductions for exemptions are permitted regardless of whether the taxpayer itemizes. However, exemption deductions are not deductions for A.G.I.

i. A deduction that may be claimed by virtually all individual taxpayers.

What is the exemption deduction, or the standard deduction? As explained above, however, certain persons are not entitled to a standard deduction. For example, a married person filing a separate return must itemize if his or her spouse does. In addition, as fully explained in Chapter 4, taxpayers cannot claim a personal exemption on their own return if they can be claimed as a dependent on another taxpayer's return.

j. A loss from this activity may not be deductible.

What are losses from rental real estate and any other activity in which the taxpayer does not materially participate? Before losses from an activity can be deducted (e.g., a loss that passes through from a partnership or a loss from renting a duplex), they must run through the gauntlet of tests prescribed by the passive loss rules covered in Chapter 12.

k. A separate tax intended to close loopholes.

What is the alternative minimum tax?

Review Question 2. Mabel, single, just reached the age of 65 and was somewhat relieved because she remembered hearing of the tax she would save as a 65-year-old senior. What tax savings can Mabel expect?

Perhaps none. The only benefit for being 65 years old is an additional standard deduction ($1,400 for unmarried taxpayers for 2009). If Mabel itemizes her deductions rather than claiming the standard deduction, she receives no benefit. If she does not itemize, her standard deduction for 2009 is $7,100 (the basic standard deduction of $5,700 plus the extra $1,400).

Review Question 3. Dick and Jane just learned that they are expecting their first child. What tax benefits can they expect after Junior is born?

Many. First are the dependency exemption deduction ($3,650 for 2009) and the child tax credit ($1,000 for 2009). In addition, Dick and Jane can look forward to a credit for any job-related child care expenses that they pay.

Review Question 4. Are deductions of a sole proprietor deductible *for* or *from* adjusted gross income? (Hint: see lines 23 through 27 on Page 1 of Form 1040 and Schedule C in Appendix B of this book.)

The trade or business expenses of a sole proprietor or someone who is self-employed are deductible for A.G.I. Note that these are not shown as one of the deductions for A.G.I. on Page 1 of Form 1040. Instead, they are netted against the sole proprietor's income on Schedule C, and this net profit is included in the taxpayer's total income reported on Page 1 of Form 1040.

Review Question 5. A sole proprietor's income generally is subject to self-employment tax. Is the deduction for one-half of the self-employment tax deducted for or from adjusted gross income? Is it reported on Schedule C or Form 1040?

This is a deduction for A.G.I. and is reported as a deduction for A.G.I. on page 1 of Form 1040 (and not Schedule C).

INTRODUCTION TO PROPERTY TRANSACTIONS

The tax provisions governing property transactions play a very important part in our tax system. Obviously, their major purpose is to provide for the tax treatment of transactions involving a sale, exchange, or other disposition of property. However, the basic rules covering property transactions can also impact the tax liability in other indirect ways. For example, the amount of the deduction granted for a charitable contribution of property may depend on what the tax result would have been had the property been sold rather than donated. As this example suggests, a basic knowledge of the tax treatment of property transactions is helpful in understanding other facets of taxation. For this reason, an overview of property transactions is presented here. Chapters 14, 15, 16, and 17 examine this subject in detail.

The tax consequences of any property transaction may be determined by answering the following three questions:

1. What is the amount of gain or loss *realized*?

2. How much of this gain or loss is *recognized*?

3. What is the *character* of the gain or loss recognized?

Each of these questions is considered in the following sections.

GAIN OR LOSS REALIZED

A realized gain or loss results when a taxpayer sells, exchanges, or otherwise disposes of property. In the simple case where property is purchased for cash and later sold for cash, the gain or loss realized is the difference between the purchase price and the sale price, adjusted for transaction costs. The determination of the realized gain or loss is more complicated when property other than cash is received, when liabilities are involved, or when the property was not acquired by purchase. As a result, a more formal method for computing the gain or loss realized is used. The formulas for computing the gain or loss realized are shown in Exhibits 3-10, 3-11, and 3-12. As these exhibits illustrate, the gain or loss realized in a sale or other disposition is the difference between the *amount realized* and the *adjusted basis* in the property given up.

EXHIBIT 3-10
Computation of Amount Realized

	Amount of money received (net of money paid)
Add:	Fair market value of any other property received
	Liabilities discharged in the transaction (net of liabilities assumed)
Less:	Selling costs
Equals:	**Amount realized**

EXHIBIT 3-11
Determination of Adjusted Basis

Basis at time of acquisition:
  For purchased property, use cost
  Special rules apply for the following methods of acquisition:
    Gift
    Bequest or inheritance
    Nontaxable transactions
Add: Capital improvements, additions
Less: Depreciation and other capital recoveries
Equals: **Adjusted basis in property**

EXHIBIT 3-12
Computation of Gain or Loss Realized

Amount realized from sale or other disposition
Less: Adjusted basis in property (other than money) given up
Equals: **Gain or loss realized**

Amount Realized. The amount realized is a measure of the economic value received for the property given up. It generally includes the amount of any money plus the fair market value of any other property received, reduced by any selling costs.[44] In determining the amount realized, consideration must also be given to any liabilities from which the taxpayer is relieved or which the taxpayer incurs. From an economic standpoint, when a taxpayer is relieved of debt, it is the same as if cash were received and used to pay off the debt. In contrast, when a taxpayer assumes a debt (or receives property that is subject to a debt), it is the same as if the taxpayer gave up cash. Consequently, when a sale or exchange involves the transfer of liabilities, the amount

---

[44]   § 1001(b).

realized is increased for the net amount of any liabilities discharged or decreased for the net amount of any liabilities incurred.

Adjusted Basis. The adjusted basis of property is similar to the concept of "book value" used for accounting purposes. It is the taxpayer's basis at the time of acquisition—usually cost—increased or decreased by certain required modifications.[45] The taxpayer's basis at the time of acquisition, or original basis, depends on how the property was acquired. For purchased property, the taxpayer's original basis is the property's cost. When property is acquired by gift, inheritance, or some form of tax-deferred exchange, special rules are applied in determining the original basis. Once the original basis is ascertained, it must be increased for any capital improvements and reduced by depreciation and other capital recoveries. The adjusted basis represents the amount of investment that can be recovered free of tax.

Example 19. This year, L sold 100 shares of M Corporation stock for $41 per share for a total of $4,100. He received a settlement check of $4,000, net of the broker's sales commission of $100. L had purchased the shares several years ago for $12 per share for a total of $1,200. In addition, he paid a sales commission of $30. L's realized gain is $2,770, computed as follows:

Amount realized ($4,100 − $100)	$4,000
Less: Adjusted basis ($1,200 + $30)	− 1,230
Gain realized	$2,770

Example 20. During the year, T sold his office building. As part of the sales agreement, T received $20,000 cash, and the buyer assumed the mortgage on the building of $180,000. T also paid a real estate brokerage commission of $7,000. T originally acquired the building for $300,000 in 1990, but since that time had deducted depreciation of $230,000 and had made permanent improvements of $10,000. T's gain realized is computed as follows:

Amount realized:		
Cash received	$ 20,000	
Liability assumed by buyer	+180,000	
Selling expenses	−7,000	
		$193,000
Less: Adjusted basis		
Original cost	$300,000	
Depreciation claimed	−230,000	
Capital improvements	+10,000	
		− 80,000
Gain realized		$113,000

GAIN OR LOSS RECOGNIZED

The gain or loss *realized* is a measure of the economic gain or loss that results from the ownership and sale or disposition of property. However, due to special provisions in the tax law, the gain or loss reported for tax purposes may be different from the realized gain or loss. The amount of gain or loss that affects the tax liability is called the *recognized* gain or loss.

---

[45] §§ 1011 through 1016.

Normally, all realized gains are recognized and included as part of the taxpayer's total income. In some instances, however, the gain recognition may be permanently excluded. For example, an individual is generally allowed to exclude up to $250,000 of gain realized on the sale of a personal residence ($500,000 for married taxpayers). Other gains may be deferred or postponed until a subsequent transaction occurs.

> **Example 21.** M exchanged some land in Oregon costing $10,000 for land in Florida valued at $50,000. Although M has realized gain of $40,000 ($50,000 − $10,000), assuming certain requirements are satisfied, this gain will not be recognized, but rather postponed. This rule was adopted because the taxpayer's economic position after the transaction is essentially unchanged. Moreover, the taxpayer has not received any cash or wherewithal with which she could pay any tax that might result.

Chapter 15 contains a discussion of the more common types of property transactions in which the recognition of an individual taxpayer's realized gains are postponed.

Any loss realized must be specifically allowed as a deduction before it is recognized. Individuals generally are allowed to deduct *three* types of losses. These are:

1. Losses incurred in a trade or business (e.g., an uncollectible receivable of an accrual basis taxpayer)

2. Losses incurred in an activity engaged in for profit (e.g., sale of investment property such as stock at a loss)

3. Casualty and theft losses

Losses in the first two categories generally are deductions for adjusted gross income. Casualty and theft losses from property used in an individual's trade, business, or income-producing activity also are allowed as deductions for adjusted gross income. However, casualty and theft losses from personal use property are classified as itemized deductions and are deductible only to the extent they exceed $100 per casualty or theft and 10 percent of A.G.I. Other than casualty and theft losses, all other losses from dispositions of personal use assets are *not* deductible. For example, if a taxpayer sold his personal residence for a loss, the loss would not be deductible. The rules governing the deductibility of losses in the first three categories are covered in Chapter 10. The special rules governing the deduction of "capital" losses are introduced below and covered in greater detail in Chapter 16.

CHARACTER OF THE GAIN OR LOSS

From 1913 through 1921, all includible income was taxed in the same manner. Since 1921, however, Congress has provided special tax treatment for "capital" gains or losses. As a result, in determining the tax consequences of a property transaction, consideration must be given to the character or nature of the gain or loss—that is, whether the gain or loss should be classified as a *capital* gain or loss or an *ordinary* gain or loss. Any *recognized* gain or loss must be characterized as either an ordinary or a capital gain or loss.

Capital Gains and Losses. Although capital gains and losses arise in numerous ways, they normally result from the sale or exchange of a *capital asset.* Any gain or loss due to the sale or exchange of a capital asset is considered a capital gain or loss.

Capital assets are defined in § 1221 of the Code as being anything *other* than the following:

1. Inventory, or other property held primarily for sale to customers in the ordinary course of a trade or business

2. Depreciable property or real property used in a trade or business of the taxpayer

3. Trade accounts or notes receivable

4. Certain copyrights, literary, musical, or artistic compositions, and letters or memoranda held by the person whose personal efforts created them, and certain specified other holders of these types of property

5. U.S. government publications acquired other than by purchase at the price at which they are sold to the general public

The term *capital assets*, therefore, includes most passive investments (e.g., stocks and bonds) and most personal use assets of a taxpayer. However, property used in a trade or business is not a capital asset but is subject to special tax treatment, as discussed later in this chapter.

Treatment of Capital Gains. Except for a short period between 1913 and 1922, the tax law consistently has taxed gains from the sale of certain "capital assets" at rates that are substantially lower than those that apply to other income. Most recently, the special advantage is justified on the grounds that it encourages greater investment and savings. Regardless of the rationale, the hard fact is that the rules necessary to carry out the objective create an incredible layer of complexity to the tax laws. To illustrate, simply consider that capital gains qualifying for special treatment could now be taxed at one of five different rates (28%, 25%, 15%, 10% or 0%).

Holding Period. The exact treatment of a capital gain or loss depends primarily on how long the taxpayer held the asset or what is technically referred to as the taxpayer's *holding period*. The holding period is a critical element in determining which of the rates will apply. As might be expected, the longer the holding period is, the lower the applicable tax rate will be. A *short-term* gain or loss is one resulting from the sale or disposition of an asset held *one year or less*. A *long-term* gain or loss occurs when an asset is held for *more than one year*. However, after this initial classification, individuals must subdivide the long-term group into additional subgroups: (1) the 28% group for long-term capital gains resulting from the sales of *collectibles* (e.g., antiques, coins, stamps) and *qualified small business stock* (note that only 50% of this gain is taxed if the holding period exceeds 60 months, making the effective tax rate 14%); (2) the 25% group for long-term capital gains (and only gains) from the sale of depreciable real estate (e.g., office buildings, warehouses, apartment buildings) held for more than one year but only to the extent of the depreciation claimed on such property; and (3) the 15% group for other (most) long-term capital gains.

The effect of the rules is to require taxpayers to assign their capital gains and losses into one of four different groups and net the amounts to determine the net gain or loss in each group as shown below.

	Short-term	Long-term		
Holding period (months)	≤ 12	Collectibles > 12 & § 1202 stock > 60	Realty > 12	> 12
	Ordinary	28%	25%	15%
Gains	$xx,xxx	$x,xxx	Gains only	$xx,xxx
Losses	(xxx)	(x,xxx)	—	(x,xxx)
Net gain or loss	????	????	Gain only	????

As a practical matter, the capital gains of most individuals arise from the sales of stocks and bonds and mutual fund transactions. Rarely do individuals have gains from collectibles, § 1202, stock or depreciable realty. Consequently, for most individuals, the classification and netting process is much easier than it might appear.

Applicable Capital Gains Rates. Generalizations about the treatment of capital gains and losses are difficult because the actual treatment can be determined only after the various groups (i.e., the four groups above) are combined, or netted, to determine the overall net gain or loss during the year. The details of this netting process are quite complex and left to Chapter 16. Suffice it to say here that the treatment of the net gains of each group—*before any netting between groups*—can be summarized as follows:

1. A net short-term capital gain (NSTCG) generally receives no special treatment and is taxed as ordinary income at the taxpayer's regular tax rate (up to 35%).

2. A net 28% capital gain (N28CG) is taxed at a maximum rate of 28%.

3. A net 25% gain (N25CG) from dispositions of realty is taxed at a maximum rate of 25% (generally only to the extent of any depreciation claimed). The balance of any gain is part of the 15% group.

4. A net 15% gain (N15CG) is taxed at a maximum rate of 15%. However, if the taxpayer's tax bracket (determined by *including* the net 15% gain) is 15% or less, the net gain in this group is taxed at a rate of 0%.

In applying these rules, it should be emphasized that they operate to set only the maximum rate at which the particular type of gain will be taxed. If the taxpayer's tax using the regular rates would be lower, the regular rates are used. For example, if the taxpayer is in the 15% tax bracket and has a 28% gain, the 15% rate would apply instead of the 28% rate.

Example 22. During the year, T, who is in the 35% tax bracket, reported the following capital gains and losses.

	Short-term	Long-term 28%	Long-term 15%
Gains	$10,000	$4,000	$10,000
Losses	(4,000)	—	(3,000)
	$ 6,000	$4,000	$ 7,000

In this case, T has a NSTCG of $6,000, a N28CG of $4,000, and a N15CG of $7,000. As explained in Chapter 16, no further netting of these transactions occurs. T's NSTCG of $6,000 receives no special treatment and is taxed as ordinary income. T's N28CG is taxed at 28% while his N15CG is taxed at 15%.

Dividends Taxed at Capital Gain Rates. Beginning in 2003 and through 2010, most dividends received are taxed at the same rate that historically has been reserved for long-term capital gains rates.[46] Currently, the rate is 15% and 0% for dividends that would otherwise be taxed at an ordinary rate of 15% or lower. The qualifying dividend is not subject to the capital gain and loss netting process. As a result, the dividends are subject to capital gains treatment regardless of whether the taxpayer has other capital gains or losses. The details related to calculating the tax on these dividends are presented in Chapter 16.

---

[46] § 1(h)(11).

Example 23. During 2008, S, single, sold stock he had held for several years. He sold 100 shares of L for a $500 long-term capital loss and 200 shares of G for a $3,200 long-term capital gain. S also received qualified dividends of $370 for the year. S is single and has no dependents. Assume her taxable income including the above transactions is $85,320. The following calculations demonstrate the application of the favorable 15 percent capital gains rate.

Gain on Evergreen Solar	$3,200
Loss on Gateway	(500)
Net capital gain	$2,700
Dividend income	370
Amount subject to 15% capital gains rate	$3,070
S's taxable income is taxed as follows:	
Amount subject to 15% capital gains rate	$3,070
Amount treated as ordinary income	
($85,320 − $3,070)	$82,250
S's tax is calculated as follows:	
Tax on ordinary income of $82,250 (see inside front cover)	$16,750
Tax on gains and dividends at 15% ($3,070 × 15%)	461
Total tax	$17,211

Treatment of Capital Losses. While capital gains receive favorable treatment, such is not the case with capital losses. As can be seen in *Example 17* above, capital losses are first netted with capital gains within the same group. A net capital loss from a particular group can then be combined with net capital gains from the other groups. As a general rule, the long-term groups are netted together before considering any short-term items. If after netting all of the groups together, the taxpayer has an overall net capital loss, the loss is deductible up to an annual limit of $3,000. The deductible capital loss is a deduction for adjusted gross income. Any losses in excess of the annual $3,000 limitation are carried forward to the following year where they are treated as if they occurred in such year. In effect, an unused capital loss can be carried over for an indefinite period.

Example 24. During the year, B reported the following capital gains and losses.

		Long-term	
	Short-term	**28%**	**15%**
Gains	$10,000	$3,000	$5,000
Losses	(18,000)	(4,000)	(3,000)
	($8,000)	($1,000)	$2,000

B's only other taxable income included his salary of $50,000. He had no other deductions for A.G.I. After netting all of his gains and losses, B has a net capital loss of $7,000. T may deduct only $3,000 of the net capital loss in determining his A.G.I. Therefore, his A.G.I. is $47,000 ($50,000 − $3,000). The unused capital loss of $4,000 ($7,000 − $3,000) is carried forward to future years when it is treated as if it arose in the subsequent year. In such case, the loss can be used against other capital gains or ordinary income just as it was this year.

Details of capital gain and loss treatment and the capital loss carryover rules are discussed in Chapter 16.

Corporate Taxpayers. The taxation of capital gains for corporate taxpayers differs somewhat from that for individuals. Most important, the capital gains of a corporation normally receive no special treatment but are taxed as ordinary income. In addition, the capital losses of a corporation can never offset ordinary income but can be carried back three and forward five years to offset other capital gains. There are a number of other differences which are considered in a full discussion of a corporation's capital gains and losses in Chapter 19.

TRADE OR BUSINESS PROPERTY

Depreciable property and real property used in a trade or business are not capital assets, but are subject to several special provisions. Nevertheless, gain on the sale of these assets may ultimately be treated as capital gain while losses may be treated as ordinary losses. These rules are quite complex and considered in Chapter 17.

✓ *CHECK YOUR KNOWLEDGE*

Try the following true-false questions.

Review Question 1. An individual always receives preferential treatment for his or her capital gains.

False. An individual can receive special treatment only for long-term capital gains. Short-term capital gains are treated just like ordinary income.

Review Question 2. J is interested in the stock market. This year she realized a $1,000 short-term capital gain and an $8,000 capital loss from stock she held for two years. She will report a $1,000 short-term capital gain and carry over the $8,000 long-term capital loss.

False. She first nets the short-term gain of $1,000 against her $8,000 15% loss, resulting in an overall long-term capital loss of $7,000. She may deduct $3,000 of this loss as a deduction for A.G.I. The remaining loss is carried over to the following year, when it will be treated as if she had realized a long-term (28%) capital loss of $4,000.

Review Question 3. K makes $500,000 a year and plays the stock market. So far this year she has realized a 15% capital gain of $3,000. It is now December 31. Should K sell stock and recognize a $3,000 15% loss?

Who knows? If she recognizes a $3,000 loss, the loss is offset against the gain and therefore reduces income that would have been taxed at a 15 percent rate. This would produce a tax benefit from the loss of only $450 ($3,000 × 15%). If she waits and uses the loss against ordinary income, it will produce a tax benefit of $1,050 (35% × $3,000), or $600 ($1,050 − $450) more. However, if she postpones the loss until some subsequent year hoping to use it to offset income taxed at a higher rate, she will lose the time value of the $450.

Review Question 4. A corporation normally receives no special treatment for its long-term capital gains.

True. The long-term capital gains of a corporation normally are treated in the same manner as ordinary income.

Review Question 5. John Doe is the typical American taxpayer. He is married, has a dog and two kids. He also owns two cars: a brand new Ford and a 1996 Chevrolet. He bought the Ford for $17,000 and the Chevy for $10,000. Both of the cars were used for

personal purposes. This year John and his family moved to New York and decided they did not need the cars, so he sold them. He sold the Chevy for only $3,000. The story on the Ford was different. The Ford happened to be a Mustang convertible, and because Mustangs were in demand and were on back order, a car nut was willing to give him $19,000, a $2,000 premium for not having to wait. How will these sales affect John's taxable income? Explain whether the taxpayer has a gain or loss, its character, and in the case of a loss whether it is deductible for or from A.G.I.

John reports a capital gain of $2,000. The first step is to determine John's gain or loss *realized.* In this case, the determination is simple. On the sale of the Chevy, John realized a loss of $7,000 ($3,000 − $10,000), and on the sale of the Mustang he realized a gain of $2,000 ($19,000 − $17,000). The second step is to determine whether he *recognizes* the gain and loss realized. John must recognize the gain. As a general rule, all income is taxable unless the taxpayer can point to a specific provision that specifically exempts the income from tax. In this case, there is no exclusion. On the other hand, the $7,000 loss is not deductible. Although all income is normally taxable, only those items specifically authorized are deductible. Only three types of losses are deductible: (1) losses incurred in carrying on a trade or business; (2) losses incurred in an activity engaged in for profit (e. g., investment losses); and (3) casualty and theft losses. In this case, the loss on the sale of the Chevy is purely personal, and therefore no deduction is allowed. Thus John is not allowed to net the loss against the gain but must report only the gain of $2,000. While this may seem like a surprising result, understand that tax is a one-way street: as a general rule, all income is taxable and only those expenses and losses specifically allowed are deductible. The final step is determining the character of the gain, that is, whether the gain is capital gain or ordinary income. In order for a taxpayer to have a capital gain, there must be a sale or exchange of a capital asset. The Code defines a capital asset as essentially everything but inventory and real or depreciable property used in a trade or business. In this case, the car is not used in business and it does not represent inventory, so it is a capital asset. As a result, John reports a capital gain of $2,000.

Review Question 6. Indicate whether the following assets are capital assets.

a. 2,000 boxes of Frosted Flakes held by a grocery store
b. A crane used in the taxpayer's bungee-jumping business
c. A warehouse owned by Wal-Mart
d. IBM stock held for investment
e. The personal residence of Jane Doe

The Code generally defines a capital asset as essentially everything but inventory, business receivables, and real or depreciable property used in a trade or business. Based on this definition, the Frosted Flakes are not a capital asset since they are held as inventory by the grocery; the crane is not a capital asset since it is depreciable property used in a business; and the warehouse is not a capital asset since it is real property used in a business. The personal residence and IBM stock are both capital assets since they are neither inventory nor property used in a trade or business.

TAX PLANNING CONSIDERATIONS

CHOICE OF BUSINESS FORM

One of the major decisions confronting a business from a tax perspective concerns selecting the form in which it conducts its operations. A taxpayer could choose to operate a business as a sole proprietorship, a partnership, a limited liability company, an S corporation, or a regular C corporation. Each of these entities has its own tax characteristics that make it more or less suitable for a particular situation. The following discussion highlights a number of the basic factors that should be considered.

Perhaps the most important consideration in choosing a business form is the outlook for the business. A business that expects losses will typically opt for a business form different from the one that expects profits. A key advantage of a conduit entity (i.e., partnership or S corporation) applies in years in which a business suffers losses. Like income, losses flow through to the owners of the entity and generally can be used to offset other income at the individual level. In contrast, losses suffered by a regular C corporation are bottled up inside the corporate entity and can benefit only the corporation. Losses of a regular corporation generally are carried back two years and carried forward 20 years to offset income that the corporation has in prior or subsequent years.

A profitable business may also benefit from choosing the proper form of organization. To illustrate, consider a business that is generating taxable income of $1 million per year. If the taxpayer conducts the business as a sole proprietorship or through one of the conduit entities, the top tax rate applied to the income is 35 percent. Similarly, if a C corporation is used to operate the business, the top rate is 35 percent. However, for most corporations—those with taxable incomes not exceeding $10 million—the top rate is 34 percent. Moreover, tax savings may also be generated at lower levels of income. This possibility can be seen in the tax rate schedules for corporations and individuals. A quick comparison reveals that the first $50,000 of income of a corporate taxpayer is taxed at a 15 percent rate, whereas married taxpayers filing jointly receive the benefits of a 15 percent (or lower) rate on a maximum of $67,900 (for 2009). Obviously, the tax-wise individual might try to structure the activities so that the best of both worlds could be obtained. Consider a business that produces taxable income of $90,000. If a corporation is used, the company could pay a deductible salary of $50,000 to the owner (assuming it is a reasonable amount), leaving $40,000 of taxable income in the corporation. By so doing, the maximum tax rate paid on the income would be 15 percent. Had the business been operated as a sole proprietorship or an S corporation, $22,100, the amount of taxable income in excess of $67,900, would have been taxed at a 25 percent rate (married filing jointly) or 10 percentage points higher. This may seem appealing, but it is a very simplistic analysis and leaves vital elements out of the equation. For example, this scheme completely ignores the problem of double taxation; it assumes that the taxpayer will be able to withdraw the $34,000 ($40,000 − $6,000 corporate income tax) left in the corporation at a later time in a deductible fashion so as to avoid the second tax. Unfortunately, doing so is not as easy as it may appear, and this plan as well as any other requires careful analysis. Suffice it to say here, however, that careful planning at the outset of a new business can save the taxpayer substantial taxes in the future.

A possible disadvantage of partnerships and S corporations concerns the treatment of certain fringe benefits. As explained in Chapter 6, the Code contains a host of fringe benefits that generally are deductible by the employer and nontaxable to the employee. For example, a corporation is entitled to deduct the costs of group-term life insurance provided

to an employee, and the benefit (i.e., the payment of the premiums) is not treated as taxable compensation to the employee but is tax-free. Note that if the employee purchases the insurance directly, it is purchased with compensation that has been previously taxed. As a result, the employee acquires the benefit with after-tax dollars. The favorable tax treatment of fringe benefits is generally available only to employees of a business. Unfortunately, partners and shareholders in S corporations who work in the business are not considered employees for this purpose and consequently cannot obtain many of the tax-favored fringe benefits. In contrast, shareholders in regular C corporations who work in the business are treated as employees and are therefore able to take advantage of the various benefits. Consideration should also be given to payroll and self-employment taxes.

ITEMIZED DEDUCTIONS VERSUS STANDARD DEDUCTION

A typical complaint of many taxpayers is that they have insufficient deductions to itemize and therefore cannot benefit from any deductions they have in a particular year. Nevertheless, with a little planning, not all of those deductions will be wasted. Taxpayers in this situation should attempt to bunch all their itemized deductions into one year. By so doing, they may itemize one year and claim the standard deduction the next. By alternating each year, total deductions over the two-year period are increased. This could be accomplished simply by postponing or accelerating the payment of expenses. Cash basis taxpayers have this flexibility because they are entitled to deduct expenses when paid.

> **Example 25.** X, a widow age 61, sold her home and moved to an apartment. Due to the sale of the house, she anticipates that the only itemized deduction she would have in the future would be charitable contributions to her church as follows.

	2008	2009
Charitable contributions	$5,700	$5,700

> If the pattern above continues, X will not receive any tax benefit from her charitable contributions since they do not exceed the standard deduction for single taxpayers, $5,700 (2009). However, what would happen if X simply shifted the payment of the charitable contributions from one year to the other by paying it either earlier or later. In such case, total itemized deductions in one year would be $10,400 ($5,700 + $5,700) and she could itemize, while in the other year she could claim the standard deduction. As a result, she would obtain total deductions over the two-year period of $16,100 ($10,400 + $5,700), or 4,700 ($16,100 − $11,400) more than if she merely claimed the standard deduction in both years.

EMPLOYEE BUSINESS EXPENSES

Most employee business expenses are typically paid by the employer, either through direct payment or reimbursement according to the accountable plan rules. Under these rules, employees must "adequately account" to their employers for their expenses by submitting a record, with receipts and other substantiation and return in excess advance or allowance, if any.[47] When this is done, it is as if the employee had no expense at all. Essentially, it is the employer's deduction. This approach, as set forth in the Regulations, is equivalent to treating the expenses as deductible for A.G.I.[48] Note that the net effect on A.G.I. is zero.

---

[47] Regs. § 1.62-2 and § 1.162-17. See also Chapter 8.

[48] § 62(b) AND Reg. § 1.62-2.

On the other hand, if an employer requires employees to incur some business expenses, the employee can claim them only to the extent he or she itemizes and has miscellaneous itemized deductions in excess of 2 percent of A.G.I. The result is the same if an employee does not adequately account for an expense under the accountable plan rules. The amount received from the employer is included in gross income and the expense is reported as a miscellaneous itemized deduction. When this occurs, the employee may receive little or no tax benefit from the expenses.

In reviewing the employee's compensation package, employers might consider changing their reimbursement policies. If an employer adopts more generous reimbursement policies in lieu of compensation increases, the employees may benefit.

> **Example 26.** E, single, is an employee with gross income of $50,000. She typically has annual employee business expenses of $1,000 that are not reimbursed. Since E does not itemize, she derives no tax benefit from the expenses.

> If, instead of the above arrangement, E received a salary of $49,000 and the $1,000 of expenses were reimbursed, she would be in the same economic position before tax. However, she would pay $250 ($1,000 × 25% marginal tax on her salary) less in Federal income taxes.

PROBLEM MATERIALS

DISCUSSION QUESTIONS

3-1 *Taxable Entities.* List the classes of taxable entities under the Federal income tax. Identify at least one type of entity that is not subject to the tax.

3-2 *Double Taxation.* It has been stated that corporate earnings are subject to double taxation by the Federal government. Elaborate.

3-3 *Fiduciary.* In some regards, the fiduciary is a conduit for Federal income tax purposes. Explain.

3-4 *Partnership and S Corporation Returns.* The partnership and S corporation tax returns are often referred to as information returns only. Explain.

3-5 *Income from Partnerships.* Y is a general partner in the XYZ Partnership. For the current calendar year, Y's share of profits includes his guaranteed compensation of $55,000 and his share of remaining profits, which is $22,000. What is the proper income tax and payroll tax (F.I.C.A. or self-employment tax) treatment of each of the following to Y for the current calendar year?
a. The guaranteed compensation of $50,000
b. The remaining income share of $22,000

3-6 *Income from S Corporations.* K is the president and chief executive officer of KL, Inc., an S corporation that is owned equally by individuals K and L. K receives a salary of $83,000, and her share of the net income, after deducting executive salaries, is $50,000. What is the proper income tax and payroll tax (F.I.C.A. or self-employment tax) treatment of each of the following to K for the current calendar year?
a. The salary, assuming it is reasonable in amount
b. The net income of $50,000 that passes through to K
c. The $3,600 that the company paid for group employee medical insurance for K and her family

3-7 *Tax Formula.* Reproduce the tax formula for individual taxpayers in good form and briefly describe each of the components of the formula. Discuss the differences between the tax formula for individuals and that for corporations.

3-8 *Gross Income.* How is gross income defined in the Internal Revenue Code?

3-9 *Deductions.* Distinguish between deductions *for* and deductions *from* adjusted gross income.

3-10 *Standard Deduction.* What is the standard deduction? Explain its relationship to itemized deductions. Which taxpayers are entitled to additional standard deductions?

3-11 *Itemized Deductions.* List seven major categories of itemized deductions. How and when are these reduced? Is the standard deduction reduced? If so, under what circumstances?

3-12 *Employee Business Expenses.* Expenses incurred that are directly related to one's activities as an employee are trade or business expenses. True or False?

3-13 *Additional Standard Deduction.* H and W are married and are 74 and 76 years of age, respectively. They also paid real property taxes on their home of $1,500. The couple does not itemize. Assuming they have gross income of $40,000 for 2009 and file a joint return, determine their taxable income.

3-14 *Exemptions.* Differentiate between personal exemptions and dependency exemptions. Which taxpayers are denied a personal exemption?

3-15 *Credits.* There are numerous credits that are allowed to reduce a taxpayer's Federal income tax liability. List at least four such credits.

3-16 *Credits.* Credits of equal amount affect persons in different tax brackets equally, whereas deductions of equal amount are more beneficial to taxpayers in higher tax brackets. Explain.

3-17 *Prepayments.* What is meant by the concept of "wherewithal to pay" for tax purposes? How do prepayments of an individual's income taxes in the form of withholding and quarterly estimates represent the application of this concept?

3-18 *Alternative Minimum Tax.* What is the alternative minimum tax? Explain what is meant by *alternative* and *minimum* in this context.

3-19 *Amount Realized.* What is meant by "the amount realized in a sale or other disposition"? How is the amount realized calculated?

3-20 *Adjusted Basis.* Describe the concept of adjusted basis. How is the basis in purchased property determined?

3-21 *Gain or Loss Realized.* Reproduce the formula for determining the gain or loss realized in a sale or other disposition of property.

3-22 *Gain or Loss Recognized.* Differentiate between the terms "gain or loss realized" and "gain or loss recognized."

3-23 *Losses.* Which losses are deductible by individual taxpayers?

3-24 *Capital Assets.* Define the term "capital asset."

3-25 *Holding Period.* The determination of the holding period is important in determining the treatment of capital gains and losses. What is the difference between a long-term holding period and a short-term holding period?

3-26 *Capital Gains.* Briefly explain the favorable treatment given to capital gains and when such treatment applies.

3-27 *Capital Losses of Individuals.* There are "limitations" on the capital loss deduction for individuals. Identify these limitations.

3-28 *Capital Losses of Corporations.* What is the limitation on the deduction for capital losses of a corporate taxpayer?

3-29 *Carryover of Excess Capital Losses.* Excess capital losses of individuals may be offset against gains for other years. Specify the carryover and/or carryback period for such excess losses.

❓ *YOU MAKE THE CALL*

3-30 Shortly after Murray began working in the tax department of the public accounting firm of Dewey, Cheatham and Howe, he was preparing a tax return and discovered an error in last year's work papers. In computing the gain on the sale of the taxpayer's duplex, the preparer had failed to increase the amount realized by the $50,000 mortgage assumed by the buyer. Apparently, the mistake was overlooked during the review process. Upon discovering the mistake, Murray went to his immediate supervisor, Norm (who actually prepared last year's return), and pointed out the error. Norm, knowing that the client would probably flip if he found out he had to pay more tax, told Murray "let's just wait and see if the IRS catches it. Forget it for now." What should Murray do?

PROBLEMS

3-31 *To Whom Is Income Taxed?* In each of the following separate cases, determine how much income is to be taxed to each of the taxpayers involved:
   a. Alpha Partnership is owned 60 percent by W and 40 percent by P, who agree to share profits according to their ownership ratios. For the current year, Alpha earned $12,000 in ordinary income. The partnership distributed $3,000 to W and $2,000 to P.
   b. Beta Trust is managed by T for the benefit of B. The trust is required to distribute all income currently. For the current year, Beta Trust had net ordinary income of $5,500 and made cash distributions to B of $7,000.
   c. Gamma Inc., a C corporation, is owned and operated by its two equal owners, H and K. This year the corporation reported earned income—before any distributions to its owners—of $24,000. On May 4, the corporation declared a dividend, distributing $1,350 to H and $1,350 to K.

3-32 *Selecting a Form of Doing Business.* Which form of business—sole proprietorship, partnership, S corporation, limited liability company, or regular corporation—is each of the following taxpayers likely to choose? An answer may include more than one business form.
   a. Edmund and Gloria are starting a new business that they expect to operate at a net loss for about five years. Both Edmund and Gloria expect to have substantial incomes during those years from other sources.
   b. Robin would like to incorporate her growing retail business for nontax reasons. Because she needs all of the net profits to meet personal obligations, Robin would like to avoid the corporate "double tax" on dividends.

3-33 *Income from C Corporations.* M is the president and chief executive officer of MN, Inc., a corporation that is owned solely by M. During the current calendar year, MN, Inc. paid M a salary of $80,000, a bonus of $22,000, and dividends of $30,000. The corporation's gross income is $350,000, and its expenses excluding payments to M are $225,000.

   a. Compute the corporation's taxable income and determine its gross income tax.

   b. Assuming M's only other income is interest income of $12,500, determine M's adjusted gross income.

   c. Does this situation represent double taxation of corporate profits? Explain.

3-34 *Income from Partnerships.* J is a one-fourth partner in JKLM Partnership. The partnership had gross sales of $880,000, cost of sales of $540,000, and operating expenses excluding payments to partners of $145,000 for the current calendar year. Partners' compensation for services of $90,000 ($45,000 to J) were paid, and distributions of $120,000 ($30,000 to J) were made for the year.

   a. Determine the partnership's net income for tax reporting purposes.

   b. Determine the amount of income J must report from the partnership for the year.

   c. Determine how much of the income in (b) is self-employment income.

3-35 *Income from Fiduciaries.* G created a trust for the benefit of B to be managed by T. For the current year, the trust had gross income of $45,000, income-producing deductions of $1,900, and cash distributions to B of $12,500.

   a. Determine the taxable income of the trust.

   b. Assuming B's only other income is interest of $22,300, determine B's adjusted gross income.

3-36 *Tax Treatment of Various Entities.* Office Supplies Unlimited is a small office supply outlet. The results of its operations for the most recent year are summarized as follows:

Gross profit on sales	$95,000
Cash operating expenses	43,000
Depreciation expense	16,500
Compensation to owner(s)	20,000
Distribution of profit to owner(s)	5,000

In each of the following situations, determine how much income is to be taxed (i.e., to be included along with any other income in calculating taxable income) to each of the taxpayers involved.

   a. The business is a sole proprietorship owned by T.

   b. The business is a partnership owned by R and S with an agreement to share all items equally. S is guaranteed a salary of $20,000 (see above).

   c. The business is a corporation owned equally by U and K. K is employed by the business and receives a salary of $20,000 (see above).

3-37 *Gross Income.* The following represent some of the more important items of income for Federal tax purposes. For each, indicate whether it is fully includible in gross income, fully excludable from gross income, or partially includible and partially excludable.

   a. Alimony received from a former spouse

   b. Interest from state and local governments

   c. Money and other property inherited from a relative

   d. Social security benefits

   e. Tips and gratuities

   f. Proceeds of life insurance received upon the death of one's spouse

3-38 *Classifying Deductions.* The following represent some of the more important deductions for Federal tax purposes. For each, indicate whether it is deductible for A.G.I. or as an itemized deduction.

   a. Alimony paid to one's former spouse

   b. Charitable contributions

    c. Trade or business expenses of a self-employed person

    d. Expenses of providing an apartment to a tenant for rent

    e. Interest incurred to finance one's principal residence

    f. Reimbursed trade or business expenses of an employee

    g. Unreimbursed trade or business expenses of an employee

3-39 *Determining Adjusted Gross Income and Taxable Income.* Fred and Susan are married and file a joint income tax return. Neither is blind or age 65. They have two children whom they support, and the following income and deductions for 2009:

Gross income.	$57,200
Deductions for A.G.I.	1,200
Total itemized deductions.	8,900
Credits and prepayments	3,050

Determine Fred and Susan's adjusted gross income and taxable income for the calendar year 2009.

3-40 *Tax Formula.* The following information is from the 2009 joint income tax return of Gregory and Stacy Jones, both of good sight and under 65 years of age.

Gross income.	$67,200
Adjusted gross income	58,350
Taxable income.	29,250
Number of personal exemptions	2
Number of dependency exemptions	2

Determine the amount of the Jones's deductions for A.G.I. and the amount of their itemized deductions.

3-41 *Tax Formula.* Complete the following table of independent cases for Zac Williams for 2009. Zac is 31 years old and is single. He has perfect eyesight. He does not own a car, truck, motorcycle or motor home. He rents an apartment, and it is not located in a federally declared disaster area.

	A	B	C
Gross income.	$50,000	$???	$???
Deductions for A.G.I.	(???)	(8,000)	(7,000)
Adjusted gross income (A.G.I.)	$42,000	$78,000	???
Itemized deductions	(???)	(4,650)	(7,350)
Standard deduction.	(???)	(???)	(???)
Exemptions	2	1	1
	(???)	(???)	(???)
Taxable income.	$25,700	$???	$63,150

3-42 *Worldwide Income Subject to Tax.* T, a U.S. citizen, has income that was earned outside the United States. The income was $20,000, and a tax of $2,000 was paid to the foreign government. Determine the general treatment of this income and the tax paid under the following circumstances:

    a. The tax paid was on income earned on foreign investments, and the U.S. tax attributable to this income is $2,800.

    b. Same as (a), except the U.S. tax attributable to this income is $1,800.

    c. Same as (a), except the income is from services rendered while absent from the United States for 13 successive months.

3-43   *Alternative Minimum Tax.* L is single, has no dependents, and uses the cash method and the calendar year for tax purposes. The following information was derived from L's records for 2009:

Taxable income (regular income tax) $74,200
AMT adjustments and preferences   70,200

Although L has substantial gross income and deductions, she does not itemize. Calculate L's regular income tax using the tax rates for 2009 and her alternative minimum tax, if any.

3-44   *Asset Classification.* For each of the assets in the list below, designate the appropriate category using the symbols given:

C - Capital asset
T - Trade or business asset (§ 1231)
O - Other (neither capital nor § 1231 asset)

a.   Personal residence
b.   Stock in Xerox Corporation
c.   Motor home used for vacations
d.   Groceries held for sale to customers
e.   Land held for investment
f.   Land and building held for use in auto repair business
g.   Trade accounts receivable of physician's office
h.   Silver coins held primarily for speculation

3-45   *Gain or Loss Realized.* During the current year, W disposed of a vacant lot which he had held for investment. W received cash of $12,000 for his equity in the lot. The lot was subject to a $32,000 mortgage that was assumed by the buyer. Assuming W's basis in the lot was $23,000, how much is his realized gain or loss?

3-46   *Adjusted Basis.* M owns a rental residence that she is considering selling, but she is interested in knowing her exact tax basis in the property. She originally paid $39,000 for the property. M has spent $8,000 on a new garage, $2,500 for a new outdoor patio deck, and $4,500 on repairs and maintenance. M has been allowed depreciation on the unit in the amount of $7,500. Based on this information, calculate M's basis in the rental residence.

3-47   *Gain or Loss Realized, Adjusted Basis.* This year S sold her rental house. She received cash of $6,000 and a vacant lot worth $30,000. The buyer assumed the $36,000 mortgage loan outstanding against S's property. S had purchased the house for $52,000 four years earlier and had deducted depreciation of $12,000. How much are S's amount realized, her adjusted basis in the house sold, and her gain or loss realized in this transaction?

3-48   *Capital Gain and Loss.* Individual D is in the 35% tax bracket. This year he executed the following transactions.

Transaction	Sales Price	Adjusted Basis	Holding Period
Sale of 100 shares of XYZ	$2,000	$1,000	15 months
Sale of land held for investment.	9,000	3,000	19 months
Sale of silver held for speculation	5,000	7,000	23 months
Sale of personal jewelry	4,000	6,000	60 months

Determine the tax consequences (e.g., gain, loss, applicable tax rates) of these transactions.

3-49 *Excess Capital Loss.* This year, T, an individual taxpayer, had a short-term capital gain of $4,000 and a capital loss of $9,000 from stock he held for four years. How much is T's allowable capital loss deduction for the year? What is the treatment of the short-term gain?

3-50 *Individual's Tax Computation.* Richard Hartman, age 29, single with no dependents, received a salary of $32,670 in 2009. During the year, he received $1,300 interest income from a savings account and a $1,500 gift from his grandmother. At the advice of his father, Richard sold stock he had held as an investment for five years, for a $3,000 gain. He also sustained a loss of $1,000 from the sale of land held as an investment and owned for four months. Richard had itemized deductions of $5,250. For 2009 compute the following for Richard:
   a. Gross income
   b. Adjusted gross income
   c. Taxable income
   d. Income tax before credits and prepayments (use the appropriate 2009 tax rate schedule located on the inside front cover)
   e. Income tax savings that would result if Richard made a deductible $2,000 contribution to a qualified Individual Retirement Account

3-51 *Tax Treatment of Income from Entities.* The G family—Mr. G, Mrs. G, and G Jr.— owns interests in the following successful entities:

   1. X Corporation is a calendar year regular corporation owned 60 percent by Mr. G and 15 percent by G Jr. During the year, it paid salaries to Mr. G of $80,000 to be its president and to G Jr. of $24,000 to be a plant supervisor. The company earned a net taxable income of $75,000, and paid dividends to Mr. G and G Jr. in the amounts of $42,000 and $10,500, respectively.
   2. Mrs. G owned a 60 percent capital interest in a retail outlet, P Partnership. The partnership earned a net taxable income of $60,000 and made distributions during the year of $72,000. The profit and the distributions were allocated according to relative capital interests.
   3. Mr. G and G Jr. each own 25 percent interest in H Corporation, an electing S Corporation. The corporation is a start-up venture and generated a net tax loss of $28,000 for the calendar year. No dividend distributions were made by H. Both Mr. G and G Jr. have bases in their H Corporation stock of $30,000.
   4. G Jr. is the sole beneficiary of G Trust created by Mrs. G's father. The trust received dividends of $16,000 and made distributions of $4,500 to G Jr.

Determine the amount of income or loss from each entity that is to be reported by the following:
   a. Mr. and Mrs. G on their joint calendar year tax return
   b. G Jr. on his calendar year individual return
   c. X Corporation
   d. P Partnership
   e. H Corporation
   f. G Trust

3-52 *Comprehensive Taxable Income Computation.* Indy Smith, single, is an anthropology professor at State University. The tax records that he brought to you for preparation of his return revealed the following items.

Income

Salary from State University	$68,150
Part-time consulting	5,000
Dividend income	1,250
Reimbursement of travel to Denver by State University	200

Expenses

Interest on personal residence	$ 9,800
Travel expenses related to consulting	1,000
Tax return preparation fee	500
Safe deposit box to hold bonds	50
Travel and lodging to present academic paper in Denver related to his teaching position	450

In addition, Indy claims a dependency exemption for his father for whom he provides 60 percent support (including 60 percent of housing costs). Compute Indy's final tax liability for calendar year 2009.

TaxCut **3-53** *Comprehensive Taxable Income Computation.* Eli and Lilly have been happily married for 30 years. Eli, 67, is a research chemist at Pharmaceuticals Inc. Lilly, 64, recently retired but stays busy managing the couple's investments, including a duplex. The majority of the couple's income is derived from Eli's employment, from which he received a salary of $95,000 this year. Other income includes interest on corporate bonds of $5,600 and interest on State of Illinois bonds of $1,000. In addition, rents collected from the duplex were $10,000 while rental expenses (e.g., maintenance, utilities, depreciation) were $6,000. During the year, the company transferred Eli to a new division located in nearby suburb about 55 miles north of his old office. As a result, the couple decided to move so that Eli would not have such a long commute. They paid deductible moving expenses of $2,000. The couple also paid the following expenses: unreimbursed medical expenses, $7,400; interest on the home mortgage, $11,400; property taxes on the home, $3,000; charitable contributions, $4,000; and rental of safe deposit box, $100. Determine the couple's taxable income for 2009.

3-54 *Alternative Minimum Tax.* H and W are married and filed a joint return for 2009. The couple has five children between the ages of 3 and 13. Their records for the current year reveal the following:

Salary income (their only income)	$165,000
State and local taxes (property and income)	30,000
Other itemized deductions	$5,000

Using the 2009 tax rates, compute the alternative minimum tax, if any.

3-55 *Losses.* This year, B and J formed a partnership to operate a bar and grill. B was the brains behind the venture and J supplied the bulk of the financing. B contributed $30,000 to the partnership, receiving a 30 percent interest while J contributed $70,000 for a 70 percent interest. B received 30 percent of the profits and losses and J received 70 percent. During the year, B worked his fingers to the bone, running the business. J did little, sitting back and watching his investment. For the year, the partnership reported a $30,000 loss (revenues $60,000, deductible expenses $90,000). Can B and J use their share of the loss as a deduction to offset other income they might have on their own individual tax return (Form 1040) such as the salary income of their spouses? Explain.

TAX RETURN PROBLEMS

CONTINUOUS TAX RETURN PROBLEMS   See Appendix D, Part 1.

RESEARCH PROBLEMS

3-56   *Using the Internal Revenue Code.* Locate a copy of the *Internal Revenue Code of 1986.* Read §§ 61 through 65, 67, 151, and 152. Read the titles of §§ 71 through 135, 161, and 162.

    a.   Describe how Congress defined "gross income."

    b.   Why is the "exemption deduction" properly called a deduction from adjusted gross income?

    c.   A taxpayer is self-employed and incurs an ordinary and necessary expense in his business endeavor. What is the authority for deducting the expense? Why is it considered a deduction *for* adjusted gross income?

    d.   A taxpayer pays alimony to her former husband. Within limits, it is deductible *for* adjusted gross income. Why?

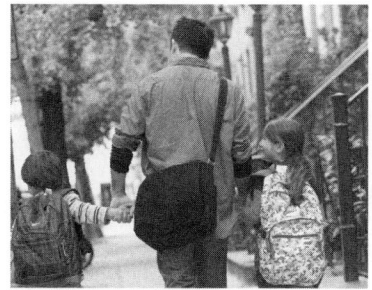

PERSONAL AND DEPENDENCY EXEMPTIONS; FILING STATUS; DETERMINATION OF TAX FOR AN INDIVIDUAL; FILING REQUIREMENTS

LEARNING OBJECTIVES

Upon completion of this chapter you will be able to:

- Identify the various requirements that a taxpayer must meet in order to claim a personal or dependency exemption

- Explain the phase-out of the deduction for personal and dependency exemptions

- Apply the rules to determine the taxpayer's filing status

- Compute the tax liability of an individual taxpayer using the tax rate schedules and the tax tables

- Explain the special approach used in computing the tax liability of certain children

- Describe the filing requirements for individual taxpayers and the role of the statute of limitations as it applies to the filing of tax returns

- Explain when taxes must be paid and the penalties that apply for failure to pay on a timely basis

CHAPTER OUTLINE

As seen in Chapter 3, numerous factors must be considered in the determination of an individual's net tax liability. Beginning in this chapter and continuing through Chapter 18, a detailed examination of these factors is conducted. This chapter is devoted to five particular concerns of individual taxpayers:

1. Personal and dependency exemptions;

2. Child tax credit;

3. Filing status;

4. Calculation of the tax liability using the tax rate schedules and tax tables; and

5. Filing requirements.

PERSONAL AND DEPENDENCY EXEMPTIONS

Since the inception of the income tax, policymakers have recognized the need to protect from tax some minimum amount of income that could be used for the support of the taxpayer and those who depend on him. The device used to accomplish this objective is the deduction allowed for exemptions. There are two types of exemptions for which deductions are allowed: personal exemptions and exemptions for a child or other dependent.[1] Taxpayers may deduct the *exemption amount* for each of their exemptions. The exemption amount for 2009 is $3,650.[2] Each type of exemption is discussed below.

---

[1]   §§ 151(a), 151(b), and 151(c).

[2]   Since 1985 the exemption amount has been increased to reflect price level changes based on changes in the consumer price index. The exact amount is announced by the IRS in the fall of the preceding year. For instance, the exemption amount for 2010 will be announced by December 15, 2009. §§ 1(f) and 151(d)(3). If the exemption amount had been adjusted for inflation since 1948, when it was $600, it would have been about $5,288 for 2008 (calculated using the Bureau of Labor Statistics inflation calculator based on the Consumer Price Index, http://data.bls.gov/cgi-bin/cpicalc.pl). Also see Steurle, "Decline in the Value of the Dependent Exemption," 62 *Tax Notes* 109 (October 4, 1993).

PERSONAL EXEMPTIONS

There are *two* types of personal exemptions:

1. Exemption for the taxpayer
2. Exemption for the taxpayer's spouse

Each individual taxpayer normally is entitled to one personal exemption. When a *joint return* is filed by a married couple, *two* personal exemptions may be claimed. This occurs not because one spouse is the dependent of the other, but because the husband and wife are each entitled to his or her own personal exemption. If a married individual files a *separate return*, however, a personal exemption may be claimed for his or her spouse only if the spouse has no gross income and is not claimed as a dependent of another taxpayer.[3]

Disallowance of Personal Exemption. A taxpayer is denied a personal exemption if he or she qualifies as a dependent of another taxpayer (see discussion below).[4] This rule prevents two taxpayers (e.g., a child and his or her parent) from benefiting from two exemptions for the same person.

Example 1. J is 21 years of age and a full-time college student. J receives a partial scholarship and works part-time, but the majority of his support is received from his parents. Assuming J is eligible to be claimed as a dependent on his parents' return, he is not entitled to a personal exemption deduction on his own return. This rule applies *regardless* of whether J's parents actually claim an exemption for him.

EXEMPTIONS FOR DEPENDENTS

For as long as most remember, an individual qualified as a taxpayer's dependent if he or she met one set of rules. Ironically, in an attempt toward simplicity, Congress added a second set of rules under which an individual might be considered a dependent. Beginning in 2005, § 152 now defines a dependent as either:

1. A qualifying child, or
2. A qualifying relative.

EXEMPTION FOR QUALIFYING CHILD

An individual is considered a *qualifying child* and can be claimed as a dependent of the taxpayer if he or she satisfies all of the following tests.[5]

1. *Relationship Test.* The individual and the taxpayer must meet one of the following relationship tests:

   ▸ Natural child, stepchild, adopted child, certain foster children
   ▸ A sibling or step-sibling
   ▸ A descendant of one of the above

---

[3] § 151(b).

[4] § 151(d)(2).

[5] § 152(c).

Note that the scope of these rules goes far beyond the conventional definition of a taxpayer's "child." For example, a taxpayer's brother or sister is considered his or her child as are his nieces or nephews. Similarly, a taxpayer's "children" include a grandchild as well as great grandchildren and other descendants.

2. *Residence Test.* The "child" must have the *same principal place of abode* (i.e., residence) as the taxpayer for more than one half of the taxable year. For this purpose, temporary absences are permissible if due to special circumstances such as education, illness, business, vacation, or military service. Note that a child could live more than half of the taxable year with more than one person where several people, including the child, live together. For example, the child could live with his mother, grandmother and grandfather. Thus this test could be met with respect to more than one person.

3. *Age Requirement.* The "child" must also meet one of the conditions concerning age:

   ▸ Has not reached age 19 by the close of the taxable year.
   ▸ Has not reached age 24 *and* is considered a full-time student at a qualifying educational institution. For this purpose, "full-time" is whatever is considered full-time under the rules and regulations of the institution. The individual must meet the full-time condition for any part of five calendar months during the calendar year.
   ▸ Is permanently and totally disabled at any time during the year. The age limitation does not apply to these individuals.
   ▸ Starting in 2009, the qualifying child must be younger than the taxpayer.

4. *Joint Return Test.* The "child" must not have filed a joint return with his or her spouse except to claim a refund (i.e., the tax due was zero before prepayments).

5. *Citizenship or Residency Test.* The "child" must be a U.S. citizen, resident or national, or a resident of Canada or Mexico.

6. *Not Self-Supporting Test.* To be a "qualifying child" the "child" may not be self-supporting; that is, the child must not have provided more than one-half of his or her own support. For this purpose, scholarships received from an educational institution are not considered an amount spent on support.

Tie Breaker Rules. Application of the tests above could result in an individual being a "qualifying child" for more than one taxpayer. For example, if a 10-year-old child lived with his father, grandmother and uncle in the same residence during the year, the father, grandmother, or uncle could potentially claim the child as a dependent since the child meets the relationship, age and residence test with respect to each. Such a situation is not surprising in an age when family structures are often unconventional due to divorce and remarriage, absentee parents, childbearing by unmarried individuals, and multi-generational households. When a child is a qualifying child for more than one taxpayer and the parties cannot agree as to who will claim an exemption, the following tie-breaker rules apply.[6]

   ▸ If only one of the taxpayers is the child's parent, the parent claims the exemption for the child.
   ▸ If both taxpayers are the child's parents and they do not file a joint return, the parent with whom the child resided for the longest period of time during the tax year claims the exemption for the child. Note that this tie-breaker rule must be used. The parents cannot agree between themselves as to whom will claim the exemption.

---

[6]   §152(c)(4).

▸ If the child resides with both parents for the same period of time during the tax year and the parents do not file a joint return, the parent with the highest adjusted gross income claims the exemption for the child.

▸ If none of the taxpayers are the child's parent, the taxpayer with the highest adjusted gross income for the tax year claims the exemption for the child.

Example 2. For the current year, M and D, mom and dad, provide a home in which they live with their son, P, and P's daughter, G. P is unmarried, 23 years of age and a full-time student. P earned $6,000 for the year, which is less than 50% of his total support. M and D may claim an exemption for P—he is their qualifying child since he meets all of the tests (age, residence and relationship). Under the tie-breaking rules, P, as parent, would be able to claim an exemption for his daughter G; however, P cannot claim G as a dependent because P is, himself, a dependent. In this case, M and D could claim an exemption for their granddaughter G because she is a qualifying child with respect to them.

EXEMPTION FOR QUALIFYING RELATIVE

The second type of dependent is a *qualifying relative*—generally a relative or member of the taxpayer's household that depends on the taxpayer for support. In contrast to the definition for qualifying children, this term permits exemptions for a broader class of individuals but only if the taxpayer provides for their support and the prospective dependent meets an income test.

Technically, an individual is considered a *qualifying relative* only if he or she is *not* a qualifying child and meets the following requirements each of which is discussed in detail below.[7]

1. *Support Test.* The taxpayer must provide more than 50 percent of the dependent's total support.

2. *Gross Income Test.* The dependent's gross income must be less than the exemption amount.

3. *Relationship or Member of the Household Test.* The dependent must be a relative of the taxpayer or a member of the taxpayer's household for the entire taxable year.

4. *Joint Return Test.* The dependent must not have filed a joint return with his or her spouse.

5. *Citizenship or Residency Test.* The dependent must be a U.S. citizen, resident or national, or a resident of Canada or Mexico.

Although an individual could conceivably be a qualifying relative and a qualifying child, the Code makes it clear that in such case the individual is treated as a qualifying child, and therefore, he or she cannot be claimed as a dependent by someone under the qualifying relative rules.

Support Test. To satisfy the support requirement, the taxpayer must provide more than half of the amount spent for the dependent's total support.[8] Total support includes not only amounts expended by others on behalf of the dependent but also any amounts spent by the dependent. Note that only the amount *actually spent* for support is relevant. Income and other funds available to the dependent for spending are ignored unless they are spent.

---

[7] § 152(d).

[8] § 152(d)(1)(c).

Example 3. During the year, C paid $10,000 to maintain her father, F, in a nursing home that provides all of his needs. No other amounts were spent for his support. C made these payments, even though her father could afford them since he has cash in the bank and tax-exempt bonds valued at $200,000. Although F has funds available for providing his own support, they are not considered in applying the support test because the funds were not spent. Consequently, the support test is satisfied.

Support is generally measured by the cost of the item to the individual providing it. However, when support is provided in a noncash form, such as the use of property or lodging, the amount of support is the fair market value or fair rental value.

What constitutes an item of support is not always clear. If, for example, a child receives a stereo or car, are these items considered support, or do only necessities qualify? The Regulations provide some guidance as to the nature of support, indicating that it includes food, shelter, clothing, medical and dental care, education, recreation, and transportation.[9] Support is not limited to these items, however. Examination of the numerous cases and rulings reveals a hodgepodge of qualifying expenditures as well as some that are not. For example, the costs for boats, life insurance, and lawn mowers are not considered support. Additionally, the value of any services performed for the dependent by the taxpayer is ignored.[10] Exhibit 4-1 presents a sampling of those items that constitute support.

The determination of support also is complicated by several items accorded special treatment. For example, scholarships and fellowships received by the taxpayer's child or stepchild are not considered support items. Accordingly, such amounts are not treated as being provided by either the taxpayer or the dependent.[11]

EXHIBIT 4-1
Partial List of Support Items

Automobile	Lodging
Care for a dependent's pet	Medical care
Charitable contributions by or on behalf of dependent	Medical insurance premiums
	Singing lessons
Child care	Telephone
Clothing	Television
Dental care	Toys
Education	Transportation
Entertainment	Utilities
Food	Vacations
Gifts	

Example 4. J was the recipient of an athletic scholarship that covered 100% of her tuition, books, supplies, room, and board. In addition, J was paid a small cash allowance. J's parents also provided her with $4,000 cash to be used for clothing, entertainment, and miscellaneous expenses.

The scholarship package, which was related to J's continued scholastic activity, was valued at $19,500 per year. Nevertheless, assuming the other four tests are met, J's parents are entitled to a dependency exemption, since the scholarship is not included in her support and she is not self-supporting.[12]

---

[9] Reg. § 1.152-1(a)(2)(i).

[10] *Markarian v. Comm.*, 65-2 USTC ¶9699, 16 AFTR2d 5785, 352 F.2d 870 (CA-7, 1965).

[11] Reg. § 1.152-1(c). Note that G.I. Bill benefits are not treated as scholarships and therefore are included as support items provided by the recipient.

[12] Any part of a scholarship providing benefits other than tuition, fees and supplies, is *includible* in the recipient's gross income to the extent of those benefits. See Chapter 6 for a discussion of taxable scholarships.

Although social security benefits generally are not taxable income to the recipient, they are considered as support provided by the person covered by social security. Thus, social security benefits are included in determining support to the extent they are spent for support.[13] State welfare payments are considered provided by the state, and therefore are not treated as provided by the parent or any other taxpayer. This is true even though the parent is entrusted to oversee the prudent expenditure of the funds.[14]

Example 5. F received support during the current year from various sources, including amounts contributed by his son, S. The amounts spent toward F's support were provided as follows:

F's social security benefits	$ 7,500
Taxable interest income	900
Amount provided by S.	4,100
Total.	$12,500

S is not entitled to a dependency exemption for F because he did not provide more than 50% of F's total support ($4,100 is not greater than 50% of $12,500).

Example 6. This year K received social security benefits of $8,000, $5,500 of which was immediately deposited in a savings account. The amounts spent toward K's support were provided as follows:

K's social security benefits spent.	$ 2,500
Taxable interest income	600
Amount provided by K's brother, B	4,000
Total.	$ 7,100

Assuming the other tests are met, B is entitled to a dependency exemption for K since he provided more than one-half of her support expenditures ($4,000 is > 50% of $7,100).

In many instances, an individual who is not self-supporting is supported by more than one taxpayer. Generally, no dependency exemption is allowed for such persons because no *one* individual provides more than 50 percent of the total support provided. However, an exemption may be allowed under what is referred to as a "multiple support agreement."

Multiple Support Agreements. A dependency exemption for a qualifying relative may be assigned to a taxpayer under a multiple support agreement if all of the following tests are met:[15]

---

[13]   Reg. § 1.152-1(a)(2)(ii).

[14]   See Rev. Rul. 71-468, 1971-2 C.B. 115 and *N. Williams*, T.C. Memo 1996-126. A similar result was reached related to state payments for the care of a mentally retarded child. See *Trail*, T.C. Memo 1993-221, *aff'd* at 73 AFTR2d ¶ 94-931 (CA-5, 1994).

[15]   § 152(c).

1. No one person contributed over half the support of the individual.

2. Over half the support was provided by a group, all of whose members are qualifying relatives of the individual.

3. The citizenship, joint return, and gross income requirements are met by the individual.

4. The dependency exemption is assigned by agreement to a group member *who contributed more* than 10 percent of the total support.

The assignment is effective only if each of the members contributing more than 10 percent signs a declaration to the effect that he or she will not claim the exemption. This declaration is made on Form 2120 (see Appendix), which is then filed with the return of the taxpayer claiming the exemption.

Example 7. M is single and received her support of $12,000 for the current year from the following sources:

	Amount	Percentage
Social security benefits	$ 4,000	33.33%
Taxable interest income	800	6.67
From D, M's daughter	4,700	39.17
From S, M's son	1,500	12.50
From G, M's grandchild	1,000	8.33
	$12,000	100.00%

Together, D, S, and G contribute more than 50% of M's support for the year ($7,200 > 50% of $12,000). If a multiple support agreement is executed, either D or S may be allowed the exemption deduction. G is not eligible since he did not contribute more than 10% of the total support. Also, note that S may claim M as a dependent even though D provided more of M's support.

Gross Income Test. The second test that must be satisfied before an individual (other than a qualifying child) may be claimed as a dependent concerns his or her gross income. A dependency exemption generally is not allowed for a person whose gross income equals or exceeds the exemption amount ($3,650 for 2009).[16] In applying this test, the technical definition of "gross income" must be heeded.[17] It does not include items that are excluded from income. Accordingly, a person whose only sources of income are excluded from gross income (e.g., social security and municipal bond interest) may qualify as a dependent.

It also should be noted that gross income is not always synonymous with includible gross receipts. Regulation § 1.61-3 indicates that gross income for a merchandising business generally means the total sales less the cost of goods sold *plus* any income from investments or other sources. The importance of this distinction between gross receipts and gross income is demonstrated in the following example.

Example 8. T provides 60% of the support for his single brothers, F and R, for the 2009 calendar year. F's sole source of income is from the sale of fireworks. During the year, he sold fireworks costing $4,000 for $6,500. R's sole source of income is

---

[16] § 151(c)(1)(A). Note that there is no relief from the gross income test for qualifying relatives. Under prior law, this relief was reserved for children of the taxpayer.

[17] See Chapters 5 and 6 for detailed discussion of "gross income."

derived from rental property. During the year, he collected rents of $4,200 while incurring expenses of $1,700 for repairs, maintenance, and interest. Although F and R each earned $2,500 (F: $6,500 − $4,000 = $2,500; R: $4,200 − $1,700 = $2,500), F's gross income was $2,500, whereas R's was $4,200. As a result, T can only claim an exemption for F, since F's *gross income* was less than the $3,650 exemption amount for 2009.

Relationship or Member of the Household Test. The third of the five hurdles that must be cleared before an individual can be claimed as a dependent concerns the individual's relationship to the taxpayer. Regardless of the amount of support that the taxpayer provides for another person, no exemption is allowed unless the prospective dependent is properly related to the taxpayer.[18] Apparently the authors of the dependency rules believed that the tax law should not grant an exemption unless there is some obligation on the part of the taxpayer to support an individual. Such an obligation normally exists between relatives or others who are members of the taxpayer's household. Therefore, to qualify as a dependent, an individual must satisfy one the qualifying relationship tests below. All of these are *familial* (i.e., related by blood, marriage, or adoption) except one. These are:

1. A child or descendant of a child (other than one who would be considered a "qualifying child" under the tests discussed earlier)

2. A brother, sister, stepbrother, or stepsister

3. The father or mother, or an ancestor of either (e.g., a grandparent)

4. A stepfather or stepmother

5. A niece or nephew[19]

6. An aunt or uncle[20]

7. A son-in-law, daughter-in-law, father-in-law, mother-in-law, brother-in-law, or sister-in-law

8. Any person who lives in the taxpayer's home and is a member of the taxpayer's household for the entire *taxable* year. Even though such a person is not legally related to the taxpayer (i.e., a familial relative), he or she is treated the same as one who satisfies one of the legal relationships as long as he or she lives with the taxpayer the entire taxable year; for this purpose, temporary absences due to illness, school, vacation, business, or military service are ignored; in addition, a person cannot be claimed as a dependent if the relationship with the taxpayer violated local law (e.g., cohabitation).[21]

A relationship created by marriage does not cease upon divorce or the death of the spouse. Thus, for tax purposes, a divorce would not terminate an individual's relationship with his or her mother-in-law.[22] Additionally, if a dependent dies before the close of the tax year, the taxpayer may still claim a dependency exemption.

---

[18] § 152(a). Note: Recall that there is no dependency exemption for a spouse. The exemption for a spouse is the *personal* exemption.

[19] A niece or nephew must be a daughter or son of a brother or sister of the taxpayer. § 152(a)(6).

[20] An aunt or uncle must be a sister or brother of the father or mother of the taxpayer. § 152(a)(7). For example, the person married to your mother's sister would be her brother-in-law, but he would not qualify as your uncle for purposes of this definition. Technically, such a person would be your "uncle-in-law," a relationship not defined in Code § 152.

[21] § 152(d)(2)(h).

[22] Reg. § 1.152-2(d).

Example 9. This year F provided all the support for several individuals, none of whom had income in excess of the exemption amount. Each person and his or her status as a relative is shown below:

1. S, F's 25-year-old son, living in Los Angeles and attending UCLA. S is a relative; a son is a familial relative and such persons need not live in the home.

2. B, F's 29-year-old brother who moved in with F on November 1 after leaving the military. B is a relative; a brother is a familial relative and such persons need not live in the home.

3. C, F's 27-year-old cousin who moved in with F on October 1 after being unemployed for 10 months. C is not a relative; a cousin is not considered a familial relative and, therefore, qualifies only if he lives with the taxpayer the entire taxable year.

4. BL, the brother of F's former wife. BL is a relative; BL is F's brother-in-law, a familial relative; such a relationship continues to exist whether F is divorced or his wife dies.

5. Z, a friend who has been living with F since December 1 of the prior year. Z is a "relative"; a person who lives with the taxpayer the *entire* taxable year qualifies as a relative even though such person is not related by blood or marriage.

Joint Return Test. The dependent must not have filed a joint return with his or her spouse. This requirement is discussed further below.

Citizenship or Residency Test. The dependent must be a U.S. citizen, resident or national, or a resident of Canada or Mexico. Additional exceptions exist as noted below.

PROVISIONS COMMON TO ALL DEPENDENCY EXEMPTIONS

As is apparent from the discussion above, there are several important differences in the definitions of a qualifying child and a qualifying relative. For example, there is no gross income test or support test applicable to a "child" of the taxpayer. In a sense, these conditions are assumed to be met where the individual is the child of the taxpayer. Notwithstanding these differences, it is important to note that—as may be apparent–there are some rules common to both types of dependents. Each of these is considered in greater detail below. Exhibit 4-2 also compares the two provisions.

No Joint Return. A taxpayer normally cannot claim a dependency exemption for a married individual if such person files a joint return.[23] This is true for both a qualifying child and a qualifying relative. This rule appears to reflect a presumption that married taxpayers usually rely on themselves for support rather than others. Note, however, that if a joint return is filed solely for a refund (i.e., the tax is zero and all withholding is refunded), the return is ignored and the individual may be claimed as a dependent (assuming the other tests are met).[24] Also observe that the test is met as long as a joint return is *not* filed. If the married individual files a separate return, he or she may still be claimed as a dependent. In certain situations, parents of newlyweds and others may find it beneficial for their child to file a married, separate return.

Example 10. B and C were married on December 21, 2009. B, a budding 25-year-old attorney, earned $48,000 for the year. C, age 23, is a full-time graduate student.

---

23 § 151(c)(2).

24 Rev. Rul. 54-567, 1954-2 C.B. 108.

Because C was fully supported by her parents, she was eligible to be claimed as a dependent on her parents' return. However, C's parents may not claim C as a dependent if B and C elect to file a joint return. The family must determine whether they are better off if: (l) B and C file a joint return and C claims her exemption on their joint return; or (2) B and C each file married filing separately and they relinquish C's exemption to her parents. A partial analysis would suggest the first alternative is far superior. If a joint return is filed, all of B's income would be taxed at 15% or less (see inside front cover of text for rates). Alternatively, the filing of separate returns would cause a substantial portion of B's taxable income to be taxed at 25%. In this case, it would appear that the additional tax caused by filing separate returns would more than offset any savings to be derived from shifting the exemption to C's parents.

Example 11. D and E were married on December 28, 2009. During 2009, D, age 22, attended State University full time. In addition, she worked part-time, earning $10,500 for the year. E, age 21, was also a full-time student, fully supported by his parents. E had no income. In this case, E's parents are entitled to claim an exemption for E even if D and E elect to file a joint return. The joint return requirement would not be violated because the couple owes no tax (the couple's standard deduction eliminates their taxable income). Consequently, under the IRS view, they would be filing merely to obtain a refund of any withholding and not filing an actual return.

It should be emphasized that the fact that a person files his or her own tax return does not bar another taxpayer (who otherwise meets all the necessary tests) from claiming him or her as a dependent. This is true as long as the dependent does not file a joint return for any reason other than to claim a refund of the entire amount of taxes withheld. Otherwise, the joint return test would not be met and the dependency exemption would be denied.

Citizenship or Residency Test. A dependent must be a citizen or national (e.g., an American Samoan) of the United States or a resident of the United States, Canada, or Mexico. In addition, an adopted child of a citizen qualifies, even though not a resident, if he or she was a member of the taxpayer's household for the entire taxable year. For example, if a taxpayer's employment results in his relocation to London where he adopts a British child, this rule enables the taxpayer to claim the child as a dependent even though the child is not a U.S. citizen or resident.

Taxpayer Not a Dependent. A person who is a dependent cannot claim others as dependents. For example, if a child is a dependent of his or her parents, the child cannot claim his or her own children as dependents.

Social Security Number. In order to claim an exemption for a dependent, the taxpayer must list the dependent's Social Security number on the tax return. If the number is not listed or is listed incorrectly, the exemption may be disallowed and a $50 penalty may be imposed. More importantly, the taxpayer's filing status (head of household, surviving spouse) or child credit could be affected. Since it usually takes about two weeks to obtain a social security number, obtaining one by the extended due date of the return normally does not present a problem.[25]

---

[25] The year that this requirement became effective the number of exemptions dropped 7 million below what had been expected, resulting in about $2.8 billion in additional tax revenue. Interestingly, more than 48 percent of the drop was attributable to single taxpayers. See IRS Pub. 1500 (August 1991).

EXHIBIT 4-2
Qualifying Child vs. Qualifying Relative

Test	Qualifying Child	Qualifying Relative
Relationship	Yes *(child and siblings, their descendants)*	Yes *(familial & certain nonrelatives)*
Residence	Yes *(> ½ taxable year)*	No *(but see support)*
Age	Yes *(< 19; < 24 & full-time student)*	No *(but see income)*
Tie-breaker	Yes *(parent first)*	No *(but see multiple support agreement)*
Support	No *(not self supporting)*	Yes *(>½ spent)*
Income	No	Yes *(but not child if < 19; < 24 & full-time student)*
Joint return	Cannot file joint return	Cannot file joint return
Citizenship	Yes	Yes

CHILDREN OF DIVORCED OR SEPARATED PARENTS

If a married couple with children is divorced or separated, special rules may apply in determining who claims exemptions for the children.[26] These rules operate when the couple is:

- ► Legally separated under a decree of divorce or separate maintenance
- ► Separated under a written separation agreement; or
- ► Lived apart at all times during the last six months of the calendar year.

In these situations, if over half of a child's support is provided by one parent or collectively by both parents and the child is in custody of one or both parents for more than half of the year, the parent with custody for the greater portion of the year may claim the exemption. Thus, the custodial parent ordinarily receives the exemption regardless of the amount paid by either parent.

In certain situations, the divorced couple may be better served if the noncustodial parent claims the exemption. Consequently, if the conditions above are met, the custodial parent may surrender his or her right to the exemption to the noncustodial parent. To accomplish this, the release must be evidenced in a signed declaration that the custodial parent will not claim the exemption. For this purpose, the custodial parent may file Form 8332. The noncustodial parent should attach the form or statement to his or her return.

PHASE-OUT OF PERSONAL AND DEPENDENCY EXEMPTIONS

Since 1989 Congress has reduced the benefits that high-income taxpayers receive from their personal and dependency exemptions. Under § 151(d), taxpayers must reduce their deduction for personal and dependency exemptions by 2 percent for each $2,500 or fraction thereof ($1,250 for married persons filing separate returns) by which a taxpayer's A.G.I. exceeds the applicable threshold. These thresholds depend on the taxpayer's filing status, and the amounts are adjusted for inflation annually. The phase-out is scheduled to expire after 2009.

---

[26]   § 152(e).

Filing Status	Threshold A.G.I.	
	2009	2008
Single individuals (not surviving spouse or head of household).............	$166,800	$159,950
Married filing jointly or surviving spouse..............................	250,200	239,950
Head of household	208,500	199,950
Married filing separately..	125,100	119,975

For 2009, the amount of the reduction is itself reduced by two-thirds. Thus the final reduction is 1/3 of that initially computed. The reduction in the exemption deduction may be computed as follows:[27]

$$\frac{\text{A.G.I} - \text{Threshold}}{\$2,500 \ (\text{or} \ \$1,250)} = \frac{\text{Factor}}{(\text{round-up})} \times \frac{2}{\text{percentage points}} = \frac{\text{Tentative}}{\text{reduction}} \times 1/3 = \frac{\text{Final}}{\text{Reduction}}$$

Example 12. H and W are married with four children. They are entitled to claim six exemptions. In 2009, their A.G.I. is $291,200. Their normal exemption deduction in 2009 before reduction is $21,900 (6 × $3,650). After reduction, their exemption would be $19,520 as computed below.

Total exemption deduction before reduction		
(6 × $3,650 for 2009)		$21,900
Computation of exemption reduction		
A.G.I...	$ 291,200	
Phase-out threshold for married filing jointly...............	(250,200)	
Excess	$ 41,000	

$$\frac{\$41,000 \ \text{excess}}{\$2,500} = \ 16.4, \ \text{rounded to} \ 17 \times 2\% = 34\% \times 1/3 = 11.333\%$$

Reduction (exemption amount $21,900 × 11.333%)	(2,481)
Exemption deduction allowed	$19,419

H and W are required to reduce their total exemption deduction by approximately 11.333%. As a result, the original exemption deduction of $21,900 ($3,650 × 6) is reduced by $2,481 to $19,419.[28] Because of their high income, the couple is allowed about 89% of their normal exemption deduction.

Note that in 2008 and 2009, the maximum one-third reduction in the exemption is reached if A.G.I. exceeds the threshold by more than $122,500. For example, if a married couple's A.G.I. exceeds $372,700 ($250,200 threshold + $122,500), their total deduction for exemptions would be subject to the maximum reduction. This maximum reduction is one-third of the exemption deduction: ($372,701 − $250,200 = $122,501) / $2,500 = 49.0004, rounded up to 50 × 2 = 100% reduction, then multiplied by one-third. For each exemption, the maximum reduction for 2009 would be $1,167 ($3,650 × 1/3), producing a minimum exemption of $2,333.

---

[27] § 151(d)(3)(E).

[28] In 2007 and 2008, the IRS calculation of the reduction on the Deduction for Exemptions Worksheet accompanying the instructions for Form 1040 manipulated the mathematical terms so that the reduction would be the tentative reduction divided by 1.5 as seen below:

$2,481 reduction in exemption deduction = ($21,900 × 34% = $7,140)/3

CHILD TAX CREDIT

Although most credits are covered in Chapter 13, the child tax credit is addressed briefly here because it is so closely tied with exemptions.[29] Under § 24, the amount of the child tax credit is $1,000 for each *qualifying child*.[30] For example, if a taxpayer had four children, the potential credit would be $4,000 ($1,000 × 4). The definition of a qualifying child for purposes of the child credit piggybacks on the uniform definition of a child used in determining a taxpayer's dependency exemption (discussed earlier in this chapter). In other words, a *qualifying child* for the child credit is a *qualifying child* as that expression is defined for determining a taxpayer's dependents but with certain modifications. A qualifying child for the child credit is any person who meets the following conditions.

▸ The individual is a *qualifying child* as defined in § 152 relating to dependents (age, relationship, residence tests).

▸ The individual has not attained the age of 17 by the close of the calendar year.

▸ The individual is a U.S. citizen.

To summarize, a taxpayer normally can claim the $1,000 credit for each child under age 17. Also note that as mentioned above, if a divorced or separated taxpayer waives his or her right to an exemption, the child credit is also waived and transferred to the noncustodial spouse.

Example 13. M and D are the proud parents of a 16-year-old daughter, C. The parents file jointly, reporting gross income of $37,475 for 2009. After claiming a standard deduction of $11,400 and three exemptions of $3,650 each, their taxable income is $15,125. Their tax on $15,125 is $1,513. After claiming their child tax credit of $1,000 for C, the couple's gross income tax before prepayments is $513.

Phase-Out of Credit. Like many other tax benefits, the child tax credit is phased out for higher income taxpayers. Specifically, the allowable credit is reduced by $50 for each $1,000 (or fraction thereof) of A.G.I. in excess of specified thresholds. The thresholds are $75,000 for unmarried taxpayers and $110,000 for married taxpayers filing jointly ($55,000 for those filing separately).[31]

Example 14. R and S have two daughters, L and M (both under age 17). R and S are married and file jointly, reporting A.G.I. of $117,100 for 2009. The child tax credit for two qualifying children is generally $2,000, but R and S must reduce their credit by $400 ($50 × 8, since $117,100 exceeds $110,000 by $7,000 and a fraction) to $1,600.

Refundable Child Tax Credit. As a general rule, most credits are limited to the taxpayer's tax liability for the year. For example, if the taxpayer's tax liability before the child credit is $5,000 and the child credit is $3,000, the taxpayer's regular tax usually would be reduced to $2,000. If the taxpayer's regular tax liability before the credit is $3,000 and the child credit is $4,000, the credit would reduce the tax to zero and *normally* the $1,000 balance of the credit would not be used and the taxpayer would not receive a

---

[29] § 24.

[30] §§ 24(c)(1)(C) and 32(c)(3)(B).

[31] § 24(b). For purposes of this phase-out, adjusted gross income is increased by the amount of the foreign earned income exclusions under §§ 911, 931, and 933.

refund of the unused credit. However, the law permits a portion of the unused child credit to be refunded. In other words, in the situation above, all or a portion of the unused credit of $1,000 would be refunded. The amount of the refundable credit depends on several variables, including the number of children, the taxpayer's earned income, other credits and some additional factors. The actual calculation of the amount of refundable credit can be found in Chapter 13 in the discussion of refundable credits.

✔ CHECK YOUR KNOWLEDGE

Try these 10 true-false questions concerning exemptions. If the statement is false, explain why. Assume all tests are met unless otherwise implied.

Review Question 1. All individuals are entitled to claim a personal exemption.

False. An individual who may be claimed as a dependent on another taxpayer's return cannot claim a personal exemption. This prohibits two different taxpayers from claiming two separate exemptions for the same person.

Review Question 2. Certain people who are normally considered relatives (e.g., cousins) do not qualify as relatives for purposes of the exemption tests.

True. A cousin is not a familial relative.

Review Question 3. An individual, such as a cousin, can qualify as a "relative" even though he or she is not a familial relative.

True. An individual who lives in the taxpayer's home the entire taxable year is treated as a relative even though such person and the taxpayer would not be "related" under the statutory definition.

Review Question 4. T takes care of his mom. He satisfies the support test if he provides more than 10 percent of her total support.

False. A taxpayer must generally provide more than 50 percent of an individual's support in order to claim the individual as a dependent. However, an individual who provides more than 10 percent of a person's support may be able to claim a dependency exemption under a multiple support agreement.

Review Question 5. In determining whether T provides more than 50 percent of his mom's support, her savings of over $100,000, and any earnings from them, are not counted except to the extent they are actually spent.

True. Funds available for an individual's support are ignored in applying the support test. Only amounts spent (or the value of support items provided, such as lodging) are considered.

Review Question 6. T's mom has no income other than social security benefits of $5,000 and interest from City of Duluth bonds of $6,000. T may claim an exemption for her mom.

True. A dependency exemption normally cannot be claimed for an individual if such person's gross income exceeds the exemption amount. For this purpose, gross income includes only income that is subject to tax. In this case, T's mom's income from social security is excluded as is the interest from the municipal bonds.

Review Question 7. T's 25-year-old son lives with him. This year he earned $5,000 from his paper route. T may not claim an exemption for his son.

True. T is not a qualifying child since he fails the age test (not less than 19 nor a full-time student less than 24). He also is not a qualifying relative because he fails the gross income test since he earns more than the exemption amount and is neither less than 19 nor a full-time student less than 24. Had T been a full-time student less than 24, he would have qualified as either a qualifying child or a qualifying relative.

Review Question 8. In the case of a divorced couple with children, the custodial parent normally receives the exemption for the children even if the noncustodial parent provides all of the child support.

True. The custodial parent is entitled to the exemption unless he or she releases it to the noncustodial parent. This generally follows from the uniform definition of a child that requires a child to have lived with the taxpayer for more than one-half of the taxable year.

Review Question 9. H and W are married with three children ages 15, 16, and 17. The couple can normally claim a child tax credit of $3,000.

False. The child tax credit is generally available for dependent children less than 17 years old. Therefore the couple can usually claim a credit of $2,000 ($1,000 × 2).

FILING STATUS

EVOLUTION OF FILING STATUS

The tax rates that are applied to determine the taxpayer's tax liability depend on the taxpayer's filing status. From 1913 to 1948, there was only one set of tax rates that applied to individual taxpayers. During this period, each taxpayer filed a separate return, even if he or she were married. For example, if both a husband and wife had income, each would file a separate return, reporting their respective incomes. This system, however, proved inequitable due to the differing state laws governing the ownership of income (or property).

In the United States, the rights that married individuals hold in property are determined using either the common law or community property system. There are ten community property states: Alaska, Arizona, California, Idaho, Louisiana, Nevada, New Mexico, Texas, Washington, and Wisconsin. In a community property state, income generated through the personal efforts of either spouse is generally owned *equally* by the community (i.e., the husband and wife). In common law states, income belongs to the spouse that earns the income. The differing treatments of income by community property and common law states produced the need for a special rate schedule for married taxpayers.

Married Status. The category of married couples filing jointly and its unique rate schedule were added to the law because of an inequity that existed between married couples in community property states and non-community property jurisdictions (separate or common law property states). As noted above, earnings derived from personal services performed by married persons in community property states generally are owned jointly by the two spouses. Accordingly, both husband and wife in a community property state would file returns showing one-half of their earned income, even though only one may

have been employed. Note that the total income of the couple would be split equally between the husband and wife regardless of who earned the income. If a couple in a non-community property state relied on one spouse's earnings, the employed spouse filed a return showing the entire amount of those earnings.

Since the tax rates are progressive, a married couple in a non-community property state would bear a larger tax burden than one in a community property state if only one spouse was employed outside the home or one spouse earned substantially more than the other. To eliminate this inequity, Congress elected to grant the benefits of income splitting to all married couples. This was accomplished by authorizing a new tax schedule for married persons filing jointly. A joint return results in the same amount of tax as would be paid on two "married, filing separate" returns showing half the total income of a married couple.

> **Example 15.** L and M are married and reside in California with their two children. L is an executive with a major corporation and M works in the home. Under state law, L's salary of $70,000 is owned equally by L and M. Each may file a separate return and report $35,000 of the salary.

> **Example 16.** S and T are married and reside in Virginia with their two children. S is an executive with a major corporation and T works in the home. S earns a salary of $70,000. If S were to file a separate return, she would report the entire $70,000 salary on that return. Since the tax rate schedules for individuals are progressive, S would pay a higher tax than the total paid by L and M in *Example 15*. Consequently, the total tax burden on S and T would be greater than that on L and M. By filing a joint return, S and T are placed in a position equivalent to that of L and M.

Head-of-Household Status. Introduction of the joint return in 1948 was not viewed by the public as merely a solution to a problem caused by differing state laws. Many saw it as a tax break for those who had family obligations. As a result, single parents and other unmarried taxpayers with dependents tried to persuade Congress that they should be entitled to some tax relief due to their family responsibilities. Their arguments were based on the fact that they suffered a greater tax burden than single-earner married couples. In 1957, a tax reduction was allowed in the form of a new tax rate schedule for taxpayers who qualify as a *head of household*. The rates were designed to be lower than the original rates, which applied to all taxpayers, but *higher* than the rates for married persons filing jointly.

Single Status. The most recent change in the overall tax rate structure was the addition of a separate tax rate schedule for single persons. This change was made because a single person was paying a higher rate of tax on the same income than married persons filing jointly and heads of households. The reduced rates for single taxpayers still are higher than those for a head of household, but lower than those in the original rate structure. As a result of this final change, the original tax rate structure that once applied to all taxpayers now applies only to married persons filing separately.

Summary. The Federal income tax on individuals is based on four tax rate schedules. Taxpayers must file under one of the following classifications, listed in order from lowest to highest in tax rates:

1. Married filing jointly (including surviving spouses)

2. Head of household

3. Single

4. Married filing separately

The 2009 tax rate schedules for these classifications are reproduced on the inside front cover of this text.[32]

MARRIED INDIVIDUALS

Marital status is determined on the last day of an individual's taxable year. A person is married for tax purposes if he or she is married under state law, regardless of whether he or she is separated or in the process of seeking a divorce.[33]

Joint Return. A husband and wife generally may file a return using the rates for married persons filing jointly.[34] If a joint return is filed, husband and wife are jointly and severally (individually) liable for any tax, interest or penalties related to *that* joint return. As a result, one spouse may be held liable for paying the entire tax, even though the other spouse earned all the income. For this reason, a spouse should be cautious in signing a joint return. However, under the *innocent spouse rule*, a spouse will not be held liable for tax and penalties attributable to misstatements by the other spouse in two instances. The first provision allows relief if the innocent spouse establishes that he or she did not know and had no reason to know of the understatement, that it is inequitable to hold him or her liable for the deficiency, and that he or she elected the benefits of this provision within two years after the date collection activities began. The second provision limits the liability of a spouse to only the portion of the deficiency properly allocable to him or her if he or she is no longer married to, is legally separated from, or is no longer living with the spouse with whom the joint return was filed.[35]

Surviving Spouse. To provide relief in those situations where a spouse dies and must continue to support the couple's children, the law permits use of the joint return rates for a short period. A so-called *surviving spouse* may use the lower rates in the first or second taxable year after the year of his or her spouse's death. Technically, a taxpayer qualifies as a surviving spouse if he or she meets two tests. First, the spouse must have died within the two taxable years preceding the current taxable year. Second, the taxpayer must provide over half the cost of maintaining a home in which he or she and a *dependent* son, stepson, daughter, or stepdaughter live.[36] In determining whether the child is a dependent, the following modifications are made when applying the qualifying individual or qualifying relative tests.

- ▸ For purpose of determining whether the child is a dependent under the "qualifying relative" standard, the gross income test is ignored.
- ▸ In applying either test, the fact that the individual files a joint return is ignored.
- ▸ In applying either test, the fact that a dependent is ineligible to have dependents is ignored.

Remarriage terminates surviving spouse status. Of course, a joint return can be filed with the new spouse.

---

32   The 2009 tax tables had not been issued by the IRS at the date of publication of this text. However, the 2008 tax tables are reproduced in Appendix A.

33   Special rules apply to a taxpayer whose spouse dies during the year. See §§ 7703(a)(1) and 6013(a)(2).

34   § 6013(a). However, a special rule applies if the spouse is a nonresident alien. See § 6013(g). Also, both spouses must have the *same* taxable year.

35   § 6015(b) and (c).

36   § 2(a).

Example 17. H and W were married and had two children, S and D. In 2009, H died. After H's death, W continued to provide a home and all the support of S and D. As a result, W is entitled to claim S and D as dependents. For the year of death, 2009, W normally will file a joint return with her deceased husband, H. In the following two years, 2010 and 2011, W may file as a surviving spouse since she provides a home for a dependent child. As a surviing spouse, she may use the same rates as married persons filing jointly. In subsequent years, W may file as a head of household if she meets all the other requirements.

Separate Returns. Normally, it will be advantageous for married persons to file a joint return because it is simpler to file one return than it is to file two, and the tax will be as low or lower than the tax based on the rules for married persons filing separately. In some situations, a taxpayer may prefer to file a separate return. For example, a person may wish to avoid liability for the tax on the income—especially any unreported income—of his or her spouse. Similarly, a husband and wife who are separated and are contemplating divorce may wish to file separate returns.

Separate returns may be to the taxpayers' advantage in certain circumstances. Although rare, use of the separate rate schedules may result in a lower total tax than by using the rates applicable to a joint return. Filing of separate returns may also prove beneficial when the filing of a joint return would prevent another taxpayer (e.g., a parent) from claiming a dependency exemption deduction for either the husband or the wife *(see Example 10 above).* State income tax laws may also make filing separately beneficial.

HEAD OF HOUSEHOLD

Head-of-household rates may be used if the taxpayer satisfies two conditions. First, the taxpayer must be unmarried (and not a surviving spouse) or considered unmarried (i.e., an abandoned spouse) on the last day of the tax year. Second, the taxpayer must provide more than one-half of the cost of maintaining as his or her home a household which is the principal place of abode for more than one-half the year of

1. A qualifying child, or
2. A dependent familial relative[37]

As might be expected, the same individuals that are considered "relatives" for exemption purposes generally qualify as relatives when applying the head-of-household rules (e.g., children, grandchildren, parents, grandparents). However, there is an exception. Even though a person who is not truly related to the taxpayer but who lives in the taxpayer's home for the entire taxable year is treated as a relative for purposes of the dependency exemption, such is not the case here. In order for the taxpayer to qualify for

EXHIBIT 4-3
Relatives for Dependency and Head-of-Household Tests

Relative	For Dependency Exemption	For Head-of-Household Test
Qualifying child	Yes	Yes
Familial relative	Yes	Yes
Other individuals—person who lives in taxpayer's home entire taxable year	Yes	No

[37] § 2(b)(1).

head-of-household status, the individual living in the home must be a familial relative.[38] Exhibit 4-3 gives a listing of those who are normally considered relatives for purposes of meeting both the head-of-household and dependency rules. Note that they are all the same except for the nonfamilial relative.

An individual normally enjoys head of household status *only* if he or she is the taxpayer's dependent *and* lives in the taxpayer's household. Two exceptions exist to this general rule.

1. A parent must be a dependent but need not live in the taxpayer's home; however, the taxpayer still must pay more than half of the cost of keeping up a home for his or her mother or father.

For example, the taxpayer qualifies if he or she paid more than half the cost of the parent's living in a nursing home and the parent is a dependent.

Example 18. D, an unmarried individual, lives in Seattle and pays more than half of the cost of maintaining a home in Reno for her dependent parents. Although her parents do not live with her in Seattle, D qualifies for the head-of-household rates.

2. An *unmarried qualifying child* of the taxpayer need not be a dependent. This exception permits a divorced parent to qualify as head-of-household even though the former other parent claims the exemption for the child.

Example 19. R is divorced and maintains a household for herself and her 10-year-old daughter. Although R is the custodial parent, she allows her former husband to claim the exemption for the child. R still qualifies for the head-of-household rates.

Example 20. M is divorced. At the beginning of the year, M's son, S, started medical school and moved in with his mom to save money. M pays all of the cost of maintaining the home and also provides more than one-half of S's support. S is 25 years old and earned $46,000 during the year. M cannot claim head of household because S is neither a qualifying child nor a qualifying relative. S is not a qualifying child because he is too old. To be a qualifying child, S must be less than 19 or a full-time student less than 24. S is also not a qualifying relative since his income is too high (i.e., $46,000 exceeds the amount of the personal exemption).[39]

It should be noted that a person for whom a dependency exemption is claimed solely under a multiple support agreement (e.g., the taxpayer did not provide over half the cost of maintaining the home) is not considered a qualifying relative and the agreement *cannot* qualify the taxpayer as a head of household. In addition, a nonresident alien cannot be a head of household.[40]

Costs of Maintaining a Home. In determining whether a taxpayer qualifies for head-of-household status, it is necessary to determine whether he or she pays more than half of the cost of maintaining a home for the taxable year. This determination must also be made for surviving spouse filing status. The costs of maintaining the home include the costs for

---

[38] §§ 2(b)(3), 152(a)(9), and 152(c).

[39] Prior to 2005, M would have qualified for head of household treatment since the child of a taxpayer was not required to be a dependent.

[40] *Supra*, footnote 36.

the mutual benefit of the occupants and include such expenses as property taxes, mortgage interest, rent, utilities, insurance, repairs, upkeep, and *food* consumed on the premises. The cost of maintaining a home does not include clothing, educational expenses, medical expenses, or transportation.[41]

Abandoned Spouse Provision. Without a special provision, an individual whose spouse has simply abandoned him or her might be forced to file using the high rates for married individuals filing separately. Aware of this problem, Congress has provided that a married individual who files a separate return may file as head of household if he or she qualifies as an *abandoned spouse*. To qualify, the individual must provide more than half the cost of maintaining a home that houses him or her and a child for whom a dependency exemption deduction is *either* claimed or could be claimed by the taxpayer except for the fact that the exemption was assigned to the noncustodial parent.[42] The child must live in the home with the taxpayer for more than half the taxable year and the taxpayer's spouse must not live in the home at any time during the last six months of the year. If each of these requirements is met, an abandoned spouse qualifies as a head of household.

Example 21. M and N are married with six children. In October, M stormed out of the house, saying he would never return. N was hopeful that M would return and consequently had not taken action to obtain a divorce by the end of the year. Although M and N are eligible to file a joint return, M indicated that he would not. Consequently, N's filing status is married filing separately. She does not qualify as an abandoned spouse since her husband lived in the home during the last six months of the year. In the following year, however, N could qualify and file as head of household.

Single. Single filing status is defined by exception. A single taxpayer is anyone who is unmarried and does not qualify as a head of household or surviving spouse. Even though single rates are somewhat lower, they may not be used by married persons filing separately.[43]

Marriage Tax Penalty. A well-known tax phenomenon faced by couples contemplating marriage is the possibility of a marriage tax penalty. Whether matrimony is for better or for worse on the couple's tax return depends on a number of factors, such as how much each earns as well as whether either individual brings dependents into the marriage.

Joint filing originally was intended as a benefit to married couples. Prior to 1969, the joint return schedule was designed to tax one-half of total marital income at the tax rates applicable to single individuals. The resultant tax was then doubled to produce the married couple's tax liability. Note that this procedure produces a perfect split of a single earner's income between two spouses so that it is taxed at a lower marginal rate. While this approach is quite beneficial for married taxpayers, single taxpayers felt that they were paying an unjustifiable "singles penalty." To illustrate, consider the situation of a single taxpayer with taxable income of $24,000. In 1965, this taxpayer owed $8,030 of income tax, with the last dollar of income taxed at a 50 percent marginal tax rate. A married couple with the same 1965 taxable income owed only $5,660 (more than $2,000 less) and faced a marginal tax rate of only 32 percent.

In 1969 Congress attempted to alleviate the singles penalty by enacting a new (and lower) rate schedule for single taxpayers. While this action did reduce (but not eliminate) the singles penalty, it also created a marriage penalty for certain individuals as shown in the example below.

---

[41]   Reg. § 1.2-2(d).

[42]   § 2(c) and § 7703(b). An adopted child of the taxpayer is considered a son or daughter for this test.

[43]   Single filing status is referred to in Code § 1(c) as "Unmarried individuals (Other Than Surviving Spouses and Heads of Households)."

Example 22. H is currently single and his only source of income is his salary of $90,000. He is considering marrying his girlfriend, W. As shown below, for 2009 his tax as a single taxpayer after considering his standard deduction and one exemption is $16,350. If H marries W and W has no taxable income, their tax on a joint return with its wider brackets and double the standard deduction and exemption amounts would be $10,200 or $6,150 less ($16,350 − $10,200). Observe that in this situation where there is one earner, there is a singles penalty. In other words, for the same amount of income ($90,000), those who are single pay more than those who are married. But now consider what happens if W also has a $90,000 salary, the same as H. If W and H remain single, they both will pay a tax of $16,350 for a combined total of $32,700. However, if they marry, their combined taxable income remains the same at $161,300 (2 × $80,650) but their tax on a joint return is $33,427.50 or $727.50 more. Here where there are two high-income earners both with about the same income, there is a marriage tax penalty.

Filing Status	2009 H One earner Single	2009 H & W One earner Married	2009 H & W Two earners Married
Gross income of H.	$90,000	$90,000	$ 90,000
Gross income of W	—	—	$ 90,000
Gross income.	$90,000	$90,000	$ 180,000
Standard deduction.	($ 5,700)	($11,400)	($ 11,400)
Exemption(s)	($ 3,650)	($ 7,300)	($ 7,300)
Taxable income	$80,650	$71,300	$ 161,300
Tax	$16,350.00	$10,200.00	$ 33,427.50

	H Single	H & W Married	H & W Married
Tax	$16,350.00	$10,200.00	$33,427.50
Tax for two singles (2 × $16,350)			(32,700.00)
Singles penalty ($16,350 − $10,200)		$ 6,150.00	
Marriage penalty ($33,427.50 − $32,700.00) . .			$ 727.50

As a general rule, if a couple marries and only one spouse has income (or there is a large disparity between their incomes), marriage will be beneficial due to the splitting effect (i.e., the married, one earner effect above). In contrast, if a couple marries and they have similar incomes, there may be a marriage tax penalty (i.e., the married, two earners effect above).

Tax Reform and the Marriage Penalty. One of the goals of the changes made in 2001 was to reduce the marriage penalty. The specific provisions are summarized as follows:

▸ The standard deduction for a married couple was increased to an amount which is exactly double that for a single individual.

▸ The tax brackets were adjusted in a way to reduce the marriage penalty. First, the 10 percent bracket for married couples ($16,700) is double that for single individuals ($8,350). Next, the 15 percent bracket was adjusted to an amount which is double that for single taxpayers. Note, however, that the higher tax brackets were not adjusted and will remain in the same proportions that they were before for married compared to unmarried persons (retaining an element of marriage penalty).

EXHIBIT 4-4
Determination of Filing Status

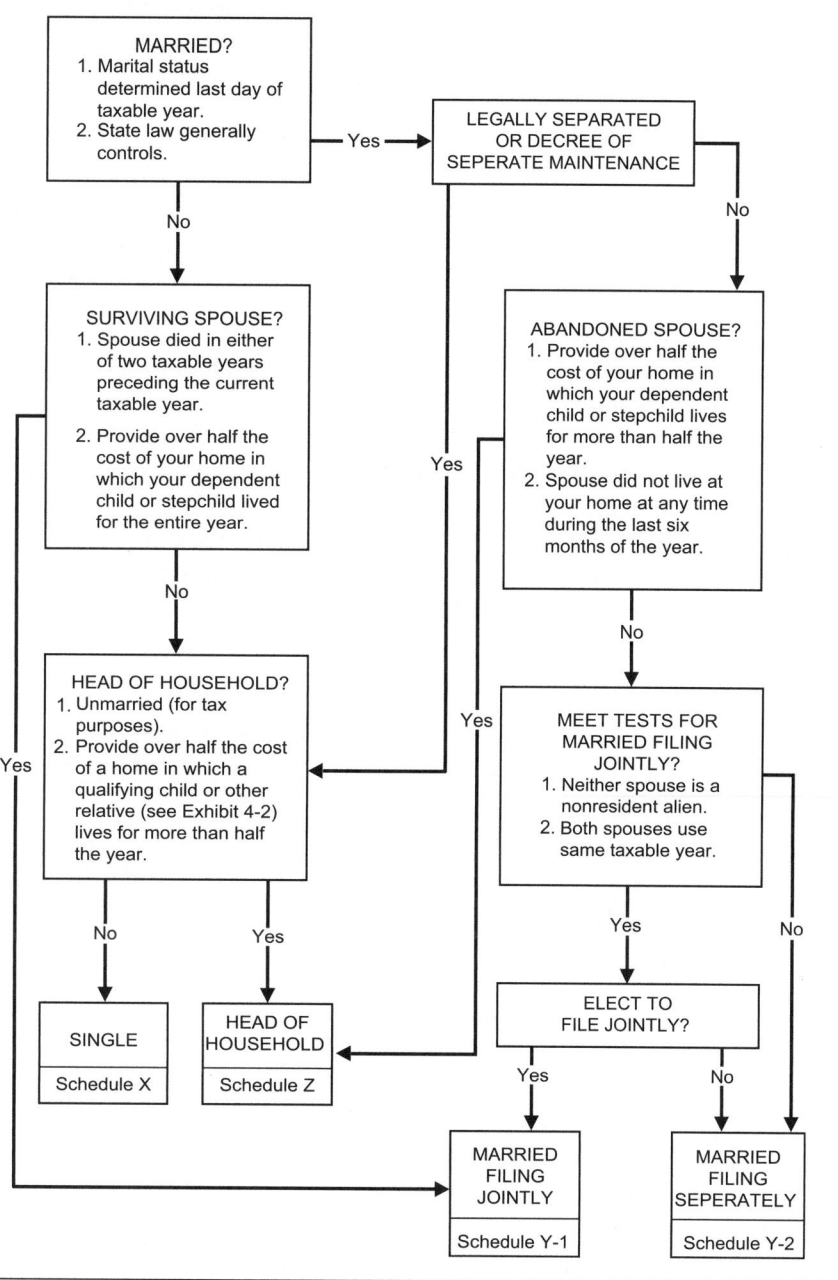

✔️ *CHECK YOUR KNOWLEDGE*

Review Question 1. List the available rate schedules in the order of their progressivity (highest to lowest tax rates).

Married filing separately, single, head of household, and married filing jointly (including surviving spouses).

Review Question 2. H died in 2007, survived by his wife, W, and two young children, S and D. What rate schedule may W use in 2009 assuming she has not remarried?

She should be able to file as a surviving spouse and use the joint return rate schedule for the two taxable years after her husband's death (2008 and 2009). A taxpayer qualifies as a surviving spouse if his or her spouse has died in either of the two taxable years preceding the current year (i.e., 2007 or 2008 in this case) and he or she provides over half the cost of a home in which he or she and a dependent child live. In this case, H died in 2007, and it appears that W provides a home in which she and her dependent children live.

Review Question 3. Q, divorced, is alive and well in Los Angeles. She has a 19-year-old daughter who attends school full-time at Arizona State. Q provides all her daughter's support, including payment of her dorm bill each month. Can Q file as a head of household? What additional questions must be asked before this question can be answered?

An individual can normally file as a head of household if he or she provides over *one-half* the cost of maintaining a home in which a qualifying child or a dependent familial relative lives for more than *one-half* of the taxable year. In this case, it is not completely clear whether the half-and-half test is met. As a general rule, the relative must live in the home of the taxpayer one-half of the year. Here Q's daughter may only live in Q's home during the summer months, and it would therefore appear that Q could not qualify. However, temporary absences due to special circumstances such as those due to education, business, vacation, and military service are ignored. Since the daughter's absence is temporary, the test is satisfied. Note that Q's daughter need not be a dependent since this requirement is relaxed in the case of an unmarried child of the taxpayer.

COMPUTATION OF TAX FOR INDIVIDUAL TAXPAYERS

Once filing status and taxable income have been determined, the tax computation for most individuals is fairly straightforward. The gross tax is computed using the tax tables or the tax rate schedules. This amount is then reduced by any tax credits available to the taxpayer and any tax prepayments in arriving at the tax due or the refund. Children under age 18 with unearned income and all persons claimed as dependents are subject to special rules in the computation of their income tax.

TAX TABLES

The vast majority of individuals must determine their tax using *tax tables*, which are provided by the IRS along with the instructions for preparing individual income tax returns. The tables are derived directly from the rate schedules to simplify compliance and reduce taxpayer errors. The tax for any particular range of taxable income is determined by using the midpoint of the range and the appropriate rate schedule. For example, the tax in the 2008 tables for a single taxpayer with taxable income of $19,010 is $3,053 which is the tax computed on $23,025 (see Exhibit 4-5 for an excerpt and Appendix A for the complete 2008 Tax Tables). The tables cover taxpayers in each filing status with taxable incomes less than $100,000. A taxpayer who qualifies generally is required to use the tax tables.[44]

---

[44] § 3.

EXHIBIT 4-5

Excerpts From Tax Tables for 2008

23,000 – 25,000

If line 43 (taxable income) is—		And you are—			
At least	But less than	Single	Married filing jointly*	Married filing separately	Head of a household
		Your tax is—			
23,000					
23,000	23,050	3,053	2,651	3,053	2,881
23,050	23,100	3,060	2,659	3,060	2,889
23,100	23,150	3,068	2,666	3,068	2,896
23,150	23,200	3,075	2,674	3,075	2,904
23,200	23,250	3,083	2,681	3,083	2,911
23,250	23,300	3,090	2,689	3,090	2,919
23,300	23,350	3,098	2,696	3,098	2,926
23,350	23,400	3,105	2,704	3,105	2,934
23,400	23,450	3,113	2,711	3,113	2,941
23,450	23,500	3,120	2,719	3,120	2,949
23,500	23,550	3,128	2,726	3,128	2,956
23,550	23,600	3,135	2,734	3,135	2,964
23,600	23,650	3,143	2,741	3,143	2,971
23,650	23,700	3,150	2,749	3,150	2,979
23,700	23,750	3,158	2,756	3,158	2,986
23,750	23,800	3,165	2,764	3,165	2,994
23,800	23,850	3,173	2,771	3,173	3,001
23,850	23,900	3,180	2,779	3,180	3,009
23,900	23,950	3,188	2,786	3,188	3,016
23,950	24,000	3,195	2,794	3,195	3,024
24,000					
24,000	24,050	3,203	2,801	3,203	3,031
24,050	24,100	3,210	2,809	3,210	3,039
24,100	24,150	3,218	2,816	3,218	3,046
24,150	24,200	3,225	2,824	3,225	3,054
24,200	24,250	3,233	2,831	3,233	3,061
24,250	24,300	3,240	2,839	3,240	3,069
24,300	24,350	3,248	2,846	3,248	3,076
24,350	24,400	3,255	2,854	3,255	3,084
24,400	24,450	3,263	2,861	3,263	3,091
24,450	24,500	3,270	2,869	3,270	3,099
24,500	24,550	3,278	2,876	3,278	3,106
24,550	24,600	3,285	2,884	3,285	3,114
24,600	24,650	3,293	2,891	3,293	3,121
24,650	24,700	3,300	2,899	3,300	3,129
24,700	24,750	3,308	2,906	3,308	3,136
24,750	24,800	3,315	2,914	3,315	3,144
24,800	24,850	3,323	2,921	3,323	3,151
24,850	24,900	3,330	2,929	3,330	3,159
24,900	24,950	3,338	2,936	3,338	3,166
24,950	25,000	3,345	2,944	3,345	3,174
25,000					
25,000	25,050	3,353	2,951	3,353	3,181
25,050	25,100	3,360	2,959	3,360	3,189
25,100	25,150	3,368	2,966	3,368	3,196
25,150	25,200	3,375	2,974	3,375	3,204
25,200	25,250	3,383	2,981	3,383	3,211
25,250	25,300	3,390	2,989	3,390	3,219
25,300	25,350	3,398	2,996	3,398	3,226
25,350	25,400	3,405	3,004	3,405	3,234
25,400	25,450	3,413	3,011	3,413	3,241
25,450	25,500	3,420	3,019	3,420	3,249
25,500	25,550	3,428	3,026	3,428	3,256
25,550	25,600	3,435	3,034	3,435	3,264
25,600	25,650	3,443	3,041	3,443	3,271
25,650	25,700	3,450	3,049	3,450	3,279
25,700	25,750	3,458	3,056	3,458	3,286
25,750	25,800	3,465	3,064	3,465	3,294
25,800	25,850	3,473	3,071	3,473	3,301
25,850	25,900	3,480	3,079	3,480	3,309
25,900	25,950	3,488	3,086	3,488	3,316
25,950	26,000	3,495	3,094	3,495	3,324

26,000 – 28,000

If line 43 (taxable income) is—		And you are—			
At least	But less than	Single	Married filing jointly*	Married filing separately	Head of a household
		Your tax is—			
26,000					
26,000	26,050	3,503	3,101	3,503	3,331
26,050	26,100	3,510	3,109	3,510	3,339
26,100	26,150	3,518	3,116	3,518	3,346
26,150	26,200	3,525	3,124	3,525	3,354
26,200	26,250	3,533	3,131	3,533	3,361
26,250	26,300	3,540	3,139	3,540	3,369
26,300	26,350	3,548	3,146	3,548	3,376
26,350	26,400	3,555	3,154	3,555	3,384
26,400	26,450	3,563	3,161	3,563	3,391
26,450	26,500	3,570	3,169	3,570	3,399
26,500	26,550	3,578	3,176	3,578	3,406
26,550	26,600	3,585	3,184	3,585	3,414
26,600	26,650	3,593	3,191	3,593	3,421
26,650	26,700	3,600	3,199	3,600	3,429
26,700	26,750	3,608	3,206	3,608	3,436
26,750	26,800	3,615	3,214	3,615	3,444
26,800	26,850	3,623	3,221	3,623	3,451
26,850	26,900	3,630	3,229	3,630	3,459
26,900	26,950	3,638	3,236	3,638	3,466
26,950	27,000	3,645	3,244	3,645	3,474
27,000					
27,000	27,050	3,653	3,251	3,653	3,481
27,050	27,100	3,660	3,259	3,660	3,489
27,100	27,150	3,668	3,266	3,668	3,496
27,150	27,200	3,675	3,274	3,675	3,504
27,200	27,250	3,683	3,281	3,683	3,511
27,250	27,300	3,690	3,289	3,690	3,519
27,300	27,350	3,698	3,296	3,698	3,526
27,350	27,400	3,705	3,304	3,705	3,534
27,400	27,450	3,713	3,311	3,713	3,541
27,450	27,500	3,720	3,319	3,720	3,549
27,500	27,550	3,728	3,326	3,728	3,556
27,550	27,600	3,735	3,334	3,735	3,564
27,600	27,650	3,743	3,341	3,743	3,571
27,650	27,700	3,750	3,349	3,750	3,579
27,700	27,750	3,758	3,356	3,758	3,586
27,750	27,800	3,765	3,364	3,765	3,594
27,800	27,850	3,773	3,371	3,773	3,601
27,850	27,900	3,780	3,379	3,780	3,609
27,900	27,950	3,788	3,386	3,788	3,616
27,950	28,000	3,795	3,394	3,795	3,624
28,000					
28,000	28,050	3,803	3,401	3,803	3,631
28,050	28,100	3,810	3,409	3,810	3,639
28,100	28,150	3,818	3,416	3,818	3,646
28,150	28,200	3,825	3,424	3,825	3,654
28,200	28,250	3,833	3,431	3,833	3,661
28,250	28,300	3,840	3,439	3,840	3,669
28,300	28,350	3,848	3,446	3,848	3,676
28,350	28,400	3,855	3,454	3,855	3,684
28,400	28,450	3,863	3,461	3,863	3,691
28,450	28,500	3,870	3,469	3,870	3,699
28,500	28,550	3,878	3,476	3,878	3,706
28,550	28,600	3,885	3,484	3,885	3,714
28,600	28,650	3,893	3,491	3,893	3,721
28,650	28,700	3,900	3,499	3,900	3,729
28,700	28,750	3,908	3,506	3,908	3,736
28,750	28,800	3,915	3,514	3,915	3,744
28,800	28,850	3,923	3,521	3,923	3,751
28,850	28,900	3,930	3,529	3,930	3,759
28,900	28,950	3,938	3,536	3,938	3,766
28,950	29,000	3,945	3,544	3,945	3,774

29,000 – 31,000

If line 43 (taxable income) is—		And you are—			
At least	But less than	Single	Married filing jointly*	Married filing separately	Head of a household
		Your tax is—			
29,000					
29,000	29,050	3,953	3,551	3,953	3,781
29,050	29,100	3,960	3,559	3,960	3,789
29,100	29,150	3,968	3,566	3,968	3,796
29,150	29,200	3,975	3,574	3,975	3,804
29,200	29,250	3,983	3,581	3,983	3,811
29,250	29,300	3,990	3,589	3,990	3,819
29,300	29,350	3,998	3,596	3,998	3,826
29,350	29,400	4,005	3,604	4,005	3,834
29,400	29,450	4,013	3,611	4,013	3,841
29,450	29,500	4,020	3,619	4,020	3,849
29,500	29,550	4,028	3,626	4,028	3,856
29,550	29,600	4,035	3,634	4,035	3,864
29,600	29,650	4,043	3,641	4,043	3,871
29,650	29,700	4,050	3,649	4,050	3,879
29,700	29,750	4,058	3,656	4,058	3,886
29,750	29,800	4,065	3,664	4,065	3,894
29,800	29,850	4,073	3,671	4,073	3,901
29,850	29,900	4,080	3,679	4,080	3,909
29,900	29,950	4,088	3,686	4,088	3,916
29,950	30,000	4,095	3,694	4,095	3,924
30,000					
30,000	30,050	4,103	3,701	4,103	3,931
30,050	30,100	4,110	3,709	4,110	3,939
30,100	30,150	4,118	3,716	4,118	3,946
30,150	30,200	4,125	3,724	4,125	3,954
30,200	30,250	4,133	3,731	4,133	3,961
30,250	30,300	4,140	3,739	4,140	3,969
30,300	30,350	4,148	3,746	4,148	3,976
30,350	30,400	4,155	3,754	4,155	3,984
30,400	30,450	4,163	3,761	4,163	3,991
30,450	30,500	4,170	3,769	4,170	3,999
30,500	30,550	4,178	3,776	4,178	4,006
30,550	30,600	4,185	3,784	4,185	4,014
30,600	30,650	4,193	3,791	4,193	4,021
30,650	30,700	4,200	3,799	4,200	4,029
30,700	30,750	4,208	3,806	4,208	4,036
30,750	30,800	4,215	3,814	4,215	4,044
30,800	30,850	4,223	3,821	4,223	4,051
30,850	30,900	4,230	3,829	4,230	4,059
30,900	30,950	4,238	3,836	4,238	4,066
30,950	31,000	4,245	3,844	4,245	4,074
31,000					
31,000	31,050	4,253	3,851	4,253	4,081
31,050	31,100	4,260	3,859	4,260	4,089
31,100	31,150	4,268	3,866	4,268	4,096
31,150	31,200	4,275	3,874	4,275	4,104
31,200	31,250	4,283	3,881	4,283	4,111
31,250	31,300	4,290	3,889	4,290	4,119
31,300	31,350	4,298	3,896	4,298	4,126
31,350	31,400	4,305	3,904	4,305	4,134
31,400	31,450	4,313	3,911	4,313	4,141
31,450	31,500	4,320	3,919	4,320	4,149
31,500	31,550	4,328	3,926	4,328	4,156
31,550	31,600	4,335	3,934	4,335	4,164
31,600	31,650	4,343	3,941	4,343	4,171
31,650	31,700	4,350	3,949	4,350	4,179
31,700	31,750	4,358	3,956	4,358	4,186
31,750	31,800	4,365	3,964	4,365	4,194
31,800	31,850	4,373	3,971	4,373	4,201
31,850	31,900	4,380	3,979	4,380	4,209
31,900	31,950	4,388	3,986	4,388	4,216
31,950	32,000	4,395	3,994	4,395	4,224

Example 23. William W. Bristol was single for 2008 and had no dependents. Bill's only income was wages of $27,410 and taxable interest of $350. Since his itemized deductions totaled only $1,650, Bill claims the $5,450 standard deduction allowed for 2008. Federal income tax of $2,820 was withheld from Bill's salary. Bill's taxable income and tax for 2008 are calculated as follows:

Salary			$27,410
Taxable interest			+350
Equals:	Adjusted gross income		$27,760
Less:	Standard deduction for 2008	$5,450	
	Personal exemption for 2008	3,500	−8,950
Equals:	Taxable income		$18,810
Tax on $18,810 from Tax Table for 2008 (See Appendix A)			$ 2,423
Less:	Income tax withheld		−2,820
Equals:	Tax due or (refund)		($ 397)

A completed Form 1040EZ for William W. Bristol, based on the information in this example, is shown in the Appendix at the end of the chapter.

Example 24. Clyde F and Delia C. Cooper were married during all of 2008 and had income from the following sources:

Salary, Clyde		$33,445
Federal income tax withheld	$1,170	
Part-time salary, Delia		23,600
Federal income tax withheld	780	
Interest from City Savings		950
Interest from U.S. Government		550

Clyde and Delia are the sole support for their two children, ages 2 and 7. During 2008 they paid job-related child care expenses of $3,500 and made deductible contributions of $4,000 to their Individual Retirement Accounts ($2,000 each). Their itemized deductions for the year do not exceed their standard deduction for 2008 of $10,900. The Coopers' taxable income and tax for 2008 are calculated as follows:

Salary ($33,445 + $23,600)		$ 57,045
Plus: Taxable interest ($950 + $550)		+1,500
Less: Contributions to IRAs		−4,000
Equals: Adjusted gross income		$ 54,545
Less: Standard deduction for 2008	$10,900	
Exemptions for 2008 ($3,500 × 4)	14,000	−24,900
Equals: Taxable income		$ 29,645
Tax on $30,245 for 2008 (See Appendix A)		$ 3,641
Less: Child care credit (.20 × $3,500)		−700
Child tax credit (2 × $1,000)		−2,000
Equals: Net tax		$ 941
Less: Income tax withheld ($1,170 + $780)		−1,950
Equals: Tax due or (refund)		($ 1,009)

A completed Form 1040A based on this information is included in the Appendix at the end of the chapter.

TAX RATE SCHEDULES

A taxpayer who is unable to use the tax tables uses the tax rate schedules in computing his or her income tax. These schedules contain the rates provided in § 1 of the Internal Revenue Code. The 2008 tax rate schedules are included, along with the 2008 tax tables, in Appendix A. The 2009 tax rate schedules are summarized in Exhibit 4-6. For future reference, the tax rate schedules for 2009 are also reproduced on the inside front cover of this text.

A typical example illustrating the use of the tax rate schedules is given below.

> **Example 25.** R, single, has taxable income of $175,000 for 2009. R's gross tax liability is $42,892.50, computed using the rate schedules as follows:
>
> | | |
> |---|---:|
> | Tax on $171,550 . . . . | $41,754.00 |
> | Plus: Tax on income above $160,850 | |
> | [($175,000 − $171,550 = $3,450) × 33%] . . . . | 1,138.50 |
> | Tax liability . . . . | $42,892.50 |

Tax Reform and the Tax Rates. As noted above, one of the major changes made by the Bush administration in 2001 was to cut the tax rates for individual taxpayers. Before the change, there were five brackets: 15%, 28%, 31%, 35% and 39.6%. The new law created the six brackets that currently exist: 10%, 15%, 25%, 28%, 33% and 35%. The lower brackets are scheduled to remain through 2010 when they revert back to the former rates. Note that all of the tax brackets (i.e., their widths) are adjusted for inflation annually.

SPECIAL TAX COMPUTATION RULES

Unfortunately, the computation of the income tax is not always as straightforward as shown in *Example 25* above. For certain individuals, special rules must be followed.

Persons Claimed as Dependents. As one might deduce from the brief introduction to tax rates, one of the most fundamental principles of tax planning concerns minimizing the marginal tax rate that applies to the taxpayer's income. The significance of this principle is easily understood when it is recognized that Federal marginal tax rates have at times exceeded 90 percent. Even with the reduction of marginal rates to their current levels, minimizing the tax rate can provide benefits.

Historically, one of the most popular techniques to minimize the tax rate has been to shift income to a lower bracket taxpayer such as a child. As discussed in Chapter 5, this could be accomplished most easily by giving the child income-producing property. For example, a parent might establish a savings account for a child. In this way, the income would be taxed to the child at his or her low rate rather than the parents' high rate. In addition, this strategy—absent any special rules—takes advantage of the personal exemption and standard deduction available to a child.

EXHIBIT 4-6
Individual Tax Rate Schedules for 2009

2009 Single:

If taxable income is				
Over	But not over	The Tax is	% on + Excess	Of the Amount over
$0	$8,350	0.00	10%	0
$8,350	$33,950	835.00	15%	$8,350
$33,950	$82,250	4,675.00	25%	$33,950
$82,250	$171,550	16,750.00	28%	$82,250
$171,550	$372,950	41,754.00	33%	$171,550
$372,950		108,216.00	35%	$372,950

2009 Married Filing Jointly:

If taxable income is				
Over	But not over	The Tax is	% on + Excess	Of the Amount over
$ 0	$ 16,700	$0.00	10%	$ 0
16,700	67,900	$1,670.00	15	16,700
67,900	137,050	$9,350.00	25	67,900
137,050	208,850	$26,637.50	28	137,050
208,850	372,950	$46,741.50	33	208,850
372,950		$100,894.50	35	372,950

2009 Head of Household:

If taxable income is				
Over	But not over	The Tax is	% on + Excess	Of the Amount over
$0	$11,950	0.00	10%	0
$11,950	$45,500	1,195.00	15%	$11,950
$45,500	117,450	6,227.50	25%	$45,500
$117,450	$190,200	24,215.00	28%	$117,450
$190,200	$372,950	$44,585.00	33%	$190,200
$372,950		$104,892.50	35%	$372,950

2009 Married, Filing Separate [§1(d)]:

If taxable income is				
Over	But not over	The Tax is	% on + Excess	Of the Amount over
$0	$8,350		10%	0.00
$8,350	$33,950	$835.00	15%	$8,350.00
$33,950	$68,525	$4,675.00	25%	$33,950.00
$68,525	$104,425	$13,318.75	28%	$68,525.00
$104,425	$186,475	$23,370.75	33%	$104,425.00
$186,475		$50,447.25	35%	186,475.00

Congress has long recognized the tax-saving potential inherent in such plans. For this reason, it is not surprising that it has taken steps to limit the opportunities. These are:

1. **Personal exemption.** A taxpayer who can be claimed as a dependent on another taxpayer's return is not entitled to a personal exemption. This rule effectively prohibits all children from claiming a personal exemption. Observe that *without this rule*, a child could currently receive up to $3,650 (2009) income tax-free due to the exemption.

2. **Standard deduction.** The standard deduction available to a taxpayer who can be claimed as a dependent on another taxpayer's return is limited to the *greater* of $950 or $300 plus his or her earned income—but not to exceed the standard deduction amount ($5,700 for single taxpayers in 2009). Without this rule, a child could receive unearned income such as interest of up to $5,700 tax-free.

3. **Kiddie tax.** As explained further below, the investment income (technically referred to as unearned income) of most children is generally taxed as if the parent received it to the extent it exceeds $1,900.[45] Absent this provision, affectionately known as the *kiddie tax*, a parent could shift up to $33,950 of taxable income to the child in 2009, who would pay taxes at a rate of 15 percent or less.

The effect of these provisions is to severely limit the success of any schemes designed to shift income to children.

Example 26. V, age 15, lives at home and may be claimed as a dependent on her parents' return. Several years ago, V's grandfather died, leaving her with a tidy sum to help send her to college. For 2009 V received interest income of $3,225. Her taxable income is computed as follows:

Adjusted gross income		$3,275
Less: Standard deduction	$950	
Personal exemption	+0	−950
Taxable income		$2,325

Note that, in computing V's taxable income, her standard deduction is limited to $950 (the larger of $300 plus her earned income, $300, or $950). The limitation is imposed because she is eligible to be claimed as a dependent on another taxpayer's return. For the same reason, she is not allowed to claim her own personal exemption deduction. In addition, a portion of her income is subject to the kiddie tax as explained below.

Example 27. Assume the same facts in *Example 26*, except that V also earns $2,000 from a part-time job. V's taxable income is determined as follows:

Adjusted gross income:		
Earned income	$ 2,000	
Interest income	+3,225	$ 5,225
Less: Standard deduction ($2,000 earned income + $300)	$ 2,300	
Personal exemption	+0	−2,300
Taxable income		$ 2,925

---

[45] § 1(g). The annual threshold is adjusted for inflation and is twice the standard deduction for dependents.

As in *Example 26*, because V is a dependent, she is not allowed to claim her personal exemption deduction, nor may she claim the full standard deduction of $5,700. Note, however, that her standard deduction has increased because of her earned income. Her standard deduction is now $2,300 (the *larger* of $300 plus her earned income of $2,000, or $950). In effect, V is able to shelter income from tax with the standard deduction to the extent it is earned from personal services (plus another $300).

Kiddie Tax. The *kiddie tax* extends to children who at the close of the taxable year are either under 19 or are full-time students under the age of 24. However, the kiddie tax does not apply to the student group if their earned income exceeds one-half of the amounts spent on their support. For this purpose, scholarships received by a child are not included in the individual's total support. In addition, the kiddie tax does not apply if the child files a joint return or has no living parents.

The kiddie tax rules are triggered only when the affected child has *net unearned income*. For this purpose, unearned income generally includes investment income such as dividends, interest, capital gains, rents, royalties and income received from a trust. Net unearned income is unearned income in excess of $1,900 in 2009.[46] In short, most "children" who have unearned income exceeding the annual threshold, $1,900 in 2009, must compute their tax using a special procedure. The effect of this calculation is that the first $950 of unearned income is offset by the standard deduction and the second $900 of unearned income is taxed at the child's rates (currently 10 percent). Any unearned income exceeding $1,900 is taxed at the parents' top rates.

Example 28. J is 17 years old. In 2009, he received interest income from a savings account and earned income from his paper route. The table below shows several sample calculations of J's taxable income assuming various amounts of earned and unearned income. In addition. the amount taxed at his rates and his parents' rates is computed.

	A	B	C	D
Unearned income	$1,950	$ 500	$1,950	$ 3,200
Earned income	350	750	700	5,700
Total	$2,300	$1,250	$2,650	$ 8,900
Standard deduction: Greater of $950 or earned income + $300 not to exceed $5,700 standard deduction	−950	−1,050	−1,000	−5,700
Personal exemption	—	—	—	—
Taxable income (a)	$1,350	$ 200	$1,650	$ 3,200
Taxed at parents' rates Unearned income > $1,900 (b)	$ 50	$ 0	$ 50	$ 1,300
Taxed at child's rates [(a) − (b)]	$1,300	$ 200	$1,600	$ 1,900

In case B, there is no net unearned income because J's unearned income was less than $1,900. J has net unearned income in cases A, C, and D. In each case, the amount taxed at his parents' rate is the amount by which the child's unearned income exceeded $1,900. Any other income is taxed at the regular rates for the child.

---

[46] § 1(i)(4).

When the child has net unearned income, the tax must be computed as if such income had been the parents' income. The child is required to pay the tax computed using his or her parents' rates except in rare cases where the tax computed in the normal manner is greater (in which case the higher tax must be paid). The tax computation cannot be completed until the parents' taxable income is known.

Although the thrust of the kiddie tax is to tax income that would be taxed at a 10 or 15 percent rate at a higher rate, determination of the child's actual tax is somewhat complicated.[47] The tax is computed on Form 8615 using the following approach:

Taxable income from parents' return...................................	$xxx
Add: Net unearned income of child (children)...........................	+xxx
Equals: Total income taxed at parents' rate.............................	$xxx
Tax on total income taxed at parents' rate.............................	$xxx
Minus: Tax on parents' income	−xxx
Equals: Parental tax on child's net unearned income	$xxx
Add: Tax on child's remaining taxable income at child's rate	+xxx
Equals: Total tax on child's taxable income	$xxx

The first step in this process requires the calculation of the parental tax. This is accomplished by combining the income of the parents with the net unearned income of the child and then calculating the total tax on this combined income as if the parents had reported all the income. Then, by subtracting the tax on the parents' income (from the parents' return), the amount of tax that the parents would have paid on the child's net unearned income is determined. This *parental tax* is, therefore, the tax that the parents would have paid on the net unearned income had they reported it directly.

The final part of the calculation involves determining the tax on the child's remaining taxable income at the child's tax rate of 10 percent (or higher). This tax is added to the parental tax to arrive at the child's total tax.

In those situations where the parents are divorced, the parental tax is computed using the taxable income of the custodial parent (or joint income if he or she has remarried). Where the parents file separate returns, the tax is computed using the greater of the parents' two taxable incomes.

In computing the tax on the parent *including* the child's net unearned income, such income is not considered when computing any of the parents' deductions or credits (e.g., the deduction for miscellaneous itemized deductions, which is limited to the amount that exceeds two percent of adjusted gross income).

Where there is more than one child under 18 with net unearned income, the parental tax must be computed using the net unearned income of all children. As shown below, the tax so computed is then allocated pro rata based on each child's relative contribution to total net unearned income.

$$\frac{\text{Child's net unearned income}}{\text{All children's net unearned income}} \times \text{Parental tax} = \text{Child's share of parental tax}$$

---

[47] If the child has dividend income or long-term capital gains, such income continues to be taxed at the favorable rates at the parents' level. See Form 8615.

Example 29. During 2009, T, age 15, received $5,300 in interest from a savings account created for him in 2004 by his now deceased grandfather. Similarly, his sister, V, age 6, had $2,400 of interest income. Since T and V are under 19 and have net unearned income of $3,400 ($5,300 − $1,900) and $600 ($2,500 − $1,900), respectively, their tax must be computed in the special manner. The children's parents had income of $105,000. In addition, due to special medical problems of the father, they incurred $12,875 of medical expenses. The couple also has other itemized deductions of $10,000. T's tax is computed as follows:

1. Tax on parents computed in the normal manner:

Adjusted gross income	$105,000
Deductions:	
Medical expenses [$12,875 − (7.5% × $105,000 = $7,875)]	−5,000
Other itemized deductions	−10,000
Exemptions (4 × $3,650)	−14,600
Taxable income computed in the normal manner	$ 75,400
Tax [$9,350 + 25% ($75,400 − $67,900 = $7,500)]	$ 11,225

2. Tax on parents including net unearned income of all children:

Parents' taxable income computed in the normal manner	$ 75,400
Net unearned income of children:	
($3,400 + $600)	+4,000
Taxable income including net unearned income	$79,400
Tax [$9,350 + 25% ($79,400 − $67,900 = 11,500)]	$ 12,225

3. Parental tax:

Tax on parents including net unearned income	$ 12,225
−Tax on parents computed in the normal manner	−11,225
= Parental Tax	$ 1,000

4. T's share of parental tax [$1,000 × ($3,400 ÷ $4,000)] = $ 850

5. Tax on T excluding net unearned income:

Interest income	$ 5,200
− Net unearned income	−3,400
− Standard deduction (as limited for dependents)	−950
− Exemption deduction (none for dependents)	−0
Taxable income	$ 850
Tax (10% × $850)	$ 85

6. Total tax on T:

Tax on T excluding net unearned income	$ 85
+ Parental Tax	+850
= T's total tax	$ 935

Note that in this case the total parental tax of $1,000 is simply the product of the net unearned income of $4,000 ($3,400 + $600) and the parents' marginal tax rate of 25%. Also note that the parents' deduction for medical expenses is computed without including the net unearned income of the children (i.e., the percentage limitation is based on $105,000 rather than $109,000).

Election to Report Child's Income on Parents' Return. In order to simplify the return filing process, parents may elect to include on their own return the unearned income of a child if certain conditions are satisfied.[48] Note that this is contrary to the normal procedure where the child files his or her own return and pays the tax computed with respect to the parents' rates. This election eliminates the hassle of filing separate returns for each child. However, the election can only be made where the child is under age 18, his or her income is more than $950 and less than $9,000 in 2008, and it consists *solely* of interest and dividends. The election is not available if estimated taxes have been paid or taxes have been withheld on dividend or interest income (i.e., the child is subject to back-up withholding).

Although making the election may make it easier to file, it may not be wise. Inclusion of the child's income, increases the parents' A.G.I. and therefore may reduce the deductions and credits that are phased-out based on A.G.I.

DETERMINATION OF NET TAX DUE OR REFUND

Once the tax is determined using the tax tables, tax rate schedules, or the special tax computation procedures described above, it is reduced by the amount of any credits or prepayments. The primary prepayments are the Federal income tax withheld from the taxpayer's salary or wages by an employer, quarterly estimated tax payments, and the estimated tax paid when an extension of time to file a return is requested. Estimated tax payments and extensions of time to file are discussed later in this chapter.

Numerous credits are allowed in computing the Federal income tax. The credit most frequently encountered on an uncomplicated income tax return is the child care credit. This and other credits are discussed in detail in Chapter 13.

✓ CHECK YOUR KNOWLEDGE

Review Question 1. What are the top and bottom tax rates for individuals?

It depends on the year. For 2009, the lowest rate is 10 percent and the highest rate is 35 percent (on taxable income over $372,950 for Married Filing Jointly, Single or Head of Household).

Review Question 2. Several years ago Grandma gave her grandchild K, now 17, $20,000 to be used for her college education. All of the money was invested in stock. This year K's dad, acting on her behalf, sold some of the stock for a $4,050 short-term capital gain. K's parents are in the 35 percent tax bracket.

---

[48]   § 1(g)(7). The parents use Form 8814 for this purpose. If the child file his or her own return, the child uses Form 8615 to compute the tax.

a. Compute K's taxable income and K's tax.

Income (unearned)	$4,050
Standard deduction:	
Greater of $900 or $300 plus earned income	−950
Exemption	0
Taxable income.......................................	$3,100

K's personal exemption and standard deduction are limited since she can be claimed as a dependent on her parent's return. Consequently, she is not entitled to an exemption, and her standard deduction is $950 since she has no earned income. K is also subject to the kiddie tax since she is less than 19. In computing K's tax, the amount of unearned income in excess of $1,900 is $2,150 ($4,050 − $1,900), which must be taxed at her parents' rates while the remainder is taxed at her rates. Thus her tax is $848 [(35% × $2,150) + ($950 × 10%)].

b. Assume there were no kiddie tax. How much unearned income could be shifted to a dependent child and taxed at the child's 15 percent or lower rate rather than the parents' rate?

The 10 percent bracket for 2009 extends from taxable income of $1 to $8,350 and the 15 percent bracket extends from $8,351 to $33,950 for single taxpayers. Plus, another $950 escapes tax all together due to the child's standard deduction.

FILING REQUIREMENTS

Individual taxpayers with extremely low levels of income are not required to file a Federal income tax return. In general, a taxpayer is not required to file an income tax return for the year if his or her gross income is less than the *total* of his or her standard deduction (including the additional amount for the elderly but not the blind) *plus* personal exemptions (but not dependency exemptions).[49] These taxpayers generally are not liable for any Federal income tax. The filing requirement is based on gross income, so taxpayers who have gross incomes exceeding specified thresholds *must* file even if they owe no Federal income tax. A partial list of filing requirements for 2009 and how they are computed is illustrated in Exhibit 4-7.

In addition to the general requirement for filing (gross income is at least as much as the taxpayer's standard deduction + personal exemptions), certain individuals *must* file returns. These include:

---

[49] § 6012(a)(1).

EXHIBIT 4-7
Gross Income Filing Requirements for 2009

	Personal Exemption	+	Standard Deduction	+	Elderly Standard Deductions	=	2009 Gross Income
Single person < 65	$3,650		$ 5,700		—		$ 9,350
Single person ≥ 65	3,650		5,700		$1,400		10,750
Head of household < 65	3,650		8,350		—		12,000
Head of household ≥ 65	3,650		8,350		1,400		$13,400
Married filing jointly, both < 65	7,300		11,400		—		18,700
Married filing jointly, both ≥ 65	7,300		11,400		2,200		20,900
Married filing separately	3,650						3,650
Surviving spouse < 65	3,650		11,400		—		15,050
Surviving spouse ≥ 65	3,650		11,400		1,100		16,150
Dependents							Special Rules

1. Any taxpayer who has self-employment income of $400 or more

2. An individual who is claimed as a dependent on another taxpayer's return *and* who has unearned income at least equal to his or her minimum standard deduction (i.e., generally $950, but increased by the additional amount for elderly or blind taxpayers)[50]

3. Any person who receives any advance payments of earned income credit

Form 1040. The individual taxpayer is required to file Form 1040, along with related forms and schedules. A complicated return involves many forms and schedules in addition to the Form 1040, whereas a simpler return may require only a few or no attached schedules.

Two simplified forms are provided for taxpayers with uncomplicated tax calculations. The Form 1040EZ is available for taxpayers who are single or married filing jointly and have no dependents. To qualify, the taxpayer's income normally must consist only of salaries and wages plus interest income of $1,500 or less. The only allowable deductions on this form are the personal exemption amount and the standard deduction.

The Form 1040A is available for a large number of taxpayers who do not itemize their deductions and have no income other than salaries and wages, dividends, interest, and unemployment compensation. This form provides for deductions for individual retirement account (IRA) contributions, personal and dependency exemptions, and the earned income credit.

Example 30. Jeremy S. Allen, a registered nurse, and Shelly R. Allen, an air traffic controller, are married and file a joint income tax return for 2008. They are the sole support of their three children: William, Susan, and Gregory (all under age 17). The following information is from their records for 2008:

---

50   § 6012(a)(1)(C)(i). As stated earlier, certain children under the age of 19 are not required to file a tax return *if* their parents *elect* to include the child's income on their return and pay the appropriate additional tax.

Salaries and wages, Jeremy		$32,875
Federal income tax withheld	$1,700	
Salaries and wages, Shelly		44,900
Federal income tax withheld	2,400	
Interest income—Mercantile National Bank		1,800
Interest income—U.S. Government Bonds		700
Interest income—Ben Franklin Savings		500
Itemized deductions are as follows:		
Unreimbursed prescription drugs		200
Hospitalization insurance		700
Unreimbursed fees of doctors, hospitals, etc		2,100
Real estate taxes on residence		1,200
State income taxes paid		3,400
Interest paid on original home mortgage		8,500
Investment interest		400
Charitable contribution—First Church		1,300
Charitable contribution—Home State University		200
Preparation of prior year's tax return		275

The Allens' adjusted gross income is $80,775 ($32,875 + $44,900 + $3,000 interest income) since there were no deductions for A.G.I. The deductible amount of their itemized deductions is $15,000, summarized as follows:

Medical expenses exceeding $6,021	
[$3,000 < (7.5% × $80,775 = $6,058)]	$ 0
Deductible taxes ($1,200 + $3,400)	4,600
Qualifying home mortgage interest	8,500
Investment interest	400
Charitable contributions	1,500
Miscellaneous itemized deductions	
exceeding $1,616 [$275 < (2% × $80,775 = $1,616)]	0
Total itemized deductions	$15,000

The Allens' taxable income, gross tax, and tax refund for 2008 are determined as follows:

Adjusted gross income			$ 80,775
Less:	Itemized deductions	$ 15,000	
	Personal and dependency		
	exemptions ($3,500 × 5)	+17,500	−32,500
Equals: Taxable income			$ 48,275
Gross Tax (from 2008 Tax Table)			$ 6,439
Less:	Prepayments ($1,700 + $2,400)		−4,100
	Child tax credit (3 × $1,000)		−3,000
Equals: Tax due or (refund)			($ 661)

The Allens' completed 2008 tax return is shown in the Appendix at the end of the chapter. It consists of a Form 1040 plus Schedules A and B.

The more common tax forms and schedules used by individual taxpayers are listed in Exhibit 4-8. Copies of these forms are contained in Appendix B at the end of the text.

EXHIBIT 4-8
List of Common Forms and Schedules Used by Individual Taxpayers

Form 1040	**U.S. Individual Income Tax Return**

Accompanying Schedules:

Schedule A	Itemized deductions
Schedule B	Interest and dividend income
Schedule C	Profit (or loss) from business or profession
Schedule D	Capital gains and losses
Schedule E	Supplemental income schedule (rents, royalties, etc.)
Schedule F	Farm income and expenses
Schedule R	Credit for the elderly
Schedule SE	Computation of social security self-employment tax

Accompanying Forms:

Form 2106	Employee business expenses
Form 2210	Underpayment of estimated tax by individuals
Form 2441	Credit for child and dependent care expenses
Form 3800	General business credit
Form 3903	Moving expense adjustment
Form 4562	Depreciation
Form 4684	Casualties and thefts
Form 4797	Supplemental schedule of gains and losses
Form 6251	Alternative minimum tax computation
Form 6252	Computation of installment sale income
Form 8582	Passive activity losses
Form 8615	Computation of tax for children under age 18 who have investment income of more than $1,700
Form 8814	Parents' election to report child's interest and dividends

Other Common Forms:

Form 1040A	U.S. Individual Income Tax Return
Form 1040EZ	Income tax return for single filers with no dependents
Form 4868	Application for automatic extension of time to file

DUE DATES FOR FILING RETURNS

The day on which a Federal return must be filed with the IRS depends upon what type of return is involved. Generally the tax returns must be filed on or before the due dates, which are as follows:[51]

---

[51] § 6072(a).

Type of Return	Due Date
Annual Individual Income Tax Returns	Fifteenth day of the fourth month following the close of the tax year (April 15 for calendar year individuals)
Annual C Corporation and S Corporation Income Tax Returns	Fifteenth day of third month following the close of the tax year (March 15 for calendar year corporations)
Annual Partnership, Estate, and Trust Income Tax Returns	Fifteenth day of the fourth month following the close of the year (April 15 for calendar year entities)
Estate Tax Returns	Nine months after the date of the descedent's death
Gift Tax Returns	April 15 (All gift tax returns are for a calendar year)

Any return that is mailed via the U.S. Postal Service is deemed to be delivered when mailed, so any return postmarked on or before the above due dates is timely filed. If any of these due dates fall on Saturday, Sunday, or a legal holiday, the return must be filed on the succeeding day that is not a Saturday, Sunday, or legal holiday.

Extension of Time to File. The Internal Revenue Code provides extensions of time for filing returns. The extension must be requested on or before the due date of the return. Currently, there is an *automatic* six-month extension for filing the individual income tax return (Form 1040). Thus the extended due date for calendar year individuals is October 15. If the taxpayer desires to use the six-month extension, he or she simply fills out Form 4868 and mails it to the IRS by the original due date along with a check covering the estimated balance due. It should be noted that an extension of time to file is not an extension of time to pay. There is *no extension* of time to pay the tax due.[52] The penalty for failing to pay the tax due is discussed below.

The extensions for other taxpayers are designed so that the extended due date is one month before the extended due date for individuals. Thus C corporations and S corporations are entitled to a six-month extension for filing their returns, resulting in an extended due date for calendar year corporations of September 15. Partnerships and trusts are entitled to a five-month extension, resulting in an extended due of September 15 if the calendar year is used.

Interest. Whenever a taxpayer fails to pay the amount of tax owed by the due date of the return, interest is charged. To encourage payment, the rate is 3 percent higher than the Federal short-term rate. For the first quarter of 2009, the annual interest rate charge on such a deficiency is 5 percent (2% + 3%), compounded daily on the unpaid balance. Interest is generally charged from the day the tax is due (e.g., the due date of the return) and continues until the tax is paid.[53]

---

[52] Reg. § 1.6081-4(a).

[53] § 6601(a). The rate is based on the federal short-term rate. Generally, the government pays interest to taxpayers in the case of overpayments, beginning on the due date for the tax (usually the due date for the tax return). The rate of interest is the same as that on underpayments for noncorporate taxpayers. See § 6621.

PENALTIES

Around April 15, it is not uncommon to hear procrastinating taxpayers ask what happens if they neither file their returns nor pay their taxes on time. When either of these occurs, taxpayers not only have to pay interest but also penalties. There are three types of penalties that may apply:[54]

1. A penalty for *failure-to-file a return* by the due date;

2. A penalty for *failure-to-pay* at least 90 percent of the *tax* by the due date; and

3. A penalty for *failure to pay estimated taxes* during the course of the year.

If the taxpayer owes nothing or is entitled to a refund, these penalties do not apply even if he or she does not file a return. On the other hand, if the taxpayer has an amount due, any one or all three of these penalties could be imposed. In addition, since these penalties are technically additions to and part of the total tax liability, any interest that must be paid effectively includes *interest on the penalties*. Finally, if the taxpayer wants to obtain a refund, there are time limits for claiming it. Each of these possibilities is discussed below.

Failure-to-File. Taxpayers who do not file their returns by the due date (e.g., April 15) or fail to obtain a proper extension on such date are subject to the *failure-to-file penalty*. Under § 6651, the penalty is 5 percent of the amount of tax due for each month the return is not filed.[55] The penalty cannot exceed a maximum of 25 percent (e.g., 5% × 5 months). For this purpose, any fraction of a month is counted as a full month. To illustrate how harsh this rule can be, consider a taxpayer who owes $10,000 and his return is postmarked one day late. Even though the return is only one day late, the failure-to-file penalty is 5 percent for an entire month on the amount due or $500 (5% × 1 month × $10,000 amount due)!

To deal with the administrative costs of handling small penalties, a minimum penalty exists. If the return is more than 60 days late, the minimum penalty is $135 or 100% of the tax due, whichever is less.[56] For example, a taxpayer who owes $300 and files her return on June 16 would normally owe a penalty of $45 (5% × 3 months × $300) but the minimum penalty is $135 (the lesser of $135 or the tax due of $300).

Taxpayers who fail to file their returns may not be penalized in certain situations. The penalty is not imposed if the failure was due to reasonable cause and not willful neglect. In addition, since the penalty is based on the amount due no penalty results if there is no amount due. Because of this rule taxpayers who are entitled to a refund are not penalized for filing late since there is no amount due.

Failure-to-Pay Penalty. Filing a return is not enough to avoid penalty. Section 6651 also imposes a *failure-to-pay* penalty if a taxpayer does not pay at least 90 percent of the total tax on or before the due date of the return.[57] In other words, the IRS does not assess a penalty if an extension of time to file is properly obtained and the tax due is less than 10 percent of the total tax shown on the return (i.e., gross tax after credits but before any withholding and estimated tax payments). The penalty can also be avoided if the failure is due to reasonable cause and not willful neglect. If the taxpayer does not meet either test, the *failure-to-pay* penalty is one-half of 1 percent (.5% or .005) per month (or any fraction of a

---

[54] Technically, the Internal Revenue Code does not refer to these as penalties but as "additions to the tax." See §§ 6651 and 6654.

[55] § 6651(a)(1). If the failure to file is fraudulent, the penalty is 15 percent per month up to a maximum of 75 percent. § 6551(f).

[56] § 6651(a)(1)

[57] § 6651(a)(2)

month) up to a maximum 25 percent of the amount due.[58] Note that if the taxpayer files an extension and pays 90 percent of the tax by the due date, the taxpayer must still pay interest on any tax due but avoids both the failure-to-pay and failure-to-file penalties.

Example 31. As the time approached for filing his tax return, W was too busy to file. Accordingly, on April 15 he requested an automatic extension of time to file until October 15. W estimated that his total tax would be $6,000, and he had prepaid taxes of $5,300 in the form of withholding. Therefore, when he filed his request for an extension, he paid $700 ($6,000 − $5,300). By filing a timely extension, he is treated as filing a return and avoids the failure-to-file a return penalty. When he finally did file his return on June 15, W's earlier estimate proved wrong and the return showed a total tax of $7,000 and a tax due of $1,000 [$7,000 total tax due − $6,000 ($5,300 withholding + $700 payment with the extension)]. W is required to pay a penalty for failure-to-pay since the total paid by the due date, $6,000 is less than 90 percent of the tax due, $6,300 (90% × $7,000). The amount of the penalty is based on the total amount due that was unpaid on April 15, $1,000 ($7,000 − $6,000 paid) and not the amount short of the 90 percent requirement ($300). In addition, assuming the current rate of interest on underpayments is 10%, W must pay interest of about $17 ($1,000 amount due at 10% annually, compounded daily until June 15 for 61 days).

Interaction of Failure-to-Pay and Failure-to-File Penalties. When both the failure-to-file and failure-to-pay penalties apply, the penalty for failure-to-file to file is reduced by the amount of the penalty for failure to pay.

Example 32. K forgot to file her Federal tax return for the most recent calendar year. When she finally filed the return on November 1 (7 months late), her return showed a gross tax of $5,200 and a tax due after withholding of $600. Assuming the current rate of interest on underpayments is 10%, K must pay not only her tax due of $600 but also late penalties of $156 and interest on the tax and penalties of $41, for a total of $797, as computed below.

Tax due.		$600
Penalties:		
Failure to pay ($600 × .005 × 7)		21
Failure to file:		
Failure-to-file penalty ($600 × .05 × 5)	$150	
Reduced by failure-to-pay penalty		
($600 × .005 × 5).	(15)	135
Total tax and penalties		$756
Interest on tax and penalties ($756 × 10% × 199/365).		41
Total due		$797

Note that the minimum failure-to-file penalty is not triggered here since the penalty of $135 computed in the normal manner exceeds the minimum penalty of $100 (the lesser of the total tax due, $600, or $100).

Estimated Tax Payments. The last of the three "late" penalties is the penalty for failure to pay estimated taxes.[59] This penalty should be distinguished from the *failure-to-file* and *failure-to-pay* penalties that begin to run as of the due date of the return. The

---

[58] § 6651(a)(2)

[59] § 6654

estimated tax penalty applies if the taxpayer fails to pay sufficient taxes *during the year*. In essence, the law sets forth a series of intermediate due dates for estimated tax payments during the tax year.

The estimated tax penalty is a product of the "pay-as-you-go" system for collection of taxes. Under this system, taxpayers are required to prepay Federal income taxes periodically during the year. Prepayments are made through withholding from certain types of income (e.g., salary and wages) and by making estimated tax payments. Failure to make adequate payments during the year results in a penalty that is computed much like interest.

As a practical matter, estimated tax penalties do not affect the vast majority of individuals. For those receiving only salaries and wages, withholding is usually sufficient to cover the required payments. However, those taxpayers with other income may need to make up the shortfall by making estimated tax payments. Regardless of the causes, if the amount of taxes paid during the year is insufficient, the penalty may apply.

Imposition of the Estimated Tax Penalty. Individual taxpayers avoid the estimated tax penalty if total prepayments (estimated taxes and withholding) equal or exceed the *required annual payment*, which is the lesser of:[60]

1. 90% of the tax shown on the return, or

2. 100% of the tax shown on the return for the individual for the preceding year. If A.G.I. in the prior year exceeded $150,000, the payment must be 110% of the prior year's tax.

3. The annualized income installment

For this purpose, the tax due includes the self-employment tax as well as the alternative minimum tax and certain other taxes. If the total amounts paid are less than the amount due, an *underpayment* exists and the penalty must be calculated and paid as explained below. However, there is no estimated tax penalty if the underpayment is less than $1,000.[61]

> **Example 33.** For 2008, T, a single individual, reported an adjusted gross income of $165,000, a taxable income of $140,000, and a tax liability (after credits) of $40,000. In 2009 his tax liability is $60,000. Under the general rules T must have paid the lesser of 90% of the current year's tax, $54,000, or 100% of last year's tax, $40,000, to avoid the underpayment penalty. However, because T's adjusted gross income exceeded $150,000 in the prior year, 2008, he is subject to the 110% rule regarding his estimated tax payments for the current year, 2009. As a result, he can avoid underpayment penalties with respect to 2009 only if he pays the lesser of the following:
>
> | | |
> |---|---:|
> | 1. 90% of the current year's tax of $60,000 . . . . | $54,000 |
> | 2. 110% of last year's tax of $40,000 . . . . | 44,000 |
>
> Thus, if T pays at least $44,000 on a timely basis during 2009, he will not be subject to any penalty for failing to pay estimated taxes.

The required payment is due in four equal installments or 25 percent on each due date. Although it is convenient to say that the payments are made on a quarterly basis, this

---

[60] § 6654(d)

[61] § 6654(e)(1)

is not quite the case. For calendar year taxpayers, the amounts are due on April 15, June 15, September 15, and January 15.

Whether the payments are adequate is determined at the end of each "quarter." For this purpose, withholding is treated as if it occurred proportionately throughout the year. For example, if a taxpayer had withholding of $3,650, he or she would be treated as if $10 was withheld each day. At the end of each quarter, the payments to date are compared to the amount required to be paid. If the proper amount has not been paid, an underpayment exists and a penalty must be paid.

The penalty is assessed on the amount of the underpayment at the same rate as the interest that is charged on tax deficiencies. This penalty is separate from the failure-to-pay penalty as well as the interest which is charged. As noted earlier, interest and the failure-to-pay penalty apply to underpayments of tax due as of the due date of the return (e.g., April 15, 2010). In contrast, the estimated tax penalty is charged from the date each estimated tax installment was due (e.g., April 15, June 15, September 15 of *2009* and January 15, 2010) until the tax is paid (or, if the tax is paid late, the due date of the return).

Example 34. For 2008 and 2009 G's gross tax was $12,000 and $16,000, respectively. G's withholding for 2009 was $6,500 and his estimated tax payments were $1,500 on April 15 and June 15 and $500 on September 15 and January 15. G's underpayment is determined as follows:

	Payment Due Date			
	4/15	6/15	9/15	1/15
Percentage due....................	25%	50%	75%	100%
90% of current year's tax				
($16,000 × .90 × percentage due) ..	$ 3,600	$ 7,200	$ 10,800	$ 14,400
100% of prior year's tax				
($12,000 × percentage due)	$ 3,000	$ 6,000	$ 9,000	$ 12,000
Payments to date:				
Withholding.....................	$ 1,625	$ 3,250	$ 4,875	$ 6,500
Estimated tax payments	+1,500	+3,000	+3,500	+4,000
Total	$ 3,125	$ 6,250	$ 8,375	$ 10,500

G's payments are adequate for the first quarter and the second quarter, since the payments up to each date exceed the lesser of the two required amounts (the prior year's tax in both cases). As of the third payment date, G is underpaid by $625 ($9,000 − $8,375); and as of the last payment date, he is underpaid by $1,500 ($12,000 − $10,500). The penalty is computed based on these amounts from the due date until the day they are paid (or April 15, if earlier).

Assuming the current rate of penalty is 10% and G does not pay his tax early, G's penalty would be $58, which is the penalty on $625 from September 15 through January 15 [$625 × .1 × 122 days/365 days) = $21] *plus* that on $1,500 from January 15 through April 15 [$1,500 × (.1 × 90 days/365 days) = $37].

The penalty for failure to make adequate estimated tax payments is calculated on Form 2210 (see Appendix for a sample form). Unless a taxpayer can reduce the penalty by applying the annualized income installment or otherwise, he or she may simply let the IRS calculate this penalty and assess a deficiency for it. In addition, the IRS may waive the underpayment penalty in the event of a casualty or unusual circumstances where it might be inequitable to impose the additional tax. The IRS may also waive the penalty for retired taxpayers who are at least age 62 or disabled where the underpayment was due to reasonable cause rather than willful neglect.

Annualized Income Installment. If income for a year is earned disproportionately during the year, the taxpayer may be able to avoid penalty for one or more of the first three payments under the *annualized income installment* method.[62] Under this method, no penalty is imposed when the payment to date exceeds the tax which would be due on the income for the months preceding the payment date determined on an annualized basis.

Example 35. F, a calendar year individual, is engaged in a seasonal business that earns most of its income during the fourth quarter. F is able to demonstrate that the income was earned as follows:

	Payment Due Date			
	4/15	6/15	9/15	1/15
Months preceding payment	3	5	8	12
Net income earned for the months preceding the payment	$10,000	$18,000	$25,000	$50,000
Annualized amount [Net income × (12/months to date)].	$40,000	$43,200	$37,500	$50,000

To apply this exception, the tax on the annualized income is determined. There is an underpayment only if the estimated tax payments are less than the appropriate portion of the tax on the annualized income.

The required payment for April 15 is the fraction 3 months ÷ 12 months times the tax on $40,000. If the tax on $40,000 is $8,000, F has no underpayment for the first payment so long as she paid $2,000 ($8,000 × 3/12) or more. If she had paid less, the underpayment would be the amount by which $2,000 exceeded the payments. A similar process would be followed for each quarter.

To apply the annualized income installment calculations, a taxpayer completes a worksheet that accompanies the Form 2210. If this method is used to the benefit of the taxpayer for one payment, it must be used for *all* four payments.

Other Penalties. As mentioned in Chapter 2, many other penalties exist to ensure proper compliance with the tax laws. For example, the Code provides for an accuracy-related penalty of 20 percent of the amount of understatement due to negligence or intentional disregard of the rules (e.g., failing to report income), or substantial valuation misstatements.[63] In addition, severe penalties, both civil and criminal, exist for fraud.[64]

CLAIM FOR REFUND

The vast majority of taxpayers actually overpay their taxes and are entitled to a refund. For example, the IRS reported in 2005 that of the 134.3 million returns filed about 101.9 million (about 75 percent) claimed a refund. On average, this represented a refund of $2,287 per return. While most people routinely file their returns and receive their refund checks, others procrastinate. Unfortunately, some people assume it makes no difference how late they file if they wish to recover a refund. That can be a costly mistake. As a general rule, the Code requires taxpayers to file a tax return to claim a refund within two years of paying the tax, deemed to be April 15 in most cases.[65] Taxpayers who file a timely return, but subsequently realize that they overpaid, have a bit longer—three years from the due date of the return.

---

[62] § 6654(d).

[63] § 6653 (a)(1)

[64] § 6653(b)

[65] See § 6511 and § 6513

Example 36. With April 15, 2007 just a few days away, C made a few quick calculations regarding his 2006 tax liability and determined that his tax was $12,000. Knowing that he had $14,000 withheld and did not owe any tax, C did not file a return. C continued to put off filing a return until one day he received a letter from the IRS. In the letter dated November 2009, the IRS explained that based on information available to it C owed a tax of $1,500. In response, C finally filed a correct return on May 1, 2010, showing that he did in fact owe $12,000 in tax and the government should refund him his overpayment of $2,000. C is not entitled to any of the $2,000 refund. Since C did not file a timely return on April 15, 2007, the time for filing a refund claim expired two years from the date the tax was paid, April 15, 2009. By procrastinating, C lost his entire refund. Had he filed a timely return, the date for claiming the refund would have been three years after the return was filed or April 15, 2010.

The two year rule applies if the taxpayer did not file a return.[66] If a return was filed, a claim for a refund can be filed by the later of three years from the date of filing the original return (April 15 if filed before such date), or two years from the time the tax was paid. In situations where a return has been filed, the claim for refund usually arises from the filing of an amended individual income tax return (i.e., Form 1040X—see Appendix).

Example 37. K filed a timely return for 2008 on March 12, 2009. The total tax on the return was $5,500, and after withholdings of $4,700, K owed $800. K's return was audited and she was required to pay a deficiency of $200 on June 3, 2010. K may file a claim for refund for any part of the tax of $5,700 ($5,500 on the original return plus the additional tax of $200) until April 12, 2012 (three years from the date filed). A claim for up to $200 could be filed up until June 3, 2012 (two years from the date the $200 was paid).

EXHIBIT 4-9
Interest and Penalties

Description	Violation	Amount
Interest on underpayments	Insufficient payment on due date; applies to tax and penalties	3% + Fed short-term rate until paid
Failure to file	Tax return or extension not filed by due date	5% per month of amount due (maximum 25%) If more than 60 days late, minimum penalty is the smaller of $100 or 100% of the tax due
Failure to file (fraud)	Tax return or extension not filed by due date because of fraud	15% per month of amount due (maximum 75%)
Failure to pay tax	Fail to pay 90% of tax due on due date	0.5% per month of amount due (maximum 25%)
Failure to pay estimated taxes	Failure to pay 25% of required annual payment on 4/15, 6/15, 9/15 or 1/15	3% + Fed short-term rate until paid
Accuracy Related Fraud	Negligence or disregard of rules or regulations	20% of tax underpayment 75% of tax underpayment
Claim for refund	Filed later that 2 years after tax paid or 3 years after return filed	Loss of refund

66 *Comm. v. Lundy,* 116 116 S. Ct. 647, 77 AFTR2d 406, 96-1 USTC 50,035 (USSC, 1996).

STATUTE OF LIMITATIONS

Even in the administration of the Federal tax laws, all things must finally come to an end. As the U.S. Supreme Court has stated:

> Congress has regarded it as ill advised to have an income tax system under which there would never come a day of final settlement and which required both a taxpayer and the Government to stand ready forever and a day to produce vouchers, prove events, and recall details of all that goes into an income tax contest.[67]

Accordingly, there are certain time periods within which the IRS must take action *against* a taxpayer. If the Service does not take action within the prescribed time period, it is *barred* from pursuing the matter further. Technically the period in which an action must be commenced is called the Statute of Limitations. If the Statute of Limitations runs (expires) without any action on the part of the IRS, then the government is prohibited from assessing additional taxes for the expired periods.

Under the general rule, the IRS has three years from the date a return is filed to assess an additional tax liability against the taxpayer. If the tax return is filed before its due date, the three-year period for assessment begins *on* the due date.

> **Example 38.** R, a calendar year taxpayer, files a 2009 income tax return (due April 15) on March 8, 2010. The IRS will be prevented from assessing R additional taxes for 2009 any time after April 15, 2013.

> **Example 39.** Refer to *Example 38*. If R files a 2009 income tax return on October 15, 2010, the IRS may assess additional taxes for 2009 at any time through October 15, 2013.

There are several important exceptions to the three-year time period for assessing additional taxes. First, if the taxpayer has filed a false or a fraudulent return with the intention to *evade* the tax, then the tax may be assessed (or a proceeding may be initiated in court without assessment) at *any time* in the future. Similarly, if the taxpayer fails to file a return, the Statute of Limitations will not begin to run. Interestingly, a willful failure to file, a negligent failure to file, or an innocent failure to file are all treated the same. Thus, under any of these circumstances there is no limit to the time in which the IRS may make an assessment or begin a court proceeding against the taxpayer.

In the case of a *substantial omission of income* from a tax return, the Statute of Limitations is extended to six years. A substantial omission is defined as an omission of income in excess of 25% of the gross income *reported* on the return.[68] If the omission of gross income was committed with the intent of evading the tax, however, the assessment period would be unlimited.

> **Example 40.** T, a calendar year taxpayer, unintentionally failed to include $8,000 of dividends in his 2008 tax return filed on April 15, 2009. If the $8,000 omitted is more than 25% of the gross income reported on T's 2008 return, the IRS may assess an additional income tax liability against him at any time until after April 15, 2015.

[67] *Rothensies v. Electric Storage Battery Co.*, 47-1 USTC ¶9106, 35 AFTR 297, 329 U.S. 296, 301 (USSC, 1946).

[68] § 6501(e).

The periods within which assessments must be made are summarized in Exhibit 4-10, which follows.

EXHIBIT 4-10

Periods Within Which Assessments Must Be Made

Circumstances of Return	Period of Assessment
Normal return had been filed	Three years from date of filing or due date, whichever is later
Return filed with substantial omission of gross income	Six years from date of filing or due date, whichever is later
No return is filed	No time limit
False or fraudulent return	No time limit

INDEXATION AND THE FEDERAL INCOME TAX

Inflation has significant effects on a progressive tax rate structure stated in terms of a *constant* dollar. Taxpayers whose *real* incomes remain constant will have increasing levels of income, stated in terms of *nominal* dollars. Accordingly, their incomes will *creep up* into higher tax brackets. As an illustration, assume a taxpayer who earned $100,000 in 2007 is entitled to an annual raise at least equal to any increase in the Consumer Price Index (approximately four percent increase in 2007). Although his 2008 salary will creep up to $104,000, his before tax income in terms of 2007 prices remains at $100,000. At first glance, the taxpayer is as well off in 2008 as he was in 2007. Note, however, that the salary increase will be taxed at his marginal tax bracket, in which case he would have less after-tax income in real terms in 2008 than he had in 2007. Over time, this *bracket creep*, as it has been labeled, results in a larger portion of the taxpayer's earnings being paid to the Federal government. In effect, unlegislated tax increases occur.

For many years, Congress simply ignored the bracket creep phenomenon, choosing instead to allow the hidden tax increases to occur. As might be expected, this was a very palatable approach to politicians, particularly considering the alternative. The concerns of the few who objected were mollified in part by tax reduction packages enacted in 1981 and 1986. Both the Economic Recovery Tax Act of 1981 and the Tax Reform Act of 1986 directly reduced tax rates. These specific tax rate adjustments have since been followed by a permanent remedy for bracket creep: indexation.

Congress began adding the concept of indexation to the tax law in 1985. In 1986 it specified the amounts of the standard deduction, exemption amounts, and tax brackets for 1987 and 1988 (and the exemption amount for 1989). Thereafter, each of these amounts and many others have been annually adjusted for price level changes as measured by the Consumer Price Index.[69]

---

[69]   See §§ 1(f), 1(g)(4), 639(c)(4), and 151(d)(3).

✔️ CHECK YOUR KNOWLEDGE

Review Question 1. Z, age 16, earned $2,000 from umpiring baseball games and refereeing soccer matches during the year. Z—rather Z's parents—wants to know whether he is required to file a tax return since this was his only income.

A taxpayer normally is not required to file a return if his or her income is less than the sum of the personal exemption amount and the standard deduction. However, this general rule does not apply to an individual who can be claimed as a dependent on another return since he or she is not entitled to claim a personal exemption and the standard deduction may be limited. In this case, all of Z's income is earned income and is therefore offset by his standard deduction of $2,300 (in 2009 the greater of $950 or $300 plus earned income). Consequently, it seems that there is no need for him to file a return. However, even though he is not subject to the income tax, he still must consider self-employment taxes (assuming the income is self-employment income). A return is required if a taxpayer has self-employment income of at least $400. As a result, Z must file a return.

Review Question 2. After spending three years on the auditing staff of a large accounting firm, Norm took a job as controller of a small construction company. On the first day of the job, Norm looked around his new office and noticed a bunch of tax forms on the corner of his desk. One looked like the 1040 for his boss, and the others were corporate and partnership returns related to the company. At first he panicked. But then he realized that it was only the end of February and he had until April 15 to figure out what needed to be done. Should Norm relax?

Doubtful. Although returns for calendar year individuals and partnerships are normally due on April 15, the returns for C corporations or S corporations are due on March 15.

Review Question 3. As always, April 15 arrived and T had not even begun to prepare his tax return. Not to worry, he thought. He could simply file for an extension.

a.   Assume T does not file for an extension and simply files his return late. Are there any penalties?

Maybe. A failure-to-file as well as a failure-to-pay penalty may be imposed. Both penalties apply only if there is a tax due. If T is entitled to a refund, there is no penalty. The failure-to-file penalty is 5 percent per month on the balance due, not to exceed 25 percent.

b.   How long is the extension?

An automatic extension of six months until October 15 is available.

c.   Is an extension for time to file the return also an extension of time to pay the tax?

No. If T does not pay a sufficient amount of his tax by April 15, he faces penalties and interest imposed on the balance due.

d.   Assuming T's gross tax liability before withholding is $10,000, how much must he pay by April 15 in order to avoid penalty?

T must pay 90 percent of the gross tax, or $9,000, by April 15. Otherwise, a penalty of ½ of 1 percent per month is imposed (up to a maximum of 25 percent) on the entire underpayment from the due date of the return (April 15).

e. Assume that T's net tax due for the year is $10,000 and he never files a return or a proper extension. What is the maximum failure-to-file and failure-to-pay penalty that can be assessed (ignore any potential fraud penalty and interest)?

The maximum failure-to-file and failure-to-pay penalty in this case is $4,750 (47.5% × $10,000). The failure-to-file penalty is 5 percent per month up to a maximum of 25 percent reduced by .5 percent per month for any month in which the failure-to-pay penalty also applies. Thus, the maximum failure-to-file penalty when the failure-to-pay penalty also applies is 22.5 percent [(5 × 5% = 25%) − (5 × .05 = 2.5%)]. The maximum failure-to-pay penalty is .5 percent per month up to a maximum of 25 percent. Adding the two penalties together produces a maximum penalty for failure to file the return and failure to pay the tax of 47.5 percent (22.5% + 25%) of the amount due.

f. If T fails to pay his tax and he is subject to penalties, how does interest work? Must he pay interest on just the tax due or on both the tax and the penalties?

He pays interest not only on the tax due but also on the penalties since the penalties are considered an additional tax.

Review Question 4. Penalties for failing to file a return and failing to pay at least 90 percent of the tax due by the due date must be distinguished from penalties for failure to adequately make estimated tax payments during the year (underpayment penalties). Try the following true-false questions concerning estimated tax payments.

a. T finally filed her 2008 tax return and is now worrying about 2009. As a general rule, an individual taxpayer must pay 22.5 percent of her 2009 tax (even though she has no idea what it will be) 15 days after the end of each quarter (i.e., April 15, July 15, October 15, and January 15).

False. Although it is true that the taxpayer must normally pay 90 percent of the current tax due during the year (or 22.5 percent per installment), the installments are due on April 15, June 15, September 15, and January 15. Notwithstanding the fact that these payments are not truly paid on a quarterly basis, most people refer to them as "quarterly" estimated tax payments.

b. In lieu of paying 90 percent of their tax liability, individual taxpayers may avoid the underpayment penalty by paying 90 percent of last year's tax liability.

False. Penalty can be avoided if the taxpayer pays 90 percent of the current year's tax or 100 percent of last year's tax. However, the 100 percent rule is increased to 110 percent if the taxpayer's adjusted gross income in the prior year exceeded $150,000.

c. T earns a salary but also does some tinkering in the stock market. In October she realized that she should have paid estimated taxes throughout the year given what her income was going to be. Asking her employer to withhold an extra $36,500 in taxes during October, November, and December will help solve T's estimated tax problems for April, June, and September.

True. Withholding is treated as being paid ratably throughout the year. Therefore the additional $36,500 is not simply applied to the later due dates. Instead, T is treated as having paid $100 per day each day of the year. For example, she is treated as having paid an additional $10,500 (105 × $100) on April 15.

Review Question 5. T filed her 2008 tax return on March 15, 2009. The IRS is barred from assessing a deficiency after

  a. March 15, 2011
  b. March 15, 2012
  c. March 15, 2013
  d. April 15, 2012
  e. April 15, 2013

d. The statue of limitations runs out on April 15, 2012, three years from the later of the due date or the date of filing.

APPENDIX

TAX RETURN ILLUSTRATIONS

The following pages provide realistic examples of uncomplicated tax returns for individual taxpayers. The information from *Examples 23, 24, and 30* of this chapter is used.

Form **1040EZ**

Department of the Treasury—Internal Revenue Service

Income Tax Return for Single and Joint Filers With No Dependents (99) **2008**

OMB No. 1545-0074

Label

(See page 9.)

Use the IRS label.

Otherwise, please print or type.

Presidential Election Campaign (page 9)

Your first name and initial	Last name	Your social security number
William W.	Bristol	187 52 5034
If a joint return, spouse's first name and initial	Last name	Spouse's social security number

Home address (number and street). If you have a P.O. box, see page 9.   Apt. no.

651 South Hampton

City, town or post office, state, and ZIP code. If you have a foreign address, see page 9.

Blue Springs, MO 64015

▲ You **must** enter your SSN(s) above. ▲

Checking a box below will not change your tax or refund.

Check here if you, or your spouse if a joint return, want $3 to go to this fund . . . ▶ ☐ **You**   ☐ **Spouse**

Income

Attach Form(s) W-2 here.

Enclose, but do not attach, any payment.

1	Wages, salaries, and tips. This should be shown in box 1 of your Form(s) W-2. Attach your Form(s) W-2.	1	27,410
2	Taxable interest. If the total is over $1,500, you cannot use Form 1040EZ.	2	350
3	Unemployment compensation and Alaska Permanent Fund dividends (see page 11).	3	
4	Add lines 1, 2, and 3. This is your **adjusted gross income.**	4	27,760
5	If someone can claim you (or your spouse if a joint return) as a dependent, check the applicable box(es) below and enter the amount from the worksheet on back. ☐ **You** ☐ **Spouse** If no one can claim you (or your spouse if a joint return), enter $8,950 if **single**; $17,900 if **married filing jointly.** See back for explanation.	5	8,950
6	Subtract line 5 from line 4. If line 5 is larger than line 4, enter -0-. This is your **taxable income.** ▶	6	18,810

Payments and tax

7	Federal income tax withheld from box 2 of your Form(s) W-2.	7	2,820
8a	**Earned income credit (EIC)** (see page 12).	8a	
b	Nontaxable combat pay election. 8b		
9	Recovery rebate credit (see worksheet on pages 17 and 18).	9	
10	Add lines 7, 8a, and 9. These are your **total payments.** ▶	10	2,820
11	**Tax.** Use the amount on **line 6 above** to find your tax in the tax table on pages 28–36 of the booklet. Then, enter the tax from the table on this line.	11	2,423

Refund

Have it directly deposited! See page 18 and fill in 12b, 12c, and 12d or Form 8888.

12a	If line 10 is larger than line 11, subtract line 11 from line 10. This is your **refund.** If Form 8888 is attached, check here ▶ ☐	12a	397

▶ b Routing number   X X X X X X X X   ▶ c Type: ☐ Checking   ☐ Savings

▶ d Account number   X X X X X X X X X X X X X X X X X

Amount you owe

13	If line 11 is larger than line 10, subtract line 10 from line 11. This is the **amount you owe.** For details on how to pay, see page 19. ▶	13	

Third party designee

Do you want to allow another person to discuss this return with the IRS (see page 20)? ☐ **Yes.** Complete the following. ☑ **No**

Designee's name ▶	Phone no. ▶ ( )	Personal identification number (PIN) ▶	

Sign here

Joint return? See page 6.

Keep a copy for your records.

Under penalties of perjury, I declare that I have examined this return, and to the best of my knowledge and belief, it is true, correct, and accurately lists all amounts and sources of income I received during the tax year. Declaration of preparer (other than the taxpayer) is based on all information of which the preparer has any knowledge.

Your signature	Date	Your occupation Restaurant Manager	Daytime phone number (816) 229-1207
Spouse's signature. If a joint return, **both** must sign.	Date	Spouse's occupation	

Paid preparer's use only

Preparer's signature ▶	Date	Check if self-employed ☐	Preparer's SSN or PTIN
Firm's name (or yours if self-employed), address, and ZIP code ▶		EIN	
		Phone no. ( )	

For Disclosure, Privacy Act, and Paperwork Reduction Act Notice, see page 37.

Cat. No. 11329W

Form **1040EZ** (2008)

Form
1040A

Department of the Treasury—Internal Revenue Service

U.S. Individual Income Tax Return (99) **2008**   IRS Use Only—Do not write or staple in this space.

OMB No. 1545-0074

Label
(See page 17.)

Use the IRS label.
Otherwise, please print or type.

Presidential Election Campaign ▶ Check here if you, or your spouse if filing jointly, want $3 to go to this fund (see page 17) ▶ ☐ **You** ☐ **Spouse**

Your first name and initial	Last name
Clyde F.	*Cooper*
If a joint return, spouse's first name and initial	Last name
Delia C.	*Cooper*

Home address (number and street). If you have a P.O. box, see page 17. *1234 Fine Street*   Apt. no.

City, town or post office, state, and ZIP code. If you have a foreign address, see page 17. *Desirable, OK 66987*

Your social security number: 234 56 7850
Spouse's social security number: 345 67 8901

▲ You **must** enter your SSN(s) above. ▲

Checking a box below will not change your tax or refund.

Filing status
Check only one box.

1 ☐ Single
2 ☑ Married filing jointly (even if only one had income)
3 ☐ Married filing separately. Enter spouse's SSN above and full name here. ▶
4 ☐ Head of household (with qualifying person). (See page 18.) If the qualifying person is a child but not your dependent, enter this child's name here. ▶
5 ☐ Qualifying widow(er) with dependent child (see page 19)

Exemptions

6a ☑ **Yourself.** If someone can claim you as a dependent, **do not** check box 6a.

b ☑ **Spouse**

c **Dependents:**

(1) First name Last name	(2) Dependent's social security number	(3) Dependent's relationship to you	(4) ✓ if qualifying child for child tax credit (see page 20)
Gary Cooper	777 99 6451	*Son*	☑
Debra Cooper	564 99 8765	*Daughter*	☑
			☐
			☐
			☐
			☐

If more than six dependents, see page 20.

Boxes checked on 6a and 6b: **2**
No. of children on 6c who:
• lived with you: **2**
• did not live with you due to divorce or separation (see page 21)
Dependents on 6c not entered above
Add numbers on lines above ▶ **4**

d Total number of exemptions claimed.

Income

Attach Form(s) W-2 here. Also attach Form(s) 1099-R if tax was withheld.

If you did not get a W-2, see page 23.

Enclose, but do not attach, any payment.

7	Wages, salaries, tips, etc. Attach Form(s) W-2.	7	*57,045*
8a	**Taxable** interest. Attach Schedule 1 if required.	8a	*1,500*
b	**Tax-exempt** interest. **Do not** include on line 8a. 8b		
9a	Ordinary dividends. Attach Schedule 1 if required.	9a	
b	Qualified dividends (see page 24). 9b		
10	Capital gain distributions (see page 24).	10	
11a	IRA distributions. 11a	**11b** Taxable amount (see page 24). 11b	
12a	Pensions and annuities. 12a	**12b** Taxable amount (see page 25). 12b	
13	Unemployment compensation and Alaska Permanent Fund dividends.	13	
14a	Social security benefits. 14a	**14b** Taxable amount (see page 27). 14b	
15	Add lines 7 through 14b (far right column). This is your **total income.** ▶	15	*58,545*

Adjusted gross income

16	Educator expenses (see page 29). 16		
17	IRA deduction (see page 29). 17	*4,000*	
18	Student loan interest deduction (see page 31). 18		
19	Tuition and fees deduction. Attach Form 8917. 19		
20	Add lines 16 through 19. These are your **total adjustments.**	20	*4,000*
21	Subtract line 20 from line 15. This is your **adjusted gross income.** ▶	21	*54,545*

For Disclosure, Privacy Act, and Paperwork Reduction Act Notice, see page 78.   Cat. No. 11327A   Form **1040A** (2008)

Form 1040A (2008)   Page **2**

Tax, credits, and payments	**22**	Enter the amount from line 21 (adjusted gross income).	22	*54,545*

23a Check if: { ☐ **You** were born before January 2, 1944, ☐ Blind } **Total boxes** { ☐ **Spouse** was born before January 2, 1944, ☐ Blind } **checked** ▶ 23a ☐

b If you are married filing separately and your spouse itemizes deductions, see page 32 and check here ▶ 23b ☐

c Check if standard deduction includes real estate taxes (see page 32) ▶ 23c ☐

24 Enter your **standard deduction** (see left margin).	24	*10,900*
25 Subtract line 24 from line 22. If line 24 is more than line 22, enter -0-.	25	*43,645*
26 If line 22 is over $119,975, or you provided housing to a Midwestern displaced individual, see page 32. Otherwise, multiply $3,500 by the total number of exemptions claimed on line 6d.	26	*14,000*
27 Subtract line 26 from line 25. If line 26 is more than line 25, enter -0-. This is your **taxable income.** ▶	27	*29,645*
28 **Tax,** including any alternative minimum tax (see page 33).	28	*3,641*

Standard Deduction for—

• People who checked any box on line 23a, 23b, or 23c **or** who can be claimed as a dependent, see page 32.

• All others:

Single or Married filing separately, $5,450

Married filing jointly or Qualifying widow(er), $10,900

Head of household, $8,000

29 Credit for child and dependent care expenses. Attach Schedule 2.	29	*700*	
30 Credit for the elderly or the disabled. Attach Schedule 3.	30		
31 Education credits. Attach Form 8863.	31		
32 Retirement savings contributions credit. Attach Form 8880.	32		
33 Child tax credit (see page 37). Attach Form 8901 if required.	33	*2,000*	
34 Add lines 29 through 33. These are your **total credits.**		34	*2,700*
35 Subtract line 34 from line 28. If line 34 is more than line 28, enter -0-.		35	*941*
36 Advance earned income credit payments from Form(s) W-2, box 9.		36	
37 Add lines 35 and 36. This is your **total tax.** ▶		37	*941*
38 Federal income tax withheld from Forms W-2 and 1099.	38	*1,950*	
39 2008 estimated tax payments and amount applied from 2007 return.	39		
40a **Earned income credit (EIC).**	40a		
b Nontaxable combat pay election. 40b			
41 Additional child tax credit. Attach Form 8812.	41		
42 Recovery rebate credit (see worksheet on pages 53 and 54).	42		
43 Add lines 38, 39, 40a, 41, and 42. These are your **total payments.** ▶		43	*1,950*

If you have a qualifying child, attach Schedule EIC.

Refund

Direct deposit? See page 55 and fill in 45b, 45c, and 45d or Form 8888.

44 If line 43 is more than line 37, subtract line 37 from line 43. This is the amount you **overpaid.**		44	*1,009*
45a Amount of line 44 you want **refunded to you.** If Form 8888 is attached, check here ▶ ☐		45a	*1,009*

▶ b Routing number ▐x▐x▐x▐x▐x▐x▐x▐x▐ ▶ **c** Type: ☐ Checking ☐ Savings

▶ d Account number ▐x▐x▐x▐x▐x▐x▐x▐x▐x▐x▐x▐x▐x▐x▐x▐x▐x▐

46 Amount of line 44 you want **applied to your 2009 estimated tax.** 46	

Amount you owe

47 **Amount you owe.** Subtract line 43 from line 37. For details on how to pay, see page 56. ▶		47	
48 Estimated tax penalty (see page 57). 48			

Third party designee

Do you want to allow another person to discuss this return with the IRS (see page 57)? ☐ **Yes.** Complete the following. ☑ **No**

Designee's name ▶ _____ Phone no. ▶ ( ) Personal identification number (PIN) ▶ ☐☐☐☐☐

Sign here

Joint return? See page 17.

Keep a copy for your records.

Under penalties of perjury, I declare that I have examined this return and accompanying schedules and statements, and to the best of my knowledge and belief, they are true, correct, and accurately list all amounts and sources of income I received during the tax year. Declaration of preparer (other than the taxpayer) is based on all information of which the preparer has any knowledge.

Your signature	Date	Your occupation	Daytime phone number
		Professional Model	( )
Spouse's signature. If a joint return, **both** must sign.	Date	Spouse's occupation	
		Programmer	

Paid preparer's use only

Preparer's signature ▶	Date	Check if self-employed ☐	Preparer's SSN or PTIN
Firm's name (or yours if self-employed), address, and ZIP code ▶		EIN	
		Phone no.	( )

Form **1040A** (2008)

Schedule 2
(Form 1040A)

Department of the Treasury—Internal Revenue Service

Child and Dependent Care Expenses for Form 1040A Filers (99) **2008**

OMB No. 1545-0074

Name(s) shown on Form 1040A

CLYDE F & CORDELIA C COOPER

Your social security number

234 : 56 : 7890

Part I

Persons or organizations who provided the care

You **must** complete this part.

1

(a) Care provider's name	(b) Address (number, street, apt. no., city, state, and ZIP code)	(c) Identifying number (SSN or EIN)	(d) Amount paid (see instructions)	
HAPPY TRAILS PRESCHOOL	*2391 BRONCO STREET DESIRABLE, OK 66789*	*44-5678656*	*3,500*	

(If you have more than two care providers, see the instructions.)

Did you receive **dependent care benefits?**

No ──────► Complete only Part II below.

Yes ──────► Complete Part III on the back next.

Caution. If the care was provided in your home, you may owe employment taxes. If you do, you must use Form 1040. See **Schedule H** and its instructions for details.

Part II

Credit for child and dependent care expenses

2 Information about your **qualifying person(s).** If you have more than two qualifying persons, see the instructions.

(a) Qualifying person's name		(b) Qualifying person's social security number			(c) Qualified expenses you incurred and paid in 2008 for the person listed in column (a)
First	Last				
GARY	*COOPER*	*777*	*99*	*6451*	*1,750*
DEBRA	*COOPER*	*564*	*99*	*8765*	*1,750*

3 Add the amounts in column (c) of line 2. **Do not** enter more than $3,000 for one qualifying person or $6,000 for two or more persons. If you completed Part III, enter the amount from line 27. — **3** — *3,500*

4 Enter your **earned income.** See the instructions. — **4** — *33,445*

5 If married filing jointly, enter your spouse's earned income (if your spouse was a student or was disabled, see the instructions); **all others,** enter the amount from line 4. — **5** — *23,600*

6 Enter the **smallest** of line 3, 4, or 5. — **6** — *3,500*

7 Enter the amount from Form 1040A, line 22. **7** *54,545*

8 Enter on line 8 the decimal amount shown below that applies to the amount on line 7.

If line 7 is:			If line 7 is:		
Over	But not over	Decimal amount is	Over	But not over	Decimal amount is
$0—15,000		.35	$29,000—31,000		.27
15,000—17,000		.34	31,000—33,000		.26
17,000—19,000		.33	33,000—35,000		.25
19,000—21,000		.32	35,000—37,000		.24
21,000—23,000		.31	37,000—39,000		.23
23,000—25,000		.30	39,000—41,000		.22
25,000—27,000		.29	41,000—43,000		.21
27,000—29,000		.28	43,000—No limit		.20

8 × *.20*

9 Multiply **line 6** by the decimal amount on line 8. If you paid 2007 expenses in 2008, see the instructions. — **9** — *700*

10 Enter the amount from Form 1040A, line 28. — **10** — *3,641*

11 **Credit for child and dependent care expenses.** Enter the **smaller** of line 9 or line 10 here and on Form 1040A, line 29. — **11** — *700*

For Paperwork Reduction Act Notice, see Form 1040A instructions.   Cat. No. 10749I   Schedule 2 (Form 1040A) 2008

Form **1040**

Department of the Treasury—Internal Revenue Service

U.S. Individual Income Tax Return **2008** (99) IRS Use Only—Do not write or staple in this space.

For the year Jan. 1–Dec. 31, 2008, or other tax year beginning , 2008, ending , 20

OMB No. 1545-0074

Label
(See instructions on page 14.)
Use the IRS label. Otherwise, please print or type.

Presidential Election Campaign ▶

Your first name and initial	Last name
Jeremy S.	*Allen*
If a joint return, spouse's first name and initial	Last name
Shelly R.	*Allen*

Home address (number and street). If you have a P.O. box, see page 14. **Apt. no.**
8473 Smithson Place

City, town or post office, state, and ZIP code. If you have a foreign address, see page 14.
Boring, OR 97832

Your social security number: 123 : 45 : 9875

Spouse's social security number: 456 : 85 : 2447

▲ You **must** enter your SSN(s) above. ▲

Checking a box below will not change your tax or refund.

Check here if you, or your spouse if filing jointly, want $3 to go to this fund (see page 14) ▶ ☐ **You** ☐ **Spouse**

Filing Status

Check only one box.

1. ☐ Single
2. ☑ Married filing jointly (even if only one had income)
3. ☐ Married filing separately. Enter spouse's SSN above and full name here. ▶
4. ☐ Head of household (with qualifying person). (See page 15.) If the qualifying person is a child but not your dependent, enter this child's name here. ▶
5. ☐ Qualifying widow(er) with dependent child (see page 16)

Exemptions

If more than four dependents, see page 17.

6a. ☑ **Yourself.** If someone can claim you as a dependent, **do not** check box 6a
  b. ☑ Spouse
  c. **Dependents:**

(1) First name Last name	(2) Dependent's social security number	(3) Dependent's relationship to you	(4)☑ if qualifying child for child tax credit (see page 17)
William Allen	789 : 65 : 4321	*Son*	☑
Susan Allen	456 : 65 : 9876	*Daughter*	☑
Gregory Allen	321 : 72 : 9347	*Son*	☑
	: :		☐

  d. Total number of exemptions claimed

Boxes checked on 6a and 6b: **2**

No. of children on 6c who:
• lived with you: **3**
• did not live with you due to divorce or separation (see page 18):

Dependents on 6c not entered above:

Add numbers on lines above ▶ **5**

Income

Attach Form(s) W-2 here. Also attach Forms W-2G and 1099-R if tax was withheld.

If you did not get a W-2, see page 21.

Enclose, but do not attach, any payment. Also, please use Form 1040-V.

7	Wages, salaries, tips, etc. Attach Form(s) W-2	7	*77,775*
8a	**Taxable** interest. Attach Schedule B if required	8a	*3,000*
b	Tax-exempt interest. **Do not** include on line 8a	8b	
9a	Ordinary dividends. Attach Schedule B if required	9a	
b	Qualified dividends (see page 21)	9b	
10	Taxable refunds, credits, or offsets of state and local income taxes (see page 22)	10	
11	Alimony received	11	
12	Business income or (loss). Attach Schedule C or C-EZ	12	
13	Capital gain or (loss). Attach Schedule D if required. If not required, check here ▶ ☐	13	
14	Other gains or (losses). Attach Form 4797	14	
15a	IRA distributions 15a **b** Taxable amount (see page 23)	15b	
16a	Pensions and annuities 16a **b** Taxable amount (see page 24)	16b	
17	Rental real estate, royalties, partnerships, S corporations, trusts, etc. Attach Schedule E	17	
18	Farm income or (loss). Attach Schedule F	18	
19	Unemployment compensation	19	
20a	Social security benefits 20a **b** Taxable amount (see page 26)	20b	
21	Other income. List type and amount (see page 28)	21	
22	Add the amounts in the far right column for lines 7 through 21. This is your **total income** ▶	22	*80,775*

Adjusted Gross Income

23	Educator expenses (see page 28)	23	
24	Certain business expenses of reservists, performing artists, and fee-basis government officials. Attach Form 2106 or 2106-EZ	24	
25	Health savings account deduction. Attach Form 8889	25	
26	Moving expenses. Attach Form 3903	26	
27	One-half of self-employment tax. Attach Schedule SE	27	
28	Self-employed SEP, SIMPLE, and qualified plans	28	
29	Self-employed health insurance deduction (see page 29)	29	
30	Penalty on early withdrawal of savings	30	
31a	Alimony paid **b** Recipient's SSN ▶	31a	
32	IRA deduction (see page 30)	32	
33	Student loan interest deduction (see page 33)	33	
34	Tuition and fees deduction. Attach Form 8917	34	
35	Domestic production activities deduction. Attach Form 8903	35	
36	Add lines 23 through 31a and 32 through 35	36	
37	Subtract line 36 from line 22. This is your **adjusted gross income** ▶	37	*80,775*

For Disclosure, Privacy Act, and Paperwork Reduction Act Notice, see page 88. Cat. No. 11320B Form **1040** (2008)

Form 1040 (2008)   Page **2**

Tax and Credits	38	Amount from line 37 (adjusted gross income)		38	80,775

39a Check { ☐ **You** were born before January 2, 1944,   ☐ Blind. } **Total boxes**
if: { ☐ **Spouse** was born before January 2, 1944,   ☐ Blind. } checked ▶ 39a

b If your spouse itemizes on a separate return or you were a dual-status alien, see page 34 and check here ▶ 39b ☐

c Check if standard deduction includes real estate taxes or disaster loss (see page 34) ▶ 39c ☐

Standard Deduction for—	40	**Itemized deductions** (from Schedule A) **or** your **standard deduction** (see left margin) .	40	15,000
	41	Subtract line 40 from line 38	41	65,775
• People who checked any box on line 39a, 39b, or 39c **or** who can be claimed as a dependent, see page 34.	42	If line 38 is over $119,975, or you provided housing to a Midwestern displaced individual, see page 36. Otherwise, multiply $3,500 by the total number of exemptions claimed on line 6d	42	17,500
	43	**Taxable income.** Subtract line 42 from line 41. If line 42 is more than line 41, enter -0-	43	48,275
	44	**Tax** (see page 36). Check if any tax is from: a ☐ Form(s) 8814 b ☐ Form 4972 .	44	6,439
• All others:	45	**Alternative minimum tax** (see page 39). Attach Form 6251	45	
Single or Married filing separately, $5,450	46	Add lines 44 and 45 . . . . ▶	46	6,439

47 Foreign tax credit. Attach Form 1116 if required . . . | 47 |
48 Credit for child and dependent care expenses. Attach Form 2441 | 48 |
49 Credit for the elderly or the disabled. Attach Schedule R . | 49 |
50 Education credits. Attach Form 8863 . . . . . . | 50 |
51 Retirement savings contributions credit. Attach Form 8880 . | 51 |
52 Child tax credit (see page 42). Attach Form 8901 if required . | 52 | 3,000 |
53 Credits from Form: a ☐ 8396 b ☐ 8839 c ☐ 5695 . | 53 |
54 Other credits from Form: a ☐ 3800 b ☐ 8801 c ☐ | 54 |

Married filing jointly or Qualifying widow(er), $10,900

Head of household, $8,000

55	Add lines 47 through 54. These are your **total credits**	55	3,000
56	Subtract line 55 from line 46. If line 55 is more than line 46, enter -0- . . . . ▶	56	3,439

Other Taxes	57	Self-employment tax. Attach Schedule SE	57
	58	Unreported social security and Medicare tax from Form: a ☐ 4137 b ☐ 8919 .	58
	59	Additional tax on IRAs, other qualified retirement plans, etc. Attach Form 5329 if required .	59
	60	Additional taxes: a ☐ AEIC payments b ☐ Household employment taxes. Attach Schedule H	60
	61	Add lines 56 through 60. This is your **total tax** . . . . . . ▶	61	3,439

Payments	62	Federal income tax withheld from Forms W-2 and 1099 .	62	4,100
	63	2008 estimated tax payments and amount applied from 2007 return	63	
If you have a qualifying child, attach Schedule EIC.	64a	**Earned income credit (EIC)**	64a	
	b	Nontaxable combat pay election	64b	
	65	Excess social security and tier 1 RRTA tax withheld (see page 61)	65	
	66	Additional child tax credit. Attach Form 8812	66	
	67	Amount paid with request for extension to file (see page 61)	67	
	68	Credits from Form: a ☐ 2439 b ☐ 4136 c ☐ 8801 d ☐ 8885	68	
	69	First-time homebuyer credit. Attach Form 5405	69	
	70	Recovery rebate credit (see worksheet on pages 62 and 63) .	70	
	71	Add lines 62 through 70. These are your **total payments** . . . . . . ▶	71	4,100

Refund	72	If line 71 is more than line 61, subtract line 61 from line 71. This is the amount you **overpaid**	72	661
Direct deposit? See page 63 and fill in 73b, 73c, and 73d, or Form 8888.	73a	Amount of line 72 you want **refunded to you.** If Form 8888 is attached, check here ▶ ☐	73a	661
	▶ b	Routing number X X X X X X X X ▶ c Type: ☐ Checking ☐ Savings		
	▶ d	Account number X X X X X X X X X X X X X X X X X		
	74	Amount of line 72 you want **applied to your 2009 estimated tax** ▶ 74		

Amount You Owe	75	**Amount you owe.** Subtract line 71 from line 61. For details on how to pay, see page 65 ▶	75	
	76	Estimated tax penalty (see page 65) 76		

Third Party Designee   Do you want to allow another person to discuss this return with the IRS (see page 66)? ☐ **Yes.** Complete the following. ☑ **No**

Designee's name ▶   Phone no. ▶ (   )   Personal identification number (PIN) ▶

Sign Here
Under penalties of perjury, I declare that I have examined this return and accompanying schedules and statements, and to the best of my knowledge and belief, they are true, correct, and complete. Declaration of preparer (other than taxpayer) is based on all information of which preparer has any knowledge.

Joint return? See page 15.

Keep a copy for your records.

Your signature	Date	Your occupation	Daytime phone number
		Registered Nurse	( )
Spouse's signature. If a joint return, **both** must sign.	Date	Spouse's occupation	
		Air Traffic Controller	

Paid Preparer's Use Only

Preparer's signature ▶	Date	Check if self-employed ☐	Preparer's SSN or PTIN
Firm's name (or yours if self-employed), address, and ZIP code ▶		EIN	
		Phone no. ( )	

Form **1040** (2008)

SCHEDULES A&B (Form 1040) Department of the Treasury Internal Revenue Service (99)	**Schedule A—Itemized Deductions** (Schedule B is on back) ▶ **Attach to Form 1040.** ▶ **See Instructions for Schedules A&B (Form 1040).**	OMB No. 1545-0074 20**08** Attachment Sequence No. **07**

Name(s) shown on Form 1040

Jeremy S & Shelly R Allen

Your social security number: 123 : 45 : 9875

Medical and Dental Expenses		**Caution.** Do not include expenses reimbursed or paid by others.				
	1	Medical and dental expenses (see page A-1).	1	3,000		
	2	Enter amount from Form 1040, line 38 2 80,775				
	3	Multiply line 2 by 7.5% (.075)	3	6,058		
	4	Subtract line 3 from line 1. If line 3 is more than line 1, enter -0-.			4	0
Taxes You Paid (See page A-2.)	5	State and local (check only one box): a ☐ Income taxes, or b ☐ General sales taxes	5	3,400		
	6	Real estate taxes (see page A-5)	6	1,200		
	7	Personal property taxes	7			
	8	Other taxes. List type and amount ▶ _____	8			
	9	Add lines 5 through 8			9	4,600
Interest You Paid (See page A-5.) **Note.** Personal interest is not deductible.	10	Home mortgage interest and points reported to you on Form 1098	10	8,500		
	11	Home mortgage interest not reported to you on Form 1098. If paid to the person from whom you bought the home, see page A-6 and show that person's name, identifying no., and address ▶ _____	11			
	12	Points not reported to you on Form 1098. See page A-6 for special rules.	12			
	13	Qualified mortgage insurance premiums (see page A-6)	13			
	14	Investment interest. Attach Form 4952 if required. (See page A-6.)	14	400		
	15	Add lines 10 through 14			15	8,900
Gifts to Charity If you made a gift and got a benefit for it, see page A-7.	16	Gifts by cash or check. If you made any gift of $250 or more, see page A-7	16	1,500		
	17	Other than by cash or check. If any gift of $250 or more, see page A-8. You **must** attach Form 8283 if over $500	17			
	18	Carryover from prior year	18			
	19	Add lines 16 through 18			19	1,500
Casualty and Theft Losses	20	Casualty or theft loss(es). Attach Form 4684. (See page A-8.)			20	
Job Expenses and Certain Miscellaneous Deductions (See page A-9.)	21	Unreimbursed employee expenses—job travel, union dues, job education, etc. Attach Form 2106 or 2106-EZ if required. (See page A-9.) ▶ _____	21			
	22	Tax preparation fees	22	275		
	23	Other expenses—investment, safe deposit box, etc. List type and amount ▶ _____	23			
	24	Add lines 21 through 23	24	275		
	25	Enter amount from Form 1040, line 38 25 80,775				
	26	Multiply line 25 by 2% (.02)	26	1,616		
	27	Subtract line 26 from line 24. If line 26 is more than line 24, enter -0-			27	0
Other Miscellaneous Deductions	28	Other—from list on page A-10. List type and amount ▶ _____			28	
Total Itemized Deductions	29	Is Form 1040, line 38, over $159,950 (over $79,975 if married filing separately)? ☑ **No.** Your deduction is not limited. Add the amounts in the far right column for lines 4 through 28. Also, enter this amount on Form 1040, line 40. ☐ **Yes.** Your deduction may be limited. See page A-10 for the amount to enter. ▶			29	15,000
	30	If you elect to itemize deductions even though they are less than your standard deduction, check here ▶ ☐				

For Paperwork Reduction Act Notice, see Form 1040 instructions.   Cat. No. 11330X   **Schedule A (Form 1040) 2008**

Schedules A&B (Form 1040) 2008   OMB No. 1545-0074   Page **2**

Name(s) shown on Form 1040. Do not enter name and social security number if shown on other side.	**Your social security number**
Jeremy S & Shelly R Allen	123 45 9875

Schedule B—Interest and Ordinary Dividends

Attachment Sequence No. **08**

		Amount
Part I **Interest** (See page B-1 and the instructions for Form 1040, line 8a.)	**1** List name of payer. If any interest is from a seller-financed mortgage and the buyer used the property as a personal residence, see page B-1 and list this interest first. Also, show that buyer's social security number and address ►	
	Mercantile Bank	*1,800*
	U.S. Bonds	*700*
	Ben Franklin Savings	*500*
		1
Note. If you received a Form 1099-INT, Form 1099-OID, or substitute statement from a brokerage firm, list the firm's name as the payer and enter the total interest shown on that form.	**2** Add the amounts on line 1	**2** *3,000*
	3 Excludable interest on series EE and I U.S. savings bonds issued after 1989. Attach Form 8815	**3**
	4 Subtract line 3 from line 2. Enter the result here and on Form 1040, line 8a ►	**4** *3,000*
	Note. If line 4 is over $1,500, you must complete Part III.	Amount
Part II **Ordinary Dividends** (See page B-1 and the instructions for Form 1040, line 9a.)	**5** List name of payer ►	
		5
Note. If you received a Form 1099-DIV or substitute statement from a brokerage firm, list the firm's name as the payer and enter the ordinary dividends shown on that form.		
	6 Add the amounts on line 5. Enter the total here and on Form 1040, line 9a . ►	**6**
	Note. If line 6 is over $1,500, you must complete Part III.	

Part III **Foreign Accounts and Trusts** (See page B-2.)	You must complete this part if you **(a)** had over $1,500 of taxable interest or ordinary dividends; or **(b)** had a foreign account; or **(c)** received a distribution from, or were a grantor of, or a transferor to, a foreign trust.	Yes	No
	7a At any time during 2008, did you have an interest in or a signature or other authority over a financial account in a foreign country, such as a bank account, securities account, or other financial account? See page B-2 for exceptions and filing requirements for Form TD F 90-22.1.		✓
	b If "Yes," enter the name of the foreign country ►		
	8 During 2008, did you receive a distribution from, or were you the grantor of, or transferor to, a foreign trust? If "Yes," you may have to file Form 3520. See page B-2		✓

For Paperwork Reduction Act Notice, see Form 1040 instructions.   Schedule B (Form 1040) 2008

PROBLEM MATERIALS

DISCUSSION QUESTIONS

4-1 *Personal and Dependency Exemptions.* Distinguish between personal and dependency exemptions.

4-2 *Dependency Exemption for a Qualifying Child.* List the requirements that must be met in order for one to claim a dependency exemption for a *qualifying child.*

4-3 *Relationship.* In addition to a natural child, which other *children* are included in the definition of a *qualifying child?*

4-4 *Tie-breaking.* Determine who gets the dependency exemption for D in each of the following independent situations. Assume that the parties cannot agree if more than one person could claim the exemption and that any requirements that are not addressed (e.g., citizenship) are met. F's other support (> $3,000) is provided by S.
   a. Q provides a home in which she lives with her daughter, C, and C's son, D. C is 25 years of age and has gross income of $6,500 for the current year.
   b. R provides a home in which she lives with her son, E, and E's son, D. E is 18 years of age and has gross income of $6,500 for the current year.
   c. S provides a home in which she lives with her daughter, F, and F's daughter, D. F is 25 years of age and has gross income of $3,000 for the current year.

4-5 *Tests for Dependency Exemptions.* List and briefly describe the five tests that must be met before a taxpayer is entitled to a dependency exemption for an individual other than a qualifying child. Must all five tests be met?

4-6 *Support.* Briefly describe the concept of support. As part of your definition, include examples of support items.

4-7 *Support—Special Items.* With respect to the support test, discuss survivor's treatment of each of the following items: athletic scholarships, social security survivors' benefits paid to an orphan, and aid to dependent children paid by the state government.

4-8 *Gross Income Test.* Describe the gross income test that is applied to the dependency exemption. Must all dependents for whom a dependency exemption is claimed meet this test?

4-9 *Gross Income Test—Dependency Exemption.* M provides more than half of the support for her father, F, who is single for tax purposes. F's other support is in the form of interest income of $5,000 and social security benefits of $9,000.
   a. May M claim a dependency exemption for supporting F in the current year?
   b. Would your answer differ if F's interest income were only $1,500?

4-10 *Relationship Test—Dependency Exemption.* Assuming Q provides more than 50 percent of their support and the dependent meets the gross income, relationship, and citizenship tests, which of the following relatives may be claimed as a dependent?
   a. Widow of Q's deceased son
   b. Q's husband's brother
   c. Daughter of Q's husband's brother
   d. Q's mother's brother
   e. Q's grandmother's brother
   f. Q's great grandson

4-11   *Joint Return Test—Dependency Exemption.* K and L were married in 2009 and elected to file a joint return. K had interest income of $5,000 and a salary of $30,000 for the year. L had interest income of $2,250 and received the remainder of her support from her mother and K.

    a.   If L's mother provided more than 50 percent of L's support, can she claim a dependency exemption for L?

    b.   If not, under what circumstances could the exemption be claimed?

4-12   This year P, 25, was accepted to medical school. P is a single parent. To save money, she and her one-year-old baby, B, moved in with P's mom and dad, M and D. The four lived together from May through December. May anyone claim an exemption for B? If so, whom?

4-13   *Community Property Law.* How does the treatment of earned income differ between a community property state and a non community property (i.e., separate property) state for Federal income tax purposes? Why?

4-14   *Filing Status, Tax Schedules.* List the four sets of rate schedules that apply to individual taxpayers. Refer to them by filing status and schedule designation (e.g., Schedule Z). Which taxpayers must use the rate schedules rather than the tax rate tables?

4-15   *Determination of Marital Status.* Married taxpayers are subject to a separate set(s) of tax rates. When is marital status determined? What authority (state or federal) controls marital status?

4-16   *Exceptions—Marital Status.* In certain instances, a person who is married may use the rates for unmarried persons. In another instance, a single person may use the rates for married persons filing jointly. Elaborate.

4-17   *Head of Household—Requirements.* What are the specific requirements for head-of-household status? List at least ten relatives who may qualify the taxpayer for head-of-household filing status.

4-18   *Head of Household—Divorced Parents.* May a divorced parent with custody of a child qualify as a head of household even though his or her former spouse is entitled to the dependency exemption for the child? Explain.

4-19   *Head of Household—Taxpayer's Home.* Must the person who qualifies a taxpayer as a head of household (i.e., the taxpayer's child or other dependent) live in the taxpayer's home? Are there any exceptions to this rule?

4-20   *Costs of Maintaining Home.* Which of the following expenses are included in determining the cost of a home when determining whether a taxpayer qualifies as a head of household?

    a.   Food consumed on the premises

    b.   Transportation for a dependent to and from school

    c.   Clothing for a dependent

    d.   Property taxes on residence

    e.   Rent paid on residence

4-21   *Abandoned Spouse.* M is married and lives with her dependent son, S. M receives child support sufficient to provide 65 percent of S's support from S's father, who lived in a nearby city for the entire year. M provides more than one-half of the cost of providing the home in which she and S live.

    a.   What is M's filing status and what is the number of exemption deductions that she may claim?

    b.   How would your answers differ if M agreed to let S's father claim the dependency exemption for S?

4-22 *Tax Tables.* Are taxpayers required to use the tax tables? Which taxpayers are ineligible to use the tables?

4-23 *Limited Standard Deduction.* W is 16 years old, single, and claimed as a dependent by his parents. His 2009 adjusted gross income is $6,150, and he claims the standard deduction.
   a. If W's taxable income is $5,200, what is the character of his income, earned or unearned?
   b. If W's taxable income is $3,700, what is the character of his income, earned or unearned?
   c. If W's taxable income is $450, what is the character of his income, earned or unearned?

4-24 *Kiddie Tax.* G is 13 years old and claimed as a dependent by her parents. G's top marginal tax rate is 10 percent and her parents' is 25 percent. Calculate G's taxable income and the rate at which it will be taxed in the following instances:
   a. Interest of $1,050
   b. Interest of $1,950
   c. Interest of $900 and wages of $5,000
   d. Interest of $3,500 and wages of $500

4-25 *Filing Requirements.* Which individuals are exempted from filing a Form 1040 (or equivalent Form 1040A or Form 1040EZ)?

4-26 *Due Date.* P is a calendar year individual taxpayer with taxable income of $45,000 and a tax due of $350 for the current year.
   a. When is P's tax return due?
   b. Assuming P uses the fiscal year ending June 30, when is her annual income tax return due?

4-27 *Extensions.* Q is a calendar year individual taxpayer with taxable income of $25,000 and a tax refund of $150 for the current year.
   a. If Q is unable to file on time, she may request an automatic extension of time to file her tax return. How long is the maximum extension period?
   b. If Q is unable to complete her return by the extended due date and she has an appropriate reason, how long of an additional extension can she request?
   c. How much is Q's penalty if she fails to file an extension?

4-28 *Due Dates for Estimated Tax Payments.* R is a calendar year taxpayer whose estimated tax liability for the current year is $4,000. What are the amounts and the due dates of R's estimated tax payments?

4-29 *Amount of Estimated Tax Payments.* H is a calendar year taxpayer who estimates his Federal income tax to be $5,500 and his self-employment tax to be $4,500 for 2008. For 2007, H's Federal income tax was $4,950, and his self-employment tax was $3,975. What is the amount of estimated tax that H must pay on each due date to avoid a penalty for failure to make adequate estimated tax payments?

4-30 *Penalties and Interest.* J is a calendar year individual whose gross tax for 2009 is $10,000. J had taxes of $5,750 withheld and made estimated tax payments of $500 each due date. She submitted $1,350 along with her request for an automatic extension on April 15. The remaining $900 was paid when J's tax return was filed on July 9. J's 2008 tax totaled $9,950.
   a. Does J owe a penalty for failure to file for 2009?
   b. Does J owe a penalty for failure to pay for 2009? If so, for what period?
   c. Does J owe a penalty for failure to make adequate estimated tax payments for 2010? If so, over what period?
   d. Does J owe interest on any of the amounts paid? If so, for what period?

4-31 *Statute of Limitations.* What is the importance of the Federal Statute of Limitations to the taxpayer? To the IRS? Generally, how long is the statute of limitations on tax matters?

4-32 *Six-Year Statute of Limitations.* Under what circumstances will the regular three-year statutory period for assessments be extended to six years?

4-33 *Indexation and the Individual Income Tax.* Congress has provided for indexation of certain deductions. What items are subject to indexation? What index is to be used as an estimate of price-level changes?

PROBLEMS

4-34 *Exemption Amount.* H and W are married and file a joint return. They claim dependency exemptions for themselves and their two children, S and D. Compute the amount of their deduction for personal and dependent exemptions if their adjusted gross income is
   a. $196,400
   b. $254,500
   c. $370,000

4-35 *Exemptions.* In each of the following situations determine the proper number of personal and dependency exemptions available to the taxpayer. Unless otherwise implied, assume that all tests are satisfied.
   a. R's mother, age 85, lives in his home. R figures that including the value of the lodging, he provides support of about $6,000. The remainder of her support is paid for with her social security benefits of $4,000.
   b. This year D sent his father, F, monthly checks of $200, or $2,400 for the year. F used these checks along with $2,300 of rental income ($4,400 of rents less $2,100 of expenses) to pay all of his support.
   c. H and W are married with one daughter, D, age 7. D models children's clothing and earned $4,000 of wages this year. D also has a trust fund of $50,000 established by her grandparents. All of D's wages were saved and none were used to pay for her support. Similarly none of the funds of the trust were used to pay for D's support.
   d. Professor and Mrs. Smith participated in the foreign exchange student program at their son's high school. In December of 2007 a student, Hans, arrived from Germany, spent the spring of 2008 with the Smiths, then returned to Germany.
   e. B and C are happily married with one son, S. S, age 20, is a full-time student at the University of Cincinnati. S worked as a painter during the summer to help put himself through school. He earned wages of $4,000, $2,500 of which was used to pay for his room and board at school and $1,500 for miscellaneous living expenses (e.g., gas for his car, dates, laundry, etc.). He lived with his parents during the summer. The value of their support including meals and lodging was $5,000. He also received a National Merit Scholarship, which paid for his tuition of $8,000.

4-36 *Personal and Dependency Exemptions.* In each of the following situations determine the proper number of personal and dependency exemption deductions available to the taxpayer.
   a. A is single and 44 years of age. He provides full support for his mother, who is 67 and lives in a small retirement community in A's hometown.
   b. D and K are married and file a joint return for the year. D is 67 years of age and K is 62. They have no dependents.
   c. E and O are married and file a joint return for the year. They provide all the support for their two younger children for the entire year. E and O also provided all the support for their oldest child (age 19) for the eight months she was a full-time student. After graduating from high school, she accepted a job that paid $3,000 in salary.

Nevertheless, her parents contributed more than one-half of her support for the entire year.

4-37   *Married Dependents.* In November of this year Jim Jenkins married his college sweetheart, Kate Brown. Jim was 27 and Kate was 25. Jim had graduated two years ago. Kate was in graduate school and had one more year left. The majority of Kate's support this year was provided by her parents. Jim earned $16,250 during the year while Kate received $950 of interest from her savings account. Assume Kate's parents are in the 25 (2009) percent tax bracket and would give the couple any tax savings to be derived from claiming Kate as a dependent.

    a. May Kate's parents claim an exemption for Kate assuming the couple files a joint return?

    b. Would the couple be better off filing separate returns (and thus receiving any taxes saved by Kate's parents) or filing a joint return? Show all computations you must make to determine your answer.

4-38   *Itemized Deductions and Exemptions.* G and H are married and file a joint return for 2009. They have A.G.I. of $259,800 for the year and the following itemized deductions and personal and dependency exemptions:

State and local taxes	$ 5,300
Residence interest	14,500
Investment interest	500
Charitable contributions	6,200
Personal and dependency exemptions	4

    a. Calculate G and H's taxable income for 2008.

    b. Calculate G and H's taxable income for 2008 assuming their A.G.I. was $269,800, a $10,000 increase over (a).

    c. By what amount did taxable income increase due to this $10,000 increase in adjusted gross income? Why wasn't it $10,000?

4-39   *Multiple Support Agreements.* G's support is provided as follows:

Social security benefits	$3,600
Taxable interest income	800
Support from:	
A, G's oldest son—Cash for trip to Europe	1,600
B, G's daughter—Fair value of lodging and cash	2,300
C, G's youngest son—Cash	700
Total	$9,000

    a. Who is entitled to a dependency exemption for G in the absence of any agreement as to who gets the deduction?

    b. Who may claim a dependency exemption for G under a multiple-support agreement?

    c. How would your answer to (b) differ if A contributed $650 instead of $1,600?

4-40   *Children of Divorced Parents.* For each of the following, determine whether M or F is entitled to the dependency exemption in 2009 for their only child, S. M and F were divorced in 2006 and M has custody, except when F has visitation privileges. Together, M and F provide 100 percent of S's support.

    a. M was granted the dependency exemption under the divorce decree. F pays child support for the year totaling $1,500. Total support expenditures for S are $5,600.

    b. No mention of the dependency exemption was made in the divorce decree. F pays child support for S of $3,400, and the total support for S is $6,500.

    c. F was granted the dependency exemption in the divorce decree and he paid child support of $2,800 for the year. M signed Form 8332, indicating that she will not claim a dependency exemption for S. The total support for S for the year was $5,500.

4-41   *Filing Status and Standard Deduction.* Determine the most beneficial filing status and the standard deduction for each of the following taxpayers for 2009:

    a.   M is a 54-year-old unmarried widow whose spouse died in 2006. During all of 2009 M's 15-year-old son, for whom she claims a dependency exemption, lives with her.

    b.   S is a 67-year-old bachelor who lives in New York City. S pays more than half the cost of maintaining a home in Tampa, Florida for his 89-year-old mother. He is entitled to a dependency exemption under a multiple-support agreement executed by his brother, his sister, and himself.

    c.   R is a widower whose wife died in 2008. R maintained a household for his three dependent children during 2009 and provided 100 percent of the cost of the household.

    d.   J is divorced and has custody of his 9-year-old child. J provides more than half the cost of the home in which he lives with his child, but his ex-wife is entitled to the dependency exemption for the child for 2008.

4-42   *Head of Household.* Indicate whether the taxpayer would be entitled to file using the head-of-household rate schedule.

    a.   Y is divorced from her husband. She maintains a home in which she and her 10-year-old son live. Her ex-husband pays child support to her that she uses to provide all of the support for the child. In addition, Y has relinquished her right to claim her son as a dependent to her former spouse.

    b.   C is divorced from his wife. He provides 75 percent of the support for his mother, who lives in a nursing home. His mother receives $5,000 of interest income annually.

    c.   J's grandson, L, had a falling-out with his parents and moved in with him early this year. J did not mind because he had grown lonely since his wife died three years ago. L is 17 years old and earned $5,000 this year as a part-time grocery clerk. L's total support was $12,000.

    d.   B's wife died four years ago and he has not remarried. Last year his daughter, D, graduated from Arizona State University and moved to Hawaii. Unfortunately, D was unable to earn enough money to make ends meet and had to rely on checks from dad. B paid for D's own apartment and provided the majority of her support.

    e.   M's wife died last year. This year he maintains a home for his 25-year-old daughter, E, who is attending graduate school in a nearby city. E earned $8,000 as a teaching assistant. Nevertheless, M provided the majority of E's support.

    f.   Same as (e) except E is the taxpayer's sister.

    g.   F's husband died this year. She continues to provide a home for her two children, ages 6 and 8.

4-43   *Dependent's Personal Exemption and Standard Deduction.* K is 16 years old and is claimed as a dependent on her parents' income tax return. She earned wages of $2,800 and collected interest of $1,450 for the year. What is the amount of K's taxable income for the year?

TaxCut **4-44**   *Dependent's Personal Exemption and Standard Deduction.* B is 20 years old and is claimed as a dependent on his sister's tax return. B earned $3,000 from a part-time job during the year. What is B's taxable income?

TaxCut **4-45**   *Computation of Tax.* R and S are married and have two dependents. The couple files a joint return and claims the standard deduction. Using the taxable incomes below, compute their tax liability after credits and their effective tax rates, assuming their total income is their A.G.I.

    a. $67,700

    b. $198,850

    c. $352,700

4-46 *High-Income Taxpayer.* H and W are married and file a joint return for 2009. They have no dependents and both are under age 40. H earned a salary of $120,000. W is self-employed and earned a net profit from business of $202,200. H and W have personal itemized deductions totaling $29,800 (all subject to the 1% cutback).

    a. What are the amounts of their adjusted gross income and taxable income on their joint income tax return?

    b. Calculate the 2009 tax liability, including W's self-employment tax. Assume that the 2009 self-employment tax is 15.3 percent on income up to $106,800 (2.9% MHI with no limit).

4-47 *Tax Tables.* S earned a salary during 2008 of $56,015. She is single, claims the standard deduction, and has no dependents for the year. Her only other income was taxable interest income of $560. Determine S's taxable income and her Federal income tax. (**Note:** This tax table computation is for 2008 because the 2009 tax tables will not be available until late 2009. See Appendix for the 2008 tax tables.)

4-48 *Tax Rate Schedules.* W and T were married and filed a joint return for 2009. Their adjusted gross income for the year was $141,950. Their total itemized deductions were $12,700 and they were entitled to three personal and dependency exemptions. Neither W nor T is 65 or older and both have good sight. Determine W and T's taxable income and their Federal income tax liability before prepayments and credits for 2009.

4-49 *Application of the Kiddie Tax.* For each of the following situations, determine the child's taxable income and the amounts that would be taxed at the child's and parents' rates for the 2009 tax year.

    a. When J's rich uncle died, he left her GM corporate bonds. This year J received $1,850 of interest from these bonds, her only income. J is seven years old and her parents claim an exemption for her.

    b. L, age 13, works in his father's music store on weekends. During the year, he earned $1,200 from this job. In addition, L had $800 of interest income attributable to a gift from his grandfather. L's father claims an exemption for him.

    c. Same as (b) except L's earned income was $5,600 and interest income was $1,850.

4-50 *Computation of the Kiddie Tax.* G's great aunt gave her a certificate of deposit that matures in ten years when she is 21. The certificate pays interest of $2,200 annually. G's parents file a joint return. Their 2009 taxable income is $131,500. Compute G's tax.

4-51 *Failure-to-File Penalty.* T, overwhelmed by other pressing concerns, simply forgot to file his tax return for 2008 until July 20, 2009. When filed, T's 2008 return showed a tax due before withholding and estimated taxes of $10,000.

    a. Will T be penalized for failure to file his return if the total income taxes withheld by his employer were $11,000?

    b. Assuming T's employer withheld $9,000, what is the amount of the failure-to-file penalty, if any?

4-52 *Failure-to-Pay Penalty.* On April 13, 2010 R, a calendar year taxpayer, sat down to prepare his 2009 tax return. Realizing that he simply did not have time to accumulate all of his records, R decided to file for an extension. R's tax liability for the previous year, 2008, was $8,000. During 2009 R's employer withheld $2,500 and R paid estimated taxes of $500. R estimates that his final gross tax liability for 2009 will be $12,000.

    a. Assuming R obtains an extension to file his 2009 return, when will his return normally be due?

    b. Based on the facts above, what amount must R pay by April 15 to avoid a failure-to-pay penalty?

c. R completed and filed his return on July 20, 2010. Unfortunately, his initial estimate of his tax was low and his final tax (before withholding and estimated tax payments) was $15,000. Assuming R paid the amount determined in part (b) above, what is the amount of the failure-to-pay penalty, if any?

4-53 *Estimated Taxes and Underpayment Penalty.* K works as a salesperson for the National Hospital Supply Corporation, selling surgical and other hospital supplies. He receives a salary plus a percentage commission on sales over a certain threshold. In the current year 2009 K's tax liability before prepayments was $20,000. His 2008 tax liability was $12,000. In each year his A.G.I. was less than $150,000.

a. What is the lowest required tax installment (including withholding) that K can make and avoid the penalty for underpaying his taxes during the year? (Ignore the annualized income installment.)

b. Assume that K paid estimated taxes of $1,000 on each due date. In addition, K's employer withheld a total of $3,000 during the year. K filed and paid the balance of his liability on April 15, 2010. Assume the applicable interest rate charged on underpayments for each period in 2009 is 10 percent. Compute K's penalty, if any, for failure to pay estimated taxes. Compute the penalty for the first installment only.

c. Assume that K works solely for commissions and that he had no income through March 31, 2009 because he decided to take a winter vacation. Income for the remainder of the year was sufficient to generate a tax liability before prepayments of $20,000. What implications do these facts have on the calculation of the underpayment penalty for 2009?

4-54 *Penalties for Inadequate Estimated Tax Payments.* Z is a calendar year individual whose gross tax for 2009 is $40,000. Z had taxes of $8,000 withheld and did not make estimated tax payments. Z's tax due was paid with his timely filed return on April 15, 2010. His 2008 tax was $35,000 on adjusted gross income of $148,000.

a. Calculate Z's penalty for failure to make adequate estimated tax payments, if any.

b. Does Z owe interest on any of the amounts paid? If so, for what period?

c. Same as (a) above, except Z's adjusted gross income for 2008 was $160,000.

4-55 *Penalties and Interest.* Y filed her tax return for 2008 on April 15, 2009. Upon discovering an inadvertent error, Y filed an amended return and submitted additional tax of $1,250.

a. Does Y owe a penalty for failure to pay? If so, how much?

b. Does Y owe interest on the $1,250 paid with the amended return? If so, how much?

4-56 *Statute of Limitations.* T, a calendar year taxpayer, filed her 2008 Federal income tax return on January 29, 2009 and received a tax refund check for overpaid 2008 taxes on May 17, 2009.

a. Assuming that T did not file a false return or have a substantial omission of income, what is the last date on which the IRS may assess an additional income tax liability against her for the 2008 tax year?

b. If T unintentionally had a substantial omission of income from her 2008 return, what is the last day on which the IRS may assess her an additional 2008 income tax liability?

c. If T had never bothered to file her 2008 tax return, what is the last day on which the IRS may assess her an additional 2008 income tax liability?

TAX RETURN PROBLEMS

CONTINUOUS TAX RETURN PROBLEMS See Appendix D, Part 1

TaxCut **4-57** *Form 1040EZ.* Samuel B. White was single for 2008 and had no dependents. Sam's only income was wages of $21,150 and taxable interest of $465. Federal income tax of $930 was withheld from Sam's salary.

Calculate Sam's Federal income tax and his tax due or refund for 2008. A Form 1040EZ may be completed based on this information. Supply fictitious occupation, social security number, and address. (**Note:** Use the 2008 tax forms since the 2009 forms may not be available)

TaxCut 4-58 *Form 1040A.* Charles D. and Alice A. Davis were married during all of 2008 and had income from the following sources:

Salary, Charles	$47,100
Federal income tax withheld	1,425
Part-time salary, Alice	16,700
Federal income tax withheld	880
Interest from Home Savings	320
Interest from U.S. Government Bonds	430

Charles and Alice provide the sole support of their two children (both under age 17). During the year, they paid job-related child care expenses of $2,200. Their itemized deductions for the year are insufficient for them to itemize, but a deductible $2,000 was deposited in each of their individual retirement accounts.

Calculate the Federal income tax and the tax due (or refund) for Mr. and Mrs. Davis, assuming they file a joint return. If the 2009 tax tables are not available, use the tax rate schedules on the inside front cover of the text. A Form 1040A may also be completed. Supply fictitious information for the address, occupations, social security numbers, and children's names. (**Note:** Use 2008 tax forms since the 2009 forms may not be available)

TaxCut 4-59 *Form 1040.* William A. Gregg, a high school educator, and Mary W. Gregg, a microbiologist, are married and file a joint income tax return for 2008. Neither William nor Mary is over 50 years old, and both have excellent sight. They provide the sole support of their three children: Barry, Kimberly, and Rachel (all under age 17). The following information is from their records for 2008:

Salaries and wages, William	$34,550
Federal income tax withheld	$2,320
Salaries and wages, Mary	44,800
Federal income tax withheld	4,360
Interest income—Home Savings and Loan	690
Interest income—City Bank	220
Tax-exempt interest income	1,400
Itemized deductions as follows:	
Hospitalization insurance	320
Unreimbursed fees of doctors, hospitals, etc	740
Unreimbursed prescription drugs	310
Real estate taxes on residence	1,350
State income taxes paid	1,440
State sales taxes paid	720
Interest paid on original home mortgage	8,430
Charitable contribution—Faith Church	1,720
Charitable contribution—State University	200
Quarterly estimated taxes paid	3,500

Calculate the 2008 Federal income tax and the tax due (or refund) for the Greggs assuming they file a joint return. Form 1040, along with Schedules A and B, may be completed. Supply fictitious information for the address and social security numbers. (**Note:** Use 2008 tax forms since the 2009 forms may not be available)

RESEARCH PROBLEMS

4-60 *Nonresident Alien Spouse.* C is a citizen of the United States who resides indefinitely in Europe. C is married to N, a citizen of Greece. C has $32,000 of gross income subject to United States tax and would like to file jointly with N. Can C accomplish this goal? If so, what steps are necessary? How is the income of N treated?

   Research aids:

   Code § 6013(g) and Reg. § 1.6013-6.

4-61 Much to Ted's surprise, his employer, a major hotel chain, asked him to manage the company's premier resort property in Cabo San Lucas, Mexico for the entire calendar year. Ted accepted and was paid $110,000 in compensation for the assignment, visiting the U. S. for only two weeks during the year. Ted's only other income is interest income of $20,000. Ted is single, claims the standard deduction and has no dependents. He is a U. S. citizen. Calculate Ted's tax due and refund assuming he uses the foreign earned income exclusion rather than the foreign tax credit. Ted's tax paid to Mexico was $8,500.

   Research aids:

   Code §§ 901 and 911(a).

PART TWO

GROSS INCOME

★ ★ ★ ★ ★ CONTENTS ★ ★ ★ ★ ★

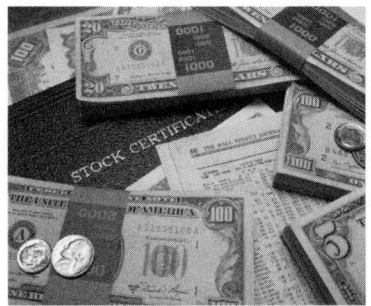

★ CHAPTER FIVE ★

GROSS INCOME

LEARNING OBJECTIVES

Upon completion of this chapter you will be able to:

► Define income for tax purposes and explain how it differs from the definitions given to it in accounting or economics

► Explain the concept of the taxable year and identify who is eligible to use fiscal years

► Apply the cash and accrual methods of accounting to determine the tax year in which items are reported

► Determine the effect of a change in accounting method

► Describe some of the special rules governing the treatment of prepaid income, interest income, interest-free loans, and income from long-term contracts

► Identify which taxpayer is responsible for reporting income and paying the taxes on such income

---

CHAPTER OUTLINE

INTRODUCTION

Determination of the final income tax liability begins with the identification of a taxpayer's gross income. Before that can be done, however, one obviously must understand what constitutes *income* for tax purposes. The primary purpose of this chapter is to examine the income concept and thus provide some general guidelines regarding what is and what is not subject to taxation. As a practical matter, income is normally easy to spot. Salary, interest, dividends, rents, gains from the sales of property, and most other items that one customarily thinks of as income are in fact income for tax purposes. In fact, these represent the bulk of all income that is reported. But what if a taxpayer is lucky enough to receive an inheritance, a gift, or a scholarship? Are these taxable? What about court-awarded damages? And if a taxpayer borrows $1,000, is there income? What happens if Publishers Clearing House gives you $10 million? Is the IRS as happy as you are? And how do hurricane victims treat their government aid? Is their relief taxable? The list of possible income items goes on and on. Fortunately, these items are more the exception than the rule. In any event, newcomers to tax should understand that there are no hard and fast rules that can be applied to every conceivable situation. The Supreme Court clearly stated the problem in a case concerning the income status of embezzled funds:

> In fact, no single conclusive criterion has yet been found to determine in all situations what is sufficient gain to support the imposition of an income tax. No more can be said in general than that all relevant facts and circumstances must be considered.[1]

Notwithstanding the Court's observations, three important generalizations developed in this chapter are

1. "Income" is broadly construed for tax purposes to include virtually any type of gain, benefit, or profit that has been realized.

2. Although the scope of the income concept is broad, certain types of income are exempted from taxation by statute, administrative ruling, or judicial decree.

3. Taxpayers who realize income may not be required to recognize and report it immediately but may be able to postpone recognition until some time in the future.

To sum up, there are three basic questions to address concerning income:

1. Did the taxpayer have income?

2. If the taxpayer had income, was it realized?

3. If the taxpayer has realized income, must it be recognized now or is it permanently excluded or perhaps temporarily deferred and reported at some future date?

The first part of this chapter examines the concept of income. Once one is sensitive to the concept of income, consideration must be given to *if and when* the income must be reported as well as *who* must report it. The latter part of the chapter focuses on the timing of income recognition and the identification of the reporting entity.

---

[1] *Comm. v. Wilcox*, 46-1 USTC ¶9188, 34 AFTR 811, 327 U.S. 404 (USSC, 1946).

GROSS INCOME DEFINED

The definition of income found in the Internal Revenue Code reflects the language of the constitutional amendment empowering Congress to impose taxes on income.[2] Section 61(a) of the Code defines *gross income* as follows:

Except as otherwise provided in this subtitle, gross income means all income from whatever source derived, including (but not limited to) the following items:

1. Compensation for services, including fees, commissions, fringe benefits, and similar items;
2. Gross income derived from business;
3. Gains derived from dealings in property;
4. Interest;
5. Rents;
6. Royalties;
7. Dividends;
8. Alimony and separate maintenance payments;
9. Annuities;
10. Income from life insurance and endowment contracts;
11. Pensions;
12. Income from discharge of indebtedness;
13. Distributive share of partnership gross income;
14. Income in respect of a decedent; and
15. Income from an interest in an estate or trust.

Despite the statute's detailed enumeration of income items, the list is not comprehensive. The items specified are only a sample of the more common types of income. Taxable income includes many other economic benefits not identified above.

As a practical matter, Code § 61 furnishes little guidance for determining whether a particular benefit should be treated as income. The statute provides no criteria or factors that could be used for assessment. For example, the general definition does not provide any clue as to whether a gift or an inheritance constitutes taxable income. Similarly, the statute is not helpful in determining whether income arises upon the discovery of buried treasure. These and similar issues, as will be seen, are often answered by reference to other, more specific, sections of the Code. On the other hand, many questions cannot be resolved by reference to the statute or the regulations. In situations where clear statutory guidance is absent, the difficult task of ascertaining how far the definitional boundary of income extends falls to the courts. To this end, the courts have utilized the meanings given income in both economics and accounting to mold a workable definition of income for tax purposes.

ECONOMIC CONCEPT OF INCOME

Economists define income as the amount that an individual could have spent for consumption during a period while remaining as well off at the end of the period as at the beginning of the period. This concept of income may be expressed mathematically as the sum of an individual's consumption during the period plus the change in the individual's net worth between the beginning and end of the period.[3] Note that an

---

[2]   See Chapter 1.

[3]   The economic definition of income given here is often referred to as the Haig-Simons definition as derived from the following works: Robert M. Haig, "The Concepts of Income—Economic and Legal Aspects," *The Federal Income Tax* (New York: Columbia University Press, 1921); Henry C. Simons, *Personal Income Taxation* (Chicago: University of Chicago Press, 1921).

increase in net worth is actually savings. Thus income can be defined as I = C + S where I is income, C is consumption and S is savings.

Example 1. K's records revealed the following assets and liabilities as of December 31, 2009 and 2010:

	12-31-09	12-31-10
Assets (fair market value)........................	$100,000	$140,000
Liabilities.....................................	(20,000)	(30,000)
Net worth	$ 80,000	$110,000

During the year, K spent $25,000 on rent, food, clothing, entertainment, and other items. From an economic perspective, K's income for 2010 is $55,000 determined as follows:

Consumption	$25,000
Change in net worth ($110,000 – $80,000)	30,000
Economic income	$55,000

There are two key aspects of an economist's definition. The first is the emphasis on a change in net worth. According to the economist, a taxpayer has income under any circumstances that cause his or her net worth to increase. Note that this view is extremely broad. Taxpayers who receive an inheritance, are the beneficiaries of a life insurance policy, discover buried treasure, or have their debts cancelled have all had an increase in net worth and would therefore have income using this definition. Some may object to this comprehensive approach. It is nevertheless consistent with § 61, which states that income includes *all* income regardless of its source.

The second and perhaps more critical aspect of the economist's definition from a tax perspective is the notion that consumption and the change in net worth must be computed using market values on an accrual basis rather than on a realization basis. For example, economists include in income any increase in the value of an individual's shares of stock during the period, even though the shares are not sold and the individual does not *realize* the increase in value. In addition, economists would include in income the rental value of one's car or home, as well as the value of food grown for personal use, since such items constitute consumption. Gifts and inheritances would also be considered income by an economist since these items would affect an individual's net worth. Although the economist's approach to income is theoretically sound, it has significant drawbacks from a practical view.

For practical application, the meaning given to income must be objective to minimize controversies. The economist's reliance on market values to measure net worth and consumption violates this premise. Few assets have readily determinable and accurate values. Valuation of most assets would be a subjective determination. For example, an individual may be able to value shares of stock by referring to an active publicized market, but how is the value of a closely held business or work of art to be computed? The difficulty in making such valuations would no doubt lead to countless disputes and administrative hassles. These practical problems of implementing the economic concept of income have caused the courts to adopt a different interpretation.

It should be pointed out, however, that the economist's approach to measuring income—the so-called net worth method—is sometimes used when the IRS decides that

the taxpayer's records do not adequately reflect income.[4] Application usually occurs where the taxpayer has not maintained records, or has falsified or destroyed any records that were kept. In these situations, the IRS reconstructs income by determining the change in net worth during the year and adding estimated living expenses.

Before leaving the economist's definition of income, a final observation is warranted. Over the years, some have argued that the income tax does not encourage savings and, therefore, the U.S. should switch to a consumption tax such as a national retail sales tax. Observe, however, that a similar result could be obtained under the current income tax law if taxpayers were given a deduction for savings. This can be demonstrated mathematically by simply manipulating the terms of the income equation above:

$$I = C + S$$

$$C = I - S$$

In light of President Bush's commitment to tax reform and simplification during his second term, it is not surprising that this concept has surfaced. Only time will tell what changes will be made.

ACCOUNTING CONCEPT OF INCOME

The principle of realization distinguishes the accountant's concept of income from that of the economist. Under this principle, accountants recognize income when it is *realized*. Income is generally considered realized when (1) the earnings process is complete, and (2) an exchange or transaction has taken place.[5] Normally, some type of *conversion* occurs that substantially changes the taxpayer's relationship to the asset. To illustrate, consider a taxpayer who discovers oil on his property. He may have "income" in the economic sense (at least to the extent that the value of his property and his net worth have increased). But he has not realized that increase in net worth and does not have income in the accounting sense until he converts his discovery into another asset (e.g., he sells the property or the oil). Observe that these two criteria provide the objective determination of value traditionally believed necessary for the work that accountants perform. As a result, accounting income usually does not recognize changes in market values of assets during a period (as would economic income) unless such changes have been realized.

INCOME FOR TAX PURPOSES: THE JUDICIAL CONCEPT

The landmark decision of the Supreme Court in *Eisner v. Macomber* in 1918 provided the first glimpse of how the concept of income would be interpreted for tax purposes.[6] In this case, the court embraced the realization principle of accounting, indicating that income must be *realized* before it can be taxed. As later decisions suggested, the primary virtue of the realization principle is not that it somehow yields a better or more theoretically precise income figure. Rather, it provides an objective basis for measuring income, eliminating the problems that would arise if income were determined using subjective valuations. In short, the realization principle is a well-entrenched part of the tax law because it makes the law so much easier to administer.

---

[4]   *Holland v. U.S.*, 54-2 USTC ¶9714, 46 AFTR 943, 348 U.S. 121 (USSC, 1954). Net worth, however, is to be determined using the tax basis in assets and not their fluctuating market values [*S. Bedeian*, 54 T.C. 295 (1970)].

[5]   "Basic Concepts and Accounting Principles Underlying Financial Statements of Business Enterprises," *Accounting Principles Board Statements No. 4* (New York: American Institute of Certified Public Accountants, 1970), ¶134.

[6]   1 USTC ¶32, 3 AFTR 3020, 252 U.S. 189 (USSC, 1920).

A second issue addressed by the *Eisner* decision concerned the scope of the income concept. How far did it reach? Did income include gifts, scholarships, court-awarded damages, a personal secretary, and other types of benefits? In essence, the Court again followed the accounting approach, stating that income was restricted to gains realized from property or personal services.

Hence, finding a $10 bill, receiving a prize or award, or profiting from a cancelled debt would not have been taxable under *Eisner*, since the benefits were obtained without any effort by the taxpayer. Later decisions, however, expanded the concept of income by rejecting the notion that only gains derived from capital or labor are recognized. The courts have taken what is often referred to as an "all-inclusive" approach; that is, *all* gains are presumed to be taxable except those specifically exempted. The Supreme Court's opinion in *Glenshaw Glass Co.* provides the definition of income that is perhaps most commonly accepted today.[7] This case involved the treatment of punitive damages awarded to Glenshaw Glass for fraud and antitrust violations of another company. In holding that such awards were income, the Court stated:[8]

> Here we have instances of undeniable accessions to wealth, clearly realized, and over which the taxpayer has complete dominion. The mere fact that the payments were extracted from wrongdoers as punishment for unlawful conduct cannot detract from their character as taxable income to the recipients.

Thus, income for tax purposes is construed to include any type of gain, benefit, profit, or other increase in wealth that has been realized and is not exempted by statute. Note that the courts have adopted key elements of both the economic and accounting definition of income: income is any increase in the taxpayer's *net worth* (i.e., wealth) that has been *realized*. Also note that, even though it all sounds very technical and precise, the rule, like so many rules in taxation, may be difficult to apply in a given situation. For example, if a tenant paints the walls of her apartment or plants some gladiolus in the garden, has the landlord realized income? Arriving at a solution for this and any particular set of facts can be quite frustrating, but one can generally take heart that these are rare and, moreover, a common sense approach generally works: if it seems as if the taxpayer is better off, there is probably income.

It should be emphasized that even though a taxpayer may have "income" that has in fact been realized, this by itself does not guarantee that it will be taxed. In tax parlance, the question still remains as to whether the taxpayer must "recognize" the income (i.e., report the income for tax purposes). There are *three* relatively common exceptions to the general rule that all income must be recognized immediately:

1. *Excluded Income.* Income that has been realized need not be recognized if it is specifically exempted from taxation by virtue of some provision in the Code. For example, as discussed in Chapter 6, interest income from state and local bonds is specifically excluded under § 103 while gifts and inheritances (which obviously increase net worth) are excluded under § 102. In these cases, the income permanently escapes tax and normally creates a difference between taxable income and financial accounting income. It should be noted that, notwithstanding the Code's all-inclusive concept of income, the tax base is far from comprehensive because of the numerous exclusions and exemptions that have crept into the law over the years.[9]

---

7   55-1 USTC ¶9308, 47 AFTR 162, 348 U.S. 426 (USSC, 1955).

8   *Ibid.*

9   For an excellent discussion of the concept of income and the notion of a comprehensive tax base see Boris Bittker, "A Comprehensive Tax Base as a Goal of Income Tax Reform," 80 *Harvard Law Review* 925 (1967).

2. *Accounting Methods.* A taxpayer may be able to defer recognition of income to a subsequent year by following some particular method of accounting (e.g., the installment sales method or the completed contract method).

3. *Nontaxable Exchanges.* Income realized on a sale or exchange may be deferred under a special nonrecognition rule. For example, a taxpayer who swaps one parcel of land costing $10,000 for another parcel worth $50,000 is not required to recognize the $40,000 gain under the like-kind exchange rules. The theory underlying nonrecognition in this and similar situations is that the taxpayer has not liquidated his investment to cash but has continued it, albeit in another form. In effect, the law is willing to defer the tax until such time when the taxpayer does in fact convert the asset to cash and has the wherewithal to pay the tax. It is important to note, however, that in these and similar cases, the gain is only *deferred*; it does not escape tax permanently as is the case with excluded income.

In summary, income for tax purposes can generally be defined as any increase in wealth (net worth) or consumption that has been realized. In addition, such income normally must be recognized unless it is specifically excluded or postponed due to an accounting rule or deferral provision. A list of some of the common types of income—both taxable and nontaxable—can be found in Exhibit 3-3 and Exhibit 3-4 in Chapter 3.

Before leaving this subject, one final observation should be made. It is important to understand that this definition of gross income is the same for all types of taxpayers. In other words, § 61 and its many interpretations not only applies to individual taxpayers but also applies equally to business entities such as C corporations, S corporations, partnerships, and LLCs as well as trusts and estates.

REFINEMENTS OF THE GROSS INCOME DEFINITION

As one might imagine, in the early years of the tax law, when there were few specific rules, people found it easy to take the position that Congress never intended to tax their particular type of "income." To support such contentions, taxpayers, never lacking for imagination, often concocted ingenious arguments explaining why they should escape tax. In one memorable case, a taxpayer who received a gift (gifts are specifically excluded from income) argued that the income from the gifted property was also exempt since the income was merely an extension of the gift. Unfortunately, the court did not accept this gift-that-keeps-on-giving theory and taxed the income. But this was typical of the development of the tax law. As the courts dealt with this and other income issues, their decisions set a number of precedents that shaped and refined the concept of income. Because of their significance, some of the principles established by early court decisions were given statutory effect; that is, the rule evolving from the decision was subsequently enacted as part of the law, or codified. For example, § 102(b) now provides that income from gifted property is not part of the gift and is fully taxable.

Other court rulings have been incorporated into the Regulations either directly or by way of reference. Several of these rulings, however, have not found their way into the Code or Regulations. Nevertheless, they provide authoritative guidance for the determination of taxable income. This section examines three major principles that are relevant to the income concept. These concern:

1. *Form of Benefit.* Must income be realized in a particular form, such as cash, before it becomes taxable?

2. *Return of Capital.* Does gross income mean gross receipts or net gain after allowance for a tax-free recovery of the taxpayer's capital investment?

3. *Indirect Economic Benefits.* Are benefits provided by an employer (such as a company car) taxable where they are not intended as compensation?

FORM-OF-BENEFIT PRINCIPLE

Many taxpayers erroneously believe that income need be reported only when cash is received. The Regulations clearly state, however, that gross income includes income realized in any form.[10] Thus, income is not limited to receipts of cash but also extends to receipts of property, services, and *any other economic benefits*. For example, taxpayers may realize income when their debts are cancelled or they purchase property at a price less than its fair market value—a so-called *bargain purchase*. In situations where income is received in a form other than cash, a cash-equivalent approach is adopted.[11] Under this method, the measure of income is its fair market value at the time of receipt.

Example 2. Several years ago on the television show *60 Minutes*, a segment was devoted to what the commentators implied was a tax travesty. In truth, it was a sad tale. According to the story, a generous employer who wanted to reward his employees for their long years of service gave them stock in the company. At that time, the stock had a value of about $100 per share. The employees, as one might guess, were extremely pleased. Unfortunately, a sudden turn of events caused the value of the shares to plummet. By the close of the year, the stock was practically worthless. Some employees still holding the stock were upset but accepted their misfortune graciously. On April 15, however, those still holding the stock found themselves in tax shock. What was the problem? As may be apparent from the discussion of the form-of-benefit principle, the employees were required to report compensation income equal to the value of stock at the time of receipt, $100 per share. This meant that many employees had to report thousands of dollars of income even though the stock was currently worthless. They had income without any way to pay the tax. Although the employees might be able to claim a deduction for worthless stock, it might not provide total relief since such loss would be a capital loss, the deduction of which is limited.

Example 3. Borrower B owed Lender L $10,000, evidenced by a note payable due in six months. If L allows B to cancel the note for a payment of $9,000, B must normally recognize gross income of $1,000.

RETURN OF CAPITAL DOCTRINE

The return of capital doctrine is best illustrated by a simple loan transaction. When a taxpayer lends money and it is later repaid, no income is recognized since the repayment represents merely a *return of capital* to the taxpayer. Although there is no statutory provision to this effect, it is a well-recognized rule. Moreover, the taxpayer's net worth has not increased (one asset, a receivable, has simply been replaced by another, cash). However, any interest on the loan that is paid to the taxpayer would be income.

Sale or Disposition. The application of the return of capital doctrine is not limited to loans. One of the first refinements made to the income concept concerned the use of the return of capital principle to determine the income from a sale of property. In 1916 the

---

[10]   Reg. § 1.61-1(a).

[11]   Reg. § 1.446-1(a)(3).

Supreme Court held that the total proceeds received on a sale were not to be treated as income.[12] Rather, the portion of the proceeds representing the taxpayer's capital (i.e., adjusted basis) could be recovered tax free. Thus, it is the return of capital doctrine that allows the taxpayer to determine the income upon a sale or disposition of property by reducing the amount realized (cash + the fair market value of other receipts such as property) by the adjusted basis of the property. Using this approach—now contained in § 1001(a)—the taxpayer's income on dispositions of property is limited to the *gain* realized.

> **Example 4.** R sold XYZ stock for $10,000. He purchased the stock for $6,000. R's realized gain is $4,000 ($10,000 amount realized − $6,000 adjusted basis) rather than the gross amount of the sales price, $10,000, since the return of capital doctrine permits him to recover his $6,000 investment tax free.

The return of capital doctrine also stands for the important proposition that gross income is not the same as gross receipts. This is reflected in Regulations, which provide that in the manufacturing, merchandising, or mining business, *gross income* means total sales less costs of goods sold.[13]

Damages. The return of capital doctrine may also apply to amounts awarded for injury inflicted upon the taxpayer.

> **Example 5.** In *Edward H. Clark*, the Clarks overpaid their taxes by about $19,000 due to a mistake made by an attorney in the preparation of their return. The attorney subsequently reimbursed the Clarks for the overpayment.[14] The Court allowed the Clarks to exclude the reimbursement since there was no economic gain but merely a recovery of their capital. In *Inaja Land Co., Ltd.*, the taxpayer received payments from the city of Los Angeles to compensate it for damages caused by the city's diversion of polluted waters into the taxpayer's fishing area.[15] The court granted an exclusion on the return of capital theory but required the taxpayer to reduce its basis in the property by the amount received.

Section 104, discussed in detail in the following chapter, specifically excludes from income the amount of any damages awarded for personal physical injury or physical sickness on the grounds that the amount received represents a return of the personal capital destroyed. In many cases, amounts are also awarded to penalize the party responsible for the wrongdoing. These so-called punitive damages are normally taxable.[16] Similarly, where the damages awarded represent reimbursement for lost profits, the amounts are considered taxable since they are merely substitutions for income.[17]

> **Example 6.** After ten consecutive losing seasons as head football coach at Trample University and a swing at his offensive line coach, Coach F was fired. Shortly thereafter, F developed an ulcer, which forced him to have surgery. It was subsequently determined that the operation had been improperly performed. F sued the university for lost wages and the court awarded him $25,000. The $25,000 is fully taxable since it represents a substitution of income. F also sued the surgeon for $200,000 for malpractice and won. If the $200,000 represents damages awarded for physical injury,

---

[12] *Doyle v. Mitchell Bros.*, 1 USTC ¶17, 3 AFTR 2979, 247 U.S. 179 (USSC, 1918). See also *Southern Pacific Company v. Lowe*, 1 USTC ¶19, 247, 3 AFTR 2989, 247 U.S. 330 (USSC, 1918).

[13] Reg. § 1.61-3(a).

[14] 40 BTA 333 (1939); See also Rev. Rul. 81-277, 1981-2 CB 14.

[15] 9 T.C. 727, (1947).

[16] § 104(a)(2); but see § 104(c) for an exception if only punitive damages can be awarded.

[17] *Phoenix Coal Co. v. Comm.*, 56-1 USTC ¶9366, 49 AFTR 445, 231 F.2d 420 (CA-2, 1956).

the amount is excluded under §104. However, if the award represents punitive damages, it is taxable.

Damages awarded to businesses are generally subject to the same tests applied to individuals. Awards or settlements for antitrust violations or patent infringements are examples of substitutions for income and thus are taxable. This is true for both actual and punitive damages. Compensation for damages to property are taxable to the extent that amounts received exceed the adjusted basis of the assets. Where the award is for damages to the goodwill of the business, the entire amount is usually taxable since the taxpayer normally does not have any recoverable basis in the goodwill.[18]

> **Example 7.** M left her car running and ran inside the bank to make a deposit. When she came back, she stopped in shock as she watched her car plunge through the front of a furniture store. The furniture store ultimately received $50,000 in damages for property for which it had a basis of $35,000. The store realized a gain of $15,000. This gain must be recognized unless certain special rules concerning involuntary conversions discussed in Chapter 15 are followed.

Other Considerations. The scope of the return of capital doctrine extends beyond situations involving damages and simple sales transactions. Numerous Code sections are grounded on this principle, and often contain detailed rules for ascertaining how a receipt should be apportioned between capital and income. For example, amounts received under a life insurance policy are not taxable on the theory that the proceeds—at least in part—represent a return of the taxpayer's premium payments.[19] Similarly, where the taxpayer purchases an annuity (i.e., an investment which makes a series of payments to the investor in the future), the return of capital doctrine provides that each payment is in part a tax-free return of capital.[20] In addition, somewhat intricate provisions exist to determine whether a corporate distribution represents a distribution of earnings (i.e., a dividend) or a tax-free return of the taxpayer's investment.[21] The special rules governing life insurance, annuities, and dividends are covered in detail in Chapter 6.

INDIRECT ECONOMIC BENEFITS

Another refinement to the otherwise all-inclusive definition of gross income concerns certain benefits provided by employers for employees. Early rulings and decisions exempted benefits conferred to employees that did not represent compensation and were provided for the convenience of the employer. For example, in 1919, the IRS ruled that lodging furnished seamen aboard ship was not taxable.[22] Similarly, in 1925, the Court of Claims held that the value of quarters provided an Army officer was not includible in income.[23] Explanations offered for exempting the lodging from income emphasized that the employee was granted the benefit solely because the employer's business could not function properly unless an employee was furnished that benefit on the employer's premises. The Court also observed that the benefits were not designed as a form of compensation for the employee, but rather were an outgrowth of business necessity. These early holdings established the view that certain benefits an employee receives indirectly from his or her employer are nontaxable. Current law grants an exclusion only

---

[18] *Raytheon Production Corp. v. Comm.*, 44-2 USTC ¶9424, 32 AFTR 1155, 144 F.2d 100 (CA-1, 1944).

[19] § 101.

[20] § 72.

[21] §§ 301 and 316.

[22] O.D. 265, 1 C.B. 71 (1919).

[23] *Jones v. U.S.*, 1 USTC ¶129, 5 AFTR 5297, 60 Ct.Cls. 552 (1925). Section 119, discussed in Chapter 6, currently provides specific rules that must be satisfied before meals and lodging may be excluded.

if the employee can demonstrate that the benefit served a business purpose of the employer other than to compensate the employee.[24]

> **Example 8.** In the following situations an employee is permitted to exclude the benefit received under the rationale discussed above.
>
> 1. An employer provides the employee with a place to work and supplies tools and machinery with which to do the work. Similarly, an employee is not taxed when his or her secretary types a letter.
>
> 2. An employer provides tuition-free, American-style schools for its overseas employees.
>
> 3. An employer provides an executive with protection in response to threats made by terrorists.
>
> 4. An employer requires its employees to attend a convention held in a resort in Florida and pays the travel costs of the employees.

It is often difficult to determine whether a particular benefit represents compensation or, alternatively, serves the business needs of the employer. For example, free parking places and similar fringe benefits provided by an employer could arguably fall into either category, depending upon the circumstances. After many years of controversy concerning the taxation of fringe benefits, Congress addressed the problem in 1984. To emphasize that fringe benefits are taxable, Congress modified the listing of typical income items found in § 61 to specifically include "fringe benefits and similar items." However, several exceptions exempting certain benefits still exist. These exceptions are discussed in Chapter 6 concerning exclusions.

✅ CHECK YOUR KNOWLEDGE

Review Question 1. After exploring the cavernous pits of his patient's mouth, Dr. Will Floss, a dentist, concluded that the gentleman had to have a root canal. Floss explained to the patient the nature of the work and that it could very well be the first in a series of expensive steps required to put his teeth back in working order. He estimated the total cost at $5,000. At that moment, the patient, a wily floor-covering dealer, immediately recalled Floss's need for new carpeting. As a result, he suggested that he would be happy to make a deal: carpeting, pad, and installation in exchange for the dental work. The two agreed, the teeth were repaired, and the carpeting was installed. Is there a tax problem here?

The issue is whether either party must report income. Many individuals think that barter transactions, exchanges of property for services or property other than cash, are not taxable. However, taxpayers who believe bartering escapes the eye of the tax collector are in for a rude awakening by the IRS. Barter transactions are fully taxable under the form-of-benefit principle. It makes no difference whether the taxpayer's net worth is increased by cash or property. In either case, the taxpayer is better off and must recognize income. Here the dentist recognizes income equal to the value of the services rendered, $5,000, and the carpet salesman has revenue equal to the value of services received.

Review Question 2. Several years ago, Intel Corporation, a leading manufacturer of computer chips in the United States, sued another chip manufacturer, American Micro, for using its patented technology. The courts awarded Intel millions of dollars for the infringement. Another situation, perhaps more well-known, was the McDonalds coffee debacle. In this case, a jury awarded 79-year-old Stella Liebeck of Albuquerque, New

---

[24]   *George D. Patterson v. Thomas*, 61-1 USTC 9310, 7 AFTR2d 862, 289 F.2d 108 (CA-2, 1960).

Mexico $200,000 in compensatory damages and another $2.7 million in punitive damages for severe burns she suffered when she spilled McDonald's coffee in her lap. (Liebeck and McDonald's ultimately settled for unknown amounts out of court.) In a comparable story, Theresa Burke and more than 8,000 other women employees of the Tennessee Valley Authority claimed unlawful discrimination in the payment of salaries on the basis of sex. The TVA had increased the salaries in certain male-dominated pay schedules, but not in certain female-dominated pay schedules. Moreover, the TVA lowered salaries in the latter. The female employees asked for and were awarded back pay, costs, and attorney's fees. Burke and the other women each received amounts in settlement according to a formula based on their length of service and rates of pay. What tax treatment might be proposed for these taxpayers?

The basic question in all of these situations is the same: does Intel, Liebeck, or Burke have taxable income? The key is recognizing that the amounts received may be taxable or nontaxable depending on the application of the return of capital doctrine and perhaps other provisions of the Code. The problem that Intel faces is demonstrating that the award for the patent infringement is not merely a replacement of lost income. It would appear that the corporation would have a difficult time overcoming a long string of cases that indicates that patent infringement awards are taxable. Nevertheless, there is no certainty in these matters without knowledge of all of the facts and a great deal of research. On the other hand, Liebeck probably had an easier time excluding her compensatory damages for her physical injury since they represent a return of her personal capital. However, the treatment of the punitive damages, although clearly taxable now, was not as clear under prior law. And what about Ms. Burke? It would seem that the knife could cut either way. On the one hand, the amounts received reimbursed her for back pay and arguably should be taxable as a substitution of income. On the other hand, the amounts could be viewed as a nontaxable reimbursement for a personal injury, sexual discrimination. If this seems difficult, it was. The courts struggled with the issue. The Sixth Circuit Court of Appeals held that the amounts were not taxable, but that decision was reversed by the Supreme Court. In 1996, Congress clarified the treatment, providing in § 104 that emotional distress does not constitute physical injury or physical sickness, thereby making damages from sex or age discrimination taxable.

Review Question 3. There is little doubt that the CEOs of Chrysler and GM, receive the use of a company car. The same can probably be said for the owners of every car dealership in the country as well as their salespeople. (If only accountants could receive such a deal!) Assume that each individual can drive the car for only 3,000 miles, after which he or she must evaluate the experience then exchange the old car for a new one and do it all over again. This is a nice arrangement: use a Jeep Grand Cherokee one month and a Chrysler Town and Country Van the next. Great benefits, but what are the tax consequences?

Once again the question concerns income. Is the value of the use of the company car taxable? Can the taxpayers argue that their use (including all personal trips) is not compensation but simply an incidental benefit that they must endure in order to evaluate the car? Does the indirect benefit rule apply? Is there a special provision that exempts fringe benefits of this nature? In a long line of cases, it has been established that the value of a car provided by an employer is compensation to the extent of the employee's personal use. The twist on the basic fact pattern—the required evaluation—may, however, suggest a different conclusion. The fringe benefit rules enacted in 1984 and discussed more fully in Chapter 6 do allow an exclusion for certain full-time automobile salespeople who use demonstration vehicles in the sales area in which the automobile dealer's sales office is located. Note that this rule applies only to salespeople. Thus an owner or executive would not qualify for an exclusion under this exception unless he or she also is considered a salesperson. There may be another escape hatch for executives and other management

personnel, however, buried in the Regulations concerning product testing.[25] These Regulations allow the employee to exclude the benefit if the employee receives goods for testing and evaluation if a laundry list of requirements is met. The key point to remember here is not necessarily knowing the specific answer to this question but recognizing that an important theory exists—the indirect benefit doctrine—that is a valuable weapon on which the taxpayer can sometimes rely to avoid taxation of what at first glance has all the characteristics of taxable income.

REPORTING INCOME: TAX ACCOUNTING METHODS

Once the taxpayer has realized an item of taxable income, he or she must determine *when* the income should be reported. This determination, however, requires an understanding of the nature of accounting periods and accounting methods that may be used for tax purposes. This section examines some of the fundamental rules of tax accounting and how they govern the timing of income recognition.

ACCOUNTING PERIODS

Taxable income is usually computed on the basis of an annual accounting period commonly known as the taxable year.[26] There are two types of taxable years: a calendar year and a fiscal year. A calendar year is a 12-month period ending on December 31, whereas a fiscal year generally is any period of 12 months ending on the last day of any month other than December.[27] Any taxpayer may use a calendar year. Fiscal years may be used only by taxpayers who maintain adequate books and records. A taxpayer filing his or her *first* return may adopt either a calendar year or a fiscal year without IRS consent simply by filing a return. After adoption, however, any change does require IRS consent.[28]

Income from Partnerships, S Corporations, Fiduciaries. Reporting income derived from an interest in a partnership, an S corporation, or an estate or trust presents a special problem. As explained in Chapter 3, income realized by a partnership or an S corporation is not taxable to either of these because they are not treated as separate taxable entities. Rather, the partnership or S corporation merely serves as a conduit through which the income flows. Consequently, partners or S shareholders report their distributive shares of the entity's income in their taxable year within which (or with which) the partnership or S corporation tax year ends. Partners or S shareholders must report their share of the income regardless of the amounts distributed to them.

Example 9. DEF Company, a fiscal year taxpayer, is a partnership owned equally by D, E, and F. For the taxable year ending September 30, 2009, the company had net income of $90,000. During the 12-month period ending on September 30, 2009, D withdrew $20,000 from his capital account. For his year ending December 31, 2009, D must report his share of partnership income, $30,000 (of $90,000), even though he only received a distribution of $20,000. Note that any income earned by the partnership from October 2009 through December 2009 is not reported until D files his 2010 tax return, which is normally due on April 15, 2011.

25   Reg. § 1.132-5(n).
26   § 441(a) and (b).
27   Reg. § 1.441-1(d) and (e). The taxpayer may elect to end the tax year on a particular day of the week rather than a date, resulting in a tax year that varies in length between 52 and 53 weeks. See Reg. § 1.441-2.
28   A request for a change is made on Form 1128. The initial selection of, or a change in, tax year may result in a short tax year, in which case the tax may have to be computed on an annualized basis. See §§ 442 and 443.

Income realized by a trust or an estate is generally taxed to the beneficiaries to the extent it is actually distributed or required to be distributed. Income that is not taxed to the beneficiaries is taxed to the estate or trust.

Limitation on Fiscal Years. One effect of allowing fiscal years for reporting is to enable certain taxpayers to *defer* the taxation of income. For instance, in *Example 9* above, the election by the partnership to use a fiscal year creates an opportunity for D. Note that D's share of the partnership's income for October 2009 through December 2009 is not reported until D files his 2010 tax return, which is normally filed on April 15, 2011. A small corporation that primarily provides personal services could obtain a similar deferral.

Example 10. G&H Inc., a law firm, is a regular C corporation owned by two attorneys, G and H. The corporation reports using a fiscal year ending on January 31. During 2009 the corporation paid G and H small salaries. Just before the close of its taxable year ending January 31, 2010, the corporation paid a bonus to G and H equal to its taxable income. By deducting the bonus, the corporation reports no income for its taxable year ending January 31, 2010, and G and H defer reporting the bonus until they file their 2010 tax return on April 15, 2011.

In 1986, Congress felt that the use of fiscal years to create deferral of income as shown above was improper. As a result, provisions were enacted that restrict the use of fiscal years by partnerships, S corporations, and so-called personal service corporations (i.e., corporations where the principal activity is the performance of services, substantially all of which are performed by employees who are also the owners of the business). Although certain exceptions enable these entities to use a fiscal year on a limited basis, as a general rule, these taxpayers normally must use the calendar year.[29]

Annual Accounting and Progressive Rates. The use of an annual accounting period in combination with other features of the taxation process causes numerous difficulties. For example, consider the effect of the tax system's use of both an annual accounting period and a progressive tax rate structure. Each year the taxpayer computes his or her taxable income for that period and applies a progressive rate structure to the income of that year. If income varies from one year to the next, taxes paid on the *total* income of those two years are likely to exceed the total taxes that would have resulted had the taxpayer earned the income equally each year. The problems that occur with so-called incoming-bunching are illustrated below.

Example 11. Taxpayer R is a salesperson whose income is derived solely from commissions. Taxpayer S earns a salary. Both taxpayers are single. In 19X1 and 19X2 R's taxable income was $80,000 and $20,000 respectively, while S had taxable income of $50,000 each year. The tax effect on R and S (rounded to the nearest dollar and using 2009 tax rates) is as follows:

	R (Single)		S (Single)	
	Taxable Income	Tax	Taxable Income	Tax
19X1	$ 80,000	$16,188	$ 50,000	$ 8,688
19X2	20,000	2,583	50,000	8,688
Total	$100,000	$18,771	$100,000	$17,376

Note that although R and S have the same total income of $100,000 for the two-year period, R's total tax bill of $18,771 exceeds S's bill of $17,376 by $1,395.

---

[29] §§ 441(i), 444, 706(b), and 1378.

As the above example demonstrates, the use of an annual accounting period may create inequities. In this particular case, R could reduce his tax bite if he could defer some of his income from one year to the next so as to split his income between years as equally as possible. In other cases, Congress has responded by enacting special provisions. For example, where a taxpayer has a loss during the year, the net operating loss rules allow the taxpayer to utilize the loss by permitting it to be carried back or forward to profitable years.[30] Without these carryback and carryover provisions, the taxpayer would receive no benefit from any losses realized.

ACCOUNTING METHODS

Once a tax year is identified, the taxpayer must determine in which period a transaction is to be reported. The year in which a particular item becomes part of the tax calculation is not a trivial matter. The time of recognition can make a substantial difference in the taxpayer's total tax liability not only because of the time value of money but also because factors affecting the tax calculations may change from year to year. For instance, tax rates may go up or down from one year to the next. Such change does not necessarily take an act of Congress. A taxpayer may simply marry, divorce, incorporate, or change from a taxable to tax-exempt entity. In such case, deferral of income to the low-rate year and acceleration of deductions to the high-rate year could produce significant savings. Similarly, Congress may completely revise the treatment of an item. For example, in 1993 Congress raised the top tax rate from 31 to 39.6 percent, eliminated the deduction for business club dues, dropped the amount of the deduction for business meals and entertainment from 80 to 50 percent, eliminated the deduction for certain moving expenses, increased the Medicare tax, increased the amount of social security benefits that are subject to tax, and raised the amount of business equipment that may be expensed from $10,000 to $17,500. Changes like these have become an annual rite in the tax area, consequently making timing critical.

The rules that determine when a particular item is reported are generally referred to as accounting methods. The Code identifies four permissible methods of accounting:[31]

1. The cash receipts and disbursements method

2. The accrual method

3. Any other method permitted by the Code (e.g., a method for a specific situation such as the completed contract method or the use of LIFO to value inventories)[32]

4. Any combination of the three methods above permitted by the Regulations

The term *accounting method* is not limited to the overall method of accounting used by the taxpayer (e.g., the cash or accrual method). It generally includes the treatment of *any particular item* if such treatment affects *when* the item will be reported. For example, the use of LIFO to value inventories would be considered an accounting method since the use of this method determines when the cost of a product will become part of cost of goods sold.

It should be emphasized that the taxpayer is not required to adopt one overall method of accounting. For example, a taxpayer with inventories generally must use the accrual method to account for inventories and related sales. However, the same taxpayer could use the cash method to report interest income or other items. This approach (referred to as the *hybrid method*) is completely acceptable as long as the taxpayer applies the same methods consistently.

---

[30]   § 172. See Chapter 10 for a discussion of the net operating loss rules.

[31]   § 446(c).

[32]   Reg. § 1.446-1(c)(1)(iii).

Taxpayers are generally allowed to select the methods of accounting they wish to use. In all cases, however, the IRS has the right to determine if the method used *clearly reflects income*, and, if not, to make the necessary adjustments.[33] For example, assume that each year a taxpayer changes the way it computes the amount of overhead that it capitalizes as part of inventory (e.g., on the basis of direct labor hours one year, machine hours the next). In such case, the IRS might require the taxpayer to use one method consistently so that income would not be distorted from year to year but would be clearly reflected.

Tax Methods versus Financial Accounting Methods. At first glance, many people— particularly accountants—would no doubt conclude that a method of accounting that conforms with generally accepted accounting principles (GAAP) would be regarded as clearly reflecting income.[34] Although this is ordinarily true, it is not always the case.[35] Conflicts sometimes exist because the objectives of the income tax system differ from that of financial accounting. The primary goal of financial accounting is to provide useful information to management, shareholders, creditors, and other interested parties. In contrast, the goal of the income tax system is to ensure that revenues are fairly collected. Due to these different goals, the tax law may disregard fundamental accounting principles. Perhaps the most obvious example can be found in the tax law's allowance of the cash method of accounting. Despite its failure to properly match revenues and expenses, the cash method is normally tolerated because from an administrative view it is simple and objective. Such administrative concerns often dictate a different approach for tax purposes. For example, an accrual basis taxpayer is often required to report prepaid income when received rather than when earned. Although this practice violates the matching principle, it ensures that the tax is imposed when the taxpayer has the cash to pay it.

The operation of differing objectives can also be seen in the use of estimates. One of the major responsibilities of financial accountants is to ensure that financial statement users are not misled. This demand normally encourages accountants to be conservative, which in turn may cause them to understate rather than overstate income. Although the government does not want taxpayers to overstate income, it certainly does not want to endorse principles that would tend toward understatement. Thus, the tax law generally does not allow taxpayers to estimate future expenses such as bad debts or warranty costs and deduct them currently, as is the case with financial accounting. Instead, the deduction is allowed only when there is objective evidence that a cost has been incurred. The government frowns on estimates of expenses, presumably because taxpayers would tend to overstate them.

Reporting of prepaid income and the treatment of estimated expenses are just two examples of where financial accounting principles deviate from tax accounting. The key point to recognize is that a particular item may be treated one way for financial accounting purposes and another way for tax purposes. As a practical matter, this may mean that two sets of books are maintained, or what is perhaps more likely, one set based on financial accounting principles to which adjustments must be made to arrive at taxable income.

CASH METHOD OF ACCOUNTING

General Rule. Virtually all individuals—as well as many corporations, partnerships, trusts, and estates—use the cash method of accounting. Its prevalence is no doubt attributable to the fact that it is easy to use. Under the cash method, taxpayers simply report items of income and deduction in the year in which they are received or paid.[36] In

---

[33] § 446(b).

[34] Reg. § 1.446-1(a)(2).

[35] For an excellent example, see *Thor Power Tool Co.*, 79-1 USTC ¶9139, 43 AFTR2d 79-362, 439 U.S. 522 (USSC, 1979).

[36] Reg. § 1.446-1(c)(1)(i).

effect, the cash method allows taxpayers merely to refer to their checkbooks to determine taxable income.

In using the cash method, items of income need not be in the form of cash but need only be capable of valuation in terms of money. Under this rule, sometimes termed the *cash equivalent doctrine*, the taxpayer reports income when the equivalent of cash is received.[37] Thus, where property or services are received, the fair market value of these items serves as the measure of income.

Due to the cash equivalent doctrine, reporting of income arising from notes and accounts receivable differs. Notes received by a cash basis taxpayer are usually considered property and hence constitute income equal to the value of the note.[38] Where a promise to pay is *not* evidenced by a note (e.g., credit sales resulting in accounts receivable), income is normally not recognized by a cash basis taxpayer until payment is received.[39] This treatment results because unsupported promises to pay normally are not considered as having a fair market value.

Constructive Receipt Doctrine. Taxpayers using the cash method of accounting have substantial control over income recognition since they may control the timing of the actual receipt of cash. If the requirement calling for *actual* receipt were strictly adhered to, the cash basis taxpayer could easily frustrate the purpose of progressive taxation. For example, taxpayers could select the year with the lowest tax rate and simply cash their salary or dividend checks or redeem their interest coupons in that year. To curtail this practice, the doctrine of constructive receipt was developed. Under this principle, a taxpayer is *deemed* to have received income even though such income has not actually been received. It should be noted that there is no corresponding doctrine for deductions (i.e., there is no constructive payment doctrine).

The constructive receipt doctrine is currently expressed in Regulation § 1.451-2(a) as follows:

> Income, although not actually reduced to the taxpayer's possession, is constructively received by him in the taxable year in which it is credited to his account, set apart for him or otherwise made available so that he could have drawn upon it during the taxable year if notice of intention to withdraw had been given. However, income is not constructively received if the taxpayer's control of its receipt is subject to substantial limitations or restrictions.

As the Regulation indicates, the taxpayer is treated as having received income when three conditions are satisfied:

1. The taxpayer has control over the amount without substantial limitations and restrictions

2. The amount has been set aside or credited to the taxpayer's account

3. The funds are available for payment by the payer (i.e., the payer's ability to make payment must be considered)

Some of the common situations to which the rule is applied are illustrated in the following examples.

---

[37]   Reg. § 1.446-1(a)(3).

[38]   *A.W. Wolfson*, 1 B.T.A. 538 (1925).

[39]   *Bedell v. Comm.*, 1 USTC ¶359, 7 AFTR 8469, 30 F.2d 622 (CA-2, 1929).

Example 12. B refereed a basketball game on Saturday night, December 31, 2009 and did not receive the check for his services until after the banks had closed. He cashed the check on January 3, 2010. B must report the income in 2009. In the case of a check, a taxpayer is deemed to have received payment in the year the check is received rather than when it is cashed.[40]

Example 13. T mailed a check on December 29, 2009, which S received in January 2010. S is not in constructive receipt of the check since it was not available to him for his immediate use and enjoyment. However, if S requested that T mail him the check so that he receives it in 2010, or if S could have received the check by merely appearing in person and claiming it, S would be deemed to have received the payment in 2009.

Example 14. When G made a deposit on January 15, 2010, the bank updated her passbook on December 31, 2009 to show that $200 of interest was credited to her account for the last quarter of 2009. G withdrew the interest on January 31. G must report the interest in 2009. Interest credited to the taxpayer's account is taxable when credited, regardless of whether it is in the taxpayer's possession, assuming that it may be withdrawn.[41]

Example 15. B Corporation mailed dividend checks dated December 20 on December 28, 2009. R, a shareholder in B, received her check on January 4, 2010. R reports the dividend income in 2010 as long as the payer customarily pays dividends by mail so that the shareholder receives it after the end of the year.[42]

Example 16. R's secretary received several checks for services that R had performed. Payments received by a taxpayer's agent are considered constructively received by the taxpayer.[43]

Example 17. A taxpayer who agrees not to cash a check until authorized by the payer has not constructively received income if the payer does not have sufficient funds in the bank to cover the check.[44]

Limitations on the Use of the Cash Method. As a method of accounting, the cash method's principal advantage lies in its simplicity and objectivity. If a taxpayer uses the cash method, taxable income is easily computed merely by referring to cash receipts and disbursements. Moreover, the amount of taxable income computed in this manner is incontrovertible—it is not open to question or dispute and is readily verifiable. Unlike the accrual method, whether income has been "earned" or expenses have been "incurred" are simply not issues under the cash method.

On other counts, the cash method scores poorly, ranking a distant second to the accrual method. From an accounting perspective, the cash method is entirely inappropriate since income and expense are recognized without regard to the taxable year in which the economic events responsible for the income or expense actually occur. Similarly, when some parties to a transaction use different methods of accounting, there may be a mismatching of income and deductions. For example, an accrual basis corporation could accrue expenses payable to a cash basis individual. In such case, the

[40] *C.F. Kahler*, 18 T.C. 31 (1952).

[41] Reg. § 1.451-2(b).

[42] *Ibid.; S.L. Avery*, 4 USTC ¶1277, 13 AFTR 1168, 292 U.S. 210 (USSC, 1934). See also *H.B. McEuen v. Comm.*, 52-1 USTC ¶9281, 41 AFTR 1169, 196 F.2d 127 (CA-5, 1952).

[43] *T. Watson*, 2 TCM 863 (1943).

[44] *A.V. Johnston*, 23 TCM 2003, T.C. Memo 1964-323.

corporation could obtain deductions without ever having to make a disbursement and, moreover, without the individual taxpayer recognizing any offsetting income.

While the above are clearly shortcomings, the major flaw found in the cash method is that it is easily abused. Taxpayers have often secured benefits by merely timing their transactions appropriately: recognizing income in one year, deductions in the next, or what is more likely, deductions in years in which the taxpayer is in a high tax bracket and income in years in which the taxpayer is in a low tax bracket.

To attack these problems, Congress has limited the use of the cash method of accounting. The following entities are normally prohibited from using the cash method:[45]

1. Regular C corporations;

2. Partnerships that have regular C corporations as partners (other than certain personal service corporations described below); and

3. *Tax shelters*, generally defined as any enterprise (other than a regular C corporation) in which interests have been offered for sale in any offering required to be registered under Federal or State security agencies.

Despite these general restrictions, Congress believed that the simplicity of the cash method justified its continued use in certain instances. For example, Congress felt that it would be costly for small businesses to switch to the accrual method. Similarly, it recognized that the accrual method would create undue complexity for farming businesses if such a method were required to account for growing crops and livestock. In addition, Congress believed that personal service corporations, which have traditionally used the cash method, should be allowed to continue their use. Accordingly, the following entities are allowed to use the cash method.[46]

1. Any corporation or partnership whose annual *gross receipts* for *all* preceding years do not exceed $5 million. This test is satisfied for any prior year only if the average annual gross receipts[47] for the three-year period ending with such year does not exceed $5 million. Once this average *exceeds* $5 million, the corporation cannot use the cash method for the following year.

2. Certain farming businesses.

3. Qualified personal service corporations. A regular C corporation is qualified if substantially all of the activities consist of performing services in eight fields, including health, law, engineering, architecture, accounting, actuarial science, performing arts, or consulting, *and* at least 95 percent of its stock is held by the employees who are providing such services.[48]

Example 18. Dr. C and Dr. D, both heart surgeons, own 100% of the stock of Cardiac Care Corporation. The corporation provides the latest in diagnostic testing and treatments, including open heart surgery and rehabilitation. Because all of the corporations's services are in the area of health and more than 95% of the stock is owned by the doctors who are providing the services, the corporation may use the cash method of accounting.

---

[45] § 448(a).

[46] § 448(b).

[47] Gross receipts include total sales (net of returns and allowances but not reduced by costs of goods sold) and amounts received for services, interest, rents, royalties, and annuities. For sales of capital assets and real or depreciable property used in trade or business, gross receipts are reduced by the taxpayer's adjusted basis in such property. See Temp. Reg. § 1.448-1T(f)(2)(iv).

[48] § 448(d)(2).

Example 19. C's Video Rentals, a regular C corporation, started business in 19X1. Since that time it has grown to 20 locations and had annual gross receipts as follows:

Year	Gross Receipts	Average Annual Gross Receipts*
19X1	$ 4,000,000	$4,000,000
19X2	2,000,000	3,000,000
19X3	6,000,000	4,000,000
19X4	10,000,000	6,000,000

$$\text{*}\frac{\text{Current } + \text{ Prior two years}}{3 \text{ (or if less, years in existence)}}$$

It initially adopted the cash method in 19X1. It was able to use the cash method through 19X4 because the average annual gross receipts for all prior years did not exceed $5 million. Note that although its gross receipts were $6,000,000 in 19X3, its *average annual* gross receipts for that year were only $4,000,000 [($4,000,000 + $2,000,000 + $6,000,000) ÷ 3]. Consequently, the cash method could be used for 19X4. It will be denied use of the cash method for 19X5 since the average annual gross receipts for 19X4 exceed $5 million [($2,000,000 + $6,000,000 + $10,000,000) ÷ 3 = $ 6,000,000].

It should be noted that the above exceptions do not apply to tax shelters. Any enterprise considered a tax shelter must use the accrual method. In addition, as discussed below, if the taxpayer maintains inventories, special rules apply.

Accounting for Inventory. As noted above, most businesses—other than large C corporations—are permitted to use the cash method. However, an important exception exists for taxpayers with inventories. According to the longstanding rule of Regulation §1.471-1 "[I]n order to reflect taxable income correctly, inventories … are necessary in every case in which the production, purchase, or sale of merchandise is an income producing factor." Regulation § 1.446-1(c)(2) adds that in any case in which it is necessary to use an inventory the accrual method of accounting must be used with regard to purchases and sales … In short, if a business sells "inventory," taxpayers must capitalize the cost of inventory purchases and can expense such costs only when the item is sold. Just as important, if not more so, businesses with inventories also must accrue and recognize income at the time of sale—regardless of when the cash is received. Both halves of the accrual requirement are significant since both effect the amount of income that the taxpayer ultimately reports in a particular year.

The reasoning behind the regulatory scheme requiring inventories is anchored in the matching principle that ensures income will be clearly reflected. The rationale was eloquently stated by the Appellate Court in *Knight-Ridder Newspapers Inc.*, a case involving whether a cash-basis corporation should inventory its costs of newsprint and ink.[49]

According to accounting wisdom the income realized from the sale of merchandise is most *clearly measured* by matching the cost of the merchandise with the revenue from its sale. In order to achieve such matching of revenue and cost, it is necessary to keep an inventory account reflecting the costs of merchandise, raw materials, and

---

[49]   84 -2 USTC ¶9827, 54 AFTR 2d 84-6120, 743 F.2d 781 (CA-11, 1984).

manufacturing expenses. These costs are not deducted immediately when paid but are deferred until the year when the resulting merchandise is sold.

To make the matching complete, the taxpayer must report income on the accrual method. That method helps to ensure that income from the sale (like the inventory costs) is reflected in the year of the sale. For example, if the sale is made on credit, the accrual method nevertheless treats the income as accrued and reflects it when the sale occurs. The prophetic skills of the accrual shaman permit it to recognize both income and deductions in the same year.

By contrast, the primal cash method is unable to achieve such a mystical joinder [matching] of inventory deductions and credit sale income. To be sure, the cash method could theoretically operate in tandem with inventories. The beast could conceivably close its eyes to deductions until the year of the sale. It could never learn, however, to prophesy future cash payments. If there were a credit sale, the beast could not grasp income and deductions simultaneously in its rugged paw. The goal of matching costs and revenues would fail.

While the inventory rule seems relatively simple and necessary to guarantee the clear reflection of income of a cash basis taxpayer, it is has led to a great deal of controversy. These issues are discussed in further detail in Chapter 10.

ACCRUAL METHOD OF ACCOUNTING

Taxpayers using the accrual method of accounting report income in the year in which it is considered earned under the so-called *all-events test.* Under this test, income is earned when all the events have occurred that fix the right to receive such income and the amount of income can be determined with reasonable accuracy.[50] As the courts have consistently observed in cases involving the all-events test, the "objective is to determine at what point in time the seller acquired an unconditional right to receive payment under the contract."[51]

> **Example 20.** S Corporation manufactures a special machine used in a process to convert oranges into orange juice. On December 15, 2009, S sold a machine to B Inc. According to the terms of the sales agreement, B was given a 30-day period for testing and acceptance. As of the end of 2009, B had not indicated its acceptance. S would not accrue the income from the sale in 2009 because it did not have an unconditional right to receive the income. The first prong of the all-events test, a fixed right to receive income, is not met. The sale was contingent on satisfaction of certain conditions—test and acceptance—and since these conditions had not been met at the close of 2009 the sale was not completed and S had no right to the income. If B subsequently rejected the machine, this would clearly mean delay or a complete loss of the sale.[52]

In most situations involving a sale of merchandise, the right becomes fixed when the goods are shipped, when the product is delivered or accepted or when title passes, as long as the method is consistently used.[53]

---

[50]   Reg. § 1.451-1(a).

[51]   *Hallmark Cards, Inc. v. CIR*, 90 T.C. 26, 33 (1988).

[52]   See *Webb Press Co. v. CIR*, 3 BTA 247 (1925) (acq.).

[53]   *Lucas v. North Texas Lumber Co.*, 2 USTC ¶484, 8 AFTR 10276, 281 U.S. 11 (USSC, 1929). See also Reg. §1.446-1(c)(1)(ii).

Example 21. In *Hallmark Cards*, the greeting card giant, a calendar year accrual basis taxpayer, shipped Valentine cards before year end but deferred income from the sales to the following year. Early shipment was necessary to deal with certain production and shipping problems related to supplying cards in a timely manner to its customers (more than 20,000 retailers at over 35,000 locations). Contracts with the customers specified that title and risk of loss passed to customers on January 1. The IRS argued that Hallmark should accrue the income when the cards were shipped since it had a fixed right to the income, therefore meeting the all-events test. Notwithstanding the fact that the items had been delivered to customers prior to year end, the Court held that Hallmark was *not* required to accrue the income upon shipment. The Court explained that "passage of title and risk of loss to buyer" did not occur under the contract until January 1 and therefore Hallmark could postpone recognition since it did not have a fixed right to the income.[54]

As the two examples above illustrate, the terms of the agreement are critical in determining whether the taxpayer has an unconditional right to the income. Other facts may also be important such as doubts concerning whether the receivable can be collected or disputes or other uncertainties relating to the amount of the liability. If the agreement requires a particular act, such as submitting a bill, and such act is viewed as simply ministerial, the requirement may be ignored in determining whether the taxpayer has a "right" to the income.

Example 22. In 1996, in *Charles Schwab Corp.*, the discount securities broker asserted that its commission income accrued on the settlement date.[55] However, the Tax Court ultimately agreed with the government that the income should be accrued on the trade date. According to the Court, the broker's "essential service" was "execution of trades," and the subsequent settlement activities were merely "of a ministerial nature."

As discussed above, the accrual method normally *must* be used in accounting for sales, purchases, and inventories if inventories are an income-producing factor. However, the taxpayer who must use the accrual method in this instance may still account for other items of income and expense using the cash method. The accrual method, as noted earlier, must be used by regular C corporations and partnerships with C corporations as partners unless one of several exceptions is satisfied.

There are several special rules relating to the accrual method of accounting that cause variations in the normal scheme. For example, dividends would normally accrue under the all-events test on the date of record. An exception exists, however, so that dividends are reported when received.[56] In addition to this exception, others exist that are discussed later in this chapter.

CHANGES IN ACCOUNTING METHODS

Taxpayers are initially given great freedom in the methods of accounting they may use. However, once a particular method has been adopted (e.g., when it is first used to account for an item), it may not be changed unless consent is granted by the IRS. Taxpayers seeking a change must apply for permission by filing Form 3115, Application for Change in Accounting Method, anytime during the tax year when the change is to become effective.[57] The IRS does not rubber-stamp these requests. Permission is granted

---

[54]   *Supra*, Footnote 51, *Hallmark Cards, Inc. v. CIR*, 90 T.C. 26, 33 (1988).

[55]   *Charles Schwab Corp. v. CIR*, 107 T.C. 282 (1996).

[56]   Reg. § 1.451-2(b), *Tar Products Corp. v. Comm.*, 42-2 USTC ¶9662, 29 AFTR 1190, 130 F.2d 866 (CA-3, 1942).

[57]   Some changes may be made automatically without consent, thereby avoiding the user fee for filing Form 3115.

only if the taxpayer is willing to make any adjustments required by the IRS. Under §481, the IRS is authorized to require adjustments if a change in method would result in the omission of income or the duplication of deductions.

> **Example 23.** T, Inc. operates a computer consulting company. It has always used the cash method to account for its income from services. In 2009, it decided that it should switch to the accrual method. At the end of 2008, T's outstanding receivables were $10,000. If T were allowed to switch to the accrual method and no adjustment were required, the $10,000 would escape taxation. The $10,000 would not be taxed in 2008 since T was on the cash basis in that year and no collections were made. Similarly, the $10,000 would not be taxed in 2009 because T is on the accrual method in that year and the income did not accrue in 2009 but rather 2008. Thus, without an adjustment, the $10,000 of income would be omitted from both the 2008 and 2009 returns, never to be taxed.

Accounting for the Adjustment. Taxpayers are normally required to report any adjustment attributable to a change in method in the year of the change and pay any additional tax due (or receive a refund).[58] In certain situations, this may create a severe hardship for the taxpayer (e.g., the required inclusion of several years' income in a single year). Moreover, taxpayers may be reluctant to change from an erroneous method of accounting to a correct method and simply wait for the IRS to detect their mistake. However, § 481(c) allows the IRS to alter this approach. The IRS has used this authority to develop a system that encourages taxpayers to switch from an erroneous method they may be using to a correct method.[59]

Under the revised approach of Revenue Procedure 97-27, the treatment of the adjustment depends primarily on whether the taxpayer voluntarily or involuntarily changes the accounting method. If the change is voluntary, the adjustment is spread over a four-year period (the year of the change and the three subsequent years). If the change is involuntary (e.g., the taxpayer is under examination and is not allowed under the rules of Revenue Procedure 97-27 to make a change) and the adjustment is positive, the entire adjustment is included in the earliest tax year under examination. However, a taxpayer may elect to use a one-year adjustment period if the entire adjustment is less that $ 25,000.

> **Example 24.** J has operated a small hardware store as a sole proprietorship since 1990. In August, 2011 the IRS audited J's 2009 tax return and determined that J had failed to use the accrual method of accounting for inventories. Instead, J had expensed all of his inventory as it was acquired. Consequently, the IRS required J to change his method of accounting. Based on a physical count and valuation of his inventory, the IRS determined that J had understated his income in prior years by $300,000. Assuming J is not allowed to voluntarily change his accounting method during the examination, he must report all $300,000 in income in 2009. Had J voluntarily made the change prior to examination or had he qualified under the special relief provisions to voluntarily make the change while under examination, he could have spread the adjustment over four years: $75,000 of income in 2009—the year of the change—and $75,000 in each of the three following years, 2010, 2011, and 2012.

> **Example 25.** During 2009, R asked for and obtained permission to change from the cash method to the accrual method. This change resulted in a negative income adjustment of $20,000. Because this adjustment is less than $25,000, R can take into account the entire adjustment in 2009.

---

[58] *Ibid.*

[59] Rev. Proc. 97-27, 1997-1, C.B. 680, as modified by Rev. Proc. 2002-19, 2002-1 C.B. 696.

Changes in accounting method are not to be confused with correction of errors. Errors such as mathematical mistakes or the improper calculation of a deduction or credit can be corrected by the taxpayer without permission of the IRS by simply filing an amended return. Alternatively, the IRS may discover the mistake and require the taxpayer to make a correction. However, if the statute of limitations has run on a return containing an error, no correction can be made. In these cases, the taxpayer's income is forever over- or understated, as the case may be.

✅ CHECK YOUR KNOWLEDGE

Review Question 1. On Sunday, December 31, 1961 in Green Bay, Wisconsin, Paul Hornung, All-American quarterback from Notre Dame, star of the Green Bay Packers and later a sports analyst, won a Corvette for being the most valuable player in the NFL championship game.[60] After the game, the editor of *Sport* magazine, the sponsor of the award, gave nothing to Hornung to evidence his ownership of the car, which was being held at a dealership in New York. Hornung picked up the car on January 3, 1962 in New York. What are the tax concerns here?

There is little question that Hornung must report income (although that was uncertain in 1961). The important issue to be resolved is when. Was Hornung in constructive receipt of the car that snowy afternoon in December 1961? Although Hornung, wanting to report the income in 1961, argued that he had received the car, the court disagreed. In a decision that should be mandatory reading for its witty analysis, the court explained that the basis of constructive receipt is unfettered control over the date of actual receipt. In this case, the facts indicated that Hornung did not have such control. He did not receive the car or even the keys or title to the car in 1961. Moreover, the car was in a dealership that was not only 1,000 miles away but was also closed. In addition, the car had not been set aside for Hornung's use and delivery was not solely up to him. Accordingly, the doctrine of constructive receipt was inapplicable.

Review Question 2. Mr. Mike, an accountant, is the proud owner of Maggie, a West Highland terrier. Shortly after Mike acquired Maggie, he discovered the need to take her to get the appropriate shots. It did not take long for Mike to pick a vet. He elected to use one of his long-time clients for whom he prepares tax returns, Nonhuman Companion Inc. that operates a chain of veterinary clinics throughout Arizona and California. Mike's visit to the vet was the first time he had actually been to his client's office. While there, he noticed that the clinic provided not only veterinarian and kennel services but also a great variety of food, toys, and pet paraphernalia for sale. To his best recollection, the corporation used the cash method of accounting. Is this the correct method?

There are two rules concerning accounting methods that come into play here. First, a corporation is normally required to use the accrual method of accounting. However, several exceptions may apply. The accrual requirement is waived if the corporation is an S corporation or its average annual gross receipts are less than $5 million for all preceding tax years. If neither of these exceptions applies, the corporation could possibly use the cash method if it is considered a personal service corporation, since it provides services in the health field. Interestingly, the IRS has addressed this question and ruled that veterinarian services fall within the definition of "personal" services (i.e., health services). Nevertheless, there could be a concern that "substantially all the activities" do not consist of performing "health" services. The second rule that operates in this situation concerns accounting for inventory. A business normally must use the accrual method to account for inventory even if it otherwise qualifies to use the cash method. The IRS has held that a

---

[60]   *Paul V. Hornung*, 47 T.C. 428 (1967).

partnership that provided veterinary services was required to switch from the cash method to the accrual method when more than 50 percent of the partnership's receipts were from merchandise (pet food, supplies, and drugs).[61]

Review Question 3. X Inc., an accrual basis calendar year taxpayer, filed a lawsuit against the U.S. government for breach of contract. X was awarded a judgment of $100,000 by the Court of Appeals for the Fifth Circuit for the alleged breach in 2008. The income was fully taxable. The government tried to appeal the decision to the Supreme Court, filing a petition for writ of certiorari. The writ and appeal were denied in 2009. No appropriation was made by the U.S. government for payment of the claim during 2008. When should X report the income?

X should accrue the income if the all-events test is met. The test is met when X has an unconditional right to the income. Here, the taxpayer's right to the income is not fixed until the Supreme Court denied the government's appeal in 2009. Such a condition is not simply ministerial in nature. In determining whether X's right was fixed, the fact that Congress did not make an appropriation for the payment of such sum in 2008 is irrelevant since the judgment became an acknowledged liability of the government in 2009.[62]

Review Question 4. In light of the decision in *Hallmark Cards, Greetings Inc.*, an accrual basis calendar year taxpayer changed the terms of its contracts for sales of Valentine cards this year so that passage of title and risk of loss to buyer did not occur under the contract until January 1. In the past, Greetings had accrued the income when the cards were shipped. Indicate whether the following statements are true or false and if false explain why.

    a. Greetings' change in the terms of its contracts constitutes a change in accounting method.
    b. Greetings must seek permission from the IRS to change its method.
    c. Any omission of income that results in Greetings' change must be reported in the year of the change

Statements (a) and (b) true. Any change which affects the time when income will be reported is considered a change in accounting method and permission must be obtained from the IRS to ensure there is not an omission of income or duplication of deduction. In this case, the change shifts incomes it normally reports in one year to the next year. Statement (c) is false. Assuming Greetings receives permission to change, it is normally permitted to spread the income adjustment over four years.

ACCOUNTING FOR INCOME: SPECIAL CONSIDERATIONS

CLAIM OF RIGHT DOCTRINE

Occasionally income may be received before the taxpayer's rights to such income have been clearly established. The tax difficulty posed in these instances concerns whether the taxpayer should report the income currently or wait until the proper claims to the income have been identified. For these situations, the courts have established a rule of law termed the *claim of right doctrine*. Under this rule, if a taxpayer actually or constructively *receives* income under a claim of right (i.e., the taxpayer claims the income is rightfully his or hers) and such income is not restricted in use, it must be included in

---

[61]   Technical Advice Memorandum 9218008.

[62]   Rev. Rul. 70-151, 1970-1 C.B. 116.

gross income.[63] In other words, earnings received must be included in income if the taxpayer has an *unrestricted claim*, notwithstanding the possibility that the income may be subsequently relinquished if the taxpayer's claim is later denied.

> **Example 26.** Television station WXYZ received $100,000 from KLM Company to air the firm's commercials during a local talk show in the month of December. During this month, the ratings dropped sharply when the star of the show quit. Shortly thereafter, KLM contacted the station, indicating that it wanted to discontinue its sponsorship and requesting return of $75,000 of the payment. In view of their interpretation of the agreement, the station continued to air the firm's commercials and retained the $100,000. KLM brought suit to recover the $75,000. Under the claim of right doctrine, WXYZ must include the entire $100,000 in income even though it may have to repay the amount or a portion thereof to KLM. The amount is included because WXYZ received the money and could use the amount without restriction.

The claim of right doctrine applies to both cash and accrual basis taxpayers. As previously discussed, income is usually reported by an accrual basis taxpayer only when all the events have occurred that fix the taxpayer's right to receive such income. However, in the case of contested income, the taxpayer's rights to such amounts have not been fixed, and under the all events test he or she would not report it. The all-events test notwithstanding, the claim of right doctrine carves out an exception to this rule for contested income the taxpayer has *received*. An accrual basis taxpayer who *receives* contested income under a claim of right without restrictions on its use must report the amount in income even though his or her rights to the income have not been fixed.[64] Alternatively, if the accrual basis taxpayer has *not received* the contested income, it will not be included because his or her rights thereto have not been fixed.[65] Thus, an *accrual basis* taxpayer's reporting of contested income depends on whether or not the taxpayer has received it.

> **Example 27.** RST, Inc, an accrual basis taxpayer, shipped parts to MNO Corporation and sent MNO a bill for $25,000. MNO used the parts and reported that they did not perform according to specifications. If MNO had paid the $25,000 and subsequently sued to recover the purchase price, RST would be required to include the $25,000 in income since the amount was received and the claim of right doctrine applies (i.e., RST has an unrestricted claim to the income). On the other hand, if MNO had not paid the $25,000, RST would not be required to accrue the income because the amount was *not* received and the all-events test has not been satisfied (i.e., RST's rights to the income have not been fixed).

The claim of right doctrine has been used in many differing instances to cause the inclusion of income in the year received. Some examples where the rule has been applied to make the income taxable are

1. Contingent legal fees that must be returned upon a reversal by an appellate court;[66]

2. Illegal income and gains (e.g., embezzled amounts);[67] and

3. Bonuses and commissions that were improperly computed and had to be subsequently repaid.[68]

---

[63] *North American Oil Consolidated v. Burnet*, 3 USTC ¶943, 11 AFTR 16, 286 U.S. 417 (USSC, 1932).

[64] *Ibid.*

[65] Reg. § 1.446-1(c)(1)(ii).

[66] *Michael Phillips v. Comm.*, 56-2 USTC ¶10,067, 50 AFTR 718, 238 F.2d 473 (CA-7, 1956).

[67] *James v. U.S.*, 61-1 USTC ¶9449, 7 AFTR2d 1361, 366 U.S. 213 (USSC, 1961).

[68] *U.S. v. Lewis*, 51-1 USTC ¶9211, 40 AFTR 258, 340 U.S. 590 (USSC, 1951).

The claim of right doctrine does not apply where the taxpayer receives the income but recognizes an obligation to repay.[69] For example, a landlord would not be required to report the receipt of a tenant's security deposit as income because the deposit must be repaid upon the tenant's departure if the apartment unit is undamaged.

In those situations where the taxpayer repays an amount that previously had been included in income, a deduction is allowed. Section 1341 provides a special rule for computing the deduction, which ensures that the tax benefit of the deduction is the equivalent to the tax paid on the income in the prior year.

PREPAID INCOME

Over the years, a web of exceptions and special rules have developed regarding the reporting of prepaid income by an *accrual basis* taxpayer. Absent these rules, the accrual basis taxpayer (in accordance with the all-events test) would defer recognition of prepaid income until it becomes earned, as is the case in financial accounting. For tax purposes, however, accrual basis taxpayers often report prepaid income in the year received. This treatment normally results from application of the claim of right doctrine, which requires income recognition when the taxpayer receives earnings under an unrestricted claim. For example, accrual basis taxpayers must report prepaid rental income when received (not when earned) since the taxpayer accepts the money under a claim of right without restrictions on its use. Unfortunately, no general rule is completely reliable to determine when prepaid income must be reported. Rather, the reporting procedure depends on the type of income received. As discussed below, special rules exist for prepaid income from rents, interest, services, warranties, goods, dues, subscriptions, and similar items. Note, however, these rules apply to *accrual basis* taxpayers only. A *cash basis* taxpayer reports all of these prepaid items of income in the year the cash is received.

Prepaid Interest, Rents, and Royalties. Several types of advance payments are included in income when received without question. For example, prepaid interest is income when received.[70] Prepaid rent and lump-sum payments, such as bonuses or advance royalties received upon execution of a lease or other agreement, are also income when received.[71] As subsequently explained, however, the term *rent* does not include payments for the use or occupancy of rooms or space where their use is ancillary to the services provided to the user of the property (e.g., hotels, motels, and convalescent homes are not considered as having received rents).[72] Because of the significant service element, these prepayments are reported using the rules applying to prepaid service income. Prepaid rents must be distinguished not only from services but also from lease or security deposits. Amounts received from a lessee that are refundable provided the lessee complies with the terms of the lease are not income since the lessor recognizes an obligation to repay.[73] The deposits become income only when the lessor becomes entitled to their unrestricted use upon the lessee's violation of the agreement.

Prepaid Service Income. Over the years, the treatment of advance payments for services—prepaid service income—has been quite controversial. Disputes between the IRS and taxpayers began when the IRS argued that the claim of right doctrine required

---

69   *Comm. v. Turney*, 36-1 USTC ¶9168, 17 AFTR 679, 82 F.2d 661 (CA-5, 1936).

70   *Franklin Life Insurance v. U.S.*, 68-2 USTC ¶9459, 22 AFTR2d 5180, 399 F.2d 757 (CA-7, 1968).

71   *South Dade Farms, Inc. v. Comm.*, 43-2 USTC ¶9634, 31 AFTR 842, 138 F.2d 818 (CA-5, 1943); *W.M. Scott*, 27 B.T.A. 951.

72   Rev. Proc. 2004-34, 2004-22 I.R.B. 991.

73   *Clinton Hotel Realty Corp. v. Comm.*, 42-2 USTC ¶9559, 29 AFTR 758, 128 F.2d 968 (CA-5, 1942).

accrual basis taxpayers to report prepayments for services as income in the year received. The IRS took this approach notwithstanding the fact that the taxpayer had not performed the services. After a great deal of litigation, the government relented and permitted limited deferral in certain circumstances. These rules were recently revised in 2004, with the issuance of Rev. Proc. 2004-34.[74]

Rev. Proc. 2004-34 now permits two acceptable methods of accounting for advanced payments for services. These are: a "full-inclusion method" and a "deferral method." The full-inclusion option is the easiest and the least desirable: all of the payments are reported in the year of receipt regardless of how the payments are reported for financial accounting purposes. In contrast, under the deferral method, taxpayers generally must report advanced payments as income in the year of receipt to the extent the payments are included in the revenues of the taxpayer's financial statements.[75] The balance of the advanced payments are deferred and reported as income in the following year. Thus, book income normally equals taxable income in the first year but may differ in subsequent years. This technique, unlike the previous approach, permits at least one year of deferral regardless of the length of the contract.

> **Example 28.** Murray Inc.—a calendar-year, accrual-method taxpayer—is in the business of providing ballroom dance lessons. On October 29 of year 1, Murray received $4,800 for a 48-month contract under which Murray would provide up to 96 lessons. Murray provides 8 lessons in year 1, 48 lessons in year 2, and 40 lessons in year 3. In its audited financial statements, the company reports the income as the lessons are provided. Therefore, for financial accounting purposes, Murray reports $400 ($4,800 × 8/96) in year 1. Similarly, under the deferral method of Rev. Proc. 2004-34, Murray would also report $400 of income for tax purposes since this procedure permits deferral equal to that reported for financial statement purposes. In year 2, for financial statement purposes, Murray would report $2,400 (48/96 × $4,800) based on the number of lessons provided. However, in year 2 for tax purposes, Murray would report the remaining balance of the advanced payment, $4,400, as income.

The advance payment rules allowing limited deferral for prepaid service income also apply to prepaid rental income if the occupancy or use of property is ancillary to the provision of services to the user of the property.[76] According to the procedure, advance payments for the use of hotel rooms or other quarters, booth space at a trade show, campsite space at a mobile home park, and recreational or banquet facilities are not considered rents but rather services. Note that this treatment permits hotels, motels and the like to enjoy the deferral provision as outlined above for services.

Advance Payments for Goods. Normally, an accrual basis taxpayer reports advance payments for sales of merchandise when they are earned (e.g., when the goods are shipped). This treatment enables the taxpayer to defer recognition of the prepayments. However, this approach is allowed only if the taxpayer follows the same method of reporting for financial accounting purposes.[77]

---

[74] Rev. Proc. 2004-34, 2004-22 IRB 991 (effective for tax years ending after 5/5/04) superseding Rev. Proc. 71-21, 1971-2 C.B. 549.

[75] If "applicable" financial statements (a certified audited financial statement used for credit purposes, reporting to shareholders, or any other substantial nontax purpose) have not been prepared, the amount of the payment earned is reported in the first year. Rev. Proc. 2004-34 (4.06), 2004-22 I.R.B. 991.

[76] Rev. Proc. 2004-34 identifies other types of prepayments that do and do not qualify as an advanced payment for which limited deferral is permitted.

[77] Reg. § 1.451-5(b). See Reg. § 1.451-4(c)(1) for certain situations where the prepayments must be reported earlier.

Example 29. C Corporation, a calendar year taxpayer, manufactures kitchen appliances. In late December 2009, it received $50,000 for kitchen appliances that it will produce and ship in May 2010. The corporation may postpone recognition of the income until 2010, assuming that such income is also reported on the financial accounting income statement in 2010.

Long-Term Contracts. Section 460 contains special rules for the reporting of income from long-term contracts. A long-term contract is defined as any contract for the manufacture, building, installation, or construction of property that is not completed within the same taxable year in which it was entered into. However, a *manufacturing* contract is still not considered long-term unless it also involves either (1) the manufacture of a unique item not normally carried in finished goods inventory (e.g., a special piece of machinery), or (2) items that normally require more than 12 months to complete. If a manufacturing contract does not qualify as a long-term contract, deferral may still be available under the rules regarding advance payments for goods discussed above. Note that contracts for services normally do not qualify for treatment as long-term contracts.

The tax law has long allowed taxpayers who enter into a long-term contract to use the percentage of completion method or the completed contract method (subject to certain limitations) to account for advance payments.[78] The percentage of completion method requires the taxpayer to recognize a portion of the gross profit on the contract based on the estimated percentage of the contract completed. In contrast, the completed contract method allows the taxpayer to defer income recognition until the contract is complete and acceptance has occurred. When available, taxpayers usually opt to use the completed contract method in order to postpone recognition of income. In some extreme cases, however, taxpayers have been able to postpone income for many years on the claim that the contract was not complete.

Over the years, Congress became concerned about the opportunities for deferral as well as the potential for abuse. Consequently, it took various steps, slowly but surely limiting the use of the completed contract method. These actions culminated with the virtual repeal of the method in 1989. As a result, long-term contracts currently entered into normally must be accounted for using the percentage of completion method.[79] However, there are two situations where the completed contract method can still be used. These include:[80]

1. *Home construction contracts.* Contracts in which 80 percent of the costs are related to buildings containing four or fewer dwelling units. Special rules apply to contracts if the buildings contain more than four units (i.e., so-called residential construction contracts).[81]

2. *Contracts of small businesses.* Construction contracts that are completed within two years of commencement and are performed by a contractor whose average annual gross receipts for the three preceding tax years do not exceed $10 million.

When using the percentage of completion method, the portion of the total contract price reported during the year and matched against current costs is computed as follows

$$\text{Total contract price} \times \frac{\text{Direct and allocable indirect costs incurred this period}}{\text{Total estimated costs of contract}}$$

---

[78] Reg. § 1.451-3.

[79] § 460(a).

[80] § 460(e).

[81] A 70 percent of completion method may be used for certain residential construction contracts.

Note that if less than 10 percent of the contract's costs have been incurred, the taxpayer may elect to defer reporting until the year in which the 10 percent threshold is reached.[82]

Example 30. In October 2009, W Corporation entered into a contract to build a hotel to be completed by May 2011. The contract price was $1 million. The company's estimated total costs of construction were $800,000. W's average annual gross receipts exceed $10 million, and it is therefore required to use the percentage of completion method. Total costs incurred during 2009 were $600,000. In 2010, the contract was completed at a total cost of $840,000. The income reported in 2009 and 2010 is computed below:

	2009	2010
Revenue recognized...........................	$ 750,000*	$ 250,000
Current costs	(600,000)	(240,000)
Total.................................	$ 150,000	$ 10,000

$$*\frac{\$600,000}{\$800,000} = 75\% \times \$1,000,000$$

Any contract for which the percentage of completion method is used is subject to the special *look-back* provisions.[83] Under these rules, once the contract is complete, annual income is recomputed based on final costs rather than estimated costs. Interest is then paid to the taxpayer if there was an overstatement of income. Conversely, the taxpayer must pay interest if income was understated.

Example 31. Same facts as in *Example 30*, above. Based on total actual costs of $840,000, W's 2009 income should have been $114,000, computed as follows:

	2009
Revenue recognized..............	$714,000*
Current costs	(600,000)
Total	$114,000

$$*\frac{\$600,000}{\$840,000} = 71.4\% \times \$1,000,000$$

Because the contract was in reality only 71.4% complete and not 75% complete, W overstated income in 2009 by $36,000 ($150,000 − $114,000). Consequently, the IRS is required to pay the taxpayer interest on the overpayment of the related tax.

Prepaid Dues and Subscriptions. Amidst much controversy concerning the reporting of prepaid income, Congress provided specific rules for the reporting of prepaid dues and subscriptions. Section 455 permits the taxpayer to elect to recognize prepaid subscription income (amounts received from a newspaper, magazine, or periodical) ratably over the subscription period. Section 456 provides that taxpayers may elect to report prepaid dues ratably over the membership period.

---

[82] § 460(b)(5).

[83] § 460(b)(2). The lookback rule is elective if the cumulative income (loss) determined using estimated contract price and cost is within 10 percent of actual.

INTEREST INCOME

The period in which a taxpayer recognizes interest income usually follows the basic tax accounting rules for cash and accrual basis taxpayers. In some cases, however, these taxpayers must observe special provisions that may cause reporting to vary from the normal pattern.

General Rules. As a general rule, cash basis taxpayers recognize interest income when received, while accrual basis taxpayers recognize the income when it is earned. As previously noted, both accrual and cash basis taxpayers that receive interest before it is earned (prepaid interest) must report the income when it is received.

Example 32. T operates a small business that manufactures pottery dishes. When one of her customers was unable to pay her bill, T accepted a $10,000 note, dated October 1, 2009, payable with 6% interest on October 1, 2010. Assuming T is a cash basis taxpayer, she will report $600 of interest income ($10,000 × 6%) when received in 2010. If T uses the accrual method, she would include $150 ($10,000 × 3/12 × 6%) in her gross income for 2009 and $450 ($10,000 × 9/12 × 6%) when received in 2010. Had the customer paid all of the interest, $600, in 2009 as a showing of good faith, T would report the entire $600 in 2009 regardless of whether she is a cash or accrual basis taxpayer.

In many instances, a taxpayer will purchase an interest-bearing instrument between payment dates. When this occurs, it is assumed that the purchase price includes the interest accrued to the date of the purchase. Thus, when the buyer later receives the interest payment, the portion accrued to the date of purchase is considered a nontaxable return of capital that reduces the taxpayer's basis in the instrument. On the other hand, the seller must include as interest income the amount accrued to the date of the purchase, regardless of the seller's method of accounting.

Example 33. S owned a $1,000, 12% AT&T bond that paid interest semiannually on November 1 and May 1. He purchased the bond at par several years ago. On September 1, 2009, S sold the bond for $1,540 including $40 of the accrued interest ($1,000 × 12% × 4/12). S must report $40 of interest income accrued to the date of sale. In addition, S will report a capital gain of $500 ($1,540 − $40 interest − $1,000 basis). The result is the same if S is a cash or accrual basis taxpayer.

Example 34. Assume B purchased for $1,540 the bond that S sold in the example above. On November 1, B receives an interest payment of $60 ($1,000 × 12% × 6/12). B treats the interest accrued to the date of purchase, $40, as a nontaxable return of basis. Thus, B's basis is reduced to $1,500 ($1,540 − $40). The remaining $20 of interest is included in B's gross income.

In practice, the broker's statement normally reflects the interest accrued to the date of the sale or purchase.

Discount. When accounting for interest income, any discount relating to the debt instrument—the excess of the face value of the obligation over the purchase price—must be considered. Discount typically results when the rate at which the instrument pays interest is less than the market rate. In such case, the discount essentially functions as a substitute for interest. Consistent with this view, the tax law attempts to ensure that the discount is treated as interest income and is normally reported currently. Special provisions have been introduced over the years to clarify the reporting of the discount income as well as to prohibit taxpayers from converting the discount income into capital gain.

Example 35. During 2007, T purchased a $10,000, 8% corporate bond for $8,000, or a $2,000 discount. In 2009 the bond matured and the taxpayer redeemed the bond for its par value of $10,000. The redemption is treated as an exchange, and the taxpayer recognizes a long-term capital gain of $2,000 ($10,000 redemption price − $8,000 basis). In this case, the taxpayer has converted the discount of $2,000, which from an economic view is ordinary interest income, to capital gain. Moreover, the taxpayer has deferred the reporting of such income from the time it accrues to the time the bond is sold. To eliminate this opptunity, the discount generally must be amortized and included in gross income as it accrues. These rules are discussed in greater detail in Chapter 16.

The tax treatment of discount depends in part on when it arises. The discount often occurs at the time the instrument is issued. For example, certain instruments such as U.S. Savings Bonds, Treasury bills, and so-called zero coupon bonds do not bear interest and are usually *issued* at discounts. Other debt obligations that do bear interest (such as corporate bonds) also may be issued at a discount, usually if the coupon rate is set lower than the current rate. Discount could also result after the instrument is issued. For example, where interest-bearing instruments are issued at par, discount may arise upon a subsequent purchase. The specific treatment of discount is examined below.

Non-Interest-Bearing Obligations Issued at a Discount. The Code provides special rules for non-interest-bearing obligations that are issued at a discount and redeemable for a fixed amount that increases over time. The instruments to which these rules would normally apply are Series E and EE U.S. Savings Bonds. Series E Bonds were issued between 1941 and 1980, having maturities up to 40 years. Beginning in 1980, these bonds were replaced by Series EE Bonds. Beginning in 2001, Series EE Bonds are inscribed with the special legend "Patriot Bonds" inspired by the tragedy of September 11, 2001. Series EE bonds earn 90 percent of five-year Treasury security yields. They do not pay interest but are sold at a discount (half their face value), and are available in denominations ranging from $50 through $10,000. They generally have maturities of 20 years. The bonds are normally redeemable at any time up until the final maturity date at a price that increases with the passage of time. No interest payments are made while the bond is held. The holder's interest income is represented by the difference between the redemption price and purchase price. Note, however, that Series EE savings bonds stop increasing in value after 20 years. Bonds issued after May 1, 2005 have a fixed rate of interest. For example, for bonds issued on or after November 1, 2008, the rate was 2.80 (down from 4.11 on November 1, 2007).

For reporting purposes, taxpayers may elect to include in income the annual increase in the redemption price of the bond.[84] In essence, this election allows a cash basis taxpayer to use the accrual method with respect to these bonds. If income is not reported on an annual basis, the taxpayer reports the entire difference between the redemption and issue prices as income when the bond is redeemed.

Example 36. S purchased Series EE Bonds with a face value of $10,000 at a cost of $8,000. The redemption price of the bonds increases during the year by $100. If S elects to report the income annually, she will include $100 in her gross income. Alternatively, S could wait until she redeems the bond to report the income. For example, if S later redeemed the bonds for $9,500, she would report $1,500 income (the difference between the redemption price of $9,500 and her cost of $8,000) at the time of redemption.

---

[84]   § 454(a).

The taxpayer may make the election to report the interest annually at any time. When the election is made, all interest previously deferred on all Series E and EE Bonds must be reported. This procedure effectively allows the taxpayer to choose the year in which the interest income is to be reported. However, once the election is made, it applies to *all* Series E and EE Bonds subsequently acquired. Should the taxpayer desire to change to reporting the income at redemption, consent from the IRS is required.[85]

As discussed in Chapter 6, certain taxpayers who cash in Series EE Bonds and use the proceeds for educational expenses may be able to exclude the interest.

Government Obligations. Special rules also govern the treatment of the discount arising upon the purchase of short-term government obligations such as Treasury bills.[86] Typically, a taxpayer purchases a short-term Treasury bill at a discount and redeems it for par value shortly thereafter. In this instance, Code § 454(b) applies to cash basis taxpayers to ensure that the gain on the redemption—in effect, the discount—is treated as ordinary interest income. Specifically, any gain realized by cash basis taxpayers from the sale or redemption of non-interest-bearing obligations issued by governmental units that have a fixed maturity date that is one year or less from the date of issue is always ordinary income. This ordinary income is reported *in the year* of sale or redemption. In contrast, accrual basis taxpayers are required to amortize the discount (i.e., include it in income) on a *daily* basis under Code § 1281(a).

> **Example 37.** On December 1, 2008, B, a cash basis calendar year taxpayer, purchased a $10,000 non-interest-bearing Treasury bill. She purchased the bill at 97 ($9,700) and redeemed the bill on March 1, 2009 at par. B recognizes a $300 gain ($10,000 − $9,700) on the redemption, and the entire gain is treated as ordinary income in 2009. The same result would occur if B had *sold* the Treasury bill for $10,000 on January 15, 2009. Note that if B were an accrual basis taxpayer, the $300 discount would have been included in income on a daily basis. Consequently, a portion of the income would be reported in 2008 and the remainder in 2009.

Original Issue Discount. When interest-bearing obligations such as corporate bonds are *issued* at a discount, a complex set of provisions operates to prevent taxpayers from not only deferring the discount income but also converting it to capital gain as depicted in *Example 35*. These rules apply only to discount that arises when the bonds are originally issued. This discount is technically referred to as *original issue discount* (OID) and is determined as follows:

Redemption price	$x,xxx
− Issue price	− xxx
= Original issue discount	$x,xxx

The thrust of the provisions is to require the holder of the bond to amortize the discount into income during the period the bond is held. A complete discussion of the treatment of OID is provided in Chapter 16.

---

[85]   As of September 1, 2004, investors are no longer able to exchange EE/E bonds for HH bonds.

[86]   Special rules also apply to Treasury Inflation-Protection Bonds (TIPs) and Treasury Inflation-Indexed Securities.

✅ *CHECK YOUR KNOWLEDGE*

Review Question 1. For financial accounting purposes, prepaid income is generally reported as it is earned. Does the same treatment apply for tax purposes? Explain the treatment of prepaid interest, rents, royalties, services, and advance payments for goods.

As a general rule, prepaid income must be reported when received. This is obviously true for cash basis taxpayers and surprisingly true for accrual basis taxpayers. The unusual treatment for accrual basis taxpayers stems from the claim of right doctrine, which requires recognition of income whenever the amount has been received and the taxpayer does not recognize an obligation to repay. This treatment applies to prepaid interest, rents, and royalties. It does not apply to prepaid service income (including prepaid rents if the property's use is secondary to the services provided) where the reporting follows that for books in the first year with the balance reported in the second year. It also does not apply to advance payments for goods, which are normally reported in the same manner as they are for financial accounting purposes (the normal accrual method).

A close look at the reporting requirements for prepaid income reveals that cash basis taxpayers report prepaid income when it is received and this approach is consistent with the cash method of accounting. In contrast, accrual basis taxpayers report—subject to certain exceptions—prepaid income as if they were on the cash basis. The table below summarizes the law's schizophrenic approach to prepaid income and—as seen in Chapter 7—prepaid expenses.

	Prepaid income	Prepaid expenses
Cash basis taxpayer	Report in year received *Consistent with cash method*	Deduct over appropriate period *Treat as if on accrual basis*
Accrual basis taxpayer	Report in year received *Treated as if on cash basis*	Deducted over appropriate period *Consistent with accrual method*

Review Question 2. After the changes made during the 1980s, some commentators pronounced the use of the completed contract method dead. Is this true? Are there any circumstances under which the completed contract method can be used?

The completed contract may be dead for large construction companies that build mammoth projects such as airplanes, stadiums, dams, office towers, and the like. But it is alive and well for the majority of construction companies. The completed contract method may be used by any home builder (regardless of size) and small construction companies (those with average annual gross receipts of less than $10 million).

Review Question 3. During the autumn of 1986, it became clear that the Reagan administration and Congress planned to cut tax rates from a top rate of 50 percent to something around 28 percent. As a result, the papers and financial press were filled with planning ideas. Some advisers suggested that people who had cash sitting in money market accounts should buy Treasury bills. Why?

An investment in Treasury bills allows the taxpayer to defer the interest until the bonds are redeemed. Consequently, many advisers suggested purchasing Treasury bills at a discount during the fall of 1986 with the idea of redeeming them when income tax rates dropped in 1987.

IDENTIFICATION OF THE TAXPAYER

A final consideration in the taxation of income concerns identification of the taxpayer to whom the income is taxed. Generally, this is not a mind-boggling task. The person who receives the income usually must pay the tax. As discussed below, however, receipt or non-receipt of income does not always govern who must report it.

INCOME FROM PERSONAL SERVICES

In the famous case of *Lucas v. Earl*, the Supreme Court was required to determine whether Mr. Earl was taxable on earnings from personal services despite a legally enforceable agreement made with his wife in 1901 that the earnings would be shared equally.[87] At the time of this decision, such agreements effectively split income between a husband and wife; this resulted in a reduced tax liability since each individual was treated as a separate taxable entity and a progressive income tax rate structure existed. The Court eliminated the usefulness of this technique, however, by holding that the income is taxable to the taxpayer who earns it. Thus, anticipatory assignments of income that one has a *right* to receive are an ineffective device to escape taxation. In explaining what has become the assignment of income doctrine, the Court gave birth to the well-known *fruit of the tree* metaphor. According to Justice Holmes, the fruit (income) must be attributed to the tree from which it grew (Mr. Earl's services).

Section 73 directly addresses the treatment of a child's earnings. This provision indicates that amounts received for the services of a child are included in the *child's* gross income. Thus, a parent or a guardian who collects income earned by a child would not report the income; rather the income would be reported by the child since he or she earned it. As discussed in Chapter 4, however, the *unearned* income of a child under age 18 may be reported on his or her parents' tax return and taxed at the parents' rates.

INCOME FROM PROPERTY

The assignment of income doctrine also applies when income from property is received. Under this rule, income from property is included in the gross income of the taxpayer who owns the property. This principle was derived from another famous case, *Helvering v. Horst*.[88] In this case, Mr. Horst clipped the interest coupons from bonds he owned and gave them to his son, who later collected them. The Supreme Court held Mr. Horst taxable since he owned and controlled the source of income (i.e., the bonds). Accordingly, income from property can be effectively assigned only if the taxpayer relinquishes ownership of the property.

UNEARNED INCOME OF CHILDREN

Perhaps the most fundamental principle in tax planning concerns minimizing the marginal tax rate that applies to the taxpayer's income. The significance of this principle is easily understood when one realizes that Federal marginal tax rates have at times exceeded 90 percent. Although the current disparity between the top and bottom rates, 25 percent (35% − 10%), is not as great as in some years, the potential for significant tax savings still exists.

---

[87] 2 USTC ¶496, 8 AFTR 10,287, 281 U.S. 111 (USSC, 1930).

[88] 40-2 USTC ¶9787, 24 AFTR 1058, 311 U.S. 112 (USSC, 1940).

Minimizing the tax rate is normally accomplished by shifting income to a lower bracket taxpayer. As discussed above, the assignment of income doctrine makes it virtually impossible for taxpayers to shift income arising from services. Opportunities do exist, however, for shifting income through transfers of property. The most popular technique in this regard has traditionally involved transferring income-producing property to a child. In this manner, not only is the tax rate applying to the income reduced, but the income also stays within the family unit, normally to be used as the parent directs.

As part of the tax overhaul in 1986, Congress took steps to reduce tax avoidance opportunities available through income shifting to a child. This was accomplished by enacting a special provision affectionately referred to as the "kiddie" tax.[89] The thrust of this rule—as explained in Chapter 4—is to tax the *unearned* income of a child under the age of 19 (or less than 24 if a full-time student) as if it were the parents' income and thus at the parents' rates. By limiting the tax to unearned rather than earned income, Congress was taking direct aim at parents and others who shifted income by making gifts of property. Accordingly, shifting techniques based on gifts of property such as bonds and rental property that produce unearned income (e.g., interest and rents) are now severely limited.

INTEREST-FREE AND BELOW-MARKET LOANS

To be successful in shifting income to another, the assignment of income doctrine generally requires that the taxpayer transfer the income-producing property itself, not merely the income from the property. Consequently, shifting income normally requires a completed gift of the property. Taxpayers, however, are understandably reluctant to forever relinquish ownership and control of the property. For this reason, taxpayers have attempted to design techniques that enable them to retain ownership of the property yet shift income.

Prior to 1984, one popular method for shifting income from one family member to another, or from a corporation to its shareholders (or employees), utilized interest-free loans. Under the typical arrangement, a father who was in the 50 percent tax bracket would make a loan to his son who was in a tax bracket far lower than his father's (or who perhaps paid no taxes at all). Upon receipt of the loan, the son (or his representative if he was a minor) would invest the funds. As a result, any income earned on the investment would be taxed to the son at a lower rate than would have been paid had the father received the income directly. This arrangement could secure substantial tax savings, particularly where there was a great disparity between the tax rates of the two family members.

The success of the tax-saving technique described above was attributable to the terms of the loan agreement. These terms required the son to repay the loan on demand *without interest*. Had the father charged interest, he would still have income attributable to the amount loaned, and no income shifting would have occurred. By not charging interest, however, the interest income that the father would have earned was successfully shifted to the son and tax savings resulted. In addition, the interest that was not charged, a valuable benefit for the son, was not considered a taxable gift. Moreover, this arrangement was extremely appealing because it did not require the father to part with the property forever. Since he had only loaned the funds to his son, he could demand repayment of the funds at any time.

The IRS did not view interest-free loans as a valid means to shift income, but rather a tax avoidance device designed to circumvent the assignment of income rules. After much unsuccessful litigation, the Service finally struck a severe blow in 1984, when the Supreme Court decided in *Dickman* that the interest-free use of the loan amount (i.e., the forgone interest) did constitute a taxable gift by the lender.[90] Despite this victory, the decision did not preclude income shifting. Instead, it merely imposed a cost on using the tax-saving technique equal to the gift tax—which could be zero if the gift of the

---

[89] § 1(i).

[90] 84-1 USTC ¶13,560, 53 AFTR2d 84-1608, 104 S.Ct. 1932 (USSC, 1984).

forgone interest was less than the amount of the annual exclusion of $13,000 (2009). As a result, the use of interest-free loans to shift income still appeared viable. However, Congress eliminated this opportunity in 1984 by enacting Code § 7872, which imputes interest income to the lender where the actual interest is considered inadequate.

Treatment of Below-Market Loans. In general, § 7872 applies to loans when the interest charged is below the current market rate of interest. As pictured below, when such a loan is made, the treatment is determined *assuming* that the borrower pays the interest to the lender at the market rate, which the lender is then deemed to transfer back to the borrower:

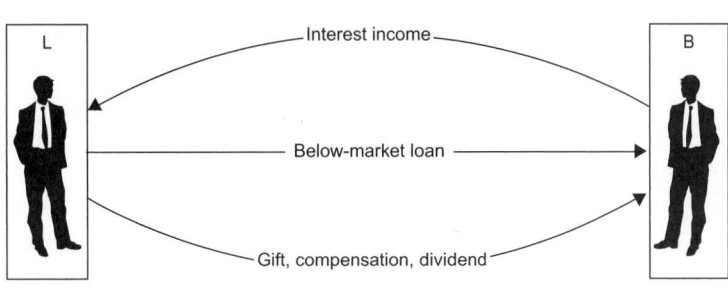

This hypothetical scenario results in the following tax consequences:

1. The borrower may be allowed a deduction for the interest hypothetically paid to the lender, while the lender reports the fictitious payment as *interest income*.

2. The lender treats the hypothetical payment to the borrower as either compensation, dividend, or gift depending on the nature of the loan. Similarly, the borrower treats the payment as either compensation, dividend, or gift as the case may be. In determining the character of the lender's hypothetical payment, the Code classifies loans into three types according to the relationship between the lender and the borrower.

    ▸ *Gift loans*—those where the forgone interest is in the nature of a gift;

    ▸ *Compensation-related loans*—those made by an employer to an employee or an independent contractor; and

    ▸ *Corporation-shareholder loans*—those made by a corporation to a shareholder.[91]

The thrust of these rules is to treat the borrower as having paid the proper amount of interest, which is funded by the lender through compensation, dividends, or gift.

Example 38. Lender L loaned $100,000 to borrowers payable on demand without interest. Assume the statutory rate of interest required to be charged is 12 percent compounded semiannually. Thus, the interest hypothetically paid by B and which must be imputed to L is $12,360. The following table shows the effect on L and B, assuming the loan is

1. A gift loan.

2. A compensation-related loan.

3. A corporation-shareholder loan.

---

[91]   In this regard, Proposed Reg. § 1.7872-4(d)(2) indicates that a payment to a shareholder-employee is presumed to be a dividend if the corporation is (1) closely held and such person owns more than 5 percent of its stock, or (2) publicly held and such person owns ½ of one percent of the stock.

	Lender L				Borrower B		
Interest Income	Gift Made	Comp. Expense	Dividend Paid	Interest Expense	Gift Received	Comp. Income	Dividend Received
(1) $12,360	$12,360			$(12,360)	$12,360		
(2) 12,360		$(12,360)		(12,360)		$12,360	
(3) 12,360			$12,360	(12,360)			$12,360

The first situation reveals the effects where the interest forgone by the lender is considered a gift (e.g., loans between family members). In this case, income shifting is prohibited since L does not avoid taxation on the income from the loan. Rather, he or she is deemed to receive an interest payment from B on the amount loaned. In addition, L is treated as having made a taxable gift to B of $360 ($12,360 gift − $12,000 annual exclusion). On the other hand, B is entitled to exclude the $12,360 gift from income. B's hypothetical interest payment may or may not be deductible, depending on whether it is treated as investment interest, business interest, or personal interest (see Chapter 11 for a discussion of interest).

The second situation assumes that the loan is made by an employer to an employee, and, thus, the hypothetical payment by the lender is considered compensation. In this case, the lender is treated as having received interest income that is offset by a deduction for compensation expense to B. Note, however, that if B is an employee, L would be responsible for employment taxes and withholding. The effect on the borrower, B, depends on whether the hypothetical interest payment is deductible. If so, there generally will be no effect since such deduction offsets B's compensation income.

The third situation demonstrates the undesirable consequences that a corporation encounters when its deemed payment is considered a dividend rather than compensation. This problem would normally arise where the loan is made to an individual who is both a shareholder and an employee of the corporation. In this situation, like the second situation above, L (a corporation) has income from the deemed payment. In contrast to the second situation, however, L receives no offsetting deduction since dividend payments are not deductible. The effect on B again depends on whether the hypothetical interest is deductible.

These provisions govern not only the treatment of gift, compensation-related, and corporate shareholder loans, but also any other type of below-market loan designed to achieve tax avoidance or affect the tax liability of the lender or the borrower.

Example 39. During the year, J joined a country club. The club requires each member to loan the club $10,000 without interest. Assuming interest rates are currently 8 percent, the club is effectively receiving annual dues of $800 from each member. More important from the member's standpoint, the dues are paid with tax-free dollars.

Had J received the $800 directly, she would be required to pay taxes. By making the loan to the club, she has effectively converted taxable income to tax-exempt income. Under Code § 7872, however, this arrangement would not be effective since J would be treated as having received the $800 income and would have no offsetting deduction for the payment to the club.

Exempt Loans. To restrict the application of § 7872 to predominantly abusive situations, Congress carved out several exceptions to the rules described above. Under the first exception, § 7872 does not apply to *gift* loans as long as the loans outstanding during the year do not exceed $10,000 *and* the borrower does not use the loan proceeds to

purchase or carry income-producing assets. Without this latter requirement, income of small amounts could still be shifted. The effect of this provision is to exempt small loans where income shifting is absent.

Congress also granted compensation-related and corporation-shareholder loans an exemption from the onerous rules of § 7872 if they do not exceed $10,000. The exemption does not apply to these loans, however, if tax avoidance is one of the principal purposes of the loan.

Interest Income Cap. Another special rule imposes a limit on the amount of imputed interest income for loans between individuals. Generally, if the amount of outstanding loans does not exceed $100,000 and their principal purpose is not tax avoidance, the deemed interest payment by the borrower to the lender is limited to the borrower's investment income. This rule follows from the theory that the amount of income shifted by the lender is limited to that which the borrower actually earns. In addition, to enable loans where tax avoidance is obviously not a motive, the lender is treated as having no imputed interest income if the borrower's investment income does not exceed $1,000. However, the lender is still deemed to have made a gift of the forgone interest.

Example 40. L has a son, B, who earns a salary and has $800 investment income. During the year, L loaned B $90,000 without interest to purchase a home. Interest imputed at the IRS rate is $14,000. L has no imputed interest income since the loan is less than $100,000 and investment income is less than $1,000. However, L is charged with a taxable gift of $2,000 ($14,000 − $12,000 exclusion). Note that if B had $7,000 of investment income, L also would have been charged with interest income of $7,000.

Loans to Qualified Continuing Care Facility. Older individuals who must enter a continuing care facility may be required to make an interest free or below-market-rate loan to the facility as a condition of admission. Absent any special rule, the § 7872 requirement to impute interest would saddle these individuals with taxable interest income without cash. Section 7872(g) creates an important exception, exempting loans made to "qualified continuing care facilities" if the contractual provisions meet certain requirements.

INCOME FROM COMMUNITY PROPERTY

In the United States, the rights that married individuals hold in property are determined using either the common law or community property system. The community property system developed in continental Europe and was adopted in several states having a French or Spanish origin. The ten states currently recognizing the community property system are Alaska, Arizona, California, Idaho, Louisiana, Nevada, New Mexico, Texas, Washington, and Wisconsin. The remaining 40 states use the common law system, which originated in England.

The community property system categorizes property into two types: separate property, which is considered belonging separately to one of the spouses, and community property, which is considered owned equally by each spouse. In general, separate property consists only of those assets owned before marriage or acquired by gift or inheritance while married. All property acquired during a marriage except by gift or inheritance is community property.

Income from separate property may be community property or separate property depending on the state of jurisdiction. In Texas, Louisiana, and Idaho, income from separate property is community property. Accordingly, for Federal tax purposes each spouse is responsible for one-half of the income. In the other seven states, income from separate

property is separate property and must be reported by the person owning the property. Income from personal services is generally treated as belonging to the community. The following example illustrates how these differing rules must be taken into account.

> **Example 41.** A husband and wife elect to file separate returns. The husband received a $30,000 salary and $1,000 of dividends on stock he had purchased prior to the couple's marriage. The husband also receives $500 of taxable interest from a certificate of deposit that he had purchased in his own name while married. The wife's income would vary depending on the state in which she lived:

	Texas	Arizona	Common Law States
Salary	$15,000	$15,000	$0
Dividends	500	0	0
Interest	250	250	0
Wife's income	$15,750	$15,250	$0

Community Income Where Spouses Live Apart. The treatment of community income can create financial problems, particularly where spouses live apart during the year and are later divorced before the end of the taxable year. For example, consider R and S, who were married but lived apart during the first half of the year before their divorce became final. Under these circumstances, the property settlement should consider the accrued tax liability that arises due to any community income. Accounting for the liability may be difficult or impossible, however, if one of the spouses has abandoned the other. In such cases, the abandoned spouse becomes liable for the tax on income earned by a spouse who cannot be located to share the financial responsibility. To eliminate these difficulties, special provisions were enacted.

Section 66 provides that a spouse will be taxed only on the earnings attributed to his or her personal services if during the year the following requirements are satisfied:

1. The two married individuals live apart at all times.

2. The couple does not file a joint return with each other.

3. No portion of the earned income is transferred between the spouses.

This rule only applies to income from personal services and not income from property.

> **Example 42.** M and N, residents of Texas, decided in November 2007 to obtain a divorce, which became final on March 31, 2009. N earns $2,000 each month and M is unemployed. N has a savings account that yielded $200 of taxable interest during the first three months of 2009. Assuming the two live apart during all of 2009 and none of the earned income is transferred between them, N will report all of the $6,000 ($2,000 × 3) attributable to her personal services and $100 of the interest. M will report his $100 share of the taxable interest.

✓ CHECK YOUR KNOWLEDGE

Review Question 1. In 1960 18-year-old Randy Hundley signed a contract to play baseball for the Chicago Cubs.[92] The contract provided for a bonus of $110,000 (a grand sum in those days) to be paid over a five-year period at a rate of $22,000 per year: $11,000 to Randy and $11,000 to his father, Cecil. The payment to Randy's father was

---

[92] *Cecil Randolph Hundley, Jr.*, 48 T.C. 339 (1967).

pursuant to an oral agreement the two had made when Randy was 16. According to the agreement, Cecil, a former semiprofessional baseball player and coach, acted as Randy's coach and business manager in exchange for 50 percent of any bonus that Randy might receive if he should obtain a baseball contract.

At about the same time that the Cubs were striking a deal with Hundley, the Philadelphia Phillies reached an agreement with Richie Allen, another future star.[93] According to this arrangement, Allen was to receive a $70,000 bonus: $30,000 paid to him over five years and $40,000 paid to his mother. How should the bonuses be treated? Should they both be treated the same?

The question in both cases is whether the child has effectively split the income between himself and his parent or merely made an anticipatory assignment of income. If the latter is true, all of the income would be taxed to the child and none to the parent. In both cases, the IRS argued that the payment to Randy's father and Richie's mother should be treated as being first made to the child and then followed by a nondeductible gift. Despite the similarity of the cases, the Court believed that the services provided by Hundley's father were instrumental in his son's success, whereas Allen's mother made no tangible contribution. As a result, Hundley was allowed to deduct the payment to his father as a business expense and, therefore, split the income between them. In contrast, no deduction was allowed to Allen and he was required to pay taxes on the entire bonus.

Review Question 2. M wants to shift income to her 19-year-old daughter (who is not a student) so that it will be taxed at the daughter's 10 percent rate rather than at M's 35 percent rate. M plans on loaning her daughter $10,000 interest-free for this purpose. Will her plan to shift income to the daughter work?

As a general rule, interest-free loans can no longer be used successfully to shift income, since interest income must be imputed to the lender. In this case, M would be treated as having received an interest payment from her daughter, thus defeating the entire plan. At first blush, some might believe that because the loan is less than $10,000, the de minimis rule operates and M is not required to impute interest; this is a typical misconception. It is true that imputation is not required if the loan is less than $10,000, but only if the borrower does not invest the loan amount in income-producing property. Of course, if the borrower does not invest in income-producing property there is no income and nothing is shifted. Therefore, the $10,000 de minimis rule does not create any opportunity. In this particular case, the $100,000 rule also would come into play. This exception provides that the maximum amount of interest to be imputed to the lender is equal to the net investment income of the borrower (zero, if net investment income is less than $1,000). This provision does provide a small opportunity. If the daughter invests the $10,000 to produce $900 of interest income, no income would be imputed to M and $900 would be successfully shifted. M would be treated as having made a gift of $900 to her daughter, but there would be no gift tax because of the annual exclusion of $12,000.

TAX PLANNING

TIMING INCOME RECOGNITION

The proper timing of income recognition can reap great benefits for the taxpayer. As a general rule, postponement of income recognition is wise since the tax on such income is deferred. The major advantage of tax deferral is that the taxpayer has continued use of the

---

[93] *Richard A. Allen*, 50 T.C. 466 (1968).

real funds that otherwise would have been used to pay taxes. Deferral of the tax is in essence an interest-free loan from the government.

When considering deferral, attention must be given to the marginal tax rates that may apply to the income. For example, taxpayers often postpone income until their retirement years, when they are usually in a lower tax bracket. Although deferral may be wise in this situation, it may be unwise where tax rates rise by operation of law or because of the taxpayer's increase in earnings. Ideally, the taxpayer should attempt to level out taxable income from one year to the next and equalize the tax rate that applies annually (to avoid the situation of R in *Example 11* and duplicate that of S).

The opportunities for most individuals to postpone income are limited, particularly in light of the constructive receipt doctrine. Several techniques do exist, however, as outlined below:

1. Installment sales of property enable the taxpayer not only to avoid the bunching of income in a single year but also to defer the tax.

2. Income on Series E and EE bonds, Treasury bills, and certain certificates of deposit may be deferred until they are redeemed.

3. Investments in Individual Retirement Accounts (IRAs), Keogh plans, and qualified retirement plans are all made with before-tax dollars (since these contributions are deductible), and earnings on these investments are not taxed until they are withdrawn.

4. Deferred compensation arrangements may be suitable, as in the case of a professional athlete, celebrity, or executive. (See Chapter 18)

INCOME-SPLITTING TECHNIQUES

As stressed earlier, the most fundamental rule in tax planning concerns minimizing the marginal tax rate that applies to the taxpayer's income. Minimizing the applicable rate is usually accomplished through use of some type of income splitting or shifting technique.

> **Example 43.** Mr. and Mrs. J pay taxes at a rate of 35% in 2009. The couple helps support Mr. J's 67-year-old retired mother, M, by giving her $5,000 annually. Such gifts do not entitle the couple to claim M as a dependent. In providing M's support through gifts, the couple is using after-tax dollars. That is, the couple would have to earn $7,692 to provide M with $5,000 in support [$7,692 − (35% of $7,692) = $5,000]. Instead, the couple could transfer income-producing property to M to provide the needed support. By so doing, the income would not be subject to tax because M could utilize her own exemption and standard deduction. In 2009, M may claim an exemption deduction of $3,650 and a standard deduction of $7,100 ($5,700 regular + $1,400 addition for unmarried 65 years of age or over) for total deductions of $10,750. Providing support in this manner would be far less expensive than making outright gifts of $5,000 annually Although this arrangement requires the couple to give up the property permanently (since any type of reversionary interest would cause the income to be taxed back to the couple), in many family situations, M would probably give the property back when she no longer needs it or when she dies. In addition, other techniques are available that can circumvent the problem of permanently departing with the property.

The above example demonstrates how income can be shifted successfully. Where income is to be shifted to children, however, the taxpayer must contend with the "kiddie" tax.

The "kiddie" tax clearly limits opportunities for shifting unearned income to children. However, it does not eliminate them. Recall that the "kiddie" tax applies generally applies to children less than 19 or those that are full-time students less than 24. However, the "kiddie" tax does not apply until unearned income exceeds $1,900 (in 2009). Consequently, for a child subject to the kiddie tax, the first $950 of unearned income bears no tax because of the standard deduction, and the next $950 is taxed at the child's rates. Although the "kiddie" tax severely curtails the amount of tax that could otherwise be saved through shifting income to children, taxpayers attempting to shift modest amounts of income are not affected.

For taxpayers wanting to shift more unearned income to their children, other techniques are available. One way of coping with the "kiddie" tax is by making investments with income that is deferred until the child is no longer subject to the tax. For example, the taxpayer could give a child Series EE savings bonds. The income from these bonds can be deferred by not electing to report the accumulated interest until after the child has turned 24 (or 19 if he or she is not a student). Interest thereafter would be reported annually. Similarly, discount bonds—those *without* original issue discount—could be purchased. In this case, the interest is not reported until the bond is sold.

The "kiddie" tax applies to unearned income and not earned income. As a result, earned income can be successfully shifted by paying the child for performing some task. Of course, shifting does not occur unless the payment is deductible by the parent. Such payments, when made by a parent directly to a child under 18, have the added benefit of not being subject to social security taxes.

EXCLUDED ECONOMIC INCOME

In arranging one's affairs, it should be observed that certain "economic" income does not fall within the definition of income for tax purposes and thus can be obtained tax-free.

Example 44. Taxpayer R received a gift from her rich uncle of $100,000, which she is considering investing in either a condominium or corporate stocks. The condominium in which she is interested is the one in which she currently lives and rents for $8,000 annually. In lieu of purchasing the condominium, she could continue to rent and invest the $100,000 in preferred stocks paying dividends of 10% annually, or $10,000 of income per year. Assume that R pays taxes at a marginal rate of 30%. The return after taxes on the preferred stock will be 7%, or $7,000. The return from the investment in the condominium is represented by the rent that she does not pay of $8,000, which is nontaxable. In essence, the condominium pays a dividend-in-kind (i.e., shelter), which is tax-exempt. Consequently, R would obtain a higher yield on her investment by purchasing the condominium. Note that income for tax purposes does not include the value of the condominium which would be considered income in the economic sense because the use of the condominium's shelter represents consumption. This same type of analysis applies to all types of investments in consumer goods that provide long-term benefits, such as washers and refrigerators.

PROBLEM MATERIALS

DISCUSSION QUESTIONS

5-1 *Economic versus Tax Concept of Income.* It has been said that the income tax discriminates against the person who lives in a rented home as compared with the person who owns his or her own residence. Comment on the truth of this assertion and why such discrimination may or may not be justified.

5-2 *Net Worth Method.* Explain the circumstances in which the economist's approach to measuring income might be used for tax purposes and what specific steps might be taken to implement such an approach.

5-3 *What Is Income?* Listed below are several items that may or may not constitute income for purposes of economics and income taxes. Indicate whether each item would be considered income for each of these purposes, including comments on why differences, if any, might exist.
   a. Beef raised and consumed by a cattle rancher.
   b. Interest received on state or local bonds.
   c. Air transportation provided by an airline to one of its flight attendants.
   d. Appreciation of XRY stock from $1,000 to $6,000 during the year.
   e. Proceeds collected from an insurance company for a casualty loss and reinvested in similar property.
   f. A loan obtained from a friend.
   g. $105 received from sale of stock purchased one year ago for $100; inflation during the past year averaged five percent.
   h. A gift received as a Christmas present.

5-4 *Cash Equivalent Doctrine.* A financial newsletter recently reported the many advantages that may be obtained from belonging to a barter club or organization. Would tax benefits be included among these advantages (e.g., no taxable income realized on the exchange of services)?

5-5 *Return of Capital Doctrine—General.* Explain the return of capital doctrine and discuss three situations in which the doctrine operates.

5-6 *Indirect Benefits.* A, an assistant manager for a department store, often is required to work overtime to help mark down merchandise for special sales. On these occasions, her employer pays the cost of her evening meal. Does the meal constitute income? Explain.

5-7 *Annual Accounting Period-Planning.* Briefly explain the notion of "income bunching" and why it is a problem.

5-8 *52-53 Week Year.* At first glance, it may appear that the "52-53 week" taxable year is one of those accounting practices that has no real world application. Using the Internet, determine if any well-known company uses the 52-53 week accounting period as its taxable year.

5-9 *Relationship between Tax and Financial Accounting Methods.* Does conformity with generally accepted accounting principles satisfy the requirement of § 446(c) that income must be clearly reflected? Explain, including some illustrations where income for tax purposes will differ from that for financial accounting purposes.

5-10 *Cash Basis Taxpayer's Receipt of Notes.* Does a cash basis taxpayer recognize income when a note is received or when collections are made?

5-11 *Constructive Receipt Doctrine.* Discuss the planning opportunities related to the cash method of accounting and how these are affected by the constructive receipt doctrine.

5-12 *Accrual Method of Accounting.* Address the following questions:
   a. When does a taxpayer using the accrual method of accounting normally report income?
   b. Under what circumstances is an accrual basis taxpayer treated like a cash basis taxpayer for purposes of reporting income?

5-13 *Change in Accounting Method.* T Corporation is considering altering the way in which it accounts for a particular item.
  a. If T wishes to make the change, how should it proceed?
  b. Explain the Section 481 adjustment and how T must account for it.

5-14 *Changing Accounting Methods: Procedures.* F files the tax returns for his three-year-old son, S. Up until this year, F had always reported the interest on S's Series EE savings bonds annually. F now wishes to report the interest income when the bonds are redeemed (e.g., when the child reaches age 18). Can F change the way he reports the interest? If so, how?

5-15 *What Is an Accounting Method?* This year, T hired a new accountant, A. As part of A's routine review procedures, A determined that T's previous accountant had improperly computed the gross profit percentage to be used in recognizing income on an installment sale. Based on the previous accountant's calculation, 40 percent of each year's receipts were to be included in income, whereas according to A's calculation the proper percentage was 50 percent. Explain what A should do upon finding the discrepancy.

5-16 *Claim of Right.* Consider the questions below.
  a. Is the application of the claim of right doctrine limited to situations that involve only contested income? Explain.
  b. Explain the difference between the claim of right and constructive receipt doctrines.

5-17 *Prepaid Rent.* In light of the tax treatment, if landlords of apartment complexes had a choice, should they characterize an initial $500 payment from their tenants as a security deposit or as a payment of the last month's rent in advance? Explain.

5-18 *Prepaid Services.* Identify several types of services where the accrual basis provider will not be permitted to defer any prepayments of income related to such services. Explain.

5-19 *Long-Term Contracts.* Indicate which method of accounting for long-term contracts—completed contract or percentage of completion—the taxpayer may use in the following situations. Assume each contract is considered a long-term contract unless otherwise implied.
  a. A contract to build an office building. The taxpayer's annual gross receipts for the past five years have exceeded $11 million.
  b. A contract to build a home to be finished next year. The taxpayer's annual gross receipts for the last five years have exceeded $11 million.
  c. A contract to build a high-rise apartment complex containing 120 units. The contractor's average gross receipts are $11 million.
  d. A contract to manufacture 15,000 seats for a football stadium. The taxpayer has several contracts for this type of seat. Average gross receipts are $12 million.
  e. A contract to manufacture a special part for NASA's space shuttles. Average annual gross receipts were $12 million.

5-20 *Taxpayer Identification—Family Trusts.* In recent years, many taxpayers have fallen victim to vendors of the so-called family trust tax shelter. Under this arrangement the taxpayer signs a contractual agreement entitling the trust to all of the taxpayer's income which is subsequently distributed to the beneficiaries of the trust. Explain how this arrangement is supposed to save taxes and why it fails.

5-21 *Income Reporting by Partnerships and S Corporations.* Absent special rules, explain how partners and shareholders in S corporations might defer the reporting of income by having their respective entities select fiscal years for reporting rather than calendar years.

5-22 *Income from Community Property.* Under what circumstances will knowledge of the community property system be relevant? Is it necessary for persons residing in common law states to understand the community property system?

5-23 *Planning—Timing Income Recognition.* Although it is generally desirable to defer income recognition and the related taxes. when would acceleration of income be preferred?

5-24 *Planning—Income Splitting.* How might R, who operates a shoe store as a sole proprietorship, reduce the taxes that are imposed on his family using income-splitting techniques?

5-25 *"Kiddie" Tax.* R has been advised that due to changes in the tax law over the years he can no longer save taxes by shifting income to his children.
   a. Explain the origin of such advice.
   b. What techniques currently exist to shift income successfully to children and other low-bracket family members?

❓ *YOU MAKE THE CALL*

5-26 In the last episode in the adventures of Dr. Will Floss, the tax-evading dentist identified earlier in this chapter, he was found exploring the cavities of his patient's mouth. As may be remembered, Dr. Floss had just made a deal with a patient whereby he exchanged a root canal for some carpet complete with pad and installation. Floss's accountant, Al, was faced with a dilemma. After dumping his records on Al's desk, Floss had proudly proclaimed that it was another great year. Al could remember his exact words: "Made over $200,000 but reported only $50,000. Not bad," said Floss. "Am I glad I talked to Dr. Moller!" Unfortunately, Al had to lower the boom on Floss's plan, explaining to him that he was required to report his barter income. However, Floss has stated flatly that he will not report the income. "If Moller doesn't report his, I'm not reporting mine," insists Floss. What should Al the accountant do about his client Floss and his friend Moller? If Floss goes to another accountant, does Al have any responsibilities?

PROBLEMS

5-27 *What Is Income?* In each of the following situations indicate whether taxable income should be recognized.
   a. Q purchased an older home for $20,000. Shortly after its purchase, the area in which it was located was designated a historical neighborhood, causing its value to rise to $50,000.
   b. R, a long-time employee of XYZ Inc., purchased one of the company's cars worth $7,000 for $3,000.
   c. I borrowed $10,000 secured by property that had an adjusted basis of $3,000 and a fair market value of $15,000.
   d. S, a 60 percent shareholder in STV Corporation, uses a company car 70 percent of the time for business and 30 percent for personal purposes. The rental value of the car is $200 per month.

5-28 *What Is Income?* In each of the following situations indicate whether taxable income should be recognized.
   a. R discovered oil on his farm, causing the value of his land to increase by $100 million.
   b. While jogging, L found a portable stereo radio valued at $200.
   c. E agreed to rent his lake cottage to F for $1,000 during the summer. After living there for two weeks, E and F agreed that E would only charge $700 if F made certain improvements.
   d. D borrowed $100,000, $20,000 each from S, T, U, V, and W. He gave them each a one-year note bearing interest at a rate of 25 percent. At the end of the year, D borrowed $200,000 from X, promising to pay him back in one year plus 30 percent interest. D used part of the $200,000 from X to pay the interest due to S, T, U, V, and W. D also convinced them to extend the original notes for another year. D has no intention of ever repaying the principal of the notes.

5-29 *What Is Income?* In each of the following situations indicate whether taxable income should be recognized.
   a. L sued her former employer for sex discrimination evidenced in his compensation policy. She was awarded $100,000, $39,000 of which represented reimbursement for mental anguish.
   b. M, a sales clerk for a department store, purchased a microwave oven from the store's appliance department. The store has a policy allowing employees a 10 percent discount. This discount results in $45 savings to M.
   c. R received a bottle of perfume and a case of grapefruit from her boss at the annual Christmas party. The items were valued at $25.

5-30 *Constructive Receipt.* When would a cash basis taxpayer recognize income in the following situations? Assume the taxpayer reports on a calendar year.
   a. R, a traveling salesperson, was out of town on payday, December 31. He picked up his check when he arrived back on January 3.
   b. C owns a bond with interest coupons due and payable on December 31. C clipped the coupons and redeemed them on January 7.
   c. R is an officer and controlling shareholder in XYZ Corporation. In December the corporation authorized bonuses for all officers. The bonus was paid in February of the following year.

5-31 *Constructive Receipt.* For each of the following situations, indicate whether the taxpayer has constructively received the income.
   a. R received a bonus as top salesperson of the year. He received the check for $20,000 at 10 p.m. on December 31 at a New Year's Eve party. All the banks were closed.
   b. On January 3, D received the check for January's rent of her duplex. The envelope was postmarked December 31.
   c. On December 25, C Corporation rewarded its top executive, E, with 100 shares of stock for a job well done. E was unable to find a buyer until March 15 of the following year.
   d. Immediately after receiving her check on December 31, Z went to her employer's bank to cash it. The bank would not cash it since the employer's account was overdrawn.

5-32 *Constructive Receipt.* For each of the following situations, indicate whether the taxpayer has constructively received the income.
   a. X Corporation declared a dividend on December 15 and mailed dividend checks on December 28. R received her check for $200 on January 4.
   b. F owns a small apartment complex. His son, S, lives in one of the units and manages the complex. Several tenants left their January rent checks with S during the last week of December. S delivered the checks to his father in January.
   c. This year, the cash surrender value of L's life insurance policy increased by $500. In order to obtain the value, L must cancel the policy.

5-33 *Changes in Accounting Method.* JB and his sons have operated a small "general store" in Backwoods, Idaho, since 1990. This year, JB hired a new accountant, who immediately told him he should be using the accrual method to account for his inventories and related sales and receivables. The receivables were primarily attributable to sales of seed to farmers as well as appliances. JB has always used the cash method of accounting, reporting all of his income when he receives it and deducting all costs when paid. According to the accountant, as of the close of the current year, JB had $70,000 in receivables outstanding (none of which had been reported in income), inventory of $130,000 (all expensed), and outstanding accounts payable for recent purchases of inventory of $20,000.

    a. If the IRS audits JB and requires him to change his method of accounting, what is the adjustment amount and when will JB report it?

    b. Same as (a) except JB voluntarily changes his method of accounting prior to the audit.

    c. If JB changes to the accrual method of accounting to account for inventories and sales, may he continue to report other items of income (e.g., interest income) and expense (e.g., supplies) using the cash method?

5-34 *Advanced Payments for Goods.* HIJ Furniture, an accrual basis company for both tax and financial accounting purposes, normally does not sell the items displayed in its showrooms, nor does it keep those items in stock. Instead, it obtains partial payment from the customer and orders the items directly from the manufacturer. During 2009, HIJ collected $60,000 with respect to furniture sales still on order at the close of the year. (The partial payments collected by HIJ do not exceed their cost for the items ordered.) Must HIJ report any of the $60,000 as income in 2009?

5-35 *Percentage of Completion.* THZ Corporation is a large construction company. This year it contracted with the city of Old York to build a new performing arts center for a price of $5,000,000. Estimated total costs of the project were $4,000,000. Annual costs incurred were as follows:

2010	$2,000,000
2011	500,000
2012	1,000,000
Total	$3,500,000

    a. What method(s) of accounting may the corporation use to report income from the project?

    b. How much income would be reported each year under the percentage of completion method?

    c. Would any interest be due to (or from) the IRS as a result of this contract? If so, compute for the first year only, assuming the taxpayer is in the 34 percent tax bracket and the interest rate is 10 percent.

5-36 *U.S. Savings Bonds.* During 2009, S purchased U.S. Government Series EE Bonds for $700. The redemption value of the bonds at the end of the year was $756. What options are available to S with respect to reporting the income from the bonds?

5-37 *Contested Income.* In 2009, GLX Company, an accrual basis taxpayer, received $10,000 for supplying running shoes to T for sale in his sporting goods store. During 2009, T claimed the shoes had defective soles and requested GLX to refund the $10,000 payment.

    a. Must GLX report any of the $10,000 as income in 2009?

    b. Had GLX not received payment in 2009, would your answer in (a) change?

5-38 *Deposits and Prepaid Rents.* Q owns several duplexes. From each new tenant she requires a $150 security deposit and $300 for the last month's rent. The deposit is refundable assuming the tenant complies with all the terms of the lease. During the year, Q collected $1,000 in deposits and $2,400 of prepaid rents for the last month of occupancy. In addition, she refunded $400 to previous tenants but withheld $300 due to damages. How much must Q include in income assuming she is an accrual basis taxpayer?

5-39 *Prepaid Service Income: Accrual Method.*
   a. LL Corporation, a calendar year and accrual basis taxpayer, is engaged in the lawn care business, providing fertilizer treatments. It sells one-, two- and three-year contracts. Each contract provides that the customer will receive four treatments (fall, winter, spring and summer). An analysis of its customer contracts revealed that it received $200,000 during the fall for a one-year contract. Each of these customers will receive one treatment in 2009 and three treatments in 2010. In its financial accounting statements, the company reports the income as services are performed. What amount of income must the corporation report in 2009 and 2010?
   b. Same as (a) above except the contracts are for two years. The customers will receive one treatment in 2009, four treatments in 2010 and three treatments in 2011.
   c. A professional basketball team that reports on the calendar year and uses the accrual method collected $700,000 in pre-season ticket sales in August and September of 2009. Of its 41-game home season, 15 games were played *prior to the end* of the year. In its financial statements, the organization reports the income as the games are played. What amount must be included in income in 2009?
   d. A posh resort hotel in Florida reports on the calendar year and uses the accrual method. During 2009, it collected $10,000 in advance payments for rooms to be rented during January and February 2010. What amount of income must be included in 2009 and 2010?

5-40 *Income from Transferred Property.* E's grandmother owns several vending machines on campus. To help him through college, she allows E to collect and keep all the receipts from the machines. During the year, E spent approximately two hours a month to collect $5,000. Who must report the income and what is the amount to be included?

5-41 *Partnership Income.* QRS, a partnership, had taxable income of $120,000 for the fiscal year ended September 30, 2009. For the first quarter ending December 31, 2009, taxable income was $30,000. During 2009, Q, a partner with a 30 percent interest in profits and losses, withdrew $1,000 per month for a total of $12,000. What is Q's taxable income from QRS for 2009?

5-42 *Reporting Interest Income.* On November 1, 2008, G received a substantial inheritance and promptly made several investments. Indicate in each of the following cases the amount of interest income that he must report and the period in which the income is properly reported, assuming that G uses (1) the cash method of accounting, or (2) the accrual method of accounting. G reports using the calendar year.
   a. G purchased a $10,000, 90-day U.S. Treasury bill at 99. The bill matured on January 30, 2009, when G redeemed it at par.
   b. G purchased $100,000 of AFN Inc. 10 percent bonds for $95,000. The bonds were issued at par in 2001. The bonds pay interest semiannually on March 1 and September 1. On March 1, 2009, G received an interest payment of $5,000.

5-43 *Interest-Free Loans.* This year Dr. W, an orthopedic surgeon, and her husband, H, an attorney, established a trust for their five-year-old daughter, D. In conjunction with setting up the trust, the couple loaned the trust $200,000 payable on demand without interest. Assuming the interest that should have been charged under the applicable rate was $23,000, explain the effect of the loan on all of the parties.

5-44 *Shareholder Advances.* In 2000, J started ACC Corporation, a construction company. J owns all of the stock of the corporation and is also its president. Like many owners of closely-held corporations, J pretty much treats the corporation's checkbook as his own. He often asks the bookkeeper to make out checks to him that he ostensibly uses for business purposes. Over time, J does repay the amounts used for personal purposes, or turns in receipts for amounts used for business. In the meantime, the bookkeeper charges these checks to a special account titled "J Suspense." Upon the accountant's review this year, he noted that the account showed a balance of $15,000 (indicating an amount due from J). Explain the tax consequences.

5-45 *Interest-Free Loans.* F is chief executive officer of CVC Corporation and has taxable income in excess of $200,000 annually. During the year, he loaned his 20-year-old son, S, $30,000, payable on demand without interest. S promptly invested the $30,000 and earned $1,200, which was his only income during the year.
   a. Assuming the interest that should have been charged under applicable rate is $3,000, compute the effect of the loan on the taxable income of both F and S.
   b. Would F be able to shift income to his son if he had made a loan of only $9,000?

5-46 *Code § 7872: Exceptions.* For each of the following independent cases, indicate the income and gift tax consequences for both the lender and the borrower.
   a. J loaned his 25-year-old son, K, $8,000 interest-free, which K used to purchase a car. K had $400 investment income from a savings account for the year.
   b. Same as (a) except K decided to invest the money in a certificate of deposit yielding $800 of interest income producing a total net investment income of $1,200 for the year.
   c. G loaned her 29-year-old daughter, D, $50,000 interest-free to help her acquire a franchise for a fast-food restaurant. All of D's funds were invested in the business and consequently she had no investment income for the year.
   d. P Corporation loaned its sole shareholder, Q, $150,000 interest-free.
   e. Same as (d) except Q owns no stock in P but is simply a key employee.

5-47 *Cash Method Eligibility.* Given the facts below, indicate whether the taxpayer may use the cash method for 2009 in the following situations.
   a. Sweatshirt Corporation, a publicly traded corporation: annual gross receipts for 2006 and previous years were $1 million annually; gross receipts for 2007 were $3 million; and for 2008, $8 million.
   b. Dewey, Cheatham, and Howe, a national public accounting firm, operated as a partnership. Annual gross receipts for the past five years have exceeded $50 million.
   c. McSwane, McMillan, and McClain, Inc., an architectural firm, operated as a regular C corporation. Annual gross receipts for the past two years have exceeded $7 million. McSwane, McMillan, and McClain own all of the stock and perform services for the firm.
   d. Buttons and Bows, Inc., an S corporation.
   e. A trust established for John Doe.
   f. Plantation Office Park, a publicly traded limited partnership: annual gross receipts have never exceeded $2 million. The partnership is a tax shelter.

5-48 *Accrual Method of Accounting.* Frank's Casing Crew and Rental Tools Inc. uses the accrual method of accounting and reports using the calendar year. The corporation sells oil pipes, leases equipment used in oil fields, and provides crews necessary to operate the leased equipment. The company's customers are primarily large oil companies. The company's contracts provide that payment is due when it sends the customer an invoice that includes all supporting documentation (i.e., job tickets, equipment tickets, and third party charges). In 2009, the company finished several jobs but did not invoice the customers until after year-end because it had not yet received a third party's invoice. When should the corporation report the income from these contracts?

5-49 *Accrual Method of Accounting.* N Corporation operates a chain of coffee shops in various locations throughout Indiana. It uses the accrual method of accounting and reports using the calendar year. In 2010, its expenses exceeded its revenue resulting in a net operating loss (NOL). Like federal law, Indiana's state law, permits corporations to carry back an NOL to prior years where it can be used to offset such year's taxable income, enabling the corporation to obtain a refund of previously paid Indiana state income taxes. (Note that state income taxes are deductible business expenses so a recovery of such expenses is taxable income.) The Indiana Department of Revenue has the right to examine any refund claim before determining whether to allow the claim and the refund amount. In 2011, the corporation filed the proper forms to carry back the NOL, seeking a refund of part of the state income taxes it had paid in previous years. In 2012, N received a refund of $100,000. When should N report the income?

5-50 *Accrual Method of Accounting.* Giant Corp. operates retail stores throughout the country. It uses the accrual method of accounting and reports using the calendar year. Each store offers film processing. Customers wanting film developed put the film in an order envelope and place the envelope in a drop box. Finished prints are produced primarily by Giant's own processing labs but also unrelated labs. The labs develop the film using highly specialized equipment and a complex chemical process, normally returning the finished prints within two days of when their couriers pick up the film. The finished prints are held for customer pick-up at the stores. Customers are not required to buy the prints unless they are completely satisfied. Store employees review the unsold prints on hand every 30 days and remind customers by phone or mail that their prints are available. Finished prints that are unclaimed after 120 days or customer rejects are discarded. Giant owns the finished prints until either a customer purchases them or they are discarded. Only a small percentage of customers do not purchase the finished prints. Upon audit, the IRS asserted that Giant should have to report the income when the stores receive the finished prints. Indicate whether the agent is correct or incorrect and explain the reasons for your answer.

5-51 *Shifting Income to Children.* Mr. and Mrs. D wish to shift income to their seven-year-old son, C, to be used for his college education. Explain whether the following would serve their goals or, alternatively, how they affect any technique designed to shift income.
   a. Paying C an allowance for making his bed and picking up his clothes.
   b. Paying C for helping to wash cars at his dad's car wash.
   c. Buying C Series EE Savings Bonds.
   d. Arranging to have Mrs. D's employer pay C part of her salary.
   e. The social security rules.
   f. The rules governing personal exemptions.

TAX RETURN PROBLEMS

CONTINUOUS TAX RETURN PROBLEMS   See Appendix D, Part 1.

CUMULATIVE PROBLEM

TaxCut **5-52** David K. Gibbs, age 37, and his wife, Barbara, age 33, have two children, Chris and Ellen, ages 2 and 12. David is employed as an engineer for an oil company, and his wife recently completed a degree in accounting and will begin working for a public accounting firm next year. David has compiled the following information for your use in preparing his tax return for 2008.
   1. For the current year, David received a salary of $50,000. His employer withheld Federal income taxes of $9,000 and the appropriate amount of FICA taxes.
   2. At the annual Christmas party, he received a card indicating that he would receive a bonus of $3,000 for his good work during the year. The bonus check was placed

in his mailbox at work on December 30. Since David was out of town for the holidays, he did not pick up the bonus check until January 2.

3. A bond issued by AM&T Inc. was sold on May 30, 2008 for $9,700, $700 of which represented interest accrued to the date of the sale. The Gibbs had purchased the bond (issued at par value of $10,000 on March 1, 1997) in 2004 for $10,000.

4. The couple has a $500 U.S. Savings Bond, which they purchased for $300 and gave to their daughter several years ago. The proper election to report the income from the bond annually was made. The bond's redemption value increased $30 this year.

5. David was an instant winner in the state lottery and won $50.

6. The Gibbs sold 100 shares of stock in JB Corporation for $10,000. They had purchased the stock on June 1, 2001 for $14,000.

7. During the year, Barbara prepared a number of tax returns for which she received $5,000. Her only deductible expense incurred in performing these services was $100 for some tax software.

8. The couple's only itemized deductions were medical expenses of $3,000, interest on their home mortgage of $7,500, and property taxes on their home of $4,000.

Compute Mr. and Mrs. Gibbs' Federal income tax liability (or refund) for 2008. If a tax return is required by your instructor, prepare Form 1040, including Schedules A and B.

RESEARCH PROBLEMS

5-53 During the year, J, a college accounting professor, received complimentary copies of various textbooks from numerous publishers. J gives some of these books to students and the school library. J also keeps some of the books for his personal use and reference. A few times during the year J sold an unwanted text to a wholesale book dealer who periodically checked with him and other professors for texts. Must J report any income related to receipt of these books?

5-54 R recently became a member of a religious order. As a member, she was subject to the organization's complete control. The organization often required its members to terminate their employment in order to work in other jobs consistent with the organization's philosophy. For example, the organization supplied personnel to missions, hospitals, and schools. The organization also requires all members to take an oath of poverty and pay over all their earnings to it. Members' living expenses are paid for by the organization out of its own funds. Is R taxed on her earnings?

5-55 In each of the following cases, indicate who is responsible for reporting the income.
a. Dr. A instructed the hospital for which he worked to pay his salary to his daughter C.
b. R, a famous entertainer, agreed to perform at a concert gratuitously (without fee) for the benefit of a charitable organization.
c. In a contest for the best essay on why education is important, T, age 25, won the right to designate a person under 17 to receive $1,000.

5-56 M owed her good friend, F, $20,000. In addition, M planned on making a charitable contribution to her church of $10,000. Instead of using cash to pay her friend and to make the contribution, M is considering transferring stock to each in the appropriate amount. The stock is currently worth $100 per share. M had purchased the 300 shares of stock several years ago for $6,000 ($20 per share). Will M realize any income if she transfers the stock rather than paying cash?

5-57 Sam Sellit is a salesperson for Panoramic Pools of St. Louis, a construction company that builds and sells prefabricated swimming pools. Over the past several years, Sam has progressed to become the top salesperson for the St. Louis franchise. Sam has done so well that he is considering purchasing his own franchise and starting a company in San Antonio. This year he contacted the home office in Pittsburgh about the possibility of opening up his own shop. The vice president in charge of expansion, Greg Grow, suggested that the two of them meet at the company's annual meeting of franchisees in

Orlando. Greg knew that Sam, although not a franchisee, would be attending because he was the top salesperson in the St. Louis office, and the company invites the top salesperson from each office as well as his or her spouse to attend the meeting.

While at the four-day meeting (Tuesday through Friday) in Orlando, Sam and his wife, Sue, met with Greg and discussed the potential venture. In addition, Greg allowed Sam and Sue to attend the parts of the meeting that were only for franchisees so that they could get a glimpse of how the company operated. Of course, while they were in Orlando, Sam and his wife visited all of the tourist attractions. On Tuesday, there were no meetings scheduled and everyone spent the day at Disney World and Epcot Center. On Thursday afternoon, no meetings were scheduled and the couple went with Greg and his wife to Sea World. Sam attended meetings for several hours on Friday while his wife played golf. The couple stayed over through Sunday and continued their sightseeing activities.

The company picked up the tab for the couple's trip, reimbursing Sam $3,500 which included the costs of air fare, meals, lodging, and entertainment. What are the tax consequences to Sam?

5-58   Large Corporation manufactures computers. Its total sales of computers last year were well over $100 million. With each computer it offers a three-year warranty, covering parts and labor. The company estimates the future costs of warranty work related to current-year sales and defers the recognition of income until such time that it expects the warranty work will be done. Currently, the corporation reports 60 percent of the warranty income in the year of sale because the majority of warranty work occurs shortly after the computer has been sold. Thirty percent of the warranty income is reported in the second year of the warranty, and the remaining 10 percent is reported in the last year of the warranty. The company's estimates were based on sophisticated statistical techniques. Such techniques have produced estimates that appear extremely accurate based on the past ten years of data. No insurance is purchased to cover the warranty risk. Upon audit this year, the IRS agent indicated that the company cannot defer the warranty income and assessed a large tax deficiency. Advise the taxpayer as to whether it should pay the additional tax or pursue the matter in court.

5-59   Several years ago, R started his own delivery company, RT Haulers Inc. (RTH). The corporation is an accrual basis taxpayer. The corporation grew quickly, in part because of the excellent service that it was able to offer. Historically, the company has accrued its income when its services were completed. If the customer objected to the manner in which the services were performed (e.g., late delivery, damaged goods), RTH gave the client a credit against any future services that it might provide. RTH is now considering changing its agreements with customers to provide for a seven day acceptance period during which the customer could reject the services, in which case the customer would not have any obligation to pay. Advise the client regarding when its income should be reported, specifically addressing how the change in terms might impact the reporting of future service revenues.

5-60   Basinger Hauling is a trucking company that does business primarily on the west coast and in Mexico and Canada. Its headquarters are in Portland, Oregon. The company generally pays its drivers a specific rate, depending on a variety of factors such as miles driven, load weight, weather, unloading, fuel costs and the like. The company treats eight percent of each driver's compensation as a reimbursement for meals and lodging. Consequently, the company does not pay employment taxes (social security and Medicare) on the portion considered a reimbursement and does not include the reimbursement on the driver's W-2 form, reporting the amount representing wage income. Advise the client regarding this practice.

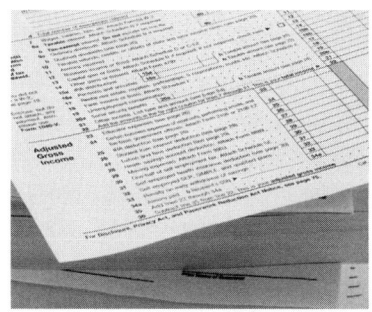

★ CHAPTER SIX ★

GROSS INCOME: INCLUSIONS AND EXCLUSIONS

LEARNING OBJECTIVES

Upon completion of this chapter you will be able to:

- ▸ Identify which items an individual taxpayer must include in the computation of gross income

- ▸ Determine which items an individual taxpayer can exclude from the computation of gross income

- ▸ Understand generally what goals Congress had in mind in passing the applicable rules and exceptions for inclusions and exclusions

- ▸ Recognize tax planning opportunities related to the more common types of income inclusions and exclusions available to individual taxpayers

CHAPTER OUTLINE

INTRODUCTION

While the tax law makes it clear that any type of gain, benefit, profit, or other increase in wealth is potentially taxable, in reality not all income is within the grasp of the IRS. As a practical matter, there are a number of special rules that must be observed before the final treatment of any particular benefit can be determined. For example, Congress has specifically exempted several types of income from tax such as interest on state and local bonds, scholarships, gifts, and inheritances. In addition, special provisions exist that clarify the treatment of a long list of possible income items such as annuities, alimony, and employee benefits. Because of these rules, the concept of income is not quite as comprehensive as perhaps suggested in Chapter 5. As a result, any particular item initially identified as "income" might ultimately fall into one of the following three categories:

► Taxable (i.e., totally includible)

► Nontaxable (i.e., excluded in full)

► Taxable in part and nontaxable in part

This chapter examines the more frequently encountered sources of income. To provide some order and logic to the presentation, the various sources of income are grouped and discussed as follows:

- ▸ Investment income (dividends, interest, annuities)
- ▸ Employee compensation and fringe benefits
- ▸ Personal transfers (gifts, inheritances, alimony)
- ▸ Transfers by unrelated individuals (life insurance, prizes, scholarships)
- ▸ Business income
- ▸ Miscellaneous items

INVESTMENT INCOME

As shown in Exhibit 6-1, the vast majority of the income reported by individuals comes in some form of employee compensation such as salaries and wages (73.3 percent of all reported income for 2003). However, as Exhibit 6-1 also shows the income of many individuals is also likely to contain some type of investment income.

EXHIBIT 6-1
Sources of Income 2006

Type of Income	Percent of Returns Showing	Percent of All Income Reported
Salaries and wages	84.09%*	68.01%
Taxable interest	45.09	2.77
Pensions, annuities, individual retirement accounts	24.61	7.17
Dividends	22.85	2.48
Qualified dividends	19.21	1.71
Net capital gain	13.03	9.04
Business or profession net income	11.71	4.11
Social Security benefits	9.93	1.80
Net capital loss	6.24	−.23
Partnership and S corporation net income	5.51	5.30
Unemployment compensation	5.33	.33
Tax-exempt interest	4.36	.91
Rent and royalty net income	4.18	.99
Business or profession net loss	3.94	−.61
Rent and royalty net loss	3.87	−.74
Farm net income less loss	1.41	−.19
Sales of property other than capital assets, net gain less loss	1.29	.05
Estate or trust net income less loss	.43	.21

* Preliminary estimates based on samples taken from 138,394,754 individual returns filed in 2006.
Source: Statistics of Income, 2006 Individual Income Tax Returns, Table 1.3, Fall 2008. Publication 1304 Internal Revenue Service, Washington, D.C. 2008.

Common examples of investment income—sometimes referred to as unearned income—include

▸ Dividends

▸ Interest

▸ Annuities

▸ Rents

For the most part, these income items present little problem for taxpayers. Each is usually fully taxable as ordinary income. In addition, to make reporting and compliance easier, those who pay dividends, interest, and annuities during the taxable year normally must report such payments to both the taxpayer and the IRS on the appropriate Form 1099. Nevertheless, special rules often apply in determining not only the amount of income that must be reported but also when it must be reported. The treatment of each is discussed below.

DIVIDENDS

Today it is not uncommon for even the smallest investor to own stock in a corporation or an interest in a mutual fund. Those who do are likely to obtain part of their investment return in the form of dividends. One of the high-profile debates surrounding the Jobs and Growth Tax Relief Reconciliation Act of 2003 concerned the taxation of dividends. The original proposal of the administration called for the complete exclusion for dividends in order to address the potential problem of double taxation. However, the final legislation did not adopt such a sweeping measure. Instead, the Act reduced the tax rates imposed on dividends to what they are for capital gains. For 2008–2010, the rate is normally 15 percent but drops to 0 percent for taxpayers whose income falls in the 10 or 15 percent ordinary income tax brackets. To emphasize, for low-bracket taxpayers (e.g., married taxpayers with taxable income less than $65,100), dividends as well as long-term capital gains are tax free![1] The reduced rate generally applies to so-called *qualified dividends*. Qualified dividends include dividends paid with respect to stock of all domestic corporations. For domestic stock, It makes no difference whether it is publicly traded or closely held. In addition, the reduced rate generally applies to dividends from foreign corporations but only if the stock is readily tradable on an established U.S. securities market. Also, to secure the special rate the taxpayer must hold the stock for more than 60 days during a 120 day window that begins 60 days before the stock goes ex-dividend. This requirement helps prevent taxpayers from exploiting the preferential treatment for dividends. To illustrate the possible injustice, consider a taxpayer who buys a stock a few days before the ex-dividend date, receives a $1,000 dividend and then sells the stock. Assuming the value of the stock drops in direct proportion to the amount of the dividend, a sale immediately after the ex-dividend date would produce a $1,000 short-term capital loss. It appears that the $1,000 dividend is offset by the $1,000 loss and the net effect is zero. However, the dividend is taxed at 15 percent and the loss may offset ordinary income that is taxed at 35 percent. In such case, the taxpayer is better-off by $200 ($350 − $150). The holding period rule requires taxpayers to be at risk for at least 61 days if they want to use this scheme.[2]

Note that this change represents a major philosophical shift that has little precedent in tax history. Dividends received by individuals have historically been taxed as ordinary income with little or no special treatment. Although a small exclusion for dividends once existed, dividends have otherwise been treated the same as ordinary income. It should also be observed that there is no special treatment for interest income.

---

[1] § 1(h)(11)

[2] The holding period is extended for preferred stock. For other special rules see §1(h)(11).

Corporate Dividends. The vast majority of all distributions made by corporations to their shareholders are considered dividends and are fully taxable as ordinary income. Technically, however, a distribution made by a corporation is treated as a *dividend* only to the extent that it is out of the corporation's current or accumulated *earnings and profits*, or *E&P* as it is commonly called.[3] Amounts not considered dividends because the distribution exceeds E&P are treated as nontaxable returns of capital to the extent of the shareholder's basis in the stock. In effect, the nondividend portion of the distribution is applied to and reduces the basis of the stock. Should the return of capital distribution exceed the shareholder's basis, the excess is capital gain. In applying these rules, all distributions by corporations are deemed to be distributions of E&P to the extent thereof.

> **Example 1.** C, Inc. distributes $100,000 to shareholders when its current E&P is $60,000 and it has no accumulated E&P. T, a 10% shareholder, has a basis in C, Inc. stock of $3,000. T receives $10,000, of which $6,000 (10% × $60,000) is from C's current E&P. Thus, T has a $6,000 taxable dividend; the $3,000 equal to his basis in the stock is a nontaxable return of investment, and the remaining $1,000 is capital gain. T's basis in the stock after the distribution will be zero.

As noted above, for individual taxpayers dividends are fully taxable as ordinary income but are taxed at favorable rates.[4]

Dividends received by corporate taxpayers are treated differently than dividend received by individuals. As explained in Chapter 3, in order to prevent multiple taxation of dividends, corporate taxpayers are entitled to a special dividends-received deduction. This special deduction (discussed more fully in Chapter 19) normally entitles the corporation to deduct 70 percent of the dividend received.[5] The favorable tax rates, 15 or 0 percent, do not apply to dividends received by a corporation.

The most critical variable in determining the treatment of a corporate distribution is the amount of the corporation's earnings and profits. The actual computation of E&P can be quite complex but the theory underlying it is relatively simple. The calculation attempts to measure the amount the corporation can pay out without impairing its capital account. In this regard, it is quite similar to the financial accounting concept of retained earnings. However, the two are not identical. Current E&P generally represents taxable income as adjusted for certain specified items.[6] Accumulated E&P is the sum of current E&P reduced by distributions. Using this information, a corporation determines the amount of its distribution that is considered a dividend (e.g., 60%) and reports this information to the shareholder on Form 1099-DIV or similar statement.

Mutual Fund Dividends. Millions of taxpayers now invest in stocks, bonds, and other securities indirectly through mutual funds. Mutual funds typically buy and sell investments realizing gains and losses as well as collect earnings from investments such as interest on bonds or dividends on stock.[7] Like corporations, mutual funds make distributions. However, the treatment of these distributions differs somewhat from regular corporate dividends in that they are generally characterized to reflect the nature of the income realized by the mutual fund. Mutual fund distributions are normally characterized as either *ordinary dividends* or *capital gain dividends*.[8] Ordinary dividends

---

[3] §§ 301 and 316.

[4] Special rules apply to the rare distribution of noncash property (e.g., land). See §§ 301(b) and (d).

[5] §§ 243 through 246. Generally, the deduction is a percentage of the dividends received from a domestic corporation determined as follows: (1) 70% when the stock ownership percentage (SOP) is less than 20%, (2) 80% when the SOP is 20% or more but less than 80%, and (3) 100% when the SOP is 80% or more.

[6] E&P is not defined in the Code. See § 312 and the related regulations.

[7] Funds are taxed like trusts, deducting income distributed and paying tax on income retained. Distributed income generally retains its character as either ordinary income or capital gain.

[8] Reg. § 1.852-4(a) and (b).

represent the individual's share of the fund's earnings from its own investments such as interest or dividends as well as any short-term gains the fund may realize. An individual reports all ordinary dividends as dividend income. The mutual fund designates the portion that represents "qualified dividend" income which is taxed at the 15 and 0 percent rates. Capital gain dividends represent the capital gains and losses actually realized by the mutual fund during the year. All capital gain dividends are treated as *long-term* capital gains. Corporate taxpayers are entitled to the dividends-received deduction for ordinary dividends but not capital gain dividends. Each fund reports the information regarding its distributions to its shareholders on Form 1099-DIV.

A few funds retain their capital gains, in which case they are required to pay tax on such amounts. Nevertheless, these gains are allocated to the shareholders who must include them in income as capital gain.[9] In such case, shareholders may claim a credit for any tax paid by the fund and increase their basis in their shares for the amount included in income less the tax paid.

Other "Dividends". There are a number of other distributions that taxpayers receive that are often called dividends. Technically, however, these are not "dividends" in the tax sense but receive special treatment. Some of these are listed below.

1. In some instances, earnings on deposits with banks, credit unions, investment companies, and savings and loan associations are referred to as dividends when they actually possess all the characteristics of interest. These dividends are reported as interest.[10]

2. Mutual insurance companies distribute amounts referred to as dividends to owners of unmatured life insurance policies. These dividends are treated as a nontaxable return of a portion of the insurance premium paid.[11]

3. Cooperatives distribute patronage dividends to cooperative members. These dividends are treated as a return of part of the original price paid for items purchased by members.[12]

4. As noted above, dividends from regulated investment companies (mutual funds) that represent gains on sales of investments from the fund are treated as long-term capital gains.[13]

Stock Dividends. From time to time, a corporation may make a distribution of its own stock. These so-called stock dividends are normally declared as a means to reduce the selling price of the stock or as simply a gesture of goodwill to the shareholders. As a practical matter, when a corporation distributes its own stock, it is not distributing an asset of the business; indeed, the corporation's assets remain completely intact and only the number of shares outstanding changes. From the shareholder's point of view, assuming all shareholders receive their proportionate shares of the stock distributed, they have essentially received nothing because their interest in corporate assets remains unchanged. Since the effect is to leave both the corporation and the shareholder in the same economic position as they held prior to the distribution, the stock dividend—a

---

[9]   § 852(b)(3)(D).

[10]   Reg. § 1.61-7(a).

[11]   § 316(b)(1).

[12]   § 1385(b).

[13]   § 1382(b).

misnomer in this case—is nontaxable.[14] On the other hand, if the distribution is structured so that the shareholder's interest does change (e.g., the shareholder can elect to take stock or cash), the stock distribution is taxable.[15]

If the distribution of stock is nontaxable, the only responsibility of the shareholder is to determine the basis of the "new" and the "old" stock. Note that only the shareholder's per-share basis is altered. Total basis for all of the stock owned remains the same. Technically, the shareholder must allocate a portion of the basis of the original stock to the distributed stock. The basis is allocated between the old and the new in proportion to the relative values of the old and new stock on the date of the distribution.[16] When the old shares are identical to the new shares (e.g., a common on common stock dividend), the basis for each share is determined simply by dividing the basis of the old stock by the total number of shares held by the shareholder after the distribution. The holding period of the old shares carries over to the new shares.[17]

> **Example 2.** V owns 100 shares of Z common with a basis of $2,200 ($22 per share). He receives 10 shares of Z common as a stock dividend. If V did not have the right to receive cash or other assets in lieu of the stock, he has no taxable income from this transaction and his $2,200 basis is allocated among the 110 shares of common for a $20 per share basis ($2,200 ÷ 110).

> **Example 3.** Q owns 100 shares of S common with a basis of $2,200. She receives 10 shares of S preferred as a stock dividend. The market value is $4,000 ($40 per share) for common and $1,000 ($100 per share) for preferred. If Q did not have the right to receive cash or other assets in lieu of the stock, she has no taxable income since her proportionate interest did not change. Her basis for the preferred stock is $440 [$1,000 ÷ ($4,000 + $1,000 = $5,000 total value) = 20% × $2,200] and her basis for the common stock is $1,760 [either ($2,200 − $440) or ($4,000 ÷ $5,000) × $2,200].

INTEREST

The second most common item of income appearing on individual tax returns is interest (see Exhibit 6-1). More than 45 percent of all returns filed in 2003 reported some type of taxable interest. As a general rule, interest income is taxable. This is true regardless of its source (a bank, business, friend, or relative) or the form of the interest-bearing instrument (savings account, bond, or note). However, there are two notable exceptions to this rule: (1) the exclusion for interest on certain state and local government obligations, and (2) the exclusion for interest on educational savings bonds.

Interest on State and Local Government Obligations. From the inception of the Federal income tax law, interest on obligations of a state, a territory, a U.S. possession, or any of their political subdivisions has been *nontaxable*.[18] From time to time and even currently this exclusion has been criticized as an unwarranted loophole. Critics often characterize this exclusion as simply a tax shelter existing primarily for the rich. In truth,

---

[14]   § 305(a).

[15]   § 305(b).

[16]   § 307(a).

[17]   § 1223(5).

[18]   § 103(a); § 103(c).

however, this treatment stems from an uncertainty about whether taxing this interest would be unconstitutional and also from political pressure exerted by the affected governments.[19] The exclusion is exceedingly beneficial to these governments because it means they can pay a lower interest rate and still attract investors, especially those investors who are subject to taxes at the highest marginal rates.

> **Example 4.** K, Inc. invests $10,000 in corporate bonds that pay 13% annually and $10,000 in state bonds that pay 9% annually. If K, Inc.'s marginal tax rate is 34%, its after-tax earnings on the corporate bonds are less than its earnings on the state bonds.

	Corporate Bonds	State Bonds
Annual interest income	$1,300	$900
Federal income tax (34%)	442	0
After-tax income	$ 858	$900

If K's marginal tax rate is 15%, however, its after-tax earnings for the corporate bonds increase to $1,105 ($1,300 − $195).

A break-even point between taxable and nontaxable rates of return may be calculated with the following formula:

$$\text{Taxable interest rate} \times (1 - \text{Marginal tax rate}) = \text{Tax-free rate}$$

Applying the numbers in the example above when K, Inc.'s tax rate is 34 percent, the breakeven point for the taxable bond is

$$13\% \times (1 - 0.34 = 0.66) = 8.58\%$$

Thus, at the 34 percent marginal tax rate, a 13 percent taxable return is equal to an 8.58 percent tax-exempt return.

The formula can be converted to compute the break-even point for the tax-exempt bond as follows:

$$\text{Tax-free rate} \div (1 - \text{Marginal tax rate})$$
$$\text{or}$$
$$9\% \div (1 - 0.34 = 0.66) = 13.6\%$$

Thus, at the 34 percent marginal tax rate, a 9 percent tax-exempt return is equal to a 13.6 percent taxable return.

A comparison of the effective yield on tax-free versus taxable investments is provided in Exhibit 6-2. Given current market conditions, the effective yield on tax-exempt securities will be difficult to match with taxable investments. For example, if a taxpayer is in the 28 percent bracket and the current yield on tax-exempt securities is five percent, the after-tax return on taxable securities would be greater as long as the yield exceeded 6.94 percent.

---

[19] The constitutional issue now seems to be moot. See *South Carolina v. Baker*, 109 S.Ct. 1355 (1988) where the Supreme Court noted that there was no constitutional prohibition barring the Federal government from taxing such interest. See also *National Life Insurance Co.*, 1 USTC ¶314, 6 AFTR 7801, 277 U.S. 508 (USSC, 1928), where the Supreme Court originally indicated that Federal taxation of *interest* paid by state and local governments was unconstitutional.

Over the years, Congress has reacted to the criticism that this exclusion subsidizes the wealthy (i.e., those subject to the highest tax rates) and has also reacted to the increasing number and complexity of financial offerings developed by state and local governments. Originally, these governments sold securities to fund public projects. More recently, however, bonds have been issued to fund business construction and other industrial development projects. When this occurs, a governmental unit retains ownership of the facilities and leases them to a business. Because the interest rate on these bonds is lower than it would be on bonds issued by the corporation, the negotiated lease payments can be lower. Congress has curtailed the tax-exempt status of these so-called industrial development bonds. With certain specified exceptions, interest on industrial development bonds is taxable income.[20]

EXHIBIT 6-2

Comparison of Taxable versus Tax-Free Investments

	If your tax-free investment is yielding:					
	4.50%	5.00%	5.50%	6.00%	6.50%	7.00%
Marginal Tax Bracket*	Your taxable equivalent yield is:					
15%	5.29%	5.88%	6.47%	7.06%	7.65%	8.24%
28%	6.25%	6.94%	7.64%	8.33%	9.03%	9.72%
31%	6.52%	7.25%	7.97%	8.70%	9.42%	10.14%
36%	7.03%	7.81%	8.59%	9.38%	10.16%	10.94%
39.6%	7.45%	8.28%	9.11%	9.93%	10.76%	11.59%

* Based on combined federal and state

In addition to the limitations imposed on industrial development bonds, there are still other restrictions intended to curb the use of state and local bonds to finance business activities. For example, tax-exempt bonds can no longer be issued to finance airplanes, gambling facilities, liquor stores, health clubs, sky boxes, or other luxury boxes. Nor can the bonds be issued to finance the acquisition of farmland or existing facilities, with certain exceptions.

Gain on Sale of Tax-Exempt Bonds. It should be noted that any exclusion on state and local obligations is for *interest* income received by the bondholder. Thus, *gain* on the sale of tax-exempt securities that does not represent interest is taxable income.[21]

Example 5. On January 1 of the current year N purchased at par a $30,000, 10-year tax exempt municipal bond, yielding 8%. On September 30 of the following year, she sold the bond for $32,000 plus accrued interest of $800. Although the accrued interest is tax-exempt, N must report $2,000 of capital gain ($32,000 − $30,000) subject to tax of up to 15%.

Educational Savings Bonds. In 1988, Congress took steps to help taxpayers finance the rising costs of higher education by offering a special tax break for those who save to meet such expenses. Code § 135 generally provides that accrued interest on Series EE savings bonds issued after 1989 is exempt from tax when the accrued interest and principal amount of such bonds are used to pay for *qualified educational expenses*

---

[20] § 103 (b).

[21] *Willcuts v. Bunn*, 2 USTC ¶640, 9 AFTR 584, 282 U.S. 216 (USSC. 1931). (See footnote 17.)

of the taxpayer or the taxpayer's spouse or dependents (but only if these relationships are satisfied in the year of the redemption). For this purpose, qualified education expenses include those for tuition or fees to attend college or certain schools offering vocational education. Costs that otherwise qualify must be reduced by any scholarships or fellowships that may be received, as well as any employer-provided assistance.

The interest exclusion is allowed only to the extent that the taxpayer uses the proceeds of the bond redemption to pay qualified educational expenses during the year that he or she redeems a bond. If the redemption proceeds received during the year exceed the amount of education expenses paid during the same year, the amount of the interest exclusion must be reduced proportionately. The amount of the exclusion may be computed as follows:

$$\frac{\text{Qualified educational expenses paid during the year}}{\text{Total redemption proceeds of qualified bonds during the year}} \times \text{Accrued interest} = \text{Exclusion}$$

Example 6. Mr. and Mrs. T purchased Series EE savings bonds in 2009 for $4,000. On June 2, 2020 they cashed in the bonds and received $10,000, $6,000 representing accrued interest and $4,000 representing their original investment. Three months later on September 2, they paid tuition of $9,000 for their dependent daughter, D, who attends a private university. In November, D received a scholarship of $1,000 for being an outstanding accounting major. Only $8,000 ($9,000 tuition − $1,000 scholarship) of D's expenses are considered qualified educational expenses. Since this amount represents only 80% ($8,000/$10,000) of the total redemption proceeds, Mr. and Mrs. T may exclude only 80% of the $6,000 accrued interest, or $4,800.

Note that to qualify for the exclusion, the savings bonds need not be transferred directly to the educational institution. The exclusion applies to interest on *any* post-1989 Series EE savings bond that is realized during the taxable year as long as the taxpayer pays sufficient qualified educational expenses during the same taxable year.

The special exclusion is designed to benefit only those who have moderate incomes. To achieve this objective, the exclusion is gradually reduced once the taxpayer's A.G.I. (as determined in the taxable year when the bonds are redeemed) reaches a certain level. The 2009 income level at which the phase-out begins depends on the taxpayer's filing status as shown below.

Filing Status	Phase-out Range Modified A.G.I.*
Single (including heads of household)	$ 69,950 − $ 84,950
Married filing jointly	$104,900 − $134,900

* Adjusted annually for inflation

The reduction of the exclusion otherwise allowed is computed as follows:

$$\frac{\text{Excess A.G.I.}}{\$15,000\ (\$30,000\text{ for joint returns})} \times \text{Otherwise excludable interest} = \text{Reduction}$$

Married taxpayers filing separately are not eligible for the exclusion. Taxpayers who are married must file a joint return to secure the exclusion.

Example 7. Mr. and Mrs. B have an A.G.I., after proper modifications, of $114,900, before the exclusion. As a result, the amount of any interest that would otherwise be nontaxable must be reduced by one third:

$$\frac{(\$114,900 \text{ A.G.I} - \$104,900 \text{ threshold} = \$10,000)}{(\$134,900 - \$104,950 = \$30,000 \text{ phase-out range})}$$

Assume the couple redeemed qualified bonds this year with accrued interest of $10,000. Only 90% of the proceeds of the bonds (i.e., interest and principal) were spent on qualifying education expenses. They could exclude $6,000 of the interest, computed as follows:

Excludable interest (90% × $10,000)	$ 9,000
Exclusion phase-out (1/3 × $9,000)	− 3,000
Amount of interest excluded.	$ 6,000

Note that the exclusion would not be available to the couple if their A.G.I. in the year they redeemed the bonds exceeded the phase-out range (e.g., $134,900 for 2009).

Without any special provision, taxpayers with high incomes might try to circumvent the income limitation to obtain the exclusion. For example, a father earning an income of $150,000 might give $10,000 to his 10-year-old daughter who would then be instructed to buy the bonds. When the daughter started college, she would redeem the bonds to pay for her tuition. Absent any restrictions, the daughter could secure 100 percent of the available exclusion since she would have little or no income. To prevent such schemes, the exclusion is available only for bonds that are *issued* to individuals who are at least 24 years old. In addition, the exclusion is available only to the original purchaser of the bond or his or her spouse. This rule prohibits gifts of qualified bonds.

Example 8. Mr. and Mrs. C have an A.G.I. of $150,000. Assume they currently hold qualified Series EE bonds with $10,000 of accrued interest. To avoid the income limitation, the bonds are given to Mr. C's father, GF, who has little income. This year, GF cashes the bonds in and pays for his grandson's tuition. The payment is sufficient to qualify the grandson as GF's dependent. Even though the redemption proceeds are used to pay for education expenses of the taxpayer's dependent, no exclusion is available for the interest since GF was not the original purchaser of the bond. Had GF originally purchased the bonds for his grandson, the exclusion would be allowed (assuming his grandson is his dependent).

ANNUITIES

An annuity is a type of investment contract normally between an individual and an insurance company. In its simplest form, the annuity contract requires the insurance company to pay a fixed amount of money to be paid to the purchaser (the annuitant) beginning at a particular date (the starting date) and continue at specific intervals for either a certain period of time or for life. Annuities are quite common in a number of situations. For example, retirees often receive their retirement benefits (i.e., their pensions) in the form of an annuity. In this case, employees and employers contribute to a retirement fund while the individual is employed. Upon retirement, the employee is usually

given the choice of receiving his or her pension in the form of a lump-sum distribution or the accumulations are used to buy an annuity. The annuity option is often selected. Annuities are also a popular investment among elderly taxpayers. These taxpayers, often fearing that they may outlive their assets, purchase an annuity that will provide a steady stream of income until they die. Indeed, the aging of the population–the graying of America–is making annuities far more popular than ever before.

When the annuity is purchased by an individual, the insurance company invests the amount received and the investment income increases the value of the account. Under the terms of the contract, the individual has the right to cancel the annuity. When this occurs, the insurance company pays the individual the value of the investment normally reduced by penalties for early cancellation referred to as surrender charges. These charges can run as high as ten percent of the amount withdrawn and are an important consideration when investing in an annuity. In most cases, however, insurance companies allow withdrawals of a certain percentage of the account annually without having to pay any surrender charge. The tax treatment of these withdrawals is discussed below.

The income earned on the investment is tax-deferred. This means the income is taxable but not during the current year when it is earned. Instead, the income is taxable at some future date when the annuitant receives cash payments. Until then, the income is automatically reinvested in full, without payment of Federal income taxes, to earn tax-deferred income. Observe that the income is not taxed currently because the individiual has not received it either directly or constructively. It is not treated as constructively received since it is not available unless the taxpayer cancels the policy–a substantial restriction on its use.

The tax deferral feature of annuities make them particularly attractive for persons considering retirement. Annuity payments are commonly scheduled to begin on retirement when the recipients' marginal tax rates are lower. Because of the lower rates, these individuals usually pay less total taxes in addition to receiving the benefits from tax deferral.

Taxation of Annuities The taxation of annuities reflects the cost recovery principle. As discussed in Chapter 5, the portion that is a return of capital is nontaxable.[22] Determination of the portion that represents income and the portion that is a nontaxable return of capital generally depends on whether the amounts are received before or after the starting date for periodic payments.

Amounts Received Before Starting Date. Cash withdrawals, including loans, before the annuity starting date are normally taxable to the extent of the earnings accumulated in the account. Amounts in excess of the earnings are treated as a nontaxable return of capital until the taxpayer's cost has been completely recovered. Additional amounts are taxable.[23]

Early Withdrawals of Annuities. To discourage investors from withdrawing funds before the starting date, a 10 percent penalty is assessed on the deferred income. The penalty is waived if the taxpayer has reached age 59½ or is disabled.[24]

---

[22] § 72(b)(1).

[23] Special rules may apply depending on the type of annuity. See Pension and Annuity Income, IRS Publication 575 (Revised 2005) p. 15.

[24] See § 72(q)(2). The penalty provision does not apply to contracts issued before August 14, 1982.

Example 9. When S was 50, he purchased an annuity from an insurance company for $10,000. The annuity was to start when S became 65. At age 55, he requested and received an $8,000 distribution from the account. At the time of the distribution, the annuity had grown by $7,000 and had a total cash value of $17,000. Since the withdrawal is before the starting date and before he reached age 59 1/2 the distribution is taxable to the extent of the accumulated earnings and a 10 percent penalty is imposed. Of the $8,000 received, $7,000 ($17,000 − $10,000) is attributable to earnings and taxable and the remaining $1,000 is a nontaxable return of capital. The penalty imposed is $700 (10% × the income recognized of $7,000).

Amounts Received on or after Starting Date. The treatment of periodic payments beginning on or after the starting date differs from that for amounts received before the starting date. In these situations, the portion that is a return of capital is the product of the exclusion ratio (investment in the contract ÷ expected return) and the amount received as shown in the following formula

$$\frac{\text{Investment in the contract}}{\text{Expected return from the contract}} \times \text{Amount received currently} = \text{Excluded portion}$$

The taxable portion is the amount received currently less the portion that is a return of capital (i.e., the excluded portion). When the annuity will be received over a stipulated number of years, the expected return from the contract is the amount to be received each year (or month) multiplied by the number of years (or months) payments are to be received.

Example 10. W invests $20,000 in a single-premium deferred annuity. At the end of 15 years, W elects to receive the $20,000 principal plus interest over the next ten years. She receives $7,000 in the current year and will receive $7,000 each of the following nine years. W's nontaxable return of capital each year is $2,000 computed as follows

$$\frac{\$20,000}{\$7,000 \times 10 \text{ years} = \$70,000} \times \$7,000 = \$2,000$$

W's taxable income each year is $5,000 ($7,000 − $2,000).

Example 11. Refer to *Example 10*. If W receives only three payments in the first year totaling $1,750 ($7,000 × 3/12), the computation remains the same except the amount received currently is $1,750 (instead of $7,000). Consequently, her nontaxable return of capital in the first year is $500 [($20,000 ÷ $70,000) × $1,750] and her taxable income is $1,250 ($1,750 − $500).

Note that the solution to *Example 10* is the same if W had simply divided the $20,000 principal by the 10 years (and to *Example 11* if W adjusted the annual amount to months). This is not true, however, when the annuity payments are received over the individual's life. For these situations, the Regulations provide several tables based on contract payment terms and the annuitant's age.[25] These tables must be used by those

---

[25] Reg. § 1.72-9.

taxpayers making post-June 1986 contributions to the annuity contract. A portion of these tables is reproduced in Exhibit 6-3.

EXHIBIT 6-3
Ordinary Life Annuities—One Life—Expected Return Multiples

Age	Multiple	Age	Multiple	Age	Multiple
21	60.9	58	25.9	95	3.7
22	59.9	59	25.0	96	3.4
23	59.0	60	24.2	97	3.2
24	58.0	61	23.3	98	3.0
25	57.0	62	22.5	99	2.8
26	56.0	63	21.6	100	2.7
27	55.1	64	20.8	101	2.5
28	54.1	65	20.0	102	2.3
29	53.1	66	19.2	103	2.1
30	52.2	67	18.4	104	1.9

When the payments will be received over the life of the annuitant, the expected return from the contract is the amount to be received each year multiplied by the multiple that corresponds to the annuitant's age in the table. It also is important to note that the portion of any annuity payment to be excluded from gross income cannot *exceed* the unrecovered investment in the contract immediately before the receipt of the payment.[26] In other words, the exclusion ratio remains the same until the investment is fully recovered at which time subsequent receipts are fully taxable. In addition, if the annuitant dies before the entire investment is recovered, the amount of the *unrecovered investment* is allowed as a *deduction* on his or her final tax return.[27] The deduction is not a miscellaneous itemized deduction subject to the 2% floor but is subject to the 1% deduction cutback.

> **Example 12.** T, 65 years old, purchased a single-premium immediate life annuity on January 1, 2009 for $11,400. It will pay $100 a month for the rest of her life (i.e., annual payment of $1,200). From Exhibit 6-3, her multiple is 20.0. T's nontaxable return of capital each year is $570 computed as follows:
>
> $$\frac{\$11,400}{\$1,200 \times 20 = \$24,000} \times \$1,200 = \$570$$
>
> T's taxable income is $630 ($1,200 − $570). The $570 is considered a return of capital until T recovers her $11,400 investment. Note that if she lives 21 years, the total amount she excludes is limited to $11,400 ($570 × 20 years = $11,400). Thus, T's taxable income for year 21 is the entire $1,200 received. In contrast, if she lives just 15 years, the total amount she excludes is $8,550 ($570 × 15 years), and the unrecovered amount of $2,850 ($11,400 − $8,550) is allowed as a deduction on T's final tax return.

As noted above, employers with qualified pension or profit-sharing plans (see Chapter 18) purchase annuity contracts for their employees' retirement. The taxable income to the employee is dependent on the employee's total *after-tax* investment in the

---

[26] § 72(b)(2). For annuities beginning before July 2, 1986, the exclusion ratio remains the same for life regardless of whether the investment is recovered and no deduction is allowed for any unrecovered investment.

[27] § 72(b)(3).

annuity. After-tax funds generally exclude contributions, for example, to certain Individual Retirement Accounts (when individuals are allowed a deduction for the contribution) and to qualified employer retirement plans (since these contributions are made from amounts that are excluded from gross income in the current year). Investments that are not from after-tax funds are ignored in determining the individual's capital investment in the annuity. In some situations, employees may not have invested any after-tax funds in the employer's plan. Consequently, their basis in the annuity contract is zero and all amounts are included in gross income when received by them. In all other instances, calculations for return of capital and taxable income are identical to the procedure outlined in the above paragraphs.

Simplified Treatment for Annuities from Qualified Plans. As a general rule, the method above must be used for purchased commercial annuities and certain other annuities. However, many, if not most annuities, come from retirement plans. The method to be used for an annuity from a qualified retirement plan depends on when the annuity started. If the annuity payments started before November 19, 1996, the method above must be used. For annuities starting after November 18, 1996, a simplified method must be used.[28]

A taxpayer using the simplified method will find the computations less onerous than those previously described for computing the exclusion ratio under § 72. Under this method, the total number of monthly annuity payments expected to be received is based on the distributee's age at the annuity starting date. Consequently, the life expectancy tables (such as Exhibit 6-3) can be ignored. Instead, Exhibit 6-4 is used, and is applicable whether the annuity is single life or joint and survivor type.[29]

EXHIBIT 6-4
Monthly Payments Table

Age of Distributee	Number of Payments
55 and under	360
56–60	310
61–65	260
66–70	210
71 and over	160

The portion of each monthly annuity payment that is nontaxable is determined using the following formula:

$$\frac{\text{Investment in the contract}}{\text{Number of monthly payments}} = \text{Nontaxable return of capital}$$

Example 13. H, an employee, retired on January 1, 2009 at the age of 65. He started receiving retirement benefits in the form of a joint and 50% survivor annuity to be paid for the joint lives of H and W (his spouse), who is 60. H contributed $52,000 (after-tax contributions) to the plan and will receive a retirement benefit of $2,000 a month. Upon

---

[28] § 74(d). The simplified method cannot be used by (1) those 75 or older on the starting date whose annuity payments are guaranteed for at least 5 years and (2) annuities from a nonqualified plan such as a private annuity.

[29] A single life annuity pays a fixed amount at regular intervals for the remainder of one person's life. A joint and survivor annuity pays a fixed amount at regular intervals to one individual for life, and on his or her death, the payments continue over the life of a designated person such as a spouse or child.

H's death, W will receive a survivor retirement benefit of $1,000 each month. The nontaxable portion of each monthly annuity payment to H is calculated as follows:

$$\frac{\$52,000 \text{ investment}}{260 \text{ payments (see Exhibit 6-4)}} = \$200 \text{ nontaxable return of capital}$$

Should H die prior to receiving his entire investment of $52,000, W will likewise exclude $200 from her $1,000 monthly payment. As explained earlier, after 260 annuity payments have been made, any additional payments will be fully taxable. Should both H and W die prior to receiving 260 payments, a deduction is allowed in the amount of the unrecovered investment in the last income tax return.

529 PLANS: QUALIFIED TUITION PROGRAMS

To help families fund the increasing costs of higher education, Congress created several tax-favored savings arrangements. The most popular plans are contained in § 529 that was enacted in 1996. There are actually two types of 529 plans: (1) prepaid tuition plans and (2) savings plans. Every state has either a prepaid tuition or a savings plan and some states have both. Similar to Educational Savings Bonds, the income from these savings programs is nontaxable if used for higher education expenses.

Prepaid Tuition Plans. Under a prepaid tuition plan, an individual buys tuition credits or certificates that can be redeemed to pay tuition at a later date. These plans enable parents to freeze the cost of future tuition to the price currently charged by the institution. States typically offer a "units" plan that allows parents to buy units of tuition (e.g., a set number of credit hours or a certain percentage of the college's tuition). Some states offer "contract" plans that permit the purchase of contracts for one to five years of tuition. Individuals normally are allowed to contribute to either arrangement in a lump sum or in installments. There is no deduction allowed for such purchases.

Without special treatment, the difference between cost of the tuition credits and the value of the credits when used would represent taxable income. However, § 529 permits taxpayers to exclude this benefit.

Example 14. Shortly after H and W had their first son, S, they decided to start saving for his college education. Betting that the costs of tuition would continue to increase, they opted for a prepaid tuition plan. They purchased 15 hours of college credit from their alma mater, State University, at a cost of $200 per hour. This year S began his freshman year at State when the cost of tuition was $350 per hour. H and W used the prepaid credits to pay for the first semester's tuition. Although H and W have income of $150 ($350 − $200) per credit, it is nontaxable.

Depending on its terms, the plan may also permit prepayment of fees, books, supplies, equipment and room and board. Prepaid tuition plans can be offered only by eligible educational institutions which include colleges and universities as well as proprietary and vocational institutions (e.g., trade schools). Prepaid tuition plans are not restricted to those residing in the state where the university is located. For example, an individual living in Illinois, can invest in a prepaid tuition plan of Indiana University. If a child does not attend the school at which the plan was established, all is not lost. The contributions may be withdrawn without penalty, assuming the funds are used at another school. If not, the 10 percent penalty would apply to any earnings. In these situations, universities provide some type of return on the individual's investment (e.g., 2 percent per year). It should be mentioned that many private universities, almost 300 (2009), have joined together so that any tuition prepaid can be used at any member college (see Independent 529 Plan at *www.independent529plan.org*).

529 College Savings Plans. A 529 savings plan (or simply a 529 plan as it is commonly called) is much different than a prepaid tuition plan. A 529 plan is simply a tax favored savings account for any person that the donor wants to name as a beneficiary. Contributions are made to 529 accounts where they normally can be invested in one or more mutual funds offered by the plan. Contributions are not deductible for federal income tax purposes. However, some states allow a deduction or a credit. The amount that can be contributed is not limited by the tax law but only by the plan itself, and these amounts can be substantial. For example, in 2009 the plan for Indiana state universities, CollegeChoice, allows contributions of up to almost $300,000 for one individual. Earnings attributable to the account are nontaxable. In other words, contributions to the plan grow tax-free for as long as money stays in the plan. Distributions from the account are nontaxable to the extent they are used to pay for qualified higher education expenses. Section 529(e)(3) defines qualified expenses as those for tuition, books, supplies, computer equipment and technology, Internet access, equipment required for enrollment or attendance and certain expenses incurred for special needs beneficiaries. Expenses for room and board also qualify if the student attends at least half-time. However, the amount cannot exceed that normally charged for housing owned or operated by the university. Amounts withdrawn which are not considered qualified are subject to 10 percent penalty. In addition, taxpayers may utilize the qualified tuition deduction ($4,000 in 2009) to deduct the amount of a distribution from a qualified tuition plan that is used for qualified expenses and is not attributable to earnings (e.g., amounts contributed). Contributions must be made by the close of the taxable year

> **Example 15.** This year, F withdrew $1,000 from a qualified tuition plan to pay her undergraduate tuition at State University. F does not claim a credit for the amount spent. If the $1,000 consists of $800 of contributions to the plan and $200 of earnings, a deduction for the $800 of contributions may be claimed for A.G.I. by F. Furthermore, the $200 of earnings is excluded from F's income.

What happens if there is a downturn in the market and the plan drops in value? If this occurs–as it did in the market crash of 2008–the contributor can deduct a loss but only if the account is liquidated; that is, everything in the account must be withdrawn. If the total withdrawals are less than the amount the individual contributed (i.e., the basis for the account), a deduction is allowed for the difference. Unfortunately, the loss is deductible only as a miscellaneous itemized deduction. In addition, the funds cannot be reinvested too soon. If the distributions are rolled over to another 529 account for that or another related beneficiary within 60 days of their withdrawal, there is not a taxable transaction and no deduction would be allowed.

In a 529 plan, the named beneficiary has no rights to the funds. The donor has complete control, deciding when withdrawals are taken and for what purpose. Most plans allow the donor to reclaim the funds at any time desired, no questions asked. However, as noted above, the earnings portion of the "non-qualified" withdrawal are subject to income tax and an additional 10 percent penalty tax. Amounts contributed can be withdrawn at any time without penalty.

In situations where an account balance is not used (e.g., student did not finish, qualified expenses did not exhaust the account balance), the unused amount can be rolled over without penalty to an account for another member of the taxpayer's family.

529 Plans versus Prepaid Tuition Plans. There are a number of differences between 529 savings plans and prepaid tuition plans. Perhaps the most important is that there is no guarantee that the amount saved in a 529 savings plan will equal the amount of tuition in the future. Poor investments in the account can produce insufficient returns or even losses. A 529 savings plan does permit the participant to use the savings at a variety of institutions, but a prepaid tuition plan may be limited by the plan's institutions. However, as noted above, many prepaid tuition plans provide a guaranteed return if a child decides not to attend

the college from which the prepaid tuition credits were purchased. Many savings plans include the ability to save for other college expenses whereas prepaid tuition plans are often limited to tuition and fees.

Gift and Estate Tax Considerations. Contributions to either a prepaid tuition plan or a 529 savings plan are considered gifts and, therefore, could be subject to the gift tax if they exceed the annual exclusion of $13,000 (2009). However, for purposes of contributions to 529 plans, a taxpayer may elect to have a contribution to a plan treated as if it had been made ratably over five years. In so doing, the amount may come under the annual exclusion. For example, a contributor could give $65,000 to a plan and treat the transfer as if he or she had made gifts of $13,000 per year over the next five years. A gift tax return must be filed for amounts contributed in excess of the exclusion. If the contributor should die before the five-year period has elapsed, the balance is included in his or her estate.

> **Example 16.** In 2009 G made a $65,000 contribution to Indiana University's qualified tuition plan for the benefit of her grandson. She elected to treat the transfer as being made over a five-year period. In 2011, G died. In 2009, 2010, and the year of death, G may exclude $13,000 annually. The remaining $21,000 [$60,000 − (3 × $13,000 = $39,000)] would be included in her gross estate.

The current gift tax law also permits an unlimited exclusion for tuition paid on someone's behalf if it is paid directly to an educational institution. This latter rule is not extended to payments made to qualified prepaid tuition plans. Consequently, only the basic $13,000 (2009) exclusion applies. For example, this prohibition bars a grandmother from prepaying a grandchild's tuition for four years (e.g., over $100,000 for some schools) and quickly removing substantial amounts from her estate tax-free.

The law also clarifies the estate tax treatment of amounts accumulated in prepaid tuition plans. Such amounts are not included in an individual's taxable estate (i.e., neither the estate of the parent nor that of the student).

Interaction with HOPE and Lifetime Learning Credits. As discussed in Chapter 13, there are two credits related to education: (1) the HOPE credit available for the first four years of college, and (2) the Lifetime Learning credit for undergraduate, graduate and other educational courses. Interestingly, the statute makes it clear that taxpayers receiving qualified tuition plan distributions are also eligible to claim either the HOPE or Lifetime Learning credit for a taxable year as long as the income portion of the distributions is not used for the same expenses for which a credit is claimed.

EMPLOYEE COMPENSATION AND OTHER BENEFITS

By far the most important source of income for individual taxpayers is compensation from their employment. As seen earlier in Exhibit 6-1, preliminary statistics from 2006 indicate that salaries and wages represent more than 68 percent of all income reported on returns. While the bulk of employee compensation consists of salaries and wages, compensation includes all payments received for personal services such as commissions, bonuses, tips, vacation pay, severance pay, jury fees, and director's fees.[30] In addition, employers typically provide a variety of fringe benefits for their employees such as health and life insurance, child care, discounts on merchandise or services, parking, and contributions to retirement plans.

Although most forms of compensation are taxable, Congress has exempted certain benefits (e.g., health insurance, group-term life insurance), hoping the exclusion would

---

[30] § 61(a)(1) and Reg. § 1.61-2(a). See Chapter 18 for the treatment of stock received for services.

encourage employers to provide such benefits for their employees. It is important to emphasize that these benefits are typically exempt not only from income tax but also from social security and medicare taxes. The power of the exclusion feature is shown in the following example.

> **Example 17.** T recently began working for B Corporation, which provides each of its employees with a number of fringe benefits. Among these benefits is payment of the premium on a health insurance policy for T and his family at an annual cost of $2,000 (a nontaxable fringe benefit). However, T may elect to receive $2,000 in cash instead. Assume that T's marginal tax rate is 15% and that he would buy the health insurance in any event. The table below compares the two options:

	Salary	Premium Payment
Amount..	$2,000	$2,000
Income tax (15% × $2,000)...........................	(300)	—
FICA (7.65% × $2,000)..............................	(153)	—
After tax...	$1,547	$2,000

> Observe that T is much better off if he elects to have the employer pay for his health care. Electing the cash option would leave T with $453 less to pay for a similar insurance policy. Moreover, the employer is probably able to secure a better insurance rate than T could individually.

As the above example demonstrates, structuring a compensation package to include nontaxable fringe benefits provides a significant advantage to an employee. In effect, the employee is able to secure a particular benefit with before-tax or pre-tax rather than after-tax dollars. Employers also benefit because not only can they deduct the cost of the benefit just like cash compensation but they normally reduce their compensation cost since they are not required to pay social security, medicare, or unemployment taxes on such amounts.

Exhibit 6-5 provides a listing of the common examples of compensation grouped by whether they are ordinarily taxable or nontaxable.

Most employee fringe benefit plans must meet rigid rules to enable the employer to deduct contributions to the plans and for employees to exclude these amounts. Basically, the plans must (1) not discriminate in favor of highly compensated employees, (2) be in writing, (3) be for the exclusive benefit of the employees, (4) be legally enforceable, (5) provide employees with information concerning available plan benefits, and (6) be established with the intent that they will be maintained indefinitely. In addition, several eligibility and benefit tests provide detailed rules that must be met to ensure that employer costs are nontaxable income for employees. Additional employment benefits involving stock option, profit-sharing, and pension plans are discussed in Chapter 18.

REIMBURSEMENT OF EMPLOYEE EXPENSES

Employers often reimburse employees for their business-related expenses. Commonly reimbursed items include expenses for transportation, out-of-town travel, entertainment, and moving expenses. Such reimbursements are generally considered taxable. However, the employee usually has an offsetting expense that is deductible for A.G.I., so the effect on the tax return is usually a wash.[31] This is not always the case, however. If the employee is over-reimbursed or reimbursed for nondeductible expenses, there is a net increase in A.G.I. The

---

[31] This is only true if the reimbursement is made pursuant to an "accountable plan." See Chapter 8 for a complete discussion.

EXHIBIT 6-5

Taxable and Nontaxable Employee Compensation

Generally included in gross income	*Generally excluded from gross income*
Salaries, wages	Premiums paid on
Commissions	• Group-term life insurance (up to $50,000 coverage)
Bonuses	• Health, accident, disability or long-term care insurance
Garnished wages	Life insurance proceeds
Tips	Meals and lodging if for employer's convenience
Director's fees	Adoption assistance
Jury fees	Educational assistance plans (undergraduate and graduate)
Severance pay	Child or dependent care
Reimbursements for	Benefits otherwise deductible by the employee (i.e., working condition fringe benefits)
Business transportation and travel	Qualified employee discounts
Business entertainment	No-additional-cost services
Indirect moving expenses	De minimus benefits
Educational expenses	Parking
Employer gifts	Use of company facilities or services
Employer awards	Qualified retirement planning services
	Supper money
	Tuition reduction by educational institutions

effects of under-reimbursements and other aspects of reporting reimbursed expenses is considered in Chapter 8.

EMPLOYER GIFTS

Although § 102(a) allows taxpayers to exclude gifts from gross income, amounts transferred from an employer to an employee in the form of cash or other property are not excludable as a gift.[32] In effect, employers are prohibited from disguising compensation as a nontaxable gift. Consequently, employers interested in providing nontaxable benefits must look to other sections of the Code that offer exclusions. For example, as discussed below, an employee can exclude certain employee achievement awards (e.g., golf clubs for productivity)[33] and certain insignificant or de minimis fringe benefits such as inexpensive holiday gifts (e.g., a turkey at Thanksgiving).[34]

EMPLOYER AWARDS

It is quite common for an employer to award an employee for some type of achievement. An employee might receive a gold watch for many years of faithful service, a gift certificate for low absenteeism, or a free dinner for a great idea dropped in the suggestion box. For many years, employees argued that such awards were gifts rather than compensation and, therefore, were not taxable. Congress addressed this problem in two ways. As discussed above, the rules governing gifts were amended to make it clear that employers generally cannot make nontaxable gifts to employees. At the same time, Congress created a special rule allowing employees to exclude awards from their employer if certain conditions are met.

---

[32] § 102(c). See Lisa B. Williams 2005-1 USTC 50,163, 95 AFTR 2d 2005-764, 120 Fed. Appx. 289 (CA-10, 2005).

[33] §§ 74(c) and 274(j).

[34] § 132(e).

Employer awards to employees, other than de minimis fringe benefits (discussed later in this chapter), are generally treated as compensation with two exceptions: if they are provided (1) for length-of-service or safety achievements, or (2) under a nondiscriminatory qualified award plan. To be nontaxable, the awards must be made with tangible personal property. No exclusion is available for cash payments, gift certificates or the equivalent. The award must be given as part of a meaningful presentation and under conditions and circumstances that do not create a significant likelihood of the payment of disguised compensation. Also, no exclusion for the length-of-service award is available if it or a similar award is made within the individual's first five years of employment with the employer. To be nontaxable, safety awards cannot have been made to more than 10 percent of a company's eligible employees. All employees are considered to be eligible except those in managerial, professional, and clerical positions.[35]

Qualifying awards are deductible by the employer and nontaxable by the employee if the amount does not exceed the statutory limits. Under these limitations, the cost of property cannot exceed $400 per employee annually for length-of-service and safety achievements or $1,600 annually for all qualified plan awards, including length-of-service and safety achievements. For example, an employee achievement award (other than a qualified plan award) that costs the employer $390 and has a fair market value of $440 would be fully excluded from the employee's gross income. Excess costs are taxable income to the extent of the *greater* of (1) the nondeductible cost to the employer due to the limitations, or (2) the property's market value in excess of the limitations. This taxable income must be reported on the employee's Form W-2.

> **Example 18.** R, Inc. pays $525 ($640 market value) J for a brooch that it awards to L in recognition of her 15 years of service to the company. No other awards are given to L during the year. R's deduction is limited to $400, and L has taxable income of $240 (the greater of $525 − $400 = $125 and $640 − $400 = $240). The $240 will appear on L's Form W-2 as taxable income.

SOCIAL SECURITY BENEFITS

When most taxpayers collect social security benefits, these benefits can be excluded from gross income. This treatment can be traced to an early IRS ruling that granted the exclusion with little explanation in 1941.[36] Interestingly, the exclusion was allowed notwithstanding the fact that there was no statutory authority for it. In 1984, however, Congress apparently felt that this gracious treatment, while proper for those whose primary source of income was social security, was not appropriate for higher-income taxpayers. As a result, it created § 86 to address its concern.

Under the 1984 legislative formula, the social security benefits of most taxpayers continued to be nontaxable. However, upper-income taxpayers could have as much as 50 percent of their social security benefits taxed. Note that the effect of this provision is to tax these amounts—at least that portion representing the taxpayer's contributions—twice; first when included as gross wages and second when included as social security benefits are received. On the other hand, the portion received representing the contribution by the employer and any earnings on the amounts contributed are not taxable at all.

The treatment created in 1984 continued until 1993 when the Clinton administration, with the backing of Congress, increased the amount that could be taxed from 50 to 85 percent.[37] The thrust of the current rules is quite simple. As long as income remains below a certain threshold, social security benefits are completely nontaxable. But as income

---

[35] See §§ 74(c) and 274(j).

[36] Rev. Rul 70-217, 1970-1 C.B. 12.

[37] § 86.

increases, the amount of social security that may be taxed increases. Unfortunately, the actual calculation of the amount that must be included in gross income is unduly cumbersome. The effect of the revised provisions is to establish two income thresholds:

	Married Filing Jointly	Married Filing Separately	Unmarried Taxpayers
Modified A.G.I. threshold #1	$32,000	$0	$25,000
Modified A.G.I. threshold #2	44,000	0	34,000

Notice that in determining whether a taxpayer's level of income warrants taxation of his or her social security benefits, an expanded notion of income referred to as *modified adjusted gross income* is used. Modified adjusted gross income is generally computed as follows:

	Adjusted gross income
+	ø of social security benefits
+	Tax-exempt income
+	Foreign earned income exclusion
	Modified A.G.I.

Taxpayers whose modified A.G.I. is less than the first threshold ($32,000 for married filing jointly) are not taxed on their social security benefits. Those whose modified A.G.I. falls between the two thresholds ($32,000 − $44,000 for married filing jointly) must include the lesser of one-half of their social security benefits or one-half of the excess of their modified A.G.I. over the specified threshold. For those taxpayers whose modified A.G.I. *exceeds* the first threshold (e.g., $32,000 for married filing jointly), the calculation can be made using the following schedules:

Married filing jointly

If modified A.G.I. is

Over	But not over	Amount taxed:
$32,000	$44,000	Step 1: Lesser of **(1)** 50% of benefits, or **(2)** 50% × (Modified A.G.I. − $32,000)
$44,000		Step 2: Lesser of **(1)** Step 1 amount, not to exceed $6,000, + 85% × (Modified A.G.I. − $44,000), or **(2)** 85% of benefits

Unmarried taxpayers

If modified A.G.I. is

Over	But not over	Amount taxed:
$25,000	$34,000	**Step 1:**
		Lesser of
		(1) 50% of benefits, or
		(2) 50% × (Modified A.G.I. − $25,000)
$34,000		**Step 2:**
		Lesser of
		(1) Step 1 amount, not to exceed $4,500, + 85% × (Modified A.G.I. − $34,000), or
		(2) 85% of benefits

Example 19. George and Mildred, happily married for 45 years, received the following income:

Dividend income $50,000
Social security benefits. 16,000

In this case, the couple's modified A.G.I. is $58,000 [$50,000 + (50% × $16,000 = $8,000)]. Because the couple's $58,000 modified A.G.I. exceeds the second threshold of $44,000, the 85% rule is triggered. Their taxable social security is $13,600, computed as follows:

Step 1 amount

Lesser of		
50% × social security of $16,000	$ 8,000	
or		
50% × ($58,000 − $32,000 = $26,000)	$13,000	
Step 1 amount		$ 8,000

Step 2 amount

Lesser of		
Step 1 amount ($8,000), not to exceed $6,000, +	$ 6,000	
85% × ($58,000 − $44,000 = $14,000)	11,900	
	$17,900	
or		
85% × benefits of $16,000	$13,600	
Step 2 amount and taxable social security benefits		$13,600

Example 20. Assume the same facts as in *Example 19* above except that dividend income amounts to $30,000. Because the couple's $38,000 modified A.G.I. [$30,000 + (50% × $16,000)] falls below the second threshold ($44,000), their taxable social security is $3,000, computed as follows:

Lesser of		
50% × social security of $16,000	$8,000	
or		
50% × ($38,000 − $32,000 = $6,000)	$3,000	
Step 1 amount and taxable social security benefits		$3,000

As indicated above, the base or threshold amount is zero for married filing separately. Consequently, married taxpayers who elect to file separately automatically expose social security benefits to taxation.

Taxpayers whose social security benefits are subject to taxation should give consideration to shifting money out of municipal bonds and into other investment vehicles such as growth stocks that do not pay dividends or into Series EE U.S. savings bonds, which generally do not produce taxable income until they are redeemed.

UNEMPLOYMENT BENEFITS

In any dynamic economy, the forces at work often leave individuals without a job. For example, in the United States, weekly unemployment claims during 2008 surged, ranging from about 300,000 to 750,000. During 2008, the unemployment rate increased from its low of 4.9% in January to a high of 7.2% in December. In order to help those workers who have lost their jobs through no fault of their own, Congress created the unemployment insurance system as part of the Social Security Act in 1935. Under this system, employers, not employees, are subject to Federal and State unemployment taxes, which they are entitled to deduct as ordinary business expenses. These taxes are then used to provide benefits for the unemployed, thus allowing them a period of time that they can seek a new job without major financial distress.

Prior to 1979, unemployment benefits received were not taxable. In 1979, however, Congress reversed direction and opted to tax such benefits. Apparently it believed that the exclusion might actually reduce the incentive to work, making unemployment more, rather than less, attractive. Currently, unemployment benefits received under a government program are fully taxable.[38]

EMPLOYEE INSURANCE

Over the years, Congress has created several exclusions for employer-provided life, health, accident, and disability insurance. The continuation for these exclusions can generally be found in the Congressional desire to ensure that all individuals are adequately protected against unforeseen hardships. As a result, it is quite common for employers to provide some type of group insurance for employees. Premiums for insurance coverage may be paid by the employer only, by the employee only, or by both the employer and employee under some shared cost arrangement. Generally, employer-paid premiums for health, accident, and disability insurance are deductible business expenses and are excluded from the employee's gross income. On the other hand, life insurance premiums paid by the employer generally are included by the employee and deductible by the employer. As may be expected, however, there are exceptions.

---

[38]   § 85(a). For 2009, $2,400 of unemployment benefits are nontaxable.

Life Insurance Premiums and Proceeds. Employer-paid life insurance premiums are nontaxable by an employee but *only* for the first $50,000 of *group-term life insurance* protection.[39] Premiums paid by an employer for any other type of life insurance are fully included in each employee's gross income. In order to qualify as group insurance, the employer's plan generally must not discriminate. The employer must provide coverage for all employees with a few permitted exceptions based on their age, marital status, or factors related to employment. Examples of employment-related factors are union membership, duties performed, compensation received, and length of service.[40] Acceptable discrimination, however, is limited by the Regulations. Thus, employers may establish eligibility requirements that exclude certain types of employees, such as those who work part-time, who are under age 21, or who have not been employed at least six months. But omitting older employees or those with longer service records generally is not permitted.

When group-term insurance protection exceeds $50,000, the employee generally must include in income the premium attributable to the amount of coverage over $50,000. The actual amount to be included is set forth in the Regulations rather than actual premiums paid. The taxable amount for each $1,000 of insurance in excess of $50,000 is based on the employee's age as of the last day of his or her tax year. These amounts (which were recently lowered by the Treasury) are shown in Exhibit 6-6.[41]

EXHIBIT 6-6
Imputed Costs of Excess Group-Term Life Insurance

Employee's Age	Includible Income per $1,000	
	Monthly	Annually
Under 25	$0.05	$ 0.60
25 to 29	0.06	0.72
30 to 34	0.08	0.96
35 to 39	0.09	1.08
40 to 44	0.10	1.20
45 to 49	0.15	1.80
50 to 54	0.23	2.76
55 to 59	0.43	5.16
60 to 64	0.66	7.92
65 to 69	1.27	15.24
70 and over	2.06	24.72
Source: Reg. § 1.79-3, effective July 1, 1999.		

Example 21. BC, Inc. provides all full-time employees with group-term insurance. Records for three of the employees show the following information. All three were employed by BC for the full year.

Employee	Age	Insurance Coverage	Coverage in Excess of $50,000
D	56	$80,000	$30,000
E	38	62,000	12,000
F	35	40,000	0

D's taxable income is $154.80 ($5.16 × $30,000 ÷ $1,000). E's taxable income is $12.96 ($1.08 × $12,000 ÷ $1,000). F has no taxable income from group-term life insurance, since the coverage does not exceed $50,000.

---

[39] § 79(a)(1). The $50,000 limit is eliminated for retired employees who are disabled.

[40] Reg. §§ 1.79-0 and 1.79-1(a)(4).

[41] Reg. § 1.79-3. Beginning in 1988, the cost of group-term life insurance that an employee must include in his or her gross income must also be treated as wages for social security withholding purposes.

As explained further within, regardless of whether life insurance is provided by the employer, proceeds received by a beneficiary on the death of the insured ordinarily are excludable from gross income.[42]

Health Insurance Benefits. As a general rule, all medical insurance benefits are excluded from income regardless of who pays the premiums.[43] Any reimbursement of medical costs simply reduces the amount of medical expenses that can be itemized (as deductions from A.G.I.—discussed in Chapter 11).[44] However, in some instances the expenses are paid in one year but reimbursement is not received until a later year. Taxpayers have a choice when this occurs. One, they may anticipate the reimbursement and not deduct any of the reimbursable expenses. This decision means the reimbursement is nontaxable when received. Alternatively, these taxpayers may choose to itemize all medical costs in the year paid even though reimbursement is expected. This decision means the reimbursement is included in gross income when received to the extent a *tax benefit* was obtained for the prior year's deduction.[45] Since only the amount of medical expenditures that exceed 7.5 percent of A.G.I. provides a tax benefit (i.e., reduces an individual's taxable income), it is possible that part of the reimbursement is nontaxable.

> **Example 22.** J pays $4,000 medical expenses in 2009 and receives reimbursement of $1,100 in 2009 and $2,900 in 2010 from the insurance company. J's 2009 A.G.I. is $20,000, and her other itemized deductions exceed the standard deduction for the year. If J chooses to deduct all unreimbursed medical expenses in 2009, her itemized deduction is $2,900 ($4,000 − $1,100 reimbursed in 2009) and her *tax benefit* is $1,400 [$2,900 − (7.5% × $20,000 A.G.I. = $1,500)]. Thus, only $1,400 of the $2,900 reimbursement received in 2010 is included in gross income. Alternatively, if J decides to forgo the deduction in 2009, she has no taxable income in 2010. In this example, the important factors in J's decision are (1) her marginal tax rates for both years, and (2) the present value to her of the tax deferral for one year.

If medical coverage is financed by the employer, any reimbursement in excess of medical expenses incurred by an employee for himself or herself, a spouse, and dependents is included in gross income.[46] These excess amounts, however, are not included if the premiums were paid by the individual.

Many businesses finance their own medical benefit plans from company funds (instead of through insurance). These companies must establish plans that do not discriminate in favor of certain officers, shareholders, or highly paid employees. If the plan is discriminatory, individuals in these three categories must report taxable income equal to any medical reimbursement they received that is not available to other employees.[47] Thus, the purpose is to encourage businesses to extend medical coverage to all of their employees.

Qualified Long-Term Care Benefits. Under prior law, benefits received under long-term care insurance policies were not necessarily excluded. Current law makes it clear

---

[42] § 101(a)(1).

[43] § 106.

[44] §§ 105(b) and 213.

[45] § 111 (a).

[46] § 105(b).

[47] § 105(h).

that insurance contracts for long-term care that provide services for chronically-ill individuals and meet a number of other requirements are considered an accident and health insurance contract. As a result, taxpayers can exclude benefits received under such policies. The amount excluded from gross income for 2009 is the greater of $260 per day or the actual cost of the care.

Under § 7702B(c), qualified long-term care services generally include necessary diagnostic, preventive, therapeutic, curing, treating, mitigating and rehabilitative services, and maintenance or personal care services that are required by a chronically-ill individual and provided pursuant to a plan of care prescribed by a licensed health care practitioner. A chronically-ill individual is generally a person who is unable to perform at least two activities of daily living (e.g., eating, toileting, transferring, bathing, dressing, and continence) for a period of at least 90 days due to a loss of some type of functional capacity.

> **Example 23.** In 2009, L, 93, broke her hip and was confined to a nursing home for 30 days. The nursing home charged L $200 per day for a total of $6,000. L's long-term care insurance policy pays 90 percent of the amount charged by the home after a 10-day waiting period. In October, L received an insurance reimbursement of $3,600 [90% × (20 days × $200). L may exclude the entire $3,600 received since it is less than the maximum allowable exclusion of $260 per day. In addition, she can deduct the unreimbursed amount of $2,400 ($6,000 − $3,600) as a medical expense subject to the 7.5 percent of adjusted gross income limitation (see Chapter 11).

Employees normally can exclude from income the value of employer-provided coverage under a long-term care plan. However, there is no exclusion if the coverage is provided through a cafeteria plan. Furthermore, long-term care services cannot be reimbursed on a tax-free basis under a flexible spending account.

Accident and Disability Insurance Benefits. As a general rule, all amounts received under an *employer-financed* accident or disability plan are taxable, with few exceptions. However, when payments are for permanent loss or use of a function or member of the body or for permanent disfigurement of the employee, employee's spouse or dependent, they are nontaxable.[48] Moreover, to be excludable, the payments must be computed with reference to the *nature* of the injury, and not on the *time* the employee is absent from work (i.e., a wage substitute).

> **Example 24.** G lost two fingers while making repairs to her automobile. She received $20,000 from her employer-provided accident insurance policy. The $20,000 is nontaxable to G because the payment was solely for loss of a function or member of the body.

In contrast with employer-financed disability plans, all disability income is *nontaxable* if the taxpayer paid for the disability coverage.[49] Consequently, those employees with long-term disabilities may incur substantial tax costs if their disability income is received from employer-financed plans.

> **Example 25.** After graduation from high school, R was employed by WW Manufacturing Company. The company's employee benefits included disability insurance. R's disability insurance premiums averaged $250 annually. After 15 years with WW, R became seriously ill. The illness left him permanently disabled. After a three-month wait, required by the insurance company, R began receiving $800 monthly disability income. Whether the $800 is taxable income depends on who paid the $250 annual premium on the

---

[48] §§ 105(a) and (c).

[49] § 104(a)(3) and Reg. § 1.104-1(d).

disability policy. If WW paid the premium, the $800 monthly disability income is taxable income. If R paid the premium, the $800 is nontaxable. If R paid a portion of the premium, for example 40%, then that portion, $320 (40% × $800), is nontaxable, and the remaining $480 is attributable to the employer's contribution and is, therefore, taxable income.

EMPLOYER-PROVIDED MEALS AND LODGING

As explained in Chapter 5, early rulings and decisions exempted certain benefits given to employees when they did not serve as compensation but rather were for the "convenience of the employer." A classic example of this principle can be found in the working relationship between many apartment owners and their managers. Typically, owners require their managers to live on the premises without charge so that they are immediately available should they be needed. While this is an obvious benefit to employees, the tax law allows employees to exclude the value of the housing because in this case it is not primarily a means of compensation but serves some overriding purpose of the employer. In 1954, Congress codified this principle for meals and lodging in § 119.

Under § 119, the value of meals and lodging provided by an employer to an employee and the employee's spouse and dependents is excluded from income if

1. Provided for the *employer's convenience*;

2. Provided on the employer's *business premises*; and

3. In the case of lodging, the employee is *required* to occupy the quarters in order to perform employment duties.[50]

Generally, meals and housing furnished to employees without charge are considered to be for the employer's convenience if a substantial noncompensatory business purpose exists.[51] The regulations provide some guidance in this regard, indicating that meals are usually considered noncompensatory if there are insufficient eating facilities in the vicinity of the employer's premises (e.g., an employee working on an oil rig in the North Sea) or the employee must be available for emergency calls during the meal period (a 911 operator). The regulations also specifically provide that meals provided to wait staff, and other food service employees are noncompensatory. Beyond the examples in the regulations, there are numerous court decisions on the subject. For example, the Tax Court found that there were substantial business reasons to provide meals and lodging to the manager of a motel who is on 24-hour call.[52] But, if the employee has the option to receive other compensation instead, the value of the meals and lodging is included in income.[53]

> **Example 26.** Z is a warden at a state prison in Northern Arizona. She must be on duty from 8:00 a.m. until 5:00 p.m. Monday through Friday. Z is given the choice of residing at the prison free of charge (value of $12,000 per year), or of residing elsewhere and receiving a cash allowance of $1,000 per month in addition to her regular salary. If she elects to reside at the prison, the value to Z of the lodging furnished by the prison will be taxable because her residence at the prison is not required in order for her to perform properly the duties of her employment.

Nontaxable meals and lodging must be furnished on the employer's premises. The term *business premises* has been interpreted to be either the primary place of business (e.g., the hotel, restaurant, or construction site) or elsewhere as long as it is near the place of business

---

[50]   § 119(a)(2) and Reg. § 1.119-1(b).

[51]   Reg. §§ 1.119-1(a)(2) and (b).

[52]   *J.B. Lindeman*, 60 T.C. 609 (1973), acq.

[53]   Reg. § 1.119-1(c)(2).

and where a significant portion of the business is conducted.[54] However, employer-owned housing located two blocks from the primary place of business, a motel, was disallowed because it was not considered to be on the employer's premises.[55] This contrasts with employer-owned housing located across the street from the primary place of business, a hotel, that was held to be on the premises.[56] Apparently, taxpayer success in this second case was based on the amount of business conducted in the home rather than its location.

Over the years, there has been a great deal of controversy about application of the exclusion where the employer did not provide the meals but rather reimbursed the employee for his or her meal cost. The landmark case in the area is *Kowalski*, which dealt with a New Jersey state trooper who was given meal allowances under the condition that he eat in his assigned duty area and remain on call.[57] In denying the exclusion, the Supreme Court explained that it applied only to meals in kind and not to cash reimbursements. Despite the apparent clarity of this decision, controversy still arises over this issue.

Interestingly, the *Kowalski* court indicated in a footnote that its decision was not intended to address the treatment of so-called supper money, the term used to describe meal money given to employees who are required to work overtime. The IRS had historically allowed taxpayers to exclude such amounts.[58] This exclusion, as discussed later in this chapter, is now preserved in the Regulations as a de minimis fringe benefit. These rules specifically allow taxpayers to exclude supper money which is provided to overtime workers on an occasional basis.[59]

> **Example 27.** F Inc., a furniture retailer, has an exhibit each year at the local home show convention. Three of F's employees are asked to put in 12-hour days during the week-long convention. To help ease their burden, F provides each of the three employees $8 per day to cover the cost of their dinner. The $56 ($8 × 7 days) each employee receives is considered "supper money" and is therefore excluded as a de minimis fringe benefit.

In addition, § 119 explains that meals provided to all employees will be excludable if provided to more than one-half of all employees for the convenience of the employer. This rule is important for employers as well since it enables employers to deduct all of such costs (e.g. the cost of a company cafeteria) and avoid employment taxes that otherwise would apply.

CHILD AND DEPENDENT CARE ASSISTANCE

A touchy issue over the years has been the treatment of child care expenses. Arguably, a taxpayer should be extended some tax relief because such costs are inevitable if he or she is to be gainfully employed. Currently, the tax law underwrites the cost of child care under these circumstances in two ways. Employees who receive reimbursements for their child care expenses or whose employer provides child care in kind (e.g., a day care facility) may exclude up to $5,000 annually.[60] In addition, the law allows gainfully employed individuals a limited credit for their child care expenses (20–35% of $3,000 – $6,000 of expenses depending on the taxpayer's income and the number of children).[61] While this might

---

54   Rev. Rul. 71-411, 1971-2 C.B. 103.

55   *Comm. v. Anderson*, 67-1 USTC ¶9136, 19 AFTR2d 318, 371 F.2d 59 (CA-6, 1966), cert. denied.

56   *J.B. Lindeman*, 60 T.C. 609 (1973), acq.

57   *Kowalski v. Comm.*, 77-2 USTC ¶9748, 40 AFTR2d 6128, 434 U.S. 77 (USSC, 1977).

58   O.D. 514, 2 C.B. 90 (1920).

59   Reg. § 1.132-6.

60   § 129(a)(1).

61   § 21.

suggest that the taxpayer may be able to secure two benefits, the law effectively prohibits this by reducing any expenses that qualify for the credit by the amount of any benefits that are excluded. In order to claim either the exclusion or the credit, a laundry list of special rules must be followed. These are discussed in connection with the child care credit in Chapter 13.

> **Example 28.** J works for the U.S. Group, Inc. J routinely drops off her two young children at a day care facility provided by her employer. This year the value of the service is worth approximately $5,000. J normally may exclude the full $5,000 from income. Had J paid $5,000 for child care which her employer reimbursed, she could also exclude the $5,000. However, in such case, the amount of her qualifying expenses for purposes of the child care credit would be zero ($5,000 expense − $5,000 exclusion). Alternatively, J could report the $5,000 as income and claim a credit equal to 20–35% of the maximum allowable expenses of $6,000. See Chapter 13 for a complete discussion.

ADOPTION ASSISTANCE PROGRAMS

To encourage adoptions, Code § 137 allows an employee an exclusion in 2009 of $12,500 per child for qualified adoption expenses paid or incurred by an employer. The exclusion begins to be phased out for taxpayers with modified A.G.I. above $182,180 and is not available once modified A.G.I. reaches $222,180. The law also provides a nonrefundable adoption credit of up to $12,500 per child adopted. A detailed discussion of the adoption credit and its interaction with the exclusion is contained in the discussion of nonbusiness credits in Chapter 13. It is worth noting here that when the adoption involves a "special needs" child, the full credit may be claimed even if there were no adoption expenses incurred.

Foster Care Payments. Under § 131, taxpayers are entitled to exclude "qualified foster care payments" made if they are eligible foster care providers. The definition of qualified payments includes payments made by either a state or local governmental agency or any "qualified foster care placement agency" that is licensed or certified by a state or local government or an entity designated by a state or local government to make payments to foster care providers. This enables payments from for-profit agencies contracting with state and local governments to provide nontaxable foster care payments to foster care providers. Prior to this change, payments made by licensed, private providers to qualified foster care providers were taxable.

EDUCATIONAL ASSISTANCE PLANS

Employers often assist their employees in furthering their education by providing them with financial assistance. To encourage such initiatives, Congress enacted § 127. This provision grants an annual exclusion of up to $5,250 for employer-provided educational assistance (i.e., tuition, fees, books, supplies and equipment). The exclusion applies to reimbursements or direct payment of expenses related to both undergraduate and graduate level courses.

SECTION 132 FRINGE BENEFITS

In 1984, Congress attempted to tackle what was a growing controversy over fringe benefits. During that time, more and more employers were finding innovative ways to reward their employees with benefits that many aggressive taxpayers argued were nontaxable fringe benefits. Congress responded to these potential abuses by inserting a clause in the definition of gross income in § 61, stating that all fringe benefits were taxable. At the same time, however, § 132 was added and it not only sanctioned the exclusion for

certain benefits that historically had escaped tax, but also created guidelines for evaluating others. It should be emphasized that the amendment to include fringe benefits as income reinforces the principle that *all* benefits are taxable unless the Code specifically excludes them. Unfortunately, this concept apparently was lost on Senator Tom Daschle who was nominated to be Secretary of Health and Human Services in 2009. During his vetting, it came to light that he had failed to report the value of a car and driver provided by his employer as income in the amounts of $73,031, $89,129 and $93,096 in 2005, 2006 and 2007, respectively. In addition, he omitted more than $80,000 of income from consulting!

An overview of the nontaxable fringe benefits now provided under § 132 is given in Exhibit 6-7. These additional employee benefits include the following:

1. Working condition fringe benefits

2. No-additional-cost services

3. Qualified employee discounts

4. De minimis fringe benefits

5. On-premises athletic facilities

6. Qualified transportation fringe benefits

7. Qualified moving expense reimbursement

8. Qualified retirement planning services

Furthermore, employees of educational institutions receive special treatment under § 117 for reduction in tuition costs.

Working Condition Fringe Benefits. This exclusion provides that fringe benefits are nontaxable to the extent that employees could deduct the costs if they reimbursed their employer or otherwise paid the costs.[62] For example, if an accounting firm paid $100 for an employee's membership dues to the AICPA and $50 for a subscription to *The Wall Street Journal*, the employee could exclude the amounts since such costs could be deducted by the employee as routine business expenses had he or she paid them directly. Similarly, many businesses furnish some of their employees with company-owned automobiles. Expenses related to the business usage of the cars are deductible by employers and are excluded from income by the employees. In contrast, personal use of the cars, which includes commuting between the employees' home and work, is taxable compensation (unless it is nontaxable under the de minimis rule discussed later in this section).[63] This income is reported as other compensation, and thus not subject to withholding taxes.[64] If, however, employees reimburse their employers for all personal use of the automobiles, there is no auto-related taxable compensation. These benefits need not be provided to all employees (i.e., they may be reserved for officers, owners, and highly paid employees).

In addition to the above exclusions, the working condition fringe allows an exclusion for payments made for education by an employer if the employee could have deducted the cost as a business expense under § 162 (e.g., the education enabled the taxpayer to improve his skills used in his business and was not necessary to meet the minimum education requirement imposed by the job). This rule supplements the exclusion for employer-provided educational assistance of $5,250 but only in those cases where the educational costs would have been deductible had they been paid by employee. For example, if an

---

[62]   Such costs would have been deductible as business expenses under § 162 or as depreciation under § 167. § 132(d); Reg. § 1.132-5.

[63]   § 61(a)(1) and Reg. § 1.61-2(d)(1).

[64]   Reg. § 1.6041-2 and Ltr. Rul. 8122017. Although not subject to withholding taxes, this income is subject to social security taxes.

EXHIBIT 6-7

Nontaxable Fringe Benefits under § 132

Type of Benefit	Conditions	Examples
No additional cost service—§ 132(b)	Company incurs no substantial additional cost Service sold in normal course of business Same-line-of-business limitations Reciprocal agreements allowed Must be nondiscriminatory	Airplane tickets Hotel rooms Telephone services
Qualified employee discount—§ 132(c)	Offered for sale in normal course of business Same-line-of-business limitation Merchandise discounts limited to employer's gross profit Service discounts limited to 20% of normal price Must be nondiscriminatory Not applicable to investment property or real estate	Retail items

Working condition fringes—§ 132(d)	Nontaxable to extent employee would
	    have deducted the cost had he or she
	    paid for the property or service
		Company car
		Club memberships
		Professional dues and subscriptions
		Seminar expenses

De minimus fringes—§ 132(e)	Benefits are so small that accounting
	    for them is unreasonable or
	    administratively impractical
		Employee picnics
		Cocktail parties
		Holiday gifts
		Occasional use of:
		    Copying machine
		    Typing services
		    Meals
		    Coffee and donuts

Qualified transportation fringes—§ 132(f)	Valuation of parking: amount a person
	    would pay in an arm's-length transaction to
	    obtain parking at the same site
	
	Available only to employees—not "partners" and "independent
	    contractors"
		Up to $230 per month:
		    Transit passes and
		    Vanpooling combined
		Up to $230 per month:
		    Parking

Qualified bicycle commuting reimbursement	Reimbursements by an employer for employee expenses related to a bicycle used regularly for commuting	Up to $20 per month Bicycle tires Repairs, storage

Moving expense reimbursement—§ 132(g)	Reimbursements or payments by an employer to an employee for
	    qualified moving expenses (i.e., those that would be deductible
	    under § 217)
		Moving expenses in connection with:
		    Beginning employment
		    Changing job locations

Athletic facilities—§ 132(j)(4)	Located on employer's premises Operated by employer Substantially all use is by employees, spouses, and children	Tennis court Golf course Gym Pool

Qualified retirement planning services—§ 132(m)(1)	Any retirement planning services
	    provided to an employee/spouse by an
	    employer maintaining a "qualified"
	    employer plan (i.e., pension plans)
		Advice and information on retirement income planning
		Does not apply to:
		    Tax preparation
		    Accounting services
		    Legal or brokerage services

employee could meet the tests for deducting the expenses related to a graduate degree (e.g., an M.B.A.), financial assistance provided by an employer could be excluded.

No-Additional-Cost Services. Some employers allow employees to use company facilities or services without charge or for a minimal maintenance fee. For example, an airline may allow its employees to fly stand-by for free because it loses nothing since the seat would have otherwise not been used. In this and similar situations, § 132(b) permits the employee to exclude the benefit as long as the company incurs *no substantial additional cost* as a result of the employee's usage. However, unlike the working condition fringe benefit, the exclusion is not allowed if the benefit discriminates in favor of officers or other highly compensated employees.

There are literally thousands of benefits that could qualify as no-additional-cost services. They range from use of company meeting rooms to free tickets in the entertainment industry for seats that would otherwise be empty. Note that the exclusion is limited to services sold in the normal course of business in which the employee works. For example, the value of a hotel room is nontaxable if used by an employee (and/or a spouse or dependent children) who works in the employer's hotel business. It is taxable, however, if the employee works for another line of business of an employer with diversified interests such as hotels and auto rentals. Those employees identified with more than one line of business (e.g., an accountant) may exclude the benefits received from all of them. The exclusion is extended to benefits provided under a written reciprocal agreement by another employer that is in the same line of business.[65] Thus, the hotel employee has nontaxable income for free use of a hotel room provided by another company that has a qualified reciprocal agreement with the employer.

Qualified Employee Discounts. It is common practice for companies to allow employees to purchase inventory items at a discount. For example, a department store may allow its employees to purchase merchandise at the selling price less a stipulated discount. Such discounts seldom result in taxable income unless they discriminate in favor of highly compensated employees.[66] The exclusion, however, is not available for discounts on investment property or on residential or commercial real estate.

The rules governing nondiscrimination, the requirement that items must be offered for sale in the normal course of business and line of business, and the rules governing coverage of spouses and dependent children discussed above for nontaxable services also pertain to nontaxable discounts. In contrast with services, however, discounts under reciprocal agreements are taxable income. The merchandise discount exclusion is limited to the employer's normal profit (i.e., the discount may not exceed the employer's gross profit). In the case of employer services, the discount may not exceed 20 percent of the price charged to customers. Any discount beyond that amount is taxable income to the employee.

Example 29. V, an employee of an auto mechanic business, has her automobile repaired by the company. Accounting records show the following information for the parts and service necessary to repair V's car:

	Normal Selling Price	Firm's Cost	V's Cost
Parts	$200	$120	$112
Service	90	81	70

V's taxable income for the parts is $8 ($120 − $112) and for the service is $2 [($90 − $70 = $20) − ($90 × 20% = $18)].

---

[65] § 132(i). The line of business limitation is relaxed in certain instances if a special excise tax is paid.

[66] § 132(c).

De Minimis Fringe Benefits. Exclusion of employee benefits also extends to items of minimal value such as the occasional use of a company's photocopy machines, other equipment, or typing services; annual employee picnics, cocktail parties, or occasional lunches; and inexpensive holiday gifts such as a turkey at Thanksgiving. No dollar amount is specified in determining what qualifies as de minimis. The general guideline is that the value of these benefits is so small that accounting for them is unreasonable or administratively impractical.[67] The exclusion also covers discounts on food served in an eating facility provided by an employer *if* (1) the facility is located on or near the employer's business premises, (2) its revenue equals or exceeds its direct operating costs, and (3) the nondiscriminatory rules discussed above are met.[68] In addition, as noted earlier, supper money—cash meal allowances—given occasionally to employees who are required to work overtime may be excluded as a de minimis fringe benefit.

Under the 1997 Act, meals provided on the employer's premises for the convenience of the employer (and excluded from an employee's income under Code § 119) are now considered a de minimis fringe benefit under Code § 132. As a result, employers will be able to deduct the entire cost of the provided meals and they no longer will be subject to the 50 percent disallowance rule that normally applies for meals and entertainment (see Chapter 8).

Employer-Provided Transportation Benefits. Historically, employers have often reimbursed employees for their costs of commuting to and from work. When Congress finally addressed the treatment of such benefits in 1984, it grandfathered the practice of excluding such items. Thus was born the "qualified transportation fringe." The components of this exclusion and their amounts in 2009 are:

- Commuting to work in a qualified commuter vehicle (i.e., a vehicle that seats at least six people, excluding the driver such as a van) and transit passes, subway tokens, vouchers; maximum total exclusion for both when summed is $230 per month.
- Qualified parking (parking on or near the employer's premises); maximum exclusion of $230 per month.
- Qualified bicycle commuting reimbursement (e.g., reimbursements for costs relating to using a bicycle for commuting such as the cost of the bicycle, repairs, and storage); maximum exclusion is $20 per month.

Amounts received in excess of these limits are included in gross income for both income and employment tax purposes.

Example 30. For each month in 2009, Employer M provides a transit pass valued at $255 to Employee D. D does not reimburse M for any portion of the pass. Because the value of the monthly transit pass exceeds the statutory limit by $25, D is subject to both income and employment taxes on the $25 excess.

Note that if an employer offers cash in lieu of free parking, those who elect to take cash are taxed while those who opt for parking are not. Also note that in determining whether an amount can be excluded, any payments made by the employee to the employer must be considered. Payments by employees for qualified transportation fringes must also be considered in determining if the value of the benefit exceeds the statutory limit.

Example 31. Employer P provides qualified parking with a value of $250 per month to its employees, but P charges the employees $30 per month. Because the net benefit of $220 ($250 − $30) is less than the exclusion amount of $230 per month, no amount is includible in the employee's gross income.[69]

---

[67] § 132(e).

[68] § 132(e)(2).

[69] Notice 94-3. p. 15.

Qualified Moving Expense Reimbursement. Section 132 also excludes reimbursements received by employees for qualified moving expenses. Such expenses, as discussed in Chapter 8, are those that would be deductible such as the cost of the moving van, transportation to the new location and certain other expenses.[70]

On-Premises Athletic Facilities. Section 132 also authorizes an exclusion for the value of the use of athletic facilities provided on the employer's premises primarily for current or retired employees, their spouses, and their dependent children. Facilities that qualify for the exclusion include gyms, golf courses, swimming pools, tennis courts, and running and bicycle paths. Resorts are not qualifying facilities. Although the athletic facility must be located on premises owned or leased by the employer, it need not be located on the employer's business premises. Because the nondiscrimination rules are not applicable to on-premises athletic facilities, they may be made available to executives only.[71]

Employer-Provided Retirement Advice. In order to help employees adequately prepare for retirement, § 132 provides that "qualified retirement planning services" are an excludable fringe benefit.[72] The exclusion is granted for retirement planning services provided to an employee and his or her spouse by an employer that maintains a qualified pension plan. For example, General Motors might pay a financial planning firm to meet with their employees regarding retirement planning. The exclusion is not intended to apply to services that may be related to tax preparation, accounting, legal, or brokerage services. In an earlier ruling, the IRS concluded that financial counseling services provided to family members of terminally ill employees and survivors of deceased employees were taxable income.[73] Presumably, the value of such services would not be taxable under current fringe benefit rules.

Qualified Tuition Reduction by Educational Institutions. A common and extremely valuable fringe benefit offered by educational institutions to their employees is a tuition reduction or tuition waiver. For example, a child of a university faculty member might pay only a portion of the tuition normally charged to other students. Since 1984, § 117(d) has blessed these arrangements and granted an exclusion for a "qualified tuition reduction." Such reductions qualify only if they are offered by a nonprofit educational institution and do not discriminate in favor of highly compensated employees. Therefore, most plans offer benefits not only to faculty but also to all other employees of the institution (e.g., advisors, librarians, secretaries, maintenance personnel). This exclusion is available to the employee, a spouse, and dependent children and is extended to these individuals even if the employee is retired, disabled, or deceased.[74]

As a general rule, the exclusion applies only to tuition waivers for undergraduate education. However, the exclusion also is extended to tuition waivers for graduate students if they are engaged in teaching or research (e.g., teaching or research assistants).[75]

It should be emphasized that the regulations indicate that only the benefit in excess of the portion representing reasonable compensation for the graduate student's services can be excluded. Moreover, the amount received for services cannot be excluded solely because all candidates for the degree are required to perform such services.

---

[70]   § 132(g).

[71]   § 132(j)(4) and Reg. § 1.132-1T(e)(5).

[72]   § 132(a)(7).

[73]   Letter Ruling 199929043.

[74]   § 117(d)(1).

[75]   § 117(d) is subject to the compensation limitation in 117(c).

Example 32. F is a doctoral student at State University. As part of her doctoral program she is required to teach one of the basic accounting courses each semester. For her efforts, she receives free tuition worth $17,000. Assuming other adjunct professors receive $3,000 for providing like services, F may only exclude $14,000. She must report $3,000 because it represents compensation for services.

MILITARY PERSONNEL

Military personnel are employees subject to most of the same provisions as nonmilitary employees. As a result, all compensation is normally taxable. However, the character and tax treatment of some military benefits differ from those of nonmilitary employee benefits. Examples of taxable compensation are active duty and reservist pay, reenlistment bonuses, lump-sum severance and readjustment pay, and retirement pay. Examples of nontaxable benefits are allowances for subsistence, uniforms, and quarters; extra allowances for housing and living costs while on permanent duty outside the United States, and family separation allowances caused by overseas duty; moving and storage expenses; compensation received by *enlisted* service members (up to the highest monthly enlisted pay plus any hostile fire or imminent danger pay received for commissioned officers) for active duty in an area designated by the President as a combat zone (e.g., Iraq); and all pay while a prisoner of war or missing in action.[76] Benefits provided to military veterans by the Veterans Administration also are nontaxable. Examples of these are allowances for education, training, and subsistence; disability income; pensions paid to veterans or family members; and grants for specially equipped vehicles and homes for disabled veterans. In addition, bonuses paid from general welfare funds by state governments to veterans are nontaxable.

Military deployed in combat zones, qualified hazardous duty areas, or certain contingency operations may deposit up to $10,000 of their pay into a special Department of Defense savings account during a single deployment. Interest accrues on the account at an annual rate of 10 percent and compounds quarterly. Although federal income earned in hazardous duty zones is tax-free, interest accrued on earnings deposited into these accounts is taxable.

REPARATIONS TO HOLOCAUST VICTIMS

Over the years, countries and businesses that benefited from forced labor or property confiscation during the Holocaust have made restitution payments to those who suffered and returned property to the rightful owners. To ensure that the victims, their heirs and estates receive the full benefit of the payments undiminished by taxes, Congress granted an exclusion for reparation payments received after January 1, 2000. In addition, confiscated property that is returned is deemed to have a basis equal to its fair market value.[77]

PERSONAL TRANSFERS BETWEEN INDIVIDUALS

While the bulk of all income is derived from the fruits of one's labor or invested capital, there are a number of items that still have significance for which special rules exist. Among these are the provisions covering the treatment of certain transfers between individuals, specifically gifts, inheritances, child support, and alimony. With the exception of alimony, each of these is nontaxable. In each case, the recipient does not include the amount in income and the payer is not entitled to a deduction.

---

[76] The TRA of 1986 consolidated existing military benefits and provided the Treasury with the authority to expand the list.

[77] § 803(a), Economic Growth and Tax Relief Reconciliation Act of 2001, P.L. 107-16

GIFTS AND INHERITANCES

Section 102 excludes the value of property received as a gift, bequest, devise, or inheritance from gross income.[78] This exclusion is normally justified on the theory that there is merely a redistribution of the donor's or decedent's after-tax income.

While gifts are nontaxable, it is not always easy to determine whether an amount received represents a gift or compensation. The problem was clearly revealed in the landmark case of *Comm. v. Duberstein*.[79] In this case, Duberstein, a businessman from Dayton, Ohio, provided the names of potential customers to Berman, an entrepreneur from New York City. The names proved to be very valuable to Berman and, to show his appreciation, he gave Duberstein a Cadillac. Although Berman's company deducted the cost of the car on its tax return as a business expense, Duberstein considered the Cadillac a gift and therefore nontaxable. The issue was ultimately reviewed by the Supreme Court, which announced its now famous distinction between gifts and compensation. According to the court, a gift is made out of a detached and disinterested generosity and not as a reward for past services or made in expectation of future services. Based on the Court's view, Berman intended the car to be remuneration for services rendered and consequently ruled that Duberstein had taxable compensation.

The exclusion for gifts does not extend to income earned on the property.[80] For example, the value of bonds inherited or received as a gift is nontaxable, but any interest income earned on the bonds by the new owner is taxable unless specifically exempted by the Code (e.g., interest on tax-exempt bonds issued by a municipality).

ALIMONY AND SEPARATE MAINTENANCE

As may be clear by now, virtually nothing is left untouched by the tax law and that includes the area of matrimonial disputes. Indeed, given the divorce rate in the United States (in 1987 about 2.4 million marriages and 1.2 million divorces), it should not be surprising that a thriving part of many tax practices relates to the tax consequences of divorce and separation. That this can be is attributable to the fact that a major element in the dissolution of many marriages is the financial arrangement of the settlement.

Typically, a divorcing couple must first split up their property and establish separate households. Under most state laws, each spouse is entitled to the property he or she brought into the marriage and an equal share of property accumulated during the marriage. In addition to the property settlement, the divorce decree may require one of the spouses to pay support for the children (i.e., child support), and in many cases make support payments— normally referred to as alimony or separate maintenance payments-to the ex-spouse. For tax purposes, the obvious questions concern the treatment of the property settlement, child support, and alimony. The general rules governing these transfers are quite straightforward:

> ▸ *Property Settlement.* The division of the property (i.e., the transfer of property from one spouse to the other in exchange for the release of that spouse's marital claim) is a nontaxable event.[81] Neither spouse has income for the property received or a deduction for the property transferred. Consistent with this approach, the basis of the property received by either spouse under the property settlement remains the same, leaving any built-in gain or loss unchanged.[82]

---

[78]   § 102(a).

[79]   60-2 USTC ¶9515, 5 AFTR2d 1626, 363 U.S. 278 (USSC, 1960).

[80]   Reg. § 1.102-1(a). Amounts paid out of an estate or trust may be taxable under certain circumstances. However, the end result should protect the exclusion for the gift or inheritance. See § 663.

[81]   § 1041(b)(2). Prior to 1985, transfers between spouses were taxable. See *U.S. v. Thomas Crawley Davis*, 62-2 USTC S ¶9509, 9 AFTR2d 1625, (USSC, 1962).

[82]   § 1041(b)(2).

▸ *Alimony.* Amounts designated as alimony (or equivalent payments) are considered a mere reallocation or sharing of the payer's income and, therefore, are taxable to the recipient and deductible by the payer.[83]

▸ *Child Support.* Amounts paid for child support, often covered in a separate agreement, are nontaxable to the recipient (regardless of how the money is used) and non-deductible to the payer.

Example 33. H and W are divorced, and W was awarded custody of their only child. Pursuant to the divorce decree, this year H transferred his various investments in stock to W worth $24,000 (basis to H of $16,000). In addition, H paid W $18,000 in alimony and $10,000 in child support. Neither H nor W is affected by the transfer of stocks. H's basis of $16,000 carries over to W so that her basis is also $16,000. Thus the built-in appreciation of $8,000 shifts to W. H is entitled to deduct all $18,000 of the alimony as a deduction for A.G.I. while W must report the $18,000 as taxable income. H is not entitled to deduct the $10,000 paid as child support, but W is allowed to exclude the $10,000 from income.

Due to the drastically different tax treatments of these transfers, characterization of a particular payment as alimony, child support, or part of the property settlement is obviously crucial in structuring a divorce settlement. As might be expected, without some rules and coordination, a paying spouse might want to call something alimony while the recipient spouse may feel that it is either child support or part of the property settlement. Moreover, the two parties, despite their failure in marriage, may be able to work out a financial arrangement that works well for both but unfairly reduces the government's rightful share. To help eliminate controversy, a number of special rules must be observed when dealing in this area. In this regard, these rules normally do not apply to divorces occurring before 1985.[84]

Alimony. Prior to 1942, there was no specific statute governing the treatment of alimony or child support. As early as 1917, however, the Supreme Court ruled that alimony did not fall within the definition of income and, consequently, the recipient avoided tax. From the payer's perspective, the payments were not deductible since there was no provision that authorized the deduction. In some cases, this treatment could produce an inequitable result. For example, consider a taxpayer who earns $150,000 and is required to pay alimony of $100,000 to his ex-wife. Assuming the taxpayer pays taxes at a rate of 50 percent, he would have only $75,000 after-tax to meet his $100,000 alimony obligation! Because alimony seriously reduced the taxpayer's ability to pay, Congress believed it was more appropriate to view the payments of alimony as simply a splitting of the payer's income. Consequently, the law was changed to make payments of alimony deductible by the payer and taxable to the recipient.

Under current law, payments qualify as alimony or separate maintenance only if[85]

1. They are made in *cash*;

2. They are made as a result of a divorce or separation under a *written decree* of separate maintenance or support;

3. They are *required* under a decree or a written instrument incident to a divorce or separation;

---

[83] § 215(a) and 71(a)(1).

[84] These rules apply to a pre-1985 divorce decree *only if* both parties expressly agree. Ltr. Rul. 8634040.

[85] § 71(a) and (b) and Reg. § 1.71-1.

4. The spouses or court do *not* elect that they be designated as not qualifying as alimony;

5. The husband and wife do not live together nor do they file a joint return together; and

6. Payments cease with the death of the *recipient*.

Payments meeting these requirements, however, are not treated as alimony if the divorce or separation agreement clearly states they are not alimony for Federal income tax purposes. Note that this provision gives the parties a great deal of flexibility in structuring the divorce.

As noted above, payments only qualify as alimony if they are in cash. However, the payments need not be made directly to the ex-spouse.[86] Specifically, the following types of payments qualify as alimony:

1. Payments made in cash, checks, and money orders payable on demand.

2. Payments of cash by the ex-husband to the ex-wife's creditors in accordance with the terms of the divorce or separation instrument such as payments of the ex-wife's mortgage (i.e., on house ex-wife owns), taxes, rent, medical and dental bills, utilities, tuition, and other similar expenses.

3. Premiums paid by the ex-husband for term or whole life insurance on the ex-husband's life made pursuant to the terms of the divorce or separation instrument, provided the ex-wife is the owner of the policy.

4. Payments of cash to a third party on behalf of the ex-wife, if they are made at the written request of the ex-wife, such as a contribution to a charitable organization.

However, the following *do not* qualify as alimony or separate maintenance payments:[87]

1. Assets transferred as a part of the property settlement, such as a home, car, stocks and bonds, life insurance policies, annuity contracts, etc.

2. Any payments to maintain property owned by the ex-husband and used by the ex-wife, including mortgage payments, real estate taxes, insurance premiums, and improvements. Such payments increase the ex-husband's equity in the property.

3. Fair rental value of residence owned by ex-husband but used exclusively by ex-wife.

4. Repayment by the ex-husband of a loan previously made to him by his ex-wife as part of the general settlement.[88]

5. Transfers of services (i.e., professional or otherwise).[89]

6. Voluntary payments not required by the divorce or separation agreement.

7. Payments made prior to a divorce or separation.

---

[86] Temp. Reg. § 1.71-1T(b).

[87] Temp. Reg. § 1.71-1T(b), Questions 5 and 6.

[88] Reg. § 1.71-1(b)(4).

[89] Temp. Reg. § 1.71-1T(b), Question 5.

Example 34. D and G are divorced. The divorce decree requires D to transfer personal assets valued at $30,000 to G, to pay G $2,400 per year until G remarries or dies, and to pay G $50,000 over a period of 12 years. During the year. D pays G the following amounts:

1. $1,000 separate maintenance, voluntarily made prior to their separation or divorce

2. $2,400 separate maintenance, made in accordance with the divorce agreement

3. $30,000 of personal assets, transferred in accordance with the divorce agreement

4. $6,000 of the $50,000 to be paid over 12 years

G's alimony is $8,400 ($2,400 + $6,000). The $1,000 separate maintenance is not alimony because it was paid voluntarily and before any divorce or separate maintenance agreement was made. The $30,000 transfer of personal assets is not alimony since it is a property settlement. Since G has taxable alimony of $8,400, D has a deduction for A.G. I. of $8,400.

Limitations on Front Loading. Absent some limitations, *both* spouses might be better off if what is really a property settlement is treated as deductible alimony. To illustrate, consider the following example.

Example 35. H and W are in the process of negotiating the terms of their divorce. It is anticipated that after the divorce, H will be in the 50% bracket while W will pay taxes at a rate of 20%. If H pays $10,000 to his wife and the amount is *not* considered alimony, the after-tax cost of the payment to the husband is $10,000 while the after-tax benefit to the wife is $10,000. On the other hand, if the payment is considered deductible alimony, H could increase the payment to W to $20,000 and it would have the same $10,000 after-tax cost as the first payment. However, in such case, W would receive $16,000 after-tax, $6,000 more even though she has to pay taxes. As a result, both H and W are inclined to characterize any payment that is made as alimony.

As the above example illustrates, depending on the tax rates of the parties, a divorcing couple may be inclined to characterize a payment as alimony regardless of its actual substance. This is particularly true for the spouse required to make the payments since the value of the alimony deductions up front is normally far greater than their value if deferred to later years.

When an arrangement like this might provide an advantage, the divorce agreement normally calls for large "alimony" payments for the first few years followed by smaller payments later. As a practical matter, however, the large payments made initially that are purportedly alimony are in all likelihood simply part of what is a disguised property settlement. To prevent this so-called front loading, Congress created special rules.[90]

The front loading rules are triggered when there is a significant drop in alimony in either the second or third year after the divorce. If such a drop occurs, the alimony is *recaptured*, that is, the payment is no longer treated as alimony. As a result, the payer must include the amount in income and the recipient who previously reported the payment as income is entitled to a deduction. Unfortunately, the actual calculation of the amount to be recaptured is quite cumbersome.

---

[90]   § 71(f).

Alimony paid in the first and second years must be recaptured in the third year if, during this three years, alimony payments decreased by more than $15,000. Amounts recaptured are included in gross income by the payor and deductible by the payee in arriving at A.G.I. To compute the recapture, the years must be considered in reverse order. Thus, the recapture formula for the second post-separation year is (1) total payments made in the second year less (2) payments made in the third year less (3) $15,000. The recapture formula for the first year is similar with one exception. In the second step, an *average* is computed of the second-year payments (less excess payments for that year, determined in the preceding computation above) plus the third-year payments.

Example 36. Alimony payments by W to H for the first three years after divorce are $25,000, $20,000, and $15,000. Since payments did not decrease by more than $15,000, no recapture is required. Both W's deductions for A.G.I. and H's taxable income are $25,000 the first year, $20,000 the second year, and $15,000 the third year.

Example 37. Alimony payments by M to F for the first three years after divorce are $50,000, $20,000, and $0. Since payments decrease by more than $15,000, recapture is required in the third year. As computed below, the recapture for the second year is $5,000 and for the third year is $27,500.

Drop from year 2 to year 3:

Total payments made in second year	$20,000
−Payments made in third year	0
Drop from year 2 to year 3	$20,000
−$15,000 allowance	(15,000)
Year 3 recapture amount	$ 5,000

Drop from year 1 to year 2:

Total payments made in first year	$50,000
−(Year 2 + year 3 payments − year 3 recapture)/2	(7,500)*
Drop from year 1 to year 2	$42,500
−$15,000 allowance	(15,000)
Recapture amount	$27,500

* ($20,000 + $0 − $5,000 = $15.000)/2 = $7,500

M's deduction for A.G.I. and F's taxable income are $50,000 the first year and $20,000 the second year. In the third year, the recaptures exceed payments: thus, M's taxable income and F's deduction for A.G.I. is $32,500 ($5,000 + $27,500).

The recapture rules do not apply for post-1984 divorce instruments if payments

1. Cease because of the death of either spouse during the three-year period;

2. Cease because the payee remarries during the three-year period;

3. Are made under a support agreement, and thus do not qualify as alimony; or

4. Are a fixed portion of income to be paid for at least three years and based on revenues from a business, from property, or from employee or self-employment compensation.

Child Support. If there are children, it is reasonable to assume that a portion of the husband's payments will be for their care and support. Amounts that qualify as child

support are nondeductible personal expenses for the husband and nontaxable income to the wife.[91] Funds qualify as child support *only* if

1. A specific amount is fixed or is contingent on the child's status (e.g., reaching a certain age);

2. Paid solely for the support of minor children; and

3. Payable by decree, instrument, or agreement.

If all three requirements are not met, the payments are treated as alimony with no part considered to be child support.[92] All other factors are irrelevant to the issue. For example, the intent of the parties involved, the actual use of the funds, and state or local support laws have no bearing on whether payments qualify as child support. Also, even though state law may be to the contrary, a minor child is anyone under age 21.[93]

Example 38. A divorce decree states that B is to pay $300 per month as alimony and support of two minor children. The agreement also states that the payments will decrease by one-third (1) if the former spouse dies or remarries, and (2) as each child reaches 21 years of age. This type of agreement meets the contingency rule for child support. Consequently, $100 per month qualifies as alimony and $200 per month qualifies as child support.

Once child support is established, no payments are considered to be alimony until all past and current child support payments are made.[94]

Example 39. A divorce decree states that H is to pay $100 per month as alimony and $200 per month as support of two minor children. The first payment was due October 1. H paid $150 in October, $300 in November, and $350 in December. These payments are allocated between child support and alimony as follows:

	Payment	Child Support	Alimony
October	$150	$150	$ 0
November	300	250	50
December	350	200	150
Total	$800	$600	$200

The above allocation is made even if H or state law stipulates that payments are to cover alimony first.

TRANSFERS BY UNRELATED PARTIES

The last section clearly revealed that the income concept can be quite broad and could, without special rules, encompass benefits normally derived from personal relationships. This section discusses a hodgepodge of provisions that are loosely associated in that the benefits are received from unrelated or third parties. These include

[91] Reg. § 1.71-1(e).

[92] See § 71(c)(2) and Temp. Reg. § 1.71-1T, Questions 16 and 17. Also, see *Arnold A. Abramo*, 78 T.C. 154 (1983) acq. and *Comm. v. Lester*, 61-1 USTC ¶9463, 7 AFTR2d 1445,366 U.S. 299 (USSC, 1961).

[93] *W.E. Borbonus*, 42 T.C. 983 (1964).

[94] Reg. § 1.71-1(e).

life insurance, prizes and awards, scholarships, cancellation of debts, and government transfer payments.

LIFE INSURANCE PROCEEDS AND OTHER DEATH BENEFITS

Life Insurance. Since its inception the tax law has contained an exclusion for life insurance proceeds received by a beneficiary after an insured person's death.[95] Congress apparently wanted to encourage individuals to buy life insurance to provide adequate resources for their survivors and, at the same time, provide tax-free funds in a time of need.

Many life insurance policies allow the beneficiary to take the life insurance proceeds in either a lump-sum payment or installments. The exclusion applies in either situation. However, the beneficiary is entitled to exclude only the face amount of the policy. Any excess (e.g., investment earnings while the proceeds were left with the insurance company) are taxable.

Example 40. This year W's husband, H, died. Under the terms of a life insurance policy, W is to receive $500,000. Alternatively, W can elect to receive $55,000 per year for the next 10 years. If W takes the lump sum payment, she can exclude the entire $500,000. If she elects to take the installment payout of $55,000 annually, $50,000 of each payment is a nontaxable return of the life insurance proceeds, but the remaining $5,000 is taxable income [$55,000 − ($500,000/10)].

Although life insurance proceeds are normally nontaxable, there are several special rules that should be observed.

Cashing-In the Policy Before Death. Some life insurance policies, notably whole-life, enable the holder to cash the policy in before the taxpayer's death. Any amount received in excess of the premiums paid is taxable. No loss is recognized if the premiums paid exceed the amount received. The 1996 tax legislation provides, however, tax-favored treatment for accelerated death benefits.

Over the past several years, many terminally-ill individuals (e.g., AIDS patients) have surrendered their life insurance policies or sold the policies to a third party in exchange for the death benefits. These death benefits would then be used to pay for medical and other expenses. Although life insurance benefits that are payable on account of death are normally nontaxable, the treatment of accelerated death benefits, often referred to as "viatical settlements," was somewhat unclear. Congress clarified their treatment by adding Code § 101(g). This section provides that accelerated death benefits (i.e., surrender of the policy to the insurer for a lump sum or sale to a third party) generally may be excluded if the individual is chronically or terminally ill. While the exclusion for terminally ill individuals is unlimited, the exclusion for a chronically ill individual (who is not also terminally ill) is restricted to the amount of long-term care services actually incurred.

An individual is considered terminally ill if he or she has been certified by a physician as having an illness or physical condition that can reasonably be expected to result in death in 24 months or less. A chronically-ill individual is generally a person who is unable to perform at least two activities of daily living (e.g., eating, toileting, transferring, bathing, dressing, and continence) for a period of at least 90 days due to a loss of functional capacity.

---

[95] § 101(a)(1). Insurance proceeds are also taxable if the policy is an investment contract with little or no *insurance risk* or the owner of the policy does not have an *insurable interest* in the insured. In addition to the insured, a spouse, dependents, business partners, and in some instances, creditors and employers are considered to possess the requisite insurable interest.

Example 41. C is 60 years old and has smoked two packs of cigarettes a day since he was a young man. Three years ago, C was diagnosed with lung cancer. His condition recently took a turn for the worse and his physician now expects that C will live less than a year. C owns a life insurance policy with a face value of $150,000. In order to pay for his medical expenses and home nursing care, C has elected to surrender the policy to his insurance provider for a lump sum of $130,000. Because C is expected to die in 24 months or less, the accelerated death benefit of $130,000 is excluded from his gross income.

Substitute for Taxable Income. In some instances, life insurance is used to protect a creditor against a bad debt loss on the death of the insured. However, the fact that the debt is offset by life insurance proceeds on the death of the insured does not cause otherwise taxable income to be nontaxable. For example, amounts equal to unreported interest due on the debt are taxable interest income.[96] Similarly, proceeds offsetting debt that was previously written off as uncollectible, or proceeds representing gain not previously reported, are included in gross income.[97]

Transfer for Valuable Consideration. If a policy is transferred to another party in exchange for valuable consideration, any *gain* from the proceeds on the insured's death is taxable income.[98] Gain is defined as the insurance proceeds less the owner's basis. Basis is the total purchase price plus all premiums paid by the subsequent owner after the transfer.

Example 42. XY Corporation purchased a $15,000 life insurance policy from S, the insured, for $7,300. The corporation made five annual premium payments of $600 each on the policy. S died at the end of the fifth year and XY collected $15,000 insurance. since XY's basis in the policy is $10,300 [($600 × 5 payments) + $7,300], its taxable income is $4,700 ($15,000 − $10,300).

There are four exceptions to *Example 43*. All gain is nontaxable if the purchaser is (1) a partner of the insured, (2) a partnership in which the insured is a partner, (3) a corporation in which the insured is a shareholder or officer, or (4) the insured.[99]

EMPLOYEE DEATH BENEFITS

Upon the death of an employee, it is not uncommon for employers to provide the employee's family with some type of compensation for their loss. For many years, $5,000 of such payments were deductible by the employer and excluded by the decedent's beneficiaries. In 1996, this exclusion was repealed, making such benefits fully taxable. Note also that beneficiaries cannot exclude these amounts as gifts.

PRIZES AND AWARDS

The tax law provides no escape for those fortunate enough to receive prizes and awards. Prizes and awards are fully taxable. This is true regardless of the reason for the award. While this was not always the case, since 1986 winners of the Nobel Prize are

---

[96] *Landfield Finance Co. v. Comm.*, 69-2 USTC ¶9680, 24 AFTR2d 69-5744, 418 F.2d 172 (CA-7, 1969), aff'g. 69-1 USTC ¶9175, 23 AFTR2d 69-601, 296 F. Supp. 1118 (DC, 1969).

[97] *St. Louis Refrigerating & Cold Storage Co. v. Comm.*, 47-2 USTC ¶9298, 35 AFTR 1477, 162 F.2d 394 (CA-8, 1947), aff'g. 46-2 USTC ¶9320, 34 AFTR 1574, 66 F. Supp. 62 (DC, 1946) and Rev. Rul. 70-254, 1970-1 C.B. 31.

[98] § 101(a)(2).

[99] § 101(a)(2)(B).

taxed the same as those who win the grand prize from Publisher's Clearinghouse. Similarly, winners of sweepstakes, lotteries, employer service awards, contests, door prizes, and raffles held by charitable organizations have taxable income to the extent the fair market value of the winnings exceeds the cost of entering the contests.[100]

Taxpayers who have won a prize or award may avoid taxation if they immediately transfer the prize or award to charity. Although this may seem unnecessary given that taxpayers are entitled to a charitable contribution deduction, the deduction is generally limited to 50 percent of the taxpayer's A.G.I. Consequently, if the taxpayer received a $100,000 award that he or she wanted to donate to charity, an outright contribution might not necessarily offset the income. This treatment is available only for prizes and awards that are made in recognition of religious, charitable, scientific, educational, artistic, literary, or civic achievements, but only if

1. The recipient was selected without any direct action on his or her part to enter the contest or proceeding;

2. The recipient is not required to perform substantial future services as a condition of receiving the prize or award; and

3. The prize or award is given by the payor to a governmental unit or tax-exempt organization as designated by the recipient.[101]

When these rules are met, the award has no impact on the winner's tax liability; it is neither taxable income nor a deductible charitable contribution.

> **Example 43.** After twenty years of medical research at the MNO Institute, E gained an international reputation for her computer studies of protein structures. As a result, she was recently awarded the Nobel Prize in Medicine. E gave the award, which amounted to $375,000, to the American Cancer Society. Because all of the conditions for exclusion are satisfied, the $375,000 prize is excludable from E's gross income.

SCHOLARSHIPS AND FELLOWSHIPS

Although scholarships and fellowships are considered to be prizes and awards, Congress has elected to specifically exempt them from the above provisions in order to promote and lower the cost of education. To this end, § 117 generally allows an exclusion of scholarships and fellowships for those individuals who are candidates under the following conditions:

- ▸ The individual is a candidate for a degree (either undergraduate or graduate).
- ▸ The degree granting organization is a qualified educational institution, that is, the organization has a faculty, curriculum, and an organized student body (e.g., obtaining a degree at correspondence schools would not qualify).
- ▸ The amount received is a scholarship. It must aid the individual in his or her pursuit of study or research and not represent compensation for services.
- ▸ The amounts received are used for tuition and related expenses, including fees, books, supplies, equipment, and other expenses that are required for either enrollment or attendance (but not room and board).

---

[100]   Reg. § 1.74-1(a)(2). For the determining the value of property won, see *Lawrence W. McCoy*, 38 T.C. 841 (1962), acq. and *Reginald Turner*, 13 TCM 462, T.C. Memo. 1954-38.

[101]   § 74(b).

> **Example 44.** C holds a Ph.D. in chemistry from the University of Michigan. This year the Gemini Foundation, a nonprofit research institution, awarded C a post-doctoral fellowship of $30,000 to do research for a semester at the University of Texas with a noted scientist. C must include the fellowship as taxable income since he is not a candidate for a degree.

As a practical matter, most scholarships easily meet these requirements. A few potential difficulties should be mentioned, however.

It should be emphasized that amounts received for room and board cannot be excluded; however, they are considered earned income for purposes of determining the individual's standard deduction, which should facilitate an offsetting deduction.

> **Example 45.** J, a junior majoring in engineering at Private University, was awarded a $10,000 scholarship during the current year. She used the funds to pay the following school-related expenses: tuition $6,000, technology fee $100, athletic fee $25, books $875, room and board $2,500, and notebooks, pencils, and other supplies, $100. J used the remaining $400 to purchase a set of software products (word processor, spreadsheet, data base, presentation) that several of her professors said would be useful in their courses. J must report $2,900 of taxable income, representing the room and board of $2,500, and the equipment that was not required of $400. Assuming J had no other sources of income, her standard deduction would be equal to her earned income, which in this case is the $2,900 spent on room and board and the suggested equipment. As a result, J's standard deduction would offset her $2,900 of taxable income.

In some situations, amounts that are characterized as scholarships may be considered compensation for services rendered or to be rendered. In such case, the amounts received are taxable even if a current employment relationship does not exist. For example, a scholarship that was awarded a beauty contest winner was considered taxable, since much like an employee, she participated in a televised pageant and was expected to perform promotional services in the future.[102]

Note, however, that amounts received by an employee may qualify for exclusion under an educational assistance plan or as a working condition fringe benefit, as discussed earlier in this chapter. Similarly, employees of educational institutions, including graduate students engaged in teaching or research activities, are entitled to exclude any tuition reductions. In addition, amounts paid for education that are related to the taxpayer's employment may be deductible if certain conditions are met, as described in Chapter 8.

CANCELLATION OF INDEBTEDNESS

When a taxpayer borrows money, no income must be recognized since there has been no increase in the taxpayer's net worth. On the other hand, if a lender reduces or cancels a taxpayer's debt, there is a corresponding increase in net worth. In such case, the taxpayer is normally required to include the amount of debt forgiveness in gross income.[103] However, in certain situations the taxpayer may be able to exclude this so-called cancellation of debt income. Some of these include:

- ▸ The cancellation represents a gift or bequest (e.g., a father forgives his son's debt).
- ▸ The cancellation occurs when the taxpayer is insolvent or bankrupt.
- ▸ The cancellation represents a renegotiation of the purchase price.
- ▸ The cancellation of student loans.
- ▸ The cancellation is of debt related to the taxpayer's principal residence.

---

[102]   Rev. Rul. 68-20, 1968-1 C.B. 55.

[103]   § 61(a)(12).

Bankruptcy or Insolvency. If the taxpayer is *solvent* at the time a debt is cancelled, there is normally no exclusion and income must be recognized to the extent of the debt forgiveness. On the other hand, if the taxpayer is *bankrupt* or *insolvent* (liabilities exceed the value of the assets), the IRS does not add to the taxpayer's financial woes with more taxable income but provides a reprieve under § 108.

When a debt is cancelled pursuant to a bankruptcy proceeding, there is no taxable income.[104] However, the taxpayer is required to reduce certain tax attributes that normally would produce tax savings in the future. For example, the taxpayer must reduce any net operating loss carryovers by the amount of debt forgiveness. As a result, the taxpayer would lose the benefit of deducting the NOL in the future. In this sense, the income is not truly excluded but rather deferred. However, any debt reduction that exceeds the attributes identified below is ignored entirely, and the related income forever escapes tax. The attributes that must be reduced are:

1. Net operating losses (NOLs) and any NOL carryovers

2. General business credit carryovers

3. Minimum tax credit

4. Capital losses (current and carryovers)

5. Basis of the taxpayer's property (generally depreciable realty)

6. Passive activity loss and credit carryovers

7. Foreign tax credit carryovers

While the attributes normally must be reduced in the order shown, the taxpayer may elect to reduce the basis of property first (i.e., shift number 5 to number 1). By so doing, the taxpayer gives up a deferred deduction (i.e., the depreciation related to the property) for perhaps an immediate deduction (e.g., an NOL as soon as income is produced).

If the taxpayer is not bankrupt when the debt is cancelled, but insolvent, the approach is generally the same as shown above.[105] However, to the extent the taxpayer becomes solvent, taxable income results. Thus, an insolvent taxpayer reduces the attributes identified above until solvency results and the balance is included in gross income.

> **Example 46.** XYZ Inc. has assets of $375,000, liabilities of $500,000, and an NOL carryover of $100,000. If creditors forgive $90,000 of debt, none of the forgiveness will generate taxable income because, as shown below, XYZ is insolvent both before and after the debt cancellation. XYZ would be required to reduce the NOL carryover by $90,000 (from $100,000 to $10,000).

	Before	After
Total assets	$ 375,000	$ 375,000
Total liabilities	(500,000)	(410,000)
Insolvent	$(125,000)	$ (35,000)

> If, on the other hand, the creditors forgive $140,000 of debt, XYZ will be solvent after the cancellation (i.e., $375,000 − $360,000 = $15,000). Consequently, the firm would report $15,000 of the forgiveness as taxable income in such case. In addition, XYZ would reduce the NOL carryover by $100,000 to zero.

---

[104] § 108(a)(1)(A).

[105] § 108(a)(1)(B).

Qualified Real Property Business Indebtedness. As explained above, if a business's debt is cancelled, the taxpayer normally must recognize income unless the business is bankrupt or insolvent. To provide relief to those engaged in the real estate business (other than corporations), Congress created a special exception. Under § 108, a taxpayer may elect to exclude the income resulting from the cancellation of indebtedness incurred or assumed in connection with real property used in a trade or business (*qualified real property business indebtedness*). This is true even though the taxpayer is neither bankrupt nor insolvent. The cancellation of debt income does not escape tax, however. The taxpayer must reduce the basis of the depreciable property for any income that is excluded. As a result, the taxpayer forgoes future deductions. The maximum amount of exclusion may not exceed the excess of the outstanding principal amount of the debt over the fair market value of the property.

Example 47. During 2001 T acquired an office building in Houston for $800,000. He borrowed $700,000 of the purchase price by giving First Bank of Houston a note payable with interest at a rate of 14%. The note was secured by the building. By 2009 the value of the building had dropped to $400,000. At that time, the balance on the note was $600,000. Instead of foreclosing and taking the property, the bank agreed it would be better to leave the real estate in the hands of T and renegotiate the terms of the note so that T could handle the payments. As a result, the bank reduced the principal of the note from $600,000 to $400,000. T may elect to exclude the cancellation of debt income of $200,000, but he must reduce the basis of the property by $200,000.

Seller Reduction of Purchaser's Debt. Another situation where § 108 allows the taxpayer to exclude cancellation of debt income relates to sales where the seller provides the financing for the buyer. If the seller/lender cancels the debt, the buyer may exclude the benefit but must reduce the basis of the property.[106] In effect, the Code treats the transaction as a renegotiation of the purchase price. Note that the result is identical to that discussed above for qualified real property business indebtedness. This rule does not apply if the buyer is bankrupt or insolvent.

Example 48. Several years ago, B purchased an apartment building from S for $1,000,000. B gave S $200,000 cash and signed a note payable to S for the $800,000 balance. The note was secured by the building. B has recently fallen on hard times and may default on the note, which has a current balance of $700,000. S, not wanting to become a landlord again and not sure that he could find another buyer, reduced the note's principal to $400,000. Since S provided the financing and B is solvent, B may exclude the $300,000 cancellation of debt income but must reduce his basis in the building by $300,000.

Cancellation of Debt on a Principal Residence. Until recently, the cancellation of debt related to a taxpayer's personal residence resulted in taxable income unless the taxpayer was bankrupt or insolvent. However, the rise in foreclosures led to a change in the law. Beginning in 2007, income realized as a result of modification of the terms of a mortgage (e.g., a restructuring) or a foreclosure on a principal residence can be excluded. The taxpayer's basis in the residence must be reduced by the amount of the exclusion. Note that the taxpayer need not be bankrupt or insolvent to take advantage of this rule. The new provision generally applies to debt of up to $2,000,000 ($1,000,000 for married

---

[106] § 108(e)(5)(A).

filing separately) used to acquire, construct or improve the taxpayer's principal residence. When the debt was the result of a refinancing, the amount of the exclusion is limited to the amount of debt that was refinanced. The rule does not apply to home equity loans or debt forgiven related to a second home, a credit card loan, a car loan or any other type of loan. The new rule applies to qualified debt forgiven in 2007 and before January 1, 2013. The exclusion is claimed on Form 982.

> **Example 49.** Several years ago, R purchased a residence for $115,000, paying $10,000 and financing the balance. R lost his job and was no longer able to make payments on the mortgage that at the time had a balance of $100,000. After discussions with the holder of the mortgage, the debt was reduced to $80,000. Although R is neither bankrupt nor insolvent, he can exclude the $20,000 cancellation of debt income. Had the lender foreclosed on the home and sold it for $80,000 in complete satisfaction of the $100,000 debt, the $20,000 of forgiveness also can be excluded.

Cancellation of Student Loans. Code § 108(f) allows individuals to exclude from income the amount of certain student loans that have been cancelled. This exclusion normally applies only if the loan is issued by the government and the forgiveness is contingent on the student's fulfilling a public service work requirement.

GOVERNMENT TRANSFER PAYMENTS

Many government transfer payments are excluded from income. For example, earlier discussion in this chapter revealed that all or a portion of Social Security benefits are excluded from income. Since medicare benefits are considered to be Social Security, they also are nontaxable. Supplementary medicare payments received as reimbursement of medical expenses deducted in a prior year are taxable, however, to the extent the taxpayer received a *tax benefit* in that year.[107]

Worker's compensation received as a result of a work-related injury is excluded from income.[108] Similar to the typical accident insurance policy discussed earlier in this chapter, worker's compensation provides the injured employee with a fixed amount for the permanent loss or use of a function or member of the body. For example, an individual who loses a hand, fingers, or hearing in a work-related accident receives a nontaxable amount, according to a schedule of payments. This exclusion is extended to compensation received by the survivors of a deceased worker. Other worker's compensation benefits are taxable unless the requirements for accident or health plans, previously discussed, are met.

Both state and Federal government transfer payments that are classified as public assistance (e.g., food stamps) or paid from a general welfare fund (e.g., welfare payments) are nontaxable.[109] Among others, these include payments to foster and adoptive parents, to individuals who are blind, to victims of crimes, for disaster relief, (e. g., hurricane or flood relief) to reduce energy costs for low-income groups, and for urban renewal relocation payments.[110]

Benefits to participants in government programs designated to train or retrain specified groups are frequently nontaxable. Whether these benefits are nontaxable or not is

---

[107] Rev. Rul. 70-341, 1970-2 C.B. 31.

[108] § 104(a)(1).

[109] Rev. Rul. 71-425 1971-2 C.B. 76.

[110] See generally § 139. Rev. Ruls. 78-80, 1978-1 C.B. 22; 74-153, 1974-1 C.B. 20; 77-323, 1977-2 C.B. 18; 74-74, 1974-1 C.B. 18; 76-144, 1976-1 C.B. 17; 78-180, 1978-1 C.B. 136; and 76-373, 1976-2 C.B. 16.

dependent upon the primary purpose of the programs. Thus, if the objective of the program is to provide unemployed or under-employed individuals with job skills that enhance their employment opportunities, amounts received are nontaxable.[111] But, if the primary purpose is to provide compensation for services, participants are government employees with taxable wages.[112]

Most government transfer payments to farmers are included in income.[113] For example, gross income from farming includes government funds received for trees, shrubs, seed, and certain conservation expenditures, and for reducing farm production.[114] If materials are received instead of cash, their fair market value is taxable income. In addition, taxpayers receiving government funds under qualifying conservation cost-sharing plans may elect to exclude the reimbursement of capital improvements. However, the capitalized cost of the projects must be reduced by the excluded amount.[115]

BUSINESS GROSS INCOME

The amount to be included in gross income for proprietorships, partnerships, and corporations is total revenues plus net sales less cost of goods sold. This same concept is applicable even if the business conducted is illegal or if the activities do not qualify as a trade or business but constitute a hobby. Many of the other includible and excludable business gross income items are discussed earlier in this chapter. Additional income items peculiar to business that deserve discussion are classified as (A) generally includible in, or (B) generally excludable from, gross income.

   A.   *Generally Includible in Gross Income*
        Agreement not to compete
        Goodwill
        Business interruption insurance proceeds
        Damages awarded
        Lease cancellation payments

   B.   *Generally Excludable from Gross Income*
        Leasehold improvements (unless made in lieu of rent)
      Contributions to capital

AGREEMENT NOT TO COMPETE AND GOODWILL

The sale of a business often contains an agreement that the seller will not compete with the buyer in the same or similar business within a particular area or distance. In such case, the seller must treat any amount assigned to the agreement as ordinary income. The purchaser may amortize (deduct) this amount over 15 years on a straight-line basis regardless of its useful life.

When the net selling price of the business exceeds the fair market value of all identifiable net assets, the business generally is considered to possess *goodwill*. That is, its potential value exceeds its net assets because of the business name, location,

---

[111]   Rev. Ruls. 63-136, 1963-2 C.B. 19; 68-38, 1968-1 C.B. 446; 71-425, 1971-2 C.B. 76; and 72-340, 1972-2 C.B. 31.

[112]   Rev. Rul. 74-413, 1974-2 C.B. 333.

[113]   Reg. § 1.61-4(a)(4).

[114]   *R. L. Harding*, 29 TCM 789, T.C. Memo. 1970-179 and Rev. Rul. 60-32, 1960-1 C.B. 23.

[115]   See § 126 and Temp. Reg. § 16A.126-1.

reputation, or other intangible factor. Goodwill is considered a capital asset and, consequently any amounts received for goodwill are normally treated as capital gain. As provided in the Revenue Reconciliation Act of 1993, acquired goodwill can be amortized ratably over a period of 15 years. If the contract includes a single amount for both goodwill *and* a noncompetition agreement, the entire amount is treated as goodwill. In negotiating the sale, the seller should consider the tradeoffs involved in an allocation of the sales price between the covenant not to compete and goodwill. As a general rule, a seller will normally prefer to allocate more of the sales price to assets that produce capital gain, such as goodwill, than to those that produce ordinary income, such as a covenant not to compete.

Example 50. On January 1 of the current year, Ralph purchased all of the assets of Ed's Bowling Alley (a sole proprietorship) for $500,000. Included in the purchase contract is $60,000 allocable to goodwill and $45,000 to a covenant that prohibits Ed from opening another bowling alley in the next five years. Ed will report $60,000 as a long-term capital gain (taxed at no more than 15%) and the $45,000 as ordinary income. On the other hand, Ralph may amortize the amount paid for goodwill over 15 years (i.e., $60,000 ÷ 15 years = $4,000 per year), and the amount paid for the covenant not to compete over 15 years, notwithstanding it has a useful life of only five years ($45,000 ÷ 15 = $3,000 per year).

BUSINESS INTERRUPTION INSURANCE PROCEEDS

Some businesses carry insurance policies that provide for the loss of the use of property and of net profits sustained when the business property cannot be used because of an unexpected event such as fire or flood. The Regulations state that the insurance proceeds are included in gross income regardless of whether they are a reimbursement for the loss of the use of property or of net profits.[116] Similarly, insurance proceeds that are to reimburse the business for overhead expenses during the period of interruption are taxable.[117]

Example 51. Jordan Manufacturing, Inc. (JMI) was the victim of arson during the current year. The fire destroyed the main office building and the company's warehouse and its contents. JMI received a check for $1.5 million from its insurance company covering the projected lost profit for six months during which operations at JMI ceased. Since the profits which were not generated would be taxed, the payment representing the lost profit is fully included in JMI's gross income.

DAMAGES AWARDED

Cash may be awarded by the courts or by insurance companies for damages suffered by businesses because of patent infringement, cancellation of a franchise, injury to a business's reputation (see later discussion concerning professional reputation), breach of contract, antitrust action, or unfair competition. The treatment of the damages depends on whether they are compensatory (i.e., those amounts making the taxpayer whole) or punitive (i.e., those amounts that serve as a penalty). Punitive damages are fully taxable.[118] On the other hand, compensatory awards may be used *first* to offset any litigation expenses or other expenditures in obtaining the award.[119] *Second*, funds that

---

[116]   Reg. § 1.1033(a)-2(c)(8).

[117]   Rev. Rul. 55-264, 1955-1 C.B. 11.

[118]   *Comm. v. Glenshaw Glass Co.*, 55-1 USTC ¶9308, 47 AFTR 162,348 U.S. 426 (USSC, 1955).

[119]   *State Fish Corp.*, 49 T.C. 13 (1967), mod'g. 48 T.C. 465 (1967).

represent a recovery of capital when damages are awarded because of a loss in value to a business's goodwill or other assets are used to offset or write down the capitalized asset costs.[120] Remaining damages generally are considered to be a reimbursement for a loss of profits and are included in gross income.[121] An exception to the latter classification occurs when compensatory damages are awarded in an antitrust suit. While the punitive damages in these cases are taxable, the compensatory damages are taxable only to the extent that losses sustained by the business resulted in a tax benefit.[122]

> **Example 52.** Several years ago, Good Corporation contracted with Bad Corporation to build a condominium project. Good later identified defects in the construction and sued Bad. This year the court awarded Good $1,000,000; $750,000 for compensatory damages and $250,000 for punitive damages. Good incurred legal fees of $150,000. Good must treat the $250,000 punitive damages as ordinary taxable income. The compensatory damages are first reduced by the costs incurred to secure the award, $150,000. The remaining $600,000 is used to reduce the basis of the property, and any excess would be taxable.

LEASE CANCELLATION PAYMENTS

Early termination of lease agreements may result in a lease cancellation payment. Either a lessor or a lessee may receive these payments, depending on which party cancelled the lease. In *Hort*, the Supreme Court held that lease cancellation funds received by a lessor are a substitute for rent.[123] Consequently, these receipts are taxable income. Amounts received by a lessee on cancellation of a lease are considered proceeds from the sale of the lease.[124] Thus, the gain is included in gross income. Whether the gain is ordinary or capital depends on the use of the property (see discussion in Chapter 16).

> **Example 53.** Alice owns a 50-unit apartment complex in Manhattan. Nancy, who rents one of Alice's units, has decided to purchase her own house. Consequently, Nancy paid Alice $1,100 in return for cancelling her lease. Alice must treat the payment as a substitute for rental income and, therefore, must include the amount as ordinary income.

> **Example 54.** This year Alice decided to convert her 50-unit apartment complex into a medical clinic for use by physicians and dentists. She paid one of her tenants $2,000 to cancel the lease. Because the lease agreement represents a capital asset to the tenants (i.e., the lease on a residence is a personal asset), the tenant will treat the $2,000 as capital gain.

LEASEHOLD IMPROVEMENTS

A lessee often makes improvements to leased real estate. These may range from minor improvements up to the construction of a building on the leased land. If these improvements are made in lieu of rent payments, they are included in the lessor's gross income.[125] Otherwise, the lessor has no taxable income either at the time the

---

[120] *Farmers' and Merchants Bank of Cattletsburg, Ky. v. Comm.*, 3 USTC ¶972,11 AFTR 619,59 F.2d 912 (CA-6, 1932) and *Thomson v. Comm.*, 69-I USTC ¶9199,23 AFTR2d 69-529,406 F.2d 1006 (CA-9, 1969).

[121] *Durkee v. Comm.*, 1950-1 USTC ¶9283,35 AFTR 1438, 162 F.2d 184 (CA-6, 1947), *rem'g.* 6 T.C. 773 (1946).

[122] § 186 and Reg. § 1.186-1.

[123] *Hort v. Comm.*, 41-1 USTC ¶9354, 25 AFTR 1207, 313 U.S. 28 (USSC, 1941).

[124] § 1241.

[125] Reg. § 1.109-1.

improvements are made or at the time the lease is terminated, even if the improvements substantially increase the property's value.[126] The lessor's only taxable income from these improvements will occur indirectly on the sale of the property to the extent the improvements result in a higher net selling price.

> **Example 55.** For the past 10 years W had leased land to X. During the current year the lease expired and W became the owner of a three-stall garage (FMV $19,000) that X had constructed on the property seven years previously. Assuming the improvements were not made in lieu of rent, the FMV of the garage is not currently included in W's gross income.

Under § 110, a retail tenant that receives cash or rent reductions from the lessor of retail space does not include such amounts in income if the cash (or equivalent) is used for qualified construction or improvement to the space. In order to qualify for the exclusion, the tenant must have a short-term lease (i.e., a lease of retail space for 15 years or less). The amount excluded cannot exceed the amount spent by the tenant for the improvement.

From time to time, lessors will make improvements on their property in order to attract lessees. If a lessor abandons a leasehold improvement in the year the lease terminates, the lessor is allowed a deduction equal to the landlord's adjusted basis of the improvement [§ 168(i)(8)]. This rule does not apply where the improvement is demolished in which case the landlord simply increases the basis of the property (§ 280B).

CONTRIBUTIONS TO CAPITAL

Cash or other property received by a business in exchange for an ownership interest are nontaxable transactions for the business. These transfers are treated as contributions to capital and not income.[127] Contributions to capital that are not in exchange for an ownership interest also are nontaxable.

MISCELLANEOUS ITEMS

As stated in the first paragraph of this chapter, gross income includes *all* income unless specifically exempted. Although this chapter is not intended to discuss every income item, some additional items are classified for discussion purposes as miscellaneous.

FEES RECEIVED

Ordinarily, fees received for services performed are included in gross income. Thus, fees paid to corporate directors, jurors, and executors are reported as miscellaneous gross income. However, if executor fees are paid regardless of whether the taxpayer performs any services, they may qualify as nontaxable gifts.[128]

ASSET DISCOVERY

Cash or other assets found by a taxpayer are taxable income even if found accidentally, with no effort expended in discovering them.[129] For example, taxpayers were held to have taxable income equal to cash found in a used piano they had purchased.[130]

---

[126] § 109.

[127] §§ 118 and 721.

[128] Rev. Rul. 57-398, 1957-2 C.B. 93.

[129] Rev. Rul. 53-61, 1953-1 C.B. 17.

[130] *Cesarini v. Comm.*, 70-2 USTC ¶9509, 26 AFTR2d 70-5107. 428 F.2d 812 (CA-6, 1970).

CAR POOL RECEIPTS

One type of earned income is nontaxable. Vehicle owners operating car pools for fellow commuters may exclude all the revenues received.[131] Car pool expenses are *personal* commuting expenses, and therefore are not deductible. If, however, the car pool activities are sufficient to qualify a taxpayer as being in a trade or business, all revenues are taxable. How much activity constitutes a trade or business is a question of fact not easily answered, but in this type of situation, the definition of trade certainly requires considerably more activity than a single automobile or small van making one round trip daily.

INCOME TAX REFUNDS

All state and local income tax refunds are nontaxable except to the extent the taxpayer received a *tax benefit* in a prior year.[132] A corporation receives a tax benefit for all business expenses, including state and local income taxes, unless the corporation incurs a net operating loss for the year of deduction. State and local income taxes paid by individuals, however, provide a tax benefit only if the taxpayer itemized these deductions in the year paid. There is no tax benefit for the expense if the standard deduction was used instead of itemized deductions. In addition, the taxable amount of a state and local income tax refund is affected by the amount of state and local sales tax that the taxpayer could have otherwise deducted. Under current law, a taxpayer is entitled to deduct the larger of state and local income taxes or state and local sales taxes (see Chapter 11). The amount of the refund is taxable only to the extent that the state income taxes deducted exceeded the amount of state sales tax that the taxpayer could have otherwise deducted.[133]

> **Example 56.** John and Lori Hansen are married and live in Kokomo, Indiana. The couple filed a joint return for 2009. Their total itemized deductions, including state income taxes withheld by their employers of $7,000, amounted to $18,100 in 2009. The couple could have deducted state and local sales taxes of $6,000 but deducted the state and local income taxes since the $7,000 amount was larger. On June 12, 2010, the Hansens received a refund from the State of Indiana for $2,500 as a result of overpaying their 2009 Indiana income taxes. Because the Hansens received a tax benefit by deducting the state income taxes on their 2009 Federal income tax return of only $1,000 ($7,000 state income tax − $6,000 state sales tax), they must include the $1,000 refund in gross income on their 2010 Federal income tax return.

TEMPORARY LIVING COSTS

If an individual receives insurance proceeds to cover temporary living costs incurred because the principal residence was destroyed or damaged by fire, flood, or other casualty, the funds are nontaxable to the extent they are offset by *extra* living costs.[134] These funds also may be excluded if the government prevented the individual from using an undamaged residence because of the existence or threat of a casualty. Extra living costs are limited to those additional costs actually incurred for temporarily housing, feeding, and transporting the taxpayer and members of the household. Typical qualifying costs are hotel or apartment rent and utilities, extra costs for restaurant meals, and additional transportation necessitated by having to live outside the immediate area of the residence.

---

[131] Rev. Rul. 55-555, 1955-2 C.B. 20.

[132] § 111(a).

[133] See *Taxable and Nontaxable Income*, IRS Publication 525 (2006), p. 20.

[134] § 123.

DAMAGES AWARDED TO INDIVIDUALS

More and more often people are suing or being sued. Each year millions of lawsuits are filed in state and federal courts. Most of these cases have financial implications. Some of these are settled out of court while others go on. In many situations, individuals receive damages compensating them for their loss (compensatory damages) and, in some, damages are awarded to penalize or punish the wrongdoer (punitive damages). Section 104(a) provides the treatment of compensatory and punitive damages.

Compensatory Damages. For many years, Section 104(a)(2) provided that damages awarded on account of personal injuries and sickness were nontaxable. Historically, the treatment was justified on the grounds that the amounts received represent a return of human capital. According to the theory, injured parties are no better off since the damages merely restored them to their original state. However, controversies arose in applying this exclusion to certain awards such as those involving age, sex, and race discrimination. Taxpayers artfully argued that these awards were related to personal injuries, hoping to qualify for an exclusion. The seriousness of the situation could be seen in a class action suit brought by hundreds of IBM employees that had been laid off who argued for the exclusion of their severance pay on the grounds that such payments were made in part to allay future claims of discrimination.

To address these concerns, § 104 was amended in 1996 to make it clear that only damages awarded on account of physical injury and sickness are not taxable.[135] In addition, § 104 explains that *emotional distress* is not considered a physical injury or sickness unless such distress had its origins from physical injury or sickness. Emotional distress includes physical symptoms such as insomnia, headaches or stomach disorders that may result from such emotional distress. According to the Committee Reports, this rule bars an exclusion for any damages received based on a claim of employment discrimination or injury to reputation accompanied by a claim of emotional distress. Thus it appears that awards made due to employment discrimination based on age, sex, race or similar factors would be fully taxable. The fact that the individual suffered emotional distress that produced physical symptoms would not enable the taxpayer to qualify for the exclusion. However, the law does explain that damages actually used to pay for medical expenses related to emotional distress are nontaxable.

> **Example 57.** In July of 2007 K filed a sex discrimination lawsuit against Statewide University after being denied promotion to associate professor with tenure. In November of 2009 the parties entered into an out-of-court settlement pursuant to which the university awarded K $80,000 in lost wages, $5,000 for medical expenses related to emotional distress and $40,000 of punitive damages. Of the $125,000 she received, only the $5,000 payment for medical expenses would be excluded from K's gross income. Amounts allocated to lost wages and punitive damages are taxable.

Punitive Damages. Historically, punitive damages normally have been taxable. At times, however, courts have reached differing opinions about the treatment of punitive damages related to cases involving damages awarded for physical injury or sickness. One theory allowed the taxpayer to exclude punitive damages related to physical injury or sickness since the compensatory damages were nontaxable. The other theory took the view that all punitive damages were taxable. Section 104(a)(2) now makes it clear that all punitive damages are taxable even if they are related to physical injury or sickness.

---

[135] But see *Marrita Murphy* 2006-2 USTC, ¶50,476, 98 AFTR 2d 2006-6088, 460 F3d 79, (CA-DC, 2006) where the appellate court recently held that this provision was unconstitutional.

TAX PLANNING

INVESTMENTS

Tax-planning strategy must be viewed in terms of each taxpayer's own financial position. When considering investments, both the after-tax return and the risk involved must be evaluated. Before-tax income frequently is lower for tax-exempt and tax-deferred investments than it is for taxable investments with the same degree of risk. Consequently, tax-exempt investments should be most attractive to those in the higher tax bracket. They may not be beneficial to those in the lower bracket. Tax-deferred investments should be most attractive to those expecting a lower tax bracket when the deferral period ends. In addition, investors must consider whether any gains will be taxed as ordinary income or capital gains (see Chapter 16), and whether capital gains will be needed to offset capital losses.

Taxpayers have a variety of investment opportunities available to them. In order to arrive at informed investment decisions, comparative evaluations are necessary. However, such evaluations must be viewed with caution. The very nature of this type of analysis means that tentative assumptions must be made about the future. For example, when comparing a possible stock purchase with an annuity purchase, assumptions must be made about (1) future cash flows for the two investments, (2) future marginal tax rates, and (3) the discount rate to be used in determining the present value of the expected cash flows. A decision should never be based on a simple nonmathematical tax comparison of the total of annual dividends plus capital gains for the stock, as opposed to the total deferred ordinary income for the annuity. A tax adviser should always remember that while taxation is a very important factor, it is just one of several that must be considered.

On the death of an insured person, life insurance companies ordinarily allow beneficiaries to receive the proceeds in one lump sum, or in installments for a stipulated period or over the beneficiary's life. Tax concerns aside, some beneficiaries may elect to leave the proceeds with the insurance company simply because they like the security of receiving a periodic payment from an established financial institution. Each installment contains a ratable portion of the proceeds plus interest. This interest is taxable income. Thus, life insurance proceeds received in installments are treated the same as annuities.

> **Example 58.** M is the sole beneficiary of her husband's $60,000 life insurance policy. She elects to receive the proceeds in monthly installments for 10 years. Her monthly installment is $500 plus interest on the unpaid principal. In the current year, she receives $6,000 plus $3,700 interest. Her taxable interest income is $3,700.

One feature of life insurance that has enticed many investors over the years is its tax-free cash build-up. Taxpayers have taken advantage of this by borrowing against the policy—in effect receiving use of the income without having to pay tax on it. To discourage the purchase of life insurance as a tax-sheltered investment vehicle, special rules have been established. As a result, taxpayers must closely scrutinize the type of insurance they purchase with respect to its tax treatment. Under the revised rules, a taxpayer who receives amounts before age 59ø, including loans, from certain single premium and other investment-oriented life insurance contracts (modified endowment contracts) is treated as receiving income first and then a recovery of basis. In addition, the recipient is subject to an additional 10 percent income tax on the amounts received that are includible in gross income. This provision affects only "modified endowment contracts" entered into on or after June 21, 1988.

An investor who desires nontaxable income may choose to purchase assets such as:

1. Qualifying state and local government bonds to obtain the full interest income exclusion

2. Stocks in companies with net income for accounting purposes, but no earnings and profits for tax purposes, to obtain the full exclusion for distributions that are treated as a return of capital

Investors who wish to defer income may choose to:

1. Exchange Series E or EE bonds that are maturing for Series HH bonds in order to continue deferring the accrued interest on the surrendered E or EE bonds

2. Purchase annuities (or to elect that life insurance proceeds be received as annuities) to obtain the deferral of all interest income until received

3. Purchase assets that are expected to appreciate, such as stocks, real estate, and collectables, to obtain the deferral of all appreciation until it is realized

If the taxpayer does not dispose of the assets, the deferral becomes permanent. That is, no one recognizes the income and the assets are inherited at their market values, including the deferred income.

EMPLOYEE BENEFITS

Company fringe benefits can provide employees with tax consequences that range from excellent savings to actual disadvantages. From a tax viewpoint, the best fringe benefits are those that are deductible by the employer and convert otherwise taxable income to nontaxable income for the recipient. For example, most employee benefits that are provided in lieu of additional salary convert taxable compensation to nontaxable benefits.

> **Example 59.** W is a new employee of Z Corporation. Her compensation package is $20,000. However, she may choose to receive (a) $20,000 salary and no benefits, or (b) $19,000 salary and Z will pay premiums of $600 for medical insurance and $400 for group-term life insurance. If W chooses the first option, she has $20,000 taxable income, but if she selects the second option, she has $19,000 taxable income.

Another very valuable type of fringe benefit is one that is nontaxable income if provided by the employer but is a nondeductible expenditure if paid by the employee. Most fringe benefits are of this type. These include premiums paid for group-term life insurance up to $50,000, qualifying meals and lodging on the premises, supper money, company parking, use of company facilities, and employee discounts. All of these benefits are deductible costs by the employer but nontaxable income to the employee when the necessary requirements discussed in this chapter are met. If, however, the employees pay these costs instead of the employer, there is no tax deduction for them.

A third type of fringe benefit includes expenditures that are deductible expenses, when paid by individuals, but are subject to restrictions. For example, health insurance premiums are deductible for employees who itemize their deductions but *only* to the extent that all qualifying medical expenditures exceed 7.5 percent of A.G.I. (see Chapter 11). Thus, employer-paid health insurance represents different tax savings to different employees.

> **Example 60.** L's compensation includes a salary of $30,000 plus employer-paid health insurance premiums of $600. L's taxable income is $30,000 since the $600 is nontaxable. If the company policy is changed so that L pays the $600 health

insurance premiums and the company increases his salary to $30,600, the tax effect on L depends on his individual tax situation.

1. If L does not itemize medical expenses, he has taxable income of $30,600 salary and no deduction for the $600.

2. If L itemizes deductions and his medical expenditures before the health insurance premiums exceed 7.5% of A.G.I., he still has taxable income of $30,600 salary but now has a deduction of $600.

Assume L has a 25% marginal tax rate. In situation 1 above, his tax benefit from employer-paid health insurance premiums is $150 ($600 × 25%). In the second situation, L appears to receive no tax benefit when his company pays the health insurance premiums. However, his A.G.I. is $600 higher when L pays the premium. Since medical expenses equal to 7.5% of A.G.I. are not deductible, this increases the nondeductible portion by $45 ($600 × 7.5%). Thus, at the 25% tax rate, his tax increases by $11.25 ($45 × 25%).

Some employer-provided benefits can be a disadvantage to employees. Recall, for example, that disability income is taxable if the premiums were paid by the employer but nontaxable if they were paid by the individual. The best tax-planning advice when employers pay disability insurance premiums is for employees to convince employers to provide another benefit and let employees pay their own disability premiums.

Considerable leeway in tax planning is available to those employees who are allowed to select their own fringe benefits. Simply looking at the cost of each benefit to the company, however, is inadequate. Each employee should carefully evaluate personal needs and the tax effect of each desirable benefit before selection is made.

EMPLOYEE VERSUS SELF-EMPLOYED

The tax advantages of many fringe benefits are available only if an employer/employee relationship exists. For example, sole proprietors are not considered employees of their proprietorships so many fringe benefits are not available to them. Similarly, partners in partnerships and members of LLCs are not considered employees and, therefore, some benefits are not available to them. In contrast, owners of C corporations can be employees of the corporation and are entitled to fringe benefits. This situation creates an incentive to operate some businesses as corporations rather than as proprietorships or partnerships or LLCs.

One of these fringe benefits, employer-furnished meals and lodging, has been of interest to closely held businesses for years. Farming represents a particularly good example of a business that requires someone to be available on the property 24 hours a day. When the working owner lives on the farm, a business deduction plus an employee exclusion for the cost of meals and lodging provided to the farmer can be significant.

Example 61. A farm owned by M has the following information for the current year:

Gross income.	$130,000
Cost of food consumed by M	2,000
Cost of lodging used by M	4,200
Salary to M.	20,000
Other farm expenses	85,000

If the farm is a proprietorship, net farming income is $25,000 ($130,000 − $20,000 − $85,000) and M has an A.G.I. of $45,000 ($25,000 + $20,000).[136] Similar results occur if the farm is a partnership, except M will report only his share of the $25,000. In contrast, if the farm is a corporation, net income is $18,800 ($130,000 − $2,000 − $4,200 − $20,000 − $85,000) and M has an A.G.I. of $20,000. Thus, M, the proprietor, has $45,000 A.G.I. compared with a combined income of $38,800 ($18,800 + $20,000) for the M Corporation and M, the employee.

Although the above example seems to result in a tax advantage for the corporate farm, such a conclusion is over-simplified. Other tax factors are important. For example, corporate net income is taxed to the corporation currently and again as dividend income to shareholders when distributed to them (see Chapter 20). Another important factor is that individuals and corporations are subject to different tax rates. Also, if farming losses occur, the results may be very unfavorable with a corporate entity. The important point to remember is that the tax advantage achieved with the corporation for meals and lodging (and other employee benefits) is just one of the necessary ingredients when evaluating whether a business should be incorporated.

DIVORCE

Insufficient attention usually is given to tax planning during separation and divorce. Of course, favorable tax results are easier to accomplish when the individuals are parting amicably, but good results still can occur amid animosity. The more disparate the husband's and wife's tax brackets, the greater the benefits to be achieved. This is because payments classified as alimony or separate maintenance are deductible by the payor and are taxable income to the recipient. In contrast, all other asset transfers are neither deductible expenses nor taxable income.

> **Example 62.** H and W are divorced. H's marginal tax rate is 35% while W's is 15%. Every $10 of alimony costs H $6.50 after taxes [$10 paid − $3.50 tax savings ($10 × 35%)] and is worth $8.50 to W after taxes [$10 received − $1.50 tax due ($10 × 15%)]. Thus, H pays $6.50 for W to receive $8.50. If W requires $425 after taxes each month, she must receive $500 if the payments qualify as alimony [$500 − ($500 × 15% = $75)] or $425 if they do not. On the surface, it seems that H would rather pay $425 a month than $500 but $500 in alimony results in an after-tax cost of $325 [$500 − ($500 × 35% = $175)] for a monthly savings of $100 ($425 − $325). Naturally, the closer the two marginal rates, the less there is in tax savings.

PROBLEM MATERIALS

DISCUSSION QUESTIONS

6-1 *Basic Concepts.* Determine whether each of the following statements is true or false. If false, rewrite the statement so that it is true. Be prepared to explain each statement.
   a. Receipts are included in gross income only if specifically listed in the Code.
   b. Tax returns show (1) gross receipts from all sources, less (2) excludable income, which equals (3) taxable income.
   c. Interest earned on tax-exempt municipal bonds is nontaxable income regardless of whether it is received by an individual or by a corporation.

---

[136] Technically, a proprietor's salary is not a farming expense but is shown in the example for comparison purposes. Thus, net income is $45,000 ($130,000 − $85,000) and M's A.G.I. is $45,000.

6-2 *Investment—Stocks versus Bonds.* C has $10,000 to invest but is uncertain whether to purchase H, Inc. stocks or tax-exempt bonds issued by the State of Illinois. List the relevant types of information that C must obtain or estimate in order to make a mathematical calculation of her after-tax return on the two investments she is considering.

6-3 *Investments—Bonds.* D, Inc. bonds are selling for $1,000 each with an interest rate of 7 percent. Tax-exempt bonds issued by the State of Kentucky are selling for $1,000 each with an interest rate of 3 percent. Which bond provides a taxpayer with the higher after-tax return when the marginal tax rate is
   a. 35 percent?
   b. 15 percent?

6-4 *Investments—Dividend Income.* Corporate distributions may qualify as dividends, return of capital, or stock dividends. Explain the tax treatment of each of these three distributions. What determines whether a distribution is a dividend, a return of capital, or a stock dividend?

6-5 *Employee Benefits.* Z, Inc. owns and operates several businesses, including six hotels and two real estate agencies. R, an employee of Z, spends three nights free of charge in one of Z's hotels in Indiana. Is the value of the lodging nontaxable to R, assuming the information below? Explain.
   a. R works for one of the real estate agencies.
   b. R tends bar in one of the hotels in Maine.
   c. R is a tax accountant in Z's corporate headquarters where the tax records of all of Z's businesses are maintained.

6-6 *Employee Benefits—Comparison.* Compare the tax treatment for each of the items listed below assuming they are paid by (1) the employer, or (2) the employee.
   a. Parking in the company lot during working hours
   b. Health insurance premiums
   c. Disability insurance premiums
   d. Meals eaten in the company cafeteria when the employee must remain on the premises for job reasons

6-7 *Employee Benefits—Meals and Lodging.* Employer-provided meals and lodging that qualify as nontaxable income can be an exceedingly valuable employee benefit.
   a. When do employer-provided meals and lodging qualify as nontaxable income?
   b. List at least 10 types of occupations in which employer-provided lodging and/or meals could qualify for the exclusion. Explain why these occupations are appropriate for the exclusion.

6-8 *Employee Benefits.* Over the years, the list of employee benefits that qualify as deductible expenses by the employer and nontaxable income for the employee has expanded. Assume Congress is interested in further expanding the list of benefits available for this special tax treatment. Prepare a list for Congress of at least three items not discussed in this chapter that would provide many employees with valuable benefits. Explain why these three would be logical additions.

6-9 *Gifts.* How can gifts to family members reduce the family's income tax liability?

6-10 *Alimony and Child Support.* A husband and wife who are obtaining a divorce disagree whether certain periodic payments should be classified as alimony or child support.
   a. What difference does it make how the payments are classified?
   b. What if the agreement states the payments are for both alimony and child support without making a specific distinction in dollar allocation between the two?

    c. List three types of compromise offers that could be made by the husband to reach an allocation that might satisfy both the husband and wife. Explain the tax consequences of each of the three possible solutions.

6-11 *Alimony.* A husband (H) and wife (W) are obtaining a divorce. He agrees to pay alimony of $25,000 in each of the two years after the divorce to enable her to attend graduate school. No alimony will be paid after the second year.

    a. What are his deductible and her taxable amount of alimony for each of the two years, and what are the tax effects in year three?

    b. How could the payment schedule be restructured to maximize his deductions?

    c. How could the payment schedule be restructured to minimize her taxable income?

6-12 *Prizes and Awards.* Contest winners must report the value of prizes won as taxable income.

    a. What arguments could the taxpayer use to convince the IRS and the courts that the values of the prizes are less than their retail selling prices?

    b. Are any prizes or awards ever nontaxable? Explain.

6-13 *Scholarships and Fellowships.* CPA firms are interested in encouraging practical research that explores accounting issues with an objective of developing better accounting methods for the profession. Assume the XY firm decides to establish a fund that will support individual research efforts. Recipients of these grants will be selected based on the quality of their past work and on a written proposal of a specific research project to be completed with funds from the XY firm. Do recipients of these grants have taxable or nontaxable income? Explain.

6-14 *Distributions from 529 Savings Plans.* During the year, G withdrew $18,000 from a 529 plan for his daughter. He used the most of the money to pay for the following costs associated with her first year of college: tuition $10,000, fees $1,000, apartment rental $3,000, computer $1,600, books $400, appliances and furniture $505 and bedding $200. How will the $18,000 be treated?

6-15 *Goodwill versus Agreement Not to Compete.* A preliminary agreement covering the sale/purchase of a dental practice includes an allocation of $40,000 to goodwill and the agreement that the seller will not practice dentistry within a five-mile radius for five years.

    a. What are the tax consequences of this $40,000 allocation?

    b. What advice should a tax adviser give the seller?

    c. What advice should a tax adviser give the buyer?

6-16 *Damages Awarded.* As the result of a newspaper article, V claims his character was damaged beyond repair, he lost his job, and he incurred medical expenses for psychiatric care. His lawsuit requested that the court award him the following amounts: $500,000 for personal injury due to slander; $30,000 in lost wages; and $5,000 for psychiatric care.

    a. What are the tax consequences to V if he is awarded the $535,000?

    b. V decides to accept an out-of-court settlement of $150,000. The newspaper and its insurer are willing to allocate the $150,000 in any manner that V requests. How should V have the amount allocated?

PROBLEMS

6-17 *Basic Concepts.* Calculate the amount to be included in gross income for the following taxpayers.

    a. T is self-employed as a beautician. Her records show

Receipts	
Services	$21,000
Product sales	3,000

Expenditures

Cost of products sold	1,800
Cost of supplies used	2,600
Utilities	2,400
Shop and equipment rent	3,600
Other expenses	1,000

b. R owns rental property. His records show

Gross rents	$6,000
Depreciation expense	4,200
Repair expense	2,100
Miscellaneous expense	300

c. S is an employee with the following tax information:

Gross salary	$15,000
Social security (FICA) taxes withheld (rounded for simplicity)	1,000
Federal income tax withheld	2,200
Health insurance premiums withheld	500
Net salary received in cash	11,300
Employer's share of social security taxes	1,000

6-18   *Investments—Cash Dividends.* Three years ago, Z purchased 50 shares of L common stock for $6,000. Although Z is married, the stocks are recorded in his name alone. The current market value of these shares totals $7,200. He and Mrs. Z file a joint return and neither of them owns any other stock. Mr. Z wants to know what effect each of the following totally separate situations has upon (1) his taxable income and (2) his basis in each share of stock.
a. L distributes a cash dividend and Z receives $330.
b. L distributes cash as a return of capital and Z receives $330.

6-19   *Investments—Stock Dividends.* A, who is single, purchased 100 shares of N Corporation common stock four years ago for $12,000. The stock has a current fair market value of $14,400. A asks how each of the following separate situations affects her (1) taxable income and (2) basis in each share of stock.
a. N distributes common stock as a dividend and A receives ten shares.
b. N distributes nonconvertible preferred stock as a dividend and A receives 10 shares. The preferred stock has a current fair market value of $100 per share.

6-20   *Investments—Cash Dividends.* D, Inc. had accumulated earnings and profits at January 1 of the current year of $20,000. During the taxable year, it had current earnings and profits of $10,000. On December 31 of the current year, D, Inc. made a cash distribution of $40,000 to its sole shareholder, G. G paid $25,000 for his stock three years ago.
a. How will G treat the $40,000 he received on December 31?
b. Assume G sold all of his stock for $36,000 on January 1 of the following year. Compute his capital gain.

6-21   *Investments—Interest.* Mr. K died at the beginning of the year. Mrs. K received interest during the year from the following sources:

Corporate bonds	$1,100
Bank savings account	200
Personal loan to a friend	500
City of Maryville bonds (issued to build a new high school)	600

In addition to the above, Mrs. K was the beneficiary of her husband's $50,000 life insurance policy. She elected to receive the $50,000 proceeds plus interest over the next 10 years. She receives $7,500 in the current year and will receive a like amount each of the following nine years. Calculate the taxable portion of the interest income received by Mrs. K during the year.

6-22   *Educational Savings Bonds Requirements.* H and W have twin sons, S and T, and two daughters, D and E. The couple purchased Series EE savings bonds, hoping to take advantage of the interest exclusion for their children's education. This year, they cashed in some of the bonds, receiving $5,000. Of this amount, $2,000 represented interest. For each of the following independent situations, indicate how much, if any, of the exclusion is allowed this year.

   a.   D enrolled at Michigan State University and paid tuition of $4,000. To help defray some of these expenses, she used an academic scholarship of $1,000.

   b.   While on her way to the first day of class, D fell and broke her leg. She withdrew from classes and received all of her money back.

   c.   S is 25 and entered the Ph.D. program at the University of Texas this year. As a teaching assistant, he receives a salary of $7,000 during the year. His parents paid $1,000 of his tuition.

   d.   H and W paid for all of T's tuition to attend Arizona State University. The couple's A.G.I. for this year was $110,000. When the couple purchased the particular bonds used to pay for T's tuition, their A.G.I. was $55,000.

   e.   E, 22, redeemed bonds this year, receiving $5,000. E used all of the proceeds to pay for her tuition. She received the bonds as a gift from her parents last year. E's A.G.I. for this year is $3,000.

6-23   *Investments—Annuities.* P is single, 65 years old, and retired. On August 1, 1990 he purchased a single-premium deferred life annuity for $40,000 using after-tax funds. This year, P received $5,000 in annuity benefits. He will receive a like amount each year for the rest of his life. (**Note:** In answering the following questions, use the information in Exhibit 6-3 of this chapter.)

   a.   Calculate P's taxable income from the annuity for the current year.

   b.   Calculate P's taxable income from the annuity for year 5.

   c.   Calculate P's taxable income from the annuity for year 22.

   d.   Assume P lives just 15 more years. Calculate the deduction that would be allowed on P's final tax return.

   e.   Assume the annuity was purchased by P and his employer jointly. P contributed $12,000 in after-tax funds, and the employer contributed $28,000. Calculate P's taxable income from the annuity for the current year.

6-24   *Annuities.* A, age 62, retired after 30 years of service as an employee of the XYZ Corporation. He started receiving retirement benefits in the form of a single life annuity on January 1 of the current year. A's total after-tax contributions to the plan amounted to $39,000, and his retirement benefit is $1,500 per month.

   a.   Determine A's nontaxable portion of each monthly payment, assuming he elects the simplified safe-harbor method.

   b.   Assume A lives another 25 years. Will there be a time period in which A will be required to fully include the monthly payments in gross income? If so, when?

6-25   *529 Savings Plan.* Z is a dependent beneficiary of a 529 savings plan established by her parents. During the current year, Z received a $20,000 distribution and used it to pay $20,000 for tuition at a private university. Z's parents contributed $60,000 to the plan and earnings from investments total an additional $20,000.

   a.   How much of the $20,000 distribution may Z exclude from gross income?

   b.   Assume Z elects to join the work force rather than attend college and the entire $80,000 accumulated in the plan is distributed to Z's parents. How much is included in the parent's gross income?

6-26 *529 College Savings Plan.* V, who is divorced, transfers $45,000 to Eastern University's 529 savings plan for the benefit of his son, W, in 2009. W received no other gifts during 2009.

    a. Compute V's taxable gift for 2009 (assume no election was made).

    b. Assume V elects to treat the contribution as a gift made over five years. Does V owe any gift taxes?

    c. Assume V dies in 2012. How much of the $45,000 contribution made in 2009 will be included in V's gross estate?

6-27 *Investments—Life Insurance.* L is 65 years old and retired. Her husband died early in the year. L was the beneficiary of his $20,000 life insurance policy. L elected to receive $5,200 annually for five years rather than receive a single payment of $20,000 immediately. Calculate L's taxable income from the first payment.

6-28 *Social Security Benefits.* X, who is single and retired, has the following income for the current year:

Taxable interest	$12,000
Dividend income	10,000
Tax-exempt bond interest	8,000
Social security benefits	7,200

    a. Compute the taxable portion of X's social security benefits.

    b. Assume the above information remains the same, except X's taxable interest amounted to $10,000. Compute the taxable portion of his social security benefits.

6-29 *Group-Term Life Insurance.* E, age 55, is Vice President of QRS, Incorporated. His salary for the year amounted to $75,000. Employees at QRS receive group-term life insurance coverage equal to twice their annual salaries. Determine E's taxable income from his group-term life insurance protection for the year.

6-30 *Employee Benefits.* Determine the (1) deductible employer amount, and (2) taxable employee amount for each of the following employer-provided benefits.

    a. Reimbursement of expenses paid by an employee to entertain a client of the business, $200.

    b. Bonus paid an employee when a sales quota was met, $300.

    c. Watches given employees at Christmas, $38 each.

    d. Free parking provided on company property, $500 market value and $220 cost per employee.

    e. Supper money of $15 paid to an employee for each of 10 nights that she worked past 6 p.m., $150.

6-31 *Employee Benefits.* Determine the (1) deductible employer amount, and (2) taxable employee (or beneficiary) amount for each of the following employer-provided benefits.

    a. A death benefit of $6,000 paid to the wife and $4,000 to the son of a deceased employee.

    b. Premiums of $700 paid on $70,000 of group-term life insurance for a 52-year-old woman employee.

    c. Ten percent employee discounts are allowed on the retail price of all merchandise purchased from the employer. During the year, sales to employees totaled $18,000 ($20,000 retail price − $2,000 discount) for merchandise that cost the employer $14,000. The employer reported the $18,000 as sales and the $14,000 as cost of goods sold.

6-32 *Employee Benefits—Medical Insurance.* F's $400 annual health insurance premium is paid by his employer. During the year, F received $870 reimbursement of medical expenses; $650 for this year's expenses and $220 for last year's expenses. Determine F's taxable income from the reimbursement in the current year if

  a. F never itemizes any medical expenses.

  b. F deducted medical expenses from his A.G.I. this year of $900 and last year of $450.

6-33 *Tax Benefit Rule.* During 2008 K had adjusted gross income of $30,000. A list of itemized deductions available to K in preparing her 2008 return is shown below:

State income taxes paid	$2,000
Property taxes on residence	600
Charitable contributions	400
Medical expenses	2,500
Interest paid on residence	1,200

K is single, and her son M, who is 8 years old, lives with her. She qualifies as a head of household. In 2009 K received $2,500 from an insurance company for reimbursement of her 2008 medical expenses. Is K required to include any of the $2,500 reimbursement in her gross income in 2009?

6-34 *Fringe Benefits versus Compensation.* P is a 46-year-old professor at Z University, a private school in the Midwest. P is married and has triplets who are freshmen at Z University. Among others, P is provided with the following fringe benefits during the current year:

> Group-term life insurance coverage of $75,000. Premium cost to Z University is $300.
> Tuition reduction of $30,000 for the triplets.

  a. How much does the group-term life insurance cost Professor P? Assume his marginal tax bracket is 31 percent.

  b. Would P be equally well off if the university simply paid him an additional $300 in compensation to cover the term insurance?

  c. Is the tuition reduction for the triplets taxable?

  d. Assuming tuition remains constant, how much will Professor P save in tuition payments by remaining on the faculty at Z University until the triplets graduate?

  e. What would be the result for the current year if the university increased Professor P's salary by $30,000 a year to pay for the triplets' tuition?

6-35 *Unemployment Compensation and Disability Income.* Mr. and Mrs. B are married filing jointly. Mrs. B was permanently disabled the entire year and Mr. B was unemployed part of the year. Both are 55 years old. Their receipts for the year were

Disability income—Mrs. B	$ 6,200
Social security income—Mrs. B	1,000
Salary—Mr. B	16,500
Unemployment compensation—Mr. B	4,500

Calculate their taxable income for the year, assuming the disability insurance premiums were paid

  a. Entirely by Mrs. B.

  b. Entirely by Mrs. B's employer.

6-36 *Damages Awarded and Disability Income.* D works for the XYZ Tool and Die Shop. On March 1, 2009 a stamping press that D was operating malfunctioned, resulting in the loss of the index finger on his right hand. D, claiming the machine was not properly maintained, sued XYZ for the following damages:

Medical expenses during D's one-week stay in the hospital..........	$ 8,000
Loss of D's finger...	50,000
Punitive damages	5,000
Total	$63,000

On April 1, 2010 the court awarded D $63,000.

a. Assuming D did not deduct the $8,000 of medical expenses he incurred in 2009, what portion of the $63,000 settlement is included in D's gross income in 2010?

b. D did not return to work for three months. During this time period, he received $3,000 in disability income payments. Assuming D paid the annual premium on the disability insurance, how much of the $3,000 is taxable income to D?

6-37 *Meals and Lodging.* Mr. and Mrs. G own and operate a small motel near Big Mountain resort area. Their only employees are two maids and one cook. The rest of the work is done by Mr. and Mrs. G. In order to be on 24-hour call, they live in a home next to the motel. The home is owned by the business. Both Mr. and Mrs. G eat most of their meals in the motel restaurant. Answer the questions below assuming the business is (1) a corporation, or (2) a partnership.

a. Are any of the costs for the meals and lodging deductible by either the business or Mr. and Mrs. G?

b. Is the value of the meals and lodging included in Mr. and Mrs. G's gross income?

c. Answer the questions in (a) and (b) again, but assume Mr. and Mrs. G paid the business for all their meals in the restaurant and for rent of the home.

6-38 *Adoption Assistance.* R and L are married and file a joint return. R is the controller of a tool and die firm and is paid a salary of $140,000. L is a grade school teacher and earns $27,500. Other income received during the current year includes $1,000 in interest on State of Indiana bonds owned by R and $2,500 in dividends on Procter & Gamble stock that L owns. R and L, who have no children of their own, incurred $9,000 in qualified adoption expenses (i.e, adoption fees, attorney fees and court costs) to adopt a 2-year-old "special needs" child. These expenses were covered by R's employer under the company's adoption assistance program.

a. Determine R and L's A.G.I. for the current year.

b. Assuming the couple elects the standard deduction, compute their taxable income for the current year.

6-39 *Transportation Fringes.* How much is includible in the employee's gross income in each of the following scenarios?

a. Employee A receives a transit pass each month from Employer X valued at $95.

b. Employer Y provides free parking each month to employee B valued at $300.

c. Employer Z provides parking each month to employee C valued at $250. Employee C pays Employer Z $40 per month for this parking fringe.

d. Employer Q reimburses employee R $15 a month for storage of his bike while at work.

6-40 *Employer-Provided Parking.* Employer G operates a factory in a rural area in which no commercial parking is available. G provides ample parking for its employees on the business premises, free of charge.

a. What guidance does the Internal Revenue Service provide for determining the value of free parking?

b. Given the facts presented above, what value would the IRS place on the free parking provided by Employer G?

6-41 *Military Compensation.* After graduating from high school last year, K, who is single, joined the U.S. Air Force. Her military compensation for 2009 is

	Cash	Market Value
Salary	$10,000	
Military housing		$2,500
Computer training on the job		1,800
Uniforms.		800
Meals on the base		3,600
Reimbursement of moving expenses	500	

Calculate K's taxable income for the year.

6-42 *Inheritances.* In each of the following independent situations. determine how much, if any, the taxpayer must include in gross income.
  a. At the beginning of this year, a taxpayer inherited rental property valued at $87,000 from his grandmother. Rental income from the property after the transfer of title totaled $6,000, and rental expenses were $5,200.
  b. A taxpayer inherited $50,000 from her employer. She was his housekeeper for ten years and was promised she would be provided for in his will if she continued employment with him until his death.
  c. A taxpayer lent $15,000 to a friend. To protect the loan, the taxpayer had his friend make him beneficiary on her $20,000 life insurance policy. Six months later the friend died and the taxpayer received $20,000 from the insurance company.

6-43 *Gifts.* In each of the following independent situations, determine how much, if any, the taxpayer must include in gross income.
  a. A taxpayer often visits her uncle in a nursing home. In addition, she manages his investment portfolio for him. To show his gratitude, he has given her stock valued at $5,000. He has also implied that if she continues these activities, he will transfer other shares of stock to her.
  b. A taxpayer saved a child's life during a fire. The child's parents gave him land valued at $5,000 to show their gratitude. They paid $2,200 for the land several years ago.
  c. Taxpayer's employer gave him $1,200 in recognition of his 20 years of service to the company. The employer deducted the $1,200 as a business expense.

6-44 *Awards.* In each of the following independent situations, determine how much, if any, the taxpayer must include in gross income.
  a. The taxpayer, a professional basketball player, was voted as the outstanding player of the year. In addition to the honor, he received an automobile with a sticker price of $16,000. He drove the car for six months and sold it for $12,000. The taxpayer's employer also gave him a gold watch worth $1,200. He wears the watch. Both donors deducted their respective costs for the automobile and the watch as business expenses. The costs of the automobile and watch were $13,500 and $800, respectively.
  b. The taxpayer was selected by the senior class as the most outstanding classroom teacher. The high school presented her with a $1,000 check in recognition of her significant accomplishments. She used the money to take a well-earned vacation to Cancun.
  c. M, Inc. gave T a watch in recognition of her 20 years of service to the company. The watch cost the employer $400.

6-45 *Child Support and Alimony.* Determine the effect on A.G.I. for the husband (H) and wife (W) in each of the following *continuous* situations. H and W are divorced and do not live in a community property state. They have three children.

a. H pays W $400 per month as alimony and support of the three children.

b. W discovers her attorney did not word the agreement correctly. H and W sign a statement that the *original* agreement is retroactively amended to hold that H pays $100 per month as alimony to W and $300 per month as support of the three children. All other language remains unchanged. What is the effect of this change on future and past payments?

c. Assume the original agreement contained the wording in (b) above. In the first year, H makes only 10 of the 12 payments for a total of $4,000. In the second year, H pays the $800 balance due for the prior year and makes all 12 payments of $400 each on time.

d. On their divorce, W was awarded an automobile. H is required to pay the loan outstanding on the car, $94 per month for 20 months. During the year, H pays $94 for 12 months. This includes $130 interest and $998 loan principal.

e. H owns the home in which W and the children live free of charge. H's mortgage payments are $360 per month for the next 20 years. During the year, his expenses on the home are $2,900 interest, $800 property taxes, $340 insurance, $280 loan principal, and $218 repairs. The rental value of the home is $425 per month.

f. In addition to the monthly alimony and support payments above, H is to pay W $30,000 over a period of 11 years. H pays $2,500 of this amount the first year and $3,600 the second year.

g. H inherits considerable property. As a result, he voluntarily increases the alimony to $150 and child support to $450 per month. He makes 12 payments of $600 each during the year.

6-46   *Alimony.* Determine the effect on A.G.I. for the husband (H) and wife (W) in each of the three years. W is to pay H alimony of $100,000 as follows:

Year	Amount
1	$56,000
2	26,000
3	18,000

6-47   *Divorce—Property Settlement.* Husband (H) and wife (W) are divorced this month. The divorce agreement states that all jointly owned property will be transferred as follows:

	Cost	Market Value	Transferred to
Home	$35,000	$65,000	W
Investments	3,000	5,000	W
Cash	7,000	7,000	H and W equally

W will occupy the home and H will rent an apartment. Determine the recognized gain or loss and the basis of the assets to H and W after the transfer. Explain.

6-48   *Divorce—Property Settlement.* H and W, who live in Michigan (a common law state), decided to end their troubled 30-year marriage. Pursuant to the divorce decree, the following assets are transferred from H to W on March 1, 2009:

	Basis to H	Market Value
Stocks (purchased by H on April 10, 2003)	$300,000	$400,000
Land (purchased by H on June 2, 2000)	200,000	500,000

In addition to the above, H transferred a life insurance policy on his life with a face value of $200,000 to W, who assumed responsibility for the annual premium.

W sold the stocks for $500,000 on November 1, 2009 and the land for $550,000 on December 1, 2009. H died on December 20, 2009.

a. Determine W's gain on the sale of the stocks and land in 2009.

b. Are any of the life insurance proceeds taxable to W? Explain.

6-49 *Accelerated Death Benefits.* T, a wife and mother of three, was diagnosed with throat cancer. Due to the complications from chemotherapy treatments, she resigned from her teaching position at a private university in Chicago on June 1. Having been certified by her medical doctor on July 7 as terminally ill, T is considering selling her life insurance policy with a face value of $200,000 to a viatical "settlement provider" (VSP) for a lump sum.

a. Assuming T has paid $15,000 in premiums, how much must she include in her gross income if she sells her policy to VSP for $150,000 on August 1?

b. Does your answer change if T lives longer than 24 months from the date of certification?

c. If T dies 8 months later, how much must VSP include in its gross income? (Assume VSP paid additional premiums of $10,000 after purchasing the policy.)

6-50 *Employee Fringe Benefits.* For each of the following independent situations, indicate whether the fringe benefit the employee receives is taxable or nontaxable. Explain your answer.

a. C is a ticket agent for North Central Airways. The airline has a nondiscriminatory policy that allows its employees to fly without charge on a standby basis only. The last week in July, C took a vacation and flew from Kansas City to San Francisco. The value of the round-trip ticket was $400.

b. Assume that C [in part (a) above] also stayed, without charge, for the entire week at a hotel in San Francisco that North Central Airways owns. The value of a week's stay in the hotel was $2,000.

c. Assume in part (a) above that C was unable to obtain an empty seat on North Central the last week in July. Consequently, utilizing the qualified reciprocal arrangement that North Central has with South Shore Airlines, C flew free to San Francisco on South Shore. The value of the round-trip ticket was $400.

d. M is a sales clerk for J-mart department store. The store has a nondiscriminatory policy whereby its employees may purchase inventory items at a discount. In June, M purchased a microwave oven for $250 that J-mart sells to its customers for $300. J-mart's gross profit rate is 20 percent.

e. F is a CPA and works for a public accounting firm. On F's behalf, the firm paid $375 in subscription fees for three professional accounting journals.

f. Officers of the XYZ Corporation are provided free parking space in a public parking garage located across the street from the firm's office building. The monthly cost of the parking space to XYZ is $300 for each officer.

6-51 *Unrelated Party Transfers.* In each of the following independent situations, determine how much, if any, the taxpayer must include in gross income.

a. Taxpayer has been very active as a volunteer hospital worker for many years. In the current year, the city named her as the Outstanding Volunteer of the Year. She later discovered that she was nominated for the award by two nurses at the hospital. The honor included a silver tray valued at $400. In addition, the two nurses collected $700 from hospital personnel and gave her a prepaid one-week vacation for two people.

b. Taxpayer, an undergraduate degree candidate, was selected as one of five outstanding sophomore students in accounting by the Institute of Management Accountants. Selection was based on an application submitted by eligible students. The winner received $15,000. Although there was no stipulation of how the money was to be used, the award was given with the expectation that the money would be used for tuition, books, and fees in the student's junior and senior years.

c. Taxpayer won the bowling league award for the highest total score over a five-week period. Taxpayer received a trophy valued at $65 and $100 cash.

    d. Taxpayer purchased church raffle tickets in her eight-year-old son's name and gave the tickets to him. One of the tickets was drawn. The prize was a $600 color television.

    e. Taxpayer receives a $20,000 grant from the National Association of Chiefs of Police to conduct a research study on crowd control. The grant stipulates that the research period is for eight months and that $8,000 of it is for travel and temporary living costs.

    f. An accounting student accepted an internship with a CPA firm and is paid $3,000. The stated purpose of the internship is to provide students with a basic understanding of how accounting education is applied. It is believed this understanding will help students in remaining course work and later job selection. Although the faculty believes internships would benefit all students, only 40 percent of the accounting majors participate in the program.

6-52 *Businesses.* In each of the following independent situations, determine how much, if any, the taxpayer must include in gross income.

    a. A taxpayer sold a beauty shop operated as a proprietorship for $60,000. The assets were valued as follows: tangible assets, $45,000; agreement not to compete, $10,000; and goodwill, $5,000. The seller's basis for the tangible assets is $45,000 but there is no basis for the other two assets.

    b. The building in which a drug store is located is damaged by fire. The store had to be closed for two weeks while repairs were made. As a result, the insurance company paid the store $50,000 for lost profits during the period and $15,000 to cover overhead expenses.

    c. E, Inc. leases land to V, Inc. The agreement states that the lease period is for five years and the annual lease payment is $1,000 per month. Under the terms of the lease, V immediately constructs a storage building on the land for $40,000. E receives $12,000 from V each year for three years. At the end of the third year, V cancels the lease and pays a cancellation penalty of $6,000. At this time, the building's market value is $30,000. Thus, in the third year, E received $18,000 cash and a building worth an additional $30,000. Determine E's taxable income from the lease for each of the three years.

    d. A corporation accepted $100,000 from an insurance company as an out-of-court settlement of a lawsuit for patent infringement.

6-53 *Debt Cancellation.* DEF, Inc. is in the van conversion business. Due to stiff competition and a declining economy in the region served by DEF, the company has incurred significant operating losses during the past year. As of December 31 of the current year, DEF's financial statements reflect the following pertinent information:

Total assets	$ 750,000
Total liabilities	1,000,000
Tax attributes	
Adjusted basis of depreciable assets	300,000
NOL carryover	100,000
Capital loss carryover	25,000

    In an attempt to rescue the company from going out of business, DEF's suppliers have agreed to forgive $180,000 of indebtedness.

    a. Assuming DEF is not in bankruptcy proceedings, what are the tax consequences to the corporation resulting from the cancellation of the debt?

    b. Would your answer to part (a) change if DEF makes an election under Code § 108 (b)(5)?

    c. Would your answer to part (a) change if the $180,000 of debt is cancelled under bankruptcy proceedings?

    d. Assume that the facts in the problem remain the same, except that DEF has total assets of $1 million and total liabilities of $750,000. What impact does the cancellation of $180,000 in debt now have on DEF?

6-54 Five years ago, J and his wife decided that it was time to quit renting and buy a new home. They had little cash. Nevertheless they shopped around and found the perfect home. Although it was beyond their price range, they could afford it by virtue of an ultra low-interest rate. Thus they bought the home for $110,000, paying $10,000 down and financing the remaining $100,000 with an adjustable rate mortgage. This year the rate was adjusted in accordance with the terms of the agreement. As a result, J was no longer able to make his mortgage payments. J considered refinancing to get a lower fixed rate but this was not an option. There was a steep penalty for refinancing. Moreover, the value of the home had actually dropped and no one was willing to refinance a mortgage that was more than the value of their home. Fortunately, the bank did not want to become the owner of the home given the current market and agreed to reduce the debt to $90,000. What are the tax consequences to J?

6-55 *Miscellaneous Items.* In each of the following independent situations, determine how much, if any, the taxpayer must include in gross income.
   a. A taxpayer's round trip mileage to and from work is 50 miles. Five fellow employees live near him and pay to ride with him. The taxpayer's records for the current year show $3,900 receipts and $3,120 automobile expenses.
   b. While walking across campus, a taxpayer found a diamond ring. She notified the authorities on campus and paid $10 for an ad in the lost-and-found section of the newspaper. When six weeks went by with no response, she had the ring appraised. It was valued at $1,200. After six more weeks with no response, she sold the ring for $850.
   c. A taxpayer was injured on the job and was out of work for most of the year. He received the following government benefits during the year: $800 in food stamps; $1,500 worker's compensation for the injury; and $1,800 in welfare payments.
   d. A taxpayer sued her neighbor for malicious slander. The court awarded her $30,000 for personal injury due to indignities suffered as a result of the slander; $3,500 in lost income; and $200 reimbursement for medical expenses incurred. The taxpayer does not itemize deductions.

6-56 *Ordinary v. Capital Gain Income.* In each of the following scenarios, determine the amount (if any) and type of income to be included in gross income by the recipient:
   a. Denise acquired all of the net assets of Mary's CPA firm. Mary operated the practice as a sole proprietorship. The purchase price includes $20,000 allocable to goodwill and $15,000 allocable to a covenant not to compete for five years.
   b. Ernie rents an apartment from Doug. Because Ernie is being transferred to another city by his employer, he paid Doug $800 to cancel his lease.
   c. Mary Ann owns an apartment complex in Jacksonville, Florida. In an effort to convert the apartment into an office building, she pays Jean, one of her tenants, $900 to cancel the apartment lease.
   d. John, who is single and lives in Detroit, had total itemized deductions in 2008 of $6,000 including $700 of state income taxes withheld by his employer. John could have deducted state and local sales taxes of $600. On May 14, 2009, John received a refund from the State of Michigan for $200 due to overpaying his Michigan income taxes in 2008.

6-57 *Miscellaneous Fringe Benefits.* In each of the following independent situations answer true if the ending sentence is correct and false if the ending sentence is incorrect.
   a. During the current year, A withdraws $2,000 from a qualified tuition plan to pay his undergraduate tuition at Ivy Tech. Of the $2,000 received, $1,600 represents contributions to the plan and $400 represents earnings. *The $400 of earnings is excluded from A's income.*
   b. B is employed at the Tire Rack Company. She works the day shift and her two children, ages 3 and 4, stay at the company's day care facility. The current year's value of this service is approximately $4,000. *B may exclude the full $4,000 from income.*

c. C works for Ever Green, Inc. During the evenings C attends State University where she is working on her undergraduate degree in Marketing. During the current year Ever Green paid C's tuition ($3,000) and her textbooks ($800) out of the company's nondiscriminatory educational assistance program. *C may exclude the full $3,800 from income.*

d. D is an employee of Night Line, Inc. where he is covered under the company's qualified pension plan. During the current year D, who is 64 years old, and his wife attended several seminars related to retirement planning that were sponsored by Night Line. The value of this service is approximately $1,500. *The $1,500 will be reported on D's Form W-2 as taxable income.*

TAX RETURN PROBLEMS

CONTINUOUS TAX RETURN PROBLEMS See Appendix D, Part 1.

CUMULATIVE PROBLEMS

TaxCut **6-58** H, age 45, and W, age 43, are married with two dependent children: M, age 18, and N, age 19. Both are full-time students at a local university. H, who is president of a local bank, is paid a salary of $150,000. He also is the sole proprietor of a jewelry store that had a net profit for 2009 of $75,000. W, a registered nurse at a large hospital, is paid a salary of $50,000. In addition to the above income, H and W received the following during 2009:

a. $3,000 cash dividend on ABC, Inc. stock, which they own jointly. They paid $25,000 for the stock three years ago and it has a current market value of $40,000. ABC, Inc. has $300,000 of current and accumulated E&P.

b. $750 in interest on State of Michigan bonds that H owns.

c. $7,000 in interest on corporate bonds that H and W purchased two years ago at face value for $100,000.

d. W received a check for $400 from her employer in recognition of her outstanding service to the hospital during the past 10 years.

e. The bank provides H with $90,000 of group term life insurance protection. The bank provides all full-time employees with group term insurance.

f. 1,000 shares of XYZ common as a stock dividend. Prior to the distribution, H and W owned 9,000 shares of common with a basis of $15,000. H and W did not have the right to receive cash or other assets in lieu of the stock.

g. Because W must be available should an emergency arise, she is required to eat her lunches in the hospital cafeteria. The value of the free meals provided by her employer during 2009 was $1,100.

h. H's grandfather passed away in February 2009, leaving H a 400-acre farm in southern Illinois valued at $500,000. H rented the land to F, a neighboring farmer, for $13,000.

i. In order to drain off the excess surface water from 10 acres, F (see h above) installed drainage pipe at a cost of $1,500.

j. W sold 50 shares of DEF stock for $100 per share. She bought the stock four years ago for $1,800.

k. H received a dividend check for $280 from the MNO Mutual Life Insurance Company. H purchased the policy in 1983, and W is the primary beneficiary.

l. H and W's only itemized deductions were interest on their home mortgage, $18,000; property taxes on their home, $4,000; and charitable contributions, $6,000.

m. The hospital withheld $11,000 of Federal income taxes on W's salary and the appropriate amount of FICA taxes. The bank withheld $30,000 in Federal income taxes from H's salary and the appropriate amount of FICA taxes. Furthermore, H's quarterly estimated tax payments for 2009 total $35,000.

Part I: Computation of Federal Income Tax. Calculate H and W's 2009 Federal income tax liability (or refund) assuming they file a joint return.

Part II: Tax Planning Ideas. H and W are very concerned about the amount of Federal income tax they now pay. Because they want to send M and N on to graduate school, they have come up with the following strategies, which they hope will reduce their family's total tax liability.

1. In 2010 M and N will begin working at the jewelry store two nights a week and on Saturdays throughout the school year and 20 hours a week during the summer months. Each child will be paid $4,500 for services during the year.
2. On January 1, 2010 H and W will sell their corporate bonds for $100,000 and invest the cash proceeds in Series EE savings bonds. H and W will use the bonds to pay for M and N's qualified educational expenses.
3. On January 1, 2010 H and W will gift their stock in ABC, Inc. to M and N equally.
4. Beginning in 2010 H will instruct the farmer who is leasing his Illinois farm to pay the $13,000 in rent directly to M and N (i.e., $6,500 each).

H and W have asked for your opinion concerning the above strategies. For each idea, explain why it will or will not reduce the family's total tax liability. Assuming H and W implement only the strategies that will reduce taxes, how much will the family save in taxes in 2010 compared to 2009 (**Note:** Calculate the 2010 tax using the tax law and rates applicable to 2009 and assume all other data from Part I above is the same.)

TaxCut **6-59** A and B are married with two children, ages 15 and 16. A, who is 45 years old, is president of Greenville Savings & Loan (a large financial institution located in Greenville, Michigan). During 2009 his salary amounted to $400,000. Additional information pertaining to A and B's financial affairs for 2009 is summarized below:

a. A and B purchased 1,000 shares of GHI, Inc. common stock on January 1, 2009 for $22,000. On May 1, 2009 A and B received 100 shares of GHI, Inc. common as a stock dividend. They did not have the right to receive cash or other assets in lieu of the stock.
b. On November 15, 2008 A and B purchased a small farm (50 acres) five miles from Greenville for $50,000. Although A and B originally planned to move to the farm when A retires, they ended up selling it on October 20, 2009 to a large real estate developer for $200.000.
c. On August 1, 2009 A and B redeemed Series EE bonds that had matured for $30,000. They originally purchased the bonds for $14,000. During the period they held the bonds, A and B never elected to include in income the annual increase in the redemption price.
d. B's father passed away on September 1, 2009. She inherited $100,000, which they deposited in a savings account at the Greenville Savings & Loan. The interest on the deposit amounted to $2,000 for the year.
e. Greenville Savings & Loan provided A with the following benefit package:

Fringe Benefit	Annual Cost to Greenville S & L
Health insurance premium	$2,400
Accident and disability premium	600
Parking space	190
Group-term life insurance of $150,000	800

f. A and B's only itemized deductions were mortgage interest on their personal residence, $40,000; state and local taxes, $30,000; and charitable contributions, $8,000.
g. The Greenville Savings & Loan withheld $100,000 of Federal income taxes on A's salary and the appropriate amount of payroll taxes. In addition, A's quarterly estimated tax payments for 2009 total $40,000.

Part I: Calculation of Taxable Income and Tax Due. Compute A and B's taxable income and Federal income tax liability for 2009 assuming they file a joint return.

Part II: Tax Planning Suggestions. Assume that A and B come to you on July 1, 2009 seeking your advice on ways in which they can reduce their 2009 Federal income tax liability. They provide you with the following additional information:

1. The real estate developer, who is interested in acquiring A and B's 50 acres, is willing to defer the purchase date to June 16, 2010. What would you recommend A and B do? Explain your answer.

2. A and B would like to get the best return possible on the money they will receive from the sale of their farm. Two options they are considering are (1) invest the proceeds in corporate bonds paying 7% annually and (2) purchase State of Michigan bonds paying 5 1/2% annually. What would you recommend A and B do? Explain your answer.

3. A and B have been informed that the Series EE bonds that mature on August 1, 2009 can be exchanged for Series HH bonds that pay interest semiannually. What would you recommend A and B do? Explain your answer.

RESEARCH PROBLEMS

6-60 *Divorce.* J and M are obtaining a divorce after ten years of marriage. They have two children. A draft of the divorce agreement and property settlement between them states that they will have joint custody of the children. They plan to live in the same general area and each child will live half of each year with each parent. Since J's A.G. I. is $40,000 and M's $15,000, he will pay her $100 per month for each child ($2,400 per year) and $500 per month for her support. The $500 ceases on his or her death, her remarriage, or when her A.G.I. equals his. In addition, J agrees to continue to pay premiums of $50 per month on his life insurance policy payable to her. All jointly owned property will be distributed as follows:

	Basis	Market Value	Transfer to
Home	$50,000	$80,000	M
Furnishings	20,000	15,000	M
Investments	10,000	30,000	J

Each will keep his or her individually owned personal items and an automobile. This is an amicable divorce and they both request your advice. Their objective is to maximize total tax benefits without making too many changes to the agreement. Use tax-planning techniques when possible in responding to the following questions.
   a. Who will be able to claim the children as dependents?
   b. What is each one's filing status for the current year if neither one remarries?
   c. Does the $500 per month qualify as alimony? Does the $50 per month qualify as alimony?
   d. J expects to make the $500 and $50 payments for three months while legally separated before the divorce. What are the tax effects during this period?
   e. What is the tax effect of the distribution of jointly owned property to J and to M?
   f. What tax planning advice could you give to J and M that would decrease their combined tax liability?

6-61 *Meals and Lodging.* H and W are married with three children. The children are 8, 10, and 15 years old. H and W are purchasing a 500-acre farm, which they will manage and operate themselves. In addition, they will employ one full-time farmer year round and several part-time people at peak times. H will be responsible primarily for management of the operations, the crops, and the dairy herd and other farm animals. W will be responsible primarily for the garden, the chickens, providing meals for the family and

farm hands, and maintaining the family home. The children are assigned farm chores to help their parents after school and on weekends.

The taxpayers prefer to operate the farm as a partnership but, after all factors are considered, are willing to incorporate the farm if it seems to provide greater benefits. Presently, they ask for detailed information about the residence on the farm and the groceries that will be purchased to feed them and their employees on the farm. Some of their specific questions are listed below.

a. What are the benefits and requirements covering meals and lodging provided by the business?

b. Is it possible to meet the requirements and obtain all or at least some of the benefits if the farm is operated as a proprietorship or partnership, or must it be operated as a corporation?

c. If full benefits are obtained, are any adjustments required for the children, for personal entertainment and meals shared with friends and relatives in the farm home, or any other personal use? If any adjustments are required, which ones, and are they made at cost or market value?

d. If full benefits are obtained, exactly what qualifies? For example, do all groceries qualify, including supplies that are not eaten, such as freezer bags to store frozen foods from the garden, soap, and bathroom supplies? Do all expenses for the home qualify, such as utilities, insurance, and repairs?

e. Should the business or should H and W own the home?

f. Is it acceptable for H and W to purchase the food and be reimbursed by the business?

6-62   *Discharge of Indebtedness.* T, who is single, purchased a new home in 1978 from the XYZ Construction Co. for $55,000. She received a 7.25 percent mortgage from the Federal Savings and Loan Association (FS&L). Currently, the home's fair market value is approximately double its original purchase price. Since interest rates have risen significantly in recent months, FS&L wants to rid itself of the low 7.25 percent mortgage. Lending to others at a much higher interest rate would clearly enhance FS&L's profits. Consequently, during the current year FS&L sent a letter to T offering to cancel the mortgage (which had a remaining principal balance of $35,000) in return for a payment of $29,000. T took advantage of the prepayment opportunity, thus receiving a discount equal to the difference between the remaining principal balance of $35,000 and the amount paid by T of $29,000, or $6,000.

a. Although T is pleased she no longer has a monthly mortgage payment, she is concerned about the possible tax consequences resulting from the discharge of indebtedness. T has come to you for your advice.

b. Assume that the fair market value of T's residence has declined to $25,000 due to the construction of a nearby land fill operation. Does this fact change your answer?

6-63   *Compensatory Damages.* T. J. Taxpayer, CLU, has owned an insurance agency in Santa Rosa, California since 1960. As an independent agent, he represented five companies selling auto, home, commercial, and life insurance. Because of his excellent reputation in the community, T. J. has built a very successful agency. Last year, T. J. applied for an agency license from the American Life Insurance Co. in order to broaden his life insurance business. In reviewing his application, American requested a credit report from Federal Credit. Federal Credit provided copies to American Life as well as other insurance companies.

The credit report contained numerous false accusations. In addition to questioning Taxpayer's integrity, the report stated that T. J. seldom returned phone calls from clients and lacked understanding of basic insurance practices and concepts. As a result, American Life denied T. J. a license to sell its life insurance. Because the report adversely affected his ability to work with existing clients and to attract new business, T. J.'s profits declined considerably.

T. J. sued Federal Credit for libel, claiming that the credit report was issued with intent to damage his business or professional reputation. The jury found that Federal

Credit had committed libel and awarded him $100,000 in compensatory damages. T. J. has heard conflicting comments from various sources about whether the $100,000 is taxable and comes to you for help. What advice would you give T. J. Taxpayer concerning the taxability of the $100,000?

6-64 *Sex Discrimination.* Alice Johnson has worked for the AMAX Corporation for ten years. In March 2007, after talking with various company employees, Alice came to the realization that there was a significant pay differential between men and women. In fact, she discovered that the corporation had modified its compensation package in 2006 whereby the salaries of employees in certain male-dominated pay schedules were increased but those in certain female-dominated pay schedules were either unchanged or reduced.

As a result, Alice Johnson brought suit (under Title VII of the Civil Rights Act of 1964) in District Court against the AMAX Corporation alleging unlawful discrimination in the payment of wages based upon gender. Alice sought back pay from the company in the amount of $10,000 to eliminate the discrimination. Rather than incur substantial costs in litigating the issue, AMAX reached an out-of-court settlement with Alice on January 15, 2009. The settlement requires AMAX to pay Alice back pay of $8,000 and to develop gender-neutral pay schedules.

Is the $8,000 subject to tax?

DEDUCTIONS AND LOSSES

★ ★ ★ ★ ★ CONTENTS ★ ★ ★ ★ ★

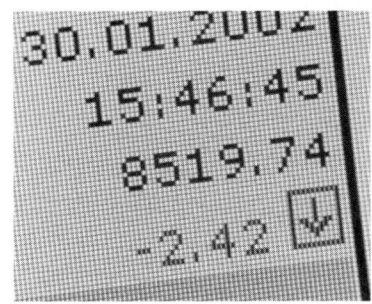

CHAPTER SEVEN

OVERVIEW OF DEDUCTIONS AND LOSSES

LEARNING OBJECTIVES

Upon completion of this chapter you will be able to:

- ► Recognize the general requirements for deducting expenses and losses
- ► Define the terms *ordinary*, *necessary*, and *reasonable* as they apply to business deductions
- ► Recognize tax accounting principles with respect to deductions and losses
- ► Explain the proper treatment of employee business expenses

- ► Describe the importance of properly classifying expenses as deductions *for* or *from* adjusted gross income
- ► Classify expenses as deductions *for* or *from* adjusted gross income
- ► Recognize statutory, administrative, and judicial limitations on deductions and losses
- ► Explain tax planning considerations for optimizing deductions

CHAPTER OUTLINE

As explained in Chapter 3, the income tax is imposed on taxable income, a quantity defined as the difference between gross income and allowable deductions.[1] The concept of gross income was explored in Chapters 5 and 6. This chapter and the following four chapters examine the subject of deductions.

There is little doubt that when it comes to taxation, the questions asked most frequently concern deductions. What is deductible? Can this expense be deducted? How much can I deduct? This is a familiar refrain around taxpaying time, and rightfully so, since any item that might be deductible reduces the tax that otherwise must be paid. Many of the questions concerning deductions are easily answered by merely referring to the basic criteria. On the other hand, many items representing potential deductions are subject to special rules. The purpose of this chapter is to introduce the general rules that are in fact used for determining the answer to that age-old question: Is it deductible?

DEDUCTION DEFINED

In the preceding chapters, the definition given for income was described as being "all-inclusive" (i.e., gross income includes *all* items of income except those specifically excluded by law). Given this concept of income, it might be assumed that a similarly broad meaning is given to the term deduction. Deductions, however, are defined narrowly. Deductions are only those *particular* expenses, losses, and other items for which a deduction is authorized.[2] The significance of this apparently meaningless definition is

---

[1]   § 63.

[2]   § 161.

found in the last word—"authorized." *Nothing is deductible unless it is allowed by the Code.* It is a well-established principle that before a deduction may be claimed the taxpayer must find some statutory provision permitting the deduction. The courts consistently have affirmed this principle, stating that a taxpayer has no constitutional right to a deduction. Rather, a taxpayer's right to a deduction depends solely on "legislative grace" (i.e., Congress has enacted a statute allowing the deduction).[3]

Although a taxpayer's deductions require statutory authorization, this does not mean that a particular deduction must be specifically mentioned in the Code. While several provisions are designed to grant the deduction for a specific item, such as § 163 for interest expense and § 164 for taxes, most deductions are allowed because they satisfy the conditions of some broadly defined category of deductions. For example, no specific deduction is allowed for the advertising expense of a restaurant owner, but the expense may be deductible if it meets the criteria required for deduction of *business expenses.*

The remainder of this chapter examines those provisions authorizing several broad categories of deductions: § 162 on trade or business expenses, § 212 on expenses of producing income, and § 165 on losses. In addition to these deduction-granting sections, several provisions that expressly deny or limit deductions for certain items are considered. The rules provided by these various provisions establish the basic framework for determining whether a deduction is allowed. Once the deductibility of an item is determined, an additional problem exists for individual taxpayers—the deduction must be classified as either a deduction *for* adjusted gross income or a deduction *from* adjusted gross income (itemized deduction). The classification process is also explained in this chapter.

DEDUCTIONS FOR EXPENSES: GENERAL REQUIREMENTS

Given that the taxpayer can deduct only those items that are authorized, what deductions does Congress in fact allow? The central theme found in the rules governing deductions is relatively straightforward: those expenses and losses incurred in business and profit-seeking activities are deductible while those incurred in purely personal activities are not. The allowance for business and profit-seeking expenses stems in part from the traditional notion that income is a *net* concept. From a conceptual perspective, income does not result until revenues exceed expenses. It generally follows from this principle that it would be unfair to tax the revenue from an activity but not allow deductions for the expenses that produced it.

In light of the Code's approach to deductions, many commentators have aptly stated that the costs of *earning* a living are deductible while the costs of living are not. Although this is a good rule of thumb, it is also an over-generalization. As will become clear, the Code allows deductions not only for the costs of producing income, but also for numerous personal expenses such as interest on home mortgages, property taxes, medical expenses, and charitable contributions. To complicate matters further, the line between personal and business expenses is often difficult to draw. For this reason, the various rules governing deductions must be examined closely.

GENERAL RULES: CODE §§ 162 AND 212

Two provisions in the Code provide the authority for the deduction of most expenses: § 162 concerning trade or business expenses and § 212 relating to expenses for the production of income. Numerous other provisions of the Code pertain to deductions. These other provisions, however, normally build on the basic rules contained in §§ 162 and 212. For this reason, the importance of these two provisions cannot be overstated.

---

3   *New Colonial Ice Co. v. Helvering*, 4 USTC ¶1292, 13 AFTR 1180, 292 U.S. 435 (USSC, 1934).

Section 162(a) on trade or business expenses reads, in part, as follows:

> In General.—There shall be allowed as a deduction all the ordinary and necessary expenses paid or incurred during the taxable year in carrying on any trade or business, including—
>
> 1) a reasonable allowance for salaries or other compensation for personal services actually rendered;
> 2) traveling expenses (including amounts expended for meals and lodging other than amounts which are lavish or extravagant under the circumstances) while away from home in the pursuit of a trade or business;
> 3) rentals or other payments required to be made as a condition to the continued use or possession, for purposes of the trade or business, of property to which the taxpayer has not taken or is not taking title or in which he has no equity.

Although § 162(a) specifically enumerates three items that are deductible, the provision's primary importance lies in its general rule: ordinary and necessary expenses of carrying on a trade or business are deductible.

Section 212 contains a general rule very similar to that found in § 162. Section 212, in part, reads as follows:

> In the case of an individual, there shall be allowed as a deduction all the ordinary and necessary expenses paid or incurred during the taxable year—
>
> 1) for the production or collection of income;
> 2) for the management, conservation, or maintenance of property held for the production of income . . .

Production of income expenses are normally those related to investments, such as investment advisory fees and safe deposit box rentals.

An examination of the language of §§ 162 and 212 indicates that a deduction is allowed under either section if it meets *four* critical requirements. The expense must have all of the following properties:

1. It must be related to carrying on a trade or business or an income-producing activity.

2. It must be ordinary and necessary.

3. It must be reasonable.

4. It must be paid or incurred during the taxable year.

It should be emphasized, however, that satisfaction of these criteria does not ensure deductibility. Other provisions in the Code often operate to prohibit or limit a deduction otherwise granted by §§ 162 and 212. For example, an expense may be ordinary, necessary, and related to carrying on a business, but if it is also related to producing tax-exempt income, § 265 prohibits a deduction. This system of allowing, yet disallowing, deductions is a basic feature in the statutory scheme for determining deductibility.

RELATED TO CARRYING ON A BUSINESS OR AN INCOME-PRODUCING ACTIVITY

The Activity. Whether an expense is deductible depends in part on the type of activity in which it was incurred. A deduction is authorized by § 162 only if it is paid or incurred in an activity that constitutes a trade or business. Similarly, § 212 permits a deduction only if it is paid or incurred in an activity for the production or collection of income. The purpose of each of these requirements is to deny deductions for expenses incurred in an activity that is *primarily personal* in nature. For example, the costs incurred

in pursuing what is merely a hobby, such as collecting antiques or racing automobiles, normally would be considered nondeductible personal expenditures. Of course, this assumes that such activities do not constitute a trade or business.

The Code does not provide any clues as to when an activity will be considered a trade or business or an income-producing activity rather than a personal activity. Over the years, however, one criterion has emerged from the many court cases involving the issue. To constitute a trade or business or an income-producing activity, the activity must be *entered into for profit*.[4] In other words, for the taxpayer's expenses to be deductible, they must be motivated by his or her hope for a profit. For this reason, taxpayers who collect antiques or race automobiles can deduct all of the related expenses if they are able to demonstrate that they did so with the hope of producing income. In such case, they would be considered to be in a trade or business. If the required profit motive is lacking, however, expenses of the activity generally are not deductible except to the extent the activity has income.

As may be apparent, the critical question in this area is what inspired the taxpayer's activities. The factors to be used in evaluating the taxpayer's motivation, along with the special provisions governing activities that are not engaged in for profit—the so-called hobby loss rules—are considered in detail later in this chapter.

A profit motive is the only requirement necessary to establish existence of an *income-producing* activity. However, the courts have imposed an additional requirement before an activity qualifies as a *trade or business*. Business status requires both a profit motive and a sufficient degree of taxpayer involvement in the activity to distinguish the activity from a passive investment. No clear guidelines have emerged indicating when a taxpayer's activities rise to the level of carrying on a business. The courts, however, generally have permitted business treatment where the taxpayer has devoted a major portion of time to the activities or the activities have been regular or continuous.[5]

> **Example 1.** C owns six rental units, including several condominiums and townhouses. He manages his rental properties entirely by himself. His managing activities include seeking new tenants, supplying furnishings, cleaning and preparing the units for occupancy, advertising, and bookkeeping. In this case, C's involvement with the rental activities is sufficiently continuous and systematic to constitute a business.[6] If the rental activities were of a more limited nature, they might not qualify as a trade or business. The determination ultimately depends on the facts of the particular situation.[7]

> **Example 2.** H owns various stocks and bonds. Her managerial activities related to these securities consist primarily of maintaining records and collecting dividends and interest. She rarely trades in the market. These activities are those normally associated with a passive investor, and accordingly would not constitute a trade or business under § 162 (they would be considered an income-producing activity under § 212).[8] On the other hand, if H had a substantial volume of transactions, made personal investigations of the corporations in which she was interested in purchasing, and devoted virtually every day to such work, her activities could constitute a trade or business.[9] Again, however, the answer depends on the facts.

---

[4]   *Doggett v. Burrett*, 3 USTC ¶1090, 12 AFTR 505, 65 F.2d 192 (CA-D.C., 1933).

[5]   *Grier v. U.S.*, 55-1 USTC ¶9184, 46 AFTR 1536, 218 F.2d. 603 (CA-2, 1955).

[6]   *Edwin R. Curphey*, 73 T.C. 766 (1980).

[7]   *Ibid.*

[8]   *Higgins v. Comm.*, 41-1 USTC ¶9233, 25 AFTR 1160, 312 U.S. 212 (UCSC, 1941).

[9]   *Samuel B. Levin v. U.S.*, 79-1 USTC ¶9331, 43 AFTR2d 79-1057, 597 F.2d 760 (Ct. Cls., 1979). But see *Joseph Moller v. U.S.*, 83-2 USTC ¶9698, 52 AFTR2d 83-633 (CA-FC, 1983) where, for purposes of the home office deduction, the court held that the taxpayer's management of his substantial investment portfolio could not be a trade or business regardless of how continuous, regular, and extensive the activities were. But see Chapter 16 and discussion of traders in securities and § 475(f)

Distinguishing between §§ 162 and 212. Prior to enactment of § 212, many investment-related expenses were not deductible because the activities did not constitute a business. The enactment of § 212 in 1942, allowing for the deduction of expenses related to production or collection of income, enabled the deduction of investment-oriented expenses. This expansion of the deduction concept to include so-called nonbusiness or investment-related expenses eliminates the need for an activity to constitute a business before a deduction is allowed. As a result, the issue of deductibility (*assuming* the other requirements are met) is effectively reduced to a single important question: Is the expense related to an activity engaged in for profit?

It may appear that the addition of § 212 completely removed the need for determining whether the activity resulting in the expense constitutes a business or is merely for the production of income. However, the distinction between business and production of income expenses remains important. For example, the classification of the expense as a deduction for or from adjusted gross income may turn on whether the expense is a trade or business expense or a production of income expense. Production of income expenses (other than those related to rents or royalties) are usually miscellaneous itemized deductions that can be deducted only to the extent they *exceed* two percent of adjusted gross income. In contrast, most business expenses are deductions for adjusted gross income and are deductible in full.

> **Example 3.** Refer to *Example 2*. In the first situation, where H is considered a passive investor, her investment related expenses (e.g., subscriptions to stock advisory services and investment newsletters) would be miscellaneous itemized deductions and deductible only to the extent they exceed 2% of adjusted gross income. In the second situation, however, the same type of expenses would be deductions for adjusted gross income since H's trading activities qualify as a trade or business.

Another reason for ascertaining whether the activity constitutes a business relates to the use of the phrase "trade or business" in other Code Sections. The phrase "trade or business" appears in at least 60 different Code Sections, and the interpretation given to this phrase often controls the tax treatment. For example, whether an activity is an active business or a passive investment affects the tax consequences related to losses (deductible or limited), bad debts (short-term capital loss versus ordinary loss), property sales (capital gain or loss versus ordinary gain or loss), expenses for offices in the home (deductible versus nondeductible), and limited expensing of depreciable property (allowed versus disallowed).[10]

The Relationship. Before an expense is deductible under §§ 162 or 212, it must have a certain relationship to the trade or business or income-producing activity. The Regulations require that business expenses be directly connected with or pertain to the taxpayer's trade or business.[11] Similarly, production of income expenses must bear a reasonable and proximate relationship to the income-producing activity.[12] Whether an expenditure is directly related to the taxpayer's trade or business or income-producing activity usually depends on the facts. For example, the required relationship for business expenses normally exists where the expense is primarily motivated by business concerns or arises as a result of business, rather than personal, needs.[13]

---

[10] See §§ 165, 166, 1221, 280A, and 179.

[11] Reg. § 1.162-1(a).

[12] Reg. § 1.212-1(d).

[13] *U.S. v. Gilmore*, 63-1 USTC ¶9285, 11 AFTR2d 758, 372 U.S. 39 (USSC, 1963).

Example 4. While driving from one business to another, T struck a pedestrian with his car. He paid and deducted legal fees and damages in connection with the accident that were disallowed by the IRS. The Court found that the expenses were not directly related to, nor did they proximately result from, the taxpayer's business. The accident was merely incidental to the transportation and was related only remotely to the business.[14]

Whether a particular item is deductible often hinges on whether the expense was incurred for business or personal purposes. Consider the case of a law enforcement officer who is required to keep in top shape to retain his employment. Is the cost of a health club membership incurred for business or personal purposes? Similarly, can a disc jockey who obtains dentures to improve his speech deduct the cost as a business expense? Unfortunately, many expenses—like these—straddle the business-personal fence and the final determination is difficult. In both of the cases above, the Court denied the taxpayers' deductions on the theory that such expenses were inherently personal.

Another common question concerns expenses paid or incurred prior to the time that income is earned. In the case of § 212 expenses, it is not essential that the activity produce income currently. For example, expenses may be deductible under § 212 even though there is little likelihood that the property will be sold at a profit or will ever produce income.[15] Deductions are allowed as long as the transaction was entered into for profit.

Example 5. B purchased a vacant lot three years ago as an investment. During the current year she paid $200 to have it mowed. Although the property is not currently producing income, the expense is deductible since it is for the conservation or maintenance of property held for the production of income.

ORDINARY AND NECESSARY EXPENSES

The second test for deductibility is whether the expense is ordinary and necessary. An expense is *ordinary* if it is normally incurred in the type of business in which the taxpayer is involved.[16] This is not to say that the expense is habitual or recurring.[17] In fact, the expense may be incurred only once in the taxpayer's lifetime and be considered ordinary. The test is whether other taxpayers in similar businesses or income-producing activities would customarily incur the same expense.

Example 6. P has been in the newspaper business for 35 years. Until this year, his paper had never been sued for libel. To protect the reputation of the newspaper, P incurred substantial legal costs related to the libel suit. Although the taxpayer has never incurred legal expenses of this nature before, the expenses are ordinary since it is common in the newspaper business to incur legal expenses to defend against such attacks.[18]

---

[14]   *Julian D. Freedman v. Comm.*, 62-1 USTC ¶9400, 9 AFTR2d 1235, 301 F.2d. 359 (CA-5, 1962); but see *Harold Dancer*, 73 T.C. 1103 (1980), where the Tax Court allowed the deduction when the taxpayer was traveling between two locations of the *same* business. Note how the subtle change in facts substantially alters the result!

[15]   Reg. § 1.212-1(b).

[16]   *Deputy v. DuPont*, 40-1 USTC ¶9161, 23 AFTR 808, 308 U.S. 488 (USSC, 1940).

[17]   *Dunn and McCarthy, Inc. v. Comm.*, 43-2 USTC ¶9688, 31 AFTR 1043, 139 F.2d 242 (CA-2, 1943).

[18]   *Welch v. Helvering*, 3 USTC ¶1164, 12 AFTR 1456, 290 U.S. 111 (USSC, 1933).

It is interesting to note that the "ordinary" criterion normally becomes an issue in circumstances that are, in fact, unusual. For example, in *Goedel*,[19] a stock dealer paid premiums for insurance on the life of the President of the United States, fearing that his death would disrupt the stock market and his business. The Court denied the deduction on the grounds that the payment was not ordinary but unusual or extraordinary.

A deductible expense must be not only ordinary, but also *necessary*. An expense is necessary if it is appropriate, helpful, or capable of making a contribution to the taxpayer's profit-seeking activities.[20] The necessary criterion, however, is rarely applied to deny a deduction. The courts have refrained from such a practice since to do so would require overriding the judgment of the taxpayer.[21] The courts apparently feel that it would be unfair to judge *currently* whether a previous expenditure was necessary at the time it was incurred.

It should be emphasized that not all necessary expenses are ordinary expenses. Some expenses may be appropriate and helpful to the taxpayer's business but may not be normally incurred in that particular business. In such case, no deduction is allowed.

> **Example 7.** W was an officer in his father's corporation. The corporation, unable to pay its debts, was adjudged bankrupt. After the corporation was discharged from its debts, W decided to resume his father's business on a fresh basis. To reestablish relations with old customers and to solidify his credit standing, W paid as much of the old debts as he could. The Supreme Court held that the expenses were necessary in the sense that they were appropriate and helpful in the development of W's business. However, the Court ruled that the payments were not ordinary because people do not usually pay the debts of another.[22]

REASONABLE EXPENSES

The third requirement for a deduction is that the expense be reasonable in amount. An examination of § 162(a) reveals that the term "reasonable" is used only in conjunction with compensation paid for services (e.g., a reasonable allowance for salaries). The courts have held, however, that reasonableness is implied in the phrase "ordinary and necessary."[23] In practice, the reasonableness standard is most often applied in situations involving salary payments made by a closely held corporation to a shareholder who also is an employee. In these situations, if the compensation paid exceeds that ordinarily paid for similar services—that which is reasonable—the excessive payment may represent a nondeductible dividend distribution.[24] Dividend treatment of the excess occurs if the amount of the excessive payment received by each employee closely relates to the number of shares of stock owned.[25] The distinction between reasonable compensation and dividend is critical because characterization of the payment as a dividend results in double taxation (i.e., it is taxable to the shareholder-employee and not deductible by the corporation).

---

[19] 39 B.T.A. 1 (1939).

[20] *Supra*, Footnote 18. See also *Comm. v. Heininger*, 44-1 USTC ¶9109, 31 AFTR 783, 320 U.S. 467 (USSC, 1943).

[21] *Supra*, Footnote 18.

[22] *Supra*, Footnote 18.

[23] *Comm. v. Lincoln Electric Co.*, 49-2 USTC ¶9388, 38 AFTR 411, 176 F.2d 815 (CA-6, 1949).

[24] Reg. § 1.162-7(b)(1).

[25] Reg. § 1.162-8.

Example 8. B and C own 70 and 30% of XYZ Corporation, respectively. Employees in positions similar to that of B earn $60,000 annually while those in positions similar to C's earn $20,000. During the year, the corporation pays B a salary of $130,000 and C a salary of $50,000. The excessive payment of $100,000 [($130,000 + $50,000) − ($60,000 + $20,000)] is received by B and C in direct proportion to their percentage ownership of stock (i.e., B's salary increased by $70,000 or 70% of the excessive payment). Because the payments are in excess of that normally paid to employees in similar positions and the excessive payment received by each is closely related to his stockholdings, the excessive payment may be treated as a nondeductible dividend.

Some of the factors used by the IRS when considering the reasonableness of compensation are:[26]

1. Duties performed (i.e., amount and character of responsibility)

2. Volume and complexity of business handled (i.e., time required)

3. Individual's ability and expertise

4. Number of available persons capable of performing the duties of the position

5. Corporation's dividend policies and history

PAID OR INCURRED DURING THE TAXABLE YEAR

Sections 162 and 212 both indicate that an expense is allowable as a deduction only if it is "paid or incurred during the taxable year." This phrase is used throughout the Code in sections concerning deductions. Use of both terms, "paid" and "incurred," is necessary because the year in which deductions are allowable depends on the method of accounting used by the taxpayer.[27] The term *paid* refers to taxpayers using the cash basis method of accounting while the term *incurred* refers to taxpayers using the accrual basis method of accounting. Accordingly, the year in which a deduction is allowed usually depends on whether the cash or accrual basis method of accounting is used. Each of these methods is discussed in detail in a later section.

EMPLOYEE BUSINESS EXPENSES

The definition of *trade or business* also includes the performance of services as an employee. In other words, an employee is considered to be in the business of being an employee. [28] As a result, the ordinary and necessary expenses incurred by an employee in connection with his or her employment are deductible under § 162 as business expenses. Examples of deductible expenses typically incurred by employees include union dues, dues to trade and professional societies, subscriptions to professional journals, small tools and supplies, medical exams required by the employer, and work clothes and uniforms as well as their maintenance (where required as a condition of employment and not suitable for everyday use).[29] Expenses such as travel, entertainment, and education may also be deducted as employee business expenses under certain conditions explained in Chapter 8.

---

[26] Internal Revenue Manual 4233, § 232.

[27] § 461(a).

[28] See *Lloyd U. Noland, Jr. v. Comm.* 59-2 USTC ¶9600, 4 AFTR 2d 5031, 269 F2d 108, (CA-4, 1959) holding that "every person who works for compensation is engaged in the business of earning his pay, and that expense which is essential to the continuance of his employment is deductible..."

[29] Rev. Rul. 70-474, 1970 C.B. 35.

As explained later in this chapter, employee business expenses—other than those that are reimbursed—are considered miscellaneous itemized deductions and thus are deductible only to the extent they exceed 2 percent of A.G.I.

ACCOUNTING FOR DEDUCTIONS

Identifying the taxable year in which a taxpayer can claim a deduction is extremely important for a number of reasons. No doubt the most important of these is the time value of money. Taxpayers normally want to claim their deductions and obtain the accompanying tax savings as soon as possible. In contrast, the government is concerned about zealous taxpayers who, in its view, prematurely deduct their expenses. When an expense is deductible generally depends on whether the taxpayer uses the cash or accrual method of accounting. However, the natural friction between taxpayers and the government over when an expense should be deducted has led to a somewhat confusingly intricate set of rules filled with exceptions. Interestingly, the effects of the various exceptions often make the accrual method look like the cash method and vice versa.

CASH METHOD OF ACCOUNTING

General Rule. For those taxpayers eligible to use the cash method (as discussed in Chapter 5), expenses are deductible in the taxable year when the expenses are actually paid.[30] However, there are numerous exceptions to this rule that are designed to restrict the flexibility a cash basis taxpayer would otherwise have in reporting deductions. Without these restrictions, a cash basis taxpayer could choose the year of deductibility simply by appropriately timing the cash payment. Before examining these restrictions, it is important to understand when the taxpayer is considered to have paid the expense.

Time of Payment. Determining when a cash basis taxpayer has paid an expense usually is not difficult. A cash basis taxpayer "pays" the expense when cash, check, property, or service is transferred. Neither a promise to pay nor a note evidencing such promise is considered payment. Consequently, when a cash basis taxpayer buys on credit, no deduction is allowed until the debts are paid. However, if the taxpayer borrows cash and then pays the expense, the expense is deductible when paid. For this reason, a taxpayer who charges expenses to a credit card is deemed to have borrowed cash and made payment when the charge is made. Thus, the deduction is claimed when the charge is actually made and not when the bank makes payment or when the taxpayer pays the bill.[31] If the taxpayer uses a "pay-by-phone" account, the expense is deductible in the year the financial institution paid the amount as reported on a monthly statement sent to the taxpayer.[32] When the taxpayer pays by mail, payment is usually considered made when the mailing occurs (i.e., dropping it in the post-office box).[33]

Restrictions on Use of Cash Method. Under the general rule, a cash basis taxpayer deducts expenses when paid. Without restrictions, however, aggressive taxpayers could liberally interpret this provision to authorize not only deductions for routine items, but also deductions for capital expenditures and other expenses that benefit future periods (e.g., supplies, prepaid insurance, prepaid rent, and prepaid interest). To preclude such an approach, numerous limitations have been imposed.

---

[30] Reg. § 1.446-1(a)(1).

[31] Rev. Rul. 78-39, 1978-1 C.B. 73.

[32] Rev. Rul. 80-335, 1980-2 C.B. 170.

[33] See Rev. Rul. 73-99, 1973-1 C.B. 412 for clarification of this general rule.

Inventories. One of the more fundamental restrictions applying to cash basis taxpayers concerns inventories. For example, if no limitation existed, a cash basis owner of a department store could easily reduce or eliminate taxable income by increasing purchases of inventory near year-end and deducting their cost. To prevent this possibility, the Regulations require taxpayers to use the accrual method for computing sales and costs of goods sold if inventories are an income-producing factor.[34] In such cases, inventory costs must be capitalized, and accounts receivable and accounts payable (with respect to cost of goods sold) must be created. The taxpayer could continue to use the cash method for other transactions, however. It is also important to note that there are two relief provisions for small business owners that allow them to elect out of the accrual method and the requirement to account for inventories. As discussed in Chapter 10, taxpayers with average gross receipts of no more than $1 million, and certain taxpayers with average annual gross receipts of more than $1 million and up to $10 million may use the cash method of accounting even when inventory is an income producing factor.[35]

Capital Expenditures. Provisions of both the Code and the Regulations limit the potential for deducting capital expenditures. As discussed later in this chapter, Code § 263 specifically denies the deduction for a capital expenditure; such costs as those for equipment, vehicles, and buildings normally are recovered through depreciation, as discussed in Chapter 9. Special rules exist requiring taxpayers to capitalize certain costs as part of their inventory under the uniform capitalization rules of § 263A. The "unicap" rules are discussed in Chapter 10.

The Regulations—at least broadly—deal with other expenditures that are not capital expenditures per se but that do benefit future periods. According to the Regulations, any expenditure resulting "in the creation of an asset having a useful life which extends *substantially beyond the close of the taxable year* may not be deductible when made, or may be deductible only in part."[36] In this regard, the courts agree that "substantially beyond" means a useful life of more than one year.[37] Perhaps the simplest example of this rule as so interpreted concerns payments for supplies. Assuming the supplies would be exhausted before the close of the following tax year, a deduction should be allowable when payment is made.

Prepaid Expenses in General. One of the most troublesome issues related to both the cash and accrual methods of accounting concerns prepaid expenses. If prepayments are made for regularly recurring expenses and the payments result in the creation of an asset having a life extending substantially beyond the taxable year of payment, the treatment historically has not always been clear. Unfortunately, the *one-year rule* described above was not necessarily applied to all expenses uniformly.

12-Month Rule. The problems with prepaid expenses became acutely apparent in *U.S. Freightways Corporation.*[38] Here an accrual basis calendar-year trucking company claimed a deduction for permits, licenses and fees paid in order for its trucks to operate legally in certain locations. In 1993, the company paid $4,308,460 for licenses, many of which expired in 1994 rather than 1993. Similarly, in 1993, the company paid premiums of $1,090,602 for liability and property insurance for the 1-year period from July 1, 1993, to June 30, 1994. Relying on the one-year rule, the corporation expensed all of the prepayments. However, the government denied the deduction, asserting that the 12-month

---

[34]   Reg. § 1.446-1(c)(2).

[35]   Rev. Proc. 2000-22, Rev. Proc. 2001-10, and Rev. Proc. 2002-28. See full discussion of inventory in Chapter 10.

[36]   Reg. § 1.446-1(a)(1).

[37]   *Martin J. Zaninovich*, 69 T.C. 605, rev'd in 80-1 USTC ¶9342, 45 AFTR2d 80-1442, 616 F.2d 429 (CA-9, 1980).

[38]   2001-2 USTC 50,731, 88 AFTR2d 2001-6703, 270 F3d 1137 (CA-7, 2001)).

rule existed solely for cash basis taxpayers and did not apply to accrual basis taxpayers. The Seventh Circuit disagreed and extended the rule to accrual basis taxpayers.

To address the confusion resulting from *U.S. Freightways* and similar cases, the government issued Regulations in early in 2004 to address the capitalization of intangibles.[39] Among these lengthy provisions is the government's own 12-month rule. Under these Regulations, taxpayers—both cash and accrual—are entitled to claim an immediate deduction for prepaid expenses (e.g. prepaid insurance) if the rights or benefits do not extend beyond the earlier of

- 12 months after the first date on which the taxpayer realizes the benefit or
- The end of the taxable year following the year in which payment was made

This rule generally is consistent with prior law that enables cash basis taxpayer to claim deductions for prepaid expenses for supplies, service and other non-capital expenditures. It should be emphasized that the rule applies to both cash and accrual taxpayers. However, as discussed below, accrual taxpayers must meet the all events and economic performance tests before a deduction can be claimed. Specific items are discussed below.

Prepaid Insurance and Prepaid Rent. Prepayments of insurance and rent follow the 12-month rule. If the 12-month rule does not apply, the prepayment must be amortized over the term for which the insurance is provided or the term of the lease.[40]

> **Example 9.** On December 1, 2009, Blue Inc., a cash basis taxpayer, paid a $12,000 insurance premium to obtain a property insurance policy with a one-year term that begins on February 1, 2010. Although the policy is only for one year, the payment does not meet the 12-month rule since the benefit attributable to the $12,000 payment extends beyond the end of the taxable year following the taxable year in which the payment was made. The corporation must capitalize the payment and amortize it over the policy period. Thus the corporation's deduction is $0 in 2009, $11,000 in 2010 and $1,000 in 2011.

> **Example 10.** Same facts as above except the policy has a term beginning on December 15, 2009. The 12-month rule applies since the benefit does not extend more than 12 months beyond December 15, 2009 (the date when the benefit is first realized by the corporation) nor beyond the close of the tax year following the year in which the payment was made (December 31, 2010). Thus the corporation may deduct the entire $12,000 prepayment in the year paid, 2009.

> **Example 11.** WRK Corporation, a cash basis taxpayer, leases space at a monthly rate of $2,000. In December of 2009, the corporation prepays its rent for the first six months of 2009 in the amount of $12,000. The corporation may deduct the entire $12,000 in 2010 since the benefits received for the prepayment do not extend beyond 12 months. (Note as discussed below accrual basis taxpayers would be required to amortize this expense over the term because the economic performance test delays deduction until the property is used.)

Other Prepayments. Perhaps the Service's current view of the proper treatment of most prepayments is best captured in a ruling concerning prepaid feed. In this ruling, the taxpayer purchased a substantial amount of feed prior to the year in which it would be used.[41] The purchase was made in advance because the price was low due to a depressed market.

---

[39]   Reg. § 1.263-(a)(4).

[40]   See Reg. 1.263(a)-4(f)(8), Examples 1, 2 and 10.

[41]   Rev. Rul. 79-229, 1979-2 C.B. 210. See also, *Kenneth Van Raden*, 71 T.C. 1083 (1979), aff'd in 81-2 USTC ¶9547, 48 AFTR2d 81-5607, 650 F.2d 1046 (CA-9, 1981).

The IRS granted a deduction for the prepayment because there was a business purpose for the advanced payment, the payment was not merely a deposit, and it did not materially distort income. Based on this ruling and related cases, prepayments normally should be deductible if the asset will be consumed by the close of the following year, there is a business purpose for the expenditure, and there is no material distortion of income.

Prepaid Interest. The Code expressly denies the deduction of prepaid interest. Prepaid interest must be capitalized and deducted ratably over the period of the loan.[42] The same is true for any costs associated with obtaining the loan. The sole exception is for "points" paid for a debt incurred by the taxpayer to purchase his or her *principal* residence. In this regard, the IRS has ruled that points incurred to refinance a home must be amortized over the term of the loan.[43] However, an Appeals Court case allowed a taxpayer to deduct the amount of points paid on refinancing a home. The proceeds were used to pay off a three-year, temporary loan that was made to allow the borrower time to secure permanent financing for the home.[44] The court stated that, since the temporary loan was merely an integrated step in securing permanent financing for the taxpayer's residence, the points were deductible currently.

> **Example 12.** K desires to obtain financing for the purchase of a new house costing $100,000. The bank agrees to make her a loan of 80% of the purchase price, or $80,000 (80% of $100,000) for thirty years at a cost of two points (two percentage "points" of the loan obtained). Thus, she must pay $1,600 (2% of $80,000) to obtain the loan. Assuming it is established business practice in her area to charge points in consideration of the loan, the $1,600 in points (prepaid interest) is deductible. However, if the house is not the principal residence of the taxpayer, then the prepaid interest must be deducted ratably over the 30-year loan period.

ACCRUAL METHOD OF ACCOUNTING

An accrual basis taxpayer deducts expenses when they are incurred. For this purpose, an expense is considered incurred when the all events test is satisfied and economic performance has occurred.[45]

All Events Test. Two requirements must be met under the all-events test: (1) all events establishing the existence of a liability must have occurred (i.e., the liability is fixed); and (2) the amount of the liability can be determined with reasonable accuracy. Therefore, before the liability may be accrued and deducted it must be fixed and determinable.

> **Example 13.** In *Hughes Properties, Inc.*, an accrual basis corporation owned a gambling casino in Reno, Nevada that operated progressive slot machines that paid a large jackpot about every four months.[46] The increasing amount of the jackpot was maintained and shown by a meter. Under state gaming regulations, the jackpot amount could not be turned back until the amount had been paid to a winner. In addition, the corporation had to maintain a cash reserve sufficient to pay all the guaranteed amounts. At the end of each taxable year, the corporation accrued and deducted the liability for the jackpot as accrued at year-end. The IRS challenged the accrual,

---

[42]   § 461(g).

[43]   Rev. Rul. 87-22, 1987-1 C.B. 146. See also Rev. Proc. 94-27, 1994-1 I.R.B. 15.

[44]   *James R. Huntsman*, 90-2 USTC ¶50,340, 66 AFTR2d 90-5020, 905 F.2d 1182 (CA-8, 1990). In an *Action on Decision* issued on February 11, 1991, the IRS ruled that although it will not appeal the *Huntsman* decision, it will not follow this decision outside the Eighth Circuit.

[45]   § 461(h).

[46]   *Hughes Properties, Inc.*, 86-1 USTC ¶9440, 58 AFTR2d 86-5015, 106 S. Ct. 2092 (USSC, 1986).

alleging that the all events test had not been met, and that the amount should be deducted only when paid. It argued that payment of the jackpot was not fixed but contingent, since it was possible that the winning combination may never be pulled. Moreover, the Service pointed out the potential for tax avoidance: the corporation was accruing deductions for payments that may be paid far in the future, and thus—given the time value of money—overstated the amount of the deduction. The Supreme Court rejected these arguments, stating that the probability of payment was not a remote and speculative possibility. The Court noted that not only was the liability fixed under state law, but it also was not in the interest of the taxpayer to set unreasonably high odds, since customers would refuse to play and would gamble elsewhere.

The all events test often operates to deny deductions for certain estimated expenditures properly accruable for financial accounting purposes. For example, the estimated cost of product guarantees, warranties, and contingent liabilities normally may not be deducted—presumably because the liability for such items has not been fixed or no reasonable estimate of the amount can be made.[47] However, the courts have authorized deductions for estimates where the obligation was certain and there was a reasonable basis (e.g., industry experience) for determining the amount of the liability.

Economic Performance Test. The condition requiring *economic performance* was introduced in 1984 due to Congressional fear that the all events test did not prohibit so-called premature accruals. Prior to 1984, the courts—with increasing frequency—had permitted taxpayers to accrue and deduct the cost of estimated expenditures required to perform certain activities *prior* to the period when the activities were actually performed. For example, in one case, a strip-mining operator deducted the estimated cost of backfilling land that he had mined for coal.[48] The court allowed the deduction for the estimated expenses in the current year even though the back filling was not started and completed until the following year. According to the court, the liability satisfied the all-events test since the taxpayer was required by law to backfill the land and a reasonable estimate of the cost of the work could be made. A similar decision involved a taxpayer that was a self-insurer of its liabilities arising from claims under state and Federal worker's compensation laws.[49] Under these laws, the taxpayer was obligated to pay a claimant's medical bills, disability payments, and death benefits. In this situation, the taxpayer was allowed to accrue and deduct the estimated expenses for its obligations even though actual payments would extend over many years. In Congress' view, allowing the deduction in these and similar cases prior to the time when the taxpayer actually performed the services, provided the goods, or paid the expenses, overstated the true cost of the expense, because the time value of money was ignored. Perhaps more importantly, Congress recognized that allowing deductions for accruals in this manner had become the foundation for many tax shelter arrangements. Accordingly, the economic performance test was designed to defer the taxpayer's deduction until the activities giving rise to the liability are performed.

The time at which economic performance is deemed to occur—and hence the period in which the deduction may be claimed—depends on the nature of the item producing the liability. A taxpayer's liabilities commonly arise in three ways, as summarized below.

1. *Liability of Taxpayer to Provide Property and Services.* When the taxpayer's liability results from an obligation to provide goods or services to a third party (e.g., perform repairs), economic performance occurs when the taxpayer provides the goods or services to the third party.

---

47 *Bell Electric Co.*, 45 T.C. 158 (1965).

48 *Paul Harrold v. Comm.*, 52-1 USTC ¶9107, 41 AFTR 442, 192 F.2d 1002 (CA-4, 1951).

49 *Crescent Wharf & Warehouse Co. v. Comm.*, 75-2 USTC ¶9571, 36 AFTR2d 75-5246, 518 F.2d 772 (CA-5, 1975).

2. *Liability for Property or Services Provided to the Taxpayer.* When the taxpayer's liability arises from an obligation to pay for services, goods, or the use of property provided to (or to be provided to) the taxpayer (e.g., consulting, supplies, and rent), economic performance occurs when the taxpayer receives the services or goods or uses the property. Note that in this case, economic performance occurs when the taxpayer *receives* the consideration bargained for, while in the situation above it occurs when the taxpayer *provides* the consideration. Under a special rule, a taxpayer may treat services or property as being provided when the taxpayer makes *payment* to the person providing the services or property *if* the taxpayer can reasonably expect the person to provide the services or property within 3½ months after the date of payment.[50]

3. *Liabilities for which Payment Represents Economic Performance.* There are a number of liabilities for which economic performance is deemed to occur only when the taxpayer actually makes payment. This rule for so-called "payment liabilities" effectively places the taxpayer on the cash basis for these liabilities. These include the following:

- Refunds and rebates
- Awards, prizes, and jackpots
- Premiums on insurance
- Provision of work to the taxpayer under warranty or service contracts
- Taxes
- Liabilities arising under a worker's compensation act or out of any tort, breach of contract, or violation of law, including amounts paid in settlement of such claims

Example 14. In 2009 C, an accrual basis corporation, contracted with P, a partnership, to drill 50 gas wells over a five-year period for $500,000. Absent the economic performance test, C could accrue and deduct the $500,000 fee in 2009 because the obligation is fixed and determinable. However, because economic performance has not occurred (i.e., the services have not been received by C), no deduction is permitted in 2009. Rather, C may deduct the expense when the wells are drilled.

Example 15. Same facts as above. Although P is obligated to perform services for C for $500,000 over the five-year period (i.e., the obligation is fixed and determinable), P cannot prematurely accrue the cost of providing these services because economic performance has not occurred. Deduction is permitted only as the wells are drilled.

Example 16. C Corporation, a calendar year, accrual method taxpayer, owns several casinos across the country. Each contains progressive slot machines. These machines provide a guaranteed jackpot that increases as money is gambled through the machine until the jackpot is won or until a maximum predetermined amount is reached. On July 1, 2009, the guaranteed jackpot amount on one of C's slot machines reaches the maximum predetermined amount of $100,000. On February 1, 2010, the $100,000 jackpot is won by B. Although the all-events test is met in 2009 when the amount of the liability becomes fixed (i.e., guaranteed) and determinable, economic performance does not occur for prizes until payment is actually made. As a result, C is not allowed to accrue the deduction in 2009 but must wait and claim the expense when it pays the jackpot in 2010. (Note this rule reverses the decision in *Hughes Properties, Inc.* However, the deduction may still be allowed under the recurring item exception discussed below.)

---

[50] § 1.461-4(d)(6)(ii).

Note that even though payment of an expense may make it ripe for accrual, other rules may require deferral of the deduction.

Example 17. On December 10, 2009, T Inc., an accrual basis calendar year taxpayer, paid a painting contractor $15,000 to paint the interior of its office building. T anticipated that the painting would be completed by February 15 of 2010. Since the painting services are to be provided within 3 ½ months after the date of payment, economic performance is deemed to have occurred when the payment is made and T may deduct the $15,000 expense in 2009.

Example 18. Kidco Products Corporation, a calendar year E accrual method taxpayer, manufactures car seats for children. On July 1, 2009 it purchased an insurance policy from INS Inc. for $360,000 under which INS must satisfy any liability arising during the next three years for any claims attributable to defects in the manufacturing. Although economic performance occurs when Kidco pays the premium, it has created an asset with a life that extends substantially beyond 2009. Under cash-basis principles, such expenses cannot be deducted currently but must be amortized. Consequently, Kidco should amortize the insurance premium over the term of the policy, deducting $60,000 ($360,000/36 × 6 months) in 2009 and the remaining $300,000 over the next 30 months.

Example 19. WNDE Corporation leases space at a monthly rate of $2,000. In December of 2009, the corporation prepays its rent for the first six months of 2010 in the amount of $12,000. If WNDE is a cash basis taxpayer, it could deduct the $12,000 in 2009 under the 12-month rule *(See Example 10 above)*. However, if WNDE uses the accrual method, economic performance for the rent does not occur until the corporation uses the property and, therefore, it cannot use the 12 month rule but must deduct the rental expense over the period it uses the property, 2010.

Economic Performance and Recurring Item Exception. To prohibit the disruption of normal business and accounting practices, certain recurring expenses are exempted from the economic performance rules. The expense may be accrued and deducted under the recurring item exception if all of the following conditions are met.[51]

1. The all-events test is satisfied.

2. Economic performance does in fact occur within eight and one-half months after the close of the taxable year or the filing of the return if earlier.

3. The item is recurring in nature, and the taxpayer consistently treats such items as incurred in the taxable year.

4. The item is immaterial or accrual in the earlier year results in a better match against income than accruing the item when economic performance occurs.

The recurring item exception does not apply to liabilities arising under a worker's compensation act or out of any tort, breach of contract, or violation of law.

Example 20. M Corporation, a calendar year, accrual method taxpayer, manufactures and sells automobile mufflers. Under the terms of an agreement with D Corporation, one of its distributors, D is entitled to a discount on future purchases (i.e., a rebate) from M based on the amount of purchases made by D from M during any calendar year. During 2009, purchases by D entitled it to future rebates of $20,000. M paid

---

[51] § 461(h)(3).

$12,000 of the rebate in January 2010 and the remaining $8,000 in October 2010. M filed its 2009 tax return on March 15, 2010. Although the all events test has been met in 2009 (i.e., the fact of the liability is fixed and the amount can be determined with reasonable accuracy), no deduction is allowed until economic performance occurs. Normally, economic performance for rebates is deemed to occur when the rebate is paid. Therefore, the expense would usually be deductible by M in 2010. However, under the recurring item exception M should be able to accrue $12,000 of the $20,000 in 2009 because all of the conditions are met: (1) the all events test is met, (2) economic performance occurs in a timely manner (i.e., the January payment occurs before the earlier of the filing of the tax return or 8½ months after the close of the year), (3) the item is recurring, and (4) accrual in the earlier year results in a better match against income. The remaining $8,000 is not eligible for the recurring item exception because economic performance (payment of the $8,000 liability) did not occur until October, which is beyond both the filing of the return and the 8½-month window.

Real Property Taxes. The addition of the economic performance test and the recurring item exception posed a problem for a great number of taxpayers who incur real property taxes.

Example 21. Oldco Corporation uses the accrual method and reports on the calendar year. It owns a warehouse in a state where the lien date (i.e., the date on which the corporation technically becomes liable) for real property taxes for 2009 is January 1, 2010. Payment is due in two installments, 40 percent due on June 1 and the remaining 60 percent due on December 1. Shortly after the close of 2009, the corporation received its bill for its 2009 taxes of $100,000, paying $40,000 on June 1 and $60,000 on December 1. For financial accounting purposes, the corporation accrues the entire $100,000 expense in 2009. For tax purposes, however, economic performance for taxes does not occur until payment is made. Therefore, accrual normally is not allowed until the payment is made (2010) unless the recurring item exception applies. In this case, the recurring item exception would apply. However, the corporation could deduct only the portion paid by the earlier of the filing of its tax return or September 15 (8½ months after the close of the taxable year). If the corporation delayed filing its return until the extended due date, September 15, it could accrue and deduct on its 2009 tax return the $40,000 paid on June 1. However, if it filed its return by March 15, none of the taxes could be accrued under the recurring item exception.

Recognizing the problem illustrated *Example 18* above, Code § 461(c) was created. Under this provision, taxpayers can elect to accrue real property taxes ratably over the period to which the taxes relate. Note that if the taxpayer makes the election, the treatment for tax purposes is consistent with that for financial accounting.

Example 22. Same facts as *Example 21*. If the corporation makes the election under § 461(c), it may accrue and deduct the entire $100,000 in 2009 because all of the taxes related to such period.

RELATIONSHIP TO FINANCIAL ACCOUNTING

As may be apparent from the discussion above, the rules for accruing expenses for tax accounting purposes do not necessarily produce the same result as those for financial accounting. Differences often occur, particularly in the treatment of estimated expenses. As noted in Chapter 5, such differences are justified given the differing goals of financial

and tax accounting. Financial accounting principles adopt a conservative approach in measuring income to ensure that income is not overstated and investors are not misled. Accordingly, financial accounting embraces the matching principle that encourages the accrual of estimated expenditures. In contrast, the objective of the income tax system is to ensure that taxable income is objectively measured so as to minimize controversy. Consistent with this view, the tax law allows a deduction only when a liability is actually fixed and economic performance has occurred. Estimates of future expenses are not sufficient to warrant a deduction for tax purposes (unless the recurring item exception should apply). Note, however, that these different accounting techniques produce differences only in *when* the expense is taken into account. The total amount of expense to be accounted for is not affected. Common examples of these so-called timing differences include:

- *Depreciation.* As discussed in Chapter 9, depreciation for tax purposes differs substantially from that for financial accounting purposes. Although the total amount of depreciation is often the same in both cases, the amount expensed in any one period may differ significantly.

- *Bad Debts.* For tax purposes, bad debts normally may be deducted only in the year they actually become worthless. In contrast, financial accounting permits use of the reserve method, which allows an estimate of future bad debts related to current year sales to be charged against current year income. The tax treatment of bad debts is discussed fully in Chapter 10.

- *Vacation Pay.* For financial accounting purposes, vacation pay accrues as it is earned by the employees. For tax purposes, however, vacation pay may be accrued and deducted only if it is paid within 2½ months following the close of the taxable year.

- *Warranty costs.* For financial accounting purposes, warranty costs are normally estimated and matched against current year sales. For tax purposes, no deduction is allowed until the warranty work is actually performed (unless the recurring item exception applies).

Timing differences should be distinguished from permanent differences. As seen throughout this text, there are a number of situations in which an expense for financial accounting purposes is not allowed as a deduction for tax purposes. For example, fines and penalties are expenses that must be taken into account in determining financial accounting income, as are expenses related to tax-exempt income. However, tax deductions for such costs are not allowed. Similarly, expenses for business meals and entertainment may be fully expensed for financial accounting but only 50 percent of such costs can be deducted for tax purposes.

The rules governing the accrual of deductions are summarized in Exhibit 7-1.

EXHIBIT 7-1

Requirements for Accrual of Deduction

Requirements

► All events test is met.

All events have occurred that fix the fact of the liability.

The amount of the liability can be determined with reasonable accuracy.

► Economic performance has occurred as follows:

Event Producing Liability	Time When Economic Performance Occurs	Example
Taxpayer obligated to provide goods or services to a third party	When the taxpayer provides the property or services	Taxpayer to perform repairs, warranty work
Goods or services provided or to be provided to the taxpayer	When taxpayer actually receives the goods or services	Taxpayer buys supplies, contracts for consulting
Property provided or to be provided to the taxpayer	When taxpayer uses the property	Taxpayer rents property
Obligations to pay refunds, rebates, awards, prizes, insurance, warranty or service contracts, taxes	When taxpayer makes payment	Refunds, rebates, etc.
Claims under worker's compensation, tort, breach of contract	When taxpayer makes payment	Taxpayer incurs product liability
Real property taxes	When taxpayer makes payment unless he or she elects special accrual rule	Real estate taxes

DEDUCTIONS FOR LOSSES

The general rules concerning deduction of losses are contained in § 165. This provision permits a deduction for any loss sustained that is not compensated for by insurance. The deductions for losses of an individual taxpayer, however, are limited to

1. Losses incurred in a trade or business

2. Losses incurred in a transaction entered into for profit

3. Losses of property not connected with a trade or business if such losses arise by fire, storm, shipwreck, theft, or some other type of casualty

Note that personal losses—other than those attributable to a casualty—are not deductible. For example, the sale of a personal residence at a loss is not deductible.

Before a loss can be deducted, it must be evidenced by a closed and completed transaction. Mere decline in values or unrealized losses cannot be deducted. Normally, for the loss to qualify as a deduction, the property must be sold, abandoned, or scrapped, or become completely worthless. The amount of deductible loss for all taxpayers cannot

exceed the taxpayer's basis in the property. Special rules related to various types of losses are discussed in Chapter 10.

CLASSIFICATION OF EXPENSES

Once the deductibility of an item is established, the tax formula for individuals requires that the deduction be classified as either a deduction *for* adjusted gross income or a deduction *from* adjusted gross income (itemized deduction).[52] In short, the deduction process requires that two questions be asked. First, is the expense deductible? Second, is the deduction for or from adjusted gross income (A.G.I.)? Additional aspects of the first question are considered later in this chapter. At this point, however, it is appropriate to consider the problem of classification.

The classification process arose with the introduction of the standard deduction in 1944. The standard deduction was introduced to simplify filing for the majority of individuals by eliminating the necessity of itemizing primarily personal deductions such as medical expenses and charitable contributions. In addition, the administrative burden of checking such deductions was eliminated. Although these objectives were satisfied by providing a blanket deduction in lieu of itemizing actual expenses, a new problem arose. The standard deduction created the need to classify deductions as either deductions that would be deductible in any event (deductions for A.G.I.), or deductions that would be deductible only if they exceeded the prescribed amount of the standard deduction (deductions from A.G.I.).

IMPORTANCE OF CLASSIFICATION

The classification problem is significant for several reasons. First, itemized deductions may be deducted only to the extent they exceed the standard deduction. For this reason, a taxpayer whose itemized deductions do not exceed the standard deduction would lose a deduction if a deduction for A.G.I. is improperly classified as a deduction from A.G.I. This would occur because deductions for A.G.I. are deductible without limitation.

A second reason for properly classifying deductions concerns the treatment of miscellaneous itemized deductions. As part of the tax overhaul in 1986, Congress limited the deduction of miscellaneous itemized deductions—defined below—to the amount that exceeds 2 percent of A.G.I. This new limitation is extremely important. Under prior law, taxpayers who itemized deductions could misclassify a deduction for A.G.I. as an itemized deduction with little or no effect, since the expense would be deductible either one place or the other. Under the current scheme, however, misclassification of a deduction for A.G.I. as a miscellaneous itemized deduction would subject the expense to the 2 percent floor, possibly making it wholly or partially nondeductible.

A third reason for properly classifying deductions concerns A.G.I. itself. Limitations on deductions such as medical expenses and charitable contributions are expressed in terms of the taxpayer's A.G.I. For example, miscellaneous itemized deductions are deductible only to the extent they exceed 2 percent of A.G.I., medical expenses are deductible only to the extent they exceed 7.5 percent of A.G.I., and charitable contributions are deductible only to the extent of various limitations (50, 30, or 20 percent) based on A.G.I.

As discussed in Chapter 3, Congress has created two relatively new limitations that are based on A.G.I. First, the amount of itemized deductions (other than for medical expenses, gambling losses, investment interest and casualty and theft losses) must be

---

[52] § 62.

reduced under the deduction cutback rule by 1 percent of a taxpayer's A.G.I. in excess of $166,800 (2009). In addition, the deduction for personal exemptions is phased out as the taxpayer's A.G.I. exceeds a threshold amount (e.g., in 2009 $250,200 for joint returns and $166,800 for a single taxpayer). Thus, the misclassification of a deduction for A.G.I. as an itemized deduction would result in a higher A.G.I. and could result in a lower deduction for itemized deductions and personal exemptions.

Adjusted gross income for Federal income tax purposes also serves as the tax base or the starting point for computing taxable income for many state income taxes. Several states do not allow the taxpayer to itemize deductions. Consequently, misclassification could result in an incorrect state tax liability.

Still another reason for properly classifying expenses concerns the self-employment tax. Under the social security and Medicare programs, self-employed individuals are required to make an annual contribution based on their net earnings from self-employment. Net earnings from self-employment include gross income from the taxpayer's trade or business less allowable trade or business deductions attributable to the income. Failure to properly classify a deduction as a deduction for A.G.I. attributable to self-employment income results in a higher self-employment tax.

DEDUCTIONS FOR A.G.I.

The deductions for A.G.I. are specifically identified in Code § 62. It should be emphasized, however, that § 62 merely classifies expenses; it does *not* authorize any deductions. Deductions *for* A.G.I. are:

1. Trade or business deductions except those expenses incurred in the business of being an employee (e.g., expenses of a sole proprietorship or self-employment normally reported on Schedule C of Form 1040)

2. Trade or business deductions of a "statutory employee," generally including traveling salespersons, full-time life insurance salespersons, agent-drivers, commission-drivers and homeworkers. Statutory employees (discussed in detail in Chapter 8) generally report both their income (i.e., wages) and their business expenses on Schedule C much like a sole proprietor.

3. Three categories of employee business deductions:

    a. Expenses that are reimbursed by an employee's employer (and the reimbursement is included in the employee's income);[53]
    b. Expenses incurred by a qualified performing artist (see below); and
    c. Expenses incurred by an official of a state or local government who is compensated on a fee basis

4. Losses from sale or exchange of property

5. Deductions attributable to rents or royalties

6. Educator expenses (K–12 teachers)

7. Deductions for reservists, performing artists, fee-basis government officials

8. Deductions for certain tuition and fees

9. Student loan interest expense

10. Deduction for certain legal expenses

---

[53] Reimbursements must be made under an "accountable plan." Chapter 8 discusses in detail the proper reporting for these reimbursements.

11. Deductions for contributions to Individual Retirement Accounts or Keogh retirement plans

12. Alimony deductions

13. Deductions for penalties imposed for premature withdrawal of funds from a savings arrangement

14. Deduction for 50 percent of self-employment tax paid by self-employed persons

15. Deduction for contributions to Medical Savings Accounts (MSAs) and Health Savings Accounts (HSAs)

16. Moving expenses

17. Deduction for 100 percent of self-employed health insurance premiums

18. Certain other deductions

All of the above are deductible for A.G.I., while all other deductions are from A.G.I. (i.e., itemized deductions).

ITEMIZED DEDUCTIONS

As seen above, only relatively few expenses are deductible for A.G.I. The predominant expenses in this category are the deductions incurred by taxpayers who are self-employed (i.e., those carrying on as a sole proprietor). All other expenses are deductible from A.G.I. as itemized deductions.

Itemized deductions fall into two basic categories: those that are *miscellaneous itemized deductions* and those that are not. The distinction is significant because miscellaneous itemized deductions are deductible only to the extent they exceed two percent of A.G.I. Miscellaneous itemized deductions are all itemized deductions *other than* the following:

1. Interest

2. Taxes

3. Casualty and theft losses

4. Medical expenses

5. Charitable contributions

6. Gambling losses to the extent of gambling gains

7. Deduction where annuity payments cease before investment is recovered

8. Certain other deductions

The miscellaneous itemized deductions category is comprised primarily of *unreimbursed* employee business expenses, investment expenses, and deductions related to taxes such as tax preparation fees. Examples of these (assuming they are not reimbursed by the employer) include:

1. Employee travel away from home (including meals and lodging)

2. Employee transportation expenses

3. Outside salesperson's expenses [unless those individuals qualify as a "statutory employee" in which case they are allowed to report their income (i.e., wages) and expenses on a separate Schedule C and avoid the two percent of A.G.I. limitation]

4. Employee entertainment expenses

5. Employee home office expenses

6. Union dues

7. Professional dues and memberships

8. Subscriptions to business journals

9. Job-seeking expenses (in the same business) or employment-seeking expenses

10. Education expenses

11. Investment expenses, including expenses for an investment newsletter, investment advice, and rentals of safety deposit boxes

12. Tax preparation fees or other tax-related advice including that received from accountants or attorneys, tax seminars, and books about taxes

With respect to item 12 above, expenses related to tax preparation and resolving tax controversies normally are reported as miscellaneous itemized deductions. However, the IRS allows taxpayers who own a business, farm, or rental real estate or have royalty income to allocate a portion of the total cost of preparing their tax return to the cost of preparing Schedule C (trade or business income), Schedule E (rental and royalty income), or Schedule F (farm income) and deduct these costs "for" A.G.I.[54] The same holds true for expenses incurred in resolving tax controversies, including expenses relating to IRS audits or business or rental activities.

SELF-EMPLOYED VERSUS EMPLOYEE

Under the current scheme of deductions for and from A.G.I., an important—and perhaps inequitable—distinction is made based on whether an individual is an employee or self-employed. As seen above, employees generally deduct all unreimbursed business expenses as itemized deductions. In contrast, self-employed taxpayers (i.e., sole proprietors or partners) deduct business expenses for A.G.I. At first glance, the difference appears trivial, particularly for those taxpayers who itemize their deductions. Recall, however, that an employee's business expenses are treated as miscellaneous itemized deductions and thus are deductible only to the extent that these and all other miscellaneous itemized deductions collectively exceed 2 percent of the taxpayer's A.G.I. Due to this distinction, deductibility often depends on the employment status of the taxpayer.

> **Example 23.** T is an accountant. During the year she earns $30,000 and pays dues of $100 to be a member of the local CPA society. These were her only items of income and expense. If T practices as a self-employed sole proprietor (e.g., she has a small firm or partnership), the dues are fully deductible for A.G.I. However, if T is an employee, none of the expense is deductible since it does not exceed the 2% floor of $600 (2% × $30,000). If T's employer had reimbursed her for the expense and included the reimbursement in her income, the expense would have been completely deductible, totally offsetting the amount that T must include in income. If T is employed, but at the same time does some accounting work on her own, part-time, the treatment is unclear.

The logic for the distinction based on employment status is fragile at best. According to the committee reports, Congress believed that it was generally appropriate to disallow deductions for employee business expenses because employers reimburse employees for those expenses that are most necessary for employment. In addition,

---

[54] Rev. Rul. 92-29, 1992-1 C.B.20.

Congress felt that the treatment would simplify the system by relieving taxpayers of the burden of record keeping and at the same time relieving the IRS of the burden of auditing such deductions.

Reimbursed Expenses. The classification and treatment of an employee's deductible business expenses can vary depending on whether they are reimbursed. If the employee is not reimbursed, the unreimbursed business expenses are deductible as miscellaneous itemized deductions. If the employee is reimbursed and he or she properly accounts to the employer according to the "accountable plan" rules, neither the amount of the reimbursement nor the expense is reported on the return.[55] The accountable plan rules, which are discussed in detail in Chapter 8, generally require employees to substantiate their expenses (e.g., provide documentation such as receipts). If the accountable plan rules are not followed or a plan does not exist, the reimbursement is treated as wages subject to employment taxes and the expense is deducted as a miscellaneous itemized deduction.

Example 24. Professor K is employed by State University in the finance department. The department has a policy of reimbursing up to $50 for each faculty member's costs of subscribing to finance journals. During the year, K spent $75 on subscriptions. He submitted the receipt for $50 of his expenses and was reimbursed by his employer. Assuming the employer's reimbursement policy meets the accountable plan requirements and K has adequately accounted for the expense, the $50 reimbursement is not included in K's wages and K claims no deduction. K may deduct the remaining $25 as a miscellaneous itemized deduction. In this situation, there is no effect on A.G.I. The transaction is a "wash" economically for K and is, therefore a "wash" on K's tax return.

Example 25. Same as above except the plan did not meet the accountable plan standard. In this case, the employer would include the reimbursement of $50 in K's wages (e.g., his W-2) and K could deduct the $50 of expenses along with the other $25 as miscellaneous itemized deductions. Of course, if K does not itemize or his miscellaneous itemized deductions do not exceed the 2 percent floor, he would not benefit from the deduction. Observe that in this situation where the accountable plan rules are not met, the transaction is not a "wash" from a tax point of view. The amount K receives is reduced by employment taxes on the $50 and he may or may not be able to deduct the $50 of his subscriptions.

Expenses of Performing Artists. Most employee business expenses were relegated to second-class status in 1986 as they became subject to the 2 percent limitation. However, one group of employees, the struggling performing artists, escaped this restriction. These actors, actresses, musicians, dancers, and the like are technically employees but exhibit many attributes of the self-employed. They often work for several employers for little income yet incur relatively large unreimbursed expenses as they seek their fortunes. For these reasons, "qualified performing artists" are permitted to deduct their business expenses *for* A.G.I. To qualify, the individual must perform services in the performing arts as an employee for at least two employers during the taxable year, earning at least $200 from each. In addition, the individual's A.G.I. before business deductions cannot exceed $16,000. Lastly, the artist's business deductions must exceed 10 percent of his or her gross service income, otherwise they too are considered miscellaneous itemized deductions.

---

[55] See Reg. § 1.62-2. Note also that the employer is not required to file an information return when there is an accountable plan..

Example 26. Z is an actress. This year she worked in two Broadway productions for two different employers, earning $7,000 from each for a total of $14,000. Her expenses, including the fee to her agent, were $2,000. She may deduct all of her expenses for A.G.I.

Self-Employed or Employee? The above discussion illustrates the importance of determining whether an individual is self-employed or is treated as an employee. However, whether an individual is self-employed or is an employee is often difficult to determine. An employee is a person who performs services for another individual subject to that individual's direction and control.[56] In the employer-employee relationship, the right to control extends not only to the result to be accomplished but also to the methods of accomplishment. Accordingly, an employee is subject to the will and control of the employer as to both what will be done and how it will be done. In the case of the self-employed person, the individual is subject to the control of another only as to the end result, and not as to the means of accomplishment. Generally, physicians, lawyers, dentists, veterinarians, contractors, and subcontractors are not employees. An insurance agent or salesperson may be an employee or self-employed, depending on the facts. The courts have developed numerous tests for differentiating between employees and self-employed persons. Each of the following situations would suggest that an employer-employee relationship exists.[57]

1. Complying with written or oral instructions (an independent contractor need not be trained or attend training sessions)

2. Regular written or oral reports on the work's status

3. Continuous relationship—more than sporadic services over a lengthy period

4. Lack of control over the place of work

5. No risk of profit or loss; no income fluctuations

6. Regular payment—hourly, weekly, etc. (an independent contractor might work on a job basis)

7. Specified number of hours required to work (an independent contractor is master of his or her own time)

8. Unable to delegate work—hiring assistants not permitted

9. Not independent—does not work for numerous firms or make services available to general public

LIMITATIONS ON DEDUCTIONS

Some provisions of the Code specifically prohibit or limit the deduction of certain expenses and losses despite their apparent relationship to the taxpayer's business or profit-seeking activities. These provisions operate to disallow or limit the deduction for various expenses unless such expenses are specifically authorized by the Code. As a practical matter, these provisions have been enacted to prohibit abuses identified in specific areas. Several of the more fundamental limitations are considered in this chapter.

---

[56]   Reg. § 31.3401(c)-1(a).

[57]   Rev. Rul. 87-41, 1987-1 C.B. 296. This Revenue Ruling actually contains 20 questions.

HOBBY EXPENSES AND LOSSES

As previously discussed, a taxpayer must establish that he or she pursues an activity with the objective of making a profit before the expense is deductible as a business or production of income expense. When the profit motive is absent, the deduction is governed by § 183 on activities not engaged in for profit (i.e., hobbies). Section 183 generally provides that hobby expenses of an individual taxpayer or S corporation are deductible only to the extent of the gross income from the hobby. Thus, the tax treatment of hobby expenses substantially differs from profit-seeking expenses if the expenses of the activity exceed the income, resulting in a net loss. If the loss is treated as arising from a profit-motivated activity, then the taxpayer ordinarily may use it to reduce income from other sources.[58] Conversely, if the activity is considered a hobby, no loss is deductible. Note, however, that hobby expenses may be deducted to offset any hobby income.

Profit Motive. The problem of determining the existence of a profit motive usually arises in situations where the activity has elements of both a personal and a profit-seeking nature (e.g., auto racing, antique hunting, coin collecting, horse breeding, weekend farming). In some instances, these activities may represent a profitable business venture. Where losses are consistently reported, however, the business motivation is suspect. In these cases all the facts and circumstances must be examined to determine the presence of the profit motive. The courts have held that the taxpayer simply is required to pursue the activity with a bona fide intent of making a profit. The taxpayer, however, need not show a profit. Moreover, the taxpayer's expectation of profit need not be considered reasonable.[59] The Regulations set out nine factors to be used in ascertaining the existence of a profit motive.[60] Some of the questions posed by these factors are:

1. Was the activity carried on in a businesslike manner? Were books and records kept? Did the taxpayer change his or her methods or adopt new techniques with the intent to earn a profit?

2. Did the taxpayer attempt to acquire knowledge about the business or consult experts?

3. Did the taxpayer or family members devote much time or effort to the activity? Did they leave another occupation to have more time for the activity?

4. Have there been years of income as well as years of loss? Did the losses occur only in the start-up years?

5. Does the taxpayer have only incidental income from other sources? Is the taxpayer's wealth insufficient to maintain him or her if future profits are not derived?

6. Does the taxpayer derive little personal or recreational pleasure from the activity?

An affirmative answer to several of these questions suggests a profit motive exists.

---

[58] The limitations imposed on losses from passive activities should not be applicable in this situation since the taxpayer materially participates in the activity. See discussion in Chapter 12 and § 469.

[59] Reg. § 1.183-2(a).

[60] Reg. § 1.183-2(b).

Presumptive Rule. The burden of proof in the courts is normally borne by the taxpayer. Section 183, however, shifts the burden of proof to the IRS in hobby cases where the taxpayer shows profits in any three of five consecutive years (two of seven years for activities related to horses).[61] The rule creates a presumption that the taxpayer has a profit motive unless the IRS can show otherwise. An election is available to the taxpayer to postpone IRS challenges until five (or seven) years have elapsed from the date the activity commenced. Making the election allows the taxpayer sufficient time to have three profitable years and thus shift the burden of proof to the IRS. This election must be filed within three years of the due date of the return for the taxable year in which the taxpayer first engages in the activity, but not later than 60 days after the taxpayer has received notice that the IRS proposes to disallow the deduction of expenses related to the hobby. The election automatically extends the statute of limitations for each of these years, thus enabling a later challenge by the IRS. It should be emphasized that this presumptive rule only shifts the burden of proof. Profits in three of the five (or two of seven) years do not absolve the taxpayer from attack.

Example 27. T enjoys raising, breeding, and showing dogs. In the past, she occasionally sold a dog or puppy. In 2008 T decided to pursue these activities seriously. During the year, she incurred a loss of $4,000. T also had a loss of $2,000 in 2009. If T made no election for any of these years (i.e., within three years of the start of the activity), the IRS may assert that T's activities constitute a hobby. In this case, the burden of proof is on T to show a profit motive, since she has not shown a profit in at least three years. If T made an election, then the IRS is barred from assessing a deficiency until five years have elapsed. Five years need to elapse to determine whether T will have profits in three of the five years and, if so, shift the burden of proof to the IRS in any litigation that may occur. If an election is made, however, the period for assessing deficiencies for all years is extended until two years after the due date of the return for the last taxable year in the five-year period.[62] In T's case, an election would enable the IRS to assess a deficiency for 2008 and subsequent years up until April 15, 2015, assuming T is a calendar year taxpayer. If an election were not made, the statute of limitations would normally bar assessments three years after the return is due (e.g., assessments for 2008 would be barred after April 15, 2012).

Deduction Limitation. If the activity is considered a hobby, the related expenses are deductible to the extent of the activity's gross income as reduced by *otherwise allowable deductions.*[63] Otherwise allowable deductions are those expenses relating to the hobby that are deductible under other sections of the Code regardless of the activity in which they are incurred. For example, property taxes are deductible under § 164 without regard to whether the activity in which they are incurred is a hobby or a business. Similarly, interest on debt secured by the taxpayer's principal or secondary residence is deductible regardless of the character of the activity. Consequently, any expense otherwise allowable is deducted *first* in determining the gross income limitation. Any other expenses are deductible to the extent of any remaining gross income (i.e., other operating expenses are taken next, with any depreciation deductions, taken last). Otherwise allowable deductions are fully deductible as itemized deductions, while other deductible expenses are considered miscellaneous itemized deductions and are deductible only to the extent they exceed 2 percent of A.G.I. (including the hobby income).

---

[61]   § 183(d).

[62]   § 183(d)(4).

[63]   § 183(b). On classification of the deductions, see Rev. Rul. 75-14, 1975-1 C.B. 90 and Senate Finance Committee Report on H.R. 3838, S. Rep. No. 99-313 (5/29/86), p. 80, 99th Cong., 2nd. Sess.

Example 28. R, an actor, enjoys raising, breeding, and racing horses as a hobby. His A.G.I. excluding the hobby activities is $68,000. He has a small farm on which he raises the horses. During the current year, R won one race and received income of $2,000. He paid $2,300 in expenses as follows: $800 property taxes related to the farm and $1,500 feed for horses. R calculated depreciation with respect to the farm assets at $6,500. As a result, R has a net loss from the activity of $6,800 ($2,000 − $2,300 − $6,500). If the activity is *not* considered a hobby but rather a trade or business, R would report the loss on Schedule C and assuming it is not a passive loss, he could use it to offset his other income. However, if the activity is considered a hobby and R itemizes deductions, he would compute his deductions as follows:

Gross income.	$2,000	
Otherwise allowable deductions:		
Taxes.	(800)	$ 800
Gross income limitation	$ 1,200	
Feed expense:		
$1,500 limited to remaining gross income		1,200
Total.		$2,000

Note that because depreciation is taken last, there is no deduction for this item.

R would include $2,000 in gross income, increasing his A.G.I. to $70,000. Of the $2,000 in deductible expenses, the property taxes of $800 are deductible in full as an itemized deduction. The remaining $1,200 is considered a miscellaneous itemized deduction. In this case, none of the $1,200 is deductible since this amount does not exceed the 2% floor of $1,400 (2% of $70,000). No deduction is allowed for the remaining feed expense of $300 ($1,500 − $1,200) due to the gross income limitation.

Example 29. Assume the same facts as in *Example 25* except that R's expense for property taxes is $2,400 instead of $800. In this case, because the entire $2,400 is deductible as an otherwise allowable deduction and exceeds the gross income from the hobby, none of the feed expense is deductible. Thus, R would include $2,000 in gross income and the $2,400 of property taxes would be fully deductible from A.G.I.

PERSONAL LIVING EXPENSES

Just as the Code specifically authorizes deductions for the costs of pursuing income—business and income-producing expenses—it denies deductions for personal expenses. Section 262 prohibits the deduction of any personal, living, or family expenses. Only those personal expenditures expressly allowed by some other provision in the Code are deductible. Some of the personal expenditures permitted by other provisions are medical expenses, contributions, qualified residence interest, and taxes. Normally, these expenses are classified as itemized deductions. These deductions and their underlying rationale are discussed in Chapter 11.

The disallowance of personal expenditures by § 262 complements the general criteria allowing a deduction. Recall that the general rules of §§ 162 and 212 permit deductions for ordinary and necessary expenses *only where a profit motive exists*. As previously seen

in the discussion of hobbies, however, determining whether an expense arose from a personal or profit motive can be difficult. Some of the items specifically disallowed by § 262 are:

1. Expenses of maintaining a household (e.g., rent, utilities)

2. Losses on sales of property held for personal purposes

3. Amounts paid as damages for breach of promise to marry, attorney's fees, and other costs of suits to recover such damages

4. Premiums paid for life insurance by the insured

5. Costs of insuring a personal residence

Legal Expenses. Legal expenses related to divorce actions and the division of income-producing properties are often a source of conflict. Prior to clarification by the Supreme Court, several decisions held that divorce expenses incurred primarily to protect the taxpayer's income-producing property or his or her business were deductible.[64] The Supreme Court, however, has ruled that deductibility depends on whether the expense arises in connection with the taxpayer's profit-seeking activities. That is, the *origin* of the expense determines deductibility.[65] Under this rule, if the spouse's claim arises from the marital relationship—a personal matter—then no deduction is allowed. Division of income-producing property would only be incidental to or a consequence of the marital relationship.

> **Example 30.** R pays legal fees to defend an action by his wife to prevent distributions of income from a trust to him. Because the wife's action arose from the marital relationship, the legal expenses are nondeductible personal expenditures.[66]

Legal expenses related to a divorce action may be deductible where the expense is for advice concerning the tax consequences of the divorce.[67] The portion of the legal expense allocable to counsel on the tax consequences of a property settlement, the right to claim children as dependents, and the creation of a trust for payment of alimony are deductible.

Contingent Attorney Fees. Over the years, there has been a great deal of controversy regarding the treatment of contingent attorney fees incurred in securing a damages award. To illustrate, assume a taxpayer receives an award of fully taxable punitive damages of $10 million and the attorney is to receive a contingent fee of 40 percent of that amount or $4 million. In this situation, the taxpayer typically asserted that the fees represent a splitting of the income and, therefore, he or she should be taxed only on the net amount received or $6 million. Conversely, the government argued that the full $10 million is included in gross income and the $4 million of attorney fees were a miscellaneous item-ized deduction subject to the two percent limitation and the one percent cutback. But more importantly, since the attorney fees were classified as miscellaneous itemized deductions, they were not allowed in computing the alternative minimum tax (AMT). As a result, an AMT often resulted. In effect, the taxpayer paid tax on $10 million when he or she had only received $6 million.

---

[64] *F.C. Bowers v. Comm.*, 57-1 USTC ¶9605, 51 AFTR 207, 243 F.2d 904 (CA-6, 1957).

[65] *Supra*, Footnote 13, Also, compare *Comm. v. Tellier*, 66-1 USTC ¶9319, 17 AFTR2d 633, 383 U.S. 687 (USSC, 1966) with *Boris Nodiak v. Comm.*, 66-1 USTC ¶9262, 17 AFTR2d 396, 356 F.2d 911 (CA-2, 1966).

[66] *H.N. Shilling, Jr.*, 33 TCM 1097, T.C. Memo 1974-246.

[67] Rev Rul. 72-545, 1972-2 C.B. 179.

Congress addressed this problem in 2004. Attorney's fees and court costs incurred for certain legal actions are deductible for A.G.I. This rule applies to most legal actions, but not necessarily all.[68] Apparently, certain types of tort actions, such as defamation, would not fall within the statute unless they occur within the employment context. By classifying these expenses as deductions for A.G.I., the AMT problem is eliminated since the AMT limitations generally apply only to certain itemized deductions.[69]

CAPITAL EXPENDITURES

A capital expenditure is ordinarily defined as an expenditure providing benefits that extend beyond the close of the taxable year. It is a well-established rule in case law that a business expense, though ordinary and necessary, is not deductible in the year paid or incurred if it can be considered a capital expenditure.[70] Normally, however, a capital expenditure may be deducted ratably over the period for which it provides benefits. For example, the Code authorizes deductions for depreciation or cost recovery, amortization, and depletion where the asset has a determinable useful life.[71] Capital expenditures creating assets that do not have a determinable life, however, generally cannot be deducted. For example, land is considered as having an indeterminable life and thus cannot be depreciated or amortized. The same is true for stocks and bonds. Expenditures for these types of assets are recovered (i.e., deducted) only when there is a disposition of the asset through sale (e.g., cost offset against sales price), exchange, abandonment, or other disposition.

As a general rule, assets with a useful life of one year or less need not be capitalized. For example, the taxpayer can write off short-lived assets with small costs such as supplies (e.g., stationery, pens, pencils, calculators), books (e.g., the Internal Revenue Code), and small tools (e.g., screwdrivers, rakes, and shovels).

Goodwill. Like land, goodwill is an example of an asset that does not have a determinable useful life. Because of this indeterminate life, acquired goodwill historically has been treated as a capitalized asset that could not be depreciated. The only way a taxpayer could receive a current tax benefit from acquired goodwill was to identify components separate and apart from goodwill that had an ascertainable value and limited useful life (e.g., client files and subscription lists). If a taxpayer was successful in establishing the requisite valuation and limited life for a goodwill component, the taxpayer could depreciate the cost of the intangible asset over its useful life using the straight-line method (known as amortization). However, in practice, taxpayers often faced challenges by the IRS, and many attempts to depreciate goodwill components were unsuccessful.

---

[68] § 62 (a)(20) extends the deduction for actions in connection with unlawful discrimination claims, certain claims against the federal government, and private causes of action under the Medicare Secondary Payer law. Unlawful discrimination actions include those that claim violations of the Civil Rights Acts of 1964 and 1991, the Congressional Accountability Act of 1995, the National Labor Relations Act, the Family and Medical Leave Act of 1993, the Fair Housing Act, the Americans with Disabilities Act of 1990, and various whistle-blower statutes.

[69] The Jobs Act does apply to cases settled prior to October 23, 2004. The Supreme Court settled the issue for these cases, reversing pro-taxpayer decisions in the Sixth and Ninth Circuits, indicating that there had been an invalid assignment of income and, therefore the legal expenses were miscellaneous itemized deductions. See *Comm. v. John W. Banks II and Comm. v. Sigitas J. Banaitis*, (combined) 2005-1 USTC ¶50,595, AFTR 2d 2005-659, (USSC, 2005), rev'g *Banks II*, 92 2003-6298, 2003-2 USTC ¶50,675,AFTR 2d, 345 F3d 373 (CA-6, 2003), and rev'g *Banaitis*, 92 AFTR 2d 2003-5834, 2003-2 USTC ¶50,638; 340 F3d 1074 (CA-9, 2003).

[70] *Supra*, footnote 18.

[71] §§ 167, 168, 169, 178, 184, 188, and 611 are examples.

Congress enacted Code § 197 to reduce the uncertainty surrounding the depreciation of goodwill and its identifiable components. Effective August 10, 1994, the cost of acquiring intangible assets (including acquired goodwill) may, at the election of the taxpayer, be amortized over a 15-year period. If the election is not made, the cost of acquiring goodwill and related intangibles must be capitalized and no amortization will be allowed.

Example 31. B has decided to purchase a newspaper business in a small town for $100,000. It can be determined that $80,000 of the purchase price is allocable to the assets of the business and $20,000 is attributable to goodwill (subscription lists and other intangibles). B may be able to recover all $100,000 of the cost through deductions for depreciation and amortization.

Capital Expenditures versus Repairs. The general rule of case law disallowing deductions for capital expenditures has been codified for expenditures relating to property. Code § 263 provides that deductions are not allowed for any expenditures for new buildings or for permanent improvements or betterments made to increase the value of property.[72] Additionally, expenditures substantially prolonging the property's useful life, adapting the property to a new or different use, or materially adding to the value of the property are not deductible.[73] Conversely, the cost of incidental repairs that do not materially increase the value of the property nor appreciably prolong its life, but maintain it in a normal operating state, may be deducted in the current year.[74] For example, costs of painting, inside and outside, and papering are usually considered repairs.[75] However, if the painting is done in conjunction with a general reconditioning or overhaul of the property, it is treated as a capital expenditure.[76]

Example 32. L operates his own limousine business. Expenses for a tune-up such as the costs of spark plugs, points, and labor would be deductible as routine repairs and maintenance since such costs do not significantly prolong the car's life. In contrast, if L had the transmission replaced at a cost of $600, allowing him to drive it for another few years, the expense must be capitalized.

Acquisition Costs. As a general rule, costs related to the acquisition of property must be capitalized. For example, freight paid to acquire new equipment or commissions paid to acquire land must be capitalized. In addition, Code § 164 requires that state and local general sales taxes related to the purchase of property be capitalized. The costs of demolition or removal of an old building prior to using the land in another fashion must be capitalized as part of the cost of the land.[77] Costs of defending or perfecting the title to property, such as legal fees, are normally capitalized.[78] Similarly, legal fees incurred for the recovery of property must be capitalized unless the recovered property is investment property or money that must be included in income if received.[79]

INDOPCO and the Long-Term Benefit Theory. Interestingly, one of the most important and widely debated tax developments to occur in recent years concerns the capital

[72] § 263(a).

[73] Reg. § 1.263(a)-1(b).

[74] Reg. § 1.162-4.

[75] *Louis Allen*, 2 BTA 1313 (1925).

[76] *Joseph M. Jones*, 57-1 USTC ¶9517, 50 AFTR 2040, 242 F.2d 616 (CA-5, 1957).

[77] § 280B.

[78] Reg. § 1.263(a)-2.

[79] Reg. § 1.212-1(k).

expenditure area. The controversy stems from a Supreme Court decision involving the treatment of costs incurred by a target company as part of a friendly takeover. In 1977, Unilever approached one of its suppliers, INDOPCO, about the possibility of a takeover to which INDOPCO agreed. During the acquisition process, INDOPCO paid an investment banking company, Morgan Stanley, about $2.2 million for advice and a fairness opinion and another $500,000 to its own legal counsel for services related to the takeover. The IRS ultimately denied deduction of the expenses (as well as amortization) on the grounds that the expenses were capital in nature. In 1992, the Supreme Court concurred with the IRS, believing that INDOPCO would receive long-term benefits from the acquisition, including the opportunity for synergy with Unilever and the future availability of Unilever's financial and business resources.[80]

The effect of the INDOPCO decision would not be so great if it were confined to costs incurred as part of a friendly takeover. However, the IRS has used the broad language of the court to capitalize any expense to which it can associate any long-term benefit. In this regard, it is important to understand that the Supreme Court indicated that the long-term benefits need not be associated with any specific identifiable asset. As long as the expenditure leads to the permanent betterment of the business as a whole, capitalization may be in order. For example, the IRS has used this approach to deny a deduction for the costs of removing asbestos insulation from equipment if the removal is part of a general plan of rehabilitation, despite the fact that the expense did not extend the life of the asset.[81] Instead, the taxpayer was required to capitalize the expenditure on the grounds that the firm would derive long-term benefits from safer working conditions and reduced risk of liability. In another ruling concerning advertising costs, the IRS, while allowing a current deduction, warned that in certain instances advertising could produce long-term benefits, in which case such expenses must be capitalized.[82] In short, the INDOPCO decision has increased the tension between taxpayers and the IRS in the capital expenditure arena.

Over time, the intensity of the controversy and the level of uncertainty produced by INDOPCO escalated to an intolerable level. In response to the criticism, the IRS issued final regulations in 2004 to reign in the scope of INDOPCO and its "long-term-benefit" theory.[83] The regulations are quite extensive. There are over 50 pages and more than 80 examples all aimed at resolving whether a particular cost related to an intangible should be capitalized. Although a full discussion of these regulations is beyond the scope of this text, they are required reading whenever a taxpayer incurs an expense related to an intangible. Specifically, the regulations address amounts paid to

- *Acquire* an intangible (e.g., purchase a customer list, lease, patent, copyright, franchise, trademark, trade name, assembled workforce, or goodwill; most of these must be amortized over 15 years under § 197)

- *Create* an intangible (e.g., costs for prepaid items such as prepaid rents and insurance, membership privileges such as membership in a trade association, rights from governmental agencies such as the exclusive rights obtained from the local government by a cable television company to serve a particular region, contract rights and contract terminations such as the rights to renew or renegotiate, licenses, and covenants not to compete)

- *Create* or enhance a separate and distinct intangible

- *Facilitate* the acquisition or creation of an intangible (e.g., legal expenses for negotiating commercial property lease, drafting agreements)

---

[80] *INDOPCO, Inc. v. Comm.*, 92-1 USTC ¶50,113, 69 AFTR2d 92-694, 503 U.S. 79 (USSC, 1992).

[81] *Norwest Corporation*, 108 T.C. No. 15 (1997).

[82] Rev. Rul. 92-80, 1992-2 C.B. 57.

[83] Reg. § 1.263(a)-4 and -5.

> ▶ *Facilitate* the acquisition of a trade or business, a change in the capital structure of a business entity, and certain other transactions (e.g., legal expenses to issue debt, payments to investment banker and outside legal counsel for evaluating alternative investments, performing due diligence, structuring the transaction, preparing SEC filings, and obtaining necessary regulatory approvals, hostile takeover defenses).

These regulations should bring to a close a period of great uncertainty that was not envisioned when the Supreme Court decided the INDOPCO case in 1992.

Environmental Remediation Costs. Under Code § 198 which took effect on August 5, 1997, a taxpayer may elect to treat certain environmental remediation expenditures that would otherwise be chargeable to a capital account as deductible in the year paid or incurred. To qualify for this special treatment, the expense must be incurred in connection with the abatement or control of hazardous substances at a qualified contaminated site. Prior to the enactment of this provision, the IRS took the view that costs incurred to clean-up the environment were controlled by the long-term benefit theory of INDOPCO and, therefore, were capital expenditures for which no deduction was allowed. The effect of § 198, then, is to override the IRS's reliance on the long-term benefit theory to deny deductions with respect to environmental remediation costs.

Elections to Capitalize or Deduct. Various provisions of the Code permit a taxpayer to treat capital expenditures as deductible expenses, as deferred expenses, or as capital expenditures. For example, at the election of the taxpayer, expenses for research and experimentation may be deducted currently, treated as deferred expenses and amortized over at least 60 months, or capitalized and included in the basis of the resulting property.[84]

BUSINESS INVESTIGATION EXPENSES AND START-UP COSTS

Another group of expenses that arguably may be considered capital expenditures are those incurred when seeking and establishing a new business, such as costs of investigation and start-up. Business investigation expenses are those costs of seeking and reviewing prospective businesses prior to reaching a decision to acquire or enter any business. Such expenses include the costs of analysis of potential markets, products, labor supply, and transportation facilities. Start-up or pre-opening expenses are costs that are incurred after a decision to acquire a particular business and prior to its actual operations. Examples of these expenses are advertising, employee training, lining up distributors, suppliers, or potential customers, and the costs of professional services such as attorney and accounting fees.

For many years, the deductibility of expenses of business investigation and start-up turned solely on whether the taxpayer was "carrying on" a business at the time the expenditures were incurred. Notwithstanding some modifications, the basic rule still remains: when the taxpayer is in the same or similar business as the one he or she is starting or investigating, the costs of investigation and start-up are wholly deductible in the year paid or incurred.[85] The deduction is allowed regardless of whether the taxpayer undertakes the business.[86] However, this rule often forces taxpayers to litigate to determine whether a business exists at the time the expenses are incurred. Prior to the

---

[84] § 174. See §§ 175 and 180 for other examples.

[85] *The Colorado Springs National Bank v. U.S.*, 74-2 USTC ¶9809, 34 AFTR2d 74-6166, 505 F.2d 1185 (CA-10, 1974).

[86] *York v. Comm.*, 58-2 USTC ¶9952, 2 AFTR2d 6178, 261 F.2d 421 (CA-4, 1958).

enactment of § 195, if the taxpayer could not establish existence of a business, the expenditures normally were treated as capital expenditures with indeterminable lives.[87] As a result, the taxpayer could only recover the expenditure if and when he or she disposed of or abandoned the business.

In 1980 Congress realized that the basic rule not only was a source of controversy but also discouraged formation of new businesses. For this reason, special provisions permitting deduction of these expenses under certain conditions were enacted.[88] Before examining these provisions, it should be emphasized that the traditional rule continues to be valid. Thus, if a taxpayer can establish that the investigation and start-up costs are related to a similar existing business of the taxpayer, a deduction is allowed.

> **Example 33.** S owns and operates an ice cream shop on the north side of the city. A new shopping mall is opening on the south side of the city, and the developers have approached her about locating a second ice cream shop in their mall. During 2009 S pays a consulting firm $1,000 for a survey of the potential market on the south side. Because S is in the ice cream business when the expense is incurred, the entire $1,000 is deductible regardless of whether she undertakes the new business.

Amortization Provision. Section 195 sets out the treatment for the start-up and investigation expenses of taxpayers who are *not* considered in a similar business when the expenses are incurred *and* who actually enter the new business. Eligible taxpayers may elect to deduct up to $5,000 of business investigation and start-up expenses in the tax year in which the business begins. If the §195 expenses exceed $5,000, the excess must be amortized over the 180-month period (15 years) beginning with the month in which the business begins.[89] If the expenses exceed $50,000, the $5,000 allowance is reduced one dollar for each dollar in excess of $50,000. Expenses for research and development, interest payments, and taxes are not considered start-up expenditures.[90] Consequently, these costs are not subject to §195 and may be deducted under normal rules.

> **Example 34.** J, a calendar year, cash basis taxpayer, recently graduated and received $10,000 from his wealthy uncle as a graduation gift. J paid an accountant $1,200 in September to review the financial situation of a small restaurant he desired to purchase. In December, J purchased the restaurant and began actively participating in its management. J may deduct $1,200 for the current year.

> **Example 35.** S, a famous bodybuilder, has decided to build his first health spa. While the facility is being constructed, a temporary office is set up in a trailer next to the site. The office is nicely decorated and contains a small replica of the facility. S hired a staff who will manage the facility but at this time are calling prospective customers. Elaborate brochures have been printed. All of these costs, including the salaries paid to the staff, the printing of the brochures, and the costs of operating the trailer such as depreciation and utilities, are start-up costs. Assuming the total start-up costs were less than $50,000, the taxpayer could expense the first $5,000 and amortize the balance over 180 months.

> **Example 36.** Same facts as above except S incorporated and the corporation incurred $23,000 of start-up and investigation expenses. The corporation was formed in July of

[87] *Morton Frank*, 20 T.C. 511 (1953).

[88] § 195(a).

[89] § 195 expenses incurred prior to October 23, 2004 are amortized over 60 months.

[90] § 195(c)(1).

this year and adopted the calendar year. In this case, the corporation could deduct $5,000 immediately and amortize the remaining balance of $18,000 over 15 years (180 months) beginning in July. This would result in amortization of $100/month for 180 months. The deduction for start-up and investigation expenses for 2009 would be $5,600 computed as follows:

First-year allowance	$5,000
Amortization ($18,000/180 = $100/month × 6 months)	600
Total deduction in first year	$5,600

In 2010, the corporation would continue to amortize the remaining expenses, resulting in a deduction of $1,200 ($100/month × 12).

Example 37. In March, 2009 LMN, LLC was formed and incurred start-up and investigation expenses of $52,000. LMN's immediate expensing allowance of $5,000 must be reduced one dollar for each dollar of § 195 expense exceeding $50,000. In this case, the allowance is reduced by $2,000 ($52,000 − $50,000) to $3,000. Thus LMN may deduct $3,000 plus amortization of the remaining $49,000, resulting in a deduction of $5,720 computed below.

First-year allowance [$5,000 − ($52,000 − $50,000 = $2,000)]		$3,000
Amortization:		
Total expense.	$52,000	
First-year allowance	(3,000)	
Amortizable balance	$49,000	
Amortization ($49,000/180 = $272/month × 10 months) . .		2,720
Total § 195 expense deduction in first year		$5,720

Note that if LMN had incurred $55,000 or more of § 195 expenses, the $5,000 immediate write-off would be reduced to zero and all $55,000 of the expenses would be amortized over 180 months.

As suggested above, the taxpayer must enter the business to qualify for amortization. Whether the individual is considered as having entered the business normally depends on the facts in each case.

If the taxpayer (who is not in a similar, existing business) does not enter into the new business, the investigation and start-up expenses generally are not deductible. The Tax Court, however, has held that a taxpayer may deduct costs as a loss suffered from a transaction entered into for profit if the activities are sufficient to be considered a "transaction."[91] The IRS has interpreted this rule to mean that those expenditures related to a *general search* for a particular business or investment are not deductible.[92] Expenses are considered general when they are related to whether to enter the transaction and which transaction to enter. Once the taxpayer has focused on the acquisition of a *specific* business or investment, expenses related to an unsuccessful acquisition attempt are deductible as a loss on a transaction entered into for profit.

Example 38. L, a retired army officer, is interested in going into the radio business. He places advertisements in the major trade journals soliciting information about businesses that may be acquired. Upon reviewing the responses to his ads, L selects two radio stations for possible acquisition. He hires an accountant to audit the books

---

[91] *Harris W. Seed*, 52 T.C. 880 (1969).

[92] Rev. Rul. 77-254, 1977-2 C.B. 63.

of each station and advise him on the feasibility of purchase. He travels to the cities where each station is located and discusses the possible acquisition with the owners. Finally, L decides to purchase station FMAM. To this end, he hires an attorney to draft the purchase agreement. Due to a price dispute, however, the acquisition attempt collapses. The expenses for advertising, auditing, and travel are not deductible since they are related to the taxpayer's general search. The legal expenses are deductible as a loss, however, since they occurred in the taxpayer's attempt to acquire a specific business.

Job-Seeking Expenses. The tax treatment of job-seeking expenses of an employee is similar to that for expenses for business investigation. If the taxpayer is seeking a job in the same business in which he or she is presently employed, the related expenses are deductible as miscellaneous itemized deductions subject to the 2 percent floor.[93] The deduction is allowed even if a new job is not obtained. No deduction or amortization is permitted, however, if the job sought is considered a new trade or business or the taxpayer's first job.

Example 39. B, currently employed as a biology teacher, incurs travel expenses and employment agency fees to obtain a new job as a computer operator. The expenses are not deductible because they are not incurred in seeking a job in the profession in which she was currently engaged. Moreover, the expenses are not deductible even though B obtained the new job. However, the expenses would be deductible if she had obtained a new job in her present occupation.

PUBLIC POLICY RESTRICTIONS

Although an expense may be entirely appropriate and helpful, and may contribute to the taxpayer's profit-seeking activities, it is not considered necessary if the allowance of a deduction would frustrate sharply defined public policy. The courts established this long-standing rule on the theory that to allow a deduction for expenses such as fines and penalties would encourage violations by diluting the penalty.[94] Historically, however, the IRS and the courts were free to restrict deductions of any type of expense where, in their view, it appeared that the expenses were contrary to public policy—even if the policy had not been clearly enunciated by some governmental body. As a result, taxpayers were often forced to go to court to determine if their expense violated public policy.

Recognizing the difficulties in applying the public policy doctrine, Congress enacted provisions specifically designed to limit its use.[95] The rules identified and disallowed certain types of expenditures that would be considered contrary to public policy. Under these provisions no deduction is allowed for fines, penalties, and illegal payments.

Fines and Penalties. A deduction is not allowed for any fine or similar penalty paid to a government for the violation of any law.[96]

Example 40. S is a salesperson for an office supply company. While calling on customers this year, he received parking tickets of $100. None of the cost is deductible because the violations were against the law.

---

[93] Rev. Rul. 75-120, 1975-1 C.B. 55, as clarified by Rev. Rul. 77-16, 1977-1 C.B. 37.

[94] *Hoover Motor Express Co., Inc. v. U.S.,* 58-1 USTC ¶9367, 1 AFTR2d 1157, 356 U.S. 38 (USSC, 1958).

[95] S. Rep. No. 91-552, 91st Cong., 1st Sess. 273-75 (1969). Note, however, that the Tax Court continues to utilize the doctrine despite Congress's attempt to restrict its use—see *R. Mazzei,* 61 T.C. 497 (1974).

[96] § 162(f).

Example 41. Upon audit of T's tax return, it was determined that he failed to report $10,000 of tip income from his job as a maitre d', resulting in additional tax of $3,000. T was also required to pay the negligence penalty for intentional disregard of the rules. The penalty—20% of the tax due—is not deductible.

Example 42. This year the Federal Drug Administration fined C Inc., a drug manufacturing company, $5,000,000 for failure to maintain adequate quality control. The fine is not deductible because the practices were in violation of Federal law.

Fines include those amounts paid in settlement of the taxpayer's actual or potential liability.[97] In addition, no deduction is allowed for two-thirds of treble damage payments made due to a violation of antitrust laws.[98] Thus, one-third of this antitrust "fine" is deductible.

Illegal Kickbacks, Bribes, and Other Payments. The Code also disallows the deduction for four categories of illegal payments:[99]

1. Kickbacks or bribes to U.S. government officials and employees if illegal

2. Payments to governmental officials or employees of *foreign* countries if such payments would be considered illegal under the U.S. Foreign Corrupt Practices Act

Example 43. R travels all over the world, looking for unique items for his gift shop. Occasionally when going through customs in foreign countries, he is forced to "bribe" the customs official to do the necessary paperwork and get him through customs as quickly as possible. These so-called grease payments to employees of foreign countries are deductible unless they violate the Foreign Corrupt Practices Act. In general, such payments are not considered to be illegal.

3. Kickbacks, bribes, or other illegal payments to any other person if illegal under generally enforced U.S. or state laws that provide a criminal penalty or loss of license or privilege to engage in business

4. Kickbacks, rebates, and bribes, although legal, made by any provider of items or services under Medicare and Medicaid programs

Those kickbacks and bribes not specified above would still be deductible if they were ordinary and necessary. The payment, however, may not be necessary and thus will be disallowed if it controverts public policy.

Kickbacks generally include payments for referral of clients, patients, and customers. However, under certain circumstances, trade discounts or rebates may be considered kickbacks.

Example 44. M, a life insurance salesperson, paid rebates or discounts to purchasers of policies. Since such practice is normally illegal under state law, the rebate is not deductible.[100]

Expenses of Illegal Business. The expenses related to an illegal business are deductible.[101] Similar to the principle governing taxation of income from whatever source

---

[97] § 162(g).

[98] Reg. § 1.162-21(b).

[99] § 162(c).

[100] *James Alex*, 70 T.C. 322 (1978).

[101] See *Max Cohen v. Comm.*, 49-2 USTC ¶9358, 176 F.2d 394 (CA-10, 1949) and *Neil Sullivan v. Comm.*, 58-1 USTC ¶9368, AFTR2d 1158, 356 U.S. 27 (USSC, 1958).

(including income illegally obtained), the tax law is not concerned with the lawfulness of the activity in which the deductions arise. No deduction is allowed, however, if the expense itself constitutes an illegal payment as discussed above. In addition, Code § 280E prohibits the deduction of any expenses related to the trafficking in controlled substances (i.e., drugs).

LOBBYING AND POLITICAL CONTRIBUTIONS

Although expenses for lobbying and political contributions may be closely related to the taxpayer's business, Congress has traditionally limited their deduction. These restrictions usually are supported on the grounds that it is not in the public's best interest for government to subsidize efforts to influence legislative matters.

Lobbying. Prior to 1962, no deduction was permitted for any type of lobbying expense. In 1962, however, Congress altered its position slightly with the addition of § 162(e), which carved out a narrow exception for certain lobbying expenses. This provision allowed a deduction for the expenses of appearing before or providing information to governmental units on legislative matters of *direct interest* to the taxpayer's business. Similarly, a deduction was permitted for expenses of providing information to a trade organization of which the taxpayer was a member where the legislative matter was of direct interest to the taxpayer and the organization. The portion of dues paid to such an organization attributable to the organization's allowable lobbying activities was also deductible. Beginning in 1994, however, these rules for deducting lobbying expenses are even more restrictive. Lobbying expenditures are now deductible only if incurred for the purpose of influencing legislation at the *local* level. Therefore, the expense of influencing national and state legislation (including the costs of hiring lobbyists to represent the taxpayer in these matters) is not deductible. This prohibition is extended to the costs of any direct communication with executive branch officials in an attempt to influence official actions or positions of such official.

The taxpayer must have a direct interest in the local legislation before lobbying expenses may be deducted. Although the definitional boundaries of the term "direct" are vague, a taxpayer is considered as having satisfied the test if it is reasonable to expect that the local legislative matter affects or will affect the taxpayer's business. However, a taxpayer does not have a direct interest in the nomination, appointment, or operation of any local legislative body.[102]

The deduction for lobbying *does not* extend to expenses incurred to influence the general public on legislative matters, elections, or referendums.[103] Expenses related to the following types of lobbying are not deductible:

1. Advertising in magazines and newspapers concerning legislation of direct interest to the taxpayer.[104] However, expenses for "goodwill" advertising presenting views on economic, financial, social, or similar subjects of a general nature, or encouraging behavior such as contributing to the Red Cross, are deductible.[105]

2. Preparing and distributing to a corporation's shareholders pamphlets focusing on certain legislation affecting the corporation and urging the shareholders to contact their representatives in Congress.[106]

---

[102]   Reg. § 1.162-20(b).

[103]   § 162(e)(2).

[104]   Rev. Rul. 78-112, 1978-1 C.B. 42.

[105]   Reg. § 1.162-20(a)(2).

[106]   Rev. Rul. 74-407, 1974-2 C.B. 45, as amplified by Rev. Rul. 78-111, 1978-1 C.B. 41.

Example 45. T owns a restaurant in Austin, Texas. Legislation has been introduced by the City Council to impose a sales tax on food and drink sold in Austin, to be used for funding a dome stadium. T places an ad in the local newspaper stating reasons why the legislation should not be passed. He goes to the City Council and testifies on the proposed legislation before several committees. He pays dues to the Austin Association of Restaurant Owners organization, which estimates that 60% of its activities are devoted to lobbying for local legislation related to restaurant owners. T may deduct the cost of travel and 60% of his dues since the local legislation is of direct interest to him. He may not deduct the ad since it is intended to influence the general public.

Political Contributions. No deduction is permitted for any contributions, gifts, or any other amounts paid to a political party, action committee, or group or candidate related to a candidate's campaign.[107] This rule also applies to indirect payments, such as the payments for advertising in a convention program and admission to a dinner, hall, or similar affair where any of the proceeds benefit a political party or candidate.[108]

EXPENSES AND INTEREST RELATING TO TAX-EXEMPT INCOME

Section 265 sets forth several rules generally disallowing deductions for expenses relating to tax-exempt income. These provisions prohibit taxpayers from taking advantage of the tax law to secure a double tax benefit: tax-exempt income and deductions for the expenses that help to produce it. The best known rule prohibits the deduction for any *interest* expense or nonbusiness (§ 212) expense related to tax-exempt *interest* income.[109] Without this rule, taxpayers in high tax brackets could borrow at a higher rate of interest than could be earned and still have a profit on the transaction.

Example 46. D, an investor in the 25% tax bracket with substantial investment income, borrows funds at 9% and invests them in tax-exempt bonds yielding 7%. If the interest expense were deductible, the after-tax cost of borrowing would be 6.75% $[(100\% - 25\% = 75\%) \times 9\%]$. Since the interest income is nontaxable, the after-tax yield on the bond remains 7%, or .25 percentage points higher than the effective cost of borrowing. Section 265, however, denies the deduction for the interest expense, thus eliminating the feasibility of this arrangement. It should be noted, however, that business (§ 162) expenses (other than interest) related to tax-exempt interest income may be deductible.

If the income that is exempt is not interest, none of the related expenses are deductible.[110]

Example 47. A company operating a baseball team paid premiums on a disability insurance policy providing that the company would receive proceeds under the policy if a player were injured. Because the proceeds would not be taxable, the premiums are not deductible even though the expenditure would apparently qualify as a business expense.[111] Note, however, that such expenses would enter into the calculation of net income for financial accounting purposes.

---

[107] § 162(e).

[108] § 276.

[109] § 265(2).

[110] § 265(1).

[111] Rev. Rul. 66-262, 1966-2 C.B. 105.

As a practical matter, it would appear difficult to determine whether borrowed funds (and the interest expense) are related to carrying taxable or tax-exempt securities. For example, an individual holding tax-exempt bonds may take out a mortgage to buy a residence instead of selling the bonds to finance the purchase price. In such case, it could be inferred that the borrowed funds were used to finance the bond purchase. Generally, the IRS will allow the deduction in this and similar cases unless the facts indicate that the primary purpose of the borrowing is to carry the tax-exempt obligations.[112] The facts must establish a *sufficiently direct relationship* between the borrowing and the investment producing tax exempt income before a deduction is denied.

> **Example 48.** K owns common stock with a basis of $70,000 and tax-exempt bonds of $30,000. She borrows $100,000 to finance an investment in an oil and gas limited partnership. The IRS will disallow a deduction for a portion of the interest on the $100,000 debt because it is presumed that the $100,000 is incurred to finance all of K's portfolio including the tax-exempt securities.[113]

> **Example 49.** R has a margin account with her broker. This account is devoted solely to the purchase of taxable investments and tax-exempt bonds. During the year, she buys several taxable and tax-exempt securities on margin. A portion of the interest expense on this margin account is disallowed because the borrowings are considered partially related to financing of the investment in tax-exempt securities.[114]

Business Life Insurance. Absent a special rule, premiums paid on insurance policies covering officers and employees of a business might be deductible as ordinary and necessary business expenses. However, to ensure that the taxpayer is not allowed to deduct expenses related to tax-exempt income (i.e., life insurance proceeds), a special provision exists. Under § 264, the taxpayer is not allowed any deduction for life insurance premiums paid on policies covering the life of any officer, employee, or any other person who may have a financial interest in the taxpayer's trade or business, if the taxpayer is the *beneficiary* of the policy. Thus, premiums paid by a business on a key-person life insurance policy where the company is beneficiary are not deductible. Note that this differs from the financial accounting treatment, where the premiums would be considered routine operating costs that should be expensed in determining net income. In contrast, payments made by a business on group-term life insurance policies where the employees are beneficiaries are deductible.

RELATED TAXPAYER TRANSACTIONS

Without restrictions, related taxpayers (such as husbands and wives, shareholders and their corporations) could enter into arrangements creating deductions for expenses and losses, and not affect their economic position. For example, a husband and wife could create a deduction simply by having one spouse sell property to the other at a loss. In this case, the loss is artificial because the property remains within the family and their financial situation is unaffected. Although the form of ownership has been altered, there is no substance to the transaction. To guard against the potential abuses inherent in transactions between related taxpayers, Congress designed specific safeguards contained in § 267.

---

[112] Rev. Proc. 72-18, 1972-1 C.B. 740, as clarified by Rev. Proc. 74-8, 1974-1 C.B. 419, and amplified by Rev. Rul. 80-55, 1980-2 C.B. 849.

[113] *Ibid.*

[114] *B.P. McDonough v. Comm.*, 78-2 USTC ¶9490, 42 AFTR2d 78-5172, 577 F.2d 234 (CA-4, 1978).

Related Taxpayers. The transactions that are subject to restriction are only those between persons who are considered "related" as defined in the Code. Related taxpayers are:[115]

1. Certain family members: brothers and sisters (including half-blood), spouse, ancestors (i.e., parents and grandparents), and lineal descendants (i.e., children and grandchildren)

2. Taxpayer and his or her corporation: an individual and a corporation if the individual owns either directly or *indirectly* more than 50 percent of the corporation's stock[116]

3. Personal service corporation and an employee-owner: a corporation whose principal activity is the performance of personal services that are performed by the employee-owners (i.e., an employee who owns either directly or indirectly *any* stock of the corporation)

4. Certain other relationships involving regular corporations, S corporations, partnerships, estates, trusts, and individuals

In determining whether a taxpayer and a corporation are related, the taxpayer's direct and indirect ownership must be taken into account for the 50 percent test. A taxpayer's indirect stock ownership is any stock that is considered owned or "constructively" owned but not actually owned by the taxpayer. Section 267 provides a set of constructive ownership rules, also referred to as *attribution rules*, indicating the circumstances when the taxpayer is considered as owning the stock of another. Under the constructive ownership rules, a taxpayer is considered owning indirectly[117]

1. Stock owned directly or indirectly by his or her family as defined above

2. His or her proportionate share of any stock owned by a corporation, partnership, estate, or trust in which he or she has ownership (or of which he or she is a beneficiary in the case of an estate or trust)

3. Stock owned indirectly or directly by his or her partner in a partnership

In using these rules, the following limitations apply: (1) stock attributed from one family member to another *cannot* be reattributed to members of his or her family, and (2) stock attributed from a partner to the taxpayer *cannot* be reattributed to a member of his or her family or to another partner.[118]

> **Example 50.** H and W are husband and wife. HB is H's brother. H, W, and HB own 30, 45, and 25% of X Corporation, respectively. H is considered as owning 100% of X Corporation, 30% directly and 70% indirectly (25% through HB and 45% through W, both by application of attribution rule 1 above). W is considered as owning 75% of X Corporation, 45% directly and 30% indirectly through H by application of attribution rule 1 (note that HB's stock cannot be attributed to H and reattributed to W). HB is considered as owning 55% of X Corporation, 25% directly and 30% indirectly through H by application of attribution rule 1 and the reattribution limitation.

---

[115]   § 267(b).

[116]   A partner and a partnership in which the partner owns more than a 50 percent interest are treated in the same manner. See § 707(b).

[117]   § 267(c).

[118]   § 267(c)(5).

Losses. The taxpayer is not allowed to deduct the loss from a sale or exchange of property directly or indirectly to a related taxpayer (as defined above).[119] However, any loss disallowed on the sale may be used to offset any gain on a subsequent sale of the property by a related taxpayer to an unrelated third party.[120]

Example 51. A father owns land that he purchased as an investment for $20,000. He sells the land to his daughter for $15,000, producing a $5,000 loss. The $5,000 loss may not be deducted because the transaction is between related taxpayers. If the daughter subsequently sells the property for $22,000, she will then realize a $7,000 gain ($22,000 sales price − $15,000 basis). However, the gain may be reduced by the $5,000 loss previously disallowed, resulting in a recognized gain of $2,000 ($7,000 realized gain − $5,000 previously disallowed loss). If the daughter had sold the property for only $19,000, the realized gain of $4,000 ($19,000 − $15,000) would have been eliminated by the previous loss of $5,000. The $5,000 loss previously disallowed is used only to the extent of the $4,000 gain. The remaining portion of the disallowed loss ($1,000) cannot be used. Had the father originally sold the property for $19,000 to an outsider as his daughter subsequently did, the father would have recognized a $1,000 loss ($19,000 sales price − $20,000 basis). Note that the effect of the disallowance rule does not increase the basis of the property to the related taxpayer by the amount of loss disallowed.

The results of these transactions are summarized below.

Original sale between related parties

Sales price	$ 15,000
Adjusted basis	(20,000)
Disallowed loss	($ 5,000)

Subsequent sale

	1	2
Sales price	$ 22,000	$ 19,000
Adjusted basis	(15,000)	(15,000)
Realized gain (loss).........................	$ 7,000	$ 4,000
Usage of disallowed loss....................	(5,000)	(4,000)
Recognized gain	$ 2,000	$ 0

Example 52. S owns 100% of V Corporation. She sells stock with a basis of $100 to her good friend T for $75, creating a $25 loss for S. T, in turn, sells the stock to V Corporation for $75, thus recouping the amount he paid S with no gain or loss. The $25 loss suffered by S, however, is not deductible because the sale was made *indirectly* through T to her wholly owned corporation.

Unpaid Expenses and Interest. Prior to enactment of § 267, another tax avoidance device used by related taxpayers involved the use of different accounting methods by each taxpayer. In the typical scheme, a taxpayer's corporation would adopt the accrual basis method of accounting while the taxpayer reported on a cash basis. The taxpayer could lend money, lease property, provide services, etc., to the corporation and charge the corporation for whatever was provided. As an accrual basis taxpayer, the corporation

---

[119]   § 267(a)(1).

[120]   § 267(d).

would accrue the expense and create a deduction. The cash basis individual, however, would report no income until the corporation's payment of the expense was actually received. As a result, the corporation could accrue large deductions without ever having to make a disbursement and, moreover, without the taxpayer recognizing any offsetting income. The Code now prohibits this practice between "related taxpayers" as defined above. Code § 267 provides that an accrual basis taxpayer can deduct an accrued expense payable to a related cash basis taxpayer *only* in the period in which the payment is included in the recipient's income.[121] This rule effectively places all accrual basis taxpayers on the cash method of accounting for purposes of deducting such expenses.

> **Example 53.** B, an individual, owns 100% of X Corporation, which manufactures electric razors. B uses the cash method of accounting while the corporation uses the accrual basis. Both are calendar year taxpayers. On December 27, 2009 the corporation accrues a $10,000 bonus for B. However, due to insufficient cash flow, X Corporation was not able to pay the bonus until January 10, 2010. The corporation may not deduct the accrued bonus in 2009. Rather, it must deduct the bonus in 2010, the year in which B includes the payment in his income.

> **Example 54.** Assume the same facts as above, except that B owns only a 20% interest in X. In addition, X is a large law firm in which B is employed. The results are the same as above because B and X are still related parties: a personal service corporation and an employee-owner.

PAYMENT OF ANOTHER TAXPAYER'S OBLIGATION

As a general rule, a taxpayer is not permitted to deduct the payment of a deductible expense of another taxpayer. A deduction is allowed only for those expenditures satisfying the taxpayer's obligation or arising from such an obligation.

> **Example 55.** As part of Q's rental contract for his personal apartment, he pays 1% of his landlord's property taxes. No deduction is allowed because the property taxes are the obligation of the landlord.

> **Example 56.** P is majority stockholder of R Corporation. During the year, the corporation had financial difficulty and was unable to make an interest payment on an outstanding debt. To protect the goodwill of the corporation, P paid the interest. The payment is not deductible, and P will be treated as having made a contribution to the capital of the corporation for interest paid.

An exception to the general rule is provided with respect to payment of medical expenses of a dependent. To qualify as a dependent for this purpose, the person needs only to meet the relationship, support, and citizen tests.[122] If the taxpayer pays the medical expenses of a person who qualifies as a dependent under the modified tests, the expenses are treated as if they were the taxpayer's expenses and are deductible subject to limitations applicable to the taxpayer.

---

[121] § 267(a)(2).

[122] § 213(a)(1).

SUBSTANTIATION

The Code requires that taxpayers maintain records sufficient to establish the amount of gross income, deductions, credits, or other matters required to be shown on the tax return.[123] As a practical matter, record keeping requirements depend on the nature of the item. With respect to most deductions, taxpayers may rely on the "*Cohan* rule."[124] In *Cohan*, George M. Cohan, the famous playwright, spent substantial sums for travel and entertainment. The Board of Tax Appeals (predecessor to the Tax Court) denied any deduction for the expenses because the taxpayer had no records supporting the items. On appeal, however, the Second Circuit Court of Appeals reversed this decision, indicating that "absolute certainty in such matters is usually impossible and is not necessary."[125] Thus, the Appeals Court remanded the case to make some allowance for the expenditures. From this decision, the "*Cohan* rule" developed, providing that a reasonable estimation of the deduction is sufficient where the actual amount is not substantiated. In 1962, however, Congress eliminated the use of the *Cohan* rule for travel and entertainment expenses and established rigorous substantiation requirements for these types of deductions. Substantiation for other expenses, however, is still governed by the *Cohan* rule. Despite the existence of the *Cohan* rule, records should be kept documenting deductible expenditures since estimates of the expenditures may be substantially less than actually paid or incurred.

TAX PLANNING CONSIDERATIONS

MAXIMIZING DEDUCTIONS

Perhaps the most important step in minimizing the tax liability is maximizing deductions. Maximizing deductions obviously requires the taxpayer to identify and claim all the deductions to which he or she is entitled. Many taxpayers, however, often overlook deductions that they are allowed because they fail to grasp and apply the fundamental rules discussed in this chapter. To secure a deduction, the taxpayer needs only to show that the expense paid or incurred during the year is ordinary, necessary, and related to a profit-seeking activity. Notwithstanding the special rules of limitation that apply to certain deductions, most deductions are allowed because the *taxpayer* is able to recognize and establish the link between the expenditure and the profit-seeking activity. The taxpayer is in the best position to recognize that an expenditure relates to his or her trade or business, not the tax practitioner. Practitioners typically lack sufficient insight into the taxpayer's activities to identify potential deductions. Thus, it is up to the taxpayer to recognize and establish the relationship between an expenditure and the profit-seeking activity. Failure to do so results in the taxpayer's paying a tax liability higher than what he or she is required to pay.

The taxpayer should maximize not only the absolute dollar amount of deductions, but also the value of the deduction. A deduction's value is equal to the product of the amount of the deduction and the taxpayer's marginal tax rate. Because the taxpayer's marginal rate fluctuates over time, the value of a deduction varies depending on the period in which the deduction is claimed. When feasible, deductions should normally be accelerated or deferred to years when the taxpayer is in a higher tax bracket. In timing deductions, however, the time value of money also must be considered. For example, in periods of

---

[123] Reg. § 1.6001-1(a).

[124] *Cohan v. Comm.*, 2 USTC ¶489, 8 AFTR 10552, 39 F.2d 540 (CA-2, 1930).

[125] *Ibid.*

inflation, the deferral of a deduction to a high-bracket year may not always be advantageous, since a deduction in the future is not worth as much as one currently.

An individual taxpayer's timing of itemized deductions is particularly important in light of the standard deduction and the floor on miscellaneous itemized deductions. Many taxpayers lose deductions because their deductions do not exceed the standard deduction in any one year. These deductions need not be lost, however, if the taxpayer alternates the years in which he or she itemizes or uses the standard deduction. For example, in those years where the taxpayer itemizes, all tax deductible expenditures from the prior year should be deferred while expenditures of the following year should be accelerated. By so doing, the taxpayer bunches itemized deductions in the current year to exceed the standard deduction. In the following year, the taxpayer would use the standard deduction. Itemized deductions are considered in detail in Chapter 11.

Maximizing deductions also requires shifting of deductions to the taxpayer who would derive the greatest benefit. For example, if two sisters are co-obligors on a note, good tax planning dictates that the sister in the higher tax bracket pay the deductible interest expense. In this case, either sister may pay and claim a deduction.

TIMING OF DEDUCTIONS

In the previous section, the importance of maximizing the absolute amount of deductions was emphasized. However, because of the time value of money it is equally important to consider the timing of deductions.

> **Example 57.** R, who pays Federal, state, and local taxes equal to 50% of his income, makes a cash expenditure of $10,000. If the $10,000 is deductible immediately, R will realize a tax benefit of $5,000 ($10,000 × 50%). Moreover, because the tax savings were realized immediately, the present value of the benefit is not diminished. On the other hand, if R is not able to deduct the $10,000 for another five years, the benefit of the deduction is substantially reduced. Specifically, assuming the annual interest rate is 10%, the present value of the $5,000 tax savings decreases to $3,105 ($5,000 × [1 ÷ (1 + 0.10)5]), a decrease of almost 38%.

As the above example illustrates, accelerating a deduction from the future to the present can substantially increase its value. Awareness of the provisions permitting acceleration of deductions allows taxpayers to arrange their affairs so as to reap the greatest rewards. For example, a taxpayer may choose an investment that the tax law allows him or her to deduct immediately rather than an investment that must be capitalized and deducted through depreciation over the asset's life.

EXPENSES RELATING TO TAX-EXEMPT INCOME

Although expenses related to tax-exempt income are not deductible, expenses related to tax-deferred income are deductible.[126] For example, income earned on contributions to Individual Retirement Accounts is not taxable until the earnings are distributed (usually at retirement). If the taxpayer borrows amounts to contribute to his or her Individual Retirement Account, interest paid on the borrowed amounts may be deductible (if the general rules for deductibility are met) because the income to which it relates is only tax-deferred, not tax-exempt.

---

[126] *Hawaiian Trust Co., Ltd. v. U.S.*, 61-1 USTC ¶9481, 7 AFTR2d 1553, 291 F.2d 761 (CA-9, 1961). See also Letter Rul. 8527082 (April 2, 1985).

"POINTS" ON MORTGAGES

"Points" paid to secure a mortgage to acquire or improve a principal residence normally are deductible in the year paid or incurred. In some cases, however, the points are not paid out of independent funds of the taxpayer but are withheld from the mortgage proceeds. For example, where a lender is charging two points on a $50,000 loan, or $1,000 (2% of $50,000), the $1,000 is withheld by the lender as payment while the remaining $49,000 ($50,000 − $1,000) is advanced to the borrower. The Tax Court has ruled that in these situations, the taxpayer has not prepaid the interest (as represented by the points) and thus must amortize the points over the term of the loan.[127] To avoid this result and obtain a current deduction, the taxpayer should pay the points out of separate funds rather than having them withheld by the lender. This requirement will be met if the cash paid by the borrower up to and at the closing (including down payments, escrow deposits, earnest money, and amounts paid at closing) is at least equal to the amount deducted for points.[128] In this regard, the IRS has ruled that points paid by the seller on behalf of a borrower will be treated as paid directly from the funds deposited by the borrower.[129] Thus, the borrower will be entitled to a deduction. However, in determining the basis of the residence, the borrower must subtract the amount of seller paid points from the purchase price.

HOBBIES

Several studies suggest that the factor on which the hobby/business issue often turns is the manner in which the taxpayer carries on the activity.[130] For business treatment, it is imperative that the taxpayer have complete and detailed financial and nonfinancial records. Moreover, such records should be used in decision making and in constructing a profit plan. The activity should resemble a business in every respect. For example, the taxpayer should maintain a separate checking account for the activity, advertise where appropriate, obtain written advice from experts and follow it, and acquire some expertise about the operation.

Although the taxpayer is not required to actually show profits, profits in *three* of *five* consecutive years create a substantial advantage for the taxpayer. Where the profit requirement is satisfied, it is presumed that the activity is not a hobby and the IRS has the burden of proving otherwise. For this reason, the cash basis taxpayer might take steps that could convert a loss year into a profitable year. For example, in some situations it may be possible to accelerate receipts and defer payment of expenses. However, the taxpayer should be cautioned that arranging transactions so nominal profits occur has been viewed negatively by the courts.

PROBLEM MATERIALS

DISCUSSION QUESTIONS

7-1 *General Requirements for Deductions.* Explain the general requirements that must be satisfied before a taxpayer may claim a deduction for an expense or a loss.

---

[127] *Roger A. Schubel*, 77 T.C. 701 (1982).

[128] Rev. Proc. 92-12, 1992-3, I.R.B. 27.

[129] Rev. Proc. 94-27, 1994 I.R.B. 15, 6.

[130] See, for example, Burns and Groomer, "Effects of Section 183 on the Business Hobby Controversy," *Taxes* (March 1980) pp. 195–206.

7-2 *Deduction Defined.* Consider the following:
 a. It is often said that income can be meaningfully defined while deductions can be defined only procedurally. Explain.
 b. The courts are fond of referring to deductions as matters of "legislative grace." Explain.
 c. Although deductions may only be defined procedurally, construct a definition for a deduction similar to the "all inclusive" definition for income.
 d. Will satisfaction of the requirements of your definition ensure deductibility? Explain.

7-3 *Business versus Personal Expenditures.* Consider the following:
 a. If the taxpayer derives personal pleasure from an otherwise deductible expense, will the expense be denied? Explain.
 b. Name some of the purely personal expenses that are deductible, and indicate whether they are deductions for or from A.G.I.

7-4 *Business versus Investment Expenses.* Two Code sections govern the deductibility of ordinary and necessary expenses related to profit-motivated activities. Explain why two provisions exist and the distinction between them.

7-5 *An Employee's Business.* Is an employee considered as being in trade or business? Explain the significance of your answer.

7-6 *Year Allowable.* The year in which a deduction is allowed depends on whether the taxpayer is a cash basis or accrual basis taxpayer. Discuss.

7-7 *Classification of Expenses.* F is a self-employed registered nurse and works occasionally for a nursing home. G is a registered nurse employed by a nursing home. Their income, exemptions, credits, etc. are identical. Explain why a deductible expense, although paid in the same amount by both, may cause F and G to have differing tax liabilities.

7-8 *Above- and Below-the-Line Deductions.* At a tax seminar, F was reminded to ensure that he properly classified his deductions as either above- or below-the-line. After the seminar, F came home and scrutinized his Form 1040 to determine what the instructor meant and why it was important. Despite his careful examination of the form, F could not figure out what the instructor was talking about or why it was important. Help F out by explaining the meaning of this classification scheme.

7-9 *Performing Artists.* V hopes to become a movie star someday. Currently, she accepts bit parts in various movies, waiting for her break. What special tax treatment may be available for V?

7-10 *Classification of Deductions.* J and K are both single, and each earns $30,000 of income and has $2,000 of deductible expenses for the current year. J's deductions are for A.G.I. while K's deductions are itemized deductions.
 a. Given these facts, and assuming that the situation of J and K is identical in every other respect, will their tax liabilities differ? Explain.
 b. Same as (a) except their deductions are $5,000.

7-11 *Constructive Distributions.* D owns all of the stock of DX Inc., which manufactures record jackets. Over the years, the corporation has been very successful. This year, D placed his 16- and 14-year-old sons on the payroll, paying them each $10,000 annually. The boys worked on the assembly line a couple of hours each week. Explain D's strategy and the risks it involves.

7-12 *Disguised Distributions.* E owns all of the stock of EZ Inc., which operates a nursery. During the past several years, the company has operated at a deficit and E finally sold all of his stock to C. C drew a very low salary before he could turn things around. Now the business is highly profitable, and C is paying himself handsomely. As C's tax adviser, what counsel if any should be given to C?

7-13 *Income and Expenses of Illegal Business.* B is a bookie in a state where gambling is illegal. During the year, he earned $70,000 accepting bets. His expenses included those for rent, phone, and utilities. In addition, he paid off a state legislator who was a customer and who obviously knew of his activity.
a. Discuss the tax treatment of B's income and expenses.
b. Same as (a) except B was a drug dealer.

7-14 *Permanent and Timing Differences.* Financial accounting and tax accounting often differ in the manner in that certain expenses are treated. Identify several expenditures that, because of their treatment, produce permanent or timing differences.

7-15 *Capital Expenditures.* Can a cash basis taxpayer successfully reduce taxable income by purchasing supplies near year-end and deducting their cost?

7-16 *Independent Contractor versus Employee.* Briefly discuss the difference between an independent contractor (self-employed person) and an employee and why the distinction is important.

7-17 *Hobby Expenses.* Discuss the factors used in determining whether an activity is a hobby and the tax consequences resulting from its being deemed a hobby.

7-18 *Public Policy Doctrine.* A taxpayer operates a restaurant and failed to remit the sales tax for August to the city as of the required date. As a result, he must pay an additional assessment of 0.25 percent of the amount due. Comment on the deductibility of this payment.

7-19 *Constructive Ownership Rules.* Explain the concept of constructive ownership and the reason for its existence.

7-20 *Expenses Relating to Tax-Exempt Income.* Discuss what types of expenses relating to tax exempt income may be deductible.

7-21 *Substantiation.* Explain the Cohan rule.

PROBLEMS

7-22 *General Requirements for Deduction.* For each of the following expenses identify and discuss the general requirement(s) (ordinary, necessary, related to business, etc.) upon which deductibility depends.
a. A police officer who is required to carry a gun at all times lives in New York. The most convenient and direct route to work is through New Jersey. The laws of New Jersey, however, prohibit the carrying of a gun in the car. As a result, he must take an indirect route to the police station to avoid New Jersey. The indirect route causes him to drive ten miles more than he would otherwise. The cost of the additional mileage is $500. (**Note:** commuting expense from one's home to the first job site generally is a nondeductible personal expense.)
b. The current president of a nationwide union spends $10,000 for costs related to reelection.
c. The taxpayer operates a lumber business. He is extremely religious and consequently is deeply concerned over the business community's social and moral responsibility to society. For this reason, he hires a minister to give him and his employees moral and spiritual advice. The minister has no business background although he does offer solutions to business problems.

d. The taxpayer operates a laundry in New York City. He was recently visited by two "insurance agents" who wished to sell him a special bomb policy (i.e., if the taxpayer paid the insurance "premiums," his business would not be bombed). The taxpayer paid the premiums of $500 each month.

7-23 *Accrual Basis Deductions.* In each of the following situations assume the taxpayer uses the accrual method of accounting and indicate the amount of the deduction allowed.

a. R sells and services gas furnaces. As part of his sales package, he agrees to turn on and cut off the buyer's furnace for five years. He normally charges $80 for such service, which costs him about $50 in labor and materials. Based on 2009 sales, R sets up a reserve for the costs of the services to be performed, which he estimates will be $9,000 over the next five years.

b. At the end of 2009, XYZ, a regular corporation, agreed to rent office space from ABC Leasing Corp. Pursuant to the contract, XYZ paid $10,000 on December 1, 2009 for rent for all of 2010.

c. RST Villas, a condominium project in a Vermont ski resort, reached an agreement with MPP Pop-Ins providing that MPP would provide maid services in 2010 for $20,000. RST transferred its note payable for $20,000 at the end of 2010 to MPP on December 1, 2009.

7-24 *Economic Performance.* KKO Printing, a calendar year, accrual method taxpayer, leases a number of copying machines. In conjunction with the lease, it typically purchases a one-year maintenance contract covering service on the machines. On July 20, 2009, KKO paid $6,000 for a one-year service contract that runs from July 1, 2009 through June 30, 2010. Ignoring the recurring item exception, when may KKO deduct the expense?

7-25 *Recurring Items.* M Corporation is an accrual basis taxpayer and uses the calendar year for both financial accounting and tax purposes. The corporation manufactures car stereo equipment and provides a one-year warranty. Based on an analysis of its sales for 2009, it estimates that its warranty expense for equipment sold in 2009 will be $500,000. For financial accounting purposes, M plans to accrue the expense in 2009. The corporation is in the process of finishing its 2009 tax return, which it plans on filing by the extended due date, September 15, 2010. According to the company's latest figures, as of August 31, it had incurred $200,000 in parts and labor costs in honoring warranties on 2009 sales. How should the corporation treat the $500,000 estimated warranty cost on its 2009 tax return?

7-26 *Accrual of Real Property Taxes.* M Corporation owns a chain of hamburger restaurants located all across the country. In one state where the company has several outlets, it paid real property taxes of $12,000 for the period October 1, 2008 through September 30, 2009 on January 10, 2010. M is an accrual basis taxpayer and uses a calendar year-end for reporting.

a. When is the corporation entitled to a deduction for the real estate taxes assuming it has not made an election under § 461(c) and the recurring item exception does not apply?

b. Same as (a) except the corporation makes an election under § 461(c).

7-27 *Accrual versus Cash Method of Accounting.* D operates a hardware store. For 2009, D's first year of operation, D reported the following items of revenue and expense:

Cash receipts	$140,000
Purchase of goods on credit	90,000
Payments on payables	82,000

By year-end, D had unsold goods on hand with a value of $25,000.

     a. Using the cash method of accounting, compute D's taxable income for the year.

     b. Using the accrual method of accounting, compute D's taxable income for the year.

     c. Which method of accounting is required for tax purposes? Why?

7-28 *Prepaid Interest.* In each of the following cases, indicate the amount of the deduction for the current year. In each case, assume the taxpayer is a calendar year, cash basis taxpayer.

     a. On December 31, P, wishing to reduce his current year's tax liability, prepaid $3,000 of interest on his home mortgage for the first three months of the following taxable year.

     b. On December 1 of this year, T obtained a $100,000 loan to purchase her residence. The loan was secured by the residence. She paid two points to obtain the loan bearing a 6 percent interest rate.

     c. Same as (b) except the loan was used to purchase a duplex, which she will rent to others. The loan was secured by the duplex.

7-29 *Prepaid Rent.* This year F, a cash basis taxpayer, secured a ten-year lease on a warehouse to be used in his business. Under the lease agreement he pays $12,000 on September 1 of each year for the following twelve months' rental.

     a. Assuming F pays $12,000 on September 1 for the next 12 months' rental, how much, if any, may he deduct? How would your answer change if F were an accrual basis taxpayer?

     b. In order to secure the lease, F also was required to pay an additional $12,000 as a security deposit. How much, if any, may he deduct?

7-30 *Prepaid Expenses.* D, a cash basis taxpayer, operates a successful travel agency. One of her more significant costs is a special computer form on which airline tickets are printed as well as stationery on which itineraries are printed. Typically, D buys about a three-month supply of these forms for $2,000. Knowing that she will be in a lower tax bracket next year. D would like to accelerate her deductions to the current year.

     a. Assuming that D pays $12,000 on December 15 for forms that she expects to exhaust before the close of next year, how much can she deduct?

     b. Same as above except D purchases the larger volume of forms because D's supplier began offering special discounts for purchases in excess of $3,000.

7-31 *Expenses Producing Future Benefits.* B took over as chief executive officer of Pentar Inc., which specializes in the manufacture of cameras. As part of his strategy to increase the corporation's share of the market, he ran a special advertising blitz just prior to Christmas that cost more than $1,000,000. The marketing staff estimates that these expenditures could very well increase the company's share of the market by 10 percent over the next three years. Speculate on the treatment of the promotion expenses.

7-32 *Capital Expenditure or Repair.* This year, Dandy Development Corporation purchased an apartment complex with 100 units. At the time of purchase, it had a 40 percent vacancy rate. As part of a major renovation, Dandy replaced all of the carpeting and painted all of the vacant units. Discuss the treatment of the expenditures.

7-33 *Identifying Capital Expenditures.* K, a sole proprietor, made the following payments during the year. Indicate whether each is a capital expenditure.

     a. Sales tax on the purchase of a new automobile

     b. Mechanical pencil for K

     c. Mops and buckets for maintenance of building

     d. Freight paid on delivery of new machinery

     e. Painting of K's office

    f.   Paving of dirt parking lot with concrete

    g.   Commissions to leasing agent to find new office space

    h.   Rewiring of building to accommodate new equipment

7-34   *Hobby Expenses—Effect on A.G.I.* C is a successful attorney and stock car racing enthusiast. This year she decided to quit watching the races and start participating. She purchased a car and entered several local races. During the year, she had the following receipts and disbursements related to the racing activities:

Race winnings	$3,000
Property taxes	2,800
Fuel, supplies, maintenance	1,000

Her A.G.I. exclusive of any items related to the racing activities is $100,000.

    a.   Indicate the tax consequences assuming the activity is not considered to be a hobby.

    b.   Assuming the activity is treated as a hobby, what are the tax consequences?

    c.   Assuming the activity is deemed a hobby and property taxes are $4,000, what are the tax consequences?

    d.   What is the critical factor in determining whether an activity is a hobby or a business?

    e.   What circumstances suggest the activity is a business rather than a hobby?

7-35   *Hobby-Presumptive Rule.* In 2008 R, a major league baseball player, purchased a small farm in North Carolina. He grows several crops and maintains a small herd of cattle on the farm. During 2008 his farming activities resulted in a $2,000 loss, which he claimed on his 2008 tax return, filed April 15, 2009. In 2009 his 2008 return was audited, and the IRS proposed an adjustment disallowing the loss from the farming activity, asserting that the activity was merely a hobby.

    a.   Assuming R litigates, who has the burden of proof as to the character of the activity?

    b.   Can R shift the burden of proof at this point in time?

    c.   Assume R filed the appropriate election for 2008 and reported losses of $3,000 in 2009 and profits of $14,000 in 2010, $5,000 in 2011, and $6,000 in 2012. What effect do the reported profits have?

7-36   *Hobby Losses and Statute of Limitations.* Assume the same facts as in *Problem 7-35*. When does the statute of limitations bar assessment of deficiencies with respect to the 2008 tax return?

7-37   *Investigation Expenses.* H currently operates several optical shops in Portland. During the year he traveled to Seattle and San Francisco to discuss with several doctors the possibility of locating optical shops adjacent to their practices. He incurred travel costs to Seattle of $175 and to San Francisco of $200. The physicians in Seattle agreed to an arrangement and H incurred $500 in legal fees drawing up the agreement. The physicians in San Francisco, however, would not agree, and H did not pursue the matter further.

       In the following year, H decided to enter the ice cream business. He sent letters of inquiry to two major franchisers of ice cream stores and subsequently traveled to the headquarters of each. He paid $400 for travel to Phoenix for discussions with X Corporation and $500 for travel to Los Angeles for discussions with Y Corporation. He also paid an accountant $1,200 to evaluate the financial aspects of each franchise ($600 for each evaluation). H decided to acquire a franchise from Y Corporation. He paid an attorney $800 to review the franchising agreement.

    a.   Discuss the tax treatment of H's expenses associated with the attempt to expand his optical shop business.

> **b.** Discuss the tax treatment of the expenses incurred in connection with the ice cream business, assuming H acquires the Y franchise and begins business.
>
> **c.** Same as (b). Discuss the treatment of these costs if H abandons the transaction after being informed that there is no franchise available in his city.

7-38   *Investigation Expenses.* P incurred significant expenses to investigate the possibility of opening a Dowell's Hamburgers franchise in Tokyo, Japan. Her expenditures included hiring a local firm to perform a feasibility study, travel, and accounting and legal expenses. Her 2009 expenditures total $25,000. With respect to this amount:

> **a.** Assuming this was P's first attempt at opening a business of her own, how much may she deduct in 2009 if she decides not to acquire the franchise?
>
> **b.** Assuming this was P's first attempt at opening a business of her own, how much may she deduct in 2009 if she decides to acquire the franchise?
>
> **c.** Assuming P was already in the fast-food business (she owns a Dowell's franchise in Toledo, Ohio), how much may she deduct in 2009 to acquire the franchise?

7-39   *Capital Expenditures.* Consider the following:

> **a.** A corporate taxpayer reimbursed employees for amounts they had loaned to the corporation's former president, who was losing money at the racetrack. Comment on the deductibility of these payments as well as those expenditures discussed in *Example 7* of this chapter (relating to payments of debts previously discharged by bankruptcy) in light of the rules concerning capital expenditures.
>
> **b.** How are expenditures such as land and investment securities recovered?
>
> **c.** How are the costs of expenditures for goodwill recovered?
>
> **d.** Distinguish between a capital expenditure and a repair.

7-40   *Classification of Deductions.* M works as the captain of a boat. His income for the year is $20,000. During the year, he purchased a special uniform for $100. Indicate the amount of the deduction and whether it is for or from A.G.I. for the following situations:

> **a.** M's boat is a 50-foot yacht, and he operates his business as a sole proprietorship (i. e., he is self-employed).
>
> **b.** M is an employee for Yachts of Fun Inc.
>
> **c.** M is an employee for Yachts, which reimbursed him $70 of the cost (included in his income on Form W-2).

7-41   *Computing Employee's Deductions.* T is employed as a supervisor in the tax department of a public accounting firm in Manhattan. She recently took the job after working on the tax staff at a commercial tax preparation firm. She lives in a condominium on the upper east side. Every day she takes the subway to and from work. She loves living in New York. T's total income for the year consisted of compensation of $80,000 and alimony of $2,100. During the year, she incurred the following expenses:

AICPA dues	$ 400
New York State Society of CPAs dues	315
State of New York CPA license	345
Subscriptions to tax journals	225
Continuing education course on new tax law	600
New business suits	700
Cleaning of suits	389
Legal fee for preparation of will ($230 related to tax planning)	1,500
Legal fee to collect alimony	250
Job hunting expenses (resumes and employment agency fee)	150
Subway expenses	456
Safe deposit box (holds investment documents)	90
Annual fee on brokerage account	130
Qualified residence interest	6,000

T's employer reimbursed her $100 for the AICPA dues (included in her income).

a. Compute T's taxable income.

b. Assuming T expects her expenses to be about the same for the next several years, what advice can you offer?

7-42 *Computing Employee's Deductions.* Z, a single taxpayer, is employed as a nurse at a local hospital. Z's records reflect the following items of revenue and expense for 2009:

Gross wages	$20,000
Expenses:	
Employee travel expenses, not reimbursed	1,100
Cost of commuting to and from work, reimbursed (included in gross wages)	520
Charitable contributions	700
Interest and taxes on personal residence	3,900
Nurse's uniform, reimbursed (included in gross wages)	250

a. What is Z's A.G.I.?

b. What is Z's total of itemized deductions?

7-43 *Interest.* Mr. E operates a replacement window business as a sole proprietorship. He uses the cash method of accounting. On November 1, 2009 he secured a loan in order to purchase a new warehouse to be used in his business. Information regarding the loan and purchase of the warehouse is shown below. All of the costs indicated were paid during the year.

Term	20 years
Loan origination fee	$ 2,000
Points	6,000
One year's interest paid in advance	20,000
Legal fees for recording mortgage lien	500

What amount may E deduct in 2009?

7-44 *Insurance.* Hawk Harris owns and operates the Waterfield Mudhens, a franchise in an indoor soccer league. Both Hawk and the corporation are cash basis, calendar year taxpayers. During 2009 the corporation purchased the following policies:

Policy Description	Cost	Date Paid
Two-year fire and theft effective 12/1/09	$2,400	12/15/09
One-year life insurance policy on Jose Greatfoot, star forward; the corporation is beneficiary; effective 11/1/09	1,000	11/1/09
One-year group-term life insurance policy covering entire team and staff; effective 1/1/09	9,000	1/15/09

One-year policy for payments
of overhead costs should
the team strike and attendance
fall; effective 11/1/09   3,600   9/1/09

In addition to the policies purchased above, the corporation is unable to get insurance on certain business risks. Therefore, the corporation has set up a reserve—a separate account—to which it contributes $5,000 on February 1 of each year.

How much may the corporation deduct for 2009?

7-45 *Life Insurance.* The Great Cookie Corporation is owned equally by F and G. Under the articles of incorporation, the corporation is required to purchase the stock of each shareholder upon his or her death to ensure that it does not pass to some undesirable third party. To finance the purchase, the corporation purchased a life insurance policy on both F and G, naming the corporation as beneficiary. The annual premium is $5,000. Can the corporation deduct the premiums?

7-46 *Business Life Insurance.* L, 56, has operated her sole proprietorship successfully since its inception three years ago. This year she has decided to expand. To this end, she borrowed $100,000 from the bank, which would be used for financing expansion of the business. The bank required L to take out a life insurance policy on her own life that would serve as security for the business loan. Are the premiums deductible?

7-47 *Public Policy-Fines, Lobbying, etc.* M is engaged in the construction business in Tucson. Indicate whether the following expenses are deductible.
  a. The Occupational Safety and Health Act (OSHA) requires contractors to fence around certain construction sites. M determined that the fences would cost $1,000 and the fine for not fencing would be only $650. As a result, he did not construct the fences and paid a fine of $650.
  b. M often uses Mexican quarry tile on the floors of homes that he builds. To obtain the tiles, he drives his truck across the border to a small entrepreneur's house and purchases the materials. On the return trip he often pays a Mexican customs official to "expedite" his going through customs. Without the payment, the inspection process would often be tedious and consume several hours. This year he paid the customs officials $200.
  c. M paid $100 for an advertisement supporting the administration's economic policies, which he felt would reduce interest rates and thus make homes more affordable. In addition, he paid $700 for travel to Washington, D.C. to testify before a Congressional Committee on the effects of high interest rates on the housing industry. While there, he paid $100 to a political action committee to attend a dinner, the proceeds from which went to Senator Q.

7-48 *Limitations on Business Deductions.* This is an extension of *Problem 7-22(d)*. In that problem, you are asked to determine if the case contains expenditures that are ordinary, necessary, and reasonable under the provisions of Code § 162. Assume the positive criteria of § 162 are met (i.e., the expenditures are ordinary, necessary, and reasonable). Are there any additional provisions in § 162 that will cause the expenditures to be disallowed?

7-49 *Related Taxpayers—Sale.* E sold stock to her son for $8,000. She purchased the stock several years ago for $11,000.
  a. What amount of loss will E report on the sale?
  b. What amount of gain or loss will the son report if he sells the stock for $12,000 to an unrelated party?
  c. If the son sells for $10,000?
  d. If the son sells for $4,000?

7-50 *Related Taxpayers—Different Accounting Methods.* G, a cash basis, calendar year taxpayer,—owns 100 percent of XYZ Corporation. XYZ is a calendar year, accrual basis taxpayer engaged in the advertising business. G leases a building to the Corporation for $1,000 per month. In December, XYZ accrues the $1,000 rental due. Indicate the tax treatment to XYZ and G assuming the payment is

    a. Made on December 30 of the current year; or

    b. Made on April 1 of the following year.

    c. Would your answers above change if G owned 30 percent of XYZ?

7-51 *Constructive Ownership Rules.* How much of RST Corporation's stock is B considered as owning?

Owner	Shares Directly Owned
B	20
C, B's brother......................................	30
D, B's partner......................................	40
E, B's 60-percent-owned corporation	100
Other unrelated parties............................	10

7-52 *Expenses of Another Taxpayer.* B is the only child of P and will inherit the family fortune. P, who is in the 28 percent tax bracket, is willing to give B and his wife $500 a month. Comment on the advisability of P paying the following directly in lieu of making a gift.

    a. Medical expenses of B, who makes $20,000 during the year; P (the father) provides 55 percent of B's support.

    b. Interest and principal payments on B's home mortgage, on which B and his wife are the sole obliges.

    c. Same as (b) except that P is also an obligee on the note.

7-53 *Losses.* This year was simply a financial disaster for Z. Indicate the effects of the following transactions on Z's taxable income. Ignore any limitations that may exist.

    a. After the stock market crash, Z sold her stock and realized a loss of $1,000.

    b. Z sold her husband's truck for $3,000 (basis $2,000) and her own car for $5,000 (basis $9,000). Both vehicles were used for personal purposes.

    c. Z's $500 camera was stolen.

    d. The land next to Z's house was rezoned to light industrial, driving down the value of her home by $10,000.

7-54 *Planning Deductions.* X, 67, is a widow, her husband having died several years ago. Each year, X receives about $30,000 of interest and dividends. Because the mortgage on her home is virtually paid off, her only potential itemized deductions are her contributions to her church and real estate taxes. Her anticipated deductions are:

Year	Contribution
2009	$2,000
2010	3,000
2011	1,000

What tax advice can you offer X?

7-55 *Timing Deductions.* T currently figures that Federal, state, and local taxes consume about 30 percent of his income at the margin. Next year, however, due to a tax law change his taxes should increase to about 40 percent and remain at that level for at least five or six years. Assuming T buys a computer for $4,000 and he has the option of

deducting all of the cost this year or deducting it ratably through depreciation over the next five years, what advice can you offer?

7-56 *Classification and Deductibility.* In each of the following independent situations, indicate for the current taxable year the amounts deductible *for* A.G.I., *from* A.G.I., or *not deductible* at all. Unless otherwise stated, assume all taxpayers use the cash basis method of accounting and report using the calendar year.

  a. M spent $1,000 on a life insurance policy covering her own life.

  b. G is an author of novels. His wife attempted to have him declared insane and have him committed. Fearing the effect that his wife's charges might have on him and his book sales, G paid $11,000 in legal fees, resulting in a successful defense.

  c. Taxpayer, a plumber employed by XYZ Corporation, paid union dues of $100.

  d. Q Corporation paid T, its president and majority shareholder, a salary of $100,000. Employees in comparable positions earn salaries of $70,000.

  e. L operates a furniture business as a sole proprietorship. She rents a warehouse (on a month-to-month basis) used for storing items sold in her store. In late December, L paid $2,000 for rental of the warehouse for the month of January.

  f. M is a self-employed security officer. He paid $100 for uniforms and $25 for having them cleaned.

  g. N is a security officer employed by the owner of a large apartment complex. He pays $150 for uniforms. In addition, he paid $15 for having them cleaned. His employer reimbursed him $60 of the cost of the uniforms (included in his income on Form W-2).

  h. K owns a duplex as an investment. During the year, she paid $75 for advertisements seeking tenants. She was unable to rent the duplex, and thus no income was earned this year.

  i. P paid $200 for subscriptions to technical journals to be used in his employment activities. Although P was fully reimbursed by his employer, his employer did not report the reimbursement in P's income.

7-57 *Classification and Deductibility.* In each of the following independent situations, indicate for the current taxable year the amounts deductible *for* A.G.I., *from* A.G.I., or *not deductible* at all. Unless otherwise stated, assume all taxpayers use the cash basis method of accounting and report using the calendar year.

  a. O paid the interest and taxes of $1,000 on his ex-wife's home mortgage. The divorce agreement provided that he could claim deductions for the payments.

  b. P paid an attorney $1,500 in legal fees related to her divorce. Of these fees, $600 is for advice concerning the tax consequences of transferring some of P's stock to her husband as part of the property settlement.

  c. R paid $10,000 for a small warehouse on an acre of land. He used the building for several months before tearing it down and erecting a hamburger stand.

  d. H and his wife moved into the city and no longer needed their personal automobiles. They sold their Chevrolet for a $1,000 loss and their Buick for a $400 gain.

  e. C is employed as a legal secretary. This year he paid an employment agency $300 for finding him a new, higher-paying job as a legal secretary.

  f. X operates his own truck service. He paid $80 in fines for driving trucks that were overweight according to state law.

  g. T, an employee, paid $175 to an accountant for preparing her personal income tax returns.

7-58 *Classification and Deductibility.* In each of the following independent situations, indicate for the current taxable year the amounts deductible for A.G.I., from A.G.I., or not deductible at all. Unless otherwise stated, assume all taxpayers use the cash basis method of accounting and report using the calendar year.

  a. B sold stock to his mother for a $700 loss. B's mother subsequently sold the stock for $400 less than she had paid to B.

b. Same as (a) but assume the mother sold the stock for $500 more than she had paid to B.

c. D operates three pizza restaurants as a sole proprietorship in Indianapolis. In July he paid $1,000 in air fares to travel to Chicago and Detroit to determine the feasibility of opening additional restaurants. Because of economic conditions, D decided not to open any additional restaurants.

d. T owns and operates several gun stores as a sole proprietorship. In light of gun control legislation, he traveled to the state capital at a cost of $80 to testify before a committee. In addition, he traveled around the state speaking at various Rotary and Kiwanis Club functions on the pending legislation at a cost of $475. T also placed an advertisement in the local newspaper concerning the merit of the legislation at a cost of $50. He pays dues to the National Rifle Association of $100.

e. D is employed as a ship captain for a leisure cruise company. He paid $1,000 for rent on a warehouse where he stores smuggled narcotics, which he sells illegally.

f. M, a plumber and an accrual basis taxpayer, warrants his work. This year he estimates that expenses attributable to the warranty work are about 3 percent of sales, or $3,000.

g. G, a computer operator, pays $75 for a subscription to an investment newsletter devoted to investment opportunities in state and municipal bonds.

7-59 *Employee Business Expenses: Planning.* J is employed as a salesman by Bigtime Business Forms Inc. He is considering the purchase of a new automobile that he would use primarily for business. Are there any tax factors that J might consider before purchasing the new car?

TAX RETURN PROBLEMS

CONTINUOUS TAX RETURN PROBLEMS See Appendix D, Part 1.

CUMULATIVE PROBLEMS

TaxCut **7-60** Tony Johnson (I.D. No. 456-23-7657), age 45, is single. He lives at 5220 Grand Avenue, Brooklyn, NY 10016. Tony is employed by RTI Corporation, which operates a chain of restaurants in and around New York City. He has supervisory responsibilities over the managers of four restaurants. An examination of his records for 2009 revealed the following information.

1. During the year, Tony earned $33,000. His employer withheld $2,200 in Federal income taxes and the proper amount of FICA taxes. Tony obtained his current job through an employment agency to which he paid a $150 fee. He previously was employed as a manager of another restaurant. Due to the new job, it was necessary to improve his wardrobe. Accordingly, Tony purchased several new suits at a cost of $600.

2. On the days that Tony works, he normally eats his meals at the restaurants for purposes of quality control. There is no charge for the meals, which are worth $2,000.

3. He provides 60 percent of the support for his father, age 70, who lived with Tony all year and who has no income other than social security benefits of $7,000 during the year. Tony provided more than one-half of the cost of maintaining the home.

4. Dividend income from General Motors Corporation stock that he owned was $350. Interest income on savings was $200.

5. Tony and other employees of the corporation park in a nearby parking garage. The parking garage bills RTI Corporation for the parking. Tony figures that his free parking is worth $1,000 annually.

6. Tony subscribes to several trade publications for restaurants at a cost of $70.

7. During the year, he paid $200 to a bank for a personal financial plan. Based on this plan, Tony made several investments, including a $2,000 contribution to an individual retirement account, and also rented for $30 a safety deposit box in which he stores certain investment related documents.

8. Tony purchased a new home, paying three points on a loan of $70,000. He also paid $6,000 of interest on his home mortgage during the year. In addition, he paid $650 of real property taxes on the home. He has receipts for sales taxes of $534.

9. While hurrying to deliver an important package for his employer, Tony received a $78 ticket for violating the speed limit. Because his employer had asked that he deliver the package as quickly as possible, Tony was reimbursed $78 for the ticket, which he paid.

Compute Tony's taxable income for the year. If forms are used for the computations, complete Form 1040 and Schedule A. (Use 2008 tax forms since the 2009 forms may not be available.)

TaxCut 7-61 Wendy White (I.D. No. 526-30-9001), age 29, is single. She lives at 1402 Pacific Beach Ave., San Diego, CA 92230. Wendy is employed by KXXR television station as the evening news anchor. An examination of her records for 2008 revealed the following information.

1. Wendy earned $150,000 in salary. Her employer withheld $22,000 in Federal income taxes and the proper amount of FICA taxes.

2. Wendy also received $10,000 in self-employment income from personal appearances during the year. Her unreimbursed expenses related to this income were: transportation and lodging, $523; meals, $120; and office supplies, $58.

3. Wendy reports the following additional deductions: home mortgage interest, $6,250; charitable contributions, $1,300; state and local income taxes, $3,100; and employment-related expenses, $920.

Compute Wendy's taxable income for 2008 and her tax due (including any self-employment tax). If forms are used for the computations, complete Form 1040, Schedule A, Schedule C, and Schedule SE. Use the 2008 forms since the 2009 forms may not be available.

Reminder: FICA and self-employment taxes are composed of two elements: social security (old age, survivor, and disability insurance) and Medicare health insurance (MHI). In 2008, social security is paid at a rate of 6.2 percent (12.4 percent for self-employed individuals) on the first $106,800 of earned income; MHI is paid at a rate of 1.45 percent (2.9 percent for self-employed individuals) on all earned income.

RESEARCH PROBLEMS

7-62 T and two associates are equal owners in LST Corporation. The three formed the corporation several years ago with the idea of capitalizing on the fitness movement. After a modest beginning and meager returns, the corporation did extremely well this year. As a result, the corporation plans on paying the three individuals salaries that T believes the IRS may deem unreasonable. T wonders whether he can avoid the tax consequences associated with an unreasonable compensation determination by paying back whatever amount is ultimately deemed a dividend.

a. What would be the effect on T's taxable income should he repay the portion of a salary deemed a dividend?

b. Would there be any adverse effects of adopting a payback arrangement?

Partial list of research aids:

Vincent E. Oswald, 49 T.C. 645.
Rev. Rul. 69-115, 1969-1 C.B. 50.

7-63 C, a professor of film studies at State University, often meets with her doctoral students at her home. In her home, C has a room that she uses solely to conduct business related to the classes she teaches at the university. In the room she and her students often review the movies the students have made to satisfy requirements in their doctoral program. Can C deduct expenses related to her home office?

7-64 R moved to St. Louis in 2008 and purchased a home. After living there for a year, his family had grown and required a much larger home. On August 1, 2009 they purchased their dream house, which cost far more than their first home. Shortly before he closed on the new residence, he put his first house on the market to sell. After two months had passed, however, he had received no offers. Fearing that he would be unable to pay the debt on both homes, R decided to rent his old home while trying to sell it. Surprisingly, he was able to rent the house immediately. However, in order to secure the party's agreement to rent monthly, he was required to perform a few repairs costing $500. Seven months after he had rented the home, R sold it. During the rental period, R paid the utilities and various other expenses. R has come to you for your advice on how these events in 2009 would affect his tax return.

7-65 In November 2009 B, employed as a life insurance salesperson for PQR Insurance Company in Newark, New Jersey, purchased a personal computer for use in his work. B has come to you for help in deciding how to handle this purchase on his 2009 tax return. He, of course, wants to expense the full price of the computer under Code § 179.

B relates the following salient information to you with respect to this purchase:

1. B files a joint return with his wife, L. They have a combined A.G.I. of $65,000 before considering this item. They have sufficient qualified expenditures to itemize deductions on Schedule A, but they have no miscellaneous itemized deductions.
2. B paid $3,000 for the laptop computer, which will be used 100 percent for business use.
3. B bought the computer to analyze client data. He figures this will help him increase his sales because he can analyze the results of various insurance options at the client's home or office (all personalized, of course).
4. PQR does not provide B with company-owned computing equipment. In fact, they refused to pay for B's computer because the expense of providing computers for all of PQR's agents would be too great.

How should B treat this purchase on his 2009 tax return?

7-66 On January 28, 2009 S comes to you for tax preparation advice. She has always prepared her own return, but it has become somewhat complicated and she needs professional advice.

During your initial interview, you discover that S is a teacher at a high school in Chicago, Illinois. She is also the coach of the golf team. In 2007 S decided she wanted to be a professional golfer. So, when she was 32 years old, she began a part-time apprenticeship program with the Professional Golfers' Association of America (PGA), where she was an unpaid assistant to the pro at a local country club. Then, in 2007 she became a member of the PGA and began her professional career.

S has not made much money as a professional golfer. In fact, her expenses exceeded her income in both 2007 and 2008 ($4,000 loss in 2007; $3,500 loss in 2008). Believing she was actively engaged in a trade or business (she kept separate records for her golf activities, practiced about 10 hours each week, and worked with a pro whenever she could), S deducted her golf-related expenses on Schedule C and reported her losses from this activity on her prior returns.

The IRS has challenged S's 2007 and 2008 loss deductions, calling them nondeductible "hobby" losses. Is the IRS correct in this matter? Would she win if the matter is taken to court? What planning steps can S take to ensure that any future losses are deductible trade or business losses?

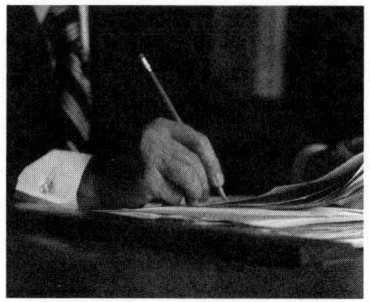

★ CHAPTER EIGHT ★

EMPLOYEE BUSINESS EXPENSES

LEARNING OBJECTIVES

Upon completion of this chapter you will be able to:

- Discuss the rules governing the deduction of several common expenses incurred by employees and self-employed persons

- Recognize when educational expenses are deductible

- Explain the rules concerning the deduction of moving expenses

- Describe when expenses of maintaining a home office are deductible

- Distinguish between deductible transportation expenses and nondeductible commuting costs

- Understand the differences between deductible travel expenses and deductible transportation costs

- Determine when entertainment expenses can be deducted

- Describe the 50 percent limitation on the deduction of meals and entertainment

- Explain the special record-keeping requirements for travel and entertainment expenses

- Discuss the two types of reimbursement arrangements: accountable and nonaccountable plans

CHAPTER OUTLINE

Over the years, many rules have been developed to govern the deductibility of specific business expenses. These rules normally augment the general requirements of § 162 (identified in Chapter 7) by establishing additional criteria that must be satisfied before a deduction may be claimed. As a practical matter, the primary purpose of many of these rules is to prohibit taxpayers from deducting what are in reality personal expenditures. For example, consider a taxpayer who uses a room at home to work or a taxpayer who takes a customer to lunch. In both cases, the expenses incurred very well may be genuine business expenses and deductible under the general criteria. On the other hand, such expenses could simply be *disguised* personal expenditures. As these examples suggest, some of the expenses that are likely to be manipulated are those often incurred by employees in connection with their employment duties. Such common employee expenses as those for travel and entertainment, education, moving, and home offices have long been the source of controversy. Of course, such costs are incurred by a self-employed person as well as by employees and raise similar problems. This chapter examines the special provisions applicable to these items.

EDUCATION EXPENSES

Historically, the tax law has taken the view that most education expenses are personal and, therefore, not deductible. For example, an art appreciation course for the taxpayer's cultural enrichment is purely personal in nature. Consequently, its cost is not

deductible.[1] Similarly, no deduction is granted for expenses of a college education as a business expense on the theory that they are costs of preparing the taxpayer to enter a new business—not the costs of carrying on a business. Therefore, such general education expenses are nondeductible capital expenditures for which no amortization is allowed. Other education expenses, however, such as those incurred by an accountant to attend a seminar on a new tax law, are considered essential costs of pursuing income and are deductible like other ordinary and necessary business expenses. To ensure that deductions are permitted only for education expenses that serve current business objectives and are not personal or capital in nature, special tests must be met.

The Regulations allow a deduction if the education expenses satisfy *either* of the following conditions *and* are not considered personal or capital in nature, as discussed below.[2]

1. The education maintains or improves skills required of the taxpayer in his or her employment or other trade or business.

2. The education meets the express requirements imposed by either the individual's employer or applicable law, and the taxpayer must meet such requirements to retain his or her job, position, or rate of compensation.

Education expenses that meet either of these conditions are still not deductible if they are considered personal or capital expenditures under either of the following two tests:[3]

1. The education is necessary to meet the minimum educational requirements of the taxpayer's trade or business.

2. The education qualifies the taxpayer for a new trade or business.

REQUIREMENTS FOR DEDUCTION

Maintain Skills. For the expense to qualify under the first criterion, the education must be related to the taxpayer's present trade or business and maintain or improve the skills used in such business. The taxpayer must be able to establish the necessary connection between the studies pursued and the taxpayer's current employment. For example, a personnel manager seeking an M.B.A. degree was allowed to deduct all of her education expenses when she ingeniously related each course taken to her job (e.g., a computer course enabled her to be more effective in acquiring information from and communicating with computer personnel).[4] In contrast, the U.S. Tax Court denied the deductions of a research chemist's cost of an M.B.A., indicating that courses such as advanced business finance, corporate strategy, and business law were only remotely related to the skills needed for his job.[5]

Refresher and continuing education courses ordinarily meet the skills maintenance test.

> **Example 1.** T repairs appliances. To maintain his proficiency, he often attends train-ing schools. The costs of attending such schools are deductible because the education is necessary to maintain and improve the skills required in his job.

---

[1]   As discussed below, beginning in 2002, § 222 permits a deduction for qualified expenses.

[2]   Reg. § 1.162-5(a).

[3]   Reg. §§ 1.162-5(b)(2) and (3).

[4]   *Frank S. Blair, III*, 41 TCM 289, T.C. Memo 1980-488.

[5]   *Ronald T. Smith*, 41 TCM 1186, T.C. Memo 1981-149.

Required by Employer or Law. Once the minimum education requirements are met to obtain a job, additional education may be required by the employer or by law to retain the taxpayer's salary or position. Costs for such education are deductible as long as they do not qualify the taxpayer for a new trade or business.

> **Example 2.** This year, R took a new job as a high school instructor in science. State law requires that teachers obtain a graduate degree within five years of becoming employed. Expenses for college courses for this purpose are deductible even though they lead to a degree since such education is mandatory under state law.

New Trade or Business. If education prepares the taxpayer to enter a new trade or business, no deduction is permitted. In this regard, a mere change of duties usually is not considered a new business.[6] For example, a science teacher may deduct the cost of courses enabling him or her to teach art since the switch is a mere change in duties. The taxpayer becomes qualified for a new occupation if the education enables the taxpayer to perform substantially different tasks, regardless of whether the taxpayer actually uses the skills acquired.

> **Example 3.** R was hired as a trust officer in a bank several years ago. His employer now requires that all trust officers must have a law degree. R may not deduct the cost of obtaining a law degree because the degree qualifies him for a new trade or business.[7] No deduction is allowed even though it is required by his employer and R does not actually engage in the practice of law.

Minimum Education. Expenses of education undertaken to gain entry into a business or to meet the minimum standards required in a business are not deductible. These standards are determined in light of the typical conditions imposed by the particular job. For example, the Tax Court denied a $21,000 deduction for the cost of a Northwestern University "MBA" because the degree not only enabled her to meet the minimum education requirements for her position at Merrill Lynch and Raymond James but also prepared her for a new trade or business.[8] In contrast, the Tax Court permitted a salesman for a dental manufacturing company to deduct the cost of his Pepperdine MBA.[9] In this case, the Court found that the employer did not have a minimum education requirement and that the MBA did not qualify the taxpayer for a new trade or business or a promotion. As these two recent cases suggest, if the government can demonstrate that the employer has a minimum education requirement either to begin the job or obtain a promotion, it will deny the deduction for any education that enables the taxpayer to meet such requirement.

The minimum education requirement also operates to prohibit the deduction of such expenses as those for a review course for the bar or C.P.A. exam and fees to take such professional exams.[10] Similarly, education expenses related to a pay increase or promotion may not be deductible under this rule if the increase or promotion was the primary objective of the education. However, as discussed below, a special provision allows a deduction for qualified tuition expenses.

TRAVEL AS A FORM OF EDUCATION

Prior to 1986, travel in and of itself was considered a deductible form of education when it was related to a taxpayer's trade or business. For example, an instructor of Spanish could

---

6   Reg. § 1.162-5(b)(3).

7   Reg. § 1.162-5(b)(3)(ii), Ex.1.

8   *Will M. McEuen III*, TC Summary Opinion 2004-107. See also *Veronica L. Foster*, TC Summary Opinion 2008-22.

9   *Daniel Allemeir* TC Memo 2005-207.

10   Rev. Rul. 69-292, 1969-1 C.B. 84.

travel around Spain during the summer to learn more about the Spanish culture and improve her conversational Spanish. In such case, the travel cost would have been deductible since it was related to the taxpayer's trade or business. In 1986, Congress became concerned that many taxpayers were using this rule to deduct what were essentially the costs of a personal vacation. Moreover, Congress believed that any business purpose served by traveling for general education purposes was insignificant. To eliminate possible abuse, no deduction is allowed simply because the travel itself is educational.[11] Deductions are allowed for travel only when the education activity otherwise qualifies and the travel expense is necessary to pursue such activity. For example, a deduction for travel would be allowed where a professor of French literature travels to France to take courses that are offered only at the Sorbonne.

TYPES AND CLASSIFICATION OF EDUCATION DEDUCTIONS

Education expenses normally deductible include costs of tuition, books, supplies, typing, transportation, and travel (including meals, lodging, and similar expenses). Typical education expenses are for college or vocational courses, continuing professional education programs, professional development courses, and similar courses or seminars.

The costs of transportation between the taxpayer's place of work and school are deductible. If the taxpayer goes home before going to school, however, the expense of going from home to school is deductible, but only to the extent that it does not exceed the costs of going directly from work. The cost of transportation from home to school on a nonworking day represents nondeductible commuting.

Unreimbursed educational expenditures of an employee are treated as miscellaneous itemized deductions subject to the 2 percent floor. In contrast, if an employer reimburses an employee for such expenses under an *accountable plan* (discussed later in this chapter), the reimbursement is excludable from gross income. Any reimbursement not made under an accountable plan must be included in the employee's gross income, and qualifying deductions must be treated as miscellaneous itemized deductions. Finally, education expenses incurred by a self-employed person are deductible *for* A.G.I.

DEDUCTION FOR QUALIFIED TUITION AND RELATED EXPENSES

The general rules governing the deduction of education expenses normally prohibit taxpayers from deducting the costs of obtaining a college education since such expenses are considered personal (i.e., incurred to meet minimum education requirements). However, to help subsidize the increasing cost of higher education, Congress created a special provision. Section 222 allows a deduction for *qualified tuition and related expenses* incurred in connection with enrollment or attendance at an *eligible educational institution*. (Note: this deduction expires after 2009 and at this writing it is uncertain whether it will be extended.) Normally, the amount of the deduction is $4,000 and is available to all taxpayers since it may be claimed for A.G.I. However, the deduction can be reduced or eliminated depending on the taxpayer's filing status and adjusted gross income as follows:

A.G.I. Joint Returns	A.G.I. Other Taxpayers	Amount of Deduction
$ 0–$130,000	$ 0–$65,000	$4,000
$130,001–$160,000	$65,001–$80,000	$2,000
>$160,000	>$80,000	$ 0

Note that there is no phase-out of the deduction, but rather a cliff effect. If A.G.I. exceeds the applicable dollar limit, the deduction is either reduced or disallowed in its entirety. The deduction can be claimed for expenses of the taxpayer, the taxpayer's spouse,

---

[11]   § 274(m)(2).

and the taxpayer's dependents. Consistent with this approach, the law prohibits taxpayers who are eligible to be claimed as dependents from claiming the deduction. In addition, married taxpayers must file jointly in order to claim the deduction. Finally, to prohibit a double benefit, the deduction is not allowed if the taxpayer or any other person claims the Hope Scholarship credit or the Lifetime Learning credit (see below) with respect to that individual for that particular year. Moreover, it the taxpayer receives distributions from a 529 plan or an educational savings account that are nontaxable (see below), the deduction must be reduced by such amounts.[12]

Only qualified tuition and related expenses may be deducted. This definition normally encompasses the tuition and fees charged by most universities. It should be noted, however, that fees for course-related books, supplies, and equipment normally do not qualify unless—according to the IRS—the fees must be paid *to the institution* as a condition of enrollment or attendance. For example, a student activity fee, a special technology or lab fee charged by a university should qualify. On the other hand, qualified expenses do not include the cost of: insurance, medical expenses (including student health fees), room and board, transportation, or similar personal, living, or family expenses. This is true even if the fee must be paid to the institution as a condition of enrollment or attendance. In addition, qualified tuition and related expenses generally do not include expenses that relate to any course of instruction or other education that involves sports, games or hobbies, or any noncredit course unless the course is part of the student's degree program. Note that both undergraduate and graduate courses qualify and it makes no difference whether the course is part of a program that leads to a degree.

Only qualified expenses paid to *eligible educational institutions* are deductible. An eligible education institution is defined as any accredited post secondary institution that offers credit toward a bachelor's degree, an associate's degree or other recognized post-secondary credential. Thus tuition for most colleges and universities as well as junior colleges qualify. Some vocational institutions (e.g., trade schools) and proprietary for-profit organizations may qualify as well.

> **Example 4.** In August 2009, Mr. and Mrs. Smith paid the tuition for their son's attendance at State University to obtain a graduate degree in accounting. Tuition was $1,900. In December 2008, the Smiths paid the tuition for the second semester of $2,300. The second semester began in January 2009. Mr. and Mrs. Smith have an A.G.I.of $121,000. The son is a graduate student and, consequently, the expenses do not qualify for the Hope Scholarship credit discussed below. In addition, because their A.G.I. exceeds $120,000, the couple is not entitled to claim the Lifetime Learning credit. While the credits are not available, a deduction is allowed since the expenses are paid during the year and are for education for such year or education that begins within three months after the close of the year. The deduction is limited to $4,000 and may be claimed for A.G.I.

> **Example 5.** This year R started law school. He is a part-time student and has a part-time job. He paid tuition of $12,000 for the year. He may deduct $4,000 of the tuition for A.G.I. Alternatively, he could elect to use the Lifetime Learning credit of $2,000 ($10,000 maximum qualified expenses × 20%). However, as noted above, he can either deduct the expenses or claim the credit but not both. If his marginal rate was 25%, the $4,000 deduction would be worth only $1,000 so in this case, he would be better off claiming the credit.

RELATIONSHIP TO EDUCATION CREDITS AND QUALIFIED PREPAID TUITION

In addition to the deduction for education expenses, the Code provides other benefits for education related expenses. There are two credits related to education: (1) the Hope

---

[12] See *Tax Benefits for Higher Education*, IRS Publication 970 (Rev. 2006, p. 33).

Scholarship credit, and (2) the Lifetime Learning credit. Special benefits are also extended to Educational Savings Accounts and Qualified Tuition Programs (§ 529 plans). These credits and tax-favored savings arrangements, discussed in detail in Chapters 13 and 18, are designed to help middle America fund the ever-increasing cost of higher education.

The Hope Scholarship credit and the Lifetime Learning credit are both available for education expenses paid on behalf of the taxpayer, the taxpayer's spouse, or a dependent. For 2009 and 2010, Hope Scholarship credit is 100 percent of the first $2,000 of education expenses and 25 percent of the next $2,000 of expenses for each student. Thus the maximum credit is $2,500 [(100% × $2,000 = $2,000) + (25% × $2,000 = $500)] per year per student. The Hope Scholarship credit generally can be claimed only for the first four years of post-secondary education (e.g., college). The Lifetime Learning credit can be claimed for 20 percent of up to $10,000 of qualified tuition and fees annually. Thus the maximum credit per taxpayer return would be $2,000. In contrast to the Hope Scholarship credit, the Lifetime Learning is available for virtually any type of education for an unlimited number of years. For any one particular student, a taxpayer could elect *either* the Hope credit or a Lifetime Learning credit but not both. Note that the Hope credit is per child and not per taxpayer. The Lifetime Learning credit is per return. As noted above, if the taxpayer elects either credit, the deduction is not allowed. Both credits are phased out for high-income earners. Under the phase-out rules, the Hope credit for married taxpayers filing joint returns is eliminated if their A.G.I. exceeds $180,000 in 2009 ($90,000 for other taxpayers). The Lifetime Learning credit is eliminated for joint filers when their A.G.I. exceeds $120,000 ($60,000 for other taxpayers).

The tax law also provides favorable treatment for two savings arrangements: (1) Educational Savings Accounts (Coverdell Accounts described in §530) and (2) Qualified Tuition Programs (so-called § 529 plans). Contributions to these plans are not deductible. However, income on amounts contributed are nontaxable when earned. In addition, amounts distributed from the plans are nontaxable if such amounts are used for certain expenses for higher education. As noted above, to prevent a double benefit, taxpayers cannot deduct qualified education expenses that have been used to figure the tax-free portion of a distribution from an education savings account or a 529 plan.[13]

It is important to note that the law prevents taxpayers from trying to double dip; that is, the law specifically prohibits taxpayers from claiming both a deduction and a credit for the same education expenses. For example, if a CPA spends $300 to attend a continuing education course, he could claim a deduction of $300 as a business expense under § 162, qualified tuition under § 222, or as the basis for the Lifetime Learning credit of $60. Observe, however, that due to limitations, differing phase-out amounts, definitions of qualifying expenditures, and the interaction with other educational provisions such as the exclusion for educational assistance of § 127 and the working condition fringe benefit rules of § 132, a single expense could be covered by multiple provisions and results in mind-boggling complexity.

> **Example 6.** J recently completed his undergraduate degree at the University of Texas and took a job with a brokerage firm in Dallas. The firm agreed to reimburse him for a portion of the cost of an M.B.A. program. In January, J enrolled as a part-time student in the M.B.A. program at a local university. This year he paid tuition of $22,250 and the firm reimbursed him $8,250 of this amount. In addition, J withdrew $1,000 from an Educational Savings account to help pay the tuition. He paid for the remaining $13,000 from a student loan.
>
> Under the educational assistance rules of § 127 (see Chapter 6), J could exclude $5,250 reimbursement for the coursework (both undergraduate and graduate courses

---

[13]   The reduction is normally equal to the amount of earnings that are nontaxable because they were used to pay qualified education expenses. However, for 529 plans, the amount representing the recovery of contributions to the program that are used for education expenses could be deducted subject to the $4,000 limitation. See footnote 12

qualify) and neither he nor his employer would be required to pay FICA or Medicare taxes on this amount. J also could exclude $1,000 withdrawn from the Educational Savings Account since it was used for qualified higher education expenses. Note that J could not deduct the amount for which he was reimbursed or the withdrawal since both were excluded. The treatment of the remaining $16,000 ($22,250 − $5,250 − $1,000) is not clear. In order to exclude the $3,000 balance reimbursed by his employer as a working condition fringe benefit under § 132, the expense must qualify as a deductible business expense under § 162. The IRS might take the position that none of the remaining amount paid is deductible under § 162 since J has not met the minimum education requirement of the brokerage firm and, therefore, the $3,000 reimbursement would not qualify for exclusion. In any event, J could deduct $4,000 as a qualified tuition expense under § 222. (Observe, that to exclude the $3,000 reimbursement as a working condition fringe under § 132, the item must be deductible under § 162—not § 222.) J could utilize the Lifetime Learning credit instead of the deduction. If it is assumed that he could not exclude the additional reimbursement under §132 and he did not deduct *any* amount under § 222, he could claim a Lifetime Learning credit of $2,000 (20% × up to $10,000). Whether J utilizes the amount paid as a basis for claiming the credit or as a deduction under § 222 depends on any phase-outs and his tax bracket. However, he cannot use the expenses for claiming both the deduction and the credit. Also note that the new § 222 deduction is a deduction for AGI and not a miscellaneous itemized deduction subject to the 2% floor.

DEDUCTION FOR EXPENSES OF PRIMARY AND SECONDARY SCHOOL TEACHERS

(Note: This deduction expires in 2009 and at this writing it is uncertain whether it would be extended.) In 2002, the Bush administration reached out to the teaching profession by creating a special deduction. The deduction originated from a 1996 National Education Association study which found that the average kindergarten–12th grade teacher spent approximately $400 per year out of their personal funds for unreimbursed classroom supplies (e.g., a first grade teacher may incur expenses for the decoration of his or her classroom). Although such expenses were deductible, because they were miscellaneous itemized deductions, it was unlikely that most teachers could deduct such expenses. In supporting the deduction, President Bush asserted that if a businessperson could deduct a meal, "a teacher certainly ought to be able to deduct the cost of pencils or a Big Chief tablet." To this end, §62(a)(2)(D) allows a deduction of up to $250 per year for unreimbursed business expenses incurred in connection with books, supplies, computer equipment, other equipment and supplementary materials used in the classroom. The deduction is for A.G.I. and, therefore, all qualifying teachers benefit. Qualifying teachers are defined as "eligible educators" who for at least 900 hours during a school year is a kindergarten–12th grade teacher, instructor, counselor, principal or aide. The educator is eligible only if he or she works at a school that provides elementary or secondary education (kindergarten–12th grade).

✓ CHECK YOUR KNOWLEDGE

For each of the following situations, indicate whether the expenditures are deductible as education expenses.

Review Question 1. Last June, D graduated magna cum laude from the University of Virginia. This fall he entered Johns Hopkins Medical School, paying tuition of thousands of dollars.

The costs of medical school are not deductible under § 162 as business expenses for two reasons. First, the education is necessary to meet the minimum educational requirements to become a doctor. Second, the education qualifies the taxpayer to carry on a new trade

or business. Nevertheless, D could deduct a portion under § 222 as qualified tuition or claim the Lifetime Learning credit, but not both.

Review Question 2. H, a practicing tax accountant, is taking a series of correspondence courses to become a certified financial planner.

As may be clear by now, very little is black or white in the tax law; here is yet another case. The IRS would probably take the position that the expenses are not deductible because the education qualifies the taxpayer to carry on a new trade or business. From the accountant's perspective, however, the course work simply improves or maintains the skills that he is already using in his business. It would appear that the education does not necessarily enable the taxpayer to do anything that he could not do before except to hold himself out as a certified financial planner. The accountant would deduct the expense. In addition, the Lifetime Learning credit and qualified tuition deduction may also be available if the courses are taken at an eligible educational institution (e.g., as part of a university sponsored program).

Review Question 3. Ms. McClain, an elementary school teacher, took a sabbatical to Ireland, where she studied the art of storytelling.

Whether her expenses are deductible ultimately depends on the facts and circumstances. As noted above, changes made in 1986 aimed to eliminate deductions for travel that were primarily personal in nature. In this case, the taxpayer appears to be pursuing that which might not be available at home. Assuming she spent a reasonable amount of time studying and researching, the expense would be deductible. In contrast, consider an architect who travels all over Europe simply taking pictures of classic architectural styles that he may incorporate in his work. Without more, a court would probably view his trip as merely a disguised vacation and deny a deduction for his travel expenses. As in the previous question, the Lifetime Learning credit and qualified tuition deduction may also be available if the courses are taken at an eligible educational institution (e.g., as part of a university sponsored program).

MOVING EXPENSES

For many years, moving expenses were viewed as nondeductible personal expenses. In 1964, however, Congress revised its position, believing that moving expenses necessitated by the taxpayer's employment should be regarded as a deductible cost of earning income. To this end, Code § 217 was enacted, expressly authorizing a deduction for moving expenses. Section 217 allows self-employed individuals and employees to deduct moving expenses incurred in connection with beginning employment or changing job locations. To ensure that the deduction is allowed only for moves required by the taxpayer's employment, the taxpayer must satisfy *both* a distance test and a time test in order to qualify for the deduction.

DISTANCE REQUIREMENT

The thrust of § 217 is to allow a taxpayer to deduct moving expenses only if there is a change in job location *and* the new location is sufficiently far away that it essentially requires the taxpayer to uproot and move his or her residence. This idea is captured in a somewhat misleading 50-mile distance test. The taxpayer does not satisfy the requirement simply by moving 50 miles to a new residence in connection with a new job location. If this were the case, the taxpayer could meet the requirement by simply moving his office down the hall and at the same time moving his residence 50 miles. Instead, the distance test is constructed to determine if the taxpayer's commute to the new job site *without the*

move would have increased at least 50 miles. Technically, the condition is satisfied if the distance between the old residence and the new job site is at least 50 miles greater than the distance between the old residence and the old job site. Note that both distances are measured from the taxpayer's *former residence*. Thus, if the taxpayer's old commute was four miles, the new commute (absent a move) would have to be at least 54 miles ($54 - 4 = 50$) before the test is satisfied.

> **Example 7.** During the year, R was promoted to district sales manager, requiring her to move from Tucson to Phoenix. To determine whether the 50-mile test is met, the distances shown below must be compared.

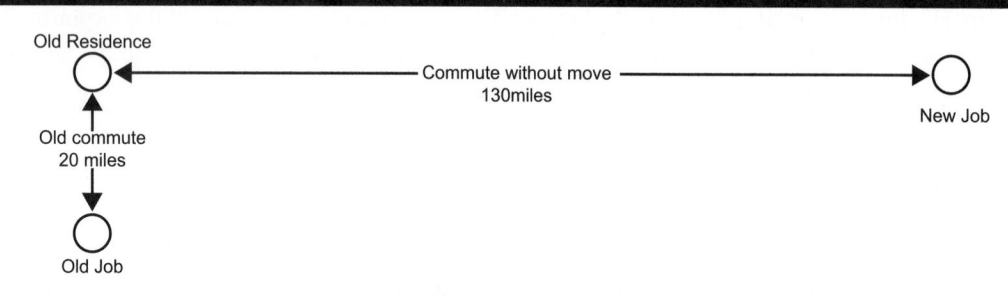

Since the distance between R's old residence and new job (AC = 130 miles) exceeds the distance between R's old residence and old job (AB = 20 miles) by at least 50 miles ($130 - 20 = 110$), the distance requirement is satisfied. In this case, it is quite clear that if the taxpayer had not moved, her commute would have increased significantly (110 miles). Consequently, § 217 grants her a deduction for the costs of moving her residence to a place where the commute is more reasonable. In applying the test, note that the location of the new residence is irrelevant.

If the taxpayer has no old job site, the distance test is satisfied if the new job site is 50 miles from the old residence.[14]

TIME TEST

If taxpayers were not required to maintain employment at the new job site for a minimum amount of time, they could move from place to place, taking temporary jobs in each location to justify the deduction of what in effect are personal travel expenses. To prohibit this possibility, the second test generally requires the taxpayer to work for a *sustained period* of time upon arrival at the new job location. This condition is met if the taxpayer is a *full-time* employee in the area of the new job location for at least 39 weeks during the 12-month period immediately following arrival.[15] Alternatively, the taxpayer may satisfy the test by being an employee or self-employed on a *full-time* basis for at least 78 weeks during the 24-month period after arrival. Note, however, that—like the first test—39 of these 78 weeks must be during the first 12-month period. In either case, the taxpayer need not work for the same employer or for 39 weeks in a row. The time requirement is waived if the taxpayer dies, becomes disabled, is involuntarily dismissed, or is transferred by the new employer.[16]

> **Example 8.** N, an accountant, left his job in Boston to take a new job with a firm in Orlando. After working for the firm for eight months, he became dissatisfied and quit to open his own practice as a sole proprietor. Due to the poor economy, N closed the

---

[14]   § 217(c)(1).

[15]   § 217(c)(2).

[16]   § 217(d).

business after six months and moved to Denver. N may not deduct his expenses of moving to Orlando. since he was employed for only 32 weeks (eight months) during the 12-month period after arrival in Orlando, he does not meet the 39-week test for employees. Similarly, he does not meet the alternative 78-week test since he was employed or self-employed only 56 weeks (14 months) of the 24-month period in Orlando after his arrival. Whether the costs of moving to Denver are deductible depends on whether either of the tests can be satisfied.

In many instances, taxpayers do not know by the end of the tax year whether they will be able to satisfy the time test. Accordingly, the law permits the taxpayer to claim the deduction on the assumption that the test will be satisfied. If the test is subsequently failed, the taxpayer must increase income in the year of failure by the amount of the previous deduction. In lieu of claiming the deduction prior to satisfaction of the test, the taxpayer may wait until the test is satisfied and file an amended return for the year of the moving expense.

DEDUCTIBLE MOVING EXPENSES

For many years, taxpayers were allowed to deduct a variety of moving expenses. These included not only direct expenses such as the cost of moving the taxpayer's personal belongings and the cost of traveling to the new location but also a limited amount of indirect expenses. For example, a taxpayer could deduct expenses for house-hunting trips, temporary living at the new location, and expenses related to disposing of the taxpayer's former residence. In 1993, however, Congress eliminated the deduction for all indirect moving expenses. Currently, only direct moving expenses are deductible. They are:[17]

1. Costs of moving household goods and personal belongings; and

2. Costs of traveling from the old location to the new location.

Costs of Moving Household Goods and Personal Belongings. This category of direct moving expenses includes the following:[18]

- ▸ Packing, crating, and transporting the taxpayer's personal possessions (e.g., the cost of hiring a moving company or renting a truck)
- ▸ Storage and insurance of goods and personal effects while "in-transit" (i.e., any consecutive 30-day period after the day the items are moved from the former home and before they are delivered to the new home)
- ▸ Connecting and disconnecting utilities required by the moving of the taxpayer's appliances
- ▸ Moving a pet
- ▸ Shipping a car

Losses sustained on dispositions of memberships in clubs, expenses of refitting rugs and drapes, mortgage prepayment penalties (although these are usually deductible as interest), and similar expenses are not deductible.

Costs of Traveling. Once the taxpayer's furniture and other items are out the door, the taxpayer's household must follow. Only the costs of moving a taxpayer's family members (including pets) are deductible. Those for such nonfamily members as servants, chauffeurs, governesses, or nurses do not qualify. The following travel expenses are deductible:

---

[17] §§ 217(b)(1)(A) and (B).

[18] Reg. § 1.217-2(b)(3).

▸ Transportation costs. The taxpayer may use actual expenses (i.e., the costs of oil, gasoline, tolls, and parking—but not those for general repairs or maintenance) or 24 cents per mile in 2009.

▸ Lodging expenses. The taxpayer may deduct the costs of lodging incurred in traveling to the new location. No deduction is allowed for any meal expenses related to the move.[19]

Nondeductible Expenses. As noted above, in 1993 Congress eliminated the deduction for so-called "indirect" moving expenses. As a result, expenses for the following are no longer deductible:

▸ House-hunting trips

▸ Temporary living at the new job location (e.g., an apartment or motel)

▸ Sale, purchase, or lease of a residence (e.g., appraisals, attorney's fees, points, or payments to a lessor to cancel a lease)

▸ Meals

Example 9. S, who was employed as a professional basketball player by the Los Angeles Lakers, was traded to the Miami Heat during the year. Although he had lived in Los Angeles for years, S decided he would move permanently to Miami. Prior to the move, S and his wife made several trips to Miami to look for a new home. After finding just the right one, they hired a moving company to pack and move all their personal belongings. During the summer, the entire family made the long trek to Miami. Upon arrival, however, complications arose and they were not able to move in immediately. They ended up staying at a hotel for three weeks before they were able to take possession. S incurred the following expenses in making the move:

Costs of traveling to Miami to look for a house	$ 900
Costs of moving van (including costs of $500 for packing and crating)	15,000
Costs of storage in Miami	1,000
Transportation costs (3,000 miles @ 24 cents per mile)	720
Three-week hotel stay (meals and lodging)	3,000
Real estate commission on sale of former residence	30,000

S is allowed to deduct only the direct expenses related to the move: the van, storage, and transportation, for a total of $16,720 ($15,000 + $1,000 + $720). The indirect expenses, house-hunting, temporary living, and selling expenses are not deductible. However, S may treat the costs of selling his home as a reduction in the amount realized on the sale of the home, decreasing any gain realized or increasing any loss realized. Note that if S's new employer reimburses S for any of the expenses, he must include the reimbursement in income.

CLASSIFYING AND REPORTING THE MOVING EXPENSE DEDUCTION

Moving expenses of an employee or a self-employed person are deductible for A.G.I. All moving expenses are reported on Form 3903.

In many cases, the employer will either pay the moving expenses directly or reimburse the employee for such expenses. When the latter occurs, the employee excludes the payment from gross income as a qualified fringe benefit under § 132. However, the exclusion is allowed only to the extent that the moving expenses meet the requirements for deductibility. It is not unusual for the employer to pay for a number of moving

---

[19] § 217(b)(1)(B).

expenses that are not deductible (e.g., house-hunting and temporary living expenses); in such case, these amounts are included in the employee's W-2 as other income. Similarly, no exclusion is allowed for any moving expenses actually deducted by the employee in the prior year.

✔ CHECK YOUR KNOWLEDGE

Review Question 1. After 15 years with the firm, J was finally promoted to partner. The substantial raise that came along with the promotion enabled him to build the house of his dreams. The new home is nestled in the woods near Lake Lemon, 60 miles from his old condo in the city. His new commute is 58 miles. Will J be able to deduct his moving expenses?

No. The distance requirement focuses on what would have happened to the taxpayer's commute had he not moved. As a general rule, J's commute absent the move must have increased by at least 50 miles. In other words, the distance between the old home and the *new job site* must exceed the distance between the old home and the *old job site* by at least 50 miles. Note that in order to satisfy this requirement there normally must be a change in job location. In this case, his commute without the move does not increase since the job location did not change. Therefore, his moving expenses are not deductible.

Review Question 2. Mitch's three grueling years in law school finally paid off. This year he graduated from Harvard and took a job with a firm in Memphis for $80,000 a year. He does not itemize his deductions. Can he deduct any of his moving expenses?

Yes. Deduction of moving expenses normally requires the taxpayer to change job sites. However, if the taxpayer is not currently employed and has no former job site, the distance test is met if the new job site is at least 50 miles from the taxpayer's old residence. Also note that because moving expenses are deductible for A.G.I., Mitch can claim the deduction even though he does not itemize.

Review Question 3. Grandma and Grandpa retired this year and moved from Detroit to Florida at a cost of $15,000. Both took part-time jobs at a local fast-food restaurant. Can they deduct their moving expenses?

No. In order to meet the time test, the taxpayer must be employed on a *full-time* basis for 39 weeks of the 12-month period immediately following arrival at the new location.

Review Question 4. Indicate whether the following moving expenses are deductible.

  a. Rental of moving truck
  b. Boxes to pack household items
  c. Brake job for car while en route to new location
  d. 55 cents per mile for each mile driven to the new job location
  e. Meals on the three-day, 900-mile trip to the new location
  f. Trip to look for a new house after the new job was secured but before the move

Only (a) and (b) are deductible. Unusual costs incurred in traveling to the new location such as repairs are not deductible. In lieu of deducting actual transportation expenses, 24 cents per mile is allowed. Meals and house-hunting trips are not deductible.

HOME OFFICE EXPENSES

It is currently estimated that more than 39 million Americans—39 percent of the labor force—work at home either full or part time. However, simply working at home does not automatically enable a taxpayer to write off the costs of owning or renting. Very narrow standards must be met before a deduction is permitted.

At one time, expenses relating to use of a portion of the taxpayer's home for business purposes were deductible without limitation when they were merely appropriate and helpful in the taxpayer's business. In 1976, however, Congress felt that the appropriate and helpful test was insufficient to prevent the deduction of what were really personal expenses. For example, under the helpful test, a university professor who was provided an office by his employer could convert personal living expenses into deductions by using a den or some other room in his residence for grading papers. In such a situation, it was unlikely that any additional expense was incurred due to the business use. To prevent the deduction of disguised personal expenses, Congress enacted § 280A, severely limiting the deduction of expenses related to the home. Section 280A generally disallows deduction of any expenses related to the taxpayer's home except those otherwise allowable, such as qualified residence interest and taxes, and those for *certain* business and rental use (the exception for rental use is discussed in Chapter 12).

REQUIREMENTS FOR DEDUCTIBILITY

Under the business use exception, a deduction is allowed for a home office if a portion of the home is "exclusively" used on a "regular" basis for any of three types of business use:[20]

1. As the principal place of business for *any* business of the taxpayer;

2. As a place of business used regularly by patients, clients, or customers in meeting or dealing with the taxpayer in the normal course of his or her trade or business; or

3. In connection with the taxpayer's trade or business when the office is located in a separate structure.

Beyond these basic requirements applicable to all taxpayers, there is one additional test that must be met if the taxpayer is an employee. Employees are entitled to claim a home office deduction only if the home office is for the *convenience of the employer.* Each of these prerequisites is considered below.

Exclusive Use. Under prior law, a taxpayer might write off his whole kitchen just because he opened his briefcase there. The exclusive use requirement was intended to put an end to such shenanigans. A deduction is allowed only when the space in the home is devoted solely to business use. The authors of § 280A apparently did not believe a deduction should be allowed where the space was used for both personal and business purposes. The exclusive use requirement does not mean that the home office must be physically separated from the remainder of the home. It is not necessary that the portion of the room be marked off by a permanent partition. It is sufficient if the home office activities are confined to a particular space in a room that is used only for business purposes.[21] To what extent, if any, the IRS will permit personal activities to be carried on

---

[20]   § 280A(c).

[21]   *George Weightman*, 42 TCM 104, T.C. Memo 1981-301.

in the home office (e.g., making personal phone calls, reading for pleasure, taking care of investments as well as business) is not clear. In any event, the taxpayer should be reminded that the key word is *exclusive*. Two exceptions to the exclusive use test, storage and daycare use, are discussed below.

Regular Use. Section 280A also requires the home office to be used on a regular basis. Fortunately, the Code and Regulations have not adopted precise rules that require the taxpayer to punch a time clock every time he or she steps into the home office. Currently, there is no requirement to keep track of the hours spent in the office. The little guidance that does exist on the issue can be found in IRS publications. The Service does not specifically define *regular* but does explain that occasional or incidental use does not meet the regular use test even if that part of the home is used for no other purpose.[22]

Convenience of the Employer. As noted above, if the taxpayer is an employee, he or she must jump one additional hurdle before claiming the home office deduction. An employee must work at home for the *convenience of the employer*. To meet this condition, the home office must be more than appropriate and helpful. The U.S. Tax Court has suggested that satisfaction of this test requires the taxpayer to show that he or she was unable to do the work performed at home at the employer's office.[23] For example, the Second Circuit has held in *Weissman* that this standard is met if the employer does not provide the employee with space to properly perform his or her employment duties.[24] In this case, a college professor who shared an office and did extensive research at home satisfied the test because in the Court's view the home office was necessitated by lack of suitable working space on campus.

Principal Place of Any Business. A taxpayer satisfies the first business use test if the home office is the principal place of business for *any* business of the taxpayer. Most taxpayers, as employees, fail this test since their only business is that of being an employee and the principal location of that business is at the employer's office. This rule is not foolproof, however. In one decision, the court held that the principal place of business of a taxpayer employed as a concert musician was his home practice room rather than where he gave performances.[25] In contrast, employees who have a *second* business (e.g., selling cosmetics or vitamins) or self-employed persons who operate these activities out of their home normally satisfy the first business use test as long as they can show that the home is in fact the principal place of business.

For years, taxpayers and the IRS squabbled over when a home office constituted a taxpayer's *principal* place of business.[26] The leading case was the Supreme Court's 1993 decision in *Nader E. Soliman*.[27] Soliman was an anesthesiologist who worked for three hospitals. However, none of the hospitals provided him an office so he spent 10 to 15 hours a week at his home office doing his billing and scheduling. To Soliman's chagrin, the IRS denied his deductions for his home office expenses. Upon review, the U. S. Tax Court was more sympathetic, allowing the deductions on the grounds that the home office was essential to Soliman's business, he had spent substantial time there, and there was no other location available to perform the office function of the business. Although the Fourth Circuit agreed with the U.S. Tax Court, the Supreme Court did not.

---

[22] § 280A(c)(1). See *Business Use of Your Home*, IRS Publication 587 (2007), p. 3.

[23] *Robert Chauls*, 41 TCM 234, T.C. Memo 1980-471.

[24] *Weissman v. Comm.*, 85-1 USTC ¶9106, 55 AFTR2d 85-539, 751 F.2d (CA-2, 1984).

[25] *Drucker v. Comm.*, 83-2 USTC ¶9550, AFTR2d 83-5804 (CA-2, 1983); but see *Popov v. Comm.*, T.C. Memo 1998-374.

[26] For example, see *Rudolph Baie*, 74 T.C. 105 (1980).

[27] *Comm. v. Soliman*, 93-1 USTC ¶50,014 (USSC, 1993), rev'g Nader E. Soliman, 94 T.C. 20 (1990).

The high court stated that it is not sufficient that the work done in the home office is essential to the business. The court explained that to satisfy the principal place of business test, the home office must be the most important place of business as compared to all the other locations where the taxpayer carries on business. In determining whether the home office is the *most important place of business*, the court identified two factors that should be considered: (1) the relative importance of the functions performed at each of the business locations, and (2) the amount of time spent at each location. In this case, the court believed that the hospital, where Soliman performed his services and treated patients, was his most important place of business.

As might be expected, a huge backlash erupted after the *Soliman* decision since it operated to deny the home office deduction to millions of taxpayers. Most affected were those who performed essential business functions in their homes but who spent most of their time at the locations of their clients and customers (e.g., salespeople, consultants, repair people, personal trainers, caterers, etc.). In response, Congress acted in 1997 to restrict the scope of *Soliman*. Although the tests of *Soliman* can still apply, the taxpayer may now meet the principal place of business test if both of the following conditions are met:

1. The office is used by the taxpayer to conduct *administrative and management activities* of a trade or business; and

2. There is no other fixed location of the trade or business where the taxpayer conducts *substantial* administrative and management activities of the trade or business.

Under the new test, taxpayers who manage or administer their businesses out of a home office should be allowed a deduction even if the taxpayer conducts substantial non-administrative or nonmanagement business activities at a fixed location of the business outside the home. For example, this new approach would allow taxpayers like the doctor in *Soliman* a deduction for their home office expenses even though they conduct significant activities away from home at a fixed location (e.g., surgery at a hospital). Similarly, outside salespeople who spend the majority of their time calling on customers can claim the deduction if they use their home office to conduct administrative activities such as receiving orders, setting up appointments, or writing-up orders. In some cases, taxpayers may have an office available to perform administrative activities but opt to perform these tasks at home. In such case, the test is still met assuming the taxpayer does not actually perform substantial management or administrative activities at the other location. At all times, however, it must be emphasized that in the case of an employee, the *convenience of the employer test* must still be met. For this reason, an *employee* may be denied the deduction of expenses for a home office used for administrative activities if suitable space is available for performing such duties at the employer's office.

> **Example 10.** T is a manufacturer's representative. He promotes the products of several companies, selling to both wholesalers and retailers all over the state of Ohio. None of the companies he represents provide him an office, so he maintains an office at home. T spends an average of 30 hours a week visiting customers and 12 hours a week working in his home office. Under the *Soliman* rule, T would not be allowed to deduct the costs of maintaining a home office since his clients' premises would be his most important place of business.[28] Using the revised approach, however, T could claim the deduction since he conducts management activities in the home and there is

---

[28] Notice 93-12, 1993-1 C.B. 202; see also, Rev. Rul. 94-24, 1994-1 C.B. 87 for how the IRS will apply the *Soliman* tests.

no other fixed location where he conducts substantial management activities related to his business.

It should be emphasized that taxpayers who cannot qualify for the home office deduction under the principal place of business test may still find relief if they meet one of the other—more liberal—tests discussed below (i.e., regularly meet with clients or separate structure tests).

Trade or Business. No deduction is permitted for home office expenses if the activities to which they relate do not constitute a business.[29]

Example 11. B, an engineer, regularly uses a room in his home exclusively for evaluating his investments. No deduction is permitted since the activity does not constitute a business.

Meeting Place. The second exception for business use is less restrictive than the first. Under this exception, the home office qualifies if clients regularly meet with the taxpayer there. Interestingly, in *John W. Green*, the taxpayer ingeniously argued that this exception should be satisfied where he regularly received phone calls in his home office. Although a majority of the U.S. Tax Court agreed with the taxpayer, the decision was reversed on appeal. The Appellate Court believed that the statute required that the taxpayer *physically* meet with clients in the home office.[30]

Separate Structure. The third exception for business use is the least restrictive of the three. If a separate structure is the site of the home office, it need be used only in connection with the taxpayer's work (e.g., a converted detached garage or barn).

AMOUNT DEDUCTIBLE

If the taxpayer qualifies for the home office deduction, an allocable portion of expenses related to the home may be deducted. The allocation of expenses generally must be based on square footage. Typical expenses include utilities, depreciation, insurance, security systems, repairs (e.g., furnace repair), interest, taxes, and rent. It should be emphasized that the home office deduction is limited to the gross income from the home business as reduced by allowable deductions. This computation is very similar to that for determining deductible hobby expenses. The taxpayer may deduct expenses equal to the extent of gross income reduced by (1) expenses allowable without regard to the use of the dwelling unit (e.g., interest—assuming it is a primary or secondary residence—and taxes), and (2) business or rental expenses incurred in carrying on the activity other than those of the home office (e.g., supplies and secretarial expenses).[31] Any home office expenses that are not deductible due to this limitation may be carried over and used to offset income from the business which led to the deduction, even if the taxpayer does not use the unit in the business in subsequent years.

When the taxpayer is self-employed (i.e., a sole proprietor), all of the taxpayer's expenses, including those attributable to the home office, are deductible for A.G.I. In contrast, if the taxpayer is an employee, the *otherwise allowable* expenses (e.g., interest and taxes) are deductible in full as itemized deductions. The other business expenses, including the home office expenses, are considered miscellaneous itemized deductions and are subject, along with other miscellaneous itemized deductions, to the 2 percent

---

[29] S. Rep. No. 94-938, 94th Cong., 2d Sess. 147-49 (1976).

[30] 78 T.C. 428 (1982).

[31] See § 280A(c)(5).

floor. All expenses for business use of a home office must be reported on Form 8829 (see Appendix B for a sample form).

Example 12. K maintains a qualifying home office. During this year, she earned only $2,000 from the home office activities. Her expenses included the following: interest and taxes allocable to the home office, $600; secretarial services, miscellaneous supplies and postage, $900; and expenses directly related to the home office including insurance, utilities, and depreciation, $1,700. K's potential deduction is $2,000 computed as follows:

Gross income...............................	$2,000	
Otherwise allowable deductions:		
Interest and taxes	(600)	$ 600
Other business expenses................	(900)	900
Gross income limitation	$ 500	
Home office expenses:		
$1,700 limited to remaining gross income..		500
Total potential deduction		$2,000

Whether the $2,000 of deductible expenses are deductible for or from A.G.I. depends on whether K is self-employed or an employee. If K is self-employed, the entire $2,000 is deductible for A.G.I. If the taxpayer is an employee, the $600 of interest and taxes allocable to the home office are deductible as itemized deductions and would be subject to the 2% cutback provision. The remaining $1,400 is considered a miscellaneous itemized deduction subject (along with other miscellaneous itemized deductions) to the 2% floor. Of course, any miscellaneous itemized deductions exceeding the 2% floor are still subject to the 2% cutback provision. The home office expenses that are not deductible this year, $1,200 [($600 + $900 + $1,700 = $3,200) − $2,000], may be carried over to the following years to be offset against future home office income.

DAYCARE AND STORAGE USE

The home office rules for taxpayers who use their home as a daycare center or as a place to store inventory or product samples of a home-based business receive special attention from the Code. In both cases, the normal rules apply except that the exclusive use test is relaxed.

Daycare Use. If a portion of the taxpayer's home doubles as both a living space and a daycare center it would appear that no deduction would be allowed since the exclusive use test would not be satisfied. When the home is used as a daycare center, however, the exclusive use test does not apply.[32] Instead, the expenses attributable to the room are prorated between personal and daycare use based on the number of hours of use per day. Thus, if the taxpayer uses a family room for daycare 40 percent of the time, 40 percent of the expenses allocable to that room would be deductible. A portion of the home qualifies for this special treatment if the taxpayer uses the home to provide daycare services for children, individuals over age 65, or those who are physically or mentally incapable of taking care of themselves.

Storage Use. If the taxpayer regularly uses part of the home to store product samples or goods sold at retail or wholesale *and* the home is the sole fixed location of that

---

[32] § 280A(c)(4).

business, expenses related to the storage space are deductible.[33] More important, the space need not be used exclusively for this purpose. However, the space should be a specific area (e.g., a particular part of a basement or closet).

RESIDENTIAL PHONE SERVICE

For many years, taxpayers who used their home phone for business or income-producing purposes deducted a portion of the basic charge for local service on the grounds that it was business-related. In 1988, however, Congress saw the issue differently. Apparently, in 1988, it believed that the cost of basic phone service to a taxpayer's residence would have been incurred in any event—without regard to any business that the taxpayer might otherwise conduct. As a result, a taxpayer may not deduct any charge (including taxes) for local phone service for the *first* phone line provided to any residence. Presumably, the same rationale would apply to cell phones, in which case only the costs associated with a second telephone number would be deductible. The taxpayer may still deduct the costs of long-distance phone calls or optional phone services such as call waiting or call forwarding, when such costs are related to business. In addition, taxpayers may deduct the costs of additional phone lines into the home that are used for business (e.g., a separate line for a fax machine or modem).

✓ CHECK YOUR KNOWLEDGE

Review Question 1. Indicate whether the following taxpayers would be allowed to deduct expenses attributable to a home office.

a. T is on the tax staff of a public accounting firm. From time to time, he brings home returns and does a little work in his home office. In addition, he does most of his technical reading in the home office.

   T would not be allowed a deduction since he does not meet the principal place of business or convenience of the employer tests. He fails the first of these tests since his principal place of business is his employer's office. He fails the convenience of the employer test since the employer provides him an office and he could do at the office what he does at home. His work at home appears to be for his own convenience.

b. R is a decorator. She works out of an office in her home. She spends about 10 hours per week visiting her client's homes and another 10 visiting businesses that carry furniture and home accessories. The remainder of her 40-hour week is spent at her home office doing sketches, ordering, keeping books, and the like.

   R may deduct her home office expenses since she conducts management activities in the home and there is no other fixed location used by her to perform substantial management activities related to her business.

c. J operates a floral shop in town. He grows the plants for his shop in a greenhouse behind his home.

   Even though the principal place of J's business is arguably at J's shop, J would still qualify for the deduction under the separate structure exception.

Review Question 2. With the kids starting college, income from their regular jobs was not enough, so this year N and her husband started a small blind and drapery

---

[33] § 280A(c)(2).

operation. They run it out of an office in their home. N orders the fabric and sews the drapes while her husband installs. In their first year of business, the couple had gross income of $2,000. Interest and taxes allocable to the home office were $600. Various supplies and equipment, including a file cabinet, table, Rolodex, sewing machine, and scissors, cost $1,000. Depreciation, utilities, insurance, and similar expenses allocable to the home office were $900. According to their friend Norm, they should be able to deduct all $1,900 since they are all ordinary and necessary business expenses. Is Norm correct? How much can they deduct?

Norm is only partially right. Section 280A limits the deduction of home office expenses. Home office expenses are essentially deductible to the extent of net income from the business before taking into account the home office expenses (other than the interest and taxes). The home office expenses cannot create a loss from the activity. As a result, the couple can deduct $400 ($2,000 − $1,000 − $600), and the couple's net income from the business after the home office deductions is zero. Note that § 280A limitations do not apply to the $1,000 of expenses for items directly used in the business. These costs relate directly to the business (rather than the home) and, therefore, are fully deductible (or depreciable, as explained in Chapter 9).

TRANSPORTATION EXPENSES

If there ever was a contest for the most popular tax deduction or at least the one that arouses the most attention, it would be easy to pick the winner. Virtually everyone who tumbles out of bed each morning and makes the daily trip to work has the same question at tax time: can I deduct the costs of getting there and getting back? In a world where commuting is routine for millions of taxpayers, it would seem that the answers would be clear-cut. But this is not necessarily the case.

Before examining the deduction for transportation expenses, the distinction between transportation expenses and travel expenses should be explained. In tax jargon, transportation and travel are not synonymous. Travel expenses are broadly defined to include not only the costs of transportation but also related expenses such as meals, lodging, and other incidentals when the taxpayer is in a travel status. As discussed below, the taxpayer is in travel status when he or she is *away from home overnight* on business.[34] In contrast, transportation expenses are defined narrowly to include only the actual costs of transportation—expenses of getting from one place to another while in the course of business when the taxpayer is *not* away from home overnight.[35] Transportation expenses normally occur when the taxpayer goes and returns on the same day. The most common transportation expense is the cost of driving and maintaining a car, but the term also includes the cost of traveling by other forms of transportation such as bus, taxi, subway, or train.[36]

> **Example 13.** M is an architect in Cincinnati. At various times during the year, he drove to Cleveland to inspect one of his projects. He often ate lunch and dinner in Cleveland before returning home. M is allowed to deduct only the costs of transportation. The costs of the meals are not deductible since he was not away from home overnight. Had he spent the night in Cleveland and returned the next day, the costs of meals and lodging as well as transportation would be deductible.

---

[34]   § 162(a)(2).

[35]   Reg. § 1.62-1(g).

[36]   *Ibid.*

The deduction for transportation is allowed under the general provisions of §§ 162 and 212. Therefore, to qualify for deduction, the transportation expense must be ordinary, necessary, and related to the taxpayer's trade or business or income-producing activity. Personal transportation, of course, does not qualify for deduction. Like many other expenses, however, the boundary between business and personal transportation is often difficult to identify. Some of the common problem areas are discussed below.

DEDUCTIBLE TRANSPORTATION VERSUS NONDEDUCTIBLE COMMUTING

The cost of transportation or commuting between the taxpayer's home and his or her place of employment may appear to be a necessary business expense. It is settled, however, that commuting expenses generally are nondeductible personal expenses. This rule derives from the presumption that the commuting expense arises from the taxpayer's *personal preference* to live away from the place of business or employment. The distance is irrelevant.[37] Moreover, this presumption persists even though there often is no place to live within walking distance of employment, much less one that is suitable or within the taxpayer's means. The fact that the taxpayer is forced to live far away from the place of employment is irrelevant and does not alter the personal nature of the expenses.

> **Example 14.** In *Sanders v. Comm.*, the taxpayers were civilian employees working on an Air Force base.[36] Despite the fact that they were not allowed to live on the base next to their employment and could only live elsewhere and commute, the transportation costs were not deductible. The Court found it impossible to distinguish between these expenses and those of a suburban commuter, both being personal in origin.

> **Example 15.** In *Tauferner v. Comm.*, the taxpayer worked at a chemical plant that was located 20 miles from any community due to the dangers involved.[39] The taxpayer was denied deductions for his commuting even though he lived in the nearest habitable spot. Arguably, the nature of his job—not personal convenience—produced additional transportation costs. Nevertheless, the Court did not believe that such hardship changed the personal character of the expenses.

While the costs of commuting normally are not deductible, there are several exceptions. These exceptions are discussed below.

Commuting with Tools and Similar Items. The fact that the taxpayer hauls tools, instruments, or other equipment necessary in pursuing business normally does not cause commuting expenses to be deductible. The Supreme Court has ruled that only the *additional* expenses attributable to carrying the tools are deductible.[40] The IRS determines the taxpayer's "additional expenses" by applying the so-called "same mode" test.[41] Under this test, a deduction is allowed for the extra cost of commuting by one mode with the tools over the cost of commuting by the same mode without the tools. Thus, a carpenter who drives a truck would not be allowed a transportation deduction simply by loading it with tools since carrying the tools created no additional expense. The fact that tools may have caused the carpenter to drive a truck, which is more expensive than some other type of transportation, is irrelevant under the IRS view. The courts, however, have rejected this test in certain cases.[42]

---

37   *Roger A. Green*, TC Summary Opinion 2008-80.

38   71-1 USTC ¶9260, 27 AFTR2d 71-832, 439 F.2d 296 (CA-9, 1971).

39   69-1 USTC ¶9241, 23 AFTR2d 69-1025, 407 F.2d 243 (CA-10, 1969).

40   *Fausner v. Comm.*, 73-2 USTC ¶95-15, 32 AFTR2d 73-5202, 413 U.S. 838 (USSC, 1973).

41   Rev. Rul. 75-380, 1975-2 C.B. 59.

42   *J.F. Grayson*, 36 TCM 1201, T.C. Memo 1977-304. See also *H.A. Pool*, 36 TCM 93, T.C. Memo 1977-20.

Example 16. M plays third trumpet in the Dallas orchestra. During the year, his employer indicated that they did not need the third trumpet and that M would have to switch to his second instrument, the tuba, to retain his job. If, in order to transport the tuba, M had to change from driving to work in a small car costing $3 per day to driving to work in a van costing $5 per day, the IRS would not allow a deduction for the additional cost. Under the same mode test, the cost of driving the van with the tuba is the same as without the tuba. The courts, however, may allow a deduction for the $2 increase in cost. On the other hand, if M rented a trailer to carry the tuba at a cost of $2 per day, the IRS would allow the deduction because the cost of driving the van with the tuba is now $2 more than without the tuba.

The IRS view on the treatment of local transportation is summarized in Exhibit 8-1.

EXHIBIT 8-1

When Are Local Transportation Expenses Deductible?

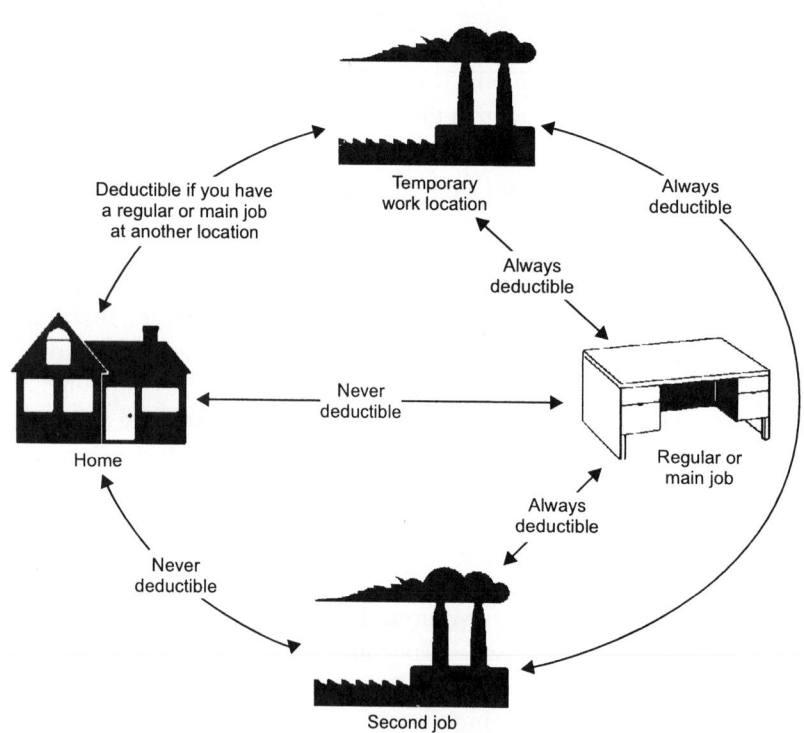

Home: The place where you reside. Transportation expenses between your home and your main or regular place of work are personal commuting expenses.

Regular or main job: Your principal place of business. If you have more than one job, you must determine which one is your regular or main job. Consider the time you spend at each, the activity you have at each, and the income you earn at each.

Temporary work location: A place where your work assignment is realistically expected to last (and does in fact last) one year or less. Unless you have a regular place of business, you can only deduct your transportation expenses to a temporary location *outside* your metropolitan area.

Second job: If you regularly work at two or more places in one day, whether or not for the same employer, you can deduct your transportation expenses of getting from one workplace to another. You cannot deduct your transportation costs between your home and a second job on a day off from your main job.

Source: *Travel, Entertainment, Gift and Car Expense,* IRS Publication 463 (Rev. 2005), p. 14.

Commuting between Two Jobs. The transportation cost of going from one job to a second job is deductible.[43] The deduction is limited to the cost of going *directly* from one job to the other.

Example 17. R works for X Corporation on the morning shift and for Y Corporation on its afternoon shift. The distances he drives are diagrammed below.

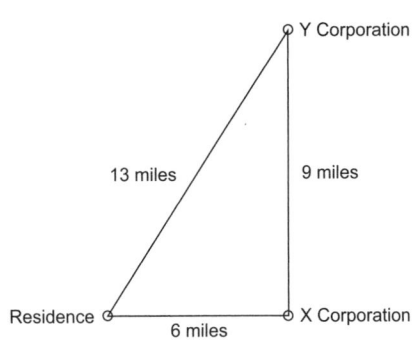

If R leaves X and goes home to eat lunch before going to Y, he actually drives 19 miles to get to Y, or 10 more miles than if he had driven directly (19 − 9). However, only the cost of driving directly, 9 miles, is deductible.

Commuting to a Temporary Assignment. Individuals are often assigned to work at a location other than where they regularly work. When a taxpayer commutes to a *temporary work location*, the commuting expenses are deductible transportation costs if either of the following tests are satisfied:

1. The temporary assignment is *within* the general area of the taxpayer's employment and he or she otherwise has a *regular* place of business (e.g., an office);[44] or

2. The temporary assignment is *outside* the general area of the taxpayer's employment (i.e., his or her tax home).[45]

Example 18. C is an auditor for a public accounting firm that has its office in downtown Chicago. C works about 30% of the time in her employer's office, and the remaining 70% is spent at various clients' offices around the city. C may deduct the costs of commuting between her residence and a client's office because the client's office is a temporary work location and C otherwise has a regular place of business (i. e., her employer's office).

Example 19. M is a carpenter. He works for a construction company that builds houses in subdivisions in various areas of Houston. Most of his assignments are located within about 25 miles of downtown Houston. During the year, M worked at two different locations, one on the north side of Houston and the other on the west side. Although M is assigned to temporary work locations, he is not allowed to deduct any of his commuting expenses because he does not otherwise have a regular place of business.

---

43   *Supra*, Footnote 39.

44   Rev. Rul. 99-7, 1999-1 C.B. 361.

45   *Ibid.*

Example 20. Assume the same facts as above except that M was temporarily assigned to a job in Galveston, 60 miles from Houston. He drove to Galveston daily and returned home in the evenings. Under these circumstances, M may deduct the cost of driving the entire 120-mile round trip from his home to Galveston. Observe that when the temporary assignment is beyond the general vicinity of employment, the taxpayer need not have a regular place of business.[46] The following diagram illustrates this approach.

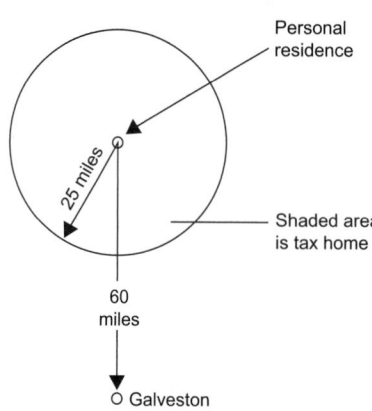

The IRS draws an important distinction between temporary and regular work locations. A work location is temporary if employment at the location is realistically expected to last and does in fact last for one year or less.[47] In contrast, a work location is considered a *regular* place of business if—as one might expect—the taxpayer performs services there on a regular basis. According to the IRS, a taxpayer may have more than one regular place of business even though he or she does not perform services at that location every week or on a set schedule. When the taxpayer commutes to these different locations on a "regular" basis, the costs of commuting would not be deductible because such locations are not temporary.

Example 21. Dr. T, a podiatrist, has an office on both the north side and south side of Indianapolis. In addition, she performs services at a clinic and a hospital with which she is associated. T may not deduct the costs of transportation between her residence and these various locations because each is considered a regular place of business and not a temporary work location. As discussed below, however, the costs of going between two business locations (e.g., a clinic and a hospital) are deductible.

Transportation between Job Sites. While the transportation costs between a taxpayer's home and the first and last job sites generally are considered nondeductible commuting expenses, transportation costs between two job sites are deductible.[48] Accordingly, once the taxpayer arrives at the first job site any business travel thereafter usually is deductible.

Example 22. R is employed as a tax accountant and works primarily in his employer's office downtown. R drives 34 miles round-trip from his home to the office. After arriving at work one day, R drove 6 miles to a client's office and returned to his employer's office. In this case, R may deduct the cost of driving 12 miles.

---

[46] See *Estate of David B. Lease, Deceased*, TC Summary Opinion 2008-11.

[47] *Ibid.*

[48] Rev. Rul. 55-109, 1955-1 C.B. 261 and Rev. Rul. 99-7, 1999-1 C.B. 361.

Example 23. Assume R drives 17 miles to work in the morning. In the afternoon, he drives 15 miles to a client's office where he conducts some business. From the client's office he drives 9 miles home. In this situation, R may deduct the cost of driving 15 miles because transportation between two job sites is deductible. In addition, it appears that he may deduct the cost of driving 9 miles since transportation between the taxpayer's residence and a temporary work location (i.e., the client's office) is deductible.

Although transportation expenses between the taxpayer's home and work normally are not deductible, the rule concerning travel between job sites creates a favorable exception for taxpayers who maintain a separate trade or business at home. For these taxpayers, the transportation from the first job site—the home—and the second job site in the same trade or business would be deductible.

Example 24. V is a landscape engineer and works out of his home. Transportation costs from his home to a client's place of business are deductible since the expenses are incurred in traveling from his principal place of business to a job site.[49]

COMPUTING CAR EXPENSES

Deductions relating to driving and maintaining a car may be computed using actual expenses or a standard mileage rate (automatic mileage method). Under either method, if the car is used for both business and personal purposes, only the car expenses attributable to business or income production are deductible.

Actual Expenses. Actual car expenses normally deducted include the costs for gas, oil, repairs, insurance, depreciation, interest on loans to purchase the car (other than that of an employee), taxes, licenses, garage rent, parking fees, and tolls. Calculating actual expenses usually requires determining the portion of the nondeductible expenses attributable to personal use. Under the actual expense method, the total actual expense is allocated based on mileage.

Example 25. R, self-employed, drove 20,000 miles during the year: 16,000 on business and 4,000 for personal purposes. Total actual expenses were as follows:

General expenses:	
Gas	$1,200
Maintenance (oil, repairs)	200
Insurance	1,100
Interest expense	600
Depreciation	1,900
Total	$5,000

Other business expenses:	
Tolls incurred on business trips	$ 10
Parking fees when calling on clients	90
Total	$ 100

---

[49]   See *Raymond Garner*, 42 TCM 1181, T.C. Memo 1981-542, and *Joe J. Adams*, 43 TCM 1203, T.C. Memo 1982-223. See also, *Charles Walker*, 101 T.C. 36 (1993) and Rev. Rul. 94-47, 1994-2 C.B. 18.

Since R used the car 80% (16,000 ÷ 20,000) for business, he may deduct 80% of the general expenses, $4,000 (80% × $5,000). In addition, he may deduct the entire $100 cost for the parking and tolls since they were incurred solely for business purposes, for a total deduction of $4,100. Note that the nonbusiness portion of the interest expense would not be deductible, assuming it is not attributable to a loan secured by his first or second home. If R were an employee, *none* of the interest would be deductible because business interest of an *employee* is not deductible.

Standard Mileage Rate. The automatic mileage method allows a deduction of 55 cents per mile (2009) for *all* business miles driven during the year.[50] The business portion of expenses for interest (if self-employed), state and local property taxes, parking, and tolls also may be added to the amount computed using the mileage rate. Other expenses such as depreciation, insurance, and maintenance are built into the mileage rate and cannot be added.

Example 26. Same facts as in *Example 25*. R's deduction using the standard mileage rate would be $9,380, as computed below.

Business mileage (16,000 × $0.55)	$8,800
Interest ($600 × 80%)	480
Parking and tolls	100
Total	$9,380

Note that in arriving at the deduction, gas, maintenance, insurance, and depreciation are not added to the amount computed using the standard rate since they are built into the rate. Conversely, interest (if self-employed), parking, and tolls are added since they are not included in the rate.

Taxpayers who lease their cars may also use the standard mileage rate. If a taxpayer elects to use the rate for a leased car, it must be used for the entire lease period.[51]

The standard mileage rate may be used *only* if it is adopted in the first year the car is placed in service. In addition, the following conditions must be satisfied:[52]

1. The car must not be one of two or more cars being used simultaneously in a business, such as in a fleet operation. When a taxpayer alternates in using different cars on different occasions, the cars are treated as one and the mileage is combined.

2. The car must not be for hire, such as a taxi.

3. Additional first-year depreciation or depreciation using an accelerated method must not have been claimed in a prior year.

If these conditions are met, the taxpayer may switch methods from year to year. However, use of the standard mileage method precludes the taxpayer from using the Modified Accelerated Cost Recovery System (MACRS) for computing depreciation in a subsequent year, and depreciation must be computed under one of the alternative methods (e.g., straight-line).[53] Note that selecting the actual method in the first year generally *prohibits* the taxpayer from ever using the standard mileage rate for that automobile.

---

50 Rev. Proc. 2008-72, IRB 2008-50.

51 Prop. Reg. § 1.274-5(g).

52 *Ibid.*

53 *Supra*, footnote 47.

Taxpayers who use the standard mileage rate are required to reduce the adjusted basis of their automobiles just as if they had claimed depreciation. The rate per mile varies by year as shown below.[54]

Year	Depreciation Per Mile
2008	21¢
2007	19¢
2005–2006	17¢
2003–2004	16¢
2001–2002	15¢
2000	14¢
1994–1999	12¢

CLASSIFICATION OF TRANSPORTATION AND TRAVEL EXPENSES

The *unreimbursed* transportation and travel expenses of an employee are treated as miscellaneous itemized deductions subject to the 2 percent floor. In contrast, if an employee is reimbursed for such expenses under a qualified arrangement known as an *accountable plan* (discussed later in this chapter), the reimbursement is excludable from gross income. Any reimbursement not made under such a plan must be included in the employee's gross income, and any qualifying deductions must be treated as miscellaneous itemized deductions. If the expenses are incurred by a self-employed person, the expenses are deductible for A.G.I. An employee reports the expenses on Form 2106, a copy of which is reproduced in the last section of this chapter.

Travel and transportation expenses related to property held for the production of income are also considered miscellaneous itemized deductions unless the income is rents or royalties, in which case the deductions would be for A.G.I. In addition, the deduction for meals may be limited to 50 percent of their cost. This limitation is discussed in detail with entertainment expenses later in this chapter.

TRAVEL EXPENSES

Section 162 of the Code provides for the deduction of travel expenses while "away from home" in the pursuit of a trade or business.[55] A similar deduction is allowed for travel expenses connected with income-producing activities not constituting a business.[56] The definition of travel expenses is not as narrow as that of transportation expenses. Travel expenses include not only the costs of transportation but also the costs of meals (but limited to 50 percent of actual costs, as discussed later), lodging, cleaning and laundry, telephone, and other similar expenses related to travel.[57] Whether these additional expenses such as meals and lodging are deductible depends on whether the taxpayer is considered "away from home."

AWAY-FROM-HOME TEST

The taxpayer must be *away from home* before travel expenses are deductible. The "away from-home" test poses two questions: for what period does the taxpayer need to be away from home, and where is the taxpayer's home for tax purposes? With respect to the first question, the Supreme Court has ruled that the away-from-home test generally

[54] For previous rates see *Travel, Entertainment, Gift and Car Expenses*, IRS Publication 463 (Rev. 2007) p. 25.

[55] *Supra*, Footnote 34.

[56] §§ 212(1) and (2).

[57] Reg. § 1.162-2(a).

requires the taxpayer to be away from home *overnight*.[58] Later interpretations of this decision have indicated that the taxpayer will be considered to be "overnight" when it is reasonable for the taxpayer to stop for needed sleep or rest. A trip where the taxpayer leaves and returns the same day is not travel and, consequently, only the transportation cost would be deductible. Meals eaten during the trip, lodging, etc., would not be deductible.

The second and more critical aspect of the away-from-home test concerns the determination of the taxpayer's *tax home*. The IRS and the Tax Court have defined the term *tax home* to mean the business location of the taxpayer or the general vicinity of the taxpayer's employment, regardless of the location of the taxpayer's personal residence.[59] The Court of Appeals in several circuits, however, has held that "home" should be interpreted in the normal fashion (i.e., as the place where the taxpayer normally maintains his or her residence;[60] *see Example 28*). The interpretation problems usually arise when taxpayers live in one location but also conduct substantial business at another location where they often stay because it is impractical to return to the residence. To illustrate, consider a construction worker who lives with his family in Milwaukee but obtains a job to work on the construction of a nuclear power plant near Chicago. During the week, he stays in a motel in Chicago and eats his meals. The issue here is the location of the taxpayer's tax home. If the taxpayer normally works in Chicago, the IRS would take the position that the taxpayer's tax home is in Chicago and deny the deductions for meals and lodging. On the other hand, if the taxpayer normally works in Milwaukee and takes a job in Chicago, he may be able to secure a deduction for his Chicago expenses if he could demonstrate that the Chicago job is only a *temporary* assignment. The IRS permits taxpayers to deduct travel expenses incurred away from the principal place of business if an assignment away from home is temporary and not indefinite. Under § 162(a), assignments in a single location lasting a year or more are not temporary but indefinite.[61] Consequently, if a taxpayer anticipates an assignment to last more than a year or it actually exceeds one year, none of the taxpayer's travel expenses are deductible (not even those for the first 12 months).

> **Example 27.** D is employed as an engineer, living and working in Kansas city. D's employer assigned her to a job in El Paso that D expected to complete in five months. In reality, D lived and worked in El Paso for ten months before completing the job and returning to Kansas city. Because she realistically expected the assignment to last for one year or less and it in fact did not exceed this period, D may deduct her travel expenses for the entire ten months. What would be the result if at the end of four months it became clear that D's stay in El Paso would exceed a year? In such case, the IRS takes the position that she would be able to treat the first four months as temporary and deduct her expenses for those months. However, the expenses for the remainder of the job assignment would not be deductible.

> **Example 28.** In *Joseph Cornelius*,[62] Mr. Cornelius, a computer system administrator, lived and worked in Austin, Texas. In 2001, his employer closed its Austin office and he became unemployed. Subsequently, he was offered work by a systems company on an "as needed" basis and was immediately assigned to work on a client in Boulder, Colorado. The assignment lasted from March, 2002 to April 2003. While in Boulder, he stayed in a hotel and shared a condominium. After Boulder, he took another assignment

---

[58] *U.S. v. Correll*, 68-1 USTC ¶9101, 20 AFTR2d 5845, 389 U.S. 299 (USSC, 1967).

[59] G.C.M. 23672, 1943 C.B. 66, superseded by Rev. Rul. 74-291, 1974-1 C.B. 42.

[60] For example, see *Rosenspan v. U.S.*, 71-1 USTC ¶9241, 27 AFTR2d 71-707, 438 F.2d 905 (CA-2, 1971).

[61] *Supra*, Footnote 44 and Rev. Rul 93-86, 1993-2 C.B. 71. Federal employees providing services related to investigating or prosecuting a Federal crime are not subject to this rule. See § 162(a), last sentence.

[62] TC Summary Decision 2008-42.

in New Jersey that lasted from April 2003 to July 2005. While in New Jersey he lived in a hotel and shared an apartment. During the time he was on both assignments, he continued to rent his apartment in Austin and periodically returned to visit family and friends. On his 2002 and 2003 tax returns, Mr. Cornelius deducted expenses for meals and lodging while on assignment on the theory that he was away from home on business temporarily. However, upon audit, the IRS denied the deductions and assessed deficiencies of $16,445 and $19,420 for the two years in question. At trial, the Court understood how Mr. Cornelius could believe his assignments to be "temporary," as that word is commonly used. Still, it denied the deductions since both assignments exceeded a year and by law could not be considered temporary. Moreover, deductions for traveling back and forth between Austin and Boulder and Austin and New Jersey were treated as being for personal purposes and disallowed.

If the taxpayer has no principal place of employment, the tax home is normally his regular place of abode.[63] However, if the taxpayer has no permanent place of residence, the courts have consistently denied the taxpayer's deductions for meals and lodging since there is no "home" to be away from. This rule has been applied to itinerant construction workers and salespeople whom the courts view as being *at home* wherever their work may take them.[64]

The purpose of the away-from-home provision is to reduce the burden of the taxpayer who, because of business needs, must maintain two places of abode and consequently incurs additional and duplicate living expenses. The rule is based on the principle that a taxpayer normally lives and works in the same general vicinity. Thus, when taxpayers choose to live in an area other than where they work, the resulting expenses normally are considered personal. This rule often is difficult to apply in particular situations. For this reason, the deduction of travel expenses ultimately depends on the facts.

> **Example 29.** C works at a testing laboratory in a remote mountain area of New Mexico, 70 miles from his home. His residence, however, is the closest place to the laboratory to live. C normally commutes to work but sometimes stays at the testing facilities' quarters overnight when he works overtime. In this situation, the IRS would not allow a deduction for travel expenses since C's tax home is at the testing laboratory, and when staying there he is not away from home. Some Appellate Courts, however, may permit the deduction for meals and lodging since he is away from his residence.[65]

COMBINED BUSINESS AND PLEASURE TRAVEL

As discussed above, travel costs are deductible only while away from home in pursuit of business or income-producing activities. When traveling away from home, however, taxpayers often combine business with pleasure with the hope that they can deduct what is really a personal vacation. With an eye to this possibility, the Regulations provide special guidance as to how much can be deducted in this situation. The rules governing combined business and pleasure travel differ depending on whether the taxpayer is traveling inside or outside of the United States.

Domestic Travel. The taxpayer who travels within the United States (all 50 states and the District of Columbia) may deduct *all* of the costs of travel to and from the destination if the trip is *primarily* for business.[66] If the trip is primarily for business, the

---

[63]   Criteria exist for determining whether a taxpayer has a regular place of abode. See Rev. Rul. 73-529, 1973-2 C.B. 37.

[64]   *George H. James v. U.S.*, 62-2 USTC ¶9735, 10 AFTR2d 5627, 308 F.2d 204 (CA-9, 1962).

[65]   For example, see *Lee E. Coombs*, 79-2 USTC ¶9719, 45 AFTR2d 80-444, 608 F.2d 1269 (CA-9, 1979).

taxpayer will not lose all or even a part of the deduction merely because he or she takes a personal side-trip or extends the trip for a short vacation. However, the costs of any personal side-trips are not allowed. Travel which is primarily for personal purposes is not deductible even though some business is conducted. Note that the taxpayer either deducts *all* of the *to-and-from* travel expenses or deducts *none* of them—there is no allocation. Of course, any travel expenses (e.g., meals and lodging) directly related to business upon arriving at the destination qualify.

> **Example 30.** F, a CPA, flew from Dallas to Denver to attend a conference. The air fare was $500. Meals and lodging for the three days she attended were $150 and $230, respectively. Upon conclusion of the meeting, F drove to the mountains and skied for two days before returning home. The travel to the mountains, including meals and lodging, cost $600. F may deduct all of the air fare, $500, because costs of transportation are fully deductible without allocation when the trip is primarily for business. In addition, F may deduct 50% of the meal costs, $75 (50% × $150), and $230 for lodging because these travel expenses are directly related to business. The expenses of $600 for the ski trip are nondeductible personal expenses.

> **Example 31.** Assume the same facts as in *Example 29*, except that F skied for five days. Here the trip may be treated as primarily personal thus preventing any deduction of the $500 air fare. Fifty percent of the expenses for meals and all of the lodging costs while at the convention on business are still deductible.

Obviously the most troublesome question concerning domestic travel is whether the nature of the trip is primarily business or pleasure. The Regulations, Rulings, and reported decisions offer little guidance—saying only that the answer depends on the facts and circumstances in each case. Among the factors normally considered, the amount of time devoted to business as compared to personal activities is often decisive. Another factor emphasized is the type of location where the business occurs (e.g., a resort hotel or a more businesslike setting). As might be expected, the IRS casts a doubtful eye on deductions for meetings in resort areas, believing that the alleged business trip is merely a disguised vacation. In this regard, Congress took action concerning travel expenses related to nonbusiness conventions (e.g., investment and tax seminars), completely disallowing their deduction after 1986.[67] However, if it can be clearly shown that the expenses were incurred for *business* purposes, the deduction is not disallowed merely because the meeting occurs at a resort.

> **Example 32.** This year, Dr H, a surgeon, attended a week-long course on arthroscopic surgery in Miami. His wife accompanied him and attended a seminar on personal financial planning. H may deduct his costs of transportation as well as the travel expenses incurred after arriving in Miami because the expenses are related to business. None of his wife's expenses are deductible because they relate not to her trade or business but to investments and taxes.

Travel Expense of Spouse and Dependents. The IRS has always taken a dim view of taxpayers who combine business travel with pleasure and in the process deduct the cost of taking their families with them. For years, the Service attacked this abuse with a long-standing regulation that denied the deduction of a family member's travel expenses unless the taxpayer could demonstrate that the family member's presence served a bona fide business purpose.[68] Apparently this ammunition was incapable of adequately policing the

---

[67] § 274(h)(7). For an interesting case, *see Carl Jones*, 131 TC 3 (2008), where the taxpayer was denied travel deductions incurred to take a course on day trading.

[68] Reg. § 1.162-2(c); Rev. Rul. 55-57, 1955-1 C.B. 315.

problem. Consequently, Congress provided the IRS more help with new legislation in 1994.[69] Currently, no deduction is allowed for any travel expenses paid or incurred with respect to a spouse, dependent, or other individual accompanying the taxpayer (or an officer or employee of the taxpayer) on business unless (1) the individual is an employee of the person paying or reimbursing the expenses, (2) the travel of such individual has a bona fide business purpose, and (3) such expenses are otherwise deductible. The rule does not apply to deductible moving expenses.

> **Example 33.** T is the owner and president of TDI Corporation, which owns seven car dealerships in and around Des Moines. This year General Motors held a meeting for all of its dealers in Maui, and T took his wife and 18-year-old daughter. TDI reimbursed T for all of his traveling expenses including those of his wife and daughter. TDI is not allowed to claim a deduction for the travel expenses of T's wife and daughter unless they are both employees of the company and it can establish that their presence had a bona fide business purpose. Note that T and TDI may be able to overcome the first requirement by employing both his wife and daughter. Satisfying the second test is more difficult. In this regard, the regulations provide that performance of incidental services does not cause a family member's expenses to qualify. The courts, however, have allowed a deduction for a spouse's expenses when the facts have shown that the spouse's presence enhanced the image of the taxpayer or the spouse acted as a business assistant.[70]

Foreign Travel. When the taxpayer travels outside the United States, the travel expenses must satisfy more stringent requirements for deduction. Generally, the costs of transportation to and from the foreign destination and other travel expenses must be allocated between business (or income-producing activities) and personal activities. If the travel is *primarily* business, the costs of transportation are fully deductible without allocation if *one* of the following conditions is satisfied:[71]

1. *Travel outside the United States does not exceed one week* (seven consecutive days). In counting the days out of the United States, the day of departure from the United States is excluded while the day of return to the United States is included. (For example, leaving on Sunday and returning on the following Sunday is exactly seven days.)

2. *More than 75 percent of the days on the trip were devoted to business.* A day is treated as a business day if during any part of the day the taxpayer's presence is required at a particular place for a business purpose. Moreover, the day is considered a business day even though the taxpayer spends more time during normal working hours on nonbusiness activity than on business activity. Weekends, holidays, or other "standby" days that fall between the taxpayer's business days are also considered business days. However, such days are not business days if they fall at the end of the taxpayer's business activities and the taxpayer merely elects to stay for personal purposes. The day of departure and the day of return are both treated as business days.

3. Taxpayer has no substantial control over arranging the business trip.

4. Personal vacation is not a major consideration in making the trip.

---

[69] § 274(m).

[70] See *Fraser Wilkins*, 72-2 USTC ¶9707, 30 AFTR2d 72-5639, 348 F. Supp. 1282 (D.Ct. Neb., 1972); *Pierre C. Warwick*, 64-2 USTC ¶9864, 14 AFTR2d 5817, 236 F. Supp. 761 (D.Ct. Va., 1974).

[71] § 274(c); Reg. § 1.274-4.

If the travel is not primarily for business or fails to satisfy one of the above conditions, an *allocation* of the to-and-from travel expenses must be made. In such cases, the deductible travel expenses are determined by the following allocation formula:

$$\frac{\text{Business days on trip}}{\text{Total days on trip}} \times \frac{\text{Total}}{\substack{\text{to-and-from} \\ \text{Travel Expenses}}} = \frac{\substack{\text{Deductible} \\ \text{to-and-from}}}{\text{Travel Expenses}}$$

A deduction for the to-and-from travel expenses is not allowed if the trip is primarily personal. However, travel costs (e.g., meals and lodging) directly related to business upon arriving at the destination are deductible.

> **Example 34.** B, an executive, arranged a trip to Japan primarily for business. He left Chicago for Tokyo on July 1 and returned on July 20. During his trip, he spent 15 days on business (including the two travel days) and five days sight-seeing. His air fare was $1,000 and his lodging plus 50% of the meal costs totaled $100 per day. Unless B can show that a personal vacation was not a major consideration for the trip, he must allocate his expenses because none of the other conditions are satisfied. In such case, B may deduct $2,250 [(15 business days ÷ 20 total days = 75%) × $3,000 total expenses]. If B had returned July 8 or spent one less day sight-seeing, no allocation would be required since he would have been out of the United States less than a week or would have spent more than 75% of his time on business activities.

Luxury Water Travel. When lawmakers lowered the boom on entertainment and meal expenses in 1986, they also took a swipe at unhurried business people who travel by cruise ships, ocean liners, and other luxury water transportation. As a general rule, deductions for transportation by water are limited to *twice* the highest per diem amount allowed to Federal employees while away from home but serving in the 48 contiguous states.[72] For example, the highest Federal per diem for travel from October 1, 2008 through September 30, 2009 was $424 so the daily limit on luxury water travel would be $848.

> **Example 35.** To conduct a business meeting in London, T traveled by ocean liner, taking five days at a total cost of $3,000. Assuming the top per diem rate for Federal employees serving in the United States is $200 per day, T's deduction is limited to $2,000 ($200 × 2 × 5).

FOREIGN CONVENTIONS

Notwithstanding the restrictions imposed on deductions related to foreign travel, substantial abuse existed until 1976. Most of this abuse involved travel to foreign conventions, seminars, cruises, etc., which if properly scheduled amounted to government-subsidized vacations. To eliminate this possibility, specific safeguards were enacted. Currently, no deduction is allowed for travel expenses to attend a convention, seminar, or similar meeting *outside* of North America *unless* the taxpayer establishes the following:[73] (1) the meeting is directly related to the active conduct of his or her trade or business, and (2) it is as reasonable to hold the meeting outside North America as within North America. North America includes the United States, its possessions, Canada, Mexico, the Trust Territory of the Pacific Islands, Bermuda and qualifying Caribbean countries.

> **Example 36.** B, a professor of international business, traveled to Spain to present a paper on tax incentives for exports at the International Accounting Convention. Since

---

[72] § 274(m)(1).

[73] See § 274(h)(1), (3), and (6).

it is as reasonable to hold an international meeting in Spain as in North America, and presentation of the paper is directly related to B's business, she may deduct her travel expenses subject to the normal rules for travel outside the United States.

CRUISE SHIPS

No deduction is allowed for the cost of attending a meeting conducted on a cruise ship unless the following requirements are met:[74] (1) the ship is a vessel registered in the United States and it sails *only* between ports in the United States or its possessions; (2) the meeting is directly related to the taxpayer's business; and (3) certain detailed information regarding the cruise is submitted with the return. For qualifying cruises, the maximum deduction is $2,000 per calendar year for each taxpayer. An employer, however, may deduct the cost of sending an individual to a foreign convention or on any type of cruise if the amount is included in the employee's income.

✔️ *CHECK YOUR KNOWLEDGE*

Review Question 1. Try the following true-false questions. F is director of sales for QVS in Los Angeles but chooses to live 90 miles away in Santa Barbara. Each day he drives to and from work. Once in a while he will leave the office to call on a customer and then return. F may not deduct his cost to commute but can deduct the cost of driving to make calls.

True. As a general rule, commuting is not deductible regardless of the distance traveled. However, the cost of going from one job site to another site is deductible.

Review Question 2. A taxpayer must have a regular work location in order to deduct the costs of commuting to a temporary work assignment outside his tax home.

False. In order to deduct the cost of commuting to a work location *within* the taxpayer's tax home, the taxpayer must have a regular place of business. The same requirement does not apply to commuting outside the taxpayer's tax home.

Review Question 3. The costs of depreciation and insurance for an automobile vary significantly depending on the type of car and driver. Consequently, these items are not reflected in the standard mileage rate; however, the taxpayer can add the appropriate amount of depreciation and insurance expense to the amount computed using the standard rate in computing deductible automobile expenses.

False. Depreciation and insurance are included in the rate.

Review Question 4. T is the district manager for Mississippi Catfish, a fast-food chain with more than 100 stores. He lives in New Orleans. On Monday he traveled to Baton Rouge and returned the same day. On Tuesday he traveled to Houston, spent the night, and returned on Wednesday. T may deduct the costs of lunch both in Baton Rouge and in Houston.

False. In order to deduct the costs of meals and lodging, the taxpayer must be in a travel status (i.e., away from home overnight). Thus T cannot deduct the cost of lunch on his day trip to Baton Rouge. He is allowed to deduct the cost of his lunch while in Houston since he was there overnight.

---

[74] § 274(h)(2).

Review Question 5. This year, Dr. F, an ophthalmologist, attended a four-day meeting of his professional organization in Cancun. He remained another three days to lie on the beach and fish. Dr. F may deduct 4/7 of his airfare.

False. If the trip is primarily for business, the taxpayer is allowed to deduct all of the transportation costs to and from the destination.

ENTERTAINMENT EXPENSES

Perhaps no single deduction has created as much controversy as that for entertainment expenses. The difficulty lies in the fact that there is no simple way to distinguish entertainment expenses incurred out of business necessity from those incurred for personal purposes. The problem is the "dual personality" of entertainment. Entertainment can be purely for fun and amusement. Or it can be used to break the ice with a potential customer, to relax, or to create an engaging atmosphere for closing the sale or getting the contract. Over the years, Congress and various administrations have continually struggled to devise the proper test that would prohibit taxpayers from deducting what might be a personal expenditure.

The Kennedy administration was the first to have some success in limiting the entertainment deduction. In 1961, President Kennedy recommended abolishing the deduction for entertaining customers at parties, nightclubs, etc., as well as disallowing the deduction for country club dues. Although Kennedy's suggestions were not enacted, Congress did move to make it more difficult to deduct entertainment expenses with the enactment of Code § 274. This provision—discussed below—still stands as the major hurdle that must be overcome before entertainment expenses may be deducted. Under § 274, entertainment expenses must not only satisfy the normal criteria for business and income-producing expenses but also several additional requirements, including certain record keeping standards. Despite these additional conditions, the so-called *Kennedy rules* still were viewed by many to be inadequate.

President Carter's administration ventured into the battle over entertainment deductions in 1977, blasting the taxpayer's right to deduct the cost of what is now the infamous "three-martini lunch." The Carter attacks were generally unsuccessful, however. It was not until President Reagan's term that the entertainment deduction was drastically curtailed. Present law now presumes that virtually every entertainment and meal expense contains a personal element that is not deductible. As discussed below, only 50 percent of the cost of allowable meals and entertainment is currently deductible.

DEDUCTION REQUIREMENTS

To be deductible, an entertainment expense must first survive the gauntlet of tests applied to all potential deductions by § 162. That is, the expense must be reasonable, ordinary, and necessary, and incurred in carrying on a trade or business.

Example 37. D is a sales representative of M Corporation, a manufacturer of cookware. Twice a month, she takes buyers from the leading retail department stores to lunch where they discuss the corporation's new products. Business meals are customary, appropriate, and helpful in commissioned sales and thus are deductible.

As a practical matter, most entertainment expenses satisfy the ordinary and necessary tests with little difficulty. It is the additional requirements of § 274 that provide the greatest obstacles.

The restrictions contained in § 274 apply to any expense related to an activity customarily considered to provide entertainment, amusement, or recreation.[75] The

---

[75] § 274(a)(1).

provision applies to expenses for entertaining guests such as those for the following: food, liquor, sporting events, movie and theater productions, social, athletic and country clubs, yachts, hunting and fishing trips, and company-provided vacations. Business gifts also are governed by this provision.[76] It should be emphasized that expenses ostensibly for other purposes also are subject to the requirements of § 274 if they are of an entertaining nature.

Example 38. A national magazine desiring publicity often sends the company president flying in a hot air balloon emblazoned with the corporation's logo. Although the expense is for advertising, § 274 applies since the activity constitutes entertainment.

As might be expected, when the IRS questions the taxpayer about his or her deductions for entertainment, the auditor does not ask whether the taxpayer had a good time. Unfortunately, the agent is concerned with whether the taxpayer has satisfied either of two principal tests. Under § 274, no deduction is allowed unless the taxpayer can adequately substantiate that the entertainment expense is *either* "directly related to" or "associated with" the taxpayer's business or falls within one of ten exceptions.

Directly-Related-to Expenses. The Regulations set forth what the taxpayer must establish for an entertainment expenditure to be considered *directly related* to the taxpayer's business or income-producing activity. Expenses are treated as directly related under the so-called *general test* if the taxpayer shows all of the following:[77]

1. More than a general expectation of deriving some income or other specific benefit (other than goodwill) existed as a result of making the expenditure; no resulting benefit must be shown, however.

2. Business was actually discussed or engaged in during the entertainment.

3. The combined business and entertainment was principally characterized by business.

Business Benefit. Prior to the enactment of § 274, entertainment deductions were liberally granted where they were shown to promote the customer's goodwill. Section 274 rejects this prior standard. Under current law, the taxpayer must have more than just a general expectation of deriving some income or some specific business benefit. Although this standard is hardly the epitome of clarity, it is clear that the likelihood of a benefit must be greater than a remote possibility.

Example 39. T, an insurance salesperson, sees his old college chum, C, in a bar. T buys his buddy a few drinks and then takes him to a ball game, using an extra ticket T has. Before the night is over, T mentions that if C ever needs insurance he should give T a call. In this case, T's prospect of a business benefit is slight, too distant, and thus not directly related. It simply creates goodwill, which is insufficient to obtain a deduction. However, T may be able to benefit from hindsight. If C later calls him about insurance, T could rightfully claim the deduction.

Actively Engage in Business. Under the general test, the taxpayer must actually discuss or engage in business. This means that at some point during the entertainment—at halftime, during the intermission, between innings—the taxpayer must forsake the merriment of the moment and get down to business, negotiating, dealing, or bargaining

[76]   § 274(d).
[77]   Reg. § 1.274-2(c)(3).

with respect to a bona fide business transaction. Since this is obviously difficult to police, the Regulations have given the IRS two helpful presumptions.[78] First, it is presumed that no business can take place if the taxpayer is not present. If the taxpayer is at home mowing the lawn while the client is enjoying the game using tickets given to him by the taxpayer, the implication is that no business can take place. (In such case, the taxpayer may be able to deduct the cost of the tickets as a business gift as discussed below.) Second, it is presumed that no business can take place where there are substantial distractions. The Regulations insist that such distractions are present at night clubs, sporting events, social gatherings, cocktail lounges, theaters, and wherever the taxpayer meets with a group including not only business associates but others. Despite these presumptions, a deduction is still allowed if the taxpayer can establish to the contrary that he or she actively engaged in the discussion of business. As a practical matter, most taxpayers take advantage of this latitude, claiming the deduction and hoping that they will never be called upon to justify it.

Principal Character Is Business. During the entertainment, business must predominate. This does not mean that the taxpayer must spend more time on business than enjoying the activity. It does mean that the business aspects must be more than incidental. As above, the Regulations rest on the rebuttable presumption that the primary character of certain activities—those on a hunting or fishing trip, a yacht or pleasure boat—is not business.

The Regulations also specify several other situations where the entertainment expense will be considered directly related. For example, entertainment is directly related if it is provided in a clear business setting—a setting where the guest recognizes the taxpayer's business motive (e.g., a hospitality room provided by a book publisher at a convention of accounting professors).[79] Expenditures for entertainment provided for those who render services for the taxpayer also are regarded as directly related. For example, a vacation trip awarded by a manufacturer to the retailer selling a number of its products qualifies.[80]

Associated-with Expenses. It is often difficult to qualify the entertainment under the directly-related-to test, generally due to the presumption regarding distractions or simply because the taxpayer could not squeeze in any business during the show or game. However, the entertainment may still qualify for deduction if it satisfies the *associated-with test.* Entertainment expenses are considered *associated with* the taxpayer's business if the entertainment is immediately before or after a substantial business discussion.[81] The key distinction between associated-with and directly-related-to expenses concerns when the business activity occurs. The associated-with test allows the business to occur immediately preceding or following the entertainment while the directly-related-to standard requires business during the entertainment. Note that to satisfy the "immediately preceding or following" requirement it is sufficient that the entertainment merely takes place on the same day as business. In some cases, the entertainment may be on the day before or after the business activity.

Example 40. B operates a chain of sporting goods stores in Dallas. Before school begins each fall, he invites area coaches to one of his stores, where he presents his new lines of equipment. Immediately afterward, he takes them to a Cowboys football game. B may deduct the costs of tickets to the game since there was substantial business activity immediately before the entertainment. Note that due to the distractions

---

[78]   Reg. § 1.274-2(c)(7).

[79]   Reg. § 1.274-2(d)(4).

[80]   Reg. § 1.274-2(d)(5).

[81]   *Supra,* Footnote 71; Reg. § 1.274-2(d).

presented by the game no deduction would be permitted if B merely took the coaches to the game and discussed business there.

Business Meals. For many years, taxpayers were allowed to deduct the cost of meals with business associates regardless of whether they satisfied the directly-related-to or associated-with requirements. More importantly, the costs could be deducted even if business was not discussed. The effect of these rules was to allow a deduction for entertaining that created goodwill. In 1986, Congress believed that this favorable treatment was no longer justified and therefore tightened the rules.

Currently, expenses for meals, like other entertainment expenses, are not deductible unless they satisfy the directly-related-to or associated-with tests.[82] Under these criteria, the business meal is not deductible unless there is a substantial and bona fide business discussion either before, after, or during the meal.[83] In addition, the taxpayer or an employee of the taxpayer normally must be present at the meal.[84] For example, if the taxpayer merely reserves a table for dinner at a restaurant for a customer, but neither the taxpayer nor one of his or her employees attends the dinner, no deduction is allowed. For purposes of this rule, an independent contractor who performs significant services for the taxpayer such as an attorney or accountant is considered an employee.

A common question regarding the deduction for business meals concerns the costs of the taxpayer's own meals. From a purely theoretical view, the cost would presumably be a nondeductible personal expense since the taxpayer has to eat in any event. In *Richard A. Sutter*, the U.S. Tax Court took just such a view in disallowing a taxpayer's deduction for his own meals at business lunches.[85] The Court said:

> We think the presumptive nondeductibility of personal expenses (the taxpayer's meals) may be overcome only by clear and detailed evidence as to each instance that the expenditure in question was *different from or in excess* of that which would have been made for the taxpayer's personal purposes (emphasis supplied).

Despite the Court's holding, the IRS has been quite gracious. The Service permits the taxpayer to deduct the *entire cost* of his or her own meal except in abusive situations where it is evident that a substantial amount of personal expenditures are being deducted.[86] Where abuse is apparent, the IRS would invoke the *Sutter* rule and allow a deduction only to the extent it exceeds the amount the taxpayer would normally spend.

Another common question concerns the costs of entertaining those who are not directly involved in the business activities to which the entertainment relates. The portion of any entertainment expense attributable to the customer's and the taxpayer's spouses is deductible where the purpose is business rather than personal or social.[87] For example, when the taxpayer entertains a business client and it is impractical to entertain the client without the spouse, the expenses of both the taxpayer's spouse and the client's spouse are deductible. Any expenses of other persons not closely connected with those who attended the business discussion are not deductible.

ENTERTAINMENT FACILITIES

For many years, the costs of owning and maintaining such status symbols as airplanes, luxury skyboxes, yachts, and hunting and fishing lodges could be subsidized by deducting

---

[82] An individual who is away from home on business and eats alone need not satisfy these tests.

[83] §§ 274(a) and (b).

[84] § 274(k)(1)(B).

[85] 21 T.C. 170 (1953).

[86] Rev. Rul. 63-144, 1963-2 C.B. 129.

[87] Reg. § 1.274-2(d)(4).

them as entertainment expenses. Typically, taxpayers would deduct expenses like depreciation, utilities, maintenance, insurance, and salaries (e.g., that of the yacht's captain) that were allocable to business usage of the property. In 1978, however, Congress imposed severe restrictions. Currently, costs such as those listed above that are related to *any entertainment facility* are not deductible.[88] Additional special rules apply to expenses incurred in using a luxury skybox.[89]

These rules governing entertainment facilities do not prohibit the deduction of out-of-pocket expenses incurred while at the entertainment facility. Expenses for such items as food or beverage would be deductible, assuming they meet the directly-related-to or associated-with tests. In addition, the various exceptions of § 274 discussed below may enable an employer to deduct expenses connected with entertainment facilities. For example, an employer may deduct the costs of vacation condominiums, swimming pools, tennis courts, and similar facilities if such entertainment facilities are provided primarily for employees.[90]

Club Dues. For years, the tax law contained an exception to the facility rule that allowed taxpayers to deduct their dues or fees paid for a membership in country clubs, etc., if the club was primarily used for business. In the never-ending attack on entertainment expenses, Congress eliminated the deduction for club dues in 1993. Currently no deduction is allowed for the cost of membership in any club organized for business, pleasure, recreation, or any other social purpose.[91] The new rule extends not only to country club dues but to all types of clubs, including luncheon, social, athletic, airline, and hotel clubs. The prohibition does not apply to dues paid to civic organizations, such as the Kiwanis or Rotary Club, or to professional organizations, such as the bar association, as long as the principal purpose of the organization is not entertainment. Note that specific expenses incurred at a club such as a business meal continue to be deductible to the extent that they satisfy any other applicable requirements.

EXCEPTIONS TO DIRECTLY-RELATED-TO AND ASSOCIATED-WITH TESTS

In certain innocent situations, entertainment and meal expenses need not meet either the directly-related-to or associated-with requirements. These include expenses for the following:[92]

1. Food and drink furnished on the business premises primarily for employees (e.g., costs of a holiday office party)

2. Recreational or social activities, including facilities primarily for employees (e. g., a summer golf outing, a company health club, an annual picnic)

3. Entertainment and meal expenses for an employee if the employee reports their value as taxable compensation (e.g., a company-provided vacation for the top salesperson)

4. Entertainment and meal expenses at business meetings of employees, stockholders, and directors (e.g., refreshments at a directors' meeting)

---

88 § 274(a)(1)(B); Reg. § 1.274-2(e)(2).

89 § 274(l)(2).

90 § 274(e)(5).

91 § 274(a)(3).

92 § 274(e)(1)-(9).

5. Costs of items made available to the general public (e.g., soft drinks at a grand opening, free ham to the first 50 customers)

6. Costs of entertainment and meals sold to customers (e.g., costs of food sold at an event)

FIFTY PERCENT LIMITATION ON ENTERTAINMENT AND MEAL EXPENSES

Opponents of the deduction for entertainment and meal expenses have long argued that, despite their business relationship, such expenses are inherently personal and should not be deductible. These same critics typically declare that business persons should not be able to live high-on-the-hog at the expense of the government. In 1986 the critics got their way, cutting the deduction to 80 percent of the actual cost. In 1993, they did it again, slashing the deduction even further.[93]

Currently, § 274(n) generally limits the amount that can be deducted for meals and entertainment to 50 percent of their actual cost. In effect, 50 percent of the cost is disallowed. For employees whose entertainment expenses are *not reimbursed*, the 50 percent limitation is applied before the 2 percent floor for itemized deductions.

> **Example 41.** B, an employee, pays $3,000 for business entertainment for which he is not reimbursed. B's A.G.I. is $50,000 for the year and he has no other miscellaneous itemized deductions. B's deduction is $500, computed as follows:

Total unreimbursed entertainment expenses...................	$ 3,000
Less 50% reduction (50% × $3,000)........................	(1,500)
Miscellaneous itemized deductions...........................	$ 1,500
Less 2% of A.G.I. (2% × $50,000).........................	(1,000)
Itemized deduction	$ 500

Expenses subject to the 50 percent limitation include the costs of taxes, tips, and parking related to a meal or an entertainment activity. In contrast, the costs of transportation to and from the activity are not subject to limitation.

> **Example 42.** B is the agent of G, who recently signed a lucrative contract with the Milwaukee Bucks. After successfully negotiating G's contract, B and G took a cab to a local restaurant where they toasted their success. After dinner, they walked to a nearby nightclub. For the night, B spent $207 for the following:

	Limited Expenses	Other
Meal	$120	
Tax	12	
Tips.......................................	30	
Cover charge..............................	38	
Cab.......................................		$7
Total	$200	$7

---

[93] § 274(n). Taxpayers subject to the hours of work limitations of the Department of Transportation (e.g., pilots and flight attendants, truck operators) and workers at remote seafood processing facilities (e.g., Alaskan whale boat captains) may deduct a greater portion.

The cost of the cab ride, $7, is not subject to limitation and thus can be deducted in full. Of the remaining $200, only $100 is deductible (50% of $200).

It should be emphasized that the percentage reduction rule applies to meals while away from home overnight on business as well as the traditional quiet business meal. The 50 percent limitation does not apply in several situations, thus allowing the taxpayer to deduct the meal or entertainment in full. These exceptions are discussed below.

Reimbursed Expenses. When the taxpayer is reimbursed for the meal or entertainment, the limitation is imposed on the party making reimbursement, not the taxpayer.[94]

Example 43. N, a sales representative for Big Corporation, took a customer to lunch after he secured a large order. He paid $30, for which he was totally reimbursed. N includes the $30 in income and may deduct the entire $30. The corporation can deduct only $15 (50% of $30).

If an employee has a reimbursement or expense allowance arrangement with the employer, but under the arrangement the full amount of business expenses is not reimbursed, special problems arise. These problems are considered along with record keeping requirements later in this chapter.

Excludable Fringe Benefit. The 50 percent limitation does not apply where the food or beverage provided is excludable as a de minimis employee fringe benefit (e.g., holiday turkeys, hams, fruitcakes, etc., given to employees, subsidized cafeterias, or to meals provided on the employer's premises for the convenience of the employer).[95]

Code § 274(e) Exceptions. The percentage reduction rule generally is not imposed on entertainment and meal costs which are exempted from the directly-related-to and associated-with tests noted above.[96] For example, there is no reduction required for the deductible costs of an annual employee Christmas party, summer golf outings, or company-provided vacations treated as compensation. Similarly, the costs of promotional items made available to the general public (e.g., 100 baseball tickets given by a radio to the first 100 callers) or the salaries of comedians paid by a nightclub are not subject to the 50 percent limitation.

Charitable Sporting Event. The costs of tickets to a sporting event are not subject to the reduction rule if the event is related to charitable fund-raising.[97] Specifically, the event must be organized for the primary purpose of benefiting a tax-exempt charitable organization, must contribute 100 percent of the proceeds to the charity, and must use volunteers for substantially all work performed in putting on the event. For example, the cost of tickets to attend a golf or tennis celebrity tournament sponsored by the local chapter of the United Way would normally satisfy these requirements and would be fully deductible. Tickets for high school, college, or other scholastic events (e.g., a football game or theater tickets) do not qualify for this exception on the grounds that volunteers do not do all the work (e.g., coaches, their assistants, and other paid individuals provide substantial work such as coaching and recruiting).

---

[94]   §§ 274(n)(2) and 274(e)(3).

[95]   § 274(n)(2)(B).

[96]   § 274(n)(2).

[97]   § 274(n)(2)(C).

LIMITATIONS ON DEDUCTIONS FOR TICKETS

In the entertainment fracas of 1986, lawmakers also struck a blow at the deductible costs of tickets. This deduction is limited to the face value of the ticket (e.g., 50% of the normal ticket price).[98] This rule is aimed at amounts paid to a ticket scalper in excess of the regular price of the ticket. Such excess is not deductible. The rule also makes nondeductible any fee paid to a ticket agency for arranging tickets. Note, however, that this rule does not apply to tickets to qualified charitable fundraisers.

BUSINESS GIFTS

In hopes that their generosity will someday be rewarded, taxpayers often make gifts to customers, clients, and others with whom they have a business relationship. Such business connected gifts are deductible under the general rules of § 162. Under prior law, taxpayers wanting to create goodwill could shower their business associates with gifts and deduct these instruments of goodwill. Moreover, the recipient of such bounty could arguably exclude the presents. Currently, § 274(b) curbs such practice by limiting the deduction for business gifts to $25 per donee per year.[99] For this purpose, the following items *are not* considered gifts:

1. An item costing $4 or less imprinted with the taxpayer's name (e.g., pens)

2. Signs, display racks, or other promotional materials to be used on the business premises of the recipient

Incidental costs such as engraving, mailing, and wrapping are not considered part of the cost of an item for purposes of the $25 limit. However, husband and wife are treated as *one* recipient for purposes of the $25 limitation.

> **Example 44.** J, a saleswoman of hospital supplies, computes her deduction for business gifts during the year in the following manner.

Description of Gift	Amount	Deduction
H, head of purchasing at St. Jude hospital:		
Perfume	$10	
Solar calculator	30	
Total	$40	$25
Dr. Z:		
Box of golf balls	$18	
Gift wrap	2	
Total	$20	20
Total business gift deduction		$45

Assuming J is an employee, she may deduct the $45 as a miscellaneous itemized deduction.

---

[98] § 274(1)(1).

[99] § 274(b).

Employee Achievement Awards. When a business expresses its gratitude for an employee's performance with a gift, special rules allow amounts greater than $25 to be transferred. The effect of these rules is to allow an employer to make and deduct gifts of up to $1,600 to an employee who is allowed to *exclude* the amount of the gift. The Code generally allows an employer to deduct up to $400 per employee for an *employee achievement award.*[100] An employee achievement award is defined as an item of tangible personal property (e.g., a television or watch, not cash or a gift certificate) transferred to the employee for *length of service* or for *safety* achievement. To help ensure that such awards are not merely disguised compensation, the award must be transferred as part of a meaningful presentation. When the employer has a qualified plan in effect—a nondiscriminatory written plan where the average annual award to all employees does not exceed $400—a deduction of up to $1,600 for a particular award is allowed.

TRAVEL AND ENTERTAINMENT RECORD KEEPING REQUIREMENTS

Travel and entertainment expenses (including business gifts) are not deductible unless the taxpayer properly substantiates the expenses.[101] The *Cohan* rule permitting a deduction for an unsupported but reasonable estimation of an expense does not apply in regard to travel and entertainment.[102]

Section 274(d) specifically requires the taxpayer to substantiate each of the following five elements of an expenditure:

1. Amount
2. Time
3. Place
4. Business purpose
5. Business relationship (for entertainment only)

In most cases, each item must be supported by adequate records such as a diary, account book, or similar record, *and* documentary evidence including receipts or paid bills. Where adequate records have not been maintained, the taxpayer's personal statement will suffice—but only if there is other corroborating evidence, such as the testimony of the individual who was entertained.[103] Congress has indicated that oral evidence would have the least probative value of any evidence and has also authorized the IRS to ask certain additional questions concerning substantiation on the return (see Part II, lines 19–21 of Form 2106, discussed below). In addition, the legislative history makes it clear that the IRS and the courts will invoke the negligence and fraud penalties in those cases where the taxpayer claims tax benefits far in excess of what can be justified.

A receipt is necessary only for lodging expenses and any other expenses of $75 or more. Cancelled checks, without other evidence, may not be sufficient. In the well-known blizzard case of 1975, the importance of properly substantiating each element of the expense was made clear.[104] In this case, the taxpayer did not keep a diary or other record of his substantial travel and entertainment expenses, but he presented the District Court

---

[100]   § 274(j).

[101]   § 274(d).

[102]   Reg. § 1.274-5T(a)(4).

[103]   Reg. § 1.274-5(c)(3).

[104]   *Cam F. Dowell, Jr. v. U.S.*, 75-2 USTC ¶9819, 36 AFTR2d 75-6314, 522 F.2d 708 (CA-5, 1975), *vac'g. and rem'g.* 74-1 USTC ¶9243, 33 AFTR2d 74-739, 370 F. Supp. 69 (D.Ct. Tex., 1974).

with over 1,700 bills, chits, and memos, as well as 20 witnesses. The District Court allowed the deduction holding that the virtual "blizzard" of bills, etc., met the required tests. The Appellate Court, however, disagreed, indicating that the District Court did not determine whether the elements of each expense were substantiated. Lacking sufficient information on the specific purpose of each expenditure, deductions were denied. A written statement of the purpose is unnecessary, however, where the business purpose or business relationship is obvious from other surrounding facts.

In lieu of substantiating the *amount* of meals and lodging expenses while away from home on business, employees and self-employed individuals may elect to compute the deduction using a standard daily allowance rate. For example, in 2009 the standard meal and incidental expense rate (M&IE rate) is usually $39 per day and is reduced by the 50 percent limit on meals. The standard lodging rate is $70 per day. These rates vary depending on location and time of year. For example, for 2009 the lodging rate in Indianapolis is $94 per day ($44 M&IE) while in Manhattan it is $360 (for 10/1/08–12/31/09) ($64 M&IE).[105]

✔ CHECK YOUR KNOWLEDGE

Review Question 1. P, the public defense attorney of South City, occasionally takes all of his staff to lunch. Q, an attorney in private practice, occasionally takes all of her staff to lunch. Can P and Q deduct the costs of the meals?

Too bad, P. This question illustrates the relatively rare situation when the taxpayer's entertainment expenses may fail the ordinary and necessary criterion or perhaps be considered lavish or extravagant. Q, the attorney in private practice, would have no trouble deducting her expenses. However, the IRS denied (with the U.S. Tax Court's support) a public defender's deduction since public defenders do not commonly take their staffs to lunch!

Review Question 2. To illustrate the problems with entertainment expenses, consider the case of Danville Plywood Corporation,[106] a custom manufacturer of plywood. In 1981, Danville sponsored a four-day excursion for 116 people to the Super Bowl in New Orleans. The so-called Super Bowl Sales Seminar cost $103,444 including tickets, airfare, food, and lodging. On its 1981 tax return, the corporation claimed a deduction for the entire amount, euphemistically calling it "advertising expense." The list of attendees included 55 customers, 37 of their spouses, and two of their children. The remainder consisted of a few employees of the corporation and their spouses, as well as the owner, a few of his friends, and two of his children. According to the corporation, the goal of the seminar was to have discussions with the customers over a period of days in order to ascertain how Danville could do a better job as well as cut down on the travel expenses its salespeople incurred on customer visits. In the past, customers had rarely participated in plant visits so the corporation thought some type of sales meeting held in conjunction with a sporting event might boost attendance. In preparation for the trip, the company instructed its employees regarding some new products and provided other information that they were to share with the customers during the Super Bowl or

---

[105] Rev. Proc. 2008-59, 2008-41 IRB. See also *Travel Resource section, Per Diem Rates tab in www.gsa.gov.* Note also that a standard meal and snack rate exists for day care providers. See Rev. Proc. 2003-22, 2003-1 CB 577.

[106] *Danville Plywood Corp. v. U.S.* 65 AFTR 2d 90-982, 899 F2d 3, 90-1 USTC ¶50,161 (CA-FC, 1990) aff'g 63 AFTR 2d 89-1036, 16 Cl Ct 584, 89-1 USTC ¶9248 (Cl Ct, 1989). Contrast with *Townsend Industries, Inc. v. U.S..* 92 AFTR 2d 2003-6096 342 F3d 890 (CA-8, 2003) rev'g 90 AFTR 2d 2002-6588 (Southern D. Ct. IA, 2002), where a fishing trip for employees had "a bona fide business purpose" for the trip and it enabled informal conversation about employer's business.

a side trip to the French Quarter. The company also arranged a display showing some of its products in an area adjacent to the lobby of the hotel where everyone stayed. However, when Danville invited its guests, the letter made no reference to business meetings of any kind, nor did the company reserve rooms where business could be conducted. The corporation did hold a dinner in the hotel for all of its guests, but other individuals were also present. Danville had sponsored a similar trip to the 1980 Super Bowl and had deducted about $98,000. Was Danville able to deduct the expenses of all of the attendees?

Unfortunately, Danville got sacked on this play and none of the costs were deductible. In denying the deduction, the court emphasized that the expenses not only had to meet the tests of § 162 (i.e., ordinary and necessary business expenses) but also had to pass the rigorous requirements of § 274. The court found little difficulty in concluding that these tests were not met. It found incredible the corporation's attempt to deduct not only the expenses of the president's children but also those of the customers, explaining that their presence did not serve a bona fide business purpose. The court felt similarly about the president's friends as well as the spouses of both the customers and the employees. With respect to the customers and employees, it noted that there was little if any business discussed—a few idle conversations at most. Moreover, the letters to the customers never mentioned the possibility of business discussions or meetings. Nor were meeting rooms reserved for such purpose. In addition, the court believed that such trips were not commonplace in the industry. Based on these observations, the court concluded that the central focus of the trip was entertainment, not business. Unfortunately, it appears that Danville could have won this contest if it had a better game plan. For example, the deduction may have been secured if only the company's correspondence had properly explained the business nature of the weekend and it had actually conducted a business meeting in a separate room devoted to such purpose. No doubt, it also did not sit well with the IRS that the corporation was so aggressive that it deducted the expenses of the children and the friends. Simply bypassing these deductions may have saved the day.

Review Question 3. Although there appears to be one test after another that taxpayers must meet before they deduct entertainment expenditures, there are some basic requirements. Describe them.

The entertainment must be either directly related or associated with business. This means that a taxpayer must discuss business either before, after, or during the entertainment activity.

Review Question 4. D, an attorney in Indianapolis, is an avid Hoosier fan. Somehow he managed to obtain season tickets to the IU basketball games. From time to time, he is unable to attend a game, so he calls a client and surprises him or her with a pair of tickets. Can D deduct the cost of the tickets for his clients?

D can continue to make his friends happy. As a general rule, no deduction is allowed unless the taxpayer or his representative (e.g., an employee) is present, since business cannot take place. However, D could deduct up to $25 as a business gift.

Review Question 5. E runs an advertising firm and is constantly taking people to lunch. Just yesterday he took the ad director at Channel 12 to dinner at his favorite gourmet restaurant. They both had drinks, salad, prime rib, dessert, and coffee: a total of $30 each. When E eats alone, he typically eats a value meal at the local fast-food place. Can E deduct the cost of his client's meal? Can he deduct the entire cost of his own meal or only the amount in excess of what he normally spends?

E can eat, drink, and be merry. As long as E and his friend discussed business in between bites or the meal followed or preceded a business meeting, he can deduct the entire $60 subject to the 50 percent limitation.

Review Question 6. This year F was admitted to the partnership of her accounting firm. Not only was F required to contribute $50,000 to the partnership but she was also required to join a country club. She joined the plush Meridian Lakes Country Club at a cost of $25,000. In addition, she must pay monthly dues of $300. Assuming F uses the club exclusively for business, can she deduct the membership and dues?

Sorry, F, but it is the price of being a partner. The Code denies a deduction for the costs of both the membership and the club dues.

Review Question 7. True or False: Taxpayers are generally allowed to deduct only 50 percent of their unreimbursed travel and entertainment expenses.

False. Do not be fooled. A typical mistake is to lump travel and entertainment together. Only meals and entertainment expenses are subject to the 50 percent rule. Travel (other than meals) is not subject to the limitation.

Review Question 8. G&H, a public accounting firm, provides continuing education for its tax staff at a resort in Florida. During the week, the employees spend hour upon hour in seminars devoted to the tax law. The firm pays for the meals and lodging of the participants. Is G&H entitled to deduct the entire costs of the meals or only 50 percent?

The 50 percent limitation normally applies to the costs of all meals and entertainment. However, the limitation does not apply if any of the various exceptions contained in § 274 (e) apply. One of these concerns business meetings of employees. Consequently, the firm is allowed to deduct 100 percent of the meal costs.

Review Question 9. This year the School of Business at X University created an annual award of $100 given to three staff members (e.g., secretaries) for outstanding performance during the year. The School's bookkeeper is uncertain as to whether taxes are to be withheld on such awards. How should the awards be handled?

Unfortunately, what appears to be an award of $100 is probably closer to $60 since the award is fully taxable and both income and employment taxes must be withheld. No exclusion is available since the award is given in cash and is not for length of service or safety.

REPORTING BUSINESS EXPENSES AND LOSSES

SOLE PROPRIETORS AND SELF-EMPLOYED PERSONS

Sole proprietors and self-employed persons are not treated as separate taxable entities. Rather, their income and expenses are compiled and reported simply as a part of their individual return. This information is reported on Schedule C or C-EZ of Form 1040. Page 1 of Schedule C appears below. An examination of Schedule C reveals that it is relatively straightforward and self-explanatory. The net income or loss as reported on line 31 of Schedule C is transferred to Page 1 of Form 1040 and is added to the taxpayer's income. The net income or loss on Schedule C also is used in the computation of self-employment tax. Accordingly, the net amount on Schedule C must also be transferred to Schedule SE.

**SCHEDULE C
(Form 1040)**

Department of the Treasury
Internal Revenue Service (99)

Profit or Loss From Business

(Sole Proprietorship)

▶ **Partnerships, joint ventures, etc., generally must file Form 1065 or 1065-B.**

▶ **Attach to Form 1040, 1040NR, or 1041.** ▶ **See Instructions for Schedule C (Form 1040).**

OMB No. 1545-0074

2008

Attachment
Sequence No. **09**

Name of proprietor

Social security number (SSN)

A Principal business or profession, including product or service (see page C-3 of the instructions)

B Enter code from pages C-9, 10, & 11
▶

C Business name. If no separate business name, leave blank.

D Employer ID number (EIN), if any

E Business address (including suite or room no.) ▶ ---
City, town or post office, state, and ZIP code

F Accounting method: **(1)** ☐ Cash **(2)** ☐ Accrual **(3)** ☐ Other (specify) ▶ ------------------------------

G Did you "materially participate" in the operation of this business during 2008? If "No," see page C-4 for limit on losses ☐ Yes ☐ No

H If you started or acquired this business during 2008, check here . . . . ▶ ☐

Part I Income

1	Gross receipts or sales. **Caution.** See page C-4 and check the box if:	
	● This income was reported to you on Form W-2 and the "Statutory employee" box on that form was checked, or	
	● You are a member of a qualified joint venture reporting only rental real estate income not subject to self-employment tax. Also see page C-4 for limit on losses. ▶ ☐	**1**
2	Returns and allowances	**2**
3	Subtract line 2 from line 1	**3**
4	Cost of goods sold (from line 42 on page 2)	**4**
5	**Gross profit.** Subtract line 4 from line 3	**5**
6	Other income, including federal and state gasoline or fuel tax credit or refund (see page C-4)	**6**
7	**Gross income.** Add lines 5 and 6 ▶	**7**

Part II Expenses. Enter expenses for business use of your home **only** on line 30.

8	Advertising	**8**	**18** Office expense		**18**
9	Car and truck expenses (see page C-5)	**9**	**19** Pension and profit-sharing plans		**19**
10	Commissions and fees	**10**	**20** Rent or lease (see page C-6):		
11	Contract labor (see page C-5)	**11**	**a** Vehicles, machinery, and equipment		**20a**
12	Depletion	**12**	**b** Other business property		**20b**
13	Depreciation and section 179 expense deduction (not included in Part III) (see page C-5)	**13**	**21** Repairs and maintenance		**21**
			22 Supplies (not included in Part III)		**22**
			23 Taxes and licenses		**23**
			24 Travel, meals, and entertainment:		
			a Travel		**24a**
14	Employee benefit programs (other than on line 19)	**14**	**b** Deductible meals and entertainment (see page C-7)		**24b**
15	Insurance (other than health)	**15**	**25** Utilities		**25**
16	Interest:		**26** Wages (less employment credits)		**26**
a	Mortgage (paid to banks, etc.)	**16a**	**27** Other expenses (from line 48 on page 2)		**27**
b	Other	**16b**			
17	Legal and professional services	**17**			

28	**Total expenses** before expenses for business use of home. Add lines 8 through 27 ▶	**28**
29	Tentative profit or (loss). Subtract line 28 from line 7	**29**
30	Expenses for business use of your home. Attach **Form 8829**	**30**
31	**Net profit or (loss).** Subtract line 30 from line 29.	
	● If a profit, enter on both **Form 1040, line 12,** and **Schedule SE, line 2,** or on **Form 1040NR, line 13** (if you checked the box on line 1, see page C-7). Estates and trusts, enter on **Form 1041, line 3.**	**31**
	● If a loss, you **must** go to line 32.	
32	If you have a loss, check the box that describes your investment in this activity (see page C-8).	
	● If you checked 32a, enter the loss on both **Form 1040, line 12,** and **Schedule SE, line 2,** or on **Form 1040NR, line 13** (if you checked the box on line 1, see the line 31 instructions on page C-7). Estates and trusts, enter on **Form 1041, line 3.**	**32a** ☐ All investment is at risk.
		32b ☐ Some investment is not at risk.
	● If you checked 32b, you **must** attach **Form 6198.** Your loss may be limited.	

For Paperwork Reduction Act Notice, see page C-9 of the instructions.   Cat. No. 11334P   **Schedule C (Form 1040) 2008**

STATUTORY EMPLOYEES

Before examining the reporting requirements for employees, attention must be given to a subset of workers commonly referred to as *statutory employees*. These are individuals who work in four occupational groups (described below) and are not otherwise employees under the usual common law tests. Rather, under a specific statutory provision, they are treated as employees for purposes of FICA (and sometimes FUTA) and are subject to favorable rules concerning the reporting of their income and deductions.[107] Statutory employees include.[108]

- ▸ Life insurance salespersons who work full-time for a single life insurance company selling life insurance or annuity contracts.

- ▸ Traveling salespersons who work full-time for one person to solicit orders for merchandise from customers for resale or supplies for use by the customers in their businesses (e.g., a manufacturers representative, salesmen that regularly call on customers and get paid a commission)

- ▸ Agent-drivers or commission-drivers that distribute meat, vegetable, fruit or bakery products, beverages (other than milk) or laundry or dry cleaning services (e.g., a delivery man that distributes bakery products)

- ▸ Individual who work off the premises of the person for whom the services are performed (e.g., at home or the home of another) according to furnished specifications on material provided and the products are returned to the principal (e.g., garment workers who make clothing, quilts, bedspreads and similar items at home and return them to the person for whom they performed the work; people who address envelopes at home or provide typing or transcribing services).[109]

To be considered statutory employees, these individuals also must perform all of the work (no delegation of a significant portion), have no substantial investment in facilities (vehicles excluded) and have a regular and recurring relationship with the business for which they are providing services.

Statutory employees report their income and expenses in a unique manner. They receive a Form W-2 that reports their wages or commissions. In recognition of their special treatment, box 13 of the W-2 for "Statutory Employee" is checked. The wages or commissions earned by the statutory employee that are reported on the W-2 are subject to FICA taxes but withholding of income taxes is optional. More significant is the manner in which a statutory employee reports the W-2 income and related expenses. They are not considered employees subject to the normal rules governing the reporting of deductions.[110] Even though a statutory employee receives a W-2, he or she reports that income and the related expenses on Schedule C. The net amount is not subject to self-employment taxes as is normally the case since the employer withheld FICA. By reporting the expenses in this fashion, a statutory employee effectively deducts these expenses for A.G.I. and avoids the need to itemize deductions as well as the floor on miscellaneous itemized deductions (MIDs). Avoiding classification as MIDs is extremely important in light of the alternative minimum tax (AMT), which denies deductions for MIDs, making the taxpayer more vulnerable to the AMT (see Chapter 13).

Although statutory employee status provides substantial benefits, unfortunately employers do not always cooperate. Sometimes they are reluctant to check the magic box

---

[107]   § 3121(d).

[108]   See reference in § 3509(d)(3)concerning withholding to the workers identified in § 3121(d)(3).

[109]   For an example of the reach of this rule, *see Laverne S. VanZant* TCS 2007-195.

[110]   Statutory employees are not considered employees for purposes of § 62 that identifies the deductions that are for A.G.I. See IRS acknowledgement in Rev. Rul. 90-93, 1990-2 CB 33 concerning a full-time life insurance salesman.

on the W-2, making the individual reluctant to claim the benefits of being a statutory employee for risk of an audit. Nevertheless, this is not a choice the employer has and it seems that the statutory employee should be able to report the W-2 correctly.

EMPLOYEES

Both the treatment and reporting of an employee's business expenses vary significantly depending on whether the expenses are reimbursed. As explained in Chapter 7, employee business expenses that are *not* reimbursed are treated as miscellaneous itemized deductions, and are therefore deductible only to the extent that total miscellaneous itemized deductions exceed 2 percent of A.G.I. In addition, such deductions would be subject to the deduction cutback. On the other hand, expenses reimbursed under an accountable plan (discussed below) are *not deductible* by the employee, *but* the reimbursement is excludable from his or her gross income. In such case, there is no effect on the taxpayer's return. This latter treatment normally applies to most employee expense accounts, including those arrangements where the employer reimburses an employee for a particular expense as well as those where the employer gives the employee a fixed allowance (e.g., a per diem amount such as $15 per day for meals and $25 per day for lodging). It should be emphasized, however, that even though an expense may appear to be reimbursed in the normal sense, it may not be treated as reimbursed for determining whether the expense is deductible from A.G.I. or the reimbursement is excludable from gross income.

Accountable and Nonaccountable Plans. Since 1989, an employee's business expenses are treated as reimbursed only if his or her employer has a reimbursement or allowance arrangement that qualifies as an *accountable plan.* An arrangement generally qualifies as an accountable plan if the employee properly substantiates the expenses to the employer, and, in the case of advances or allowances, is required to return to the employer any amount in excess of that which is substantiated.[111] If the arrangement does not meet the accountable plan requirements, it is considered a *nonaccountable plan.* As might be expected, the tax treatment of payments under the two different plans differs drastically.

Reimbursements or advances made under an accountable plan are treated far more favorably than those under a nonaccountable plan. Amounts paid under an accountable plan are normally excluded from gross income, not reported on the employee's Form W-2, and are exempt from employment taxes (i.e., social security and unemployment). In contrast, reimbursements and advances made under a nonaccountable plan must be reported in the employee's gross income, included on Form W-2, and are subject to employment taxes. More importantly, the expenses for which the employee is reimbursed under a nonaccountable plan must be claimed as miscellaneous itemized deductions subject to the 2 percent floor. In contrast, in the case of an accountable plan, consistent with the fact that the reimbursement is not included in income, the expense is not deducted—at least in the normal sense. Instead, the expense, like the reimbursement, is not reported. As the IRS puts it, there is "no deduction since [the employee's] expenses and reimbursements are equal." In effect, the employer claims the deduction rather than the employee.

Under either plan, the employee normally summarizes employee business expenses on Form 2106 (shown on pp. 8–51 and 8–52). When this form is properly completed, expenses not considered reimbursed flow to Schedule A and are deducted as miscellaneous itemized deductions. The reporting of employee business expenses is summarized in Exhibit 8-2, which follows.

---

[111] Temp. Reg. § 1.62-2T.

EXHIBIT 8-2
Reporting Travel, Transportation, Meal, and Entertainment Expenses and Reimbursements

Type of Reimbursement or Other Expense Allowance Arrangement	Employer *Reports on Form W-2*	Employee *Shows on Form 2106*	Employee *Claims on Schedule A*
1. Accountable *Adequate accounting and excess returned*	*Not reported*	*Not shown*	*Not claimed*
2. *Per diem or mileage allowance (up to government rate)* *Adequate accounting and excess returned*	*Not reported*	*All expenses and reimbursements only if excess expenses are claimed. Otherwise, form is not filed*	*Expenses the employee can prove and which exceed the reimbursements received*
3. *Per diem or mileage allowance (exceeds government rate)* *Adequate accounting up to the government rate only and excess not returned*	*Excess reported as wages in Box 1. Amount up to the government rate is reported only in a Box 13—it is not reported in Box 1*	*All expenses, and reimbursements equal to the government rate, only if expenses in excess of the government rate are claimed.[1] Otherwise, form is not filed*	*Expenses the employee can prove and which exceed the government rate[2]*
4. Nonaccountable *Adequate accounting or return of excess either not required or required but not met*	*Entire amount is reported as wages in Box 1.[3]*	*All expenses[1]*	*Expenses the employee can prove[2]*
5. *No reimbursement*	*Normal reporting of wages, etc.*	*All expenses[1]*	*Expenses the employee can prove[2]*

[1] These amounts are subject to income tax withholding and to all employment taxes such as FICA and FUTA.

[2] Any allowable expense is carried to line 20 of Schedule A and deducted as a miscellaneous itemized deduction.

[3] These amounts are subject to the applicable limits including the 50 percent limit on meals and entertainment expenses and the two percent of adjusted gross income limit on the total miscellaneous itemized deductions.

Source: Travel, Entertainment, Gift and Car Expense, IRS Publication 463 (Rev. 2008), p. 31.

Under an accountable plan, an employee who substantiates his or her expenses and returns any excess reimbursement reports neither the reimbursements nor the expenses because there is a complete wash. See Exhibit 8-2 Item 1.) *However*, if the employee fails to return any excess reimbursement, a different accounting is required. In this case, the excess reimbursement is treated as *if* paid under a nonaccountable plan. Therefore, the employer must report the *excess* in the employee's Form W-2 as well as pay the related employment taxes. On the other side, the employee must include the excess in gross income. (See Exhibit 8-2, Item 3).

Example 45. R is a sales representative for C Corporation and has an expense account arrangement. Under this arrangement, R fills out an expense report every two weeks, documenting all of his expenses, and submits it for reimbursement. This year R submitted travel expenses of $5,000, all of which were reimbursed. Assuming this is an accountable plan and R has properly substantiated expenses of $5,000, there is nothing included on his Form W-2 and none of the expenses are reported on his return. In effect, there is no effect on R because the reimbursement and expenses wash. (See Exhibit 8-2 Item 1.)

Example 46. Assume the plan in *Example 44* was not properly structured and did not require R either to substantiate his expenses or to return any excess reimbursement. In this case, the arrangement would be a nonaccountable plan. Consequently, the $5,000 reimbursement would be included as income in R's Form W-2 and he could deduct the $5,000 as a miscellaneous itemized deduction. In this case, the income and deduction do not necessarily wash (e.g., if R does not itemize), and R ends up with taxable income that economically he does not have. (See Exhibit 8-2 Item 4. The Form 2106 shown on pp. 8–51 and 8–52 reveals how this information would be reported.)

As the above examples illustrate, most employers should opt to establish reimbursement arrangements that meet the accountable plan requirements so that employees are not unduly penalized. Nevertheless, as noted above, even if the employer has an accountable plan, the employee must still substantiate any expenses and return any reimbursements in excess of the expenses substantiated to avoid unfavorable treatment.

Substantiation. A plan generally satisfies the substantiation requirement if the employee meets the normal rules for substantiation of expenses. For example, travel and entertainment expenses must be substantiated under the special rules of § 274(d) discussed earlier in this chapter. Note that an employee whose reimbursement is based on some type of fixed allowance (e.g., a per diem for meals and lodging or a mileage allowance) is *deemed* to have substantiated the amount of his or her expenses up to the amount set by the IRS for per diem, mileage, or other expense allowances.[112] Generally, the only expense substantiation for such plans is the number of business miles traveled and the number of days away from home spent on business. Due to this rule, employees who receive allowances within the IRS guidelines will have no reimbursements in excess of their substantiated expenses and, therefore, will not have any excess to return.

Example 47. K works as an accountant for a public accounting firm in Tampa. This year she attended a continuing education course in Jacksonville. The firm gives its employees a meal allowance of $12 per diem, which is within the IRS guidelines. K attended the course for five days. When she returned from the trip, she submitted

---

[112]   See Temp. Regs. §§ 1.62-2T(e)(2) and 1.274-5T(g).

her expense report requesting reimbursement for meals of $60 (5 × $12). In reality, K, wanting to save as much as she could, spent only $40 on meals. Although K has actually received $20 more than she spent ($60 − $40), she does not have to return the excess because she is deemed to have substantiated expenses of $60.

If an employee has expenses that the employer did not reimburse, the employee should file Form 2106 to claim a deduction for the unreimbursed expenses. Proper completion of this form results in the unreimbursed expenses being claimed as miscellaneous itemized deductions on Schedule A. (See Exhibit 8-2 Item 2.)

Example 48. Under an accountable plan, T is reimbursed 40 cents per mile for all business miles driven. For the year, he received $1,000. After consulting his records, T determined that his actual expenses exceed 40 cents per mile for a total of $1,200. None of the reimbursement is included on T's Form W-2 because this is an accountable plan and the allowance does not exceed the government rate. T should report the $1,200 of expenses on lines 1–6 of Form 2106. The $1,000 reimbursement is entered on line 7 and subtracted from the $1,200 expense amount to leave $200. The $200 (the amount for which T did not receive a reimbursement) flows through to Schedule A and is treated as a miscellaneous itemized deduction. (See line 10 of Form 2106 and Exhibit 8-2, Item 2).

Example 49. J's employer pays her a flat $100 per month to cover her car expenses. The employer does not have an accountable plan. Thus the employer must include the $100 as income in J's Form W-2, and J may deduct her car expenses as miscellaneous itemized deductions. (See Exhibit 8-2, Item 4.)

In certain instances, the employer may give the employee a per diem allowance that exceeds the Federal government allowable rate (e.g., 60 cents per mile instead of the allowable standard mileage rate). In such cases, special reporting rules apply.[113] Similarly, special allocation rules must be observed when the amount of the reimbursement covers only a portion of the employee's expenses.[114]

TAX PLANNING CONSIDERATIONS

MOVING EXPENSES

Upon retirement, many individuals move to another location. Normally, the moving expenses would not be deductible. If the taxpayer can obtain a *full-time* job at the new location, however, the costs of moving become deductible. In this regard, the taxpayer must be sure to satisfy the 39- or 78-week test.

TRAVEL AND ENTERTAINMENT EXPENSES

The rules governing deductions for combined business and pleasure travel permit some vacationing on business trips without jeopardizing the deduction. As long as the trip is primarily for business, the entire cost of traveling to the business/vacation destination is deductible. Although the expenses of personal side-trips are not allowed, these expenses may be incidental to the major costs of getting to the desired location. For example, a taxpayer living in New York can deduct a major portion of the cost of a vacation in

---

[113] *Supra*, Footnote 101, p. 11.
[114] Reg. § 1.62-1(f).

Form **2106**

Department of the Treasury
Internal Revenue Service (99)

Employee Business Expenses

▶ See separate instructions.

▶ **Attach to Form 1040 or Form 1040NR.**

OMB No. 1545-0074

2008

Attachment
Sequence No. **129**

Your name	Occupation in which you incurred expenses	Social security number
R. Employee	Sales representative	456-78-9102

Part I   **Employee Business Expenses and Reimbursements**

Step 1   **Enter Your Expenses**

		Column A Other Than Meals and Entertainment		Column B Meals and Entertainment	
1	Vehicle expense from line 22c or line 29. (Rural mail carriers: See instructions.)	**1**			
2	Parking fees, tolls, and transportation, including train, bus, etc., that **did not** involve overnight travel or commuting to and from work .	**2**			
3	Travel expense while away from home overnight, including lodging, airplane, car rental, etc. **Do not** include meals and entertainment	**3**	5,000		
4	Business expenses not included on lines 1 through 3. **Do not** include meals and entertainment	**4**			
5	Meals and entertainment expenses (see instructions)	**5**			
6	**Total expenses.** In Column A, add lines 1 through 4 and enter the result. In Column B, enter the amount from line 5	**6**	5,000		

Note: *If you were not reimbursed for any expenses in Step 1, skip line 7 and enter the amount from line 6 on line 8.*

Step 2   **Enter Reimbursements Received From Your Employer for Expenses Listed in Step 1**

7	Enter reimbursements received from your employer that were **not** reported to you in box 1 of Form W-2. Include any reimbursements reported under code "L" in box 12 of your Form W-2 (see instructions)	**7**	-0-		

Step 3   **Figure Expenses To Deduct on Schedule A (Form 1040 or Form 1040NR)**

8	Subtract line 7 from line 6. If zero or less, enter -0-. However, if line 7 is greater than line 6 in Column A, report the excess as income on Form 1040, line 7 (or on Form 1040NR, line 8) . .	**8**	5,000		
	Note: *If **both columns** of line 8 are zero, you cannot deduct employee business expenses. Stop here and attach Form 2106 to your return.*				
9	In Column A, enter the amount from line 8. In Column B, multiply line 8 by 50% (.50). (Employees subject to Department of Transportation (DOT) hours of service limits: Multiply meal expenses incurred while away from home on business by 80% (.80) instead of 50%. For details, see instructions.)	**9**	5,000		
10	Add the amounts on line 9 of both columns and enter the total here. **Also, enter the total on Schedule A (Form 1040), line 21** (or on **Schedule A (Form 1040NR), line 9**). (Reservists, qualified performing artists, fee-basis state or local government officials, and individuals with disabilities: See the instructions for special rules on where to enter the total.) . . . ▶	**10**	5,000		

For Paperwork Reduction Act Notice, see instructions.   Cat. No. 11700N   Form **2106** (2008)

Form 2106 (2008) R. Employee | Page **2**

Part II Vehicle Expenses

Section A—General Information (You must complete this section if you are claiming vehicle expenses.)

			(a) Vehicle 1	**(b)** Vehicle 2
11	Enter the date the vehicle was placed in service	11	/ /	/ /
12	Total miles the vehicle was driven during 2008	12	miles	miles
13	Business miles included on line 12	13	miles	miles
14	Percent of business use. Divide line 13 by line 12	14	%	%
15	Average daily roundtrip commuting distance	15	miles	miles
16	Commuting miles included on line 12	16	miles	miles
17	Other miles. Add lines 13 and 16 and subtract the total from line 12.	17	miles	miles

18 Was your vehicle available for personal use during off-duty hours? ☐ Yes ☐ No
19 Do you (or your spouse) have another vehicle available for personal use? ☐ Yes ☐ No
20 Do you have evidence to support your deduction? ☐ Yes ☐ No
21 If "Yes," is the evidence written? ☐ Yes ☐ No

Section B—Standard Mileage Rate (See the instructions for Part II to find out whether to complete this section or Section C.)

22a Multiply business miles driven **before** July 1, 2008, by 50.5¢ (.505) . **22a**
  b Multiply business miles driven **after** June 30, 2008, by 58.5¢ (.585) . **22b**
  c Add lines 22a and 22b. Enter the result here and on line 1 . **22c**

Section C—Actual Expenses

			(a) Vehicle 1		**(b)** Vehicle 2	
23	Gasoline, oil, repairs, vehicle insurance, etc.	23				
24a	Vehicle rentals	24a				
b	Inclusion amount (see instructions)	24b				
c	Subtract line 24b from line 24a	24c				
25	Value of employer-provided vehicle (applies only if 100% of annual lease value was included on Form W-2—see instructions)	25				
26	Add lines 23, 24c, and 25	26				
27	Multiply line 26 by the percentage on line 14	27				
28	Depreciation (see instructions)	28				
29	Add lines 27 and 28. Enter total here and on line 1	29				

Section D—Depreciation of Vehicles (Use this section only if you owned the vehicle and are completing Section C for the vehicle.)

			(a) Vehicle 1		**(b)** Vehicle 2	
30	Enter cost or other basis (see instructions)	30				
31	Enter section 179 deduction and special allowance (see instructions)	31				
32	Multiply line 30 by line 14 (see instructions if you claimed the section 179 deduction or special allowance)	32				
33	Enter depreciation method and percentage (see instructions)	33				
34	Multiply line 32 by the percentage on line 33 (see instructions)	34				
35	Add lines 31 and 34	35				
36	Enter the applicable limit explained in the line 36 instructions	36				
37	Multiply line 36 by the percentage on line 14	37				
38	Enter the **smaller** of line 35 or line 37. If you skipped lines 36 and 37, enter the amount from line 35. Also enter this amount on line 28 above	38				

Form **2106** (2008)

Florida—the cost of getting there—by properly scheduling business in Miami. In those situations where vacation time exceeds time spent on business, the taxpayer must be prepared to establish that the trip would not have been taken *but for* the business need.

When traveling, the taxpayer may also be able to deduct the expenses of a spouse if a business purpose for the spouse's presence can be established. Even where a spouse's travel expenses are clearly not deductible, only the *incremental* expense attributable to the spouse's presence is not allowed. When an automobile is used for transportation, there is no incremental expense. In the case of lodging, the single room rate would be fully deductible and only the few extra dollars added for a double room rate, if any, would not be deductible.

The importance of adequate records for travel and entertainment expenses cannot be over-emphasized. However, the *actual* cost of travel expenses need not be proved when a per diem or a fixed mileage allowance arrangement exists between the employee and the employer. In these situations, the other elements of the expense—time, place, and business purpose—must still be substantiated by the employer and employee. Moreover, the taxpayer must substantiate the cost of travel where the employee is "related" to the employer (an employee is considered related when he or she either owns more than 10 percent of a corporate employer's stock or is the employer's spouse, brother, sister, ancestor, or lineal descendant). Notwithstanding the relaxation of the substantiation requirements for travel costs, it is advisable to maintain receipts and other records to substantiate the other elements of the expenditure.

The taxpayer should get in the habit of contemporaneously recording the required elements for each expenditure. Although a bothersome task, this must be done to secure deductions for travel and entertainment expenses. *Each* element of each expenditure must be established.

With respect to vehicle expenses, the taxpayer cannot simply deduct the expenses and hope that he or she will never be asked to produce evidence supporting the deduction. Form 2106 (Part II, line 21) specifically asks whether the taxpayer has proper written evidence. Thus, failure to maintain such documentation would mean that the taxpayer could not answer this question in the affirmative, increasing the probability of audit. Of course, indicating that such evidence exists when it in fact does not could subject the taxpayer to negligence or fraud penalties.

PROBLEM MATERIALS

DISCUSSION QUESTIONS

8-1   *Requirements for Education Expenses.* J has been told that, as a practical matter, most education expenses are considered nondeductible personal expenses. Under what conditions. if any, may J deduct expenses for education?

8-2   *Education: Degrees, Promotion, and Employer Assistance.* Y is currently employed as the manager of a fast-food restaurant, earning $29,000. In order to improve her upward mobility in the company, Y decides that she should go to college and earn her degree.
   a.   Can Y deduct any of the cost of obtaining her bachelor's degree in business?
   b.   Same as above, except Y already has her bachelor's degree and now decides to take courses which could lead to her receiving an M.B.A.
   c.   What is the effect on Y if her employer pays for her education costs this year of $6,000? Answer for both a bachelor's degree and an M.B.A.

8-3   *Expenses of Education.* F, vice president of sales for a large corporation, is in the executive M.B.A. program at the University of Michigan. F lives in Chicago and travels to Ann Arbor and Detroit to take certain courses.

a. F's employer reimburses F for the tuition, which is $8,000 per year. Explain how F will treat the reimbursement and the expense. What if F was not reimbursed?
    Indicate whether the following expenses incurred by F would be deductible:
b. Meals and lodging when he stays overnight
c. Transportation costs from Chicago and back
d. Books
e. Secretarial fees for typing term projects
f. Copying expenses
g. Value of vacation time used to take classes
h. Tutor

8-4 *Qualifying Educational Expenses.* Indicate whether education expenses would be deductible in the following situations:
a. J is currently an elementary school teacher. State law requires beginning teachers to have a bachelor's degree and to complete a master's degree within five years after first being hired. This year he took two courses toward the master's degree.
b. R is a full-time engineering student and has a part-time job as an engineer with a firm that will employ him as an engineer when he graduates.
c. C is an airline pilot and is presently taking lessons to become a helicopter pilot.
d. H retired from the finance department of the Army and now is getting his M.B.A. He plans to get a job with a financial institution.

8-5 *Moving Expenses.* Address the following:
a. What two tests must be satisfied before moving expenses may be deducted?
b. What moving expenses are deductible?
c. Are moving expenses deductible *for* or *from* adjusted gross income?

8-6 *Moving Expenses: Real Estate Commissions.* B's employer transferred him during the year. As a result, B sold his home in North Dakota and moved to New York, where he lives in an apartment. He does not plan to move into a new home. B's real estate commissions were $6,000. B has asked how he should treat the real estate commissions.

8-7 *Home Office Expenses.* The enactment of the restrictive rules related to home office deductions caused many commentators to conclude that the home office deduction had been essentially eliminated. Which particular requirement(s) of § 280A prompted such a conclusion?

8-8 *Computing Car Expenses.* Briefly answer the following:
a. With respect to a business car, can the taxpayer claim depreciation in addition to the expense determined using the standard mileage rate?
b. Can a taxpayer switch to the automatic mileage method after using MACRS to compute depreciation? If so, when does the car become fully depreciated?

8-9 *Transportation vs. Travel.* Explain the distinction between transportation expenses and travel expenses.

8-10 *U.S. Travel vs. Foreign Travel.* Compare and contrast the rules governing travel in the United States to those rules governing travel outside of the United States.

8-11 *Limitations on Entertainment and Meals.* T is employed by KL Publishing Corporation. He is a sales representative with responsibility for college textbook sales in Alabama, Florida and Georgia. T lives in Atlanta. For each of the following situations, indicate whether T's or the corporation's deduction for entertainment or meals would be limited, and if so, how?
a. T flew to Birmingham on a Tuesday night. After checking in at the hotel, he caught a cab to his favorite restaurant where he ate by himself. The cost of the meal was

$20, including a $1 tax and a $3 tip. The cost of the cab ride was $10. The next day he called on a customer.

b. Same as (a), except that T's employer reimbursed him under an accountable plan for all of his costs.

c. Same as (a), but further assume that T's A.G.I. for the year was $30,000 and that he has other miscellaneous itemized deductions of $700.

d. At the year-end Christmas party for employees, the corporation gave T a 10-pound, honey-baked ham, costing $40. The cost of the party (excluding the ham), which was held at a local restaurant, was $300.

e. During the annual convention of college marketing professors in New Orleans, the corporation rented a room in the convention hotel for one night and provided hors d'oeuvres. The room cost $200 while the food and drink cost $1,000.

8-12 *Statutory Employees.* L was an education consultant for ALS. Her duties required her to visit schools, collect data and input the data into a software template provided by ALS. Upon completion, she e-mailed the information to ALS. Is she a statutory employee? Regardless of your answer, explain the benefits of being so classified.

8-13 *Entertainment Expenses.* Distinguish between entertainment expenses that are considered "directly related to" the taxpayer's business and those that are "associated with" the taxpayer's business.

8-14 *Business Meals.* Can the taxpayer deduct the cost of his or her own meal when he or she pays for the lunch of a customer and no business is discussed?

8-15 *Entertainment Facilities.* Under what circumstances are expenses related to an entertainment facility deductible?

8-16 *Substantiation of Travel and Entertainment Expenses.* What information must the taxpayer be prepared to present upon the audit of his or her travel and entertainment expenditures? Does the taxpayer need to maintain records if he or she has a per diem arrangement with the employer?

8-17 *Foreign Convention.* Dr. B recently learned that a world famous plastic surgeon will be making a presentation concerning her area of expertise at a convention of physicians in Switzerland. If B attends, can she deduct the costs of airfare, meals, lodging, and registration? Explain.

8-18 *Cruise Ship Seminars.* The American Organization of Dental Specialists is offering a seven-day seminar on gum disease aboard a cruise ship. Dr. D, a dentist. would like to attend. If D attends, can he deduct his expenses?

8-19 *Reporting Reimbursements.* R is regional sales manager for a large steel manufacturing corporation. His job requires him to travel extensively to call on customers and salespeople. As a result, he incurs substantial expenses for airfare, hotel, meals, and entertainment, for which he is reimbursed. Under what conditions may R simply ignore reporting the reimbursements and the expenses for tax purposes?

8-20 *Reporting Employee Business Expenses.* T is a salesperson for Classy Cosmetics Inc. During the year, she incurred various business expenses for which she was reimbursed under an accountable plan. Discuss the problems T encounters when reporting the reimbursements and expenses in the following situations, assuming an adequate accounting was made.

a. T was reimbursed $3,800 for expenses totaling $3,000.

b. T was on a per diem of $25 per day for lodging and $15 per day for meals. She received $2,000 under the per diem arrangement for expenses totaling $2,200.

8-21 *Per Diem Arrangement.* A1 was recently hired by a public accounting firm as a staff accountant. When A1 is out of town on business (e.g., staff training or an audit at a client's place of business), the firm gives him $12 a day for dinner. A1 normally spends $5 and banks the rest. What are the tax consequences?

8-22 *Substantiation Requirements.* Indicate whether each of the following is required in order to properly substantiate a deduction:
   a. Purpose of an entertainment expenditure
   b. Date of entertainment expenditure
   c. Receipt for business meal with client, which cost $15
   d. Receipt for lodging at Motel Cheap, which cost $12
   e. Description of what the taxpayer wore on the day he lunched with client
   f. Diary detailing information normally required for substantiation of entertainment expenses
   g. Canceled check for $12 for tickets to baseball game that was attended with customer
   h. Social security number of client entertained

YOU MAKE THE CALL

8-23 The unfortunate experience of Danville Plywood Corporation and its deduction for the Super Bowl trip described earlier in this chapter raises another issue. The corporation booked what clearly seemed to be entertainment expenses as advertising expenses, perhaps with the hope that the expense would be forever buried. Assume that you were the accountant on the job, noted this, and proposed a reclassification entry to the client who objected. What action should you take?

PROBLEMS

8-24 *Education Expenses.* Indicate the amount, if any, of deductible education expenses in each of the following cases. Comment briefly on your answer and state whether the deduction is deductible *for* or *from* adjusted gross income:
   a. C is employed as a plumber, but is training to become a computer programmer. During the year, he paid $500 for tuition and books related to a college course in programming.
   b. E is a licensed nurse. During the year, she spent $300 on courses to become a registered nurse.
   c. R paid a $75 fee to take the C.P.A. exam and $800 for a C.P.A. review course. R currently is employed by a public accounting firm.
   d. R is an IRS agent. This year, he began taking courses toward a law degree emphasizing tax. Tuition and books cost $1,000.
   e. H is a high school instructor teaching European history. On a one-year sabbatical leave from school, he traveled to Europe, taking slides which he planned on using in his classes. The trip cost $7,000, including $1,000 for meals.

8-25 *Moving Expenses.* In May of the current year. M found a new job, forcing him to move from Tulsa to Seattle. On June 1, the moving company picked up all of M's possessions. M and his family stayed in a hotel on June 1, left the morning of June 2, and arrived in Seattle on June 4. They incurred the following expenses.
   1. Airfare and meals for him and his wife while traveling to Seattle to look for a new house, $260 and $50 respectively. They failed to find a home. Consequently, they moved into an apartment, from which they continued their search.
   2. Lodging in Tulsa on the day they moved out of their house, $70.
   3. Expenses on the way to Seattle included meals, $80, and lodging, $100.
   4. Mileage to Seattle, 2,000 miles.
   5. Car repair on trip to Seattle, $175.
   6. Moving van, $4,000.

7. Storage charges for furniture that would not fit in the apartment: $3 per day for the period June 5–July 31.
8. Temporary living expenses for period June 5–July 31: apartment, $10 per day; meals, $20 per day; and cleaning and laundry, $25.
9. Realtor's commission on sale of old home. $1,000.

Compute M's moving expense deduction (Form 3903 may be helpful).

8-26 *Home Office.* In each of the following independent situations, indicate whether the taxpayer is entitled to deduct expenses related to the home office:
  a. C, a dermatologist employed by a hospital, also owns several rental properties. He regularly uses a bedroom in his home solely as an office for bookkeeping and other activities related to management of the rental properties.
  b. R, an attorney employed by a large law firm, frequently brings work home from the office. She uses a study in her home for doing this work as well as paying bills, sorting coupons and conducting other personal activities.
  c. M is a research associate employed by the Cancer Research Institute. His duties include designing and carrying out experiments, reviewing data, and writing articles and grant proposals. His employer furnishes M a laboratory but due to insufficient space cannot provide an office for him. Thus, for about three hours each day, M uses a portion of his bedroom (where he and his wife sleep) to do the writing, reviewing, and other related activities.
  d. T is a self-employed tax consultant. He has an office downtown and a home office. He occasionally meets with his clients in the home office since it is often more convenient for the clients to meet there.
  e. S, an artist, converted a detached garage to a studio for painting. She sells her paintings at her own gallery located in town.
  f. D has four toddlers. Since her home is virtually a nursery already, she decided to turn her family room into a daycare center.

8-27 *Home Office.* R is considering purchasing a home priced somewhat over her budget. Her brother has suggested that converting a room to a home office would enable her to deduct a substantial part of the costs related to the home, thus making the purchase feasible. R is a sales manager for X Corporation, which transfers its middle management employees frequently.
  Comment on the following advice given to R by her brother:
  a. Establishing a home office is an effective method for reducing the costs of home ownership by the amount of the tax benefits received.
  b. There are no disincentives for claiming the home office deduction.

8-28 *Home Office Computations.* T is employed as a law professor at State University. Outside of her university work she teaches continuing education courses for attorneys and occasionally provides legal services. T does all her work for these outside pursuits in her home office. Income and expenses relating to these were

Income:	
Fees for services	$2,000
Expenses:	
Depreciation on home office furniture and computer	400
Miscellaneous supplies, books, etc	500
Expenses attributable to home office:	
Depreciation	500
Insurance and utilities	700
Taxes	300
Interest	700

Determine the tax consequences resulting from T's part-time activities.

8-29 *Deductible Moving Expenses.* Indicate whether the following expenses qualify as deductible moving expenses:
   a. Costs of meals and lodging while en route to new location.
   b. Insurance on household and personal effects being transported—an option provided by the moving company.
   c. Costs of driving the family car to new location.
   d. Costs of storing items that would not fit in apartment at the new location; the apartment served as a temporary residence until a home was purchased.
   e. Costs of new carpeting and wallpaper to prepare old home to be sold.
   f. Real estate commission on sale of former residence.
   g. Loss on sale of residence.
   h. Payment of six months' rent to settle lease obligation at old location; the lease had six more months to run.
   i. Cost of appraisal of new home required as part of loan application.

8-30 *Moving Expenses: Time Test.* On September 1, 2009, L left her former employment in Indianapolis to seek her fortune in Cincinnati. Indicate whether L could deduct the cost of her moving expenses to Cincinnati under the following conditions.
   a. L found a teaching job with the public school system for which she worked ten months, September through June. After school was out, L took a three-month vacation. She then decided to leave Cincinnati and move to Atlanta.
   b. Same as (a) except L found a job as a substitute teacher and was considered self-employed.
   c. L moved to take a new position as product manager with P&G Corporation. After working three months, she and her new employer had a falling out over what she considered unethical advertising. She quit her job and moved to New York.

8-31 *Moving Expenses: Distance Test.* P is an accountant for L Corporation. This year, his employer moved from its downtown Manhattan location to a new office in New Jersey. As a result, P decided to move to be closer to the office.
   a. Assuming P did not change jobs, is he allowed to deduct any moving expenses?
   b. Regardless of your answer to (a), indicate whether P satisfies the distance test in light of the following information:
      – Old office building to new building: 60 miles
      – Old home to new home: 65 miles
      – New home to old office: 51 miles
      – Old home to old office: 30 miles
      – New home to new office: 15 miles
      – Old home to new office: 58 miles

8-32 *Standard Mileage Rate.* R, self-employed, leases her car. She elects to compute her deduction for car expenses using the standard mileage rate. Indicate whether the following expenses may be deducted in addition to expenses computed using the standard rate:
   a. Depreciation
   b. Interest on car loan
   c. Insurance
   d. Parking while calling on customers
   e. Parking tickets incurred while on business
   f. Major overhaul
   g. Personal property taxes on car
   h. Tolls

8-33 *Transportation Expenses.* Indicate the amount, if any, deductible by the taxpayer in each of the following cases. (Ignore the floor on miscellaneous itemized deductions.)

a. R works in downtown Denver, but chooses to live in the mountains 90 miles away. During the year, he spent $2,700 for transportation expenses to and from work.

b. Q, a high school basketball coach, liked to scout his opposition. On one Friday afternoon, he left school and drove 40 miles to attend the game of the team he played next. On the way, he stopped for a meal ($5). He watched the game and returned home.

c. R, a carpenter, commutes to work in a truck. He drives the truck in order to carry the tools of his trade. During the year, R's total transportation costs were $5,000. R estimates that his costs of transportation without the tools would have been $4,000, since he otherwise would have taken public transportation.

d. G, an attorney, works downtown. She is on retainer, however, with a client who has offices two miles from her home. G often stops at the client's office before going to work. The distance between these locations is as follows: home to office, 20 miles; home to client, 2 miles; and client to office, 22 miles. During the year, G drove directly to work 180 days and via the client's office 50 days.

8-34 *Transportation to Temporary Assignments.* For each of the following cases, indicate the number of business miles driven by the taxpayer. (Ignore the floor on miscellaneous itemized deductions.)

a. K is employed as a salesperson for Midwest Surgical Supply Company. The company's offices are in downtown Chicago. K's sales territory is the northwest side of Chicago and the adjacent suburbs. During Monday through Thursday, K drives directly from her residence to call on various customers. She sees each customer about once a month. On Friday of each week, she goes directly from her home to her office downtown to turn in orders, attend the weekly sales meeting, and do any other miscellaneous work. A portion of K's trip diary appears below.

		Odometer Reading		
Date	Destination	Begin	End	Mileage
3-17	Springmill Clinic	470	482	12
	Dr. J	482	485	3
	Home	485	500	15
3-18	Office	500	530	30
	Home	530	560	30

b. F, an electrician, works for EZ Electrical. He lives and works in the Los Angeles area. For 200 days of this year, he was assigned to do the wiring on a 30-story office building in downtown Los Angeles. His mileage from his home to the building was 20 miles. For 50 days during the year, he was assigned to a job in San Diego. Most of F's assignments are 20 miles closer than San Diego. F commuted 70 miles from his home to San Diego.

8-35 *Travel Expenses.* Indicate the amount, if any, deductible by the taxpayer in each of the following situations. (Ignore the floor on miscellaneous itemized deductions.)

a. P, a steelworker, obtained a job with XYZ Corporation to work on a nuclear reactor 200 miles from his residence. P drove to the site early on Monday mornings and returned home late Friday nights. While at the job site he stayed in a boarding house. P anticipates that the job will last for eight months. During the year, he traveled 4,000 miles in going to and from the job. Other expenses while away from home included the following: meals, $1,000; lodging, $900; and laundry, $75.

b. Same as (a), except P anticipates the job to last for more than a year.

c. W plays professional football for the Minnesota Vikings. He has an apartment in St. Paul but he and his wife's permanent personal residence is in Tucson. During the season, W usually stays in St. Paul. In the off-season he returns to Tucson. Expenses for the year include travel between St. Paul and Tucson, $2,000; apartment in St. Paul, $1,800; meals while in St. Paul, $900.

d. R took a trip to New York primarily for business. R's husband accompanied her. She spent two weeks on business and one week sight-seeing in the city. Her train fare was $400 and meals and lodging cost $30 and $50 per day, respectively. R's husband incurred similar expenses.

e. L flew from Cincinnati to Chicago for $300 round-trip. She spent one day on business and four days shopping and sight-seeing. Her meals and lodging cost $30 and $50 per day, respectively.

8-36 *Car Expense Computation.* E, a salesperson for T Corporation, incurred the following expenses for transportation during the year:

Gas and oil	$ 1,200
Repairs	200
Insurance	700
Interest on car loan	400
Depreciation	2,000
License	100

In addition, he spent $70 on parking while calling on customers. E drove the car 20,000 miles during the year, 18,000 for business.

a. Compute E's deduction, assuming the standard mileage rate is elected.

b. Compute E's deduction, assuming he claims actual expenses.

8-37 *Travel Outside of the United States.* S, an executive for an automotive company, traveled to Paris this year for business meetings with a European subsidiary. Prior to the trip, she thought that the meetings presented an ideal opportunity for her to vacation in Paris as well as to conduct business. For this reason, she scheduled the trip. S's airfare to Paris was $1,000 and her daily meals and lodging were $30 and $50 respectively. Given the additional facts below, indicate the amount, if any, of the deduction that S may claim.

a. S's trip was primarily business. She spent two days on business (including travel days) and four days sight-seeing.

b. Her itinerary revealed the following:

Thursday May 1:	Depart New York, arrive Paris
Friday, May 2:	Business 9–11 a.m.; remainder of day sight-seeing in Paris
Saturday and Sunday, May 3–4:	Tour French countryside
Monday and Tuesday, May 5–6:	Business 9–5
Wednesday–Sunday, May 7–11:	Tour Germany
Monday, May 12:	Business 9–5
Tuesday, May 13:	Depart Paris, arrive New York

c. Same as (a) except the travel was to Paris for the International Car Exposition, a foreign convention.

d. Same as (a) except the business meetings took place on a luxury liner cruising the Caribbean.

e. Same as (a) except S had no control over arranging the trip.

f. Same as (a) except the trip was primarily personal.

8-38   *Entertainment Expenses.* R is president of X Corporation, a company that manufactures and distributes office supplies. During the year, he and the company incurred various expenses relating to entertainment. In each of the following situations, indicate the amount of the deduction for entertainment expenses. Briefly explain your answer and classify the deduction as either *for* or *from* adjusted gross income. (Assume all the substantiation requirements are satisfied.)

   a.   R and his wife took a potential customer and his wife to a night club to hear a popular singer. Tickets for the event cost $10 each. R was unable to discuss any business during the evening.

   b.   After agreeing in the afternoon to supply S's company with typing paper, R took S to a baseball game that evening. Tickets were $8 each. X Corporation reimbursed R $16 for the tickets under an accountable plan.

   c.   R and S, a client, went to lunch at an expensive restaurant. R paid the bill for both his meal, $30, and S's meal, $40. No business was discussed during lunch.

   d.   X Corporation purchased a vacation condominium for use primarily by its employees. Expenses relating to the condominium, including depreciation, maintenance, utilities, interest, and taxes, were $7,000.

   e.   R joined an exclusive country club this year. The membership fee, which is not refundable, was $1,000. In addition, R paid annual dues of $3,600. During the year, R used the club 100 days, 70 days for entertainment directly related to business and 30 days for personal use.

   f.   R gave one of the company's best customers a $100 bottle of wine.

   g.   X Corporation gave one of its retailers 1,000 golf balls ($1 each) to distribute for promotional purposes. X Corporation's name was imprinted on the balls.

8-39   *Convention and Seminar Expenses.* Dr. F, a pediatrician, is employed at a hospital located in Chicago. He also operates his own practice. During the year, he attended the following seminars and conventions. In each case, he incurred expenses for registration, travel, meals, and lodging. Indicate whether such expenses would be deductible assuming he attended.

   a.   "The Care and Feeding of Newborns," a seminar in Honolulu sponsored by the American Family Medical Association.

   b.   While Dr. F was attending the meeting above, his wife attended a concurrent seminar entitled "Tax Planning for Physicians and their Spouses."

   c.   "The Economics of a Private Practice: Make Your Investment Count," sponsored by the American Management Corporation in Chicago.

   d.   "Investing and Inside Information," sponsored by the National Association of Investment Specialists in Orlando.

CUMULATIVE PROBLEM

TaxCut   **8-40**   George (445-42-5432) and Christina Campbell (993-43-9878) are married with two children, Victoria, 7, and Brad, 2. Victoria and Brad's social security numbers are 446-75-4389 and 449-63-4172, respectively. They live at 10137 Briar Creek Lane, Tulsa, OK 74105. George is the district sales representative for Red Duck, a manufacturer of sportswear. His principal job is to solicit orders of the company's products from department stores in his territory, which includes Oklahoma and Arkansas. The company provides no office for him. Christina is a maker of fine quilts which she sells in selected shops in the surrounding area. The couple uses the cash method of accounting and reports on the calendar year. Their records for the year reveal the following information:

1. George received a salary of $65,000 and a bonus of $5,000. His employer withheld Federal income taxes of $5,000 and the proper amount of FICA taxes.

2. Christina's income and expenses of her quilting business, Crazy Quilts, include

Quilt sales	$7,000
Costs of goods sold	600
Telephone (long-distance calls)	100

Christina makes all of the quilts at home in a separate room that is used exclusively for her work. This room represents 10 percent of the total square footage of their home. Expenses related to operating the entire home include utilities, $2,000; and insurance, $500. Depreciation attributable solely to the home office is $800. Christina computes her deduction relating to use of her car using actual expenses, which included gas and oil, $900; insurance, $300; and repairs, $100. The car is fully depreciated. Her daily diary revealed that, for the year, she had driven the car a total of 20,000 miles, including the following trips:

Trip Description	Miles
Home to sales outlets and return	10,000
Between sales outlets	2,000
Miscellaneous personal trips	8,000

3. George incurs substantial expenses for travel and entertainment, including meals and lodging. He is not reimbursed for these expenses. This is the second year that George has used the standard mileage rate for computing his automobile expenses. During the year he drove 50,000 miles; 40,000 of these were directly related to business. Expenses for parking and tolls directly related to business were $90. Total meal and lodging costs for days that he was out of town overnight were $600 and $1,200, respectively. Entertainment expenses were $400.

4. This is George's second marriage. He has one child, Ted (age 11), from his first marriage to Hazel, who has custody of the child. He provides more than 50 percent of the child's support. The 2003 divorce agreement between George and Hazel provides that George is entitled to the exemption for Ted. George paid Hazel $4,800 during the year, $1,600 as alimony and the remainder as child support. Ted's Social Security number is 122-23-3221.

5. The couple's other income and expenses included the following:

Dividends (IBM stock owned separately by George)	$ 400
Interest on redeemed Treasury bills	700
Interest on City of Reno bonds	566
Interest paid on home mortgage	10,000
Real property taxes on home	900
Safety deposit box fee	50

6. Both taxpayers elect to give to the Presidential campaign fund.

Compute the couple's tax liability for the year. If forms are used, complete Form 1040 for the year, including Schedules A, B, C, SE, and Form 2106.

RESEARCH PROBLEMS

8-41   *Travel Away from Home.* M is a traveling salesperson who lives with his family in Cincinnati. His sales territory consists of Indiana, Illinois, and Kentucky. Most of his business, however, is in the Louisville area. For this reason, he normally travels to Louisville weekly and spends three or four days there living in a hotel. He also spends considerable time traveling throughout his territory. M completes the paperwork and other tasks incidental to his work at his home in Cincinnati. M's wife has a good job in Cincinnati and consequently M has never considered moving to Louisville. May M deduct the costs of traveling between his residence in Cincinnati and Louisville (including the costs of meals and lodging while in Louisville)?

8-42   *Business Gifts.* R is product manager for a large pharmaceutical company. At the annual Christmas party, he handed out $50 gifts (checks from his personal account) to each of the 10 employees that work in his division under his supervision. R's group had been highly successful during the year and he felt that each person contributed to the division's profitability. He also gave his secretary $100. What amount, if any, may R deduct?

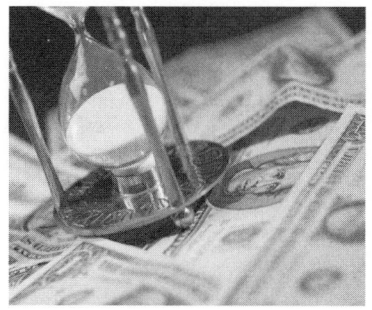

★ CHAPTER NINE ★

CAPITAL RECOVERY: DEPRECIATION, AMORTIZATION, AND DEPLETION

LEARNING OBJECTIVES

Upon completion of this chapter you will be able to:

- Identify the various depreciation methods and accounting conventions available under the Modified Accelerated Cost Recovery System (MACRS)

- Make recommendations concerning the selection of an appropriate depreciation method and accounting convention

- Compute a taxpayer's depreciation deduction under each of the various depreciation methods and accounting conventions

- Explain the depreciation rules for listed property

- Identify property eligible for the election to currently expense rather than depreciate its cost

- Determine the current depletion deduction for various assets

- Explain the options available in selecting the appropriate tax treatment of research and experimentation expenditures

- Recognize tax planning opportunities related to depreciation, amortization, and depletion deductions

CHAPTER OUTLINE

The concept of capital recovery originated with the basic premise that income does not result until revenues exceed the capital expended to produce such revenues. For example, consider the situation where a taxpayer purchases an asset at a cost of $1,000 and subsequently sells it. Generally, the sale produces no income unless the asset is sold for a price exceeding $1,000. This result derives from the principle that the taxpayer first must *recover* his or her $1,000 of capital invested (basis) before he or she can be considered as having income. Here, the recovery occurs as the taxpayer offsets the basis of the asset against the amount realized on the sale. This same principle operates when an asset, instead of being sold and providing a readily identifiable benefit, provides benefits indirectly (e.g., a machine used for many years as part of a process to manufacture a product). In this case, the cost of the asset or the capital invested is *recovered* by offsetting (deducting) the asset's cost against the revenues the asset helps to produce. Thus, in the absence of a sale or other disposition of an asset, capital recovery usually occurs when the taxpayer is permitted to deduct the expenditure. Certain capital expenditures such as research and experimental costs are recovered in the year of the expenditure since the tax law allows immediate deduction. For other types of capital expenditures, the taxpayer is allowed to deduct or recover the cost over the years for which the asset provides benefits.

This chapter examines the various cost allocation methods allowed by the Code. These are depreciation, amortization, and depletion. Although each of these methods relates to a process of allocating the cost of an asset over time, different terms for the same process are used because each method relates to a different type of property. Depreciation concerns *tangible property*, amortization concerns *intangible property*,

and depletion concerns *natural resources.* Tangible property means any property having physical existence (i.e., property capable of being touched such as plant, property, and equipment). Conversely, intangible property has no physical existence but exists only in connection with something else, such as the goodwill of a business, stock, patents, and copyrights. There are two types of tangible property: real property and personal property. Real property (or *realty*) is land and anything attached to the land such as buildings, curbs, streets, fences, and other improvements. Personal property is property that is not realty and is usually movable. The concept of personal property or *personalty* should be distinguished from property that a person owns and uses for his or her benefit—usually referred to as *personal-use* property.

In addition to the cost recovery methods mentioned above, this chapter discusses the tax treatment of other capital expenditures such as those for research and experimentation, and certain expenses of farmers.

DEPRECIATION AND AMORTIZATION FOR TAX PURPOSES

GENERAL RULES FOR DEPRECIATION DEDUCTIONS

The Code allows as a depreciation deduction a reasonable allowance for the exhaustion, wear and tear, and obsolescence of property that is either used in a trade or business or held for the production of income.[1] This rule makes it clear that not all capital expenditures for property are automatically eligible for depreciation. Rather, like all other expenditures, only those that satisfy the initial hurdles can be deducted.

Exhaustion, Wear and Tear, and Obsolescence. Only property that wears out or becomes obsolete can be depreciated. As normally construed, this requirement means that depreciation is allowed only for property that has a *determinable life.*[2] Property such as land that does not wear out and that has no determinable life cannot be depreciated. Similarly, works of art cannot be amortized or depreciated since they normally have an indefinite life. In contrast, intangible assets with definite lives, such as patents, copyrights, and licenses that cover a fixed term, can be amortized.

Business or Income-Producing Property. Like other expenses, no deduction is allowed for depreciation unless the property is used in a trade or business or an income-producing activity. Property used for personal purposes cannot be depreciated. In many instances, however, a single asset may be used for *both* personal purposes and profit-seeking activities. In these cases, the taxpayer is permitted to deduct depreciation on the portion of the asset used for business or production of income.

Example 1. N is a salesperson who uses his car for both business and personal purposes. He purchased the car this year for $18,000. During the year, N drove the car 50,000 miles: 40,000 miles for business and 10,000 miles for personal purposes. Under these circumstances, 80% (40,000 ÷ 50,000) of the cost of the car is subject to depreciation in the current year. Note that the business-use percentage may vary from year to year. If so, the depreciation allowed each year will vary accordingly.

Property held for the production of income, even though not currently producing income, may still be depreciated. For example, a duplex held out for rental that is temporarily vacant may still be depreciated for the period during which it is not rented.

---

[1]   § 167(a).

[2]   Reg. §§ 1.167(a)-2 and 1.167(a)-3.

Similarly, if the taxpayer's trade or business is suspended temporarily, rather than indefinitely, depreciation can be continued despite the suspension of activity.

Depreciable Basis. The basis for depreciation is the adjusted basis of the property as used for computing gain or loss on a sale or other disposition.[3] This is usually the property's cost. Where property used for personal purposes *is converted* to use in business or the production of income, the basis for depreciation purposes is the lesser of the fair market value or the adjusted basis at the time of conversion.[4] This ensures that no deduction is claimed for declines in value while the property was held for personal purposes.

Example 2. R purchased a home computer for $1,000 while attending college. He used it solely for personal purposes. After graduation, R went into the consulting business and began using the computer for business purposes. At the time he converted the computer to business use, its value was $400. R may compute depreciation using a basis of $400 (the lesser of the adjusted basis, $1,000, or its value, $400, at the time of conversion).

Commencement of Depreciation. The date on which depreciation begins can be quite important. Depreciation may not begin until an asset is *placed in service*. This is not necessarily the time when the asset is purchased. According to the Regulations, an asset is placed in service when it is in a "state of readiness and availability for the assigned function" of the activity.[5] For those assets acquired for a new business, the depreciation period starts when the business begins.

Example 3. In 1981, William and Lois Walsh[6] leased a building and immediately began making substantial repairs and improvements to prepare it to open as a restaurant. Although the restaurant did not open until 1982, the couple claimed depreciation deductions in 1981 that were denied by the IRS. At trial, the taxpayers asserted that their restaurant business began in 1981 when they acquired assets for use in the restaurant and executed a lease for the premises. Although the taxpayers purchased the assets in 1981, the court denied the taxpayers' 1981 depreciation deductions. According to the court, the restaurant had not yet begun to function as a going concern and to perform those activities for which it was organized. For this reason, the assets had not been placed in service until the restaurant opened in 1982.

HISTORICAL PERSPECTIVE

Prior to 1981, taxpayers could compute depreciation using either of two approaches: (1) the facts-and-circumstances method or (2) the Class Life System. Depreciation methods such as straight-line, declining balance, and sum-of-the-years'-digits were available for most assets under each system. The facts-and-circumstances method enabled taxpayers to choose useful life and salvage value estimates for depreciable assets based on their experience and judgment of all surrounding facts and circumstances. There were no predetermined or prescribed guidelines. Conflicts often arose between taxpayers and the IRS over useful life selections because taxpayers were motivated to employ short useful lives in order to maximize the present value of tax savings from depreciation deductions.

---

[3]   § 167(g).

[4]   Reg. § 1.167(g)-1.

[5]   Reg. §§ 1.46-3(d)(1) and § 1.167(a)-11(e)(1)(i).

[6]   William J. Walsh, TC Memo 1988-242.

As an alternative to the facts-and-circumstances system, the Class Life System became part of the law in 1971. It was developed primarily to minimize IRS-taxpayer conflicts over useful life estimates. The system prescribed depreciable life ranges for numerous categories of assets. For example, office furniture and fixtures could be depreciated using lives from 8 years to 12 years under the Class Life System.[7] Taxpayers electing this system were not challenged by the IRS. However, IRS-taxpayer conflicts were not eliminated because many taxpayers continued to employ the facts-and-circumstances system, seeking depreciable lives that were shorter than those available with the Class Life System.

In 1981, the facts-and-circumstances system and Class Life System were all but eliminated for assets placed in service after 1980. In the Economic Recovery Tax Act of 1981 (ERTA), Congress substantially revised the method for computing depreciation by enacting Code § 168 and the Accelerated Cost Recovery System (ACRS). Altered several times since 1981, the current version of this system is known as the Modified Accelerated Cost Recovery System (MACRS). An alternative to MACRS, called the Alternative Depreciation System (ADS), is also available.

A major benefit of MACRS and ADS is the elimination of previous areas of dispute between taxpayers and the IRS. Under these systems, the taxpayer is required to choose from a small set of predetermined options regarding depreciable life and depreciation method. Salvage value is ignored in all cases. Thus, depreciation calculations are more uniform for all taxpayers.

It should be emphasized, however, that some assets may not be depreciated using either of these systems. For this reason, the facts-and-circumstances approach and the Class Life System have continuing validity in certain instances.

MODIFIED ACCELERATED COST RECOVERY SYSTEM

AN OVERVIEW OF MACRS

Once it is determined that property is eligible for depreciation, the amount of the depreciation deduction must be computed. Under current law, taxpayers are required to calculate depreciation for most property using the Modified Accelerated Cost Recovery System (MACRS) or what is sometimes referred to as the General Depreciation System or GDS. As suggested earlier, MACRS is a radical departure from traditional approaches to depreciation. Under MACRS, useful lives for assets are termed *recovery periods* and are prescribed by statute. Regardless of the effects of nature and outside forces, each asset is deemed to have a particular useful life of 3, 5, 7, 10, 15, 20, 27.5, or 39 years. In addition, salvage value is ignored under MACRS. By assuming there is no salvage value, taxpayers can depreciate the basis of each asset to zero. With these rules, possibilities for abuse using unrealistic values for useful life and salvage value are essentially eliminated. Finally, certain assumptions—so-called *accounting conventions*—exist regarding about how much depreciation is allowed for the year of acquisition and disposition (e.g., a half-year or something more or less).

The basic machinery of MACRS that is used to compute depreciation can be summarized as follows:

   1. The system establishes eight classes or categories of property (e.g., three-year property).

---

[7]   Rev. Proc. 77-10, 1977-1 C.B. 548.

2. For each class of property, a specific useful life and depreciation method are prescribed (e.g., for three-year property the useful life is three years and either the 200 percent declining-balance or straight-line method must be used).

To actually compute depreciation, taxpayers must first determine when the asset is placed in service, whether the property is subject to MACRS, then—based on the property's classification—determine the applicable method, recovery period, and accounting convention. These elements of the depreciation calculation are discussed below.

PROPERTY SUBJECT TO MACRS

Taxpayers generally must use MACRS to compute depreciation for all *tangible* property, both real and personal, new or used.[8] MACRS is not used to amortize *intangible* assets such as patents or copyrights, which are amortized using the straight-line method. In addition, MACRS may not be used with respect to the following property:[9]

1. Property depreciated using a method that is not based on years (e.g., the units-of production or income forecast methods)

2. Automobiles if the taxpayer has elected to use the standard mileage rate (such an election precludes a depreciation deduction)

3. Property for which special amortization is provided and elected by the taxpayer in lieu of depreciation (e.g., amortization of pollution control facilities)

4. Certain motion picture films, video tapes, sound recordings, and public utility property

5. Generally, any property that the taxpayer—or a party related to the taxpayer— owned or used (e.g., leased) prior to 1987

As a practical matter, MACRS is mandatory for all tangible property. But as explained below, the taxpayer has several alternatives under MACRS, including the option to elect out entirely and use the Alternative Depreciation System. In addition, in lieu of depreciation, the taxpayer may be allowed to expense up to $250,000 (2009) annually of certain assets placed in service during the year. Observe, however, that there are no elections available enabling the taxpayer to use the facts-and-circumstances method typically used for financial accounting purposes. Exhibit 9-1 identifies the depreciation methods and accounting conventions available under the MACRS and ADS systems.

---

[8] § 168(a).

[9] § 168(f).

EXHIBIT 9-1

Depreciation Methods and Accounting Conventions Under MACRS and ADS

8 MACRS Property Classes	Modified Accelerated Cost Recovery System (MACRS): Use MACRS Property Class Life	Alternative Depreciation System (ADS): Use ADS Life	Accounting Convention[1]
3-year, 5-year, 7-year, 10-year[2]	Choices: 200% DB, 150% DB, or SL[3]	SL	Half-year or mid-quarter
15-year, 20-year	Choices: 150% DB or SL	Choices: 150% DB or SL	Half-year or mid-quarter
Residential rental real estate	27.5 years SL	40 years SL	Mid-month
Nonresidential real estate	39 years SL	40 years SL	Mid-month

Notes:

(1) Taxpayers do *not* have the option of choosing either the half-year or mid-quarter convention. As explained later in this chapter, either the half-year or mid-quarter convention is *required* depending on the timing of asset purchases during the year.

(2) Under certain conditions, $250,000 (2009) immediate expensing under Code § 179 is available for most 3-, 5-, 7-, and 10-year assets (i.e., depreciable tangible personal property).

(3) Abbreviations:
DB = declining balance
SL = straight-line

CLASSES OF PROPERTY

As indicated in Exhibit 9-1, all property subject to MACRS is assigned to one of eight classes.[10] Classification is important because the recovery periods, methods, and accounting conventions to be used in calculating depreciation can vary among the different classes of property. Property is assigned to a particular class based on its *class life* as prescribed in Revenue Procedure 87-56.[11] This Revenue Procedure, an excerpt of which is provided in Exhibit 9-2, specifies not only the class lives of various assets but also the recovery periods to be used for both MACRS and ADS. Note that the "General Depreciation System" column of Exhibit 9-2 pertains to MACRS. Exhibit 9-3 provides examples of property in each of the eight MACRS property classes.

In examining Exhibit 9-2, it is important to emphasize that many classes of assets and their descriptions are omitted. Only by examining Revenue Procedure 87-56 can one truly appreciate its scope. Nevertheless, it is impossible to identify the useful life of every asset. For this reason, as can be seen in Exhibit 9-2, Revenue Procedure 87-56 divides assets into two major categories: *Specific Depreciable Assets Being Used in All Business Activities* (such as computers and automobiles) and *Depreciable Assets Used in the Following Activities*. Thus if a particular asset is not assigned a recovery period—a common occurrence, its life is determined by the activity in which it is used.

---

[10] § 168(e).

[11] 1987-2 C.B. 674, as modified by Rev. Proc. 88-22, 1988-1 C.B. 785. For class lives, see *How to Depreciate Property*, IRS Publication 916, (Rev. 2006) p. 101.

EXHIBIT 9-2

Excerpt from Revenue Procedure 87-56

Asset Class	Description of Assets Included	Class Life (in years)	Recovery Periods (in years)	
			General Depreciation System	Alternative Depreciation System
SPECIFIC DEPRECIABLE ASSETS USED IN ALL BUSINESS ACTIVITIES, EXCEPT AS NOTED:				
00.11	**Office Furniture, Fixtures, and Equipment:** Includes furniture and fixtures that are not structural components of a building. Includes such assets as desks, files, safes, and communications equipment. Does not include communications equipment that is included in other classes	10	7	10
00.12	**Information Systems:** Includes computers and their peripheral equipment	6	5	5
00.13	**Data Handling Equipment, except Computers:** Includes only typewriters, calculators, adding and accounting machines, copiers, and duplicating equipment	6	5	6
00.21	**Airplanes (airframes and engines), except Those Used in Commercial or Contract Carrying of Passengers or Freight, and All Helicopters (Airframes and Engines)**	6	5	6
00.22	**Automobiles, Taxis**	3	5	5
00.23	**Buses**	9	5	9
00.241	**Light General Purpose Trucks:** Includes trucks for use over the road (actual unloaded weight less than 13,000 pounds)	4	5	5
00.242	**Heavy General Purpose Trucks:** Includes heavy general purpose trucks, concrete ready mix trucks, and ore trucks, for use over the road (actual unloaded weight 13,000 pounds or more)	6	5	6

EXHIBIT 9-2

Excerpt from Revenue Procedure 87-56 (continued)

Asset Class	Description of Assets Included	Class Life (in years)	Recovery Periods (in years) General Depreciation System	Alternative Depreciation System
	DEPRECIABLE ASSETS USED IN THE FOLLOWING ACTIVITIES:			
01.1	**Agriculture:** Includes machinery and equipment, grain bins, and fences but no other land improvements, that are used in the production of crops or plants, vines, and trees; livestock; the operation of farm dairies, nurseries, greenhouses, sod farms, mushroom cellars, cranberry bogs, apiaries, and fur farms; the performance of agriculture, animal husbandry, and horticultural services .	10	7	10
01.11	**Cotton Ginning Assets**	12	7	12
01.21	**Cattle, Breeding or Dairy**	7	5	7
01.4	**Single-Purpose Agricultural or Horticultural Structures**	15	10	15
15.0	**Construction** Includes assets used in construction by general building, special trade, heavy and marine construction contractors, operative and investment builders, real estate subdividers and developers, and others except railroads	6	5	6
20.1	**Manufacture of Grain and Grain Mill**	17	10	17
27.0	**Printing, Publishing, and Allied Industries**	11	7	11
36.0	**Manufacture of Electronic Components, Products, and Systems**	6	5	6
37.11	**Manufacture of Motor Vehicles**	12	7	12
39.0	**Manufacture of Athletic, Jewelry and Other Goods:** Includes assets used in the production of jewelry; musical instruments; toys and sporting goods; motion picture and television films and tapes; pens, pencils, office and art supplies, brooms, brushes, caskets, etc.	12	7	12
45.0	**Air Transport**	12	7	12
48.2	**Radio and Television Broadcastings:** Includes assets used in radio and television broadcasting, except transmitting towers	6	5	6
48.42	**CATV-Subscriber Connection and Distribution Systems**	10	7	10
79.0	**Recreation** . . . . Includes assets used in the provision of entertainment services on payment of a fee or admission charge, as in the operation of bowling alleys, billiard and pool establishments, theaters, concert halls, and miniature golf courses. Does not include amusement and theme parks and assets which consist primarily of specialized land improvements or structures, such as golf courses, sports stadia, race tracks, ski slopes, and buildings which house the assets used in entertainment services	10 10	7 7	10 10
80.0	**Theme and Amusement Parks**	12.5	7	12

Example 4. FunSpot Inc. operates a chain of bowling alleys all over New Jersey. During the year, it purchased furniture, computers, automatic pin-setters, bowling balls and shoes. In determining the recovery period of these assets, the only assets to which a specific life has been assigned are the furniture (Asset Class .11, 7 years) and the computers (Asset Class .12, 5 years). The life of the pin-setters, bowling balls and shoes would be determined based on the activity in which they are used, (Asset Class 80.0, 7 years).

CALCULATING DEPRECIATION

Under MACRS, depreciation is a function of *three* factors: the recovery period, the method, and the accounting convention.

Recovery Periods. As seen in Exhibit 9-1, recovery periods run various lengths of time depending on the class of property.[12] In examining the different classes, several features should be observed. First, certain property is assigned to a class without regard to its class life. The most notable example of this is cars, which are assigned to the five-year class (see asset class 00.22 in Exhibit 9-2). Note also that the current structure provides different recovery periods for real property, depending on whether it is residential (27.5 years) or nonresidential (39 years) real estate. As a result, when a building is used for both residential and nonresidential purposes (e.g., a multilevel apartment building with commercial space on the bottom two floors) it must be classified as one or the other. For this purpose, realty qualifies as residential real estate if 80 percent of the gross rents are for the dwelling units.[13]

EXHIBIT 9-3

Examples of MACRS Property

MACRS Property Class	Examples
3 years	Special tools, race horses, tractors, and property with a class life of 4 years or less
5 years	Automobiles, trucks, computers and peripheral equipment (such as printers, external disk drives, and modems), typewriters, copiers, R&E equipment, and property with a class life of more than 4 years and less than 10 years
7 years	Office furniture, fixtures, office equipment, most machinery, property with a class life of 10 years or more but less than 16 years, and property with no assigned class life
10 years	Single-purpose agricultural and horticultural structures, assets used in petroleum refining and manufacturing of tobacco and certain food products, and property with a class life of 16 years or more but less than 20 years
15 years	Land improvements (such as sidewalks, roads, parking lots, irrigation systems, sewers, fences, and landscaping), service stations, billboards, telephone distribution plants, and property with a class life of 20 years or more but less than 25 years
20 years	Municipal sewers and property with a class life of 25 years or more
27.5 years	Residential rental real estate, including apartment buildings, duplexes, etc.
39 years	Nonresidential real estate, including office buildings, warehouses, factories, and farm buildings

[12] § 168(c).

[13] § 168(e)(2).

Depreciation Method. The depreciation method to be used—like the recovery period—varies depending on the class of the property. A closer look at Exhibit 9-1, however, reveals that the variation is actually between real and personal property. Real property is depreciated using the straight-line method, while personal property is depreciated using either straight-line or a declining balance method. If a declining-balance depreciation method is elected, a switch to straight-line is made in the first year in which a larger depreciation would result. *Example 5* illustrates this procedure, and the IRS depreciation tables presented later in this chapter incorporate the switch to straight-line.

Accounting Conventions. For assets placed in service or disposed of during the year, an assumption is made regarding the amount of depreciation that is allowed for the year (e.g., a half-year).[14] These assumptions are referred to as depreciation or accounting conventions. The conventions apply only in the years of acquisition and disposition. The applicable convention generally depends on the type of property: realty or personalty. As discussed further below, they are:

Type of Property	Convention
Real property	Mid-month convention
Tangible personal property	Half-year convention
Tangible personal property	Mid-quarter convention

Half-Year Convention. The half-year convention applies to all property *other than* nonresidential real property and residential rental property. From a practical perspective, the half-year convention applies to *all depreciable tangible personal property.* Under the half-year convention, one-half year of depreciation is allowed regardless of when the asset is placed in service or sold during the year (e.g., ½ × the annual depreciation as normally computed).[15] Since only one-half year's depreciation is allowed in the first year, the recovery period is effectively extended one year so that the remaining one-half may be claimed.

Example 5. On March 1, 2009 T purchased a car to be used solely for business for $10,000. It was his only acquisition during the year. The car had an estimated useful life of four years and an estimated salvage value of $2,000. Although these estimates might be used for financial accounting purposes, under MACRS, salvage value is ignored and T is required to use the recovery period, depreciation method, and accounting convention prescribed for five-year property, the class to which cars are assigned under MACRS. T elects to compute his depreciation using the 200% declining-balance method (switching to straight-line where appropriate), a five-year recovery period, and the half-year convention. The 200% declining-balance rate would be 40% (200% × straight-line rate, 15 or 20%). The declining balance method would be used until 2012, when a switch to straight-line maximizes the depreciation deduction. Due to the half-year convention, the cost is actually recovered over six years rather than the five-year recovery period. Depreciation would be computed as follows:

---

[14] § 168(d).

[15] § 168(d)(4).

Year	Depreciation Method	Basis for Depreciation Computation	Rate	Depreciation
2009	200% D.B.	$10,000	20%*	$ 2,000
2010	200% D.B.	8,000	40%	3,200
2011	200% D.B.	4,800	40%	1,920
2012	200% D.B.	2,880	40%	1,152**
2013	S.L.	1,730	1.0/1.5	1,152***
2014	S.L.	1,730	0.5/1.5	576
				$ 10,000

* Half-year allowance (40% × ½ = 20%).

** Note that straight-line depreciation is the same ($2,880 × 2/5).

*** Declining-balance depreciation would have been $692 ($1,730 × 40%); since straight-line depreciation over the remaining 1.5 years is $1,152 and greater than $692, the switch to straight-line is made.

Example 6. Same facts as above except the property was sold on December 20, 2011. In computing depreciation for personal property in the year of sale or disposition, the half-year convention must also be used. Thus, depreciation for 2011 would be $960 ($4,800 × 40% × ½).

To simplify the computation of depreciation, the IRS provides optional tables as shown in Exhibit 9-4 to Exhibit 9-7.[16] The percentages (or rates) shown in the tables are the result of combining the three factors used in determining depreciation—method, rate, and convention—into a single, composite percentage to be used for each class of property.[17]

EXHIBIT 9-4

MACRS Accelerated Depreciation Percentages Using the Half-Year Convention for 3-, 5- and 7-Year Property

Recovery Year	Property Class		
	3-Year	5-Year	7-Year
1	33.33%	20.00%	14.29%
2	44.45	32.00	24.49
3	14.81	19.20	17.49
4	7.41	11.52	12.49
5		11.52	8.93
6		5.76	8.92
7			8.93
8			4.46

Source: Rev. Proc. 87-57, Table 1.

Appendix C has additional depreciation tables.

---

[16] Rev. Proc. 87-57, 1987-2 C.B. 687.

[17] Depreciation percentages in the tables are rounded to one-hundredth of a percent for recovery property with a recovery period of less than 20 years, and one-thousandth of a percent for all other property. See Rev. Proc. 87-57 *supra*.

Example 7. The depreciation rates shown in Exhibit 9-4 for 5-year property for the year that it is placed in service and for the following year is determined as follows:

Year 1

Straight-line rate (1/5)	20%
× Declining-balance rate	× 200%
200% declining-balance rate	40%
× Half-year allowance.	× ½
Depreciation rate per table	20%

Year 2

Basis of asset remaining (100% − 20%).	80%
× 200% declining-balance rate	× 40%
Depreciation rate per table	32%

In studying *Example 7* above, note how the table percentage for the second year, 32 percent, is derived. This percentage takes into account the requirement of the declining-balance method that the annual rate must be applied to the cost of the asset less previous depreciation [i.e., the second-year percentage of 32 percent is the product of the annual rate of 40 percent and the balance of the asset not yet depreciated, 80% (100% − 20%)]. Similarly, the percentages given for declining-balance methods also incorporate a switch to the straight-line method whenever the straight-line rate would yield a higher depreciation amount. Because these various considerations are already reflected in the tables, depreciation is computed by simply applying the appropriate percentage to the *unadjusted basis* of the property. The general formula for computing depreciation can be expressed as follows.

Unadjusted basis of the property × Recovery percentage = Annual depreciation

Example 8. Same facts as in *Example 5*. Depreciation computed using the table in Exhibit 9-4 would be the same as above, computed as follows:

Year	Unadjusted Basis	×	Accelerated Recovery Percentage	Annual Depreciation
2009	$10,000		20.00%	$ 2,000
2010	10,000		32.00	3,200
2011	10,000		19.20	1,920
2012	10,000		11.52	1,152
2013	10,000		11.52	1,152
2014	10,000		5.76	576
			100.00%	$10,000

Example 8 illustrates the basic steps necessary to compute annual depreciation. These steps are as follows:

1. Identify the *depreciable basis* of the asset (generally its cost): $10,000 in *Example 8*

2. Determine the MACRS *property class:* five-year property in *Example 8*

3. Identify the *depreciation convention* (either half-year or mid-quarter for personal property; mid-month for real estate): half-year convention in *Example 8*

4. Determine the *recovery period* and *method.* See Exhibit 9-1 for a summary of the available choices: five-year 200 percent declining balance in *Example 8*

5. Locate the *appropriate table* based on the depreciation convention, recovery period, and method: Exhibit 9-4 for *Example 8* (Note the depreciation convention is already reflected in the table percentages for the year of acquisition, but *not* for the year of disposition.)

6. Choose the *table percentages* relating to the recovery period of the asset: five-year property percentages for *Example 8* (i.e., 20 percent, 32 percent, etc.).

7. Multiply the table percentages by the depreciable (cost) basis of the asset to *compute annual depreciation* amounts: $10,000 multiplied by 20 percent provides $2,000 of depreciation for 2009 in *Example 8*

When using the depreciation tables, a special adjustment must be made if there is a disposition of the property before its cost is fully recovered. As noted above, under the half-year convention the taxpayer is entitled only to a half-year of depreciation in the year of disposition. Therefore, where the half-year convention applies and the property is used for only a portion of the disposition year, only one-half of the amount of depreciation determined using the table is allowed.

Example 9. Same facts as *Example 8* except the taxpayer sold the property on December 1, 2011. Since the taxpayer did not hold the property the entire taxable year and the half-year convention is in effect, only one-half of the amount of depreciation using the table is allowed. Therefore, depreciation for 2011 would have been $960 ($10,000 × 19.2% × ½). Note that this is the same result as obtained in *Example 6* above.

Mid-Month Convention. This convention applies only to real property (i.e., nonresidential real property and residential rental property).[18] Under the mid-month convention, one-half month of depreciation is allowed for the month the asset is placed in service or sold and a full month of depreciation is allowed for each additional month of the year that the asset is in service.[19] For example, if a calendar year taxpayer places a building in service on April 3, the fraction of the annual depreciation allowed is 8.5/12 (half-month's depreciation for April and eight months' depreciation for May through December).

Example 10. The first-year depreciation rate for residential rental realty that is placed in service in April is determined as follows:

Straight-line rate (1/27.5)	3.636%
× Mid-month convention	× 8.5/12
Depreciation rate per table	2.576%

Due to the mid-month convention, the recovery period must be extended one month to claim the one-half month of depreciation that was not claimed in the first month. For example, the entire cost of residential rental property is recovered over 331 months (27½ years is 330 months + 1 additional month to claim the half-month of depreciation not claimed in the first month). As a result, depreciation deductions are actually claimed over either 28 or 29 years depending on the month in which the property was placed in

---

[18] § 168(d)(2).

[19] § 168(d)(4)(B).

service. This can be seen by examining the composite depreciation percentages for real property reflecting the mid-month convention given in Exhibit 9-5 and Exhibit 9-6.

EXHIBIT 9-5

MACRS Depreciation Percentages for Residential Rental Property

Month Placed in Service	Recovery Year					
	1	2	3–26	27	28	29
1	3.485%	3.636%	3.636%	3.636%	1.970%	0.000%
2	3.182	3.636	3.636	3.636	2.273	0.000
3	2.879	3.636	3.636	3.636	2.576	0.000
4	2.576	3.636	3.636	3.636	2.879	0.000
5	2.273	3.636	3.636	3.636	3.182	0.000
6	1.970	3.636	3.636	3.636	3.485	0.000
7	1.667	3.636	3.636	3.637	3.636	0.152
8	1.364	3.636	3.636	3.637	3.636	0.455
9	1.061	3.636	3.636	3.637	3.636	0.758
10	0.758	3.636	3.636	3.637	3.636	1.061
11	0.455	3.636	3.636	3.637	3.636	1.364
12	0.152	3.636	3.636	3.637	3.636	1.667

Source: IRS Publication No. 534. Appendix C of this book has additional depreciation tables.

EXHIBIT 9-6

MACRS Depreciation Percentages for

Nonresidential Real Property Placed in Service after May 12, 1993

Month Placed in Service	Recovery Year		
	1	2–39	40
1	2.461%	2.564%	0.107%
2	2.247	2.564	0.321
3	2.033	2.564	0.535
4	1.819	2.564	0.749
5	1.605	2.564	0.963
6	1.391	2.564	1.177
7	1.177	2.564	1.391
8	0.963	2.564	1.605
9	0.749	2.564	1.819
10	0.535	2.564	2.033
11	0.321	2.564	2.247
12	0.107	2.564	2.461

Source: IRS Publication No. 534.

Appendix C of this book has additional depreciation tables.

Example 11. S purchased a duplex as an investment for $110,000 on July 17, 2009. Of the $110,000 cost, $10,000 is allocated to the land. The estimated useful life of the duplex is 30 years—the same period as her mortgage—and the estimated salvage value is $15,000. Despite these estimates, under MACRS salvage value is ignored and S is required to use the recovery period, depreciation method, and convention prescribed for residential rental property, the class to which the duplex is assigned. Therefore, S uses a 27.5-year life, the straight-line method, and the mid-month convention. Using the table in Exhibit 9-5, depreciation for the first year would be $1,667 ($100,000 × 1.667%).

When using the depreciation tables, an adjustment must be made if there is a disposition of the real property before its cost is fully recovered. This adjustment is similar to that required where the half-year convention applies, but not identical. In the year of disposition, the taxpayer may deduct depreciation only for those months the property is used by the taxpayer. In addition, under the mid-month convention, the taxpayer is entitled to only a half-month of depreciation for the month of disposition.

> **Example 12.** Same facts as *Example 11* except the taxpayer sold the property on May 22, 2010. Depreciation for 2010 would be $1,363 ($100,000 × 3.636% × 4.5/12).

Mid-Quarter Convention. The mid-quarter convention applies only to *personal property*. However, it applies only if more than 40 percent of the aggregate bases of all personal property placed in service during the taxable year is placed in service during the last three months of the year.[20] Property placed in service and disposed of during the same taxable year is not taken into account. Also not taken into account is any amount immediately expensed under § 179 (discussed below) or property used for personal purposes. If the 40 percent test is satisfied, the mid-quarter convention applies to *all* personal property placed in service during the year (regardless of the quarter in which it was actually placed in service).

> **Example 13.** During the year, K Company, a calendar year taxpayer, acquired and placed in service the following assets:
>
> | Assets | Acquisition Date | Cost |
> |---|---|---|
> | Office furniture............................ | March 28 | $20,000 |
> | Machinery................................ | October 9 | 80,000 |
> | Warehouse............................... | February 1 | 90,000 |
>
> Of the total *personal* property placed in service during the year, more than 40% [$80,000 ÷ ($20,000 + $80,000)] occurred in the last quarter (i.e., October through December). As a result, K must use the mid-quarter convention for computing the depreciation of both the furniture and the machinery.

When applicable, the mid-quarter convention treats all personal property as being placed in service in the middle of the quarter of the taxable year in which it was actually placed in service.[21] Therefore, one-half of a quarter's depreciation—in effect one-eighth (½ × ¼) or 12.5 percent of the annual depreciation—is allowed for the quarter that the asset is placed in service or sold. In addition, a full quarter's depreciation is allowed for each additional quarter that the asset is in service. For example, personal property placed in service on March 3 would be treated as having been placed in service in the middle of the first quarter and the taxpayer would be able to claim 3½ quarters—3.5/4 or 87.5 percent—of the annual amount of depreciation. The percentages of the annual depreciation allowed under the mid-quarter convention for a year in which an asset is placed in service are

	Quarter Placed in Service			
	First January–March	Second April–June	Third July–September	Fourth October–December
Percentage of annual depreciation allowed ..	87.5%	62.5%	37.5%	12.5%

---

[20]   § 168(d)(3).

[21]   *Ibid.*

The above chart illustrates that where an asset is placed in service in the first quarter and the mid-quarter convention applies, the taxpayer is allowed to deduct 87.5 percent of the annual depreciation. In contrast, for personal property placed in service during the fourth quarter only 12.5 percent of the annual depreciation may be deducted. Note that the recovery period must be extended by one year so that the balance of the depreciation not claimed in the first year may be deducted. Composite depreciation percentages to be used for 3-year and 5-year property where the mid-quarter convention applies are provided in Exhibit 9-7. Appendix C has depreciation tables for all categories of personal property under the mid-quarter convention.

EXHIBIT 9-7

**MACRS Accelerated Depreciation Percentages Using the
Mid-Quarter Convention for 3- and 5-Year Property**

3-Year Property:

	Quarter Placed in Service			
Recovery Year	1	2	3	4
1	58.33%	41.67%	25.00%	8.33%
2	27.78	38.89	50.00	61.11
3	12.35	14.14	16.67	20.37
4	1.54	5.30	8.33	10.19

5-Year Property:

1	35.00	25.00	15.00	5.00
2	26.00	30.00	34.00	38.00
3	15.60	18.00	20.40	22.80
4	11.01	11.37	12.24	13.68
5	11.01	11.37	11.30	10.94
6	1.38	4.26	7.06	9.58

Source: Rev. Proc. 87-57. Appendix C has additional depreciation tables.

Example 14. In 2009 T, a calendar year taxpayer, purchased five trucks to use in his business at a cost of $20,000 each. These purchases were his only acquisitions of personal property during the year. Four of the trucks were purchased in December while the other truck was purchased in January. Since more than 40% of the property placed in service during the year was placed in service in the last quarter ($80,000 ÷ $100,000 = 80%), the mid-quarter convention applies in computing depreciation. Thus, the depreciation allowed on the truck purchased in January would be limited to 87.5% of a full year's depreciation, and the depreciation allowed on the three trucks purchased in December would be limited to 12.5% of a full year's depreciation. Since a full year's depreciation would be 40% of cost (straight-line rate of 20% per year × 200% declining-balance = 40%), the depreciation for the January purchase would be limited to 35% of cost (40% × 87.5%), or $7,000 (35% × $20,000). Similarly, the depreciation for the December purchases would be limited to 5% of cost (40% × 12.5%), or $4,000 (5% × $80,000). Total depreciation under the mid-quarter convention is limited to $11,000 ($4,000 + $7,000). These amounts are easily computed using the tables in Exhibit 9-7.

Note that had the mid-quarter convention not applied, the depreciation percentage would have been 20%—reflecting the half-year allowance for 5-year property (40% × ½ = 20%), or $20,000 ($100,000 × 20%). Due to the timing of the acquisitions, T's depreciation for the year is reduced by $9,000 ($20,000 − $11,000).

When using the depreciation tables, a special adjustment must be made if there is a disposition of the property before its cost is fully recovered. This adjustment is similar to that for the half-year and mid-month conventions. As noted above, under the mid-quarter convention, the taxpayer is entitled to only one-half of a quarter's depreciation—in effect one-eighth ($\frac{1}{2} \times \frac{1}{4}$) or 12.5 percent of the annual depreciation—for the quarter that the asset is sold. In addition, a full quarter of depreciation is allowed for each quarter that the asset is in service. For example, if property was sold on August 2, the taxpayer could claim 2½ quarters—2.5/4 or 62.5 percent—of the annual amount of depreciation. The percentages of annual depreciation allowed under the mid-quarter convention for the year an asset is sold are

	Quarter Property Sold			
	First January–March	*Second* April–June	*Third* July–September	*Fourth* October–December
Percentage of annual depreciation allowed ..	12.5%	37.5%	62.5%	87.5%

Example 15. Same facts as in *Example 14* above, except the truck acquired in January 2009 was sold on August 9, 2011. Since T did not hold the property the entire taxable year and the mid-quarter convention is in effect, only 62.5% of the amount of depreciation using the table is allowed. Therefore, using the table in Exhibit 9-7, T's depreciation for this truck would have been $1,950 ($20,000 × 15.6% × 62.5%).

OTHER METHODS

The accelerated depreciation methods prescribed by MACRS are normally desirable since they allow taxpayers to recover their costs more rapidly than the straight-line method. However, there may be circumstances where the slower-paced straight-line method may be more advantageous. For example, if the taxpayer is currently in the 10 or 15 percent tax bracket, he or she may want to defer depreciation deductions to years when he or she is in a higher tax bracket. By doing this, the taxpayer may be able to maximize the present value of the tax savings from depreciation deductions (depending upon the taxpayer's discount rate).

Perhaps a more common reason for using straight-line depreciation concerns the alternative minimum tax (AMT). As discussed briefly in Chapter 3 and in detail in Chapter 13, the AMT is an alternative system for computing the tax, using certain modifications. For AMT purposes, depreciation is generally computed using a method slower than MACRS (e.g., 150% rather than 200% declining balance). This difference can lead to an AMT liability. To avoid this, taxpayers often elect to use a straight-line method for regular tax purposes. If a taxpayer elects to use the straight-line method in lieu of the accelerated method, two different approaches are available: straight-line under MACRS, or straight-line under ADS.

MACRS Straight-Line. Although it may seem inconsistent, the *Modified Accelerated Cost Recovery System* offers taxpayers a straight-line method of depreciation.[22] If the taxpayer so elects, the straight line method is used in conjunction with all of the other rules that normally apply under MACRS; that is, the taxpayer simply uses the straight-line method (in lieu of the accelerated method) along with the applicable recovery period and accounting convention. The depreciation percentages to be used where the taxpayer elects the straight-line method are contained in Exhibit 9-8 (half-year convention property) for 3-, 5-, and 7-year property. Appendix C has straight-line depreciation tables for all categories of personal property under the half-year convention. The depreciation

---

[22] § 168(b)(3)(C).

percentages for the straight-line method when the mid-quarter convention applies can be found in Revenue Procedure 87-57.[23]

Example 16. On June 1, 2009 L purchased 5-year property (to which the half-year convention applies) for $50,000. Using the table in Exhibit 9-8, depreciation for the year would be $5,000 ($50,000 × 10%). Depreciation for 2010 would be $10,000 (20% × $50,000). If L sold the property on January 22, 2011, depreciation would be $5,000 ($50,000 × 20% × ½).

EXHIBIT 9-8

MACRS and ADS Straight-Line Depreciation Percentages Using the Half-Year Convention for 3-, 5-, and 7-Year Property

Recovery Year	Property Class		
	3-Year	5-Year	7-Year
1	16.67%	10.00%	7.14%
2	33.33	20.00	14.29
3	33.33	20.00	14.29
4	16.67	20.00	14.28
5		20.00	14.29
6		10.00	14.28
7			14.29
8			7.14

Source: Rev. Proc. 87-57

Appendix C has additional depreciation tables.

The election to use the straight-line method is made annually by class (recall the straight-line method must be used for realty). For example, if in 2009 the taxpayer makes the election for 7-year property, *all* 7-year property placed in service during the year must be depreciated using the straight-line method. The election does not obligate the taxpayer to use the straight-line method for any other class. Similarly, the taxpayer need not use the straight-line method for such class of assets placed in service in the following year.

Alternative Depreciation System. The Alternative Depreciation System (ADS) is an option for taxpayers.[24] This system is similar to MACRS in two ways: salvage value is ignored, and the same averaging conventions must be followed. The major differences between MACRS and ADS are the longer recovery periods provided by ADS for most assets and in some cases, slower rates of depreciation. The recovery period to be used for ADS is normally the property's class life. The class life—which is usually longer than the MACRS life—is used unless no class life has been prescribed for the property or a specific class life has been designated in Code § 168. For example, as shown in Exhibit 9-2, the ADS class life for copiers (asset class 00.13) is six years, whereas the MACRS life is five years. Thus, depreciation under ADS would be computed using a six-year life, whereas depreciation for MACRS would be computed using a five-year life. The recovery periods to be used for ADS are summarized in Exhibit 9-9.

Taxpayers electing ADS for real property are restricted to straight-line depreciation. Thus, an office building (nonresidential real property) would be depreciated using straight-line and a 40-year recovery period under ADS. The ADS depreciation percentages for real property are found in Exhibit 9-10.

---

[23] 1987-2 C.B. 687.

[24] § 168(g).

In contrast, either straight-line or 150 percent declining balance depreciation may be chosen for depreciable tangible personal property. The ADS straight-line depreciation percentages for such property, which in fact have class lives of three, five and seven years, are the same as those for MACRS straight-line and can be found in Exhibit 9-8.

EXHIBIT 9-9

Alternative Depreciation System Recovery Periods

General Rule: Recovery period is the property's class life unless
1. There is no class life (see below), or
2. A special class life has been designated (see below).

Type of Property	Recovery Period
Personal property with no class life	12 years
Nonresidential real property with no class life	40 years
Residential rental property with no class life	40 years
Cars, light general-purpose trucks, certain technological equipment, and semiconductor manufacturing equipment	5 years
Computer-based telephone central office switching equipment	9.5 years
Railroad track	10 years
Single-purpose agricultural or horticultural structures	15 years
Municipal wastewater treatment plants, telephone distribution plants	24 years
Low-income housing financed by tax-exempt bonds	27.5 years
Municipal sewers	50 years

EXHIBIT 9-10

ADS Straight-Line Depreciation Percentages for Real Property Using the Mid-Month Convention

Month Placed in Service	Recovery Year		
	1	2–40	41
1	2.396%	2.500%	0.104%
2	2.188	2.500	0.312
3	1.979	2.500	0.521
4	1.771	2.500	0.729
5	1.563	2.500	0.937
6	1.354	2.500	1.146
7	1.146	2.500	1.354
8	0.938	2.500	1.562
9	0.729	2.500	1.771
10	0.521	2.500	1.979
11	0.313	2.500	2.187
12	0.104	2.500	2.396

Source: Rev. Proc. 87-57, Table 13.

Taxpayers have as many as four options for depreciating personal property—straight line or accelerated depreciation over the MACRS recovery period, or straight line over a longer ADS recovery period. Accelerated depreciation options are 200 percent or 150 percent declining balance. For example, the ADS option for a copier consists of straight-line over six years. The MACRS alternatives allow for a five-year write-off using either 200 percent or 150 percent declining balance or straight line. Which of these four choices would be best for depreciating the copier? In general, the taxpayer should select

the depreciation method that maximizes the present value of tax savings from depreciation deductions. For taxpayers who expect their future marginal tax rate to either remain constant or decline, the fastest depreciation method over the shortest time period will maximize the present value of tax savings from depreciation.

The mechanics of the election to use ADS—except for real property—are identical to those of MACRS discussed above. Except for real property, the taxpayer may elect to use ADS on a class-by-class, year-by-year basis.[25] For realty, the election is made on a property-by-property basis. In addition, the taxpayer *must* use ADS straight-line for depreciating the following:[26]

- Certain "listed property" that is not used predominately for business (see discussion below)
- Foreign use property (i.e., property used outside the U.S. more than half of a taxable year)
- Property leased to a tax-exempt entity
- Property leased to foreign persons (unless more than 50 percent of the income is subject to U.S. tax)
- Property financed by the issuance of tax-exempt bonds (i.e., tax-exempt bond-financed property).

ADS is also used for computing depreciation for purposes of the alternative minimum tax (discussed in Chapter 13) and a corporation's earnings and profits (discussed in Chapter 20).

CHANGES IN DEPRECIATION

There are many situations where the taxpayer incorrectly computes depreciation, resulting in too much or too little depreciation. For example, a corporation may discover it mistakenly classified an asset initially and the wrong recovery period was used. Similarly, the IRS may change the recovery period of an asset. In 2003, the Service ruled that the life of canopies at gas stations that protect the pumps and customers from inclement weather are 5-year rather than 15-year property.[27] When the taxpayer is entitled to additional depreciation, the IRS permits a change in accounting method and the taxpayer may deduct all of the unclaimed depreciation for years that are closed by the statute of limitations as well as open years. This is normally done through a § 481(a) adjustment that reduces income in the year of the change (a single year adjustment).[28] If the adjustment increases the taxpayer's income, the increase is normally spread over four years.

☑ CHECK YOUR KNOWLEDGE

Review Question 1. Indicate whether the following statements concerning tax depreciation are true or false.

a. During the year, Mr. L purchased a computer that he uses to track how his stocks and bonds are doing. L can depreciate the computer even though it is not used in a trade or business.

---

[25] § 168(g)(7).

[26] § 168(g)(1).

[27] Rev. Rul. 2003-54, 2003-23 I.R.B. 982.

[28] Rev. Proc. 96-31, 1996-1 C.B. 714. But see *Brookshire Brothers Holding, Inc.*, 320 F.3d 507 (CA-5, 2003) where the court held that it was not a change in accounting method and the government was barred from reducing depreciation in closed years. See also *Green Forest Manufacturing Inc.*, T.C. Memo 2003-75.

True. An asset generally may be depreciated to the extent that it is used in a trade or business or an income-producing activity. Since the computer is used to monitor investments, an income-producing activity, it is depreciable. Thus if L uses the computer 30 percent of the time to monitor his stocks and bonds and 70 percent for playing solitaire (i.e., personal use), 30 percent of the cost of the computer could be depreciated.

b. Land and goodwill are never depreciable or amortizable since neither has a determinable life.

False. Assets without a determinable life normally cannot be depreciated or amortized. Under normal circumstances, neither of these assets would be considered as having a determinable life and, therefore, neither could be depreciated. However, § 197 of the Code creates a specific exception to this rule for goodwill, allowing taxpayers to amortize goodwill over 15 years. Land normally is not depreciable.

c. This year Z Corporation purchased a new car to be used in its business. For financial accounting purposes, the company computed depreciation assuming the car had an estimated useful life of three years and an approximate salvage value of $1,000. In computing depreciation for tax purposes, the company will also use a three-year life and a salvage value of $1,000.

False. The computation of tax depreciation ignores the asset's actual useful life and salvage value. For tax purposes, a car is deemed to have a five-year life and salvage value is always ignored. Note that because different depreciation methods are used annual depreciation for financial accounting will normally differ from tax depreciation.

Review Question 2. In November of this year, Park and Ride Inc., a calendar year taxpayer, purchased five new vans to use in its limousine service for $100,000. In February, the company closed on the acquisition of a new maintenance facility. Indicate whether the following are true or false.

a. Assuming the cost of the maintenance facility was $50,000, the corporation must use the mid-quarter convention to depreciate the facility.

False. The mid-quarter convention applies only to personal property and not realty. The mid-month convention must be used in computing depreciation for realty. The mid-quarter convention must be used for the vans.

b. Assuming the cost of the maintenance facility was $500,000, the corporation must use the *half-year* convention in depreciating the vans.

False. The mid-quarter convention applies if more than 40 percent of the *personal property* placed in service during the year is placed in service during the last three months. For purposes of making this calculation, only personal property—the vans—is considered and the realty (i.e., the maintenance facility) is ignored. Moreover, any personal property that is expensed under § 179 (discussed below) is also ignored. In this case, all of the personal property was placed in service during the last quarter of the year and, therefore, the corporation must use the mid-quarter convention.

Review Question 3. During the year, C Corporation purchased equipment that qualifies as five-year property. Due to other purchases of personal property during the year, the mid-quarter convention must be used in computing depreciation. Compute the first-and second-year depreciation rates that should be used assuming the asset was placed in service in February. Check your answers by using the table in Exhibit 9-7.

The depreciation rates are 35 percent for the first year and 26 percent for the second year, which are computed as follows:

Year 1:

	Straight-line rate (1/5)	20%
×	Declining-balance rate	× 200%
	200 percent declining-balance annual rate.	40%
	Mid-quarter percentage	× 87.5%
		35%

Year 2:

	Basis of asset remaining (100% − 35%).	65%
×	200 percent declining-balance annual rate.	× 40%
	Depreciation rate per table	26%

Review Question 4. On February 15 of this year, K Corporation purchased a warehouse for $250,000 ($50,000 allocable to the land). For financial accounting purposes, the building is treated as having a 40-year life and a salvage value of $20,000.

a. Compute the depreciation deduction for the year.

Depreciation for the year is $4,494 as computed below. Note that the useful life and the salvage value that are used for financial accounting purposes are irrelevant for tax purposes.

	Unadjusted basis of the building	$200,000
×	Recovery percentage for month placed in service (February)	× 2.247%
	Depreciation.	$ 4,494

b. Assuming the corporation sold the building on March 10 of the following year, compute the depreciation deduction for the year.

	Unadjusted basis of the building	$ 200,000
×	Recovery percentage for second year	× 2.564%
×	Mid-month convention in year of disposition.	× 2.5/12
	Depreciation.	$ 1,068

LIMITED EXPENSING ELECTION: CODE § 179

When Congress introduced ACRS in 1981, it also created § 179. This provision allows taxpayers (other than estates or trusts) to *elect* to treat the cost of qualifying property as a currently deductible expense rather than a capital expenditure subject to depreciation. Initially, the maximum amount that could be expensed under § 179 was $5,000. Over the years, Congress has gradually increased that amount and in 2009 it is $250,000 (adjusted annually for inflation). This measure was intended primarily to stimulate investment; however, its corollary effect was to eliminate the need for maintaining depreciation records where the taxpayer's annual acquisitions were not substantial.

Although the maximum amount that can be expensed by a taxpayer is $250,000 for 2009, two limitations may restrict the amount that the taxpayer may otherwise expense:

1. *Acquisitions of Eligible Property Exceeding $800,000* (2009). When the aggregate cost of *qualifying* property placed in service during the year exceeds $800,000 (in 2009), the $250,000 amount must be reduced $1 for each $1 of cost in excess of $800,000. For example, taxpayers purchasing $810,000 of property could expense up to $240,000 [$250,000 − ($810,000 − $800,000 = $10,000)] of the cost while taxpayers purchasing in excess of $1,050,000 ($800,000 + $250,000) could not benefit from § 179 at all.

2. *Taxable Income Limitation.* The deduction under § 179 cannot exceed the amount of taxable income derived from all of the taxpayer's trades or businesses (including wage income).[29] Any amount that cannot be deducted can be carried over indefinitely to following years to be used against future income. The $250,000 maximum amount that can be expensed in subsequent years is not increased by the carryover amount, however. Rather than carry over the amount that could not be expensed because of the taxable income limitation, the taxpayer has the option of not reducing the property's basis by the carryover amount so it can be depreciated along with the rest of the property's cost.

As explained later in this chapter, additional limitations on the use of § 179 apply in the case of luxury automobiles, sports utility vehicles (SUVs) and "listed" property.

The taxpayer may elect to expense all or a portion of an asset so long as the total amount expensed does not exceed the dollar limitation. If only a portion of an asset is expensed, the remaining portion is subject to depreciation.

Example 17. T Corporation purchased 5-year property for $100,000 and 7-year property for $300,000 during the current year. Both assets are eligible to be expensed subject to the limitations of § 179. Assume T expects its future marginal tax rate to remain constant. To maximize the present value of the tax savings from limited expensing and depreciation deductions, T should expense $250,000 of the 7-year property rather than the 5-year property since the cost of the 5-year property could be recovered more quickly, thus resulting in higher depreciation deductions in the current year. Assuming T elects to expense $250,000 of the 7-year property, its deduction for such property would be $257,145 computed as follows:

	Original cost.	$ 300,000	
−	Expensed portion	− 250,000	$ 250,000
	Remaining depreciable basis.	$ 50,000	
×	Depreciation percentage	× 14.29%	
	Depreciation deduction.	$ 7,145	7,145
	Total deduction.		$ 257,145

In addition to the deductions for the 7-year property, the taxpayer could claim a deduction for *depreciation* of the 5-year property.

Assume these two assets were the only depreciable assets T purchased during the year. Further assume that the five-year property was purchased in August (the third quarter of the year) and the seven-year property was purchased in November (the fourth quarter of the year). If immediate expensing had *not* been elected, T would be

---

[29] Taxable income is computed with § 1231 gains and interest from working capital but not deductions allowable for § 179, one half of self-employment tax, net operating loss carrybacks or carryforwards and deductions suspended under other Code sections (e.g., passive losses, partnership or S corporation losses limited for lack of basis). Note that taxable income presumably reflects depreciation for the § 179 property without considering § 179. [See § 179(b)(3)(C) and Reg. § 1.179-2(c)(1) and -(2)(c)(5)].

required to use the mid-quarter convention for both assets since more than 40 percent of the cost was placed in service during the fourth quarter [$300,000 is 75% of $400,000 ($100,000 + $300,000)]. Because T expenses $250,000 of the $300,000 asset, the cost of the asset placed in service in the fourth quarter is deemed to be $50,000, not $300,000. Thus, the mid-quarter convention is avoided and the taxpayer can maximize depreciation for the year using the half-year convention.

Eligible Property. Only property that satisfies certain requirements is eligible for expensing. To qualify, the property may be new or used and must be:[30]

1. Recovery property;

2. Property that would have qualified for the investment credit (e.g., most property other than buildings and their components);

3. Property used in a trade or business, as distinguished from property held for the production of income; and

4. Property acquired by purchase from someone who is generally not a "related party" under § 267 (e.g., gifted or inherited property usually does not qualify nor would property acquired from a spouse or parent).

Certain property is designated as *ineligible* for expensing. Such property includes:

1. Property used predominantly to furnish lodging or in connection with furnishing lodging unless the business is a hotel or motel that provides accommodations used primarily by transients. Presumably, this rule prohibits taxpayers who provide long-term rentals (e.g., apartments, duplexes, etc.) from expensing such items as furniture and appliances.

2. Air conditioning and heating units;

3. Property that is primarily used by a tax-exempt organization; and

4. Property used outside the U.S. (But there are a number of exceptions).

Recapture. Without any special rule, taxpayers could use an asset in business for a short period (e.g., one day), expense it for tax purposes, then convert it to nonbusiness use. To prohibit this possible abuse, a special rule applies. If the property is converted to *nonbusiness* use *at any time*, the taxpayer must *recapture* the benefit derived from expensing.[31] For this purpose, a sale does not trigger recapture. Recapture requires the taxpayer to *include* in income the difference between the amount expensed and the MACRS deductions that would have been allowed for the actual period of business use.

Example 18. On January 1, 2009 F purchased a computer for $5,000. He used it for business for one year, then gave it to his teenage son as a graduation present and bought himself another computer. F may expense the entire $5,000 cost of the computer. However, in 2010 he must recapture and include in income the difference between the expensed amount and the deduction computed under MACRS, $4,000 [$5,000 expensed − MACRS deduction of $1,000 ($5,000 × 20%)]. Note that the net effect in this case is to allow F a deduction equal to what he otherwise could have claimed under MACRS, $1,000.

---

[30] §§ 179(d)(1) and (2).

[31] § 179(d)(10).

ADDITIONAL FIRST-YEAR (BONUS) DEPRECIATION

The sagging economy recently prompted Congress to turn to a tool that it often has used for stimulation: additional first-year or so-called bonus depreciation. Effective for property placed in service in 2008 and 2009, taxpayers may claim an additional first-year depreciation deduction equal to 50% of the adjusted basis of new qualified property.[32] Bonus depreciation is in addition to any amount expensed under § 179 and regular depreciation.[33] Bonus depreciation is scheduled to expire in 2010 (2011 for certain long-lived and transportation property).

Qualified Property. Section 168(k)(2) provides that qualified property is generally all newly acquired depreciable property—other than buildings. Only new property qualifies. Used property does not qualify. In other words, to qualify, the property's first or original use must commence with the taxpayer after December 31, 2007 and before January 1, 2010. For this purpose, capital expenditures incurred to recondition or rebuild property meet this requirement. In contrast, the cost of reconditioned or rebuilt property acquired by the taxpayer is considered used property and does not qualify. Technically, qualified property includes:

- Property eligible for MACRS depreciation with a recovery period of 20 years or less (business and investment property);
- Certain water utility property (as defined in Code § 168(e)(5));
- Computer software (except software acquired in connection with the acquisition of a business unless such software is available to the general public and is not substantially modified); and
- Qualified leasehold improvement property. A qualified leasehold improvement is an interior improvement made under a lease of commercial property (such as an office building or warehouse), and placed in service more than three years after the building was first placed in service. Certain structural improvements do not qualify, and neither do expansions.

In light of these rules, certain property is not eligible. Bonus depreciation cannot be used for residential and nonresidential real estate since the lives of these properties (27.5 and 39 years respectively) exceed 20 years. Intangibles are not subject to MACRS and, thus, do not qualify for the additional allowance. Section 197 intangibles such as goodwill, covenants not to compete, and customer lists acquired in connection with the purchase of a business also would not be eligible. In addition, property that must be depreciated using the alternative depreciation system (ADS) does not qualify. As discussed below, under the special depreciation limitations of § 280F for so-called listed property (e.g., automobiles), ADS is required if qualified business used does not exceed 50 percent. Similarly, ADS must be used for tangible property (e.g., a machine) used predominantly outside of the U.S. However, if the taxpayer merely elects to use ADS for certain property, bonus depreciation can still be claimed

Computation of Bonus Depreciation. There is no limitation on the amount of bonus depreciation that may be claimed. Taxpayers may claim bonus depreciation for all *qualified* property. In addition, taxpayers may claim both bonus depreciation and § 179 expensing. When both amounts are claimed for the same property, the bonus depreciation is equal to 50 percent of the adjusted basis of the property *after the reduction for the amount expensed under § 179*. The effect is to reduce the amount of bonus depreciation that may be claimed since the basis is smaller. Regular depreciation is computed after the basis of the property is reduced by both the § 179 amount and the 50 percent additional allowance.

---

[32] § 168(k)

[33] Bonus depreciation can be used for purposes of the alternative minimum tax but not in computing the earnings and profits of a corporation.

Example 19. In March 2009, X Corporation purchased two heavy-duty machines. Each machine cost $300,000. The corporation elected to expense $250,000 of the cost of one machine and take advantage of the additional 50 percent allowance for both machines. The machinery is 5-year property. Regular depreciation, § 179 expense and bonus depreciation for the first year would be computed as shown below.

	Machine #1		Machine #2	
Adjusted basis	$300,000		$300,000	
§ 179 expensed portion	(250,000)	$250,000	—	
Remaining depreciable basis	$50,000		$300,000	
Additional allowance	× 50%		× 50%	
Bonus depreciation	$25,000	25,000	$150,000	$150,000
Remaining depreciable basis	$25,000		$150,000	
Regular depreciation	× 20%		× 20%	
Regular depreciation	$5,000	5,000	$30,000	30,000
Total deduction		$280,000		$180,000

A comparison of the *bonus depreciation* for both machines reveals different amounts deducted even though the costs of the machines were the same. This occurs because of the special ordering rule. The rule requires that the property's basis for computing bonus depreciation must first be reduced by any amount expensed under § 179.

The full amount of bonus depreciation may be claimed regardless of whether the mid-quarter convention applies. Note also that a taxpayer may elect *not* to claim the additional 50 percent allowance. This may be done simply by computing depreciation in the normal fashion.

Bonus Depreciation and § 179 Compared. Bonus depreciation and § 179 expensing allowance are subject to special limitations that are similar but not identical. Bonus depreciation

- is not limited to the taxable income from the business;
- does not phase-out based on the amount of property placed in service during the year;
- is allowed for investment property and § 179 applies only to business property;
- can be claimed on purchases from related parties while § 179 cannot;
- can be used by estates and trusts which are not allowed to elect § 179;
- cannot be used for used property while § 179 can.

LIMITATIONS FOR AUTOMOBILES

Over the years, Congress has become more and more concerned about taxpayers who effectively use the benefits of the tax law to reduce the cost of what are essentially personal expenses. For example, a taxpayer may justify the purchase of a luxury rather than standard automobile on the grounds that the government is helping to defray the additional cost through tax deductions and credits allowed for the purchase. In 1984 Congress enacted Code § 280F to reduce the benefits of depreciation and limited expensing for certain automobiles and other properties that are often used partially for personal purposes. In addition, the record keeping requirements for travel and entertainment were tightened and extended to certain property used for personal purposes.

Section 280F sets forth a special set of limitations for *passenger automobiles.* A passenger automobile is defined as any four-wheeled vehicle manufactured primarily for use on public streets, roads, and highways that weighs 6,000 pounds or less unloaded. For purposes of § 280F, the term *passenger automobiles* does not include vehicles for hire, such as taxis, rental trucks, and rental cars.[34] Ambulances and hearses directly used in a trade or business are also unaffected by the § 280F limitations. Temporary regulations create certain exceptions to the definition of passenger automobile. Excluded is any "qualified nonpersonal use vehicle" defined as any vehicle which, by reason of its nature (i.e., design or modification), is not likely to be used more than a *de minimis* amount for personal purposes.[35] This category would include police and fire vehicles, ambulances, qualified moving vans, and delivery and utility repair trucks.

For passenger automobiles, § 280F generally imposes a ceiling on the amount of annual depreciation and first-year expensing deductions. The *maximum* depreciation and/or § 179 expense for autos is shown in Exhibit 9-11. The limits for a particular auto are determined by the year the auto is placed in service by the taxpayer. Thus, annual limits for autos placed in service in 2009 are found in the 2009 column in Exhibit 9-11.[36] For example, in 2009 the deduction for depreciation and § 179 expensing cannot exceed $2,960 for the year placed in service and $4,800 for the second year of service. If the taxpayer uses bonus depreciation in 2008 or 2009, the first year deduction amounts for passenger vehicles as well trucks and vans are increased by $8,000. However, the later year amounts are not changed. For example, if bonus depreciation is used, the first year amount for passenger automobile is $10,960 ($2,960 + $8,000).

The 2009 limitations under § 280F restrict the annual depreciation amounts for autos costing $14,800 or more (assuming 200 percent declining-balance depreciation was claimed). The $14,800 amount reflects the $2,960 first-year depreciation limitation ($14,800 × 20% regular depreciation rate for five-year property).

---

[34] § 280F(d)(5).

[35] Regs. § 1.274-5T(k)(2)).

[36] Rev. Proc. 2008-22, 2008-12 IRB 658.

EXHIBIT 9-11

Section 280F Depreciation Limits for Autos

	Limits for Autos Based on Year Placed in Service		
	2009	2008	2007
First year of service	$2,960*	$2,960*	$3,060
Second year of service	4,800	4,800	4,900
Third year of service	2,850	2,850	2,850
Thereafter	1,775	1,775	1,775

*Increase by $8,000 to $10,960 if bonus depreciation claimed.

Where the car is used less than 100 percent of the time for business—including the portion of time the car is used for production of income purposes—the maximum amounts given above must be reduced proportionately.

Example 20. T purchased a car for $20,000 in 2009. She used it 60% of the time for business purposes and 20% of the time traveling to her rental properties. Depreciation and limited expensing may not exceed $2,368 (80% × $2,960) for the first year, $3,840 (80% × $4,800) for the second year, and so on.

If the property's basis has not been fully deducted by the close of the normal recovery period (i.e., normally the extended recovery period of six years), a deduction for the *unrecovered basis* is allowed in subsequent years. Deductions for the property's unrecovered basis are limited to $1,775 (2009) annually until the entire basis is recovered.

Example 21. On December 1, 2009 R purchased a new automobile for $18,000 which he uses solely for business. R's regular depreciation for the first year initially is $3,600 but is limited to $2,960 as shown below:

Original cost...	$18,000	
Depreciation percentage	× 20%	
Depreciation before limitation		$3,600
Limitation		$2,960

The calculation of regular depreciation for the first year and subsequent years is summarized below.

In examining the schedule below, note that the recovery period is extended from six to eight years due to the limitations. Also, understand that the unadjusted depreciable basis used for computing depreciation is $18,000 for each year even though only $2,960 of the depreciation was deducted in the first year.

	1 2009	2 2010	3 2011	4 2012	5 2013	6 2014	7 2015	8 2016
Unadjusted basis.........	$18,000	$18,000	$18,000	$18,000	$18,000	$18,000	$18,000	$18,000
Depreciation Percentage ..	20.00%	32.00%	19.20%	11.52%	11.52%	5.76%		
MACRS depreciation	$ 3,600	$ 5,760	$ 3,456	$ 2,074	$ 2,074	$ 1,037	$ 1,775	$ 1,775
Limit...................	$ 2,960	$ 4,800	$ 2,850	$ 1,775	$ 1,775	$ 1,775	$ 1,775	$ 1,775
Deduction...............	$ 2,960	$ 4,800	$ 2,850	$ 1,775	$ 1,775	$ 1,037	$ 1,775	$ 1,028
Cumulative depreciation .	$ 2,960	$ 7,760	$10,610	$12,385	$14,160	$15,197	$16,972	$18,000
Adjusted basis...........	$15,040	$10,240	$ 7,390	$ 5,615	$ 3,840	$ 2,803	$ 1,028	0

Trucks, Vans, and SUVs. Responding to criticisms that the limitations for passenger automobiles did not fairly reflect the higher price that must be paid for trucks and vans, the IRS created a separate set of limitations for these vehicles as shown in Exhibit 9-12.

EXHIBIT 9-12

Section 280F Depreciation Limits for Trucks and Vans

Year	2009	2008	2007
1	$3,060*	$3,160*	$3,260
2	4,900	5,100	5,200
3	2,950	3,050	3,050
Thereafter	1,775	1,875	1,875

*Increase by $8,000 to $11,960 if bonus depreciation claimed.

For this purpose, a vehicle qualifies as a truck or van if it is built on a truck chassis. Since most Sport Utility Vehicles (SUVs) are built on a truck chassis these higher limits would apply, assuming these vehicles do not have a gross vehicle weight exceeding 6,000 pounds. If the weight exceeds 6,000 pounds, special rules apply as discussed below.

Leasing. Without any special rule, the taxpayer could lease a car and circumvent the limitations on depreciation since the restrictions would appear to apply only to the deduction for depreciation and not lease payments. For instance, in *Example 21* above, the taxpayer might lease the car for $400 per month and claim a deduction of $4,800 for the year—far in excess of the amount allowed for depreciation after the first year. To prohibit this possibility, lessees may deduct the amount of the lease payment (applicable to business or income-producing use)—but must *include* certain amounts in income to bring their deductions for use of the car in line for owners. In practice, these inclusion amounts are not actually added to income but simply reduce the deduction for the lease payment.

The amount that the taxpayer must include in income is generally based on the automobile's fair market value and is determined in the following manner.[37]

1. Using the value of the automobile for the taxable year in which the auto is first used under the lease, identify the annual inclusion amount from the table found in Exhibit 9-14. Note that for the last year of the lease, the dollar amount for the preceding year is used unless the lease term begins and ends in the same year.

2. Prorate the dollar amount for the number of days of the lease term included in the taxable year.

3. Multiply the prorated dollar amount by the business and investment use for the taxable year.

Taxpayers who lease trucks and vans do not use the tables above for passenger automobiles but must use separate tables designed specifically for these two categories.

Example 22. On April 1, 2008, M, a calendar year taxpayer, signed a three-year lease on a new passenger automobile with a value of $26,800. For 2008 and 2009, M used the car exclusively in his business. During 2010 and 2011, his business use dropped to 40%. The amounts that M must include in income for 2008 through 2011 are computed as follows:

Tax Year	Dollars Amount	Proration	Business Use%	Inclusion Amount
2008	$ 58	275/365	100%	$ 44
2009	126	366/366	100%	126
2010	188	365/365	40%	75
2011	188	90/365	40%	22

Observe that dollar amounts are based on the value of the car in the first year of the lease. Subsequent declines in the car's value are ignored. Also note that in computing the inclusion amount for 2011, the $188 amount for the preceding year (2010) is used instead of $223 per the table because the lease did not begin and end in the same year.

---

[37] § 280F(c) and Reg. § 1.280F-7(a). Note that these limitations do not apply to cars leased for 30 or fewer days or to lessors who regularly engage in the auto-leasing business.

EXHIBIT 9-14

Leased Passenger Automobile (that are not Trucks and Vans):
Income Inclusion Amounts for Automobile Leases Beginning in 2008

Fair Market Vale of Passenger Automobile		Tax Year During Lease				
Over	Not Over	1st	2nd	3rd	4th	5th & Later
$18,500	$19,000	20	42	62	73	84
19,000	19,500	22	47	71	83	94
19,500	20,000	25	53	78	93	106
20,000	20,500	27	58	87	102	117
20,500	21,000	30	63	95	112	128
21,000	21,500	32	69	103	122	139
21,500	22,000	34	75	111	131	151
22,000	23,000	38	83	123	146	167
23,000	24,000	43	94	139	165	190
24,000	25,000	48	105	155	185	212
25,000	26,000	53	115	172	204	235
26,000	27,000	58	126	188	223	257
27,000	28,000	63	137	204	243	279
28,000	29,000	68	148	220	262	302
29,000	30,000	73	159	236	282	324
30,000	31,000	78	170	252	301	347
31,000	32,000	83	181	268	321	368
32,000	33,000	88	192	284	340	391
33,000	34,000	93	202	301	359	414
34,000	35,000	98	213	317	379	436
35,000	36,000	103	224	333	398	459
36,000	37,000	108	235	349	418	481
37,000	38,000	113	246	365	437	503
38,000	39,000	118	257	381	457	525
39,000	40,000	123	268	397	476	548
40,000	41,000	128	279	413	495	571
41,000	42,000	133	289	430	515	593
42,000	43,000	137	301	446	534	615
43,000	44,000	142	312	462	553	638
44,000	45,000	147	323	478	573	659
45,000	46,000	152	333	495	592	682
46,000	47,000	157	344	511	611	705
47,000	48,000	162	355	527	631	727
48,000	49,000	167	366	543	650	750
49,000	50,000	172	377	559	670	772
50,000	51,000	177	388	575	689	794
·						
·						
·						
240,000	and up	1,142	2,507	3,720	4,459	5,148

Source: Rev. Proc. 2008-22, 2008-12 IRB 658. This table extends to values of $240,000 and up.

Deducting SUVs. As noted above, a truck or van—including an SUV or minivan—is *not* treated as a passenger automobile subject to annual depreciation limits if it has *a gross vehicle weight* (GVW) of more than 6,000 pounds. "GVW" is the weight of the vehicle plus its maximum load (typically printed on the inside of the driver's door).[38] This exception was created for taxpayers who need to use large vehicles in their businesses such as farmers, construction workers and others—but not white-collar professionals. However, without further limitations, any taxpayer would be able to expense "heavy" SUVs (assuming they were used for business). When the limited expensing amount was raised to $100,000 ($250,000 in 2009), this enabled taxpayers to deduct the entire cost of a qualified SUV. For example, the taxpayer could expense the entire cost of a Porsche Cayenne or a Hummer H2 that weigh about 7,000 pounds and cost more than $100,000, assuming they were used entirely for business. Believing that many of these SUVs were in reality luxury automobiles, Congress decided to close what had become the so-called Hummer loophole.

As revised, §179 now limits the first-year write-off for vehicles considered SUVs. The maximum amount that can be expensed in the first year is limited to $25,000. Taxpayers may still claim regular depreciation for the balance. Note that the $25,000 amount is not reduced for personal use (as are the other limitations as seen in Example 20).

The $25,000 allowance applies only to SUVs as defined in §179(b)(6)(B). This provision defines an SUV as any four-wheeled vehicle that is primarily designed or that can be used to carry passengers over public streets, roads, or highways and that weighs more than 6,000 pounds unloaded gross weight and not more than 14,000 pounds gross vehicle weight. Thus heavier vehicles, weighing 14,000 pounds or more (e.g., refrigerated trucks) are not subject to the $25,000 limitation. Similarly, to ensure that the $25,000 limitation does not apply to heavy pickup trucks, vans and small buses (and thereby allowing the taxpayer to expense up to $250,000 of their cost), the following vehicles are not considered SUVs.

- A vehicle designed to have a seating capacity of more than nine persons behind the driver's seat.
- A vehicle equipped with a cargo area of at least six feet in interior length which is an open area or is designed for use as an open area but is enclosed by a cap and is not readily accessible directly from the passenger compartment.
- A vehicle having an integral enclosure, fully enclosing the driver compartment and load carrying device, and does not have seating rearward of the driver's seat.
- A vehicle having no body section protruding more than 30 inches ahead of the leading edge of the windshield.

Note that the exceptions would permit deductions for large pick-up trucks weighing more than 6,000 pounds under the cargo area exception or because it as no seats behind the driver. Similarly, cargo vans should qualify under the exception.

Example 23. In 2009, T purchased a Lexus LX 470 for $65,000. The SUV has a GVW exceeding 6,000 pounds and is used 100% for business. In such case, the § 179 deduction is $25,000, the bonus depreciation is $20,000 [50% × ($65,000 − $25,000 = $40,000)] and regular depreciation would be $4,000 [20% × ($65,000 − $45,000 = $20,000)] for a total deduction of $49,000 ($25,000 + $20,000 + $4,000). If T were in the 35% tax bracket, the deduction would save him $17,150. Note that the limitation on the § 179 deduction is $25,000 and there is no limit on depreciation since the SUV is not a passenger automobile because it weighs more than 6,000 pounds.

[38] PLR 9520034.

Example 24. Same facts as in *Example 23* except the SUV is used 80% of the time for business. There is no reduction for the $25,000 allowance as is required for the luxury automobile limitations. Thus the § 179 amount is still $25,000. However, depreciation must be adjusted for personal use, reducing bonus depreciation to $16,000 [50% × $32,000 (80% × ($65,000 − $25,000 = $40,000))] and regular depreciation to $4,800 [20% × $24,000 ($65,000 − $25,000 − $16,000)] for a total deduction of $45,800 ($25,000 + $16,000 + $4,800).

Below is a list of some SUVs with GVWs more than 6,000 pounds:

SUV	
BMW X5	Land Rover Discovery
Cadillac Escalade	Land Rover Range Rover
Chevrolet Suburban	Lexus LX 470
Chevrolet Tahoe	Lexus GX 470
Dodge Durango	Lincoln Navigator
Ford Expedition	Mercedes-Benz M Class
Ford Excursion	Mercedes-Benz G 500
Hummer H2	Porsche Cayenne
Hummer H1	Toyota Land Cruiser
GMC Yukon	Toyota Sequoia

LIMITATIONS FOR PERSONAL USE

Section 280F also restricts the amount of depreciation that may be claimed for so-called listed property that is not used predominantly—more than 50 percent—for business. If the property is not used more than 50 percent *for business* in the year it is placed in service, the following restrictions are imposed:[39]

1. Limited expensing under § 179 is not allowed.

2. MACRS may *not* be used in computing depreciation. Property not qualifying must be depreciated using the straight-line method of ADS and the asset's class life (except in the case of certain property such as automobiles and computers, where the life to be used is specifically prescribed as five years).

Note that these restrictions are imposed if the property is not used primarily for business in the *first* year. Subsequent usage in excess of 50 percent does not permit the taxpayer to amend the earlier return or later use accelerated depreciation or limited expensing. On the other hand, if qualified usage initially exceeds 50 percent but subsequently drops to 50 percent or below, benefits previously secured must be relinquished. The recapture of these benefits is discussed below. Exhibit 9-15 identifies the depreciation methods available for listed property.

These restrictions apply only to *listed property*. Listed property includes the following:[40]

1. Passenger automobiles (as defined above)

2. Any other property used as a means for transportation (e.g., motorcycles and trucks)

---

[39] § 280F(b).

[40] § 280F(d)(4).

3. Any property generally used for purposes of entertainment, recreation, or amusement (e.g., yacht, photography equipment, video recorders, and stereo equipment) *unless* used exclusively at a regular business establishment (e.g., at the office or at a home office) or in connection with the taxpayer's principal trade or business

4. Any computer or peripheral equipment *unless* used exclusively at a regular business establishment

5. Any cellular telephones and similar communications equipment

Example 25. K, self-employed, purchased a car for $20,000 in 2009. She uses her car 40% of the time for business and the remaining time for personal purposes. Since the property is a car, the limitations on depreciation are first reduced in light of the personal usage. In the first year, depreciation would initially be limited to $1,184 ($2,960 maximum allowed × 40% business use). In addition, since the car is listed property and is not used more than 50% for business, K must use ADS to compute depreciation. Thus, no bonus depreciation is allowed. Therefore, depreciation in the first year is $800 ($20,000 cost × 40% business use = $8,000 × 10% ADS rate).

Qualified Business Use. In determining whether the property is used more than 50 percent for business, only *qualified business use* is considered.[41] Generally, qualified business use means any use in a trade or business of the taxpayer.[42] Thus, for this test *only*, use in an activity that does not constitute a trade or business is ignored (e.g., use of a computer to monitor the taxpayer's investments does not count toward the 50 percent threshold since the activity is not a business).[43] Additionally, an employee's use of his or her own property in connection with employment is not considered business use unless it is for the *convenience of the employer* and is *required as a condition of employment.*[44] According to the Regulations, these two requirements generally have the same meaning for § 280F as they have for § 119 relating to the exclusion for meals or lodging.[45] Given this interpretation, a mere statement by the employer expressly requiring the employee to use the property is insufficient. Ordinarily, the property is considered required only if it enables the employee to properly perform the duties of his or her employment.

Example 26. T is employed by X, a newspaper company, to deliver papers in a rural area where the homes are widely scattered. The company does not provide T with a car and does not require T to own a car for employment. Since the car enables T to properly perform his duties and is for the convenience of X, T's use should qualify for purposes of the 50% test even though he is not explicitly required to own a car.

Example 27. J is a budget analyst in the accounting department of a large construction firm. She owns a personal computer that is identical to the one she uses at work. Instead of staying late at the office, J occasionally brings home work for which she uses her computer. J's use of her computer for her work is not qualified business use.

---

[41]   § 280F(b)(1) and (2).

[42]   § 280F(d)(6).

[43]   Temp. Reg. § 1.280F-6T(d)(2).

[44]   § 280F(d)(3).

[45]   Temp. Reg. § 1.280F-6T(a)(2).

EXHIBIT 9-15

Depreciation Methods Available for Listed Property

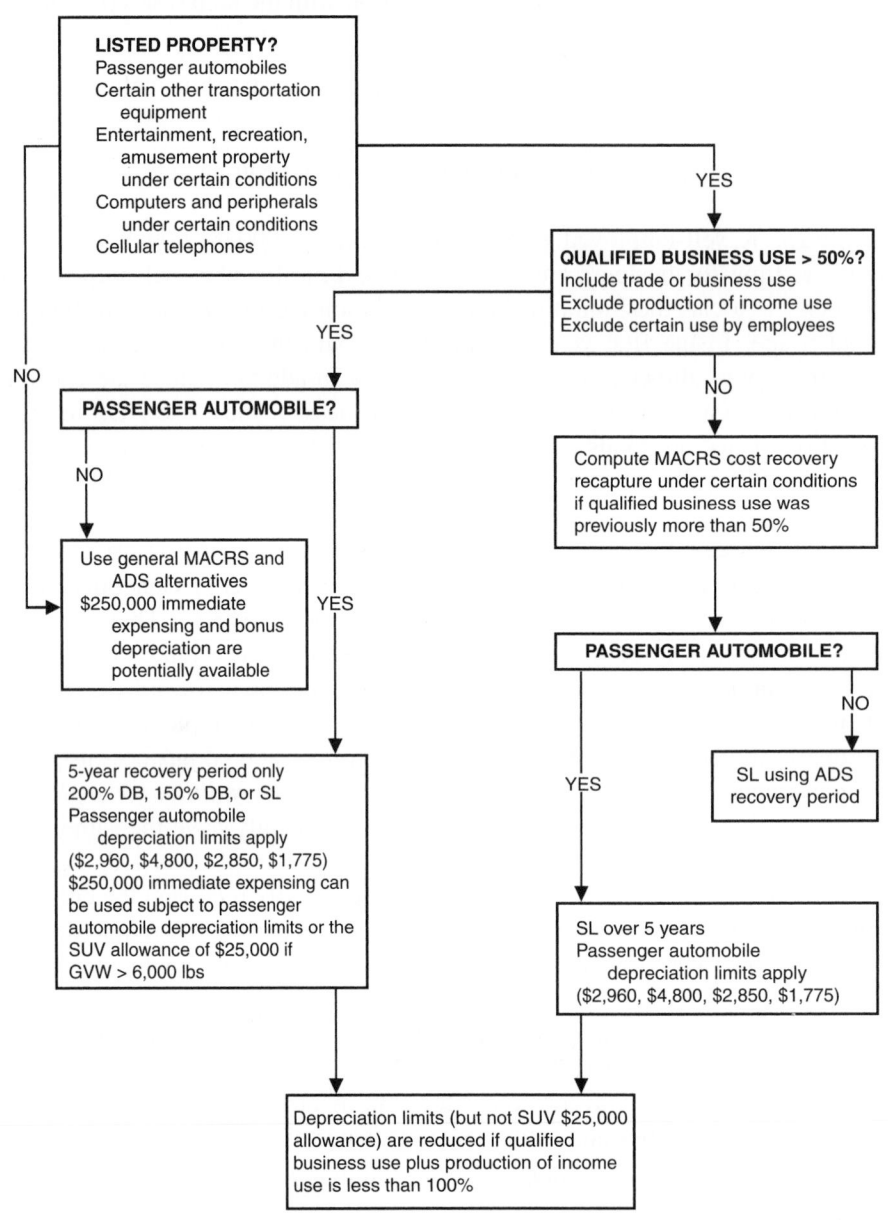

The IRS takes a very narrow view regarding what satisfies the convenience-of-the-employer and condition-of-employment tests. In one instance, the Service held that a professor's use of her home computer for writing related to her research—which was required for continued employment—did not satisfy the tests.[46] Although the Service agreed that the use of the computer was related to her work, it found no evidence that employees who did not use home computers were professionally disadvantaged. The Service also felt that her employer did not explicitly require use of the home computer before she was hired. Apparently, the Service will require taxpayers to demonstrate that the work could not properly be performed without the computer or at least that they will

---

[46] Letter Ruling 8615024.

be professionally disadvantaged if they do not use the computer. In addition, under the IRS view, taxpayers will be obliged to show that use of the computer was mandatory and not optional.

The reach of this and other rulings goes farther than it first appears. As brought out by the Service, a literal interpretation of the statute indicates that if an employee does not satisfy the convenience-of-the-employer and condition-of-employment tests, *none* of the employee's use is treated as business use. This view does *not* mean that the employee is merely relegated to using ADS for depreciation. Rather, with no business use, the employee is prohibited from claiming any deductions relating to the listed property. Only time will tell whether this interpretation is consistent with Congressional intent.

In those cases where qualified business use exceeds 50 percent, any usage for the production of income or other business purposes is included in determining the percentage of the asset that may be depreciated using MACRS. Similarly, if business use is 50 percent or less, the usage for production of income or other nonqualified business purposes is still included in determining the percentage of the asset that may be depreciated using ADS. Note that depreciation is still allowed where the 50 percent test is not met, assuming there is business or investment usage.

> **Example 28.** V, a financial consultant, purchased a car for $20,000. She uses the car 25% of the time for business and 55% for production of income activities that do not qualify as a business. V must use ADS since business usage is only 25%. Although the time spent for the production of income cannot be counted toward the 50% test, it may be considered in the depreciation computation. Thus, V's depreciation would be $1,600 [$20,000 × (55% + 25%) × 10%]. It should be noted that where the listed property is an automobile, the limitations on depreciation also apply. Here the depreciation limitation is $2,368 [(55% + 25%) × $2,960]; note that the production of income usage is considered in making the proper reduction]; thus it does not restrict the amount of the depreciation deduction. Had the usage percentages been reversed (i.e., 55% for business), the depreciation and limited expensing deduction would still have been limited to $2,368.

Employer-Provided Cars. The qualified business use rules directly address the problems of the company-owned car and other company-owned property used by employees. In the case of automobiles, employers typically provide company-owned cars to their employees principally for use in the employer's business. Normally, however, the employee also uses the car for personal purposes if only to commute to work. Under prior law, the employer claimed deductions and credits for the car without limitation (i.e., 100 percent of the car's basis was taken into account) while employees were required to treat the personal use as compensation. In most cases, the compensation income was avoided as long as the employee reimbursed the company for the value of the personal use, which the company in turn reported as income. Section 280F now prescribes specific rules governing depreciation where listed property is used by someone *other than* the owner—such as an employer-provided automobile. The following discussion examines these rules as they apply to employer-provided automobiles; however, such rules extend to other listed property as well.

Where an employee uses an automobile, an *employer* is able to secure 100 percent qualified business use—and thus depreciate the entire cost of the automobile—in one of four ways.[47]

1. The employee's actual business usage is disregarded and the *entire value* of using the vehicle is included in the employee's income.

---

[47] Temp. Reg. § 1.280F-6T(d)(4)(iv).

2.   The employee's actual business usage is combined with inclusion of the value of any personal use by the employee as income.

3.   The employee's actual business usage is combined with a reimbursement arrangement where the employee reimburses the employer for any personal use (i.e. a fair rent is paid).

4.   The use falls under one of four exceptions.

Conditions 2 and 3 cannot be applied to qualify the use of a person owning greater than a 5 percent interest in the business (e.g., the company president, who is also a 30 percent shareholder). In this case, the employer can depreciate the car based only on the employee's actual business usage.

Before looking at several examples of these rules, it should be noted that each requires a valuation of the vehicle's use to the employee. The value can be determined using a facts-and-circumstances approach (e.g., considering such variables as geographic location, make and model, etc.) or one of several safe harbors provided by Temporary Regulations.[48] For example, the Regulations provide a table (i.e., a lease value table) based on the car's total value which provides values for personal use. Another alternative that can be used to value personal use under certain circumstances is the standard mileage allowance.

> **Example 29.**   During the 2009, X Corporation provided T, an employee, with a new car costing $10,000. T drove the company car 15,000 miles, 9,000 miles or 60% for business purposes, and 6,000 miles or 40% for personal purposes. X Corporation may use any of the first three alternatives to account for the car.
>
> *Alternative No. 1.* Under this full inclusion method, the employee's actual use is disregarded and the employee must include 100% of the value of the car's use in income, $8,250 (15,000 × 55 cents—the standard mileage rate for 2009)[49] just as if it were salary (i.e., X Corporation includes it on T's Form W-2 and withholds income and FICA taxes). Therefore, all of T's use qualifies and X may depreciate 100% of the car using MACRS. T may then deduct any substantiated business use as a miscellaneous itemized deduction subject to the 2% floor. One advantage of this method for the employer is that it shifts all of the substantiation burden to the employee.
>
> *Alternative No. 2.* Under this partial inclusion method, only T's personal use is treated as income, or $3,300 (6,000 × 55 cents). X could depreciate the car in the same manner as above. T may be better off under this method since the amount of compensation is reduced. This may have an effect on the amount of deductions or credits T may otherwise claim (e.g., the 2% floor on miscellaneous itemized deductions would be smaller due to the lower amount of income). In this case, X must be able to substantiate the employee's actual business use.
>
> *Alternative No. 3.* Under the rental reimbursement method, T would pay X Corporation for his personal use, $3,300. X could depreciate the car in the same manner as above. T would be worse off in this situation. Each dollar of reimbursement costs T one dollar, while inclusion of the value of the personal use costs the employee only the tax on the value. Again, X must be able to substantiate the employee's actual business use.
>
> *Five Percent Owner.* If T owns 5% or more of the business (i.e., X Corporation), the only alternative is to compute depreciation using T's actual business mileage. In

---

[48]   Temp. Reg. § 1.61-2T(d)(2)(iii).

[49]   See Chapter 8 for discussion of standard mileage rate.

this case, X could depreciate 60% of the car using MACRS. Had T's business usage been 50% or less, X would be required to use ADS to compute depreciation.

Additional rules for determining qualified business usage exist for other situations. For example, leasing the property to a 5 percent owner of the business or a related person is not considered qualified business use. Similarly, special rules are provided for aircraft.

Recapture Provisions. If the 50 percent test is satisfied in the year property is placed in service but failed prior to the time when the cost of the asset would be completely recovered using the listed property recovery rules, the taxpayer is required to relinquish the benefits of MACRS. Technically, the taxpayer must recompute the depreciation in the prior years using ADS and include in income the excess of the depreciation actually claimed over the ADS amounts. Depreciation in future years is computed using the straight-line method.

Example 30. In 20X1 G purchased a car for $10,000 and used it entirely for business. Depreciation for 20X1 was $2,000 ($10,000 × 20%). In 20X2 G's business usage dropped to 40%. Since G's business usage is no longer greater than 50%, he must recapture the benefits of accelerated depreciation. Depreciation using the straight-line method in 20X1 would have been $1,000 ($10,000 × 10%). Thus, G must include $1,000 ($2,000 original depreciation—$1,000 straight-line depreciation) in income in 20X2. Depreciation for 20X2 and all subsequent years must be computed using the straight-line method.

Recordkeeping Requirements. Not only has Congress severely restricted tax benefits for listed property, it also has imposed strict record keeping requirements for such property. The substantiation rules contained in Code § 274(d), which were formerly reserved solely for travel and entertainment expenses, now extend to expenses related to "listed property." For listed property, the taxpayer is required to substantiate the following:[50]

1. The amount of each expenditure related to the property, including the cost of acquisition, maintenance, and repairs

2. The date of the use of the property

3. The amount of each business or investment use as well as total use [the number of miles—in the case of a car or other means of transportation—or the amount of time that the property was used for other listed property (e.g., a computer)]

4. The purpose of the use of the property

In those cases where the overall use of the property for a taxable year can be definitely determined without entries, nonbusiness use need not be recorded. For example, in the case of a car, total miles can be determined by comparing the odometer readings at the beginning and the end of the taxable year. Consequently, the taxpayer needs to make entries only for business and investment use.

---

[50] Temp. Reg. § 1.274-5T(b)(6).

☑️ *CHECK YOUR KNOWLEDGE*

Review Question 1. This year Y purchased new property. Indicate whether the following questions are true or false.

a.   Assuming the property is a duplex that Y rents to others, she may not expense any of the cost.

True. Only eligible property may be expensed. As a general rule, only personal property such as machinery and equipment are eligible. Buildings are normally not eligible.

b.   Assuming the property is machinery costing $270,000, Y may expense $250,000, and the $20,000 balance may be carried over to the following years to be expensed to the extent the maximum amount is not used in such years.

False. Y may expense $250,000, and the balance is subject to depreciation

c.   Assuming the property is a $20,000 passenger automobile that is used 70 percent for business, Y may deduct $14,000.

False. Depreciation and expensing for automobiles are limited. The maximum amount of depreciation or expense claimed in the year the automobile is placed in service is limited to $2,072 ($2,960 × 70%). In 2008 and 2009, if bonus depreciation is used, this amount could be increased to $7,672 [80% × ($2,960 + $8,000)]. This amount could be deducted for the current year, and the remaining balance could be depreciated beginning next year.

d.   Assuming the property is a $40,000 car that is used 30 percent for business, Y may deduct $888 ($2,960 × 30%).

True. If the property is listed property and qualified business use does not exceed 50 percent, the taxpayer is not allowed to expense any of the car and must use straight-line depreciation. Therefore, Y's potential deduction is $1,200 ($40,000 × 30% × 10%) but is limited to $888. Note that in 2008 and 2009 the basic limitation is increased by $8,000 to $10,960 if bonus depreciation is used. However, if the property is depreciated using ADS, which is required in this case, bonus depreciation is not permitted. Thus the answer would be the same.

e.   If the property is listed property, such as a passenger automobile or a computer, and the property is not used more than 50 percent of the time for business, the restrictions of § 280F do not affect the total amount of cost deducted but simply alter the time when it is deducted.

True. The total depreciation is not changed. If the property is restricted and qualified business use does not exceed 50 percent, the taxpayer is simply forced to use the straight-line method in lieu of the accelerated methods of MACRS and the expensing allowance of § 179 that are normally available.

OTHER CONSIDERATIONS

Anti-Churning Rules. In some cases, a taxpayer's depreciation deductions under MACRS would be higher than those that the taxpayer may currently have. For this reason, Congress believed that some taxpayers would engage in transactions that might enable them to secure the advantages of MACRS.

Example 31. In 1980 H acquired an apartment building as an investment that she chose to depreciate using the straight-line method over 35 years. H made this decision

because the use of accelerated depreciation caused a portion of any gain from the sub-sequent sale of such property to be treated as ordinary income rather than favorable capital-gain. With the elimination of favorable capital-gain treatment in 1986, there no longer was any disincentive to use the accelerated method. Therefore, H created a plan to benefit from the change. She sold the property to her son, who immediately leased it back to her. The rental payments to be paid by H were structured in light of the higher depreciation deductions (27.5-year life instead of 35 years) that her son would be able to take as the new owner of the property.

Sales, exchanges, and other dispositions of assets such as that illustrated above are referred to as "churning" transactions—exchanges of used property solely to obtain the benefits of MACRS.

The thrust of the anti-churning rules is to preclude the use of MACRS for property placed in service prior to the enactment of either version of MACRS, unless the property is transferred in a transaction where not only the owner changes but also the user.[51] In *Example 31* the anti-churning rules prohibit H's son from using MACRS since ownership did not truly change.

There are three sets of rules designed to police churning. For practical purposes these provisions should be given close review whenever the taxpayer is involved in a leasing or nontaxable transaction. For example, a taxpayer would typically be subject to the anti-churning rules in the following situations:

1. Sale followed by immediate leaseback

2. Like-kind exchange

3. Formation and liquidation of a corporation or partnership, including transfers of property to and distributions from these entities

Expensing Costs of Qualified Film and Television Productions. Over the years, production of American film projects has migrated to foreign locations often lured by tax and other incentives offered by foreign countries. To encourage producers to bring feature film and television production projects back to the U.S., Congress created § 181 in 2004. Section 181 allows immediate deduction for costs of qualified film or television productions. To qualify, one condition requires that at least 75 percent of the total compensation expended on the production is for services performed in the U.S.. The special expensing allowance is limited to smaller productions in that it does not apply if the aggregate production costs exceed $15 million. In other words, if the total costs exceed $15 million, none can be expensed. Instead the amount must be capitalized and amortized. The $15 million amount is increased to $20 million if a significant amount of the production expenditures are incurred in areas eligible for designation as a low-income community or eligible for designation by the Delta Regional Authority as a distressed county or isolated area.

Property Leased to Tax-Exempt Entities. For a variety of reasons, tax-exempt enti-ties, such as schools, hospitals, or government organizations, lease property from taxable entities rather than purchase it. One incentive for this type of transaction is that the taxable entity can benefit from depreciation deductions, whereas the tax-exempt entity cannot. Thus, a tax plan might be devised under which a taxable lessor and a tax-exempt lessee "share" the tax benefits of the depreciation deductions. This would be accomplished through discounted lease payments. The taxable lessor would be willing to accept discounted lease payments "in exchange" for receiving all of the tax benefits from depreciation deductions. To reduce the incentive for this type of tax plan, depreciation of

---

[51]   § 168(e)(4).

"tax-exempt use property"—most property leased to a "tax-exempt entity"—must be depreciated using ADS with special rules to determine the applicable recovery period.[52] This rule applies regardless of the tax planning motives of the lessor and lessee. The result of the rule is to lower the present value of the tax savings from the depreciation deductions. There are several types of leasing transactions that are exempted from the rule. For example, the rule does not apply to "short-term leases."

AMORTIZATION

As previously discussed, MACRS does not apply to intangible property. Therefore, intangibles are subject to the rules existing prior to enactment of ACRS and MACRS. Generally, intangibles are amortized using the straight-line method over their estimated useful life. Special amortization and depreciation rules apply to certain expenditures, however.

GOODWILL AND COVENANTS NOT TO COMPETE

As mentioned in Chapter 6, buyers of a going concern often pay an amount in excess of the fair market value of the concern's tangible assets. This excess purchase price normally is attributable to intangible assets such as goodwill and/or a covenant not to compete. The tax treatment for such intangible assets was changed dramatically by the Revenue Reconciliation Act of 1993 for acquisitions occurring after August 10, 1993. Acquisitions taking place on or before August 10, 1993 continue to be treated under prior law, which held that goodwill could not be amortized because it was considered as having an unlimited life. Thus, recovery of a taxpayer's basis in goodwill could occur only when the business was subsequently sold or abandoned. In contrast, a covenant not to compete usually has an ascertainable life because the seller typically agrees to refrain from conducting similar business or some other activity for a certain number of years. As a result, prior law held that any cost attributable to the covenant may be amortized over the appropriate period using the straight-line method.

Under prior law, taxpayers attempted to allocate the purchase price to assets other than goodwill since goodwill could not be amortized. In this regard, accountants were quite creative, assigning the purchase price to a variety of intangibles such as covenants not to compete, favorable contracts, customer lists, accounting control systems, and a long list of other items. As long as the taxpayer was able to establish that the intangible was separate and distinct from goodwill and had a determinable useful life, the taxpayer was entitled to amortize the cost. For example, a taxpayer might allocate a substantial portion of the purchase price of a business to a covenant not to compete and amortize the cost over three years, producing a significant benefit where otherwise there would be no benefit at all if the cost were allocated to goodwill.

Post–August 10, 1993 Acquisitions. As might be expected, the IRS did not sit idly by and allow taxpayers to do as they pleased. In case after case, the IRS challenged the taxpayer's allocation, and there was a great deal of controversy and litigation. To put an end to the disputes and clear up the uncertainty, Congress enacted § 197. Effective for acquisitions after August 10, 1993 all "Section 197 intangibles" must be amortized over 15 years. (A taxpayer may elect to have the rules of § 197 apply to intangibles acquired after July 15, 1991.) Much like MACRS, § 197 forces the taxpayer to use the 15-year period even if the useful life is actually more or less than 15 years. Section 197 intangibles include a number of items such as goodwill, going-concern value, covenants

---

[52] § 168(g)(1)(C).

not to compete, information bases such as customer or subscription lists, know-how, customer-based intangibles, governmental licenses and permits (e.g., liquor licenses, taxicab medallions, landing or takeoff rights, regulated airline routes, television or radio licenses), franchises, trademarks, and trade names.

To further prohibit the deduction of an intangible obtained as part of an acquisition, special rules govern disposition. No loss is allowed on the disposition of an intangible if the business retains other intangible assets acquired in the same or a series of related transactions. Instead, any remaining basis is reallocated among the bases of other § 197 intangibles. Although losses are not recognized, the same treatment does not apply to gains.

If § 197 intangibles are sold at a gain, the gain is recognized. The tax character of the entire gain is ordinary income if the intangible is held one year or less. Gains from sales of intangibles held more than one year are treated as gains from sales of § 1245 property. As explained in Chapter 17, gains from dispositions of § 1245 property are "recaptured" and treated as ordinary income up to the amount of amortization on the intangible deducted through the time of sale. Any excess gain is a § 1231 gain.

> **Example 32.** Buyer allocates $150,000 to intangible assets in a purchase. Under § 197 Buyer would claim $10,000 per year for 15 years as an amortization deduction. The deduction would not be affected by breaking the $150,000 into separate portions for goodwill, a covenant not to compete, or any other specifically identified intangibles.
>
> Assume that the purchase occurred on January 1, 2009. Buyer will claim a $10,000 deduction every year for 15 years through 2023. Assume that Buyer allocates $105,000 to goodwill and the remaining $45,000 to a covenant not to compete that would expire on January 1, 2012. From 2009 through 2011. Buyer claims an annual amortization deduction of $3,000 ($45,000/15) on the covenant and $7,000 ($105,000/15) on the goodwill. Note that the covenant not to compete is amortized over 15 years regardless of its economic life. On January 1, 2012, Buyer will have an unrecovered basis of $36,000 on the covenant, which has expired [$45,000 − $9,000 amortization ($3,000 amortization per year for three years)]. However, Buyer must add the $36,000 unrecovered basis to the basis of goodwill and continue to deduct $10,000 per year as amortization of the goodwill.

A number of anti-churning rules exist to prohibit taxpayers from creating and amortizing goodwill and going-concern value. Other intangibles are not covered by these rules.

FIVE-YEAR ELECTIVE AMORTIZATION

To accomplish certain economic and social objectives, Congress has enacted various optional five-year (60-month) amortization procedures from time to time over the last 40 years. During certain periods, a five-year amortization election (in lieu of regular depreciation) has been available for expenditures made in connection with child care facilities (§ 188), pollution control facilities (still an option under § 169), railroad rolling stock (§ 184), and rehabilitation of low-income housing [§ 167(k)]. In 2006, Congress passed legislation allowing five-year amortization of costs of creating or acquiring musical works or copyrights (§167(g)).

LEASEHOLD IMPROVEMENTS

Taxpayers often lease property and improve the property while leasing it. In this situation, the lessee is entitled to recover the investment in the improvement.[53] After 1986, the

---

[53]   § 168(i)(8); also see § 178(a) when the lease permits renewals.

cost of any leasehold improvement made by a lessee is normally depreciated in the normal manner without regard to the term of the lease. However, under §168(e)(6), property owners are allowed to depreciate improvements they make for tenants, such as interior walls or lighting fixtures, over 15 years rather than the current 39 years. This special rule applies to property placed in service before 2010. They must use the straight-line method. Similarly, tenants who make their own improvements receive the same benefit. Any unrecovered cost at the end of the lease term would increase the taxpayer's basis for determining gain or loss. The recovery of the costs of acquiring a lease is determined under special rules in Code § 178.

DEPLETION

A taxpayer who invests in natural resources that are exhausted over time is entitled to recover his or her capital investment. Depletion is the method of recovering this cost and is similar to depreciation.[54] Depletion usually is claimed for investments in oil, gas, coal, copper, and other minerals. Land is not subject to depletion.

To qualify for depletion, the taxpayer must have an economic interest in the mineral deposits.[55] Typically, both the owner of the land who leases the property and the operator to whom the land is leased have the requisite interest since they both receive income from the severance or extraction of the minerals.

COMPUTING THE DEPLETION DEDUCTION

Taxpayers generally are permitted to compute their depletion deduction using either the cost or percentage (statutory) depletion method. The taxpayer computes both cost and percentage depletion and is required to claim the higher amount.[56]

Cost Depletion. Using cost depletion, the taxpayer recovers the actual investment (adjusted basis in the natural resource) as the mineral is produced. The following formula is used:[57]

$$\frac{\text{Annual cost}}{\text{depletion}} = \frac{\text{Unrecovered adjusted basis}}{\text{Estimated recoverable units}} \times \frac{\text{Number of units sold}}{\text{during the year}}$$

This formula generally matches the cost of the investment against the revenues produced.

Example 33. A coal producer, T, paid $150,000 to acquire the mineral rights in a property which contains coal. He estimates that 90,000 tons of coal are recoverable from the property. During the year, 58,000 tons of coal were produced and 30,000 were sold. T's cost depletion would be $50,000 computed as follows:

$$\frac{\$150,000 \text{ basis}}{90,000 \text{ units}} \times \frac{30,000}{\text{units sold}} = \frac{\$50,000}{\text{depletion}}$$

Similar to depreciation, total cost depletion can never exceed the taxpayer's adjusted basis in the property.

---

[54]   § 611.

[55]   Reg. § 1.611-1(b).

[56]   § 613(a); Reg. § 1.611-1(a).

[57]   Reg. § 1.611-2(a).

Percentage Depletion. For large oil and gas producers, cost depletion is the only depletion method allowed. However, both cost depletion and percentage depletion are available to small "independent" oil and gas producers as well as royalty owners.[58] Both cost depletion and percentage depletion are also allowed for *all* producers of certain types of minerals (e.g., gold, silver, gravel).

Under the percentage depletion method, the taxpayer's depletion deduction is computed *without reference* to the taxpayer's cost of the investment. Rather, percentage depletion is based on the amount of income derived from the property.[59] For this reason, the taxpayer may deduct percentage depletion in excess of the adjusted basis of the investment. Thus, the taxpayer is entitled to a deduction for percentage depletion as long as the property continues to generate income.

To compute percentage depletion, a percentage specified in the Code (see Exhibit 9-16) is applied to the *gross* income from the property. The resulting product is the amount of percentage depletion unless limited. For oil and gas properties, percentage depletion is generally limited to the taxpayer's *taxable* income before depletion. Percentage depletion is limited to 50 percent of the taxpayer's taxable income from mineral properties. Gross income is the value of the natural resource when severed from the property before any processing. Taxable income from the property is the difference between income and operating expenses including overhead.

EXHIBIT 9-16
Summary of Various Percentage Depletion Rates

Natural Resource	Percentage Rate
1. Gravel, sand, and other items	5
2. Shale and clay used for sewer pipes; or brick and clay, shale, and slate used for lightweight aggregates	7.5
3. Asbestos, coal, sodium chloride, etc.	10
4. Gold, silver, oil and gas, oil shale, copper, and iron ore from deposits in the United States	15
5. Sulfur and uranium and a series of minerals from deposits in the United States	22
6. Metals, other than those subject to 22% or 15% rate	14

Example 34. Assume the same facts in *Example 33* and that the 30,000 tons sold were sold for $10 per ton (gross income of $300,000). Further, operating expenses attributable to the coal operation were $260,000. Percentage depletion is computed as follows:

Gross income	$300,000
Statutory percentage for coal	× 10%
Percentage depletion before limitation	$ 30,000

Taxable income limitation:

Gross income	$300,000
Less: Operating expenses	− 260,000
Taxable income before depletion	$ 40,000
Limitation percentage	× 50%
Percentage depletion limit	$ 20,000
Percentage depletion allowable	$ 20,000

---

[58] § 613A(c).

[59] § 613.

In this situation, T would use cost depletion of $50,000 as computed in *Example 33* because it exceeds allowable percentage depletion.

Example 35. Assume the same facts in *Example 34* except that barrels of oil are being produced, rather than tons of coal. Cost depletion computations are the same as in *Example 33*. Percentage depletion is computed as follows:

Gross income.	$300,000
Statutory percentage for oil	× 15%
Percentage depletion before limitation	$ 45,000
Gross income.	$300,000
Less: Operating expenses	− 260,000
Taxable income before depletion.	$ 40,000
Percentage depletion limit	$ 40,000
Percentage depletion allowable.	$ 40,000

T would use cost depletion of $50,000 (computed in *Example 33*) rather than percentage depletion of $40,000 because cost depletion is larger.

Whether percentage or cost depletion is used, the taxpayer must reduce the property's basis (but not below zero) by the amount of depletion claimed. Note that once the basis of the property is reduced to zero, only percentage depletion may be claimed (when the taxpayer is permitted to take percentage depletion), and *no* adjustment is made to create a negative basis.

RESEARCH AND EXPERIMENTAL EXPENDITURES

At first glance, it may appear that the proper tax treatment for research and development expenses requires their capitalization as part of a project's cost. This approach seems appropriate since these costs normally yield benefits only in future periods. Under this theory, the capitalized costs could be recovered over the period during which the project provides benefits or when the project is disposed of or abandoned. Upon closer examination, however, it becomes apparent that this approach is fraught with problems. Since it is difficult to establish any direct relationship between costs of research and development and the actual period benefited, it may be impossible to determine the appropriate period for recovery. For example, establishing a useful life for a scientific discovery that has numerous applications and which continually contributes to later research would be guesswork at best. A similar problem exists for unsuccessful efforts. Although a particular effort may not prove fruitful, it may at least indicate what does not work and thus lead to other, perhaps successful, research. In such case, it is not clear whether the costs should be written off or capitalized as part of the subsequent project.

Due to the administrative difficulties inherent in these determinations, the IRS historically granted research and experimental costs favorable treatment by generally allowing the taxpayer to deduct the expenses as incurred or to capitalize the expenses and amortize them over whatever period the taxpayer desires. Although this approach encountered difficulties in the courts, Congress eliminated the problems with enactment of special provisions in 1954.

RESEARCH AND EXPERIMENTAL EXPENDITURES DEFINED

The Code provides separate rules for research and experimental costs.[60] It should be emphasized that the provisions apply to research and *experimental* costs, not to research and development costs. The term *experimental* was used instead of *development* to limit the special treatment to laboratory costs.[61] Qualified costs generally include those incident to the development or improvement of a product, a formula, an invention, a plant process, an experimental or pilot model, or similar property. Research and experimental costs do *not* include expenditures for ordinary testing or inspection of materials or products for quality control, efficiency surveys, management studies, consumer surveys, advertising, or promotion. Costs of obtaining a patent, such as legal fees, qualify. However, the costs of acquiring an existing patent, model, or process are not considered research and experimental costs. Expenditures for depreciable property do not qualify but the depreciation allowable on the property is eligible for special treatment.

ALTERNATIVE TAX TREATMENTS

Three alternative methods may be used to account for research and experimental expenditures. The expenses may be deducted as they are paid or incurred, deferred and amortized, or capitalized. Immediate deduction usually is the preferred method since the present value of the tax benefit is greater using this method. Deferral may be preferable in two instances, however. If the taxpayer's income is low in the current year, the tax benefit of the deduction might be increased by deferring the deduction to high-income years when the taxpayer is in a higher marginal tax bracket. Deferral also may be better if an immediate deduction creates or adds to a net operating loss since such losses may be carried over and used only for a limited period of time. The general rule for selecting the best alternative is to choose the one that maximizes the present value of the tax savings from the research and experimental expenditures.

Expense Election. The taxpayer can elect to deduct all research and experimental expenditures currently.[62] Note, however, that expenditures for depreciable property cannot be expensed currently.[63] If the taxpayer adopts this method in the first tax year in which research and experimental expenses are incurred, the method must be used for all such expenditures in all subsequent years, unless permission is secured to change methods of part or all of the expenditures.[64] The IRS does not need to approve the method the taxpayer adopts initially. Consent is required, however, if the taxpayer wishes to change methods.

Deferral Option. Research and experimental expenditures may be deferred and amortized at the election of the taxpayer.[65] The expenses must be amortized ratably over a period not less than 60 months beginning in the period in which benefits from the expenditures are first realized. It should be emphasized that costs of depreciable property are not deferred expenses; rather, the depreciation expense must be capitalized and amortized over 60 months. Also, if the taxpayer elects to defer the expenditures and a patent is subsequently obtained, the cost must be amortized over the life of the patent,

---

[60] § 174.

[61] Reg. § 1.174-2(a).

[62] § 174(a).

[63] § 174(c).

[64] § 174(a)(2).

[65] § 174(b).

20 years (17 before June 8, 1995). If the deferral method is initially elected, the taxpayer must use this method for all future expenses in subsequent tax years unless permission to change methods is obtained.[66]

Election to Capitalize. A taxpayer who does not elect either to amortize research and experimental expenditures over 60 months or to deduct them currently must capitalize them. Capitalizing the expenditure increases the basis of the property to which the expense relates. No deduction is permitted for the capital expenditure until the research project is considered worthless or abandoned. A disposition of the research project such as a sale or an exchange enables the taxpayer to offset the capitalized expenditures—the basis of the project—against any amount realized.

Example 36. L Corporation, a drug manufacturer, is an accrual basis, calendar year taxpayer. During 2009 the corporation performed research to improve various cold and flu medications. On December 1, 2009 a new cold and flu product line was successfully introduced on the market. In connection with this project, L incurred the following costs:

Lab equipment (5-year property)	$50,000
Salaries	90,000
Laboratory materials	5,000

If L Corporation elects to expense the research and experimental costs, it may deduct $105,000 in 2009 as follows:

MACRS depreciation on lab equipment (20% of $50,000)	$ 10,000
Salaries	90,000
Laboratory materials	5,000
Total deductions	$105,000

Note that only the depreciation on the lab equipment may be deducted as a research and experimental cost, not the entire cost of the equipment. If L Corporation elects to defer the expense, its monthly amortization beginning December 1, 2009 would be

$$\frac{\$105,000}{60} = \$1,750$$

Alternatively, L could capitalize all the expenses as an asset (including the $10,000 of depreciation) and receive no deduction until a later disposition or abandonment.

OTHER RELATED PROVISIONS

Several other provisions exist relating to the treatment of research and experimental expenditures, such as a tax credit for research and experimentation. Generally, the credit is 20 percent of the current year's expenditures after adjustments (see Chapter 13).[67] Taxpayers electing the credit are generally required to reduce their research and experimentation expenses by 50 percent of the credit for purposes of computing the amount to either be expensed, deferred, or capitalized.[68] Special rules also exist for contributions of research property by corporations (see Chapter 11).[69]

---

[66] § 174(b)(2).

[67] § 41.

[68] § 280C(c).

[69] § 170.

EXPENSES OF FARMERS AND RANCHERS

Special provisions exist for certain types of expenditures incurred by those engaged in farming and ranching. The rules examined below generally differ from the treatment of expenses that normally would be considered capital expenditures subject to depreciation.

EXPENSES RELATED TO LIVESTOCK

Costs of acquiring animals used for breeding, dairy, work, or sport are treated as capital expenditures and are depreciable under MACRS unless such animals are primarily held for sale and would be appropriately included in inventory. If a farmer raises his or her own livestock, however, expenses incurred such as feed normally can be deducted as paid, assuming the taxpayer uses the cash basis method of accounting.[70] This rule is in sharp contrast to that applying to other self-production costs. Costs incurred by farmers and others in constructing their own equipment and buildings must be capitalized and depreciated.

SOIL AND WATER CONSERVATION, FERTILIZER, LAND CLEARING

Farmers often incur expenses for soil and water conservation. Examples of these expenses are the costs of leveling or terracing the soil to control the flow of water, irrigation and drainage ditches, ponds, dams, eradication of brush, and planting windbreaks. Although normal tax rules would require these expenses to be capitalized, Code § 175 permits a deduction when such expenses are paid or incurred as long as such expenses are consistent with a conservation plan approved by the Soil Conservation Service of the Department of Agriculture. To encourage these practices and still restrict the availability of this benefit, the Code requires that the taxpayer be engaged in the business of farming. In addition, the annual deduction for these expenses is limited to 25 percent of the taxpayer's gross income from farming. This limitation prohibits a taxpayer from using the deductions to reduce nonfarm income. Expenditures exceeding this limitation may be carried over to subsequent years.

Like soil and water conservation expenditures, Code § 180 provides that the cost of fertilizer, lime, and other materials used to enrich farmland can be deducted in the year paid or incurred by those engaged in the business for farming. There is no limitation imposed on the amount of the deduction.

Taxpayers engaged in the farming business must capitalize expenses of clearing land in preparation for farming. These expenses include any cost of making the land suitable for farming such as those for removing and eradicating brush or tree stumps and the treating or moving of earth. Routine brush clearing and other ordinary maintenance related to the land may be expensed, however.

DEVELOPMENT EXPENSES

Expenses incurred in the development of farms and ranches prior to the time when production begins may be capitalized or expensed at the election of the taxpayer.[71] Examples of these expenses are costs of cultivation, spraying, pruning, irrigation, and management fees.

The expensing of development and other farm-related costs prior to the period in which the farm begins to produce income provides an attractive device for high-bracket

---

[70] Reg. § 1.162-12

[71] *Ibid.*

taxpayers—who have no interest in farming—to shelter their income from other nonfarm sources. These and other tax advantages offered by farming in the 1960s brought such an influx of "urban cowboys" to the farming industry that several farm groups protested and demanded protection. Congress first responded to these groups in 1969. Currently, this provision prohibits the immediate expensing of any amount attributable to the planting, cultivation, maintenance, or development of any citrus or almond grove. Any of these development costs that are incurred in the first four years of the grove's life must be capitalized.

Congress adopted additional safeguards in 1976. Section 447 generally requires that corporations (and partnerships having a corporate partner) engaged in the business of farming must use the accrual method of accounting. Since this provision was intended to protect small farmers and family-owned farms, the following are not treated as corporations: (1) S corporations; (2) family-owned corporations (at least 50 percent of the stock is owned by family members); and (3) any corporation that did not have gross receipts exceeding $1 million in any prior year. In addition, farming syndicates may deduct the costs of feed, seed, fertilizer, and similar farm supplies only as they are actually used.[72] A farming syndicate generally is defined to include partnerships and S corporations where the sale of their interests is specifically regulated by state or local securities laws, or more than 35 percent of their losses during any period are allocated to limited partners or persons who do not actively participate in the management of the business.

In 1986 the prohibition against the deduction of prepaid farming expenses was extended to all farmers that prepay more than 50 percent of their expenses such as feed, seed, and fertilizer.[73] Farmers cannot deduct such expenses until the items are consumed or used. Several exceptions exist, however.

TAX PLANNING CONSIDERATIONS

DEPRECIATION AND AFTER-TAX CASH FLOW

Many taxpayers, when analyzing an investment, fail to consider the tax aspects. For example, a taxpayer who looks solely to the cash flow projections of investing in a rental property might overlook the effect of depreciation. The depreciation deduction does not require an outlay of cash, but does produce a tax benefit.

Example 37. In January of the current year, L purchased a duplex for $80,000, which she rented to others. Of the $80,000 purchase price, $70,000 was allocable to the building and $10,000 was allocable to the land. L financed the purchase with a $5,000 downpayment and a mortgage calling for monthly payments of interest and principal of $400. During the year, L rented the property for $7,000. Expenses for the year were as follows:

Mortgage interest	$ 4,000
Taxes	1,200
Insurance	500
Maintenance and utilities	300
Depreciation (MACRS: $70,000 × 3.485%)	2,440
Total expenses	$ 8,440

---

[72]   § 464.

[73]   § 464(f).

The net taxable loss from the real property would be

Rental income	$ 7,000
Less: Rental expenses	− 8,440
Net taxable loss	$ 1,440

Note that the taxable loss contains depreciation expense of $2,440, a noncash expenditure. Assuming L is in the 28 percent tax bracket, the net cash flow from the project would be computed as follows:

Cash inflow:			
Rental income			$7,000
Tax saving from loss ($1,440 × 28%)			403
Total cash inflow			$7,403
Cash outflow:			
Total expenses		$ 8,440	
Less: Depreciation		− 2,440	
		$ 6,000	
Debt service			
Mortgage payments ($400 × 12)	$ 4,800		
Less: Interest (included in expenses above)	− 4,000	+ 800	
Total cash outflow			(6,800)
After-tax cash flow			$ 603

Therefore, L has a positive cash flow of $603 on the project notwithstanding the taxable loss that she suffered of $1,440.

Under certain circumstances, limitations are imposed on the deduction of losses from rental property. These limitations are discussed in Chapter 12.

ACCELERATING DEPRECIATION WITH COST SEGREGATION

Prior to 1981, some taxpayers used a technique called "component depreciation" to accelerate real estate depreciation deductions. These taxpayers separated the costs of their depreciable buildings into various components with useful lives shorter than the rest of the building. For example, structural components such as wiring, plumbing, and roofing were depreciated over periods of 10 or 15 years rather than the much longer periods typically associated with the useful life of the building shell.

While the introduction of ACRS and MACRS prohibited component depreciation, it did not eliminate a similar but different technique referred to as "cost segregation." In 1997, the Tax Court, in a the seminal case on cost segregation, *Hospital Corporation of America (HCA)*, permitted HCA for purposes of depreciation to segregate the costs of components constituting real property (§ 1250 property) and tangible personal property (§ 1250 property).[74] As a result, HCA was able to depreciate a long list of improvements as 5-year property rather than 39-year property, producing huge tax savings. Shortly after the *HCA* decision, the IRS grudgingly acquiesced and announced that cost segregation did not constitute component depreciation.[75] As a result, this subtle distinction permitted what has become the widespread use of cost segregation.

---

[74] 109 TC 21 (1997)

[75] AOD 1999-008 9/08/1999 and Announcement 99-116, 1999-52 I.R.B. 763. See also Reg. § 1.446-1T and CCA 199921045

The importance of cost segregation cannot be overemphasized. Consider the benefits of reclassifying $100,000 of property from a 39 to a 5 year recovery period. Depreciation as 39-year property using the required straight-line method produces an annual deduction of about $2,600 per year for 39 years. In contrast, depreciation as 5-year property using double declining balance results in the entire cost being deducted over six years ($20,000, $32,000, $19,200, $11,500, $11,500 and $5,760). Reclassifying $100,000 from 39 to 5-year property produces about $16,000 in net-present-value savings, assuming a 5% discount rate and a 35% marginal tax rate. It is no wonder that a whole niche business involving cost segregation has developed.

Examples of assets that taxpayers should segregate from the cost of the building and depreciate over five or seven years include movable partitions, computers, separate fire protection systems, manufacturing equipment and built-in desks and cabinets. Properties reclassified from 39 to 5 year property in *HCA* included carpeting, vinyl wall and floor coverings, electrical distribution system and a number of other items. A rule of thumb for identifying these separate depreciable assets is to assess whether the items would be removed if the business were to relocate. If so, the removable assets can have their own depreciation schedules.

Land improvements represent another set of costs that should be separated since they can be depreciated over 15 years. These include parking lots, landscaping, sewers and irrigation systems.

To segregate costs successfully, taxpayers or their advisers should work closely with building contractors to document the costs of fast-depreciating assets. Early involvement with the contractor or architect could even lead to building designs that maximize the number of separate depreciable assets while not reducing the productive use of the building.

GOODWILL AMORTIZATION RULE BENEFITS BUYERS AND SELLERS

Prior to August 10, 1993 the goodwill portion of the cost of acquiring a business provided no tax benefit to the buyer until the buyer later sold the business because the basis assigned to goodwill could not be amortized. Now that goodwill can be amortized over 15 years, its value is greater because the present value of a series of tax deductions received throughout a 15-year period is higher than the present value of a single deduction received many years in the future (assuming constant or declining marginal tax rates over time). Buyers and sellers will share this increase in value as they negotiate purchase/sale prices of their businesses.

Typically, buyers and sellers have some flexibility regarding the allocation of purchase price between goodwill (a capital asset that produces capital gain for the seller) and other intangibles. Two factors encourage increased allocations to goodwill. First, the seller will recognize capital gain income instead of ordinary income (assuming the allocation choice is between goodwill and a covenant not to compete). Second, for buyers concerned about earnings per share, goodwill may be preferable to payments for a covenant not to compete due to the treatment of goodwill under generally accepted accounting principles (GAAP). Under GAAP, goodwill normally is not amortized unless it is found to be impaired. Thus, as long as there is no reduction in the value of goodwill, no amortization is required. In contrast, the covenant may be amortized over its economic life. Buyers not concerned about GAAP should be indifferent between allocations to goodwill versus a covenant not to compete because *all* intangibles are amortizable over 15 years for tax purposes. Thus, at best, increased allocations to goodwill could benefit both buyers and sellers of businesses. At worst, increased goodwill allocations will neither help nor harm buyers or sellers.

PROBLEM MATERIALS

DISCUSSION QUESTIONS

9-1   *Requirements for Depreciation.* Indicate the basic requirements that must be satisfied before property may be depreciated.

9-2   *Depreciation and Amortization: Eligible Property.* Indicate whether a taxpayer could claim deductions for depreciation or amortization of the following property:
   a.   Land used in the taxpayer's farming business.
   b.   A duplex—the taxpayer lives in one half while he rents the other half out.
   c.   The portion of the taxpayer's residence that she uses as a home office.
   d.   The taxpayer's former residence, which he listed for rental temporarily until he is able to sell it. The residence was listed in late November and was not rented as of the end of the taxable year.
   e.   A mobile home that the taxpayer initially purchased and used while he was in college and this year began renting to several students.
   f.   The costs attributable to goodwill and a covenant not to compete.
   g.   An automobile used for business. The taxpayer accounts for his deductible car expenses using the standard mileage rate.

9-3   *Definitions: Cost Allocation Methods and Types of Property.* Explain the terms depreciation, amortization, and depletion. Include in your discussion an explanation of tangible and intangible property as well as personal and real property.

9-4   *Depreciation Systems.* Briefly describe the depreciation systems (e.g., MACRS) for computing tax depreciation that one may encounter in practice.

9-5   *Ineligible Property.* What types of property are not depreciated using MACRS? How can the taxpayer avoid MACRS?

9-6   *Depreciation Methods and MACRS Statutory Percentages.*
   a.   Indicate the first-year depreciation percentage applicable to office furniture and show how it is determined.
   b.   Same as (a) except the property is an apartment building.

9-7   *MACRS and Straight-Line Depreciation.* Assuming a taxpayer desires to use the straight-line method of depreciation, what alternatives, if any, are available?

9-8   *Alternative Depreciation System.* Typically, all depreciation is computed using MACRS. However, Code § 168 also establishes an alternative depreciation system (ADS). As a practical matter, when will use of ADS be most likely?

9-9   *Depreciating Recovery Property.* During the year, X purchased land and a building for a total of $500,000 and furniture for the building for $100,000. He intends to lease the building. Indicate whether the following factors are taken into account in computing the depreciation of these assets.
   a.   Each asset's useful life as estimated by the taxpayer in light of industry standards.
   b.   Salvage value.
   c.   The month in which the property was placed in service.
   d.   The use of the building by the lessee.
   e.   The taxpayer is a corporation.
   f.   The property is used for investment rather than business use.
   g.   The acquisition cost of the building including the land.
   h.   The lessee.

9-10 *Half-Year Convention.* Indicate whether the following statements are true or false regarding the half-year convention.

    a. Depreciation can be claimed for the *entire* year if the asset has been in service for more than six months.

    b. The half-year convention applies to *all* property placed in service during the year.

    c. The half-year convention applies *both* in the year of acquisition and the year of disposition of the asset.

    d. The convention must be considered when expensing an asset under Code § 179.

9-11 *Acquiring a Business.* L has worked as a salesperson in the outdoor advertising business for ten years. This year he decided to go into business for himself. To this end he purchased all of the assets of Billboards Unlimited Corporation for $2 million. The value of the tangible assets such as the office building, furniture, and equipment was $1.4 million. Explain how L will recover the cost of his investment.

9-12 *Luxury Cars.* Indicate whether the following statements are true or false. If false, explain why.

    a. W purchased a new car used solely for business for $12,000. The limitations imposed by Code § 280F on deductions related to automobiles do not alter what W could claim in the year of acquisition.

    b. P Corporation is a distributor of hospital supplies. During the year, it purchased a $20,000 car for its best salesperson. Section 280F does not alter the total amount of depreciation deducted while P owns the car. Section 280F alters only the timing of the depreciation deductions.

9-13 *Leasing and Luxury Automobiles.* D is a manufacturer's representative for several different companies. His sales territory covers all of Indiana, Kentucky and Ohio. Recently, he decided it was time to get rid of his old car, which had just passed the 100,000-mile mark. Many of his friends have told him that he should lease his next car rather than buy it. Assuming D plans on using the car exclusively for business, briefly discuss the tax factors that should be considered in making the decision.

9-14 *Listed Property.* Indicate whether the following statements are true or false. If false, explain why.

    a. J is a part-time photographer. This year she purchased a camera that cost $1,000 for her videocassette recorder. Thirty percent of her usage was for business while the remainder was personal. J may use the accelerated depreciation recovery percentages of MACRS.

    b. P, a proprietor of a lighting store, purchased computer equipment for $10,000 which he uses 50 percent of the time for business. Under Code § 280F, the maximum deduction for depreciation and limited expensing in the first year is $500, while without § 280F the deduction would be $5,000.

    c. C purchased computer equipment that he uses 60 percent of the time for managing his investments and 35 percent of the time in connection with a mail-order business he operates out of his home. C may claim straight-line depreciation deductions based on 95 percent of the cost of the asset.

    d. G is employed as a research consultant for RND Corporation, a research institute. G uses the company's computer at the office but often takes home work, which she does on her home computer. G's use of her home computer for work done for her employer is considered qualified business use.

    e. T is a college professor who uses a computer, for which he properly claims deductions, to write textbooks in his home office. It is unnecessary for T to maintain records on business usage of the computer.

9-15 *Employer-Provided Automobiles.* WS Corporation, a large clothing manufacturer, provides a company car for each of its salespeople. Indicate whether the following statements are true or false. If false, explain why.

   a. An employee must generally include the value of any personal use of the automobile as income; however, he or she is allowed to depreciate the car to the extent of any business use and to deduct any other business-related operating expenses.

   b. This year B, an employee, used a new company-owned vehicle 55 percent of the time for personal purposes and 45 percent of the time for business. The corporation can only depreciate 45 percent of the car, and, since qualified business use is less than 50 percent, it cannot use limited expensing and must use straight-line depreciation.

   c. This year C, an employee, used a company car, driving it 50,000 miles: 40,000 for business and 10,000 for personal purposes. Under the arrangement with C, the company includes $27,500 (50,000 × 55 cents) in C's W-2 as additional income. C may deduct any business expenses incurred related to operation of the car.

   d. Assuming WS charges all of its employees the standard mileage rate for each mile of personal use, the corporation may ignore any personal use of the cars by its salespeople and depreciate 100 percent of the cost of the cars.

   e. WS Corporation also provides a car for its chief executive officer, C, who owns 10 percent of the company's stock. All of C's use is for business except for commuting to work, which represents 60 percent of the car's use. C reimburses the company for the personal use. WS may claim accelerated depreciation for the car based on 40 percent of the car's cost.

9-16 *Amortization.* How are the costs of patents, copyrights, and goodwill recovered?

9-17 *Leasing Restrictions.* Address the following:

   a. Construct a numerical example illustrating why a tax-exempt entity would rather lease than buy.

   b. R acquired a ten-year ground lease on three acres on which it constructed a small office building. Explain how R will recover its cost of the building.

9-18 *Depreciation—Allowed or Allowable.* R inherited her mother's personal residence in 1979 and converted it to rental property. Her basis for depreciation was $100,000. The residence had an estimated useful life of 30 years. This year, R sold the residence for $170,000. During the time R held the property, she never claimed a deduction for depreciation on the residence. What amount of gain will R report upon the sale?

9-19 *Salvage Value.* How is salvage value used in computing the depreciation deduction using MACRS?

9-20 *Depreciable Basis and Limited Expensing.* Explain how the taxpayer's depreciable basis may be affected by the amount expensed under the limited expensing election of § 179.

9-21 *Anti-Churning Rules.* Explain the purpose of the anti-churning rules and when they normally will apply.

9-22 *Component versus Composite Depreciation.* Answer the following:

   a. Distinguish component depreciation from composite depreciation.

   b. May the taxpayer use either method? Explain.

9-23 *Mid-Quarter Convention.* T Company, a calendar year taxpayer, purchased $300,000 of equipment on December 3 of this year.

   a. Under what circumstances will the mid-quarter convention apply in computing depreciation of the equipment?

    b.   Assume that T can purchase the equipment at any time during the year. How will T time the acquisitions if it wants to maximize the firm's depreciation deductions for the year?

9-24   *Determining Recovery Periods: Special Considerations.* During the year, the WJ LLC opened a gas station that also had a convenience food store. The controller is trying to determine how these new items should be depreciated for tax purposes.

    a.   After reading *Iowa 80 Group and Subs v. U.S.* 95 AFTR 2d 2005-2367, 371 F. Supp. 2d 1036 (D.Ct. Southern District of Iowa, 2004), explain the alternatives that might be available and how the court ruled. For fun, see http://www.iowa80truckstop.com/tour1.htm

    b.   What happened in *Iowa 80* on appeal?

    c.   What can you conclude about using the standard procedures for determining depreciation outlined in this chapter?

9-25   *Depletion.* Address the following:

    a.   Briefly describe how cost and percentage depletion are computed and determine which is used in a particular year.

    b.   Assuming the taxpayer has completely recovered her depletable cost basis (e.g., her basis is zero), is she entitled to further depletion deductions?

9-26   *Farming Expenses.* N plans on stepping down from his position as president of a large energy company in five years. At that time, he and his wife would like to move to the country where they would retire and perhaps operate a small dairy farm. N has spotted some land through which a sparkling creek runs. His accountant has suggested that he purchase the land now and begin to operate it despite initial losses. Explain the rationale behind the accountant's advice.

PROBLEMS

9-27   *Depreciation of Converted Personal-Use Property.* F purchased a mobile home to live in while at college. The home cost $50,000. When he graduated, he left the home in the trailer park and rented it. At the time he converted the home to rental property, it had a fair market value of $15,000.

    a.   What is F's basis for depreciation?

    b.   F now lives 75 miles away from his alma mater. Can he deduct the cost of traveling back to check on his rental property (including those trips on which he also attended a football game)?

9-28   *MACRS Accelerated Depreciation.* In 2009 T, a calendar year taxpayer, decided to move her insurance business into another office building. She purchased a used building for $700,000 (excluding the land) on March 15. T also purchased new office furniture for the building. The furniture was acquired for $200,000 on May 1. Compute MACRS depreciation. Ignore first-year expensing and bonus depreciation. MACRS depreciation tables are located in the Appendix.

    a.   Compute T's depreciation deduction for 2009.

    b.   Compute T's depreciation deduction for 2010.

    c.   Assuming that T sold the office building and the furniture on July 20, 2011, compute T's depreciation for 2011.

    d.   Answer (a), (b), and (c) above assuming that the furniture was purchased on October 20.

9-29   *Mid-Quarter Convention.* Q Corporation anticipates purchasing $300,000 of office furniture and fixtures (seven-year property) next year. This will be Q's only personal property acquisition for the year. Q Corporation management is willing to purchase and place the property in service any time during the year to accelerate its depreciation deductions. In addition, management wants to depreciate the property as rapidly as

possible. MACRS depreciation tables are located in the Appendix. Ignore limited expensing.

  a. Compute depreciation for the first two years of ownership assuming *all* of the property is purchased and placed in service on February 2.

  b. Compute depreciation for the first two years of ownership assuming *all* of the property is purchased and placed in service on December 6.

  c. Compute depreciation for the first two years of ownership assuming $177,000 (59%) of the property is purchased and placed in service on February 2 and $123,000 (41%) is purchased and placed in service on December 6.

  d. Based on the results of (a) through (c) above, what course of action do you recommend for Q Corporation?

9-30 *MACRS Straight-Line Depreciation.* G Corporation operates a chain of fast-food restaurants. On February 7, 2009 the company purchased a new building for $1,000,000 (excluding the land). In addition, on May 5, 2009 G purchased a used stove for $5,000 and refrigeration equipment for $30,000 (both seven-year property). G does not elect to use the limited-expensing provision. The company does elect to compute depreciation using the straight-line method under MACRS. MACRS depreciation tables are located in Appendix. Ignore limited expensing and bonus depreciation.

  a. Why might G elect to use the straight-line method?

  b. Assuming G elects to use the straight-line method and a seven-year recovery period for depreciating the stove applies, can it use MACRS accelerated recovery percentages for the refrigeration equipment? For the building?

  c. Compute G's depreciation for the stove and building in 2009 assuming it elects the straight-line method for the seven-year property.

  d. Compute the depreciation for the stove and building in 2010.

  e. If G does not dispose of either the stove or building, what is the final (i.e., last year's) depreciation deduction for the stove and the building?

  f. Assuming G disposes of both the stove and the building on October 18, 2010, what is the depreciation for each of these assets in 2010?

9-31 *ADS Depreciation.* P retired several years ago to live on a small farm. To supplement his income, he cuts wood and sells it in the nearby community. This year he purchased a used light duty truck to haul and deliver the wood. He used the truck 20 percent of the time for business. Assuming the truck cost $9,000, compute P's depreciation for the year.

9-32 *Section 179 Election.* Although K is currently a systems analyst for 3L Corporation, her secret desire is to write a best-selling novel. To this end, she purchased a computer for $3,000 this year. She used the computer only for writing her novel. Can she deduct the entire cost of her computer this year even though she has not yet received any income from the novel? Next year?

9-33 *Limitations on § 179 Expensing.* In each of the following situations, indicate whether T may elect to use the limited-expensing provisions of § 179. Assume the acquisition qualifies unless otherwise indicated.

  a. T is a corporate taxpayer.

  b. This year, T purchased a $600,000 building and $50,000 of equipment.

  c. T suffered a net operating loss of $40,000 this year before consideration of the § 179 deduction.

  d. T purchased the asset on the last day of the taxable year.

9-34 *Limited-Expensing Election: Eligible Property.* For each of the following assets, indicate whether the taxpayer may elect to expense a portion or all of the asset's cost.

  a. A $40,000 car used 75 percent of the time for business purposes and 25 percent of the time for personal purposes.

  b. A home computer used by the taxpayer to maintain records and perform financial analyses with respect to her investments.

    c. An apartment building owned by a large property company.

    d. A roll-top desk purchased by the taxpayer's father, who gave it to the taxpayer to use in her business.

9-35 *Limited-Expensing Election Calculations.* N, a single taxpayer, purchased duplicating equipment to use in his business. He purchased the equipment new on June 3 of the current year for $300,000. N elects to expense the maximum amount allowable with respect to the equipment.

    a. What portion of the cost of the equipment may N expense for this year?

    b. Compute N's depreciation deduction for the current year.

    c. Answer parts (a) and (b) assuming that the cost of the equipment was $840,000.

9-36 *Leasing Automobiles.* On May 27, 2008 J signed a three-year lease on a new Corvette with a list price of $40,000. His lease payments are $600 a month beginning on June 15. Assuming J is self-employed and uses the car exclusively for business, how does the lease affect his taxable income in 2008 and 2009?

9-37 *Section 280F Calculations.* In the current year, H purchased a new automobile for $30,000. The first-year expensing election is not made. Use the most current limits from Exhibit 9-11 in responding to the questions below.

    a. Assuming the car is used solely for business, prepare a depreciation schedule illustrating the amount of annual depreciation to which H is entitled assuming he holds the car until the entire cost is recovered.

    b. Assume the same facts as (a) except the car is used 80 percent of the time for business and 20 percent of the time for personal purposes. Compute the current year's depreciation deduction.

    c. Same as (b) except the car is used 70 percent of the time for business, 10 percent of the time for production of income activities, and 20 percent of the time for personal purposes.

    d. Same as (a) except the car is used 40 percent of the time for business and 60 percent of the time for personal purposes.

9-38 *SUV Limitations.* On March 7, 2009, C, an attorney, purchased an SUV for $40,000. The SUV had a gross vehicle weight exceeding 6,000 pounds. She expects to use the vehicle 80 percent of the time for business. C wishes to maximize her deductions related to the vehicle. Ignore bonus depreciation.

    a. Compute C's depreciation and § 179 expense for 2009.

    b. Same as (a) except the SUV cost $30,000.

    c. Assume C plans to purchase a pickup truck rather than the SUV. She plans to buy a pickup truck that is available in three body styles (regular cab, extended cab and crew cab) and three bed lengths (5.5-foot, 6.5-foot and 8-foot). The truck has a gross vehicle weight exceeding 6,000 pounds. What tax advice may be appropriate, assuming C plans to use the truck like the SUV?

    d. Would the answer to (a) change if the vehicle weighed more than 14,000 pounds? If so, how?

9-39 *Section 280F Calculations.* M purchased a new automobile for $30,000. The first year expensing election is not made. The car is used solely for business. M is in the 25 percent tax bracket. The present value factors for a 10 percent discount rate are as follows: year 1, .91; 2, .83; 3, .75; 4, .68; 5, .62; 6, .56; 7, .51; 8, .47; 9, .42; 10, .39; 11, .35; 12, .32; 13, .29; 14, .26; 15, .24; 16, .22; 17, .20.

    a. Prepare a depreciation schedule.

    b. Compute the total tax savings M will receive throughout the recovery period from depreciation deductions.

    c. Using an after-tax discount rate of 10 percent, compute the present value of tax savings from depreciation deductions under § 280F.

    d. Using an after-tax discount rate of 10 percent, compute the present value of tax savings from depreciation deductions under MACRS as if § 280F were repealed.

e. Compare the results of (b) and (c) above. What impact does discounting have in assessing the tax benefits of depreciation?

f. Compare the results of (c) and (d) above. What is the discounted after-tax cost of the § 280F limitations for this taxpayer?

9-40 *Research and Experimental Expenditures.* ABC Corporation is developing a new process to develop film. During the year, the company had the following expenditures related to research and development:

Salaries	$60,000
Laboratory equipment (5-year property)........................	30,000
Materials and supplies	10,000

Compute ABC's deduction for research and experimental expenditures under each of the alternative methods.

9-41 *Depletion.* DEF Company produces iron ore. It purchased a property for $100,000 during the year. Engineers estimate that 50,000 tons of iron ore are recoverable from the property. Given the following information, complete DEF's depletion deduction and undepleted cost basis for each year.

Year	Units Sold (tons)	Gross Income	Taxable Income before Depletion
1	15,000	$300,000	$124,000
2	20,000	400,000	50,000
3	10,000	250,000	90,000

9-42 *Depletion.* Assume the same facts in *Problem 9-41* except that barrels of oil are being produced rather than tons of iron ore. Compute DEF's depletion deduction and undepleted cost basis for each year.

CUMULATIVE PROBLEMS

9-43 David and Lauren Hammack are married with one child, Jim, age 12. The couple lives at 2006 Rolling Drive, Indianapolis, IN 46222. David is a product manager for G&P Corporation, a food company. Lauren operates a clothing store as a sole proprietorship (employer identification number 35-1234567). The couple uses the cash method of accounting except where the accrual method is required. They report on the calendar year.

David earned a salary of $60,000 during the year. G&P also provides health insurance for David and his family. Of the total insurance premium, the company paid $750. Income taxes withheld from David's salary were $7,000. The couple paid $9,000 in estimated taxes in four equal installments during the year. Last year's tax liability was $5,000.

Lauren's father died on June 20. As a result, Lauren received $40,000 as beneficiary of a life insurance policy on her father. In addition, her father's will provided that she receive all of his shares of IBM stock. The stock was distributed to her in October when it was worth $30,000.

On August 1 of this year, the couple purchased a six-month Treasury Bill for $9,700. They redeemed it on February 1 of the following year for its face value, $10,000. In addition, the couple purchased a previously issued AT&T bond with the face value of $1,000 for $890 on June 1. The bond pays interest at 6 percent per year on January 1 and July 1. On July 1 they received an interest payment of $30, which was also reported on Form 1099-INT, sent to them shortly after year-end. The couple plans on reporting any accrued market discount in taxable income when they sell or redeem the bond, in some future year.

Each year, Lauren travels to Paris to attend the annual fashion shows for buyers. When scheduling her trip for this year, Lauren decided to combine business with pleasure.

On Thursday, March 6, Lauren departed for Paris, arriving on Friday morning. Friday afternoon was devoted to business discussions with several suppliers. Since the shows began on Monday, she spent the weekend touring Paris. After attending the shows Monday through Wednesday, she returned to Indianapolis on Thursday, arriving late that night. The cost of her round-trip air fare to Paris was $500. Meals were $30 per day and lodging was $100 per day for Friday through the following Wednesday.

In addition to running her own shop, Lauren teaches an M.B.A. course in retailing at the local university. She received a $5,400 salary for her efforts this year. The university withheld $429 in FICA taxes, but did not make additional tax withholdings related to the salary. The school is ten miles from her office. Normally, she goes home from her office to get dinner before she goes to the school to teach (16 miles from her home). According to her log, she made 80 trips from home to school. In addition, the log showed that she had driven 20,000 miles related to her clothing business. She uses the standard mileage rate to compute her automobile expenses.

Lauren's records, which she maintains for her business using the cash method of accounting, reveal the following additional information:

Sales.	$120,000
Cost of goods sold.	(50,000)
Gross profit	$ 70,000
Advertising.	6,000
Insurance.	1,400
Rent	9,000
Wages	15,000
Employment taxes.	2,000

The insurance included (1) a $200 premium paid in September for coverage of her car from October through March of the following year; and (2) a $1,200 payment for fire insurance for June 1 through May 31 of the following year. Similarly, rent expense includes a $4,500 payment made on November 1 for rent from November through April. She has a five-year lease requiring semiannual rental payments of $4,500 on November 1 and May 1.

During the year, David purchased a new automobile for $30,000, which he uses 60 percent of the time for business (i.e., "qualified business usage" is 60 percent). His actual operating expenses, excluding depreciation, were $3,000.

In addition to the information provided earlier in this problem, the couple paid the following amounts during the year:

State income taxes	$5,500
County income taxes	500
Real estate taxes.	2,400
Mortgage interest on their home	3,600
Charitable contributions	2,000

David and Lauren's social security numbers are 445-54-5565 and 333-44-5789, respectively. Their son Jim's social security number is 464-57-4681.

Compute David and Lauren's tax liability for the year. Make all computations (including any special elections required) to minimize the Hammacks' tax liability based on *current* tax law. If a tax return is to be prepared for this problem, complete the following forms: 1040 (including Schedules A, C, and SE), and 2106. There is no alternative minimum tax liability. (**Note:** If the § 280F limitations apply to any auto depreciation, you should use the most current numbers from Exhibit 9-11.)

9-44 Michelle Kay purchased a small building on February 1 of the current year for $650,000. In addition, she paid $15,000 for land. Ms. Kay obtained a $640,000 mortgage for the acquisition. She and five of her employees use the property solely to store and sell a variety of gift items under the business name of "Michelle's Gifts." The following information pertains to the business:

Sales.	$950,000
Cost of goods sold.	625,000
Wages for employees ($20,000 each)	100,000
Payroll taxes for five employees	?
Depreciation.	?
Advertising.	25,000
Mortgage interest	60,000
Legal services	20,000
Real estate taxes.	4,000
Fire insurance	3,000
Meals and entertainment	2,500

During the year, Ms. Kay purchased the following assets for the business. She wants to depreciate all business assets as rapidly as the law allows.

	Cost	Month/Day of Acquisition
Personal computer	$14,000	March 31
Printer for computer	2,000	April 2
Office furniture and fixtures	20,000	April 29
Machinery (7-year property).	30,000	May 12

Michelle Kay was divorced from Benjamin Kay two years ago. The divorce decree stipulates that Benjamin Kay would receive the dependency exemption for their son, Eric (now 12 years old), even though Eric lives full-time with Ms. Kay in a home she maintains. During the year, Ms. Kay provided 25 percent of Eric's support and Mr. Kay provided 75 percent. Ms. Kay received $15,000 of alimony and $10,000 of child support from Mr. Kay during the year. Ms. Kay's social security number is 333-46-2974. Her address is 567 North Hollow Drive, Grimview, IL 48124. For business purposes, her employer ID number is 66-2869969. She uses the cash method of accounting for all purposes.

Unrelated to her business, Ms. Kay paid the following amounts during the year:

Estimated federal income taxes.	$16,000
State income taxes	3,500
County income taxes	1,500
Real estate taxes.	2,000
Mortgage interest on her home	5,600
Charitable contributions	2,900
Deductible contribution to individual retirement account (Note: This is a deduction for A.G.I. It is one of the 'adjustments to income' on page 1 of Form 1040.).	2,000
Health insurance for Ms. Kay.	1,000

Compute Ms. Kay's tax liability for the year based on *current* tax law. (**Hint:** Ms. Kay's adjusted gross income is less than $100,000.) If a tax return is to be prepared for this problem, complete the following forms: 1040 (including Schedules A, C, and SE) and 4562. There is no alternative minimum tax liability. For grading purposes, attach a sheet to Schedule C showing supporting calculations for payroll taxes.

RESEARCH PROBLEMS

9-45 *Depreciation.* S is a land developer. During the year, he finished construction of a complex containing a new shopping mall and office building. To enhance the environment of the complex, substantial landscaping was done including the planting of many trees, shrubs, and gardens. In addition, S acquired a massive sculpture that served as the focal point of the complex. S also purchased numerous pictures, which were hung in the shopping center and office building. Can S claim depreciation deductions for any of the items noted above?

9-46 *Amortization.* During the year, the metropolis of Burnsberg accepted bids from various cable television companies for the right to provide service within its city limits. The accepted bid was submitted by Cabletech Inc. in the amount of $500,000. For this amount, the city granted the company a license to operate for 10 years. The terms of the agreement further provided that the company's license would be renewed if the city was satisfied with the services provided. May Cabletech amortize the cost of the license?

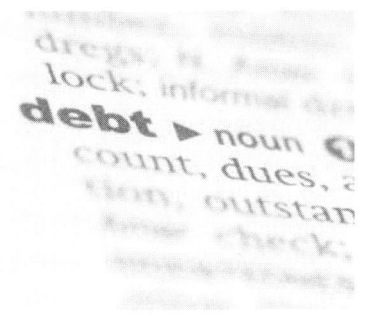

CHAPTER TEN

CERTAIN BUSINESS DEDUCTIONS AND LOSSES

LEARNING OBJECTIVES

Upon completion of this chapter you will be able to:

- Determine when a deduction is allowed for a bad debt

- Understand the different tax treatment for business and nonbusiness bad debts

- Explain what constitutes a deductible casualty or theft loss

- Compute the amount of the deduction for casualty and theft losses

- Determine the net operating loss deduction and explain how it is treated

- Explain the basic tax accounting requirements for inventories

- Identify the costs that must be capitalized as part of inventory and the role of the uniform capitalization rules in making this determination

- Explain how inventory costs are assigned to costs of goods sold using the FIFO and LIFO assumptions

- Compute ending inventory using double-extension dollar-value LIFO

- Apply the lower of cost or market rule in valuing ending inventory

CHAPTER OUTLINE

The rules governing the treatment of expenses and losses discussed in Chapter 7 set forth the general requirements that must be met if the taxpayer wishes to claim a deduction. As already seen, the basic test—whether the item was incurred in carrying on business or profit-seeking activities—is often just the initial hurdle in obtaining a deduction. Other provisions in the Code may impose additional conditions or limitations that must be considered. This chapter examines some of the special rules that relate to certain business losses and expenses of the taxpayer, including the provisions for bad debts, casualty losses, the net operating loss deduction, and inventories.

BAD DEBTS

Loans are made for a variety of reasons. Some are made in connection with the taxpayer's trade or business while others are made for purely personal purposes. People also make loans hoping to make a profit. Regardless of the motive, with the extension of credit comes the possibility—as every lender knows—that the loan will never be repaid. When the borrower, in fact, cannot repay the loan, the taxpayer has what is termed a *bad debt* and may be entitled to a deduction. For tax purposes, a bad debt is considered a special form of loss subject to the specific rules of Code § 166. This provision governs the treatment of all types of bad debts: those that arise from the sale of goods or services such as accounts receivable, as well as those resulting from a direct loan of money. Moreover, § 166 applies regardless of the form of the debt (e.g., a secured or unsecured note receivable or a mere oral promise to repay).[1]

---

[1]   Notes issued by a corporation (with interest coupons or in registered form) that are considered capital assets in the hands of the taxpayer are treated as worthless securities, as discussed in Chapter 12.

TREATMENT OF BUSINESS VERSUS NONBUSINESS BAD DEBTS

The tax treatment of a bad debt vastly differs depending on whether it is a *business* or *nonbusiness* bad debt. Business bad debts generally may be deducted without limitation. In contrast, nonbusiness bad debts are deductible only as *short-term* capital losses and are therefore subject to the limitation on deductions of capital losses (i.e., to the extent of capital gains plus $3,000).[2] Congress provided this distinctive treatment for nonbusiness bad debts in part to ensure that investments cast in the form of loans are handled in virtually the same manner as other investments that become worthless. As a general rule, an investment in a company's stock or bonds that becomes worthless also receives capital loss treatment.

Another difference between business and nonbusiness bad debts concerns the method allowed to claim a deduction. For some debts, it may be apparent that a portion of the loan will become uncollectible but determination of the exact amount must await final settlement. In the case of a nonbusiness bad debt, there is no deduction for partial worthlessness.[3] A deduction is postponed until the ultimate status of the debt is determined.

> **Example 1.** R loaned his neighbor $5,000 in 2008. During 2009 his neighbor declared bankruptcy, and it is estimated that R will recover no more than 20 cents on the dollar or a maximum of $1,000 from the debt. Although R can establish that he has a bad debt of at least $4,000 ($5,000 − $1,000), no deduction is permitted in 2009 since the debt is nonbusiness, and it is partially worthless. If in 2010 R settles for $500, he will realize a loss of $4,500. Assuming he has no capital gains or other capital losses, he may deduct $3,000 of this loss as a *short-term* capital loss and carry over the remaining $1,500 ($5,000 − $3,000 − $500) to the following year. On the other hand, if the debt had arisen from R's *business*, R could deduct $4,000 in 2009 based on his estimate of the uncollectible amount, and the $500 remainder of the loss in 2010, all against ordinary income.

Because of their significantly different treatments, the determination of whether a particular debt is a business or nonbusiness bad debt has produced substantial controversy.

Business Bad Debts. Business bad debts are defined as those that arise in connection with the taxpayer's trade or business.[4] To qualify, the loan must be closely related to the taxpayer's business activity. Simply making a loan to a business associate does not make the loan business-related; it must support the business activity. Common business bad debts include the following:

1. Uncollectible accounts receivable (for accrual basis taxpayers only)

2. Loans to suppliers to ensure a reliable source of materials

3. Loans to customers, clients, and others to preserve business relationships or nurture goodwill

4. Loans to protect business reputation

5. Loans or advances to employees

6. Loans by employees to protect their employment

7. Loans made by taxpayers in the business of making loans

---

[2]   § 166(d)(1)(B). See Chapter 16 for a detailed discussion of capital gains and losses.

[3]   Reg. § 1.166-5(a)(2).

[4]   § 166(d)(2).

It is important to note that C corporations are not subject to the nonbusiness bad debt rules.[5] All loans made by a C corporation are deemed to be related to its trade or business. Thus, any bad debt of a corporation is considered to be a *business* bad debt.

Nonbusiness Bad Debts. A nonbusiness bad debt is defined as any debt other than one acquired in connection with the taxpayer's trade or business.[6] From a practical perspective, nonbusiness bad debts are simply those that do not qualify as business bad debts.

The most common nonbusiness bad debts are losses on personal loans, such as those made to friends or relatives. As suggested above, however, nonbusiness bad debt treatment also extends to loans that are made to make a profit and that essentially function as investments. For example, a loan to an acquaintance to start a new business is in effect an investment and thus a nonbusiness debt. Similarly, a loan to a business to protect an investment in such enterprise would be considered a nonbusiness debt. For instance, an investor may loan funds to a struggling corporation in which he owns stock, hoping that the infusion of cash might sustain it and save the original investment.

Although the dividing line between business and nonbusiness bad debts usually is clear, controversy typically arises in several common situations. One troublesome area involves taxpayers who frequently make loans to make a profit but who do not make such loans their full-time occupation. In such cases, the Service takes the view that the taxpayers are not in the business of making loans and thus any bad debts are not business bad debts. These situations can become even more difficult when the taxpayer devotes substantial time and energy to establishing and developing the business.

> **Example 2.** In *Whipple v. Comm.*, Whipple had made sizable cash advances to the Mission Orange Bottling Co., one of several enterprises that he owned.[7] He spent considerable effort related to these enterprises but received no type of compensation, either salary, interest, or rent. When these advances subsequently became worthless, Whipple deducted them as a business bad debt. The Supreme Court held that the loans made by the shareholder to his closely held corporation were nonbusiness bad debts even though Whipple had worked for the company. According to the Court:
>
> > Devoting one's time and energies to the affairs of a corporation is not of itself, and without more, a trade or business of the person so engaged. Though such activities may produce income, profit or gain in the form of dividends—this return is distinctive to the process of investing—as distinguished from the trade or business of the taxpayer himself. When the only return is that of an investor, the taxpayer has not satisfied his burden of demonstrating that he is engaged in a trade or business.

Despite the Court's holding in *Whipple*, taxpayers have achieved limited success where they have shown that they were in the business of organizing, promoting, and financing businesses.

The other prominent area of controversy concerns a situation common to many new struggling corporations: loans made to corporations by employees who are also shareholders. Here, the issues are similar to that above. Is the taxpayer making the loan to protect an investment or to protect his or her job (i.e., the business of being an employee)? When employee-shareholders have been able to show that a loan was made to protect their jobs rather than their investment, they have been able to secure business bad debt treatment.

---

[5]   § 166(d)(1).

[6]   § 166(d)(2).

[7]   63-1 USTC ¶9466, 11 AFTR2d 1454, 373 U.S. 193 (USSC, 1963).

Although the deduction is normally unlimited, in the case of an employee, the loss is considered an employee business expense and therefore treated as a miscellaneous itemized deduction subject to the 2% floor.[8]

GENERAL REQUIREMENTS

To be deductible, the debt must not only be partially or totally worthless but must also represent a bona fide debt and have a basis.[9]

Bona Fide Debt. A debt is considered bona fide if it arises from a true debtor-creditor relationship. For this relationship to exist, there must be a promise to repay a fixed and determinable sum, and the obligation must be enforceable under local law.

The question of whether there is valid debtor-creditor relationship usually arises when it appears that the taxpayer made the loan with little expectation of being repaid. This is typically the case when there is a close relationship between the taxpayer and the borrower. For example, loans to relatives or friends are likely to be viewed as nondeductible gifts rather than genuine debts. Such treatment is most likely where the lender makes little attempt to enforce repayment of the loan—a common occurrence when the borrower is a child or parent. In a similar fashion, advances to a closely held corporation that are not repaid may be considered nondeductible contributions to capital. On the other hand, loans made by a corporation may be something other than what they purport to be. For example, a loan to a shareholder may be treated as a disguised dividend distribution while a loan to an employee could be considered compensation.

To determine whether a bona fide debtor-creditor relationship exists requires an assessment of all of the facts and circumstances related to the debt. Besides the relationship of the parties, factors typically considered are (1) whether the debt is evidenced by a note or some other written instrument (in contrast to a mere oral promise to repay that has not been reduced to writing); (2) whether the debt is secured by collateral; (3) whether the debt bears a reasonable interest rate; and (4) whether a fixed schedule for repayment has been established.

Basis. A taxpayer may deduct a loss from a bad debt only if he or she has a basis in the debt.[10] For this reason, cash basis taxpayers who normally do not report income until it is received are not entitled to deductions for payments they cannot collect. Their loss is represented by the unrecovered expenses incurred in providing the goods or services. Conversely, accrual basis taxpayers who engage in credit transactions usually report income as it is earned. Accordingly, they may deduct bad debts for those amounts previously included in income. Uncollectible loans (as distinguished from accounts receivable) made by either cash or accrual basis taxpayers may be deducted, assuming the taxpayer has a basis for the loan.

Example 3. R is an orthodontist and uses the cash method of accounting. This year he completed some dental work for B for $3,000, which he never collected. In addition, he loaned $1,000 to a material supplier who left the country. Assuming both debts are worthless, R may deduct only the loan to the supplier for $1,000. No deduction is allowed for the uncollected $3,000 since R does not report the amount as income until he collects it and, therefore, has no basis in the debt. However, any expenses incurred in doing the dental work (i.e., materials. etc.) are deductible.

---

[8] *Graves v. Comm.*, 2007-1 USTC ¶50,252, 99 AFTR 2d 2007-950, 220 Fed. Appx. 601 (CA-9, 2007). Note that miscellaneous itemized deductions are not deductible for purposes of the alternative minimum tax in which case the taxpayer may not benefit from the deduction.

[9] Reg. §§ 1.166-1(c) and (e).

[10] Reg. §§ 1.166-1(d) and (e).

Worthlessness. Whether a debt is worthless ultimately depends on the facts. The Regulations indicate that a taxpayer does not have to undertake legal action to enforce payment or obtain an uncollectible judgment with respect to the debt to prove its worthlessness.[11] It is sufficient that the surrounding circumstances suggest that legal action would not result in recovery. Among the circumstances indicating a debt's worthlessness are the debtor's bankruptcy or precarious financial position, consistent failure to pay when requested, or poor health or death. As noted above, a *business* bad debt need not be totally worthless before a deduction is allowed. When events occur which suggest that the debt will not be recoverable in full, a deduction for partial worthlessness is granted.

DEDUCTION METHODS

As a general rule, deductions for bad debts must be claimed using the specific charge-off method.[12] This method—often called the direct write-off method—allows a deduction only in the year when the debt actually becomes worthless. The reserve method, which allows deductions for estimated bad debts and is typically used for financial accounting purposes, was repealed for all businesses except certain financial institutions and service businesses by the Tax Reform Act of 1986.

The direct write-off method provides some flexibility in accounting for business bad debts. When the facts indicate that a specific debt is *partially* worthless, the portion considered uncollectible may be deducted, but only if such portion is actually written off the taxpayer's books for financial accounting purposes.[13] Any remaining portion of the debt that later becomes worthless can be deducted in subsequent years. Using this approach, taxpayers need not wait until the debt becomes totally worthless before any deduction is claimed. Alternatively, taxpayers can wait until the debt becomes totally worthless and claim the entire deduction at that time. Note that when the debt is totally worthless (in contrast to partially worthless), there is no requirement that the debt actually be written off the taxpayer's books.

> **Example 4.** K Company is a major supplier of lumber to homebuilders. One of its customers, which owed the company $10,000, fell on hard times in 2009 and declared bankruptcy. Because this event suggests that the debt is partially worthless, a deduction is permitted. K estimated that it would recover $7,000 of the debt, and therefore claimed a $3,000 bad debt deduction in 2009. The $3,000 amount was also charged off the taxpayer's books as required. In 2011 K Company actually received $1,000 and deducted the remainder of the loss, $6,000 ($10,000 − $3,000 previously deducted − $1,000 actually received). Alternatively, K may opt to claim no deduction for 2009 and deduct the entire $9,000 loss in 2011. Note that when the debt becomes totally worthless in either case, the taxpayer is not required to write the debt off its books for financial accounting purposes. The company should take heed, however. If the IRS later determines that the debt is partially worthless, no deduction would be allowed since the debt was not written off on the books.

Experience Method for Service Businesses. Although the 1986 Act ostensibly eliminated the reserve method of accounting for bad debts, it provided an equivalent—but not identical—technique for service businesses. If a business uses the *accrual method* to account for income from services, the business is not required to accrue any amount that, *based on experience*, it knows will not be collected.[14] Businesses can take advantage of

---

[11] Reg. §§ 1.166-2(a) and (b).

[12] § 166(a).

[13] Reg. § 1.166-3(a).

[14] § 448(d)(5).

this exception only if they do not charge interest or a late charge on the amount billed. The experience method is available only for businesses that (1) have average annual gross receipts of less than $5,000,000 or (2) perform services in the following eight areas: health, law, engineering, architecture, accounting, actuarial science, performing arts, or consulting.

As a practical matter, the actual use of this technique may be limited, since most service businesses are allowed and often do use the cash method rather than the accrual method of accounting. Service businesses usually are exempt from the rule requiring use of the accrual method,[15] falling under the exceptions for sole proprietorships, S corporations, qualifying partnerships, personal service corporations, or taxpayers with gross receipts that generally do not exceed $5 million.

✓ CHECK YOUR KNOWLEDGE

Review Question 1. Over the years Dr. D has done extremely well financially and has made a number of investments. Several years ago, her good friend T started a small amusement park with such attractions as a water slide and a miniature golf course. Needing some venture capital, T convinced D to lend the new business $50,000, which he would repay to D in three years with 15 percent interest. This year the note came due and T was unable to repay because his business had failed. How will D treat the bad debt?

D's loan did not arise during the ordinary course of business but rather was in the nature of an investment. Therefore, the debt is considered a nonbusiness bad debt and is deductible as a short-term capital loss (limited annually to $3,000 plus capital gains).

Review Question 2. T worked for P Corporation for 25 years. When the company began struggling this year, she worked without pay. The company finally went out of business this year, owing T six months of back pay. Does T have a business or nonbusiness bad debt?

Neither. Although most taxpayers would believe that they have a deductible loss, such is not the case. As a cash basis taxpayer, which T no doubt is, no deduction is allowed because she has no basis in her debt. Had she reported the income (i.e., had she been on the accrual basis), the IRS would be happy to allow a bad debt deduction.

Review Question 3. At the close of current year, Z Corporation, a lumber company, estimated that based on current year sales about $30,000 of its accounts receivable would be uncollectible. Therefore, in accordance with generally accepted accounting principles, the company adjusted its reserve account, charging bad debt expense for $22,000. May Z claim a $22,000 bad debt deduction for tax purposes?

For most businesses, the reserve method is not permitted for tax purposes. Since 1986 the law has generally required the use of the direct write-off method. Under this method, a taxpayer can claim a deduction for a bad debt only when the debt actually becomes totally or partially worthless. This requirement is relaxed for service businesses that are allowed to use a method based on their experience. Consequently, since Z is not a service business, it is not allowed to deduct $22,000 but only the amount that represents debts that are actually worthless.

---

[15] Subject to certain exceptions, § 448 requires corporations, partnerships with corporate partners, or tax shelters to use the accrual method of accounting.

CASUALTY AND THEFT LOSSES

GENERAL RULES

Unfortunately, as everyone knows, disaster may strike at any moment. Hurricanes hit, volcanoes erupt, and rivers overflow. Thieves steal, and people are mugged. The list of possible calamities is endless. Luckily, Congress has recognized that when such events occur they may seriously impair a taxpayer's ability to pay taxes. For this reason, taxpayers are generally allowed to deduct losses arising from casualty or theft. The special rules governing this deduction are the subject of this section.

The Code generally provides that an individual's losses arising from casualty or theft are deductible regardless of the activity in which the losses are incurred. An individual's casualty and theft losses related to profit-seeking activities may be deducted under the general rules, which provide that losses incurred in a trade or business or a transaction entered into for profit are deductible.[16] In addition, § 165(c)(3) expressly allows a deduction for losses related to property used for *personal* purposes where the loss arises from fire, storm, shipwreck, theft, or other casualty.

A deduction is allowed only for casualty losses related to property owned by the taxpayer; no deduction is allowed for damages the taxpayer may be required to pay for inflicting harm upon the person or property of another.[17] Further, the casualty must damage the property itself. A casualty that indirectly reduces the resale value of the property normally does not create a deductible loss (e.g., a mud slide near the taxpayer's residence).[18] Any expenses of cleanup, or similar expenses such as repairs to return the damaged property to its condition prior to the casualty, are usually deductible as part of the casualty loss. Incidental expenses that arise from the casualty, such as the cost of temporary housing or a rental car, are considered personal expenses and are not deductible as part of the casualty loss.

CASUALTY AND THEFT DEFINED

Casualties. The Code permits a deduction for losses arising not only from fire, storm, or shipwreck, but also from other casualties. While the terms *fire*, *storm*, and *shipwreck* are easily construed and applied, such is not the case with the phrase "other casualty." Interpretation and application of this phrase is a continuing subject of conflict. The courts and the IRS generally have agreed that to qualify as a casualty the loss must result from some *sudden, unexpected, or unusual event, caused by some external force*.[19] Losses deductible under these criteria include those resulting from earthquakes, floods, hurricanes, cave-ins, sonic booms, and similar natural causes.[20] On the other hand, losses resulting from ordinary accidents or normal everyday occurrences (e.g., breakage due to dropping) are not considered unusual and consequently are not deductible.[21] Similarly, no deduction is allowed for losses due to a gradual process, since such losses are not sudden and unexpected.[22] For this reason, losses suffered because of rust, corrosion, erosion, disease, insect infestation, or similar types of *progressive deterioration*, generally are not deductible. Unfortunately, the casualty criteria are vague, and the taxpayer may be forced to litigate to determine if his or her

---

[16]   §§ 162 and 212.

[17]   *Robert M. Miller*, 34 TCM 528, T.C. Memo 1975-110.

[18]   *Pulvers v. Comm.*, 48 T.C. 245, aff'd. in 69-1 USTC ¶9272, 23 AFTR2d 69-678, 407 F.2d 838 (CA-9, 1969).

[19]   *Matheson v. Comm.*, 2 USTC ¶830, 10 AFTR 945, 54 F.2d 537 (CA-2, 1931).

[20]   *Your Federal Income Tax*, IRS Publication 17 (Rev. Nov. 96), p. 190.

[21]   *Diggs v. Comm.*, 60-2 USTC ¶9584, 6 AFTR2d 5095, 281 F.2d 326 (CA-2, 1960).

[22]   *Supra*, Footnote 18.

loss is sufficiently sudden or unusual to qualify. For example, the IRS has ruled that termite damage does not occur with the requisite swiftness to be deductible.[23] The courts, however, have found the necessary suddenness to be present in several termite cases and have allowed a deduction for the resulting losses.[24]

Thefts. Losses of business or personal property due to theft are deductible. The term *theft* includes, but is not limited to, larceny, embezzlement, and robbery.[25] If money or property is taken as the result of kidnapping, blackmail, threats, or extortion, it also may be a theft. Seizure or confiscation of property by a foreign government does not constitute a casualty or theft loss but may be deductible if incurred in profit-seeking activities.[26] Losing or misplacing items is not considered a theft but may qualify as a casualty if it results from some sudden, unexpected, or unusual event.[27]

> **Example 5.** H slammed a car door on his wife's hand, dislodging the diamond from her ring, never to be found. The Tax Court held that the loss was deductible as an "other" casualty.[28]

LOSS COMPUTATION

The loss computation is the same whether the casualty or theft relates to property connected with profit-seeking activities or personal use.[29] As explained below, however, limitations on the amount of deductible loss may differ depending on the property's use.

The *amount* of the loss is the difference between the fair market value immediately before the casualty and the fair market value immediately after the casualty as reduced by any insurance reimbursement. Of course, when the property is completely destroyed or stolen, the loss is simply the fair market value of the property as reduced by any insurance reimbursement. Although appraisals are the preferred method of establishing fair market values, costs of repairs to restore the property to its condition immediately before the casualty may be sufficient under certain circumstances.[30]

For many years, a controversy existed concerning the deductibility of insured casualty losses for which taxpayers chose not to file a claim. The problem typically arises when taxpayers avoid filing a claim for fear that their insurance coverage may be cancelled or its cost may increase. When this occurs, the Treasury is effectively acting as an insurance company, partially subsidizing the taxpayer's loss. In 1986 Congress eliminated the controversy for *nonbusiness* property by providing that no deduction is permitted for casualty losses of insured property unless a timely insurance claim is filed.[31]

The amount of the deductible loss generally is limited to the lesser of the property's adjusted basis or fair market value (decline in value if a partial casualty).[32] The lesser of these two amounts is then reduced by any insurance reimbursements. There are two exceptions to this general rule, however. First, for property used in a trade or business or for the production of income that is *completely* destroyed or stolen, the deductible loss is the property's adjusted basis reduced by insurance reimbursements. Second, losses to property *used for personal* purposes are deductible only to the extent they exceed a $100

---

23 Rev. Rul. 63-232, 1963-2 C.B. 97.

24 *Rosenberg v. Comm.*, 52-2 USTC ¶9377, 42 AFTR 303, 198 F.2d 46 (CA-8, 1952).

25 Reg. § 1.165-8(d).

26 *W.J. Powers*, 36 T.C. 1191 (1961).

27 Rev. Rul. 72-592, 1972-2 C.B. 101.

28 *John P. White*, 48 T.C. 430 (1967).

29 Reg. § 1.165-7(a).

30 Reg. § 1.165-7(a)(2)(ii).

31 § 165(h)(4)(E).

32 Reg. § 1.165-7(b)(i).

floor. (Note that this amount is increased to $500 for 2009 but is scheduled return to $100 in 2010.) The $100 floor does not apply to property used in a trade or business or for the production of income. The $100 floor applies to each event, not each item. Further, if spouses file a joint return, they are subject to a single $100 floor. If spouses file separately, each one is subject to a $100 floor for each casualty.[33]

In 1982, Congress added a further limitation on the deduction for casualty or theft losses of property used for personal purposes. In addition to the $100 floor on personal losses, only total losses (after reduction by the $100 floor) in excess of 10 percent of adjusted gross income are deductible.[34] This limitation does not apply to property used in a trade or business or an income-producing activity. The computation of the casualty and theft loss deduction is summarized in Exhibit 10-1.

EXHIBIT 10-1

Computation of Casualty and Theft Loss Deduction

Smaller of
1. Decline in value; or
2. Adjusted basis*

Less:
- Insurance reimbursement
- $100 floor/casualty if personal
- 10% of A.G.I. if personal

Equals: Deductible casualty loss

* Adjusted basis, not decline in value, is used used if business or income property is completely destroyed or stolen.

Example 6. R had four casualties during the year:

Casualty	Property	Adjusted Basis	Before Casualty	After Casualty
1. Accident	Business car	$ 3,000	$ 9,000	$ 5,000
2. Robbery	Ring	500	800	0
	Suit	95	75	0
3. Tornado	Residence	50,000	60,000	57,000
4. Fire	Business computer	3,000	4,000	0

(Fair Market Value: Before Casualty, After Casualty)

R received a $600 insurance reimbursement for his loss on the residence. The deductible loss for each casualty is as follows:

1. The loss for the business car is $3,000 [lesser of the decline in value $4,000 ($9,000 − $5,000) or the adjusted basis of $3,000]. The deduction is *for* A.G.I. unless it is related to R's business as an employee, in which case the deduction would be an itemized deduction.

2. The loss for the ring and suit is $475. The loss for the ring is $500 [lesser of decline in value of $800 ($800 − $0) or the adjusted basis of $500]. The loss for the suit is $75 [lesser of decline in value of $75 ($75 − $0) or the adjusted basis of $95]. The total loss attributable to the robbery is $575 ($500 + $75). This loss

[33] Reg. § 1.165-7(b)(4)(iii).

[34] § 165(h)(2). The 10 percent floor is waived for losses in federally declared disasters (§ 165(h)(3)).

must be reduced by the $100 floor to $475 ($575 − $100). Note that the $100 floor is applied to the event, not to each item of loss. The loss, subject to the ten percent overall limitation, is deductible *from* A.G.I.

3. The loss on the residence is $2,300 [lesser of decline in value of $3,000 ($60,000 − $57,000) or the adjusted basis of $50,000, reduced by the insurance reimbursement of $600 and the $100 floor]. The loss, subject to the ten percent overall limitation, is deductible *from* A.G.I. Assuming R's A.G.I. is $20,000, $775 is deductible [$2,300 + $475 − $2,000 (10% × $20,000)].

4. The loss for the computer is $3,000. Since the computer is used for business and is completely destroyed, the loss is the adjusted basis of the property regardless of its fair market value. The loss is deductible *for* A.G.I.

CASUALTY GAINS AND LOSSES

When the claims for some casualties are settled, the insurance reimbursement may exceed the taxpayer's adjusted basis for the property resulting in a gain. As discussed in Chapter 15, the Code provides some relief in this case, permitting the taxpayer to postpone recognition of the gain if the insurance proceeds are reinvested in similar property. When the gain must be recognized, however, Code § 165(h) sets forth special treatment.

Under § 165(h), all gains and losses arising from a casualty unrelated to business or a transaction entered into for profit—*personal casualty gains and losses*—must first be netted. For this purpose, the personal casualty loss is computed after the $100 floor but before the 10 percent limitation. If personal casualty gains exceed personal casualty losses, each gain and each loss is treated as a gain or loss from the sale or exchange of a capital asset. The capital gain or loss would be long-term or short-term depending on the holding period of the asset. In contrast, if losses exceed gains, the net loss is deductible as an itemized deduction to the extent it exceeds 10 percent of the taxpayer's A.G.I.

Example 7. This year T had three separate casualties involving personal use assets.

Casualty	Property	Adjusted Basis	Fair Market Value Before Casualty	Fair Market Value After Casualty
1. Accident	Personal car	$ 12,000	$ 8,500	$ 6,000
2. Robbery	Jewelry	1,000	4,000	0
3. Hurricane	Residence	60,000	80,000	78,000

T received insurance reimbursements as follows: (1) $900 for repair of the car; (2) $3,200 for the theft of her jewelry; and (3) $1,500 for the damages to her home. If T does not elect (under § 1033) to purchase replacement jewelry, her personal casualty gain exceeds her personal casualty losses by $300, computed as follows:

1. The loss for the car is $1,500 [(lesser of $2,500 decline in value or the $12,000 adjusted basis = $2,500) − $900 insurance recovery − $100 floor].

2. The loss from the residence is $400 [(lesser of $2,000 decline in value or the $60,000 adjusted basis = $2,000) − $1,500 insurance recovery − $100 floor].

T must report each separate gain and loss as a gain or loss from the sale or exchange of a capital asset. The classification of each gain and loss as short-term or long-term depends on the holding period of each asset.

Example 8. Assume the same facts as in *Example 7* except the loss for the personal car was not insured. In this case the loss on the car is $2,400 and the personal casualty losses exceed the gain by $600 ($2,400 + $400 − $2,200). T must treat the $600 net loss as an itemized deduction subject to the limitation of 10% of A.G.I.

YEAR DEDUCTIBLE

A casualty loss usually is deductible in the taxable year in which the loss occurs.[35] A theft loss is deductible in the *year of discovery*. If a claim for reimbursement exists and there is a reasonable prospect of recovery, the loss must be reduced by the amount the taxpayer *expects* to receive.[36] If later receipts are less than the amount originally estimated and no further reimbursement is expected, an amended return is *not* filed. Instead, the remaining loss is deductible in the year in which no further reimbursement is expected. If the casualty loss deduction was reduced by the $100 floor in the prior year, the remaining loss need not be further reduced. However, the remaining loss is subject to the 10 percent limitation of the later year.

Example 9. G's diamond bracelet was stolen on December 4, 2009. Her loss was $700 before taking into account any insurance reimbursement. She expects the insurance company to reimburse her $400 for the loss. In 2009 G may deduct $200 ($700 loss less the expected reimbursement of $400 and reduced by the $100 floor) subject to the 10% limitation for 2009. If G actually receives only $300 in the following year, she may deduct an additional $100 (the difference between the expected reimbursement of $400 and the $300 received) subject to the 10% limitation for 2010. If the reimbursement was greater than that expected, the excess is included in gross income.

A special rule exists for the reporting of casualty losses sustained within an area designated by the President as a "disaster area." This rule permits the taxpayer to accelerate the tax relief provided for casualty losses by electing to deduct the disaster loss in the taxable year immediately preceding the year of the disaster loss.[37] In addition, the loss is not subject to the 10 percent floor.

Example 10. F, a calendar year taxpayer, suffered a loss in a "disaster area" from a flood on March 4, 2009. F may elect to deduct the loss on his 2008 return. If he has not filed the 2008 return by the casualty date, he may include the loss on the original 2008 return. If the 2008 return has been filed prior to the casualty, an amended return or refund claim is required. Alternatively, F could claim the loss on his 2009 return.

✓ *CHECK YOUR KNOWLEDGE*

Review Question 1. While acting like a couch potato and channel surfing one rainy day, S felt a drop on the end of his nose. Then, all of a sudden, water started gushing out of the ceiling. S later determined that squirrels had eaten a hole in his roof. Can S claim a casualty loss deduction for any damage caused by the squirrels? What must S demonstrate before he can claim a casualty loss deduction?

In order to claim a deduction for an "other casualty," S must establish that the damage is sudden, unexpected, and unusual. As can be imagined, these standards are often difficult

---

[35] Reg. § 1.165-7(a).

[36] Reg. § 1.165-1(d)(2)(i).

[37] § 165(i).

to apply. In this case, the IRS has ruled that no deduction was allowed since it is common knowledge that squirrels are destructive and because the roof holes caused by the rodents were not unexpected or unusual.[38]

Review Question 2. In 2003 B purchased a music box as a Christmas present for his wife at a cost of $1,000. This year the box was stolen. It turned out that the music box was an antique worth more than $5,000. Because of the deductible on his homeowner's insurance policy, B received only $400 for his loss.

a. Before considering *any* limitation, what is the amount of B's casualty loss deduction?

In the case of a casualty of personal use property, a taxpayer is generally allowed to deduct the lesser of the property's value or basis as reduced by any insurance reimbursement. As a result, B is allowed to deduct a loss of $600 ($1,000 − $400).

b. After B found out that his loss in the eyes of the tax law was only $600, he went crazy. He said it was ridiculous to allow a deduction of only $600 when in fact his economic loss was really $4,600 ($5,000 − $400). Is B right or wrong?

B's belief that he has a $4,600 loss rather than a $600 loss is based on the value of the property. It is true that he has had an economic loss of $4,600, but he never had to recognize the increase in value from $1,000 to $5,000 as income for tax purposes. Therefore, the loss is measured from his basis.

c. Answer (a) assuming the music box had been worth only $700.

In this case, the deduction would be $300 [(lesser of fair market value, $700, or basis, $1,000) − $400]. Note that B would probably believe this is unfair since he paid $1,000 for the box and was reimbursed only $400. However, the starting point for measuring the loss is the value; Congress did not want to allow a deduction for the loss in value that is not attributable to the casualty since to do so would allow the taxpayer to deduct a personal expense.

d. Even though B has a casualty loss, he will probably not receive any tax relief. Why?

Despite the loss, the deduction for *personal* casualty losses is subject to two limitations. The amount of the casualty (as measured above) must exceed the $100 floor per casualty and 10 percent of the taxpayer's A.G.I. After the 10 percent floor was added to the law in 1982, reported casualty loss deductions fell by 97 percent. Because of this limitation, a personal casualty loss must be almost catastrophic before a taxpayer receives any tax relief.

e. Answer (a) and (c) assuming that B was in the business of selling music boxes.

If the property is used in a trade or business, the taxpayer is entitled to a deduction equal to the basis of the property reduced by an insurance reimbursement. Consequently, in (a), where the box is worth $5,000 and has a basis of $1,000, the deduction would be $600 (adjusted basis $1,000 − insurance reimbursement $400). The same rationale provided for the solution in (b) above

---

[38] Ltr. Rul. 8133097.

applies here. The deduction is limited since the taxpayer has never recognized the appreciation as income. In (c), where the box is worth $700 and has a basis of $1,000, the taxpayer is also allowed a deduction for $600 (rather than $300 as was the case when the property was used for personal purposes). Note that even though the value of the property is less than its basis, the business taxpayer is allowed to deduct the entire basis in the property. This treatment is allowed since the taxpayer would have been able to deduct the $1,000 in any event because the property is used in a trade or business. For example, the taxpayer would be able to claim a deduction when the property was sold or if the property was depreciable, through depreciation.

Review Question 3. Checkers Pizza delivers. This year one of its cars was stolen. Does the $100 floor and 10 percent of A.G.I. limitation apply in determining the amount of its casualty loss?

The $100 floor and 10 percent rule do not apply to casualties of property used in a trade or business or an income-producing activity. These limitations apply only to casualties of personal use property.

Review Question 4. During 2009, the Smiths' house was destroyed by a hurricane. As a result, the Smiths moved into a motel until their home was rebuilt six months later. The cost of their motel stay was $2,700. May the couple deduct the $2,700 cost as a casualty loss?

No deduction is allowed. This is considered an incidental personal expense and is not deductible as part of the casualty loss.

NET OPERATING LOSSES

As someone once said, life is not always a bed of roses. This chapter, at least in part, is a testimonial to that. Debts do go bad, lightning may strike, and casualties can happen. Perhaps taxpayers can take some consolation in that in both of these cases, the government shares in the taxpayer's misfortune and provides some relief. Unfortunately, this section also dwells on the negative. For some taxpayers, income does not always exceed deductions. Businesses are not always profitable and catastrophic events may give rise to large expenses. In those lean or rotten years, the taxpayer may actually have a negative taxable income, usually referred to as a loss. When this happens, as might be expected, the taxpayer to his or her joy does not have to pay taxes. More importantly, the taxpayer may be able to use the loss to reduce his or her tax in a previous or subsequent year. This section examines this possibility.

In a year during which the taxpayer's deductions exceed gross income, the taxpayer is allowed to use the excess deductions to offset taxable income of prior or subsequent years.[39] Technically, the excess of deductions over income, as modified for several complex adjustments, is referred to as the taxpayer's *net operating loss* (NOL).[40] The Code generally permits the taxpayer to carry back the NOL two years and forward 20 years to redetermine taxable income.[41]

---

[39] § 172.

[40] § 172(c).

[41] § 172(b)(1). Pre-1998 NOLs are carried back three and forward 15 years. NOLs arising in 2001 and 2002 and those of a small business attributable to federally declared disasters may be carried back five rather than two years. For an NOL arising in 2008, businesses with less than $15 million in gross receipts may elect to carry it back either 3, 4 or 5 years, instead of the normal 2-year carryback period.

Allowance of the net operating loss deduction reduces the inequity that otherwise exists due to the use of an annual reporting period and a progressive tax rate structure. For example, consider a situation involving two taxpayers, R and S, who over a two-year period have equivalent taxable incomes of $100,000 each. R earned $50,000 each year while S earned $300,000 in the first year and had a loss of $200,000 in the second year. Without the NOL provisions, S would *not* be able to offset his $200,000 loss against his $300,000 income and consequently would pay a substantially greater tax than R. Such a result clearly would be unfair since both taxpayers had identical taxable incomes over the two-year period. The NOL provision partially eliminates this inequity by allowing a loss in one year to offset income in other years.

CARRYBACK AND CARRYFORWARD YEARS

As mentioned above, an NOL resulting in the current year is generally carried back two years and forward 20 years. The loss is first carried back to the second prior year (i.e., the earliest year first) and taxable income is recomputed for that year. If any loss remains after reducing that year's tax liability to zero, the remaining loss is carried to the first prior year. If a loss still remains, the taxpayer carries it forward to the first year after the loss and so on up to the 20th year following the loss year. For example, a loss occurring in 2009 would be applied to taxable income of these years as follows: 2007, 2008, 2010, 2011, . . . , 2029, 2030.

The taxpayer may *elect* to forego the carryback period and carry forward the loss instead.[42] The election is made simply by attaching a statement to the tax return for the year to indicate the taxpayer's intention of forgoing the carryback period. This election must be made by the due date of the return (including extensions) in which the net operating loss is reported. The election *cannot* be subsequently claimed or revoked by filing an amended return. This election normally is appropriate only where the taxpayer expects future profits. If future profits are anticipated, the taxpayer must determine whether carrying the loss back or forward will yield the greater tax benefit. This decision is often difficult since the taxpayer may be unable to predict the future with any certainty.

When the taxpayer carries the loss back to a prior year, the loss deduction is claimed on an amended return for the earlier year (Form 1040X). For this purpose, the statute-of-limitations period for returns of the earlier years normally is extended to three years after the due date (including extensions) of the return in which the loss is reported.[43] Alternatively, the loss may be claimed using Form 1045 (Form 1139 for corporations) for a so-called quick refund. This form must be filed *after* the return of the loss year is filed and *within* one year after the *close* of the loss year. If the taxpayer fails to file Form 1045, an amended return (Form 1040X) may still be filed.

> **Example 11.** B, a calendar year taxpayer, reported a loss for 2009. He filed his 2009 return April 15, 2010. Under normal conditions, B must file an amended return for 2007 (the year to which the loss is carried) by April 15, 2011 (three years after April 15, 2008, the due date for the 2007 return). The Code, however, extends the period for filing an amended return for 2007 until April 15, 2013, three years after the due date of the return for the loss year. Alternatively, B may claim the loss using Form 1045 by filing the form before December 31, 2010, one year after the close of the loss year.

---

[42] § 172(b)(3)(c).

[43] § 6511(d)(2).

Where the taxpayer carries the loss forward, the loss deduction is claimed on the subsequent year's normal return (Form 1040).

If the taxpayer has losses occurring in two or more years, the loss occurring in the earliest year is used first. When the loss from the earliest year is absorbed, the losses from later years may be claimed.

NET OPERATING LOSS COMPUTATION

The term *net operating loss* (NOL) is defined as the excess of the deductions allowed over gross income, computed with certain modifications.[44] The purpose of the modifications is twofold. First, the net operating loss provisions are designed to permit a taxpayer a deduction for his or her true *economic* loss. Thus, certain artificial deductions that do not require cash outlays (such as the deductions for personal and dependent exemptions) are added back to negative taxable income. Second, the net operating loss provisions were enacted to provide relief only in those cases where there is a business or casualty loss. As a practical matter, a net operating loss is caused by one of the following:

- ▸ Loss from operating a sole proprietorship (e.g., a loss on Schedule C)
- ▸ Loss from rental operations in which the taxpayer actively participates subject to certain limitations
- ▸ Share of an S corporation or partnership loss
- ▸ A casualty or theft loss

Since the NOL provisions generally allow only for the carryback or carryforward of losses attributable to business or casualty, restrictions are imposed on the amount of nonbusiness expenses that may be deducted in computing the NOL. As will be seen, it is these limitations on the deduction of nonbusiness expenses and losses that make the computation of the NOL deduction so complex.

The net operating loss deduction of an individual taxpayer is computed by making the following modifications in computing taxable income:[45]

1. Any net operating loss deduction carried forward or carried back from another year is not allowed.

2. The deduction for personal and dependent exemptions is not allowed.

3. Deductions for capital losses and nonbusiness expenses are limited as explained below.

To determine the extent of any deduction for capital losses and nonbusiness expenses, gross income must be classified into *four* categories: (1) capital gains from business; (2) other income from business; (3) capital gains not from business; and (4) other income not from business. With income so classified, the following rules are applied with respect to nonbusiness expenses and capital losses in the following order:[46]

---

44   *Supra*, Footnote 39.

45   § 172(d)(1) through (4).

46   § 172(d)(4).

1. Nonbusiness capital losses may be deducted to the extent of any nonbusiness capital gains; thus, any excess is added back to taxable income.

2. Nonbusiness expenses may be deducted to the extent of any nonbusiness income, including any excess of nonbusiness capital gains over nonbusiness capital losses (as determined in step l); thus, any excess is added back to taxable income.

3. Business capital losses may be deducted to the extent of any business capital gains; any excess business capital losses may be deducted to the extent of any excess of nonbusiness capital gains over nonbusiness capital losses and nonbusiness expenses (as determined in step 2).

A general formula for computing the NOL deduction is set forth in Exhibit 10-2. As may be surmised from the previous discussion and the formula, the critical first step when actually calculating the deduction is classifying income and deductions and gains and losses as either business or nonbusiness. Exhibit 10-3 identifies and classifies the most common items appearing on tax returns.

EXHIBIT 10-2
Computation of Net Operating Loss

Taxable loss shown on return

Add back:
* Exemptions

* Nonbusiness deductions
    Less:
        Nonbusiness ordinary income
        Nonbusiness net capital gain

* Nonbusiness capital losses
    Less:
        Nonbusiness capital gains

* Business capital losses
    Less:
        Nonbusiness net capital gains
        Less: (Nonbusiness deductions − nonbusiness income)

Equals: Net Operating Loss Deduction

EXHIBIT 10-3

Calculation of Net Operating Loss Deduction: Classification of Business and Nonbusiness Income and Expenses

Business income	Nonbusiness income
Salaries and wages	Interest income
Schedule C income	Dividends
Rental income	Pension income
Farm income	Annuity income
Partnership and S corporation income if not passive	Partnership and S corporation income if passive
Gains from sale of business assets	Gain from sale of capital assets not used in business (such as stocks)

Business deductions	Nonbusiness expenses
Schedule C expenses	Standard deduction
Rental expenses	Itemized deductions including medical, interest, taxes, contributions
Farm expenses	
Partnership and S corporation loss if not passive	Partnership and S corporation loss if passive
Casualty or theft losses (business and personal)	IRA contribution
Loss on sale of § 1244 stock	Contribution to self-employed retirement plan
Miscellaneous itemized deductions for business	Alimony
Moving expenses	

Example 12. In 2009 G quit his job and opened a car repair shop. G's filing status is married, filing jointly, and he reported the following income and deductions for the year:

Income

Business income	$40,000
Salary from previous job	10,000
Business capital gains—long term	7,000
Business capital losses—long term	(2,000)
Nonbusiness capital gains—long term	5,000
Nonbusiness capital losses—long term	(3,000)
Interest income on nonbusiness investments	1,000

Expenses

Business expenses	70,000
Casualty loss on personal car	5,100
Interest on home mortgage	8,000

Taxable income is computed as follows:

Net business loss ($40,000 − $70,000)		($30,000)
Salary		10,000
Interest earned		1,000
Net long-term capital gain		7,000
Adjusted gross income (loss)		($12,000)
Less: Itemized deductions		
Casualty loss	$5,000*	
Mortgage interest paid	8,000	(13,000)
Less: Personal exemptions ($3,650 × 2)		(7,300)
Taxable income (loss)		($32,300)

* $5,100 − $100 floor. Note that the 10 percent limitation does not apply since A.G.I. is a negative number.

Following the format of Exhibit 10-2, G's net operating loss for 2009 is computed as follows:

Taxable income (loss)			($32,300)
Modifications			
Add back:			
Personal exemptions			7,300
Excess nonbusiness expenses:			
Mortgage interest		$8,000	
Nonbusiness income:			
Interest	$1,000		
Nonbusiness net capital			
gain ($5,000 − $3,000)	+ 2,000	(3,000)	5,000
Net operating loss for 2008			($20,000)

Computation of the real dollar loss or economic loss results in a similar deduction:

Business loss	($30,000)
+ Salary	10,000
+ Business capital gains	5,000
− Casualty loss	(5,000)
Net operating loss	($20,000)

Note that the nonbusiness income (capital gains of $2,000 and interest income of $1,000) is not considered in this computation of economic loss since it is offset by nonbusiness expenses.

RECOMPUTING TAXABLE INCOME FOR YEAR TO WHICH NET OPERATING LOSS IS CARRIED

Once the net operating loss deduction is computed, it is carried to the appropriate year and used in the recomputation of taxable income for that year. The net operating loss deduction is a deduction *for* A.G.I. As a result, the deduction may have an effect on the amount of the deduction for certain items such as medical expenses, which are based on the taxpayer's A.G.I. All expenses based on A.G.I. except charitable contributions must be *recomputed* in determining the revised taxable income.[47] The net operating loss deduction also may have an effect on any tax credits originally claimed. For example, if a year 2011 net operating loss deduction completely eliminates the taxable income of 2009, any credit originally claimed in 2009 becomes available for use in another year.

After the effect on the tax of the earliest year is computed, the amount of any loss remaining to be carried forward must be determined. In other words, a computation is required to determine how much of the net operating loss is absorbed in the year to which it is carried and how much may be carried to subsequent years. Although this calculation is somewhat similar to that explained above, additional nuances exist making the computation somewhat complex. For this reason, further reference should be made to the Regulations and Form 1045.

---

[47] Reg. § 1.172-5(a)(3)(ii).

✔ CHECK YOUR KNOWLEDGE

During 2009, C. D. opened his own computer store, specializing in sales of multimedia. He operated the business as an S corporation. Upon his first crack at computing his taxable income for the year, C. D. determined that he had a negative taxable income of $15,000.

Review Question 1. Assuming C. D. has a net operating loss for the year, how is it treated?

An NOL is generally carried back two years and forward 20 years. The 2009 loss is carried back to the second prior year (i.e., the earliest year, 2007), where taxable income is recomputed and a refund claim is filed. If any loss remains after reducing the taxable income of 2007 to zero, the loss is carried forward to the first prior year (i.e., 2008). If a loss still remains, C. D. may carry it forward for up to 20 years, after which any remaining loss expires and is lost. Alternatively, C. D. may elect not to carry the loss back but to carry the loss forward for 20 years. Carrying forward the loss may make more sense if he expects to be in a tax bracket in the future that is higher than past years. In such case, the loss would produce greater benefit.

Review Question 2. A review of C.D.'s tax return reveals that his negative taxable income of $15,000 includes several items of income and deductions. For example, his only income other than that related to his business was interest and dividends of $5,000. Indicate whether the following deductions would be allowed in computing C. D.'s net operating loss deduction and, if so, how much could be used.

a. Personal exemption
b. Dependency exemption
c. Net loss from S corporation operations (sales less operating expenses)
d. Casualty loss to personal residence from earthquake damage
e. Interest expense on the mortgage on his personal residence of $7,000
f. Net capital loss $8,000 ($3,000 used to offset ordinary income and $5,000 carried over)

In computing his net operating loss deduction, C. D. must make certain adjustments to negative taxable income to arrive at the taxpayer's true economic loss that the law allows to be carried over. No deduction is allowed for personal or dependency exemptions since these are artificial deductions. Therefore, the exemption deduction must be added back to negative taxable income. The net loss from his business (i.e., the S corporation) does reduce taxable income in calculating the NOL, so there is no adjustment. The casualty loss is also allowable in computing the NOL. Nonbusiness expenses such as mortgage interest and taxes are considered personal expenses and can be deducted only to the extent of nonbusiness income. Therefore, only $5,000 of the $7,000 expense is deductible, requiring an addback of $2,000. Finally, a capital loss can generally be used only to offset capital gains. Thus the $3,000 deduction attributable to the capital loss is not allowed and must be added back.

INVENTORIES

As might be expected, taxpayers who buy or produce merchandise for subsequent sale are not allowed to deduct the costs of the merchandise *at the time* the goods are produced or purchased. Instead, such costs normally must be capitalized (i.e., inventoried) and deducted when the goods are sold. The following example illustrates what might occur if taxpayers were not required to capitalize the costs of inventory.

Example 13. C Corporation began business in 2009 and purchased 10,000 gizmos at $10 each for a total of $100,000. In 2009 the corporation sold 6,000 gizmos for $120,000. In 2010 the corporation made no further purchases and sold the remaining 4,000 gizmos for $80,000. Gross profit reported with and without inventories is computed below:

	No Inventories		Inventories	
	2009	2010	2009	2010
Sales.	$120,000	$80,000	$120,000	$80,000
Cost of good sold:				
Beginning inventory.	—	—	—	$40,000
+ Purchases	$100,000	—	$100,000	—
– Ending Inventory	—	—	(40,000)	—
Costs of goods sold (4,000 @ $10)	$100,000	—	$ 60,000	$40,000
Gross profit	$ 20,000	$80,000	$ 60,000	$40,000

Although the total income for the two-year period is the same under either method ($100,000), the time when it is reported differs significantly. The use of inventories produces higher income and higher taxes in the first year because only the costs of goods actually sold are deducted.

As the preceding example shows, the lack of inventories causes a mismatching of revenues and expenses and with it the possibility of widely fluctuating incomes. Without inventories, the income reported in any one year would in most cases represent a distorted picture—not a clear reflection—of how well the firm was doing. Perhaps what is more crucial, at least from the Treasury's point of view, is that taxpayers would be able to postpone the payment of taxes if inventories were not required. Note in *Example 13* that absent inventories, the taxpayer is able to defer $40,000 ($60,000 – $20,000) of income and the corresponding tax from 2009 to 2010. Congress recognized these possibilities at an early date and in 1918 took corrective action that is still intact today. Currently, Code § 471 provides the following:

> Whenever in the opinion of the Secretary the use of inventories is necessary in order clearly to determine the income of any taxpayer, inventories shall be taken by such taxpayer on such basis as the Secretary may prescribe as conforming as nearly as may be to the best accounting practice in the trade or business and as most clearly reflecting income.

With the enactment of § 471, Congress delegated its rulemaking authority concerning inventories to the IRS. The IRS has responded with a number of regulations indicating when inventories are necessary as well as what methods are acceptable for tax purposes.

The Regulations require taxpayers to maintain inventories whenever the production, purchase, or sale of merchandise is an income-producing factor.[48] As a practical matter, this means virtually all manufacturers, wholesalers, and retailers must keep track of inventories while service businesses are usually exempt. Note that inventories are required regardless of the taxpayer's method of accounting. Cash basis taxpayers must account for inventories as do accrual basis taxpayers. However, the mandatory use of the

---

[48] Reg. § 1.471-1 and Reg. § 1.446-1(a)(4)(i).

accrual method for purchases and sales does not prohibit taxpayers from using the cash method to account for other items such as advertising costs or interest income.[49]

EXCEPTIONS TO THE INVENTORY REQUIREMENT

While the inventory rule seems relatively straightforward, it has led to a significant amount of controversy. To understand the problem, it is necessary to recall that where inventory exists, the taxpayer not only must capitalize inventory costs, it also must accrue income from credit sales. The difficulty stems from the requirement that only those items representing merchandise *inventory* must be capitalized. In contrast, under Regulation §1.162-3 materials and supplies that are considered *incidental* to the primary function of the business may be expensed currently. In contrast, *nonincidental* materials and supplies can be deducted only as they are consumed—much like inventory. Therefore, according to these rules, if a taxpayer can successfully argue that items are merely incidental materials or supplies, the items can be expensed immediately and the taxpayer may defer recognition of income from their sale until cash is received. On the other hand, if the IRS can prove that the items are inventory, the items must be capitalized and the income from their sale must be accrued. Note how much is at stake in the definition of inventory. If the items are considered incidental, the taxpayer wins the entire battle: deductions now and income in the future. If the items are nonincidental, the IRS secures a partial victory in that nonincidental items cannot be deducted immediately but only as they are consumed; however, income is still deferred. But if the items are considered inventory, the IRS has won the entire war since such characterization not only prevents an immediate write-off of the items' costs but also forces the taxpayer to accrue income currently. The difficulty is that there is no clear definition of inventory.

The problem is particularly acute with service providers. In *Wilkinson-Beane*, a mortuary provided funeral services, including supplying the caskets.[50] The taxpayer did not separately bill for the caskets but merely charged a flat fee for the services. Consistent with this approach, the taxpayer did not treat the caskets as inventory even though the costs represented 15.1 percent of total cash receipts. Unfortunately for the taxpayer, the court held that the caskets must be capitalized and any income forthcoming from the services to be accrued. A different approach was taken in the recent decision in *Osteopathic Medical Oncology and Hematology P.C.*[51] In this situation, the taxpayer provided chemotherapy treatment for cancer patients. In so doing, it used certain drugs. The IRS argued that the drugs were inventory and, therefore, the taxpayer could not expense the drugs and had to report the income when the treatments were provided (rather than when the cash was received—usually much later). However, the Tax Court sided with the taxpayer, ruling that the drugs were not inventory but rather an indispensable and inseparable part of the service of treating patients.

Due to the growing controversy about the definition of inventory and the ensuing problems, the government reacted. In 2000, the IRS began to relax its position on the mandatory use of inventories and at the same time the mandatory use of the accrual method. In a series of Revenue Procedures, the IRS has carved out two major exceptions, allowing taxpayers with inventories to escape the clutch of the accrual method. As may be grasped from the discussion above, the exceptions are of huge importance primarily because they permit the taxpayers—at least small businesses—to defer income.

1. *Gross Receipts of $1,000,000 or Less.* Taxpayers with average annual gross receipts of $1,000,000 or less are not required to use the accrual method for

---

[49]   Reg. § 1.446-1(c)(1)(iv).

[50]   70-1 USTC ¶9173, 25 AFTR 2d 70-418 420 F.2d 352 (CA-1, 1970).

[51]   113 T.C. 376.

inventories. This does not mean that taxpayers can simply expense inventory purchases. Instead, as discussed above, the items must be accounted for as nonincidental materials and supplies and expensed as they are used or consumed. While the treatment of inventory *costs* is essentially the same whether the costs are treated as inventory or nonincidental materials and supplies, the treatment of *income* significantly differs. Taxpayers who fall under this exception need not recognize accounts receivable income until they collect the receivables. In other words, they may defer the recognition of income until they receive payment for the merchandise.[52]

2. *Gross Receipts Less Than $10,000,000.* The above rule carves out a special exception only for small businesses: taxpayers with gross receipts of $1,000,000 or less. Revenue Procedure 2002-28 extends the same rule discussed above to taxpayers with average annual gross receipts exceeding $1,000,000 but less than $10,000,000 but only if they are not in certain industries, including manufacturing, wholesale, retail and information industries (e.g., newspapers, books, periodicals, database publishers and sound recording industries) or meet certain other exceptions. These businesses also need not use the accrual method for purchases and sales but inventory must be accounted for as nonincidental materials and supplies and expensed as they are used or consumed. Note that this rule does not override § 448 discussed above. Farming businesses, C corporations having gross receipts exceeding $5,000,000 and partnerships with a tainted C corporation partner do not qualify for this exception. This rule should benefit small businesses primarily in service businesses.[53]

Example 14. Golf Accessories Inc. (GAI) sells a variety of items for golfers, such as golf balls, tees, headcovers, ball marks, towels, clothing, training tapes and devices. The company sells direct to the public through its Internet site as well as to golf shops around the country. It has average annual gross receipts (e.g., sales) of $700,000. GAI began the year with $80,000 of merchandise on hand. During the year it purchased $300,000 of new merchandise, and at the end of the year had $70,000 on hand. Sales during the year were $650,000 but at the end of the year it had $40,000 of receivables outstanding. It also collected $15,000 of the receivables outstanding from the prior year. Because GAI averages gross receipts of less than $1,000,000 it need not use the accrual method to account for purchases and sales. As a result, it has revenues of $625,000 ($15,000 + $650,000 − $40,000) and costs of good sold of $310,000 ($80,000 + $300,000 − $70,000). Note that under the exception GAI is able to defer the $40,000 of income from the uncollected receivables until it is collected next year—a very valuable benefit. Also note that the inventory costs were still capitalized and could not be expensed until the items were sold or consumed.

Example 15. Same facts as above except GAI Inc. had average annual gross receipts of $4,000,000. Under these revised circumstances, the company would not qualify for the first exception since its gross receipts exceed $1,000,000. Moreover, it also would not qualify for the second exception even though its gross receipts are less than $10,000,000 since it is in one of the prohibited businesses of retail and wholesale trade.

---

[52] Rev. Proc. 2000-22, 2000-1 C.B. 1008 *modified* and *superseded* by Rev. Proc. 2001-10, I.R.B. 2001-2, 272. Note that Rev. Proc. 2001-10 eliminated the book conformity requirement.

[53] Rev. Proc. 2002-28, 2002-18 I.R.B. 2002-18, 815 clarifying and implementing Notice 2001-76, I.R.B. 2001-52, 613. See Rev. Proc. 2002-28 for exceptions where the principal business activity is the provision of services or fabrication or modification of or property to meet customer specifications.

Example 16. Same facts as in *Example 14* above except that GAI Inc. had average annual gross receipts of $8,000,000 and provided heating and air conditioning services. GAI meets the requirements of the second exception in that it is in the business of providing services and its gross receipts are less than $10,000,000. It would appear that GAI could avoid use of the accrual method and defer income from credit sales. However, if GAI is a C Corporation, it must still use the accrual method in accounting for purchases and sales because its gross receipts exceed $5,000,000.

INVENTORY ACCOUNTING IN GENERAL

A close reading of § 471 reveals that Congress has given the IRS two criteria to be followed in determining what inventory accounting methods are acceptable for tax purposes: (1) the method should conform as nearly as possible to the best accounting practice used in the taxpayer's trade or business; and (2) the method should clearly reflect income. Because of these requirements, the tax rules for inventory are quite similar to those used for financial accounting. Nevertheless, it is important to recognize that the IRS is the ultimate authority on determining what method represents the "best accounting practice" as well as what method most clearly reflects income. Consequently, as will be seen, taxpayers are sometimes required to adopt methods that vary from generally accepted accounting principles and cause differences between book income and taxable income.

There are three steps that must be followed in accounting for inventories and computing costs of goods sold: (1) identifying what costs (e.g., direct and indirect) are to be inventoried or capitalized; (2) evaluating the costs assigned to the ending inventory and determining whether reduction is necessary to reflect lower replacement costs (i.e., lower of cost or market); and (3) allocating the costs between ending inventory and costs of goods sold (e.g., specific identification, FIFO, LIFO). Each of these steps is discussed below.

COSTS TO BE INVENTORIED

The first step in determining costs of goods sold and ending inventory is identifying the costs that should be capitalized as part of inventory. Without guidance, taxpayers no doubt would be inclined to expense as many costs as possible. However, over the years, the IRS with help from Congress has established strict guidelines concerning what can be deducted currently (i.e., period costs) and what must be capitalized (i.e., product costs). The most recent development in this continuing debate was the enactment of the *uniform capitalization rules* (unicap) in 1986. As discussed below, the unicap provisions narrow further what the taxpayer is able to treat as a period cost.

As a general rule, the costs that must be capitalized depend on whether the taxpayer manufactures the goods (e.g., a producer of razor blades) or purchases the items for later resale (e.g., a wholesaler or a retailer such as a department store). When merchandise is bought for resale, the taxpayer must capitalize as a cost of inventory the invoice price less trade discounts plus freight and other costs of acquisition. Cash discounts may be deducted from the inventory cost or reported as a separate income item. In addition, certain retailers and wholesalers are subject to the unicap rules that require capitalization of particular indirect costs as discussed below. For manufactured items, inventory cost includes costs of raw materials, direct labor, and certain indirect costs. The unicap rules apply to all manufacturers.

Many of the problems concerning inventory involve the treatment of indirect costs. Various methods have been devised to account for these costs. For example, under the *prime costing* method only the costs of direct materials and direct labor are capitalized; all indirect costs are expensed. Another method, often advocated by cost accountants, is the *variable* or *direct costing* approach. This method capitalizes only those costs varying with production and expenses all fixed costs. Despite the acceptance of these methods for managerial and internal reporting, the IRS has outlawed their use.

Determining which costs should be included in inventory has been a continuing source of irritation in the tax law. Prior to 1973, questions were often resolved on a case-by-case method, resulting in confusion and inconsistency. In 1974, the IRS addressed the problems by issuing regulations requiring all manufacturers to use the *full absorption costing method*.[54] The full absorption method requires the capitalization of direct costs of material and labor as well as the capitalization of certain indirect expenses. However, retailers and wholesalers were not subject to the full absorption rules, and, therefore, were not required to capitalize any indirect costs. The full-absorption rules seemed to work but apparently not well enough and were essentially replaced in 1986 by the enactment of § 263A containing *the uniform capitalization rules* (UNICAP).

The UNICAP rules attempt to provide standard guidelines regarding the capitalization of expenditures for all types of taxpayer and all types of activities. The UNICAP rules apply to *all* manufacturers. In addition, they apply to any retailers and wholesalers (resellers) if their average annual gross receipts for the past three years exceed $10 million. For tax purposes, the UNICAP rules generally replace the full-absorption costing method. However, in practice, many manufacturers continue to use the full-absorption method modified to meet the UNICAP requirements. UNICAP requires more expenses to be capitalized than full-absorption so it is sometimes referred to as the super-absorption method. To be clear, for covered taxpayers, UNICAP requirements must be met and traditional full-absorption methods often used for financial accounting purposes do not meet these standards unless modified.

Section 263A requires the capitalization of direct material, direct labor costs, and, most important, any indirect costs that, in the words of the Regulations, "directly benefit or are incurred by reason of the performance of a production or resale activity."[55] The effect of these rules is to require taxpayers to capitalize many costs that they may have otherwise deducted. The Regulations require covered taxpayers to categorize all costs into three categories and treat them as follows.

	Category	Treatment
1.	Production and resale activities	Capitalize
2.	General administration	Do not capitalize (expense)
3.	Mixed service costs (benefit both production/resale and administration)	Allocate between production and administration

As seen in the more detailed breakdown in Exhibit 10-4, the Regulations classify costs as (1) those that benefit only production and resale activities (must capitalize); (2) those that benefit only policy and management functions (do not capitalize); (3) those that benefit both production and resale activities and policy and management functions, referred to as mixed service costs (capitalized by using any reasonable basis to allocate costs between production and policy functions). In addition, interest expense is subject to special rules.

---

[54] Reg. § 1.471-11. Absorption costing is currently used for financial statement purposes.

[55] Reg. § 1.263A-1T(b)(2)(ii).

Taxpayers are required to develop reasonable bases for cost allocations. In this regard, the Regulations provide several straightforward allocation techniques.[56]

A threshold question with respect to UNICAP (as well as the special deduction for domestic production activities discussed below) is whether a taxpayer is a manufacturer. If the taxpayer is a manufacturer, § 263A applies regardless of the size of the taxpayer's business. If the taxpayer is not a manufacturer, § 263A only applies if the taxpayer's average gross receipts are greater than $10 million. In this regard, gross receipts includes those from all sources, not merely gross receipts from the sale of inventory. Because of the differing treatment between the two groups, a major concern is whether the manufacturing activities of a business are sufficient to cause it to be treated as a manufacturer. For example, are businesses that assemble some products that they sell considered manufacturers? Is a grocery store that uses a portion of its space to prepare foods for consumption on the premises or for takeout considered a manufacturer? As these examples suggest, a clear distinction between manufacturers and resellers does not always exist.

---

[56]   For example, Reg. § 1.263A-3(d) for a discussion of the simplified resale method and the same method using used in conjunction with the historic absorption ratio.

EXHIBIT 10-4

Capitalizable Costs for Uniform Capitalization

Direct costs	Unicap
Direct material	C
Direct labor	C
Indirect costs	
Repairs/maintenance (equipment and facilities)	C
Utilities (equipment and facilities)	C
Rent (equipment and facilities)	C
Indirect labor	C
Indirect material and supplies	C
Small tools and equipment	C
Quality control and inspection	C
Taxes other than income taxes	C
Depreciation and depletion for books	C
Depreciation and depletion: excess tax	C
Insurance (facilities, contents, equipment)	C
Current pension costs	C
Past service pension costs	C
Bidding expenses—successful bids	C
Engineering and design	C
Warehousing, purchasing, handling and general and administrative related to such functions	C
Policy and Management	
Marketing, selling, advertising, and distribution	E
Bidding expenses-unsuccessful bids	E
Research and experimental expenses	
Losses	E
Depreciation on idle equipment or facilities	E
Income taxes	C
Strike costs	E
Interest	*
Mixed Service Costs	
Administrative/coordination of production or resale	C
Personnel department	C
Purchasing department	C
Materials handling and warehousing	C
Accounting and data servicing departments	C
Data processing	C
Security services	C
Legal department providing services to production	C
Overall management and policies	E
General business planning	E
Financial accounting	E
General financial planning	E
General economic analysis and forecasting	E
Internal audit	E
Shareholder and public relations	E
Tax department	E

C: Capitalize
E: Expense currently

* Capitalized if the produced property has a life of 20 years or more, if the property has an estimated production period of more than two years, or if the production period exceeds one year and the cost exceeds $1 million. Does not apply to property acquired for resale.

ALLOCATING INVENTORIABLE COSTS

After total product costs for the year have been identified, these costs along with the cost of beginning inventory must be allocated between the goods sold during the year and ending inventory. If each item sold could be identified (e.g., a car or jewelry) or all items had the same cost, there would be little difficulty in determining the cost of items sold and those still on hand. As a practical matter, these conditions rarely exist. Consequently, the taxpayer must make some assumptions regarding which costs should be assigned to costs of goods sold. Like financial accounting, the tax law does not require the cost flow assumption to be consistent with the physical movement of goods. There are several acceptable approaches for allocating costs: specific identification, first-in first-out (FIFO), last-in first-out (LIFO), and weighted averaged.

Example 17. K Corporation's inventory records revealed a beginning inventory of 300 units acquired at a cost of $3 per unit. This year the corporation purchased 400 units for $4 per unit, and it sold 500 units for $5,000. Gross profit using FIFO and LIFO are computed below:

	FIFO	LIFO
Sales (500 units @ $10)	$5,000	$5,000
Costs of goods sold:		
Beginning inventory (300 @ $3)	$ 900	$ 900
Purchase (400 @ $4)	1,600	1,600
Goods available	$2,500	$2,500
Ending inventory:		
FIFO (200 @ $4)	(800)	
LIFO (200 @ $3)		(600)
Costs of goods sold	$1,700	$1,900
Gross profit	$3,300	$3,100

If K uses FIFO it is assumed that goods are used in the order that they are purchased (i.e., the first goods in are the first goods to be sold). Thus, the ending inventory consists of the most recent purchases, $800 (200 at $4 per unit). The effect of FIFO is to assign the oldest costs to costs of goods sold. In contrast, LIFO assumes that the last goods purchased are the first sold. As a result, under LIFO the most recent costs are assigned to costs of goods sold and the oldest costs to ending inventory. Thus, ending inventory under LIFO is $600 (200 at $3).

The preceding example illustrates the principal advantage of LIFO. In periods of rising prices, LIFO matches current costs against current revenue. From a financial accounting perspective, it can be reasoned that this produces a better measure of current income since both revenues and costs are stated on a comparable price basis, thereby reducing the inflationary element of earnings.[57] From a tax perspective, LIFO appears preferable because taxable income is typically lower and the corresponding tax is reduced. In effect, taxable income is not "overstated" by fictitious gains. Interestingly, LIFO became part of

---

[57] Arguably, income results only to the extent that the sales price exceeds what it will cost to buy a replacement item for the merchandise sold. LIFO approximates this approach.

the tax law in 1939 for just this reason—to help businesses reduce the "paper profits" that conventional methods were yielding and that were being taxed at wartime rates of close to 80 percent.

It must be noted, however, that the advantage of LIFO is lost to the extent that sales in any one year exceed purchases (*see Example 17* above). In this case, the lower prices of goods purchased in previous periods are charged to costs of goods sold. This dipping into the past LIFO layers creates inventory profits, the specific problem that LIFO was designed to address. In a worst case scenario, a company that adopted LIFO in 1942 might unexpectedly liquidate all of its LIFO layers, matching 1942 costs with 2009 revenues. This would no doubt lead to an unforeseen tax liability with little "real" income to pay the tax. This is a significant risk when LIFO is used. At the same time, it may represent an opportunity. Companies may be able to create income, if desirable, by liquidating LIFO layers (e.g., to absorb an expiring net operating loss).

DOLLAR VALUE LIFO

As a practical matter, applying the LIFO procedure to specific goods can be quite cumbersome and costly. In contrast to the simple one-item example above, most firms have hundreds or thousands of individual inventory items, and the number of units purchased and sold each period may amount to hundreds of thousands or more. Pricing each separate unit at the oldest costs and properly accounting for the liquidation of any LIFO layers might be a recordkeeping nightmare. Moreover, the major advantage of LIFO could be lost if old LIFO layers had to be liquidated because a specific item was discontinued or replaced. To address the problems of specific-goods LIFO, variations of LIFO have been developed. Perhaps the most widely used version of LIFO is the dollar-value method.

The dollar-value method reaches the desired result—eliminating the inflationary element of earnings attributable to inventory—in a unique way. Ending inventory is priced using the prices at the time LIFO was originally adopted (base-year). This value is then compared to beginning inventory to determine if there is a real increase or decrease in the pool of dollars invested in inventory. If there is no real change (i.e., ending inventory at base-year prices is the same as beginning inventory at base-year prices), the effect is to charge costs of goods sold with an amount reflecting current prices. On the other hand, if there is a real increase in inventory in terms of base-year dollars, the increase is valued at current prices and added to beginning inventory as a separate LIFO layer to determine ending inventory.

> **Example 18.** T Corporation had an ending inventory on December 31, 2008 of 10,000 units at a cost of $20,000. During the year, T sold the original units and purchased another 10,000 units for $24,000. On December 31, 2009 ending inventory valued at current prices was $24,000. In such case, costs of goods sold would be $20,000, computed as follows:

Beginning inventory	$20,000
Purchases	24,000
Ending inventory	(24,000)
Costs of goods sold	$20,000

But what if, as the facts suggest, prices have increased by 20%? If so, the real amount invested in inventory has not changed ($24,000 ÷ 120% = $20,000). Consequently, valuing ending inventory at current-year prices of $24,000 (as above) effectively assigns the oldest costs of $20,000 to costs of goods sold, resulting in an inflationary

profit of $4,000. Dollar-value LIFO eliminates this artificial gain—the objective of LIFO—by restating ending inventory at base-year prices. In this case, ending inventory would be restated at $20,000 ($24,000 ÷ 120%). This restatement would yield a cost of goods sold of $24,000, and would properly match current-year costs against current-year revenues.

The important difference between dollar-value and specific-goods LIFO is that increases and decreases in inventory are measured in terms of dollars rather than physical units. This approach allows goods to be easily combined into pools and effectively treated as a single unit. Consequently, the likelihood of liquidating LIFO layers is reduced.

Although there are various methods of dollar-value LIFO, the most frequently used is the *double-extension method*.[58] The steps to be used in applying the double-extension method are summarized in Exhibit 10-5 and applied to the following example.

EXHIBIT 10-5
Double-Extension Dollar-Value LIFO Computation of Ending Inventory

Step 1. *Extension #1.* Value ending inventory at current-year prices (actual cost of most recent purchases, average cost, or other acceptable method).

Step 2. *Extension #2.* Value ending inventory at base-year prices.

Step 3. Compute current-year quantity increase or decrease by comparing beginning and ending inventories at base-year prices.

> Ending inventory at base-year price (Step 2)
> − Beginning inventory at base-year price
> Curent-year quantity increase (decrease) at base-year price

Step 4. Calculate current-year price index.

$$\text{Index} = \frac{\text{Ending inventory at current-Year price (Step)}}{\text{Ending inventory at base-year price (Step 2)}}$$

Step 5. Compute the quantity increase or decrease to be added to or subtracted from beginning inventory.

    a. For a quantity increase: convert the increase measured at base-year prices (Step 3) to current year's prices using the current-year price index (Step 4).

$$\begin{array}{c}\text{Quantity increase at} \\ \text{Base-year price} \\ \text{(Step 3)}\end{array} \times \begin{array}{c}\text{Index} \\ \text{(Step 4)}\end{array} = \begin{array}{c}\text{New} \\ \text{LIFO} \\ \text{layer}\end{array}$$

    b. For a quantity decrease: a current-year decrease consumes the layer(s) of inventory in LIFO fashion (i.e., the decrease must be subtracted from the most recently added layer). Previous layers are peeled off at the prices at which they were added.

Step 6. Ending LIFO inventory is the beginning inventory increased by the new LIFO layer [Step 5 (a)] or decreased by any liquidation of LIFO layers [Step 5(b)].

---

[58] Taxpayers may use the link-chain method or certain simplified procedures. See Code §§ 472(f) and 474 and the applicable regulations.

Example 19. In 2009 T Corporation elected to value inventories using double-extension dollar-value LIFO. Beginning inventory for 2008 consisted of the following:

Date	Pool Items	Ending Quantity	Current Cost Per Unit	Total at Current Cost
1-1-09	A	3,000	$3	$ 9,000
	B	4,000	6	24,000
Total base-year cost				$33,000

Inventory information for 2009–2011 and the computation of ending inventory using the steps in Exhibit 10-5 are shown below.

Steps 1 and 2: Double extend ending inventory.

Date	Pool Items	Ending Quantity	Ending Inventory at Current-Year Prices		Ending Inventory at Base-Year Prices	
			Current Cost Per Unit	Total at Current Cost	Base-Year Cost Per Unit	Total at Base-Year Cost
12-31-09	A	2,000	$ 4	$ 8,000	$3	$ 6,000
	B	5,000	7	35,000	6	30,000
				$ 43,000		$ 36,000
12-31-10	A	6,000	$ 5	$ 30,000	$3	$ 18,000
	B	7,000	9	63,000	6	42,000
				$ 93,000		$ 60,000
12-31-11	A	4,000	$ 6	$ 24,000	$3	$ 12,000
	B	5,000	10	50,000	6	30,000
				$ 74,000		$ 42,000

Step 3: Determine quantity increase (decrease) at base-year price.

	2009	2010	2011
Ending inventory base-year price	$36,000	$60,000	$42,000
Beginning inventory base-year price..........	(33,000)	(36,000)	(60,000)
Quantity increase at base-year price..........	$ 3,000	$24,000	($18,000)

Step 4: Calculate current-year price index.

$$\text{Index} = \frac{\text{Ending inventory at current-year price}}{\text{Ending inventory at base-year price}}$$

	2009	2010	2011
	$43,000 / $36,000	$93,000 / $60,000	Decrease: use index at which units were added
	1.19	1.55	1.55

Step 5: Compute quantity increase or decrease to be added to or subtracted from beginning inventory.

	2009	2010	2011
Quantity increase at base-year price	$ 3,000	$24,000	($18,000)
× Index	×1.19	×1.55	×1.55
= Increase or decrease to beginning inventory	$ 3,570	$37,200	($27,900)

Step 6: Compute ending inventory.

	2009	2010	2011
Base-year..............................	$33,000	$33,000	$33,000
2009 layer.............................	3,570	3,570	3,570
2010 layer.............................	—	37,200	9,300*
Total ending inventory....................	$36,570	$73,770	$45,870

* $37,200 − $27,900 = $9,300

THE LIFO ELECTION

Taxpayers may elect to use LIFO by filing Form 970 with the tax return for the year in which the change is made. Unlike most other changes in accounting method, prior approval by the IRS is not required. Conversely, the LIFO election cannot be revoked unless consent is obtained. As explained below, the lower of cost or market procedure may not be used with LIFO. Consequently, in the year LIFO is elected, all previous write-downs to market must be restored to income. For many years, the IRS required that all of the income due to the change had to be reported in the year of the change. In 1981, Congress expressed its disfavor with this view and enacted Code § 472(d). This provision allows the taxpayer to spread the adjustment equally over three years, the year of the change and the two following years. Nevertheless, if substantial write-downs have been made, there may be a considerable cost to elect LIFO.

Another ramification of the LIFO election concerns the *conformity requirement.* Under § 472(c), taxpayers who use LIFO for tax purposes must also use LIFO in preparing financial reports to shareholders and creditors. Failure to comply with this rule terminates the LIFO election and requires the taxpayer to change the method of accounting for inventory. As a result, taxpayers not conforming may be forced to give back any income tax savings previously obtained with LIFO.

The conformity requirement appears to have stifled the use of LIFO, presumably because during periods of rising prices it produces lower income and earnings per share than other inventory methods. This is true notwithstanding the tax savings that are available with LIFO and the relaxation of the rule over the years. The Regulations now permit the taxpayer to disclose income using an inventory method other than LIFO if the disclosure is made in the form of a footnote to the balance sheet or a parenthetical on the face of the balance sheet.[59] No comparative disclosures are allowed on the face of the income statement.

---

[59] Reg. § 1.472-2(e).

LOWER OF COST OR MARKET

In certain instances, the value of an inventory item may have dropped below the cost allocated to such items. When this occurs, financial accounting has traditionally abandoned the historical cost principle and allowed businesses to write-down their inventories to reflect the decline in value. The tax law has adopted a similar approach. Under the Regulations, taxpayers may value inventory at either (1) cost, or (2) the lower of cost or market.[60] However, the lower of cost or market approach may not be used if the LIFO method is used. Note that the lower of cost or market procedure deviates from the normal rule that losses are not deductible until they are realized.

In the phrase the *lower of cost or market*, "market" generally means replacement cost, or in the case of manufactured products, reproduction cost. When the rule is applied, the value of each similar item must be compared to its cost, and the lower is used in computing ending inventory.

Example 20. J's inventory records reveal the following:

Item	FIFO Cost	Market	Lower of Cost or Market
A	$ 3,100	$ 3,500	$ 3,100
B	5,100	3,000	3,000
C	6,000	7,500	6,000
	$14,200	$14,000	$12,100

If J elects to value inventories at cost, the inventory value is $14,200. Alternatively, if the lower of cost or market approach is elected, the inventory is valued at $12,100. This value is used because unsimilar items cannot be aggregated for tax purposes. For financial accounting purposes, J could combine the various items. Consequently, a difference may arise between book and taxable income.

The approach used above is that prescribed in the Regulations for normal goods. Note that these rules only allow a write-down to replacement cost. What if the firm believes that it will ultimately sell the item for less than what it would cost to replace it? Financial accountants refer to estimated sales price less costs of disposition as net realizable value. For tax purposes, a write-down below this value is allowed only for what are often referred to as "subnormal" goods.[61]

Subnormal goods are those items in inventory that cannot be sold at normal prices because of damage (e.g., a dent in a file cabinet), imperfections (e.g., a thousand sweatshirts with the logo improperly spelled), shop wear, changes of style, odd or broken lots, and so on. The Regulations allow the taxpayer to value these "subnormal" goods at a bona fide selling price less direct costs of disposition. However, this lower value is acceptable *only* if the goods are actually offered for sale at such price 30 days after the

---

[60] Reg. § 1.471-2(c).

[61] See Reg. § 1.471-2(c). Note that reduction of net realizable value by an allowance for a normal profit margin is not allowed for tax purposes.

inventory date (e.g., cars with severe hail-damage are actually on the lot with a sales price slashed below replacement cost within 30 days of when inventory is taken).

> **Example 21.** In the landmark decision of *Thor Power Tool Co.*,[62] the taxpayer manufactured power tools consisting of 50 to 200 parts. Thor followed the common practice of producing additional parts at the same time it manufactured the original tool. This practice helped the company to avoid expensive retooling and special production runs as replacement parts were actually required. When accounting for these spare parts, the company initially capitalized their costs and—consistent with GAAP—subsequently wrote them down to reflect the decline in their expected sales price. The Supreme Court ultimately denied the write-down because Thor could not show that the parts (i.e., the excess inventory) were a subnormal good, and even if they had, the company had not actually offered the parts for sale at the lower price. The effect of this decision is to prohibit companies from writing down the value of slow-moving inventory.

QUALIFIED PRODUCTION ACTIVITIES DEDUCTION

Over the years, Congress has adopted a number of measures that it hoped would attract, create and maintain manufacturing jobs in the U.S. For the most part, these provisions were designed to encourage businesses to increase its exports. Most of these approaches, however, resulted in a permanent reduction of U.S. tax and were held to constitute an illegal export subsidy under the U.S. trade agreements with the World Trade Organization. Congress addressed the problem with a different tactic in the *American Jobs Creation Act of 2004* (Jobs Act) with the creation of § 199.

In short, the law now provides direct tax breaks for domestic production activities. The focus has shifted to what companies are doing in the United States, not what they are exporting or moving overseas. Section 199 allows taxpayers to claim a special deduction relating to production and manufacturing activity undertaken in the U.S. and Puerto Rico, regardless of whether the items are exported. When fully effective in 2010, eligible taxpayers will be able to claim a deduction equal to 9 percent of the taxpayer's *qualified production activities income* (QPAI) or if less, the taxpayer's taxable income (modified A.G.I. in the case of an individual). The deduction percentage normally allowed is phased in as follows:

Year	Deduction Percentage
2005–2006	3%
2007–2009	6
2010 and thereafter	9

All taxpayers are entitled to the deduction (C corporations, S corporations, partnerships, sole proprietorships, estates and trusts). For individual taxpayers, the deduction is for A.G.I. but is not deductible in computing self-employment tax. The effect of the deduction is to reduce a corporation's effective tax rate by about 3 percent ($35\% \times 9\% = 3.15\%$).

---

[62] 79-1 USTC ¶9139, 43 AFTR2d 79-362, 439 U.S. 522 (USSC, 1979).

Limitations on Deduction. There are two critical limitations impacting the deduction. QPAI cannot exceed the taxable income limitation and the § 199 deduction itself cannot exceed 50 percent of the employer's wages.

Taxable Income Limitation. As noted above the deduction is generally 9 percent of QPAI or if smaller, the taxpayer's taxable income. For individual taxpayers, A.G.I. with certain modifications is substituted for taxable income. The taxable income limitation normally applies when a taxpayer has current losses from activities other than production sufficient to offset production income or no current income because of a carryback or carryforward of losses. In such case, the taxpayer receives no benefit from the manufacturing deduction, either currently or by an increase in its NOL carryback or carryforward.

For pass-through entities, the taxable income limitation is determined at the owner or beneficiary level. Therefore, partnerships, S corporations, trusts and estates must separately state the amount of QPAI that flows through to the owners or beneficiaries.

W-2 Wages Limitation. The § 199 deduction itself cannot exceed 50 percent of the W-2 wages of the employer for the taxable year. W-2 wages are defined as the sum of wages and elective deferrals [e.g., contributions to 401(k) plans that must be reported on Form W-2]. Fiscal year taxpayers use the W-2 wages for the calendar year that ends within the taxpayer's fiscal year Wages include production and non-production employees, as well as key executive officers and staff, in-house counsel, and research and marketing staff. Only wages that are related to domestic production gross receipts are considered in computing the limitation. In addition, in a concession to the film industry, any compensation for services performed in the U.S. by actors, directors and producers is considered W-2 wages.

> **Example 22.** H and W are married and file a joint return. Each owns and operates a separate business. H has a tax practice with 10 employees. W's business manufactures handcrafted baskets, pottery, ceramics and matching accessories. W's business has about 25 employees directly involved in production and 10 others including herself that are involved in administration, accounting, marketing and similar support functions. Without a special rule, W could count the wages paid by H to his employees in determining the wage limitation. However, § 199 makes it clear that in determining the wage limitation, only the wages related to domestic production gross receipts are considered. Thus only the wages paid to W's employees are taken into account since the wages paid to H's employees are not related to production activities. Also note that the wages of not only those involved directly in the manufacturing process are counted but also those paid to support personnel. Finally observe that the result would be the same if both activities were carried on within a single C or S corporation or partnership.

With respect to partnerships, S corporations and other flow-through entities, the partners, S shareholders and beneficiaries are treated as having paid qualified wages in an amount equal to that owner's allocable share of the wages paid by the entity.

Wages do not include the Schedule C earnings of sole proprietors or the Schedule F earnings of farmers. In addition, wages do not include payments made to partners in partnerships for services rendered (so-called guaranteed payments). In light of this rule, it would appear that "one-person" sole proprietorships do not qualify for the deduction because the income from such businesses is not paid to the owner in the form of wages. This may encourage "one-person" operations to be conducted in the form of an S corporation that pays its owner/sole-employee wages.

Example 23. Red Flag Inc. manufactures and sells flags of all types. For 2009, it has qualified production activities income (QPAI) of $2,000,000 and taxable income of only $500,000 due to losses from rental activities. The § 199 deduction normally would be $120,000 (6% × $2,000,000) but due to the taxable income limitation the deduction is restricted to $30,000 (6% × $500,000 taxable income). The deduction is limited to 6% of the lesser of QPAI or taxable income. Moreover, the deduction cannot exceed 50% of wages paid.

Example 24. Organic Farms Inc. has QPAI and taxable income of $10,000,000 in 2012 (when the deduction percentage is completely phased in to 9%). Organic's W-2 wage expense for the year is $1,500,000. The normal deduction would be $900,000 (9% of $10,000,000) but is limited to $750,000 (50% × wages of $1,500,000).

Example 25. Carl's Custom Cabinets operates as a single member LLC. Carl produces all of the cabinets himself and has no employees. The LLC reports Schedule C net income of $100,000. The amount of the § 199 deduction is zero since CarlŌs LLC paid no wages. If the $100,000 net income included a $20,000 payment to an independent contractor, the deduction would still be zero since he paid no W-2 wages. The same result would occur if Carl's business was engaged in farming rather than cabinetry.

Qualified Production Activities Income (QPAI). QPAI and the § 199 deduction are computed in the following manner:

	Domestic production gross receipts
−	Allocable costs of goods sold
−	Directly allocable deductions
−	Ratable allocation of other deductions not directly allocable to another class of income
=	Qualified production activities income (QPAI) not to exceed taxable income
×	(6% in 2007–2009, 9% in 2010 and thereafter)
=	Qualified production activities deduction not to exceed 50% of W-2 wages

The starting point for computing QPAI is "domestic production gross receipts" (DPGR). DPGR means the gross receipts derived from the following:[63]

1. Any lease, rental, license, sale, exchange, or other disposition of:
   - *Qualifying production property* (QPP) that is manufactured, produced, grown or extracted by the taxpayer in whole or in significant part within the U.S. According to the Regulations, the qualifying activities also include constructing, building, installing, manufacturing, developing or improving property. QPP includes tangible personal property, computer software and certain sound recordings. Production includes farming, food storage, and food processing.
   - Certain *qualified films* produced by the taxpayer, including copyrights, trademarks and other intangibles created in production of the film.
   - Electricity, natural gas and potable (drinking) water produced in the U.S.

2. Construction performed in the U.S. (including not only erection but also substantial renovation of residential or nonresidential buildings); and

3. Engineering or architectural services performed in the U.S. for construction projects in the U.S.

---

[63] §199(c)(4). For purposes of § 199, the term United States includes Puerto Rico (§ 199(d)(8)). Thus DPGR attributable to activities in Puerto Rico qualify.

Example 26. XBX Corporation sells a CD-ROM disk in a plastic case that contains a video game to be played on a computer. XBX also provides technical support. The CD-ROM and the case are tangible personal property but the computer game on the disk is considered computer software. If the disk was manufactured in China, the case was manufactured in Mexico and the software was developed in California, the proceeds of the sale must be allocated between qualified DPGR (the software) and nonqualified gross receipts (the CD-ROM and the case). Note also that computer software qualifies even though it might not be be operated on a computer (e.g., a video game for a video game player (e.g., Playstation, Xbox, Gameboy)). In addition, observe that in selling the game the company has also sold a service (technical support), the price of which is embedded in the total price of the item. Receipts from services do not qualify as DPGR. A special de minimis rule permits the taxpayer to ignore the receipts attributable to the services if they are less than five percent of the receipts received from the property.

Example 27. Same facts as in *Example 26* except the game may be played on demand online for a fee. According to the Regulations, such fees are not considered qualified DPGR. As might be expected, businesses question whether such interpretation is appropriate since the software is produced in the same way but simply delivered differently.

Note that the definition of DPGR is quite broad, extending the benefits of § 199 to a wide variety of activities. In fact, some of these activities normally are not associated with manufacturing. For example, § 199 blesses receipts from engineering and architectural services, publishing and related advertising, motion picture production, television production, musical recording production, traditional or cable broadcasting, home construction, the writing of machine-readable computer code and meat packing. However, § 199 identifies certain gross receipts that do not qualify, including those from the

1. Sale of food and beverages prepared by the taxpayer at a retail establishment (e.g., restaurants); but, wholesale sales of such prepared items do qualify.

2. Transmission or distribution of electricity, natural gas, or potable (drinkable) water.

3. Property leased, licensed, or rented by the taxpayer for use by any related person.

De Minimus 5% Rule. One major simplification addresses the calculation of DPGR where the taxpayer has receipts from both qualifying and nonqualifying activities (e.g., U.S. and foreign production or manufacturing and services). If the taxpayer earns less than five percent of total gross receipts from nonqualifying activities (including interest, dividends, royalties and all other nonqualifying receipts), it may treat all of its gross receipts as domestic production gross receipts and no allocation is required. The reverse is also true. If less than five percent of total gross receipts are from domestic production activities, all of the taxpayer's gross receipts may be treated as non-DPGR. This rule enables taxpayer to avoid the complex provisions of § 199. In this regard, it should be emphasized that § 199 is not optional.

DPGR: Item-By-Item Determination. In many cases, a product represents the combination of several components only some of which may be qualified property (e.g., manufactured in the U.S). For example, televisions, cars, computers or similar products may consist of components manufactured in the U.S. or elsewhere. In these situations, DPGR must be determined on an item-by-item basis and not by division, product line or transaction.[64] Generally this requires that the taxpayer drill down and perform an analysis of each component of the property to determine its origin even though doing so

---

[64]   Reg. § 1.199-3(d)(1)

can be unduly burdensome and costly. This approach is often referred to as the "shrinkback rule" because the taxpayer must "shrink back" the product to the largest component that does qualify. The government believes that if this approach was not used, taxpayers might otherwise receive benefits for gross receipts that do not qualify.

Example 28. Since 1930 CH Inc. has operated a shoe manufacturing business in Maine. Historically, everything was "made in the U.S.A." However, last year, CH hired a new CEO who brought in new ideas, including changes in the company's traditional manufacturing practices. Under the new approach, the company continues to manufacture leather and rubber soles but imports the shoe's uppers (the parts of the shoe above the sole). CH manufactures shoes for sale by sewing or otherwise attaching the soles to the imported uppers. In determining CH's DPGR from the shoe sales, the gross receipts from the sale of the entire shoe would not qualify. However, under the shrinkback rule, the soles would be considered the item and the sales receipts allocable to the soles would qualify as DPGR.

Expense Allocation. After DPGR is determined, allocable costs are subtracted to arrive at QPAI. As may be seen in the formula, if a taxpayer is in a "manufacturing" business, the taxpayer's QPAI theoretically will equal its taxable income. Indeed, for many businesses, particularly small ones, this should be the case. For example, if a company only manufactures envelopes in the U.S., its taxable income and QPAI should be the same. since all of its taxable income relates to manufacturing. This also would be the case for a contractor that only builds homes in the U.S. Similarly, an architectural firm whose sole source of income is from providing architectural services should have identical amounts of taxable income and QPAI. On the other, because this is often not the case, the key to calculating the correct deduction amount is a proper allocation of items of gross receipts, expense, losses, and deductions for determining QPAI.

The Regulations contain three methods for allocating expenses. Two of these are simplifed methods for small businesses while the third applies to all other taxpayers (or small businesses if they choose).

1. *Small Business Simplified Overall Method.* Taxpayers with gross receipts less than $5 million may allocate all costs, including costs of goods sold, based on gross receipts. This also applies to taxpayers with gross receipts less than $10 million if they are eligible to use cash-method of accounting.

2. *Simplified Deduction Method.* Taxpayers with less than $25 million gross receipts may allocate non-costs of good sold expenses based on gross receipts.

3. *Section 861 method.* This method uses the principles relating to determining the source of taxable income for purposes of the foreign tax credit (i.e., whether taxable income derives from activities within or outside the United States). The § 861 method is mandatory for taxpayers with greater than $25 million gross receipts; it is voluntary for other taxpayers.

Example 29. G Inc. manufactures razor blades in a plants in Columbus, Ohio and Munich, Germany. The blades from both factories are sold all over the world. Gross receipts from the sales of blades from the Columbus operation qualify as DPGR for purpose of calculating the production deduction since they are derived from the sale of qualifying production property—tangible personal property (the razor blades)—that is manufactured by the taxpayer, G, entirely in the U.S. Note that all of the gross receipts qualify as domestic notwithstanding the fact that a portion could be attributable to sales in foreign countries (e.g., Canada and Mexico).

Example 30. Same facts as above. For the current year, the company reported taxable income of $4,000,000. Total wages for all employees were $6,000,000. The company's records reveal the additional information below. Based on this information the production deduction is $2,400,000 computed as follows:

Qualifying domestic production gross receipts.	$15,000,000	
Allocable costs:		
Costs of good sold $4,000,000		
Directly allocable expenses. 3,000,000		
Indirect expenses 1,000,000		
Total allocable costs	(8,000,000)	
Qualified production activities income.	$7,000,000	
Taxable income before the production deduction	$4,000,000	
Lesser of QPAI $7,000,000 or taxable income $4,000,000	$4,000,000
2009 rate	× 6%
Tentative production deduction	$2,400,000
Wage limitation (50% × $6,000,000 wages)	$3,000,000
Production deduction	
(lesser of tentative production deduction or wage limitation)	$2,400,000

Note that the production deduction is permitted for AMT purposes. However, the taxable income limitation is based on AMTI rather than taxable income.

Unresolved Issues. Unfortunately, the artificial simplicity of the examples above masks the many obstacles that make application of § 199 troublesome. To appreciate the difficulty, simply consider the basic requirements that must be met in order to secure the deduction: *qualified property must be manufactured, produced, grown, or extracted by the taxpayer in whole or in significant part within the U.S.* At the start, § 199 provides no definition of manufacturing or production. Does assembly of vacuum cleaners or conversion of orange concentrate into orange juice constitute production? What about mixing water and concentrate to produce soft drinks or French Vanilla coffee? When McDonald's sells a hamburger is it providing a service or is it combining inputs to manufacture a product? While the Regulations address some of these issues, many are still unresolved.

Still another complication involves the complexity in distinguishing between qualified and nonqualified gross receipts and the problem of allocating expenses between them. The already famous "Starbucks footnote" found in the Conference Report acknowledges the difficulty.

Example 31. Coffee Inc. operates a chain of coffee shops all over the world. It buys coffee beans and roasts and packages them at its own central processing facility. It distributes the packages of roasted coffee to its own retail stores which the stores brew for selling to customers. In addition, the stores sell the packaged coffee directly to consumers and to other retail stores. How are the gross receipts from a single sale of coffee classified? How much is attributable to the qualifying production activity, the roasting of the beans, and how much is attributed to the nonqualifying activity, the processing in the retail establishment. An even more daunting question concerns how the various costs of operating the company are to be allocated between these activities. According to the footnote, only the sales receipts attributable to the off-site roasting function can be taken into account in computing QPAI. The balance of the

receipts is not qualified. Note also that the rule creates an incentive for a company like Starbucks to increase the amount that its factory charges its retail store in order to increase the amount of factory gross receipts and thus increase the deduction.

There are many other issues worthy of consideration but are beyond the scope of this overview. The Regulations issued in October 2005 do provide guidance on how to solve some of these problems but not all. In any event, it should be emphasized that § 199 can have a major impact not simply on the accounting systems that must be designed to capture the required information but also on how a company structures itself and conducts its business.

TAX PLANNING CONSIDERATIONS

CASUALTY AND THEFT LOSSES

Much of the controversy surrounding casualty losses results from insufficient documentation of the loss. For this reason, taxpayers should give careful attention to accumulating the evidence necessary to establish the deduction. Such evidence would include, where appropriate, pictures, eyewitnesses, police reports, and newspaper accounts. The taxpayer also should gather evidence regarding the value of the property damaged or destroyed. In situations where an item is not repaired or replaced, an appraisal may be the only method of adequately valuing the loss.

In some cases, a taxpayer may suffer a casualty loss and in seeking insurance reimbursement incur appraisal costs. Even if the casualty loss is not deductible due to the 10 percent limitation, the appraisal costs are deductible as a cost of preparing the tax return and are therefore claimed as a miscellaneous itemized deduction.

Taxpayers often measure the amount of their casualty losses by the amount paid for repairs that are necessary to bring the property back to its condition before the casualty. This method of measuring may be inappropriate, however, if the repairs do not restore the property to its same condition before the casualty. In such case, an additional loss representing the decline in value should be claimed.

The rules for determining the deductible casualty loss have important implications for the amount of insurance that a taxpayer should maintain.

> **Example 32.** T purchased a home in Boston for $70,000 15 years ago. This year, the home burned to the ground and the taxpayer received a $70,000 reimbursement from the insurance company. The cost of rebuilding the house was $200,000. Although T's economic loss was $130,000 ($200,000 − $70,000), none of the loss is deductible as a casualty loss. The casualty loss deduction is the *lesser* of the decline in value, $200,000, or the taxpayer's adjusted basis, $70,000, less the insurance reimbursement. Since the insurance reimbursement of $70,000 completely offset T's basis, there is no deductible loss.

BAD DEBTS

It is not uncommon for family members or friends to make loans to each other that are never repaid. This often occurs when a son or daughter is embarking on a business venture in which a parent is willing to invest. If the taxpayer wishes to claim a deduction if the debt is not paid, steps should be taken upon making the loan to ensure that the loan is not considered a gift. For example, the taxpayer should document the transaction in such a way that it is clear that both parties intend that repayment of the loan will occur. The best

method of documenting the parties' wishes is to have a formal note drafted. Such a note would lend support to the argument that a debtor-creditor relationship existed between the parties. The note also should have a definite payment schedule, and each payment should be made on time. Collateral could be included as well. In addition, the note should call for a reasonable amount of interest. Failure to charge adequate interest could cause the imputed interest rules discussed in Chapter 5 to operate.

> **Example 33.** In 2009 F loaned his friend K $10,000 to start a chocolate chip cookie business. The business struggled along, requiring K to ask F for another $5,000, which he gladly loaned her. The business failed after six months. If F documented the loans and sought repayment, he may claim a deduction for a nonbusiness bad debt. If he failed to do so, any deduction may be disallowed.

NET OPERATING LOSSES

When a taxpayer suffers a net operating loss, a decision must be made whether to carry the loss back or elect to carry it forward only. Due to the time value of money, a carryback is usually more advantageous since an immediate tax refund can be obtained. However, this gain must be weighed against the future benefits to be obtained by a carryforward. If the taxpayer expects to be in a higher tax bracket in the future, the present value of the higher savings may be greater than the value of an immediate refund.

PROBLEM MATERIALS

DISCUSSION QUESTIONS

10-1 *Business vs. Nonbusiness Bad Debts.* R is employed as the chief executive officer of XYZ Corporation. Believing the company's future to be bright, he has acquired 75 percent of XYZ's stock. During the year, R loaned XYZ $10,000. Explain the tax consequences assuming XYZ is unable to repay all or a portion of the loan.

10-2 *Bad Debt Requirements.* Under what circumstances, if any, is a cash basis taxpayer allowed to claim a deduction for a bad debt? An accrual basis taxpayer?

10-3 *Identifying Bad Debts.* For each of the following situations, indicate whether the taxpayer would be able to claim a deduction for a bad debt.
   a. Several years ago, F advanced $30,000 to his wholly owned corporation, which was experiencing financial difficulties. Last year he loaned it another $10,000. No notes were executed and no payments have been made. During the current year, the company declared bankruptcy.
   b. E quit his old job as a salesperson to become a sales manager for K Corporation this year. As part of his arrangement with K, he was to receive a $10,000 bonus if the company reached $1 million in sales for the year. Sales for the year were $900,000, and K Corporation did not pay E a bonus.
   c. B and C each own 50 percent of ABC Incorporated. Over the years, ABC made loans to C. When C died he was penniless. He owed the company $20,000.

10-4 *Is There a Bad Debt?* Several years ago, R's son, S, got into the restaurant business. R loaned S $10,000 to help him get the business going. No note was signed nor was any interest charged. The business was initially a huge success but as time passed, it began having financial problems. This year the son's business failed.
   a. Can R claim a bad debt deduction? If so, is the debt a business or nonbusiness bad debt and how much is the deduction?
   b. Same as (a) except R obtained a signed note from his son.

10-5 *Bad Debt of Related Party.* H loaned her son $10,000 to enter the car repair business. If the son subsequently abandons the business and does not repay the loan, what are the tax consequences to H?

10-6 *Casualty Losses.* Explain the rationale underlying the rules (lower of basis or value with certain exceptions) for computing the amount of the deduction for a casualty loss.

10-7 *Casualty Losses.* During the year, R had various losses. Explain whether each of the following would qualify as a casualty loss.
    a. Loss of stove due to electrical fire.
    b. Damage to water pipes from freezing temperatures in Southern California.
    c. Loss of tree from Dutch elm disease.
    d. Ruined carpeting from clogged sewer line.
    e. Hole in his suit from cigarette ashes he dropped; ruined shirt from pen leaking.
    f. Damage to both his and his neighbor's car while R's son drove R's car.
    g. Luggage and contents seized by a foreign government during a European vacation.

10-8 *Theft Loss Calculation.* If taxpayers could plan their taxes to account for thefts of their own personal use property (e.g., theft of their stereo and television), would they want the burglar to take all the property at once or take some property the first time and return for more later?

10-9 *Net Operating Losses in General.* Comment on each of the following:
    a. The purposes of the net operating loss deduction.
    b. The rationale underlying the complex calculation of the net operating loss deduction.
    c. How a net operating loss occurring in 2009 is utilized (i.e., the carryover process).

10-10 *Inventoriable Costs: § 263A.* HHG operates a chain of retail appliance stores. The company has grown tremendously over the past several years. It expects that its gross receipts will exceed $10 million this year. What are the implications of this growth for the company's method of accounting for inventories?

10-11 *LIFO vs. FIFO.* During the 1970s, there was a tremendous shift from the FIFO method of inventory to LIFO. Nevertheless, not every company shifted to the LIFO method. Discuss why some might shift to LIFO although others might not.

PROBLEMS

10-12 *Treatment of Bad Debts.* AAA Computer Company, an accrual basis corporation, installed a new computerized accounting system for a customer and billed him $1,500 in June, 2009. When aging its accounts receivable at year-end, the company found that the customer was experiencing financial difficulties.
    a. Assuming the company estimated that only $1,000 of the account would be collected, what is the amount of the bad debt deduction, if any, that it can claim in 2009?
    b. Would the answer to (a) change if the debt were a nonbusiness bad debt?
    c. In 2010 the company actually collected $200 and the remainder of the debt was worthless. What is the amount of the bad debt deduction, if any, that it can claim in 2010?

10-13 *Bad Debts and Accounting Methods.* Dr. D, a dentist, performed a root canal for a patient and charged him $300. The patient paid $100, then left town, never to be seen again. What is the amount of bad debt deduction, if any, that D may claim assuming that she is a cash basis taxpayer?

10-14 *Uncollectible Loan.* Several years ago, L loaned his old high-school friend B $5,000 to help him start a new business. Things did not go as well as B planned, and late in 2009 B declared bankruptcy. L expects to collect 40 cents on the dollar. In 2010 all of B's affairs were settled and L received $1,000. What are the tax consequences to L in 2009 and 2010?

10-15 *Personal Casualty.* When the waters of the Mississippi began to overflow their banks and flood the surrounding area, M was forced to leave her home and head for higher ground. On December 2, she returned to her home to find that it had been vandalized as well as damaged from the flood. After cleaning up, she determined that the following items had been stolen or damaged:

Item	Adjusted Basis	FMV Before	FMV After	Insurance Reimbursement
Fur coat	$6,000	$7,000	$0	$7,000
Computer	4,000	3,000	0	Uninsured
Couch	1,200	800	See below	500
Van	7,000	5,000		

The couch had been damaged and M had it reupholstered for $700. The insurance company reimbursed her for the amounts shown on December 27. Under M's insurance policy, the company did not reimburse her for loss on the car until 45 days had passed. M expected to recover $4,000 but, after several delays, finally received a check for $2,000 on April 25, 2010. While she was waiting for reimbursement for her van, she rented a car at a total cost of $700. Although M received value for the coat, she did not replace it. In addition to the losses shown above, her real estate broker advised that even though her house had not been damaged by the flood, the value had dropped by $20,000 since it was evident that it was located in an area prone to flooding.

a. Compute M's casualty loss deduction, assuming her A.G.I. in 2009 was $18,000 and in 2010, $20,000.

b. Assume the loss occurred on January 2, 2010 and the location was officially designated a disaster area by the President. Explain when the loss could be deducted.

10-16 *Casualty Loss: Business and Investment Property.* H is a private detective. While sleuthing this year, his car was stolen. The car, which was used entirely for business, was worth $7,000 and had an adjusted basis of $12,000. H received no insurance reimbursement for his car. Also this year, his office was the victim of arson. The fire destroyed only a painting that had a basis of $1,500 and was worth $3,000. H received a reimbursement of $800 from his insurance company for the painting. H suffered yet another misfortune this year as his rental property was damaged by a flood, the first in the area in 70 years. Before the casualty, the property—which had greatly appreciated in value—was worth $90,000 and afterward only $40,000. The rental property had an adjusted basis of $30,000. He received $20,000 from the insurance company, the maximum amount for which homes in a flood plain could be insured. Compute H's casualty loss deduction assuming his A.G.I. is $30,000. Can a casualty loss create a net operating loss?

10-17 *Casualty Gains and Losses.* This year, C's jewelry, which cost $10,000, was stolen from her home. Luckily, she was insured and the insurance company reimbursed her for its current value, $19,000. In addition, while she was on vacation all of her camera equipment was stolen. The camera equipment had cost her $3,500 and was worth $3,100. She received no reimbursement since she carried a large deductible on such items. C's A.G.I. for the year was $15,000.
    a. What is the effect of the casualty losses on C's taxable income?
    b. Same as above except the jewelry was worth $11,000.

10-18 *Casualty and Theft Loss Computation.* In each of the following cases, compute the taxpayer's casualty loss deduction (before percentage limitations) and indicate whether it is deductible *for* or *from* adjusted gross income.
    a. While G was at the theater, his house (adjusted basis $60,000, fair market value $80,000) was completely destroyed by fire. The fire also completely destroyed both his skiing equipment (cost $300, fair market value $90) and a calculator (adjusted basis $110, fair market value $80) used for business. He was reimbursed for $30,000 with respect to the house.
    b. B owned a duplex which she rented. A tornado demolished the roof but did not damage the remainder of the duplex. The duplex's value before the tornado was $45,000 and after the tornado was $40,000. B's adjusted basis in the property was $30,000. The President declared the entire city a "disaster area."
    c. Assume the same facts in (b) except that instead of B's duplex being partially damaged it was her personal cabin cruiser, and she received a $2,000 reimbursement from the insurance company.
    d. L backed his car out of the garage and ran over his 10-speed bicycle (cost $400, fair market value $300). The bicycle is worthless.

10-19 *NOL Items.* Indicate whether the following items can create a net operating loss for an individual taxpayer.
    a. Business capital loss
    b. Nonbusiness bad debt
    c. Casualty loss
    d. Interest expense on mortgage secured by primary residence
    e. Employee business expenses
    f. Contribution to Individual Retirement Account
    g. Alimony
    h. Personal exemption

10-20 *Items Considered in Computing an NOL.* Indicate whether the following items are considered in computing the net operating loss deduction for an individual.
    a. Salary
    b. Capital gain on the sale of investment property
    c. Interest income
    d. Interest on a mortgage on a primary residence

10-21 *Net Operating Loss Computation.* R, a single taxpayer, operates a bicycle shop. For the calendar year 2009 he reports the following items of income and expense:

Gross income from business	$150,000
Business operating expenses	210,000
Interest income from investments	7,000
Casualty loss	4,000
Interest expense on home mortgage.	9,000
Long-term capital gains (nonbusiness).	3,000
Long-term capital loss (nonbusiness)	5,000
Long-term capital gains (business)	1,000

The casualty loss represented the uninsured theft of R's personal auto worth $4,100 ($9,000 adjusted basis).

a. Compute R's net operating loss for 2009.

b. Assuming R carries the loss back to 2007, when must the corrected return for 2007 be filed?

10-22 *Net Operating Loss Computation.* V, married with two dependents, owns a hardware store. For the current year, her records reveal the following:

Gross income from sales	$180,000
Business operating expenses	230,000
Royalties from investment	6,000
Nonbusiness expenses	9,000
Long-term capital gain (nonbusiness)	5,000
Long-term capital gain (business)	3,000
Long-term capital loss (business)	3,500

What is V's net operating loss?

10-23 *Valuing Inventories.* Chapters Inc., a large publishing house, prints a variety of titles, some of which are best sellers and others of which are duds. Because it is very difficult for Chapters to estimate with any accuracy which books will be successful, and because the marginal cost of printing an additional book is small, it typically prints 5,000 more copies than it expects to sell. Books that are not sold within a year of release are stored. The company's experience has shown that 95 percent of the books stored are never sold. Consequently, the company writes off any excess copies once they are delivered to storage. This practice appears permissible for financial accounting purposes. Can the same procedure be used for tax purposes?

10-24 *Applying Lower of Cost or Market.* Fitness Galore specializes in selling physical fitness equipment. The company's inventory at the close of this year revealed the following:

Mercandise	Cost	Replacement Cost
Weight machines	$40,000	$43,000
Stationary bicycles	10,000	8,000
Stair climbers	24,000	27,000

a. Compute the company's inventory assuming it uses the lower of FIFO cost or market.

b. Assume the company adopts LIFO next year. Explain the tax consequences.

10-25 *Double Extension Dollar-Value LIFO.* Unwound Sound has recently engaged an accountant to evaluate its inventory procedures and determine whether it should change from using FIFO to LIFO to account for inventories. The company's inventory records for 2008 and 2009 are shown below. Assume that the company had adopted double-extension dollar-value LIFO in 2008, and compute the ending inventory for:

a. 2008

b. 2009

	1-1-08		12-31-09	
Inventory Pool	Units	Cost Per Unit	Units	Cost Per Unit
Records	5,000	$2	3,000	$2
Tapes	4,000	3	6,000	4
Compact discs	2,000	6	5,000	7

	12-31-09	
Inventory Pool	Units	Cost Per Unit
Records	2,000	$3
Tapes	3,000	5
Compact discs	4,000	7

10-26 *LIFO Pooling.* As shown in *Problem 10-25* above, the inventory of Unwound Sound consists of records, tapes, and compact discs. Over the last 15 years, the components of the company's inventory have changed dramatically. Whereas once the company only carried records, now it also carries tapes and CDs. Unwound Sound expects that in the very near future it will discontinue selling records. Assuming the company uses LIFO, explain the advantages of having one single pool containing all three items rather than three different pools.

10-27 *Accounting for Inventories.* VE Trucking Inc., an S Corporation and a cash-basis taxpayer, buys and transports sand and gravel for its customers, primarily contractors and developers. The contractors and developers use the materials in the construction of foundations for streets, houses, buildings and other construction projects. Normally, a customer contacts VE and orders a load of sand or gravel which VE subsequently buys from another source. VE then picks up the materials and delivers them to the customer's job site. VE bills the customer a flat sum, representing the costs of the materials and transportation. To determine the amount of the charge, the total cost is marked up for a reasonable profit. Because VE acquires and delivers the sand and gravel to its customers during the same business day, it does not possess any sand and gravel at the beginning or end of its business day. VE has been very profitable over the past ten years, averaging annual earnings of about $4,000,000 on annual revenues of about $15,000,000.
   a. Must VE use the accrual method? If so, will the accrual method have any impact given that VE has no materials at the beginning and end of each business day?
   b. Same as (a) except VE has average annual gross receipts of $8,000,000.
   c. Same as (b) except VE is a C corporation
   d. Same as (a) except VE has average annual gross receipts of $700,000.

10-28 *Production Deduction.* For each of the following situations, explain how the facts affect application and determination of the § 199 deduction related to qualified production activities.
   a. BAH is a strategic management and technology consulting firm that provides advisory services to companies around the world.
   b. AMZ Corporation sells books and other products over the Internet throughout the world. All of its products that are purchased for resale are manufactured or produced by U.S. companies in the U.S.
   c. MSFT Inc. distributes software written by its employees.

d. RYL Corporation, located in Detroit, is a construction company that primarily builds residential homes. It also is in the business of selling and assembling prefabricated steel buildings used primarily by businesses. The materials for these metal buildings are supplied by another corporation. RYL simply pours the foundation and bolts the materials in place. In addition, RYL's engineers and architects provide consulting services. One of RYL's subsidiaries is in the remodeling business.

e. CSC is currently a single member limited liability company operated by Jim Smith. The LLC has seven employees. It is in the advertising business, producing commercials for television, radio, the Internet, and print media.

f. PNA Inc. operates several restaurants in Houston. Its menu consists primarily of soup and sandwiches. The company's baked products such as bread and cookies are also popular. In fact, PNA has its own central baking operation that produces bread and other pastry items that are sold to some of the finest restaurants in the area.

10-29 *Domestic Production Gross Receipts.* OMG owns and operates grocery stores throughout the greater metropolitan area of Chicago. In addition to its retail outlets, it has its own bakery, ice-making, meat-processing and egg-farming businesses. Answer the following questions concerning the company's domestic production gross receipts (DPGR).

a. OMG is primarily a reseller. Will it qualify for the § 199 deduction?

b. Many of OMG's stores have their own bakery that bakes bread, cakes, donuts and similar items that are sold at the store to its retail customers. Do the receipts qualify as DPGR?

c. Many of the stores have arrangements to provide fresh baked goods daily to area restaurants. Would receipts from sales to these wholesale customers qualify as DPGR?

d. Many of the baked goods sold to retail customers at OMG stores such as bread are baked off-site at a central baking facility and transported to their stores. Would receipts from sales to its retail customers qualify as DPGR?

e. In some instances, dough may be made or bread may be partially baked at a central baking facility and then transported to the stores for final baking. Would receipts from sales to its retail customers qualify as DPGR?

f. OMG has a construction division that builds the company's stores as well as strip malls in which the stores are located and serve as anchors. It leases the space in the strip malls to other businesses. Does OMG have any qualifying DPGR from these activities?

RESEARCH PROBLEMS

10-30 R has had several minor automobile accidents in the last two years. During the current year, R demolished his car (value, $7,000; adjusted basis, $8,000) when he ran into a telephone pole. He used the car solely for business. R decided not to report the accident to the insurance company and claim his reimbursement because he believes his insurance rates will be raised if he does. Will R's deduction of his unreimbursed casualty loss be allowed?

10-31 T, a cash basis taxpayer, paid a swimming pool contractor, C, the sum of $10,000 in advance for improvements that C agreed to make to T's personal residence. C performed part of the contract and then ceased activity, leaving much of the work uncompleted.

T seeks your advice concerning whether she may claim a deduction for a bad debt.

10-32 Ten years ago Mac and Beth left the stress of city life and moved to a beautiful home near Davenport overlooking the Mississippi River. Mac took a job as a dealer at a local riverboat gambling casino while Beth became a full-time mom. The couple was happily raising their four children until 2008, the year of the great flood. Their home, although several miles from the river, suffered thousands of dollars of water damage. Other

homes in their small subdivision that were on somewhat lower ground had far worse damage. Mac and Beth and their neighbors were quite shocked that this could happen to them since they lived in an area where it had not flooded for over 100 years. But then some were calling this the 100-year flood. After cleaning up, several of the owners decided to move, not willing to take any more chances. Unfortunately, those people who were able to sell their homes sold them for far less than what they thought they were worth, presumably because they lived in what was now perceived as a flood-prone area. Although Mac was not planning on selling his home, he did decide it was time to refinance his mortgage, the second time in 18 months. As part of the process, he got an appraisal that revealed that the value of his home had dropped substantially from the last time it was appraised. In 2005, when he refinanced for the first time, it appeared that he had made a great investment since he had purchased the house for $150,000 and the house was appraised at a value of $225,000. However, the most recent appraisal revealed that the house was worth only $120,000. What is the amount of the couple's casualty loss deduction, if any?

10-33   In 1986, Michael Malone, a professor of computer science and a specialist in digital technology, realized that it was only a short time before the computer would change the way people lived. Although he was 49 and quite happy with his $70,000 annual salary, he decided that this was an opportunity he just could not pass up. In 1986, he formed a new corporation, investing virtually all of his accumulated wealth, $200,000, in exchange for 51 percent of its stock. Three other individuals contributed additional cash for the remaining 49 percent of the stock. In the first few years of operation, the corporation was immensely successful. In 1988 Mike retired from the university and turned all of his attention to the business. All went well. In fact, things went so well that, by 1995, Mike turned over the supervision of everyday operations to several trusted employees; he began spending more time at the golf course and less time at the office. He was completely content working 20 hours a week and drawing an annual salary of $70,000. That income combined with his pension from the university of $20,000 a year was more than enough to keep him happy. During 2007, however, the competition in the computer business became fierce and the corporation had cash flow problems. As a result, Michael loaned the corporation $150,000 to keep it afloat. Unfortunately, the corporation was not able to survive and declared bankruptcy in 2009. How should Michael treat the worthless loan?

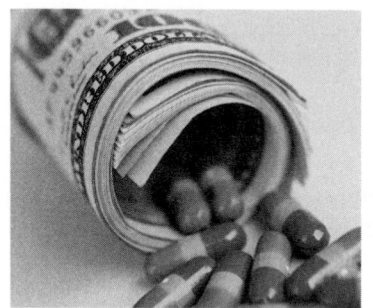

CHAPTER ELEVEN

ITEMIZED DEDUCTIONS

LEARNING OBJECTIVES

Upon completion of this chapter you will be able to:

▸ Identify the personal expenses that qualify as itemized deductions

▸ Explain the rules regarding deductible medical expenses and compute the medical expense deduction

▸ Distinguish between deductible taxes and nondeductible fees or other charges

▸ Explain the rules regarding deductible state income taxes, including the proper treatment of such taxes by married persons filing joint or separate returns

▸ Distinguish between currently deductible and nondeductible interest expenses

▸ Explain the requirements for the deductibility of charitable contributions and compute the contribution deduction

▸ Identify the personal expenditures that qualify as either miscellaneous itemized deductions or other itemized deductions

▸ Explain the cutback rule applicable to certain itemized deductions of high-income taxpayers and compute their total deduction allowed

CHAPTER OUTLINE

Although the vast majority of deductions are those for trade or business expenses, a taxpayer's deductions are not confined to these alone. As noted in Chapter 7, since 1942 Congress has also allowed taxpayers to deduct expenses relating to profit-seeking activities—thus creating a *second* category of so-called investment or nonbusiness expenses. In addition, despite the fact that Code § 262 expressly prohibits the deduction of personal expenditures, Congress has created various exceptions. As a result, a *third* category of deductible expenses exists, which contains such personal items as medical expenses, casualty losses, interest on home mortgages, taxes on real and personal property, charitable contributions, and tax return preparation costs. The last four chapters have focused primarily on business expenses. This chapter continues the discussion of the three types of deductions by examining the specific statutory and administrative authority relating to personal itemized deductions. As defined in Chapter 3, these personal expenses are deducted by a taxpayer only if (1) they exceed the available standard deduction, or (2) the taxpayer is not eligible for the standard deduction.

Before considering these deductions in detail, it should be emphasized that a particular type of expense (e.g., interest) does not necessarily receive the same treatment in all situations. More often than not, the expense is treated differently depending on whether it is business, investment, or personal in nature. For example, the deductibility of interest expense generally depends on whether it is related to a loan that was used to make a business, investment, or personal expenditure. In contrast, real property taxes are deductible regardless of whether the property is used for business, investment, or personal purposes. The character of the expense may also affect the deduction's

classification. Generally, trade or business expenses (other than the unreimbursed expenses of an employee) and expenses related to producing rents or royalties are deductions *for* A.G.I., while other expenses are *itemized deductions* which may or may not be subject to the 2 percent floor.

MEDICAL EXPENSES

IN GENERAL

Deductible medical expenses include amounts paid for the diagnosis, cure, relief, treatment, or prevention of disease of the taxpayer, his or her spouse, and dependents.[1] The status of a person as the taxpayer's spouse or dependent must exist *either* at the time the medical services are rendered *or* at the time the expenses are paid.[2] A spousal relationship does not exist if the taxpayer is legally separated from his or her spouse under a decree of separate maintenance because the two parties are not considered married.[3] For purposes of dependency status, however, *both* the gross income test and the joint return test are waived.[4]

> **Example 1.** T pays all the medical expenses of his mother, M, during the current year. Although M had gross income in excess of the exemption amount ($3,650 in 2009) for the current year, all other dependency tests are met by T. Even though T cannot claim M as a dependent, he will be allowed to deduct all medical expenses paid on her behalf (assuming T itemizes his deductions and they exceed the percentage limitations imposed on medical deductions).

Medical expenses for children of divorced parents are deductible by the parent who pays for them, regardless of which parent is entitled to the dependency exemption. Additionally, if a taxpayer is entitled to a dependency exemption under a multiple support agreement, the taxpayer will be allowed to deduct any medical expenses which he or she actually pays on behalf of the claimed dependent.[5]

Medical expenses also include payments for treatment affecting any part or function of the body,[6] expenditures for certain medicines and drugs,[7] expenses paid for transportation primarily *for* and *essential* to the rendition of the medical care,[8] and payments made for medical care insurance for the taxpayer, his or her spouse, and dependents.[9] Again, the term *dependent* includes any person who would otherwise qualify as the taxpayer's dependent even though the gross income or separate return tests are not met, and any person claimed as a dependent under a multiple support agreement.

---

[1]   See §§ 213(a) and 213(d)(1).

[2]   Reg. § 1.213-1(e)(3).

[3]   § 143(a).

[4]   See Reg. § 1.213-1(a)(3)(i) and Chapter 4 for a discussion of the dependency tests.

[5]   See § 213(d)(5) and Reg. § 1.213-1(a)(3)(i). Medical expenses taken into account under § 21 in computing a credit for the care of certain dependents are not allowed to be treated as deductible medical expenses. See § 213(e) and Reg. § 1.213-1(f) and Chapter 13 for a discussion of the tax credit allowed under § 21.

[6]   § 213(d)(1)(A) and Reg. § 1.213-1(e)(1)(i).

[7]   § 213(d)(2) and Reg. § 1.213-1(e)(2).

[8]   § 213(d)(1)(B) and Reg. § 1.213-1(e)(1)(iv).

[9]   § 213(d)(1)(C) and Reg. § 1.213-1(e)(4).

Partial lists of deductible and nondeductible medical expenses are presented in Exhibits 11-1 and 11-2. The most recent addition to the list of nondeductible medical expenses involves cosmetic surgery or other similar procedure. Cosmetic surgery is defined as any procedure that is directed at improving the patient's appearance and does not meaningfully promote the proper function of the body or prevent or treat disease. Thus, the costs of face lifts, liposuction, hair transplants, and other similar elective procedures undertaken primarily to improve the taxpayer's physical appearance are not deductible. However, deductions are allowed for procedures necessary to ameliorate a congenital deformity, a personal injury arising from an accident or trauma, or a disfiguring disease.

EXHIBIT 11-1
Partial List of Deductible Medical Expenses[10]

Fees paid for doctors, surgeons, dentists, osteopaths, ophthalmologists, optometrists, chiropractors, chiropodists, podiatrists, psychiatrists, psychologists, and Christian Science practitioners

Fees paid for hospital services, therapy, nursing services (including nurse's meals while on duty), ambulance hire, and laboratory, surgical, obstetrical, diagnostic, dental, and X-ray services

Meals and lodging provided by a hospital during medical treatment, and meals and lodging provided by a center during treatment for alcoholism or drug addiction

Medical and hospital insurance premiums

Medicines and drugs, but only if prescribed by doctor (includes vitamins, iron, and pills or other birth control items)

Special foods and drinks prescribed by doctor, but only if for the treatment of an illness

Special items, including braces for teeth or limbs, false teeth, artificial limbs, eyeglasses, contact lenses, hearing aids, crutches, wheelchairs, and guide dogs for the blind or deaf

Smoking cessation programs

Transportation expenses for needed medical care, including air, bus, boat, railroad, and taxi fares

EXHIBIT 11-2
Partial List of Nondeductible Expenditures[11]

Accident insurance premiums

Bottled water

Care of a normal and healthy baby by a nurse*

Cosmetic surgery (with limited exceptions)

Diaper service

Funeral and burial expenses

Health club dues

Household help*

Illegal operation or treatment

Maternity clothes

Social activities, such as dancing lessons, for the general improvement of health, even though recommended by doctor

Toothpaste, toiletries, cosmetics, etc.

Trip for general improvement of health

Vitamins for general health

* **Note:** A portion of these expenditures may qualify as expenses for the child or dependent care tax credit allowed under § 21. See Chapter 13 for further discussion of this credit.

---

[10]   See *Your Federal Income Tax*, IRS Publication 17 (Rev. 2008), p. 143.

[11]   *Ibid.*

WHEN DEDUCTIBLE

In computing the medical expense deduction for a given tax year, the taxpayer is allowed to take into account *only* those medical expenses *actually paid* during the taxable year, regardless of when the illness or injury that occasioned the expenses occurred, and regardless of the method of accounting used by the taxpayer in computing his or her taxable income (i.e., cash or accrual).[12] Consequently, if the medical expenses are incurred but not paid during the current tax year, the deduction for such expenses will not be allowed *until* the year of payment. The IRS has ruled, however, that the use of a bank credit card to pay for medical expenses *will* qualify as payment in the year of the credit card charge regardless of when the taxpayer actually repays the bank.[13]

The *prepayment* of medical expenses does not qualify as a current deduction unless the taxpayer is required to make the payment as a condition of receiving the medical services.[14] Accordingly, the IRS has ruled that a taxpayer's nonrefundable advance payments required as a condition for admission to a retirement home or institution for future lifetime medical care are deductible as expenses in the year paid.[15]

> **Example 2.** As a prerequisite for prenatal care and the delivery of her child, M prepays $3,150 to her doctor on November 15, 2009. Even though much of the prenatal care and the delivery of the child does not occur until 2010, M will be allowed to treat the prepayment as a medical expenditure in 2009.

DEDUCTION LIMITATIONS

The medical expense deduction was created by Congress with the stated social objective of providing individual taxpayers relief from a heavy tax burden during a period of medical emergency and thereby encouraging the maintenance of a high level of public health. However, the deduction was designed to provide relief for only those expenditures in excess of a normal or average amount. Currently, the medical expense deduction is allowed only to the extent medical expenditures exceed 7.5 percent of the taxpayer's adjusted gross income. This limitation ensures that only extraordinary medical costs will result in a deduction.

In addition to the percentage limitation imposed on the medical expense deduction, it is important to note that most of the everyday type of expenditures incurred by an individual for items incident to his or her general health and hygiene are excluded from the definition of qualifying medical expenses. For example, medicine and drug expenditures are deductible only if they are for insulin and *prescribed* drugs.[16] Over-the-counter medicines and drugs such as aspirin, cold remedies, skin lotions, and vitamins are not deductible. Other nondeductible expenditures are listed in Exhibit 11-2.

---

[12] Reg. § 1.213-1(a)(1).

[13] Rev. Rul. 78-39, 1978-1 C.B. 73.

[14] See *Robert S. Basset*, 26 T.C. 619 (1956). Absent such a prohibition, a taxpayer could maximize the tax benefits of medical deductions simply by timing the year of payment.

[15] Rev Rul. 75-303, 1975-2 C.B. 87.

[16] § 213(b) and Reg. § 1.213-1(b)(2)(i).

Example 3. F had adjusted gross income of $30,000 for 2009 and paid the following medical expenses:

Doctors	$ 500
Dentist	600
Hospital	1,300
Medical insurance premiums	800
Medicines and drugs:	
Prescription drugs	300
Nonprescription medicines	150

Assuming F is not reimbursed for any of the medical expenditures during 2009, her medical expense deduction is computed as follows:

Medical insurance premiums	$ 800
Fees paid doctors and dentist	1,100
Hospital costs	1,300
Prescription drugs only	300
Total medical expenses taken into account	$3,500
Less: 7.5% of $30,000 (A.G.I.)	−2,250
Allowable medical deduction for 2009	$1,250

SPECIAL ITEMS AND EQUIPMENT

The term *medical care* includes not only the diagnosis, treatment, and cure of disease, but the mitigation and prevention of disease as well. Thus, a taxpayer's expenditures for special items such as contact lenses, eyeglasses, hearing aids, artificial teeth or limbs, and ambulance hire would also qualify as medical expenditures.[17] Similarly, the cost of special equipment (e.g., wheelchairs and special controls or other equipment installed in an auto for use by a physically handicapped person) purchased *primarily* for the prevention or alleviation of a physical or mental defect or illness will be allowed as medical deductions. If the purchase of special equipment qualifies as a medical expenditure, the cost of its operation and maintenance is also a deductible medical expense.[18]

Capital expenditures generally are not deductible for Federal income tax purposes (i.e., depreciation is allowed only for property or equipment used in a taxpayer's trade or business or other income-producing activity). However, if a capital expenditure would otherwise qualify as a medical expense (i.e., it is incurred primarily for medical care), it will not be disqualified as a deduction. If the capital expenditure is for the permanent improvement or betterment of property such as the taxpayer's home, *only* the amount of the expenditure which *exceeds* the increase in value of the property improved will qualify as a medical expense.[19]

---

[17] Reg. § 1.213-1(e)(1)(ii). The IRS has ruled that the costs to acquire, train, and maintain a dog that assists a blind or deaf taxpayer are deductible medical expenses (see Rev. Rul. 55-216, 1955-1 C.B. 307 and Rev. Rul. 68-295, 1968-1 C.B. 92). In the Committee Reports for the Technical and Miscellaneous Revenue Act of 1988, Congress indicated its approval of this IRS position and stated that similar costs incurred with respect to a dog *or* other service animal used to assist individuals with *other physical disabilities* would also be eligible for the medical expense deduction.

[18] *Supra,* Footnote 10.

[19] Reg. § 1.213-1(e)(1)(iii).

Example 4. After suffering a heart attack, T is advised by his physician to install an elevator in his residence rather than continue climbing the stairs. If the cost of installing the elevator is $18,000 and the increase in the value of his residence is determined to be only $7,000, the difference of $11,000 will be deductible by T as a medical expense in the year paid. Annual operating costs (i.e., utilities) and maintenance of the elevator also qualify as deductible medical expenses.

In two specific situations, any increase in value of the improved property is ignored (or deemed to be zero) for purposes of measuring the medical expense deduction. First, if permanent improvements are made to property *rented* by the taxpayer, the *entire* costs are deductible (subject to the 7.5% floor).[20] Likewise, the entire cost of certain home-related capital expenditures incurred by a physically handicapped individual qualifies as a medical expense. Qualifying costs include expenditures for (1) constructing entrance or exit ramps to the residence; (2) widening doorways at entrances or exits to the residence; (3) widening or otherwise modifying hallways and interior doorways to accommodate wheelchairs; (4) railings, support bars, or other modifications to bathrooms to accommodate handicapped individuals; (5) lowering of or other modifications to kitchen cabinets and equipment to accommodate access by handicapped individuals; and (6) adjustment of electrical outlets and fixtures.

SPECIAL CARE FACILITIES

Expenses paid for emergency room treatment or hospital care of the taxpayer, his or her spouse, or dependents qualify for the medical deduction.[21] However, the deductibility of expenses for care in an institution other than a hospital depends upon the medical condition of the individual *and* the nature of the services he or she receives. If the *principal reason* an individual is in an institution (such as a nursing home or special school) is the availability of medical care, the *entire cost* of the medical care qualifies as a medical expenditure. This includes the cost of meals and lodging as well as any tuition expenses of special schools.[22]

Example 5. T enrolled his dependent son, S, in a special school for children with hearing impairments. If the principal reason for S's attendance at the school is his medical condition *and* the institution has the resources to treat or supervise training of the hearing impaired, the entire cost of S's attendance at the school qualifies as a medical expense. This includes tuition, meals and lodging, and any other costs that are incidental to the special services furnished by the school.

If an individual's medical condition *is not* the principal reason for being in an institution, only that part of the cost of care in the institution which is attributable to medical care will qualify as a medical expense.[23]

Example 6. T placed her dependent father, F, in a nursing home after F suffered a stroke and partial paralysis. Of the $6,000 total nursing home expenses, only $2,500 is attributable to the medical care and nursing attention furnished to F. If F is not in

---

[20] Rev. Rul. 70-395, 1970-2 C.B. 65.

[21] This includes the cost of meals and lodging incurred as an in-patient of a hospital. See Reg. § 1.213-1 (e)(1)(v).

[22] Reg. § 1.213-1(e)(1)(v)(a). See also *Donald R. Pfeifer*, 37 TCM 817, T.C. Memo 1978-189; *W.B. Counts*, 42 T.C. 755 (1963); Rev. Rul. 78-340, 1978-2 C.B. 124; and Rev. Rul. 58-533, 1958-2 C.B. 108.

[23] Reg. § 1.213-1(e)(1)(v)(b). This *excludes* meals and lodging and any other expenses not directly attributable to the medical care or treatment.

the nursing home for the principal reason of the medical and nursing care, only $2,500 will be deductible by T.

LONG-TERM CARE COSTS

As life expectancy has increased and the population aged, more and more people have incurred costs related to long-term care. Costs of long-term care include expenses not only for medicine and medical treatment but also a variety of services (e.g., help in eating, dressing, using the bathroom, bathing, taking medications, going places, grooming and the like). Prior to 1996, it was unclear whether the costs of long-term care qualified as a medical expense. The IRS commonly challenged such costs as personal and denied their deduction. Tax legislation passed in 1996 clarified the treatment of such expenses by providing that the costs for qualified long-term care services provided to a chronically-ill taxpayer (or his or her spouse or dependents) that are not reimbursed, as well as the premiums paid for long-term care insurance that meets certain requirements, are eligible for deduction as medical expenses.

Qualified long-term care services generally include necessary diagnostic, preventive, therapeutic, curing, treating, mitigating and rehabilitative services, and maintenance or personal care services that are required by a chronically-ill individual and provided pursuant to a plan of care prescribed by a licensed health care practitioner. A chronically-ill individual is generally a person who is unable to perform at least two activities of daily living (e.g., eating, toileting, transferring, bathing, dressing, and continence) for a period of at least 90 days due to a loss of functional capacity.

The amount deductible for insurance premiums is subject to limitations, but also is adjusted annually for inflation. The limits for 2009 are as follows:

Age before close of tax year	Limitation
40 or less	$ 320
More than 40 but less than 50	600
More than 50 but less than 60	1,190
More than 60 but less than 70	3,180
More than 70	3,980

Amounts paid to relatives for long-term care services normally are not eligible for deduction unless such person is a licensed professional with respect to the services that he or she is providing.

In addition, § 7702B allows an income exclusion for long-term care benefits received by an individual. For 2009, the exclusion from gross income is the greater of $280 per day or the actual cost of the care.

MEDICAL TRAVEL AND TRANSPORTATION

Expenses paid for transportation to and from the office of a doctor or dentist or to a hospital or clinic usually are deductible as medical expenses. This includes amounts paid for bus, taxi, train, and plane fares, as well as the out-of-pocket expenses for use of the taxpayer's personal vehicle (i.e., gas and oil, parking fees, and tolls). If the taxpayer uses his or her personal automobile for medical transportation and does not want to calculate actual expenses, the IRS allows a deduction. For 2009, the deduction is 24 cents a mile *plus* parking fees and tolls paid while traveling for medical treatment.[24]

Travel costs include *only* transportation expenses and the cost of lodging. For these expenses to qualify as a medical deduction, a trip beyond the taxpayer's locale *must* be

---

[24]   Rev. Proc. 2008-72, 2008-50 I.R.B.

"primarily for and essential to medical care."[25] Meal costs are deductible only if provided by a hospital or similar institution as a necessary part of medical care. Thus, meals consumed while en route between the taxpayer's home and the location of the medical care are not deductible.

If an individual receives medical treatment as an outpatient at a clinic or doctor's office, the cost of lodging while in the new locality may be deductible—but not the cost of meals. The cost of lodging will qualify as a medical expense if (1) the lodging is not lavish or extravagant under the circumstances; and (2) there is no significant element of personal pleasure, recreation, or vacation in the travel away from home. If deductible, the amount of lodging costs includible as a medical expense may not exceed *$50* for *each night* for each individual.[26] It is important to note that travel costs of a companion (including parents or a nurse) are included as medical expenses if the individual requiring medical treatment could not travel alone, or if the companion rendered medical treatment en route.[27] Thus, the lodging costs of such a person while in the new locality should also be treated as a part of any medical expenses (subject to the $50 per night limitation).

> **Example 7.** At the advice of a doctor, T travels with his three-year-old daughter, D, from Lincoln, Nebraska to Houston, Texas. D has a rare blood disease and a hospital in Houston is the nearest facility specializing in treatment of her disorder. The transportation costs and lodging for both T and his daughter while en route to and from Houston are deductible. If they stay at a nearby hotel while D receives treatment as an outpatient, the costs of lodging (but not meals) incurred in Houston—up to $100 per night—are also deductible.

MEDICAL INSURANCE COSTS AND REIMBURSEMENTS

Amounts paid for medical care insurance for the taxpayer, his or her spouse, and dependents qualify as medical expenses. If premiums are paid under an insurance contract which offers coverage beyond medical care (e.g., coverage for loss of life, limb, or sight, or loss of income), only the portion of the premiums paid that is attributable to medical care is deductible. To be deductible, however, the medical care portion of the premiums paid must either be separately stated in the contract itself, or included in a separate bill or statement from the insurer.[28]

Taxpayers receiving reimbursements for medical expenses in the *same year* in which the expenses were paid must reduce any medical expense deduction to a net amount. However, if the reimbursement is for medical expenses in a prior year, the income tax treatment of the reimbursement depends upon whether the taxpayer claimed a medical expense deduction for the year in which the expenses were actually paid. If no medical expense deduction was taken in the year in which the expenses were paid (e.g., taxpayer used the standard deduction or total medical expenses did not exceed the required percentage of A.G.I.), any reimbursement for such expenses will not be included in gross income. If the taxpayer claimed a deduction for the medical expenses in the prior year, however, the reimbursement must be included in gross income to the extent of the *lesser* of: (1) the previous medical expense deduction, or (2) the excess of the taxpayer's itemized deductions over his or her standard deduction. The inclusion in gross income of all or a part of the reimbursement is in accordance with the tax benefit rule.

---

[25] See § 213(d)(2), Reg. § 1.213-1(e)(1)(iv), and *Comm. v. Bilder*, 62-1 USTC ¶9440, 9 AFTR2d 1355, 369 U.S. 499 (USSC, 1962).

[26] § 213(d)(2).

[27] See Rev. Rul. 75-317, 1975-2 C.B. 57.

[28] Reg. § 1.213-1(e)(4). Participants in the Federal Medicare program are entitled to treat as medical care insurance premiums the amounts withheld for voluntary doctor-bill insurance.

Example 8. T has adjusted gross income of $30,000 for 2009. During the year, T pays the following medical expenses:

Hospitalization insurance premiums	$1,900
Doctor and dental bills	800
Eyeglasses	175
Medical transportation	25

T's medical expense deduction is computed as follows:

Total medical expenses	$2,900
Less: 7.5% of $30,000 (A.G.I.)	− 2,250
Medical expense deduction for 2009	$ 650

T's itemized deductions (including the $650 medical expense deduction) for 2009 exceeded his standard deduction by $1,500. In 2009, T received $400 as a reimbursement from his insurance company. T must include the *entire* $400 in gross income for 2010. If T had received the $400 reimbursement in 2009, his medical expense deduction would have been limited to $250.

Example 9. Assume the same facts as in *Example 8* except that the medical expense reimbursement was $900 instead of $400. If the reimbursement was received in 2010, T would be required to include only $650 in gross income—the amount of the medical expenses included in his itemized deductions. If the amount by which T's itemized deductions exceeded his standard deduction was *less* than $650 for 2009, he would include in gross income for 2010 only so much of the reimbursement represented by the prior year's itemized deductions in excess of the standard deduction amount. However, if T had used the standard deduction in 2009, none of the $900 reimbursement would be included in 2010 gross income because T received no tax benefit in 2009.

The situations illustrated in *Examples 8 and 9* occur quite often because taxpayers are *not required* to reduce a current year's medical expense deduction by *anticipated* insurance reimbursements. Notice that this can result in a taxpayer receiving reimbursements early in the next tax year and not being required to pay income taxes on the reimbursement until April 15 of the following year.

HEALTH SAVINGS ACCOUNTS AND MEDICAL SAVINGS ACCOUNTS

During the past ten years, Congress has taken several steps to make health care more affordable. Chief among these was the creation of Medical Savings Accounts (also known as Archer MSAs) and Health Savings Accounts (HSAs).[29] These accounts enable individuals to pay for unreimbursed medical expenses on a before tax basis. For those familiar with flexible spending accounts for medical expenses (now used by many employers and their employees), MSAs and HSAs are virtually identical without the use it or lose it rule. For those familiar with Individual Retirement Accounts, MSAs and HSAs are quite similar.

Example 10. In 2009, H set up an HSA for his family. H can contribute up to $5,950 to the HSA and claim the amount as a deduction for A.G.I. Any amounts withdrawn from the account that are used to pay for medical expenses are nontaxable. As a result,

---

[29] See §§ 220 and 223

income funneled through HSAs to pay medical expenses is never subject to tax. Amounts not withdrawn from the HSA can earn income and such income normally is not taxable as long as it remains in the account or is withdrawn to pay medical expenses. In order to obtain this favorable tax treatment, H has a health insurance policy that meets several requirements. The policy has a high "deductible," meaning that he must pay for the first $2,300 of medical expenses incurred by his family (i.e., the individual must report medical expenses to the plan and pay $2,300 before the insurance starts paying). The policy also limits the total costs that H could incur to $11,600 thus providing his family with catastrophic protection. Most importantly for H, because the plan has such a high deductible, the cost of the plan is much less than most and he is able to afford coverage that he otherwise might not be able obtain.

Congress first introduced MSAs in 1996 as an experiment, restricting both the number that could be created and those who were eligible to use them. After a lukewarm reception, a bipartisan effort expanded the concept of MSAs and created HSAs which debuted in 2004. HSAs are a vast improvement over MSAs and very well may become an important tool in the fight against the rising costs of health care.[30] The plans are intended to hold down costs by giving consumers a tax incentive to shop for the best price for health services and to forgo procedures they do not need. At this point, it is difficult to determine whether this theory will work. However, recent reports suggest that there is growing interest in HSAs as more and more employers are offering them to their employees in lieu of traditional plans.[31] As interest in HSAs grow, interest in MSAs has dropped. For this reason, the following discussion focuses on HSAs.

Section 223 permits individuals to deduct for A.G.I. a limited amount of contributions to an HSA. Similarly, § 106(b) allows individuals to exclude limited contributions to such accounts made on their behalf by their employers. Amounts contributed to the HSA may be invested and the earnings are nontaxable. Distributions from the account are nontaxable as long as they are used for medical expenses that normally would be deductible under § 213 other than those for health insurance.

Note that no deduction is allowed for expenses paid for with dollars out of the HSA. However, the deduction for amounts *contributed* and the exclusion for amounts distributed essentially provide the same benefit. The end result of these rules effectively enables an individual to pay for medical expenses not covered by insurance with dollars that have never been subject to tax. Observe that if the taxpayer pays for unreimbursed medical expenses using dollars that do not come from the HSA, they normally are not deductible due to the 7.5 percent limitation. In such case, the payments are effectively made with after-tax dollars.

> **Example 11.** Assume M is in the 30% tax bracket with an adjusted gross income of $60,000. He is covered by health insurance that pays for most but not all of his medical expenses. During the year, M contributed $1,000 to an HSA. Later during the year he withdrew the entire $1,000 to pay for medical expenses related to knee surgery that were not covered by his insurance. As shown by the following analysis (ignoring exemptions and the standard deduction and assuming M itemized deductions), by using an HSA, M saves $300, the tax that otherwise would have been paid on the amounts used to pay for the unreimbursed medical expenses.

---

[30]   MSAs are available only to employees of certain small businesses and to self-employed persons and the number of MSAs were restricted. HSAs are available to all individuals and the required health plan is far more flexible.

[31]   Individuals covered by other medical insurance plans are not eligible for HSAs

	Employee Pays	HSA Pays	
Income	$60,000	$60,000	
Deduction for contribution to HSA	—	(1,000)	
Adjusted gross income	$60,000	$59,000	
Medical expense deduction			
[$1,000 − (7.5% × $60,000)]	0	—	
Income	$60,000	$59,000	
Tax @ 30%	(18,000)	(17,700)	
Cost of medical expense	(1,000)	—	(HSA pays)
After-tax income	$41,000	$41,300	

Another advantage of contributions provided by an employer to an HSA is that they are not subject to FICA or FUTA taxes.

Penalty for Distributions Not Used for Medical Expenses. If the taxpayer withdraws amounts from the HSA and uses them for something other than qualified medical expenses before age 65 (or death or disability), a penalty equal to 10 percent of the amount withdrawn is imposed. Amounts withdrawn after age 65 are not subject to penalty but will be taxed as ordinary income to the extent they are not used to pay for medical expenses.

Eligible Individuals. HSAs may be established only by eligible individuals. A person is eligible if he or she is:

- Covered under a high deductible health plan (HDHP). A HDHP is a plan that for 2009 has an annual deductible of at least $1,150 and an annual limitation on out-of-pocket expenses (other health care premiums) not greater than $5,800. These limits are doubled to $2,300 and $11,600 for family coverage.
- Not covered by any other health care plan that is not an HDHP
- Not eligible for Medicare (i.e., has not reached the age of 65)
- Not claimed as a dependent on another person's tax return

Deductible Contributions. In 2009, annual contributions to HSAs are generally limited to $3,000 for singles and $5,950 for families. Individuals from age 55–64 are entitled to make "catch-up" contributions up to $1,000.

EXHIBIT 11-3

Health Savings Accounts High Deductible Health Plan (HDHP) Requirements and Contribution Limitations 2009

	Individual	*Family*
Minimum Deductible	$1,150	$2,300
Maximum Out-Of-Pocket Expenses	5,800	11,600
Maximum Contribution deduction	3,000	5,950

Treatment of HSAs at Death. If the taxpayer dies before using the amount in the HSA, the treatment of the balance for both income tax and estate tax purposes depends on who is the beneficiary of the account.[32]

- *Surviving spouse as beneficiary.* If the surviving spouse is the beneficiary, the surviving spouse has no income and treats the account as his or her own.

---

[32] § 223(f)(8)

- *Beneficiary other than surviving spouse.* If the surviving spouse is not the beneficiary but another person is the beneficiary (e.g., a son or daughter), the account stops being an HSA, and the beneficiary must include in taxable income the fair market value of the HSA in the year of the owner's death. Such person would be able to exclude from gross income the amount of any qualified medical expenses for the decedent that are paid by the beneficiary within one year after the date of death as well as deduct any estate taxes that may be paid that are attributable to such amounts.
- *Estate.* If no beneficiary is named or the estate is the beneficiary, the value of the HSA is included on the decedent's final income tax return; however, such amount is *not* reduced by final medical expenses of the decedent paid after death.

Upon death, any balance in the HSA is included in the decedent's gross estate subject to estate taxes. Such amount would be subject to estate taxes unless it passes to the surviving spouse and therefore, qualifies for the marital deduction.

Recordkeeping and Filing Requirements. Taxpayers with HSAs must file Form 8889 with their Form 1040 if there was any activity in the HSA during the year. Activity includes both distributions (e.g., to pay medical expenses) as well as contributions by the taxpayer or spouse or the employer of either. In addition, HSA owners must keep records sufficient to show that: (1) any distributions were used exclusively for qualified medical expenses; (2), the qualified medical expenses had not been previously paid or reimbursed from another source; and (3) the medical expenses had not been taken as an itemized deduction in any year.

HEALTH INSURANCE COSTS OF SELF-EMPLOYED TAXPAYERS

Self-employed individuals are allowed to treat the amounts paid for health insurance on behalf of a self-employed individual, his or her spouse, and dependents as a deductible business expense.[33] A more than two percent owner-employee of S Corp. stock can deduct 100% of the amount paid for medical insurance for himself, spouse and dependents [§ 162 (l)(5)]. The deduction is allowed in determining adjusted gross income (i.e., a deduction *for* A.G.I.) rather than being treated as an itemized medical expense deduction subject to the 7.5 percent floor. No deduction is allowable to the extent it *exceeds* the taxpayer's net earnings from self-employment.[34] Thus, the deduction cannot create a loss. More important, the deduction does not reduce the income base for which the taxpayer is liable for self-employment taxes.

> **Example 12.** K, a self-employed individual, paid $2,600 for health insurance for himself, his wife, and their two children. K had no employees during the year. K is entitled to deduct the entire $2,600 in determining adjusted gross income, provided the deduction does not exceed his net earnings from self-employment, and his A.G.I. before the deduction is at least $2,600.[35]

Absent a special rule, self-employed individuals who are also employees might be tempted to opt out of an employer-provided medical insurance plan. By so doing, the 7.5 percent floor on medical expenses could be avoided and taxpayers could deduct a portion of what normally would be nondeductible premium payments. To prevent this

---

[33] § 162(l).

[34] § 162(l)(2)(A).

[35] § 162(l)(3).

course of action, the deduction is not allowed if a self-employed individual or spouse is eligible to participate in a health insurance plan of an employer.[36]

PERSONAL CASUALTY AND THEFT LOSSES

As discussed in Chapter 10, Congress has provided for a deduction of losses related to property used for *personal* purposes where the loss arises from fire, storm, shipwreck, or other casualty, or theft.[37] Like the medical expense deduction, the deduction for personal casualty and theft losses is designed to provide relief for only extraordinary losses. Thus, an individual taxpayer's deduction for personal casualty and theft losses is allowed only to the extent such losses exceed $100 per occurrence *and* the sum of all losses (after reduction by the $100 floor) for a given tax year exceeds 10 percent of the taxpayer's adjusted gross income. These deduction limitations were discussed and illustrated in Chapter 10.

YEAR DEDUCTIBLE

A personal casualty loss is generally deductible in the taxable year in which the loss occurs. Recall, however, that a theft loss is deductible only in the year of discovery. If a claim for insurance reimbursement (or any other potential recovery) exists and there is a reasonable prospect of recovery, the loss must be reduced by the amount *expected* to be received.[38] If later receipts are *less* than the amount originally estimated and no further reimbursement is expected, an amended return is not filed. Instead, the remaining loss is deductible in the year in which no further reimbursement is expected. Most important, if the casualty loss deduction claimed in the prior year was reduced by the $100 floor and exceeded the 10 percent A.G.I. limitation, the remaining loss is not further reduced. However, the remaining loss is subject to the 10 percent limitation of the later year.[39]

REPORTING CASUALTY LOSSES

Individual taxpayers are required to report and compute casualty losses on Form 4684,[40] which is to be filed with Form 1040. The casualty loss deduction, if any, is reported with other itemized deductions on Schedule A, Form 1040.

TAXES

Code § 164 is the statutory authority that permits taxpayers to deduct several types of taxes for Federal income tax purposes. If the taxes are related to an individual taxpayer's trade or business or income-producing activity, the deduction is generally allowed in arriving at adjusted gross income. However, both the IRS and the courts have taken the position that state, local, and foreign *income* taxes are deductible by an individual taxpayer *from* his or her adjusted gross income—even though it could be argued that such taxes are related to his or her trade or business. Likewise, if *property* taxes are related to personal use property (e.g., residence, car, etc.), such taxes are generally deductible only if the individual itemizes his or her deductions. As discussed below, for tax years 2008 and 2009 individual taxpayers who do not itemize their deductions are allowed to increase

---

36 § 162(l)(2)(B).

37 § 165(c)(3) For 2009, the floor is raised to $500 and is scheduled to revert to $100 in 2010. Special rules apply to casualties and thefts occurring in Federally declared disaster areas.

38 Reg. § 1.165-1(d)(2)(i).

39 *See Example 9* of Chapter 10.

40 See Appendix B for a sample of this form.

their standard deduction by a limited amount of their real property taxes. If taxes are deductible by taxpayers other than individuals, the deductions simply reduce gross income to taxable income.[41]

The types of taxes specifically allowed as deductions under § 164 are:

1. State, local, and foreign real property taxes;

2. State and local personal property taxes;

3. State and local general sales taxes;

4. State, local, and foreign income, war profits, and excess profit taxes; and

5. The generation-skipping transfer tax.[42]

The generation-skipping transfer tax is imposed on income distributions from certain trusts. Discussion of this tax is beyond the scope of this text. However, each of the other types of deductible taxes is discussed in detail below.

GENERAL REQUIREMENTS FOR DEDUCTIBILITY

A tax is deductible *only* if (1) it is imposed on the taxpayer's income or property; and (2) it is paid or incurred by the taxpayer in the taxable year for which a deduction is being claimed. Even if these two requirements are met, deductions for certain Federal, state, and local taxes are expressly denied. Exhibit 11-4 contains a list of nondeductible taxes.

In addition to the nondeductible taxes listed in Exhibit 11-4, deductions for *fees* (whether or not labeled as taxes) paid by taxpayers usually are denied *unless* the fees are incurred in the taxpayer's trade or business or for the production of income. Fees paid or incurred in connection with a trade or business, if ordinary and necessary, are deductible as business expenses under § 162. Similarly, fees related to the production of income generally are deductible expenses under § 212.[43]

EXHIBIT 11-4
Nondeductible Taxes[44]

Nondeductible Federal taxes:
Federal income taxes (including those withheld from an individual's pay)
Social security or railroad retirement taxes withheld from an individual by his or her employer (includes self-employment taxes)
Social security and other employment taxes paid on the wages of the taxpayer's employee who performed domestic or other personal services
Federal excise taxes or customs duties unless they are connected with the taxpayer's business or income-producing activity
Federal estate and gift taxes

Nondeductible state and local taxes:
Motor vehicle taxes (unless they qualify as ad valorem taxes on personal property)
Inheritance, legacy, succession, or estate taxes
Gift taxes
Per capita or poll taxes
Cigarette, tobacco, liquor, beer, wine, etc., taxes

---

[41] See the later section in this chapter entitled "Reporting Deductions for Taxes."

[42] § 164(a).

[43] See Chapter 7 for a discussion of the requirements that must be met in order to deduct business and nonbusiness expenses of this nature.

[44] See § 275, Reg. § 1.164-2, and *Your Federal Income Tax*, IRS Publication 17 (Rev. 2008), p. 149.

The IRS distinguishes a "tax" from a "fee" by looking to the *purpose* of the charge.[45] If a particular charge is imposed upon the taxpayer for the purpose of *raising revenue* to be used for public or government purposes, the IRS will consider the charge to be a tax. However, if the charge is imposed because of either *particular acts or services* received by the taxpayer, such charge will be considered as a *fee*. Thus, fees for driver's licenses, vehicle registration and inspection, license tags for pets, hunting and fishing licenses, tolls for bridges and roads, parking meter deposits, water bills, sewer and other service charges, and postage fees are not deductible *unless* related to the taxpayer's trade or business, or income-producing activity.[46]

Since most individual taxpayers use the cash receipts and disbursements method of accounting for tax purposes, the following discussion of income and property tax deductions concentrates on cash-basis taxpayers and the requirement that taxes be *paid* in the year of deduction. Bear in mind throughout this discussion, however, that accrual method taxpayers are allowed a deduction for taxes in the tax year in which the obligation for payment becomes fixed and determinable (i.e., the all-events test is met).

INCOME TAXES

Most state, local, or foreign income taxes paid or accrued by a taxpayer are deductible in arriving at taxable income. For individual taxpayers, however, a deduction for state and local income taxes is allowed only if the taxpayer itemizes his or her deductions. Furthermore, as explained below, in lieu of deducting state and local income taxes, taxpayers can deduct state and local sales taxes (i.e., deduct either but not both).

Although the income taxes may be related solely to the individual's business income (e.g., income from a sole proprietorship or partnership), or income from rents and royalties, these taxes are considered personal in nature. Since income taxes paid to a foreign country or a U.S. possession may either be deducted as an itemized deduction or claimed as a credit against the U.S. income tax, an individual who does not itemize deductions should elect to claim foreign income taxes as credits.[47]

Cash-basis taxpayers are allowed to deduct state and local income taxes *paid* during the taxable year, including those taxes imposed on interest income that is exempt from Federal income taxation. Amounts considered paid during the taxable year include:

1. State and local income or foreign taxes withheld from an individual's salary by his or her employer;

2. Estimated payments made by the taxpayer under a pay-as-you-go requirement of a taxing authority; and

3. Payments made in the current year on an income tax liability of a prior year.

Example 13. During 2009, Z, a cash basis taxpayer, had $1,500 of Illinois state income taxes withheld by her employer. In 2009, she paid the remaining $450 in state income taxes due on her 2008 Illinois tax return, and also paid $300 in estimated state income tax payments during 2009. If Z itemizes her deductions for Federal income tax purposes, she is entitled to a $2,250 ($1,500 + $300 + $450) state income tax deduction for 2009.

---

[45] See § 275 and Reg. § 1.164-2.

[46] *Your Federal Income Tax*, IRS Publication 17 (Rev. 2008), p. 150.

[47] § 27.

If a cash basis taxpayer receives a refund of state, local, or foreign income taxes in the current year, the refund must be included in the current year's gross income to the extent a deduction in an earlier tax year provided a tax benefit.[48]

> **Example 14.** Assume the same facts as in *Example 13*. While preparing her 2009 Illinois state income tax return in early 2010, Z determined she had overpaid the state tax liability by $375. She received a refund of the entire overpayment on August 10, 2010. If Z claimed the total $2,250 state income taxes paid as a deduction on her 2009 Federal income tax return and her itemized deductions exceeded the standard deduction amount by at least $375, she must include the entire refund in gross income on her 2010 Federal income tax return.

In determining the amount of the refund that must be included in income, the IRS further explains that the amount is limited to the excess of the tax deducted for the year over the state and local sales taxes that the taxpayer chose not to deduct for that same year.[49]

> **Example 15.** In preparing his 2008 income tax return, H elected to deduct $12,000 of state income tax instead of $11,000 of state sales tax. During 2009, H received a refund of his state income tax of $2,500. The amount of state income tax refund that H must include in gross income for 2009 is $1,000 ($12,000 − $11,000) since he could have deducted the state sales tax.

DEDUCTION FOR STATE AND LOCAL GENERAL SALES TAX

Taxpayers are currently allowed to deduct state and local sales and use taxes instead of state and local income taxes.[50] The sales tax deduction was elimated in 1986 but was resurrected in 2004 when states without income taxes but high sales taxes wanted equitable treatment. Although scheduled to expire at the end of 2007, Congress extended the deduction for both 2008 and 2009.

The sales tax deduction is classified as an itemized deduction but not a miscellaneous itemized deduction. It is subject to the itemized deduction cutback discussed in a later part of this chapter. In addition, the deduction for state and local sales and use taxes is not allowed for alternative minimum tax purposes.

Only "general" sales taxes are deductible. Section 164(b)(5)(B) defines a general sales tax as a tax imposed at one rate with respect to the sale at retail of a broad range of classes of item. In determining whether a tax is a "general" sales tax, the fact that it does not apply to food, clothing, medical supplies and motor vehicles, or applies at a different rate is disregarded. If other items are taxed at a different rate, such taxes are not deductible. If the rate of tax on a motor vehicle exceeds the general rate, the excess is disregarded. If the amount of the general sales tax is separately stated, to the extent it is paid by the consumer, the amount is treated as a tax imposed on and paid by the consumer.

Taxpayers may deduct their actual sales taxes as substantiated by accumulated receipts or use IRS-published tables. These tables are contained in Appendix A of this text. The tables take into account the number of exemptions, "available" income (A.G.I.

---

[48]   § 111. Special rules apply when married taxpayers file separate state or Federal income tax returns. See *Your Federal Income Tax*, IRS Publication 17 (Rev. 2008), p. 147.

[49]   These basic rules for inclusion must be modified in several other situations. For example, when a taxpayer receives a state income tax refund for 2008 and the last estimated tax payment of the 2008 state taxes was made in 2009, the portion of the refund attributable to the 2009 payment reduces the deduction for state income taxes. A special calculation is also required if the taxpayer was subject to the deduction cutback or had to pay the alternative minimum tax. See *Taxable and Nontaxable Income,* IRS Publication 525 (2008), pp. 21 and 22.

[50]   See § 165(b)(5). According to the IRS, the sales tax deduction was claimed on approximately 11.2 million tax returns filed in 2006. Only time will tell if Congress decides to continue its current extension of this deduction.

increased by any tax-exempt income such as social security and tax-exempt interest) and rates of state and local general sales taxation. Since sales tax rates vary from state to state (and even by localities within a state), there are 51 different tables for the 50 states and the District of Columbia. The tables extend to available income as high as $200,000.

The tables include only general *state* sales taxes and do not include any additional *local sales taxes*. A special calculation must be made to determine the amount of local sales taxes that may be added to the table amount. In addition to the amount determined using the table, taxpayers may add the taxes on cars, motorcycles, motor homes, recreational vehicles, sport utility vehicles, trucks, vans, and off-road vehicles, aircraft, boats, homes (including mobile and prefabricated), or home-building materials, if the tax rate was the same as the general sales tax rate. Tax commentators have suggested that the sales taxes on other high-priced unusual purchases such as expensive furniture, high-definition plasma televisions or the like arguably could be added. However, the IRS limits the additions to those noted above.[51] Special rules apply when a taxpayer lives in more than one state during the year. A portion of the tables appears below.

2008 Optional State and Certain Local Sales Tax Tables

Income At least	Income But less than	Alabama 4.0000% 1	2	3	4	5	Over 5	Arizona 5.6000% 1	2	3	4	5	Over 5	Arkansas 6.0000% 1	2	3	4	5	Over 5	California¹ 7.2500% 1	2	3	4	5	Over 5	Colorado 2.9000% 1	2	3	4	5	Over 5
$0	$20,000	201	246	278	303	324	354	205	234	253	267	279	295	287	334	366	390	410	438	246	280	303	320	334	354	96	110	120	127	133	142
20,000	30,000	310	377	423	460	491	535	350	397	429	453	472	500	469	544	594	633	665	709	423	480	518	547	571	603	161	184	200	212	222	235
30,000	40,000	364	442	495	538	574	625	427	484	522	551	575	608	563	652	712	758	796	849	518	587	633	668	696	736	195	223	242	256	268	285
40,000	50,000	411	497	557	604	644	701	494	560	604	637	664	702	644	746	813	866	909	969	601	681	734	774	806	852	225	257	279	295	308	327
50,000	60,000	453	546	612	663	707	769	556	629	678	715	745	788	717	830	905	963	1010	1077	678	767	825	870	907	958	253	288	312	330	345	366
60,000	70,000	491	591	661	717	764	830	612	693	747	787	821	867	784	907	988	1051	1103	1175	748	846	910	960	1000	1056	278	317	343	363	379	402
70,000	80,000	527	634	708	767	817	888	667	754	812	856	892	942	848	979	1067	1135	1191	1269	815	922	991	1045	1088	1149	302	344	372	393	411	436
80,000	90,000	560	673	751	814	866	941	718	811	873	920	959	1012	907	1047	1141	1213	1272	1355	879	992	1067	1124	1171	1236	325	370	399	422	441	467
90,000	100,000	592	710	792	857	912	991	766	866	932	982	1023	1080	962	1111	1210	1287	1350	1437	939	1060	1140	1201	1251	1320	347	394	425	450	470	497
100,000	120,000	633	759	846	915	973	1056	831	938	1009	1063	1107	1169	1036	1196	1302	1384	1452	1546	1019	1150	1236	1302	1356	1430	375	426	460	486	507	537
120,000	140,000	690	825	919	994	1057	1146	920	1039	1117	1176	1225	1292	1138	1312	1429	1518	1592	1695	1131	1275	1370	1443	1502	1584	415	471	508	536	560	593
140,000	160,000	740	883	983	1062	1129	1224	1000	1128	1212	1276	1328	1401	1227	1414	1539	1635	1714	1825	1230	1386	1488	1567	1631	1720	450	510	550	581	606	641
160,000	180,000	790	941	1047	1131	1201	1301	1079	1217	1307	1376	1433	1511	1316	1516	1650	1752	1837	1955	1330	1497	1608	1692	1761	1856	485	550	592	625	652	690
180,000	200,000	835	994	1104	1192	1266	1371	1152	1298	1394	1467	1527	1610	1397	1609	1749	1858	1948	2072	1420	1599	1716	1805	1879	1980	517	586	631	666	694	734
200,000 or more		1060	1254	1390	1497	1587	1715	1522	1711	1836	1931	2008	2116	1801	2070	2250	2387	2501	2660	1885	2117	2269	2385	2481	2613	681	768	826	871	908	959

Example 16. A family of four living in Arizona has available income of $51,800 for 2008. If the election is made to claim a deduction for their general sales taxes rather than state and local income taxes, the family will be allowed a deduction of $715. If the taxpayers paid a sales tax of $450 on a new truck purchased in 2008, the sales tax table amount would be increased to $1,165 ($715 + $450). Note that the 2008 Optional Sales Tax Table is used here because the 2009 tables were not available at the publication date of this text.

Since the addition of the sales tax deduction in 2004, the taxpayers in the seven states that do not impose an income tax—Alaska, Florida, Nevada, South Dakota, Texas, Washington and Wyoming—have an additional itemized deduction. As a result, taxpayers in these states, who may not have been able to itemize their deductions, now may be able to itemize. For taxpayers in the other 43 states, which levy at least some form of state or local income tax, they will be forced to make a decision about whether an election should be made.

PROPERTY TAXES

Personal property taxes paid to a state, local, or foreign government are deductible *only* if they are *ad valorem* taxes.[52] Ad valorem taxes are taxes imposed on the *value* of property. Quite often, state and local taxing authorities impose a combination tax and fee

---

[51] 164(b)(5)(H)

[52] § 164(b)(1) and Reg. § 1.164-3(c).

on personal property. In such cases, only that portion of the charge based on value of the property will qualify as a deductible tax.[53]

> **Example 17.** State A imposes an annual vehicle registration charge of 60 cents per hundredweight. X, a resident of the state, paid $24 in 2009 for the registration of his personal automobile. Since this charge is not based on the value of the auto, X has not paid a deductible tax.

> **Example 18.** State B imposes an annual vehicle registration charge of 1% of value plus 50 cents per hundredweight. Y, a resident of the state, owns a personal use automobile having a value of $10,000 and weighing 4,000 pounds. Of the $120 [(1% × $10,000) + (50¿ × 40 hundredweight)] total registration charge paid by Y, only $100 would be deductible as a personal property tax.

Real property (real estate) taxes are generally deductible only if imposed on property owned by the taxpayer and paid or accrued by the taxpayer in the year the deduction is claimed. If real property taxes are imposed on jointly held real estate, each owner may claim his or her portion of the taxes. For example, if cash basis, married taxpayers file separate Federal income tax returns and real property taxes are imposed on jointly held real estate, each spouse may claim *half* of the taxes paid.

If real estate is sold during the year, the deduction for real estate taxes *must be apportioned* between the buyer and seller according to the number of days in the year each held the property, regardless of which party actually paid the property taxes.[54] The taxes are apportioned to the seller up to (but not including) the date of sale, and to the buyer beginning with the date of sale.

> **Example 19.** The real property tax year in Colorado County is April 1 to March 31. X, the owner on April 1, 2009 of real property located in Colorado County, sells the real property to Y on June 30, 2009. Y owns the real property from June 30, 2009 through March 31, 2010. The real property tax is $730 for the county's tax year April 1, 2009 to March 31, 2010. For purposes of § 164(a), $180 (90 ÷ 365 × $730 = $180 taxes for April 1, 2009 through June 29, 2009) of the real property tax is treated as imposed on X, the seller. The remaining $550 (275 ÷ 365 × $730 = $550 taxes for June 30, 2009 through March 31, 2010) of such real property tax is treated as imposed on Y, the purchaser.[55]

When both buyer and seller of real property are cash-basis taxpayers and only one of the parties *actually* pays the real property taxes for the period in which both parties owned the property, *each* party to the transaction is entitled to deduct the portion of the real property taxes based on the number of days he or she held the property. As a practical matter, real property taxes are usually allocated during the closing process, and the details are provided in the closing statement for real property sales. A taxpayer need only acquire the closing statement to ascertain the proper allocation and how the sales price has been affected by the allocation.

Unless the actual real property taxes are apportioned between buyer and seller as part of the sale/purchase agreement, adjustments for the taxes must be made to determine the amount realized by the seller, as well as the buyer's cost basis of the property.[56] The treatment of the adjustments depends upon which party actually paid the real estate taxes.

---

[53] § 164(b)(2)(E). States known to include some ad valorem tax as part of auto and boat registration fees are Arizona, California, Colorado, Indiana, Iowa, Maine, Massachusetts, Nevada, New Hampshire, Oklahoma, Washington, and Wyoming.

[54] § 164(d) and Reg. § 1.164-6(b).

[55] Reg. § 1.164-6(b)(3), *Example 1.*

[56] Reg. § 1.164-6(d); Reg. § 1.1001-1(b); and Reg. § 1.1012-1(b). A similar result should occur if buyer and seller are using different accounting methods.

Example 20. Assume that buyer and seller are both cash basis, calendar year taxpayers, and real estate taxes for the entire year are to be paid at the end of the year. Real property is sold on October 1, 2009 for $30,000, and B, the buyer, pays the real estate taxes of $365 on December 31, 2009. The real estate taxes attributable to and deductible by B are $92 (92 ÷ 365 × $365). The remaining $273 ($365 −$92) of the taxes will be apportioned to and deductible by S, the seller. As a result of this apportionment, the seller must increase the amount realized from the sale to $30,273, and the buyer will have an adjusted cost basis for the property of $30,273.

Example 21. Assume the same facts as in *Example 20*, except that the real property taxes are payable in advance for the entire year and that S, the seller, paid $365 in January 2009. The real estate taxes are apportioned in the same manner, and the buyer, B, will be entitled to deduct $92. However, B must adjust his cost basis of the property to $29,908 ($30,000 purchase price − $92 taxes paid by seller). The seller, S, is entitled to deduct $273 of the taxes and reduce his amount realized from the sale to $29,908.

Real property taxes assessed against local benefits of a kind tending to increase the value of the property assessed (e.g., special assessments for paved streets, street lights, sidewalks, drainage ditches, etc.) are not deductible.[57] Instead, the property owner simply adds the assessed amount paid to his or her cost basis of the property. However, if assessments for local benefits are made for the purpose of maintenance or repair, or for the purpose of meeting interest charges with respect to such benefits, they are deductible.[58] If an assessment is in part for the cost of an improvement and in part for maintenance, repairs or for interest charges, only *that* portion of the tax assessment relating to maintenance, repairs, or interest charges will be deductible. Unless the taxpayer can show the allocation of the amounts assessed for the different purposes, *none* of the amount paid is deductible.[59]

Standard Deduction Increase for Real Property Taxes. With the *Housing Assistance Act of 2008*, Congress added a new twist to the general tax treatment of real property taxes. As a general rule, taxpayers are allowed an itemized deduction for real property taxes (e.g., the property taxes paid with respect to a personal residence). However, many homeowners who pay property taxes are not able to itemize and take the deduction because their itemized deductions do not exceed the standard deduction. This is particularly true for retired homeowners. Retirees have often paid off the mortgages on their homes and no longer itemize because they no longer have deductible mortgage interest. Yet they still have property taxes. To help these homeowners, the new law allows all taxpayers to increase their standard deduction.

Taxpayers now may increase the standard deduction for a limited amount of real property taxes paid – up to $500, or in the case of joint filers, $1,000. The rule applies to virtually all real property taxes paid and is not limited to those related to the taxpayer's personal residence. Property taxes paid on a vacation home would qualify. However, taxes that are deductible for A.G.I. (e.g., incurred in a trade or business or income producing activity) are not taken into account. In addition, at the time of this writing, it is not clear whether foreign real property taxes would be included. The special rule applies for tax years 2008 and 2009.

---

[57]   § 164(c)(1), Reg. § 1.164-2(g), and Reg. § 1.164-4(a).

[58]   § 164(c)(1) and Reg. § 1.164-4(b)(1).

[59]   Reg. § 1.164-4(b)(1).

Example 22. H and W are married and file a joint return. They are both age 65. In 2009, they pay $1,400 in state and local real property taxes. However, their other itemized deductions (e.g., charitable contributions, mortgage interest, and state income taxes) are not sufficient to itemize. So they claim the standard deduction. Under the 2008 Housing Act, their 2009 standard deduction will equal $14,600: the $11,400 basic standard deduction for joint filers plus $2,200 in additional standard deductions as marrieds who are both age 65 ($1,100 each) plus a $1,000 real property tax standard deduction. The balance of the real property taxes, $400, is not deductible since the couple did not itemize their deductions.

Example 23. Same facts as in *Example 22*, except H and W also have charitable contributions and mortgage interest on their residence of $20,000. In this case, their itemized deductions would be $21,400 ($20,000 + $1,400 of real property taxes). Since their itemized deductions of $21,400 would exceed the standard deduction as increased to $14,600, the couple would itemize their deductions. Note that if the taxpayer itemizes, the real property taxes are claimed as an itemized deduction.

Also note that the new rule does not make the real property taxes deductible for A.G. I., but merely increases the standard deduction. In addition, it should be noted that the standard deduction is not allowed as a deduction for computing the alternative minimum tax. Consequently the additional standard deduction for real property taxes, as a part of the standard deduction is not deductible for alternative minimum tax purposes. The alternative minimum tax rules are discussed in detail in Chapter 13.

REPORTING DEDUCTIONS FOR TAXES

Deductible state and local taxes are reported on different forms depending on the taxpaying entity claiming the deduction. Corporations report their deductions for these taxes on Form 1120. Fiduciaries (trusts and estates) report deductible taxes on Form 1041. Partnerships and S corporations report deductible taxes on Forms 1065 and 1120S, respectively. Individuals report deductible taxes on Form 1040, but the particular schedule used depends upon whether the taxes are business expenses or personal itemized deductions.

An individual's deduction for taxes (other than income taxes) related to his or her trade or business is reported on Schedule C of Form 1040 (Schedule F for farmers and ranchers). Deductible taxes (other than income taxes) related to rents and royalties are reported on Schedule E. All other deductible taxes, including state and local general sales taxes or state and local income taxes on business income or income from rents or royalties, are reported by an individual taxpayer on Schedule A of Form 1040.

INTEREST EXPENSE

Interest expense is an amount paid or incurred for the use or forbearance of money.[60] Under the general rule of Code § 163(a), all interest paid or accrued on indebtedness within the taxable year is allowed as a deduction. As with most general rules in the tax law, however, there are limitations imposed on the deduction of certain interest expense as well as the complete disallowance of deductions for interest related to certain items. These restrictions are discussed below.

LIMITATIONS ON DEDUCTIONS OF INTEREST EXPENSE

Prior to 1987, interest expense for most taxpayers was totally deductible. As part of the tax reform package of 1986, however, Congress substantially limited the deduction for interest. Over the years, Congress became concerned that by allowing a deduction for all interest expense the tax system encouraged borrowing and, conversely, discouraged savings. This problem was exacerbated by the fact that the "economic" income arising from the ownership of housing and other consumer durables is not subject to tax. For example, when a taxpayer purchases a residence, the return on the investment—the absence of having to pay rent for the item—is not subject to tax. Had the taxpayer invested in assets other than housing or other durables, the return (e.g., interest or dividends) would have been fully taxable. In those situations where the investment is financed by borrowing, allowing a deduction is equivalent to allowing a deduction for expenses related to tax-exempt income—which is expressly prohibited under Code § 265. The net result of this system is to provide an incentive to consume rather than save.

In rethinking the approach to interest in 1986, Congress believed that it would not be advisable to impute income on investments in durables and tax it. However, Congress did feel that it was appropriate and practical to address situations where consumer expenditures are financed by borrowing. Accordingly, Congress enacted rules that prohibit the deduction for personal interest (other than certain home mortgage interest and interest on certain education loans). As a result, interest expenses on personal auto loans, credit card purchases, etc., are no longer deductible.

In eliminating the deduction for personal interest, Congress effectively established *six* categories of interest expense, each of which is subject to its own special set of rules. The different categories of interest expense are (1) personal interest, (2) qualified residence interest, (3) trade or business interest, (4) investment interest, (5) passive-activity interest, and (6) qualified student loan interest. As explained in detail below, interest (other than qualified residence interest) is classified according to how the loan proceeds are *spent*. Consequently, taxpayers are required to determine the nature of an expenditure from loan proceeds before the amount of the interest deduction can be determined.

Personal Interest. Today, taxpayers are not allowed to deduct any *personal interest*. Personal interest is defined as all interest arising from personal expenditures *except* the following:[61]

1. Interest incurred in connection with the conduct of a trade or business (other than the performance of services as an employee);

2. Investment interest;

---

[60]   *Old Colony Railroad v. Comm.*, 3 USTC ¶880, 10 AFTR 786, 284 U.S. 552 (USSC, 1936).

[61]   § 163(h)(1).

3. Qualified residence interest;

4. Interest taken into account in computing the income or loss from passive activities;

5. Interest on qualified education loans; and

6. Interest related to payment of the estate tax liability where such tax is deferred.

The effect of these rules is to severely limit the deduction for interest on consumer debt. For example, if a taxpayer borrows $3,000 from the bank and uses it to take a Caribbean cruise, none of the interest on the loan is deductible. Similarly, interest and finance charges would not be deductible on the following:

1. Automobile loans;

2. Furniture and appliance loans;

3. Credit card debt;

4. Life insurance loans;

5. Loans from qualified pension plans [including § 401(k) plans]; and

6. Delinquent tax payments and penalties.

It should be emphasized that interest incurred by an *employee* in connection with his or her trade or business is treated as consumer interest and is not deductible. In contrast, interest incurred by a self-employed person in his or her trade or business is fully deductible.

Example 24. K sells cosmetics for Fantastic Faces, Incorporated. Her job involves calling on department stores all over the state of Ohio and soliciting their orders. She uses her car entirely for business. Interest on her car loan for the year was $2,000. Since K is an employee, none of the interest is deductible.

Example 25. R is a real estate agent working for Bungalow Brokers. All of his compensation is based on the number of homes he sells during the year. He uses his car entirely for business. Under the employment tax rules (§ 3508), real estate agents and direct sellers are not considered employees where their remuneration is determined by sales. Since R would not be considered an employee, all of the interest on his car loan would be deductible.

Example 26. P is a reporter for the *News-Gazette*. She purchased a portable computer for $1,000, charging it on her bank credit card. She uses the computer entirely for business. Finance charges attributable to the purchase are $25. Even though the finance charges are incurred in connection with P's business, they are not deductible since she is an employee.

Qualified Residence Interest. The elimination of the deduction for personal interest in 1986 did not extend to interest on most home mortgages. As a general rule, interest on any debt *secured* by a taxpayer's first or second home is deductible. The interest is normally deductible whether the interest is on an original, second, or refinanced mortgage. Moreover, the interest is deductible regardless of how the taxpayer uses the money as long as the debt is *secured* by a mortgage on his or her primary or secondary residence. Unfortunately, tucked behind these seemingly simple rules are several complex restrictions.

Qualifying Indebtedness. Technically, only "qualified residence interest" is deductible. There are two types of qualified residence interest:[62]

1. Interest on *acquisition indebtedness:* Interest on debt that is incurred in acquiring, constructing, or improving a qualified residence *and* that is secured by such residence.

2. Interest on *home equity indebtedness:* Interest on debt secured by a qualified residence to the extent that the debt does not exceed the property's fair market value reduced by its acquisition debt.[63]

Note that in both cases, the crucial element in determining whether the interest qualifies is whether the debt is secured by a residence. Unsecured debt and debt secured by other property does not qualify even though the debt proceeds may be used to acquire a personal residence.

> **Example 27.** J borrowed $50,000 from her pension plan and $10,000 from her father to buy a new home. None of the interest on the debt is deductible because neither of the debts is secured by the residence. This is true even though the borrowed amounts were used to buy a residence.

Also observe that in the case of both acquisition and home equity debt, the debt must be secured by a *qualified* residence. A qualified residence is the taxpayer's principal home and one other residence of the taxpayer.[64] This rule effectively allows taxpayers to deduct the interest on only two homes: their first home and a second of their choosing. A taxpayer with more than two homes must designate which is the second home when the return is filed. Different homes can be selected each year.

> **Example 28.** After winning the New York State lottery, T retired from her job and purchased a home in Tampa, Florida. She also purchased a motor home and a condominium in Vail, Colorado. All purchases were debt-financed and secured by the property. Within certain dollar limitations, T can treat the interest paid on her home in Tampa *and* the interest paid on *either* the motor home *or* the condominium as qualified residence interest.

> **Example 29.** Assume the same facts as above except that T converted the condominium into rental property at the advice of her tax accountant. In this case, the condominium will not qualify as T's secondary residence.[65]

In determining the deductibility of interest on a second home, special rules must be considered if the taxpayer *rents* it out. These rules are examined in conjunction with vacation homes discussed later in this chapter. If the second home is not rented out, no personal use is actually needed in order to meet the qualified residence test.

Congress also took steps to ensure that a taxpayer could not convert nondeductible interest into qualified residence interest simply by pitching a tent on the property and calling it a second home (e.g., vacant land or a car). In determining whether the debt is incurred with respect to a qualified residence, the term *residence* includes a vacation home,

---

[62] § 163(h)(3).

[63] Interest relating to home equity loans is not deducitble for purposes of the alternative minimum tax unless the loan proceeds are used for improvements. See § 56(e).

[64] § 163(h)(4).

[65] This does not mean that a taxpayer's interest expense on rental property is not deductible. As discussed later, however, losses from rental property (including interest expense) may be subject to deduction limitations.

condominium, mobile home, boat, or recreational vehicle as long as the property contains basic living accommodations (i.e., sleeping space, toilet, and cooking facilities).

Limitations on Deductible Amount. To prevent taxpayers from taking undue advantage of the deductibility of home mortgage interest, Congress imposed limits on the maximum amount of debt qualifying under either definition. The aggregate amount of debt that can be treated as acquisition indebtedness for any taxable year cannot exceed $1 million ($500,000 in the case of a married individual filing a separate return),[66] whereas the aggregate amount of debt that will be treated as home equity indebtedness for any taxable year cannot exceed $100,000 ($50,000 if married and filing separately).[67] Collectively, the total amount of debt in any one year on which the interest paid or accrued will be treated as qualified residence interest cannot exceed $1.1 million.

> **Example 30.** During the current year, T purchases a principal residence in Boston for $900,000 and a vacation home in Tampa for $500,000. Mortgages secured by both properties total $1.3 million. T may treat *only* the interest paid on $1 million of acquisition indebtedness as qualified residence interest. In addition, he may treat $100,000 of the loans as home equity indebtedness and, therefore, the related interest is deductible as qualified residence interest. Whether interest on the balance of the debt, $200,000, is deductible depends on how the funds are used.

> **Example 31.** C purchased his present residence several years ago at a cost of $1.9 million. The present balance on his home mortgage is $800,000 and the property is valued at $2.5 million. This year, C borrowed $300,000 secured by a second mortgage on his home. Even though the total indebtedness does not exceed $1.1 million, C may deduct the interest on the $800,000 unpaid acquisition indebtedness and the interest on only $100,000 of the home equity mortgage. Any excess interest paid during the year will be treated as personal interest.

It is important to note that the interest paid on qualifying home equity indebtedness is allowed as a deduction *regardless* of how the taxpayer uses the loan proceeds. Thus, the obvious reason for the $100,000 limit on qualifying home equity debt is to impose a limit on the amount of an interest deduction the taxpayer may claim on loan proceeds used for personal purposes.

> **Example 32.** K purchased her present residence 10 years ago at a cost of $70,000. The present balance on her home mortgage is $40,000 and the property is appraised at a value of $150,000. This year, K borrowed $80,000 secured by a second mortgage on her home. She used the loan proceeds to purchase new clothes and a new automobile, and to take a vacation to Hawaii. The interest on the $80,000 loan is deductible since it is qualified residence interest. The fact that K used the loan proceeds for personal purposes is irrelevant. Also note that K's original cost of $70,000 is not used to limit the amount of her $80,000 home equity loan.

Refinancing. As mortgage interest rates rise and fall, homeowners often refinance their original home loans to get a better rate. During the past 25 years, refinancing has been quite common as the rates on 30-year fixed mortgages have been as high as about 18 percent in 1982 and as low as about 4 percent in 2009. Any attempt to refinance acquisition

---

[66] Any qualified residence indebtedness incurred before October 14, 1987—whether it is acquisition debt, home equity debt, or a combination of both—is to be treated as acquisition debt and is not subject to the $1 million limitation. If the property is later refinanced, however, the new indebtedness is subject to this limitation. § 163(h)(3)(D).

[67] § 163(h).

indebtedness should be undertaken with caution. A qualifying residence's acquisition debt is *reduced* by principal payments and *cannot be increased* unless the loan proceeds are used for home improvements. Thus, the acquisition debt can be refinanced only to the extent that the principal amount of the refinancing does not exceed the principal amount of the acquisition debt immediately before the refinancing.[68] The interest paid on any excess refinanced debt will not be treated as acquisition indebtedness. However, any excess may be treated as home equity indebtedness. As noted above, the total qualifying indebtedness (acquisition and home equity) cannot exceed the value of the residence.

> **Example 33.** In 1970, G purchased her California bungalow for $25,000. The house is now worth $350,000. G paid off the mortgage on the home several years ago. This year, G mortgaged her house for $120,000 and subsequently loaned the money to her grandson to enable him to buy his first home. None of the loan qualifies as acquisition debt because the balance of acquisition debt refinanced was zero. However, G may deduct interest on $100,000 of the loan, which qualifies as home-equity debt.

> **Example 34.** R purchased his present residence in 1998 for $250,000 and borrowed $210,000 on a 11% mortgage secured by the property. In 2009, R refinanced the balance of his mortgage, $190,000, by securing a new mortgage of $230,000 at 6%. Unless R used the additional loan proceeds to substantially improve the residence, only $190,000 of the new mortgage constitutes acquisition indebtedness, and the corresponding interest is therefore deductible. In addition, the $40,000 balance of the debt may be treated as home-equity debt. In such case, the interest on the entire $230,000 mortgage would be deductible as qualified residence interest.

Qualified Mortgage Insurance. Many individuals who purchase homes are required to buy mortgage insurance. The insurance is intended to provide funds to pay off the mortgage balance or help meet the payments on a mortgage as they fall due in the case of the individual's death or disability. Mortgage insurance is typically required when the loan has a loan to value ratio of 80 percent or greater (i.e., the down payment is less than 20% of the home's value). Such insurance is often called private mortgage insurance (PMI) for conventional loans, because a private institution rather than the federal government backs the loan.

Under the Tax Relief and Health Care Act of 2006, taxpayers were allowed to deduct premiums paid in 2007 for qualified mortgage insurance.[69] Congress extended this deduction through the year 2010 by the Mortgage Forgiveness Debt Relief Act of 2007. Premiums on mortgage insurance provided by VA, FHA, RHA, and private mortgage insurance normally qualify. In addition, the insurance qualifies only if it is on acquisition indebtedness on a qualified residence.

The deduction is subject to phase-out. The phase-out begins when the taxpayer's A.G.I. exceeds $100,000 and is complete once A.G.I. is greater than $109,000. For example, a taxpayer with $1,500 of qualified premiums and A.G.I. of $103,000 will be limited to a deduction of $1,000 [$1,500 – ($3,000/$9,000 × $1,500 = $500)].

Trade or Business Interest. While the taxpayer normally cannot deduct interest of a personal nature, interest related to a trade or business expenditure is totally deductible. Perhaps the most common example of business interest is that arising from loans used to acquire fixed assets such as buildings and equipment that are used in the business. Business interest also includes that attributable to loans used to acquire an interest in an S corporation or a partnership in which the taxpayer materially participates. Recall, however,

---

[68] § 163(h)(3)(B).

[69] § 163(h)(4)(E)(i).

that interest incurred in connection with performing services as an employee is not considered business interest, and thus is considered nondeductible personal interest.

As explained below, the fact that a business incurs interest expense does not necessarily mean that such interest is classified as business interest. If interest expense incurred by a business arises from an investment considered unrelated to the business, it will not be business interest (e.g., a closely held corporation purchases stock on margin).

Investment Interest. The fourth category of interest expense subject to limitation is investment interest. This limitation is imposed on taxpayers, other than regular corporations, who have paid or incurred interest expense to purchase or carry investments.[70] Common examples include interest on loans to purchase unimproved land and interest incurred on margin accounts used to purchase stocks and other securities. Congress imposed the investment interest limitation to eliminate what it perceived was an unfair advantage to certain wealthy investors. For example, consider the taxpayer who borrows to acquire or carry investments that produce little or no income currently but pay off handsomely when the investment is sold. This is commonly the hoped-for result with investments in such assets as growth stock or land. Without any restrictions, the taxpayer would be able to claim an immediate deduction for interest expense yet postpone any income recognition until the property was ultimately sold. Moreover, the income that the taxpayer would realize on the sale would normally be favorable capital gain. Congress apparently felt that this mismatching of income and expense was unwarranted and reacted by limiting the taxpayer's deduction for investment interest to the taxpayer's current investment income.

Before examining the investment interest limitation, the definition of investment interest should be clarified. *Investment interest* is generally any interest expense on debt used to finance property held for investment. It does not include, however, qualified residence interest or any interest related to a passive activity. As discussed in Chapter 12, interest related to a passive activity is allocated to the passive activity and is taken into account in computing the activity's income or loss. As a result, such interest is effectively limited by the passive-loss rules. Note, however, that any interest incurred by a passive activity that is related to its portfolio income (i.e., interest and dividend income) would normally be considered investment interest subject to the investment interest limitation. Because rental activities are usually treated as a passive activity, interest expense allocable to a rental activity is normally subject to the passive-loss rules.

The annual deduction for investment interest expense is limited to the taxpayer's *net investment income*, if any, for the tax year.[71] Any investment interest that exceeds the limitation and is disallowed may be carried forward until it is exhausted. Operationally, the disallowed interest is carried forward to the subsequent year, where it is combined with current year interest and is once again subject to the net investment income limitation. (Note that a sale of the financed property does not trigger the allowance of any disallowed interest.)

Net Investment Income. Net investment income is the excess of the taxpayer's investment income over investment expenses. For this purpose, *investment income* is generally defined as the gross income from property held for investment. Common examples of investment income include:

1. Interest;

2. Royalties;

---

[70]   § 163(d).

[71]   § 163(d)(1).

3. Ordinary income from the recapture of depreciation or intangible drilling costs under §§ 1245, 1250, and 1254;

4. Portfolio income under the passive loss rules; and

5. Income from a trade or business in which the taxpayer did not materially participate (but which is not a passive activity, e.g., a working interest in an oil or gas property).

Note that income from rental property and income from a passive activity (other than portfolio income) are not considered investment income. As noted above, any interest expense incurred in rental or passive activities is allocated to those activities and is used in computing the passive income or loss of such activity.[72] For example, mortgage interest on rental property would be deductible only to the extent of passive income. It is also important to note that qualified dividends (i.e., those taxed at a rate of 15 percent) and a net long-term capital gain from the disposition of an asset producing investment income (e.g., stocks or bonds) normally is not included in investment income. However, a taxpayer currently facing a limitation on the deduction for investment interest expense because of a limited amount of investment income may elect to include all or a part of the dividends or gain as investment income. Basically, such an election results in the dividends or the net capital gain being taxed as ordinary income in order to increase the electing taxpayer's ordinary deduction for investment interest expense.

Investment expenses are generally all those deductions (except interest) that are directly connected with the production of the investment income. Any investment expenses that are considered miscellaneous itemized deductions are considered only to the extent they exceed the 2 percent floor. For this purpose, the 2 percent floor is first absorbed by all other miscellaneous expenses.

Example 35. G's records for 2009 revealed the following information:

Salary	$ 40,000
Dividends and interest	3,500
Share of partnership income:	
Partnership ordinary income	700
Portfolio income:	
Dividends	50
Interest	80
Rental income from duplex	15,000
Rental expenses	(14,000)
Adjusted gross income	$ 45,330
Qualified residence interest	$ 8,000
Real estate taxes on home	4,000
Property tax on land held for investment	1,000
Miscellaneous itemized deductions:	
Safety deposit box rental	50
Financial planner	1,500
Fee to maintain brokerage account	100
Unreimbursed employee business expenses	725

G is a limited partner in the partnership and thus treats the partnership as a passive activity. G also paid $7,700 of interest expense on the land held for investment. G's net investment income is computed as follows:

---

[72] § 163(d)(4)(E). See Chapter 12 for a detailed discussion of the passive loss rules.

Investment income:		
Dividends and interest............................	$3,500	
Partnership income:		
Portfolio income:		
Dividends..................................	50	
Interest...................................	80	
Total investment income............................		$3,630
Investment expenses:		
Property tax on land.............................	$1,000	
Safe deposit box rental	50	
Financial planner	1,500	
Fee to maintain brokerage account	100	

Miscellaneous itemized deductions disallowed			
2% floor (2% × $45,330).......................	$ 907		
Unreimbursed employee business expenses..........	(725)		
Investment expenses classified as			
miscellaneous itemized deductions disallowed......		(182)	
Total investment expenses		(2,468)	
Net investment income.............................		$ 1,162	

For 2009, G may deduct $1,162 of investment interest expense (*not* subject to the itemized deduction cutback rule). The balance of $6,538 ($7,700 −$1,162) is carried over to the next year, 2010, and is treated as if it were paid in 2010. There is no limit on the carryover period. Note that in computing investment expenses, only investment expenses exceeding the 2% floor are allowed. In computing the disallowed portion, investment expenses are deemed to come last. Also note that rental income is not considered investment income.

Passive Activity Interest. Deductions attributable to so-called *passive activities* (e.g., those in which a taxpayer does not participate in a material fashion) are subject to special rules. Interest expense incurred by a passive activity itself (e.g., a limited partnership), or by investment in a passive activity, is treated as a deduction relating to the passive activity and is limited by the passive loss rules.[73] The passive activity loss rules are discussed in Chapter 12.

Interest on Student Loans. One of several measures enacted by Congress to help taxpayers finance the cost of higher education concerns the treatment of interest on student loans. As noted earlier, without a special rule, interest paid on loans to help pay college tuition and the like would be nondeductible personal interest. Currently, § 221 authorizes a deduction for interest on qualified educational loans. The maximum amount of interest that can be deducted annually is limited to $2,500.

---

[73]   § 163(d)(3)(B).

If the interest qualifies for deduction, it is deductible *for* adjusted gross income. Therefore taxpayers are not required to itemize in order to benefit from the deduction. (It is also true that the deduction would not be subject to the two-percent cutback; however, those taxpayers subject to the cutback would not be able to deduct the expense due to the phase-out rules discussed below.)

Like many of the relief provisions created by the new law, the deduction for interest on qualified educational loans is not extended to high-income taxpayers. To accomplish this objective, the maximum deduction is phased out once the taxpayer's A.G.I. (computed with certain modifications) exceeds $120,000 for joint returns ($60,000 for other returns). The reduction occurs over a $30,000 income range for married filing jointly ($15,000 for all others), producing a complete phase-out as follows:

Student Loan Interest Deduction Phase-Out

$$\text{Reduction of deductible Portion of student loan interest} = \text{Deductible Amount of Interest (\$2,500 maximum in 2009)} \times \frac{\text{Modified A.G.I.} - \text{threshold}}{\text{Income range}}$$

	Modified A.G.I. Phase-Out Begins	Modified A.G.I. Phase-Out Complete
Married filing jointly	$120,000	$150,000
Other taxpayers	60,000	75,000

For this purpose, modified A.G.I. is A.G.I. before the exclusions for (1) foreign earned income and housing; (2) income from American Samoa, Guam and the Northern Mariana Islands; and after the exclusions for (1) Series EE savings bonds interest used to pay for education; (2) employer provided adoption benefits; (3) social security; (4) the deduction for contributions to IRAs; and (5) the deduction for losses on passive activities.

> **Example 36.** In 2009, S, single, graduated from Notre Dame with a law degree. During the year, she paid student loan interest of $5,000 and reported adjusted gross income before consideration of the interest of $66,000. Since S's adjusted gross income exceeds the $60,000 threshold for single taxpayers by $6,000 (40% of the $15,000 range), the maximum allowable deduction is reduced in 2009 to $1,500 [$2,500 − ($6,000/$15,000 × $2,500 = $1,000)]. Therefore, S may deduct $1,500 of the $5,000 interest for adjusted gross income.

Only interest on qualified education loans is deductible. Such loans are defined as any debt (other than a loan from a related party) incurred to pay qualified educational expenses for the taxpayer, the taxpayer's spouse, or other individuals who were the taxpayer's dependents at the time the debt was incurred. No deduction is allowed for interest paid by the taxpayer if the taxpayer is claimed as a dependent on another's return. For example, a child who pays interest on his student loans could not deduct the interest if his parents claim an exemption for him. Married taxpayers must file a joint return to claim the deduction.

Interest is deductible only if the education is furnished to an eligible student. An eligible student is generally one who is enrolled in a degree, certificate, or other program leading to a recognized credential at an eligible institution of higher education. In addition, the student must have been attending at least half-time (i.e., one-half of the normal full-time work load for the course of study that the student is pursuing).

Qualified educational expenses include the costs of attendance at an eligible educational institution. They include tuition, fees, room and board, and related expenses, such as books and supplies. Such amounts must be reduced by any amounts excluded under § 127 concerning employer educational assistance plans, § 135 concerning interest excluded on Series EE bonds, or § 530 excluding distributions from education IRAs (see discussion in Chapter 6).

CLASSIFICATION OF INTEREST EXPENSE

The different rules for different types of interest expense force taxpayers to classify and allocate their interest expense among appropriate categories. The classification procedure established by the Treasury is very straightforward in principle. Under the Temporary Regulations, interest is generally classified according to how the loan proceeds are spent—that is, the character of the expenditure determines the character of interest.[74] The type of collateral that may secure the loan is irrelevant in the classification process—except in the case of the qualified residence interest which is deductible regardless of how loan proceeds are spent.[75]

> **Example 37.** This year, T pledged IBM stock held as an investment as collateral for a loan which he uses to purchase a personal car. Any interest expense on the loan is considered nondeductible personal interest since the debt proceeds were used for personal purposes. The fact that the debt is secured by investment property is irrelevant. If the loan were secured by T's primary residence, the interest could be deductible as qualified residence interest.

The classification scheme demands that the taxpayer trace how any loan proceeds were used. To simplify this task, specific rules exist for debt proceeds that are (1) deposited in the borrower's account, (2) disbursed directly by the lender to someone other than the borrower, or (3) received in cash.

Proceeds Deposited in the Borrower's Account. In most cases, taxpayers borrow money, deposit it in an account, and write checks for various expenditures. Since money is fungible (that is, one dollar cannot be distinguished from another) it would be impossible without special rules to determine how the loan proceeds were spent, and therefore, how the related interest should be allocated. The Temporary Regulations create such rules.[76]

The first presumption created by the Regulations concerns the treatment of interest on funds that have not been spent. To the extent borrowed funds are deposited and not spent, interest attributable to such a period is considered *investment interest* regardless of whether the account bears interest income.[77]

> **Example 38.** On November 1, K borrowed $1,000 which she intends to use to fix up her boat. She deposited the $1,000 in a separate account. No expenditures were made during the remainder of the year. In this case, K is subject to the interest allocation rules since the interest expense is considered attributable to an investment, and is therefore, investment interest.

---

[74] Temp. Reg. § 1.163-8T.

[75] Temp. Reg. § 1.163-8T(c)(1). For purposes of the alternative minimum tax, however, qualified housing interest is deductible only if the debt is spent on the residence. See Chapter 13 for further discussion.

[76] Temp. Reg. § 1.163-8T(c)(4).

[77] *Ibid.*

Example 39. Same as above except K makes several personal expenditures during the next three months. Interest must be allocated between investment interest and personal interest.

Example 40. A borrows $100,000 on January 1 and deposits it in a separate account where it remains until April 1 when he purchases an interest in a limited partnership for $20,000. On September 1, R purchases a new car for $30,000. Interest expense attributable to the $100,000 is allocated in the following manner:

	Debt Proceeds		
Period	Investment Interest	Passive Interest	Personal Interest
1/1–3/31	$100,000		
4/1–8/31	80,000	$20,000	
9/1–12/31	50,000	20,000	$30,000

Commingled Funds. In most situations, a taxpayer has one account in which all amounts are deposited. When this occurs, all expenditures from the account after the loan is deposited are deemed to come first from the borrowed funds.

Example 41. On October 1, B borrowed $1,000 to purchase a snowplow attachment for the front of his truck. He plans to make some extra money this winter by plowing driveways and parking lots. B deposited the $1,000 in his only checking account. On October 20, he bought the attachment for $1,500. Prior to October 20, he wrote $700 in checks for groceries and other personal items. Of the $1,000 loan, $700 is deemed to have been spent for personal items while the remaining $300 is allocated to the snow plow. Consequently, B may deduct only the interest expense on $300.

If proceeds from more than one loan are deposited into an account, expenditures are treated as coming from the borrowed funds in the order in which they were deposited (i.e., first-in, first-out).

Example 42. Dr. T has a personal checking account with a current balance of $3,000. On November 1, T obtained a $1,000 one-year Loan (Debt A) from her bank, which it credited to her personal account. She planned to use the loan to purchase a small copier for her dental practice. After shopping, T determined she would need additional funds. Therefore, on November 30 she obtained another $1,000 loan (Debt B). On December 12, T wrote a check for $800 to pay for her husband's Christmas present, a diamond ring. On December 19, she wrote a check for $2,100 to purchase the copier. These transactions are summarized as follows:

Date	Transaction	
11/1	Borrowed (Debt A)	$1,000
11/30	Borrowed (Debt B)	1,000
12/12	Purchased ring	(800)
12/19	Purchased copier	(2,100)

For purposes of determining the deduction for the interest on the loan, $800 of Debt A is deemed to be used for personal purposes (i.e., the ring purchase) and $200 toward the copier. All of Debt B is used for the copier. Thus, interest attributable to $800 of

Debt A is nondeductible personal interest while that attributable to $200 is totally deductible. All of the interest on Debt B is deductible business interest. This may be summarized as follows:

Expenditure	11/1 Debt A $1,000		11/30 Debt B $1,000		Other
	Personal	Business	Personal	Business	
$ 800 ring	$800				
2,100 copier		$200		$1,000	$900

Fifteen-Day Rule. In lieu of allocating the debt proceeds in the above manner, an alternative method is available. A borrower can elect to treat any expenditure made within 15 days after the loan proceeds are deposited as having been made from the proceeds of that loan.

Example 43. C borrowed and deposited $5,000 in his checking account on December 1. On December 2, he wrote a check for $6,000 for his estimated income taxes. On December 10, he wrote a check for $5,000 for furniture for his business. Under the normal allocation rule, the entire $5,000 proceeds from the debt would be considered spent for personal purposes. Under the 15-day rule, however, C may treat the $5,000 as used to purchase the furniture since the proceeds were spent within 15 days of deposit.

Loan Proceeds Received Indirectly. In many transactions, a borrower incurs debt without receiving any loan proceeds directly. For example, if the taxpayer borrowed $100,000 from a bank to purchase a building, the bank typically disburses the $100,000 directly to the seller rather than to the borrower. Similarly, the borrower may purchase the building and assume the seller's $100,000 mortgage. In this and similar situations, the borrower is treated as having received the proceeds and used them to make the expenditure for the property, services, or other purpose.[78]

Loan Proceeds Received in Cash. When the borrower receives the loan proceeds in cash, the taxpayer may treat any cash expenditure made within 15 days after receiving the cash as made from the loan. If the loan proceeds are not spent within 15 days, however, the loan is deemed to have been spent for personal purposes.

Debt Repayments, Refinancings, and Reallocations. Loans that are used for several purposes present a unique problem when a portion of the loan is repaid. In this case, repayments must be applied in the following order:[79]

1. Personal expenditures;

2. Investment expenditures and passive activity expenditures (other than rental real estate in which the taxpayer actively participates);

3. Rental real estate expenditures;

4. Former passive activity expenditures; and

5. Trade or business expenditures.

---

[78]   Temp. Reg. § 1.163-8T(c)(3).

[79]   *Ibid.*

Example 44. R borrows $10,000, $6,000 of which is used to purchase a personal automobile and $4,000 of which is used to invest in land. On June 1 of this year she paid $7,000 on the loan. Of the $7,000 repayment, $6,000 reduces the portion of the loan allocated to personal expenditures and the remaining $1,000 reduces the portion allocated to investment.

If the taxpayer refinances an old debt, interest on the new debt is characterized in the same way as that on the old debt.

Example 45. In 2008, S borrowed $10,000 at an annual interest rate of 14%. He used $8,000 to purchase a new boat and $2,000 to purchase a computer to use in his business. This year, he borrowed $6,000 from another bank at 10% to pay off the balance of the old loan. At the time the original loan was paid off, $4,000 of the $6,000 balance was allocated to the boat purchase and $2,000 was allocated to the computer purchase. The new debt will be allocated in the same manner as the old debt.

If the taxpayer borrows to finance a business asset, the debt must be recharacterized whenever the asset is sold or the nature of the use of the asset changes.

Example 46. Several years ago B, a traveling salesperson, borrowed $12,000 to buy a car that he used entirely for business. This year, B gave his car to his wife who uses it solely for personal use. The loan and interest thereon must be reclassified.

Computation and Allocation of Interest Expense. The special rules governing the taxpayer's deduction for interest expense do not affect its computation. Interest is computed in the normal manner. However, allocation of the interest expense among the different categories does present certain difficulties. As a general rule, interest expense accruing on a debt for any period is allocated in the same manner as the debt. Interest which accrues on interest—that is, compound interest—is allocated in the same manner as the original interest.[80]

Example 47. On January 1, R borrowed $100,000 at an interest rate of 10%, compounded semiannually. She deposited the loan in a separate account and on July 1 used the funds to purchase a yacht. On December 31, R paid the accrued interest of $10,250, computed as follows:

Period	Principal		Rate		Time		Interest
1/1–6/30	$100,000	×	10%	×	6/12	=	$ 5,000
7/1–12/31	105,000	×	10%	×	6/12	=	5,250
							$10,250

Under the allocation rules, R's loan is classified as an investment loan from January 1 through June 30 and, therefore, the interest accruing for that period of $5,000 is investment interest. In addition, the interest expense which accrues on this $5,000 from July 30 through December 31 of $250 ($5,000 × 10% × 612) is considered investment interest for a total of $5,250. This $250 of "compound interest" accruing from July 31 through December 31 is allocated to the investment category even though the original loan has been assigned to a new category for the same period. The remaining $5,000 of interest expense accruing from July 1 through December 31 ($100,000 × 10% × 612) is personal interest.

---

[80] Temp. Reg. § 1.163-8T(c)(2).

To simplify the allocation of interest expense, the taxpayer may use a straight-line method. Using this technique, an equal amount of interest is allocated to each day of the year. For this purpose, the taxpayer may treat a year as consisting of twelve 30-day months.

> **Example 48.** Assume the same facts as in *Example 47* above, except that R elects to allocate the interest expense on a straight-line basis, treating the year as consisting of twelve 30-day months. As a result, interest expense of $5,125 (180/360 × $10,250) would be investment interest while the remaining $5,125 of interest expense would be personal interest.

WHEN DEDUCTIBLE

The taxpayer's method of accounting generally controls the timing of an interest expense deduction. Accrual method taxpayers generally may deduct interest over the period in which the interest accrues, regardless of when the expense is actually paid. However, cash-basis taxpayers must *actually* pay the interest before a deduction is allowed. Many situations arise in which the "actual payment" requirement imposed on cash-basis taxpayers delays the timing of a deduction. Other situations concern measurement of the amount of interest actually paid. The most common of these situations are briefly discussed below.

Interest Paid in Advance. If interest is paid in advance for a time period that extends beyond the end of one tax year, *both* accrual method and cash-basis taxpayers generally are required to spread the interest deduction over the tax years to which it applies.[81] An important exception is made for cash-basis individual taxpayers who are required to pay interest "points" in connection with indebtedness incurred to *purchase* or *improve* the taxpayer's principal residence (i.e., taxpayer's home).[82] The term *points* is often used to describe charges imposed on the borrower under such descriptions as "loan origination fees," "premium charges," and "maximum loan charges." Such charges usually are stated as a percentage (point) of the loan amount. If the payment of any of these charges is *strictly* for the use of money *and* actual payment of these charges is made out of *separate funds* belonging to the taxpayer, an interest deduction is allowed in the year of payment.[83]

> **Example 49.** R borrowed $15,000 from State Bank to make improvements on his home. The loan is payable over a 10-year period, and the bank charged R a loan origination fee of $300 (2 points). If R pays the $300 charge from separate funds, it is currently deductible as an interest expense (assuming R itemizes his deductions). However, if the $300 charge is added to the amount of the loan, R has not currently paid interest. Instead, R will be required to treat the charge as note-discount interest (see discussion below).

Note-Discount Interest. Taxpayers often sign notes calling for repayment of an amount greater than the loan proceeds actually received. This occurs when the creditor subtracts (withholds) the interest from the face amount of the loan and the taxpayer receives the balance, or when the face amount of the note simply includes add-on interest. In either case, cash-basis taxpayers are not allowed a deduction until the tax year in which

---

[81]   § 461(a).

[82]   § 461(g).

[83]   See *Roger A. Schubel*, 77 T.C. 701 (1982), and *James W. Hager*, 45 TCM 123, T.C. Memo 1982-663. Note, however, that this interest deduction is subject to the rules regarding qualified residence interest.

the interest is actually paid. Accrual-method taxpayers are allowed to deduct the interest over the tax years in which it accrues.

Graduated Payment Mortgages. A creature of the high interest rate mortgage market of recent years, graduated payment mortgages provide for increasing payments in the early years of the mortgage until the payments reach some level amount. Under these plans, the payments in the early years are less than the amount of interest owed on the loan. The unpaid interest is added to the principal amount of the mortgage and future interest is computed on this revised balance. As should be expected, cash-basis taxpayers may deduct *only* the interest actually paid in the current year; the increases in the principal balance of the mortgage are treated much the same as note-discount interest.

Installment Purchases. Individual taxpayers who purchase personal property or pay for educational services under a contract calling for installment payments in which carrying charges are separately stated but the interest charge cannot be determined are allowed to *impute* an interest expense. The imputed expense is allowed whether or not a payment is actually made during the tax year, and is computed at a rate of 6 percent of the *average unpaid balance* of the contract during the year.[84] The average unpaid balance is the sum of the unpaid balance outstanding on the first day of each month of the tax year, divided by 12 months.[85] Credit card and revolving charge account finance charges are generally much greater than 6 percent. Fortunately, these charges are usually stated separately at a *predetermined* interest rate (e.g., finance charge of 1ø% of unpaid monthly balance). Recall, however, that this type of interest expense is generally personal interest and thus nondeductible!

WHERE REPORTED

Like the deductions for taxes, the appropriate tax form or schedule on which deductible interest is reported depends upon the entity entitled to the deduction and the nature of the indebtedness to which the interest relates. A corporation's deductible interest is reported on its annual tax return Form 1120. Estates and trusts report interest deductions on Form 1041; partnerships and S corporations claim interest deductions on Forms 1065 and 1120S, respectively. Individuals claiming a deduction for interest expense must report the amount on the appropriate schedule of Form 1040. If the interest is related to business indebtedness—and the business is self-employment—the individual will claim his or her deduction on Schedule C (Schedule F for farmers and ranchers). Interest on debt incurred in connection with the production of rents or royalties is reported on Schedule E. Deductible interest on indebtedness incurred for personal use must be reported as an itemized deduction on Schedule A (with the exception of qualifying student loan interest which is deductible for A.G.I.). However, any individual who has refinanced his or her home, or is otherwise subject to the limitations imposed on qualified residence interest, should see IRS Publication 936 for instructions in computing the home mortgage interest deduction.

An individual's current deduction for investment interest expense should be calculated on Form 4952 (see Appendix B), and any disallowed deduction reported as a carryover amount. The deductible amount from Form 4952 should be transferred to and claimed as a deduction on the individual's Schedule E, Form 1040, if the interest relates to the production of royalties; otherwise, the deductible amount is reported on Schedule A. Partnerships and S corporations are not allowed to deduct investment interest expense in determining income or loss. Instead, these conduit entities are required to set out and separately report each partner's or shareholder's share of *both* investment interest expense *and* net investment

---

[84]   § 163(b)(1).

[85]   *Ibid.*

income for the current year. Each partner or shareholder must claim his or her deduction subject to the previously described limitations. Recall, however, that a partner that is a regular corporation will not be subject to the investment interest expense limitation.

CHARITABLE CONTRIBUTIONS

To encourage the private sector to share in the cost of providing many needed social services, Congress allows individuals, regular corporations, estates, and trusts deductions for charitable contributions (or gifts) of money or other property to certain qualified organizations. Partnerships and S corporations are not allowed to deduct charitable contributions. Instead, these conduit entities pass the contributions through to the partners and shareholders who must claim the deduction on their own Federal income tax returns.[86]

Code § 170 contains the rules regarding deductions for charitable contributions made by individuals and regular corporations. Code § 642(c) sets forth the rules regarding the amount and timing of charitable contribution deductions claimed by estates and trusts. The rules related to the measurement, timing, and qualification of contribution deductions claimed by individuals and corporations are discussed below. A discussion of the percentage limitations imposed on current deductions by individual taxpayers is also included. The specific rules regarding limitations imposed on a corporation's annual charitable contribution deduction are discussed in Chapter 19.

DEDUCTION REQUIREMENTS

Individual taxpayers are allowed a deduction for contributions of cash or other property *only if* the gift is made to a qualifying donee organization. Additionally, individuals are required to actually pay cash or transfer property before the close of the tax year in which the deduction is claimed. An exception to the payment requirement is made in the case of contribution deductions which, due to deduction limitations, have been carried over from prior years. The deduction limitations and carryover rules are discussed later in this chapter.

In addition to these basic considerations, Congress added two extremely important limitations in 2007 that will have widespread effect. First, no deduction is allowed for contributions of cash, check or any other type of monetary gift unless the taxpayer has some type of bank record such as a cancelled check, credit card statement or receipt from the charity verifying the contribution. Note that this rule applies to any contribution of money, regardless of amount. Thus, there is no de minimis exception to the new substantiation requirements for gifts of cash to charity.[87] Second, a charitable contribution for clothing and household goods will be permitted only if the items are "in good used condition or better." In this regard, the IRS is authorized to deny deductions for items of minimal value (e.g., used socks and underwear). Unfortunately, the new law provides no guidance as to what is good condition for used items or how the new rule might be enforced.[88]

Qualifying Donees. To be deductible, contributions of cash or other property must be made to or for the use of one of the following:[89]

---

[86]   See §§ 702(a)(4) and 1366(a)(1).

[87]   Section 170(f)(17), introduced by the Pension Protection Act of 2006. As a result of these requirements, taxpayers are likely to make more contributions by check.

[88]   See § 170(f)(16) and other limitations applying to such items as "taxidermy property," conservation easements and certain other property

[89]   See § 170(c).

1. A state, a U.S. possession, a political subdivision of a state or possession, the United States, or the District of Columbia, if the contribution is made solely for public purposes;

2. A community chest, corporation, trust, fund, or foundation that is organized or created in, or under the laws of, the United States, any state, the District of Columbia, or any possession of the United States *and* is organized and operated exclusively for religious, charitable, scientific, literary, or educational purposes or for the prevention of cruelty to children or animals;

3. A war veterans' organization;

4. A nonprofit volunteer fire company or civil defense organization;

5. A domestic fraternal society operating under the lodge system, but only if the contribution is to be used for any of the purposes stated in item 2 above; and

6. A nonprofit cemetery company, if the funds are to be used solely for the perpetual care of the cemetery as a whole, and not for a particular lot or mausoleum crypt.

If the taxpayer has not been informed by the recipient organization that it is a qualifying donee, he or she may check its status in the *Cumulative List of Organizations* (IRS Publication 78). This publication contains a frequently updated listing of organizations which have applied to and received tax-exempt status from the IRS. To be a qualifying donee, however, the organization is not required to be listed in this publication.

Disallowance Possibilities. Direct contributions to needy or worthy individuals are not deductible. In addition, contributions to qualifying organizations must not be restricted to use by a specific person; if so, deductions generally are disallowed.

Example 50. F contributed cash of $10,000 to his son, S. S is a missionary for a church that is a qualified organization, and the gift proceeds were used exclusively by S to further the charitable work of the church. F is not entitled to a charitable contribution deduction since the gift was not made to a qualifying donee. Similarly, F would be denied a deduction if he made the gift to the church but restricted the use of the funds only for his missionary son.[90]

A taxpayer's contribution to a qualified organization that is motivated by the taxpayer's expectation and receipt of a significant economic benefit will not be deductible as a charitable contribution. The receipt of an unexpected and indirect economic benefit as a result of the gift should not disqualify the taxpayer's deduction, however.

Example 51. T donated two parcels of land to a nearby city for use as building sites for new public schools. The location of the building sites was such that the city had to construct two access roads through the taxpayer's remaining undeveloped land in order to make use of the gifted property. Construction of the access roads significantly enhanced the value of T's remaining acreage, and as a result, his charitable contribution deduction may be denied.[91]

Apparently, because Congress does not believe that the benefit received by a taxpayer is of great significance, 80 percent of the amount paid by a taxpayer to a college or university that either directly or indirectly entitles the taxpayer to purchase tickets to the

---

[90] *White v. U.S.*, 82-1 USTC ¶9232, 49 AFTR2d 82-364, 514 F. Supp. 1057 (D.Ct. Utah, 1981). For a similar result, see *Babilonia v. Comm.*, 82-2 USTC ¶9478, 50 AFTR2d 82-5442 (CA-9, 1982).

[91] See *Ottawa Silica Co. v. U.S.*, 83-1 USTC ¶9169, 51 AFTR2d 83-590, 699 F.2d 1124 (CA-Fed. Cir., 1983) where, under similar circumstances, the taxpayer's claimed contribution deduction was disallowed.

institution's athletic events is allowed as a deduction.[92] However, any amount actually paid for the tickets will not be deductible.

LIMITATIONS ON DEDUCTIONS

Unlike the requirement that an individual's medical expenses and casualty losses *exceed* some minimum percentage of adjusted gross income (referred to as the *floor* amount) *before* any deductions are allowed, deductions for charitable contributions are subject to *ceiling* limitations (i.e., not to *exceed* a percentage of A.G.I.). Generally, an individual's current deduction for charitable contributions is limited to 50 percent of the taxpayer's adjusted gross income. A 30 percent ceiling limitation is imposed on an individual's contributions of *certain appreciated property*, and a 20 percent overall limitation is imposed on an individual's contributions to *certain qualifying organizations*.

Under the general rule, the amount of a taxpayer's charitable deduction (before any percentage limitation) is the *sum* of money *plus* the fair market value of any property other than money which is contributed to a qualifying donee. However, both the gift of property to certain organizations and the gift of certain types of property other than money may result in a deduction of an amount *less than* the property's fair market value. These exceptions to the general rule are explained below, followed by a discussion of the various percentage limitations imposed on an individual's deduction for charitable contributions.[93]

Contributions Other Than Money or Property. No charitable contribution deduction is allowed for the value of time or services rendered to a charitable organization.[94] Likewise, no deduction is allowed for any "lost income" associated with the rent-free use of a taxpayer's property by a qualifying charity. However, *unreimbursed* (out-of-pocket) *expenses* incurred by the taxpayer in rendering services to a charitable institution or allowing rent-free use of property by such an organization *qualify* as charitable contributions.[95] For example, a taxpayer is allowed a deduction for the cost and upkeep of uniforms required to be worn while performing the charitable services, but only if the uniforms are not suitable for everyday use. Similarly, a taxpayer is generally allowed to deduct amounts paid for transportation to and from his or her home to the place where the charitable services are performed.[96] This includes the costs for gasoline, oil, parking, and tolls incurred by a taxpayer using his or her own vehicle in connection with the charitable services. In lieu of deducting the actual expenses for gasoline and oil, a taxpayer is allowed to use a standard mileage rate in calculating the cost of using an automobile in charitable activities. In 2009, the rate is 14 cents per mile.[97] In either case, no deduction is allowed for insurance, depreciation, or the costs of general repairs and maintenance.

---

[92] See § 170(m).

[93] Regular corporations are subject to an overall limitation of 10 percent of taxable income, determined without regard to certain deductions. See Chapter 19 for more details.

[94] Reg. § 1.170A-1(g).

[95] *Ibid.*

[96] The Tax Reform Act of 1986 added § 170(k) to the Code to disallow a deduction for travel expenses related to charitable services where there is a significant element of personal pleasure, recreation, or vacation in such travel.

[97] See § 170(j) and Rev. Proc. 2008-72, I.R.B. 2008-50.

Example 52. T is the scoutmaster of a local troop of the Boy Scouts of America. During the current year, T incurred the following expenses in rendering his services to this charitable organization:

Cost and upkeep of uniforms	$ 80
Gasoline and oil expenses	200
Parking and tolls	30
Estimated value of rent-free use of den in home	1,000
Estimated value of services (500 hours @ $50 per hour)	25,000
Total	$26,310

T is entitled to a $310 charitable contribution deduction for his out-of-pocket expenses ($80 + $200 + $30) incurred in rendering the charitable services as a scoutmaster. No deduction is allowed for the estimated value of his services or the rent-free use of his home.

Example 53. Assume the same facts as in *Example 52*, except that T drove his automobile 3,000 miles in connection with the charitable services. If he did not keep records of the actual expenses for gasoline and oil, T could use the standard mileage rate of 14 cents per mile. In this case, he will be allowed to deduct $530 [(3,000 miles × 14¢ per mile for charitable use of auto = $420) + $30 for parking and tolls + $80 related to uniforms].

Fair Market Value Determination. The IRS defines fair market value as "the price at which the property would change hands between a willing buyer and a willing seller, neither being under any compulsion to buy or sell and both having reasonable knowledge of relevant facts."[98] Determination of this amount usually means the taxpayer must make an educated guess or incur the cost of an independent appraisal. Since the IRS requires that the taxpayer attach a statement to his or her return when a deduction exceeding $500 is claimed for a charitable gift of property (Form 8283, Noncash Charitable Contributions), many taxpayers seek independent appraisals to support their claimed deductions. Independent appraisals are *required*—and the donee must *attach* a summary of the appraisal to his or her return—if the claimed value of the contributed property exceeds $5,000.[99] Appraisal fees are not deductible as contributions. However, they are deductible by individuals as miscellaneous itemized deductions (subject to the 2% floor).[100]

Ordinary Income Property. The term *ordinary income property* is used to describe any property which, if sold, would require the owner to recognize gain *other than* long-term capital gain. For example, ordinary income property includes a donor/taxpayer's property held primarily for sale to customers in his or her trade or business (i.e., inventory items), a work of art created by the donor, a manuscript prepared by the donor, letters and memoranda prepared by or for the donor, and a capital asset held by the taxpayer for not more than one year (i.e., short-term capital gain property). Musical compositions can be treated as capital assets for purposes of determining the character of the gain or loss on a sale or exchange but are considered ordinary income property for purposes of determining the amount of the contribution. Thus a contribution of song by the composer would

---

[98] Reg. § 1.170-1(c)(1).

[99] § 6050L. A donee charity that sells or otherwise disposes of such property within two years of the donation *must* report the disposition (and amount received, if any) to the IRS and the donor.

[100] Under § 212(3), individuals are allowed to deduct expenses associated with the determination of their tax liability. This includes appraisal fees paid in valuing property contributions.

normally result in a deduction equal to the song's basis which is usually little or nothing.[101] The term also includes property which, if sold, would result in the recognition of ordinary income under any of the depreciation recapture provisions.[102]

The charitable deduction (without regard to any percentage limitations) for the gift of ordinary income property is equal to the property's fair market value *reduced* by the amount of ordinary income that would be recognized if the property had been sold at its fair market value (this amount is often called the *ordinary income potential*).[103]

> **Example 54.** F donated 100 shares of IBM stock to his church on December 15, 2009. F had purchased the stock for $9,000 on August 7, 2009 and it was worth $12,000 on the date of the gift. Since F would have recognized a short-term capital gain if the stock had been sold on December 15, 2009 (i.e., holding period not more than one year), the stock is ordinary income property. As a result, F's charitable contribution deduction is limited to $9,000 ($12,000 fair market value − $3,000 ordinary income potential).

In most cases, the charitable deduction for ordinary income property will be limited to the taxpayer's adjusted basis in the property since its fair market value is reduced by the *unrealized appreciation* in value (fair market value − adjusted basis), which would not result in long-term capital gain if the property were sold. There are, however, three important instances when this would not be the case. First, the charitable deduction for *any property* which, if sold, would result in a *loss* (i.e., adjusted basis > fair market value) is limited to the property's fair market value.

> **Example 55.** J donated 1,000 shares of Intel stock to the University of Alabama that he purchased several years ago for $40,000 but that were now worth only $15,000. J may claim a charitable contribution deduction only for the stock's fair market value of $15,000. Note that the property does not qualify as either capital gain property or ordinary income property (since he would have recognized a capital loss on the sale). J would have been better off had he sold the property, recognized the loss and donated the proceeds from the sale.

Second, any depreciable property held by the taxpayer for more than one year and used in his or her trade or business is *§ 1231 property*. The amount of gain from the sale of such property that exceeds any depreciation recapture is referred to as "§ 1231 gain." Potential § 1231 gains are treated as long-term capital gains for purposes of measuring a taxpayer's charitable contribution deduction.[105] As such, any unrealized appreciation in the value of property that is attributable to § 1231 gain will not be considered ordinary income potential for purposes of the limitation described above.

The remaining exception entitles C corporations to increase their deduction for contributions of certain ordinary income items by one-half of the unrealized ordinary income in the property. The enhanced deduction, which is limited to twice the property's basis, is available for contributions of the following:[104]

- Contributions of inventory or depreciable property used in business that is used by the charitable organization for the care of children, the ill, or the needy. For example, gifts of drugs and medical supplies by pharmaceutical companies to a

---

[101] See §§ 170(e)(1)(A) and 1221(b)(3).

[102] See § 170(e)(1), Reg. §§ 1.170A-4(b)(1) and (b)(4).

[103] § 170(e)(1). For an application of this rule, see *William Glen*, 79 T.C. 208 (1982).

[105] Reg. § 1.170A-4(b)(4).

[104] §170(e)(3).

charity would qualify. Gifts of food inventory (by any entity) and book inventory to schools also qualify but are subject to additional rules.

- Contributions of "scientific property or apparatus" constructed or assembled by the taxpayer that is held as inventory and is donated within two years of its manufacture to an educational institution for use in research or for research training in physical or biological sciences. For example, a computer manufacturer's contribution of computers to a university for use in research or by its students in computer science courses would qualify.
- Contributions of computer software, computers, peripheral equipment, and fiber optic cable for computer use to a school, organizations formed to support elementary and secondary education and certain public libraries.

Example 56. ELI Corporation manufactures insulin and gives $1,000,000 of the drug (basis $700,000) to hospitals around the country to be used for charitable purposes. Normally, the deduction would be limited to the property's adjusted basis of $700,000. However, because the hospitals will use it for the care of children and those who are needy, the deduction is $850,000 [$700,000 + $150,000 (50% × ($1,000,000 − $700,000 = $300,000 unrealized ordinary income))] If the basis had been $100,000, the tentative deduction would be $550,000 ($100,000 + $450,000 (50% × $900,000) but it would be limited to $200,000 (2 × adjusted basis of $100,000).

Capital Gain Property. Any property which, if sold by the donor/taxpayer, would result in the recognition of a long-term capital gain or § 1231 gain is *capital gain property*.[106] A taxpayer is generally allowed to claim the fair market value of such property as a contribution deduction. There are two important exceptions to this rule, however. *First*, if capital gain property is contributed to or for the use of a private nonoperating foundation [as defined in § 509(a) such as the Gates Foundation], the donor must *reduce* the contribution deduction by the *entire* amount of any long-term capital gain or § 1231 gain that would be recognized if the property were sold at its fair market value.[107] In effect, this exception treats the contribution of capital gain property to private nonoperating foundations exactly like contributions of ordinary income property, since the donor must reduce the contribution deduction to the basis of the property.

Example 57. G donates land worth $10,000 to a private nonoperating foundation on November 17, 2009. G had purchased the land for $4,000 on August 23, 2005. G's charitable contribution deduction must be reduced to $4,000 ($10,000 fair market value − entire $6,000 appreciation).

It is important to note that this limitation *generally* does not apply to donations of capital gain property to public charities.

Example 58. Assume the same facts as in *Example 57*, except that G donated the land to her alma mater, State University (a public charity). G's charitable contribution would be $10,000 because the reduction requirement applies only to contributions to private foundations.

The *second* exception to the general rule that taxpayers are allowed to claim a deduction for the fair market value of contributed capital gain property involves

---

[106] § 170(e)(1).

[107] § 170(e)(1)(B)(ii). An exception is provided for contributions of publicly traded stock to private foundations. Taxpayers making such contributions are allowed to deduct the full fair market value of such stock.

contributions of tangible personalty.[108] If tangible personalty is contributed to a public charity (i.e., a university, museum, church, etc.) and the property is put to an *unrelated use* by the donee organization, the charitable contribution must be reduced by the entire amount of the property's unrealized appreciation in value (i.e., to the property's basis). For purposes of this limitation, the term *unrelated use* means that the property could not be used by the public charity in its activities for which tax-exempt status had been granted. For example, if antique furnishings are donated to a local museum that either stores, displays, or uses the items in its office in the course of carrying out its functions, the use of such property is a related use.[109] Thus, if the taxpayer can reasonably anticipate that the tangible personalty donated to the charitable organization will be put to a related use, this limitation will not be applicable.[110]

> **Example 59.** J contributes a painting to the local university. He had purchased the painting in 1993 for $10,000, and it was appraised at $60,000 on the date of the gift. The painting was placed in the university's library for display and study by art students. J's charitable contribution will be measured at $60,000 (the painting's fair market value) since the property was not put to an unrelated use. This is true even if the university later sells the painting.

> **Example 60.** R donates her gun collection to the YWCA (a public charity). R had paid $8,000 for the collection 10 years ago, and the guns were appraised at $18,000 on the date of the gift. The YWCA immediately sold the collection for $18,000 to a local gun dealer. Although the property had appreciated by $10,000, R's charitable contribution must be reduced to $8,000 (the property's basis) since the property was not (and most likely could not be) put to a related use.

Fifty Percent Limitation. An individual's deduction for contributions made to public charities may not exceed 50 percent of his or her adjusted gross income for the year.[111] This "ceiling" deduction limitation applies to contributions made to the following types of public charities:[112]

1. A church or a convention or association of churches;

2. An educational organization that normally maintains a regular faculty and curriculum;

3. An organization whose principal purposes or functions are providing medical or hospital care (hospitals) or medical education or medical research (medical schools);

4. An organization that receives support from the government and is organized and operated exclusively to receive, hold, invest, and administer property for the benefit of a college or university;

5. A state, a possession of the United States, or any political subdivision of any of the foregoing, or the United States or the District of Columbia;

---

[108] As described in Chapter 9, tangible personalty is all tangible property *other than* realty (i.e., land, buildings, structural components).

[109] Reg. § 1.170A-4(b)(3). Under § 170(e)(7), if tangible personal property worth more than $5,000 is contributed and later sold by the charity, the donor may be required to include certain amounts in income.

[110] Reg. § 1.170A-4(b)(3)(ii).

[111] § 170(b) and Reg. § 1.170A-8(b).

[112] § 170(b)(1).

6. An organization that normally receives a substantial part of its support from a government unit (described in item 5 above) or from the general public; and

7. Certain types of private foundations discussed below.

Private foundations are organizations that, by definition, do not receive contributions from the general public. Examples of well-known private foundations include the Ford, Carnegie, Cullen, and Mellon Foundations. For charitable deduction purposes, private foundations are classified as either operating or nonoperating foundations. Contributions to *all* private operating foundations are subject to the 50 percent ceiling limitation.[113] The 50 percent limit also applies to contributions to certain private, nonoperating foundations if the organizations:

1. Distribute the contributions they receive to public charities and private operating foundations *within* 2ø months following the year the contributions were received; or

2. Pool all contributions received into a common fund, and distribute *both* the income and the principal from the fund to public charities.

An individual's contributions of cash and ordinary income property to public charities, private operating foundations, and the above described nonoperating foundations that exceed the 50 percent limitation are carried forward and deducted in subsequent years. The carryover rules are discussed in a later section of this chapter. Contributions of capital gain property *and* contributions to private nonoperating foundations (other than those described above) are subject to *either* the 30 percent or 20 percent limitation. These limitations are discussed below.

Thirty Percent Limitation. There are *two* situations in which the 30 percent limitation may apply. The first situation involves the following types of contributions:

1. Contributions for the *use* of any charitable organization;

2. Contributions to veterans' organizations, fraternal societies, and not-for-profit cemetery companies; *and*

3. Contributions to most private nonoperating foundations.

The annual deduction for these contributions is limited to the *lesser of*:

1. Thirty percent of adjusted gross income, *or*

2. An amount equal to 50 percent of adjusted gross income, *reduced* by contributions qualifying for the 50 percent limitation.[114]

Example 61. R has adjusted gross income of $50,000 for the current year and contributes $5,000 cash to his church and $20,000 cash to the Veterans of Foreign Wars. R's deduction for the contribution to his church will not be limited because it does not exceed 50% of A.G.I. (i.e., $5,000 < $25,000). However, only $15,000 of the contribution to the veterans' organization will be allowed as a deduction for the current year because this donation is subject to the 30% limitation.

---

[113] See § 4942(j) for the requirements for classification as a private operating foundation. For all practical purposes, an operating foundation is recognized as a public charity.

[114] See § 170(b)(1)(C).

Contribution to church............................	$ 5,000

Plus: Lesser of
  (1)   30% × $50,000 = $15,000
         or
  (2)   50% × $50,000 = $25,000, reduced
         by $5,000 gift to church = $20,000

	15,000
Total contribution deduction..........................	$20,000

Example 62. Assume the same facts in *Example 61*, except that the contribution to the church was $20,000 and the contribution to the veterans' organization was $8,000. Again, the contribution to the church will not be limited because it does not exceed 50% of A.G.I. However, the contribution to the veterans' organization will be limited to $5,000, computed as follows:

Contribution to church............................	$20,000

Plus: Lesser of
  (1)   30% × $50,000 = $15,000
         or
  (2)   50% × $50,000 = $25,000, reduced
         by $20,000 gift to church = $5,000

	5,000
Total contribution deduction..........................	$25,000

Note that it is not the 30% of A.G.I. Limitation that causes R's contribution to the veterans' organization to be limited. Instead, it is the fact that the overall limitation on the annual contribution deduction amount is 50% of adjusted gross income, and the contribution to the public charity is considered first.

The *second* situation in which the 30 percent limitation may apply involves contributions of capital gain property. The annual deduction allowed for contributions of capital gain property that have not been reduced by the unrealized appreciation will generally be limited to 30 percent of the taxpayer's adjusted gross income.[115] As in the first situation discussed above, these contributions subject to the 30 percent limit are considered only after the amount of contributions allowed under the 50 percent limitation has been determined. Contributions in excess of the 30 percent limit can be carried forward and deducted in subsequent years.

Example 63. K has adjusted gross income of $30,000 for the 2009 tax year. The only contribution made by K in 2009 consisted of stock worth $10,000, which she had purchased for $4,000 in 2005. The stock was given to her church. Although the contribution does not exceed 50% of her adjusted gross income, K's deduction is limited to $9,000 (30% × $30,000 A.G.I.) since the stock is capital gain property. The $1,000 excess contribution can be carried over to subsequent years.

---

[115]   § 170(b)(1)(C)(i).

Example 64. Assume the same facts as in *Example 63*, except that K's 2009 adjusted gross income is $40,000 and she also gave $14,000 cash to her church. In this case, her deduction for the gift of the stock is limited to $6,000 (50% × $40,000 A.G.I. = $20,000 − $14,000 cash contribution) since the 50% overall limitation is applied before the 30% limitation. The remaining $4,000 ($10,000 fair market value of stock − $6,000 deduction allowed) will be carried forward to subsequent years.

When capital gain property has been contributed, the 30 percent limitation can be avoided if the taxpayer *elects* to reduce his or her claimed deduction for the capital gain property by the property's unrealized appreciation.[116] This may result in a larger deduction in the current year since the reduced amount will be subject to a higher ceiling limitation (i.e., 50 percent of A.G.I. rather than 30 percent). It is important to note that this election, if made, applies to all contributions of capital gain property made during the year.

Example 65. T has adjusted gross income of $50,000 for the current year and contributes stock worth $23,000 to the American Heart Association (a public charity). T had purchased the stock for $19,000 two years earlier. Assuming this is T's only contribution for the current year, he can either claim his deduction subject to the 30% limitation and carry over any excess, or *elect* to reduce the claimed deduction by the capital gain property's unrealized appreciation and forgo any carryover. T's deduction choices are:

1. $15,000 current deduction (30% × $50,000 A.G.I.) and $8,000 ($23,000 − $15,000) contribution carryover; or

2. $19,000 current deduction ($23,000 − $4,000 unrealized appreciation) and no carryover.

Obviously, the decision to reduce a current deduction by the property's unrealized appreciation *or* to claim the deduction subject to the 30 percent limit and carry over any excess amount will depend on several factors. Among the factors to be considered are:

1. The difference between the capital gain property's fair market value and its adjusted basis to the taxpayer (i.e., unrealized appreciation);

2. The taxpayer's current marginal income tax bracket compared to his or her anticipated future marginal tax rates; and

3. The expected remaining life of the taxpayer and his or her anticipated future contributions.

Twenty Percent Limitation. The 50 percent ceiling limitation imposed on an individual's annual charitable contribution deduction is an "overall" limitation. The 30 percent limitation applies to most contributions of capital gain property and to contributions of cash and ordinary income property contributed to nonqualifying private nonoperating funds. However, a more severe restriction is imposed on deductions for contributions of capital gain property to such private nonoperating foundations. In addition to the required *reduction* of the contribution by any unrealized appreciation in

---

[116] § 170(b)(1)(c)(iii).

value, the deduction allowed for contributions to *private charities* (i.e., organizations not included in the seven categories listed earlier) is limited to the *lesser of*:

1. Twenty percent of adjusted gross income; or

2. An amount equal to 50 percent of adjusted gross income, and reduced by contributions qualifying for the 50 percent and 30 percent limitations, including any amount in excess of the 30 percent limitation.[117]

Like excess contributions to public charities, any contributions to private nonoperating foundations that exceed the 20 percent limitation are carried forward and deductible subject to the 20 percent limit, in subsequent years.[118]

> **Example 66.** D contributed $8,000 to his church (a public charity) and land worth $15,000 to a private nonoperating foundation in 2009. D had purchased the land for $11,000 in 2004. His adjusted gross income for the year is $20,000. D's contribution deduction for 2009 is $10,000 [$8,000 contribution to church + $2,000 of the eligible $11,000 contribution to private foundation ($15,000 market value − $4,000 unrealized "appreciation" = $11,000)]. The deduction allowed for the contribution to the private foundation is limited to the *lesser of*:
>
> 1. $4,000 (20% × $20,000 A.G.I.); or
>
> 2. $2,000 [(50% × $20,000 A.G.I. = $10,000) − $8,000 contribution qualifying for the 50% limitation].
>
> Note that D's total contribution deduction of $10,000 does not exceed 50 percent of his current adjusted gross income. If D had contributed $10,000 or more to his church, *none* of the $11,000 contribution to the private foundation would have been allowed. In either case, the excess contributions can be carried over to subsequent years.

CONTRIBUTION CARRYOVERS

An individual's contributions that exceed either the 20 percent limitation, the 30 percent limitation, or the 50 percent overall limitation may be carried over for five years.[119] All excess contributions due to the 20 and 30 percent limitations will *again* be subject to these limitations in the carryover years.[120] Although contribution carryovers are treated as having been made in the year to which they are carried, contributions *actually* made in the carryover year must be claimed before any carryover amounts are deducted.[121]

> **Example 67.** In 2009, D contributes $10,000 cash to State University (a public charity). Her adjusted gross income for 2009 is $15,000. D's contribution deduction for 2009 is limited to $7,500 (50% × $15,000 A.G.I.) and she may carry over the remaining $2,500 to 2010. If she does not make contributions in 2010 that exceed the 50% limitation, D can claim the $2,500 carryover as a deduction. If the contributions actually made in 2010 exceed 50% of D's 2010 adjusted gross income, she must carry over the 2010 excess contributions *and* the $2,500 carryover from 2009.

---

[117] § 170(b)(1)(B)(i).

[118] § 170(d)(1).

[119] § 170(d)(1)(A) and Reg. § 1.170A-10(a).

[120] Reg. § 1.170A-10(b)(2).

[121] Reg. § 1.170A-10(c)(1).

Example 68. Assume the same facts as in *Example 67*, except that D's contribution was a capital gain property worth $10,000 instead of cash. Her 2009 deduction would be limited to $4,500 (30% × $15,000 A.G.I.) and she would have a $5,500 contribution carryover. Since this carryover resulted from the 30% limitation, it will be subject to the 30% limit in any carryover year. Thus if D has adjusted gross income of $10,000 and does not make contributions in 2010, she can claim a deduction of $3,000 (30% × $10,000 A.G.I.) and carry over the remaining $2,500.

All charitable contribution carryovers are applied on a first-in, first-out basis in determining the amount of any carryovers deductible in the current year.[122] Since such carryovers will expire if not deducted within five succeeding tax years, taxpayers obviously should limit actual contributions until the carryovers are used.

MISCELLANEOUS ITEMIZED DEDUCTIONS

As discussed in Chapter 7, two major changes regarding miscellaneous itemized deductions were introduced into the tax laws in 1986. Perhaps the most significant change involves the inclusion in this category of all *unreimbursed* employee business expenses. Prior to 1987, an employee's unreimbursed travel and transportation expenses were allowed as deductions in arriving at adjusted gross income. Since 1986, *both* unreimbursed employee expenses *and* those not reimbursed under an accountable plan must be treated as miscellaneous itemized deductions.[123] Additionally, an employee's unreimbursed costs for business entertainment and meals (whether or not incurred in connection with travel) must first be reduced by a 50 percent disallowance since only 50 percent of these costs qualify for deduction.[124] It is also important to remember that interest on any indebtedness to finance an employee's business expenses is treated as *nondeductible* personal interest expense.

The second major change involves the introduction of a deduction *floor* on the total of all expenses in this category similar to the approach taken for medical and casualty loss deductions. After 1986, miscellaneous itemized deductions are deductible only to the extent they *exceed* 2 percent of A.G.I.[125] The obvious intent of this change in the law is to limit the number of taxpayers who will be able to deduct miscellaneous itemized deductions—and thereby reduce the administrative cost of policing such deductions. Exhibit 11-5 contains a partial list of items qualifying as miscellaneous itemized deductions.

---

[122]   Reg. § 1.170A-10(b)(2).

[123]   Reg. § 1.62-2.

[124]   § 274(n).

[125]   § 67(a).

EXHIBIT 11-5
Partial List of Miscellaneous Itemized Deductions

Reimbursed employee expenses under
    A nonaccountable plan

Unreimbursed employee expenses for
    Travel away from home (lodging and 50% of meals)
    Transportation expenses
    Entertainment expenses (after 50% reduction)
    Home office expenses
    Outside salesperson's expenses
    Professional dues and memberships
    Subscriptions to business journals
    Uniform costs, cleaning, and maintenance expenses
    Union dues

Investment expenses for
    Investment advice
    Investment newsletter subscriptions
    Management fees charged by mutual funds
    Rentals of safe deposit boxes

Qualifying education expenses

Job seeking expenses (in the same business)

Tax determination expenses for
    Appraisal costs incurred to measure deductions for medical expenses
        (capital improvements), charitable contributions, and casualty losses
    Tax return preparation fees
    Tax advice, tax seminars, and books about taxes

Example 69. T has $40,000 of adjusted gross income in 2009. His unreimbursed employee business expenses and other miscellaneous itemized deductions include:

Unreimbursed business travel expenses	$ 90
Subscription to *The Wall Street Journal*	110
Professional dues	250
Safe deposit box rental	50
Tax return preparation fee	250
Total	$750

Since T's total miscellaneous itemized deductions of $750 do not exceed $800 (2% × $40,000 A.G.I.), he will not be able to claim any deduction for these expenses.

OTHER ITEMIZED DEDUCTIONS

The final category of itemized deductions includes certain personal expenses and losses that cannot be classified in any of the other categories discussed thus far. Some of the items in this category—referred to as "Other Miscellaneous Itemized Deductions"—are discussed in other chapters.

1. Unrecovered investment in an annuity where the taxpayer's death prevents recovery of the entire investment. As discussed in Chapter 6, this deduction is allowed on the taxpayer's final tax return.

2. Impairment-related work expenses of persons with disabilities.

3. Amortizable premium on bonds purchased before October 23, 1986. Amortization of bond premium is discussed in Chapter 16.

4. Gambling losses to the extent of gambling winnings.

It is important to note that each of these items may be subject to its own unique set of limitations (e.g., gambling losses). Unlike miscellaneous itemized deductions, however, these deductions *are not* subject to the two percent limit.

DEDUCTION CUTBACK RULE

As mentioned in Chapter 3, the total itemized deductions of certain high-income taxpayers are subject to another limitation. Basically, in 2008 and 2009, taxpayers must reduce total itemized deductions otherwise allowable (*other than* medical expenses, casualty and theft losses, investment interest, and gambling losses) by one percent of their A.G.I. in excess of $166,800 ($83,400 for married individuals filing separately).[126] However, this reduction cannot exceed 26.67 percent of the deductions. Again, this ensures that taxpayers subject to the cutback rule can deduct at least 73.33 percent of their so-called "one-percent" deductions. Consequently, a taxpayer's itemized deductions are never completely phased out.

Exhibit 11-6 identifies the itemized deductions that are subject to the cutback rule. Again, it is important to note that a taxpayer's medical expenses, investment interest expense, casualty and theft losses, and gambling losses are not subject to this limitation.

EXHIBIT 11-6
Itemized Deductions Subject to Cutback Rule

Taxes paid, including
>   State, local, and foreign income taxes
>   State and local general sales taxes
>   State, local, and foreign real property taxes
>   State and local personal property taxes

Mortgage interest on personal residences
Charitable contributions
Miscellaneous itemized deductions (in excess of 2% of A.G.I.)

Example 70. Z is single and has adjusted gross income of $316,800 for the current year. Z has the following itemized deductions: medical expenses ($5,100 after the 7.5% limitation), real estate taxes paid ($3,000), state income taxes ($7,400), home mortgage interest ($10,300), charitable contributions ($2,500), and miscellaneous itemized deductions ($800 after the 2% limitation). The amount of itemized deductions that Z may deduct for the current year is computed as follows:

---

[126] § 68. These threshold amounts were $159,950 and $79,975 respectively, for 2008, and they are adjusted annually for inflation. Prior to 2006, these deductions were subject to a three-percent cutback. However, § 68 (f) provides that for 2006 and 2007 the cutback is only 2/3 of the 3%, resulting in a 2% cutback or a maximum 53.34%. The cutback is reduced in 2008 and 2009 to 1/3 of the 3%, resulting in a 1% cutback or a maximum of 26.67%. The cutback is scheduled to expire after 2009.

Itemized deductions subject to cutback:

Taxes paid ($3,000 + $7,400)	$ 10,400	
Home mortgage interest	10,300	
Charitable contributions	2,500	
Miscellaneous itemized deductions	800	
Deductions subject to 1% cutback rule		$24,000

Tentative cutback:

Adjusted gross income	$316,800	
Threshold amount	(166,800)	
Excess A.G.I.	$150,000	
Times: 1%	×1%	
Tentative cutback	$ 1,500	

Cutback limit:

Itemized deductions subject to cutback.	$ 24,000	
Times: 26.67%	×26.67%	
Maximum cutback	$ 6,400	

Cutback: *Lesser* of tentative cutback or maximum cutback .	(1,500)

Amount deductible after 1% cutback.	$22,500
Plus: Itemized deductions not subject to cutback	
(medical expenses)	5,100
Total deduction for itemized deductions	$27,600

Example 71. Assume the same facts as in *Example 70* above, except that Z's adjusted gross income for the current year is $2,966,800.

Total itemized deductions subject to cutback.	$24,000

Tentative cutback:

Adjusted gross income	$2,966,800	
Threshold amount	(166,800)	
Excess A.G.I.	$2,800,000	
Times: 1%.	×1%	
Tentative cutback	$ 28,000	

Cutback limit:

Itemized deductions subject to cutback.	$ 24,000	
Times: 26.67%.	×26.67%	
Maximum cutback	$ 6,400	
Cutback: *Lesser* of tentative cutback or maximum		
cutback		(6,400)

Amount deductible after maximum cutback	$17,600
Plus: Itemized deductions not subject	
to cutback (medical expenses)	5,100
Total deduction for itemized deductions	$22,700

Note that in this case Z's tentative cutback ($28,000) exceeds the maximum cutback ($6,400). Thus, Z is allowed to deduct at least 73.33% ($24,000 × 73.33% = $17,600) of the itemized deductions subject to the cutback rule.

It should be obvious from the above examples that relatively few taxpayers will suffer drastic cutbacks in their itemized deductions. However, those taxpayers with adjusted gross incomes above the annual threshold amount will find that they face another complexity in computing their itemized deductions.

TAX PLANNING CONSIDERATIONS

MAXIMIZING PERSONAL DEDUCTIONS

Each year the taxpayer must choose between taking the standard deduction and itemizing actual deductions. If the standard deduction is chosen, then legitimate itemized deductions are lost. If the taxpayer chooses to itemize actual deductions, then the standard deduction is lost. One technique used to minimize the loss of personal deductions is to shift actual itemized deductions from one year to another (to the extent allowed by law) so that they are high in one year and low in the next.

Example 72. S is single and has itemized deductions that are expected to be constant in 2009 and 2010 as follows:

Mortgage interest	$ 400
Dental expense (deductible portion)	1,400
State and local taxes	350
Charitable contributions	1,350
Total	$3,500

S cannot itemize actual deductions in 2009 or 2010 because actual deductions are less than the standard deduction for single status (assumed to be $4,000 in each year for illustration purposes). Over the two-year period, S will deduct $8,000 for personal expenses by claiming the standard deduction. However, if S were able to shift $1,000 of elective dental expenses from 2010 into 2009, and to accelerate the 2010 charitable contribution into 2009, then she would receive a greater tax benefit in the two-year period for personal expenses. Actual expenses in each year would be:

	2009	*2010*
Mortgage interest	$ 400	$ 400
Dental expense (deductible portion)	2,400	400
State taxes	350	350
Charitable contributions	2,700	0
Total	$5,850	$1,150

Although actual personal expenses still total $7,000 over the two-year period, S now has itemized deductions of $5,850 in 2009 and a standard deduction of $4,000 in 2010. During the two-year period S will deduct $9,850 for personal expenses and will receive $1,850 more in deductions than if personal expenses had not been shifted.

Personal expenses should be shifted into years when adjusted gross income is lower. Not only will the 7.5 percent medical expense threshold and the two percent miscellaneous expense threshold be lower, but the effect of the one percent cutback on itemized deductions may be less. If adjusted gross income is under the prevailing threshold amount in the year that the itemized deductions are bunched, the one percent cutback rule will be avoided altogether.

MEDICAL EXPENSES

The dependency exemption under a multiple support agreement should be assigned to the taxpayer who pays the medical expenses of the dependent. The medical expenses are deductible only by the family member entitled to the dependency exemption and only if that family member actually pays on behalf of the claimed dependent. Medical expenses paid by other family members on behalf of the dependent will not be allowed as deductions.

Often expenditures incurred in the care of an ill or handicapped child may qualify for either a medical expense deduction or for the child care credit (discussed in Chapter 13). When this happens, the tax liability should be computed under each alternative to determine which is more advantageous. Usually the choice depends on the taxpayer's marginal tax rate as compared to the credit percentage rate. The choice will also depend on the 7.5 percent threshold and whether the taxpayer is itemizing or taking the standard deduction.

> **Example 73.** In 2009, T and W spend $2,000 for care of their handicapped child. The $2,000 qualifies both as a medical expense and for the child care credit. T and W have other medical expenses that exceed the 7.5% threshold amount. T and W file a joint tax return, and their marginal tax rate is 31%. The applicable percentage for the child care credit is 20%. If T and W are able to itemize deductions, they will receive a $620 tax benefit ($2,000 × 31%) for claiming the expenditure as a medical expense, whereas they will receive only a $400 tax benefit ($2,000 × 20%) if they claim the expenditure for the child care credit. If T and W are not able to itemize deductions or if they cannot exceed the 7.5% medical expense threshold amount, then the expenditure should be claimed for the child care credit.

CHARITABLE CONTRIBUTIONS

When a taxpayer makes noncash donations of property having a fair market value lower than the adjusted tax basis, it may be more advantageous to sell the property and donate the proceeds. If the property is held for investment, the sale will yield a deductible capital loss in addition to the charitable deduction. No loss will result, however, if the property itself is donated. To recognize a loss when selling depreciated property, the property must be held for investment or business use rather than for personal use.

> **Example 74.** T owns 100 shares of X Corporation stock that he bought for $5,000 in 2007. The stock currently has a fair market value of $2,000. If T donates the stock to a qualified charity, he will only be entitled to a $2,000 charitable deduction. If T sells the stock and donates the $2,000 proceeds to a qualified charity, he will be entitled to a $3,000 capital loss as well as a $2,000 charitable deduction.

MISCELLANEOUS DEDUCTIONS

Because certain miscellaneous itemized deductions are deductible only to the extent that they aggregately exceed 2 percent of the adjusted gross income, it is important that expenses that can be properly classified into another, nonlimited category be identified

and separated. For example, if a taxpayer supplements his or her regular salary with self-employed consulting income, it may be proper to deduct some of the cost of professional publications, professional journals, and educational expenses on Schedule C rather than as a miscellaneous itemized deduction.

Some unreimbursed employee business expenses that are not presently deductible because of the 2 percent limit might be converted into deductible reimbursed employee business expenses by agreement with the employer.

> **Example 75.** K incurs $500 of unreimbursed employee business expenses each year for subscriptions to professional journals. Her miscellaneous itemized deductions do not exceed the 2 percent limit; she is therefore unable to deduct any of this expense. K's employer agrees, as part of next year's compensation increase, to reimburse her for this $500 of employee business expenses. In effect, K is using pre-tax dollars for the professional subscriptions and the result is equivalent to $500 of increased wages offset by a fully deductible $500 of employee business expenses.

PROBLEM MATERIALS

DISCUSSION QUESTIONS

11-1 *Medical Expenses and Dependency Status.* Under what circumstances is a taxpayer entitled to deduct medical expenses attributable to other people?

11-2 *Medical Expenses.* F and M are the divorced parents of three minor children. M, the custodial parent, has proposed to F that the current child-support payments be increased in order to pay the expected dental costs of having braces put on their oldest son's teeth. F's tax advisor has suggested that F agree to pay these costs directly to the dentist rather than increasing the support payments. From a tax perspective, why has F's advisor made this suggestion?

11-3 *Medical Expenses.* K and her two brothers currently provide more than half the support of their mother. For the past several years, they have taken turns claiming a dependency exemption deduction for their mother under a multiple support agreement. This year, K will be entitled to the exemption, and her mother needs money for cataract surgery and new eyeglasses. K's accountant has suggested that she can double up on the tax benefits by directing her share of her mother's support toward these expenses. How is this possible?

11-4 *Medical Expenses.* For the past several years, L's total itemized deductions have barely exceeded his standard deduction amount, and this pattern is not expected to change in the near future. L is currently faced with elective surgery to repair a hernia, and the procedure is not covered under his health insurance policy. Strictly from a tax perspective, and assuming that this ailment is not life-threatening, what advice would you give to L concerning the timing of the surgery?

11-5 *Prepaid Medical Expenses.* What is the requirement imposed on taxpayers who wish to deduct prepaid medical expenses? What potential abuse is prevented by this requirement?

11-6 *Medical Deductions—Percentage Limitation.* The only medical expenditures made by taxpayer T during 2009 were for prescription drugs costing $1,800 and new eyeglasses costing $250. If T has adjusted gross income of $20,000 for the year and itemizes his deductions, how much, if any, medical expense deduction will he be allowed?

11-7 *Medical Travel Expenses.* W resides in Gary, Indiana and suffers from chronic bronchitis. At the advice of her doctor, W spends three months each year in Flagstaff, Arizona. Under what circumstances would W be entitled to claim the costs incurred for these trips as deductible medical expenses? If deductible, which costs?

11-8 *Casualty Losses.* Taxpayer F has adjusted gross income of $20,000 during the current year and he asks you the following questions regarding the deductibility of damages to his home caused by a recent hurricane. (**Hint:** See Chapter 10 for discussion of limitations on casualty loss deductions.)
   a. If F does not have home insurance, how much must his loss be before any deduction is available?
   b. If F repairs the damage himself, what amount can he deduct for the value of his time?
   c. If the area in which he resides is declared a disaster area, what options are available to F as to when and how to claim a deduction for the casualty loss?

11-9 *Taxes versus Fees.* What is the distinction between a deductible tax and a fee? If an individual taxpayer paid appraisal fees in connection with the determination of his personal casualty loss and charitable contribution deductions, would these payments be deductible?

11-10 *Deductible Income Taxes.* Which income taxes are deductible by an individual taxpayer? Does it make any difference whether the taxes are paid directly by the taxpayer as opposed to being withheld from his or her salary and paid by an employer to the appropriate taxing authority?

11-11 *Filing Status and State Income Taxes.* If married taxpayers file separate state or Federal income tax returns, how is the Federal tax deduction for state income taxes determined?

11-12 *State and Local Sales Tax Deduction.* Your brother has called you for advice concerning the deductibility of the $1,460 state sales taxes that he paid on the purchase of his new Ford F250 truck. What other information would you need from you brother to properly answer his question?

11-13 *Personal Property Taxes.* What is an ad valorem tax? What difference does it make to a taxpayer if he or she pays a tax on nonbusiness property and the tax is based on weight or model year as opposed to value?

11-14 *Real Estate Tax Apportionment.* How are real estate taxes apportioned between the buyer and seller in the year real property is sold? What effect does the apportionment have on the seller if the buyer pays the real estate taxes for the entire year?

11-15 *Special Tax Assessments.* Under what circumstances can a property owner claim a deduction for a special tax assessment?

11-16 *Personal Interest.* What is the current limitation imposed on the deductions of personal interest? What impact do you suppose this restriction might have on debt-financed consumer purchases?

11-17 *Deductible Interest.* Your neighbor has come up with an excellent tax plan and he asks you for advice on structuring his scheme. He plans to give each of his five children a $10,000 promissory note, due in 20 years and bearing interest at 10 percent per year. The interest will be paid annually and he plans to claim a $5,000 interest expense deduction. Do you see any flaws in this plan? What advice would you give to your neighbor?

11-18 *Classifying Interest Expenses.* The local bank has just introduced a new loan program entitled "Home Equity Credit Line" under which individuals can either borrow funds or finance credit card purchases based on the equity they have in their homes. What is the tax incentive offered by this arrangement?

11-19 *Investment Interest Expense.* What is the investment interest expense limitation? Which taxpayers are not subject to this limitation? What is the purpose of the limitation?

11-20 *Types of Interest Expense.* D is a spender, not a saver. In fact, he spends money he doesn't even have. This year he borrowed more than $50,000 and paid interest of close to $7,000. D was shocked when his accountant told him that only certain types of interest were deductible.
   a. Identify the different types of interest expense and explain the treatment of each.
   b. How will D classify the interest expense that he paid?

11-21 *Charitable Contribution Requirements.* What are the basic requirements imposed on an individual taxpayer's deduction for charitable contributions?

11-22 *Contributions of Ordinary Income Property.* What is ordinary income property? Does this contribution deduction limitation apply to all taxpayers? Explain.

11-23 *Contributions of Capital Gain Property.* Under what circumstances must a taxpayer reduce his or her contribution deduction by the unrealized appreciation in value of capital gain property donated to a qualifying charity? How might this limitation be avoided?

11-24 *Contribution Deduction Percentage Limitations.* What are the percentage limitations imposed on an individual taxpayer's annual charitable contribution deduction? In what order must these percentage limitations be applied to current contributions?

11-25 *Contribution Carryovers.* Which excess contributions may be carried forward by an individual taxpayer? For how many years? In determining the amount of his or her contribution deduction for the current year, how must the taxpayer treat the carryovers from prior years?

11-26 *Miscellaneous Itemized Deductions.* E's employer has offered her the option of a $50 monthly pay raise or a reimbursement plan to cover her current subscriptions to professional journals ($200) and her dues to professional organizations ($350). E files a joint return with her husband, and they expect their adjusted gross income to be $50,000 for the upcoming year. Assuming that their only miscellaneous itemized deductions are from E's subscriptions and professional dues, is this a good offer? Explain.

11-27 *Deduction Cutback Rule.* Explain the difference between the tentative cutback and the maximum cutback amounts related to the total deduction allowed for itemized deductions. Which itemized deductions are not subject to the cutback rule?

PROBLEMS

11-28 *Medical Expense Deduction.* R, an unmarried taxpayer, has adjusted gross income of $20,000 for 2009. During the year, he paid the following amounts for medical care: $300 for prescription medicines and drugs, $600 for hospitalization insurance, and $1,100 to doctors and dentists. R filed an insurance reimbursement claim in December 2009 and received a check for $1,200 on January 24, 2010.
   a. Assuming R itemizes deductions, determine the deduction allowed for the medical expenses paid in 2009.

b. What effect does the insurance reimbursement have on R's deduction for 2009? How should the reimbursement be treated in 2010 if R's itemized deductions for 2009 (including the medical expense deduction) were $4,500 greater than his standard deduction?

c. How should the reimbursement be treated in 2010 if R's itemized deductions for 2009 were $400 greater than his standard deduction?

11-29 *State Income Taxes.* During 2009, K paid $500 in estimated state income taxes. An additional $400 in state income taxes was withheld from her salary by K's employer and remitted to the state. K also received a $200 refund check during 2009 for excess state income taxes paid in 2008. She had claimed a deduction for $750 of state income taxes paid in 2008. K uses the cash method of accounting and has adjusted gross income of $50,000 for the year.

a. If K itemizes her deductions, how much may she claim as a deduction for state income taxes on her 2009 Federal tax return?

b. If K's itemized deductions for 2008 were $1,900 greater than her standard deduction, how must the $200 refund be treated for Federal income tax purposes?

11-30 *General Sales Tax Deduction.* Rob and Lisa are married and file a joint return for 2008. They have three dependent children ages 7, 9, and 12 and the family lived in Orlando Florida for the entire year. For each of the questions below, assume that the couple has A.G.I. of $87,900 and no other available income.

a. Using the 2008 optional sales tax tables located in Appendix A of this text, determine the couple's state sales tax deduction for 2008.

b. How would your answer in (a) above change if Rob and Lisa also paid $1,250 sales tax on the purchase of a new car and an additional $350 on the purchase of new furniture?

c. Assume that the family lived in Georgia rather than Florida for the entire year. Also assume that Rob and Lisa paid $3,200 in state income taxes in 2008. How does this additional information change your answer to (b) above?

11-31 *Real Estate Tax Apportionment.* S sells her home located in Blue Springs, Missouri, on March 1, 2009. Blue Springs assesses real property taxes at the beginning of each calendar year for the entire year, and the property tax becomes a personal liability of the owner of real property on January 1. The tax is payable on April 1, 2009. Buyer B paid $80,000 for the home on March 1, 2009 and also paid the $1,200 real estate taxes on April 1. Both S and B are cash basis, calendar year taxpayers.

a. How much of the $1,200 in real estate taxes is deductible by S? What adjustment must S make to the amount she realized from the sale?

b. How much of the $1,200 in taxes is deductible by B? How will he treat any of the taxes paid which are attributable to S?

11-32 *Interest Expense Limitations.* Indicate in each of the following cases the amount of interest expense, if any, that the taxpayer is allowed to deduct.

a. During the year, H used his bank credit card to purchase a new stereo for his teen-age daughter. Finance charges for the year were $70.

b. Over the years, G has consistently borrowed against her insurance policies because of their low rates. This year, she paid interest of $1,100 on the loans.

c. D lives and works in Birmingham. He owns a house there as well as a summer home at Hilton Head and a condominium at Sun Valley. He paid interest expense of $6,000 on loans on each unit.

d. B owns a home in Denver that she purchased in 1998 for $95,000. The current balance on B's mortgage loan is $60,000 and the property is worth $150,000. During the year, B obtained a second mortgage on her home, receiving $20,000 which she used to pay off her two outstanding car loans. Interest on the first mortgage was $4,000 while interest on the second mortgage was $1,000.

    e. M is a heavy trader of stocks and bonds, using his margin account frequently. This year, interest expense charged on his margin purchases was $5,200. M's investment income was $2,400.

    f. R is an employee of a television repair shop. He uses his own truck solely for business, making customer service calls. During the year, he paid $1,450 interest on a loan on his truck.

11-33   *Investment Interest Expense.* R, a cash basis, single taxpayer, paid $17,000 of investment interest expense during 2009. R uses the calendar year for tax purposes and reports the following investment income: $1,500 interest income, and $3,500 dividends.

    a. How much of the investment interest expense is deductible by R in 2009?

    b. What must R do with any investment interest expense deduction which is disallowed for 2009?

11-34   *Investment Interest Expense Limitation.* L is an engineer. This year, she borrowed $300,000 and purchased 40 acres south of Houston. For the year, L paid interest of $30,000 on the loan. Her tax records revealed the following additional information:

Income:

Salary	$50,000
Qualifying dividends	8,000
Share of partnership income:	
Ordinary loss	(3,000)
Portfolio income:	
Interest	1,000
Rental income	8,000
Expenses:	
Rental expenses	7,000
Qualified residence interest	10,000
Property tax on land	5,000
Investment publications	400
Professional dues, licenses, and subscriptions	1,100

    The items noted concerning the partnership result from L's limited partnership interest in Country Homes, a real estate development. The rental income is derived from a four-unit apartment complex that is currently filled with tenants with one-year leases. The related rental expenses include $2,000 of interest expense on the debt to acquire the apartments. Compute L's deduction for investment interest expense this year, assuming that she includes the qualifying dividends in the calculation of net investment income.

11-35   *Interest Expense—Note Discount.* Taxpayer T signed a note for $2,000 on August 30, 2009, agreeing to pay back the loan in 12 equal installments beginning September 30, 2009. The 12 percent interest charge ($2,000 × 12% = $240) was subtracted from the face amount of the note and T received $1,760, all of which was used to purchase furniture for his business. T uses the calendar year as his taxable year.

    a. If T is a cash-basis taxpayer and he makes the four payments scheduled for 2009, what is his deduction for interest on the note in 2009? In 2010?

    b. Would your answers to (a) change if T were an accrual method taxpayer? Explain.

11-36   *Charitable Contributions.* Determine the amount of the charitable deduction (without regard to percentage limitations) allowed in each of the following situations:

    a. Rent-free use of building for three months allowed for the United Way fund drive. The building normally rents for $900 per month, and the owner paid $1,100 for utilities during this period.

    b. Gift of General Motors stock valued at $9,000 to State University. Taxpayer purchased the stock five months ago for $11,000.

c. Donation of stamp collection valued at $4,000 to local museum for display to the general public. Taxpayer had paid $1,000 for the stamps many years ago.

d. Gift of paintings to local hospital to be placed on the walls of a remodeled floor. The paintings were painted by the donor and were appraised at $20,000.

e. Donation of Civil War relics to American Heart Association to be sold at its current fund-raising auction. Taxpayer paid $1,000 for the relics ten years ago and an expert appraiser valued them at $7,000 on the day of the gift.

11-37 *Contribution Deductions—Percentage Limitations.* J contributed $10,000 to the University of Southern California and a long-term capital asset worth $10,000 (basis of $5,000) to a private nonoperating foundation during 2009. Assuming his adjusted gross income for the year is $24,000, answer the following:

a. What is the amount of J's contribution deduction for 2009?

b. How must any excess contributions be treated?

c. If J had come to you for advice before making the gifts, what advice would you have offered?

11-38 *Contribution Deductions—Percentage Limitations.* During 2009 R donated land to her church (a public charity) to be used as a building site for a new chapel. R had purchased the land as an investment in 2001 at a cost of $10,000. The land was appraised at a fair market value of $30,000 on the date of the gift. Assuming R's adjusted gross income for 2009 is $60,000, answer the following:

a. If R made no additional charitable contributions during 2009, what is the amount of her contribution deduction for the year?

b. If R contributed cash of $20,000 to her church in addition to the land, what is the amount of her charitable contribution deduction for 2009?

c. Calculate the amount of R's excess contributions from (a) and (b) and explain how these amounts are to be treated.

11-39 *Contribution Deductions—Percentage Limitations.* T, a single taxpayer, had adjusted gross income of $20,000 for 2009. During the year, T contributed cash of $1,000 and Xerox Corporation stock worth $10,000 to his church (a public charity). T inherited the stock during 2006 when it was valued at $8,000.

a. Calculate T's total contribution deduction for 2009.

b. How must any excess contributions be treated?

c. If T does not anticipate being able to itemize his deductions in any future years, what might he do in 2009 to increase his current contribution deduction?

11-40 *Miscellaneous Itemized Deductions.* R, single, has the following miscellaneous itemized deductions for the current year:

Unreimbursed employee business expenses	$1,350
Professional dues and subscriptions.................	650
Job-seeking expenses	800
Tax return preparation fee	250
Safe-deposit box rental (for stocks and bonds)	50

Assume that R itemizes his deductions for the current year.

a. What is the amount of R's deduction for the above items if his adjusted gross income is $70,000 for the current year?

b. What is the amount of R's deduction for these items if his adjusted gross income is $100,000 for the current year?

TaxCut 11-41 *Deduction Cutback Rule.* H and W are married and file a joint return for the current year. They have the following itemized deductions (after any percentage limitations) for the year:

Medical and dental expenses	$8,000
Real estate taxes on home	3,500
Deductible interest on home mortgage	9,000
State income taxes paid	5,500
Charitable contributions	4,000
Miscellaneous itemized deductions	2,500

Determine H and W's itemized deductions, assuming the following levels of adjusted gross income for the current year:
a. $100,000
b. $566,800
c. $3,500,000

TaxCut 11-42 *Calculating Itemized Deductions.* Robert and Jean Snyder have an adjusted gross income of $30,000 for 2009. Their expenses for 2009 are:

Prescription drugs	$ 300*
Medical insurance premiums	900
Doctor and dental bills paid	1,400*
Eyeglasses for Robert	155
Hospital and clinic bills paid	450*
Property taxes paid on home	900
State income taxes paid:	
Remaining 2008 tax liability	125
Withheld from wages during year	1,850
State and local sales taxes paid:	
Amount paid on new automobile	800
Amount paid on new wide screen television	280
Personal property taxes paid	100
Interest on home mortgage**	4,750
Interest paid on personal auto loan	1,100
Interest paid on credit card purchases	400
Interest paid on E.F. Hutton margin account***	120
Cash contributions to church	2,000
Fair market value of Hightech Corp. stock contributed to church (purchased for $1,000 three years ago)	5,000
Labor union dues paid by Robert	200
Qualifying education costs paid by Jean	300
Safe deposit box rental (for stocks and bonds)	50
Fee paid accountant for preparation of 2008 state and Federal tax returns	350

*These amounts are net of insurance reimbursements received during 2009.
**This mortgage was created at the time the home was purchased.
***This investment interest expense is related to the production of $1,500 of net investment income.

The Snyders drove their personal automobile 500 miles for medical and dental treatment and an additional 1,000 miles in connection with charitable services performed for their church. Assuming Robert and Jean are both under age 40, lived in Virginia for the entire year, and plan to file a joint income tax return, determine their total itemized deductions. If a tax form is used for the computations, complete Schedule A (Form 1040).

RESEARCH PROBLEM

11-43   Sam Simpson transferred stock, real estate, and his principal residence to his former wife, Shirley, under the terms of the property settlement agreement. In exchange, Shirley agreed to pay Sam $250,000 down and another $750,000 at 10 percent per year for 10 years. Can Shirley deduct any of the interest she expects to pay over the next 10 years? Explain.

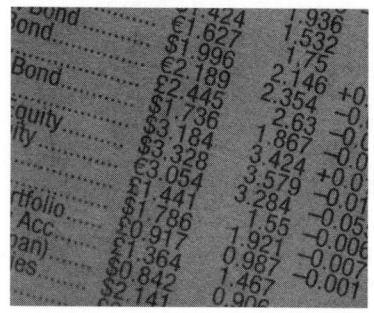

CHAPTER TWELVE

DEDUCTIONS FOR CERTAIN INVESTMENT EXPENSES AND LOSSES

LEARNING OBJECTIVES

Upon completion of this chapter you will be able to:

▸ Discuss the basic rules governing the deduction of investment expenses

▸ Explain the limitations imposed on the deduction of losses incurred in an activity in which a taxpayer does not materially participate (i.e., passive losses)

▸ Understand the special treatment for interest expense related to a passive activity

▸ Discuss the restrictions imposed on deductions related to vacation homes

CHAPTER OUTLINE

Since 1942 Congress has generally allowed taxpayers to deduct expenses and losses incurred in connection with investment activities. As explained in Chapter 7, Code § 212 currently authorizes the deduction of investment-oriented expenses. This provision specifically allows a deduction for expenses incurred for the production or collection of income or for the management, conservation, or maintenance of property held for the production of income. Deductible investment expenses typically include such items as fees paid to rent a safety deposit box to hold securities, cost of financial advice, and travel expenses incurred in managing property. Expenses incurred in operating rental property such as those for maintenance, depreciation, utilities, and insurance are also deductible under § 212. Similarly, deductions for interest expense incurred by taxpayers to finance their investments also are deductible under § 212, although certain restrictions apply (as discussed in Chapter 11). Most important, the law generally allows the deduction of losses flowing through to the taxpayer from investments in partnerships and S corporations. Specific investment expenses incurred by the taxpayer are normally classified as miscellaneous itemized deductions and are subject to the two percent limitation and the deduction cutback. However, expenses related to property held for the production of rents or royalties are deductible *for* A.G.I. In addition, losses flowing from a partnership or S corporation are generally deductible for A.G.I.

For many years, the general rules adequately governed the deduction of most investment expenses and losses. In time, these rules became insufficient to police growing abuse. As a result, Congress enacted special provisions to restrict investment-type deductions where it found the general rule to be lacking. This chapter examines four additional measures: the at-risk rules, the passive activity limitations, the restrictions on the deduction for interest expense related to passive activities, and the provisions related to the rental of vacation homes.

INTRODUCTION TO TAX SHELTERS

Historically, the tax law has generally allowed taxpayers to use deductions from one activity to offset the income of another. Similarly, most credits could be used to offset tax attributable to income from any of the taxpayer's activities.

> **Example 1.** R earns $50,000 annually working as vice president of marketing at Plentiful Products, Inc. Over the years, he has accumulated a modest portfolio of stocks which generates dividends of about $10,000 a year. In addition, he is a 10% limited partner in a partnership that owns an apartment complex consisting of 200 units. During the year, the apartment complex had operating expenses that exceeded rental income, creating a $100,000 loss. Prior to 1987, R could use his share of the loss, $10,000, to offset his other income, both salary and dividends. Assuming R's marginal tax rate was 30%, the loss produced tax savings of $3,000.

The above example illustrates the essentials of what is now a well-publicized phenomenon: under prior law, an individual could reduce his or her tax liability—even eliminate it—by investing in "tax shelters" that produced losses which could be offset against other income. The attraction of such losses for taxpayers wishing to avoid taxes was so great that the tax shelter business grew into a thriving industry.

A tax shelter is simply an investment which takes advantage of certain tax rules to enhance its rate of return. Like any investment, there is an outlay of cash (or credit) for something that hopefully will yield income year after year and produce gain on its disposition. The ultimate reward or potential loss is usually commensurate with the risk that the investor is willing to assume. It is the tax treatment of the various pieces of the investment that converts an ordinary investment to a potential tax shelter. For example, in the broadest sense, an investment in municipal bonds may be considered a type of tax

shelter because the return paid on the investment—the interest—is tax exempt. In the real world, however, the term *tax shelter* is usually not associated with tax-exempt bonds—tax-favored probably would be a more appropriate label. The words "tax shelter" typically conjures up images of complex investments that—as in *Example 1*—throw off losses to "shelter" the investor's other income.

STRUCTURE OF THE TAX SHELTER

In the heyday of the industry, a tax shelter was organized as a limited partnership. From a tax perspective, the partnership form is the perfect structure for the shelter because it is not a separate taxable entity. Instead, a partnership acts as a conduit, enabling the tax benefits produced by the activity to flow through to the investing partners. Operating losses from the partnership's business flow through to the partners who may be able to offset the losses against their other income. Long-term capital gains realized by the partnership flow through, retaining their favorable character to be reported by the partners on their own returns. Special credits generated by the partnership's activity (e.g., the rehabilitation and low-income housing credits) might pass through to the partners to be used to reduce the tax on other taxable income. Observe the vital role that the flow-through characteristic of a partnership plays in a tax shelter. Such results could not be obtained with a C corporation. A C corporation, which is a separate taxable entity, pays taxes on its own income which may be taxed again when distributed to the shareholders as a dividend. More important, at least in a tax shelter sense, the losses of a C corporation can only be used by the corporation to offset its own income and, therefore, produce no benefits to the investing shareholders. For these reasons, tax shelters are not organized as C corporations. Indeed, it is not surprising that as tax shelters became more popular, the IRS tried to halt their growth by arguing that tax shelters posing as limited partnerships were not really partnerships but—because of their limited liability and their close resemblance to a corporation—were corporations. However, the government had little success with this theory and had to devise other techniques to eliminate the perceived abuse.

Promoters of tax shelters historically used limited partnerships—rather than general partnerships—as the vehicle of choice. The promoter, the one who put the deal together and got a fee for his efforts, normally acted as the general partner. To lure an investor, the promoter had to limit an individual's exposure to risk. By structuring the investment as a "limited" partnership, individuals could invest and limit the possibility of financial loss to the amount of their investment. Any liability in excess of that borne by the limited partners was the responsibility of the general partner. This ceiling on an individual's exposure was an extremely attractive feature in the promotion of tax shelters, paving the way for otherwise wary investors to make a financial commitment to the activity.

ELEMENTS OF A TAX SHELTER

Most tax shelters are constructed to offer three basic benefits: tax deferral, conversion of ordinary income into capital gain, and leverage. Each of these characteristics on its own can produce significant benefits. But when the three are combined into a single package, the result is almost too good to be true.

Deferral. Deferral is one of the most important tools in tax planning. Postponing the time at which taxes must be paid is the equivalent of an interest-free loan from the government. To illustrate, consider a taxpayer who can defer the payment of $10,000 of taxes for a five-year period. Assuming an after tax rate of return of ten percent, the

present value of the tax payment is only $6,210 [$10,000 × (1/(1.10)^5]. In this case, postponing payment of tax saves $3,790, a decrease of almost 38 percent!

A typical tax shelter achieves deferral through a mismatching of revenues and expenses. Mismatching occurs because of the timing of income and deductions. Normally a tax shelter produces deductible expenses prior to the period in which the investment produces income in sufficient amounts to offset the deductions. In the appropriately structured tax shelter, taxpayers may be able to use these excess deductions, in effect losses from the shelter, to offset income from other sources thus producing immediate benefits. Most tax shelters were built around this same modus operandi: deduct expenses now while the gain accrues and is not taxed until later. This approach, "deduct now, pay later," is still the foundation of many current tax planning ideas.

> **Example 2.** R, S, and T formed a partnership for the purpose of breeding cattle. Each contributed $15,000 for a one-third interest. The partnership uses the cash to purchase a herd of cattle consisting primarily of cows, heifers and a few bulls. The partnership's only cash expenses during the year were the costs for breeding and maintaining the cattle totaling $45,000. No income was produced since none of the cattle were sold. Assuming the partnership uses the cash method of accounting and ignoring depreciation, the partnership has a loss of $45,000 which is allocated equally among R, S and T. As a result, R, S and T each have a $15,000 deduction for the losses attributable to their investment in the partnership, and this loss can be offset against income from other sources. Assuming each is in the 50% tax bracket (federal, state and local), each saves taxes of $7,500 ($15,000 × 50%).

Note in the above example that the tax savings occur because the cash method of accounting results in a mismatching of expenses and revenues. Had the partnership been required to use the accrual method or simply prohibited from deducting the expenses until the partnership *sold* the cattle, revenue and expenses would have been properly matched—at least in the financial accounting sense—and no tax savings would result (unless the cattle are later sold at a loss). It also should be emphasized that the taxes saved in this situation are not permanently avoided but only *deferred* until the future when the cattle are sold.

> **Example 3.** Refer to the situation in *Example 2* where expenses during the first year of operations were $45,000, producing a $45,000 deductible loss. Now assume that the cattle that were born and raised are sold for $45,000 on the first day of the next accounting period. If there were no other expenses, the partnership would have income of $45,000, each partner reporting $15,000. Since each partner is in the 50% tax bracket each pays taxes of $7,500. Note that the taxes paid in this period are the same as the taxes saved in the prior period. Thus, the taxpayer has not escaped $7,500 in taxes; nevertheless, the taxpayer has benefited since he deferred payment of the tax for one year. In addition, the taxpayer has benefited even though he had no gain or loss on the transaction as a whole ($45,000 income was equal to the $45,000 cost of breeding and raising). Of course, whether the taxpayers are happy with the result depends on the return that they could have otherwise received had the $45,000 been invested elsewhere.

The cattle example typifies the classic tax shelter but there were many more. Taxpayers could invest in partnerships created to explore for oil and gas, produce a movie or broadway show, buy art masters from which lithographs and prints could be made, or lease equipment (e.g., railroad boxcars, barges, cable TV systems, houseboats, executive jets and any other item someone might be willing to rent). Perhaps the shelter of all shelters is real estate. Here the partnership buys an office or apartment building

for which current depreciation deductions can be claimed even though the value of the building is holding or increasing. Despite their differences, all tax shelters had one common thread: claim deductions this year for expenses that add value that will not be taxed until next year.

While deferral is a huge advantage, the opportunities increase dramatically when the element of conversion can be added to the mix.

Conversion. The second element of the successful tax shelter involves conversion. Conversion is a two-step process. The first step concerns the treatment of deductions arising from the tax shelter activity. These expenses are deductible and reduce ordinary operating income that would otherwise be taxed at ordinary tax rates. The second step is where the conversion takes place. When the tax shelter activity is sold, any gain on the sale is taxed as long-term capital gain, which is taxed at the far more favorable capital gain rates.

Example 4. Recall *Example 3* where the cattle were purchased, bred and raised at a cost of $45,000. Assume now that the cattle are sold after they were held for more than two years—the holding period necessary for cattle if gain is to qualify for long-term capital gain treatment. Given this additional fact, the $45,000 gain would be treated as long-term capital gain and thus each partner would (using the tax rates in effect today) pay taxes at a capital gains rate of 20%, producing a tax of $3,000 (20% × $15,000) for each of the partners. Contrast the tax paid on the gain, $3,000, with the $7,500 of taxes saved from deducting the costs (50% × $15,000 share of the loss = $7,500). Most important, note that there was no real economic gain on the transaction: the cattle cost $45,000 to raise and then were sold for $45,000. However, because of the difference between the tax rates applying to ordinary income and capital gains, each partner is better off by $4,500 ($7,500 − $3,000). Note that in the previous example the $7,500 of taxes initially saved by each partner were entirely recouped by the government when the cattle were sold. In this situation, however, the government recoups only $3,000 of the original savings because the ordinary income was converted to capital gain. Thus, in this case, the taxpayer has not only benefited from deferral—deductions now, income later—but also earned $4,500 from the conversion of ordinary income into capital gain.

Leverage. The third element of most tax shelters is leverage. In physics, a strategically placed lever provides a mechanical benefit, enabling people to lift more than they would be able to with their own physical strength. The principle is the same in the world of finance. In investing, borrowing money enables an individual to obtain a larger return than otherwise could be obtained. For example, assume an individual purchases land for $100,000, $10,000 of her own money and $90,000 borrowed from a lender. If the investment is sold a year later for $120,000, there has been a 20 percent return on the total $100,000 investment. But for the individual investor, after paying back the lender $90,000 and $10,000 for the use of the money (i.e., interest), the $20,000 remaining means that she has doubled her money, a return of 100 percent! In tax terminology, the term *leverage* means that by borrowing money, a taxpayer can obtain a disproportionately large benefit from a small investment. The most common use, sometimes referred to as "tax leverage" concerns depreciation. For example, a tax shelter partnership might purchase a railroad boxcar for $25,000 down and finance the balance with a $75,000 note (i.e., the leverage). The law allows depreciation on the entire $100,000 not just the $25,000—creating much larger depreciation deductions than could have been obtained had depreciation been allowed only on the amount not borrowed.

Example 5. Assume the same facts as in the previous examples concerning the cattle breeding tax shelter except that the partnership acquired the original herd using an initial investment of $5,000 each—$15,000 total—and $30,000 of funds borrowed from the bank for which the partners are personally liable. Note the result when the taxpayer leverages a small investment with borrowed funds: each taxpayer receives a deductible loss providing a tax saving of $7,500 ($45,000 deduction × 1/3 = $15,000 × 50%) which is more than his $5,000 original investment!

Note in the example above that by using leverage the taxpayers are able to generate $45,000 of deductions for an investment of only $15,000. In the language of tax shelters, this means that the taxpayers got a 3:1 write-off, $3 of deduction for each $1 invested. If the taxpayer is in the 50 percent tax bracket, a $3 deduction produces a benefit of $1.50 in tax savings at a cost of $1—clearly a miracle. When tax shelters were at the peak of their popularity, some investments boasted far greater benefits, 5:1, 10:1 and higher.

While the principle of leverage can work miracles, it can also spell disaster. If a taxpayer invests in a tax shelter where the write-off is 10:1, this means that the deal is highly leveraged—a large amount is being borrowed. If the investment goes sour, the lender still must be repaid. In such cases, the cost of the deductions could result in a severe financial loss. However, tax shelter promoters usually solved this problem by using a magical tool: *nonrecourse financing*.

A nonrecourse note is a loan for which the borrower bears no liability for the debt. If the borrower defaults on the loan, the lender can foreclose on the property (i.e., the collateral). However, if the funds derived from foreclosure and sale of the property are not sufficient to satisfy the loan obligation, the lender is out of luck—there is no recourse against the borrower. In a partnership, if the financing for the tax shelter activity was provided using nonrecourse debt (e.g., an office building or other real estate), the investing partners were only liable for the debt to the extent of their investment. As might be imagined, promoters took advantage of this phenomenon. In the most outrageous deals, the promoter would overstate the value of the investment and then act as the banker, providing the financing, all nonrecourse. The investors' cash investment would cover any real costs of the promoter and the nonrecourse financing simply served to create deductions.

Example 6. P put together a limited partnership to create deductible losses for the investors. Ten doctors invested $10,000 each for a partnership interest. The partnership used the $100,000 to buy a building from P for $1,000,000. The partnership signed a nonrecourse note to P for $900,000, payable with interest only for 20 years and a balloon payment of $900,000 at the end of the term. Before consideration of depreciation, operation of the office building broke even. The partnership proceeded to depreciate the property (a noncash expenditure), producing net losses that could be passed through and deducted by the partners. At the end of 20 years, the partnership might default on the note. In this case, P would take back his property and each partner would have received essentially $100,000 of deductions at a cost of $10,000. If the partners were in the 50% tax bracket, the deductions would be worth $50,000 and the arrangement would have provided a terrific return on the partners' investments. On the other side of the deal, P would pocket the $100,000 for his trouble. Note that the value of the building could have been whatever the partnership wanted to set, $1 million, $1.5 million, $2 million, or whatever, since the debt was nonrecourse and no one was ever going to pay!

In order to prevent what it considered the harmful and excessive use of tax shelters, Congress took action—albeit indirect—with enactment of the at-risk rules in 1976 and

the passive loss rules in 1986. Perhaps fearing that it would alienate certain constituencies, Congress opted not to eliminate or limit the provisions on which shelters are built (e.g., special benefits for low-income housing and rehabilitation of old and historic buildings). Instead, the new legislation, placed limitations on the losses created by these special provisions.

AT-RISK RULES

As can be seen in *Example 6*, the linchpin that held many tax shelters together was nonrecourse financing. From the outset, the government believed that investors should not be entitled to deductions unless they actually incurred a cost—something that was not necessarily present when a tax shelter was structured with nonrecourse financing. Consequently, to eliminate the possibility of artificial deductions, as part of the Tax Reform Act of 1976, Congress enacted § 465 and the so-called at-risk rules. Section 465 generally limits the deductions of individuals and closely held businesses to the amount which they could actually lose from the investment—the amount at-risk. Consequently, to secure the deduction, investors generally must commit personal funds to the venture's activities or be personally liable for debt incurred by the venture in carrying on its activities. The at-risk rules were subsequently amended in the Revenue Act of 1978 and the Tax Reform Act of 1986.

Initially, the at-risk rules were limited to four specific types of activities: (1) holding, producing, or distributing motion picture films or tapes; (2) farming; (3) leasing personal property; and (4) oil and gas exploration and development. As the list suggests, all of these were ripe for sheltering income. In 1978, legislation extended the rules to cover all other activities with one blatant omission: real estate. Real estate was added in 1986 but a huge exception was created in 1987. This exception essentially allowed real estate ventures to escape the at-risk limitations when they were financed using funds from a third-party commercial lender. Consequently, as the law currently reads, the at-risk rules apply to all trade or business or the production of income activities operated by individuals and closely held businesses. Real estate placed in service before 1987 (e.g., an office building or an apartment complex) is exempt as is a separate activity that involves the leasing of equipment by a closely held C corporation. It is important to realize that the at-risk rules cover *any* trade or business or investment activity. Unlike the passive loss rules discussed below, they are not limited to those investments that produce portfolio income or loss, or to those that produce passive income or loss.

AT-RISK COMPUTATION

Under § 465(a), the at-risk provisions limit the deduction of losses incurred in an activity to the amount *at-risk* in the activity at the close of the tax year. Any loss in excess of the amount at-risk cannot be deducted in the current year but can be carried forward and used when there is an increase in the amount at-risk. The following formula can be used to compute the amount at-risk (see Form 6198):

	Beginning at-risk balance
+	Contributions of cash and property (adjusted basis)
+	Increases in recourse debt (taxpayer is personally liable and the lender has no interest in the venture)
+	Increases in debt for which the taxpayer has pledged property which is not used in the activity as security
+	Increases in qualified nonrecourse debt related to realty
+	Income (taxable and tax-exempt)
−	Cash or property withdrawals or distributions
−	Nondeductible expenses related to tax-exempt income
−	Decreases in qualified nonrecourse debt related to realty
−	Decreases in recourse debt (T/P personally liable)
−	Losses
=	Amount at-risk

Observe that the calculation attempts to measure the amount of the taxpayer's economic investment that could be lost from the activity. Accordingly, a taxpayer's at-risk basis includes cash and other assets committed to the activity. Similarly, adjustments are made for income that is retained within the activity and not distributed since such amounts represent additional investments that might be lost. In addition, the at-risk amount includes amounts borrowed for use in the activity for which the taxpayer is personally liable for repayment—recourse debt—as well as amounts borrowed for which the taxpayer has pledged property as security (other than property used in the activity). Finally, as discussed further below, Congress appeased the real estate industry by including in the amount at-risk certain nonrecourse debt related to the holding of real property. Note that while the taxpayer's at-risk basis increases as these items increase, conversely, the at-risk amount is reduced as these items decrease (e.g., amounts are withdrawn, losses are incurred, recourse debt is reduced).

Example 7. This year, G started a business, designing web pages and providing connections to the Internet. He operated the business as a sole proprietorship. His first step was to purchase a server from a computer manufacturer for $100,000. He gave the company $10,000 cash and agreed to pay the manufacturer $90,000 over the next 10 years. In addition, he put up 20 shares of stock that he owned in his father's business worth $20,000 as collateral. The company agreed to accept the stock and equipment as security for the loan. G also borrowed $150,000 from the local bank. The bank required S to sign a note for the loan for which he is personally liable for repayment. During the year, he contributed another $50,000 of his own money to keep the business running. The first year the business turned a small profit of $30,000 and G left the money in the business for working capital. G's at-risk basis includes, the $50,000 of his own money contributed to the business, the $10,000 used to purchase the equipment, the $20,000 of stock that he pledged to secure the equipment loan, the debt of $150,000 for which he is personally obligated, and the $30,000 of income that he left in the business for a total of $260,000. It does not include the $90,000 to be paid to the manufacturer since the note is nonrecourse and the property is used in the business. Note that the pledged property is included since the property is not used in the business as is the case with the equipment.

In the second year of operations, the business turned sour and produced a loss of $10,000. In addition, G withdrew $50,000 for personal use. He also made a $20,000 payment on the principal of the loan. Since G's at-risk basis is $260,000 the loss is not limited and G may use the loss to offset his other income (assuming he satisfies the passive loss rules discussed later in this chapter). G must adjust his beginning

at-risk basis of $260,000 by reducing it for the loss of $10,000, the distribution of $50,000 and the $20,000 payment of the debt, leaving an at-risk basis of $180,000.

While the at-risk rules went a long way to eliminate abusive tax shelters, one industry was able to escape—real estate. After much controversy, the real estate lobby convinced Congress to provide relief for real estate deals to the extent that they used arm's length, third-party commercial financing (e.g., savings and loan provides loan and charges interest at a reasonable market rate). Consequently, a taxpayer's at-risk amount includes so-called qualified nonrecourse financing. Section 465(b)(6) sets forth the specific requirements.

1. The financing is secured by the real property used in the activity.

2. No person is personally liable for the debt (nonrecourse debt).

3. The amounts are borrowed from a person who is regularly engaged in the lending business (e.g., a commercial lender such as a bank or savings and loan or a federal, state, or local governmental unit).

4. The lender is not related to the taxpayer. Note that financing made by a lending institution that has an equity interest in the venture is permissible if the loan is commercially reasonable and similar to those made to unrelated parties.

5. The lender is not the seller of the property or the promoter of the deal (i.e., receives a fee for the taxpayer's investment) or related to the seller or promoter.

Example 8. J was one of 10 investors to contribute $100,000 to Silver Queen Partnership. Each investor received a 10% partnership interest. The partnership used the cash and $900,000 borrowed from First National Bank to purchase an office building for $1,000,000. The debt was secured by a mortgage on the building and was payable over 20 years with interest at 7%, the current market rate. None of the partners were personally liable on the obligation. This year J's share of the partnership's loss was $200,000. J's at-risk amount is $190,000, including the $100,000 cash contribution and 10% of the $900,000 nonrecourse loan. The loan is considered qualified nonrecourse financing since it was borrowed from an unrelated commercial lender and not the seller. Although J's share of the loss is $200,000, her deduction is limited to the amount she has at-risk, $190,000, and the balance is carried over. Her at-risk basis is reduced to zero and she may not deduct the $10,000 carryover until her amount at-risk increases.

Despite the at-risk rules, wily tax shelter promoters were able to structure investments that could avoid them. As might be expected, many of these deals involved real estate since real estate was effectively exempt if the financing was properly structured. To the chagrin of Congress, the tax shelters industry continued to grow. Perhaps one of the most revealing testimonials of the popularity of tax shelters can be found on the cover of the February 1986 issue of *Money* magazine. The cover pictured three highly successful individuals, and indicated that each had made more than a million dollars but paid no taxes. In light of this and other similar reports, it is not surprising that taxpayer confidence in the fairness of the tax system had badly eroded. Many taxpayers had come to believe that tax was paid only by the naive and the unsophisticated. This belief, in turn, was leading to noncompliance and providing incentives for expansion of the tax shelter market, often diverting investment capital from productive activities to those principally or exclusively servicing tax avoidance goals. Consequently, Congress took aim at tax shelters again in 1986 and enacted yet another hurdle to be cleared before losses could be deducted: the passive loss rules of § 469. These rules go beyond the at-risk provisions,

placing far-reaching restrictions on when deductions, losses, and credits of a passive activity can be used to offset the income of another activity. Although these restrictions were designed principally for losses from a limited partnership interest, they also limit losses from rental activities, as well as losses from any trade or business in which the taxpayer does not materially participate.

PASSIVE ACTIVITY LOSS LIMITATIONS

GENERAL RULE

The thrust of § 469 is to divide a taxpayer's income into three types: (1) wages, salaries, and other income from activities in which the taxpayer materially participates (e.g., income from an S corporation that the taxpayer owns and operates); (2) portfolio income (e.g., interest, dividends, capital gains and losses); and (3) passive income—the sort deemed to be produced by most tax shelters and rental activities. Expenses related to passive activities can be deducted only to the extent of income from *all* such passive activities. Any excess expenses of these passive activities—the passive activity loss— may not be deducted against portfolio income or wages, salaries, or any other income from activities in which the taxpayer materially participates. Losses that cannot be used are held in suspension and carried forward to be used to offset passive income of future years.[1] Suspended losses from a passive activity can be used in full to offset portfolio or active income *only* when the taxpayer disposes of his or her entire interest in the activity. Upon disposition, any current and suspended losses (including any loss realized on the disposition) are used to offset income in the following order:[2]

1. Any gain on the disposition of the interest

2. Any *net* income from all passive activities (after taking into account any suspended losses)

3. Any other income or gain (i.e., active and portfolio income)

Observe that this special ordering rule requires the taxpayer to use up the suspended losses against gain on the disposition and any passive income (net of any passive losses) before offsetting such losses against active or portfolio income. Without this rule, a taxpayer would use all of the suspended loss against active income, thus freeing up the passive gain on the disposition to absorb other passive losses.

> **Example 9.** T owned and operated her own construction company as a sole proprietorship. For the year, the company had net income of $120,000. T has a substantial portfolio that produced dividends of $15,000 and a short-term capital loss from the sale of stock of $7,000. In addition, her investment in LP1, a limited partner-ship, produced a passive loss. T's share of the loss was $30,000. Her investments in LP2 and LP3, two other limited partnerships, generated passive activity income. T's share of the income was $5,000. Under the capital gain and loss provisions, T may deduct $3,000 of the capital loss and carry over the remaining $4,000. The $30,000 passive loss is deductible only to the extent of passive income, which is $5,000. In

---

[1]   Suspended losses are carried forward to the following year, where they are treated as if they were incurred in such year. Temp. Reg. § 1.469-1T(f)(4)(B). Special limitations apply to farm losses of noncorporate taxpayers that receive subsidies (§ 461(j)).

[2]   § 469(g). To date, Regulations have not been issued on dispositions, leaving many unanswered questions. See Erickson, "Passive Activity Disposition," *The Tax Adviser* (May 1989), p. 338. See TAM 9742002 where the taxpayer did not have to offset current and suspended losses from sold activities with passive income from only those activities that produced net incomes.

effect, income and loss from the passive activities are netted, and the net loss attributable to LP1, $25,000, is carried over to the following year.

Example 10. Same facts as above. T held on to her investment in LP1 until this year, when she sold her entire interest, producing a gain of $40,000. Total suspended losses attributable to her investment in LP1 were $70,000. Net income from LP2 was $30,000 for the year while LP3 produced a net loss of $10,000. T may deduct the entire $70,000 loss: $40,000 against the gain, $20,000 against the net passive income from LP2 and LP3 ($30,000 − $10,000), and $10,000 against any other income.

As a practical matter, many taxpayers will have investments in several passive activities, some that produce income and some that produce losses. If the taxpayer has losses from more than one activity, the suspended loss for *each* activity must be determined in the event that the taxpayer subsequently disposes of one of the activities. The suspended loss of each activity is determined by allocating the total loss disallowed for the year, including any suspended losses, pro rata among the loss activities using the following formula:[3]

$$\text{Total disallowed loss for year} \times \frac{\text{Loss for this activity}}{\text{Total losses from all activities with losses}} = \frac{\text{Suspended loss}}{\text{for this activity}}$$

Note that this fraction simply represents the percentage of losses attributable to a particular activity. For example, if a loss from a particular activity represents 10 percent of all losses, 10 percent of the disallowed loss is allocated to such activity and carried over to the following year. Alternatively, it could be said that the particular activity absorbs 10 percent of any passive income. In effect, each loss activity absorbs this fraction of any passive income from other activities.

Example 11. T owns an interest in three passive activities: A, B, and C. For 2009, activity B reports income of $2,000 while activities A and C report losses of $10,000, $6,000 from A and $4,000 from C. T is allowed to deduct the passive losses from A and C to the extent of the passive income from B. Thus he may deduct $2,000 of the losses. The remaining loss of $8,000 cannot be used to offset T's income from other sources (e.g., wages, dividends, or interest income) but must be suspended and carried forward to the following year. The suspended loss of $8,000 must be allocated between the loss activities pro rata. Since 60% ($6,000/$10,000) of the net loss was attributable to A, the suspended loss for A is $4,800 (60% × $8,000). Similarly, the suspended loss for C is $3,200 [($4,000/$10,000) × $8,000]. Alternatively, the loss activities could be viewed as absorbing the passive income. Using this approach, the suspended losses would be computed somewhat differently but with the same result.

	A	C	Total
Loss for the year	$ (6,000)	$ (4,000)	$ (10,000)
Loss absorbed:			
$2,000 × ($6,000/$10,000)...............	1,200	—	1,200
$2,000 × ($4,000/$10,000)...............	—	800	800
Suspended loss........................	$ (4,800)	$ (3,200)	$ (8,000)

These losses are carried over and treated as if they were a deduction in the following year.

---

[3] Temp. Reg. § 1.469-1T(f)(2).

Example 12. Assume the same facts as in *Example 11*. The income and loss for 2010 of the three activities is shown below.

Activity	Current Net Income (Loss)	Carryforward from Prior Years	Total
A	$ (5,200)	$ (4,800)	$ (10,000)
B	12,000	—	12,000
C	(1,800)	(3,200)	(5,000)
Total	$ 5,000	$ (8,000)	$ (3,000)

The total passive loss disallowed in 2010 is $3,000. The $3,000 disallowed loss is allocated among the activities with total losses (taking into account both current operations and losses suspended from prior years) as follows:

Activity	Total Disallowed Loss	×	Percentage of Total Loss	=	Allocable Portion of Loss
A	$3,000	×	$10,000/($10,000 + $5,000)	=	$2,000
C	3,000	×	5,000/($10,000 + $5,000)	=	1,000

In making the allocation, the disallowed loss is allocated based on an activity's net loss *including* suspended losses (e.g., $10,000 for A) rather than the loss that actually occurred in the current year (e.g., $5,200 for A).

Example 13. J has three passive activities: R, S, and T. The suspended losses and current income and losses for each activity for 2009 are shown below. In addition, J sold activity S for a $10,000 gain in 2009. Because there has been a complete disposition of S, J is able to deduct all of the suspended losses for S as shown below.

	R	S	T
Suspended loss.............................	$ (9,000)	$(12,000)	$(15,000)
Current income (loss)	(5,000)	(6,000)	(7,000)
Total	$(14,000)	$(18,000)	$(22,000)
Gain on disposition of S		10,000	
Excess loss of S deducted against other income		$ (8,000)	

J must first offset the suspended and current losses of $18,000 from activity S against the $10,000 gain on the sale of S. The next step is to offset the $8,000 balance of losses against any net passive income for the year. In this case, the activities have no income, and thus none of the loss is absorbed by passive income. At this point, the remaining loss of $8,000 is no longer considered passive and can be used to offset any active or portfolio income that J may have.

Example 14. K has three passive activities: X, Y, and Z. The suspended losses and current income and losses for each activity for 2009 are shown below. In addition, in 2009, K sold activity Y for a $21,000 gain. K is able to deduct all of the suspended losses of Y as shown below.

	X	Y	Z
Suspended loss..........................	$ (7,000)	$(10,000)	$(18,000)
Current income (loss)......................	(8,000)	(6,000)	8,000
Total..................................	$(15,000)	$(16,000)	$(10,000)
Gain on disposition of Y.....................	—	21,000	—
	$(15,000)	$ 5,000	$(10,000)
Loss absorbed:			
$5,000 × ($15,000/$25,000)...............	3,000		
$5,000 × ($10,000/$25,000)...............			2,000
Suspended loss..........................	$(12,000)		$ (8,000)

K must first offset Y's current and suspended losses of $16,000 against the $21,000 gain on the sale. Note that the balance of the gain ($5,000) is considered passive income that can be combined with the net losses (the sum of current income or loss and suspended losses) from the other passive activities for the year.[4]

Rules similar to those for passive losses apply to tax credits produced by passive activities (e.g., the low-income housing credit, rehabilitation credit, research credit, and jobs credit). Passive credits can be used *only* to offset any tax attributable to passive income. Any unused credit may be carried forward to the next taxable year to offset future taxes arising from passive income. In contrast to passive losses, however, credits being carried over are not fully triggered when a passive activity is sold. In the year of disposition, like any other year, the credit can be used only if there is tax attributable to passive income (including gain on the sale of the activity). If the credit cannot be used, it can continue to be carried over to offset tax from other passive activities. However, the credit is subject to its own rules concerning carryover and expiration.

Example 15. T invested in a limited partnership that rehabilitated a historic structure. In 2009, T sold his interest, realizing a gain of $5,000. At that time, T had suspended losses of $20,000 and credits of $10,000. T is able to use $5,000 of the losses to offset the gain and the other $15,000 to offset other active or portfolio income. None of the credit can be used, however, because there is no income from the passive activity. Had T sold the property for a gain of $50,000, he would have had $30,000 of passive income. Assuming T is in the 28% tax bracket, he could have used $8,400 ($30,000 × 28%) of the credit. The remaining credit of $1,600 may be carried over to offset tax that may arise from passive income.

TAXPAYERS SUBJECT TO LIMITATIONS

The passive loss rules apply to individuals, estates, trusts, personal service corporations, and certain closely held C corporations.[5] Partnerships and S corporations are not subject to the limitations per se. However, their activities flow through to the owners who are subject to limitation.

---

[4]   § 469(g)(1)(A) and Temp. Reg. § 1.469-2T(c)(2)(i)(A)(2).

[5]   § 469(a)(2).

The passive loss rules generally do not apply to regular C corporations. Presumably, their immunity is based on the theory that individuals generally do not benefit from losses locked inside the corporate form. Congress, however, did not want taxpayers to be able to circumvent the passive loss rules merely by incorporating. Absent a special rule, a taxpayer could utilize corporate immunity to shelter income derived from personal services. Taxpayers would simply incorporate as a personal service corporation and acquire tax shelter investments at the corporate level. The losses produced by the tax shelters would offset not only the service income but also income from any investments made at the corporate level. Consequently, the passive loss rules apply to *personal service corporations* (PSC). A PSC is one where the principal activity is the performance of personal services and such services are primarily performed by employee-owners who, *in the aggregate*, own more than 10 percent of the stock of the corporation either directly or indirectly (e.g., through family members). Common examples of personal service corporations are professional corporations such as those of doctors, accountants, attorneys, engineers, actors, architects, and others where personal services are performed.

Without additional restrictions, any taxpayer—not just one who derives income from services—could incorporate his or her portfolio and offset the investment income with losses from tax shelters. To prohibit this possibility, the passive loss rules also apply in a limited fashion to all closely held C corporations (i.e., a regular C corporation where five or fewer individuals own more than 50 percent of the stock either directly or indirectly). Note that some personal service corporations that might escape the tests above may still be subject to the rules due to their status as closely held corporations. A closely held corporation may not use passive losses to offset its portfolio income. However, such corporations may offset losses from passive activities against the income of any active business carried on by the corporation.[6]

> **Example 16.** R and his two brothers own Real Rustproofing Corporation. This year the corporation suffered a loss from operations of $10,000. In addition, it received interest income from short-term investments of working capital of $20,000. The corporation also had a passive loss from a real estate venture of $30,000. In determining taxable income, the passive activity limitation rules apply since the corporation is closely held (i.e., five or fewer individuals own more than 50%). As a result, none of the loss can be deducted since the loss cannot offset portfolio income of the corporation and the corporation did not have any income from operations. Had the corporation had $50,000 of operating profit, the entire loss could be deducted since passive losses can be used by a closely held corporation to offset active income—but not portfolio income.

PASSIVE ACTIVITIES

Assuming the taxpayer is subject to the passive activity rules, the most important determination is whether the activity in which the taxpayer is engaged is *passive*. The characterization of an activity as passive generally depends on the level of the taxpayer's involvement in the activity, the nature of the activity, or the form of ownership. Section 469(c) provides that the following activities are passive:

1. Any activity (other than a working interest in certain oil and gas property) that involves the conduct of a trade or business in which the taxpayer *does not materially participate*; and

2. *Any* rental activity regardless of the level of the taxpayer's participation.

---

[6] § 469(e)(2).

Given these definitions, several questions must be addressed to determine whether a particular endeavor of the taxpayer is a passive activity.

1. What is an activity?
2. Is the activity a rental or nonrental activity?
3. What is material participation?

Unfortunately, none of these questions are easily answered. An exceedingly complex set of Regulations exists that, in large measure, creates intricate definitions designed to prohibit wily taxpayers from deducting their passive losses. The basic rules are considered below.

DEFINITION OF AN ACTIVITY

The definition of an activity serves as the foundation for the entire structure of the passive loss rules. Virtually all of the important determinations required in applying the passive loss rules are made at the activity level. Perhaps the most significant of these concerns the taxpayer's level of participation. As discussed later in this chapter, if the taxpayer participates for more than 500 hours per year in a nonrental activity, he or she is deemed to materially participate in the activity, and the activity is therefore not passive. As the following example illustrates, this 500-hour test requires an unambiguous definition of an activity.

> **Example 17.** Mr R. Rock owns and operates 10 restaurants in 10 different cities. In addition, in each of those 10 cities he owns and operates 10 movie theaters. R spends 80 hours working in each restaurant during the year for a total of 800 hours. R spends 70 hours working in each movie theater for a total of 700 hours. If *each* restaurant and each movie theater are treated as separate activities, it would appear that R would not be treated as a material participant in any one of the businesses because he devoted only a minimum amount of his time during the year, 80 or 70 hours, to each. On the other hand, if all the restaurants are aggregated and deemed a *single activity*, R's total participation in all the restaurants, 800 hours would, in fact, be considered material. A similar conclusion could be reached for the movie theaters. In addition, if the restaurants are adjacent to the movie theaters (or in fact are concession stands in the theaters), it might be appropriate to treat the restaurant operation and the movie theater operation as a single activity.

The definition of an activity is not only important for the material participation test, but it is also significant should there be a disposition. As noted above, a complete disposition of an activity enables a taxpayer to deduct any suspended losses of the activity.

> **Example 18.** Same facts as in *Example 17* above. Also assume that there are suspended losses for each restaurant. If each restaurant is treated as a separate activity, a sale of one of the restaurants would enable R to deduct the suspended loss for that restaurant. In contrast, if the restaurant is not considered a separate activity, none of the loss would be recognized on the tax return for the year of sale.

Examples 17 and 18 demonstrate not only the importance of the definition of an activity but also the problems inherent in defining what constitutes an activity.

The authors of § 469 obviously anticipated the difficulty in defining an activity and therefore provided no working definition in the Code. As a result, the formidable task of defining an activity fell in the laps of those who write the Regulations. Defining an activity would not be difficult if all taxpayers were engaged in a single line of business

at one location. As a practical matter, this is not always the case. Some taxpayers, such as Mr. Rock in *Example 17*, are involved in several lines of business at multiple locations. Consequently, any definition of an activity had to consider such situations. In fixing the scope of an activity, the Treasury feared that a narrow definition would allow taxpayers to generate passive income at will that could be used to offset passive losses. For example, if Mr. Rock were able to treat each restaurant as a separate activity, he could easily manipulate his participation at each restaurant to obtain passive or active income as he deemed most beneficial. To combat this problem, the IRS initially designed a broad definition that generally required a taxpayer to aggregate various endeavors into a single activity. By establishing a broad definition that treats several undertakings as a single activity, the IRS made the material participation test easier to meet, resulting in active rather than passive income. Unfortunately, the initial definition was quite complicated, as evidenced by the Temporary Regulations, which contained 196 pages of intricate rules and examples devoted to the subject.[7] In a refreshing change of direction, however, the IRS allowed these Temporary Regulations to expire, creating a far simpler approach all contained in only four pages![8]

Appropriate Economic Unit. Under the final regulations, taxpayers are required to treat one or more trade or business activities or one or more rental activities as a single activity if the activities constitute an *appropriate economic unit* for measuring gain or loss.[9] Whether two or more activities constitute an appropriate economic unit (AEU) is determined by taking into account all of the relevant facts and circumstances. Five factors are to be given the greatest weight in making the determination. These are as follows:

1. Similarities and differences in *types* of business;

2. The extent of common control;

3. The extent of common ownership;

4. Geographical location; and

5. Interdependencies between activities (e.g., they have the same customers or same employees, are accounted for with a single set of books, purchase or sell goods between themselves, or involve products or services that are normally provided together).

A taxpayer may use *any* reasonable method of applying the relevant facts and circumstances.

Example 19. C operates several businesses as a sole proprietor. These include a bakery and a movie theater at a shopping mall in Santa Fe and a bakery and a movie theater in Albuquerque. Reasonable groupings, depending on the facts and circumstances. may be as follows:

- ▸ A single activity
- ▸ A movie theater activity and a bakery activity
- ▸ A Santa Fe activity and an Albuquerque activity
- ▸ Four separate activities

---

[7]   Temp. Reg. § 1.469-4T(a)(2).

[8]   Reg. § 1.469-4.

[9]   Reg. § 1.469-4(c)(1).

Consistency Requirement. To ensure that taxpayers do not bounce from one grouping to another to fit their needs, a consistency requirement is imposed. Once the activities have been grouped in a particular manner, the grouping may not be changed unless the original grouping was clearly inappropriate or there has been a material change in the facts and circumstances that makes the original grouping inappropriate.[10] For instance, in *Example 19* above, once one of the groupings is selected, the taxpayer is required to continue using the grouping unless a material change in the facts and circumstances makes it clearly inappropriate.

In addition, to prevent a taxpayer from misusing the facts-and-circumstances approach, the IRS has the power to regroup activities if the taxpayer's grouping fails to reflect one or more appropriate economic units and one of the primary purposes of the taxpayer's grouping is to circumvent the passive loss rules.[11]

Activities Conducted through Conduit Entities. As a practical matter, many taxpayers will conduct activities through a partnership or an S corporation. In this case, the grouping is done at the partnership or S corporation level. Partners and S corporation shareholders then determine whether they should aggregate the entity activities with those they conduct directly or through other partnerships or S corporations.[12]

Grouping of Rental and Nonrental Activities. Rental activities and nonrental activities normally may *not* be grouped together and treated as a single activity. This rule is consistent with the basic provision that all rental activities are passive regardless of the taxpayer's participation. Therefore, it makes sense that rental and nonrental activities should not be aggregated. The practical significance of the rule is to prohibit taxpayers from sheltering active income with passive rental losses. Nevertheless, the Regulations do carve out an exception, allowing aggregation of rental and nonrental activities whenever either activity is *insubstantial* in relation to the other or the owners of the business activity have the same proportionate ownership interest as they have in the rental activity (e.g., 40% in one and 40% in the other).[13]

> **Example 20.** PB&K, an accounting firm, operates its practice out of an office building that it owns. The firm occupies two floors of the building and leases the other three floors to third parties. This year, 90% of the firm's income is from its accounting practice and 10% is from rental of the office space. Because the rental operation is insubstantial in relation to the nonrental operation, the rental and nonrental operations are aggregated into a *single nonrental* activity. Note that in this case any net loss on the rental activity is effectively combined with the income of the accounting operation.

> **Example 21.** H and W, husband and wife, equally own Sliders, an S corporation that owns and operates 25 restaurants throughout the Midwest. Sliders is quite profitable. Several years ago, the company decided it should buy an airplane to enable it travel easily to its various locations. On the advice of their attorney, H formed Airmax, a single member LLC that purchased and leases out the plane. Sliders rents the plane on a long-term basis from Airmax. The S corporation pays the LLC a fair rent for use of the plane but because of depreciation and interest, the LLC annually reports a net rental loss from its operations. The LLC does not provide any services with respect to

---

[10] Reg. § 1.469-4(g). In Notice 2008-64, 2008-31 IRB 268, the IRS proposed that taxpayers should be required to report any changes in groupings on the return.

[11] Reg. § 1.469-4(h).

[12] Reg. § 1.469-4(j).

[13] Reg. § 1.469-4(d).

providing the plane so it is considered a rental activity and therefore is deemed to be passive. Absent any special rule, H would not be able to offset the losses of Airmax against the income from Sliders. However, under the Regulations, H may elect to group the LLC rental activity and the S corporation restaurant business as a single activity. This grouping election is permitted because the LLC and the S corporation have identical ownership. Alternatively, had there not been identical ownership, H may have been able to group the airplane leasing activity with the restaurant business assuming the rental activity is insubstantial to the restaurant activity.

It should also be noted that the rental of real property and the rental of personal property cannot be grouped unless the personal property is provided in connection with the real property.[14]

Example 22. T owns a small apartment building with eight units that he rents completely furnished. In addition, the building contains a small room with coin-operated laundry facilities. As a general rule, the laundry rental and apartment rental cannot be aggregated because the rental of real property cannot be grouped with the rental of personal property. In this case, however, the rental income and laundry income can be grouped since the personal property is provided in connection with the real property.

Rental and nonrental operations normally must be separated because they are subject to different rules. For example, rental activities are always passive, whereas nonrental activities are passive only if the taxpayer does not materially participate in such activities. In addition, owners of rental real estate are normally entitled to deduct up to $25,000 of rental losses annually without limitation, whereas there is no comparable rule for nonrental activities. Although rentals and nonrental activities are usually separated, certain exceptions may allow aggregation. As discussed above, if either activity is insubstantial to the other, aggregation can occur or if the owners own the same proportionate interest in each activity, they may be grouped.

RENTAL VERSUS NONRENTAL ACTIVITIES

Under the general rule described above, all rental activities are deemed to be passive, *regardless* of whether the taxpayer materially participates. Congress adopted this view based on the belief that there is seldom any significant participation in rental activities. Therefore, it created a presumption that all rental activities would be passive. For this purpose, a rental activity is defined as any activity whereby a taxpayer receives payments that are principally for the use of property owned by the taxpayer (e.g., apartments or equipment).

Observe that this blanket rule effectively classifies many rental activities as passive even though an owner might render significant services in connection with the rental. For example, renting video tapes would be considered passive under the general rule even though the owner might perform substantial services. This approach would be unfair to those who participate yet suffer losses. Moreover, the rule creates a huge planning opportunity for those seeking passive income given that many rental businesses are profitable. Recognizing these problems, the authors of the Regulations identified six situations where what is normally a rental is to be treated as a nonrental activity.[15]

---

[14] Reg. § 1.469-4(e).

[15] Temp. Reg. § 1.469-1T(e)(3)(ii).

1. *1–7 Days Rental.* The activity is not a rental if the average rental period is seven days or less. Under this exception, short-term rentals of such items as cars, hotel and motel rooms, or videocassettes are not considered rental activities.

2. *8–30 Days Rental.* The activity is not a rental if the average rental period is 30 days or less and significant services are performed by the owner of the property. In determining whether *significant services* are provided, consideration is given to the type of service performed and the value of the services relative to the amount charged for the use of the property. In this regard, the Regulations indicate that telephone service and cable television are to be ignored as are those services commonly provided in connection with long-term rentals of commercial and residential property (e.g., janitorial services, repairs, trash collection, cleaning of common areas, and security services provided by landlords of shopping malls and centers). Unfortunately, the Regulations provide few other clues as to what constitutes significant services.

Example 23. T owns and rents a resort condominium in Florida. He provides telephone, cable, trash removal, cleaning of the common areas, and daily maid and linen service. The cost of the maid and linen services is less than 10% of the amount charged to tenants occupying the apartments. In determining whether significant services are provided, the telephone, cable, trash, and cleaning services are disregarded. Moreover, according to the Regulations, the maid and linen services would not be considered significant in this case. Because there are no significant services under the Regulations' view, the activity would be considered a rental (*assuming* the average rental use exceeds seven days) and, therefore, a passive activity.

3. *Extraordinary Services.* The activity is not a rental if extraordinary personal services are provided by the owner of the property. Services are considered extraordinary if the use of the property is merely incidental to the services performed.

Example 24. Nathan Hale Military Academy, a private college preparatory school, provides housing for its students. The school's rental of such facilities would be considered incidental to the educational services provided and thus be treated as a nonrental activity.

4. *Incidental Rentals.* The activity is not a rental activity if the rental of the property is merely incidental to the nonrental activity.

The Temporary Regulations identify two situations when this rule applies.[16]

- *Investment Property.* An activity is not considered a rental if the rental property is held primarily for investment. Two tests must be met. First, the principal purpose for holding the property must be for the expectation of gain from appreciation due to market changes and not due to improvements to the property. Second, the gross rental income from the property is insignificant; that is, the rent must be less than two percent of the lesser of (1) the unadjusted basis of the property or (2) the fair market value of the property.

---

[16]   Temp. Reg. § 1.469-1T(e)(3)(vi)(B).

Example 25. S owns land that she is holding for future appreciation. She purchased the land for $500,000 and it is currently worth $800,000. To defray the costs of holding the land, she leases it to a rancher for grazing his cattle. The rent is $9,000 per year. Since the rent is less than $10,000 (2% of the lesser of the basis of the property $500,000 or its fair market value of $800,000), the two percent test is met. Because S is holding the property primarily as an investment and her rental income is insignificant (it is less than the two percent threshold), the rental is considered incidental and would not be automatically treated as a rental activity for purposes of the passive loss rules. On the other hand, if S bought the land intending to build a shopping center on it, the rental would not be considered incidental since the land is not considered held primarily for appreciation. In such case, the activity is deemed to be a rental.

- *Property Normally Used in a Trade or Business.* A rental is not considered a rental activity if the property is normally used by the taxpayer in a business and occasionally is rented to others when it is not needed in the business. The property qualifies as business property only if (1) the property is used in the business during the current year (or two of the last five) and (2) the two percent test is met (i.e., gross rental income from the property is less than two percent of the lesser of the unadjusted basis of the property or the fair market value of the property).

Example 26. P, a farmer, owns land that he uses for farming. This year a nearby country club, Roaring Fork Golf and Country Club, is hosting the U.S. Open. P rented a portion of his land to the club to be used for a parking lot for the month of June for $3,000. The allocable cost of the land is $200,000 and it is currently worth $500,000. The rental income is considered incidental and not passive since the property is normally used in P's farming business and the $3,000 rent is less than $4,000 (2% of the lesser of the basis of the property $200,000 or its fair market value of $500,000). The result would be the same if P had rented the property to another farmer or for some other purpose.

5. *Nonexclusive Use.* The activity is not a rental activity if the taxpayer customarily makes the property available during defined business hours for the nonexclusive use of various customers. For example, this exception would apply to a golf course that sells annual memberships but which is also open to the public on a daily basis.

6. *Property Made Available for Use in a Nonrental Activity.* The activity is not a rental activity if the taxpayer owns an interest in a partnership, S corporation, or joint venture to which the property is rented. For example, if T rents equipment to a partnership in which he is a partner, the rental is treated as a nonrental activity.

Similarly, rental of property to a C corporation in which the taxpayer materially participates is not considered a rental.

Example 27. Mr. F, an attorney, owns and operates F&H Corporation, a law firm. This year F and his wife leased a building that they owned jointly to F&H Inc. The corporation was the sole tenant. Mr. F would like to treat the rent as passive and use it to absorb the couple's passive activity losses. Unfortunately, the regulations provide that rental to a C corporation in which the taxpayer materially participates is a nonrental activity. Therefore, the amounts received for leasing the building are not considered passive income.[17]

---

[17] See *Remy Fransen, Jr.*, 99-2 USTC ¶50,882 (CA-5, 1999), aff'g 98-2 USTC ¶50,776 (D.C., E.D. La., 1998) where the Court upheld the validity of Reg. § 1.469-2(f)(6), recharacterizing the activity as active and not passive. See also *Schwalbach*, 111 T.C. No. 9 (1998).

As noted above, any activity constituting a "rental" is a passive activity. Note, however, that those activities not classified as rentals (i.e., nonrental activities) may still be considered passive. Whether a *nonrental* activity is a passive activity depends on whether the taxpayer has materially participated in the activity.

MATERIAL PARTICIPATION

Material participation serves a crucial role in the application of the passive loss rules. It is the criterion that distinguishes between "passive" and "active" nonrental activities. The Code provides that an individual meets the material participation test only if he or she is involved in the operation of the activity on a regular, continuous, and substantial basis. Without further guidance, applying this nebulous criterion would essentially be left to the subjective interpretation of the taxpayer. However, the Regulations establish objective standards that look to the actual number of hours spent in the activity.

Under the regulatory scheme, a taxpayer materially participates in an activity if he or she meets one of seven tests.[18]

1. *More Than 500 Hours.* An individual materially participates if he or she spends more than 500 hours in the activity during the taxable year. Apparently the authors of the Regulations believed that this threshold (e.g., about 10 hours per week) appropriately distinguished those who truly were involved in the business from mere investors. Note that the work of a spouse is counted if it is work typically done by owners. For example, if B owned an S corporation that suffered losses (e.g., a football team), he would materially participate if he devoted more than 500 hours to the activity. However, if he spent only 300 hours and hired his wife as a receptionist who spent 250 hours, the test is not met because her work is not normally done by owners.

2. *Substantially All of the Participation.* The individual and his or her spouse materially participate if they are the sole participants or their participation constitutes substantially all of the participation of all individuals (including nonowners and nonemployees) who participate in the activity. This test, as well as the next, takes into account the fact that not all businesses require 500 hours to operate during the year. For example, if S operates a snow removal service by himself and spends only 50 hours in the activity this year because of light snow, the test is met because he was the sole participant.

3. *More Than 100 Hours and Not Less Than Anyone Else.* An individual materially participates if he or she participates for more than 100 hours and no other individual spends more time on the activity. For example, assume that S, above, occasionally hires E to help him remove snow. If S spent 160 hours and E 140, S qualifies because he spent more than 100 hours and not less than anyone else. Had S spent only 60 and E 40, S arguably would not qualify under either this or the previous test.

4. *Significant Participation in Several Activities.* An individual materially participates if his or her total participation in all *significant participation activities* (SPAs) exceeds 500 hours. A significant participation activity is

---

[18]   Temp. Reg. § 1.469-5T(a).

defined as a trade or business in which the taxpayer participates more than 100 hours, but fails the other six tests for material participation. Thus a taxpayer must spend more than 100 hours in each activity and greater than 500 in all. The rule derives from the view that an individual who spends more than 500 hours in several different activities should be treated the same as those who spend an equivalent amount of time on a single activity.

Example 28. T spends 140 hours overseeing his car wash, 160 hours supervising his quick-lube operation, and 499 hours managing his gas station. Each activity qualifies as a SPA because T spends more than 100 hours in each. More importantly, T is treated as materially participating in each because the total hours in all SPAs exceeds 500. However, if T spent two more hours in his gas station, then he would not be a material participant in either the car wash or quick-lube business. This occurs because the gas station would no longer be a SPA since the activity by itself satisfies the more-than-500-hours test. As a result, T's total hours in all SPAs, 300 (160 + 140), would not exceed the 500-hour benchmark. Obviously, this is a strange result.

The Regulations provide what at first glance is a curious treatment of SPAs. As expected, losses from SPAs failing to meet the 500-hour test are passive and generally not deductible. However, income from SPAs failing to meet the 500-hour test is *not* passive. Note that the IRS obtains the best of both worlds when a taxpayer is unable to combine his or her SPAs to get over the 500-hour threshold: passive loss but not passive income. This "heads I win, tails you lose" approach was designed to prevent taxpayers from creating passive income that could be used to absorb passive losses by spending small amounts of time in unrelated activities that are profitable.[19]

5. *Prior Participation.* An individual materially participates if he or she has materially participated (by tests 1 through 4) in an activity for five of the past ten years. This test prevents the taxpayer from moving in and out of material participation status. For example, D and son are partners in an appliance business that D started 30 years ago. D has essentially retired, leaving the day-to-day operations to his son. Without a special rule, D could tailor his participation year by year to obtain passive or nonpassive income as fits his needs.

6. *Prior Participation in a Personal Service Activity.* An individual materially participates in a personal service activity if he or she has materially participated in the activity for at least three years. Like the previous test, this rule eliminates the flexibility those working for personal service businesses have in tailoring their participation to obtain passive or nonpassive income as they need. For example, if a general partner in a law firm retired and converted her interest to a limited partnership interest, she would still be treated as a material participant in that law firm.

7. *Facts and Circumstances.* An individual materially participates if, based on the facts and circumstances, he or she participates in the activity on a regular, continuous, and substantial basis.

---

[19]   See Reg. § 1.469-2T(f)(2).

Rental Real Estate Exception. An extremely important exception to the passive activity rules is carved out in § 469(i) for rental real estate activities of the small investor. In many cases, the rental real estate held by a taxpayer is a residence that is used part-time, was formerly used, or may be used by the taxpayer in the future. Relief was provided for this type of rental real estate because it is often held to provide financial security to individuals with moderate incomes. In such a case, these individuals share little common ground with the tax shelter investors. The relief is provided solely to individuals and certain trusts and estates. Regular C corporations are ineligible.

Under the exception, a taxpayer who *actively* participates (in contrast to materially participates) may deduct up to $25,000 of losses attributable to rental real estate annually. The $25,000 allowance is reduced by 50 percent of the excess of the taxpayer's A.G.I. over $100,000. This relationship may be expressed as follows:

$$\text{Reduction in } \$25{,}000 \text{ allowance} = 50\% \,(\text{A.G.I} - \$100{,}000)$$

Based on this formula, high-income taxpayers (i.e., those with A.G.I. of $150,000 or more) cannot take advantage of this provision. A.G.I. for this purpose is computed without regard to contributions to individual retirement accounts, taxable social security, and any net passive losses that might be deductible. Any portion of the rental loss that is not deductible may be carried over and deducted subject to the same limitations in the following years.

Example 29. L moved to a new home this year. Instead of selling his old home, L decided to rent it out to supplement his income. During the first year, rents were $3,000 while expenses including maintenance, depreciation, interest, utilities, and taxes were $10,000. L's A.G.I. is $40,000. L may deduct the $7,000 loss for A.G.I. Had L's A.G.I. been $140,000, he could have deducted only $5,000 and carried over $2,000 to the following year. This computation is illustrated below.

Loss allowance		$ 25,000
Phase-out:		
A.G.I.	$ 140,000	
Threshold	(100,000)	
Excess A.G.I.	$ 40,000	
Rate	× 50%	
Phase-out		(20,000)
Maximum loss allowed		$ 5,000

It should be emphasized that the taxpayer can use this exception only if the property is considered rental real estate. It cannot be used for losses from rental of personal property. More important, the real estate is not considered a "rental" activity where the rental period is either 1 to 7 days or between 8 and 30 days and significant services are performed.[20] For example, consider the typical investor who owns a vacation condominium. If the average rental of the condominium is 1 to 7 days, the condominium is not considered rental property and the $25,000 exception does not apply. The result is the same if the average rental period is between 8 and 30 days and significant services

---

[20] For an excellent discussion of this topic and issue see Bomyea and Marucheck, "Rental of Residences," *The Tax Adviser* (September 1990), p. 543.

are provided. Note that even though the $25,000 exception is not available in either case, all is not necessarily lost. In both situations, the condominium is treated as a nonrental activity. In such case, the taxpayer will be able to deduct all losses if there is material participation.[21]

> **Example 30.** M lives in Orlando, where she practices law. M owns a condominium, which she rents out on a daily basis to tourists. M runs ads in the local newspaper, makes arrangements for the rental, and cleans the unit as needed. In this case, it appears that the activity is not a rental business because of the short-term rental. As a result, the $25,000 exception for rentals does not apply. However, M still may be able to deduct a loss. Since the property by definition is not a rental activity due to the short-term rental period, it is—by default—a nonrental activity. Accordingly, the loss would be deductible if she materially participates in the activity. For example, if M spent more than 100 hours in the activity and more than anyone else or met any of the other six material participation tests, the loss would be deductible.

As noted above, the Code draws a distinction between material and active participation. The primary difference concerns the taxpayer's degree of involvement in operations. For example, a taxpayer is actively involved if he or she participates in management decisions such as approving new tenants, deciding on rental terms, approving capital or repair expenditures, or if he or she arranges for others to provide services such as repairs. In all cases, the taxpayer is not treated as actively participating in the activity if less than a 10 percent interest is owned. On the other hand, the taxpayer is not presumed to actively participate if the interest is 10 percent or more. The above standard still must be satisfied.

Real Estate Professional Exception. Under the basic rules described above, taxpayers who are engaged in the rental real estate business (e.g., owners of warehouses, shopping centers, or office buildings) cannot deduct losses from such business activities since the law presumes that virtually all long-term rental real estate activities are passive. Note that this treatment occurs regardless of the amount of time and energy spent by the taxpayer in such activities. The level of the taxpayer's participation is irrelevant. After much debate, however, Congress finally agreed in 1994 that the passive loss rules were aimed at passive investors in real estate and not those who were in the real estate business. For this reason, it took steps to enable these individuals to deduct losses arising from these activities. This special relief is granted only if the individual can pass certain tests that effectively establish that he or she is truly in the real estate business.

Generally, an individual can take advantage of the exception for real estate professionals if he or she spends more than half of their working hours in the real estate business and the number of hours spent exceeds 750. Technically an individual is *eligible* to deduct losses from rental real estate if both of the following conditions are met:[22]

1. Services representing more than 50 percent of the total personal services performed by the individual in all trades or businesses during the tax year are performed in *real property trades or businesses* in which the taxpayer materially participates during the year. For this purpose, real property trades or businesses include real property development, redevelopment, construction, acquisition, conversion, rental, operation, management, leasing, and brokerage. In the case of

---

[21] See *Steven D. Rapp*, T.C. Memo 1999-249, 78 TCM 175 and *Walter A. Barniskis*, T.C. Memo 1999-258, 78 TCM 226.

[22] § 469(c)(7). For an interesting example, see *Edward C. Hanna* T.C. Summary Opinion 2006-57.

a closely held C corporation, this test is met if more than 50 percent of the gross receipts of such corporation are derived from real property businesses in which the corporation materially participates.

2. The individual performs more than 750 hours of services in *real property trades or businesses in which he or she materially participates.*

If a joint return is filed, the special relief is available if either spouse separately satisfies the requirements. Note that for this purpose, the couple *cannot* aggregate their hours.

Observe that satisfaction of these two tests merely opens the door for possible deduction of losses. In order to treat the losses as nonpassive, the taxpayer must still meet the material participation requirements (e.g., spend more than 500 hours in the activity). For this purpose, each activity is normally treated as a separate activity. However, the taxpayer may elect to aggregate such activities.[23] In most cases, it would seem that those who are eligible and who elect to aggregate their real property businesses should be able to meet the material participation tests. It should also be emphasized that personal services as an *employee* in a real property business are not treated as performed in the real property business unless the individual owns at least 5 percent of the business.

> **Example 31.** G graduated from the Vanderbilt law school in 1961 and has been practicing his trade ever since. Over the years, however, he has accumulated a number of properties. As a result, he is increasingly spending more time being a real estate magnate and less time being a lawyer. Currently, he owns, operates, and manages a small shopping center and several duplexes. Each of these rental activities produces a loss, primarily due to depreciation. According to G's detailed diary of how he spends his time, he worked 40 hours a week for 50 weeks during the year for a total of 2,000 hours. Assuming G elects to aggregate his interests in each of the rental real estate activities and treat them as a single activity, the majority, 1,100 hours, was devoted to his real estate ventures. The other 900 hours related to his law practice. In this case, G meets both tests that enable him to treat the rental operations as nonrental activities: (1) more than 50% of his personal services were performed in real property businesses, and (2) his 1,100 hours of service in these businesses exceeded the 750-hour threshold. Although the rental taint is removed, this does not necessarily mean G is allowed to deduct the losses. He must still satisfy the material participation tests. Whether this final requirement is met depends on whether G elects to aggregate all of the activities. If so, his 1,100 hours of participation is greater than the 500 hours required and he would be entitled to deduct all of the losses.

RECHARACTERIZED PASSIVE INCOME

As is evident throughout the passive loss Regulations, the IRS was concerned that taxpayers might create passive income which could be used to absorb otherwise nondeductible passive losses. Nowhere is this more evident than in the recharacterization rules. In certain situations, income that is characterized under the general rules as passive is recharacterized under a special rule and treated as active. An example of the type of recharacterization that can occur was discussed earlier in connection with SPAs. As noted in that discussion, income from SPAs that fail to meet the 500-hour test would normally be treated as passive, but under the special recharacterization rule it is treated

---

[23] The aggregation election is made by filing a statement with the taxpayer's *original* income tax return for the taxable year pursuant to Reg. § 1.469-9(g). The statement must contain a declaration that the taxpayer is a qualifying taxpayer for the taxable year and is making the election pursuant to § 469(c)(7). Merely, aggregating the rental operations on Schedule E is not sufficient. For an excellent example of what not to do, see *Karl Jahina, et ux. v. Commissioner*, TC Summary Opinion 2002-150.

as active. There are several other situations when this might occur. Consequently, before it can be concluded that income is passive, the recharacterization rules must be considered. These rules operate to convert the following types of income to nonpassive (i.e., active) or portfolio income rather than passive income.[24]

1. *Significant Participation Activities:* Income from "significant participation activities" that fail to meet the 500-hour test is nonpassive.

2. *Rental of Nondepreciable Property:* Income from rental activities is active if less than 30 percent of the basis of the property rented is depreciable (e.g., rental of land). This rule makes not only rental income nonpassive but also gain on a sale of the activity or property used in it. However, losses are passive.

3. *Developer Sales of Rental Property:* Rental income, including gain on the sale of rental property, if (1) gain on the sale is included in income during the taxable year; (2) rental of the property commenced less than 24 months before the date of disposition; and (3) the taxpayer performed sufficient services that enhanced the value of the rental property.

4. *Self-Rented Property:* Income from rental of property to an activity in which the taxpayer materially participates, other than related C corporations.

5. *Licensing of Intangible Property:* Royalty income from a pass-through entity that the taxpayer acquired after the entity created the intangible property.

6. *Equity-Financed Lending Activity:* Income from the trade or business of lending money if certain conditions are satisfied.

Example 32. Dr. S owns a dental practice that he operates through a corporation, Family Dentistry, Inc. He also has substantial passive losses derived from two rental properties, an apartment and shopping center. Hoping to generate some passive income to absorb such losses, he purchased a building and leased it to his corporation for $25,000 this year. The corporation uses the building to house the doctor's dental practice. The self-rental rule treats the rental income received by Dr. S as portfolio income since S materially participates in the corporation to which the property is rented.[25]

In a similar move, S and his brother, B, formed an LLC to establish a trailer park. The LLC purchased the land for $300,000 and made depreciable improvements on the land of $100,000. Any rental income derived from the park is treated as portfolio income rather than passive income since the basis of the depreciable property (unadjusted for depreciation) is less than 30% of the basis of all the property used in the rental activity ($100,000/$400,000 = 25%). Any gain on the sale of the partnership interest would also be treated as portfolio income. Note that this recharacterization rule is usually triggered when the bulk of the rental property's cost is in the land rather than the improvements.

PASSIVE-ACTIVITY INTEREST EXPENSE

One aspect related to the passive loss rules that requires special attention is the treatment of interest expense. As discussed in Chapter 11, Congress has imposed severe limitations on the deduction of interest. Interest expense incurred by a taxpayer to finance an investment in a passive activity is subject to the passive loss rules and is not

---

[24] Temp. Reg. § 1.469-2T(f).

[25] *Krukowski*, 114 T.C. 366 (2000).

considered investment interest. Similarly, interest expense incurred by an activity that is considered passive (e.g., a partnership if the taxpayer is a limited partner) is subject to the passive loss rules.[26]

> **Example 33.** Dr. P borrowed $50,000 and invested it by acquiring an interest in a limited partnership that produces movies. Interest on the loan for the year is $5,000. P can deduct the interest only to the extent of any passive income that he may have.

> **Example 34.** Assume the partnership above incurs interest expense related to loans obtained to acquire equipment used in its operations. The interest is treated as a normal deduction and is used in arriving at the partnership's net income or loss for the year. This year, the partnership suffered a net loss including deductions for interest expense. Dr. P is allowed to deduct his share of the loss only to the extent he has passive income from other activities.

✔ CHECK YOUR KNOWLEDGE

Try the following true-false questions.

Review Question 1. This year T's tax records revealed that he had income consisting of a salary of $90,000, dividends of $10,000, and a capital gain from the sale of stock of $5,000. In addition, he received a Schedule K-1 from a partnership in which he is a limited partner. According to the K-1, his share of the partnership's loss for the year was $50,000. T can deduct $15,000 of this loss (i.e., to the extent of his passive dividend and capital gain income).

False. While a taxpayer is entitled to deduct passive losses to the extent of passive income, passive income does not include dividends, interest, capital gains, and the like, which are considered portfolio income.

Review Question 2. A passive loss that cannot be deducted in the current year is generally suspended. The suspended loss is deductible only in the year in which the property to which the loss relates is sold, since the sale affirms the fact that the taxpayer has actually suffered an economic loss.

False. The above is true for the most part, but suspended passive losses are not frozen to thaw only when the taxpayer sells his or her interest. Passive losses that cannot be deducted in a particular year are carried over to the following year and treated as if they occurred in that subsequent year. Accordingly, the suspended loss can be deducted to the extent that the taxpayer has passive income in the following year. In addition, the taxpayer is allowed to deduct the suspended losses whenever the property to which the loss relates is sold.

Review Question 3. A capital gain from the sale of stock in an S corporation in which the taxpayer does not materially participate is considered portfolio income.

False. Capital gains are normally considered portfolio income, but when such gain arises from the sale of the taxpayer's interest in a passive activity, it is treated as passive income.

Review Question 4. The passive loss rules do not apply to regular C corporations since the losses do not flow through and are not available to the individual shareholders.

---

[26] § 163(d)(3)(B).

False. The passive loss rules do apply to personal service corporations and closely held corporations (i.e., corporations where five or fewer individuals own more than 50 percent of the stock). Personal service corporations must play by the same rules applicable to individuals. Closely held corporations, however, are allowed to offset passive losses against income from operations *other than* portfolio income.

Review Question 5. Moe, Larry, and Curly pooled all of their savings to start a new restaurant, Stooges. Stooges is operated as an S corporation, and its stock is owned equally by the threesome. In its first year, the restaurant produced a loss. Depending on the circumstances, Moe may be able to deduct his share of the loss this year while Larry and Curly may not be able to deduct their shares.

True. Whether a deduction is allowed for the loss depends on whether the taxpayer materially participates in the activity. Moe may be actively involved on a daily basis, and Larry and Curly may be passive investors. In such a case, only Moe would be able to deduct the loss currently.

Review Question 6. D operates a small bed-and-breakfast motel. Most of his customers rent rooms for one or two days. D's operation is not considered a rental activity for purposes of the passive-loss rules.

True. An activity is not considered a rental for purposes of the passive-loss rules if the average period of customer use is seven days or less.

Review Question 7. T owns a duplex and rents it out. She normally signs six-month leases with her tenants. Any loss related to the rental is considered a passive loss and is not deductible regardless of T's participation.

True. This activity is considered a rental since the average period of customer use exceeds 30 days and T does not provide any extraordinary services. Losses on long-term rental real estate are normally not deductible except to the extent of passive income unless the taxpayer can qualify under one of two exceptions. First, she is permitted to deduct up to $25,000 of losses from rental real estate if she actively participates and her adjusted gross income is less than $150,000. In addition, a special exception allows individuals who spend more than 50 percent of their time in real property businesses and more than 750 hours in such businesses to treat the activities as nonrental and deduct any losses if they materially participate in such activities.

Review Question 8. Several years ago, Q purchased an interest in a limited partnership. This year his share of the partnership's loss was $10,000. Assuming Q's adjusted gross income is $80,000, he may deduct the loss since it is less than $25,000.

False. The loss would be treated as a passive loss since Q does not materially participate in the partnership activity. The de minimis exception that enables a taxpayer to deduct up to $25,000 of passive losses annually applies only to losses from rental real estate activities in which the taxpayer actively participates.

Review Question 9. B opened her first Planet Jupiter Cafe five years ago in Aspen. Now she has five restaurants, each located in a different resort. Since each store is located in a separate city, she must treat each store as a separate activity.

False. A taxpayer is required to treat one or more activities as a single activity if the activities constitute an appropriate economic unit (AEU). The Regulations give the taxpayer a great deal of flexibility in determining what constitutes an AEU. Thus, the taxpayer could

treat each as a separate activity, combine all and treat as a single activity, or use some other grouping that may be appropriate under the Regulations.

Review Question 10. B is a college professor who recently got involved in a mail-order smoke alarm business. This year he spent about 100 hours in the activity, taking orders and arranging to fill them. B materially participates in the business.

True. Under the general rule, a taxpayer is considered a material participant if he or she spends more than 500 hours in the activity during the year. Although B does not meet the general rule, he does meet an alternative test; that is, his participation constitutes substantially all of the participation in the activity. Therefore the activity is not a passive activity.

Review Question 11. G owns two businesses, a convenience grocery store and a dry cleaners. For the last several years, the grocery has not done as well as G had hoped and she has lost money. This year, G did not play as much golf as usual and spent about 400 hours trying to turn the business around. She spent about 300 hours at the cleaners. Each business has a number of full-time employees. G may offset any loss attributable to the grocery store against the profits from her dry cleaners.

True. The restaurant and the dry cleaners are considered significant participation activities since G spends more than 100 hours in each. If the total participation in all SPAs exceeds 500 hours, the taxpayer is deemed to materially participate in each of the activities. In this case, the total participation in all SPAs exceeds the 500-hour threshold, and G is therefore deemed to materially participate in each of the activities. Thus, she can use the loss in the grocery activity to offset the income from the cleaning business.

Review Question 12. Same as above, except G spends 100 hours at the cleaners, 300 hours at the grocery, and the remaining time at the beach. G may offset any loss attributable to the grocery against the profits from her dry cleaners.

False. In this case, G's combined participation in the SPAs does not exceed 500 hours. This is the "heads we win, tails you lose" situation: the loss is passive, the income is nonpassive, and the two cannot be combined.

Review Question 13. J borrowed $100,000 to purchase an interest in the Lockwood Limited Partnership, which operates several apartment complexes. This year J paid $8,000 interest on the loan to acquire his interest. In addition, J's share of the partnership's losses was $10,000. J has no passive income. The loss is a passive loss and cannot be deducted, but the interest is treated as investment interest and is deductible to the extent of J's investment income.

False. J simply treats the $8,000 of interest expense as another operating expense of the partnership, increasing the loss from $10,000 to $18,000. None of the loss, including the interest, is deductible.

RENTAL OF RESIDENCE (VACATION HOME RENTALS)

Section 280A imposes restrictions on the deduction of expenses related to rental of a residence if the taxpayer is considered as using the residence primarily for personal purposes rather than for making a profit. These restrictions are aimed at the perceived abuse existing in the area of vacation home rental. Prior to the enactment of § 280A,

many felt that personal enjoyment was the predominant motive for purchasing a vacation home. Any rental of the vacation home served merely to minimize the personal expense of ownership and not to produce income.

BASIC RULES

In 1976, Congress prescribed an objective method for ascertaining the purpose of the rental activity as well as the amount of the deduction. According to this approach, the expenses incurred by the taxpayer in owning and operating the home (e.g., interest, taxes, maintenance, utilities, and depreciation) must first be allocated between personal use and rental use. The deductibility of the expenses allocated to each then depends on whether the home is considered the taxpayer's *residence or rental property*. This latter determination is made based on the owner's personal use and the amount of rental activity.[27]

1. *Nominal Rentals:* If the residence is rented out fewer than 15 days, all rental income is excluded from gross income and no deduction is allowed for rental expenses. Otherwise allowable deductions, such as those for qualified residence interest, real estate taxes, and casualty losses may be deducted *from* A.G.I.

2. *Used as a "Residence":* If the taxpayer uses the vacation home for more than 14 days or 10 percent of the number of days the property is actually rented out, whichever is greater, the home is treated as his or her residence and deductions are restricted as explained below. A typical taxpayer caught by this rule is the owner of a vacation home who uses it for more than two weeks and rents it out to defray the cost.

    a. *Expenses Allocable to the Rental Use:* These expenses are deductible to the extent of gross income less otherwise allowable deductions. Any deductions in excess of gross income can be carried over and deducted to the extent of any future income. These expenses are deductible *for* A.G.I. since they are related to rental use. Note that the passive-loss rules do not apply since the property is used as a residence and not a rental.

    b. *Expenses Allocable to Personal Use:* Since these expenses are considered personal, they may be deducted only if they are specifically authorized by the Code. Allocable property taxes are deductible without limitation as an itemized deduction since such expenses are fully deductible regardless of the activity in which they are incurred. Interest expense *may* be deductible as an itemized deduction. Allocable interest is normally qualified residence interest since the home—*in this case*—is considered the taxpayer's residence (e.g., because it is used more than 14 days). However, if the home is not the primary or secondary residence of the taxpayer (e.g., the taxpayer has several vacation homes), no deduction would be available. The other operating expenses are not deductible.

3. *Used as "Rental Property":* If the taxpayer does not use the property extensively (i.e., more than the greater of 14 days or 10 percent of the number of days rented out), then the property is effectively treated as rental property.

    a. *Expenses Allocable to the Rental Use:* These expenses are deductible subject only to the restrictions on passive losses. If the property's average rental period is either (1) 1–7 days or (2) 8–30 days *and* significant services are provided, the property is not rental property under the passive loss rules.

---

[27] §§ 280A(c)(5) and 280A(d) through (g).

Thus, the treatment of any loss depends on whether the taxpayer materially participates in this "nonrental activity." If the taxpayer materially participates, any loss would not be passive and would therefore be fully deductible. (See *Example 20* earlier in this chapter.) If the property is considered a rental (e.g., perhaps under the facts-and-circumstances test or if the rental is 8–30 days and no significant services are provided) and the taxpayer is considered as having met the active participation standard, the taxpayer may qualify for the rental exception under the passive loss rules. This would allow the taxpayer to deduct up to $25,000 in losses annually. Any deductions would be for A.G.I.

b. *Expenses Allocable to Personal Use:* As noted above, since these expenses are personal, they may be deducted only if they are specifically authorized by the Code. In this case, property taxes would continue to be fully deductible. On the other hand, none of the interest expense would be deductible as qualified residence interest since the vacation home is not considered a "residence" (because the taxpayer did *not* use it more than 14 days). However, the excess interest expense would be treated as investment interest and could be deducted to the extent of investment income. Other operating expenses would not be deductible.

This treatment is summarized in Exhibit 12-1.

EXHIBIT 12-1
Vacation Homes—Summary of § 280A Rules

Character of vacation home:	Residence	Rental property
Characterization:		
Personal use exceeding the greater of	Yes	No
1. 14 days, or		
2. 10 percent of days rented out		
Expenses allocable to rental use:	Limited to gross income by § 280A	Limited by passive-loss rules Rental exception may apply
Expenses allocable to personal use:		
Taxes	Deductible	Deductible
Interest	Qualified residence interest	Investment interest
Other	Not deductible	Not deductible

For purposes of the owner use test, the number of days a unit is rented out does not include any day the unit is used for personal purposes. The unit is generally treated as used for personal purposes on any day where the owner or a member of his or her family uses it for any portion of the day for personal purposes or the unit is rented at less than a fair rental.[28] A day on which the taxpayer spends at least two-thirds of the time at the unit (or if less than two-thirds then at least eight hours) on repairs is not counted as a personal day. This is true even though individuals who accompany the taxpayer do not perform repairs or maintenance.[29]

---

[28] § 280A(d)(2).

[29] Prop. Reg. § 1.280A-1(e)(4) and § 280A(d)(2).

Example 35. In 1985, Floyd Toups and his wife purchased a vacation home for $120,000. The unit was one of 155 individually owned "cottages" located at Callaway Gardens, a favorite vacation resort in Pine Mountain, Georgia, about 70 miles south of Atlanta. The units were marketed and managed by a development company that received 50% of the net rental income for its services. Each owner was entitled to rent-free use of the cottage for no more than 14 days during the year. On their 1988, 1989, and 1990 returns, the Toupses took the position that the cottage, which was generating losses, was a *nonrental* activity since the average period of customer use of the cottage was seven days or less, and accordingly the Toupses deducted the losses on their Schedule C on the grounds that they materially participated in the activity. However, the IRS disagreed and assessed deficiencies exceeding $3,000 for each year. In the Tax Court, the Toupses attempted to justify their position, explaining that they had spent 341 hours each year in activities related to the rental of the unit. They listed 13 activities, which they believed supported their claim. According to the couple they (1) provided funds for the purchase; (2) prepared an annual budget; (3) prepared a cash flow analysis; (4) provided a rental agency for renting their unit; (5) marketed the resort and rental of the cottage; (6) met with other owners; (7) established rental rates for the cottages with other owners; (8) inspected the cottage and common areas at least twice a year; (9) reviewed monthly reports received from the rental agent; (10) reviewed other correspondence from the rental agent; (11) reviewed advertising brochures about the resort received from the rental agent; (12) received and deposited net revenues received from the rental; and (13) issued checks for expenses of the cottage. The Tax Court agreed that the property was not "rental property" under the passive-loss rules and, therefore, did not qualify for the $25,000 allowance available for rental real estate. Unfortunately, the court did not agree with the taxpayers' claim that they materially participated in the activity. The court found that the activities of the taxpayer did not constitute material participation because they were not involved in the day-to-day operation of their cottage or in its management. The activities of the taxpayers were considered to be activities of an investor, and therefore their losses were passive.[30]

ALLOCATION OF EXPENSES

As discussed above, the treatment of expenses incurred in operating a vacation home varies depending on whether the expenses are allocated to rental or personal use. Consequently, the critical first step in applying the vacation home rules is allocation of the expenses. Once expenses are properly allocated between rental and personal use, the appropriate limitations can be applied.

Vacation home expenses can be classified as either direct and indirect. Direct expenses are those that are *not* related to the general operation or maintenance of the unit but which are incurred to obtain tenants.[31] For example, advertising, brokers' fees, office supplies, and depreciation on office equipment used in the rental activity are considered directly related to the rental. These direct expenses reduce gross rental receipts to arrive at gross rental income. All other expenses are considered indirect expenses—including otherwise allowable deductions such as interest and taxes—and must be allocated *between* personal and rental use.

In allocating the expenses between personal and rental use, two different methods are used. Under the so-called *Bolton* approach, otherwise allowable deductions such as interest and taxes are assumed to *accrue daily* regardless of use.[32] Consequently, the

[30] *Floyd A. and Joanna Toups*, 66 T.C.M. 370, T.C. Memo 1993-359.

[31] Prop. Reg. § 1.280A-3(d)(2).

[32] *Dorance D. Bolton*, 77 T.C. 104 (1982), aff'd. at 82-2 USTC ¶9699, 51 AFTR2d 83-305 (CA-9, 1982).

fraction for allocating these items to the rental use was:

$$\text{Otherwise allowable deduction} \times \frac{\text{Number of rental days}}{365} = \text{Portion attributable to rental use}$$

In contrast, expenses such as utilities, maintenance, and depreciation are considered a *function of use.* As a result, the fraction used for allocating these items to the rental use was:

$$\text{Operating expenses} \times \frac{\text{Number of rental days}}{\text{Rental + Personal days}} = \text{Portion attributable to rental use}$$

The method of allocating expenses and their treatment is summarized in Exhibit 12-2 below.

Note that the court's approach in *Bolton* (which uses a denominator of 365 rather than total personal and rental days used) allocates less interest and taxes to the rental portion and, therefore, more to the residential or personal portion. This approach enables the taxpayer to deduct a larger amount of expenses allocable to the rental. At the same time, this method increases the amount of the itemized deduction for interest and taxes. The end result is that a larger deduction can be secured using the *Bolton* approach. Unfortunately, the IRS continues to oppose *Bolton* so taxpayers must proceed with caution.[33] The example below follows *Bolton*.

> **Example 36.** A owns a condominium in a ski resort. During the year, A uses the condominium as a secondary residence for 30 days and rents it out for 90 days. The condominium is not used the remainder of the year. During the year, A's rental agent, R, collected rents of $5,000. The agent's standard fee was 30% of rents; therefore the charge was $1,500 and R sent Form 1099 to A showing net rental income of $3,500.

EXHIBIT 12-2
Vacation Homes—Expense Allocation Rules

Type of Expense	Personal Use	Rental Use
Directly related (advertising, brokers' fees)	None allocated	Gross rental receipts – Directly related expenses Sch. E Gross rental income
Otherwise allowable (qualified residence interest, taxes, etc.)	Itemized deduction*	– Otherwise allowable Sch. E Limit on indirect rental expenses
Indirect (maintenance, depreciation, utilities, etc.)	Not deductible	– Indirect expenses Sch E**

* **Interest allocated to personal use:**
   (1) if the property is treated as a residence, deductible as qualified residence interest;
   (2) if not a residence, the interest may be deductible as investment interest to the extent of investment income.
   Taxes allocated to personal use are fully deductible in either case.

****Indirect expenses allocated to rental use:**
   (1) if the property is treated as a residence, such expenses are limited to remaining rental income;
   (2) if not a residence but a rental, passive loss rules apply unless not considered a rental (i.e., average customer use does not exceed seven days);
   (3) if rental for passive loss purposes, limited to passive income and $25,000 allowance may be available;
   (4) if not a rental for passive activity purposes, loss deductible if materially participate

---

[33] § 280A(e). The IRS continues to take the position that all expenses should be allocated based on use. See *Residential Rental Property*, IRS Publication 527 (2006), p. 8.

Total expenses for the entire year include maintenance and utilities of $1,000, interest of $6,200, taxes of $1,100, and $2,000 depreciation on the entire cost of the unit.

A's use for 30 days is more than 14 days, the greater of 14 or 9 days (10% of the 90 days rented). Therefore, the unit is treated as a residence. For this reason, expenses attributable to the rental are deductible to the extent of gross income as reduced by otherwise allowable deductions (the interest and taxes). Deductions are computed and deducted in the *following order:*

Gross rental receipts...	$ 5,000
Deduct directly related expenses (brokerage fee)	−1,500
Gross rental income	$ 3,500
Deduct allocable portion of otherwise allowable deductions:	
Interest and taxes [$7,300 × (90 ÷ 365)]......................	−1,800
Gross income limitation	$ 1,700
Deduct allocable portion of deductions other than those otherwise allowable and depreciation:	
Utilities and maintenance [$1,000 × 90 ÷ (30 + 90)]	− 750
Gross income limitation	$ 950
Deduct allocable portion of depreciation:	
Depreciation [$2,000 × 90 ÷ (30 + 90)] = $1,500 but limited to $950 balance of gross income	− 950
Net income...	$ 0

All of the above deductions are *for* A.G.I. The balance of interest and taxes not allocated to the rental use, $5,500 ($7,300 − $1,800), is deductible if the taxpayer itemizes deductions. Note that the interest in this case is qualified residence interest since the unit is treated as A's residence. The deduction for maintenance and utilities is not limited by gross income since all of these expenses attributable to the rental activity are deductible. The $250 ($1,000 − $750) remaining balance of maintenance and utilities would not be deductible in any case since it represents the expenses attributable to personal use. Of the remaining depreciation balance of $1,050 ($2,000 − $950), $550 ($1,500 − $950) attributable to the rental is not deductible due to the gross income limitation but may be carried over to subsequent years. The other $500 of depreciation is not deductible since it is the portion attributable to personal use. Also note that only the $950 of depreciation allowed is treated as a reduction in the basis of A's condominium.

Example 37. Assume the same facts as in *Example 34*, except that A used the condominium for 10 days rather than 30. Also assume that the rental is on a three-month basis to locals and no services are provided. In such case, the condominium would be treated as rental property rather than as a residence since A stayed less than 14 days. In addition, the $25,000 rental exception of the passive loss rules would apply since there is a long-term rental and no significant services are provided. A's deduction would be computed as follows:

Gross rental receipts.	$ 5,000
Deduct directly related expenses (brokerage fee)	−1,500
Gross rental income	$ 3,500
Deduct allocable portion of otherwise allowable deductions	
($7,300 × 90 ÷ 365)	−1,800
Deduct allocable portion of utilities and maintenance	
[$1,000 × 90 ÷ (90 + 10)].	− 900
Deduct allocable portion of depreciation	
($2,000 × 90 ÷ (90 + 10)].	−1,800
Loss	$ (1,000)

In this case, a loss is created that may offset any other income of the taxpayer under the $25,000 rental loss exception. In contrast to *Example 34* above, however, the balance of the interest expense, $5,500 ($7,300 − $1,800), would not be deductible as qualified residence interest since the property does not qualify as a residence. Nevertheless, the taxpayer may be able to deduct the amount as investment interest to the extent of any net investment income that he or she may have from other investments. Lacking investment income, the taxpayer would be better off using the condominium more, in order that he could qualify it as a second residence and deduct the interest. The balance of the other expenses would not be deductible.

The vacation home rules, as discussed above, could operate to eliminate legitimate deductions for those taxpayers who convert their personal residence for rental during the year. In these cases, the owner usually uses the residence for more than 14 days and thus deductions are limited. However, § 280A(d) provides relief for taxpayers in these situations. The provision accomplishes this goal by not counting as personal use days any days of personal use during the year immediately before (or after) the rental period begins (or ends). This rule, often referred to as the *qualified rental period exception*, applies only if the rental period is at least a year (or if less than a year, the house is sold at the end of the rental period).

> **Example 38.** B lived in her home from January through July. In August, she moved into a condominium and decided to convert her old home to rental property. B was able to find a tenant who leased the old home for a year. Under the normal rules of § 280A, B's deductions related to the old home would be limited to gross income since her personal use exceeded 14 days. The relief measure of § 280A(d) removes this limitation because the seven months of personal use preceding the one-year rental period are not counted as personal use days. As a result, B would treat the lease as a rental activity and could deduct expenses subject to the passive loss rules, possibly qualifying for the $25,000 exception.

✓ CHECK YOUR KNOWLEDGE

Review Question 1. During the Olympics held in Atlanta during 1996, many Georgians left town and rented their homes out for the two weeks the games were in town. It was rumored that some of the mansions were rented for more than $100,000 during this time. How would these temporary landlords treat the income?

Under § 280A, if the home is rented out for less than 15 days, all of the rental income is excluded and none of the expenses allocable to the rental period are deductible. Consequently, these temporary landlords received a real windfall because they were allowed to exclude all of the income.

Review Question 2. T owns a condominium in Vail. This year his rental agent was able to rent it out for 100 days (most guests stayed for six days). Unfortunately, he was able to use the condo for personal purposes for only one week in January because of a skiing accident in which he broke his shoulder. Interest expense and taxes allocable to the personal use were $500. The net loss attributable to the rental during the remainder of the year was $4,000. What amount can T deduct? Is the property considered rental property subject to the passive loss rules?

Since the personal use was nominal (i.e., not more than the greater of ten percent of the number of days rented or two weeks), the property is not considered a residence. Moreover, it is not considered rental property under the passive loss rules since the average rental period was less than eight days. Thus, it is considered a nonrental activity with the treatment dependent on whether T materially participates in the activity. Since he does not materially participate, the loss is a passive loss and is not deductible unless he has other passive income. The interest attributable to the period of personal use is not qualified residence interest since the unit did not qualify as a residence. Instead the interest is treated as investment interest and is deductible to the extent of investment income.

Review Question 3. W owns a condominium in St. John in the Caribbean. She rented it out for seven months (one month at a time) during the year but used it personally for the entire month of January. Can W treat the activity as a rental activity and take advantage of the $25,000 de minimis exception that would allow her to deduct a loss from the property?

No. If a taxpayer uses a home for more than two weeks or 10 percent of the number of days the unit is rented, she treats the home as a residence. In this case, the taxpayer used the home 31 days for personal purposes, thereby exceeding the threshold and converting the property to a residence. Any interest is deductible as qualified residence interest, assuming this is a first or second home. On the other hand, rental expenses can be deducted only to the extent of rental income. The excess expenses may be carried over and deducted in subsequent years to the extent the unit generates income. The passive loss rules do not apply, and the $25,000 allowance is not available.

PROBLEM MATERIALS

DISCUSSION QUESTIONS

12-1   *Tax Shelters and the Solution.* In 1982, T purchased for $10,000 an interest in Neptune III, a limited partnership created by Dandy Development Company to finance and build a 25-story office building in downtown Houston. T, who was in the 50 percent tax bracket, hoped that this investment would significantly cut her taxes.

    a. Explain the features of the investment that during that period made such investments attractive and might produce the benefits desired by T.

    b. Explain what steps Congress took in 1986 to eliminate the benefits of investments in such activities as Neptune III. Comment in some detail on the approach used by Congress to accomplish its objective.

    c. What steps might you have suggested had you been advising Congress on the restriction of tax shelter?

12-2   *Effect of Code § 469.* D owns and operates several ski rental shops in Vail, Aspen, Beaver Creek, and Steamboat Springs. Over the years, the shops have had their ups and downs, with profits in some years, losses in others. Recently, D has spent less and less time at the shop, letting his employees do most of the work.

    a. What is the significance should the business be characterized as a passive activity?

b. Should D worry about his business being treated as a passive activity? When is an activity considered passive?

c. Does the fact that D's business is a rental operation have any bearing on the nature of the activity?

d. What are the aggregation or grouping rules and why might they be important in D's case?

12-3 *Taxpayers Subject to § 469.* Dr. R has been quite successful over the years. She left St. James hospital in 1981 and started her own sports medicine practice, The Sports Institute Inc., a regular C corporation. After building this operation into a thriving practice, she branched out. In 1990, she and a good friend opened their own restaurant, The Diner, a partnership. In 1993, her college roommate persuaded R to invest and buy stock in a new venture, Compatible PCS, a corporation that manufactured personal computers. Compatible PCS was owned by R and three other individuals and operated as a regular C corporation until this year, when it converted to S status. Dr. R's other investments include a single family house that she rents out, a limited partnership interest in an oil and gas operation, and a limited partnership interest in a business that develops land into shopping centers. Explain how R is affected by the passive loss rules.

12-4 *Definition of an Activity and Planning.* D owns several businesses, including an indoor soccer facility, a gas station adjacent to the soccer facility (he bought it with the intention of someday expanding the soccer facility), and a fast-food restaurant across the street from the soccer facility. Within the soccer facility, he has rented space to a local soccer retail store. He also rents space in the facility to another company, which operates a small bar and restaurant. In any one year, each business may be profitable or may have losses. For simplicity, assume each business is operated as a sole proprietorship.

a. Assuming one of the businesses is profitable, would D prefer passive or active income?

b. Assuming one of the businesses has losses, would D prefer a passive or active loss?

c. Discuss the passive loss rules, how they might apply to D, and what planning might be considered. Identify as many questions as possible that might be asked in determining how the passive loss rules apply to D.

12-5 *Aggregating Activities.* Aggregation of activities may be required for purposes of the material participation tests.

a. Explain the general rules concerning aggregation and their purpose.

b. Explain when this rule is beneficial and when it is detrimental for the taxpayer.

12-6 *Rental Activities and Material Participation.* T owns a 10-unit apartment complex. He not only manages the apartments but also performs all of the routine maintenance and repairs as well as keeping the books. Most of the leases that he signs with tenants are for one year. This year the complex produced a loss of $30,000. How will T treat the loss, assuming his adjusted gross income from other sources is $90,000?

12-7 *Recharacterization.* Briefly explain the purpose of the recharacterization rules and why they must not be overlooked when dealing with passive activities.

12-8 *Credits from a Passive Activity.* P is considering rehabilitating a home in a historic neighborhood. She hopes to qualify for both the rehabilitation credit and the low-income housing credit.

    a. Assuming she qualifies, explain how she will compute the amount of credit that she may claim.

    b. P's accountant has explained the limitations that apply to losses and has indicated to P that any losses on the rental that are denied currently will ultimately be allowed once P sells the property. Can the same be said of credits?

12-9 *Grouping Activities.* Urged by their accountants to reduce their tax liability, a group of orthopedic surgeons invested in real estate that produced passive losses. Prior to 1986, these losses did in fact serve as tax shelters. After 1986, however, the passive loss rules significantly restricted the tax benefits of the investments. Consequently, the accountants prodded the doctors to form a partnership to acquire and operate X-ray equipment. The doctors do not participate in the X-ray partnership, and, therefore, any income produced by the partnership is passive income. Most of the income from operation of the partnership is derived from services provided to the doctors themselves. Will this scheme successfully produce passive income that can be used to absorb passive losses?

12-10 *Interest Expense.* This year Dr. Z purchased a 20 percent interest in a partnership that is building an office building in downtown Dallas. To finance the acquisition, he used his line of credit at the bank and borrowed $100,000. As a result, he paid $10,000 in interest during the year.

    a. How will Dr. Z treat the interest expense?

    b. After the building was completed, the partnership secured permanent financing. This year the partnership paid mortgage interest of $700,000, of which $14,000 represented Dr. Z's allocable share. How will Dr. Z treat the interest?

PROBLEMS

12-11 *Identifying Activities.* For each of the following situations, indicate the number of activities in which the taxpayer participates.

    a. S owns and operates an ice cream store in Southwoods Mall. He is also a camera buff and owns a camera shop in the same mall.

    b. T owns a small "strip" shopping center that houses 10 businesses, including T's own video store. This year T received $40,000 in income from renting out space in the shopping center and grossed $60,000 from her video store.

    c. O owns five greeting card stores spread all around Denver.

    d. P owns 10 gas stations throughout the state of Georgia. Each station not only sells gas but also sells groceries. Seven of the stations derive 60 percent of their income from gas sales and 40 percent from food sales. Two of the stations derive 55 percent of their income from food sales and 45 percent from gas sales. One station also provides auto repair services and derives one-third of its income from each operation.

    e. E owns a beer distributorship and ten liquor stores throughout Minneapolis. Sixty percent of the distributorship sales are to the liquor stores.

12-12 *Combining Activities.* T owns a 70 percent interest in each of three partnerships: a radio station (WAKO), a minor league baseball team (the Harrisville Hippos), and a video and film company (Dynamite Productions) that produces short subjects for television, including advertisements. In any particular year, one business may be profitable while another may be unprofitable. Each business is at a different location. Each business also prepares its own financial statements and has its own management, although T participates extensively in the management of all three partnerships. Any financing needed for the three partnerships is usually obtained from Second National,

a local bank. The radio station broadcasts all of the Hippo games, and the production company often prepares material for local television spots on the Hippos. Occasionally, some employees in one partnership assist the other partnership in periods of peak activity or emergency. Explain how the passive loss rules apply to T in this case.

12-13 *Material Participation.* During the week, A is a mild-mannered reporter for the local paper. On the weekends, he is a partner with his brother-in-law, B, in a small van-conversion operation in Elkhart. The two typically work seven or eight hours on most Saturdays during the year. This year, the partnership suffered a loss of $10,000.
   a. How will A treat the loss?
   b. What planning might you suggest?

12-14 *Participation Defined.* Three recent Purdue graduates—C, D, and E—formed their own lawn treatment company. Each of the three participates on a part-time basis because each is otherwise employed on a full-time basis. In this, their first year of operations, C spent 40 hours, D spent 70 hours, and E contributed 80 hours. E's wife also kept the books for the partnership. Explain whether C, D, and E satisfy the material participation test.

12-15 *Material Participation.* F is an accountant with a large C.P.A. firm. She also has an interest in two partnerships: a night club and a family-owned drugstore. F maintains the accounting records for each partnership, spending 200 hours working for the night club and 400 hours for the drugstore.
   a. How will F treat any losses that the partnerships might have?
   b. How will F treat any income that the partnerships might have?

12-16 *Material Participation.* In 1986, H started his own replacement window business, Sting Construction, an S corporation. Up until 1999 H had been the sole shareholder. In 1999 he sold 90 percent of his stock to J and K, who continued the business. From time to time, H still provides advice to J and K. This year, H spent 300 hours working for the company. J and K each devoted 1,500 hours to the business. Unfortunately, the corporation suffered a loss this year because of a downturn in the economy. How will H treat the loss?

12-17 *Rental or Nonrental Activities.* Indicate whether the following are rental or nonrental activities.
   a. P owns an airplane. She has an arrangement with a flying club at a small airport to lease the plane out on a short-term basis to its students. Most of the time the plane is rented for two to three hours.
   b. Q owns a condominium in Aspen that he rents out during the year. The average stay is one week. Q has arranged to provide daily maid and linen service for the unit. In addition, his monthly condominium fee pays for maintenance of the common areas.
   c. S and his wife, T, own White Silver Sands, a posh resort on the coast of Florida. As part of its package, the resort provides everything a vacationer could want (daily maid service, free use of the golf, tennis, and pool facilities, an on-site masseuse, etc.). The average stay is two weeks.
   d. Z owns a duplex near the University of Texas that she normally rents out to students on a long-term basis. The average stay is nine months. Z provides typical landlord services such as repairs and maintenance.
   e. B owns Quiet Quarters, a retirement home for the elderly. The home's staff includes a physician and several nurses.

    f.   C owns and operates Body Beautiful, a fitness club. The club has over 1,000 members. who have use of the club daily from 6 a.m. to 11 p.m.

    g.   D owns a 200-acre parcel of land on the outskirts of Lubbock. The land is worth $700,000 (basis $200,000). During the year, D leased the land to a local car enthusiast who used it as a raceway. D collected rents of $5,000.

12-18 *Passive Activities.* G is the head chef for Half-Way Airlines, making a salary of $70,000 a year. In addition, his portfolio income is about $20,000 a year. Over the years, G has made numerous investments and has been a participant in many ventures. Indicate whether the passive activity rules would apply in each of the following situations:

    a.   A $10,000 loss from G's interest in Flimsy Films, a limited partnership. G is a limited partner.

    b.   A $5,000 loss from G's interest as a shareholder in D's Bar and Grill, an S corporation. G and his wife operate the bar. Each spent 300 hours working there in the current year.

    c.   G and his friend, F, are equal partners in a partnership that produces and markets a Texas-style barbecue sauce. G leaves the management of the day-to-day operations to F. However, G spent 130 hours working in the business during the current year. For the year, the partnership had income of $15,000. Assume that this is G's only investment.

    d.   Same as (c) except G has an ownership interest in three other distinctly different activities (e.g., construction and consulting). He spends 130 hours in each of the four activities.

    e.   G is a 10 percent partner in a restaurant consulting firm. The firm operates the business on the bottom floor of a three-story building it owns. The firm leases the other two floors to a law firm and a real estate company. The consulting side of the business reported a $100,000 profit from consulting, $5,000 in interest income, and had a loss from the rental operation.

    f.   G is the sole owner of Try, Inc., a regular C corporation that produces G's special salad dressing. The corporation had an operating profit of $4,000. In addition, Try, Inc. had interest income of $5,000 and a $7,000 loss from its investment in a real estate limited partnership in which it was a limited partner.

12-19 *Passive-Activity Limitations.* M is a successful banker. Two years ago, M's 27-year-old son, J, asked his dad to become his partner in opening a sporting goods store. M agreed and contributed $50,000 for a 50 percent interest in the partnership. J operates the store on his own, receiving little advice from his father. Information regarding M's financial activities reveals the following for the past two years:

Year	Salary	Interest Income	Partnership Income (Loss)
2009	$100,000	$20,000	$(40,000)
2010	100,000	20,000	12,000

All parties are cash basis, calendar year taxpayers. Answer the following questions.

    a.   How did M's investment in the partnership affect his A.G.I. in 2009?

    b.   How did M's investment in the partnership affect his A.G.I. in 2010?

    c.   Would your answer to (b) change if the partnership had a loss in 2010 and the income shown was from M's interest as a limited partner in a real estate venture?

    d.   On January 1, 2011, M sold his interest in the partnership to his son for a $40,000 gain. What effect?

12-20   *Passive-Activity Limitations: Rental Property.* L, single, is the chief of surgery at a local hospital. During the year, L earned a salary of $120,000. L owns a four-unit apartment building that she rents out unfurnished. The current tenants have one-year leases, which expire at various times. This year, the property produced a loss of $30,000 due to accelerated depreciation. L is actively involved in the rental activity, making many of the decisions regarding leases, repairs, etc.
   a. How much of the loss may L deduct?
   b. Would the answer to (a) change if L materially participated?

12-21   *Rental Real Estate.* M and H are real estate moguls. Together they have created a number of partnerships that own more than 50 shopping malls as well as a few office buildings, apartments, and warehouses. Most of their lease agreements with their mall tenants are tied to the tenant's gross receipts. Unfortunately, with the downturn in the economy, several of the mall projects have produced substantial losses. How will M and H treat their share of the losses?

12-22   *Suspended Losses.* When tax shelter activity was at its highest, G was one of its biggest proponents. Currently, she still owns an interest in several limited partnerships. She is now considering what she should do in light of the passive loss rules. To help her make this decision, she has put together her best guess as to the performance of her investments over the next two years. These are shown below.

Activity	2009	2010
X	$(7,000)	$(2,000)
Y	(3,000)	(9,000)
Z	6,000	1,000

   a. Determine the amount of suspended loss for each activity at the end of 2009 and 2010.
   b. Assume the same facts as in (a) above, except assume that in 2010 G sells the Y activity for a $4,000 gain. Explain the effect of the disposition on any suspended losses G might have, including the amount of suspended losses to be carried forward to 2011.

12-23   *Characterizing Income.* Indicate whether the income in the following situations is passive or nonpassive:
   a. Ten years ago, T purchased a strip of land for $300,000. Shortly thereafter, he built an office building on the land for $100,000. He currently leases the entire building to a large corporation on a ten-year lease for $90,000 annually. This year he sold the building for $700,000.
   b. Q owns a real estate development business that she operates as an S corporation. In 2008, she purchased a vacant lot for $100,000. Q proceeded to put in roads, sewers, and other amenities at a cost of $50,000. Shortly thereafter, she contracted for the construction of a warehouse at a cost of $1 million. Upon completion of the building in September 2008, Q began leasing the space. It was completely leased by June 2009. In December 2010, she sold the property for $2 million.
   c. T owns 100 percent of the stock of Z Corporation, an S corporation that operates a construction company. This year T purchased and leased a crane to the corporation. T received total rents of $10,000.
   d. X operates a travel agency and an office supply store to which she devotes 300 and 100 hours, respectively. The travel agency produced a profit of $10,000 while the office supply business sustained a loss of $40,000.

12-24   *Rental versus Nonrental Activities.* Identify rental activities that would not be considered "rental activities" for purposes of the passive loss rules.

12-25 *Vacation Home Rental.* S owns a condominium in Florida, which he and his family use occasionally. During the year, he used the condominium for 20 days and rented it for 40 days. The remainder of the year, the condominium was vacant. S compiled the following information related to the condominium for the entire year:

Rental income	$1,000
Expenses:	
Interest on mortgage	3,650
Maintenance.	900
Depreciation	6,000

    a. Compute the tax effect of the rental activity on S.

    b. Assuming S only used the condominium personally for ten days, compute the tax effect.

    c. Assuming S only rented the condominium for 14 days, compute the tax effect.

12-26 *Vacation Home-Personal Use Days.* Indicate the number of personal use days in each of the following situations:

    a. Saturday morning, March 3, S drove to Vail to replace a water heater in his vacation home. He arrived in Vail at 9 a.m. and skied until late afternoon, when he retired to his condominium at 6 p.m. After dinner, he worked on replacing the water heater until midnight, when he went to sleep. The following morning he awoke and went skiing until 5 p.m., when he returned home.

    b. Same as (a) except S's wife and family accompanied him. S's family also skied but did not perform any repairs or maintenance related to the vacation home.

    c. T owns a duplex, which he rents. On February 1 of this year, the one-year lease of the tenant living upstairs expired and she moved. Unable to rent the upstairs unit, T moved in on December I and remained through the end of the year.

12-27 *Participation in Real Estate.* When D reached age 60 several years ago, he decided to cut back on the number of hours he devoted to his dental practice. He figured that the income from a mini-warehouse, a trailer park, and a duplex that he owned would sufficiently supplement the income that he derived from his practice. Unfortunately, this year all of these rental activities produced losses. Assuming D has no passive income, indicate whether each of the following statements is true or false. If false, explain why.

    a. D is not allowed to deduct the losses since rental real estate activities are considered passive regardless of the taxpayer's participation.

    b. D is allowed to deduct the losses if most of his working hours are spent managing the real estate properties.

    c. Assuming D works 700 hours managing the properties and his wife spends 200 hours helping him, the couple will be able to deduct the losses on their joint return.

12-28 *At-Risk Computation.* Ajax Construction builds apartments and condominiums. It has developed a unique construction technique. It created forms in the shape of a U in which concreted is poured. The U forms are then inverted and set on top of each other to form the walls and floors of a building. A crane is needed to hoist a U out of the concrete forms and stack it on top of another U. The owners of Ajax Construction, A and B, formed the AB Partnership to purchase the crane and other heavy equipment that would be rented to Ajax and other parties. The partnership is formed on January 1, 2008 by equal partners A and B who each contribute $100,000. The AB Partnership reports on a calendar year and is engaged in activities subject to §465. The following transactions occurred during 2008 and 2009:

7/01/2008	AB Partnership borrows $120,000 from a bank using a recourse note.
10/01/2008	AB Partnership acquires equipment at a cost of $400,000 by giving a nonrecourse note to the vendor.
12/01/2008	AB Partnership reduces the recourse note balance to $30,000 and the nonrecourse note balance to $380,000.
12/31/2008	AB Partnership reports a taxable loss of $420,000 for 2008.
12/31/2008	Partners A and B each withdraw $40,000 from the partnership.
4/01/2009	Partners A and B each contribute $50,000 to the partnership.
12/31/2009	AB Partnership reports taxable income of $120,000

a. Computer partner A's amount at risk on 12/31/2008.
b. Compute partner A's amount at risk on 12/31/2009.

12-29 *At-Risk: Real Estate.* Kingsmill is a limited partnership. The partnership has three equal partners and it deals exclusively in rental real estate. S is the only general partner. On January 1, all three capital accounts were zero. No changes in the accounts occurred during the year. The partnership incurred losses of $75,000 during the year. As of the close of the year, the partnership had liabilities in the form of $20,000 of accounts payable and a $30,000 nonrecourse mortgage obtained from a commercial lender.
a. What losses can the partners claim as deductions on their returns for the year?
b. Would the result be the same if the partnership were engaged in equipment leasing rather than rental real estate?

PART FOUR

ALTERNATIVE MINIMUM TAX AND TAX CREDITS

★ ★ ★ ★ ★ CONTENTS ★ ★ ★ ★ ★

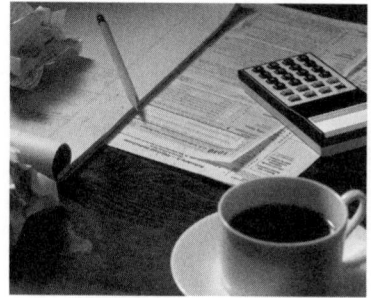

CHAPTER THIRTEEN

THE ALTERNATIVE MINIMUM TAX AND TAX CREDITS

LEARNING OBJECTIVES

Upon completion of this chapter you will be able to:

▶ Explain the tax policy reasons underlying the Alternative Minimum Tax (AMT) system

▶ Understand the conceptual framework of the AMT system and understand the terminology necessary to communicate AMT issues or concerns to a tax professional

▶ Determine the amount of AMT adjustments, preferences, and exemptions, and calculate the alternative minimum taxable income, the tentative minimum tax, and the AMT

▶ Complete Form 6251, Alternative Minimum Tax—Individuals

▶ Explain the tax policy reasons for enacting recent tax incentives in the form of tax credits rather than deductions

▶ Distinguish between nonrefundable tax credits subject to dollar limitations and refundable tax credits, which have no such limitations

▶ Understand the components of the general business credit and be able to calculate the amount of credit allowable with respect to separate components

▶ Identify and calculate the nonbusiness tax credits, including the child tax credit, the dependent care credit, the educational tax credits, the earned income credit, and the minimum tax credit

▶ Understand and apply the tax credit carryover, carryback, and recapture rules

CHAPTER OUTLINE

INTRODUCTION

As may be abundantly clear at this point, the U.S. tax system is replete with rules whose purpose is not simply to raise revenue but also to shape the behavior of its citizens.[1] These so-called tax incentives—*or tax preferences*—are sprinkled throughout the Code, and they come in several forms. There are exclusions, deductions, and credits that stimulate economic activity and/or modify social behavior. For example, accelerated depreciation stimulates the acquisition of machinery and equipment, and percentage depletion boosts investment in natural resources. Research is encouraged through a quick write-off as well as a credit. There are also credits to attract investment in low-income housing and the rehabilitation of old buildings. Still other credits exhort taxpayers to use certain fuels, buy electric cars, and hire certain people. Even more tax benefits await those who invest in empowerment zones, enterprise communities, and small corporations.

Unfortunately, using the Code to solve some of the country's ills has created problems of its own. As the number of tax preferences began to grow, astute tax advisers and promoters saw an opportunity. They began to structure business and investment deals—all perfectly legal—that took advantage of the favorable treatment extended to

---

[1]   See "Goals of Taxation" discussion in Chapter 1.

particular investments. In fact, tax professionals did their jobs so well that it was not unusual to find wealthy individuals with large economic incomes who paid little or no income tax. Indeed, in 1966, it was determined that 154 individuals with adjusted gross incomes in excess of $200,000 were able to completely escape tax by using the various incentives. Although the revenue lost from these high-income, no-tax individuals was slight, concerns started to surface. By the late 1960s, Congress recognized that an increasing number of people were losing faith in the system, believing that it was unfairly tipped in favor of the rich. Finally, amidst cries that only the poor and middle class paid taxes, the Johnson administration responded.

In 1969, legislation was enacted to guarantee that all wealthy individuals paid at least some amount of Federal income tax. The method adopted, however, was circuitous. Instead of repealing the tax preferences that created the opportunities, Congress chose to add another layer of taxation: the minimum tax. Since 1969, the minimum tax has come a long way, steadily growing in scope and importance. The first part of this chapter takes a look at these complex provisions.

The second part of this chapter is devoted to the world of credits. Over the years, Congress has established a number of credits that attempt to accomplish a variety of objectives. In addition to the business credits noted above, there are also several credits reserved for individuals. For example, there are credits to aid individuals with child care, help the elderly and disabled, and encourage individuals to get off welfare and go to work. Each of the common credit provisions is discussed below.

ALTERNATIVE MINIMUM TAX

POLICY OBJECTIVES

Since its enactment in 1969, the minimum tax has gone through a virtual metamorphosis. Substantial revisions occurred in 1976, 1978, 1981, and 1982, and a complete overhaul took place in 1986. Throughout, however, the rationale behind the tax has remained virtually unchanged. The policy underlying the minimum tax was well-summarized in the following excerpt from the Senate Finance Committee Report on the Tax Reform Act of 1986:

Reasons for Change

The committee believes that the minimum tax should serve one overriding objective: to ensure that no taxpayer with substantial economic income can avoid significant tax liability by using exclusions, deductions, and credits. Although these provisions may provide incentives for worthy goals, they become counterproductive when taxpayers are allowed to use them to avoid virtually all tax liability. The ability of high-income individuals and highly profitable corporations to pay little or no tax undermines respect for the entire tax system and, thus, for the incentive provisions themselves. In addition, even aside from public perceptions, the committee believes that it is inherently unfair for high-income individuals and highly profitable corporations to pay little or no tax due to their ability to utilize various tax preferences.[2]

Guided by these goals, Congress revised the AMT to ensure that the tax liability is at least a minimum percentage of a broad-based concept of income, less related expenses and certain personal or unavoidable expenditures. The intent of the legislation is to increase tax levies on certain wealthy taxpayers.

Under the current AMT rules, taxpayers must make a completely separate tax calculation to determine the *tentative minimum tax*; if the tentative minimum tax is greater than the regular tax liability, the taxpayer will have to pay the higher amount. The

---

[2] Senate Finance Committee Report. H.R. 3838, Page 518, U.S. Government Printing Office, May 29, 1986.

upshot of these rules is that the separate tax calculations force taxpayers to keep a separate set of books just to compute the AMT.

OVERVIEW OF AMT

The AMT applies to all of the separate taxable entities: individuals, estates, trusts, and regular C corporations. Partnerships and S corporations are not subject to the AMT per se; but if either has items of AMT significance, such items flow through to the partners or shareholders, who must consider them in calculating their own AMT. Consequently, these flow-through entities, like any other taxpayer, cannot ignore the AMT. The Taxpayer Relief Act of 1997 significantly impacted the AMT system. One ramification is discussed here and the others have been integrated with their related rules discussed later in this chapter. In an attempt at simplification, the new law exempts "small corporations" from the AMT for taxable years beginning after December 31, 1997.[3] For this purpose, a small corporation is one that has less than $5,000,000 in average annual gross receipts for the first three-taxable year period (or portion thereof) of the corporation beginning after December 31, 1993. Subsequent to the first three-taxable year period the corporation's average gross receipts for all three-taxable-year periods ending before the current taxable year cannot exceed $7,500,000.[4]

The basic formula for computing the AMT, like the basic formula for determining taxable income, is relatively uncomplicated. As can be seen from Exhibit 13-1, the calculation starts with the taxpayer's final taxable income computed in the normal fashion.[5] This amount, regular taxable income, is increased by any *tax preferences* and further modified—increased or decreased—by certain *adjustments* (see Exhibits 13-3 and 13-5 for a list and brief explanation). The resulting amount is termed *alternative minimum taxable income* (AMTI). However, AMTI is not the amount subject to tax. AMTI is further reduced by an *exemption* to arrive at the tax base or "taxable excess." The appropriate rate is then applied to produce the gross AMT. This amount is reduced by an available AMT foreign tax credit to yield the *tentative minimum tax*. Finally, the tentative minimum tax is compared to the regular tax and the taxpayer pays the higher. Technically, the excess of the tentative minimum tax over the regular tax is the AMT, but as can be seen from the formula, the effect is to require the taxpayer to pay the higher amount.[6] It is important to observe that, in computing the AMT, the general business tax credits normally cannot be used to reduce the tentative minimum tax (TMT).[7] This can be quite a surprise for taxpayers who have a large general business credit that wipes out their regular tax liability but does nothing to shield them from the AMT. Lastly, to prevent more individual taxpayers from paying the AMT, the non-business credits can offset both the regular tax and the AMT.[8]

---

[3] § 55(e).

[4] See § 448 and Chapter 5. This test is the same as the one applied in determining whether a corporation must use the accrual method of accounting. Note that once a corporation is classified as a small corporation, special rules apply when the gross receipts exceed $7,500,000 because the corporation will lose its status as a small corporation [§ 55(e)].

[5] § 55(b)(2).

[6] § 55(a).

[7] The empowerment zone credit can offset 25 percent of the tentative minimum tax as authorized by § 38(c)(2)(A).

[8] For tax years 2000 through 2009, most of the nonrefundable personal credits may be offset against the regular tax and the AMT. The credits include the following: credit for the elderly and disabled, adoption expense credit, child tax credit, credit for interest paid or accrued on certain home mortgages of low-income persons, credit for higher education expenses (the Hope and Lifetime Learning credits), credit for elective deferrals and IRA contributions (saver's credit), non-business energy property credit for energy-efficient improvements to a principal residence, residential energy efficient property credit for photovoltaic, solar hot water, and fuel cell property added to a residence and first-time home buyer credit for the District of Columbia.

EXHIBIT 13-1

The Alternative Minimum Tax Formula

Start with:	Regular taxable income		$ xxx,xxx
Plus/Minus:	AMT adjustments (see Exhibit 13-3)	±	xx,xxx
Equals:	AMT adjusted taxable income		$ xxx,xxx
Plus:	Sum of tax preference items (see Exhibit 13-5)	+	xx,xxx
Equals:	Alternative minimum taxable income (AMTI)		$ xxx,xxx
Less:	Exemption amount (adjusted for phase-out)	−	xx,xxx
Equals:	AMT base (taxable excess)		$ xxx,xxx
Times:	AMT rate.	×	xx%
Equals:	Gross alternative minimum tax		$ xx,xxx
Less:	AMT foreign tax credit.	−	x,xxx
Equals:	Tentative minimum tax (TMT)		$ xx,xxx
Less:	Regular tax liability	−	x,xxx
Equals:	Alternative minimum tax.		$ xx,xxx

The last concern that is not revealed in the AMT formula concerns some Congressional largess. In an attempt to protect taxpayers from being taxed under both the regular tax system and the AMT system, Congress introduced the minimum tax credit. As explained later, the minimum tax credit provision essentially allows the alternative minimum tax paid in one year to be used (with some modifications) as a credit in subsequent years against the taxpayer's regular tax liability.

Example 1. K is single and has taxable income of $92,500, on which she is required to pay a regular income tax of $19,620. In computing her regular taxable income, she utilized regular tax incentives that resulted in $55,000 of AMT adjustments (including her personal exemption) and $35,000 of AMT tax preference items. K's alternative minimum taxable income is $182,500 ($92,500 + $55,000 + $35,000).

As might be suspected, it is not the AMT formula that causes problems. The difficulty lies in the determination of the various adjustments and preferences that must be computed to arrive at AMTI. The next several sections examine each of the items entering into the AMT calculation.

AMT RATES AND EXEMPTIONS

Tax Rates. Until 1993, the AMT was computed with two flat rates, one rate for corporations and a different rate for noncorporate taxpayers. But the increase in individual tax rates by the Revenue Reconciliation Act of 1993 (RRA) apparently necessitated a change in this approach for individuals, estates, and trusts. Consequently, these

entities must use a two-tier rate system. Today, the rates for individuals, estates, and trusts are:

If the AMT base is

Over	But not over	Tax liability is	Of the amount over
$ 0	$ 175,000	26%	$ 0
175,000	—	$45,500 + 28%	175,000

In addition, to help ensure that taxpayers are not snared by the AMT due to the new lower rates on capital gains, Congress conformed the AMT and regular tax. The new lower rates for unrecaptured § 1250 gain (25%) and long-term capital gains (15%) now apply for AMT purposes.[9] In contrast, the rate for corporate taxpayers is a flat 20 percent.

AMT Exemptions. In order to shield taxpayers with small amounts of tax preferences from the AMT, the Code provides an exemption. As shown in Exhibit 13-2, the exemption amount varies depending on the entity and, in the case of an individual, his or her filing status. Although the exemption is designed to reduce the reach of the AMT, the substantial reduction in the regular tax rates in 2001 without corresponding cuts in the AMT rates have resulted in more and more taxpayers paying the AMT, the exemption notwithstanding. Consequently, in the last several years Congress has enacted specific legislation, on an annual basis, to increase the exemption to minimize the AMT's impact.[10]

The exemption provides little or no protection for high income taxpayers. Presumably, Congress did not want high income taxpayers to benefit from the exemption. Consequently, the law provides that the exemption is reduced as the taxpayer's income increases. Specifically, the exemption amount for each taxpayer is reduced (but not below zero) by 25 cents for each $1 of AMTI exceeding a certain threshold. These thresholds are identified in Exhibit 13-2. Note that the phase-out rule completely eliminates the exemption as AMTI increases beyond a certain amount. For example, the $70,950 (2009) exemption for married taxpayers is completely eliminated when AMTI reaches $415,000 [($433,800 − $150,000 = $283,800) × .25 = $70,950]. The various points at which the phase-out is complete are also shown in Exhibit 13-2.

EXHIBIT 13-2
Alternative Minimum Tax Exemptions and Phase-Out Levels for 2002–2009

Taxpayer	Exemption Amount		Phase-Out Begins	Phase-Out Complete
	2002*	2009	2009	2009
Married filing jointly	$45,000	$70,950	$150,000	$433,800
Single individuals[11]	33,750	46,700	112,500	299,300
Married filing separately	22,500	35,475	75,000	216,900
Estates & Trusts	22,500	22,500	75,000	165,000
C Corporations	40,000	40,000	150,000	310,000

* For 2010, the exemption amounts are scheduled to decline to 2002 levels shown above, but it is anticipated that tax legislation enacted in 2010 will extend the higher exemption amounts through 2009 or beyond.

[9]   § 55(b)(3).

[10]   § 55(d).

[11]   § 59(j). The exemption amount for children subject to the "kiddie tax" is earned income plus $6,700. The phase-out range is the same as that for single individuals. Rev. Proc. 2008-66, I.R.B. 2008-45.

Example 2. Assume the same facts as in *Example 1.* Since K is single, her initial AMT exemption is $46,700. However, because K's $182,500 AMTI exceeds the $112,500 threshold for single individuals by $70,000, her exemption amount must be reduced by $17,500 ($70,000 × 0.25). Thus, the allowable exemption for the year is $29,200 (46,700 − 17,500).

K's AMT is $20,238, computed as follows:

Regular taxable income	$ 92,500
Plus: AMT adjustments	+ 55,000
AMT adjusted taxable income	$147,500
Plus: AMT preference items	+ 35,000
AMTI	$182,500
Less: Exemption amount [$46,700 − 25% ($182,500 − $112,500)]	− 29,200
AMTI base	$153,300
Times: AMT rate	× 26%
Gross AMT	$ 39,858
Less: AMT foreign tax credit	− 0
Tentative AMT	$ 39,858
Less: Regular tax liability	−19,620
AMT	$ 20,238

ADJUSTMENTS AND TAX PREFERENCE ITEMS IN GENERAL

Once taxable income is determined, the search for AMTI can begin. As noted above, there are two types of modifications that must be made to regular taxable income to arrive at AMTI: adjustments and preferences. Although both of these modifications serve a similar purpose (i.e., provide a more "realistic" measure of the taxpayer's economic income), they are not identical. *Preferences* generally require only an add-back to income. For example, one tax preference item requires the taxpayer to add back certain private activity bond income that was excluded from regular tax gross income under § 103. In contrast, *adjustments* generally call for the complete substitution of some special AMT treatment for the regular tax treatment. For instance, instead of using the regular tax rules to compute depreciation, the taxpayer must use the slower-paced methods for the AMT. Note that, when this occurs, depreciation for regular tax purposes may be more or less than AMT depreciation, resulting in either a positive or a negative adjustment. In short, AMT adjustments may increase or decrease taxable income whereas preferences only increase taxable income.

Another important distinction between adjustments and preferences concerns their effect on the taxpayer's basis in property. Adjustments, such as those for AMT depreciation, usually cause the property's basis for AMT purposes to differ from that for regular tax purposes. Consequently, when the taxpayer later disposes of the property, gain or loss for AMT purposes will normally not be the same as the gain or loss reported for regular tax purposes.[12] As might be imagined, this system effectively requires the taxpayer to maintain a separate set of records for AMT purposes. These separate records are used to compute the annual adjustments as well as the adjustment when the asset is subsequently sold. Note that adjustments can generally be thought of as timing

---

[12] § 56(b)(1)(F).

differences between regular taxable income and AMTI. In early years the adjustment normally produces an increase in AMTI. In later years, however, the trend reverses and a negative adjustment is required, actually reducing AMTI.

Although adjustments affect a property's basis, preferences do not. This approach makes accounting for preferences somewhat easier than it is for adjustments. In many cases, only a side calculation is necessary to determine the preference. The preference amount is then simply added to taxable income in the determination of AMTI. Generally, tax preference items are analogous to permanent differences between the regular tax and the minimum tax.

AMT ADJUSTMENTS

AMT adjustments can be classified into four groups. As shown in Exhibit 13-3, not all adjustments apply to all taxpayers; some apply to all taxpayers while others apply only to individuals or only to corporations.[13] In addition, there are special adjustments concerning losses from tax shelters. Although all of the adjustments are listed in Exhibit 13-3, only the more common adjustments are discussed below.

AMT ADJUSTMENTS APPLICABLE TO ALL TAXPAYERS

Depreciation. For AMT purposes, depreciation of property *placed in service after 1986* must be computed using the Alternative Depreciation System (ADS) with an exception for personal property discussed below.[14] This substitution of ADS for the taxpayer's normal method (e.g., MACRS) creates a difference between AMT depreciation and regular tax depreciation, and an adjustment must be made. The amount of the AMT adjustment is merely the difference between regular tax and AMT depreciation, which may be positive or negative as illustrated below.

As discussed in Chapter 9, depreciation under ADS is computed using the straight-line method, the appropriate convention, and the ADS life (the class life for personal property and 40 years for real property). While this same approach generally applies for AMT purposes, there is an exception for tangible personal property. ADS must be applied using a 150 percent declining-balance rate over the class life of the property for personal property placed in service prior to 1999. For personal property placed in service after 1998, Congress simplified the depreciation system and the AMT adjustments by allowing the MACRS recovery periods to be used for AMT purposes. The 150 percent declining-balance method does not apply to assets for which the taxpayer has elected the straight-line method for regular tax purposes. The allowable methods of depreciation for regular tax and AMT purposes are shown in Exhibit 13-4. The exhibit reveals that there are four methods of depreciation available for regular tax purposes, two of which are also suitable for AMT purposes. Two observations should be made that are not obvious from this table. The first concerns realty: note that even though the straight-line method must be used for both AMT and regular tax purposes, an adjustment is still necessary since the AMT class life is longer than the normal recovery period (40 years vs. 27.5 or 39 years).[15] The second concerns avoidance of the AMT adjustment. Observe that the taxpayer can avoid the AMT adjustment by electing regular tax depreciation, which uses a slower rate (150% declining-balance or straight-line).[16]

---

[13] § 56.

[14] § 56(a)(1).

[15] § 168(g)(2)(C)(iii).

[16] The Tax Reform Act of 1997 allows AMT depreciation to be computed using the same recovery periods as are used for regular tax purposes. For property placed in service prior to 1999, the AMT required tangible personal property to be depreciated over the longer Alternative Depreciation System class life of the property. See §56(a)(1)(A)(i).

EXHIBIT 13-3
AMT Adjustments

Applicable to All Taxpayers		Brief Explanation
§ 56(a)(1)	Depreciation	Use ADS or 150% DB
§ 56(a)(2)	Mining exploration and development costs	Capitalize and amortize over 10 years
§ 56(a)(3)	Income reported on the completed contract method	Use percentage completion
§ 56(a)(4)	Alternative tax net operating loss deduction	Recompute with AMT rules
§ 56(a)(5)	Pollution control facilities	MACRS with straight line method
§ 56(a)(6)	Gains or losses on asset dispositions	Differing AMT basis
§ 56(a)(7)	Alcohol fuel credit	Do not include as income

Applicable Only to Individuals		
§ 56(b)(1)(A)	Itemized deductions	No taxes, misc. itemized deductions; adjust interest, adjust medical
§ 56(b)(1)(E)	Standard deduction	Not allowed
§ 56(b)(1)(E)	Personal dependent exemptions	Not allowed
§ 56(b)(1)(D)	Income tax refunds	Do not include
§ 56(b)(2)	Circulation and research expenditures	Capitalize and amortize
§ 56(b)(3)	Incentive stock options	Include spread (FMV − option price)

Applicable Only to Corporations		
§ 56(c)	ACE (adjusted current earnings)	Add 75% (ACE − AMTI)

Specialized Tax Shelter Loss Adjustments		
§ 56(b)	Passive activity losses	Recompute with AMT rules
§ 56(a)	Farm shelter losses	Deduct in following year, if income

EXHIBIT 13-4

Allowable Depreciation Methods for AMT and Regular Tax Purposes for Property Placed in Service after 1998

Method	Depreciable Life	Regular Tax	AMT	AMT-ACE
200% DB	Recovery period	✓		
150% DB	Recovery period	✓	✓	✓
Straight line	Recovery period	✓		
Straight line	Class life	✓	✓	✓

Example 3. T placed an asset costing $100,000 in service on February 5, 2009. Assume the asset is "3-year property" and has an ADR class life of 3 years. The effect on the minimum tax is computed below assuming that the 150 percent declining-balance method was used for AMT purposes.

	2009	2010	2011	2012
Regular tax deduction (200%)	$ 33,330	$ 44,450	$ 14,810	$ 7,410
AMT deduction (150%).	− 25,000	− 37,500	− 25,000	− 12,500
Effect of adjustment on AMTI.	$ 8,330	$ 6,950	($10,190)	($5,090)
	increase	increase	decrease	decrease

Note that in the first two years regular depreciation exceeds what is allowed for AMTI—requiring the taxpayer to increase AMTI—a positive adjustment. In the third year, however, the trend reverses itself, and AMT depreciation is greater than what was actually deducted for regular tax purposes. Consequently, the taxpayer is allowed to decrease AMTI—a negative adjustment. Also note that the differences in regular and AMT depreciation cause the property's basis for AMT purposes to be different from the regular tax basis. Accordingly, if the property is sold, the amount of gain or loss for AMT and regular tax purposes may differ.

Recognizing the burdensome task of maintaining one set of depreciation books for each tax system, Congress took steps to coordinate the two. As shown in Exhibit 13-4, taxpayers may eliminate the AMT adjustment by electing the appropriate method for regular tax purposes.[17] For example, the taxpayer could, for regular tax purposes, elect to use the 150 percent declining balance method, which would be the same as AMT depreciation. Alternatively, if the taxpayer elects to use the ADS life and the straight-line method for regular tax purposes, that same method must be used for the AMT. Either approach eliminates the AMT adjustment.

Example 4. Assume the same facts as in *Example 3* above, except T elects to use the 150 percent modification. In this case, the need for an AMT adjustment is eliminated, as shown below.

	2009	2010	2011	2012
Regular tax depreciation (150%, ADS life)	$ 25,000	$ 37,500	$ 25,000	$ 12,500
AMT depreciation (150%, ADS life)	− 25,000	− 37,500	− 25,000	− 12,500
AMT adjustment	$ 0	$ 0	$ 0	$ 0

Section 179 Limited Expensing. Given the elaborate scheme to curtail accelerated depreciation deductions for AMT purposes, it is surprising that the election to expense property under § 179 does not give rise to an AMT adjustment. Currently, first-year § 179 expensing deductions are allowed for both AMT and regular tax purposes.[18]

---

[17] §§ 168(g)(7) and 56(a)(1)(A)(ii).

[18] See Footnote 2, *supra*, page 552, note 5.

Mining Exploration and Development Costs. For regular tax purposes, mining exploration and development costs related to mineral property are currently expensed. For AMT purposes, however, such costs must be capitalized and amortized ratably over a 10-year period.[19]

Long-Term Contracts. As explained in Chapter 5, for regular tax purposes, taxpayers normally must use the percentage of completion method to account for long-term contracts. However, the Code carves out two exceptions. The completed contract method may be used to account for home construction contracts and by small contractors who have gross receipts less than $10 million. AMT treatment is similar, but it is not identical. For AMT purposes, there is no exception for small contractors. Consequently, the percentage of completion method must be used for computing AMTI in all cases except in accounting for home construction contracts.[20]

Pollution Control Facilities. While taxpayers are permitted to amortize expenditures related to pollution control facilities over 60 months for regular tax purposes, the AMT requires use of ADS.[21]

Alternative Tax Net Operating Loss (ATNOL) Deduction. An ATNOL is allowed as a deduction for minimum tax purposes.[22] The procedure for computing the ATNOL parallels its cousin, the regular tax NOL, but the ATNOL must be determined taking into consideration all of the AMT adjustments and tax preference items. In addition, the amount of the ATNOL is *limited* to 90 percent of the AMTI determined without regard to this deduction. Note, however, as part of the Job Creation and Worker Assistance Act of 2002, taxpayers are entitled to deduct 100 percent of the AMT NOLs generated in 2001 or 2002 as well as any AMT NOLs that are carried forward into 2001 or 2002. Also, an election to forgo the NOL carryback period for regular tax purposes is likely to control the treatment for the ATNOL.[23]

AMT ADJUSTMENTS APPLICABLE ONLY TO INDIVIDUALS

All of the adjustments applicable only to individual taxpayers are listed in Exhibit 13-3. Each of these is discussed below. But first it is important to note that the IRS, while routinely taking the position that the AMT and the regular tax system are two distinct and separate systems, has issued regulations governing the computation of AMTI for noncorporate taxpayers. These regulations provide that, in determining the AMTI of noncorporate taxpayers, all references to the taxpayer's A.G.I. or modified A.G.I. in determining the amount of items of income, exclusion, or deduction in the AMT system must be treated as references to the taxpayer's modified A.G.I. as determined for regular tax purposes.[24] For example, in the AMT system the medical expense deduction is subject to a 10 percent limitation just as the regular tax medical expense deduction is limited to a 7½ percent limitation. The important but apparently inconsistent point is that the limitation for the AMT system is not subject to 10 percent of AMTI (as it should be if the AMT were a separate system), but rather the regulation specifies that the AMT limitation will be subject to 10 percent of the taxpayer's regular tax system A.G.I. The purported

---

[19]   §§ 616 and 617; but see Footnote 52, *infra,* for the election under § 59(e) that allows taxpayers to avoid an AMT adjustment with respect to these expenditures.

[20]   § 56(a)(3).

[21]   § 169 and § 56(a)(5).

[22]   § 56(a)(4).

[23]   *Branum v. Comm.*, 94-1 USTC ¶50, 163, (CA-5, 1994).

[24]   Reg. § 1.55-1(e).

goal of the regulations is to reduce the complexity and to ease the record keeping burdens that are imposed on noncorporate taxpayers under a completely separate and parallel system that would require a computation of a separate adjusted gross income for alternative minimum tax purposes.

Itemized Deductions. For the most part, itemized deductions allowed for regular tax purposes are also allowed for AMT purposes (sometimes referred to as alternative minimum tax deductions, or ATIDs). However, there are several important exceptions and modifications. These adjustments differ from those above (e.g., depreciation) in that they serve to increase the tax base as permanent adjustments instead of merely altering the timing of the item.

Two itemized deductions are totally disallowed for AMT purposes:[25]

1. Miscellaneous itemized deductions (MIDs). For example, unreimbursed employee business expenses and tax preparation expenses are not allowed for the AMT.[26]
2. Itemized deductions related to the payment of any tax. For example, state, local, and foreign income taxes and real and personal property taxes are not allowed as deductions for AMT purposes.

In computing the itemized deductions allowed for AMT purposes, the limitations for regular tax purposes normally apply (e.g., the 10% limitation on personal casualty losses or the 50% limitation for charitable contributions). However, the 2 percent cutback rule that applies to certain itemized deductions *does not* apply for AMT purposes.[27] In addition, as noted below, special rules exist for medical expenses and interest.

ATIDs generally include the following:[28]

1. Medical expenses, but *only in excess* of 10 percent of taxpayer's regular tax A.G.I.
2. Interest expense, but only for:
   a. Qualified housing interest
   b. Investment interest expense to the extent of net investment income
3. Charitable contributions
4. Theft, casualty, and wagering losses
5. Estate tax deductions resulting from reporting income in respect of a decedent under § 691
6. Impairment-related work expenses
7. Bond premium amortization deductions

The above list is self-explanatory with the exception of the amount of interest that will be allowed as an ATID. Several new terms and concepts regarding the deduction for interest were developed and incorporated into the alternative minimum tax system. *Qualified housing interest* is interest paid or accrued on indebtedness incurred after June 30, 1982, in acquiring, constructing, or substantially rehabilitating property that is a principal residence (within the meaning of Code § 121) or qualified dwelling, including a

---

[25] § 56(b)(1)(A).

[26] Beginning in 1998, employee business expenses relating to service as an official of a state or local government or political subdivision thereof are deductible for A.G.I. provided the official is compensated on a fee basis. Thus, these expenses become deductible for the AMT system.

[27] § 56(b)(1)(F).

[28] See § 67(b) for a complete list of itemized deductions that are allowed as ATIDs. Also note that a standard deduction is not allowed for AMT purposes.

secondary residence.[29] For indebtedness incurred *before* July 1, 1982, a deduction can be taken for interest paid or accrued on a debt that, at that time, was secured by a qualified dwelling without regard for the purpose or use of the proceeds of the indebtedness. The essence of these rules is that interest on second mortgages on homes—home equity loans—established after 1982 is not deductible for AMT purposes as qualified housing interest *unless* the proceeds are used to improve the principal residence.

When interest rates fall, taxpayers often refinance their homes, and a question arose about the interest paid on a loan (new loan) the proceeds of which were used to pay off the original qualified housing indebtedness (old loan). The TRA of 1986 resolved the issue by allowing an interest expense deduction for AMT purposes on the new loan used to refinance the principal residence, but only to the extent that the new loan does not exceed the outstanding balance of the old loan.[30]

Investment interest expense is allowed as an ATID, but only to the extent of qualified *adjusted* net investment income.[31] The adjustment in computing the net investment income is required for AMT purposes as a result of including a portion of the tax-exempt interest income from specified private activity bonds (SPAB) as a tax preference item that increases the AMTI (see *Example 10* for details relating to the tax-exempt income preference item). If exempt interest income from SPABs is included as a preference item for AMT purposes, the interest expense incurred with respect to it will be allowed as a deduction for AMT purposes. These adjustments for tax-exempt income and its related interest expenses are also allowed in computing the "adjusted" net investment income for AMT purposes.

Circulation and Research Expenditures. For regular tax purposes, § 173 allows newspapers, magazines and other periodicals to immediately deduct circulation expenditures (i.e., costs incurred to establish, maintain, or increase circulation). However, for AMT purposes, circulation expenditures must be capitalized and amortized over a three year period. The same rule applies to research and experimental expenditures, except the amortization period is ten years.[32] However, the Revenue Reconciliation Act of 1989 repealed the AMT adjustment for research expenses of individuals who materially participate in the activity in which research expenses are incurred.[33] As with other adjustments that create a disparity between basis for regular tax and basis for AMT, *separate records must be maintained* to determine the allowable amortization deduction in subsequent years or the gain or loss on disposition or abandonment.

Gains from Incentive Stock Options (ISOs). For regular tax purposes, the bargain element of ISOs (i.e., the difference between the fair market value of the stock and the option price) is *not* required to be included in income either at the time the option is granted or when the option is exercised.[34] However, an income adjustment may be required for the AMT. Assuming the stock acquired is not subject to substantial risk of forfeiture, the adjustment to AMTI is equal to the amount by which the value of the share

---

[29]   A qualified dwelling is a house, apartment, condominium, or mobile home (not used on a transient basis). Qualified dwelling for AMT is a narrow definition and differs from that of Code § 280A(f)(1), which broadly defines a dwelling unit as a house, apartment, condominium, mobile home, boat, or similar property.

[30]   § 56(e)(1). See the Tax Reform Act of 1986.

[31]   See Chapter 11 for a discussion of the investment interest deduction limitation.

[32]   § 56(b)(2)(A)(ii). See Footnote 52, *infra*, for an optional tax accounting method for research and experimental expenditures.

[33]   § 56(b)(2)(D). The repeal is effective for taxable years beginning after December 31, 1990.

[34]   See Chapter 18 for a discussion of ISOs and § 83.

at the time of exercise exceeds the option price. If the stock is disposed of in the option year, however, this income adjustment is not required because the income attributable to the bargain element will be reported under the regular tax system in the same year.

> **Example 5.** D receives an incentive stock option to purchase 1,000 shares of her employer's stock at $50 per share. Three years after the receipt of the option, D exercises her option when the stock is selling for $70 per share. When D exercises the option, she has an AMT adjustment of $20,000 ($70,000 − $50,000).

Since the AMT adjustment amount computed above increases the AMTI, an upward basis adjustment in the stock of an equal amount is allowed for AMT purposes. This disparity in the stock's basis for regular tax and the AMT requires an *extra set of books* to determine the amount of gain recognized upon a subsequent disposition of the stock for AMT purposes.

> **Example 6.** Assume the same facts as in *Example 5* and that D holds the stock until it further increases in value to $85,000. If D sells the stock for $85,000, she has a $35,000 gain for regular tax purposes ($85,000 − $50,000). However, for AMT purposes, the gain is $15,000 ($85,000 - AMT basis of $70,000). To reflect the difference in the regular tax and AMT gain, D makes a negative adjustment to AMTI of $20,000 ($35,000 regular tax gain - $15,000 AMT gain) which potentially reduces her tentative AMT in the year of the sale.[35]

Standard Deduction Not Allowed. Individuals are not permitted to take into account the standard deduction in computing the alternative minimum taxable income.[36]

Personal Exemptions. Personal exemptions authorized under § 151 are not allowed as deductions in computing the AMTI.[37]

Adjustment to Income for Tax Refunds. Generally, taxpayers who itemize deductions must report a refund of a prior year's state or local income tax as gross income in the year of receipt.[38] However, since itemized deductions for all tax expenditures are not allowed for AMT purposes, the refund or recovery in *all cases* is excluded from AMTI.

ADJUSTMENT APPLICABLE ONLY TO CORPORATIONS

The only adjustment applicable solely to corporate taxpayers[39] is the adjustment based on a corporation's adjusted current earnings—commonly referred to as the *ACE adjustment.*[40] The ACE adjustment, like the minimum tax itself, was the Congressional

---

[35] Taxpayers that have exercised ISOs, properly reported the income for AMT purposes and paid an AMT in the year of exercise, traditionally have looked to the minimum tax credit to reduce the regular tax imposed on the gain from the sale of the stock for regular tax purposes. The AMT rules were designed so that the gain in the regular tax system makes the regular tax larger than the tentative minimum tax and allows the minimum tax credit to reduce the regular tax imposed in excess of the tentative minimum tax. This approach works when the stock appreciates in value but it is flawed if the stock is disposed of after it has decreased in value. There may not be a gain on the disposition in the regular tax system and the taxpayer will not benefit from the minimum tax credit. This situation has been addressed by Congress and is discussed later in this chapter under the refundable minimum tax credit rules.

[36] § 56(b)(1)(E).

[37] *Ibid.*

[38] See § 56(b)(1)(D) and Chapter 6 for an exception based on the tax benefit rule.

[39] Recall, however, that small corporations are exempt from the AMT system. *See supra*, Footnote 3.

[40] This adjustment *does not* apply to certain corporations, including S corporations, regulated investment companies, real estate investment trusts, or real estate mortgage investment conduits. § 56(g)(6).

response to what seemed an increasingly frequent phenomenon: corporations were reporting substantial earnings for financial accounting purposes yet paying little or no income tax. Curiously, this occurred despite the existence of the AMT. To address the problem, Congress created the ACE adjustment. This special adjustment is designed to ensure that all corporations pay some minimum tax on economic income.

In theory, the ACE adjustment is relatively simple. It requires a corporation to compare its economic income to taxable income to determine the amount of economic income, if any, that escaped tax. Part of this elusive income is then included in the corporation's AMTI. Technically, the ACE adjustment is equal to 75 percent of the difference between *adjusted current earnings* and AMTI.[41] In this calculation, adjusted current earnings essentially serve as a substitute for economic income. The actual computation of adjusted current earnings is quite technical. It begins with AMTI, to which a laundry list of adjustments are made.[42] A discussion of the various adjustments is beyond the scope of this text. Suffice it to say that their collective purpose is to yield the corporation's economic income so its true ability to pay tax can be determined.

Example 7. T Corporation has AMTI of $200,000 without regard to the ACE adjustment. T's adjusted current earnings are determined to be $400,000. T's regular income tax liability is $41,750. T has an ACE adjustment of $150,000, AMTI of $350,000, a tentative AMT of $70,000, and AMT of $28,250, computed as follows:

AMTI before ACE	$ 200,000
Plus: Ace adjustment [($400,000 − $200,000) × 75%]	+ 150,000
AMTI	$ 350,000
Less: Exemption amount (completely phased out)	− 0
AMTI base	$ 350,000
Times: AMT rate	× 20%
Gross AMT	$ 70,000
Less: AMT foreign tax credit	− 0
Tentative AMT	$ 70,000
Less: Regular tax liability	− 41,750
AMT	$ 28,250

This portion of the alternative minimum tax system has been crafted to make certain the AMT is imposed on corporate taxpayers having an economic ability to pay.

SPECIAL TAX SHELTER LOSS ADJUSTMENTS

Certain losses that may be deductible for regular tax are *denied* for purposes of the AMT. Specifically, tax shelter farm losses and passive-activity losses allowed as deductions for regular tax purposes must be recomputed under the AMT system, taking into account all of the AMT tax accounting rules.[43] Clearly, a separate set of books will be required for each activity. The amount of the AMT adjustment required by the statute is the difference between the loss allowed for the regular tax system and the loss allowed under the AMT system.

---

[41] § 56(g)(1).

[42] § 56(g)(4).

[43] These rules are specified in §§ 56 and 57.

Tax Shelter Farm Losses. Noncorporate taxpayers and personal service corporations are not allowed to deduct losses from a tax shelter farm activity in computing AMTI.[44] For the AMT system, the disallowed loss will be treated as a deduction allocable to such activity in the *first* succeeding taxable year, and will be allowed to offset income from that activity in any succeeding year. Under this rule, each farm is treated as a separate activity. In the year that the taxpayer disposes of his or her entire interest in any tax shelter farm activity, the amount of previously disallowed loss related to that activity is allowed as a deduction for the year under the AMT system.

Passive-Activity Losses. As discussed in Chapter 12, there are limitations on the use of losses from passive activities to offset other income of the taxpayer for regular tax purposes.[45] For AMT purposes, similar rules apply, except for AMT purposes a loss generated from a passive activity must be recomputed to reflect the AMT rules. This means that depreciation, certain intangible drilling and development costs, certain percentage depletion, and other adjustments and preferences must be reflected in computing the loss for AMT purposes.[46] Because of the differences in the treatment of such items, the amount of suspended losses relating to an activity may differ for minimum tax and regular tax purposes and may require that two sets of books be kept in order to track the passive-loss carryover on each activity.[47]

> **Example 8.** C has $200,000 of salary income, $50,000 of gross income from passive activities, and $170,000 of deductions from passive activities for the current year. C's passive activity loss is $120,000 for regular tax purposes. Because the recomputed expenses for AMT purposes are only $130,000, the passive-activity loss is $80,000 for AMT purposes. For regular tax purposes, the taxpayer has taxable income of $200,000 and a suspended passive loss in the amount of $120,000 ($170,000 passive deductions − $50,000 passive income). For minimum tax purposes, the taxpayer has AMTI of $200,000 and a suspended passive loss of $80,000 ($130,000 − $50,000).

As illustrated in the example above, the recomputed passive loss using the AMT rules can be significantly different from the regular tax passive loss with respect to an activity. In fact, in some situations it is possible to have a regular tax passive-loss amount *and* an AMT passive income amount on the same activity!

> **Example 9.** Assume that taxpayer C in the example above had passive-activity deductions of $80,000 for regular tax purposes and $40,000 for minimum tax purposes. C would have regular taxable income of $200,000 and a suspended passive loss of $30,000 ($80,000 − $50,000) for regular tax purposes. For AMT purposes, C has alternative minimum taxable income of $210,000 [$200,000 salary + ($50,000 − $40,000)] and no suspended passive loss for minimum tax purposes.

TAX PREFERENCE ITEMS

Since tax preference items are required to be identified and computed for both corporate and noncorporate taxpayers, all the current preference items are listed in Exhibit 13-5; however, only the most common items are explained below.[48]

---

[44] § 58(a).

[45] See Chapter 12 for a discussion of passive losses.

[46] § 58(b).

[47] P.L. 99-514, Tax Reform Act of 1986, Conference Committee Report, Act § 701.

[48] § 57 sets forth all of the tax preference items and the specifics of each calculation.

EXHIBIT 13-5
AMT Tax Preference Items

Percentage depletion in excess of cost basis on certain mineral properties
Certain intangible drilling and development costs
Specified tax-exempt interest
Exclusion for gain on sale of certain small business stock

Excess Depletion. The amount of the preference item is the excess (if any) of the percentage depletion claimed for the taxable year over the adjusted basis of the property at the end of the taxable year (determined without regard to the depletion deduction for the taxable year).[49] This computation must be made for each unit of property.

Intangible Drilling and Development Costs. In general, the amount of the tax preference is equal to the intangible drilling costs (IDC) incurred and deducted on productive oil, gas, and geothermal wells reduced by the sum of:

1. The amount allowed as if the IDCs had been capitalized and amortized over a ten-year period, and
2. Sixty-five percent of the net income for the year from these properties.[50]

If the intangible drilling and development costs are capitalized and amortized in accord with special rules contained in § 59(e), they are not treated as a preference item.[51]

Private Activity Bond Interest. This preference item pertains to interest income on specified private activity bonds (SPABs) issued after August 7, 1986.[52] The term *private activity bond* means any bond issued if 10 percent of the proceeds of the issue is used for private business use in any trade or business carried on by any person that is not a governmental unit. Where interest income on SPABs is includible in AMTI under the above rule, the regular tax rule of Code § 265 (denying deductions for expenses and interest relating to tax-exempt income) does not apply, and expenses and interest incurred to carry SPABs are deductible for minimum tax purposes.

Example 10. Taxpayer P is required to include in AMTI $10,000 of otherwise tax-exempt interest income on SPABs as a preference item. She incurred $900 of interest expense on a temporary loan in order to purchase the bonds. Code § 265 disallows a deduction of this $900 for regular tax purposes, but it is deductible for minimum tax purposes.

Gain on the Sale of Qualified Small Business Stock. As explained in detail in Chapter 16, the Revenue Reconciliation Act of 1993 created a special incentive to encourage taxpayers to invest in the stock of qualified small businesses (i.e., stock of a C corporation with gross assets of $50 million or less at the time the stock was issued and that was held by the original owner for more than five years prior to sale). Under this

---

[49] § 57(a)(1). This preference was repealed for certain independent producer and royalty interest owners of oil and gas properties for taxable years beginning after 1992.

[50] § 57(a)(2)(E)(ii). The CNEPA of 1992 repealed this preference item for taxpayers (other than certain integrated oil and gas companies) for years beginning after December 31, 1992. However, the repeal of the excess IDCs preference "may not result in more than a 40 percent reduction in the amount of the taxpayer's AMTI computed as if the present-law excess IDC preference had not been repealed."

[51] Code § 59(e) was enacted to provide relief to taxpayers that are subject to the AMT, but through proper planning want to maximize the regular tax deductions and at the same time minimize the impact of the AMT. This section provides an election to capitalize "qualified expenditures" and deduct them ratably over a 10-year period (three years in the case of circulation expenditures). Qualified expenditures include IDCs, circulation, research and experimentation, and mining exploration and development costs.

[52] § 57(a)(5)(C)(iv).

special rule, a taxpayer is entitled to exclude 50 percent of the gain on the sale of the stock. However, what Congress gives with the right hand it takes away with the left. Seven percent of this exclusion (or 3.5% of the entire gain) is treated as a tax preference item.[53]

> **Example 11.** On October 31, 2009, J sold qualified small business stock and recognized a gain of $80,000. Only 50 percent of the gain, $40,000, is subject to regular tax, and the remaining $40,000 is excluded. For AMT purposes, J has a tax preference of $2,800 (7% × $40,000).

ALTERNATIVE MINIMUM TAX COMPUTATIONS

Before the alternative minimum tax calculations can be made, the taxpayer's current taxable income and Federal income tax liability must first be determined. As shown in Exhibit 13-1, a taxpayer's AMT liability is the excess of the tentative minimum tax over the regular tax liability. To further examine this interaction, a factual situation is presented below in *Example 12*, where the taxpayer's regular tax liability is determined. The same facts are then used to compute the ATIDs in *Example 13* and the taxpayer's AMT liability in *Example 14*.

> **Example 12.** T is a married taxpayer filing a joint return for 2009. He had the following items of income, expenses, and regular tax liability for the year:

Income:		
Salary	$88,000	
Interest	12,000	
Adjusted gross income		$100,000[(1)]
Itemized deductions:		
Medical expenses [$9,500 total − (7.5% of $100,000 A.G.I.)]	$ 2,000	
Real property taxes on home	12,000	
Real property taxes on mountain range property	8,000	
Personal property taxes	4,000	
Interest expense:		
Residence interest	20,000[(2)]	
Investment interest on mountain range property ($12,000 total, but limited to)	4,000[(3)]	
Charitable contributions	10,000	
Casualty loss [$13,000 total − (10% of A.G.I.)]	3,000	
Miscellaneous itemized deductions [$11,000 total − (2% of A.G.I.)]	9,000	
Total itemized deductions		− 72,000
Personal exemptions (2 × $3,650)		− 7,300
Taxable income		$ 20,700
Regular tax		$ 2,270

[(1)] Although not required to be included in his taxable income, T exercised an incentive stock option for $20,000 when the fair market value of the stock was $80,000.

[(2)] Residence interest includes $18,000 of qualified housing interest (interest on mortgage to acquire home) and $2,000 of interest on a home equity loan to buy a boat.

[(3)] The mountain range property was acquired as a speculative investment and was 90 percent debt-financed. Recall that interest on investment indebtedness is allowed as a deduction under § 163(d) to the extent of net investment income. Net investment income = $12,000 interest − $8,000 property taxes = $4,000. Thus the $12,000 interest expense is limited to $4,000.

---

[53] § 57(a)(7), as amended by the Tax Increase Prevention and Reconciliation Act of 2005. The rule is applicable for tax years beginning before 2011.

Example 13. Refer to *Example 12*. T's 2009 alternative tax itemized deductions (ATIDs) and the resulting AMT adjustments are determined as follows:

	Allowed ATIDs for AMT	Allowed Itemized Deductions for Regular Tax	AMT Adjustments
Medical expenses (in excess of 10% of A.G.I.)	$ 0*	$ 2,000	$ 2,000
Itemized deductions for taxes (not allowed)	0	24,000	24,000
Qualified housing interest......................	18,000	18,000	0
Home equity loan.............................	0	2,000	2,000
Other qualified interest (limited to net investment income, = $12,000).......................	12,000**	4,000	(8,000)**
Casualty losses	3,000	3,000	0
Charitable contributions	10,000	10,000	0
Miscellaneous itemized deductions (not allowed) ...	0	9,000	9,000
Totals	$ 43,000	$ 72,000	$ 29,000

*$9,500 does not exceed 10% of $100,000, or $10,000.

**The real property taxes on the investment mountain property are not deductible for AMT purposes. § 56(b)(1)(C)(v).

Note that the computations for ATIDs are similar to those in *Example 12* for itemized deductions except (1) the reduction in medical expenses is 10% of the regular tax A.G.I. rather than 7.5%, (2) deductions for state and local taxes are not allowed, (3) the miscellaneous itemized deductions are not allowed, (4) the interest on the home equity loan to purchase the boat is not allowed and (5) in the calculation of net investment income, the real property taxes on the mountain property are excludable for AMT purposes. The differences between the ATIDs allowed for AMT purposes and the itemized deductions allowed for regular tax purposes result in AMT adjustments. These adjustments are added back to T's regular taxable income to arrive at AMT adjusted taxable income and are reported on Form 6251, Computation of Alternative Minimum Tax for Individuals.

Example 14. Refer to *Examples 12 and 13*. T's alternative minimum tax (AMT) 2009 is computed as follows:

Regular taxable income		$ 20,700
Plus:	Net adjustment for itemized deductions	+ 29,000[(1)]
	Net adjustment for exercise of ISO	+ 60,000[(2)]
	Adjustment for personal exemptions	+ 7,300
AMT adjusted taxable income		$117,000
Plus:	Tax preference items	+ 0
Alternative minimum taxable income (AMTI)		$117,000
Less:	Exemption amount (married filing jointly)	− 70,950
AMT base (taxable excess)		$ 46,050
Times:	AMT rate	× 26%
Gross alternative minimum tax		$ 11,973
Less:	AMT foreign tax credit	− 0
Tentative minimum tax		$ 11,973
Less:	Regular tax liability	− 2,270
AMT liability for 2009		$ 9,703

[(1)] Regular tax itemized deductions	$72,000
ATIDs allowed for AMT	(43,000)
Disallowed itemized deductions increase in the AMTI	$29,000
[(2)] Stock FMV when ISO exercised	$80,000
Option price	(20,000)
Excess is AMT adjustment that increases AMTI	$60,000

Since the tentative minimum tax of $11,973 *exceeds* his $2,270 regular tax liability (computed in *Example 12*), T must pay the difference of $9,703 for 2009 because of the alternative minimum tax. Note that T must pay a total of $11,973 in taxes for 2009 ($2,270 regular income tax + $9,703 alternative minimum tax).

The previous example illustrates an unfortunate consequence of the strict application of the AMT provisions. The tax benefits of longstanding regular-tax incentive provisions such as home ownership (e.g., deductibility of interest and real property taxes) and medical expenses are either decreased or totally eliminated by the AMT. Although Congress continues to support the objectives of these incentives, their use by individuals to avoid all or most of their Federal income tax liability is not the intent of the law. Recent changes to the AMT are an attempt to minimize such perceived abuses. As illustrated in *Example 14*, because of the limited definition of ATIDs and the decreasing Federal income tax rates, it is possible that many unsuspecting individuals (like T) will be subject to the AMT.[54] Consequently, tax planning to avoid or minimize the AMT is becoming more important for a growing number of taxpayers. As an adjunct to planning for the impact of the AMT, it should be remembered that each taxpayer has the responsibility to maintain adequate records to support the accuracy of the amounts of tax preferences and adjustments used in the AMT computation [as required by Reg. § 1.57-5(a)].

A completed Form 6251, based on the facts from *Examples 12, 13, and 14*, is contained in Exhibit 13-6. The 2008 form is used because the 2009 form was not available at the publication date of this text.

With all of the potential complexity and extra reporting work required by the AMT provisions, it is noteworthy that Congress once made an attempt to make another area of

---

[54] *N. Holly v. Comm.*, T.C. Memo 1998-55.

EXHIBIT 13-6

Taxable income before subtracting the exemption amounts.

Form **6251**

Department of the Treasury
Internal Revenue Service (99)

Alternative Minimum Tax—Individuals

▶ See separate instructions.

▶ Attach to Form 1040 or Form 1040NR.

OMB No. 1545-0074

2008

Attachment Sequence No. **32**

Name(s) shown on Form 1040 or Form 1040NR
MR. AND MRS. T

Your social security number
324 ¦ 91 ¦ 0070

Part I — Alternative Minimum Taxable Income (See instructions for how to complete each line.)

1	If filing Schedule A (Form 1040), enter the amount from Form 1040, line 41 (minus any amount on Form 8914, line 2), and go to line 2. Otherwise, enter the amount from Form 1040, line 38 (minus any amount on Form 8914, line 2), and go to line 7. (If less than zero, enter as a negative amount.)	**1** 28,000
2	Medical and dental. Enter the **smaller** of Schedule A (Form 1040), line 4, **or** 2.5% (.025) of Form 1040, line 38. If zero or less, enter -0-	**2** 2,000
3	Taxes from Schedule A (Form 1040), line 9	**3** 24,000
4	Enter the home mortgage interest adjustment, if any, from line 6 of the worksheet on page 2 of the instructions	**4** 2,000
5	Miscellaneous deductions from Schedule A (Form 1040), line 27	**5** 9,000
6	If Form 1040, line 38, is over $159,950 (over $79,975 if married filing separately), enter the amount from line 11 of the **Itemized Deductions Worksheet** on page A-10 of the instructions for Schedule A (Form 1040)	**6** ( )
7	If claiming the standard deduction, enter any amount from Form 4684, line 18a, as a negative amount	**7** ( )
8	Tax refund from Form 1040, line 10 or line 21	**8** ( )
9	Investment interest expense (difference between regular tax and AMT)	**9** (8,000)
10	Depletion (difference between regular tax and AMT)	**10**
11	Net operating loss deduction from Form 1040, line 21. Enter as a positive amount	**11**
12	Interest from specified private activity bonds exempt from the regular tax	**12**
13	Qualified small business stock (7% of gain excluded under section 1202)	**13**
14	Exercise of incentive stock options (excess of AMT income over regular tax income)	**14** 60,000
15	Estates and trusts (amount from Schedule K-1 (Form 1041), box 12, code A)	**15**
16	Electing large partnerships (amount from Schedule K-1 (Form 1065-B), box 6)	**16**
17	Disposition of property (difference between AMT and regular tax gain or loss)	**17**
18	Depreciation on assets placed in service after 1986 (difference between regular tax and AMT)	**18**
19	Passive activities (difference between AMT and regular tax income or loss)	**19**
20	Loss limitations (difference between AMT and regular tax income or loss)	**20**
21	Circulation costs (difference between regular tax and AMT)	**21**
22	Long-term contracts (difference between AMT and regular tax income)	**22**
23	Mining costs (difference between regular tax and AMT)	**23**
24	Research and experimental costs (difference between regular tax and AMT)	**24**
25	Income from certain installment sales before January 1, 1987	**25** ( )
26	Intangible drilling costs preference	**26**
27	Other adjustments, including income-based related adjustments	**27**
28	Alternative tax net operating loss deduction	**28** ( )
29	**Alternative minimum taxable income.** Combine lines 1 through 28. (If married filing separately and line 29 is more than $214,900, see page 8 of the instructions.)	**29** 117,000

Taxable income before exemptions ($21,000 + $7,000 = $28,000)

Part II — Alternative Minimum Tax (AMT)

30 Exemption. (If you were under age 24 at the end of 2008, see page 8 of the instructions.)

IF your filing status is ...	AND line 29 is not over ...	THEN enter on line 30 ...
Single or head of household	$112,500	$46,200
Married filing jointly or qualifying widow(er)	150,000	69,950
Married filing separately	75,000	34,975

30 70,950

2009 Exemption

If line 29 is **over** the amount shown above for your filing status, see page 8 of the instructions.

31	Subtract line 30 from line 29. If more than zero, go to line 32. If zero or less, enter -0- here and on lines 34 and 36 and skip the rest of Part II	**31** 46,050
32	• If you are filing Form 2555 or 2555-EZ, see page 9 of the instructions for the amount to enter. • If you reported capital gain distributions directly on Form 1040, line 13; you reported qualified dividends on Form 1040, line 9b; **or** you had a gain on both lines 15 and 16 of Schedule D (Form 1040) (as refigured for the AMT, if necessary), complete Part III on the back and enter the amount from line 55 here. • All others: If line 31 is $175,000 or less ($87,500 or less if married filing separately), multiply line 31 by 26% (.26). Otherwise, multiply line 31 by 28% (.28) and subtract $3,500 ($1,750 if married filing separately) from the result.	**32**
33	Alternative minimum tax foreign tax credit (see page 9 of the instructions)	**33** 11,973
34	Tentative minimum tax. Subtract line 33 from line 32	**34** 11,973
35	Tax from Form 1040, line 44 (minus any tax from Form 4972 and any foreign tax credit from Form 1040, line 47). If you used Schedule J to figure your tax, the amount from line 44 of Form 1040 must be refigured without using Schedule J (see page 11 of the instructions)	**35** 2,270
36	**AMT.** Subtract line 35 from line 34. If zero or less, enter -0-. Enter here and on Form 1040, line 45	**36** 9,703

For Paperwork Reduction Act Notice, see page 12 of the instructions.   Cat. No. 13600G   Form **6251** (2008)

the Federal tax laws more orderly—the part specifying credits against the tax liability. The remainder of this chapter is devoted to the tax incentives provided by the tax credit provisions. However, at the risk of upsetting what otherwise is an orderly presentation of the various credits, it seems only appropriate that the special minimum tax credit should be considered before we leave the AMT.

MINIMUM TAX CREDIT

One significant feature of the AMT system is that many taxpayers are required to pay the AMT long before they would have had to pay the regular income tax from certain investments. For example, taxpayers with substantial investments in depreciable personal property are *denied* the tax reduction benefits of MACRS for purposes of computing the AMT.[55] Likewise, a taxpayer who exercises an ISO must recognize income for AMT purposes to the extent the fair market value of the stock exceeds its option price, but for regular income tax purposes the taxpayer does not recognize income until the stock acquired with the ISO is sold. Without some form of relief, a taxpayer could be subject to the AMT in one year and the regular tax in a later year on the same item.

In order to limit the possibility of double taxation under the two tax systems, Congress introduced an AMT credit. Basically, the AMT paid in one year may be used as a credit against the taxpayer's *regular* tax liability in subsequent years. The credit may be carried forward indefinitely until used; however, the credit cannot be carried back *nor*, until recently, could it be used to offset any future AMT liability.[56]

> **Example 15.** In 2009, J paid an alternative minimum tax, and his AMT credit after making the appropriate adjustments was $20,000. In 2009, J's regular tax liability before considering the minimum tax credit, is $45,000 and his *tentative* minimum tax is $40,000. Since J's regular tax exceeds his tentative minimum tax, there is no AMT for 2010. In computing his final tax liability, J is entitled to use the minimum tax credit against his regular tax liability but only to the extent that it does not create an AMT (i.e., bring his regular tax liability below his tentative minimum tax). Consequently, he may use $5,000 of the credit, reducing his regular tax liability to $40,000, as shown below. The remaining $15,000 of the minimum tax credit may be carried forward indefinitely.

Regular tax liability		$45,000
Minimum tax credit:		
Limitation		
Regular tax	$ 45,000	
Tentative minimum tax	− 40,000	
Allowable minimum tax credit		− 5,000
Total tax due		$40,000

Note that the minimum tax credit effectively converts the AMT from a permanent out-of-pocket tax to a prepayment of regular tax to the extent the AMT is attributable to deferral or timing preferences and adjustments rather than to exclusion items.[57]

For noncorporate taxpayers, the minimum tax credit for any year is the amount of the taxpayer's *adjusted net minimum tax* for all tax years after reduction for the minimum tax credit utilized for all such prior years. The adjusted net minimum tax, generally the amount of the minimum tax credit, is the difference between the AMT actually paid and

---

[55]   Recall that depreciable personal property placed in service after 1986 can be depreciated using either the 150 percent declining balance or the ADS straight-line method over the asset's class life for AMT purposes.

[56]   § 53(a). See next section for discussion of AMT refundable credit.

[57]   § 53(d)(1)(B)(iv) authorizes corporate taxpayers to use the entire minimum tax liability as the minimum tax credit.

the amount of AMT that would have been paid if only exclusion items were taken into account. The exclusion items are listed below.

1. Itemized deductions or standard deduction

2. Personal exemptions

3. Percentage depletion treated as a preference

4. Tax-exempt interest treated as a preference

5. The preference amount computed on the sale of the § 1202 stock.

Example 16. J is married and files a joint return for the current year on which she reports $79,200 of taxable income and claims the standard deduction. In computing her taxable income, J excluded $56,000 of tax-exempt interest from SPABs, which creates a $56,000 AMT preference item, and she claimed a $100,000 deduction for research expenses from an activity in which she does not materially participate, which creates a $90,000 AMT adjustment for research and experimental expenditures. J's minimum tax credit to be carried forward is $29,678, as computed below.

The amount of AMT actually required to be paid is $38,924, determined as follows:

Regular taxable income			$ 79,200
Plus:	AMT adjustment for research expenses		+ 90,000
	AMT adjustment for personal exemptions		+ 7,300
	AMT adjustment for standard deduction		+ 11,400
	AMT preference item for SPAB income		+ 56,000
AMTI			$243,900
Less:	Exemption amount [$70,950 − $23,475 phase-out		
	($243,900 − $150,000 = $93,900 × 0.25)]		− 47,475
AMT base			$196,425
Tentative minimum tax [$45,500 + 28% ($196,425 − $175,000)]			$ 51,499
Less:	Regular tax liability for 2009		− 12,575
AMT liability for current year			$ 38,924

The amount of AMT that would have been required to be paid if only exclusion items were taken into account is determined as follows:

Regular taxable income			$ 79,200
Plus:	AMT adjustment for personal exemptions		+ 7,300
	AMT adjustment for standard deduction		+ 11,400
	Tax preference item for SPAB income		+ 56,000
AMTI			$153,900
Less:	Exemption amount (no phase-out		
	[$70,950 − $975 phaseout ($153,900 − $150,000 =		
	$3,900 × .25)]		− 69,975
AMT base			$ 83,925
Times:	AMT rate		× 26%
Tentative AMT			$ 21,821
Less:	Regular tax liability		− 12,575
AMT using only exclusions			$ 9,246

The minimum tax credit is computed as follows:

AMT liability for current year.	$ 38,924
AMT using only exclusion items.	− 9,246
Minimum tax credit	$ 29,678

The $29,678 minimum tax credit may be carried forward and used to offset (reduce) the regular tax liability in subsequent years.

AMT REFUNDABLE TAX CREDIT

As part of the Tax Relief and Health Care Act of 2006, Congress created an AMT refundable credit. The relief provided by this credit is intended primarily for individuals who had minimum tax credits but could not use them. This problem normally occurred when individuals exercised ISOs at a profit and subsequently sold the stock when the price had significantly declined. Taxpayers in these situations normally paid an AMT on the profit in the year of the exercise, producing an AMT credit. However, because of the diminution in value of the stock at the time of the sale, little or no gain was recognized for regular tax purposes and the AMT credit could not be used. As a result, such individuals ended up with large minimum tax credits that they may not be able to use for many years to come.

> **Example 17.** During the height of the bull market in 2000, T was working for a high-tech company. While there, she exercised an ISO to buy her employer's stock worth $1,000,000 for $9,000. As a result, T had an AMT adjustment of $991,000 and paid an AMT of $277,000. This in turn created a minimum tax credit (MTC) of $277,000. Consistent with the AMT rules, T's AMT basis in the acquired stock was $1,000,000 ($9,000 cost plus the $991,000 adjustment). In 2002, the company went bankrupt. For regular tax purposes, the worthless stock is deemed to have been sold for $0 (basis $9,000), resulting in a long-term capital loss of $9,000. For AMT purposes, the rules are the same but because her basis is $1,000,000, she has an AMT capital loss of $1,000,000. Unfortunately, she has no AMT capital gains and all she can deduct for AMT purposes in the current year is the same amount that she can deduct for regular tax purposes, $3,000.[58] Although the MTC of $277,000 can be used to offset the regular tax in excess of the TMT in subsequent years, she may receive little or no benefit from the MTC in the future.

To address the problem illustrated above, Congress created a special credit. Beginning in 2007, § 53(e) generally allows taxpayers that have long-term unused minimum tax credit carryovers to claim a *refundable* AMT credit for each taxable year prior to 2013. For taxable years after 2007 the AMT refundable credit amount each year is the greater of:

A. 50 percent of the long term unused minimum tax credit for the year, or
B. The amount (if any) of the AMT refundable credit determined for the taxpayer's preceding year.

---

[58]   See *Merlo v. Comm.*, 126 TC 205 (2006).

The long-term unused minimum tax credit for a tax year is the portion of the MTC available at the beginning of the third tax year immediately preceding the current year. For example, for the tax year 2009, the available credit would be that which existed at the beginning of 2006. In applying the rules, the credits are treated as allowed on a FIFO basis. Note also that the credit is available for only individual taxpayers. In addition, because it is refundable, this credit reduces both the AMT liability and the regular tax liability and the remainder of the credit amount being paid to the taxpayer as a refund.

Example 18. Refer to the facts in the previous example and assume that T has a MTC carryover at the beginning of 2005 of $277,000. In addition, assume that T is married to H, has two children in college, files a joint return and takes the standard deduction. The couple's only income is T's salary of $124,300 from which T's employer withheld $18,000 in federal income tax. The couple's regular tax liability for 2008 is $17,538 and they have no AMT liability for the year and no other credits are allowable. As a result, T's AMT refundable credit amount is $138,500 (50% x $277,000). In this case, $17,538 (the amount of the couple's regular tax) is treated as a nonrefundable credit and the remaining $120.962 is treated as a refundable credit. T's refund for the year will also include the $18,000 of federal income tax that she had withheld from her salary, for a total refund of $138,962.

Example 19. Refer to the facts in previous two examples to compute the AMT refundable credit for 2009. Assume that the couple's only income is T's salary of $124,300 from which T's employer withheld no federal income tax. The couple's regular tax liability for 2009 is $16,950 and they have no AMT liability for the year and no other credits are allowable. The couple's AMT refundable credit amount is $138,500 as computed below. The AMT refundable credit amount is the greater of:

A.   50% of the long-term unused minimum tax credit for the year $138,500 (50% × $277,000) or

B.   The amount of the credit for the preceding year, $138,500 in 2008.

In 2009 $16,950 is treated as a nonrefundable credit and the $121,550 is treated as a refundable credit, providing a refund to the couple of $121,550.

✓ CHECK YOUR KNOWLEDGE

Review Question 1. After completing his tax return for the year, C has a regular tax liability of $30,000, a tentative minimum tax of $45,000, and an alternative minimum tax of $15,000. How much does C actually owe the IRS?

C owes $45,000 in taxes, consisting of a regular tax liability of $30,000 and an AMT liability of $15,000.

Review Question 2. True-False. Jack is a professional golfer, earning more than $800,000 on the tour this year. After deducting expenses, taxable income for the year is $400,000. He and his wife are entitled to a $70,950 (2009) exemption in computing their alternative minimum tax liability.

False. The exemption phases out once their AMTI exceeds $150,000 and is completely phased out when AMTI reaches $433,800. Based on the size of his earnings, it would appear that his AMTI exceeds $433,800 so that the exemption would provide no benefit.

Review Question 3. True-False. In determining AMTI, the taxpayer begins with taxable income and then adds back all of the deductions allowed by so-called loopholes. There are no negative adjustments.

False. Although the effect of the AMTI is to fill in the loopholes, adjustments may be positive or negative (e.g., when AMT depreciation exceeds regular tax depreciation). All tax preference items are positive.

Review Question 4. True-False. In 2009, Steelco Corporation acquired several new copying machines for its offices and depreciated them under MACRS, using the 200 percent declining-balance method and a five-year recovery period. For AMT purposes, Steelco must use the straight-line method and a six-year class life. (**Hint:** See Revenue Procedure 87-56 contained in Exhibit 9-2).

False. Steelco may use the recovery period of five years, but is only allowed to use 150 percent declining-balance in computing depreciation for personal property for AMT purposes.

Review Question 5. Fred and Ethel are married with two children. Fred is a partner in a public accounting firm. Ethel recently retired as a traveling salesperson for an athletic shoe manufacturer. After completing their return, Fred and Ethel realized that they may have to pay the alternative minimum tax. Indicate whether an adjustment is required for AMT purposes for the following items that the couple reported for regular tax purposes.

  a. Personal exemptions for Fred and Ethel
  b. Dependent exemptions for their children
  c. Social security benefits that were nontaxable, $10,000
  d. Contribution to individual retirement account, $2,000
  e. Fred's membership dues to the Indiana C.P.A. Society reimbursed by his employer, $200
  f. Straight-line depreciation on their newly acquired duplex, which they are currently renting out, $6,000
  g. State income taxes, $10,000
  h. Property taxes on their personal residence, $4,000
  i. Tax-exempt interest from City of Indianapolis bonds used to finance its downtown mall, $2,000 (the bonds were issued after August 7, 1988)
  j. State income tax refund, $500
  k. Interest on the mortgage on their personal residence, $22,000
  l. Interest on a second mortgage on their residence (proceeds used to add a porch), $3,600
  m. Ethel's unreimbursed travel and entertainment expenses related to her employment, $1,000
  n. Alimony to Fred's ex-wife, Luci, $4,000

An adjustment is required for (a) and (b) (exemptions not allowed), (f) (40- vs. 39-year life), (g) and (h) (taxes), (i) (private activity bond), (j) (no AMT income for tax refunds), and

(m) (miscellaneous itemized deduction). No adjustment is required for (c), (d), (e) (reimbursed employee business expense deductible for A.G.I.), (k) (qualified housing interest), (l) (home equity loan used for improvement to house is qualified housing interest), or (n) (no adjustment required).

Review Question 6. GHI Construction Corporation, a calendar year taxpayer, specializes in building warehouses. Its annual gross receipts average about $8 million. The corporation began work on a building in November 2009 and finished construction in February 2010. The contract was approximately 40 percent complete as of the close of the year. For regular tax purposes, the corporation uses the completed contract method. Consequently, it reported all of the income from the contract, $100,000, in 2010.

a.   What is the amount of the AMT adjustment for 2009, if any?

GHI must use the percentage of completion method for AMT purposes. Therefore, the AMT adjustment would be a positive $40,000 (40% of $100,000).

b.   Assume that the AMT attributable to the above contract was $8,000 (20% × $40,000) and that GHI paid this amount as AMT when it filed its 2009 tax return. In 2010, GHI reported the entire $100,000 profit for regular tax purposes. Is the $40,000 of profit earned in 2009 taxed twice, once under the AMT system when it is included as a $40,000 adjustment in 2009 and once under the regular tax system when it is included in the $100,000 reported in 2010?

No. The AMT paid in 2009 may be credited against the regular tax in 2010. The minimum tax credit ensures that the income is not taxed twice. Note that in this case the AMT effectively operates to accelerate the income tax paid on a portion of the $100,000 profit.

INCOME TAX CREDITS

One reason tax credits are popular is that a credit is viewed as providing a more equitable benefit than a comparable deduction. This is because a credit is a direct reduction of the tax liability, while a deduction merely reduces the amount of taxable income. This difference is illustrated in *Example 20*.

Example 20. Hi is in the 36% tax bracket, and Lo is in the 15% tax bracket. A credit of $100 is worth the *same* to both taxpayers since it reduces the tax liability of each by $100. On the other hand, a deduction of $100 provides a *different* benefit for each: $36 (36% × $100) for Hi and only $15 (15% × $100) for Lo.

The results from *Example 20* can be generalized for tax policy as (1) all taxpayers receive the *same dollar benefit* from credits, regardless of marginal tax rates; (2) taxpayers with higher marginal tax rates benefit more from tax deductions than do those with lower marginal rates; and (3) taxpayers receive more benefit from tax credits than from tax deductions of the same amount. In addition, the argument has been made that credits are of more benefit to those with lower incomes. This is based on the reasoning that the $100 tax saved has more relative value for those with low incomes than it has for those with high incomes. However, this line of reasoning is questionable since taxable income is just one inexact measure of a person's economic situation.

OVERVIEW OF TAX CREDITS

In recent years, the number of tax credits has been significantly increased by Congress. Most of them have been enacted into law to achieve a specified social, economic, or political goal. These goals range from encouraging taxpayers to engage in scientific research (the research credit) and the conservation of energy (energy tax credits) to providing compensatory tax reductions for those individuals who may carry greater burdens than others (credits for the elderly and for individuals with low earned incomes).

As the table in Exhibit 13-7 illustrates, the credit provisions are divided into *six* major groups. Technically these are all subparts of Part IV - Credits Against Tax contained in Subchapter A of the Code. Subpart A consists of nonrefundable individual tax credits and Subpart B contains certain other nonrefundable credits. All of these nonrefundable credits may be used to reduce the tax liability, but *only* to the extent of the "regular tax liability." Subpart C contains the *refundable* credits. Subpart D consists of 13 separate credits, which are combined to form the "general business credit." The minimum tax credits are contained in Subpart G. And finally, the credit to holders of clean renewable energy bonds is in Subpart H. A quick look at the Exhibit reveals that Congress has gone wild on credits. While some of the credits have widespread applicability, many apply to a very limited group of taxpayers.

Limitation on Nonrefundable Credits. The nonrefundable credits may be used to reduce only the taxpayer's regular tax liability as that quantity is defined in §26. Under § 26, a taxpayer's "regular tax liability" does not include (1) the alternative minimum tax (§ 55); (2) the additional tax imposed on distributions from certain annuities [§ 72(m)]; (3) the additional tax imposed on distributions from educational IRAs [§ 530(d)]; (4) the accumulated earnings tax (§ 531); (5) the personal holding company tax (§ 541); (6) the tax on certain capital gains of S corporations (§ 1374); or (7) the tax on passive income of S corporations (§ 1375). Thus, the nonrefundable credits cannot be used to offset penalty taxes imposed by the Code (e.g., personal holding company tax, accumulated earnings tax, etc.). The practical impact of defining the "regular tax liability" in this manner is that the regular tax credits cannot offset the alternative minimum tax. Note, however that for taxable years 2002 through 2009 Congress generally has authorized the nonrefundable personal credits to offset the AMT as well as the regular tax liability.[59]

For taxpayers to whom two or more credits apply, generally the Code specifies an ascending order for the use of nonrefundable credits. Nonrefundable credits are to be used to reduce the § 26 tax liability in the following order: §§ 21, 22, 25A, 25, 25B, 24, 27, 23, 29, 30, 30A, 38 and 53.[60] This order is important because some of the credits may be carried forward or back and utilized in different tax years, while others "fall through the cracks" (i.e., provide no tax benefit) if they exceed the § 26 tax liability in the year they originate.

---

[59] *Huntsberry v. Comm.*, 83 T.C. 742. But see Footnote 8 for an amendment to § 26(a) that allows personal credits to offset the AMT for the years 2000 through 2009

[60] The order in which credits are absorbed can be pieced together by reading §§ 25(e), 23(b), 25B(g) and 53(c).

EXHIBIT 13-7

Table of Tax Credits

	Code Section	Specific Credit	Termination Date
Subpart A:	§ 21	Child and Dependent Care Credit	None
	§ 22	Credit for the Elderly	None
	§ 23	Credit for Adoption Expenses	None
	§ 24	Child Tax Credit	None
	§ 25	Credit for Interest on Certain Home Mortgages	None
	§ 25A	HOPE and Lifetime Learning Credits	None
	§ 25B	IRA Contribution Credit	None
	§ 25C	Residential Energy Property Credit	12/31/2010*
	§ 25D	Residential Alternative Energy Credit	12/31/2016
Subpart B:	§ 27	Possession and Foreign Tax Credit	None
	§ 30	Credit for Qualified Electric Vehicle	12/31/2006*
	§ 30B	Alternative Motor Vehicle Credit	12/31/2010
	§ 30C	Alternative Motor Vehicle Refueling Property Credit	12/31/2009
	§ 30D	New Qualified Plug-In Electric Drive Motor Vehicles	12/31/2014
Subpart C:	§ 31	Credit for Taxes Withheld on Wages	None
	§ 32	Earned Income Credit	None
	§ 33	Credit for Taxes Withheld at Source on Nonresident Aliens and Foreign Corporations	None
	§ 34	Credit for Certain Uses of Gasoline and Special Fuels	None
	§ 35	Health Insurance credit	None
Subpart D:	§ 38	General Business Credit (including)	
		1. Alcohol Fuels Credit (§ 40)	12/31/2010
		2. Research Credit (§ 41)	12/31/2009*
		3. Low-Income Housing Credit (§ 42)	None
		4. Enhanced Oil Recovery Credit (§ 43)	None
		5. Disabled Individual Access Credit (§ 44)	None
		6. Renewable Electricity Production (§ 45)	None
		7. Indian Employment Credit (§ 45A)	12/31/2009*
		8. Employer Social Security Credit (§ 45B)	None
		9. Credit for Clinical Testing of Certain Drugs (§ 45C)	None
		10. New Markets Tax Credit (§ 45D)	12/31/2009
		11. Small Employer Pension Plan Start Up Costs (§ 45E)	12/31/2010
		12. Employer Provided Child Care Credit (§ 45F)	12/31/2010
		13. Railroad Track Maintenance Credit (§ 45G)	12/31/2010
		14. Credit for production of low sulfur diesel fuel (§ 45H)	None
		15. Credit for producing oil and gas from marginal wells (§ 45I)	None
		16. Credit for production from advanced nuclear power facilities (§ 45J)	None
		17. Credit for producing fuel from a non-conventional source (§ 45K)	12/31/2010
		18. New Energy Efficient Home Credit (§ 45L)	12/31/2009
		19. Energy Efficient Appliance Credit (§ 45M)	12/31/2010
		20. Mine Rescue Team Training Credit (§ 45N)	12/31/2009
		21. Agricultural Chemical Security Credit (§ 45O)	12/31/2012
		22. Differential Wage Payment Credit (§ 45P)	None
		23. Carbon Dioxide Sequestration (§ 45Q)	None
		24. Rehabilitation Credit (§ 47)	None
		25. Energy Credit (§ 48)	12/31/2016
		26. Qualifying Advanced Coal Project Credit (§ 48A)	None
		27. Qualifying Gasification Project Credit (§48B)	None
		28. Work Opportunity Credit (§ 51)	8/31/2011
		29. Empowerment Zone Employment Credit (§ 1396)	12/31/2009
Subpart G:	§ 53	Credit for Prior Year Minimum Tax Liability	None
	§ 53(e)	AMT Refundable Credit	12/31/2012
Subpart H:	§ 54	Credit to holders of Clean Renewable Energy Bonds	12/31/2009

* May be extended by tax legislation enacted in 2009.

Refundable Credits. Refundable credits—listed in Exhibit 13-7 under Subpart C—are accounted for *after* the nonrefundable ones and may be applied against *any* income tax imposed by the Code-including the penalty taxes. As the name suggests, refundable credits may result in the taxpayer receiving a refund check for an amount in excess of any Federal taxes paid or withheld. In a sense, these credit provisions may result in a "negative income tax."

Due to the magnitude and relative importance of the business credits, they are examined first. A discussion of the tax credits available only to individual taxpayers immediately follows.

GENERAL BUSINESS CREDIT

As shown in Exhibit 13-7, the general business credit actually consists of a variety separate credits that are commonly available to business. Each of these credits is separately computed under its own set of rules. The various credits are then combined to determine the current year's total business credit. The credits are combined in order to determine an overall limitation on the amount of credit that can be used.

In order to prevent taxpayers from using business credits to avoid paying all income taxes, the general business credit is limited each year by the taxpayer's *net regular tax liability*. The net regular tax liability is the § 26 tax liability reduced by the credits allowed in §§ 21 through 30A. In addition, taxpayers with a net regular tax liability exceeding $25,000 are subject to an additional limitation. The business credit is limited to $25,000 *plus* 75 percent of the net regular tax liability in excess of $25,000.[61] It should also be recalled that the business credits normally are not allowed to offset the AMT. Generally, credits arising in tax years beginning after December 31, 1997 that are unused because of these limits can be carried back one year and then forward 20 years, applied on a first-in, first-out basis.[62]

> **Example 21.** In 2009, F has a potential general business credit of $92,000 and a net regular tax liability of $100,000. The maximum allowable business credit for 2009 is $81,250 [$25,000 + (75% × $75,000 = $56,250)]. The unused credit of $10,750 ($92,000 − $81,250) is subject to the carryover rules.

When the general business credit is limited and two or more components of the credit are applicable, special ordering rules as specified in § 38(d) apply to determine which credits will be utilized currently and which credits will be subject to the carryback and carryover rules.

The common rules for computing the separate components of the general business credit beginning with the investment tax credit, are detailed in the following sections.

INVESTMENT CREDIT

In 1962, Congress enacted the investment tax credit in hopes of stimulating the economy by encouraging taxpayers to purchase certain assets—generally tangible personal property used in a trade or business. Although application of the provision became quite difficult, the essence of the law was simple. It allowed a credit equal to a particular percentage of the cost of the property. For example, taxpayers who purchased equipment at a cost of $100,000 might be entitled to a credit equal to 10 percent of the cost, or $10,000—but only as long as they met a host of requirements.

---

[61] § 38(c)(1). Married taxpayers filing separate returns are limited to $12,500 plus 75 percent of the tax liability in excess of $12,500 [§ 38(c)(4)].

[62] § 39(a). Note that credits arising in years prior to 1998 generally could be carried back three years and then forward for 15 years.

Since its enactment, the investment tax credit has had a tortuous history, in the law one year and out the next. It most recently was part of the Code in 1985 before it fell victim to the Tax Reform Act of 1986. In order to partially offset the significant loss of Federal tax revenues resulting from the 1986 tax rate reductions, Congress terminated the regular investment tax credit for assets placed in service after December 31, 1985. However, Congress allowed certain portions of the old credit to continue as the investment credit (IC). Under current law, the IC is made up of distinct parts: (1) the credit for rehabilitation expenditures and, (2) the energy credit. Each part of the IC is computed separately under its own specific rules. The actual amount of each part of the IC is the function of two factors: the taxpayer's basis in property qualifying for the credit, and the rate of the credit. The two components of the IC—the rehabilitation and energy credits—are discussed below.[63]

Rehabilitation Investment Credit. The Economic Recovery Tax Act of 1981 grafted onto the regular investment credit an additional tax credit designed to encourage the restoration of buildings constructed prior to 1936. The credit represents a unique tax incentive for the restoration of old buildings.

With an emphasis on urban renewal, the rehabilitation investment credit is limited to substantial *rehabilitation expenditures* (excluding the purchase price) of *commercial buildings* and *historic structures*.[64] *Substantial* is defined to mean qualifying expenditures that exceed the greater of (1) the property's basis, or (2) $5,000. To prevent destruction of these buildings, the amended legislation requires that:

1. Fifty percent or more of the existing external walls of the buildings is retained in place as external walls;

2. Seventy-five percent or more of the external walls of the building is retained in place as internal or external walls; and

3. Seventy-five percent or more of the existing internal structural framework of the building is retained in place.

If these requirements are met, the credit is available for qualified expenditures on *both* nonresidential real property and residential rental property or an addition or improvement to either type of property. However, if the rehabilitation credit is taken, the property *must* be depreciated under the straight-line method over the MACRS recovery period or the alternative depreciation system.[65]

The rate of rehabilitation credit is:

Rate	Type of Structure
10%	Commercial building originally placed in service prior to 1936
20	All certified historic structures[66]

Example 22. On January 3, 2009, R purchases a commercial building that was constructed in 1920. In addition to the $300,000 of the purchase price allocated to the building, the entire core of the building is renovated at a cost of $600,000. R's rehabilitation credit is $60,000. computed as follows:

---

[63] Credits for qualifying advanced coal projects and for qualifying gasification projects were added to the energy credit in 2005 but are of limited application and are not discussed in this chapter.

[64] § 47(a).

[65] § 47(c)(2)(B).

[66] § 47(c)(3). The designation as a certified historic structure is made by the Secretary of the Interior.

Qualified investment	$600,000
Rate of credit	× 10%
Current credit (before limitations)	$ 60,000

In some instances, rehabilitation expenditures also qualify for the energy investment credit (discussed below). When this occurs, taxpayers *must choose* between the two credits because both credits cannot be claimed for the same expenditure.[67]

Energy Investment Credit. Recognizing the need for energy conservation, Congress added the *energy credit* provisions to the Code. The objective of this credit is to encourage taxpayers to decrease energy consumption or change the type of energy used.

The credit is 10 percent for qualified microturbine property and 30 percent for solar energy property, qualified fuel cell property and qualified small wind energy property.[68] "Energy property" for which the credit is allowed includes subject to a number of limitations:

- Equipment that uses solar energy to generate electricity, to heat or cool (or provide hot water for use in) a structure, to provide solar process heat and in certain cases to illuminate a room
- Equipment used to produce, distribute, or use energy from a geothermal deposit
- Qualified fuel cell property or qualified microturbine property
- Qualified small wind energy property

Example 23. S is the owner of a deluxe print shop. In March 2009, S installed four solar panels to heat water to be used in a photographic development process. The panels, pumps, valves, storage tanks, control system, and installation cost a total of $80,000. S's energy tax credit is $8,000.

Qualified investment	$80,000
Rate of credit	× 30%
Current credit (before limitations)	$ 2,400

Basis Reduction of Qualified Property. At one time, taxpayers were allowed to take a full 10 percent IC or any applicable energy tax credit and still recover their entire cost basis of qualifying property under ACRS. In 1986, Congress decided that this treatment was too liberal with respect to rehabilitation property and required the basis of the property to be reduced by the amount of IC taken with respect to the property.[69] A similar rule requires that the basis of energy property be reduced by *one-half* of the amount of the IC taken on such energy property.[70]

Example 24. Refer to the facts in *Example 22*, where R's rehabilitation credit is $60,000. R purchased the property for $300,000 and incurred $600,000 of rehabilitation expenditures. R's basis in the rehabilitated property is $840,000 ($300,000 + $600,000 − $60,000).

---

[67]   § 48(a)(2).

[68]   § 48.

[69]   § 50(c)(1). Note that for determining the amount and character of gain on the disposition of the property, the downward basis adjustment is treated as a deduction allowed for depreciation. Accordingly, the amount of the basis adjustment will be subject to the § 1245 depreciation recapture rules discussed in Chapter 7.

[70]   § 50(c)(3).

Example 25. Refer to the facts in *Example 23*, where S's energy tax credit is $8,000. S purchased the solar property for $80,000. S's basis in the energy property is $76,000 ($80,000 − $4,000).

The investment credit calculations discussed here provide the background for computing the recapture of IC on early dispositions required by the Code.[71] The amount of IC recapture should be an economic consideration in planning the disposition of any asset upon which the IC was claimed.

IC Recapture. When taxpayers place qualified investment property into service, they claim the full amount of IC regardless of how long they intend to use the property. However, if an asset ceases to be qualified property during a five-year period (due to a sale or other disposition, or a change in the purpose or use of the asset), taxpayers are required to recapture a portion of the "unearned" IC. The recapture percentages illustrated in Exhibit 13-8 must be used to calculate the amount of unearned credit that is recaptured as an additional tax in the year of early disposition. As a general rule, 20 percent of the credit is "earned" for each full year the property is held. For example, a qualified rehabilitation property placed in service on December 20, 2008 qualified for the rehabilitation credit in 2008 and was taken on the taxpayer's return for the year. However, none of the credit was *earned* until December 21, 2009. On that date, 20 percent of the credit allowed in 2008 was earned and thus no longer subject to recapture.

EXHIBIT 13-8
Itc Recapture Percentages[72]

If qualified property ceases to be qualified property—	The recapture percentage is:
Before one full year, after placed in service	100%
After one year, within two full years	80
After two years, within three full years	60
After three years, within four full years	40
After four years, within five full years	20

Example 26. Assume that the commercial building (acquired on January 3, 2009) in *Example 22* was sold by R on September 1, 2010. The IC recapture is computed as follows:

Property	IC Claimed	×	Recapture Percentage	=	Amount Recaptured
Commercial bldg.	$60,000	×	80%	=	$48,000

This amount is reported on Form 4255 and is treated as an additional tax imposed on the taxpayer in the year in which an early disposition occurs. Because the building's basis was originally decreased by the entire credit claimed, its basis is increased by the amount of the recapture for purposes of computing the gain or loss to be recognized on the sale.[73]

---

[71] § 50(a).

[72] § 50(a)(1)(B).

[73] § 50(c)(2). A similar rule applies to energy property, but only one-half of the amount of recapture is added to the basis of the property.

In addition to sales and exchanges (including like-kind exchanges), dispositions generally include gifts, dividend distributions from corporations, cessation of business usage, and involuntary conversions.[74] Even though the recaptured IC is referred to as an "other tax" on Form 1040, the amount recaptured will not be treated as a tax for purposes of determining the amount of nonrefundable tax credits allowed under § 26.[75]

The recapture rules do not apply to transfers by reason of death or to assets transferred in certain corporate acquisitions.[76] The recapture rules also will not apply to transfers of property between spouses, even if the transfer is made incident to divorce.[77] Finally, property is not treated as ceasing to be qualified property when a mere change in the form of conducting the trade or business occurs, so long as the property continues to be qualified property in the new business and the taxpayer retains a substantial interest in this trade or business.[78]

IC Carryovers. Like the other components of the general business credit, the IC allowed in tax years beginning after December 31, 1997 but not utilized because of the tax liability limitation can be carried forward for 20 years. Finally, in determining the extent to which an investment credit is used in a taxable year, the regular investment credit is deemed to be used *before* the rehabilitation credit and the energy credit.[79]

WORK OPPORTUNITY CREDIT

For many years Congress has tried to spur employment by granting businesses a tax credit for hiring new workers that otherwise had a hard time finding employment. Since 1979, businesses have been able to claim the credit if they hire individuals from certain targeted groups. The targeted groups have been most recently redefined to include:[80]

- ▸ Recipients of a state law providing assistance for needy families with minor children,
- ▸ Qualified veterans,
- ▸ Qualified ex-felons,
- ▸ High-risk youth,
- ▸ Vocational rehabilitation referrals,
- ▸ Qualified summer youth employees,
- ▸ Qualified food stamp recipients, or
- ▸ Qualified SSI recipients.
- ▸ A long term family assistance recipient.
- ▸ Unemployed veterans
- ▸ Disconnected youth

To be eligible, each individual must obtain certification from a designated local agency, specifying that the individual meets the established criteria and therefore qualifies as a member of one of the targeted groups.

Amount of Credit. The work opportunity tax credit is 40 percent of the first $6,000 of first-year wages paid to a qualified individual.[81] Thus, the maximum credit is $2,400

---

[74]   Reg. § 1.47-2.

[75]   § 50(a)(5)(C).

[76]   § 50(a)(4).

[77]   § 50(a)(5)(B).

[78]   § 50(a)(4) and Reg. § 1.47-3(f).

[79]   See § 38(d).

[80]   §§ 51(d) and 51(c)(4).

[81]   See § 51(i) for other limitations based on the number of hours worked.

for each new employee. Note that, without any restriction, the employer would be able not only to claim a credit for the wages paid to the employee but also to deduct those wages. However, employers who elect to take the credit must reduce their wage expense by the amount of the credit; this eliminates the potential windfall. Note also that, as part of the general business credit, the § 38 rules limiting the amount of the credit ($25,000 + 75% of the tax liability in excess of $25,000) are applicable, as are the one-year carryback and 20-year carryover rules.

Special Rule for Qualified Summer Youth Employees. Employers are allowed to claim the jobs credit for wages paid for the summer employment of teenagers that are members of economically disadvantaged families. These individuals must be 16 or 17 years of age on the hiring date and must not have worked previously for the employer. To qualify for the credit, the services must be attributable to any 90-day period between May 1 and September 15. The summer youth employment credit is 40 percent of the first $3,000 of eligible wages, for a maximum credit of $1,200 per youth.[82] If a summer youth employee continues to work after the 90-day period, his or her wages may qualify for the general targeted jobs credit previously discussed. However, certification of this employee as a member of a second target group must be determined as of the date of the second certification rather than on the basis of the employee's original certification as a qualified summer youth employee. In addition, the $6,000 wage limit for the targeted job credit must be reduced by the qualified summer wages.

Example 27. On July 29, 2009, the owners of a farm hired 10 youths that were certified as qualified summer employees to help harvest crops. The owners paid the youths $150 a week for eight weeks (through September 22). The amount of targeted jobs credit in 2009 without regard to additional certifications is $4,200, computed in the following manner:

Qualifying wages ($150 × 10 youths × 7 weeks)	$10,500
Percent of credit	× 40%
Amount of credit	$ 4,200

The wage expense deduction attributable to the youths' salaries would be $7,800, computed as follows:

Total wages paid ($150 × 10 youths × 8 weeks)	$12,000
Reduced by allowable credit	− 4,200
Allowable wage expense	$ 7,800

Note that the eighth week does not qualify for the credit since it occurs after the September 15 cutoff date.

Special rules for a long term family assistance recipient. The former Welfare to Work Credit has been combined with the Work Opportunity Credit. For individuals that receive assistance for more than 18 months under a State program funded under part A of Title IV of the Social Security Act, the credit amount for the first year of employment is up to 40% on the first $10,000 of wages. Also, an additional 50% credit is

---

[82] § 51(d)(12)(B).

available for wages paid up to $10,000 in the second year of employment. The maximum credit per new employee over the two year period is $9,000.[83]

ALCOHOL FUEL CREDIT

The fourth component of the general business credit is the alcohol fuel credit. To foster the production of gasohol, an income tax credit for alcohol and alcohol-blended fuels applies to fuel sales and uses before January 1, 2011. The alcohol fuel credit is computed and reported on Form 6478. Generally, for 2009 and 2010 the credit is $0.45 per gallon of alcohol used in a qualified alcohol mixture or as a straight alcohol fuel.[84] Although taxpayers are entitled to a credit, they must include an amount equal to the credit claimed in income.[85]

RESEARCH AND EXPERIMENTAL (R&E) CREDIT

The fifth component of the general business credit is the research credit—commonly referred to as the R&E credit. Created in 1981 and amended several times since, the R&E credit provisions generally allow taxpayers a credit equal to 20 percent of their *incremental* expenditures that constitute either (1) qualified research expenditures or (2) basic research payments.[86] The method for identifying what qualifies as an incremental expenditure is considered in detail below, as are the types of qualifying research. First, however, the relationship of the R&E credit and the deduction for R&E must be addressed.

Impact of R&E Credit on Current Deductions. The research credit is the second part of Congress's two-prong approach for stimulating research. The first part of this plan, as might be recalled from Chapter 9, allows taxpayers either to deduct research and experimental expenditures immediately or capitalize the expenditures and amortize them over 60 months. As might be expected, taxpayers are not allowed to have their research cake and eat it too—they must reduce their R&E deduction for the amount of R&E credit determined for the year.[87] For those taxpayers who normally expense R&E costs, this means that their deduction for R&E is simply smaller. For those taxpayers who capitalize and amortize the costs, the amount capitalized is reduced. Note that if the credit is not utilized by the taxpayer within the 20-year carryover period, a deduction equal to the amount of the expiring credit is allowed in the year following the expiration of the tax credit carryover period.[88]

Without additional rules, the cutback of the deduction for the credit could prove unduly harsh for taxpayers subject to the AMT, which generally does not allow the use of credits. For this reason taxpayers are allowed to *elect* to claim a reduced credit.[89] This election effectively enables the taxpayer to trade a credit that is not allowed to reduce the AMT for a deduction that could be used to reduce the AMT.

---

[83] 51(e).

[84] § 40. A similar credit applies to small ethanol producers.

[85] § 87.

[86] § 41(a).

[87] § 280C(c).

[88] § 196. The deduction allowed is 50 percent of the expired R&E credits attributable to taxable years beginning before 1990.

[89] § 280C(c)(3).

Qualified Research Expenditures. The R&E credit is allowed for both in-house research and contract (outside) research. *Qualified research expenditures* are those incurred in carrying on a trade or business for in-house research expenses (e.g., wages, supplies, rental of equipment, overhead) and 65 percent of *contract research expenses* (those paid to any person other than an employee of the taxpayer for qualified research).[90] To be eligible for the credit, the expenditures must meet the same criteria that must be met for their deduction. As a general rule, these criteria extend special treatment only for research and development in the experimental or laboratory sense. This includes (1) the development of an experimental or pilot model, plant process, formula, invention, or similar property, and (2) the improvement of such types of property already in existence.[91] In addition, the expenditures must be technological in nature *and* must relate to establishing a new or improved function, or improving the performance, reliability, or quality of a product.[92] Finally, the credit is *denied* for certain expenditure items,[93] including:

1. Research undertaken outside the United States

2. Research conducted in the social sciences or humanities

3. Ordinary testing or inspection of materials or products for quality control

4. Market and consumer research

5. Research relating to style, taste, cosmetic, or seasonal design

6. Advertising and promotion expenses

7. Management studies and efficiency surveys

8. Computer software for internal use of the taxpayer

9. Research to locate and evaluate mineral deposits, including oil and gas

10. Acquisition and improvement of land and of certain depreciable or depletable property used in research (including the annual depreciation deduction)

Amount of Credit. The 20 percent credit is extended only to taxpayers who increase their research activities. As shown in the formula in Exhibit 13-9, this is accomplished by allowing a credit only for qualified research expenditures for the current year that exceed the taxpayer's base amount.[94] The base amount is a fixed percentage of the taxpayer's average gross receipts for the four previous years.[95] As a result, those taxpayers who continually increase their research benefit the most from this special incentive.

The fixed-base percentage is computed differently for firms with a history of doing research than for firms that do not have such a history. For taxpayers reporting both qualified research expenses and gross receipts during each of at least three years from 1984 to 1988, the "fixed-base percentage" is the ratio that its total qualified research expenses for the 1984 to 1988 period bears to its total gross receipts for this period, subject to a maximum ratio of 16 percent. "Start-up companies" and those taxpayers not meeting the

---

[90] § 41(b)(4). The trade or business requirement may be met by certain start-up companies even though they are not currently in business.

[91] Reg. § 1.174-2(a).

[92] § 41(d)(1)(B).

[93] § 41(d)(4).

[94] § 41(a)(1).

[95] § 41(c).

R&E expenditures and gross receipt requirements above are assigned a fixed-base percentage of 3 percent for the first five years in which qualified research expenditures are incurred.[96]

EXHIBIT 13-9
Calculation of R&E Credit

R&E Credit = 20% × (qualified R&E expenditures − base amount)

Base amount = Fixed-base percentage × Average gross receipts for four previous years

$$\text{Fixed} - \text{base percentage*} = \frac{\text{Total research expenses}(1984 - 1988)}{\text{Total gross receipts}(1984 - 1988)}$$

*Subject to special rules for start-up companies and limited to a maximum of 16 percent.

Example 28. Assume R Corporation reported the following research expenditures and gross receipts:

	1986	1987	1988
Research expenditures	$ 90,000	$100,000	$110,000
Gross receipts	700,000	900,000	800,000

	2005	2006	2007	2008	2009
Research expenditures......	$120,000	$130,000	$ 140,000	$ 150,000	$ 180,000
Gross receipts	700,000	800,000	1,000,000	1,100,000	1,200,000

R Corporation's R&E credit for 2009 is computed as follows:

1. Fixed-base percentage = $300,000/$2,400,000 = .125
2. Base amount = .125 × $3,600,000/4 = $112,500
3. Qualified R&E expenditures for 2009 = $180,000
4. R&E Credit = 20% × ($180,000 − $112,500) = $13,500

Note that R's fixed-base percentage is based on the research activity and gross receipts during 1984–1988, whereas the average annual gross receipts number is based on receipts for the four previous years, 2005–2009 ($700,000 + $800,000 + $1,000,000 + $1,100,000 = $3,600,000). Also note that in 2009, R must reduce its current deduction for research expenditures by $13,500, or if the deferred asset method of accounting is used, the $180,000 R&E costs must be reduced to $166,500 ($180,000 − $13,500) before being capitalized and amortized over a period of not less than 60 months.

Basic Research Expenditures. The second category of expenditures qualifying for the research credit is the *incremental* amount of *basic research payments* made to universities and other qualified organizations.[97] Basic research means any original investigation for the advancement of scientific knowledge not having a specific

---

[96] Special rules apply to start-up companies after the sixth taxable year in which they incur qualified research expenditures. See § 41(c)(3)(B).

[97] § 41 (e)(2)

commercial objective. The term "basic research payment" means any amount paid in cash during the taxable year by a corporation to a qualified organization for basic research, but only if such payment is made pursuant to a written agreement and the basic research is to be performed by the qualified organization. Qualified organizations include educational institutions, certain scientific research organizations, and certain grant organizations.

The R&E credit applies to the *excess* of corporate cash expenditures in a year over the qualified organization base period amount. The qualified organization base period amount is the *sum* of (l) the minimum basic research amount, plus (2) the maintenance-of-effort amount. The *maintenance-of-effort amount* prevents the corporation from shifting its historical charitable contribution to any qualifying educational organization over to a creditable basic research payment. It is an amount equal to the *average* nondesignated university contributions paid by the corporation during the base period, increased by the cost of living adjustment for the calendar year over the amount of nondesignated university contributions paid by the taxpayer during that year. Any portion of the basic research payment that does not exceed the qualified organization base period amount will be treated as contract research expenses for computing the incremental qualified research expenditures discussed above under "qualified research expenditures" above.[98]

Alternative Incremental Credit. For taxable years beginning after June 30, 1996, a taxpayer may make an election to compute the research credit utilizing three tiers of reduced fixed base percentages and reduced credit rates.[99] This election may be beneficial for companies that have average gross receipts increasing at a faster rate than the increases in qualified research expenditures. This election is mentioned here only to round out the discussion of this credit but further analysis of the election is beyond the scope of this text.

Alternative Simplified Credit for Qualified Research Expenses. The Tax Relief and Health Care Act of 2006 allows taxpayers, at their election, to compute the research credit under a third method. This method is referred to as the alternative simplified credit. Under this approach, a taxpayer can claim an amount equal to 12 percent of the amount by which qualified research expenses exceed 50 percent of the average qualified research expenses for the three preceding tax years. If the taxpayer has no qualified research expenses for any of the preceding three tax years, then the credit is equal to six percent of the qualified research expenses for the current tax year. As with the alternative incremental credit, an election to calculate the research credit using the alternative simplified credit is effective for all succeeding tax years unless revoked with the consent of the IRS.[100]

Credit Limitations. As part of the general business credit, the tax liability limitation ($25,000 + 75% of the tax liability in excess of $25,000) applies, as do the one-year carryback and 20-year carryover rules. Additional limitations are imposed in an effort to prevent the research credit from being exploited by tax shelter promoters. For individuals with ownership interests in unincorporated businesses (i.e., partners of a partnership), trust or estate beneficiaries, or S corporation shareholders, any allowable pass-through of the credit cannot exceed the *lesser of* (1) the individual's net regular tax liability limitation discussed earlier, or (2) the amount of tax attributable to the individual's taxable income resulting from the individual's interest in the entity that earned such credit.

---

[98]   § 41(e)(1)(B).

[99]   § 41(c)(4). These percentages were increased for years beginning after 2006.

[100] § 41(c)(5).

The final unique characteristic of the R&E credit is applicable to changes in business ownership. Special rules apply for computing the credit when a business changes hands, under which qualified research expenditures for periods prior to the change of ownership generally are treated as transferred with the trade or business that gave rise to those expenditures.[101]

LOW-INCOME HOUSING CREDIT

The next component of the general business credit is the low-income housing credit. This credit is available for low-income housing that is constructed, rehabilitated, or acquired after 1986. The credit is claimed over a 10-year period, with an annual credit of approximately 9 percent of the qualifying basis of low-income units placed in service. If federal subsidies are used to finance the project, the credit is limited to approximately 4 percent.[102] For property placed in service after 1987, the exact percentage is determined by the IRS on a monthly basis. The percentages for any month are calculated to yield, over a 10-year credit period, amounts of credit that have a present value equal to (1) 70 percent of the qualified basis of new buildings that are not federally subsidized for the tax year, and (2) 30 percent of the qualified basis of existing buildings and new buildings that are federally subsidized.[103]

> **Example 29.** In January 2009, H, an individual, constructed and placed in service a qualified low-income housing project. The qualified basis of the project was $1 million. The 70% present value credit for buildings placed in service in January 2009 is 5.49%.[104] Thus, the annual credit that H could claim is $54,900.

Each year, the sum of allowed low-income housing credits is subject to a nationwide cap. The cap amount is allotted among all of the states so that each state will have a cap on the amount of low-income housing credits it can authorize. A credit allocation from the appropriate state credit authority must be received by the owner of the property eligible for the low-income housing credit. The credit is available on a per-unit basis; thus, a single building may have some units that qualify for the credit and some that do not. In order to qualify, a low-income housing project must meet a host of exacting criteria throughout a 15-year compliance period.[105]

DISABLED ACCESS CREDIT

Another component of the general business credit is the disabled access credit. This credit was established in 1994 primarily as a relief measure for those businesses that are required under the Americans with Disabilities Act of 1990 to make improvements that make existing facilities accessible to the disabled. Under Code § 44, an eligible small business can elect to take a nonrefundable tax credit equal to 50 percent of the amount of the eligible access expenditures for any taxable year that exceed $250 but do not exceed $10,250. An eligible small business is defined as one having gross receipts for the preceding taxable year that did not exceed $1,000,000, or having no more than 30 full-time employees during the preceding taxable year. Eligible access expenditures are defined as amounts paid or incurred by an eligible small business to comply with

---

[101] § 41(f)(3).

[102] § 42(b)(1).

[103] § 42(b)(2)(B). A formula for making such computations is provided in Rev. Rul. 88-6, 1988-1 C.B. 3.

[104] Rev. Rul. 2009-1, IRB 2009-2.

[105] See §§ 42(g) and 42(l).

applicable requirements of the Disabilities Act. Eligible access expenditures generally include amounts paid or incurred for the following:

1. Removing architectural, communication, physical, or transportation barriers that prevent a business from being accessible to, or usable by, individuals with disabilities

2. Providing qualified interpreters or other effective methods of making aurally delivered materials available to individuals with hearing impairments

3. Providing qualified readers, taped texts, and other effective methods of making visually delivered materials available to individuals with visual impairments

4. Acquiring or modifying equipment or devices for individuals with disabilities

5. Providing other similar services, modifications, materials, or equipment

In cases where the eligible business is being conducted as a partnership or an S corporation, the dollar limitations are applied at both the entity and the owner level. Any portion of the unused general business credit attributable to the disabled access credit may not be carried back to any taxable year ending before 1990.

> **Example 30.** J, a sole proprietor, had gross receipts of $700,000 last year and incurred $5,250 of eligible access expenditures this year. J's disabled access credit for this year is $2,500 [($5,250 − $250) × 50%].

As is the case with other components of the general business credit, the depreciable basis of assets acquired subject to the credit using access expenditures must be reduced by the amount of credit claimed with respect to those expenditures. Alternatively, any current deduction attributable to the access expenditures must be reduced by the amount of credit claimed.[106]

EMPOWERMENT ZONE EMPLOYMENT CREDIT

To help rebuild distressed urban and rural areas, the RRA of 1994 created several tax incentives. The hope is that these incentives will encourage businesses to locate in these areas and hire individuals who live there. The goal is carried out in § 1396, which authorizes the Secretary of Housing and Urban Development and the Secretary of Agriculture to identify 95 *enterprise communities* and 29 *empowerment zones* where the tax benefits will be offered. The regions must meet certain criteria concerning population, size (urban areas cannot exceed 20 square miles and rural areas cannot exceed 1,000 square miles), and poverty (a minimum rate of 20 percent).[107]

Businesses that operate within the designated areas are entitled to a variety of benefits. Perhaps the most important of these is the empowerment zone employment credit (EZEC). All employers located in an empowerment zone are entitled to a 20 percent credit for the first $15,000 of wages paid to full-time as well as part-time employees who are residents of the empowerment zone. The maximum credit per employee is $3,000 per year. If an employer is entitled to both a work opportunity credit (WOC) and an EZEC, the first $6,000 of wages paid qualify for the higher WOC of 40 percent, and the next $9,000 qualify for the EZEC of 20 percent. Thus, the payment of $15,000 of wages could enable the employer to claim a credit as high as $4,200 ($6,000 × 40% = $2,400) + ($9,000 × 20% = $1,800). Of course, the employer's deduction for wages must be reduced by the amount of credits allowed.

---

[106] § 44(c)(7).

[107] §§ 1391(a), 1391(g) and 1396.

Like the WOC, the EZEC is part of the general business credit and is consequently subject to the tax liability limitation as well as the carryback and carryover rule. Unlike the WOC, the EZEC can offset 25 percent of the employer's AMT liability.

CREDIT FOR EMPLOYER-PROVIDED CHILD-CARE

To encourage employers to provide quality child care for its employees, Congress established a special credit in 2002. The credit is considered a part of the general business credit.

Under new § 45F, employers may claim a credit equal to 25 percent of the cost of qualified child care expenditures and 10 percent of qualified child care resource and referral expenditures. The maximum total amount of credit is limited to $150,000 per year. In addition, the basis of any property is reduced by the amount of credit claimed. Similarly, any other deduction or credit must be reduced by the amount of credit claimed.

Qualifying expenditures include the costs of (1) building, acquiring, rehabilitating or expanding property that is used as part of a *qualified child care facility* of the taxpayer for its employees, (2) operating such facilities, and (3) a contract with a qualified child care facility. A qualified child care facility is a facility whose principal use is to provide child care assistance and meets the requirements of all applicable laws and regulations of the state and local government in which it is located, including the licensing requirements applicable to a child care facility. The definition does not include a facility which is the principal residence of the taxpayer, any employee of the taxpayer, or the operator of the facility. Thus day care centers will be qualified only if they are separate and distinct from the operator's personal residence.

In addition, expenses incurred in providing child-care resource and referral services are eligible for a 10 percent credit. Usage of a facility cannot favor high-income earners, and at least 30 percent of the children in the center must be children of employees. Finally, if the facility is no longer used as a child care center or there is a disposition of the taxpayer's interest (e.g., the taxpayer sells the property), § 45F(d)(2) requires the taxpayer to recapture (i.e., pay back to the government) a percentage of the tax savings from prior years as shown below.

If the Recapture Event Occurs in Years	Percentage Recapture
1–3	100%
4	85
5	70
6	55
7	40
8	25
9–10	10
11	0

OTHER COMPONENTS OF THE GENERAL BUSINESS CREDIT

There are several other credits that make up the general business credit:

▸ *Indian Employment Credit.* Added by the RRA of 1994 to encourage the hiring of Native Americans, the Indian employment credit (authorized in § 45A) generally entitles employers conducting businesses located on Indian reservations to claim a credit of 20 percent for up to $20,000 of wages and insurance benefits paid to employees who are members of an Indian tribe and who work and live on the reservation. This credit is set to expire after 2009.

▸ *Employer Social Security Credit.* This credit represents a relief measure (or perhaps a peace offering) for the restaurant industry, which presumably was detrimentally impacted by the 1994 cut in the deduction for business meals from 80 to 50 percent. Section 45B allows employers operating food and beverage establishments to claim a credit against their income tax liability for their FICA obligation (7.65%) on tips in excess of those treated as wages for purposes of satisfying the minimum wage provisions. To prevent a double benefit, no deduction is allowed for any FICA taxes taken into account in determining the credit.

▸ *Renewable Electricity Production Credit.* Section 45 provides a credit for taxpayers who produce electricity from qualified wind energy or certain other renewable resources from facilities placed in service after 2003.

▸ *Enhanced Oil Recovery Credit.* This is a special credit directed at owners of oil and gas properties requiring secondary or tertiary methods of production.

▸ *Orphan Drug Credit.* The credit for qualified clinical testing expenses for certain drugs for rare diseases or conditions has been made a permanent part of the general business credit. The credit is equal to 50 percent of the qualified clinical testing expenses for the taxable year.

▸ *Credit for Plan Start-up Costs of Small Employers.* Small employers with no more than 100 employees receive a tax credit for some of the costs of establishing new retirement plans. The credit equals 50 percent of the start-up costs incurred to create or maintain a new employee retirement plan. The credit is limited to $500 in any tax year and it may be claimed for qualified costs incurred in each of the three years beginning with the tax year in which the plan becomes effective [Code § 45E(b).]

▸ *Alternative Motor Vehicle Credit.* Perhaps the credit of greatest interest to individuals is that for purchases of personal or business automobiles. Section 30B offers an incentive to purchase energy efficient cars. The alternative motor vehicle credit is available for purchases of four types of vehicles:
  • Hybrid vehicle. These vehicles generally run on a combination of conventional fuels and energy from batteries (e.g., the Toyota Prius or Ford Escape). Depending on the fuel efficiency of the car, the credit for fuel economy ranges from $400–$2,400 and the conservation credit is $250–$1,000. According to Toyota, the tax credit for a Toyota Prius would range anywhere from $2,500 to $3,000.
  • Advanced lean burn technology vehicle. These vehicles use conventional internal combustion engines but utilize direct fuel injection to obtain greater efficiency. The credit is the same as for hybrid vehicles above.
  • Alternative fuel vehicle. These vehicles can burn only select fuels such as natural gas, hydrogen, electricity or a liquid that is 85 percent methanol. The credit is a percentage of the additional costs of energy efficient components and is capped based on weight. For example, a vehicle weighing under 8,500 pounds could qualify for a credit of up to $4,000.

- Fuel cell vehicle (FCV). The credit can be as much as $12,000 for vehicles powered by fuel cells. However the cost of these vehicles can be well over $100,000. FCVs are propelled by electric motors that are somewhat like batteries. Fuel cells create their own electricity through an electrochemical reaction between hydrogen and oxygen taken from the air.

▶ *Energy Efficient Appliance Credit.* Manufacturers can qualify for a credit for producing energy efficient dishwashers, clothes washers, and refrigerators. The credit depends on the type of appliance and how much energy it saves. The maximum tax credit is $100 per dishwasher or clothes washer, and $175 per refrigerator. Appliances eligible for the credit include only those produced by the taxpayer during the calendar year in the U.S. that exceed the average amount of production by the taxpayer in the U.S. during the three prior calendar years. Details are contained in § 45M. Currently, the credit is available only for two years (i.e., property placed in service after 2005 and before 2011).

▶ *Savers Credit.* Section 25B allows low and middle-income taxpayers a nonrefundable tax credit of up to $2,000 of qualified retirement savings contributions. This credit is discussed in Chapter 18.

▶ *Non-business Energy Property Credit.* Section 25C allows individuals to claim annual nonrefundable credits for amounts spent to make energy improvements to their homes. The credit is generally 30% of amounts paid for "qualified energy efficient improvements" and "residential energy property expenditures." The credit is available for expenses for such items as insulation, exterior doors and windows (including skylights), and properly coated metal as well as certain energy efficient heating and air conditioning units. However, the total non-business energy credits claimed by taxpayers during 2009 and 2010 cannot exceed $1,500. Expenses must be made on or in connection with a dwelling unit located in the U.S., owned and used by the taxpayer as his principal residence and originally placed in service by the taxpayer. Currently, the credit is available for expenditures made before 2011.

▶ *Residential Energy Efficient Property Credit.* Section 25D also allows individuals annual nonrefundable credit for the purchase of property for their homes that is energy efficient. Qualifying property includes certain photovoltaic property (i.e., property that uses solar power to generate electricity in a home), solar-powered water heaters and certain fuel cell property. Each of the credits is generally 30% of the cost of the property up to a maximum of $2,000. The credit is set to expire in 2016.

In addition to those credits that make up the general business credit, there are still other credits available to business, but they are of limited applicability and are not discussed in this text. The foreign tax credit available to both businesses and individuals, is discussed briefly below.

GENERAL BUSINESS CREDIT CARRYOVER RULES

Recall that the carryback period is one year and the carryforward period is 20 years for business credits incurred in years beginning after 1997. If the business credit carryover cannot be used within the stipulated time period, the credit expires. Without special rules, this would be a double loss for taxpayers who claimed the full investment tax credit percentages or other credits and who decreased the basis of property for MACRS computations. Not only have they lost the credit but they also were unable to depreciate the full cost of the assets. Because of this possibility, taxpayers are allowed to take a deduction equal to the amount of the previous reductions from basis stipulated by the expired IC or

other credits. This deduction may be taken in the year *following* the expiration of the tax credit carryover period.[109]

> **Example 31.** Q originally claimed an IC of $10,000 and reduced the basis in the assets by $5,000. After the expiration of the carryforward period, an unused IC of $3,000 expires. In the first taxable year after the expiration of the credit carryover period, Q may deduct $1,500 (½ of $3,000). This amount equals the original decrease in basis for the expired investment credit.

FOREIGN TAX CREDIT

The new emphasis on the global economy and global investing is making the treatment of foreign income and foreign taxes a concern for far more taxpayers than ever before. As explained in Chapter 3, U.S. citizens (including U.S. corporations) and resident aliens must pay U.S. taxes on their worldwide income: income earned in the United States as well as income from foreign sources. In many cases, they pay not only U.S. taxes but also foreign taxes on the same income. To alleviate the burden of two taxes on the same income, § 27 generally allows taxpayers to claim a credit for income taxes paid or accrued to a foreign country. Alternatively, taxpayers may elect to claim a deduction for the taxes. Also note that if the taxpayer elects to use the $91,400 (2009) earned income exclusion (see Chapter 3), any foreign taxes paid on such income cannot be claimed as a credit.

Although the taxpayer is normally allowed a credit for any foreign taxes paid, the amount of the credit may be limited in some cases. As a general rule, the credit for the foreign taxes cannot exceed the U.S. tax that would otherwise be paid on the same income. For example, assume a U.S. taxpayer earns $10,000 while living abroad and pays a foreign tax on such income of $3,000. If the U.S. tax on such income is only $2,000, the taxpayer's credit is limited to $2,000, and she consequently pays a foreign tax of $3,000 and no U.S. tax because her $2,000 U.S. tax liability is reduced to zero by the $2,000 FTC. Note that, without the limitation, the United States could effectively lose $1,000 of taxes on other U.S. income that it would otherwise receive. As this example illustrates, the limitation is generally triggered when the foreign tax rate exceeds the U.S. tax rate. The actual limitation is computed using the following formula:

$$\frac{\text{Foreign source taxable income}}{\text{Worldwide taxable income*}} \times \text{U.S. tax before credits} = \text{Foreign tax credit limitation}$$

*U.S. source taxable income + Foreign source taxable income + Personal exemptions

Any unused foreign tax credits may be carried back two years and carried forward five years. However, the credits may be carried over only to years where the foreign tax credit limitation has not been exceeded.

> **Example 32.** This year Mr. and Mrs. T took their financial consultants' advice on global investing. As a result, they received $10,000 of dividends from several foreign stocks. The couple's taxable income including the dividends was $92,700, producing a tax before credits of $15,550. The maximum foreign tax credit would be computed as follows:
>
> $$\frac{\$10,000}{\$92,700 + \$7,300 = \$100,000} \times \$15,550 = \$1,550$$

---

[109] § 196.

One caveat is in order before leaving the foreign tax credit. Although the above rules normally apply, taxpayers must be careful. Not only are the rules complex (they are applied separately to different classes of income), but tax treaties with a particular country may provide special rules for income earned in that country by U.S. citizens. Such treaties must be examined when dealing with foreign income.

NONBUSINESS CREDITS

In addition to the numerous business credits discussed thus far, there are several non-business credits available to individual taxpayers only. These credits include (1) the child tax credit, (2) the child and dependent care credit, (3) the HOPE and Lifetime learning credits, (4) the credit for adoption expenses, (5) the credit for the elderly, (6) the credit for interest on certain home mortgages, and (7) the earned income credit and other refundable credits. Each of these credits is discussed below.

CHILD TAX CREDIT

Section 24 currently allows most taxpayers to claim a special credit of $1,000 for each qualifying child. The amount of the credit is $1,000 per qualifying child for 2009. As a general rule, the credit is nonrefundable. Importantly, however, a portion of the credit may be refundable. The refundable child tax credit is discussed later in this Chapter along with other refundable credits.

In order to be considered a qualifying child, the individual in question must meet the following conditions:

▶ The individual must be the child of the taxpayer. For this purpose, a stepson or stepdaughter or an eligible foster child qualifies as a child. Descendants of these individuals are also treated as a qualifying child.

▶ The child must not have attained the age of 17 before the close of the taxable year.

▶ The taxpayer is eligible to claim a dependency exemption for the child.

▶ The child is a citizen, or a national of the U.S., or a resident of the U.S.

Like many of the other tax relief provisions contained in the Code, the benefits of the credit are not extended to wealthy individuals. To accomplish this policy objective, the credit is reduced by $50 for each $1,000 (or part thereof) of adjusted gross income (computed with certain modifications) exceeding the following levels of income for 2009.

EXHIBIT 13-10

2009 Child Tax Credit Phase-out

Taxpayer	Phase-out begins When Modified A.G.I. Exceeds	Phase-Out Ends when Modified A.G.I. Exceeds			
		One child	Two children	Three children	Four children
Single	$ 75,000	$ 86,000	$ 98,000	$ 110,000	$122,000
Married filing jointly	$110,000	$121,000	$133,000	$145,000	$157,000

Modified A.G.I. is A.G.I. determined before any exclusion for foreign earned income and foreign housing costs and income from certain possessions. These thresholds are not indexed for inflation. In order to claim the credit, the taxpayer must disclose the TIN of each qualifying child on the return and the taxable year of the taxpayer must include a 12 month period.

> **Example 33.** H and W are married with three children. At the close of 2008, the children, X, Y, and Z, were ages 12, 16 and 18 respectively. H and W claim a dependency exemption for each of the children. This year H and W reported adjusted gross income of $114,200. H and W may claim a child credit for X and Y since they are both dependents and did not attain the age of 17 before the close of the year. The amount of the credit is limited to $1,750 determined as follows:

Tentative credit for each child		$1,000
Qualifying children.		× 2
Total credit before phase-out.		$2,000
Reduction:		
Adjusted gross income	$114,200	
Threshold for joint return.	(110,000)	
Excess adjusted gross income.	$ 4,200	
Reduction [($4,200/$1,000 = 4.2 rounded up to 5) × $50]		(250)
Child credit allowed for children		$1,750

The amount of the child tax credit that can be claimed by a taxpayer for any taxable year shall not exceed the excess of the sum of the § 26 regular tax liability plus the AMT over the sum of the credits allowed by the Child and Dependent Care Credit (§ 21), the Credit for the Elderly (§ 22), the Credit for Interest on Certain Home Mortgages (§ 25), the HOPE and Lifetime Learning credit (§ 25A) and the foreign tax credit (§ 27). The nonrefundable portion of the child tax credit may be claimed against both reguar and AMT tax liability.

CHILD AND DEPENDENT CARE CREDIT

The emergence of the working wife and two-earner couples during the post-World War II era produced a new tax issue. The dilemma concerned the treatment of the costs for the care of children and other dependents. The question posed was whether taxpayers who were forced to pay such costs in order to work should be entitled to deduct them as business expenses. Early court cases denied a deduction for these expenses on the grounds that they were personal in nature. In the court's view, the expenses stemmed from a personal choice by married couples to employ others to discharge their domestic duties, a purely personal expense. Congress, however, became sensitive to the issue in the

late 1960s and responded with a limited deduction in 1971. After several alterations and amendments, the deduction received a complete makeover and was converted into a credit in 1976—a far better deal for those who did not itemize. It now appears that, almost 20 years after its creation, the credit is a permanent part of the tax law, presumably justified as both a relief measure for those who have differing abilities to pay and as a stimulant that reduces the costs of entering the work force.

As the statute is now drawn, taxpayers are able to claim a credit for a portion of their child and dependent care expenses if they meet two requirements: (1) the taxpayer maintains a household for a qualifying individual and (2) the expenses—so-called *employment-related expenses*—are incurred to enable the taxpayer to be gainfully employed.[110] Each of these requirements and the computation of the credit are discussed below.

Qualifying Individual. What many believe is simply a credit for child care actually has a far broader scope. True to its name, the *child and dependent care credit* is available not only to those who have children but also to those who take care of other dependents, such as an aging parent or other relative. A taxpayer (or in the case of divorced parents, only the custodial parent) can claim the credit only if he or she maintains a household for one of the following individuals:[111]

▶ A dependent under the age of 13 (e.g., taxpayer's child)

▶ An incapacitated dependent

▶ An incapacitated spouse

Note that the year in which a dependent turns 14 is an important factor in determining the applicability of the credit. First, if the individual becomes 13 during the year, he or she normally qualifies only for the part of the year he or she was under 13. Second, once the individual reaches age 14, expenses do not qualify unless the individual is incapable of self-care.

Employment-Related Expenses. Only certain expenses that enable the taxpayer to be gainfully employed or *seek* gainful employment qualify for the credit.[112] The work can be either full-time or part-time, but it must be work. Volunteer work for a nominal salary does not constitute gainful employment. For example, expenses for a baby-sitter while the taxpayer works at a church or hospital do not qualify. Note, however, that expenses incurred when one spouse works and the other attends school on a full-time basis are eligible.

Only certain types of expenses qualify as employment-related expenses. The expenses generally must be for the care of the qualifying individual (e.g., the cost of a baby-sitter). In this regard, the costs of household services qualify if the expenses are attributable at least in part to the care of a qualifying individual. Thus the IRS generally takes the position that the costs of a maid, nanny, or cook can qualify, but not those of a gardener or chauffeur. Eligible expenses normally do not include amounts paid for food, clothing, or entertainment. Similarly, the costs of transportation to a place for care do not qualify unless the qualifying individual is incapacitated. In addition, educational expenses incurred for a child in the first or higher grade level do not qualify. Observe, however, that the costs of pre-school or nursery school are eligible for the credit.

---

[110] § 21.

[111] §§ 21(b)(1) and 21(e)(5).

[112] § 21(b)(2).

As a general rule, expenses for services both inside and outside the home qualify for the credit. However, there are several notable exceptions for the outside services:

- Care provided by a dependent care facility (e.g., a day care center) qualifies only if the facility provides care for more than six individuals.[113]
- Services outside the home for qualifying individuals other than a dependent under 13 (e.g., nursing home services for a spouse or an over-13-year-old dependent who is incapable of self-care) are eligible only if the individual spends at least eight hours a day in the employee's household.[114]
- Overnight camps do not qualify (day camps, however, can qualify).[115]

A final note on eligible expenses concerns payments made to relatives. Can the credit be claimed if the taxpayer simply pays his mother to baby-sit while he works? Payments to individuals do qualify as long as the individual is not a dependent of the taxpayer.[116] Thus payments to a child's grandparents would probably qualify since the grandparents normally are not dependents. Conversely, payments to a child's older brothers or sisters normally would not qualify since such individuals would be dependents. However, payments to the taxpayer's child can qualify if the child is not a dependent and is at least 19 years of age.

Computation of the Credit. The credit is generally computed by multiplying the applicable percentage times employment-related expenses. A general formula for the calculation is shown in Exhibit 13-11.

Applicable Percentage. The applicable percentage begins at 35 percent but is reduced (but not below 20 percent) by one percentage point for each $2,000 (or fraction thereof) that the taxpayer's adjusted gross income exceeds $15,000. For example, the rate for a taxpayer with an A.G.I. of $17,001 is 33 percent, one point reduction for the first $2,000 over $15,000 and another point reduction for the fractional part of the next $2,000. Based on this scheme, taxpayers with adjusted gross incomes exceeding $43,000 have a rate of 20 percent.[117]

EXHIBIT 13-11

Computations of the Child and Dependent Care Credit

	Employment-related expenses
	Lesser of:
	1. Amount paid,
	2. Earned income or imputed earned income if full-time student or incapacitated spouse, or
	3. $3,000 (if one qualifying individual) or $6,000 (if more than one)
×	Applicable percentage (20–35%)
=	Child and dependent care credit

---

113   § 21(b)(2)(C).

114   § 21(b)(2)(B).

115   Last sentence of § 21(b)(2)(A).

116   § 21(e)(6).

117   § 21(a)(2).

Limitations on Employment-Related Expenses. The Code imposes several limitations on the amount of expenses eligible for the credit. The first limitation simply sets a maximum dollar amount of expenses that may be taken into account in computing the credit. These amounts are based on the number of qualifying individuals: $3,000 for one qualifying individual and $6,000 for two or more individuals.[118] Thus, the maximum credits would be $1,050 (35% × $3,000) and $2,100 (35% × $6,000). As explained below, however, these amounts may be reduced. The computation of the credit requires a three-step approach, as illustrated in the following example.

Example 34. F is a widower and maintains a household for his two small children. He incurs $5,000 of employment-related expenses and reports A.G.I. of $27,300 for the current year. F's child care credit is determined as follows:

Step 1: Determining the applicable percentage:

Adjusted gross income	$27,300
Less: Ceiling on 35% rate	(15,000)
Adjusted gross income over $15,000 limit	$12,300

Divided by $2,000 and rounded up: ($12,300 ÷ $2,000) = 6.15%
　Rounded up to 7%

Maximum rate	35%
Percentage reduction	(7%)
Allowable percentage	28%

Step 2: Determine the allowable employment-related expenses:

Lesser of $5,000 paid or $6,000 limit	$ 5,000

Step 3: Determine the dependent care credit:

Allowable employment-related expenses	$ 5,000
Times: Applicable percentage	× 28%
Dependent care credit	$ 1,400

Earned Income Limitation. In addition to the $3,000 and $6,000 limitations, employment-related expenses are limited to the individual's earned income for the year.[119] For this purpose, earned income generally includes such items as salaries, wages, and net earnings from self-employment, but not investment income such as dividends and interest.

The earned income limitation is a bit more cumbersome for married couples. If an individual is married, a joint return is required to claim the credit, and the amount of the exclusion may not exceed the lesser of the taxpayer's earned income or the earned income of the taxpayer's spouse.[120] In addition, in determining the lesser earned income for

---

[118] § 21(c).

[119] § 21(d)(1).

[120] § 21(e)(2) and 21(d)(2).

married couples, special rules apply if one spouse is either a *full-time student*[121] or an incapacitated person. The student or incapacitated spouse will be deemed to have earned income of $250 a month if there is one qualified dependent or $500 a month if there are two or more qualified dependents for each month a taxpayer is incapacitated or is a full-time student. This deemed income does not increase A.G.I. when determining the applicable percentage. These rules are illustrated in the following example.

> **Example 35.** B and G are married, have one dependent child, age 9, incur employment-related expenses of $2,700, and have A.G.I. of $22,500 for the current taxable year. G is employed full-time and earns $27,000 a year. B returned to graduate school and was a full-time student for 10 months during the year. He was not employed during the year.

> ***Step 1:*** The applicable percentage is determined to be 31% [35% − ($22,500 − $15,000 = $7,500 ÷ $2,000 = 3.75%, rounded up to 4%)].

> ***Step 2:*** The allowable employment-related expenses are $2,500. This is determined by the lesser of three amounts: (1) the $2,700 spent, (2) the $3,000 limit, and (3) B's deemed earned income of $2,500 ($250 for one dependent × 10 months).

> ***Step 3:*** Determine the dependent care credit:

> | | |
> |---|---:|
> | Allowable employment-related expenses | $2,500 |
> | Applicable percentage (35% − 4%) | × 31% |
> | Dependent care credit | $ 775 |

Filing Requirements for the Child and Dependent Care Credit. In order to claim the credit for taxable years beginning after 1996, married couples must file a joint return and the taxpayer ID numbers of *both* the day care service provider and of the child must be disclosed on the return.

Relationship to Other Credits. The child and dependent care credit is nonrefundable and is used to offset the tax liability determined under § 26. It is the *first* credit to be used in reducing an individual's tax liability, and there is no carryover or carryback available for unused credits.

Relationship to Dependent Care Assistance Programs. Congress has addressed the problem of child and dependent care in two ways: the child care credit and the exclusion for dependent care assistance. As mentioned in Chapter 6, since 1981 employers have been allowed to establish qualified dependent care assistance plans.[122] These plans allow employers a current deduction for contributions to the plans and allow employees to exclude from gross income up to $5,000 of payments (e.g., reimbursements) received under the plan to the extent that the expenses would qualify as employment-related expenses for purposes of the child and dependent care credits. If the taxpayer elects to exclude a reimbursement for care, the limit on the amount of employment-related expenses that qualify for the credit ($3,000 or $6,000) is reduced dollar for dollar by the

---

[121] § 21 (d)(2). For this purpose, a full-time student is defined exactly the same as for the dependency test (i.e., for at least five months, partial months count as full months).

[122] See § 129 and the discussion in Chapter 6.

amount excluded.[123] Whether the taxpayer is better off using the exclusion or the credit requires careful analysis of the taxpayer's situation, and some tax planning may be in order.

> **Example 36.** H and W are married with two children. H works full-time as an accountant, and he estimates his earnings for the year will be $50,000. W is employed part-time and estimates her earnings will be $20,000 for the year. H and W estimate that they will incur $4,000 of qualified employment-related expenses for the year. H and W are in the 28 percent tax bracket.
>
> At the beginning of H's employer's plan year, H has a decision to make. He can elect to have $1,000 excluded from his gross income in accordance with his employer's qualified dependent care assistance plan, which will be distributed to him as a reimbursement for qualified expenses, or he can elect to have the $1,000 included in his gross income as part of his salary. If the couple elects not to exclude the reimbursement, the child care credit is $800 (20% × $4,000), and they must pay taxes of $280 on the $1,000 of income, a net benefit of $520 ($800 − $280). On the other hand, if the couple elects to exclude the reimbursement, they pay no income tax on the $1,000 reimbursement, and their credit and net benefit is $800, computed as follows:

Employment-related expenses	$4,000
Dollar limit: maximum allowable expenses for two individuals	$6,000
Reduction for employer-provided dependent care excluded from income	(1,000)
Limit on expenses eligible for credit.	$5,000
Amount of credit (20% × lesser of $4,000 or $5,000)	$ 800

Note that only the dollar limit eligible for the credit is reduced by the excluded income. The employment-related expenses total of $4,000 is still eligible for the credit.

EDUCATION CREDITS

A major thrust of the Tax Reform Act of 1997 was to provide tax incentives to help reduce the cost of higher education and life-long learning. The law added six different provisions directed at this policy objective. Unfortunately, these rules often conflict and can be quite complex.

Taxpayers planning for the cost of educational programs or college degrees now must consider the following tax incentives:

- ► The exclusion for interest on Series E bonds.[124]
- ► The deductibility of certain interest on student loans.[125]

---

[123] § 21(c).

[124] See § 135 and Chapter 6.

[125] § 222. With respect to tax incentives directed toward students, also see § 117 (exclusion for scholarships and fellowships) and § 127 (employer paid educational expenses).

- ▸ Participation in qualified state tuition programs (529 plans).[126]
- ▸ Distributions from regular IRAs to pay educational expenses.[127]
- ▸ Establishing an education IRA.[128]
- ▸ The HOPE scholarship credit.[129]
- ▸ The Lifetime Learning credit.[130]

Section 25A contains two credits, the HOPE Scholarship credit and the Lifetime Learning credit, that are directly aimed at subsidizing the costs of pursuing undergraduate and graduate degrees as well as vocational training. While there are two credits, for any one particular student, a taxpayer could elect either the HOPE credit or a Lifetime Learning credit but not both. Like most of the other tax incentives created in 1997, these credits are phased out at specific income levels and, therefore, are not available to high income or wealthy taxpayers. The following discussion first looks at each credit individually and then at requirements common to each credit.

HOPE Scholarship Credit. The HOPE Scholarship credit (sometimes referred to as the American Opportunity Credit) was born out of Congressional desire to enable all students to continue to pursue their education once they have completed high school. The credit is allowed for qualified tuition and certain related expenses for post secondary education furnished to an eligible student. For 2009 and 2010, a taxpayer may elect to claim a credit for 100 percent of the first $2,000 of qualifying expenses and 25 percent of the next $2,000 of expenses for each student. Thus the maximum credit is $2,500 per year per student (e.g., the taxpayer whose triplets enroll at the local state college could claim a maximum credit for the year of $7,500). In its initial form, the HOPE credit could be used only for the first two years of post-secondary education. However, to help underwrite the cost of a college education, Congress extended eligibility in 2009 to four taxable years. In addition, 40 percent of the credit is refundable unless the taxpayer could be subject to the kiddie tax (i.e., the child is a full-time student less than 24 and whose earned income does not exceed one-half his or her support).

The credit is available only for expenses paid on behalf of the taxpayer, the taxpayer's spouse, or a dependent. In the case of a dependent's expenses, the eligible student is not entitled to claim a credit if he or she is claimed as a dependent by the parent or another taxpayer. Instead, if a parent or other taxpayer claims a student as a dependent, any qualified tuition and related expenses paid by the student are treated as paid by the parent and the parent benefits from the credit![131]

The credit is generally available only for expenses paid during the taxable year for education that begins during such year.[132] For this purpose, education that begins during the first three months of the next year is treated as having started in the previous year. This special three-month rule allows a credit for prepaid expenses. Observe that these rules require careful planning to take advantage of the full credit. Because the credit is tied to the taxable year rather than the typical academic year (i.e., a year that begins with

[126] § 529.
[127] § 72(t).
[128] § 530.
[129] § 25A.
[130] *Ibid.*
[131] § 25A(g)(3).
[132] § 25A(b)(1)(A).

the fall semester and ends with the spring semester), taxpayers may lose some of the credit's benefits without taking advantage of the prepayment privilege.

> **Example 37.** H is a typical high school graduate who enrolled for the 2009 fall semester of a local two-year community college. He plans to finish in the spring semester of 2011. The school charges $2,000 tuition per semester. Assuming H elects to claim the credit in 2009 and 2010, he can claim a total credit for the two years of $4,500 ($2,000 for fall 2009 + $2,500 for spring and fall of 2010. In such case, he does not benefit from the entire $5,000 ($2,500 per year) credit available. In order to avoid this result, H should prepay his 2010 tuition in December of 2009. Since prepayments qualify for the credit as long as the education occurs within the first three months of the following year, he would be eligible for the full $2,500 credit in 2009. He should also prepay in 2010 his tuition for the spring 2011 semester so that he will have paid at least $4,000 in 2010.

Note that qualifying expenses paid with loan proceeds are eligible for both credits in the year the expenses are paid, not when the loan is repaid.

Eligible Student. Expenses qualify for the credit only if they are for an eligible student. An eligible student is one who is enrolled in a program leading to a degree, certificate or other recognized educational credential at an eligible education institution. In addition, the student must carry one-half the load that a normal full-time student carries for at least one academic period per year. For example, if a student goes part-time during the spring semester (i.e., presumably one academic period) and carries one-half the full time load, his expenses for the summer and fall semesters will qualify even if he takes less than one-half the full time load during these later periods. Note also that the credit is not available for students that have been convicted of a federal or state felony offense consisting of the possession or distribution of a controlled substance.

Qualified Tuition and Expenses. Qualified tuition and related expenses include tuition and fees required for the enrollment or attendance at an eligible institution. Expenses also include course materials. However, expenses that do not directly relate to the student's education such as student activity fees, athletic fees, insurance expenses, transportation, or other expenses unrelated to an individual's academic course of instruction do not qualify for either credit. Similarly, expenses related to courses involving sports, games, or hobbies do not qualify unless such course is part of the individual's degree program. In addition, neither the HOPE credit nor the Lifetime Learning credit is available for expenses incurred to purchase books or for room and board.

For both the HOPE credit and the Lifetime Learning credit, the amount of qualifying expenses must be reduced by amounts covered by excludable scholarships or educational assistance plans.[133] However, amounts withdrawn from a qualified prepaid tuition plan and used to pay eligible expenses qualify for the credit.

Eligible Institutions. Only expenses paid to eligible institutions qualify for the credit. While most colleges and universities would be considered eligible, other providers of courses may also qualify. Technically, an eligible institution includes accredited post-secondary educational institutions offering credit toward a bachelor's degree, an associate's degree, or another recognized post-secondary credential. Certain proprietary institutions and post-secondary vocational institutions also are eligible. The bright line test is whether the institution is eligible to participate in Department of Education student aid programs.

---

[133] § 25(g)(2).

Phase-out for High Income Taxpayers. The HOPE credit (like the Lifetime Learning credit discussed below) is not extended to high income taxpayers. To accomplish this objective, the total maximum credit allowed for all eligible students is phased out once the taxpayer's modified adjusted gross income exceeds certain thresholds. For 2009 and 2010, the thresholds for the HOPE credit differ from those for the Lifetime Learning Credit. For the HOPE credit, the phase-out begins at $160,000 for joint returns and $80,000 for other returns. The reduction occurs over a $20,000 *income range* for joint filers and $10,000 for other taxpayers. If the taxpayer is married, a joint return must be filed to claim the credits. The formula for determining the phase-out and the levels at which a complete phase-out occurs is shown below.

EXHIBIT 13-12

Phase-Out of HOPE and the Lifetime Learning Credits for 2009-2010

$$\text{Reduction of total allowable credits} = \text{Allowable credits} \times \frac{\text{Modified A.G.I.}^* - \text{threshold}}{\text{Income range}}$$

Credit	Taxpayer	Modified A.G.I.* Phase-out begins	Modified A.G.I.* Phase-out complete
HOPE	Married filing joint	$160,000	$180,000
	Other taxpayers	80,000	90,000
Lifetime Learning	Married filing joint	$96,000	$116,000
	Other taxpayers	48,000	58,000

* Modified A.G.I. is A.G.I. increased by income earned outside the U.S. which normally is excluded under § 911. The income phase-out threshold amounts are indexed annually for inflation.

Example 38. M, a single mother, has modified A.G.I. of $81,000. In 2009, M's daughter, D, begins studying for her bachelor's degree as a full-time student at City University. On September 1, M pays $5,000 in qualified tuition for D's first semester. Without the income limitations, M would be entitled to the maximum HOPE credit of $12,500 (100% of $2,000 plus 25% of $2,000). However, taking into account the income limitations, M's credit is reduced as shown below.

$$\text{Reduction of total allowable credits} = \$2,500 \times \frac{\$81,000 - \$80,000}{\$10,000} = \$250$$

Thus, M is entitled to a $2,250 ($2,500–$250) HOPE credit.

Lifetime Learning Credit. In addition to the HOPE credit, § 25A creates the Lifetime Learning credit. This credit can be claimed for 20 percent of qualified tuition and fees incurred during the taxable year on behalf of the taxpayer, the taxpayer's spouse, or any dependents. Up to $10,000 of qualified tuition and fees per taxpayer return are eligible for the credit (i.e., the maximum credit per return is $2,000). For any one particular student, a taxpayer could elect either the HOPE credit or a Lifetime Learning credit but not both.

In contrast to the HOPE credit, a taxpayer may claim the Lifetime Learning credit for a unlimited number of taxable years. Also in contrast to the HOPE credit, the maximum amount of the Lifetime Learning credit that may be claimed on a taxpayer's return is not related to the number of students in the taxpayer's family. The key variable is the amount of qualified expenses incurred during the year and not the number of eligible individuals.

Qualified Tuition and Related Expenses for Lifetime Learning Credit. Qualified tuition and fees for purposes of the Lifetime Learning credit are defined in the same manner as for the HOPE credit but with several important additions. As noted above, the HOPE credit is available only for four taxable years and ceases after the year the student has completed four years of post-secondary education. In contrast, the Lifetime Learning credit—true to its name—applies not only to these same expenses but also such expenses incurred in any taxable year during the taxpayer's lifetime. For example, the Lifetime Learning credit would be applicable to expenses incurred in obtaining an undergraduate degree (all four years or whatever is required) or a graduate degree (e.g., a law degree, a medical degree, an M.B.A., and similar graduate degrees). In addition, the definition of qualified tuition and expenses is expanded for the Lifetime Learning credit to include any course of instruction at an eligible educational institution to acquire or improve job skills of the taxpayer. Thus expenses need not be incurred in a degree program but could be simply a continuing education course (e.g., a C.P.A. takes a course on the new tax law). Note, however, that for the course to qualify it must be provided by a qualifying educational institution (e.g., one that is eligible to participate in student aid programs of the Department of Education).

Like the HOPE credit, the amount of qualifying expenses for the Lifetime Learning credit must be reduced by amounts covered by scholarships or educational assistance plans (assuming such amounts are excludable from gross income). Expenses taken into account for the HOPE credit cannot be taken into account for the Lifetime Learning credit.

These credits are automatically available to the taxpayer unless the taxpayer elects not to take the credit with respect to the qualified tuition and related expenses of an individual for any taxable year. Previously, the taxpayer had to elect to claim the credit.[134]

Interaction of HOPE Credit, Lifetime Learning Credit, Education IRAs and Series EE Savings Bonds. Special rules exist to prohibit the taxpayer from obtaining multiple benefits from the credits and nontaxable withdrawals from education individual retirement accounts. For each eligible student in each taxable year, the taxpayer must elect one of the three tax benefits: (1) the HOPE credit, (2) the Lifetime Learning credit, or (3) the exclusion from gross income for withdrawals from education IRAs. The election is separate for each student. Thus a parent could elect the HOPE credit for one child, the Lifetime Learning credit for another child, and the exclusion for IRA withdrawals for a third child. Any educational expenses taken into account for purposes of the credits or the IRA withdrawal cannot again be taken into account in determining the exclusion for interest on Series EE savings bonds that are used to pay for educational expenses.

CREDIT FOR ADOPTION EXPENSES

To encourage adoptions, § 23 provides a maximum nonrefundable credit of $12,150 (2009) per child for qualified adoption expenses paid or incurred by the taxpayer. Qualified adoption expenses are reasonable and necessary adoption fees, court costs, attorney's fees and other expenses that are directly related to the legal adoption of an eligible child. An eligible child is an individual (1) who has not attained age 18 as of the time of the adoption, or (2) who is physically or mentally incapable of caring for himself or herself. No credit is allowed for expenses incurred (1) in violation of state or federal law, (2) in carrying out any surrogate parenting arrangement, or (3) in connection with the adoption of a child of the taxpayer's spouse. The credit is phased out ratably for taxpayers with modified adjusted gross income above $182,180, and is fully phased out at $222,180

---

[134] § 25A(e), as amended by the 2001 Tax Act, makes the credits applicable to the taxpayer unless the taxpayer *elects out* of the credit provisions.

of modified A.G.I. For these purposes modified A.G.I. is computed by increasing the taxpayer's A.G.I. by the amount otherwise excluded from gross income of citizens or residents living abroad.

The $12,150 limit is a per child limit, not an annual limitation. If adoption expenses are paid during a tax year prior to the tax year in which the adoption is final, the credit is allowed for the year the adoption is made final. If adoption expenses are paid during or after the tax year in which the adoption is finalized, the credit is allowed for the tax year in which the expense is paid. For example, in the case of an adoption which is finalized in 2009, if a taxpayer pays or incurs $3,500 of otherwise allowable qualified adoption expenses with respect to the child in year 2008 and $9,500 of otherwise allowable qualified adoption expenses with respect to that same child in 2009, then the taxpayer would receive a $3,500 credit with respect to expenses incurred in 2008 and a $8,650 credit with respect to expenses incurred in 2009 (both credits are allowed on the 2009 tax return).

When the adoption credit is attributable to amounts chargeable to a capital account (e.g., the costs of constructing an elevator at the taxpayer's house to accommodate a wheelchair that is required as a condition of the adoption), the taxpayer is not allowed additional basis in the house to the extent of the adoption credit allowed. An ordering rule specifies that qualified adoption expenditures not chargeable to a capital account (the legal fees) are allowed for the credit before any amounts that are chargeable to a capital account.

A special rule applies to the adoption of a child with special needs. "Special needs" include the child's ethnic background, age, or membership in a minority or sibling group, or the presence of such factors such as medical conditions or physical, mental or emotional handicaps. In the case of a special needs child, $12,150 is allowed as an adoption credit regardless of whether the taxpayer has qualified adoption expenses. The credit for a special needs child is only allowed if the adoption becomes final and the credit is only allowed in the year in which the adoption becomes final.[135]

Interaction with the Exclusion for Qualified Adoption Expenses. A companion but separate $12,150 exclusion from gross income is also available to employees for qualified adoption expenses paid by the employer in accordance with a qualified adoption assistance program.[136]

Adoption expenses paid or reimbursed under an adoption assistance program may not be taken into account in determining the adoption credit. A taxpayer may, however, satisfy the requirements of the adoption credit *and* the exclusion with different expenses paid or incurred by the taxpayer and the employer, respectively. For example, in the case of an adoption that costs $14,000 with $7,000 of expenses paid by the taxpayer and $7,000 paid by the taxpayer's employer under an adoption assistance program, the taxpayer may qualify for the adoption credit and the exclusion.

There are special rules that apply to the adoption of foreign children, with no credit allowed until the year in which the adoption is final.

In order to claim the adoption credit, married couples must file a joint return and include the child's taxpayer I.D. number on the tax return claiming the adoption credit.[137] Recall that this credit can be used to offset the tentative minimum tax. If the credit is limited, it can be carried over for five years.

---

[135] § 23(a)(3).

[136] § 137.

[137] § 23(f).

CREDIT FOR THE ELDERLY AND PERMANENTLY DISABLED

A nonrefundable tax credit is available to certain taxpayers who are either 65 years of age or older or are permanently and totally disabled.[138] The credit is 15 percent of an individual's earned and investment income that does not exceed the taxpayer's appropriate § 22 amount.[139] The maximum § 22 amount is:

1. $5,000 for single individuals

2. $5,000 for a joint return where only one spouse is at least 65 years old

3. $7,500 for a joint return where both spouses are 65 years or older

4. $3,750 for a married individual filing separately

The maximum amount from above is then reduced by excludable pension and annuity income received during the year, including social security and railroad retirement benefits, and by one-half of the taxpayer's A.G.I. that exceeds:

1. $7,500 for unmarried individuals

2. $10,000 if married filing jointly

3. $5,000 if married filing separately

Example 39. P is single, 65 years old, and has A.G.I. of $8,300 from interest and dividends. During the taxable year, she also received social security of $1,500. Her credit for the elderly is computed as follows:

Maximum § 22 amount		$5,000
Less: Social security received	$1,500	
50% of A.G.I. over $7,500 ($8,300 − $7,500 = $800 × 50%)	+400	(1,900)
Section 22 amount available for credit		$3,100
Multiply by rate		× 15%
Amount of credit		$ 465

There are a number of additional special rules, and because these rules are quite complicated, individuals are allowed to file their return with a request that the IRS compute their tax liability and tax credit. However, few people are able to take advantage of the credit for the elderly since social security receipts commonly exceed the maximum § 22 amount.

The credit for the elderly or permanently disabled is limited to the § 26 tax liability reduced by the child and dependent care credit. Like the child and dependent care credit, this credit is nonrefundable and may not be carried back or forward.

CREDIT FOR INTEREST ON CERTAIN HOME MORTGAGES

In order to help provide financing for first-time home buyers, Congress has created several special programs. One of these allows state and local governments to issue

---

[138] Limited rules apply to taxpayers who are under 65 years old if they are certain governmental retirees subject to the Public Retirement System and elect to have this section apply [see § 22(c)].

[139] § 22(a).

mortgage credit certificates (MCCs).[140] Taxpayers who receive such certificates are allowed to claim a nonrefundable credit for a specified percentage of interest paid on mortgage loans on their principal residence. Each certificate must specify the principal amount of indebtedness that qualifies for the credit as well as the applicable percentage rate of the credit. The credit percentage may differ with each certificate but must be between 10 and 50 percent. If the credit exceeds 20 percent, the maximum credit is limited to $2,000. Of course, the amount of the taxpayer's interest deduction must be reduced by the amount of the credit claimed during the year. Any credit that cannot be used may be carried over for three years.

> **Example 40.** After saving for years, R and his wife, W, decided to buy their first house. In order to finance the purchase, R applied for and received from the state an MCC. The certificate specifies that the rate is 15% and the maximum loan amount is $70,000. The couple purchased a house for $75,000 and obtained a loan of $65,000 from a savings and loan. For the year, R and W paid interest of $5,000 on the loan. They may claim a credit of $750 ($5,000 × 15%). In addition, they may deduct interest of $4,250 ($5,000 − $750).

While the credit can provide a significant benefit, it is not available to everyone. Under the MCC program, state and local governments are limited in the volume of credits they may dispense and in the individuals to whom they may be issued. Taxpayers are eligible to receive a certificate only if they meet certain narrowly defined criteria. For example, the purchaser's income cannot generally exceed 115 percent of the area's median gross income, the price of the home cannot exceed 90 percent of the average purchase price of homes in the area, and the homes may be available only in targeted areas. Still other constraints exist that restrict the credit's use.

REFUNDABLE CREDITS

Refundable credits are those credits that are recoverable even though an individual has no income tax liability in the current year. They are treated as payments of taxes. Included in this category are the credit for taxes withheld at the source (§ 31), the earned income credit (§ 32), the credit for tax withheld at the source on nonresident aliens and foreign corporations (§ 33), the gasoline and special fuels credit (§ 34) and the AMT refundable credit (§ 53(e)).

Refundable credits may be used to offset all taxes imposed by the Code, including penalty taxes. This result is accomplished by combining all the refundable credits and accounting for them after all the nonrefundable credits have been used to offset the § 26 tax liability.

TAX WITHHELD AT THE SOURCE

The first and most important of the refundable credits is styled "Credit for Tax Withheld on Wages" and obviously includes the amount withheld by an employer as a tax on wages earned.[141] However, the credit has broader application with respect to certain taxes withheld by the payor at the source of payment, including:

1. Tax on pensions and annuities withheld by the payor

2. Overpaid FICA taxes (in cases where a taxpayer has two or more employers in the same year)

---

[140] § 25.

[141] §§ 31(a) and 3401.

3.   Amounts withheld as backup withholding in cases where the taxpayer fails to furnish a taxpayer identification number to the payor of interest or dividends[142]

4.   Quarterly estimated tax payments

EARNED INCOME CREDIT

In 1975, Congress introduced the earned income credit to eliminate some of the disincentives that discouraged low-income taxpayers with children from working.[143] The credit was specifically designed to alleviate the increasing burden of social security taxes. In many cases, income taxes were not a concern for these low-income taxpayers since they were protected by personal and dependent exemptions as well as the standard deduction. However, they were not exempt from social security taxes. Consistent with its purpose, the credit is refundable (e.g., the taxpayer would receive the credit amount even if he or she is not required to pay income taxes since it is viewed as a refund of the social security taxes).

Since its creation, the earned income credit has been the subject of a great deal of Congressional tinkering. The most recent round of adjustments was introduced by the Clinton administration in 1993. These changes not only increased the benefits of the credit but also expanded its coverage. Beginning in 1994, the credit may apply even if the taxpayer does not have children.

Computation of the Credit. The starting point for determining the credit is determination of the taxpayer's earned income. As might be expected, *earned income* consists of wages, salaries, tips, and other employer compensation plus earnings from self-employment included in gross income for the taxable year. Taxpayers may elect to treat combat zone compensation that is otherwise excluded from gross income under § 112 as earned income.[144] Earned income does not include pension and annuity income even if provided by an employer for past services. Amounts received similar to compensation that are excluded are not treated as earned income. For example, excludable dependent care benefits, the value of meals and lodging furnished for the convenience of the employer, excludable educational assistance benefits and salary deferrals [contributions to a § 401(k) plan] are not included in earned income.

The initial credit is computed by multiplying the earned income of the taxpayer (limited by a ceiling amount) by a statutory percentage; however, this initial credit amount is phased out as the taxpayer's income increases above a phase-out amount. As can be seen from Exhibit 13-13, the maximum amounts of earned income that qualify for the credit as well as the statutory credit percentages vary depending on the number of children the taxpayer has.[145] Observe that the credit for an individual with no children is essentially designed to give the taxpayer back the FICA taxes on the first $5,970 wages (7.65% rate × $5,970). The maximum credits for eligible individuals for 2009 are shown in Exhibit 13-13.

---

[142]   §§ 31(c) and 3406.

[143]   § 32(a).

[144]   § 32(c)(2)(B)(vi).

[145]   § 32(b)(1).

EXHIBIT 13-13
Earned Income Credit: Credit Percentages and Maximum Credits

Number of Qualifying Children	Credit Percentage	Ceiling on Earned Income	Maximum Credit
0	7.65%	$ 5,970	$ 457.00
1	34.00	8,950	3,043.00
2	40.00	12,570	5,028.00
3 or more	45.00	12,570	5,656.50

As noted above, the credit begins to phase out once the taxpayer's income increases above the phase-out amount. The credit is reduced if *either* the earned income or the A.G.I. of the taxpayer exceeds certain specified amounts shown in Exhibit 13-14.[146]

The phase-out is computed by multiplying the applicable phase-out rate by the excess of A.G.I. or earned income (whichever is greater) over the phase-out amounts. The credit can be computed using the following formula:

Maximum credit
  Applicable percentage × earned income (not to exceed the ceiling amounts)
− Reduction
  Applicable percentage × (larger of earned income or A.G.I. − Phase-out amount)
= Earned income credit

For example, the maximum 2009 earned income credit for a taxpayer with one child is $3.043 ($8,950 × 34%). This credit is completely eliminated when the taxpayer's modified A.G.I. or earned income exceeds $35,463 [15.98% × ($35,463 − $16,420 = $19,043) = $3,043]. The levels at which the credit is completely phased out are shown in Exhibit 13-14.

EXHIBIT 13-14
Earned Income Credit: Phase-Outs

Qualifying Children	Phaseout Percentage	Other than Joint Filers		Joint Filers	
		Threshold Phaseout Starts at	Completed Phaseout Level	Threshold Phaseout Starts at	Completed Phaseout Level
0	7.65%	$ 7,470	$13,440	$12,470	$18,440
1	15.98	16,420	35,463	21,420	40,463
2 or more	21.06	16,420	40,295	21,420	45,295

Example 41. D and M are married, file a joint return for 2009, and maintain a household for their dependent son, who is three years old. D has earned income of $20,000 and M has none. The couple own investments that produce $1,475 of includible

---

[146] Rev. Proc. 2008-66, IRB 2008-45.

income for the year and have an A.G.I. of $21,475 ($20,000 + $1,475). The earned income credit is computed as follows:

Maximum credit (34% × $8,950)		$3,043
Less:	Reduction for A.G.I. over $19,540	
	($21,475 − $19,540 = $1,935 × 15.98%)	− 309
Earned income credit		$2,734

To help taxpayers compute the credit, the IRS provides a worksheet and an earned income credit table to aid taxpayers in determining the correct amount of the earned income credit. The worksheet and table are included with the instructions for completing Form 1040 and Form 1040A (see the Appendix B for a copy of the 2008 Table).[147]

As a refundable credit, qualified individuals may receive tax refunds equal to their earned income credit even in years when they have no tax liability.[148]

> **Example 42.** Y has earned income and A.G.I. of $10,000, has three exemptions (including two qualified children), and files as head of household. As a result, she has no income tax liability for the year. However, she is entitled to a tax refund equal to the earned income credit of $4,000 ($10,000 × 40%) plus any taxes (other than FICA taxes) withheld from her wages. She may also qualify for a refundable child tax credit (see the next section and *Example 43*).

Eligibility Requirements. Because the earned income credit was a mechanical calculation under the former rules, some wealthy taxpayers inadvertently qualified for the earned income credit in years in which they reported a small amount of earned income. To preclude such taxpayers from taking advantage of the earned income credit, a major change was made. The earned income credit is now disallowed for taxpayers that have too much investment income. Taxpayers are not allowed to claim the earned income credit if they have more than $3,100 of disqualified income.[149] The definition of disqualified income includes:

- ▶ Interest
- ▶ Dividends
- ▶ Tax-exempt interest
- ▶ The net income from rents or royalties not derived in ordinary course of a trade or business
- ▶ Capital gain net income
- ▶ The excess of aggregate passive income over aggregate passive losses

Finally, in an attempt to cut down on fraud and abuse relating to this credit, the taxpayer identification number required to be disclosed on the return means a Social Security number issued to an individual by the Social Security Administration.

Until 1993, the earned income credit was available only to taxpayers who had children. In a major change, the RRA of 1993 extended the earned income credit to certain individuals without children. In so doing, the act significantly broadened the availability of the credit. In either situation, if the taxpayer is married a joint return must be filed as a

---

[147] § 32(f) Note that the earned income credit table prepared annually by the IRS reflects the credit based on a midpoint of each $25 increment of an income range.

[148] The taxpayer is required to reduce his or her earned income credit by the amount of the alternative minimum tax imposed on that individual.

[149] See § 32(i) and Rev. Proc. 2008-66, IRB 2008-45.

requirement to obtain the EIC.[150] The eligibility requirements for taxpayers with and without children are set forth below.

Taxpayers without Children. Taxpayers without a qualifying child are eligible to claim the credit if the taxpayer meets three conditions:[151]

1. The taxpayer (or the spouse of the taxpayer) must be at least 25 years old and not more than 64 years old at the end of the taxable year.

2. The taxpayer is not a dependent in the same year the credit is claimed.

3. The taxpayer has a principal residence in the United States for more than one-half of the taxable year.

Taxpayers with Children. Taxpayers are entitled to claim the credit if they have a qualifying child. The child need not be a dependent but must meet the following tests:

1. *Relationship.* The individual must be a child, stepchild, foster child, a legally adopted child of the taxpayer, or a descendant of any such individual. A married child does not meet this test unless the taxpayer can claim the child as a dependent.

2. *Age.* The child must be either (1) less than 19 years old at the close of the calendar year, (2) less than 24 years old and a full-time student at the close of the calendar year, or (3) permanently and totally disabled any time during the year.

3. *Residency.* The child must share the same principal place of abode as the taxpayer for more than one-half of the taxable year, and that abode must be located in the United States.

Assuming all of the above requirements are met and the taxpayer properly identifies the child on the return (i.e., name, age, taxpayer identification number), the credit is allowed.

REFUNDABLE CHILD TAX CREDITS

Taxpayers who qualify for the regular child credit may also qualify for a refundable Child Tax Credit which is authorized in § 24(d). Any amount allowed as a refundable credit will reduce the Child Tax Credit (CTC) that would otherwise be allowed under § 24.

One of the principal policy goals of the Child Tax Credit for low-income taxpayers is to offset not only the taxpayer's regular income tax but also the employee's share of FICA (or for those who are self-employed, one-half of the taxpayer's self-employment tax). To accomplish this goal, a portion of the Child Tax Credit was made refundable.

The overall limit on the amount of the CTC that will be refundable is the amount of the CTC determined as if the tax liability limitation did not apply. Recall that the CTC is limited to an amount not to exceed the excess of the sum of the § 26 regular tax liability plus the AMT over the sum of the credits allowed by the Child and Dependent Care Credit (§ 21), the Credit for the Elderly (§ 22), the credit for Interest on Certain Home Mortgages (§ 25), the HOPE and Lifetime Learning credit (§ 25A) and the foreign tax credit (§ 27). Generally this limitation will be equal to the full CTC computed by multiplying the per child amount by the number of qualifying children.

---

[150] § 32(d).

[151] § 32(c)(1)(A)(ii).

The amount of the refundable Child Tax Credit is the lesser of:

1. The child credit allowed without regard to the tax liability limitation of § 26, or

2. The amount by which the nonrefundable personal credits allowed would increase if the tax liability limitation were increased by 15 percent of the taxpayer's earned income in excess of $12,550.

Referred to as the 15 percent rule, the CTC is refundable to the extent that the nonrefundable personal credits allowed would increase if the tax liablity limitation was increased by 15 percent of the taxpayer's earned income in excess of $12,550. For purposes of computing earned income as applicable to the refundable CTC, combat pay excludable from gross income under §112, is treated as earned income.

Taxpayers with three or more children may calculate the refundable portion of the credit using the excess of their social security taxes (i.e., the taxpayer's share of the FICA taxes and one-half of self-employment taxes) over the earned income credit if this calculation results in a greater amount than computed under the 15 percent rule.

Example 43. D, a single parent, is raising two children at home and earns a salary in 2009 of $22,000. The CTC is the only nonrefundable personal tax credit that D is entitled to.

Income	$22,000
Standard deduction	(8,350)
Personal exemptions	(10,950)
Taxable income	$ 2,700
Tax on $2,700	$ 270
Earned income credit [$5,028 − (21.06% × ($22,000 − $16,420))]	$ 3,853
FICA paid (7.65% × $22,000)	$ 1,683

The refundable portion of the CTC is the lesser of:

1. CTC determined as if the tax liability limitation did not apply = $2,000 (2 × $1,000),
    or

2. the amount by which the nonrefundable personal credits would increase if the tax liability were increased by 15 percent of the earned income over $12,550, or $1,418 [15% × ($22,000 − $12,550)].

If D's tax liability were increased by $1,418, D's tax liability would be $1,688 ($1,418 + $270) and the amount of nonrefundable credits would go from $270 to $1,688. This is an increase of $1,418 which is D's allowable refundable portion of the CTC for 2009.

Thus D's refundable portion of the CTC is $1,418. D's nonrefundable CTC is $582 and will be allowed to reduce her regular tax liability.

D's total tax refund is $5,271, computed as follows:

Tax liability		$ 270
Less: CTC		(582)
Tax liability before refundable credits		$ 0
Less: Refundable credits:		
CTC	$1,418	
EIC	3,853	(5,271)
Total refund		$5,271

Example 44. H and W have three children and earned income of $30,000. For 2009 their tax liability would be $160. The CTC is the only nonrefundable personal credit that H and W are entitled to.

Income	$30,000
Standard deduction	(11,400)
Personal exemptions	(18,250)
Taxable income	$ 350
Tax on $1,600	$ 35
Earned income credit [$5,657 − $1,807 (21.06% × ($30,000 − $21,420))]	$ 3,850
FICA paid (7.65% × $30,000)	$ 2,295

The refundable portion of the CTC is the lesser of:

1. CTC determined as if the tax liability limitation did not apply = $3,000
   or
2. the amount by which the nonrefundable personal credits would increase if the tax liability were increased by 15 percent of the earned income over $12,550, or $2,618 [15% × ($30,000 − $12,550)].

If H & W's tax liability were increased by $2,618, their nonrefundable CTC would also increase by $2,618; therefore, $2,618 of the CTC will be a refundable credit.

Since H and W have at least three children, they should compute the excess of their FICA taxes over their EIC and compare it to $2,618. In this case, there is no excess and H and W will be able to treat $2,618 as the refundable portion of their CTC. Thus their nonrefundable CTC is $382 ($3,000 − $2,618).

H and W's total refund is $5,146, computed as follows:

Tax liability		$ 35
Less: CTC		(582)
Tax liability before refundable credits		$ 0
Less: Refundable credits:		
CTC	$2,618	
EIC	3,850	(6,468)
Total refund		$6,468

Although the total amount of the child credit is the same whether or not part of it is treated as a refundable credit, it is advantageous for taxpayers to claim a refundable credit rather than a nonrefundable child credit. As noted above, nonrefundable credits are subtracted from the total tax for the year and may *only* reduce the regular tax and the AMT tax to zero; any excess is not refunded. In contrast, refundable credits are treated as tax payments, and are added to the amounts of federal income taxes that have been withheld and any estimated tax payments that have been made. If this sum is more than the total tax due, the excess is refunded.

OTHER REFUNDABLE CREDITS

Three other refundable credits are allowed. Code § 33 allows as a credit the amount of tax withheld at the source for nonresident aliens and foreign corporations. Code § 34 provides an income tax credit for the amount of excise tax paid on gasoline, where the gasoline is used on a farm, for other nonhighway purposes, by local transit systems, and by operators of intercity, local, or school buses. Finally, Code § 35 provides that an overpayment of taxes resulting from filing an amended return will be treated as a refundable credit.

PROBLEM MATERIALS

DISCUSSION QUESTIONS

13-1 *Alternative Minimum Tax.* It has been said that a taxpayer must maintain a second set of books to comply with the AMT system. Why is the extra set of books necessary?

13-2 *Alternative Minimum Tax.* The AMT requires taxpayers to keep an extra set of books for several adjustment items. What action can a taxpayer take to minimize the recordkeeping requirements with respect to depreciation deductions?

13-3 *Alternative Minimum Tax.* Assume a taxpayer has a regular tax liability of $25,000, a tentative AMT of $28,000, and an AMT of $3,000 for the current year. How much does the taxpayer actually owe the IRS?

13-4 *Alternative Minimum Tax.* A taxpayer has an AMT liability of $50,000 and a general business credit of $50,000. He is not concerned about paying the AMT because he thinks the general business credit can be used to offset the AMT. Is he correct? What if the taxpayer were a corporation?

13-5 *Alternative Minimum Tax.* Is it safe to assume that only wealthy individuals who have low taxable incomes are subject to the alternative minimum tax? Are any taxpayers

whose marginal rates exceed 26 percent subject to the alternative minimum tax? Explain.

13-6   *Alternative Minimum Tax.* G will be subject to the alternative minimum tax in 2009 but not in 2010. G's property tax on her residence is due November 15, 2009. If she defers payment of the property tax until 2010, she must pay a 5 percent penalty. When should G pay the property tax? Explain.

13-7   *Alternative Minimum Tax.* Some interest expense can be taken as an itemized deduction for regular tax purposes but different rules control the interest expenses allowable as an AMT itemized deduction. Explain the differences in these rules and note which rules are more restrictive.

13-8   *Alternative Minimum Tax.* Is the § 179 (first-year expensing) deduction allowed as a deduction for the AMT system?

13-9   *Credits vs. Deductions.* Assume taxpayers have a choice of deducting $1,000 for A.G.I. or taking a $250 tax credit for the current year. Which taxpayers should choose the deduction? Why?

13-10 *Rehabilitation and Energy Credits.* A taxpayer purchased an old train station, which was placed in service in 1935, for $20,000. He plans to tear the building down and erect a new office building for $100,000. Will any of this qualify for the rehabilitation or energy investment credit? What tax advice could you give the taxpayer for his consideration in maximizing these credits?

13-11 *Rehabilitation and Energy Credit.* When a taxpayer claims a rehabilitation credit, what impact does the credit have on the basis of the property for cost recovery purposes? What is the impact on the basis when a business energy credit is claimed? What if the disabled access credit is claimed?

13-12 *IC Recapture.* Explain two possible consequences if a taxpayer claims an investment credit on property and then makes an early disposition of the property.

13-13 *Minimum Tax Credit.* If a taxpayer pays an AMT in the current year, what consequences does that payment have on the AMT liability that may be owed in subsequent years? What impact does the payment of the AMT in the current year have on the regular tax liability in subsequent years?

13-14 *Dependent Care Credit.* A husband and wife both work and employ a babysitter to watch the children during their work hours. How much of the babysitter's salary qualifies for the child and dependent care credit if:
   a. The babysitter performs cooking and cleaning services while she is watching the children.
   b. The babysitter also performs services around the house including gardening, bartending, and chauffeuring.

13-15 *Earned Income Credit.* A husband and wife with A.G.I. and earned income of $7,000 maintained a household for their son but were unable to claim him as a dependent because he was 20 years old and earned $3,500. Can the son or his parents qualify for the earned income credit? Explain.

13-16 *Research Credit.* An entrepreneur works in a garage during 2008 doing research for a new patent. He spends $15,000 on the research in 2008. In January 2009, he forms an S corporation and applies for the patent, which is granted in 2009. How much credit for research expenditures will the taxpayer be allowed and in what year?

13-17 *Work Opportunity Credit.* The purpose of the work opportunity credit is to encourage the employment of certain groups of people with high unemployment rates. The credit has not quite achieved the desired objectives. What changes should be made to the present credit to increase its effectiveness?

PROBLEMS

13-18 *Alternative Minimum Tax—Computation.* T is single and has taxable income of $56,550 and a regular tax liability of $10,325 for the current year. T uses the standard deduction for regular tax purposes and has $60,000 of positive adjustments (excluding the adjustment for the standard deduction) for AMT purposes.
  a. Determine T's tentative minimum tax and her AMT.
  b. Determine the amount that T actually has to pay the IRS this year.

13-19 *Alternative Minimum Tax—Computation.* V and W are married and file a joint return for the current year. They have no other dependents and they take the standard deduction. V and W's taxable income is $94,250 and their regular tax liability is $15,938. They have $60,000 of AMT preference items and $32,050 of AMT positive adjustments. Determine V and W's tentative AMT and their AMT liability.

13-20 *AMT and Qualified Small Business Stock.* T is an avid investor, always looking for that one stock that will make him rich and famous. On January 4, 1997, BC Corporation, a fast food chain, went public, and T thought this could be the one. He purchased 10,000 shares of stock for $100,000. One of the benefits from buying this initial offering was that BC's stock was eligible for treatment as qualified small business stock. After enduring the ups and downs of the market, T sold 5,000 shares of the stock for $250,000 on January 9, 2009.
  a. Determine the gain recognized on the sale of the BC stock and the amount included in T's regular taxable income.
  b. Determine the amount of tax preference or adjustment, if any, that T must take into account in computing his alternative minimum tax.

13-21 *Alternative Minimum Tax—Charitable Contribution Preference.* During the year, J contributed stock to the local university. He had purchased the stock in 1984 for $10,000, and it was appraised at $60,000 on the date of gift. The stock was sold shortly after the contribution was made, and a painting was purchased by the university with the proceeds from the sale. The university placed the painting in its Art Building for display and study by art students. J's A.G.I. in the year of contribution is $300,000.
  a. Determine J's allowable charitable contribution deduction for the regular tax system.
  b. Based solely on these facts, determine any AMT adjustments or preference items that apply to J.

13-22 *Alternative Minimum Tax—Computation.* B is single and reports the following items of income and deductions for the current year:

Salary	$ 50,000
Net long-term capital gain on sale of investment property	200,000
Medical expenses	17,500
Casualty loss	4,500
State and local income taxes	15,000
Real estate taxes	20,000
Charitable contributions (all cash)	15,000
Interest on home mortgage	12,000
Interest on investment loans (unimproved real property)	10,000

The only additional transaction during the year was the exercise of an incentive stock option of her employer's stock at an option price of $12,000 when the stock was worth $100,000. Compute B's tax liability and AMT, if any.

13-23   *Alternative Minimum Tax.* Refer to the facts in *Problem 13-22* and assume B holds the stock acquired by exercising her ISO for two years and sells it for $105,000. Determine the amount of gain that must be reported for regular tax purposes and the gain that must be reflected in the AMT calculations in the year the stock was sold.

13-24   *Alternative Minimum Tax—Cost Recovery Adjustment.* In 2009, T placed a light-duty truck in service at a cost of $40,000. T uses the applicable MACRS method of depreciation for all his assets and does not elect the § 179 first-year expensing option. Identify and calculate the minimum tax adjustment that must be made for AMT purposes in 2009.

13-25   *Alternative Minimum Tax—Cost Recovery.* Refer to the facts in *Problem 13-24*, but assume the truck that was placed in service this year at a cost of $40,000 was a heavy-duty truck. Identify and calculate the minimum tax adjustment that must be made for AMT purposes in 2009.

13-26   *Alternative Minimum Tax—Cost Recovery Adjustment.* In January 2009, A purchases residential rental property for $200,000, excluding the cost of the land. For regular tax purposes, the 2009 depreciation on the building is $6,970. For AMT purposes, depreciation is $4,792. Determine the AMT adjustment for cost recovery for 2009 and 2010.

13-27   *Alternative Minimum Tax—Computation.* O is married to G and they file a joint return for 2009. O and G have A.G.I. of $70,000. One of the deductions from gross income was $50,000 of percentage depletion. Cost depletion on their gold mine was zero because the cost basis of the property was reduced to zero by prior years' depletion deductions. They do not itemize deductions. Determine O and G's tax liability for 2009.

13-28   *Alternative Minimum Tax.* T is an unmarried entrepreneur. In 2003, he purchased several rental properties and leased them to tenants on long-term leases. In 2009, T has $100,000 of rental losses on his real estate activities in which he actively participates and income of $100,000 from his brokerage business. T also has a $25,000 general business credit carryover from 2008. Determine T's tax liability for 2009, assuming he does not itemize his deductions.

13-29   *Minimum Tax Credit.* Refer to the facts in *Problem 13-22* and determine the minimum tax credit, if any, that is available to offset the regular tax liability in 2010.

13-30   *General Business Credit—Limited by Tax Liability.* K's tax liability before credits is $35,000. She earned a general business credit of $40,000. Determine K's tax liability after credits and any general business credit carryback or carryforward that may exist.

13-31   *Energy Credit.* In May of the current year, J invested $60,000 in a solar system to heat water for a production process.
  a.   Determine the amount of business energy credit available to J.
  b.   Determine the basis of the energy property that J must use for cost recovery purposes.

13-32   *Rehabilitation Credit.* During the current year, T incurred $300,000 of qualified rehabilitation expenditures with respect to 75-year-old property. Prior to these expenditures, T had a $100,000 cost basis in the depreciable building.
  a.   Determine the amount of rehabilitation credit available to T.
  b.   Determine the basis of the rehabilitated property that T must use for cost recovery purposes.

13-33   *Rehabilitation Credit—Computation.* During the current year, K incurred $200,000 of qualified rehabilitation expenditures with respect to property constructed in 1930. The entire block where his property is located has been designated as a Certified Historical District.
  a.   Determine the amount of credit allowable to K if his structure is recognized as a historical structure.
  b.   Assuming that K paid $180,000 for his building in the current year and that he would claim MACRS depreciation, calculate his adjusted basis in the building at the end of the year. Assume that the property was placed in service in July of the current year.

13-34   *IC Recapture.* Assume D claimed a business energy credit of $30,000 for property placed in service on December 18, 2006 and that D sold this property on January 7, 2007. Determine the amount, if any, of IC recapture that D should report as an additional tax in 2009.

13-35   *IC Recapture.* Assume L claimed rehabilitation credit of $80,000 on property placed in service on February 18, 2006 and that L exchanged this rehabilitated property for like-kind property (a § 1031 exchange) on March 17, 2009. Determine the amount of IC recapture that L should report as an additional tax in 2009, if any.

13-36   *Research and Experimentation Credit.* M, a sole proprietor, has been in business only two years but is very successful. He has average annual gross receipts of $150,000 for this period and incurred $40,000 in qualified R&E expenses this year.
  a.   Determine M's R&E credit for the current year.
  b.   Determine the current deduction for R&E expenditures that M is entitled to, assuming he elects to deduct R&E expenditures currently.

13-37   *Disabled Access Credit—Computation.* P Corp. had gross receipts of $500,000 last year and incurred $9,000 of eligible access expenditures to build a wheelchair ramp this year.
  a.   Determine P's disabled access credit.
  b.   Determine the basis of the wheelchair ramp that will be eligible for cost recovery deductions.

13-38   *Child Tax Credit.* H and W are married with three children. At the close of 2009, the children, A, B, and C, were ages 2, 6, and 8, respectively. H and W claim a dependency exemption for each of the children. This year H and W reported adjusted gross income of $125,000. Determine the allowable child tax credit for H and W.

13-39   *Child Tax Credit.* M is a single mom raising one child, age 16, at home. M may claim a dependency exemption for her child. This year M earned $70,000 as salary and had investment income of $12,500. Determine the allowable child tax credit for M.

13-40 *Dependent Care Credit.* V and J are married and file a joint return for the current year. Because they both work, they had to pay a babysitter $5,200 to watch their three children (ages 7, 8, and 9). V earned $17,000 and J earned $21,200 during the year. They do not have any other source of income nor do they claim any deductions for adjusted gross income. Determine the allowable dependent care credit for V and J.

13-41 *Dependent Care Credit.* M and B are married, have a son three years old, and file a joint return for the current year. They incurred $500 a month for day care center expenses. During the year, B earned $23,000 but M did not work outside the home. They do not have any other source of income nor do they claim any deductions for adjusted gross income. Determine the allowable dependent care credit for the year if:
   a. M enrolled as a full-time student in a local community college on September 6 of the current year.
   b. M was in school from January through June, and from September through December of the current year.

13-42 *Dependent Care Credit.* C is a single parent raising a son who is eight years old. During the current year, C earned $19,500 and paid $3,000 to a sitter to watch her son after school. Determine C's dependent care credit for the current year.

13-43 *HOPE Scholarship Credit.* D is a single dad and has modified A.G.I. of $52,000. This year D's son begins studying for his bachelor's degree as a half-time student at Arapahoe County Community College. On September 1, D pays $2,500 in qualified tuition for his son's first semester. Determine the amount of HOPE credit available to D.

13-44 *HOPE Scholarship Credit.* H and W are married and have twins who are attending the State University as freshmen this year. State University is on the semester system and charges $1,000 tuition per semester. H and W pay State University $2,000 this year. H and W have adjusted gross income of $83,000.
   a. Determine the allowable HOPE Scholarship credit for H and W.
   b. If H and W ask your advice in terms of maximizing the HOPE Scholarship credit, what advice would you give them?

13-45 *Earned Income Credit.* R is 43, divorced, and maintains a household for his 7-year-old dependent daughter. R was laid off in 2008 and his unemployment benefits have run out. During 2009, he worked at part-time jobs earning $5,500. He has no other sources of income.
   a. Determine R's allowable earned income credit.
   b. Determine R's tax payment due or his refund, assuming that nothing was withheld from his wages and that he did not make any quarterly estimated tax payments.

13-46 *Earned Income Credit.* S, who is 24 and a single parent, maintains a household for her 3-year-old dependent daughter and her 10-month-old son. S earned $16,000 during this calendar year. S has no other source of income and does not itemize her deductions.
   a. Determine S's allowable earned income credit.
   b. Determine S's tax payment due or her refund, assuming that $200 was withheld from her wages and that she did not make any quarterly estimated tax payments.

13-47 *Additional Child Tax Credit.* H and W have four children and earned $24,000 for 2009. H and W paid $1,836 in FICA taxes but neither had any income tax withheld from their wages. Determine the amount of refund they should receive from the IRS.

13-48 *Integrative Credit Problem.* J, who is 32 and a single parent, maintains a household for his six-year-old dependent son. J earned $20,000 and paid $3,000 in child care payments during the calendar year. J did not have any Federal income tax withheld from his check. Determine the amount of J's refund from the IRS, if any, or the amount that J must pay the IRS, if required.

13-49   *Credit for the Elderly.* P and D are 66 years old, married, and file a joint return. The only sources of income they have are dividend income of $14,000 and social security of $2,500.

    a.   Determine the allowable credit for the elderly for the current year.

    b.   Determine the tax payable or refund due, assuming that no withholding was made on the dividends and that no quarterly estimated payments were made.

CUMULATIVE PROBLEMS

TaxCut   **13-50**   R and S, married and the parents of two children ages 10 months and 6 years, file a joint return. R is a college professor of civil engineering and teaches at State University. R applied for a one-year visiting professorship with International Engineering Corporation (IEC) and was selected for the position. The visiting professor position was available from July 1 to May 31 of the following year and required R to relocate his family from Detroit to Los Angeles at a total cost of $6,500 during the last week in June. IEC reimbursed R only $5,000 for these expenses. R rented his Detroit home for the last six months of the calendar year at a net loss of $6,000 for regular tax purposes. Due to the longer life of the residential real property for AMT purposes, and therefore a smaller cost recovery deduction, the net loss for AMT purposes was only $4,000.

      S was employed by the government and was able to get a temporary transfer to Los Angeles. S earned $12,000 for the calendar year. During the calendar year, R and S paid $6,000 in child care expenses.

      R and his family incurred expenses of $2,500 a month to rent a furnished apartment (assume $1,000 a month was attributable to R and $1,000 a month was attributable to S) for the last six months of the calendar year. R and his family incurred expenses of $800 a month for food during the last six months of the year (assume 25% of the food is specifically attributable to R and that 25% is attributable to S). In addition, R incurred transportation expenses, parking fees, and laundry expenses of $2,500, and he spent $1,200 on lunches on work days during the last half of the year. S incurred transportation expenses of $500 and took her lunch to work with her. R earned $25,000 from State University for teaching half of the calendar year and $60,000 from IEC for practicing half of the year. Together, R and S had $12,000 of Federal income tax withheld from their paychecks.

During the year, R and S also incurred the following expenses:

Unreimbursed medical expenses	$7,000
Charitable contribution of stock to State University (adjusted basis $1,000)	5,000
State and local income taxes	4,000
Real estate taxes on lake property	3,000
Real estate taxes on principal residence (one-half year)	2,000
Interest on principal residence (one-half year)	4,800

The couple also had these additional income items:

State tax refund from previous year	$1,500
Interest income from private activity bonds	7,000

      R and S have a minimum tax credit carryover from last year of $5,000. Determine R and S's tax liability for the year.

RESEARCH PROBLEMS

13-51   *Rehabilitation Credit.* Taxpayer S, a real estate developer, rehabilitated an old commercial building and was entitled to an investment credit based on the rehabilitation expenses incurred. Prior to placing the new offices into service, S is approached by P, who is interested in purchasing the building. As an inducement to get

P to buy the property, S offers to transfer the IC to P. That is, S agrees not to claim the credit on his tax return with the expectation that P can claim the credit instead. Will P be allowed to take credit on her tax return in the year she places the office building into service?

13-52 *Dependent Care Credit.* B is a single parent and his child is enrolled in a public school. The school administrators have scheduled a supervised trip to Dearborn, Michigan for one full week for the students to see Greenfield Village and the Henry Ford Museum. Total trip cost per student is $800. If B pays for his child to make the trip, will he be entitled to a child care credit for the expenditures? If so, how much of the costs will qualify?

13-53 *Alternative Minimum Tax.* This year T was the victim of his company's restructuring and downsizing. Midway through the year his employer, ABC Corporation, offered him early retirement on the condition that he would provide consulting services when needed. The offer proved so lucrative that T accepted. T ended up working for the company for the first six months of the taxable year and earned $50,000 during this period. Prior to his retirement he exercised an incentive stock option he had received several years earlier. At the time he exercised the option, the market price of the stock was $140,000 and the purchase price under the option was $50,000. After he retired, T began a new business of building toys for disabled children. He materially participated in the business and incurred a loss of $60,000, which he properly reported on Schedule C of his Form 1040 tax return. T is married and files a joint return with his wife. The couple paid $18,000 in qualified housing interest and $6,000 in real estate taxes, and made a $25,000 cash contribution to Children's Hospital during the year. Determine T's regular tax liability and AMT, if any.

13-54 *Child Care Credit.* K recently divorced and decided to go back to school full-time to get her Masters of Taxation at Central University. She has a four-year-old child who attends nursery school at a cost of $4,000 per year. As a single parent, K finds it difficult just to get by. However, she maintains her home using her alimony payments, some dividend and interest income, and her child support. She also works as a volunteer for 10 hours a week at the library and receives $15 per week. This year she attended school for 11 months. Is K eligible for the child care credit?

PROPERTY TRANSACTIONS

★ ★ ★ ★ ★ CONTENTS ★ ★ ★ ★ ★

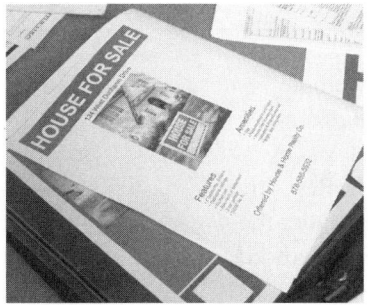

CHAPTER FOURTEEN

PROPERTY TRANSACTIONS: BASIS DETERMINATION AND RECOGNITION OF GAIN OR LOSS

LEARNING OBJECTIVES

Upon completion of this chapter you will be able to:

▶ Understand the concepts of realized and recognized gain or loss from the disposition of property

▶ Explain the process of determining gain or loss required to be recognized on the disposition of property, including computation of the following:

 ▶ Amount realized from a sale, exchange, or other disposition

 ▶ Effect of liabilities assumed or transferred

 ▶ Adjusted basis of property involved in the transaction

▶ Identify the most common types of adjustments to basis of property

▶ Define an installment sale and identify taxpayers eligible to use the installment method of reporting gain

▶ Compute the amount of gain required to be recognized in the year of installment sale and the gain to be reported in any subsequent year

▶ Explain the limitations imposed on certain installment sales, including

 ▶ The imputed interest rules

 ▶ Related-party installment sales

 ▶ Gain recognition on the disposition of installment obligations

 ▶ Required interest payments on deferred Federal income taxes

▶ Identify various transactions in which loss recognition is prohibited

CHAPTER OUTLINE

Section 61(a)(3) of the Code provides that gross income includes gains derived from dealings in property. Similarly, § 165 allows a deduction, subject to limitations, for losses incurred in certain property transactions. The term *dealings in property* includes sales, exchanges, and other types of acquisitions or dispositions of property. This chapter examines the determination of the amount of gains and losses from dealings in property. Specific rules regarding gain recognition are addressed, as are the gain-deferral possibilities associated with certain installment sales. Various limitations on the deductibility of losses also are addressed.

Other topics dealing with property transactions are examined in the next three chapters. Chapter 15 deals with certain nontaxable exchanges. Chapter 16 covers the special treatment accorded gains and losses from sales or exchanges of capital assets. The unique rules governing the disposition of property used in a trade or business, including depreciable property, are examined in Chapter 17.

DETERMINATION OF GAIN OR LOSS

INTRODUCTION

Determining the gain or loss realized in a property transaction is usually a simple computation. It is the mathematical difference between the amount realized in a sale or other disposition and the adjusted basis of the property surrendered (See Exhibit 14-1). The amount realized is a measure of the consideration received in the transaction. It represents the economic value *realized* by the taxpayer.

EXHIBIT 14-1

Computatin of Gain or Loss Realized

	Amount realized (See Exhibit 14-3)
−	Adjusted basis
=	Gain or loss realized

Sale or other disposition essentially refers to any transaction in which a taxpayer realizes benefit in exchange for property. It is not necessary that there be a sale transaction or that cash be received for gain or loss to be realized by the taxpayer surrendering property other than cash.

The adjusted basis of purchased property is generally cost, plus or minus certain adjustments. Computing gain or loss realized is similar to determining gain or loss for accounting purposes, and adjusted basis is similar in concept to book value. However, the adjusted basis of a property will not always be, and frequently is not, equal to its book value for accounting purposes.

In effect, the adjusted cost, or adjusted basis, of a given property is the amount that can be recovered tax-free upon its disposition. For example, if property is sold for exactly its cost, as adjusted, there is no gain or loss realized. This concept is referred to as the *recovery of capital or recovery of basis* principle. If a taxpayer receives more than the adjusted basis in exchange for property, gain is realized only to the extent of that excess. The adjusted basis is recovered tax-free. The following examples illustrate this concept:

Example 1. K transferred 30 acres of land to ZX Company for $42,000 cash. K had purchased the 30 acres five years earlier for $35,000, which is his adjusted basis. As a result of this "sale or other disposition," K has a realized gain of $7,000 ($42,000 − $35,000). His $35,000 basis in the land is recovered tax-free.

Example 2. In 2007, L purchased 300 shares of W Corporation stock for $3,600 cash, including brokerage fees. When the market outlook for W Corporation's product began to weaken in 2009, L sold her shares for $3,100. The broker deducted a commission of $48 and forwarded $3,052 cash to her. L has a realized loss on this transaction of $548 ($3,052 − $3,600) in 2009.

Example 3. R transferred 200 shares of C Corporation stock worth $4,000 and $2,000 cash for an auto he will use for personal purposes. The C Corporation stock had been purchased two years earlier for $4,600. R realizes a loss of $600 [($6,000 − $2,000) − $4,600] on the "sale or other disposition" of the stock.

GENERAL RULE OF RECOGNITION

Any gain or loss realized must be recognized unless some provision of the Internal Revenue Code provides otherwise. A *recognized gain* is reported on a tax return. For example, a gain on the sale of stock generally is recognized in full in the year of sale (i.e., the gain is reported on a tax return, included in gross income, and considered in determining the tax liability for the year). In determining taxable income, the recognized gain is either offset against losses for the year or included in the computation of taxable income.[1]

A *recognized loss* also is generally given its full tax effect in the year of realization. Depending on the type of loss, it may be either offset against gains or deducted against

---

[1] Capital gains must be offset by capital losses, and only net capital gains are included in taxable income. See the discussion of capital gains and losses in Chapter 16.

other forms of income in determining taxable income. Some losses, however, are not deductible[2] and others are limited.[3] For example, losses on the sale of property used for personal purposes are disallowed. Certain other losses are deferred to later tax years. Some examples of nontaxable exchanges are listed in Exhibit 14-2.

EXHIBIT 14-2
Partial List of Nontaxable Exchanges

Types of Transaction	Action Required	Tax Result
Casualty, theft, condemnation (involuntary conversion)	Reinvest in similar property	Gain may be deferred see Chapter 15 and § 1033
Like-kind exchange	Exhchange directly for like-kind property	Gain or loss is deferred* see Chapter 15 and § 1031
Formation of a corporation or subsequent stock issues	Transfer property in exchange for stock by controlling shareholders	Gain or loss is deferred* see § 351
Corporate reorganizations	Examples include mergers, consolidations divisions, recapitalizations	Gain or loss is deferred* see § 368
Partnership formation	Transfer property in exchange for a partnership interest	Gain or loss is deferred* see § 721

* When gain or loss is deferred, the deferral is only until the replacement property is sold or otherwise transferred (i.e., the deferred gain or loss is recognized along with any subsequent gain or loss when the replacement property is sold).

COMPUTING AMOUNT REALIZED

The amount realized from a sale or other disposition of property includes the amount of money received plus the fair market value of any other property received in a transaction. Other property includes both tangible and intangible property.

Example 4. P received $20,000 and a motor home worth $80,000 in exchange for a sailing yacht that she had used for personal enjoyment. P's amount realized on the disposition of the yacht is $100,000 ($20,000 + $80,000).

The amount realized also includes any debt obligations of the buyer, and if the contract provides for inadequate interest or no interest, interest must be imputed and the sales price reduced accordingly.

Example 5. Y sold his vintage Dodge automobile to C for $10,000 and a note payable from C to Y for $15,000 plus interest compounded monthly at 9%. Y's amount realized in this transaction is $25,000, the down payment plus the value of C's note.

---

[2] Losses on certain sales to related parties are disallowed under § 267, and losses on the sale of personal use property are not allowed under § 165(c).

[3] The deduction for capital losses is limited under § 1211(b).

Example 6. Z sold a parcel of real estate for $100,000. Her basis in the land was $60,000. The sales contract called for $10,000 to be paid upon transfer of the property and the remaining $90,000 to be paid in full two years later.

Since no interest was provided for in the contract, interest must be imputed on the buyer's $90,000 obligation (in this case, 9% interest, compounded semiannually, is used).[4] Accordingly, the sales price is reduced to $85,471 [$10,000 cash down payment + $75,471 (the discounted present value of the $90,000 payment in two years)]. Z will report an amount realized of $85,471 and a gain realized of $25,471 ($85,471 − $60,000 basis). When Z collects the $90,000, she must report interest income of $14,529 ($90,000 face value − $75,471 present value on date of sale).

The amount realized also includes the amount of any existing liabilities of the seller discharged in the transaction. Specifically, it includes any debts assumed by the buyer and any liabilities encumbering the property transferred that remain with the property in the buyer's hands.[5] Exhibit 14-3 illustrates the computation of *both* the amount realized and the gain or loss realized from the sale or other disposition of property.

EXHIBIT 14-3

Computation of Amount Realized and Gain or Loss Realized

Amount realized:		
Amount of money received		$xxx,xxx
Add:	Fair market value of other property received	+ x,xxx
	Liabilities discharged:	
	Liabilities assumed by the buyer	+ xx,xxx
	Liabilities encumbering the property transferred	+ x,xxx
Less:	Selling expenses	− xx,xxx
	Amount of money given up	− x,xxx
	Liabilities incurred:	
	Liabilities assumed by the taxpayer	− xx,xxx
	Liabilities encumbering the property received	− x,xxx
Equals:	Amount realized.	$xxx,xxx
Less:	***Adjusted basis*** in property other than money given up	− xx,xxx
Equals:	***Gain or loss realized***	$xxx,xxx

Example 7. B purchased a rental house for $40,000 in 2002. She paid $8,000 down and signed a mortgage note for the balance. During the years she owned the property, B deducted depreciation totaling $16,000 and made principal payments on the note of $4,000, leaving a mortgage balance of $28,000.

During 2009, B sold the house for $62,000. The buyer paid $34,000 cash and assumed the $28,000 mortgage liability. B's amount realized is $62,000 ($34,000 cash + $28,000 relief of liability), and her adjusted basis is $24,000 ($40,000 cost reduced by $16,000 depreciation). Her gain realized is therefore $38,000 ($62,000 amount realized − $24,000 adjusted basis).

Any expenses of selling the property reduce the amount realized. Selling costs include many costs, paid by the seller, associated with offering a property for sale and transacting the sale. For example, selling costs include advertising expenses, appraisal fees, sales

---

[4]   The actual rate is determined with reference to current market rates and is announced periodically by the IRS. For transactions involving $2.8 million or less, the rate cannot exceed 9 percent compounded semiannually.

[5]   Reg. § 1.1001-2. Also, see the following discussion of the effect of liabilities in property transactions.

commissions, legal fees, transfer taxes, recording fees, and mortgage costs of the buyer paid by the seller.

BASIS DETERMINATION RULES

The adjusted basis of property may be determined in several ways, depending on how the property is acquired and whether any gain or loss is being deferred in the transaction. Various methods of acquiring property and their specific basis determination rules are discussed below.

PROPERTY ACQUIRED BY PURCHASE

Cost Basis. In a simple purchase transaction, basis is the cost of the property acquired. Cost is the amount of money paid and the fair market value of any other property transferred in exchange for a given property.[6] The cost basis includes any payments made by the buyer with borrowed funds and any obligations (i.e., promissory notes) of the buyer given to the seller or any obligations of the seller assumed by the buyer in the exchange.[7]

Any costs of acquiring property are included in basis. For stock and securities, commissions, transfer taxes, and other acquisition costs are included. For other property, many types of acquisition costs, including commissions, legal fees related to purchase, recording fees, title insurance, appraisals, sales taxes, and transfer taxes, are added to basis.[8] Any installation and delivery costs also are part of basis.

> **Example 8.** C purchased a new machine for his auto repair business during 2009. He paid $16,500 for the machine, $8,500 of which was made possible by a bank loan. In addition, C paid state sales taxes of $660, delivery charges of $325, and installation charges of $175. C's cost basis in the equipment is $17,660 ($16,500 purchase price + $660 sales taxes + $325 delivery charges + $175 installation charges).

Periodic operating costs such as interest and taxes are generally deducted in the year paid. However, a taxpayer may elect to *capitalize* (i.e., include in basis) certain taxes and interest related to unproductive and unimproved real property or related to real property during development or improvement rather than take a current tax deduction.[9]

> **Example 9.** T purchased a small parcel of unimproved land near a lake known for its excellent fishing. She uses the property as a weekend retreat and plans someday to build a log cabin. T annually pays $150 for local property taxes but does not itemize deductions. T should elect to capitalize the property taxes paid each year as a part of her basis in the land.

Identification Problems. Generally, the adjusted basis of property sold or otherwise transferred is easily traced to the acquisition of the property and certain subsequent events. However, identification of cost may be difficult if a taxpayer has multiple homogeneous assets. For example, if a taxpayer owns identical shares of stock in a corporation that were acquired in more than one transaction and sells less than his or her entire investment in

---

[6]   Reg. § 1.1012-1(a).

[7]   § 1001 and *Crane v. Comm.*, 47-1 USTC ¶9217, 35 AFTR 776, 331 U.S. 1 (USSC, 1947).

[8]   § 1012 and Reg. § 1.1012-1(a).

[9]   § 266 and Reg. § 1.266-1(b)(1).

that stock, it is necessary to identify which shares are sold. For tax purposes, the owner must use the *first-in, first-out* (FIFO) method of identification if it is impossible to identify which shares were sold. Specific identification of the shares sold is appropriate if the shares can be identified.[10]

> **Example 10.** K purchased the following lots of G Corporation stock:
>
> | 50 shares | Purchased 1/10/06 | Cost $5,500 |
> | 75 shares | Purchased 8/15/06 | Cost $9,000 |
> | 40 shares | Purchased 6/18/08 | Cost $4,600 |
>
> K sold 60 shares of her G Corporation stock in 2009 for $8,700. Unless she can specifically identify the shares sold, her basis will be determined using the FIFO method. Therefore, her basis in 50 shares sold is $5,500 and her basis in 10 shares sold is $1,200 [10 shares × $120 ($9,000 ÷ 75 shares)]. Her total gain is $2,000.

> **Example 11.** Assuming the same facts in *Example 10*, the gain would be different if K could specifically identify the shares sold. If she directed her broker to deliver to the buyer the shares purchased on 8/15/06, referring to them by certificate number and date of purchase, her gain would be $1,500 [$8,700 sale price − $7,200 ($120 basis per share × 60)].

PROPERTY ACQUIRED BY GIFT

Generally, the basis of property received by gift is the same as the basis was to the donor.[11] This basis is *increased* by that portion of the gift tax paid by the donor, which is attributable to the appreciation in the property's value, if any, up to the date of the gift. A property's taxable value is its fair market value on the date of gift reduced by any gift tax exclusion, marital deduction or charitable deduction taken on the gift. The appreciation is measured by the difference between the taxable value of the property and the donor's adjusted basis in the property immediately before the gift.[12] The appropriate increase in basis for a given property is determined using the following formula:[13]

$$\frac{\text{Fair market value date of gift} - \text{Donor's basis date of gift} = \text{Appreciation}}{\text{Taxable gift}} \times \text{Gift taxes paid}$$

In making the adjustment for the gift tax, the amount of increase cannot exceed the amount of the tax. Also observe that there is an adjustment for gift tax only if the property had appreciated in the donor's hands at the time of the gift.

> **Example 12.** On March 7, 2007, Eve received 10 acres of undeveloped land as a gift from her Uncle Oral. On the date of the gift, the land had a value of $112,000 and Oral's adjusted basis in the land was $82,000. On his gift tax return, Oral reported a taxable gift of $100,000 (fair market value $112,000 − annual exclusion $12,000) and paid gift taxes of $41,000. Since Eve received the land, she has held it for investment. Now she is thinking about selling the property. If Eve sells the property, her basis in the land, including an adjustment for gift taxes, is $94,300 as determined below.

---

[10] Reg. § 1.1012-1(c).

[11] § 1015(a).

[12] See § 1015(d)(6) and Reg. § 1-1015-5(c)(3). For gifts made before 1977, the entire amount of the gift taxes paid could be used for the gift tax adjustment, but the adjusted basis could not exceed the property's taxable value at the time of the gift.

[13] See § 1015(d)(2) and Reg. § 1-1015-5(c)(3), Example 1. If there is more than one gift on the annual gift tax return, the gift tax is allocated among the gifts proportionately based on the amount of the taxable gift.

Appreciation at date of gift:

Fair market value of property	$112,000
Adjusted basis	(82,000)
Appreciation	$ 30,000

Donee's basis calculation:

Donor's adjusted basis	$ 82,000
Gift tax attributable to appreciation	
Gift tax $41,000 × ($30,000 appreciation at date of gift / $100,000 taxable gift). .	12,300
Donee's adjusted basis.	$ 94,300

If Eve sells the land for $154,300, her taxable gain would be $60,000 ($154,300 − $94,300). If Eve sells the land for $74,300, her deductible loss would be $20,000 ($74,300 − $94,300). Note that since the property had appreciated as of the date of the gift, the basis for determining gain and loss is the same.

Loss Limitation Rule. If the fair market value of the property *at the time of the gift* is less than the donor's basis (i.e., it has a built-in loss), special rules must be applied to determine the basis for the donee. The special rule is designed to prevent shifting of the loss to the taxpayer (e.g., a family member), who would obtain the greatest benefit. Perhaps the clearest expression of the rules in this case is as follows: the basis for *determining gain* is the donor's basis, while the basis for *determining loss* is the lower of either (1) the donor's basis or (2) the property's fair market value at the date of the gift.[14] Due to the way the rule for determining loss is stated, the donee will not recognize any gain or loss if the property is disposed of for any amount that is *less than* the donor's basis *but greater than* the value of the property at the date of the gift. These rules are illustrated in the following examples.

Example 13. S received 200 shares of X Corporation stock as a gift from his uncle. The stock had a basis to the uncle of $32,000 and a fair market value on the date of the gift of $29,000. Gift taxes of $1,400 were paid on the transfer.

This year, S sold all of the shares for $24,000. His loss realized on the sale is $5,000 ($24,000 sale price − $29,000 fair market value at date of gift). Note that S was not permitted to add any of the $1,400 gift taxes to his basis since such adjustments are allowed only if the taxable value is more than the donor's basis on the date of the gift (i.e., the property appreciated in the donor's hands).

Example 14. Assuming the same facts as in *Example 13*, if S's stock had been sold for $36,000, his realized gain would have been $4,000 ($36,000 sales price − $32,000 gain basis). There is no adjustment for gift taxes paid because the property did not appreciate in the donor's hands.

Example 15. Assuming the same facts as in *Example 13*, if S had sold his stock for $31,000 he would not realize gain or loss on the sale. His basis for gain is $32,000 (the donor's basis) and his basis for loss is limited to $29,000 (fair market value on the date of the gift). Since the $31,000 sales price does not exceed the gain basis and is not less than his loss basis, neither gain nor loss is realized on the sale.

Application of these special rules illustrates *three* important points. First, *any gain* realized by the donee on a subsequent sale of the property is limited to the amount of gain that the donor would have realized had he or she sold it at the donee's sales price. Second,

---

[14] § 1015(a). It also should be noted that total depreciation claimed using the gain basis for computation cannot exceed the property's fair market value at date of gift. Reg. § 1.167(g)-1.

any loss allowed on a subsequent sale of the property is limited to the decline in the property's value that occurs while owned by the donee. Third, although the payment of a gift tax may be required as a result of the gift, the donee is not allowed to adjust the donor's basis in the property by any gift taxes paid because there is no appreciation in value of the property in the donor's hands (i.e., the taxable value of the property at the time of the gift is less than the donor's basis).

PROPERTY ACQUIRED FROM A DECEDENT

The adjusted basis of property acquired from a decedent generally is its fair market value on the date of the decedent's death.[15] This also is the value used in determining the taxable estate for estate tax purposes.[16] The fiduciary (executor or administrator) of the estate may, however, *elect* to value the estate for estate tax purposes six months after the date of death.[17] This election is available only if (1) the estate is required to file a Federal estate tax return (Form 706), and (2) the alternate valuation reduces *both* the gross estate and the Federal estate tax.[18] If the fiduciary elects to use this alternate valuation date, the fair market value on the later date must also be used as the income tax basis to the heir or estate.[19]

> **Example 16.** D inherited some gold jewelry from his grandmother several years ago. The fair market value of the jewelry on the date of her death was $4,000 and its adjusted basis to the grandmother was $3,050. If D sells the jewelry this year for $4,350, his realized gain will be $350 ($4,350 sale price − $4,000 basis).

> **Example 17.** If D, from the previous example, sells the jewelry for $3,000, he will have a realized loss of $1,000 ($3,000 − $4,000).

Exceptions to this basis rule are provided for *income in respect of a decedent* under § 691[20] and for certain property acquired by the decedent by gift. Income in respect of a decedent (often referred to as IRD) includes all items of income that the decedent had earned or was entitled to as of the date of death, but which were not included in the decedent's final income tax return under his or her method of accounting. For example, if a cash basis individual performed all the services required to earn a $3,000 consulting fee but had not collected the fee before his or her death, the $3,000 would be income in respect of a decedent. All IRD items are includible in the decedent's gross estate at fair market value for Federal estate tax purposes. Whoever receives the right to collect these items of income must report them in the same manner as the decedent would have been required to report them had he or she lived to collect the income. As a result, IRD items generally are fully included in the gross income of the recipient when received.[21]

If appreciated property was acquired by the decedent by gift within one year before his or her death and the property passes *back* to the donor or the donor's spouse, the recipient's adjusted basis is the decedent's adjusted basis.[22]

---

[15]   § 1014(a).

[16]   § 2031(a).

[17]   § 2032(a).

[18]   § 2032(c).

[19]   § 1014(a)(2).

[20]   § 1014(c).

[21]   § 691(a)(1).

[22]   § 1014(e).

Example 18. H transferred a parcel of lake-front real estate to his elderly grand-mother when the property had an adjusted basis to H of $3,000 and a fair market value of $40,000. No gift taxes were paid on the transfer.

H's grandmother died three months after the gift and left the lake-front property to H in her will. H's basis in the property is $3,000 (the rules used for gifted property apply rather than those for inherited property). If his grandmother had lived for more than a year after the gift was made, H's basis would have been determined under the general rule for property acquired from a decedent.

Another exception is provided in the case of real property subject to special use valuation for Federal estate tax purposes. In such cases, the basis to the heir is the special value used for estate tax purposes. This special use valuation applies only to certain real property used in a trade or business and held by the heir more than 10 years.[23]

PROPERTY ACQUIRED IN A NONTAXABLE EXCHANGE

Most nontaxable exchanges provide deferral, rather than permanent nonrecognition of gain or loss. The mechanism for such deferral is typically an adjustment to the basis in some replacement property.[24] This adjustment is a reduction in basis in the case of a deferred gain and an increase in basis in the case of a deferred loss.

The specific rules for determining the basis of property acquired in nontaxable trans-actions, along with the requirements of each nontaxable transaction, are discussed in vari-ous parts of this text. Several such transactions are discussed in the next chapter. The following example illustrates one such transaction:

Example 19. T exchanged a five-acre residential lot for a 100-acre tract of farmland. He realized a $70,000 gain on the exchange because the farmland was worth $90,000 and his basis in the residential lot was $20,000. Since T met all the requirements for nonrecognition of gain in a like-kind exchange under § 1031, his basis in the farmland is $20,000 ($90,000 fair market value − $70,000 deferred gain).

PROPERTY CONVERTED FROM PERSONAL USE TO BUSINESS USE

Losses on the disposition of personal use properties are clearly not deductible. Absent some provision to the contrary, business owners could simply convert personal use assets to business use before disposing of them in order to generate business deductions for losses on their sale. Accordingly, when property is converted from personal use to trade or business use, its basis is limited for determining realized loss and for depreciation pur-poses. For each of those purposes, fair market value on the date of conversion is used as the property's basis if it is less than its adjusted basis.[25]

Example 20. J owned a single-family home that had been her personal residence for five years. When J discontinued use of the house as her residence, she converted it to rental property. J's original basis in the property was $90,000, and the property was worth $70,000 on the date of conversion. J must determine any depreciation using the fair market value of $70,000, since it is less than her $90,000 adjusted basis. If the property is later sold, J's *gain basis* will be the original $90,000 adjusted basis reduced by the depreciation allowed after the conversion. Her *loss basis* will be the lower fair market value on the date of conversion, $70,000, reduced by the allowed

---

[23] § 2032A(b).

[24] See, for example, § 1031(d), dealing with like-kind exchanges.

[25] Reg. §1.167(g)-1.

depreciation. Note that if J was hoping to deduct her loss of $20,000 on the property by converting it to business use, she is out of luck since the basis for loss is $70,000. Also observe the similarity to the basis rules that would have applied if J had received the residence as a gift (see *Examples 13, 14*, and *15*).

PROPERTY CONVERTED FROM BUSINESS USE TO PERSONAL USE

Once property is converted from business use to personal use, it is treated as personal use property. Any loss on the disposition of such property would, therefore, be disallowed; and, in the event that the property was subsequently converted back to business use, the limitations discussed above would apply.

> **Example 21.** W has a photocopier used exclusively for business. The copier cost $4,000 and depreciation of $1,800 has been allowed, making its basis $2,200. If W converts the copier to personal and family use and later sells it for $500, no loss will be deductible. Of course, if W had immediately sold the copier at a loss rather than converting it to personal use, he would have a business loss.

ADJUSTMENTS TO BASIS

Regardless of the method used in determining a property's basis initially, certain adjustments are made to that basis. Generally, the adjustments can be broken down into three groups. Basis is *increased* by *betterments* or *improvements*[26] and *reduced* by *depreciation allowed* or *allowable*[27] and by *other capital recoveries.*[28]

Depreciation reduces basis regardless of whether it is actually deducted by the taxpayer. The *allowable depreciation* is determined using the straight-line method if no method is adopted by the taxpayer.[29]

Various types of *capital recoveries* also reduce a property's adjusted basis. The following are some of the specific items that reduce basis:

1. Certain dividend distributions that are treated as a return of basis[30]

2. Deductible losses with respect to property, such as casualty loss deductions[31]

3. Credits for rehabilitation expenditures related to older commercial buildings and certified historic structures[32]

Numerous other events have an impact on a property's adjusted basis. Many of them are discussed in the remaining chapters of this text, which deal with specific types of transactions.

Exhibit 14-4 summarizes the rules for determining a property's adjusted basis.

EFFECT OF LIABILITIES ON AMOUNT REALIZED

Mention has been made of the fact that the amount realized in a sale or other disposition of property includes the amount of any liabilities of the seller assumed by the

---

[26]   § 1016(a)(1).

[27]   § 1016(a)(2).

[28]   See following examples.

[29]   § 1016(a)(2).

[30]   § 1016(a)(4).

[31]   See Reg. § 1.1016-6 and Rev. Rul. 74-206, 1974-1 C.B. 198.

[32]   See §§ 46(a), 48(q), and 1016(a)(22).

buyer plus any liabilities encumbering the transferred property that remain with the property.[33] The amount realized from a transaction is reduced by any liabilities assumed by the seller plus any liabilities encumbering property received in the transaction that remain with the property. The basis of any property received includes the portion of the cost represented by the liabilities assumed by the seller or encumbering the property.[34]

> **Example 22.** B exchanges a vacant lot with an adjusted basis of $20,000 for a mountain cabin worth $75,000. B's vacant lot has a fair market value of $50,000 and is subject to a $15,000 mortgage. The mountain cabin B receives is subject to a mortgage of $40,000. B assumes the $40,000 mortgage on the mountain cabin and the other party to the exchange assumes the $15,000 mortgage on the vacant lot.
>
> B's amount realized on this exchange is $50,000 ($75,000 fair market value of cabin received + $15,000 mortgage on vacant lot assumed by the other party − $40,000 mortgage on the mountain cabin assumed by B). If this exchange does not qualify for tax deferral, B has a realized and recognized gain of $30,000 ($50,000 amount realized − $20,000 adjusted basis of the vacant lot given up); and his basis in the mountain cabin is $75,000 (i.e., its fair market value).

EXHIBIT 14-4
Determination of Adjusted Basis

Method of Acquisition	Basis	Exceptions
General Rule		
Acquired by purchase	Purchase cost	See special rules
Special Rules		
Acquired by gift	Donor's basis + gift tax paid adjustment, if any	If fair market value at date of gift is less than donor's basis use fair market value to determine loss
Acquired from a decedent	Fair market value at date of death (or alternate valuation date, if elected)	1. Income in respect of a decedent 2. Property given to the decedent by the donor/heir within one year of decedent's death 3. Property subject to special § 2032A
Converted from personal use	Adjusted basis before conversion	For determining loss and depreciation, use fair market value date of conversion if lower than original adjusted basis
Acquired in a nontaxable exchange	Fair market value less any gain not recognized or plus any loss deferred	

Note: The basis as determined under any of the above methods is subject to adjustments as provided by other provisions of the Code. Basis is increased by betterments or improvements and reduced by depreciation allowed or allowable and by other capital recoveries.

---

[33] Reg. § 1.1001-2(a)(1).

[34] *Crane v. Comm.*, 47-1 USTC ¶9217, 35 AFTR 776, 331 U.S. 1 (USSC, 1947). Such liabilities are not included if they are contingent or not subject to valuation. Rev. Rul. 78-29, 1978-1 C.B. 62.

Example 23. D, the other party to the exchange in *Example 22*, had an adjusted basis in her mountain cabin of $65,000. D's amount realized on the exchange is $75,000 ($50,000 fair value of vacant lot received + $40,000 mortgage assumed by B − $15,000 mortgage on the vacant lot). If the exchange does not qualify for tax deferral, D has a realized and recognized gain of $10,000 ($75,000 amount realized − $65,000 adjusted basis in the mountain cabin given up); and her basis in the vacant lot is $50,000 (i.e., its fair market value).

The amount realized on a sale or exchange of property is affected by liabilities even though neither the buyer nor the seller is personally obligated for payment.[35] The rationale for such treatment is that the owner benefits from the nonrecourse liabilities as owner of the property because his or her basis in the property, or some other property, is properly increased because of the liability.[36]

CONCEPTS RELATED TO REALIZATION AND RECOGNITION

SALE OR OTHER DISPOSITION

Realization of gain or loss occurs upon any sale or other disposition of property. Whether such an event has occurred generally is not difficult to ascertain. A typical sale or exchange obviously constitutes a sale or other disposition, but other transactions in which the taxpayer surrenders property other than cash also may be so classified. The timing of such realization is determined according to the taxpayer's method of accounting. Under the accrual method, realization generally occurs when a transaction is closed and the seller has an unqualified right to collect the sales price.[37] Under the cash method, the taxpayer realizes gain or loss upon the receipt of cash or cash equivalents.[38] In any case, a sale is consummated and realization occurs if beneficial title or possession of the burdens and benefits of ownership are transferred to the buyer.[39]

Transactions Involving Certain Securities. Generally, a sale or other disposition occurs any time a taxpayer surrenders property in exchange for some consideration. Accordingly, if a taxpayer exchanges securities of one type for securities of another type, a taxable event has occurred.[40]

Example 24. F exchanged X Corporation 12% bonds with a face value of $100,000 for Z Corporation 9% bonds with a face value of $120,000. Each group of bonds was worth $105,000 at the time of the exchange. If the X Corporation bonds that F exchanged had a basis of $100,000, he has a $5,000 gain on the exchange.

Several exceptions to this scheme do exist. In some instances, the exchange of *substantially identical* bonds of state or municipal governments has been declared a nontaxable transfer.[41] The condition of being substantially identical is usually

---

[35]   *Ibid.*

[36]   See *Tufts v. Comm.*, 83-1 USTC ¶9328, 51 AFTR2d 1983-1132, 461 U.S. 300 (USSC, 1983) for an excellent discussion of nonrecourse liabilities and their impact on basis.

[37]   See *Alfred Scully*, 20 TCM 1272, T.C. Memo 1961-243 (1961), and Rev. Rul. 72-381, 1972-2 C.B. 581.

[38]   See, for example, *Comm. v. Union Pacific R.R. Co.*, 36-2 USTC ¶9525, 18 AFTR 636, 86 F.2d 637 (CA-2, 1936).

[39]   *Ibid.*

[40]   Rev. Rul. 60-25, 1960-1 C.B. 283, and Rev. Rul. 78-408, 1978-2 C.B. 203.

[41]   *Motor Products Corp. v. Comm.*, 44-1 USTC ¶9308, 32 AFTR 672, 142 F.2d 449 (CA-6, 1944), and Rev. Rul. 56-435, 1956-2 C.B. 506.

determined in terms of rate of return and fair market value. If the bonds received do not meet this test, the exchange may be taxable.[42]

It is clearly established that converting bonds into stock under a conversion privilege contained in the bond instrument does not result in the recognition of gain.[43] Similarly, the conversion of stock into some other stock of the same corporation pursuant to a right granted under the stock certificate does not result in recognition of gain or loss.[44]

Transfer Related to Taxpayer's Debt. When property is transferred to a creditor, the transfer may or may not be a disposition. The mere granting of a lien against property to secure a loan is not a disposition.[45] The transfer of property in satisfaction of a liability, however, is a taxable disposition.[46] Similarly, the loss of property in a foreclosure sale[47] and the voluntary transfer of mortgaged property to creditors in satisfaction of debt[48] are dispositions of property.

> **Example 25.** M purchased a commercial property for $20,000, paying $4,000 down and signing a note secured by a mortgage for the $16,000 difference. Three years later, when M had reduced the balance on the note to $7,000, the lender accepted 300 shares of T Corporation stock in satisfaction of the obligation. The T Corporation stock had a fair market value of $7,000 and an adjusted basis to M of $5,000. By transferring the stock to satisfy the liability, there is a disposition of the stock and M has a $2,000 realized gain. Note that this result is the same as if M had sold the stock for $7,000 cash and paid the balance on the note.

> **Example 26.** K purchased a warehouse for use in her business for $30,000, paying $5,000 down and signing a nonrecourse note (K is not personally liable) secured by a mortgage lien for the $25,000 difference. Over a three-year period, K's business suffered a decline and as a result she was able to make payments of only $3,000 on the note. During the same three-year period, K deducted depreciation of $12,000, thereby reducing her basis in the warehouse to $18,000.
>
> After the three years, K reduced the size of her business substantially and voluntarily transferred the warehouse to the lender. Upon the transfer, K's amount realized from the discharge of the remaining indebtedness is $22,000 ($25,000 original note − $3,000 payments). Since her basis in the warehouse was $18,000, K has a $4,000 realized gain on the disposition of the property.

Abandonment. The abandonment of property used in a business or income-producing activity, whether depreciable or not, results in realization of loss to the extent of the property's adjusted basis. A loss deduction is allowed if the taxpayer takes action that demonstrates that he or she has no intention of retrieving the property for use, for sale, or other disposition in the future.[49]

---

[42]   See *Emery v. Comm.*, 48-1 USTC ¶9165, 36 AFTR 741, 166 F.2d 27 (CA-2, 1948), and Rev. Rul. 81-169, 1981-25 I.R.B. 17. Also, see *Mutual Loan and Savings Co. v. Comm.*, 50-2 USTC ¶9420, 39 AFTR 1034, 184 F.2d 161 (CA-5, 1950) for an example of nonrecognition where the state Supreme Court held the new bonds with a lower interest rate to be a mere continuation of the original issue.

[43]   Rev. Rul. 57-535, 1957-2 C.B. 513.

[44]   Ltr. Rul., 2-23-45, ¶76,130 P-H Fed. 1945.

[45]   See *Dorothy Vickers*, 36 TCM 391, T.C. Memo 1977-90.

[46]   *Carlisle Packing Co.*, 29 B.T.A. 514 (1933), and Rev. Rul. 76-111, 1976-1 C.B. 214 (1976).

[47]   *O'Dell & Sons Co., Inc.*, 8 T.C. 1165 (1947).

[48]   *Estate of Delman*, 73 T.C. 15 (1979).

[49]   Reg. §§ 1.165-2 and 1.167(a)-8.

Example 27. While working in a logging operation, R's truck became unoperational, and it was clear that the cost of having the truck moved to a repair site exceeded its value. R abandoned the truck with no intention of seeking its return. If R has a $2,500 adjusted basis in the truck, he is entitled to an abandonment loss deduction of $2,500.

Demolition. No deduction is allowed for expenses related to the demolition of a building or for a loss where the adjusted basis of the building exceeds any salvage value. Both the cost of the demolition and any disallowed loss are added to the basis of the land on which the building stood.[50]

Example 28. T purchased a rezoned commercial lot with a small house for $75,000. The structure was worth $2,000. In order to expedite construction of a new car wash, T simply razed the house at a cost of $1,500. No deduction is allowed for the loss of the house or the razing cost, and T's basis in the vacant lot is $76,500 ($73,000 lot + $2,000 house + $1,500 demolition costs).

Spousal Transfers. The transfer of property to one's spouse while married or as a result of dissolution of the marriage does not constitute a taxable event. This is true even if the transfer is in exchange for the release of marital rights under state law or for some other consideration. This rule applies to *any* transfer made to one's spouse during the marriage or within *one year* after the marriage is terminated. It also applies to later transfers to a former spouse if the transfers are made incident to the divorce (e.g., under a provision of the divorce decree).[51] In a consistent manner, the basis of the transferred property for the transferee (recipient) is the same as the transferor's basis.[52]

It is important to note that this nonrecognition provision applies to all transfers between spouses—including the sale of property at a fair market price. Additionally, the transferor is required to provide the transferee with records needed to determine the basis and holding period of the property.[53]

Example 29. H and W were divorced this year. Under the terms of their agreement, H received marketable securities with a basis of $16,000 and a value of $10,000. W received the house with a basis of $80,000, valued at $96,000 and subject to a mortgage of $60,000. No gain or loss is recognized by either party regardless of who owned the property before the transfer. H and W have bases in their separate properties of $16,000 and $80,000, respectively.

Example 30. Under an option provided in their divorce agreement, W (from the previous example) sold the house to H six months later (subject to the mortgage obligation) for $36,000. W still recognizes no gain and H's basis in the residence is $80,000.

Gift or Bequest. A transfer of property by gift or bequest generally does not constitute a sale or other disposition. Accordingly, there is no gain or loss recognized by the donor or decedent, respectively. An exception exists, however, in the case of a sale of property at a price below its fair market value. In such a *part-gift* and *part-sale*, the donor recognizes gain *only* to the extent the sales price exceeds the adjusted basis of the property transferred.[54]

---

[50]   § 280B.

[51]   §§ 1041(a) and (c).

[52]   § 1041(b)(2).

[53]   Temp. Reg. § 1.1041-1T(e).

[54]   Reg. § 1.1015-4(d).

Example 31. M sold her personal automobile to her brother for $4,000. She had a basis of $12,000 in the auto which was worth $6,000 on the date of sale. M has made a gift of $2,000 in this part-sale/part-gift transaction and she recognizes no gain or loss.

Example 32. Assume the same facts above, except that M's basis in the auto had been reduced to $3,000 from depreciation deductions allowed in prior years. Although M has still made a $2,000 gift in this transaction, she must now recognize a $1,000 gain on the sale ($4,000 amount realized − $3,000 adjusted basis).

If the donee/buyer pays some cash and assumes debt of the donor/seller, or takes the property subject to encumbrances, the amount of the liabilities must be included by the donor/seller in the amount realized from the transaction.[55] Even if no cash changes hands, the part-gift and part-sale rules apply if there are liabilities associated with the transfer. Accordingly, if the donee assumes liabilities that exceed the donor's basis in the transferred property, the donor has taxable gain to the extent the liabilities exceed such basis.[56] Also, the donee/purchaser will take as his or her basis in the property acquired the *greater* of the basis under the gift rules or the purchase (cost) basis.

Example 33. F gave a duplex rental unit to her grandson for his 18th birthday so he could develop property management skills. The duplex had a basis to F of $22,000 and a fair market value on the date of the gift of $40,000. The property was subject to a mortgage of $25,000, for which the grandson is now responsible. F has an amount realized on the gift transaction of $25,000 (transfer of the mortgage). Since the adjusted basis of the duplex was $22,000, F has a $3,000 taxable gain. If no gift taxes were paid, the grandson's basis in the duplex will be $25,000, the greater of the basis under the gift rules ($22,000) or the purchase (cost) basis.

Example 34. If the property in the previous example had been subject to a mortgage of only $8,000, the general rule would have applied, and F would not have recognized gain or loss. The exception only applies when the discharged liabilities exceed the adjusted basis of the gifted property. Note also that the grandson's basis in the duplex would be $22,000, the same basis F had in the property.

Transfer of Property to Charities. The transfer of property to a charity generally is not treated as a sale or other disposition. Accordingly, no gain or loss is realized or recognized. However, an exception is provided for *bargain sales* of property to charities that result in a charitable contribution deduction to the seller. In such a case, the adjusted basis of the transferred property must be allocated between the sale portion and the contribution portion based on the fair market value of the property—and any resulting gain must be recognized.[57]

Example 35. P sold land to her church for $30,000. P had an adjusted basis in the land of $25,000. The land was appraised at $50,000 at the time of the bargain sale. P is entitled to a charitable contribution deduction of $20,000 ($50,000 fair market value − $30,000 sale price). She also has taxable gain of $15,000 on the sale ($30,000 amount realized − the $15,000 pro rata share of the adjusted basis allocable to the sale portion [($30,000 sale price ÷ $50,000 fair market value) × $25,000 basis]).

---

[55] *Reginald Fincke*, 39 B.T.A. 510 (1939).

[56] *Levine Est. v. Comm.*, 80-2 USTC ¶9607, 46 AFTR2d, 80-5349, 634 F.2d 12 (CA-2, 1980).

[57] § 1011(b); Reg. § 1.1011-2(a).

A charitable contribution of encumbered property is also treated as a bargain sale. The amount realized includes the amount of cash and the fair market value of any other property received plus the amount of the liabilities transferred. Accordingly, the property's adjusted basis must be allocated between the sale portion (represented by the amount realized) and the contribution portion.[58] This is true even if no cash or other property is received by the taxpayer.[59]

> **Example 36.** E made a gift of land to his alma mater. The land had a fair market value of $50,000 and was subject to a $22,000 mortgage which was assumed by the university. If the land is a long-term capital asset, E is entitled to a charitable contribution deduction of $28,000 ($50,000 fair market value reduced by the $22,000 mortgage).[60]
>
> Additionally, E's $20,000 adjusted basis in the property must be allocated between the contribution of $28,000 and the amount realized of $22,000. The basis allocated to the sale portion is $8,800 [$20,000 basis × ($22,000 amount realized ÷ $50,000 fair market value)]. The result of the bargain sale is a taxable gain to E of $13,200 ($22,000 amount realized − $8,800 allocated basis).

ALLOCATIONS OF PURCHASE PRICE AND BASIS

Properties purchased in a single transaction are often sold separately. In such a situation, the total basis must be allocated between the various items in order to determine gain or loss on the independent sales. Generally, relative fair market values at the time of acquisition are used to allocate the total basis among the various properties.[61] Similarly, allocation is necessary when a single sale involves properties acquired at different times in separate transactions. It may be necessary to allocate the sales price to individual assets; in such a situation, the relative fair market values on the date of sale are used for the allocation. Generally, an allocation in the sale agreement between buyer and seller will sufficiently establish the relative values unless it is shown that such assigned values were arbitrary or unreasonable.[62]

> **Example 37.** T purchased a commercial lot in 2002 for $30,000 and built a warehouse on the site in 2003 at a cost of $60,000. During the six years he used the warehouse in his business, T deducted depreciation of $32,000. The property was sold this year for $110,000. T must allocate the $110,000 sale price between the building and the land to determine the gain or loss on each. If $40,000 is allocated to the land and $70,000 is allocated to the building based on relative fair market values, T has a gain of $10,000 ($40,000 − $30,000) and $42,000 [$70,000 − ($60,000 − $32,000)], respectively, on the properties.

Sale of a Business. When a business operated as a sole proprietorship is sold, the sale is treated as a sale of each of the individual assets of the business. Accordingly, allocations of sales price and basis must be made to the individual assets of the business.[63] The various gains and losses have separate impact, according to their character, on the taxable income of the owner.

---

[58] See Reg. § 1.1011-2(a).

[59] *Winston Guest*, 77 T.C. 9 (1981) and Rev. Rul. 81-163, 1981-1 C.B. 433.

[60] See Chapter 11 for a discussion of charitable contributions involving long-term capital gain property.

[61] See, for example, *Fairfeld Plaza, Inc.*, 39 T.C. 706 (1963), and Rev. Rul. 72-255, 1972-1 C.B. 221.

[62] See *John B. Resler*, 38 TCM 153, T.C. Memo 1979-40.

[63] See Rev. Rul. 55-79, 1955-1 C.B. 370, and *Williams v. McGowan*, 46-1 USTC ¶9120, 34 AFTR 615, 152 F.2d 570 (CA-2, 1945).

Example 38. F has owned and operated a convenience store for 12 years. F's increased interest in her grandchildren and in fishing prompted her to sell the store and retire. The sales agreement with the buyer allocated the total sales price to the individual assets as follows:

	Value per Sales Agreement	F's Adjusted Basis
Inventory	$16,000	$18,000
Furniture and fixtures	14,000	6,000
Leasehold and leasehold improvements	20,000	3,000
Goodwill	0	0
Total	$50,000	$27,000

F has a $2,000 loss on the sale of inventory, and gains on the furniture and fixtures of $8,000 and on the leasehold and improvements of $17,000, each of which has its separate impact on taxable income.

The sale of an interest in a partnership or in a corporation that operates a business is generally treated as the sale of such interest, rather than of the underlying assets. Therefore, no allocation is necessary and gain or loss is recognized on the sale of the interest. For each type of entity, major exceptions to this treatment exist and are discussed in a later chapter.[64]

INSTALLMENT SALE METHOD

The general rule of Federal taxation is that all gains or losses are recognized in the year of sale or exchange. This rule could place a severe burden on taxpayers who sell their property for something other than cash, particularly deferred payment obligations. Without some relief, taxpayers would be required to pay their tax liability before obtaining the sale proceeds with which they could pay the tax. If the tax is substantial, a requirement to pay before sufficient cash collections occur might necessitate the sale of other assets the taxpayer wished to retain.

Because of the potential hardship placed on taxpayers from reporting gain without the corresponding receipt of cash, Congress enacted the installment sale method of reporting in 1926. The installment method has been significantly modified over the years, with each modification further restricting *both* the types of gains and the taxpayers eligible for its use. The eligibility requirements are discussed below.

GENERAL RULES

The installment method is used to report *gains*—not losses—from qualifying installment sales of property. An *installment sale* is defined as any sale of property whereby the seller will receive at least one payment after the close of the tax year in which the sale occurs. Unfortunately, not all gains from installment sales qualify for installment reporting.

---

[64] See Chapter 19 for a discussion of corporate taxation, and Chapter 22 for partnership taxation.

Ineligible Sales. Currently, use of the installment method is denied for reporting gains from sales of the following:[65]

1. Property held for sale in the ordinary course of the taxpayer's trade or business (e.g., inventories)

2. Stocks or securities that are traded on an established securities market

In addition, the portion of any gain from the sale of depreciable property that must be reported as ordinary income under the depreciation recapture rules is not eligible for installment reporting. These rules are discussed in Chapter 17.

Mandatory Reporting Requirement. Generally, gains from eligible sales *must* be reported under the installment method regardless of the taxpayer's method of accounting.[66] Thus, the installment method is considered to be *mandatory* rather than elective. However, Congress recognized the fact that for some taxpayers the installment method of reporting would not be the relief measure that it was intended to be. Consequently, taxpayers are allowed to *elect out* of the installment method simply by reporting the entire gain in the year of sale.[67]

ELECTION OUT OF INSTALLMENT REPORTING

There are various reasons why a taxpayer might wish to elect not to use the installment method of reporting gain from the sale of property. Such reasons might include the following:

1. The taxpayer's income in the year of sale is quite low and income is expected to be higher in subsequent years.

2. The taxpayer might have a large capital loss with which to absorb the capital gain in the year of sale.

3. The taxpayer might have an expiring net operating loss.

4. It might be necessary for the taxpayer to report the gain in order to utilize a tax credit carryover.

5. The burden of complying with the installment sale rules might outweigh the advantage of the installment reporting of the gain.

If a taxpayer *elects not to use* the installment method for a given sale, the amount of gain must be computed under his or her usual method of accounting (i.e., cash or accrual) and reported in the year of sale.[68] A cash basis taxpayer must use the *fair market value* of any installment obligation received in determining the amount realized from the installment sale.[69] On the other hand, an accrual basis taxpayer must account for an installment obligation at its *face value* in computing the amount realized.[70]

---

[65]   §§ 453(b), (i), and (l). See § 453(l)(2) for certain limited exceptions.

[66]   § 453(a).

[67]   See § 453(d) and Temp. Reg. 15a.453-1(d)(2)(ii).

[68]   *Ibid.*

[69]   § 1001(b).

[70]   Rev. Rul. 79-292. 1979-2 C.B. 287.

Example 39. S, a cash basis taxpayer, sold land to B on December 15, 2009. S received $100,000 cash and a note from B payable in five equal annual installments of $80,000 (i.e., face value), bearing a 9% interest rate. The note has a fair market value of $300,000 and S has a $75,000 basis in the land. If S elects not to use the installment method, his gain to be reported in 2009 is computed as follows:

Amount realized:		
	Cash received	$100,000
	FMV of installment obligations	300,000
		$400,000
	Less: Basis of land	(75,000)
	Gain to be reported in 2009	$325,000

In addition to the interest income that S will recognize when the installment payments are collected, he must recognize additional income on the collection of each installment payment as follows:

Amount realized (installment payment)	$ 80,000
Less: Basis in each installment	
($300,000 FMV of note ÷ 5 installments)	(60,000)
Ordinary income to be reported	$ 20,000

Example 40. Assume the same facts as in *Example 39*, except that S is an accrual basis taxpayer. His gain to be reported in the year of sale is computed as follows:

Amount realized:		
	Cash received	$100,000
	Face value of installment obligations	400,000
		$500,000
	Less: Basis in land	(75,000)
	Gain to be reported in 2008	$425,000

In this case, S will not be required to report any income other than the interest received as each of the payments are collected because his basis in each installment obligation is $100,000 (i.e., its face amount).

GAIN REPORTED UNDER THE INSTALLMENT METHOD

The following *six* factors must be taken into account by a taxpayer using the installment method of reporting gain:

1. The gross profit on the sale
2. The total contract price
3. The gross profit percentage
4. The payments received in the year of sale
5. The gain to be reported in the year of sale
6. The gain to be reported in the following years

Determining Gross Profit. A taxpayer's gross profit is nothing more than the total gain that will be reported (excluding interest) from the installment sale. It is determined by subtracting the *sum* of the seller's adjusted basis and expenses of sale from the selling price:[71]

Selling price	$xxx,xxx
Less: Adjusted basis in property plus selling expenses	− xx,xxx
Gross profit on sale	$ xx,xxx

Determining the Total Contract Price. The total contract price is the total amount of cash (excluding interest) that the seller expects to collect from the buyer over the term of the installment sale. It is usually equal to the selling price less any liabilities of the seller that are transferred to the buyer. However, if the liabilities assumed by the buyer *exceed* the seller's adjusted basis in the property and the selling expenses, the excess must be treated as a *deemed payment* received in the year of sale. Because a deemed payment is treated as cash collected in the year of sale, it must be added to the contract price.[72]

Determining Gross Profit Percentage. The taxpayer's gross profit percentage is the percentage of each dollar received that must be reported as gain. It is equal to the gross profit divided by the total contract price.[73]

$$\frac{\text{Gross profit}}{\text{Total contract price}} = \text{Gross profit percentage}$$

Determining Payments Received in Year of Sale. Payments received in the year of sale include the following:[74]

1. Money received at the time of closing the sale, including any selling expenses *paid* by the buyer

2. Deemed payments (i.e., excess of seller's liabilities transferred over the property's adjusted basis plus selling expenses)

3. The fair market value of any third-party obligations received at the time of closing and the fair market value of any other property received

4. Installment payments received in the year of sale, excluding interest income

Gain Reported in Year of Sale. Gain reported in the year of sale is computed as follows:

$$\frac{\text{Gross profit}}{\text{Total contract price}} \times \text{Payments received} = \text{Recognized gain}$$

---

[71]   Temp. Reg. § 15a.453-1(b)(2)(v).

[72]   § 453A(a)(2) and Temp. Reg. § 15a.453-1(b)(2)(ii).

[73]   § 453(c) and Temp. Reg. § 15a.453-1(b)(2)(i).

[74]   Temp. Reg. § 15a.453-1(b)(3)(i).

Gain Reported in Following Years. Gain to be reported in the years following the year of sale equals the taxpayer's gross profit percentage multiplied by the principal payments received on the purchaser's note in that year.

Example 41. T sold a 70-acre tract of land that she had held as an investment on March 1, 2009. The facts concerning the sale are as follows:

Sales price:		
Cash payment............................	$120,000	
Mortgage assumed by buyer.................	200,000	
Buyer's notes payable to T	480,000	$800,000
Less: Selling expenses...........................	$ 50,000	
T's basis in land	250,000	(300,000)
Gross profit on sale.............................		$500,000

The contract price is $600,000 ($800,000 sales price − $200,000 debt assumed by buyer). Assuming the $120,000 payment is the only payment received in 2009, T's gain to be reported for the year is computed as follows:

$$\frac{\$\,500,000(\text{gross profit})}{\$\,600,000(\text{contract price})} \times \$\,120,000 = \$\,100,000 \text{ gain to be recognized}$$

As T collects the remaining $480,000 of the total contract price, she will report the remaining $400,000 gross profit from the sale (i.e., $480,000 × 5/6 gross profit percentage = $400,000).

Example 42. Assume the same facts as in *Example 41*, except that T's basis in the land is only $100,000. In this case, the gross profit on the sale is $650,000 [$800,000 − ($50,000 + $100,000)]. T's payments received in the year of sale are computed as follows:

Cash payment.......................................		$120,000
Plus: deemed payment received:		
Mortgage assumed by buyer.....................	$200,000	
Less: Selling expense	(50,000)	
T's basis in land..............................	(100,000)	50,000
Total payments received in 2009......................		$170,000

The total contract price is $650,000 ($800,000 selling price − $200,000 mortgage transferred + $50,000 excess of mortgage assumed over T's basis in property and selling expenses). T's gain to be reported in 2009 is computed as follows:

$$\frac{\$\,650,000(\text{gross profit})}{\$\,650,000(\text{contract price})} \times \$\,170,000 \text{ payments} = \$\,170,000$$

Note that the excess of the mortgage transferred over T's basis in the land and the selling expenses (i.e., the deemed payment) causes the gross profit percentage to become 100%. This adjustment to *both* the total contract price and the payments received in the year of sale must be made to ensure that the entire gain from the sale is ultimately reported by the seller. As a result, all payments received by T in subsequent years (excluding interest) will be reported as gain from the sale [$650,000 total gross profit − $170,000 gain reported in year of sale = $480,000 gain to be reported in subsequent years ($480,000 buyer's notes × 100%)].

LIMITATIONS ON CERTAIN INSTALLMENT SALES

As mentioned earlier, the installment sales provisions have been modified over the years to limit or stop perceived taxpayer abuse of what was intended to be simply a relief from immediate taxation of all gain from deferred payment sales. These modifications have created the following problem areas:

1. Imputed interest rules

2. Related-party rules

3. Gain recognition on dispositions of installment note

4. Required interest payments on deferred taxes

Each of these problem areas is discussed below.

Imputed Interest Rules. Without some limitation, a taxpayer planning a deferred payment sale of a capital asset could require the buyer to pay a higher sales price in return for a lower than prevailing market rate of interest on the deferred payments, thereby converting into capital gain what would have been ordinary (interest) income. The imputed interest rules were designed to prevent just such a scheme. Under these rules, any deferred payment sale of property with a selling price exceeding $3,000 must provide a *reasonable* interest rate.[75] Thus, in a deferred payment sale providing little or no interest, the selling price must be *restated* to equal the sum of payments received on the date of the sale and the discounted present value of the future payments. The difference between the face value of the future payments and this discounted value (i.e., the imputed interest) generally must be reported as interest income under the accrual method of accounting, regardless of the taxpayer's regular accounting method.[76]

If the sales contract does not provide for interest equal to the *applicable Federal rate* (AFR), interest will be imputed at that rate.[77] The AFR is the interest rate the Federal government pays on borrowed funds, and the actual rate varies with the terms of the loan. Loans are divided into short-term (not over three years), mid-term (over three years but not over nine years), and long-term (over nine years).[78]

> **Example 43.** S, a cash basis taxpayer, sold land held as an investment on July 1, 2009 for $1 million cash and a non-interest-bearing note (face value of $4 million) due on July 1, 2011. At the time of the sale, the short-term AFR was 10% (compounded semiannually). Because the sales contract did not provide for interest of at least the AFR, the selling price must be restated and interest must be imputed at 10% (compounded semiannually).

Sale price:	
Cash payment	$1,000,000
Present value of $4,000,000 note due July 1, 2011 (0.8227 × $4,000,000) . .	3,290,800
Recomputed sale price	$4,290,800

---

[75] See §§ 483 and 1274.

[76] See §§ 1272(a), 1273(a), and 1274(a). Also see §§ 483 and 1274(c) for various exceptions to this requirement.

[77] § 1274(d)(1).

[78] These three Federal rates are published monthly by the IRS.

S must use this recomputed sale price in determining the total contract price, gross profit percentage, gain to be reported in the year of sale, and gain to be reported (excluding interest) when the $4 million deferred payment is received. In addition, S must report $164,540 of imputed interest income in 2009, computed as follows:

Period	Present Value	×	10% Compounded Semiannually	=	Imputed Interest
7/1/09 to 12/31/09	$3,290,800	×	0.05	=	$164,540

S must also compute and report her imputed interest for 2010 and 2011. When the $4 million note payable is collected on July 1, 2011, S will report only the gain on the sale remaining after that portion reported in 2009.

Related-Party Sales. Generally, installment sales between related parties are subject to the same rules as other such sales *except* (1) when the related-party purchaser resells the property before payment of the original sales price;[79] and (2) when the property sold is depreciable property.[80] The primary purpose of the *resale* rule is to prevent a related-party seller from deferring his or her gain on the first sale while the related-party purchaser enjoys the use of proceeds from its resale.

Example 44. M plans to sell a capital asset (basis $40,000) to B, an unrelated party, for $200,000. Instead of selling the asset to B, she sells it to her son, S, for $10,000 cash and a $190,000 note due in five years and bearing a reasonable interest rate. Shortly after his purchase, S sells the asset to B for $200,000.

Without the resale rule, M would report a gain of $8,000 in the year of sale, computed as follows:

$$\frac{\$200,000 - \$40,000}{\$200,000} \times \$10,000 = \$8,000$$

M would have a deferred gain of $152,000 ($160,000 gross profit − $8,000 gain reported in year of sale). More importantly, S would have a cost basis of $200,000 in the asset and report no gain on the subsequent resale to B. The net result of the two transactions is a $152,000 deferred gain and the immediate use of the sales proceeds by a family member.

Under the resale rule, any proceeds collected by the related-party purchaser on the subsequent sale are treated as being collected by the related-party seller. Consequently, M must report her $152,000 deferred gain when S resells the property, even though she has not yet collected the $190,000 note.

For purposes of the resale rule, the term *related party* includes the spouse, children, grandchildren, and parents of the seller.[81] Any controlled corporation, partnership, trust, or estate in which the seller has an interest is also considered related under these rules.[82] It is also important to note that the resale rule does not apply when the second sale occurs (1) more than two years after the first sale, or (2) after the death of the related-party seller.[83]

The installment method is generally not allowed to be used to report a gain on the sale of depreciable property to an entity controlled by the taxpayer.[84] This rule is designed to

---

[79] § 453(e).

[80] § 453(g).

[81] §§ 453(f) and 267(b).

[82] §§ 453(f) and 318(a).

[83] § 453(e)(2).

[84] *Supra*, Footnote 80.

prevent a related-party seller from deferring gain on a sale that will result in the purchaser's being able to use a higher (cost) basis to claim depreciation deductions. For this purpose, a *controlled entity* is a partnership or corporation in which the seller owns a more than 50 percent direct or indirect interest. Indirect ownership includes any interest owned by the seller's spouse and certain other family members.[85] It is important to note that this rule is based on a presumption that the related-party installment sale is motivated by tax avoidance. Thus, the related-party seller can use the installment method of reporting the sale if he or she can establish that tax avoidance *was not* the principal motive of the transaction. This makes such a sale subject to a facts and circumstances review and approval of the Internal Revenue Service.

Dispositions of Installment Obligations. After deciding to report a deferred payment sale under the installment method, rather than *electing out*, sellers ordinarily collect the payments in due course and report the remaining gain in full. However, if this process is interrupted by a sale, gift, or other transfer of some or all of the installment obligations, rules require that any unreported gain be reported at the time of the transfer. Consequently, if an installment obligation is satisfied at other than its face value or is distributed, transmitted, sold, or otherwise disposed of, the taxpayer is generally required to recognize gain or loss.

The amount of gain or loss is the difference between the obligation's basis and *either* the amount realized, if the obligation is satisfied at an amount other than its face value because it is sold or exchanged, *or* its fair market value when distributed, transmitted, or disposed of, if the transfer is not a sale or exchange.[86] The obligation's basis is its face amount less the amount of gain that would have been reported if the obligation had been satisfied in full.[87]

Taxable dispositions include most sales and exchanges. Also included are gifts, transfers to trusts, distributions by trusts and estates to beneficiaries, distributions from corporations to shareholders, net proceeds from the pledge of an installment obligation, and cancellation of the installment obligation.

The obvious purpose of the disposition rules is to prevent the seller from *either* shifting the income to another taxpayer (e.g., by gift) *or* enjoying the use of the sales proceeds prior to gain recognition (e.g., by pledging an installment obligation for borrowed funds). However, there are several exceptions to the requirement of immediate gain recognition. Transfers of installment obligations upon the death of the seller, transfers incident to divorce, transfers to or distributions from a partnership, certain transfers to controlled corporations, and certain transfers incident to corporate reorganization are among the exceptions to these rules.[88]

Required Interest Payments on Deferred Taxes. Another rule designed to reduce the benefits of installment reporting for certain taxpayers is the requirement to pay interest to the government on the deferred taxes. This rule applies if *two conditions* are met. First, the taxpayer must have outstanding installment obligations from the sale of property (other than farming property) for more than $150,000. Second, the outstanding obligations from such sales must exceed $5 million at the close of the tax year.[89] Only the deferred taxes attributable to the installment obligations in *excess* of $5 million are subject to this annual interest payment. The interest must be calculated using the tax underpayment rate in § 6621.

---

[85]   §§ 1239(b) and (c).

[86]   § 453B(a).

[87]   § 453B(b).

[88]   See §§ 453B(c), (d), and (g).

[89]   § 453A.

Example 45. T has $9 million of installment obligations outstanding on December 31, 2009. These obligations arose from the sale of a vacant lot located in the downtown area of Chicago. T's gross profit percentage on the installment sale was 40%. Assuming the underpayment rate in § 6621 is 10% and T's 2009 marginal tax rate is 35%, the required interest payment on the deferred taxes is computed as follows:

Outstanding installment obligations	$9,000,000
Less: Amount not subject to rule	(5,000,000)
Excess installment obligations	$4,000,000
Times: Gross profit percentage	× 40%
Deferred gross profit	$1,600,000
Times: T's marginal tax rate	× 35%
Deferred Federal income taxes	$ 560,000
Times: § 6621 underpayment rate	× 10%
Required interest payment	$ 56,000

Because taxpayers are allowed to have up to $5 million of installment obligations outstanding without being subject to the required interest payment rule, it is apparent that only those taxpayers with one or more substantial installment sales need be concerned with this rule.

REPORTING GAIN ON INSTALLMENT SALES

Taxpayers reporting gain on the installment sale method should attach Form 6252, Computation of Installment Sale Income, to the tax return for the year of sale and each subsequent year in which a payment is collected. A sample of this form is contained in Appendix B.

DISALLOWED LOSSES

Various limitations exist regarding gain and loss recognition in certain property transactions. Several such limitations have already been discussed. Recall that any losses on the sale of personal use assets are disallowed. Similarly, losses on the sale of property acquired by gift are limited to the decline in its value subsequent to the transfer by gift. This results because the basis for determining loss is the fair market value on the date of gift, if that fair market value is less than the donor's basis (which would otherwise be the donee's basis).[90] Likewise, a loss on the disposition of property that has been converted from personal use to business use is limited to the decline in its value subsequent to the conversion. In determining any loss on such a disposition, the adjusted basis is the lesser of the taxpayer's adjusted basis or the fair market value on the date of conversion.[91]

There are several other limitations on the deductibility of losses arising from sales or other dispositions of property. As discussed in Chapter 7, losses incurred in sales between related taxpayers are not deductible. Also, certain losses incurred from the sale of stock or securities will not be allowed as a deduction.

---

[90]   § 1015(a).

[91]   Reg. § 1.165-9(b).

WASH SALES

A *wash sale* occurs when a taxpayer sells stock or securities at a loss and reinvests in substantially identical stock or securities within 30 days before or after the date of sale. Any loss realized on such a wash sale is not deductible.[92] In essence, a taxpayer who has a wash sale has not had a *change* in economic position—thus the transaction resulting in a loss is ignored for tax purposes. The loss is, however, taken into consideration in determining the adjusted basis in the new shares.[93]

> **Example 46.** C, a calendar year taxpayer, owns 400 shares of X Corporation stock (adjusted basis of $9,000), all of which he sells for $5,000 on December 28, 2009. On January 7, 2010. C purchases another 400 shares of X Corporation stock for $5,500. C's realized loss of $4,000 in 2009 will not be deductible because it resulted from a wash sale. Instead, his basis in the 400 shares purchased in 2010 is increased to $9,500 ($5,500 purchase price + $4,000 disallowed loss).

The *numbers* of shares purchased and sold are not always the same. When the number of shares reacquired is less than the number sold, the deduction for losses is disallowed only for the number of shares purchased.[94]

> **Example 47.** Assume the same facts as in *Example 46*, except that C purchased only 300 shares of X Corporation stock for $4,125. Because C replaced only 300 of the shares previously sold at a loss, only 75% (300 ÷ 400) of the $4,000 realized loss is disallowed. Consequently, C will report a $1,000 loss ($4,000 × 25%) in 2009 and will have a basis of $7,125 ($4,125 purchase price + $3,000 disallowed loss) in the 300 shares purchased.

When the number of shares repurchased is greater than the number of shares sold, none of the loss is deductible and the basis in a number of shares equivalent to the number of shares sold is affected by the disallowed loss.[95]

Any loss also will be disallowed if the "substantially equivalent" stock or securities are acquired by certain related parties. For example, the U.S. Supreme Court held that the wash sale provisions apply if replacement stock is acquired by a taxpayer's spouse *and* they file a joint return for the tax year of the loss.[96]

SALES BETWEEN RELATED PARTIES

The Code places numerous limitations on gain or loss recognition from transactions between certain related parties. The purpose of such restrictions is to prevent related taxpayers from entering into various property transactions solely for the tax reduction possibilities. For example, a father could sell land to his daughter at a loss, deduct the loss, and the property would still remain within the family unit. Similarly, a taxpayer could sell depreciable property to her spouse and report a long-term capital gain on their joint return. For many years thereafter, she and her husband could claim ordinary deductions for depreciation on this higher basis. To control such potentially abusive situations, Congress enacted Code §§ 267 and 1239.

---

[92] § 1091(a).

[93] § 1091(d).

[94] Reg. § 1.1091-1(c).

[95] Reg. § 1.1091-1(d).

[96] *Helvering v. Taft*, 40-2 USTC ¶9888, 24 AFTR 1976, 311 U.S. 195 (USSC, 1940).

Section 267 disallows deductions for any losses that result from the sale or exchange of property between related parties.[97] Such losses may, however, be used by the related purchaser to offset any gain realized from a subsequent disposition of the property.[98] For purposes of § 267, related parties include the following:[99]

1. Members of an individual's family—specifically, brothers and sisters (including by half blood), spouses, ancestors (i.e., parents and grandparents), and lineal descendants (i.e., children and grandchildren)

2. A corporation owned more than 50 percent in value by the taxpayer (directly or indirectly)

3. Two corporations owned more than 50 percent in value by the taxpayer (directly or indirectly) if either corporation is a personal holding company or a foreign personal holding company in the tax year of the transaction

4. Various partnership, S corporation, grantor, fiduciary, and trust relationships with regular corporations and individual taxpayers

Example 48. M sells stock (adjusted basis of $10,000) to her daughter, D, for its fair market value of $8,000. D sells the stock two years later for $11,000. M's $2,000 loss is disallowed as a deduction. However, D's realized gain of $3,000 ($11,000 sales price − $8,000 cost basis) is reduced by the $2,000 previously disallowed loss, and she will report only $1,000 of gain.

Note the similarity between the results in *Example 48* and the situation that would result if D had received the stock as a gift from M. First, D's basis for gain would be $10,000 (M's basis) if the stock had been received as a gift; its subsequent sale for $11,000 would have resulted in the same $1,000 recognized (reported) gain. Although the disallowance of a loss deduction might discourage many related-party transactions, some taxpayers prefer to sell rather than give property to a related party in order to avoid paying state or Federal gift taxes.

Section 1239 provides that any gain realized from the sale of depreciable property between specified related parties will be taxed as ordinary income.[100] In effect, this statute precludes the possibility that any gain on the sale might be taxed as a long-term capital gain since the sale results in a higher basis in the depreciable property to a related party. Furthermore, recall that such related-party sales of depreciable property are not eligible for installment sale treatment.[101] Transactions subject to § 1239 treatment are discussed in Chapter 19 (Corporate Taxation) and Chapter 22 (Partnership Taxation).

TAX PLANNING CONSIDERATIONS

GIFT VERSUS BEQUEST

In devising a plan for transferring wealth from one family member to another, several considerations related to the income tax, the transfer taxes, and the wishes of the parties involved must be evaluated. If there is a desire to transfer properties, there

---

[97]   § 267(a)(1).

[98]   § 267(d).

[99]   See §§ 267(b) and (c).

[100]   § 1239(a).

[101]   § 453(g).

are relative advantages and disadvantages to lifetime transfers as opposed to testamentary transfers (transfers by will). Some of the specific factors that should be considered are as follows:

1. The income tax rate of each individual (decedent and heirs) relative to the estate and gift tax rates.

2. Whether the property is highly appreciated. If so, a testamentary transfer may be preferred since the property's basis to the heirs or the estate will be its fair market value at date of death or alternate valuation date. If the property is gifted, its basis will be the donor's basis increased by a fraction of any gift taxes paid. If the property has declined in value, only the *original owner* (donor) can benefit from any tax loss by disposing of the property to an unrelated party, due to the basis for determination of loss under § 1015(a).

3. Whether the property is expected to appreciate rapidly in the foreseeable future. If so, a current gift might be considered because the amount subject to gift taxes would be the current market value. If the property were held until death, the higher fair market value at that time would be used in calculating estate taxes. This action is, of course, speculative in nature.

4. Whether the transferee is likely to hold the property for a long period of time. If so, the basis considerations are not as important as they would be if the property were to be sold immediately upon its receipt.

5. Whether the property is income-producing property. If the property produces income, and the owner (donor) is in a high income tax bracket, a lifetime transfer could result in the profits being taxed at a lower tax rate to another family member. If the donee is in a significantly lower income tax bracket, substantial income tax savings can be accomplished.

These factors, as well as the health of the parties involved and other personal considerations, must all be considered. It is possible that the personal factors will outweigh the tax factors, or that significant amounts of taxes cannot be saved.

CHARITABLE TRANSFERS INVOLVING PROPERTY OTHER THAN CASH

Taxpayers who are considering making major charitable transfers and who have property other than cash that they would consider transferring must consider both the effects of any gain or loss if property is sold and the effects of any allowable charitable deduction. If a property has declined in value, its owner may benefit from selling the property and deducting the loss and later contributing the cash proceeds to the charity.

Planning can be even more important when the property is appreciated, since in certain instances a charitable deduction is allowed equal to the fair market value of the property. This is true when the property is long-term capital gain property that is used in the exempt function of the charity, is intangible, or is real estate (see Chapter 11). In such a case, the taxpayer will avoid paying tax on the property's unrealized appreciation and still receive full benefit from the charitable deduction.

CHANGES IN THE USE OF PROPERTY

A taxpayer who converts business property to personal use when its value is less than its adjusted basis should consider selling the asset in order to trigger a deduction for the loss. Also, a taxpayer who buys property that he or she intends to use in a business should think carefully before using the asset for personal purposes. For example, a taxpayer who purchases a new auto and drives it for personal purposes for two years before converting

it to business use must use the fair value upon conversion—if less than adjusted basis—in determining both depreciation and any loss on disposition.

SALES TO RELATED PARTIES

Care must be exercised to avoid the undesirable effects of transactions between related parties. If a loss on the sale of property to a related party is disallowed, the tax benefit of a loss deduction is permanently lost unless the value of the property subsequently increases. The only way to generate a tax deduction for the loss is for the original owner to sell the property to an unrelated party. Also, characterizing gain on the sale of depreciable property as ordinary income under § 1239 should normally be avoided.

USE OF INSTALLMENT SALES

Installment sale treatment provides an excellent opportunity for deferring the tax on gain (other than depreciation recapture) when a taxpayer is willing to accept an installment obligation in exchange for property. Actually, installment reporting may provide such attractive tax deferral and tax savings possibilities that the taxpayer is induced to accept an installment obligation, even though he or she would not do so otherwise. In short, this is a tax variable that must be considered by a prudent taxpayer in planning sales of property.

A taxpayer may benefit in at least two ways from the installment method. First, benefits accrue from the deferral of the tax. The time value of money works to the taxpayer's benefit, assuming the sales contract provides for a fair rate of interest. The second benefit from installment reporting is the spreading of the gain over more than one tax year. If the gain on a sale is unusual and moves the taxpayer into a higher tax bracket, spreading the gain over several years tends to allow the overall gain to be taxed in lower tax brackets.

It is important to remember, however, that taxpayers may face several limitations on certain installment sales. First, if a reasonable interest rate is not provided in the deferred payment sale, the seller will be required to impute interest at the appropriate Federal rate. Second, a taxpayer unaware of the rules relating to related-party sales may find that he or she is required to report all the gain on such a sale long before the actual collection of cash from the installment obligations. Third, taxpayers with installment obligations must be informed of the rules requiring immediate gain recognition on certain dispositions of such obligations. These rules include treating borrowed funds as collections on the installment notes if such notes are used as collateral for a loan. Finally, taxpayers with significant amounts of installment obligations outstanding at the end of a particular tax year (i.e., in excess of $5 million) may find that the required interest payment on the deferred income taxes is greater than the interest currently being collected.

PROBLEM MATERIALS

DISCUSSION QUESTIONS

14-1 *Realization versus Recognition.* In a few sentences, distinguish realization from recognition.

14-2 *Return-of-Capital Principle.* What is the return-of-capital principle?

14-3   *Computing Amount Realized.* Reproduce the formula for computing the amount realized in a sale or exchange.

14-4   *Impact of Liabilities.* What impact do liabilities assumed by the buyer or liabilities encumbering property transferred have on the amount realized? How are they treated if both parties to the transaction incur new liabilities?

14-5   *Cost Basis.* How does one determine cost basis for property acquired? How is this basis affected if property other than money is transferred in exchange for the new property?

14-6   *Gift Basis.* Reproduce the formula for the general rule for determining basis of property acquired by gift.

14-7   *Gift Basis Exception.* When does the general rule for determining basis of property acquired by gift *(Question 14-6)* not apply?

14-8   *Basis of Inherited Property.* The basis of property acquired from a decedent is generally fair market value at date of death. What are the two exceptions to this rule (do not include property subject to special-use valuation)?

14-9   *Basis Adjustments.* List the three broad categories of adjustments to basis.

14-10   *Transfers Pursuant to Divorce.* In general, do transfers of property in a divorce action result in the realization of gain or loss? Under what circumstances might gain recognition be required?

14-11   *Part-Sale/Part-Gift.* When does a bargain sale to a donee (part-gift) result in gain to the donor? Does the assumption of the donor's liabilities by the donee have any impact? Explain.

14-12   *Bargain Sales.* How is a bargain sale of property to a charitable organization treated for tax purposes?

14-13   *Allocating Sales Price.* Allocations are generally necessary when a sole proprietorship is sold as a unit. What method is normally used for such allocation? What impact does the sales agreement have if it allocates the price to the individual assets?

14-14   *Installment Sales Method—General Rules.* What is the purpose of the installment sale method of reporting gains? Is it an elective provision? How does one elect out of the installment sale method? What sales do not qualify for installment sale treatment?

14-15   *Installment Sales Method—Key Terms.* Explain how each of the following factors related to an installment sale is determined.
    a.   Gross profit on deferred payment sale
    b.   Total contract price
    c.   Gross profit percentage
    d.   Payments received in the year of sale
    e.   Gain to be reported in the year of sale

14-16   *Imputed Interest Rules.* Under what circumstances must a taxpayer impute interest income from an installment sale? How is the applicable Federal rate (AFR) determined?

14-17   *Related-Party Installment Sales.* Under what circumstances will a taxpayer be faced with the related-party installment sale rules? Explain how a resale of the property by the related

party purchaser before the seller has collected the balance of the installment obligation affects the seller.

14-18 *Dispositions of Installment Obligations.* Your neighbor has $30,000 of installment obligations from a recent sale of land held for investment. He asks you for advice concerning his planned gift of these obligations to his children to be used for their future college expenses. An examination of Form 6252 attached to his most recent tax return reveals a gross profit percentage of 60 percent and a reasonable market rate of interest related to these installment obligations. What tax advice would you give regarding this plan?

14-19 *Wash Sale.* What is a wash sale? How is a wash sale treated for tax purposes?

14-20 *Timing of Recognition.* Under what circumstances is a realized gain actually recognized? What event generally controls the timing of gain recognition?

PROBLEMS

14-21 *Sale Involving Liabilities.* C sold a cottage in which his basis was $32,000, for cash of $12,000 and a note from the buyer worth $28,000. The buyer assumed an existing note of $30,000 secured by an interest in the property.
   a. What is C's amount realized in this sale?
   b. What is C's gain or loss realized on this sale?

14-22 *Exchange Involving Liabilities.* D exchanged a mountain cabin for a leisure yacht and $30,000 cash. The yacht was worth $25,000 and was subject to liabilities of $10,000, which were assumed by D. The cabin was subject to liabilities of $32,000, which were assumed by the other party.
   a. How much is D's amount realized?
   b. Assuming D's basis in the cabin was $42,000, what is his gain or loss realized?

14-23 *Identification of Stock Sold.* T purchased the following lots of stock in Z Corporation:

50 shares	1/12/00	Cost $1,200
100 shares	2/28/05	Cost $3,000
75 shares	10/16/06	Cost $2,500

T sold 75 shares on January 16, 2009 for $2,800. His only instruction to his broker, who actually held the shares for T, was to sell 75 shares.
   a. How much gain or loss does T recognize on this sale?
   b. How could this result be altered?

14-24 *Sale of Property Acquired by Gift.* J received 1,000 shares of Exxon stock as a gift from her grandmother in 2005, when the stock was worth $50,000. The stock had a basis to the grandmother of $10,000, and gift taxes of $16,000 were paid on the $40,000 taxable value of the gift.
   a. How much gain does J recognize when she sells the stock for $80,000 (net of commissions) during the current year?
   b. What would be your answer if the sale price were $35,000 (net of commissions)?
   c. What would be your answer if the sale price were $19,000 (net of commissions)?

14-25 *Sale of Property Acquired by Gift.* In 2006, F gave his son, S, 100 shares of IBM stock, which at that time were worth $30,000. F paid a gift tax on the transfer of $5,000. Assuming F had purchased the stock in 2002 for $40,000, what are the tax consequences to S if he sells the stock for the following amounts?
   a. $25,000
   b. $37,000
   c. $45,000

14-26 *Sale of Inherited Property.* D inherited two acres of commercial real estate from her grandmother, who had a basis in the property of $52,000, when it had a fair market value of $75,000. For estate tax purposes, the estate was valued as of the date of death, and estate and inheritance taxes of $8,250 were paid by the estate on this parcel of real estate.
  a. How much gain or loss will be realized by D if she sells the property for $77,000?
  b. What would be your answer if the sale price were $66,000?

14-27 *Basis of Inherited Property.* H inherited a parcel of real estate from his father. The property was valued for estate tax purposes at $120,000, and the father's basis was $45,000 immediately before his death. H had given the property to his father as a gift six weeks before his death. The proper portion of the gift taxes paid by H are included in his father's basis.
  a. What is H's basis in the real estate?
  b. What would be your answer if H had given the property to his father two years before his father's death?

14-28 *Basis of Converted Property.* K converted his 2003 sedan from personal use to business use as a delivery vehicle in his pizza business. The auto had an adjusted basis to K of $4,200 and a fair market value on the date of the conversion of $2,400. K properly deducted depreciation on the auto of $900 over two years before the auto was sold.
  a. How much is K's gain or loss if he sells the auto for $800?
  b. What would be your answer if the auto were sold for $3,500?

14-29 *Part-Sale/Part-Gift.* G sold a personal computer to his son for $2,000. The computer was worth $3,000, and G had a basis in the unit of $2,200. G has made a gift of $1,000 in this part-sale/part-gift.
  a. How much gain, if any, must G recognize on this sale?
  b. Would your answer differ if G's basis had been $1,700?

14-30 *Bargain Sale to Charity.* F sold a parcel of land to the city to be used as a location for a new art museum. The land had a market value of $70,000 and was sold for $40,000. F's adjusted basis in the property was $35,000. How much is F's charitable contribution deduction on this transfer? How much gain does F recognize on this sale?

14-31 *Installment Sale.* On July 1, 2009, G sold her summer cottage (basis $70,000) for $105,000. The sale contract provided for a payment of $30,000 at the time of sale and payment of the $75,000 balance in three equal installments due in July 2010, 2011, and 2012. Assuming a reasonable interest rate is charged on this deferred payment sale, compute each of the following:
  a. Gross profit on the sale
  b. Total contract price
  c. Gross profit percentage
  d. Gain to be reported (excluding interest) in 2009
  e. Gain to be reported (excluding interest) in 2010
  f. Gain to be reported in 2009 if G elects not to use the installment method

14-32 *Imputed Interest on Installment Sale.* On January 1, 2009, S sold a 100-acre tract of land for $200,000 cash and an $800,000 non-interest-bearing note due on January 1, 2012. On the date of sale, the land had a basis of $400,000. Assuming the applicable Federal rate is ten percent compounded semiannually, calculate the following:
  a. Gain, excluding interest, to be reported in 2009
  b. The imputed interest to be reported by S for 2009
  c. Gain, excluding interest, to be reported in 2012

14-33 *Wash Sale.* R purchased 500 shares of Y Corporation common stock for $12,500 on August 31, 2008. She sold 200 shares of this stock for $3,000 on December 21, 2009. On January 7, 2010, R purchased an additional 100 shares of Y Corporation common stock for $1,600.

    a. What is R's realized loss for 2009?

    b. How much of the loss realized can R report in 2009?

    c. What is R's adjusted basis in the 100 shares purchased on January 7, 2010?

14-34 *Related-Party Sale.* J sold 2,000 shares of T Corporation stock, in which he had an adjusted basis of $3,000, to his brother, F, for $1,200.

    a. How much of the realized loss is recognized (reported) by J?

    b. How much gain or loss to F if he subsequently sells the stock for $1,000? For $2,000?

14-35 *Property Settlements.* H was divorced from W this year. H was required to transfer stock, which was his separate property, to W in satisfaction of his obligation for spousal support. The stock was worth $5,700 and had an adjusted basis to H of $2,900.

    a. How much gain, if any, does H recognize on the transfer?

    b. How much gain or loss does W recognize? What is her basis in the property received?

14-36 *Property Tax Allocation.* J purchased a rental property during the current year for $45,000 cash. He was required to pay all of the property taxes for the year of sale, and under the law of the state $47 is allocable to the period before J purchased the property (see Chapter 11).

    a. How much is J's property tax deduction if the total payment made during the tax year of acquisition is $700?

    b. What is J's adjusted basis in the property?

14-37 *Sales of Inherited Properties.* Each of the following involves property acquired from a decedent. None of the properties include income in respect of a decedent. Determine the gain or loss for each.

Case	Decedent's Basis	Death Taxes Paid	Fair Market Value(*)	Sales Price
A	$3,000	$600	$4,000	$6,000
B	6,000	600	4,000	5,000
C	6,000	400	4,000	3,000

* Date of decedent's death.

14-38 *Nontaxable Dividends.* M owned 300 shares of X Corporation common stock, in which her basis was $6,000 on January 1, 2009. With respect to her stock, during 2009 M collected dividends of $600 and tax-free distributions of $400. What is M's basis in the stock as of December 31, 2009?

RESEARCH PROBLEMS

14-39   *Gain Realized from Transferred Debt.* H owns a small office building and commercial complex, which he purchased for $175,000 in 2003. H invested $20,000 and signed a nonrecourse note secured by an interest in the property for the difference. The note provided for 9 percent interest, compounded annually and payable quarterly.

After six years, H decided his property was not as good an investment as he had originally thought. He found a buyer who offered him $1,000 cash for the property, subject to the existing liabilities. H eventually accepted the offer and sold the property. During the six years he owned the property, H made timely interest payments and no payments of principal. He was allowed depreciation deductions of $34,000, using the straight-line method of depreciation and a 39-year recovery period.

Required:

1.   How much is H's gain or loss realized on this sale?
2.   Would your answer differ if H's building was only worth $150,000 and instead of selling the building he had voluntarily transferred it to the obligee on the note?

Partial list of research aids:

> Reg. § 1.1001-2.
> *Crane v. Comm.*, 47-1 USTC ¶9217, 35 AFTR 776, 331 U.S. 1 (USSC, 1947).
> *Tufts v. Comm.*, 83-1 USTC ¶9328, 51 AFTR2d 1983-1132, 461 U.S. 300 (USSC, 1983).
> *Millar v. Comm.*, 78-2 USTC ¶9514, 42 AFTR2d 78-4276, 577 F.2d 212 (CA-3, 1978).

14-40   *Bargain Sale to Charity.* K sold a mountain cabin for $55,000 to State University (her alma mater) for use in an annual fund-raising auction. The cabin was worth $85,000. K had purchased the cabin five years earlier as an investment for $40,000, and no depreciation has been allowed.

Required:

1.   What is K's charitable contribution deduction and her gain or loss realized on this bargain sale?
2.   Would your answers differ if the property were a painting instead of a mountain cabin?

Research aids:

> § 170(e)(1).
> § 1011(b).
> Reg. §§ 1.170A-4(a)(2) and (c)(2).
> Reg. § 1.1011-2.

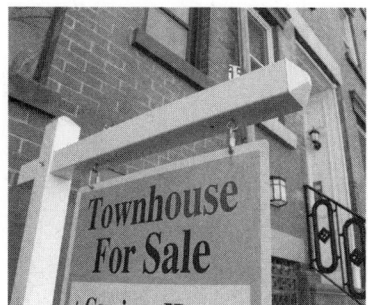

CHAPTER FIFTEEN

NONTAXABLE EXCHANGES

LEARNING OBJECTIVES

Upon completion of this chapter you will be able to:

▸ Understand the rationale for deferral of gains and losses on certain property transactions

▸ Explain how gain or loss deferral is accomplished through adjustment to basis of the replacement property

▸ Apply the nonrecognition rules to the following transactions:

  ▸ Sale of a taxpayer's principal residence

▸ Involuntary conversion of property

▸ Like-kind exchange of business or investment property

▸ Identify other common nontaxable transactions

▸ Recognize tax planning opportunities related to the more common types of gain-deferral transactions available to individual taxpayers

CHAPTER OUTLINE

INTRODUCTION

"If I could show you a perfectly legal way to pyramid your wealth to $1 million without paying tax, would you be interested?" Although this sounds like it came straight out of the con artist's guide to tax scams, its source is far more reputable.[1] More important, the assertion is entirely true. If a taxpayer is able to make the right investments—obviously a big if—the Internal Revenue Code is willing to lend a helping hand. The key to this wonderland without taxes can be found in the provisions concerning nontaxable exchanges, the subject of this chapter.

By now, the basic recipe for determining the tax treatment of any sale or exchange is fairly familiar. Whenever a taxpayer disposes of property, three questions must be addressed: (1) what is the gain or loss *realized*, (2) how much of this realized gain or loss is *recognized*, and (3) what is its character. This chapter focuses on the second of these questions, examining a handful of property transactions—such as the sale of a residence or a like-kind exchange—where all or at least a portion of the gain or loss realized is not recognized.

As a general rule, any gain or loss realized on a sale or other disposition of property must be recognized unless an exception is specifically provided. For the most part, this means taxpayers must include all of their realized gains and losses in determining their taxable income. However, there are a number of transactions that the Code has singled out for *nonrecognition*. In many cases, the property sold or exchanged is replaced with new property. For example, a taxpayer might trade in an old business car for a new one. When this occurs, any gain or loss realized is usually not taxed—at least immediately—on

---

[1] Robert J. Bruss, "Real Estate Exchange Provides a Way to Build Net Worth," *The Palm Beach Post*, February 19, 1989, p 57H.

the theory that the taxpayer's economic situation has not changed sufficiently to warrant taxation. Nonrecognition is deemed appropriate since the taxpayer has not liquidated her investment to cash but has continued it, albeit in another form. In substance, the taxpayer's investment has remained intact. For these situations, Congress is willing to allow a taxpayer to postpone the tax (or perhaps defer the deduction for a loss) until such time when the taxpayer does in fact convert the asset to cash and has the wherewithal to pay the tax.

When the recognition of a gain or loss is deferred, it is normally recognized later, when the replacement property from the deferred transaction is sold in a taxable transaction. This deferral is usually achieved by building the gain or loss not recognized into the basis of the replacement property.

> **Example 1.** D exchanged a vacant lot in San Jose that had been held for investment for unimproved farmland near Fresno. The city lot had cost $35,000 fifteen years earlier and had not been improved. Both the city lot and the rural property were worth $120,000. D recognizes no gain on the exchange and his basis in the farmland is $35,000.[2] Of course, if D later sells the farm for $130,000, his recognizable gain will be $95,000, the gain on the farm of $10,000 plus the gain deferred from the city lot of $85,000.

It is important to observe that nonrecognition can take one of two forms: permanent exclusion or temporary deferral. The world of permanent exclusions, first introduced in Chapter 6, is relatively small. It includes such items as interest paid on state and local government bonds, insurance proceeds paid on account of death, gifts, inheritances, scholarships, child support, and a number of fringe benefits. On the other side of the ledger, losses and expenses that are personal in nature (other than casualty losses) are generally disallowed. Note that if nonrecognition is permanent, the gain or loss never affects taxable income.

One instance in which the permanent exclusion of gain is allowed in property transactions is upon the sale of one's principal residence. This benefit, which was widely expanded by the *Taxpayer Relief Act of 1997*, allows a taxpayer who has owned and used his or her residence for two years to simply avoid tax on part or all of any gain.

> **Example 2.** F, an elderly widow, sold her personal residence of 30 years for $92,000 (basis $21,000) and moved into a rented unit in a retirement community. Under Code § 121, F is allowed to exclude her gain of $71,000 from gross income. Since the gain is excluded, F will never be required to pay tax on the gain from that residence.[3]

TYPES OF NONTAXABLE EXCHANGES

There are several types of nontaxable exchanges allowed under the Internal Revenue Code. Three are discussed in detail in this chapter. The sale of a personal residence is covered initially. Separate discussions of the deferral of gain on involuntary conversions and the deferral of gain or loss on like-kind exchanges follow. Then several other types of nontaxable transactions are discussed briefly.

---

[2] See discussion of § 1031 following.

[3] See discussion of § 121 following.

SALE OF A PERSONAL RESIDENCE

While one's home may be one's castle, in the United States it is also a tax shelter. The tax law contains several provisions that encourage home ownership. Two of these, the deductions for interest and property taxes, were discussed in Chapter 11. A third, considered in detail below, concerns the sale of a residence. The effect of these provisions, whether intended or not, is to provide what is clearly a tax bonanza. If an individual sells a residence, any gain may be totally excluded from income up to $250,000 ($500,000 for certain married persons filing jointly) if the taxpayer qualifies under § 121. Gain in excess of the limit will generally be recognized.

> **Example 3.** T sold his principal residence for $400,000 on July 22, 2009. He has lived in the home since 1997. His basis in the property was $225,000 and his realized gain on the sale is $175,000 ($400,000 − $225,000). T may exclude all of the $175,000 in gain from his taxable income.

COMPUTATION OF BASIS OF RESIDENCE AND GAIN OR LOSS REALIZED

The calculation of the gain recognized on the sale of the house begins in the normal fashion. It starts with the sales price, which is then reduced by selling expenses to determine the amount realized. The sales price is usually easy to determine. Selling expenses are generally those costs paid to bring about the sale of the property. Although they are not directly deductible, they do reduce the potential gain. A few of the more common selling expenses incurred when selling a home are:

Realtor's commission	Legal fees
Advertising	Title fees (abstracts, certificate, opinion)
Surveys	Transfer taxes
Buyer's points paid by the seller	Mortgage title insurance
Inspection fees (termites, radon, etc.)	Escrow fees

Gain or Loss Realized. The amount of the gain or loss realized is merely the difference between the amount realized and the adjusted basis. In computing the basis of the home, improvements the owner has made should be included. These include anything that adds value to the house and prolongs its useful life. Some of these are:

Additions (rooms, porch, deck)	Flooring (carpeting, tile, vinyl)	Driveway, walks
Roof, siding, insulation	Fences	Curtains
Appliances, attic fan, grill	Air conditioning, furnaces,	Well
Landscaping, sprinkling system	water heaters	Mailbox, house numbers
Garage	Alarm system	Septic system
Basement improvement	Basketball goal post	Sewer assessment
Shed	Solar or geothermal heating	Smoke detector

Gain or Loss Recognized. The next concern, and no doubt the most important, is the determination of the amount of the gain or loss to be recognized. Losses are not subject to any special provision. Accordingly, since a personal residence is not held for either trade or business or investment purposes, any recognized loss is not deductible.[4] While losses are not deductible, gains receive far more favorable treatment. As explained below, if certain requirements are met, most homeowners will be able to exclude all or at least part of their gain.

---

[4]   § 165(c).

SECTION 121 EXCLUSION OF GAIN

On the sale of a principal residence, § 121 generally allows a taxpayer to exclude any gain realized up to a maximum of $250,000 ($500,000 for married taxpayers). Any realized gain in excess of this threshold is taxable as capital gain. This relief provision applies to taxpayers of all ages and as frequently as every two years. To obtain this special treatment, taxpayers must meet several requirements as discussed below.

Principal Residence. The exclusion applies only to the sale of the taxpayer's *principal* residence. Most taxpayers have one residence, and if they move, they simply change their principal residence. However, it is sometimes difficult to determine which residence is the *principal residence* for taxpayers with multiple residences. This is a facts and circumstances determination. Some of the factors to be considered are the amount of time each residence is used, the taxpayer's place of employment, where other family members live, the addresses used (for things like tax returns, driver's licenses, car and voter registration, bills and correspondence), and the location of banks, religious organizations and recreational clubs.[5]

The exclusion only applies if the property is a *residence.* A residence not only includes a conventional home but also a condominium, a cooperative apartment, a mobile home, and a fully equipped recreational vehicle (e.g., plumbing, kitchen, sleeping facilities) notwithstanding that it is a means of transportation.[6] The residence also includes the land on which the residence sits and any gain attributable to the land is eligible for exclusion.[7] Land adjacent to the home qualifies if it is regularly used by the owner as part of the residential property, and it is sold along with the home or within two years before or after the sale of the home.[8]

It is not that uncommon for the seller of a home to also sell property that is technically not part of the residence such as furniture, lawn equipment, pool table, hot tub, or similar property. Unless such personalty is treated as a fixture under local law it is not considered part of the residence and, therefore, is not eligible for the exclusion. In most cases, however, sales of such items would result in nondeductible losses.

Ownership and Use Tests. The § 121 exclusion is applicable to the sale of a residence only if the residence was *owned* by the taxpayer and *used* as his or her principal residence for at least two of the five years preceding its sale.[9] Observe that the five year window permits taxpayers to use the exclusion even though the property is not owned or used by the taxpayer at the time of the sale. The taxpayer merely needs to meet both tests at some time during the five year period.

The ownership and use requirements are two separate tests. Normally, the period of ownership is not an issue.[10] However, whether the taxpayer *uses* the property as a *principal residence* for the requisite two years during the five-year window can be a bit more troubling. Whether this test is met depends on the fact and circumstances. In this regard, recall that an individual can only have one principal residence at any given time.

---

[5]   Reg. § 1.121-1.

[6]   See Reg. § 1.121-1(b)(1) and (e)(2), § 280A(f)(1)(A); Prop Reg § 1.280A-1(e)(7), Ex (2) and *Ronald Haberkorn* 75 T.C. 259 (1980). See also *Richard Dougherty,* T.C. Memo 1994-597, T.C. Memo ¶94597 where a 32-foot charter cruiser that berthed six was considered a home.

[7]   But see where a taxpayer who moved his house and sold the land was not entitled to the exclusion for the land. See also IRS Publication 523 (2005) p. 3.

[8]   Reg. § 1.121-1(b)(3).

[9]   § 121(a).

[10]   See Reg. § 1.121-1(c)(3) allowing the exclusion where the residence is owned by grantor trusts and disregarded entities such as a single member LLC.

Example 4. Y purchased a home in Miami 1988 and lived in it until she took a new job in Orlando on April 30, 2005. From May 1, 2005 until the Miami house was sold on May 1, 2009, it was used by Y only on occasional days off since she lived in a rented apartment in Orlando. In determining whether the exclusion is available, Y has met the ownership test because she owned it for two of the five years prior to its sale. However, she fails the use test because she did not use the house as her principal residence for two of the five years before its sale. Since she did not meet both tests, she does not qualify for the § 121 exclusion.

If, taking into account all facts and circumstances, the house, and not the apartment, had been Y's principal residence, she would have qualified. She would have to be able to demonstrate that she lived in the house, with only temporary visits to the apartment.

In applying the use test, short temporary absences, such as for vacation or other seasonal absence are counted as periods of use. For this purpose, temporary rental of the property is ignored.

Example 5. T purchased his home in South Bend in 1999. He used the house as his principal residence until January 31, 2007, when he moved to Chicago. Upon moving, T rented his house to tenants until April 18, 2009, when he sold it. T is eligible for the exclusion because he has owned and used the house as his principal residence for at least two of the five years preceding the sale.

Example 6. B owned and used her house in Houston as her principal residence from 1989 to the end of 2003. On January 4, 2004, she moved to Denver. Shortly thereafter, B's son moved into the house in March 2004 and used the residence until it sold on July 1, 2009. B may not exclude gain from the sale because she did not use the property as her principal residence for at least two years out of the five years preceding the sale. Use by the son is not counted as the mother's use.

Maximum Exclusion. The maximum amount excludable with respect to any sale or exchange is $250,000. This amount is doubled to $500,000 for most married taxpayers filing joint returns. In such cases, the ownership requirement only needs to be met by one spouse. So if either spouse meets the ownership test and both spouses meet the use test, the $500,000 exclusion applies.[11] However, if only one spouse satisfies the use test, the exclusion is allowable but limited to $250,000 (or the sum of the amount excludable by each spouse individually).

Example 7. H and W sold their jointly owned and occupied family residence on June 3, 2009, for $650,000. Their basis in the property, that they had owned for thirty years, was $125,000, so their gain was $525,000. If H and W file a joint return for their calendar year 2009, they may exclude $500,000 of the gain and must recognize a long-term capital gain of $25,000.

Example 8. Q purchased a home for use as her principal residence in 1993. On March 31, 2006, Q was transferred by her employer, so she moved away, rented an apartment and left her residence unused. When Q sells the residence at a gain of $200,000 on March 1, 2009, she may exclude the entire gain. During the five years preceding the sale—March 1, 2004 to February 28, 2009—Q *owned* the property for all five years and *used* it as her principal residence for 25 months (i.e., more than the requisite two years).

---

[11] § 121(b)(1) and (2).

Example 9. L purchased a residence for use as his principal residence for $123,000 on July 12, 2007. Presented with an attractive offer on the property, L sold the residence on February 2, 2009 for $198,000 (net of selling costs). L must report a long-term capital gain of $75,000 since L does not meet the two of five year tests.

Example 10. F purchased a new personal residence in 1989 for $40,000 and lived in it until June 30, 1998. The house was rented out until January 1, 2006, with depreciation of $8,500 being claimed. On January 2, 2006, F moved back into the house and occupied it as her principal residence until February 5, 2009, when it was sold for $280,000. Since F owned and lived in the home for at least two of the five years preceding the sale, she may exclude up to $250,000 of gain (see subsequent discussion of depreciation recapture).

FREQUENCY LIMITATION: ONE SALE EVERY TWO YEARS

The benefits of the § 121 exclusion are so great that without some prohibition taxpayers might utilize the provision in unintended ways. One could easily envision a taxpayer selling one principal residence and excluding the gain, buying and selling another residence and excluding the gain, and continuing this pattern, using the exclusion as a tax shelter. To restrict this possibility, the Code imposes a limitation on the frequency with which the exclusion may be used. The exclusion cannot be used for sales occurring within two years of its last use. In other words, the law allows the exclusion for one sale every two years. To ensure that this rule does not unfairly penalize taxpayers who may be forced to sell their homes before the two-year period has elapsed, special rules concerning sales for unforeseen circumstances exist and are discussed below.[12]

Example 11. M purchased a residence for use as her principal residence for $70,000 on January 2, 2004, and lived in it until March 15, 2006. On March 16, 2006, M rented the original residence and purchased and moved into another residence costing $85,000. Upon retiring, M sold the original residence for $90,000 on December 31, 2007, and excluded most of her gain on the sale (see subsequent discussion of depreciation recapture). Even though M would otherwise be eligible to exclude any gain on the sale of the other residence on March 16, 2008, due to this one sale every two years rule, M will not be eligible until January 1, 2010 (see subsequent discussion related to electing out of § 121).

EXCEPTIONS TO OWNERSHIP, USE AND FREQUENCY TESTS

At times, taxpayers may be forced to sell their homes due to events beyond their control. For example, an individual may be forced to take a job in another location or move because of health reasons. In these and similar situations, taxpayers may run afoul of the ownership and use requirement or the frequency limitation. Without relief, any realized gain on the sale of the house would be *fully* taxable notwithstanding the fact that there was nothing the taxpayer could do to avoid the sale. Recognizing this problem, § 121 provides some relief.[13] Taxpayers who fail the two-year ownership and use requirement or the one-sale-every-two-year rules may qualify for a *portion* of the exclusion if the sale were due to unforeseen circumstances. In many cases the reduced exclusion would be more than sufficient to offset any appreciation that occurred.

---

[12]   § 121(b)(3).

[13]   § 121(c).

Computation of the Reduced Exclusion. The portion of the exclusion allowed is the percentage of the required 24 months for which the taxpayer satisfies the ownership and use test or if lower the number of months used since the last sale.[14]

$$\text{Exclusion} \atop (\$250,000 \text{ or } \$500,000) \quad \times \quad \frac{\text{Lesser of time owned and used or time since last sale}}{24 \text{ months}} \quad = \quad \text{Reduced} \atop \text{Exclusion}$$

Example 12. H and W have one son, S, who was recently diagnosed to have a rare disease. After living in their home only six months, the couple sold their home in Kansas City and moved to Memphis to obtain special treatment only available at St. Jude's Children's Research Hospital. H and W do not meet the ownership and use test since they did not own and use the home as their principal residence for two of the five years prior to the sale. However, because the sale is due to unforeseen circumstances, they qualify for a reduced exclusion of $125,000 [(6/24 = 25%) × $500,000].

This rule is often misconstrued. Taxpayers are *not* entitled to a portion of the exclusion just because they meet the ownership and use test for a few months. For example, if a taxpayer owns and uses the home for only 8 of the 24 months required, he or she is *not* automatically entitled to one-third of the exclusion. The reduced exclusion is granted only if the sale is due to unforeseen circumstances. If a taxpayer simply decides to sell before meeting the tests (e.g., because of market conditions) and without cause, the entire gain is taxable.

Unforeseen Circumstances. The Code provides that the reduced exclusion is available only if due to:[15]

- Change in place of employment
- Health concerns
- Unforeseen circumstances

Change in place of employment. Under a safe harbor provided by the Regulations, the reduced exclusion is available due to a change in employment if the new place of business is at least 50 miles farther from the old residence than was the old job.[16] This is the same test that must be met to deduct moving expenses (the taxpayer's new commute without the move would exceed the old commute by more than 50 miles). If the taxpayer was not employed and moves to obtain employment, the distance between the new job and the residence sold must be at least 50 miles.

The tests regarding employment can be met by the:

- Taxpayer
- Taxpayer's spouse
- Member of the taxpayer's household
- Co-owner of the residence

Health Reasons. A reduced exclusion is also allowed for sales due to health reasons (i.e., the sale enables the taxpayer "to obtain, provide, or facilitate the diagnosis, cure mitigation, or treatment of diseases, illness or injury").[17] If a physician recommends a change of location for health reasons, the test should be met. In contrast, sales that are merely beneficial to the general health or well-being of an individual do not qualify.

---

[14] § 121(c)(1).

[15] § 121(c)(2).

[16] Reg. § 1.121-3(c)(2).

[17] Reg. § 1.121-3(d).

Unforeseen Circumstances. If an event occurs that could not reasonably have been anticipated *before* purchasing the residence, the reduced exclusion can be used. According to the Regulations, unforeseen circumstances include:[18]

- Involuntary conversion of the residence
- Natural or man-made disasters
- Acts of war or terrorism resulting in a casualty to the residence
- Death
- Unemployment so as to qualify for unemployment compensation
- Change in employment or self-employment status that results in the taxpayer's inability to pay housing costs and reasonable basic living expenses for the taxpayer's household
- Divorce
- Multiple births resulting from the same pregnancy

If a safe harbor is not met, the reduced exclusion may still be available.[19] The Regulations identify a number of other factors to be considered.

> **Example 13.** F purchased a personal residence on March 15, 2008 for $125,000. F must have been living right—he was transferred by his employer to his favorite city, received a big raise, and sold his house in two weeks time for $200,000 (on September 15, 2009). Even though F did not meet the two of five years test, he may exclude his entire $75,000 gain. Because the sale was related to a change of place of employment, F can exclude up to $187,500 [$250,000 × (18 months/24 months)].

EXHIBIT 15-1
Section 121 Exclusion Basics

Taxpayer Qualifies If

- The residence was *owned* and *used as a principal residence* for two of the five years preceding the sale
    and
- No gain was excluded under § 121 in a qualifying sale made within the two years preceding the sale

Maximum Amount Excluded

- Generally $250,000
- $500,000 for married taxpayers filing jointly if either spouse meets the ownership test and both spouses meet the use test
- A fraction of these amounts is allowed if the sale is related to a change in the taxpayer's work location, health, or other qualifying unforeseen circumstances

---

[18]   Reg. § 1.121-3(e).

[19]   In PLR 200403049, the IRS found that hostilities between the taxpayers and their neighbors concerning a household member released from rehabilitation qualified as unforeseen circumstances for purposes of § 121.

Effects of Marriage. In applying the two of five year test, a widow or widower (who has not remarried) selling a residence is treated as having owned and occupied a residence for the period of time it was owned and occupied by his or her deceased spouse.[20]

> **Example 14.** R married S on November 27, 2007, and moved into a home that had been owned and occupied by S since 1997. S died on March 15, 2008, leaving the residence to R. Since R is deemed to have owned and lived in the residence since 1997, she qualifies for the $250,000 exclusion when the residence is sold on February 12, 2009.

Homes owned by one spouse before marriage or held as separate property during a marriage could also present problems in applying the two of five year rule. To prevent inequities, if a property is transferred to a spouse or former spouse in a transaction that is tax-free under § 1041 (e.g., in a divorce), the transferee is deemed to have owned the residence for the period of time it was owned by the transferor.

> **Example 15.** D lived in a residence owned as separate property by his spouse, E, for the duration of their four-year marriage. Upon their divorce, D received the residence. Fifteen months after the divorce, D married G and sold the residence (on December 24, 2009), realizing a gain of $280,000. D lived in the residence four years and is deemed to have owned the residence all of the five years preceding the sale. He may, therefore, exclude gain of $250,000 and recognize long-term capital gain of $30,000. D and G cannot exclude $500,000 since G does not meet the residential use test with respect to the residence.

When a spouse dies, the exclusion normally would be limited to that for single taxpayers, $250,000. However, the law provides relief in these situations. A surviving spouse (who has not remarried) qualifies for the $500,000 exclusion if the following conditions are satisfied:

1. All the requirements for the larger exclusion were met at the time of death (i.e., at least one spouse meets the two year ownership test and both spouses meet the two year use test) and

2. The sale occurs within two years of the date of death.

Incapacitated Taxpayers. A taxpayer who purchases a residence and is soon forced to move to a rest home or similar facility may never be able to meet the time requirement for the § 121 exclusion. Fortunately, if a person in this situation lives in the residence for at least one year, he or she will be treated as having lived in that residence during any period of time that he or she has lived in a licensed facility for incapacitated individuals.[21] Thus, anyone who purchases a home, lives in it one year, and spends at least a year in a rest home while still owning the home will meet all the tests for § 121.

Involuntary Conversions. For purposes of § 121, an involuntary conversion of a qualifying residence is treated as the sale of that residence.[22] Thus, a person who meets the ownership and use tests can exclude at least a portion of any gain from the destruction, theft, or condemnation of his or her residence. Involuntary conversions are discussed in detail later in this chapter.

Depreciation Recapture. In some situations, a residence qualifying for the Section 121 exclusion may have been used as a rental property or business property (e.g., the taxpayer

---

[20] § 121(e)(1) and (2).

[21] § 121(d)(9).

[22] § 121(d)(5)(A).

had a home office). In such case, the taxpayer may have depreciated the property. To be able to depreciate a property, resulting in a basis reduction, and subsequently exclude any gain is to good to be true. Realizing this, Congress requires that the gain be recognized to the extent of any depreciation allowed after May 6, 1997.[23]

> **Example 16.** P purchased a home for use as a residence in 1992 for $60,000 and made improvements costing $18,000 in 2005. On June 30, 2008, P retired, moved out and converted the house to rental property. Between that date and the day the property was sold for $200,000, September 30, 2009, P claimed depreciation of $3,600, making the basis in the property $74,400 [$60,000 + $18,000 − $3,600]. P's realized gain is $125,600 ($200,000 − $74,400). P must recognize $3,600 of the gain and may exclude the remaining $122,000 under § 121.

> **Example 17.** Assume the same facts as in the prior example, except the sales price is $77,000. P's gain is $2,600 ($77,000 − $74,400). Since the gain realized is less than the depreciation claimed after May 6, 1997, none of the gain may be excluded under § 121. P must, therefore, recognize a $2,600 gain (i.e., the lesser of the gain realized or the depreciation claimed).

When only a portion of a dwelling was used for business purposes, including use as an office in the home, gain is recognized only to the extent of the depreciation recapture that is required.[24] Any additional gain qualifies for the exclusion.

> **Example 18.** B purchased a residence for use as his principal residence for $125,000 in 1991. After the children moved out, he converted a bedroom (ten percent of the residence) to a business office. Depreciation of $1,350 was claimed over three years before the residence was sold during the current year for $375,000. The total gain realized is $251,350 [$375,000 − ($125,000 − $1,350)]. One way to look at the sale would be to treat the sale as that of two separate properties.

	Business 10%	Personal 90%
Sales price	$ 37,500	$ 337,500
Adjusted basis	(11,150)*	(112,500)
Gain	$ 26,350	$ 225,000

> * $125,000 × 10% − $1,350

> Fortunately, the IRS chose not to require this two separate sales approach, and B is required to recognize gain of only $1,350. The remaining gain of $250,000 ($251,350 − $1,350) qualifies for exclusion since B owned and occupied the residence for the required period.

Rental and Other Nonqualified Use. Before 2009, individuals who owned rental property could convert it to a personal residence in order to exclude all or a portion of their gain on a subsequent sale.

> **Example 19.** J, a resident of Illinois, purchased a vacation home in Florida in 1998 for $120,000. After many years of renting it out, he moved into the home on December 19, 2005 and made it his personal residence. At the time of conversion, he had deducted depreciation of $20,000 on the property. After living in the home for the

---

[23]   § 121(e)(6).

[24]   Temp. Reg. § 1.121-2.

required two years, he sold the residence on December 29, 2008 for $210,000. J realizes a gain of $110,000 [$210,000 − (120,000 − $20,000 = $100,000)]. He must recognize gain of $20,000 due to the depreciation recapture rule. However, prior to 2009, the remaining $90,000 was excluded under § 121.

To eliminate the possibility described above, § 121 was amended in 2008. Currently, any gain allocable to periods of nonqualified use after 2008 is not eligible for exclusion. The portion of the gain attributable to nonqualified use is computed as follows:

$$\frac{\text{Gain realized}}{\text{(net of depreciation)}^{25}} \times \frac{\text{Aggregate periods of nonqualified use}}{\text{Total time owned}} = \text{Taxable Gain}$$

The key factor in determining the amount of gain that could be taxed is the taxpayer's nonqualified use. Nonqualified use is generally any period during which the property is not used as the principal residence of the taxpayer or spouse (or former spouse). For this purpose, the numerator does not include nonqualified use prior to 2009. On the other hand, the denominator is the total time owned, including that before 2009. Periods during which the property is vacant or used by relatives are considered periods of nonqualified use. Note also that if the property appreciates in value after a taxpayer makes the property his or her principal residence, the gain is still potentially taxable even though the appreciation occurred while the taxpayer used the property as a personal residence.

> **Example 20.** B, single, was a long-time resident of Cincinnati. On January 1, 2009, he purchased a condominium in South Carolina for $400,000. He used the condo as rental property for two years. He claimed $20,000 of depreciation deductions, reducing his basis in the home to $380,000. On January 1, 2011, B moved to Florida and moved into the condo converting it to his principal residence. After living there for three years, on January 1, 2014 B sold the condo for $700,000 and moved out. His gain realized would be $320,000 [($700,000 − ($400,000 − $20,000 = $380,000)]. The $20,000 of gain attributable to the depreciation is included in income.[26] Of the remaining $300,000 gain (the amount remaining after depreciation), 40 percent of the gain (2/5), or $120,000 is allocated to nonqualified use and is taxable as long-term capital gain. The remaining 60 percent of the gain, $180,000, is attributable to qualified use and can be excluded.

> **Example 21.** R bought an investment property on January 1, 2007 and rented it until January 1, 2010 when he began occupying it as his principal residence for the next three years. He sold the property on January 1, 2013, realizing a gain. The two years prior to January 1, 2009 are disregarded for determining nonqualified use (but included for purposes of the ownership test). Thus he has one year of nonqualified use (disregard 2007 and 2008) and six years of total ownership. Thus, 16.67 percent (1/6) of the gain (after accounting for depreciation) is taxable.

Although the above examples measure use in terms of years, presumably the regulations will require taxpayers to keep track of their use and its type in terms of months or perhaps days.

The nonqualified use rule was aimed at taxpayers that purchase rental property, rent the property out and then convert it to a personal residence. That is, the rule is designed for taxpayers that formerly used their residence as rental property. For this reason, nonqualified use that occurs after the taxpayer's last use of the property as a principal

---

[25] § 121(b)(4)(D) provides that the gain potentially ineligible for the exclusion is the gain remaining after applying depreciation recapture rule.

[26] Gain attributable to the depreciation would be taxed at a maximum rate of 25 percent (unrecaptured straight-line depreciation on § 1250 property). See Chapter 17.

residence and is within five years prior to the sale is disregarded. This rule allows homeowners to move out of their principal residence and convert it to nonqualified use property (e.g., rental) and still be eligible for the full exclusion assuming the other requirements of § 121 are met.

> **Example 22.** T purchased a home in Nantucket on June 1, 2009. She used it as her personal residence for two years until June 1, 2011 and then converted it to rental property. On June 1, 2014, she sold the home. The nonqualified rental use is disregarded since it occurred after T had used it as her residence and within five years prior to the sale. While she would be required to recognize income to the extent of any depreciation deducted, the remaining gain would be eligible for the exclusion. Note that the special rule gives taxpayer up to three years to sell the home after moving out without having the exclusion reduced. Had T sold her home on June 1, 2015, she would not have qualified for the exclusion because she did not use it as her personal residence for 2 of the last 5 years.

In identifying nonqualified use, certain periods when the homeowner did not live in the residence are ignored. These include absences due to government service (e.g., service in the military, intelligence community or U.S. Foreign Service), change of employment, health conditions and other unforeseen circumstances.

> **Example 23.** Before shipping off to military duty in Europe, H purchased a home in Maryland. He rented the property for the five years that he was stationed overseas. The rental use is not considered nonqualified use since it was attributable to military service.

Sale After a Like-Kind Exchange. The $250,000 or $500,000 exclusion is so attractive that without certain restrictions, it could be easily abused. For example, owners of rental property might be interested in exchanging a rental property for another rental property in a tax-deferred exchange (see subsequent coverage in this chapter), later converting the replacement property to a principal residence, and then (after at least two years) selling the replacement property and taking advantage of the exclusion. This possibility remains, but the § 121 exclusion will not apply to a property unless five years have passed since the like-exchange occured.

> **Example 24.** B owned a duplex that he rented to college students. He purchased it for $240,000 in 1991. Depreciation of $98,000 was claimed, so B's basis is $142,000. On November 16, 2007, B exchanged the duplex for a residential property worth $450,000 that was used as rental property. In October 2007, the tenant moved out and B moved into the residence. Under the general rule, B would qualify for the § 121 exclusion in October 2009. However, the special rule for like-kind exchange property applies. As a result, B will not qualify until November 16, 2012 (five years after the exchange).
>
> If B sells the property, after November 15, 2012, for $490,000, the gain realized is $348,000 [$490,000 − ($240,000 − $98,000)]. B can exclude $250,000. However, if the sale had occurred earlier, none of the gain is excludable.

Interaction of Sections 121 and 1031. Occasionally, a like-kind exchange may involve property that not only qualifies for tax-deferral under the like-kind exchange provisions of Section 1031 but also qualifies for the residence exclusion of Section 121. For example, a taxpayer may have used a house as a principal residence from 2003 through 2007, rented out the house from 2008 through 2009 and then exchanged the house for cash and new property that will be rented. The IRS has provided guidance for the tax consequences of such exchanges.[27]

---

[27] Rev. Proc. 2005-14 IRB No. 2005-7.

Electing Out. Taxpayers may find themselves in a position where they may have two or more residence sales within a two year period. However, as noted above, the exclusion cannot be used within two years of its last use. In such case, a taxpayer normally wants to apply the exclusion to the sale producing the most gain. Section 121 provides such flexibility by allowing a taxpayer to elect not to have § 121 apply to an otherwise qualifying sale. The election is made by reporting the gain on the tax return for the year of the sale.[28] Presumably (unless future guidance provides otherwise) the election can be made on an amended return.

> **Example 25.** S purchased her first residence in Chicago on May 1, 2003. She lived there until she was transferred by her employer to Phoenix on August 1, 2006. She did not immediately sell her Chicago residence but decided to rent it to an old friend. In Phoenix, she purchased a second residence which she occupied beginning on September 1, 2006. On December 15, 2008, S sold the second residence in Phoenix, realizing a gain of $5,000. Then on January 31, 2009, she sold her original Chicago residence at a gain of $177,000 ($2,000 of which is attributable to depreciation allowed). Only $175,000 can qualify for exclusion due to the depreciation claimed.
>
> Both residences meet the two of five years ownerships and use tests. If S excludes the $5,000 gain from the second residence in 2008, she cannot exclude the $175,000 gain from the original residence in 2009 because of the one sale every two years rule. It would, therefore, be in her best interest to elect out of the benefits of § 121 exclusion with respect to the $5,000 gain, in order to take advantage of the § 121 exclusion with respect to the $175,000 gain.

✔️ CHECK YOUR KNOWLEDGE

Review Question 1. True-False. Helen excluded $250,000 of gain from the sale of her primary residence which was sold on August 4, 2007. Helen cannot exclude her $23,000 gain from the sale of another primary residence on November 1, 2009, even though she has owned and used this home for more than two years.

False. Since more than two years transpired from the first sale to the second sale, Helen qualifies to exclude gain on both sales. The fact that the sale was in the second tax year after the original sale is not determinative.

Review Question 2. True-False. Mick purchased a residence on March 1, 2005 and lived in it until July 31, 2006. He rented it from August 1, 2006 until June 30, 2008 (claiming depreciation of $7,000), and then lived in it again from July 1, 2008 until it was sold on June 1, 2009. Mick cannot exclude any of his gain of $40,000 under § 121.

False. Mick qualifies for the § 121 exclusion because he lived in the residence more than two years during the five years preceding the sale (i.e., June 1, 2004 to May 31, 2009). Specifically, he lived there 28 (17 + 11) months. However, Mick can only exclude $33,000, since the first $7,000 of the $40,000 gain must be recognized due to the depreciation claimed.

Review Question 3. Lin purchased a residence on June 1, 2008, for $235,000. On December 1, 2009, she sold the residence for $295,000, so she could move to a nearby city where she was transferred by her employer. How much gain, if any, may Lin exclude under § 121?

---

[28] See § 121(f) and I.R.S. Publication 523, p.2.

All $60,000. Even though Lin did not meet the two of five years ownership and use requirements, she qualifies for a reduced exclusion limit since the sale is related to a change in the place of employment. The reduced limit if $187,500 [$250,000 × (18 months/24 months)].

Review Question 4. J and K were married on June 1, 2008, and K moved into the home that J had owned and occupied for ten years. On September 1, 2009, J and K sold the residence, recognizing a gain of $295,000. How much of the gain may J and K exclude on their joint return for 2009?

Only $250,000. In order to qualify for the increased $500,000 exclusion, both husband and wife must have used the residence for two of the five years preceding the sale. K only lived there for 15 months.

Review Question 5. After living together for ten years, L and M finally married on June 1, 2008. After their marriage, the couple continued to live in L's home. L never retitled the property and held it separately primarily for estate planning purposes. On September 1, 2009, L sold the residence, recognizing a gain of $360,000. How much of the gain may L and M exclude on their joint return for 2009?

All $360,000. In order to qualify for the increased $500,000 exclusion, only one spouse must have owned the residence for two of the preceding five years, but both husband and wife must have used the residence for two of the five years. They must file a joint return, but there is no requirement that the property be jointly owned or that they be married during the two years that they lived there.

INVOLUNTARY CONVERSIONS

Taxpayers occasionally lose their property from casualty or theft or are forced to sell their property because of some type of condemnation proceeding. When an *involuntary conversion* like this occurs, the taxpayer usually receives some form of compensation such as insurance proceeds or a condemnation award. In some cases, the compensation may actually cause the taxpayer to realize a gain from the "loss." Without any special rule, the tax resulting from this gain could produce a real hardship since the taxpayer typically uses the compensation received to acquire a replacement property. Recognizing that taxpayers may not have the wherewithal to pay the tax in this situation—which was totally beyond their control—Congress provided some relief. Special rules allow taxpayers to defer any gain realized from an involuntary conversion if they acquire qualified replacement property within a specified period of time.

Example 26. J operates a fishing boat in Miami. Unfortunately, the boat was totally destroyed when Hurricane Charley hit the Florida coast. J's basis in the boat was $40,000 (cost of $60,000 less depreciation of $20,000). Luckily, J was insured. He filed an insurance claim and received $75,000 based on the fair market value of the boat. As a result, he realized a gain of $35,000 ($75,000 − $40,000). J may defer the entire gain if he reinvests at least $75,000 in similar-use property within the allowable period.

INVOLUNTARY CONVERSION DEFINED

An involuntary conversion is defined in the Code as the compulsory or involuntary conversion of property "as a result of its destruction in whole or in part, theft, seizure, or requisition or condemnation or threat or imminence thereof."[29] The terms *destruction* and

---

[29] § 1033(a).

theft have the same basic meaning as when they are used for casualty and theft losses. The IRS has ruled, however, that the destruction of property for purposes of § 1033 need not meet the *suddenness* test, which has been applied to casualty loss deductions.[30]

Typical involuntary conversions involve accidents, natural disasters, and other events beyond the control of the taxpayer. This has been found to include damages caused by other parties such as poisoning of cattle by contaminated feed and destruction of crops and soil by chemicals.[31] In each case, the taxpayer was allowed to defer recognition of gain upon the receipt of damages by reinvesting in qualified property.

Seizure, Requisition, or Condemnation. It is not as simple to determine what qualifies as a "seizure, or requisition or condemnation" as it is to identify theft or destruction. The property must be taken without the taxpayer's consent and the taxpayer must be compensated.[32]

Not all types of forced dispositions will qualify. For example, the courts have found that a foreclosure sale[33] and a sale after continued insistence by a Chamber of Commerce[34] did not constitute involuntary conversions. Similarly, the IRS has ruled that the condemnation of rental properties due to structural defects or sanitary conditions does not constitute an involuntary conversion since the sale was made to avoid making property improvements necessary to meet a housing ordinance.[35] Generally, a transfer must be made to an authority that has the power to actually condemn the property, and the property must be taken for a public use.

In the case of the conversion of part of a single economic unit, § 1033 applies not only to the condemned portion, but also to the part not condemned if it is *voluntarily sold*. When a truck freight terminal was rendered virtually useless because the adjoining parking lot for the trucks was condemned, a single economic unit was found to exist and § 1033 applied to the sale of the terminal as well as the condemnation of the parking area.[36] In a similar situation when a shopping center was partially destroyed by fire and the owner chose to sell the entire shopping center rather than reconstruct the destroyed portion, the IRS ruled that no conversion existed with respect to the remaining portion since the undamaged portion could still be used and the damaged portion repaired. The fire insurance proceeds, but not the sale proceeds, qualified for deferral under § 1033.[37]

Threat or Imminence of Condemnation. The possibility of a condemnation may very well cause a taxpayer to sell property before the actual condemnation occurs. For example, a farming corporation may discover that its property is being considered as the site for a new airport and sell the property. Section 1033 extends deferral to these *voluntary* sales to someone other than the condemning authority if they are due to the *threat or imminence* of condemnation. It should be emphasized that newspaper reports, magazine articles, or rumors that property is being considered for condemnation are not sufficient.[38] Threat or imminence exists only after officials have communicated that they intend to condemn the property and the owner has good reason to believe they would.

[30]   Rev. Rul. 59-102, 1959-1 C.B. 200.

[31]   Rev. Rul. 54-395, 1954-2 C.B. 143 and Ltr. Rul. 9615041.

[32]   See, for example, *Hitke v. Comm.*, 62-1 USTC ¶9114, 8 AFTR2d 5886, 296 F.2d 639 (CA-7, 1961).

[33]   See *Cooperative Publishing Co. v. U.S.*, 40-2 USTC ¶9823, 25 AFTR 1123, 115 F.2d 1017 (CA-9, 1940), and *Robert Recio*, 61 TCM 2626, T.C. Memo. 1991-215.

[34]   *Davis Co.*, 6 B.T.A. 281 (1927), acq. VI-2 C.B. 2.

[35]   Rev. Rul. 57-314, 1957-2 C.B. 523.

[36]   *Harry Masser*, 30 T.C. 741 (1958), acq. 1959-2 C.B. 5; Rev. Rul. 59-361, 1959-2 C.B. 183.

[37]   Rev. Rul. 78-377, 1978-2 C.B. 208, distinguishing Rev. Rul. 59-361, Footnote 27.

[38]   Rev. Rul. 58-557, 1958-2 C.B. 402.

Example 27. LSA Corporation has owned a department store in downtown Indianapolis for more than 50 years. The property has a value of about $2 million and a basis of only $400,000 (since the building is completely depreciated). Recently, the corporation learned that the city fathers, in an attempt to revive the downtown area, plan to build a new mall that may result in the condemnation of the building. Fearing that interest rates may rise before the city gets around to condemning the property, the corporation sold the building to another investor, who wanted to try to preserve the building as a historic structure. The corporation quickly used the sales proceeds to build another store in a nearby suburb. Unfortunately, the corporation's sale may not qualify for deferral since it has not been officially notified that the building will be condemned. The threat or imminence does not exist merely because the city is considering plans that may lead to condemnation. Nevertheless, the corporation may be able to produce evidence that clearly suggests otherwise.

As noted above, the sale to a third party after the threat exists is permissible.[39] If the third party realizes gain when the property is later sold to the condemning authority, the new transaction may also qualify for involuntary conversion treatment if the proceeds are reinvested in qualified property after the condemnation of the property, even though the threat existed before the property was acquired.[40]

Example 28. T has owned and operated a successful automobile dealership for many years. This year he received legal notice from the City of New Orleans indicating that it planned to condemn his showroom and car lot for use as the site of a new convention center in approximately five years. As a result, T began searching for an acceptable new location. After finding a suitable location, T sold the old property to a person who could use it for just four or five years.

T's sale and reinvestment qualifies for involuntary conversion treatment and his gain can be deferred so long as all other requirements are met. When the property is finally purchased by the city, the new owner can also qualify for involuntary conversion treatment if he or she realizes a gain and the proceeds are reinvested in qualifying property within the replacement period.

REPLACEMENT PROPERTY

To qualify for deferral of gain on an involuntary conversion, the taxpayer must reinvest in property that is *similar or related in service* or *use* to the property that is converted.[41] The IRS and taxpayers often disagree as to what qualifies as replacement property. It is clear, however, that the new property must replace the converted property, and therefore, property that was already owned by the taxpayer will not qualify.[42]

Generally, the replacement property must serve the same functional use as that served by the converted property. This *functional use* test requires that the character of service or use be the same for both properties.

Example 29. N has successfully owned and operated a bowling alley for many years. This year the bowling alley was destroyed by fire, and N replaced it with a billiard parlor. The billiard parlor is not qualified replacement property since services provided by each are not functionally equivalent. Although they both

---

[39] *Creative Solutions, Inc. v. U.S.*, 63-2 USTC ¶9615, 12 AFTR2d 5229, 320 F.2d 809 (CA-5, 1963); Rev. Rul. 81-180, 1981-2 C.B. 161.

[40] Rev. Rul. 81-181, 1981-2 C.B. 162.

[41] § 1033(a).

[42] § 1033(a)(1)(A)(i).

provide recreational services, the IRS believes bowling balls and billiard balls are not the same.[43]

When tangible trade or business personalty is destroyed in a Presidentially declared disaster area, the taxpayer is given more flexibility. The destroyed property may be replaced with *any* tangible trade or business personalty.[44]

A different and more liberal test has been applied to rental properties involved in involuntary conversions. This test is the *taxpayer use* test, which basically requires that the replacement property be used by the taxpayer/lessor as rental property regardless of the lessee's use.[45]

> **Example 30.** Several years ago J purchased 30 acres of land and built a large warehouse that he leased to an appliance store. This year the warehouse site was condemned, and J used the proceeds to purchase a gas station that he currently leases to an oil company. The gas station is qualified replacement property since both properties are rental properties. The fact that the tenants use the properties for different purposes is irrelevant. From the owner's perspective each property is being used in the same way.

Control of Corporation. The replacement property in an involuntary conversion may be controlling stock in a corporation owning property that is "similar or related in use or service."[46] Control consists of owning at least 80 percent of all voting stock plus at least 80 percent of all other classes of stock.[47]

Condemned Real Estate. Congress provided special relief in the situation where real property is condemned by an outside authority. A more liberal interpretation of "similar or related in use" is allowed for the replacement of condemned real property if it is held by the taxpayer for use in a trade or business or for investment. The Code provides that the *like-kind* test shall be applied.[48] This is the test used for § 1031 like-kind exchanges. As explained later in this chapter, these rules allow nonrecognition whenever a taxpayer exchanges real estate for real estate regardless of the real estate's use. Thus, if the taxpayer's unimproved real estate (e.g., raw land) is condemned and replaced with improved real estate (e.g., shopping center), deferral would be granted.

Conversion of Livestock. Section 1033 includes certain special provisions related to sales of livestock. Livestock sold because of disease[49] or solely because of drought, flood or other weather-related conditions[50] are considered involuntarily converted. Furthermore, if livestock are sold because of soil contamination or environmental contamination and it is not feasible for the owner to reinvest in other livestock, then other farm property, including real property, will qualify as replacement property.[51]

---

[43]   Rev. Rul. 76-319, 1976-2 C.B. 242.

[44]   § 1033(h).

[45]   Rev. Rul. 71-41, 1971-1 C.B. 223.

[46]   § 1033(a)(2)(A).

[47]   § 1033(a)(2)(E)(i).

[48]   § 1033(g)(1). The similar or related in use test must be applied if the real property is destroyed or the replacement property is stock in a controlled corporation.

[49]   § 1033(d).

[50]   § 1033(e).

[51]   § 1033(f).

Property Acquired from a Related Party. Congress was concerned that the replacement property would conveniently be acquired from a related party. In order to prevent this, C corporations, partnerships with C corporations as partners, and other taxpayers deferring gains in excess of $100,000, will not be allowed the deferral under § 1033 if the replacement is purchased from a related party. For this purpose, a related party includes certain close family members and most entities where there is more than 50 percent control.[52]

REPLACEMENT PERIOD

The taxpayer is entitled to deferral only if reinvestment in the replacement property occurs within the proper time period. The replacement period usually begins on the date of disposition of the converted property; but in the case of condemnation or requisition, it begins at the earliest date of threat or imminence of the requisition or condemnation. The replacement period ends on the last day of the second taxable year after the year in which a gain is first realized,[53] but may be extended by the IRS if the taxpayer can show reasonable cause for being unable to replace within the specified time limit.[54] In the case of condemned real property used in a trade or business or held for investment, the replacement period is extended. The extension is one year, causing the replacement period to remain open until the end of the third taxable year after the first year in which gain is first realized.[55] These time periods are diagrammed below.

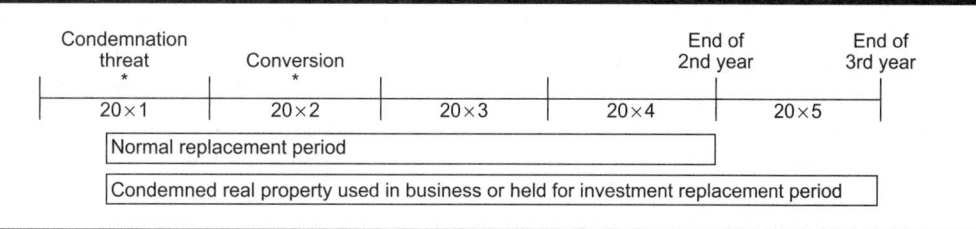

Example 31. E's rental house was condemned for public use by the county during 2008. Her basis in the residence was $32,000 and the county paid her $46,000. E's replacement period begins the day of the condemnation, or threat thereof. The replacement period normally ends at the close of the second taxable year after the year of the conversion. However, in the case of realty that has been held for productive use in business or for investment and which has been condemned, the replacement period is extended to the close of the third taxable year. In this case, the replacement period ends on December 31, 2011.

Example 32. If the residence in the previous example had been used as E's personal residence, the replacement period would end on December 31, 2010. As noted above, the replacement period is extended only for real estate held for productive use in a trade or business or for investment, so the usual two-year rule applies.

Earlier reference was made to specific provisions dealing with replacement property upon the destruction of one's principal residence. A special reinvestment period is also provided. When the destruction is in a Presidentially declared disaster area, the

---

52   § 1033(i).

53   § 1033(a)(2)(B).

54   Reg. § 1.1033(a)-2(c)(3).

55   § 1033(g)(4).

reinvestment period is extended to the last day of the fourth year following the year in which gain is first realized.[56]

> **Example 33.** U's principal residence was destroyed in an earthquake. U's insurance policy included limits of $100,000 for the residence, $40,000 for contents, and an additional $20,000 for U's prized musical instruments. U realized gains on the residence and musical instruments and a small loss on the contents. The region affected by the earthquake was declared a disaster area by the President and U's insurer paid the maximum amounts under the policy. U may defer his gain on the structure and musical instruments by reinvesting $120,000 in similar (residence or contents) property. The reinvestment must take place by the end of U's fourth taxable year after receiving the insurance settlement.

ELECTION REQUIRED

As a general rule, taxpayers are allowed to elect whether or not they want to defer any gain realized from an involuntary conversion. The election is made simply by not reporting any of the deferred gain on the tax return for the year in which the gain is realized. However, deferral of gain is mandatory if the property is converted directly into property that is similar or related in use.[57]

> **Example 34.** G owned 100 acres of land next to an airport. He had farmed the land for 25 years. All of that changed this year when the city condemned G's land to expand the airport. Pursuant to the condemnation agreement, the city transferred similar farmland to G. In this case, nonrecognition is mandatory since there was a direct conversion into similar property. Had the city paid G for the land, G would have had the option to elect deferral or recognize any gain realized.

The return for the year of conversion must include detailed information relating to the involuntary conversion,[58] and if the taxpayer has not yet reinvested when the return is filed, he or she is required to notify the IRS when replacement property has been acquired or that no replacement will occur.[59] If after an election has been made under § 1033 *and* the taxpayer fails to reinvest all of the required amount within the allowable period, the tax return for the year (or years) in which gain was realized must be *amended to include the recognized gain* and the tax deficiency must be paid.[60]

Statute of Limitations. The statute of limitations is extended for involuntary conversions when the taxpayer elects to defer his or her gain but has not replaced the property by the time the return for the year of the conversion is filed. The IRS may audit the transaction and assess a deficiency any time within three years after the taxpayer notifies the IRS that he or she has replaced the converted property or has failed to replace the property triggering the recognition of gain.[61]

---

[56]   § 1033(h)(1)(B).

[57]   § 1033(a).

[58]   Reg. § 1.1033(a)-2(c)(2).

[59]   Reg. § 1.1033(a)-2(c)(5).

[60]   Special rules extend the statute of limitations. § 1033(a)(2)(C): Reg. § 1.1033(a)-2(c)(5).

[61]   § 1033(a)(2)(C).

AMOUNT OF GAIN RECOGNIZED

No gain is recognized by an electing taxpayer on an involuntary conversion if the amount reinvested in replacement property equals or exceeds the amount realized from the converted property (i.e., the taxpayer does not "cash out" on the transaction). If the amount reinvested is less than the amount realized, the taxpayer has "cashed out" on the transaction and *must* recognize gain to the extent of the amount *not* reinvested (see Exhibit 15-2).[62] No gain is recognized in a direct conversion.[63]

The *amount reinvested* is the *cost* of the replacement property. The property may not have been acquired by gift, inheritance, or any other method resulting in other than a cost basis.[64] The cost basis would include the amount of any debt incurred in the purchase.

The taxpayer will determine his or her basis in property acquired in an involuntary conversion by taking into consideration the deferred gain. In the case of a direct conversion, the basis of the replacement property is the same as the basis in the converted property. In conversions into money and other property, the basis in the replacement property is its cost *reduced* by the amount of gain realized but not recognized (see Exhibit 15-2).[65]

EXHIBIT 15-2

Involuntary Conversion:

Computation of Recognized Gain and Basis of Replacement Property

1. Gain realized

	Amount realized (net proceeds)
Less:	Adjusted basis
	Gain (loss) realized

2. Gain recognized

	Amount realized
Less:	Cost of replacement property
	Gain recognized (not to exceed gain realized)*

3. Basis of replacement property

	Cost of replacement property
Less:	Gain not recognized
	Adjusted basis of replacement property

*If this amount is negative, the taxpayer has reinvested more than the amount realized and no gain is recognized.

Example 35. M owned a rented industrial equipment warehouse that was adjacent to a railway. The warehouse was destroyed by fire on January 15, 2009, and M received $240,000 from her insurance carrier on March 26, 2009. Her basis in the warehouse was $130,000. M constructed a wholesale grocery warehouse on the same site since the predicted demand for such space was superior to equipment storage. The new warehouse was constructed at a cost of $280,000 and was completed May 7, 2010.

---

[62] § 1033(a)(2)(A).

[63] § 1033(a)(1).

[64] Reg. § 1.1033(a)-2(c)(4).

[65] § 1033(b); Reg. § 1.1033(b)-1.

Leased (rental) property is subject to the more liberal *taxpayer use* test, rather than the *functional use* test that is applied to other properties. Therefore, the new warehouse meets the similar or related in use test since it is rental property to M.

As calculated below, M reports no gain on her 2009 return since she reinvested a sufficient amount within the reinvestment period, which ends December 31, 2011. She is required to give the IRS the details of the conversion with her 2009 return and provide a description of the replacement property when it is completed. The basis in the replacement property is $170,000 (cost of $280,000 − the gain not recognized of $110,000).

Amount realized....................................	$ 240,000
Less: Adjusted basis	(130,000)
Gain (loss) realized	$ 110,000
Amount realized..	$ 240,000
Less: Cost of replacement property......................	(280,000)
Gain recognized (not to exceed gain realized).................	None
Cost of replacement property..............................	$ 280,000
Less: Gain not recognized	(110,000)
Adjusted basis of replacement property	$ 170,000

Example 36. Assume the same facts as in *Example 30*, except that M reinvested $200,000. In this case she would be required to recognize a gain since she did not reinvest all of the insurance proceeds of $240,000. As a result, her recognized gain would be $40,000 and her basis in the replacement property would be $130,000, calculated as follows:

Amount realized...	$ 240,000
Less: Cost of replacement property.......................	−200,000
Gain recognized (not to exceed gain realized).................	$ 40,000
Cost of replacement property..............................	$ 200,000
Less: Gain not recognized ($110,000 − $40,000)	−70,000
Adjusted basis of replacement property	$ 130,000

Conversion of Personal Residence. Section 1033 also applies to the involuntary conversion of a principal residence. Taxpayers that qualify may elect to use § 121 instead of, or along with, § 1033 for the involuntary conversion of a personal residence.[66]

---

[66]   § 121(d)(4).

✓ CHECK YOUR KNOWLEDGE

Over the last several years, Rock and Roller Blades Inc. opened two new roller skating rinks to capitalize on the in-line skating craze. In February 2008, however, one of the rinks was destroyed by fire. At that time, the building had a basis of $300,000. The insurance proceeds awarded to the company amounted to $360,000.

Review Question 1. If the corporation uses the insurance proceeds to build a new indoor soccer facility, will the soccer facility be considered qualified replacement property?

Probably not. In order to qualify for deferral, the replacement property must be similar to or related in service or use to the converted property. This generally means that the replacement property must provide the same functional use as the converted property. Based on the IRS ruling that a billiard parlor is not functionally equivalent to a bowling alley, it would appear that a soccer facility does not provide the same services as a roller rink.

Review Question 2. By what date must the calendar year corporation invest in qualified replacement property?

The corporation must reinvest by the close of the second taxable year following the year in which the conversion takes place, in this case December 31, 2011. The extended replacement period for business or investment realty only applies if the property is condemned.

Review Question 3. Assuming the corporation immediately erects another roller rink at the cost of $390,000 and elects to defer any gain realized, the company's gain (or loss) recognized will be:

    a. $60,000
    b. $30,000
    c. $90,000
    d. $0
    e. $30,000 loss
    f. None of the above

The answer is (d). As shown in the following computations, the corporation is allowed to defer the entire gain realized since it reinvested all of the insurance proceeds.

Amount realized.	$ 360,000
Less: Adjusted basis	−300,000
Gain (loss) realized	$ 60,000
Amount realized.	$ 360,000
Less: Cost of replacement property	−390,000
Gain recognized (not to exceed gain realized)	None

Review Question 4. Same facts as in Question 3. The basis of the replacement property is:

    a. $300,000
    b. $390,000
    c. $370,000
    d. $0
    e. $360,000
    f. None of the above

The answer is (f). The basis is $330,000, determined as follows:

Cost of replacement property	$ 390,000
Less: Gain not recognized	−60,000
Adjusted basis of replacement property	$330,000

LIKE-KIND EXCHANGES

Section 1031 of the Code provides that a taxpayer may exchange certain types of property *in kind* without the recognition of a taxable gain or loss. Specifically, no gain or loss is recognized when qualifying property is exchanged *solely* for other qualifying property that is of like-kind.

> **Example 37.** E traded in his automobile that was worth $4,500 and was used entirely for business purposes and also paid $15,000 cash for a new auto worth $19,500. E's basis in the old auto was $8,200, based on an original cost of $16,000 less depreciation of $7,800. E recognizes no gain or loss on the transaction since it is a qualifying like-kind exchange. His basis in the new auto is $23,200 ($8,200 basis of trade-in + $15,000 cash paid).

If property other than like-kind property—commonly called *boot*—is received in the exchange, a gain may be recognized.[67] Losses, however, are never recognized.

In order for a transaction to qualify as a nontaxable exchange, it must meet four separate requirements:

1. Both the property exchanged and the property received must be held for business or investment purpose.

2. Both the items exchanged and received must not be specifically excluded from § 1031 treatment.

3. The properties are like-kind.

4. There must be an exchange.

Each of these requirements are discussed below.

QUALIFIED PROPERTY

Holding Purpose. In order to qualify for like-kind exchange treatment, a property must be held *either* for use in a trade or business *or* for investment. A qualified exchange may, however, involve the transfer of investment property for trade or business property, or vice versa.[68] No personal use properties qualify.

It is important to note that it is the taxpayer's purpose for holding that is critical. The purposes or plans of the other party to the exchange are irrelevant. For example, if the taxpayer held the property exchanged for business or investment, the taxpayer has met the holding-purpose requirement even if the other party plans to sell the property, has a contract to sell it before the exchange, or is helped by the taxpayer in finding a buyer.

---

[67] § 1031(b).

[68] Reg. § 1.1031(a)-1(a).

Excluded Properties. Certain properties are specifically excluded from like-kind exchange treatment. These are:[69]

- Inventory or other property held primarily for sale
- Stocks, bonds, or notes
- Other securities or evidences of indebtedness
- Partnership interests
- Interest in trusts (e.g., the beneficiary's interest)
- Livestock of different sexes

Whether an item is inventory (i.e., held primarily for sale to customers in the ordinary course of a trade or business) is discussed in Chapter 16. Several courts have interpreted the phrase *held for sale* to include any property that is acquired in an exchange only to be resold shortly thereafter.[70]

> **Example 38.** K exchanged a parcel of real estate held for investment for another parcel and immediately offered the parcel received for sale. The parcel was sold on the installment basis. Since K held the new property for sale rather than for use in a trade or business or for investment, the entire gain realized on the exchange must be recognized at the time of the exchange.

LIKE-KIND PROPERTY

The term like-kind is not defined in the Code. However, the Regulations provide that "the words like-kind have reference to the nature or character of the property and not to its grade or quality."[71] This interpretation has been applied to allow exchanges of realty for realty and personalty for personalty. Exchanges of realty for personal property (nonrealty) or vice versa, are not considered exchanges of like-kind property and are fully taxable.

Real Estate. Generally, any exchange of realty for realty will meet the like-kind test. It is immaterial whether the real property is improved or unimproved.[72] No distinction is made between improved or unimproved, productive or unproductive, or similar differences since these relate to the grade or quality of the property and are to be specifically ignored. The IRS has ruled that a lease of real property with a remaining term of at least 30 years will be treated as real property for purposes of determining whether a like-kind exchange has occurred.[73] Accordingly, a realized loss from the exchange of property that had declined in value for a lease interest in that property with a life of 30 years or more resulted in a nondeductible (nonrecognized) loss.[74] Recall that condemned real estate in an involuntary conversion is also subject to the like-kind test.

Tangible Depreciable Personalty. In determining the meaning of "like-kind" for personalty, the IRS, with some support, has adopted a much narrower interpretation than

---

[69] § 1031(a)(2).

[70] Ethel Black, 35 T.C. 90 (1960); *George M. Bernard*, 26 TCM 858, T.C. Memo. 1967-176.

[71] Reg. § 1.1031(a)(1)(A).

[72] Reg. § 1.1031(a)-1(b). It is also important to note that § 1250 may supersede § 1031 and cause the recognition of gain. Effectively, § 1250 property (generally depreciable realty) must be acquired in an amount at least as great as the § 1250 recapture potential—§ 1250(d)(4)(C). See Chapter 17 for a discussion of § 1250 recapture of depreciation.

[73] Rev. Rul. 76-301, 1976-2 C.B. 241.

[74] *Century Electric Co. v. Comm.*, 51-2 USTC ¶9482, 41 AFTR 205, 192 F.2d 155 (CA-8, 1951).

its view toward realty.[75] This stems from the fact that personality includes a far greater variety of assets than realty. From the Service's perspective, adoption of a lenient "like-kind" test for personality would enable exchanges that violate the spirit of § 1031 (e.g., a car for a horse, a railroad boxcar for an airplane). As noted earlier, deferral is granted on the theory that the taxpayer's economic position has not changed sufficiently to warrant taxation. In the government's opinion, this principle would be seriously undermined if taxpayers were permitted to exchange any type of personality. Thus, a restrictive approach is understandable. Unfortunately, this approach (i.e., determining whether replacement property represents a continuing interest or a conversion to a wholly new endeavor) is very subjective and difficult to implement.

Notwithstanding support for its position, the IRS became concerned about what it believed could be endless debate over what personality was like-kind. Consequently, the government issued new Regulations in 1991.[76] These Regulations put taxpayers on alert that the government would continue to take its narrow view of whether one item of personality is considered the equivalent of another, but, at the same time, offered safe harbors that would provide the taxpayer with some certainty.

Under the current Regulations, personal property qualifies for § 1031 treatment if the properties are either:

1. Like-kind or

2. Like-class.

The definition of "like-kind" remains the same, nebulous as it may be. In contrast, the *like-class* definition offers a more practical approach to determine if properties have the requisite similarity. The like-class definition utilizes a two class system: (1) General Asset Classes and (2) Product Classes. If the properties are within the same General Asset Class or the same Product Class, they are considered like-class and, therefore, like-kind for § 1031 purposes. Note that if the properties meet the like-class standard, they are considered like-kind regardless of whether the exchanged properties would be considered like-kind under general § 1031 standards. The like-class system is significant in that it provides taxpayers the certainty they need before engaging in a transaction. This is particularly true given the absence of authority on like-kind characterizations for personal property.

The General Asset Classes are identified and defined in Revenue Procedure 87-56. There are 13 classes of assets, as shown in Exhibit 15-3. If two assets fall in the same class, they are considered like-class. For instance, a computer, printer, monitor, and modem used in a trade or business would qualify as like-class properties since they are all part of the information systems class (General Asset Class .12). Note that these classes are quite narrow. For example, an automobile and a light-duty truck would not be considered like-class since they are not in the same Class. Recall, however, that these classes serve only as safe harbors in which taxpayers have guaranteed like-kind treatment.[77]

If a General Asset Class is not provided for a particular asset, the Product Classes are to be used to determine if the exchanged properties are like-class. Observe that it is possible—but not likely—that the properties may be in two different General Asset

---

[75] In *California Federal Life Insurance Co.*, 50 AFTR 2d 82-5271, 680 F2d 85, 82-2 USTC ¶9464 (CA-9, 1982), aff'g 76 TC 107 (1981) the courts upheld the government's argument that Swiss francs and U.S. double-eagle gold coins were not like-kind. In explaining its holding, the Ninth Circuit noted that it was Congressional concern for lenient interpretation of the like-kind standard that prompted it to amend § 1031 to say that livestock of different sexes are not like-kind. According to the Ninth Circuit, in so acting, Congress was suggesting that personal property was to be accorded different treatment.

[76] Reg. § 1.1031(a)-2(b)(1).

[77] PLR 200450005 provides that sport utility vehicles (SUVs) and passenger automobiles are like-kind. Note, however, that for depreciation purposes heavy SUVs are not subject to the depreciation limitations applicable to passenger automobiles under § 280F.

EXHIBIT 15-3
General Asset Classes: Revenue Procedure 87-56

Asset Class	Class Number
1. Office furniture, fixtures, and equipment	.11
2. Information systems (computers and peripheral equipment)	.12
3. Data handling equipment, except computers	.13
4. Airplanes and helicopters (airframes and engines), except those used in commercial or contract carrying of passengers or freight	.21
5. Automobiles, taxis	.22
6. Buses	.23
7. Light general-purpose trucks	.241
8. Heavy general-purpose trucks	.242
9. Railroad cars and locomotives	.25
10. Tractor units for use over the road	.26
11. Trailers and trailer-mounted containers	.27
12. Vessels, barges, tugs, and similar water-transportation equipment, except those used in marine construction	.28
13. Industrial steam and electric generation and/or distribution systems	.4

Classes but in the same Product Class. In such case, the items are not like-class since the Product Classes cannot be used if the properties can be found in the General Asset Classes which were designed by the government.

Assets are within the same Product Class if they have the same four-digit product code as listed in the *North American Industrial Classification System* (NAICS) *Manual* published by the Department of Commerce.

As noted above, if the property does not qualify as like-class under the safe harbors created by the Regulations, it may still be treated as like-kind. The IRS historically has allowed like-kind exchange treatment for personal property when the properties were substantially the same. The courts have ruled that livestock used in a trade or business, but not held for sale, may qualify as like-kind. However, the Code does explain that livestock of different sexes are not like-kind.[78] While it may be obvious that a bull is not a cow, the treatment of bullion-type coins (e.g., decorative gold coins) has created a great deal of controversy. For some investors, collecting and trading gold and silver coins is a popular investment strategy. The IRS has ruled that an exchange of gold bullion held for investment for silver bullion held for the same purpose is not a like-kind exchange since gold and silver are intrinsically different minerals.[79] On the other hand, bullion-type coins of different countries constitute like-kind property.[80] Currency exchanges are not like-kind exchanges. Similarly, legal tender coins (currency) are not of like-kind with bullion-type noncurrency coins.[81]

Intangibles. The like-class rules apply only to tangible depreciable personalty. There are no like classes for intangible personal property. Whether intangibles such as patents and copyrights are like-kind depends on the nature of the property to which the rights relate. For example, copyrights on two novels are like-kind; but a copyright on a novel

---

[78] § 1031(e). Apparently, if male calves could be exchanged for female calves, a breeding herd of females could be built up more quickly and sold for capital gain treatment.

[79] Rev. Rul. 82-166, 1982-2 C.B. 190.

[80] Rev. Rul. 76-214, 1976-1 C.B. 218.

[81] Rev. Rul. 79-143, 1979-1 C.B. 264; *California Federal Life Insurance Co. v. Comm.*, 82-2 USTC ¶9464, 50 AFTR2d 82-5271, 680 F.2d 85 (CA-9, 1982), aff'g. 76 T.C. 107 (1981). It is interesting that the Revenue Ruling states that U.S. gold coins are currency, while the courts in these cases state that they are more like "other property" than "money."

and a copyright on a song are not like-kind.[82] Similarly, the IRS has ruled that the contracts of professional athletes are like-kind.

Multiple Property Exchanges. In some cases an exchange may involve more than one property. When this occurs, as in an exchange of one business for another, the Regulations provide a somewhat complex set of rules. The effect of these rules is that the various assets are matched with those of the same kind or class. Note that if two businesses are exchanged, the IRS guidelines provide that the goodwill and going concern values of similar businesses are not considered like-kind properties."[83]

Property Outside the United States. Generally, real property located outside the U.S. is not like-kind with respect to real property located within the U.S. Similarly, personal property used predominately outside the U.S. is not like-kind with respect to personalty used predominantly within the U.S. In determining where property is predominately used, the two years before the exchange are considered for the property given up and the two years after the exchange are considered for the property received.[84]

RECEIPT OF PROPERTY NOT OF A LIKE-KIND (BOOT)

As a general rule, an exchange is nontaxable only if property is exchanged *solely* for like-kind property. But in many cases, taxpayers wanting to make an exchange do not have like-kind property of equal values. Consequently, one of the parties typically throws in cash or some other non-like-kind property—commonly called *boot*—to equalize the values exchanged. Fortunately, the receipt of boot does not totally disqualify the transaction. Instead, § 1031(b) provides that the taxpayer must recognize any gain realized to the extent of any boot received. For these purposes, *boot* includes any money received in the exchange *plus* the fair market value of any property that is either nonqualified or not like-kind. Under § 1031(c), the receipt of boot does not cause the recognition of any realized losses in such an exchange.[85]

Example 39. J transferred a vacant lot held as an investment and worth $8,000 to another party in exchange for a similar lot worth $6,000. J received $2,000 cash in addition to the new lot. J's basis in her old lot was $5,500. J's realized gain is $2,500 ($8,000 amount realized − $5,500 basis). If she holds the new lot as an investment, J still must recognize gain on this exchange in the amount of $2,000 because she received *cash boot* of $2,000.

Example 40. If J's basis in the property given up in the prior example had been $6,500, her realized gain would have been $1,500 ($8,000 amount realized − $6,500 basis). Although she received $2,000 of boot, J's recognized gain is $1,500 (recognized gain is *never* more than the realized gain).

Example 41. If J's basis in the vacant lot exchanged in the previous two examples had been $9,000, she would have a realized loss of $1,000 and a recognized loss of zero. Losses in like-kind exchanges are never recognized.

Liabilities as Boot. In many exchanges, a taxpayer transfers property encumbered by indebtedness (e.g., land subject to a mortgage) or has liabilities assumed as part of the

---

[82] Reg. § 1.1031(a)-2(c)(3), *Examples 1* and 2.

[83] Reg. § 1.1031(a)-2(c)(2).

[84] § 1031(h).

[85] If a note is received as boot, the gain may be reported using the installment sales rules. See § 453(h)(6) and (7).

exchange agreement. When a taxpayer is relieved of a liability, the tax law takes the view that such relief is the economic equivalent of receiving cash and paying off the liability. In essence, the party assuming the liability is treated as having paid cash for the property. Consistent with this view, any liabilities from which the taxpayer is relieved in a like-kind exchange are treated as boot received (or boot paid in the case of the party assuming the debt).[86] Note that without these rules, taxpayers could mortgage property shortly before the exchange, receive cash, and then transfer the property along with liability without having to recognize any gain. The treatment of liability relief as boot thwarts such plans.

> **Example 42.** Wanting to move his business out of the city, R exchanged his downtown warehouse encumbered by a mortgage of $200,000 for a new suburban building worth $700,000. R's basis in the warehouse was $600,000. As a result, R realized a gain of $300,000 ($700,000 + $200,000 = $900,000 amount realized − $600,000 basis). Although R received only the building, the relief of the $200,000 liability is treated as boot received. Therefore, R must recognize a gain of $200,000.

Relief and Assumption of Liabilities. If both parties to the exchange assume a liability (e.g., the taxpayer is relieved of a liability of $100,000 but also incurs a liability of $90,000), the process becomes a bit more confusing. In this case, the taxpayer first nets the assumption and the relief. If the taxpayer has net relief (i.e., net decrease in liabilities), such amount is treated as boot received, which in turn may trigger gain recognition.[87] If the taxpayer has net incurred (i.e., net increase in liabilities), such amount is treated as boot paid and no gain is recognized. Note that liabilities are the only type of boot paid or received that can be netted. Other types of boot are not netted. But what if a taxpayer receives cash and incurs liabilities? Can the taxpayer offset any cash received (and the gain that goes with it) by any liabilities incurred? And what if a taxpayer is relieved of liabilities? Can the taxpayer offset any liability relief by giving cash? The Regulations have addressed these possibilities. A taxpayer cannot offset boot received by liabilities incurred. However, liability relief can be offset by boot given (since the taxpayer could presumably pay off the debt with the boot, thereby reducing the liability relief).[88] These various situations are addressed in the next three examples.

> **Example 43.** S exchanged a tractor worth $11,000 for a lighter duty tractor worth $9,000, both held for use in his landscaping business. The tractor given up was subject to a secured obligation of $8,000 and S incurred a liability secured by the new tractor of $6,000. S's basis in the tractor given up was $6,500, his cost of $13,500 less depreciation allowed of $7,000. S's realized gain on this exchange is $4,500, computed as follows:

Fair market value of property received	$ 9,000
Plus: Liabilities encumbering the property transferred.	+8,000
Less: Liabilities assumed by tax payer	−6,000
Amount realized.	$ 11,000
Less: Adjusted basis of property given up.	−6,500
Gain realized	$ 4,500

---

[86]   § 1031(d).

[87]   See Reg. §§ 1.1031(b)-1(c) and 1.1031(d)-2. It is important to note that liabilities incurred in anticipation of a like-kind exchange will not qualify for this netting treatment. See Prop. Reg. § 1.1031(b)-1(c).

[88]   Reg. 1.1031(d)-2, Ex. 2.

S's recognized gain is $2,000 since his net liability relief ($8,000 liability relief − $6,000 liability assumed) is treated as boot.

Example 44. Use the facts in *Example 43*, but assume that instead of receiving a $9,000 tractor and incurring a $6,000 liability, S received a tractor worth $7,500 and paid $4,500 cash. S's realized gain is $4,500 computed as follows:

Fair market value of property received	$ 7,500
Plus: Liabilities encumbering the property transferred.	+8,000
Less: Amount of money given up	−4,500
Amount realized.	$ 11,000
Less: Adjusted basis of property given up.	−6,500
Gain realized	$ 4,500

S's recognized gain is $3,500, the amount of his liability relief ($8,000) less the other boot paid ($4,500 cash).

Example 45. If S had received a tractor worth $3,000 and incurred no liabilities and paid no cash in the transaction, his realized gain is still $4,500, computed as follows:

Fair market value of property received	$ 3,000
Plus: Liabilities encumbering the property transferred.	+8,000
Amount realized.	$ 11,000
Less: Adjusted basis of property given up.	−6,500
Gain realized	$ 4,500

The amount of boot received is $8,000, the amount of his liability relief. The recognized gain is $4,500, since the gain is recognized to the extent of boot received, but never more than the gain realized.

BASIS IN PROPERTY RECEIVED

Exhibit 15-4 presents two ways of computing the basis of property received in a like-kind exchange. The first method (Method 1), prescribed by the Code, is based on the notion that the like-kind property received in the exchange is merely a continuation of the taxpayer's investment in the like-kind property given up. Thus, the basis of the property received should be the same as the property given up—a so-called *substituted* basis. This basis is *increased* by any gain recognized and by any additional consideration given or to be paid in the future, or *decreased* by the fair market value of any boot received and by any liabilities transferred.[89] The second method is derived from the basis determination method used for replacement property in involuntary conversions and sales of principal residences. Under this method, the fair market value of the like-kind property received (i.e., its cost if purchased) is *reduced* by a deferred gain or *increased* by deferred loss in determining its basis. This adjustment is made so that if the newly acquired property is later sold, any realized gain or loss that is not recognized (deferred amount) from the previous like-kind exchange will be automatically considered in the computation of the realized gain or loss. Under either method, the basis of any boot received is its fair market value.

---

[89] § 1031(d).

EXHIBIT 15-4
Basis of Property Received in a Like-Kind Exchange

Method 1:

Adjusted basis of property given up.			$xxx,xxx
Plus:	Gain recognized	$xx,xxx	
	Boot paid	x,xxx	
	Liabilities assumed by the taxpayer.	xx,xxx	
	Liabilities encumbering the property received	xx,xxx	+xx,xxx
			$xxx,xxx
Less:	Boot received.	$xx,xxx	
	Liabilities assumed by the other party (transferee)	xx,xxx	
	Liabilities encumbering the property transferred	xx,xxx	−xx,xxx
Basis of property received			$xxx,xxx

Method 2:

Fair market value of like-kind property received.		$xxx,xxx
Less:	Deferred gain (realized gain − recognized gain)	−xx,xxx
Plus:	Realized loss (deferred)	+xx,xxx
Basis of property received		$xxx,xxx

Example 46. J operates a charter flight business out of Ft. Lauderdale. This year he put together a deal with one of his flying buddies whereby he traded his old plane, with a basis of $40,000, for another smaller plane worth $53,000 and a hangar to park it in, worth $7,000. J's realized gain is $20,000 [($53,000 + $7,000 = $60,000) − $40,000]. Since the hangar is realty, it is treated as boot. Thus, J must recognize a gain of $7,000 (lesser of the gain realized or boot received). The basis of the boot received, the hangar, is its fair market value of $7,000. J's basis in the new plane is $40,000, computed as follows:

Method 1:

Adjusted basis of property given up.	$ 40,000
Plus: gain recognized	7,000
Less: boot received.	−7,000
Basis of property received	$ 40,000

Method 2:

Fair market value of like-kind property received.	$ 53,000
Less: Deferred gain ($20,000 − $7,000).	−13,000
Basis of property received	$ 40,000

At first glance, the basis calculations may not make sense. In the substituted basis computation, the basis of the new property is initially the same as the property given up, $40,000. However, any gain recognized, in this case $7,000, must be added to

ensure that upon subsequent sale of the property such gain is not taxed again. The sum of these two amounts ($40,000 + $7,000 = $47,000) represents the basis for the like-kind property and the boot received. A portion of this total is then allocated to the boot by subtracting the value of the boot, $7,000. In effect, the basis assigned to the boot is its $7,000 value, leaving the remaining $40,000 to be assigned to the like-kind property. Note how a subsequent sale of the like-kind property for its $53,000 value would cause the taxpayer to recognize the previously postponed gain of $13,000 ($53,000 − $40,000). This same result is accomplished in a much more obvious manner in the second calculation, where the deferred gain is simply subtracted from the value of the property. The following example is a comprehensive review of the like-kind exchange rules.

Example 47. E exchanged a rental house for T's rental condominium. E's house was worth $36,000 and her adjusted basis was $27,000. The house was not subject to any liabilities. T's condominium was worth $82,000 and was subject to a mortgage of $54,000. T also transferred $8,000 worth of Alpha Corp. stock to E in order to equalize the transaction. T's adjusted basis in his condominium and the Alpha stock were $64,000 and $5,600, respectively. The gains realized by E and T are computed as follows:

E		
Fair market value of property received		
Rental condominium (like-kind property)		$ 82,000
Alpha Corp. stock (boot received)		+8,000
		$ 90,000
Less: Liabilities (mortgage) assumed by taxpayer		−54,000
Amount realized		$ 36,000
Less: Adjusted basis of rent house given up		−27,000
Gain realized		$ 9,000

T		
Fair market value of rental house received		$ 36,000
Plus: Liabilities discharged (assumed by E)		+54,000
Amount realized		$ 90,000
Less: Adjusted basis of properties given up:		
Rental condominium	$64,000	
Alpha Corp. stock (boot paid)	5,600	−69,600
Gain realized		$ 20,400

E's gain recognized is $8,000, the amount of boot (stock) received. The amount of boot received by T is $54,000 (the amount of liabilities discharged), which is reduced by his boot paid of $8,000 (fair market value of Alpha stock). Therefore, T's net liabilities discharged are $46,000. T's recognized gain, however, is $20,400, since recognized gain never exceeds realized gain. T's recognized gain consists of $2,400 ($8,000 fair market value − $5,600 basis) for the taxable exchange of the Alpha stock, and the remaining $18,000 is attributable to the exchange of his house.

E and T's bases in their like-kind property received are determined as follows:

		E's Condominium	T's House
Adjusted basis of like-kind property given up		$27,000	$64,000
Plus:	Gain recognized	+8,000	+20,400
	Boot paid	+0	+5,600
	Liabilities assumed	+54,000	+0
Less:	Boot received.	−8,000	−0
	Liabilities discharged.	−0	−54,000
Basis of property received		$81,000	$36,000

E's basis in the Alpha Corp. stock is $8,000, its fair market value.[90] E and T could have computed their bases in the like-kind property received by using the alternative method (Method 2) discussed previously.

	E	T
Fair market value of like-kind property received:		
Rental house.		$ 36,000
Rental condominium	$ 82,000	
Less: Deferred gain	−1,000	−0
Basis of like-kind property received.	$ 81,000	$ 36,000

EXCHANGE REQUIREMENT

Generally, the determination of whether an exchange has occurred is not difficult. All that is required is a reciprocal transfer of qualifying properties. An exchange of one real estate investment for another would normally qualify. Similarly, a trade-in of a business auto along with some cash for another auto is a qualifying exchange. However, an argument can be made for collapsing seemingly independent transactions that might appear to be an exchange in substance.[91]

> **Example 48.** B, a traveling salesperson, "sold" his business auto to a car dealership for $3,200 cash. Shortly thereafter, he purchased another auto from the same dealer for $12,000 cash. The IRS could collapse the *two* transactions (sale and purchase) between the same parties in *one* like-kind exchange. Thus, if B's basis in the old vehicle was $6,000, his loss would be disallowed, and his basis in the new auto would be $14,800 ($12,000 fair market value of new auto + $2,800 deferred loss).

Three-Corner Exchanges. It is not always easy for two parties with properties of equal value, both of which are suitable to the other party, to get together. Even so, it may be possible for a taxpayer who cannot find an exchange partner to qualify for like-kind treatment through a three-corner exchange.

Several forms of multiple-party exchanges have qualified for like-kind exchange treatment. The IRS has ruled that when three property owners entered into an exchange in which each gave up and received qualifying property, like-kind exchange treatment was

---

90 Reg. §§ 1.1031(d)-1(c) and 1.1031(d)-1(d).

91 Rev. Rul. 61-119, 1961-1 C.B. 395.

appropriate.[92] However, a three-corner exchange must be part of a single, integrated plan.[93]

> **Example 49.** X, Y and Z each own rental property. They exchange the properties as follows:
>
> X gets Y's property, Y gets Z's property, and Z gets X's property. X, Y, and Z pay or receive boot in order to equalize the difference in the values of the properties.
>
> This three-party transaction qualifies as a like-kind exchange under §1031. Each party receiving boot must recognize gain up to the amount of the boot received.

Perhaps a more common situation involves a taxpayer who is willing to "sell" property but does not want to recognize gain. In this situation, the interested buyer purchases like-kind property identified by the "seller" and then exchanges it for the seller's property.

> **Example 50.** C owned rental property worth $70,000 (adjusted basis of $34,000), which she was willing to dispose of only if she could do so without recognizing any gain. B wanted to purchase C's property, but in order that C might defer her potential gain of $36,000, he agreed to purchase another rental property of equal value that was suitable to C. As long as she receives no boot, C would recognize no gain and her basis in the replacement property would be $34,000 ($70,000 fair market value of property received − $36,000 deferred gain). B will not qualify for § 1031 treatment since he purchased the property specifically for the exchange and thus never held it for business use or investment.[94] However, B will not have any realized gain or loss as a result of the transaction since his amount realized of $70,000 (fair market value of rental property received from C) is equal to his cost basis of the property given up.

Delayed Exchanges. The property to be accepted by the taxpayer in a like-kind exchange need not be received *simultaneously* with the transfer of his or her property. Delayed exchanges are popularly referred to as *Starker* exchanges, after a 1979 case in which a taxpayer transferred significant real property in exchange for a promise by a corporation to deliver the replacement property over five years.[95] These exchanges qualify currently for tax deferral only if specific timing requirements are met. In order to qualify for nonrecognition treatment, the property to be acquired must be:

1. Identified within 45 days after the date the taxpayer surrenders his or her property; and

2. Received within 180 days of the transfer, but no later than the due date (including extensions) of the tax return for the year of transfer.[96]

> **Example 51.** R has agreed to purchase any real property worth $120,000 that is acceptable to S if S will immediately transfer his commercial parking lot, which is adjacent to R's store, to R. S agrees to the plan. S later identifies a duplex worth $120,000 and directs R to purchase it for him. This delayed exchange will qualify under § 1031 if the duplex is specified as the replacement property within 45 days

---

92   Rev. Rul. 57-244, 1957-1 C.B. 247; Rev. Rul. 73-476, 1973-2 C.B. 300.

93   Rev. Rul. 75-291, 1975-2 C.B. 332; Rev. Rul. 77-297, 1977-2 C.B. 304.

94   *Biggs v. Comm.*, 81-1 USTC ¶9114, 47 AFTR2d 81-484, 632 F.2d 1171 (CA-5, 1980).

95   *Starker v. U.S.*, 79-2 USTC ¶9541, 44 AFTR 2d 79-5525, 602 F.2d 1341 (CA-9, 1979).

96   § 1031(a)(3).

and is transferred to S within 180 days of the transfer of the parking lot to R. Note how the taxpayer has effectively sold the property for $120,000 cash and then reinvested the cash without having to pay tax.

Delayed exchanges are frequently expedited by an escrow company that holds money that is to be used to purchase a property for the transferor. It is possible that a property would be identified within 45 days but, due to circumstances beyond the taxpayer's control, cannot be acquired. To prevent this misfortune, the taxpayer may identify one or more additional properties within the 45-day period to be acquired if the acquisition of the first property cannot be completed.[97]

Related-Party Exchanges. For many years, related parties used a clever device to reduce gain on the sale of appreciated property. At the heart of the scheme were the substituted basis rules applied in like-kind exchanges. These rules effectively enabled the taxpayer to create a high basis for what otherwise was low-basis property that the taxpayer planned to sell.

> **Example 52.** T owns all of the stock of D Corporation, which is planning to sell 100 acres of land for $700,000 (basis $100,000). Accordingly, D anticipates that it will recognize a gain of $600,000. To minimize the gain on the sale, however, T transfers one of his real estate investments worth $700,000 (basis $500,000) to the corporation in exchange for the land and subsequently sells the land. T's gain on the sale of the land is only $200,000 ($700,000 − $500,000) since the like-kind exchange rules enabled him to substitute the higher basis of his realty, $500,000, as the basis for the land.

To put an end to the so-called basis-swapping illustrated in *Example 47*, Congress created a special rule. If a taxpayer exchanges property with a *related party* and either taxpayer disposes of the transferred property within two years, the like-kind exchange rules do not apply to the original exchange and any deferred gain must be recognized in the year of the subsequent disposition.[98] For this purpose, the definition of a related party is the same as that used for the loss disallowance rules of §§ 267 and 707(b)(1), which generally includes the taxpayer's family (spouse, brothers, sisters, ancestors, lineal descendants) and certain entities (e.g., corporations and partnerships) in which the taxpayer owns more than a 50 percent interest.

> **Example 53.** Assume the same facts as in *Example 47* above. Under current law T's plan would not work since T and his corporation are considered related parties and he sold the property within two years of the exchange. As a result, both T and D must recognize their deferred gains on the original exchange in the year of the sale. T recognizes a gain of $200,000 ($700,000 − $500,000) and D recognizes a gain of $600,000 ($700,000 − $100,000). T recognizes no gain on the sale itself because his basis in the land is now treated as $700,000 (i.e., his cost) since the original transaction became taxable. Note that T's plan would have worked had T been patient and sold the land more than two years after the exchange.

TREATMENT MANDATORY

Like-kind exchange treatment is mandatory. Therefore, no gain or loss is recognized on any transaction that meets the like-kind exchange requirements even if the taxpayer desires otherwise. Since the provision applies to losses as well as gains, like-kind

---

[97]   Reg. § 1.1031(k)-1. Also see Rev. Proc. 2000-37, 2000 I.R.B. 40, where the IRS provides a safe harbor for exchanges that occur through an intermediary in a reverse order.

[98]   § 1031(f).

treatment may work to the disadvantage of a taxpayer, and it may be to his or her benefit to avoid exchange status.

> **Example 54.** This year B swapped her rental property in Malibu worth $200,000 (basis $230,000) for rental property in Vail worth $175,000 and cash of $25,000. B has realized a loss of $30,000 ($200,000 − $230,000). Although she received boot of $25,000, none of the loss is recognized. In this case, B would probably be better off selling the Malibu property and purchasing the Vail property so that she could recognize her loss.

HOLDING PERIOD

The holding period of like-kind property received in a § 1031 exchange includes the holding period of the property given up on the exchange.[99] This also applies to the holding period of replacement property in an involuntary conversion. However, the holding period of any property received as boot in a § 1031 exchange *begins* on the date of its receipt. In effect, when boot received is property other than money (or liability relief), it is treated as if the taxpayer received money (equal to the property's fair market value) and used it to purchase the property. Consequently, the property's holding period starts on the day of the exchange *and* the basis of the property is its fair market value.

✔️ CHECK YOUR KNOWLEDGE

Review Question 1. This year H retired. He decided to continue to live in Chicago but wanted to get rid of his rental property (fair market value $240,000, basis $140,000) and buy a condominium in Florida. H is now entertaining an offer to sell the property to a real estate mogul who loves the property and is hot to buy. What would you advise?

Without good advice, most taxpayers would sell the property, recognize a $100,000 gain, and pay a capital gains tax of up to $25,000, leaving them with as little as $72,000 to invest. There is a much better approach. H is a perfect candidate for a delayed like-kind exchange. He could "sell" the property and have the buyer transfer the funds to an escrow agent, who would hold the money while H identifies the property in Florida he wants. He must do this within 45 days after the sale. As long as he closes on the new property within 180 days of the transfer (but no later than the due date of the return for the year of the transfer, including extensions), the like-kind exchange provisions will apply and H does not have to recognize the gain!

Review Question 2. At the outset of this chapter, it was indicated that there is a way to pyramid one's wealth to $1 million without ever having to pay tax. How could this be done?

The first step is to make wise investments (typically real estate). If the investor desires to sell after the property has appreciated, he or she may "sell" the property using the delayed like-kind exchange technique just as H did in the previous question. The effect is to invest in replacement property without having to pay any tax. If H can continue to invest successfully, he never has to pay tax along the way to $1 million (and beyond). Note that H does not necessarily have to find a property of equal value, assuming the amount escrowed is reinvested in like-kind property. As long as all of the cash is used and none passes to H, he does not recognize any gain. Thus, H could effectively use the property as a down payment for new property and use additional leverage to accelerate the process.

---

[99] § 1223(1).

Note that the property must be qualifying property. Since like-kind exchange treatment does not apply to stocks and bonds, this scheme would not work with respect to stock market investments.

Review Question 3. True-False. This year D swapped her billiard parlor building for a bowling alley building. The transaction qualifies as a like-kind exchange.

True. Although the properties are not considered similar or related in use according to the functional use test applied to involuntary conversion rules, the two investments are considered like-kind property since they are both realty.

Review Question 4. True-False. During the year, E exchanged her personal residence for a rental house. The swap qualifies as a like-kind exchange.

False. The properties exchanged must be held for productive use or investment. In this case, E is not holding her home for investment, and therefore the exchange is taxable.

Review Question 5. True-False. Under the like-kind exchange rules, a taxpayer must receive cash before any gain realized is recognized.

False. Although this may appear to be true, the taxpayer is taxed whenever boot is received. Any property other than the like-kind property received is treated as boot. For example, the boot could take the form of stock, a note, or even liability relief.

Review Question 6. True-False. This year, F swapped her investment land for a friend's land and $10,000 of cash. As a result, F realized a $20,000 loss. F may recognize a loss of $10,000.

False. Losses are never recognized on a like-kind exchange even if the taxpayer receives boot.

Review Question 7. True-False. G sold her rental property in Galveston for $100,000 and realized a $25,000 gain. Two months later, she used the $100,000 plus an additional $50,000 to purchase another rental property on Padre Island for $150,000. G does not recognize gain since she has not liquidated her investment but continued it in another rental property.

False. Although G seems to have met the spirit of the law, there must, as a general rule, be a direct exchange in order to qualify for nonrecognition under the like-kind exchange provisions. Note that G could have postponed the gain had she taken advantage of the delayed like-kind exchange rules or had she simply had the buyer of her property buy the Padre Island property and then done an exchange.

Review Question 8. During the year, Fred traded one of his buddies a tractor used solely in his construction business for another tractor for the same use. On the date of the trade, the old tractor had an adjusted basis of $3,000. He received in exchange $500 in cash and a smaller tractor with a fair market value of $2,800. Fred should recognize a gain on the exchange of:

 a. $800
 b. $500
 c. $300
 d. $0
 e. None of the above

The answer is (c). Fred realized a gain of $300 [($2,800 + $500 = $3,300) − $3,000]. Since he received boot of $500, he must recognize the lesser of the gain realized, $300, or the boot received, $500.

Review Question 9. Assuming the same facts as above, the basis of the new tractor to Fred would be:

    a. $3,300
    b. $3,000
    c. $2,800
    d. $2,300
    e. None of the above

The answer is (c), as determined below.

Method 1:

Adjusted basis of property given up.	$3,000
Plus: Gain recognized	300
Less: Boot received	−500
Basis of property received	$2,800

Method 2:

Fair market value of like-kind property received.	$2,800
Less: Deferred gain	−0
Basis of property received	$2,800

OTHER NONTAXABLE TRANSACTIONS

CHANGES IN FORM OF DOING BUSINESS

Several provisions in the Internal Revenue Code are intended to allow mere changes in the form of carrying on a continuing business activity without the recognition of gain or loss. Section 721, for example, allows the transfer of property to a partnership in exchange for a partnership interest without the recognition of taxable gain or loss. Section 351 allows a similar treatment when property is transferred to a corporation solely in exchange for its stock by persons possessing control, and § 355 provides for nontaxability in certain corporate reorganizations. These specific topics are addressed in subsequent chapters.

CERTAIN EXCHANGES OF STOCK IN SAME CORPORATION

No gain or loss is recognized by the shareholder who exchanges common stock for common stock or preferred stock for preferred stock in the same corporation under § 1036. The exchange may be voting stock for nonvoting stock, and it is immaterial whether the exchange is with another shareholder or with the issuing corporation.[100] If the exchange is not solely in kind, the rules of § 1031(b) (applicable to like-kind exchanges) are applied to determine the amount of any gain recognized.[101]

---

[100] Reg. § 1.1036-1(a).

[101] Reg. § 1.1036-1(b).

CERTAIN EXCHANGES OF U.S. OBLIGATIONS

Gain may be deferred in the case of certain exchanges of U.S. obligations between the taxpayer and the U.S. Government. Section 1037 applies to exchanges of bonds of the government issued under Chapter 31 of Title 31 (the Second Liberty Bond Act). The Treasury regulations for § 1037 discuss the application of this section.

REPOSSESSION OF REAL PROPERTY

Section 1038 provides that the seller of real property will recognize a gain on the repossession of real property only to the extent the sum of the money and other property besides the repossessed realty received exceeds the gain from the transaction previously reported. This provision applies only to repossessions to satisfy debt obligations received in exchange for the sold property (e.g., foreclosure for nonpayment of mortgage). Such purchase-money obligations must be secured by an interest in the property. If any part of these obligations has previously been deducted as a bad debt, the amount of such deductions is included in income in the year of the repossession.

CERTAIN EXCHANGES OF INSURANCE POLICIES

Section 1035 allows the deferral of gain on the exchange of a life insurance contract for another insurance policy. Additionally, it allows certain exchanges involving annuity contracts and endowment contracts.

TAX PLANNING CONSIDERATIONS

CURRENT RECOGNITION VERSUS DEFERRAL

A basic concept in tax planning, as discussed in earlier chapters, is the deferral of tax payments. Each of the provisions discussed in this chapter (as it relates to gains) is a perfect example of such a deferral. A taxpayer is usually better off by deferring any gain—unless he or she expects to be in a much higher effective tax bracket in the later year when the deferred gain would be recognized. Of course, a taxpayer is *always* better off if he or she can avoid tax altogether, as is the case under § 121. However, if a loss is deferred under § 1031, taxes are accelerated. Thus, if the adjusted basis of business or investment property being disposed of exceeds its fair market value, the nonrecognition treatment of § 1031 should be avoided.

CURRENT GAIN RESULTING IN FUTURE REDUCTIONS

In each case of deferred gain, the mechanism is a reduced basis in the replacement property. If this replacement property is depreciable property, the depreciation deductions will also be smaller. It may be advantageous to report a large gain *currently* if the tax cost is low, and reap the benefit of the larger depreciation deductions in later years.

> **Example 55.** W plans to dispose of a building that would result in capital gain if sold, and acquire similar property in a different location. W could defer gain by arranging an exchange, but his basis in the new property would be low. W also has a large capital loss carryforward that he has been deducting at the rate of $3,000 per year.
>
> If W sells the property, the gain would offset the capital loss carryforward and he would pay no tax. His basis in the new building would be its cost, resulting in larger future depreciation deductions.

IMPORTANCE OF CAPITAL BUDGETING IN DECISION MAKING

In any decision of whether to defer taxes when subsequent tax years are affected, capital budgeting techniques are appropriate in making the decision. When considering possible investment opportunities, a taxpayer must *compare* current investment requirements and tax effects with the future returns from the investment and their tax effects. Some form of present-value analysis will help the taxpayer to make a sound decision. A similar analysis should be applied in deciding the appropriateness of entering into any nontaxable (tax-deferred) transaction.

PROBLEM MATERIALS

DISCUSSION QUESTIONS

15-1 *Repair versus Improvement.* H owned her personal residence for ten years before she had to incur a cost of $4,000 due to a leaking roof. Is this roof maintenance a nondeductible repair or a capitalized improvement? Explain.

15-2 *Principal Place of Residence.* V lived in Milwaukee and worked in Chicago for many years. Finally, V rented an apartment in Chicago, where she stayed on weeknights. Weekends and holidays were spent in Milwaukee. Where is V's *principal* place of residence for purposes of § 121?

15-3 *Section 121 Exclusion.* List the two principal requirements that must be met before one can qualify for the § 121 exclusion upon the sale of a residence.

15-4 *Limit on Amount of Exclusion.* What is the maximum amount of gain that can be excluded under § 121?

15-5 *Loss on Sale of Personal Assets.* Y sold his principal residence and realized a $12,000 loss. What is the proper tax treatment of this loss?

15-6 *Conversion of Residence.* Y purchased a property to be used as a rental on September 15, 1998. Y moved into this house on May 1, 2009 so it would qualify for the § 121 exclusion.
  a. Can the residence eventually qualify for the § 121 exclusion?
  b. If so, how long must Y live in it before the gain can qualify for the exclusion?
  c. Can the entire gain be excluded?

15-7 *Two of Five Years Test.* F sold her primary residence on June 2, 2008, and excluded her $22,500 gain. She purchased and moved into another primary residence on August 5, 2008. On what date can F first qualify for the § 121 exclusion with respect to the second residence?

15-8 *One Sale Every Two Years Rule.* G sold a qualifying residence on June 2, 2008, and excluded his $22,500 gain on his calendar year 2008 return. G had previously purchased and moved into another residence on December 7, 2007. On what date may G first qualify for the § 121 exclusion with respect to the second residence?

15-9 *Sale Due to Unanticipated Events.* S purchased her dream home on April 17, 2008 for $120,000. Then, much to her surprise, she was given a promotion and transferred by her employer. So she sold the home on January 2, 2009, for $170,000.
  a. Does S qualify for the exclusion of gain under § 121?
  b. If so, what is the maximum amount S can exclude?
  c. Under what other circumstances might S be able to qualify for this partial exclusion?

15-10 *Conversion of Rental Property.* R lives in the suburbs of Miami. Several years ago, he bought a condo on the beach. He rented the condo out for several years. During this time, the property appreciated substantially. He is now considering selling his suburban home, converting the condo into his personal residence and then selling it to take advantage of the exclusion for gains on the sale of a personal residence. What advice would you give R?

15-11 *Marriage and § 121.* D gave E a one-half interest in D's home of 10 years as a wedding gift. E moved into the home after the wedding. Eighteen months later, on December 2, 2009, the residence was sold at a gain of $314,500. How much of the gain may be excluded by D and E on their joint return for 2009?

15-12 *Divorce and § 121.* F and G lived in a home that was F's separate property during the duration of their five-year marriage. Upon their divorce, G received title to the property. How much, if any, of the $200,000 gain may G exclude upon the sale of the house one year later?

15-13 *Death of a Spouse and § 121.* X and Y were married on November 14, 2009, after which Y moved into the home that had been owned and occupied by X for more than 30 years. Upon X's death, Y inherited the home that had cost $40,000 and was worth $300,000. How much gain must Y recognize when she sells the home one year after X's death for $315,000?

15-14 *Condemnation.* What is required in order to have "threat or imminence" of condemnation?

15-15 *Replacement Property under § 1033.* How does the concept of "similar or related in service or use" differ between an owner/user of property and an owner/lessor?

15-16 *Replacement Period.* B's beauty salon was destroyed by fire on April 21, 2009. The building was covered by current value insurance, and B realized a gain of $70,000. When must B reinvest in order to defer this gain under § 1033?

15-17 *Making the § 1033 Election.* How does a taxpayer elect to defer gain under § 1033 in involuntary conversions?

15-18 *Interaction of §§ 121 and 1033.* G and H had an amount realized of $800,000 and a gain of $520,000 in 2008 on the insurance recovery from the fire that totally destroyed their residence of ten years. May the taxpayers use both the residence exclusion and the involuntary conversion rules to avoid gain recognition?

15-19 *Ineligible Property.* Property "held for sale" is not eligible for like-kind exchange treatment. Elaborate.

15-20 *Real Property under § 1031.* K proposes to exchange a downtown office building she holds as rental property for a 450-acre ranch in Virginia that she would operate as a horse ranch. Will this transaction qualify for like-kind exchange treatment?

15-21 *Personal Property under § 1031.* What constitutes personal property of "like-kind"?

15-22 *Boot.* What is the meaning of "boot" in § 1031 like-kind exchanges?

15-23 *Liabilities.* Are liabilities discharged always treated as boot received in a like-kind exchange under § 1031? Explain.

15-24 *Basis of Property Received.* How is the basis in the property received in a like-kind exchange under § 1031 determined? What is the basis in any boot received?

15-25   *§ 1031 Elective or Mandatory.* Is like-kind exchange treatment elective with the taxpayer? If not, how could such treatment be avoided if the taxpayer was so inclined?

15-26   *Holding Period.* In the current year, R received a rental house and 300 shares of IBM common stock in exchange for a vacant lot he had held as an investment since April 16, 2005. When does the holding period for the rental house begin? For the IBM stock?

PROBLEMS

15-27   *Calculation of Gain Realized.* M, single. purchased a residence on May 1, 1994 for $195,000. M lived in the residence until June 1, 2000 and from December 1, 2006, until it was sold on May 6, 2009. In between, the property was rented. The following information was derived from M's records:

Purchase closing costs.................................	$ 1,450
Depreciation claimed while the property was rented..........	12,250
Addition of family room (January 2005)...................	23,500
Painting of interior (April 2007).........................	4,200

The property sold for $289,000, and M incurred realtor's commissions of $16,340 and other closing costs of $2,300. The depreciation claimed after May 6, 1997 was $12,250.

   a.   How much is M's basis in the residence at the time of the sale?

   b.   How much is M's gain realized on the sale?

   c.   How much is M's gain recognized?

   d.   How would the answer to "c" differ if any of the rental period had been after December 31, 2008?

15-28   *Section 121 Exclusion.* P and Q, who are married, sold their residence of 19 years on February 12, 2009. The house had cost $120,000 and improvements of $22,000 had been made. The house sold for $750,000. Selling costs of $37,500 were incurred and deferred maintenance costs of $4,500 were paid weeks before the sale. P and Q have taxable income not including this gain of $70,000 on their joint return for the year.

   a.   How much is P and Q's gain realized on this sale?

   b.   How much of that gain, if any, must be recognized? How will it be taxed?

15-29   *Section 121 Exclusion.* Four years ago C bought a sail boat for $225,000. Immediately after the purchase he moved in and it became his principal residence. He keeps the sail boat in a slip near Sarasota but often sails off for weeks at a time. This year he decided to sell the boat. In preparation for sale, he made improvements costing $22,300 and repairs totaling $32,000. He sold the boat for $345,000. How is this sale treated on C's income tax return for the calendar year of sale?

15-30   *Section 121 Exclusion with Depreciation.* V owned a house that cost $200,000 in which she lived from July 1, 1996 until June 30, 2008. From July 1, 2008 until September 30, 2008, the home was rented, and depreciation of $8,000 was claimed. How will the sale of the residence for $325,000 on October 1, 2009 be treated?

15-31   *Limitation on Amount Excluded.* In each of the following situations, determine the maximum amount that may be excluded under § 121.

   a.   H and W sold their home on October 31, 2009. The home was owned as separate property and lived in by W for six years. H lived in the home since they were married three years ago.

   b.   K owned a rental property which she rented to J for several years. Upon marrying J on June 1, 2008, K moved into the house. The house was sold on August 1, 2009. and J and K file a joint return for 2009.

   c.   L, an unmarried individual, purchased and moved into a residence on March 15, 2008 for $650,000. One June 16, 2009, L sold the residence for $825,000 because she was transferred to a new work location.

15-32 *Sale of Principal Residence—Costs.* U received and accepted an offer to purchase her principal residence for $78,000 on March 12 and completed the sale on May 8 (all in the current year). She later purchased a replacement residence. Specify whether each of the following is properly classified as a nondeductible expense, a selling expense, an addition to the basis of the residence that was sold, or none of these.

    a. New garage built during February of the current year at a cost of $12,500 because the city requires that every residence that is sold in the subdivision have a garage.

    b. Real estate transfer taxes of $780 assessed by the city government.

    c. Steam cleaning of carpets for $125 on April 22 and paid for upon completion.

    d. Painting interior of residence completed and paid for in February.

    e. Commissions of $4,680 paid to listing and selling real estate brokers.

15-33 *Sale Due to Unanticipated Events.* Q purchased a new residence on April 17, 2007 for $720,000. Upon receiving a very lucrative offer of employment, Q moved to another city and sold the residence on January 17, 2009, for $1,000,000. How much gain must Q recognize on this sale?

15-34 *Sale of Principal Residence.* During the current year, H and W ended their stormy marriage of 20 years. They had jointly owned a residence valued at $330,000 with a basis of $95,000. As part of their divorce settlement, H sold his interest in the home to W for $165,000. Assuming that there were no selling costs or fixing-up expenses, answer the following:

    a. How much gain must H recognize?

    b. What is W's basis in the residence?

15-35 *Rental Use.* K purchased a house for $200,000 on May 1, 2000. She rented the house to tenants from May 1, 2000 to May 1, 2009 and deducted depreciation of $50,000. On May 1, 2009, she moved into the home and used it as her residence until May 1, 2011. On April 30, 2015, she sold the home for $400,000. What is the amount gain recognized on the sale of the home?

15-36 *Involuntary Conversion.* The business office of K, a real estate broker, was destroyed by fire on August 22, 2009.

    a. By what date must K reinvest to avoid recognizing gain from the insurance proceeds received as a result of the fire?

    b. What type of property must K purchase to avoid recognition?

    c. Would your answers differ if, rather than being destroyed by fire, the office building had been condemned by the state for highway right of way?

15-37 *Involuntary Conversion.* L owned a leased warehouse that was totally destroyed by fire on October 31, 2009. The building had a basis to L of $45,000 and his insurance paid the replacement cost of $75,000. L completed construction of a new warehouse on the same land on December 2, 2011 at a cost of $80,000.

    a. How much gain must L recognize on this conversion?

    b. What is L's basis in the replacement warehouse?

    c. Summarize L's reporting requirements.

    d. How would your answers to parts (a), (b), and (c) differ if L had invested only $65,000 in the replacement property?

15-38 *Involuntary Conversion.* Complete the following table involving certain involuntary conversions in which the taxpayer elects to defer gain. The property is converted into cash and the cash is invested in qualifying replacement property in each case. Each case is independent of the others.

Case	Amount Realized	Adjusted Basis	Amount Reinvested	Gain Recognized	Basis in Replacement
A	$3,000	$1,600	$1,200	$	$
B	3,000	1,300	1,400	$	$
C	6,000	4,000	5,500	$	$
D	7,500	3,400	7,900	$	$
E	8,400	9,000	8,700	$	$

15-39 *Involuntary Conversion Replacement Period.* For each of the following involuntary conversions, state the beginning date and the ending date of the permissible replacement period.

    a. The city of Lemon Tree announced plans to condemn D's rental property on March 15, 2008 and completed condemnation proceedings on June 12, 2009 for $330,000.

    b. Assume the same facts as in part (a), except that the property was D's principal residence.

    c. A fire destroyed G's bike shop on November 7, 2008. G received an insurance settlement on April 12, 2009.

15-40 *Involuntary Conversion—Condemned Real Estate.* The city of Orange Grove condemned T's automobile parts warehouse for use as a community park. Plans to condemn the property were announced on June 14, 2008, instituted on December 12, 2008, and completed on May 1, 2009. T's basis in the warehouse was $235,000, and the condemnation award was $366,000.

    a. Describe the type of property with which T must replace this warehouse in order to qualify for involuntary conversion treatment.

    b. Specify the reinvestment period during which T must reinvest in order to qualify for involuntary conversion treatment.

    c. Determine the amount of gain that T must recognize and T's basis in the replacement property, which costs $387,000.

15-41 *Involuntary Conversion—Destroyed Residence.* B's residence and contents were totally destroyed when a nearby gas main burst. The gas company paid B $90,000 for the building (with a basis of $65,000) and $35,000 for the contents as follows:

	Fair Value	Adjusted Basis
Clothing, personal effects..............................	$10,000	$22,000
Furniture and fixtures	8,000	16,500
Appliances, utensils, etc.	7,000	11,000
Art collection	10,000	4,500

    a. What requirements must be met for B to defer all of his gain under § 1033?

    b. How would your answer differ if the loss had been caused by a fire which was a Presidentially declared disaster and the payments were made by B's insurer (the art collection was not separately listed in the insurance policy)?

15-42 *Interaction of §§ 121 and 1033.* B's home was totally destroyed by fire on May 22, 2009. B, an unmarried individual, received $1,050,000 for the house which had cost $700,000 five years earlier.

    a. How much gain may B exclude under § 121?

    b. Can B defer the remaining gain, if any, under § 1033? If so, how much is the minimum amount that B must reinvest in order to exclude all of the gain?

    c. Assuming that B reinvests $760,000 in another personal residence, what is the amount of gain B must recognize and what is his basis in the replacement residence?

15-43 *Like-Kind Exchange.* F traded in an automobile that was used 100 percent of the time for business for a new auto for the same use. F had fully depreciated the old auto. The auto received was worth $12,000 and F paid $5,000 cash in addition to giving up her old auto.
    a. How much gain must F recognize on the trade-in?
    b. What is F's adjusted basis in the new auto?

15-44 *Like-Kind Exchange.* T transferred his farmland (100 percent business) to V in exchange for a parcel of unimproved urban real estate held by V as an investment. The farm was valued at $400,000 and was subject to a mortgage obligation of $260,000. T's basis in the farm was $340,000. The urban real estate was valued at $450,000 and was subject to a mortgage of $310,000.
    a. How much gain must T recognize on this exchange?
    b. What is T's basis in the urban real estate received?

15-45 *Like-Kind Exchange.* Refer to *Problem 15-44*. Assume that V had a basis of $360,000 in the urban real estate transferred to T.
    a. How much gain must V recognize on the exchange?
    b. What is V's basis in the farm property received?

15-46 *Like-Kind Exchange.* B exchanged undeveloped land worth $245,000 with C for developed land worth $225,000 and DEF corporation stock worth $20,000. B's adjusted basis in the land was $176,000. C's adjusted bases in the land and stock were $243,000 and $17,500, respectively.
    a. How much gain or loss must B recognize in this exchange, and what are his bases in the land and stock received?
    b. How much gain or loss must C recognize in this exchange, and what is her basis in the land received?

15-47 *Like-Kind Exchange.* F exchanged undeveloped land worth $45,000 with G for land worth $42,000 and a personal automobile worth $3,000. F's adjusted basis in the land was $36,000. G's adjusted bases in the land and automobile were $39,500 and $2,500, respectively.
    a. How much gain or loss must F recognize in this exchange, and what are his bases in the land and automobile received?
    b. How much gain or loss must G recognize in this exchange, and what is her basis in the land received?

15-48 *Like-Kind Exchange: Installment Reporting.* D entered into an agreement on December 15, 2008 under which he will immediately receive an apartment complex worth $300,000 and an installment obligation of the buyer for $200,000 with interest at 12 percent annually. D is to give up another apartment complex in which he has a basis of $320,000.
    a. What is the minimum gain that D must recognize on this exchange in 2008?
    b. How much gain must D report when he receives his first principal installment of $20,000 (plus accrued interest) in 2009?

15-49 *Like-Kind Exchanges.* Complete the following table for exchanges that qualify for like kind exchange treatment under § 1031.

Case	Adjusted Basis of Property Given Up	FMV of Property Received	Cash Boot Received	Cash Boot Paid	Gain or Loss Recognized	Basis of Property Received
A	$3,000	$2,500	$ 0	$ 0	$	$
B	5,000	5,000	0	1,000	$	$
C	4,000	6,000	1,000	0	$	$
D	7,000	5,900	600	0	$	$
E	5,000	4,000	2,500	0	$	$
F	3,000	3,200	200	0	$	$
G	4,000	3,600	500	0	$	$

RESEARCH PROBLEMS

15-50 *Exchange of Businesses.* T has owned and operated a taxi service (T's Taxi) for many years, but he now wishes to move to a new city. If T sells his business, he will have a substantial gain. Through a business broker, T has arranged to exchange his business for a limousine service (U's Limos) in the other city. In order to strike the deal, U insists that T sign a covenant-not-to-compete that U and T value at $25,000. The balance sheets (representing fair market values) of the two businesses are as follows:

	T's Taxi	U's Limos
Automobiles	$700,000	$750,000
Computers and data handling equipment	60,000	30,000
Covenant-not-to-compete	25,000	
Goodwill	65,000	60,000
Totals	$850,000	$840,000

In order to equalize the transaction, U will pay T $10,000 cash. T's bases are as follows: in the automobiles, $675,000; in the computers, etc., $65,000; and in the covenant and goodwill, $0. T has asked you to determine the tax effect of this proposed exchange before he completes it.

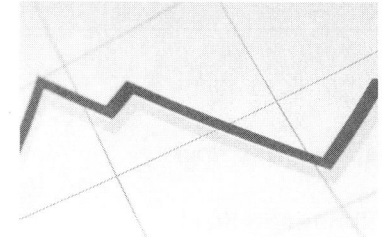

CHAPTER SIXTEEN

PROPERTY TRANSACTIONS: CAPITAL GAINS AND LOSSES

LEARNING OBJECTIVES

Upon completion of this chapter you will be able to:

- Define a capital asset and use this definition to distinguish capital assets from other types of property

- Explain the holding period rules for classifying a capital asset transaction as either short-term or long-term

- Apply the capital gain and loss netting process to a taxpayer's capital asset transactions

- Understand the differences in tax treatment of an individual's capital gains and losses

- Explain the differences in tax treatment of the capital gains and losses of a corporate taxpayer versus those of an individual taxpayer

- Identify various transactions to which capital gain or loss treatment has been extended

- Discuss the tax treatment of investments in corporate bonds and other forms of indebtedness

CHAPTER OUTLINE

The final piece of the property transaction puzzle concerns the treatment of the taxpayer's recognized gains and losses. In the infancy of the tax law, solving this puzzle was relatively easy. Taxpayers who sold or otherwise disposed of property needed only to determine their gain or loss realized and how much, if any, they had to recognize. The actual treatment of the gain or loss recognized—or more precisely, the rate at which it was taxed—was identical to that for other types of income. The simplicity of treating all income and loss the same was short-lived, however, lasting a mere eight years, from 1913 to 1921. Since 1921, the taxation of property transactions has been complicated by the additional need to determine not only the amount of the taxpayer's gain but also its character. Virtually all of this complication can be traced to one source: Congress's desire to provide some type of preferential treatment for capital gains.

Whether capital gains should be taxed more leniently than wages and other types of income is the subject of what seems to be a never-ending debate. When the first income tax statute was enacted, there was nothing in the definition of income to indicate that gains on dealings in property were taxable. Seizing on the omission, taxpayers relied on somewhat abstract tax theory and ingeniously argued that a gain on a sale of property (e.g., a citrus grove) was not the same as income derived from such property (e.g., sale of the fruit) and should not be taxed at all. Moreover, taxpayers who sold property and reinvested in similar property argued that they had not altered their economic position and that taxation was therefore not appropriate. While detractors cried "nonsense!" champions of favorable treatment offered additional justification, explaining that capital gain is often artificial, merely reflecting increases in the general price level. Perhaps the most defensible argument can be found in the Ways and Means Committee Report that

accompanied the Revenue Act of 1921. As the following quotation shows, Congress believed that the progressive nature of the tax rates was unduly harsh on capital gains, particularly when the rate (at that time) could be as high as 77 percent.

> The sale of . . . capital assets is now seriously retarded by the fact that gains and profits earned over a series of years are under present law taxed as a lump sum (and the amount of surtax greatly enhanced thereby) in the year in which the profit is realized. Many of such sales . . . have been blocked by this feature of the present law. In order to permit such transactions to go forward without fear of a prohibitive tax, the proposed bill . . . adds a new section [providing a lower rate for gains from the sale or dispositions of capital assets].[1]

Although the top rate is currently much lower than it has been historically, the bunching effect is still cited as one of the major justifications for lower rates for capital gains. Proponents also reason that taxing capital gains at low rates encourages taxpayers to make riskier investments and also helps stimulate the economy by encouraging the mobility of capital. Without such rules, taxpayers, they believe, would tend to retain rather than sell their assets.

Of course, opponents of special treatment are equally vocal in their objections to the benefits extended capital gains. They reject the proposition that capital gain should not be taxed. They maintain that income is income regardless of its form. Opponents also doubt the stimulus value of preferential treatment and complain about the uneven playing field that such treatment creates. Finally, opponents offer one argument for which there is no denial. As will become all too clear in this and the following chapter, the special treatment reserved for capital gains and losses creates an inordinate amount of complexity in the tax law.

Despite the various objections, Congress has generally sided with those in favor of preferential treatment. But, as history shows, there is little agreement on exactly what that treatment should be. From 1922 to 1933, taxpayers were given the option of paying a flat 12.5 percent tax on their capital gains and the normal rate on ordinary income. From 1934 to 1937, the treatment was altered to allow an exclusion for capital gains ranging from 20 to 80 percent, depending on how long the asset was held. After some tinkering with the exclusion in 1938, Congress moved again in 1942. This time it replaced the exclusion with a deduction equal to 50 percent of the gain. The 50 percent deduction—increased in 1978 to 60 percent—made capital gains the most popular game in town for almost 45 years. In 1986, however, Congress had a complete change of heart. After lowering the top rate on ordinary income to 28 percent, it apparently believed that special treatment for capital gains was no longer needed. Accordingly, favorable capital gain treatment was repealed. This period of low rates, however, proved to be only temporary, as Congress raised the top rate to 31 percent in 1991 and 39.6 percent in 1993. The increase prompted Congress to resurrect favorable treatment for capital gains, in this case providing that the gains of an individual would be taxed at a maximum rate not to exceed 28 percent. In 2003, Congress decided, once again, to improve the tax advantage extended to capital gains. Under the new rules, capital gains qualifying for special treatment can be taxed at one of four different rates (28 percent, 25 percent, 15 percent, 10 percent, or 0 percent).

The current rates applying to capital gains, like their predecessors, can produce substantial savings. The table below illustrates the benefit of the 15 percent capital gains rate. It should be emphasized that the 15 percent rate is 0 percent for 2008 through 2010 for taxpayers whose gains would be taxed at 15 or 10 percent if they were ordinary income.

---

[1] House Rep. No. 350, 67th Cong. 1st Sess., pp. 10–11, as quoted in Seidman, *Legislative History of the Income Tax Laws, 1938–1961*, 813 (1938).

Ordinary Rate	Capital Gains Rate	Differential Rate	Percentage Savings
35.0%	15%	20.0%	57.14%
33.0	15	18.0	54.55
28.0	15	13.0	46.43
25.0	15	10.0	40.00
15.0	0	15.0	100.00
10.0	0	10.0	100.00

As is apparent, capital gain treatment is extremely desirable. But as the remainder of this chapter explains, this favorable treatment is not extended to just any gain. The taxpayer must jump through a few hoops, turn a couple of cartwheels, and clear innumerable hurdles before he or she reaches the pot of gold at the end of the capital gains rainbow.

GENERAL REQUIREMENTS FOR CAPITAL GAIN

A gain or loss is considered a capital gain or loss and receives special treatment only if each of several factors is present. The asset being transferred must be a *capital asset* and the disposition must constitute a *sale or exchange*. In addition, the exact treatment of any net gain or loss can be determined only after taking into consideration the *holding period* of the property transferred. Each of these factors is discussed below.

CAPITAL ASSETS

DEFINITION OF A CAPITAL ASSET

In order for a taxpayer to have a capital gain or loss, the Code generally requires a sale or exchange of a *capital asset*. Obviously, the definition of a capital asset is crucial. Sales involving property that qualifies as a capital asset are eligible for a reduced tax rate while sales of assets that have not been so blessed may not be as lucky.

The Internal Revenue Code takes a roundabout approach in defining a capital asset. Instead of defining what a capital asset is, the Code identifies what is not a capital asset. Under § 1221, all assets are considered capital assets unless they fall into one of five excluded classes. The following are *not* capital assets:

1. Inventory or property held primarily for sale to customers in the ordinary course of a trade or business

2. Accounts and notes receivable acquired in the ordinary course of a trade or business for services rendered or from the sale of inventory

3. Depreciable property and land used in a trade or business

4. Copyrights, literary, musical,[2] or artistic compositions, letters or memoranda, or similar property held by the creator, or letters or memoranda held by the person for whom the property was created; in addition, such property held by a taxpayer whose basis is determined by reference to the creator's basis (e.g., acquired by gift), or held by the person for whom it was created

5. Publications of the United States Government that are received from the Government by any means other than purchase at the price at which they are

---

[2] Beginning May 18, 2006 taxpayers may elect to treat musical compositions or copyrights in musical works as capital assets but only for sales or exchanges of such items and not charitable contributions. See §1221(b)(3).

offered to the public, and which are held by the taxpayer who received the publication or by a transferee whose basis is found with reference to the original recipient's basis (e.g., acquired by gift)

Before looking at some of these categories, one should appreciate the statutory scheme and the rationale behind it.

As noted above, the Code starts with the very broad premise that all property held by the taxpayer is a capital asset. Thus the sale of a home, car, jewelry, clothing, stocks, bonds, inventory, and plant, property, and equipment used in a trade or business would produce, *at least initially*, capital gain or loss since all assets are by default capital assets. However, § 1221 goes on to alter this general rule with several significant exceptions. It specifically excludes from capital asset status inventory, property held for resale, receivables related to the sales of services and inventory, and certain literary properties. As may be apparent, the purpose of these exclusions, as the Supreme Court has said, "is to differentiate between the 'profits and losses arising from the everyday operation of business' on the one hand ... and 'the realization of appreciation in value accrued over a substantial period of time' on the other."[3] In essence, the statute is generally drawn to deny capital gain treatment for income from regular business operations. Income that is derived from the taxpayer's routine personal efforts and services is also treated as ordinary income and in effect receives the same treatment as wages, interest, and all other types of income.

Based on the above analysis, it might seem strange that § 1221 also excludes from capital asset status a class of assets that most people would consider capital assets: the fixed assets of a business (depreciable property and land used in a business). Although it is true that these assets are not "pure" capital assets, as will be seen in Chapter 17, these assets can, if certain tests are met, sneak in the back door and receive capital gain treatment. Also observe that this rule does not exclude intangibles from capital asset treatment even though they may be amortizable. For example, goodwill is a capital asset even though it may be amortized.

One final note: it should be emphasized that the classification of an asset as a capital asset may affect more than the character of the gain or loss on its sale. For example, the amount of a charitable contribution deduction also may be affected in certain instances. For example, generally the amount of a charitable contribution of property is its value but only if its sale would have produced long-term capital gain. Otherwise the amount of the contribution is normally the adjusted basis of the property. For this reason, whether the contributed property is a capital asset is critical. For example, authors and artists can deduct only the adjusted basis of art objects or manuscripts (usually little or nothing) because such assets are not capital assets.[4]

INVENTORY

The inventory exception has been the subject of much litigation and controversy. Whether property is held primarily for sale is a question of fact. The Supreme Court decided in *Malat v. Riddell*[5] that the word "primarily" should be interpreted as used in an ordinary, everyday sense, and as such, means "principally" or of "first importance." As a practical matter, such interpretations provide little guidance. In many cases, it simply boils down to whether the court views the taxpayer as a "dealer" in the particular property or merely an investor. Unfortunately, the line of demarcation is far from clear.

The determination of whether an item is inventory or not frequently arises in the area of sales of real property. In determining whether a taxpayer holds real estate, or a particular tract of real estate, primarily for sale, the courts seem to place the greatest

---

3   *Malat v. Riddell*, 66-1 USTC ¶9317, 17 AFTR2d 604, 383 U.S. 569 (USSC, 1966).

4   See § 170(e)(1) and Chapter 11 for a discussion of these charitable contribution limitations.

5   *Supra*, Footnote 2.

emphasis on the frequency, continuity, and volume of sales.[6] Other important factors considered by the courts are subdivision and improvement,[7] solicitation and advertising,[8] purpose and manner of acquisition,[9] and reason for and method of sale.[10]

COPYRIGHTS, ARTISTIC WORKS, LETTERS AND SIMILAR ITEMS

Should authors and artists be entitled to favorable capital gains treatment on the sale of their works? Should the sale of game show formats like Jeopardy or scripts for television or radio programs produce capital gain to their creators? Prior to 1950, sale of such works were granted lucrative tax treatment even though the property was attributable to the creator's personal efforts.[11] However, amidst growing concerns about the extension of low rates to such transactions, Congress reacted. Section 1223(3) now bars capital asset status to "a copyright, a literary, musical, or artistic composition, a letter or memorandum, or similar property" if the property was created by the taxpayer's personal efforts. In the case of letters, memoranda, and similar property, the disqualification also applies to the person for whom the work was prepared or produced.[12] In addition, a person receiving these items by gift from the creator or the person for whom the work was created is denied capital gain treatment.

The term similar property includes theatrical productions, radio programs, newspaper cartoon strips, manuscripts, diaries, corporate archives, financial records and other property eligible for copyright protection.[13] It is important to emphasize, however, that this provision does not include patents, inventions or other designs that may be protected only under patent law. Thus inventors get favorable capital gain for their creative genius!

Surprisingly, in 2006, Congress created an exception to this rule, allowing taxpayers to elect to treat musical compositions or copyrights in musical works sold as capital assets. This exception extends favorable capital gain treatment not only to the creators of musical compositions (i.e., song writers) but also those who acquire and sell them. This election is available for compositions or copyrights sold or exchanged in a taxable year beginning after May 17, 2006 and before January 1, 2011. It should be noted that musical compositions are not treated as capital assets for purposes of the charitable contributions rules. Thus the deduction for contributions of compositions is not the value but rather the basis of the property, which is usually little or nothing.

> **Example 1.** J is an amateur artist who loved to paint desert landscapes. This year she sold one of her paintings through an art dealer in Santa Fe for $2,000. J has ordinary income on the sale because artistic compositions such as paintings are not capital assets. The result would be the same had J painted the picture for her daughter, D, and D sold the picture. Even though D did not paint the picture herself, it was prepared for her and capital asset status is denied for both the creator and the one for whom it was prepared.

---

6   See, for example, *Houston Endowment, Inc. v. U.S.*, 79-2 USTC ¶9690, 44 AFTR2d 79-6074, 606 F.2d 77 (CA-5, 1979) and *Reese v. Comm.*, 80-1 USTC ¶9350, 45 AFTR2d 80-1248, 615 F.2d 226 (CA-5, 1980).

7   See, for example, *Houston Endowment, Inc.*, and *Biedenharn Realty Co., Inc. v. U.S.*, 76-1 USTC ¶9194, 37 AFTR2d 76-679, 526 F.2d 409 (CA-5, 1976).

8   See, for example, *Houston Endowment, Inc.*

9   See, for example, *Scheuber v. Comm.*, 67-1 USTC ¶9219, 19 AFTR2d 639, 371 F.2d 996 (CA-7, 1967), and *Biedenharn Realty Co., Inc. v. U.S.*

10   See, for example, *Voss v. U.S.*, 64-1 USTC 9290, 13 AFTR2d 834, 329 F.2d 164 (CA-7, 1964).

11   For examples, see *Julius H. Marx* 29 T.C. 88 (1957) and *Jack Benny* 25 T.C. 197 (1955).

12   This expansion was added in 1969 to prevent public officials (e.g., Presidents, Congressmen) from deducting the value of the memorabilia they had collected in office and then contributed to libraries, universities and museums.

13   Reg. § 1.1221-1(c)(1) and (2).

Example 2. B returned from a trip around the world and decided to write a book. This year she died and her son, S, inherited the manuscript which he sold several years later for a gain of $10,000. S would have long-term capital gain because the manuscript is a capital asset since S's basis is not determined in reference to B's basis but is automatically fair market value as of the date of death.

FEDERAL PUBLICATIONS

Publications of the U.S. government (e.g., the Congressional Record) that are given to a taxpayer by the government are not capital assets. This provision was enacted in 1976 primarily to prohibit Presidents, Congressmen, Cabinet members and others from securing charitable contribution deductions for gifts to libraries and museums of items that they collected while working for the government. By denying capital asset treatment for these items, the amount of the contribution is limited to the taxpayer's basis rather than its value.[14] As a result, little or no deduction is available for the contributions.

DISPOSITION OF A BUSINESS

The treatment of the sale of a business depends on the form in which the business is operated and the nature of the sale. If the business is operated as a sole proprietorship, the sale of the proprietorship business is not, as one taxpayer argued, a sale of a single integrated capital asset.[15] Rather, it is treated as a separate sale of each of the assets of the business. Accordingly, the sales price must be allocated among the various assets and gains and losses determined for each individual asset. Any gain or loss arising from the sale of inventory items and receivables would be treated separately as ordinary gains and losses. Gains and losses from the sale of depreciable property and land used in the business would be subject to special treatment discussed in Chapter 17 and may qualify for capital gain treatment. Finally, gains and losses from capital assets would of course be treated as capital gains and losses.

If the business is operated in the form of a corporation or partnership, the sale could take one of two forms: (1) a sale of the owner's interest (e.g., the owner's stock or interest in the partnership) or (2) a sale of all the assets by the entity followed by a distribution of the sales proceeds to the owner. An owner's interest—stock or an interest in a partnership—is a capital asset. Consequently, a sale of such interest normally produces capital gain or capital loss (although there are some important exceptions for sales of a partnership interest). On the other hand, a sale of assets by the entity would be treated in the same manner as the sale of a sole proprietorship, a sale of each individual asset.

✓ CHECK YOUR KNOWLEDGE

Review Question 1. Lois Price operates an office supply store, Office Discount, and owns the property listed below. Indicate whether each of the following assets is a capital asset. Respond yes or no.

a. Refrigerator in her home used solely for personal use
b. The building that houses her business
c. A picture given to her by a well-known artist
d. 100 shares of Chrysler Corporation stock held as an investment
e. Furniture in her office
f. A book of poems she has written

---

[14] See § 170(e)(1). The addition of this rule overturned the holding in Rev. Rul. 75-342 1997-2 CB 341 that such assets were capital assets.

[15] *Williams v. McCowan*, 46-1 USTC ¶9120, 34 AFTR 615, 152 F.2d 570 (CA-2, 1945); Rev. Rul. 55-79, 1955-1 C.B. 370.

    g. The portion of her home used as a qualifying home office

    h. 1,000 reams of paper held for sale to customers

    i. Goodwill of the business

The following are capital assets: (a), (d), and (i). The other assets are not capital assets, including inventory (item h), real or depreciable property used in a trade or business (items b, e, g), literary or artistic compositions held by the creator (item f), or property received by gift from the creator (item c). Note that the Code does not exclude intangible assets from capital assets status. For example, internally generated (i.e., not previously purchased) goodwill that is sold as part of a sale of a business is treated as a capital asset.

Review Question 2. Slam-Dunk Corporation manufactures collapsible basketball rims in Houston, Texas. Because of its tremendous growth, Mr. Slam and Ms. Dunk, the owners of the company, brought in a highly skilled executive to manage it, the famous Sam Jam. As part of the employment agreement, the company agreed to buy Sam's house if it should terminate his contract. Slam and Dunk did not get along with Sam and his creative management techniques. Consequently, the corporation dismissed Sam after two years and purchased his house at Sam's original cost of $300,000. Needing the cash, the corporation decided to unload the house immediately. Unfortunately, in the depressed housing market of Houston, the corporation sold the house for only $200,000. Explain the tax problems associated with the sale by the corporation. What important issue must be resolved and why?

In this situation, the corporation has realized a loss of $100,000. The critical issue is determining whether the loss is an ordinary or capital loss. The treatment, as explained below, is quite different. If the loss is ordinary, the corporation may deduct the entire loss in computing taxable income. In contrast, if the loss is a capital loss, the corporation can deduct the loss only to the extent of any capital gains that it has during the year or a three-year carryback and five-year carryforward period. The determination turns on the definition of a capital asset.

SALE OR EXCHANGE REQUIREMENT

Before capital gain or loss treatment applies, the property must be disposed of in a "sale or exchange." In most cases, determining whether a sale or exchange has occurred is not difficult. The requirement is met by most routine transactions and as a practical matter is often overlooked. Nevertheless, there are a number of situations when a sale or exchange does not actually occur but the Code steps in and creates one, thus converting what might have been ordinary income or loss to capital gain or capital loss. Several of these are considered below.

WORTHLESS AND ABANDONED PROPERTY

When misfortune strikes, leaving the taxpayer with worthless property, the taxpayer normally has a loss equal to the adjusted basis of the property. Note, however, that the loss in these situations does not technically arise from a sale or exchange, leaving the taxpayer to wonder how the loss is to be treated.

Worthless Securities. The Code has addressed this problem with respect to worthless securities (e.g., stocks and bonds). In the event that a qualifying security becomes worthless at any time during the taxable year, the resulting loss is treated as having arisen from the sale or exchange of a capital asset on the last day of the taxable

year.[16] Losses from worthlessness are then treated as either short-term or long-term capital losses depending on the taxpayer's holding period.

> **Example 3.** After receiving a hot tip, N bought 200 shares of Shag Carpets, Inc. for $2,000 on November 1, 2008. Just three months later, on February 1, 2009, N received a shocking notice that the company had declared bankruptcy and her investment was worthless. Because of the worthlessness, N is treated as having sold the stock for nothing on the last day of her taxable year, December 31, 2009. Because the sale is deemed to occur on December 31, 2009 (and not February 1), N is treated as if she actually held the stock for more than a year. As a result, she reports a $2,000 long-term capital loss.

The sale or exchange fiction applies only to qualifying securities. To qualify, the security must be (1) a capital asset and (2) a security as defined by the Code. Under § 165, the term *security* means stock, stock rights, and bonds, notes, or other forms of indebtedness issued by a corporation or the government. When these rules do not apply (e.g., property other than securities), the taxpayer suffers an ordinary loss. Whether a security actually becomes worthless during a given year is a question of fact, and the burden of proof is on the taxpayer to show that the security became worthless during the year in question.[17]

Worthless Securities in Affiliated Corporations. The basic rule for worthless securities is modified for a corporate taxpayer's investment in securities of an affiliated corporation. If securities of an affiliated corporation become worthless, the loss is treated as an ordinary loss and the limitations that normally apply if the loss were a capital loss are avoided.[18] A corporation is considered affiliated to a parent corporation if the parent owns at least 80 percent of the voting power of all classes of stock and at least 80 percent of each class of nonvoting stock of the affiliated corporation. In addition, to be treated as an affiliated corporation for purposes of the worthless security provisions, the defunct corporation must have been truly an operating company. This test is met if the corporation has less than 10 percent of the aggregate of its gross receipts from passive sources such as rents, royalties, dividends, annuities, and gains from sales or exchanges of stock and securities. This condition prohibits ordinary loss treatment for what are really investments.

> **Example 4.** Toy Palace Corporation is the parent corporation for more than 100 subsidiary corporations that operate toy stores all over the country. Each subsidiary is 100 percent owned by Toy Palace. This year the store in Chicago, TPC Inc., declared bankruptcy. As a result, Toy Palace's investment in TPC stock of $1 million became totally worthless. Toy Palace is allowed to treat the $1 million loss as an ordinary loss since TPC was an affiliated corporation (i.e., Toy Palace owned at least 80 percent of TPC's stock and TPC was an operating corporation). Observe that without this special rule, Toy Palace would have a $1 million capital loss that it could deduct only if it had capital gains currently or within the three-year carryback or five-year carryforward period.

Abandoned Property. While the law creates a sale or exchange for worthless securities, it takes a different approach for abandoned business or investment property. When worthless property (other than stocks and securities) is abandoned, the

---

[16] § 165(g).

[17] *Young v. Comm.*, 41-2 USTC ¶9744, 28 AFTR 365, 123 F.2d 597 (CA-2, 1941). Code § 6511(d) extends the statute of limitations from three years to seven years because of the difficulty of determining the specific tax year in which stock becomes worthless.

[18] § 165(g)(3).

abandonment is not considered a sale or exchange.[19] Consequently, any loss arising from an abandonment is treated as an ordinary loss rather than a capital loss, a much more propitious result. Note, however, that the loss is deductible only if the taxpayer can demonstrate that the business or investment property has been truly abandoned and not simply taken out of service temporarily.

CERTAIN CASUALTIES AND THEFTS

Still another exception to the sale or exchange requirement involves *excess* casualty and theft gains from the involuntary conversion of *personal use assets*. As discussed in Chapter 10, § 165(h) provides that if personal casualty or theft gains *exceed* personal casualty or theft losses for any taxable year, each such gain and loss must be treated as a gain or loss from the sale or exchange of a capital asset. Each separate casualty or theft loss must be reduced by $100 before being netted with the personal casualty or theft gains.

Example 5. T had three separate casualties involving personal-use assets during the year:

| | | | Fair Market Value | |
| | | Adjusted | Before | After |
Casualty	Property	Basis	Casualty	Casualty
1. Accident	Personal car	$12,000	$ 8,500	$ 6,000
2. Robbery	Jewelry	1,000	4,000	0
3. Hurricane	Residence	60,000	80,000	58,000

T received insurance reimbursements as follows: (1) $900 for repair of the car; (2) $3,200 for the theft of her jewelry; and (3) $21,500 for the damages to her home. Assuming T does not elect (under § 1033) to purchase replacement jewelry, her personal casualty gain exceeds her personal casualty losses by $300, computed as follows:

1. The loss for the car is $1,500 [(lesser of $2,500 decline in value or the $12,000 adjusted basis = $2,500) − $900 insurance recovery − $100 floor].

2. The gain for the jewelry is $2,200 ($3,200 insurance recovery − $1,000 adjusted basis).

3. The loss from the residence is $400 [(lesser of $22,000 decline in value or the $60,000 adjusted basis = $22,000) − $21,500 insurance recovery − $100 floor].

T must report each separate gain and loss as a gain or loss from the sale or exchange of a capital asset. The classification of each gain and loss as short-term or long-term depends on the holding period of each asset.

It is important to note that this exception *does not* apply if the personal casualty losses exceed the gains. In such case, the *net* loss, subject to the 10 percent limitation, is deductible *from* A.G.I. Recall, however, that casualty and theft losses are among those itemized deductions that are not subject to the deduction cutback rule imposed on high-income taxpayers. (See Chapter 11 for a discussion of this cutback rule.)

Example 6. Assume the same facts in *Example 5* except the insurance recovery from the hurricane damage to the residence was only $11,500. In this case, the loss from the hurricane is $10,400 ($22,000 − $11,500 − $100), and the personal casualty losses exceed the gain by $9,700 ($1,500 + $10,400 − $2,200). T must treat the $9,700 net loss as an itemized deduction subject to the 10% of A.G.I. limitation, but not subject to the cutback rule.

---

[19] Reg. §§ 1.165-2 and 1.167(a)-8.

OTHER TRANSACTIONS

There are still other situations where the sale or exchange requirement is an important consideration. For example, foreclosure, condemnation, and other involuntary events are treated as sales even though they may not qualify as such for state law purposes. Similarly, as discussed in greater detail later in this chapter, the collection of the face value of a corporate bond (i.e., bond redemption) at maturity is treated as a sale or exchange.

HOLDING PERIOD

The exact treatment of a capital gain or loss depends primarily on how long the taxpayer held the asset or what is technically referred to as the taxpayer's *holding period*. The holding period is a critical element in determining which of the various tax rates will apply. As might be expected, the longer the holding period is, the lower the applicable tax rate will be. A *short term* gain or loss is one resulting from the sale or disposition of an asset held *one year or less*.[20] A *long-term* gain or loss occurs when an asset is held for *more than one year*.

In computing the holding period, the day of acquisition is not counted but the day of sale is. The holding period is based on calendar months and fractions of calendar months, rather than on the number of days.[21] The fact that different months contain different numbers of days (i.e., 28, 30, or 31) is disregarded.

> **Example 7.** P purchased 10 shares of EX, Inc. on March 16, 2009. Her gain or loss on the sale is short-term if the stock is sold on or before March 16, 2010, but long-term if sold on or after March 17, 2010.

> **Example 8.** T purchased 100 shares of FMC Corp. stock on February 28, 2009. His gain or loss will be long-term if he sells the stock on or after March 1, 2010.

The holding period runs from the time property is acquired until the time of its disposition. Property is generally considered *acquired* or *disposed* of when title passes from one party to another. State law usually controls the passage of title and must be consulted when questions arise.

STOCK EXCHANGE TRANSACTIONS

The holding period for securities traded on a stock exchange is determined in the same manner as for other property. The trade dates, rather than the settlement dates, are used as the dates of acquisition and sale.

Generally, both cash and accrual basis taxpayers must report (recognize) gains and losses on stock or security sales in the tax year of the trade, even though cash payment (settlement) may not be received until the following year. This requirement is imposed because the installment method of reporting gains is not allowed for sales of stock or securities that are traded on an established securities market.[22]

> **Example 9.** C, a cash basis calendar year taxpayer, sold 300 shares of ARA stock at a gain of $5,000 on December 29, 2009. The settlement date was January 3, 2010. C must report the gain in 2009 (the year of trade).

---

[20]   § 1222.

[21]   Rev. Rul. 66-7, 1966-1 C.B.188.

[22]   § 453(k)(2). See Chapter 14 for a detailed discussion of the installment sale method.

SPECIAL RULES AND EXCEPTIONS

Section 1223 contains a number of special provisions that must be used for determining the holding period of certain properties. The rules address the holding period of property acquired (1) in a tax-deferred exchange; (2) by gift; (3) by inheritance; (4) in a wash sale; (5) as a stock dividend; or (6) by exercising stock rights or options.

Property Acquired in Tax-Deferred Transaction. The holding period of property received in an exchange *includes* the holding period of the property given up in the exchange if the basis of the property is determined by reference, in whole or in part, to the basis in that property given up (e.g., a substituted basis in a like-kind exchange).[23] This rule applies only if the property exchanged is a capital asset or a § 1231 asset (e.g., real or depreciable property used in a trade or business) at the time of the exchange. For this purpose, an involuntary conversion–where the taxpayer normally purchases replacement property for that which was involuntarily converted—is treated as an exchange.[24]

As suggested above, this rule commonly can be found operating when there is a like-kind exchange. For example, if a taxpayer purchased land on May 16, 1981 and swapped it for other land in 2010, the taxpayer's holding period for the new land would begin in 1981 since the basis of the new land is the same as the old land, $50,000, (i.e., the basis of the new land was "determined by reference" to the property given up). Normally, if any gain or loss is deferred, the holding period of the replacement property includes the holding period of the property that was converted or exchanged.

> **Example 10.** In 2008, the city of Milwaukee condemned 10 acres of M's farm land (a § 1231 asset) in order to build an exit for an interstate highway. M had acquired the land on May 1, 1995 for $20,000. M received $120,000 for the land and therefore realized a gain of $100,000. On July 7, 2010, M replaced the property by purchasing new land for $120,000. As a result, he was able to defer all of the realized gain, producing a basis for the new property of $20,000 ($120,000 cost less $100,000 deferred gain). Since an involuntary conversion is treated as an exchange, M's holding period begins on the date that he acquired the original property, May 1, 1995.

Property Acquired by Gift. Another exception provides that if a taxpayer's basis in property is the same basis as another taxpayer had in that property, in whole or in part, the holding period will include that of the other person.[25] Therefore, the holding period of property acquired by gift generally will include the holding period of the donor. This will not be true, however, if the property is sold at a loss and the basis in the property for determining the loss is fair market value on the date of the gift. If the donee's basis is fair market at the date of the gift, the donee's holding period begins on the date of the gift.

> **Example 11.** G received a gold necklace from her elderly grandmother as a birthday gift on August 31, 2009. The necklace was worth $5,200 at that time and had a basis to the grandmother of $1,300. Grandmother had bought the necklace in 1976. Contrary to her grandmother's wishes, G sold the family heirloom for $5,000 on December 13, 2009. G will recognize a gain of $3,700 ($5,000 − $1,300). Her holding period began in 1976 since her $1,300 basis is determined (under § 1015) by reference to her grandmother's basis, *and* her holding period includes the time the necklace was held by her grandmother.

---

[23]   § 1223(1).

[24]   § 1223(1)(A).

[25]   § 1223(2).

Example 12. If G's grandmother had a basis in the necklace of $6,000, G's basis for determining loss would be $5,200, the fair market value at the date of the gift (see discussion in Chapter 14). Because G's basis is *not* determined by reference to her grandmother's basis, the grandmother's holding period is not added to G's holding period and the holding period begins on the date of the gift. Since G only held the necklace for three months, she will have a $200 short-term capital loss ($5,200 basis − $5,000 sales price).

Property Acquired From a Decedent. A special rule is provided for the holding period of property acquired from a decedent. The holding period formally begins on the date of death. However, the Code provides that, if the heir's basis in the property is its fair market value under § 1014 and the property is subsequently sold after the decedent's death, the property is deemed to have a long-term holding period.[26]

Example 13. P sold 50 shares of Xero Corp. stock for $11,200 on July 27, 2009. The stock was inherited from P's uncle who died on May 16, 2009, and it was included in the uncle's Federal estate tax return at a fair market value of $12,000. Since P's basis in the stock ($12,000) is determined under § 1014, the $800 loss on the sale will be a capital loss from property deemed to be held more than 12 months. This would be the case even if P's uncle had purchased the stock within days of his death. The decedent's prior holding period is irrelevant.

Other Holding Period Rules. There are various other provisions that contain special rules for determining holding periods. The holding period of stock acquired in a transaction in which a loss was disallowed under the "wash sale" provisions (§ 1091) is added to the holding period of the replacement stock.[27] Also, when a shareholder receives stock dividends or stock rights as a result of owning stock in a corporation, the holding period of the stock or stock rights includes the holding period of the stock already owned in the corporation.[28] The holding period of any stock acquired by exercising stock rights, however, begins on the date of exercise.[29]

The holding period of property acquired by exercise of an option begins on the day after the option is exercised.[30] If a taxpayer sells the property acquired by option within one year after exercising the option, then he or she will have a short-term gain or loss.

Example 14. N owned an option to purchase ten acres of land. She had owned the option more than one year when she exercised it and purchased the property. Her holding period for the property begins on the day after she exercises the option. Had she sold the option, her gain or loss would have been long-term. If she had sold the property immediately, her gain or loss would have been short-term.

The holding period of a commodity acquired in satisfaction of a commodity futures contract includes the holding period of the futures contract. However, the futures contract must have been a capital asset in the hands of the taxpayer.[31]

---

[26]   § 1223(9).

[27]   § 1223(3); Reg. § 1.1223-1(d).

[28]   § 1223(5); Reg. § 1.1223-1(e).

[29]   § 1223(6); Reg. § 1.1223-1(f).

[30]   See, for example, *Helvering v. San Joaquin Fruit & Inv. Co.*, 36-1 USTC ¶9144, 17 AFTR 470, 297 U.S. 496 (USSC, 1936), and *E.T. Weir*, 49-1 USTC ¶9190, 37 AFTR 1022, 173 F.2d 222 (CA-3, 1949).

[31]   § 1223(8); Reg. § 1.1223-1(h).

TREATMENT OF CAPITAL GAINS AND LOSSES

The Taxpayer Relief Act of 1997 and the amendments of the Jobs and Growth Tax Relief Reconciliation Act of 2003 significantly cut the tax rates on capital gains but not without introducing an inordinate amount of complexity. The adventure begins below.

THE PROCESS IN GENERAL

The first step in determining the treatment of a taxpayer's capital gain or loss is identifying the applicable holding period. Once the holding period is determined, the gain or loss can normally be assigned to an appropriate group to determine its taxation. Historically, there have only been two groups: short-term and long-term. However, beginning in 1997, the law made the classification process a bit more cumbersome, producing the following groups for individual taxpayers.

- *Short-Term group.* Gains and losses from properties held not more than one year
- *Long-Term group.* Generally gains and losses from properties held more than one year. However, individual taxpayers must subdivide the long-term group into additional subgroups according to the rate at which they are to be taxed. The long-term group includes:

   1. The 28% group (28CG and 28CL)
      - Capital gains and losses from collectibles (e.g., works of art, antiques, gold and silver bullion, etc.)[32]
      - Capital gains from qualified small business stock (taxable portion of § 1202 gains discussed below)

   2. The 25% group (25CG)
      - Capital *gains* (and only gains) from the sales of depreciable real estate (e.g., office buildings, warehouses, apartment buildings) that are held for more than 12 months but only to the extent of any unrecaptured straight-line depreciation on such property. (See Chapter 17 for discussion of depreciation recapture.)

   3. The 15% group (15CG and 15CL)
      - Capital gains and losses from the dispositions of other capital assets held more than 12 months.

The effect of the rules is to require taxpayers to assign their capital gains and losses into one of four different groups and net the amounts to determine the net gain or loss in each group as shown below.

	Short-Term	Long-Term		
Holding period (months)	≤12 Ordinary	Collectibles & § 1202 stock > 12 28%	Realty > 12 25%	> 12 15%
Gains	$xx,xxx	$x,xxx	Gains only	$xx,xxx
Losses	(xxx)	(x,xxx)	—	(x,xxx)
Net gain or loss	????	????	Gain only	????

The capital gains of most individuals arise from sales of stocks and bonds and mutual fund transactions. Rarely do individuals have gains from collectibles, § 1202 stock, or

---

[32]   § 1(h)(1)(C) and (h)(4).

depreciable realty. Consequently, for most individuals, the classification and netting process is much easier.

NETTING PROCESS

Generalizations about the treatment of capital gains and losses are difficult because the actual treatment can be determined only after the various groups (i.e., the four groups above) are combined, or netted, to determine the overall net gain or loss during the year. This process is described below.[33]

Netting Within Groups. The first step in the netting process is to combine the gains and losses within each group to produce one of the following:

1. Net short-term capital gain or net short-term capital loss (NSTCG or NSTCL).

2. Net 28% capital gain or net 28% capital loss (N28CG or N28CL).

3. Net 15% capital gain or net 15% capital loss (N15CG or N15CL).

Note that the first step requires no netting in the 25% group since this group initially contains only gains.

Netting Between Groups. The second step requires the combination of the net capital loss positions in any particular group against any net capital gain positions. The treatment of these different groups is explained below.

1. *Short-Term Capital Gains and Losses.* A NSTCG receives no special treatment and is taxed as ordinary income. If a NSTCL results, it may be used to offset net gains of the long-term group in the following order: (1) the net 28% gain; (2) any 25% gain; and (3) the net 15% gain. Any remaining NSTCL not absorbed by the capital gains in the groups above is deductible subject to limitations on the deduction of capital losses discussed below.

2. *28% Group.* A N28CG is taxed at a maximum 28%.[34] Any net loss in the 28% group (N28CL) is applied in the following order: (1) 25% gain; (2) net 15% gain; and (3) NSTCG. Any remaining N28CL that is not absorbed is deductible subject to limitations on the deduction of capital losses discussed below.

3. *25% Group.* The 25% group generally includes *only* capital *gains* from the sales of depreciable real estate held for more than 12 months. Such gains are only included to the extent of any unrecaptured straight-line depreciation on such property. The net 25% capital gain (N25CG) is taxed at a maximum rate of 25%.[35] Note that there can be no net loss in the 25% group.

4. *15% Group.* A N15CG is taxed at a maximum of 15%. However, if the taxpayer's tax bracket (determined by *including* the N15CG) is only 10 or 15%, the net gain falling into these brackets is taxed at 0%.[36] Any N15CL is applied in the following order: (1) the net 28% gain; (2) any 25% gain; and (3) any NSTCG. Any remaining N15CL not absorbed is deductible subject to limitations on the deduction of capital losses discussed below.

---

[33] § 1(h)(1).

[34] § 1(h)(1)(C). Note that 28% gains are taxed at the lower rates (10%, 15%, 25%), if such brackets are not filled by the taxpayer's other taxable income.

[35] § 1(h)(1)(B).

[36] § 1(h)(1)(D) and (E). Note that this is not the case with 28% gains, which would be taxed at the normal 10 or 15% rate.

It should be noted that the three *long-term* groups (the 28%, 25% and 15% groups) are always netted together before taking into accounting any short-term items. Also observe that Congress has generally given taxpayers the best possible treatment of net capital losses in that a NSTCL offsets the net capital gain from the highest taxed group, then the next highest taxed and so on.

Example 15. During the year, T, who is in the 35 percent tax bracket, reported the following capital gains and losses.

	Short-Term	Long-Term 28%	Long-Term 15%
Gains	$10,000	$5,000	$8,000
Losses	(4,000)	(1,000)	(1,000)
Net	$ 6,000	$4,000	$7,000

In this case, T first nets the items within each group. She nets the $10,000 STCG and $4,000 STCL to arrive at a NSTCG of $6,000; she nets a $5,000 28CG and a $1,000 28CL to produce a N28CG of $4,000; and she nets the $8,000 15CG and the $1,000 15CL, resulting in a N15CG of $7,000. No further netting of these groups can occur since each group contains a positive amount. T's NSTCG of $6,000 receives no special treatment and is taxed as ordinary income. T's N28CG is taxed at 28% while her N15CG is taxed at 15%.

Example 16. This year, L, who is in the 28% tax bracket, reported the following capital gains and losses:

	Short-Term	Long-Term 28%	Long-Term 15%
Gains	$10,000	$5,000	$8,000
Losses	(15,000)	(1,000)	(1,000)
Net	($5,000)	$4,000	$7,000
Netting	5,000	(4,000)	(1,000)
Net	$ 0	$ 0	$6,000

Here L has a NSTCL of $5,000 which is netted *first* against N28CG of $4,000, reducing it to zero. The remaining NSTCL of $1,000 would next be offset against N25CG, if any. In this case, there is no N25CG, therefore the remaining NSTCL of $1,000 is offset against the N15CG of $7,000, reducing it to $6,000 which would be taxed at a rate of 15%.

Example 17. This year, X, who is in the 35% tax bracket, reported the following capital gains and losses:

	Short-Term	Long-Term 28%	Long-Term 25%	Long-Term 15%
Gains	$14,000	$1,000	$1,000	$6,000
Losses	(4,000)	(9,000)	—	(1,000)
Net	$10,000	($8,000)	$1,000	$5,000
Netting	(2,000)	8,000	(1,000)	(5,000)
Net	$ 8,000	$ 0	$ 0	$ 0

Here X has a N28CL of $8,000 which is netted first against the 25CGs of $1,000, reducing this group to zero. X next uses the remaining $7,000 N28CL to offset his $5,000 N15CG, reducing it to zero. The remaining N28CL of $2,000 ($7,000 − $5,000) is offset against NSTCG, producing a NSTCG of $8,000 which is treated as ordinary income. Note that the effect of the rules is to net the long-term groups before considering any short-term items. Absent these rules, X would prefer to use the N28CL loss against the NSTCG which would leave $5,000 to be taxed at 15% and $2,000 to be taxed as ordinary income, a far more beneficial result. X must net the long-term groups first.

Treatment of Capital Losses. While capital gains receive favorable treatment, such is not the case with capital losses. As can be seen above, capital losses are first netted with capital gains within the same group (rather than reducing ordinary income). A net capital loss from a particular group can then be combined with net capital gains from the other groups. If after netting all of the groups together, the taxpayer has an overall net capital loss, the loss is deductible against ordinary income. This deduction is limited to the lesser of (1) $3,000 ($1,500 in the case of a married individual filing a separate return) or (2) the net capital loss. In either case, the capital loss deduction cannot exceed taxable income before the deduction.[37] The deductible capital loss is a deduction *for* adjusted gross income. Any losses in excess of the annual $3,000 limitation are carried forward to the following year where they are treated as if they actually occurred in such year. In effect, an unused capital loss can be carried over for an indefinite period.[38] However, should the taxpayer die, any unused capital loss is normally lost.

If the netting process results in a NSTCL and either a N28CL or N15CL or both, the NSTCL is applied first toward the maximum $3,000 limit. For example, if the taxpayer has a NSTCL of $5,000 and a N15CL of $4,000, the NSTCL is used first. Any NSTCL in excess of the $3,000 limit along with any other unused losses may be carried forward to subsequent years indefinitely. In this case, the NSTCL carryover retains its character to be treated just as if it had occurred in the subsequent year. The N15CL or N28CL are both carried over as N28CLs. In other words, any long-term capital loss carryover is carried over as a 28CL. In the example above, $3,000 of the $5,000 NSTCL would be used first against ordinary income and the $2,000 remaining would be carried over as a STCL while the $4,000 N15CL would be carried over as a 28CL. In the absence of a NSTCL or, if after deducting any existing NSTCL, the taxpayer has not reached the annual $3,000 limit for the capital loss deduction, the taxpayer uses any other net capital losses (e.g., the excess of N15CL over N28CG and N25CG or the excess of N28CL

---

[37] § 1212(b).

[38] Reg. § 1.211-1(b)(4)(i).

over 25 CG and N15CG) to reduce ordinary income up to the $3,000 limit.[39] In this regard, the order in which the remaining net capital losses are used is irrelevant since any remaining losses (i.e., the long-term losses) are carried over as a N28CL which is treated as if it occurred in the subsequent year.

Example 18. During the year, B reported the capital gains and losses revealed below. B's only other taxable income included his salary of $50,000. He had no other deductions for A.G.I. The combination of gains, losses, and ordinary income is shown in the following table.

	Short-Term	Long-Term 28%	Long-Term 15%
Gains	$ 10,000	$ 5,000	$ 9,000
Losses	(18,000)	(7,000)	(6,000)
Net	($ 8,000)	($ 2,000)	$ 3,000
Netting (long-term against long-term)		2,000	(2,000)
		$ 0	$ 1,000
Netting (long-term against short-term)	1,000		(1,000)
	($ 7,000)		$ 0
Deduction	3,000		
Carryover	($ 4,000)		

B first nets the long-term items, that is, the N28CL of $2,000 is netted against the N15CG of $3,000. This produces a N15CG of $1,000 ($3,000 − $2,000). B then combines the $8,000 NSTCL and the remaining N15CG of $1,000, leaving a NSTCL of $7,000. In determining his A.G.I., B may deduct only $3,000 of the NSTCL. Therefore his A.G.I. is $47,000 ($50,000 − $3,000). The unused NSTCL of $4,000 ($7,000 − $3,000) is carried forward to future years as a STCL where it is treated as if it arose in the subsequent year.

Example 19. This year, Q reported the capital gains and losses as shown below. He had no other deductions for A.G.I. The combination of gains, losses, and ordinary income is revealed in the following table.

	Short-Term	Long-Term 28%	Long-Term 15%
Gains	$ 1,000	$ 5,000	$ 4,000
Losses	(2,000)	(3,000)	(9,000)
Net	($ 1,000)	$ 2,000	($ 5,000)
Netting (long-term against long-term)	0	(2,000)	2,000
Net	($ 1,000)	$ 0	($ 3,000)
Deduction	1,000		2,000
Carryover	$ 0		($ 1,000)

Here Q has a NSTCL of $1,000 and a net $5,000 N15CL. He first combines the long-term groups, using $2,000 of the $5,000 N15CL to offset the N28CG of $2,000, reducing it to zero. The remaining $3,000 normally would be netted against 25CG if there were any. No further netting is allowed. Therefore, J first uses the NSTCL of

---

$1,000 and then $2,000 of the $3,000 N15CG remaining toward the $3,000 offset against ordinary income. The remaining N15CL of $1,000 is carried over and is treated as a *28CL*. It should be emphasized that the N15CL of $1,000 does not retain its character but becomes a capital loss in the 28% group. Note that the carryover rule is quite favorable. If next year J had $1,000 of N28CG and $1,000 of N15CG, the carryover would wipe out the N28CG, leaving the most favorable gain to be taxed.

Example 20. W's records for 2008 and 2009 revealed substantial ordinary income and the following capital gains and losses:

		Long-Term	
	Short-Term	28%	15%
2008 gains	$ 1,000	$ 5,000	$ 4,000
2008 losses	(2,000)	(9,000)	(9,000)
	$ (1,000)	$ (4,000)	$ (5,000)
2009	$10,000	$12,000	$15,000

In 2008, there can be no further netting. Therefore, W first uses the NSTCL of $1,000 against ordinary income and then uses $2,000 of the $9,000 in long-term losses, leaving a long-term capital loss carryover of $7,000. Note that it makes no difference which long-term loss is used (i.e., the 28% loss or the 15% loss) since all long-term capital loss carryovers are treated as 28CLs.

In 2009, W treats the $7,000 long-term capital loss carryover as a N28CL. As a result, W would report a N28CG of $5,000 ($12,000 − the $7,000 loss carryover), N15CG of $15,000 and a NSTCG of $10,000.

DIVIDENDS TAXED AT CAPITAL GAIN RATES

In negotiations related to the *Jobs and Growth Tax Relief Reconciliation Act of 2003*, Congress and the Bush administration considered a number of alternative statutory schemes to reduce or eliminate the double taxation of corporate dividends.

The result was surprising. Beginning in 2003, qualifying dividends are taxed at capital gains rates:[40] 15 percent generally and in 2008–2010, 0 percent for dividends that would otherwise be taxed at an ordinary rate of 15 percent or lower. Qualified dividends are not included in the capital gain and loss netting process but are simply added to the net capital gain for purposes of computing the tax. As a result, the dividends are taxed at capital gains rates regardless of whether the taxpayer has other capital gains or losses.[41]

Qualified dividends are dividends from domestic corporations or qualified foreign corporations but only if the stock meets a holding period requirement.[42] *Qualified foreign corporations* generally include those that are incorporated in possessions of the United States, those subject to a treaty with the U.S. (involving the exchange of tax information by the governments) and others, the stocks of which are traded on a U.S. stock exchange (certain foreign corporations that are not subject to U.S. tax are not included). The holding period test requires the taxpayer to hold the stock for more than 60 days during a 120 day window that begins 60 days before the stock goes ex-dividend.

---

[40] § 1(h)(11).

[41] Like other long-term capital gains, dividends qualifying for capital gain treatment are not investment income for purposes of the investment interest limitation. However, a taxpayer can elect to treat the dividends as investment income and forego the capital gain treatment. See § 1(h)(11)(D)(i).

[42] § 1(h)(11)(B).

This requirement helps prevent taxpayers from exploiting the preferential treatment for dividends. To illustrate the possible injustice, consider a taxpayer who buys a stock a few days before the ex-dividend date, receives a $1,000 dividend and then sells the stock. Assuming the value of the stock drops in direct proportion to the amount of the dividend, a sale immediately after the ex-dividend date would produce a $1,000 short-term capital loss. It appears that the $1,000 dividend is offset by the $1,000 loss and the net effect is zero. However, the dividend is taxed at 15 percent and the loss may offset ordinary income that is taxed at 35 percent. In such case, the taxpayer is better-off by $200 ($350 − $1500). The holding period rule requires taxpayers to be at risk for at least 61 days if they want to use this scheme.[43]

CORPORATE TAXPAYERS

The capital gains and losses of corporate taxpayers are treated a bit differently from those of individual taxpayers. Corporations separate all of their capital gains and losses into only two groups: short-term and long-term (holding period of more than one year). Unlike individuals, there is no further subdividing of the long-term group. Items within the groups are then netted, producing one of the following: NLTCG, NLTCL, NSTCG or NSTCL. If the taxpayer has a NSTCG and a NLTCG, no further netting is allowed. However, if the taxpayer has either a NSTCL and NLTCG or a NSTCG and a NLTCL, these results can be combined to produce a final position. This can be illustrated as follows:

	Short-Term	Long-Term	Result
Holding period (months)	≤ 12	> 12	
Gains	$xx,xxx	$xx,xxx	
Losses	(xxx)	(x,xxx)	
Net gain or loss	????	????	
Possibilities	NSTCG	NLTCG	No further netting
	NSTCG	NLTCL	NLTCL or NSTCG
	NSTCL	NLTCG	NSTCL or NLTCG
	NSTCL	NLTCL	No further netting

A corporate taxpayer receives no special treatment for either a NSTCG or NLTCG.[44] They are treated just like ordinary income. If after netting, the corporation has a NSTCL or a NLTCL, such losses receive special treatment. Unlike an individual taxpayer, a corporation is not allowed to offset capital losses against ordinary income. A corporate taxpayer's capital losses can be used only to reduce its capital gains.[45] Any excess losses are first carried back to the three prior years as *short-term capital losses* and offset against any net short-term capital gains and then any net long-term capital gains. Absent any capital gains in the three prior years, or if the loss carried back exceeds any capital gains, the excess may be carried forward for five years.[46] If the loss is not used at the end of the five year period, it is lost.

Example 21. An examination of C Corporation's records for 2009 revealed $200,000 of net ordinary taxable income, a long-term capital loss of $9,000 and a short-term capital gain of $2,000. The corporation nets the loss against the gain to produce a NLTCL of $7,000. The corporation cannot offset the loss against

---

[43] The holding period is extended for preferred stock. For other special rules see § 1(h)(11).

[44] For tax years ending after May 22, 2008 and beginning before May 22, 2009, NLTCGs from the sale of certain timber by a C Corporation are taxed at a maximum rate of 15 percent. See § 1201(b).

[45] § 1212(a).

[46] *Ibid.*

ordinary income and, therefore, reports $200,000 of taxable income (undiminished by the NLTCL). Instead the NLTCL is carried back to the third prior year, 2006, as a STCL where it can be used to first offset any NSTCG and then any NLTCG. If there are no capital gains in 2006, the corporation would carryover the loss, now a STCL of $7,000, to 2007 to use against capital gains. This process would continue until the loss is entirely used or it expires at the end of 2014. Note that when the loss is used in prior years, an immediate refund can be obtained.

CALCULATING THE TAX

Section 1(h) provides a special tax calculation to ensure that an individual's capital gains will not be taxed at a rate greater than the applicable preferred rate (i.e., in 2009 the 28%, 25%, 15%, 10% or 0% rate). This calculation can only reduce the tax, not increase it.

> **Example 22.** H and W are married. For 2009, their sole source of income was a 15CG of $88,600 from the sale of assets held four years. Their taxable income is computed as follows:

15CG	$88,600
Standard deduction	(11,400)
Exemption deduction (2 × $3,650)	(7,300)
Taxable income	$69,900

The 10% and 15% tax brackets for taxpayers filing jointly in 2009 extend to $67,900 at which point any dollar of income in excess of that amount is taxed at 25%. Since all of the couple's income is from capital gain, however, none of it is taxed at the 15% or 25% ordinary brackets. The effect of the special capital gains calculation is to tax the portion of the N15CG that falls into the 10% and 15% bracket at a 0% rate and the portion that falls into the 25% bracket at 15%. Therefore, $67,900 of the N15CG is taxed at 0% and the remaining $2,000 ($69,900 − $67,900) is taxed at 15%. The total tax is $300 [($67,900 × 0% = $0) + ($2,000 × 15% = $300)].

It may be clear from the above example that whenever an individual's *ordinary* taxable income exceeds the amount that would be taxed at 10 or 15 percent (e.g., $67,900 in 2009 for a joint return, $45,500 for head of household and $33,950 for single), none of the N15CG is taxed at 0 percent. In such case, the taxpayer computes the tax liability by first calculating the regular tax on ordinary taxable income and adding to that a tax of 15 percent on the N15CG. On the other hand, if ordinary taxable income does not exceed the amount that is taxed at 10 or 15 percent, a portion of the N15CG is taxed at the 0 percent rate until the 10 and 15 percent brackets are exhausted. A similar approach applies for N25CGs and N28CGs.

Before proceeding, it is important to understand some statutory terms. The first term is *net capital gain*—the excess of the net long-term capital gain over the net short-term capital loss for a year. If there is no net short-term capital loss, the net capital gain is simply the net gain from the 15 percent group, the 25 percent group, and the 28 percent group combined. If there is a short-term loss, it is the excess of the combined long-term gains minus the net short-term capital loss. The second term is *adjusted net capital gain*—the net capital gain reduced (but not below zero) by the 25 percent gain and the net 28 percent gain (reduced by any net short-term capital loss).

The actual steps to compute the capital gains tax are built into Schedule D of Form 1040. They are also summarized in Exhibit 16-1.

EXHIBIT 16-1
Tax Computation Involving Capital Gains

Step 1.   Calculate the regular income tax using the regular rates on the taxpayer's taxable income

Step 2.   Determine the tax on the *ordinary income*

    a.   Select the greater of—

        ▸ Ordinary taxable income (taxable income − net capital gain), or

        ▸ The lesser of—

        ▸ The maximum amount that would be taxed at 15 percent, or

        ▸ Taxable income − the adjusted net capital gain

    b.   Compute the regular income tax on this amount

Step 3.   Determine the tax on the *net capital gain* by adding the following together

    a.   *Tax on 0 Percent Gains*—0 percent of the portion of the adjusted net capital gain that would have been taxed at 10 or 15 percent when added to ordinary income [i.e., the lesser of (1) the adjusted net capital gain or (2) the maximum amount that would normally be taxed at 10 or 15 percent minus the amount of ordinary income].

    b.   *Tax on 15 Percent Gains*—15 percent of (the adjusted net capital gain minus any 0 percent gains).

    c.   *Tax on 25 Percent Gains*—The lesser of

        ▸ 25 percent of the 25 percent gains, or

        ▸ If less, (1) 10 or 15 percent (respectively) of the amount of the 25 percent gains that, when added to ordinary income and any 0 percent gains, would be taxed at 10 or 15 percent*, plus (2) 25 percent of any remaining 25 percent gains.

    d.   *Tax on 28 Percent Gains*—The lesser of

        ▸ 28 percent of the 28 percent gains, or

        ▸ If less, (1) 10 or 15 percent (respectively) of the amount of the 28 percent gains that, when added to ordinary income, any 0 percent gains, and any 25 percent gains, would be taxed at 10 or 15 percent**, plus (2) 28 percent of any remaining 28 percent gains.

Step 4.   Add the tax on the ordinary income (Step 2) to the tax on the net capital gain (Step 3) to get the total capital gains tax.

Step 5.   The final tax is the lesser of the taxes computed in Step 1 and Step 4.

---

 * This is the amount that would otherwise be taxed at 10 or 15 percent when added to ordinary income and any 0 percent gains (or stated differently, it is the maximum amount that would be taxed at 10 or 15 percent minus the amount of ordinary income and the amount of 0 percent gains).

**This is the amount that would otherwise be taxed at 10 or 15 percent when added to ordinary income, any 0 percent gains, and any 25 percent gains (or, stated differently, it is the maximum amount that would be taxed at 15 percent minus the amount of ordinary income and the amount of 0 percent gains).

Example 23. J and K are married and file a joint return for 2009. They have taxable income of $82,900, including a N15CG of $15,000. Thus they have ordinary taxable income of $67,900. Their tax is computed as follows:

Step 1:	Regular tax on $82,900 = $13,100

Regular tax on $82,900:

Tax on $67,900 (10% and 15% brackets)		$ 9,350
Plus: Tax on excess at 25%		
[($82,900 − $67,900) × 25%]		+3,750
Equals: Total tax		$13,100

Step 2a:	Ordinary income = $67,900 ($82,900 − $15,000)
Step 2b:	Regular tax on ordinary income of $67,900 = $9,350
Step 3:	Tax on the net capital gain = $2,250

    a. Tax on 0% Gains = 0% of zero (All of the net capital gain would have been taxed at a rate exceeding 15% since V's ordinary income plus 25% gains and 28% gains equaled or exceeded $65,100—the limit of the 15% bracket)

    b. Tax on 15% Gains = 15% × $15,000 = $2,250

    c. Tax on 25% Gains = 25% of zero

    d. Tax on 28% Gains = 28% of zero

Step 4:	Total capital gains tax = $11,600 ($9,350 + $2,250)
Step 5:	The final tax is $11,600. The *savings* is $1,500 ($13,100 − $11,600). Note that this $1,500 is the 10% difference (25% − 15%) on the $15,000 gain.

Example 24. V is single for 2009 and has taxable income for the year of $100,000 including the following:

Loss from stock held 11 months	($2,000)
Gain from stamps held for investment 3 years	3,000
Gain from land held 9 years	16,000
Loss from stock held 2 years	(3,000)

V would summarize his gains and losses as follows:

	Short-Term	Long-Term 28%	Long-Term 15%
	($2,000)	$3,000	$16,000
	—	—	(3,000)
	($2,000)	$3,000	$13,000
Netting	2,000	(2,000)	—
	$ 0	$1,000	$13,000

The loss is a STCL since it was held for not more than a year. The gain on the sale of the stamps is treated as a 28CG since it is a collectible. Collectibles are treated as 28CGs even though they may have been held more than 12 months. The gain and loss from the land and stock are both classified as 15% items since they were held more than 12 months. Thus V's overall capital gain is $14,000, consisting of a N28CG of $1,000 and a N15CG of $13,000. V's tax is computed as follows:

Step 1: Regular tax on $100,000 = $21,720

Tax on $82,250 (10%, 15% and 25% bracket)	$16,750
Plus: Tax on excess at 28% [($100,000 − $82,250) × 28%]	4,970
Equals: Total tax	$21,720

Step 2a: Ordinary income = $86,000 ($100,000 − $14,000)

Step 2b: Regular tax on ordinary income of $86,000 = $17,800

Tax on $82,250	$16,750
Plus: Tax on excess at 28% [($86,000 − $82,250) × 28%]	1,050
Equals: Total tax	$17,800

Step 3: Tax on the net capital gain = $2,230 ($280 + $1,950)

    a. Tax on 0% Gains = 0% of zero (All of the net capital gain would have been taxed at a rate exceeding 15% since V's ordinary income exceeded $31,850—the limit of the 15% bracket)

    b. Tax on 15% Gains = 15% × $13,000 = $1,950

    c. Tax on 25% Gains = 25% of zero

    d. Tax on 28% Gains = 28% × $1,000 = $280

Step 4: Total capital gains tax = $20,030 ($17,800 + $2,230)

Step 5: The final tax is $20,030 (the lesser of *Step 1* or *Step 4*). The difference between the regular tax and the capital gains tax is $1,690 ($21,720 − $20,030). Note that this $1,690 is the 13% difference (28% − 15%) on $13,000 (13% × $13,000 = $1,690). There is no capital gain difference on the 28 percent gain since the ordinary rate and the capital gain rate are the same.

Example 25. Same as *Example 22*, except V's total taxable income is $35,000.

Step 1: Regular tax on $35,000 = $4,938

Tax on $33,950	$4,675
Plus: Tax on excess at 25% [($35,000 − $33,950) × 25%]	263
Equals: Total tax	$4,938

Step 2a: Ordinary income = $21,000 ($35,000 − $14,000)

Step 2b: Regular tax on $21,000 = $2,733 ($8,350 × 10% + $12,650 × 15%)

Step 3:   Tax on the net capital gain = $257 ($0 + $7 + $250)

    a.   Tax on 0% Gains = $0 [$12,950 × 0%—The N15CG is taxed at 0% to the extent the limit on the 15% tax bracket exceeds the ordinary income ($33,950 − $21,000 = $12,950)]

    b.   Tax on 15% Gains = $7 [($13,000 − $12,950 = $50) × 15%—The adjusted net capital gain reduced by the portion taxed at 0% multiplied by 15%]

    c.   Tax on 25% Gains = 25% of zero

    d.   Tax on 28% Gains = 25% × $1,000 = $250 [Since ordinary income plus the 0% gains, 15% gains, and 25% gains are more than the limit on the 15% tax bracket ($21,000 + $12,950 + $50 > $33,950) but less than the top of the 25% bracket amounts, the 28% gains are taxed at 25%.]

Step 4:   Total capital gains tax = $2,990 ($2,733 + $257)

Step 5:   The final tax is $2,990 (the lesser of *Step 1* or *Step 4*). The difference between the regular tax and the capital gains tax is $1,948 ($4,938 − $2,990). Note that this savings of $1,948 is the sum of the 15% difference (15% − 0%) on $12,950 or $1,943 and the 10% difference (25% − 15%) on $50 ($13,000 − $12,950) or $5. Observe that there is no difference on the 28% gain that was taxed at the ordinary income rate.

REPORTING CAPITAL GAINS AND LOSSES

Individual taxpayers report any capital gains or losses on Schedule D of Form 1040.[47] This form is designed to facilitate the netting process, with one part used for reporting short-term gains and losses and another part used to report long-term transactions. A third part of the form is available for the second step of the netting process in the event the taxpayer has either NSTCGs and NLTCLs *or* NLTCGs and NSTCLs.

Regular corporations must report capital gains and losses on Schedule D of Form 1120 in much the same manner as individual taxpayers. Partnerships and S corporations must also report capital gains and losses on a separate schedule (Schedule D of Form 1065 for partnerships and Schedule D of Form 1120S for S corporations). However, these conduit entities are limited to the *first* step of the netting process. Each owner (partner or S corporation shareholder) must include his or her share of the results from the entity with the appropriate capital transactions being netted on the owner's Schedule D, Form 1040.

✓ CHECK YOUR KNOWLEDGE

Review Question 1. For 2009, Ms. Reyes earned a salary of $70,000 from her job as an art curator. In addition, she sold stock, realizing the following capital gains and losses:

15CG	$10,000
15CL	(7,000)
STCL	(11,000)

In 2010, she changed jobs, becoming a tax accountant and earning a salary of $300,000. In addition, she realized a 15CG of $12,000.

Compute Ms. Reyes's adjusted gross income for 2009 and 2010 and indicate the amount, if any, that is eligible for preferential treatment as long-term capital gain.

---

[47]   See Appendix for a sample of this form.

Her adjusted gross incomes for 2009 and 2010 are $67,000 and $307,000, respectively. After netting her capital gains and losses in 2009, Ms. Reyes has a net capital loss of $8,000, all of which is short-term. The deduction for capital losses of an individual is generally limited to $3,000. As a result, her adjusted gross income is $67,000 ($70,000 − $3,000). She is entitled to carry over the remainder of her short-term loss of $5,000. In 2010, she nets the $5,000 short-term capital loss against her $12,000 15CG to produce a N15CG of $7,000. The $7,000 is combined with her other $300,000 of salary income to produce an adjusted gross income of $307,000. Of this amount, her N15CG of $7,000 is taxed at a preferred rate of 15 percent.

Review Question 2. True-False. This year Mr. and Mrs. Simpson retired. The couple's only income was a capital gain from the sale of stock held three years. Assuming the Simpsons file a joint return, all $100,000 of their taxable income is taxed at a rate of 15 percent.

False. The tax computation operates to ensure that the 15CG is taxed at 0 percent to the extent that ordinary income does not absorb the 10 and 15 percent brackets. For 2009 the 15 percent bracket for a joint return extends to taxable income of $67,900. Therefore, $67,900 is taxed at a 0 percent rate and the remaining $32,100 is taxed at a 15 percent rate.

The Simpsons should have considered making the sales in two separate years (perhaps 2009 and 2010) if they have no other income in either year. That would allow them to double the benefit of the 0 percent rate.

Review Question 3. True-False. An individual taxpayer is generally entitled to deduct any capital loss recognized during the current year to the extent of any capital gains recognized plus $3,000. Any capital loss in excess of this amount retains its character and may be used in subsequent years until it is exhausted.

True.

CAPITAL GAIN TREATMENT EXTENDED TO CERTAIN TRANSACTIONS

The Internal Revenue Code contains several special provisions related to capital asset treatment. In some instances the concept of capital asset is expanded and in others it is limited. Some of the provisions merely clarify the tax treatment of certain transactions.

PATENTS

Section 1235 provides that certain transfers of patents shall be treated as transfers of capital assets held for more than one year. This virtually assures that a long-term capital gain will result if the patent is transferred in a taxable transaction, because the patent will have little, if any, basis since the costs of creating it are usually deducted under §174 (research and experimental expenditures) in the tax year in which such costs are incurred. Any transfer, other than by gift, inheritance, or devise, will qualify as long as *all substantial rights* to the patent are transferred. All substantial rights have been described as all rights that have value at the time of the transfer. For example, the transfer must not limit the geographical coverage within the country of issuance or limit the time application to less than the remaining term of the patent.[48]

---

[48]   Reg. § 1.1235-2(b).

The transferor must be a *holder* as defined in § 1235(b). The term *holder* refers to the creator of the patented property or to an individual who purchased such property from its creator if such individual is neither the employer of the creator nor related to such creator.[49]

The sale of a patent will qualify for § 1235 treatment even if payments are made over a period that ends when the purchaser's use of the patent ceases or if payments are contingent on the productivity, use, or disposition of the patent.[50] It also is important to note that §§ 483 and 1274, which require interest to be imputed on certain sales contracts, do not apply to amounts received in exchange for patents qualifying under § 1235 that are contingent on the productivity, use, or disposition of the patent transferred.[51]

> **Example 26.** K, a successful inventor, sold a patent (in which she had a basis of zero) to Bell Corp. The sale agreement called for K to receive a percentage of the sales of the property covered by the patent. All of K's payments received in consideration for this patent will be long-term capital gain regardless of her holding period.

LEASE CANCELLATION PAYMENTS

Section 1241 allows the treatment of payments received in cancellation of a lease or in cancellation of a distributorship agreement as having been received in a sale or exchange. Therefore, the gains or losses will be treated as capital gains or losses if the underlying assets are capital assets.[52]

INCENTIVES FOR INVESTMENTS IN SMALL BUSINESSES

Congress has frequently provided incentives for investment in general or for specific investments. The Subchapter S election, for example, was intended to remove any impediment for small business owners who were not incorporating because they believed there was a double tax on corporate profits. Other incentives provide special treatment upon the disposition of certain business interests. The following sections deal with various prominent examples.

LOSSES ON SMALL BUSINESS STOCK: § 1244

Losses on dispositions (e.g., sale or worthlessness) of corporate stock are generally classified as capital losses. For a year in which a taxpayer has no capital gains, the deduction for capital losses would be limited to $3,000 annually. In contrast, a loss on the disposition of a sole proprietorship would be recognized upon the disposition of the assets used in the business. Losses on the sale of many (if not most) of the assets would be treated as ordinary losses, thereby avoiding (or partially avoiding) the $3,000 limit. Similarly, proper planning could result in ordinary loss treatment upon the disposition of interests in businesses operated in the partnership form.

---

[49] For definition of "relative," see § 1235(d).

[50] § 1235(a).

[51] §§ 483(d)(4) and 1274(c)(4)(E). See Chapter 14 for a discussion of the imputed interest rules.

[52] See Chapter 17 for treatment if the asset is a § 1231 asset.

Without special rules, the limitation on deductions for capital losses might discourage investment in new corporations. For example, if an individual invested $90,000 in stock of a new corporate venture, deductions for any loss from the investment, absent offsetting gains, would be limited to $3,000 annually.[53] Thus, where the stock becomes worthless it could take the investor as long as 30 years to recover the investment. This restriction on losses also is inconsistent with the treatment of losses resulting from investments by an individual in his or her sole proprietorship or in a partnership. In the case of a sole proprietorship or a partnership, losses generally may be used to offset the taxpayer's other income without limitation. For example, assume a sole proprietor sank $150,000 into a purchase of pet rocks that he ultimately sold for only $100,000. In such case, he would have an ordinary loss of $50,000, all of which could be used to offset other ordinary income. Assume the same individual invested $150,000 in a corporation that had the same luck. If the taxpayer could at best sell the stock for $100,000, he would realize a capital loss of $50,000. Obviously the sole proprietor is in a much better position. To eliminate these problems and encourage taxpayers to invest in small corporations, Congress enacted § 1244 in 1958.

Under § 1244, losses on "Section 1244 stock" generally are treated as ordinary rather than capital losses.[54] Ordinary loss treatment normally is available *only to individuals* who are the original holders of the stock. If these individuals sell the stock at a loss or the stock becomes worthless, they may deduct up to $50,000 annually as an ordinary loss. Taxpayers who file a joint return may deduct up to $100,000 regardless of how the stock is owned (e.g., separately or jointly). When the loss in any one year exceeds the $50,000 or $100,000 limitation, the excess is considered a capital loss.

> **Example 27.** T, married, is one of the original purchasers of RST Corporation's stock, which qualifies as § 1244 stock. She separately purchased the stock two years ago for $150,000. During the year, she sold all of the stock for $30,000, resulting in a $120,000 loss. On a joint return for the current year, she may deduct $100,000 as an ordinary loss. The portion of the loss exceeding the limitation, $20,000 ($120,000 − $100,000), is treated as a long-term capital loss.

Stock issued by a corporation (including preferred stock issued after July 18, 1984) qualifies as § 1244 stock only if the issuing corporation meets certain requirements. The most important condition is that the corporation's total capitalization (amounts received for stock issued, contributions to capital, and paid-in surplus) must not exceed $1 million at the time the stock is issued.[55] This requirement effectively limits § 1244 treatment to those individuals who originally invest the first $1 million in money and property in the corporation.

> **Example 28.** In 2007, F provided the initial capitalization for MNO Corporation by purchasing 700 shares at a cost of $1,000 a share for a total cost of $700,000. In 2009, G purchased 500 shares at a cost of $1,000 per share or a total of $500,000. All of F's shares otherwise qualify as § 1244 stock. Only 300 of G's new shares qualify for § 1244 treatment, however, since 200 of the 500 purchased caused the corporation's total capitalization to exceed $1 million.

---

[53] A taxpayer can offset any capital losses against capital gains, if any.

[54] § 1244(a).

[55] § 1244(c)(3)(A).

QUALIFIED SMALL BUSINESS STOCK (§ 1202 STOCK)

As part of the *Revenue Reconciliation Act of 1993*, Congress created a new tax incentive to stimulate investment in small business. By virtue of this special rule, individuals who start their own C corporations or who are original investors in C corporations (e.g., initial public offerings) may be richly rewarded for taking the risk of investing in such enterprises.

Exclusion. Under § 1202, noncorporate investors (i.e., individuals, partnerships, estates, and trusts) are allowed to exclude a portion of the gain on the sale of *qualified small business stock* (QSB stock or § 1202 stock) held for more than five years.[56] The exclusion is normally 50 percent of the gain. However, that amount is increased to 75 percent for stock acquired after February 17, 2009 and before January 1, 2011. The balance of this gain is treated as a 28 percent gain. The effect of this provision is to impose a maximum effective tax of 14 percent (50% × 28% maximum capital gain rate) on the gains from such investments,[57] a far lower rate than the 35 percent that may apply to other types of income received by the taxpayer.

> **Example 29.** On October 31, 2002, N purchased 1,000 shares of Boston Cod Corporation for $10,000. The stock was part of an initial public offering of the company's stock that was designed to raise $30 million to open another 200 fast fish restaurants. On December 20, 2009, N sold all of her shares for $50,000. As a result, she realized a capital gain of $40,000, her only gain or loss during the year. Since N was one of the original investors and the stock qualified as § 1202 stock at the time of its issue (assets at that time were less than $50 million), she is entitled to exclude 50 percent of her gain, or $20,000. The maximum tax on the $20,000 gain is $5,600 ($20,000 × 28%). Note that if the taxpayer is in a bracket lower than 28% (e.g., 25%, 15% or 10%), the gain would be taxed at that rate.

In the netting process, only the § 1202 gain remaining after the exclusion is taken into account.

> **Example 30.** Assume the same facts as above, but assume that in addition to the $40,000 gain on § 1202 stock, N also has other long-term capital gains of $10,000 and short-term capital losses of $5,000. N first applies the 50% exclusion and then nets the remainder with the other capital gains and losses. Therefore, N's net capital gain for the year is $25,000 [($40,000 − $20,000 = $20,000) + $10,000 − $5,000].

> **Example 31.** Assume N has a gain on § 1202 stock of $40,000 and a short-term capital loss of $23,000. N first applies the 50% exclusion and then nets the remaining gain with the capital loss. As a result, N has a net capital loss of $3,000 ($20,000 − $23,000).

Rollover Provision. An individual who realizes a gain on the sale of QSB stock held for more than six months can defer recognition of the gain by reinvesting in other QSB stock within 60 days of the sale. Note that the stock qualifies for the rollover provision if it is held more than six months (not five years). The individual must recognize gain to the extent that the amount reinvested is less than the sales price of the original stock. If the taxpayer uses the rollover provision, the basis in the newly

---

[56] Special rules apply for computing the exclusion on the sale of stock in a specialized small business investment company (see following discussion).

[57] § 1h. Recall that the § 1202 gain on the sale of qualified small business stock is excluded from the adjusted net capital gain. Therefore, the 15 percent rate does not apply.

acquired QSB stock is reduced by the deferred gain. The holding period of the new QSB stock includes the holding period of the old QSB stock.

> **Example 32.** D purchased Netbrowser stock two years, for $10,000. The stock qualified as § 1202 stock. After rising dramatically, the stock started to fall so D sold it for $14,000 before he lost all of his profit. He realized a $4,000 gain on the sale. D wanted to preserve the special treatment for § 1202 stock so 45 days after the sale, he reinvested in MMX Inc., another issue of § 1202 stock, for $15,000. D recognizes no gain on the sale since his holding period of two years exceeded the required six months and he reinvested all $10,000 received from the sale of § 1202 stock. His basis in the replacement stock is $11,000 ($15,000 − $4,000) and the two-year holding period of the old stock attaches to the new. Had D reinvested only $13,000, he would have recognized a gain of $1,000 ($14,000 − $13,000) and have a basis in the replacement stock of $10,000 ($13,000 − deferred gain of $3,000). Note that this rollover provision enables the taxpayer to move in and out of positions in QSB stock so long as QSB is repurchased.

§ 1202 Requirements. Stock qualifies as § 1202 stock if it is issued after August 10, 1993 and meets a long list of requirements.

1. At the time the stock is issued, the corporation issuing the stock must be a *qualified small business*. A corporation is a qualified small business if:
   - The corporation is a domestic C corporation
   - The corporation's gross assets do not exceed $50 million at the time the stock was issued (i.e., cash plus the fair market value of contributed property measured at the time of contribution plus the adjusted basis of other assets)

2. The seller is the original owner of the stock (i.e., the stock was acquired directly from the corporation or through an underwriter at its original issue)

3. During substantially all of the seller's holding period of the stock, the corporation was engaged in an active trade or business other than the following:
   - A business involving the performance of providing services in the fields of health, law, engineering, architecture, accounting, actuarial science, performing arts, consulting, athletics, financial services, brokerage services, or any other business where the principal asset is the reputation or skill of one or more of its employees
   - Banking, insurance, financing, leasing, or investing
   - Farming
   - Businesses involving the production or extraction of products eligible for depletion
   - Business of operating a hotel, motel, or restaurant

4. The corporation generally cannot own:
   - Real property with a value that exceeds 10 percent of its total assets unless such property is used in the active conduct of a trade or business (e.g., rental real estate is not an active trade or business)
   - Portfolio stock or securities with a value that exceeds 10 percent of the corporation's total assets in excess of its liabilities

Note that the active trade or business requirement and the prohibition on real estate holdings severely limit the exclusion. These conditions effectively grant the exclusion to corporations engaged in manufacturing, retailing, or wholesaling businesses.

The new provision also imposes a restriction, albeit a liberal one, on the amount of gain eligible to be excluded on the sale of a particular corporation's stock. The

maximum amount of gain that may be excluded on the sale of one corporation's stock is the *larger* of:

1. $10 million, reduced by previously excluded gain on the sale of such corporation's stock; or

2. 10 times the adjusted basis of all qualified stock of the corporation that the taxpayer sold during the tax year.

This exclusion is extremely attractive, but it should be remembered that whatever Congress gives it can also take away. And that is exactly what Congress has done with § 1202 stock. For purposes of the alternative minimum tax, § 57 provides that 7% of the amount excluded from gross income under § 1202 (i.e., 3.5% of the total gain) is a tax preference item. In addition, the excluded gain is generally not considered investment income for purposes of determining the investment interest limitation.

ROLLOVER OF GAIN ON CERTAIN PUBLICLY TRADED SECURITIES

Another creature of the 1993 Act encourages investment in small businesses owned by disadvantaged taxpayers. Individuals and C corporations that recognize gain on the sale of publicly traded securities are allowed to defer recognition of such gain if they reinvest the proceeds from the sale in common stock or a partnership interest in a *specialized small business investment company* (SSBIC).[58] The reinvestment must occur within 60 days of the sale. An SSBIC is generally any corporation or partnership licensed by the Small Business Administration under § 301 of the Small Business Investment Act of 1958 (as in effect on May 13, 1993). This typically includes investment companies that finance small businesses owned by disadvantaged taxpayers.

The maximum amount of gain that a taxpayer may exclude per year is generally limited to $50,000 (or, if smaller, $500,000 reduced by any previously excluded gain). These limits are increased to $250,000 and $1 million, respectively, for C corporations. Note that the special deferral privilege is not available for partnerships, S corporations, estates, or trusts.

The operation of the deferral provision is virtually identical to the rollover rules for gains on the sale of a residence and involuntary conversions. As a general rule, the taxpayer must recognize gain to the extent that the sales proceeds are not properly reinvested. Any gain deferred reduces the basis of the stock acquired.

> **Example 33.** G sold 4,000 shares of IBM stock for $200,000, realizing a long-term capital gain of $40,000. Less than a week later, G used the entire $200,000 plus additional cash of $15,000 to purchase an interest in the P Partnership, an SSBIC. G may exclude the gain of $40,000 since she reinvested at least $200,000 in qualified property within 60 days. Her basis in the partnership interest would be $175,000 ($215,000 cost − $40,000 deferred gain).

DEALERS AND DEVELOPERS

Since property held primarily for sale to customers in the ordinary course of a trade or business (or inventory) is generally excluded from the definition of a capital asset, any gain or loss on the sale of inventory is generally treated as ordinary gain or loss. For taxpayers who would otherwise benefit from capital gain treatment, this is an obstacle. In certain instances, Congress has provided special relief.

---

[58]   § 1202(g).

DEALERS, INVESTORS AND TRADERS OF SECURITIES

With the arrival of the Internet and the ease in which individuals can buy and sell securities (e.g., computerized trading, day traders), the need for taxpayers and practitioners to understand the potential problems has significantly increased. Important differences in the tax treatment exist, depending on whether the taxpayer is an investor, trader or dealer.[59]

Dealers. A dealer is a taxpayer who purchases securities from customers or sells securities to customers in the ordinary course of business. The securities held by a dealer represent inventory held primarily for resale. Dealers are distinguished from traders in two ways: (1) they have customers and (2) their income is primarily based on a mark-up on the buying and selling of securities, rather than obtaining profit from price fluctuations. Dealers report ordinary income or ordinary loss from their business transactions, using the mark-to-market provisions discussed below.

The difficulty with the tax treatment of dealers is that they not only hold stocks and bonds for sale to customers as part of their regular business operations, but they also invest in stocks and bonds for their own account. As may be apparent, the potential for abuse is great. Since long-term capital gain and ordinary loss are generally preferred, securities dealers have the natural tendency to classify the assets to provide the greatest tax benefit. On the other hand, the IRS wants to do just the opposite. To eliminate the potential controversy and prohibit taxpayers from using their hindsight, Congress enacted § 1236. This provision simply requires the dealer to indicate that a particular security is held for investment (and is therefore a capital asset) by the end of the day on which it was acquired. If the security is not properly identified on a timely basis, the dealer must characterize any gain or loss as ordinary.

Investors. In contrast to dealers, investors are not conducting a trade or business. Their income is normally derived from the price movement of the securities as well as dividends and interest. Most individuals are investors. The basic rules discussed in this chapter concerning capital gains and losses (including the wash sales provisions) apply to investors. Investors report their gains and losses on Schedule D. On the expense side, because investors are not carrying on a trade or business, their expenses may be restricted in some way. For example, the investment interest provisions of § 163(d) limit the deduction of investment interest to investment income. Similarly, the home office deduction is not extended to investors since it is allowed only for those carrying on a trade or business. Likewise, § 179 concerning limited expensing is allowed only for property used in a business. Moreover, any expenses that are deductible are treated as investment expenses and characterized as miscellaneous itemized deductions subject to the 2% limitation as well as the 2% cutback rule. And perhaps the most significant problem for investors is the elimination of the deduction of these expenses for purposes of the alternative minimum tax (AMT).

Traders. The tax treatment of a trader's transactions can differ significantly from those of an investor. For this reason, it is important to draw the distinction. Unfortunately, there is not a clear line of demarcation between the two. A trader is one whose stock and security transactions are so regular and continuous as to rise to the level of a trade or business. In this regard, the distinguishing factors are the individual's intent and the frequency or regularity of trades.

Although traders are treated as conducting a business, they do not have inventory and do not have clients. Therefore, their gains and losses on the sales of securities are still treated as capital gains and capital losses and reported on Schedule D, the same as an investor. Similarly, dividend and interest income are still treated as investment income, reported on Schedule B. But expenses are treated much differently. Traders may deduct

---

[59] For an excellent discussion, see Robison and Mark, "On-Line Transactions Intensify Trader vs. Investor Question," *Practical Tax Strategies* (February, 2001).

their expenses such as margin account interest, management fees, home office expenses and others as deductions for A.G.I. on Schedule C. This solves the limitations associated with miscellaneous itemized deductions, the 2% cutback rule and the AMT. Notwithstanding the fact that traders are in a trade or business they are not subject to self-employment tax. Dividends, interest from securities and gain or loss from the sale of capital assets, are not considered self-employment income. In addition to these rules, traders are entitled to special treatment not extended to investors: the use of the mark-to-market rules.

Traders and Mark-to-Market Provisions. Traders are given an important option unavailable to investors. Taxpayers who are considered traders (but not investors) may take advantage of the mark-to-market (MTM) rules of § 475. Under the MTM rules, traders who make the § 475(f) election are deemed to have sold all of their stocks and securities for their fair market value on the last business day of the taxable year. As a result, traders must recognize all gains and losses as of that date. Traders report their gains and losses on Schedule C. Due to the deemed sale, the basis of the securities is increased to fair market value and used as the basis for subsequent transactions. Although making the MTM election eliminates the opportunity to defer income beyond year end, it offers at least one huge advantage. Section 475(d)(3) provides that the gains and losses recognized on the deemed sales are treated as ordinary income or ordinary losses. This rule is extremely important since it allows traders (who make the election) to avoid the limitation on the deduction of capital losses.[60] By making the election, losses can be used to offset all other taxable income without limitation. Moreover, as business losses, they could add to or create a net operating loss that can be carried back two years and forward for twenty years. Also, the wash sales rules do not apply.

Although the MTM election converts capital losses to ordinary losses, it also converts capital gains to ordinary income. As a practical matter, this is of little significance since the income of most traders would be short-term capital gain which is treated as ordinary income. However, traders who want to preserve the possibility of long-term capital gain treatment for certain securities may do so by taking advantage of another special rule. Section 475(f)(1)(B) permits a trader to segregate trader transactions from investor transactions by using separate accounts for each.

For the § 475(f) election to be effective for a particular tax year, a statement must be filed with the IRS no later than the due date (without extensions) for the tax return for the immediately preceding year. Thus, an election for 2008 must be filed no later than the due date of the 2007 return, April 15, 2008. The election is a change in accounting method so those rules (see Chapter 5) must be observed.

SUBDIVIDED REAL ESTATE

The dealer vs. investor debate also raises its ugly head for taxpayers selling land. Is the land held for investment or primarily for resale?

It is not uncommon for a taxpayer to hold land for investment for many years and then subdivide or improve it just before selling it. If the subdivision and improvements are significant, the property will probably be deemed to be held primarily for sale to customers in a trade or business. If the activities are minor, the land probably retains its character as a capital asset. As was pointed out earlier in this chapter, the determination usually is made based on the frequency, continuity, and volume of sales, but development activities are also very important.

---

[60]   To appreciate the mark-to-market election, see L.S. Vines 126 T.C. 279 (2006).

In an attempt to prevent disputes, Congress created a safe harbor that guarantees capital gain treatment where there is a limited amount of subdivision activity. This rule allows the taxpayer, as someone once said, to subdivide and conquer the ordinary income problem. Under § 1237, real estate is not treated as held primarily for sale if all of the following conditions are met:[61]

1. The tract of land has been held at least five years prior to the sale (except in the case of inheritance).

2. The taxpayer has made no substantial improvements to the property that increase the value of the lots sold while the property was owned.

3. The parcel sold, or any part thereof, had not previously been held by the taxpayer primarily for resale.

4. No other real property was held by the taxpayer primarily for sale during the year of the sale.

Even if the requirements are met, the taxpayer may still be required to report a portion of the gain as ordinary income. If five or fewer lots are sold from the same tract of land, the entire gain is capital gain. However, in the year that the sixth lot is sold, all lots sold in that year and later years become the target of § 1237(b). This special rule provides that 5 percent of the sales price (not gain) is ordinary income.[62] In addition, any selling expenses reduce the ordinary income portion of the gain (limited to the amount of ordinary income), rather than the amount treated as capital gain.[63]

> **Example 34.** Twenty years ago X bought 100 acres 20 miles south of Tulsa for $100,000. This year he retired and decided to sell the land. In order to sell the property, he subdivided it into 10 lots of 10 acres each. This year X sold 5 lots for $310,000 and paid a real estate commission of $10,000. As a result, he recognized a gain of $250,000 ($310,000 − $10,000 − $50,000 basis). Since he sold only 5 lots, the gain on each sale is treated as long-term capital gain. Had X sold 6 lots for the same total price, 5% of his selling price, $15,500 (5% × $310,000), would be considered ordinary income and he could reduce this amount by the selling expenses of $10,000, for net ordinary income on the sale of $5,500.

Note that § 1237 applies to property that has been subdivided, but it is of no help where significant improvements have been made to the property.

OTHER RELATED PROVISIONS

NONBUSINESS BAD DEBTS

Bad debt losses from nonbusiness debts are deductible as short-term capital losses. Nonbusiness bad debts are deductible only in the year they become totally worthless since no deduction is allowed for partially worthless debts.[64] These rules and others related to the allowable deduction for bad debts were discussed in Chapter 10.

---

[61] § 1237(a).

[62] § 1237(b)(1).

[63] § 1237(b)(2).

[64] See § 166(d) and related discussion in Chapter 10.

FRANCHISE AGREEMENTS, TRADEMARKS, AND TRADE NAMES

Section 1253 includes specific guidelines for the treatment of both the transferee and the transferor of payments with respect to franchise, trademark, and trade name agreements. The transfer of such rights is *not* treated as the sale or exchange of a capital asset by the transferor *if* he or she retains significant power, right, or continuing interest with respect to the property.[65] Capital gain and loss treatment also is denied for periodic payments that are contingent on the productivity, use, or sale of the property.[66]

"Significant power, right, or continuing interest" is defined in the Code by example. Some of the characteristics listed in the Code as indicative of such power, right, or interest retained by the transferor of the franchise are as follows:[67]

1. The right to terminate the franchise at will;

2. The right to disapprove any assignment;

3. The right to prescribe quality standards;

4. The right to require that the transferee advertise only products of the transferor;

5. The right to require that the transferee acquire substantially all of his or her supplies or equipment from the transferor; and

6. The right to require payments based on the productivity, use, or sale of the property.

The transferee is allowed current deductions for amounts paid or accrued that are contingent on the productivity, use, or sale of the property transferred.[68] Other payments must be at least partially deferred. They generally are amortized over 15 years.[69]

> **Example 35.** M, Inc. and R enter into a franchise agreement that allows R to operate a hamburger establishment using the trade name and products of M, Inc. According to the contract, M, Inc. has retained all six rights that are listed above. R is required to pay M $50,000 upon entering the contract and 2% of all sales. The term of the contract is 25 years with provision for renewals. R must also pay for any supplies provided by M. Both the $50,000 payment and the percentage royalty payment are ordinary income to M, Inc.
>
> R may treat the royalty payments to M, Inc. as ordinary deductions incurred in his trade or business. The initial fee of $50,000 is amortized equally over 10 years beginning with the year in which the payment is made.

SHORT SALES

Investors who believe that the price of a security will fall rather than rise may bank on their belief by using short sales. Selling short essentially means selling shares that are not actually owned. To accomplish this, the seller typically borrows shares from a broker, sells such shares, and agrees to return an equivalent number of substantially identical shares to the broker within a certain period of time. For example, an investor may sell 100 shares of borrowed stock for $100 per share, or $10,000. If the stock price falls to

---

65   § 1253(a).

66   § 1253(c).

67   § 1253(b)(2).

68   § 1253(d)(1).

69   § 197(d)(1)(F).

$80 per share, the investor can purchase 100 shares in the market for $8,000, replace the 100 borrowed shares, and have a tidy profit of $2,000. Of course, if the price goes up to $110, it costs the investor $11,000 to *cover* the short position and a loss is realized.

The tax consequences of short sales are triggered at the time the seller replaces the borrowed shares (i.e., the short position is closed or covered). No gain or loss is recognized until this time.[70] The character of the gain or loss realized depends on whether the asset involved (normally stock) is a capital asset. Determination of the holding period is more confusing. If the replacement securities have been held for a year or less before the *short sale* or are acquired after the sale, the gain or loss realized on closing the position is short term.[71] Moreover, if the taxpayer does not use such stock to replace the borrowed shares, the holding period of such securities starts again, beginning on the date the short position was closed.[72] If the replacement property has been held for more than a year prior to the short sale, the gain or loss recognized on closing is long-term, regardless of the holding period of the actual shares used to close the short position.

> **Example 36.** On March 15, 2007, T purchased 100 shares of S stock for $4,000. On February 15, 2008, T sold 100 shares of S stock short for $5,000. On June 15, 2008, T closed out her short position by delivering the March 15, 2007 shares. Because T held the replacement shares less than one year before she shorted the stock (March 15, 2007 to February 15, 2008), she reports a $1,000 short-term capital gain.

> **Example 37.** Same facts as *Example 34*, except T closed out her position by purchasing 100 new shares on June 15, 2008 for $6,500. In addition, she sold the original shares on August 15, 2008 for $7,000. T reports a capital loss of $1,500 ($5,000 − $6,500) upon covering her short position, and it is short-term since she held substantially identical stock less than a year before she shorted the stock (March 15, 2007 to February 15, 2008). In addition, T reports a *short-term* capital gain on the sale of the original stock of $3,000 ($7,000 − $4,000) even though she has held the stock for more than one year (March 1, 2007 to August 15, 2008). The holding period for the original stock begins again on the date the short sale was closed by virtue of the fact that she owned such stock less than one year before the short sale.

Constructive Sale Treatment for Appreciated Financial Positions. For many years, investors often wanted to lock in their gain positions without having to recognize them for tax purposes. To accomplish this, an investor would sell stock short and close out the position at a later time. This was referred to as selling short against the box. The tax benefit of this technique was eliminated in 1997. Now, if a taxpayer undertakes a short sale or similar disposition of property that he or she owns, the taxpayer must treat the short sale as the disposition of the underlying property and recognize gain as if the underlying property had been sold.[73]

> **Example 38.** P owns 200 shares of BDF Corporation that was purchased at a cost of $24 per share. On November 14 of the current year, P sold 50 shares of BDF short for $50 per share. P is treated as selling the shares for $2,500 on November 14 and must recognize a gain of $1,300 ($2,500 − $1,200).

---

[70]   Reg. § 1.1233-1(a)(1).

[71]   § 1233(b).

[72]   *Ibid.*

[73]   § 1259.

This rule does not apply if the transaction is closed within 30 days after the close of the year of the short sale or similar disposition.

OPTIONS

Options of one variety or another have become commonplace in the business and investment world. They can be used in a variety of ways (e.g., an option to buy a house or buy land), but they are probably best known as a technique—sometimes a speculative one—to invest in the stock and commodities markets. The popularity of options has skyrocketed since the Chicago Board Options Exchange began organized trading in listed options in 1973. Currently, listed options on hundreds of securities can be bought and sold just like the securities themselves. One need only glance at the daily quotes in the *Wall Street Journal* or similar financial resource on the Internet to appreciate this everyday phenomenon. This growth in the use of options requires tax advisers to have some appreciation of how they work and how they are taxed.

For some, however, options are shrouded in a cloud of mystery, an esoteric investment tool too sophisticated for the common investor. In reality, the basic operation of options is not that complicated. An option simply gives the holder the right to buy or sell a specific asset at a certain price by a specified date. A taxpayer who owns an option may either exercise the option, sell the option, or allow it to expire. The tax treatment of these actions is just as straightforward as the operation of the option itself.

Treatment of Option Buyer. If the taxpayer exercises the option, the amount paid for the option is treated as a capital expenditure and added to the taxpayer's basis for the property. If the taxpayer sells the option or allows it to expire, the tax treatment depends on the nature of the underlying property.[74] In other words, if the taxpayer sells the option, the sale is treated as a sale of the option property. Therefore, any gain or loss recognized is a capital gain or loss only if the option property is a capital asset.

Example 39. On May 1, J purchased for $500 an option to buy 100 shares of Wells Fargo common stock at a price of $100 per share at any time before August 2nd. On August 1, when Wells Fargo was trading at $130 per share, J exercised his option and bought 100 shares for $10,000. Although J is immediately better from his purchase, he has no income. The basis of his stock is $10,500 (the $500 cost of the option + the $10,000 cost of the stock) and the holding period begins on August 2nd.

Example 40. On January 2, Compaq common stock was trading at what K thought was a bargain price of $65 per share. Consequently, K purchased for $700 an option to buy 100 shares of Compaq at a price of $80 on or before March 15. After the corporation reported its earnings, the stock value jumped, and by March 1 the price was bouncing between $95 and $100 per share. The value of K's option had also increased, and he sold it for $3,000. Since the option property, the stock, is a capital asset, K reports a short-term capital gain of $2,300 ($3,000 − $700).

Example 41. Same facts as *Example 38*, except Compaq's earnings were disappointing and the value of the stock as well as the value of K's option decreased. On March 15, the stock was trading at $60 per share and K decided to let the option expire. K recognizes a short-term capital loss of $700.

---

[74] § 1234(a). Note that the lapse of an option is treated as a sale or exchange [§ 1234(b)].

Options are generally billed as a way to secure a potentially large profit from a relatively small investment with a known risk. The option buyer knows in advance that the most that can be lost is the amount paid for the option. There are generally two types of options: puts and calls. A *call* is simply the shorthand term given to an option that gives the holder the right to purchase a particular security at a fixed price. All of the discussion and examples above deal with call options. For example, if an individual believes the price of IBM will rise from $50 to $70 over the next several months, she might purchase a call that enables her to buy 1,000 shares at a price far lower than the $50,000 that would be required to actually buy the stock. The ultimate tax treatment of the call depends, as explained above, on whether the taxpayer sells or exercises the option or allows it to lapse.

Treatment of Option Writer (Seller). In any option agreement, there are two parties, the party who buys the option and the person who "writes," or sells, the option. Individuals who write, or sell, call options obligate themselves to deliver a certain number of shares at a particular price in exchange for the payment of some amount referred to as the call premium. If the call is written by a person who owns the underlying stock (a "covered" call), the individual can deliver such stock if the call is exercised. If the writer does not own the stock (a "naked" call), the stock must be purchased to meet the obligation—a very risky situation. Writers of covered calls generally view the call premium as an additional source of income or as a hedge against a possible decline in the value of the stock. If the buyer exercises the call, the writer of the option adds the premium to the amount realized in determining the gain or loss realized on the stock sold. The gain or loss is long-term or short-term depending on the holding period of the underlying stock. If the buyer allows the call to expire, the writer of the call treats the premium received for the option as a short-term capital gain regardless of the actual holding period.[75] The gain is reported at the time the option expires.

> **Example 42.** After discussing it with her broker, W decided to write call options on her 100 shares of Colgate that she bought several years ago for $3,000. She deposited the stock with her broker and instructed him to write a call that allows an investor to purchase 100 shares of Colgate at $40 per share at a premium of $5 per share. Within a few business days, W's account was credited with $500 for writing the call. If the call is not exercised, W has a $500 short-term capital gain. If the call is exercised, W sells her stock and realizes a long-term capital gain of $1,500 ($4,000 + $500 − $3,000).

Puts. To understand puts, one has to mentally shift gears. Puts are the exact opposites of calls. Whereas a buyer of a call buys the right to purchase stock at a fixed price, a buyer of a put buys the right to sell stock at a fixed price. As in short sales, the buyer of a put typically believes that the price of the underlying stock will drop. If the put is sold, the taxpayer reports a short-term capital gain or loss regardless of the holding period. If the put is exercised (i.e., the taxpayer does in fact sell the underlying stock), the amount realized on the sale is decreased by the premium paid for the put. If the put lapses, a loss is allowable as of the date the option expires. As a practical matter, most puts are bought with the intention of selling them.

> **Example 43.** After seeing reports on television that the airline industry was falling on hard times, P believed the current $47 price on Boeing stock would fall. He immediately called his broker and bought a put at a price of $200 on March 4. The put enables him to sell 100 shares of the stock at a price of $45 per share before

---

[75] If the writer of the call is in the trade or business of granting options, the gain would be ordinary rather than capital gain. § 1234(b).

August 24. The price did in fact fall and bottomed at $40 per share. As a result, his put, that is, his right to sell the stock at $45, became more valuable, and he sold the put for $500. P must report a short-term capital gain of $300 ($500 − $200).

CORPORATE BONDS AND OTHER INDEBTEDNESS

Investments in corporate bonds and other forms of indebtedness present several unique problems that must be considered by taxpayers who choose this form of investment. Under the general rules, mere collection of principal payments does not constitute a sale or exchange and, therefore, a capital gain or capital loss cannot result. However, the Code creates an exception for certain forms of debt. This special rule provides that any amounts received by the holder on retirement of any debt are considered as amounts received in exchange for the debt.[76] Consequently, capital gain or loss is normally recognized when the debt is redeemed or sold for more or less than the taxpayer's basis in the debt.

> **Example 44.** B purchased a $1,000, 10% bond issued by Z Corporation for $990. Assuming the bond is held to maturity and redeemed by the corporation, B will recognize a capital gain of $10. If B had sold the bond prior to redemption for $995, he would recognize a capital gain of $5.

A second and more difficult problem to be considered concerns the *interest element* that may be inherent in the purchase price of a corporate bond. For example, if the rate at which a bond pays interest—the stated rate—is less than the current market rate, the bond will sell for less than its face value, or at a discount. In this case, the *discount* effectively functions as a substitute for interest income. Conversely, if the stated rate exceeds the market rate, the bond will sell for more than its face value, or at a premium. Here, the *premium* essentially reduces the amount of interest income. Without special rules, the proper amount of interest income would not be captured and reported in a timely manner.

> **Example 45.** Several years ago when interest rates were 10%, T purchased a $10,000, 8% corporate bond for $8,000, or a $2,000 discount. This year the bond matured and T redeemed the bond for its par value of $10,000. Under normal accounting procedures, the redemption is treated as an exchange and the taxpayer would recognize a long-term capital gain of $2,000 ($10,000 − $8,000). In this case, the taxpayer would have converted the discount of $2,000, which from an economic view is ordinary interest income, to capital gain. Moreover, this income would be deferred until T sold the bond.

The example above illustrates the problems that the special tax rules governing bond transactions address. The provisions ensure that any premium or discount is not treated as part of the capital gain or loss realized on disposition of the bond, but rather is treated as an *adjustment* to the taxpayer's interest income received from the bond. In addition, the Code provides rules for determining how much of the premium or discount will affect interest income and *when* the additional interest income (in the case of discount) or the interest expense (in the case of premium) will be reported.

The Code provides a separate set of rules governing the treatment of premium and discount. In the case of discount, the rules differ depending on when the discount arises. One set applies when the bonds were *originally issued* at a discount (the "original issue discount" provisions) and another set applies if the discount arises when the bonds are purchased later in the open market (the "market discount" rules). The rules governing premium are the same regardless of when the premium arises.

---

[76]   § 1271.

ORIGINAL ISSUE DISCOUNT

When corporate bonds are *issued* at a price less than the stated redemption price at maturity (i.e., the bond's face value), the resulting discount is referred to as *original issue discount*, or more commonly OID. The amount of OID is easily computed as follows:

	Redemption price (face value).............................	$x,xxx
−	Issue price	− xxx
=	Original issue discount	$x,xxx

The OID provisions generally require the holder of the bond to amortize the discount and include it in income during the period the bond is held.[77] For purposes of computing the gain or loss on disposition of the bond, the holder must increase the basis of the bond by the amount of any amortized discount. Any gain or loss on the disposition of the bond normally is capital gain. However, if at the time of issue there was an intention to call the bond before maturity, any gain on the bond is treated as ordinary income to the extent of any unamortized discount.[78]

Before examining the amortization methods, it should be emphasized that the Code furnishes a de minimis rule that may exempt the debt from the OID amortization requirements. OID is considered to be zero when the bond discount is less than one-fourth of one percent of the redemption price at maturity multiplied by the number of complete years to maturity.[79] This may be expressed as follows:

	Redemption price at maturity.........................	$x,xxx
×	Percentage..	× 0.25%
×	Number of complete years to maturity	×x
=	De minimis amount	$x,xxx

In most cases, new bond issues do not create OID because the stated interest rate is set near the market rate so that the amount of discount that arises, if any, does not exceed the de minimis amount. As a result, no amortization is required.

For bonds issued after July 1, 1982, the discount is amortized into income using a technique similar to the effective interest method used in financial accounting.[80] To determine the includible OID, the OID attributable to an accrual period must be computed. This is done by multiplying the *adjusted issue price* at the beginning of the *accrual period* by the *yield to maturity* and reducing this amount by any interest payable on the bond during the period. The adjusted issue price is the bond's original issue price as increased for previously amortized OID. The accrual period is generally the six-month period ending on the anniversary date of the bond (date of original issue) and six months before such date. The yield to maturity must be determined using present value techniques or may be found in bond tables designed specifically for this purpose.[81]

Once the OID attributable to the entire bond period is computed, this amount is allocated ratably to each day in the bond period. The bondholder's includible OID is the

---

[77]   §§ 1271–1275.

[78]   § 1271(a)(2).

[79]   § 1273(a)(3).

[80]   § 1272(a). For bonds issued after July 1, 1982, and before January 1, 1985, the accrual period is one year.

[81]   Given the issue price, the redemption price, and the number of periods to maturity, the yield to maturity may be approximated by reference to appropriate present-value tables.

sum of the daily portions of OID for each day during the taxable year that the owner held the bond.

Example 46. On July 1, 2009, R purchased 100 newly issued 30-year, 8% bonds with a face value of $1,000 for $800 each or $80,000. The bonds pay interest semiannually on July 1 and December 31. The OID rules apply since the $200 discount per bond exceeds the de minimis amount of $75.

Redemption price at maturity	$ 1,000
× Percentage	×0.25%
× Number of complete years to maturity	×30
= De minimis amount	$ 75

Using present value calculations, the annual yield to maturity for this bond is 10.14% (or 5.07% semiannually). The OID that R must include in income in 2009 and 2010 for all of the bonds is computed in the aggregate as follows:

	7/1–12/31 2009	1/1–6/30 2010	10/1–12/31 2010
Adjusted issue price	$80,000	$80,056*	$80,115
Semiannual yield	× 5.07%	× 5.07%	× 5.07%
Total effective interest	$ 4,056	$ 4,059	$ 4,062
Less: Interest received	− 4,000	− 4,000	− 4,000
Includible OID	$ 56	$ 59	$ 62

* $100,000 × 4% = $4,000
*$80,000 + $56 = $80,056

R would include the amount of OID in income in addition to the interest income actually received. Note that the issuer of the bond would include in its annual deduction for interest expense the amount of OID that must be amortized.

Example 47. Assume the same facts as above, except that R sells all of the bonds for $85,000 on July 1, 2010. Assuming there was no intention to call the bonds when issued, R will report a capital gain of $4,885 ($85,000 − $80,115).

Additional computations are required when the purchase price exceeds the original issue price as increased by OID amortized by previous holders. As a practical matter, the issuer of the bond is obligated to provide the taxpayer a Form 1099-OID, Statement of Original Issue Discount, disclosing the amount of interest income to be reported annually. For those who do not receive such a form, the IRS provides a special publication with the necessary information.

For bonds issued before July 2, 1982, the OID is generally included in the income of the holder ratably over the term of the bond (i.e., a straight-line method is used).[82]

Example 48. Assume the bond in *Example 44* was issued prior to July 2, 1982. The original issue discount included annually would be $667 ($20,000 ÷ 30).

---

[82]   § 1272(a); for bonds issued before May 28, 1969, special rules apply. See § 1272(b).

Although the OID rules are to apply to virtually all debt instruments, there are several notable exceptions:[83]

1. U.S. Savings Bonds (which are treated as discussed in Chapter 5)

2. Tax-exempt state and local obligations (although the discount income is not included as taxable income, the taxpayer increases the basis of the instrument)

3. Debt instruments that have a fixed maturity date not exceeding one year [unless held by certain parties identified in § 1281(b), including accrual basis taxpayers]

4. Obligations issued by individuals before March 2, 1984

5. Nonbusiness loans between individuals of $10,000 or less.

In 1984, the coverage of the OID rules was substantially extended to help curb abuses that occurred when a taxpayer sold property and received a note in exchange. The application of the OID rules in this area was discussed in Chapter 14 in conjunction with unstated interest.

MARKET DISCOUNT

As previously noted, without special rules, amortization of discount would not be required where the security was treated as having no OID (e.g., where the discount on the bond when originally issued was small). For example, if a bond having a $10,000 face value bearing 10 percent interest over a 30-year term was issued for $9,500, there would be no OID since the discount is less than $750 (0.25% × 30 × $10,000). In subsequent years, however, interest rates might rise, causing the bond to sell at a substantially greater discount (i.e., lower value), say $8,000 (e.g., if rates rose to 14 percent the bond's price might fall to $8,000). In such case, an investor could purchase the bond and ultimately report the built-in appreciation as capital gain—the $2,000 rise from the discounted price to face value at maturity—notwithstanding the fact that a portion of the increase in value actually represents interest income. Moreover, the investor could borrow amounts to purchase the investment and obtain an immediate deduction for interest on the debt, although the income from the bond was deferred until it was redeemed or sold. This highly publicized and extremely popular investment technique was foreclosed by the Deficit Reduction Act of 1984 for newly issued bonds.

Changes made in 1993 make the rules applicable to *all* bonds purchased after April 30, 1994. Code § 1276 provides that any gain on the disposition of a bond is treated as ordinary income to the extent of any accrued *market discount*. Market discount, in contrast to OID, is measured at the time the purchaser acquires the bond. Hence, market discount is the excess of the stated redemption price over the basis of the bond immediately after *acquisition*.[84] Like OID, market discount is considered to be zero if it is less than one-fourth of one percent of the stated redemption price multiplied by the number of complete years to maturity after acquisition. The portion of market discount that is considered ordinary income upon disposition of the bond is computed assuming the discount accrues ratably over the number of days from the purchase of the bond to the bond's maturity date.

> **Example 49.** On January 1, 2008, T purchased a bond issued in 2007 having a face value of $10,000 for $8,000. The bond matures four years later on January 1, 2012. The market discount on the bond is $2,000, the difference between the stated redemption price of $10,000 and the taxpayer's $8,000 basis in the bond immediately after acquisition (assuming there was no OID). The $2,000 is deemed

---

[83] §§ 1272(a)(2) and 1274(c)(2).

[84] § 1277(a)(2). If the bond also has OID, the market discount is reduced by the amortized portion of OID.

to accrue on a daily basis over the 1,460 days remaining on the bond's term. Assuming T sells the bond for $9,000 on January 2, 2009, her gain is $1,000, of $500 of which is ordinary interest income [$2,000 × (365 ÷ 1,460)] and the remaining $500 is long-term capital gain.

In lieu of using the daily method of computing the accrued market discount, the taxpayer may use the effective interest method similar to that used for amortizing OID. In addition, the taxpayer may elect to report accrued market discount in taxable income annually rather than at the date of disposition. If this election is made, the taxpayer increases the basis of the bond by the amount of market discount included in income.

Congress also enacted provisions limiting the taxpayer's interest deduction on loans to purchase market discount bonds. Section 1277 requires the taxpayer to defer the deduction for interest expense until that time when income from the bond is reported.

CONVERSION TRANSACTIONS

The original issue discount and market discount provisions exist in order to prevent taxpayers from converting ordinary interest income into capital gain when the interest element is in the form of a discount. In certain instances, taxpayers may still be able to avoid this treatment by structuring the transactions somewhat differently. Congress refers to these as *conversion transactions*.

Conversion transactions are certain investments on which the return is attributable to the time value of money, or for which the sales price of the investment is known at the time the investment is made. Upon the sale or disposition of such investments, any gain is treated as ordinary income, rather than capital gain, to the extent of a return on the investment calculated at 120 percent of the applicable federal rate.[85] Any gain in excess of the ordinary income or any loss realized on the investment is treated as capital gain or loss, assuming the contract is a capital asset to the taxpayer.

BOND PREMIUM

The treatment of premium depends in part on whether the interest income on the bond is taxable.[86] When the interest income is taxable, the taxpayer *may* elect to amortize and deduct the premium as interest expense and concomitantly reduce the basis in the bond. The interest expense in this case is considered investment interest and is, therefore, deductible as an itemized deduction to the extent of net investment income. If the taxpayer does not elect to amortize the premium, the unamortized premium is simply included as part of the taxpayer's basis in the bond and thus decreases the gain or increases the loss on disposition of the bond.

If the interest income on the bond is tax-exempt, the premium *must* be amortized and the bond's basis decreased. No deduction is allowed for the amortized premium since it merely represents an adjustment in the amount of nontaxable income received by the holder. In other words, no deduction for the premium is allowed since it represents interest expense related to producing tax-exempt income. Note that by requiring amortization of the premium, the taxpayer is prohibited from securing a deduction for the premium in the form of a capital loss or a reduced gain on the disposition of the bond.

Example 50. V purchased a $1,000 tax-exempt bond for $1,100. If V holds the bond to maturity, all of the premium will be amortized and his basis in the bond will be $1,000. Therefore, on redemption of the bond for $1,000, no gain or loss is

---

[85] § 1258.

[86] § 171.

recognized. However, if amortization of the premium was not required, V would report a capital loss of $100 on redemption of the bond.

The method to be used for amortizing premium depends on when the bond was issued. If the bond was issued before September 28, 1985, the premium is amortized using the straight-line method over the number of months to maturity. Premium on bonds issued on or after that date must be amortized based on the bond's yield to maturity determined when the bond was issued.

TAX PLANNING CONSIDERATIONS

TIMING OF CAPITAL ASSET TRANSACTIONS

A taxpayer with investments that he or she may wish to sell should pay careful attention to the timing of those sales, particularly near the end of a year. Since the netting process takes into consideration only the sales for the year under consideration plus any capital loss carryovers, the year into which a particular transaction falls may have significant impact on the total amount of taxes paid. The taxpayer must also consider market conditions, since he or she may believe that waiting to sell a particular asset may cost more than paying any additional tax.

Strictly from a tax planning perspective, a taxpayer should consider timing the recognition of year-end capital gains and losses using the following strategy:

1. *No Capital Gains or Losses Currently*—recognize up to $3,000 STCL or LTCL to take advantage of the annual capital loss deduction.

2. *Currently Have STCG*—recognize either STCL or LTCL to offset the STCG and more, if possible, to take advantage of the capital loss deduction.

3. *Currently Have LTCG*—recognize either LTCL or STCL to offset the LTCG and more, if possible, to take advantage of the capital loss deduction.

4. *Currently Have STCL*—if less than $3,000, recognize more STCL or LTCL to take advantage of the capital loss deduction. If more than $3,000, recognize either STCG or LTCG to offset the STCL in excess of $3,000.

5. *Currently Have LTCL*—if less than $3,000, recognize more LTCL or STCL to take advantage of the capital loss deduction. If more than $3,000, recognize either STCG or LTCG to offset the LTCL in excess of $3,000.

The current tax rate differential between ordinary income and capital gains for noncorporate taxpayers (including flow-through entities) makes it far more important to distinguish between ordinary income and capital gain. Taxpayers should carefully plan in order to secure the benefit of this rate differential, which can be as great as 20 percent (35% − 15%).

SECTION 1244 STOCK

The importance of § 1244 should not be overlooked when making an investment.

Example 51. Dr G is extremely successful and consequently is often approached by friends, promoters, and others asking her to make an investment in one deal or another. If G loans $30,000 to a friend to start a business which ultimately fails, the loss would be governed by the worthless-security rules and thus treated as a capital loss. In such case, Dr. G's annual loss deduction is limited to the extent of her

capital gains plus $3,000. If G has no capital gains (which are not necessarily easily found), it could take her as long as ten years to deduct her loss. However, if the investment had been in the form of § 1244 stock, the entire $30,000 loss would be deductible in the year incurred.

Under § 1244, the taxpayer is allowed to deduct up to $50,000 ($100,000 in the case of a joint return) of loss *annually*. Any loss in excess of this amount is treated as a capital loss and is subject to limitation. In light of these rules, a taxpayer who anticipates a loss on § 1244 stock that exceeds the annual limitation should attempt to limit the loss recognized in any one year to $50,000 (or $100,000).

Example 52. C, a bachelor, invested $200,000 in Risky Corporation several years ago, receiving 1,000 shares of § 1244 stock. It now appears that Risky, true to its name, will fail and that C will receive at best $100,000 for his investment. If C sells all of his shares this year, $50,000 of the loss is completely deductible as an ordinary loss under § 1244, while the remaining $50,000 of the loss would be a capital loss of which only $3,000 could be deducted (assuming he has no capital gains). C should sell half of his shares this year and half of his shares next year. By so doing, his loss for each year will be $50,000. In such case, neither loss would exceed the annual limitation, and therefore both would be deductible in full.

PROBLEM MATERIALS

DISCUSSION QUESTIONS

16-1 *Capital Asset Defined.* Define a capital asset. How would you describe the way a capital asset is defined?

16-2 *Sale of a Business.* How is the sale of an operating business treated? Discuss the sale of sole proprietorships, partnerships, and corporations in general.

16-3 *Holding Period.* Explain the holding period requirements that must be met to secure favorable capital gain treatment. How does one determine the holding period for purchased property?

16-4 *Holding Period.* What is the rule for determining the holding period for property acquired by gift?

16-5 *Holding Period.* What is the holding period of property acquired from a decedent?

16-6 *Holding Period—Stock Exchange Transactions.* T placed an order with her stock broker to sell 100 shares of Kent Electronics, Inc. stock on December 23, 2009. Because the sale order was received after the close of the market on the 23rd, the sale was executed at 9:00 A.M. on December 30, 2009. T received a settlement check from the brokerage house on January 5, 2010. What is the date of sale and what is the last date of T's holding period?

16-7 *Holding Period—Worthless Securities.* D purchased 1,000 shares of H, Inc. for $4,450 in a speculative investment on October 25, 2008. Weeks later, on January 5, 2009, D received notice that the H, Inc. stock was worthless. What are the amount and character of D's loss in 2009?

16-8 *Capital Gain and Loss Netting Process.* Describe the three possible results of the capital gain and loss netting process. How are the gains treated for tax purposes?

16-9 *Capital Gains Tax.* D is single and has taxable income for the current year of $72,000, including a $7,000 capital gain on the sale of stock held for two years. Describe how D will determine the tax on his income for the year.

16-10 *Capital Loss Deduction: Individuals.* How is the capital loss deduction limited for individual taxpayers?

16-11 *Capital Gains and Losses: Corporations.* The tax rules governing a corporation's capital gains and losses differ somewhat from those for an individual.
  a. Explain how a corporation treats capital gains and losses and how this treatment differs from that of an individual.
  b. Some commentators are fond of saying that corporations rarely have capital gains and losses to worry about. Why might this be true?

16-12 *Capital Loss Carryover.* Capital losses in excess of the annual limit can be carried forward to the subsequent year. How long may losses be carried forward by individual taxpayers? What is the character of the loss carryover and what happens if net losses from each of the groups (short-term, 28 percent, and 15 percent) are carried forward?

16-13 *Patents.* What is necessary for a patent to qualify for capital gain or loss treatment under § 1235?

16-14 *Ordinary v. Capital Loss Treatment.* What are the tax consequences to P, a bachelor, of a $70,000 loss occurring on June 1 of the current year attributable to the following:
  a. An uncollectible nonbusiness loan to XYZ Corporation
  b. Worthless bonds of XYZ Corporation acquired on November 30 of the prior year
  c. The sale of XYZ stock qualifying as § 1244 stock when acquired two years ago

16-15 *Section 1244 Stock.* When is a taxpayer's stock considered § 1244 stock? Why is the designation significant?

16-16 *Fifty Percent Exclusion.* S purchased qualified small business stock in U Corp. on October 27, 2009 for $35,000 with hopes to later qualify for the 50 percent exclusion.
  a. What two major requirements must U Corp. meet throughout S's holding period?
  b. What is the first day on which S may sell the stock and qualify for the 50 percent exclusion?
  c. What is the rollover provision and why is it important?

16-17 *Rollover of Gain on Sales of Publicly Traded Securities.* Q sold common stock in K Corp., a publicly traded corporation, for $140,000, realizing a gain of $60,000.
  a. How much must Q reinvest in a corporation or partnership that is licensed by the Small Business Administration under § 301(d) of the Small Business Investment Act of 1958 (as in effect on May 13, 1994) in order to defer all of the $60,000 gain?
  b. By what day must Q reinvest to qualify for this gain rollover (deferral)?

16-18 *Dealers, Traders and Investors.* In September 2008, R decided to try his luck in the stock market. Using a recent inheritance and borrowing funds on margin, he started investing. On a tip, one of his purchases was 10,000 shares of Overpriced Corp. He paid $70 per share at a total cost of $700,000. By December, 2008, the stock price had slipped to $30 per share. The prices of his other investments also were falling. All of this was happening and he was paying interest on his margin account as well.
  a. Would R be considered a dealer? Why or why not?
  b. If R is a dealer, how could R guaranteed that a particular investment will not be subject to capital gain or loss treatment?

    c. If R is an investor, how will his gains or losses be treated for tax purposes? His expenses?

    d. If R is a trader, how will his gains or losses be treated for tax purposes? His expenses?

    e. What is the mark-to-market election? Is R eligible for the mark-to-market election?

    f. If R can make the election, when must it be made and what effect will it have? Explain the effect of the election on any unrealized gains and losses he may have, expenses that he may incur such as margin interest and home office costs, and other concerns such as self-employment taxes and the alternative minimum tax.

16-19   *Dealers in Securities.* How does a dealer in securities guarantee that a particular "investment" will qualify for capital gain or loss treatment?

16-20   *Original Issue Discount—Deep Discount Bonds.* Financial consulting services often advise investment in so-called *deep discount bonds* (e.g., a $1,000 par value bond maturing in 10 years with coupon rate of six percent that sells at a discounted price of $400). Explain how such an investment could provide any tax savings in light of the original issue discount rules.

16-21   *Bond Premium.* This year, G purchased a $1,000 bond for $1,100. The bond matures in 2015 and pays interest at a rate of 10 percent. Interest is paid semiannually on February 1 and August 1. Explain the treatment of the premium on the bond if the bond was issued by:

    a. General Motors

    b. City of Sacramento

PROBLEMS

16-22   *Identifying Capital Assets.* Which of the following items are capital assets?

    a. An automobile held for sale to customers by Midtown Motors, Inc.

    b. An automobile owned and used by Sherry Hartman to run household errands

    c. An automobile owned and used by Windowwashers, Inc.

    d. The private residence of Robert Hamilton

    e. Letters from a famous U.S. President written to Jane Doe (Jane Doe has the letters.)

    f. A warehouse owned and used by Holt Packing Company

    g. Gold bullion

    h. A country and western ballad written by W. Nelson.

16-23   *Identifying Capital Assets.* Which of the following properties are capital assets? Briefly explain your answers.

    a. A house built by a home-building contractor and used by her as her principal residence

    b. A house, 80 percent of which is used as a residence and 20 percent of which is used to store business inventory

    c. The same house in (b) above, used as stated for 10 years, and now used exclusively as a residence

    d. Undeveloped land held for investment by a real estate broker

    e. Stock held for investment by a stock broker

16-24 *Capital Gain Netting Process.* D sold the following capital assets during 2009:

Description	Date Acquired	Date Sold	Sales Price	Adjusted Basis
100 shares XY Corp.	1/10/87	1/12/09	$14,000	$1,000
50 shares LM Inc.	9/14/08	1/12/09	1,900	4,000
140 shares CH Corp.	11/20/08	4/10/09	3,400	3,000
Gold necklace	4/22/95	6/30/09	5,000	1,300
Personal auto	5/10/03	8/31/09	4,000	6,500

Explain the effects of the transactions above on D's taxable income and final tax liability.

16-25 *Calculation of Capital Gains Tax.* Refer to the facts in *Problem 16-24* above. Assuming D, single, also has taxable income of $77,000 (net of her standard deduction and exemption), compute her tax liability.

16-26 *Capital Gain Netting Process.* Each of the following situations deals with capital gains and losses occurring during the current year for an individual taxpayer. For each case, determine the change in adjusted gross income and the maximum tax to be imposed on any gain.

	Note:	N15CG(L) = Net 15 percent capital gain or (loss)
		NSTCG(L) = Net short-term capital gain or (loss)

Case	N15CG(L)	NSTCG(L)
A	$1,200	$1,200
B	1,600	(1,000)
C	(1,200)	1,800
D	4,500	(800)
E	2,400	1,800

16-27 *Gain and Losses on Property Acquired by Gift.* In each of the following independent situations, assume that the taxpayer received the capital asset as a gift on March 19, 2009, that the donor had held the property since 2005, and that the property was sold during 2009. No gift taxes were payable on the transfer. Determine the gain or loss recognized in each case.

Case	Date of Sale	Sales Price	Donor's Basis	FMV Date of Gift
A	4/19	$1,000	$ 400	$ 600
B	6/3	1,000	1,400	1,200
C	11/20	1,000	900	1,100

16-28 *Capital Gains and Losses.* K, a single individual, earned salaries and wages of $59,000 and interest $2,000 and dividends of $1,700 for the current year. In addition, K sold the following capital assets:

100 shares of GHJ common stock, held 14 months	$3,400 gain
1955 Ford pickup, used five years for personal purposes. . . .	4,500 gain
30 acres of land, held three years for investment.	6,200 loss

    a. Compute K's net capital gain or loss.
    b. Compute K's adjusted gross income.

16-29 *Capital Gains and Losses.* L, a single individual, earned salaries and wages of $57,000 and interest of $3,000 and dividends of $3,700 for the current year. In addition, L sold the following capital assets:

10 shares LMN common stock, held ten months	$1,400 gain
1990 Dodge sedan, used four years for personal purposes . .	2,600 loss
10 acres of land, held six years for investment.	9,200 loss

    a. Compute L's overall capital gain or loss.
    b. Compute L's adjusted gross income.

16-30 *Capital Gains Tax.* During her calendar year 2009, G, a single individual with no dependents, had the following capital gains and losses:

Asset	Gain/Loss	Holding Period
200 shares of Western Airlines	$1,400 loss	11 months
Land held for appreciation	12,300 gain	8 years
Silver vases held for appreciation	1,800 loss	15 months

    a. Assuming G's taxable income (properly calculated) is $34,000, calculate G's gross tax.
    b. Same as above, except G's taxable income is $75,000.

16-31 *Capital Gains Tax.* R is a single, calendar year taxpayer. During 2009, R recognized a $20,000 15 percent capital gain from the sale of stock held for three years. Calculate R's tax liability (before credits and prepayments) for each of the following levels of taxable income, assuming that the net capital gains have been included in the taxable income numbers.
    a. $43,950
    b. $102,250
    c. $600,000

16-32 *Capital Gains Tax.* H and J are married, calendar year taxpayers who elect to file jointly. They have no dependents and do not itemize their deductions. Their income and deductions for 2009 are summarized below.

Salaries and wages.	$105,500
Interest income	16,900
Qualifying dividends received	4,500
Short-term capital loss	5,000
Long-term capital gains (held > 12 months)	20,000

Determine H and J's tax liability (before credits and prepayments).

16-33 *Effective Tax Rate on Net Capital Gains.* T is an unmarried, calendar year taxpayer. He provides more than one-half the support of his elderly mother, who is living in a nearby nursing home. T's income and deductions for 2009 are summarized below.

Salary	$152,500
Interest income	14,550
Itemized deductions (all subject to the 3% cutback rule).	12,800
Personal and dependency exemptions.	2

   a. Calculate T's taxable income and income tax liability (before credits and prepayments) for the year.

   b. How would your answers to (a) above change if T also had a $20,000 capital gain during the year from the sale of stock held 15 months?

   c. Is the additional income tax from the capital gain limited to $3,000 ($20,000 × 15%)? If not, explain why.

16-34 *Tax Treatment of Dividends as Capital Gain.* P and H, married, cash basis, calendar year taxpayers who file a joint return have the following income and expenses for 2009:

Salaries and wages.	$91,400
Qualifying dividends	4,000
Long-term capital gains	5,000
Short-term capital gains or (losses).	0
Itemized deductions	31,700
Dependents—None	

   a. Calculate the federal income tax for P and H for the year.

   b. How would you answer differ if P and H also had short-term capital losses of $10,000?

16-35 *Netting Process and Capital Losses.* T, an unmarried taxpayer, sold the following capital assets during her calendar year 2009:

	Date Acquired	Date Sold	Sales Price	Adjusted Basis
100 shares CZ Corp.	1/10/09	9/17/09	$14,000	$18,000
75 shares PC, Inc.	7/6/09	9/17/09	5,200	4,300
Silver coins (held as a collector)	12/2/04	11/20/09	2,000	5,000

Complete each of the following requirements based on T's taxable income of $37,000 before capital gains and losses:

   a. T's net 15 percent capital gain or loss

   b. T's net 28 percent capital gain or loss

   c. T's net short-term capital gain or loss

   d. T's capital loss deduction in arriving at adjusted gross income

   e. T's capital loss carryover to 2010 (describe amount and character)

   f. How would your answers to (d) and (e) differ if T's basis in the PC stock had been $1,000?

16-36 *Capital Loss and Carryover.* N earned a salary of $59,000 and interest and dividends of $6,500 for the current year. N also has the following capital gains and losses for the current year:

30 shares MNO common stock, held ten months	$ 400 gain
50 shares NOP common stock, held four years.............	3,600 loss
Long-term capital loss carryforward from prior year	11,600 loss
10 acres of land, held six years for investment..............	9,200 gain

   a. Compute L's overall capital gain.
   b. Compute L's adjusted gross income.

16-37 *Capital Gains and Losses.* Each of the following independent cases involves capital gains and losses occurring during the calendar year for an unmarried individual taxpayer.

> **Note:** N15CG(L) = Net 15 percent capital gain or (loss)
> NSTCG(L) = Net short-term capital gain or (loss)

Case	N15CG(L)	NSTCG(L)
A	$1,200	$(4,300)
B	(5,000)	200
C	(1,200)	(2,300)
D	(7,000)	200
E	(5,000)	(200)

   a. Determine the amount deductible in arriving at adjusted gross income in each case for the current year.
   b. Which, if any, of the above case(s) generate(s) a capital loss carryover to the following year? Give the amount and character.

16-38 *Capital Loss Deduction and Capital Loss Carryover.* W, an unmarried calendar year individual, had numerous capital asset transactions during the years listed. Determine the amount deductible in each year and the amount and character of any carryover.

Year	N15CG(L)	NSTCG(L)
2009	$(8,000)	$1,000
2010	(1,500)	(2,000)
2011	0	(4,000)
2012	2,000	(3,000)

16-39 *Capital Loss Deduction and Capital Loss Carryover.* M, an unmarried calendar year individual, had numerous capital asset transactions during the years listed. Determine the amount deductible in each year and the amount and character of any carryover.

Year	N15CG(L)	NSTCG(L)
2009	$1,000	$(5,000)
2010	(6,000)	0
2011	3,000	(3,000)
2012	(3,000)	(3,000)

16-40 *Capital Loss Carryovers.* For her calendar year 2008, H, a single individual with no dependents, had unused short-term capital losses of $10,000. For 2009, her gains and losses were as follows:

Asset	Amount	Holding Period
Corporate stock............................	$ 1,400 loss	11 months
Land held for appreciation	14,300 gain	8 years
Miniature dolls held as a collector	1,800 gain	25 months

After completing the netting process, how much are H's 15 percent gains and 28 percent gains?

16-41 *Requirements for § 1244 Stock.* During the year, X, who is single, sold stock and realized a loss. For each of the following situations, indicate whether § 1244 would apply to the taxpayer's stock loss. Unless otherwise indicated, Code § 1244 applies.

a. The stock was that issued to X when she incorporated her business several years ago.

b. The stock was that of General Motors Corporation and was purchased last year.

c. X inherited the stock from her grandfather, who had started the company ten years ago.

d. X is a corporate taxpayer.

e. X acquired her stock interest in 2003. The other four owners had acquired their interest for $250,000 each in 1998.

f. The loss was $60,000.

16-42 *Section 1244 Stock Computation.* S is a bachelor. During the year, he sold stock in X Corporation that qualifies as § 1244 stock at a loss of $70,000. In addition, S sold stock in Y Corporation, realizing a $4,000 15 percent capital gain. Compute the effect of these transactions on S's A.G.I.

16-43 *Short Sales.* K purchased 400 shares of Intel common five years ago for $7,000. During the current year, she sold short 200 shares for $17,500. Her plan is to either buy new shares to cover the short sale or deliver 200 of the original shares in one year. Assuming the stock drops, and as planned, K purchases 200 shares for $16,000 to cover the short sale, how are these transactions treated for tax purposes?

16-44 *Worthless Securities.* Several years ago, T was persuaded by his good friend W to invest in her new venture, Wobbly Corporation. T purchased 100 shares of Wobbly stock from W for $60,000. He also purchased Wobbly bonds, which had a face value of $20,000 for $18,000. This year, Wobbly declared bankruptcy and T's investment in Wobbly became worthless. What are the tax consequences to T?

16-45 *Sale of Stock.* B owned 50 percent of the stock in a small incorporated dress shop. The business was successful for several years until a new freeway diverted nearly all of the traffic away from the location. The shop was moved, but to no avail, and the stock continued to quickly decline in value. Other than small interest payments, the income of the business came exclusively from sales of women's apparel.

The total paid-in capital of the corporation was $250,000, all in the form of cash. B's basis in the stock was always $125,000. In an attempt to prevent further losses, the shop was sold to a larger competitor during 2009. B received $50,000 for all of her stock.

a. How will B report the loss on the joint return she files with her husband for 2009?

b. How would your answer to (a) differ if the stock became totally worthless rather than being sold in 2009?

16-46 *Worthless Securities.* Y purchased 30 shares of BCD Corporation common stock on March 2, 2008, for $2,475. On February 26, 2009, Y was notified by her broker that the stock was worthless.

    a. What are the amount and character of Y's loss?

    b. Could this loss qualify as an ordinary deduction under § 1244? Explain.

16-47 *Fifty Percent Gain Exclusion.* E purchased qualified small business stock in P, Inc. on October 27, 2002 for $75,000. The stock continued to qualify until E sold it for $400,000 on December 15, 2009.

    a. How much is E's gain realized upon this sale?

    b. How much of this gain may E exclude from gross income?

    c. What is the maximum amount of tax that E could pay on this gain (assuming no change in tax rates)?

    d. How could E avoid recognizing the gain realized?

16-48 *Rollover of Gain on Sale of Publicly Traded Securities.* R sold common stock in L Corp., a publicly traded corporation, on March 13, 2009 for $160,000, realizing a gain of $40,000. On April 1, 2009, R reinvested $200,000 in M Partnership, a partnership licensed by the Small Business Administration under § 301(d) of the Small Business Investment Act of 1958 (as in effect on May 13, 1993).

    a. How much gain must R recognize on the sale of the L Corp. stock?

    b. What is R's basis in his interest in M Partnership?

16-49 *Combining the Exclusion and Rollover.* Y sold common stock in X Corp., a publicly traded corporation, on October 1, 2003 for $200,000, realizing a gain of $35,000. On October 15, 2003, Y reinvested $250,000 in N, Inc., a corporation licensed by the Small Business Administration under § 301(d) of the Small Business Investment Act of 1958 (as in effect on May 13, 1993), the stock of which is qualified small business stock. On December 1, 2009, Y sold all of the N, Inc. stock for $625,000.

    a. How much is Y's gain realized on the sale of the N, Inc. stock?

    b. How much of this gain is excludable from gross income?

16-50 *Lease Cancellation Payment.* L rents a house to T for $450 per month under a two-year lease. When T is transferred, he offers L $675 to terminate the lease. If L accepts, what is the tax treatment of the transaction to L and T?

16-51 *Franchise Agreements.* J entered into a franchise agreement with Box, Inc. under which J will operate a fast food restaurant bearing the trademark and using the products of Box. Box retained "significant power, right and continuing interest" related to the franchise agreement.

    J made an initial payment under the contract of $40,000, which entitles him to the rights under the contract for 15 years with indefinite extensions at the agreement of both parties. J also is required to pay for all supplies used plus a royalty of 1.5 percent of gross sales. J's sales were $112,000 during the first year. All of the payments described, totaling $41,680, were made during the current year.

    a. How will J report these payments on his cash basis tax return for the current year?

    b. How would Box, Inc. treat the payments from J on its return for the current year? The corporation reports on the cash basis.

16-52 *Original Issue Discount.* On January 1, 2009, B purchased from XYZ Corporation a newly issued, $1 million, 30-year, 4 percent bond for $300,000. The bond produces a semiannual yield to maturity of 7 percent. Interest is paid semiannually on January 1 and July 1. What is B's income with respect to the bond in 2009 and 2010?

16-53 *Market Discount.* D purchased a $10,000, 7 percent bond, for $6,350, on January 1, 2008. The bond was issued at par on January 1, 2007 and matures January 1, 2012. On January 1, 2009, D sold the bond for $8,000. What is D's income from the sale?

16-54 *Conversion Transaction.* J purchased a non-interest-bearing financial instrument on June 1, 2008 for $60,000. It was purchased subject to a contract that allows J to redeem the instrument for $66,000 on May 31, 2009, but it may not be redeemed early. The applicable federal rate is 5 percent throughout J's holding period. What are the amount and character of J's gain recognized in 2009?

16-55 *Comprehensive Capital Gain Problem.* P is an unmarried full-time investor with no dependents. Her income for the year 2009 is as follows:

Taxable interest income	$25,750
Excludable municipal bond interest	8,600
Qualifying dividends	11,650
Consulting fees	6,400
Social security benefits	8,400

Although P does not have sufficient deductions to itemize, her records reveal the following:

Investment expenses	$ 850
Expenses related to consulting	1,200

In addition to the above, P recognized the following gains and losses during the year:

Loss on sale of 100 shares of A, Inc., held three years	$(1,200)
Loss on sale of personal automobile	(1,800)
Sales price of 100 shares of B Corp., sold short	8,200
(This short sale was closed the following year with newly purchased shares costing $9,600. P owned no B Corp. stock at the time of the short sale.)	
Gain on sale of unimproved land held as an investment for six years	45,000

Calculate P's adjusted gross income, taxable income, and gross income tax based on the above for 2009. Begin by calculating P's self-employment tax.

16-56 *Investors vs. Traders.* M has a large portfolio of stocks. It seems that she is always buying and selling one stock or another. During the year, she realized gains of $300,000 and losses of $500,000 on sales of stocks that she held for less than a year. At the end of the year, she had unrealized gains of $150,000 and unrealized losses of $375,000. In managing her portfolio, she paid $12,000 of investment expenses. She also has paid $10,000 in margin interest. She conducts all of these activities online in her home office. This year she purchased a new computer for $3,000. Explain the tax treatment of her income and expenses (including how they would be reported (e.g., forms) as well as any related effects (e.g., self-employment taxes, alternative minimum tax) if she is considered:
a. An investor.
b. A trader who has not made the § 475(f) mark-to-market election.
c. A trader who has made the § 475(f) mark-to-market election.

RESEARCH PROBLEMS

16-57 *Transfer of Patents.* G has just completed a successful invention of a new automotive fuel conservation device. He is willing to sell his patent rights for all areas of the United States east of the Rocky Mountains.

In the current year, G entered into an agreement with a marketing firm, giving it exclusive rights to market his invention anywhere east of the Rockies. In exchange, he received a principal sum and is to receive royalties based on sales volume.

Is G entitled to capital gain treatment on this sale under § 1235? Would it make any difference if the transferee of the patent was given exclusive rights to the patent and was given the right to "sublease" the patent?

Research Aids:

Kueneman v. Comm., 80-2 USTC ¶9616, 46 AFTR2d 80-5677, 628 F.2d 1196 (CA-9, 1980).
Klein Est v. Comm., 75-1 USTC ¶9127, 35 AFTR2d 75-457, 507 F.2d 617 (CA-7, 1974).
Rouverol v. Comm., 42 T.C. 186 (1964), non. acq., 1965-2 C.B. 7.

16-58 *Sale of Subdivided and Improved Real Property.* D, a full-time physician, has owned 15 acres of unimproved suburban real estate for 10 years. The property was originally purchased for $30,000 and has been held solely for investment. D is now interested in selling the property and has several alternatives. She has come to you for advice concerning the tax treatment of these alternatives. What is the proper tax treatment of each of the following?

a. A sale of the entire acreage to an unrelated party in a single transaction for $150,000.

b. Recording the property with the county as 30 single residential lots, adding roads and improvements at a cost of $100,000, and selling the lots for $25,000 each.

c. Recording the property with the county as 30 single residential lots, and then selling them to an unrelated developer in a single transaction for $190,000.

d. Recording the property with the county as 30 single residential lots and then selling them for $190,000 in a single transaction to a partnership in which D is a 40 percent partner. The partnership then adds roads and improvements at a cost of $100,000 and sells the lots for $25,000 each.

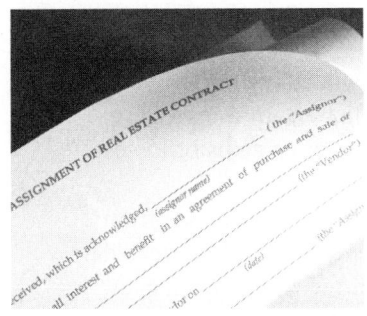

★ CHAPTER SEVENTEEN ★

PROPERTY TRANSACTIONS: DISPOSITIONS OF TRADE OR BUSINESS PROPERTY

LEARNING OBJECTIVES

Upon completion of this chapter you will be able to:

▶ Trace the historical development of the special tax treatment allowed for dispositions of trade or business property

▶ Apply the § 1231 gain and loss netting process to a taxpayer's § 1231 asset transactions

▶ Determine the tax treatment of § 1231 gains and losses

▶ Explain the purpose of the depreciation recapture rules

▶ Compute depreciation recapture under §§ 1245 and 1250

▶ Explain the additional recapture rule applicable only to corporate taxpayers

▶ Identify tax planning opportunities related to sales or other dispositions of trade or business property

---

CHAPTER OUTLINE

INTRODUCTION

As is no doubt clear by now, the treatment of property transactions is a complex story that seeks to answer three questions: (1) What is the gain or loss realized? (2) How much is recognized? and (3) What is its character? This chapter, the final act in the property transaction trilogy, addresses the problems in determining the character of gains or losses on the dispositions of *property used in a trade or business.*

In an uncomplicated world, it might seem logical to assume that gains or losses from property dispositions—be it stock, equipment, buildings, or whatever—would be treated just like any other type of income or deduction. But, as shown in the previous chapter, treating all items alike apparently was not part of the grand plan. Congress forever changed the process with the institution of preferential treatment for capital gains in 1921. Since that time taxpayers have been required to determine not only the gain or loss realized and recognized but also whether a disposition involved a capital asset. It is important to understand that these rules did not simply tip the scales in favor of capital gain. In the interest of fairness and equity, they also established a less than friendly environment for capital losses. The limitations on the deductibility of capital losses is clearly a major disadvantage, particularly considering that ordinary losses are fully deductible. The end result of Congress's handiwork was the creation of a system in which the preferred result is capital gain treatment for gains and ordinary treatment for losses. This chapter contains the saga of what happens when Congress attempts to provide taxpayers with the best of both worlds.

SECTION 1231

The road to tax heaven—capital gain and ordinary loss—begins at § 1231 (in tax parlance properly pronounced as "twelve thirty-one"). While § 1231 can be a completely bewildering provision, its basic operation is relatively simple. At the close of the taxable year, the taxpayer nets all gains and losses from so-called § 1231 property (e.g., land and depreciable property used in a trade or business). If there is a net gain, it is treated as a long-term capital gain. If there is a net loss, it is treated as an ordinary loss. In short, § 1231 allows taxpayers to have their cake and eat it, too. Unfortunately, this is accomplished only with a great deal of complexity, much of which makes sense only if the historical events that shaped § 1231 are considered.

HISTORICAL PERSPECTIVE

At first glance, it seems that the productive assets of a business—its property, plant, and equipment—would be perfect candidates for capital gain treatment and would therefore be considered capital assets. Indeed, that was exactly the case initially. From 1921 to 1938, real or depreciable property used in business was in fact treated as a capital asset. At that time, the classification of such property as a capital asset seemed not only appropriate but desirable—particularly as the economy grew during the early 1920s and taxpayers were realizing gains. However, the opposite became true with the onset of the Great Depression. As the economy deteriorated, businesses that had purchased assets at inflated prices during the booming 1920s found themselves selling such properties at huge losses during the depression-plagued 1930s. To make matters worse, the tax law treated such losses as capital losses, severely limiting their deduction. But Congress apparently had a sympathetic ear for these concerns. Hoping that a change would help stimulate the economy, Congress enacted legislation that removed business properties from the list of capital assets. The legislative history to the Revenue Act of 1938 provides some insight into Congressional thinking, explaining that "corporations will not, as formerly, be deterred from disposing of partially obsolescent property,

such as machinery or equipment, because of the limitations imposed ... upon the deduction of capital losses."[1] With the 1938 changes in place, business got the ordinary loss treatment it wanted but at the same time was saddled with ordinary income treatments for its gains.

Although these rules worked well during the Depression years as businesses were reporting losses, they produced some unduly harsh results once the country moved to a wartime economy. By 1942, the build-up for World War II had the economy humming and inflation had once again set in. Businesses that earlier had sold assets for 10 cents on the dollar now found themselves realizing gains. Of course, under the 1938 changes these gains no longer benefited from preferential treatment but were taxed at extraordinarily high tax rates (88 percent for individuals and 40 percent for corporations). The shipping industry was particularly hard hit by the new treatment. Shippers not only had gains as the enemy destroyed their insured ships but also profited when they were forced to sell their property to the government for use in the war. Other businesses that had their factories and equipment condemned and requisitioned also felt the sting of higher ordinary rates. Although these companies could have deferred their gains had they replaced the property under the involuntary conversion rules of § 1033, qualified reinvestment property was in short supply, making § 1033 virtually useless. Understanding the plight of business, Congress once again came to the rescue. In 1942, Congress enacted legislation generally reinstating capital gain treatment but preserving ordinary loss treatment.

The changes in 1942 stemmed primarily from a need to provide relief for those whose property was condemned for the war effort. But in the end they went much further. For consistency, capital gain treatment was extended not only to condemnations of a business property but to other types of involuntary conversions as well. Under the new rules, casualty and theft gains from business property and capital assets also received capital gain treatment. In addition, the new legislation unexpectedly extended capital gain treatment to regular sales of property, plant, and equipment. Apparently, Congress felt that capital gain treatment was also appropriate for taxpayers who were selling out in anticipation of condemnation or simply because wartime conditions had made operations difficult. While Congress thought capital gain treatment was warranted for these gains, it also knew that other businesses had not profited from the war and were still suffering losses from their property transactions. Accordingly, it acted to preserve ordinary loss treatment. The end result of these maneuvers was the enactment of § 1231, an extremely complex provision that provides taxpayers with the best of all possible tax worlds: capital gain and ordinary loss.

The product of Congressional tinkering in 1942 still remains today. To summarize, real and depreciable property used in a trade or business is specifically denied capital asset status. But this does not necessarily mean that such property will be denied capital gain treatment. As explained at the outset, § 1231 generally extends capital gain treatment to gains and losses from these assets if the taxpayer realizes a net gain from all § 1231 transactions. On the other hand, if there is a net loss, ordinary loss treatment applies. But this summary lacks a great deal of precision. The specific rules of § 1231 are described below.

SECTION 1231 PROPERTY

The special treatment of § 1231 is generally granted only to certain transactions involving assets normally referred to as *§ 1231 property*.[2] Section 1231 property includes a variety of assets, but among them the most important is *real or depreciable property that is used in the taxpayer's trade or business* and that is held for more than

---

[1]   House Ways and Means Committee, H.R. Rep. 1860, 75th Cong., 3d Sess. (1938).

[2]   As explained below, § 1231 also applies to involuntary conversions of pure capital assets held more than one year that are used in a trade or business or held for investment. Involuntary conversions by theft or casualty of personal assets are not included under § 1231 but are subject to a special computation.

one year.[3] This definition takes in most items commonly identified as a business's fixed assets, normally referred to as its property, plant, and equipment. For example, the reach of § 1231 includes depreciable personal property used in business, such as machinery, equipment, office furniture, and business automobiles. Similarly, realty used in a business, such as office buildings, warehouses, factories, and farmland, is also considered § 1231 property.

The Code specifically excludes the following assets from § 1231 treatment:

1. Property held primarily for sale to customers in the ordinary course of a trade or business, or includible in inventory, if on hand at the close of the tax year;

2. A copyright; a literary, musical, or artistic composition; a letter or memorandum; or similar property held by a taxpayer whose personal efforts created such property or by certain other persons; or

3. A publication of the United States Government received from the government other than by purchase at the price at which the publication is offered to the general public.[4]

Note that the excluded assets are also excluded from the definition of a capital asset. As a result, gains or losses on the disposition of inventory, property held primarily for resale, literary compositions, and certain government publications always yield ordinary income or ordinary loss.

One of the critical conditions for § 1231 treatment requires that the property be used in a trade or business. Although this test normally presents little difficulty, from time to time it has created problems, particularly for those with rental property. As an illustration, consider the common situation of a taxpayer who sells rental property such as a house, duplex, or apartment complex. Is the property sold a capital asset or § 1231 property? If a taxpayer sells rental property at a gain, the gain would normally receive capital gain treatment regardless of whether the property is a capital asset or § 1231 property. On the other hand, if the taxpayer sells the rental property at a loss, § 1231 treatment is usually far more desirable. Although the Code does not provide any clear guidance on the issue, the courts have generally held that property used for rental purposes is considered as used in a trade or business and is therefore eligible for § 1231 treatment.[5]

OTHER § 1231 PROPERTY

From time to time, Congress has been convinced that particular industries deserve special tax relief. As a result, it has added a number of other properties to the § 1231 basket. Those eligible for capital gain and ordinary loss are:

1. Timber, coal, and iron ore to which § 631 applies;[6]

2. Unharvested crops on land used in a trade or business and held for more than one year;[7] and

3. Certain livestock.[8]

---

[4] § 1231(b)(1).

[5] See, for example, *Mary Crawford*, 16 T.C. 678 (1951) A. 1951-2 C.B. 2, and *Gilford v. Comm.*, 53-1 USTC ¶9201, 43 AFTR 221, 201 F.2d 735 (CA-2, 1953).

[6] § 1231(b)(2).

[7] § 1231(b)(4).

[8] § 1231(b)(3).

Timber. Under § 631, the mere cutting of timber by the owner of the timber, or by a person who has the right to cut the timber and has held the timber or right more than one year, is to be treated, at his or her election, as a sale or exchange of the timber that is cut during the year. The timber must be cut for sale or for use in the taxpayer's trade or business. In such case, the taxpayer would report a § 1231 gain or loss and potentially receive capital gain treatment for what otherwise might be considered the taxpayer's inventory—a very favorable result. It may appear that the timber industry has secured an unfair advantage, but timber's eligibility is arguably justified on the grounds that the value of timber normally accrues incrementally as it grows over a long period of time.

The amount of gain or loss on the "sale" of the timber is the fair market value of the timber on the first day of the taxable year minus the timber's adjusted basis for depletion. For all subsequent purposes (i.e., the sale of the cut timber), the fair market value of the timber as of the beginning of the year will be treated as the cost of the timber. The term *timber* not only includes trees used for lumber and other wood products, but also includes evergreen trees that are more than six years old when cut and are sold for ornamental purposes (e.g., Christmas trees).[9]

> **Example 1.** B owned standing timber that he had purchased for $250,000 three years earlier. The timber was cut and sold to a lumber mill for $410,000 during 2008. The fair market value of the standing timber as of January 1, 2008 was $320,000. B has a § 1231 gain of $70,000 if he makes an election under § 631 ($320,000 fair market value of the timber on the first day of the taxable year less its $250,000 adjusted basis for depletion). The remainder of his gain on the *actual* sale of the timber, $90,000 ($410,000 selling price − $320,000 new "cost" of the timber), is ordinary income. Any expenses incurred by B in cutting the timber would be deductible as ordinary deductions.

An election under § 631 with respect to timber is binding on all timber owned by the taxpayer during the year of the election *and* in all subsequent years. The IRS may permit revocation of such election because of significant hardship. However, once the election is revoked, IRS consent must be obtained to make a new election.[10]

Section 631 also applies to the sale of timber under a contract providing a retained economic interest (i.e., a taxpayer sells the timber, but keeps the right to receive a royalty from its later sale) for the taxpayer in the timber. In such a case, the transfer is considered a sale or exchange. The gain or loss is recognized on the date the timber is cut, or when payment is received, if earlier, at the election of the taxpayer.[11]

Coal and Iron Ore. When an owner disposes of coal or domestic iron ore under a contract that calls for a retained economic interest in the property, the disposition is treated as a sale or exchange of the coal or iron ore. The date the coal or ore is mined is considered the date of sale and since the property is § 1231 property, the gain or loss will be treated under § 1231.[12]

The taxpayer may not be a co-adventurer, partner, or principal in the mining of the coal or iron ore. Furthermore, the coal or iron ore may not be sold to certain related taxpayers.[13]

---

[9]   § 631(a).

[10]   *Ibid.*

[11]   § 631(b).

[12]   § 631(c).

[13]   §§ 631(c)(1) and (2).

Unharvested Crops. Section 1231 also addresses the special situation where a farmer sells land with unharvested crops sitting upon the land. In this case, it seems logical that the farmer should allocate the sales price between the crops and the land to ensure ordinary income or loss for the sale of the farmer's inventory and capital gain or ordinary loss on the sale of the land. While this may be the theoretically correct result, Congress wanted to eliminate potential controversy over the allocation. Accordingly, for administrative convenience it brought the entire transaction into the § 1231 fold in 1951. Currently, whenever land used in a trade or business and unharvested crops on that land are sold at the same time to the same buyer, the gain or loss is subject to § 1231 treatment as long as the land has been held for more than a year.[14] It is worth noting that the benefits of § 1231 were not extended to farmers free of charge. At the same time, Congress eliminated the current deduction for production expenses. The law now provides that any expenses related to the production of crops cannot be deducted currently but must be capitalized as part of the basis of the crops.[15] Such treatment, in a year when land and crops are sold, reduces the farmer's capital gain on the sale rather than any other ordinary income.

Example 2. F sold 100 acres of land that she used in her farming business just days before the corn on the land was harvested. For the "package" deal, she received $600,000, including an estimated $70,000 for the unharvested crops that she figured had cost her $20,000 to produce. F had purchased the land many years ago for $200,000. In determining the character of her gain, F is not required to allocate the sales price between the crops and the land since she sold both at the same time to the same buyer, therefore qualifying for § 1231 treatment. As a result, she reports a § 1231 gain of $380,000 computed as follows:

Sales price	$600,000
Adjusted basis ($200,000 + $20,000)	−220,000
§ 1231 gain	$380,000

Note that in the year of the sale F has effectively turned the $50,000 ($70,000 − $20,000) profit from the sale of her crops from ordinary income into potential capital gain.

Livestock. As a general proposition, livestock that are used for breeding and other income producing purposes are depreciable assets much like machinery and equipment and therefore qualify for § 1231 treatment. In many situations, however, livestock are used for these purposes for only a short period of time and then sold. If this is the farmer's or rancher's normal practice, the IRS is inclined to argue that the animals are held primarily for resale, in which case the law specifically denies § 1231 treatment. To help end this controversy, Congress specifically made all livestock (other than poultry) used for draft, breeding, dairy, or sporting purposes eligible for § 1231 treatment as long as they are held for over a year.[16] In the case of cattle and horses, however, the holding period is extended to two years. Note that this treatment is extremely beneficial since the taxpayer effectively gets capital gain from animals pulled out of the breeding process and sold. Moreover, the farmer or rancher is allowed to deduct the costs of raising such animals currently against ordinary income. The extension of the holding period for cattle and horses was in part, an attempt to cut back on the benefits of this favorable treatment.

---

[14]   § 1231(b)(4).

[15]   § 268.

[16]   § 1231(b)(3).

SECTION 1231 NETTING PROCESS

The treatment of § 1231 gains or losses ultimately depends on the outcome of a netting process that is far more complicated than outlined earlier.[17] As can be seen from the flowchart in Exhibit 17-1, the taxpayer must first identify all of the gains and losses that enter into the netting process. As might be expected, these include gains and losses from what has been described above as § 1231 property. In addition, the § 1231 hodgepodge includes *involuntary conversions* of certain *capital assets*. Surprisingly, gains or losses recognized from casualties, thefts, or condemnations of capital assets that are used in a trade or business or held for investment are part of the § 1231 netting process. Involuntary conversions of capital assets that are held for *personal use* are not considered under § 1231 but are subject to special rules.

After identifying all of the § 1231 transactions, the taxpayer must segregate the § 1231 gains and losses arising from casualty and theft from those attributable to sale, exchange, and condemnation. The end result is that there are two sets of § 1231 transactions:

1. Involuntary conversions due to casualty and theft of:
   - § 1231 property
     - Real and depreciable property used in business and held more than one year
     - Timber, coal, iron ore, unharvested crops, and livestock
   - Capital assets
     - Used in a trade or business or held for investment in connection with business and held more than one year

2. Sales and exchanges of:
   - § 1231 property
     - Real and depreciable property used in business
     - Timber, coal, iron ore, unharvested crops and livestock

   Involuntary conversion due to condemnation of:
   - § 1231 property
     - Real and depreciable property used in business and held more than one year
     - Timber, coal, iron ore, unharvested crops, and livestock
   - Capital assets
     - Used in a trade or business or held for investment in connection with business and held more than one year

---

[17] § 1231(a).

EXHIBIT 17-1
Section 1231 Netting Process

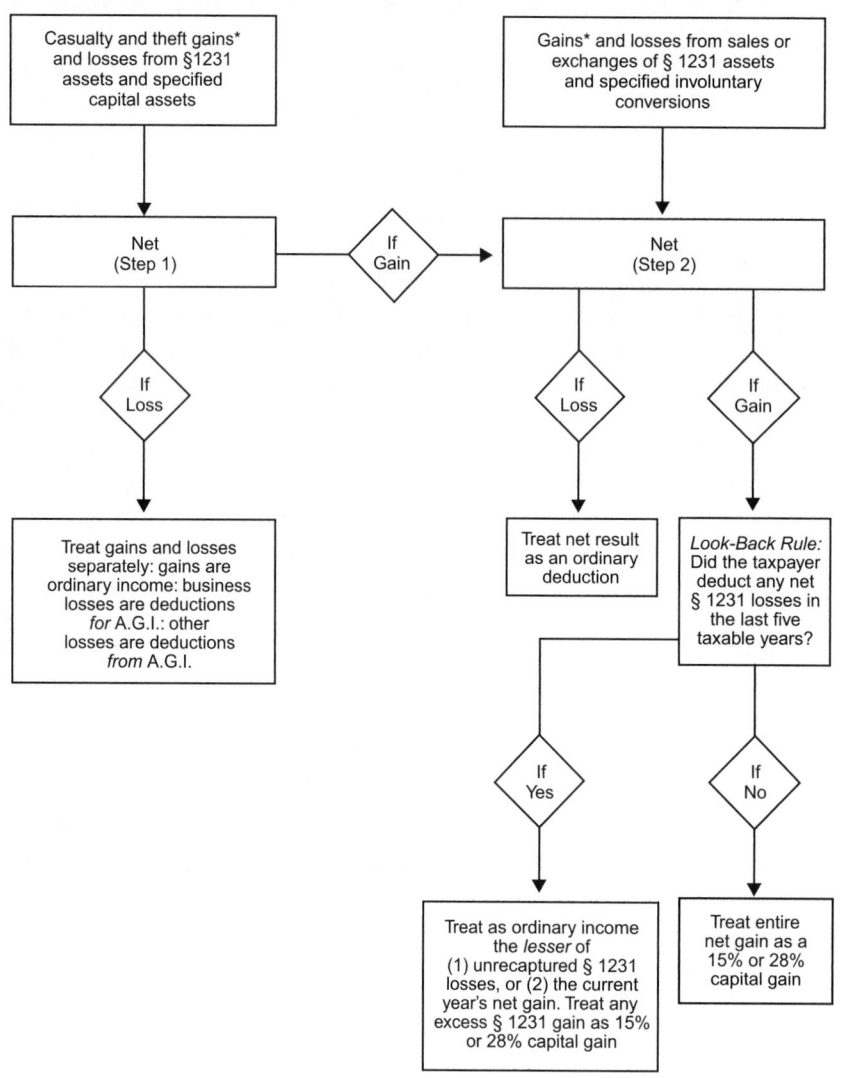

* Gains remaining after reduction for any depreciation recapture

Within each of these two categories, each gain and loss must be assigned to one of the three *potential* long-term capital gain groups and netted just as if they had been 28%, 25% or 15% capital gains or losses (see Chapter 16). This means that each § 1231 gain or loss is assigned to one of the following three categories: (1) 15% group for § 1231 gains and losses (15G or 15L); (2) 25% group for unrecaptured § 1250 depreciation related to gains from § 1231 assets (25G discussed below); and (3) 28% group for gains and losses from collectibles (28G or 28L). Once all of the appropriate transactions have been poured into the § 1231 process, the netting process can begin. There are three steps.

1. First, all of the gains and losses in the first category of § 1231 transactions (casualties and thefts) are netted. Specifically, gains and losses within the 15% and 28% groups are netted to arrive at one of the following: (1) a net gain or loss on 15% § 1231 assets (N15G or N15L); and (2) a net gain or loss on 28% § 1231

assets (N28G or N28L). Any net loss positions are then combined with the net gain positions using the rules discussed for netting the three groups for capital asset transactions:

▸ A N28L first offsets 25G, then N15G.

▸ A N15L first offsets a N28G, then 25G.

▸ There can be no net loss in the 25G group since this group contains only gains.

This netting process is summarized as follows:

	Section 1231 Gains and Losses from Casualty and Theft		
	Collectibles	Unrecaptured Depreciation	Other
	28%	25%	15%
Gains	$x,xxx	Gains only	$xx,xxx
Losses	(x,xxx)	–	(x,xxx)
Net gain or loss	????	Gain only	????
Possibilities:			
1.	N28G	25G	N15G
2.	N28G	25G	N15L
3.	N28L	25G	N15G
4.	N28L	25G	N15L

If the netting process results in a net gain position(s) (e.g., a N28G, N25G, and a N15G) the net gains from casualties and thefts become § 1231 gains and become part of the second category of other § 1231 transactions (each assigned to either the 28%, 25%, or 15% groups).

Example 3. During the year, T, who is in the 35% tax bracket, reported the following § 1231 gains and losses from casualties of § 1231 assets (including casualties of capital assets used in a trade or business) and netted them as shown below.

	Section 1231 Gains and Losses		
	Collectibles	Unrecaptured Depreciation	Other
	28%	25%	15%
Gains	$10,000	$4,000	$2,000
Losses	(4,000)	—	(7,000)
Net gain or loss	$ 6,000	$4,000	($5,000)
Netting	(5,000)	—	5,000
To Section 1231 Other	$ 1,000	$4,000	$ 0

In this case, T has a N28G of $1,000 and a N25G of $4,000. Since the end results are net gains, each of these net gains is assigned to its appropriate group in the second category of other § 1231 transactions.

If a net loss results, the casualty and theft gains and losses are removed from the § 1231 process and treated separately. The gains are treated as ordinary income, and the losses on business use assets are deductible for A.G.I. Any other casualty and theft losses are deductible from A.G.I.

2. The second step of the process is to combine any net casualty or theft gains from the first step with the gains or losses in the second set of § 1231 transactions. In this regard, the net casualty and theft gains must be assigned to the appropriate group (15%, 25%, or 28% group) in the second category of § 1231 transactions (sales and exchanges of § 1231 assets and certain condemnations). For example, if the taxpayer had a net 15% gain from § 1231 casualties, this gain would become a 15% gain in the second category of § 1231 transactions. These transactions are then netted just as if they had been 28%, 25%, or 15% capital gains or losses to determine if there is a net gain or loss.

3. The third and final step in the § 1231 netting process is to characterize the gain or loss resulting from netting the transactions in the second step. If the net result is a loss, the net loss is treated as an ordinary deduction for adjusted gross income. It is not treated as a capital loss. If the net result is a gain (e.g., a N25G and a N15G), these gains are normally treated as capital gains and become part of the capital gain and loss netting process.

The § 1231 netting process is illustrated in Exhibit 17-1 and the following examples.

Example 4. During the current year, D sold real estate used in her business for $45,000. She had purchased the property several years ago for $36,000. D also sold a business car (held for more than 15 months) at a loss of $1,200. D's gain on the real estate is computed as follows:

Selling price	$45,000
Less: Adjusted basis	(36,000)
Gain realized and recognized	$ 9,000

D nets the gain and loss as follows:

15% Gain from sale of § 1231 asset	$ 9,000
15% Loss from sale of § 1231 asset	(1,200)
Net 15% § 1231 gain for year	$ 7,800

D's net 15% § 1231 gain of $7,800 is treated as a 15% capital gain. If she had other capital gains or losses during the year, they will be subject to the capital gain and loss netting process discussed in Chapter 16.

Example 5. During the year R, a sole proprietor, sold a business computer for $32,000. His basis at the time of the sale was $44,000. He also sold land used in his business at a gain of $1,400 and had an uninsured theft loss of works of art used to decorate his business offices (i.e., capital assets held in connection with a trade or business). R had purchased the artwork for $1,500 and it was valued at $5,000 before the burglary. All of the assets were acquired more than 12 months ago.

R nets his gains and losses as follows:

Step 1: The net loss from the casualty is $1,500 (adjusted basis). Since R has a net 15% casualty loss, it is not treated as a § 1231 loss. Instead, the loss is treated as an ordinary loss (which is fully deductible for A.G.I. since the art works were business property).

Step 2: Combine gains and losses from sales of § 1231 assets:

15% loss from sale of business computer.	($12,000)
15% gain from sale of business land	1,400
Net § 1231 loss for year	($10,600)

Step 3: A net § 1231 loss is treated as an ordinary deduction. Thus, R's $10,600 loss can be used to offset other ordinary income.

Note that the theft loss of the works of art is included in the first step of the netting process even though these items are capital assets. This loss would have offset, dollar for dollar, any casualty or theft gains (net of depreciation recapture) from § 1231 assets as well as any casualty or theft gains from other capital assets held in connection with R's business. Also note that the current year's deductible § 1231 loss may result in a change in the character of any net § 1231 gains in the next five years due to the look-back rule.

LOOK-BACK RULE

For many years, taxpayers took advantage of the § 1231 netting process. For example, assume a taxpayer in the 35 percent tax bracket currently owns two § 1231 assets, both held for 15 months. One asset has a built-in gain of $10,000 and the other has a built-in loss of $9,000. If both assets are sold during the year, the loss offsets the gain and the taxpayer pays a capital gain tax of $150 [($10,000 − $9,000 = $1,000) × 15%]. If the taxpayer had sold the assets in different years, the loss would *not* have reduced the gain, and the tax after both transactions would have been $1,500 in one year ($10,000 × 15%) and $3,150 ($9,000 × 35%) of savings in the other year, for a net tax savings of $1,650 ($3,150 − $1,500). As might be imagined, taxpayers carefully planned their transactions to maximize their tax savings.

In an effort to prevent taxpayers from cleverly timing their § 1231 gains and losses to ensure that § 1231 losses reduced ordinary income and not potential capital gain, Congress enacted the so-called *look-back* rule in 1984. Under this rule, a taxpayer with a net § 1231 gain in the current year must report the gain as ordinary income to the extent of any *unrecaptured* net § 1231 losses reported in the past five taxable years.[18] In recapturing the § 1231 gains, recapture occurs in the following order: 28% gains, 25% gains, and 15% gains. Unrecaptured net § 1231 losses are simply the *net* § 1231 losses that have occurred during the past five years that have not been previously recaptured (i.e., the excess of net § 1231 losses of the five preceding years over the amount of such loss that has been recaptured in the five prior years).

Example 6. Assume the same facts in *Example 5* and that R's 2008 net § 1231 loss of $10,600 is the only loss he has deducted in the past five years. In 2009, R has a net 15% § 1231 gain of $15,000. R is subject to the look-back rule since in the prior year he reported a § 1231 loss of $10,600 that has not been recaptured. He must report $10,600 of ordinary income and $4,400 of net 15% § 1231 gain. Should R have a § 1231 gain in the following year, he will not be subject to the look-back rule again since he has recaptured all prior year's net § 1231 losses.

---

[18] § 1231(c).

APPLICABILITY OF LOWER RATES

Five potential tax rates apply to long-term capital gains; six, to ordinary income, which includes short-term capital gains. How can the calculation of the capital gains tax, including any § 1231 gain, be completed in such a way as to arrive at a single right answer?

Caution must be exercised so as to complete the netting process in the prescribed order, as elaborated so far in this chapter and in Chapter 16.

- ▸ The first step is to complete the § 1231 netting process.

  - If there is a net § 1231 loss, that loss must be treated as an ordinary loss and it is left out of the capital gain and loss netting process entirely.
  - If there is a net § 1231 gain, it is treated as a long-term capital gain and is entered into the capital gain and loss netting process in the next step. In order to do this, a determination must be made as to which part of the gain, if any, is 25% gain, and which part, if any, is 15% gain.

- ▸ Netting of capital gains and losses occurs in each of the various groups of assets.

  - Short-term gains are netted against short-term losses and long-term gains are netted against long-term losses.
  - Within the long-term netting process, gains and losses are further broken down in the various sub-groups with 15% gains and losses, and 28% gains and losses being netted. Since there are no 25% losses, the 25% gains are not reduced.
  - The net gains and losses from these three groups are netted against one another as prescribed in Chapter 16 (e.g., 28% losses are first offset against 25% gains, then 15% gains, and 15% losses are first offset against 28% gains, then 25% gains).

- ▸ Short-term gains and losses are netted/combined with long-term gains and losses. Short-term losses are first netted against 28% gains, then 25% gains, and finally 15% gains. Net long-term losses are netted against short-term gains.

- ▸ The net results are subject to the capital gains tax.

  - Short-term gains are treated like ordinary income
  - Long-term gains are subject to tax at the appropriate specified capital gains rates (0%, 10%, 15%, 25%, and 28%)
  - Losses are subject to the $3,000 annual limit with the excess being carried forward.

Numerous possibilities exist, therefore, for any net § 1231 gain. Perhaps, the gain would be offset by capital losses, receiving no favorable treatment at all. However, if the § 1231 gain survives the netting process to be included in a net capital gain, it is subject to the preferred rates right along with any other long-term capital gains with surviving unrecaptured § 1250 gain being treated as 25% gain and any other surviving gain treated as 15% gain.

✔ CHECK YOUR KNOWLEDGE

Review Question 1. Indicate whether the following gains and losses are § 1231 gains or losses or capital gains and losses or neither. Make your determination prior to the § 1231 netting process and assume any holding period requirement has been met.

a. Gain on the sale of General Motors stock held as a temporary investment by Consolidated Brands Corporation.

b. Gain on the sale of a four-unit apartment complex owned by Lorena Smith. This was her only rental property.

c. Loss on the sale of welding machinery used by Arco Welding in its business.

d. Loss on theft of welding machinery used by Arco Welding in its business.

e. Gain on sale of diamond bracelet by Nancy Jones.

f. Income from sale of electric razors by Razor Corporation, which manufactures them.

g. Gain on condemnation of land on which Tonya Smith's personal residence is built.

h. Gain on condemnation of land owned by Tonya Smith's business.

i. Loss on sale of personal automobile.

Answer. The § 1231 hodgepodge contains not only gains and losses from § 1231 property but also those from involuntary conversions by casualty, theft, or condemnation of capital assets that are used in a trade or business or held as an investment in connection with a trade or business.

a. The sale of the GM stock is not included in the § 1231 pot since it is a sale of a capital asset and not an involuntary conversion.

b. The rental property is generally considered property used in a trade or business and thus § 1231 property even if the owner owns only a single property.

c. The welding machinery is depreciable property used in a business and is therefore considered § 1231 property.

d. The theft of the welding machinery is also a § 1231 transaction. Note, however, that in processing the § 1231 gains and losses, the casualties must be segregated from the sales.

e. The sale of the diamond bracelet produces capital gain since it is a pure capital asset and not trade or business property.

f. The razors are inventory and are therefore neither capital assets nor § 1231 property.

g. The condemnation of the land near the residence is considered a personal involuntary conversion gain. Since the land is not held in connection with a trade or business, it does not qualify as § 1231 property, but it is a capital asset.

h. The condemnation of the land held for business does enter into the § 1231 hodgepodge as a regular § 1231 gain.

i. Although the personal automobile is a capital asset, no loss is allowed from the sale.

Review Question 2. During his senior year at the University of Virginia, Bill decided that he never wanted to leave Charlottesville. After some thought, he opened his own hamburger joint, Billy's Burgers. That was 20 years ago and Bill has had great success, owning a number of businesses all over Virginia and North Carolina. Not believing in corporations, Bill and his wife, Betty, operate all of these as partnerships.

a. Information from the partnerships and his own personal records revealed the following transactions during the current year:

1. Sale of one of 50 apartment buildings that one of their partnerships owns: $50,000 gain (ignore depreciation)

2. Sale of restaurant equipment: $20,000 loss

Assuming both assets have been held for several years, how should Bill and Betty report these transactions on their current year return?

Answer. Under § 1231, the taxpayer generally nets gains and losses from the sale of § 1231 property. If a net gain results, the gain is treated as a long-term capital gain, while a net loss is treated as an ordinary loss. For this purpose, § 1231 property generally includes real or depreciable property used in a trade or business. In this case, both the apartment complex and the restaurant equipment are § 1231 property and both are in the 15 percent group. As a result, the couple should net the gain and loss and report a 15 percent capital gain of $30,000.

    b.   The couple's records for the following year revealed several gains and losses:

        1.   Office building burned down: $20,000 loss

        2.   Crane for bungee jumping business stolen: $35,000 gain (assume no depreciation had been claimed)

        3.   Parking lot sold: $14,000 loss

        4.   Exxon stock sold: long-term capital loss of $10,000

        5.   Condemnation of Greensboro land held for use in the business: $15,000 gain.

Assuming each of the assets was held for several years, determine how much 15 percent capital gain or loss as well as the amount of ordinary income or loss that Bill and Betty will report for the year.

Answer. The § 1231 netting process requires the taxpayer to separate § 1231 casualty gains and losses from other § 1231 transactions (sometimes referred to as regular § 1231 items). The casualty loss on the office building and the casualty gain on the crane are both considered § 1231 15 percent casualties since they involve § 1231 property (i.e., real or depreciable property used in business). Note that the condemnation—even though it is an involuntary conversion—is not treated as a § 1231 casualty. The casualty items are netted to determine whether there is a net gain or loss. Here, there is a net casualty 15 percent gain of $15,000 ($35,000 − $20,000). This net gain is then combined with any "regular" § 1231 items, in this case the $14,000 loss on the sale of the parking lot (real property used in a business) and the $15,000 gain on the condemnation of the land (a capital asset). Note that both "regular" § 1231 items are also in the 15 percent group. After netting these items, the partnership has a net gain of $16,000. This $16,000 net § 1231 gain is treated as a 15 percent capital gain and is combined with $10,000 15 percent capital loss on the sale of the stock. The end result is a $6,000 15 percent capital gain. This process can be summarized as follows (see also Exhibit 17-3):

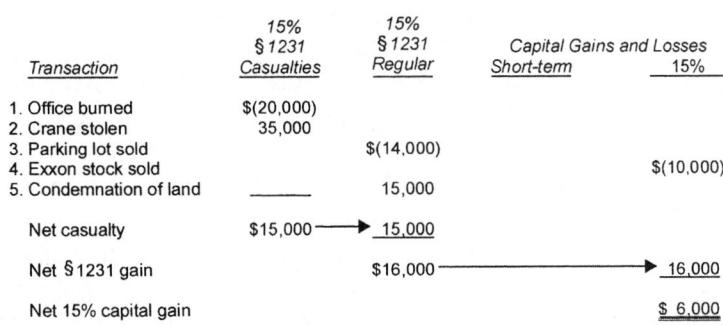

Transaction	15% §1231 Casualties	15% §1231 Regular	Capital Gains and Losses Short-term	15%
1. Office burned	$(20,000)			
2. Crane stolen	35,000			
3. Parking lot sold		$(14,000)		
4. Exxon stock sold				$(10,000)
5. Condemnation of land		15,000		
Net casualty	$15,000 ⟶	15,000		
Net §1231 gain		$16,000 ⟶		16,000
Net 15% capital gain				$ 6,000

c. Same as in (b), except Bill and Betty reported a net § 1231 loss of $3,000 in the previous year.

Answer. In this case, the look-back rule applies, causing $3,000 of the net 15 percent § 1231 gain to be treated as ordinary income. As a result, the couple's 15 percent capital gain from the § 1231 netting process is $13,000 and their net 15 percent capital gain is only $3,000.

DEPRECIATION RECAPTURE

HISTORICAL PERSPECTIVE

For many years, taxpayers have taken advantage of the interaction of § 1231 and the depreciation rules to secure significant tax savings. Prior to 1962 there were no substantial statutory restrictions on the depreciation methods that could be adopted. Consequently, a taxpayer could quickly recover the basis of a depreciable asset by selecting a rapid depreciation method such as declining balance and using a short useful life. If the property's value did not decline as quickly as its basis was being reduced by depreciation deductions, a gain was ensured if the property was disposed of at a later date. The end result could be quite beneficial.

Example 7. During the current year, T purchased equipment for $1 million. After two years, T, using favorable depreciation rules, had claimed and deducted $600,000 of depreciation, leaving a basis of $400,000. Assume that the property did not truly depreciate in value and T was able to sell it in the third year for its original cost of $1 million. In such case T would report a gain of $600,000 ($1,000,000 − $400,000). Except for time value of money considerations, it appears that the $600,000 gain and the $600,000 of depreciation are simply a wash. However, the depreciation reduced ordinary income that would be taxed at ordinary rates while the gain would be a § 1231 gain and likely taxed at capital gain rates. As an illustration of the savings that could be achieved, assume that the law at this time provided for a top capital gain rate of 20% and the taxpayer's ordinary income was taxed at a 40%. In this case the depreciation would offset ordinary income and provide tax savings of $240,000, but the $600,000 gain on the sale would be treated as a capital gain and produce a tax of only $120,000. Thus, even though the taxpayer has had no economic gain or loss with respect to the property—he bought

and sold the equipment for $1,000,000—he was able to secure a tax benefit of $120,000 ($240,000 − $120,000).

The above example clearly illustrates how taxpayers used rapid depreciation and the favorable treatment of § 1231 gains to effectively convert ordinary income into capital gain. In fact, this strategy—deferring taxes with quick depreciation write-offs at ordinary rates and giving them back later at capital gains rates—was the foundation of many tax shelter schemes.

Legislation to limit these benefits came in a number of forms, but the most important was the enactment of the so-called *depreciation recapture* rules. These rules strike right at the heart of the problem, generally treating all or some portion of any gain recognized as ordinary income, based on the amount of depreciation previously deducted. Thus, in the above example, the taxpayer's $600,000 gain, which was initially characterized as a § 1231 gain, is treated as ordinary income because of the $600,000 of depreciation previously claimed. In this way, all of the tax savings initially given away by virtue of the ordinary depreciation deductions are recaptured. In this regard, it may be useful to think of a gain as consisting of two parts: the gain attributable to depreciation and the gain attributable to holding the asset (resulting from appreciation and inflation). "Depreciation gains" normally are treated as ordinary income while "holding gains" are § 1231 gains and potentially taxed as long-term capital gains. Unfortunately, much like § 1231 in general, the recapture rules can become quite complex. The operations of the specific provisions are discussed below.

WHEN APPLICABLE

Before specific recapture rules are examined, there are two very important points to keep in mind. First, depreciable assets held for one year or less do not qualify for § 1231 treatment. Thus, any gain from the disposition of such assets is always reported as ordinary income. Second, the depreciation recapture rules *do not apply* if property is disposed of at a *loss*. Remember that losses from the sale or exchange of depreciable assets are treated as § 1231 losses if the property is held more than a year. In addition, casualty or theft losses of such property are included in the § 1231 netting process. Any loss from a depreciable asset held one year or less is an ordinary loss regardless of whether it was sold, exchanged, stolen, or destroyed.

TYPES OF DEPRECIATION RECAPTURE

There are essentially *three* depreciation recapture provisions in the Code. These are:

1. Section 1245 Recapture—commonly called the *full recapture rule*, and applicable primarily to depreciable personalty (rather than realty)

2. Section 1250 Recapture—commonly called the *partial recapture rule*, and applicable to most depreciable realty if a method of depreciation other than straight-line was used

3. Section 291 Recapture—commonly called the *additional recapture rule*, and applicable *only* to corporate taxpayers

These depreciation recapture provisions affect the character—not the amount—of the gain. Losses are not affected. Each of these recapture rules is discussed below.

FULL RECAPTURE—§ 1245

The recapture concept was first introduced with the enactment of § 1245 by the Revenue Act of 1962. Section 1245 generally requires any gain recognized to be reported as ordinary income to the extent of *any* depreciation allowed on § 1245 property after 1961.

Definition of § 1245 Property. The recapture of depreciation under § 1245 applies only to *§ 1245 property*, normally *depreciable personal property*.[19] Because the definition of personal property itself is so broad, § 1245 generally covers a wide variety of depreciable assets such as:

- Machinery and equipment used in production of goods and services
- Office furniture and equipment
- Automobiles, vans, trucks, and other transportation equipment
- Livestock used for breeding or production
- Intangibles such as patents, copyrights, trademarks, and goodwill that have been amortized under § 197 or otherwise.

Essentially the amortization is treated the same as depreciation, just like any portion of the cost of a depreciable asset that is expensed under § 179 is treated as depreciation allowed.[20] It is important to understand that § 1245 applies only if the property is depreciable or amortizable. Consequently, it pertains only to property that is used in a trade or business and property held for the production of income. For example, livestock that are considered inventory are not subject to depreciation and are therefore not § 1245 property, although any gain or loss from the disposition of inventory is ordinary income.

Although the above definition is usually sufficient, § 1245 property actually includes a number of other assets besides depreciable personalty, including the following:[21]

1. Property used as an integral part of manufacturing, production, or extraction, or in furnishing transportation, communications, electrical energy, gas, water, or sewage disposal services.

   a. However, any portion of a building or its structural components is not included.

   b. A research facility or a facility for the bulk storage of commodities related to an activity listed above is included.

2. A single-purpose agricultural or horticultural structure (e.g., greenhouses).

3. A storage structure used in connection with the distribution of petroleum or any primary product of petroleum (e.g., oil tank).

4. Any railroad grading or tunnel bore.

5. Certain other property that is subject to a special provision allowing current deductibility or rapid amortization (e.g., pollution control facilities and railroad rolling stock).

Operation of § 1245. Section 1245 generally requires any gain recognized to be treated as ordinary income to the extent of *any* depreciation allowed.[22] To state the rule in another way: any gain on the disposition of § 1245 property is ordinary income to the extent of the *lesser* of the gain recognized or the § 1245 recapture potential, generally the depreciation claimed and deducted. Although both statements say the same thing, the latter helps focus attention on two points and eliminates some misconceptions. First, a taxpayer is never required to report more income than the amount of gain realized regardless of the amount of depreciation claimed and deducted (i.e., regardless of the

---

[19]   § 1245(a)(3).

[20]   See § 197(f)(7) for intangibles and § 1245(a)(3)(D) for expensed property and certain other properties subject to unique expensing rules.

[21]   The definition parallels that of § 38 property, which qualified for the investment tax credit. § 48(a)(1).

[22]   § 1245(a).

amount of recapture potential). For example, if the taxpayer realizes a gain of $10,000 and has deducted depreciation of $15,000, the taxpayer reports only $10,000 of income, all of which would be ordinary. Note that the depreciation recapture rules do not affect the amount of gain or loss, only the character of any gain to be recognized. Second, using the term *recapture potential* helps emphasize that sometimes the amount that must be recaptured may include more than mere depreciation.

Section 1245 *recapture potential* includes *all* depreciation or amortization allowed (or allowable) with respect to a given property—regardless of the method of depreciation used. This is why § 1245 is often called the full recapture rule. Recapture potential also includes adjustments to basis related to items that are expensed (e.g., under § 179 expense election) or where tax credits have been allowed under various sections of the Code.[23]

To summarize, determining the character of gain on the disposition of § 1245 property is generally a three-step process:

1. Determine the amount of gain to be recognized, if any.

2. The gain is ordinary income to the extent of the *lesser* of the gain recognized or the § 1245 recapture potential (all depreciation allowed or allowable).

3. Any recognized gain in excess of the recapture potential retains its original character, usually § 1231 gain.

Recall that there is no § 1245 depreciation recapture when a property is sold at a loss, so any loss is normally a § 1231 loss.

> **Example 8.** T owned a printing press that he used in his business. Its cost was $6,800 and T deducted depreciation in the amount of $3,200 during the three years he owned the press. T sold the press for $4,000 and his realized and recognized gain is $400 ($4,000 sales price − $3,600 adjusted basis). T's recapture potential is $3,200, the amount of depreciation taken on the property. Thus, the entire $400 gain is ordinary income under § 1245.

> **Example 9.** Assume the same facts as in *Example 8*, except that T sold his press for $7,000. In this case, T's realized and recognized gain would be $3,400 ($7,000 − $3,600). The ordinary income portion under § 1245 would be $3,200 (the amount of the recapture potential), and the remaining $200 of the gain is a § 1231 gain. Note that in order for any § 1231 gain to occur, the property must be sold for more than its original cost since all of the depreciation is treated as ordinary income.

> **Example 10.** Assume the same facts as in *Example 8*, except that the printing press is sold for $3,000 instead of $4,000. In this case, T has a loss from the sale of $600 ($3,000 − $3,600 adjusted basis). Because there is a loss, there is no depreciation recapture. All of T's loss is a § 1231 loss.

Exceptions and Limitations. In many ways, § 1245 operates much like the proverbial troll under the bridge. It sits ready to spring on its victim whenever the proper moment arises. Section 1245 generally applies whenever there is a transfer of property. However, § 1245 does identify certain situations where it does not apply, most of which are nontaxable events. For example, there is no recapture on a transfer by gift or bequest since both of these are nontaxable transfers.[24]

---

[23]   See § 1245(a)(2) for a listing of these adjustments and their related Code sections, including the basis adjustment related to the earned portion of any investment credit.

[24]   §§ 1245(b)(1) and (2). Recapture of depreciation under § 1245 is required, however, to the extent § 691 applies (relating to income in respect to a decedent).

In involuntary conversions and like-kind exchanges, the depreciation recapture under § 1245 is limited to the *gain recognized*.[25] Similarly, in nontaxable business adjustments such as the formation of partnerships, transfers to controlled corporations, and certain corporate reorganizations, § 1245 recapture is limited to the gain recognized under the controlling provisions.[26] In any situation where recapture is not triggered, it is generally not lost but carried over in some fashion.

PARTIAL RECAPTURE—§ 1250

As originally enacted in 1961, the concept of recapture as set forth in § 1245 generally applied only to personalty. Gains derived from dealing in realty were not subject to recapture. In 1963, however, Congress eliminated this omission by enacting § 1250, a special recapture provision that applied to most buildings. Since 1963, § 1245 has generally been associated with depreciation recapture for personal property while § 1250 served that role for buildings. Although the two provisions are similar, § 1250 is far less damaging. Specifically, § 1250 calls for the recapture of only a *portion* of any *accelerated* depreciation allowed with respect to *§ 1250 property*. Note that while §§ 1250 and 1245 are essentially the same—they both convert potential capital gain into ordinary income—§ 1250 differs from § 1245 in several important ways: (1) it applies only if an accelerated method is used; (2) it does not require recapture of all the depreciation deducted but only a portion—generally only the *excess of accelerated depreciation over what straight-line would have been*; and (3) it applies to a different type of property, *buildings and their components*, rather than personal property. These basic concepts are illustrated in the following example and discussed further below.

> **Example 11.** T purchased an office building in 1979 for $600,000. In 1979, depreciation generally was computed using either the straight-line or accelerated method based on the estimated useful life of the property and estimated salvage value, all determined by the taxpayer. T depreciated the building over its estimated useful life of 40 years, using an accelerated method and no salvage value. This year, T sold the building for $900,000. At the time of sale, accelerated depreciation actually deducted was $500,000. Straight-line depreciation using the same facts would have been $300,000. The building is § 1250 property since it is realty acquired after 1969. As determined below, T recognizes a gain of $800,000, $200,000 is recaptured as ordinary income under § 1250 and the $600,000 balance is § 1231 gain.

Amount realized		$900,000*
Adjusted basis		
Cost	$600,000	
Depreciation (accelerated)	(500,000)	
Adjusted basis		(100,000)
Gain on sale		$800,000
Depreciation recapture under § 1250		
Accelerated depreciation actually deducted	$500,000	
Hypothetical straight-line depreciation	(300,000)	
Section 1250 recapture reported as ordinary income		$200,000
Section 1231 gain		$600,000

* A separate allocation and calculation would be required to determine any gain or loss on the land and is ignored here for simplicity.

---

[25]　§ 1245(b)(4).

[26]　§ 1245(b)(3). See Chapter 19 for further discussion of nontaxable business adjustments.

Note that under the partial recapture rule of § 1250 only the excess of the actual amount of accelerated depreciation deducted ($500,000) over what the straight-line depreciation would have been ($300,000), a difference of $200,000, is recaptured. This excess is treated as ordinary income. Had the property been § 1245 property, all $500,000 would have been recaptured. Also observe that under § 1250 none of the straight-line depreciation, $300,000 is recaptured. However, this unrecaptured depreciation on § 1250 property is taxed at a maximum rate of 25% as discussed below.

As noted in the example, § 1250 does not recapture the straight-line depreciation. In enacting § 1250 Congress wanted to ensure that ordinary income treatment would be applied only to what were truly excess depreciation deductions. Gain not attributable to excess depreciation was considered attributable to a rise in price levels and was eligible for relief provided for capital gains and not subject to recapture.

Section 1250 Property. Section 1250 property is generally any real property that is depreciable and is not covered by § 1245.[27] For the most part, § 1250 applies to all of the common forms of real estate such as office buildings, warehouses, apartment complexes, and low-income housing. As a practical matter, sales of these properties rarely produce recapture because the law has required the straight-line method for depreciation since 1986. However, Section 1250 property also includes 15- and 20-year realty which is depreciated using the 150 percent declining balance and, therefore, is capable of creating excess depreciation. This category includes such assets as multi-purpose agricultural structures (e. g., barns), land improvements (roads, sidewalks, fences, landscaping, shrubbery, docks), gas stations, convenience stores and more. As explained earlier, nonresidential real estate (e.g., warehouses and office buildings) placed in service after 1980 and before 1987 for which an accelerated method was used is covered by the full recapture rule of § 1245.[28]

Depreciation of Real Property. Section 1250 applies only if an accelerated method of depreciation is used. If the straight-line depreciation method is used, § 1250 does not apply and there is no depreciation recapture for noncorporate taxpayers.[29] For this reason, a critical first step in determining the relevance of § 1250 is determining how the taxpayer has depreciated the realty.

Realty Placed in Service before 1987. Prior to 1987, taxpayers could choose to use either an accelerated or straight-line method to compute depreciation for realty. This was an extremely important decision. It affected not only the amount of depreciation the taxpayer claimed but also the character of any gain on a subsequent disposition of the property. For example, a taxpayer could accelerate depreciation deductions but only at the possible expense of recapture. Alternatively, the taxpayer could accept the slower-paced straight-line method and avoid the § 1250 recapture rules. But the Tax Reform Act of 1986 ended this flexibility and at the same time simplified the law. Taxpayers who place realty in service *after 1986* must use the straight-line method for residential and nonresidential realty. As a result, the recapture rules of § 1250 do not apply to residential and nonresidential realty acquired after 1986. However, much of the existing inventory of real property was acquired before 1987 and may therefore be subject to § 1250, depending on the depreciation method used.

---

[27]   § 1250(c).

[28]   It is important to note, however, that such properties are § 1250 property if the optional straight-line method is used. § 1245(a)(5).

[29]   As explained within, corporate taxpayers are still required to recapture 20 percent of any straight-line depreciation under § 291. Also, any unrecaptured straight-line depreciation is taxed at a maximum rate of 25 percent.

Realty Placed in Service from 1981 through 1986. For real property acquired between the beginning of 1981 and the end of 1986, the taxpayer could either use the accelerated depreciation method allowed under ACRS or elect an optional straight-line method. In most cases, a taxpayer would select the accelerated method. If an accelerated method is used for *residential* realty acquired during 1981 through 1986, § 1250 applies, requiring recapture of the excess depreciation. However, as noted earlier, if an accelerated method is used for *nonresidential* realty acquired during 1981 through 1986, the property is considered § 1245 and the full recapture rule applies.

By the close of 2005, realty acquired during 1981 through 1986 became fully depreciated since the lives were 15, 18 or 19 years during this time. As a result, there is no § 1250 recapture for residential realty since there is no excess depreciation (i.e., total accelerated depreciation would be identical to total straight-line depreciation). Similarly, there is no § 1250 recapture for nonresidential realty if the straight-line method was used. However, to reiterate, if the accelerated method was used in depreciating nonresidential realty acquired during these tainted years, 1981–1986, § 1245 applies and all of the accelerated depreciation is recaptured.

Realty Placed in Service before 1981. All depreciable real property acquired before 1981 is classified as § 1250 property. For such property acquired before 1981 (non-ACRS property), taxpayers were required to estimate useful lives and salvage values. Although various methods could be used, there were restrictions.[30] In those situations where an accelerated method was used, § 1250 applies subject to certain limitations. As discussed further below, none of the excess depreciation produced by realty for years after 1963 and before 1970 is subject to recapture. In the case of *low-income housing* and other *residential* real estate, excess depreciation resulting after 1969 and before 1976 is no longer recaptured. After 1975, excess depreciation on low-income housing is exempt from recapture if the property is held more than 16 2/3 years.

Summary of § 1250 Application. The significance of § 1250 has declined considerably over the years. Subject to certain unusual situations (e.g., certain low-income housing, certain Liberty Zone property, etc.), the following general observations can be made about the current status of § 1250:

- For residential and nonresidential realty acquired after 1986, there is no § 1250 recapture because the straight-line method must be used for such property and no excess depreciation results.
- For *residential* realty acquired during 1981–1986 there is no § 1250 recapture since these assets are fully depreciated and there is no excess depreciation.
- For *nonresidential* realty acquired during 1981–1986 for which the straight-line method was used, there is no recapture under § 1250, but § 1245 requires full-recapture if an accelerated method was used for the property.
- The reach of § 1250 is usually limited to realty acquired during 1970–1980. And much of this property, which at this point is 27–37 years old, has turned over and in the hands of the new buyer § 1250 does not apply.

Although the traditional recapture rules of § 1250 may not apply, gains on § 1250 property are not guaranteed the benefits of favorable capital gain rates. As explained further below, such gains may be taxed at a rate of up to 25 percent to the extent of any unrecaptured straight-line depreciation

---

[30]   § 167(j).

Operation of § 1250. The two critical factors in determining the amount, if any, of *§ 1250 recapture* are the gain realized *and* the amount of *excess depreciation*. Excess depreciation refers to depreciation deductions in excess of that which would be deductible using the straight-line method. For property held one year or less, all depreciation is considered excess depreciation.[31]

As a general rule, § 1250 requires recapture of the excess depreciation, that is, the excess of accelerated over straight-line. Consequently, even if the taxpayer uses an accelerated method to compute the amount of depreciation deducted on the return, the hypothetical amount of straight-line depreciation must still be computed in order to determine the excess of accelerated over straight-line when the property is sold. In determining the hypothetical amount of straight-line depreciation, the taxpayer uses the same life and salvage value, if any, that were used in computing accelerated depreciation.[32] Because of this approach, a taxpayer who uses the straight-line method would have no excess depreciation and no recapture. Because the § 1250 recapture rule applies only to any excess depreciation claimed by a taxpayer, it is sometimes referred to as the partial recapture rule. However, it should be emphasized that beginning in 1997, the unrecaptured § 1250 depreciation (e.g., the straight-line depreciation) on § 1250 property held more than 12 months is subject to a special 25 percent tax rate (assuming it survives the § 1231 netting process).

Determining the taxation of any gain recognized on the disposition of § 1250 property is a four-step process:

1. Determine the amount of gain to be recognized, if any.

2. The gain is ordinary income to the extent of the *lesser* of the gain recognized or the § 1250 recapture potential (generally the excess depreciation allowed).[33]

3. Any recognized gain in excess of the recapture potential is usually treated as § 1231 gain.

4. Any gain recognized on § 1250 property held more than 12 months that is due to depreciation that is not recaptured and which survives the applicable netting processes is taxed at a maximum rate of 25 percent to the extent of any unrecaptured depreciation. Any additional gain is generally 15 percent gain.

Two other considerations should be noted. If § 1250 property is held for a year or less, all depreciation (not just the excess) is recaptured.[34] In addition, there is no § 1250 depreciation recapture when a property is sold at a loss, so any loss is normally a § 1231 loss.

Unrecaptured § 1250 Gain. As may be apparent from step 3 above, under § 1250, taxpayers are required to recapture depreciation only if an accelerated method is used to depreciate the property. Consequently, individual taxpayers never recapture depreciation on § 1250 property if the straight-line method is used. Without some special rule, any gain attributable to straight-line depreciation for § 1250 property held more than 12 months would normally qualify for taxation at a 15 percent rate. Congress felt this treatment was too generous and created a special rule for *unrecaptured § 1250 gain.* The unrecaptured § 1250 gain is the lesser of (1) the gain recognized, or (2) the depreciation allowed after each (the gain recognized and the depreciation allowed) is reduced by any § 1250

---

[31] § 1250(b).

[32] § 1250(b)(5).

[33] See § 1250(a) and discussion following dealing with recapture of only a portion of the excess depreciation for certain properties.

[34] § 1250(b)(1).

recapture. The resulting amount will equal the amount of straight-line depreciation that was claimed or would have been claimed had the straight-line method been used (or, if less, the gain recognized minus the § 1250 recapture).

> **Example 12.** About 10 years ago, F purchased some residential rental property for $100,000. This year he sold the property for $110,000. He had claimed straight-line depreciation of $30,000 over this time, resulting in a basis of $70,000 (do not attempt to verify this amount). As a result, F recognized a gain of $40,000. Since the property is realty and a straight-line depreciation method was used there is no § 1250 recapture. Consequently, the entire gain is a § 1231 gain. However, the § 1231 gain will be treated as a 25% gain to the extent of any straight-line depreciation claimed. Therefore, $30,000 of the gain is a 25% § 1231 gain while $10,000 is a 15% § 1231 gain (i.e., in the capital gain netting process these will be 15% and 25% long-term gains, respectively). If F had sold the property for $90,000, he would have had a gain of $20,000, all of which would have been a 25% gain (i.e., the lesser of the gain realized, $20,000, or the unrecaptured straight-line depreciation, $30,000).

> **Example 13.** Same facts and $110,000 sales price from *Example 12* above, except that F also has a $400 gain on the sale of K Corporation stock held 26 months. F is single and has taxable income, excluding these transactions, of $85,250. F's tax would be computed as follows (using the 2009 tax rates for single taxpayers):

Regular tax on $85,250:		
Tax on $82,250.	$16,750	
Tax on excess at 28%		
[($85,250 − $82,250 = $3,000) × 28%]	840	
		$17,590
Tax on 15% gains (15% × $10,400)		1,560
Tax on 25% gains (25% × $30,000)		7,500
Total tax		$26,650

Combined Results. The net gain from the disposition of § 1250 property can be treated as ordinary income subject to the regular tax rate, 15 percent capital gain, and/or 25 percent capital gain (and rarely 28 percent capital gain). Each step in the netting and tax calculation processes has been covered. *Examples 14 through 17* and *Comprehensive Example 19* illustrate how they work in combination.

> **Example 14.** During the current year, L sold a small office building for $38,000. The building cost $22,000 in 1980, and she had deducted depreciation of $12,000 using an accelerated method ($10,000 was assigned to the land and was not depreciable). Straight-line depreciation would have been $10,600. L's gain recognized on the sale is $28,000 ($38,000 amount realized − $10,000 adjusted basis). Of that amount, $1,400 ($12,000 − $10,600 = $1,400 excess depreciation) is ordinary income under § 1250 and the remainder, $26,600, is § 1231 gain. Of the $26,600 § 1231 gain, the unrecaptured depreciation of $10,600 ($12,000 − $1,400) is a 25% gain. The $16,000 excess of the amount realized over the original basis is 15% gain.

> **Example 15.** M purchased a rental duplex during 1986 for $60,000 (not including any value assigned to land). He deducted $60,000 depreciation using the 19-year realty ACRS tables. Depreciation using the straight-line recovery percentages for 19-year realty would have resulted in total depreciation of $60,000 (the duplex is fully depreciated under each method).

On January 3 of the current year M sold the property for $87,000. His gain is reported as follows:

Sales price		$87,000
Less: Adjusted basis		
Cost	$60,000	
Depreciation allowed	(60,000)	(-0-)
Gain to be recognized		$87,000
Accelerated depreciation claimed and deducted		$60,000
Straight-line depreciation (hypothetical)		(60,000)
Excess depreciation subject to recapture		$ -0-
Character of gain:		
Ordinary income (partial recapture)		$ -0-
§ 1231 gain subject to 25% rate		60,000
§ 1231 gain subject to 15% rate		27,000
Total gain recognized		$87,000

First, observe that the property is residential property (rather than nonresidential property) so it is subject to §1250 that requires recapture of the excess of accelerated depreciation over straight line. In this case, however, there is no excess depreciation since the rental property is fully depreciated. Thus, without a special rule, the gain not recaptured under § 1250 might be subject to the 15% capital gains rate. However, the depreciation that has not been recaptured, $60,000, is carved out and is considered a 25% § 1231 gain. Also observe that the $60,000 of 25% § 1231 gain is the amount of straight-line depreciation. The remaining gain (i.e., the amount above the original cost) of $27,000 is a 15% § 1231 gain.

Example 16. Assume the same facts as in *Example 15*, except that M elected to recover his basis in the duplex using the 19-year straight-line method. Consequently she still recognizes gain of $87,000 computed as follows:

Sales price			$87,000
Less:	Adjusted basis		
	Cost	$60,000	
	Depreciation (straight-line)	(60,000)	
			(-0-)
Gain			$(87,000)

None of the gain is subject to § 1250 recapture since M used straight-line depreciation (a requirement after 1986). However, the amount representing the unrecaptured depreciation (i.e., the straight-line depreciation) of $60,000 is considered a 25% § 1231 gain and the $27,000 balance is considered a 15% § 1231 gain.

Example 17. Assume the same facts as in *Example 15*, except that the property is an office building rather than a duplex. In this case, because the property is nonresidential real property and the accelerated method was used, the asset is treated as § 1245 property rather than § 1250 property. Thus, M is subject to full rather than partial depreciation recapture. All of the $60,000 depreciation is recaptured and treated as ordinary income. The balance of the gain, $27,000 is treated as a 15% § 1231 gain.

History of § 1250. Over the years, § 1250 has been changed frequently, with a general trend toward an expanded scope. The rules explained above apply only to

depreciation allowed on nonresidential property after 1969 and residential property (other than low-income housing) after 1975. Only a *portion* of any other excess depreciation on § 1250 property is included in the recapture potential. The following percentages are applied to the gain realized in the transaction or the excess depreciation taken during the particular period, whichever is less:

1. For all excess depreciation taken after 1963 and before 1970, 100 percent less 1 percent for each full month over 20 months the property is held.[35] Any sales after 1979 would result in no recapture of pre-1970 excess depreciation since this percentage, when calculated, is zero.

2. For all excess depreciation taken after 1969 and before 1976, as follows:

    a. In the case of low-income housing, 100 percent less 1 percent for each full month the property is held over 20 months.
    b. In the case of other residential rental property (e.g., an apartment building) and property that has been rehabilitated [for purposes of § 167(k)], 100 percent less 1 percent for each full month the property is held over 100 months.[36]

All sales from this group of real property after August 1992 will have no recapture of excess depreciation claimed before 1976.

3. For excess depreciation taken after 1975 on low-income housing and property that has been rehabilitated [for purposes of § 167(k)], 100 percent less 1 percent for each full month the property is held over 100 months.[37]

In summary, 100 percent of the excess depreciation allowed with respect to § 1250 property after 1975 is subject to recapture unless it falls into one of the above categories. Any gain recognized to the extent of any unrecaptured depreciation will be considered 25% gain. The rules for the various categories are set forth in § 1250(a).

Exceptions and Limitations under § 1250. Generally, the exceptions and limitations that apply under § 1245 also apply under § 1250. Thus, gifts, inheritances, and most nontaxable exchanges are allowed to occur without triggering recapture.[38] This exception is extended to any property to the extent it qualifies as a principal residence and is subject to deferral of gain under § 1034 or nonrecognition of gain under § 121.[39] In such nontaxable exchanges, the excess depreciation (that is not recaptured) taken prior to the nontaxable exchange on the property transferred carries over to the property received or purchased.[40] Similarly, in the case of gifts and certain nontaxable transfers in which the property is transferred to a new owner with a carryover basis, the excess depreciation carries over to the new owner.[41] In the case of inheritances in which basis to the successor in interest is determined under § 1014, no carryover of excess depreciation occurs.[42]

Certain like-kind exchanges and involuntary conversions may result in the recognition of gain solely because of § 1250 if insufficient § 1250 property is acquired. Since not all real property is depreciable, it is possible that the replacement property would not be

---

[35] § 1250(a)(3).

[36] § 1250(a)(2).

[37] § 1250(a)(1).

[38] §§ 1250(d)(1) through (d)(4).

[39] § 1250(d)(7).

[40] Reg. §§ 1.1250-3(d)(5) and (h)(4).

[41] Reg. §§ 1.1250-3(a), (c), and (f).

[42] Reg. § 1.1250-3(b).

§ 1250 property and would still qualify for nonrecognition under the appropriate rules of §§ 1033 or 1034. In such situations, gain will be recognized to the extent the amount that would be recaptured exceeds the fair market value of the § 1250 property received (property purchased in the case of an involuntary conversion).[43]

> **Example 18.** D completed a like-kind exchange in the current year in which he transferred an apartment complex (§ 1250 property) for rural farmland (not § 1250 property). The apartment had cost D $175,000 in 1980 and depreciation of $89,000 has been taken under the 200% declining-balance method. D would have deducted $62,000 under the straight-line method.
>
> The farm land was worth $200,000 at the time of the exchange. There were no improvements on the farm property. D's realized gain on the exchange is $114,000 ($200,000 amount realized − $86,000 adjusted basis in property given up). If there had been no § 1250 recapture, then D would have had no recognized gain. Because the property acquired was not § 1250 property, § 1250 supersedes (overrides) § 1031. D has a recognized gain of $27,000 [($89,000 − $62,000), the amount of excess depreciation], which is all ordinary income under § 1250.

Exhibit 17-2 provides an overview of the handling of sales and exchanges of business property. Exhibit 17-3 provides a chart that may be useful in summarizing property transactions. Note that for purposes of this Exhibit 17-3, no distinction is made between 15%, 25% and 28% § 1231 gains and losses or 15%, 25% and 28% capital gains and losses. A comprehensive example of sales and exchanges of trade or business property is presented below.

EXHIBIT 17-2
Stepwise Approach to Sales or Exchange of
Trade or Business Property—An Overview

Step 1: Determine the amount of gain to be recognized, if any. There is no recapture in the case of losses.

Step 2: Calculate any depreciation recapture on the disposition of § 1245 property and § 1250 property sold or exchanged at a taxable *gain* during the year.

Step 3: For any remaining gain (after recapture) on depreciable property held for more than one year, add to other § 1231 gains and losses and complete the § 1231 netting process.

▶ The § 1231 gain must be broken down into the portions that qualify as 15%CG and 25%CG (and rarely 28%CG).

Step 4: Complete the netting process for capital assets, taking into consideration the net § 1231 gain, if any.

▶ The § 1231 gain is combined with other long-term capital gains and losses (with separate netting for 15%CG, 25%CG, and 28%CG. Then the long-term capital gain or loss is combined with the short-term capital gain or loss.

---

[43]   § 1250(d)(4)(C). A similar rule is provided for rollovers (deferral) of gains from low-income housing under § 1039 [see § 1250(d)(8)].

Example 19. Ted and Carol Smith sold the following assets during the current year:

Description	Holding Period	Selling Price	Adjusted Basis	Recognized Gain (Loss)
Land and building (straight-line depreciation) Cost, $13,000 Depreciation allowed, $4,000	3 years	$14,000	$9,000	$5,000
Photocopier Cost, $2,500 Depreciation allowed, $500	14 months	2,600	2,000	600
Business auto Cost, $4,000 Depreciation allowed, $2,080	2 years	1,800	1,920	(120)

In determining the tax consequences of these sales, the Smiths must start with gains and losses from § 1231 transactions. The ultimate treatment of the gains, the character of the gain and any possible depreciation recapture must be considered.

- On the sale of the land and the building, there is no depreciation recapture for the building since straight-line depreciation was used. However, there is unrecaptured depreciation of $4,000 which is accounted for as a 25% § 1231 gain. The balance of the gain on the land and building, $1,000, is a 15% § 1231 gain.
- On the sale of the photocopier, $500 of the § 1231 gain of $600 is recaptured and treated as ordinary income. The balance of the gain, $100, is a 15% § 1231 gain.
- On the sale of the automobile, there is no recapture since it is sold at a loss. The $120 loss is treated as a 15% § 1231 loss. This information can be summarized as follows:

	Section 1231 Gains and Losses		
	Collectibles	Unrecaptured Depreciation	Other
	28%	25%	15%
Land and building		$4,000	$1,000
Photocopier			100
Automobile....................			(120)
Capital gains from § 1231........	$0	$4,000	$ 980

In this situation, the Smiths net the various groups, resulting in net gains in each of the groups as shown above. These amounts are then combined with the appropriate capital gain groups to determine the final treatment. Note that if the Smiths had unrecaptured § 1231 losses, they would first offset the 28% gains, then 25% gains, and finally 15% gains. The information is summarized in Exhibit 17-3.

EXHIBIT 17-3
Summary of Property Transactions

Recognized Gains (Losses)	Depreciation Recapture	Section 1231 Casualty and Theft*	Section 1231 Other *	Capital Gains/Losses Long-term* Short-term	Ordinary Income (Loss)
	§1245 Full recapture Personalty	Casualty and theft	Sale or exchange	Sale or exchange	
		1. §1231 property	§1231 property	Capital assets	
	§1250 Partial recapture Realty	Real or depreciable property used in business Timber, coal, iron ore, livestock, unharvested crops	Real or depreciable property used in business Timber, coal, iron ore, livestock, unharvested crops	All property except inventory, property held for resale, real and depreciable property used in trade or business, literary com- positions, and government publications	
	§291 Corporations only 20% straight-line				
		2. Capital assets used in trade or business or held for invest- ment in connection with business more than a year	Condemnation 1. §1231 property 2. Capital assets used in trade or busi- ness or held for invest- ment in connection with business more than a year		
$x,xxx		$x,xxx $(x,xxx)	$x,xxx $(x,xxx)	$x,xxx $x,xxx $(x,xxx) $(x,xxx)	$x,xxx
		Net loss			$(x,xxx)
		Net gain → $x,xxx			
			Net loss		$(x,xxx)
			Net gain		
			Look-back rule: Recaptured gains Unrecaptured gains → $x,xxx	$x,xxx	$x,xxx
				$x,xxx $x,xxx → $x,xxx Overall CG or NCL	

* These catagories must be subdivided into 15%, 25% and 28% groups.

Example 20. Assume that the Smiths, from the previous example, had the following capital asset transactions during the same year:

Description	Holding Period	Selling Price	Adjusted Basis	Description of Gain or (Loss)
100 shares XY Corp.	4 months	$ 3,200	$4,200	$(1,000) STCL
100 shares GB Corp.	3 years	3,200	4,600	(1,400) LTCL
1 acre vacant land	5 years	12,000	5,000	7,000 LTCG

Taking into consideration the § 1231 gains from *Example 18*, the Smith's summarize their transactions as follows.

| | Short-Term | Capital Gains and Losses | | |
| | | Collectibles | Unrecaptured Depreciation | Other |
	Ordinary	28%	25%	15%
Capital gains from § 1231		$0	$4,000	$ 980
XY stock loss	(1,000)			
GB stock loss				(1,400)
Vacant land gain				7,000
	$(1,000)	$0	$4,000	$6,580
Netting	1,000		(1,000)	
Total	$ 0	$0	$3,000	$6,580

Ted and Carol Smith would report a $3,000 N25CG and a $6,580 N15CG.

A Form 4797 and Schedule D containing the information from *Examples 18* and *19* are included in Exhibit 17-4 which follows. In using the forms, it should be pointed out that neither the Form 4797 nor Schedule D Parts I, II, and III (i.e., the form for reporting capital gains and losses) require the taxpayer to distinguish 25% gains from 28% or 15% gains. The 25% distinction comes into play only when the taxpayer computes the tax as can be seen on Schedule D, Part IV, Lines 25 and 47. The tax is computed assuming the taxpayers have taxable income of $126,830 (including the capital gains).

ADDITIONAL RECAPTURE—CORPORATIONS

Corporations generally compute the amount of § 1245 and § 1250 ordinary income recapture on the sales of depreciable assets in the same manner as do individuals. However, Congress added Code § 291 to the tax law in 1982 with the intent of reducing the tax benefits of the accelerated cost recovery of depreciable § 1250 property available to corporate taxpayers. For sales or other taxable dispositions of § 1250 property, corporations must treat as ordinary income 20 percent of any § 1231 gain *that would have been* ordinary income if § 1245 rather than § 1250 had applied to the transaction.[44] The effect of this provision is to require the taxpayer to recapture 20 percent of any straight-line depreciation that has not been recaptured under some other provision. Technically, the amount that is treated as ordinary income under § 291 is computed in the following manner:

Amount that would be treated as ordinary income under § 1245	$xx,xxx
Less: Amount that would be treated as ordinary income § 1250	(x,xxx)
Equals: Difference between recapture amounts	$xx,xxx
Times: Rate specified in § 291	×20%
Equals: Amount that is treated as ordinary income	$xx,xxx

---

[44] § 291(a)(1).

EXHIBIT 17-4

Completed Form 4797

Form **4797**	**Sales of Business Property**	OMB No. 1545-0184
Department of the Treasury Internal Revenue Service (99)	(Also Involuntary Conversions and Recapture Amounts Under Sections 179 and 280F(b)(2)) ▶ Attach to your tax return. ▶ See separate instructions.	20**08** Attachment Sequence No. **27**

Name(s) shown on return	Identifying number
TED AND CAROL SMITH	467-42-6030

1 Enter the gross proceeds from sales or exchanges reported to you for 2008 on Form(s) 1099-B or 1099-S (or substitute statement) that you are including on line 2, 10, or 20 (see instructions) . . . . | **1** |

Part I **Sales or Exchanges of Property Used in a Trade or Business and Involuntary Conversions From Other Than Casualty or Theft—Most Property Held More Than 1 Year** (see instructions)

2	**(a)** Description of property	**(b)** Date acquired (mo., day, yr.)	**(c)** Date sold (mo., day, yr.)	**(d)** Gross sales price	**(e)** Depreciation allowed or allowable since acquisition	**(f)** Cost or other basis, plus improvements and expense of sale	**(g) Gain or (loss)** Subtract (f) from the sum of (d) and (e)
	AUTO	3-1-03	10-2-06	1,800	2,080	4,000	(120)

3	Gain, if any, from Form 4684, line 45 . . .	**3**	
4	Section 1231 gain from installment sales from Form 6252, line 26 or 37	**4**	
5	Section 1231 gain or (loss) from like-kind exchanges from Form 8824	**5**	
6	Gain, if any, from line 32, from other than casualty or theft.	**6**	5,100
7	Combine lines 2 through 6. Enter the gain or (loss) here and on the appropriate line as follows:	**7**	4,980

Partnerships (except electing large partnerships) and S corporations. Report the gain or (loss) following the instructions for Form 1065, Schedule K, line 10, or Form 1120S, Schedule K, line 9. Skip lines 8, 9, 11, and 12 below.

Individuals, partners, S corporation shareholders, and all others. If line 7 is zero or a loss, enter the amount from line 7 on line 11 below and skip lines 8 and 9. If line 7 is a gain and you did not have any prior year section 1231 losses, or they were recaptured in an earlier year, enter the gain from line 7 as a long-term capital gain on the Schedule D filed with your return and skip lines 8, 9, 11, and 12 below.

8	Nonrecaptured net section 1231 losses from prior years (see instructions)	**8**	
9	Subtract line 8 from line 7. If zero or less, enter -0-. If line 9 is zero, enter the gain from line 7 on line 12 below. If line 9 is more than zero, enter the amount from line 8 on line 12 below and enter the gain from line 9 as a long-term capital gain on the Schedule D filed with your return (see instructions)	**9**	4,980

Part II **Ordinary Gains and Losses** (see instructions)

10 Ordinary gains and losses not included on lines 11 through 16 (include property held 1 year or less):

11	Loss, if any, from line 7	**11**	( )
12	Gain, if any, from line 7 or amount from line 8, if applicable	**12**	
13	Gain, if any, from line 31	**13**	500
14	Net gain or (loss) from Form 4684, lines 37 and 44a	**14**	
15	Ordinary gain from installment sales from Form 6252, line 25 or 36	**15**	
16	Ordinary gain or (loss) from like-kind exchanges from Form 8824.	**16**	
17	Combine lines 10 through 16	**17**	500

18 For all except individual returns, enter the amount from line 17 on the appropriate line of your return and skip lines a and b below. For individual returns, complete lines a and b below:

a If the loss on line 11 includes a loss from Form 4684, line 41, column (b)(ii), enter that part of the loss here. Enter the part of the loss from income-producing property on Schedule A (Form 1040), line 28, and the part of the loss from property used as an employee on Schedule A (Form 1040), line 23. Identify as from "Form 4797, line 18a." See instructions . . | **18a** | |

b Redetermine the gain or (loss) on line 17 excluding the loss, if any, on line 18a. Enter here and on Form 1040, line 14 | **18b** | 500 |

For Paperwork Reduction Act Notice, see separate instructions.	Cat. No. 13086I	Form **4797** (2008)

EXHIBIT 17-4

Completed Form 4797—Continued

Form 4797 (2008)   *TED AND CAROL SMITH*   Page **2**

Part III   Gain From Disposition of Property Under Sections 1245, 1250, 1252, 1254, and 1255
(see instructions)

19	(a) Description of section 1245, 1250, 1252, 1254, or 1255 property:	(b) Date acquired (mo., day, yr.)	(c) Date sold (mo., day, yr.)
A	*LAND/BUILDING*	7-14-0	11-21-06
B	*PHOTOCOPIER*	6-12-05	8-31-06
C			
D			

	These columns relate to the properties on lines 19A through 19D. ▶		Property A	Property B	Property C	Property D
20	Gross sales price (**Note:** See line 1 before completing.) .	20	14,000	2,600		
21	Cost or other basis plus expense of sale	21	13,000	2,500		
22	Depreciation (or depletion) allowed or allowable. . .	22	4,000	500		
23	Adjusted basis. Subtract line 22 from line 21.	23	9,000	2,000		
24	Total gain. Subtract line 23 from line 20	24	5,000	600		
25	**If section 1245 property:**					
a	Depreciation allowed or allowable from line 22 . . .	25a		500		
b	Enter the **smaller** of line 24 or 25a	25b		500		
26	**If section 1250 property:** If straight line depreciation was used, enter -0- on line 26g, except for a corporation subject to section 291.					
a	Additional depreciation after 1975 (see instructions) .	26a				
b	Applicable percentage multiplied by the **smaller** of line 24 or line 26a (see instructions)	26b				
c	Subtract line 26a from line 24. If residential rental property or line 24 is not more than line 26a, skip lines 26d and 26e	26c				
d	Additional depreciation after 1969 and before 1976. .	26d				
e	Enter the **smaller** of line 26c or 26d	26e				
f	Section 291 amount (corporations only)	26f				
g	Add lines 26b, 26e, and 26f.	26g	0			
27	**If section 1252 property:** Skip this section if you did not dispose of farmland or if this form is being completed for a partnership (other than an electing large partnership).					
a	Soil, water, and land clearing expenses	27a				
b	Line 27a multiplied by applicable percentage (see instructions)	27b				
c	Enter the **smaller** of line 24 or 27b	27c				
28	**If section 1254 property:**					
a	Intangible drilling and development costs, expenditures for development of mines and other natural deposits, and mining exploration costs (see instructions) . . .	28a				
b	Enter the **smaller** of line 24 or 28a	28b				
29	**If section 1255 property:**					
a	Applicable percentage of payments excluded from income under section 126 (see instructions)	29a				
b	Enter the **smaller** of line 24 or 29a (see instructions) .	29b				

Summary of Part III Gains. Complete property columns A through D through line 29b before going to line 30.

30	Total gains for all properties. Add property columns A through D, line 24	30	5,600
31	Add property columns A through D, lines 25b, 26g, 27c, 28b, and 29b. Enter here and on line 13	31	500
32	Subtract line 31 from line 30. Enter the portion from casualty or theft on Form 4684, line 39. Enter the portion from other than casualty or theft on Form 4797, line 6	32	5,100

Part IV   Recapture Amounts Under Sections 179 and 280F(b)(2) When Business Use Drops to 50% or Less
(see instructions)

			(a) Section 179	(b) Section 280F(b)(2)
33	Section 179 expense deduction or depreciation allowable in prior years.	33		
34	Recomputed depreciation (see instructions)	34		
35	Recapture amount. Subtract line 34 from line 33. See the instructions for where to report . .	35		

Form **4797** (2008)

EXHIBIT 17-5

Completed Schedule D

SCHEDULE D (Form 1040) Department of the Treasury Internal Revenue Service (99)	**Capital Gains and Losses** ▶ Attach to Form 1040 or Form 1040NR. ▶ See Instructions for Schedule D (Form 1040). ▶ Use Schedule D-1 to list additional transactions for lines 1 and 8.	OMB No. 1545-0074 20**08** Attachment Sequence No. **12**

Name(s) shown on return	Your social security number
TED AND CAROL SMITH	467 42 6030

Part I   Short-Term Capital Gains and Losses—Assets Held One Year or Less

(a) Description of property (Example: 100 sh. XYZ Co.)	(b) Date acquired (Mo., day, yr.)	(c) Date sold (Mo., day, yr.)	(d) Sales price (see page D-7 of the instructions)	(e) Cost or other basis (see page D-7 of the instructions)	(f) Gain or (loss) Subtract (e) from (d)
1 100 SHS XY CORP	6-1-06	10-15-06	3,200	4,200	(1000)

2 Enter your short-term totals, if any, from Schedule D-1, line 2	**2**	
3 **Total short-term sales price amounts.** Add lines 1 and 2 in column (d)	**3**	3,200

4 Short-term gain from Form 6252 and short-term gain or (loss) from Forms 4684, 6781, and 8824	**4**	
5 Net short-term gain or (loss) from partnerships, S corporations, estates, and trusts from Schedule(s) K-1	**5**	
6 Short-term capital loss carryover. Enter the amount, if any, from line 8 of your **Capital Loss Carryover Worksheet** on page D-7 of the instructions	**6** (	)
7 **Net short-term capital gain or (loss).** Combine lines 1 through 6 in column (f)	**7**	(1000)

Part II   Long-Term Capital Gains and Losses—Assets Held More Than One Year

(a) Description of property (Example: 100 sh. XYZ Co.)	(b) Date acquired (Mo., day, yr.)	(c) Date sold (Mo., day, yr.)	(d) Sales price (see page D-7 of the instructions)	(e) Cost or other basis (see page D-7 of the instructions)	(f) Gain or (loss) Subtract (e) from (d)
8 100 SHS XY CORP	6-1-03	11-1-06	3,200	4,600	(1,400)
VACANT LAND	6-1-01	12-1-06	12,000	5,000	7,000

9 Enter your long-term totals, if any, from Schedule D-1, line 9	**9**	
10 **Total long-term sales price amounts.** Add lines 8 and 9 in column (d)	**10**	15,200
11 Gain from Form 4797, Part I; long-term gain from Forms 2439 and 6252; and long-term gain or (loss) from Forms 4684, 6781, and 8824	**11**	4,980
12 Net long-term gain or (loss) from partnerships, S corporations, estates, and trusts from Schedule(s) K-1	**12**	
13 Capital gain distributions. See page D-2 of the instructions	**13**	
14 Long-term capital loss carryover. Enter the amount, if any, from line 13 of your **Capital Loss Carryover Worksheet** on page D-7 of the instructions	**14** (	)
15 **Net long-term capital gain or (loss).** Combine lines 8 through 14 in column (f). Then go to Part III on the back	**15**	10,580

For Paperwork Reduction Act Notice, see Form 1040 or Form 1040NR instructions.   Cat. No. 11338H   **Schedule D (Form 1040) 2008**

EXHIBIT 17-5

Schedule D—Continued

Schedule D (Form 1040) 2008 *TED AND CAROL SMITH* Page **2**

Part III **Summary**

16 Combine lines 7 and 15 and enter the result.	**16**	*9,580*

If line 16 is:
- A **gain**, enter the amount from line 16 on Form 1040, line 13, or Form 1040NR, line 14. Then go to line 17 below.
- A **loss**, skip lines 17 through 20 below. Then go to line 21. Also be sure to complete line 22.
- **Zero**, skip lines 17 through 21 below and enter -0- on Form 1040, line 13, or Form 1040NR, line 14. Then go to line 22.

17 Are lines 15 and 16 **both** gains?
☐ **Yes.** Go to line 18.
☐ **No.** Skip lines 18 through 21, and go to line 22.

3,000

18 Enter the amount, if any, from line 7 of the **28% Rate Gain Worksheet** on page D-8 of the instructions . . . . ▶ | **18** |

19 Enter the amount, if any, from line 18 of the **Unrecaptured Section 1250 Gain Worksheet** on page D-9 of the instructions . . . . ▶ | **19** |

20 Are lines 18 and 19 **both** zero or blank?
☐ **Yes.** Complete Form 1040 through line 43, or Form 1040NR through line 40. Then complete the **Qualified Dividends and Capital Gain Tax Worksheet** on page 38 of the Instructions for Form 1040 (or in the Instructions for Form 1040NR). **Do not** complete lines 21 and 22 below.
☐ **No.** Complete Form 1040 through line 43, or Form 1040NR through line 40. Then complete the **Schedule D Tax Worksheet** on page D-10 of the instructions. **Do not** complete lines 21 and 22 below.

21 If line 16 is a loss, enter here and on Form 1040, line 13, or Form 1040NR, line 14, the **smaller** of:

- The loss on line 16 or
- ($3,000), or if married filing separately, ($1,500) } . . . . | **21** ( )

Note. When figuring which amount is smaller, treat both amounts as positive numbers.

22 Do you have qualified dividends on Form 1040, line 9b, or Form 1040NR, line 10b?
☐ **Yes.** Complete Form 1040 through line 43, or Form 1040NR through line 40. Then complete the **Qualified Dividends and Capital Gain Tax Worksheet** on page 38 of the Instructions for Form 1040 (or in the Instructions for Form 1040NR).
☐ **No.** Complete the rest of Form 1040 or Form 1040NR.

Schedule D (Form 1040) 2008

Example 21. This year K Corporation sold residential rental property for $500,000. The property was purchased for $400,000 in 1986. Assume that K claimed ACRS depreciation of $140,000 (i.e., do not attempt to verify this estimate). Straight-line depreciation would have been $105,000. K Corporation's depreciation recapture and § 1231 gain are computed as follows:

Step 1:	Compute realized gain:			
	Sales price			$500,000
	Less:	Adjusted basis		
		Cost	$400,000	
		ACRS depreciation	(140,000)	(260,000)
	Realized gain			$240,000
Step 2:	Compute *excess* depreciation:			
	Actual depreciation			$140,000
	Straight-line depreciation			(105,000)
	Excess depreciation			$ 35,000
Step 3:	Compute § 1250 depreciation recapture:			
	Lesser of realized gain of $240,000			
	or			
	Excess depreciation of $35,000			
	§ 1250 depreciation recapture			$ 35,000
Step 4:	Compute depreciation recapture if § 1245 applied:			
	Lesser of realized gain of $240,000			
	or			
	Actual depreciation of $140,000			
	Depreciation recapture if § 1245 applied			$140,000
Step 5:	Compute § 291 ordinary income:			
	Depreciation recapture if § 1245 applied			$140,000
	§ 1250 depreciation recapture			(35,000)
	Excess recapture potential			$105,000
	Times: § 291 rate			× 20%
	§ 291 ordinary income			$ 21,000
Step 6:	Characterize recognized gain:			
	§ 1250 depreciation recapture			$ 35,000
	Plus:	§ 291 ordinary income		21,000
	Ordinary income			$ 56,000
	Realized gain			$240,000
	Less:	Ordinary income		(56,000)
	§ 1231 gain			$184,000

Note that without the additional recapture required under § 291, K Corporation would have reported a § 1231 gain of $205,000 ($240,000 total gain − $35,000 § 1250 recapture). If the property had been subject to § 1245 recapture, K Corporation would have only a $100,000 § 1231 gain ($240,000 − $140,000 § 1245 recapture). Section 291 requires that the corporation report 20% of this difference ($205,000 − $100,000 = $105,000 × 20%), or $21,000, as *additional* recapture.

Note that this is 20% of the straight-line depreciation that is normally not recaptured on the disposition of nonresidential or residential real estate.

Example 22. Assume the same facts as in *Example 21*, except that the property is an office building rather than residential realty *and* straight-line depreciation was elected. An individual taxpayer would report the entire gain of $205,000 [$500,000 − ($400,000 basis − $105,000 straight-line depreciation)] as a § 1231 gain. However, the corporate taxpayer must recapture $21,000 (20% × $105,000 depreciation) as ordinary income under § 291. The remaining $184,000 ($205,000 − $21,000) would be a § 1231 gain.

OTHER RECAPTURE PROVISIONS

There are several other recapture provisions that exist. They include the recapture of farmland expenditures,[45] recapture of intangible drilling costs,[46] and recapture of gain from the disposition of § 126 property (relating to government cost-sharing program payments for conservation purposes).[47] Another type of recapture is investment credit recapture.[48] This is discussed in detail in Chapter 13.

✓ CHECK YOUR KNOWLEDGE

Review Question 1. True-False. This year T sold equipment for $6,000 (cost $15,000, depreciation $10,000), recognizing a gain of $1,000 ($6,000 − $5,000). To ensure that all of the ordinary deductions obtained from depreciation are recaptured, T must report ordinary income of $10,000 and a capital loss of $9,000, ultimately producing net income of $1,000.

False. This novel approach may seem consistent with Congressional intent, but it is incorrect. Under § 1245 any gain realized is treated as ordinary income to the extent of any depreciation allowed. As a result, the entire $1,000 is ordinary income. It may be useful to think of the depreciation recapture as an adjustment to the depreciation claimed. Depreciation of $10,000 was claimed, but the value of the equipment dropped by $9,000 ($15,000 cost − $6,000 sales price). T claimed an ordinary depreciation deduction of $10,000, and recognized ordinary income of $1,000, for a net ordinary deduction of $9,000.

Review Question 2. True-False. This year L sold a machine and recognized a small gain. Assuming L claimed straight-line depreciation, there is no depreciation recapture.

False. The machine is § 1245 property since it is depreciable personalty. Under the full recapture rule of § 1245, all depreciation is subject to recapture regardless of the method used.

Review Question 3. Several years ago Harry purchased equipment at a cost of $10,000. Over the past three years he claimed and deducted depreciation of $6,000. Assuming that Harry sold the equipment for (1) $7,000, (2) $13,000, or (3) $1,000, determine the amount of gain or loss realized and its character (i.e., ordinary income or § 1231 potential capital gain).

---

[45] § 1252.

[46] § 1254.

[47] § 1255.

[48] § 47.

	1	2	3
Amount realized..............................	$ 7,000	$13,000	$ 1,000
Adjusted basis ($10,000 − $6,000)................	− 4,000	− 4,000	− 4,000
Gain (loss) recognized	$ 3,000	$ 9,000	$(3,000)

The equipment is § 1245 property since it is depreciable personalty. As a result, the full recapture rule operates and any gain recognized is ordinary income to the extent of any depreciation deducted. In the first case, the entire $3,000 is ordinary income (the lesser of the gain recognized, $3,000, or the recapture potential, $6,000). In the second situation, $6,000 is ordinary income (the lesser of the gain recognized, $9,000, or the recapture potential, $6,000) and $3,000 is § 1231 gain. In the final case, § 1245 does not apply because the property is sold at a loss. Therefore, Harry has a § 1231 loss that is potentially an ordinary loss. Its ultimate treatment depends on the outcome of the § 1231 netting process.

Review Question 4. True-False. In 1990, Sal purchased an office building to rent out. This year she sold the building, recognizing a large gain. The entire gain is a § 1231 gain since there is no recapture under either § 1245 or § 1250.

True. The office build is § 1250 property. The recapture rules of § 1250 apply only when the taxpayer uses an accelerated method, in which case the excess of accelerated depreciation over straight-line is treated as ordinary income. However, since 1987 taxpayers have been required to use the straight-line method in computing depreciation on real estate. As a result, § 1250 is inapplicable and Sal's gain retains its original § 1231 character. Nevertheless, the gain will not be treated as a 15 percent gain to the extent of any unrecaptured § 1250 depreciation (i.e., all of the straight-line depreciation) but rather 25 percent gain.

Review Question 5. True-False. In 1997, Z Corporation purchased an office building to rent out. This year the corporation sold the building, recognizing a large gain. The entire gain is a § 1231 gain since there is no recapture under either § 1245 or § 1250.

False. There is no recapture under § or § 1250. However, under § 291, corporate taxpayers are required to recapture up to 20 percent of any straight-line depreciation. The 25 percent rate does not apply to corporate taxpayers.

Review Question 6. True-False. In 1986, the Rose Partnership purchased a new office building to use as its headquarters. This year the partnership sold the building, recognizing a gain of $100,000. The partnership claimed and deducted accelerated depreciation of $40,000. Straight-line depreciation would have been $40,000. The partnership will report ordinary income of zero and § 1231 gain of $100,000.

False. This would be true if the building were § 1250 property, but § 1250 does not apply. Nonresidential real estate such as this office building that was acquired from 1981 through 1986 is treated as § 1245 property and is subject to the full recapture rule if accelerated depreciation was used. In this case, the taxpayer opted for accelerated depreciation, so $40,000 is ordinary income and the remaining $60,000 is a 15% § 1231 gain.

Review Question 7. In 1984, the Daisy Partnership purchased a new apartment complex to rent out. This year the partnership sold the building, recognizing a gain of $100,000. The partnership claimed and deducted straight-line depreciation of $35,000.

Accelerated depreciation would have been $40,000. The partnership will report ordinary income of $35,000 and § 1231 gain of $65,000.

False. In contrast to question 6, the property is residential real estate and is consequently treated as § 1250 property. The partial recapture rule of § 1250 applies only if the taxpayer actually uses an accelerated method. In this case the taxpayer used straight-line, so the recapture rules of § 1250 are not triggered. As a result, the entire $100,000 gain is a § 1231 gain. However, the gain will be a 25 percent gain to the extent of any unrecaptured § 1250 gain (i.e., the $35,000 straight-line depreciation).

RELATED BUSINESS ISSUES

INSTALLMENT SALES OF TRADE OR BUSINESS PROPERTY

As discussed in Chapter 14, gains on sales of trade or business property may be deferred using the installment sale method. However, depreciation recapture does not qualify for installment sale treatment. Thus, ordinary income from depreciation recapture must be reported in the year of sale—*regardless* of whether the seller received any payment in that year.[49] Consequently, only the § 1231 gain from such sales will qualify for installment gain deferral.

Example 23. During the year, K sold a rental house for $90,000. According to the terms of the sale, K received $30,000 down and the balance in two equal installments of $30,000 over the next two years. K had purchased the house in 1986 for $60,000 and deducted $20,000 of accelerated depreciation. Had she used the straight-line method, the straight-line depreciation would have been $15,000. K realizes a gain of $50,000 and has $5,000 of § 1250 recapture, computed as follows:

Amount realized.	$90,000
Adjusted basis ($60,000 − $20,000)	−40,000
Gain realized	$50,000
Accelerated depreciation on residential real estate acquired before 1987	$20,000
Hypothetical straight-line depreciation	−15,000
Excess depreciation	$ 5,000

K must report all of the depreciation recapture, $5,000, as ordinary income in the year of the sale. In addition, she must report $15,000 of the remaining gain of $45,000 as a § 1231 gain under the installment sale rules for the year of sale, computed as follows:

$$\frac{\text{Remaining gain, } \$45,000}{\text{Contract price, } \$90,000} \times \$30,000 \text{ Payment received} = \$15,000 \text{ Gain recognized}$$

Note that in computing the gross profit ratio, only the remaining gain is used in the numerator and not the entire $50,000 gain realized, as would normally be the case.

---

[49] § 453(i). See Chapter 14 for a detailed discussion of installment reporting.

INTANGIBLE BUSINESS ASSETS

Historically, many purchased intangible assets were not subject to amortization for tax purposes. This was because the life of the assets was indefinite and the amortization deduction was indeterminable. However, § 197 currently allows the amortization (over 15 years) of most *purchased* intangibles acquired after August 11, 1993. No amortization is allowed, of course, for intangibles *developed* by the taxpayer.

For years, conventional thinking was that goodwill and similar intangibles were capital assets. A taxpayer who purchased or developed goodwill and similar intangibles generally recognized capital gain (or loss) to the extent the proceeds of the sale of a business were allocated to them.

All this became much more complex with the passage of § 197. Section 197(e) stipulates that upon the sale or disposition of § 197 assets, they are to be treated as depreciable property.

Private Letter Ruling [PLR] 200243002 brought clarity to this change. Under this ruling, intangible assets that are not subject to amortization are still treated as capital assets. This applies to assets placed in service on or before August 11, 1993, and any self developed goodwill and other intangibles (with no basis). However, intangibles purchased after August 11, 1993 (i.e. amortizable "§ 197 intangibles") are to be treated as depreciable assets and upon sale they are subject to § 1245 and § 1231 treatment.

Under § 1245, any gain recognized will be ordinary income to the extent of amortization allowed. Any remaining gain or loss will be subject to the netting process under § 1231 and whatever treatment is required after the netting process.

DISPOSITIONS OF BUSINESS ASSETS AND THE SELF-EMPLOYMENT TAX

Gains and losses on the disposition of business assets do not increase or decrease self-employment income. So, even though gains are ordinary income for income tax purposes to the extent of depreciation recapture under § 1245 and § 1250, these amounts are not included in self-employment income.

TAX PLANNING CONSIDERATIONS

TIMING OF SALES AND OTHER DISPOSITIONS

Timing the sale of trade or business properties is very important and, from a tax perspective, can be critical. In the simplest case, if a taxpayer has a tax loss or is in a lower tax bracket, any contemplated sales at a gain should be considered to take advantage of the favorable tax result under § 1231. If tax rates are particularly high in the current year, loss transactions should be considered. Any net § 1231 loss is treated as an ordinary deduction for A.G.I. and avoids the $3,000 deduction limit imposed on net capital losses.

In addition, a net § 1231 gain qualifies as a long-term capital gain. For high-income taxpayers with no capital asset transactions or with a net capital gain in the current year, the net § 1231 gain qualifies for the maximum capital gains tax rate of 15 percent. The benefit can be even greater for a taxpayer with substantial capital losses for the year. Because the losses in excess of $3,000 would otherwise be suspended, any net § 1231 gain that would be offset by these losses can be currently recognized at no additional tax cost.

If a taxpayer has recognized or could recognize a § 1231 gain for the year and benefit from § 1231 treatment, additional sales of § 1231 property at a loss should be

avoided. Because such losses must be netted against the gains, the favorable treatment of the gains is lost.

The look-back rule must be considered whenever a taxpayer is contemplating the timing of sales of § 1231 gain and loss assets. If no § 1231 losses have been recognized in the past five years, the gain assets should be sold in the current year to receive the favorable treatment of net § 1231 gains. The loss assets can then be sold in the next year and be treated as ordinary losses. This plan will not work, however, if the loss assets are sold first.

Finally, the timing of casualty and theft gains and losses should be considered. Obviously, a taxpayer cannot control the timing of such losses—not legally, anyway. However, the § 1033 gain deferral rules discussed in Chapter 15 may offer some tax planning opportunity. Because this deferral provision is generally elective, the taxpayer should consider existing § 1231 gains or losses before making a decision to defer gain. For example, a taxpayer with substantial capital losses may decide not to defer a capital gain or § 1231 gain under § 1033 even though the involuntarily converted asset is to be replaced. Immediate recognition of the gain will not have any negative tax consequences because it can be offset by the existing capital losses. The replacement property will have a higher (cost) basis for future depreciation. This plan is much more important to corporate taxpayers because excess capital losses can be carried forward only five years.

SELECTING DEPRECIATION METHODS

The accelerated cost recovery system provides taxpayers with several choices of depreciation methods and conventions. For example, a taxpayer with depreciable personalty may elect to use the straight-line method and either the class life or a longer alternative life. For real estate, an alternative 40-year life may be used.

Effect of Recapture. Generally, a taxpayer should adopt the most rapid method of depreciation available because this results in a deferral of income taxes. Unless tax rates are expected to change significantly in the near future, the tax benefits produced by large depreciation deductions currently allow the taxpayer the use of the money that would otherwise have been used to pay income taxes. In addition, the availability of the like-kind exchange and involuntary conversion provisions eliminates the risk of depreciation recapture when the taxpayer plans to continue in business. It is also important to remember that, for noncorporate taxpayers, there is no depreciation recapture possibility for real estate placed in service after 1986. Because only the straight-line depreciation method can be used, there will be no excess depreciation. However, the unrecaptured § 1250 depreciation is taxed at 25 percent.

Section 179. As discussed in Chapter 9, any § 179 expense amount is treated as depreciation allowed. As a result, the comments above may also apply in deciding whether to claim the option to expense the cost of qualifying property. If more than one qualifying asset is placed in service during the year and their total cost exceeds the annual limit (or reduced limit), the taxpayer must select the assets to be expensed. Obviously, only the assets not expected to be sold should be considered for this option. Given the time value of money, however, it seems unlikely that any taxpayer should forgo the § 179 expense option—unless the additional record keeping is considered to outweigh the current tax benefit.

INSTALLMENT SALES

Installment sales provide an excellent tax deferral possibility. Caution must be exercised, however, if trade or business property is to be sold under a deferred-payment arrangement. Because any depreciation recapture must be reported as income in the year of sale regardless of the amount of money received, taxpayers should require a cash down payment sufficient to pay any income taxes resulting from the depreciation recapture.

SALES OF BUSINESSES

The sale of a business typically involves some recognition of intangible assets, whether it be goodwill, or some similar asset, or other assets such as customer lists. The buyer is generally entitled to amortize the intangibles over 15 years. The seller may have ordinary income, capital gain, and/or § 1231 gain.

The IRS generally is required to recognize agreements between the buyer and the seller as to the value of the various assets in the sale of a business so long as they are reasonable. Thus in negotiating the value of the underlying assets, the buyer should consider the possible deductions related to the purchased assets. For depreciable assets and purchased intangibles, the deductions come in the form of depreciation and amortization. With respect to these assets, the buyer should also evaluate the effects of the depreciation recapture of the assets if they are to be sold in a short period of time.

DISPOSITIONS OF BUSINESS ASSETS AND THE SELF-EMPLOYMENT TAX

Gains on the disposition of business assets do not increase self-employment income. Similarly, losses do not reduce self-employment income. Generally speaking, foregoing allowable depreciation is not really optional since the basis of the depreciable assets must be reduced by depreciation allowed or allowable. So a taxpayer who does not feel like he or she needs the deduction, and realizes that the resulting gain if the asset is sold at a gain will be depreciation recapture, should claim it anyway!

> **Example 24.** D purchased a machine for $4,000 in the current year. The machine qualifies for expensing under § 197. D is uncertain as to whether she should claim the entire $4,000 since she expects to sell the machine for $3,200 the next tax year. Her dilemma involves the fact that the $4,000 is an ordinary deduction and the $3,200 is an ordinary gain. Why not just depreciate the machine? The reason is that by claiming the entire amount, she defers the tax on $3,200 for a year—assuming no change in her marginal tax rate.

Taxpayers paying self-employment tax should normally depreciate assets as rapidly as possible since the depreciation allowed will reduce the self-employment tax, but the future gain on the disposition of the asset is not includible in self-employment income.

> **Example 25.** D, in the prior example, can deduct the full $4,000, reducing her income tax and her self-employment tax. However, when she sells the machine the next year, the gain is subject only to income tax (as ordinary income).

PROBLEM MATERIALS

DISCUSSION QUESTIONS

17-1   *Section 1231 Assets.* What are § 1231 assets? What is the required holding period? Does the § 1231 category of assets include § 1245 and § 1250 assets as well? Elaborate.

17-2   *Excluded Assets.* What type of property is excluded from § 1231 treatment?

17-3   *Section 1231 Netting Process.* Briefly describe the § 1231 netting process. Are personal use assets included in this process?

17-4   *Net § 1231 Gains.* What is the appropriate tax treatment of net § 1231 gains? Are they offset by short-term capital losses? Can they be offset by capital loss carryovers from prior years?

17-5   *Net § 1231 Losses.* What is the appropriate tax treatment of net § 1231 losses? Are they subject to any annual limitation? Can they be used to create or increase a net operating loss for the year?

17-6   *Certain Casualty or Theft Gains and Losses.* Which casualty or theft gains and losses are included in the § 1231 netting process? What is the proper treatment of a net casualty or theft gain? What is the proper treatment of a net casualty or theft loss?

17-7   *Section 1231 Look-Back Rule.* Describe how the § 1231 look-back rule operates. Why do you think Congress enacted such a rule?

17-8   *Section 1245 Property.* What category of trade or business property is subject to § 1245? What depreciable real property has been included in this category?

17-9   *Full Depreciation Recapture—§ 1245.* What is meant by § 1245 recapture potential? Why is this rule sometimes called the full recapture rule? What is the lower limit of § 1245 recapture?

17-10 *Section 1245 Recapture Potential.* During the current year Z sold a vacuum used in his pool-cleaning business. The vacuum had cost $3,600 three years ago, and he had expensed the entire amount under § 179.
   a.   How much is the § 1245 recapture potential with respect to this vacuum?
   b.   If the vacuum was sold for $900, what is the character of the gain?

17-11 *Asset Classification.* When will the sale or other disposition of depreciable equipment be subject to both § 1231 and § 1245? What is the appropriate treatment of any loss from the sale of such equipment?

17-12 *Section 1245 Property.* F gave property with § 1245 recapture potential to his daughter, D. Will F be required to recapture any of the depreciation previously claimed? How must D characterize any gain she might recognize on a subsequent disposition of the property?

17-13 *Section 1245 Recapture Potential.* What happens to the § 1245 recapture potential when property is disposed of in a like-kind exchange?

17-14 *Section 179 Expense Treatment.* Explain the proper tax treatment of any gain recognized on the disposition of an asset that the taxpayer had earlier elected to expense under § 179. Does this mean that any amounts ever deducted under § 179 will always be subject to recapture? Explain.

17-15 *Section 1250 Property.* Is land included in the definition of § 1250 property? Is any real property depreciated under the straight-line method included in this definition?

17-16 *Section 1250 Property.* Is nonresidential real estate acquired after 1980 always § 1250 property? Explain.

17-17 *Section 1250 Property.* Why will depreciable real property placed in service after 1986 never be subject to § 1250 recapture? How is the unrecaptured depreciation treated?

17-18 *Section 1250 Recapture Potential.* Why is § 1250 sometimes called the partial recapture rule? Will the § 1250 recapture potential ever simply disappear? Explain.

17-19 *Section 1250 Recapture Potential.* This year Y sold a duplex that she had rented out for several years. The house had cost $40,000 20 years earlier and depreciation expense of $27,000 has been claimed. Straight-line depreciation would have been $24,500.
  a. How much is the § 1250 recapture potential with respect to the duplex?
  b. If the duplex was sold for $75,000, what is the character of Y's gain and how is it taxed?

17-20 *Additional Recapture—§ 291.* Briefly describe the additional depreciation recapture rule of § 291.
  a. Which taxpayers are subject to this rule?
  b. Compare this to the special rate for unrecaptured depreciation on § 1250 property for individual taxpayers.

17-21 *Section 291 Recapture.* Can a corporation that has always elected to use the straight-line depreciation method for all real property ever be subject to additional recapture under § 291? Explain.

17-22 *Reporting § 1231 Transactions.* What tax form does a taxpayer use to report the results of § 1231 transactions? How is any depreciation recapture reported on this form?

17-23 *Planning § 1231 Transactions.* Under what circumstances should a taxpayer with an involuntary conversion gain from business property consider not electing to defer the gain under § 1033?

17-24 *Planning § 1231 Transactions.* A taxpayer plans to trade in depreciable property in order to acquire new property but is quite disappointed to find that his old equipment is worth less than its unrecovered cost basis. He is currently in the top marginal tax bracket and has no capital gains or losses or other § 1231 transactions for the year. What tax advice would you offer this taxpayer concerning the planned exchange?

17-25 *Installment Sales and Depreciation Recapture.* Briefly describe how recapture is reported when either § 1245 property or § 1250 property is disposed of in an installment sale. What tax planning should a taxpayer undertake concerning such sales?

PROBLEMS

17-26   *Characterizing Assets.* Indicate whether the following gains and losses are § 1231 gains or losses or capital gains and losses or neither. Make your determination prior to the § 1231 netting process.

    a.   Printing press used in A's business; held for three years and sold at a loss.

    b.   Goodwill sold as part of the sale of B's business

    c.   Vacant lot used five years as a parking lot in C's business; sold at a gain

    d.   House, 80 percent of which is D's home and 20 percent of which is used as a place of business; held 15 years and sold at a gain

    e.   Camera used in E's business; held for 10 months and sold at a gain

    f.   Land used by F for 10 years as a farm and sold at a loss

    g.   Personal residence sold at a loss

17-27   *Section 1231.* During the year H sold the following assets, both of which had been held for several years:

Asset	Gain (Loss)
Vacant land held for investment	$52,000
Equipment used in his business	(12,000)

    Determine how much capital gain or loss as well as the amount of ordinary income or loss that H will report for the year. At what rate will the gain, if any, be taxed?

17-28   *Section 1231 Netting.* G operates the Corner Bar and Grill as a sole proprietorship. During the year he sold the following assets, all of which had been held for several years:

Asset	Gain (Loss)
IBM stock	$(12,000)
Land and building used in the business	34,000
Equipment used in the business	(3,000)

    The building had been acquired in 1993. Straight-line depreciation claimed and deducted with respect to the building was $8,000. Straight-line depreciation on the equipment was $4,000. Determine how much capital gain or loss as well as the amount of ordinary income or loss that G will report for the year and explain how they will be taxed.

17-29   *Involuntary Conversions and § 1231.* Assume the same facts as in *Problem 17-28.* In addition, G's records revealed the following information:

    ▸ A portion of the grill's parking lot was condemned by the city when it decided to expand the adjacent street. G pocketed the cash and recognized a gain of $5,000.

    ▸ A pool table was destroyed as part of a barroom brawl. G realized a casualty loss of $2,000.

    Determine how much capital gain or loss as well as the amount of ordinary income or loss that G will report for the year. At what rate will the recognized gain, if any, be taxed?

17-30 *Section 1231 Hodgepodge.* For 30 years Rae has operated The General Store, a hardware store in Columbus. Rae runs the business as a sole proprietorship. During the year, she recognized the following gains and losses from assets held several years:

1. Uninsured warehouse burned down: $10,000 loss

2. Equipment stolen: $190,000 gain (ignore depreciation)

3. Parking lot sold: $120,000 gain

4. IBM stock sold: capital loss of $70,000

5. Condemnation of land: $1,000 gain

Determine how much capital gain or loss as well as the amount of ordinary income or loss that Rae will report for the year. At what rate will the gain, if any, be taxed?

17-31 *Section 1231 Lookback.* J has recognized the following § 1231 gains and losses in the current year (2009) and since the inception of his business:

Year	Net § 1231 Gain (Loss)
2009	$50,000
2008	12,000
2007	(35,000)
2006	0
2005	65,000
2004	(13,000)

How will J treat the $50,000 gain for the current year?

17-32 *Section 1231—Timber.* A owns timber land that she purchased in 1991. During 2009, the timber was cut and A elected § 631 treatment for the gain. Her cost assignable to the timber was $25,000 and its fair market value on January 1, 2009 was $40,000. The actual sales price of the cut timber when it was sold in 2008 was $55,000.
a. How much is A's gain or loss recognized and what is its character?
b. Can A deduct the costs of cutting the timber?

17-33 *Section 1231—Unharvested Crops.* This year L sold her farmland, which she had owned for 20 years. L had made minor improvements to the farm and had used straight-line depreciation to depreciate them. No personal property was sold with the farm.

The sales price was $80,000 and L's adjusted basis was $36,000. The unharvested crops on the land represented $8,000 of the sales price, and L had spent $3,200 in producing the crop to the point of sale.
a. How does L report the gain or loss from the sale of the farm?
b. If L has no other sales of trade or business property or of capital assets, how much of the gain is included in her taxable income?

17-34 *Section 1245 Recapture.* During the current year, D sold a drill press he had used in his wood shop business for three years. D had purchased the press for $820 and had deducted depreciation of $476. Straight-line depreciation would have been $410. Determine the amount and character of gain or loss to D under each of the following circumstances below:
a. The press is sold for $500.
b. The press is sold for $100.
c. The press is sold for $900.

17-35   *Section 1245 Recapture.* This year N sold three different pieces of equipment used in her business:

Description	Holding Period	Sales Price	Cost	Depreciation Allowed
Processing machine	3 years	$1,200	$1,400	$600
Work table	4 years	1,600	1,300	500
Automatic stapler	2 years	500	900	300

What are the amount and character of N's gain or loss from these transactions?

17-36   *Section 1245 Recapture.* Fill in the missing information for each of the three independent sales of § 1245 assets identified below. Enter a dollar amount or n/a (for not applicable) in each blank space.

	Assets		
	A	B	C
Sales price	$105	$ 90	$ ____
Cost	100	125	100
Depreciation allowed.	30		30
Depreciation recapture			20
§ 1231 gain or (loss)		(10)	

17-37   *Basis Reductions.* Dr. T purchased a treadmill for use in his cardiology practice for $13,000 on August 14, 2007. T claimed § 179 expense of $10,000 and depreciation of $429 in 2007. The depreciation for 2008 and 2009 is $735 and $524, respectively. T sold the treadmill on January 13, 2009 for $3,500,
  a.   What are the amount and character of T's gain on the sale?
  b.   What would be your answer if the unit had been sold for $13,500?

17-38   *Section 1250 Recapture.* Fill in the missing information for each of the three independent sales of § 1250 assets identified below. Enter a dollar amount or n/a (for not applicable) in each blank space.

	Assets		
	X	Y	Z
Sales price	$100	$ ____	$200
Cost	135	100	100
Depreciation allowed.	55		30
Straight-line depreciation		20	
Depreciation recapture	0	10	
§ 1231 gain or (loss)		30	120

17-39   *Real Property Acquired after 1986.* V sold an office building in the current year that she had purchased for $60,000 in 2007. Depreciation of $4,127 was claimed before the building was sold for $75,000.
  a.   What are the amount and character of V's gain on this sale?
  b.   At what rate will the gain be treated?

17-40 *Depreciation Recapture.* K purchased a warehouse on January 18, 1986 for $50,000 ($10,000 allocable to the land and $40,000 allocable to the building). The property was 19-year realty and was depreciated using the 175 percent declining balance method and mid-month convention. The unit was sold on January 15, 2008 for $120,000 ($30,000 allocable to the land and $90,000 allocable to the building). At the time the property was sold, the building was fully depreciated (i.e., K deducted depreciation of $40,000 while holding the property).

    a. How much is K's gain and what is its character? At what rate will the gain be treated?

    b. If K had used the optional straight-line method and a 19-year life under ACRS, the depreciation deductions would have been the same, $40,000. What would be the amount and character of K's gain using this method? At what rate will the gain be treated?

    c. What would be your answer to (b) if K were a corporation?

17-41 *Depreciation Recapture.* Happy Acres operates a small organic farm. In 2009, it sold some of its land including a barn for $500,000. The company purchased the property in 2002 for $300,000. The barn is used for multiple purposes (storage of hay, tractors, equipment, animals). For MACRS, multi-purpose agricultural buildings are considered 20-year property and are depreciated using the 150% declining balance method (§ 168(b)(2)(A)). Assume accelerated depreciation deducted was $125,000 and straight-line depreciation would have been $105,000. For the following questions, ignore the land.

    a. Compute the amount of gain realized and its character.

    b. What amount of the gain, if any, is taxed at 25 percent?

    c. What would your answer to (a) be if the company is a corporation?

17-42 *Depreciation Recapture.* JWP Development, an LLC, built a hotel in downtown Chicago in 1980 at a cost of $700,000. It depreciated the building using an accelerated method over a useful life of 40 years. This year it sold the building for $1,000,000. At the time of the sale, the company had deducted accelerated depreciation of $400,000. Straight-line depreciation on the building would have been $150,000. (Do not try to verify these amounts.)

    a. What is the amount of the company's gain and what is its character?

    b. What amount of the gain, if any, will be taxed at a 25 percent rate?

    c. If the company had used the straight-line method, what would be the amount and character the gain? At what rate would the gain be treated?

    d. What would be your answer to (a) if JWP were a corporation?

17-43 *Installment Sales and Recapture.* Assume the same facts as in Problem 17-42 except that Z sold the property under an installment contract with $100,000 down and $100,000 in each of the next nine years along with reasonable interest. How much gain would Z report in the year of sale and the following year and what is its character?

17-44 *Unrecaptured § 1250 Gain.* B purchased a small warehouse for $45,000 in 2005. This year he sold the property for $62,000. He had deducted straight-line depreciation of $6,500 on the property prior to the sale. What is the amount of gain, if any, and how will it be taxed?

17-45 *Twenty-five Percent Gains.* V had the following gains and losses for the current year:

§ 1250 recapture	$2,000
Net § 1231 gains	6,000
Net short-term capital loss	(3,000)

V's § 1231 gain was from a building that was held 15 years. The total depreciation allowed was $5,000. How much are V's *15 percent gains* and *25 percent gains*, respectively?

17-46 *Section 1231 Gain and Look-Back Rule.* R sold land and a building used in farming for many years at a gain of $30,000 during 2009. No other sales or dispositions of § 1231 assets were made during the year. The § 1250 depreciation recapture for the building was zero and the unrecaptured depreciation was $1,000.
  a. How is R's gain to be reported if he had a net § 1231 gain of $10,000 in 2006, a net § 1231 loss of $12,000 in 2007, and no § 1231 transactions in 2008?
  b. How would your answer to (a) differ if the sale of the property had resulted in a loss of $7,500?

17-47 *Section 1231 and Depreciation Recapture.* Fill in the missing information for each of the separate sales of § 1231 assets indicated below. Enter a dollar amount or n/a (for not applicable) in each blank space.

	Land	Building	Machine	Machine
Sales price	$100	$ ___	$90	$ ___
Cost	140	100	125	100
Depreciation allowed.	0	30	___	30
Straight-line depreciation	0	20	___	___
Depreciation recapture	___	___	___	___
§ 1231 gain or (loss)	___	30	(10)	5

17-48 *Depreciation Recapture and the § 1231 Netting Process.* T had three § 1231 transactions during the current year. All of the assets were held for several years.
  a. Theft of electric cart used on business premises. The cart was worth $600, originally cost $800, and had an adjusted basis of $425.
  b. Sale of equipment used in manufacturing. The equipment sold for $5,500, originally cost $8,000, and had an adjusted basis of $4,250.
  c. Sale of land and a small building used for storage. The property was sold for $60,000, originally cost $56,000, and had an adjusted basis of $42,500. Straight-line depreciation was claimed on the building.

Determine the amount of ordinary income or loss and capital gain or loss that T must report from these transactions for the current year.

17-49 *Section 1231 Transactions.* K has the following business assets that she is interested in selling in either 2009 or 2010.

	Fair Market Value	Basis
Manufacturing equipment.	$220,000	$400,000
Factory building	350,000	220,000
Land used for factory	450,000	120,000

Straight-line depreciation of $60,000 was claimed on the factory. K has never sold any other § 1231 assets.

   a. What are the tax results if K sells the land and building in 2009 and the equipment in 2010?
   b. What are the tax results if K sells the equipment in 2009 and the land and building in 2010?
   c. What are the tax results if K sells all the assets in 2009?

17-50 *Comprehensive Problem for Capital Asset and Trade or Business Property Transactions.* T owned a number of apartment units and sold several properties related to that trade or business during the current year as follows:

Description	Holding Period	Sales Price	Cost	Depreciation Allowed	Method
Apartment unit, including land (straight-line depreciation = $2,400)	3 years	$65,000	$24,000	$3,000	DB
Lawn tractor	5 years	1,000	3,000	2,600	SL
Spray painter	2 years	500	1,400	600	SL

During a severe winter storm, T also lost a depreciable motor scooter used in his business. The scooter, which was owned by T for two years and used exclusively in the business, had cost $2,600 and had an adjusted basis of $1,750.

In addition, T sold several capital assets during the current year as follows:

Description	Holding Period	Sales Price	Adjusted Basis
100 shares LM Corp.	16 months	$2,000	$1,000
75 shares PL, Inc.	8 months	1,600	6,000
Silver ingots	6 years	2,600	6,000

Assuming T has never deducted § 1231 losses before, calculate the following amounts based on the above information:
   a. The amount of § 1245 recapture and § 1250 recapture, if any.
   b. The net § 1231 gain or loss.
   c. The capital gain or loss and the rate at which it is taxed.
   d. The net short-term capital gain or loss.
   e. The overall impact of the above transactions on T's adjusted gross income.

17-51 *Netting Gains and Losses.* G had the following gains and losses for the current calendar year:

DFG Corporation stock held 3 years	$4,000
Gold held 6 years.	(5,000)
Sale of business building:	
§ 1250 recapture	1,500
§ 1231 gain.	7,000

Depreciation of $7,500 had been claimed on the building. What is the character of these gains in calculating the capital gains tax?

17-52 *Capital Gains Tax.* C, an unmarried head of household, has the following gains and losses for the current taxable year:

GHJ, Inc. stock held 16 months	($3,000)
Land held for investment 15 years	4,000
Sale of business real estate held 15 years:	
§ 1250 recapture	1,800
Net § 1231 gain	7,250

Depreciation claimed on the real estate was $7,800. C's taxable income (properly calculated and including the information above) is $121,900. How much is C's income tax for the current calendar year?

17-53 *Comprehensive Problem with Sales of Business Use Assets.* O and P are married. They have no dependents and elect to file jointly for the current year. They recently decided to retire, sell their home, and try renting for a while. Their income and related transactions for the year follow:

Ordinary income from business	$ 45,200
Interest income	10,100
Sale of personal residence of 20 years:	
Sales price	$760,000
Selling costs	43,000
Adjusted basis	195,000
Sale of business:	
§ 1245 recapture	15,000
§ 1250 recapture	26,000
§ 1231 gain	90,000
Gain on sale of stock held 5 years	16,000
Itemized deductions (after 2 percent cutback)	23,400

O and P had claimed depreciation on the § 1245 property and the § 1250 property in the amount of $25,000 and $56,000, respectively. Calculate O and P's adjusted gross income, taxable income, and gross income tax for the current year.

17-54 *Sections 1231 and 1245 Property.* The terms § 1231 property and § 1245 property are often used interchangeably. However, there are times when a specific asset can be classified as (1) *both* § 1231 and § 1245 property; (2) only § 1231 property; or (3) only § 1245 property. Based on the values assigned to the letters below, indicate the appropriate classification for each of the following mathematical expressions.

$$\text{Let} \quad \begin{aligned} X &= \text{asset's original cost} \\ Y &= \text{depreciation claimed} \\ Z &= \text{asset's adjusted basis} \\ T &= \text{amount realized on sale} \end{aligned}$$

a. If T Z, asset is § _____ property.
b. If $T > X$, asset is § _____ property.
c. If $X > T < Z$, asset is § _____ property.
d. If $Y > T > Z$, asset is § _____ property.

17-55 *Section 1231 and § 1250 Property.* It is possible that (1) *both* § 1231 and § 1250 apply to the sale of depreciable real property, (2) only § 1250 applies, or (3) only § 1231 applies. Based on the values assigned to the letters below, indicate which Code sections apply for each of the following mathematical expressions.

> Let X = asset's original cost
> Y = depreciation claimed
> Z = asset's adjusted basis
> T = amount realized on sale
> S = amount of straight-line depreciation

    a. If $Y > S$ and T Z, § _____ applies.
    b. If $Y > S$ and $T > X$, § _____ applies.
    c. If $Y = S$, § _____ applies.
    d. If $Y > S$ and $(T-Z)$ $(Y-S)$, § _____ applies.

17-56 *Sale of Property Converted from Personal Use—Comprehensive Problem.* L owned and used a house as her personal residence since she purchased it in 2004 for $110,000. On February 11, 2007, when it was worth $85,000, L moved out and converted the property into a rental property. She rented the house until December 15, 2009, when it was sold for $104,500.
    a. Determine L's depreciation deductions for the rental property from the time it was converted in 2007 until it was sold in 2009. Ignore land value.
    b. What are the amount and character of L's gain or loss to be recognized from the sale?

17-57 *Sale of Property Converted to Personal Use—Comprehensive Problem.* Z purchased a computer system with peripherals for $14,500 on August 12, 2006. The system was used exclusively in his business. In October 2009, when the computer was worth $8,200, Z closed the business and began using the unit for personal purposes.
    a. Determine Z's depreciation deductions for the computer system from the time it was purchased until it was converted to personal use, assuming that he elected the maximum § 179 expensing option for other assets placed into service in 2006.
    b. Assume the computer system was sold for $5,400 on May 15, 2009 rather than being converted to personal use. What are the amount and character of Z's loss?

RESEARCH PROBLEMS

17-58 *Capital Assets versus § 1231 Assets.* R inherited a residence that had been used exclusively by her grandmother as a principal residence for 30 years. Upon receiving the property, R immediately offered the property for rent and rented to several tenants. After several months, R encountered an interesting potential business venture that would require a substantial capital investment. After an agonizing decision, she proceeded to sell her inherited rental unit. The unit was sold at a loss and R deducted the loss under § 1231. Since she had no § 1231 gains, the loss was deducted as an ordinary deduction. Is the treatment R chose the appropriate treatment for the loss? Does the character of the property to her grandmother carry over to R, resulting in disallowance of the loss or capital loss treatment?

Research aids:
> *Campbell v. Comm.*, 5 T.C. 272 (1945).
> *Crawford v. Comm.*, 16 T.C. 678 (1951), acq. 1951-2 C.B. 2.

17-59 *Business Use of Personal Residence.* J purchased a home in March 1989 for $120,000. Twenty percent of its cost was attributable to the land. From the date of purchase until March 2005, 20 percent of the house was used as a home-office, the costs of which were properly deducted annually (including depreciation). The home was used exclusively as J's residence from April 2005 until the house was sold for $325,000 on November 15, 2009.

    a. J used the straight line method and the normal useful life of 32.5 years. What amount of depreciation did he claim over the 15-year period that the property was used as a home-office?

    b. Is there any depreciation recapture to be reported if gain is reported on the sale?

    c. Is there depreciation recapture to be reported if all or part of the gain is excluded?

PART SIX

EMPLOYEE COMPENSATION AND RETIREMENT PLANS

★ ★ ★ ★ ★ CONTENTS ★ ★ ★ ★ ★

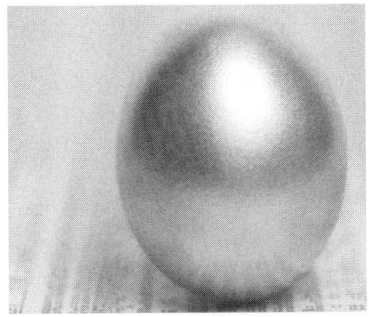

CHAPTER EIGHTEEN

EMPLOYEE COMPENSATION AND RETIREMENT PLANS

LEARNING OBJECTIVES

Upon completion of this chapter you will be able to:

▶ Distinguish between taxable and nontaxable employee fringe benefits

▶ Determine the tax consequences of the issuance and exercise of both nonqualified and qualified stock options

▶ Explain the advantages and disadvantages of nonqualified deferred compensation arrangements, including

  ▶ The deferral of both the employee's recognition of income and the employer's deduction

  ▶ The economic risk associated with unfunded arrangements

▶ Specify the two basic tax benefits of qualified retirement plans

▶ Distinguish between a defined benefit plan and a defined contribution plan

▶ Calculate the limitations on annual contributions to the various types of qualified plans

▶ Compute the annual amount of deductible contribution to an Individual Retirement Account

▶ Describe the characteristics of a Simplified Employee Pension

CHAPTER OUTLINE

INTRODUCTION

For a large majority of individual taxpayers, compensation received for services rendered as an employee is the most significant, if not the only, source of taxable income. Because of this significance, the topic of taxation of employee compensation is of primary interest to the tax-paying public. Employee compensation consists not only of cash wage and salary payments but an incredible variety of compensation "packages" designed to accommodate the needs and desires of employer and employee alike.

The tax consequences to both the employer and employee of various types of employment compensation are examined in this chapter. Because the concept of compensation includes provisions for employee retirement income, the chapter also includes a discussion of the numerous types of retirement income plans available to both employees and self-employed taxpayers.

TAXATION OF CURRENT COMPENSATION

Under the broad authority of § 61, a taxpayer's gross income includes all compensation for services rendered including wages, salaries, fees, fringe benefits, sales commissions, customer tips, and bonuses. Compensatory payments may be made in a medium other than cash. For example, payment for services rendered may be made with property, such as marketable securities. In such cases, the fair market value of the property is the measure of the gross compensation income received.[1]

Payment for services performed by Taxpayer A for Taxpayer B could consist of services performed by Taxpayer B for Taxpayer A. For example, a lawyer might agree to draft a will for a carpenter, who in turn agrees to repair the lawyer's roof. As a result of such a *service swap*, both taxpayers must recognize gross income equal to the value of the services received.[2]

STATUTORY FRINGE BENEFITS

As a general rule, any economic benefit bestowed on an employee by his or her employer that is intended to compensate the employee for services rendered represents gross income. This is true whether the benefit is in the form of a direct cash payment or an indirect noncash benefit that nonetheless improves the recipient's economic position.

Certain indirect or *fringe benefits*, however, are excludable from gross income under specific statutory authority. The following is a list of nontaxable fringe benefits and the authority for their exclusion from income. The details of these exclusions are discussed in Chapter 6.

1. Employer payment of employee group-term life insurance premiums (up to $50,000 of coverage)—§ 79

2. Employer contributions to employee accident or health plans—§ 106

3. Amounts paid to an employee under an employer's medical expense reimbursement plan—§ 105(b)

4. Employee meals or lodging furnished for the convenience of the employer—§ 119

5. Amounts received under an employer's group legal services program—§ 120

6. Amounts received under an employer's educational assistance program—§ 127

7. Amounts received under an employer's dependent care assistance program—§ 129

8. No-additional-cost services, qualified employee discounts, working condition fringes, and de minimis fringes—§ 132

The length of the above list demonstrates Congressional tolerance for the use of innovative fringe benefits to attract employees. Employers who want to design the most flexible compensation package for employees who have differing compensation needs may use a *cafeteria plan* of employee benefits. Under a cafeteria plan, an employee is allowed to choose among two or more benefits consisting of both cash and statutory nontaxable benefits.[3]

---

[1]   Reg. § 1.61-2(d).

[2]   *Ibid.*

[3]   § 125.

DEFERRED COMPENSATION

Deferral of compensation can be accomplished under a variety of methods that includes both "qualified" and "nonqualified" plans. A qualified plan is one that meets the requirements of Code § 401(a) and offers the employer a current deduction for money set aside for the eventual benefit of the employee. In this manner, the employees are not taxed on the amount set aside until it is distributed to them, and the income earned on the funds is exempt from tax. A nonqualified plan, on the other hand, does not possess all the specialized tax benefits, but offers a plan that is easier to administer and allows for discrimination among employees. Some of the more popular types of each of these plans are listed in Exhibit 18-1.

The purpose of deferred compensation plans is to allow employees to receive income at a later date when, presumably, they will have much less income. The employee's tax objective in participating in such an arrangement is to ensure that they will be taxed only when payments are received under the plan or agreement. The employer's tax objective is to offer a vehicle that will attract and compensate key personnel while obtaining a current tax deduction for any funds set aside for these employees.

Changes in the tax law, specifically the 1986 Tax Reform Act, reduced some of the glamour of deferred arrangements through its repeal of the capital gains differential and compression of the individual-corporate tax rate structure. However, subsequent legislation has reinstated a modest resurgence in plan activity due to the prospects of a widening capital gain differential and a probable increase in tax rates. Nevertheless, while the 1986 Act reduced the tax benefits of qualified plans, it is still possible to achieve both deferral of taxation and capital gains treatment on the eventual distribution of funds to the employee. However, most deferred compensation arrangements are not ordinarily utilized as vehicles to recharacterize the form of income.

EXHIBIT 18-1
Types of Deferred Compensation Plans

Qualified Plans

Defined Contribution Plans
Defined Benefit Plans
Money Purchase Plans
Stock Bonus Plans
Employee Stock Ownership Plans
Cash or Deferred Arrangements (401k)
Simplified Employee Plans
Individual Retirement Accounts
Incentive Stock Options
SIMPLE Plans

Nonqualified Plans

Restricted Stock
Deferred Payments
Rabbi Trusts
Secular Trusts
Nonqualified Stock Options

While numerous deferred compensation arrangements focus on tax benefits, most qualified plans are flexible and have a wide range of purposes other than reducing an

employee's tax liability. For example, a retirement benefit program can have a substantial psychological impact on an employee's morale because it offers an effortless program of saving for the future. In addition, a nonqualified deferred compensation arrangement can be tailored to attract and compensate new executives for benefits they may have forfeited when they left their former employer. Finally, both qualified and nonqualified deferred compensation plans can provide other benefits, such as disability guarantees, death benefits, income security, and plan loans, to safeguard and preserve the well-being of the company's most valued asset—its employees.

RECEIPT OF PROPERTY FOR SERVICES

From a corporate employer's point of view, any form of employee compensation that somehow strengthens that employee's commitment to the corporation is highly desirable. One such type of compensation is a payment made in the capital stock of the corporation itself. Such payment converts the employee into a stockholder and gives him or her an equity interest in the future prosperity of the corporation.

When stock in the corporate employer is used to compensate employees, it is typical for the employment contract to provide that the employee must continue to work for the corporation for some stated time period before he or she is given unrestricted ownership of the stock. If the employee leaves the job before the period expires, the stock received will be forfeited. In this situation, the tax consequences of the compensatory payment to both employee and employer are governed by § 83.

GENERAL RULE OF § 83

If in connection with the performance of services, property of any type is transferred to any person other than the person for whom such services are performed, § 83(a) provides that the fair market value of such property shall be included in the gross income of the person performing such services. If the recipient made any payment for the property, only the excess of the property's value over the amount of such payment is includible gross income. Such inclusion shall occur in the first taxable year in which the rights of the person having the beneficial interest in such property are *transferable* or are not subject to a *substantial risk of forfeiture*, whichever is applicable. If the property received for services is not immediately transferable by the recipient or is subject to risk of forfeiture, it is referred to as *restricted property.*

Regulation § 1.83-3(c)(1) explains that a substantial risk of forfeiture exists when the ownership of the transferred property is conditioned, directly or indirectly, upon the future performance (or refraining from performance) of substantial services by the recipient. The Regulation also states that the existence of a substantial risk of forfeiture can only be determined by examining the facts and circumstances of the specific situation.

Section 83(h) entitles the taxpayer for whom services were performed and who transferred property as compensation to a deduction equal to the fair market value of the property. The deduction must be taken in the taxable year in which (or with which) ends the taxable year in which the value of the property is recognized as gross income to the recipient.

Example 1. Corporation M is on a fiscal year ending June 30. On November 1, 2006, the corporation gave employee E, a calendar year taxpayer, 100 shares of its own stock worth $100 per share as compensation for E's services to Corporation M. If E leaves M's employ for any reason during the three-year period beginning on November 1, 2006, he must return the shares. On November 2, 2009, E is still employed and the risk of forfeiture of the stock lapses. On this date the stock is worth $120 per share. For his taxable year 2009, E must include $12,000 in gross income;

his tax basis in his shares will also be $12,000. Corporation M has a deduction of $12,000 for its fiscal year ending June 30, 2010.

The Regulations make it clear that a deduction is available to the transferor of the property only if the transfer is an expense meeting the deductibility requirements of § 162 or § 212. If the transfer constitutes a capital expenditure, it must be capitalized rather than deducted.[4]

Example 2. Refer to the facts in *Example 1*. If the shares were transferred to E because E performed organizational services for Corporation M, the corporation must capitalize the $12,000 amount included in E's gross income.

THE § 83(B) ELECTION

Section 83(b) gives a taxpayer who has performed services for *restricted* property an interesting option. Within 30 days of the receipt of the property, the taxpayer may choose to include its fair market value in his or her current year's gross income. This election accelerates the recognition of gross income to the taxpayer. However, the election could be beneficial if the property were rapidly appreciating in value and consequently would have a higher fair market value on the date the risk of forfeiture or other restrictions are scheduled to lapse.

Example 3. In 2006, employee Z receives property worth $10,000 as payment for services rendered. The property is subject to a substantial risk of forfeiture, but Z elects to include the $10,000 value in her 2007 gross income. In 2009, when the risk of forfeiture lapses, the property is worth $25,000. However, Z has no gross income attributable to the property in 2009. Z will have a $10,000 basis in her stock, and Z's employer has a $10,000 deduction for its taxable year that includes December 31, 2007.

The election is not without risk. If the property depreciates during the forfeiture period, the election leads to a larger gross income inclusion as well as acceleration of tax recognition. And more costly still, if the property is in fact forfeited, the taxpayer receives no deduction for the original gross income inclusion.[5] Obviously, the decision to use the § 83(b) election requires a careful analysis of both the current and expected future value of the property, current and future marginal tax rates, and the nature of the restriction involved.

QUALIFIED RETIREMENT PLANS FOR CORPORATIONS

Historically, Congress has viewed with favor the establishment of employer retirement plans as part of a total compensation package offered to employees. The existence of an employer designed and administered plan encourages the young employee to think seriously about his or her retirement years and offers the employee a most convenient way to provide financially for such retirement.

Congress provided an extremely attractive set of tax benefits available to *qualified* employer retirement plans as part of the Internal Revenue Code of 1954. Since the enactment of the 1954 Code, the scope of the benefits has been periodically expanded, and Congress has made different forms of qualified plans available to an ever-increasing number of individual taxpayers. Before examining the various types of qualified plans

---

4 Reg. § 1.83-6(a)(4).

5 § 83(b)(1).

and the specific features of each, it will be useful to analyze the two basic tax benefits associated with qualified plans for employees—the tax-free nature of employer contributions and the tax-free growth of these contributions.

TAX BENEFITS OF QUALIFIED PLANS

When an employer makes a current contribution to a *qualified* retirement plan on behalf of an employee, §§ 402(a) and 403(a) provide that the value of the contribution is not includible gross income to the employee, even though the employee has obviously received additional compensation in the form of the contribution. In contrast, if the contribution was made by the employer to a *nonqualified* retirement plan in which the employee had a vested interest, the employee would have additional gross income equal to the value of the contribution. As a result, the net amount saved toward retirement by the employee participating in a nonqualified plan is less than the amount saved by the employee participating in a qualified plan.

The second major benefit of qualified retirement plans is that the earnings generated by employer contributions are nontaxable. Sections 401(a) and 501(a) provide that a trust created to manage and invest employer contributions to a qualified retirement plan is exempt from tax.

The effect of these two benefits on the total amount of savings available to an employee at retirement is illustrated in Exhibit 18-2. The exhibit compares two retirement plans, A and B. The plans are identical in every respect but one—A is a nonqualified personal savings plan while B is a qualified employer's trust. The exhibit is based on the following assumptions:

1. The employer will make an annual $10,000 contribution to the plan on behalf of the employee.

2. The employee has a 25 percent marginal tax rate. Therefore, the net amount saved by the employee in Plan A is only $7,500 ($10,000 − $2,500 tax on the current compensation represented by the contribution). The net amount saved in Plan B is $10,000.

3. Funds invested in both plans can earn a 12 percent before-tax return. The earnings from Plan A are taxable to the employee so that the plan's after-tax rate of return is 9 percent. Plan B is in the form of a qualified trust and therefore its earnings are tax-exempt.

EXHIBIT 18-2
Comparison of Nonqualified versus
Qualified Retirement Plans' Year-End Values of Employer Contributions

	Nonqualified Plan A	Qualified Plan B
Year 1................................	$ 7,500	$ 10,000
Year 2................................	15,675	21,200
Year 15................................	220,208*	372,800**

* $7,500 × 29.361 (factor for the sum of an annuity of $1.00 at 9% for 15 years)
** $10,000 × 37.280 (factor for the sum of an annuity of $1.00 at 12% for 15 years)

The difference in the amounts available to an employee after 15 years of participation in either plan is dramatic. It is not difficult to understand why qualified retirement plans have become such an attractive fringe benefit to employees concerned with providing

for their retirement years. However, before the analysis presented in Exhibit 18-2 is complete, it is necessary to examine the general rule as to the taxability of benefits paid out of a qualified plan upon an employee's retirement.

When an employee begins to withdraw funds from a nonqualified retirement savings plan, such funds represent *after-tax* dollars, and he or she will not be taxed on these funds a second time. In comparison, benefits received by an employee out of a qualified plan funded solely by employer contributions are fully taxable to the employee. It is important to understand that the retirement dollars available under Plan A of Exhibit 18-2 are excludable (as a return of capital), while the retirement dollars available under Plan B are fully includible in the recipient's gross income.

TAXABILITY OF QUALIFIED PLAN LUMP-SUM DISTRIBUTIONS

If an employee who has made no contributions to the employer's qualified retirement plan receives a distribution from the plan, the employee has no investment in the distribution and therefore must include the entire amount in adjusted gross income.[6] When the distribution is made by a series of payments (i.e., an annuity), the taxability of the distribution is spread over a number of years.[7] If the distribution is made in a lump sum, all the retirement income is taxed in one year.[8] Given the progressive rate structure of the Federal income tax, the normal tax on a large lump sum distribution could be prohibitive.

To mitigate this problem, Congress provided two relief provisions that benefit the recipient of a lump-sum distribution from a qualified retirement plan. First, an employee could treat the portion of a distribution attributable to the employee's participation in the retirement plan prior to 1974 as long-term capital gain.[9] The Tax Reform Act of 1986 generally repealed such capital gain treatment. However, a taxpayer who was age 50 before January 1, 1986 may elect to utilize this relief provision. In such case, the long-term capital gain portion of a distribution will be taxed at a flat 20 percent rate.[10] Note that in 2001, individuals who turned 65 before the close of the year would be eligible for this special treatment.

A second relief provision is a special procedure for computing the amount of current tax on a lump sum distribution. Prior to the Tax Reform Act of 1986, the procedure involved a 10-year forward averaging computation; for distributions made after December 31, 1986, the averaging period has been reduced to five years.[11] A taxpayer who was age 50 before January 1, 1986 may elect to use the 10-year forward averaging computation based on 1986 income tax rates for distributions received after 1986.[12]

While the original intent of the averaging rules was to prevent a bunching of income, Congress felt that taxpayers now have more control in determining the year that benefits are received. In addition, the averaging rules were perceived to be overly burdensome and the responsibility for this burden lay directly with the taxpayer. As a result, the special five-year averaging option under § 402(d) was repealed under the Small Business Job Protection Act of 1996. The repeal is effective for tax years beginning after December 31, 1999.

Under pre-2000 law, the averaging computation could be elected only for lump sum distributions received on or after the taxpayer had reached $59\frac{1}{2}$ years of age, and a

---

[6]   If the employee has made contributions to the plan, he or she will have an investment in the plan, which may be recovered tax-free under the rules of § 72.

[7]   § 402(a).

[8]   § 402(e)(1).

[9]   § 402(a)(2), repealed by the Tax Reform Act of 1986.

[10]   Tax Reform Act of 1986, Act § 1122(h)(3).

[11]   § 402(e).

[12]   Tax Reform Act of 1986, Act § 1122(h)(5).

taxpayer could only make one such election.[13] Note that those who were born before 1936 continue to be eligible for ten-year averaging even after the five-year averaging is repealed.

ADDITIONAL TAXES ON PREMATURE OR EXCESS DISTRIBUTIONS

Congress intended for the tax-favored status of qualified plans to serve as an inducement for taxpayers to provide for a source of retirement income. Therefore, if a taxpayer makes a premature withdrawal from a qualified plan, a 10 percent penalty tax is imposed on the amount of the distribution included in the taxpayer's gross income.[14] However, the Code does permit penalty-free withdrawal from IRAs before age $59\frac{1}{2}$ if any of the distributions are:

- ► On account of death or permanent disability.

- ► In the form of annuity payments over the taxpayer's lifetime.

- ► For medical expenses of the individual, his or her spouse and dependents that exceed 7.5 percent of A.G.I.

- ► For medical insurance of the individual, his or her spouse and dependents (without regard to the 7.5% of A.G.I. floor) if the individual has received unemployment compensation for at least 12 weeks, and the withdrawal is made in the year such unemployment compensation is received or the following year.

- ► For qualified education expenses. For this purpose, the term qualified higher education expenses is defined in § 529(e)(3) and generally means tuition, fees, books, supplies, and equipment required for enrollment or attendance at an eligible educational institution. It also includes the reasonable costs of room and board. In order to qualify, the expenses must be for education furnished to the taxpayer, the taxpayer's spouse, or any child or grandchild of the taxpayer or the taxpayer's spouse at an eligible education institution. Such expenses are reduced by amounts excluded from gross income that are used for such education.

- ► For first-time homebuyer expenses. The penalty waiver applies only to the first $10,000 withdrawn during the taxpayer's lifetime. The withdrawals must be used within 120 days of withdrawal to acquire, construct, or reconstruct a home that is the principal residence of the individual, his or her spouse, or any child, grandchild, or ancestor of the individual or spouse. Acquisition costs include any usual settlement, financing, or other closing costs. Although the name of the law suggests that it applies only to the purchase of a taxpayer's first home (and therefore is a once-in-a-lifetime opportunity), such is not the case. A first time homebuyer is defined as an individual (or if married, such individual's spouse) who had no present ownership interest in a principal residence during the two-year period ending on the date of acquisition. Thus, as long as the taxpayer has not owned a home in the past two years, withdrawals may be made from an IRA to help pay for the "new" home even though it is not the taxpayer's first home.

- ► To reservists called to active duty for at least 179 days.

ROLLOVER CONTRIBUTION

There are many situations in which taxpayers receive lump-sum distributions from qualified plans prior to retirement. For example, a taxpayer who quits his job with his current employer to accept a position with a new employer may have a right to a distribution

---

[13] § 402(e)(4)(B).

[14] § 72(t).

from his current employer's qualified plan. Any taxpayer who receives a qualified plan distribution but does not need additional disposable income can exclude the distribution from gross income (and thus avoid both the income tax and any penalty tax on the distribution) by making a *rollover contribution* of the distributed funds. A rollover contribution must be made into another qualified employer plan, a Keogh plan, or an IRA, and it must be made within 60 days of the receipt of the distribution.[15] Note that in the case of a withdrawal, an employer is normally required to withhold 20 percent of the distribution as an estimated tax payment. However, withholding can be avoided if the amount is rolled directly into another qualified retirement plan, Keogh plan, or an IRA on a timely basis.[16] Failure to observe these rules can create a severe hardship and may lead to a penalty.

> **Example 4.** T is 45 years old. This year his employer laid-off 200 employees and, unfortunately, T lost his job. T decided to take a lump-sum distribution from his retirement plan of $200,000. Absent a direct rollover, T's employer will withhold $40,000 (20% × $200,000) and T will receive $160,000. Note that in order to avoid taxation on the $200,000 as well as the ten percent early withdrawal penalty, T must rollover the entire $200,000 to a qualified plan, even though he only received $160,000. Consequently, he would have to find an additional $40,000 to go along with the $160,000 to avert a catastrophe!

PLAN LOANS

Plan participants can avoid making taxable withdrawals from qualified plans while indirectly utilizing their retirement funds by borrowing money from their qualified plans. There is a very complex limit on the amount of a plan loan. In very general terms, a plan loan to a participant is limited to the lesser of (1) one-half the participant's vested accrued benefit (but not less than $10,000) or (2) $50,000. Any amount of a loan in excess of this limit is considered a taxable distribution.[17] Currently, owners of any small business (those with fewer than 100 employees) are generally permitted to make participant loans.

> **Example 5.** R and S are members of P's small business qualified plan. R has accrued vested benefits of $14,000, and S has accrued vested benefits of $80,000. R can borrow up to $10,000 even though this amount exceeds 50% of his vested benefits. If S, on the other hand, borrows $62,000 from the fund, $22,000 will be treated as a taxable distribution to her because this exceeds 50% of her benefits (which is more severe than the $50,000 ceiling violation).

In order to avoid being treated as a taxable distribution, a loan must be repaid in quarterly installments with interest within five years of the loan. However, if a taxpayer uses the loan to purchase a principal residence, any reasonable repayment period is allowed. The treatment of the interest expense depends on how the loan proceeds were used and whether the taxpayer is a key employee. If the plan loan is secured by the residence, the interest is qualified residence interest and is fully deductible as an itemized deduction. If the loan is used for investment purposes, the interest is considered investment interest and is normally deductible to the extent of any investment income. Unlike regular employees, key employees are not allowed to deduct any interest on plan loans.

---

[15] § 402(a)(5).

[16] § 3405(c)(2).

[17] § 72(p).

TYPES OF QUALIFIED PLANS

Qualified plans fall into two basic categories, defined benefit plans and defined contribution plans. A *defined benefit plan* is one designed to systematically provide for the payment of definitely determinable benefits to retired employees for a period of years or for life. The focus of the plan is on the eventual retirement benefit to be provided. The amount of the benefit is usually based on both an employee's compensation level and years of service to the company. Defined benefit plans are commonly referred to as pension plans. The current amount of employer contributions that are required to fund future pension benefits under a given plan must be determined actuarially.[18]

Defined contribution plans provide for annual contributions to each participating employee's retirement account. Upon retirement, an employee will be entitled to the balance accumulated in his or her account. Defined contribution plans are designed to allow employees to participate in the current profitability of the business. Generally, in profitable years, an employer will make a contribution to a qualified trust and such contribution will be allocated to each employee's retirement account. However, contributions may be made to a qualified profit sharing plan without regard to current or accumulated profits of the employer corporation.[19] Although the employer may have the discretion as to the dollar amount of an annual contribution, such contributions must be recurring and substantial if the plan is to be qualified.[20]

While most defined contribution plans constitute "profit sharing plans," other types of defined contribution arrangements exist. These arrangements include *money purchase plans*, *stock bonus plans*, and *employee stock ownership plans*. Each of these is briefly discussed below.

In an effort to encourage small businesses to establish qualified retirement plans, Congress enacted a special credit as part of the 2001 Tax Act. The credit is 50 percent of up to $1,000 (i.e., $500 maximum credit) of the administrative and retirement education costs incurred during the first three years of the plan to create or maintain the plan. The special credit is only available to businesses that did not employ, in the previous year, more than 100 employees with compensation of at least $5,000.

Money Purchase Plans. A money purchase plan is a defined contribution plan that is treated like a defined benefit plan. The employer's annual contribution is determined by a specific formula that involves either a percentage of compensation of covered employees or a flat dollar amount. Under a money purchase plan, unlike a defined benefit plan, a definite pension amount is not guaranteed. Rather, a participant's retirement benefit will be determined by his or her vested account balance at retirement.

Because an employee's account balance will be fashioned according to a definite formula under a money purchase plan, a certain amount of flexibility is permitted in structuring the plan's contribution formula.

Example 6. Under a company's money purchase plan formula, an employer is required to contribute to the plan 3% of an employee's compensation plus an extra 1% for each year of prior service up to a maximum of 10%. Thus, an employee with 12 years of service would receive a contribution equal to 13% [3 + (12 limited to 10)] of his covered compensation. A new employee would receive only 3%.

Note that under a money purchase plan an employer is required to make a contribution. If an employer fails to make these required contributions under the plan, the

---

[18]   Reg. § 1.401-1(b)(1)(i).

[19]   § 401(a)(27).

[20]   Reg. § 1.401-1(b)(1)(ii).

employer will be subject to certain excise taxes. This minimum funding standard does not apply to stock bonus or profit-sharing plans.[21]

Stock Bonus Plans. A stock bonus plan is another type of deferred compensation arrangement in which the employer establishes a plan in order to contribute shares of the company's stock. A stock bonus plan is subject to the same requirements as a profit sharing plan; therefore, a stock bonus plan must have a predetermined formula for allocating and distributing the stock among the employees. All benefits paid from the plan must be distributed in the form of the employer company's stock. An exception is made for fractional shares distributed from the plan, which may be paid in the form of cash.[22]

Employee Stock Ownership Plans. Another variety of qualified plans is the Employee Stock Ownership Plan (ESOP). As the name suggests, the major purpose of the ESOP legislation was to encourage stock ownership by all employees by giving employers and employees a host of tax incentives. Supporters of ESOPs believe in the fundamental principle that ownership of a business by its employees can help cure many of the ills of a market-based economy. A major proponent of this principle, former Senator Russell Long now deceased, endlessly extolled the virtues of ESOPs, saying that they could eliminate all of what is wrong with capitalism. According to Long and his followers, ESOPs increase worker productivity, improve labor relations, promote economic justice, provide a source of low-cost capital and are basically a savior for our economic system. On the other hand, critics of ESOPs say such claims are merely snake oil. Regardless of the view, ESOPs are now plentiful and have been a part of the system for more than 25 years.

Technically, an ESOP is a defined contribution plan. Like other qualified plans, a company that wants an ESOP first establishes a trust to which it makes annual contributions. The employer contributes either cash or its own stock. If the employer contributes cash, the ESOP uses the cash to purchase stock or securities of the sponsoring employer (rather than stocks or bonds of other companies). Regardless of how the stock or securities are obtained, they are then allocated to individual employee accounts within the trust using some type of formula. For example, the allocation may be in proportion to the employee's compensation or according to years of service or some combination of compensation and years of service. As a result, the company's employees—rather than outsiders—wind up owning a portion or all of the company. Any income earned by the ESOP is treated like that in other plans; that is, the income is completely tax-exempt. When the employee retires, he or she typically sells his or her shares of stock back to the trust and receives cash.

The tax benefits of this arrangement, once huge, have been whittled back by Congress over the years. Nevertheless, ESOPs still offer significant advantages. If the employer contributes stock, it receives a deduction for the value of the stock contributed.[23] Since it costs the employer little or nothing to issue the stock, the employer increases its cash flow by the taxes saved from the deduction. If the employer contributes cash that is subsequently used by the ESOP to purchase stock from the employer, the same benefit is obtained.

Example 7. This year P Corporation established an ESOP. Under the terms of the plan, P transferred 30,000 shares of unissued stock valued at $90,000 to the trust. Under § 1032, the issuance of the stock is nontaxable to P. However, P is entitled to a deduction for the value of the stock contributed, $90,000. Assuming P's marginal rate

---

[21]   § 412(h)(1).

[22]   Regs. § 1.401-1(b)(1)(iii).

[23]   § 1032.

is 34 percent, the contribution provides tax savings of $30,600 ($90,000 × 34%) with little or no cash drain.

The deductibility of contributions to an ESOP becomes even more attractive in the case of a *leveraged* ESOP. In a leveraged ESOP, the ESOP typically borrows money from a lender (e.g., a bank) and uses the cash to purchase the sponsoring corporation's stock. In subsequent years, the company makes contributions to the ESOP that are used to repay the interest and principal on the loan. When the contributions are used to pay the loan, such contributions are deductible. Observe that the effect is to allow the company to deduct the payments of not only the interest but also the principal. This feature makes the ESOP a very attractive form of debt financing for the employer. Similarly, the Code allows the company to deduct any dividends paid on ESOP stock which are used to repay the loan or which are passed through to the employees (a special feature of ESOPs).

Another significant benefit of the ESOP—no doubt the one that attracts the most attention—is the tax-free rollover permitted by § 1042. If the conditions of this provision are met, a shareholder who sells stock to an ESOP and who has owned the stock for at least three years may defer recognition of any gain realized on the sale by reinvesting in other stocks or bonds. This enables a retiring owner to get out of the business at the cost of one capital gains tax (rather than two taxes in most cases) that is deferred until the replacement property is sold.

SIMPLE Plans. As a general rule, retirement plan coverage is lower for small employers than among medium and larger employers. Congress believed that one of the reasons for this result stemmed from the complexity of the rules relating to establishment of tax-qualified retirement plans as well as the high costs associated with complying with those rules. In an effort to encourage small employers to adopt retirement plans for its employees, Congress created a simplified retirement plan option known as SIMPLE (the Savings Incentive Match Plan for Employees).[24]

Under a SIMPLE plan, employers with 100 or fewer employees and no other employer-sponsored retirement plan are permitted to establish a savings incentive match plan for their employees. Deductible contributions may be made either to individual IRA accounts established for each employee or to accounts established as part of a 401(k) plan. One of the key benefits of adopting a SIMPLE plan is that those plans which satisfy the SIMPLE plan contribution requirements are not required to satisfy the nondiscrimination and top-heavy requirements that other qualified plans must continue to meet.

Under a SIMPLE plan, an employer generally must either match elective employee contributions dollar-for-dollar up to 3 percent of compensation or make a 2 percent of compensation contribution on behalf of each eligible employee. The limitation on employee contributions is reflected in the table below. Contributions to a SIMPLE account are deductible by the employer and excluded from the employee's income. Distributions are generally taxed under the rules applicable to IRAs. All employees with W-2 income of at least $5,000 annually must be allowed to participate.

The annual contribution limit to a SIMPLE plan is as follows:

Year	Amount
Prior to 2002	$ 6,000
2002	7,000
2003	8,000
2004	9,000
2005–2006	10,000
2007–2008	10,500
2009	11,500

---

[24] §§ 1421 and 1422 of the Small Business Job Protection Act of 1996 amending § 401(k) and § 408(p).

Catch-up Contributions. A SIMPLE plan can permit participants who are age 50 or over at the end of the calendar year to make catch-up contributions. The catch-up contribution limit for 2008 and 2009 is $2,500. The amount of a catch-up contribution that a participant can make for a year cannot exceed the lesser of the following amounts:

- The catch-up contribution limit; or
- The excess of the participant's compensation over the salary reduction contributions that are not catch-up contribution.

QUALIFICATION REQUIREMENTS

In order for a retirement plan to be *qualified* and therefore eligible for preferential tax treatment, it first must comply with a long list of requirements set forth in §§ 401 through 415. These requirements are extremely complex and can prove burdensome to the employer wishing to establish a qualified plan for his or her employees. The rigorous requirements are intended to ensure that a qualified retirement plan operates to benefit a company's employees in an impartial and nondiscriminatory manner.

The current requirements for plan qualification came into the law in 1974 with the enactment of the Employees Retirement Income Security Act (ERISA). Prior to ERISA, many qualified plans were designed to benefit only those employees who were officers of the company, shareholders, or highly compensated executives. Since the passage of ERISA, such discriminatory plans are no longer qualified.

EXISTENCE OF A QUALIFIED TRUST

Under § 401 and the accompanying Treasury Regulations, contributions made as part of a qualified plan must be paid into a domestic (U.S.) trust, administered by a trustee for the exclusive benefit of a company's employees. The plan must be in written form and its provisions must be communicated to all employees. The plan must be established by the employer. Any type of employer—sole proprietor, partnership, trust, or corporation—may establish a plan.

ANTI-DISCRIMINATION RULES

A retirement plan will not qualify if the contributions to or benefits from the plan discriminate in favor of the *prohibited group*. The prohibited group is defined as employees who are highly compensated or who are officers or shareholders of the company. If a plan provides for contributions or benefits to be determined under an equitable and reasonable formula, the fact that the prohibited group receives a greater dollar amount of contributions or benefits than employees in the nonprohibited group will not constitute discrimination.[25]

The Small Business Job and Protection Act of 1996 substantially simplified the definition of a "highly compensated employee." Currently, a highly compensated employee is a 5 percent owner during the current or prior year, or an employee with compensation during the prior year over $110,000 (2009). Employers may also elect to limit the pool of highly compensated employees to anyone who satisfies the basic definition and is in the top 20 percent of employees by compensation.[26]

---

[25]   §§ 401(a)(4) and (5).

[26]   § 414(q).

An important aspect of the statutory antidiscrimination rules for qualified plans is the fact that such plans may be integrated with public retirement benefits.[27] Under the integration rules, the calculation of plan benefits may take into account the extent to which an employee is covered by social security or a state retirement program. In effect, an employer can credit a portion of its social security contribution toward the amount it is required to contribute to the qualified plan. Without any limitations, integration could be used to pay substantially more benefits to a highly compensated employee. For example, assume H owns a corporation that has two employees, H who earns $150,000 and L who earns $20,000. Also assume that the corporation's qualified plan contribution rate was 6.2 percent of compensation. Using integration and ignoring current limitations, the corporation would not be required to contribute any amounts for L since all of its required contribution is met by its payment for L's social security. On the other hand, it would contribute 6.2 percent for H for every dollar above the social security wage base, $102,000 in 2008. As might be expected, special rules exist to prohibit such abuse. Nevertheless, integration can be used in a limited fashion to increase the benefits to highly compensated employees at the expense of other employees.

SCOPE OF PLAN PARTICIPATION AND COVERAGE

A qualified retirement plan must provide that a substantial portion of a company's employees are eligible to participate in the plan. Specifically, any employee who has reached age 21 must be eligible to participate after completing one year of service for the employer.[28] The plan may not exclude an employee from participation on the basis of a maximum age.[29]

In addition to these *minimum* and *maximum* age and service conditions, a qualified plan must meet complex minimum coverage requirements. A qualified plan must satisfy one of the following three minimum coverage tests: the *percentage test*, the *ratio test*, or the *average benefits test*.[30]

Under the percentage test, a plan must benefit 70 percent or more of all of the employer's non-highly compensated employees. For this test, all eligible employees are considered to benefit under the plan. A plan that has no coverage requirements or highly compensated employees will automatically satisfy this test.

> **Example 8.** P Corporation has two divisions, R and S. P Corporation adopts a plan that covers only the employees of division S. If R division has 2 highly compensated and 20 non-highly compensated employees and S division has 18 highly compensated and 80 non-highly compensated employees, P satisfies the percentage test. This is because the plan covers 80% [80% of (20 + 80)] of the nonhighly paid employees.

The ratio test requires that the plan benefit a classification of employees that does not allow more than a reasonable difference between the percentage of an employer's highly compensated employees who are covered and a similarly computed percentage for non-highly compensated employees. In other words, the ratio test allows the percentage test to be proportionately reduced.

> **Example 9.** Assume the same facts as *Example 8*. Because only 90% of the highly compensated employees are covered (18 of 20), only 90% of the percentage test must

---

[27]   § 401(a)(5).

[28]   § 410(a)(1). The plan may defer participation for two years if it provides immediate 100 percent vesting.

[29]   § 410(a)(2).

[30]   § 410(b)(1).

be met. Thus, the plan would meet the ratio test if as few as 63% of the non-highly compensated employees are covered (90% of 70%).

A plan will satisfy the average benefits test if (1) it benefits employees under a classification that the IRS finds does not discriminate and (2) the average benefit percentage for non-highly compensated employees is at least 70 percent of the average benefit percentage for highly compensated employees. The average benefit percentage, with respect to any group of employees, is the sum of all employer contributions and benefits under the plan provided to the group, expressed as a percentage of pay for all group members. An employer may compute the average benefit percentage based on either the current plan year or on a rolling average of three plan years that includes the current year. Once the employer makes this choice, it must obtain IRS consent to revoke it.[31]

The 50/40 Rule. While this rule is not a separate coverage rule, the 50/40 rule deserves attention because of the significance of the law involved. Basically, a plan will lose its qualification unless on each day of the plan year, it benefits the lesser of (1) 50 employees or (2) 40 percent of all employees of the employer. The 50/40 requirement applies separately to each qualified plan, and the Regulations exempt certain plans from this rule.[32]

VESTING REQUIREMENTS AND FORFEITURES

Once an employee is participating in an employer-sponsored retirement plan, he or she may not be entitled to any benefits under the plan for a certain period of time. After the requisite period of time, the employee's benefits *vest* and become nonforfeitable regardless of his or her continued employee status.

Under a qualified plan, vesting for non-top heavy employees must occur according to one of two statutory schedules designed to guarantee that an employee obtains a right to plan benefits within a reasonable time.[33] These two schedules are often referred to as "Cliff" vesting and "Graded" vesting.

Cliff Vesting. This schedule derived its name from the tendency, before ERISA, of some employers to push off the employment "cliff" (terminate) those employees just about to become vested in the retirement plan. Effective for years beginning after 1988, plans are no longer permitted to be more restrictive than five-year cliff vesting. Beginning in 2002, the cliff vesting must be complete within three years. Under three-year cliff vesting, an employee would not be entitled to any vesting before completing three years of service. At the end of the third year, the employer would have to vest the employee 100 percent in his or her accrued benefit attributable to employer contributions.[34]

Graded Vesting. The second permissible non-top heavy vesting schedule is graded vesting. Under such a schedule, employees must become proportionately vested over a two- to six-year vesting period. Under six-year graded vesting, a plan must provide at a minimum the following:

[31] § 410(b)(2)(C).

[32] § 401(a)(26) and Prop. Regs. § 1.401(a)(26)-2.

[33] § 411(a)(2).

[34] § 411(a)(2)(A).

20%	vesting after two years service;
40%	vesting after three years service;
60%	vesting after four years service;
80%	vesting after five years service; and
100%	vesting after six years service.

Under this schedule, the potential for discrimination diminishes because vesting occurs at a more gradual rate and, after three years of service, all employees are entitled to some vesting.[35]

If an employee leaves the job before some or all of the retirement benefits have vested, he or she forfeits the right to such benefits. Previous employee contributions toward these forfeited benefits are not returned to the employer, but instead transfer to remaining plan participants in a nondiscriminatory manner.[36]

FUNDING AND CONTRIBUTION LIMITATIONS

Qualified retirement plans must be *funded*. Consequently, an employer is required to make current payments into a qualified trust. For a defined benefit plan, an actuarially determined minimum current contribution is required by statute.[37] For a defined contribution plan, the annually determined contribution must be *paid* to the trustee. Because of these rules, an employer must back up its promises to the employees with actual plan contributions.

The Code limits the amount of contributions or benefits that are provided for employees. If these amounts should be exceeded, the plan will terminate.[38] In addition, § 404 establishes a limit on the amount that an employer may deduct. Sometimes the deductibility issue may have an impact on the amount that an employer may contribute on behalf of an employee.

Defined Contribution Plans. Under a defined contribution plan, the maximum contribution that can be made to the account of an employee is limited to the lesser of the following:

1. $46,000 (in 2008); or

2. 100 percent of the employee's compensation (subject to limits described in Exhibit 18-3 below).

EXHIBIT 18-3
Maximum Annual Inflation-Adjusted Dollar Amounts

Plan Type	2008	2009
Defined Benefit Plan	$185,000	$195,000
Defined Contribution Plan	46,000	49,000
Annual Compensation Limit	230,000	245,000
Cash or Deferred (401k)	15,500	16,500
Highly Compensated Employees	105,000	110,000
SIMPLE Contribution Limit	10,500	11,500

---

35 § 411(a)(2)(B).

36 Rev. Rul. 71-149, 1971-1 C.B. 118.

37 § 412.

38 §§ 415(a) and (b).

Example 10. S is a participant in Summa Inc.'s qualified profit sharing plan. If S's annual salary is $275,000, her employer can make a maximum annual contribution for 2009 on her behalf of $49,000 (the *lesser* of $49,000 or 100% of S's first $245,000 of compensation).

Example 11. If S's current salary is $35,000, the annual contribution is limited to $35,000 (the *lesser* of $49,000 or 100% of S's compensation).

Defined Benefit Plans. Under a defined benefit plan, the maximum annual benefit that can accrue to a participant is limited to the lesser of the following:[39]

1. $195,000 for 2009; or

2. 100 percent of the participant's average compensation for his or her three most highly compensated consecutive years of service with the employer.

Section 401(a)(17) was amended in 1993 to reduce the annual compensation limit to $150,000. Proposed regulations provide illustrations of how these new compensation limits affect *average compensation* for defined benefit plans.[40]

The limit is indexed annually for inflation, and adjustments to this figure are to be made if benefit payments are to begin before or after Social Security retirement age. Adjustments will be downward if payments begin before Social Security retirement age and upward if they begin after that age. The amount of the adjustment is determined actuarially based upon a straight-life annuity.[41] The current limitation is $195,000 for 2009.

TOP HEAVY PLANS

Section 416 contains additional requirements for qualified status of retirement plans that are deemed to be "top heavy." A *top heavy plan* is one in which more than 60 percent of the cumulative benefits provided by the plan are payable to *key employees*. Key employees include officers of the employer and highly compensated owner-employees. If a top heavy plan exists, § 416 provides an extra measure of assurance that the plan does not discriminate against non-key employees. To maintain qualified status a top heavy plan *must provide* a more rapid vesting schedule (generally 100% vesting after three years of service) and a minimum benefit to *all* employees regardless of social security or similar public retirement benefits.

DEDUCTIBILITY OF CONTRIBUTIONS BY EMPLOYER

Section 404(a) allows a deduction for employer contributions to qualified retirement plans if the contributions represent an ordinary and necessary business expense. In addition, § 404 contains complex rules that limit the dollar amount of the annual deduction. (Note that the statutory limitations on employer deductions are independent of the previously discussed limitations on the amount of contributions.) For example, the deduction for an employer's contribution to a qualified profit sharing plan is subject to a general limitation of 25 percent of total annual compensation paid to participating employees.[42] If an employer makes a contribution that exceeds this percentage limitation,

---

[39] § 415(b)(1)(A).

[40] Prop. Regs. § 1.401(a)(17)-1(b).

[41] § 415(b)(2)(B).

[42] § 404(a)(3).

the excess may be carried forward and deducted in succeeding years (subject to the percentage limitation for each succeeding year).[43]

DETERMINATION LETTERS

At this point, it should be obvious to the beginning tax student that the qualification rules for employer-sponsored plans are many and complex. As a result, employers are well advised to request a determination letter from the IRS before a plan is put into effect. Such determination letter is a *written approval* of the plan verifying that the plan, as described to the IRS, complies with all requirements for qualified status. If a plan treated by an employer as qualified is disqualified in an IRS audit, the employer could be liable for a considerable amount of unwithheld income and payroll taxes on employer contributions.

QUALIFIED PLANS FOR SELF-EMPLOYED INDIVIDUALS

Unincorporated taxpayers who earn money through self-employment are often precluded from retirement benefits afforded employees. To mitigate this result, Keogh (H.R. 10) plans were developed whereby contributions to such a plan are tax deductible, earnings accrue tax-free, and the self-employed individual is not taxed on any of the benefits until retirement. While Keogh plans provide substantial benefits, there are specific requirements that must be followed.

A self-employed individual who establishes an employer qualified retirement plan for his employees is not an employee eligible for participation in the plan. Self-employed individuals include sole proprietors and the partners in a business partnership. These taxpayers, however, may use the *Keogh* rules to obtain the tax benefits of a qualified plan.[44] A Keogh plan must benefit both the self-employed taxpayer and his or her employees in a nondiscriminatory manner under the wide range of rules for qualified plans previously discussed. In addition, the top heavy rules of § 416 apply to Keogh plans.[45]

To be eligible for a Keogh plan, the sole proprietor or partner must be an individual who satisfies one of the following conditions:[46]

1. Has "earned income" for the taxable year;

2. Would have had "earned income" for the year, but the trade or business being carried on had no net profits; or

3. Has been self-employed for any prior taxable year.

Generally, net earnings from self-employment will be the gross income from the trade or business less any related deductions; plus any distributive share of income or loss (if any) from a partnership. More specific definitions that are required for the tax computations are found in Exhibit 18-4.

---

43 *Ibid.*

44 See § 410(c)(1). It is interesting to note that retirement plans for self-employed individuals often are referred to as Keogh *or* H.R. 10 plans. Actually, the descriptions are interchangeable since H.R. 10 designated the legislative bill introduced by Congressman Keogh and passed by Congress in 1962.

45 § 416(i)(3).

46 § 415(c)(1)(B).

EXHIBIT 18-4
Special Definitions for KEOGH Plans

Earned Income	Self-employment income reduced by the self-employment tax deduction *and* the amount of the allowable Keogh deduction.
Net Earnings from Self-Employment	Earnings from self-employment without regard to the self-employment tax deduction or the allowable Keogh deduction.
Modified Net Earnings from Self-Employment	Net earnings from self-employment reduced by the self-employment tax deduction.
Self-Employment Tax Deduction	One-half of the self-employment taxes due for the year.

CONTRIBUTION LIMITATIONS

Annual contributions to Keogh plans are generally subject to the same limitations that apply to employer plans. For a defined contribution plan, the annual contribution by a self-employed taxpayer is limited to the lesser of $49,000 (2009) or 100 percent of *earned income*.[47] As seen in Exhibit 18-4, the definition of earned income includes the deduction for the allowable Keogh contribution, so the computation is a circular one.[48] The computation of the allowable contribution can best be expressed in the following formula:

$$\begin{array}{rl} & \text{Net Earnings from Self-Employment (NE)} \\ - & \underline{\text{Self-Employment Tax Deduction}} \\[1em] & \text{Modified Net Earnings from Self-Employment (MNE)} \\ - & \underline{\text{Allowable Contribution (AC)}} \\[1em] & \text{Earned Income (EI)} \\ \times & \underline{100\%} \\[1em] = & \underline{\text{Allowable Contribution (AC)}} \end{array}$$

The results of this formula can now be restated in the form of the equation found in Exhibit 18-5. Notice that the solution to this equation demonstrates that the actual limit on a self-employed taxpayer's annual contribution to a defined contribution Keogh plan is just 50 percent of *modified net earnings*. For individuals who have self-employment income but no liability for employment taxes (e.g., they have exceeded the maximum FICA through other employment), the allowable contribution will be 50 percent of their *net earnings* from self-employment not to exceed the dollar limit for the year.

---

[47] §§ 415(c)(1) and (3)(B).

[48] § 401(c)(2).

EXHIBIT 18-5
Circular Computation of Allowable KEOGH Contribution

$$AC = 1.00(EI) = 1.00(MNE - AC) = 1.00MNE - 1.00AC$$
or
$$2.00AC = MNE$$
thus
$$AC = [MNE/2.00 = .50MNE (50\% \text{ of MNE})]$$

Example 12. During the current year, Mr. T earned $75,924 and paid $7,848 in self-employment taxes. The maximum contribution T can make to his defined contribution plan is 100% of $72,000 [$75,924 − ($\frac{1}{2}$ of $7,848)] less the contribution itself. Therefore, the maximum contribution is $36,000 [100% of ($75,924 − $3,924 − $36,000)]. Note that this contribution is actually 50% of the modified net earnings of $72,000.

A different limitation applies to a Keogh plan if it is purely a discretionary profit sharing plan as opposed to the defined contribution plan discussed above. In this case, § 404(a)(3) limits the deductible contribution to only 15 percent of *modified net earnings* from self-employment. Once again, because the computation is a circular one, a calculation similar to Exhibit 18-5 would be necessary. While the computation is not illustrated, the results of such a determination indicate that the actual limit is 13.043 percent of *modified net earnings* (net earnings if no self-employment taxes are paid) from self-employment. For those self-employed individuals who desire to make a deductible contribution equal to the maximum, a defined contribution plan that combines a discretionary profit sharing plan with a money purchase plan that requires an annual contribution can be established.

QUALIFIED PLANS FOR EMPLOYEES

Since the establishment of employer-qualified plans as part of the Internal Revenue Code of 1954, Congress has expanded the scope of the law to provide similar plans for individual taxpayers who are not covered by an employer plan or who wish to supplement their employer plan.

CASH OR DEFERRED ARRANGEMENTS [§ 401(K) PLANS]

Cash or deferred arrangements (CODAs), also known as salary reduction plans or 401(k) plans, have attained enormous popularity because these plans offer all the tax advantages of a qualified retirement plan and allow employees to make tax excludable contributions to the plan from their own funds. Contributions made on behalf of the employee can come in the form of bonuses paid to the employee, additional salary, or an agreement by the employee to reduce his or her normal salary.[49]

One of the major benefits of a CODA is the flexibility it offers an employee. For example, a plan may be designed to allow an employee to defer up to 6 percent of his or her compensation. If the employee elects, he can defer 6 percent, or any smaller amount

---

[49] Regs. § 1.401(k)-1(a).

such as 1, 2, or 3 percent. This gives employees greater control of their taxable income in as much as they may choose annually how much they want in salary and how much they want to place in trust. In addition, loans from the trust are available to the plan participants.

The amount that an employee may elect to defer under a CODA many not exceed $15,000 for 2006 as shown in the table below.[50] While this figure is adjusted annually for inflation, it must be reduced by contributions to other retirement plans such as tax sheltered annuities and simplified employee plans. Any amounts in excess of this limit must be included in the individual's gross income. Furthermore, the limitations apply to the plan year and not to the calendar year of the individual. Thus, a CODA on a noncalendar year could theoretically allow an employee on a calendar year to defer up to $27,000 ($14,000 + $13,000), for example, in a single year.

Section 401(k) Plan Contributions Limitations

Year	Amount
2001	$10,500
2002	11,000
2003	12,000
2004	13,000
2005	14,000
2006	15,000
2007 and 2008	15,500
2009	16,500

Employer Contributions. One of the major benefits of a CODA to an employer is that it provides a low-cost method of financing retirement benefits to the employee. Thus, amounts that would have been paid in salaries or wages can now be directed toward the retirement plan. The offsetting administrative expenses of initiating and operating the plan should be relatively low so that they do not detract from its overall benefits. When establishing a CODA, contributions made to the trust should be treated as employer contributions as opposed to employee contributions. This is necessary to ensure the exclusion from income that is available only to contributions made by the employer.[51]

> **Example 13.** An employee's election form to fund a CODA should not state that she elects to contribute $5,000 of her salary to a CODA. Instead, the election should request that the employer reduce her salary by $5,000 in exchange for the employer's agreement to fund a CODA by the amount of $5,000.

An employer is entitled to take a deduction for a contribution to a CODA of up to 25 percent of an employee's compensation. This 25 percent limit is reduced by the employee's active contribution. Compensation for this purpose is net compensation after considering the employee's contribution.

> **Example 14.** E, an employee of Z Corporation, desires to make an elective contribution of $8,000 to a qualified CODA. If E's compensation for the year is $110,000, the available contribution that Z Corporation can make for the year is determined as follows:

---

[50] § 402(g)(5).

[51] § 414(h)(1).

Compensation	$110,000
Less: E's contribution	(8,000)
Net Compensation	$102,000
Employer limit	× 25%
Maximum Contribution	$ 25,500
Less: E's contribution	(8,000)
Available Contribution.	$ 17,500

Catch-up Adjustment for Individuals Over Age 50. Beginning in 2002, taxpayers who are over the age of 50 are permitted to make additional elective deferrals in excess of the otherwise permissible limits in order to compensate for the increased limits. These additional amounts can be contributed to § 401(k) plans, § 403(b) plans, SEPs, and SIMPLE plans. These additional deferrals may be made without regard to the qualification requirements or limitations that usually apply to these provisions. The amount of the catch-up adjustments (by year) are illustrated in the table below:

Year	§ 401(k)	§ 403(b)	SEPs	SIMPLE	IRAs
2008	5,000	5,000	5,000	2,500	1,000
2009	5,500	5,500	5,500	2,500	1,000

Plan Requirements. In order to secure the benefits of a CODA, specific requirements must be satisfied. While a detailed explanation is beyond the scope of this coverage, a synopsis of these rules summarizes their features.[52]

1. A CODA must meet the qualification requirements of a profit sharing or stock bonus plan including its participation and coverage requirements.

2. A CODA must provide for an election by each eligible participant to have their employer make payments to a qualified trust or directly to them in cash.

3. Amounts held under a qualified CODA are restricted as to when the funds may be distributed to the employee, and the employee's right to those benefits must be nonforfeitable.

4. Under complicated rules, amounts available for tax deferral may not discriminate in favor of highly compensated employees.[53]

Roth 401(k) Plans. Beginning in 2006, taxpayers may create a Roth 401(k), 403(b) or similar plans. Amounts contributed to such plans (i.e., salary reductions), like those to Roth IRAs, would not be deferred but would be reported on a participant's Form W-2. For most purposes, these Roth 401(k) plans are identical to Roth IRAs with certain limited

---

[52]   § 401(k)(2) and (3).

[53]   Regs. § 1.401(k)-1(a)(4)(iv).

differences. For example distributions for first-time home-buyers before age $59\frac{1}{2}$ are not permitted tax-free. In addition, there is no income limitation imposed on a Roth 401(k). Taxpayers may establish Roth 401(k) plans regardless of their adjusted gross income.

INDIVIDUAL RETIREMENT ACCOUNTS

Prior to 1974, the benefits of qualified retirement plans were generally limited to employees of companies that opted to incur the expense of establishing plans. In 1974, however, Congress decided to provide an incentive for retirement savings in situations where there was no employer-provided plan and created the Individual Retirement Account (IRA). Since their creation, IRAs have been immensely popular.

The basic operation of a conventional IRA then and now mirrors that for employer-provided plans. Under the IRA provisions, an individual is generally entitled to make an annual tax-deductible contribution to the IRA. The contribution is a deduction for A.G.I., making it available to those who do not itemize deductions as well as those who do. Contributions are then invested and the income earned on such investments is not taxable currently. However, when amounts are withdrawn from the IRA they are fully taxable (both the earnings and the amounts representing the contributions). From an investment perspective, the tremendous advantages of the IRA relative to a traditional savings arrangement are the same as discussed earlier for employer-provided retirement plans. As explained above, the benefits of an IRA can be traced to two key factors: (1) the amounts invested are before-tax, providing a greater initial investment and (2) the tax is deferred until the amounts are withdrawn, resulting in greater earnings over the life of the investment.

The popularity of the IRA and the need to stimulate savings for retirement has caused Congress to expand the IRA concept over the years. Currently, there are three types of savings arrangements that bear the IRA name. They are:

1. The traditional or conventional IRA (discussed above).

2. The Roth IRA

3. The Educational IRA

Unfortunately, even though each of these savings vehicles is called an IRA, their treatment can be quite different.

TRADITIONAL IRA

The traditional IRA is currently the most common type of IRA since they have been in existence since 1974. Individuals are permitted to make three types of contributions to a traditional IRA.

1. Deductible contributions

2. Nondeductible contributions

3. Rollover contributions (i.e., contributions of amounts withdrawn from other qualified retirement plans)

Deductible Contributions to a Traditional IRA. As a general rule, an individual who is not covered by an employer-sponsored retirement plan can deduct contributions to a traditional IRA of up to $5,000 per year (in 2008 and 2009). The contribution limit increases as illustrated in the table below. However, the deduction cannot exceed the

taxpayer's compensation for the year.[54] In addition, taxpayers over $70\frac{1}{2}$ cannot make contributions to a traditional IRA.

Increase in IRA Contribution Limit

Year	Amount
2002–2004	$3,000
2005–2007	4,000
2008 and thereafter	5,000

Similar to the § 401(k) rules discussed earlier, individuals age 50 and over are permitted to make additional annual IRA contributions in the following amounts:

- $500 for years 2002–2005 and
- $1,000 for 2006 and thereafter.

Example 15. H and W are married with two kids, Z and K. H's mom, M, also lives with the family. This year, Z, 14, received $500 of interest income from a savings account and earned $1,500 from sacking groceries at the local supermarket. K, 17, earned $5,000 delivering pizzas. M, age 75, earned $7,000 from a part-time job at a fast-food restaurant and had $40,000 of interest and dividends. Since Z's earned income is only $1,500, the maximum amount that he can deduct for contributions to an IRA is limited to $1,500 (his compensation). In contrast, K is able to contribute and deduct the maximum amount of $5,000 (2009) since she has compensation of at least $5,000. On the other hand, M cannot make contributions to an IRA since she is more than $70\frac{1}{2}$ years old.

Example 16. Assume the same facts as *Example 15* except that M is 55 years old. In this case, her contribution to an IRA is limited to $6,000 for 2009. This includes the $5,000 that was available because of her compensation, as well as the $1000 additional *catch-up adjustment* due to her age.

Deduction Phase-out Rules for Plan Participants. If a taxpayer or his or her spouse is an active participant in an employer-sponsored retirement plan *and* has A.G.I. in excess of a specified *applicable dollar amount*, the maximum deductible amount is phased out.[55] The applicable dollar amounts differ depending on which of following four categories the taxpayer is in:

1. Files jointly and is an active participant in an employer-sponsored plan.

2. Files jointly, is not active in another employer-sponsored plan but has a spouse that is active in an employer-sponsored plan.

3. Files married filing separately and is active in an employer-sponsored plan.

4. Files as a single or head of household taxpayer and is active in another employer-sponsored plan.

The applicable dollar amounts at which the phase-out begins and the IRA deduction ends are shown for each group in Exhibit 18-6. Note that the applicable dollar amounts increase over the next several years (except in the latter two cases). Also observe that if

---

54 § 219(b)(l).

55 § 219(g) and (g)(3)(B).

A.G.I. exceeds the applicable dollar amount by more than $10,000, none of the contribution is deductible. For excess A.G.I. amounts between $0 and $10,000, the phase-out is proportional. For example, if the excess A.G.I. is $4,000, the taxpayer loses 40 percent of the $5,000 deduction or $2,000. The amount of the phase-out can be computed using the following formula:

$$\frac{\text{A.G.I.} - \text{Applicable Dollar Amount}}{\$10,000} \times \text{IRA Deduction} = \text{Reduction in Dedcutible Allowance}$$

EXHIBIT 18-6
Applicable Dollar Amount Phase-out Ranges

	Married Joint Active Participant Phase-out	Single or Head of Household Active Participant Phase-out	Married Inactive but Active Spouse Phase-out	Married Separate Active Participant Phase-out
2009	$89,000–$109,000	$55,000–$65,000	$166,000–$176,000	$0–$10,000
2008	$85,000–$105,000	$53,000–$63,000	$159,000–$169,000	$0–$10,000

Example 17. Q, a single taxpayer, is a salesperson for C Corporation. She actively participates in her employer's qualified retirement plan. In 2008, her compensation and A.G.I. were $28,000. Even though she participates in her employer's plan, her maximum deductible contribution is $4,000 since her A.G.I. does not exceed the applicable dollar amount of $53,000. In 2009, her compensation and A.G.I. were $59,000. Since she participates in an employer plan and her A.G.I. exceeds the applicable dollar amount of $55,000, the amount that she can deduct is subject to the phase-out rules. Her maximum deductible IRA contribution for 2009 is $3,000 [$5,000 (2009 amount) − $2,000 as calculated below].

$$\frac{\$59,000 \text{ A.G.I.} - \$55,000 \text{ Applicable Dollar Amount}}{\$10,000} = 40\% \times \$5,000 (2009 \text{ amount})$$
$$= \text{Reduction in Deductible Allowance in the amount of } \$2,000$$

Example 18. T, a single taxpayer, is an accountant for a small corporation. He received compensation of $70,000 in 2009. T's employer does not maintain a retirement plan. Since T is not an active participant in a qualified plan, he is not subject to the phase-out rules and can deduct contributions to a traditional IRA of up to $5,000.

Special Rules for Married Couples. Traditional IRAs provide a special rule for married couples where one spouse is the major breadwinner. Each spouse may make a deductible IRA contribution of up to $5,000 (2009) provided the couple's combined compensation exceeds the amount of the contributions. In effect, this allows a married couple to contribute up to $10,000 even though only one spouse works (assuming the working spouse has A.G.I. of at least $10,000).

Example 19. H and W are married. H had compensation income of $22,000 while W had no compensation and stayed at home taking care of the family's children. Although W had no compensation for the year, she may make a deductible IRA contribution of $5,000 to her own account in addition to H's contribution to his account since their combined compensation of $22,000 exceeded their total contributions for the year of $10,000.

As noted above, if one spouse is an active participant in an employer-provided plan but the other spouse is not, the nonworking spouse may still contribute to a traditional deductible IRA but the nonworking spouse's contribution is subject to phase-out if the couple's A.G.I. exceeds $166,000 in 2009. The active participant's phase-out begins at $89,000 for 2009.

Example 20. H and W are married. W is covered by a qualified plan sponsored by her employer. H is not employed. The couple files a joint return for 2009 reporting A.G.I. of $135,000. Even though H is married to an active participant in a qualified plan, he may make a deductible IRA contribution of $5,000 since the applicable dollar amount for the spouse of an active participant begins at $166,000. On the other hand, W may not make a deductible IRA contribution since the couple's adjusted gross income exceeds the $89,000 applicable dollar amount for married plan participants in 2009 by more than $10,000.

Example 21. Assume the same facts as the *Example 20* above except that the couple's A.G.I. is $195,000. In this case, neither spouse could make a deductible contribution because their A.G.I. exceeds the applicable dollar amounts ($166,000 and $89,000) by more than $10,000 for each spouse.

Nondeductible IRA Contributions to a Traditional IRA. Individuals are permitted to make *nondeductible* contribution to their IRAs. These contributions can be made only to the extent that the maximum deduction for IRA contributions is not claimed (i.e., $5,000 or 100 percent of compensation).[56] Note that there is no phase-out or compensation income limitation that applies to nondeductible contributions.

Example 22. G, single, had compensation and A.G.I. for 2009 of $64,000. G is covered by his employer's qualified plan. Since G's A.G.I. exceeds the threshold by $9,000 ($64,000 − $55,000) his maximum deductible contribution is $500 [$5,000 − (90% × $5,000)]. However, he is still permitted to make nondeductible contributions of $4,500 ($5,000 − 500).

Excess Contributions. Since the earnings generated by contributions into an IRA are tax deferred, taxpayers might be tempted to contribute amounts in excess of the contribution limit. To prohibit this possibility, a 6 percent penalty tax is imposed on any excess contribution left in an IRA after the close of the taxable year.

Rollover Contributions. As alluded to earlier, one reason for establishing an IRA is for the purpose of *rolling over* a lump-sum distribution from a qualified retirement plan. In addition, individuals who receive distributions from an IRA may also make rollovers of distributions into another IRA. By rolling over a distribution to an IRA, the taxpayer avoids taxation as well as any early withdrawal penalty.

Rollovers generally take one of two forms: (1) the distribution is paid to the plan participant who then must roll the distribution into an IRA within 60 days; or (2) the

---

[56]   § 408(o).

distribution is paid directly to the IRA. Failure to transfer the funds to an IRA within the 60-day period makes the distribution taxable and also subject to the early withdrawal penalty. Note that by having the distribution paid directly to the IRA, the participant avoids the provision that requires the employer to withhold 20 percent of the distribution as an estimated tax payment. It should also be noted that taxpayers who choose to roll over a lump-sum distribution forego the right to use any beneficial capital gain or forward averaging rules for computing the tax on the distribution when it is ultimately withdrawn from the IRA.

Withdrawals from a Traditional IRA. Income earned in an IRA is tax-exempt, regardless of the deductibility of the contributions to the IRA.[57] When funds are withdrawn from an IRA, an amount of the withdrawal proportionate to any unrecovered nondeductible contributions in the account is not subject to tax; the balance of the withdrawal is fully includible in gross income.[58]

> **Example 23.** In the current year, taxpayer A, age 61, withdrew $9,000 from his IRA, after which the account balance was $26,000. A has made $1,500 of unrecovered nondeductible contributions to the IRA. The nontaxable portion of the withdrawal is $386, computed as follows:
>
> $$\frac{\underset{\text{(nondeductible contributions)}}{\$1,500}}{\underset{\text{(account balance before withdrawal)}}{\$26,000 + \$9,000}} \times \$9,000 \text{ withdrawal} = \$386$$
>
> For subsequent years, A's unrecovered nondeductible contribution balance is $1,114 ($1,500 − $386).

Distribution Requirements. Without special rules, IRA owners might postpone distributions for as long as possible hoping to take advantage of tax deferral to build their estate. However, the law requires taxpayers to take the entire IRA balance or start taking periodic distributions from their IRAs no later than April 1 of the year following the year in which the taxpayer reaches age $70\frac{1}{2}$. The minimum distribution is generally based on either the life expectancy of the taxpayer or the joint life expectancies of the taxpayer and his or her spouse or another designated beneficiary. The actual calculation of required distribution is somewhat complex and beyond the scope of this text. However, it is important to note that if the distributions received are less than the required distribution amount, a penalty equal to 50 percent of the shortage may apply. Special rules apply to IRAs that are inherited. Note that Roth IRAs are not subject to these distribution requirements.

The 2008 Recovery Act provides a one year suspension of the minimum distribution rules for 2009. Thus, no minimum distribution is required for calendar year 2009 from:

1. Defined contribution plans, as described in §§ 401(a), 403(a), or 403(b);

2. Eligible deferred compensation plans under § 457(b) which are maintained by a state, a political subdivision of a state, or any state agency; and

3. Individual retirement plans. The next required minimum distribution will be for calendar year 2010.

---

[57] § 408(c).

[58] § 408(d).

ROTH IRAS

The 1997 Tax Act created a nondeductible IRA called the Roth IRA. Under this plan honoring Senator Roth of Delaware, individuals may make nondeductible contributions of up to $5,000 annually. However, the $5,000 maximum contribution limit is reduced to the extent of any contributions to another IRA in the same taxable year. In addition, the maximum annual contribution that can be made to a Roth IRA is phased out for single individuals with A.G.I. between $105,000 and $120,000 and for joint filers with A.G.I. between $166,000 and $176,000. The increase in contribution limits for the Roth IRA closely follows the traditional IRA over the next several years.

A Roth IRA is an IRA which is designated at the time of establishment as a Roth IRA. The major benefits of a Roth IRA are that distributions from a Roth IRA are generally not taxable, and unlike a deductible or nondeductible IRA, contributions to a Roth IRA may be made even after the individual for whom the account is established reaches the age of $70\frac{1}{2}$.

Technically, only qualified distributions are nontaxable. A qualified distribution is any distribution that:

- Is made after the taxable five-year period beginning with the first taxable year in which the individual made a contribution to a Roth IRA and

- Meets *one* of the following conditions:

    1. Is made on or after the date on which the individual attains age $59\frac{1}{2}$

    2. Is made to a beneficiary (or to the individual's estate) on or after the death of the individual

    3. Is attributable to the individual being disabled

    4. Is a distribution for first-time homebuyer expenses (see earlier discussion)

    5. Is used for certain education expenses

Distributions from a Roth IRA that are *not* qualified distributions are includible in income to the extent they are not attributable to contributions. In addition, these distributions are subject to the 10 percent early withdrawal tax that also applies to other IRAs. An ordering rule applies for purposes of determining what portion of a distribution is not a qualified distribution and is includible in income. Under the ordering rule, distributions from a Roth IRA are treated as made from contributions *first*. For purposes of determining the amount of contributions, all of an individual's Roth IRAs are treated as a single Roth IRA. Thus, no portion of a distribution from a Roth IRA is treated as attributable to earnings until the total of all distributions from a Roth IRA exceeds the sum of all contributions as well as rollover contributions. In effect, a taxpayer can make withdrawals of previous *contributions* without penalty or tax at any time—even within the mandatory five-year holding period.

> **Example 24.** L first opened a Roth IRA at his bank on November 1, 2007, making a contribution of $4,000. He continued to make $5,000 contributions in 2008, 2009, 2010, and 2011. On May 1, 2011, L celebrated his 65th birthday, retired and took a distribution of $11,000 from his Roth IRA to take a trip to Europe. Under the ordering rule, the $11,000 withdrawal represents his contributions in 2007 ($4,000), 2008 ($5,000), and 2009 ($2,000) and, therefore, is neither taxable nor subject to the 10 percent penalty that otherwise applies to distributions during the five-year holding

period. Note that he can begin withdrawing distributions in excess of previous contributions (without penalty) once the five-year holding period requirement is met in 2012. Observe that the five-year holding period begins in 2007, the first taxable year that L contributed to the Roth IRA.

Conversion of Traditional IRA to Roth IRA. The lure of tax-free earnings and tax-free distributions forever is so strong that individuals who have traditional IRAs may want to convert them to Roth IRAs. Graciously, Congress has blessed such conversions. The law permits individuals to convert traditional IRAs to Roth IRAs if certain requirements are met.

Generally, individuals, other than those who are married and file separately, are entitled to convert their traditional IRAs if their modified adjusted gross income (MAGI), exclusive of the sum being converted, is $100,000 or less. Technically, the conversion is accomplished by transferring the assets from a traditional IRA and reinvesting them (within 60 days) in a Roth IRA. This is normally referred to as a "conversion contribution." There is no minimum or maximum amount that must be converted. Most importantly, on conversion any previously untaxed amounts in the traditional IRA are taxable as ordinary income. The 10% penalty for withdrawal before age $59\frac{1}{2}$ does not apply. After conversion, the taxpayer's A.G.I. includes the taxable portion of the conversion for all purposes (e.g., exemption phase-out, 2% floor on miscellaneous itemized deductions, 7.5% floor on medical expenses). The conversion must be completed by December 31 of the year in question.

> **Example 25.** C, single, age 48, has an A.G.I of $70,000 for 2009. As of May 1, he had accumulated $200,000 in his traditional IRA that he is wants to convert. C's A.G.I. for conversion purposes is $70,000, the amount of his A.G.I. before considering any taxable income resulting from the conversion. The amounts in the IRA represent deductible contributions, nontaxable earnings and funds from a prior rollover from his 401(k) plan. Assuming C converts the traditional IRA, he will have taxable income of $70,000. There is no penalty for early withdrawal.

Beginning in 2010, the A.G.I. limitation is eliminated. In 2010, any amount that is taxable as a result of the conversion is spread equally and reported in the following two years, 2011 and 2012. Also beginning in 2010, married taxpayers filing separately may convert amounts from a traditional IRA to a Roth IRA.

CREDIT FOR CONTRIBUTIONS TO PLANS BY LOW-INCOME INDIVIDUALS

To encourage low and middle-income taxpayers to save for their retirement, the 2001 Tax Act created a nonrefundable credit for contributions to certain retirement saving plans (§ 25B). Credits are available for contributions to § 401(k) plans, § 403(b) plans, § 457 state and local government plans, SIMPLE plans, SEP plans, traditional IRAs, and Roth IRAs. The credit is in addition to the deduction to which the taxpayer is normally entitled. The amount of the credit is generally equal to 50 percent of the individual's retirement savings contributions not to exceed $2,000. Thus the maximum credit is $1,000 (50% × $2,000). On a joint return, the maximum credit would be $2,000, however, the credit decreases as the taxpayer's income increases. The allowable credit percentage is a function of the taxpayer's modified adjusted gross as follows:

MODIFIED ADJUSTED GROSS INCOME CREDIT DETERMINATION (2009)

Joint Return		Head of Household		All Others		
Over	Not Over	Over	Not Over	Over	Not Over	Percentage
$ 0	$33,000	$ 0	$24,750	$ 0	$16,500	50%
33,000	36,000	24,750	27,000	16,500	18,000	20%
36,000	55,500	27,000	41,625	18,000	27,750	10%
55,500		41,625		27,750		0%

The credit is *not* available to the following individuals:

1. Individuals who have not attained the age of 18 by the close of the tax year;

2. Individuals for whom a dependency exemption my be claimed; and

3. Full-time students.

Example 26. T, single, graduated from college last year and took a job with a national accounting firm. His adjusted gross income for the year was $24,000. If T contributes $5,000 to a Roth IRA, he may claim a credit of $200 for 2009 (10% credit percentage × $2,000 ceiling amount). Had T been a full-time college student for the year, he would not have been eligible for the credit.

EDUCATION IRAS (COVERDELL EDUCATION SAVINGS ACCOUNTS)

In an effort to encourage savings and provide a vehicle to promote higher education, the Tax Reform Act of 1997 created a special type of IRA known as an education IRA or Coverdell Education Savings Account (CESA).[59] Although the creation of such an account has nothing to do with retirement planning, as the name might suggest, the tax treatment of this arrangement is very similar to that for nondeductible contributions to traditional or Roth IRAs—thus its classification as an IRA.

Currently, taxpayers may make *nondeductible* contributions of up to $2,000 in cash per year into a CESA for certain qualified beneficiaries. A CESA is a trust account that is created for the purpose of paying *qualifying higher education* expenses. A qualified beneficiary is any individual under the age of 18 years, or any special needs child regardless of age. Qualifying higher education expenses include tuition, fees, books, supplies and equipment required for enrollment that are incurred during the taxable year for a student who attends an eligible education institution. The term also includes amounts contributed to a prepaid tuition plan. In certain circumstances, *room and board* are also included in these expenses. An eligible educational institution means any post-secondary education courses (e.g., undergraduate or graduate courses) as well as the cost of elementary, secondary, private and parochial schools.

Similar to retirement IRAs, earnings on the amounts contributed to a CESA are not taxed as they accumulate. Withdrawals from a CESA are totally nontaxable to the extent that they are used exclusively for the purpose of paying qualifying higher education expenses. Furthermore, no contribution may be made during a taxable year in which a contribution is made by *anyone* to a qualified prepaid tuition program on behalf of the same beneficiary. Note also that for any year in which an exclusion from gross income is claimed with respect to distribution from an education IRA, neither a Hope credit nor a Lifetime Learning credit may be claimed with respect to education expenses incurred during that year on behalf of the same beneficiary.

---

[59]   § 530.

Contribution Limit. The $2,000 annual contribution limit, computed at the donor level, is phased out ratably for contributors with A.G.I. (computed with certain modifications) between $95,000 and $110,000 ($190,000 and $220,000 for contributors filing joint returns). The term "Modified A.G.I." means A.G.I. increased by income earned outside the U.S. that normally is excluded under § 911. Individuals with modified A.G.I. greater than the upper phase-out range are not allowed to make contributions to an education IRA established on behalf of any other individual.

EXHIBIT 18-7
Phase-out for CESAs

$$\frac{\text{Reduction of the}}{\$2,000 \text{ Contribution}} = \$2,000 \text{ Contribution} \times \frac{\text{Modified A.G.I.} - \text{threshold}}{\text{Income Range}}$$

	Modified A.G.I. Phase-out begins	Modified A.G.I. Phase-out complete
Married filing jointly:	$190,000	$220,000
Other taxpayers:	$ 95,000	$110,000

Multiple CESAs for a Single Beneficiary. Taxpayers contributing more than $2,000 per year to an a CESA for a single beneficiary are subject to a penalty. Section 4973 imposes a six percent excise tax on excess contributions. An excess contribution consists of two parts:

1. The amount by which contributions to all CESAs for a single beneficiary exceed $2,000, plus

2. The amount contributed during the year to a qualified tuition plan.

Note that this rule prohibits a taxpayer from contributing to both a qualified tuition plan and a CESA without penalty. These rules do not appear to prohibit parents from contributing $2,000 to a CESA for one child while the grandparents contribute to a prepaid tuition plan. Moreover, there is no rule requiring that the person contributing be related to the beneficiary. Similarly, there is no restriction on the number of CESAs an individual may establish as long as each has a different beneficiary.

Distributions. Distributions from a CESA that are used to pay qualifying education expenses are generally nontaxable. In reality, this general rule is a bit more complex. Technically, distributions from a CESA are deemed to consist of a proportionate part of both the original contributions and the earnings on such contributions. Distributions representing contributions are always nontaxable. Distributions of earnings are excludable from gross income only to the extent that the distribution does not exceed qualified higher education expenses incurred by the beneficiary during the year the distribution is made. In effect, all of the earnings on a CESA are nontaxable as long as they are used for qualified education expenses. Distributions of earnings in excess of qualified expenses cause a ratable portion of the entire distribution to be taxable. In addition, an excise tax of 10 percent is imposed on the portion not used for education.

Rollovers. If any balance remains in a CESA at the time a beneficiary becomes 30 years old, such amount *must* be distributed, and the amount representing the account's earnings will be taxable. In addition, the distribution will be subject to a 10 percent penalty tax because the distribution was not for educational purposes. Prior to the time the beneficiary reaches 30, the 1997 Act allows tax-free (and penalty-free) transfers and

rollovers of account balances from one CESA benefiting one beneficiary to another education IRA benefiting a different beneficiary (as well as redesignations of the named beneficiary), provided that the new beneficiary is a member of the family of the old beneficiary. For this purpose, a family member includes the beneficiary's spouse or a familial relative described in the rules governing dependency exemptions. These would include a child, sibling, parent and certain other individuals. For example, if the taxpayer's son did not fully utilize the amount in the CESA, the unused balance could be converted to an account for his daughter or his grandchild.

Gift and Estate Tax Treatment. Contributions made to CESAs are considered completed gifts and qualify for the annual exclusion. Distributions are not treated as gifts nor is a rollover to another beneficiary and, therefore, not subject to gift tax. Amounts in a CESA are not includible in the estate of any individual. If a beneficiary dies and the interest passes to a spouse, the spouse simply becomes the beneficiary of the CESA. If the interest passes to someone other than a spouse, the CESA terminates at death and the account balance is includible in the beneficiary's income (e.g., a child).

SIMPLIFIED EMPLOYEE PENSIONS

The concept of a Simplified Employee Pension (SEP) was added to the law in 1978 to provide employers with a way to avoid the fearsome complexities involved in establishing and maintaining a qualified retirement plan. By following the relatively simple rules of § 408(k), which are designed to prevent discrimination in favor of the prohibited group, an employer may establish a SEP. This qualified plan allows the employer to make contributions directly into an employee's existing IRA, thereby avoiding the necessity of a qualified trust.

The annual limit on SEP contributions is the lesser of 25 percent of employee compensation (subject to compensation limits) or $49,000 (2009). Employer contributions to a SEP are excludable from an employee's gross income.[60]

RETIREMENT PLANNING USING NONQUALIFIED DEFERRED COMPENSATION

For many years employers have designed total compensation packages for valued employees that combined both a current compensation element and a *deferred* compensation element. A *nonqualified* deferred compensation arrangement typically is one in which the employee is compensated for current services rendered by the employer's promise to pay a certain amount at some future date. Although nonqualified deferred compensation plans do not receive the favorable tax treatment given to qualified plans, such arrangements are often attractive to employers because of their flexibility. Many employers find that what may be lost in tax benefits is more than made up in the savings derived from not having to comply with restrictive rules concerning the discrimination, participation, vesting, and funding that apply to qualified plans. The two questions that must be answered about a deferred compensation arrangement are:

1. When is the employee taxed on deferred compensation that is earned currently but will be received in a later year?

2. When is the employer entitled to a business deduction for deferred compensation that will be paid in a later year?

---

[60]   § 402(h).

Note that if a plan is a qualified plan, an employer is entitled to a current deduction for contributions and the employee is taxed on such contributions only when they are distributed. For nonqualified plans, however, the timing of the deduction and income is not quite as clear.

In order to completely answer the first question, an examination of the constructive receipt doctrine is necessary. To thoroughly answer the second, an examination of funded and unfunded plans is required.

CONSTRUCTIVE RECEIPT

The Regulations state that income (both current and deferred) is to be included in gross income for the taxable year in which it is actually or constructively received by the taxpayer.[61] Thus for a cash basis taxpayer, all items that constitute gross income (whether in the form of cash, property, or services) are to be included for the taxable year in which they are actually or constructively received. Consequently, the question to be resolved is whether deferred compensation is constructively received in the taxable year when it is authorized or in the year of actual receipt.

A mere promise to pay, not represented by notes or secured in any way, is not regarded as a receipt of income under the cash receipts and disbursements method. This should not be construed to mean that under the cash receipts and disbursements method income may be taxed only when realized in cash. Income, although not actually received, is constructively received by an individual in the taxable year during which it is credited to his account or set aside for him so that he may draw upon it at a later date.[62] Thus, under the doctrine of constructive receipt, a taxpayer may not deliberately turn his back upon income, nor may a taxpayer, by a private agreement, postpone receipt of income from one year to another.

Income is not constructively received if the taxpayer's control of its receipt is subject to substantial limitations or restrictions. Consequently, if a corporation credits its employees with bonus stock, but the stock is not available to those employees until some future date, the mere crediting on the books of the corporation does not constitute constructive receipt. In most cases, speculating whether an employer would have been willing to relinquish a payment earlier or determining a taxpayer's control over funds is not an easy task. As a result, in each case involving a deferral of compensation (especially nonqualified plans), the determination of whether the constructive receipt doctrine is applicable must be made on a fact-and-circumstances basis.

> **Example 27.** T, a football player, entered into a two-year contract to play football for the California Cauliflowers. In addition to his salary, as an inducement for signing the contract, T would be paid a signing bonus of $150,000. Although T could have demanded and received his bonus at the time of signing the contract, T's attorneys suggested that the $150,000 be transferred to an escrow agent to be held for five years and then paid to T over the next five years as an annuity. If T should die, the escrow account would become part of his estate. Because the bonus is set aside for T, the $150,000 bonus must be included in T's gross income in the year in which the club unconditionally paid the amount to the escrow agent. The employer's obligation for payment terminated when the amount of the bonus was fixed at $150,000 and irrevocably set aside for T's sole benefit.[63]

---

61   Regs. § 1.451-1(a).

62   Regs. § 1.451-2(a).

63   Rev. Rul. 55-527, 1955-2 C.B. 25.

TREATMENT OF NONQUALIFIED DEFERRED COMPENSATION PLANS

Persuaded by corporate scandals at companies such as Enron, the *American Jobs Creation Act of 2004* imposes new restrictions and limitations on the design of nonqualified deferred compensation plans.[64] Under the new law, in order for deferred compensation to be excluded from gross income, the deferred compensation plan must meet specific guidelines. These guidelines include: (1) a distribution requirement, (2) an acceleration of benefits requirement, and (3) certain election requirements.

Restrictions on Distributions. Under Code § 409A(a)(2)(A), a nonqualified deferred compensation plan may not permit distributions from the plan earlier than:

- The participant's separation from service, as determined by the IRS, subject to a special rule for separation from service of any "specified employee";
- The date the participant becomes "disabled";
- The participant's death;
- A time specified, or a schedule fixed, under the plan at the date of the deferral of the compensation;
- To the extent allowed by the IRS, a change in the ownership or effective control of the corporation, or in the ownership of a substantial portion of the corporation's assets; or
- The occurrence of an "unforeseeable emergency" as defined in §409A(a)(2)(B)(ii).

Additionally, specified employees (referred to as "key employees") of publicly traded corporations generally may not receive their distributions earlier than six months after separation. A key employee is defined as an officer with compensation greater than $150,000 in 2008 (adjusted for inflation and limited to 50 employees); 5 percent owners; and 1 percent owners with compensation greater than $170,000. Furthermore, taking a distribution with a "haircut" (i.e., forfeiture of a portion of the account balance in exchange for access to the plan account) is no longer a distribution option.

Acceleration of Benefits. Section 409A does not permit a plan to allow for the acceleration of benefits. However, under the anticipated IRS regulations, a nonqualified deferred compensation plan would not violate the prohibition on accelerations in certain limited situations. For example, a plan could provide that upon separation from service of a participant, account balances less than $10,000 will be automatically distributed (except in the case of specified key employees).

Election Requirements. Under the new law, the flexibility of a participant to change his or her deferral elections generally must be made in the tax year preceding the year in which the services are performed, or within 30 days of becoming eligible for plan partici-pation. If the award is performance-based (e.g., an incentive bonus), the election must be made no later than six months before the end of the performance period.

In addition to the above rules, a deferred compensation plan may not provide that the deterioration in the financial status of the employer will trigger payment of the deferred compensation. Offshore Rabbi trusts and Rabbi trusts that are convertible into Secular trusts (protecting the assets from general creditors) are also prohibited under the new law.

Effective Date of New Rules. The new rules generally apply to amounts deferred after December 31, 2004. If a plan fails to meet the requirements, or is not operated in accordance with any of these three requirements, all compensation earned and deferred

---

[64] § 409A.

must be included in income for the first tax year that the nonqualified deferred compensation plan fails to meet the requirements, to the extent not subject to a "substantial risk of forfeiture" and not previously included in gross income.[65] A 20 percent penalty will also be imposed on the amount required to be included in income. Interest will also be assessed on the underpayment, at the underpayment rate plus one percentage point. Any compensation that becomes taxable will be subject to income tax withholding.

UNFUNDED DEFERRED COMPENSATION PLANS

If an employer contractually promises to pay deferred compensation to an employee and does not set aside current funds in some type of trust arrangement, the employee is put in the position of an unsecured creditor of the employer. If the employee is a cash basis taxpayer and does not have any current right to payment under the deferred compensation plan, there is no constructive receipt of the compensation and thus no current taxable income to the employee. The employee will not be taxed until the year in which the deferred compensation is actually paid.[66]

From the employer's point of view, such unfunded arrangements are attractive because they do not require any current cash outflow from the business. However, neither a cash basis nor an accrual basis employer may take a deduction for deferred compensation until the deferred amount is includible in the employee's gross income.[67]

FUNDED DEFERRED COMPENSATION PLANS

Employees who agree to a nonqualified deferred compensation arrangement normally prefer that their employers secure the promise of future compensation by transferring current funds into an independent trust for the employee's benefit. While these employees desire the protection of a funded plan, they do not wish to subject those funds to current taxation. Therefore, innovative methods have been devised to allow deferral of an employee's income under a funded method by making the employee's interest in those funds forfeitable. To this end, an employer can establish one of many types of trusts. Two of the more common nonqualified arrangements are the *Rabbi trust* and the *Secular trust*. The rules of § 83, discussed earlier in the chapter, apply to these funded deferred compensation plans.[68]

Rabbi Trusts. Rabbi trusts are so named because the first IRS ruling that approved this arrangement involved a fund established by a congregation for its rabbi. In the typical Rabbi trust arrangement, the rights of employees are forfeitable, so an employee will not recognize taxable income until he or she actually receives a distribution from the trust. If a deferred compensation arrangement provides that employees' rights in the retirement fund eventually become nonforfeitable (i.e., vested), an employee must recognize taxable income in the year his or her rights vest. In both cases, the employer will receive a deduction only in the taxable year in which the deferred compensation is includible in the gross income of the employee.[69]

Example 28. As part of a deferred compensation arrangement, employer X agrees to place $10,000 annually into a trust account for employee Y. Y's rights to the trust funds are forfeitable until he completes 10 years of service for X. In the year in which

[65] § 409A(a)(1)(A)(i).
[66] Rev. Rul. 69-649, 1969-2 C.B. 106.
[67] Rev. Rul. 69-650, 1969-2 C.B. 106.
[68] § 402(b).
[69] § 404(a)(5).

Y's risk of forfeiture lapses, the value of the trust funds is included in Y's gross income. Subsequent payments into the fund by X are fully taxable to Y.[70]

A disadvantage of the Rabbi trust is that if the employer gets into financial difficulty, the trust assets are subject to the claims of the employer's creditors. In addition, any income that is generated by the trust will be taxable to the employer.

Secular Trusts. Designed in 1988, the Secular trust is a variation of the Rabbi trust.[71] Under a Secular trust, the employee receives a vested interest in the full amount of the transfer to the trust. Because the employee has a nonforfeitable interest, the employee is taxed immediately on the transfer of funds to the trust even though he or she has not actually received the funds. In return for the transfer, the employer receives an immediate deduction. The advantage of this arrangement is that the trust assets are not subject to the claims of the employer's creditors. The disadvantage, of course, is that the funds are immediately taxable to the employee. A Secular trust differs from a Rabbi trust, because the assets of the Rabbi trust will not be protected from the creditors of the employer in the event of bankruptcy.

STOCK OPTIONS

As an alternative to the payment of compensation in the form of corporate stock, corporate employers may issue *options* to purchase stock at a specified price to employees whom the company wants to retain. As a general rule, stock options have no value on the date they are issued because the option price is equal to or greater than the market price of the stock. Consequently, the options will have value to the recipient (and become a cost to the employer) *only if* the market price of the shares increases.

If an option has no value upon date of grant to an employee, the employee obviously has not received taxable income. However, in certain unusual cases options may have a value at date of grant. If such value can be determined with reasonable accuracy under criteria provided in Regulation § 1.83-7(b)(2), the value represents compensation income to the recipient of the option. If an option is actively traded on an established market, it is deemed to have an ascertainable value at date of grant.[72]

Example 29. Corporation C grants employee D an option to purchase 100 shares of C common stock for $11 a share at any time over the next ten years. If C stock is selling at $9 per share, D's option has no readily ascertainable value. Therefore, D has no taxable income at date of grant, and a zero-tax basis in the option. If, however, D's option is actively traded on an established market and as a result can be valued at $5, D has received taxable compensation of that amount, and will have a $5 basis in the option.

OPTION EXERCISE

When the owner of a stock option that had no ascertainable value at date of grant exercises the option, the difference between the option price and the market price (bargain element) of the stock purchased represents ordinary income to the owner. If the option had an ascertainable value at date of grant, so that the recipient recognized taxable income upon receipt of the option, no additional income is recognized when the option is exercised.[73]

---

[70]   Reg. § 1.402(b)-1(b).

[71]   PLR8841023.

[72]   Reg. § 1.83-7(b)(1).

[73]   Reg. § 1.83-7(a).

Example 30. In 2006, employee M received certain stock options as part of her compensation from Corporation Q. At date of grant, the options had no ascertainable value. However, in 2009 M exercised the options and purchased 1,000 shares of Q stock, market value $90 per share, for the option price of $60 per share. In 2009 M must recognize $30,000 of ordinary income ($30 per share bargain element × 1,000 shares). M's tax basis in her shares is $90,000.

From the employer's point of view, the value of a stock option can be taken as a deduction under the previously discussed rule of § 83(h). Generally, an employer will receive a deduction at date of grant if the option has a readily ascertainable value. If the option has no value at date of grant, the deduction will equal the income recognized by the owner of the option when the option is exercised.

INCENTIVE STOCK OPTIONS

In the past, Congress has experimented with a variety of *qualified stock options—* options afforded preferential tax treatment under § 421. Currently there is only a single type of qualified option, the Incentive Stock Option (ISO) of § 422A.[74]

Under § 421(a), the exercise of an ISO will not result in any income recognition to the owner. Correspondingly, the corporate employer who issued the option will never receive any deduction for the spread between option and market price at date of exercise. If and when the stock received upon exercise is sold, the employee will realize capital gain equal to the difference between the option price and selling price. The difference in tax consequences between a nonqualified stock option and an ISO is presented in the example below.

Example 31. Employee T was granted an option in 2003 to purchase one share of his corporate employer's stock at any time within the two succeeding calendar years. At the time the option was granted, the option price was $150 and the market price was $140. Assume that T exercised the option in 2005 when the stock had a market price of $200, and the stock acquired was sold in 2009 for $375. The tax consequences for each tax year would be as follows:

	Nonqualified Stock Option	*Incentive Stock Option*
2003	None	None
2005	Market price of $200 − $150 option price = $50 ordinary income and $200 basis in purchased stock ($150 cost + $50 income recognized). Employer deduction = $50	No income and $150 basis in purchased stock
2009	Sale price of $375 − $200 basis = $175 capital gain	Sale price of $375 − $150 basis = $225 capital gain

It should be noted that § 83 will apply to a tax-free transfer of an incentive stock option in determining a taxpayer's AMTI. Under § 83(a), the taxpayer will include in AMTI the excess of the stock's fair market value at the first time it is transferable over the amount paid for the stock under the option. See Chapter 13 for a discussion of the alternative minimum tax (AMT).

---

[74] The rules of § 422A apply to options granted on or after January 1, 1976 and outstanding on January 1, 1981.

HOLDING PERIOD REQUIREMENTS

For the beneficial rule of § 421(a) to apply, an individual may not dispose of the stock purchased upon exercise of the ISO within two years from the date of the granting of the option and within one year from the date of exercise.[75] Additionally, the individual must be an employee of either the corporation granting the ISO or a parent, subsidiary, or successor corporation from the date of grant until the day three months before the date of exercise.[76]

If an individual violates the holding period requirement by disposing of his or her stock too quickly after purchase, § 421(b) provides that the *compensation income* (ordinary income) the individual did not recognize at date of exercise must be recognized in the year of disposition. Any gain so recognized increases the cost basis of the stock.[77] In such a situation the employer will be entitled to a corresponding deduction.

> **Example 32.** Beta Corporation grants an ISO to employee Z on November 1, 2003. The option allows Z to purchase 500 shares of Beta stock at $3 per share. Z exercises the option on December 1, 2008, when Beta stock is selling for $7 per share. Z sells his 500 shares on March 1, 2009 for $9 per share. Because of the premature disposition (less than one year from date of exercise), Z must recognize $2,000 ordinary income [500 shares × $4 bargain price ($7 market price − $3 option price)] and a $1,000 capital gain in 2009. Additionally, Beta Corporation may claim a $2,000 deduction in 2009.

If the amount realized on a premature sale is less than the value of the stock at date of exercise, only the excess of the amount realized over the option price is recognized as ordinary income.[78]

> **Example 33.** Refer to the facts in *Example 32*. If Z sold his Beta stock for $6 rather than $9 a share, his ordinary income (and Beta's deduction) would be limited to $1,500 [500 shares × $3 bargain price ($6 selling price − $3 option price)].

QUALIFICATION REQUIREMENTS

An employee stock option must meet a number of statutory requirements set forth in § 422A(b) to qualify as an ISO. The primary requirements are as follows:

1. The option is granted pursuant to a plan that specifies the total number of shares that may be issued under options and the class of employees eligible to receive the options. The shareholders of the corporation must approve the plan within twelve months before or after the date the plan is adopted.

2. The options are granted within ten years of the date of adoption or the date of shareholder approval, whichever is earlier.

3. The option price is not less than the market value of the stock at date of grant.

4. The option must be exercised within ten years of date of grant.

5. The option can only be exercised by the recipient employee during his or her lifetime and can only be transferred at the employee's death.

---

[75]   § 422A(a)(1).

[76]   § 422A(a)(2).

[77]   Reg. § 1.421-5(b)(2).

[78]   § 422A(c)(2).

6. The recipient of the option does not own stock possessing more than 10 percent of the total combined voting power of all classes of stock of the employer corporation or of its parent or subsidiary corporation.[79]

A major restriction on the use of ISOs is the statutory requirement that the value of stock with respect to which ISOs are *exercisable* shall not exceed $100,000 per calendar year per employee. For purposes of this requirement, the value of the stock is determined at date of grant.[80]

Example 34. In calendar year 2008, Corporation Q granted Employee F an ISO to purchase 1,000 shares of Q stock with a current aggregate value of $200,000. In calendar year 2009, Corporation Q granted Employee F a second ISO to purchase 1,200 shares of Q stock with a current aggregate value of $300,000. If Employee F decides to exercise any of her ISOs in 2009, she may only purchase 500 (500/1,000 × $200,000 = $100,000 limit) shares through exercise of her 2007 option or 400 shares through exercise of her 2009 option (400/1,200 × $300,000 = $100,000 limit).

Exclusion from Wages. The *American Jobs Creation Act of 2004* eliminated the uncertainty as to employer withholding obligations upon the exercise of statutory stock options. The Act provides a specific exclusion from the FICA/FUTA payroll tax withholding obligations for remuneration on account of the transfer of stock pursuant to the exercise of an incentive stock option or under an employee stock purchase plan, or any disposition of such stock.[81] The new law also provides that federal income tax withholding is not required on a disqualifying disposition of stock acquired from ISO and employee stock purchase plans (ESPP), nor when compensation is recognized in connection with an ESPP discount.

NONQUALIFIED STOCK OPTIONS

A Nonqualified Stock Option (NQSO), also referred to as a nonstatutory stock option, is generally any option that does not meet the statutory requirements in the Code to be treated as an Incentive Stock Option (ISO). NQSOs are often used as implements of deferred compensation because the corporation can avail itself of a tax deduction without a cash outlay and the options themselves can be issued with more flexible terms than ISOs. The only major disadvantage of using an NQSO is the potential for income recognition to the employee. That potential is, in turn, dependent upon whether the option has a readily ascertainable fair market value.

Readily Ascertainable Fair Market Value. If an option is actively traded on an established exchange (e.g., American Stock Exchange or Chicago Board of Options Exchange), it is deemed to have a readily ascertainable fair market value. An option that is not traded on an established exchange will not have a readily ascertainable fair market value unless it can be measured with reasonable accuracy. The Regulations support this presumption with detailed conditions for determining value.[82]

Determining value is important because, if the option has a readily ascertainable fair market value at the time of grant, the employee will be taxed immediately. Any gain or loss that accrues after the time of the grant will be recognized as capital gain or loss on the disposition of the underlying stock. When gain is recognized, the employee's basis in the

---

[79]   § 422A(c)(6) waives this requirement in certain cases.

[80]   § 422A(b)(7).

[81]   §§ 3121(a)(22), 3306(b)(19), 421(b), and 423(c).

[82]   Regs. § 1.83-7(b)(2).

stock includes any amounts paid for the stock plus the amount that was recognized as ordinary income at the time of the grant. The corporate employer takes a deduction in the same year (and for the same amount) income is recognized by the employee.[83] It is important to notice that the result of these options is conditioned on establishing a value for the option and not establishing a value for the stock of the corporation.

No Readily Ascertainable Fair Market Value. If an option does not have a readily ascertainable fair market value, the transaction will remain "open," and the employee will not be taxed when the option is granted. Instead, the employee recognizes ordinary income when the option is exercised. The amount of income to be recognized is the spread between the value of the stock purchased and the price paid at the date of exercise. Any appreciation in the stock after the exercise date will be recognized as capital gain. The corporate employer takes a corresponding tax deduction in the same year and to the extent of ordinary income recognized by the employee.

> **Example 35.** On January 1, 2009, R Corporation grants S, an employee, the option to purchase 1,000 shares for $12 per share on or before August 15, 2010. At the time of the grant, R stock is valued at $20 per share. On June 3, 2010, when the value of R stock is $35, S exercises the option and acquires the stock for $12,000 (1,000 × $12). On November 1, 2010, S sells the stock for $48,000 (1,000 × $48). If the option granted has no readily ascertainable fair market value, S will recognize $23,000 ($35,000 − $12,000) of ordinary income and a $13,000 ($48,000 − $35,000) capital gain, both in 2010. R takes a deduction of $23,000 in 2010. If on the other hand, the option has a readily ascertainable value (for example $8 per share), S must recognize $8,000 of ordinary income in 2009 (the grant date) and a capital gain of $28,000 in 2010 (the sale date). R will take an $8,000 deduction in 2009.

STOCK APPRECIATION RIGHTS

Occasionally, NQSOs can create a problem for employees when they generate taxable income without providing resources to pay the tax. Unfortunately, when this occurs, some employees find it necessary to sell the stock to raise the capital, and this defeats the purpose of providing equity compensation. To ameliorate this dilemma, some employers wrap an NQSO with a Stock Appreciation Right (SAR).

An SAR is a type of right (similar to an option) that entitles the employee to a cash payment equal to the difference between the fair market value of one share of the common stock of the corporation on the date of the *exercise* of the SAR over its fair market value on the date it was *granted*. An employee need not own any stock of the corporation to receive an SAR, and SARs are granted without cost to the employee. An SAR cannot be exercised before one year after it was granted and must be exercised by the fifth year, or the SAR will be deemed exercised and cash will be paid to the employee. An SAR is not included in taxable income until the year the right is exercised. The IRS has ruled that an employee who receives an SAR will not be in constructive receipt of income in the year it was granted.[84]

TAX PLANNING CONSIDERATIONS

The area of employment compensation and retirement planning offers tremendous opportunity for creative tax planning. During a taxpayer's productive years, he or she

---

[83] Regs. § 1.421-6(c), (d), (e), and (f).

[84] Rev. Rul. 80-300. 1980-2 C.B. 165.

needs to be able to analyze and appreciate the tax consequences of the various types of compensation alternatives that may be offered. The taxpayer must be aware of the tradeoff between types of compensation that will be taxed currently and fringe benefits that may not be taxable upon receipt. Sophisticated forms of compensation such as § 83 property and incentive stock options should be considered in designing a specialized compensation package.

Taxpayers should also appreciate the necessity for long-range retirement planning. An understanding of the different tax consequences of qualified and nonqualified retirement plans is essential to effective planning for post-employment years. Exhibit 18-8 contains a comparison of the plans discussed in this chapter.

PLANNING FOR RETIREMENT INCOME

One of the central features of an individual's financial plan should be a provision for some source of retirement income. As the life span of the average American lengthens, the number of prospective retirement years increases. As a result, many individuals realize that some amount of current investment is necessary in order to ensure that their retirement years can be a period of financial security.

In analyzing a particular retirement plan, two basic questions must be answered:

1. Are payments into the plan deductible for Federal income tax purposes by the taxpayer?

2. To what extent are retirement benefits received from a plan includible in the recipient taxpayer's gross income?

ADVANTAGES OF IRAS

IRAs used to be among the best retirement saving plans around until Congress clipped some of their more generous features in 1986. Today they are still a useful part of many retirement portfolios; however, some limitations will apply.

Prior to 1987, IRAs were available to anyone who had not reached the age of $70\frac{1}{2}$. Contributions were allowable up to the $3,000 annual limit and were fully tax deductible. Today, these rules apply to only two types of people:

▸ Those who are not eligible for an employer-sponsored retirement plan; or
▸ Those whose incomes fall below specified levels.

For individuals with company retirement plans, deductible IRAs are still available, provided certain tests can be satisfied. The first test of IRA deductibility is income. A taxpayer may still make a fully deductible IRA contribution as long as A.G.I. does not exceed certain levels. Exhibit 18-8 provides a list of eligible individuals and the limitations on IRA deductions.

> **Example 36.** H and W have A.G.I. of $169,000 and file a joint tax return. Their table amount indicates they are entitled to a partial deduction. To determine their deduction, subtract their A.G.I. from the limit for that particular row ($176,000 − $169,000 to get $7,000). Next, divide that amount ($7,000) by $10,000 to get a percentage ($7,000/$10,000 = 70%). This is the percentage of the IRA base, $5,000, that may be deducted. Accordingly, H and W may deduct $3,500.
>
> *Note* that the taxpayers may still *contribute* the full $5,000, but cannot deduct the extra $1,500.

EXHIBIT 18-8

IRA Deductions for Active Participants in Qualified Plans for 2006 and 2007

A.G.I. Before IRA Deduction	Single or Head of Household	Filing Jointly or Widower	Married, Filing Separately
$ 0–$ 10,000	full	full	partial
$10,000–$ 55,000	full	full	NONE
$55,000–$ 65,000	partial	full	NONE
$65,000–$176,000	NONE	partial	NONE
$176,000 +	NONE	NONE	NONE

* Locate income and filing status. If the word *full* appears, a $5,000 deduction is available in 2008; if *NONE* appears, no deduction is available; and if *partial* appears, a prorated amount is deductible.

SPOUSAL IRAS

Holding a job is not a prerequisite to opening and deducting an IRA. A nonworking spouse may start a *spousal IRA*, as long as both taxpayers file jointly and the combined total of both spouse's earned income equals $10,000. When these two requirements are met, each spouse may make contributions to an IRA. Together, they may contribute as much as $10,000 in any single year. No more than $5,000 of that amount, however, may go to either account. If the combined total earned income is less than $10,000, the deduction is not lost. The combined total of the IRA's is limited to the amount of combined income (limited to $5,000 per spouse).

WHAT IS AN ACTIVE PARTICIPANT?

As discussed earlier, an individual may not be eligible for a deductible IRA if he or she is an active participant or eligible to participate in a pension or profit sharing plan. As a general rule, the IRS considers a taxpayer an active participant in a defined plan if the plan's guidelines state that the taxpayer is covered, even if they decline to participate. As a result, just being eligible for a plan makes the taxpayer an active participant.

If an individual is not sure if he is an active participant, he can look at his W-2 form, provided by his employer. It provides a box for the taxpayer's employer to check. If this box is blank, additional research may be necessary. Exhibit 18-9 provides aid in determining whether a taxpayer is eligible to participate.

EXHIBIT 18-9
Active Participation

Participation in any of the following plans can make a taxpayer an active participant and not eligible to deduct IRA contributions.

- Qualified pension, profit sharing, or stock bonus plans, including Keogh plans
- Qualified annuity plans simplified employee pension plans (SEPs)
- Retirement plans for Federal, state, or local government employees
- Certain union plans [so-called § 501(c)(18) plans]
- Tax-sheltered annuities for pubic school teachers and employees of charitable organizations.
- § 401(k) plans

MAKING A NONDEDUCTIBLE CONTRIBUTION TO AN IRA

Even if a taxpayer is not eligible, for whatever reason, to make deductible contributions to an IRA, a nondeductible contribution is available. Whether a taxpayer should make a nondeductible IRA contribution depends on the circumstances. Some of the following pros and cons should be considered before a taxpayer makes a decision.

The most obvious pro is that even though a taxpayer may not deduct his or her annual IRA contribution, the earnings from IRA investments accumulate and compound tax-deferred. This means a faster fund build-up compared to a taxable savings account. (See Exhibit 18-10 for a similar comparison.)

The most obvious con is that once money is put into an IRA, it is locked in until the taxpayer attains the age $59\frac{1}{2}$. Otherwise, the taxpayer is subject to pay a 10 percent penalty for early withdrawal. The penalty applies to the deductible portion of the IRA contribution and to any earnings that may have accumulated tax-deferred in the account. However, no penalty applies when nondeductible contributions are withdrawn.

Many investment counselors suggest tax-free bonds as a reasonable alternative to making a nondeductible IRA contribution. The earnings from the bonds are tax-free and are not subject to a penalty if the taxpayer needs to withdraw any of the money. Moreover, a taxpayer is not limited to investing $5,000 ($10,000 for spousal IRAs).

Bonds, however, come with two potential drawbacks. First, a taxpayer can possibly get locked into the bonds until maturity. If interest rates rise, the value of the bonds generally declines, and a taxpayer would potentially have to sell the bonds at a loss. Second, depending on the market, the yields on bonds are sometimes low compared to the after-tax yields of other securities. So, potentially, bonds can be a very poor investment.

EXHIBIT 18-10
Comparison of Corporate Retirement Plans

Description	Corporate Plan	Keogh [HR 10]	Roth or Traditional IRA	SEP	CODA (401(k))	Funded	
						Rabbi	Secular
Qualified	Yes	Yes	Yes	Yes	Yes	No	No
Participation	21 years old or > 1 year = 100% vested	21 years old or > 1 year = 100% vested	Limited by AGI	21 years old or 3 out of 5 year's service	1 year's service	No Requirements	
Limitations	100% | $44,000 or 100% of $220,000 | 100% average.	100% | $44,000 or 13.043% of $220,000 | 100% average.	$4,000 or 100% Earned Income	$44,000 or 15% Earned Income	$15,000 (for 2006)	No limitations if paid as reasonable compensation	
Vesting	3 years Cliff or 6 years Graded	3 years Cliff or 6 years Graded	100%	100%	100% of employee's contribution	Subject to claims of creditors	100%
Premature Distributions	Rollover or 10% Penalty	Rollover or 10% Penalty	Rollover or 10% Penalty	Rollover or 10% Penalty	Rollover or 10% Penalty	Taxable only if not previously taxed	
Lump-Sum 5/10 Year Averaging Available	Yes	Yes	No, taxed as Ordinary Income or Tax free	No, taxed as Ordinary Income	Yes	Not available: in some cases funds previously taxed	
Date Plan Must Be Established	By last day of plan year	By last day of plan year	Regular tax due date	Regular tax due date	By last day of plan year	By last day of plan year	
Required Date to Contribute	Extended due date	Extended due date	Regular due date	Regular due date	Extended due date	Year end	
Employee Loans from the Plan	Yes	None: Owner-Employees	None	None	Limited	Yes, but very risky	Yes

PROBLEM MATERIALS

DISCUSSION QUESTIONS

18-1   *Taxation of Barter Transactions.* Your friend who is a practicing dentist tells you that he filled a tooth for a friend's child "for no payment" because the friend had prepared the dentist's income tax return for the previous year. Must the dentist recognize taxable income because of this arrangement? Explain.

18-2   *Taxation of Fringe Benefits.* Define the term *fringe benefit*. As a general rule are fringe benefits taxable?

18-3   *Taxation of Fringe Benefits.* Every year, Employer E gives each employee the choice of a turkey or ham as a Christmas "gift." Is the value of this fringe benefit taxable to

the employees? Would your answer be different if each employee received a Christmas bonus of $500 cash?

18-4 *Fringe Benefits—Cafeteria Plans.* What is a cafeteria plan of employee benefits?

18-5 *Reasons for Stock Options.* How does a corporation benefit from compensating valuable employees with shares of stock in the corporation rather than a cash wage or salary?

18-6 *Receipt of Restricted Property for Services.* What factors should a taxpayer consider when deciding to make an election under § 83(b) with regard to restricted property?

18-7 *ISO Plans.* An ISO (incentive stock option) allows the recipient both a deferral of income and a conversion of ordinary income into capital gain. Explain.

18-8 *Funded versus Unfunded Deferred Compensation Arrangements.* Why would an employee normally prefer a funded rather than an unfunded deferred compensation arrangement? Which would the employer normally prefer?

18-9 *Deferred Compensation and the Constructive Receipt Doctrine.* Explain the doctrine of constructive receipt as it relates to a cash basis employee who has a deferred compensation arrangement with his or her employer.

18-10 *Tax Advantages of Qualified Retirement Plans.* Discuss the tax advantages granted to qualified retirement plans.

18-11 *Defined Benefit versus Defined Contribution Plans.* Differentiate between a defined benefit retirement plan and a defined contribution retirement plan.

18-12 *Retirement Plan Qualification Requirements.* Any employee of Trion Ltd. Partnership can participate in the company's pension plan after they have been employed by Trion for 36 consecutive months. Can Trion's plan be a qualified retirement plan? Discuss.

18-13 *The Meaning of Vested Benefits.* Explain the concept of vesting as it relates to qualified retirement plans. How does it differ from the concept of participation?

18-14 *Profit-Sharing Plans versus Pension Plans.* Many small, developing companies will choose to establish a qualified profit-sharing plan rather than a pension plan. Why?

18-15 *Spousal IRAs.* Discuss the purpose of a spousal IRA (individual retirement account).

18-16 *Lump-Sum Distribution Rollovers.* Why might an employee who receives a lump-sum distribution from a qualified retirement plan choose to roll over the distribution into an IRA? What are the negative tax consequences of doing so?

18-17 *Roth IRAs versus Traditional IRAs.* In 1998, Congress provided taxpayers wanting to establish an IRA a choice. Taxpayers may now use either a Roth IRA or a traditional IRA or both.
   a. Identify the major differences between Roth IRAs and traditional IRAs.
   b. Identify circumstances when a Roth IRA may be preferred over a traditional IRA and vice versa.

18-18 *Education IRAs.* One of the tax incentives created for higher education in 1998 was the Education IRA.
   a. Explain how an education IRA works.
   b. Compare an education IRA to a qualified prepaid tuition and how it relates to the Hope and Lifetime Learning credits.

PROBLEMS

18-19 *Receipt of Restricted Property for Services.* D, a calendar year taxpayer, is an employee of M Corporation, also on a calendar year for tax purposes. In 2009, M Corporation transfers 100 shares of its own common stock to D as a bonus for his outstanding work during the year. If D quits his job with M within the next three years, he must return the shares to the corporation. At date of transfer, the shares are selling on the open market at $35 per share. Three years later, when the risk of forfeiture lapses, the stock is selling at $100 per share.

     a. Assume D does not make the election under § 83(b). How much income must he recognize in 2009 because of his receipt of the stock? In 2012 when his restriction lapses?

     b. Assume D does elect under § 83(b). How much income must he recognize in 2009? In 2012?

     c. Refer to questions (a) and (b). In each case how much of a deduction may M Corporation claim and in which year should the deduction be taken?

18-20 *Tax Consequences of a Nonqualified Stock Option Plan.* In 2009, Z Corporation grants a nonqualified stock option to employee M. The option allows M to purchase 100 shares of Z Corporation stock for $20 per share at any time during the next four years. Because the current market value of Z stock is $22 per share, the option has a readily ascertainable value of $200 ($2 per share bargain element × 100 shares) at date of grant. M exercises the option in 2010 when the market value of the Z stock has increased to $28 per share.

     a. How much income does M recognize in 2009 because of the receipt of the option?

     b. How much income does M recognize in 2011 upon exercise of the option?

     c. What amount of deduction is available to Corporation Z because of the option granted to M? In what year is the deduction claimed?

18-21 *Tax Consequences of a Nonqualified Stock Option Plan.* In 2009, X Corporation grants a nonqualified stock option to E, a valued employee, as additional compensation. The option has no value at date of grant, but entitles E to purchase 1,000 shares of X stock for $20 per share at any time during the next five years. E exercises the option in 2010, when X Corporation's stock is selling on the open market at $48 per share.

     a. How much income does E recognize in 2009 because of her receipt of the option?

     b. How much income does E recognize in 2010 upon exercise of the option?

     c. What amount of deduction is available to X Corporation because of the option granted to E? In what year is the deduction claimed?

18-22 *Nonqualified Stock Option Plans.* Refer to the facts in *Problems 18-20* and *18-21*. In each case, what tax basis does the employee have in the purchased corporate stock?

18-23 *Incentive Stock Options (ISO) versus Nonqualified Stock Options.* Refer to the facts in *18-21.* If the stock option issued by X corporation had been an ISO rather than a nonqualified option, how much income would E recognize in 2010 upon option exercise?

18-24 *Incentive Stock Option Plans.* In May 2008, employee N exercised an ISO that entitled him to purchase 50 shares of Clay Corporation common stock for $120 a share. The stock was selling on the open market for $210 per share. N sold the 50 shares in 2011 for $390 per share.

     a. How much income must N recognize in 2008 upon exercise of the option?

     b. How much income must N recognize in 2011 upon sale of the Clay stock?

18-25 *Incentive Stock Options—Early Disposition of Stock.* Refer to the facts in *Problem 18-24.* What would be the tax consequences if N sold the Clay stock in August 2008 for $250 per share? For $190 per share?

18-26 *Tax Computation on Lump Sum Distributions.* T participated in his employer's qualified profit sharing plan from 1981 until his retirement at age 64 in the current year. T made no contributions to the plan. In the current year, T received a lump sum distribution of $75,000 from the plan.
  a. How much of the distribution is taxable to T in the current year?
  b. Assuming T is single with no dependents, does not itemize deductions, and has only $13,000 of other taxable income (including exemptions and the standard deduction), use the five-year forward averaging method to compute his current-year tax liability.

18-27 *Tax Computation on Lump-Sum Distributions.* In the current year, Mrs. Z, age 61, retired after a 35-year career with the same corporate employer. She received her entire $51,000 account balance from her employer's qualified profit sharing plan. In the current year, Mrs. Z and her husband will file a joint return on which they will report $21,000 of other taxable income (net of all deductions and exemptions). If Mrs. Z elects five-year averaging, compute the tax liability on the joint return.

18-28 *Qualified Pension Plan—Maximum Annual Benefits.* During his last three years as president of R Corporation, G was paid $200,000 in 2007, $230,000 in 2008, and $280,000 in 2009 as total compensation for his services. These were the three highest compensation years of his employment. What is the maximum retirement benefit payable to G from the corporation's qualified pension plan (a defined benefit plan)?

18-29 *Qualified Profit Sharing Plans—Maximum Annual Contribution.* In the current year, Mr. W, a corporate vice president, earned a base salary of $350,000. His corporate employer maintains a qualified retirement plan that provides for an annual contribution equal to 10 percent of each employee's base level of compensation. Based on these facts. compute the maximum current-year contribution to Mr. W's retirement account.

18-30 *Additional Taxes on Plan Distributions.* In the current year, Mr. L, age 51 and in perfect health, resigns as President of Meta Industries, Inc. Mr. L receives a $300,000 lump sum distribution from Meta's qualified retirement plan. Before consideration of this distribution, Mr. L's taxable income for the year is over $200,000. If Mr. L decides not to "roll over" the contribution into another qualified plan or IRA, compute the net after-tax amount of the distribution that Mr. L will be able to spend.

18-31 *Maximum Annual Contributions to Keogh Plans.* H is a self-employed business person with several employees. He has established a profit-sharing plan for himself and his employees. The annual net earned income from his business is $132,000. What is the maximum amount of a deduction available to H for his contribution to the plan for the year?

18-32 *Maximum Annual Contributions to IRAs.* H and W file a joint tax return. W is a lawyer with current-year earned income of $65,000. H works part-time as a landscape architect and earned $22,000 in the current year.
  a. Assume that W is an active participant in the firm's qualified profit-sharing plan. How much may W and H contribute to their IRAs for the current year? How much of the contribution is deductible?
  b. Assume neither H nor W is an active participant in a qualified retirement plan. How does this assumption change your answers to (a) above?

18-33 *Maximum Deductible Contributions to IRAs.* In the current year, Ms. A, a single taxpayer, contributed $1,400 to her IRA. She also is an active participant in her employer's qualified money purchase pension plan. Ms. A's adjusted gross income

(before any deduction for her IRA contribution) is \$29,640. How much of the IRA contribution is deductible in 2009?

18-34 *Taxability of IRA Distributions.* Taxpayer B, age 66, makes his first withdrawal of \$8,800 from his IRA in the current year and uses the money to make a down payment on a sailboat. At the end of the year, B's IRA balance is \$36,555. During previous years, B had made nondeductible contributions to the IRA totaling \$13,400. Based on these facts, what amount of the \$8,800 withdrawal must B include in current-year gross income?

18-35 *Simplified Employee Pensions.* Z is an employee of a company that has established a SEP. Z's current-year salary is \$18,000.
  a. How much may Z's employer contribute to her IRA during 2009?
  b. May Z make any additional deductible contribution herself to her IRA?

RESEARCH PROBLEMS

18-36 *Current versus Deferred Compensation.* Roy Hartman is a 55-year-old executive of the Robco Oil Tool Corporation. The corporation does not have any type of qualified pension or profit-sharing plan, nor does it intend to adopt one in the near future. However, in an effort to ensure the continuing services of Mr. Hartman, Robco Corporation has offered him a choice between two different compensation arrangements. One pays \$40,000 additional annual salary; and the other provides for \$50,000 a year deferred compensation for 10 years beginning when Roy retires at age 65. Currently, Hartman's marginal tax rate is 31 percent. Roy does not expect to be in a lower tax bracket within his last 10 years of employment or after retirement. Since he does not need the \$28,800 which would remain after paying current taxes on the \$40,000 additional annual salary, Mr. Hartman asks you to evaluate his alternative compensation proposals. Assuming a 10 percent pre-tax return on savings will prevail over the entire 20-year period (10 years before and 10 years after retirement), and assuming that he would save the entire \$28,800 annual after-tax salary under the \$40,000 additional annual compensation arrangement, which alternative would you recommend? Why?

18-37 *Qualified Retirement Plans.* Shelly Carol is the sole shareholder of Gills Corporation. The corporation has been in business since 1989 manufacturing dog food. Profits have averaged about \$300,000 per year for the past five years. Shelly projects that with the purchase of additional manufacturing equipment costing \$700,000, he can double his production of dog food, resulting in additional profits of \$200,000. Unfortunately, Shelly does not have the funds readily available to make the additional capital purchases, so in order to implement the plan he intends to borrow the entire \$700,000.

Required:
1. How can Gills Corporation achieve its goal of financing the capital improvements while providing an incentive benefit to its employees?

2. Assume that Gills Corporation's payroll is approximately \$600,000 and that Shelly intends to set aside \$100,000 for the benefit of the employees. Compare the plan selected in (1) above with an ordinary pension or profit-sharing plan.

3. What are some of the disadvantages that Shelly should consider in using the plan established in (1)?

Research aids
§ 401(a)(28)(C)
§ 404(a)(3)
§ 404(a)(9)
§ 409(h)
§ 4975(e)(7)

PART SEVEN

CORPORATE TAXATION

★ ★ ★ ★ CONTENTS ★ ★ ★ ★ ★

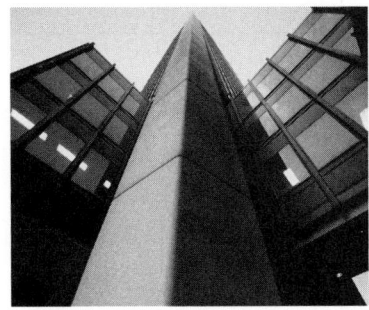

★ CHAPTER NINETEEN ★

CORPORATIONS: FORMATION AND OPERATION

LEARNING OBJECTIVES

Upon completion of this chapter you will be able to:

- Define a corporation for Federal income tax purposes

- Compare and contrast corporate and individual taxation

- Compute the corporate income tax, including the tax for personal service corporations

- Describe the corporate tax forms and filing requirements

- Explain the basic tax consequences of forming a new corporation, including:

  - Determination of the gain or loss recognized by the shareholders and the corporation

  - Determination of the basis of the shareholder's stock in the corporation and the corporation's basis in the property received

- Describe the requirements for qualifying a transfer to a corporation for tax-free treatment

- Understand the effects of transferring liabilities to an existing corporation

CHAPTER OUTLINE

INTRODUCTION

As discussed in Chapter 3, there are several types of taxable entities. The individual taxpayer has already been discussed at length. Various aspects of the corporate entity are covered in this chapter and the next two chapters. S corporations, partnerships, and fiduciaries are covered in later chapters.

WHAT IS A CORPORATION?

A corporation is an artificial "person" created by state law. The state may impose restrictions on the issuance of shares and the type of business conducted. The state also specifies the requirements for incorporation, such as the filing of articles of incorporation, the issuance of a corporate charter, and the payment of various fees (e.g., franchise taxes).

Federal tax law provides that a tax will be imposed upon the taxable income of every corporation. For this purpose, a *corporation* is a business entity organized under a Federal or state statute, if the statute refers to the entity as incorporated or as a corporation, body corporate, or body public.[1] This definition includes entities such as insurance companies, state-statute authorized joint-stock companies or associations, banks with any FDIC-insured deposits, businesses wholly owned by state or political subdivisions, and business entities, such as publicly traded partnerships, that are treated

---

[1] § 7701(a)(3).

as corporations. The regulations also classify a list of specified foreign entities as corporations.

ASSOCIATIONS

Historically, an association that was not treated as a corporation under state or Federal law (e.g., a partnership) could be classified as a corporation for Federal income tax purposes and thus be inadvertently exposed to the disadvantages of the regular (C) corporate form of doing business. The aspects that were addressed in determining whether an association should be classified and taxed as a corporation included:[2]

1. Continuity of life,

2. Centralized management,

3. Limited liability, and

4. Free transferability.

If three of these four characteristics were satisfied, an entity would be taxed as a corporation, even if the entity was treated differently under state law. For example, a limited liability partnership (LLP) or a limited liability company (LLC) could be treated as a corporation for tax purposes if it had, along with limited liability, two of the other three characteristics (e.g., centralized management and no restrictions on the transfer of interests).

It is important to note what could happen to any anticipated tax benefits if an organization was unexpectedly classified as an association. For example, if the owners of a real estate business expected losses in the early years of operations, the corporate tax entity would not be the best choice of business form unless the organization qualified for and elected S corporation status. If the business was treated as a partnership or an S corporation, the losses flowed through to the owners and could be deductible on their personal tax returns, subject to the passive activity loss rules. However, if the entity was classified as an association and was thereby taxable as a regular corporation, the losses simply accumulated at the corporate level in the form of net operating loss carryovers, the tax benefit of which expired at the end of 20 years.[3] Obviously, if the organization's owners did not think that the business was a corporation, they certainly would not file the required election to be treated as an S corporation for Federal income tax purposes. Thus, unless the organization qualified as a partnership for tax purposes, any anticipated tax benefits would *either* be lost or, at best, unduly delayed.

Naturally, the above classification rules led to a great number of conflicts between the IRS and taxpayers. To simplify this process, the IRS issued regulations in 1998 that replace the old rules for classifying entities with a "check-the-box" system.[4] Under the new rules, an entity organized as a corporation under state law, or an entity classified under the Code as a corporation, will be treated as a corporation and will not be allowed to make an election. However, any other business entity (e.g., an LLC) that has at least two members may elect to be treated as a corporation or a partnership for tax purposes (an entity with only one member will be treated as a corporation or a sole proprietorship). In general, existing entities will continue to operate as they are as long as there is a reasonable basis for the current classification. These rules greatly simplify the process of selecting the form of business in which the owners wish to operate.

---

2   Reg. § 301.7701-2.

3   See § 172(b)(1)(B).

4   Reg. § 301.7701-1.

An important exception to the classification rules, however, is the so-called *publicly traded partnership* (PTP). A partnership meeting the definition of a PTP will be treated *and* taxed as a regular corporation. Basically, a partnership is a PTP if it (1) is a limited partnership, (2) was organized after December 17, 1987 and (3) has interests that are traded on an established securities market or are readily tradeable on a secondary market. Certain exceptions exist for PTPs in existence on December 17, 1987 and for those with income consisting primarily of interest, dividends, rental income from real property and gains from the sale of such property, gains from the sale of capital or § 1231 assets, and income and gains from development, mining or production, refining, transportation, or marketing of any mineral or natural resource (see Chapter 22 for further discussion).

LIMITED LIABILITY COMPANIES

The "check-the-box" rules eliminate the need for LLCs to create artificial features (e.g., limits on centralized management, restrictions on transferability, limits on life of the entity) to receive the desired entity classification. Under a default system, a newly formed LLC will automatically be classified as a partnership if it has at least two members unless it affirmatively elects to be taxed as a corporation. Thus, LLCs can easily and effectively provide limited liability to their members while still being treated as a partnership for Federal tax purposes.

SHAM CORPORATIONS

In some instances, the IRS will ignore the fact that an entity is considered a corporation as defined by its state law. This may happen when a corporation's only purpose is to reduce taxes of its owners or to hold title to property. If the corporation has no real business or economic function, or if it conducts no activities, it may be a "sham," or "dummy," corporation.[5] Generally, as long as there is a business activity carried on, a corporation will be considered a separate taxable entity.[6]

> **Example 1.** M owns a piece of real estate. To protect it from his creditors, M forms X Corporation and transfers the land to it in exchange for all of X Corporation's stock. The only purpose of X Corporation is to hold title to the real estate, and X Corporation conducts no other business activities. It is properly incorporated under state law. The IRS is likely to designate X Corporation as a sham corporation and to disregard its corporate status. Any income and expenses of X Corporation will be considered as belonging to M.
>
> If X Corporation had conducted some business activities (such as leasing the property and collecting rents), it is likely that it will not be considered a sham corporation.

Generally the IRS, but not the taxpayer, is allowed to disregard the status of a corporation. The courts have frequently agreed that if a taxpayer has created a corporation, he or she should not be allowed to ignore its status (i.e., in order to reduce taxes). However, the Supreme Court has ruled that a taxpayer could use a corporate entity as the taxpayer's agent in securing financing.[7] Thus, under certain conditions, taxpayers may use a corporation for a business purpose and not have it treated as a corporation for Federal tax purposes.

---

[5]   See *Higgins v. Smith*, 40-1 USTC ¶9160, 23 AFTR 800, 308 U.S. 473 (USSC, 1940).

[6]   *Moline Properties, Inc.*, 43-1 USTC ¶9464, 30 AFTR 1291, 319 U.S. 436 (USSC, 1943).

[7]   *Jesse C. Bollinger*, 88-1 USTC ¶9233, 61 AFTR2d 88-793, 108 S.CT. 1173 (USSC, 1988).

COMPARISON OF CORPORATE AND INDIVIDUAL INCOME TAXATION

A corporation's taxable income is computed by subtracting various deductions from its gross income. Although this appears to be the same basic computation as for individual taxpayers, there are numerous important differences. In order to highlight these differences, Exhibits 19-1 and 19-2 contain the tax formulas for corporate and individual taxpayers.

GROSS INCOME

The definition of gross income is the same for both corporations and individuals.[8] However, there are some differences in the exclusions from gross income. For example, capital contributions to a corporation (i.e., purchase of corporate stock by shareholders) are excluded from gross income.[9]

EXHIBIT 19-1

Tax Formula for Corporate Taxpayers

Income (from whatever source)	$xxx,xxx
Less: Exclusions from gross income	−xx,xxx
Gross income	$xxx,xxx
Less: Deductions	−xx,xxx
Taxable income	$xxx,xxx
Applicable tax rates	xx%
Gross tax	$ xx,xxx
Less: Tax credits and prepayments	−x,xxx
Tax due (or refund)	$ xx,xxx

---

[8] § 61(a).

[9] § 118(a).

EXHIBIT 19-2

Tax Formula for Individual Taxpayers

Total income (from whatever source)...............................				$xxx,xxx
Less: Exclusions from gross income....................................				−xx,xxx
Gross income...				$xxx,xxx
Less: Deductions for adjusted gross income				−xx,xxx
Adjusted gross income				$xxx,xxx
Less:	1.	The larger of		
		a.	Standard deduction.................	$x,xxx	
			or	*or*	−x,xxx
		b.	Total itemized deductions............	$x,xxx	
	2.	Number of personal and dependency		
		exemptions × exemption amount		−x,xxx
Taxable income...				$xxx,xxx
Applicable tax rates				
(from Tables or Schedules X, Y, or Z)				xx%
Gross income tax				$ xx,xxx
Plus:		Additional taxes (e.g., self-employment taxes and		+x,xxx
		recapture of tax credits)		
Less:		Tax credits and prepayments........................		−x,xxx
Tax due (or refund)				$ xx,xxx

DEDUCTIONS

Corporations have no "Adjusted Gross Income." Thus, for corporations there are no "deductions for A.G.I." or "deductions from A.G.I." All corporate expenditures are either deductible or not deductible. All allowable deductions are subtracted from gross income in arriving at taxable income.

Although corporations are considered to be "persons" under the tax law, they are not entitled to the following "personal" deductions that are available for individuals:

1. Personal and dependency exemptions

2. Standard deduction

3. Itemized deductions

All activities of a corporation are considered to be business activities. Therefore, corporations usually deduct all their losses since they are considered business losses.[10] In addition, corporations do not have to reduce their casualty losses by either the $100 statutory floor or by 10 percent of adjusted gross income. (Corporations have no A.G.I., as mentioned.)

Corporations do not have "nonbusiness" bad debts, since all activities are considered business activities. All bad debts of a corporation are business bad debts.[11]

---

[10]   § 165(a). Like individuals, certain corporations are subject to the passive-loss rules discussed in Chapter 12.

[11]   § 166.

Several deductions are available only for corporations.[12] These are deductible in addition to the other business deductions and include the dividends-received deduction and the amortization of organizational expenditures.

DIVIDENDS-RECEIVED DEDUCTION

No doubt the most salient tax aspect of operating a business in the corporate form is that double taxation occurs when corporate profits are distributed in the form of dividends to the shareholders. The corporation is not allowed a deduction for the dividends paid, and an individual shareholder is not entitled to an exclusion. Therefore, when one corporation is a shareholder in another corporation, *triple* taxation might occur. To alleviate this, Congress provided corporations with a deduction for dividends received.[13]

Generally, the dividends-received deduction (DRD) is 70 percent of the dividends received from taxable domestic (U.S.) corporations.[14] However, a corporation that owns at least 20 percent—but less than 80 percent—of the dividend-paying corporation's stock is allowed to deduct 80 percent of the dividends received.[15] In addition, members of an *affiliated group* are allowed to deduct 100 percent of the dividends that are received from another member of the same group. A group of corporations is generally considered affiliated when at least 80 percent of the stock of each corporation is owned by other members of the group.[16]

Taxable Income Limitation. The 70 percent dividends-received deduction may not exceed 70 percent of the corporation's taxable income computed without the deduction for dividends received, net operating loss carrybacks or carryforwards, and capital loss carrybacks.[17] However, if the dividends-received deduction adds to or creates a net operating loss for the current year, the 70 percent of taxable income limitation does not apply.

Like the dividends-received deduction percentage, the taxable income limitation percentage becomes 80 rather than 70 percent if the dividend-paying corporation is at least 20 percent owned by the recipient corporation. In the unlikely event a corporation receives dividends subject to *both* the 70 and 80 percent rules, a special procedure must be followed. First, the 80 percent limitation is applied by treating the "70 percent dividends" as other income. The 70 percent limitation is then applied by treating the "80 percent dividends" as if they had not been received.[18]

Exhibit 19-3 contains a format for the computation of the 70 percent dividends-received deduction, and *Example 2*, *Example 3*, and *Example 4* illustrate this computational procedure.[19]

---

[12]   § 241.

[13]   §§ 243 through 246.

[14]   § 243(a)(1).

[15]   § 243(c).

[16]   §§ 243(a)(3), 243(b)(5), and 1504.

[17]   § 246(b)(2).

[18]   § 246(b)(3).

[19]   To apply the 80 percent rules, simply substitute 80 for 70 percent in this exhibit and accompanying examples.

EXHIBIT 19-3
Computation of Corporate Dividends-Received Deduction

Step 1: Multiply the dividends received from taxable domestic (U.S.) corporations by 70 percent.* This is the *tentative* dividends-received deduction (DRD).

Step 2: Compute the tentative taxable income for the current year, using the tentative DRD (from Step 1):

Total revenues (including dividend income)
Less: Total expenses
Equals: Taxable income (before DRD)
Less: Tentative DRD (Step 1)
Equals: Tentative taxable income (loss)

If the tentative taxable income is *positive*, the taxable income limitation may apply. Go to Step 3.

If the tentative taxable income is *negative*, there is no taxable income limitation. The dividends-received deduction is the amount computed in Step 1.

Step 3: Compute the taxable income limitation:
Taxable income (before DRD) (Step 2)
Add: Any net operating loss carryovers from other years that are reflected in taxable income
Add: Any capital loss carrybacks from later years that are reflected in taxable income
Equals: Taxable income, as adjusted
Multiply by 70 percent
Equals: Taxable income limitation

Step 4: Compare the tentative DRD (Step 1) to the taxable income limitation (Step 3). Choose the *smaller* amount. This is the corporate dividends-received deduction.

* To apply the 80 percent rules, simply substitute 80 for 70 percent in Steps 1 and 3 above.

Example 2. R Corporation has the following items of revenue and expenses for the year:

Dividends received from domestic corporations	$40,000
Revenue from sales	60,000
Cost of goods sold and operating expenses	54,000

The dividends-received deduction is computed as follows:

Step 1: $40,000 dividends received
×70%

$28,000 *tentative* DRD

Step 2:

Dividend income	$ 40,000
Revenue from sales	+60,000
Total revenues	$100,000
Less: Total expenses	−54,000
Taxable income (before DRD)	$ 46,000
Less: Tentative DRD	−28,000
Tentative taxable income	$ 18,000

Since tentative taxable income is positive, the taxable income limitation may apply. Go to Step 3.

Step 3: Compute the taxable income limitation:

Taxable income (before DRD)	$46,000
Multiply by 70%	×70%
Taxable income limitation.	$32,200

Step 4: Compare the tentative DRD ($28,000) to the taxable income limitation ($32,200). Choose the *smaller* amount ($28,000). In this case, R Corporation's dividends-received deduction is $28,000 (not subject to limitation).

Example 3. Assume the same facts as in *Example 2* except that the revenue from sales is $50,000. The dividends-received deduction is computed as follows:

Step 1: $40,000 dividends received
×70%
$28,000 *tentative* DRD

Step 2:

Dividend income	$40,000
Revenue from sales	+50,000
Total revenues.	$90,000
Less: Total expenses	−54,000
Taxable income (before DRD)	$36,000
Less: Tentative DRD (Step 1).	−28,000
Tentative taxable income	$ 8,000

Since tentative taxable income is *positive*, the taxable income limitation may apply. Go to Step 3.

Step 3: Compute the taxable income limitation:

Taxable income (before DRD)	$36,000
Multiply by 70%	×70%
Taxable income limitation.	$25,200

Step 4: Compare the tentative DRD ($28,000) to the taxable income limitation ($25,200). Choose the smaller amount ($25,200). In this case, R Corporation's dividends-received deduction is $25,200 (limited to 70% of taxable income).

Example 4. Assume the same facts as in *Example 2* except that the revenue from sales is $41,000. The dividends-received deduction is computed as follows:

Step 1: $40,000 dividends received
                 ×70%

                 $28,000 *tentative* DRD

Step 2:

Dividend income	$40,000
Revenue from sales	+41,000
Total revenues...................................	$81,000
Less: Total expenses	−54,000
Taxable income (before DRD).......................	$27,000
Less: Tentative DRD	−28,000
Tentative taxable income	($1,000)

Because the tentative taxable income (loss) is *negative*, there is no taxable income limitation. The dividends-received deduction is $28,000.

The taxable income limitation discussed above *does not* apply to dividends received from affiliated corporations that are subject to the 100 percent dividends-received deductions.[20]

Other Restrictions on Dividends-Received Deduction. The dividends-received deduction will be limited if the purchase price of the stock was debt-financed or the stock was refinanced and any portion of the debt remains unpaid during the period dividends are received on that stock.[21] In taxable years before 1984, a corporation could increase its cash flow and decrease its tax liability by purchasing stock with borrowed funds. Under prior law, the interest paid on the debt was fully deductible, whereas the dividends were only partially taxable because of the dividends-received deduction. Currently, corporations must reduce the dividends-received deduction if the stock was debt-financed. The dividends-received deduction for debt-financed stock equals the 70 percent deduction multiplied by the percentage of the stock price that is *not* debt-financed.[22]

Example 5. T Corporation purchased 100 shares of XYZ stock for $100,000. T borrowed $60,000 of the purchase price. Therefore, the corporation used $40,000 of its own funds or 4% of the purchase price. The dividends-received deduction for dividends from XYZ will be limited to 28% (70% × 40%). As T Corporation *reduces* the debt, the dividends-received deduction will increase. For instance, if T reduces the debt to $50,000 before the next dividends are received from XYZ, the dividends-received deduction *increases* to 35% (70% × 50% of stock price no longer debt-financed). When the debt is retired, the dividends-received deduction is restored to the full 70%.

The dividends-received deduction may also cause a reduction in the basis of the stock. If a corporation receives an *extraordinary dividend* within the first two years that the stock is owned, the basis of the stock must be reduced by the nontaxable portion of the extraordinary dividend.[23] An extraordinary dividend is any dividend that equals or

---

20 § 246(b)(1).

21 § 246A.

22 § 246A(a)(1); 80 percent in the case of any dividends received from a 20 percent or more owned corporation. This limitation does not apply to dividends that are eligible for the 100 percent dividends-received deduction.

23 § 1059(a).

exceeds 10 percent of the taxpayer's basis of common stock, or 5 percent of the basis of preferred stock.[24] If the taxpayer can prove the fair market value of the stock, then the taxpayer can use such value instead of basis to determine if the dividend is extraordinary.

> **Example 6.** P Corporation purchases 100 shares of Y Corporation common stock on January 1, 2009 for $100,000. On December 31, 2009 Y Corporation declares and pays a $30,000 dividend to P. Since the dividend exceeds 10% of the basis of the stock, it is an extraordinary dividend. P Corporation must reduce its basis of the Y Corporation stock by $21,000 (70% × $30,000), the amount of the dividends-received deduction.

ORGANIZATIONAL EXPENDITURES

When a corporation is formed, various expenses directly related to the organization process are incurred, such as attorneys' fees, accountants' fees, and state filing charges. Although some of the attorneys' and accountants' fees may be ordinary and necessary business expenses which do not benefit future periods (and are therefore deductible), most of these expenditures will benefit future periods and are therefore capitalized as *organizational expenditures.* These organizational expenditures are intangible assets that have value for the life of the corporation.

Generally, assets with indefinite lives may not be amortized for Federal income tax purposes. However, Congress has given corporations the option of expensing some of the organization expenditures and amortizing the remainder. The amount that can be expensed is limited to $5,000 reduced by the amount of the expenditures over $50,000. The amortizable amount is amortized over 180 months.[25] The 180-month period starts in the month in which the corporation begins business.

The Regulations give the following examples of organizational expenditures:[26]

1. Legal services incident to the organization of the corporation, such as drafting the corporate charter, by-laws, minutes of organizational meetings, and terms of original stock certificates

2. Necessary accounting services

3. Expenses of temporary directors and of organizational meetings of directors or stockholders

4. Fees paid to the state of incorporation

The Regulations also give several examples of items that are *not* considered organizational expenditures, such as costs of issuing stock.[27] The costs of issuing stock are considered to be selling expenses, and therefore are reductions in the proceeds from selling the stock. They reduce stockholders' equity and do not create any tax deduction.

> **Example 7.** N Corporation was formed and began business on July 1, 2009 and incurred and paid qualifying organizational expenditures of $8,600. N Corporation has chosen to use the calendar year for tax purposes. On its first tax return (2009),

---

[24] Amounts distributed to corporate shareholders on certain preferred stock or as part of a partial liquidation or non-pro rata redemption that are treated as dividends are also considered extraordinary dividends. See Chapter 20 for a discussion of redemptions and partial liquidations.

[25] See § 248.

[26] Reg. § 1.248-1(b)(2).

[27] Reg. § 1.248-1(b)(3).

N Corporation will expense $5,000 and claim an amortization deduction of $120, computed as follows:

$$\frac{\text{Organizational expenditures}}{180 \text{ months}} = \text{Amortization per month}$$

$$\frac{\$3,600}{180 \text{ months}} = \$20 \text{ Amortization per month}$$

$$\$20 \times 6 \text{ months in 2009 (July–December)} = \underline{\underline{\$120}}$$

The amortization deduction for organizational expenditures for 2010 will be $240 ($20 per month × 12 months).

An election to amortize organizational expenditures is made by attaching a statement to the corporation's first tax return.[28] If the election is not made, the organizational expenditures may not be amortized.

NET OPERATING LOSS

Corporations, like individuals, are entitled to deduct net operating loss carryovers in arriving at taxable income. As discussed in Chapter 8, numerous modifications are considered in computing an individual's net operating loss. However, only two modifications are considered in computing a corporation's net operating loss. These two modifications are the net operating loss deductions[29] and the dividends-received deduction.[30] Net operating loss deductions for each year are considered separately. Therefore, the net operating loss deductions for other years are omitted from the computation of the current year's net operating loss. The modification relating to the dividends-received deduction is that the 70 percent (or 80 percent) taxable income limitation is ignored (i.e., the dividends-received deduction is allowed in full).

A corporate net operating loss may be carried back two years and carried forward 20 years.[31] The loss is first carried back to the earliest year. Any unabsorbed loss is carried to the first prior year, the first year after the loss was created, and then forward until the loss is completely used or the 20-year period expires.

A corporation may elect not to carry the loss back.[32] If a corporation makes this election, the loss would be carried forward for 20 years. No loss would be carried back. This election is irrevocable.[33]

Example 8. T Corporation had the following items of revenue and expense for 2009:

Revenue from operations	$42,000
Dividends received from a less than 20% owned corporation	40,000
Expenses of operations	63,000

---

[28] Reg. § 1.248-1(c).
[29] § 172(d)(1).
[30] § 172(d)(5).
[31] § 172(b)(1).
[32] § 172(b)(3)(C).
[33] *Ibid.*

T Corporation's net operating loss for 2009 is computed as follows:

Revenue from operations		$42,000
Dividend income		40,000
Total revenue		$82,000
Less:	Total expenses	−63,000
Less:	Dividends-received deduction (ignore	
	the taxable income limitation)	−28,000
Net operating loss (negative taxable income)		($9,000)

The 2009 net operating loss is carried back two years to 2007. If T Corporation's taxable income for 2007 is $3,000, the 2009 net operating loss is treated as follows:

2007 taxable income	$3,000
Less: NOL carryback	−9,000
NOL carryover to 2008	($6,000)

A corporate net operating loss is carried back by filing either Form 1120X (Amended U.S. Corporation Income Tax Return) or Form 1139 (Corporation Application for Tentative Refund). T Corporation should receive a refund of its 2007 income tax paid.

CHARITABLE CONTRIBUTIONS

A corporation's charitable contribution deduction is much more limited than the charitable contribution deductions of individuals. As with individuals, the charitable contributions must be made to qualified organizations.[34] The amount that can be deducted in any year is the amount actually donated during the year plus, *if the corporation is on the accrual basis*, any amounts that are authorized during the year by the board of directors, provided the amounts are actually paid to the charity by the 15th day of the third month following the close of the tax year.[35]

> **Example 9.** C Corporation donated $3,000 cash to United Charities (a qualified charitable organization) on June 3, 2009. On December 20, 2009 the board of directors of C Corporation authorized a $2,500 cash donation to United Charities. This $2,500 was actually paid to United Charities on March 12, 2010. C Corporation uses the calendar year as its accounting period.
>
> If C Corporation is a *cash basis* corporation, only the $3,000 contribution to United Charities made in 2009 may be deducted in 2009. The additional $2,500 authorized contribution may not be deducted until 2010.
>
> If C Corporation is an *accrual basis* corporation, then $5,500 ($3,000 + $2,500) may be deducted in 2009.
>
> *Note:* If the $2,500 donation authorized on December 20, 2009 had been paid after March 15, 2010, the $2,500 contribution deduction would not be allowed until 2010.

Contributions of Ordinary Income Property. The amount deductible when property is contributed generally is the fair market value of the property at the time it is donated.

---

[34] § 170(c).

[35] §§ 170(a)(1) and (2).

There are, however, several exceptions to this general rule. One exception involves donations of *ordinary income property*.[36] The Regulations define ordinary income property as property that would produce a gain *other than* long-term capital gain if sold by the contributing corporation for its fair market value. The charitable contribution deduction for ordinary income property generally may not exceed the corporation's basis in the property.

> **Example 10.** G Corporation donates some of its inventory to a church. The inventory donated is worth $5,000 and has an adjusted basis to G Corporation of $2,000. G Corporation's deduction for this contribution is $2,000, its adjusted basis in the inventory.

There is an exception that permits corporate taxpayers to claim contribution deductions in excess of the basis of the ordinary income property. A corporation is allowed to deduct its basis *plus* one-half of the unrealized appreciation in value (not to exceed twice the basis) of any inventory item donated to a qualifying charity and used solely for the care of the ill, the needy, or infants.[37] This rule also applies in two other situations: (1) the gift to a college or university of a corporation's newly manufactured scientific equipment if the donee is the original user of the property and at least 80 percent of its use will be for research or experimentation;[38] and (2) computer equipment donated to a primary or secondary school (i.e. grades K through 12), provided the property is not more than two years old.[39] In either case, the corporation is required to obtain a written statement from the charity indicating that the use requirement has been met.

Contributions of Capital Gain Property. As discussed in Chapter 11, there are limitations on an individual's deduction for contributions of appreciated property (property which has increased in value). In *two* situations, a corporation also is limited in the amount of deduction when appreciated long-term capital gain property is contributed.[40] The *first* situation is when tangible personal property donated to a charity is put to a use that is not related to the charity's exempt purpose. The *second* situation in which a limitation will apply is the donation of appreciated property to certain private foundations. The limitation applied in these cases is that the fair market value of the property must be reduced by the unrealized appreciation (i.e., the deduction is limited to the property's adjusted basis). For other types of capital gain property, the contributions deduction is the fair market value of the property.

> **Example 11.** L Corporation donated a painting to a university. The painting was worth $10,000 and had an adjusted basis to L Corporation of $9,000. If the painting is placed in the university for display and study by art students, this is considered a use related to the university's exempt purpose.[41] The limitation mentioned above would not apply, and L Corporation's charitable contribution deduction would be $10,000, the fair market value of the painting.
>
> If, however, the painting is immediately sold by the university, this is considered to be a use that is not related to the university's exempt purpose. L Corporation's contribution deduction would be limited to $9,000, its basis in the painting ($10,000 fair market value − $1,000 unrealized appreciation).

36   Reg. § 1.170A-4(b)(1).

37   § 170(e)(3).

38   § 170(e)(4).

39   § 170(e)(6).

40   § 170(e)(1).

41   Reg. § 1.170A-4(b)(3).

Annual Deduction Limitations. In addition to the limitations based on the type of property contributed, there is a maximum annual limitation. The limitation is 10 percent of the corporation's taxable income before certain deductions.[42] The 10 percent limitation is based on taxable income without reduction for charitable contributions, the dividends-received deduction, net operating loss carrybacks, and capital loss carrybacks. Amounts contributed in excess of this limitation may be carried forward and deducted in any of the five succeeding years.[43] In no year may the total charitable contribution deduction exceed the 10 percent limitation. In years in which there is both a current contribution and a carryover, the current contribution is deductible first. At the end of the five-year period, any carryover not deducted expires.

Example 12. M Corporation has the following for tax year 2009:

Net income from operations	$100,000
Dividends received (subject to 70% rules)	10,000
Charitable contributions made in 2009	8,000
Charitable contribution carryforward from 2008	5,000

M Corporation's contribution deduction for 2009 is limited to $11,000, computed as follows:

Net income from operations	$100,000
Dividends received	+10,000
Taxable income without the charitable contribution deduction and the dividend-received deduction	$110,000
Multiply by 10% limitation	×10%
Maximum contribution deduction for 2009	$ 11,000

Taxable income for the year will be $92,000, computed as follows:

Net income from operations		$100,000
Dividends received		+10,000
		$110,000
Less: Special corporate deductions:		
Charitable contributions (maximum)	$ 11,000	
Dividends received (70% of $10,000)	+7,000	
Total special deductions		−18,000
M Corporation's 2009 taxable income		$ 92,000

Example 13. Based on the facts in *Example 12*, M Corporation has a $2,000 charitable contribution carryover remaining from 2008. The first $8,000 of the $11,000 allowed deduction for 2009 is considered to be from the current year's

---

[42] § 170(b)(2).

[43] § 170(d)(2).

contributions, and the $3,000 balance is from the 2008 carryover. Thus, the remaining (unused) $2,000 of the 2008 contributions must be carried over to 2010.

CAPITAL GAINS AND LOSSES

Like individuals, corporate taxpayers receive special treatment for capital gains and losses. The definition of a capital asset, the determination of holding period, and the treatment of net short-term capital gains are the same for corporations as they are for individuals. Prior to 1988, corporate taxpayers could obtain favorable treatment for their net long-term capital gains by electing to tax such gains at an alternative rate. For example, in 1986, the alternative tax rate was 28 percent while the top rate applying to ordinary income was 46 percent. Beginning in 1988, however, a corporation's net long-term capital gain is taxed in the same manner as ordinary income. Although such treatment suggests that there is no reason to distinguish capital gains and losses from ordinary income, such is not the case. Like an individual, a corporation's deduction for capital losses is limited.

Net capital losses of corporations may *only* be used to offset corporate capital gains.[44] A corporation is never permitted to reduce income from operations or investment by a capital loss. As a result, corporations may not deduct their excess capital losses for the year. Instead, a corporation may carry back the excess capital losses for three years and forward for five years,[45] and use them to offset capital gains in those years. The losses are *first* carried back three years. They may reduce the amount of capital gains reported in the earliest year. Any amount not used to offset gain in the third previous year can offset gain in the second previous year and then the first previous year. If the sum of the capital gains reported in the three previous years is less than the capital loss, the excess is carried forward. Losses carried forward may be used to offset capital gains recognized in the succeeding five tax years. Losses unused at the end of the five-year carryforward period expire.

> **Example 14.** B Corporation has income, gains, and losses as follows:
>
> | | 2006 | 2007 | 2008 | 2009 |
> |---|---|---|---|---|
> | Ordinary income | $100,000 | $100,000 | $100,000 | $100,000 |
> | Net capital gain (or loss) | 4,000 | 3,000 | 2,000 | (10,000) |
> | Total income | $104,000 | $103,000 | $102,000 | $ 90,000 |
>
> B reported taxable income in years 2006, 2007, and 2008 of $104,000, $103,000, and $102,000, respectively, since net capital gains are added into taxable income. In 2008, B must report $100,000 taxable income because capital losses are nondeductible. However, B Corporation is entitled to carry the net capital loss back to years 2006, 2007, and 2008 and file a claim for refund of the taxes paid on the capital gains for each year. Because the 2009 capital loss carryback ($10,000) exceeds the sum of the capital gains in the prior three years ($9,000), B has a $1,000 capital loss carryforward. This loss carryforward can be used to offset the first $1,000 of capital gains recognized in years 2010 through 2014.

Corporations treat all capital loss carrybacks and carryovers as short-term losses. At the present, this has no effect on the tax due and it is often immaterial whether the carryover is considered long-term or short-term. However, if Congress ever reinstates special

---

[44] § 1211(a).

[45] § 1212(a).

treatment for corporate long-term capital gains, keeping short-term and long-term carry-overs separate will once again have meaning.

SALES OF DEPRECIABLE PROPERTY

Corporations generally compute the amount of § 1245 and § 1250 ordinary income recapture on the sales of depreciable assets in the same manner as do individuals. As discussed in Example 17, however, Congress added Code § 291 to the tax law in 1982 with the intent of reducing the tax benefits of the accelerated cost recovery of depreciable § 1250 property available to corporate taxpayers. As a result, corporations must treat as ordinary income 20 percent of any § 1231 gain which would have been ordinary income if Code § 1245 rather than § 1250 had applied to the transaction. In effect, a corporation must recapture 20 percent of the straight-line depreciation claimed on residential or nonresidential realty. Similar rules apply to amortization of pollution control facilities and intangible drilling costs incurred by corporate taxpayers.

> **Example 15.** C Corporation sells residential rental property for $500,000 in 2009. The property was purchased for $400,000 in 1986, and C claimed ACRS depreciation of $120,000. Straight-line depreciation would have been $65,000. C Corporation's depreciation recapture and § 1231 gain are computed as follows:

Step 1:	Compute realized gain:		
	Sales price		$500,000
	Less: Adjusted basis		
	Cost	$400,000	
	ACRS depreciation	−120,000	−280,000
	Realized gain		$220,000
Step 2:	Compute *excess* depreciation:		
	Actual depreciation		$120,000
	Straight-line depreciation		−65,000
	Excess depreciation		$ 55,000
Step 3:	Compute § 1250 depreciation recapture:		
	Lesser of realized gain of $220,000		
	or		
	Excess depreciation of $55,000		
	§1250 depreciation recapture		$ 55,000
Step 4:	Compute depreciation recapture if § 1245 applied:		
	Lesser of realized gain of $220,000		
	or		
	Actual depreciation of $120,000		
	Depreciation recapture if §1245 applied		$120,000

Step 5:	Compute § 291 ordinary income:		
	Depreciation recapture if § 1245 applied		$120,000
	§ 1250 depreciation recapture		−55,000
	Excess recapture potential.		$ 65,000
	Multiplied by § 291 rate		×20%
	§ 291 ordinary income.		$ 13,000
Step 6:	Characterize recognized gain:		
	§ 1250 depreciation recapture		$ 55,000
	Plus: § 291 ordinary income		+13,000
	Ordinary income		$ 68,000
	Realized gain.		$220,000
	Less: Ordinary income		−68,000
	§ 1231 gain.		$152,000

TRANSACTIONS BETWEEN CORPORATIONS AND THEIR SHAREHOLDERS

As discussed in Chapter 7, no deduction is allowed for a loss incurred in a transaction between related parties.[46] A corporation may be subjected to this rule. For example, a loss on the sale of the property from a corporation to a shareholder who owns more than 50 percent of the corporation is nondeductible. In such case, the unrecognized loss must be suspended and may be used by the shareholder to offset gain when the property is sold. A corporation also may be subjected to the prohibition of deductions for *accrued* but *unpaid* expenses incurred in transactions between related parties. For example, an accrual basis corporation will be denied a deduction for accrued expenses payable to cash basis related parties *until* the amount actually is paid.[47] In calculating ownership, stock owned by family members and other entities owned by the taxpayer are included.[48] With respect to the matching of income and deduction provisions only, the Tax Reform Act of 1986 expanded the definition of a related party in the case of a *personal service corporation* to include any employee that owns any of the corporation's stock. For this purpose, a personal service corporation is one where the principal activity of the corporation is the performance of personal services *and* such services are substantially performed by employee-owners. This rule applies to firms engaged in the performance of services in the fields of health, law, engineering, architecture, accounting, actuarial science, performing arts, or consulting.

The sale of property at a *gain* between a corporation and its controlling shareholders is not affected by the disallowance rules. Instead, the gain is *reclassified* as ordinary income rather than capital or § 1231 gain if the property is depreciable by the purchaser.[49] For purposes of this rule, a controlling shareholder is defined the same as under the disallowed loss rule (i.e., more than 50 percent ownership).[50] In addition, sales of

---

[46] § 267(a)(1).

[47] § 267(a)(2).

[48] §§ 267(b) and (c).

[49] § 1239(a).

[50] § 1239(c).

depreciable property between a corporation and a more than 50 percent shareholder generally are ineligible for the installment method.[51]

DEDUCTION ATTRIBUTABLE TO DOMESTIC PRODUCTION

In an attempt to make U.S. corporations more competitive in the world market, Congress has enacted a special deduction for corporations engaged in production activities within the United States. The deduction is 9 percent times the lesser of *qualified production activity income* or taxable income. Qualified income is gross receipts from domestic production less cost of goods sold, direct expenses allocated to this income and a ratable share of indirect expenses allocated to this income. The deduction may not exceed 50 percent of the taxable wages paid during the year.

COMPUTATION OF CORPORATE INCOME TAX

For many years the maximum individual tax rate exceeded the maximum corporate tax rate. The Tax Reform Act of 1986 reversed this situation. This led many advisers to consider entities other than corporations. The Revenue Reconciliation Act of 1993 raised the maximum individual rate, making it once again greater than the maximum corporate rate. This may have the effect of encouraging the formation of corporations. The corporate tax rates for 1993 and subsequent years are as follows:[52]

Taxable Income	Tax Rate
$ 1–50,000	15%
50,001–75,000	25
75,001–10,000,000	34
More than $10,000,000	35

CORPORATE SURTAX

In an effort to restrict the tax benefit of the lower graduated rates to small corporate businesses with taxable incomes of $100,000 or less, a 5 percent *surtax* is imposed on corporate taxable income in excess of $100,000, up to a maximum surtax of $11,750—the net "savings" of having the first $75,000 of corporate income taxed at the lower rates rather than at 34 percent. For corporations with taxable income in excess of $15 million, an additional surtax is imposed equal to the lesser of $100,000 or 3 percent of the taxable income in excess of $15 million.[53] The purpose of this additional surtax is to eliminate the tax "savings" arising from taxing the first $10 million at 34 percent rather than 35 percent (i.e., 1% of $10 million = $100,000 additional surtax).

---

[51]   § 453(g). The sale can qualify for installment treatment if the taxpayer can prove absence of tax avoidance motive.

[52]   § 11(b).

[53]   *Ibid.*

Example 16. L corporation has taxable income of $120,000 for its 2009 calendar year its tax liability is computed as follows:

15%	×	$50,000	=	$ 7,500
25%	×	25,000	=	6,250
34%	×	45,000	=	15,300

Tax liability before surtax	$29,050
Plus: 5% surtax on $20,000 ($120,000 − $100,000)	+1,000
Total tax liability for 2009	$30,050

Example 17. P Corporation has taxable income of $335,000 for its 2009 tax year. Its tax liability is computed as follows:

15%	×	$ 50,000	=	$ 7,500
25%	×	25,000	=	6,250
34%	×	260,000	=	88,400

Tax liability before surtax	$102,150
Plus: 5% surtax on $235,000	+11,750
Total tax liability for 2009	$113,900

Note that the 5% surtax on the $235,000 income in excess of $100,000 completely offsets the benefit of the lower graduated tax rates of 15 and 25%.

Example 18. R Corporation has taxable income of $20 million for its 2009 tax year. Its tax liability is computed as follows:

15%	×	$ 50,000	=	$ 7,500
25%	×	25,000	=	6,250
34%	×	9,925,000	=	3,374,500
35%	×	10,000,000	=	3,500,000

Tax liability before surtaxes			$6,888,250
Plus:	5% surtax		11,750
	3% surtax on $3,333,333		100,000
Total tax liability for 2009			$7,000,000

Note that the combined effect of the 5 and 3% surtaxes results in a flat tax rate of 35% for corporations with taxable income of $18,333,333 or more.

Taking the 5 percent and 3 percent surtaxes into account, a corporate tax rate schedule applicable to *most* corporations would be as follows:

Taxable Income		Tax Rate
$ 1–$ 50,000		15%
50,001– 75,000		25
75,001– 100,000		34
100,001– 335,000		39
335,001– 10,000,000		34
10,000,001– 15,000,000		35
15,000,001– 18,333,333		38
More than $18,333,333		35

This rate structure is not available to so-called personal service corporations or to certain related corporations. The specific rules applicable to these corporations are discussed below.

PERSONAL SERVICE CORPORATIONS

As described earlier, a personal service corporation (PSC) is a corporation where the principal activity is the performance of services in the fields of health, law, engineering, architecture, accounting, actuarial science, the performing arts, or consulting, *and* substantially all of the stock is owned by employees, retired employees, or their estates.[54] Apparently concerned that PSCs were being used to shield income from the employee-owners' higher individual tax rates, Congress denied the benefits of the lower tax rates to such corporations for taxable years after 1987. As a result, the taxable income of a PSC is subject to a flat rate of 35 percent.[55]

ALTERNATIVE MINIMUM TAX

As discussed in Chapter 13, corporations are subject to the alternative minimum tax. This tax is computed at a 20 percent rate on alternative minimum taxable income (AMTI) in excess of $40,000.[56] The $40,000 exemption is reduced by 25 percent of the amount of AMTI in excess of $150,000.[57] Consequently, the exemption is completely eliminated for AMTI in excess of $310,000.

Corporations are required to use many of the tax preferences and adjustments that individuals use in arriving at AMTI. However. there is one very important additional adjustment for corporations. The adjustment is 75 percent of the difference between adjusted current earnings (ACE) and alternative minimum taxable income.[58] In general, adjusted current earnings will equal current earnings and profits. The adjustment will be added to taxable income in arriving at AMTI.[59]

In an attempt at simplification, the Taxpayer Relief Act of 1998 exempts small corporations from the AMT. All corporations are exempt their first year of existence. In its second year, a corporation is exempt if its gross receipts for the first year were less than $5,000,000. Starting in its third year, the corporation is exempt if its average annual gross

---

[54] § 448(d)(2).

[55] § 11(b)(2). Note that a PSC is not subject to the 5 or 3 percent surtax since it does not benefit from the lower corporate tax rates.

[56] See §§ 55(b)(1)(B) and (d)(2).

[57] § 55(d)(3)(A).

[58] § 56(g).

[59] See Chapter 13 for a detailed discussion of the required adjustments and tax preferences used in computing the alternative minimum tax.

receipts for all prior three year periods are less than $7,500,000. Once a corporation fails this test, it may not claim exemption as a small corporation even if its gross receipts decline to less than $7,500,000. A corporation that fails to meet the $7.5 million gross receipts test becomes subject to the corporate AMT only with respect to preferences and adjustments that relate to transactions and investments entered into after the corporation loses its status as a small corporation. For example, if a corporation fails the test in 2008, it is not required to calculate AMT depreciation for assets placed in service in previous years but only for those placed in service in 2009 (i.e., the year in which they become subject to the AMT).

TAX CREDITS

Most of the same tax credits available to individuals are also available to corporations. However, corporations are not entitled to the earned income credit, the child care credit, or the credit for the elderly.[60]

ACCOUNTING PERIODS AND METHODS

A corporation is generally allowed to choose either a calendar year or fiscal year for its reporting period.[61] However, a personal service corporation (PSC) must use a calendar year for tax purposes unless it can satisfy IRS requirements that there is a business purpose for a fiscal year.[62] Special rules apply to deductions for year-end payments made by a fiscal year PSC to its employee-owners.[63] Like PSCs, S corporations generally must use a calendar year for tax purposes.[64]

Unlike individuals, most corporations are denied the use of the cash method of accounting for tax purposes. There are three basic exceptions, however. The cash method may be used by the following:

1. Corporations with average annual gross receipts of $5 million or less in all prior taxable years

2. S corporations

3. Personal service corporations[65]

CORPORATE TAX FORMS AND FILING REQUIREMENTS

Corporations are required to report their income and tax liability on Form 1120. Page 1 of this form contains the summary of taxable income and tax due the Federal government or the refund due the corporation. There are separate schedules for the computation of cost of goods sold, bad debt deduction, compensation of officers, dividends-received deduction, and tax computation.

In addition to the computational schedules, Form 1120 also has several schedules that contain additional information. For example, Schedule L requires the corporation to

---

[60] §§ 32 and 22.
[61] § 441.
[62] § 441(i).
[63] § 280H.
[64] § 1378(b). But see § 444 for an exception, and Chapter 23 for further discussion.
[65] § 448.

provide a balance sheet as prepared for book purposes as of the beginning and end of the year. Form 1120 also contains two schedules of reconciliation, Schedules M-1 and M-2.

Schedule M-1 is a reconciliation of income per books and income per tax return. Both permanent and timing differences will appear in this schedule. For corporations with total assets greater than $10 million, Schedule M-3 is used instead of Schedule M-1.

Schedule M-2 reconciles opening and closing retained earnings. This schedule uses accounting rather than tax data. Corporations without any special transactions will show an increase in retained earnings for net income and a decrease for distributions (i.e., dividends) as the major items in Schedule M-2. The use of these schedules is illustrated in an example of a corporate tax return presented later in this chapter.

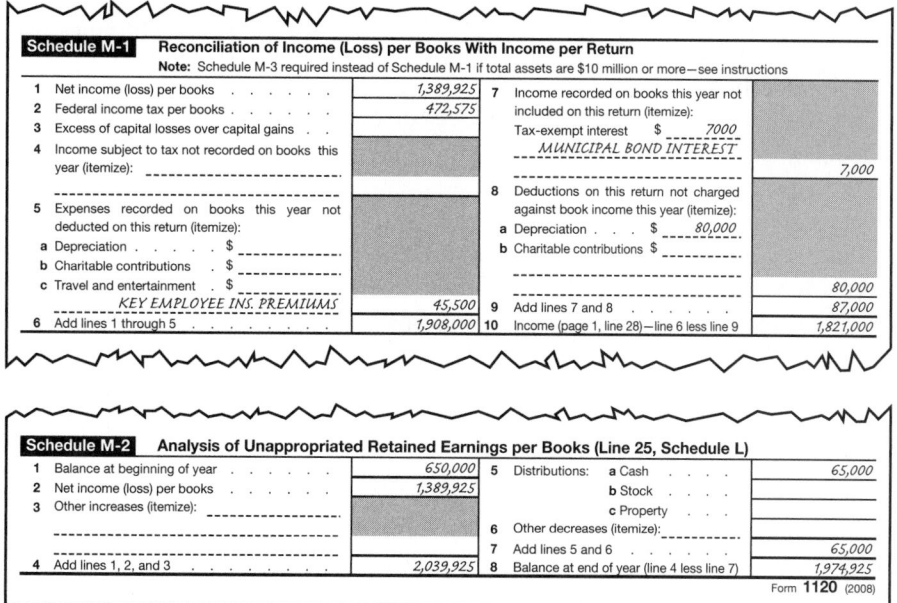

FILING REQUIREMENTS

Form 1120 is required to be filed by the 15th day of the third month following the close of the corporation's tax year.[66] As mentioned previously, a corporation is permitted to elect either a calendar or fiscal year. The decision generally is unaffected by the tax years of its shareholders.[67] The selection is made by filing the first return by the appropriate due date. For calendar year corporations, the due date is March 15. The return must be signed by an officer or other authorized person.[68]

Corporations may obtain an automatic six-month extension of time to file the tax return.[69] The extension covers only the return—not the tax due. The request for extension (Form 7004) must be accompanied by the full amount of estimated tax due. The extension can be terminated by the government on ten days' notice.

---

[66] § 6072(b).

[67] Although a regular corporation's selection of a calendar or fiscal year is not affected by the tax years of its shareholders, a corporation electing to be treated as a conduit (flow-through) entity under Subchapter S of the Code generally is required to use the calendar year for tax purposes. See Chapter 23 for greater details.

[68] § 6062.

[69] § 6081(b).

ESTIMATED TAX PAYMENTS

Corporations are required to file and pay estimated tax (including any estimated AMT liability).[70] The estimates are due the 15th day of the 4th, 6th, 9th, and 12th months of the tax year. For a calendar year corporation, the payment dates for estimated taxes are April 15, June 15, September 15, and December 15. One-fourth of the estimated tax due is to be paid on each payment date.

To avoid a penalty for underpayment of the estimated tax, at least 100 percent of the corporation's tax due for the year must be paid as estimated taxes. Specifically, the corporation must pay *one-fourth* of this amount—25 percent (100% ÷ 4) of the tax shown on its return—by the due date of each installment.[71] However, the underpayment penalty is normally not imposed where the installment for any period is:

1. At least 25 percent of the tax shown on the prior year's return (if such return was for 12 months and showed a tax liability); or

2. Equal to 100 percent or more of the tax due for each quarter based on annualized taxable income.[72]

A so-called *large* corporation—one with taxable income of $1 million or more in any of its three preceding taxable years—is not allowed to use exception (1) above *except* for its first estimated tax payment of the year.[73] In addition, a corporation whose tax liability for the year is less than $500 is not subject to the underpayment penalty.[74] If a corporation does not qualify for any of the exceptions, its underpayment penalty is computed on Form 2220.

EXAMPLE OF CORPORATE TAX RETURN

The next few pages contain an illustration of a corporation's annual Federal income tax return (Form 1120). This return is based on the following information:

R Corporation is a calendar year, accrual method taxpayer, which operates as a men's clothing store. John Beyond owns 100 percent of R Corporation's stock and is employed as the company's only officer. The corporation had the following items of income and expense for the current year:

---

[70] § 6655.

[71] § 6655(b).

[72] See §§ 6655(d) and (e) for these exceptions.

[73] § 6655(d)(2).

[74] § 6655(f).

Gross sales	$3,900,000
Sales returns	20,000
Inventory at beginning of year	120,000
Purchases	1,100,000
Inventory at end of year	140,000
Salaries and wages:	
Officers	400,000
Other	150,000
Rent expenses	120,000
Interest expense	50,000
Interest income:	
Municipal bonds	7,000
Other	10,000
Charitable contributions	79,000
Depreciation	110,000
Dividend income	30,000
Advertising expenses	50,000
Professional fees paid	20,000
Taxes paid (state income and payroll taxes)	40,000
Premiums paid on key employee life insurance policy	45,500

R Corporation timely paid $600,000 in estimated income tax payments based on its prior year's tax liability of $595,200. All dividends received by the corporation qualify for the 70 percent dividends-received deduction. The corporation declared and paid dividends of $65,000 to its sole shareholder. Additional information is provided in the balance sheets in Schedule L.

R Corporation's 2009 tax liability is $612,000 ($1,800,000 × 34%).

Note: The sample corporate tax return is shown on 2008 tax forms because the 2009 forms were not available at the publication date of this text.

Form **1120**		**U.S. Corporation Income Tax Return**				OMB No. 1545-0123

Department of the Treasury
Internal Revenue Service

For calendar year 2008 or tax year beginning _____ , 2008, ending _____ , 20 _____

▶ **See separate instructions.**

2008

A Check if:

1a Consolidated return (attach Form 851) ☐
b Life/nonlife consolidated return . . ☐
2 Personal holding co. (attach Sch. PH) . ☐
3 Personal service corp. (see instructions) . ☐
4 Schedule M-3 attached ☐

Use IRS label. Otherwise, print or type.

Name
R. CORPORATION

Number, street, and room or suite no. If a P.O. box, see instructions.
123 JONES AVENUE

City or town, state, and ZIP code
ANYWHERE, U.S.A. 98765

B Employer identification number
74 0987650

C Date incorporated
1-1-2006

D Total assets (see instructions)
$ 2,184,925

E Check if: **(1)** ☐ Initial return **(2)** ☐ Final return **(3)** ☐ Name change **(4)** ☐ Address change

Income	**1a**	Gross receipts or sales `3,900,000` **b** Less returns and allowances `20,000` **c** Bal ▶	**1c**	3,880,000
	2	Cost of goods sold (Schedule A, line 8)	**2**	1,080,000
	3	Gross profit. Subtract line 2 from line 1c	**3**	2,800,000
	4	Dividends (Schedule C, line 19)	**4**	30,000
	5	Interest	**5**	10,000
	6	Gross rents	**6**	
	7	Gross royalties	**7**	
	8	Capital gain net income (attach Schedule D (Form 1120))	**8**	
	9	Net gain or (loss) from Form 4797, Part II, line 17 (attach Form 4797) . .	**9**	
	10	Other income (see instructions—attach schedule) . . . . ▶	**10**	
	11	**Total income.** Add lines 3 through 10 . . . . ▶	**11**	2,840,000
Deductions (See instructions for limitations on deductions.)	**12**	Compensation of officers (Schedule E, line 4) . . . . ▶	**12**	400,000
	13	Salaries and wages (less employment credits)	**13**	150,000
	14	Repairs and maintenance	**14**	
	15	Bad debts	**15**	
	16	Rents	**16**	120,000
	17	Taxes and licenses	**17**	40,000
	18	Interest	**18**	50,000
	19	Charitable contributions	**19**	79,000
	20	Depreciation from Form 4562 not claimed on Schedule A or elsewhere on return (attach Form 4562) . .	**20**	110,000
	21	Depletion	**21**	
	22	Advertising	**22**	
	23	Pension, profit-sharing, etc., plans	**23**	50,000
	24	Employee benefit programs	**24**	
	25	Domestic production activities deduction (attach Form 8903)	**25**	
	26	Other deductions (attach schedule) . . . . . . *PROFESSIONAL FEES* . . .	**26**	20,000
	27	**Total deductions.** Add lines 12 through 26 . . . . ▶	**27**	1,019,000
	28	Taxable income before net operating loss deduction and special deductions. Subtract line 27 from line 11 . .	**28**	1,821,000
	29	**Less: a** Net operating loss deduction (see instructions) . . . . . **29a** `21,000`		
		b Special deductions (Schedule C, line 20) **29b**	**29c**	21,000
Tax, Refundable Credits, and Payments	**30**	**Taxable income.** Subtract line 29c from line 28 (see instructions)	**30**	1,800,000
	31	**Total tax** (Schedule J, line 10)	**31**	612,000
	32a	2007 overpayment credited to 2008 . . **32a**		
	b	2008 estimated tax payments . . . . **32b** `600,000`		
	c	2008 refund applied for on Form 4466 . . **32c** ( ) **d** Bal ▶ **32d** `600,00`		
	e	Tax deposited with Form 7004 . . . . **32e**		
	f	Credits: **(1)** Form 2439 **(2)** Form 4136 **32f**		
	g	Refundable credits from Form 3800, line 19c, and Form 8827, line 8c . . . **32g**	**32h**	600,000
	33	Estimated tax penalty (see instructions). Check if Form 2220 is attached . . . . ▶ ☐	**33**	
	34	**Amount owed.** If line 32h is smaller than the total of lines 31 and 33, enter amount owed	**34**	
	35	**Overpayment.** If line 32h is larger than the total of lines 31 and 33, enter amount overpaid	**35**	
	36	Enter amount from line 35 you want: **Credited to 2009 estimated tax** ▶ Refunded ▶	**36**	

Sign Here

Under penalties of perjury, I declare that I have examined this return, including accompanying schedules and statements, and to the best of my knowledge and belief, it is true, correct, and complete. Declaration of preparer (other than taxpayer) is based on all information of which preparer has any knowledge.

John Beyond — Signature of officer | 3-14-10 Date | PRESIDENT Title

May the IRS discuss this return with the preparer shown below (see instructions)? ☐ **Yes** ☐ **No**

Paid Preparer's Use Only

Preparer's signature	▶ *Sherry L. Hartman*	Date 3-12-10	Check if self-employed ☐	Preparer's SSN or PTIN 454-24-9464
Firm's name (or yours if self-employed), address, and ZIP code	▶ ROY W. HARTMAN & DAUGHTERS 11318 KINGSLAND BLDV, SEALY, TX		EIN 74 2735841	
			Phone no.	

For Privacy Act and Paperwork Reduction Act Notice, see separate instructions.   Cat. No. 11450Q   Form **1120** (2008)

Form 1120 (2008)   Page **2**

Schedule A   Cost of Goods Sold (see instructions)

1	Inventory at beginning of year	120,000
2	Purchases	1,100,000
3	Cost of labor	
4	Additional section 263A costs (attach schedule)	
5	Other costs (attach schedule)	
6	**Total.** Add lines 1 through 5	1,220,000
7	Inventory at end of year	140,000
8	**Cost of goods sold.** Subtract line 7 from line 6. Enter here and on page 1, line 2	1,080,000

9a Check all methods used for valuing closing inventory:

    (i) ☐ Cost

    (ii) ☑ Lower of cost or market

    (iii) ☐ Other (Specify method used and attach explanation.) ▶ ------------------------------

b Check if there was a writedown of subnormal goods   ▶ ☐

c Check if the LIFO inventory method was adopted this tax year for any goods (if checked, attach Form 970)   ▶ ☐

d If the LIFO inventory method was used for this tax year, enter percentage (or amounts) of closing inventory computed under LIFO   **9d**

e If property is produced or acquired for resale, do the rules of section 263A apply to the corporation?   ☐ Yes   ☑ No

f Was there any change in determining quantities, cost, or valuations between opening and closing inventory? If "Yes," attach explanation   ☐ Yes   ☑ No

Schedule C   Dividends and Special Deductions (see instructions)

		(a) Dividends received	(b) %	(c) Special deductions (a) × (b)
1	Dividends from less-than-20%-owned domestic corporations (other than debt-financed stock)	30,000	70	21,000
2	Dividends from 20%-or-more-owned domestic corporations (other than debt-financed stock)		80	
3	Dividends on debt-financed stock of domestic and foreign corporations		see instructions	
4	Dividends on certain preferred stock of less-than-20%-owned public utilities		42	
5	Dividends on certain preferred stock of 20%-or-more-owned public utilities		48	
6	Dividends from less-than-20%-owned foreign corporations and certain FSCs		70	
7	Dividends from 20%-or-more-owned foreign corporations and certain FSCs		80	
8	Dividends from wholly owned foreign subsidiaries		100	
9	**Total.** Add lines 1 through 8. See instructions for limitation			
10	Dividends from domestic corporations received by a small business investment company operating under the Small Business Investment Act of 1958		100	21,000
11	Dividends from affiliated group members		100	
12	Dividends from certain FSCs		100	
13	Dividends from foreign corporations not included on lines 3, 6, 7, 8, 11, or 12			
14	Income from controlled foreign corporations under subpart F (attach Form(s) 5471)			
15	Foreign dividend gross-up			
16	IC-DISC and former DISC dividends not included on lines 1, 2, or 3			
17	Other dividends			
18	Deduction for dividends paid on certain preferred stock of public utilities			
19	**Total dividends.** Add lines 1 through 17. Enter here and on page 1, line 4 ▶	30,000		
20	**Total special deductions.** Add lines 9, 10, 11, 12, and 18. Enter here and on page 1, line 29b ▶			21,000

Schedule E   Compensation of Officers (see instructions for page 1, line 12)

Note: *Complete Schedule E only if total receipts (line 1a plus lines 4 through 10 on page 1) are $500,000 or more.*

(a) Name of officer	(b) Social security number	(c) Percent of time devoted to business	Percent of corporation stock owned		(f) Amount of compensation
			(d) Common	(e) Preferred	
1 JOHN BEYOND, PRESIDENT	451-54-6184	100 %	100 %	%	400,000
714 ENDEL CIRCLE		%	%	%	
ANYWHERE, U.S.A. 98765		%	%	%	
		%	%	%	
		%	%	%	

2	Total compensation of officers	400,000
3	Compensation of officers claimed on Schedule A and elsewhere on return	
4	Subtract line 3 from line 2. Enter the result here and on page 1, line 12	400,000

Form **1120** (2008)

Form 1120 (2008)   Page **3**

Schedule J   Tax Computation   (see instructions)

1	Check if the corporation is a member of a controlled group (attach Schedule O (Form 1120)) ▶ ☐		
2	Income tax. Check if a qualified personal service corporation (see instructions) ▶ ☐	**2**	
3	Alternative minimum tax (attach Form 4626)	**3**	612,000
4	Add lines 2 and 3	**4**	612,000
5a	Foreign tax credit (attach Form 1118)	**5a**	
b	Credit from Form 8834	**5b**	
c	General business credit (attach Form 3800)	**5c**	
d	Credit for prior year minimum tax (attach Form 8827)	**5d**	
e	Bond credits from Form 8912	**5e**	
6	**Total credits.** Add lines 5a through 5e	**6**	0
7	Subtract line 6 from line 4	**7**	612,000
8	Personal holding company tax (attach Schedule PH (Form 1120))	**8**	
9	Other taxes. Check if from: ☐ Form 4255 ☐ Form 8611 ☐ Form 8697 ☐ Form 8866 ☐ Form 8902 ☐ Other (attach schedule)	**9**	
10	**Total tax.** Add lines 7 through 9. Enter here and on page 1, line 31	**10**	612,000

Schedule K   Other Information   (see instructions)

		Yes	No
1	Check accounting method: a ☐ Cash b ☐ Accrual c ☑ Other (specify) ▶ HYBRID		
2	See the instructions and enter the:		
a	Business activity code no. ▶ 448110		
b	Business activity ▶ MEN'S CLOTHING STORE		
c	Product or service ▶ CLOTHING		
3	Is the corporation a subsidiary in an affiliated group or a parent-subsidiary controlled group?		✓
	If "Yes," enter name and EIN of the parent corporation ▶		
4	At the end of the tax year:		
a	Did any foreign or domestic corporation, partnership (including any entity treated as a partnership), or trust own directly 20% or more, or own, directly or indirectly, 50% or more of the total voting power of all classes of the corporation's stock entitled to vote? For rules of constructive ownership, see instructions. If "Yes," complete (i) through (v).		✓

(i) Name of Entity	(ii) Employer Identification Number (if any)	(iii) Type of Entity	(iv) Country of Organization	(v) Percentage Owned in Voting Stock

		Yes	No
b	Did any individual or estate own directly 20% or more, or own, directly or indirectly, 50% or more of the total voting power of all classes of the corporation's stock entitled to vote? For rules of constructive ownership, see instructions. If "Yes," complete (i) through (iv).	✓	

(i) Name of Individual or Estate	(ii) Identifying Number (if any)	(iii) Country of Citizenship (see instructions)	(iv) Percentage Owned in Voting Stock
JOHN BEYOND	451-54-6184	USA	100%

Form **1120** (2008)

Form 1120 (2008)

Page **4**

| **Schedule K** | *Continued* |

5 At the end of the tax year, did the corporation:

			Yes	No

a Own directly 20% or more, or own, directly or indirectly, 50% or more of the total voting power of all classes of stock entitled to vote of any foreign or domestic corporation not included on **Form 851,** Affiliations Schedule? For rules of constructive ownership, see instructions . If "Yes," complete (i) through (iv). [No: ✓]

(i) Name of Corporation	(ii) Employer Identification Number (if any)	(iii) Country of Incorporation	(iv) Percentage Owned in Voting Stock

b Own directly an interest of 20% or more, or own, directly or indirectly, an interest of 50% or more in any foreign or domestic partnership (including an entity treated as a partnership) or in the beneficial interest of a trust? For rules of constructive ownership, see instructions . If "Yes," complete (i) through (iv). [No: ✓]

(i) Name of Entity	(ii) Employer Identification Number (if any)	(iii) Country of Organization	(iv) Maximum Percentage Owned in Profit, Loss, or Capital

6 During this tax year, did the corporation pay dividends (other than stock dividends and distributions in exchange for stock) in excess of the corporation's current and accumulated earnings and profits? (See sections 301 and 316.) . . . . [No: ✓]

If "Yes," file **Form 5452,** Corporate Report of Nondividend Distributions.

If this is a consolidated return, answer here for the parent corporation and on Form 851 for each subsidiary.

7 At any time during the tax year, did one foreign person own, directly or indirectly, at least 25% of **(a)** the total voting power of all classes of the corporation's stock entitled to vote or **(b)** the total value of all classes of the corporation's stock? . . . . . [No: ✓]

For rules of attribution, see section 318. If "Yes," enter:

(i) Percentage owned ▶ _____ and **(ii)** Owner's country ▶ _____

(c) The corporation may have to file **Form 5472,** Information Return of a 25% Foreign-Owned U.S. Corporation or a Foreign Corporation Engaged in a U.S. Trade or Business. Enter the number of Forms 5472 attached ▶ _____

8 Check this box if the corporation issued publicly offered debt instruments with original issue discount . . . . ▶ ☐

If checked, the corporation may have to file **Form 8281,** Information Return for Publicly Offered Original Issue Discount Instruments.

9 Enter the amount of tax-exempt interest received or accrued during the tax year ▶ $ _____ *7,000*

10 Enter the number of shareholders at the end of the tax year (if 100 or fewer) ▶ _____ *1*

11 If the corporation has an NOL for the tax year and is electing to forego the carryback period, check here . . . . . . ▶ ☐

If the corporation is filing a consolidated return, the statement required by Regulations section 1.1502-21(b)(3) must be attached or the election will not be valid.

12 Enter the available NOL carryover from prior tax years (do not reduce it by any deduction on line 29a.) ▶ $ _____

13 Are the corporation's total receipts (line 1a plus lines 4 through 10 on page 1) for the tax year **and** its total assets at the end of the tax year less than $250,000? . . . . [No: ✓]

If "Yes," the corporation is not required to complete Schedules L, M-1, and M-2 on page 5. Instead, enter the total amount of cash distributions and the book value of property distributions (other than cash) made during the tax year. ▶ $

Form **1120** (2008)

Form 1120 (2008) Page **5**

Schedule L — Balance Sheets per Books

Assets	Beginning of tax year (a)	Beginning of tax year (b)	End of tax year (c)	End of tax year (d)
1 Cash		30,000		320,000
2a Trade notes and accounts receivable	180,000		210,000	
b Less allowance for bad debts	( )	180,000	( )	210,000
3 Inventories		120,000		140,000
4 U.S. government obligations				100,000
5 Tax-exempt securities (see instructions)				104,425
6 Other current assets (attach schedule)				
7 Loans to shareholders				
8 Mortgage and real estate loans				
9 Other investments (attach schedule)		200,000		970,500
10a Buildings and other depreciable assets	420,000		420,000	
b Less accumulated depreciation	(50,000)	370,000	(80,000)	340,000
11a Depletable assets				
b Less accumulated depletion	( )		( )	
12 Land (net of any amortization)				
13a Intangible assets (amortizable only)				
b Less accumulated amortization	( )		( )	
14 Other assets (attach schedule)				
15 Total assets		900,000		2,184,925

Liabilities and Shareholders' Equity	(a)	(b)	(c)	(d)
16 Accounts payable		150,000		110,000
17 Mortgages, notes, bonds payable in less than 1 year				
18 Other current liabilities (attach schedule)				
19 Loans from shareholders				
20 Mortgages, notes, bonds payable in 1 year or more				
21 Other liabilities (attach schedule)				
22 Capital stock: a Preferred stock				
b Common stock	10,000	10,000	10,000	10,000
23 Additional paid-in capital		90,000		90,000
24 Retained earnings—Appropriated (attach schedule)				
25 Retained earnings—Unappropriated		650,000		1,974,925
26 Adjustments to shareholders' equity (attach schedule)				
27 Less cost of treasury stock	( )		( )	
28 Total liabilities and shareholders' equity		900,000		2,184,925

Schedule M-1 — Reconciliation of Income (Loss) per Books With Income per Return

Note: Schedule M-3 required instead of Schedule M-1 if total assets are $10 million or more—see instructions

1 Net income (loss) per books	1,389,925	7 Income recorded on books this year not included on this return (itemize):		
2 Federal income tax per books	472,575	Tax-exempt interest $ 7000		
3 Excess of capital losses over capital gains		MUNICIPAL BOND INTEREST		7,000
4 Income subject to tax not recorded on books this year (itemize): _____		8 Deductions on this return not charged against book income this year (itemize):		
		a Depreciation . . . $ 80,000		
5 Expenses recorded on books this year not deducted on this return (itemize):		b Charitable contributions $		
a Depreciation . . . . $				80,000
b Charitable contributions . $				
c Travel and entertainment . $				
KEY EMPLOYEE INS. PREMIUMS	45,500	9 Add lines 7 and 8		87,000
6 Add lines 1 through 5	1,908,000	10 Income (page 1, line 28)—line 6 less line 9		1,821,000

Schedule M-2 — Analysis of Unappropriated Retained Earnings per Books (Line 25, Schedule L)

1 Balance at beginning of year	650,000	5 Distributions: a Cash		65,000
2 Net income (loss) per books	1,389,925	b Stock		
3 Other increases (itemize): _____		c Property		
		6 Other decreases (itemize): _____		
		7 Add lines 5 and 6		65,000
4 Add lines 1, 2, and 3	2,039,925	8 Balance at end of year (line 4 less line 7)		1,974,925

Form **1120** (2008)

CORPORATE FORMATION

When a corporation is formed, property generally is transferred to the corporation and the transferors receive stock in exchange for their property. If the fair market value of the stock received is more than the transferor's adjusted basis in the property transferred, that person has a *realized gain*. Without any special provisions in the Code, this realized gain would be recognized.[75] However, Congress did not wish to prevent or discourage incorporation because of tax reasons. Moreover, this treatment was justified since the taxpayer had not "cashed in" but continued to have an indirect interest in and control over the property transferred. Therefore, Congress enacted Code § 351 permitting the nonrecognition of gain or loss on incorporation.

Section 351(a) provides that:

No gain or loss shall be recognized if *property* is transferred to a corporation by *one or more persons solely* in exchange for *stock* in such corporation and immediately after the exchange such person or persons are in *control* of the corporation. (Emphasis added.)

This nonrecognition treatment is mandatory and not optional. Thus, if the transferor meets all the requirements, neither gain nor loss will be recognized. Only by failure to meet prescribed conditions will there be recognition of gain or loss.

TRANSFER OF PROPERTY

The first requirement in § 351(a) is that *property* must be transferred to a corporation. The Code states that property does not include services rendered.[76] From this it is inferred that property includes money,[77] real property, and tangible and intangible personal property.

A person who receives stock in exchange for services is required to recognize income from services rendered. In this case, the corporation is entitled to deduct the amount as an expense or capitalize it depending on the nature of services rendered.

Example 19. T incorporates his grocery store. He transfers all the assets for stock. The corporation issues additional stock to S, an attorney, in payment of her fee for legal services rendered in connection with the incorporation. T has neither gain nor loss recognized. S, however, is required to report the value of the stock as income. Note that this is the economic equivalent of paying S cash for her services followed by her investment of the amount received in stock of the corporation. The corporation must capitalize the value of the stock issued to S as an organization expense.

The rule that property but not services can be transferred under § 351 is generally applied to persons who transfer both. Such transferors are required to allocate the stock received between the property and services transferred and report the value of the stock received for services as income. Although the shareholder who contributes services is required to report some income, he or she can generally count *all* of the shares received in the determination of control.

---

[75] § 1001(c).

[76] § 351(d)(1).

[77] Rev. Rul. 69-357, 1969-1 C.B. 101.

BY ONE OR MORE PERSONS

For purposes of § 351(a), the term *persons* includes individuals, trusts, estates, partnerships, associations, corporations, or any combination of these.[78] Examples of transactions that might qualify for nonrecognition under § 351 include:

1. Starting a new business

2. Incorporating a business already in existence

3. The formation of a subsidiary corporation by an existing corporation

4. Additional contributions to an existing corporation by an existing shareholder or a new shareholder

SOLELY FOR STOCK

Section 351 generally applies only if the transferor receives *solely* stock in exchange for property. The stock received by the transferor must be issued by the transferee (new) corporation. This requirement ensures that nonrecognition is granted only where the transferor has a continuing interest in the assets transferred. Stock may be common or preferred, voting or nonvoting, participating or nonparticipating. Stock rights and warrants are not considered stock since these represent only the right to obtain an equity interest.[79] In addition, preferred stock that is redeemable or whose dividend varies with interest rates or commodity prices is not considered stock.

CONTROL

One of the conditions imposed by § 351 is that the transferors be in *control* of the corporation immediately after the transfer. Under § 368(c), control exists if the transferor(s) own at least 80 percent of the total voting power and at least 80 percent of the total number of shares of all other classes of stock.[80]

The phrase *"immediately after the exchange"* has raised several questions. The first question is *when* to measure control. Transfers by two or more transferors do not have to be simultaneous to fall under this nonrecognition provision provided the transfers are part of one transaction. Therefore, control is measured at the conclusion of the intended transaction and not after each transfer. Another question that has been raised is whether the transferor must obtain control with the transfer or simply have control afterward. The wording of § 351(a) indicates that the transferor(s) must simply have control *after* the exchange.

> **Example 20.** B owns all the outstanding stock of R Corporation. In the current year, he transfers real estate to the corporation as an additional capital contribution. B does not receive any additional stock from the corporation. The transfer qualifies, therefore, under § 351. B has control of R Corporation *after* the transfer. He did not have to acquire control as a result of the transfer. B did not receive anything other than stock, but the fact that he did not receive anything is immaterial.

The final question raised by the phrase "immediately after the exchange" concerns the *loss of control* after the transfer. Is it necessary for the transferors to maintain control of the corporation or is it sufficient if they have control momentarily? There is no

---

[78] Reg. § 1.351-1(a)(1).

[79] Reg. § 1.351-1(a)(1)(ii).

[80] See Rev. Rul. 59-259, 1959-2 C.B. 115, for specific rules regarding voting power.

specified length of time for which the transferor must maintain control. Instead, the courts have looked at whether the loss of control is an integral part of the initial transfer.[81] As long as the transaction in which control is lost is not arranged and enforceable prior to the transfer, the receipt of the corporation's stock should be nontaxable. The subsequent transfer of stock and loss of control will be considered a separate transaction.

RECEIPT OF BOOT

Although § 351(a) states that the transferor(s) may receive only stock, § 351(b) deals with the receipt of property other than stock (e.g., money). This cash and other nonqualified property is referred to as *boot*. The receipt of boot does *not* invalidate the § 351(a) nonrecognition treatment. Section 351(a) still applies to the extent that stock is received. However, any realized gain must be recognized to the extent that boot is *received* by the transferor.[82] This treatment is similar to the receipt of nonqualifying property in a like-kind (§ 1031) exchange.

The amount of gain recognized is the lesser of the realized gain or the fair market value of the boot received. The receipt of boot does not cause the recognition of loss.[83] The gain recognized may be either long- or short-term. The nature of the gain is determined by the property transferred to the corporation. If the property was a capital asset in the hands of the transferor, the gain is capital. If the property was ordinary income property, the gain is ordinary.

> **Example 21.** T transfers land to X Corporation in return for all of the common stock and $5,000 cash. T had purchased the land three years ago as a speculative investment for $40,000. At the time of transfer, the land was worth $100,000. The stock received is worth $95,000. The corporation plans on subdividing and selling the property.
>
> T's realized and recognized gains are computed as follows:
>
> | | | |
> |---|---|--:|
> | Value of the stock received | | $ 95,000 |
> | Plus: Boot (cash) received | | +5,000 |
> | | | |
> | Amount realized | | $100,000 |
> | Less: T's adjusted basis in the land | | −40,000 |
> | | | |
> | Realized gain | | $ 60,000 |
> | | | |
> | Gain recognized equals *lesser* of | | |
> | **a.** | Realized gain | $ 60,000 |
> | | or | |
> | **b.** | Boot received | $ 5,000 |

Thus, T's recognized gain is $5,000.

The gain is a long-term capital gain because the land was a capital asset in the hands of T. The fact that the land will be inventory to the corporation is immaterial. If no boot had been received by T, no gain would have been recognized.

---

[81]   *American Bantam Car Co.*, 11 T.C. 397; *aff'd.*, 49-2 USTC ¶9471, 38 AFTR 820, 177 F.2d 513 (CA-3, 1949).

[82]   § 351(b)(1).

[83]   § 351(b)(2).

ASSUMPTION OF LIABILITIES

Transfers to a corporation often include the transfer of liabilities as well as assets. Normally, the relief of a liability is treated the same as if cash had been received and the liability paid off. In a transaction otherwise qualifying under § 351, such treatment would result in the taxpayer receiving boot and having to recognize gain. However, for § 351 transactions, Code § 357(a) carves out a special *exception.*

The general rule of § 357(a) states that the assumption of the transferor's liability by the transferee corporation will not be considered *boot.* Therefore, under the general rule of this special exception, the assumption of liabilities by the transferee corporation will not cause recognition of gain.

However, there are two exceptions to this general rule. First, if the reason for the transfer of any of the liabilities is *tax avoidance*, then the total amount of the liabilities transferred will be considered as boot received.[84]

> **Example 22.** K transferred land to a corporation in exchange for all of its common stock, worth $85,000. The land cost $40,000 and had a fair market value of $100,000. The day before the § 351 transfer, K mortgaged the land, receiving $15,000. The corporation assumed the $15,000 mortgage. The loan and its transfer were principally entered into to avoid tax. K's realized gain is computed as follows:
>
> | | |
> |---|---|
> | Fair market value of stock received | $ 85,000 |
> | Plus: Liabilities assumed by transferee corporation | +15,000 |
> | Amount realized | $100,000 |
> | Less: Basis in land transferred | −40,000 |
> | Realized gain | $ 60,000 |

Because the primary purpose of the transfer was tax avoidance, the liabilities assumed by the transferee corporation are treated as boot received.

Gain recognized equals *lesser* of

a.	Realized gain	$60,000
	or	
b.	Boot received	$15,000

Thus, K's recognized gain is $15,000.

The second exception to the general rule concerning the assumption of liabilities operates when the amount of the liabilities transferred *exceeds* the adjusted basis of all property (including money) transferred. This situation produces a recognized gain, computed as follows:

Liabilities assumed by the transferee corporation	$xx,xxx
Minus: Adjusted basis of all property transferred (by that transferor) including money	−xx,xxx
Equals: Recognized gain	$xx,xxx

---

[84] § 357(b).

Example 23. N transfers land to a corporation in exchange for all of its common stock (worth $50,000). N's adjusted basis in the land is $10,000 and has a fair market value of $90,000. The land is subject to a $40,000 mortgage, which the corporation assumes. N's recognized gain is computed as follows:

Liabilities assumed by transferee corporation	$40,000
Minus: Adjusted basis in property transferred.	−10,000
Recognized gain	$30,000

If tax avoidance is not the motivation, and the basis of the assets equals or exceeds the amount of the liabilities, the transferor will not be treated as having received boot.

EFFECT OF § 351 ON THE TRANSFEREE CORPORATION

Section 1032 provides that a corporation will not recognize gain or loss when it issues its own stock in exchange for money or other property. Therefore, gain or loss is not recognized by the transferee corporation in a § 351 transfer.

BASIS TO SHAREHOLDERS

Following a transfer to which § 351 applies, the transferors (shareholders) must determine the basis of the stock and property received. To preserve the gain or loss not recognized on the transfer, the shareholder's basis in any stock received is generally the same as the basis of the property transferred (i.e., a substituted basis). Technically, the basis of the stock and other property received by a shareholder is determined under § 358, computed as follows:

Basis of property transferred		$xxx,xxx
Plus:	Gain recognized by transferor	+x,xxx
Less:	Money received by transferor.	−x,xxx
	Fair market value of any other property (except stock)	
	received by transferor.	−x,xxx
	Liabilities assumed by transferee corporation	−xx,xxx
Equals:	Shareholder's (transferor's) basis in stock received	$xxx,xxx

If several classes of stock are received, the total basis is allocated among the several classes based on the relative fair market value of the stock. The shareholder's basis in any other property (boot) received is its fair market value.[85] The holding period of the stock will include the holding period of the assets transferred to the corporation if the transferred property would have produced a capital or § 1231 gain on sale.[86] Otherwise, the holding period starts with the date of transfer.

Example 24. J owns MNO, Inc. In the current year, he transfers land and building to the corporation in return for 50 shares of common stock and 10 shares of preferred stock. The corporation also assumes mortgage of $40,000. J's adjusted basis in the land is $10,000 and $90,000 in the building. The land and building together have a

---

85   § 358(a)(2).
86   § 1223.

current fair market value of $200,000. The common stock has a fair market value of $120,000, and the preferred stock has a value of $40,000.

J's basis in the stock received is

Basis of property transferred		$100,000
Less:	Liabilities assumed by transferee corporation	−40,000
J's basis in the stock received		$ 60,000

The $60,000 total basis is allocated based on the relative fair market value of the stock. Thus, J's basis in each class of stock is computed as follows:

Common Stock :

$$\$60{,}000 \text{ total basis} \times \frac{\$120{,}000 \text{ value of common stock}}{\$160{,}000 \text{ value of all stock}} = \$45{,}000 \text{ basis}$$

Preferred Stock :

$$\$60{,}000 \text{ total basis} \times \frac{\$40{,}000 \text{ value of preferred stock}}{\$160{,}000 \text{ value of all stock}} = \$15{,}000 \text{ basis}$$

BASIS TO TRANSFEREE CORPORATION

The transferee corporation must also determine the basis of the property it has received from the transferor(s). This is computed under § 362 as follows:

Transferor's basis in property	$xx,xxx
Plus: Gain recognized to transferor on transfer	+x,xxx
Equals: Transferee corporation's basis in property received	$xx,xxx

If the corporation receives assets under §§ 351 or 118 with a built-in loss, then the corporation's basis in the assets will be their fair market value. As an alternative, the transferor can elect to reduce his or her stock basis by the built-in loss instead of the corporation taking the lower basis.

DEPRECIATION RECAPTURE

If the transferor has no recognized gain in a § 351 transfer, then there will be no recapture of depreciation.[87] However, the transferee corporation is responsible for recapturing depreciation when the asset is later sold or disposed of in a taxable transaction. If there is gain recognized in a § 351 transfer, the depreciation recapture provisions apply to the recognized gain.

Exhibit 19-4 contains a summary of the computations required in a § 351 transfer. A comprehensive example of § 351 transfers follows Exhibit 19-4.

---

[87] §§ 1245(b)(3) and 1250(d)(3).

EXHIBIT 19-4
Computation in a § 351 Transfer

Step 1: Compute the amount realized by the transferor [§ 1001(b)].

Fair market value of stock received			$xxx,xxx
Plus:	Amount of money received	$xx,xxx	
	Fair market value of other property received	xx,xxx	
	Liabilities assumed by transferee corporation	xx,xxx	+xx,xxx
Less:	Amount of money given up (paid)	$xx,xxx	
	Expenses of transfer	x,xxx	
	Liabilities assumed by the transferor	x,xxx	−xx,xxx
Equals:	Amount realized		$xxx,xxx

Step 2: Compute gain realized by transferor [§ 1001(a)].

Amount realized		$xxx,xxx
Less:	Adjusted basis in property transferred	−xx,xxx
Equals:	Gain realized	$ xx,xxx

Step 3: If any *boot* was *received*, compute transferor's gain recognized [§ 351 (b)].
Gain recognized equals *lesser* of
  a. Gain realized,
     or
  b. Boot received
  If no boot was received, then there is no gain recognized by the transferor.

Step 4: Compute shareholder's basis in stock received (§ 358).

Basis of property plus any money transferred			$ xx,xxx
Plus:	Gain recognized by transferor		+x,xxx
Less:	Money received by transferor	$ x,xxx	
	Fair market value of any other property (except stock) received by transferor	x,xxx	
	Liabilities assumed by transferee corporation	x,xxx	−x,xxx
Equals:	Shareholder's (transferor's) basis in stock received		$ xx,xxx

The shareholder's basis in any other property (boot) received is its fair market [see § 358(a)(2)].

Step 5: Compute the transferee corporation's basis in the property transferred to it (§ 362).

Transferor's basis in property		$ xx,xxx
Plus:	Gain recognized to transferor on transfer	+xx,xxx
Equals:	Transferee corporation's basis in property received	$ xx,xxx

Example 25. R and S pooled their assets to form a new corporation, T Incorporated. R transferred the following:

1. Land (adjusted basis of $54,000, fair market value of $75,000).

2. A mortgage of $52,000 which the land was subject to.

3. Cash of $7,000.

S transferred the following:

1. Patent (adjusted basis of $24,000, fair market value $31,000)

R received the following:

50 shares of T Corporation stock, fair market value* $30,000

S received the following:

50 shares of T Corporation stock, fair market value* $30,000
$1,000 cash

*The value of the T Corporation stock is computed as follows:

R's investment:

Land, FMV		$75,000
Less: Mortgage		(52,000)
Cash paid		7,000

S's investment:

Patent, FMV		31,000
Less: Cash received		(1,000)
Value of T Corporation stock		$60,000

Step 1: Compute amount realized.

		R	S
FMV of stock received		$30,000	$30,000
Plus: Money received		0	1,000
Liabilities assumed by transferee corporation		52,000	0
Less: Amount of money given up		(7,000)	0
Amount realized		$75,000	$31,000

Step 2: Compute gain realized.

		R	S
Amount realized		$75,000	$31,000
Less: Adjusted basis in property transferred		(54,000)	(24,000)
Gain realized		$21,000	$ 7,000

Step 3: Compute gain recognized.

Gain recognized equals lesser of

		R	S
a.	Gain realized	$21,000	$ 7,000
b.	Boot received	0	1,000
Gain recognized is		$ 0	$ 1,000

Step 4: Compute shareholder's basis in property received.

		R	S
Basis of property and money transferred ($54,000 + $7,000)		$61,000	$24,000
Plus: Gain recognized		0	1,000
Less: Money received,		0	(1,000)
Less: Liabilities assumed by the transferee		(52,000)	0
Shareholder's basis in stock received		$ 9,000	$24,000

Step 5: Compute corporation's basis in property received.

		R	S
Transferor's basis in property		$54,000	$24,000
Plus: Gain recognized to transferor on transfer		0	1,000
Basis in land received		$54,000	
Basis in patent received			$25,000

CAPITAL CONTRIBUTIONS

MADE BY SHAREHOLDERS

A corporation recognizes neither gain nor loss on the issuance or sale of its stock.[88] It is immaterial whether the stock is a newly authorized issue, previously unissued stock, or treasury stock that the corporation had previously acquired. If it is treasury stock that was purchased for a price different from its sale price, the difference is merely an increase or decrease in the stockholders' equity. If it is a new sale of stock, the discount or premium also is a stockholders' equity adjustment. The contingent liability associated with issuing par value stock at a discount has no counterpart in tax.[89] The sale of stock at a discount is treated as the issuance of stock for the amount received. This provision, however, does not prevent a corporation deducting as an expense the value of stock issued for services. However, no gain or loss is recognized.

The provision against recognizing gain or loss afforded a corporation applies only to the issuance or sale of the corporation's own stock. Sale or exchange of stock in another corporation will be treated as any other sale or exchange of an asset. The difference between cost and sale price will produce realized gain or loss. This general rule applies to stock acquired as a short-term investment as well as stock in related corporations.

In addition to the exclusion of gain or loss on the issuance of stock, contributions to capital are excluded from the corporation's income.[90] This exclusion applies to contributions from shareholders and nonshareholders. Although nonshareholder contributions are not as frequent as shareholder contributions, communities occasionally donate land and/or buildings in return for the relocation of a corporation's facilities.

MADE BY NONSHAREHOLDERS

There are special rules for contributions by nonshareholders.[91] Property contributed by a nonshareholder will have a *zero* basis. This prevents a corporation from obtaining a tax deduction either through depreciation or expense for the property. The provision was placed in the law because the value of the property is not treated as income to the corporation. This provision also guarantees that any amount received by the corporation upon sale of the property will be a taxable gain. The exclusion from income applies only to the receipt of property by the corporation as a contribution to capital, however.

If the property received by the corporation is money, the above rule does not apply. It is impossible to assign a zero basis to cash. Instead, the corporation is required to reduce the basis of property purchased using the cash by the amount of the contribution.[92] If the corporation does not acquire property with the contributed cash within 12 months, it is required to reduce the basis of property it already owns by the amount of the contribution.

---

[88]   § 1032.

[89]   In many states, it is *illegal* for a corporation to issue its own stock below par value.

[90]   § 118.

[91]   § 362(c)(1).

[92]   § 362(c)(2).

PROBLEM MATERIALS

DISCUSSION QUESTIONS

19-1 *What Is a Corporation?* Although an entity may be a corporation under state law, what characteristics must the entity possess to be treated as a corporation for Federal tax purposes? What difference will it make in the Federal tax classification if the entity possesses *all* or only a few of these characteristics?

19-2 *Disregard of Corporate Form.* Why might the IRS try to disregard the corporate status of an entity that meets the state law requirements for a corporation? Under what circumstances might shareholders try to use the corporate form but attempt to disregard it for Federal tax purposes?

19-3 *Corporate vs. Individual Taxation.* What are the differences in income tax treatment of corporations and individuals for the items below?
  a. Dividends received
  b. Classification of deductions
  c. Casualty losses
  d. Charitable contribution limitations
  e. Capital loss deduction
  f. Capital loss carryovers and carrybacks
  g. Gain on sale of depreciable realty

19-4 *Dividends-Received Deduction.* Why is a corporation allowed a dividends-received deduction? Under what circumstances is the recipient corporation allowed an 80 percent rather than the usual 70 percent dividends-received deduction?

19-5 *Limitations on Dividends-Received Deduction.* What are the limitations imposed on a corporation's dividends-received deduction? Under what circumstances can one of these limitations be disregarded?

19-6 *Charitable Contribution Carryovers.* Under what circumstances must a corporation carry over its qualifying contributions to subsequent years? If contributions are made in the current prior year, which contributions are deducted first? Why do you suppose Congress imposes this ordering of contribution deductions?

19-7 *Five-Percent Surtax.* Which corporations are subject to the five percent surtax? What is the marginal tax rate on the last dollar of taxable income of a corporation with taxable income of $170,000? What is the flat tax rate imposed on a corporation with taxable income of $335,000?

19-8 *Property Requirement of § 351.* What constitutes property for purposes of § 351? If an individual receives stock for both property and services, what are the tax consequences?

19-9 *What Are Transferring Persons?* What types of entities are "persons" for purposes of § 351? When might such "person" or "persons" make use of the § 351 nonrecognition provision?

19-10 *Solely for Stock.* What is considered stock for purposes of § 351? Why do you suppose Congress imposes as a requirement for nonrecognition treatment the receipt of only stock by the transferor?

19-11 *Control Requirement.* What is the control requirement for purposes of § 351? What is the meaning of the term "immediately" when used to qualify the control requirement?

19-12 *Taxable § 351 Transfers.* Under what circumstances may a transferor be subject to gain recognition even though his or her transfer is subject to § 351?

19-13 *Transfer of Liabilities.* Unlike Code § 1031 transactions (like-kind exchanges), the transfer (discharge) of a liability generally is not treated as boot for purposes of Code § 351. Explain.

19-14 *Transfer of Liabilities and Tax Avoidance.* A transferor is considering whether to receive some cash in addition to stock when she transfers appreciated property to a corporation, or to mortgage the property for a similar amount of money and then transfer the property and the liability to the corporation. What difference will either alternative make?

19-15 *Basis of Stock Received.* How does a shareholder determine basis in stock received in a § 351 transfer? If both common stock and preferred stock are received, how is basis in each determined?

19-16 *Corporation's Basis.* What is the corporation's basis in property received in a § 351 transfer? If due to his current tax situation a transferor will not incur additional income taxes on any gain recognized, would it benefit the corporation to have a partially taxable § 351 transfer? Explain.

19-17 *Depreciation Recapture.* How do the depreciation recapture rules (i.e., §§ 1245, 1250, 291) apply to a § 351 transfer?

PROBLEMS

19-18 *Comparison of Corporate vs. Individual Taxation.* In each of the situations below, explain the tax consequences if taxpayer T were either a corporation or a single individual.

   a. For the current year, T has gross income of $60,000, including $10,000 dividends from Ford Motor Company. Without regard to taxable income, how much of the dividend income will be subject to tax?

   b. During the current year, T sustains a total loss of an asset. The asset was valued at $2,000 shortly before the loss and had an adjusted basis of $2,700. If the casualty loss were incurred by T as an individual, it would be a personal rather than business loss. Without regard to any taxable income limitation, what is the measure of the casualty loss deduction?

   c. During 2009, T had $8,000 of long-term capital gains and $3,000 of short-term capital gains. During 2008, the only prior year with capital asset transactions, T had a short-term capital loss of $6,000. How much of T's 2009 gross income will consist of capital gains?

   d. T's taxable income for 2009, before any deduction for charitable contributions, is $50,000. If T were an individual, adjusted gross income would be $60,000. If T made cash contributions of $40,000 during the year, what is the maximum amount that could be claimed as a deduction for 2009?

19-19 *Dividends-Received Deduction.* K Corporation has the following items of revenue and expense for the current year:

Sales revenue, net of returns	$100,000
Cost of sales	30,000
Operating expenses	40,000
Dividends (subject to 70% rules)	20,000

    a. What is K Corporation's dividends-received deduction for the current year?

    b. Assuming that K Corporation's operating expenses were $72,000 instead of $40,000, what is its dividends-received deduction for the current year?

19-20 *Dividends-Received Deduction.* During 2009 R Corporation (a cash method, calendar year taxpayer) has the following income and expenses:

Revenue from operations	$170,000
Operating expenses	178,000
Dividends (subject to 70% rules)	40,000

    a. What is R Corporation's 2009 dividends-received deduction?

    b. Assuming R Corporation's 2009 tax year has not yet closed, what would be the effect on its dividends-received deduction if R accelerated to 2009 $5,000 of operating expenses planned for 2010?

19-21 *Organizational Expenditures.* G Corporation incurred and paid $6,800 of qualifying organizational expenditures in 2009. Assuming G Corporation makes an election under § 248 to expense and amortize these costs, what is the maximum amount that may be deducted for each of the following years if G Corporation adopts a calendar tax year?

    a. For 2009, during which G Corporation began business on September 1?

    b. Calendar year 2010?

    c. Calendar year 2014?

19-22 *Charitable Contributions Deductions.* T Corporation has the following for tax year 2009:

Net income from operations	$600,000
Dividends received (subject to 70% rules)	100,000

    a. What is T Corporation's maximum charitable contribution deduction for 2009?

    b. Assuming T Corporation made charitable contributions of $68,000 during 2009 and had a $10,000 charitable contribution carryover from 2007, how much of its 2008 contributions will be carried over to 2010?

19-23 *Computation of Corporate Tax Liability.* L Corporation had taxable income of $150,000 for 2008. What is L Corporation's 2008 income tax liability before credits or prepayments?

19-24 *Corporate Tax Computation.* T Corporation had the following items of income for its calendar year 2009:

Net income from operations	$150,000
Dividends received (subject to 70% rules)	10,000
Charitable contributions	30,000
Net operating loss carryover from 2008	30,000
Long-term capital gains	8,000
Long-term capital losses	6,000
Short-term capital gains	3,000
Capital loss carryover from 2008	9,000

    a. Compute T Corporation's 2009 income tax liability before credits or prepayments.

    b. What is the nature and amount of any carryovers to 2010?

19-25   *Corporate Formation.* Individuals J and R form the JR Corporation. J transfers land with a basis of $50,000 and a fair market value of $100,000. R transfers all the depreciable property from his former business, which has a basis of $80,000 and a fair market value of $70,000. In order to be an equal shareholder, R also transfers cash of $30,000 to the corporation. J and R each receive 100 shares of JR Corporation stock.

    a. What is J's realized gain or loss? Recognized gain or loss?
    b. What is R's realized gain or loss? Recognized gain or loss?
    c. What basis will J have in the JR Corporation stock?
    d. What basis will JR Corporation have in the land?
    e. What basis will R have in the JR Corporation stock?
    f. What basis will JR Corporation have in the depreciable property?

19-26   *Corporate Formation.* Individuals K, L, and M form the KLM Corporation. K transfers land with a basis of $30,000, with fair market value of $100,000, and which is subject to a $20,000 mortgage in exchange for 80 shares of KLM common stock. L transfers $50,000 cash and equipment with a basis of $25,000 and fair market value of $40,000 in exchange for 90 shares of KLM common stock. M transfers $18,000 cash and renders services incident to the organization of KLM Corporation in exchange for 30 shares of its common stock.

    Net of the mortgage transferred by K and assumed by the corporation, KLM issued 188 shares of common stock in exchange for money and other property with a net fair market value of $188,000 [$80,000 from K ($100,000 fair market value of land − $20,000 mortgage) + $90,000 from L ($50,000 cash + $40,000 fair market value of equipment) + $18,000 cash from M]. The additional 12 shares of common stock issued to M were in exchange for services.

    a. What is K's realized and recognized gain?
    b. What basis will K have in the KLM stock?
    c. What basis will KLM Corporation have in the land?
    d. How much gain must L recognize?
    e. What basis will L have in the KLM stock?
    f. What basis will KLM Corporation have in the equipment?
    g. How much income, if any, must M recognize?
    h. What basis will M have in the KLM stock?
    i. Assume that KLM Corporation incurred and paid $6,800 of organizational costs, in addition to its payment of stock in exchange for M's services incident to organization. If the corporation begins business on October 1, 2009, adopts a calendar tax year, and elects to expense and amortize its organizational expenditures, what amount can KLM Corporation deduct for 2009?

19-27   *Transfer of Liabilities.* Each of the transfers below qualifies as a § 351 transaction, and in each case the transferee corporation assumes liabilities involved in the transfer. For each transfer, compute the transferor shareholder's recognized gain, the transferor's basis in any stock or securities received, and the transferee corporation's basis in any property received.

    a. T transfers land with a basis of $60,000 and subject to a mortgage of $20,000 in exchange for stock worth $55,000.
    b. A transfers machinery with a basis of $4,000 and subject to a mortgage of $9,000 in exchange for stock worth $6,000. The $9,000 mortgage was created two weeks before the transfer and A used the loan proceeds to take her husband on a vacation trip to Europe.
    c. Assume the same facts in (b) except that the $9,000 liability is the balance remaining on a five-year $40,000 mortgage loan created to acquire the machinery transferred by A.
    d. X transfers equipment with a basis of $30,000 and subject to a liability of $10,000 in exchange for stock worth $80,000 and a $20,000 security (bond) maturing in 10 years and paying 15 percent interest annually.

RESEARCH PROBLEMS

19-28 *Corporate Formation.* T, an individual taxpayer, plans to incorporate his farming and ranching activities currently operated as a sole proprietorship. His primary purpose of incorporating is to transfer a portion of his ownership in land to his son and daughter. T believes that gifts of stock rather than land will keep his business intact. T's current thought is to incorporate and immediately transfer 40 percent of the corporate stock to his two children. In fact, he has promised his children that he would make the stock gifts as soon as the corporation is created. What potential tax problems might result if T pursues his current plans? Would it make any difference if T received all voting stock and had the new corporation transfer nonvoting stock to the children?

Research aid:

Rev. Rul. 59-259, 1959-2 C.B. 115.

19-29 *Admission of New Shareholder.* RST Corporation is currently owned by three individuals, R, S, and T. The corporation has a net worth of $750,000 and has 500 shares (1,000 shares authorized) of common stock outstanding. R owns 200 shares (40 percent), and S and T each own 150 shares (30 percent). Individual E owns land worth $90,000 which the corporation could use as a new plant site. However, E is not interested in selling the land now because it would result in a large capital gain tax. E is willing to transfer the land to the corporation in exchange for 60 shares of its common stock or securities of equivalent value, but only if the transfer will be nontaxable. How would you advise the parties to structure the transaction?

Research aids:

Rev. Rul. 73-472, 1973-2 C.B. 115.
Rev. Proc. 76-22, 1976-1 C.B. 562.
Reg. § 1.351-1(a)(1)(ii).

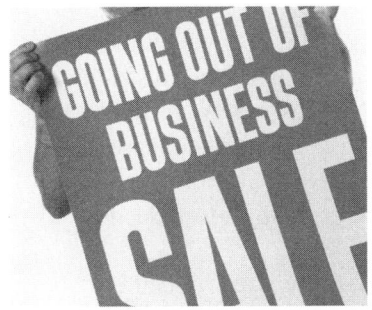

CHAPTER TWENTY

CORPORATE DISTRIBUTIONS, REDEMPTIONS AND LIQUIDATIONS

LEARNING OBJECTIVES

Upon completion of this chapter you will be able to:

▸ Determine the tax consequences of dividend distributions to shareholders and the distributing corporation

▸ Compute a corporation's earnings and profits

▸ Identify the more common types of constructive dividends

▸ Explain the tax consequences of taxable and nontaxable stock dividends

▸ Define a redemption and distinguish it from other types of nonliquidating distributions

▸ Explain the tax consequences of a redemption to a shareholder and the distributing corporation

▸ Define a liquidation and determine its tax consequences to shareholders and the liquidating corporation

▸ Discuss the special rules that apply when a corporation liquidates a subsidiary

CHAPTER OUTLINE

INTRODUCTION

The life cycle of a corporation starts with its formation. This is followed by a period of operation and growth. During the growth stage, the corporation generally makes distributions to its shareholders, called *dividends.* Shareholders not only expect to receive dividends, but also expect their stock to appreciate in value. Following the growth phase, the corporation enters a period of maturity. In the maturity stage profits may stabilize, but eventually business may start to decline. A decline may force the corporation to redeem stock, reorganize, or possibly liquidate.

This chapter deals with the Federal income tax aspects of corporate dividends, redemptions of stock, and liquidations as they relate to both the shareholders and the corporations.

DIVIDENDS

A distribution by a corporation of cash or property to a shareholder is income to the shareholder to the extent it is a *dividend.*[1] A dividend is defined as a distribution by a corporation out of either its accumulated earnings and profits since 1913 (the inception of corporate income tax) or its earnings and profits for the current year.[2] If the distribution exceeds the corporation's earnings and profits, the excess is treated as a nontaxable reduction of the shareholder's basis in his or her stock. If the distribution exceeds both the corporation's earnings and profits and the shareholder's adjusted basis in his or her stock, the excess is treated as a gain on the sale of the shareholder's stock.

> **Example 1.** J purchased 100 shares of M Corporation common stock on January 1, 2002 for $1,000. On February 3, 2009, M Corporation distributed to J $5,000 with respect to its stock, of which $2,300 is a dividend. (The amount of M Corporation's earnings and profits allocable to J is $2,300.)
>
> J is required to include this $2,300 of dividend income in gross income. The remaining $2,700 is applied first to reduce the $1,000 basis of J's stock to zero, and the rest ($1,700) is treated as a gain on the sale of his stock. It will be a long-term capital gain since he has held the stock as an investment for more than one year. J still has the 100 shares of stock, but his basis is reduced to zero.

EARNINGS AND PROFITS

The term *earnings and profits* (also referred to as "E&P") is not defined in either the Internal Revenue Code or the Regulations. Instead, the effect of certain transactions on earnings and profits is described.[3] From an examination of these transactions, however, it is possible to create a general definition of earnings and profits. Basically, corporate earnings and profits equal taxable income *increased* by nontaxable income and *decreased* by nondeductible expenses. Although earnings and profits are similar to retained earnings as used in financial accounting, there are often significant differences between the two. These differences are caused by differences in the treatment of various items (e.g., stock dividends) for financial accounting purposes as opposed to the items' tax treatment. Therefore, the computation of earnings and profits should be completely independent of any computation of retained earnings.

---

[1]   § 301.

[2]   § 316(a).

[3]   § 312.

As mentioned previously, earnings and profits generally consist of taxable income plus nontaxable income minus nondeductible expenses. Exhibit 20-1 contains a partial list of the adjustments that must be made to determine earnings and profits for a taxable year.

Although most are self-explanatory, several items in Exhibit 20-1 require further clarification. For example, while there is an adjustment for tax-exempt interest income, there is no adjustment for the portion of a gain that is realized but not recognized in a like-kind exchange. A gain on the sale of assets affects earnings and profits only to the extent that the gain is recognized.[4]

Depreciation. The use of accelerated depreciation is not permitted in computing earnings and profits.[5] The corporation generally must use the straight-line method. Specifically, depreciation for E&P purposes must be computed under the Alternative Depreciation System (ADS), using the straight-line method and the property's class life. Because taxable income reflects any accelerated methods used, an adjustment in determining earnings and profits is to *add* to taxable income the excess of the accelerated depreciation over straight-line. In the later years of the asset's class life, the corporation would be required to *subtract* from taxable income the excess of straight-line depreciation over accelerated depreciation.

Example 2. N Corporation uses the 150% declining balance method to compute the depreciation on its warehouse. (Assume that all other assets are depreciated using the straight-line method and that there are no other adjustments to earnings and profits.) The depreciation claimed on the warehouse for the current year (2009) was $7,350. Straight-line depreciation using ADS on the warehouse would have been $5,000. N Corporation's taxable income for 2009 was $19,000. Earnings and profits for 2009 are computed as follows:

Taxable income for 2009		$19,000
Plus: Excess of accelerated over straight-line depreciation:		
Accelerated depreciation	$7,350	
Straight-line depreciation	(5,000)	+ 2,350
Earnings and profits for 2009		$21,350

---

4   § 312(f)(1).

5   § 312(k)(1).

EXHIBIT 20-1

Partial List of Adjustments Used in Computing Current Earnings and Profits

Taxable Income

Plus:

Tax-exempt interest income

Deferred gain on installment sales

Dividends-received deduction

Excess of accelerated depreciation over straight-line depreciation

Excess of ACRS depreciation over straight-line depreciation [§ 312(k)(3)]

Excess of LIFO cost of goods sold over FIFO cost of goods sold

Four-fifths ($\frac{4}{5}$) of deduction for immediate expensing of assets under § 179 taken during
the current year [§ 312(k)(3)(B)]

Excess of depletion taken over cost depletion

Increases in cash surrender value of life insurance when the corporation is the beneficiary
(directly or indirectly)

Proceeds of life insurance when the corporation is the beneficiary (directly or indirectly)

Net operating loss deductions carried over from other years

Federal income tax refunds

Recoveries of bad debts and other deductions, but only if they *are* not included in taxable
income under the tax benefit doctrine

Income based on the percentage-of-completion rather than the completed contract method

In the year they are reflected in taxable income: charitable contribution carryovers, capital loss
carryovers, and other timing differences (since they reduced E&P in the year that
they originated)

Minus:

Federal income taxes

Nondeductible expenses:

Penalties and fines

Payments to public officials not reflected in taxable income

Expenses between related parties not deductible under § 267

Interest expense related to the production of tax-exempt income

Life insurance premiums when the corporation is the beneficiary (directly or indirectly)

Travel, entertainment, and gift expenses that do not meet the substantiation
requirements of § 247(d)

Fifty percent of meals and entertainment disallowed as a deduction under § 274(n)

Other expenses disallowed to the corporation as the result of an IRS audit

Nondeductible losses between related parties under § 267

Charitable contributions in excess of the 10 percent limitation

Excess capital losses for the year that are not deductible

Gains on sales of depreciable property to the extent that accelerated depreciation or
ACRS exceeds the straight-line depreciation method used for computing increases in E&P

Gains on sales of depletable property to the extent that depletion taken exceeds cost depletion

One-fifth ($\frac{1}{5}$) of any immediate expensing deduction under §179 taken during the previous
four years [§ 312(k)(3)(B)]

Foreign taxes paid that have been treated as credits on the corporations tax return

Equals: **Current Earnings and Profits**

> *Note:* This exhibit does not include the effect of corporate distributions and dividends on E&P,
> which is discussed later in the chapter.

Code § 179 Expense. If a corporation has elected the immediate expensing option of § 179, E&P adjustments are made for the year in which the asset is expensed and also for the four following years.[6] The effect of a § 179 election on earnings and profits is that the amount expensed is an earnings and profits deduction in equal installments over the five-year period.

> **Example 3.** X Corporation elected to expense a $5,000 asset under § 179 in 2009. X Corporation's taxable income for 2009 was $20,000. Although the entire $5,000 deduction is reflected in X Corporation's taxable income, the amount that affects E&P is $1,000 per year for five years. Therefore, taxable income must be adjusted as follows (assume there are no other adjustments to earnings and profits):
>
> | | |
> |---|---:|
> | 2009 Taxable income | $20,000 |
> | Plus: $\frac{4}{5}$ of immediate expensing deduction ($\frac{4}{5}$ of $5,000) | 4,000 |
> | 2009 Earnings and profits | $24,000 |
>
> In 2010, through 2013, $1,000 per year ($\frac{1}{5}$ of the 2009 immediate expensing deduction) is subtracted when computing E&P.

Adjustments to More Accurately Reflect Income. Over the years, Congress has required additional adjustments to be made in the computation of a corporation's earnings and profits in an attempt to have E&P more accurately reflect the corporation's current economic gain or loss.[7] One of the most important of these adjustments affects corporations using the LIFO method of inventory valuation. These firms must adjust E&P for the *difference* between the inventory as valued by LIFO and the value the inventory would have if FIFO had been used.[8]

Another similar adjustment applies to corporations that use the installment method for any asset sale. The corporation's E&P must include the full amount of the gain in the year of sale as if the corporation had not used the installment method.[9]

DISTRIBUTIONS FROM EARNINGS AND PROFITS

A special approach has been designed for determining whether a distribution is made out of E&P and therefore treated as a dividend. This approach treats E&P as consisting of two distinctly separate pools of earnings from which distributions may be made: current E&P and accumulated E&P. Using this approach, the law creates a presumption that any distribution made during the year is deemed to come *first* from any current E&P that may exist.[10] If distributions during the year *exceed* current E&P, the distribution is treated as having been paid from any accumulated E&P. Note that under this "two-pot" process, it is possible for a distribution to be a taxable dividend out of current E&P even though the corporation has a deficit in accumulated E&P that, in fact, exceeds current E&P. In addition, a distribution may be treated as a taxable dividend even though it is distributed at a time during the year when the firm had a current loss. This result can occur because current E&P is computed at the close of the taxable year, without reduction for any distributions.

---

[6]   § 312(k)(3)(B).

[7]   § 312(n).

[8]   § 312(n)(5).

[9]   § 312(n)(6).

[10]   Reg. § 1.316-2(a).

Example 4. T Corporation distributed $10,000 cash on February 1 and $10,000 on November 1. The corporation has $25,000 of current earnings and profits and $15,000 of accumulated earnings and profits. The entire $20,000 distributed is a taxable dividend from current earnings and profits, since distributions are considered to come first from current earnings and profits and then from accumulated earnings and profits.

Example 5. Assume the same facts as in *Example 4* except that there is a deficit in accumulated earnings and profits of $15,000. The $20,000 distributed is still a taxable dividend since there are current earnings and profits of $25,000. Accumulated earnings and profits will still have a deficit of $15,000.

Example 6. R Corporation made a $15,000 distribution to its shareholders on December 31. R Corporation has $3,000 earnings and profits for the current year and $18,000 accumulated earnings and profits. The entire $15,000 distribution is a taxable dividend. Accumulated earnings and profits are reduced to $6,000 as a result of the distribution.

In applying this basic scheme to determine whether a distribution is in fact a dividend, the following additional rules must be observed:[11]

1. Current E&P is allocated among *all* distributions made during the year on a pro rata basis, as follows:

$$\frac{\text{Amount of the distribution}}{\text{Total current distributions}} \times \frac{\text{Amount of}}{\text{current E\&P}} = \frac{\text{Distribution's share}}{\text{of current E\&P}}$$

Example 7. During the current year, P Corporation distributed $12,000 to its shareholders on March 1 and an other $12,000 to its shareholders on October 1. Current E&P was only $10,000. Each distribution would be treated as consisting of $5,000 of current E&P [($12,000 ÷ $24,000) × $10,000]. The balance of each distribution would be deemed to come from any accumulated E&P that may exist at the time of the distribution.

2. Accumulated E&P is allocated among distributions made during the year in *chronological order.*

Example 8. Same facts as in *Example 7*. In addition, the corporation had accumulated E&P of $7,000. Earnings and profits are allocated as follows:

	$12,000 March Distribution	$12,000 October Distribution	Total
Current earnings and profits [allocated pro rata to all distributions: ($12,000 ÷ $24,000) × $10,000 current E&P = $5,000]	$ 5,000	$5,000	$10,000
Accumulated earnings and profits (allocated in chronological order: first to the March distribution and then to the October distribution)	7,000	0	7,000
Taxable dividend	$12,000	$5,000	$17,000

The entire amount of the March distribution ($12,000) is a taxable dividend, but only $5,000 of the October distribution is a taxable dividend to the shareholders. The

---

[11]   Reg. § 1.316-2.

remaining $7,000 of the October distribution is a return of capital to the shareholders and will first be applied to reduce their bases in their stock. Any amount in excess of their stock bases will be treated as a gain from the sale of their stock.

This allocation process becomes especially important if there is a change of ownership during the year, since each shareholder is concerned with how much of each distribution he or she receives is taxable as dividends. However, the *total* amount of taxable dividends is not affected by the allocations.

3. If there is a deficit in current E&P for the year (e.g., a current operating loss), it is treated as occurring *ratably* during the year (unless it can be shown that the loss did not occur evenly during the year).[12] Accordingly, the loss is allocated on a daily basis against any accumulated E&P.

Example 9. T Corporation distributed $10,000 to its shareholders on February 1 and $10,000 to its shareholders on October 1. T Corporation had a $6,000 loss for its current calendar tax year and accumulated earnings and profits from prior years of $20,000. The $6,000 loss is assumed to have occurred evenly throughout the year (assume $500 per month). The tax treatment of the distributions is determined as follows:

February distribution: Since there are no current earnings and profits, the distribution is presumed to come from accumulated earnings and profits. Accumulated earnings and profits as of February 1 are considered to be $19,500 [$20,000 − $500 (one month of the current loss)]. The entire February distribution of $10,000 is a taxable dividend since accumulated earnings and profits are applied chronologically.

The balance in accumulated earnings and profits after the February distribution is $9,500 ($20,000 − $500 − $10,000).

October distribution: Since there are no current earnings and profits, the next step is to look at accumulated earnings and profits. Accumulated earnings and profits as of October 1 are $5,500 [$9,500 remaining after the February 1 distribution − $4,000 (8 months of current loss @ $500 per month from February through September)]. Therefore, $5,500 of the October distribution is a taxable dividend to the shareholders. The remaining $4,500 is a return of capital to the shareholders. After the October 1 distribution, the balance in accumulated earnings and profits is zero.

At the end of the year, the balance in accumulated earnings and profits is a deficit of $1,500 (the remaining 3 months of current loss at $500 per month).

CASH DIVIDENDS

Shareholders are required to include in income the amount of any distribution that is a dividend. If the distribution is cash, the amount of the distribution is simply the amount of the cash. As demonstrated in the above examples, earnings and profits are reduced by the amount of the cash distribution, but not below zero.[13]

PROPERTY DIVIDENDS

Corporations make distributions of property as well as distributions of cash. Code § 317(a) defines property as "money, securities, and any other property," but excludes

---

[12]   *Ibid.*

[13]   § 312(a)(1).

from the definition stock and stock rights in the distributing corporation. Special rules must be followed when a property distribution is made. Basically, the thrust of the property distribution rules is to treat the corporation and shareholders as if the corporation had sold the property and distributed to the shareholders the cash proceeds from the sale.

Code § 311 provides that a corporation must recognize gain—*but not loss*—upon the distribution of property other than its own obligations.[14] Thus, when a corporation distributes property that has a value exceeding its basis, gain must be recognized. In contrast, a corporation is not allowed to recognize loss on a distribution of property whose value is less than its basis. This rule prohibits a corporation and its shareholders from circumventing the gain recognition requirement by distributing loss property that would offset the gain on appreciated property. When the corporation distributes appreciated property and recognizes gain, its E&P is first increased by the gain and then reduced by the fair market value of the property distributed.[15] In contrast, if the corporation distributes depreciated property, no loss is recognized and the corporation decreases its E&P by the basis of the property distributed.[16]

Both corporate and noncorporate shareholders that receive a distribution of property report the fair market value of the property as a dividend to the extent it is out of the corporation's E&P.[17] The shareholder's basis in the property is also its fair market value.[18]

> **Example 10.** P Corporation distributed land worth $100,000 (basis $20,000) and equipment worth $30,000 (basis $45,000) to its sole shareholder, individual X. The corporation must recognize the $80,000 ($100,000 − $20,000) gain realized on the distribution of the land. Although P also realizes a loss on the distribution of the equipment, the loss is not recognized. Assuming the corporation has adequate E&P, X reports a dividend of $130,000 (the fair market values of the property, $100,000 + $30,000). X's basis in the land and equipment is $100,000 and $30,000, respectively. The net effect of the distribution on the corporation's E&P is to decrease it by $65,000 ($80,000 gain − $100,000 value of the land − $45,000 basis of the equipment).

Adjustments for Liabilities. The above discussion ignores the possibilities that the property may be distributed subject to a liability or that the shareholder may assume a liability in conjunction with the property distribution. In such case, the rules regarding the amount of the distribution and the adjustment to E&P must be modified to account for any liabilities.[19] When a liability is distributed in connection with property, the amount of the distribution is decreased by the liability. Similarly, the reduction in E&P is decreased (i.e., E&P is increased by the amount of the liability). There is no adjustment to the basis of the property to the shareholder.

CONSTRUCTIVE DIVIDENDS

In addition to actual distributions of cash and property, a shareholder can be charged with the *constructive receipt* of a dividend. For example, excessive salaries to the shareholder or a member of the shareholder's family can be treated as a dividend. The

---

[14]   §§ 311(a) and (b).

[15]   § 312(b).

[16]   § 312(a)(3).

[17]   § 301(b)(1).

[18]   § 301(d).

[19]   § 301(b)(2).

corporation is limited to deducting only those salaries that are reasonable. The amount in excess of the reasonable standard will be considered a constructive dividend. Other transactions that have given rise to constructive dividends are:

1. Loans to shareholders where there is no intent to repay the amounts loaned

2. Bargain purchases and rentals of corporate property by shareholders

3. Excess payment for corporate use of shareholder property

4. Payment of shareholder's loans or expenses by the corporation

5. Personal use by shareholder of corporate assets

As indicated by the above types of transactions, constructive dividends usually arise in closely held corporations, especially those with only one or two shareholders. Constructive dividends are not planned by the corporations. They usually arise in an IRS audit as the result of lack of formality in dealing with the corporate entity and a lack of transactions at "arm's length" (for fair market value). Therefore, it is possible for a shareholder to be considered as having received a dividend even though the corporation did not declare one.

As with other dividends, the corporation must have sufficient earnings and profits for a constructive dividend to be taxable to the shareholders. Also, the dividends-received deduction is available to corporate shareholders with respect to constructive dividends.

STOCK DIVIDENDS AND STOCK RIGHTS

Occasionally, a corporation may want to pay a dividend but does not have sufficient cash or property to distribute. In this situation, the corporation may declare a dividend of its stock or of rights to acquire its stock.

Stock Dividends. As a general rule, a shareholder does not have any income as the result of receiving a distribution of the distributing corporation's own stock.[20] Instead, the shareholder simply allocates the basis of his or her old stock between the old stock and the new stock. There are several exceptions to this general rule, however. If the shareholder is given a choice between receiving stock or receiving property or money, the distribution will be taxable.[21] It does not matter which form of distribution the shareholder actually selects. The ability to select makes the distribution taxable. In fact, the ability of *any* of the shareholders to select property or stock will make the distribution taxable to all of the shareholders.[22]

Another case in which a stock dividend will be taxable is if the distribution is *disproportionate*.[23] The Code defines *disproportionate* in this situation as the receipt of cash or other property by some shareholders with an increase in the proportionate interests of other shareholders in the corporation. The determination as to whether or not a distribution is disproportionate is made at the end of the distribution or series of distributions and is made based on the result of the transactions.

Distributions of preferred stock to common stockholders are covered by the general rule of nontaxability. However, a distribution or a series of distributions that results in some shareholders receiving common and others receiving preferred is a taxable transaction.[24] In addition, any distribution (e.g., common stock) to a preferred stockholder

---

[20]   § 305(a).

[21]   § 305(b)(1).

[22]   Reg. § 1.305-2.

[23]   § 305(b)(2).

[24]   § 305(b)(3).

is taxable.[25] A special rule applies for distributions of convertible preferred stock. The distribution will be taxable unless it can be shown that the result will not be disproportionate[26] (see above for definition of disproportionate).

Taxable stock dividends can be either actual or deemed dividends.[27] Actual dividends require distributions of stock. Deemed-dividend transactions include changes in conversion ratios, changes in redemption price, an excess redemption price over issue price, or any other transaction that increases the proportionate ownership of one or more shareholders. Deemed dividends can be totally unintentional. For example, in a corporate reorganization the issuance of preferred stock with a redemption value greater than its current issue price is a possible taxable stock dividend.[28]

Nontaxable Stock Dividends. If the taxpayer receives a nontaxable distribution of stock, the basis of the shares received is determined by allocation. The basis of the shares upon which the dividend is received is allocated between the old stock and the new stock based on their relative fair market values at the time of distribution.[29] If the shares received are identical to the shares owned (i.e., both the old and new stock are the same class of common stock), the allocation can be accomplished simply by dividing the basis of the old stock by the total number of shares owned after the distribution. If the type of shares received differs from the shares originally owned (e.g., old stock was common stock and new stock is preferred stock), the allocation of basis between the old stock and new stock is computed based on relative fair market value. The holding period of the new stock includes the holding period of the old stock.[30]

Example 11. Q owned 100 shares of common stock of V Corporation. His basis in the V Corporation stock was $1,300 ($13 per share). Q received a stock dividend of 25 additional shares of V Corporation common stock in a nontaxable distribution. Q's $1,300 basis in the old stock is allocated between his old stock (100 shares) and his new stock (25 shares) as follows:

$$\frac{\text{Basis in old stock}}{\text{Number of shares after distribution}} \times \frac{\$1,300}{125 \text{ shares}} = \underline{\$10.40} \text{ per share}$$

Q's basis in his stock is still $1,300, which is $10.40 per share, since he now has 125 values of V Corporation common stock.

Example 12. Assume the same facts as in *Example 11* except that Q received 25 shares of preferred stock instead of common stock. On the date of distribution, the fair market value of V Corporation common stock was $15 per share and the fair market value of V Corporation preferred stock was $5 per share. Q's $1,300 basis in his stock is allocated between the old stock and the new stock as follows:

Step 1: Determine fair market value of stock:

Fair market value of Q's common stock (100 shares × $15).........	$1,500
Fair market value of Q's preferred stock (25 shares × $5)	125
Total fair market value of Q's stock	$1,625

---

[25] § 305(b)(4).

[26] § 305(b)(5).

[27] § 305(c).

[28] See Rev. Rul. 83-119, 1983-2 C.B. 57.

[29] Reg. § 1.307-1.

[30] § 1223(5).

Step 2: Compute basis in each type of stock based on relative fair market value:

(a) $\dfrac{\text{Fair market value of Q's common stock}}{\text{Total fair market value of Q's stock}} \times \text{Old basis} = \begin{array}{c}\text{New basis in}\\\text{common stock}\end{array}$

$\dfrac{\$1,500}{\$1,625} \times \$1,300 = \underline{\underline{\$1,200}}$ $\begin{array}{c}\text{New basis in}\\\text{common stock}\end{array}$ ($12 per share)

(b) $\dfrac{\text{Fair market value of Q's preferred stock}}{\text{Total fair market value of Q's stock}} \times \text{Old basis} = \begin{array}{c}\text{New basis in}\\\text{preferred stock}\end{array}$

$\dfrac{\$125}{\$1,625} \times \$1,300 = \underline{\underline{\$100}}$ $\begin{array}{c}\text{Basis in}\\\text{preferred stock}\end{array}$ ($4 per share)

A nontaxable stock dividend *does not affect* the earnings and profits of the distributing corporation.[31]

Taxable Stock Dividends. The recipient shareholder must treat a taxable distribution of stock the same as a property distribution. If the stock distribution is taxable, the shareholder must report dividend income equal to the *lesser* of the fair market value of the stock received or the distributing corporation's earnings and profits.[32] The basis of the stock received is the amount of income reported.[33] The holding period of the shares received would start on the date of distribution. The basis of the original stock is not affected by a taxable stock dividend. Taxable stock dividends have the same effect on the earnings and profits of a corporation as property dividends. However, the distributing corporation does not recognize gain or loss from taxable distribution of its stock.

Stock Rights. Instead of stock, corporations may distribute stock rights to their shareholders. The taxation of the receipt of stock rights is governed by the same general principles as stock dividends.[34] In determining whether the distribution is taxable, it is often easier to assume that the stock that can be acquired by exercise of the rights was distributed instead of the rights. If the distribution of the stock to which the stock rights apply would have been taxable, the rights are taxable. If a distribution of the related stock would not have been taxable, the rights are not taxable.

Example 13. N Corporation had 100 shares of common stock and 100 shares of nonvoting preferred stock outstanding. The corporation distributed rights to acquire a new issue of nonvoting preferred stock to all of its existing shareholders. The common shareholders have received a nontaxable distribution, whereas the preferred shareholders have received a taxable distribution. Since the distribution of the new preferred stock to the common shareholders would have been nontaxable, the rights received by the common shareholders are nontaxable. However, since preferred shareholders receive only taxable stock dividends, the rights received by the preferred shareholders also are taxable.

Nontaxable Stock Rights. If the stock rights are not taxable, there is a basis allocation similar to the one for stock dividends.[35] The basis of the old stock is allocated between the old stock and the new rights based on the relative fair market values at the

---

[31]   § 312(d)(1).

[32]   Reg. § 1.305-1(b)(1); Code §§ 301(b) and 316(a).

[33]   § 301(d).

[34]   § 305(a).

[35]   § 307(a).

date of distribution. There is no allocation of basis to the rights if the shareholder allows them to lapse[36] (and consequently no recognized loss on the lapse of the rights). Therefore, although the allocation uses the fair market values as of the date of distribution, the actual allocation generally is not made until the rights are sold or exercised.

Example 14. T Corporation distributed nontaxable stock rights to its shareholders on January 3. C received 100 rights on the 100 shares of common stock he purchased three years ago for $1,000. On the date of distribution, T Corporation's common stock had a value of $15 per share and the rights had a value of $5 each. On March 1, C sold the rights for $7 each. The stock had a value of $17 per share on March 1. C allocates the basis of his old stock between the stock and the rights based on their relative fair market values as of January 3, the date of the distribution. The March 1 value of the stock is irrelevant. The basis allocation is computed as follows:

Step 1:	Fair market value of C's common stock (100 × $15)	$1,500
	Fair market value of C's stock rights (100 × $5)	500
	Total fair market value of stock and stock rights	$2,000

$$(a) \quad \frac{\text{Fair market value of C's common stock}}{\text{Total fair market value of stock and stock rights}} \times \text{Old basis}$$

$$= \frac{\$1,500}{\$2,000} \times \$1,000 = \underline{\$750} \quad (\$7.50 \text{ per share})$$

$$(b) \quad \frac{\text{Fair market value of C's stock rights}}{\text{Total fair market value of stock and stock rights}} \times \text{Old basis}$$

$$= \frac{\$500}{\$2,000} \times \$1,000 = \underline{\$250} \quad (\$2.50 \text{ per stock right})$$

C's gain on the sale of his stock rights is computed as follows:

Selling price of stock rights (100 × $7)	$700
Less: Basis in stock rights	−250
Gain on sale of stock rights	$450

Example 15. Assume the same facts as in *Example 14* except that C does not sell the stock rights, but allows them to lapse on June 1. Since the stock rights lapsed, rather than being exercised or sold, there is no basis allocated to them. C has no recognized loss (since the rights have no basis) and the basis of the old shares remains $1,000.

If the taxpayer sells or exercises his or her rights, basis is allocated to the rights. The holding period of the rights includes the holding period of the old stock.[37] The fair market value of stock rights is frequently small in relation to the value of the stock on which it was distributed. As a result, an allocation of basis between the old stock and the new rights would produce a very small basis in the stock rights. For this reason, there is an

---

[36] Reg. § 1.307-1(a).

[37] § 1223(5).

exception to the rule regarding allocation of basis. If the fair market value of the stock rights is *less than* 15 percent of the value of the stock at the date of distribution, no basis is *required* to be allocated to the rights.[38] The basis of the rights is zero and the basis of the old stock remains unchanged. However, even though the basis of the rights is zero, the holding period of the rights includes the holding period of the old stock.[39] If a taxpayer wishes, he or she may elect to allocate basis to the rights even though there is no requirement to allocate basis to the rights under this 15-percent rule.[40] This election to allocate is made by filing a statement with the taxpayer's tax return for the year in which the rights are received. The election applies to all the stock rights received in the distribution and is irrevocable

> **Example 16.** Assume the same facts as in *Example 14* except that the fair market values of the stock and rights on January 3 were $19 and $1, respectively. Since the value of the rights ($100) is less than 15% of the value of the stock (15% of $1,900 = $285), no allocation is required. C would have a $700 gain on the sale of the stock rights since their basis was zero. The gain would be long-term since the holding period of the rights includes the holding period of the stock.

> **Example 17.** Assume the same facts as in *Example 16* except that C elects to allocate basis between the stock and the stock rights. The basis of the rights is computed as follows:

$$\frac{\text{Fair market value of stock rights}}{\text{Fair market value of stock and stock rights}} \times \text{Old basis}$$

$$= \frac{(100 \text{ rights} \times \$1)}{(100 \text{ rights} \times \$1) + (100 \text{ shares} \times \$19)} \times \underline{\underline{\$1,000}} \text{ Old basis}$$

$$\frac{\$100}{\$2,000} \times \$1,000 = \underline{\underline{\$50}} \text{ basis in stock rights}$$

In this situation, the sale of the rights for $700 would result in a $650 gain.

Taxable Stock Rights. The taxable receipt of stock rights, like a taxable stock dividend, is treated as a property dividend by the shareholder. The shareholder would have dividend income equal to the lesser of the fair market value of the rights on date of receipt or the distributing corporation's earnings and profits.[41] The rights would have a basis equal to the fair market value[42] and the holding period starts on the date of distribution. If the rights lapse, the taxpayer will have a loss equal to the basis of the rights. Stock rights have the same effect on a corporation's earnings and profits as stock dividends. Additionally, the corporation does not recognize gain or loss from taxable distributions of its stock rights.

NONDEDUCTIBILITY OF DIVIDENDS TO CORPORATION

A corporation is not permitted a deduction for distributions to its shareholders with respect to its stock. It does not matter whether the distribution is cash, property, stock, or stock rights. As mentioned in Chapter 19, this produces "double taxation." The shareholders are taxed individually on dividends (distributed corporate earnings and

[38] § 307(b)(1).

[39] § 1223(5).

[40] § 307(b)(2) and Reg. § 1.307-2.

[41] Reg. § 1.305-1(b)(1): Code §§ 301(b) and 316(a).

[42] § 301(d).

profits), but the distributing corporation may not take a corresponding deduction for the dividends.

STOCK REDEMPTIONS

Corporations occasionally will acquire their own shares. Sometimes the acquisition is motivated by a desire to eliminate an issue of stock. In these cases, the corporation might cancel the stock after its acquisition. Alternatively, the corporation might reacquire its own shares in order to issue the shares as additional compensation to hire or retain qualified employees or to acquire additional assets or even a whole business. The stock may be kept as treasury stock until needed. Such an acquisition is called a *stock redemption*. A redemption is defined in the Code as the acquisition by a corporation of its own stock from its shareholders in exchange for cash or other property, regardless of whether the shares are canceled, retired, or held as treasury stock.[43]

IN GENERAL

The taxation of the acquisition of the shares from an existing shareholder could take either of two forms. It could be treated as a sale of stock, with the corporation treated as an independent purchaser. This generally would result in a capital gain or loss for the shareholder. Alternatively, the sales price could be treated as a distribution. In this situation, the shareholder would have dividend income to the extent of the corporation's earnings and profits. Generally, the key factor as to whether a stock redemption is treated as a sale or a dividend distribution is whether or not the shareholder's proportionate interest in the corporation is significantly reduced.

As a general rule, if a shareholder's interest is basically the same or nearly the same after a redemption, the redemption is treated as a distribution. The tax treatment is based on whether the distribution is of cash or other property. The taxability of cash and property dividends was discussed previously in this chapter.

There are *five* situations in which stock redemptions are treated as a sale by the shareholder instead of as a dividend distribution. These five situations are as follows:

1. Redemptions not equivalent to dividends [§ 302(b)(1)]

2. Substantially disproportionate redemptions of stock [§ 302(b)(2)]

3. Terminations of shareholders' interests [§ 302(b)(3)]

4. Redemptions from noncorporate shareholders in partial liquidation [§ 302(b)(4)]

5. Distributions in redemption of stock to pay death taxes (§ 303)

In the above five situations, a shareholder recognizes gain or loss equal to the difference between the redemption proceeds and the basis of the stock surrendered.

REDEMPTIONS NOT EQUIVALENT TO DIVIDENDS

The Code states that a stock redemption is treated as a sale or exchange of the shareholder's stock "if the redemption is not essentially equivalent to a dividend."[44] The Regulations refer to *dividend equivalency* as meaning that the redemption has "the same effect as a distribution without any redemption of stock."[45] Several cases have helped to

---

[43] § 317(b).

[44] § 302(b)(1).

[45] Reg. § 1.302-2(a).

further clarify this provision. The most significant litigation over this issue was *U.S. v. Davis*,[46] decided by the Supreme Court in 1970. The case involved the redemption of all of the corporation's outstanding preferred stock from the sole shareholder (directly and indirectly)[47] of the corporation. The Court ruled that the redemption was a distribution and not a sale. In reaching this decision, the Court rejected the taxpayer's argument that since there was a business purpose for the issuance and redemption of the preferred stock, the transaction was not equivalent to a dividend. Instead, the Court decided that to meet the requirement of § 302(b)(1), there must be a meaningful reduction in the shareholder's interest in the corporation. There are *no other* relevant considerations. One of the outgrowths of this decision is that no redemption from a sole shareholder will qualify as being "not equivalent to a dividend." A sole shareholder remains a 100 percent owner after *any* redemption. Therefore, there can never be a meaningful reduction in a sole shareholder's interest.

Following the decision in *Davis,* it was generally felt that the "not essentially equivalent to a dividend" exception was effectively canceled. Subsequent litigation has shown that this is not so. Taxpayers have been successful in those cases in which they were able to convince the court that there was a meaningful reduction in their interest in the corporation. Unfortunately, no precise definition of "meaningful reduction" has emerged from the litigation. Consequently, all subsequent taxpayers must prove the significance of the reduction based on the facts and circumstances of each specific case.

When a stock redemption is determined to be essentially equivalent to a dividend, the shareholder's basis in the stock redeemed is *added* to the basis of the stock that was not redeemed.[48]

> **Example 18.** R owned 1,000 shares (100%) of the common stock of T Corporation. (T Corporation had no other classes of stock outstanding.) R's basis in the stock was $20,000 ($20 per share). T Corporation redeemed 500 shares of R's common stock for $15,000. Since R owned 100% of T Corporation, both before and after the redemption, the redemption was essentially the same as a dividend. (There was no meaningful reduction in R's interest in the corporation.) R, therefore, has a distribution of $15,000, a taxable dividend if T Corporation has sufficient earnings and profits. R's basis of $10,000 ($20 per share) in the 500 shares redeemed is added to the basis in his remaining 500 shares. After the redemption. R's basis in his remaining 500 shares is $20,000 ($40 per share).

SUBSTANTIALLY DISPROPORTIONATE REDEMPTIONS

A stock redemption is treated as a sale if it is *substantially disproportionate.*[49] In order for a redemption to be substantially disproportionate with respect to a shareholder, the shareholder must, after the redemption, own less than 80 percent of the voting stock owned prior to the redemption and own less than 80 percent of the common stock owned prior to the redemption.[50] By requiring the shareholder's ownership of both *voting* and *common stock* to be less than 80 percent of his or her former ownership, the law prevents redemption of solely preferred stock from meeting the § 302(b)(2) requirements. Redemptions of preferred stock may qualify only if there is also a redemption of common stock. In addition to the above requirements, a shareholder is not eligible for sale or exchange treatment unless the shareholder's ownership of voting stock after the redemption is less than

---

[46]   70-1 USTC ¶9289. 25 AFTR 2d 70-827. 397 U.S. 301 (USSC. 1970).

[47]   The provisions regarding constructive ownership of stock are discussed later in this chapter.

[48]   Reg. § 1.302-2(c).

[49]   § 302(b)(2).

[50]   § 302(b)(2)(C).

50 percent of the total voting stock.[51] Basically, satisfaction of these three mathematical tests provides a safe harbor for qualifying a redemption as not equivalent to a dividend (i.e., sale or exchange treatment).

Example 19. M owned 100 shares of Q Corporation's voting common stock. M's basis in this stock was $500 ($5 per share). Q Corporation had 200 shares of common stock (its only class of stock) issued and outstanding. The corporation redeemed 40 shares of M's stock for $300. The tax treatment of the redemption is determined as follows:

Test 1: Does M own less than 80% of the voting stock that she owned prior to the redemption?

Before the redemption M owned 50% of the voting stock. $\left(\dfrac{100}{200}\right)$

After the redemption M owned 37.5% of the outstanding voting stock. $\left(\dfrac{60}{160}\right)$

$$\dfrac{\text{M's percentage interest in the voting stock after the redemption}}{\text{M's percentage interested in the voting stock prior to the redemption}} = \dfrac{37.5\%}{50\%} = \underline{75\%}$$

(**Alternative Computation:** 80% of 50% = 40%; therefore, Test 1 is met because 37.5% is less than 40%.)

Test 2: Does M own less than 80% of the common stock that she owned prior to the redemption? Since the voting stock in this example is the same as the common stock, Test 2 is a repetition of Test 1. Therefore, Test 2 is also met.

Test 3: Is M's ownership of voting stock after the redemption less than 50% of the total voting stock? (This is measured in voting *power* if different classes of stock have unequal voting rights.)

$$\dfrac{\text{Number of shares of voting stock owned by M after the redemption}}{\text{Total number of shares of voting stock after the redemption}} = \dfrac{60}{160} = \underline{37.5\%}$$

37.5% is less than 50% of the voting stock, so Test 3 is met.

(**Alternative Computation:** 160 shares × 50% = 80 shares; therefore, Test 3 is met since 60 shares is less than 80 shares.)

All three tests must be met in order for a stock redemption to be "substantially disproportionate." Since all three tests are met in this example, the redemption of 40 shares of M's stock meets the requirements of § 302(b)(2) and is, therefore, treated as a sale or exchange of the stock. M's gain is computed as follows:

Proceeds from redemption.	$300
Less: M's basis in the 40 shares redeemed (40 × $5)	(200)
Gain from redemption	$100

The gain will be long-term or short-term depending on how long the stock was held.

Note: All computations regarding ownership after the redemption were made using 160 shares, the number of shares outstanding after 40 of the 200 originally outstanding shares had been redeemed by Q Corporation.

---

[51]   § 302(b)(2)(B).

Example 20. X owned 150 of the 200 outstanding shares of W Corporation's voting common stock. (W Corporation has no other classes of stock.) The corporation redeemed 100 shares of X's stock. The tax treatment of the redemption is determined as follows:

Test 1: Does X own less than 80% of the voting stock that he owned prior to the redemption?

Before the redemption X owned 75% of the voting stock. $\left(\dfrac{150}{200}\right)$

After the redemption X owned 50% of the voting stock. $\left(\dfrac{50}{100}\right)$

$$\frac{50\%}{75\%} = \underline{\underline{67\%}}$$

67% is less than 80%, so Test 1 is met.

Test 2: Does X own less than 80% of the common stock that he owned prior to the redemption? Since the voting stock in this example is the same as the common stock, Test 2 is a repetition of Test 1. Therefore, Test 2 is also met.

Test 3: Is X's ownership of voting stock after the redemption less than 50% of the total voting stock?

$$\frac{50\%}{100\%} = \underline{\underline{50\%}}$$

Exactly 50% is not less than 50%. Therefore, Test 3 is not met.

Because *all three tests* must be met in order for a stock redemption to be "substantially disproportionate," the redemption is treated as a distribution, not a sale. Any proceeds from the redemption are treated as a dividend to the extent of earnings and profits, and X's basis in the 100 shares redeemed is added to the basis in his remaining 50 shares.

To prevent abuses in cases of multiple redemptions, the law requires that the tests be applied at the end of the series of redemptions if the redemptions are all part of one plan. Without this limitation, it would be possible to meet the substantially disproportionate rules after each redemption while leaving the redeeming shareholders' relative interests unaffected at the close of the intended transactions.[52]

Example 21. A, B, and C each owned 50 shares ($\frac{1}{3}$) of F Corporation's common stock. There are no other classes of stock. On January 2, pursuant to an overall plan, the corporation redeemed 40 shares of stock from A. On February 1, pursuant to the same plan, the corporation redeemed 40 shares from B. Finally, on March 3, the corporation redeemed 40 shares from C. Independently, each redemption is disproportionate. However, combining the series, A, B, and C each end up with the same $\frac{1}{3}$ ownership of F Corporation. Consequently, the redemptions are not substantially disproportionate.

TERMINATION OF A SHAREHOLDER'S INTEREST

The third case in which a redemption can qualify as a sale is if the redemption completely terminates the shareholder's interest.[53] A *complete termination* requires the

---

[52] § 302(b)(2)(D).

[53] § 302(b)(3).

corporation to redeem all of the shares that the stockholder owns. If a shareholder is completely terminating his or her interest in a corporation in which various close relatives own stock, special rules apply to the termination of the shareholder's interest.[54] These special rules regarding constructive ownership of stock are discussed later in this chapter.

REDEMPTION FROM NONCORPORATE SHAREHOLDER IN PARTIAL LIQUIDATION

The fourth case in which a redemption can qualify as a sale is a redemption from a noncorporate shareholder in partial liquidation.[55] A *partial liquidation* is a distribution that is not essentially equivalent to a dividend, determined at the corporate level rather than at the shareholder level.[56] To qualify, the distribution must be made in accordance with a plan of partial liquidation and made either in the year the plan is adopted or in the following year.

The Code specifically provides that a distribution in partial liquidation shall include (but not be limited to) distributions attributable to the termination of a business.[57] To satisfy this test, the distribution must be the result of the corporation ceasing to conduct a trade or business that had been in existence for at least five years prior to the distribution. The corporation, following the distribution, must be conducting a trade or business that also has been in existence for at least five years. Neither the continuing nor the terminated business may have been acquired during the five-year period in a transaction in which a gain or loss was recognized.[58] This provision was included to prevent the corporation from purchasing a business in order to convert a dividend into a partial liquidation.

There is no exact definition of a "trade or business." The Regulations state that a trade or business consists of a group of activities that includes every step in the process of earning income.[59] Owning investment assets or real estate used in a trade or business is not a trade or business by itself. The Regulations are helpful but do not eliminate all the questions as to what constitutes a trade or business.

REDEMPTIONS OF STOCK TO PAY DEATH TAXES

The fifth provision in the Code that classifies a redemption as a sale rather than as a distribution deals with the redemption of stock to pay death taxes.[60] This provision only applies to stock included in a decedent's gross estate and was designed to provide a way to obtain cash needed for the administration of an estate. It permits the redemption of stock in an amount equal to the taxes imposed as a result of decedent's death and to the funeral and administration expenses deductible by the estate.[61] There is no restriction in the law that the redemption proceeds actually be used to pay taxes or expenses. The limitation refers simply to the maximum amount that can be redeemed under the provision. The tax treatment of any amount redeemed in excess of the amount of the above expenses is determined by applying the rules previously discussed regarding taxability of stock redemptions.

In order to be eligible to redeem stock using this provision, the value of the stock that the decedent owned in the redeeming corporation must exceed 35 percent of the value of

---

[54]   § 302(c)(2).

[55]   § 302(b)(4).

[56]   § 302(e)(1).

[57]   § 302(e)(2).

[58]   § 302(e)(3).

[59]   Reg. § 1.355-1(c).

[60]   § 303(a).

[61]   Ibid.

the decedent's gross estate reduced by expenses and losses of the estate.[62] This condition effectively limits the use of this exception to estates of which the stock of the redeeming corporation is a substantial part. It is also possible to use this provision when two or more corporations comprise a substantial part of a decedent's estate. In this situation, if 20 percent or more of the value of the outstanding stock of each of two or more corporations is included in the decedent's gross estate, the corporations are treated as a single corporation for the purpose of determining the 35 percent requirement.[63]

CONSTRUCTIVE OWNERSHIP OF STOCK

As demonstrated above, one of the primary factors distinguishing a stock redemption qualifying for sale or exchange treatment from a dividend distribution is whether there has been a change in the taxpayer's proportionate interest in the corporation. Ownership in a corporation refers to both *actual* and *constructive* ownership.[64]

Under the rules of constructive ownership of stock, a taxpayer is considered to own not only those shares of stock he or she personally owns, but also to own those shares of stock owned by certain relatives and entities in which the taxpayer has an interest. The only family members considered relatives for these constructive ownership rules are the taxpayer's spouse, children, grandchildren, and parents.[65] Excluded from the list are siblings (i.e., brothers and sisters) and grandparents.

> **Example 22.** F, an individual, owns 60% of the stock of G Corporation. The remaining 40% is owned by S, F's son. F is considered to own 100% of G Corporation, 60% directly and 40% by the application of the constructive ownership rules.

> **Example 23.** H is married to W. They have one son, C, and a grandchild, G. H owns 100 shares of ABC Corporation. Either W or C can be considered to constructively own H's stock. G is not considered to be a constructive owner of H's stock, since an individual is not considered to constructively own his or her grandparent's stock.

Under the constructive ownership rules (also called the *attribution rules*), a person is deemed to own a proportionate share of the stock owned by a partnership, estate, or trust in which he or she has an interest.[66] Partnerships, estates, and trusts are also deemed to own the stock owned by persons who have an ownership interest in them.[67]

> **Example 24.** Y and Z are equal (50% each) partners in the YZ Partnership. The YZ Partnership owns 300 shares of A Corporation. Since Y and Z each own one-half of the partnership, they are each considered to constructively own one-half of the 300 shares of A Corporation owned by the YZ Partnership, or 150 shares each.

> **Example 25.** Assume the same facts as in *Example 24* except that the 300 shares of A Corporation stock are owned by Y instead of by the partnership. Since a partnership is considered to constructively own all of the stock of its partners, the YZ Partnership is deemed to own the entire 300 shares of A Corporation stock. Z

---

[62]   § 303(b)(2)(A).

[63]   § 302(b)(2)(B).

[64]   § 318.

[65]   § 318(a)(1).

[66]   §§ 318(a)(2)(A) and (B).

[67]   §§ 318(a)(3)(A) and (B).

does not constructively own any of the stock unless Y and Z are related family members.

In order for there to be attribution (constructive ownership) between a shareholder and a corporation, the shareholder must own, actually or constructively, at least 50 percent of the value of the corporation's stock.[68] Once this requirement is met, a shareholder is deemed to own a proportionate share of the stock owned by the corporation.

> **Example 26.** C Corporation is owned 60% by B and 40% by W. C Corporation owns 1,000 shares of Z Corporation stock. B constructively owns 600 (1,000 shares × 60%) shares of the Z Corporation stock. W does not constructively own any shares of Z Corporation stock since he does not own at least 50% of C Corporation.

A corporation is deemed to own all of the stock owned by shareholders who have a 50 percent or more interest in the corporation.[69]

There are rules against *double* attribution. Specifically, stock may not be attributed to a family member from a family member and then reattributed to another family member.[70] In addition, stock attributed to an entity from an owner may not then be attributed to another owner.[71] These rules prevent attribution between unrelated individuals.

> **Example 27.** P has two children, R and S. R owns 100 shares of H Corporation. Therefore, P constructively owns R's 100 shares of H Corporation. Without the rules against double attribution, the 100 shares could be reattributed from P to S, resulting in sibling attribution, which is not authorized by the definition of relatives.

Complete Termination of Interest. The stock attribution rules could make it very difficult for a redemption by a family-owned corporation to qualify as a complete termination of interest under § 302(b)(3). Any constructively owned stock would prevent the shareholder from qualifying as having completely terminated his or her interest. To eliminate this problem, the Code permits the redeeming shareholder to ignore the family attribution rules (but not attribution from other entities) in determining whether there has been a complete termination of the shareholder's interest.[72] To qualify for this provision, the shareholder must not have any interest in the corporation after the redemption other than that of a creditor. Specifically, the shareholder may not be an officer, director, or even an employee of the corporation. In addition, the shareholder must not acquire one of the prohibited interests in the corporation during the 10 years following the redemption. This provision makes it much easier for a shareholder to qualify a redemption as a complete termination of interest.

REDEMPTIONS THROUGH RELATED CORPORATIONS

As stated earlier, a stock redemption is defined as the acquisition by a corporation of its own stock. The limitations on sale treatment discussed thus far could be avoided by an individual who controls two or more corporations. Instead of having a corporation redeem its stock, the shareholder could *sell* the stock of one controlled corporation to another controlled corporation. To prevent this type of transaction from avoiding the redemption

---

[68] § 318(a)(2)(C).

[69] § 318(a)(3)(C).

[70] § 318(a)(5)(B).

[71] § 318(a)(5)(C).

[72] § 302(c)(2).

limitations, Code § 304 reclassifies the "sale" of one controlled corporation's stock to another controlled corporation as a stock redemption.[73] Two different transactions are included in the reclassification provision. First, the sale of stock of a corporation controlled by one or more persons to another corporation controlled by the *same persons* is reclassified as a redemption.[74] Control is defined as ownership of either 50 percent or more of the combined voting power or 50 percent or more of the value of the outstanding stock.[75] The second reclassified transaction is the sale of stock of a parent corporation to its controlled subsidiary.[76]

> **Example 28.** A, B, and C, unrelated individuals, each own equal shares of T Corporation's outstanding stock. These same individuals own 100% of V Corporation's stock. If either A, B, or C sells shares of T Corporation to V Corporation, the transaction will be treated as a stock redemption.

> **Example 29.** Individual D owns all of the stock of P Corporation. P Corporation owns all of the stock of S Corporation. If D sells some of her P Corporation stock to S Corporation, the transaction will be treated as a stock redemption.

The fact that a transaction is reclassified as a stock redemption does not mean that the shareholder will be denied sale treatment. Instead, it requires that the selling shareholder meet one of the special rules relating to stock redemptions in § 302 (i.e., being not essentially equivalent to a dividend, substantially disproportionate, a complete termination of an interest, or a partial liquidation from a noncorporate shareholder) to qualify for sale treatment. In measuring the change in ownership under § 302, the stock of the issuing corporation—not the purchasing corporation—is used.[77] In addition, stock owned by attribution is counted.

> **Example 30.** Individual G owns 80 of the 100 shares of X Corporation and 90 of the 100 shares of Y Corporation. G "sells" 10 shares of X Corporation stock to Y Corporation. Since G controls both corporations, the transaction is reclassified as a redemption. Before the transaction, G owns 80% of X Corporation. After the transaction, G owns 79% of X, computed as follows:

Actual ownership (70 × 100 shares)	70%
Constructive ownership:	
(90% ownership of Y corporation ×	
Y Corporation's 10% ownership of × Corporation).	9%
Total direct and indirect ownership	79%

Since G's ownership of X Corporation has only declined from 80% to 79%, the redemption does not meet any of the tests for sale treatment. Consequently, G must treat the "sale" proceeds as a dividend.

If the transaction is treated as a dividend rather than a sale, the amount of dividend income is measured by the earnings and profits of *both* the issuing corporation and the purchasing corporation.[78] This deemed dividend is considered as having been paid first

---

[73]   § 304.

[74]   § 304(a)(1).

[75]   § 304(c)(1).

[76]   § 304(a)(2).

[77]   § 304(b)(1).

[78]   § 304(b)(2).

from the E&P of the purchasing (acquiring) corporation to the extent thereof, and then from the E&P of the issuing corporation.

> **Example 31.** Assume the same facts as in *Example 30*. Since the transaction is treated as a dividend, it is considered to come from Y Corporation's E&P first and then, if necessary, from X Corporation's E&P.

EFFECT OF REDEMPTIONS ON REDEEMING CORPORATION

In a stock redemption, the stockholders are concerned with whether the redemption is treated for tax purposes as a sale or as a distribution. The redeeming corporation, however, is concerned with whether or not it has income on the redemption and what effect there is on earnings and profits.

Gain or Loss. The tax effect of redemption distributions on the corporation is identical to that arising from property distributions discussed earlier. As previously explained, the corporation must recognize gain—but not loss—on the distribution of property.[79]

Effect of Redemption on E&P. The E&P of a corporation must be adjusted to reflect any redemption distributions. First, if the corporation must recognize gain on the distribution under § 311, E&P must be increased for the gain. The amount of the reduction of E&P on account of the distribution depends on whether the distribution qualifies for sale treatment. If the distribution does not qualify for sale treatment but rather is treated as a dividend, the rules discussed earlier for cash and property dividends must be followed. If the redemption qualifies for sale treatment, only a portion of the distribution is charged against E&P. In such case, E&P is reduced by the redeemed stock's proportionate share of E&P but not by more than the amount of the redemption distribution.[80]

> **Example 32.** B Corporation had the following capital accounts on January 2:
>
> | | |
> |---|---|
> | Common stock.............................. | $100,000 |
> | Paid-in capital in excess of par.................... | 300,000 |
> | Earnings and profits .... | 500,000 |
>
> The common stock outstanding consisted of 1,000 shares of $100 par value stock. On January 2, B Corporation redeemed 100 shares for $700 per share (a total of $70,000). The corporation therefore redeemed 10% of its stock (100 ÷ 1,000). Of the $70,000 paid for the shares, B Corporation must charge $50,000 to its earnings and profits (10% × $500,000). The remaining $20,000 is charged to the capital accounts [$10,000 to common stock (10% × $100,000) and the remaining $10,000 to paid-in capital in excess of par].
>
> ***Note:*** This example assumes that this redemption meets the requirements for sale or exchange treatment.

---

[79]   § 311.

[80]   § 312(n)(7).

COMPLETE LIQUIDATIONS

INTRODUCTION

As discussed earlier in the chapter, in a partial liquidation or stock redemption the corporation redeems only a portion of its stock. In these situations, the corporation continues to operate all or part of its business. In other situations, however, a corporation may wish to terminate its existence by liquidating completely. A complete liquidation of a corporation occurs when, under a plan of complete liquidation, the corporation redeems *all* of its stock using a series of distributions.[81] In addition, the corporation must be in a status of liquidation throughout the life of the liquidation. The Regulations state that a status of liquidation exists when a corporation ceases to be a going concern and is engaged in activities whose sole function is the winding up of the business affairs.[82] There is one set of rules that governs most liquidations and one special set of rules that governs liquidations of a subsidiary.

COMPLETE LIQUIDATIONS: THE GENERAL RULES

Shareholder Gain or Loss. When a shareholder receives a liquidating distribution, the treatment of the shareholder—except where a parent liquidates a subsidiary—is governed solely by Code § 331. This rule provides that shareholders treat property received in liquidation of a corporation as full payment for their stock. Therefore, the shareholder must recognize gain or loss equal to the difference between the *net* fair market value of the property received (fair market value of the assets received less any liabilities assumed by the shareholder) and the basis of the stock surrendered. Special rules must be followed where a shareholder receives an installment note arising from a sale by the corporation within the 12-month period after the corporation has adopted a plan of liquidation.[83] If the stock was purchased at different times and for different amounts, the gain or loss is computed on each separate lot. The gain or loss normally is capital gain or loss since the shareholder's stock is usually a capital asset.

Basis to Shareholder. When a shareholder uses the general rule of § 331 to determine gain or loss on the liquidation, the shareholder's basis in the property received in the liquidation is its fair market value on the date of distribution.[84]

Example 33. K owned 100 shares of stock in L Corporation. K's adjusted basis in the stock was $400. L Corporation completely liquidated and distributed to K $200 cash and office equipment worth $700 in exchange for his stock. K's recognized gain is computed as follows:

Cash received by K	$200
Fair market value of property distributed to K	700
Amount realized	$900
Less: K's adjusted basis in his stock	(400)
Realized gain	$500

---

[81] § 346(a).

[82] Reg. § 1.332-2(c).

[83] § 453(h).

[84] § 334(a).

K's entire realized gain of $500 is recognized under § 1001(c). K's basis in the cash received is, of course, $200. K's basis in the office equipment received is $700, its fair market value on the date of distribution.

Gain or Loss to the Liquidating Corporation. A corporation generally must recognize gain *and* loss on the distribution of property as part of a complete liquidation.[85] The gain or loss is computed as if such property were sold to the shareholder for its fair market value.

Example 34. Sleepwaves Corporation, a waterbed retailer, fell on hard times and decided to dissolve the business. During the year, the corporation adopted a plan of liquidation and completely liquidated. The furniture that the corporation was unable to move in their going-out-of-business sale was distributed to its sole shareholder. This inventory was worth $5,000 (basis $1,000). In addition, the corporation distributed land held for investment worth $8,000 (basis $10,000). The corporation must recognize $4,000 of ordinary income ($5,000 − $1,000) on the distribution of the inventory and a $2,000 capital loss ($8,000 − $10,000) on the distribution of the land.

If the shareholder assumes a corporate liability or takes the property subject to a liability, the fair market value of the property is treated as being no less than the liability.[86] Therefore, where the liability exceeds the value of the property, gain must be recognized to the extent the liability exceeds the basis of the property.

Example 35. T Corporation's only asset is a building with a basis of $100,000 and which is subject to a liability of $400,000. The low basis is attributable to accelerated depreciation. The property is currently worth $250,000. During 2009, T distributed the land to its sole shareholder, R. T Corporation must recognize a gain of $300,000 ($400,000 liability − $100,000 basis). Had the liability been $200,000, T would have ignored the liability and recognized a gain of $150,000 ($250,000 value − $100,000 basis).

The treatment of distributions in liquidation differs from that of nonliquidating distributions in that the corporation is normally allowed to recognize loss on a liquidating distribution. This is not true for all liquidating distributions, however. As with nonliquidating distributions, Congress was concerned that taxpayers might use the loss recognition privilege to circumvent the gain recognition rule. To prohibit possible abuse, § 336(d) provides two exceptions concerning the treatment of losses.

The first exception prohibits the deduction of the loss if certain conditions are satisfied. Section 336(d)(1) provides that the liquidating corporation cannot recognize any loss on the distribution of property to a *related party* if the distribution is either (1) non-pro rata or (2) the property was acquired by the corporation during the five-year period prior to the distribution, either in a nontaxable transfer under § 351 (relating to transfers to a controlled corporation) or as a contribution to capital. For this purpose, a related party is the same as that defined in Code § 267 (e.g., an individual who owns either directly or constructively more than 50 percent of the distributing corporation).

Example 36. J is the sole shareholder of Z Corporation. In anticipation of the corporation's liquidation, J contributed a dilapidated warehouse to the corporation, with a built-in loss of $100,000 (value $200,000, basis $300,000). Shortly thereafter, Z Corporation distributed the warehouse along with land worth $90,000 (basis

---

[85] § 336.

[86] § 336(b).

$20,000). Absent the special rule, the corporation would recognize a loss of $100,000, which would offset the $70,000 gain on the land that it must recognize ($90,000 − $20,000). Under the exception, however, no loss is recognized since the distribution is to a related party, J, and the property was acquired as a contribution to capital within five years of the liquidation.

The second provision concerning losses limits the amount of loss that can be deducted—assuming the loss is not disallowed entirely under the related-party rule above. Under § 336(d)(2), the amount of loss recognized by a liquidating corporation on the sale, exchange, or distribution of any property acquired in a § 351 transaction or as a contribution of capital is reduced. This rule applies only if the principal purpose for the acquisition was the recognition of a loss by the corporation in connection with the liquidation. It is generally presumed that any property acquired in the above manner during the period starting two years prior to the date on which a plan of liquidation is adopted was acquired for the purpose of recognizing a loss. When the tax-avoidance motive is found, the rule effectively limits the loss deduction to the decline in value that occurs while the property is in the hands of the corporation. In other words, any built-in loss existing at the time of contribution is not deductible. To ensure that any built-in loss is not deducted, the Code provides a special computation. For purposes of determining the *loss* on the disposition of the tainted property, the basis of such property is reduced (but not below zero) by the amount of the built-in loss (i.e., the excess of the property's basis over its value at the time the corporation acquired it). By reducing the basis, any subsequent loss recognized is reduced.

Example 37. R, S, T, and U own the stock of Q Corporation. Knowing that the corporation planned to liquidate, R contributed land to the corporation with a built-in loss of $100,000 (value $200,000, basis $300,000) in exchange for shares of Q stock that qualified for nonrecognition under § 351. During the liquidation, the corporation sold the property for $160,000. Under the general rule, the corporation would recognize a loss of $140,000 ($160,000 amount realized − $300,000 carryover basis). However, since the property was acquired in a § 351 exchange and the principal purpose of the transaction was to recognize loss on the property in liquidation, the special rule applies. The loss recognized is limited to that which occurred in the hands of the corporation $40,000 ($200,000 value at contribution − $160,000 amount realized). In other words, the loss computed in the normal manner, $140,000, must be reduced by the built-in loss of $100,000. Technically, Q Corporation would compute the loss by reducing its basis in the property by the amount of built-in loss as follows:

Amount realized.			$160,000
Adjusted basis:			
Carryover basis		$ 300,000	
− Basis reduction:			
Carryover basis.	$300,000		
−Value at contribution.	−200,000		
Built-in loss		−100,000	
Adjusted basis			(200,000)
Loss recognized			($ 40,000)

LIQUIDATION OF A SUBSIDIARY

A parent corporation generally recognizes no gain or loss on property it receives from the liquidation of a subsidiary corporation.[87] In order to qualify to use this provision (Code § 332), the parent corporation must own at least 80 percent of the voting power and this stock must have a value at least equal to 80 percent of the total value of the subsidiary corporation's stock.[88] For purposes of these computations, nonvoting preferred stock is excluded.[89] This minimum amount of stock must be owned on the date of adoption of the plan of liquidation and at all times thereafter until the liquidation is completed. All of the property of the subsidiary must be distributed in complete cancellation of the subsidiary's stock within three years following the close of the tax year in which the first distribution takes place.[90] It also is important to note that Code § 332 is not elective. If the above conditions are met, no gain or loss is recognized.

Effect on Subsidiary. Under § 337, a subsidiary recognizes no gain or loss on the distribution of its assets to its parent in a liquidation under § 332.[91] This rule only applies to property transferred to the parent corporation in the liquidation. Property transferred to minority shareholders will result in the recognition of gain but not loss.[92]

Ordinarily, when one taxpayer is indebted to another and the debt is canceled, the indebted taxpayer has income to the extent of the debt due to the relief of the indebtedness. Section 337(b) contains an exception to this general rule. The exception states that when a subsidiary corporation is indebted to its parent corporation and the subsidiary liquidates under § 332, no gain or loss is recognized when the subsidiary transfers property to the parent to satisfy the debt.

Basis of Assets—General Rule. When a subsidiary is liquidated by its parent corporation, the basis of the assets transferred from the subsidiary to the parent must be determined. Generally, the basis of each of the assets transferred is the same for the parent corporation as it had been for the subsidiary.[93] This rule applies not only to property transferred in cancellation of the subsidiary's stock, but also to property transferred in order to satisfy the subsidiary's debt to the parent.[94] The amount of the parent's investment in the subsidiary's stock is ignored. The parent's basis is determined solely by the subsidiary's basis.

Example 38. T Corporation had assets with a basis of $1 million and no liabilities. P Corporation bought all of the stock of T Corporation for $1.2 million. Several years later, when T Corporation's assets had a basis of $800,000, P Corporation liquidated T Corporation in a tax-free liquidation under § 332. P Corporation's basis in the assets received from T Corporation is $800,000, the same basis as T Corporation had in the assets. The $400,000 difference between the basis of the assets and P Corporation's basis in the stock of T Corporation is lost.

---

[87]   § 332.

[88]   §§ 332(b)(1) and 1504(a)(2).

[89]   § 1504(a)(4).

[90]   § 332(b)(3).

[91]   § 337(a).

[92]   §§ 337(a) and 336(d)(3).

[93]   § 334(b)(1).

[94]   §§ 337(b)(1) and 334(b)(1).

Example 39. Assume the same facts as in *Example 38* except that P Corporation had paid $700,000 (instead of $1,200,000) for T Corporation's stock. P Corporation's basis in the assets received from T Corporation is still $800,000, the same as T Corporation's basis in the assets. In this example, rather than losing a $400,000 investment, P Corporation received a $100,000 tax-free increase in its basis in T Corporation and its assets ($800,000 basis in T Corporation's assets − $700,000 basis that P Corporation had in T Corporation's stock).

As demonstrated above, this carryover of the basis of assets from a subsidiary to its parent can be either beneficial *(Example 39)* or detrimental *(Example 38)* to the parent corporation.

Basis of Assets—Exception. The carryover basis rule was challenged in the case of *Kimbell-Diamond Milling Co. v. Commissioner:*[95] In this case, Kimbell-Diamond's plant was destroyed by fire. The corporation wished to purchase replacement property to avoid recognizing gain on the involuntary conversion. The only plant that they wanted was owned by a corporation that would not sell. To acquire the asset, Kimbell-Diamond purchased the corporation's stock and then liquidated the corporation. Kimbell-Diamond used the basis of the assets of the liquidated corporation as its basis for the assets. The amount that Kimbell-Diamond paid for the stock of the corporation was *much less* than the liquidated corporation's basis in the assets, so that by using the carryover basis, Kimbell-Diamond received much larger depreciation deductions (and therefore had much smaller taxable income) than if it had actually purchased the plant. Upon review, however, the IRS reclassified the transaction as a purchase of assets, rather than a purchase of stock followed by a separate liquidation. The Tax Court agreed with the IRS that the two transactions should be treated as one. This decision created the *Kimbell-Diamond* exception. Under this exception, if the original purpose of the stock acquisition was to acquire assets, the purchaser's basis in the assets acquired was the cost of the stock rather than the liquidated corporation's basis.

Congress incorporated the Kimbell-Diamond exception into the Internal Revenue Code,[96] effectively allowing an acquiring corporation such as Kimbell-Diamond to select the basis to be used for the subsidiary's assets: either a basis equal to the purchase price of the assets or the same basis as that of the subsidiary. As might be expected, many acquiring corporations attempted to take advantage of this latitude provided by the Code. Consequently, to curb potential abuses, Congress enacted § 338 in 1982. Although § 338 is still a codification of the *Kimbell-Diamond* exception, its requirements are much more specific than the previous law.

Code § 338—Purchase of Assets. To qualify for a purchase price basis offered under § 338, the parent corporation must purchase stock having at least 80 percent of the voting power and at least 80 percent of the value of all stock (except nonvoting, nonparticipating, preferred stock).[97] To qualify as a purchase, the stock may not be acquired from a related party, in a transaction that qualifies under Code § 351, or in any transaction that will result in the purchaser using a carryover basis.[98] This acquisition of control may occur in a series of transactions; however, no more than 12 months may elapse between the first purchase and the acquisition of the required 80 percent control.[99]

---

[95] 14 T.C. 74 (1950), aff'd., 51-1 USTC ¶9301, 40 AFTR 328, 187 F2d 718 (CA-5, 1951).

[96] The Kimbell-Diamond exception was formerly § 334(b)(2).

[97] § 338(d)(3).

[98] § 338(h)(3).

[99] § 338(d) and (h).

If the parent corporation meets the purchase requirement, it must elect to treat the acquisition as an asset purchase by the 15th day of the ninth month following the month of acquisition.[100] The election, once made, is irrevocable. Failure to make the election results in the parent being treated as having purchased stock and thus prohibits the subsidiary from adjusting the basis of its assets. After the election, the subsidiary generally increases or decreases the basis of its assets to their fair market value.

Code § 338 does not require a liquidation. As a result, both the parent and the subsidiary may continue to exist. Section 338 takes a *two-step* approach to achieve the basis step-up. First, the subsidiary is treated as having sold in a single transaction all of its assets at fair market value on the close of the acquisition date. Any gain or loss realized on this hypothetical sale must be recognized *and* reported on the subsidiary's final tax return. Second, the subsidiary is treated as a new corporation that is deemed to have purchased all of the assets of the old subsidiary (i.e., the acquired or target corporation) on the day after the date the parent obtained the necessary control. For purposes of determining the subsidiary's new basis in its assets, the deemed purchase price is generally equal to the price the parent corporation paid for the subsidiary's stock adjusted for ownership less than 100 percent (i.e., the portion not owned by the parent) as well as liabilities of the subsidiary and other relevant items.[101] Note that in increasing the purchase price of the stock for liabilities of the subsidiary, such liabilities include the tax liability attributable to income arising from the deemed sale.

> **Example 40.** During 2009, P Corporation purchased all of the stock of T Corporation for $1 million. T's only asset is land with a basis of $200,000. It had no liabilities. Assuming P makes the appropriate election under § 338, T is deemed to have sold its assets, in this case the land, for its fair market value, $1 million. Thus, T must recognize a gain of $800,000 ($1,000,000 − $200,000). The tax liability arising from the deemed sale is $272,000 ($800,000 × 34%). After the hypothetical sale and repurchase, P's basis in the land is $1,272,000, its purchase price of the stock ($1 million) increased by the liability arising on the deemed sale of $272,000. Note that P, as the new owner of T, bears the economic burden of the tax liability. Consequently, assuming the value of the land is truly $1 million, P would no doubt desire to reduce the purchase price of the stock by the liability that arises with a § 338 election; that is, it probably would try to buy the stock for $728,000 ($1,000,000 − $272,000). If P did buy the stock for $728,000, presumably the gain on the deemed sale would still be $800,000, since the land is considered sold for its value of $1 million. In such case, the tax liability would still be $272,000 and the basis of the land under § 338 would be $1 million ($728,000 purchase price of the stock + $272,000 tax liability). Note that the effect of these rules is to reduce the value of the target subsidiary by an amount equal to the tax liability that would arise if § 338 is elected.

Under § 338, the subsidiary is considered to have purchased all of its assets from itself at the deemed price. The subsidiary must increase or decrease the basis of its assets so that its new basis in its assets equals the deemed purchase price. The method of allocating the basis among the assets is outlined by the Regulations.[102]

Allocation of Deemed Purchase Price. The temporary regulations under Code § 338 provide that the deemed purchase price of the stock is to be allocated to the

---

[100]   § 338(g).

[101]   § 338(a). § 338(b) provides that the basis is the sum of the grossed-up basis of stock purchased during the 12-month acquisition and the basis of stock not purchased during the period, adjusted as necessary.

[102]   § 338(b)(3).

subsidiary's assets using the "residual value" approach.[103] Under this technique, assets must be grouped into seven classes for purposes of making the allocation:

1. *Class I:* Cash, demand deposits, and other cash equivalents
2. *Class II:* Certificates of deposit, U.S. government securities, readily marketable securities, and other similar items
3. *Class III:* Accounts receivable;
4. *Class IV:* Inventory;
5. *Class V:* All assets other than those in Classes I, II, III, or IV, such as accounts receivable, inventory, plant, property, and equipment
6. *Class VI:* Section 197 intangibles other than goodwill or going concern value
7. *Class VII:* Intangible assets in the nature of goodwill and going-concern value

According to the system, the purchase price is first allocated to Class I assets in proportion to their relative fair market values as determined on the date following the acquisition. Because Class I assets are either cash or cash equivalents, the basis assigned to them is their face value. Once this allocation is made, any excess of the purchase price over the amount allocated to Class I assets is allocated to Class II assets, again based on relative fair market values. Any excess purchase price remaining after making the allocation to Class II assets is allocated to Class III assets based on relative values. Then amounts are allocated to Classes IV, V and VI in order. Any excess of purchase price over amounts allocated to Classes I, II, III, IV, V and VI is allocated to Class VII assets based on relative fair market values. In allocating such excess to Class II through Class VI assets, the amount allocated *cannot exceed the fair market value* of the asset. Thus, any purchase price which remains after the allocation to Class I, II, III, IV, V and VI assets is assigned to Class VII assets—hence the reason for calling this method the *residual* value approach. By limiting the allocation to Class I, II, III, and IV, V and VI assets to the assets' fair market values, the rules generally seek to ensure that corporate taxpayers allocate the proper amount to goodwill.

For the purpose of these allocation rules, the temporary regulations provide that the fair market value of the asset is its gross value computed without regard to any mortgages, liens, or other liabilities related to the property. These rules are illustrated in the following example.

Example 41. P Corporation purchases from an unrelated person 100% of the stock of T Corporation on June 1, 2009. Assume the purchase price adjusted for all relevant items is $100,000. T's assets at acquisition date are as follows:

	Basis	Fair Market Value
Cash	$10,000	$10,000
Accounts receivable	20,000	20,000
Inventory	25,000	55,000
Total	$55,000	$85,000

The purchase price is first allocated to cash in the amount of $10,000. This leaves $90,000 to be allocated. Since there are no Class II assets, the allocation is to Class III. Thus $20,000 is allocated to the accounts receivable. If the residual approach was not required, the taxpayer might allocate all of the remaining $70,000 to the inventory, despite the fact that its value is only $55,000. If this were allowed, the subsequent sale of the inventory would result in a loss. However, since the remaining purchase price ($70,000) exceeds the fair market value of the Class IV assets, the

---

[103] Temp. Reg. § 1.338-6T.

basis of the assets in this class is their fair market value, $55,000 for the inventory. This leaves $15,000 of the purchase price which has not been allocated. It is all assigned to goodwill since there are no Class VII intangibles.

If the parent corporation owns less than 100 percent of the subsidiary, the deemed price must be "grossed up" to take into account the minority interest. The adjustment for a minority interest results in a deemed purchase price called the "grossed-up basis." This grossed-up basis is obtained by multiplying the actual purchase price of the stock by a ratio, the numerator being 100 percent and the denominator equal to the percentage of the subsidiary stock owned by the parent.[104] This computation can be expressed as follows:

$$\text{Grossed-up basis} = \frac{\text{Parent corporation's basis in the subsidiary's stock on the acquisition date}}{} \times \frac{100\%}{\text{Percentage of subsidiary's stock held by parent on the acquisition date}}$$

Example 42. P Corporation purchased 90% of the outstanding stock of T Corporation for $900,000. T Corporation had only one asset, land with a basis of $900,000. Assume there are no liabilities or other relevant items that affect the deemed purchase price. Since P owns less than 100% of T, a grossed-up basis must be calculated. The result is $1 million [$900,000 purchase price × (100 ÷ 90, the percentage of T owned by P)]. If P elects § 338, T's basis for the land is $1 million. Note, however, that it is likely that the Regulations require the deemed sales price to be increased by any liabilities of the subsidiary. In such case, the deemed purchase price here would include the tax liability resulting from the fact that P purchased less than 100% of the stock, which in turn causes T to recognize income.

Section 338 not only entitles the subsidiary to a stepped-up basis for its assets, it also treats the subsidiary as a new corporation in every respect. As a result, the subsidiary may adopt any tax year it chooses, unless it files a consolidated return with the parent corporation, in which case it must adopt the parent's tax year. It may adopt new accounting methods if it desires. MACRS depreciation may be used for all of the hypothetically purchased property—the antichurning rules being inapplicable since the old and new subsidiary are considered unrelated. The new subsidiary acquires none of the other attributes of the old subsidiary. The earnings and profits of the old subsidiary are eliminated and any net operating loss carryovers of the old subsidiary are unavailable to the new subsidiary.

In most situations, the target subsidiary has some assets that have appreciated in value (i.e., fair market value exceeds the asset's basis) and other assets where the value is less than the asset's basis. In such cases, the acquiring corporation, desiring the highest possible basis for the assets, might first purchase the appreciated property, then purchase the subsidiary's stock and liquidate the subsidiary under § 332. By so doing, the acquiring corporation would obtain the best of both worlds: a basis for the appreciated property equal to its fair market value and a carryover basis for the other assets. In the latter case, the basis is higher than it would have been had the assets themselves been purchased or the stock purchased followed by an election under § 338. To prohibit the acquiring corporation from effectively selecting the basis that is most desirable for each separate asset, the Code contains the so-called consistency provisions. According to these rules, an acquiring corporation is required to use a carryover basis for purchased assets unless a § 338 election is made for the acquired corporation. The consistency period begins one year before the date of the first acquisition that comes within § 338 and ends one year

---

[104] § 338(b)(2). This approach is modified when the parent holds stock not acquired during the 12-month period.

after the acquisition date (i.e., the date on which the corporation obtains 80 percent control).

> **Example 43.** P Inc. purchased 60% of T Corporation's stock on March 7, 2009 and the remaining 40% on December 4, 2009. The consistency period runs from March 7, 2008 through December 4, 2010. If P acquires any assets of T during this period, it will be required to use carryover basis unless a § 338 election is made.

As mentioned above, § 338 is an elective provision. If the election is not made and the subsidiary is liquidated, § 332, the general rule for the nontaxable liquidation of a subsidiary, applies. If § 332 is used, the parent corporation carries over the subsidiary's basis for its assets, whereas under § 338 the basis of the assets is their deemed purchase price (based upon the parent corporation's investment in the subsidiary).

PROBLEM MATERIALS

DISCUSSION QUESTIONS

20-1   *Dividends.* Define the term *dividend.*

20-2   *Earnings and Profits.* What are "earnings and profits"? Are earnings and profits the same as "retained earnings"? Why or why not?

20-3   *Earnings and Profits.* In addition to taxable income, what types of items affect earnings and profits?

20-4   *Earnings and Profits.* How does the use of an accelerated method of depreciation affect a corporation's earnings and profits?

20-5   *Earnings and Profits.* How does the § 179 immediate expensing option affect a corporation's earnings and profits?

20-6   *Distributions.* Is it possible for a distribution to be a taxable dividend even if there is a deficit in accumulated earnings and profits? If so, how?

20-7   *Cash Dividends.* What is the amount of distribution when cash is distributed?

20-8   *Property Dividends.* What is the amount of the distribution when property other than cash is distributed?

20-9   *Property Dividends and Liabilities.* What effect does a liability have on the amount and basis of property distributed if the property is subject to the liability?

20-10   *Constructive Dividends.* What are constructive dividends? When do they arise?

20-11   *Effect of Property Dividend on the Corporation.* In what situations must a corporation recognize income as a result of a distribution?

20-12   *Effect of Property Dividends on Earnings and Profits.* How do property dividends affect earnings and profits?

20-13   *Stock Dividends.* What is a stock dividend?

20-14   *Stock Dividends.* In what situations may a stock dividend be taxable? When is it not taxable?

20-15 *Stock Dividends.* How is the shareholder's basis in a stock dividend determined?

20-16 *Stock Dividends.* How do stock dividends affect earnings and profits?

20-17 *Stock Rights.* What are stock rights? How does their tax treatment differ from stock dividends?

20-18 *Dividends.* What is the effect of a dividend on the distributing corporation's taxable income?

20-19 *Stock Redemptions.* What is a stock redemption?

20-20 *Stock Redemptions.* List the situations in which a stock redemption will be treated as a sale of stock.

20-21 *Constructive Ownership.* What is constructive ownership of stock? How may stock be constructively owned?

20-22 *Effect of Redemption on Redeeming Corporation.* How do stock redemptions affect the redeeming corporation? In what situations must gain or loss be recognized when stock is redeemed? How do stock redemptions affect earnings and profits?

20-23 *Complete Liquidations.* What is a complete liquidation?

20-24 *Code § 331.* Generally explain the treatment of the shareholders in a complete liquidation.

20-25 *Code § 336.* Generally explain the treatment of the liquidating corporation in a complete liquidation.

20-26 *Liquidation of a Subsidiary.* What conditions must be met in order for § 332 to apply to the liquidation of a subsidiary?

20-27 *Liquidation of a Subsidiary—Basis.* What is the general rule for determining the parent corporation's basis in the assets received from its liquidated subsidiary?

20-28 *Kimbell-Diamond Exception.* What is the *Kimbell-Diamond* exception?

20-29 *Code § 338—Purchase of Assets.* When does § 338 apply to the liquidation of a subsidiary? How does it differ from the general rule for determining basis in the liquidation of a subsidiary?

PROBLEMS

20-30 *Dividends.* A's basis in his 50 shares of Q Corporation stock is $3,000. A purchased the Q Corporation stock in 2004. On November 11, 2009, Q Corporation distributed $8,000 to A with respect to the Q Corporation stock. The portion of Q Corporation's earnings and profits allocable to A is $3,500. What is the tax treatment of the $8,000 distribution to A?

20-31 *Earnings and Profits.* D Corporation's taxable income for the year was computed as follows:

Gross income from operations.....................		$1,000,000
Less: Operating expenses.................		(900,000)
Net income from operations.....................		$ 100,000
Dividend income		20,000
Long-term capital gain	$15,000	

Less: Capital loss carryover		(7,000)	8,000

Income before special deductions.			$ 128,000
Net operating loss carryover	$ 9,000		
Dividends-received deduction	16,000		
Total of special deductions.			(25,000)
Taxable income			$ 103,000

Additional information:
1. The corporation received $5,000 in tax-exempt interest income.
2. Included in operating expenses is depreciation of $130,000. Straight-line depreciation of the depreciable assets would have been $50,000.

Compute the earnings and profits of D Corporation for the current year.

20-32 *Earnings and Profits.* V Corporation's taxable income for the year included the following items:
1. A $12,000 charitable contributions deduction. Actual charitable contributions made by V Corporation were $20,000, but only $12,000 was deductible this year due to the 10 percent charitable contributions limitation.
2. An 80 percent dividends-received deduction of $8,000. The amount of dividend income received by V Corporation was $10,000.
3. Percentage depletion of $4,000 was deducted by V Corporation. Cost depletion would have been $800.
4. $2,000 of assets purchased by V Corporation this year were expensed using the § 179 immediate expensing option.
5. MACRS depreciation of $1,500 was taken on a new heavy-duty truck (five-year property) purchased this year. The cost of the automobile was $10,000.

Compute the effect of the above items on V Corporation's current earnings and profits.

20-33 *Distributions.* For each of the following independent situations, compute the amount of dividend income to the shareholder as a result of the distribution(s), and specify the source of each distribution (current and/or accumulated earnings and profits).

Distributions

	April 1	October 1	Current E&P	Accumulated E&P
a.	$5,000	$5,000	$15,000	$10,000
b.	9,000	9,000	15,000	10,000
c.	2,000	4,000	7,000	(20,000)
d.	6,000	2,000	0	11,000
e.	3,000	5,000	(12,000)	30,000
f.	3,000	2,000	1,000	0
g.	1,000	3,000	(6,000)	8,000

20-34 *Cash and Property Dividends.* A Corporation is owned by J (an individual) and B Corporation. A Corporation declared and paid the following dividends: $10,000 cash and a printing press with a fair market value of $10,000 and an adjusted basis of $6,000. A Corporation's current and accumulated earnings and profits exceed $20,000. Consider each alternative independently.
   a. If B Corporation received the cash and J received the printing press, how much dividend income would each report?
   b. If J received the cash and B Corporation received the printing press, how much dividend income would each report?

    c. What are the tax consequences to A Corporation of the distribution?

    d. What is the effect of the distribution on corporate earnings and profits?

20-35 *Property Dividends—Installment Obligations.* G Corporation distributed installment notes with a face value of $20,000 to its shareholders. The gross profit percentage of the notes was 20 percent, and the fair market value of the notes was $18,000 when they were distributed. Compute G Corporation's recognized gain on the distribution of the installment notes.

20-36 *Stock Dividends.* P owns 100 shares of Z Corporation common stock, which she purchased in 2001 for $50 a share. Z Corporation declared and paid a 100 percent stock dividend to all common stockholders. At the date of record, the selling price of a share of common stock was $200. Immediately following the distribution, the stock was selling for $225 per share.

    a. How much income must P recognize on the receipt of the 100 shares of common stock as a dividend?

    b. What is the basis of the dividend shares?

    c. Assume that P received the dividend on June 1 and sold 50 shares of stock (25 new and 25 old) on July 1 for $150 per share. What is P's recognized gain or loss? Is it long-term or short-term?

20-37 *Stock Dividends.* R owns 50 shares of A Corporation common stock, which he purchased in 2004 for $100 per share. On January 1 of the current year, A Corporation declared a dividend of one share of new preferred stock for each share of common. The shares were distributed on March 1. On that date, the common stock was selling for $150 per share and the preferred stock had a value of $50 per share.

    a. How much income must R recognize on the receipt of the preferred stock?

    b. What is R's basis in the preferred stock?

    c. On June 1, R sells 25 shares of common stock for $175 per share and 25 shares of preferred stock for $75 per share. What is R's recognized gain or loss? Is it long-term or short-term?

20-38 *Stock Dividends.* N owns 200 shares of M Corporation preferred stock. She purchased the stock for $200 per share in 2006. On February 1 of the current year, the corporation declared and paid a 50 percent stock dividend. At date of declaration, the preferred stock was selling for $220 per share. Immediately following the distribution (June 1), the preferred stock was selling for $150 per share.

    a. How much income will N have as a result of the dividend?

    b. What is her basis of the dividend shares?

    c. If N sells 25 shares of the old and 25 shares of the new for $180 per share on August 1, what is her recognized gain or loss? Is it long-term or short-term?

20-39 *Stock Rights.* Y Corporation's profits had taken a deep dive in recent years. To encourage purchase of its stock, the corporation issued one stock right for each share of outstanding common stock. The rights allow the holder to purchase a share of stock for $1. The common stock was selling for $1.50 when the rights were issued (June 1). The value of the stock rights on June 1 were $0.50 each. A owns 1,000 shares of common stock for which he paid $20 per share 10 years ago, and therefore received 1,000 stock rights. A sold 100 rights on July 1 for $175. He exercised 100 rights on August 1 when the stock was selling for $1.80 per share. The remaining rights lapsed on December 30.

    a. How much dividend income must A recognize?

    b. How much gain or loss must A recognize on the July 1 sale of the stock rights? Is it long-term or short-term?

    c. What is A's recognized loss when the remaining rights lapse?

    d. What is the basis of the original 1,000 shares on December 31?

20-40 *Stock Redemptions.* B owned 100 shares (100%) of the common stock of C Corporation. C Corporation has no other classes of stock outstanding. B's basis in his 100 shares was $3,000 ($30 per share). C Corporation redeemed 20 of B's shares for $1,000.

    a. What is B's recognized gain or loss on the redemption? What is the character of B's recognized gain or loss?

    b. What is B's basis in his remaining shares of C Corporation stock?

20-41 *Stock Redemptions.* W has owned 500 shares of X Corporation's 1,000 outstanding shares of voting common stock since 1998. X Corporation has no other classes of stock outstanding. W's basis in her 500 shares was $1,500 ($3 per share). X Corporation redeemed 200 shares of W's stock for $800.

    a. Is this redemption treated as a sale or a distribution?

    b. What is W's recognized gain or loss on the redemption? What is the character of W's recognized gain or loss?

    c. What is the basis of W's remaining shares after the redemption?

20-42 *Stock Redemptions.* Assume the same facts as in *Problem 20-41* except that X Corporation redeemed 100 shares of W's stock instead of 200 shares. Answer the above questions a, b, and c for this situation.

20-43 *Stock Redemptions.* T Corporation is owned by the following unrelated individuals:

K	60 shares
L	20 shares
M	10 shares
N	10 shares
Total	100 shares

If T Corporation redeems 30 shares owned by K, will the transaction qualify as a sale? Why or why not?

20-44 *Stock Redemptions—Constructive Ownership.* Use the same facts as in *Problem 20-43*. Would this redemption qualify as a sale if L is K's son? Why or why not?

20-45 *Constructive Ownership of Stock.* Q, an individual, owns 20 percent of A Corporation. Mrs. Q owns 60 percent of A Corporation and 50 percent of BC Partnership. R, Q's daughter, owns 30 percent of BC Partnership and 10 percent of A Corporation. What is Q's ownership (directly and indirectly) in A Corporation and BC Partnership, if the constructive ownership rules of § 318 apply?

20-46 *Constructive Ownership of Stock.* D is a 30 percent partner in DE Partnership. DE Partnership owns 10 percent of F Corporation. Using the § 318 constructive ownership rules, what percentage of F Corporation is D considered to own?

20-47 *Constructive Ownership of Stock.* G owns 200 shares of H Corporation stock. G is a 50 percent partner in GJ Partnership. Using the § 318 constructive ownership rules, how many shares of H Corporation is the GJ Partnership considered to own?

20-48 *Liquidations—General Rule (§§ 331 and 336).* S, an individual, owns all of the stock of B Corporation. S purchased the stock 10 years ago for $300,000. S decided to completely liquidate B Corporation, and all of the assets of B Corporation were distributed to S. The balance sheet for B Corporation immediately prior to the liquidation was as follows:

	Basis	Fair Market Value
Cash	$ 40,000	$ 40,000
Marketable securities	40,000	80,000
Equipment $300,000		
Less: Accumulated depreciation .... (150,000)	150,000	200,000
Land	520,000	880,000
Total assets	$750,000	$1,200,000
Retained earnings.......................	$450,000	$ 0
Common stock.........................	300,000	1,200,000
Total equity.........................	$750,000	$1,200,000

a. What is S's recognized gain or loss?
b. What is S's basis in the assets received?
c. How much, if any, income or loss will B Corporation recognize as a result of the liquidation?

20-49 *Liquidations (§ 332).* Assume the same facts as in *Problem 20-48* except that the stock is owned by S, Inc.
a. How much, if any, gain or loss must S, Inc. recognize?
b. What is the basis of the assets received by S, Inc.?
c. How much, if any, income must B Corporation recognize as a result of the liquidation?

20-50 *Section 338 Election.* Assume the same facts as in *Problem 20-48* except that all the stock was purchased by Z Corporation during the past 12 months for $1 million. Assume Z makes a § 338 election and pays taxes at a 34 percent rate.
a. What is Z's recognized gain or loss?
b. What, if any, income must B recognize?
c. What is the total basis of the assets to B after the election?

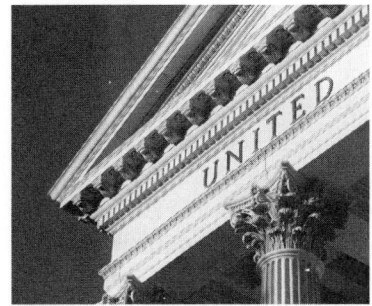

CHAPTER TWENTY ONE

TAXATION OF CORPORATE ACCUMULATIONS

LEARNING OBJECTIVES

Upon completion of this chapter you will be able to:

▸ Understand the rationale for the two corporate penalty taxes: the accumulated earnings tax and the personal holding company tax

▸ Identify the circumstances that must exist before the accumulated earnings tax will apply

▸ Recognize when earnings have accumulated beyond the reasonable needs of the business

▸ Explain how the accumulated earnings tax is computed

▸ Indicate when the personal holding company tax applies

▸ Apply the stock ownership and income tests to determine if a corporation is a personal holding company

▸ Explain how the personal holding company tax is computed and how it might be avoided

---

CHAPTER OUTLINE

INTRODUCTION

In addition to the regular tax, a corporation may be subject to two penalty taxes—the *accumulated earnings tax* and the *personal holding company tax*. As the label "penalty" suggests, the primary goal of these taxes is not to raise revenues but rather to prohibit certain activities. The objective of the accumulated earnings tax and the personal holding company tax is to discourage individual taxpayers from using the corporate entity solely for tax avoidance. These taxes contend with potential abuse by imposing limitations on the amount of earnings a corporation may retain without penalty. The rationale for these taxes is readily apparent when some of the opportunities for tax avoidance using the corporate structure are considered.

Perhaps the best illustration of how the corporate entity could be used to avoid taxes involves the 70 percent dividends-received deduction. As discussed in Chapter 1, this deduction is available only to corporate taxpayers. Nevertheless, individuals could take advantage of the deduction by establishing a corporation and transferring their dividend-paying stocks to it. By so doing, all dividend income would be taxable to the corporation instead of the individual. Using this arrangement, the corporation would pay tax on dividends at an effective rate of 10.5 percent or lower [$35\% \times (100\% - 70\%)$] in 2006. Most individual taxpayers with taxable dividend income would reap substantial tax savings from this arrangement since all individual marginal rates are 15 percent or higher. This is but one of the alluring features of the corporate entity.

Another corporate advantage that individuals previously used to avoid taxes concerned the difference between individual and corporate tax rates. Until the current year, because the highest individual tax rate exceeded the top corporate tax rate, individuals operating a business in the corporate form could benefit by leaving earnings in the corporation and reinvesting at this lower tax rate. The savings obtained by utilizing this disparity, the dividends-received deduction, and other advantages of the corporate entity, illustrate that individuals could achieve wholesale tax avoidance if not for some provision denying or discouraging such plans.

The two penalty taxes were developed to battle avoidance schemes such as those above by attacking their critical component: the accumulation. This can be seen by examining the two previous examples. The fate of both tax savings schemes rests on whether the shareholder can reduce or totally escape the second tax normally incurred when the income is ultimately received. In other words, the success of these arrangements depends on the extent to which double taxation is avoided. Herein lies the role of corporate accumulations. As long as the earnings are retained in the corporation, the second tax is avoided and the taxpayer is well on the way to obtaining tax savings. To foil such schemes, Congress enacted the accumulated earnings tax and the personal holding company tax. Both taxes are imposed on unwarranted accumulations of income—income that normally would have been taxable to the individual at individual tax rates if it had been distributed. By imposing these taxes on unreasonable accumulations, Congress hoped to compel distributions from the corporation and thus prevent taxpayers from using the corporate entity for tax avoidance.

Although these penalty taxes are rarely incurred, each serves as a strong deterrent against possible taxpayer abuse. However, with the reduction in the tax rate on dividends to 15 percent, imposition of these penalties or change in corporate behavior is even less likely. This chapter examines the operation of both the accumulated earnings tax and the personal holding company tax.

Mitigation of the double tax penalty and any resulting tax savings are not achieved solely through corporate accumulations. The effect of double taxation can be reduced or avoided in other ways. The most common method used to avoid double taxation is by making distributions that are deductible. Typical deductible payments include compensation for services rendered to the corporation, rent for property leased to the corporation by the shareholder, and interest on funds loaned to the corporation. All of

these payments are normally deductible by the corporation (thus effectively eliminating the corporate tax) and taxable to the shareholder. Avoidance of the double tax penalty does not ensure tax savings, however. All of these payments are taxable to the shareholder; thus, savings through use of the corporate entity may or may not result. For example, savings could occur if the payments are made to shareholders after they have dropped to a tax bracket lower than the one in which they were when the earnings were initially realized by the corporation. In addition, even if the shareholder's tax bracket remains unchanged, deferral of the tax could be beneficial.

> **Example 1.** L operates a home improvement company, specializing in kitchen renovations. He is in the 35% bracket in 2009. Assume that he incorporates his business in 2009 and it earns $100,000, of which $50,000 is paid to him as a salary and $50,000 is accumulated. In 2009 L saves $10,000 [(35% − 15%) × $50,000] in taxes on the $50,000 not distributed. However, if the $50,000 accumulated is distributed to L as a salary in 2014 when he is still in the 35% bracket, the $10,000 of taxes originally saved is lost. Although no taxes have been saved, L continues to benefit because he has been able to postpone the $10,000 in tax for five years. Assuming his after-tax rate of return is 10%, the present value of the $10,000 tax is reduced to $6,209—a savings of $3,791, or almost 38%. Note that the savings would have increased if the distribution had been made to L when his tax bracket dropped below 35%.

ACCUMULATED EARNINGS TAX

The accumulated earnings tax, unlike most taxes previously discussed, is not computed by a corporation when filing its annual income tax return. There is no form to file to determine the tax. Normally, the issue arises during an audit of the corporation. Consequently, the actual tax computation is made only after it has been determined that the penalty must be imposed.

AN OVERVIEW

The accumulated earnings tax applies whenever a corporation is "formed or availed of" for what is generally referred to as the *forbidden purpose*, that is, "for the purpose of avoiding the income tax with respect to its shareholders ... by permitting earnings and profits to accumulate instead of being ... distributed."[1] Whether a corporation is in fact being used for the forbidden purpose and thus subject to penalty is an elusive question requiring a determination of the taxpayer's *intent*. Without guidance from the law, ascertaining the taxpayer's intent might prove impossible. However, the Code states that the required intent is deemed present whenever a corporation accumulates earnings beyond its reasonable needs unless the corporation can prove to the contrary by a preponderance of evidence.[2] The problems concerning intent are considered in detail below.

Not all corporations risk the accumulated earnings tax. The Code specifically exempts tax-exempt corporations, personal holding companies, and passive foreign investment companies.[3] In addition, the tax normally does not apply to an S corporation since it does not shield shareholders from tax. An S corporation's earnings are taxed to its shareholders annually.

---

[1]   § 532(a).

[2]   § 533(a).

[3]   § 532.

If it applies, the accumulated earnings tax is imposed on the annual increment to the corporation's total accumulated earnings, not on the total accumulated earnings balance. This annual addition is referred to as *accumulated taxable income*. The tax is 15 percent of the corporation's accumulated taxable income.[4] This tax does not replace any other taxes (e.g., the corporate income tax or the alternative minimum tax) but is imposed in addition to these taxes.

> **Example 2.** In an audit of P Corporation, it was determined that the company had accumulated earnings beyond the reasonable needs of its business. In addition, the corporation's accumulated taxable income was $150,000. Since evidence of the forbidden purpose is present and the corporation has accumulated taxable income, the accumulated earnings tax must be paid. P Corporation's accumulated earnings tax is $22,500 ($150,000 × 15%).

In short, the corporation actually pays the accumulated earnings tax only if the forbidden purpose is found and it has accumulated taxable income. The following sections examine the determination of the taxpayer's intent and the computation of accumulated taxable income.

INTENT

The accumulated earnings tax is imposed only if the corporation is formed or used for the purpose of avoiding income tax on its shareholders by accumulating earnings.[5] Unfortunately, the Code provides no objective, mechanical test for determining whether a corporation is in fact being used for the forbidden purpose. As a result, application of the accumulated earnings tax rests on a subjective assessment of the shareholders' intent. The Code and regulations offer certain guidelines for making this assessment. Section 533 provides that a corporation is deemed to have been formed or used for the purpose of avoiding tax on its shareholders in two situations:

1. If the corporation has accumulated earnings beyond the reasonable needs of the business; or

2. If the corporation is a mere holding or investment company.

The first situation is the most common cause of an accumulated earnings tax penalty. Consequently, avoidance of the accumulated earnings tax normally rests on whether the corporation can prove that its balance (i.e., the amount in excess of the $250,000 or $150,000 threshold) in accumulated earnings and profits is required by the reasonable needs of the business. Before discussing what constitutes a "reasonable need" of the business, it should be noted that other circumstances may indicate that the forbidden purpose does or does not exist.

According to the Regulations, the following factors are to be considered in determining whether the corporation has been used to avoid tax:[6]

1. Loans to shareholders or expenditures that benefit shareholders personally;

2. Investments in assets having no reasonable connection with the corporation's business; and

3. Poor dividend history.

---

[4]   § 531.

[5]   § 532(a).

[6]   § 1.533-1(a)(2).

Although these factors are not conclusive evidence, their presence no doubt suggests improper accumulations.

In determining whether the requisite intent exists, the courts have considered not only the criteria mentioned above but also whether the corporation's stock is widely held. As a general rule, the accumulated earnings tax does not apply to publicly held corporations. Publicly held corporations normally are protected since the number and variety of their shareholders usually preclude the formation of a dividend policy to minimize shareholder taxes. Nevertheless, the tax has been applied to publicly held corporations in which management was dominated by a small group of shareholders who were able to control dividend policy for their benefit.[7] Moreover, in 1984, Congress eliminated any doubts as to whether publicly held corporations are automatically exempt from the penalty tax. Section 532(c) currently provides that the tax be applied without regard to the number of shareholders of the corporation. Thus, the tax may be imposed on a publicly held corporation if the situation warrants.

While publicly held corporations usually are immune from the penalty tax, closely held corporations are particularly vulnerable since dividend policy is easily manipulated to meet shareholders' desires. Indeed, it may be a formidable task to prove that the corporation was not used for tax avoidance in light of the *Donruss* decision.[8] In that case, the Supreme Court held that the tax avoidance motive need not be the primary or dominant motive for the accumulation of earnings before the penalty tax is imposed. Rather, if tax avoidance is but one of the motives, the tax may apply.

As a practical matter, it is difficult, if not impossible, to determine the actual intent of the corporation and its shareholders. For this reason, the presumption created by § 533(a) looms large in virtually all accumulated earnings tax cases. Under this provision, a tax avoidance purpose is deemed to exist if earnings were accumulated beyond the reasonable needs of the business.[9] As might be expected, most of the litigation in this area has concerned what constitutes a reasonable need of the business. In fact, many cases do not even mention intent, implying that the accumulated earnings tax will be applied in all cases in which the accumulation exceeds business needs. Except in the unusual case in which a corporation's intent can be demonstrated, a corporation should be prepared to justify the accumulations based on the needs of the business.

REASONABLE NEEDS OF THE BUSINESS

The Code does not define the term "reasonable needs of the business." Instead it states that the reasonable needs of the business include the *reasonably anticipated needs* of the business.[10] The Regulations clarify the term reasonably anticipated needs.[11] First, the corporation must have specific, definite, and feasible plans for the use of the accumulation. The funds do not have to be expended in a short period of time after the close of the year. In fact, the plans need only require that the accumulations be expended within a *reasonable* time in the future. However, if the plans are postponed indefinitely, the needs will not be considered reasonable. As a general rule, the plans

---

[7]   See *Trico Products*, 42-2 USTC ¶9540, 31 AFTR 394, 137 F.2d 424 (CA-2, 1943). In *Golconda Mining Corp.*, 58 T.C. 139 (1972), the Tax Court held that the tax applied where management controlled 17 percent of the outstanding stock of a publicly held corporation but the Ninth Circuit reversed, suggesting the tax should be applied solely to closely held corporations, 74-2 USTC ¶9845. 35 AFTR2d 75-336, 507 F.2d 594 (CA-9, 1974). Tax applied to publicly held corporation in *Alphatype Corporation v. U.S.* 76-2 USTC ¶9730, 38 AFTR2d 76-6019 (Ct. Cls., 1976). In Rev. Rul. 73-305, 1975-2 C.B. 228 the IRS confirmed its position that it will apply the tax to publicly held corporations.

[8]   *U.S. v. Donruss*, 69-1 USTC ¶9167, 23 AFTR2d 69-418, 393 U.S. 297 (USSC, 1969).

[9]   § 533(a).

[10]   § 537(a)(1).

[11]   Reg. § 1.537-1(b).

must not be vague and uncertain. If the plans are based on specific studies containing dollar estimates and are approved by the board of directors, the corporation is in a better position to prove that the plans qualify as reasonable business needs.

In addition to reasonably anticipated needs, the Code and Regulations identify certain specific reasons for accumulations that are considered to be reasonable needs of the business.[12] Several of these reasons are discussed below.

Stock Redemptions from an Estate. A corporation is allowed to temporarily accumulate earnings in order to redeem the stock of a deceased shareholder in conjunction with Code § 303 (discussed in Chapter 20).[13] The accumulations may commence *only after* the death of a shareholder. The fact that a shareholder dies after accumulations have been made and the corporation redeems his or her stock under § 303 is ignored in evaluating pre-death accumulations.[14] If the shareholder owned stock in two or more corporations, each corporation is entitled to accumulate only a portion of the total redeemable amount unless the estate's executor or administrator has indicated that more shares of one of the corporations will be offered for redemption than will those of another corporation.[15] The requirements of § 303 (relating to redemption of stock to pay death taxes) must be met in order for this provision to apply.

Product Liability Loss Reserves. The Code also allows accumulations to cover product liability losses.[16] Product liability is defined as damages for physical or emotional harm as well as damages and loss to property as a result of the use of a product sold, leased, or manufactured by the taxpayer.[17] The amount accumulated can cover both actual and reasonably anticipated losses.

Business Expansion or Plant Replacement. Perhaps the most common reason for accumulating earnings that the Regulations specifically authorize is for *bona fide* expansion of business or replacement of plant.[18] This provision includes the purchase or construction of a building.[19] It also includes the modernization, rehabilitation, or replacement of assets.[20] However, this provision does not shield a corporation which has not adequately specified and documented its expansion needs.[21]

Acquisition of a Business Enterprise. A second reason offered in the Regulations for accumulating earnings is for the acquisition of a business enterprise through the purchase of stock or assets.[22] This provision appears to encourage business expansion, since the Regulations state that the business for which earnings can be accumulated includes any line of business the corporation wishes to undertake, and not just the line of business previously carried on.[23] However, this provision for accumulation is limited by the statement in the Regulations that investments in properties or securities that are

---

[12]   See § 537(a) and (b), and Reg. § 1.537-2.

[13]   § 537(b)(1).

[14]   § 537(b)(5).

[15]   Reg. § 1.537-1(c)(3).

[16]   § 537(b)(4).

[17]   § 172(f).

[18]   Reg. § 1.537-2(b)(1).

[19]   *Sorgel v. U.S.*, 72-1 USTC ¶9427, 29 AFTR2d 72-1035, 341 F. Supp. 1 (D. Ct. Wisc., 1972).

[20]   *Knoxville Iron*, 18 TCM 251, T.C. Memo 1959-54.

[21]   *I.A. Dress Co.*, 60-1 USTC ¶9204, 5 AFTR2d 429, 273 F.2d 543 (CA-2, 1960), aff&g. 32 T.C. 93; *Herzog Miniature Lamp Works, Inc.*, 73-2 USTC ¶9593, 32 AFTR2d 73-5282, 273 F.2d 543, (CA-2, 1973).

[22]   Reg. § 1.537-2(b)(2).

[23]   Reg. § 1.537-3(a).

unrelated to the activities of the business of the corporation are unacceptable reasons for accumulations.[24] The statements in the Regulations raise a question as to the validity of accumulations for diversification. On one hand the corporation can acquire an enterprise or expand its business into any field. On the other hand the acquisition should be related to the corporation's activities. This apparent conflict in the Regulations is reflected in court decisions. A corporation that manufactured automobile clutches was permitted to accumulate income to acquire a business that would make use of the corporation's metal-working expertise, whereas a corporation in the printing business was not permitted to accumulate income to acquire real estate.[25] The extent to which a corporation can diversify is uncertain. It appears that diversification into passive investments is unacceptable whereas diversification into an operating business, no matter how far removed from the original line of business, is acceptable.

Retirement of Indebtedness. The Regulations also provide for the accumulation of earnings to retire business indebtedness.[26] The debt can be to either a third party or a shareholder as long as it is a bona fide business debt.

Investments or Loans to Suppliers or Customers. The Regulations state that earnings may be accumulated to provide for investments or loans to suppliers or customers.[27] However, loans to shareholders, friends and relatives of shareholders, and corporations controlled by shareholders of the corporation making the loan indicate that earnings are possibly being accumulated beyond reasonable business needs.[28]

Contingencies. Although the Regulations do not specifically allow accumulations for contingencies, they do imply approval of such accumulations as long as the contingencies are not unrealistic.[29] Unfortunately, the distinction between realistic and unrealistic contingencies is difficult to define. However, the more specific the need, the more detailed the cash estimate, and the more likely the occurrence, the easier it will be to prove the accumulation is reasonable.

Redemption of Stock. As noted above, accumulations to redeem stock from a decedent's estate under § 303 constitute a reasonable need of the business. This provision does not cover any other stock redemption. Several cases have held that a redemption may be a reasonable need provided the redemption is for the benefit of the corporation and not the shareholder.[30] For example, the redemption of a dissenting minority shareholder's stock can be for the corporation's benefit whereas the redemption of a majority shareholder's stock would be for the shareholder's benefit. It might also be possible to prove that the redemption was necessary to reduce or eliminate disputes over management or conduct of the business.

Working Capital. Another reason mentioned in the Regulations for a reasonable accumulation of earnings and profits is the need for working capital.[31] This is one of the

---

[24]   Reg. § 1.537-2(c)(4).

[25]   *Alma Piston Co.*, 22 TCM 948, T.C. Memo 1963-195; *Union Offset*, 79-2 USTC ¶9550, 44 AFTR2d 79-5652. 603 F.2d 90 (CA-9, 1979).

[26]   Reg. § 1.537-2(b)(3).

[27]   Reg. § 1.537-2(b)(5).

[28]   Reg. §§ 1.537-2(c)(1), (2), and (3).

[29]   Reg. § 1.537-2(c)(5).

[30]   See *John B. Lambert & Assoc. v. U.S.*, 38 AFTR2d 6207 (Ct. Cls., 1976); *C.E. Hooper, Inc. v. U.S.*, 38 AFTR2d 5417, 539 F.2d 1276 (Ct. Cls.,1976); *Mountain State Steel Foundries, Inc. v. Comm.*, 6 AFTR2d 5910, 284 F.2d 737 (CA-4, 1960); and *Koma, Inc. v. Comm.*, 40 AFTR 712, 189 F.2d 390 (CA-10, 1951).

[31]   Reg. § 1.537-2(b)(4).

primary justifications corporations use for the accumulation of earnings. A corporation is permitted to retain earnings to provide necessary working capital. Initially, the courts tried to measure working capital sufficiency by using rules of thumb. A current ratio of 2.5 to 1 generally meant that the corporation had not accumulated income unreasonably.[32] The courts considered a current ratio more than 2.5 to 1 an indication of unreasonable accumulation.

In the 1965 case of *Bardahl Mfg. Corp.*, the Tax Court utilized a formula to compute the working capital needs of a corporation.[33] Under this approach (called the *Bardahl* formula), the working capital needed for one operating cycle is computed. This amount in essence represents the cash *needed* to meet expenses incurred during the operating cycle—the period required for a business to convert cash into inventory, sell the merchandise, convert the customer's accounts receivable into cash, and pay its accounts payable. This necessary working capital is then compared to actual working capital. If necessary working capital is greater than actual working capital, an accumulation of earnings to meet the necessary working capital requirements is justified. If actual working capital is greater than the working capital needed, the corporation must show other reasons for the accumulation of earnings in order to avoid the accumulated earnings tax.

The initial step of the *Bardahl* formula is to calculate the inventory, accounts receivable, and accounts payable cycle ratios. These ratios are computed as follows:

1. *Inventory cycle ratio* $= \dfrac{\text{Average inventory}}{\text{Cost of goods sold}}$

2. *Accounts receivable cycle ratio* $= \dfrac{\text{Average accounts receivable}}{\text{Net sales}}$

3. *Accounts payable cycle ratio* $= \dfrac{\text{Average accounts payable}}{\text{Purchases}}$

The ratios resulting from these calculations represent the cycle expressed as a percentage of the year. In other words, if the accounts receivable cycle ratio is 10 percent, then it normally takes about 36 days ($10\% \times 365$) to collect a receivable once it has been generated by a sale.

Instead of using the *average* inventory and the average receivables, a corporation can use *peak values* if it is in a seasonal business. If the corporation uses peak values for the other ratios, it may be required to use peak payables.

Once computed, the three ratios are combined. The result represents the number of days—expressed as a fraction of the year—during which the corporation needs working capital to meet its operating expenses. The operating cycle ratio is computed as follows:

$$\begin{array}{l}\text{Inventory cycle ratio}\\ +\text{Accounts receivable cycle ratio}\\ \underline{-\text{Accounts payable cycle ratio}}\\ = \text{Operating cycle ratio}\end{array}$$

The operating cycle ratio is multiplied by the *annual operating expenses* to compute the necessary working capital. Operating expenses are defined as the cost of goods sold plus other annual expenses (i.e., general, administrative, and selling expenses). The operating expense category does not include depreciation since depreciation does not require the use of cash. However, the category can include income taxes if the corporation pays estimated taxes and will make a tax payment during the next operating cycle.[34] Other expenses should be included if they will require the expenditure of cash during the next operating cycle.

32 *J Scripps Newspaper*, 44 T.C. 453 (1965).

33 *Bardahl Mfg. Corp.*, 24 TCM 1030, T.C. Memo 1965-200.

34 *Empire Steel*, 33 TCM 155, T.C. Memo 1974-34.

The required working capital computed by the *Bardahl* formula is compared to actual working capital to determine if there have been excess accumulations. Since the computed working capital is based on accounting data, it is normally compared to actual working capital (current assets − current liabilities) computed from the corporation's financial statements. There are exceptions to this rule. Financial statements are not used if they do not clearly reflect the company's working capital. The Supreme Court authorized the use of fair market value instead of historical cost to value a firm's current assets in *Ivan Allen Co.*[35] The assets in question were marketable securities that had appreciated. The decision is broad enough to permit the Internal Revenue Service to determine actual working capital based on current value any time there is a significant difference between cost and market.

Any corporation whose actual working capital does not exceed required working capital (per the *Bardahl* formula) should be exempt from the accumulated earnings tax. If the actual working capital exceeds required working capital, the excess is considered an indication of unreasonable accumulations. This excess is compared to the reasonable needs of the business (other than working capital) to determine if the accumulations are unreasonable. To the extent that the corporation has needs, it may accumulate funds. If all of the excess working capital is not needed, the tax is imposed. The tax is based on the accumulated taxable income and not the excess working capital.

> **Example 3.** K owns and operates K's Apparel, Inc. (KAI). After hearing that a friend's corporation was recently slapped with an accumulated earnings tax penalty, she asked her accountant to determine the vulnerability of her own business. The following is a balance sheet and income statement for 2008 and 2009 for KAI.

Balance Sheet

	2008	2009
Current Assets:		
Cash	$ 55,000	$ 67,000
Marketable securities	10,000	8,000
Accounts receivable (net)	45,000	55,000
Inventory	30,000	20,000
Total Current Assets	$ 140,000	$ 150,000
Property, plant, and equipment (net)	300,000	425,000
Total Assets	$ 440,000	$ 575,000
Current Liabilities:		
Notes payable	$ 5,000	$ 4,000
Accounts payable	50,000	30,000
Accrued expenses	8,000	16,000
Total Current Liabilities	$ 63,000	$ 50,000
Long-term debt	37,000	40,000
Total Liabilities	$ 100,000	$ 90,000
Stockholders' Equity:		
Common stock	10,000	10,000
Earnings and profits	330,000	475,000
Total Liabilities and Stockholders' Equity	$ 440,000	$ 575,000

---

[35] *Ivan Allen Co. v. U.S.*, 75-2 USTC ¶9557, 36 AFTR2d 75-5200, 422 U.S. 617 (USSC, 1975).

Income Statement

Sales.......................................	$ 400,000	$ 500,000
Cost of goods sold:		
Beginning inventory.........................	$ 40,000	$ 30,000
Purchases..................................	300,000	320,000
Ending inventory	(30,000)	(20,000)
Total..................................	$ 310,000	$ 330,000
Gross profit	$ 90,000	$ 170,000
Other expenses:		
Depreciation...............................	$ 40,000	$ 55,000
Selling expenses	10,000	15,000
Administrative	20,000	50,000
Total..................................	$ 70,000	$ 120,000
Net income before taxes......................	$ 20,000	$ 50,000
Income tax expense	(2,000)	(5,000)
Net income...................................	$ 18,000	$ 45,000

In addition to this information, K indicated that at the end of 2009 the securities were worth $15,000 more than their book value, or $23,000. K also estimates that her reasonable needs for the current year 2009 amount to $20,000.

Under the *Bardahl* formula, her working capital needs are determined as follows:

Step 1: Operating cycle expressed as a fraction of the year (in thousands):

$$\text{Inventory cycle} = \frac{\text{Average inventory}}{\text{cost of goods sold}} = [(30 + 20) + 2] \;\div\; 330 = 0.0758$$

$$+ \;\;\text{Receivable cycle} = \frac{\text{Average receivables}}{\text{Sales}} = [(45 + 55) + 2] \;\div\; 500 = 0.1000$$

$$- \;\;\text{Payables cycle} = \frac{\text{Average payables}}{\text{Purchases}} = [(50 + 30) + 2] \;\div\; 320 = (0.1250)$$

= Operating cycle expressed as percentage of the year	= 0.0508

Step 2: Computation of operating expenses:

Operating expenses:	
Cost of goods sold	$330,000
Selling expenses	15,000
Administrative expenses.................	50,000
Taxes	5,000
Total operating expenses...................	$400,000

Step 3: Working capital needs:

Operating expenses (Step 2)...................	$400,000
× Operating cycle (Step 1)......................	× 0.0508
= Working capital needs........................	$ 20,320

K's working capital needs, $20,320, must be compared to actual working capital using the assets' fair market value. Any excess of actual working capital over required working capital must be compared to the current year's needs to determine if unwarranted accumulations exist. Assuming the marketable securities are actually worth $23,000, the comparison is made as follows:

	Actual working capital:		
	Current assets		
	($150,000 + $15,000).........	$165,000	
−	Current liabilities	(50,000)	
=	Actual working capital.........		$115,000
−	Required working capital (Step 3)		(20,320)
=	Excess working capital		$ 94,680
−	Reasonable needs		(20,000)
=	Accumulations beyond current needs........		$ 74,680

The accumulated earnings tax focuses on whether the corporation has accumulated liquid assets beyond its reasonable needs that could be distributed to shareholders. In this case, actual working capital exceeds required working capital and other needs of the business by $74,680, implying that the accumulated earnings tax applies. If so, the actual penalty tax is computed using accumulated taxable income, as explained below.

COMPUTATION OF THE ACCUMULATED EARNINGS TAX

The purpose of the accumulated earnings tax is to penalize taxpayers with unwarranted accumulations. To accomplish this, a 15 percent tax is imposed on what the Code refers to as accumulated taxable income. Accumulated taxable income is designed to represent the amount that the corporation could have distributed after funding its reasonable needs. In essence, the computation attempts to determine the corporation's dividend-paying capacity. Exhibit 21-1 shows the formula for computing accumulated taxable income.[36]

---

[36] § 535.

EXHIBIT 21-1

Accumulated Taxable Income[37]

Taxable income:

Plus:	1.	The dividends-received deduction
	2.	Any net operating loss deduction that is reflected in taxable income
	3.	Any capital-loss carryovers from other years that are reflected in taxable income
Minus:	1.	Federal income taxes for the year, but not the accumulated earnings tax or the personal holding company tax
	2.	The charitable contributions for the year in excess of the 10 percent limitation
	3.	Any net capital loss incurred during the year reduced by net capital gain deductions of prior years that have not previously reduced any net capital loss deduction
	4.	Any net capital gain (net long-term capital gain − the net short-term capital loss) for the year minus the taxes attributable to the gain and any net capital losses of prior years that have not reduced a net capital gain deduction in determining the accumulated earnings tax

Equals: *Adjusted taxable income*

Minus:	1.	Accumulated earnings credit (see Exhibit 21-2)
	2.	Dividends–paid deduction (see Exhibit 21-3)

Equals: *Accumulated taxable income*

The computation of accumulated taxable income begins with an imperfect measure of the corporation's ability to pay dividends-taxable income. To obtain a more representative measure of the corporation's dividend-paying capacity, taxable income is modified to arrive at what is often referred to as *adjusted taxable income*.[38] For example, the deduction allowed for dividends received is added back to taxable income since it has no effect on the corporation's ability to pay dividends. The same rationale can be given for the net operating loss deduction. In contrast, charitable contributions in excess of the 10 percent limitation may be deducted in determining adjusted taxable income since the corporation does not have the nondeductible amount available to pay dividends. For the same reason, Federal income taxes may be deducted in computing adjusted taxable income.

The deduction for capital gains stems from the assumption that these earnings are used to fund the corporation's needs and consequently may be accumulated with impunity. Capital losses are deductible since these amounts are unavailable for payment of dividends and are not reflected in taxable income. As shown in Exhibit 21-1, however, the deductions for capital gains as well as capital losses must be modified.

Prior to 1984, corporations were entitled to reduce taxable income not only by the amount of their net capital gains (reduced by related taxes) but also by the full amount of their net capital losses, depending on whether a net capital gain or loss occurred. Consequently, there was an advantage in recognizing capital gains in one year and capital losses in another year in order to avoid netting and thus permit both gains and losses to be deducted in full. For example, if the corporation had a capital loss of $1,000 this year and a capital gain of $5,000 next year (ignoring taxes), both could be deducted in full each year in computing adjusted taxable income. However, if they occurred in the same year, the deduction would be limited to $4,000. To eliminate this

---

[37] § 535. Several additional adjustments are required for computing accumulated taxable income of a holding or investment company.

[38] This term is not found in the Code; it is used here solely for purposes of exposition.

planning opportunity, corporations are now required to reduce their net capital losses by any net capital gain deductions that have been used to arrive at adjusted taxable income in prior years. Under these rules, it is immaterial in what order or in what year gains and losses are recognized. In effect, taxable income is reduced only by the overall net gain or loss that the corporation has recognized to date.

Example 4. T Corporation has the following income and deductions for 2009:

Income from operations	$150,000
Dividend income (from less than 20% owned corporations)	40,000
Charitable contributions	25,000

T Corporation computes its taxable income as follows:

Income from operations		$150,000
Dividend income		40,000
Income before special deductions		$190,000
Special deductions:		
Charitable contribution (limited)	$ 19,000	
Dividend-received deduction	28,000	
Total special deductions		(47,000)
Taxable income		$143,000

T Corporation's Federal income taxes for 2009 are $39,020. T Corporation's adjusted taxable income is computed as follows:

Taxable income		$143,000
Plus: Dividend-received deduction		28,000
		$171,000
Minus the sum of		
Federal income taxes	$39,020	
Actual charitable contributions for the year minus the charitable contribution deduction reflected in taxable income ($25,000 − $19,000)	6,000	(45,020)
Equals: Adjusted taxable income		$125,980

Two additional deductions are permitted in computing accumulated taxable income: the accumulated earnings credit and the dividends-paid deduction. The deduction allowed for dividends is consistent with the theory that the tax should be imposed only on income that has not been distributed. The accumulated earnings credit allows the taxpayer to accumulate without penalty $250,000 or an amount equal to the reasonable needs of the business, whichever is greater.

ACCUMULATED EARNINGS CREDIT

In creating the accumulated earnings tax, Congress realized that a corporation should not be penalized for keeping enough of its earnings to meet legitimate business

needs. For this reason, in computing accumulated taxable income, a corporation is allowed—in effect—a reduction for the amount out of current year's earnings necessary to meet such needs. This reduction is the *accumulated earnings credit*.[39] Note that despite its name, the credit actually operates as a deduction. As a practical matter, it is this credit that insulates most corporations from the accumulated earnings tax.

Specifically, the credit is the greater of two amounts as described in Exhibit 21-2 and discussed further below. Generally, however, the credit for the current year may be determined as follows:

Reasonable business needs (or $250,000 if larger)	$xxx,xxx
Less: Beginning Accumulated E&P.	(xx,xxx)
Accumulated earnings credit	$xxx,xxx

EXHIBIT 21-2
Accumulated Earnings Credit[40]

The accumulated earnings credit is the greater of

1. *General Rule:* Earnings and profits for the taxable year that are retained to meet the reasonable needs of the business, minus the net capital gain for the year (reduced by the taxes attributable to the gain),

   or

2. *Minimum Credit:* $250,000 ($150,000 for personal service corporations) minus the accumulated earnings and profits of the corporation at the close of the *preceding* taxable year, adjusted for dividends paid in the current year *deemed* paid in the prior year.

Part 1 of Exhibit 21-2 contains the general rule authorizing accumulations. It permits corporations to accumulate earnings to the extent of their reasonable needs without penalty.[41] In determining the amount of the earnings and profits for the taxable year that have been retained to meet the reasonable needs of the business, it is necessary to consider to what extent the accumulated earnings and profits are available to cover these needs.[42] In effect, prior accumulations reduce the amount that can be retained in the current year. If the corporation's accumulated earnings and profits are sufficient to meet the reasonable needs of the business, *none* of the current earnings and profits will be considered to be retained to meet the reasonable needs of the business.

Part 2 of Exhibit 21-2 is the so-called *minimum credit*.[43] For most corporations the amount of the minimum credit is $250,000. For personal service corporations, the minimum credit is $150,000. Personal service corporations are corporations that provide services in the area of health, law, engineering, architecture, accounting, actuarial science, performing arts, or consulting. The lower credit for personal service corporations reflects the fact that their capital needs are relatively small when compared to retail or manufacturing businesses.

To determine the amount of the minimum credit available for the current year, the base amount, $250,000 ($150,000), must be reduced by the accumulated earnings and profits at the close of the preceding tax year. For purposes of this computation, the accumulated earnings and profits at the close of the preceding year are reduced by the

[39] § 535(c).

[40] § 535(c)(1).

[41] *Ibid.*

[42] Reg. § 1.535-3(b)(1)(ii).

[43] § 535(c)(2).

dividends that were paid by the corporation within 2 ½ months after the close of the preceding year.[44]

Example 5. X Corporation, a calendar year retail department store, had current earnings and profits for 2009 of $75,000. Its accumulated earnings and profits at the close of 2008 were $200,000. X Corporation has paid no dividends for five years. X Corporation's taxable income for 2009 included a net capital gain of $20,000. [The taxes related to this net capital gain were $6,800 (34% × $20,000).] The reasonable needs of X Corporation are estimated to be $240,000. The amount of X Corporation's current earnings and profits that are retained to meet reasonable business needs is computed as follows:

Estimated reasonable needs of X Corporation.	$ 240,000
Less: Accumulated earnings and profits as of 12/31/08	(200,000)
Extent to which current earnings and profits are needed to cover the	
reasonable needs of the business.	$ 40,000

Even though the current earnings and profits are $75,000, only $40,000 of the current earnings and profits are needed to meet the reasonable needs of the business.

The accumulated earnings credit is the greater of

1. Current earnings and profits to meet the		
reasonable needs of the business		$ 40,000
Minus: Net capital gain.	$20,000	
Reduced by the taxes attributable to the gain	(6,800)	(13,200)
General rule credit		$ 26,800
or		
2. $250,000		$ 250,000
Minus: Accumulated earnings		
and profits as of 12/31/08		(200,000)
Minimum credit.		$ 50,000

X Corporation's accumulated earnings credit is $50,000, the greater of the general rule credit ($26,800) or the minimum credit ($50,000).

Example 6. Assume the same facts as in *Example 5*, except that X Corporation is an engineering firm. The general rule credit would still be $26,800, but the minimum credit would be computed as follows:

$150,000	$ 150,000
Minus: Accumulated earnings	
and profits as of 12/31/08	(200,000)
Minimum credit (the minimum credit	
cannot be a negative number)	$ 0

In this situation the accumulated earnings credit is $26,800, the greater of the general rule credit ($26,800) or the minimum credit ($0).

Two aspects of the accumulated earnings credit deserve special mention. First, the minimum credit has a very limited role. Since the $250,000 (or $150,000 for service

---

[44] § 535(c)(4).

corporations) is reduced by the prior accumulations, the minimum credit will always be zero for firms that have greater than $250,000 of accumulated earnings. In other words, accumulations in excess of $250,000 must be justified by business needs.

The second aspect involves capital gains. As discussed previously, capital gains (net of related taxes) are subtracted from taxable income in arriving at adjusted taxable income. Therefore, a corporation can accumulate all of its capital gains without the imposition of the accumulated earnings tax. At the same time, however, capital gains are subtracted from business needs in arriving at the general credit (see Exhibit 21-2). As a result, a capital gain may cause accumulations of ordinary income to be subject to the special tax even though the capital gain itself escapes penalty. In effect, the computations are based on the assumption that business needs are funded first from capital gains and then from income from operations.

DIVIDENDS-PAID DEDUCTION

Exhibit 21-1 indicated that both the accumulated earnings credit and the dividends-paid deduction are adjustments in computing accumulated taxable income. Exhibit 21-3 lists the types of dividends that constitute the dividends-paid deduction.

EXHIBIT 21-3
Dividends-Paid Deduction[45]

1. Dividends paid during the taxable year, [46]
2. Dividends paid within 2½ months after the close of the taxable year, [47]
3. Consent dividends, [48] plus
4. Liquidating distributions, [49]

    Equals: **Dividends-Paid Deduction**

To qualify for the dividend deduction, the distribution must constitute a "dividend" as defined in § 316.[50] As previously discussed, § 316 limits dividends to distributions out of current earnings and profits and accumulated earnings and profits since 1913. Property distributions qualify only to the extent of their adjusted basis.[51]

Throwback Dividends. The dividends-paid deduction includes not only dividends paid during the year, but also so-called *throwback dividends*, dividends paid during the 2½ months following the close of the tax year.[52] Amounts paid during the 2½-month period *must* be treated as if paid in the previous year.[53] This treatment is mandatory and not elective by the shareholders or the corporation.

Consent Dividends. In addition to actual dividends paid, the corporation is entitled to a deduction for consent dividends.[54] Sometimes a corporation may have a large amount of accumulated earnings, but insufficient cash or property to make a dividend

---

[45]   §§ 561 through 565.

[46]   § 561(a)(1).

[47]   § 563(a).

[48]   § 565.

[49]   § 562(b)(1).

[50]   § 562(a).

[51]   Reg. § 1.562-1(a).

[52]   § 563.

[53]   § Reg.1.563-1.

[54]   § 565.

distribution. In order to avoid the accumulated earnings tax, the corporation may obtain a dividends-paid deduction by using consent dividends—so called because the shareholders consent to treat a certain amount as a taxable dividend on their tax returns even though there is no distribution of cash or property. Not only are the shareholders deemed to receive the amount to which they consent, but they also are treated as having reinvested the amount received as a contribution to the corporation's capital.

To qualify a dividend as a consent dividend, the shareholders must file a consent form (Form 972) with the corporate income tax return. The consents must be filed by the due date (including extensions) of the corporate tax return for the year in which the dividend deduction is requested. Only shareholders who own stock on the last day of the tax year need file consent forms. On the forms, each shareholder must specify the amount of the consent dividend and then include this amount as a cash distribution by the corporation on his or her individual income tax return. Consent dividends are limited to the amount that would have qualified as a dividend under Code § 316 had the dividend been distributed in cash.[55] Only shareholders of common and participating preferred stock may consent to dividends.[56]

Liquidating Distributions. If the distribution is in liquidation, partial liquidation, or redemption of stock, the portion of the distribution chargeable to earnings and profits is included in the dividend deduction.[57] For partial liquidations and redemptions, this is the redeemed stock's proportionate share of accumulated E&P. For complete liquidations, any amount distributed within the two years following the adoption of a plan of liquidation and that is pursuant to the plan is included in the dividends-paid deduction, but not to exceed the corporation's current earnings and profits for the year of distribution.[58]

PERSONAL HOLDING COMPANY TAX

As mentioned earlier in this chapter, the accumulated earnings tax is not the only penalty tax applicable to corporations. Congress has also enacted the personal holding company tax. This tax evolved in 1934 from the need to stop the growing number of individuals who were misusing the corporate entity despite the existence of the accumulated earnings tax. The personal holding company tax was designed to thwart three particular schemes prevalent during that period.

The first two schemes specifically aimed to take advantage of the disparity between individual and corporate tax rates. At that time, the maximum individual tax rates were approximately 45 percentage points higher than the maximum corporate rates. A typical plan used to take advantage of this differential involved the formation of a corporation to hold an individual's investment portfolio. This plan allowed an individual's interest and dividends to become taxable to the corporation rather than to the individual and consequently to be taxed at the lower corporate rates. Another, somewhat more sophisticated, technique enabled the transfer of an individual's service income to a corporation. The blueprint for this plan required the formation of a corporation by an individual (e.g., movie star) who subsequently became an employee of the corporation. With the corporation in place, parties seeking the individual's services were forced to contract with the corporation rather than with the individual. The individual would then perform the services, but the corporation would receive the revenue. Finally, the corporation would pay the individual a salary that was less than the revenue earned.

---

[55]   Reg. § 1.565-2(a).

[56]   § 565(f).

[57]   § 562(b)(1).

[58]   § 562(b)(1)(B).

Through this plan, the individual succeeded in transferring at least some of the revenue to the corporation, where it would be taxed at the lower corporate rates.

The final scheme was not specifically designed to take advantage of the lower corporate rates. Instead, its attraction grew from the practical presumption that all corporate activities are business activities. Given this presumption, an individual would transfer his or her personal assets (e.g., a yacht, race car, or vacation home) along with other investments to the corporation. Under the veil of the corporation, the expenses relating to the personal assets, such as maintenance of a yacht, would be magically transformed from nondeductible personal expenses to deductible business expenses which could offset the income produced by the investments. In short, by using the corporate form, individuals were able to disguise their personal expenses as business expenses and deduct them.

Although the Internal Revenue Service tried to curb these abuses using the accumulated earnings tax, such attempts often failed. These failures normally could be attributed to the problem of proving that the individuals actually intended to avoid taxes. Aware of this problem, Congress formulated the personal holding company tax, which could be applied without having to prove that the forbidden purpose existed. In contrast to the accumulated earnings tax, which is imposed only after a subjective assessment of the individual's intentions, the personal holding company tax automatically applies whenever the corporation satisfies two objective tests.

Not all corporations that meet the applicable tests are subject to the penalty tax, however. The Code specifically exempts certain corporations. These include S corporations, tax-exempt corporations, banks, life insurance companies, surety companies, foreign corporations, lending and finance companies, and several other types of corporations.[59]

If the personal holding company tax applies, the tax is 15 percent of undistributed personal holding company income.[60] Like the accumulated earnings tax, the personal holding company tax is levied in addition to the regular tax.[61] The personal holding company tax differs from the accumulated earnings tax however, in that the corporation is required to compute and remit any personal holding tax due at the time it files its annual return. Form 1120-PH is used to compute the tax and must be filed with the corporation's annual Form 1120. In those cases where both the accumulated earnings tax and the personal holding company tax are applicable, only the personal holding company tax is imposed.[62]

PERSONAL HOLDING COMPANY DEFINED

The personal holding company tax applies only if the corporation is considered a personal holding company (PHC). As might be expected in light of the schemes prevalent at the time the tax was enacted, a corporation generally qualifies as a personal holding company if it is closely held and a substantial portion of its income is derived from passive sources or services. Specifically, the Code provides that a corporation is deemed to be a personal holding company if it satisfies both of the following tests.[63]

1. *Ownership*—At any time during the last half of the taxable year, more than 50 percent of the value of the corporation's outstanding stock is owned by five or fewer individuals.[64]

---

59   § 542(c).

60   § 541.

61   *Ibid.*

62   § 532(b)(1).

63   § 542.

64   § 542(a)(2).

2. *Passive income*—At least 60 percent of the corporation's adjusted ordinary gross income consists of personal holding company income (PHCI).[65]

Before each of these tests is examined in detail, the distinction between the personal holding company tax and the accumulated earnings tax should be emphasized. The accumulated earnings tax applies only when it is proven that it was the shareholder's intention to use the corporation to shield income from individual tax rates. In contrast, application of the personal holding company tax requires only that two mechanical tests be satisfied. As a result, a corporation may fall victim to the personal holding company tax where there was no intention to avoid tax by misusing the corporation. For example, consider a closely held corporation in the process of liquidating. During liquidation, the corporation may have income from operations and passive income from temporary investments (investments made pending final distributions). If the passive income is substantial—60 percent or more of the corporation's total income—the corporation will be treated as a personal holding company subject to the penalty tax even though there was no intention by the shareholders to shelter the passive income. As this example illustrates, the mechanical nature of the personal holding company tax, unlike the subjective nature of the accumulated earnings tax, presents a trap for those with the noblest of intentions.

PHC OWNERSHIP TEST

As indicated above, the first part of the two-part test for personal holding company status concerns ownership. Apparently it was Congressional belief that the tax-saving schemes described above succeeded primarily in those cases where there was a concentration of ownership. For this reason, the ownership test is satisfied only if five or fewer individuals own more than 50 percent of the value of the corporation's outstanding shares of stock at any time during the last half of the taxable year.[66] As a quick study of this test reveals, a corporation having less than ten shareholders always meets the ownership test since there will always be a combination of five or fewer shareholders owning more than 50 percent of the stock (e.g., $100\% \div 9 = 11\%$; $11\% \times 5 > 50\%$). Thus, it becomes apparent that closely held corporations are extremely vulnerable to the tax.

In performing the stock ownership test, the shareholder's *direct and indirect* ownership must be taken into account.[67] Indirect ownership is determined using a set of constructive ownership rules designed specifically for the personal holding company area.[68] According to these rules, a taxpayer is considered owning indirectly the following:

1. Stock owned directly or indirectly by his or her family, including his or her brothers, sisters, spouse, ancestors, and lineal descendents;[69]

2. His or her proportionate share of any stock owned by a corporation, partnership, estate, or trust in which he or she has ownership (or of which he or she is a beneficiary in the case of an estate or trust);[70] and

3. Stock owned indirectly or directly by his or her partner in a partnership.[71]

---

[65] § 542(a)(1).

[66] § 542(a)(2).

[67] *Ibid.*

[68] § 544.

[69] § 544(a)(2).

[70] § 544(a)(1).

[71] § 544(a)(2).

In using these rules, the following guidelines must be observed: (1) stock attributed from one family member to another cannot be reattributed to yet another member of the family,[72] (2) stock attributed from a partner to the taxpayer cannot be reattributed to a member of his or her family or to yet another partner,[73] (3) stock on which the taxpayer has an option is treated as being actually owned,[74] and (4) convertible securities are treated as outstanding stock.[75] In addition, Code § 544 contains other rules that may affect an individual's stock ownership.

INCOME TEST

Although the stock ownership test may be satisfied, a corporation is not considered a personal holding company unless it also passes an income test. In general terms, this test is straightforward: at least 60 percent of the corporation's income must be derived from either passive sources or certain types of services. Unfortunately, the technical translation of this requirement is somewhat more complicated. According to the Code, at least 60 percent of the corporation's adjusted ordinary gross income must be *personal holding company income*.[76] This relationship may be expressed numerically as follows:

$$\frac{\text{Personal holding company income}}{\text{Adjusted ordinary gross income}} \geq 60\%$$

As will be seen below, the definition of each of these terms can be baffling. However, the general theme of each term and the thrust of the test should not be lost in the complexity. Personal holding company income is generally passive income, while adjusted ordinary gross income is just that, ordinary gross income with a few modifications. Performing the income test is, in essence, a matter of determining whether too much of the corporation's income (adjusted ordinary gross income) is passive income (personal holding company income).

> **Example 7.** K, a high-bracket taxpayer, wished to reduce her taxes. Upon the advice of an old friend, she transferred all of her stocks and bonds to a newly formed corporation of which she is the sole owner. During the year, the corporation had dividend income of $40,000 and interest income of $35,000. In this case, the corporation is treated as a personal holding company because both the stock ownership test and the income test are satisfied. The stock ownership test is met since K owned 100% of the stock in the last half of the year. The income test is also met since all of the corporation's income is passive income—or more specifically, its personal holding company income, $75,000 ($40,000 dividends + $35,000 interest) exceeds 60% of its adjusted ordinary gross income, $45,000 (60% of $75,000).

The technical definitions of adjusted ordinary gross income and personal holding company income are explored below.

ADJUSTED ORDINARY GROSS INCOME

The first quantity that must be determined is adjusted ordinary gross income (AOGI).[77] As suggested above, the label given to this quantity is very appropriate since

---

[72] § 544(a)(5).

[73] *Ibid.*

[74] § 544(a)(3).

[75] § 544(b).

[76] § 542(a)(1).

[77] § 543(b)(2).

the amount which must be computed is just what the phrase implies; that is, it includes only the ordinary gross income of the corporation with certain adjustments. In determining AOGI, the following amounts must be computed: (1) gross income, (2) ordinary gross income, and (3) the adjustments to ordinary gross income to arrive at AOGI. Therefore, the starting point for the calculation of AOGI is gross income.

Gross Income. The definition of gross income for purposes of the personal holding company provisions varies little from the definition found in § 61. Accordingly, gross income includes all income from whatever source except those items specifically excluded. In addition, gross income is computed taking into consideration cost of goods sold. The only departure from the normal definition of gross income concerns property transactions. Only the net gains from the sale or exchange of stocks, securities, and commodities are included in gross income.[78] Net losses involving these assets do not reduce gross income. Similarly, any loss arising from the sale or exchange of § 1231 property is ignored and does not offset any § 1231 gains.

Ordinary Gross Income. In applying the income test, capital-gain type items are ignored and consequently have no effect on whether the corporation is treated as a personal holding company. Therefore, since the quantity desired is adjusted "ordinary" gross income, the second step of the calculation requires the removal of capital-gain type items from gross income. As seen in Exhibit 21-4, all capital gains and § 1231 gains are subtracted from gross income to arrive at ordinary gross income.[79] It should be noted that this amount, "ordinary gross income," is not simply a subtotal in arriving at AOGI. As discussed below, ordinary gross income (OGI) is an important figure in determining whether certain types of income are treated as personal holding company income.

EXHIBIT 21-4
Ordinary Gross Income[80]

Gross income		
Minus:	a.	Capital gains
	b.	(b) Section 1231 gains
Equals: **Ordinary gross income (OGI)**		

Adjustments to OGI. For many years, OGI generally served as the denominator in the income-test fraction shown above. In 1964, however, modifications were necessary to discourage the use of certain methods taxpayers and their advisors had forged to undermine the income test. The popular schemes capitalized on the fact that $1 of gross rental income could shelter 60 cents of passive personal holding company income. This particular advantage could be obtained even though the rental activity itself was merely a break-even operation. Consequently, a taxpayer could easily thwart the income test and reap the benefits of the corporate entity by investing in activities that produced substantial gross rents or royalties, notwithstanding the fact that these activities were not economically sound investments.

Example 8. Refer to the facts in *Example 7.* Absent special rules, K could circumvent the income test by purchasing a coin-operated laundry which generated gross rents of more than $50,000 (e.g., $51,000) and transferring it to the corporation.

---

[78] Prop. Reg. § 1.543-12(a). Also see Reg. §§ 1.542-2 and 1.543-2.

[79] § 543(b)(1).

[80] *Ibid.*

In such case, assuming the rents would not be treated as personal holding income, the personal holding company income would still be $75,000 (dividends of $40,000 + interest of $35,000). However, when the laundry rents are combined with the personal holding company income to form the new AOGI, personal holding company income would be less than 60% of this new AOGI [$75,000 60% × ($40,000 + $35,000 + $51,000) = $75,600]. Although the laundry business might not show a profit, this would be irrelevant to K since she would have gained the advantage of the dividends-received deduction and avoided personal holding company status.

To deter the type of scheme illustrated above, the calculation now requires rental and royalty income to be reduced by the bulk of the expenses typically related to this type of income: depreciation, interest, and taxes. This requirement reduces the ability of the activities to shelter income. For instance, in *Example 8* above, K would be required to reduce the gross rental income by depreciation, interest, and taxes—which would severely curtail the utility of purchasing the laundry business.[81] The specific modifications that reduce ordinary gross income to arrive at adjusted ordinary gross income are shown in Exhibit 21-5.[82] Exhibit 21-6 and Exhibit 21-7 illustrate the adjustments required to be made to gross income from rents and mineral, oil, and gas royalties for purposes of computing adjusted ordinary gross income.

EXHIBIT 21-5
Adjusted Ordinary Gross Income[83]

Ordinary gross income (OGI)

Minus:
- **a.** Depreciation, property taxes, interest expense, and rents paid related to gross rental income. These deductions may not exceed gross rental income. (Gross rental income is income for the use of corporate property and interest received on the sales price of real property held as inventory.)
- **b.** Depreciation and depletion, property and severance taxes, interest expense, and rents paid related to gross income from mineral, oil, and gas royalties. These deductions may not exceed the gross income from the royalties.
- **c.** Interest on tax refunds, on judgments, on condemnation awards, and on U.S. obligations (only for a dealer in the obligations).

Equals: *Adjusted ordinary gross income* **(AOGI)**

EXHIBIT 21-6
Adjusted Income from Rents[84]

Gross rental income

Minus:
- **a.** Depreciation
- **b.** Property taxes
- **c.** Interest expense
- **d.** Rents paid

Equals: **Adjusted income from rents**

---

[81] Under current law, it is also likely that the rents would be treated as PHCI, thus further spoiling the plan.

[82] § 543(b)(2).

[83] § 543(a)(1).

[84] § 543(a)(1).

EXHIBIT 21-7

Adjusted Income from Mineral, Oil, and Gas Royalties[85]

Gross income from mineral, oil, and gas royalties (including production payments and overriding royalties)

Minus:	**a.**	Depreciation
	b.	Property and severance taxes
	c.	Interest expense
	d.	Rents paid

Equals: **Adjusted income from mineral, oil, and gas royalties** [86]

PERSONAL HOLDING COMPANY INCOME (PHCI)

Following the computation of AOGI, the corporation's personal holding company income must be measured to determine whether it meets the 60 percent threshold. Although personal holding company income can be generally characterized as passive income and certain income from services, the Code identifies eight specific types of income which carry the personal holding company taint.[87] These are listed in Exhibit 21-8. Selected items of PHCI are discussed below.

Dividends, Interest, Royalties, and Annuities. The most obvious forms of PHCI are those usually considered passive in nature: dividends, interest, royalties, and annuities.[88] Generally, identification and classification of these items present little problem. The most noteworthy exception concerns royalties. Mineral, oil, gas, copyright, and computer software royalties generally are included in this category of PHCI. However, as seen in Exhibit 21-8, items b, c, and d, these royalties are not treated as PHCI if certain additional tests are satisfied.

---

[85]   *Ibid.*

[86]   § 543(b)(4).

[87]   § 543.

[88]   § 543(a)(1).

EXHIBIT 21-8

Personal Holding Company Income (PHCI)

Dividends, interest, royalties (except mineral, oil, or gas royalties, copyright royalties, and certain software royalties), and annuities.

Plus: **a.**   Adjusted income from rents, *but* the adjusted income from rents is not added to PHCI *if*

    1.   The adjusted income from rents is 50 percent or more of AOGI, and

    2.   The dividends paid, the dividends considered paid, and the consent dividends equal or exceed

        i.   PHCI computed without the adjusted income from rents

        ii.   Minus 10 percent of OGI.

  b.   Adjusted income from mineral, oil, and gas royalties, *but* the adjusted income from these royalties is not added to PHCI *if*

    1.   The adjusted income from the royalties is 50 percent or more of AOGI,

    2.   PHCI computed without the adjusted income from these royalties does not exceed 10 percent of OGI, and

    3.   The § 162 trade or business deductions equal or exceed 15 percent of AOGI.

  c.   Copyright royalties, *but* the copyright royalties are not added to PHCI *if*

    1.   The copyright royalties are 50 percent or more of OGI,

    2.   PHCI computed without the copyright royalties does not exceed 10 percent of OGI, and

    3.   The § 162 trade or business deductions related to the copyright royalties equal or exceed 25 percent of

        i.   The OGI minus the royalties paid, plus

        ii.   The depreciation related to the copyright royalties.

  d.   Software royalties, *but* these are not added to PHCI *if*

    1.   The royalties are received in connection with the licensing of computer software by a corporation which is actively engaged in the business of developing, manufacturing, or production of such software,

    2.   The software royalties are 50 percent or more of OGI,

    3.   Research and experimental expenditures, § 162 business expenses, and § 195 start-up expenditures allocable to the software business are generally 25 percent or more of OGI computed with certain adjustments, and

    4.   Dividends paid, considered paid, and the consent dividends equal or exceed

        i.   PHCI computed without the software royalties and certain interest income

        ii.   Minus 10 percent of OGI.

  e.   Produced film rents, but the produced film rents are not added to PHCI if the produced film rents equal or exceed 50 percent of OGI.

  f.   Rent (for the use of tangible property) received by the corporation from a shareholder owning 25 percent or more of the value of the corporation's stock. This rent is only included in PHCI if PHCI computed without this rent and without the adjusted income from rents exceeds 10 percent of OGI.

  g.   Income from personal service contracts *but only if*

    1.   Someone other than the corporation has the right to designate who is to perform the services or if the person who is to perform the services is named in the contract, and

    2.   At some time during the taxable year, 25 percent or more of the value of the corporation's outstanding stock is owned by the person performing the services.

  h.   Income of estates and trusts taxable to the corporation.

Equals: **Personal holding company income (PHCI)**

Example 9. B Corporation has three stockholders. Its income consisted of

Gross income from a grocery	$52,000
Interest income	38,000
Capital gain	6,000

B Corporation's OGI (see Exhibit 21-4) is $90,000, computed as follows:

Gross income ($52,000 + $38,000 + $6,000)	$96,000
Minus: Capital gains	(6,000)
OGI	$90,000

In this example, AOGI is the same as OGI since the amounts which are subtracted from OGI to arrive at AOGI are zero (see Exhibit 21-5).

B Corporation's PHCI is $38,000, the amount of the interest income (see Exhibit 21-8). Since the corporation's PHCI ($38,000) is not 60 percent or more of its $90,000 AOGI ($90,000 × 60% = $54,000), it does not meet the income requirement.

Although B Corporation meets the stock ownership requirement since it has only three shareholders, it does not meet *both* the ownership requirement and the income requirement. As a result, it is not a personal holding company and is not subject to the personal holding company tax.

Example 10. Assume the same facts as in *Example 9* except that B Corporation had received $88,000 of interest income.

B Corporation's OGI and AOGI would be computed as follows:

Gross income ($52,000 + $88,000 + $6,000)	$146,000
Minus: Capital gains	(6,000)
OGI (also AOGI)	$140,000

B Corporation's PHCI is now $88,000, the amount of the interest income. Since the corporation's $88,000 of PHCI is more than 60% of the $140,000 AOGI ($140,000 × 60% = $84,000), it meets the income requirement.

Since B Corporation meets both the ownership requirement and the income requirement, *it is* a personal holding company.

Adjusted Income from Rents. Rental income presents a special problem for the personal holding company provisions. Normally, rents—generally defined as compensation for the use of property—represent a passive type of income. However, for many corporations, most notably those involved in renting real estate and equipment, rental operations are not merely a passive investment but represent a true business activity. If all rental income were considered personal holding income, closely held corporations involved in the rental business could not escape PHI status. To provide these corporations with some relief, rental income is not treated as PHCI under certain circumstances.

The amount of rental income potentially qualifying as PHCI is referred to as the *adjusted income from rents*.[89] As seen in Exhibit 21-6, adjusted income from rents consists of the corporation's gross rental income reduced by the adjustments required for

---

[89]   § 543(b)(3).

determining AOGI—depreciation, property taxes, interest expense, and rental payments related to such income (e.g., ground lease payments). The corporation's adjusted income from rents is treated as PHCI unless it can utilize the relief measure suggested above. Specifically, adjusted income from rents is PHCI unless: (1) it is 50 percent or more of the corporation's AOGI, and (2) the corporation's dividends during the taxable year as well as dividends paid within the first 2½ months of the following year *and* consent dividends are not less than the amount by which nonrental PHCI (e.g., dividends and interest) exceeds 10 percent of OGI.[90]

These relationships may be expressed as follows:

1. Adjusted income from rents $\geq$ (50% $\times$ AOGI); *and*

2. Dividends $\geq$ [nonrental PHCI $-$ (10% $\times$ OGI)].

As the latter expression indicates, when rents represent a substantial portion of OGI relative to nonrental PHCI (as typically would be the case where a corporation is truly in the rental "business"), no dividends are required. In other words, as long as nonrental income is not a major portion of the corporation's total income—does not exceed 10 percent of the corporation's OGI—dividends are unnecessary. Otherwise, a corporation in the rental business is forced to make dividend distributions to avoid penalty.

> **Example 11.** D Corporation had four shareholders in 2009 and therefore met the stock ownership requirement. The following information is available for D Corporation for 2009:
>
> | | |
> |---|---:|
> | Interest income | $ 10,000 |
> | Gross rental income | 25,000 |
> | Depreciation, property taxes, and interest expense related to rental income | 24,000 |
> | Maintenance and utilities related to rental income | 3,000 |
> | Dividends paid during 2008 | 8,000 |
>
> OGI (Exhibit 21-4) is $35,000 ($10,000 + $25,000). AOGI (see Exhibit 21-5) is computed as follows:
>
> | | |
> |---|---:|
> | OGI | $ 35,000 |
> | Minus: Depreciation, property taxes, and interest expense related to rental income | (24,000) |
> | AOGI | $ 11,000 |
>
> D Corporation's adjusted income from rents is computed as follows (see Exhibit 21-6):
>
> | | |
> |---|---:|
> | Gross rental income | $ 25,000 |
> | Minus: Depreciation, property taxes, and interest expense related to rental income | (24,000) |
> | Adjusted income from rents | $ 1,000 |

Note that in determining AOGI and adjusted income from rents, the maintenance and utility expenses are ignored. Such expenses are also not taken into account in determining gross income or OGI. The next step is to determine if the adjusted income from rents is to be added to PHCI. It is *not* added to PHCI if *both* of the following tests are met.

---

[90]   *Ibid.*

Test 1. (50% test): Is the adjusted income from rents 50% or more of AOGI?

The adjusted income from rents ($1,000) is not 50% or more of AOGI ($11,000), so Test 1 is *not* met.

The adjusted income from rents is excluded from PHCI only if *both* Test 1 and Test 2 are met. Since Test 1 is not met, the adjusted income from rents *is* included in PHCI, and there is no need to go on to Test 2. However, Test 2 is done here for illustrative purposes.

Test 2. (10% test): Does the total of the dividends paid, the dividends considered paid, and the consent dividends equal or exceed PHCI (computed without the adjusted income from rents) reduced by 10% of OGI? This test can also be expressed as:

Dividends ≥ [nonrental PHCI − (OGI × 10%)]. Nonrental PHCI is $10,000 (interest income). OGI × 10% = $35,000 × 10% = $3,500. Therefore, nonrent PHCI ($10,000) minus OGI × 10% ($3,500) is $6,500. Since the total dividends ($8,000) were more than $6,500, Test 2 is met.

However, as mentioned above, *both* Test 1 and Test 2 must be met if the adjusted income from rents is to be excluded from PHCI. Therefore, the adjusted income from rents *is part of PHCI*.

D Corporation's PHCI is computed as follows (see Exhibit 21-8):

Interest income	$10,000
Adjusted income from rents	1,000
PHCI	$11,000

D Corporation's $11,000 PHCI is more than 60% of the $11,000 AOGI. In this example, in fact, PHCI is 100% of AOGI since all of the income is personal holding company income. D Corporation, therefore, meets *both* the ownership requirement and the income requirement, and thus is a personal holding company.

The rules relating to mineral, oil, gas, copyright, and software royalties are very similar to those discussed above for rents. See Exhibit 21-7 and Exhibit 21-8, items b, c, and d.

Income from Personal Service Contracts. The shifting of service income to a corporation by highly compensated individuals, such as actors and athletes, is sharply curtailed by the personal holding company provision. The PHC provisions attack the problem by treating service income as PHCI under certain conditions. Generally, amounts received by a corporation for services provided are treated as PHCI if the party desiring the services can designate the person who will perform the services and that person owns 25 percent or more of the corporation's stock[91] (see Exhibit 21-8, item g).

Example 12. T Corp., a producer of motion pictures, wanted RK to act in a new movie it was producing. Assume that RK's services could be obtained only by contracting with his wholly owned corporation, RK Inc. Accordingly, a contract is drafted providing that RK Inc. will provide the services of RK to T Corp. for $500,000. All of the income is PHCI to RK Inc. since RK owns at least 25% of the corporation *and* he is actually designated in the contract to perform the services.

Given the general rule, it would appear that virtually all service corporations are likely candidates for the PHC tax. This problem was considered in Revenue Ruling

---

[91] § 543(a)(7).

75-67.[92] According to the facts of the ruling, a corporation's primary source of income was attributable to the services of its only employee, a doctor, who also owned 80 percent of the corporation's stock. In this case, all the facts suggested that the income would be PHCI. The only question was whether the doctor's patients formally designated him as the one to perform the services. Although a formal designation was lacking, it was implicit since the doctor was the only employee of the corporation and the patients never expected someone other than the doctor to perform the services. Despite evidence to the contrary, the IRS ruled that the income was not PHCI on the theory that there was no indication that the corporation was obligated to provide the services of the doctor in question. In addition, the ruling emphasized that the services to be performed were not so unique as to prohibit the corporation from substituting someone else to perform them. The Service also relied on the uniqueness rationale in situations involving a CPA who had incorporated his or her practice and a musical composer who had incorporated his or her song-writing activities.[93] Apparently, as long as the services are not so unique as to preclude substitution and there is no formal designation of the individual who will perform the services, a service business can escape PHC status.

COMPUTATION OF THE PHC TAX

The personal holding company penalty tax is 15 percent of the *undistributed personal holding company income*. Undistributed personal holding company income is defined as adjusted taxable income minus the dividends-paid deduction.[94] The computation of adjusted taxable income and undistributed PHCI is shown in Exhibit 21-9.

EXHIBIT 21-9
Undistributed Personal Holding Company Income[95]

Taxable income

Plus:
- **a.** Dividends-received deduction.
- **b.** Net operating loss deduction (but not a net operating loss of the preceding year computed without the dividends-received deduction).
- **c.** The amount by which the § 162 (trade or business) deductions and the § 167 (depreciation) deductions related to rental property exceed the income produced by the rental property, unless it can be shown that the rent received was the highest possible and that the rental activity was carried on as a bona fide business activity.

Minus:
- **a.** Federal income taxes (but not the accumulated earnings tax or the personal holding company tax).
- **b.** The amount by which actual charitable contributions exceeds the charitable contributions deduction reflected in net income.
- **c.** Net capital gain reduced by the taxes attributable to the net capital gain.

Equals: ***Adjusted taxable income***

Minus: *Dividends-Paid Deduction*

Equals: ***Undistributed Personal Holding Company Income***

---

[92]   Rev. Rul. 75-67, 1975-1 C.B. 169.

[93]   Rev. Rul. 75-290, 1975-1 C.B. 172; Rev. Rul. 75-249, 1975-1 C.B. 171; and Rev. Rul. 75-250, 1975-1 C.B. 179.

[94]   § 545(a). The term "adjusted taxable income" is not found in the Code.

[95]   § 545.

Like the computation of accumulated taxable income, the calculation attempts to determine the corporation's dividend-paying capacity. As a practical matter, the tax is rarely paid because of a deduction allowed for "deficiency dividends," which can be made once it has been determined the PHC tax applies.

Dividends-Paid Deduction. The dividends-paid deduction for personal holding companies is similar to the one for the accumulated earnings tax. It includes the following types of distributions:

1. Dividends paid during the taxable year;

2. Throwback dividends: dividends paid within 2½ months after the close of the taxable year (but subject to limitation as discussed below);

3. Consent dividends;

4. Liquidating distributions; and

5. Deficiency dividends.

Note that this list of qualifying distributions is identical to that provided in Exhibit 21-3 for the accumulated earnings tax, except for the special deficiency dividend. In addition, personal holding companies are entitled to a dividend carryover, which is not available for accumulated earnings tax purposes.[96]

Throwback Dividends. As in the accumulated earnings tax computation, a personal holding company is allowed a deduction for throwback dividends (i.e., dividends paid within 2½ months after the close of the taxable year).[97] However, the PHC throwback dividend differs from that for the accumulated earnings tax in two ways. First, it is included in the dividends-paid deduction only if the corporation makes an election at the time the corporate tax return is filed to treat the dividends as applying to the previous year.[98] Second, the amount treated as a throwback dividend is limited to the smaller of the following:[99]

1. Twenty percent of the dividends actually paid during the taxable year in question; or

2. Undistributed PHCI (computed without the dividends paid during the 2½-month period).

Consent Dividends. The rules for consent dividends are the same for personal holding companies as for the accumulated earnings tax.[100] As mentioned previously, a consent dividend is an amount that a shareholder agrees to consider as having been received as a dividend even though never actually distributed by the corporation. Consent dividends are limited to shareholders who own stock on the last day of the tax year. Their shares must be either common stock or participating preferred stock. Consent dividends do not include preferential dividends. A shareholder who consents to a dividend is treated as having received the amount as a cash dividend and contributing the same amount to the corporation's capital on the last day of the year.

---

[96] § 561(a)(3).

[97] § 563.

[98] § 563(b).

[99] *Ibid.*

[100] § 565.

Dividend Carryover. A personal holding company is also entitled to a dividend carryover as part of its dividends-paid deduction.[101] If the dividends paid in the two prior years exceed the adjusted taxable incomes (see Exhibit 21-9) for those years, the excess may be used as a dividend carryover (and therefore as part of the dividends-paid deduction) for the year in question.

Deficiency Dividends. Once a determination has been made that a corporation is subject to the personal holding company tax, the tax can still be abated by the use of a *deficiency dividend.*[102] Following the determination of the personal holding company tax, the corporation is given 90 days to pay a deficiency dividend. A deficiency dividend must be an *actual cash dividend* which the corporation elects to treat as a distribution of the personal holding company income for the year at issue, and it is taxable to the shareholders. It does not reduce the personal holding company income of any year other than the year at issue. A deficiency dividend effectively reduces the amount of the penalty tax. However, interest and penalties are still imposed as if the deduction were not allowed. Thus, the corporation may be able to escape the tax itself—but not any interest or penalties related to such tax. It should also be noted that the deficiency dividend is available *only* to reduce the personal holding company tax. This escape is not available to those corporations subject to the accumulated earnings tax.

Example 13. C Corporation determined that it was a personal holding company and had to file Form 1120-PH. Its records for 2009 reveal the following:

Gross profit from operations.	$ 150,000
Dividend income	400,000
Interest income	350,000
Long-term capital gain	30,000
Gross income.	$ 930,000
Compensation	(30,000)
Selling and administrative.	(100,000)
	$ 800,000
Dividends-received deduction	(280,000)
Charitable contributions	(80,000)
Taxable income.	$ 440,000
Federal income tax @ 34%	$ 149,600

Charitable contributions actually made during the year were $90,000, but are limited to $80,000 (10% × $800,000 taxable income before the deductions for contributions and dividends received). C paid dividends of $20,000 in 2009 and $10,000 during the first 2½ months of 2010, which it *elects* to throw back to 2009 in computing the dividends-paid deduction. The personal holding company tax is computed as follows:

---

[101] § 564.

[102] § 547.

	Taxable income	$ 440,000
+	Dividends-received deduction	280,000
−	Excess charitable contributions	(10,000)
−	Federal income taxes	(149,600)
−	Long-term capital gain net of tax [$30,000 − (34% × $30,000)]	(19,800)
	Adjustable taxable income	$ 540,600
−	Dividends paid deduction:	
	2009	(20,000)
	2010 Throwback (Limited to 20% of 2009 dividends)	(4,000)
	UPHCI	$ 516,600
	Times: PHC tax rate	× 15%
	PHC tax	$ 77,490

C Corporation's tax liability for 2009 is $227,090 ($149,600 regular tax + $77,490 PHC tax). The PHC tax could be avoided by paying a deficiency dividend equal to UPHCI ($516,600). However, the payment of the dividend would not eliminate any penalties or interest that might be assessed on the $77,490 PHC tax due if Form 1120-PH is not filed in a timely manner.

TAX PLANNING

ACCUMULATED EARNINGS TAX

For taxpayers wanting to use the corporate form to shield their income from individual taxes, the accumulated earnings tax represents a formidable obstacle. Although there is an obvious cost if the tax is incurred, that cost may be far more than expected. This result often occurs because the imposition of the tax for one year triggers an audit for all open years. In addition, the IRS usually takes the position that the negligence penalty of Code § 6653 should be imposed whenever the accumulated earnings tax is applicable. Moreover, in contrast to the personal holding company tax which can normally be averted using the deficiency dividend procedure, the accumulated earnings tax, once levied, cannot be avoided. At the time of the audit, it is too late for dividend payments or consent dividends!

Despite the potential cost of the tax, the rewards from avoidance—or at least the deferral—of double taxation are often so great that the shareholders are willing to assume the risk of penalty. Moreover, many practitioners believe that with proper planning the risk of incurring the accumulated earnings tax is minimal, particularly since the tax is not self-assessed but dependent on the audit lottery. In addition, it is possible to shift the burden of proof to the IRS. The discussion below examines some of the means for reducing the taxpayer's exposure to the accumulated earnings tax.

Liquid Assets and Working Capital. Normally, the accumulated earnings tax is not raised as an issue unless the corporation's balance sheet shows cash, marketable securities, or other liquid assets that could be distributed easily to shareholders. The absence of liquid assets indicates that any earnings that have been retained have been reinvested in the business rather than accumulated for the forbidden purpose. It is a rare occasion, however, when such assets do not exist. Consequently, most IRS agents routinely assess whether the level of the corporation's working capital is appropriate by applying the *Bardahl* formula.

The courts have made it clear that the *Bardahl* formula serves merely as a guideline for determining the proper amount of working capital. In *Delaware Trucking Co., Inc.*, the court held that the amount needed using the *Bardahl* formula could be increased by 75 percent due to the possibility of increased labor and other operating costs due to inflation.[103] Nevertheless, in those instances where working capital appears excessive, the Internal Revenue Manual directs agents to require justification of such excess. Therefore, the corporation should closely control its working capital to ensure that it does not exceed the corporation's reasonable needs.

One way to reduce working capital is to increase shareholder salaries, bonuses, and other compensation. Since these payments are deductible, double taxation is avoided. This technique also has the benefit of reducing taxable income, which in turn reduces the accumulated earnings tax should it apply. However, this method of reducing working capital may not be feasible if the compensation paid exceeds a reasonable amount. To the extent that the compensation is unreasonable, the payments are treated as dividends and double taxation results. In addition, if the unreasonable compensation is not pro rata among all shareholders, the dividend will be considered preferential and no deduction will be allowed for the dividend in computing adjusted taxable income.

Another method for reducing working capital is for the corporation to invest in additional assets. However, the taxpayer must be careful to avoid investments that are of a passive nature or that could be considered unrelated to the corporation's existing or projected business. With respect to the latter, the courts have ruled that the business of a controlled subsidiary is the business of the parent while the business of a sister corporation normally is not the business of its brother.[104]

Reasonable Needs. The courts have accepted a variety of reasons as sufficient justification for the accumulation of earnings. On the one hand, the needs deemed reasonable have been both certain and well-defined, such as the repayment of corporate debt. On the other hand, the courts have approved needs as contingent and unknown as those arising from possible damage from future floods.

One contingency that seemingly could be asserted by all corporations as a basis for accumulating funds is the possibility of a business reversal, depression, or loss of major customer. Interestingly, the courts have often respected this justification for accumulations, notwithstanding the fact that it is a risk assumed by virtually all business entities. Acceptance of this need, however, appears to be dependent on the taxpayer's ability to establish that there is at least some chance that a business reversal could occur that would affect the taxpayer. For example, in *Ted Bates & Co.*, the corporation was in the advertising business and received 70 percent of its fees from only five clients.[105] In ruling for the taxpayer, the court held that the corporation was allowed to accumulate amounts necessary to cover its fixed costs for a period following the loss of a major client. Much of the court's opinion was based on its view that the advertising business was extremely competitive and the possibility of losing a client was not unrealistic. A similar decision was reached where a manufacturer sold all its products to one customer and had to compete with others for that customer's business. The court believed that accumulations were necessary to enable the corporation to develop new markets if it lost its only customer. Relying on a possible downturn in business as a basis for accumulations has not always sufficed. In *Goodall*, the company accumulated earnings in light of the prospect that military orders would be lost.[106] The court upheld the

---

[103]   32 TCM 104, T.C. Memo 1973-29.

[104]   For example, see *Latchis Theatres of Keene, Inc. v. Comm.*, 54-2 USTC ¶9544, 45 AFTR 1836, 214 F.2d 834 (CA-1,1954).

[105]   24 TCM 1346, T.C. Memo 1965-251.

[106]   *Robert A. Goodall Estate v. Comm.*, 68-1 USTC ¶9245, 21 AFTR2d 813, 391 F.2d 775, (CA-8.1968).

penalty tax, indicating that even if the loss occurred, it would not have a significant effect because the corporation's business was expanding.

Although the courts have sustained various reasons for accumulations, a review of the cases indicates that the taxpayer must demonstrate that the need is realistic. This was made clear in *Colonial Amusement Corp.*[107] In this case, the corporation's accumulations were not justified when it wanted to construct a building on adjacent land and building restrictions existed that prohibited construction.

In establishing that a need is realistic, a taxpayer's self-serving statement normally is not convincing. Proper documentation of the need is critical. This is true even when the need is obvious and acceptable. In *Union Offset*, the corporation stated at trial that its accumulations were necessary to retire outstanding corporate debt, a legitimate business need.[108] To the taxpayer's dismay, however, the Tax Court still imposed the tax because the corporation had failed to document in any type of written record its plan to use the accumulations in the alleged manner. In this case, a simple statement in the Board of Directors' minutes concerning the proposed use of the funds would no doubt have saved the taxpayer from penalty.

S Corporation Election. In those cases where it is difficult to justify accumulations, the shareholders may wish to elect to be treated as an S corporation. Since the earnings of an S corporation are taxed to the individual shareholders rather than the corporation, S corporations cannot be used to shelter income and thus are immune to the accumulated earnings tax. However, the election insulates the corporation only prospectively (i.e., only for that period for which it is, an S corporation). Prior years open to audit are still vulnerable. In addition, the S election may raise other problems. The shareholders will be required to report and pay taxes on the income of the corporation even though it may not be distributed to them. As a result, cash flow problems may occur. Further, because the corporation has accumulated earnings and profits, the excess passive income tax specifically designed for C corporations that have elected S status may apply. In addition, the corporation may be subject to the built-in gains tax.[109] For these reasons, an S election should be carefully considered.

PERSONAL HOLDING COMPANY TAX

The personal holding company tax, like the accumulated earnings tax, is clearly a tax to be avoided. Unfortunately, the personal holding company tax differs from the accumulated earnings tax in that it is not reserved solely for those whose intent is to avoid taxes. Rather, it is applied on a mechanical basis, regardless of motive, to all corporations that fall within its purview. For this reason, it is important to closely monitor the corporation's activities to ensure that it does not inadvertently become a PHC.

One important responsibility of a practitioner is to recognize potential personal holding company problems so that steps can be taken to avoid the tax or the need to distribute dividends. This responsibility not only concerns routine operations but extends to advice concerning planned transactions that could cause the corporation to be converted from an operating company to an investment company. For example, a corporation may plan to sell one or all of its businesses and invest the proceeds in passive type assets. Similarly, a planned reorganization may leave the corporation holding stock of the acquiring corporation. Failure to identify the possible personal holding company difficulty which these and other transactions may cause can lead to serious embarrassment.

---

[107]   7 TCM 546.

[108]   79-2 USTC ¶9550, 603 F.2d 90 (CA-9, 1979).

[109]   See Chapter 23 for a discussion of these special taxes that may be imposed on S corporations.

Although the thrust of most tax planning for personal holding companies concerns how to avoid the tax, there are certain instances when a planned PHC can provide benefits. Both varieties of personal holding companies, the planned and the unplanned, are discussed below.

PHC Candidates. All corporations could fall victim to the PHC tax. However, some corporations are more likely candidates than others. For this reason, their activities and anticipated transactions should be scrutinized more carefully than others.

Potential difficulties often concern corporations that are involved in rental activities and those that have some passive income. In this regard, it should be noted that the term "rent" is defined as payments received for the use of property. As a result, "rental companies" include not only those that lease such items as apartments, offices, warehouses, stadiums, equipment, vending machines, automobiles, trucks, and the like, but also those that operate bowling alleys, roller and ice skating rinks, billiards parlors, golf courses, and any other activity for which a payment is received for use of the corporation's property. All of these corporations are at risk since each has rental income which could be considered passive personal holding company income unless it satisfies the special two-prong test for rental companies.

There are several other types of corporations that must be concerned with PHC problems. Investment companies—corporations formed primarily to acquire income producing assets such as stock, bonds, rental properties, partnership interests, and similar investments—clearly have difficulties. Corporations that derive most of their income from the services of one or more of their shareholders also are vulnerable. In recent years, however, the Service has taken a liberal view toward the professional corporations of doctors, accountants, and several others. Another group of corporations that are probable targets of the PHC tax includes those that collect royalty income. The royalty income might arise from the corporation's development and licensing of a product (e.g., patent on a food processor or franchises to operate a restaurant). Other logical candidates for the PHC tax are banks, savings and loans, and finance companies since the majority of their income is interest income from making loans and purchasing or discounting accounts receivable and installment obligations. Banks and savings and loans need not worry, however, since they are specifically excluded from PHC status. Finance companies are also exempt from the penalty tax, but only if certain tests—not discussed here—are met. Consequently, those involved with finance companies should review their situation closely to ensure such tests are satisfied.

Avoiding PHC Status. In general, if a corporation is closely held and 60 percent of its income is derived from passive sources or specified personal services, the PHC tax applies. Thus, to avoid the PHC tax *either* the stock ownership test or the income test must be failed.

Stock Ownership Test. The stock ownership test is satisfied if five or fewer persons own more than 50 percent of the stock. This test is the most difficult to fail since it requires dilution of the current shareholders' ownership. Moreover, dilution is very difficult to implement in practice due to the constructive ownership rules. The rules make it virtually impossible to maintain ownership in the family since stock owned by one family member or an entity in which the family member has an interest is considered owned by other family members. Therefore, to fail the ownership test, sufficient stock must be owned by unrelated parties to reduce the ownership of the five largest shareholders to 50 percent or less. Unfortunately, it is often impossible to design an arrangement that meets these conditions yet is still desirable from an economic viewpoint.

Passive Income Test. The corporation is deemed to satisfy the passive income test if 60 percent of its adjusted ordinary gross income (AOGI) is personal holding company income (PHCI)—income from dividends, interest, annuities, rents, royalties, or specified shareholder services. The potential for failing this test is perhaps more easily seen when this test is expressed mathematically:

$$\frac{PHCI}{AOGI} \geq 60\%$$

The steps that can be taken to fail this test fall into three categories: (1) increasing operating income or AOGI, (2) reducing PHCI, and (3) satisfying the exceptions to remove the PHC taint from the income.

Increasing Operating Income. One way to fail the 60 percent test is to increase the denominator in the income test fraction, AOGI, without increasing the numerator. This requires the corporation to increase its operating income without any corresponding increase in its passive income. Obtaining such an increase is not easy since it is essentially asking that the corporation generate more gross income. This does not necessarily mean that sales must increase, however. The corporation might consider increasing its profit margin. Although this could reduce sales, the resulting increase in gross income could be sufficient to fail the test. Alternatively, the corporation might consider expanding the operating portion of the business. Expansion not only in increases AOGI but also may have the effect of reducing PHCI if the investments generating the PHCI are sold to invest in the expansion.

Reducing Personal Holding Income. Failing the income test normally is accomplished by reducing personal holding company income. It is sometimes asserted that merely reducing PHCI is not sufficient since both the numerator and the denominator in the test fraction are reduced by the same amounts. (This occurs because AOGI includes PHCI.) A mathematical check of this statement shows that it is incorrect and that a simple elimination of PHCI aids the taxpayer.

Example 14. Z Corporation has $100,000 of AOGI, including $70,000 of interest income that is PHCI. Substituting these values into the test fraction reveals that the corporation has excessive passive income.

$$\frac{PHCI}{AOGI} = \frac{\$70,000}{\$100,000} = 70\%$$

If Z Corporation simply reduces its interest income by $30,000, the corporation would fail the income test despite the fact that both the numerator and the denominator are reduced by the same amounts.

$$\frac{PHCI}{AOGI} = \frac{\$40,000}{\$70,000} = 57.1\%$$

One way a corporation could eliminate part of its PHCI is by paying out as shareholder compensation the amounts that otherwise would be invested to generate PHCI. Alternatively, the corporation could eliminate PHCI by switching its investments into growth stocks where the return is generated from capital appreciation rather than dividends. Of course, the taxpayer would not necessarily want to switch completely out of dividend-paying stocks since the advantage of the dividends-received deduction would be lost.

The corporation could also reduce its PHCI by replacing it with tax-exempt income, capital gains, or § 1231 gains. This would have the same effect as simply eliminating the PHCI altogether.

Example 15. Same as *Example 14* above except the corporation invests in tax-exempt bonds which generate $20,000 of tax-exempt, rather than taxable, interest. In addition, the corporation realizes a $10,000 capital gain instead of taxable interest. The effect of replacing the taxable interest of $30,000 with capital gains of $10,000 and tax-exempt income of $20,000 would produce results identical to those above. This derives from the fact that the tax-exempt interest and capital gains are excluded from both the numerator, PHCI, and the denominator, AOGI, creating fractions identical to those shown above.

Removing the PHC Taint. In some situations, income which is normally considered PHCI (e.g., rental income) is not considered tainted if certain tests are met. For example, the Code provides escape hatches for rental income; mineral, oil, and gas royalties; copyright royalties; and rents from the distribution and exhibition of produced films. Although additional tests must be met to obtain exclusion for these types of income, there is one requirement common to each. *Generally*, if a corporation's income consists predominantly (50 percent or more) of only one of these income types, exclusion is available. More importantly, this condition can normally be obtained without great difficulty. To satisfy the 50 percent test, the taxpayer should take steps to ensure that a particular corporation receives only a single type of income. This may require forming an additional corporation that receives only one type of income, but by so doing the 50 percent test is met and the PHC tax may be avoided.

With proper control of their income, these corporations will have no difficulty in satisfying the income test since at least 50 percent of their AOGI is from one source. For corporations with rental income, however, dividends equal to the amount that their nonrental PHC income exceeds 10 percent of their OGI still must be paid. Note, however, that if a corporation has little or no nonrental PHC income, no dividends are necessary to meet the test. Also note that each additional dollar of gross rents, unreduced by expenses, decreases the amount of dividend that must be paid.

Example 16. G Corporation has $60,000 of OGI, including $53,000 of rental income and $7,000 of dividend income. In this case, dividends of only $1,000 are necessary since nonrental PHCI exceeds the 10% threshold by only $1,000 [$7,000 − (10% of OGI of $60,000)]. If the taxpayer wants to avoid distributing dividends, consideration should be given to increasing gross rents. Note how an increase of $10,000 in gross rents to $63,000 would increase OGI and concomitantly eliminate the need for a dividend. This increase in gross rents would be effective even if the typical adjustments for depreciation, interest, and taxes reduce the taxpayer's net profit to zero or a loss. This is true because such adjustments are not included in determining OGI, but only AOGI. Thus, an incentive exists for the corporation to invest in breakeven or unprofitable activities as a means to eliminate the dividend.

Reducing the PHC Tax with Dividends. If the tests for PHC status cannot be avoided, the penalty can be eliminated or minimized by the payment of dividends. Although a similar opportunity exists for the accumulated earnings tax, the treatment of dividends differs in several important respects.

On the one hand, the PHC tax requires quicker action than the accumulated earnings tax. For accumulated earnings tax purposes, all dividends paid within the 2½-month period after the close of the taxable year are counted as paid for the previous year. However, for purposes of the PHC tax, the after-year-end dividends are limited to 20 percent of the amount actually paid during the year. Thus, if no dividends are paid during the year, then none can be paid during the 2½-month period. On the other hand, the PHC tax can almost always be avoided through payment of a deficiency dividend, which is not available for the accumulated earnings tax. The deficiency dividend may

come at a high price, however. As previously mentioned, any interest and penalties that would have been imposed had the penalty tax applied must be computed and paid as if the PHC tax were still due.

Planned Personal Holding Companies. Treatment of a corporation as a personal holding company is normally considered a dire consequence. Yet, in certain cases, PHC status may not be detrimental and at times can be beneficial. Two of these situations are outlined below.

Certain taxpayers seeking the benefits of the corporate form are unable to avoid characterization as a personal holding company. For example, an athlete or movie celebrity may seek the benefits reserved solely for employees, such as group-term life insurance, health and accident insurance, medical reimbursement plans, and better pension and profit-sharing plans. In these situations, if the individual incorporates his or her talents, the corporation will be considered a PHC since all of the income for services will be PHCI. This does not mean that the PHC tax must be paid, however. The PHC tax is levied only upon undistributed PHCI. In most cases, all of the undistributed PHCI can be eliminated through the payments of deductible compensation directly to the individual or deductible contributions to his or her pension plan. As a result, the individual can obtain the benefits of incorporation without concern for the PHC tax. This technique was extremely popular prior to 1982, when the benefits of corporate pension plans were significantly better than those available to the self-employed (i.e., Keogh plans).

Over the years, personal holding companies have been used quite successfully in estate planning in reducing the value of the taxpayer's estate and obtaining other estate tax benefits. Under a typical plan, a taxpayer with a portfolio of securities would transfer them to a PHC in exchange for preferred stock equal to their current value and common stock of no value. The exchange would be tax free under Code § 351. The taxpayer would then proceed to give the common stock to his or her children at no gift tax cost since its value at the time is zero. The taxpayer would also begin a gift program, transferring $10,000 of preferred stock annually to heirs, which would also escape gift tax due to the annual gift tax exclusion. There were several benefits arising from this arrangement.

First and probably foremost, any appreciation in the value of the taxpayer's portfolio would accrue to the owners of the common stock and thus be successfully removed from the taxpayer's estate, avoiding both gift and estate taxes. Second, the corporation's declaration of dividends on the common stock would shift the income to the lower-bracket family members. Dividends on the preferred stock would also be shifted to the extent that the taxpayer has transferred the preferred stock. The dividends paid would in part aid in eliminating any PHC tax. Third, the taxpayer's preferred stock in the PHC would probably be valued at less than the value of the underlying assets for estate and gift tax purposes. Although the IRS takes the position that the value of the stock in the PHC is the same as the value of the corporation's assets, the courts have consistently held otherwise. The courts have normally allowed a substantial *discount* for estate and gift tax valuation, holding that an investment in a closely held business is less desirable than in the underlying shares since the underlying securities can easily be traded in the market while the PHC shares cannot.[110]

---

[110] For example, see *Estate of Maurice Gustane Heckscher*, 63 T.C. 485 (1974). Also, See Chapter 26 for possible limitations on this estate planning technique.

PROBLEM MATERIALS

DISCUSSION QUESTIONS

21-1   *Double Taxation.* List four approaches that corporations use to avoid the effects of double taxation.

21-2   *Accumulated Earnings Tax.* What is the purpose of the accumulated earnings tax?

21-3   *Accumulated Earnings Tax.* What is the accumulated earnings tax rate? Why do you suppose Congress chose this particular tax rate?

21-4   *Accumulated Taxable Income.* What is the difference between accumulated taxable income and taxable income?

21-5   *Accumulated Earnings Credit.* What is the accumulated earnings credit? How does it affect the accumulated earnings tax?

21-6   *Dividends-Paid Deduction.* What constitutes the dividends-paid deduction for purposes of the accumulated earnings tax?

21-7   *Throwback Dividend.* What is a throwback dividend?

21-8   *Consent Dividends.* What is a consent dividend? What is its purpose?

21-9   *Intent of Accumulations.* What situations are considered to indicate the intent of a corporation to unreasonably accumulate earnings?

21-10   *Reasonable Needs.* List six possible reasons for accumulating earnings that might be considered reasonable needs of the business.

21-11   *Reasonable Needs—The Bardahl Formula.* What is the *Bardahl* formula? How is it used?

21-12   *Personal Holding Company Tax.* What is the purpose of the personal holding company tax?

21-13   *Personal Holding Company.* What requirements must be met by a corporation in order for it to be a personal holding company?

21-14   *Ownership Requirement.* What is the ownership requirement for personal holding companies? What constructive ownership rules apply?

21-15   *Income Requirement.* What is the income requirement for personal holding companies? What terms must be defined in order to determine if a corporation meets the income requirement?

21-16   *Income Requirement.* What tests must be met in order to determine whether the adjusted income from rents is included in personal holding company income?

21-17   *Computing the Personal Holding Company Tax.* How is the personal holding company penalty tax computed?

21-18   *Adjusted Taxable Income.* How does adjusted taxable income differ from taxable income?

21-19 *Dividends-Paid Deduction.* How does the dividends-paid deduction for personal holding company tax purposes differ from the dividends-paid deduction for accumulated earnings tax purposes?

21-20 *Deficiency Dividends.* What is a deficiency dividend? What is its purpose? What effect does it have on the personal holding company tax?

PROBLEMS

21-21 *Computing the Accumulated Earnings Tax.* Z Corporation had accumulated taxable income of $180,000 for the current year. Calculate Z Corporation's accumulated earnings tax liability.

21-22 *Computing Adjusted Taxable Income.* R Corporation has the following income and deductions for the current year:

Income from operations	$200,000
Dividend income (from less than 20% owned corporations)	60,000
Charitable contributions	40,000

Compute R Corporation's adjusted taxable income.

21-23 *Minimum Accumulated Earnings Tax Credit.* B Corporation, a calendar year manufacturing company, had accumulated earnings and profits at the beginning of the current year of $60,000. If the corporation's earnings and profits for the current year are $270,000, what is B Corporation's minimum accumulated earnings tax credit?

21-24 *Accumulated Earnings Tax Credit.* Assume the same facts in *Problem 21-23* above, except that B Corporation has estimated reasonable business needs of $170,000 at the end of the current year.
  a. Compute B Corporation's accumulated earnings tax credit for the current year.
  b. Would your answer differ if B Corporation was an incorporated law practice owned and operated be one person? If so, by how much?

21-25 *Computing the Accumulated Earnings Tax.* T Corporation had accumulated earnings and profits at the beginning of 2009 of $300,000. It has never paid dividends to its shareholders and does not intend to do so in the near future. The following facts relate to T Corporation's 2009 tax year:

Taxable income	$200,000
Federal income tax	61,250
Dividends received (from less than 20% owned corporations)	40,000
Reasonable business needs as of 12/31/09	356,850

  a. What is T Corporation's accumulated earnings tax?
  b. If T Corporation's sole shareholder wanted to avoid the accumulated earnings tax, what amount of consent dividends would be required?

21-26 *Dividends-Paid Deduction.* J Corporation, a small oil tool manufacturer, projects adjusted taxable income for the current year of $200,000. Its estimated reasonable business needs are $500,000; and the corporation has $380,000 of prior years' accumulated earnings and profits as of the beginning of the current year. Using this information, answer the following:
  a. Assuming no dividends-paid deduction, what is J Corporation's accumulated earnings tax for the current year?
  b. If J Corporation paid $50,000 of dividends during the year, what is J Corporation's accumulated earnings tax liability?

    c. If J Corporation's shareholders are willing to report more dividends than the $50,000 actually received during the year, what amount of consent dividends is necessary to avoid the accumulated earnings tax?

    d. If the corporation's shareholders are not interested in paying taxes on hypothetical dividends, what other possibility is available to increase the dividends-paid deduction?

21-27 *Working Capital Needs—The* Bardahl *Formula.* X Corporation wishes to use the Bardahl formula to determine the amount of working capital it can justify if the IRS agent currently auditing the company's records raises the accumulated earnings tax issue. For the year under audit, X Corporation had the following:

Annual operating expenses	$285,000
Inventory cycle ratio	.41
Accounts receivable cycle ratio	.61
Accounts payable cycle ratio	.82

    a. How much working capital can X Corporation justify based on the above facts?

    b. If X Corporation's turnover ratios are based on annual averages, what additional information would you request before computing working capital needs based on the *Bardahl* formula?

21-28 *Working Capital Needs—Bardahl Formula.* B owns and operates BKA Inc., which is a retail toy store. One Wednesday morning in January 2010, she noticed in the *Wall Street Journal's* tax column an anecdote about a small corporation that was required to pay the accumulated earnings tax. Concerned, B presented the following information to her tax advisor to evaluate her exposure as of the end of 2009.

Balance Sheet

	2008	2009
Current Assets:		
Cash	$ 15,000	$ 30,000
Marketable securities (cost)	10,000	23,000
Accounts receivable (net)	55,000	45,000
Inventory	30,000	50,000
Property, plant, and equipment (net)	500,000	552,000
Total Assets	$610,000	$700,000
Current Liabilities:		
Accounts payable	$ 13,000	$ 31,000
Long-term debt	147,000	119,000
Common stock	50,000	50,000
Earnings and profits	400,000	500,000
Total Liabilities and Equity	$ 610,000	$ 700,000

Income Statement

Sales.....................................		$400,000
Cost of goods sold:		
Beginning inventory......................	$ 30,000	
Purchases.............................	220,000	
Ending inventory	(50,000)	
Total.............................		(200,000)
Gross profit		$200,000
Other Expenses:		
Depreciation...........................	$ 70,000	
Selling expenses and administrative.........	25,000	
Interest	5,000	
Total		(100,000)
Net income before taxes....................		$100,000
Income taxes		(25,750)
Net income...............................		$ 74,250

B noted that the market value of the securities was $40,000 as of December 31, 2009. In addition, B estimates the future expansion of the business (excluding working capital) will require $25,000. Determine whether the accumulated earnings tax will apply to B.

21-29 *Personal Holding Company—Income Requirement.* K Corporation is equally owned and operated by three brothers. K Corporation's gross income for the current year is $80,000, which consists of $10,000 of dividend income, interest income of $40,000, and a long-term capital gain of $30,000.
   a. Calculate ordinary gross income.
   b. Calculate adjusted ordinary gross income.
   c. Is K Corporation a personal holding company?

21-30 *Personal Holding Company—Rent Exclusion.* T Corporation has gross income of $116,000, which consists of gross rental income of $86,000, interest income of $20,000, and dividends of $10,000. Depreciation, property taxes, and interest expense related to the rental property totaled $16,000. Assuming T Corporation has seven shareholders and has no dividends-paid deduction, answer the following:
   a. What is T Corporation's ordinary gross income?
   b. Adjusted ordinary gross income?
   c. Does the rental income constitute personal holding company income?
   d. Is T Corporation a personal holding company?

21-31 *Personal Holding Company Income.* V Corporation is equally owned by two shareholders. The corporation reports the following income and deductions for the current year.

Dividend income	$30,000
Interest income	15,000
Long-term capital gain	10,000
Rental income (gross)....................................	80,000
Rental expenses:	
Depreciation...	10,000
Interest on mortgage.................................	9,000
Property taxes	3,000
Real estate management fees	8,000

    a. Calculate ordinary gross income.

    b. Calculate adjusted ordinary gross income.

    c. Calculate adjusted income from rentals.

    d. Calculate personal holding company income.

    e. Is V Corporation a personal holding company?

    f. If V Corporation paid $3,000 of dividends to each of its two shareholders during the current year, how would this affect your answers to (d) and (e) above?

21-32 *Items of PHC Income.* Indicate whether the following would be considered personal holding company income.

    a. Income from the sales of inventory

    b. Interest income from AT&T bond

    c. Interest income from State of Texas bond

    d. Dividend income from IBM stock

    e. Long-term capital gain

    f. Short-term capital gain

    g. Rental income from lease of office building (100% of the corporation's income is from rents)

    h. Fees paid to the corporation for the services of Jose Greatfoot, internationally known soccer player.

21-33 *PHC Income Test.* All of the stock of C Corporation is owned by B. Next year, the corporation expects the following results from operations:

Sales.	$500,000
Costs of goods sold.	200,000
Other operating expenses	40,000
Interest income	10,000

What is the maximum amount of dividend income that the corporation can have without being classified as a personal holding company?

21-34 *Computing the Personal Holding Company Tax.* P Corporation is owned by five individuals. For the current year P had the following:

Taxable income.	$200,000
Federal income tax	60,750
Dividends received (from less than 20% owned corporations).	40,000
Long-term capital gain	10,000

Compute P Corporation's personal holding company tax assuming that P meets the income test, P did not pay dividends, and the long-term capital gain was taxed at 34 percent.

21-35 *Personal Holding Company—Dividend Deduction.* H, a personal holding company, anticipates having undistributed personal holding company income of $120,000 before any dividend deduction for 2009. The company wishes to distribute all of its income to avoid the penalty. Because of cash flow problems, it wishes to pay as much of this dividend as it can in the 2½ months after the close of the tax year.

    a. What is the *maximum* amount that H can distribute during 2010 to accomplish its task if dividends of $50,000 were paid during 2009?

    b. What is the *minimum* amount that H must distribute during 2009 and still be able to defer until 2010 the payment of any additional dividends?

21-36   *Personal Holding Company—Service Income.* J, an orthopedic surgeon, is the sole owner of J Inc. The corporation employs surgical nurses and physical therapists in addition to J. The nurses assist Dr. J on all operations, and the therapists provide all follow-up treatment. J Inc. bills all clients for all services rendered and pays the employees a stated salary. Will any of J Inc.'s fee be personal holding company income?

21-37   *PHC Dividends—Paid Deduction.* Indicate whether the following distributions would qualify for the personal holding company dividends—paid deduction for 2009. Assume that the corporation is a calendar year taxpayer.
  a. Cash dividends paid on common stock in 2009.
  b. Dividend distribution of land (value $20,000, basis $5,000) paid on common stock in 2009.
  c. Cash dividends paid on common stock March 3, 2010.
  d. Cash dividends paid on common stock in 2008.
  e. Consent dividend; the 2009 corporate tax return was filed on March 3, 2010; the consents were filed on May 15, 2010.
  f. Cash dividend paid in 2012 shortly after it was determined that the corporation was a personal holding company.
  g. The corporation adopted a plan of liquidation in 2007 and the final liquidating distribution was made during 2009.

21-38   *Accumulated Earnings Tax Dividends-Paid Deduction.* Indicate whether the distributions identified in *Problem 21-37* would qualify for the accumulated earnings tax dividends-paid deduction for 2009.

21-39   *Understanding the PHC Tax.* Indicate whether the following statements regarding the personal holding company tax are true or false.
  a. The PHC tax is self-assessed and, if applicable, must be paid in addition to the regular income tax.
  b. An S corporation or partnership may be subject to the PHC tax.
  c. A corporation that can prove that its shareholders did not intend to use it as a tax shelter is not subject to the PHC tax.
  d. A publicly traded corporation normally would not be subject to the PHC tax.
  e. A corporation that derives virtually all of its income from leasing operations does not risk the PHC tax, even though such income is normally considered passive.
  f. Federal income taxes reduce the base on which the PHC tax is assessed.
  g. Long-term capital gains are not subject to the PHC tax.
  h. A corporation that consistently pays dividends normally would not be subject to the PHC tax.
  i. Throwback dividends are available to reduce the corporation's potential liability without limitation.
  j. Corporations without cash or property that they can distribute cannot benefit from the dividends-paid deduction.
  k. The PHC tax is not truly a risk because of the deficiency dividend procedure.
  l. A corporation may be required to pay both the accumulated earnings tax and the personal holding company tax in the same year.

21-40   *Understanding the Accumulated Earnings Tax.* Indicate whether the statements in *Problem 21-39* are true or false regarding the accumulated earnings tax.

RESEARCH PROBLEMS

21-41   H Corporation is owned and operated by William and Wilma Holt. The corporation's principal source of income for the past few years has been net rentals from five adjacent rent houses located in an area that the city has condemned in order to expand

its freeway system. The Holts anticipate a condemnation award of approximately $400,000, and a resulting gain of $325,000. Although convinced that they will have the corporation reinvest the proceeds in other rental units, the Holts would like to invest the corporation's condemnation proceeds in a high-yield certificate of deposit for at least three years. They have come to you for advice.

a. What advice would you give concerning the reinvestment requirements of Code § 1033?

b. If H Corporation will have substantial interest income in the next few years, could the § 541 tax be a possibility?

c. If the Holts have considered liquidating the corporation and reinvesting the proceeds in rental units, what additional information would you need in order to advise them?

21-42 Stacey Caniff is the controlling shareholder of Cotton, Inc., a textile manufacturer. She inherited the business from her father. In recent years earnings have fluctuated between $0.50 and $3.00 per share. Dividends have remained at $0.10 per share for the past ten years with a resulting increase in cash. On audit, the IRS agent has raised the accumulated earnings tax issue. In your discussion with Stacey, she has indicated that the dividends are so low because she is afraid of losing the business (as almost happened to her father during the Depression), of decreased profitability from foreign competition, and of the need to modernize if OSHA were to enforce the rules concerning cotton dust. Evaluate the possibility of overcoming an accumulated earnings tax assessment.

PART EIGHT

FLOW-THROUGH ENTITIES

★ ★ ★ ★ ★ CONTENTS ★ ★ ★ ★ ★

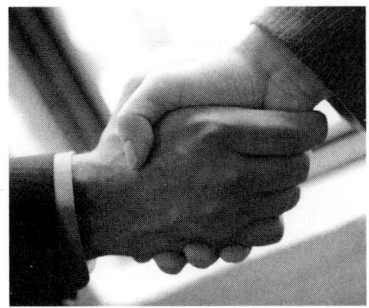

CHAPTER TWENTY-TWO

TAXATION OF PARTNERSHIPS AND PARTNERS

LEARNING OBJECTIVES

Upon completion of this chapter you will be able to:

- Define the terms *partner* and *partnership* for federal income tax purposes
- Distinguish between the entity theory and the aggregate theory of partnerships
- Analyze the tax consequences of forming a new partnership
- Determine the tax basis of a partnership interest
- Compute partnership taxable income or loss and identify any separately computed items of partnership income, gain, loss, deduction, or credit
- Explain how the tax consequences of partnership operations are reported on the tax returns of the partners and how the partners' bases in their partnership interests are adjusted to reflect these tax consequences

- Identify the tax consequences of various transactions between a partner and a partnership
- Determine the tax consequences of both current and liquidating distributions from a partnership
- Analyze the tax consequences of a sale of a partnership interest to both the seller and purchaser
- Apply the family partnership rules to partnership interests created by gift
- Recognize a termination of a partnership and summarize the tax consequences of the termination to the partners

CHAPTER OUTLINE

When two or more parties agree to go into business together, they must first decide which form of business to use. Should the business be incorporated or should it operate as a partnership? Although the corporate form predominates for large companies, it is certainly not appropriate for all businesses. Consequently, partnerships are widely used throughout the business world.

Partnerships come in a wide assortment of shapes and sizes. For example, two accountants may form a professional partnership through which to conduct their business, or a family may organize a partnership to manage real estate or operate a corner delicatessen. In contrast, two international corporations may form a partnership to develop a new product or to conduct research. Partnerships may also be used as investment vehicles. For instance, hundreds or thousands of people may invest in partnerships that drill for oil, construct office buildings, or make movies. For whatever reason, when two or more parties decide to pool their resources in order to carry on a profit-making activity, they often choose to do so as partners in a partnership.

The federal tax consequences of business activities that meet the statutory definition of a partnership are governed by the provisions of Subchapter K of the Internal Revenue Code (§§ 701 through 777). This chapter begins with an analysis of this definition and a brief introduction to several other important concepts that underlie Subchapter K. The chapter also includes discussions of the formation and operation of a partnership, the mechanics by which partnership income or loss is allocated to and taken into account by each partner, and the tax consequences of common transactions between partners and partnerships. The more advanced topics of current and liquidating partnership distributions and dispositions of partnership interests are also introduced.

DEFINITIONS

WHAT IS A PARTNERSHIP?

The Uniform Partnership Act defines a partnership quite simply as "an association of two or more persons to carry on as co-owners a business for profit."[1] This basic definition is expanded in the Code to include a syndicate, group, pool, joint venture, or any other unincorporated organization.[2] For an organization to constitute a partnership, it must have at least two partners. Note that there are no restrictions on either the maximum number of partners or on the type of entity that may be a partner. Individuals, corporations, trusts, estates, and even other partnerships may join together as partners to carry on a profit-making activity.

As a practical matter, determining whether an organization qualifies as a partnership is rarely a problem. For example, any organization formed under the Uniform Partnership Act or the Uniform Limited Partnership Act should expect to be treated as a partnership. However, as explained in Chapter 19, certain unincorporated organizations may or may not be treated as partnerships for tax purposes. Under the "check the box" regulations, all business entities incorporated under a state law providing for a separate corporation, a joint stock company, an insurance company, a bank, or certain foreign entities will be classified as corporations for federal tax purposes.[3] All other business entities, known as associations, which are not automatically defined as a corporation can *elect* to be taxed as a corporation. Any association, including any limited liability company having two or more owners and that does not make the election, will be treated as a partnership.[4]

A foreign entity in which all owners have limited liability will be treated as a corporation. A foreign entity in which one or more owners have unlimited liability will be treated as a partnership unless it makes the election to be taxed as a corporation.[5]

Other treasury regulations clarify that certain arrangements are not treated as partnerships for federal tax purposes. A joint undertaking is not a partnership if the only joint activity is the sharing of expenses. For example, if two adjacent property owners share the cost of a dam constructed to prevent flooding, no partnership exists. Similarly, joint ownership of property is not a partnership if the co-owners merely rent or lease the property and provide minimal services to the lessees. In such case, the co-owners are not actively conducting a trade or business. If, however, these co-owners provide substantial tenant services, they may elevate their passive co-ownership to active partnership status.[6]

ELECTING OUT OF SUBCHAPTER K PARTNERSHIPS

Section 761(a) allows certain unincorporated organizations that potentially constitute partnerships for federal tax purposes to be excluded from the application of the statutory rules of Subchapter K. An organization may elect out of the statutory rules governing the taxation of partners and partnerships if it is formed for (1) investment purposes only and not for the active conduct of a business, or (2) the joint production,

---

[1] Uniform Partnership Act, § 6(1).

[2] § 761(a).

[3] Reg. §§ 301.7701-1(b) and 301.7701-4.

[4] A limited liability company with only one owner cannot be considered a partnership for tax purposes. Instead, such an entity will be treated as either a corporation or sole proprietorship.

[5] See Reg. §§ 301.7701-1(b) and 301.7701-4.

[6] Reg. § 1.761-1(a).

extraction, or use of property. The members of such an organization must be able to compute their separate incomes without the necessity of computing partnership taxable income (i.e., income for the organization as a whole). The election is made by attaching a statement to a properly filed Form 1065 (U.S. Partnership Return of Income) for the first taxable year for which the organization desires exclusion from Subchapter K. The statement must identify all members of the organization and indicate their consent to the election.[7]

GENERAL AND LIMITED PARTNERSHIPS

There are two types of partnerships: *general* partnerships and *limited* partnerships. The two differ primarily in the nature of the rights and obligations of the partners; the major differences can be summarized as follows:

1. General partnerships are owned solely by general partners, whereas limited partnerships must have at least one general partner and one or more limited partners.

2. General partners have *unlimited liability* for partnership debt, whereas limited partners are usually liable only to the extent of their capital contributions to the partnership.

3. General partners participate in the management and control of the partnership business, whereas limited partners are not allowed to participate in such business.[8]

4. General partners are subject to self-employment taxes on partnership business earnings even if they do not perform services for the partnership, whereas limited partners are not.

Two other types of entities that are usually taxed as partnerships are limited liability companies (LLC) and limited liability partnerships (LLP). In an LLC, all members (i.e., owners) have limited liability. Generally, the partners in an LLP have better liability protection than general partners, but more liability exposure than limited partners. LLP partners usually have unlimited liability, except any particular partner is not personally liable for claims arising from a tort that was committed by a different partner. Nevertheless, the partner committing the tort is personally liability for the claims resulting from his or her actions.

All references throughout the text are to general partners and general partnerships unless otherwise stated.

ENTITY AND AGGREGATE THEORIES

Most rules governing the taxation of partnerships are based on either the entity or aggregate theory of partnerships.[9] According to the *entity theory*, partnerships should be regarded as entities distinct and separate from their owners. As such, partnerships may enter into taxable transactions with partners, may hold title to property in their own names, are not legally liable for debts of partners, are required to file annual returns

---

[7]   Reg. § 1.761-2(b)(2).

[8]   A limited partner who takes part in the control of the partnership business may become liable to the creditors of the partnership by doing so. Revised Uniform Limited Partnership Act (1976), § 303(a).

[9]   For an interesting historical discussion of the development of these conflicting theories, see Arthur B. Willis, John S. Pennell, and Philip F. Postlewaite, *Partnership Taxation* (Colorado Springs, CO.: Shepard's/ McGraw-Hill, Inc.), Chapter 4.

(Form 1065) that report the results of operations, and can make tax elections concerning partnership activities that apply to all partners.

In contrast, the *aggregate theory* views a partnership as a collection of specific partners, each of which indirectly owns an undivided interest in partnership assets. Under this theory, the partnership itself has no identity distinct from that of its partners. The fact that a partnership is a pass-through rather than a taxable entity, functioning only as a conduit of income to the partners, is a clear reflection of the aggregate theory. The aggregate theory also prevents the recognition of gain or loss on several types of transactions between partners and their partnerships.

The inconsistent application of the entity and aggregate theories throughout Subchapter K certainly complicates the taxation of partners and their partnerships. In extreme cases, a single Code section may contain elements of both theories. In spite of this confusion, taxpayers and their advisers who can determine which theory underlies a particular rule of partnership tax law will gain valuable insight into the proper application of that rule to a specific fact situation.

FORMING A PARTNERSHIP

The first step in the formation of any partnership is the drafting of a partnership agreement by the prospective partners. A *partnership agreement* is a legal contract stipulating the rights and obligations of the co-owners of the business. Ideally a partnership agreement should be drafted by a competent attorney, should be in writing, and should be signed by each partner. However, even oral partnership agreements between business associates have been respected as binding contracts by the courts.[10]

A partner's *interest in a partnership* is an intangible asset—an equity interest in the partnership business, the exact nature of which is defined in the partnership agreement. Under the typical agreement, each partner has a specified interest in partnership cash and property. The dollar amount of such interest at any time is reflected by the balance in each partner's *capital account* in the equity section of the partnership balance sheet. In addition to his or her capital interest, each partner has an interest in any income or loss generated by the partnership's activities. This interest is usually expressed as a *profit-and-loss sharing ratio* among the partners. If the partners consent, the terms of their agreement may be modified with respect to a particular taxable year at any time before the unextended due date by which the partnership return for such year must be filed.[11]

Partners may certainly agree to share profits and losses in different ratios. They may also agree that these ratios will be independent of the relative amounts of capital to which the partners are entitled.

> **Example 1.** Doctors J and K decide to form a general partnership to carry on a medical practice. Both individuals contribute $50,000 of cash to the partnership so that both have an initial capital account balance of $50,000. The partnership will use the cash to purchase equipment and supplies and to lease office space. Doctor J has been in local practice for several years and has an established reputation, while Doctor K recently graduated from medical school. Consequently, the partnership agreement provides that Doctor J will be allocated 65% of profits and losses, while Doctor K will be allocated 35%. The agreement stipulates that J and K will renegotiate this profit-and-loss sharing ratio after three years.

---

[10] See, for example, *Elrod*, 87 T.C. 1046 (1986).

[11] § 761(c).

CONTRIBUTIONS OF PROPERTY

Partners may make initial contributions to partnership capital in the form of cash, property, or a combination of both. When a partner transfers property to a partnership in exchange for an ownership interest, § 721 provides that neither the partner nor the partnership recognizes any gain or loss on the exchange.[12] The partner's tax basis in the transferred property carries over to become the partnership's basis in the property (i.e., a *carryover* basis).[13] The tax basis in the transferring partner's newly acquired partnership interest equals the basis of the transferred property plus any amount of cash contributed to the partnership (i.e., a *substituted* basis).[14] Tax professionals who specialize in the partnership area have coined the term *inside basis* to refer to the tax basis of assets owned by a partnership. In contrast, the term *outside basis* refers to the tax basis of a partner's interest in a partnership. Although neither term is used in the Code or Regulations, they provide a descriptive and easy way to differentiate between these two basis concepts.

The partnership's holding period for contributed assets includes the holding period of the assets in the hands of the contributing partner.[15] If the assets were either capital assets or § 1231 assets to the contributing partner, the partner's holding period for these assets becomes the holding period for his new partnership interest.[16] If the contributed assets were not capital or § 1231 assets, the partner's holding period for his interest begins on the date the interest is acquired.

> **Example 2.** A contributes § 1231 assets with a fair market value of $25,000 and an adjusted basis of $15,500, and B contributes $25,000 cash to the AB Partnership. The capital accounts on the partnership books are credited to reflect the equal $25,000 contributions of each partner. A does not recognize any gain on the exchange of the appreciated business assets for his interest in the AB Partnership. However, A's initial outside basis in his partnership interest is only $15,500. A's holding period for this interest includes the period of time for which A owned the contributed § 1231 assets. Even though the partnership recorded the contributed assets on its books at their $25,000 fair market value, the partnership's inside basis in these assets is only $15,500. B's initial tax basis in her partnership interest is $25,000, and her holding period for this interest begins on the date of contribution.

The above example illustrates two important points. First, a partner's outside basis is not necessarily equal to the balance in his or her capital account on the partnership's financial books and records. The partnership book capital accounts reflect the economic value of contributions to the partnership, while the partners' outside bases in their partnership interests reflect the tax basis of their respective contributions. Second, the tax rules governing contributions to partnerships result in an initial equilibrium between the partners' aggregate outside bases and the total inside basis of partnership assets. In *Example 2*, A and B have aggregate outside bases of $40,500. The AB Partnership has total inside basis in its assets of $40,500 ($25,000 cash + $15,500 carryover basis of its § 1231 assets). This equilibrium reflects the aggregate theory of partnerships under

---

[12] This nonrecognition rule does not apply to gain realized on transfer of appreciated stocks and securities to an investment partnership. § 721(b). Also, special rules—beyond the scope of this text—apply to transfers to partnerships with foreign persons and transfers of intangibles to foreign partnerships. See §§ 721(c) and 721(d).

[13] § 723. If contributed property is depreciable, the partnership will continue to use the cost recovery method and life used by the contributing partner. § 168(i)(7).

[14] § 722.

[15] § 1223(2).

[16] § 1223(1).

which A and B are considered to own indirect interests in AB's assets. However, it is possible that during the partnership's existence the aggregate outside basis will differ at times from the total inside basis.

A partner may have a divided holding period in his or her partnership interest in two circumstances. If a divided holding period occurs, the portion of a partnership interest to which a holding period relates is based on the relative fair market values of the properties contributed.[17] This will occur if the partner acquired portions of the partnership interest at different times.[18]

> **Example 3.** R purchased a 10% interest in Z Partnership for $10,000 on January 1, 2009. She purchased another 5% interest in Z for $5,000 on November 1, 2009. As of January 1, 2010, R has a one-year holding period in two-thirds of her partnership interest ($10,000/$15,000), and a two-month holding period for one-third ($5,000/$15,000) of her interest.

A partner will also have a divided holding period in his or her partnership interest if the partner contributed more than one property for the partnership interest, and these properties had different holding periods in the hands of the partner.[19]

> **Example 4.** E contributes cash of $2,000 and a capital asset (basis = $1,000; value = $2,000) held for five years for a 25% interest in Partnership Y. The portion of E's interest attributable to the cash, 50% [$2,000/($2,000 + $2,000)], will have a holding period beginning the day after the contribution. The portion of his interest attributable to the capital asset (50%) has a five-year holding period.

EFFECT OF PARTNERSHIP LIABILITIES ON BASIS

When a partnership borrows money, the general partners typically have unlimited liability for repayment of the debt to the partnership's creditors. If the partnership itself is unable to repay its debts, each partner must contribute personal funds to satisfy the unpaid balance. As a result, a partner's economic investment in a partnership consists not only of the contribution of cash or property reflected in his or her capital account, but also of the share of partnership debt for which the partner might ultimately be held responsible.

Section 752(a) acknowledges this responsibility by providing that any increase in a partner's share of the liabilities of a partnership or any assumption of a partnership debt by a partner is treated as a contribution of money to the partnership. This constructive cash contribution increases the partner's outside basis in his or her partnership interest. Conversely, § 752(b) provides that any decrease in a partner's share of the liabilities of a partnership or any assumption of a partner's debt by a partnership is treated as a distribution of money from the partnership to the partner. This constructive cash distribution reduces the partner's outside basis.[20]

> **Example 5.** M and N are equal partners in the M&N Partnership. On January 1 of the current year, both M and N had a $25,000 outside basis in their partnership interests, and the partnership had no debt on its balance sheet. On January 31, the partnership borrowed $15,000 from a local bank and used the funds to buy business assets. Because this transaction increased M and N's respective shares of the

---

[17]   Reg. § 1.1223-3(b)(1).

[18]   Reg. § 1.1223-2(a); for transfers of partnerships interests after September 20, 2000.

[19]   Reg. § 1.1223-3(a)(2).

[20]   § 733.

partnership's liabilities by $7,500, each was considered to have contributed this amount of cash to the partnership. As a result, their outside bases as of January 31 increased to $32,500.

On June 1, the partnership repaid $6,000 of the outstanding debt. Because this payment decreased M and N's respective shares of partnership debt, each was considered to have received a $3,000 cash distribution from the partnership. As a result, their outside bases as of June 1 decreased to $29,500.

		M	N
January 1 outside basis		$25,000	$25,000
Plus: Increase in share of partnership debt on 1/31		7,500	7,500
Less: Decrease in share of partnership debt on 6/1		(3,000)	(3,000)
June 1 outside basis		$29,500	$29,500

Note that in the above example, the inclusion of partnership debt in the partners' outside bases maintained the equilibrium between inside and outside basis. Between January 1 and June 1, M and N's aggregate outside bases increased by a net amount of $9,000. During this same period, the basis of partnership assets also increased by $9,000 ($15,000 debt proceeds − $6,000 cash distribution).

Partner's Share of Partnership Liabilities. The combined result of § 752(a) and (b) is that on any particular date, a partner's outside basis includes a share of the various debts reflected on the partnership balance sheet as of that date. The Treasury Regulations under § 752 provide a lengthy and complex set of rules for determining a partner's share of partnership liabilities. Under these regulations, each partner's share of any specific debt depends on the classification of the debt itself and whether the partner is a general or limited partner. All partnership debts are classified as either recourse or nonrecourse. A debt is *recourse* if the creditor can look to the personal assets of any general partner to satisfy the unpaid portion of the debt in the event the partnership does not have sufficient assets for repayment. A debt is *nonrecourse* if the creditor cannot look beyond the assets of the partnership for repayment.

A partner's share of recourse debt equals the portion of such debt for which that partner bears the *economic risk of loss*.[21] Because limited partners generally bear no responsibility for the repayment of partnership liabilities, they have no risk of loss with respect to partnership recourse debt. Consequently, no amount of such debt is apportioned to any limited partner. The extent to which general partners are deemed to bear the economic risk of loss for partnership recourse debt is generally determined by using the results from a hypothetical *constructive liquidation scenario*.[22] The basic idea behind these rules is to consider which partners would have to actually satisfy these liabilities if the absolute worst scenario imaginable (i.e., all liabilities are due but all partnership assets are worthless) happened to the partnership. The following transactions are assumed to occur, simultaneously, at the end of the partnership's taxable year:

1. All liabilities must be paid immediately in full.

2. All partnership assets, including cash, are assumed to have a fair market value of zero.

---

[21] Reg. § 1.752-2(a).

[22] Reg. § 1.752-2(b). In so-called straight-up partnerships in which the partners' profit-and-loss sharing ratios correspond to the ratios of their respective capital account balances, the application of this analysis has the same result as an apportionment based on loss-sharing ratios.

3. All partnership assets are sold for no consideration, which results in a recognized loss for each asset equal to the asset's adjusted basis.

4. These losses are allocated to the partners according to the loss sharing ratios in the partnership agreement.

5. The partners reduce their respective capital accounts by the amount of the losses.

6. The partnership liquidates. Consequently, any partner having a negative capital account after step five is deemed to make a cash contribution to the partnership, equal to this negative amount, so that his or her ending capital account will be zero.

7. The partnership is deemed to use this cash to pay off the recourse liabilities of the partnership.

8. Any remaining cash is deemed to be distributed to partners that have positive capital account balances.

The amount of cash that is deemed to be contributed to the partnership under step six is the partner's share of the recourse liabilities.

Example 6. Individuals W and X are general partners and individuals Y and Z are limited partners in the WXYZ Partnership. Partnership losses are allocated 20% to W, 30% to X, and 25% respectively to Y and Z. As of December 31 of the current year, the partnership has $100,000 of recourse debt. The partnership's balance sheet as of December 31 is as follows:

	Basis	Fair Market Value
Cash	$ 50,000	$ 50,000
Inventory	75,000	200,000
Machinery and equipment	75,000	150,000
	$200,000	$400,000
Recourse liabilities	$100,000	$100,000
W, capital	20,000	60,000
X, capital	30,000	90,000
Y, capital	25,000	75,000
Z, capital	25,000	75,000
	$200,000	$400,000

If the assets were worthless and sold for no consideration, a $200,000 loss would be recognized. In allocating this loss to the partners, the limited partners cannot have a negative capital account since they have limited liability. Therefore, whereas Y and Z would otherwise each be allocated $50,000 of loss ($200,000 × 25%), each is limited to a loss allocation of $25,000. The remaining $150,000 of loss is allocated to W and X based on their relative loss sharing ratios, as follows:

W: $150,000 × 20%/(20% + 30%) = $60,000

X: $150,000 × 30%/(20% + 30%) = $90,000

After allocation of these losses, the capital accounts are as follows:

	W	X	Y	Z
Capital, 12/31	$ 20,000	$ 30,000	$25,000	$25,000
Loss allocation	(60,000)	(90,000)	(25,000)	(25,000)
	$(40,000)	$(60,000)	-0-	-0-

The WXYZ Partnership is now assumed to liquidate. W and X must contribute $40,000 and $60,000 to the partnership, respectively, to restore their capital accounts to zero. This $100,000 is then used to pay the $100,000 recourse liability. Therefore, W and X are allocated $40,000 and $60,000 of the recourse liability, respectively, while Y and Z are not allocated any of the liability.

If a partnership defaults on the repayment of a nonrecourse debt and partnership assets are insufficient to satisfy the debt, the creditor cannot look to the personal assets of any partner for satisfaction. Therefore, no partner—general or limited—bears any economic risk of loss with regard to partnership nonrecourse debt. As a result, separate rules are provided for the allocation of nonrecourse debt. In general, the Regulations provide that nonrecourse debt is apportioned to all partners based on their profit-sharing ratios. However, an exception is provided to this rule if a partner has contributed property to the partnership encumbered with nonrecourse debt that has a built-in gain. In this case, the contributing partner is first allocated nonrecourse debt to the extent of the lower of 1) the built-in gain on the contributed property, or 2) the excess of the non-recourse debt over the adjusted basis of the contributed property. Any remaining debt is then allocated to all the partners based on their profit-sharing ratios.[23] This apportionment rule reflects the fact that such debt will be repaid from partnership profits and that both general and limited partners alike will pay tax on their allocated shares of such profits.

> **Example 7.** Individuals G and H are general partners and individuals I and J are limited partners in the GHIJ Partnership. Partnership profits are allocated 10% to G, 20% to H, and 35% respectively to I and J. As of December 31 of the current year, the partnership has $100,000 of nonrecourse debt. This $100,000 debt is attached to property that was contributed by G. At the time of contribution, the property had an adjusted basis to G of $80,000 and a fair market value of $120,000. The first $20,000 of the $100,000 debt is allocated to G as follows:
>
> Lower of
>
> 1. the built-in gain on the property, $40,000 ($120,000 – **$80,000),**
>
>   *or*
>
> 2. the excess of the non-recourse debt over the adjusted basis of the contributed property, $20,000 ($100,000 – **$80,000)**

The remaining $80,000 of nonrecourse debt is allocated based on the profit sharing ratios.
In summary, the $100,000 nonrecourse debt is allocated as follows:

	G	H	I	J
Built-in gain	$20,000	$ 0	$ 0	$ 0
Profit ratio	8,000	16,000	28,000	28,000
	$28,000	$16,000	$28,000	$28,000

---

[23] Reg. § 1.752-3(a); these regulations also include the concept of minimum gain for allocations of nonrecourse debt, but that discussion is beyond the scope of this book.

Consequently, G, H, l, and J may include $28,000, $16,000, $28,000, and $28,000 of the debt respectively in the outside bases of their partnership interests.

Liabilities Transferred to the Partnership. A partner who contributes property to a partnership in exchange for an ownership interest may negotiate for the partnership to assume a recourse liability of the partner as part of the exchange transaction. Similarly, the property contributed to the partnership may be subject to a nonrecourse liability. In both cases, the rules of § 752 have an impact on the computation of the contributing partner's outside basis.

Any debt from which the contributing partner is relieved of personal liability reduces that partner's basis in his or her new partnership interest. However, this outside basis is also increased by any amount of such debt apportioned to the contributor in his or her capacity as partner. Because this decrease and increase occur simultaneously as the result of a single transaction, only the net increase or decrease is taken into account in computing the contributing partner's basis.[24] The net increase or decrease for the contributing partner's basis can be computed as: amount of liability transferred $\times$ (100% $-$ partner's percentage share of debt).

Example 8. Individual T contributes business assets with an adjusted basis of $50,000 to a partnership in exchange for a 25% general interest in partnership capital, profits, and losses. As part of the contribution, the partnership assumes $12,000 of T's business recourse debt, relieving T of personal liability. The partnership has no other debts. Although T is relieved of the $12,000 debt in her individual capacity, she continues to bear the economic risk of loss for 25% of the debt in her capacity as general partner. Accordingly, T's outside basis in her partnership interest immediately subsequent to her contribution is $41,000 ($50,000 basis of contributed property $-$ $9,000 *net* relief of debt).

Basis of contributed property		$50,000
Less:	Relief of personal liability	(12,000)
Plus:	Liability for debt as general partner	
	(25% $\times$ $12,000)	3,000
T's outside basis in partnership interest		$41,000

A partnership's assumption of a contributing partner's debt has tax consequences not only to the contributor but to the other partners as well. The outside bases of the noncontributing partners will increase by the amount of newly assumed debt apportioned to them and decrease by the amount of existing partnership debt apportioned to the newly admitted partner.

Example 9. Individual L contributes business assets with a fair market value of $23,600 and adjusted basis of $10,000 to a partnership in exchange for a one-third general interest in partnership capital, profits, and losses. As part of the contribution, the partnership assumes $3,600 of L's business recourse debt, relieving L of personal liability. Consequently, L's contribution has a net value of $20,000 ($23,600 $-$ $3,600) and a net basis of $6,400 ($10,000 $-$ $3,600). The partnership has $6,000 of existing debt as of the date of contribution. Immediately after the contribution, the partnership has the following balance sheet:

---

[24] Reg. § 1.752-1(f).

	Inside Basis	Fair Market Value
Contributed assets	$10,000	$23,600
Existing assets.	30,000	46,000
	$40,000	$69,600
Assumed debt	$ 3,600	$ 3,600
Existing debt	6,000	6,000
Capital: Partner L (33.3%)	6,400	20,000
Partner M (33.3%).	12,000	20,000
Partner N (33.3%)	12,000	20,000
	$40,000	$69,600

L's outside basis in his new partnership interest is $9,600 ($10,000 basis of contributed property − $2,400 ($3,600 × 66.7%) net relief of the assumed debt + $2,000 ($6,000 × 33.3%) assumption of one-third of existing partnership debt).

Prior to L's admission to the partnership, partners M and N each had $15,000 of outside basis in his partnership interest. This basis number represented a one-half interest in the $24,000 net inside basis of existing partnership assets plus one-half of the $6,000 of existing partnership debt. Upon L's admission, M and N are each apportioned $1,200 of the assumed debt. However, they are each relieved of $1,000 of existing debt. Subsequent to L's admission, their outside bases have each increased to $15,200 ($15,000 + $200 net increase in share of partnership liabilities).

Note that in *Example 9*, the inclusion of $9,600 of total partnership debt in the partners' outside bases maintains the equilibrium between the $40,000 aggregate outside basis (L's $9,600 basis + M's $15,200 basis + N's $15,200 basis) and the $40,000 total inside basis of the partnership assets.

CONTRIBUTION OF SERVICES

The nonrecognition rule of § 721 does not apply when an incoming partner contributes personal services to a partnership in exchange for an ownership interest. The tax consequences of such an exchange to both parties depend on whether the service partner receives an interest in partnership *capital* or merely an interest in the *future profits* of the partnership business.

Receipt of a Capital Interest. If a service partner receives an interest in the existing capital of a partnership, the partner must recognize ordinary compensation income to the extent of the value of such interest.[25] The amount of income recognized becomes the partner's initial outside basis in the interest received.[26]

Example 10. G agrees to perform services for the AB Partnership in exchange for a 20% interest in partnership capital, profits, and losses. On the date that C is admitted to the partnership, the net value of the partnership assets is $250,000. The value of C's newly acquired interest is $50,000 (20% of $250,000), which equates to the value of the assets that C would receive if the partnership were to immediately liquidate and

---

[25] Reg. § 1.721-1(b)(1). The partnership can usually deduct the value of the capital interest given for services as an ordinary business expense. A complete analysis of the tax consequences of this payment by the partnership is beyond the scope of this chapter.

[26] Reg. § 1.722-1.

distribute its assets to each partner based on their relative capital account balances. C must recognize $50,000 of compensation income on the exchange and will have a $50,000 outside basis in her partnership interest.

Receipt of a Profits Interest. The partners in an established partnership may be reluctant to give up any part of their equity in existing partnership assets (i.e., a capital interest) as compensation to a newly admitted service partner. These partners might be more willing to give the service partner an interest in the future profits of the business— profits partially attributable to the new partner's efforts on behalf of the partnership.

Example 11. J agrees to perform services for the GHI Partnership in exchange for a 25% interest in future partnership profits and losses. On the date that J is admitted to the partnership, the net value of the partnership's assets is $800,000. However, J is not given an initial capital account and has no legal interest in these assets. If the partnership were to immediately liquidate and distribute its assets to the partners based on their relative capital account balances, J would receive nothing. If the partnership generates income subsequent to J's admission, J will be entitled to 25% of such income.

The tax consequences to a service partner who receives nothing more than an interest in future partnership profits have been the subject of heated debate among tax experts for many years. The courts have also struggled with this issue with confusing and inconclusive results.[27] Currently, the uneasy consensus of opinion is that a service partner does not recognize current income upon the receipt of a profits interest because the interest has no immediate liquidation value. Consequently, the service partner's initial basis in the interest is zero. The partner will, of course, recognize income to the extent of his or her share of future partnership profits.

PROPOSED REGULATIONS CHANGE RULES FOR SERVICES

Proposed regulations issued in 2005 provide that an employer that transfers a capital partnership interest to a service provider would not have to recognize gain or loss on the transaction.[28] Under the proposed regulations, service providers would still recognize income on the receipt of a capital interest (but not a profits interest) and the employer would receive a compensation deduction for the value of the interest (unless the payment is an organization expense). However, this conclusion is reached in a slightly different fashion than existing law. The proposed regulations provide that the value of the partnership interest is its current liquidation value immediately after the transaction. Profits interest would have no liquidation value, so service providers receiving a profits interest would have no income.

OPERATING THE PARTNERSHIP

Section 701, the first section in Subchapter K, states that "a partnership as such shall not be subject to the income tax imposed by this chapter. Persons carrying on business as partners shall be liable for income tax only in their separate or individual capacities." Even though partnerships are not taxable entities, they are required to file an annual information return, Form

---

[27] See *Sol Diamond*, 56 T.C. 530 (1971), *aff'd* 74-1 USTC ¶9306, 33 AFTR2d 74-852, 492 F.2d 286 (CA-7, 1974), *William G. Campbell*, 59 TCM 236, T.C. Memo 1990-162, *rev'd* 1991-2 USTC ¶50,420 (CA-8, 1991), and Rev. Proc. 93-27, 1993-2 C.B. 343.

[28] Prop. Reg. §§ 1.721-1(b) and 1.83-3(e).

1065 (U.S. Partnership Return of Income).[29] Basically, this return shows the computation of partnership taxable income and how such income is allocated to each partner. Form 1065 is due by the 15th day of the fourth month following the close of the partnership taxable year.[30]

In order to compute its annual taxable income, a newly formed partnership must make a number of initial elections, including the adoption of both an accounting method (or methods) by which to compute income and the partnership taxable year. The fact that these important elections are made by the partnership itself rather than by each partner is a very practical application of the entity theory of partnerships.[31] As a general rule, partnerships are free to elect the cash receipts and disbursements method, the accrual method, or a hybrid method of accounting for tax purposes.[32] As explained in the next section of the chapter, they have much less flexibility in the choice of a taxable year.

THE PARTNERSHIP'S TAXABLE YEAR

Income generated by a partnership is included in the taxable income of a partner for the partner's year in which the partnership's taxable year ends.[33] If partnerships had no restrictions as to their choice of taxable year, this simple timing rule could be used to achieve a significant deferral of income recognition.

> **Example 12.** R and S, calendar year individuals, decide to operate a business as equal partners. The RS Partnership begins business on February 1, 2009. During its first year of operations the partnership generates $3,000 of taxable income each month. If the partnership could adopt a fiscal year ending January 31, its $36,000 of first-year income ($33,000 of which was earned in 2009) would be included in the partners' 2010 tax returns because 2010 is the partners' taxable year in which the partnership's fiscal year ends. For each subsequent year that the RS Partnership remains in existence, eleven months of income earned in one calendar year would not be taxed at the partner level until the following calendar year.

Subchapter K contains a set of complex rules designed to minimize the potential for income deferral through use of a partnership. A partnership must adopt the taxable year used by one or more partners who own more than a 50 percent aggregate interest in partnership capital and profits. If no such *majority interest taxable year* exists, the partnership must adopt the taxable year used by its principal partners (those partners owning at least a 5 percent interest in partnership capital or profits).[34] If the principal partners use different taxable years, the partnership must adopt a taxable year resulting in the least aggregate deferral of income to the partners. The taxable year resulting from the application of these rules is known as the "required taxable year."

Under the *least aggregate deferral method*,[35] all year-ends that any of the partners have must be tested, and the one that produces the least amount of deferral for the partners as a group is the required tax year. The deferral for each partner is computed as the time from the year-end being tested until the next year-end of the partner. The months of deferral are then weighted by each partner's profits interest. The least aggregate deferral method is illustrated by the following example:

---

[29] § 6031.

[30] § 6072. Partnerships may apply for a six month extension of time to file. The IRS is considering reducing the extension of time for partnership returns from six months to five months.

[31] § 703(b).

[32] § 446(c). Section 448(a) limits the use of the cash method for a partnership that (1) is a tax shelter, or (2) has a C corporation as a partner. However, § 448(b) provides several important exceptions to this restrictive limitation.

[33] § 706(a).

[34] § 706(b)(1)(A).

[35] Reg. § 1.706-1(b)(3).

Example 13. M and N are equal corporate partners in the MN Partnership. M has a year-end of March 31 and N has a year-end of November 30. Since M and N each own 50% of the partnership, no partner, or group of partners, that have the same year-end own a more than 50% interest in the partnership. MN Partnership has two principal partners, but the principal partners do not have the same year end. Therefore, the least aggregate deferral method must be used. The two months that must be tested are March and November.

Test of March 31 Year-End

Partner	Year-End	Profit Interest	×	Months of Deferral	Weighted Deferral
M	3/31	50%	×	0	0.0
N	11/30	50%	×	8	4.0
				Aggregate Deferral	4.0

Test of November 30 Year-End

Partner	Year-End	Profit Interest	×	Months of Deferral	Weighted Deferral
M	3/31	50%	×	4	2.0
N	11/30	50%	×	0	0.0
				Aggregate Deferral	2.0

Therefore, the required year end is November 30 since it produces the least amount of deferral for the partners as a group.

If the partners wish to use a year different from the "required tax year," the Code offers relief from these mechanistic rules by allowing a partnership to adopt any taxable year (without reference to the taxable years of its partners) if it can convince the IRS that there is a valid business purpose for such year.[36] The IRS will generally agree that a partnership has a *business purpose* for adopting a taxable year that conforms to its natural business year. For example, a partnership operating a ski resort might have a natural business year that ends on April 30. The IRS should allow this partnership to adopt this fiscal year for tax purposes, regardless of the taxable years used by the various partners. A partnership can also use a different year-end from its required year-end if it meets the 25 percent test. This test holds that a partnership may change its tax year if at least 25 percent of the taxpayer's annual gross receipts are recognized in the last two months of the tax year to which the partnership wishes to change, and this 25 percent test is met for three consecutive years.[37]

ORGANIZATION COSTS AND SYNDICATION FEES

Any costs incurred to organize a partnership, such as legal fees for drafting the partnership agreement and filing fees charged by the state in which the partnership is formed, must be capitalized and are not deductible as ordinary and necessary business expenses. The partnership may elect to expense up to $5,000 of these *organization costs* and to amortize the remainder over a period of 180 months, beginning with the month in which the partnership begins business.[38] The $5,000 amount to be expensed must be reduced (but not below zero)

---

[36] § 706(b)(1)(B).

[37] Rev. Proc. 2002-39, 2002-22 I.R.B. 1046, provides guidelines for changing from the required tax year because of the business purpose test and the 25 percent gross receipts test. Also see Rev. Rul. 87-57, 1987-2 C.B. 117 for other examples of circumstances that may or may not be considered valid business purposes.

[38] § 709(b).

by the amount of organizational costs in excess of $50,000. Any *syndication fees* connected with the issuance and marketing of partnership interests must also be capitalized. These fees may not be amortized and will remain as an intangible asset on the partnership books until the partnership is liquidated.[39]

COMPUTATION OF PARTNERSHIP TAXABLE INCOME

Partnership taxable income is computed in the same manner as the taxable income of an individual.[40] However, a partnership must make a separate accounting of any item of income, gain, deduction, loss, or credit that is potentially subject to special treatment at the partner level.[41] Separately stated items include capital gains and losses, § 1231 gains and losses, investment income and expenses, net rental income or loss, and charitable contributions. As a result, partnership taxable income is the net of all items that are not separately stated, which can be narrowly defined as gross receipts from services or gross profits from sales of inventory less deductible business expenses incurred by the partnership during the year. This net number is computed on page 1 of Form 1065 and is labeled *ordinary income (loss)*. In contrast, all separately stated items are listed as such on page 3, Schedule K of Form 1065. (Appendix contains a copy of Form 1065 and accompanying Schedule K.)

The character of any item of partnership income, gain, deduction, or loss is determined with reference to the activities of the partnership rather than the activities of the individual partners.[42] For example, gain on the sale of land held by a partnership as an investment for two years is long-term capital gain. This characterization holds even if some of the partners to whom the gain will be taxed are real estate developers in whose hands the land would have been inventory. Similarly, the gain is long-term even if some of the partners have owned their partnership interests for less than one year.[43]

Section 724 contains three exceptions to the general rule that tax characteristics are determined at the partnership level.

1. In the case of unrealized receivables contributed to the partnership by a partner, any gain or loss recognized when the partnership disposes of the receivables must be treated as ordinary gain or loss.

2. In the case of inventory contributed to the partnership by a partner, any gain or loss recognized on disposition within the five-year period subsequent to contribution must be treated as ordinary gain or loss.

3. In the case of a capital asset contributed to the partnership by a partner, any loss recognized on disposition within the five-year period subsequent to contribution must be treated as capital loss to the extent the basis of the asset exceeded its fair market value at date of contribution.

Example 14. Three years ago, D exchanged land that he held as an investment ($50,000 fair market value and $65,000 basis) and an inventory asset from his sole proprietorship ($20,000 fair market value and $18,000 basis) for an interest in the DEF Partnership. Both assets had a carryover basis to the partnership under § 723. Both contributed assets were used in the partnership business, and therefore were characterized as § 1231 assets at the partnership level. During the current year, the

---

[39] § 709(a).

[40] § 703(a).

[41] § 702(a). Reg. § 1.702-1(a)(8)(ii) explains that each partner must be able to take into account separately his or her distributive share of any partnership item that results in an income tax liability different from that which would result if the item were not accounted for separately.

[42] § 702(b).

[43] Rev. Rul. 67-188, 1967-1 C.B. 216.

partnership sold both assets, realizing a $22,000 loss on the sale of the land and a $3,500 gain on the sale of the former inventory asset.

Because the sales took place within the five-year period subsequent to contribution, the partnership must recognize $15,000 of the loss on the land sale (excess of $65,000 contributed basis over $50,000 contributed value) as capital loss and the $7,000 remainder as § 1231 loss. The partnership must recognize the entire gain on the sale of the former inventory as ordinary income. If the sales had taken place after the expiration of the five-year period, both the recognized loss and gain would have been § 1231 in nature.[44]

REPORTING OF PARTNERSHIP ITEMS BY PARTNERS

Partners must take into account their distributive shares of partnership taxable income and any separately stated partnership items in computing their taxable incomes.[45] This passthrough of partnership items to the partners is deemed to occur on the last day of the partnership's taxable year. Consequently, the passthrough items are included in each partner's return for the partner's taxable year within which the partnership year ends.[46]

Each partner's distributive share of every partnership item is reported on a Schedule K-1 for that partner. Partnerships must include a copy of each Schedule K-1 with the annual partnership return filed with the IRS. A second copy is transmitted to each partner. Upon receipt, partners must incorporate the information reported on the Schedule K-1 into their tax returns.

> **Example 15.** Individual A and Corporation B are calendar year taxpayers and equal partners in the AB Partnership, which uses a September 30 fiscal year end for tax purposes. During December 2009, each partner received a Schedule K-1 showing the following results of partnership operations from October 1, 2008 through September 30, 2009.
>
> | | |
> |---|---:|
> | Ordinary income from business activities (partnership taxable income) | $42,300 |
> | Dividend income | 2,300 |
> | Net long-term capital loss | (4,000) |
> | Investment interest expense | (5,500) |
> | Charitable contributions | (1,900) |

Individual A will include his $42,300 share of ordinary business income on Schedule E, his $2,300 share of dividend income on Schedule B, and his $4,000 share of the long-term capital loss on Schedule D of his 2009 Form 1040. Per § 163(d), A's $5,500 share of investment interest expense is deductible only to the extent of his net investment income for 2009. Furthermore, the deductible portion of the interest expense and A's $1,900 share of the charitable contribution must be reported as itemized deductions on Schedule A, Form 1040.

Corporation B will include both its $42,300 share of ordinary business income and its $5,500 share of investment interest expense on page 1, and its $4,000 share of long-term capital loss on Schedule D of its 2009 Form 1120. [Corporations are not subject to the § 163(d) limitation.] B will include its $2,300 share of dividend income on Schedule C (Dividends and Special Deductions) and will compute an

---

[44]   § 704(c) also requires a special allocation of both loss and gain among the partners. This allocation rule is discussed in a later section of the chapter.

[45]   § 702(a). Section 772(a) provides a simplified reporting system for certain electing *large* partnerships. Large nonservice partnerships with 100 or more members can elect to reduce the number of items that must be separately reported to their numerous partners. See §§ 771 through 777.

[46]   § 706(a).

appropriate dividends-received deduction. B's $1,900 share of the charitable contribution may be deducted on page 1 of Form 1120 to the extent that the corporation's total charitable contributions for 2009 do not exceed 10% of taxable income.

ADJUSTMENTS TO PARTNER'S BASIS

A partner's distributive share of annual partnership income is determined without reference to actual cash distributions made by the partnership to its partners. If a partner's share of annual partnership income exceeds any cash received from the partnership during the year, the undistributed income will be recorded as an increase in that partner's capital account balance (his or her equity in the partnership) at year-end. On the other hand, in a year in which a partnership operates at a loss, a partner's share of such loss will be recorded as a capital account decrease.

The fluctuating nature of a partnership investment is also reflected in the basis of the partner's interest in the partnership. Outside basis is *increased* by a partner's distributive share of both taxable and nontaxable partnership income.[47] Outside basis is *decreased* by distributions made by the partnership to the partner and by the partner's distributive share of partnership losses and nondeductible current expenditures.[48] These basis adjustments are made in the above order at the end of the partnership taxable year.[49] Even if cash distributions representing advances or draws against a partner's share of current income are made at various dates throughout the year, the effect of these distributions on basis is determined as of the last day of the year.[50]

> **Example 16.** M owns a 40% interest in the capital, profits, and losses of the KLMN Partnership. Both M and KLMN use a calendar year for tax purposes. At the beginning of the current year, M's outside basis in her partnership interest was $35,000. During the year, M received four cash distributions of $5,000 each as advances against her share of current-year income. At the end of the year, the partnership has $20,000 of nonrecourse debt. M's Schedule K-1 for the current year showed the following distributive shares:
>
> | | |
> |---|---:|
> | Ordinary income | $33,000 |
> | Tax-exempt interest income | 4,000 |
> | Net long-term capital gain | 8,100 |
> | Nondeductible penalty | (1,700) |
> | Nondeductible 50% business meals and entertainment | (600) |

As of the last day of the current year, M's outside basis is increased by $8,000 ($20,000 × 40%) for her share of the debt and by $45,100 (her share of partnership taxable and tax-exempt income), decreased by the $20,000 of cash distributions made during the year, and decreased by $2,300 (her share of the partnership nondeductible current expenses). Consequently, M's outside basis as of the first day of the next taxable year is $65,800.

PARTNERS' DISTRIBUTIVE SHARES

The income or loss generated by a business conducted in partnership form is measured and characterized at the partnership level, then allocated to the various

---

[47]   § 705(a)(1).

[48]   § 705(a)(2).

[49]   Reg. § 1.705-1(a).

[50]   Reg. § 1.731-1(a)(1)(ii).

partners for inclusion on their income tax returns. Each partner's *distributive share* of any item of partnership income, gain, loss, deduction, or credit is determined by reference to the partnership agreement.[51] Consequently, the partners themselves can decide exactly how the profits or losses from their business are to be shared. The sharing arrangement as specified in the partnership agreement can be an equal allocation of profits and losses to each partner or a more elaborate arrangement under which different items of gain or loss are shared in different ratios among different categories of partners.

Although partners certainly have a great deal of flexibility in determining the allocation of partnership income and loss, § 704(b) warns that such allocations must have *substantial economic effect* if they are to be respected by the Internal Revenue Service. If the IRS concludes that the allocation of any partnership item lacks substantial economic effect, it may reallocate the item among the partners. Such reallocation will be based upon the partners' true economic interests in the partnership, as determined by the IRS upon examination of all relevant facts and circumstances.

SUBSTANTIAL ECONOMIC EFFECT

Treasury regulations provide an intricate set of rules for determining whether partnership allocations meet the substantial economic effect test of § 704(b). The basic objective of the regulations is to "ensure that any allocation is consistent with the underlying economic arrangement of the partners. This means that in the event there is an economic benefit or economic burden that corresponds to an allocation, the partner to whom the allocation is made must receive such economic benefit or bear such economic burden."[52] The economic benefit or burden of an allocation equates to the impact of the allocation on a partner's interest in partnership capital. In other words, an allocation of income or loss for tax purposes must correspond to an allocation of dollars to or from a partner's capital account on the partnership books.

The regulations attempt to ensure this correspondence through a three-pronged test for economic effect.[53] Any allocation for tax purposes will have economic effect only if the following three conditions are met:

1. The allocation is reflected in the partners' capital accounts for book purposes.

2. Upon liquidation of the partnership, liquidating distributions of cash and property are made to the partners based upon the balances in their capital accounts.

3. Partners with deficit balances in their capital accounts upon liquidation are unconditionally required to restore such deficit balance to the partnership. (This obligation may be expressly stated in the partnership agreement or imposed by state law.)[54]

Example 17. The RST Partnership agreement provides that taxable income or loss will be allocated 50% to R and 25% respectively to S and T. The agreement provides that this allocation will be reflected in the partnership capital accounts, that liquidating distributions will be based on capital account balances, and that any partner with a deficit capital account balance must restore the deficit immediately prior to liquidation.

---

51 § 704(a).

52 Reg. § 1.704-1(b)(2)(ii)(a).

53 The additional requirement that economic effect be *substantial* is discussed in Reg. § 1.704-1(b)(2)(iii). Any discussion of this difficult regulation is beyond the scope of an introductory text.

54 Reg. § 1.704-1(b)(2)(ii)(c).

For the current year, the RST Partnership generated $48,000 taxable income, $24,000 of which was reported as R's distributive share on his Schedule K-1 and $12,000 of which was reported as S and T's respective distributive shares on their Schedules K-l. Each partner's capital account was increased by the amount of income reported as his distributive share for tax purposes. Because the allocation meets the three-pronged test, it has economic effect and should be respected by the IRS.

Note that in the above example, the taxable income allocated to each partner matched the increase in each partner's capital account balance for the year. Moreover, upon liquidation of the partnership, the partners will receive an amount of dollars (or property) equal to the balances in their capital accounts. Contrast this result with that in the following example.

Example 18. The XYZ partnership agreement provides that taxable income or loss will be allocated 50% to X and 25% respectively to Y and Z. The agreement states that for book purposes income will be allocated equally to each partner. For the current year, the XYZ Partnership generated $48,000 of taxable income, $24,000 of which was reported as X's distributive share on his Schedule K-l and $12,000 of which was reported as Y and Z's respective distributive shares on their Schedules K-l. However, each partner's capital account on the partnership books was increased by $16,000.

In this example, the allocation of taxable income fails to reflect the allocation of dollars to the partners. Because this tax allocation obviously lacks economic effect, the IRS can reallocate the taxable income to the partners based upon its determination of how the partners actually intend to share the economic benefit of the income. The facts of this simple example indicate that X, Y, and Z intend to share the dollars generated by their partnership business equally. Consequently, the IRS will allocate $16,000 of current-year taxable income to each partner.

ALLOCATIONS WITH RESPECT TO CONTRIBUTED PROPERTY

When a partner contributes property to a partnership and the value of such property is more or less than the contributing partner's tax basis in the property, subsequent allocations of taxable income, gain, loss, and deduction with respect to the contributed property will lack substantial economic effect within the meaning of § 704(b).

Example 19. M contributed an asset (fair market value $20,000, adjusted basis $14,000) and N contributed $20,000 cash to M&N Partnership in exchange for a one-half interest in partnership capital, profits, and losses. The asset contributed by M was recorded on the partnership books at $20,000 but had a carryover tax basis to the partnership of $14,000. The capital accounts for both M and N were credited with the $20,000 values of their respective contributions. Three months after its formation, the partnership sold the contributed asset for $20,000. For tax purposes, the partnership recognized a $6,000 gain on sale. For book purposes, the partnership realized no gain and made no entry to either partner's capital account.

Because of the initial difference between the contributed *value* and the contributed *basis* of the asset in the above example, the taxable gain on the sale is not equal to the gain realized for book purposes. Consequently, any allocation of the taxable gain to the partners does not have substantial economic effect because the allocation cannot be reflected in book capital accounts.

Section 704(c) solves this problem by mandating a special allocation rule for items of income, gain, loss, and deduction attributable to contributed assets. Essentially, any difference between the amount of the item for tax purposes and for book purposes at the time of contribution must be allocated to the contributing partner when the partnership disposes of the asset. The remainder of the item is allocated for both tax and book purposes according to the sharing ratios specified in the partnership agreement. The application of this special rule to the $6,000 taxable gain recognized in *Example 19* results in an allocation of the entire $6,000 gain to contributing partner M. Note that this amount of gain equals the deferred gain that M was not required to recognize upon the contribution of the appreciated asset to the partnership.

> **Example 20.** O contributed an asset (FMV $20,000, adjusted basis $26,000) and P contributed $20,000 cash to O&P Partnership in exchange for a one-half interest in partnership capital, profits, and losses. The asset contributed by O was recorded on the partnership books at $20,000 but had a carryover tax basis to the partnership of $26,000. The capital accounts for both O and P were credited with the $20,000 values of their respective contributions. Seven months after its formation, the partnership sold the contributed asset for $17,000. For tax purposes, the partnership recognized a $9,000 loss on sale, while for book purposes it realized only a $3,000 loss (the decline in the value of the asset subsequent to its contribution to the partnership). The first $6,000 of the tax loss must be allocated to contributing partner O. The remaining $3,000 loss is allocated equally between O and P.

Section 704(c) affects the allocation of depreciation deductions attributable to contributed property as well as allocations of gains and losses recognized by the partnership upon disposition of the property. These depreciation deductions are first allocated to the noncontributing partners in an amount equal to their allocable share of book depreciation (depreciation computed on the contributed value of the property). Any remaining tax depreciation is allocated to the partner who contributed the property.

> **Example 21.** D contributed a depreciable asset (fair market value $60,000, adjusted basis $48,000) and E contributed $120,000 cash to DEF Partnership in exchange for a one-third and a two-thirds interest respectively in partnership capital, profits, and losses. The partnership will depreciate the asset over five years on a straight-line basis. In each year, tax depreciation on the contributed asset is $9,600 (20% of the $48,000 contributed basis), while book depreciation is $12,000 (20% of the $60,000 contributed value). One-third and two-thirds of the book depreciation is allocated to D and E respectively. Each year noncontributing partner E is allocated the first $8,000 of tax depreciation (her two-thirds share of the $12,000 book depreciation). The remaining $1,600 of the annual tax depreciation is allocated to contributing partner D.

RETROACTIVE ALLOCATIONS

In addition to the substantial economic effect requirement of § 704(b) and the special allocation rule of § 704(c), the determination of each partner's annual distributive share of partnership income, gain, loss, deduction, or credit must take account of any change in the partner's equity interest in the partnership during the year.[55] This *varying interest rule* was enacted to prevent retroactive allocations of partnership items to new partners who were admitted to the partnership after the items were recognized or incurred.

---

[55]   § 706(d)(1).

Example 22. K and L have been equal partners in the calendar year cash basis K&L Partnership since 2001. On November 1 of the current year, M contributed $100,000 cash in exchange for a one-third interest in partnership capital. The partnership generated a $108,000 operating loss for the current taxable year. The maximum amount of this loss that can be allocated to M under the revised partnership agreement among K, L, and M is $18,049, the portion of the loss attributable to the last 61 days of the year during which M owned an interest in the partnership.

BASIS LIMITATION ON LOSS DEDUCTIBILITY

Under § 704(d), a partner's distributive share of partnership loss is deductible only to the extent of the partner's outside basis in his or her partnership interest as of the end of the partnership year in which the loss was incurred. Any nondeductible portion of a current year loss is carried forward indefinitely into future years and can be deducted if and when sufficient outside basis is restored. This loss limitation rule is applied only after a partner's basis has been increased by any distributive share of current-year partnership income and decreased by any distributions made to the partner for the year.[56]

Example 23. F is a partner in the calendar year DEFG partnership. At the beginning of the current year, F's outside basis in her partnership interest was $14,500. During the year, F received a $3,000 cash distribution from DEFG. At the close of the year, Schedule K-1 showed that her distributive share of the partnership's current-year operating loss was $20,000, while her shares of current-year dividends and long-term capital gains were $3,400 and $1,300 respectively. F will increase her outside basis by $4,700 (her share of partnership income) and decrease it by the $3,000 cash distribution. Under § 704(d), F may deduct her allocated partnership loss only to the extent of her $16,200 remaining outside basis, thereby reducing her year-end basis to zero. The $3,800 nondeductible portion of F's loss will carry forward into subsequent taxable years.

F's January 1 outside basis	$ 14,500
Plus: Allocated share of income	4,700
Less: Distributions	(3,000)
Deductible share of allocated loss	(16,200)
F's December 31 outside basis	-0-
F's loss carryforward	$ 3,800

If a partner is allocated a distributive share of more than one type of loss and the partner's outside basis is insufficient to absorb the aggregate amount of losses, the § 704 (d) limitation is applied proportionately to each type of loss.[57]

Example 24. Refer to the facts in *Example 23*, but assume that F is allocated a $6,000 § 1231 loss in addition to the $20,000 operating loss. F's currently deductible amounts of each type of loss are computed as follows:

Operating loss: ($20,000 ÷ $26,000) × $16,200 = $12,462

§ 1231 loss: ($6,000 ÷ $26,000) × $16,200 = $3,738

---

[56] Reg. § 1.704-1(d)(2).

[57] Reg. § 1.704-1(d)(2).

The nondeductible $7,538 operating loss and $2,262 § 1 231 loss are carried forward into subsequent years.

TRANSACTIONS BETWEEN PARTNERS AND PARTNERSHIPS

Under the entity theory, a partner and a partnership are separate and distinct entities that can transact with each other at arm's length. This perspective is adopted in § 707(a), which states that "if a partner engages in a transaction with a partnership other than in his capacity as a member of such partnership, the transaction shall, except as otherwise provided in this section, be considered as occurring between the partnership and one who is not a partner." Because of this general rule, a partner can assume the role of unrelated third party when dealing with the partnership. For example, a partner can lend money to or borrow money from a partnership, rent property to or from a partnership, buy property from or sell property to a partnership, or provide consulting services to a partnership as an independent contractor. The tax consequences of all the above transactions will be determined as if the partnership were dealing with a nonpartner.[58]

The major exception to the general rule of § 707(a) concerns partners who work in the partnership business on a regular and ongoing basis. The point was made earlier in the chapter that general partners are considered self-employed individuals, rather than employees of their partnership. Consequently, partners cannot be paid a salary or wage by the partnership, even if they perform exactly the same duties as nonpartner employees. However, partners who work in a partnership business certainly expect to be compensated for their time and effort. The tax consequences of compensatory payments made by partnerships to partners in their capacities as such are governed by § 707(c). The annual amounts of such payments are typically determined with reference to the extent and nature of the services performed, without regard to the income of the partnership for that year. Such *guaranteed payments* must be recognized as ordinary income by the recipient partner. The partnership will either deduct the guaranteed payment as a § 162 business expense or capitalize it to an appropriate asset account as required by § 263.[59]

> **Example 25.** P has a one-third interest in the calendar year OPQ Partnership. Unlike partners O and Q, P works in the partnership business on a full-time basis. The partnership agreement provides that for the current year P will receive a monthly guaranteed payment of $4,000 from the partnership. The partnership business generates $175,000 of annual income before consideration of P's guaranteed payment.
>
> Based on the nature of the work performed by P, the partnership may claim a current deduction for the guaranteed payment; accordingly its net income for the year is $127,000 ($175,000 − $48,000 total guaranteed payments), and each partner's one-third distributive share is $42,333. P will report total partnership income for the year of $90,333 ($48,000 guaranteed payment + $42,333 distributive

---

[58] Under § 267(a)(2), a payment made by an accrual basis taxpayer to a cash basis related party may not be deducted by the payor until the taxable year in which the payee includes the payment in gross income. Per § 267(e), a partnership and any partner are related parties for purposes of this matching rule. The rule does not apply to § 707(c) guaranteed payments.

[59] Guaranteed payments can also be made with respect to a partner's capital account. Such payments are functionally equivalent to interest, always represent ordinary income to the recipient partner, and will be either deducted or capitalized by the partnership.

share), while O and Q will each report only their $42,333 distributive shares of income.

> **Example 26.** Assume the same facts as in *Example 25*, except that the OPQ Partnership generates only $30,000 of annual income before consideration of P's guaranteed payment. In this case, the deduction of the payment results in an $18,000 net *loss* of which each partner's distributive share is $6,000. P will report total partnership income for the year of $42,000 ($48,000 guaranteed payment − $6,000 loss), while O and Q will each report only their $6,000 distributive shares of loss.

From an economic perspective, a guaranteed payment received by a partner is functionally equivalent to a salary received by an employee. Nonetheless, for tax purposes several important differences distinguish the two. An employer is required by law to withhold federal, state, and local income taxes and employee payroll taxes from an employee's salary. Guaranteed payments are not subject to any similar withholding requirement. At the end of each calendar year, employees receive a Form W-2 on which gross annual compensation and various withheld amounts are summarized. Guaranteed payments are reported only as a line item on the recipient partner's Schedule K-1 issued by the partnership. Finally, while cash basis employees must recognize salary payments as gross income in the year the payments are received, guaranteed payments are deemed to be paid to partners on the last day of the tax year, regardless of when they are actually paid during the year.[60]

> **Example 27.** Refer to the facts in *Example 26*, but assume the OPQ Partnership is on a fiscal year ending September 30. As a result, P actually received three $4,000 guaranteed payments in October, November, and December of the prior calendar year and only nine $4,000 payments during the current calendar year. Notwithstanding, P will report the entire $48,000 of guaranteed payments in the current year because all twelve months of guaranteed payments are deemed to be paid on September 30. Note that this result holds regardless of the amount of any renegotiated guaranteed payment that P may receive during the last three months of the current year.

SALES BETWEEN PARTNERS AND CONTROLLED PARTNERSHIPS

Section 707(b) defines two situations in which the general rule of § 707(a) is overridden and the tax consequences of transactions between partners and partnerships are not determined as if the transaction were negotiated at arm's length between independent parties. Both situations involve a sale of property between (1) a partnership and any person owning more than a 50 percent interest in either partnership capital or profits, or (2) two partnerships in which the same persons own more than a 50 percent interest in either capital or profits.[61] If such a sale results in a recognized loss to the seller, such loss is disallowed. If the purchaser of the property subsequently disposes of the property at a gain, the originally disallowed loss may be used to offset such gain.[62]

> **Example 28.** T owns a 60% interest in the TV Partnership. During the current year, T sells investment land to TV for $100,000; T's basis in the land is $145,000.

---

[60] Reg. § 1.707-1(c).

[61] Percentage ownership is determined with reference to the constructive ownership rules of § 267(c) other than paragraph (3) of such section. § 707(b)(3).

[62] § 707(b)(1). Note the similarity to the more general loss disallowance rule of § 267(a)(1).

T may not recognize his $45,000 loss realized on the sale, and TV will take a $100,000 cost basis in the land. If the partnership subsequently sells the land for more than $100,000, T's $45,000 disallowed loss may be used to offset the amount of taxable gain the partnership must recognize. If the partnership sells the land for less than $100,000, T's disallowed loss will have no effect on the amount of the taxable loss the partnership will recognize.

If a sale of property between a partner and a related partnership results in a recognized gain, and the property is *not* a capital asset in the hands of the purchaser, the gain must be characterized as ordinary income.[63]

Example 29. Refer to the facts in *Example 28*, but assume that T's basis in the investment land was $70,000. If the TV Partnership uses the land in its trade or business, rather than holding it as a capital asset, T's $30,000 recognized gain on the sale must be characterized as ordinary income.

PARTNERSHIP DISTRIBUTIONS

This next section of this chapter is an analysis of the broad set of rules applicable to partnership distributions to which the specialized provision of § 751(b) does not apply. (Any discussion of disproportionate distributions is beyond the scope of this chapter.) All partnership distributions can be classified as either current or liquidating. A *current distribution* reduces a partner's interest in partnership capital but does not extinguish the interest. In other words, subsequent to the receipt of a current distribution, a partner is still a partner. In contrast, a *liquidating distribution* extinguishes the recipient partner's entire equity interest in the partnership. An ongoing partnership may make liquidating distributions to any of its partners who terminates an interest. When a partnership itself terminates, it will make a final liquidating distribution to all its partners.

The aggregate theory of partnerships predominates in the sections of Subchapter K (§§ 731–737) devoted to distributions. Under this theory, a partner's interest in a partnership represents an indirect ownership interest in partnership assets. Therefore, a partner who receives a distribution of cash or property is merely converting his or her indirect interest in partnership assets to direct ownership of the distributed assets. This change in ownership form should not be a taxable event and should have no effect on the tax basis of the distributed assets. This theoretical foundation is clearly discernible in the set of rules explained in the following paragraphs.

CURRENT DISTRIBUTIONS

Cash Distributions. Partners may withdraw cash from their partnerships at various times throughout the partnership's taxable year in order to meet their personal short-term liquidity needs or as advance payments of their anticipated distributive shares of current-year partnership income. Partners may also receive periodic cash distributions as guaranteed payments for ongoing services rendered to the partnership. Finally, partners may receive constructive cash distributions in the form of reductions in their respective shares of partnership liabilities.[64]

Regardless of the nature of a current cash distribution, § 731(a) provides that the recipient partner does not recognize gain upon its receipt. The cash distribution is instead treated as a nontaxable return of capital that reduces the recipient's outside basis in his or

---

[63] An almost identical (and therefore redundant) gain characterization rule can be found in § 1239(a).

[64] § 752(b).

her partnership interest.[65] However, the basis of a partnership interest can never be reduced below zero. Consequently, a partner who receives a cash distribution in excess of outside basis must recognize the excess as gain derived from sale of the partnership interest.[66]

Guaranteed payments and other cash distributions representing advances against the recipient's share of current-year partnership income are taken into account as of the last day of the partnership year.[67] This timing rule minimizes the possibility that distributions will trigger gain recognition at the partner level.

Example 30. Partnership WXYZ and 25% partner Z both use a calendar year for tax purposes. At the beginning of the current year, Z's outside basis was $50,000, and partnership debt totaled $60,000 ($15,000 of which was properly included in Z's outside basis). On July 7, the partnership made a $75,000 cash distribution to Z. As of the last day of the year, partnership debt totaled $80,000. Partnership income for the current year consisted of $109,000 ordinary income and a $5,600 capital loss. Z's outside basis at the end of the year is computed as follows:

Basis on January 1		$ 50,000
Increased by:	25% share of ordinary income	27,250
	25% share of $20,000 increase in partnership debt	5,000
Decreased by:	July 7 cash distribution	(75,000)
	25% share of capital loss	(1,400)
Basis on December 31		$ 5,850

The effect of the July 7 distribution is determined as if the distribution had occurred on the last day of the partnership year. Because Z's outside basis is first increased by his distributive share of partnership income and his share of WXYZ's increased debt load, the distribution is treated as a nontaxable return of capital.

If the $75,000 distribution had not been a guaranteed payment or advance against income, its tax effect would have been determined on July 7. Assuming that the partnership debt on this date was still $60,000, Z must recognize a $25,000 capital gain equal to the excess of the distribution over his $50,000 basis. Subsequent to the distribution, Z's outside basis would have been reduced to zero.

Property Distributions. As a general rule, a current distribution of partnership property to a partner does not cause gain or loss recognition at either the partnership or the partner level.[68] The recipient partner simply takes a *carryover* basis in the distributed property and reduces the outside basis in her partnership interest by a corresponding amount.[69]

Example 31. S receives a current distribution of property from the STUV Partnership. At date of distribution, the property has a fair market value of $14,000 and an inside basis to the partnership of $7,500. Immediately prior to the distribution, S's outside basis in her partnership interest was $12,000. Neither the partnership nor

---

[65]   § 733.

[66]   § 731(a)(1). This gain is capital gain per § 741.

[67]   Reg. § 1.731-1(a)(1)(ii).

[68]   § 731(a) and (b). Section 731(c) provides that certain marketable securities are treated as money rather than property for purposes of § 731(a). Consequently, the distribution of such securities by a partnership may trigger gain recognition to the recipient partner. Discussion of this special rule is beyond the scope of this text.

[69]   §§ 732(a)(1) and 733.

S recognizes a gain on the distribution. S's basis in the property becomes $7,500 and her outside basis is reduced to $4,500 ($12,000 − $7,500).

Note that in the above example, the $7,500 inside basis of the distributed property (i.e., the carryover basis) was preserved by shifting $7,500 of S's outside basis to the property. If the recipient partner's outside basis is less than the inside basis of the distributed property, the distribution is referred to as a *substituted* basis transaction. In such a situation, the basis of the distributed property in the hands of the partner is limited to his or her outside basis amount.[70]

Example 32. Refer to the facts in *Example 31*. If S's predistribution outside basis had been only $6,000, S's basis in the distributed property would be $6,000 and her postdistribution outside basis would be zero ($6,000 − $6,000). Note that S simply substitutes her outside basis as the basis in the distributed asset.

If a partnership distribution consists of multiple assets and the recipient partner's outside basis is less than the aggregate inside bases of the assets, the outside basis must *first* be reduced by any amount of cash included in the distribution. The remaining basis is allocated between two categories of noncash assets in the following order of priority:

1. To any unrealized receivables and inventory (Category 1) in an amount not to exceed the basis of these assets in the hands of the partnership.[71]

2. To any other distributed properties (Category 2).

Basis is allocated to multiple assets within either of these two categories under a *basis decrease formula*. The basis decrease is first allocated to property with unrealized depreciation (i.e., inside basis greater than fair market value) to the extent of the unrealized depreciation in each property.[72]

Example 33. J receives a current distribution from the JKL Partnership consisting of the following:

	JKL Basis	FMV
Cash	$4,000	$4,000
Accounts receivable	0	3,000
Inventory	2,000	2,900
Capital asset 1	1,000	1,500
Capital asset 2	3,000	1,000

Immediately prior to the distribution, J's outside basis in his partnership interest was $8,000. This basis must first be reduced by the $4,000 cash distribution. The $4,000 remaining basis is allocated to the Category 1 assets in an amount not to exceed JKL's inside basis:

	Partner J's Basis
Unrealized receivables	$ 0
Inventory	2,000

---

[70] § 732(a)(2).

[71] An unrealized receivable is any right to payment for goods or services provided to customers in the ordinary course of business that has not been recognized by the partnership as ordinary income. Reg. § 1.732-1(c)(1) and § 751(c).

[72] § 732(c)(3)(A).

Because J's $2,000 remaining outside basis is less than the aggregate inside bases of the Category 2 assets distributed, the basis decrease formula must be used to allocate this amount to the two capital assets received. First, the amount of the basis decrease is computed to be $2,000 by subtracting J's remaining outside basis amount ($2,000) from the aggregate inside bases ($1,000 + $3,000 = $4,000) of these assets. The $2,000 basis decrease is then allocated to any of these assets with unrealized depreciation; in this case only Capital asset 2. Thus J's basis in Capital asset 2 is $1,000 ($3,000 − $2,000). J's resulting basis in each of these assets is reflected below:

	Inside Basis	FMV	Unrealized Depreciation	Partner J's Basis
Capital asset 1	$1,000	$1,500	$ 0	$1,000
Capital asset 2	3,000	1,000	2,000	1,000

Subsequent to this distribution, J's outside basis in his partnership interest has been reduced to zero.

If more than one of the distributed assets from the same category has depreciated in value, the basis decrease is allocated based on relative depreciation.

Example 34. Assume the same facts in *Example 33* above, except that the fair market value of Capital asset 1 is $500 instead of $1,500. In this case, the basis decrease is allocated between the two capital assets based on relative depreciation. J's basis in each of these assets is determined as follows:

	Inside Basis	FMV	Unrealized Depreciation
Capital asset 1	$1,000	$ 500	$ 500
Capital asset 2	3,000	1,000	2,000

	J's Basis
Capital asset 1:	
$1,000 carryover basis − $400 [($500/$2,500) × $2,000 basis decrease] =	$ 600
Capital asset 2:	
$3,000 carryover basis − $1,600 [($2,000/$2,500) × $2,000 basis decrease] =	1,400

Finally, if the required basis decrease exceeds the unrealized depreciation of the assets, any further decrease is allocated in proportion to the assets relative bases (as previously adjusted).[73]

Example 35. Assume the same facts as in *Example 34* above, except that the total amount of the required basis decrease is $2,800 instead of $2,500. In this case, the bases of Capital assets 1 and 2 would first be reduced by the existing depreciated amount to $500 and $1,000, respectively. The $300 remaining basis decrease would be allocated between these assets in proportion to these reduced bases. J's basis in each of the capital assets would be computed as follows:

	JKL Basis	Depreciation	Reduced Basis	$300 Basis Decrease	J's Basis
Capital asset 1	$1,000	$ 500	$ 500	$100 [($500/$1,500) × $300]	$400
Capital asset 2	3,000	2,000	1,000	200 [($1,000/$1,500) × $300]	800

---

[73]   § 732(c)(3)(B).

There is one exception to the rule that the partnership does not recognize gain or loss on partnership distributions. The IRS has recently ruled that gain may be recognized if appreciated property is given to a partner to satisfy a guaranteed payment obligation. For example, if a partner has an $80,000 guaranteed payment and the partnership uses property with a basis of $60,000 and fair market value of $80,000 to satisfy this obligation, the partnership must recognize gain of $20,000.[74]

LIQUIDATING DISTRIBUTIONS

Cash Distributions. When a partner's entire interest in a partnership is extinguished upon receipt of a liquidating cash distribution, the partner will recognize capital gain to the extent of any amount of cash in excess of the outside basis in his partnership interest. Conversely, if the cash distribution is less than outside basis, the partner may recognize the amount of unrecovered basis as capital loss.

> **Example 36.** C receives a liquidating distribution of $20,000 cash from the ABC Partnership. (This distribution equals the $20,000 value of C's capital account as of the date of distribution.) Because she is no longer a partner, C is relieved of $13,000 of partnership debt. C's total cash distribution is $33,000 ($20,000 actual cash + $13,000 constructive cash in the form of debt relief).
>
> If C's outside basis immediately prior to distribution is $24,500, she must recognize a $8,500 capital gain equal to the excess of the $33,000 cash distribution over this basis.
>
> If C's outside basis immediately prior to distribution is $35,000, she may recognize a $2,000 capital loss equal to the excess of this basis over the $33,000 cash distribution.

Property Distributions. Liquidating distributions of property generally do not result in gain or loss recognition to either partnership or partner, except as noted in footnote 68 above. When a partnership distributes property as a liquidating distribution, the recipient partner's outside basis (reduced by any amount of cash included in the distribution) is allocated to the distributed property.[75] In most cases, this substituted basis rule defers the recognition of any economic gain or loss realized by the partner upon liquidation.

> **Example 37.** M receives a liquidating distribution of $6,000 cash and a partnership § 1231 asset with a fair market value of $25,000 and a $14,600 inside basis to the partnership.
>
> Assume M's predistribution outside basis is $40,000. This basis is reduced by the $6,000 cash distribution and the remaining $34,000 basis is substituted as the basis of the distributed asset to M. Neither M nor the partnership recognizes gain or loss because of the distribution.
>
> Assume M's predistribution outside basis is $9,000. This basis is reduced by the $6,000 cash distribution and the remaining $3,000 basis is substituted as the basis of the distributed asset to M. Neither M nor the partnership recognizes gain or loss because of the distribution.
>
> Assume M's predistribution outside basis is only $4,000. M must recognize the $2,000 cash distribution in excess of basis as capital gain. The distributed asset will have a zero basis to M.

---

[74]   Rev. Rul. 2007-40, 2007-25 IRB 1426.

[75]   § 732(b).

If a liquidating distribution includes multiple assets, the recipient partner's outside basis (reduced by any cash distributed) is allocated between two categories of noncash assets in the following order of priority:

1. To any unrealized receivables and inventory (Category 1) in an amount not to exceed the basis of these assets in the hands of the partnership.

2. To any other distributed properties (Category 2).

Unlike the current (nonliquidating) distribution rules that limit the distributee partner's bases in *any* assets to the distributing partnership's inside basis (i.e., a carryover basis), only the bases of unrealized receivables or inventory (Category 1 assets) are subject to this rule in a liquidating distribution. If the distributee partner's outside basis exceeds the partnership's inside basis of any unrealized receivables or inventory distributed, the remaining outside basis must be assigned to any asset received from Category 2.[76] If the partner does not receive any Category 2 assets, then the excess of the outside basis over the inside basis of the Category 1 assets is recognized as a loss by the partner.[77] However, if Category 2 assets are received, the partner can never recognize a loss.

Example 38. R receives a liquidating distribution from the RST Partnership that consists of the following:

	RST Basis	FMV
Cash	$2,500	$2,500
Accounts receivable	0	2,000
Inventory	3,000	4,000
Capital asset	5,000	9,000

R's predistribution outside basis in his partnership interest was $12,000. This basis must first be reduced by the $2,500 cash distribution. The $9,500 remaining basis is allocated to the Category 1 assets in an amount not to exceed RST's inside basis:

	Partner R's Basis
Unrealized receivables	$ 0
Inventory	3,000

The $6,500 remaining basis is allocated to the capital asset (Category 2 asset), even though this substituted basis exceeds the RST Partnership's $5,000 inside basis. In addition, neither R nor the RST Partnership recognizes gain or loss because of the distribution.

Example 39. N receives a liquidating distribution from the MNOP Partnership that consists of the following:

	MNOP Basis	FMV
Cash	$ 700	$ 700
Accounts receivable	0	800
Inventory asset 1	1,000	1,300
Inventory asset 2	2,100	2,500

Immediately prior to the distribution, N's outside basis is $4,000. This basis must first be reduced by the $700 cash distribution. Only $3,100 of the $3,300 remaining basis is allocable to the Category 1 assets.

---

[76] § 732(c).

[77] § 731(a)(2).

	Partner N's Basis
Unrealized receivables...................	$ -0-
Inventory asset 1........................	1,000
Inventory asset 2........................	2,100

N may recognize her $200 unrecovered outside basis as a capital loss.

Note that in *Example 39* partner N received a liquidating distribution with a total fair market value of $5,300 so that she realized an economic gain upon termination of her partnership interest. The Subchapter K rules governing the tax consequences of partnership property distributions ensure that a partner's economic gain or loss with respect to the distribution is deferred until subsequent disposition of the property.

Example 40. Refer to the facts in *Example 39*. Although N recognized a $200 tax loss upon receipt of the liquidating distribution, she realized a $1,300 economic gain ($5,300 value of assets received in excess of $4,000 basis in N's liquidated partnership interest). However, N's basis in the distributed assets is only $3,100. If N were to sell the unrealized receivables and inventory for their aggregate value of $4,600, she would recognize a $1,500 taxable gain.

This result is consistent with the aggregate theory of partnerships under which N has not severed her interest in the MNOP Partnership until she no longer owns any interest in partnership *assets*. When N finally sells the distributed MNOP assets, her $1,500 recognized gain on sale netted against her $200 recognized loss upon distribution equates to her $1,300 economic gain attributable to the termination of her partnership interest.

Finally, when a partner receives more than one Category 2 asset in a liquidating distribution, his or her remaining outside basis must be allocated between the assets using one of the following:

1. *Basis decrease formula*—where the sum of the bases of the distributed Category 2 assets *exceeds* the distributee partner's outside basis remaining after reduction for any cash received and basis allocated to any unrealized receivables or inventory (Category 1 assets).

2. *Basis increase formula*—where the sum of the bases of the distributed Category 2 assets is *less* than the distributee partner's outside basis remaining after reduction for any cash received and basis allocated to any unrealized receivables or inventory (Category 1 assets).

Example 41. After reduction for a distribution of cash and the required allocation of basis to unrealized receivables and inventory received in a liquidating distribution from the RST Partnership, partner T's remaining outside basis of $25,000 must be allocated to the following capital assets:

	RST's Basis	*FMV*
Capital asset 1........................	$10,000	$20,000
Capital asset 2........................	30,000	10,000

Because T's $25,000 remaining outside basis is less than the aggregate bases of the Category 2 assets, the basis decrease formula must be used. First, the amount of the basis decrease is computed to be $15,000 by subtracting T's outside basis amount ($25,000) from the aggregate inside bases ($40,000) of these assets. The $15,000

basis decrease is then allocated to any of the assets with unrealized depreciation; in this case only Capital asset 2. T's basis in each of these assets is reflected below:

	Inside Basis	FMV	Unrealized Depreciation	Partner T's Basis
Capital asset 1	$10,000	$20,000	$ 0	$10,000
Capital asset 2	30,000	10,000	20,000	15,000

Note that even though the depreciation in value of Capital asset 2 is $20,000, the total basis decrease is only $15,000. Thus, the $30,000 inside basis in that asset is reduced to $15,000 in T's hands.

If more than one of the distributed assets from the same category has depreciated in value, the basis decrease is allocated based on relative depreciation.

Example 42. Assume the same facts in *Example 41* above, except that the fair market value of Capital asset 1 is $5,000 instead of $20,000. In this case, the $15,000 total basis decrease is allocated between the two capital assets based on relative depreciation as follows:

J's Basis

Capital asset 1:
  $10,000 carryover basis − $3,000 [($5,000/$25,000) × $15,000 basis decrease] = $ 7,000
Capital asset 2:
  $30,000 carryover basis − $12,000 [($20,000/$25,000) × $15,000 basis decrease] = 18,000

Example 43. After reduction for a distribution of cash and the required allocation of basis to unrealized receivables and inventory received in a liquidating distribution from the RST Partnership, partner T's remaining outside basis of $25,000 must be allocated to the following capital assets:

	RST's Basis	FMV
Capital asset 1.............................	$10,000	$20,000
Capital asset 2.............................	5,000	25,000

Because the aggregate bases of the Category 2 assets is *less* than T's remaining outside basis, the basis *increase* formula must be used. First, the amount of the basis increase is computed to be $10,000 by subtracting the aggregate inside bases ($15,000) of these assets from T's outside basis amount ($25,000). The $10,000 basis increase is then allocated to the assets based on relative unrealized appreciation. T's basis in each of these assets is reflected below:

	Inside Basis	FMV	Unrealized Appreciation	Basis Increase
Capital asset 1	$10,000	$20,000	$10,000	$3,333
Capital asset 2	5,000	25,000	20,000	6,667

T's basis in Capital asset 1 will be $13,333 ($10,000 carryover basis + $3,333 basis increase) and his basis in Capital asset 2 will be $11,667 ($5,000 carryover basis + $6,667 basis increase). Note that the total of T's bases in these assets ($13,333 + $11,667 = $25,000) equals his $25,000 remaining predistribution outside basis.

If only one of the assets in *Example 43* above had unrealized appreciation, it would have been allocated all of the basis increase up to its total fair market value. In the event that the basis increase exceeded the unrealized appreciation, any remaining basis increase amount would be allocated between the assets based on relative fair market values.

Closing of Partnership Year. When a partner's entire interest in a partnership is liquidated, the partnership taxable year closes with respect to that partner.[78] As a result, the partner may have to include a proportionate share of more or less than 12 months of partnership income in his or her taxable year in which the liquidation occurs.

Example 44. The BCD Partnership and partner B both use a calendar year for tax purposes. On September 30, 2009, B received a liquidating distribution from BCD that terminated his interest in the partnership. BCD's taxable year closed with respect to B on September 30. As a result, B will include his proportionate share of BCD's income from January 1 through September 30 (nine months) in his 2009 tax return. BCD's taxable year does not close with respect to the remaining partners, who will include their proportionate shares of BCD's income for the full calendar year on their respective returns.

Example 45. Refer to the facts in *Example 44*. If BCD uses a fiscal year ending May 31 for tax purposes, two partnership years (June 1, 2008 through May 31, 2009 and the short year June 1, 2009 through September 30, 2009) ended within partner B's 2009 taxable year. As a result, B will include his proportionate share of BCD's income from June 1, 2008 through May 31, 2009 (12 months) and from June 1, 2009 through September 30, 2009 (four months) in his 2009 tax return.

In *Example 44* and *Example 45*, B's outside basis in his partnership interest immediately prior to the receipt of his liquidating distribution should reflect his distributive share of BCD's income or loss through September 30, 2009.[79] Therefore, B cannot determine the tax consequences of the distribution itself until he receives his final Schedule K-1 from the BCD Partnership.

SECTION 736 PAYMENTS

The amount of a liquidating distribution paid to a partner who is terminating an interest in an ongoing partnership should theoretically equal the partner's proportionate interest in the value of the partnership assets. In reality, partners may negotiate for and partnerships may agree to pay liquidating distributions in excess of such amount. In such case, § 736 provides that only the portion of the total distribution attributable to the partner's interest in partnership assets is subject to the statutory rules dealing with partnership distributions. The remainder of the distribution (labeled a *§ 736(a) payment*) is not subject to the normal distribution rules. Instead, § 736(a) payments that are determined without regard to the income of the partnership are classified as *guaranteed payments*. Section 736(a) payments determined with reference to partnership income are classified as *distributive shares* of such income.

Example 46. R, a 20% general partner in the RSTU Partnership, retired from the partnership business during the current year. As of the date of R's retirement, the partnership had the following balance sheet:

---

[78] § 706(c)(2)(A)(ii).

[79] § 705(a).

	Inside Basis	FMV
Cash	$ 50,000	$ 50,000
Business assets	65,000	90,000
	$115,000	$140,000
Debt	$ 5,000	$ 5,000
Capital: R	22,000	27,000
Other partners	88,000	108,000
	$115,000	$140,000

Even though R's capital account balance was only $27,000, the other partners agreed to pay R $40,000 cash in complete liquidation of his equity interest. The additional $13,000 payment was in grateful recognition of R's long years of faithful service to the business.

The total liquidating payment to R consisted of $41,000 ($40,000 actual cash + $1,000 relief of 20% of the partnership debt). R's 20% interest in the value of partnership assets was $28,000 (as evidenced by the $27,000 value of his capital account and 20% share of the partnership debt). Therefore, only $28,000 of the liquidating payment is treated as a distribution. If R's outside basis in his partnership interest was $23,000, R must recognize a $5,000 capital gain equal to the excess of the cash distribution over this basis.

The $13,000 § 736(a) payment to R was determined without regard to partnership income. Consequently, it is classified as a guaranteed payment, which R must recognize as ordinary income and the partnership may deduct as a current expense.

Payments for Unrealized Receivables and Unspecified Goodwill. Section 736 contains a special rule concerning liquidating payments made with respect to a partner's interest in certain partnership assets. Payments made with respect to unrealized receivables must be considered § 736(a) payments rather than distributions.[80] Payments made with respect to goodwill are similarly classified unless the partnership agreement specifies that a withdrawing partner will be paid for his or her share of goodwill. Prior to the enactment of the Revenue Reconciliation Act of 1993, this special rule applied to liquidating payments made to any partner by any partnership. The 1993 Act limited its application to payments made to *general* partners by partnerships in which capital is not a material income-producing factor.[81]

Example 47. E is a 10% general partner in the Beta Partnership, a professional service partnership in which capital is not a material income-producing factor. During the current year, E had a serious disagreement with the other partners and decided to withdraw from the partnership. As of the date of E's withdrawal, the partnership had the following balance sheet:

---

[80] § 751(c) provides that, for § 736 purposes, the term *unrealized receivables* includes only zero basis accounts receivable and not § 1245, § 1250, or other types of ordinary income recapture.

[81] § 736(b)(3). Capital is not a material income-producing factor if substantially all of the partnership's income consists of fees, commissions, or other compensation for personal or professional services performed by individuals.

	Inside Basis	*FMV*
Cash	$ 35,000	$ 35,000
Accounts receivable	0	24,000
Business assets	100,000	145,000
	$135,000	$204,000
Debt	$ 15,000	$ 15,000
Capital: E	12,000	18,900
Other partners	108,000	170,100
	$135,000	$204,000

After considerable negotiation, the other partners agreed to pay E $20,000 cash in complete liquidation of her equity interest. The partners determined that this was a fair price for E's 10% capital interest because the partnership business has considerable goodwill and going concern value that is not recorded as an asset on its balance sheet. The Beta Partnership agreement does not provide for specific payments with respect to partnership goodwill.

The total liquidating payment to E consisted of $21,500 ($20,000 actual cash + $1,500 relief of 10% of the partnership debt). E's 10% interest in the value of the recorded partnership assets was $20,400 (as evidenced by the value of her $18,900 capital account and 10% share of the partnership debt). However, the $2,400 payment made with respect to E's 10% interest in Beta's unrealized receivables must be classified as a § 736(a) payment. Consequently, only $18,000 of the liquidating payment ($20,400 − $2,400) is treated as a distribution. If E's outside basis in her partnership interest was $13,500, E must recognize a $4,500 capital gain equal to the excess of the cash distribution over this basis.

The $3,500 § 736(a) payment to E represents the value of her 10% interest in Beta's accounts receivable and unspecified goodwill. Because the payment was determined without regard to partnership income, it is classified as a guaranteed payment, which E must recognize as ordinary income and Beta may deduct as a current expense.

DISPOSITIONS OF DISTRIBUTED PROPERTY

If a partner who received either a current or liquidating distribution of partnership unrealized receivables subsequently collects the receivables or disposes of them in a taxable transaction, that partner must recognize the excess of the amount realized over the zero basis in the receivables as ordinary income.[82] Similarly, if a partner sells inventory distributed from a partnership within five years of the date of distribution, any gain or loss recognized must be characterized as ordinary gain or loss.[83] A partnership's holding period for a distributed asset is included in the recipient partner's holding period.[84]

---

[82]   § 735(a)(1). This paragraph provides that both gain or loss realized on a partner's disposition of partnership unrealized receivables is characterized as ordinary gain or loss. Except in unusual circumstances, such receivables will have a zero basis in the hands of a distributee partner; consequently, their disposition can only trigger gain recognition.

[83]   § 735(a)(2).

[84]   § 735(b).

Example 48. Two years ago, G received a current distribution of land from the EFG Partnership, which operates a real estate development business. The land was an inventory asset to EFG and took a carryover basis of $140,000 in G's hands. G held the land as an investment and sold it in the current year for $200,000. Because she sold the land within five years of the date of its distribution by EFG, G must recognize her gain as ordinary income, even though the land was a capital asset in her hands.

BASIS ADJUSTMENTS TO PARTNERSHIP PROPERTY

Under the general rules governing the tax consequences of partnership distributions, no gain or loss is recognized at either the partnership or the partner level and distributed assets simply take a carryover basis in the hands of the recipient partner. However, in certain circumstances, a partner may be required to recognize either capital gain or loss because of a distribution. In other cases, the inside basis of a distributed partnership asset does not carry over to the recipient partner.

These exceptions to the general rules can be viewed as anomalies that violate the aggregate theory of partnerships. Subchapter K provides a mechanism to correct these anomalies in the form of an adjustment to the inside basis of undistributed partnership property. Specifically, if a partnership has a *§ 754 election* in effect, it is allowed to *increase* the basis of partnership property by (1) any amount of gain recognized by a partner as the result of a distribution, and (2) any reduction of the inside basis of a distributed partnership asset in the hands of the recipient partner.[85]

Example 49. Partner L received a current distribution from the LMNO Partnership that consisted of $5,000 cash and partnership inventory with an inside basis of $1,500. Because L's predistribution outside basis was only $3,600, L recognized a $1,400 capital gain and took a zero basis in the distributed inventory. If LMNO has a § 754 election in effect, it may increase the inside basis in its remaining assets by $2,900 ($1,400 gain recognized by L + $1,500 reduction in the basis of the distributed inventory).

In *Example 49*, $1,400 of the positive basis adjustment counterbalances the current gain recognized at the partner level by decreasing the amount of future gain the partnership will recognize on a sale of assets (a $1,400 basis increase is equivalent to a $1,400 decrease in gain potential). The remaining $1,500 positive basis adjustment to LMNO's assets compensates for the $1,500 lost basis in the distributed inventory.[86]

A partnership with a § 754 election in effect is required to *decrease* the basis of partnership property by (1) any amount of loss recognized by a partner as the result of a distribution, and (2) any increase in the basis of a distributed partnership asset in the hands of the recipient partner.[87]

Example 50. Partner E received a liquidating distribution of $5,000 cash from the EFGH Partnership. Because E's predistribution outside basis was $7,000, E recognized a $2,000 capital loss. Partner F received a liquidating distribution from EFGH consisting of a capital asset with an inside basis of $10,000. Because F's predistribution outside basis was $14,500, F took a $14,500 substituted basis in the distributed asset.

If EFGH has a § 754 election in effect, it must decrease the basis in its remaining assets by $6,500 ($2,000 loss recognized by E + $4,500 increase in the basis of the distributed capital asset).

---

[85]   § 734(b)(1).

[86]   The rules for allocating a § 734(b) basis adjustment to specific partnership assets are found in § 755 and the regulations thereunder.

[87]   § 734(b)(2).

In *Example 50*, $2,000 of the negative basis adjustment counterbalances the current loss recognized at the partner level by decreasing the amount of future loss the partnership will recognize on a sale of assets (a $1,400 basis decrease is equivalent to a $1,400 decrease in loss potential). The remaining $4,500 negative basis adjustment to EFGH's assets compensates for the $4,500 additional basis in the distributed capital asset.

The optional basis adjustment is allocated to the same asset class in which the distributed property falls. For purposes of this adjustment, the partnership's assets are divided into two property classes:

1. Capital assets and § 1231 property (i.e., capital gain property), and

2. All other assets (i.e., ordinary income property).

However, any loss resulting from the distribution of cash, unrealized receivables, and inventory, must be allocated to the partnership's capital gain property. Further, any gain recognized from the distribution of cash must also be allocated to the capital gain property.

For allocations of increases in basis within a class, the increase must be allocated first to any properties in that class with unrealized appreciation. If more than one property has unrealized appreciation, the increase is allocated in proportion to each asset's unrealized appreciation. However, in no case can the allocated increase for an asset exceed that asset's unrealized appreciation. If any increase remains after this allocation, it is allocated to properties within that class in proportion to their fair market values.

The rules are similar for a decrease in basis. The decrease must be allocated first to any properties in that class with unrealized depreciation. If more than one property has unrealized depreciation, the decrease is allocated in proportion to each asset's unrealized depreciation. However, in no case can the allocated decrease for an asset exceed that asset's unrealized depreciation. If any decrease remains after this allocation, it is allocated to properties within that class in proportion to their adjusted bases. The adjusted bases used for this allocation include any adjustments already made as part of the overall allocation process.[88] In no case can the adjusted basis for an asset be reduced below zero. If the bases of all assets within a class have been reduced to zero, any remaining decreases are suspended until the partnership acquires property in that class.[89]

It is important to note that the rules for increases and decreases are similar, except that any remaining adjustment after the initial allocations are based on relative *fair market values* for increases, but on relative *adjusted bases* for decreases.

Example 51. Refer to the facts in *Example 49*. The § 734 adjustment was $2,900: $1,400 for the gain from the cash distribution and $1,500 due to the reduction in basis for the distributed inventory. The $1,400 for the gain must be allocated to capital gain property. Since inventory is an ordinary asset, the $1,500 for the inventory basis must be allocated to the ordinary income class.

Assume that LMNO Partnership owns the following two capital assets:

	Adjusted Basis	FMV	Unrealized Appreciation
Capital Asset A	$1,000	$3,000	$2,000
Capital Asset B	1,000	1,000	-0-

Since the only capital asset with unrealized appreciation is asset A, its basis is increased by $1,400 to $2,400.

---

88   Reg. § 1.755-1(c)(2).

89   Reg. § 1.755-1(c)(4).

Alternatively, assume that LMNO Partnership owns the following two capital assets:

	Adjusted Basis	FMV	Unrealized Appreciation
Capital Asset A	$1,000	$2,200	$1,200
Capital Asset B	1,000	1,800	800

The $1,400 basis increase is allocated to the assets based on the relative unrealized appreciation. Therefore, asset A receives a basis increase of $840 ($1,200/$2,000 × $1,400). Asset B receives a basis increase of $560 ($800/$2,000 × $1,400). Note that these basis increases are allowed because neither exceeds the unrealized appreciation for the respective asset. Asset A's basis is increased from $1,000 to $1,840, and asset B's basis is increased from $1,000 to $1,560.

Example 52. Refer to the facts in *Example 50*. The § 734 adjustment was $6,500: $2,000 for the loss recognized and $4,500 for the increase in basis of the capital asset. This results in a $6,500 decrease in the basis of capital assets, because all losses due to distributions are allocated to capital assets, as are adjustments due to the distribution of capital assets.

Assume that LMNO Partnership owns the following two capital assets:

	Adjusted Basis	FMV	Unrealized Depreciation
Capital Asset A	$12,000	$ 4,000	$8,000
Capital Asset B	10,000	12,000	-0-

Since the only capital asset with unrealized depreciation is asset A, its basis is decreased by $6,500 to $5,500.

The Section 754 Election. A partnership will adjust the inside basis of its assets as the result of a distribution to a partner only if it has a § 754 election in effect for the year of the distribution. A partnership makes a § 754 election simply by attaching a statement to that effect to its Form 1065 for the first taxable year for which the election is to be effective. Once made, the election applies for all subsequent years unless the Internal Revenue Service agrees to its revocation.[90]

Substantial Basis Reduction. Even if a § 754 election is not in effect, the rules discussed above will apply if there is a substantial basis reduction to partnership property as the result of a distribution. A substantial basis reduction occurs if the sum of 1) the partner's loss on the distribution, and 2) the basis increase to the distributed properties is more than $250,000.[91]

Example 53. Partner B has a basis of $4,000,000 in her partnership interest in Partnership AB. Partnership AB does not have a § 754 election in effect. She receives a liquidating distribution of land from the partnership having a fair market value of $3,500,000 and a basis of $1,800,000. She will recognize no gain or loss on the distribution. Her basis in the land will be $4,000,000 and the basis in her partnership interest will be reduced to zero. Since the basis of the land has increased by more than $250,000 (by $2,200,000, from $1,800,000 to $4,000,000) a substantial basis

---

[90]   Reg. § 1.754-1.

[91]   See § 734(d)(1). These rules apply for distributions made after October 22, 2004. Different rules apply to electing investment partnerships. A discussion of these rules is beyond the scope of this text.

reduction has occurred. Therefore, Partnership AB will have to reduce the basis of its other properties by $2,200,00 according to the rule § 755.

DISPOSITIONS OF PARTNERSHIP INTERESTS

The most common way for a partner to dispose of a partnership interest is through a liquidating distribution from the partnership itself. There are, however, a number of other types of dispositions, each of which has a unique set of tax consequences to both partner and partnership.

SALES OF PARTNERSHIP INTERESTS

Partnership agreements typically place restrictions on the partners' right to sell their equity interests in the partnership to third parties. For example, an agreement might provide that a partner must offer his or her interest to the partnership itself or to the existing partners before offering it to a third-party purchaser. The agreement may also provide that a prospective purchaser must be approved by the general partners or by a majority of all partners. Because of such limits on transferability, partnership interests are considered illiquid assets.

When a partner sells his or her entire interest in a partnership, the partnership's taxable year closes with respect to that partner.[92] The selling partner's outside basis in the partnership interest immediately prior to sale includes his or her distributive share of partnership income or loss through date of sale. The tax consequences of the sales transaction itself to both seller and purchaser are governed by specific rules in Subchapter K.

Tax Consequences to Seller. Upon sale of a partnership interest, the seller recognizes gain or loss to the extent the amount realized exceeds or is less than the outside basis of the interest. Section 741 contains a general rule that such gain or loss is capital in nature. This rule reflects the entity theory under which a partnership interest represents the partner's equity in the partnership as a whole rather than a proportionate interest in each specific asset owned by the partnership. Literally in mid sentence, § 741 shifts to the aggregate theory by cautioning that the general rule is inapplicable to the extent provided in § 751(a). This subsection applies only if the partnership owns unrealized receivables or inventory, which for convenience' sake tax practitioners have simply labeled *hot assets*.

Hot Assets. The term *unrealized receivables* includes zero basis trade accounts receivable generated by a cash basis partnership. The term also includes the § 1245 and § 1250 ordinary income recapture potential inherent in depreciable partnership assets.[93] All partnership unrealized receivables are deemed to have a zero tax basis.[94] The term *inventory* includes not only stock in trade and property held primarily for sale to customers in the ordinary course of business, but also any other property that is not a capital asset or a § 1231 asset to the partnership.[95]

---

[92] § 706(c)(2)(A)(i). Refer to the discussion of the closing of a partnership year with respect to a partner at 77, *supra*.

[93] § 751(c). The term *unrealized receivables* also includes many esoteric types of ordinary income recapture potential, such as § 1254 recapture of intangible drilling and development costs of oil and gas wells and mining development and exploration expenditures.

[94] Reg. § 1.751-1(c)(5).

[95] § 751 inventory also includes any partnership property that would be inventory if held by a selling or distributee partner [§ 751(d)(2)].

Example 54. The accrual basis MNO Partnership owns the following assets:

		Tax Basis	FMV
Cash		$ 7,000	$ 7,000
Accounts receivable		29,000	27,000
Stock in trade.		330,000	410,000
Equipment cost	$100,000		
Accumulated depreciation	(30,000)	70,000	80,000
Other 1231 assets.		250,000	390,000
Total		$686,000	$914,000

If MNO were to sell its equipment for market value, it would recognize a $10,000 gain, all of which would be recaptured as § 1245 ordinary income. Consequently, the partnership has $10,000 of unrealized receivables.

Both MNO's accounts receivable and stock in trade are inventory assets because accounts receivable are not a capital or § 1231 asset to the partnership.[96]

Under § 751 (a) the amount of gain or loss for the hot assets (unrealized receivables and inventory) is determined by assuming that these assets are sold by the partnership in a fully taxable transaction for cash in an amount equal to the fair market value of the properties. The partner selling his partnership interest is allocated the portion of the ordinary income that would have been allocated to him if these assets had actually been sold by the partnership.[97]

Example 55. K sold her 10% interest in the KLM Partnership to P for $45,000 cash. KLM used the cash method of accounting and had the following balance sheet as of the date K sold her interest. K's outside basis in her interest was $35,500.

	Inside Basis	FMV
Cash	$ 40,000	$ 40,000
Accounts receivable	0	30,000
Stock in trade.	90,000	100,000
Section 1231 assets (no recapture).	225,000	300,000
	$355,000	$470 000
Debt	$ 20,000	$ 20,000
Capital: K	33,500	45,000
Other partners	301,500	405,000
	$355,000	$470,000

At date of sale, the partnership had both unrealized receivables of $30,000 (zero basis accounts receivable) and $100,000 of inventory.

If the hot assets were sold by the partnership at fair market value the partnership would recognize $40,000 of ordinary income ($130,000 fair market value − $90,000 basis). Ten percent of this income, or $4,000, would be allocated to K. Therefore, on the sale of her partnership interest K must recognize $4,000 of ordinary income under § 751(a).

Subsequent to the application of § 751(a), the amount realized on the sale of K's partnership interest has been reduced to $34,000 ($47,000 total amount realized − $13,000 attributable to hot assets). K's outside basis in her partnership interest has

---

[96] Accounts receivable of a cash basis partnership are both an unrealized receivable and an inventory item for purposes of § 751.

[97] Reg. § 1.751-1(a)(2).

been reduced to $26,500 ($35,500 predistribution basis − $9,000 basis allocated to hot assets). Under the general rule of § 741, K recognizes a $7,500 capital gain on the sale of her partnership interest.

These computations can be summarized as follows:

	Total	Hot Assets [§ 751(a)]	Other (§ 741)
Amount realized	$ 47,000	$13,000	$ 34,000
Adjusted basis	(35,500)	(9,000)	(26,500)
Recognized gain/loss	$ 12,500	$ 4,000	$ 7,500
		Ordinary Income	Capital Gain

In addition to the recognition of ordinary income if the partnership has hot assets, the seller of a partnership interest may also have special tax treatment in three other situations: collectibles gain, § 1250 capital gain, and residual long-term capital gain or loss.

First, if at the time of the sale of a partnership interest (which has been held for more than one year) the partnership holds collectibles with unrealized appreciation, the gain attributable to this appreciation is taxed at 28 percent.[98] A collectible includes any work of art, rug, antique, metal, gem, stamp, coin, or alcoholic beverage.[99]

> **Example 56.** H and G are individuals that have been equal partners in HG for the last three years. The partnership owns gems that qualify as collectibles that have an adjusted basis of $500 and a fair market value of $1,100. H sells her interest in HG to I. As a result, $300 of H's gain from the sale will be characterized as collectibles gain (50% of the $600 gain that HG would have realized if it sold its collectibles in a fully taxable transaction).

Second, unrecaptured § 1250 gain is taxed at a 25 percent maximum rate. Unrecaptured § 1250 gain is the capital gain that would be treated as ordinary income if § 1250(b)(1) required all depreciation to be recaptured as ordinary income. If a partner sells an interest in a partnership, and the partnership has unrecaptured § 1250 gain, then the partner must take into account his or her portion of that gain in computing the tax results.[100]

> **Example 57.** Assume in *Example 56* above that HG also owns residential rental property. At the time of H's sale, the property had a fair market value of $110,000 and adjusted basis of $60,000. The property's original cost basis was $100,000. Straight-line depreciation of $40,000 had been claimed on the property. At the time of H's sale, one must compute what H's share of unrecaptured § 1250 gain would be if the property was sold. Since the property is realty and straight-line depreciation was used there would be no § 1250 recapture. Consequently, the entire gain ($50,000) would be a § 1231 gain. However, the § 1231 gain would be treated as a 25% gain to the extent of any straight-line depreciation claimed ($40,000). H's share of the 25% gain is $20,000. Consequently, of the total gain recognized by H on the sale of his partnership interest, $20,000 will be 25% gain due to the § 1250 unrecaptured gain.

The collectibles gain and § 1250 unrecaptured gain that are allocable to a partner that has sold his or her partnership interest are together known as the look-through capital gain.[101] The residual long-term capital gain or loss is computed as follows:

---

[98] § 1(h)(6)(B).

[99] § 408 (m)(3).

[100] Reg. § 1.1(h)-1(b)(3)(ii).

[101] § 1(h)(1)(D); Reg. § 1.1(h)-1(b)(1).

Residual long-term capital gain/loss =
§ 741 long-term capital gain or loss (after application of § 751)
— Look-through capital gain or loss.

Example 58. G and H are individuals that have been equal partners in Partnership B for the last two years. B owns collectibles with a basis and fair market value of $3,000 and $5,000, respectively. G sells his interest in partnership B to R and has a total recognized gain of $500. After the application of the § 751 hot assets rules, assume that G recognizes ordinary income of $2,000 and § 741 long-term capital loss of $1,500 (i.e., the pre-look through long-term capital loss). G's share of the collectibles gain (i.e., the look-through capital gain) is $1,000 [($5,000 − $3,000) × 50%].

Total gain	$ 500
§ 751 Hot asset ordinary income	(2,000)
Pre-look through long-term capital loss.	(1,500)
Gain from collectibles	1,000
Residual long-term capital loss	$(2,500)

To summarize, G has $2,000 of ordinary income, $1,000 collectibles gain taxed at 28%, and a $2,5000 capital loss.

Tax Consequences to Purchaser. Section 742 states that the basis of a partnership interest acquired other than by contribution shall be determined under the normal basis rules provided in §§ 1011 and following. Thus, the purchaser of a partnership interest takes a *cost* basis in the interest. The *cost basis* includes the amount of cash and the value of any noncash property paid to the seller plus the amount of any partnership liabilities assumed by the purchaser in his or her role as a new partner.

The fact that a purchaser is given a cost basis in the partnership interest rather than in a proportionate share of partnership assets reflects the entity theory of partnerships. Section 743(a) reinforces this perspective by specifying that the basis of partnership property shall not be adjusted as the result of a transfer of an interest in a partnership by sale or exchange. This general rule typically results in an imbalance between a purchasing partner's outside basis and the inside basis of his or her proportionate share of partnership assets.

Example 59. P purchased a 10% interest in the accrual basis KLM Partnership from K for $45,000 cash. As of the date of sale, the partnership had the following balance sheet:

	Inside Basis	FMV
Cash	$ 40,000	$ 40,000
Accounts receivable	30,000	30,000
Stock in trade	90,000	100,000
Depreciable assets	225,000	300,000
	$385,000	$470,000
Debt	$ 20,000	$ 20,000
Capital: K (replaced by P).	36,500	45,000
Other partners	328,500	405,000
	$385,000	$470,000

P's cost basis in his new partnership interest is $47,000 ($45,000 cash + 10% of KLM's debt). The transaction between P and K had no effect on the basis of the

partnership assets, so that P's aggregate inside basis in 10% of KLM's assets is only $38,500.

The imbalance between P's outside and inside bases in *Example 59* has several negative implications for P. If the partnership sells its entire stock in trade for $100,000, P will be allocated $1,000 of ordinary income (the excess of the $10,000 value of 10 percent of the stock in trade over its $9,000 basis), even though P indirectly paid $10,000 to acquire his share of this asset. Similarly, P will be allocated tax depreciation computed on the $22,500 inside basis of 10 percent of KLM's depreciable assets, even though P indirectly paid $30,000 to acquire his share of these assets.

Special Basis Adjustment for Purchaser. Strict adherence to the entity theory is relaxed if a purchaser acquires an interest in a partnership with a § 754 election in effect.[102] In this case, § 743(b) provides that any excess of the purchaser's outside basis over the inside basis of his or her proportionate share of partnership assets becomes a *positive* adjustment to that partner's inside basis.[103] Conversely, any excess of a purchaser's inside basis in his or her proportionate share of partnership assets over outside basis becomes a *negative* adjustment to that partner's inside basis.

Any positive or negative adjustment to the inside basis of the partnership property must be allocated to specific assets in such a manner as to reduce the difference between the fair market value and the tax basis of the asset. For purposes of this adjustment, the partnership's assets are divided into two property classes:[104]

1. Capital assets and § 1231 property (i.e., capital gain property), and

2. All other assets (i.e., ordinary income property).

The allocation of the optional basis adjustment between these two classes is based on the gain or loss that would be allocated to the transferee partner based on a hypothetical sale of all the partnership's assets. Therefore, it is possible that a positive adjustment could be made to the capital assets and a negative adjustment to the other assets, or vice-versa.

The adjustment to the ordinary income class is the amount of income, gain, or loss allocated to the transferee partner from the hypothetical sale of all ordinary income property at fair market value for cash. The adjustment to the capital asset class is then the difference in the total adjustment less the adjustment to the ordinary income class. However, any decrease in basis adjustment for the capital asset class cannot reduce the basis of the capital assets below zero. Once the basis of the capital assets is reduced to zero, any remaining negative adjustment must be used to reduce the basis of ordinary income property.[105]

The adjustment to each class must then be allocated to assets within that class. Generally, the adjustment to each item of ordinary income property equals the amount of income, gain, or loss allocated to the transferee partner in a hypothetical sale of the item. The adjustment for each item in the ordinary income class is determined as shown below.

Example 60. G sells his 25% interest in the JJG Partnership to D on March 15, 2009. JJG Partnership previously made a § 754 election. D paid $50,000 to G and assumed G's share of partnership liabilities. JJG's balance sheet at the date of sale is as follows:

[102] The § 754 election is discussed at Footnote 88, *supra*.
[103] § 743(b)(1).
[104] § 755.
[105] Reg. § 1.755-1(b).

	Inside Basis	FMV
Cash......................................	$ 40,000	$ 40,000
Accounts receivable	20,000	15,000
Inventory	42,000	50,000
Building..................................	70,000	85,000
Land	20,000	40,000
	$192,000	$230,000
Debt	$ 30,000	$ 30,000
Capital: G (replaced by D)	40,500	50,000
Other partners....................	121,500	150,000
	$192,000	$230,000

Since the JJG Partnership has a § 754 election in effect, D is entitled to a $9,500 basis adjustment [the excess of his $57,500 outside basis over the $48,000 inside basis of his 25% share of JJG's assets ($192,000 × 25%)]. Note that his outside basis is computed as the $50,000 cash payment plus 25% of the partnership's debt. The $9,500 is labeled as a § 743(b) adjustment.

The § 743(b) adjustment is allocated between classes and among properties based on the allocations of income, gain, or loss that the transferee partner would receive from a hypothetical sale of all partnership assets.

Allocation Between Classes:

	D's Allocable Share (25%)		
Ordinary Income Property	Adjusted Basis	FMV	Gain/(Loss)
Accounts receivable	$ 5,000	$ 3,750	$(1,250)
Inventory	10,500	12,500	2,000
Total	$ 15,500	$ 16,250	$ 750

Capital Gain Property	Adjusted Basis	FMV	Gain/(Loss)
Building	$ 17,500	$ 21,250	$ 3,750
Land	5,000	10,000	5,000
Total	$ 22,500	$ 31,250	$ 8,750

Therefore, the § 743(b) adjustment is allocated $750 to the ordinary income property and $8,750 to the capital gain property.

Allocation Within Classes:

If a hypothetical sale occurred, D would be allocated a loss of $1,250 from the sale of the receivables and a gain of $2,000 from the sale of the inventory. D would also be allocated a gain of $3,750 for the building and a gain of $5,000 for the land. Therefore, these amounts are D's basis adjustment for each of these assets.

To summarize, D's allocation of the inside basis of JJG's assets is as follows:

	Inside Basis	25% of Basis	§ 743(b) Adjustment	Adjusted Inside Basis
Cash	$40,000	$10,000	$ 0	$10,000
Accounts receivable	20,000	5,000	(1,250)	3,750
Inventory	42,000	10,500	2,000	12,500
Building	70,000	17,500	3,750	21,250
Land	20,000	5,000	5,000	10,000
				$57,500

Note that D's total outside basis of $57,500 is now equal to his allocation of the inside basis of the partnership's assets.

Effect of the Adjustment. A § 743(b) special basis adjustment belongs only to the purchasing partner and has no effect on the other partners. Although any benefit of a § 743(b) basis adjustment accrues only to the purchasing partner, the burden of record keeping for the adjustment falls upon the partnership. This disparity is one reason partnerships may be reluctant to make the § 754 election necessary to activate § 743(b). If a partner has a special basis adjustment with respect to an asset disposed of by the partnership in a taxable transaction, the adjustment will be taken into account in calculating that partner's distributive share of gain or loss.

> **Example 61.** If the JJG Partnership in the previous example sells its inventory for $50,000 and recognizes $8,000 of ordinary income, D's 25% share of that is $2,000. However, D's $2,000 special basis adjustment in the inventory reduces his distributive share of the partnership ordinary income to zero.

If a partner has a special basis adjustment with respect to a depreciable or amortizable asset, the adjustment will generate an additional cost recovery deduction for that partner.[106] Therefore, D can depreciate the $3,750 step-up in basis for the building in *Example 60*.

Substantial Built-in Loss. Even if a § 754 election is not in effect, the rules discussed above will apply if there is a substantial built-in loss to the partnership immediately after the transfer of the partnership interest. A substantial built-in loss occurs if the partnership's basis in its assets exceeds the fair market value of those assets by more than $250,000.[107]

> **Example 62.** Partner M sells his 20% partnership interest for $500,000 at a time when the MN partnership has a basis and fair market value in it is assets of $3,000,000 and $2,500,000, respectively. Since the basis of the partnership's assets exceeds the fair market value by more than $250,000 [by $500,000 [($3,00,000 − $2,500,000)], a substantial built-in loss exists. Therefore, even if Partnership MN does not have a § 754 election in effect, the partnership must reduce the acquiring partner's share of the basis in its assets by $100,000, the proportional amount of the $500,000 built-in loss according to §755.

Special Rule for Built-in-Losses. If the seller of a partnership interest had previously contributed built-in-loss property to the partnership, special rules apply. As explained earlier, if a partner contributes property with built-in losses, § 704(c) requires that when the property is sold, any recognized loss must be allocated to that contributing partner to the extent of the built-in loss, with any remaining loss allocated per the partnership agreement. However, § 704(c)(1)(C) requires that in determining the amount of items allocated to other (non-contributing partners), the basis of the property is assumed to be its fair market value at the time of contribution.[108]

> **Example 63.** Partner L contributes land to equal partnership LO with a basis of $100 and a fair market value of $80. Therefore, the land has a built-in loss of $20. If the partnership sold the land for $80, the $20 loss would be allocated to L.
>
> Assume that L sells his partnership interest to M for $80. L would recognize a loss of $20 from the sale of his partnership interest. Under previous law, M would "step

---

[106] A § 743(b) basis adjustment to depreciable property is considered a newly purchased asset placed in service in the year in which the adjustment arises. Prop. Reg. § 1.168-2(n).

[107] See § 743(d)(1). These rules apply for distributions made after October 22, 2004.

[108] This provision does not apply to contributions of property made before October 23, 2004.

into the shoes" of L and the first $20 loss from the future sale of the land would be allocated to M. Section 704(c)(1)(C) now requires that the basis of the land be treated as $80 (its fair market value on the date of contribution) for purposes of allocating any tax items to partners M and O. Thus, if the land was later sold by the partnership for $70, the basis of the land would be $80 (not $100). The sale would create a $10 loss ($70 amount realized less $80 basis), none of which is a built-in loss. The $10 loss would be allocated equally to partners M and O.

The purpose of this rule is to prevent the partners from benefiting from a double loss. If L recognizes a loss of $20 on the sale of the partnership interest and M could recognize another loss of $20 when the land was sold, a double benefit would be created.

GIFTS OF PARTNERSHIP INTERESTS AND FAMILY PARTNERSHIPS

Dispositions of partnership interests by gift generally have no income tax consequences to either donor or donee, although the donor may be liable for a gift tax on the transfer. The donee will take a basis in the partnership interest as determined under § 1015.

Transfers of partnership interests by gift usually involve donors and donees who are members of the same family, and therefore often result in the creation of *family partnerships*. Such partnerships can be an effective way to divide the income from a family business among various family members. To the extent the income can be allocated and taxed to individuals in the lower marginal tax brackets, family partnerships can also achieve a significant tax savings.

Not surprisingly, the tax laws restrict the use of family partnerships as income shifting devices. If the income earned by a partnership is primarily attributable to the individual efforts and talents of its partners, any allocation of that income to nonproductive partners would be an unwarranted assignment of earned income. Accordingly, a family member generally cannot be a partner in a personal or professional service business unless he or she is capable of performing the type of services offered to the partnership's clientele.[109]

A family member can be a partner in a business in which capital is a material income-producing factor.[110] In contrast to a service partnership, the mere ownership of an equity interest in a capital intensive partnership entitles a partner to a share of partnership income. Under the general rules of § 704, a partner's allocable share of income does not have to be in proportion to his or her interest in partnership capital as long as the allocation has substantial economic effect. However, § 704(e)(2) provides that in the case of any partnership capital interest *created by gift*, the income allocable to such interest cannot be proportionally greater than the income allocated to the donor's capital.

Example 64. M creates a partnership with his son S and daughter D by giving each child an equity interest in his business. M is in the highest marginal tax bracket, while his children are in the 15% marginal tax bracket. The initial MSD Partnership balance sheet appears as follows:

Contributed business assets	$300,000	

Capital:	M	$200,000
	S	50,000
	D	50,000
		$300,000

---

[109] See *Comm. v. Culbertson*, 337 U.S. 733 (USSC, 1949).

[110] § 704(e)(1). Capital is a material income-producing factor if the operation of the partnership business requires substantial inventories or a substantial investment in plant, machinery, or equipment. Reg. § 1.704-1(e)(1)(iv).

If S and D's interests had not been created by gift, the partnership agreement could allocate any amount of partnership income to S and D as long as the allocation had substantial economic effect. Because the interests were created by gift, the maximum percentage of income allocable to S and D respectively is 16.7% ($50,000 donee's capital ÷ $300,000 total capital of both donor and donees).

Section 704(e)(2) also requires that any allocation of income with respect to donor and donee partners take into account the value of services rendered to the partnership by the donor. This statutory requirement prevents a donor partner from forgoing reasonable compensation from the partnership in order to maximize the amount of income shifted to the donee partners.

> **Example 65.** Refer to the facts in *Example 64*. If M performs services for MSD during its first taxable year that are reasonably worth $25,000, he must be compensated for the services before any amount of partnership income may be allocated to S and D. If the partnership earns $145,000 of operating income during its first year, the maximum amount of such income allocable to S and D respectively is $20,000 [16.7% of ($145,000 operating income − $25,000 compensation to M)].

Note that the restrictions illustrated in *Example 64* and *Example 65* technically apply to any partnership interest created by gift, regardless of any familial relationship between donor and donee. Realistically, these restrictions most frequently apply to family partnerships. In order to prevent families from circumventing these restrictions, the statute states that a partnership interest purchased from a family member is considered to have been acquired by gift.[111]

DEATH OF A PARTNER

When an individual partner dies, his or her partnership interest passes to a *successor in interest* in the partnership.[112] The partner's gross estate for federal estate tax purposes includes the fair market value of the partnership interest at date of death, and the decedent's successor takes an outside basis in the interest equal to such fair market value.[113] Because the death of a partner causes a closing of the partnership's tax year with respect to that partner, items of income, gain, loss, deduction, or credit attributable to the deceased partner's interest up to date of death will be included on the final tax return of the decedent. Any amounts for the remainder of the partnership's tax year must be reported by the deceased partner's successor in interest.[114]

> **Example 66.** Individual Z, who owned a 40% interest in the capital, profits, and loss of the calendar year XYZ Partnership, died on November 3 of the current year. Under the terms of Z's will, all his assets (including his interest in XYZ) passed to his estate. Because the partnership's tax year closes with respect to Z on the date of his death, XYZ's income or loss attributable to this interest from January 1 to November 3 will be included in Z's final tax return. Income or loss attributable to this 40% interest for

---

[111] § 704(e)(3). For purposes of this rule, a partner's family members include a spouse, ancestors, and lineal descendants.

[112] The successor in interest is named under the decedent partner's will or determined by reference to state intestacy laws if the decedent died without a will.

[113] § 1014(a). Any imbalance between a successor in interest's outside basis and inside basis in the partnership assets is remedied if the partnership has a § 754 election in effect. In such case § 743(b) permits a special adjustment with respect to the inside basis of the partnership assets.

[114] § 706(c)(2)(A)(ii). Prior to 1998, the death of a partner did not cause the partnership's tax year to close with respect to the deceased partner. As a result, income or loss attributable to the interest for the entire year was usually included on the tax return of the successor in interest.

the remainder of the year must be included in the first fiduciary income tax return filed on behalf of Z's estate.

PARTNERSHIP TERMINATION

One of the important legal characteristics of the partnership form of business is *limited life*. Under state law, a partnership is dissolved whenever any partner ceases to be associated in the carrying on of the partnership business.[115] From a legal perspective, a partnership's identity, and therefore its existence, is dependent upon the continued association of a particular group of partners. This perspective is consistent with the aggregate theory of partnerships. Nevertheless, it would be totally impractical to require a partnership to close its taxable year and make a final accounting of its business activities every time an existing partner left or a new partner joined the partnership.

Section 708(a) adopts the entity theory by providing that a partnership does not terminate for tax purposes simply because it may be dissolved under state law. In other words, a partnership shall continue in existence as an entity for purposes of Subchapter K even if the association of partners changes. Section 708(b) provides that a partnership shall terminate for tax purposes *only if*:

1. No part of any business, financial operation, or venture is being conducted by the partnership (*natural termination*), or

2. Within a 12-month period there is a sale or exchange of 50 percent or more of the total interest in partnership capital and profits (*technical termination*).

TECHNICAL TERMINATIONS

When a partnership ceases to conduct any type of economic activity, its termination for federal tax purposes marks the natural end of its life as a business entity. In contrast, a partnership that is terminated because of a sale or exchange of more than a 50 percent interest may be conducting a vital, ongoing business. Moreover, the partners who were not involved in the sale or exchange may be unaware that the terminating transaction even occurred!

Only sales or exchanges of partnership interests can trigger a technical termination. Other types of dispositions, such as gifts or transfers at death, are ignored. Similarly, changes in the relative ownership interests of partners because of contributions to or distributions from a partnership cannot result in termination. Sales or exchanges will not cause termination unless *at least* a 50 percent cumulative interest in both capital and profits changes hands within a 12-month period.

Example 67. Partners A, B, and C have owned equal interests in the capital and profits of the ABC Partnership since 1999.

- ▶ On January 12, 2008, A sold her one-third interest to new partner D.
- ▶ On July 8, 2008, B sold 10% of his interest to new partner E.
- ▶ On November 22, 2008, C gave his one-third interest to new partner F.
- ▶ On January 9, 2009, F exchanged this interest for stock in a new corporation; the exchange was nontaxable under § 351.

The January 12 sale did not terminate the ABC Partnership because only a 33.3% interest in capital and profits was sold. The July 8 sale did not terminate the

[115] Uniform Partnership Act, § 29.

partnership because at that point in time only a 43.3% cumulative interest in capital and profits had been sold within a 12-month period. The November 22 gift did not enter into the termination calculation. The January 9 exchange did result in a termination of the ABC Partnership; within the 12-month period beginning on January 12, 2008, a cumulative 76.6% interest in the partnership was sold or exchanged. If F had delayed his exchange until after January 11, 2009, the transaction would have not triggered a termination.

In determining whether a cumulative 50 percent interest has been sold or exchanged within the crucial 12-month time period, multiple transfers of the *same interest* are counted only once.[116] In *Example 67*, if D (rather than F) had exchanged his one-third interest for corporate stock on January 9, 2009, the exchange would not have resulted in a technical termination.

EFFECT OF TERMINATION

Upon termination, a partnership's taxable year closes with respect to all its partners. If the partnership and any partner use different taxable years, a bunching of more than 12 months of income may occur.

> **Example 68.** The QRS Partnership uses a calendar year for tax purposes, while corporate partner A uses a fiscal year ending June 30. The partnership terminated on March 31, 2009 and closed its taxable year on that date. Because two partnership years (calendar year 2008 and the short taxable year from January 1–March 31, 2009) ended within its fiscal year ending June 30, 2009, Q must include its distributive share of 15 months of partnership income in its taxable income for the year.

Pursuant to a natural termination, a partnership typically will wind up its affairs and distribute all remaining cash and assets to the partners in complete liquidation of their interests.[117] In a technical termination, the partnership contributes all of its assets and liabilities to a new partnership in exchange for an interest in the new partnership. The terminated partnership then distributes interests in the new partnership to the purchasing partner and all other remaining partners.[118] The result of the application of these rules is that the technical termination does not automatically result in adjustments to the bases of the partnership assets because no assets are treated as being distributed.[119]

PROBLEM MATERIALS

DISCUSSION QUESTIONS

22-1 *Partnership versus Corporation.* List both tax and nontax advantages or disadvantages of operating a business as a partnership rather than as a corporation.

22-2 *General versus Limited Partners.* Distinguish between the legal rights and responsibilities of a general partner and a limited partner.

---

[116] Reg. § 1.708-1(b)(2).

[117] Reg. § 1.708-1(b)(1).

[118] Reg. § 1.708-1(b)(1)(iv).

[119] A complete analysis of the potential tax consequences of technical terminations is beyond the scope of an introductory text.

22-3 *Aggregate versus Entity Theory.* How does the aggregate theory of partnerships differ from the entity theory of partnerships? Give a specific example of a Subchapter K rule that reflects each theory.

22-4 *Contributions of Property.* True or false: neither a partner nor a partnership ever recognizes gain or loss on the contribution of property in exchange for a partnership interest. Explain your conclusion.

22-5 *Partnership Liabilities as Basis.* What is the economic rationale for including a portion of partnership recourse debt in the partners' bases of their partnership interests? What is the rationale for the inclusion of nonrecourse debt?

22-6 *Contributions of Services.* Distinguish between the tax consequences to a partner who contributes services in exchange for a capital interest in a partnership and one who contributes services in exchange for an interest in future profits.

22-7 *Organization Costs versus Syndication Fees.* Compare the tax treatment of partnership organization costs to that of syndication fees.

22-8 *Partnership Taxable Year.* What choices are available to a business partnership when selecting a taxable year?

22-9 *Basis Adjustments.* Indicate whether each of the following occurrences increases, decreases, or has no effect on a general partner's basis in his partnership interest. Assume all liabilities are recourse liabilities.
   a. The partnership borrows cash that will be repaid in two years.
   b. The partnership earns tax-exempt interest on municipal bonds.
   c. The partnership generates an operating loss for the year.
   d. The partnership distributes cash to its partners.
   e. The partnership incurs a nondeductible penalty.
   f. The partnership makes a principal payment on a mortgage secured by partnership property.
   g. The partnership recognizes a long-term capital gain on the sale of marketable securities.

22-10 *Partners' Transactions with Partnerships.* Give three examples of a transaction between a partnership and a partner that will be treated as a transaction between the partnership and a nonpartner for tax purposes. Does such arm's length treatment reflect the aggregate or the entity theory of partnerships?

22-11 *Partners as Employees.* May a general partner be an employee of the partnership for federal tax purposes? Explain your conclusion.

22-12 *Current versus Liquidating Distributions.* Explain the difference between a current distribution and a liquidating distribution from a partnership.

22-13 *Current Distributions.* Is the statement that a partner never recognizes a loss upon the receipt of a current distribution true or false? Explain your conclusion.

22-14 *Liquidating Distributions.* Under what circumstances will a partner recognize a capital loss upon the receipt of a liquidating distribution?

22-15 *Closing of Partnership Year.* Partner Z received a liquidating distribution from a calendar year partnership on April 3 of the current year. Explain why Z could not determine the tax consequences of the distribution until the end of the year.

22-16 *Partnership Goodwill.* Explain the difference in tax consequences to both partner and partnership of liquidating payments with respect to (1) specified and (2) unspecified partnership goodwill.

22-17 *Sale of a Partnership Interest.* Is the statement that the sale of an interest in a partnership owning hot assets can result in either ordinary gain or loss recognition true or false? Explain your conclusion.

22-18 *Sale of a Partnership Interest.* Does the fact that a partner recognizes capital gain or loss on the sale of an interest in a partnership with no hot assets reflect the entity or aggregate theory of partnerships?

22-19 *Tax Consequences to Purchaser.* Explain why the outside basis in a purchased interest in a partnership without a § 754 election in effect is usually different than the purchaser's proportionate share of the inside basis of partnership assets. Does this result reflect the entity or aggregate theory of partnerships?

22-20 *Family Partnerships.* In what ways does the tax law restrict the use of a family partnership as a device to shift income to individuals in the lower marginal tax brackets?

22-21 *Death of a Partner.* How is any partnership income, gain, loss, deduction, or credit attributable to a deceased partner's interest allocated between that partner's final tax return and that of the successor in interest? Assume for purposes of your answer that death occurred on August 15th and that both the partnership and the deceased were calendar year taxpayers.

22-22 *Partnership Terminations.* Distinguish between the dissolution of a partnership under state law and the termination of a partnership for federal tax purposes.

PROBLEMS

22-23 *Formation—No Liabilities.* J and G form the JG Partnership and contribute the following business assets:

Asset	Fair Market Value	Basis	Contributed by
Land	$60,000	$30,000	J
Inventory	50,000	28,000	G
Auto	10,000	14,000	G

J and G will share profits and losses equally.
a. Calculate each partner's realized and recognized gain or loss.
b. Calculate each partner's basis in his or her partnership interest.
c. Calculate the partnership's basis in each asset.

22-24 *Formation—No Liabilities.* The A-E Partnership is being formed by five individuals who each contribute assets in exchange for a 20 percent capital and profit/loss interest. Calculate the following for each partner: (1) recognized gain or loss, (2) each partner's basis in his or her partnership interest, (3) the partnership's basis for each asset, and (4) the holding period of the partnership interest for the partner and the assets for the partnership. Assume all contributed assets will be used in the partnership's trade or business.
a. A contributes business furniture with a market value of $10,000. The furniture cost $16,000 when purchased four years ago, and A's adjusted basis in the furniture is $5,000.
b. B contributes business equipment with a market value of $10,000. The equipment cost $20,000 when purchased two years ago, and B's adjusted basis in the equipment is $12,000.

    c. C contributes business inventory with a market value of $10,000. The inventory cost $9,000 when purchased 16 months ago.

    d. D and E contribute $10,000 cash each.

22-25 *Formation—Liabilities.* Refer to *Problem 22-24*, but assume that D and E made the following contributions *instead* of cash. How do these new facts change your answers for each partner?

    a. D contributes land with a market value of $16,000. The land was acquired 10 months ago for $9,000 cash and a $6,000 note payable (recourse debt). The $6,000 note payable is also transferred to the partnership.

    b. E contributes land with a market value of $18,000. E received the land three years ago as a gift from a relative and has a basis of $5,000. In addition, E transfers an $8,000 mortgage (nonrecourse debt) on the land to the partnership.

22-26 *Partner's Holding Period.* Individuals X and Y contributed $50,000 each to the equal Z Partnership on January 1, 2009. On July 1, 2009, X contributed land with an adjusted basis of $10,000 and fair market value of $25,000 to Z for an increased interest in the partnership. X had owned the property as an investment for six months. On October 1, 2009, Y contributed land with an adjusted basis of $30,000 and fair market value of $25,000 to Z for an increased interest in the partnership. Y, a dealer in real property, had owned the land for three years. As of December 31, 2009, what are the partners' holding period in their partnership interests?

22-27 *Allocation of Recourse Debt.* Individuals A and B are general partners and individual L is a limited partner in the ABL Partnership. Partnership losses are allocated 40 percent to A, 35 percent to B, and 25 percent to L. As of December 31 of the current year, the partnership has $50,000 of recourse debt. The partnership's balance sheet as of December 31 is as follows:

	Basis	Fair Market Value
Cash	$ 25,000	$ 25,000
Receivables	50,000	75,000
Land	25,000	40,000
	$100,000	$140,000
Recourse liabilities	$ 50,000	$ 50,000
A, capital	20,000	36,000
B, capital	20,000	36,000
L, capital	10,000	18,000
	$100,000	$140,000

How would the $50,000 of recourse debt be allocated to A, B, and L?

22-28 *Relief of Debt in Excess of Basis.* Corporation C contributed land used in its business to the Beta Partnership in exchange for a 40 percent general interest in partnership capital, profits, and loss. The land had a $320,000 basis to the corporation and an appraised fair market value of $850,000, and was subject to a $635,000 recourse mortgage. Beta assumed the mortgage in the exchange transaction; as of the date of the exchange, Beta had no other liabilities.

    a. What are the tax consequences to Corporation C of its contribution of the land to Beta? What initial basis does Corporation C have in its partnership interest?

    b. How would your answers to (a) change if the $635,000 mortgage were nonrecourse rather than recourse?

c. How would your answers to (a) change if Beta had $200,000 of other recourse liabilities on its books as of the date of Corporation C's contribution of the land?

22-29 *Receipt of Partnership Interest for Services.* In return for services rendered to the AX Partnership, T receives a 20 percent unrestricted interest in partnership capital. On the day T receives her interest, the partnership owned the following assets:

	Basis	Fair Market Value
Inventory	$ 5,000	$10,000
Equipment	10,000	14,000
Land	15,000	21,000
Building	40,000	50,000
Totals	$70,000	$95,000

Assuming the partnership has no liabilities and that before T's admission it is owned 60 percent by partner A and 40 percent by partner X, answer the following questions:
a. How much compensation income must be reported by T?
b. What is T's basis in the partnership interest received?

22-30 *Required Taxable Year.* F, G, and H are partners in the FGH Partnership. F, G, and H have profit-sharing ratios of 30 percent, 50 percent, and 20 percent, respectively. F has a year-end of December 31, G of February 28, and H of September 30. What is the required year-end for FGH Partnership?

22-31 *Computation of Partnership Taxable Income.* N is a 10 percent general partner in the KLMN Partnership. The partnership's records for the current year show the following:

Gross receipts from sales	$ 670,000
Cost of sales	(500,000)
Operating expenses	(96,000)
Net income from rental real estate	48,000
Dividend income	10,000
Business meals and entertainment	(6,700)
Section 1231 loss	(13,500)

N's outside basis in his partnership interest was $125,000 at the beginning of the year. During the year, partnership recourse liabilities increased by $55,000; the partnership has no nonrecourse liabilities. KLMN made no distributions during the year to its partners.
a. Calculate the partnership's taxable income (Form 1065, page 1) for the current year.
b. Calculate N's basis in the partnership at the end of the year.

22-32 *Organization and Syndication Costs.* The Sigma Limited Partnership was organized during May and June of the current year. During these two months, the partnership paid $25,000 to a law firm to draft the partnership agreement and $13,000 to a CPA to set up an accounting system for the partnership business. The partnership also paid a $2,500 filing fee to the state of Illinois and $18,000 to advertise and market the sale of limited interests to potential investors. Sigma began business in August of the current year and properly adopted a fiscal year ending September 30 for tax purposes. Based on these facts, what portion of the above expenses may be expensed and amortized on Sigma's first Form 1065?

22-33 *Contributed Property—Allocations.* At the beginning of the current year, S contributed depreciable business property (market value $90,000 and basis $67,200)

and T contributed investment land (market value $180,000 and basis $145,000) to form the ST Partnership. S has a one-third interest and T has a two-thirds interest in partnership capital, profits, and loss.

    a. The ST Partnership will depreciate the property contributed by S on a straight-line basis over six years. Compute the amount of first year tax depreciation on the property and allocate the depreciation between partners S and T.

    b. Assume the partnership sells the property contributed by S on the first day of the partnership's third taxable year. The amount realized on sale is $65,000. Compute the taxable gain or loss recognized on the sale and allocate the gain or loss between partners S and T.

    c. How would your answer to (b) change if the amount realized on sale had been $54,000 rather than $65,000?

    d. During its fourth taxable year, the ST Partnership sells the land contributed by T for $200,000. Compute the taxable gain recognized on sale and allocate the gain between partners S and T.

22-34 *Sale of Contributed Property—Allocations.* Two years ago, X contributed property, which was part of his proprietorship inventory, to the D Partnership in exchange for a one-third partnership interest. At the date of contribution, the property had a basis of $120,000 and a value of $145,000. The property was used in the partnership's business as a nondepreciable § 1231 asset. The partnership sold the property for $160,000 in the current year.

    a. Calculate the amount and character of the taxable gain recognized on the sale allocable to X.

    b. How would the answer for (a) change if the sale occurred six years rather than two years after contribution?

    c. How would the answer for (a) change if the property had been sold for $100,000 rather than $160,000?

22-35 *Retroactive Loss Allocations.* On September 1 of the current year, Corporation M contributed $125,000 cash to the calendar year, accrual basis Topper Partnership. For the current year, Topper recognized a $180,000 net operating loss; $82,000 of this loss had accrued as of August 31. In June of the current year, Topper sold marketable securities, recognizing a $63,000 capital gain.

    a. If Topper does not make an interim closing of its books on August 31, what is the maximum amount of current-year net operating loss and capital gain that can be allocated to Corporation M? Explain your conclusion. (In answering the question, you may assume that any allocation will have substantial economic effect.)

    b. If Topper does make an interim closing of its books on August 31, what is the maximum amount of current-year net operating loss and capital gain that can be allocated to Corporation M? Explain your conclusion. (In answering the question, you may assume that any allocation will have substantial economic effect.)

22-36 *Losses—Section 704(d).* Z has a 60 percent interest in the capital, profits, and losses of the Zeta Partnership. Both Z and Zeta are calender year taxpayers. At the beginning of the current year, Z's basis in her partnership interest was $100,000. For the current year, Zeta incurred a $200,000 ordinary loss from its business operation, earned $14,600 of dividend and interest income on its investments, and recognized a $62,000 capital gain on the sale of a partnership capital asset. On March 12 of the current year, Z received a $15,000 cash distribution from Zeta. Assume that there was no change in the amount of Zeta's liabilities during the current year.

    a. How much of the $200,000 operating loss may Z deduct on her current-year tax return? In answering this question, ignore any impact of the at-risk or passive activity loss limitations.

    b. Calculate Z's basis in her partnership interest at the end of the year.

22-37 *Losses—Section 704(d).* Corporation Q owns a 50 percent interest in the capital, profits, and loss of the QRST Partnership. Both Q and QRST are calendar year taxpayers.

At the beginning of the current year, Q's outside basis in its partnership interest was $30,000. For the current year, the partnership earned $14,000 of tax-exempt interest on its investment in municipal bonds, incurred a $106,000 ordinary loss from its business operation, and recognized a $42,000 capital loss on the sale of a partnership capital asset. QRST made no distributions to partners during the year and did not change the amount of partnership debt on its books. Based on these facts, how much of the partnership's operating loss and capital loss may Corporation Q deduct in the current year? (In answering this question, assume that Q has sufficient current-year capital gains against which to deduct any amount of partnership capital loss.)

22-38 *Transactions between Partners and Partnerships.* A calendar year, accrual basis partnership rents property from a calendar year, cash basis partner, paying an arm's-length rent of $4,000 per month. The December rent payment for the current year was not received by the partner until January 5 of the subsequent year. The partnership pays this same partner a guaranteed payment for services rendered to the partnership of $10,000 per month. The December guaranteed payment was not received by the partner until January 10 of the subsequent year.

    a. In what year should the partnership deduct the December rent payment, and in what year should the partner include this payment in gross income?

    b. In what year should the partnership deduct the December guaranteed payment, and in what year should the partner include this payment in gross income?

22-39 *Guaranteed Payments.* B and G are partners in the DR Partnership. B oversees the daily operations of the business and therefore receives compensation of $50,000, regardless of the amount of the partnership's net income. In addition, his distributive share of profits and losses is 50 percent.

    a. If the partnership had $75,000 ordinary income before any payments to partners, determine the amount and character of B's total income.

    b. Same as (a), but assume the partnership had $30,000 ordinary income before payments to partners.

    c. Same as (a), except assume the partnership had $25,000 ordinary income and $50,000 long-term capital gain before payments to partners.

22-40 *Sale to Related Partnership—Loss.* V, a 60 percent partner, sells land to the partnership for $8,000. V's basis in the land is $9,000.

    a. Determine (1) V's recognized loss and (2) the partnership's basis in the land after the transaction.

    b. What are the tax consequences to the partnership if it sells the land six months later for (1) $7,500, (2) $8,600, or (3) $9,300?

    c. How would your answers to (a) and (b) differ if V were a 40 percent partner?

22-41 *Sale to Related Partnership—Gain.* During the current year, Corporation J sold investment land with a $400,000 basis to the Kappa Partnership for a selling price of $525,000. Determine the amount and character of Corporation J's recognized gain on the sale under each of the following sets of assumptions.

    a. Corporation J owns a 75 percent interest in the capital, profits, and loss of Kappa, and Kappa also holds the land as an investment asset.

    b. Corporation J owns a 35 percent interest in the capital, profits, and loss of Kappa, and Kappa uses the land in its business operation.

    c. Corporation J owns a 75 percent interest in the capital, profits, and loss of Kappa, and Kappa uses the land in its business operation.

22-42 *Contribution of Inventory with Built-in Gain.* V is a 40 percent partner in the TUV Partnership. V is a dealer in computer equipment, and V contributes computers to TUV that the partnership will use in its business operations. The computers have a basis to V of $10,000 and a fair market value of $16,000. What are the tax consequences to V and to TUV under the following circumstances?

    a. TUV sells the computers six months later for $15,000. Assume the basis is the same.

    b. TUV sells the computers six years later for $3,000. Assume the basis is zero at that time.

    c. What would your answer be if the facts are the same as in part a, except that TUV also is a dealer in computer equipment?

22-43 *Contribution of Capital Asset with Built-in Loss.* W is a 20 percent partner in the WXY Partnership. W has owned a parcel of land as an investment for three years. W contributes this land to WXY. WXY is a dealer in land. The land has a basis to W of $120,000 and a fair market value of $100,000. What are the tax consequences to W and to WXY under the following circumstances?

    a. WXY sells the land six months later for $100,000.

    b. WXY sells the land six months later for $90,000.

    c. WXY sells the land six years later for $90,000.

    d. WXY sells the land six years later for $150,000.

22-44 *Current Distributions—Proportionate.* X is a 50 percent partner in XY, a calendar year partnership. X had a basis in her partnership interest of $10,000 at the beginning of the year. On October 1, she and the other partner withdrew $15,000 cash each as an advance against their anticipated share of partnership income for the year. The partnership's ordinary, taxable income for the year was $60,000.

    a. How much gain or loss must X recognize on October 1?

    b. What is X's distributive share of partnership taxable income for the year, and what is her basis in her partnership interest at the end of the year?

    c. How would the answers to (a) and (b) change if partnership taxable income had been $6,000 instead of $60,000?

22-45 *Current Distribution—Proportionate.* During the current year, partner J received a proportionate distribution from HIJK Partnership, consisting of $13,000 cash and land (an investment asset to the partnership). The land had a basis to the partnership of $20,000 and FMV of $33,000. Prior to the distribution, J's basis in his partnership interest was $40,000. The distribution had no effect on J's profit and loss sharing ratio.

    a. How much gain or loss must J recognize because of this distribution? What basis will J have in the land? What basis will J have in his partnership interest after the distribution?

    b. Does the partnership recognize any gain on the distribution of the appreciated land to J?

    c. How would the answer to (a) change if J's basis in his interest prior to distribution had been $25,000 rather than $40,000?

22-46 *Current Distribution of Inventory.* C received a current proportionate distribution consisting of partnership inventory with an inside basis of $25,000 and a FMV of $31,000. C's predistribution outside basis in his partnership interest was $22,500.

    a. How much gain or loss must C recognize because of this distribution?

    b. What basis will C take in the distributed inventory and what will be C's postdistribution outside basis?

    c. How would your answers to (a) and (b) change if C's predistribution outside basis had been $29,000 rather than $22,500?

22-47 *Dispositions of Distributed Inventory.* Refer to the facts in *Problem 22-46*.

    a. What will be the tax consequences to C if he sells the distributed inventory for $30,000 in the first year following the distribution?

    b. How does your answer to (a) change if C waits for six years and then sells the distributed inventory for $40,000?

22-48 *Optional Adjustment to Basis—Current Proportionate Distribution.* Refer to *Problem 22-46(b)* and *(c)*. The partnership has a § 754 election in effect. Determine the § 734(b) basis adjustment for the partnership assets.

22-49 *Basis of Distributed Property—Current Distribution.* R receives a current distribution from the RST Partnership consisting of the following:

	Inside Basis	Fair Market Value
Cash	$10,000	$10,000
Accounts receivable	0	7,500
Inventory	4,000	5,000
Capital Asset 1	5,000	4,000
Capital Asset 2	8,000	6,000

Immediately prior to the distribution, R's outside basis in her partnership interest was $22,000. What are R's bases in the distributed assets, and what is her basis in his partnership interest after the distribution?

22-50 *Liquidating Distribution—Proportionate.* Immediately prior to its termination, the FN Partnership owned the following assets:

	Inside Basis	Fair Market Value
Cash	$ 40,000	$40,000
Equipment	100,000	70,000
Accumulated depreciation	(60,000)	
Capital asset	10,000	30,000

F, a 50 percent owner, receives one-half of all the assets in complete liquidation of her partnership interest. F's outside basis in this interest is $45,000.
a. Calculate F's basis for each asset received in the distribution.
b. How would your answer to (a) change if F's outside basis in her partnership interest is $95,000?

22-51 *Basis of Distributed Property—Liquidating Distribution.* After reduction for a distribution of cash and the required allocation of basis to unrealized receivables and inventory received in a liquidating distribution from the HIJ Partnership, Partner J has an outside basis of $100,000. J also receives the following capital assets as part of the liquidating distribution:

	Inside Basis	Fair Market Value
Capital asset 1	$25,000	$60,000
Capital asset 2	50,000	20,000

What basis does J have in the capital assets?

22-52 *Section 734 Basis Adjustment.* Partner F received a liquidating distribution of $9,000 cash from the EFG Partnership. F's predistribution outside basis was $12,000. Assume that EFG has a § 754 election in effect. Partnership EFG owns the following assets after the distribution to F:

	Inside Basis	Fair Market Value
Cash	$20,000	$20,000
Inventory	12,000	15,000
Capital asset M	14,000	10,000
Capital asset N	10,000	8,000

a. What is F's gain or loss from the distribution?
b. What are the § 734 basis adjustments for the partnership's remaining assets?

22-53 *Payments to a Retiring Partner.* The balance sheet of RST Partnership shows the following:

	Inside Basis	Fair Market Value
Cash............................	$120,000	$120,000
Accounts receivable	20,000	20,000
Inventory	105,000	112,000
§ 1231 assets......................	4,000	57,000
	$249,000	$309,000
Liabilities........................	$ 9,000	$ 9,000
R, capital	80,000	100,000
S, capital........................	80,000	100,000
T, capital........................	80,000	100,000
	$249 000	$309,000

During the current year, partners S and T agree to liquidate R's interest in the partnership for $115,000 cash. Capital is a material income-producing factor to the RST Partnership and the partnership has no unrecorded goodwill. R's basis in his interest (including his one-third share of partnership liabilities) is $83,000.

  a. What are the tax consequences to R of the cash distribution from the partnership?
  b. What are the consequences to the partnership of the liquidating distribution?

22-54 *Section 754 Election and Partnership Distributions.* Refer to the facts in *Problem 22-53.* What are the tax consequences to the continuing partnership if a § 754 election is in effect for the year in which R's interest is liquidated?

22-55 *Sale of a Partnership Interest.* Refer to the facts in *Problem 22-53.* Assume that U, an unrelated party, will purchase R's interest in RST Partnership for a lump sum payment of $115,000.

  a. What are the tax consequences of the sale to R?
  b. Compute U's basis in his newly purchased partnership interest.
  c. What is the effect of U's purchase of R's partnership interest on the inside basis of partnership assets if RST Partnership does not have a § 754 election in effect?

22-56 *Consequences of a § 754 Election to a Purchasing Partner.* Refer to the facts in *Problem 22-55.* What are the tax consequences to new partner U and to RST Partnership if a § 754 election is in effect for the year in which U purchases R's partnership interest?

22-57 *Sale of Partnership Interest with Hot Assets.* T, a general partner in the accrual basis TUV Partnership, sells her one-third partnership interest to D at the end of the current year for $50,000 cash. The partnership's balance sheet at the end of the year is as follows:

	Basis	FMV		Basis	FMV
Cash...........	$61,000	$ 61,000	T, capital	$30,000	$ 50,000
Inventory	21,000	39,000	U, capital	$30,000	$ 50,000
Land	8,000	50,000	V, capital	$30,000	$ 50,000
	$90,000	$150,000		$90,000	$150,000

  a. What is T's gain or loss from this sale?
  b. What basis does D have in her partnership interest?

    c. If the partnership sells the land for $50,000 immediately after D purchases her interest, what is the tax effect to D?

    d. What should D request that the partnership do to prevent the result in part (c) from occurring?

    e. Instead of inventory, assume that the partnership owns collectibles with a basis of $21,000 and fair market value of $39,000. Also, assume that instead of land, the partnership owns a building with a basis of $8,000, fair market value of $50,000, depreciation claimed of $30,000 (of which $20,000 would have been straight-line depreciation). What is T's gain or loss on the sale?

22-58   *Section 754 Election.* Based on the facts from *Problem 22-57*, what would the tax result be to D upon the sale of the land if the partnership had a § 754 election in effect?

22-59   *Dispositions of Partnership Interests.* K owns a limited interest in the Kappa Investment Partnership. The interest has a FMV of $50,000 and a basis to K of $37,000. No amount of partnership debt is included in this basis number. What are the tax consequences to K in each of the following situations?

    a. K exchanges the interest for a general interest in Kappa that is worth $50,000.

    b. K exchanges the interest for investment land worth $50,000.

    c. K dies and bequeaths the interest to her nephew.

    d. K exchanges the interest for newly issued stock in Gamma Inc. Immediately after the exchange, K owns 12 percent of Gamma's outstanding stock.

    e. K determines that the value of the interest is not $50,000 but is zero. Consequently, she abandons the interest.

22-60   *Dispositions of Partnership Interests Holding Built-In Loss Property.* C and D create the equal CD Partnership in 2008. C contributes cash of $1,000 and D contributes land (holding period is 5 years) having a basis of $1,400 and a fair market value of $1,000. What are the tax consequences to the partners in the following independent situations? Assume that the partnership has not made a § 754 election.

    a. The partnership sales the land for $800 on January 15, 2009.

    b. D sells his partnership to E for $900 on March 15, 2009.

    c. After D sells the partnership interest to E, the partnership sells the land for $800.

22-61   *Partnership Termination.* At the beginning of 2009, Beta Partnership was owned by four equal partners. On June 8, 2009, Partner A sold her one-fourth interest to B, one of the other three partners. On November 19, 2009, new partner G contributed cash and property in exchange for a 55 percent interest in partnership capital and profits. On March 31, 2010, G sold a 30 percent interest to a new partner P. Beta and all its partners use the calendar year for tax purposes.

    a. Do any of the capital transactions described above terminate the Beta partnership?

    b. What is the effect of any termination on Beta's taxable year?

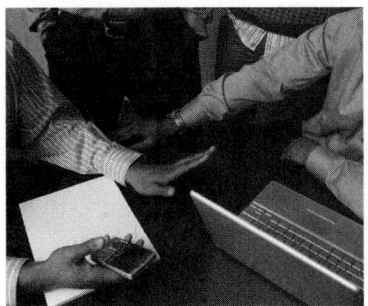

CHAPTER TWENTY THREE

S CORPORATIONS

LEARNING OBJECTIVES

Upon completion of this chapter you will be able to:

▸ Identify the requirements necessary to attain S corporation status

▸ Recognize the actions that terminate S status

▸ Compute the taxable income or loss for an S corporation and the impact of S corporate operations on shareholders' taxable income

▸ Recognize transactions between shareholders and their S corporations that are subject to special treatment

▸ Determine the shareholders' basis in the S corporation stock and debt, and understand the significance for loss deductions and distributions

▸ Determine the appropriate taxable year for an S corporation

▸ Explain the unique concepts relevant to family members

▸ Calculate gain or loss for the S corporation and its shareholders when asset distributions are made and the S corporation (1) has no AE&P or (2) has AE&P

▸ Calculate the special taxes on excessive passive income and on built-in gains

▸ Understand how dispositions of S corporate stock differ from those of C corporate stock

▸ Compare the four business organizations—proprietorships, partnerships, S corporations, and C corporations (see Exhibit 11-6)

CHAPTER OUTLINE

INTRODUCTION

Congress added Subchapter S to the Internal Revenue Code in 1958, giving birth to a unique tax entity: the S corporation. The S corporation passes taxable income, losses and other items to its owners, similar to a partnership. However, this entity has all of the nontax (and some tax) characteristics of a corporation. In providing this distinctive treatment, Congressional intent was to allow small businesses to have "the advantages of the corporate form of organization without being made subject to the possible tax disadvantages of the corporation."[1] As this statement suggests, Congress recognized that many taxpayers who normally would incorporate their businesses to secure limited liability were reluctant to do so because of the possibility of double taxation. Accordingly, one of the major objectives of the Subchapter S legislation was to minimize taxes as a factor in the selection of the form of business organization. To accomplish this objective, a complete set of special rules were designed, most of which are contained in Subchapter S.

Although the treatment of S corporations resembles that of partnerships, this goal was not achieved under the 1958 legislation. As originally written, the rules governing S corporations (or Subchapter S corporations as they were initially called) bore little resemblance to partnership rules. Many of these differences were eliminated, however, with the substantial modifications introduced by the Subchapter S Revision Act of 1982. Under the revised rules, Federal income tax treatment of S corporations and their shareholders is similar to that of partnerships and their partners. The S corporation generally is not subject to the corporate *Federal income tax*. Rather, like a partnership, the S corporation is merely a conduit. The income, deductions, gains, losses, and credits of

---

[1]   S. Rept. No. 1622, 83rd Cong., 2d Sess., 119 (1954).

the S corporation flow through to its shareholders. An S corporation, however, may be subject to a special tax, such as the tax on excessive passive income or on built-in gains.

Even though the Federal income tax treatment of an S corporation resembles that of a partnership, this entity is subject to many rules that apply to regular corporations. For example, since an S corporation is formed in the same manner as a regular corporation (defined as "C" corporations), the basic rules governing organization (i.e., the nonrecognition rules contained in § 351 concerning transfers to a controlled corporation discussed in Chapter 19) of all corporations also apply to S corporations. Similarly, redemptions of an S corporation's stock, as well as liquidation and reorganization of an S corporation, generally are subject to the rules applying to regular corporations. As a practical matter, however, each provision must be closely examined to determine whether special treatment is provided for S corporations.

S CORPORATION ELIGIBILITY REQUIREMENTS

The special tax treatment provided for S corporations is available only if the corporation is a *small business corporation* and its shareholders *consent* to the corporation's election to be taxed under Subchapter S. A small business corporation must:[2]

1. Be an *eligible domestic* corporation;

2. Not have more than 100 *eligible* shareholders; and

3. Have only *one class of stock* outstanding.

The corporation must meet all of these requirements when it files its S corporation election and at all times thereafter. Failure at any time to qualify as a small business corporation terminates the election, and as of the date of termination, the corporation is taxed as a regular corporation (hereafter referred to as a C corporation).[3]

The phrase *small business corporation* may be a misnomer. As the requirements for this status indicate, the sole restriction on the size of the corporation is the limitation imposed on the *number* of shareholders. Corporations are not denied use of Subchapter S due to the amount of their assets, income, net worth, or any other measure of size. In addition, the S corporation is not required to conduct an active business. Merely holding assets does not bar the corporation from Subchapter S.

ELIGIBLE CORPORATIONS

Subchapter S status is reserved for *eligible domestic corporations.*[4] Thus, foreign corporations do not qualify. In addition, certain types of domestic corporations are considered ineligible. These ineligible corporations include insurance companies, banks that use the reserve method of accounting for bad debts, corporations electing the special possessions tax credit under Code § 936 and domestic international sales corporations (DISCs).[5]

It should be emphasized that only corporations or entities that are considered corporations may take advantage of Subchapter S. As a practical matter, this is rarely an issue. A limited liability company (LLC) or other unincorporated entity can qualify as an S corporation if it elects to be treated as a corporation under the check-the-box regulations (see

---

[2] § 1361. For S corporations' taxable years beginning before January 1, 2005, the limit was 75.

[3] § 1362(d)(2). As discussed later, however, a corporation may avoid loss of its election by applying for "inadvertent termination" relief.

[4] § 1361(b); Reg. 301.7701-5(b) includes any U.S. territory as well as states.

[5] § 1361(b)(2).

Chapter 19).[6] Under these rules, the entity could only be considered an S corporation if it opts to be taxed as a corporation *and* subsequently makes a valid S election. In other words, an LLC that elects to be treated as a corporation is treated as a C corporation until the corporation files an S election.

Although there once was a restriction about ownership of subsidiaries, S corporations may own stock in *C corporations* without limitation. Thus, S corporations have the freedom to structure their ownership in C corporations to meet the needs of their organization. For example, an S corporation may establish a wholly owned C corporation as a subsidiary to hold a risky business, thereby protecting the assets of the parent. However, S and C corporations cannot file a consolidated return.[7] Thus, the C corporation must file Form 1120 and the S corporation must file Form 1120S.

> **Example 1.** D Inc., an S corporation, is interested in purchasing T Inc., a C corporation. T operates a hazardous waste disposal business that is quite profitable but also quite risky. D would like to structure the acquisition in such a way that it does not expose its current business to the risks associated with T's operation. D may own as little or as much of T stock that it wants since there are no rules prohibiting an S corporation from owning the stock of a C corporation.

While S corporations may own stock of C corporations, the reverse is not allowed. As discussed below, S corporations generally are not allowed to have any corporate shareholders. However, an S corporation may own the stock of another corporation, and treat the wholly-owned corporation as a qualified subchapter S subsidiary (QSub).

Qualified Subchapter S Subsidiary (QSub). A QSub is a corporation that is 100 percent owned by an S corporation (i.e., the parent) that elects to treat the subsidiary as a QSub.[8] The QSub is a corporation that exists as a disregarded entity for Federal income tax purposes, but is a separate corporation for most other purposes. By electing to treat the subsidiary as a QSub, the parent corporation agrees to report all of the income and deductions of the QSub along with its own tax items. Note that if a parent S corporation acquires all of the stock of an existing corporation (C or S), it must treat the subsidiary as if it were liquidated for tax purposes when it elects QSub status for the subsidiary.[9] Alternately, the parent S corporation could treat the subsidiary corporation as a C corporation, regardless of the amount of stock it owned. To elect QSub status, the parent files the election on Form 8869. If the parent elects to treat the subsidiary as a QSub, the subsidiary's income and deductions are included in the parent company's tax return (Form 1120S). If the parent does not elect QSub status, the subsidiary's income and deductions should be reported separately on the subsidiary's Form 1120.

SHAREHOLDER REQUIREMENTS

Subchapter S imposes several restrictions on S corporation shareholders. Not only is the total number of shareholders limited to 100, but certain parties are prohibited from owning stock of the corporation.

Type of Shareholder. The stock of an S corporation may be owned only by:

1. Individuals who are citizens or resident aliens of the United States,

2. Estates,

---

[6]   Rev. Proc. 2004-48, 2004-32 I.R.B.

[7]   § 1504(b)(8).

[8]   § 1361(b)(3)(B).

[9]   Use Form 8869. The liquidation is nontaxable under §§ 332 and 337.

3. Certain trusts, and

4. Charitable organizations, pension trusts (not IRAs), and employee stock ownership plans.

Nonresident aliens (i.e., generally foreign citizens residing outside the United States), C corporations, other S corporations, partnerships, and most trusts are *not* allowed to hold stock in an S corporation.

Over the years, rules prohibiting trusts as shareholders have proved unduly inflexible, often intruding on sensible planning. This prohibition has been particularly troublesome in the estate and retirement planning area. For example, an individual may not want to leave the shares of his or her S corporation outright to a young child in his or her will but rather in trust for the benefit of a child. Without special rules, this obviously prudent action would be barred. Consequently, the current provisions allow some freedom in using trusts.

Eligible Trusts. The list of trusts that are eligible shareholders and a brief description of each follows below. In examining the list, note the concern for the shareholder limitation issue and how the shareholders are counted when an eligible trust holds shares.[10]

Grantor Trusts. A grantor trust is a trust that is disregarded under the trust taxation rules because of the power, control and benefits retained by the individual who established the trust (i.e., the grantor). All of the income of a grantor trust (e.g., a revocable trust that is used to avoid probate) is normally taxed to the grantor rather than the trust. If the grantor dies, the S shares normally have to be distributed to the beneficiaries within two years after the death. The grantor is treated as the shareholder for tax purposes. (See Chapter 26 for a discussion of these trusts.)

Beneficiary Controlled Trust or Deemed Grantor Trust. A deemed grantor trust is similar to the grantor trust, except the income of the trust is taxed to the beneficiary (rather than the grantor) because of the power that the beneficiary holds over trust property. The beneficiary is treated as the shareholder for tax purposes.

Qualified Subchapter S Trust (QSST). A QSST is a trust that has *only one* current income beneficiary (who must be a U.S. citizen or resident) to whom all of the income of the trust must be distributed annually and for which a proper election to be treated as a QSST has been filed in a timely manner. The trust's beneficiary (or legal guardian thereof) must file an election to include all of the trust's share of the S corporation's income, deductions and other tax items directly on the beneficiary's return as if he or she were the shareholder of the trust's stock. The beneficiary must file this election within two months and 16 days from the date the trust acquires the stock.[11] (If the trust owns shares on the date the corporation elects to become an S corporation, the beneficiary must file this election within two months and 16 days after the corporation files its S election. In practice the two elections are often made concurrently.) In addition to this election, there are certain other restrictions on the QSST.

The trust may not be able to distribute any of its income or property to any person other than the current income beneficiary during his or her lifetime. In addition, the trust must distribute (or be required to distribute) all of its income to this beneficiary annually. Note that failure to adhere to these rules properly results in the trust becoming an ineligible shareholder and thus causing loss of the S election.

---

[10]   § 1361(c)(2).

[11]   Inexplicably, this is one day longer than the grace period in which an S corporation has to file a timely S election.

In practice, the QSST election is often misunderstood. The result has been a multitude of private letter rulings allowing a corporation's S election to take effect, or continue in effect, after a trust has acquired the stock and the beneficiary has failed to make a timely QSST election. Accordingly, the IRS has issued an expedited relief rule for a QSST election that is no more than 24 months late.[12] A trust that qualifies for this provision applies to the IRS Center where the corporation files its returns. Thus it avoids the need for a ruling request and user fee. If the QSST election is not filed within the 24-month period, the corporation must apply for inadvertent termination or inadvertent invalid election relief. Relief is sought from the National Office of the IRS in the form of a letter ruling request, which must be accompanied by a user fee.

For all purposes of subchapter S, the beneficiary of the QSST is treated as the shareholder. This treatment applies to consents, allocations of income, other items, and the 100-shareholder limit.

Electing Small Business Trust (ESBT). In contrast to the QSST that has only a single beneficiary, an *ESBT* can have more than one potential current beneficiary (PCB). The trustee can have the right to accumulate or distribute income to any of the PCBs. The trustee must file a timely election for the trust to qualify. A price is paid for use of this trust since all of the income flowing from the S corporation to the trust is taxed to the trust itself (i.e., there is no deduction for distributions of the trust) and such income is taxed at the highest marginal rate (35 percent for ordinary income in 2008). In addition, the ESBT must pay tax on any capital gains in the same manner as an individual taxpayer who is in the highest marginal tax bracket. This rule applies both to any capital gains passing through from the S corporation to the trust and to any gain recognized by the trust on the disposition of the S corporation stock. However, a distribution from the trust to a beneficiary is tax-free to the beneficiary and is nondeductible to the trust. In counting shareholders, each PCB is considered to be a shareholder in the S corporation. Thus each PCB must be a U.S. citizen or resident. There may not be enough PCBs to cause the number of shareholders to exceed 100, although with the family attribution rules this situation is not likely to be a frequent cause of concern. However, for administrative purposes, such as consents to the corporation's various elections, the trustee is treated as the shareholder.

Testamentary Trusts. A testamentary trust is one that is created by the decedent's last will and testament. A testamentary trust may only be an eligible shareholder for two years unless it also qualifies under one of the other trust rules. The estate is treated as the owner of the stock in the case of one or more testamentary trusts that are established (e.g., if three trusts are created, the estate is considered the single owner).

Charitable Organizations, Pension Trusts, and Employee Stock Ownership Plans. For taxable years beginning after 1997, these organizations (generally tax-exempt) can be shareholders in S corporations. However, individual retirement accounts are not allowed to hold stock in an S corporation.[13]

Charitable organizations and pension trusts may find S corporations unappealing since they must include their share of income from the S corporation as unrelated business taxable income (UBTI). Thus these organizations would be subject to income tax on their income from the S corporation. However, the S corporation will usually make sufficient cash distributions to enable all shareholders to pay their income taxes on their portions of the S corporation's income. In contrast, these organizations are not subject to taxation on

---

[12] Rev. Proc. 2003-43, 2003-23 I.R.B. 998.

[13] There is an extremely narrow exception for certain IRAs that held stock in banking corporations on October 22, 2004. Under a special rule, these IRAs (and no others) are permitted shareholders. See §1361(c)(2)(A).

interest or dividend income derived from an investment in a C corporation. In addition, they are normally not taxable on gains from the disposition of stock or securities of a C corporation. However, gain from disposition of S corporation stock is UBTI to the charity. Employee Stock Ownership Plans (ESOPs) may also view investment in an S corporation unattractive since they may lose some special tax breaks to which they are entitled if they own stock in a C corporation. However, the combination of ESOP ownership and S corporation status may be quite attractive for a few corporations with broad-based participation in the ESOP.

Voting Trusts. A voting trust is a trust created primarily to hold the shares and exercise the voting power of the stock transferred to it. For a voting trust, each beneficiary is treated as a shareholder.

Number of Shareholders. As a general rule, a corporation does not qualify as an S corporation if the number of shareholders exceeds 100 at any moment during the taxable year. For purposes of counting the number of shareholders in an S corporation, members of a single family are subject to some rather broad attribution rules, which treat a family unit as a single shareholder. Specifically, the law permits six generations of descendants from common ancestors to elect to be treated as a single shareholder, but only for purposes of the shareholder count.[14] Moreover, the six generation limit applies only on the date the corporation files its S election or the date the first family member acquires stock in the corporation, whichever is later. Thereafter the number of generations is limitless. There is no requirement that members of each generation must be living. Thus it is possible to have extended generations of second, third and fourth cousins all be treated as one shareholder. A spouse (or former spouse) of any of the lineal family members is also included in this attribution. However, any of these individuals that holds stock at the time a corporation files an election for S status would have to consent to the election in his or her individual capacity. As a practical matter, few S corporations are troubled by this requirement.

When a permissible trust is a shareholder of the S corporation, the number of shareholders counted depends on the type of trust. As discussed above, all qualifying trusts, *except* ESBTs and voting trusts, represent one shareholder. For ESBTs and voting trusts, each beneficiary is counted as a shareholder.

When stock is held in the name of a nominee, agent, guardian, or custodian, the beneficial owner of the stock is treated as the shareholder.

Example 2. XYZ Bank and Trust, a corporation, holds legal title to stock in an S corporation. The XYZ corporation holds the stock for the benefit of R, a minor child. In this case, R, the beneficial owner, is treated as the shareholder rather than XYZ whether the trust qualifies as a QSST, an ESBT, or a deemed grantor trust. As a result, the S corporation is not denied the benefits of Subchapter S because of a corporate shareholder.

Example 3. F holds stock in an S corporation as custodian for his two minor children. For purposes of counting shareholders, F is ignored and the children are counted as two separate shareholders.

ONE CLASS OF STOCK

In order to minimize the problems of allocating income of the S corporation among shareholders, the corporation is allowed only one class of stock outstanding. Stock that is authorized but unissued does not invalidate the election. For example, an S corporation may have authorized but unissued preferred stock. Similarly, stock rights, options, or convertible debentures may be issued without affecting the election. A corporation that has

---

[14]   See §1361(c)(1) and §1361(c)(1)(B)(ii).

issued a second class of stock may qualify if the stock is reacquired and cancelled or held as Treasury stock.

Outstanding shares generally must provide identical distribution and liquidation rights to all shareholders. However, differences in *voting rights* are expressly authorized by the Code.[15] This exception enables control of the organization to be exercised in a manner that differs from stock ownership and income allocation.

> **Example 4.** R organized MND, an S corporation. MND issued two classes of common stock to R: class A voting and class B nonvoting stock. The rights represented by the stock are identical except for voting rights, and thus do not invalidate the S election. Shortly after the organization of the corporation, R gives the class B nonvoting stock to her two children. Although R has shifted income and future appreciation of the stock to her children (assuming certain other requirements are satisfied), she has retained all of the voting control of the corporation.

Debt as a Second Class of Stock. In the past, the second class of stock issue has arisen where the IRS or the courts have stepped in and reclassified an S corporation's debt as stock. Reclassification might occur when the corporation is thinly capitalized (e.g., the debt to equity ratio exceeds 4:1). If this were to happen to an S corporation, the result would be particularly disastrous since the S corporation might be considered as having two classes of stock, resulting in loss of its S election. To provide S corporations and their shareholders with some certainty in this area, Congress created a safe-harbor for debt meeting certain requirements. Under these rules, an S corporation's *straight debt* will not be classified as a second class of stock if:[16]

1. The interest rate and interest payment dates are not contingent on either the corporation's profits, management's discretion, or similar factors;

2. The debt instrument is written and cannot be converted into stock; and

3. The creditor is an individual, estate or trust, (but only if the trust is a grantor trust, QSST or ESBT) that is eligible to hold stock in an S corporation, or any person that is actively and regularly engaged in the business of lending money (e.g., a bank).

Straight debt is defined as any written unconditional promise to pay on demand, or on a specified date, a certain sum of money. Also included as straight debt are any short-term unwritten advances from a shareholder less than $10,000 in the aggregate—if treated as debt by the parties, and if expected to be repaid in a reasonable period of time.[17]

Whether an S corporation has more than one class of stock is determined by the corporate charter, articles of incorporation, bylaws, applicable state law, and binding agreements relating to distributions and liquidation. Unintended unequal distributions will generally not cause a second class of stock, unless they are pursuant to a plan to circumvent the one class of stock rule. The corporation must also correct the situation by making a catch-up distribution or taking some other action to place all shares on an equal footing. For example, excessive compensation paid to an owner-employee may be recharacterized as a distribution by the IRS. However, regulations for § 1361 hold that this type of distribution normally will not result in a second class of stock.[18] The Regulations also permit unequal distributions that occur in states that require the S corporation to withhold state taxes from distributions made to some or all of its shareholders, but only if there

---

[15]   § 1361(c)(4).

[16]   § 1361(c)(5).

[17]   Reg. 1.1361-1(l)(4)(ii)(B).

[18]   Reg. § 1.1361-1(1)(2)(vi), Example 3.

is a compensating distribution to shareholders who are not subject to the state withholding. Generally, the facts and circumstances of each situation will be considered.

ELECTION OF S CORPORATION STATUS

A corporation that qualifies as a small business corporation is taxed according to the rules of Subchapter S only if the corporation elects to be an S corporation. This election exempts the business from the corporate income tax and all other Federal income taxes normally imposed on corporations except for (1) the tax on excessive passive investment income, (2) the tax on built-in gains, and (3) the investment tax credit recapture tax, which may happen when the corporation has claimed a rehabilitation credit and then disposes of the rehabilitated property. The S corporation may also be required to pay a tax on LIFO recapture income, but that tax is part of the income tax imposed on a C corporation immediately before it converts to become an S corporation. In addition, the corporation is exempt from the personal holding company tax and the accumulated earnings tax. Although the S corporation generally avoids taxation as a regular corporation, most rules governing regular corporations such as those concerning organization, redemptions, and liquidations apply.

MAKING THE ELECTION: MANNER AND PERIOD OF EFFECT

In order for a corporation to be taxed according to the rules of Subchapter S, the corporation must file an election on Form 2553. The effective date of the election, as well as the required shareholder consents that must be evidenced on the form, generally depend on when the election is filed. The election must be filed with the IRS center where the S corporation files its tax returns.

Time of the Election. To be effective for the corporation's current taxable year, the election must be filed within two months and 15 days of the beginning of the corporation's taxable year.[19] Note that well-meaning shareholders or tax professionals trying to ensure a prompt election might file an election before the corporation has actually started its first taxable year. Unfortunately, an election cannot be made before the corporation is in existence and any election filed before such date would be invalid. Since the election must be filed in a particular time period—neither too early nor too late—the starting date is critical. For this purpose, the first taxable year starts on the earliest date that the corporation (1) issues shares; (2) acquires property; or (3) commences business.[20] Once the tax year begins, the election may be filed any time on or before the two months and 15 days deadline. For many years, there was no relief for taxpayers who filed a late election even if there were good reasons for the failure. However, the IRS is now allowed to treat a late election as being timely filed if there is reasonable cause.[21]

> **Example 5.** J and B decided to start a publishing corporation in 2008. The corporation issued shares on December 13, 2008 in exchange for $20,000. On January 15, 2009, the corporation opened a bank account and deposited the $20,000. On February 1, 2009, the corporation started operations. In this case, the corporation is considered to have started business on December 13, 2008 (the earliest of the dates that it issued shares, acquired property or commenced business). Consequently, the election is due on or before February 27, 2009 to be treated as timely filed. If the start date was

---

[19]   §§ 1362(b)(1)(B) and (b)(2) and Reg. § 1.1362-6(a)(2)(ii).

[20]   Reg. § 1.1362-6(a)(2)(ii)(c).

[21]   § 1362(b)(5).

May 1, the election is due on or before July 15. Note that in all of these examples, the third month and the start of the 15-day count begins on the same numerical day as the year began (i.e., February 13, July 1 plus 14 days yields the critical date).

If the corporation does not file a timely election or secure recognition of a late election, it will be considered a C corporation for the taxable year in question and the S election will be effective for the following tax year. Failure to make a timely election can be a crucial blunder. For instance, any losses that occurred during the C year would not flow through and any distributions could be treated as fully taxable dividends. However, since enactment of the legislation specifically enabling the acceptance of late elections, such mistakes have not been quite as costly.

Under current law, the IRS has been reasonable, if not outright lenient, in granting late elections. In 2003, the IRS authorized its Service Centers to accept S elections that are up to a year and six months late as long as the extended due date of the return for the first year of desired S status has not passed and the corporation states a "reasonable cause" for the lateness of the election.[22] The election must include the consent of every person who has been a shareholder from the first day of the first year for which the election is to be effective until the day the corporation files the election with the Service Center. Each shareholder must state that he or she has not filed a tax return that is inconsistent with the corporation's S status.

In 2007, the IRS issued Rev. Proc. 2007-62,[23] which adds to the possibilities for validating late S elections without resorting to a ruling request and user fee. This Revenue Procedure allows the corporation to file Form 2553 along with Form 1120S for the desired S year with the service center. To qualify, the corporation must not have already filed a tax return for the year, and there must be no violations of Subchapter S, except for the failure to file a timely Form 2553.

If the corporation has already filed Form 1120S for its first intended S year, it may file Form 2553 with the Service Center any time up to the day that the election is two years late. In this case all shareholders must state that they have filed returns that are consistent with the S election.

> **Example 6.** This year J and B formed a calendar year corporation on May 1, 2009. Unfortunately, J and B were unaware that they needed to file the S election by July 15 (i.e., two months and 15 days after May 1) and their error was not discovered until they visited an accountant in January 2010. Under the current approach, the IRS would accept an election up to September 15, 2010, the extended due date of the return for the first year it desired S status. If the corporation has not already filed its Form 1120S for 2009, it should file its Form 2553 and 1120S simultaneously. If the corporation has already filed Form 1120S, it may file Form 2553 with the Service Center on or before July 15, 2011 (two years after the due date). If the corporation does not meet these qualifications it must apply to the IRS National Office for relief. This request must be in the form of a letter ruling request and requires payment of the user fee.

If an S corporation does not meet these criteria and still wishes to validate a late election, it must apply to the National Office of the IRS for a private letter ruling—a process that can be a very costly (e.g., the IRS fee for the ruling, currently $11,500, plus the expense of the accounting or law firm that prepares the ruling request). The IRS frequently grants favorable rulings on these requests. The fee is reduced to $625 if the corporation has no more than $250,000 of gross receipts. If the corporation has between $250,000 and $1,000,000 gross receipts the fee is $2,100.[24]

---

[22]   Rev. Proc. 2003-43, 2003-23 I.R.B. 998.

[23]   Rev. Proc. 2007-62, 2007-41 I.R.B. 786.

[24]   See Rev. Proc. 2009-1, 2009-1 I.R.B. 1, Appendix A for the most recent schedule of user fees.

It should also be noted that the law instructs the IRS to accept a timely filed but defective election (e.g., second class of stock outstanding) if the reason for the defect is inadvertent. Inadvertence is a higher standard than reasonable cause and only the National Office of the IRS can approve a defective election.[25]

Shareholder Consent. In order for the election to be valid, the corporation must secure and file the consents of the shareholders along with the election. Consent to the election must be obtained not only from *all* shareholders holding stock (voting and nonvoting) at the time of election, but also from former shareholders who have held stock during the earlier portion of that taxable year.[26] The consent of former shareholders is required since they will be allocated a share of the income, losses, and other items applicable to the time they held the stock. The IRS may grant an extension for filing the consent for one or more shareholders if reasonable cause can be shown.[27] If a *former* shareholder will not or does not sign the consent, the election is effective for the following taxable year. Similarly, if the corporation fails to meet any of the Subchapter S requirements during the pre-election portion of the year, the election is effective for the following taxable year.

> **Example 7.** At the beginning of 2009, D, E, and F owned the stock of GHI Corporation, a calendar year taxpayer. On February 15, 2009, F sold all of her shares in GHI to C. On March 1, 2009 an S corporation election is desired. In order for the election to be effective for 2009, all shareholders on the date of election (C, D, and E), as well as any shareholders in the pre-election portion of the year (F), must consent. Failure to obtain F's consent would cause the election to become effective for 2010. Consent is required from both C and D even if they are family members and qualify as one shareholder for purposes of the maximum shareholder limit.

Election Effective for Subsequent Years. Elections made after the first two months and 15 days of the current taxable year are effective for the following taxable year.[28] When the election becomes effective in the following taxable year, only shareholders holding stock on the date of election must consent. The consent of shareholders who acquire stock after the election is not required.

> **Example 8.** On November 1, 2009, J Corporation filed an S election on Form 2553, including all of the shareholder consents. The election was to be effective for its next taxable year beginning on January 1, 2010. Unknowing to those handling the incorporation, one of the consenting shareholders, V, was a Canadian citizen, living in Vancouver. On December 15, 2009, the corporation discovered the problem and V agreed to sell all of his stock to one of the other shareholders. Since the corporation had a nonresident alien shareholder on the date that the election was filed, the election is not valid. The fact that the problem was corrected before the year in which the election was to be effective is irrelevant. Note, however, that if the corporation recognized the error, it could cure it by filing another Form 2553 by March 15, 2010. As an alternative, the corporation could file—at a cost—a ruling request asking the IRS to accept the inadvertently invalid election. Such requests are granted frequently.

---

[25] § 1362(f).

[26] §§ 1362(a)(2) and (b)(2)(B)(ii).

[27] Reg. § 1.1362-6(b)(3)(iii).

[28] § 1362(b)(3).

TERMINATION OF THE ELECTION

An election to be taxed as an S corporation is effective until it is terminated. The election may be terminated when the corporation:[29]

1. Revokes the election;

2. Fails to satisfy the requirements; or

3. Receives excessive passive income.

Revocation. The S corporation election may be revoked if shareholders holding a *majority* of the shares of stock (voting and nonvoting) consent.[30] A revocation filed by the fifteenth day of the third month of the taxable year (e.g., March 15 for a calendar year corporation) normally is effective for the current taxable year.[31] In contrast, if the revocation is filed after this two months and 15-day period has elapsed, it usually becomes effective for the following taxable year.[32] In both situations, however, a date on or after the date of revocation may be specified for the termination to become effective.[33]

> **Example 9.** A calendar year S corporation is owned equally by C, D, and E. On February 12, 2009, C and D consent to revoke the S corporation election. Since C and D own a majority of the outstanding shares of stock, the election is effective beginning on January 1, 2009, unless the revocation specifies February 12, 2009 or some later date.

> **Example 10.** Same as *Example 9* above except the revocation was made on May 3, 2009. The election is effective for the following taxable year beginning January 1, 2010. If the revocation had specified, however, that the termination was to become effective May 3, 2009, the S corporation year would end on May 2, 2009.

> **Example 11.** An S corporation has 100 shares of outstanding stock, 75 owned by J and 25 owned by B. On June 1 of this year, J sold 60 of her 75 shares to D. Since D owns a majority of the outstanding shares, he may cause the corporation to revoke the election, even if J and B are opposed to the revocation. However, the corporation must file the revocation. A statement filed by a shareholder is insufficient to revoke the election.

Failure to Meet the Eligibility Requirements. If the S corporation fails to satisfy any of the Subchapter S requirements at any time, the election is terminated on the date the disqualifying event occurs.[34] In such case, the corporation is treated as an S corporation for the period ending the day before the date of termination. This often causes the corporation to have two short taxable years: one as an S corporation and one as a C corporation. As a result, the corporation must allocate income and loss for the entire year between the two years. The tax returns for both the short S year and short C year are due two months and 15 days after the end of the C short year, and may be extended for an additional six months.[35]

---

[29] § 1362(d).

[30] § 1362(d)(1)(B).

[31] § 1362(d)(1)(C)(i).

[32] § 1362(d)(1)(C)(ii).

[33] § 1362(d)(1)(D).

[34] § 1362(d)(2).

[35] § 1362(e)(6)(B).

Example 12. C, D, and E own a calendar year S corporation. On June 3 of this year, E sold her stock to a corporation. The S corporation's year ends on June 2. The same result would be obtained if the sale had been to a partnership or to an individual who became the 101st shareholder. The S short year includes January 1 through June 2. The C short year is June 3 through December 31. Both returns are due on March 15 of the next year, although they may be extended to September 15.

Unless the S election termination occurs on the first day of the corporation's tax year, the termination year is split into two short periods. There are some special rules governing the allocation of income between the two short periods. The two methods that the corporation may use are the pro-rata allocation and the interim closing method.

Using the pro-rata method, each item required to be reported to the shareholders is assigned equally to each day in the entire tax year.[36] If the corporation uses the interim closing method it must separately account for activities during the S and C portions of the year.[37]

Example 13. On March 14, 2009, X Corporation terminates its S election. S uses the calendar year for tax purposes. Its income and loss items for 2009 occurred during the following periods.

	S Short Year	C Short Year	Total
Ordinary income	$80,000	$40,000	$120,000
Long-term capital gain	16,000	0	16,000
Dividend income (X holds 20% stock in payor)	0	5,000	5,000

If the corporation uses the interim closing method, it will report $80,000 of ordinary income and $16,000 of long-term capital gain to the shareholders, who will include these items on their 2009 tax returns. X would include $45,000 income, less a 70% dividends-received deduction of $3,500, on its Form 1120 for the C short year ending December 31, 2009. If the corporation pro rates all of the items, the allocation would be as follows:

	S Short Year (73/365)	C Short Year (292/365)	Total
Ordinary income	$24,000	$96,000	$120,000
Long-term capital gain	3,200	12,800	16,000
Dividend income	1,000	4,000	5,000

The corporation must use the pro-rata method unless it elects to use the interim closing, or there is a change of ownership of 50 percent or more of the corporation's shares within the S termination year.[38] The election is filed with the corporation's Form 1120 for the C short year. The election must be accompanied by consents of all persons who are shareholders at any time during the S short year, as well as all shareholders on the first day of the C short year.[39]

---

[36]   § 1362(e)(1).

[37]   § 1362(e)(3).

[38]   § 1362(e)(6)(D).

[39]   Reg. § 1.1362-6(a)(5).

The corporation must annualize its income and tax for the C short year. This is accomplished by grossing up the income as if it were earned ratably for a year of 365 days (366 in a leap year), and then apportioning the tax for the number of days in the C short year.

> **Example 14.** Refer to *Example 13*, above. Assume that the corporation elects to use the interim closing method. X would report the following annualized income and tax:

Ordinary income	$40,000
Dividend income	5,000
Less dividends received deduction	(3,500)
Taxable income	$41,500
Annualization	(365/292)
Annualized taxable income	$51,875
Tax on $51,875	$ 7,969
Annualization	(292/365)
Annualized tax	$ 6,375

When termination is *inadvertent*, the Code authorizes the IRS to allow a corporation to continue its S status uninterrupted if the disqualifying action is corrected.[40] It is possible, for example, that if stock is transferred to an ineligible shareholder, the IRS might allow the corporation to correct the violation and continue its S status uninterrupted. Inadvertent termination relief can only be granted to a corporation that applies to the IRS National Office and pays the user fee for a letter ruling.

> **Example 15.** On the advice of his attorney, a majority shareholder transferred his S corporation shares to an ineligible trust. Neither the attorney nor the shareholder were knowledgeable about the specific rules of Subchapter S. When the shareholder discovered the transfer terminated the S corporation election, the trust transferred the stock to the previous shareholder. The IRS has ruled, under similar circumstances, that the S election was not lost since the termination of the S status was inadvertent, it occurred as the result of advice from counsel, and it was corrected as soon as the violation of S status was discovered.[41]

The same inadvertent termination rules apply to defective (not late) S corporation elections. The corporation must apply for a ruling, disclosing the defect and agreeing to treat the corporation as an S corporation. All shareholders must sign the ruling request, under penalties of perjury. Any of the Subchapter S rules may be violated and cause termination or a defective election. However, a disproportionately high number of these violations have come from the failure to make timely QSST or ESBT elections. Accordingly the IRS has authorized the Service Centers to accept these elections up to two years late, in which case the corporation may avoid the ruling request and user fee.[42]

Excessive Passive Income. Without special rules relating to passive income, owners of C corporations might convert to S status to avoid problems they face as a C corporation. To illustrate, consider the retiring owner of a C corporation who causes the corporation to sell all of its operating assets. After paying the corporate level tax on the

---

[40]   § 1362(f).

[41]   Rev. Rul. 86-110, 1986-38 I.R.B. 4. Also, see Ltr. Ruls. 8550033 and 8608006.

[42]   Rev. Proc. 2003-43, 2003-23 I.R.B. 998.

sale, the owner could distribute the after tax proceeds in liquidation, resulting in yet a second tax at the shareholder level. The owner could then take what is left of the original sales price after paying two taxes (one by the C corporation and one by the shareholder on the liquidation) and invest it. Alternatively, the owner could opt not to liquidate and elect S status. Using this latter approach, the tax on the liquidation is avoided, the owner has more capital to invest, yet the investment income is taxed only once—the same as it would have been taxed if the owner held the investments personally. Moreover, the owner need not be concerned with the accumulated earnings tax or the personal holding company tax since these penalty taxes are reserved solely for C corporations. To foil this plan and others, Congress created two provisions that are triggered when evidence of this scheme are present. In short, if an S corporation has E&P accumulated while it was a C corporation (i.e., evidence of conversion) and too much passive income (i.e., investment income), the S corporation will have to pay a corporate level tax and could lose its S election. A later section examines the passive investment income tax.

Under the passive income test, the election is terminated if the corporation has:[43]

1. Passive investment income exceeding 25 percent of its gross receipts for three consecutive years, *and*

2. C corporation accumulated earnings and profits (AE&P) at the end of each of the three consecutive years.

If both of these conditions are satisfied, the termination becomes effective at the beginning of the first year following the end of the three-year period.[44]

As reflected in the second condition above, the excessive passive income test applies only to corporations that were C corporations prior to becoming S corporations. An S corporation might also have earnings and profits if it absorbed a former C corporation in a tax free reorganization, liquidation or QSub election. In addition, the test applies to these former C corporations only if they have AE&P from C years. Accordingly, corporations that have never been C corporations as well as corporations that have distributed all AE&P cannot lose their S election because of passive investment income.

Passive investment income generally is defined as gross receipts from royalties, rents, dividends, interest (including tax-exempt interest but excluding interest on notes from sales of inventory and interest derived from a lending business), annuities, and gains on sales or exchanges of stock or securities.[45] For this purpose, rents are not considered passive income if the corporation provides significant services (e.g., room rents paid to a hotel) or if the rents are received in the ordinary course of a rental business.[46] In computing total gross receipts, costs of goods sold, returns and allowances and deductions are ignored. Before 2007, receipts from the sale or exchange of stocks and securities were included to the extent of gains [i.e., gross receipts = amount realized − adjusted basis = gain (but not loss)]. In contrast, receipts from the sale or exchange of capital assets other than stocks and securities are included only to the extent of net gains (i.e., capital gains less capital losses).[47]

> **Example 16.** OBJ, an S corporation, was a C corporation for several years before it elected to be taxed under Subchapter S beginning in 2008. For 2008 and 2009 the corporation had excessive passive income. In addition, at the close of 2008 and 2009, OBJ reported a balance in its AE&P that was attributable to its years as a

---

[43]   § 1362(d)(3).

[44]   § 1362(d)(3)(A)(ii).

[45]   § 1362(d)(3)(D).

[46]   Reg. § 1.1362-2(c)(5)(ii)(B)(2).

[47]   §§ 1362(d)(3)(C) and 1222(9).

C corporation. OBJ's income and expenses for 2010 are shown below. No distributions from its AE&P were made during the year. The corporation's passive investment income and total gross receipts, based on its reported items, are determined as follows:

	Reported	Gross Receipts	Passive Income
Sales................................	$200,000	$200,000	$ 0
Cost of goods sold......................	(150,000)	0	0
Interest income	30,000	30,000	30,000
Dividends.............................	15,000	15,000	15,000
Rental income (passive).................	40,000	40,000	40,000
Rental expenses	(28,000)	0	0
Gain on sale of stock ($20,000 − $5,000)....	15,000	15,000	0
Loss on sale of stock ($10,000 − $12,000) ..	(2,000)	0	0
Total...........................		$300,000	$85,000
25% of gross receipts		$ 75,000	

Because OBJ's passive investment income exceeds 25% of its gross receipts for the third consecutive year and it also has a balance of AE&P at the end of each of those years, the election is terminated beginning on January 1, 2011.

Even though a corporation may avoid having its election terminated by failing the excessive passive income test once every three years, a corporation still may be required to pay a tax on its excessive passive investment income. This tax is explained in detail later in this chapter.

ELECTION AFTER TERMINATION

When the election is terminated, whether voluntarily through revocation or involuntarily through failure to satisfy the Subchapter S or passive income requirements, the corporation normally may not make a new election until the fifth taxable year following the year in which the termination became effective.[48] The five-year wait is unnecessary, however, if the IRS consents to an earlier election. Consent usually is given in two instances: (1) when the corporation's ownership has changed such that more than 50 percent of the stock is owned by persons who did not own the stock at the time of termination, or (2) when the termination was attributable to an event that was not within the control of the corporation or its majority shareholders.[49] A corporation must apply to the IRS National Office for an early re-election. It must request a ruling and pay the user fee.

Example 17. KLZ, an S corporation, was wholly owned by G. The corporation revoked its S election effective on July 17, 2007. KLZ may not make an election until 2012 unless it obtains permission from the IRS. Permission to reelect S status prior to 2012 would ordinarily be denied unless persons other than G acquired more than 50% of the KLZ stock.

---

[48] § 1362(g).

[49] Reg. § 1.1362-5(a).

OPERATING THE S CORPORATION

Once an S election is effective, a corporation officially becomes an S corporation and is subject to a special set of rules governing the measurement and reporting of its income. Under the provisions of Subchapter S, S corporations, like partnerships, are pass-through entities. While S corporations may pay taxes in certain situations (e.g., the passive investment income tax or the built-in gains tax discussed below), they primarily serve as conduits. Items of income, expense, gain, loss, and credit are measured at the S corporation level and then passed through to shareholders who report them on their own returns.[50] The focus of this section is on three questions:

- ► What items at the corporate level must be reported to the shareholder?
- ► How much of each item is reported to each shareholder?
- ► When does the shareholder report the items on his or her own tax return?

DETERMINING S CORPORATION NET INCOME

S corporations generally compute net income, gains, and losses in a manner similar to a partnership. The following discussion examines some of the more important aspects that should be considered in measuring S corporation income, particularly the differences between S corporations and partnerships.

Elections. Consistent with the partnership provisions, most special elections that must be made in determining the amount of income are made at the S corporation level and not by the shareholder.[51] Among the elections that must be made by the corporation are the corporation's overall method of accounting (e.g., cash or accrual), the inventory method (e.g., FIFO or LIFO), depreciation methods, § 179 limited expensing, the installment method (election out), and deferral of gain on involuntary conversions. The exceptions to this general approach are the same as those for partnerships and affect few taxpayers.

Payments to a Shareholder-Employee. The treatment of payments to an S shareholder who works for the corporation is markedly different from that of a partner who works for the partnership. S corporation shareholders who work for the corporation are treated as *employees*. As a result, salary paid to a shareholder-employee as well as payroll taxes related to the salary are deductible by the S corporation. In contrast, a partner who works for a partnership is not considered an employee and the payment received for work for the partnership is not technically considered a salary. As discussed in Chapter 22, compensation paid to partners is referred to as a guaranteed payment. Like salaries, partnerships normally deduct guaranteed payments. However, unlike salaries, guaranteed payments are not subject to withholding or payroll taxes.[52] Instead, a partner's compensation is treated as self-employment income.

> **Example 18.** H and W own their own company. This year the company made net income of $60,000 before consideration of any payments to H and W. Assume that H and W each receive a salary of $10,000 for total salary payments of $20,000. If the business is an S or C corporation, the salary is subject to withholding taxes and the

---

[50]   § 1366(a).

[51]   § 1363(c).

[52]   Reg. § 1.707-1(c), Rev. Rul. 56-675, 1956-2 CB 459 and Rev. Rul. 69-180, 1969-1 CB 256.

corporation must pay FICA and unemployment taxes on it. If, however, the business is a partnership, there are no payroll taxes for owner compensation and partnership net income is $40,000 ($60,000 − $20,000), which is usually self-employment income and is subject to self-employment tax at the partner level. In addition, the salaries of $20,000 (i.e., guaranteed payments in the context of a partnership) would be subject to self-employment taxes.

A comparison of the two business forms reveals the following:

	Partnership	S Corporation
Net income before compensation	$60,000	$60,000
Guaranteed payment or salary	(20,000)	(20,000)
Employer FICA tax (7.65% × $20,000).	0	(1,530)
Federal unemployment tax (6.2% × $7,000 × 2).	0	(868)
Flow-through income	$40,000	$37,602
Add guaranteed payment or salary	20,000	20,000
Withheld FICA tax (7.65% × $20,000)		(1,530)
Self-employment tax (15.3% × $60,000 × .9235)	(8,478)*	0
Net income after taxes	$51,522	$56,072

* The partner claims a deduction for 50% of these taxes.

As this example demonstrates, the S corporation is preferred to the partnership if capital is to be retained in the business. This derives from the fact that the partners are subject to self-employment tax on their portions of partnership income, whether or not it is distributed. The S corporation and its shareholders, by contrast, are only subject to the FICA tax on money actually distributed to the shareholders as compensation.

Employment Taxes and Undercompensation. It is important to note that, unlike partnerships, no self-employment income passes from an S corporation to its shareholders. In the S corporation setting, the only amounts subject to employment taxes are the salaries paid. In light of this treatment, owners of S corporations are tempted to undercompensate themselves in order to avoid social security and other payroll taxes. To illustrate, consider the example above. In this situation, the owners took only $20,000 in salary, paying employment taxes of $3,928 ($1,530 + $1,530 + $868). This is far less than the $8,478 in self-employment tax that the owners would pay if they were partners in a partnership even though the amounts paid in both cases were identical ($20,000). The difference is due to the fact that the net income of the S corporation, $37,602, is not subject to employment taxes. However, there is another mitigating factor that reduces this difference. Each partner is allowed a deduction for A.G.I. for one-half of the self-employment tax paid on partnership income. Indeed, it would appear that the owners could avoid all employment taxes using an S corporation by not paying themselves any salary but simply distributing the profits. As might be expected, the IRS, with the support of the courts, frowns on this technique. In situations when this occurs, that is, when shareholders are undercompensated for their services, the Service generally recharacterizes all or a part of any distributions as compensation thereby securing the applicable payroll taxes.[53]

Social Security Benefit Cutback. With the graying of America, the treatment of payments to S corporation owners is also becoming an increasingly important issue for social security purposes. An individual who retires before "normal" retirement age, must

---

53 See Rev. Rul. 74-44, 1974-1 C.B. 287, *Radtke v. U.S.*, 90-1 USTC ¶50,113 and *Spicer Accounting, Inc., v. U. S.*, 918 F.2d 90 (CA-9, 1990).

reduce his or her social security benefits if he or she earns income above a certain level. In 2009, the *normal retirement* age is 66 years of age. A person who is at least 62 but has not reached normal retirement age by the end of 2009 will be required to reduce his or her social security benefit by $1 for each $2 of earned income in excess of $14,160. After normal retirement age, an individual may receive full social security benefits regardless of the amount of earned income. For this reason, some owners of S corporations are tempted to take distributions from an S corporation rather than salary for services rendered. In a number of cases involving such attempts, however, the courts have upheld the Social Security Administration's bid to reclassify the distributions as wages.[54]

Employee Benefits. One of the most important differences concerning the taxation of C corporations, partnerships, and S corporations is the treatment of fringe benefits provided to the owners (e.g., health and accident insurance, group-term life insurance). The taxation of a number of these benefits depends on whether the individual is an "employee" of the business. If the individual is an employee, the employer normally is allowed to deduct the cost of the benefit and its value is never subject to income or employment taxes. On the other hand, if the individual is not an employee, the benefit is usually considered compensation deductible by the employer but is subject to income and employment taxes to the payees.

It is not always clear as to whether or not a self-employed person is considered an "employee" for fringe benefit purposes. In the case of C corporations, an owner who works for the business is considered an employee. Therefore, shareholder-employees of C corporations enjoy the best of all possible worlds: the corporation is allowed to deduct the cost of these benefits yet their value to the shareholder-employees is never subject to income or employment taxes. In contrast, a partner (much like a sole proprietor) is normally not considered an employee of the business. Consequently, several of the key fringe benefits provided by partnerships to their partners are considered compensation (i.e., guaranteed payments) that are deductible by the partnership but subject to income and self-employment taxes to the partners. Unfortunately, the treatment of these key fringe benefits by an S corporation for the most part mirrors that for partnerships rather than that for C corporations.[55]

In determining the treatment extended to S corporations, shareholder-employees are divided into two groups: those who own more than 2 percent of the stock and those who own 2 percent or less.[56] The treatment for the two groups is summarized below.

Shareholders Owning 2 Percent or Less. For those S shareholders who own 2 percent or less, the treatment follows the C corporation rules: the benefits are deductible by the corporation and nontaxable (both income and employment) to the employee.

Shareholders Owning More than 2 Percent. More-than-2 percent shareholders are treated much like partners.[57] The fringe benefits requiring employee status are considered compensation: the benefits are deductible by the corporation but are included in the shareholder's gross income.[58] Unlike a partnership where these benefits are subject to self-employment tax, the value of health insurance provided to an S corporation employee is not subject to FICA or FUTA.[59] Note also that while the more-than-2

[54] *Ludeking v. Finch*, 421 F.2d 499 (CA-8, 1970).

[55] § 1372(a)(1) and (2).

[56] § 1372(a) and (b).

[57] § 1372(a)(2).

[58] Rev. Rul. 91-26, 1991-1 C.B. 184, § 162(a) (subject to the capitalization rules of § 263), and § 61(a), respectively.

[59] Announcement 92-16, 1992-5 I.R.B. 53.

percent shareholder is required to include the benefit in income, he or she is also entitled to treat such amount as if he or she paid for the benefit. For example, in the case of medical insurance premiums paid by the S corporation on behalf of a more-than-2-percent shareholder, the shareholder is entitled to deduct 100 percent of the premiums as a deduction for A.G.I.[60]

In determining whether an individual owns more than 2 percent of an S corporation's stock, the constructive ownership rules of § 318 are applied.[61] For example, § 318 provides that an individual is deemed to own the stock of his or her spouse, children, parents or grandchildren. This rule prevents an owner (e.g., a husband) from employing a family member that does not own stock (e.g., a wife) in order to provide tax-free fringe benefits from the corporation to the family unit.

There are currently six fringe benefits which are nontaxable to owners of C corporations but which are treated as compensation to partners and more-than-2 percent shareholders. They are:

- ▸ Group-term life insurance (§ 79)
- ▸ Amounts received under accident and health (medical reimbursement) plans (§ 105)
- ▸ Premiums on employer-paid accident and health insurance (§ 106)
- ▸ Meals and lodging provided by the employer (§ 119)
- ▸ Value of transit passes (but this qualifies as a de minimis fringe if not greater than $21 per month) [§ 132(f)(5)(E)]
- ▸ Parking provided by the employer (except that provided away from the business such as at a client's) [§ 132(f)(5)(E)]

The value of all of these is included in the shareholder-employee's Form W-2 as noncash compensation. Premiums on accident and health insurance are not subject to FICA tax.

The remaining fringe benefits are eligible for exclusion not only by shareholder-employees of C corporations but also to partners and, therefore, more-than-2 percent shareholders of S corporations. In effect, the statutes governing these particular benefits specifically explain that, for purpose of the given exclusion, partners are considered employees, thereby enabling exclusion not only for partners but also all S corporation shareholders. These include:

- ▸ Child and dependent care assistance (§ 129)
- ▸ Educational assistance plans (§ 127)
- ▸ No additional cost services [§ 132(b)]
- ▸ Qualified employee discounts [§ 132(c)]
- ▸ Working condition fringe benefits [§ 132(d)]
- ▸ De minimis fringes [§ 132(e)]
- ▸ Company dining room [§132(e)]
- ▸ On-premise athletic facilities [§132(h)]
- ▸ Employee achievement awards [§74(c)]

Subdivision of Real Estate. Under the "subdivide and conquer" rules of § 1237, *individual* taxpayers are ensured capital gain rather than ordinary income treatment when they subdivide and sell land if they meet a number of requirements. To qualify, the land must be held more than five years (unless inherited); there must be no substantial improvements to the property; and the parcel sold, or any part thereof must not have

---

60   §§ 162(l) and 106, respectively.

61   § 1372(b). See Chapter 20 for discussion of § 318.

previously been held by the taxpayer primarily for resale. An S corporation (as well as a partnership) is treated in the same manner as an individual and is entitled to this special treatment.[62]

Section 291 Recapture. In most cases, an S corporation is not subject to the special rules of § 291 that require the recapture as ordinary income 20 percent of any straight-line depreciation claimed on residential or nonresidential real estate (see Chapter 19 for an example). However, an S corporation that was a C corporation for any of the three immediately preceding taxable years is subject to the special depreciation recapture rules of § 291(a)(1).[63]

Accounting Methods. Certain entities are prohibited from using the cash method of accounting, and consequently are required to use the accrual method. The cash method normally cannot be used by a C corporation unless its annual gross receipts average $5 million or less for the past three years, or it is a qualified personal service corporation. In contrast, an S corporation can use the cash method (unless it is required to maintain inventories to clearly reflect income).[64]

Charitable Contributions. Charitable contributions made by an S corporation are treated as if they are made directly by the shareholder. Consequently, unlike C corporations, an S corporation that uses the accrual method of accounting is not entitled to deduct accrued contributions.[65] Like an individual, contributions made by an S corporation can be deducted by the shareholders only in the tax year in which the contribution is made. Similarly, the special rule allowing C corporations to deduct the adjusted basis plus one-half of the foregone gross profit of inventory contributed to a organization for the care of the needy, the ill, or infants is not available to S corporations, except for the temporary allowance for all taxpayers as a result of the Katrina relief legislation.[66]

Qualified Production Activities Income Deduction. The deduction for Qualified Production Activities Income (QPAI) is allowed to all tax entities. However, for the S corporation, this deduction is to be computed at the shareholder level.[67]

REPORTING S CORPORATION INCOME

Once an S corporation identifies and measures the relevant items of income, deduction and credit, such items must be passed through to the shareholders for reporting on their own returns. The approach used is similar to that used by partnerships. Consistent with the conduit concept, the items normally retain their character when they are allocated to the shareholders. For example, charitable contributions made by the S corporation flow through and are reported as charitable contributions by the shareholders subject to all the special tax rules that apply to individuals. The amounts allocated to the shareholders are based on their percentage of stock owned during the year. Unlike partnerships, Subchapter S contains no provision for special allocations among owners. This can be a disadvantage if special allocations are desirable.

---

[62] § 1237(a).

[63] See § 1363(b)(4).

[64] § 448. However, see Rev. Proc. 2001-10, which allows any taxpayer with no more than $1 million gross receipts to use the cash method. Also see Rev. Proc. 2002-28, which allows certain taxpayers with up to $10 million gross receipts to use the cash method.

[65] See § 1363, which incorporates the rules of § 702 that disallow the deduction of charitable contributions to partnerships.

[66] § 170(e)(3)(A). Also see Rev. Rul. 2000-43, 2000-41 I.R.B. 333.

[67] §199(d)(1).

To accomplish the pass-through, the S corporation must file an annual information return, Form 1120S. Indeed, the similarity between the taxation of S corporations and partnerships becomes readily apparent when Forms 1120S and 1065 are compared. (See Exhibit 23-1 for an illustration of Form 1120S.) There are some differences in computing the net ordinary income on page one of the two tax forms, however. Unlike Form 1065, Form 1120S has a section for computing any taxes due on excessive passive investment income and Schedule D built-in gains (both are discussed in a later section of this chapter).

All income, expenses, gains, losses, and credits that may be subject to special treatment by one or more of the shareholders are reported separately on Schedule K, which is filed with Form 1120S.[68] Schedule K-1 is then prepared for the shareholders' use. (See Exhibit 23-1 for an illustration. Also see Exhibit 23-2 for a summary of items.) Again, these schedules are quite similar to the schedules applicable to partnerships and partners. There are differences, including the following:

- ▸ There are no guaranteed payments on the S corporation schedule.
- ▸ There is no self-employment income on the S corporation schedule.
- ▸ There are no reconciliations of capital accounts on the S corporation schedule.
- ▸ There is no allocation of liabilities on the S corporation schedule.

Finally, the S corporation schedule includes a section for reporting distributions. These are divided into two categories: (1) distributions from earnings of the S corporation, and (2) if it has been operated as a C corporation in previous years, distributions from earnings of the C corporation. (Distributions are discussed in a later section of this chapter.)

Filing Requirements. Form 1120S, with the attached Schedule K-1s, must be filed for the S corporation on or before the 15th day of the third month following the close of its taxable year. An automatic extension of six months may be obtained. Thus a calendar year S corporation's normal due date is March 15 but may be extended until September 15. In order to obtain the extension, the corporation must file Form 7004 on or before March 15 (or two months and 15 days after the close of the corporation's fiscal year). In contrast, partnership returns are due on the 15th day of the fourth month following the close of the taxable year (e.g., April 15 for a calendar year partnership). So even though an S corporation is treated much like a partnership, its return is due at the same time as a C corporation return.

In addition to attaching the Schedule K-1s to Form 1120S, the S corporation is required to provide shareholders with Schedule K-1 by the due date of the return. The shareholder need not attach the K-1 to his or her Form 1040.

---

[68] § 1366(a)(1)(A).

EXHIBIT 23-1
Forms 1120S

Form **1120S**	**U.S. Income Tax Return for an S Corporation**	OMB No. 1545-0130
Department of the Treasury Internal Revenue Service	► Do not file this form unless the corporation has filed or is attaching Form 2553 to elect to be an S corporation. ► See separate instructions.	**2008**

For calendar year 2008 or tax year beginning , 2008, ending , 20

A S election effective date *1-1-08*	Use IRS label. Other-wise, print or type.	Name *T COMPANY*	**D** Employer identification number *88 : 9138761*
B Business activity code number *(see instructions)* *448110*		Number, street, and room or suite no. If a P.O. box, see instructions. *8122 SOUTH 8TH STREET*	**E** Date incorporated *1-1-08*
C Check if Sch. M-3 attached ☐		City or town, state, and ZIP code *NORFORLK, VA 23508*	**F** Total assets *(see instructions)* $ *322,000*

G Is the corporation electing to be an S corporation beginning with this tax year? ☑ Yes ☐ No If "Yes," attach Form 2553 if not already filed

H Check if: **(1)** ☐ Final return **(2)** ☐ Name change **(3)** ☐ Address change

(4) ☐ Amended return **(5)** ☐ S election termination or revocation

I Enter the number of shareholders who were shareholders during any part of the tax year . . . . ► *1*

Caution. *Include only trade or business income and expenses on lines 1a through 21. See the instructions for more information.*

Income

1a Gross receipts or sales *470,000* **b** Less returns and allowances *-0-* **c** Bal ►		**1c**	*470,000*
2 Cost of goods sold (Schedule A, line 8)		**2**	*300,000*
3 Gross profit. Subtract line 2 from line 1c		**3**	*170,000*
4 Net gain (loss) from Form 4797, Part II, line 17 (attach Form 4797)		**4**	
5 Other income (loss) (see instructions—attach statement)		**5**	
6 **Total income (loss).** Add lines 3 through 5. . . . . . . ►		**6**	*170,000*

Deductions (see instructions for limitations)

7 Compensation of officers *$ 24,000 + $ 700 EMPLOYEE BENEFITS*		**7**	*24,700*
8 Salaries and wages (less employment credits)		**8**	*48,000*
9 Repairs and maintenance		**9**	*12,000*
10 Bad debts		**10**	
11 Rents		**11**	
12 Taxes and licenses *$ 3,000 PROPERTY TAXES + $ 6,000 PAYROLL TAXES*		**12**	*9,000*
13 Interest		**13**	*3,300*
14 Depreciation not claimed on Schedule A or elsewhere on return (attach Form 4562) . . .		**14**	*15,000*
15 Depletion **(Do not deduct oil and gas depletion.)**		**15**	
16 Advertising		**16**	
17 Pension, profit-sharing, etc., plans		**17**	
18 Employee benefit programs. *LIFE INSURANCE COVERAGE* . . .		**18**	*1,400*
19 Other deductions (attach statement) *$ 2,500 UTILITIES & PHONE + $ 1,100 OFFICE EXPENSE*		**19**	*6,700*
20 **Total deductions.** Add lines 7 through 19 *+ $ 3,100 INSURANCE EXPENSE* . . . ►		**20**	*120,000*
21 **Ordinary business income (loss).** Subtract line 20 from line 6		**21**	*49,900*

Tax and Payments

22a Excess net passive income or LIFO recapture tax (see instructions) .	**22a**		
b Tax from Schedule D (Form 1120S)	**22b**		
c Add lines 22a and 22b (see instructions for additional taxes) . .		**22c**	*NONE*
23a 2008 estimated tax payments and 2007 overpayment credited to 2008	**23a**		
b Tax deposited with Form 7004	**23b**		
c Credit for federal tax paid on fuels (attach Form 4136) . . .	**23c**		
d Add lines 23a through 23c		**23d**	*NONE*
24 Estimated tax penalty (see instructions). Check if Form 2220 is attached . . . . ► ☐		**24**	
25 **Amount owed.** If line 23d is smaller than the total of lines 22c and 24, enter amount owed .		**25**	*NONE*
26 **Overpayment.** If line 23d is larger than the total of lines 22c and 24, enter amount overpaid .		**26**	
27 Enter amount from line 26 **Credited to 2009 estimated tax** ► Refunded ►		**27**	*NONE*

Sign Here ► *adolph Z.T* Signature of officer | *3-10-09* Date ► | *PRESIDENT* Title |

Under penalties of perjury, I declare that I have examined this return, including accompanying schedules and statements, and to the best of my knowledge and belief, it is true, correct, and complete. Declaration of preparer (other than taxpayer) is based on all information of which preparer has any knowledge.

May the IRS discuss this return with the preparer shown below (see instructions)? ☐ Yes ☐ No

Paid Preparer's Use Only	Preparer's signature ►	Date	Check if self-employed ☐	Preparer's SSN or PTIN
	Firm's name (or yours if self-employed), address, and ZIP code ►		EIN	
			Phone no. ( )	

For Privacy Act and Paperwork Reduction Act Notice, see separate instructions. Cat. No. 11510H Form **1120S** (2008)

EXHIBIT 23-1

Continued

Form 1120S (2008)   Page **2**

Schedule A   Cost of Goods Sold (see instructions)

1	Inventory at beginning of year	1	12,000
2	Purchases	2	302,000
3	Cost of labor	3	
4	Additional section 263A costs (attach statement)	4	
5	Other costs (attach statement)	5	
6	**Total.** Add lines 1 through 5	6	314,000
7	Inventory at end of year	7	14,000
8	**Cost of goods sold.** Subtract line 7 from line 6. Enter here and on page 1, line 2	8	

9a Check all methods used for valuing closing inventory: (i) ☐ Cost as described in Regulations section 1.471-3

    (ii) ☑ Lower of cost or market as described in Regulations section 1.471-4

    (iii) ☐ Other (Specify method used and attach explanation.) ▶ ---

  b Check if there was a writedown of subnormal goods as described in Regulations section 1.471-2(c) . . . . . . ▶ ☐

  c Check if the LIFO inventory method was adopted this tax year for any goods (if checked, attach Form 970) . . . . ▶ ☐

  d If the LIFO inventory method was used for this tax year, enter percentage (or amounts) of closing
inventory computed under LIFO . . . . | **9d** | |

  e If property is produced or acquired for resale, do the rules of section 263A apply to the corporation? . . . ☐ Yes ☑ No

  f Was there any change in determining quantities, cost, or valuations between opening and closing inventory? . ☐ Yes ☑ No
If "Yes," attach explanation.

Schedule B   Other Information (see instructions) | Yes | No

1 Check accounting method: **a** ☐ Cash   **b** ☑ Accrual   **c** ☐ Other (specify) ▶ ----------------------

2 See the instructions and enter the:
  a Business activity ▶ ____*RETAIL SALES*____   **b** Product or service ▶ *MEN'S CLOTHING*

3 At the end of the tax year, did the corporation own, directly or indirectly, 50% or more of the voting stock of a domestic
corporation? (For rules of attribution, see section 267(c).) If "Yes," attach a statement showing: **(a)** name and employer
identification number (EIN), **(b)** percentage owned, and **(c)** if 100% owned, was a QSub election made? . . . | | ✓ |

4 Has this corporation filed, or is it required to file, a return under section 6111 to provide information on any reportable
transaction? . . . . | | ✓ |

5 Check this box if the corporation issued publicly offered debt instruments with original issue discount . ▶ ☐
If checked, the corporation may have to file **Form 8281,** Information Return for Publicly Offered Original Issue Discount
Instruments.

6 If the corporation: **(a)** was a C corporation before it elected to be an S corporation **or** the corporation acquired an
asset with a basis determined by reference to its basis (or the basis of any other property) in the hands of a
C corporation **and (b)** has net unrealized built-in gain (defined in section 1374(d)(1)) in excess of the net recognized
built-in gain from prior years, enter the net unrealized built-in gain reduced by net recognized built-in gain from prior
years . . . . ▶ $ ----------------------------

7 Enter the accumulated earnings and profits of the corporation at the end of the tax year. $_____

8 Are the corporation's total receipts (see instructions) for the tax year **and** its total assets at the end of the tax year
less than $250,000? If "Yes," the corporation is not required to complete Schedules L and M-1 . . . . | | ✓ |

Schedule K   Shareholders' Pro Rata Share Items | | Total amount |

	1	Ordinary business income (loss) (page 1, line 21)			1	49,900
	2	Net rental real estate income (loss) (attach Form 8825)			2	
	3a	Other gross rental income (loss)	3a			
	b	Expenses from other rental activities (attach statement)	3b			
Income (Loss)	c	Other net rental income (loss). Subtract line 3b from line 3a			3c	
	4	Interest income			4	
	5	Dividends: **a** Ordinary dividends			5a	2,000
		b Qualified dividends	5b	2,000		
	6	Royalties			6	
	7	Net short-term capital gain (loss) (attach Schedule D (Form 1120S))			7	
	8a	Net long-term capital gain (loss) (attach Schedule D (Form 1120S))			8a	1,000
	b	Collectibles (28%) gain (loss)	8b			
	c	Unrecaptured section 1250 gain (attach statement)	8c			
	9	Net section 1231 gain (loss) (attach Form 4797)			9	
	10	Other income (loss) (see instructions) . . Type ▶			10	

Form **1120S** (2008)

EXHIBIT 23-1

Continued

Form 1120S (2008)

Page **3**

	Shareholders' Pro Rata Share Items (continued)		Total amount	
Deductions	**11** Section 179 deduction *(attach Form 4562)*	**11**	*7,000*	
	12a Contributions	**12a**		
	b Investment interest expense	**12b**		
	c Section 59(e)(2) expenditures **(1)** Type ▶_____ **(2)** Amount ▶	**12c(2)**		
	d Other deductions *(see instructions)* . . . Type ▶	**12d**		
Credits	**13a** Low-income housing credit (section 42(j)(5))	**13a**		
	b Low-income housing credit (other)	**13b**		
	c Qualified rehabilitation expenditures (rental real estate) *(attach Form 3468)*	**13c**		
	d Other rental real estate credits *(see instructions)* Type ▶ _____	**13d**		
	e Other rental credits *(see instructions)* . . Type ▶ _____	**13e**		
	f Alcohol and cellulosic biofuel fuels credit *(attach Form 6478)*	**13f**		
	g Other credits *(see instructions)* . . . . . Type ▶*REHABILITATION CRERDIT*	**13g**	*2,000*	
Foreign Transactions	**14a** Name of country or U.S. possession ▶_____			
	b Gross income from all sources	**14b**		
	c Gross income sourced at shareholder level	**14c**		
	Foreign gross income sourced at corporate level			
	d Passive category	**14d**		
	e General category	**14e**		
	f Other *(attach statement)*	**14f**		
	Deductions allocated and apportioned at shareholder level			
	g Interest expense	**14g**		
	h Other	**14h**		
	Deductions allocated and apportioned at corporate level to foreign source income			
	i Passive category	**14i**		
	j General category	**14j**		
	k Other *(attach statement)*	**14k**		
	Other information			
	l Total foreign taxes (check one): ▶ ☐ Paid ☐ Accrued	**14l**		
	m Reduction in taxes available for credit *(attach statement)*	**14m**		
	n Other foreign tax information *(attach statement)*			
Alternative Minimum Tax (AMT) Items	**15a** Post-1986 depreciation adjustment	**15a**		
	b Adjusted gain or loss	**15b**		
	c Depletion (other than oil and gas)	**15c**		
	d Oil, gas, and geothermal properties—gross income	**15d**		
	e Oil, gas, and geothermal properties—deductions.	**15e**		
	f Other AMT items *(attach statement)*	**15f**		
Items Affecting Shareholder Basis	**16a** Tax-exempt interest income	**16a**		
	b Other tax-exempt income	**16b**		
	c Nondeductible expenses	**16c**		
	d Property distributions *LAND: FMV = $ 10,000 + $ 12,000 CASH*	**16d**	*22,000*	
	e Repayment of loans from shareholders	**16e**		
Other Information	**17a** Investment income *DIVIDENDS*	**17a**	*2,000*	
	b Investment expenses	**17b**		
	c Dividend distributions paid from accumulated earnings and profits	**17c**		
	d Other items and amounts *(attach statement)*			
Reconciliation	**18** **Income/loss reconciliation.** Combine the amounts on lines 1 through 10 in the far right column. From the result, subtract the sum of the amounts on lines 11 through 12d and 14l .	**18**	*45,900*	

Form **1120S** (2008)

EXHIBIT 23-1

Continued

Form 1120S (2008)   Page **4**

Schedule L — Balance Sheets per Books

		Beginning of tax year		End of tax year	
	Assets	**(a)**	**(b)**	**(c)**	**(d)**
1	Cash				
2a	Trade notes and accounts receivable				
b	Less allowance for bad debts	( )		( )	
3	Inventories				
4	U.S. government obligations				
5	Tax-exempt securities (see instructions)				
6	Other current assets (attach statement)				
7	Loans to shareholders		*FIRST*		
8	Mortgage and real estate loans		*YEAR*		
9	Other investments (attach statement)		*CORPORATION*		
10a	Buildings and other depreciable assets				
b	Less accumulated depreciation	( )		( )	
11a	Depletable assets				
b	Less accumulated depletion	( )		( )	
12	Land (net of any amortization)				
13a	Intangible assets (amortizable only)				
b	Less accumulated amortization	( )		( )	
14	Other assets (attach statement)				
15	Total assets				322,000
	Liabilities and Shareholders' Equity				
16	Accounts payable				
17	Mortgages, notes, bonds payable in less than 1 year				
18	Other current liabilities (attach statement)				
19	Loans from shareholders				
20	Mortgages, notes, bonds payable in 1 year or more				
21	Other liabilities (attach statement)				
22	Capital stock				
23	Additional paid-in capital				
24	Retained earnings				
25	Adjustments to shareholders' equity (attach statement)				
26	Less cost of treasury stock		( )		( )
27	Total liabilities and shareholders' equity				322,000

Schedule M-1 — Reconciliation of Income (Loss) per Books With Income (Loss) per Return

Note: Schedule M-3 required instead of Schedule M-1 if total assets are $10 million or more—see instructions

1	Net income (loss) per books	45,900	5	Income recorded on books this year not included on Schedule K, lines 1 through 10 (itemize):	
2	Income included on Schedule K, lines 1, 2, 3c, 4, 5a, 6, 7, 8a, 9, and 10, not recorded on books this year (itemize):		a	Tax-exempt interest $	
3	Expenses recorded on books this year not included on Schedule K, lines 1 through 12 and 14l (itemize):		6	Deductions included on Schedule K, lines 1 through 12 and 14l, not charged against book income this year (itemize):	
a	Depreciation $		a	Depreciation $	
b	Travel and entertainment $				
			7	Add lines 5 and 6	
4	Add lines 1 through 3	45,900	8	Income (loss) (Schedule K, line 18). Line 4 less line 7	45,900

Schedule M-2 — Analysis of Accumulated Adjustments Account, Other Adjustments Account, and Shareholders' Undistributed Taxable Income Previously Taxed (see instructions)

		(a) Accumulated adjustments account	(b) Other adjustments account	(c) Shareholders' undistributed taxable income previously taxed
1	Balance at beginning of tax year	0		
2	Ordinary income from page 1, line 21	49,900		
3	Other additions $2,000 DIVIDENDS	3,000		
4	Loss from page 1, line 21 + $1,000 CAP GAIN			
5	Other reductions	(7,000 charitable)	( )	
6	Combine lines 1 through 5	(45,900)		
7	Distributions other than dividend distributions	22,000		
8	Balance at end of tax year. Subtract line 7 from line 6	23,900		

Form **1120S** (2008)

EXHIBIT 23-1
Continued

671108

Schedule K-1
(Form 1120S)
Department of the Treasury
Internal Revenue Service

2008

For calendar year 2008, or tax
year beginning _____ , 2008
ending _____ , 20___

Shareholder's Share of Income, Deductions, Credits, etc. ► See back of form and separate instructions.

☐ Final K-1   ☐ Amended K-1   OMB No. 1545-0130

Part III	Shareholder's Share of Current Year Income, Deductions, Credits, and Other Items

	Part I	Information About the Corporation

A Corporation's employer identification number
88 9138761

B Corporation's name, address, city, state, and ZIP code

T COMPANY

8122 SOUTH 8TH STREET

NORFOLK, VA 23508

C IRS Center where corporation filed return
MEMPHIS, TN

	Part II	Information About the Shareholder

D Shareholder's identifying number
467–63–5052

E Shareholder's name, address, city, state, and ZIP code

ADOLF Z.T

1291 MAPLE STREET

NORFOLK, VA 23508

F Shareholder's percentage of stock
ownership for tax year . . . . _____ 100 %

#	Description		#	Description
1	Ordinary business income (loss) 49,900		13	Credits
2	Net rental real estate income (loss)			*Rehabilitation Credit = 2,000*
3	Other net rental income (loss)			
4	Interest income			
5a	Ordinary dividends			
5b	Qualified dividends 2,000		14	Foreign transactions
6	Royalties 2,000			
7	Net short-term capital gain (loss)			
8a	Net long-term capital gain (loss) 1,000			
8b	Collectibles (28%) gain (loss)			
8c	Unrecaptured section 1250 gain			
9	Net section 1231 gain (loss)			
10	Other income (loss)		15	Alternative minimum tax (AMT) items
11	Section 179 deduction		16	Items affecting shareholder basis
12	Other deductions CHARITABLE CONTRIBUTIONS = 7,000			*$ 22,000 property distributions*
			17	Other information INVESTMENT INCOME = 2,000

* See attached statement for additional information.

For IRS Use Only

For Paperwork Reduction Act Notice, see Instructions for Form 1120S.   Cat. No. 11520D   Schedule K-1 (Form 1120S) 2008

EXHIBIT 23-2
Separately and Nonseparately Stated Items

For each of the following items of income, deduction, loss, and credit, and "X" in the appropriate column indicates whether the item is includible in an S corporation's combined ordinary income or loss (reported on Form 1120S, page 1; Schedule K, line 1; and Schedule K-1, line 1) or whether the item must be separately stated (reported on Schedules K and K-1, and lines 2 and following).

		Combined Ordinary Income or (Loss) (Form 1120S, p.1)	Separately Stated Item (Schedule K)	Reason
a.	Sales	X		No special shareholder treatment
b.	Income or loss from rental activities		X	Passive income for § 469 purposes
c.	Dividends		X	Investment (portfolio) income
d.	Taxable interest		X	Investment (portfolio) income
e.	Tax-exempt interest		X	May affect shareholder interest deductions (§ 265), or tax on social security benefits
f.	Cost of sales	X		No special shareholder treatment
g.	State and local taxes	X		Generally, no special shareholder treatment
h.	Net long-term capital gain or loss		X	Requires netting at shareholder level
i.	Net short-term capital gain or loss		X	Requires netting at shareholder level
j.	Net gain from sales of collectibles		X	Requires netting at shareholder level
k.	Net unrecaptured § 1250 gain		X	Requires netting at shareholder level
l.	Gain from sales of qualified small business stock		X	Requires netting at shareholder level
m.	Charitable contribution		X	Subject to A.G.I. limitation of shareholder
n.	Foreign income		X	Required for foreign tax credit computation at shareholder level
o.	Foreign taxes		X	Subject to election to credit or deduct
p.	Medical expenses		X	Includible by shareholder; deductible by shareholder subject to A.G.I. limitation; deductible by S corporation
q.	Investment interest		X	Subject to investment interest limitation
r.	MACRS or ACRS on plant and equipment	X	X	Subject to AMT tax liability at shareholder level[a]
s.	Section 179 expensing		X	Subject to § 179 shareholder limit
t.	Research and experimentation expenditures		X	Subject to special election by shareholder
u.	Work opportunity credit		X	Subject to tax liability limitation at shareholder level
v.	Recovery of a bad debt		X	Subject to § 111 determination at shareholder level
w.	Advertising	X		No special shareholder treatment
x.	Repairs and maintenance	X		No special shareholder treatment
y.	Expenses for production of income (§ 212)		X	Miscellaneous itemized deduction at shareholder level
z.	QPAI information		X	Deductions claimed at shareholder level

[a] Any preference or adjustment resulting from the use of accelerated depreciation must be separately reported, along with any § 179 expense.

ALLOCATIONS TO SHAREHOLDERS

All S corporation items (except distributions) are allocated among the shareholders based on their *ownership percentage* of the outstanding stock on each day of the year.[69] Thus, a shareholder owning 20 percent of the outstanding stock all year is deemed to have received 20 percent of *each item*. The allocation rate can be changed only by increasing or decreasing the percentage of stock ownership. This precludes shareholders from dividing net income or losses in any other manner. Of course, a certain amount of special allocation can be achieved through salaries and other business payments to owners. If there is no change in stock ownership during the year, each item to be allocated is multiplied by the percentage of stock owned by each shareholder. In contrast, actual distributions of assets are assigned to the shareholder who receives them.

Example 19. M owns 100 of an S corporation's 1,000 shares of common stock outstanding. Neither the number of shares outstanding nor the number owned by M has changed during the year. The S corporation items for its calendar year are allocated to M, based on her 10% ownership interest, as follows:

	Totals on Schedule K	M's 10% on Schedule K-1
Ordinary income (from Form 1120S, page 1)............	$70,000	$7,000
Net capital gain	2,000	200
Charitable contributions	4,000	400

If the ownership of stock changes during the year, there are two methods for determining the allocations for those shareholders whose interests have changed. These are (1) the *per day allocation method* and (2) the *interim closing of the books* method. Generally, the per day allocation method must be used. However, the S corporation may elect to use either method if:

1. A shareholder's ownership interest is *completely* terminated;

2. There is a disposition by one shareholder of *more than* 20 percent of the outstanding shares of the corporation within 30 days; or

3. The corporation issues shares to one or more new shareholders and the new shares are at least 25 percent of the number previously outstanding.

Per Day Allocation. This method assigns an equal amount of the S items to each day of the year.[70] When a shareholder's interest changes, the shareholder *must* report a pro rata share of each item for each day that the stock was owned. For this purpose, the seller is deemed to own the stock on the day of the sale. This computation may be expressed as follows:

$$\frac{\text{Percentage of}}{\text{shares owned}} \times \frac{\text{Percentage of}}{\text{year stock was owned}} = \frac{\text{Portion of}}{\text{item to be reported}}$$

Example 20. Assume the same facts as in *Example 19*, except that M sold all of her shares on August 7 to T. Because the S corporation uses the calendar year, M has held 100 shares for 219 days, or 60% of the year (219 ÷ 365). (The day of sale is considered an ownership day for the seller, M.) Thus M is allocated 6% (60% × 10%)

---

[69]   §§ 1366(a) and 1377(a).

[70]   § 1377(a)(1).

of each corporate item while T is allocated 4% (40% × 10%). Based on the per day allocation method, M's and T's shares of the S corporation items are as follows:

	Totals on Schedule K	10 Percent to M & T	M's Portion (10% × 219/365)	T's Portion (10% × 146/365)
Ordinary income	$70,000	$7,000	$4,200	$2,800
Net capital gain	2,000	200	120	80
Charitable contributions	4,000	400	240	160

The per day allocation method also is applicable for a shareholder whose stock interest varies during the year; however, the computation is more complex.

Example 21. Assume the same facts as in *Example 20*, except M only sold 20 shares on August 7 to T. Thus, she owned 10% of the business the first 219 days and 8% the remaining 146 days. Based on the per day allocation method. M's and T's shares of the S corporation items are as follows:

	Totals Schedule K	1/1–8/7 (10% × 219/365)	8/8–12/31 (8% × 146/ 365)	M's Schedule K-1	T's Schedule K-1 (2% × 146/365)
Ordinary income	$70,000	$4,200	$2,240	$6,440	$560
Net capital gain	2,000	120	64	184	16
Charitable contributions .	4,000	240	128	368	32

Interim Closing of the Books. As noted above, the per day method must be used unless there is either (1) a complete termination of a shareholder's interest, (2) a disposition of more than 20 percent of the outstanding stock of the corporation by one shareholder within a 30-day period, or (3) issuance of shares to persons who were not previously shareholders equal to at least 25 percent of the number previously outstanding. In any of these situations, the corporation may elect to use the interim closing of books method instead of the per day allocation method.[71] If the corporation elects, the year is divided into two short taxable years for allocation purposes and all owners report the actual dollar amounts that were accumulated while they owned their shares. A valid election must be filed by the corporation with Form 1120S. All parties who are affected by the transaction must consent to the election. This election does not require the corporation to file separate returns for each portion of the year.

Example 22. Assume the same facts as in *Example 20*, except the interim closing of books method is elected. since M sells *all* of her shares on August 7 to T, the S corporation's year ends the day before on August 6. Corporate records show the following amounts for the first 219 days, for the last 146 days, and M's share for the first 219 days.

	First 219 days	Last 146 days	M's 10% on Schedule K-1	T's 10% on Schedule K-1
Ordinary income (from Form 1102S, page 1)	$15,000	$55,000	$1,500	$5,500
Net capital gain	1,000	1,000	100	100
Charitable contributions	0	4,000	0	400

---

[71] § 1377(a)(2).

The computations for M's share are the amounts for the first 219 days *multiplied* by her 10% ownership interest. T's share are the amounts for the last 146 days *multiplied* by his 10% ownership interest. The combined amounts for M and T equal the amount for M in *Example 19*.

It is also possible for an S corporation to have an ordinary loss for part of the year and ordinary income for the remaining period.

LOSSES OF THE S CORPORATION

One of the most common reasons a corporation elects Subchapter S status is because of the tax treatment for corporate losses. Recall that the C corporation's benefits are limited to those available from carrying the losses to another year to offset its own income. Refunds may be obtained to the extent *prior* year income is offset while losses carried to future years reduce the taxes due in those years. Frequently, these carryover benefits provide little or no value to the corporation. For example, many businesses report losses in the first few years so the carryback privilege is useless. In addition, many new businesses are never successful. But, even those that are successful receive no tax benefit from their losses currently—generally when the need is the greatest.

The pass-through feature of S corporations can be a significant advantage when a corporation has a net loss. Based on the flow-through concept, shareholders include their distributive shares of the S corporation's losses in their taxable income currently. Thus, the deduction for losses is transferred to the shareholder and generally results in tax savings for the current year. Even if a shareholder is unable to use the loss currently, carryover provisions may provide the shareholder with tax benefits in the near future.

Limitations. Each shareholder's deductible share of net losses may not exceed that shareholder's basis in the corporation's stock and the basis in any debt that the corporation owes to the shareholder. (Shareholder basis is discussed in more depth later in this chapter.) Any losses that exceed a shareholder's basis may be carried forward indefinitely to be used when the shareholder's basis is increased.[72] When basis is insufficient and there is more than one item that reduces basis, the flow-through of each item is determined in a pro rata manner.[73] In addition, any income items that increase basis flow through to the owner before any items that reduce basis, including distributions on stock.[74]

Example 23. G owns 200 of an S corporation's 1,000 shares of common stock outstanding and has a basis of $10,000 at the beginning of the year. Neither the number of shares outstanding nor those owned by G has changed during the year. The S corporation items for its calendar year are allocated to G, based on his 20% ownership interest, as follows:

	Totals on Schedule K	G's 20% on Schedule K-1
Ordinary loss (from Form 1120S, page 1).........	($70,000)	($14,000)
Net capital loss	(5,000)	(1,000)
Section 1231 gain	10,000	2,000

---

[72] § 1366(d)(2). Losses may also be subject to limitation under § 465 at-risk rules and § 469 passive activity rules.

[73] Reg. § 1.1366-2(a)(4).

[74] §§ 1366(d)(1) and 1367(a). After positive adjustments, basis is reduced by distributions and nondeductible items, before separately stated deductions and losses. See discussion below.

G's share of the S corporation's losses is limited as follows:

	Basis	Loss Carryover
G's beginning basis	$10,000	
Section 1231 gain	2,000	
Limitation on losses	$12,000	
Ordinary loss*	(11,200)	$2,800
Net capital loss**	(800)	200
G's ending basis	$ 0	

* ($14,000/$15,000 × $12,000)
**($1,000/$15,000 × $12,000)

Because G's basis is less than the $15,000 total loss, G may report ordinary loss of only $11,200 and net capital loss of $800. The remaining ordinary loss of $2,800 and net capital loss of $200 are carried forward to be used at the end of the first year that G's basis increases.

The above allocation of losses is applicable to all losses and separate deductions (e.g., investment interest and state income taxes) for owners of both the S corporation and the partnership.

Carryovers from C Corporation Years. Generally, no carryovers from a C corporation may be used during the years it is taxed as an S corporation (or vice versa). For example, a C corporation with a net operating loss may not use it to offset income in an S year. There is one exception: C corporate NOL carryforwards may be used to offset the S corporation's built-in gains (discussed later in this chapter).[75] The S years are counted, however, when determining the expiration period of the carryover. Thus, a carryback of two years means two fiscal or calendar years regardless of whether the corporation was a C corporation or an S corporation.[76]

DETERMINING SHAREHOLDER BASIS

A shareholder's basis in his or her stock as well as any debt owed to the shareholder is critical for three principal purposes. First, upon a sale of stock, shareholders must know the basis of the stock to compute gain or loss on the sale. Second, the treatment of distributions depends on the basis of a shareholder's stock. Third, shareholders must know their stock basis as well as their debt basis in loss years since losses are deductible only to the extent of the basis in their stock and debt.

BASIS IN S CORPORATE STOCK

Conceptually, the computation of a shareholder's stock basis is similar to that for a partner's interest in a partnership. Both calculations are designed to ensure that there is neither double taxation of income nor double deduction of expenses. Consider a typical situation where two individuals form a business. Assume both parties contribute $10,000

---

[75] § 1374(b)(2).

[76] §§ 1371(b) and 1362(e)(6)(A).

for a 50 percent interest in an S corporation which immediately takes the money and invests it in land that it subsequently sells for $22,000. In this case, the S corporation has income of $2,000 ($22,000 − $20,000) and each shareholder reports his $1,000 share. Note that the shareholders report their share of the S corporation's income even if they receive no distributions from the S corporation. However, to ensure that an S corporation's income is not taxed again when it is distributed, each shareholder must keep track of his or her investment, that is, basis in the S corporation. In this case, each shareholder has an original basis equal to the amount contributed to the S corporation, $10,000. Upon the reporting of S corporation income, each shareholder adjusts basis in the S corporation interest for his or her share of income, increasing it from $10,000 to $11,000. When a shareholder actually receives the $1,000 share of the income, the distribution is treated as tax-free to the extent of basis. Each shareholder would then reduce basis by $1,000 back to the original basis of $10,000. The end result is that the shareholders have reported and received income that has been subject to only one tax. The same rationale can be applied to situations involving tax-exempt income, deductible losses and nondeductible expenses to ensure the proper result is reached.

The steps for calculating a shareholder's stock basis are shown and compared to that for a partner in Exhibit 23-3.[77] Generally, both computations begin with the owner's initial investment, increased by items of taxable and tax-exempt income then decreased by distributions, nondeductible expenditures,[78] deductible expenses and losses in that order. As may be apparent in Exhibit 23-3, the primary difference between the two calculations is that an S corporation shareholder does not include a proportionate share of corporate debt to other lenders. In addition, as illustrated later, the treatment of the distribution of noncash property differs from that of a partnership.

---

[77] § 1367.

[78] With respect to the order of nondeductible and deductible expenditures, there is no special rule for partnerships and in absence of sufficient basis, presumably a pro rata portion of each type of expenditure is deducted as shown in *Example 23*. In contrast, S corporation shareholders must use the order shown unless they make a special election to reverse the order and agree to carry forward any disallowed expenses which exceed basis to reduce basis in future years. See Reg. § 1.1367-1(g).

EXHIBIT 23-3
Adjustments to Ownership Basis

Shareholder's Basis in S Corporation Stock	Partner's Basis in Partnership Interest
Original Basis	**Original Basis**
Cost	Generally same as S unless received in
Substitute for property contributed in § 351 exchange Donor's basis	exchange for property contributed to partnership where partner assumed or reduced liabilities
Inherited basis (estate tax value from deceased shareholder)	
Increased by	**Increased by**
Taxable income (ordinary or separately stated)	Same
Tax-exempt income	Same
Decreased (but not below zero) by	**Decreased (but not below zero) by**
Distributions of cash	Same
Distributions of property at fair market value	Partnership basis of distributed property (in most cases)
Nondeductible expenses (unless election)*	Same
Losses (ordinary and separately stated)	Same
No Effect	**Additional Effect**
Increase in corporate liabilities	Increase partner's basis for share of liabilities
Decrease in corporate liabilities	Decrease partner's basis for share of liabilities

*Nondeductible expenses must be used to offset basis before deductible items unless the shareholder files a special election to reverse the order. Reg. § 1.1367-1(g).

BASIS IN S CORPORATION DEBT

If a shareholder's portion of the corporation's losses exceeds his or her stock basis, the shareholder must next turn to debt basis to determine whether or not any loss passing through from the corporation may be deductible. Unlike a partnership, in which a partner increases basis for his or her portion of the organization's debt to outsiders, a shareholder in an S corporation must actually loan money to the corporation in order to receive debt basis. This issue has been frequently litigated by shareholders with little success. The loan must represent an actual economic outlay on the shareholder's part, rather than a mere paper shuffling of debt instruments.[79] The loan must be made directly by the shareholder, rather than indirectly through a related party.[80] A shareholder guarantee of the corporation's debt to the lender does not create shareholder basis.[81] Thus there must be a debt directly from the corporation to the shareholder, based on the shareholder's economic outlay. Quite logically, the shareholder's basis, before any adjustments, is the amount loaned by the shareholder.

A shareholder's basis in the loan is adjusted *only* (1) when the actual indebtedness itself changes due to additional loans or repayment of loans, (2) when corporate net losses exceed the shareholder's basis in S stock, and (3) to restore any basis reduction due to the

---

[79] *Wilson*, T.C. Memo. 1991-544.

[80] *Hitchins*, 103 T.C. 40 (1994).

[81] *Raynor*, 50 T.C. 762 (1968).

prior flow-through of net losses. The application of these latter two rules is somewhat tricky. As a general rule, losses first reduce the shareholder's stock basis (but not below zero). (Note that nondeductible expenses reduce basis before deductible expenses and losses unless a special election is made.) If there is insufficient stock basis to absorb the loss, the loss is deducted to the extent of the shareholder's debt basis. If there is insufficient stock and debt basis, the loss is carried over and used once there is sufficient basis to absorb the loss.

Example 24. An S corporation incurs a net operating loss of $30,000 in 2009. L, its sole shareholder, has a basis in the stock of $24,000 and a note due him from the corporation totals $10,000.

	Stock Basis	Debt Basis
Balance 12/31/2008	$24,000	$10,000
Loss to extent of stock basis	(24,000)	
Loss to extent of debt		(6,000)
Balance 12/31/2009	$ 0	$ 4,000

The $30,000 loss flows through to L, first to the extent of his $24,000 stock basis and the remaining $6,000 because of the $10,000 note owed to him.

If the 2009 loss had been $36,000, only $34,000 would be deductible by L, reducing his basis in both stock and debt to zero. The remaining $2,000 loss would be carried forward indefinitely until a positive basis adjustment occurs in stock or debt.

As the corporation earns income, the shareholder restores stock and debt basis. Debt basis is increased only for income in excess of current year distributions and deductible and nondeductible expenses and losses.[82] Thus if there are no distributions or losses during the year, the basis of the debt is increased first. However, in years where there are distributions and/or losses, the effect is to first allocate income to the stock's basis equal to the amount of any current year losses and distributions with any excess to the debt. While these rules are obviously confusing, failure to properly understand their operation may cause the shareholder to inadvertently have gain on the repayment of any corporate debt.

Example 25. Refer to *Example 24*. The S corporation has net income of $3,000 in 2010 and $8,000 in 2011. There were no losses or distributions in either of these years.

	Stock Basis	Debt Basis
Balance 12/31/2009	$ 0	$ 4,000
2010 net income	0	3,000
2011 net income	5,000	3,000
Balance 12/31/2011	$5,000	$10,000

---

[82] § 1367(b)(2).

In 2010, the excess of income over distributions and losses is $3,000 ($3,000 − $0 − $0) and, therefore, the basis of the note is increased by $3,000. In 2009, the excess of income over distributions and losses is $8,000 ($8,000 − $0 − $0). Consequently, the basis of the debt is increased first by $3,000 to its original $10,000 face amount ($7,000 + $3,000). The remaining income of $5,000 ($8,000 − $3,000) is used to increase the basis of the stock.

Example 26. The records of X, an S corporation, reveal the information below for 2009 and 2010. In addition, at the beginning of 2009, X's sole shareholder had a basis of $10,000 in her stock and $12,000 in the loan she had made to the corporation during 2008.

	2009	2010
Tax-exempt income	$ 5,000	
Loss	(30,000)	
Income		$21,000
Distribution		14,000

In 2009, the shareholder first increases the basis in her stock by the tax-exempt income of $5,000, resulting in a stock basis of $15,000. The $30,000 loss is then applied: first to the extent of her stock basis, $15,000, and then to the extent of her debt basis, $12,000. The remainder of the loss, $3,000, is carried over to 2010. These calculations are shown below:

	Stock Basis	Debt Basis
Begin 2009	$10,000	$12,000
Tax-exempt income	5,000	
Loss $30,000	(15,000)	(12,000)
End 2009	$ 0	$ 0
Loss in excess of basis		$ 3,000

In 2010, the corporation reports taxable income of $21,000 and distributes $14,000. The $21,000 income is applied in the following order:

	Stock Basis	Debt Basis
Begin 2010	$ 0	$ 0
2010 income	$21,000	
2010 distribution	(14,000)	7,000
Loss from 2009		(3,000)
End 2010	$ 0	$ 4,000

The shareholder deducts $27,000 of the 2009 loss in 2009 and carries the remaining $3,000 forward. In 2010, the shareholder reports $21,000 of income and deducts the remaining $3,000 of the 2009 loss.

After a shareholder's basis in the indebtedness is reduced, repayments of the debt in excess of basis result in taxable income. If the debt is a note, bond, or other written debt instrument, the shareholder recognizes capital gain to the extent the payment exceeds

basis.[83] If the debt is an *open* account, the shareholder recognizes ordinary income.[84] This ordinary income can be recharacterized as capital gain by converting the open account to a capital contribution; no gain is recognized for this conversion, even if the open account has been reduced by net losses (i.e., its basis is less than its face or market value).[85]

In accounting for repayments, the following rules must be followed:[86]

1. Only the bases of loans outstanding at the close of the year are reduced.

2. Only loans outstanding at the beginning of the year are restored.

The operation of these rules generally favors the taxpayer. Observe that the basis of any loan that is completely paid off during the year may be increased for income earned during the year but is not reduced for losses.

Example 27. J owns all of the stock of H, an S corporation. At the beginning of 2009, J had a basis in his S stock of $13,000 and a loan outstanding to the corporation of $10,000. On July 1, the corporation paid J the $10,000 it owed to him on the loan. As of July 1, the corporation's books and records revealed a loss of $15,000. The loss for the entire year was $20,000. J recognizes no gain on repayment of the loan since his basis is $10,000. Even though the losses suffered by the corporation at the date of the repayment, $15,000, and at the close of the year, $20,000, exceeded J's stock basis, there is no reduction in the basis of the loan since only the basis of a loan outstanding at the close of the year is reduced. However, J can only deduct $13,000 of the loss, the amount equal to his stock basis.

Example 28. Assume the same facts above except that the corporation repaid the loan on June 1 of the following year, 2010. In this case, J's basis in the loan at the beginning of 2010 would be $3,000 computed as follows:

	Stock Basis	Debt Basis
Begin 2009	$13,000	$10,000
Loss for year $20,000	(13,000)	(7,000)
End 2009	$ 0	$ 3,000

If the corporation had no income for 2010, J would report a gain on the repayment of $7,000 ($10,000 − $3,000). On the other hand, if the corporation had income for the year of $6,000 *and* no distributions were made, the basis of the loan would be increased by the income of $6,000 to $9,000 and the gain on the repayment would be $1,000 ($10,000 − $9,000). Notice that in this latter case the basis of the loan is increased by income for the entire year even though the loan is paid off during the year. This follows from the rule that calls for loans outstanding at the first of the year to be restored.

---

[83] § 1232 and Rev. Rul. 64-162, 1964-1 C.B. 304.

[84] Rev. Rul. 68-537, 1968-2 C.B. 372 and *Cornelius v. U.S.*, 74-1 USTC ¶9446, 33 AFTR2d 74-1331, 494 F.2d 465 (CA-5, 1974).

[85] §§ 108(e)(6) and (d)(7)(C). The holding period of the capital asset (the note) begins with the creation of the note—not the date of the unwritten loan.

[86] Reg. § 1.1367-2(d).

RELATIONSHIP BETWEEN AN S CORPORATION AND ITS SHAREHOLDERS

The S corporation is a legal entity, distinctly separate from its owners. As a result, transactions between an S corporation and its shareholders are treated as though occurring between unrelated parties unless otherwise provided. Of course, these transactions must be conducted in an arm's-length manner, based on market values that would be used by unrelated parties.

TRANSACTIONS BETWEEN S CORPORATIONS AND THEIR SHAREHOLDERS

Owners may engage in *taxable transactions* with their S corporations. For example, shareholders may lend money, rent property, or sell assets to their S corporations (or vice versa). With few exceptions, owners include the interest income, rent income, or gain or loss from these transactions on their tax returns. Meanwhile, the S corporation is allowed a deduction for the interest, rent, or depreciation expense on assets purchased (if applicable).

Example 29. During the year, K received the following amounts from an S corporation in which she owns 30% of the stock outstanding:

1. $2,750 interest on a $25,000 loan made to the corporation;

2. $3,600 rental income from a storage building rented to the corporation; and

3. $6,300 for special tools sold to the corporation; the tools were acquired for personal use two years ago for $5,800.

Assume that the S corporation's net ordinary income, excluding the above items, is $40,000, and the depreciation deduction for the tools is $900. K's income is computed as follows:

	S Corporation	Shareholder K
Ordinary income (before items below)	$40,000	
Gain on sale of tools ($6,300 − $5,800)		$ 500
Depreciation of tools	(900)	
Interest	(2,750)	2,750
Rent	(3,600)	3,600
Ordinary income:		
Corporation	$32,750	
K ($32,750 × 30%)		9,825

There is a restriction, however, on when an S corporation may deduct expenses owed but not paid to a shareholder, regardless of the amount of stock owned. An accrual basis business (whether an S corporation or partnership) may not deduct expenses owed to a cash basis owner until the amount is paid.[87]

Example 30. Assume the same facts as in *Example 29*, except that $2,000 of the $2,750 interest is accrued but not paid at the end of 2009, the S corporation is on the

---

[87] §§ 267(a)(2) and 267(e). This same restriction applies to a C corporation only if a cash basis shareholder owns more than 50 percent of its stock. § 267(b)(10).

accrual basis, and K is on the cash basis. The corporation paid K the accrued interest of $2,000 on January 15, 2010. Because K is a shareholder the corporation cannot deduct the $2,000 of accrued interest in 2009 but must wait until it pays the amount. Consequently, the corporation will deduct the interest when it is paid in 2010. K will report the payment when she receives it in 2010.

Two special rules governing related-party transactions affect all business forms. Both are discussed in Chapter 22. *First*, realized *losses* on sales between related parties are disallowed.[88] This is not a deferral; therefore, there is no carryover of basis or holding period. However, if this property is later sold at a gain, the gain is offset by the previously disallowed losses.[89] *Second*, recognized gains on sales between related parties of *property* that will be *depreciable* to the new owner are taxed as ordinary income.[90] A related party is defined as one who owns directly or indirectly more than 50 percent of the business when losses are disallowed or when depreciable property is involved. (See the discussion and examples in Chapter 22 regarding these transactions and the definitions of related parties.) A *third* restriction, affecting transactions between partners and their 50 percent owned partnerships, is *not* applicable to either S or C corporations. For these partners, recognized gains on sales of capital assets that will not be capital assets to the partnership are taxed as ordinary income.[91] In contrast, shareholders may sell capital assets to their more than 50 percent owned S or C corporations and the gain is capital, as long as the assets will not be depreciable property to the corporation. Note that this rule may favor the S corporation over the partnership or LLC for certain activities such as real estate development.

SELECTING A TAXABLE YEAR

Shareholders report their shares of S corporation income, deductions, and credits in their tax years in which the corporation's year ends regardless of when distributions of assets are actually made.[92] This timing requirement makes the selection of a year-end for the owners and the business an important tax planning decision. Under current law, an S corporation normally must use the calendar year. Fiscal years are available but only if very strict conditions are met.

Currently an S corporation may have as its taxable year:

- ► A calendar year.
- ► A fiscal year if it is a natural business year.
- ► A fiscal year if its majority shareholders are on the same year.
- ► A fiscal year under the special election of § 444.

Calendar Years. An S corporation is allowed to have a calendar year.[93] No permission is needed to adopt the calendar year. As will become evident, the severe requirements that must be met to obtain a fiscal year force the vast majority of S corporations to use the calendar year.

---

[88]   §§ 267 and 707(b)(1).

[89]   § 267(d).

[90]   § 1239.

[91]   § 707(b)(2).

[92]   § 1366(a); § 706 provides a similar rule for partnerships.

[93]   § 1378.

Natural Business Year. Section 1378 permits an S corporation to adopt a fiscal year if it "establishes a business purpose to the satisfaction of the Secretary." In this regard, the IRS has indicated that it will allow a fiscal year only in the case of a *natural business year.* An S corporation can qualify for use of a fiscal year end if it considered to have a "natural business year-end." There are two general categories of the natural business year end for S corporations: fiscal year-ends that meet a "25 percent gross receipts test" and fiscal year ends that meet an "annual business cycle" or "seasonal business" test. Year-ends qualifying under the gross receipts test can be adopted automatically by the S corporation. The other category requires permission of the IRS.

Automatic Adoption. A corporation that is electing S status, or a corporation that already has an S election in effect may automatically retain, adopt or change to a natural business year-end if it meets the "25 percent" test for its gross receipts of the past four years. To determine if this test is met, the corporation selects its desired year end (for example June 30) and determines its receipts for the two months ended on June 30 (May and June), and for the twelve months ending on that date in its most recent history (e.g., July through June). If the gross receipts for the final two months (e.g., May and June) exceed 25 percent of its gross receipts for the twelve months ending on that date (e.g., July through June), the S corporation meets the test. The S corporation must meet the test for its past three years ending on that date. A corporation that qualifies under this test may claim its fiscal year without receiving permission for the IRS, although it must file Form 1128 if it is changing its year.[94]

Annual Business Cycle or Seasonal Business Tests. An S corporation may also qualify to apply for a natural business year-end under the annual business cycle test, or the seasonal business test. The annual business cycle test is for a corporation that has a "peak" period of receipts. The seasonal business test exists when there is a period of inactivity due to the nature of the business. Thus a retailer with peak sales during December holiday periods may qualify for the business cycle test, and a ski resort may qualify for the seasonal business test. However, the S corporation may not automatically claim a year-end based on either of these tests, but must apply to the National Office of the IRS and pay a ruling request fee.[95]

> **Example 31.** An S corporation is organized November 1, 2009. Its net ordinary income for the first 14 months is as follows:
>
> | | |
> |---|---:|
> | November 1, 2009–December 31, 2009 | $ 20,000 |
> | January 1, 2010–October 31, 2010 | 200,000 |
> | November 1, 2010–December 31, 2010 | 40,000 |
>
> All shareholders report on the calendar year. If the S corporation's year-end also is December 31, the owners have includible income of $20,000 in 2009 and $240,000 ($200,000 + $40,000) in 2010. If, however, the S corporation meets the natural business year requirements and receives permission for an October 31 year-end, the owners have no includible income in 2009 but have includible income of $220,000 ($20,000 + $200,000) in 2010. The $40,000 will be combined with the net income or loss for the first ten months in 2011 and reported in 2011.

Majority Ownership Year. Consistent with its concern about deferral, the IRS permits an S corporation to adopt a tax year that is identical to that of owners holding a majority of the corporation's stock.[96] For example, if an individual who operated a farm

---

[94] See Rev. Proc. 2002-37, 2002-22 I.R.B. 1030, § 5.06, Rev. Proc. 2002-38, 2002-22 I.R.B. 1037, § 5.05 and Rev. Proc. 2002-39, 2002-22 I.R.B. 1046, § 5.03(3).

[95] See Rev. Proc. 2002-39, 2002-22 I.R.B. 1046 for details.

[96] Rev. Proc. 2002-37, § 5.05 and Rev. Proc. 2002-38, § 5.06.

used a March 31 year-end, his wholly owned S corporation could use the same year-end since it conformed to the year of its majority owner. However, as a practical matter, this option is seldom used since most shareholders are individuals and certain trusts and they rarely use a fiscal year (e.g., trusts must use a calendar year).

Section 444 Year. A partnership or an S corporation may elect to adopt or change its tax year to any fiscal year that does not result in a deferral period longer than three months—or, if less, the deferral period of the year currently in use.[97] This election requires the electing partnership or S corporation to make a single deposit on or before May 15 of each year computed on the deferred income at the highest tax rate imposed on individual taxpayers *plus* one percent (for 2008, 35% + 1% = 36%).[98] This deposit does *not* flow through to the shareholders. In essence, the partnership or S corporation must maintain a non-interest-bearing deposit of the income taxes that would have been deferred without this requirement. Since this option eliminates some tax benefits of income deferral and has burdensome compliance requirements, few S corporations make the election. The deposit is refunded if the S corporation's income declines in the future.

Since restrictions on C corporation year-end choices are much more lenient than those for S corporations, an election by a fiscal year C corporation to become an S corporation also may require a change in the corporate year-end. This new year is applicable to all future years, even if the Subchapter S election is cancelled and the business reverts to a C corporation.

FAMILY OWNERSHIP

Many of the benefits available to family businesses from *income splitting* are dependent on which organizational form is selected. Some income splitting, however, may be achieved by employing relatives in the business regardless of the organizational form. For example, owners may hire their children to work for them. All reasonable salaries are deductible business expenses and includible salary income to the children. In addition to the tax benefits, some owners believe this provides personal advantages, including encouraging the children to take an interest in the business at an early age.

In some instances, family businesses are formed primarily for tax reasons. The most common example includes both a parent and one or more otherwise dependent children as owners. The basic tax rate structure provides considerable incentive for this type of arrangement when the child is at least 20 years of age.[99]

Rules similar to those affecting the family partnership (discussed in Chapter 22) are applicable to family S corporations.[100] Thus, if reasonable compensation is not paid for services performed or for the use of capital contributed by a family member, the IRS may reallocate S corporation income or expenses.[101] Unlike the partnership, this rule extends to all family members, including those who are *not* owners and when there is no donee/donor relationship.

---

[97] § 444 and Temp. Reg. § 1.444-1T(b). Partnerships and S corporations in existence before 1987 are allowed to continue their fiscal years even if the deferral period exceeds three months (i.e., the fiscal year is "grandfathered").

[98] § 7519 and Temp. Reg § 1.7519-2T(a)(4)(ii).

[99] Recall that many of the income-splitting advantages involving passive income are not available with children under 18 years of age.

[100] § 1366(e) and Reg. § 1.1366-3(a).

[101] Family member, as defined by the Code, is the same for the partnership and the S corporation. §§ 704(e)(3) and 1366(e).

Example 32. This year, Dr. F created LME Corporation, an S corporation whose business is leasing medical equipment. He gave all of the stock in LME to his son and daughter. For the year, LME has $20,000 of net rental income. If Dr. F performs services for LME and is not adequately compensated, the IRS may adjust the income of the parties to force Dr. F to include reasonable compensation in his income, and reduce LME's income accordingly. The IRS is not required to make this adjustment.

CURRENT DISTRIBUTIONS OF CORPORATE ASSETS

The treatment of distributions by an S corporation borrows from the rules applying to distributions from partnerships and C corporations. Normally, distributions from an S corporation, like those from a partnership, represent accumulated income that has been previously taxed to its owners. Accordingly, this income should not be taxed again when it is distributed. Consistent with this approach, most distributions by an S corporation are considered nontaxable to the extent of the shareholder's stock basis. Any distribution in excess of the shareholder's stock basis is treated as gain from the sale of the underlying stock, producing capital gain.

Problems arise if the retained earnings of an S corporation consist of any C corporation earnings and profits (i.e., AE&P as discussed in Chapter 20). As might be expected, when this occurs, clarification is required regarding how the S and C corporation rules interact. Consequently, one of the first questions that must be considered before the treatment of a distribution can be determined is whether an S corporation has AE&P. Beyond this first concern, however, still other considerations may be relevant. For example, special rules can operate if the S corporation distributes property (i.e., assets other than cash) or the distribution occurs shortly after the S corporation election terminates. Each of these issues and several others are examined below.

THE E&P QUESTION

As noted above, the treatment of an S corporation distribution can depend on whether the corporation has any AE&P. Normally a corporation that has been an S corporation since its inception will not have AE&P since it never operated as a C corporation.[102] Nevertheless, AE&P could be found in the retained earnings of a lifelong S corporation if a C corporation was merged or liquidated into the S corporation. An election to treat a subsidiary corporation as a QSub is a deemed liquidation of the subsidiary, governed by Code §§ 332 and 337. Accordingly, any AE&P of the subsidiary becomes AE&P of the parent S corporation.

An S corporation is far more likely to have AE&P if it operated as a C corporation before it elected S status. This is not at all uncommon. For example, it is estimated that due to substantial changes made by the Tax Reform Act of 1986, about 500,000 C corporations made S elections. Many of these converted C corporations are alive and operating today. There are also many other C corporations that for one reason or another have opted for S status. In these cases, AE&P is likely to exist. In any event, whether the corporation has always been an S corporation or is a converted C corporation, it is crucial to ascertain whether the corporation has AE&P. This determination often requires a long detailed study.

---

[102] Prior to 1983, it was possible for an S corporation to generate AE&P while it was an S corporation. Starting in 1997, an S corporation's C earnings and profits do not include any AE&P that was produced while it was an S corporation prior to 1983. See § 1311 of the Small Business Jobs Protection Act. (P.L. 104-88).

S CORPORATIONS WITH NO AE&P

All cash distributions by S corporations that have no AE&P are nontaxable unless they exceed the shareholder's basis in the stock.[103] It should be emphasized that the shareholder's stock basis is the critical variable in measuring the taxability of the distribution. The basis of any debt is irrelevant in this regard.

In determining whether a distribution exceeds the shareholder's stock basis, all distributions are deemed to be made on the last day of the tax year. For this purpose, the basis in the stock is increased for all positive adjustments before accounting for distributions. Like partnerships, distributions reduce the owner's basis before consideration of losses.[104] If the shareholder owns stock on the last day of the taxable year, all of the basis adjustments are made on the last day of the corporation's taxable year (or on the last day of ownership for a shareholder whose interest completely terminates). The general approach used by S corporations in accounting for distributions is illustrated below.

	Original basis (purchase, formation, inherited, gift, etc.)
+	Additional capital contributions
+	Separately stated income items (taxable and tax-exempt)
+	Nonseparately stated income items (taxable and tax-exempt)
−	Distributions
−	Nondeductible, non-capital, expenses
−	Separately and nonseparately stated deduction and loss items
=	Ending basis of stock

Example 33. D and F have been equal owners of an S corporation for five years. D has a basis in his stock of $40,000 while F's stock basis is $10,000. The corporation's records for the year revealed the following:

Ordinary taxable income	$50,000
Tax-exempt income	10,000
Nondeductible portion of meals and entertainment	2,000
Capital loss (not fully deductible by shareholder)	30,000

---

[103] § 1368(b).

[104] Prior to 1997, distributions of S corporations were the final item absorbed (i.e., distributions were after losses and separately stated items of deductible and nondeductible expenses).

During the year, the corporation distributed $100,000, $50,000 to D and $50,000 to F. Based on these facts, the distribution to D would be nontaxable while the distribution to F would result in a capital gain of $10,000 as determined below.

	D's Share		F's Share	
	Taxable Income	Basis	Taxable Income	Basis
Beginning basis		$40,000		$ 10,000
Positive adjustments:				
Exempt income		5,000		5,000
Ordinary taxable income	$25,000	25,000	$25,000	25,000
Basis before $50,000 distribution to each		$70,000		$40,000
Nontaxable portion of distribution		(50,000)		(40,000)
Taxable portion of distribution (capital gain)	0	—	10,000	—
Basis before negative adjustments		$20,000		$ 0
Negative adjustments:				
Nondeductible meals and entertainment		(1,000)		—
Capital loss		(15,000)		—*
Ending basis		$ 4,000		$ 0

* The capital loss would be allowed to F in any future year if F's basis were to increase.

In determining the treatment of the distributions, the stock basis for each shareholder is first adjusted for all positive adjustments before accounting for the distribution. In this case, the positive adjustments boost D's basis to $70,000 so that his $50,000 distribution is completely tax-free. After accounting for the distribution, D reduces his basis for his share of the nondeductible expenses and then the capital loss. The reduction to basis for the capital loss is made even though D is not able to fully deduct the loss on his own return. Any portion of the capital loss that D cannot deduct is carried over to subsequent years until it is exhausted.

The distribution to F results in a capital gain of $10,000 since his basis after positive adjustments, $40,000, is insufficient to absorb the entire $50,000 distribution. Note also that F cannot deduct any of the capital loss since losses are deductible only to the extent of the shareholder's basis. However, the capital loss carries over until such time that F has sufficient basis to enable its flow-through. Contrast the treatment of the capital loss with that of the nondeductible portion of meals and entertainment. There is no requirement that F must carry over the nondeductible expenses and reduce his basis. When it is known that distributions will exceed a shareholder's basis, the recognition of capital gain can be avoided if the shareholder increases his or her stock basis before the year ends. This may be done by (1) contributing capital to the S corporation, or (2) having debt owed this shareholder converted to capital.

S CORPORATIONS WITH AE&P

The distribution rules for S corporations that have AE&P—regardless of the amount—are far more complex than those for S corporations without AE&P. This derives from the fact that the distributions that are out of an S corporation's earnings that were accumulated while it was a C corporation (C AE&P) are treated much differently from those out of its earnings accumulated while it was an S corporation. Distributions out of the S corporation's AE&P are treated as dividends and are fully taxable as ordinary

income to the shareholder. In contrast, distributions out of the S corporation's earnings accumulated while it was an S corporation are generally nontaxable to the extent of the shareholder's stock basis. As a result, the source of the distribution is extremely important. This distinction—and a special concern about a potential abuse—requires the corporation to break down its retained earnings into several components. It is important to remember that while each of these components have its own special characteristics, all of them are simply part of the S corporation's total earnings that have been accumulated and not distributed over the years. There are four corporate level equity accounts. They are referred to as (1) the accumulated adjustments account (AAA); (2) previously taxed income (PTI); (3) AE&P; and (4) the other adjustments account (OAA). The treatment of the distributions from such accounts, as discussed below, can be summarized as follows:

Order	Source	Description	Treatment	Effect on Basis
1.	AAA	All S corps to the extent of AAA	Nontaxable unless exceeds shareholder's stock basis	Reduces stock basis to the extent thereof
2.	PTI	Distributions to shareholders who have personal pre-1983 PTI accumulations	Nontaxable unless exceeds shareholder's stock basis	Reduces stock basis to the extent thereof
3.	AE&P	S corps that have C AE&P	Ordinary dividend income	No effect
4.	OAA	All remaining distributions from S corp's tax-exempt income	Nontaxable unless exceeds shareholder's stock basis	Reduce basis to the extent thereof
5.	Paid-in Capital	All remaining distributions	Nontaxable unless exceeds shareholder's stock basis	Reduce basis to the extent thereof

Accumulated Adjustments Account. The *accumulated adjustments account* (AAA) is the initial reference point for determining the source of a distribution and therefore its treatment. All distributions are assumed to first come out of AAA to the extent thereof. While neither the name of the account nor its acronym are descriptive, this account generally represents post-1982 income of the S corporation that has been taxed to shareholders but has not been distributed. Consequently, distributions from the account are a *nontaxable* return of the shareholder's basis in his or her stock. Distributions from the AAA that exceed the shareholder's stock basis are capital gain.[105]

The AAA is a corporate-level equity account that must be maintained if the S corporation has accumulated E&P from years when it was operated as a C corporation.[106] The AAA is the cumulative total of the S corporation's post-1982 income and gains (other than tax-exempt income) as reduced by all expenses and losses (both deductible and nondeductible other than those related to tax-exempt income) and any distributions deemed to have been made from the account. The specific formula for computing the balance in the AAA is shown in Exhibit 23-4. Note that the adjustments to the AAA are similar to those made by shareholders to their basis in their stock with some exceptions:[107]

---

[105] § 1368(b).

[106] § 1368(c).

[107] § 1368(e)(1).

1. Tax-exempt income increases the shareholder's stock basis but has no effect on the AAA. These items are posted to the OAA discussed below.

2. Expenses and losses related to tax-exempt income decrease the shareholder's stock basis but have no effect on the AAA. [However, other nondeductible expenditures reduce the AAA as they do the shareholder's stock basis (e.g., the 50 percent of meal and entertainment expenses that is not deductible, fines, and penalties).]

3. The various adjustments to the AAA (other than distributions) can create either a positive or negative balance in the AAA account. In contrast, the shareholder's stock basis can never be negative.

4. The ordering rules for the AAA are somewhat different than for basis. The corporation adjusts for income, then subtracts deductions and losses (but *only* to the extent of income items) before it calculates the balance available for distributions. In a year in which the corporation has deductions and losses in excess of income items, it reduces the AAA for this excess (called the "net negative adjustment") *after* reduction for distributions.

EXHIBIT 23-4

Accumulated Adjustments Account Computations

Beginning Balance (S Years Beginning after 1982)

Add income items:
    Taxable income
    Separately stated gains and income (not including tax-exempt income)
Less losses and deductions (not to exceed income items above)
    Nondeductible losses and expenses (excluding expenses relating to tax-exempt income)
    Ordinary loss
Less distributions (to extent of beginning balance plus income less losses and deductions)
Less losses and deductions, to the extent they exceed income items (the net negative adjustment)

Equals AAA end of the year

Example 34. In 1985, T formed ABC Inc. and operated it as a calendar year C corporation until 1992, when it elected to be treated as an S corporation. T has owned 100% of the stock since the corporation's inception. T's basis in his stock at the beginning of 2009 was $10,000. Other information related to the S corporation for 2009 is shown below.

Net ordinary income	$50,000
Charitable contribution	9,000
Tax-exempt interest income	10,000
Expenses related to tax-exempt interest income	1,000
Disallowed portion of meal expenses	2,000
Cash distributions	20,000
Beginning accumulated adjustments account	10,000

The first five items listed above flow through to T. Of these, T must include the $50,000 of ordinary taxable income on his 2009 tax return. In addition, T is allowed

to report the $9,000 charitable contribution made by the corporation as an itemized deduction on his return.

    T's basis and the balances in the AAA and OAA accounts at the end of the year are computed in the following manner:

	Basis	AAA	OAA
Beginning balance.........................	$10,000	$10,000	$ 0
Positive adjustments:			
Taxable income	50,000	50,000	0
Tax-exempt income.....................	10,000	0	$10,000
Basis before distributions	$70,000	—	—
Negative items to AAA:			
Disallowed meal expense.................	—	(2,000)	
Charitable contributions		(9,000)	
AAA before distribution.....................		$49,000	
Less distribution...........................	(20,000)	(20,000)	
Basis and AAA after distribution	$50,000	$29,000	
Negative items to basis:			
Disallowed meal expense.................	(2,000)		
Expenses related to tax-exempt income.........	(1,000)		(1,000)
Charitable contribution	(9,000)		
Final balances.............................	$38,000	$29,000	$ 9,000

Note that for purposes of the determining the treatment of the distribution, the shareholder's stock basis is determined after the positive adjustments but before the negative adjustments. In contrast, the AAA balance available for distributions is determined after the nondeductible and deductible items (including losses) but only to the extent of the positive adjustments. Also observe that the $9,000 ($38,000 − $29,000) difference between the increase in T's basis in his stock and the corporation's AAA is attributable to the tax-exempt interest income of $10,000 less the $1,000 of expenses related to this income, neither of which affects the AAA. These items are reflected in the OAA account.

As noted above, distributions from the AAA are nontaxable to the shareholder unless they exceed the shareholder's stock basis. However, it is rare for shareholders to receive distributions from the AAA that exceed the basis in their stock. Most of the time, the aggregate basis of the shareholders will equal or exceed the AAA (e.g., *see Example 34* above). Note also that the AAA is a corporate-level account and is unaffected by either shareholder transactions or shareholder basis in the stock. Therefore, if a shareholder sells stock, new shareholders are entitled to distributions from the AAA, which will be reductions of basis. On rare occasions a distribution from the AAA will exceed a shareholder's stock basis. In such case, the excess is treated as a gain from the sale of stock.

    Previously Taxed Income. The second account from which a distribution may come consists of undistributed income that has been previously taxed for S years before 1983, commonly referred to as previously taxed income (PTI).[108] As a practical matter, this account may be viewed as the AAA for years prior to 1983. The balance in this account represents taxable income that was earned by the corporation while it was an S corporation prior to 1983 and which has not been distributed to shareholders. Distributions from this account, like those from the AAA, are considered to be a nontaxable return of the shareholder's basis in his or her stock. Unlike AAA, PTI is

---

[108] § 1368(c).

considered a personal account and is nontransferable. Therefore buyers of a shareholder's interest do not obtain any of that shareholder's PTI.

Accumulated E&P of C Years. The third account from which a distribution may come represents earnings and profits accumulated in years when the corporation was a C corporation. Distributions from AE&P are taxable as dividend income. There is no schedule or reconciliation of AE&P on Form 1120S.

Other Adjustments Account. Schedule M-2 of Form 1120S creates a fourth classification, entitled *other adjustments account* (OAA). The OAA represents post-1982 tax-exempt income and expenses related to such income and other items that do not flow into the AAA. Thus, the OAA is used to show amounts that affect shareholder bases but not the AAA.

Schedule M-2. Schedule M-2 on page 4 of Form 1120S is a reconciliation of the beginning and ending balances in these corporate accounts: the AAA, the OAA, and shareholders' undistributed taxable income previously taxed (i.e., PTI). Interestingly, the M-2 does not reflect the ordering rules (i.e., distributions before losses and other expenses); nor does the M-2 provide for any reconciliation of AE&P.

Example 35. Same facts as in *Example 34* above. The corporation's Schedule M-2 for the year would appear as follows:

Schedule M-2	Analysis of Accumulated Adjustments Account, Other Adjustments Account, and Shareholders' Undistributed Taxable Income Previously Taxed (see instructions)		
	(a) Accumulated adjustments account	**(b)** Other adjustments account	**(c)** Shareholders' undistributed taxable income previously taxed
1 Balance at beginning of tax year . . .	10,000		
2 Ordinary income from page 1, line 21 . .	50,000		
3 Other additions		10,000	
4 Loss from page 1, line 21	( )		
5 Other reductions	(11,000)	(1,000)	
6 Combine lines 1 through 5	49,000	9,000	
7 Distributions other than dividend distributions	20,000		
8 Balance at end of tax year. Subtract line 7 from line 6	29,000	9,000	

Form **1120S** (2008)

Source of Distribution. As discussed above, the treatment of a distribution depends on its source. For this purpose, distributions are presumed to flow out of the various accounts in the following order with the treatment as described.[109]

1. *Accumulated Adjustments Account (AAA).* Distributions are first considered distributions out of the AAA and, therefore, are nontaxable to extent of the shareholder's stock basis. Any amount received out of the AAA that is in excess of the shareholder's basis is treated as a sale of the underlying stock, resulting in capital gain.

2. *Previously Taxed Income (PTI).* Distributions of PTI are nontaxable to the extent of the shareholder's stock basis with any excess treated as capital gain.

3. *Accumulated Earnings and Profits (AE&P).* Distributions of AE&P are treated as dividends income just as if distributed from a C corporation and, therefore, are fully taxable as dividend income to the shareholder.

4. *Other Adjustments Account (OAA).* Distributions out of the OAA are nontaxable to the extent of the shareholder's stock basis with any excess treated as capital gain.

---

[109] § 1368(c).

5. *Remaining Distributions.* Distributions in excess of the amounts in the accounts described above (i.e., the other accounts are exhausted) are treated as returns of the shareholder's capital and are nontaxable to the extent of the shareholder's stock basis. Any excess is treated as capital gain.

Note that all of the distributions above reduce the shareholder's stock basis except amounts out of the corporation's AE&P.

Example 36. J and W have been equal owners of a calendar year S corporation for several years. It has been operated as a C and an S corporation in the past. Balances at the beginning of the year are shown below in the schedule. Operations for the year show $12,000 net ordinary income, $2,000 tax-exempt interest income, and $24,000 cash distributions. Based on the approach described above, the $24,000 cash distribution exhausts (1) all of the $18,000 AAA, (2) all of the $4,000 PTI, and (3) $2,000 ($24,000 − $18,000 − $4,000) of the AE&P. The balances at the end of the year are determined as follows:

	Corporate Accounts				Stock Basis	
	AAA	PTI	AE&P	OAA	J	W
Beginning balances.........	$ 6,000	$4,000	$3,000	$ 0	$10,000	$6,000
Net ordinary income	12,000				6,000	6,000
Tax-exempt interest income..				2,000	1,000	1,000
Cash distributions:..........						
AAA....................	(18,000)				(9,000)	(9,000)
PTI....................		(4,000)			(2,000)	(2,000)
AE&P.................			(2,000)		0	0
Ending balances	$ 0	$ 0	$1,000	$2,000	$6,000	$2,000

Both J and W have $6,000 net ordinary income (from S operations) and $1,000 dividend income (from AE&P). Note that J and W recognize dividend income because tax-exempt income does not increase AAA. Also note that there is no longer any need to maintain an account for PTI once the corporation has distributed its PTI.

Example 37. Refer to *Example 36*. Operations for the following year show net ordinary income of $9,400 and cash distributions of $16,000. The balances at the end of this year are determined as follows:

	Corporate Accounts				Stock Basis	
	AAA	AE&P	OAA		J	W
Beginning balances	$ 0	$1,000	$2,000		$6,000	$2,000
Net ordinary income	9,400				4,700	4,700
Cash distributions:.........						
AAA..................	(9,400)				(4,700)	(4,700)
AE&P.................		(1,000)			0	0
OAA.................			(2,000)		(1,000)	(1,000)
Remaining (basis)				(3,600)	(1,800)	(1,000)
Remaining gain to W				(800)		
Ending balances	$ 0	$ 0	$ 0		$3,200	$ 0

Both J and W have $4,700 net ordinary income and $500 dividend income (from AE&P). In addition, W has $800 capital gain since the distributions that reduce basis exceed her basis in the stock by $800. Because this S corporation no longer has AE&P, any future distributions will be nontaxable unless they exceed a shareholder's basis in the stock. Note that in this case there is no PTI component because the S corporation has no PTI.

DISTRIBUTIONS OF PROPERTY

Although most distributions consist solely of cash, an S corporation may distribute property. Rules governing property distributions of an S corporation are a unique blend of both the partnership and C corporation provisions.

Like C corporations, the amount of any property distributed by an S corporation is the fair market value of the property less any associated liabilities. Also like a C corporation, an S corporation must recognize gain—but not loss—on the distribution of property. Any gain recognized by the S corporation on the distribution passes through to be reported by the shareholders. In addition, this gain increases each shareholder's stock basis. Upon receipt of the distribution, the shareholder reduces his or her basis by the fair market value of the property received (but not below zero). Any amount in excess of the shareholder's basis is capital gain. The shareholder's basis in the property is its fair market value. The treatment of property distributions is identical to the approach described above for cash distributions.[110]

Example 38. After using the following equipment for four years of its five-year MACRS life, an S corporation distributes it to H, its sole owner.

Asset	Cost	Accumulated Depreciation	Basis	Fair Market Value
Equipment	$10,000	$7,900	$2,100	$4,300

H's stock basis, after all adjustments except the equipment distribution, is $1,800.

	Includible Income	Stock Basis
H's basis, before		$1,800
S gain recognized (§ 1245: $4,300 FMV – $2,100 basis)	$2,200	2,200
Balance		$4,000
Tax-free distribution		(4,000)
Taxable distribution	$300	
H's basis, after		$ 0

H must also recognize a $300 capital gain since the $4,300 FMV of the equipment exceeds his $4,000 stock basis. His basis in the equipment becomes $4,300.

SPECIAL RULES RELATING TO SOURCE OF DISTRIBUTIONS

While the normal rules for the sourcing of distributions usually is favored by shareholders, this is not always the case. For example, recall that an S election is terminated if an S corporation has excess passive income and AE&P for three consecutive years. In this

---

[110] Under current IRS instructions to Form 1120S, both property and cash reduce PTI.

situation and others, the corporation may want to purge itself of its AE&P to avoid losing its election. Note, however, that under the normal rules, the corporation must distribute all of its AAA before it can begin distributing its AE&P. Fortunately, the law provides possible relief and makes a special election available to the corporation to alter the source of the distribution. Section 1368(e)(3) allows the corporation to make the so-called *bypass election*. As shown in Exhibit 23-5, this election enables the corporation to bypass AAA and treat accumulated E&P as being distributed before AAA.[111] The corporation files the election by attaching an appropriate statement to a timely filed or extended return. The election applies only to the year covered by the return. Thus, if AE&P remain at the beginning of the next year, the balance will again be behind the corporation's AAA.

When an S corporation has PTI and needs to eliminate AE&P, the election under § 1368(e)(3) is not sufficient. The corporation must also exhaust PTI before it can start distributing AE&P. The Regulations make this possible by allowing the corporation to elect to bypass PTI when determining the treatment of its distributions.[112] If the corporation elects to bypass both AAA and PTI (as shown in Exhibit 23-5), AE&P is deemed to be the first item distributed by the S corporation.

In many cases, an S corporation identifies the need to distribute its AE&P after the close of the taxable year—normally a time when it would be too late to take action. However, the Regulations rescue the corporation in this situation with a very valuable tool: the deemed dividend election.[113] When every shareholder who receives a distribution during the year consents to this election, the corporation is treated as having made a distribution of its AE&P on the last day of its taxable year. The shareholders must first include the deemed dividend in their income and then are treated as having contributed the amount to the corporation as a contribution to capital increasing the basis in their stock. The bypass and deemed dividend elections require the consent of all "affected shareholders" (those who have received distributions or deemed distributions during the tax year).

EXHIBIT 23-5
Sources of Distributions

Distribution Order	Normal Treatment	AAA and PTI Bypass Elections	Post-Termination Transition Period
1	AAA	AE&P	AAA
2	PTI	AAA	CE&P
3	AE&P	PTI	AE&P
4	OAA	OAA	Unspecified return of capital

POST-TERMINATION TRANSACTIONS

Distributions. When a corporation election terminates its S election, the entity is immediately treated as a C corporation. Without special rules, this transition could be particularly severe. Recall that distributions for a C corporation are dividends to the extent of E&P. This is true even though the C corporation may have undistributed nontaxable income from S years. This could create a special hardship on a person who had been a shareholder during the corporation's final S corporation year and who had received an allocation of income from the corporation attributable to that period. In such a situation, the shareholder would not be able to withdraw money from the corporation, even to the extent necessary to pay taxes on his or her portion of the S corporation's taxable income, without the possibility of dividend treatment. To address this problem, special rules allow

---

[111] Reg. § 1.1368-1(f)(2).

[112] Reg. § 1.1368-1(f)(4).

[113] Reg. § 1.1368-1(f)(3).

a shareholder to treat distributions as being from the AAA during the post-termination transition period (PTTP).

The PTTP begins the day after the S corporation's final tax year and lasts at least one year and perhaps longer.[114] During the PTTP, cash—but not property—distributions are deemed to come from AAA to the extent thereof.[115] But this is where the normal pattern of distributions ends. Any PTTP distributions in excess of AAA are *not* considered as having come from PTI or OAA but rather current or accumulated E&P. As shown in Exhibit 23-5, any distributions during the PTTP in excess of AAA would be fully taxable as dividends to the extent of the corporation's E&P. Note that this special ordering rule for distributions during the PTTP is deemed to occur unless the corporation elects not to have it apply. Also observe that a distribution during the PTTP is only treated as coming from the AAA if it is received by a person who was a shareholder on the corporation's final day as an S corporation.[116]

Losses. In some cases, a shareholder who had sustained losses prior to the termination of an S election may have lacked sufficient basis to deduct those losses. Without some relief, those losses would provide no tax benefit after the termination since the corporation is no longer an S corporation but a C corporation. However, the Code enables shareholders to secure those losses by allowing them to increase their stock basis during the PTTP.[117] Note that a loan during this period does not create basis for prior losses. Only increases in stock basis can secure losses. For example, shareholders could cancel any corporate debt owed to them and treat the cancellation as a contribution to capital with a corresponding increase in basis. Similarly, a shareholder could exchange the debt for additional stock. A shareholder could also increase the stock's basis by simply contributing additional cash or property to the capital of the corporation.

TAXES IMPOSED ON THE S CORPORATION

S corporations, like partnerships, normally are considered nontaxable entities. Unlike partnerships, however, S corporations may be required to pay one of the following taxes:

1. Excessive passive investment income tax

2. Tax on built-in gains

3. LIFO recapture tax

TAX ON EXCESSIVE PASSIVE INCOME

When Congress revised Subchapter S in 1982, it was concerned that C corporations with a potential accumulated earnings tax or personal holding company tax, particularly those that are mere holding companies (i.e., those whose principal assets are investment properties such as stocks, securities, and real estate projects), would attempt to escape these penalty taxes by electing to be treated as S corporations. Subchapter S can provide a refuge for these corporations since S corporations normally are exempt from both penalty taxes. To guard against this possibility, Congress enacted two provisions. First, as previously explained, when a corporation has AE&P *and* excessive passive income in three

---

[114] § 1377(b).

[115] § 1371(e).

[116] Reg. § 1.1377-2(b).

[117] § 1366(d)(3).

consecutive years, the corporation's S election is terminated.[118] Second, an S corporation must pay a special tax on its passive income if (1) it has AE&P at the close of its tax year, *and* (2) passive investment income exceeds 25 percent of its gross receipts that year.[119] Note that this tax, as well as the termination provision for excessive passive income (discussed early in this chapter), only applies to corporations that have AE&P from C corporation years at the end of the taxable year. Consequently, the tax is not imposed on corporations that have distributed all of their AE&P or that have never been C corporations.

The tax on excessive passive income is equal to the maximum corporate rate for the year (35 percent in 2008) multiplied by *excess net passive income* (ENPI). ENPI is computed as follows:

$$\text{ENPI} = \text{Net passive income} \times \frac{\text{Passive investment income} - 25\% \text{ of gross receipts}}{\text{Passive investment income}}$$

In computing the tax, several rules must be observed.

1. For any taxable year, *ENPI* cannot exceed the corporation's taxable income, computed as though it were a C corporation but before reduction for the dividends-received deduction and net operating loss deduction.[120]

2. *Passive investment income* is defined the same as it is for the termination provisions of § 1362(d) discussed previously:[121] generally gross receipts from dividends, interest (including tax-exempt interest), rents, royalties, and annuities, and gains from sales of stocks and securities (before 2007).

3. *Net passive income* is passive investment income reduced by any allowable deductions directly connected with the production of this income. These deductions include such expenses as property taxes and depreciation related to rental property but exclude such deductions as the dividends-received deduction.[122]

The amount of any tax paid reduces the amount of each item of passive investment income that flows through to shareholders. The tax is allocated proportionately based on net passive investment income.[123]

> **Example 39.** PTC is owned equally by R and S. At the close of the year, PTC, an S corporation, reports gross receipts of $200,000 and a balance in its AE&P account of $24,000. Gross receipts include $25,000 interest and $50,000 of passive rent. Deductions directly attributable to rents were $30,000, including depreciation, maintenance, insurance, and property taxes. Using this information, PTC has excess net passive investment income of $15,000 determined as follows:

---

[118] § 1362(d)(3).

[119] § 1375(a).

[120] § 1375(b)(1)(B) and Reg. § 1.1375-1(b)(1)(ii).

[121] §§ 1375(b)(3) and 1362(d)(3).

[122] § 1375(b)(2).

[123] Reg. § 1.1366-4(c).

Total gross receipts:

Gross receipts:		
	Interest..	$ 25,000
	Rent (passive)...	50,000
	Total passive gross receipts	$ 75,000
	Active gross receipts	125,000
Total gross receipts..		$200,000

Permitted passive portion (25% × $200,000).....................................	$ 50,000

Excess passive gross receipts ($75,000 − $50,000)	$ 25,000
Net Passive Income:	
Passive gross receipts...	$ 75,000
Deductions connected with rent	(30,000)
Net passive income..	$ 45,000

Excess net passive income:	
Excess passive gross receipts	$ 25,000
Divide by total passive gross receipts	75,000
Excess fraction ($25,000/$75,000)	$\frac{1}{3}$
Times net passive income..	45,000
Excess net passive income	15,000

Since the corporation has passive investment income exceeding 25% of its gross receipts ($25,000) *and* it has AE&P at the end of the taxable year, the tax on excessive passive income is imposed.

PTC's excessive passive investment income tax is $5,250 (35% × $15,000). This amount is allocated as follows:

	Interest	Rent	Total
Gross receipts	$25,000	$50,000	$75,000
Expenses	0	(30,000)	(30,000)
....	$25,000	$20,000	$45,000
Tax allocation......................	(2,916)	(2,334)	(5,250)
....	$22,084	$17,666	$39,750
To each shareholder (50%)	$11,042	$ 8,833	$19,875

TAX ON BUILT-IN GAINS

Without special rules, C corporations planning sales or distributions of appreciated property (e.g., as a dividend or in liquidation) could avoid double taxation by electing S status before making the distributions.

Example 40. R, a regular C corporation, owns land worth $50,000 (basis $10,000). If R Corporation distributes the land to its sole shareholder, D, as a dividend, the corporation recognizes a gain of $40,000 ($50,000 − $10,000) and D recognizes dividend income of $50,000. Therefore, two taxes are imposed. In contrast, compare the result that occurs if R Corporation has S status. R still recognizes a $40,000 gain. However, that gain is not taxed at the corporate level but flows through to D to be included on his tax return. In addition, D increases his basis in his stock by $40,000. On receipt of the property, D does not report any income but simply reduces the basis in his stock. As a result, there is only a *single tax* if R Corporation has S status.

To eliminate the tax-avoidance possibility of electing S status before the distribution (or a sale), Congress enacted § 1374. This section imposes a special corporate-level tax—the *built-in gains tax*—on gains recognized by an S corporation that accrued while it was a C corporation. The tax applies *only* to certain gains recognized during the 10-year period following the S election.

Under § 1374, it is presumed that *any* gain recognized on the sale or distribution of any property by a "converted" S corporation is subject to the built-in gains tax. However, the corporation may rebut this presumption and avoid the tax by proving either of the following: (1) the asset sold or distributed was not held on the date that the corporation elected S status; or (2) the gain had not accrued at the time of the election. As a practical matter, this approach requires every C corporation electing S status to have an independent appraisal of its assets on the date the S election becomes effective (i.e., the conversion date) in order to rebut the presumption. Note that for purposes of this tax, built-in gains are applicable to *all* assets, including inventory, unrealized receivables of a cash basis taxpayer, any gain on a long-term contract that has not been recognized (e.g., the taxpayer uses the completed contract method of accounting), and any goodwill.

As a general rule, the special tax applies only to S corporations having a *net unrealized built-in gain*. A net unrealized built-in gain is defined as the difference between the value and basis of all assets held on the conversion date. This difference represents the *maximum* amount that may be subject to the built-in gains tax.

Example 41. On November 3, 2008 T Corporation made an S election. The election was effective for calendar year 2009. On January 1, 2009 its balance sheet revealed the following assets:

	Adjusted Basis	Fair Market Value	Built-in Gain (Loss)
Equipment	$ 50,000	$ 75,000	$25,000
Land	30,000	70,000	40,000
Stock.	20,000	15,000	(5,000)
	$100,000	$160,000	$60,000

T Corporation's net unrealized built-in gain is $60,000. Note that the built-in loss on the stock effectively limits the taxpayer's future exposure to the built-in gains tax.

Only the *net recognized built-in gain* (NRBIG) is subject to tax.[124] According to the regulations, NRBIG is the lesser of:

1. The *Pre-Limitation Amount* (PLA). The PLA is the S corporation's taxable income as if its *only* recognized items for the year were its recognized built-in gains and losses. The S corporation must observe the C corporation rules in making this computation. However, in using the C rules, the corporation is not permitted to claim any dividends-received deduction or any loss carryforward.

2. The *Taxable Income Limit* (TIL). The TIL is the S corporation's taxable income computed in the same manner as a C corporation, including *all* of its recognized gross income and deductions for the taxable year. Again, it is not allowed to claim the dividends-received deduction or any loss carryforward. Due to this rule,

---

[124] § 1374(b).

NRBIG cannot exceed the taxable income that the corporation would have had if it had been a C corporation.

3. The *Net Unrealized Built-in Gain Limit* (NUL). In its first S corporation year, the NUL is the same as the net *unrealized* built-in gain (i.e., the maximum net built-in gain that could be recognized). In subsequent years, the NUL is the original net unrealized built-in gain reduced by all net recognized built-in gains in prior years. In this manner, the net unrealized built-in gain acts as the limiting factor on the total net recognized built-in gains that could be reported during the ten year recognition period.

The corporation computes each of these amounts and the lowest is the NRBIG for the year. After the corporation computes this amount, it is then allowed to reduce it by any unused net operating loss carryforwards from years in which it was a C corporation. The corporation applies a flat rate of 35 percent to this amount, which in turn may be offset by certain credit carryforwards from prior years.

> **Example 42.** Refer to the facts in *Example 41*. During 2009 T Corporation sold the equipment and the stock for $77,000 and $15,000, respectively. Although T recognizes a gain of $27,000 ($77,000 − $50,000) on the sale of the equipment, T's built-in gain recognized is limited to the amount accrued on the date of conversion from a C corporation to S status, $25,000. T's net recognized built-in gain that is potentially subject to tax is $20,000 (the built-in gain of $25,000 less the $5,000 built-in loss recognized.)

> **Example 43.** Refer to the facts in *Example 41 and 42*. Assume that during 2009, T Corporation's taxable income, including the equipment and stock sales, is $38,000. This figure is computed using the modified C corporation rules. At this point, the TIL is greater than the PLA of $20,000, so the PLA is treated as the taxable built-in gain. The corporation then computes its NUL. In its first S corporation year, the NUL is the same as the net unrealized built in gain, $60,000. As a result, the net realized built-in-gain (NRBIG) for the year is $20,000 (the lesser of PLA of $20,000, TIL $38,000, and NUL $60,000).
>
> If the corporation had sold the land at a gain of $40,000 instead of selling the stock, the total gain for the first S corporation year would have been $67,000 ($40,000 gain from land + $27,000 gain from equipment). However, only $60,000 of this gain would be potentially subject to the § 1374 tax because T's NUL is the maximum amount subject to the tax. Moreover, since its TIL is $38,000, the gain would be further limited to $38,000.
>
> In subsequent years, the NUL is computed by subtracting all net recognized built-in gains to date from the original net unrealized built-in gain. In this manner, the net unrealized built in gain may act as the limiting factor on the total net recognized built-in gains during the ten year recognition period.

In determining the built-in gains tax, the net recognized built-in gain (after applying all limitations) is reduced by any NOL and capital loss carryforward from C corporate years. In addition, business tax credit carryforwards arising in a C year can be used to reduce the tax.[125] Any net recognized built-in gain not subject to tax because of the TIL is carried over to the following year and treated as if it occurred in that year. The calculation of the tax is summarized below.

---

[125] § 1374(b)(2) and (3).

	Net recognized built-in gain	$ x,xxx
−	NOL and NCL carryforward from C year	(xxx)
=	Tax base	$ x,xxx
×	Top corporate tax rate	× xx%
=	Potential tax	$ x,xxx
−	Business credit and AMT carryforward from C year	(xxx)
=	Tax	$ x,xxx

Example 44. Refer to the facts in *Example 42*. Assume that T sold the land for $70,000 in its first S corporation year, but did not sell the equipment or stock. T recognizes a $40,000 gain, which is also the total PLA for the year. The TIL is $38,000 and the NUL is $60,000. Assume T also has a NOL carryforward of $3,000 from C corporation years. The corporation's built in gains tax is:

Least of:		
PLA	$40,000	
NUL	$60,000	
TIL	$38,000	$38,000
Less NOL carryforward		(3,000)
Taxable amount		$35,000
Tax rate		× 35%
Built in gains tax		$12,250

After the S corporation calculates its built-in gains tax for the year, it needs to make some additional computations:

1. If the TIL is the least of the three net recognized built-in gain measures, the corporation will need to determine its recognized built-in gain carryforward to the next year.

2. The corporation must apportion the tax as a reduction to the income items flowing through to the shareholders, as well as the year's increment to the AAA.

3. The corporation must compute its NUL for its next taxable year.

For the corporation in *Example 44* above, the calculations are shown below.

Adjustment to next year's PLA to reflect the gain carryforward arising from the TIL for the current year.

Lesser of NUL ($60,000) or PLA ($40,000)	$40,000
Subtract TIL, if less	(38,000)
Gain carryforward to add to next year's PLA	$ 2,000

Adjustment to next year's NUL:

NUL at beginning of current year	$60,000
Less net recognized built-in gain of current year	(38,000)
NUL for next year	$22,000

The corporation must then subtract its built-in gains tax from the income items that created the built-in gain in order to determine the pass-through of items to the shareholders. Assuming that the recognized built-in gain of $40,000 was a § 1231 gain, the corporation would reduce this gain by the tax of $12,250 and pass through $27,750 of § 1231 gain ($40,000 − $12,250) to its shareholders. Assuming that the corporation had a net ordinary loss of $2,000, to yield the TIL of $38,000, the corporation would pass the loss of $2,000 through to its shareholder's and the year's net addition to the AAA would be $25,750 computed as follows:

§ 1231 gain.	$40,000
Built in gains tax.	(12,250)
Ordinary loss	(2,000)
Net increment to AAA	$25,750

LIFO RECAPTURE

A corporation using the LIFO method of accounting for inventories in its last taxable year before an S election becomes effective must include in taxable income for its last C corporation year an additional amount, called the LIFO recapture amount.

The LIFO recapture amount is the excess of the inventory's value under FIFO (lower of cost or market) over its actual LIFO basis as of the end of the corporation's last C corporation taxable year.[126] The increase in tax liability is referred to as the LIFO recapture tax, although it is not a separate tax per se, and it is not imposed on the income after the corporation becomes an S corporation. This portion of the tax is payable in four equal installments, with the first installment due on the due date of the corporation's last C corporation return and the subsequent payments due on the due dates of the first three S corporation returns.[127] No interest is due if the required installments are paid on a timely basis, and there is no requirement that estimated tax payments be made with respect to any LIFO recapture tax due.[128] Finally, the inventory's basis is increased by the LIFO recapture amount. Any additional appreciation attributable to the inventory (i.e., excess of fair market value over its FIFO basis) will be subject to the built-in gains tax as the inventory is sold. However, if the corporation does not report a decrement from its initial S corporation LIFO layer during its recognition period, it will not recognize income as a built-in gain.

> **Example 45.** H Corporation converts to S corporation status for 2009. H used the LIFO method of accounting for its inventory in 2008 and had an ending LIFO inventory basis of $90,000. At the end of 2008, the inventory's actual fair market value was $175,000 and its FIFO value was $150,000. H must add the $60,000 LIFO recapture amount (FIFO value of $150,000 − $90,000 LIFO value) to its 2008 taxable income. Assuming a 35 percent corporate tax rate, H Corporation's 2008 tax liability is increased by $21,000, the LIFO recapture tax. Thus, H must pay $5,250 (one-fourth) of the LIFO recapture tax with its 2008 corporate tax return and the remaining three installments of $5,250 each must be paid with H's next three tax returns. Note also that after adjusting the inventory's basis to $150,000, there is $25,000 of remaining unrealized appreciation that may be subject to the built-in gains tax as the inventory is sold. However, the future gains will be calculated by the LIFO method.

---

[126] § 1363(d)(3).

[127] § 1363(d)(2)(B).

[128] § 6655(g)(4).

ESTIMATED TAXES

S corporations are required to pay estimated taxes for (1) excessive passive investment income taxes (§ 1375), and (2) taxes on built-in gains (§ 1374). The computations of estimated taxes generally follow the rules applicable to C corporations.[129] Shareholders should include their portions of S corporation income or loss when calculating their own estimated tax payments.[130]

DISPOSITION OF OWNERSHIP INTEREST

Based on the entity theory, sales of stock by shareholders of an S corporation result in capital gain or loss. This, of course, is identical to how stock sales of a C corporation are treated. However, the amount of the gain or loss will differ since an S shareholder's basis is adjusted for income, losses, and distributions whereas a C shareholder's basis is not. All other stock transfers also follow the rules of an exchange or gift of a capital asset. This is a significant advantage for the S (or C) corporate shareholder when compared with the complicated and often unfavorable rules of the partnership. Shareholders who sell or otherwise dispose of their stock must report their share of the S corporation's current-year items, based either on the per-day allocation method or the interim closing-of-the-books method.

WORTHLESS SECURITIES

S and C shareholders who hold worthless securities, including stock and debt, are subject to the same provisions with one exception. The S corporation's flow-through rules apply *before* the deduction for worthless stock or debt. The loss on worthless securities is treated as though it occurred on the last day of the *shareholder's* taxable year (not the S corporation's year) from the sale or exchange of a capital asset. Thus, it is possible for stock to become worthless before corporate activities are completed. In addition, if the S corporation's year ends *after* the stockholder's year ends, worthlessness could occur before the flow-through is available. This potential loss of deduction could be a serious disadvantage to shareholders.

The deduction for worthless stock is a capital loss unless the stock qualifies for ordinary loss treatment under § 1244.[131] Bad debts also are capital losses unless the shareholder can establish that they are business bad debts.[132] For example, the debts may have arisen as a result of a business transaction or the shareholder's employment status with the corporation. Business bad debts are ordinary losses. Nonbusiness bad debts are short-term capital losses.

CORPORATE LIQUIDATION

Generally, provisions governing liquidations and reorganizations for C corporations are applicable to S corporations (see Chapter 20).

---

[129] See § 6655 for estimated taxes applicable to C corporations.

[130] The Code and Regulations do not expressly provide that but the language of §§ 1366 and 6654 is broad enough to require inclusion of S corporation items. See Ltr. Ruls. 8542034 and 8544011.

[131] Compare §§ 165(g) and 1367(b)(3) with § 1244(a).

[132] Compare §§ 166(a) and (d).

TAX PLANNING

CHOICE OF ENTITY: COMPARING S CORPORATIONS, C CORPORATIONS, PARTNERSHIPS, AND LLCS

No doubt one of the most common questions asked by a taxpayer who is anticipating starting a new business or has an existing business concerns the form of organization that should be used. That decision has probably never been as confusing as it is today. For years, nontax factors, specifically the desire to limit an individual's liability, often were the key determinant in the choice of entity decision. Professional advisors, wishing to minimize the owner's personal liability, usually encouraged the owner to incorporate and secure the liability protection that the corporate entity offered. Assuming the owner took the advice, the only decision left from a tax perspective was whether the corporation would elect to be treated under the rules of Subchapter S or operate as a regular corporation subject to the rules of Subchapter C.

The limited liability company (now authorized in all 50 states) has made the choice of entity decision far more difficult. This new creature, which provides limited liability yet is taxed as a partnership, has added an important new dimension to the business organization question. Business owners who seek limited liability are no longer constrained to accept the corporate form and the C or S tax treatment that accompanies it. They may now opt for partnership tax treatment provided by limited liability companies and still obtain the protection that was formerly available only with a corporation. In short, the limited liability company has for the most part made the liability factor moot. Consequently, the decision now turns on other critical factors, which for small business owners include tax considerations.

A complete comparison of these entities and the advantages and disadvantages of operating each can fill volumes and is beyond the scope of this text. Nevertheless, Exhibit 23-6 identifies some of the key transactions in the life of a business and explains how each of the various entities would be treated.

EXHIBIT 23-6

Comparative Analysis of Business Forms

Items for Comparison	Proprietorship / Proprietor	Partnership / Partner	S Corporation / Shareholder	C Corporation / Shareholder
1. What are the restrictions on the number of owners or who may be an owner?	One owner who must be an individual	None, except there must be at least two owners	No more than 100 shareholders who must be individuals, estates, certain trusts, charities, pensions and ESOPs	None.
2. Are owners liable for business debts that they have not personally guaranteed?	Yes, except if single-member LLC	Yes, for general partners but no for limited partners or partners in an LLP, LLC members	No	No
3. What are the appropriate tax forms and schedules and who files them?	Schedules C, SE, and all supporting schedules and forms	Form 1065 and Schedules K-1 are prepared by partnership; partners report on Schedules E, SE and other supporting schedules	Form 1120S and its Schedules K-1 are prepared by corporation; shareholders report on Schedule E and other supporting schedules	Form 1120 and all supporting schedules are filed for the C corporation; shareholders report dividend income on Schedule B
4. Who is the taxpayer?	Proprietor	Partners	Shareholders except tax on built-in gains, excess passive investment income, and LIFO recapture	C corporation: its shareholders are also taxed on dividend income when corporate earnings are distributed
5. Do owners have self-employment (SE) income from the business?	Yes, the net income from Schedule C	Yes, each general partner's share of net (SE) income plus guaranteed payments; for limited partners, only guaranteed payments from services	No	No
6. Must the business's taxable year be the same as that of the majority owners?	Yes	Generally, but a different year may be used if the partnership has natural business year or pays a tax on deferred income	Same as partnership	No, any period may be used except for personal service corporation
7. Are contributions of assets for an ownership interest taxable transactions?	No	No, same as proprietorship	No, if parties to the exchange own more than 80 percent of the corporation after the contribution, but otherwise, a taxable exchange with no carryover of tax attributes	Same as S corporation

EXHIBIT 23-6

Continued

Items for Comparison	Proprietorship / Proprietor	Partnership / Partner	S Corporation / Shareholder	C Corporation / Shareholder
8. Are distributions of cash includible income to owners?	No	No, except a distribution in excess of the partner's basis in the partnership is treated as a partial sale of the ownership interest	No, unless distribution exceeds shareholder's basis or is from accumulated E&P	Yes, if from the C corporation's earnings and profits
9. Do property distributions result in taxable income to the business or the owners?	No; basis is preserved in distributed property	No, with several exceptions	Yes, S corporation must recognize realized gain—but not loss—if a nonliquidating distribution; shareholders have dividend income if the FMV of the property exceeds AAA	Yes. Corporation recognizes gain, but not loss; shareholders have dividend income to extent of property's value or E&P
10. May an owner enter into taxable transactions (sales, loans, etc.) with the business?	No	Yes, when acting in a nonpartner capacity, but subject to related-party restrictions	Yes, subject to related-party restrictions	Same as S corporation
11. May an accrual basis business deduct accrued expenses to cash basis owners?	No, not applicable	No, deductible only when paid (except see 12 below)	Not deductible until shareholder includes in income. Applies to any shareholder	Not deductible until shareholder includes in income. Applies to >50% shareholder
12. Are accrued expenses of the business includible income to cash basis owners? If yes, when?	No, not applicable	Yes, when received, except guaranteed salary and interest on capital are includible when accrued	Yes, when received	When accrued to minority shareholders, when received by majority shareholders
13. Can owners be employees of the business and be paid salaries subject to employment taxes and withholding?	No	No	Yes	Yes
14. Are fringe benefits for owner/ employees deductible expenses?	No	Yes, but partner must include in gross income	Yes, but a more than 2 percent shareholder must include in gross income	Yes

EXHIBIT 23-6

Continued

Items for Comparison	Proprietorship / Proprietor	Partnership / Partner	S Corporation / Shareholder	C Corporation / Shareholder
15. May the business use the cash method?	Yes, depending on income and type of business unless it qualifies as a tax shelter	Yes, depending on income and type of business unless it qualifies as a tax shelter or has a C corporation as a partner	Yes, depending on income and type of business unless it qualifies as a tax shelter	No, unless gross receipts do not exceed $5 million or it qualifies under "type of business" exception
16. Is the business a conduit with the original character of the items flowing through to its owners as of the last day of the business's taxable year?	Yes	Yes	Yes	No, the business is an entity and the flow-through concept is not applicable
17. How are capital gains and losses of the business treated?	As though received by the proprietor	Flow through to each partner	Same as partnership	Net capital gain includible in corporate taxable income and taxed at regular rates; net capital losses carried back 3, forward 5 years, with no deduction against ordinary income
18. How is dividend income received by the business treated?	Includible income as though received by the proprietor (may be subject to reduced rate)	Flows through to each partner as dividend income (may be subject to reduced rate)	Same as partnership	Includible income with a dividend-received deduction
19. How are charitable contributions treated?	An itemized deduction as though contributed by the proprietor	Flow through to each partner as an itemized deduction	Same as partnership	Deductions may not exceed 10 percent of taxable income before certain deductions
20. Who pays state and local income taxes on the business net income and how are they treated?	Proprietor; an itemized deduction as though paid by the proprietor	Each partner; an itemized deduction	Same as partnership, except some state and local income taxes are assessed on the S corporation	Deductible expense
21. How are tax credits treated?	Offsets proprietor's tax	Qualifying credits flow through to each partner subject to any limitations applicable at the partner level	Same as partnership	Computed at the corporate level and reduces corporate tax liability
22. How is net ordinary income treated?	Includible with proprietor's A.G.I.	Flows through to each partner	Same as partnership	Included in corporate taxable income
23. How is net ordinary loss treated?	Reduction of proprietor's A.G.I.	Flows through to each partner, potentially deductible up to that partner's basis in the partnership; any excess is carried forward	Same as partnership except that basis rules differ	Subject to carryover rules (back two years and forward 20 years or forward 20 years only) and deductible against net ordinary income

EXHIBIT 23-6

Continued

Items for Comparison	Proprietorship / Proprietor	Partnership / Partner	S Corporation / Shareholder	C Corporation / Shareholder
24. How are AMT adjustments and preferences treated?	Included on proprietor's return	Flow through to partners	Same as partnership	Included in corporation's AMTI; ACE adjustment required: small corporations exempt
25. Is § 291(a)(1) applicable?	No	No	Yes, if C corporation for any of three prior tax years	Yes
26. How are items allocated among the owners?	Not applicable	According to profit and loss ratio or may be specially allocated	According to stock ownership ratio; special rules for years of termination or dispositions	Not applicable
27. Is the basis of business assets adjusted when an ownership interest is sold?	Not applicable	Yes, if partnership has elected the optional adjustment to basis	No, unless § 338(h)(10) election is in effect	No, unless § 338(h)(10) election is in effect
28. Is basis affected by business liabilities?	Not applicable	Yes, a partner's basis includes his or her share of partnership liabilities	No, except for loans directly from shareholders	No
29. Is basis affected by business income, gains, deductions, and losses?	Not applicable	Yes, all income and gains increase basis and all expenses and losses (that flow through) decrease basis	Yes, same as partnership	No
30. What is the character of gains and losses on the sale of a business interest?	Each asset is treated as sold individually and the character of the gain or loss is dependent on that asset	Capital gain or loss except ordinary income to the extent of partner's share of unrealized receivables, depreciation recapture, or inventory. Some gain may be taxed at 25 percent or 28 percent	Capital gains and losses, except losses may qualify as § 1244 ordinary losses if the corporation meets certain requirements. Some gain may be taxed at 28 percent (but not at 25 percent).	Same as S corporation, except no 28 percent portion. Special rules apply if stock is § 1202 stock.
31. Must a reasonable salary be allocated to family members performing services for the business?	No	Yes	Yes	No

PROBLEM MATERIALS

DISCUSSION QUESTIONS

23-1   *Eligibility Requirements.* May the following corporations elect Subchapter S? If not, explain why.
  a.   A corporation is 100 percent owned by another corporation.
  b.   A corporation has 101 shareholders, including Mr. and Mrs. V and Mr. and Mrs. Z.
  c.   A family corporation is owned by a father and his three children. Since the children are under age 18, their shares are held in a trust fund.
  d.   A corporation has 1,000 shares of common stock outstanding and 500 shares of authorized but unissued preferred stock.
  e.   A corporation has 70 unrelated shareholders and 35 shareholders who are all descendants of Mr. and Mrs. A.

23-2   *Eligibility Requirements.* Y corporation's shareholders want to elect S status. Do any of the following facts about the corporation prevent the election? Why?
  a.   It has a wholly owned subsidiary.
  b.   It has 99 shareholders who own their shares solely in their own name and a married couple who own the stock jointly.
  c.   It has 10 shareholders, and one is the estate of a former shareholder. It is expected that the shares held by the estate will be distributed to three U.S. citizens and one Englishman who is a U.S. resident.
  d.   It has 73 shareholders plus L, who owns no shares but serves as custodian for shares owned by her two minor children.
  e.   What if L, in (d) above, is a nonresident alien, but the children are U.S. citizens?
  f.   It has 15 owners of common stock and no owners of its authorized preferred stock.
  g.   It has 10 owners of voting common stock and five owners of nonvoting common. Except for voting, all other rights of the two sets of common stock are identical.
  h.   A corporation was formed many years ago by X, Y and Z. Several generations later there are 210 shareholders, 150 of whom are descendants of X, Y and Z.

23-3   *Eligibility Requirements and Termination.* Refer to *Problem 23-2* and assume Y corporation made its S election in 2003. Do the following facts about the corporation terminate the election? When? Why? Can the shareholders prevent the termination?
  a.   Refer to a above. It has $5 billion in sales with various customers in the United States and $10,000 sales that it places through its subsidiary.
  b.   Refer to b above. The married couple is divorced December 29, 2009, and each receives one-half the shares in Y that were owned jointly by them prior to that date.
  c.   Refer to c above. The Englishman decides it is time to return home and moves to London, England, on March 3, 2009. He continues to own five shares of Y and gives up his residency in the United States.
  d.   Refer to f above. M exchanges her 500 shares of Y common for 700 shares of Y preferred. Although the number of shares differs, the dollar value of M's holdings remains the same.
  e.   The corporation elects to revoke its S election. Holders of 70 percent of the stock consent to the revocation. The other shareholders do not consent.
  f.   On June 5, 2009 a 20 percent shareholder transfers her stock to a C corporation she owns.
  g.   Y has $15,000 accumulated earnings and profits (AE&P) from C corporate years, and 30 percent of its gross receipts in 2008, 2009 and 2010 are from dividends and interest on investments.

23-4 *Stock Requirements.* A mother wishes to establish an S corporation with her two children. However, she is concerned about the one class of stock requirement. She does not want to provide her children with voting control but does wish to give them 60 percent of the stock. Can she achieve her wishes? Explain.

23-5 *Election.* F, M, and T are shareholders of a calendar year corporation. On February 15, 2009 they are advised they should elect Subchapter S status. All agree to the election. However, they state that they purchased a 10 percent ownership interest from V on January 4, 2009. V sold his interest because he said he never wanted to have any contact with F, M, or T again. Can the corporation make an S election for 2009? Explain.

23-6 *Election.* B, C, and D are shareholders, each owning 1,000 shares. On February 20, 2009 they are advised to elect S status for 2009. Can they make the election for all of 2009 under the following circumstances? Explain.
  a. B purchased 10 shares from R on January 5, 2009. R is hitchhiking across Europe and cannot be located until April 1, 2009.
  b. C sells 10 percent of her interest (after the election) July 7, 2009 to X. X refuses to agree to the S election and wants it terminated.

23-7 *Elections.* This year, RJ, an individual, formed ABC Corporation. ABC commenced business on April 17, 2009. The corporation issued its first shares on March 2, 2009. RJ transferred property (fair market value $100,000, adjusted basis $20,000) to the corporation on March 28, 2009 in a nontaxable § 351 exchange. ABC intends to use the calendar year for tax purposes. For the years in question ABC does not have any attribute that would disqualify it from S status.
  a. By what date must ABC make an election to be an S corporation if the election is to be in effect for the corporation's first taxable year, assuming the corporation does not utilize any relief provisions?
  b. Assume that ABC discovers, on February 15, 2010 that it has not made a timely S election for its year ended December 31, 2009. Could the corporation make an election to take effect for its taxable year beginning January 1, 2010?
  c. If the corporation made an S election for its taxable year beginning January 1, 2010, would it have any exposure to the built-in gains tax?
  d. Assume that on February 15, 2010 ABC discovered that no S election had been made. What would be needed for the corporation to make an S election to take effect for its year 2009 tax year?
  e. Assume the same facts in (b) above except that the corporation discovered that it had not made an S election as of April 15, 2012. What would be required for the corporation to make an S election for its 2010 taxable year?

23-8 *Termination of the Election.* Compare the effects of an intentional revocation, an unintentional violation of the eligibility requirements, and a termination due to the receipt of excessive passive investment income.

23-9 *Termination of the Election.* A calendar year S corporation unexpectedly receives a government contract on April 3, 2009. The profits from the contract in 2009 will be substantial. The three equal shareholders wish to revoke the election for 2009. Can they? Explain.

23-10 *Passive Investment Income.* An S corporation with AE&P of $5,000 is expected to receive 30 percent of its gross income from rents but only 18 percent of its net income from these rents. Will the excess passive investment income test be violated? Assume the S corporation's taxable year does not end for seven months and all income is earned equally over the year.
  a. Can any action be taken during the next seven months to ensure the test will not be violated?
  b. Could the corporation take any corrective action if it does not determine the nature of its gross receipts until after the end of its tax year?

23-11 *Employee-Owner.* Which of the three organizational forms—S corporation, C corporation, or partnership—treats owners who work for the business in the following manner?
  a. The owner's compensation is a deductible business expense.
  b. The owner's compensation is subject to FICA withholding.
  c. The employee benefits are deductible expenses.
  d. The employee benefits are excluded from the owner-employee's gross income.

23-12 *Schedule K-1.* Why must each shareholder of an S corporation be provided with a Schedule K-1?

23-13 *Business Income.* How is each of the following items treated by an S corporation?
  a. Dividend income
  b. Accrued rental expense to a shareholder
  c. Net capital gain
  d. Distribution of assets with a market value in excess of basis

23-14 *Family Ownership.* A taxpayer operates a retail store as an S corporation. He has a 16-year-old daughter and an 11-year-old son.
  a. Can he employ either or both of them in the business and deduct their salaries?
  b. Can they be shareholders in the S corporation?
  c. Can a trust be formed to hold the shares of stock owned by a minor child?

23-15 *Family Ownership.* A mother wants to transfer a substantial portion of her ownership in an S corporation to a trust for her son and daughter. She wants to transfer value but retain voting control. She also wants to be able to exercise some control over how the assets of the trust are distributed. However, she is willing to use an independent trustee to manage the assets.
  a. Can she transfer nonvoting stock to the children and retain voting shares without creating a second class of stock?
  b. If she transfers stock to a trust, but retains the ability to remove the shares from the trust, will she disqualify the corporation from S status?
  c. How could she create a QSST for each child? What restrictions would the trusts face? Who would pay the tax on the income of the corporation allocated to the trusts' shares?
  d. What would be the advantages of using an ESBT? Who would pay the tax on the income of the corporation allocated to the trust's shares?

23-16 *Stock and Debt Basis.* What is the significance of stock basis and debt basis to a shareholder? How does a shareholder adjust basis for the activity of an S corporation for a year? How does a shareholder obtain debt basis?

23-17 *Property Distributions.* What effect do noncash distributions have on the S corporation and on the shareholder if the S corporation has no AE&P, and:
  a. The property's market value exceeds its basis, or
  b. The property's basis exceeds its market value?

23-18 *Distributions.* When do cash distributions result in includible income to the S shareholder?

23-19 *Post-Termination Transition Period.* What is a post-termination transition period? How is it useful?

23-20 *Basic Comparison.* List the tax advantages and the tax disadvantages of an S corporation when compared with:
  a. A partnership.
  b. A C corporation.

PROBLEMS

23-21 *Termination of Election.* T, the sole shareholder and president of T, Inc., had operated a successful automobile dealership as a regular C corporation for many years. In 2006, the corporation elected S corporation status. After T's unexpected illness in 2008, the corporation sold most of its assets and retained only a small used car operation. In 2008 and 2009, T, Inc. had paid the tax on excessive passive income and had AE&P (from its C corporation years) at the end of both years. In 2010, the corporation paid no dividends and had the following income and expenses:

Interest income	$50,000
Dividend income	5,000
Gain from prior installment sale	30,000
Used car sales	40,000
Cost of sales	20,000

Is the S election terminated, and if so, when?

23-22 *Consequences of Revocation of an S Election.* In July 2009 S Inc., a calendar year corporation, revoked its S election as of August 1, 2009. The corporation's taxable income for January through December is $432,000, and the shareholders do not elect to perform an interim closing of the corporate books.
  a. What tax return(s) must S file for the year, and what are the due dates of the return (s)?
  b. Compute S's corporate taxable income for the short year for the (1) S corporation and (2) C corporation.
  c. Compute the C corporation's Federal income tax.

23-23 *Net Income from Operations.* A and B are MDs in the AB partnership. Because of limited liability considerations, their attorney has advised them to incorporate. A typical year for the MDs (who are equal partners) is as follows:

Revenues	$400,000
Operating expenses	190,000
Charitable contributions	10,000
Owner compensation	200,000

  a. Calculate AB's ordinary net income if it is taxed as (1) a partnership or (2) an S corporation.
  b. Calculate the effect on A's ordinary income if AB is taxed as (1) a partnership; (2) and S corporation; or (3) a C corporation.
  c. Ignoring limited liability considerations, should the partners incorporate? If so, should they elect S status?
  d. If A and B desire partnership tax treatment, is there any business entity that would meet their needs?

23-24 *Net Income.* A calendar year S corporation has the following information for the current taxable year:

Sales.	$180,000
Cost of goods sold.	(70,000)
Dividend income	5,000
Net capital loss	(4,000)
Salary to Z	12,000
Life insurance for Z	500
Other operating expenses	40,000
Cash distributions to owners	20,000

Assume Z is single and her only other income is $30,000 salary from an unrelated employer. She is a 20 percent owner with a $10,000 basis in the S stock at the beginning of the year. Calculate the S corporation's net ordinary income and Z's adjusted gross income and ending basis in the S corporation stock.

23-25 *Net Losses.* A calendar year S corporation has the following information for the current taxable year:

Sales.	$180,000
Cost of goods sold.	(130,000)
Net capital loss	(6,000)
Salary to Z	18,000
Charitable contributions	1,000
Other operating expenses	65,000
Dividend income	4,000

Assume Z is single and her only other income is $30,000 salary from an unrelated employer. She is a 40 percent owner with a $10,000 basis in the S stock and no corporate debt owed to her. Calculate the S corporation's net ordinary loss, Z's adjusted gross income, and the character and amount of S corporate items that flow through to her.

23-26 *Net Income/Loss and Basis.* For 2009, an S corporation reported an ordinary loss of $100,000, a net capital loss of $10,000, and a § 1231 gain of $20,000. M owns 10 percent of the stock and at the beginning of the year had a basis in her stock of $7,500. In addition, M loaned the corporation $5,000 during the year. She materially participates in the S corporation.
   a. Compute her deductible loss.
   b. The following year, the corporation reported ordinary income of $70,000 and made no distributions. How does this income affect M's basis in the stock and the debt?

23-27 *Allocations.* V owns 500 shares of stock of an S corporation with 2,000 shares outstanding. The calendar year S corporation's records show the following information:

Net ordinary income	$200,000
Net capital loss	(10,000)

Calculate V's share of the items if on March 15 he sells:
   a. 200 of his shares of stock;
   b. All 500 shares of his stock and the per-day allocation method is used; or
   c. All 500 shares of his stock and the interim closing of the books method is used. The records reveal that through March 15, net ordinary income was $60,000 and net capital loss was $ 10,000.

23-28 *Basis.* A calendar year business reports the following information as of the end of 2008 and 2009:

	2008	2009
Accounts payable to suppliers	$10,000	$11,000
Note payable to City Bank	40,000	37,000
Note payable to H	12,000	10,000
Cash distributions to owners		20,000
Net ordinary income	15,000	

H, a 30 percent owner, had a basis in the business at the end of 2008 of $9,000. Calculate H's basis in his ownership interest at the end of 2009 assuming the business is:

a. A partnership

b. An S corporation

23-29 *Deductibility of Losses by Shareholders.* B, Inc. was incorporated and its shareholders made a valid S election for B's first taxable year. At the beginning of the current year, Shareholder Z had a basis of $14,500 in his B stock and held a $10,000 note receivable from B with a $10,000 basis. For the current year Z was allocated a $32,000 ordinary loss and a $4,000 capital loss from the corporation. B did not make any distributions to its shareholders during the current year.

a. How much of each allocated loss may Z deduct in the current year?

b. What happens to any losses in excess of the limits in (a) above?

c. How much basis will Z have in his B stock and his note receivable at the end of the current year?

23-30 *Basis Adjustments—Restoration.* Refer to the facts in *Problem 23-29* above. In the next year Z is allocated $7,000 of ordinary income and $5,500 of tax-exempt income from B. B did not make any distributions to its shareholders during the year. What effect will these income allocations have on Z's basis in his B stock and note receivable?

23-31 *Losses and Basis.* J, Inc. is an S corporation that reported the following selected items as of December 31, 2009.

Ordinary loss (from Form 1120S, page 1).	$(30,000)
Long-term capital gain	500
Tax-exempt interest income.	1,000
Notes payable to banks	30,000
(1/1/09 balance = $20,000)	
Notes payable to LJ.	5,000
(1/1/09 balance = $0)	

The corporation is owned 60 percent by LJ and 40 percent by RS. At the beginning of the year, they had a basis in their *stock* of $12,000 and $10,000, respectively. How much income or loss will each of the shareholders report for 2009?

23-32 *Basis.* M, a 40 percent owner, has a basis in the S corporate stock of $15,000 and in a note receivable from the S corporation of $8,000. Compute the basis of the stock and the note and the amount of the ordinary loss and income that flow through to M in 2009 and 2010.

a. The S corporation has a net operating loss of $45,000 in 2009.

b. The S corporation has a net operating income of $20,000 in 2010.

23-33   *Basis.* A calendar year S corporation has the following information for the two years:

	2009	2010
Net ordinary income (or loss)	$(50,000)	$10,000
Dividend income	5,000	2,000

X, an unmarried 60 percent shareholder, has a basis in the stock on January 1, 2009 of $18,000 and a note receivable from the corporation for $12,000. X's only other income is salary from an unrelated business.

    a. Calculate X's basis in the stock and in the note after the above income and loss are recorded for 2009.

    b. Calculate X's basis in the stock and in the note after the above income items are recorded for 2010.

    c. Assume the corporation paid the $12,000 note on April 3, 2010. Calculate X's basis in the stock after the above income distributions are recorded for 2010, and calculate the effect on X's adjusted gross income for all 2010 items, including the payment of the note.

23-34   *Inside and Outside Basis.* XYZ is an S corporation owned equally by three shareholders. X has often disagreed with the other shareholders over business matters and now believes he should withdraw from the corporation. X's basis in his stock is $50,000. The corporation's balance sheet appears as follows:

Cash	$100,000
Accounts receivable	50,000
Land	30,000
Equipment (net)...................................	10,000
Accounts payable	30,000
Note payable to X	10,000
Shareholders' equity................................	150,000

The equipment's market value is approximately the same as its net book value, but the land is now valued at $60,000. X sells all of his stock to W for $60,000.

    How much gain must X recognize?

23-35   *Family Ownership.* K operates a small retail store as a proprietorship. Annual net ordinary income is expected to be $60,000 next year. The estimated value of her services to the business is $25,000. K's 14-year-old son is interested in the business. She is considering giving him a 30 percent ownership interest in the business. If she does this, she will be paid a salary of $25,000. K files as head of household and does not itemize deductions. Neither she nor her son has any other includible income. Ignore all payroll and self-employment taxes in the following computations.

    a. Determine next year's tax savings that will be achieved if K establishes an S corporation with her son at the beginning of the year compared with continuing the business as a proprietorship.

    b. Will K or her son have any includible income if they exchange the appreciated proprietorship assets for the 70 and 30 percent ownership interests, respectively, in the S corporation?

    c. What advice should you give K on establishing and operating the S corporation?

23-36 *Property Distributions.* M receives the following equipment from an S corporation as a distribution of profits.

Asset	Cost	Accumulated Depreciation	Basis	Fair Market Value
Equipment	$10,000	$7,900	$2,100	$2,280

The equipment was used in the business for four years of its five-year MACRS life and will be a nonbusiness asset to M. M is a 60 percent owner and has a basis in the stock of $11,000 before the property distribution. Calculate the following amounts.
a. The S corporation's recognized gain
b. M's basis in the equipment
c. The effect on M's basis in the stock
d. The effect on M's adjusted gross income

23-37 *Property Distributions.* Refer to *Problem 23-36*. Calculate the same amounts if M's basis in the S corporation, before the distribution, is $1,200 instead of the $11,000.

23-38 *Property Distribution.* J purchases 20 percent of an S corporation's stock for $50,000 when its records show the following:

	Fair Market Value	Basis
Cash	$ 40,000	$ 40,000
Inventory	60,000	45,000
Land—investment.	80,000	20,000
Other operating assets	100,000	80,000
Liabilities.	(30,000)	(30,000)
Net assets	$250,000	$155,000

Six months later, all of the land is distributed in equal plats to the shareholders. What is the effect of this distribution on J?

23-39 *Cash and Property Distributions—No AE&P.* An S corporation with no AE&P distributes $10,000 cash, land ($7,000 FMV and $4,000 basis), and desks ($3,000 FMV and $4,500 basis) to *each* of its three equal shareholders. (That is, $30,000 in cash, $21,000 in land, and $9,000 in desks was distributed in total.) One of the shareholders, T, has a basis in the stock before the distribution of $12,000 and a long-term note from the corporation of $5,000. The other two shareholders have a basis in the stock before the distribution of $40,000 and no debt from the corporation. Calculate the effect of the distribution on the A.G.I. of each of the shareholders.

23-40 *Computation of AAA and Basis.* J formed R Corporation in 1986. The corporation operated as a C corporation from 1986 until 2003, when it elected to be taxed as an S corporation. At the beginning of the current year, J had a basis in his stock of $100,000.

The corporation's balance in the AAA at the beginning of the current year was $143,000. R's records for the current year reveal the following information:

Sales.	$300,000
Cost of goods sold.	(120,000)
Miscellaneous operating expenses	50,000
Salary to J	40,000
Nondeductible portion of entertainment	4,000
Tax-exempt interest income.	13,000
Expenses related to tax-exempt interest income.	3,000
Capital gain	7,000
Capital loss.	(2,000)
Charitable contribution	5,000
Cash distribution to J.	10,000

The corporation also had AE&P from C years of $4,000.

Compute J's basis in his stock and the corporation's balance in the AAA as of the end of the taxable year. Assume J is the sole shareholder.

23-41 *Treatment of Distributions: Converted C Corporation.* Assume the same facts as in *Problem 23-40* above. Explain the tax treatment to J if he receives the following distributions during the year.
  a. $100,000
  b. $220,000
  c. $260,000

23-42 *Cash and Property Distributions—AE&P.* S, Inc. had previously been a regular C corporation, but elected to be taxed as an S corporation in 1982. It is owned equally by J and G, who have a basis in their stock of $100,000 each at the beginning of the current year. Also at the beginning of the current year, the corporation had the following balances:

Accumulated adjustments account	$50,000
Previously taxed income.	40,000
Accumulated earnings and profits.	30,000
Other adjustments account	0

During the current year, the corporation had ordinary income of $35,000 and distributed IM stock worth $75,000 to J and cash of $75,000 to G. The stock was purchased four years ago for $50,000.
  a. What are the tax effects of the distribution on the corporation?
  b. What are the consequences to each of the shareholders?

23-43 *Cash Distributions—AE&P.* A calendar year S corporation has the following balance on January 1, of the current year:

Accumulated adjustments account	$13,000
Previously taxed income.	2,000
Accumulated earnings and profits.	6,000
Other adjustments account	0

This year the S corporation records show $12,000 net ordinary income, $4,000 tax-exempt income net of related expenses, and $55,000 cash distributions. Y owns 70 percent of the stock. Her basis in the stock on January 1, was $7,000, and she has a

note receivable from the corporation of $5,000. Y is single, and her only other income is salary from an unrelated business.

a. Calculate the balances in the corporate accounts as of December 31.

b. Calculate the effect on Y's adjusted gross income for the year.

c. Calculate the basis in Y's stock and note as of December 31.

23-44 *Property Distributions—AE&P.* Assume the same facts as in *Problem 23-43* except the distribution is stock held more than one year as an investment with a market value of $55,000 and a basis of $53,000.

a. Calculate the balances in the corporate accounts as of December 31.

b. Calculate the effect on Y's adjusted gross income.

c. Calculate the basis in Y's stock and note as of December 31.

23-45 *Cash Distributions—AE&P.* D, Inc. was incorporated in 1999, and its shareholders made a valid S election for D's 2003 calendar year. At the end of the current year but before the distribution is considered, D had $19,000 of accumulated earnings and profits from 1999 through 2002, and an accumulated adjustments account of $11,000. D made only one cash distribution of $20,000 during the current year, $5,000 of which was paid to shareholder M, who owns 25 percent of D's stock. After all adjustments *except* any required for the distribution, M's basis in his stock was $18,000.

a. What are the tax consequences of the distribution to M, and what is M's basis in his D stock after the distribution?

b. What are the balances in D's accumulated earnings and profits account and accumulated adjustments account after the distribution?

23-46 *Cash Distribution—AE&P.* M and J have been equal owners of an S corporation for several years. It was operated as a C corporation its first two years and as an S corporation since then. This year it has $12,000 ordinary income, $2,000 tax-exempt interest income, $24,000 cash distributions, and the following balances at the end of the prior year:

Accumulated adjustments account	$8,000
Previously taxed income ($1,000 to M, $1,000 to J)	2,000
AE&P from C years	3,000

M's stock basis at the end of last year was $8,500 and J's was $13,000.

a. Calculate the balances in the corporate accounts as of December 31.

b. Calculate the effect on M's and J's adjusted gross income.

c. Calculate the basis in M's and J's stock as of December 31.

23-47 *Property Distribution—AE&P.* Refer to *Problem 23-46*, but assume the $24,000 distribution is of land that has a $23,000 basis.

23-48 *Excess Passive Investment Income.* A calendar year S corporation has AE&P of $15,000 from years when it was operated as a C corporation. Its records show the following:

Sales.	$100,000
Cost of goods sold.	(55,000)
Operating expenses	(15,000)
Dividend income	20,000
Rental income (passive).	40,000
Rental expenses	(25,000)

The corporation is owned equally by three brothers. Determine the tax effect on the S corporation and on each brother.

23-49   *Tax on Built-in Gains.* A corporation, organized in 1983, was operated as a C corporation until Subchapter S was elected as of January 1, 2001, when it had total assets of $240,000 FMV and $185,000 basis. Assets held on that date ($80,000 market value and $50,000 basis) are distributed in 2007 when the market value is $90,000. Calculate the tax on built-in gains if taxable income, based on computations for a C corporation, is:

a. $60,000

b. $20,000

23-50   *Tax on Built-in Gains.* On February 5, 2009 L Corporation, a cash basis calendar year C corporation, elected S status effective for January 1, 2009. On January 1, L's balance sheet revealed the following assets:

	Adjusted Basis	Fair Market Value
Inventory	$20,000	$85,000
Land	30,000	70,000
Equipment	45,000	15,000

During the current year, L sold all of its inventory for $90,000. It also sold the equipment for $9,000 (L did not claim any more depreciation on the equipment this year, so its basis at the time of sale was $45,000). L's taxable income limitation is $100,000 for the current year. Compute L Corporation's built-in gains tax.

23-51   *LIFO Recapture Tax.* T Corporation converts to S corporation status for 2009. T used the LIFO method of accounting for its inventory in 2008 and had an ending LIFO inventory basis of $540,000. The ending inventory's FIFO value was $650,000 and its fair market value was $800,000.

a.   What is T Corporation's LIFO recapture amount?

b.   Assuming its corporate tax rate is 35 percent, what is T Corporation's LIFO recapture tax?

c.   How is the LIFO recapture tax required to be paid?

23-52   *Worthless Securities.* A calendar year S corporation is bankrupt. E, a 60 percent owner for several years, will not receive any assets from the business. His basis in the stock as of January 1, 2009 was $70,000, and he has a note receivable of $25,000 from the corporation. Both are determined to be uncollectible July 1, 2009. The S corporation has a net ordinary loss during 2007 of $30,000; $20,000 before July 1 and $10,000 after July 1. E lent the corporation the $20,000 last year and $5,000 four months ago in an effort to protect his ownership interest in the business. Calculate E's adjusted gross income and capital loss carryovers if his adjusted gross income from other sources totals $120,000.

TAX RETURN PROBLEMS

23-53   *Tax Return Problem.* Individuals P and K formed P&K Corporation on March 1, 1994 to provide computer consulting services. The company has been an S corporation since its formation, and the stock ownership is divided as follows: 60 percent to P and 40 percent to K. The business code and employer identification numbers are 7389 and 24-3897625, respectively. The business office is located at 3010 East Apple Street, Atlanta, Georgia 30304. P and K live nearby at 1521 South Elm Street and 3315 East Apple Street, respectively. Their social security numbers are 403-16-5110 for P and 518-72-9147 for K.

The calendar year, cash basis corporation's December 31, 2007 balance sheet and December 31, 2008 trial balance contain the following information:

	Balance Sheet 12/31/07		Trial Balance 12/31/08	
	Debit	Credit	Debit	Credit
Cash	$ 12,000		$ 22,000	
Note receivable([1])	14,000		14,000	
Equipment([2],[3])	150,000		190,000	
Accumulated depreciation		$ 38,000		$ 63,500
Notes payable([3],[4])		94,000		17,200
Capital stock		10,000		10,000
Accumulated adjustments account . . .		34,000		34,000
Cash distributed to P			25,440	
Cash distributed to K			16,960	
Revenues				235,000
Interest income([1])				1,400
§ 1245 gain				3,500
Salary expense([5])			110,000	
Rent expense			12,000	
Interest expense			16,600	
Tax expense (property and payroll) . . .			13,800	
Repair expense			5,800	
Depreciation expense			29,200	
Health insurance expense([6])			1,600	
Property insurance expense			1,500	
Office supplies expense			3,000	
Utility expense			2,200	
Charitable contributions			500	
Totals	$ 176,000	$ 176,000	$ 464,600	$ 464,600

(1) The note receivable is from K and is due December 31, 2011. The annual interest rate is 10 percent and K paid $1,400 on December 28, 2008.

(2) Equipment was sold May 12, 2008 for $9,800. It was purchased new on May 1, 2007 for $10,000 and its basis when sold was $6,300.

(3) New equipment was purchased March 1, 2008 with $5,000 cash and a $45,000 three-year note payable. The first note payment is March 1, 2009.

(4) Notes payable are long-term except for $20,000 of the note to be paid next year.

(5) Salary expense is composed of salary of $30,000 each to P and to K and $50,000 to unrelated employees.

(6) Health insurance premiums paid were for the unrelated employees.

Prepare Form 1120S (including Schedules K, L, and M), and Schedule K-l for shareholder P. Complete all six pages, including responses to all questions. If any necessary information is missing in the problem, assume a logical answer and record it. Do not prepare Schedule K-l for shareholder K or other required supplemental forms at this time.

23-54 *Tax Return Problem.* During 2008, Lisa Cutter and Jeff McMullen decided they would like to start their own gourmet hamburger business. Lisa and Jeff believed that the public would love the recipes used by Lisa's mom, Tina Woodbrook. They also thought that they had the necessary experience to enter this business, since Jeff currently owned a fast-food franchise business while Lisa had experience operating a small bakery. After doing their own market research, they established Slattery's Inc. and elected to be taxed as an S corporation. The company's address is 5432 Partridge Pl., Tulsa, Oklahoma 74105 and its employer identification number is 88-7654321.

The company started modestly. After refurbishing an old gas station that it had purchased, the company opened for business on February 25, 2008. Shortly after business

began, however, business boomed. By the end of 2008, the company had established two other locations.

Slattery's has three shareholders who own stock as follows:

Shareholder	Shares
Lisa Cutter	500
Jeff McMullen.	200
Tina Woodbrook	300
Total outstanding	1,000

Slattery's was formed on February 1, 2008. On that date, shareholders made contributions as follows:

▸ Lisa Cutter contributed $30,000 in cash and 200 shares of MND stock, a publicly held company, which had a fair market value of $20,000. Lisa had purchased the MND stock on October 3, 1998 for $8,000.

▸ Jeff McMullen contributed equipment worth $35,000 and with a basis of $29,000.

▸ Tina Woodbrook contributed $30,000 in cash.

Assume 2008 depreciation for tax purposes is $11,500, and omit the detailed computations for depreciations from Form 4562.

The company is on the accrual basis and has chosen to use the calendar year for tax purposes. Its adjusted trial balance for *financial accounting* purposes reveals the following information:

	Debit	Credit
Cash	$270,700	
Ending inventory	16,000	
Equipment	35,000	
Land	10,000	
Building.	15,000	
Improvements to building	55,000	
Accumulated depreciation		$ 9,000
Notes payable		78,000
Accounts payable		40,000
Taxes payable		8,000
Salaries payable		20,000
Capital stock		115,000
Sales.		400,000
Gain on sale of MND stock		18,000
Dividend from MND Corporation		2,000
Cost of goods sold.	84,000	
Legal expenses	6,000	
Accounting expenses	4,000	
Miscellaneous expenses	2,100	
Premium on life insurance policy	800	
Advertising	8,600	
Utilities	8,000	
Payroll taxes	12,500	
Salary expenses	120,000	
Insurance	9,000	
Repairs.	6,500	
Charitable contributions	17,600	
Depreciation per books.	9,000	
Interest expense	200	

The company has provided additional information below.

The company took a physical count of inventory at the end of the year and determined that ending inventory was $16,000. Ten percent of the notes payable are due each year for the next ten years.

The legal costs were for work done by Slattery's attorney in February for drafting the articles of incorporation and by-laws. Accounting fees were paid in May for setting up the books and the accounting system. Miscellaneous expenses included a one-time $100 fee paid in February to the State of Oklahoma to incorporate.

The MND stock was sold for $38,000 on April. Shortly before the sale, MND had declared and paid a dividend. Slattery's received $2,000 on April 1. MND was incorporated in Delaware.

Slattery's has elected *not* to use the limited expensing provisions of Code § 179 but has otherwise claimed the maximum depreciation with respect to all assets. Any other elections required to minimize the corporation's tax liability were made.

Lisa Cutter (Social Security No. 447-52-7943) is president of the corporation and spends 90 percent of her working time in the business. She received a salary of $60,000. No other officers received compensation. Social security numbers are 306-28-6192 for Jeff and 403-34-6771 for Tina. The life insurance policy covers Lisa's life, and she has the right to name the beneficiary.

Prepare Form 1120S and other appropriate forms and schedules for Slattery's. On separate schedule(s), show all calculations used to determine all reported amounts except those for which the source is obvious or which are shown on a formal schedule to be filed with the return. If information is missing to answer a question on the return, make up an answer and circle it.

RESEARCH PROBLEMS

23-55 *Expanding an S Corporation.* L Inc., an S corporation, manufactures computers. Most of its computers are sold through individually owned retail computer stores. This year it decided it wanted to expand its operations into the retail market. To this end, it has decided to acquire Micros Unlimited, which operates a chain of computer retail stores nationwide.

If L Inc. acquires all of the stock of Micro, may it operate Micro as a C corporation? May it operate Micro as a QSub? What would be some major considerations with each form of business?

23-56 *Basis and Losses.* J and K, individuals, are equal shareholders in JK, Inc., an S corporation. For the current year, the corporation anticipates a loss of approximately $200,000. Neither shareholder has any substantial stock basis. The corporation has a $200,000 loan from First National Bank. J and K have personally guaranteed the loan. They are concerned about their ability to deduct the loss in the current year. Please advise if they have debt basis due to the current arrangement. If they do not have basis, explain how they might create basis without any outlay of additional funds.

Research aids:

   Raynor, 50 T.C. 762 (1968).
   Rev. Rul. 75-144, 1975-1 C.B. 277.

23-57 *Losses and Basis.* Q, an individual, is the sole shareholder of QR Corporation, an S corporation. In past years, Q's losses have exceeded her basis by $100,000. Now QR Corporation is insolvent and is $100,000 in debt. The lenders realize that they will have no possibility of collecting the full amount and are writing down the $100,000. After

the debt reduction, QR will not be solvent. QR's tax advisors have told Q that the write-down of debt will not result in taxable income to QR due to the insolvency exception of § 108. Q understands that tax-exempt income flows through to shareholders in S corporations and increases stock basis. She asks you to find out if any income realized by QR due to the cancellation of debt will give her basis to deduct her prior suspended losses.

Research aids:

> § 108(d)(7).
> Reg. § 1.1366-1(a)(2)(viii).

23-58   *Distribution Problems.* Dr. A has operated his medical practice as a sole proprietor. He has heard that there is no self-employment income passing through from an S corporation to a shareholder. He has also heard that distributions from corporations are not subject to social security tax. Accordingly, he intends to incorporate his medical practice. He will take no salary or other compensation for his services. Instead, he will cause the corporation to declare dividends each quarter and withdraw the profits as distributions from the corporation. He believes he will not be subject to self-employment tax or social security tax. Do you see any problems with this scheme?

Research aid:

> Rev. Rul. 74-44, 1974-1 C.B. 287.

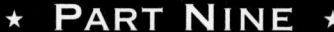

★ PART NINE ★

FAMILY TAX PLANNING

★ ★ ★ ★ ★ CONTENTS ★ ★ ★ ★ ★

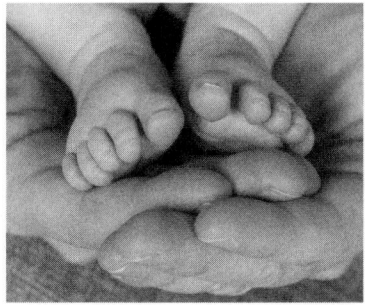

CHAPTER TWENTY FOUR

THE FEDERAL TRANSFER TAXES

LEARNING OBJECTIVES

Upon completion of this chapter you will be able to:

- Characterize the types of transfers that are subject to the Federal gift tax

- Compute a donor's total taxable gifts for the current year, including

  - Determination of all available annual exclusions

  - Calculation of any available marital or charitable deduction

- Explain the mechanics of the calculation of the gift tax, including the role of the unified credit

- List the three basic steps involved in the computation of a decedent's taxable estate

- Specify the various types of property interests that must be valued for inclusion in a decedent's gross estate

- Describe any deductions from the gross estate

- Explain the mechanics of the calculation of the estate tax, including the role of the unified credit

- Discuss the purpose of the generation skipping transfer tax

CHAPTER OUTLINE

INTRODUCTION

Since 1916 Congress has imposed taxes aimed solely at an individual's transfer of wealth: the estate tax (1916), the gift tax (1932), and the generation-skipping transfer tax (1976). As a practical matter, these taxes have produced relatively little revenue—about 1 percent of total revenues—and affected few individuals—also around 1 percent. Despite their limited impact, the taxes have survived. But that may all be coming to an end. In 2000, Congress repealed all of the transfer taxes by a wide margin but President Clinton vetoed the legislation and Congress was unable to muster sufficient votes to overturn the veto. However, with the inauguration of President Bush in 2001, the tide changed. Under the Economic Growth and Tax Relief Reconciliation Act of 2001, the estate tax—but not the gift tax—is scheduled to die. The estate tax is scheduled for phase-out and complete elimination in 2010. However, the gift tax remains with an exemption of $1,000,000 and a top rate of 35 percent. It should be emphasized that without further action by Congress, many of the rules enacted by the 2001 Act are effectively repealed beginning in 2011. In other words, in 2011, the tax law will revert to the rules that existed prior to enactment of the 2001 Act. In such case, the estate tax would be reinstated in 2011 as would all of the other rules that existed prior to the 2001 Act. Consequently, good tax planning suggests

that taxpayers should die in 2010! That said, the current sentiment of most commentators indicates that the estate tax will survive. Only time will tell.[1]

HISTORY AND OVERVIEW

The estate tax became a permanent part of the tax system in 1916. In short, it is merely an excise tax on the transfer of the decedent's *net* wealth (fair market value of total assets less debts and expenses) that passes to his or her heirs at death. For example, if a taxpayer dies with a home worth $1,000,000 and a mortgage of $200,000, he or she is potentially taxed on the net amount of $800,000. Whether or not the taxpayer is actually taxed on such amount depends in part on a number of variables including who receives the property. For example, the law currently provides deductions for transfers to a spouse or qualifying charitable organizations.

Shortly after the enactment of the estate tax it became clear that without additional rules a taxpayer could easily avoid the estate tax simply by giving away property before he or she died. As might be expected, to prevent full scale avoidance of the estate tax Congress enacted a gift tax in 1924. A unique feature of the gift tax is the fact that unlike the income tax where the current year's tax is based on the current's year's income, the gift tax is computed on the cumulative amount of gifts made by an individual during his or her lifetime. Because of the progressive transfer tax rates, this approach makes every gift more expensive in terms of tax dollars than the last. Another important characteristic of the gift tax is the annual exclusion. To eliminate the vast administrative problems that would result if the gift tax were imposed on all gifts (e.g., birthday and Christmas presents) the gift tax is imposed only on those that exceed a certain threshold, currently $13,000 (2009) per donee per year (previously $3,000 from 1932 to 1981).

Until 1976, the estate and gift tax were separate and distinct taxes. Although both taxes imposed a tax on transfers of wealth, one on lifetime transfers and one on transfers at death, they differed in several important ways. One important difference could be found in the rate structures. For many years, the gift tax rates were 25 percent less than estate tax rates, presumably to encourage taxpayers to transfer their assets during their lifetime rather than hoarding them until death. Another difference involved the amount of transfers exempted from tax. The gift tax had its own lifetime exemption of $30,000 while the estate tax exemption was $60,000. Any of the exemption for gifts that was not used during the taxpayer's lifetime could not be carried over and used at death but was lost. Another distinction concerned the tax computation. Transfers made during the taxpayer's lifetime (i.e., taxable gifts) did not enter into the calculation of the tax on the taxpayer's transfers at death (i.e., the taxable estate). However, these distinctions came to an end with the passage of the Tax Reform Act of 1976 when the two taxes were unified. Although current practice still refers to these transfer taxes as the estate tax and the gift tax, they are really part of what is a unified transfer tax system.

The unification of the estate and gift tax eliminated the differences between the two taxes, completely integrating the two systems into the one that exists today. The new law replaced the two separate rate schedules with a single, unified transfer tax rate schedule used to compute both the estate and the gift tax. Moreover, since 1976 a decedent's taxable estate is effectively treated as an individual's final taxable gift. This is accomplished by computing the estate tax on a base that includes not only the taxable estate but also any taxable gifts made during the decedent's life. The changes in 1976 also replaced the separate exemptions with a single unified credit. The credit is unified in the

---

[1]   Recent IRS statistics indicate the number of estate tax returns filed decreased from 130,000 in 2000 to 22,000 in 2006, but collections increased to $24 billion. Measured as a percent of deaths, taxable estates fell from 1.86% to .7% or seven for every thousand deaths. Net collections derived from the estate and gift taxes totaled $28 billion in 2006, representing 1.2% of total federal revenue.

sense that whatever amount is used to offset the gift tax during life is unavailable to reduce the estate tax at death. Beginning in 2004, however, the exemption for the estate tax slowly increases to $3.5 million by 2009 ($2 million for 2006-2008). In contrast, the gift tax exemption remains at $1 million.

Another change made in 1976 was the introduction of a third Federal transfer tax on generation-skipping transfers. This tax, designed to complement the gift and estate taxes, is quite complex and highly controversial. It is discussed later in this chapter.

The Economic Recovery Tax Act of 1981 (ERTA 1981) continued the restructuring of the transfer tax system begun in 1976. The most important feature of this legislation was the unlimited marital deduction. This deduction makes gifts between spouses completely nontaxable and allows the first spouse to die to leave the family wealth to the surviving spouse at no Federal transfer tax cost. Thus, after 1981, the taxable unit for the imposition of the gift or estate tax is no longer the individual but the marital unit.

PROPERTY INTERESTS

Since the estate and gift taxes concern transfers of property, understanding the two taxes requires an appreciation of the nature of property interests and the different forms of property ownership. In the United States, each of the 50 states has its own system of *property law*—statutory rules that govern an individual's right to own and convey both real and personal property during his or her lifetime. Unfortunately, the specific property laws of each state vary considerably and therefore generalizations about property laws can be dangerous. However, the various state legal systems can be divided into two basic categories: *common law systems* and *community property systems*. The common law system, derived from English laws of property ownership, focuses on individual ownership of assets, regardless of the marital status of the individual. This system has been adopted in 41 states. The community property system is a derivation of Spanish property law and is followed in nine states: Arizona, California, Idaho, Louisiana, Nevada, New Mexico, Texas, Washington, and Wisconsin. Under either system, an individual may own property alone or jointly with another. In addition, an individual may own only a partial interest in the property such as an income interest. The different forms of co-ownership and various types of partial interests are considered below.

FORMS OF CO-OWNERSHIP

The consequences of holding property jointly with another can vary substantially, depending on the type of co-ownership. There are four forms of co-ownership: (1) tenancy in common, (2) joint tenancy, (3) tenancy by the entirety, and (4) community property ownership.

Tenancy in Common. A tenancy in common exists when two or more persons hold title to property, each owning an undivided fractional interest in the whole. The percentage of the property owned by one tenant need not be the same as the other co-tenants but can differ as the co-tenants provide. The most important feature of this type of property interest is that it is treated in virtually all respects like property that is owned outright. Thus, the interest can be sold, gifted, willed, or, when there is no will, passed to the owner's heirs according to the laws of the state. Another important characteristic of a tenancy in common is the *right of partition*. This right permits co-owners who disagree over something concerning the property to go to court to secure a division of the property among the owners. In some cases, however, a physical division is impossible (e.g., 50 acres of land where each acre's value is dependent on the whole), and consequently, the property must be sold with the proceeds split between the owners.

Joint Tenancy. Under a joint tenancy arrangement, two or more persons hold title to property, each owning the same fractional interest in the property. Joint tenancy normally implies the right of survivorship (joint tenancy with right of survivorship, or JTWROS). This means that upon the death of one joint tenant, the property automatically passes to the surviving joint tenants. Consequently, the disposition of the property is *not* controlled by the decedent's will. Like tenants in common, joint tenants have the right to sever their interest in the property. This is a particularly valuable right since the tenant may wish to disinherit the other joint tenants.

Tenancy by the Entirety. A tenancy by the entirety is a JTWROS between husband and wife. The critical difference between a tenancy by the entirety and a JTWROS is that in most states a spouse cannot sever his or her interest without the consent of the other spouse. In addition, in some states the husband has full control over the property while alive and is entitled to all the income from it.

Community Property. In a community property system, married individuals own an equal, undivided interest in all wealth acquired during the course of the marriage, regardless of which spouse made any individual contribution to the marital wealth. In addition to a half interest in such "community property," a spouse may also own property in an individual capacity as "separate property." Generally, assets acquired prior to marriage and assets received by gift or inheritance are separate property. However, in all nine community property states there exists a strong legal presumption that all property possessed during marriage is community, and that presumption can only be overcome by convincing proof of the property's separate nature.

Marital Property. Before leaving the subject of joint ownership, the concept of marital property deserves attention. Except in community property states, it is a common mistake to assume that all property acquired during marriage is jointly held. State laws vary widely on this issue. In some states, only property specifically titled as JTWROS is treated as jointly held. In these and other states, it is not unusual that property acquired during marriage belongs to the husband regardless of whose earnings were used to acquire the property. In other states, each spouse is deemed to own that which can be traced to his or her own earnings. Because of the problems with marital property, transfers of such property should be evaluated carefully to ensure that the rights of either spouse are not violated.

LIFE ESTATES, REVERSIONS, AND REMAINDERS

Persons who own property outright have virtually unlimited rights with respect to their property. They can sell it, mortgage it, or transfer it as they wish. In addition, they can divide the ownership of the property in any number of ways. In this regard, it is not uncommon for property owners to transfer ownership in property to someone temporarily. During the period of temporary ownership, the beneficiary could have the right to use, possess, and benefit from the income of the property. Assuming that the beneficiary's interest is limited to the income from the property, he or she would be treated as having an *income interest*. The time to which the beneficiary is entitled to the income from the property could be specified in any terms, such as common measures of time: days, weeks, months, or years. Alternatively, the time period could be determined by reference to the occurrence of a specific event. For example, when an individual has an income interest for life, the interest is referred to as a life estate. In this case, the person entitled to the *life estate* is called the life tenant.

The owner of property has the right to provide for one or more temporary interests, subject only to the *rule against perpetuities*. This rule requires that the property pass outright to an individual within a certain time period after the transfer. Normally, ownership of the property must vest at a date no later than 21 years after the death of persons alive at the time the interest is created.

Interestingly, a few states have recently repealed the rule. For example, trusts in Alaska, Delaware, Washington D.C., Illinois, New Jersey, South Dakota, Virginia and Wisconsin can now be designed to last forever. Trusts in Utah and Wyoming can last for up to 1,000 years while those in Florida must end after 360 years.

After any temporary interests have been designated, the owner has the right to provide for the outright transfer of the property. If the owner specifies that the property should be returned to the owner or his or her estate, the interest following the temporary interest is referred to as a *reversionary interest*. If the property passes to someone other than the owner, the interest is called a *remainder interest*. The holder of the remainder interest is the *remainderman*.

Life estates, remainders, and reversions are property interests that can be transferred, sold, and willed (except for life estates) like other types of property. These interests can also be reached by creditors in satisfaction of their claims. However, a person can establish a trust with so-called *spendthrift* provisions, which prohibit the beneficiary from assigning or selling his or her interest (e.g., a life estate) or using the assets to satisfy creditors.

THE GIFT TAX

The statutory provisions regarding the Federal gift tax are contained in §§ 2501 through 2524 of the Internal Revenue Code. These rules provide the basis for the gift tax formula found in Exhibit 24-1. The various elements of this formula are discussed below.

EXHIBIT 24-1
Computation of Federal Gift Tax Liability

Fair market value of all gifts made in the current year		$xxx,xxx
Less the sum of		
Annual exclusions ($13,000 per donee in 2009)	$xx,xxx	
Marital deduction	xx,xxx	
Charitable deduction	x,xxx	−xx,xxx
Taxable gifts for current year		$xxx,xxx
Plus: All taxable gifts made in prior years		+xx,xxx
Taxable transfers to date		$xxx,xxx
Tentative tax on total transfers to date		$ xx,xxx
Less the sum of		
Gift taxes computed at current rates on prior years' taxable gifts.	$ x,xxx	
Unified transfer tax credit.	x,xxx	−xx,xxx
Gift tax due on current gifts.		$ xx,xxx

TRANSFERS SUBJECT TO TAX

Section 2511 states that the gift tax shall apply to transfers in trust or otherwise, whether the gift is direct or indirect, real or personal, tangible or intangible. The gift tax is imposed only on transfers of property; gratuitous transfers of services are not subject to tax.[2] The types of property interests to which the gift tax applies are virtually unlimited. The tax applies to transfers of such common items as money, cars, stocks, bonds, jewelry, works of art, houses, and every other type of item normally considered property. It should

---

[2]   Rev. Rul. 56-472, 1956-2 C.B. 21.

be emphasized that no property is specifically excluded from the gift tax. For example, the transfer of municipal bonds is subject to the gift tax, even though the income from the bonds is tax free.

The gift tax reaches transfers of partial interests as well. One example is a transfer of property in trust where the income interest is given to someone—the income beneficiary—for his or her life, while the trust property or remainder interest is given to another person—the remainderman—upon the income beneficiary's death. In this case, the donor would be treated as having made two separate gifts, a gift of the income interest and a gift of the remainder interest.

The application of the gift tax to both direct and indirect gifts ensures that the tax reaches all transfers regardless of the method of transfer. Direct gifts encompass the common types of outright transfers (e.g., father transfers bonds to daughter, or grandmother gives cash to grandson). On the other hand, indirect gifts are represented primarily by transfers to trusts and other entities. When a transfer is made to a trust, it is considered a gift to the beneficiaries of the trust. Similarly, a transfer to a corporation or partnership is considered a gift to the shareholders or partners. However, if the donor owns an interest in a partnership or corporation, he or she is not treated as making a gift to the extent it would be a gift to himself or herself. An individual may also be treated as making a gift if he or she refuses to accept property and the property passes to another person on account of the refusal.

Most taxpayers understand that the gift tax is imposed on transfers of property motivated by affection and generosity. However, the tax may also be imposed on a transfer of property not intended as a gift within the commonly accepted definition of the word. The tax is intended to apply to any transfer of wealth by an individual that reduces his or her potential taxable estate. Therefore, § 2512 provides that any transfer of property, in return for which the transferor receives *less than adequate or full consideration* in money or money's worth, is a transfer subject to the gift tax.

Adequate Consideration. Revenue Ruling 79-384 provides an excellent example of a transfer for insufficient consideration.[3] The taxpayer in the ruling was a father, who had made an oral promise to his son to pay him $10,000 upon the son's graduation from college. The son graduated but the father refused to pay him the promised amount. The son then successfully sued the father, who was forced to transfer the $10,000. The IRS ruled that the father had received no consideration in money or money's worth for the transfer and therefore had made a taxable gift to his son.

Revenue Ruling 79-384 illustrates two important concepts. First, *donative intent* on the part of a transferor of property is *not necessary* to classify the transfer as a taxable gift.[4] Second, anything received by the transferor in exchange for the property must be subject to valuation in monetary terms if it is to be consideration within the meaning of § 2512.[5] The father did receive the satisfaction resulting from his son's graduation, and this consideration was sufficient to create an enforceable oral contract between father and son. However, because the consideration could not be objectively valued in dollar terms it was irrelevant for tax purposes.

The question of sufficiency of consideration normally arises when transfers of assets are made between family members or related parties. When properties are transferred or exchanged in a bona fide business transaction, the Regulations specify that sufficiency of consideration will be presumed because of the arm's-length negotiation between the parties.[6]

---

3   1979-2 C.B. 12.

4   Reg. § 25.2511-1(g)(1).

5   Reg. § 25.2512-8.

6   *Ibid.*

Transfers of wealth to dependent family members that represent support are not taxable gifts. The distinction between support payments and gifts is far from clear, particularly when the transferor is not legally obligated to make the payments. Section 2503(e) specifies that amounts paid on behalf of any individual for tuition to an educational organization or for medical care shall not be considered taxable gifts to such individual. However, this rule only applies if the payments are made directly to the educational institution or the health care provider.

Payments that a divorced taxpayer is legally required to make for the *support* of his or her former spouse are not taxable gifts.[7] However, Regulation § 25.2512-8 specifies that payments made prior to or after marriage in return for the recipient's relinquishment of his or her *marital property rights* are transfers for insufficient consideration and subject to the gift tax. Section 2516 provides an exception to this rule. If a transfer of property is made under the terms of a written agreement between spouses and the transfer is (1) in settlement of the spouse's marital property rights, or (2) to provide a reasonable allowance for support of any minor children of the marriage, no taxable gift will occur. For the exception to apply, divorce must occur within the three-year period beginning on the date one year before such agreement is entered into.

Retained Interest. The final criterion of a taxable transfer is that the transfer must be complete. A transfer is considered complete only if the donor has surrendered all control over the property. For this reason, when the donor alone retains the right to revoke the transfer, the transfer is incomplete and the gift tax does not apply. For example, creation of a joint bank account is not considered a completed gift since the depositor is free to withdraw the money deposited in the account. Similarly, the donor must not be able to redirect ownership of the property in the future; nonetheless, to have a completed gift it is not necessary that the donees have received the property or that the specific donees even be identified.[8]

> **Example 1.** Donor D transfers $1 million into an irrevocable trust with an independent trustee. The trustee has the right to pay the income of the trust to beneficiaries A, B, or C *or* to accumulate the income. After 15 years, the trust will terminate and all accumulated income and principal will be divided among the surviving beneficiaries. Because D has parted with all control over the $1 million, it is a completed gift, even though neither A, B, or C has received or is guaranteed any specified portion of the money.

VALUATION

The value of a transfer subject to the Federal gift tax is measured by the fair market value of the property transferred less the value of any consideration received by the transferor. Determining fair market value can be the most difficult aspect of computing a gift tax due. Fair market value is defined in the Regulations as "the price at which such property would change hands between a willing buyer and a willing seller, neither being under any compulsion to buy or to sell, and both having reasonable knowledge of relevant facts."[9]

The determination of an asset's fair market value must be made on the basis of all relevant facts and circumstances. The Regulations under § 2512 are quite detailed and extremely useful in that they prescribe methods for valuation of a variety of assets.

---

[7]   Rev. Rul. 68-379, 1968-2 C.B. 414.

[8]   Reg. § 25.2511-2(a).

[9]   Reg. § 25.2512-1.

Example 2. Donor S transfers 10 shares of the publicly traded common stock of XYZ Corporation on June 8, 2009. On that date, the highest quoted selling price of the stock was $53 per share. The lowest quoted selling price was $48 per share. Regulation § 25.2512-2(b)(1) specifies that the fair market value of the XYZ stock on June 8, 2009 shall be the mean between the highest and lowest quoted selling price [($53 + $48) ÷ 2], or $50.50 per share.

Valuation of Income and Remainder Interests. In estate planning, it is quite common for individuals to make gifts of only a partial interest of property. These arrangements usually involve transfers to a trust such as the following:

- An individual transfers property to a trust, giving away an income interest to one beneficiary and a remainder interest to another beneficiary. In this case, the taxpayer has actually made two gifts—the income interest and the remainder interest—each of which must be valued for gift tax purposes.

- An individual transfers property to a trust, retaining the income interest and giving away the remainder interest. Here there is only a single gift of the remainder interest.

- An individual transfers property to a trust, giving the income interest to a beneficiary but providing that the remainder interest reverts or returns to the individual once the income interest has expired. In this case, the taxpayer has made a single gift of the income interest.

Gifts of income and remainder interests are valued using actuarial tables. These tables take into consideration current interest rates and, if necessary, current mortality rates. In valuing the various types of transfers, the tables assume that property transferred produces income at a certain rate, regardless of the actual amount of income that is produced.

For transfers after April 30, 1989, § 7520 requires valuations using the interest rate prevailing at the time of the transfer. Specifically, the rate to be used is 120 percent of the applicable Federal midterm rate in effect under § 1274(d)(1) for the month in which the transfer is made. These rates are published monthly. Using the appropriate rate, the values can be found in actuarial tables published by the IRS. The tables were first issued in 1989 in Notice 89-60.[10] Section 7520(c)(3) requires that the tables be revised at least once every 10 years thereafter to reflect the most recent mortality experience available. They were most recently revised in 1999 and can be found in IRS Publications 1457, 1458 or 1459.[11] These three massive volumes provide factors for interest rates of 2.2 percent to 26 percent and annuity factors for ages 0–110. The IRS issues monthly announcements indicating which of these tables applies for the month.[12] For example, the § 7520 rate for October, 2008 was 3.8 percent.[13] Table S shows the factors for determining the value of an annuity, a life estate, or a remainder interest based on a single life. Table B shows the factors for determining the value of an annuity, a life estate or a remainder interest for a term of years Selected portions of the tables can be found in Appendix A in this book.

---

[10]   1989-1 C.B. 700.

[11]   IRS Publication 1457, Actuarial Values, Aleph Volume (2001); IRS Publication 1458, Actuarial Values, Beth Volume (2001); IRS Publication 1459, Actuarial Values, Gimel Volume (2001).

[12]   These rates are published monthly. For transfers after December 31, 1970 and before December 1, 1983 the interest rate used to compute the value of reversions and other interests was six percent. The factors can be found in the appropriate table contained in Reg § 20.2031-10(f). For transfers after November 30, 1983, and before May 1, 1989, the interest rate used to compute the value of reversions and other interests was 10 percent.

[13]   Rev. Rul. 2008-49, 2008-40 IRB 1.

In examining the tables, observe that if the value of the property is split between an income interest and a remainder interest, there are two factors and the sum of those two factors equals one. In a case where the remainder factor is known but the income factor is unknown or vice-versa, the income factor can be determined as follows:

$$\text{Income factor} = 1.000000 - \text{Remainder factor}$$

Example 3. In May, 19X9, H transferred $100,000 to a trust for his son, S, and his grandson, GS. According to the terms of the trust, S is to receive the income for life and upon his death, the remainder is to be paid to GS, if living, otherwise to GS's estate. S was 40 years old at the time the trust was created. H has made two gifts. The value of S's income interest is a function of three factors determined at the time of the gift: (1) S's life expectancy, (2) the current interest rate, and (3) the value of the trust property. Assume the applicable rate for valuing the interest is five percent (120% of the May Federal mid-term rate). Using the table for valuing a remainder interest (Table S in Appendix A-1), the value of the remainder interest is $19,519 ($100,000 × .19516). The value of the income interest is $80,484 [$100,000 × (1 − .19516 = .80484)]. Note that the sum of the remainder interest and the income interest equals the total value of the property.

Example 4. In June, 19X2, M transferred $100,000 to a trust for her daughter, D. Under the terms of the trust, D is to receive the income for 20 years at which time the trust will terminate and the property will revert to M. Assume the applicable rate for valuing the interest is 5.2% (120% of the June Federal mid-term rate). In this case, the factor for the income interest must be determined by subtracting the factor for the remainder interest from 1. Using the table for valuing a term certain remainder interest (Table B in Appendix A-2), the value of D's income interest for 20 years is $63,719 ($100,000 × .637185).

The valuation of a gift of a partial interest in property is subject to special rules when the donor retains an income interest. These rules are considered in Chapter 26 in conjunction with the discussion on special estate planning techniques [e.g., grantor retained income trusts, annuity trusts, and unitrusts (GRITS, GRATS, and GRUTS)].

BASIS

The basis of an asset in the hands of a donee is calculated under the rules of § 1015. Generally, the basis of property received as a gift is the basis of the asset in the hands of the donor, increased by the amount of any gift tax paid attributable to the excess of fair market value over the donor's basis at the date of gift. This general rule applies only if the asset is sold at a gain by the donee. If the carryover basis rule would result in a realized loss upon subsequent sale, the basis of the asset will be considered the *lesser* of the carryover basis (donor's basis) *or* the asset's fair market value at date of gift. If the asset is sold at a price greater than the fair market value at date of gift but less than its carryover basis, no gain or loss is recognized.

THE GIFT TAX EXCLUSION

When the gift tax was enacted in 1932, Congress wanted to "eliminate the necessity of keeping an account of and reporting numerous small gifts." To this end, it created an annual exclusion designed to exempt gifts under a certain threshold from the gift tax.[14] The annual exclusion was initially set at $3,000 until it was raised to $10,000 in 1981 where it remained through 2001. Starting in 2002, the exclusion has been adjusted for inflation.

---

[14] § 2503(b).

For 2002-2005, the exclusion was $11,000. For 2006 through 2008, the exclusion was $12,000. For 2009 the exclusion is $13,000.

A donor is entitled to exclude $13,000 (2009) per year per donee. Note, however, that not all gifts are eligible for the annual exclusion. Congress was concerned about the problems that could arise in determining the number of exclusions when there was only a remote possibility that a donee would receive a gift (e.g., remote and contingent beneficiaries). For this reason, to qualify for the exclusion the gift must be constitute a *present* interest. Regulation § 25.2503-3 (b) defines a present interest as one that gives the donee "an unrestricted right to the immediate use, possession, or enjoyment of property or the income from property." Therefore, the annual exclusion is not available for a gift that can only be enjoyed by the donee at some future date, even if the donee does receive a present ownership interest in the gift.

> **Example 5.** Donor D gifts real estate worth $20,000 to donees M and N. M is given a *life* estate (the right to the income from the property for as long as M lives) worth $8,000. N receives *the remainder interest* (complete ownership of the property upon the death of M) worth $12,000. Although both M and N have received legal property interests, D may claim only one exclusion for his gift to M. The gift to N is a gift of a future rather than a present interest. Thus D has made a taxable gift of $12,000.

Securing the tax benefit of the annual exclusion can be difficult if the gift in question is made to a minor or an incapacitated donee. In such cases, the donor may be reluctant to give an unrestricted present interest in the donated property. Strategies for making gifts to minors or incapacitated donees is included in Chapter 26.

GIFT SPLITTING

A gift made by a married individual residing in a community property state may have two donors (husband and wife) because of state property law. Property laws in the 41 non-community property states do not produce this *two donor* result. To compensate for this difference, § 2513 provides a *gift splitting* election to a married donor.

If a donor makes the proper election on his or her current gift tax return, one-half of all gifts made during the year will be considered to have been made by the donor's spouse. Both spouses must consent to gift splitting for the election to be valid. Since evidence of the spouse's consent is necessary when gift splitting is used, a gift tax return must be filed.

> **Example 6.** In 2009, husband H gives $100,000 to his son and $100,000 to his daughter. His wife, W, makes a gift of $5,000 to their daughter. H and W elect gift splitting on their current gift tax returns. As a result, H reports a gift to the daughter of $52,500 ($50,000 + $2,500) and a gift to the son of $50,000, and will claim two $13,000 gift tax exclusions, resulting in total taxable gifts of $76,500 ($52,500 + $50,000 − $26,000). W will report exactly the same gifts and claim two $13,000 exclusions, resulting in the same amount of taxable gifts as her husband H, $76,000, for a total of $152,000.
>
> Without gift splitting, H would still be entitled to $26,000 of exclusions, but W could only claim an exclusion of $5,000 for her gift to the daughter. Without splitting, H and W would have total taxable gifts of $174,000 compared to $152,000 with splitting. By splitting, the couple is able to increase the exclusions by $22,000 ($13,000 for the gift to the son and $9,000 for the gift to the daughter).

GIFTS TO POLITICAL AND CHARITABLE ORGANIZATIONS

Code § 2501(a)(5) excludes gifts of money or other property to a political organization from the statutory definition of taxable transfers. If a gratuitous donation is made to a qualified charitable organization, § 2522 provides a deduction for such gift from the donor's taxable gifts for the calendar year. Thus, transfers made without sufficient consideration to qualifying political or charitable groups are not subject to the Federal gift tax.

THE GIFT TAX MARITAL DEDUCTION

Under § 2523, gifts to spouses are fully deductible by the donor. The marital deduction is permitted only if certain requirements are satisfied. A full discussion of these requirements is considered in conjunction with the discussion of the marital deduction for estate tax purposes.

The gift tax marital deduction allows an individual to make tax-free transfers of wealth to his or her spouse. This opportunity to equalize the wealth owned by husband and wife plays an essential role in family tax planning, a role that will be discussed in Chapter 16.

COMPUTATION AND FILING

Unlike the income tax, which is computed on annual taxable income, the Federal gift tax is computed on cumulative taxable gifts made during a donor's lifetime. This is done by adding taxable gifts for the current year to all taxable gifts made in prior years, calculating the gross tax on the sum of cumulative gifts, and subtracting the amount of gift tax calculated on prior years' gifts.[15] The transfer tax rate schedule currently in effect is reproduced in Exhibit 24-2. Consistent with the ultimate repeal of the estate tax in 2010, the maximum estate and gift tax rate is gradually reduced as follows:

Year	Top Rate
2002	50%
2003	49%
2004	48%
2005	47%
2006	46%
2007–09	45%
2010	–
2011 & later	55%

EXHIBIT 24-2
2009 Estate and Gift Tax Rates

If taxable transfer is		Tax liability	Of the amount over
Over	But not over		
$ 0	$ 10,000	18%	$ 0
10,000	20,000	$ 1,800 + 20%	10,000
20,000	40,000	3,800 + 22%	20,000
40,000	60,000	8,200 + 24%	40,000
60,000	80,000	13,000 + 26%	60,000
80,000	100,000	18,200 + 28%	80,000
100,000	150,000	23,800 + 30%	100,000
150,000	250,000	38,800 + 32%	150,000
250,000	500,000	70,800 + 34%	250,000
500,000	750,000	155,800 + 37%	500,000
750,000	1,000,000	248,300 + 39%	750,000
1,000,000	1,250,000	345,800 + 41%	1,000,000
1,250,000	1,500,000	448,300 + 43%	1,250,000
	Over 1,500,000	555,800 + 45%	

---

[15] § 2502(a). The amount of gift tax calculated on prior years' gifts is based on current gift tax rates, regardless of the rates in effect when the gifts were actually made.

Example 7. In 1995, X made his first taxable gift of $100,000 (after the exclusion). The tax (before credits) on this amount was $23,800. X made a second taxable gift of $85,000 in 2009. The tax (before credits) on the second gift is $26,200, computed as follows:

1995 taxable gift	$100,000
2009 taxable gift	+85,000
Cumulative gifts	$185,000
Tax on $185,000	$ 50,000
Less: Tax on 1995 taxable gift	−23,800
Tax on 2009 gift	$ 26,200

This cumulative system of gift taxation and the progressive rate schedule cause a higher tax on the 2009 gift, even though the 2009 gift was $15,000 *less* than the 1995 gift.

Unified Credit. Both the estate and gift tax provisions have long contained exemptions to ensure that the taxes do not apply to modest transfers of wealth. As noted earlier, prior to their unification in 1976, each tax had its own separate exemption: the estate tax provided for an exemption of $60,000 while the gift tax allowed a lifetime exemption of $30,000 for otherwise taxable gifts (i.e., those not otherwise exempt by the annual exclusion). The unification in 1976 led to the creation of the unified credit. The unified credit is a lifetime credit available for offsetting the tax on all taxable transfers (i.e., the taxes imposed on taxable gifts or the taxable estate). In 2009, the credit is $1,455,800 for the estate tax and $345,800 for the gift tax. This gift tax credit of $345,800 completely offsets the tax on $1,000,000 of taxable transfers. For example, consider a taxpayer whose first *taxable* gift is $1,000,000. The tax on the $1,000,000 taxable transfer would be $345,800. However, the credit of $345,800 would completely eliminate the tax, effectively providing an exemption from tax for transfers of up to $1,000,000.

As can be seen in Exhibit 24-3, the amount of the credit has been increased over the years. In 1976, the credit was originally set so that when it was completely phased in by 1981 it would exempt from tax transfers of up to $175,625. However, by 1981, Congress and the Reagan administration viewed that amount as inadequate. Consequently, legislation was passed to gradually increase the credit so that it would reach $192,800 in 1987 where it would exempt $600,000 of transfers from tax. The credit remained at that level for more than 10 years until Congress acted again in the Taxpayer Relief Act of 1997. Beginning in 1998, the credit began to increase gradually. However, before the increase was complete, Congress changed course and moved toward ultimate repeal of the estate tax. Beginning in 2004, the exemption amounts for the estate tax and the gift tax are no longer the same. The gift tax is not scheduled for repeal and the exemption is set permanently at the $1,000,000 level. On the other hand, the exemption for the estate tax gradually increases to $3,500,000 in 2009 before the tax is eliminated in 2010 as shown below.

EXHIBIT 24-3
Credit and Exemption Equivalent

Year	Credit		Exemption Equivalent	
	Estate Tax	Gift Tax	Estate Tax	Gift Tax
1/1/77–6/30/77	$ 6,000	Same	$ 30,000	Same
7/1/77–12/31/77	30,000	Same	120,666	Same
1978	34,000	Same	134,000	Same
1979	38,000	Same	147,333	Same
1980	42,500	Same	161,563	Same
1981	47,000	Same	175,625	Same
1982	62,800	Same	225,000	Same
1983	79,300	Same	275,000	Same
1984	96,300	Same	325,000	Same
1985	121,800	Same	400,000	Same
1986	155,800	Same	500,000	Same
1987–97	192,800	Same	600,000	Same
1998	202,050	Same	625,000	Same
1999	211,300	Same	650,000	Same
2000–01	220,550	Same	675,000	Same
2002–03	345,800	Same	1,000,000	Same
2004–05	555,800	$345,800	1,500,000	$1,000,000*
2006–08	780,800	345,800	2,000,000	1,000,000
2009	1,455,800	345,800	3,500,000	1,000,000
2010	Repealed	345,800	Repealed	1,000,000
2011 & later	345,800	345,800	1,000,000	1,000,000

* Gift tax exemption is frozen at $1,000,000 for all subsequent years and the credit is no longer unified.

The unified credit is the only credit available to offset the Federal gift tax. As noted above, the credit offsets the tax on $1,000,000 of taxable gifts. Thus, an individual may make substantial transfers of wealth before any tax liability is incurred. The unified credit must be used when available—a taxpayer may not decide to postpone use of the credit if he or she makes a taxable gift during the current year.[16]

Example 8. In 1995, Y made her first taxable gift of $350,000. The tax calculated on this gift is $104,800, and Y must use $104,800 of her available unified credit so that the actual gift tax due is reduced to zero. In 2009, Y makes her second taxable gift of $2,000,000. The tax on this gift is $592,500, computed as follows:

Taxable gift for 2009		$2,000,000
Plus: 1995 taxable gift		+350,000
Taxable transfers to date		$2,350,000
Tentative 2009 tax on total transfers to date (See Exhibit 24-2)		$ 938,300
($555,800 + 45% ($2,350,000 − $1,500,000) = $850,000). . . .		
Less: Gift taxes calculated on 1995 gift		−104,800
Tentative tax on 2009 gift		$ 833,500
Less: Remaining unified transfer tax credit:		
Total credit available for 2009	$ 345,800	
Less: Unified transfer tax credit used in 1995	−104,800	−241,000
Gift tax due on 2009 gift		$ 592,500

---

[16] Rev. Rul. 79-398, 1979-2 C.B. 338.

Filing Requirements. The Federal gift tax return, Form 709, is filed annually on a calendar year basis. The due date of the return is the April 15th after the close of the taxable year. If a calendar year taxpayer obtains any extension to file his or her Federal income tax return, such extension automatically applies to any gift tax return due. If the donor dies during a taxable year for which a gift tax return is due, the gift tax return must be filed by the due date (nine months after death) plus any extensions of the donor's Federal estate tax return.[17]

THE OVERLAP BETWEEN THE GIFT AND ESTATE TAXES

A beginning student of the Federal transfer tax system might reasonably assume that an inter vivos (during life) transfer of property that is considered complete and therefore subject to the gift tax would also be considered complete for estate tax purposes, so that the transferred property would not be included in the decedent's taxable estate. This, however, is not the case. The gift tax and the estate tax are not mutually exclusive; property gifted away in earlier years can be included in the donor's taxable estate. The relationship between the two taxes is illustrated in the following diagram:

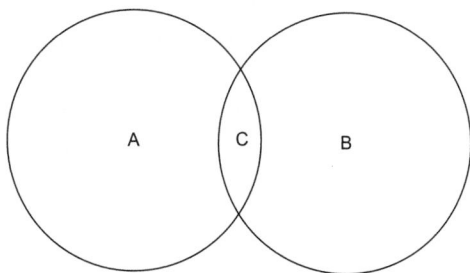

Circle A represents property transferred by the decedent during his or her lifetime and subject to the gift tax. Circle B represents the decedent's taxable estate. Overlap area C represents property already subject to a gift tax that is nevertheless included in the donor/decedent's taxable estate.

Examples of transfers that fall into the overlap area above will be presented later in the chapter. At this point, however, it is important to note that any gift tax paid on a transfer which is considered incomplete for estate tax purposes reduces the amount of estate tax payable.[18]

TRANSFERS OF PROPERTY AT DEATH

ROLE OF A WILL

Each of the 50 states gives its citizens the right to transfer the ownership of their property at death by means of a valid will. State law provides various formal requirements for valid wills, and as a result great care must be taken that a will is drafted in strict accordance with such requirements. There are few restrictions on the right of an individual to dispose of property at death in any manner he or she chooses. The most common restriction is the right under state law of a surviving spouse to receive a specified statutory share of the deceased individual's wealth. The statutory share

---

[17]   § 6075(b).

[18]   § 2001(b)(2).

rules effectively prevent an individual from completely disinheriting a surviving spouse.[19]

INTESTACY

When a person dies with no will or an invalid will, the transfer of his or her wealth is determined under the intestacy laws of the deceased's state of residence. Again, the particulars of the intestacy laws of each state are different. As a general rule, property will pass in order in prescribed shares to a decedent's surviving spouse, children and lineal descendants, parents and lineal ancestors, collateral relatives, and finally, if no relatives of any degree can be located, to the state of residence itself. For example, in Indiana if the decedent has a surviving spouse but no children, $^1/_3$ of the property generally passes to the spouse and $^1/_4$ passes to the decedent's parents. If there were two children, the spouse normally would receive $^1/_2$ while the children would receive $^1/_2$ of the property.

PROBATE

Probate is the legal process whereby a decedent's will is established as genuine and valid, and during which creditors of the decedent may submit their claims for payment from the estate. A decedent's probate estate consists of property interests owned at death that will pass under the terms of a decedent's will (or under the laws of intestacy if no valid will exists). It is extremely important for an individual engaged in estate planning to be aware of any property interests that he or she owns but which will *not* be included in the probate estate at death. A major example of such a property interest is a joint tenancy with right of survivorship (JTWROS). As previously explained, upon the death of one of the joint tenants, ownership of the asset automatically shifts to the surviving joint tenant or tenants. This is true *regardless* of the provisions of the deceased joint tenant's will. Similarly, survivor benefits, such as those from a life insurance policy or an annuity, or payments from pension and profit sharing plans, usually pass directly to the beneficiary and are not controlled by the will.

It should be apparent that those individuals who have amassed any amount of wealth and who wish to control the disposition of that wealth at death should have a validly executed will. However, there are compelling reasons why *every* responsible adult should have a will. When an individual dies intestate (without a valid will), the resulting legal and administrative complications can cause unnecessary hardship and confusion for the surviving family. Finally, one of the most critical functions of a will is to name a guardian for the decedent's minor children; failure to have a will can result in years of family discord and distress.

THE TAXABLE ESTATE

Code §§ 2001 through 2056A contain the statutory rules providing for the imposition of a tax on the transfer of the taxable estate of every decedent who is a citizen or resident of the United States. Sections 2101 through 2108 provide for an estate tax on the value of assets located within the United States owned by a nonresident alien decedent. Discussion of this latter tax is beyond the scope of an introductory text.

Computation of a decedent's taxable estate involves three basic steps:

1. Identification and valuation of assets includible in the gross estate;

---

[19] Modern statutory share laws have their origins in the English common law property concepts of the "dower" rights of a widow and the "curtesy" rights of a widower.

2. Identification of deductible claims against the gross estate and deductible expenses of estate administration; and

3. Identification of any deductible bequests out of the gross estate.

The formula for computing the estate tax is shown in Exhibit 24-4 below.

EXHIBIT 24-4
Estate Tax Formula

Gross estate (§§ 2031 through 2046)		$x,xxx,xxx
Less the sum of		
Expenses, indebtedness,		
and taxes (§ 2053)	$ xx,xxx	
Losses (§ 2054)	x,xxx	
State death taxes (§ 2058)	x,xxx	
Charitable bequests (§ 2055)	xx,xxx	
Marital deduction (§ 2056).	xxx,xxx	−xxx,xxx
Taxable estate (§ 2051)		$ xxx,xxx
Plus: Taxable gifts made		
after December 31, 1976 [§ 2001(b)]		+ xx,xxx
Total taxable transfers		$ xxx,xxx
Tentative tax on total transfers (§ 2001)		$ xxx,xxx
Less the sum of		
Gift taxes paid on post-1976 taxable gifts (§ 2001).	$ x,xxx	
Unified transfer tax credit (§ 2010).	xx,xxx	
Other tax credits (§§ 2012 through 2016)	x,xxx	−xx,xxx
Estate tax liability.		$ xx,xxx

THE GROSS ESTATE CONCEPT

Section 2031 broadly states that "the value of the gross estate of the decedent shall be determined by including to the extent provided for in this part the value at the time of his death of all property, real or personal, tangible or intangible, wherever situated." The Regulations under this section make it clear that property located in a foreign country is included in this definition.[20]

Sections 2033 through 2044 identify the various types of property that are includible in a decedent's gross estate. Section 2033 is the most commonly applied of these Code sections. It requires the inclusion of any property interest owned by the decedent at date of death. The property interests specified in § 2033 correspond to the legal concept of a decedent's *probate estate*, property interests that will pass to the beneficiaries under the terms of the decedent's will.[21] If the decedent dies without a valid will, these interests will be distributed to the decedent's heirs under the state intestacy laws.

---

[20] Reg. § 20.2031-1(a).

[21] Reg. § 20.2031-1(a)(1).

All individuals are, in a sense, on the accrual method of accounting for estate tax purposes. Any legal claim to or interest in an asset that exists at death is includible in the gross estate. For example, a cash basis taxpayer who performed substantial services and was to be paid $20,000 would not report the fee as income until collected. However, if death occurred before collection, the decedent is considered to have owned a $20,000 asset, the right to the fee which would be includible in his or her gross estate.

The concept of the gross estate is much broader than the legal probate estate. Exhibit 24-5 lists the various types of property interests and assets includible in the gross estate and the statutory authority for each inclusion. These various inclusions are discussed in more detail later in the chapter.

Although the estate tax reaches virtually all types of property interests, it does not extend to property in which the decedent owned a life estate created by another. Section 2033 does not require inclusion of such property since the decedent's only legal interest in the property terminated upon death.

> **Example 9.** Upon W's death, she transferred stock worth $300,000 in trust, giving her son, S, a life estate and the remainder to her grandson. Several years later, S died when the property was worth $900,000. However, his estate does not include the stock, since his interest terminates at his death and he is not transferring the property to the grandson.

The above example illustrates why the life estate is one of the most important devices used in estate planning. Note that the son is entitled to use the property for his life, yet the property and all of the appreciation escapes taxation in his estate. In other words, the property was taxed in the first and third generations (i.e., in their estates) but not the second generation. Congress addressed this problem by enacting the generation-skipping transfer tax, discussed later in this chapter. This special tax, however, has not eliminated all of the benefits of using the life estate for family tax planning purposes.

VALUATION OF GROSS ESTATE AND BASIS

Once an asset is identified as part of the gross estate, its fair market value at date of death must be determined. Practically, valuation of assets is the most difficult and subjective problem in computing a decedent's gross estate. Many assets, such as stock in a closely held corporation, have no readily ascertainable fair market value. Fortunately, the estate tax Regulations, like their gift tax counterparts, provide detailed guidelines to the valuation of many types of assets.[22]

In the 41 common law states, a surviving spouse may have a legally enforceable claim against assets owned by a decedent that cannot be defeated by the terms of the decedent's will. Section 2034 states that the value of property included in the decedent's gross estate is not diminished by such a claim. In the nine community property states, most property owned by a married individual is community property in which both spouses have equal interests. Only one-half the value of such community property is included in a decedent's gross estate.

Although the gross estate is normally valued as of the decedent's date of death, § 2032 allows the executor to elect an alternative valuation date of six months after death. If the election is made, the alternative valuation date must be used for every asset in the gross estate. If an asset is disposed of within six months of death, its value at date of disposition is used. This choice of two possible dates for valuation gives the executor some flexibility in minimizing the value of the gross estate and any estate tax liability.

---

[22]   Reg. § 20.2031.

EXHIBIT 24-5
Property Included in the Gross Estate

Property	Statutory Authority
Any property interest owned by the decedent at death	Section 2033
Includes	
cash	
stocks, bonds, other investment securities	
personal assets	
personal residence	
collectibles (antiques, etc.)	
investment real estate	
business interests (sole proprietorship, partnership interest)	
Certain gifts made within three years of death (limited application after 1981)	Section 2035
Assets transferred during life in which the decedent retained an income interest or control over the enjoyment of the assets or the income therefrom	Section 2036
Assets transferred during life in which the decedent retained more than a 5 percent reversionary interest and possession of which could only be obtained by surviving the decedent	Section 2037
Assets transferred during life if, at death, the decedent possessed the right to alter, amend, revoke, or terminate the terms of the transfer	Section 2038
Certain survivor benefits and annuities	Section 2039
Joint tenancies with right of survivorship	Section 2040
Assets over which the decedent held a *general* power of appointment	Section 2041
Insurance proceeds on the decedent's life if	Section 2042
1. payable to the decedent's estate; *or*	
2. the decedent possessed any incident of ownership in the policy at death.	
Assets in a QTIP trust in which the decedent had the income interest	Section 2044

BASIS

For income tax purposes, the basis of property in the hands of a person acquiring the property from a decedent is the property's fair market value at date of death or on the alternate valuation date under Code § 2032.[23] Under § 1223(11), assets acquired from a decedent are presumed to have a holding period in excess of one year. In the case of community property, the adjustment to fair market value is available for the *entire property* rather than just the one-half interest that is included in the gross estate of the decedent spouse.[24] Note that if the estate tax is repealed in 2010, the basis rule is modified

[23] § 1014(a). This rule does not apply to items of property that constitute income in respect of a decedent. §1014(c). For a complete discussion of income in respect of a decedent, see Chapter 25.

[24] § 1014(b)(6).

to limit the amount of basis increase to $1.3 million ($4.3 million in the case of a surviving spouse).

In situations in which the Federal estate tax to be imposed on a particular estate is minimal, an executor might actually elect the alternate valuation date in order to increase the valuation of assets included in the gross estate, thus achieving maximum step-up in the basis of the assets for income tax purposes. Section 2032(c) eliminates this particular tax planning option by providing that no § 2032 election may be made unless such election will decrease the value of the gross estate *and* the amount of the Federal estate tax imposed.

SPECIAL USE VALUATION: § 2032A

The requirement that property in a decedent's gross estate be valued at fair market value can create hardship if a principal estate asset is real property used in a family business. The value of such real property as it is used in the business may be considerably less than its potential selling price on the open market. As a result, an estate might be forced to sell the real estate and terminate the family business in order to pay the Federal estate tax.

Section 2032A provides that qualifying real estate used in a closely held business may be valued based on its business usage rather than market value. The requirements for qualification under this section are formidable, but can be summarized as follows:

- ▸ *Location.* The realty must be located in the United States.
- ▸ *Qualified Heir.* The realty must pass from the decedent to a "qualified heir" (generally a family member including the taxpayer's spouse, siblings, parents, grandparents and other ancestors, or children, grandchildren and other lineal descendants).
- ▸ *Qualified Farming or Business Use.* During the eight years prior to death (or disability or the time at which he begins to receive social security), there were at least 5 years when the realty was used for farming or in business and the decedent or a member of his family materially participated in the operation of the farm or business.
- ▸ *Realty and Personal Property Value (50 Percent Test).* The *adjusted value* of the real and personal property used in farming or business must be at least 50 percent of adjusted value of the gross estate. For purpose of this test and the test below, the adjusted value of the realty is the value of the property less any related debt while the adjusted value of the gross estate is the value of the gross estate less any debts related to property included in the estate.
- ▸ *Realty Value (25 Percent Test).* The adjusted value of the real property taken by itself is at least 25 percent of the adjusted value of the gross estate.

If these requirements are met, the maximum reduction from highest and best use value was originally $750,000, but is now adjusted for inflation. For 2009 the amount is $1,000,000. Note also that when special valuation is elected, the basis of the realty to the heirs is the reduced value.

> **Example 10.** F died in 2009. He owned a large farm south of a major urban center. As farming property, F's real estate was worth $4,000,000; however, developers wanting to acquire the real estate for future use as commercial and residential property had offered F $7,000,000 for the real estate. If all the qualifications of § 2032A can be met, F's real property would be valued at $6,000,000 ($7,000,000 − $1,000,000) in his gross estate, and would take an income tax basis of $6,000,000.

Recapture of Tax Savings. The estate tax savings offered by the election of qualified-use valuation is conditional upon the continued use of the qualified real property in the family farm or other business. If the heirs of the decedent dispose of the real property or discontinue its qualified use within 10 years of the decedent's death, Code § 2032A(c) requires that the heirs repay the estate tax saved by the original use of the § 2032A election.

GROSS ESTATE INCLUSIONS

The Federal estate tax is not a property tax levied on the value of property owned at death. Instead, it is a transfer tax levied on the value of any shift in a property interest that occurs because of a decedent's death. As a result, a decedent's gross estate may include assets not owned by a decedent at death, the transfer of which is not controlled by the terms of the decedent's will.

INSURANCE ON THE LIFE OF THE DECEDENT

The proceeds of an insurance policy on the life of a decedent do not come into existence until the death of the insured and are paid to the beneficiaries specified in the insurance contract, not the beneficiaries named in the decedent's will. However, § 2042 provides that such proceeds shall be included in the decedent's gross estate if either of the following is true:

1. The decedent's estate is the beneficiary, or

2. The decedent, at his or her death, possessed any incident of ownership in the life insurance policy, alone or in conjunction with any other person.

The term *incident of ownership* implies any economic interest in the policy and is broadly interpreted by the IRS. The Regulations under § 2042 list the power to change the policy's beneficiary, the right to cancel or assign the policy, and the right to borrow against the policy as incidents of ownership.[25]

> **Example 11.** In 2003, T purchased a term insurance policy on his own life. Under the terms of the policy, beneficiary B would receive $150,000 upon T's death. In 2009 T died. Immediately before T's death the policy had no value since it was term insurance. Nevertheless, the $150,000 paid to B is includible in T's gross estate.

SURVIVOR BENEFITS

Section 2039 requires that the value of an annuity or any payment receivable by a beneficiary by reason of surviving a decedent be included in the decedent's gross estate. This rule only applies to the extent that the value of the annuity or payment is attributable to contributions made by the decedent or the decedent's employer. A second condition for applicability is that the payment or annuity be payable to the decedent or that the decedent possess the right to payment at death. For example, social security death benefits paid to a decedent's family are not covered by § 2039 because the decedent had no right to the payments during his or her lifetime.

The value of an annuity includible under § 2039 is the replacement cost to the beneficiary of a comparable commercial annuity.[26]

---

[25] Reg. § 20.2042-1(c)(2).

[26] Reg. § 20.2031-8(a).

Example 12. H purchased a self and survivor annuity contract that was to pay him $1,500 a month for his life and, upon his death, $1,000 a month to his widow, W. At the date of H's death, W would have to pay $24,000 to purchase a $1,000 a month lifetime annuity for herself. Under § 2039, the value of the annuity received by W, $24,000, is includible in H's gross estate.

JOINT INTERESTS

Nonspousal Joint Tenancies. As discussed earlier in the chapter, a joint tenancy with right of survivorship is a form of equal co-ownership of an asset that causes full ownership of the asset to vest automatically in the survivor when the first joint tenant dies. The decedent's will cannot change this result; property owned in joint tenancy is not included in a decedent's probate estate. However, some portion of the value of this property may be includible in the decedent's gross estate. Under § 2040, it is necessary to determine the proportion of the decedent's original contribution toward the acquisition of the asset. This same proportion of the value of the asset at date of death must be included in the decedent's gross estate.

Example 13. Brothers A and B decided to purchase a tract of real estate as equal joint tenants with right of survivorship. A contributed $40,000 and B contributed $10,000 toward the $50,000 purchase price. At A's death, the real estate was worth $150,000. A's gross estate must include $120,000, 80% [$40,000 ÷ ($40,000 + $10,000)] of the real estate's value. If B had died before A, only $30,000, 20% of the real estate's value, would be includible in B's gross estate.

Note in *Example 13* that in the year the real estate was acquired, A made a taxable gift to B of $15,000, the difference between half the value of the asset when purchased, $25,000, and B's $10,000 contribution. In spite of this completed gift, a portion of the property is taxed in A's gross estate under the authority of § 2040 if he dies before B.

Spousal Joint Tenancies. If a husband and wife own property as joint tenants with right of survivorship, § 2040(b) contains a rule that requires 50 percent of the value of the property to be included in the gross estate of the first spouse to die, regardless of the original contribution of that spouse.

GENERAL POWERS OF APPOINTMENT

A *power of appointment* is a right to dispose of property that the holder of the power does not legally own. It is normally created by the will of a decedent in conjunction with a transfer of property in trust. Typically, the decedent's will provides for the transfer of property in trust, giving an individual a life estate and a power to appoint the remainder interest during his or her life or at death through a will. By so doing, the decedent transfers the ability to control the property's disposition to the holder of the power, even though the holder does not own the property. In effect, a power of appointment gives a person the right to fill in the blanks of another person's will.

A power of appointment may be *specific*, meaning that the holder of the power may only give the property to members of a specified eligible group of recipients which does *not* include the holder. Alternatively, the power may be *general*, so that the holder may appoint the property to himself or herself, or his or her creditors, estate, or creditors of that estate. The terms of the power should specify to whom ownership of the property will go if the holder deliberately or inadvertently fails to exercise the power.

A *general power of appointment* over property is tantamount to actual ownership of the property. If the holder appoints the property to another person, the exercise is treated

as a taxable gift per § 2514.[27] Section 2041 provides that if a decedent holds a general power over property at his or her death, the value of the property must be included in the gross estate.

> **Example 14.** P has the right to appoint ownership of certain real estate to any of P's children or grandchildren. He may exercise the right during life or by will. Upon P's death, his will appoints the property to his daughter, D. Because P held only a *specific power*, the value of the appointed property is not included in P's gross estate.

> **Example 15.** M has the right to appoint ownership of certain real estate to *himself* or any of his brothers and sisters. He may exercise the right during life or by will. However, M dies without exercising the power. The terms of the power provide that if the power is not exercised the property shall go to M's uncle. Because M possessed a *general power* of appointment, the date of death value of the property must be included in M's gross estate.

Nontaxable Powers. As indicated above, a specific power of appointment over property will not result in inclusion of the property in the holder's gross estate. There are other situations where a power does not cause taxation. If the holder's power to appoint property for his or her benefit is limited to an *ascertainable standard*, it is not a general power of appointment and inclusion is not required. A power is considered limited to a standard if appointments of property may be made solely for the holder's health, education, maintenance, or support in his or her accustomed manner of living. The language used to describe the scope of the holder's power is extremely important. For example, a power is not considered limited if it permits appointments for the holder's comfort, happiness, or well-being.

> **Example 16.** H's will provided for the transfer of $600,000 in trust, giving his wife a life estate and a power to appoint the property to herself for her support. Upon the wife's death, nothing is included in her gross estate since she does not have a general power of appointment. The power does not cause inclusion since it is limited to an ascertainable standard.

Another nontaxable power which offers great planning flexibility is the so-called five and five power. Section 2041 generally does not require inclusion if the amount that the holder can appoint for his or her use in any one year does not exceed the greater of $5,000 or five percent of the value of the property. As long as the power is drawn within these limits, the power need not be restricted in any other manner to avoid taxation. However, in the year of the holder's death, the power is considered a general power to the extent of the greater of the two amounts and thus causes inclusion in the holder's estate to that extent.

> **Example 17.** R created a $1,000,000 trust for his wife, giving her the income for life and the remainder to the children. R wanted to give his wife access to the corpus of the trust without causing it to be included in her estate. Therefore, he gave his wife the annual right to withdraw for her use any time during the year the greater of $5,000 or five percent of the aggregate value of the trust. As a result, assuming the value of the trust remained at $1,000,000, his wife could withdraw up to $50,000 (5% of $1,000,000) annually without having the entire corpus included in her estate. However, in the year of the wife's death, she must include $50,000 in her estate, the amount over which she might have exercised the power at death.

---

[27] If the holder of a general power releases the power or allows it to lapse, the transfer of ownership is still considered a taxable gift made by the holder. See §§ 2514(b) and (e).

TRANSFERS TAKING EFFECT AT DEATH

Taxpayers who are reluctant to give away property during life but who also want to minimize the tax burden on their estate have designed a variety of inter vivos gifts with "strings attached." Such gifts are subject to a condition or restriction that enables the donor to continue to benefit from or enjoy the property until death. Such a transfer may be complete for gift tax purposes. Nevertheless, for estate tax purposes it may be classified as a transfer taking effect at death, with the result that the date of death value of the property is includible in the donor's gross estate.

Code §§ 2036, 2037, and 2038 govern transfers taking effect at death. Because these three sections were added to the Code at different times, there is a confusing amount of overlap in their coverage. The sections' requirements are very complex and difficult to apply. However, a brief description of each section can give the beginning tax student an idea of their general functions.

One important rule to remember is that all three sections can only require the inclusion in a decedent's gross estate of property that was originally owned by the decedent. A second rule is that the sections are inapplicable if the transfer of the property by the decedent was for sufficient consideration.

Code § 2036. This section requires that the value of any property given away by the decedent, but to which the decedent retained the right to the property's income or the right to designate who may possess or enjoy the property, shall be included in the decedent's gross estate. Section 2036 also specifies that the retention of the voting rights of shares of stock in a controlled corporation represents a retention of enjoyment.[28]

> **Example 18.** In 2003, F made a completed gift of rental property to his son, S, subject to the condition that F was to receive the net rent from the property for the rest of his life. Upon F's death in the current year, the date of death value of the rental property must be included in F's gross estate since he retained a right to income (i.e., rentals), even though S is the owner of the property.

> **Example 19.** In the current year, M transferred assets into an irrevocable trust for the sole benefit of her grandchildren. Under the terms of the trust instrument, M reserved the right to designate which of the grandchildren should receive the annual income of the trust. Because M retained the right to designate the persons who shall possess the income from the trust assets, the value of the trust assets will be included in M's gross estate upon her death.

The IRS is very aggressive in applying § 2036. For example, in a situation in which a parent gifts a family residence to a child but continues to occupy the residence rent free, the parent is considered to have retained a beneficial interest in the residence, with the result that the value of the residence will be includible in the parent's gross estate.[29]

Code § 2037. This statute requires inclusion in a decedent's gross estate of the value of previously transferred property if two conditions are met:

1. Possession or enjoyment of the property can only be obtained by surviving the decedent,

---

[28] § 2036(b)(2) defines a controlled corporation as a corporation in which the decedent controlled (directly or indirectly) at least 20 percent of the voting power of all classes of stock.

[29] Rev. Rul. 70-155, 1970-1 C.B. 189; and *Estate of Linderme*, 52 T.C. 305 (1966).

2. The decedent owns a reversionary interest in the property, the value of which exceeds 5 percent of the value of the property. The value of the reversion is computed as of the moment immediately before death, based on actuarial tables.[30]

Regulation § 20.2037-1(e) gives the following example of the application of Code § 2037.

> **Example 20.** The decedent transferred property in trust, with the income payable to his wife for life and with the remainder payable to the decedent or, if he is not living at his wife's death, to his daughter or her estate. The daughter cannot obtain possession or enjoyment of the property without surviving the decedent. Therefore, if the decedent's reversionary interest immediately before death exceeded 5% of the value of the property, the value of the property less the value of the wife's outstanding life estate is includible in the decedent's gross estate.

Note in *Example 20* that the decedent's reversionary interest was extinguished at death and did not constitute an interest in property that would be transferred under the terms of the decedent's will. However, it is the event of the decedent's death that completes the transfer of the remainder interest in the trust to the daughter or her estate.

Code § 2038. If, on the date of death, the decedent had the power to alter, amend, or revoke the enjoyment of any property previously given away by the decedent, § 2038 requires that the date of death value of the property be included in the decedent's gross estate. Obviously, a revocable transfer falls within § 2038. However, the scope of the section is broad enough to apply to much less obvious types of powers.

> **Example 21.** Individual Z creates an irrevocable trust for the benefit of her children and names the trust department of a national bank as trustee. The only right retained by Z allows her to replace the trustee with a different trust department. Upon Z's death, Revenue Ruling 79-353[31] states that Code § 2038 applies and the value of the trust corpus must be included in Z's gross estate.

GIFTS IN CONTEMPLATION OF DEATH

For many years, Code § 2035 required that the date of death value of any gift made by the decedent during the three years prior to death, plus the amount of any gift tax paid on such gifts, be included in the decedent's gross estate. In 1981, Congress drastically altered this section so that it currently applies only to gifts of interests described in the sections governing transfers taking effect at death (§§ 2036, 2037, and 2038) and § 2042, relating to gifts of life insurance. In addition, § 2035 applies for determining the applicability of provisions such as § 2032A, concerning special use valuation (e.g., any property given away within three years of death is added back to the gross estate in applying the 50 and 25 percent tests). Notwithstanding the limited application of the general rule, § 2035(c) continues to require the inclusion in the gross estate of any gift tax paid within three years of death.

> **Example 22.** Refer to the facts in *Example 18*. Assume that one year prior to his death, F made a gift of his retained income interest in the rental property to his granddaughter, D. Section 2035 applies to the transfer of the income interest, with the

---

[30]   Reg. § 20.2037-1(c)(3).

[31]   1979-2 C.B. 325.

result that the date of death value of the rental property and any gift tax paid on the gift are included in F's gross estate.

TRANSFERS FOR INSUFFICIENT CONSIDERATION

A transfer for which the donor received consideration less than the value of the transferred property is vulnerable to the application of §§ 2035, 2036, 2037, or 2038 upon the donor's death. However, 2043 does allow the estate an offset for the consideration received.[32]

> **Example 23.** A transferred her 100 shares of stock in Famco Corporation to her daughter, D, subject to the condition that A would retain the voting rights in the shares. At date of transfer, the fair market value of the stock was $500,000, and D paid A only $300,000 cash in exchange. The transfer constituted a taxable gift of $200,000. Upon A's death, the value of the stock, $1.2 million, is includible in A's gross estate under § 2036. However, A's estate may reduce this value by $300,000, the amount of the consideration received by A.

The § 2043 consideration offset equals the value of the consideration at date of receipt. Therefore, in *Example 23* only 40 percent ($200,000 ÷ $500,000) of the value of the property was transferred without consideration, but 75 percent [($1.2 million − $300,000) ÷ $1.2 million] of the date of death value of the property must be included in the gross estate.

DEDUCTIONS FROM THE GROSS ESTATE

Not all of the value of a decedent's gross estate will be available for transfer to estate beneficiaries or other individuals. Some of the value must first be used to pay off debts of the decedent and other claims against the estate. The second step in computing an individual's taxable estate is to identify the debts and claims that are deductible against the gross estate.

EXPENSES, INDEBTEDNESS, AND TAXES

The estate tax is based on the *net* wealth that is actually transferred by the decedent. Consistent with this concept, the law permits deductions for expenses associated with death as well as costs of settling the estate and other claims against the property in the estate. As might be expected, the executor cannot spend and borrow willy-nilly and expect to deduct these items. Section 2053(a) generally allows deductions for funeral and administrative expenses, mortgages on property included in the gross estate and other personal debts owed by the decedent. Under § 2053(a), these items are deductible *only* if allowed by local law and *only* to the extent they are incurred in administering property subject to claims (i.e., creditors of the decedent can seek satisfaction of their claims from these assets). This normally encompasses those expenses relating to administering the probate estate. In addition, Section 2053(b) grants deductions for expenses incurred in administering property that is included in the gross estate but which is *not* subject to the claims of the estate's creditors. For example, expenses related to a revocable trust would be deductible even though creditors cannot seek satisfaction of their claims from the trust property. These deductions are allowed because the assets of the trust are included in the gross estate [§ 2053(b)].

---

[32]   See Reg. § 20.2043-1(a).

Funeral Expenses. Deductible funeral expenses include costs for the funeral service, clergy, mortuary, hearse, limousines, casket, cremation, pianist, singers, flowers and the like. In addition, a deduction is allowed for costs of a tombstone, monument, mausoleum crypt, or for a burial lot, either for the decedent or his family. If the decedent had acquired the burial lots prior to death, no deduction is allowed but the lots are not included in the gross estate. Deductions are also allowed for a reasonable expenditure for the future care of the lot. Transportation costs of the person bringing the body to the burial site also are deductible as funeral expenses (e.g., a corpse is flown home). Traveling expenses for beneficiaries or others to attend the decedent's funeral are not deductible (e.g., costs of flying decedent's grandchildren to the funeral are not deductible).

Administrative Expenses. Section 2053 also permits deductions for administering and settling the decedent's estate. Deductions normally include all probate costs such as those incurred in collection and preservation of probate assets (bank charges), payment of debts and distribution of property (e.g., cost of wire transfer). Common administrative expenses are fees paid to the executor or administrator of the estate, accounting and legal expenses, court costs, and appraisal fees. In addition, expenses incurred in preserving the estate, including the costs of maintaining and storing property (e.g., utility bills on the decedent's home after death) are deductible.

It should be emphasized that deductions are limited for those expenses in the administration of the estate. Those that are not "essential" to the proper settlement of the estate, but are incurred for the benefit of the heirs or others, may not be claimed as deductions. In this regard, selling expenses are deductible administrative expenses, if the assets must be sold to pay debts, expenses or taxes. Regulation § 20.2053-3(d)(2) authorizes the deduction of the expenses of selling assets of the estate only if the sale is necessary (1) to pay debts, administrative expenses or tax; (2) to preserve the estate; or (3) to effect distribution.

Example 24. In *Estate of David Smith*, a famous sculptor died and left over 425 pieces of his work.[33] The executors of his estate paid commissions in excess of $1,000,000 to a gallery for selling the decedent's work presumably to raise money to pay expenses of the estate. However, only $290,000 of those commissions were identified as attributable to sales needed to pay the decedent's debts, taxes, and other administration expenses. The Court held that only $290,000 of commissions were attributable to the estate's liquidity needs and denied a deduction for the remainder. Moreover, the court found no evidence that it was necessary to sell all of the works promptly. Presumably, such expenses could be claimed as selling expenses on the estate's income tax return. Note that *Smith* also stands for the proposition that assets cannot be valued in the gross estate at their value net of any expected selling expenses.

Adminstrative expenses incurred after death can be claimed as either a deduction on the estate tax return (Form 706) or on the estate's income tax return but not on both.[34]

The executor must be careful not to waste any deductions for administration expenses. This is a major concern when the estate owes no estate tax (e.g., due to the unlimited marital or charitable deductions or the unified credit) since the only potential benefit could be derived from deducting the expense for income tax purposes. Even if the executor properly waives the deduction for estate tax purposes, this does not ensure that an income tax benefit will be derived since the estate may have little or no income that could be reduced by

---

[33]   75-1 USTC ¶13,046, AFTR 2d 75-1594, 510 F.2d 479 (CA-2, 1975) aff'g 57 TC 650 (1972) cert. denied.

[34]   § 642(g).

the deduction. However, if the deduction exceeds income *in the year the estate terminates*, § 642(h) provides that all excess deductions pass through to the beneficiaries succeeding to the decedent's property who can then deduct them on their individual tax returns as itemized deductions. This is allowed only for the excess deductions that occur in the year of termination. If excess deductions occur in earlier years (e.g., because the estate chooses the wrong time to pay the expense) the deduction is generally lost.

Claims against the Estate. Deductions are allowed for any debts that the decedent owed at the time of death. The deduction for these items reflects the fact that the estate must pay these amounts before the property is distributed thereby reducing the amount that is transferred to the heirs by the decedent. Debts of the estate typically include unpaid mortgages or liens on property included in the gross estate, unpaid income taxes on income received by the decedent before he or she died, property taxes accrued before death as well as personal obligations of the decedent. Examples of personal liabilities are balances due on credit card accounts, utility bills, interest on mortgages accrued before death, margin accounts, and other loans outstanding at the date of death. Interest accrued after the date of death is normally not deductible on the Form 706 even if the alternate valuation date is elected.[35]

Medical expenses of the decedent are deductible as a claim against the estate. However, if such expenses are paid within one year of death, they may be claimed as income tax deduction on the final return. The expenses cannot be claimed on both returns, however.

LOSSES

Section 2054 allows deductions for casualty and theft losses occurring while the estate is being settled are deductible in computing the taxable estate. For example, the decedent's car may be stolen or his home destroyed by fire. The amount of the deductible loss is the value of the property reduced for any insurance proceeds received. If the alternate valuation date is elected, the property is valued at zero when determining the value of the gross estate. Therefore no loss deduction is allowed.

Although casualty and theft losses are also deductible for income tax purposes, there is no double deduction allowed.[36] The loss can be deducted on either the estate tax return or the estate's income tax return, but not both. In most cases, a greater benefit could be secured by deducting the expenses on the estate tax return since such expenses may be subject to limitations for income tax purposes.

STATE DEATH TAXES

In addition to the Federal estate tax, decedents must be concerned about state death taxes. Most states impose some type of death tax. These usually take the form of an inheritance tax, an estate tax or both. On the other hand very few states impose any type of gift tax. However, gifts made in contemplation of death (e.g., a deathbed transfer) are usually subject to the state's death tax.

State Inheritance Taxes. Many states and some local jurisdictions impose an inheritance tax on the right to receive property at death. Unlike an estate tax, which is imposed on the estate according to the value of property transferred by the decedent at death, an inheritance tax is imposed on the recipient of property from an estate (although it is typically paid out of the estate). The amount of an inheritance tax payable usually is directly

---

[35] Reg. § 20.2053-7.

[36] *Supra* Footnote 34.

affected by the degree of kinship between the recipient and the decedent. The inheritance tax typically provides an exemption from the tax, which increases as the relationship between the recipient (e.g., the surviving spouse, children, grandchildren, etc.) and the decedent becomes closer. For example, under the Indiana inheritance tax rules, transfers to a surviving spouse are exempt while transfers to the decedent's children under 21 are entitled to an exemption of $100,000. The rate of tax also differs depending on the relationship. For example, the Indiana rates for transfers to children range from 1 to 10 percent while transfers to nonrelatives range from 10 to 20 percent. Observe that the small exemptions, at least in Indiana, make even modest estates subject to state inheritance taxes even though they may be exempt from the Federal estate tax.

State Estate Taxes. These taxes are similar to the Federal estate tax and are based on the value of the property held by the decedent at the date of death.

Deduction for State Death Taxes. Prior to 2005, the estate was allowed a credit for state death taxes. Beginning in 2005, however, the state death tax credit was eliminated and replaced by a deduction. Note that the deduction is for state death taxes. There is no deduction for Federal estate taxes.

Technically, § 2058 allows a deduction for the amount of any estate, inheritance, legacy, or succession taxes actually paid to any state or the District of Columbia, in respect of property included in the gross estate. The amount must be actually paid to the estate, not merely estimated or accrued. Observe that many states permit a discount for prompt payment. For example, Indiana allows a five percent discount if the tax is paid within 9 months of date of death. In such case, the amount paid, not the amount assessed, is the amount of the deductible state death tax.

CHARITABLE CONTRIBUTIONS

An estate may deduct the value of any transfer of assets to a qualified charitable organization under § 2055. Qualifying organizations are specifically defined in the statute. If an individual is willing to leave his or her entire estate for public, charitable, or religious use, there will be no taxable estate.

For a charitable contribution to be deductible, it normally must consist of the decedent's entire interest in the underlying property. For example, if a decedent bequeaths a life interest in real estate to his son and the remainder interest in the property to charity, the value of the remainder interest is not deductible. Similarly, if the decedent bequeaths the interest in the real estate to a charity for a term of years (e.g., 20 years), and the remainder to his son, the value of the income interest is not deductible. However, this restriction does not apply if the transfer is in a specific statutory form: a *charitable lead trust*, where an income interest is given to the charity, or a *charitable remainder trust*, where a remainder interest is given to the charity.[37] A detailed description of such trusts is beyond the scope of this text, but they do allow a decedent to create both a charitable and a noncharitable interest in the same property and secure a deduction for the charitable interest. The restriction also is inapplicable to a charitable contribution of a remainder interest in a personal residence or farm and to certain contributions for conservation purposes.[38]

If an individual taxpayer is considering making bequests to charity upon his or her death, his or her tax adviser should certainly explore the possibility of having the individual make such charitable contributions during his or her life. Such inter vivos contributions would serve a dual purpose: the donated assets would be removed from

---

[37] § 2055(e)(2).

[38] *Ibid.*

the individual's potential taxable estate, and the donation would create a deduction for income tax purposes.

THE MARITAL DEDUCTION

Code § 2056 provides an unlimited deduction for the value of property passing to a surviving spouse. If a married taxpayer, no matter how wealthy, is willing to leave all his or her property to the surviving spouse, no transfer tax will be imposed on the estate.[39] Only upon the subsequent death of the spouse will the couple's wealth be subject to taxation. Planning for maximizing the benefit of the unlimited marital deduction is discussed in Chapter 26.

In certain instances, interests transferred to the surviving spouse are not deductible—so-called *nondeductible terminable interests*. If a decedent leaves an interest in property to his or her spouse that can or will terminate at a future date *and* if after termination another person receives an interest in the property from the decedent, the value of the interest passing to the spouse is ineligible for the marital deduction.[40] Absent this rule, the interest would escape taxation entirely, since it terminates prior to or with the death of the surviving spouse and thus is not included in his or her gross estate.

> **Example 25.** Decedent H leaves a life estate in real property to his surviving spouse, W, with the remainder after W's death left to their daughter. The interest passing to W is a terminable interest ineligible for the marital deduction. Note that without this rule barring a marital deduction, the value of the property would completely escape estate taxation since it would not be taxed in either H's estate (due to the marital deduction) or W's estate (since W's life estate terminates at her death).

The property need not pass directly to the surviving spouse to qualify for the marital deduction. Section 2056(b)(5) generally allows the deduction if the surviving spouse is entitled to annual payments of all of the income from the property for life and has a general power of appointment over the property exercisable during life or at death. In this case, the entire value of the property will be included in the estate of the surviving spouse because of his or her general power of appointment.

For many years, these two methods of leaving property to a spouse (outright or in trust with a general power of appointment to the surviving spouse) were essentially the only two techniques available if the decedent wanted to qualify the transfer for the marital deduction. This often left a married couple with a perplexing problem. Notice that in both situations, the decedent surrenders control of the property to the surviving spouse. When the surviving spouse is given a general power of appointment over the property, he or she has complete control over the ultimate disposition of the property—the same control that would have been obtained if he or she had received the property outright. Under either scenario, the surviving spouse is left with the choice of who will be the beneficiaries of the decedent's property. In other words, the decedent could not be assured that property that had been accumulated during marriage would reach the desired beneficiaries, typically the couple's children. For example, if the surviving spouse remarried, the decedent's property could end up being used for the benefit of the new spouse and new children, usually not the result desired by the decedent. Unfortunately, more suitable arrangements from a nontax point of view normally did not qualify for the marital deduction. Consequently, the tax law put taxpayers in a very awkward position, requiring them to either give up control or face higher taxes.

---

[39] No marital deduction is allowed for the value of property passing to a surviving spouse who is not a U.S. citizen unless the property is placed in a "qualified domestic trust."

[40] § 2056(b).

In 1981, Congress addressed this problem by sanctioning the marital deduction for a life estate for the surviving spouse. Observe that without this relief provision the life estate would be considered a nondeductible terminable interest. However, as explained below, the deduction is allowed only if the property (that would normally escape tax by virtue of the life estate rules) is included in the surviving spouse's estate upon his or her death. The special rules enabling this treatment are contained in § 2056(b)(7).

Under § 2056(b)(7), a marital deduction is allowed for the value of *qualifying terminable interest property* left to a surviving spouse. Qualifying terminable interest property is property from which the entire income must be paid to the spouse at least annually. During the spouse's lifetime, no one else must be able to receive any interest in the property. Upon the spouse's death, the property may pass to anyone. If the executor elects, the entire value of the property is deductible on the decedent's estate tax return. In most cases, these requirements are met by transferring property to a trust from which the spouse receives the income for life. Such arrangements are normally referred to as QTIPs, reflecting the fact that they are created to enable to the property to be considered Qualifying Terminable Interest Property.

Without further requirements, the interest described above is simply a life estate that would totally escape tax as described in *Example 25* above. However, § 2044 requires that when the surviving spouse dies, the entire value of the qualifying terminable interest property at that time must be included in the spouse's gross estate. If the surviving spouse gives away the income interest during life, § 2519 requires that the gift will consist of the entire value of the property.

> **Example 26.** H and W, husband and wife, have been married for ten years. They have three children, A, B, and C, ages 9, 7, and 4. H wants to ensure that their children receive the couple's assets after he dies. For this reason, he does not want to leave the property outright to his spouse nor does he want to leave the property in trust to her with a general power of appointment. To this end, his will provides that upon his death, all of his assets are transferred to a trust that gives W an income interest for life and the remainder interest to A, B and C upon W's death. Note that H has provided for W but has retained control over who ultimately receives the property. From a tax perspective, this normally would be considered a nondeductible terminable interest as described above and would not qualify for the marital deduction. However, if an election is made by the executor of H's estate, this otherwise nondeductible terminable interest becomes qualifying terminable interest property, that is, a QTIP, and qualifies for the marital deduction. When W dies, the value of the property at her death is automatically included in her gross estate. In this way, the property does not escape estate tax. Any estate tax that is attributable to inclusion of the property in the W's estate can be paid by her estate. However, if this is not suitable, the law requires that the tax will be paid from the property itself (e.g., the property could be sold to pay the estate tax and the property net of the estate tax would be passed to the children of H and W).

While the examples above provide some measure of the trade-offs that must be considered when planning with the marital deduction, these issues are just part of the story. Other factors that must be considered in order to effectively design marital bequests are discussed in Chapter 26.

COMPUTATION OF THE ESTATE TAX

Once the value of the taxable estate has been determined, the first step in computing the estate tax liability is to add the taxable estate to the amount of the decedent's *adjusted taxable gifts*. Adjusted taxable gifts are defined in Code § 2001(b) as the total amount of

taxable gifts (after any available exclusion or deduction) made after December 31, 1976 *other than* gifts includible in the gross estate of the decedent.

The transfer tax rates of § 2001(c) are then applied to the sum of the taxable estate plus adjusted taxable gifts. The tentative tax calculated is then reduced by any gift taxes paid or payable at current rates for gifts made after December 31, 1976. The result is the Federal estate tax liability *before* credits.

ESTATE TAX CREDITS

The major credit available to reduce the Federal estate tax is the unified credit of Code § 2010. As seen in Exhibit 24-3, the estate and gift tax credits are the same until 2004 at which time the gift tax credit is frozen at $345,800 and the estate tax credit continues to increase until the elimination of the estate tax in 2010. The mechanics of the estate tax calculation ensure that the decedent's estate benefits from the credit only to the extent that it was not used to offset any gift tax during his or her lifetime. It is important to understand that the two credits combined will shelter a maximum of $3,500,000 (2009) of transfers from the imposition of transfers from the imposition of any Federal transfer tax.

The remaining estate tax credits are:

- Foreign death tax credit
- Credit for taxes on prior transfers0
- Credit for pre-1977 gift taxes

Foreign Death Tax Credit. Section 2014 allows the estate a credit for all or part of the death taxes that must be paid to a foreign country on account of property located in that country that is included in the gross estate. The amount of the credit is limited to the lesser of (1) the foreign death tax attributable to the foreign property, or (2) the Federal estate tax attributable to the foreign property.

Credit for Tax on Prior Transfers. If two family members die within a short period of time, the same property may be included in both taxable estates and be subject to two rounds of estate taxation in rapid succession. Section 2013 provides a credit to the estate of the second decedent to mitigate this excessive taxation. The credit generally is computed as a percentage of the amount of tax attributable to the inclusion of property in the estate of the first decedent. The percentage is based on the number of years between the two deaths as follows:

0–2 years	100%
3–4 years	80%
5–6 years	60%
7–8 years	40%
9–10 years	20%

If the second decedent outlived the first by more than 10 years, no § 2013 credit is allowed.

Example 27. Individual A died in March 2006. Under the terms of his will, A left $1,000,000 in assets to his younger sister, B. B. died unexpectedly in May 2009 and the assets inherited from A were included in B's taxable estate. The amount of tax paid by A's estate that is attributable to the assets is calculated at $100,000. Since B died just over three years after A's death, 80% of the tax paid by A's estate is available to B's estate as a credit of $80,000 (80% × $100,000).

Gift Taxes Paid on Pre-1977 gifts. If a taxable gift was made prior to 1977 (i.e., prior to unification) and the gifted property is included in the transferor's gross estate

(e.g., under the rules of §§ 2036, 2037, or 2038), § 2012 allows a credit for any gift tax paid. The amount of the credit is limited to the lesser of the gift tax paid or the estate tax attributable to inclusion of the gifted property in the taxpayer's gross estate.

A COMPREHENSIVE EXAMPLE

The following example illustrates the complete computation of the Federal estate tax. In 1997, taxpayer M makes his first taxable gift to his son S. The fair market value of the property transferred is $200,000. The gift tax is computed as follows:

Value of gift	$ 200,000
Less: Annual exclusion (1997)	−10,000
Taxable gift	$ 190,000
Gift tax before credits	$ 51,600
Less: Unified credit	−51,600
Gift tax liability for 1997	$ 0

In 1998, M makes gifts to son S and daughter D. The value of each transfer is $250,000.

Value of gifts	$500,000
Less: Annual exclusions	−20,000
Taxable gifts for 1998	$ 480,000
Plus: 1997 taxable gift	+190,000
Taxable transfers to date	$670,000
Tentative tax on total transfers to date	$ 218,700
Less: Tax on 1997 gift	−51,600
Less: 1998 unified credit ($202,050 − $51,600)	−150,450
1998 gift tax liability	$ 16,650

M dies in 2009, leaving a taxable estate valued at $4 million. The estate tax is computed as follows:

Taxable estate		$4,000,000
Plus: Taxable gifts made in prior years		+670,000
Total taxable transfers		$4,670,000
Tentative tax on total transfers		
($555,800 + 45% (4,670,000 − 1,500,000 = $3,170,000)		$1,982,300
Less the sum of		
Gift taxes paid on post-1976		
taxable gifts (on 1998 gift)	$ 16,650	
Unified credit (2009)	1,455,800	−1,472,450
Estate tax liability		$509,850

PAYMENT OF THE ESTATE TAX

The Federal estate tax return, Form 706, is due nine months after the date of the decedent's death, and any tax liability shown is payable with the return. However, Congress appreciates the fact that the payment of the estate tax is often unforeseen, and has provided for a variety of relief measures for the estate with a substantial tax liability and insufficient liquidity to pay the tax nine months after death.

Section 6161 authorizes the Secretary of the Treasury to extend the time of payment of the estate tax for up to 10 years past the normal due date. To obtain an extension, the executor must show reasonable cause for the delay in payment. For example, the fact that the executor of an estate requires additional time to sell a particularly illiquid asset to generate the cash with which to pay the estate tax might be accepted as reasonable cause for an extension of the payment date for the estate tax.

Section 6166 allows an estate to pay a portion of its estate tax liability in installments if a substantial portion of the estate consists of the decedent's interest in a closely held business.[41] To be considered "closely-held" at least 20 percent of the total capital of the partnership or 20 percent of the total value of the corporation's voting stock must be included in the gross estate or the decedent is a partner in the partnership or a shareholder in the corporation and such partnership or corporation has 45 or fewer partners or shareholders (as increased by the 2001 legislation). An estate is eligible if more than 35 percent of the *adjusted gross estate* (gross estate less §§ 2053 and 2054 deductions for debts of the decedent, funeral and administrative expenses, and losses) consists of the value of such an interest. The percentage of the estate tax liability that can be deferred is based on the ratio of the value of the closely held business to the value of the adjusted gross estate.

If a decedent owned an interest in more than one closely held business, the values of the interests can be combined to meet the 35 percent test *if* the decedent's interest represents 20 percent or more of the total value of the business.

Example 28. The taxable estate of decedent X is composed of the following:

		Value
Sole proprietorship		$ 300,000
40% interest in closely held corporation		1,500,000
Other assets		2,500,000
Gross estate		$4,300,000
Less sum of		
Code §§ 2053 and 2054 deductions	$300,000	
Code § 2055 charitable deduction	500,000	−800,000
Taxable estate		$3,500,000

The decedent owned 100% of the value of the sole proprietorship and 40% of the value of the closely held corporation. The combined values of these interests, $1,800,000, represents 45% of the adjusted gross estate of $4,000,000 ($4,300,000 − $300,000). Therefore, the executor may elect to defer payment on 45% of the estate tax liability.

The tax deferred under § 6166 is payable in 10 equal annual installments. The first installment is payable five years and nine months after death. The IRS does charge the estate interest on the unpaid balance for the entire 15-year period.[42] Historically the

---

[41] § 6166(b) provides specific definition of the phrase "interest in a closely held business."

[42] See § 6601(j) for applicable interest rate.

interest rate charged on the deferred tax has been substantially less than the current market rate. Legislation in 1997 cut the rate even more. Currently, the interest rate is only two-percent of the deferred tax on the so-called *two-percent portion*. The tax on the two-percent portion is limited to the tax on the sum of $1,330,000 (as adjusted for inflation in 2009) and the exemption equivalent for the year of death less the applicable unified credit. For example, in 2009, the maximum two percent portion would be $598,500 computed as follows:

Base amount	$1,330,000
Exemption equivalent (2009)	3,500,000
Two percent portion	$4,830,000
Gross tax on two percent portion	$2,054,300
[$555,800 + (45% × ($4,830,000 − $1,500,000))]	
Unified credit (2009)	(1,455,800)
Tax on two-percent portion.	$ 598,500

In addition, the interest rate imposed on the amount of the deferred estate tax attributable to the taxable value of the business in excess of this amount ($1,330,000 + the exemption of $3,500,000 or $4,830,000 in 2009) is reduced to 45 percent of the rate applicable to underpayments of estimated taxes. No estate tax deduction is allowed for the interest paid. If the estate disposes of 50 percent or more of the value of the qualifying closely held interest, any outstanding amount of deferred estate tax must be paid immediately.

THE GENERATION-SKIPPING TRANSFER TAX

As part of the Tax Reform Act of 1976, Congress added a third type of transfer tax to the Internal Revenue Code. The *generation-skipping transfer tax* (GSTT) was designed to "plug a loophole" in the coverage of the gift and estate taxes. The original version of the GSTT was intimidatingly complex, and was criticized by tax practitioners from the moment of enactment.

The Tax Reform Act of 1986 retroactively repealed the 1976 version of the GSTT and replaced it with a new tax applicable to testamentary transfers occurring after the date of enactment and to inter vivos transfers made after September 25, 1985. Any tax actually paid under the 1976 GSTT is fully refundable.

A traditional generation-skipping transfer involves at least three generations of taxpayers. In its simplest form, a generation-skipping transfer occurs whenever there is a so-called *direct skip*, an outright transfer of wealth for the sole benefit of persons at least two generations younger than the transferor.[43]

> **Example 29.** This year Grandpa made a gift to his grandchild. Although a gift tax may be imposed on Grandpa, no gift or estate tax is imposed on the intervening generation, that is, the child's father. Therefore there is a direct skip of the estate and gift tax.

A more complicated yet equally important example involves a so-called *taxable termination* as illustrated below.

---

[43] § 2612.

Example 30. Several years ago, Mother, M, died. Her will created a trust with income to Daughter, D, for life, remainder to the grandchildren. In this case, M would pay an estate tax at the time of her death on the value of the property used to create the trust. More important, however, is the result when D dies and her interest terminates. Even though D is able to enjoy the income from the trust property for life, there is no estate tax imposed on her when she dies because her interest terminates at death. As a result, there is no estate or gift tax imposed on the second generation.

Generally, the value of property transferred in a taxable generation-skipping transaction is subject to a flat-rate tax of 45 percent (2009).[44] However, each transferor is allowed a lifetime exemption of $3,500,000 for 2009 for generation-skipping transfers of any type.[45] In addition, the tax is not imposed to the extent that the transfer is not subject to gift taxes (e.g., due to the annual exclusion or the exemption on transfers for medical or educational purposes). For example, small gifts from grandparents to grandchildren which fall within the annual exclusion would not be subject to the tax.

TAX PLANNING CONSIDERATIONS

The statutory rules of Federal gift, estate, and generation-skipping taxes have been examined in this chapter. Any individual taxpayer who desires to maximize the accumulated wealth available to family members will want to minimize the burden of these three transfer taxes. Tax planning for transfer taxes would be incomplete, however, without consideration of any interrelated Federal income taxes. Many gifts are made by transfers to a trust, and the income taxation of the trust entity and its beneficiaries may have a significant impact upon the original tax minimization plan. For this reason, the Federal income taxation of trusts, estates, and beneficiaries is discussed in the next chapter (Chapter 25). The tax planning considerations for transfer taxes and any attendant income taxes are incorporated in Chapter 26, *Family Tax Planning*.

PROBLEM MATERIALS

DISCUSSION QUESTIONS

24-1 *Interrelation of Federal Estate and Gift Taxes.* Discuss the various reasons why the Federal gift and estate taxes can be considered as a single, unified transfer tax.

24-2 *Entity for Transfer Tax Purposes.* Why can the married couple rather than each individual spouse be considered the taxable entity for transfer tax purposes?

24-3 *What Constitutes a Gift?* Businessperson B offers X $40,000 for an asset owned by X. Although X knows the asset is worth $60,000, he is in desperate need of cash and agrees to sell. Has X made a $20,000 taxable gift to B? Explain.

24-4 *Adequate Consideration.* During the current year, K offered to pay $50,000 to his only son, S, if S would agree to live in the same town as K for the rest of K's life. K is very elderly and frail and desires to have a relative close at hand in case of emergency. Does the $50,000 payment constitute a taxable gift made by K?

---

[44] § 2641.

[45] § 2631.

24-5   *When Is a Gift Complete?* Wealthy Grandmother G wants to provide financial support for her Grandson GS. She opens a joint checking account with $20,000 of cash. At any time, G or GS may withdraw funds from this account. Has G made a completed gift to GS by opening this account? At what point is the gift complete?

24-6   *Cumulative Nature of Transfer Taxes.* The Federal income tax is computed on an annual basis. How does this contrast to the computation of the Federal gift tax?

24-7   *Purpose of Unified Transfer Tax Rates.* A decedent's taxable estate can be considered the last taxable gift the decedent makes. Why?

24-8   *Incomplete Transfers.* The Federal gift tax and estate tax are not mutually exclusive. Give examples of transfers that may be treated as taxable gifts but that do not remove the transferred assets from the donor's gross estate.

24-9   *Computation of Taxable Estate.* What are the three steps involved in computing the taxable estate of a decedent?

24-10   *Probate Estate vs. Gross Estate.* How can the value of a decedent's probate estate differ from the value of his or her gross estate for tax purposes?

24-11   *Jointly Held Property.* Property held in joint tenancy with right of survivorship is often called a will substitute. In other words, if all property is held in joint tenancy, a will is unnecessary.
     a. Does joint tenancy eliminate the need for a will?
     b. Identify some of the problems that arise when property is titled in joint tenancy.

24-12   *Special Use Valuation of § 2032A.* The gross estate of decedent F consists of a very successful farming operation located 80 miles east of an expanding metropolitan area. The estate includes 2,000 acres of real estate worth $400,000 as agricultural land. However, a real estate developer is willing to pay $1.5 million for the property because of its potential for suburban development. Discuss the utility of § 2032A to F's estate.

24-13   *Powers of Appointment.* What are some *nontax* reasons for the creation of a power of appointment? What is the difference between a specific and a general power?

24-14   *Gifts in Contemplation of Death.* Discuss the scope of § 2035 concerning gifts made within three years of death after the enactment of ERTA 1981.

24-15   *Estate Tax Credits.* With the exception of the unified credit of § 2010, what is the basic purpose of the various estate tax credits?

24-16   *Due Date of Estate Tax Return and Payment.* Why is the tax law particularly lenient in authorizing extensions for payment of the Federal estate tax?

24-17   *Unified Transfer Tax Credit.* Section 2010 appears to allow a second $1,455,800 (2009) (2006-2008) credit against the Federal estate tax (in addition to the credit allowed for gift tax purposes under § 2505). Is this the case?

24-18   *Generation-Skipping Transfers.* Decedent T's will created a trust, the income from which is payable to T's invalid daughter D for her life. Upon D's death, the trust assets will be paid to T's two sons (D's brothers) in equal shares. Has T made a generation-skipping transfer? Explain.

PROBLEMS

24-19 *Gift Splitting.* During 2009, Mr. and Mrs. Z make the following cash gifts to their adult children:

Mr. Z:

to son M	$30,000
to daughter N	8,000
Total	$38,000

Mrs. Z:

to son M	$ 2,000
to daughter N	12,000
to daughter O	18,000
Total	$32,000

a. Assume Mr. and Mrs. Z do *not* elect to split their gifts per § 2513. Compute the total taxable gifts after exclusions for each.

b. How does the amount of taxable gifts change if Mr. and Mrs. Z *elect* to split their gifts?

24-20 *Computing Gift Tax Liability.* B, a single individual, made a cash gift of $200,000 his niece C in 1996. In 2009, B gives C an additional $700,000 and nephew D $900,000. Compute B's gift tax liability for the current year.

24-21 *Computing Taxable Gifts.* C, a single individual, makes the following transfers during current year:

	Fair Market Value
Cash to sister D	$13,000
Real estate:	
Life estate to brother B	28,000
Remainder to nephew N	21,000
Cash to First Baptist Church	25,000

What is the total amount of taxable gifts C must report?

24-22 *Amount of the Gift and the Annual Exclusion.* In 2009, Mr. C decided he wanted to set up trusts for his adult daughter and his grandson. To this end, he transferred $50,000 cash to a trust. The income of the trust was payable annually to his daughter, D, for 20 years with the remainder to D's son, R. For your computations, assume 120% of the applicable Federal midterm rate is 4.8 percent.

a. What is (are) the amount(s) of the taxable gift(s)?

b. Same as (a) except D is to receive the income for the rest of her life (she is age 40).

24-23 *Computing Taxable Gifts.* During 2009, L, a widower, makes the following transfers:

	Fair Market Value
Tuition payment to State College for nephew N, age 32	$ 6,000
New automobile to nephew N	9,000
Cash to a local qualified political committee	15,000

What is the total amount of taxable gifts L must report?

24-24 *Computing Taxable Gifts.* During 2009, Z, a widow, makes the following transfers:

	Fair Market Value
Real estate located in France to son J	$500,000
City of Philadelphia municipal bonds to daughter K	120,000
Payment to local hospital for medical expenses of brother-in-law M	18,000

What is the total amount of taxable gifts Z must report?

24-25 *Basis of Gifted Assets.* During the current year, L received a gift of land from his grandmother. The land had a basis to the grandmother of $100,000 and a fair market value of $250,000 on the date of the gift. A gift tax of $30,000 was paid on the transfer.
  a. If L subsequently sells the land for $300,000, how much gain or loss will he recognize?
  b. What would be the amount of L's recognized gain or loss on the sale if the land had a tax basis of $325,000 (rather than $100,000) to the grandmother?

24-26 *Marital Deduction.* F died during the current year, leaving a gross estate valued at $5 million. F's will specifically provided that no amount of her wealth was to be left to her estranged husband, G. However, under applicable state law, G is legally entitled to $1 million of his deceased wife's assets. How does the payment of $1 million affect the value of:
  a. F's *gross* estate,
  b. F's *taxable* estate?

24-27 *Gross Estate Inclusions.* Q was a cash basis taxpayer who died in the current year. On the date of Q's death, he owned corporate bonds, principal amount of $50,000, with accrued interest of $3,950. On the date of death, the bonds were selling on the open market for $54,000. Six months later the market price of the bonds had dropped to $51,500; there was $3,200 of accrued interest on the bonds as of this date. Neither market price includes any payment for accrued interest.
  a. Assuming the executor of Q's estate does not elect the alternate valuation date, what amounts should be included in Q's gross estate because of his ownership of the bonds?
  b. Assuming the executor does elect the alternate valuation date, what amounts should be included in Q's gross estate?

24-28 *Interests in Trusts Included in Gross Estate.* M's mother left property in trust (Trust A), with the income payable to M for M's lifetime and the remainder to M's daughter. At M's death, Trust A was worth $6.5 million. M's grandfather created a trust (Trust B), with the income payable to M's father for his lifetime. Upon the father's death, the remainder in Trust B was payable to M or M's estate. At M's death, his 82-year-old father was still living and Trust B was worth $2.1 million. Assuming a 5.0 percent

interest rate, what are the values of the inclusions in M's gross estate attributable to M's interests in Trust A and Trust B? (See Table S, contained in Appendix A-4.)

24-29   *Computing Gross Estate.* Upon A's death, certain assets were valued as follows:

	Fair Market Value
Probate estate	$ 750,000
Insurance proceeds on a policy on A's life. The policy has always been owned by A's niece, the beneficiary	150,000
Corpus of Trust A. A possessed the right to give the ownership of the corpus to herself or any of her family. In her will she left the corpus to cousin K.	15,000,000

Based on these facts, what is the value of A's gross estate?

24-30   *Computing Gross Estate.* Upon G's death, the following assets were valued:

	Fair Market Value
Probate estate	$ 350,000
Social security benefits payable to G's widow	38,000
Annuity payable to G's widow out of G's employer's pension plan	20,000
Corpus of revocable trust created by G for the benefit of his children 10 years prior to death. Upon G's death, the trust becomes irrevocable	1,000,000

What is the value of G's gross estate?

24-31   *Gifts Included in Gross Estate.* Donor D, age 66, makes a gift in trust for his grandchildren K and L. Under the terms of the trust instrument, D will receive the income from the trust for the rest of his life. Upon his death, the trust assets will be distributed equally between K and L. Upon the date of D's death, at age 77, the value of the trust assets is $2.5 million. What amount, if any, is included in D's gross estate?

24-32   *Gifts in Contemplation of Death.* In 2008, S made a taxable gift of marketable securities to his nephew and paid a gift tax of $14,250. In 2007, S gave an income interest in trust property to the same nephew and paid a gift tax of $5,000. S originally created the trust in 1990, retaining the income interest for life and giving the remainder to another family member. S died in 2009, when the marketable securities were worth $300,000 and the trust property was worth $972,000. Based on these facts, what amounts, if any, are included in S's gross estate?

24-33   *Gifts Included in Gross Estate.* In 1997, F transferred real estate into a trust, the income from which was payable to M during her lifetime. Upon M's death, the trust property will be distributed in equal portions among M's children. However, the trust instrument gives F the right to change the remainder beneficiaries at any time. F dies in the current year without ever having changed the original trust provisions. At date of death, the trust property is worth $3.9 million and M is 60 years old. Assuming a five percent interest rate, determine the amount, if any, to be included in F's gross estate. (See Table S, contained in Appendix A-1.)

24-34 *Gifts Included in Gross Estate.* In 1993, P transferred $500,000 of assets into an irrevocable trust for the exclusive benefit of his children. Under the terms of the trust agreement, annual income must be distributed among the children according to P's direction. When the youngest child attains the age of 25 years, the trust corpus will be distributed equally among the living children. P dies in the current year while the trust is still in existence and the corpus has a fair market value of $3,200,000. How much, if any, of the corpus must be included in P's gross estate?

24-35 *Powers of Appointment.* In 1999, donor D transferred $100,000 of assets into an irrevocable trust for the exclusive benefit of her minor grandchildren. Under the terms of the trust agreement, the grandchildren will receive the annual income from the trust, and when the youngest grandchild attains the age of 21, the trust corpus will be divided among the living grandchildren as S, D's only child, so directs. S dies in the current year while the trust is still in existence and the corpus has a fair market value of $400,000. S's valid will directs that the corpus of the trust will go entirely to grandchild Q. How much, if any, of the corpus must be included in S's gross estate?

24-36 *Including Insurance in Gross Estate.* Decedent R left a probate estate of $3,000,000. Two years prior to his death, R gave all incidents of ownership in an insurance policy on his own life to his daughter S, the policy beneficiary. Because the policy had a substantial cash surrender value, R paid a gift tax of $77,000 on the transfer. Upon death, the insurance policy paid $5,000,000 to S. What is the value of R's gross estate?

24-37 *Joint Tenancy.* In 2002, individual Q pays $500,000 for an asset and takes title with his brother R as joint tenants with right of survivorship. R makes no contribution toward the purchase price. In the current year, when the asset is worth $1.2 million, Q dies and ownership of the asset vests solely in R.
  a. What are the gift tax consequences of the creation of the joint tenancy?
  b. How much of the date of death value of the asset must be included in Q's gross estate?
  c. How much would be included in the gross estate of R if R, rather than Q, died in the current year?

24-38 *Computing Taxable Estate.* Decedent T left a gross estate for tax purposes of $8 million. T had personal debts of $60,000 and his estate incurred funeral expenses of $12,000 and legal and accounting fees of $35,000. T's will provided for $100,000 bequest to the American Cancer Society, with all other assets passing to his grandchildren. Compute T's taxable estate.

24-39 *Sections 2053 and 2054 Expenses.* Decedent D died on July 1 of the current year. D owned a sailboat valued at $85,000 as of the date of death. However, on December 1 of the current year, the boat was destroyed in a storm, and the estate was unable to collect any insurance to compensate for the loss. In December, the executor of D's estate received a $2,200 bill from the company that had stored the sailboat from January 1 through December 1 of the current year.
  a. If the executor does not elect the alternate valuation date, will the $85,000 value of the boat be included in D's gross estate? D's taxable estate?
  b. May any portion of the $2,200 storage fee be deducted on D's Federal estate tax return? On the first income tax return filed by the estate?

24-40 *Marital Deduction Assets.* J, who was employed by Gamma Inc. at the date of his death, had been an active participant in Gamma's qualified retirement plan. Under the terms of the plan, J's widow will receive an annuity of $1,500 per month for the next 20 years. The replacement value of the annuity is $145,000. In his will, J left his interest in a patent worth $50,000 to his widow; the patent will expire in eight years. To what extent will these transfers qualify for a marital deduction from J's gross estate?

24-41 *Qualified Terminable Interest Trust.* Under the will of decedent H, all his assets (fair market value of $10 million) are to be put into trust. His widow, W, age 64, will be paid all the income from the trust every quarter for the rest of her life. Upon W's death, all the assets in the trust will be distributed to the couple's children and grandchildren. During W's life, no part of the trust corpus can be distributed to anyone but W.

    a. What amount of marital deduction is available on H's estate tax return?

    b. W dies eight years after H and under the terms of H's will the trust assets are distributed. What percentage, if any, of the value of these assets must be included in W's gross estate?

24-42 *Deferring Estate Tax Payments.* Decedent X has the following taxable estate:

Sole proprietorship		$ 3,800,000
Ten percent interest in a closely held corporation		200,000
Other assets.		1,200,000
Gross estate.		$ 5,200,000
Less sum of		
§§ 2053 and 2054 deductions.	$800,000	
§ 2056 marital deduction	400,000	−1,200,000
Taxable estate		$ 4,000,000

Assume the estate tax liability on this estate is $1,400,000.

    a. How much of the liability may be deferred under § 6166?

    b. If X died in November 2009, when is the first installment payment of tax due?

24-43 *Computing Estate Tax Liability.* Decedent Z dies in 2008 and leaves a taxable estate of $5 million. During his life, Z made the following unrestricted gifts and did not elect gift splitting with his wife:

	Fair Market Value
1995: Gift of 2,000 shares of Acme stock to son S	$900,000
1997: Gift of cash to daughter D	600,000
1999: Gift of cash to wife W	700,000

Compute Z's estate tax liability after utilization of the available unified credit.

RESEARCH PROBLEMS

24-44 In 2000, JW gifted 30 percent of her stock in W Corporation to her favorite nephew, N. Although she retained a 50 percent interest in W Corporation and her husband owned the remaining 20 percent of the outstanding stock, JW was concerned that the family might eventually lose control of the firm. To reassure JW, the three stockholders agreed to restrict transferability of their stock by signing an agreement that any shareholder wishing to dispose of W Corporation stock must offer the stock to the corporation for a formula price based on the average net earnings per share for the three previous years. The corporation would then be obligated to purchase the stock at the formula price. At the time the buy-sell agreement was entered into, this formula resulted in a price very close to the stock's actual fair market value.

    JW died in the current year at a time when the value of her W Corporation stock was substantially depreciated because of certain unfavorable local economic conditions. Several independent appraisals of the stock valued JW's 50 percent interest at $650,000. However, the formula under the 2000 buy-sell agreement resulted in a value

of only $150,000 for the decedent's 50 percent interest. What is the correct value of the 50 percent interest in the corporation for estate tax purposes?

Some suggested research materials:

> Rev. Rul. 59-60, 1959-1 C.B. 237.
> *Estate of Littick*, 31 T.C. 181 (1958), acq. 1959-2 C.B. 5.
> Code § 2703.

24-45   In 2003, Mr. and Mrs. B (residents of a common law state) created two trusts for the benefit of their children. Mr. B transferred $600,000 of his own property into trust, giving the income interest to his wife for her life, and the remainder interest to the children. Mrs. B transferred $640,000 of her own property into trust, giving the income interest to her husband for his life, and the remainder interest to the children. In the current year, Mrs. B dies. How much, if any, of the current value of the corpus of the 2003 trust created by Mrs. B will be included in her gross estate?

Some suggested research materials:

> *United States v. Estate of Grace*, 69-1 USTC ¶12,609.
> 23 AFTR 2d 69-1954, 395 U.S. 316 (USSC, 1969).

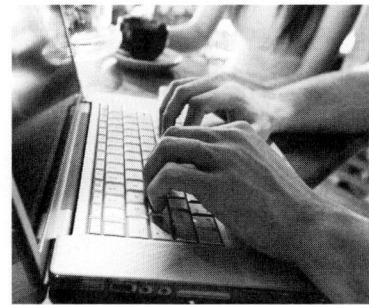

CHAPTER TWENTY FIVE

INCOME TAXATION OF ESTATES AND TRUSTS

LEARNING OBJECTIVES

Upon completion of this chapter you will be able to:

- Compute fiduciary accounting income and determine the required allocation of such income among the various beneficiaries of the fiduciary

- Identify the special rules that apply to the computation of fiduciary taxable income

- Explain the concept of income and deductions in respect of a decedent

- Compute both the taxable and nontaxable components of a fiduciary's distributable net income

- Describe the defining characteristics of a simple and a complex trust, including

  - The computation of the deduction for distributions to beneficiaries for both types of trusts

  - The distinction between tier one and tier two distributions from a complex trust

- Determine the tax consequences of fiduciary distributions to the recipient beneficiaries

CHAPTER OUTLINE

INTRODUCTION

Trusts and estates are taxable entities subject to a specialized set of tax rules contained in Subchapter J of the Internal Revenue Code (§§ 641 through 692). The income taxation of trusts and estates (commonly referred to as fiduciary taxpayers) and their beneficiaries is the subject of this chapter. Grantor trusts, a type of trust not recognized as a taxable entity and therefore not subject to the rules of Subchapter J, are discussed in Chapter 26.

THE FUNCTION OF ESTATES AND TRUSTS

ESTATES

An estate as a legal entity comes into existence upon the death of an individual. During the period of time in which the decedent's legal affairs are being settled, assets owned by the decedent are managed by an executor or administrator of the estate. Once all legal requirements have been satisfied, the estate terminates and ownership of all estate assets passes to the decedent's beneficiaries or heirs.

During its existence, the decedent's estate is a taxable entity that files a tax return and pays Federal income taxes on any income earned.[1] Normally an estate is a transitional entity that bridges the brief gap in time between the death of an individual taxpayer and the distribution of that individual's wealth to other taxpayers. However, estates as taxpayers may continue in existence for many years if the correct distribution of a decedent's wealth is in question. If the administration of a decedent's estate is unreasonably prolonged, the IRS may treat the estate as terminated for tax purposes after a reasonable amount of time for settlement of the decedent's affairs has elapsed.[2]

---

[1] § 641(a)(3).

[2] Reg. § 1.641(b)-3(a).

TRUSTS

A trust is a legal arrangement in which an individual, the *grantor*, transfers legal ownership of assets to one party, the *trustee*, and the legal right to enjoy and benefit from those assets to a second party, the *beneficiary* (or beneficiaries). Such an arrangement is usually designed for the protection of the beneficiary. Often trust beneficiaries are minor children or family members incapable of competently managing the assets themselves.

The terms of the trust, the duties of the trustee, and the rights of the various beneficiaries are specified in a legal document, the *trust instrument*. The assets put into trust are referred to as the trust *corpus*, or *principal*.

The role of the trustee is that of a fiduciary; he or she is required to act in the best interests of the trust beneficiaries rather than for his or her own interests. The position of trustee is usually filled by the professional trust department of a bank or a competent friend or family member. Professional trustees receive an annual fee to compensate them for services rendered.

The purpose of a trust is to protect and conserve trust assets for the sole benefit of the trust beneficiaries, not to operate a trade or business. A trust that becomes involved in an active, profit-making business activity runs the risk of being classified as an *association* for Federal tax purposes, with the unfavorable result that it will be taxed as a corporation rather than under the rules of Subchapter J.[3]

TRUST BENEFICIARIES

An individual who desires to establish a trust has virtually unlimited discretion as to the identity of the trust beneficiaries and the nature of the interest in the trust given to each beneficiary. For example, assume grantor G creates a trust consisting of $1 million of assets. G could specify in the trust instrument that individual I is to receive all the income of the trust for I's life, and upon I's death the assets in the trust are to be distributed to individual R. In this example, both I and R are trust beneficiaries. I owns an *income interest* in the trust, while R owns a *remainder interest* (the right to the trust principal at some future date).

A grantor can give trust beneficiaries any mix of rights to trust income or principal (trust assets) that will best accomplish the goals of the trust. In the previous example, if grantor G decided that the trust income might be insufficient to provide for I, the trust document could specify that I also will receive a certain amount of trust principal every year. Alternatively, if G believed that I might not need all the trust income annually, the trust document could provide that the trustee could accumulate income to distribute to I at some later point. As may be apparent, a trust can be a very flexible arrangement for providing for the needs of specific beneficiaries.

FIDUCIARY ACCOUNTING INCOME

There is no standard accounting system that applies to fiduciaries. The accounting income of an estate or trust is determined by reference to the decedent's valid will or the trust instrument. These documents can specify how fiduciary receipts, disbursements, and other transactions affect income, principal, or both. In other words, every fiduciary may have its own unique set of rules for the computation of accounting income, and the executor or trustee must refer exclusively to this income number in carrying out his or her duties. If a will or trust instrument is silent concerning the impact of a particular transaction on accounting income, such impact must be determined by reference to controlling state law. Most states have enacted a version of the Revised Uniform Principal

---

[3] See *Morrissey v. Comm.*, 36-1 USTC ¶9020, 16 AFTR 1274, 296 U.S. 344 (USSC, 1936), for this result.

and Income Act, a model set of fiduciary accounting rules proposed by the Uniform Commission on State Laws.

One common difference between fiduciary accounting income and taxable income is the classification of fiduciary capital gains. Typically, capital gains represent an increase in the value of the principal of the fiduciary and normally are not available for distribution to income beneficiaries. Of course, for Federal tax purposes capital gains represent taxable income. Similarly, stock dividends are often regarded as an increase in principal rather than trust income, even though the dividend may be taxable income under the Internal Revenue Code.

Trustee fees are generally deductible for tax purposes. However, for fiduciary accounting purposes such fees may be charged *either* to trust income or to trust principal.

Depreciation may or may not have an effect on fiduciary accounting income. If local law or the trust instrument requires the fiduciary to establish a reserve for depreciation, depreciation is computed in accordance with the local law or the trust instrument and subtracted in computing trust accounting income. In effect, the fiduciary transfers cash out of income (reducing the amount that can be distributed to the income beneficiary) and sets this amount aside for future replacement of the depreciable property. Note that the amount of depreciation computed for tax purposes can be quite different than the amount of depreciation for fiduciary accounting income purposes. For this reason, tax depreciation requires special treatment as described below.

Exhibit 25-1 identifies various items of income and expense and shows how they are normally allocated between income and corpus.

EXHIBIT 25-1
Fiduciary Accounting Income

Typical income items
> Interest
> Dividends
> Royalties
> Net rental income (income less expenses) from real or personal property
> Net profits from operation of a trade or business; losses are usually charged to corpus
> All or a portion of trustee commissions
> Depreciation to the extent of any required reserve

Typical corpus items
> Gain or loss on the sale or exchange of trust property (capital gains)
> Casualty losses
> Stock dividends
> All or a portion of trustee commissions

Example 1. During the year, the records of a trust revealed the following information:

Receipts:

Dividends	$10,000
Interest from municipal bonds	12,000
Long-term capital gain allocable to principal under state law	6,500
Stock dividend allocable to principal under the trust instrument	4,000
Total receipts	$32,500

Disbursements:

Trustee fee (half allocable to trust income; half allocable to principal under the trust instrument)	$ 3,000

Based on the above, the accounting income of the trust would be $20,500, computed as follows:

Dividends	$10,000
Interest from municipal bonds	12,000
	$22,000
Less: One-half of the trustee fee ($3,000 ÷ 2)	(1,500)
Trust accounting income	$20,500

If the trustee of this particular trust was required to distribute the entire amount of trust income to a particular group of beneficiaries, the trustee would make a payment of $20,500. Note that this amount bears little relationship to the *taxable income* generated by the trust's activities.

INCOME TAXATION OF FIDUCIARIES

For Federal tax purposes, fiduciaries are taxable entities.[4] Every estate that has annual gross income of $600 or more, and every trust that has either annual gross income of $600 or more *or* any taxable trust income, must file an income tax return. Furthermore, if a fiduciary has a beneficiary who is a nonresident alien, that fiduciary must file a return regardless of the amount of its gross or taxable income for the year.[5]

Form 1041, the U.S. Fiduciary Income Tax Return, must be filed by the 15th day of the fourth month following the close of the fiduciary's taxable year (see Appendix B for sample Form 1041). An estate may adopt a calendar or any fiscal taxable year. However, the taxable year of a trust must be a calendar year.[6] In the case of an estate, the first taxable year begins on the day following the date of death of the decedent.[7] In the case of a trust, the date of creation as specified in the controlling trust instrument marks the beginning of the first taxable year.

Fiduciaries generally must make quarterly estimated tax payments in the same manner as individuals. However, no estimated taxes must be paid by an estate or a grantor trust to which the residual of the grantor's estate is distributed for any taxable year ending within the two years following the decedent's death.[8] A trustee may *elect* to treat any portion of an excess estimated tax payment made by a trust as a payment of estimated tax made by a beneficiary. If the election is made, the payment is considered as having been distributed to the beneficiary on the last day of the trust's taxable year and then remitted to the government as estimated tax paid by the beneficiary on January 15th of the following year.[9]

Example 2. On April 15, 2008, Trust T made an estimated tax payment of $14,000. However, later in the year, the trustee decided to distribute all 2008 trust income to beneficiary B. Because Trust T will have no 2008 tax liability, the trustee may elect to treat the $14,000 payment as a cash distribution made to beneficiary B on December 31, 2008. Beneficiary B will report the $14,000 as part of his 2008 estimated tax payment made on January 15, 2009.

---

[4]   See §§ 7701(a)(6) and 641(a).

[5]   § 6012(a)(3), (4), and (5).

[6]   § 645. This requirement does not apply to tax-exempt and charitable trusts.

[7]   See Reg. §§ 1.443-1(a)(2), and 1.461-1(b).

[8]   § 6654(l).

[9]   § 643(g).

Section 641 (b) provides that "the taxable income of an estate or trust shall be computed in the same manner as in the case of an individual, except as otherwise provided in this part." Thus, many of the rules governing the taxation of individuals apply to fiduciaries. Before examining the specific rules unique to fiduciary income taxation, it will be useful to look at the basic approach for computing fiduciary taxable income.

Step One: Compute fiduciary accounting income and identify any receipts and disbursements allocated to principal (under either the trust instrument or state law).

Step Two: Compute fiduciary taxable income *before* the deduction for distributions to beneficiaries authorized by Code §§ 651 and 661.

Step Three: Compute the deduction for distributions to beneficiaries. This step will require a computation of fiduciary "distributable net income" (DNI).

Step Four: Subtract the deduction for distributions to arrive at *fiduciary taxable income.*

Step One, the computation of fiduciary accounting income, was discussed earlier. Detailed discussions of Steps Two and Three constitute most of the remainder of this chapter.

FIDUCIARY TAXABLE INCOME

Unless otherwise modified, the fiduciary computes its taxable income in a manner identical to that of an individual taxpayer. The major difference is the deduction granted for distributions made to beneficiaries, explained later in this chapter. In addition, § 642 contains a number of special provisions that must be followed in computing fiduciary taxable income and the final tax. These unique aspects of estate and trust taxation are considered below.

FIDUCIARY TAX RATES

The tax rates for estates and trusts for 2008 are shown in Exhibit 25-2. Note that the 10 percent rate that applies to individuals does not apply to trusts or estates. Also note that there is very little progressivity in the fiduciary rate schedule; taxable income in excess of $10,700 is taxed at the highest 35 percent rate. However, under § 1(j), any component of fiduciary taxable income consisting of net long-term capital gain or dividend income is taxed at a maximum 15 percent rate.

EXHIBIT 25-2
Income Tax Rates for Estates and Trusts

For Taxable Years Beginning in 2009

If taxable income is

Over—	But not over—	The tax is			Of the amount over—
$ 0	$ 2,300	$ 0		15%	$ 0
2,300	5,350	345.00	+	25%	2,300
5,350	8,200	1,107.50	+	28%	5,350
8,200	11,150	1,905.50	+	33%	8,200
11,150	—	2,879.00	+	35%	11,150

In determining their final tax liability, fiduciaries are subject to the alternative minimum tax provisions.[10]

STANDARD DEDUCTION AND PERSONAL EXEMPTION

Unlike individual taxpayers, fiduciaries are not entitled to a standard deduction.[11] However, a fiduciary, like an individual taxpayer, is entitled to a personal exemption. The amount of the exemption depends on the type of fiduciary. The personal exemption for an estate is $600. The exemption for a trust that is required by the trust instrument to distribute all trust income currently is $300. The exemption for any trust not subject to this requirement is $100.[12]

LIMITATIONS ON DEDUCTIBILITY OF FIDUCIARY EXPENSES

Because fiduciaries generally do not engage in the conduct of a business, the gross income of a fiduciary usually consists of investment income items such as dividends, interest, rents, and royalties. Fiduciary expenses are normally deductible under the authority of § 212, which provides for the deduction of ordinary and necessary expenses paid for the management, conservation, or maintenance of property held for the production of income. However, there are several limitations on the deduction of expenses that apply to individuals that also apply to fiduciaries.

Limitations on Deductions Related to Tax-Exempt Income. As a general rule, § 265 denies the deduction for any expenses related to tax-exempt income. In contrast, any expense that is *directly related* to taxable fiduciary income is fully deductible. For example, rent expenses are directly related to rental income and would not be subject to this limitation. Expenses that are not directly related to a particular type of income— sometimes referred to as *indirect* expenses—must be allocated proportionately between taxable and tax-exempt income.[13] For example, consider a common expenditure of trusts such as trustee commissions. These fees are viewed as relating to both taxable and tax-exempt income and, therefore, an allocation is required. Assuming 20 percent of the trust's income is tax-exempt, then 20 percent of the trustee commission would be nondeductible. On the other hand, most practitioners take the position that tax preparation

---

[10]   See § 59(c). A special computation is used that is beyond the scope of this text.

[11]   § 63(c)(6)(D).

[12]   § 642(b).

[13]   Reg. § 1.642(g)-2.

fees need not be allocated to tax-exempt income since they are only related to taxable income.

The portion of an indirect expense that is not deductible can be determined using the following formula:

$$\frac{\text{Tax exempt income}}{\text{Total trust income}} \times \frac{\text{Expenses not directly related to}}{\text{a particular type of income}} = \frac{\text{Nondeductible}}{\text{expenses}}$$

In computing the denominator of the above formula, trust accounting income does not include capital gains unless capital gains are actually included in trust accounting income.[14] In addition, the denominator is computed using gross receipts.

Example 3. This year Trust T paid trustee fees of $7,000, $5,000 allocable to income and $2,000 allocable to corpus. Its records reveal the following additional information:

	Amounts
Rental income	$70,000
Rental expenses	(30,000)
Net rental income	$40,000
Long-term capital gains allocable to corpus	$25,000
Long-term capital losses allocable to corpus	(5,000)
Net capital gain	$20,000
Sales	$20,000
Costs of goods sold	(15,000)
Gross income	$ 5,000
Interest on State of New York bonds	$10,000

To determine the amount of commissions that are not deductible, the denominator does not include the net capital gain allocable to corpus of $20,000. However, the denominator does include the gross amounts of income received and is not reduced by expenses. Thus the denominator includes the rent of $70,000, sales of $20,000, and tax-exempt interest of $10,000 for a total of $100,000. Therefore 10% ($10,000/$100,000) of the $7,000 of trustee's commissions or $700 is not deductible, and the remaining $6,300 is deductible. Note that in computing the amount of the deductible commissions, the fact that they are allocable to income or corpus for trust accounting purposes is irrelevant.

Limitation on Double Deduction of Administrative Expenses. Section 642(g) provides a second major limitation on the deductibility of fiduciary expenses. If an administrative expense is claimed as a deduction on the estate tax return of a decedent, it may not also be claimed as a deduction on an income tax return of the decedent's estate or subsequent trust. However, Regulation § 1.642(g)-2 provides that administrative expenses that could be deducted for either estate tax or income tax purposes can be divided between the two returns in whatever portions achieve maximum tax benefit.

Limitation on Miscellaneous Itemized Deductions. Section 67(a) limits certain miscellaneous itemized deductions, including the § 212 deduction for investment

---

[14]   Rev. Rul. 77-365. Other approaches may be available. For example, see *Whittemore, Jr. v. U.S.* 20 AFTR 2d 5533, 67-2 USTC ¶9670 383 F.2d 824 (CA-8, 1967).

expenses. Such itemized deductions are allowed only to the extent they exceed 2 percent of adjusted gross income. Section 67(e) provides that the deduction for expenses paid or incurred in connection with the administration of a fiduciary that would have been avoided if the property were not held by the fiduciary shall be allowable in computing the adjusted gross income of the fiduciary. In other words, fiduciary expenses such as administration fees which are incurred only because of the trust or estate form are not considered itemized deductions subject to the 2 percent floor. Unfortunately, whether an expense is unique to a trust or an estate is not always clear. Most of the controversy has concerned investment management and advisory expenses. However, in 2008, the Supreme Court resolved the matter, holding that investment management and advisory fees were miscellaneous itemized deductions.[15] According to the Court, if an expense of a trust or estate is commonly incurred by an individual, it is not unique to a trust. Applying this theory to fees for investment management, the Court believed that it would not be uncommon or unusual for individuals to hire an investment adviser. Therefore, it held that such expenses are miscellaneous itemized deductions. In this regard, the proposed regulations would require that trustee fees be unbundled so that the proper amounts may be allocated properly between trust or estate administration and investment advice. After the *Knight* decision, it appears that such expenses as the costs of accounting, tax return preparation, division of income or corpus among beneficiaries, will or trust contests or construction, fiduciary bond premiums and communications with beneficiaries regarding trust or estate matters would not be miscellaneous itemized deductions.

The computation of the limitation on miscellaneous itemized deductions can be quite cumbersome. Since adjusted gross income of the trust depends on the amount of the distribution deduction and the distribution deduction in turn depends on taxable income after taking into account the deduction for miscellaneous itemized deductions (taxable DNI as explained below), the calculation of allowable miscellaneous itemized deductions may require the use of simultaneous algebraic equations.

Deduction Cutback. Section 68 generally requires that the total of an individual's itemized deductions for the year be reduced by a percentage of the amount of adjusted gross income in excess of an inflation adjusted threshold. This requirement is expressly inapplicable to any estate or trust.[16]

Medical Expenses. Medical expenses paid by an estate or trust require special consideration. Medical expenses paid for the care of a *decedent* prior to his death that are paid by an estate within one year after death can be deducted either on the income tax return of the decedent (final Form 1040) or the estate tax return (Form 706), but not both. Medical expenses paid after the one-year period are deductible only as liabilities on the estate tax return (Form 706) if such return is actually filed. Medical expenses of *beneficiaries* that are paid by the trust or estate are treated as distributions of income to the beneficiaries and are not deductible per se on the fiduciary income tax return.

CHARITABLE CONTRIBUTIONS

Section 642(c) authorizes an unlimited charitable deduction for any amount of gross income paid by a fiduciary to a qualified charitable organization. Fiduciaries are given a great deal of flexibility as to the timing of charitable contributions; if a contribution is paid after the close of one taxable year but before the close of the next taxable year, the fiduciary may elect to deduct the payment in the earlier year.[17]

---

[15] *Michael J. Knight, Trustee of the William L. Rudkin Testamentary Trust,*, 2008-1 USTC ¶50,132, 101 AFTR 2d 2008-544, 128 S. Ct. 782 (USSC, 2008).

[16] § 68(e).

[17] § 642(c)(1). See Reg. § 1.642(c)-1(b) for the time and manner in which such an election is to be made.

If a fiduciary receives tax-exempt income that is available for charitable distribution, its deduction for any charitable contribution made normally must be reduced by that portion of the contribution attributable to tax-exempt income.[18]

> **Example 4.** During the current year, Trust T receives $30,000 of tax-exempt interest, $25,000 of taxable interest, and $45,000 of taxable dividends. The trust makes a charitable contribution of $20,000 during the year. Because 30% of the trust's income available for distribution is nontaxable, 30% of the charitable distribution is nondeductible and the trust's deduction for charitable contributions is limited to $14,000.

DEPRECIATION, DEPLETION, AND AMORTIZATION

The total allowable amount of depreciation, depletion, and amortization that may be deducted by the fiduciary (or passed through to the beneficiaries) is determined in the normal manner. A fiduciary is entitled to bonus depreciation but not allowed to expense any portion of the cost of eligible property under § 179.

Deductions for depreciation and depletion available to a fiduciary depend upon the terms of the controlling will or trust instrument. If the controlling instrument authorizes a reserve for depreciation or depletion, any *allowable* (deductible) tax depreciation or depletion will be deductible by the fiduciary to the extent of the specified reserve. If the allowable tax depreciation or depletion exceeds the reserve, the excess deduction is allocated between the fiduciary and beneficiaries based upon the amount of fiduciary income allocable to each.[19]

> **Example 5.** Trust R owns rental property with a basis of $300,000. The trust instrument authorizes the trustee to maintain an annual depreciation reserve of $15,000 (5% of the cost of the property). For tax purposes, however, the current year's depreciation deduction is $22,000. The trust instrument provides that one-half of annual trust income including rents will be distributed to the trust beneficiaries. For the current year, the trust is entitled to a depreciation deduction of $18,500 [5% of $300,000 + one-half the tax depreciation in excess of $15,000 (ø × $7,000 = $3,500)].

Note that if the controlling instrument is silent, depreciation and depletion deductions are simply allocated between fiduciary and beneficiaries on the basis of fiduciary income allocable to each. If a fiduciary is entitled to statutory amortization, the amortization deduction also will be apportioned among fiduciary and beneficiaries on the basis of income allocable to each.[20]

FIDUCIARY LOSSES

Because the function of a trust generally is to conserve and protect existing wealth rather than to engage in potentially risky business activities, it is unusual for a trust to incur a net operating loss. It is not unusual, however, for an estate or trust that owns a business interest (e.g., an interest in a partnership or an S corporation) to incur this type of loss. In any case, if a net operating loss does occur, a fiduciary may carry the loss back two years and forward for 20.[21] Capital losses incurred by a fiduciary are deductible against capital gains; a maximum of $3,000 of net capital loss may be deducted against other sources of

---

[18]   Reg. § 1.642(c)-3(b).

[19]   Reg. § 1.167(h)-1; Reg. § 1.611-1(c)(4).

[20]   Reg. § 1.642(f)-1.

[21]   §§ 172(b)(1) and 642(d).

income.[22] Nondeductible net capital losses are carried forward to subsequent taxable years of the fiduciary.[23]

Fiduciaries are also subject to the limitations imposed on passive activity losses and credits by § 469.[24] Therefore, a fiduciary may only deduct current losses from passive activities against current income from passive activities. Any nondeductible loss is suspended and carried forward to subsequent taxable years. If an interest in a passive activity is distributed by a fiduciary to a beneficiary, any suspended loss of the activity is added to the tax basis of the distributed interest.[25]

Section 469(I) normally provides for a $25,000 *de minimis* offset for losses attributable to rental real estate. However, this allowance is extended only to "natural persons" and, therefore, normally does not apply to trusts or estates. This rule prevents taxpayers from circumventing the $25,000 limitation by transferring multiple properties to multiple trusts with each claiming a $25,000 allowance. However, the provision is extended to estates for losses occurring for tax years ending less than two years after the decedent's date of death.

NOLs, Capital Losses, and Excess Deductions. Unlike the net losses of a partnership or an S corporation, fiduciary losses do not flow through to beneficiaries. An exception to this rule applies for the year in which a trust or estate terminates. If the terminating fiduciary has net operating losses, capital loss carryforwards, or current year deductions in excess of current gross income, § 642(h) provides that such unused losses and excess deductions become available to the beneficiaries succeeding to the property of the fiduciary.

> **Example 6.** D died in 2009. In 2010, the year of termination, the estate had gross income of $5,000 and legal fees of $15,000. The excess deductions of $10,000 do not create an NOL (that would carryover to the beneficiaries) since legal fees are considered a nonbusiness expense and are not deductible in computing an NOL. However, because the excess deductions occur in the year of termination, they pass through to the beneficiary who can claim the $10,000 as an itemized deduction subject to the deduction cutback rule. It should be emphasized that had this not been the year of termination, the $10,000 excess would be wasted. Due to this treatment, the fiduciary should take steps to ensure that excess deductions occur only in the year of termination. For example, a cash basis estate could postpone paying the legal fees until the final year.

Casualty losses of a fiduciary are subject to the rules pertaining to individual taxpayers. For casualty losses, the limitation of the deduction to that amount in excess of 10 percent of adjusted gross income applies, although the concept of adjusted gross income is normally not associated with trusts or estates.[26] In addition, § 642(g) prohibits the deduction by a fiduciary of any loss that has already been claimed as a deduction on an estate tax return.

INCOME AND DEDUCTIONS IN RESPECT OF A DECEDENT

The death of an individual taxpayer can create a peculiar timing problem involving the reporting of income items earned or deductible expenses incurred by the taxpayer prior to death. For example, if a cash basis individual had performed all the services

---

[22]   § 1211(b).

[23]   § 1212(b).

[24]   § 469(a)(2)(A).

[25]   § 469(j)(12).

[26]   See Form 4684 and its instructions for this computation.

required to earn a $5,000 consulting fee but had not collected the fee before death, by whom shall the $5,000 of *income in respect of a decedent* (IRD) be reported? The individual taxpayer who earned the income never received payment, but the recipient of the money, the individual's estate, is not the taxpayer who earned it. Section 691(a) gives a statutory solution to this puzzling question by providing that any income of an individual not properly includible in the taxable period prior to the individual's death will be included in the gross income of the recipient of the income, typically the estate of the decedent or a beneficiary of the estate. Common IRD items include unpaid salary or commissions, retirement income (e.g., IRA), rent income, or interest accrued but unpaid at death, and the amount of a § 453 installment obligation that would have been recognized as income if payment had been received by the decedent prior to death.

Certain expenses incurred by a decedent but not properly deductible on the decedent's final return because of nonpayment are afforded similar statutory treatment. Under § 691(b), these *deductions in respect of a decedent* (DRD) are deducted by the taxpayer who is legally required to make payment. Allowable DRD items include business and income-producing expenses, interest, taxes, and depletion.

ESTATE TAX TREATMENT AND THE § 691(C) DEDUCTION

Items of IRD and DRD represent assets and liabilities of the deceased taxpayer. As such, these items will be included on the decedent's estate tax return. Because IRD and DRD also have future income tax consequences, special provisions in the tax law apply to these items. First, even though the right to IRD is an asset acquired from a decedent, the basis of an IRD item does not become the item's fair market value at date of death. Instead, under § 1014(c), the basis of the item to the decedent carries over to the new owner. This special rule preserves the potential income that must be recognized when the IRD item is eventually collected. The character of IRD also is determined by reference to the decedent taxpayer.

Secondly, items of DRD that are deducted as administrative expenses on an estate tax return are *not* subject to the rule prohibiting a deduction on a subsequent income tax return.[27] Therefore, unlike administrative expenses of an estate that cannot be deducted on both the fiduciary income tax return (Form 1041) and the estate tax return (Form 706), DRD can be deducted on both.

Perhaps the most important reason for identifying items of IRD is the allowance of a special deduction for the recipient. To appreciate this deduction, consider the normal estate tax treatment given to a decedent's income. Such income is included *net* of any income tax that the decedent has paid. In contrast, items of IRD are included without reduction for the related income tax since the income tax on IRD is not a liability of the decedent but a liability of the recipient. Consequently, the amount of IRD income that is included in the gross estate is overstated and, therefore, the related estate tax is overstated. An heir who is the recipient of the income ends up with less than he would have had if the income had been taxed to the decedent and passed on to the heir net of the estate tax.

> **Example 7.** D died on March 7, 2009. He was in the 40% income tax bracket and the 50% estate tax bracket. At the time of his death, D's employer owed him $10,000 of income. The following analysis shows the tax consequences that result if D had collected the $10,000 before he died as compared to those which would occur if his son, his heir, collects the $10,000 (assuming he is in the 40% tax bracket).

---

[27]   § 642(g).

	D Collects Before Death	Total Tax	Heir Collects After Death	Total Tax
Income	$10,000		$10,000	
Income tax to decedent	(4,000)	$4,000	0	$ 0
Aftertax income in estate	$ 6,000		$10,000	
Estate tax at 50%	$ 3,000	3,000	$ 5,000	5,000
Income to heir	$ 0		$10,000	
Income tax to heir			$ 4,000	4,000
Total income and estate tax		$7,000		$9,000

In this case, the total income and estate tax imposed on the $10,000 if D collected the $10,000 is $7,000. In contrast, if the heir collects the $10,000 from the employer the total income and estate tax is $9,000. The $2,000 difference is attributable to the fact that the entire $10,000 is subject to estate tax in the latter case while only $6,000 ($10,000 net of the income tax of $4,000) is subject to estate tax in the first case (50% × $4,000 = $2,000).

Perhaps the best way to treat this problem is to estimate the amount of income tax that the decedent would have paid had he or she received the income and give the estate a deduction for this amount. However, because this amount would presumably be difficult to estimate, the authors of § 691 opted for an alternative that produces about the same result. Section 691(c) allows the recipient of IRD a deduction for any estate tax attributable to the income.

The deduction is a percentage of the estate tax attributable to the total *net* IRD included in an estate based on the ratio of the recognized IRD item to all IRD items. Estate tax attributable to net IRD is the excess of the actual tax over the tax computed without including the IRD in the taxable estate.

The § 691(c) deduction can be computed using the following two steps:

1. Determine the estate tax attributable to net IRD:

$$\begin{array}{rl} & \text{Estate tax actually incurred (including net IRD)} \\ - & \text{Estate tax without NIRD} \\ \hline = & \text{Total estate tax attributable to IRD} \end{array}$$

2. Recipient's deduction is based on the proportionate amount of IRD (not net IRD) that is received.

$$\frac{\text{IRD received}}{\text{Total IRD}} \times \frac{\text{Total estate tax}}{\text{attributable to IRD}} = \frac{\text{Section 691(c)}}{\text{deduction}}$$

Note that if an estate or trust is the recipient of the IRD, it is not subject to the deduction cutback for itemized deductions. In contrast, if an individual taxpayer receives the IRD, the amount is considered an itemized deduction subject to the deduction cutback.

Example 8. Taxpayer T's estate tax return included total IRD items valued at $145,000. DRD items totaled $20,000. If the *net* IRD of $125,000 had not been included in T's estate, the Federal estate tax liability would have decreased by $22,000. During the current year, the estate of T collected half ($72,500) of all IRD items and included this amount in estate gross income. T's estate is entitled to a § 691(c) deduction of $11,000. The $11,000 is not subject to the deduction cutback since such rule does not apply to estates or trusts.

THE DISTRIBUTION DEDUCTION AND THE TAXATION OF BENEFICIARIES

The central concept of Subchapter J is that income recognized by a fiduciary will be taxed *either* to the fiduciary itself or to the beneficiaries of the fiduciary. The determination of the amount of income taxable to each depends upon the amount of annual distributions from the fiduciary to the beneficiary. Conceptually, distributions to beneficiaries represent a flow-through of trust income that will be taxed to the beneficiary. Under §§ 651 and 661, the amount of the distribution will then be available as a *deduction* to the fiduciary, reducing the taxable income the fiduciary must report. Income that flows through the fiduciary to a beneficiary retains its original character; therefore, the fiduciary acts as a *conduit*, similar to a partnership in this respect.[28]

In computing the deduction for distributions, the law generally presumes that *every distribution consists of a pro rata portion of current taxable and nontaxable income that is in fact distributable*. Sections 651 and 661 refer to this quantity as *a distributable net income* (DNI) and allow the fiduciary a deduction for amounts distributed but limit the deduction to taxable DNI. It should be emphasized that whatever amount is deductible by the fiduciary is the same amount that is taxable to the beneficiaries. This follows from the fact that the deduction merely serves to allocate taxable income from the fiduciary to the beneficiary. Distributions exceeding DNI represent accumulated income of the fiduciary that has been previously taxed, or corpus. Such amounts are neither deductible by the fiduciary nor taxable to the beneficiary.

Before further examining the computation of the deduction concept and DNI, it is important to understand that a trust or estate can make distributions of either cash or property, both of which may or may not carry out DNI (i.e., taxable and nontaxable income). However, § 663(a)(1) provides that *specific* gifts or bequests properly distributed from a fiduciary to a beneficiary under the terms of the governing instrument are distributions of principal rather than of income. Correspondingly, the fiduciary does not recognize gain or loss upon the distribution of a specific property bequest.

> **Example 9.** During the current year, the Estate of Z recognized $30,000 of income, all of which is taxable. During the year, the executor of the estate distributed a pearl necklace to beneficiary B. The necklace had a fair market value of $6,000. If the will of decedent Z specifically provided for the distribution of the necklace to B, no estate income will be taxed to her. Alternatively, if there were no such specific bequest and B received the necklace as part of her general interest in estate assets, she will have received an income distribution.

The amount of income associated with a property distribution from a fiduciary depends upon the tax treatment of the distribution *elected* by the fiduciary. Section 643(e)(3) provides an election under which the fiduciary recognizes gain on the distribution of appreciated property as if the property had been sold at its fair market value. In this case, the amount of fiduciary income carried by the property distribution and the basis of the property in the hands of the beneficiary equals the property's fair market value. If the election is not made, the distribution of property produces no gain or loss to the fiduciary, and the amount of fiduciary income carried by the distribution is the lesser of the basis of such property in the hands of the fiduciary or the property's fair market value.[29] In the

---

[28]   §§ 652(b) and 662(b).

[29]   § 643(e)(2).

case where the election is not made, the basis of the property in the hands of the fiduciary will carry over as the basis of the property in the hands of the beneficiary.[30]

> **Example 10.** During the current year, Trust T distributes property to beneficiary B. The distribution is not a specific gift of property. On the date of distribution, the property has a basis to the trust of $10,000 and a fair market value of $17,000. If the trust so elects, it will recognize a $7,000 gain on the distribution, and B will be considered to have received a $17,000 income distribution and will have a $17,000 basis in the property. If the trustee does not make the election, it will not recognize any gain upon distribution of the property. B will be considered to have received only a $10,000 income distribution and will have only a $10,000 basis in the property.

When a beneficiary is entitled to a specific gift or bequest of a sum of money (a pecuniary gift or bequest), and the fiduciary distributes property in satisfaction of such gift or bequest, any appreciation or depreciation in the property is recognized as a gain or loss to the fiduciary.[31]

> **Example 11.** Under the terms of E's will, beneficiary M is to receive the sum of $60,000. E's executor distributes 600 shares of corporate stock to M to satisfy this pecuniary bequest. At the time of distribution, the stock has a fair market value of $100 a share and a basis to E's estate of $75 a share. Upon distribution, the estate must recognize a capital gain of $15,000 (600 shares × $25 per share appreciation). Note that because this distribution represents a specific bequest, it is not an income distribution to M and the § 643(e)(3) election is inapplicable. The basis of the stock to M will be its fair market value.

In any case in which the distribution of depreciated property by a trust or an estate to a beneficiary results in the recognition of loss, § 267 disallows any deduction of the loss by the trust.

COMPUTATION OF DISTRIBUTION DEDUCTION AND DNI

To calculate the distribution deduction available to a fiduciary and the amount of fiduciary income taxable to beneficiaries, it is first necessary to calculate the *distributable net income* (DNI) of the fiduciary. DNI represents the net income of a fiduciary available for distribution to income beneficiaries.

DNI has several important characteristics. First, it does not include taxable income that is unavailable for distribution to income beneficiaries. For example, in most states capital gains realized upon the sale of fiduciary assets are considered to represent a part of *trust principal* and are not considered *fiduciary income*. Such capital gains, while taxable, are not included in DNI. Secondly, DNI may include nontaxable income that is available for distribution to income beneficiaries.

At this point, it would appear that the amount of DNI is the same amount as fiduciary accounting income. However, there is an important difference between the two concepts. All expenses that are deductible *for tax purposes* by the fiduciary enter into the DNI calculation, even if some of these expenses are chargeable to principal and not deducted in computing fiduciary accounting income.

A beneficiary who receives a distribution from a fiduciary with both taxable and nontaxable DNI is considered to have received a proportionate share of each.[32]

---

[30]   § 643(e)(1).

[31]   Reg. § 1.661(a)-2(f)(1).

[32]   Reg. § 1.662(b)-1.

Example 12. Trust A has DNI of $80,000, $30,000 of which is nontaxable. During the year, beneficiary X receives a distribution of $16,000. This distribution consists of $10,000 of taxable DNI [$16,000 distribution × ($50,000 taxable DNI ÷ $80,000 total DNI)] and $6,000 of nontaxable DNI.

The amount of a fiduciary's *taxable* DNI represents *both* the maximum income that may be taxed to beneficiaries and the maximum deduction for distributions available to the fiduciary in computing its own taxable income.[33] Therefore, computing DNI is crucial to the correct computation of the taxable incomes of both beneficiary and fiduciary. Note that in *Example 12* Trust A is entitled to a deduction for distributions to beneficiaries of $10,000.

THE COMPUTATION OF DNI

Section 643 defines DNI as fiduciary taxable income before any deduction for distributions to beneficiaries, adjusted as follows:

1. No deduction for a personal exemption is allowed.

2. No deduction against ordinary income for net capital losses is allowed.

3. Taxable income allocable to principal and not available for distribution to income beneficiaries is excluded.

4. Tax-exempt interest reduced by expenses allocable thereto is included.

Example 13. A trust that is not required to distribute all income currently has the following items of income and expense during the current year:

Tax-exempt interest	$10,000
Dividends	5,000
Rents	20,000
Long-term capital gains allocable to principal	8,000
Rent expense	6,700
Trustee fee allocable to income	3,500

The trust's taxable income before any deduction for distributions to beneficiaries is $23,700, computed as follows:

Dividends		$ 5,000
Rents		20,000
Capital gain		8,000
		$33,000
Less: Rent expense	$6,700	
Trust fee allocable to *taxable* trust income*	2,500	
Exemption	100	(9,300)
Taxable income before distribution deduction		$23,700

$$* \; \$3,500 \text{ fee} \times \frac{\$25,000 \text{ taxable trust income}}{\$35,000 \text{ total trust income}}$$

---

[33] §§ 651(b) and 661(c).

The trust's DNI is $24,800, computed as follows:

Trust taxable income before distribution deduction	$23,700
Add back exemption	100
	$23,800
Exclude: Nondistributable capital gain	(8,000)
Include: *Net* tax-exempt interest ($10,000 total − $1,000 allocable to trustee fee)**.	9,000
Distributable net income (DNI).	$24,800

$$** \ \$3,500 \ fee \times \frac{\$10,000 \ tax\text{-}exempt \ income}{\$35,000 \ total \ trust \ income}$$

SIMPLE TRUSTS

Section 651 defines a *simple trust* as one that satisfies these conditions:

1. Distributes all trust income currently

2. Does not take a deduction for a charitable contribution for the current year

3. Does not make any current distributions out of trust principal

Because of the requirement that a simple trust distribute all trust income to its beneficiaries, all taxable DNI of a simple trust is taxed to the beneficiaries, based upon the relative income distributable to each.

Example 14. Trust S is required to distribute 40% of trust income to beneficiary A and 60% of trust income to B. The trust's DNI for the current year is $100,000, of which $20,000 is nontaxable. For the current year, beneficiary A must report $32,000 of trust income (40% of *taxable* DNI) and B must report $48,000 of trust income (60% of *taxable* DNI). Trust S's deduction for distributions to beneficiaries is $80,000 (i.e., taxable DNI).

In *Example 14*, the tax results would not change if the trustee had failed to make actual distributions to the beneficiaries. In the case of a simple trust, the taxability of income to beneficiaries is not dependent upon cash flow from the trust.[34]

COMPLEX TRUSTS AND ESTATES

Any trust that does not meet all three requirements of a simple trust is categorized as a *complex trust*. The categorization of a trust may vary from year to year. For example, if a trustee is required to distribute all trust income currently but also has the discretion to make distributions out of trust principal, the trust will be *simple* in any year in which principal is not distributed, but *complex* in any year in which principal is distributed.

Computing the taxable income of complex trusts and estates generally is more difficult than computing the taxable income of a simple trust. Complex trusts and estates potentially may distribute amounts of cash and property that are less than or in excess of DNI.

If distributions to beneficiaries are less than or equal to DNI, each beneficiary is required to report the amount of the distribution representing *taxable* DNI in his or her gross income. Taxable DNI remaining in the fiduciary is taxed to the fiduciary.

[34] § 652(a).

Example 15. In the current year, Trust C has DNI of $50,000, of which $20,000 or 40% is nontaxable. During the year, the trustee makes a $5,000 distribution to both beneficiary M and beneficiary N. M and N will each report $3,000 of income from Trust C [$5,000 distribution × ($30,000 taxable DNI ÷ $50,000 total DNI)]. Trust C is allowed a $6,000 deduction for distributions to beneficiaries.[35] As a result, $24,000 of taxable DNI will be reported by (and taxed to) Trust C.

Example 16. Using the same facts as in *Example 13*, assume the trust distributes $10,000. The trust is generally entitled to a deduction for amounts distributed. However, this amount is further limited to the portion of taxable DNI contained in the distribution. In this case, the amount of the distribution deduction and the amount taxable to the beneficiaries is $6,371 computed as follows:

Distributable net income	$24,800
Net tax-exempt income ($10,000 − $1,000)	(9,000)
Taxable DNI	$15,800

$$\frac{\text{Taxable DNI}}{\text{Total DNI}} \times \text{Amount distributed} = \text{Distribution deduction}$$

$$\frac{\$15,800}{\$24,800} \times \$10,000 = \$6,371$$

In this case, the trust did not distribute all of its DNI, $24,800, but only a portion, $10,000. Consequently, the calculation effectively treats a portion of the amount distributed as taxable (63.71% or $6,371) and a portion as nontaxable (36.29% or $3,629). Taxable income of the trust would be $17,329 as computed below.

Taxable income before distribution deduction	$23,700
Deduction for distributions	(6,371)
Trust taxable income	$17,329

When distributions to beneficiaries exceed DNI, the entire taxable portion of DNI will be reported as income by the beneficiaries. Amounts distributed in excess of DNI are nontaxable, representing either accumulated income that has been previously taxed or corpus.

Allocation of DNI. In those cases when distributions exceed DNI and there are multiple beneficiaries, DNI must be allocated among the beneficiaries. In determining the amount of DNI allocated to each beneficiary (and, therefore, the amount of taxable income and nontaxable income that is allocable to each), the distribution rules acknowledge that some beneficiaries' rights to income may be superior to those of others. For example, the trust agreement may provide that distributions of income must be made to certain beneficiaries each year while other beneficiaries receive distributions solely at the discretion of the trustee. In recognition of this possibility, the Code establishes a so-called tier system to allocate DNI.[36]

Under the tier system, DNI (increased for charitable contributions) is first allocated proportionately to the distributions that are *required* to be made. These mandatory distributions are commonly referred to as *first-tier* or *tier-one* distributions. After allocating DNI to first-tier distributions, *any* DNI remaining (as reduced by first-tier distributions and charitable contributions) is allocated proportionately to *second tier* or *tier-two* distributions (i.e., discretionary distributions).

---

[35] § 661(c).

[36] §§ 662(a)(1) and (2).

Example 17. This year Trust T reported taxable DNI of $60,000. During the year, the trust made required distributions of $40,000 to beneficiary R. In addition, the trustee made discretionary distributions of $40,000 to R and $20,000 to S. DNI would be allocated as follows:

	Total	R	S
Required distributions	$ 40,000	$40,000	—
Discretionary distributions	60,000	40,000	$20,000
Total distributions received	$100,000	$80,000	$20,000

	Total	R	S
DNI before contributions	$60,000		
First-tier distributions	(40,000)	$40,000	—
DNI available for charity	20,000		
Charitable distributions	(0)		
DNI for second tier	$20,000		
Second-tier distributions	(20,000)	13,333*	$ 6,667*
DNI received		$53,333	$ 6,667

$$* \text{DNI for second tier} \times \frac{\text{Beneficiary's second-tier distribution}}{\text{Total second-tier distribution}}$$

$20,000 \times \$40,000/\$60,000 = \$13,333$ to R
$20,000 \times \$20,000/\$60,000 = \$ 6,667$ to S

Observe that the first $40,000 of DNI must be allocated to R because this distribution was mandatory thus making it a first-tier distribution. The remaining $20,000 of DNI is allocated proportionally to the discretionary or second-tier distributions received by R and S. Note that all of the trust's DNI is allocated and taxed to the beneficiaries and none is taxed to the trust. In this case, R received $80,000 from the trust of which $53,333 is taxable while S received $20,000 of which $6,667 is taxable. The balance of each distribution represents either accumulated income or corpus. Although the trust distributed $100,000, its deduction for distributions is limited to its taxable DNI for the year, $60,000.

In determining the treatment of a beneficiary's distributions, the treatment of charitable contributions can be a bit confusing. On the one hand, a contribution is treated as an expense that reduces the trust's taxable income (i.e., it is reported on Line 13 of Form 1041 and not on a Schedule K-1). On the other hand, the charity itself is treated like a beneficiary in the sense that it absorbs taxable and nontaxable DNI just like any other beneficiary. It should be emphasized that the charity is not considered a beneficiary when computing the deduction for distributions to beneficiaries. Instead, the distribution is accounted for as an expense.[37]

Example 18. This year the F Trust reported $80,000 of dividend income. Pursuant to the trust instrument the trustee distributed $90,000 as follows: (1) a required distribution to beneficiary J of $50,000; (2) a charitable contribution of $30,000; and (3) a discretionary distribution to K of $10,000. Taxable DNI would be $50,000 ($80,000 − $30,000) all of which would be allocated to J as computed below.

[37] § 662(a)(2). For purposes of determining DNI available for first-tier distribution only, no charitable contribution deduction is allowed.

DNI before contributions ($50,000 + $ 30,000)	$80,000
First-tier distribution to J	(50,000)
DNI available for charity	$30,000
Charitable distribution.	(30,000)
DNI for second tier.	$ 0

Note that J would report $50,000 of DNI, all of which would be taxable. In contrast, K receives no taxable DNI since there is none available after taking into account the charitable contribution. Although the trust distributed $60,000 to J and K, its distribution deduction is limited to taxable DNI of $50,000. Trust taxable income would be $0 as calculated below.

Dividends	$80,000
Contribution	(30,000)
Distribution deduction (limited to taxable DNI)	(50,000)
Trust taxable income.	$ 0

CHARACTER OF BENEFICIARY'S INCOME

Not only must a beneficiary determine the amount of taxable income received from a trust or estate, but he or she must determine its character as well. As stated at the outset, estates and trusts generally serve as conduits to the extent they make distributions. Consequently, each distribution is deemed to contain a pro rata portion of each type of distributable income received by the trust or estate. For example, if a portion of a trust's income consisted of dividends, a portion of the distribution received by the beneficiary is considered dividend income.

To determine the composition of a distribution, the gross amount of each item of distributable income must be reduced by any deduction directly related to that item of income. Any other expenses may be allocated against whatever class of distributable income the fiduciary selects. However, charitable contributions are treated as consisting of a proportionate share of each type of distributable income.

Example 19. This year the records of the T Trust revealed the following information, resulting in DNI of $60,000:

	Income and Expenses	DNI
Rental income	$70,000	$70,000
Dividends	30,000	30,000
Long-term capital gain	50,000	
Charitable contribution	10,000	(10,000)
Rent expense.	23,000	(23,000)
Trustee commission allocable between income and corpus	7,000	(7,000)
DNI		$60,000

During the year, the trust distributed $6,000 to its only beneficiary, X. The character of the distribution is determined below.

Elements of DNI	Rents	Dividends	Total
Income	$70,000	$30,000	$100,000
Expenses:			
Rental expenses	(23,000)		(23,000)
Trustee fees		(7,000)	(7,000)
Contribution	(7,000)*	(3,000)*	(10,000)
Total DNI	$40,000	$20,000	$60,000
Percentage of DNI	67%	33%	100%

* $10,000 × $70,000/$100,000 = $7,000
  $10,000 × $30,000/$100,000 = $3,000

Since X received 10% of the DNI ($6,000/$60,000) she is deemed to receive 10% of each item of DNI. Thus she will report rental income of $4,000 (10% × $40,000) and dividend income of $2,000 (10% × $20,000). In other words, of the $6,000 of DNI received, $4,000 or 67% is rents while $2,000 or 33% is dividends. Note how the expenses were allocated in determining the composition of DNI. The rental expenses are charged against the rental income since they are directly related. In contrast, the charitable contribution is charged proportionately against each type of distributable income. On the other hand, the trustee fees may be allocated however the trustee wishes. In this case, he elects to charge the trustee fees against the dividend income. In light of the 15% tax rate that applies to dividends, the trustee should consider allocating the fees to the rental income.

A special problem arises when the trust receives qualified dividends that are taxed at a maximum rate of 15 percent (5% if in the 15% tax bracket). A calculation must be made to determine the amount of qualified dividends *retained* by the trust to be taxed at the favorable rate. The amount deemed to be retained by the trust is equal to the proportion of distributable net income (DNI) retained by the trust.

Example 20. Same facts as in *Example 19*. The total DNI was $60,000 and the trust distributed 10% of the DNI ($6,000/$60,000) to the beneficiary and retained 90% ($54,000/$60,000). Thus the qualified dividends retained by the trust are $27,000 (90% × $30,000). Alternatively, the amount could be computed by using the amount of DNI allocated to the beneficiary as follows:

Qualified dividends	$30,000	$30,000
Allocation to beneficiary		
$$\frac{\text{DNI distributed to beneficiary } \$6,000}{\text{Total DNI } \$60,000}$$	×10%	(3,000)
Allocation to trust		$27,000

Note that this method of allocating the amount of qualified dividends between the beneficiary and the trust is used solely for calculating the tax liability of the trust. The actual amount of qualified dividends to be reported on the Schedule K-1 which the beneficiary must report is not $3,000 but is $2,000 (10% × $20,000) as shown above.

REPORTING REQUIREMENTS FOR BENEFICIARIES

A beneficiary who receives a distribution from a fiduciary will receive a summary of the tax consequences of the distribution in the form of a Schedule K-1 from the executor or trustee. The K-1 will tell the beneficiary the amounts and character of the various items of income that constitute the taxable portion of the distribution.

A beneficiary also may be entitled to depreciation or depletion deductions and various tax credits because of distributions of fiduciary income. Such items are also reflected on the Schedule K-1.

If the taxable year of a beneficiary is different from that of the fiduciary, the amount of fiduciary income taxable to the beneficiary is included in the beneficiary's tax year within which the fiduciary's year ends.[38]

> **Example 21.** Estate E is on a fiscal year ending January 31. During its fiscal year ending January 31, 2009, but prior to December 31, 2008, the estate made cash distributions to beneficiary Z, a calendar year taxpayer. Because of these distributions, Z must report income of $8,000. However, this income will be reported on Z's 2009 individual tax return.

THE SEPARATE SHARE RULE

In certain circumstances, the rules governing the taxation of beneficiaries of a complex trust can lead to an inequitable result. Assume a grantor created a single trust with two beneficiaries, A and B. The grantor intended that each beneficiary have an equal interest in trust income and principal. The trustee has considerable discretion as to the timing of distributions of income and principal. Consider a year in which beneficiary A was in exceptional need of funds and, as a result, the trustee distributed $15,000 to A as A's half of trust income for the year *plus* $10,000 out of A's half of trust principal. Because B had no need of current funds, the trustee distributed neither income nor principal to B.

If the trust's DNI was $30,000 for the year, the normal rules of Subchapter J would dictate that A would have to report and pay tax on $25,000 of trust income. However, the clear intent of the grantor is that A only be responsible for half of trust income and no more. To reflect such intent, § 663(c) provides the following rule: if a single trust contains substantially separate and independent shares for different beneficiaries, the trust shall be treated as separate trusts for purposes of determining DNI. Therefore, using this separate share rule, beneficiary A's *separate trust* would have DNI of only $15,000, the maximum amount taxable to A in the year of distribution. This rule is inapplicable to estates.

A COMPREHENSIVE EXAMPLE

The AB Trust is a calendar year taxpayer. In the current year, the trust books show the following:

Gross rental income	$25,000
Taxable interest income	10,000
Tax-exempt interest income	15,000
Long-term capital gain	8,000
Trustee fee	6,000
Rent expenses	3,000
Contribution to charity	1,500
Distributions to	
Beneficiary A	20,000
Beneficiary B	20,000

---

[38] §§ 652(c) and 662(c).

Under the terms of the trust instrument the capital gain and one-third of the trustee fee are allocable to principal. The trustee is required to maintain a reserve for depreciation on the rental property equal to one-tenth of annual gross rental income. (For tax purposes, assume actual tax depreciation is $1,300.) The trustee is required to make an annual distribution to beneficiary A of $12,000 and has the discretion to make additional distributions to A or beneficiary B.

Based on these facts, the computation of the income taxable to the trust and the beneficiaries is as follows:

Step One: Compute fiduciary accounting income.

Gross rental income	$25,000
Taxable interest income	10,000
Tax-exempt interest income	15,000
	$50,000
Trustee fee charged against income	(4,000)
Rent expenses	(3,000)
Depreciation ($\frac{1}{10} \times$ $25,000)	(2,500)
Fiduciary accounting income	$40,500

Step Two: Compute fiduciary taxable income before the § 661 deduction for distributions to beneficiaries.

Gross rental income	$25,000
Taxable interest income	10,000
Long-term capital gain	8,000
	$43,000
Deductible trustee fee	(4,200)*
Deductible rent expense	(3,000)
Deductible depreciation allocable to fiduciary	(1,300)
Deductible charitable contribution	(1,050)*
Exemption	(100)
Taxable income before § 661 deduction	$33,350

* $35,000 ÷ $50,000 of gross fiduciary accounting income is taxable; thus, only 70% of both the $6,000 trustee fee and $1,500 charitable contribution is deductible.

Step Three: Compute DNI and the § 661 deduction for distributions to beneficiaries.

Taxable income from Step Two	$33,350
Add back:	
Exemption	100
Net tax-exempt income	12,750*
Subtract:	
Capital gain allocable to principal	(8,000)
Distributable net income (DNI)	$38,200

* $15,000 tax-exempt interest less 30% of the $6,000 trustee fee and $1,500 charitable contribution.

Step Four: Subtract the § 661 deduction for distributions to beneficiaries

Taxable income before deduction	$33,350
Section 661 deduction for distributions	(25,450)*
Trust taxable income	$ 7,900

Because distributions to beneficiaries exceeded DNI, the trust will deduct the entire amount of taxable DNI. $25,450 ($38,200 − $12,750).

Tax Consequences to Beneficiaries. The $40,000 cash distribution to beneficiaries exceeds the total DNI of $38,200; thus, the entire amount of DNI must be allocated to the beneficiaries.

	Total	A	B
DNI	$38,200		
Add-back charitable contribution	1,500		
DNI before charitable contribution	$39,700		
First-tier distributions	(12,000)	$12,000	—
DNI available for charity	$27,700		
Charitable distributions	(1,500)		
DNI for second tier	$26,200		
Second-tier distributions	(26,200)	7,483*	$18,717**
DNI received	(26,200)	$19,483	$18,717
Percentage of DNI received		51%	49%

$$* \text{ DNI for second tier} \times \frac{\text{Beneficiary's second-tier distribution}}{\text{Total second-tier distributions}}$$

*$26,200 × $8,000/$28,000 = $7,483 to A
**$26,200 × $20,000/$28,000 = $18,717 to B

The composition of DNI is as follows:

	Rent	Taxable Interest	Tax-Exempt Interest	Total
Gross receipts	$25,000	$10,000	$15,000	$50,000
Rent expense	(3,000)			(3,000)
Depreciation	(1,300)			(1,300)
Trustee fee *		(4,200)	(1,800)	(6,000)
Charitable contribution**	(750)	(300)	(450)	(1,500)
Total	$19,950	$ 5,500	$12,750	$38,200

* The trustee fee allocable to taxable income may be arbitrarily allocated to **any** item of taxable income. Reg. 1.652(b)-3(b).

**In the absence of a specific provision in the trust instrument, the charitable contribution is allocated proportionally to each class of income. Reg. § 1.642(c)-3(b)(2).

Each beneficiary should report the following:

	Rent	Taxable Interest	Tax-Exempt Interest	Total DNI Allocated
Beneficiary A (51%)	$10,175*	$2,805	$ 6,503	$19,483
Beneficiary B (49%)	9,775	2,695	6,247	18,717
Total	$19,950	$5,500	$12,750	$38,200

* Beneficiary A's proportionate share of DNI 51% multiplied by $19,950 total rent income included in DNI equals beneficiary A's share of rent income. This same procedure is used to determine each beneficiary's share of all other items.

A completed Form 1041 for the AB Trust and Schedule K-1 for Beneficiary A are shown on the following pages.

THE SIXTY-FIVE DAY RULE

Fiduciaries may want to avoid accumulating income since such income may be taxed at very high rates. Because DNI is often not calculated until after the close of the trust's taxable year, the amount of current distributions necessary to avoid accumulation may be unknown. To alleviate this timing problem, § 663(b) provides that a trust or an estate *may elect* that any distribution made within the first 65 days of a taxable year will be considered paid to the beneficiary on the last day of the preceding taxable year.[39] This rule allows a trustee to make distributions after the close of a year to eliminate any accumulations of DNI for that year.

---

[39]   See Reg. § 1.663(b)-2 for the manner and time for making such an election.

Form **1041**

Department of the Treasury—Internal Revenue Service

U.S. Income Tax Return for Estates and Trusts **2008**

OMB No. 1545-0092

A Type of entity (see instr.):

☐ Decedent's estate
☐ Simple trust
☐ Complex trust
☐ Qualified disability trust
☐ ESBT (S portion only)
☐ Grantor type trust
☐ Bankruptcy estate–Ch. 7
☐ Bankruptcy estate–Ch. 11
☐ Pooled income fund

For calendar year 2008 or fiscal year beginning , 2008, and ending , 20

Name of estate or trust (If a grantor type trust, see page 14 of the instructions.)

A B TRUST

Name and title of fiduciary

Number, street, and room or suite no. (If a P.O. box, see page 15 of the instructions.)

City or town, state, and ZIP code

C Employer identification number

D Date entity created

E Nonexempt charitable and split-interest trusts, check applicable boxes (see page 16 of the instr.):

☐ Described in section 4947(a)(1)
☐ Not a private foundation
☐ Described in section 4947(a)(2)

B Number of Schedules K-1 attached (see instructions) ▶

F Check applicable boxes:

☐ Initial return ☐ Final return ☐ Amended return
☐ Change in fiduciary ☐ Change in fiduciary's name

☐ Change in trust's name
☐ Change in fiduciary's address

G Check here if the estate or filing trust made a section 645 election . . . . . ▶ ☐

Income	1	Interest income	1	*10,000*
	2a	Total ordinary dividends	2a	
	b	Qualified dividends allocable to: **(1)** Beneficiaries _____ **(2)** Estate or trust _____		
	3	Business income or (loss). Attach Schedule C or C-EZ (Form 1040) . . .	3	
	4	Capital gain or (loss). Attach Schedule D (Form 1041)	4	*8,000*
	5	Rents, royalties, partnerships, other estates and trusts, etc. Attach Schedule E (Form 1040)	5	*20,700*
	6	Farm income or (loss). Attach Schedule F (Form 1040)	6	
	7	Ordinary gain or (loss). Attach Form 4797	7	
	8	Other income. List type and amount _____	8	
	9	**Total income.** Combine lines 1, 2a, and 3 through 8 . . . . ▶	9	
Deductions	10	Interest. Check if Form 4952 is attached ▶ ☐	10	
	11	Taxes	11	
	12	Fiduciary fees	12	*4,200*
	13	Charitable deduction (from Schedule A, line 7)	13	*1,050*
	14	Attorney, accountant, and return preparer fees	14	
	15a	Other deductions **not** subject to the 2% floor (attach schedule)	15a	
	b	Allowable miscellaneous itemized deductions subject to the 2% floor . . .	15b	
	16	Add lines 10 through 15b . . . . ▶	16	*5,250*
	17	Adjusted total income or (loss). Subtract line 16 from line 9 . . [**17**]		*33,450*
	18	Income distribution deduction (from Schedule B, line 15). Attach Schedules K-1 (Form 1041)	18	*22,450*
	19	Estate tax deduction including certain generation-skipping taxes (attach computation) .	19	
	20	Exemption	20	*100*
	21	Add lines 18 through 20 . . . . ▶	21	*22,550*
Tax and Payments	22	Taxable income. Subtract line 21 from line 17. If a loss, see page 23 of the instructions	22	*7,900*
	23	**Total tax** (from Schedule G, line 7)	23	*855*
	24	**Payments: a** 2008 estimated tax payments and amount applied from 2007 return . .	24a	
	b	Estimated tax payments allocated to beneficiaries (from Form 1041-T) . . .	24b	
	c	Subtract line 24b from line 24a	24c	
	d	Tax paid with Form 7004 (see page 24 of the instructions)	24d	
	e	Federal income tax withheld. If any is from Form(s) 1099, check ▶ ☐ . . .	24e	
		Other payments: **f** Form 2439 _____ ; **g** Form 4136 _____ ; Total ▶	24h	
	25	**Total payments.** Add lines 24c through 24e, and 24h . . . . ▶	25	
	26	Estimated tax penalty (see page 24 of the instructions)	26	
	27	**Tax due.** If line 25 is smaller than the total of lines 23 and 26, enter amount owed . .	27	*855*
	28	**Overpayment.** If line 25 is larger than the total of lines 23 and 26, enter amount overpaid	28	
	29	Amount of line 28 to be: **a** Credited to 2009 estimated tax ▶ ; **b** Refunded ▶	29	

Sign Here

Under penalties of perjury, I declare that I have examined this return, including accompanying schedules and statements, and to the best of my knowledge and belief, it is true, correct, and complete. Declaration of preparer (other than taxpayer) is based on all information of which preparer has any knowledge.

▶ _____ _____ ▶ _____
Signature of fiduciary or officer representing fiduciary Date EIN of fiduciary if a financial institution

May the IRS discuss this return with the preparer shown below (see instr.)? ☐ Yes ☐ No

Paid Preparer's Use Only

Preparer's signature ▶		Date	Check if self-employed ☐	Preparer's SSN or PTIN
Firm's name (or yours if self-employed), address, and ZIP code ▶			EIN
			Phone no. ( )

For Privacy Act and Paperwork Reduction Act Notice, see the separate instructions.

Cat. No. 11370H

Form **1041** (2008)

Form 1041 (2008)   Page **2**

Schedule A   **Charitable Deduction.** Do not complete for a simple trust or a pooled income fund.

1	Amounts paid or permanently set aside for charitable purposes from gross income (see page 25)	**1**	1,500
2	Tax-exempt income allocable to charitable contributions (see page 25 of the instructions)	**2**	450
3	Subtract line 2 from line 1	**3**	1,050
4	Capital gains for the tax year allocated to corpus and paid or permanently set aside for charitable purposes	**4**	
5	Add lines 3 and 4	**5**	1,050
6	Section 1202 exclusion allocable to capital gains paid or permanently set aside for charitable purposes (see page 25 of the instructions)	**6**	
7	**Charitable deduction.** Subtract line 6 from line 5. Enter here and on page 1, line 13	**7**	1,050

Schedule B   **Income Distribution Deduction**

1	Adjusted total income (see page 26 of the instructions)	**1**	33,450
2	Adjusted tax-exempt interest	**2**	12,750
3	Total net gain from Schedule D (Form 1041), line 15, column (1) (see page 26 of the instructions)	**3**	
4	Enter amount from Schedule A, line 4 (minus any allocable section 1202 exclusion)	**4**	
5	Capital gains for the tax year included on Schedule A, line 1 (see page 26 of the instructions)	**5**	
6	Enter any gain from page 1, line 4, as a negative number. If page 1, line 4, is a loss, enter the loss as a positive number . <GAIN>	**6**	<8000>
7	**Distributable net income.** Combine lines 1 through 6. If zero or less, enter -0-	**7**	38,200
8	If a complex trust, enter accounting income for the tax year as determined under the governing instrument and applicable local law **8** 40,500		
9	Income required to be distributed currently	**9**	12,000
10	Other amounts paid, credited, or otherwise required to be distributed	**10**	28,000
11	Total distributions. Add lines 9 and 10. If greater than line 8, see page 26 of the instructions	**11**	40,000
12	Enter the amount of tax-exempt income included on line 11	**12**	12,750
13	Tentative income distribution deduction. Subtract line 12 from line 11	**13**	27,250
14	Tentative income distribution deduction. Subtract line 2 from line 7. If zero or less, enter -0-	**14**	22,450
15	**Income distribution deduction.** Enter the smaller of line 13 or line 14 here and on page 1, line 18	**15**	25,450

Schedule G   **Tax Computation** (see page 27 of the instructions)

1 Tax: a	Tax on taxable income (see page 27 of the instructions)	**1a**	855
b	Tax on lump-sum distributions. Attach Form 4972	**1b**	
c	Alternative minimum tax (from Schedule I (Form 1041), line 56)	**1c**	
d	**Total.** Add lines 1a through 1c	**1d**	855
2a	Foreign tax credit. Attach Form 1116	**2a**	
b	Other nonbusiness credits (attach schedule)	**2b**	
c	General business credit. Attach Form 3800	**2c**	
d	Credit for prior year minimum tax. Attach Form 8801	**2d**	
3	**Total credits.** Add lines 2a through 2d	**3**	0
4	Subtract line 3 from line 1d. If zero or less, enter -0-.	**4**	855
5	Recapture taxes. Check if from: ☐ Form 4255 ☐ Form 8611	**5**	
6	Household employment taxes. Attach Schedule H (Form 1040)	**6**	
7	**Total tax.** Add lines 4 through 6. Enter here and on page 1, line 23	**7**	855

Other Information   Yes   No

1 Did the estate or trust receive tax-exempt income? If "Yes," attach a computation of the allocation of expenses ✓
Enter the amount of tax-exempt interest income and exempt-interest dividends ▶ $ 15,000

2 Did the estate or trust receive all or any part of the earnings (salary, wages, and other compensation) of any individual by reason of a contract assignment or similar arrangement?   ✓

3 At any time during calendar year 2008, did the estate or trust have an interest in or a signature or other authority over a bank, securities, or other financial account in a foreign country?   ✓
See page 29 of the instructions for exceptions and filing requirements for Form TD F 90-22.1. If "Yes," enter the name of the foreign country ▶

4 During the tax year, did the estate or trust receive a distribution from, or was it the grantor of, or transferor to, a foreign trust? If "Yes," the estate or trust may have to file Form 3520. See page 29 of the instructions   ✓

5 Did the estate or trust receive, or pay, any qualified residence interest on seller-provided financing? If "Yes," see page 30 for required attachment   ✓

6 If this is an estate or a complex trust making the section 663(b) election, check here (see page 30) ▶ ☐

7 To make a section 643(e)(3) election, attach Schedule D (Form 1041), and check here (see page 30) ▶ ☐

8 If the decedent's estate has been open for more than 2 years, attach an explanation for the delay in closing the estate, and check here ▶ ☐

9 Are any present or future trust beneficiaries skip persons? See page 30 of the instructions   ✓

Form **1041** (2008)

SCHEDULE D
(Form 1041)

Department of the Treasury
Internal Revenue Service

Capital Gains and Losses

▶ **Attach to Form 1041, Form 5227, or Form 990-T. See the separate instructions for Form 1041 (also for Form 5227 or Form 990-T, if applicable).**

OMB No. 1545-0092

20**08**

Name of estate or trust   *A B TRUST*

Employer identification number

Note: *Form 5227 filers need to complete **only** Parts I and II.*

Part I — Short-Term Capital Gains and Losses—Assets Held One Year or Less

(a) Description of property (Example: 100 shares 7% preferred of "Z" Co.)	(b) Date acquired (mo., day, yr.)	(c) Date sold (mo., day, yr.)	(d) Sales price		(e) Cost or other basis (see page 4 of the instructions)	(f) Gain or (loss) for the entire year Subtract (e) from (d)
1a						

b Enter the short-term gain or (loss), if any, from Schedule D-1, line 1b **1b**

2 Short-term capital gain or (loss) from Forms 4684, 6252, 6781, and 8824 . . . . **2**

3 Net short-term gain or (loss) from partnerships, S corporations, and other estates or trusts . **3**

4 Short-term capital loss carryover. Enter the amount, if any, from line 9 of the 2007 Capital Loss Carryover Worksheet . . . . **4** ( )

5 **Net short-term gain or (loss).** Combine lines 1a through 4 in column (f). Enter here and on line 13, column (3) on the back . . . . ▶ **5**

Part II — Long-Term Capital Gains and Losses—Assets Held More Than One Year

(a) Description of property (Example: 100 shares 7% preferred of "Z" Co.)	(b) Date acquired (mo., day, yr.)	(c) Date sold (mo., day, yr.)	(d) Sales price		(e) Cost or other basis (see page 4 of the instructions)	(f) Gain or (loss) for the entire year Subtract (e) from (d)
6a						*8,100*

b Enter the long-term gain or (loss), if any, from Schedule D-1, line 6b. **6b**

7 Long-term capital gain or (loss) from Forms 2439, 4684, 6252, 6781, and 8824 . . . . . . **7**

8 Net long-term gain or (loss) from partnerships, S corporations, and other estates or trusts . **8**

9 Capital gain distributions **9**

10 Gain from Form 4797, Part I **10**

11 Long-term capital loss carryover. Enter the amount, if any, from line 14 of the 2007 Capital Loss Carryover Worksheet . . . . **11** ( )

12 **Net long-term gain or (loss).** Combine lines 6a through 11 in column (f). Enter here and on line 14a, column (3) on the back . . . . ▶ **12** *8,000*

For Paperwork Reduction Act Notice, see the Instructions for Form 1041.   Cat. No. 11376V   Schedule D (Form 1041) 2008

Part III Summary of Parts I and II		(1) Beneficiaries' (see page 5)	(2) Estate's or trust's	(3) Total
	Caution: *Read the instructions **before** completing this part.*			
13 Net short-term gain or (loss)	**13**			
14 Net long-term gain or (loss):				
a Total for year	**14a**		8,000	8,000
b Unrecaptured section 1250 gain (see line 18 of the wrksht.) .	**14b**			
c 28% rate gain	**14c**			
15 Total net gain or (loss). Combine lines 13 and 14a . ▶	**15**		8,000	8,000

Note: *If line 15, column (3), is a net gain, enter the gain on Form 1041, line 4 (or Form 990-T, Part I, line 4a). If lines 14a and 15, column (2), are net gains, go to Part V, and **do not** complete Part IV. If line 15, column (3), is a net loss, complete Part IV and the **Capital Loss Carryover Worksheet,** as necessary.*

Part IV	Capital Loss Limitation

16 Enter here and enter as a (loss) on Form 1041, line 4 (or Form 990-T, Part I, line 4c, if a trust), the **smaller** of:

a The loss on line 15, column (3) **or** b $3,000 . . . .   **16** |(   )

Note: *If the loss on line 15, column (3), is more than $3,000, **or** if Form 1041, page 1, line 22 (or Form 990-T, line 34), is a loss, complete the **Capital Loss Carryover Worksheet** on page 7 of the instructions to figure your capital loss carryover.*

Part V	Tax Computation Using Maximum Capital Gains Rates

Form 1041 filers. Complete this part **only** if both lines 14a and 15 in column (2) are gains, or an amount is entered in Part I or Part II and there is an entry on Form 1041, line 2b(2), **and** Form 1041, line 22, is more than zero.

Caution: *Skip this part and complete the worksheet on page 8 of the instructions if:*

● *Either line 14b, col. (2) or line 14c, col. (2) is more than zero, or*

● *Both Form 1041, line 2b(1), and Form 4952, line 4g are more than zero.*

Form 990-T trusts. Complete this part **only** if both lines 14a and 15 are gains, or qualified dividends are included in income in Part I of Form 990-T, **and** Form 990-T, line 34, is more than zero. Skip this part and complete the worksheet on page 8 of the instructions if either line 14b, col. (2) or line 14c, col. (2) is more than zero.

17	Enter taxable income from Form 1041, line 22 (or Form 990-T, line 34) .	**17**	7,900	
18	Enter the **smaller** of line 14a or 15 in column (2) but not less than zero *LTCG*	**18** 8,000		
19	Enter the estate's or trust's qualified dividends from Form 1041, line 2b(2) (or enter the qualified dividends included in income in Part I of Form 990-T) . . .	**19**		
20	Add lines 18 and 19 *LTCG*	**20** 8,000		
21	If the estate or trust is filing Form 4952, enter the amount from line 4g; otherwise, enter -0- . ▶	**21** -0-		
22	Subtract line 21 from line 20. If zero or less, enter -0- *LTCG* . .	**22** 8,000	
23	Subtract line 22 from line 17. If zero or less, enter -0-	**23** 0	
24	Enter the **smaller** of the amount on line 17 or $2,200	**24** 2,200	
25	Is the amount on line 23 equal to or more than the amount on line 24?		
	☐ **Yes.** Skip lines 25 and 26; go to line 27 and check the "No" box.		
	☑ **No.** Enter the amount from line 23	**25** 0	
26	Subtract line 25 from line 24	**26** 2,200	
27	Are the amounts on lines 22 and 26 the same?		
	☐ **Yes.** Skip lines 27 thru 30; go to line 31. ☑ **No.** Enter the **smaller** of line 17 or line 22	**27** 7,900	
28	Enter the amount from line 26 (If line 26 is blank, enter -0-). . . .	**28** 2,200	
29	Subtract line 28 from line 27	**29** 5,700	
30	Multiply line 29 by 15% (.15) *BALANCE OF LTCG AT 15%*		**30** 855
31	Figure the tax on the amount on line 23. Use the 2008 Tax Rate Schedule for Estates and Trusts (see the Schedule G instructions)		**31** –
32	Add lines 30 and 31		**32** 855
33	Figure the tax on the amount on line 17. Use the 2008 Tax Rate Schedule for Estates and Trusts (see the Schedule G instructions)		**33** 1,840
34	**Tax on all taxable income.** Enter the **smaller** of line 32 or line 33 here and on line 1a of Schedule G, Form 1041 (or line 36 of Form 990-T).		**34** 855

661108

Schedule K-1
(Form 1041)

20**08**

Department of the Treasury
Internal Revenue Service

| Final K-1 | | Amended K-1 | OMB No. 1545-0092 |

For calendar year 2008,

or tax year beginning _____ , 2008,

and ending _____ , 20 _____

Beneficiary's Share of Income, Deductions, Credits, etc.   ▶ See back of form and instructions.

| **Part I** | **Information About the Estate or Trust** |

A   Estate's or trust's employer identification number

A B TRUST

B   Estate's or trust's name

C   Fiduciary's name, address, city, state, and ZIP code

A B TRUST

D ☐ Check if Form 1041-T was filed and enter the date it was filed
_____/_____/_____

E ☐ Check if this is the final Form 1041 for the estate or trust

| **Part II** | **Information About the Beneficiary** |

F   Beneficiary's identifying number

G   Beneficiary's name, address, city, state, and ZIP code

BENEFICIARY A

H ☐ Domestic beneficiary   ☐ Foreign beneficiary

Part III	**Beneficiary's Share of Current Year Income, Deductions, Credits, and Other Items**

1	Interest income	2,805	11	Final year deductions	
2a	Ordinary dividends				
2b	Qualified dividends				
3	Net short-term capital gain				
4a	Net long-term capital gain				
4b	28% rate gain		12	Alternative minimum tax adjustment	
4c	Unrecaptured section 1250 gain				
5	Other portfolio and nonbusiness income				
6	Ordinary business income	10,175			
7	Net rental real estate income	12,980	13	Credits and credit recapture	
8	Other rental income	12,980			
9	Directly apportioned deductions				
			14	Other information	6,503
10	Estate tax deduction				

*See attached statement for additional information.

Note. A statement must be attached showing the beneficiary's share of income and directly apportioned deductions from each business, rental real estate, and other rental activity.

For IRS Use Only

TAX PLANNING CONSIDERATIONS

The tax planning considerations for the use of trusts are discussed in Chapter 26, *Family Tax Planning*.

PROBLEM MATERIALS

DISCUSSION QUESTIONS

25-1 *Trusts and Estates as Conduits.* What does it mean to describe a fiduciary as *a conduit* of income? To what extent does a fiduciary operate as a conduit?

25-2 *Purpose of Trusts.* Trusts are usually created for nonbusiness purposes. Give some examples of situations in which a trust could be useful.

25-3 *Trust as a Separate Legal Entity.* A trust cannot exist if the only trustee is also sole beneficiary. Why not?

25-4 *Trust Expenses Allocable to Principal.* For what reason might the grantor of a trust stipulate that some amount of trust expenses be paid out of trust principal rather than trust income?

25-5 *Use of Fiduciaries to Defer Income Taxation.* Although a trust must adopt a calendar year for tax purposes, an estate may adopt any fiscal year, as well as a calendar year, for reporting taxable income. Why is Congress willing to allow an estate more flexibility in the choice of taxable year?

25-6 *Trust Accounting Income vs. Taxable Income.* Even though a trustee may be required to distribute all trust income currently, the trust may still have to report taxable income. Explain.

25-7 *Deductibility of Administrative Expenses.* Explain any options available to the executor of an estate with regard to the deductibility of administrative expenses incurred by the estate.

25-8 *Capital Loss Deductions.* To what extent may a fiduciary deduct any excess of capital losses over capital gains for a taxable year?

25-9 *Operating Losses of a Fiduciary.* How does the tax treatment of operating losses incurred by a fiduciary differ from the treatment of such losses by a partnership or an S corporation?

25-10 *Purpose of DNI.* Discuss the function of DNI from the point of view of the fiduciary and the point of view of beneficiaries who receive distributions from the fiduciary.

25-11 *Taxable vs. Nontaxable DNI.* Why is it important to correctly identify any nontaxable component of DNI?

25-12 *Charitable Deductions.* Enumerate the differences in the charitable deduction allowable to a fiduciary and the charitable deduction allowable to an individual.

25-13 *Timing Distributions from an Estate.* Why might a beneficiary of an estate prefer *not* to receive an early distribution of property from the estate?

25-14 *Simple vs. Complex Trusts.* All trusts are complex in the year of termination. Why?

25-15 *Trust Reserves for Depreciation.* Discuss the reason why a grantor of a trust would require the trustee to maintain a certain reserve for depreciation of trust assets.

25-16 *Distributions Exceeding DNI.* How are distributions in excess of distributable net income treated?

25-17 *Sixty-five Day Rule.* Explain the sixty-five day rule and what purpose it serves.

PROBLEMS

25-18 *Computation of Fiduciary Accounting Income.* Under the terms of the trust instrument, the annual fiduciary accounting income of Trust MNO must be distributed in equal amounts to individual beneficiaries M, N, and O. The trust instrument also provides that capital gains or losses realized on the sale of trust assets are allocated to principal, and that 40 percent of the annual trustee fee is to be allocated to principal. For the current year, the records of the trust show the following:

Dividend income	$38,000
Tax-exempt interest income	18,900
Taxable interest income	12,400
Capital loss on sale of securities	(2,500)
Trustee fee	5,000

Based on these facts, determine the required distribution to each of the three trust beneficiaries.

25-19 *Tax Consequences of Property Distributions.* During the taxable year, beneficiary M receives 100 shares of Acme common stock from Trust T. The basis of the stock is $70 per share to the trust, and its fair market value at date of distribution is $110 per share. The trust's DNI for the year is $60,000, all of which is taxable. There were no other distributions made or required to be made by the trust.

   a. Assume the stock distribution was in satisfaction of an $11,000 pecuniary bequest to M. What is the tax result to M? To Trust T? What basis will M have in the Acme shares?

   b. Assume the distribution did not represent a specific bequest to M, and that Trust T did not make a § 643(e)(3) election. What is the tax result to M? To Trust T? What basis will M have in the Acme shares?

   c. Assume now that Trust T did make a § 643(e)(3) election with regard to the distribution of the Acme shares. What is the tax result to M? To Trust T? What basis will M have in the Acme shares?

25-20 *Trust's Depreciation Deduction.* Under the terms of the trust instrument, Trustee K is required to maintain a reserve for depreciation equal to $3,000 per year. All trust income, including rents from depreciable trust property, must be distributed currently to trust beneficiaries.

   a. Assume allowable depreciation for tax purposes is $2,000. What is the amount of the depreciation deduction available to the trust? To the trust beneficiaries?

   b. Assume allowable depreciation for tax purposes is $7,000. What is the amount of the depreciation deduction available to the trust? To the trust beneficiaries?

25-21   *Trust Losses.* Complex Trust Z has the following receipts and disbursements for the current year:

Receipts:

Rents...	$ 62,000
Proceeds from sale of securities (basis of securities = $55,000)	48,000
Dividends	12,000
Total receipts	$122,000

Disbursements:

Rent expenses	$ 70,000
Trustee fee (100% allocable to income)....................	4,000
Total disbursements.................................	$ 74,000

The trustee made no distributions to any beneficiaries during the current year. Based on these facts, compute trust taxable income for the current year.

25-22   *Deductibility of Funeral and Administrative Expenses.* Decedent L died on May 12 of the current year, and her executor elected a calendar taxable year for L's estate. Prior to December 31, L's estate paid $4,800 of funeral expenses, $19,900 of legal and accounting fees attributable to the administration of the estate, and a $6,100 executor's fee. Before consideration of any of these expenses, L's estate has taxable income of $60,000 for the period May 13 to December 31. Decedent L's taxable estate for Federal estate tax purposes is estimated at $1,700,000.

    a.   To what extent are the above expenses deductible on L's estate tax return (Form 706) or on the estate's income tax return (Form 1041) for the current year? On which return would the deductions yield the greater tax benefit?

    b.   Assume that L was married at the time of her death and that all the property included in her gross estate was left to her surviving spouse. Does this fact change your answer to (a)?

25-23   *Amount of Distribution Taxable to Beneficiary.* During the current year, Trust H has DNI of $50,000, of which $30,000 is nontaxable. The trustee made a $10,000 cash distribution to beneficiary P during the year; no other distributions were made.

    a.   How much taxable income must P report?

    b.   What deduction for distributions to beneficiaries may Trust H claim?

25-24 *Deductibility of Trust Expenses.* Trust A has the following receipts and disbursements for the current year:

Receipts:

Nontaxable interest	$ 40,000
Taxable interest	30,000
Rents	30,000
Total receipts	$100,000

Disbursements:

Charitable donation	$ 10,000
Rent expense	6,500
Trustee fee	5,000
Total disbursements	$ 21,500

   a. What is Trust A's deduction for charitable contributions for the current year?
   b. How much of the trustee fee is deductible?
   c. How much of the rent expense is deductible?

25-25 *Computation of DNI and Trust's Tax Liability.* Trust M has the following receipts disbursements for the current year:

Receipts:

Nontaxable interest	$ 4,000
Taxable interest	25,000
Rents	11,000
Long-term capital gain allocable to principal	9,000
Total receipts	$49,000

Disbursements:

Rent expense	$ 2,400
Trustee fee	1,000
Total disbursements	$ 3,400

The trustee is required to distribute all trust income to beneficiary N on a quarterly basis.
   a. Compute Trust M's DNI for the current year.
   b. Compute Trust M's taxable income for the current year.
   c. Compute Trust M's tax liability for the current year.

25-26 *Taxation of Trust and Beneficiaries.* Trust B has the following receipts and disbursements for the current year:

Receipts:

Nontaxable interest	$10,000
Dividends	10,000
Rents	30,000
Long-term capital gain allocable to principal	15,000
Total receipts	$65,000

Disbursements:

Rent expense	$ 7,500
Trustee fee	5,000
Total disbursements	$12,500

During the year, the trustee distributes $20,000 to beneficiary C and $10,000 to beneficiary D. None of these distributions is subject to the throwback rule. The trust and both beneficiaries are calendar year taxpayers.

a. Compute Trust B's DNI for the current year.
b. Compute Trust B's taxable income for the current year.
c. How much taxable income must each beneficiary report for the current year?

25-27 *Distributions from Complex Trusts.* Under the terms of the trust instrument, the trustee of Trust EFG is required to make an annual distribution of 50 percent of trust accounting income to beneficiary E. The trustee can make additional discretionary distributions out of trust income or principal to beneficiaries E, F, or G. During the current year, the trust accounting income of $85,000 equaled taxable DNI.

a. Assume that the trustee made current distributions of $60,000 to E and $10,000 to G. How much taxable income must each beneficiary report for the current year? What is the amount of the trust's deduction for distributions to beneficiaries?

b. Assume that the trustee made current distributions of $80,000 to E and $40,000 to G. How much taxable income must each beneficiary report for the current year? What is the amount of the trust's deduction for distributions to beneficiaries?

25-28 *First- and Second-Tier Distributions.* For the current year, Trust R has DNI of $100,000, of which $25,000 is nontaxable. The trustee is required to make an annual distribution of $60,000 to beneficiary S. Also during the year, the trustee made discretionary distributions of $40,000 to beneficiary T and $30,000 to beneficiary U. None of these distributions is subject to the throwback rules. How much taxable income must each beneficiary report?

25-29 *Distribution Exceeding DNI.* In 2007 and 2008, complex Trust C had taxable DNI of $18,000 and $28,500, respectively. No distributions were made to beneficiaries in either year and the trust paid income taxes totaling $13,041 for the two years. In 2009, trust DNI was $33,000 and the trustee distributed $100,000 to beneficiary W. Explain how such distribution is taxed.

25-30 *Income in Respect of a Decedent.* Individual K is a self-employed business consultant. In the current year, K performed services for a client and billed the client for $14,500. Unfortunately, K died on October 10 of the current year, before he received payment for his services. A check for $14,500 was received by K's executor on November 18. At the date of K's death, he owed a local attorney $1,600 for legal advice concerning a child custody suit in which K was involved. K's executor paid this bill on December 15.

a. Assuming that K was a cash basis taxpayer, describe the tax consequences of the $14,500 receipt and the $1,600 payment by K's executor.
b. How would your answer change if K had been an accrual basis taxpayer?

25-31 *Income in Respect of a Decedent.* Early in 2008, Z (an unmarried cash basis taxpayer) sold investment land with a basis of $50,000 for $200,000. In payment, Z received an installment note for $200,000, payable over the next ten years. Z died on December 1, 2008. As of the date of death, Z had received no principal payments on the note. Accrued interest on the note as of December 1, 2008 was $18,000, although the first interest payment was not due until early in 2009.

a. Assuming that no election is made to avoid installment sale treatment, how much of the $150,000 gain realized by Z will be included on her final income tax return? How much of the accrued interest income will be included?

b. In 2009, the estate of Z collects the first annual interest payment on the note of $19,700, and the first principal payment of $20,000. What are the income tax consequences to the estate of these collections?

c. Assume that the amount of estate tax attributable to the inclusion of the IRD represented by the installment note and the accrued interest in Z's taxable estate is $10,000, and that there are no other IRD or DRD items on the estate tax return. Compute the § 691(c) deduction available on the estate's 2009 income tax return.

TAX RETURN PROBLEMS

25-32 The MKJ trust is a calendar year, cash basis taxpayer. The trust was created pursuant to the will of Murray Kyle Jacobs, who died on November 11, 2000. For 2009, the trust's book and records reflect these transactions:

Receipts:

Dividends (qualified)		$30,000
Gross rents		25,000
Interest:		
Bonds of the City of New York		25,000
U.S. government bonds		20,000

Capital gains:

General Motors stock received from estate of MKJ:

Sales price—December 2, 2009	$48,000	
Less: Basis (FMV on date of death)	(30,000)	18,000

Disbursements:

Trustee commissions (50% paid out of income, 50% paid out of principal)		5,300
Legal fee		28,800
Contribution—American Cancer Society (paid out of principal)		12,000
Depreciation—rental property		2,000
Real estate tax—rental property		4,000
Repairs and maintenance—rental property		4,200
Federal quarterly estimated tax payments		9,000

The legal fee was a legitimate trust expense and was incurred because of the choice of trust form. The fee was allocated by the trustee to the various income classes as follows:

Dividends	$ 0
Taxable interest	16,000
Tax-exempt interest	6,000
Rents	6,800
Total legal fee	$28,800

The propriety of this allocation is *not* in question. Under the terms of the trust instrument (i.e., Mr. Jacobs' will), the $2,000 depreciation reserve equals the available tax depreciation deduction for the year. The trust instrument also specifies that all capital gains are allocable to principal and that the trustee has discretion as to the amount of trust income distributed to Brenda Jacobs, the sole individual beneficiary, and several charities specified in Mr. Jacobs' will. During 2009, the trustee distributes $24,000 of income to Brenda and $12,000 of income to the American Cancer Society.

Required: Complete Form 1041 and Schedule D for the MKJ trust. If the 2009 forms are not available, use the 2008 forms. **Note**: If the student is required to complete a Schedule K-l for Brenda Jacobs, he or she should refer to Reg. §§ 1.661(b)-1, 1.661(c)-2, and 1.661(c)-4, and the comprehensive example in this chapter in order to determine the character of any income distributed to the beneficiary.

RESEARCH PROBLEM

25-33 In 2003, N transferred $600,000 of assets into an irrevocable trust for the benefit of her mother, M. The independent trustee, T, is required to distribute annually all income to M. The trust instrument also provides that any capital gains or losses realized upon the sale of trust assets are to be allocated to trust principal. In 2005, and 2007, the trustee sold trust assets and distributed an amount equal to the capital gain realized to M, in addition to the required distribution of trust income. During the current year, T sold certain trust securities and realized a net gain of $25,000. The trust also earned $10,000 of other income. During the year, $35,000 was distributed to M. Should the DNI of the trust for the current year include the $25,000 capital gain?

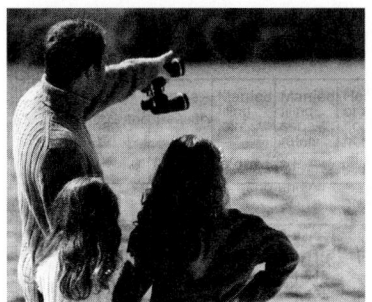

CHAPTER TWENTY SIX

FAMILY TAX PLANNING

LEARNING OBJECTIVES

Upon completion of this chapter you will be able to:

▸ Explain the concept of income shifting and the judicial constraints on this tax planning technique

▸ Describe the marriage penalty and the singles penalty and identify the taxpayer situations in which either might occur

▸ Identify different planning techniques that achieve tax savings by the shifting of income among family members

▸ Characterize a regular corporation, an S corporation, and a partnership in terms of their viability as intrafamily income-shifting devices

▸ Explain how the "kiddie tax" is computed on the unearned income of a minor child

▸ Understand the role of a trust as a vehicle for intrafamily income shifting

▸ Distinguish between a grantor trust and a taxable trust

▸ Specify the tax advantages of inter vivos gifts as compared to testamentary transfers of wealth

▸ Explain the potential tax advantages and disadvantages of the estate tax marital deduction

CHAPTER OUTLINE

INTRODUCTION

Under the United States system of taxation, individuals are viewed as the basic unit of taxation. However, most individuals who are members of a nuclear family tend to regard the family as the economic and financial unit. For example, the individual wage earner with a spouse and three children must budget his or her income according to the needs of five people rather than one individual. Similarly, the family that includes a teenager who has received a college scholarship may perceive the scholarship as a financial benefit to all its members.

The concept of family tax planning is a product of this family-oriented economic perspective. Such planning has as its goal the minimization of taxes paid by the family unit as opposed to the separate taxes paid by individual members. Minimization of the total annual income tax bill of a family results in greater consumable income to the family unit. Minimization of transfer taxes on shifts of wealth among family members increases the total wealth that can be enjoyed by the family as a whole.

Before beginning a study of family tax planning, it is important to remember that such planning is only one aspect of the larger issue of family financial planning. Nontax considerations may often be more important to a family than the tax consequences of a course of action. For example, a family that faces the possibility of large medical expenses might

be more concerned with their short-term liquidity needs than minimization of their current tax bill. A competent tax adviser must always be sensitive to the family's nontax goals and desires before he or she can design a tax plan that is truly in the family's best interests.

FAMILY INCOME SHIFTING

A general premise in tax planning holds that, given a single amount of income, two taxpayers are always better than one. This premise results from the progressive structure of the United States income tax. As one taxpayer earns an increasing amount of income, the income is taxed at an increasing marginal rate. If the income can be diverted to a second taxpayer with less income of his or her own, the diverted amount will be taxed at a lower marginal rate. In 2009, the tax rates applicable to individuals range from 10 percent on the first dollar of taxable income to 35 percent on taxable income in excess of $372,950. This 25-percentage-point spread between the lowest and highest marginal rates is a powerful incentive for individuals to adopt tax plans that incorporate some type of income-shifting technique.

A family unit composed of several individuals theoretically represents a single economic unit, which nonetheless is composed of separate taxpayers. A shift of income from one of these taxpayers to another has no effect economically. However, if the shift moves the income from a high tax bracket to a low tax bracket, the family has enjoyed a tax savings. A simple example can illustrate this basic point.

> **Example 1.** Family F is composed of a father and his 15-year-old daughter. The father earns taxable income of $90,000 a year, an amount that represents total family income. During the summer, the daughter needs $10,000 for various personal expenses. To earn the money, she agrees to work for her father for a $10,000 salary, payment of which represents a deductible expense to him.
>
> Based on this arrangement, the family saves $2,070 [$13,440 − ($10,940 + $430 = $11,370)] as computed below.

	Father Split	Daughter Split	Father No Split
Gross income	$80,000	$10,000	$90,000
Standard deduction	(8,350)	(5,700)	(8,350)
Exemptions	(7,300)	0	(7,300)
Taxable income	$64,350	$ 4,300	$74,350
Tax (head of household rates)	$10,940		$13,440
Tax (single rates)		$ 430	

Note that the father's income tax, standard deduction and exemptions are based on the fact that he would be considered a head of household and can claim an exemption for his daughter. Observe also that the fact that the daughter is a taxpayer does not prevent the father from qualifying as a head of household for filing purposes. However, because the daughter is eligible to be claimed as a dependent on her father's return she is not entitled to a personal exemption.[1]

The tax savings in the above example is attributable to two factors. First, the daughter as a taxpayer with earned income is entitled to a $5,700 standard deduction, which shelters

---

[1] § 151(d)(2).

$5,700 of the income shifted to her from any taxation at all.[2] Second, the income taxable to the daughter is subject to a 10 percent tax rate; if this income had been taxed on the father's return, it would have been subject to a 25 percent tax rate.

JUDICIAL CONSTRAINTS ON INCOME SHIFTING

The Federal courts have consistently recognized that the United States system of taxation cannot tolerate arbitrary shifting of income from one family member to another. The decisions in a number of historic cases have established clear judicial doctrine that limits the assignment of income from one taxpayer to another.

The 1930 Supreme Court case of *Lucas v. Earl*[3] involved a husband and wife who entered into a contract providing that the earnings of either spouse should be considered as owned equally by each. The contract was signed in 1901, twelve years before the first Federal income tax law was written, and was legally binding upon the spouses under California law.

The taxpayers contended that because of the contract certain attorney fees earned by Mr. Earl should be taxed in equal portions to Mr. and Mrs. Earl. However, the Supreme Court agreed with the government's argument that the intent of the Federal income tax law was to tax income to the individual who earns it, an intent that cannot be avoided by anticipatory arrangements to assign the income to a different taxpayer. The decision of the Court ended with the memorable statement that the tax law must disregard arrangements "by which the fruits are attributed to a different tree from that on which they grew."[4]

The Supreme Court followed the same logic in its 1940 decision in *Helvering v. Horst.*[5] This case involved a father who owned corporate coupon bonds and who detached the negotiable interest coupons from the bonds shortly before their due date. The father then gifted the coupons to his son, who collected the interest upon maturity and reported the income on his tax return for the year.

The Court's decision focused on the fact that ownership of the corporate bonds themselves created the right to the interest payments. Because the father owned the bonds, he alone had the right to and control over the interest income. In exercising his control by gifting the interest coupons to his child, the father realized the economic benefit of the income represented by the coupons and therefore was the individual taxable on the income.

These two cases illustrate the two basic premises of the *assignment of income doctrine*. Earned income must be taxed to the individual who performs the service for which the income is paid. Investment income must be taxed to the owner of the investment capital that generated the income. All legitimate efforts to shift income from one individual to another must take into account these judicial constraints.

JOINT FILING AND THE SINGLES PENALTY

The most obvious candidates for intrafamily income shifting are a husband and wife, one of whom has a much larger income than the other. However, since 1948 married couples have been allowed to file a joint income tax return, which reports the total income earned by the couple and taxes the income on the basis of one progressive rate schedule.[6]

---

2   § 63(c)(5).

3   2 USTC ¶496, 8 AFTR 10287, 281 U.S. 111 (USSC, 1930).

4   *Ibid.* 281 U.S. 115.

5   40-2 USTC ¶9787, 24 AFTR 1058, 311 U.S. 112 (USSC, 1940).

6   § 6013. Married individuals may choose to file separate returns, but they must use the rate schedule of § 1(d), which simply halves the tax brackets of the married filing jointly rate schedule of § 1(a). As a general rule, separate filing results in a greater tax than joint filing and such filing status is elected only for nontax reasons.

Joint filing originally was intended as a benefit to married couples. Prior to 1969, the joint filing tax rates were designed to tax one-half of total marital income at the tax rates applicable to single individuals. The resultant tax was then doubled to produce the married couple's tax liability. This perfect split and the corresponding tax savings were perceived as inequitable by unmarried taxpayers, who felt they were paying an unjustifiable "singles penalty."

To illustrate, consider the situation of a single taxpayer with taxable income of $24,000. In 1965, this taxpayer owed $8,030 of income tax, with the last dollar of income taxed at a 50 percent marginal tax rate. A married couple with the same 1965 taxable income owed only $5,660 and faced a marginal tax rate of only 32 percent.

THE MARRIAGE PENALTY

In 1969, Congress attempted to alleviate the singles penalty by enacting a new (and lower) rate schedule for single taxpayers.[7] While this action did reduce (but not eliminate) the singles penalty, it also created a marriage penalty for certain individuals. In 2001, Congress addressed the marriage tax penalty by modifying the standard deduction and the tax rates. For 2009, the standard deduction for joint returns is exactly double that of single taxpayers. Similarly, the 10 percent and 15 percent rate brackets for joint filers are exactly twice the size of the corresponding bracket for an unmarried individual ($8,350 vs. $16,700 and $33,950 vs. $67,900). The brackets for the higher rates are *not* expanded to twice the corresponding single filer tax brackets. As a practical matter, these changes will eliminate the marriage tax penalty for most individuals. Nevertheless, a penalty may still result for higher income taxpayers as shown below.

> **Example 2.** J and S are thinking about getting married and starting a family. The calculations below demonstrate what may happen if (1) J and S do not marry and J earns $90,000; (2) J and S do marry and J earns $90,000; and (3) J and S marry and both earned $90,000.

	J Single	J & S Married	J & S Married
Gross income of J	$90,000	$90,000	$ 90,000
Gross income of S	–	–	90,000
Standard deduction	(5,700)	(11,400)	(11,400)
Exemption	(3,650)	(7,300)	(7,300)
Taxable income	$80,650	$71,300	$161,300
Tax	$16,350	$ 10,200	$ 33,428
Tax for two singles ($16,350 × 2)			(32,700)
Singles penalty ($16,350 – $10,200)		$ 6,150	
Marriage penalty			$ 728

Interpretations of these results differ depending on the point of view. If J is single, he may not like the fact that his married friends who make the same income pay $6,150 less tax than he does. Obviously, he needs to find a wife! If J and S are considering getting married and S does not work, they should marry immediately since they would save $6,150 or avoid the singles penalty that J currently pays. But what happens if both individuals earn income? If each had about the same income and the amounts did not exceed about $77,850, there would be no penalty. However, if they both earn $90,000, as seen above, getting married produces an additional tax of $728—some may say a small price for marital bliss. Most individuals contemplating marriage need

---

[7]   Act. § 803(a), P.L. 91-172, Dec. 30, 1969.

not worry about the cost of marriage since the penalty normally occurs only at higher income levels.

Generally, a singles penalty may occur when *one* income can be taxed at married, rather than single, rates. A marriage penalty may occur when *two* incomes are combined and taxed at married, rather than single, rates. Today, two-income families have become the rule rather than the exception, and the marriage penalty has received considerable publicity. The recent changes by Congress will go a long way to putting an end to the controversy. Nevertheless there will be married couples who want to avoid the penalty. For these people who might entertain the notion of divorce, they should be wary. Because marital status is determined as of the last day of the taxable year,[8] couples have attempted to avoid the marriage penalty by obtaining a technically legal divorce shortly before year end. When a couple has immediately remarried and the only purpose of the divorce was to enable the husband and wife to file as single taxpayers, the IRS and the courts have had little trouble in concluding that the divorce was a sham transaction and therefore ineffective for tax purposes.[9]

Before leaving this topic, one last observation is worth noting. While the recent changes should eliminate most objections to the marriage tax penalty, this does not mean the system is neutral on marriage. Inequities between married and single taxpayers have not necessarily been resolved. No doubt singles who pay more taxes that their married counterparts who earn the same income will complain—much as their ancestors did in 1969. Only time will tell if Congress will once again provide relief and start the cycle once again.

INCOME SHIFTING TO CHILDREN AND OTHER FAMILY MEMBERS

Because a married couple is considered one rather than two taxpayers for Federal tax purposes, intrafamily income shifting usually involves a transfer of income from parents to children (or, less commonly, other family members) who are considered taxpayers in their own right.

The fact that children are taxpayers separate and distinct from their parents is recognized by § 73, which states "amounts received in respect of the services of a child shall be included in his gross income and not in the gross income of the parent, even though such amounts are not received by the child." The regulations elaborate by stating that the statutory rule applies even if state law entitles the parent to the earnings of a minor child.[10]

Because children typically will have little or no income of their own, a shift of family income to such children can cause the income to be taxed at a lower marginal rate. The income shifted from parent to child also represents wealth that is owned by the child rather than the parent. Thus, the future taxable estate of the parent will not include the accumulated income that is already in the hands of younger-generation family members.

INCOME-SHIFTING TECHNIQUES

The next section of this chapter explores a variety of techniques whereby income can be successfully shifted to family members in a lower marginal tax bracket. The circumstances of each particular family situation will dictate the specific technique to be used.

---

[8] § 7703(a).

[9] Rev. Rul. 76-255, 1976-2 C.B. 40; and *Boyter v. Comm.*, 82-1 USTC ¶9117, 49 AFTR2d 451, 668 F.2d 1382 (CA-4, 1981).

[10] Reg. § 1.73-1(a).

FAMILY MEMBERS AS EMPLOYEES

The first technique for intrafamily income shifting is for a low-bracket family member to become an employee of a family business. This technique does not involve the transfer of a capital interest in the business, so the family member who owns the business does not dilute his or her ownership by this technique.

In the simplest case in which the family business is a sole proprietorship, any family members who become employees must actually perform services the value of which equates to the amount of compensation received. This requirement implies that the employee is both capable and qualified for his or her job and devotes an appropriate amount of time to the performance of services.

> **Example 3.** F owns a plumbing contracting business as a sole proprietorship. During the current year, F employs his son S as an apprentice plumber for an hourly wage of $10. The total amount paid to S for the year is $9,000.

If the father can prove to the satisfaction of the IRS that his son performed services worth $10 per hour and that the son actually worked 900 hours during the year, the father may deduct the $9,000 as wage expense on his tax return and the son will report $9,000 of compensation income on his own return.

If, on the other hand, the IRS concludes that the son was not a legitimate employee of his father's business, the transfer of $9,000 to the son would be recharacterized as a gift. As a result, the father would lose the business deduction, and no income shift from father to son would occur.

Obviously, the legitimacy of the employment relationship between father and son can only be determined by an examination of all relevant facts and circumstances. Facts to be considered would include the age of the son, his prior work experience and technical training, and his actual participation on contracted jobs requiring an apprentice plumber.

When a family member is an employee of a family business, any required payroll taxes on his or her compensation must be paid. However, compensation paid to an employer's children under the age of 18 is not subject to Federal payroll tax.[11]

FAMILY EMPLOYEES OF PARTNERSHIPS AND CORPORATIONS

If a family member wants to work as an employee of a family business operated in partnership or corporate form, the requirement that the value of his or her services equate to the amount of compensation received does not change. If the employment relationship is valid, the partnership or corporation may deduct the compensation paid to the family member. If the family member is not performing services that justify the salary he or she is drawing from the business, the IRS may recharacterize the payment.

In the case of a partnership, the payment may be recharacterized as a constructive cash withdrawal by one or more partners followed by a constructive gift of the cash to the pseudo employee.

> **Example 4.** Brothers X, Y, and Z are equal partners in Partnership XYZ. The partnership hires S, the sister of the partners, to act as secretary-treasurer for the business. S's salary is $20,000 per year. Assume that S has no business or clerical training and performs only minimal services for the business on a very sporadic basis. As a result, the IRS disallows a deduction to the partnership for all but $5,000

---

[11] §§ 3121(b)(3)(A) and 3306(c)(5).

of the payment to the sister. The nondeductible $15,000 will be treated as a withdrawal by the partners that was transferred as a gift to the sister.

Constructive cash withdrawals from a partnership could have adverse tax consequences to the partners. If the withdrawal exceeds a partner's basis in his or her partnership interest, the excess constitutes capital gain to the partner.[12] Similarly, a constructive gift to a family member could result in an unexpected gift tax liability.

When the employer is a family corporation and a salary or wage paid to a nonshareholder family member is disallowed, the tax results can be extremely detrimental. Not only does the corporation lose a deduction, but the payment could be recharacterized as a constructive dividend to the family members who are shareholders, followed by a constructive gift to the family member who actually received the funds.[13] Thus, the corporate shareholders would have dividend income without any corresponding cash, and a potential gift tax liability.

The lesson to be learned from the preceding discussion should be clear. If an intrafamily income shift is to be accomplished by hiring a family member as an employee of a family business, the family member must perform as a legitimate employee. If the employment relationship has no substance, the unintended tax consequences to the family could be costly indeed.

FAMILY MEMBERS AS OWNERS OF THE FAMILY BUSINESS

A second technique for intrafamily income shifting is to make a low-bracket family taxpayer a part owner of the family business. By virtue of his or her equity or capital interest, the family member is then entitled to a portion of the income generated by the business. This is a more extreme technique in that it involves an actual transfer of a valuable asset. Moreover, the disposition of a partial ownership interest may cause dilution of the original owner's control of the business. These and other negative aspects of this technique will be discussed in greater detail later in the chapter.

The gratuitous transfer of an equity interest in a business will constitute a taxable gift to the original owner.

> **Example 5.** M runs a very successful business as a sole proprietorship. She wants to bring her son S into the business as an equal general partner. Under the terms of a legally binding partnership agreement, she contributes her business, valued at $1 million, to the partnership. Although the son will have a 50% capital interest in the partnership, he contributes nothing. As a result, M has made a $500,000 taxable gift to S.

Of course, if the transfer of the equity interest is accomplished by sale rather than gift, no initial gift tax liability will result. But in a typical family situation, the equity interest is being transferred to a family member without significant income or wealth, so that family member lacks the funds to purchase the interest. Also, the income tax consequences of a sale could be more expensive than gift tax consequences, depending upon the facts and circumstances. The prudent tax adviser should explore both possible methods of transfer when designing a particular plan.

---

[12] § 731(a).

[13] *Duffey v. Lethert*, 63-1 USTC ¶9442, 11 AFTR2d 1317 (D.Ct. Minn., 1963).

FAMILY PARTNERSHIPS

A family partnership can be used as a vehicle for the co-ownership of a single business by a number of family members. As a partner, each family member will report his or her allocable share of partnership income (or loss) on his or her individual tax return.[14] Therefore, through use of a partnership, business income can be shifted to family members with relatively low marginal tax brackets.

If the family partnership is primarily a service business, only a family member who performs services can receive an allocation of partnership income. In such service partnerships, the physical assets of the business (the capital of the partnership) are not a major factor of income production. Rather, it is the individual efforts and talents of the partners that produce partnership income. An attempt to allow a family member who cannot perform the appropriate services to participate in partnership income is an unwarranted assignment of earned income.

If the family partnership is one in which capital is a major income-producing factor, the mere ownership of a capital interest will entitle a family member to participate in partnership income. The determination of whether or not capital is a material income-producing factor is made by reference to the facts of each situation. However, capital is ordinarily a material income-producing factor if the operation of the business requires substantial inventories or investment in plant, machinery, or equipment.[15]

Section 704(e)(1) specifies that a family member will be recognized as a legitimate partner if he or she owns a capital interest in a partnership in which capital is a material income-producing factor. This is true even if the family member received his or her interest as a gift. However, § 704(e)(2) limits the amount of partnership income that can be shifted to such a donee partner. Under this statute, the income allocated to the partner cannot be proportionally greater than his or her interest in partnership capital.

> **Example 6.** Grandfather F is a 50% partner in Magnum Partnership. At the beginning of the current year, F gives his grandson G a 20% capital interest in Magnum (leaving F with a 30% interest). For the current year Magnum has taxable income of $120,000. The *maximum* amount allocable to G is $24,000 (20% × $120,000). If F wanted to increase the dollar amount of partnership income shifted to G, he must give G a greater equity interest in the partnership.

Section 704(e)(2) contains a second restriction on income allocation. A donor partner who *gifts* a capital interest must receive reasonable compensation for any services he or she renders to the partnership before any income can be allocated to the donee partner.

> **Example 7.** Refer to the facts in *Example 6*. During the current year, F performs services for Magnum worth $15,000 but for which he receives no compensation. Half of the $120,000 partnership income is still allocable to F and G with respect to their combined 50% capital interests; however, the maximum amount allocable to G decreases to $18,000 [($60,000 − $15,000 allocated to F as compensation for services) × 40%].

Note that in the above example, Grandfather F might be willing to forgo any compensation for the services performed for Magnum in order to increase the amount of partnership income shifted to his grandson. Unfortunately, § 704(e)(2) effectively curtails this type of indirect assignment of earned income.

---

[14] § 702(a).

[15] Reg. § 1.704-1(e)(1)(iv).

Family members are not able to avoid the dual limitations of § 704(e) by arranging a transfer of a capital interest to a lower-bracket family member by sale rather than by gift. Under § 704(e)(3), a capital interest in a partnership purchased by one member of a family from another is considered to be created by gift from the seller. In this context the term *family* includes an individual's spouse, ancestors, lineal descendants, and certain family trusts.

REGULAR CORPORATIONS

Family businesses are frequently owned as closely held corporations. There are a number of business reasons why the corporate form is popular. For example, shareholders in a corporation have limited liability so that creditors of the corporation cannot force the shareholders to pay the debts of the corporation out of the shareholders' personal assets. There are also tax benefits to the corporate form of business. The owners of the business can function as employees of the corporate entity. As employees, they may participate in a wide variety of tax-favored employee benefit plans, such as employer-sponsored medical reimbursement plans. If the family business were in sole proprietorship or partnership form, the owners of the business would be self-employed and ineligible to participate in such employee benefit plans.

The corporate form of business must be regarded as a mixed blessing from a tax point of view. The incorporation of a family business does result in the creation of a new taxable entity, separate and distinct from its owners. Business income has been shifted to the corporate taxpayer, and because corporate tax rates are progressive, a net tax savings to the business can be the result.[16]

> **Example 8.** Individual T, married, owns a sole proprietorship that produces $100,000 of net income before taxes. Ignoring the availability of any deductions or exemptions, T's 2009 tax on this income is $17,375 (married filing jointly rates). If T incorporates the business and draws a salary of $50,000, he will pay an individual tax of only $6,665. The corporation will also have income of $50,000 ($100,000 net income − $50,000 salary to T). The corporate tax on $50,000 is $7,500. Therefore, the *total* tax on the business income has decreased by $3,210 to $14,165 ($6,665 + $7,500).

The tax savings to T's business ($3,210) achieved by incorporation is certainly dramatic. However, the potential problem created by the incorporation of T's business is that the after-tax earnings of the business are now in the corporation rather than in T's pocket. If T needs or wants more than $43,335 ($50,000 salary − $6,665 tax liability) of after-tax personal income, he may certainly have his corporation pay out some of its after-tax earnings to him as a dividend. But any dividends paid must be included in T's gross income and taxed at the individual level.

This double taxation of corporate earnings paid to shareholders as dividends can quickly offset the tax savings resulting from using a corporation as a separate entity. Therefore, shareholders in closely held corporations usually become very adept in drawing business income out of their corporations as deductible business expenses rather than nondeductible dividends.

Shareholders who are also employees will usually try to maximize the amount of compensation they receive from the corporation. Section 162(a)(1) authorizes the corporation to deduct a *reasonable* allowance for salaries or other compensation paid. If the IRS determines that the compensation paid to an owner employee is unjustifiably high

---

[16] Because of the 5 percent surtax on taxable income between $100,000 and $335,000, corporations with taxable income between $335,000 and $10 million face a flat 34 percent tax rate rather than a progressive rate. Qualified personal service corporations pay a flat 35 percent of their total taxable income. § 11(b)(2).

and therefore *unreasonable*, the excessive compensation can be reclassified as a dividend. As a result, the corporation loses the deduction for the excessive compensation, and to a corresponding extent, business earnings are taxed twice.

Other types of deductible payments from corporations to shareholders include rents paid for corporate use of shareholder assets and interest on loans made to the corporation by shareholders. The arrangements between corporation and shareholder that give rise to such rent or interest payments will be subject to careful scrutiny by the IRS. If an arrangement lacks substance and is deemed to be a device to camouflage the payments of dividends to shareholders, the corporate deduction for the payments will be disallowed.

Because it is a taxpayer in its own right, a regular corporation cannot be effectively used to shift business income to low-bracket family members. If such family members are made shareholders in the corporation and have no other relationship to the corporate business (employee, creditor, etc.), the only way to allocate business earnings to them is by paying dividends on their stock. As previously discussed, dividend payments are usually considered prohibitively costly from a tax standpoint.

Closely held regular corporations do have tremendous utility in other areas of tax planning. However, for purposes of intrafamily income shifting, the S corporation is a highly preferable alternative to a regular corporation.

S CORPORATIONS

The complex set of statutory provisions that govern the tax treatment of S corporations is explained in Chapter 23. For family tax planning purposes, the most important characteristic of an S corporation is that the corporate income escapes taxation at the corporate level and is taxed to the corporation's shareholders. This characteristic makes an S corporation a very useful mechanism for intrafamily income shifting.

Section 1366(a) provides that the taxable income of an S corporation is allocated to the shareholders on a pro rata basis. Thus, any individual who is a shareholder will report a proportionate share of the corporate business income on his or her personal tax return for the year with or within which the S corporation's taxable year ends.

> **Example 9.** Individual M, married, owns a sole proprietorship with an annual net income before taxes of $200,000. Ignoring the availability of any itemized deductions or exemptions, M's personal tax on this income is $44,264 (joint return schedule). If at the beginning of 2009 M incorporates the business, gives each of his four unmarried children 20% of the stock, and has the shareholders elect S status for the corporation, the corporate income of $200,000 will be taxed in equal $40,000 amounts to the five shareholders. Ignoring other deductions or exemptions, the 2009 tax bill on the business income will be $29,915 [$5,165 on a joint return + (4 × $6,187.80 = $24,750 on a single return)]. By splitting the income, M saves $14,348.50 ($44,263.50 − $29,915).

A shareholder who is also an employee of a family-owned S corporation will not be able to divert corporate income to other shareholders by forgoing any compensation for services rendered to the corporation. Code § 1366(e) provides that if such a shareholder employee does not receive reasonable compensation from the S corporation, the IRS may reallocate corporate income to the shareholder employee so as to accurately reflect the value of his or her services.

Because shareholders of an S corporation are taxed on all the taxable income earned by the corporation, subsequent cash withdrawals of this income by shareholders are tax free.[17] However, the technical requirements for cash withdrawals from an S corporation

---

[17] § 1368(b).

are dangerously complicated. Because of the complexity of these requirements and many other tax aspects of S corporations, family tax plans involving their use should be carefully designed and monitored by the family tax adviser.

NEGATIVE ASPECTS OF OWNERSHIP TRANSFERS

A high-bracket taxpayer who desires to shift income to low-bracket family members by making such members co-owners of the taxpayer's business must reconcile himself or herself to several facts. First, the transfer of the equity interest in the business must be complete and legally binding so that the recipient of the interest has "dominion and control" over his or her new asset. A *paper* transfer by which the transferor creates only the illusion that a family member has been given an equity interest in a business will be treated as a sham transaction, ineffective for income-shifting purposes.[18]

As a general rule, the recipient of an ownership interest in a family business is free to dispose of the interest, just as he or she is free to dispose of any asset he or she owns. If the recipient is a responsible individual and supportive of the family tax planning goals, his or her legal right to assign the interest may not be a problem. But if the recipient is a spendthrift in constant need of ready cash, he or she may sell the interest to a third party, thereby completely subverting the family tax plan.

One popular technique that can prevent an unexpected and undesired disposition of an interest in a family business is a buy-sell agreement. A taxpayer can transfer an equity interest to a low-bracket family member on the condition that should the family member desire to sell the interest he or she must first offer the interest to its original owner at an independently determined market value. Such an agreement is in no way economically detrimental to the family member, yet affords a measure of protection for both the original owner and the family tax plan.

A related aspect of the requirement that the taxpayer must legally surrender the ownership of the business interest transferred is that the transfer is irrevocable. Ownership of the interest cannot be regained if future events cause the original tax plan to become undesirable. For example, an estrangement between family members could convert a highly satisfactory intrafamily income-shifting plan into a bitterly resented trap. A father who has an ill-favored son as an employee can always fire him. It is another matter entirely if the son is a 40 percent shareholder in the father's corporation.

A change in economic circumstances could also cause a taxpayer to regret a transfer of a business interest. Consider a situation in which a formerly high-income taxpayer suffers a severe financial downturn. A tax plan that is shifting income *away* from such a taxpayer could suddenly become an economic disaster.

PRESERVATION OF CONTROL OF THE BUSINESS

A taxpayer who is contemplating transferring an ownership interest in a business to one or more family members should also consider any resultant dilution of his or her control of the business. The taxpayer may be willing to part with an equity interest in order to shift business income to low-bracket family members, but may be very reluctant to allow such family members to participate in the management of the business.

A limited partnership can be used to bring family members into a business without allowing them a voice in management. A family member who owns a capital interest as a limited partner in a partnership may be allocated a share of business income, subject to the family partnership rules, and yet be precluded from participating in management of the business.

---

[18] For example, see Reg. § 1.704-1(e)(2).

If the family business is in corporate form, various classes of stock with differing characteristics can be issued. For example, nonvoting stock can be given to family members without any dilution of the original owner's voting power, and hence control, over the business. If the original owner does not want to draw any dividends out of the corporate business but is willing to have dividends paid to low-bracket family members, nonvoting preferred stock can be issued to such family members.

Unfortunately, this flexibility in designing a corporate capital structure that maximizes income-shifting potential while minimizing loss of control is not available to S corporations. To qualify for S status a corporation may have only one class of stock outstanding.[19] Thus, all outstanding shares of stock in an S corporation must be identical with respect to the rights they convey in the profits and assets of the corporation. However, shares of stock in S corporations may have different *voting rights* without violating the single class of stock requirement.[20]

SHIFTS OF INVESTMENT INCOME

In many ways the shifting of investment income to family members is simpler than the shifting of business income. Questions of forms of co-ownership and control are not as difficult to resolve if the income-producing asset to be transferred is in the form of an investment security rather than a business interest.

The simplest means to shift investment income from one taxpayer to another is an outright gift of the investment asset. Even gifts to minors who are under legal disabilities with regard to property ownership can be accomplished under state Uniform Gifts to Minors Acts. By using a custodian to hold the property for the benefit of a minor, the donor has shifted the investment income to the minor's tax return.[21]

Although gifting of investment property is a relatively simple technique, the donor must be aware that the transfer must be complete. The asset (and the wealth it represents) is irrevocably out of the donor's hands. If the donor attempts to retain an interest in or control over the asset, the gift may be deemed incomplete and the attempted income shift ineffectual.

If a donee receives an unrestricted right to a valuable investment asset, there is always the worry that he or she will mismanage it, or worse, assign it to a third party against the wishes of the donor. Because of these negative aspects of outright gifts, the private trust has become a very popular vehicle for the transfer of investment assets, especially when minor children are involved. A subsequent section of the chapter explores the use of trusts in family tax planning.

TAXATION OF UNEARNED INCOME OF MINOR CHILDREN

Tax law significantly limits the ability of parents to shift investment income to their children. Section 1(g) provides that any *net unearned income* of a minor child in excess of a $950 (2009) base is taxed at the marginal rate applicable to the income of the child's parents.[22] A minor child is one who by the close of the tax year has not obtained the age of 19 or is a full-time student less than the age of 24 who does not provide more than one-half of his or her support and who has at least one living parent on that date.

Net unearned income is generally defined as passive investment income such as interest and dividends, reduced by the $950 standard deduction available against unearned

---

[19] § 1361(b)(1)(D).

[20] § 1361(c)(4).

[21] Rev. Rul. 56-484, 1956-2 C.B. 23. However, income earned by the custodian account used for the support of the minor will be taxed to the person legally responsible for such support (i.e., the parent).

[22] In the case of parents who are not married, the child's tax is computed with reference to the tax rate of the custodial parent. If the parents file separate tax returns, the tax rate of the parent with the *greater* taxable income is used. § 1(g)(5).

income of a dependent.[23] The amount of net unearned income for any taxable year may not exceed the child's taxable income for the year. The *source* of the unearned income is irrelevant for purposes of this so-called "kiddie tax."

> **Example 10.** Several years ago grandchild G, age 15, received a gift of corporate bonds from her grandparents. G's 2009 interest income from the securities totaled $8,000. G had no other income or deductions for the year. G's parents claimed G as a dependent and reported taxable income of $500,000 on their joint return. G's taxable income is $7,050 ($8,000 gross income − an $950 standard deduction) and her net unearned income to be taxed at her parents' rate is $6,100 ($8,000 − the $950 base − an $950 standard deduction). Thus $6,100 is taxed at her parents' rates and the balance, $950, is taxed at her rates, resulting in a tax liability of $2,230 computed as follows:

Tax on unearned income at parents' rates:	
($8,000 − $1,900 = $6,100 × 35%)...............	$2,135
Tax on remaining taxable income at child's rates:	
($950 × 10%).................................	95
Tax liability.......................................	$2,230

> In this example, it is important to note that the income was interest and, therefore, subject to tax at the parents' highest tax rate. In contrast, dividend income or long-term capital gains that are shifted to a child are generally taxed at 15% (or 5%) but a special computation is required.

In certain cases parents may elect to include a dependent's unearned income on their return, rather than filing a separate return and making the "kiddie tax" calculation. As a general rule, this should not be done since the additional income increases the parents' adjusted gross income, which may reduce the amount of deductions that the parent may claim and have other unintended effects.

THE TRUST AS A TAX PLANNING VEHICLE

As discussed in Chapter 25, a private trust is a legal arrangement whereby the ownership and control of property are vested in a trustee while the beneficial interest in the property is given to one or more beneficiaries. The trustee has a fiduciary responsibility to manage the property for the sole benefit of the beneficiaries.

ADVANTAGES OF THE TRUST FORM

The use of a trust has many nontax advantages. If an individual desires to make a gift of property to a donee who is not capable of owning or managing the property, the gift can be made in trust so that a competent trustee can be selected to manage the property free from interference from the donee-beneficiary.

The trust form of property ownership is very convenient in that it allows the legal title to property to be held by a single person (the trustee) while allowing the beneficial enjoyment of the property to be shared by a number of beneficiaries. If legal ownership of the property were fragmented among the various beneficiaries, they would all have to jointly participate in management decisions regarding the property. This cumbersome and often-times impractical co-ownership situation is avoided when a trustee is given sole management authority over the property.

---

[23] § 63(c)(5).

If a donor would like to give property to several donees so that the donees have sequential rather than concurrent rights in the property, the trust form for the gift is commonly the solution.

> **Example 11.** Individual K owns a valuable tract of income-producing real estate. She would like ownership of the real estate to ultimately pass to her three minor grandchildren. She also would like to give her invalid brother an interest in the real estate so as to provide him with a future source of income. K can transfer the real estate into trust, giving her brother an income interest for a designated time period. Upon termination of the time period, ownership of the real estate will go to K's grandchildren.

TAX CONSEQUENCES OF TRANSFERS INTO TRUST

The use of the trust form can have distinct income tax advantages to a family because both the trust itself and any beneficiaries who receive income from the trust are taxpayers in their own right.

> **Example 12.** F, a high-bracket taxpayer, transfers income-producing assets into a trust of which his four grandchildren are discretionary income beneficiaries. In the current year, the trust assets generate $100,000 of income, of which the trustee distributes $24,000 to each child. The $100,000 of investment income will be taxed to five taxpayers, the four grandchildren and the trust itself.

In determining the benefit of splitting income in *Example 12*, it is important to remember that unearned income *distributed* from a trust to a beneficiary may be subject to the kiddie tax. The income will be taxed at the marginal rate applicable to the beneficiary's parents, even if the parents did not create the trust. However, if the beneficiary is not subject to the kiddie tax (e.g., a grandparent), substantial savings can be obtained.

GIFT-LEASEBACKS

A popular and controversial method for family income shifting through use of a trust involves a technique known as a gift-leaseback. Typically, a taxpayer who owns assets that he or she uses in a trade or business transfers the assets as a gift in trust for the benefit of the taxpayer's children (or other low-bracket family members). The independent trustee then leases the assets back to the taxpayer for their fair rental value. The rent paid by the taxpayer to the trust is deducted as a § 162 ordinary and necessary business expense and becomes income to the taxpayer's children because of their status as trust beneficiaries.

The IRS has refused to recognize the validity of gift-leaseback arrangements and has consistently disallowed the rent deduction to the transferor of the business assets under the theory that the entire transaction has no business purpose. However, if the trust owning the leased assets has an independent trustee and the leaseback arrangement is in written form and requires payment to the trust of a reasonable rent, the Tax Court and the Second, Third, Seventh, Eighth, and Ninth Circuits have allowed the transferor to deduct the rent paid.[24] To date, only the Fourth and Fifth Circuits have supported the government's position that gift-leaseback transactions are shams to be disregarded for tax purposes.[25]

---

[24]   See *May v. Comm.*, 76 T.C. 7 (1981), *aff'd.* 84-1 USTC ¶9166, 53 AFTR2d 84-626 (CA-9. 1984).

[25]   See *Mathews v. Comm.*, 75-2 USTC ¶9734, 36 AFTR2d 75-5965, 520 F.2d 323 (CA-5, 1975), cert. denied, 424 U.S. 967 (1976).

GIFT TAX CONSIDERATIONS

The obvious income tax advantage of a family trust, such as the one described in *Example 12* above, can be offset if the original gift of property into the trust is subject to a substantial gift tax. Thus, the first step in designing a family trust is the minimization of any front-end gift tax. If the fair market value of the transferred property is less than the taxable amount sheltered by the unified credit of § 2505, no gift tax will be paid. However, the reader should bear in mind that the use of the credit against inter vivos gifts reduces the future shelter available on the donor's estate tax return.

An essential element in the minimization of any gift tax for transfers into trust is securing the $13,000 (2009) annual exclusion (§ 2503) for the amount transferred to each beneficiary-donee. This can be difficult when certain of the donees are given only a prospective or future interest in the trust property.

> **Example 13.** Donor Z transfers $100,000 into trust. The independent trustee has the discretion to distribute income currently among Z's five children, or she may accumulate it for future distribution. Upon trust termination, the trust assets will be divided equally among the children. Because the five donees have only future interests in the $100,000, Z may not claim any exclusions in computing the amount of the taxable gift.[26]

SECTION 2503(C) AND CRUMMEY TRUSTS

One method of securing the exclusion for transfers into trust is to rely on the *safe harbor* rules of § 2503(c). Under this subsection a transfer into trust will not be considered a gift of a future interest if:

1. The property and income therefrom may be expended for the benefit of the donee-beneficiary before he or she reaches age 21; and

2. If any property or income is not so expended, it will pass to the donee-beneficiary at age 21 or be payable to his or her estate if he or she dies before that age.

One drawback to the "§ 2503(c) trust" is that the trust assets generally must go to the beneficiaries at age 21. Many parent-donors would prefer to postpone trust termination until their children-donees attain a more mature age. This goal can be accomplished through the use of a *Crummey trust.*[27]

A Crummey trust is one in which the beneficiaries are directly given only a future right to trust income or corpus. The term of the trust may extend well beyond the time when the beneficiaries reach age 21. However, the trust instrument contains a clause (the Crummey clause) that authorizes any beneficiary or his or her legal representative to make a current withdrawal of any current addition to the trust of up to $13,000. The withdrawal right is made noncumulative from year to year. As long as the beneficiary is given notification of this right within a reasonable period before it lapses for the year, the donor will be entitled to an exclusion for the current transfers into trust.[28] It should be noted that most donors anticipate that their donees will never exercise their withdrawal right; the Crummey clause is included in the trust instrument for the *sole purpose* of securing the $13,000 exclusion for gift tax purposes.

---

[26]   Reg. § 25.2503-3(c), Ex. 3.

[27]   The amusing designation comes from the court case which established the validity of the technique—*Crummey v. Comm.*, 68-2 USTC ¶12,541, 22 AFTR2d 6023, 397 F.2d 82 (CA-9, 1968). The IRS *acquiesced* to this decision in Rev. Rul. 73-405, 1973-2 C.B. 321.

[28]   Rev. Rul. 81-7, 1981-1 C.B. 27.

GRANTOR TRUSTS

In certain cases a taxpayer may desire to transfer property into trust but does not want to surrender complete control over the property. Alternatively, the taxpayer may want to dispose of the property (and the right to income from the property) for only a limited period of time. Prior to the enactment of the 1954 Internal Revenue Code there was no statutory guidance as to when the retention of powers over a trust by the grantor (transferor) would prevent the trust from being recognized as a separate taxable entity. Nor was there statutory guidance as to the tax status of a reversionary trust, the corpus of which reverted to the grantor after a specified length of time.

The judicial attitude toward these *grantor* trusts was reflected in the Supreme Court decision of *Helvering v. Clifford.*[29] This case involved a taxpayer who transferred securities into trust for the exclusive benefit of his wife. The trust was to last for five years, during which time the taxpayer as trustee would manage the trust corpus as well as decide how much, if any, of the trust income was to be paid to his wife. Upon trust termination, corpus was to return to the taxpayer while any accumulated income was to go to the wife.

In reaching its decision, the Court noted the lack of a precise standard or guide supplied by statute or regulations. As a result, the Court turned to a subjective evaluation of all the facts and circumstances of this particular short-term trust arrangement and held that "the short duration of the trust, the fact that the wife was the beneficiary, and the retention of control over the corpus by respondent all lead irresistibly to the conclusion that the respondent continued to be the owner."[30] As a result, the trust income was held to be taxable to the grantor rather than the trust or its beneficiary.

The authors of the 1954 Internal Revenue Code recognized that the uncertainty regarding the tax treatment of grantor trusts was undesirable and supplanted the subjective *Clifford* approach with a series of code sections (§§ 671 through 679) containing more objective rules as to the taxability of such trusts. The basic operative rule is contained in § 671. If §§ 673 through 679 specify that the grantor (or another person) shall be treated as the owner of any portion of a trust, the income, deductions, or credits attributable to that portion of the trust shall be reported on the grantor's (or other person's) tax return. If §§ 673 through 679 are inapplicable, the trust shall be treated as a separate taxable entity under the normal rules of Subchapter J (see Chapter 25).

REVERSIONARY TRUSTS

Section 673 provides that the grantor shall be treated as the owner of any portion of a trust in which he or she has a reversionary interest, if upon creation of the trust the value of the reversion exceeds 5 percent of the value of the assets subject to reversion.

Example 14. In the current year, grantor G transfers assets worth $500,000 into trust. Niece N, age 20, will receive the income from the trust for 15 years, after which the trust will terminate and the assets returned to G. On the date the trust is created, the reversion is properly valued at $121,000. Because the reversion is worth more than 5% of $500,000, the income will be taxed to G, even though it will be distributed to N.

---

[29] 40-1 USTC ¶9265, 23 AFTR 1077, 309 U.S. 331 (1940).

[30] *Ibid.*, 309 U.S. 332.

Example 15. If in the previous example, N had been given the income from the trust for her life, the proper value of G's reversion would only be $13,000. Because this reversionary interest is worth only 2.6% of the value of the trust assets, the trust is not a grantor trust and the income will be taxed to N.

In the case of a trust in which a lineal descendant of the grantor (child, grandchild, etc.) is the income beneficiary, and the grantor owns a reversionary interest that takes effect only upon the death of the beneficiary prior to the age of 21, the trust *will not* be considered a grantor trust.[31]

INTEREST-FREE LOANS

Through use of a reversionary trust, a taxpayer may divert income to low-bracket family members only if he or she is willing to part with control of the trust corpus for a significant period of time. For many years the use of an interest-free demand loan between family members provided an alternative to a reversionary trust. A taxpayer could loan a sum of money to a family member on a demand basis and the money could be invested to earn income for that family member. Because the loan was interest-free, the creditor-taxpayer had no income from the temporary shift of wealth and could call the loan (demand payment) at any time.

The IRS was understandably hostile to such loans and argued that the creditor was making a gift of the use of the money to the borrower and that the amount of the gift equaled the interest that the creditor would have charged an unrelated borrower. In 1984, Congress codified the IRS position by enacting Code § 7872, concerning below- market-rate-interest and no-interest loans. The thrust of this provision is to impute interest income to the creditor donor and correspondingly allow an interest deduction for the borrower-donee. Therefore, the creditor-donor is effectively treated as having received interest income and then gifting such income to the borrower. The deemed transfer is subject to the gift tax to the extent the interest exceeds the annual exclusion. As a result, interest-free loans are no longer an effective device for shifting income.

Example 16. On January 1 of the current year, father F loaned $175,000 to his daughter, S. The loan was interest free and F may demand repayment at any time. The current interest rate as determined by the IRS is 10% per annum. On December 31 of the current year, S is considered to have paid $17,500 of deductible interest to F, and F is considered to have received $17,500 of taxable interest income from S. On the same date, F is considered to have made a $17,500 gift to S which is eligible for the $13,000 annual gift tax exclusion.

POWER TO CONTROL BENEFICIAL ENJOYMENT

Section 674(a) contains the general rule that a grantor shall be treated as the owner of any portion of a trust of which the grantor, a nonadverse party, or both, controls the beneficial enjoyment. However, if the exercise of such control requires the approval or consent of an *adverse party*, the general rule shall not apply. An adverse party is defined in § 672(a) as any person who has a substantial beneficial interest in the trust that would be adversely affected by the exercise of the control held by the grantor.

Example 17. F transfers income-producing property into trust with City Bank as independent trustee. F's two children are named as trust beneficiaries. However, F retains the unrestricted right to designate which of the children is to receive annual

---

[31] § 673(b).

distributions of trust income. This is a grantor trust with the result that all trust income is taxed to F.

Example 18. Refer to the facts in *Example 17.* Assume that the trust instrument provides that the trust income will be paid out on an annual basis in equal portions to F's two children. However, F retains the right to adjust the amount of the income distributions at any time with the consent of the older child C. Because C is an adverse party with respect to the one-half of the income to which he is entitled, only the other half of the income is considered subject to F's control. As a result, only half the trust property is deemed owned by F and only half the trust income is taxable directly to him.[32]

The general rule of § 674(a) is subject to numerous exceptions contained in §§ 674(b), (c), and (d). Any tax adviser attempting to avoid the grantor trust rules should be aware of these exceptions. For example, § 674(c) provides that the power to distribute income within a class of beneficiaries will not cause the grantor trust rules to apply if the power is solely exercisable by an *independent* trustee.

Example 19. M transfers income-producing property into trust and names Midtown Bank as independent trustee. The trustee has the right to *sprinkle* (distribute) the annual income of the trust among M's three children in any proportion the trustee deems appropriate. Even though the power to control the enjoyment of the income is held by a nonadverse party, such party is independent of the grantor and the trust is not a grantor trust.

OTHER GRANTOR TRUSTS

Section 675 provides that the grantor shall be treated as the owner of any portion of a trust in respect of which he or she holds certain administrative or management powers.

Example 20. T transfers 60% of the common stock in his closely held corporation into trust with City National Bank as independent trustee. All income of the trust must be paid to T's only grandchild. However, T retains the right to vote the transferred shares. Because T has retained an administrative power specified in § 675(4), he will be taxed on the income generated by the corporate stock.

If a grantor, a nonadverse party, or both have the right to revest in the grantor the ownership of any portion of trust property, § 676 provides that such portion of the trust is considered to be owned by the grantor. Therefore, revocable trusts are grantor trusts for income tax purposes.

Under § 677, a grantor also is treated as owner of any portion of a trust the income of which *may be* distributed to the grantor or spouse without the approval of any adverse party. This rule also applies if trust income may be used to pay premiums for insurance on the life of the grantor and spouse. This provision is inapplicable if the beneficiary of the policy is a charitable organization.

Example 21. Individual J transfers income-producing assets into trust and designates Second National Bank as independent trustee. Under the terms of the trust instrument, the trustee may distribute trust income to either J's spouse or J's brother. In the current year the trustee distributes all trust income to J's brother.

---

[32] Reg. § 1.672(a)-1(b).

Because a nonadverse party (the trustee) could have distributed the trust income to J's spouse, this is a grantor trust and all income is taxed to J.

If trust income may be expended to discharge a legal obligation of the grantor, § 677 applies,[33] subject to two important exceptions. Section 682 creates an exception for *alimony trusts*. In certain divorce situations an individual who is required to pay alimony may fund a reversionary trust, the income from which will be paid to the grantor's former spouse in satisfaction of the alimony obligation. Under § 682, the recipient of the trust income rather than the grantor will be taxed on the income regardless of the applicability of any other of the grantor trust rules.

As a second exception, § 677(b) specifies that if trust income may be distributed for the support or maintenance of a beneficiary (other than the grantor's spouse) whom the grantor is legally obligated to support, such a provision by itself will not cause the trust to be a grantor trust. However, to the extent trust income is actually distributed for such purposes, it will be taxed to the grantor.

The final type of trust that is not recognized as a separate taxable entity is described in § 678. Under this provision, a person *other than* the grantor may be treated as the owner of a portion of a trust if such person has an unrestricted right to vest trust corpus or income in himself or herself. Section 678 shall not apply to the situation in which a person, in the capacity of trustee, has the right to distribute trust income to a beneficiary whom the person is legally obligated to support. Only to the extent that trust income is actually so expended will the income be taxed to the person.

> **Example 22.** Grantor G creates a trust with an independent corporate trustee and names his children and grandchildren as beneficiaries. The trust instrument also provides that G's sister S has the unrestricted right to withdraw up to one-third of trust corpus at anytime. S is considered the owner of one-third of the trust and will be taxed on one-third of the income, regardless of the fact that such income is not distributable to her.

GRANTOR TRUSTS AND THE TRANSFER TAX RULES

As a general rule, a transfer of assets into trust that is incomplete for income tax purposes, so that the grantor is taxed on trust income, is also incomplete for gift and estate tax purposes.

> **Example 23.** M transfers income-producing properties into a trust but retains the right to designate which of the specified trust beneficiaries will receive a distribution of trust income. The arrangement is a grantor trust per § 674. Under the gift tax Regulations, M has not made a completed gift of the income interest in the trust, and per § 2036 the value of the trust corpus will be included in M's gross estate upon his death.

However, it should be emphasized that the general rule does not always hold.

> **Example 24.** Grantor G transfers assets into a reversionary trust that will last only eight years. During the existence of the trust, all income must be paid to G's cousin, C. For income tax purposes, this is a grantor trust and all trust income is taxable to G. However, for gift tax purposes G has made a completed gift of the income interest to C.

---

[33] Reg. § 1.677(a)-1(d).

TRANSFER TAX PLANNING

The first part of this chapter dealt with a variety of techniques to shift income within a family group and thereby minimize the family's income tax burden. The second part of the chapter focuses on family tax planning techniques designed to reduce any transfer tax liability on intrafamily shifts of wealth. At this point, the student should be cautioned against thinking of income tax planning and transfer tax planning as two separate areas; both types of planning should be considered as highly interrelated aspects of a single integrated family tax plan.

A second aspect of transfer tax planning of which any tax adviser should be aware is that a client's nontax estate planning goals may conflict with an optimal tax-oriented estate plan. From a client's point of view, an orderly disposition of wealth that benefits the heirs in the precise manner that the client desires may be the primary planning objective, regardless of the tax cost. A client planning for his or her own death may be most concerned with his or her own emotional and psychological needs as well as those of other family members. Minimization of the Federal estate tax levied on the estate simply may not be a central concern. A tax adviser who fails to appreciate the client's priorities and who designs an estate plan that fails to reflect the client's nontax needs is not acting in the best interest of that client.

TAX PLANNING WITH INTRAFAMILY GIFTS

Before enactment of the Tax Reform Act of 1976, the Federal transfer tax savings associated with gifting assets to family members during the donor's life rather than transferring the assets at death were obvious. The gift tax rates were only 75 percent of the estate tax rates, and because of the progressive nature of both rate schedules, inter vivos gifts could shift an individual's wealth out of a high marginal estate tax bracket into a lower marginal gift tax bracket.

The Tax Reform Act of 1976 integrated the gift and estate taxes by providing a single rate schedule for both taxes and by including in the estate tax base the amount of post-1976 gifts made by a decedent.[34] Thus, any inter vivos gift made by a decedent after 1976 has the effect of boosting his or her taxable estate into a higher tax bracket.

> **Example 25.** In 2000, D made a taxable gift of $400,000, her only taxable inter vivos transfer. D dies in the current year, leaving a taxable estate of $5,000,000. The base for computing D's estate tax is $5.9 million, her taxable estate plus the $400,000 taxable gift.

Because of the integration of the gift and estate taxes, the tax benefit of inter vivos giving has been reduced but certainly not eliminated. The following advantages of making gifts have survived the integration process.

1. All appreciation in value of the transferred property that occurs after the date of gift escapes taxation in the donor's gross estate. Refer to *Example 25*. If the value of the gifted asset increased from $400,000 in 2000 to $700,000 in the current year, the $300,000 appreciation is not taxed in D's estate. It should be noted that inter vivos transfers of appreciating assets do have a potentially serious negative income tax consequence. The basis of such assets to the donee will be a carryover basis from the donor, increased by the amount of any gift tax paid attributable to the difference between the value of the gift and the

---

[34] § 2001(b).

donor's tax basis.[35] If the donor retained the property until death, the basis of the property would be stepped up to its fair market to value at date of death.[36] Thus, a transfer of the asset during life rather than at death preserves rather than eliminates pre-death appreciation in the value of the asset that will be subject to income taxation on subsequent sale.

2. Future income generated by property that the donor has transferred will be accumulated by younger generation family members rather than in the estate of the donor.

3. The availability of the annual $13,000 exclusion allows a donor to give away a substantial amount of wealth completely tax free.

4. All other factors being equal, it is cheaper to pay a gift tax rather than an estate tax. This is true because the dollars used to pay a gift tax are never themselves subject to a Federal transfer tax. However, dollars used to pay an estate tax have been included in the taxable estate and are subject to the estate tax.

For this reason, the estate tax is said to be *tax inclusive* (since the estate tax is itself taxed) while the gift tax is sometimes said to be *tax exclusive* (the gift tax itself is not taxed).

Example 26. D has $10,000,000 in assets and wants to transfer $5,500,000 to a beneficiary. Ignore the annual exclusion, the unified credit and assume a flat rate of 45%. If D dies with an estate of $10,000,000, the estate will pay a tax of $4,500,000 out of the estate's assets and $5,500,000 will be left to pass to the heirs. In contrast, if the individual had made a $5,500,000 gift before he died, he would have had to pay only a $2,475,000 tax for the privilege of transferring $5,500,000. In other words, it would cost $2,025,000 less ($4,500,000 − $2,475,000) to give $5,500,000 than to *will* such amount. In effect, if he gave $5,500,000 while he was living, he would have had $2,025,000 left to do with as he pleases. By making the gift and paying the gift tax, he is removing the gift tax amount ($2,025,000) from his estate, never to be taxed!

Example 27. W has only $1,000,000 of assets. Assume a 45% rate and ignore the unified credit and annual exclusion. If W dies and leaves the $1,000,000 to her child, W pays a tax of $450,000 and the child receives $550,000. If W had used the same $1,000,000 to make a gift and pay the tax, she could have given her child $689,655, determined as follows:

$$
\begin{aligned}
x &= \text{Amount of the gift} \\
.45x &= \text{Gift tax} \\
\\
x + .45x &= \$1,000,000 \\
1.45x &= \$1,000,000 \\
x &= \$689,655 \\
.45x &= \$310,345
\end{aligned}
$$

Thus if W makes a gift of $689,655, she will pay a gift tax of $310,345, exhausting the $1,000,000. Note that by giving, the child receives $689,655 rather than $550,000 or $139,655 more!

---

[35] § 1015.

[36] § 1014.

"FREEZING" THE VALUE OF ASSETS IN THE GROSS ESTATE

A long-range plan of inter vivos giving from older generation to younger generation family members is a basic component of most family tax plans. However, elderly individuals can be very reluctant about making substantial gifts of their wealth, even when they fully understand the tax advantages in doing so. Psychologically it is difficult to part with wealth that is the result of a lifetime of endeavor. Elderly individuals often fear that gifts of property might leave them without sufficient income or capital to provide for their future comfort and security. They may even worry that their children and grandchildren might "desert" them if the offspring were given the family wealth too soon.

For these and many other reasons it may be difficult for the tax adviser to persuade an older client to transfer existing wealth during his or her lifetime. However, the same client may be much more amenable to simply "freezing" the value of his or her current estate, so that future accumulations of wealth are somehow transferred to younger members of the family and therefore not subject to estate tax upon the client's death.

Gifts of Property. The simplest type of estate freeze is a gift. A gift of appreciating property is taxed at its current value for gift tax purposes and any future appreciation is forever removed from the estate tax base. Note, however, that this technique is not without problems. Taxpayers who want to maximize the amount of wealth that their heirs ultimately receive must balance the trade-offs between giving the property during their lifetime or willing the property at death.

If a taxpayer gives appreciating property during life, the gift removes any appreciation from the estate. However, the basis of the property to the donee will normally be the same as the donor's basis. In such case, the donee would be required to pay an income tax on a subsequent sale of the property. Note that this income tax would not have resulted had the property been retained till death due to the step-up in basis for inherited property. Moreover, if the taxpayer must pay gift tax on the transfer, the time value of any gift tax paid would be lost. In short, a gift of appreciating property normally saves transfer taxes at a rate up to 45 percent but results in an income tax of up to 15 percent (assuming the property is a capital asset) and loss of the time value of gift tax (net of estate tax). Conversely, retaining the property normally saves on income taxes but at the cost of an estate tax on the appreciation.

Example 28. In 1991, T purchased 300 acres of land on the far west side of Dallas for $100,000. While the land was truly in a remote area, T expected that it would one day be prime property since it is near an interstate highway. By 2000, it was clear that an increase in the value of the property was imminent. Assume the property will triple in value to $300,000 by the time T dies in 10 years. Also assume that the transfer tax rate is 45%, the applicable income tax rate is 15%, and the aftertax interest rate is 8%. The following is a simple comparison (ignoring present values) of what happens if (1) T gives the property now, or (2) holds it until death.

1.	Give property now before it appreciates		Tax cost
	Gift tax now ($100,000 × 45%)		$ 45,000
	Income tax to beneficiaries later due to carryover basis		
	Gift: [($300,000 − $100,000 = $200,000) × 15%]		30,000
	Value of gift tax paid today lost:		
	Gift tax ($45,000 × 8% × 10 years)	$36,000	
	Estate tax [$36,000 − (45% × $36,000)]	(19,800)	16,200
	Tax cost		$ 91,200

2.	Retain property until death	Tax cost
	Estate tax later ($300,000 × 45%)	$135,000
	No income tax later	
	Bequest ($300,000 − $300,000 = $0 × 15%).............	0
	Tax cost	$135,000

In this case, it would appear that giving the property away during T's life would produce a smaller overall tax cost than retaining it till death. However, this result is based on many assumptions and fails to consider many others. Nevertheless, the example illustrates some of the basic considerations that should be taken into account when doing estate planning.

Interests in Closely Held Businesses. For individuals who have a stake in a business, such as stock in a family-held C or S corporation or an interest in a partnership or LLC, the interest in the company is not only their lifeblood but in most cases represents a substantial portion of their estate. Indeed, the business often represents the bulk of the assets that they wish to leave to their heirs. Unfortunately, without proper planning, the costs associated with transferring such business (e.g., illiquidity, the estate, gift and generation-skipping transfer taxes, probate) can decimate the business, leaving the heirs with little or no inheritance. Over the years, practitioners have addressed these problems in a number of ways. Most of these plans are directed at valuation of the assets and how that value can be reduced and frozen. In this regard, it should not be forgotten that for estate and gift tax purposes, the minimum marginal tax rate is 45 percent, meaning that every $1,000 of reduced valuation produces $450 of savings!

Closely held businesses normally present valuation problems of monumental proportions. The difficulty lies in the fact that, unlike their publicly traded cousins, there is no market where closely held businesses are actively traded.

For its part, the government's primary contribution concerning the valuation problem is contained in the often cited Revenue Ruling 59-60. In this ruling, the IRS has identified a list of factors to be considered in valuing such businesses. These are:

1. Book value and financial condition of the corporation.

2. Earning capacity of the company.

3. Dividend paying capacity.

4. Whether the enterprise has goodwill or other intangible value.

5. The economic outlook in general and the condition and outlook of the specific industry in particular.

6. The nature of the business and the history of the enterprise from its inception.

7. Sales of stock and the size of the block of stock to be valued.

8. The market price of stocks of corporations engaged in the same or a similar line of business that are actively traded in a free and open market.

Unfortunately, the ruling provides little guidance regarding how these factors are to be used. The ruling simply states that the weight to be accorded each factor depends upon the facts of each case. While experts in business valuation (a niche industry in and of itself) utilize these and other widely accepted methods, there is no certainty that the value obtained is objective and unbiased. As a practical matter, the estate is left to its own devices to determine the value of the company and convince the IRS and/or judge that its method and value are correct.

Valuation: Premiums and Discounts. In establishing the value of an interest in a closely held company, additional value is generally attributed to the interest if it represents control. A so-called *control premium* is warranted since it enables the holder to extract more value from the firm through his or her ability to dominate management. For example, an individual with control can elect the entire board of directors, remove a director, control the business and affairs of the company, elect and remove all of the officers, fix their salaries, and control the declaration of dividends. The major valuation issue when control is present is determining how much value, if any should be assigned to the control element. This has often been the source of a great deal of controversy.

Example 29. The uncertainties of valuation are made abundantly clear in *Estate of Joseph E. Salsbury*[37]. In this case, the value of the company, particularly the amount of premium, was the primary issue. Salsbury died holding 51.8% of the stock of Salsbury Laboratories, a manufacturer of drug and health products for the poultry industry. At the time of his death, all of the stock of the corporation was owned by the decedent, members of his family, trusts for their benefit and a private charitable foundation. The IRS asserted an estate tax deficiency of $6,007,503 primarily attributable to the difference in values placed on the stock held by the decedent. The date of death values placed on the decedent's shares by the parties and the expert witnesses for the taxpayer and the IRS were worlds apart as shown below:

Value claimed on estate tax return	$ 372,152
Value asserted by the IRS in deficiency notice	11,655,000
Expert witness for the taxpayer	558,228
Expert witness for the IRS	8,748,152
Expert witness for the IRS	1,400,000

The sole issue of contention regarding the valuation was the amount that should be assigned to the control element held by the decedent. Note the difference in valuation even though these are valuation experts. Interestingly, the court ultimately held that the stock was worth $514,000.

Discounts. In contrast to a control premium, a *discount* may be available. Over the years, taxpayers have identified a number of reasons why a discount should be allowed.

It is well accepted that a discount may be appropriate when valuing large blocks of stock. When a taxpayer owns such a large block of stock that the price at which the stock would be traded in the market would *not* be representative of the value, a *blockage discount* may be claimed. Blockage discounts are available if the executor can show that the block of stock to be valued is so large in relation to the actual sales on the existing market that the stock could not be liquidated in a reasonable time without depressing the market.

---

[37] T.C. Memo 1975-33.

Discounts have also been granted for the tax consequences that could result upon a disposition of the business. For example, if a taxpayer owns stock in a C corporation, the ultimate value that the owner can extract from the company can be substantially reduced because of the double taxation problems that can occur on liquidation of the corporation.

By far the most important types of discount are those available if the taxpayer's ownership represents a minority interest or where there is lack of marketability or both. In reviewing the court decisions addressing this issue, it is not uncommon to see discounts of between 25 and 50 percent and sometimes more! With proper planning, taxpayers can successfully secure these discounts to obtain literally huge savings. For this reason, understanding the justification for these discounts and the techniques used to achieve them is extremely important.

The lack of marketability discount is based on the fact that an interest in a closely held business is generally less attractive because it is illiquid—hard to convert to cash—and more difficult to sell than an interest for which there is an active trading market. This is a particularly acute problem when the majority of interests are owned by family members. Stock that if publicly traded would be worth $1,000,000 would be worth far less because it would be unlikely to find an outside buyer to purchase the stock. Adding to the discount is the fact there would be substantial costs incurred such as underwriting expenses involved if a company were to go public.

The rationale for *minority interest discounts* is founded upon the owner's limited power to influence business decisions (e.g., control day-to-day or long-range managerial decisions, affect future earnings, control efforts for growth potential, establish executive compensation or dividend policy, or compel a sale of assets or a liquidation). As a practical matter, a discount is warranted due to the fact that an unrelated party interested in purchasing an interest in a family-owned business would not pay full value for such an interest.

> **Example 30.** D owns all of the stock of Close Corporation, which has a value of $9,000,000. If D were to die, the entire value of the stock would be included in his estate. D might be able to reduce the transfer cost substantially if he were to give one-third of the stock to his son, one-third to his daughter and die holding one-third. At first thought, it might appear that the value of the gifts would be one-third of the total or aggregate value or $3,000,000 each. However, by arguing that the each gift constitutes a minority interest, he may be able to claim a substantial discount when he makes the gifts or at death.

The IRS has not always accepted the minority discount theory, particularly when the person acquiring the interest is related. Historically, the government consistently argued that for purposes of valuing gifts and bequests of stock or partnership interests to family members, the ownership interests of the family members should be aggregated and valued as a whole.[38] Applying this approach to the example above, the IRS may take the position that no discount is allowed and the value of each gift is $3,000,000. In fact, when the IRS took this approach, using an aggregate value, it often included a control premium, and then used the increased value as the basis for assigning a value to the fraction of shares transferred.

After years of denying taxpayers minority discounts in the family setting, the IRS finally abandoned its position. In Revenue Ruling 93-12, the IRS stated that it would no longer challenge a discount solely because the transferred interest, when aggregated with interests held by family members, would be considered part of a controlling

---

[38] See Revenue Ruling 81-253 1981-2 C.B. 187 which held that no minority interest discount would be allowed for intrafamily transfers of stock in a corporation controlled by the family absent discord among the family members.

interest.[39] For example, when the taxpayer transferred all of his stock in equal gifts to each of his 11 children, the IRS ruled that the value of the gift to each is computed by considering each gift separately and not by aggregating all of the donor's holdings.[40]

Since the government's surrender in 1993, fractionalizing an owner's interest to obtain minority discounts has become virtually an indispensable part of estate planning. As explained below, corporate and partnership freezes, particularly the use of family limited partnerships, has become a staple of the estate planning industry.

Freezing the Value of the Estate: C Corporations. To freeze the transfer tax value of an interest in a C corporation, the corporation engages in a type "E" reorganization referred to as a recapitalization. The following steps are taken:

1. The owner exchanges common stock for both new voting preferred and new non-voting common which together has a value equal to his original shares of common.

2. Pursuant to the reorganization provisions of § 368(a)(1)(E), this exchange of stock is nontaxable.

3. At the time of the exchange, the preferred stock is structured to represent the majority of the value of the corporation while the common stock has little value. The preferred stock typically carried a fixed-rate, non-cumulative dividend and preferential treatment for dividends and assets upon liquidation. Other rights and privileges may be attached.

4. The owner gives the nonvoting common stock to the heirs at little or no gift tax cost since all of the value of the corporation is in the preferred stock which is held by the owner.

5. The result is that all of the future appreciation of the corporation is attributable to the common stock and shifted to the donees since the preferred stock's value is locked in at time of exchange (i.e., its value is attributable to its preferred claim on assets in the event of liquidation and its yield). Moreover, the owner has retained income security.

Example 31. F owns all of the voting common stock of C corporation with a value of $1,500,000 (basis $100,000). Approaching retirement, F wants to transfer the ownership of the business to his daughter and do so at the least possible tax cost. In addition, he wants to maintain control of the business and retain a steady stream of income for life. To this end, he exchanged his voting common stock for nonvoting common stock worth $1,000,000 and voting preferred stock with a par value set such that it is equal to $500,000. F has a non-cumulative "put" with the corporation that enables him to sell the preferred stock back to the corporation at its par value of $500,000. The preferred stock pays a non-cumulative dividend of 15 percent. The put and the dividend enable F to claim the stock is at least worth $500,000 since at any time the stock could be sold to the corporation for $500,000. F realizes a gain of $1,400,000 ($500,000 + $1,000,000 − $100,000) but under the reorganization provisions this gain is not recognized. F subsequently gives the common worth $1,000,000 ($1,500,000 total value − $500,000 value of preferred) to his daughter and pays no gift tax due to the unified credit which shelters the $1,000,000 taxable gift. If the value of the preferred is respected, F has (1) retained control of the corporation since he owns all of the voting stock, (2) ensured a steady stream of income for retirement since he can vote himself a dividend at any time, (3) frozen

---

[39] 1993-1 C.B. 202.

[40] TAM 9449001.

the value of his estate at $500,000 and (4) shifted all of the appreciation to his daughter who holds the common stock. As might be expected, in these situations, the Service was reluctant to accept the value placed on the preferred since it was unlikely that F would ever exercise his put nor would he ever vote himself a dividend.

While this plan can be used successfully, there are certain restrictions that limit its value as discussed below.

Freezing the Value of the Estate: Partnerships. Steps similar to that used in freezing the value of an interest in a family-held C corporation can be taken to freeze the value of an interest in a partnership (or LLC). In addition, a partnership could be used to freeze the value of appreciating property such as farms, ranches, timberland, and other unimproved or improved real estate. The partnership form provides an almost perfect vehicle to fractionalize interests in the property to create minority discounts. A partnership freeze normally involves recapitalizing an existing partnership or the formation of a new partnership. Family limited partnerships are the vehicle commonly used. The following steps are taken:

1. The owners of property (e.g., the senior members of the family such as parents or grandparents) normally transfer the property to a limited partnership in exchange for (1) a general partnership interest which represents growth interest and (2) a limited partnership interest which represents the frozen interest.

2. The exchange normally is nontaxable under § 721.

3. The transferors retain a small general partnership interest and transfer a large limited partnership interest.

Example 32. H and W transfer 1,000 acres of land worth $10,000,000 to a family limited partnership. In exchange H and W each receive one percent general partnership interests and 49% limited partnership interests. H and W then transfer the limited partnership interests to their children. Significant discounts are normally available for transfers of limited partnership interests. Normally there is a minority interest discount since limited partners have no control over the partnership (e.g., no voice in management and no right to force a liquidation) as well as a lack of marketability discount since such interests are usually illiquid.

Valuation Issues in Corporate and Partnership Freezes. The approach normally used to value the interest transferred in a corporate or partnership freeze is a residual one. The entire business is valued and then the value of the retained interest is identified. Any residual value is the value of the transferred interest. This method is show in the formula below.

FMV of business
− FMV of retained interest
= FMV of transferred interest and gift to heirs

For many years, planners kept the value of the transferred interest (e.g., the common stock) low by assigning valuable rights to the retained interest (e.g., the preferred stock) in order to increase the value of the retained interest. For example, in a preferred stock freeze, these included an above market-rate cumulative (and often noncumulative) dividend, conversion rights, call rights, liquidation preferences and voting rights. Even if it

was clear that it was unlikely that those rights would be exercised, the courts usually took them into account in valuing the preferred stock.[41]

Congress became concerned about assigning value to these "discretionary" rights given to the owner in that such rights probably would not be exercised. To address this problem, in 1987 Congress enacted the now infamous anti-freeze rules of §2036(c) that were so controversial that they were subsequently repealed in 1990. In their place, Congress substituted § 2701, which contains the rules currently in operation today. Section 2701 attempts to more accurately value the property that is transferred among family members when the transferor retains some interest in the business. The approach is to value certain retained discretionary rights (e.g., rights to dividends or distributions, liquidation rights, put, call, and conversion rights) at *zero* unless they meet tests that virtually guarantee their exercise. Note that if these retained rights are valued at zero, a transfer of the common stock or limited partnership interests would be treated as a gift of the full fair market value of the business.

Section 2701 generally operates only if the following conditions exist (note this is the normal pattern of a corporate or partnership freeze discussed above):

1. The taxpayer makes a transfer of an interest in a corporation or partnership.

2. The transferor controls the entity. Control is defined as ownership of at least 50 percent of the entity either directly or indirectly.

3. The transfer is made to a family member (i.e., spouse, lineal descendant of the transferor or spouse, or a spouse of such descendant).

4. The transferor retains an applicable retained right (distribution rights).

In general, the retained interests must provide for a periodic *qualified payment* (e.g., a dividend or distribution). If there is no provision for qualified payments, no value may be assigned to the retained interest, resulting in a gift of the full value of the business.

Qualified Payments. A qualified payment depends on the type of entity. For corporations, a qualified payment is any dividend payable at a fixed rate on a periodic basis on cumulative preferred stock. For partnerships, a qualified payment is a comparable payment at a fixed rate made with respect to any partnership interest. The value of the retained interest must be determined by calculating the present value of the future cash flows from the retained interest or more precisely discounting the qualified payment. No value is assigned to any other rights (put, call, conversion) attached to the stock or partnership interest. Note that if a very low payout rate is selected, there will be a lower annual cash payout required but there will also be a lower value placed on the preferred stock or retained partnership interest. In contrast, if there is a high payout rate, the value of the retained interest is greater, yielding a smaller gift. However, selecting a high payout rate in order to increase the value of the retained interest and reduce the value of the gifted interest has the effect of returning more value (e.g., dividends) to the taxpayer's estate. In any event, a minimum value is placed on the common stock or partnership interest that is transferred. At least 10 percent of the value of the business must be assigned to the gifted stock or partnership interest. This ensures that there is a gift of at least 10 percent of the value of the corporation.

> **Example 33.** This year D decided to transfer her business, a C corporation, to her children. To this end, she exchanged all of her common stock in the corporation for nonvoting common and voting preferred in a transaction qualifying as a tax-free recapitalization. After the transfer, D owned 3,000 shares of $1,000 par value voting preferred stock, each share paying a cumulative annual dividend of seven percent. In

---

[41]   Rev. Rul. 83-120, 1983-2 C.B. 170.

addition, there are 10,000 shares of nonvoting common stock outstanding. D gave all of the common stock to her daughter. Pursuant to an appraisal, the corporation's value was estimated to be $3,100,000. The value of the preferred stock must be determined by discounting the future dividends. Here the annual dividends are $210,000 ($1,000 par value × 7% = $70 per share × 3,000 shares). According to the regulations, the value is determined by assuming that the dividend is paid in perpetuity. Assuming the applicable federal rate is ten percent, the present value of a $210,000 annuity discounted at ten percent is $2,100,000 (1/.1 × $210,000). Thus the value of the preferred is $2,100,000 and the value of the common is $1,000,000 ($3,100,000 − $2,100,000). Consequently, D is treated as making a $1,000,000 gift. If D has not made any other taxable gifts during her lifetime, the entire transfer is tax-free. More important, if the corporation's value increases at a rate greater than the dividend rate of seven percent, all of the excess appreciation is attributable to the common and, therefore, out of her estate.

Family Limited Partnerships. Although the corporate or partnership freeze can be useful, the qualified payment requirement can be a difficult hurdle when trying to accomplish the taxpayer's goals. For this reason, some plans do not meet or do not attempt to meet the qualified payment rule. In such case, the gift is the full value of the interest. However, to minimize this problem, a family limited partnership (FLP) is often formed to create minority and marketability discounts that reduce the value of the transferred interests.

Example 34. H and W, husband and wife, together own all of the stock of a corporation worth $4,000,000. As part of a plan to transfer the stock to their children, they transfer all of the stock to a limited partnership in exchange for a one percent general partnership interest and a 99 percent limited partnership interest. The couple then transfers the limited partnership interest to their children, claiming minority and marketability discounts totaling 50 percent. As a result, the partnership interests transferred by each are about $1,000,000 each and totally tax free because of the unified credit.

Due to the power of the FLP, they have become extremely popular and, at the same time, frequently abused. The most flagrant situations involve transfers of publicly traded securities to FLPs and taking substantial discounts. Although the IRS retreated in their challenge of such arrangements in Revenue Ruling 93-12, it is now pursuing these with some recent successes. Only time will tell the final outcome.[42]

Sales of Property. Another technique for freezing the value of an asset in a taxpayer's estate is for the taxpayer to sell the asset to a younger generation family member.

Example 35. Grandfather G owns several acres of undeveloped real estate with a current value of $1 million. The land is located near a rapidly growing metropolitan area and its value is expected to triple over the next decade. If G sells the real estate to his granddaughter D for $1 million cash, the value of his current estate is unchanged. However, the future increase in the value of the land has been removed from G's estate and will belong to D. In addition, D's basis is at least equal to the value of the property at the time of the transfer rather than G's basis had it been gifted.

An attractive variation of the selling technique illustrated in *Example 35* is an installment sale to the granddaughter. If D does not have $1 million of cash readily available (a most realistic assumption), G could simply accept his granddaughter's bona fide installment note as payment for the land. If the note is to be paid off over 20 years, G could use the installment sale method of reporting any taxable gain on the sale. If

---

[42] For example, see *Estate of Charles Reichardt v. Comm.*, 114 T.C. 144 (2000)

G had no need for cash during the term of the note, he could forgive his granddaughter's note payments and interest as they become due. Such forgiveness of indebtedness would not change the income tax consequences of the installment sale to G and would represent a gift to D eligible for the annual $11,000 exclusion.[43]

GRITs, GRATs, and GRUTs. Another freezing technique that gained popularity over the years is the so-called *GRIT*, the acronym for *grantor retained income trust*. Under this arrangement, the grantor transfers property to a trust, retains the income for a period of years, and gifts the remainder. Under the right circumstances, substantial benefits can be obtained. If the grantor survives the term, nothing is pulled back into the grantor's estate under § 2036 since the grantor did not retain an interest until death. As a result, the taxpayer has transferred the property at the cost of a gift tax on the remainder which normally represents only a fraction of the value of the entire property. In addition, all of the appreciation in the property is out of the estate. Note, however, that if the grantor does not survive the term, the property is included in the estate at its date of death value and nothing has been accomplished.

Example 36. R owns rapidly appreciating real estate. Its current value is $3,000,000. In 2009, he transferred the property to a trust, retaining the income from the property for 10 years and giving the remainder to his son. Assume the income interest is worth $2,000,000. As a result, the remainder interest is $1,000,000 and due to the unified credit there is no gift tax on the transfer. Eleven years after the transfer R died when the property was worth $9,000,000. Under prior law, nothing would be included in R's gross estate under § 2036 since he did not have an interest in the property at the time of his death. Moreover, if the property did not in reality produce any income, the $2,000,000 assigned to the retained interest is a fiction and is never subject to income or estate taxes. Thus, if R survives the transfer by more than 10 years, he was able to transfer property worth $9,000,000 and avoid all transfer tax.

Example 37. Same facts as above except R died five years after the trust was created. In such case, all of the property is included in R's gross estate at its date of death value and nothing will have been accomplished.

Historically, the value of the retained income interest in a GRIT was determined using IRS tables that often placed a higher value on the retained income interest than was justified by the actual income generated on the property. The effect of this was to deflate the value of the gift of the remainder which could be sheltered by the donor's unified credit. As might be expected, the IRS attacked this technique primarily on the grounds that the retained income interest was undervalued. Consequently, legislation was enacted to ensure that the value of the income interest was indeed real.

Under § 2702, the value of the retained income interest is *zero* and the gifted value of the remainder is the entire value of the property unless the transfer is to a *grantor retained annuity trust (GRAT)* or a grantor retained unit trust (GRUT). When either of these is used, the value of the gift of the remainder is the value of the property less the value of the annuity or unitrust interest as shown below.

Fair market value of property
Value of income interest
FMV of remainder and gift to heirs (no exclusion since future interest)

When the transfer is made, the grantor specifies how much income will be retained [e.g., either a fixed dollar amount (i.e., an annuity trust) or a percentage of the annual asset

---

43   See Rev. Rul. 77-299, 1977-2 C.B. 343 for the IRS's negative reaction to this tax plan.

value (i.e., a unitrust)] as well as the period for which the annuity will last. If the grantor retains an annuity interest, the arrangement is referred to as a GRAT. If the grantor retains a unitrust interest, the arrangement is called a GRUT. Note that in either case the income interest-retained annuity effectively replaces the transferred property. One of the biggest differences between a GRIT and GRATs and GRUTs is that annual payments under GRATs and GRUTs *must be made* even if the trust assets do not generate sufficient income to make the payments. Trust principal may have to be invaded to meet the distribution requirement (however, a debt obligation may suffice).

> **Example 38.** In 1997, R transferred land worth $1,000,000 to a GRAT. He wanted the amount of the gift of the remainder interest to be $600,000 in order to use his unified credit (exemption equivalent of $600,000 in 1997), but no more. R is 55 and he decides to use a term of 15 years to compute the required annuity. The present value of an annuity of $1 for 15 years using the IRS tables and a discount rate of 10% is $7.6061. Thus the present value of an annuity of $52,589 ($400,000/7.6061) at 10% for 15 years is $400,000. Therefore to achieve the desired result, the annuity rate is set at 5.26% and payments of $52,589 must be paid annually, even if the property does not generate sufficient income. This departs drastically from the GRIT where no payment was required if there was in fact no income. Note that if R lives the entire term, he will receive $788,835 ($52,589 × 15) which is the original $400,000 retained income interest plus the growth on the $400,000 at 10% for 15 years. Although R's estate may contain $788,835, he will have removed any appreciation from his estate. In short, if the property appreciates (or produces income at a rate exceeding the annuity rate) all of the excess appreciation or income is removed from his estate. In addition, R could remove part of this $788,835 by embarking on a gift-giving program.

MARITAL DEDUCTION PLANNING

At first glance, it would appear that all of a decedent's property should be left to his or her spouse to avoid estate taxes. However, using the marital deduction to reduce a decedent's taxable estate to zero could result in a waste of the decedent's unified credit under § 2010. Moreover, all of the property would be taxed as part of the surviving spouse's estate to the extent it is not consumed or given away. For these reasons, an effective estate plan usually attempts to leave a *taxable estate* exactly equal to the tax shelter provided by this credit.

> **Example 39.** H and W are happily married. The couple currently has simple wills, providing that upon either's death, all of the assets of one will be left to the other. Upon the death of the survivor, all of the assets are to be passed to the children. They both had assets worth $3,500,000 for a total of $7,000,000. In 2009, H died with an estate of $3,500,000 and left it all to W who dies shortly thereafter. In this case, the estate passing to the kids shrinks by a tax liability of $1,575,000 as computed below.

	1st to Die	Surviving Spouse
Gross estate	$3,500,000	$7,000,000
Marital deduction	(3,500,000)	—
Taxable estate	$ 0	$7,000,000
Tax	$ 0	$3,030,000
Unified credit	—	(1,455,800)
Tax due	$ 0	$1,575,000

Note that with this simple, but common, arrangement H has wasted his unified credit. In contrast, had H left his estate of $3,500,000 to his children and W had done the same, both would have utilized their unified credits and neither would have paid any estate tax as shown below. As a result, the children would be better off by the taxes saved of $1,575,000! In short, with just a small amount of planning, a married couple in 2009 can pass $7,000,000 to their heirs tax-free. Note that due to the gradually increasing exemption amount, a will must be carefully drawn to ensure that the exemption is fully utilized.

	1st to Die	Surviving Spouse
Gross estate.	$3,500,000	$3,500,000
Marital deduction	—	—
Taxable estate	$3,500,000	$3,500,000
Tax	$1,455,800	$1,455,800
Unified credit	(1,455,800)	(1,455,800)
Tax due.	$ 0	$ 0

The unlimited marital deduction permits a deferral of any estate tax on the wealth accumulated by a married couple until the death of the second spouse. This deferral can be highly advantageous even if the bequest to the surviving spouse causes the wealth to be subsequently taxed at a higher marginal tax rate.

Example 40. W died in 2001 with a net estate of $1,400,000. W's will provides that all her wealth in excess of the amount sheltered by the available unified credit shall pass to her husband, H. At the time of her death, the credit shelters a taxable estate of $625,000; therefore, $775,000 of her estate is transferred to her husband and becomes a marital deduction against W's gross estate. No estate tax is due upon W's death. If H has $3.5 million of wealth in addition to his $775,000 inheritance from W, and if he outlives his wife by five years, the estate tax upon his death in 2009 is $348,750 [($555,800 + .45 × ($4,275,000 − $1,500,000 = $2,775,000) = $1,804,550) − $1,455,800 credit].[44]

If W had not left any of her estate to H, the estate tax payable on her death would have been $310,750 ($512,800 tax − $202,050 unified credit), computed at a marginal rate of 43 percent. However, because of the marital bequest, her estate was "stacked" on that of her surviving spouse. As a result, the actual tax on her estate was $348,750 computed at a marginal rate of 45 percent ($775,000 × .45).[45] But the actual tax payment was deferred for five years. Using a discount rate of 8 percent, the present value of a $348,750 tax paid at the end of five years is only $273,255 ($348,750 × 0.7835). Thus, the use of the unlimited marital deduction saved the family of H and W approximately $75,495 ($348,750 − $273,255) in estate taxes.

In addition to the deferral of tax available through use of the unlimited marital deduction; the postponement of tax until the death of the second spouse increases the length of time during which estate planning objectives can be accomplished. The surviving spouse can continue or even accelerate a program of inter vivos giving to younger generation family members. Deferral also provides the surviving spouse with the opportunity to seek advice about areas of estate planning neglected before the death of the first spouse.

---

[44] For simplicity's sake, this example assumes no appreciation in assets between the two deaths.

[45] $348,750 is the difference between $348,750 (the tax on H's estate of $2,775,000 including his inheritance from W) and zero tax (the tax on H's estate of $2,000,000 without an inheritance from W).

QUALIFYING TERMINAL INTEREST PROPERTY

Section 2056(b) denies a marital deduction for an interest in property that passes to a surviving spouse if the interest will terminate at some future date and if after termination someone other than the surviving spouse will receive an interest in the property. This restriction was designed to ensure that assets escaping taxation in the estate of the first spouse by virtue of a marital deduction do, in fact, become the property of the surviving spouse includible in that spouse's taxable estate.

Prior to the enactment of the Economic Recovery Tax Act of 1981 (ERTA 1981), a wealthy taxpayer desiring to secure the tax savings offered by the use of the marital deduction had to be willing to entrust to his or her surviving spouse the ultimate disposition of the assets passing to that spouse. Because of § 2056(b), the surviving spouse had to receive control over the transferred assets sufficient to pull the assets into that spouse's gross estate. This generally required an outright transfer of the property to the surviving spouse, or transfer in trust giving the spouse a general power of appointment. In certain situations wealthy taxpayers were reluctant to accept this condition. For example, a taxpayer with children from a previous marriage might be concerned that his surviving second wife might not leave the marital deduction assets to these children upon her death. As a result, the taxpayer might not take advantage of the marital deduction in order to leave his wealth directly to his children.

To increase the utility of the marital deduction, Congress added § 2056(b)(7) to the law as part of ERTA 1981. This paragraph allows a marital deduction equal to the value of *qualifying terminable interest property*. Such property is defined as property in which the surviving spouse is entitled to all the income, payable at least annually for life. During the life of the spouse, no one may have a power to appoint any part of the property to anyone other than the spouse.

> **Example 41.** Under the will of X, $1 million worth of assets are transferred into trust. X's surviving spouse, S, must be paid the entire trust income on a quarterly basis. During S's life, no person has any power of appointment over trust corpus, and upon S's death, trust corpus will be divided equally among X's living grandchildren. Because the assets are qualifying terminable interest property, X's estate may claim a marital deduction of $1 million.

Upon the death of the surviving spouse, the entire date of death value of the qualifying terminable interest property must be included in the surviving spouse's gross estate per § 2044. Thus, even though the property is passing to a recipient chosen by the first spouse to die, it is taxed in the estate of the second spouse.[46]

CHARITABLE GIVING

Another important tool that estate planners often use to reduce a family's tax burden is the charitable transfer. Obviously, an individual can reduce or even eliminate any estate taxes by simply leaving part or all of his or her property to a qualified charity. As explained in Chapter 24, bequests to qualified charitable organizations may be deducted from the gross estate without limitation. However, from a tax planning perspective it is usually preferable for the taxpayer to make a charitable donation during life rather than at death.

---

[46] If the surviving spouse gives away the income interest in the qualifying terminable interest property during life, § 2519 requires that the entire value of the property constitute a taxable gift. When either § 2044 or § 2519 applies, § 2207(A) allows the estate or donor to recover an appropriate amount of transfer tax from the party receiving the actual property.

While many individuals would like to make large contributions of property to a charity during their lifetime, they often delay the contribution to their deaths believing they may need the income and the property before that time. Unfortunately, these kind-hearted donors, while securing the contribution deduction for estate tax purposes, lose the income tax deduction. On the other hand, some individuals may be willing to give the property and its income to a charity temporarily but ultimately want to pass the property to their heirs. Long ago charitable organizations recognized these problems and designed a solution, the so-called split interest gift.

A split-interest gift is simply a transfer of property—typically to a trust—where part of the property is given to a charity and the other part is retained by the donor. There are two common types of charitable trusts: charitable remainder trusts, and charitable lead trusts.

Charitable Remainder Trusts. With a charitable remainder trust, an individual transfers property to a trust, leaving the income from the property to a noncharitable beneficiary (e.g., a spouse or child) typically for life, and upon the beneficiary's death, the property passes to the charitable beneficiary. The beauty of a charitable remainder trust is that the donor retains the security of a steady income stream yet is entitled to an income tax deduction for the present value of the remainder interest—a deduction that would be lost had the gift been postponed until death. In order to secure the deduction for the remainder interest, a number of special requirements must be met to ensure that the charity in fact receives something once the income interest terminates.

Charitable Lead Trusts. Charities also have an answer for individuals who wish to transfer property and its income to a charity for a period of years yet want the property returned after the term has run. The solution is referred to as a charitable lead trust. In this case, the donor receives both an income and gift-tax deduction for the present value of the income interest given to the charity. However, the income tax deduction is limited to 20 percent of A.G.I., since it is for the "use of the charity" rather than "to the" charity. No carryover is allowed.

For many years, the grantor of a charitable lead trust was not charged with the income of the trust but simply got a deduction for income given to the trust that he was never taxed on! In 1969, Congress believed that this was an "unwarranted tax advantage"—a duplication of benefits—and eliminated such favorable treatment. Currently, the trust must be a grantor trust to qualify. The effect in such case is to accelerate the deduction to the current year, yet defer the income to the year it is actually received.

Using a charitable lead trust is particularly beneficial when taxpayers want to bunch all of their charitable deductions in one year. Bunching or accelerating deductions to a particular year may be advantageous in situations when taxpayers have a particularly good year with high income and need the deduction or they simply expect to be in a lower bracket in the future. As with charitable remainder trusts, a number of requirements must be met in order to secure the deduction for the income interest.

Example 42. This year J sold his business, recognizing a large amount of income. To offset some of this income, J gave $100,000 to a charitable lead trust for his alma mater, the University of Nebraska. According to the terms of the gift, the university receives the income for the next five years after which the property is returned to J. Assuming the present value of the income over the next five years is $60,000, J receives a $60,000 deduction this year. Assume that next year, the trust earns $12,000. Because J has retained a reversionary interest that reverts too quickly, the trust is a grantor trust and J is taxed on the income of $12,000.

LIQUIDITY PLANNING

The Federal estate tax is literally a once-in-a-lifetime event. Because taxpayers do not have to pay the tax on a regular recurring basis, many individuals give little thought to the eventual need for cash to pay the tax.

When an individual dies leaving a large estate but little cash with which to pay death taxes and other expenses, serious problems can result. The family may be forced to sell assets at distress prices just to obtain cash. In a severe situation, a decedent's carefully designed dispositive plan may be shattered because of the failure to anticipate the liquidity needs of the estate.

One of the functions of a competent tax adviser is to foresee any liquidity problem of his or her client's potential estate and to suggest appropriate remedies. The remainder of this chapter covers some of the common solutions to the problem of a cash-poor estate.

SOURCE OF FUNDS

An excellent source of funds with which to pay an estate tax is insurance on the life of the potential decedent. For a relatively small cash outlay, a taxpayer can purchase enough insurance coverage to meet all the liquidity needs of his or her estate. It is absolutely vital that the insured individual does not possess any incidents of ownership in the policies and that his or her estate is not the beneficiary of the policies. If these two rules are observed the policy proceeds will not be included in the insured's estate and needlessly subjected to the estate tax.[47]

A second source of funds is any family business in which the decedent owned an interest. Under the terms of a binding buy-sell agreement, the business could use its cash to liquidate the decedent's interest. If the business is in corporate form, a redemption of the decedent's interest under § 303 can be a highly beneficial method of securing funds. If the fairly straightforward requirements of § 303 are met, the corporation can purchase its own stock from the decedent's estate without danger of the payment being taxed as a dividend. Because the estate's basis in the stock has been stepped up to its fair market value at date of death, the estate normally will realize little or no taxable gain on sale. The amount of the corporate distribution protected by § 303 cannot exceed the amount of death taxes and funeral and administrative expenses payable by the estate.[48]

In order for a redemption of stock to qualify under § 303, the value of the stock must exceed 35 percent of the value of the gross estate less § 2053 and § 2054 expenses.[49] Careful pre-death planning may be necessary to meet this requirement.

> **Example 43.** C owns a 100% interest in F Corporation, a highly profitable business with substantial cash flow. However, the value of the F stock is only 29% of the value of C's projected estate. As C's tax adviser, you could recommend that C (1) gift away other assets to reduce the estate, or (2) transfer assets into F Corporation as a contribution to capital in order to increase the stock's value.

---

[47] § 2042.

[48] § 303(a).

[49] § 303(b)(2)(A).

FLOWER BONDS

Certain issues of Treasury bonds known as *flower bonds* may be used to pay the Federal estate tax at their par value plus accrued interest.[50] Because these bonds have very low interest rates, they are obtainable on the open market at a price well below their par value. Thus, an estate can satisfy its Federal tax liability with bonds that cost much less than the amount of that liability. The bonds must be included in the decedent's estate at their par, rather than market value.[51]

PLANNING FOR DEFERRED PAYMENT OF THE ESTATE TAX

Under § 6166, an estate may be entitled to pay its Federal estate tax liability on an installment basis over a 15-year period. This provision can be a blessing for an illiquid estate. However, only estates that meet the requirements of § 6166 may use the installment method of payment. As a result, pre-death planning should be undertaken to ensure qualification.

Basically, only an amount of estate tax attributable to a decedent's interest in a closely held business may be deferred.[52] In addition, the value of the closely held business must exceed 35 percent of the gross estate minus Code § 2053 and § 2054 deductions. If a deferral of estate tax is desirable in a specific situation, the tax adviser should make certain that such requirements are met on a prospective basis.

CONCLUSION

This chapter has introduced the reader to one of the most fascinating and satisfying areas of tax practice—family tax planning. Such planning involves arrangements whereby family income can be shifted to low-bracket members so as to reduce the income taxes paid by the family unit. The use of trusts also has been discussed, and grantor trusts whose income is taxed not to the trust or its beneficiaries but to the grantor have been described.

Transfer tax planning techniques for reducing the family transfer tax burden have been introduced. Such techniques include long-range programs of inter vivos giving, asset freezes, selective use of the marital deduction, and liquidity planning. The family tax planner should never lose sight of the basic premise of family tax planning: only a plan that meets the subjective nontax goals and desires of a family as well as the objective goal of tax minimization is a truly well-designed plan.

PROBLEM MATERIALS

DISCUSSION QUESTIONS

26-1 *Assignment of Income Doctrine.* Explain the assignment of income doctrine as it relates to earned income. How does the doctrine apply to investment income?

26-2 *Income Shifting.* Assignment of income from one taxpayer to another can result in a tax savings only in a tax system with a progressive rate structure. Discuss.

---

[50] § 6312 provided the authorization for such usage. However, the section was repealed with respect to bonds issued after March 3, 1971. Bonds issued before this date and still outstanding continue to be eligible for payment of the estate tax.

[51] Rev. Rul. 69-489, 1969-2 C.B. 172.

[52] § 6166(a)(2).

26-3 *Family Employees.* List some of the factors the IRS might consider in determining whether a particular family member is a bona fide employee of a family business.

26-4 *Shareholder/Employee.* Discuss the tax consequences if the IRS determines that a family member is receiving an amount of unreasonable compensation from a family-owned corporation if that family member is a shareholder. What if the family member is not a shareholder?

26-5 *Gift of Business Interest.* An individual who transfers an equity interest in his or her business to a family member may be accomplishing an income shift to that family member. What are some nontax risks associated with such an equity transfer?

26-6 *Buy-Sell Arrangements.* How may a buy-sell agreement be utilized when an intrafamily transfer of an equity interest in a business is contemplated?

26-7 *Regular Corporation vs. S Corporation.* As a general rule, a regular corporation is an inappropriate vehicle by which to shift business income to low-bracket family members. Discuss.

26-8 *Limitation on Using S Corporations.* An S corporation may have only a single class of common stock outstanding. How does this fact limit the utility of the S corporation in many family tax plans?

26-9 *Use of Grantor Trusts.* Grantor trusts are ineffective as devices for shifting income to trust beneficiaries. However, such trusts may be very useful in achieving nontax family planning goals. Explain.

26-10 *Crummey Trusts.* What is a Crummey trust and why might a grantor prefer a Crummey trust to a § 2503(c) trust?

26-11 *Reversionary Trusts and Interest-Free Loans.* Can a trust in which the grantor has the right to receive his or her property back after a specified period of time be considered a valid trust for tax purposes so that the income is taxed to the beneficiaries rather than the grantor? Can an interest-free demand loan achieve an income shift from the lender to the debtor?

26-12 *Inter Vivos Gifts.* Why are inter vivos gifts beneficial from a transfer tax planning viewpoint?

26-13 *Limitations of Inter Vivos Gifts.* For what reasons might an elderly taxpayer be reluctant to make inter vivos gifts?

26-14 *Estate Freezes.* Define an "asset freeze" as the term relates to estate planning.

26-15 *Current vs. Testamentary Contributions.* Is it preferable to make a charitable contribution during a taxpayer's life or at his or her death under the terms of his or her will?

26-16 *Marital Deduction.* Discuss the tax benefits associated with the unlimited marital deduction of § 2056.

26-17 *Limiting Estate Taxes.* Why is it generally inadvisable for a taxpayer to plan to reduce his or her taxable estate to zero? What can be considered an "optimal" size for a decedent's taxable estate?

26-18 *Qualifying Terminable Interests.* In what circumstances would a taxpayer desire to make a bequest to a surviving spouse in the form of qualifying terminable interest property? What are the tax consequences of such a bequest?

PROBLEMS

26-19   *Using Family Employees.* F runs a carpet installation and cleaning business as a sole proprietorship. In the current year, the business generates $83,000 of net income.
   a.   Assume F is married, has three children (all under the age of 19), does not have any other source of taxable income, and does not itemize deductions. What is his current year tax liability?
   b.   Assume F can use all three children in his business as legitimate part-time employees. He pays each child $6,000 per year, but continues to provide more than one-half of their support. Compute the family's total tax bill for the current year.

26-20   *Sole Proprietorship vs. Corporation.* Single individual K owns a sole proprietorship that is K's only source of income. In the current year, the business has net income of $130,000.
   a.   If K does not itemize deductions, what is her current year tax liability?
   b.   If K incorporates the business on January 1 and pays herself a $40,000 salary (and no dividends), by how much will she have reduced the tax bill on her business income? (Assume the corporation will not be a personal service corporation.)

26-21   *Sole Proprietorship vs. Corporation.* Mr. and Mrs. C own their own business, which they currently operate as a sole proprietorship. Annual income from the business averages $400,000. Mr. and Mrs. C are considering incorporating the business. They estimate that each of them could draw a reasonable annual salary of $75,000. In order to maintain their current standard of living, they would also have to draw an additional $50,000 cash out of the business annually in the form of dividends. Based on these facts, compute the income tax savings or cost that would result from the incorporation. In making your calculation, ignore any deductions or exemptions available on the C's joint return.

26-22   *Singles Penalty.* Single taxpayer S has current year taxable income of $35,000 (after all available deductions and exemptions). His fiancé F has a taxable income of $6,000. Assuming they both itemize deductions, and that no deductions are affected by their combined adjusted gross income, should F and S marry before or after December 31? Support your conclusion with calculations.

26-23   *Marriage Penalty.* Taxpayers H and W are married and file a joint return. Both are professionals and earn salaries of $28,000 and $39,000, respectively. Assuming H and W have no other income and do not itemize deductions, compute any *marriage penalty* they will pay.

26-24   *Married vs. Head-of-Household.* Refer to the facts in *Problem 26-23*. Assume H and W are not married and H has a child by a previous marriage that entitles him to file as a head-of-household. If H and W marry, will the marriage penalty they incur be more or less than in *Problem 26-23*?

26-25   *Unearned Income of a Minor Child.* In the current year, taxpayer M receives $12,000 of interest income and earns a salary of $2,500 from a summer job. M has no other income or deductions. M is 13 years old and is claimed as a dependent on his parents' jointly filed tax return. His parents report taxable income of $200,000. Based on these facts, compute M's income tax liability.

26-26   *Sheltering Unearned Income of a Minor Child.* Taxpayer P made a gift of investment securities to his 13-year-old dependent daughter, D, under the Uniform Gift to Minors Act. The securities generate annual dividend income of $4,000. P is considering a second gift to D that would generate an additional $3,000 of investment income annually. Calculate the amount of tax savings to the family if P could employ D in his

business and pay her an annual salary of $3,000, rather than making the second gift. In making your calculation, assume P is in a 40 percent tax bracket.

26-27 *Family Partnerships.* F owns a 70 percent interest in Mako Partnership, in which capital is a material income-producing factor. On January 1 of the current year, F gives his son S a 35 percent interest in Mako (leaving F with a 35% interest). For the current year, Mako has taxable income of $200,000.

    a. Assume F does not perform any services for Mako. What is the maximum amount of partnership income allocable to S?

    b. Assume F performs services for Mako for which he normally would receive $30,000. However, F has not charged the partnership for his services. Based on these facts, what is the maximum amount of partnership income allocable to S in the current year?

26-28 *Gift of S Corporation Stock.* Grandfather G owns all 100 shares of the outstanding stock of Sigma, Inc., a calendar year S corporation. On January 1 of the current year, G gives 10 shares of Sigma stock to each of his four minor grandchildren under the Uniform Gift to Minors Act. For the current year, Sigma reports taxable income of $70,000. To whom is this income taxed?

26-29 *Gift-Leaseback.* Taxpayer B owns land used in his sole proprietorship with a tax basis of $75,000 and a fair market value of $100,000. B gives this land to an irrevocable simple trust for the equal benefit of his three children (ages 19, 20, and 21) and leases back the land from the trust for a fair market rental of $9,000 per year.

    a. Assuming that all three children are B's dependents and have no other source of income, calculate the tax savings to the family of this gift-leaseback arrangement. In making your calculation, assume B is in a 40 percent tax bracket.

    b. What are the gift and estate tax consequences of this transaction to B and his family? Assume that B has made no prior taxable gifts and that he is married.

26-30 *Use of Trusts.* Grandfather Z is in the habit of giving his 20-year-old grandchild, A, $10,000 annually as a gift. Z's taxable income is consistently over $500,000 per year, and A has no income. If Z creates a valid trust with investment assets just sufficient to yield $12,000 of income a year and specifies in the trust instrument that A is to receive the trust income annually, what will be the net tax savings to the family? (For purposes of this problem, assume that A is not a full-time student and *ignore* the fact that A may be claimed as a dependent on the return of another taxpayer.)

26-31 *Reversionary Trusts.* Grantor G transfers $100,000 of assets into a trust that will last for 10 years, after which time the assets will revert to G or his estate. During the trust's existence all income must be paid to beneficiary M on a current basis. For the current year, ordinary trust income is $18,000. To whom is this income taxed?

26-32 *Reversionary Trusts.* Refer to the facts in *Problem 26-31*. Assume that under the terms of the trust agreement the trust will last for M's lifetime. Upon M's death, the trust corpus will revert to G or his estate. On the date the trust is created, M is 18 years old. For the current year, ordinary trust income is $40,000. To whom is this income taxed?

26-33 *Irrevocable Trusts.* F transfers assets into an irrevocable trust and designates First City Bank as independent trustee. F retains no control over the trust assets. The trustee may distribute income to either of F's two adult brothers or to S, F's minor son whom F is legally obligated to support. During the year, the trustee distributed all of the trust income to one of F's brothers. To whom will the income be taxed?

26-34 *Irrevocable Trusts.* M transfers assets into an irrevocable trust and appoints National Bank independent trustee. M retains no control over trust assets. Under the terms of the trust agreement, M's sister N is given the right to determine which of M's three minor children will receive trust income for the year. N herself is not a trust beneficiary.

During the year, N directs that trust income be divided equally among M's three children. To whom will the income be taxed?

26-35 *Irrevocable Trusts.* Grantor B transfers assets into an irrevocable trust and designates Union State Bank independent trustee. B retains no control over trust assets. Under the terms of the trust instrument the trustee must use trust income to pay the annual insurance premium on a policy on B's life. Any remaining income must be distributed to B's grandson, GS. For the current year, trust income totals $60,000, of which $9,000 is used to pay the required insurance premium. To whom will the income be taxed?

26-36 *Grantor Trusts.* Although T is not a beneficiary of the ABC Trust, T does have the right under the terms of the trust instrument to appoint up to 10 percent of the trust assets to himself or any member of his family. T has never exercised this right. For the current year, the trust income of $80,000 is distributed to the income beneficiaries of the trust.
  a. To whom will the income be taxed?
  b. If T dies before exercising his right to appoint trust corpus, will the possession of the right have any estate tax consequences?

26-37 *Gift Splitting.* Every year D gives each of her nine grandchildren $15,000 in cash to be used toward their education.
  a. If D is unmarried, what is the amount of her annual taxable gift?
  b. If D is married and she and her husband elect to "gift split," what is the amount of her annual taxable gift?

26-38 *Terminable Interest Trusts.* Taxpayer Q dies in 2009 and leaves a net estate of $7 million. Under the terms of his will, $3.5 million of the estate will be put into trust. Q's widow, W, will be paid trust income annually and during W's life no person has the right to appoint any of the trust corpus. Upon W's death, the trust corpus will be divided among Q's offspring from a previous marriage. The remaining $3,500,000 of Q's estate is to be paid to unrelated friends named in Q's will.
  a. What is the amount of Q's taxable estate?
  b. What is the estate tax liability on Q's taxable estate? (Q made no taxable gifts during his lifetime.)
  c. W outlives Q by only eight years. If the value of the corpus of the trust created for W's benefit by Q is $6.3 million at the date of W's death, what amount must be included in W's gross estate?

26-39 *Inter Vivos Gifts.* Decedent T died in 2009 and left the following taxable estate:

	Fair Market Value
Investment real estate	$6,000,000
Cash and securities	3,500,000
Gross estate	$9,500,000
Less: § 2053 and § 2054 expenses	(500,000)
Taxable estate	$9,000,000

After payment of all death taxes, the estate will be divided equally among T's five surviving married children.
  a. If T has never made any inter vivos gifts, compute the estate's Federal estate tax liability (before credit for any state death tax paid).
  b. How much tax could have been saved if T had made cash gifts equal to the maximum annual exclusion under § 2503 to each of his children and their spouses in each of the 10 years preceding his death?

26-40   *Power of Giving.* W is thinking about the possibility of dying in the next ten years. She currently has an estate of $5,000,000. Assuming W is in the 45% transfer tax bracket, how much more could she give to her child if she made a gift to her child rather than dying with the entire $5,000,000? Ignore the annual exclusion and the unified credit.

26-41   *Liquidity Planning.* Decedent D left the following taxable estate:

	Fair Market Value
Life insurance proceeds from policy on D's life (D owned the policy at his death)	$4,500,000
Real estate.	1,300,000
Stock in Acme Corporation (100% owned by D)	650,000
Gross estate.	$6,450,000
Less: § 2053 and § 2054 expenses	(450,000)
Taxable estate.	$6,000,000

a.   If D has never made any inter vivos gifts and dies in 2009, what is the estate's Federal estate tax liability (before credit for any state death tax paid)?

b.   How much tax could have been avoided if D had not been the owner of the life insurance policy?

c.   Can the Acme stock qualify for a § 303 redemption? What if the life insurance proceeds were not included in the gross estate?

RESEARCH PROBLEMS

26-42   In 2001, P, a resident of St. Louis, Missouri, created an irrevocable trust for the benefit of his teenage son, S, and his brother, B. The independent trustee, T, has discretionary power to use the trust income for the "payment of tuition, books, and room and board at any institution of higher learning that S chooses to attend." After an 11-year period, the trust will terminate with any accumulated income payable to S and the trust corpus payable to B. In the current year, S received an income distribution of $7,000 from the trust, which he used to attend a state-supported school, the University of Missouri. To whom will the $7,000 of trust income be taxed?

Some suggested research aids:

§ 677 and accompanying regulations

Morrill, Jr. v. United States, 64-1 USTC ¶9463, 13 AFTR2d 1334, 228 F.Supp. 734 (D.Ct. Maine, 1964).

Braun, Jr., 48 TCM 210, T.C. Memo 1984-285.

26-43   Decedent D died on January 19, 2004. Under the terms of D's will, D's sister S, age 57, is to receive $500,000 as a specific bequest. The remainder of D's estate will be distributed to D's various grandchildren. On June 8, 2006, S decides to join a religious community and take a vow of poverty. She makes written notification to the executor of D's estate that she will not accept her bequest from her late sister, and that the $500,000 should be added to the amount to be distributed to the grandchildren. What are the transfer tax consequences of S's action?

Suggested research aid:

§ 2518

★ APPENDICES ★

★ ★ ★ ★ ★ CONTENTS ★ ★ ★ ★ ★

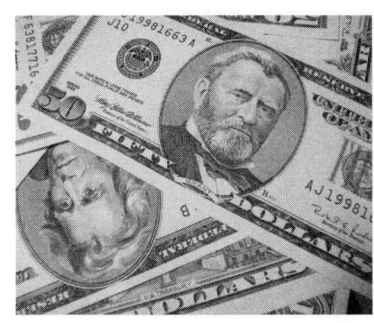

★ APPENDIX A ★

TAX RATE SCHEDULES AND TABLES

		Page Nos.
A-1 | 2008 Income Tax Rate Schedules. . . . . | A-2
A-2 | 2008 Income Tax Tables. . . . . | A-3
A-3 | Unified Transfer Tax Rate Schedule . . . . | A-15
A-4 | Estate and Gift Tax Valuation Tables. . . . . | A-16
A-5 | Optional State Sales Tax Tables. . . . . | A-21

2008 Tax Rate Schedules

The Tax Rate Schedules are shown so you can see the tax rate that applies to all levels of taxable income. Do not use them to figure your tax. Instead, see the instructions for line 44 that begin on page 36.

Schedule X—If your filing status is Single

If your taxable income is: Over—	But not over—	The tax is:	of the amount over—
$0	$8,025	.... 10%	$0
8,025	32,550	$802.50 + 15%	8,025
32,550	78,850	4,481.25 + 25%	32,550
78,850	164,550	16,056.25 + 28%	78,850
164,550	357,700	40,052.25 + 33%	164,550
357,700	....	103,791.75 + 35%	357,700

Schedule Y-1—If your filing status is Married filing jointly or Qualifying widow(er)

If your taxable income is: Over—	But not over—	The tax is:	of the amount over—
$0	$16,050	.... 10%	$0
16,050	65,100	$1,605.00 + 15%	16,050
65,100	131,450	8,962.50 + 25%	65,100
131,450	200,300	25,550.00 + 28%	131,450
200,300	357,700	44,828.00 + 33%	200,300
357,700	....	96,770.00 + 35%	357,700

Schedule Y-2—If your filing status is Married filing separately

If your taxable income is: Over—	But not over—	The tax is:	of the amount over—
$0	$8,025	.... 10%	$0
8,025	32,550	$802.50 + 15%	8,025
32,550	65,725	4,481.25 + 25%	32,550
65,725	100,150	12,775.00 + 28%	65,725
100,150	178,850	22,414.00 + 33%	100,150
178,850	....	48,385.00 + 35%	178,850

Schedule Z—If your filing status is Head of household

If your taxable income is: Over—	But not over—	The tax is:	of the amount over—
$0	$11,450	.... 10%	$0
11,450	43,650	$1,145.00 + 15%	11,450
43,650	112,650	5,975.00 + 25%	43,650
112,650	182,400	23,225.00 + 28%	112,650
182,400	357,700	42,755.00 + 33%	182,400
357,700	....	100,604.00 + 35%	357,700

A-2   2008 Income Tax Tables

2008 Tax Table

See the instructions for line 44 that begin on page 36 to see if you must use the Tax Table below to figure your tax.

Example. Mr. and Mrs. Brown are filing a joint return. Their taxable income on Form 1040, line 43, is $25,300. First, they find the $25,300–25,350 taxable income line. Next, they find the column for married filing jointly and read down the column. The amount shown where the taxable income line and filing status column meet is $2,996. This is the tax amount they should enter on Form 1040, line 44.

Sample Table

At least	But less than	Single	Married filing jointly *	Married filing separately	Head of a household
			Your tax is—		
25,200	25,250	3,383	2,981	3,383	3,211
25,250	25,300	3,390	2,989	3,390	3,219
25,300	25,350	3,398	2,996	3,398	3,226
25,350	25,400	3,405	3,004	3,405	3,234

If line 43 (taxable income) is— At least	But less than	Single	Married filing jointly *	Married filing separately	Head of a household
			Your tax is—		
0	5	0	0	0	0
5	15	1	1	1	1
15	25	2	2	2	2
25	50	4	4	4	4
50	75	6	6	6	6
75	100	9	9	9	9
100	125	11	11	11	11
125	150	14	14	14	14
150	175	16	16	16	16
175	200	19	19	19	19
200	225	21	21	21	21
225	250	24	24	24	24
250	275	26	26	26	26
275	300	29	29	29	29
300	325	31	31	31	31
325	350	34	34	34	34
350	375	36	36	36	36
375	400	39	39	39	39
400	425	41	41	41	41
425	450	44	44	44	44
450	475	46	46	46	46
475	500	49	49	49	49
500	525	51	51	51	51
525	550	54	54	54	54
550	575	56	56	56	56
575	600	59	59	59	59
600	625	61	61	61	61
625	650	64	64	64	64
650	675	66	66	66	66
675	700	69	69	69	69
700	725	71	71	71	71
725	750	74	74	74	74
750	775	76	76	76	76
775	800	79	79	79	79
800	825	81	81	81	81
825	850	84	84	84	84
850	875	86	86	86	86
875	900	89	89	89	89
900	925	91	91	91	91
925	950	94	94	94	94
950	975	96	96	96	96
975	1,000	99	99	99	99

1,000

At least	But less than	Single	Married filing jointly *	Married filing separately	Head of a household
1,000	1,025	101	101	101	101
1,025	1,050	104	104	104	104
1,050	1,075	106	106	106	106
1,075	1,100	109	109	109	109
1,100	1,125	111	111	111	111
1,125	1,150	114	114	114	114
1,150	1,175	116	116	116	116
1,175	1,200	119	119	119	119
1,200	1,225	121	121	121	121
1,225	1,250	124	124	124	124
1,250	1,275	126	126	126	126
1,275	1,300	129	129	129	129

If line 43 (taxable income) is— At least	But less than	Single	Married filing jointly *	Married filing separately	Head of a household
			Your tax is—		
1,300	1,325	131	131	131	131
1,325	1,350	134	134	134	134
1,350	1,375	136	136	136	136
1,375	1,400	139	139	139	139
1,400	1,425	141	141	141	141
1,425	1,450	144	144	144	144
1,450	1,475	146	146	146	146
1,475	1,500	149	149	149	149
1,500	1,525	151	151	151	151
1,525	1,550	154	154	154	154
1,550	1,575	156	156	156	156
1,575	1,600	159	159	159	159
1,600	1,625	161	161	161	161
1,625	1,650	164	164	164	164
1,650	1,675	166	166	166	166
1,675	1,700	169	169	169	169
1,700	1,725	171	171	171	171
1,725	1,750	174	174	174	174
1,750	1,775	176	176	176	176
1,775	1,800	179	179	179	179
1,800	1,825	181	181	181	181
1,825	1,850	184	184	184	184
1,850	1,875	186	186	186	186
1,875	1,900	189	189	189	189
1,900	1,925	191	191	191	191
1,925	1,950	194	194	194	194
1,950	1,975	196	196	196	196
1,975	2,000	199	199	199	199

2,000

At least	But less than	Single	Married filing jointly *	Married filing separately	Head of a household
2,000	2,025	201	201	201	201
2,025	2,050	204	204	204	204
2,050	2,075	206	206	206	206
2,075	2,100	209	209	209	209
2,100	2,125	211	211	211	211
2,125	2,150	214	214	214	214
2,150	2,175	216	216	216	216
2,175	2,200	219	219	219	219
2,200	2,225	221	221	221	221
2,225	2,250	224	224	224	224
2,250	2,275	226	226	226	226
2,275	2,300	229	229	229	229
2,300	2,325	231	231	231	231
2,325	2,350	234	234	234	234
2,350	2,375	236	236	236	236
2,375	2,400	239	239	239	239
2,400	2,425	241	241	241	241
2,425	2,450	244	244	244	244
2,450	2,475	246	246	246	246
2,475	2,500	249	249	249	249
2,500	2,525	251	251	251	251
2,525	2,550	254	254	254	254
2,550	2,575	256	256	256	256
2,575	2,600	259	259	259	259
2,600	2,625	261	261	261	261
2,625	2,650	264	264	264	264
2,650	2,675	266	266	266	266
2,675	2,700	269	269	269	269

If line 43 (taxable income) is— At least	But less than	Single	Married filing jointly *	Married filing separately	Head of a household
			Your tax is—		
2,700	2,725	271	271	271	271
2,725	2,750	274	274	274	274
2,750	2,775	276	276	276	276
2,775	2,800	279	279	279	279
2,800	2,825	281	281	281	281
2,825	2,850	284	284	284	284
2,850	2,875	286	286	286	286
2,875	2,900	289	289	289	289
2,900	2,925	291	291	291	291
2,925	2,950	294	294	294	294
2,950	2,975	296	296	296	296
2,975	3,000	299	299	299	299

3,000

At least	But less than	Single	Married filing jointly *	Married filing separately	Head of a household
3,000	3,050	303	303	303	303
3,050	3,100	308	308	308	308
3,100	3,150	313	313	313	313
3,150	3,200	318	318	318	318
3,200	3,250	323	323	323	323
3,250	3,300	328	328	328	328
3,300	3,350	333	333	333	333
3,350	3,400	338	338	338	338
3,400	3,450	343	343	343	343
3,450	3,500	348	348	348	348
3,500	3,550	353	353	353	353
3,550	3,600	358	358	358	358
3,600	3,650	363	363	363	363
3,650	3,700	368	368	368	368
3,700	3,750	373	373	373	373
3,750	3,800	378	378	378	378
3,800	3,850	383	383	383	383
3,850	3,900	388	388	388	388
3,900	3,950	393	393	393	393
3,950	4,000	398	398	398	398

4,000

At least	But less than	Single	Married filing jointly *	Married filing separately	Head of a household
4,000	4,050	403	403	403	403
4,050	4,100	408	408	408	408
4,100	4,150	413	413	413	413
4,150	4,200	418	418	418	418
4,200	4,250	423	423	423	423
4,250	4,300	428	428	428	428
4,300	4,350	433	433	433	433
4,350	4,400	438	438	438	438
4,400	4,450	443	443	443	443
4,450	4,500	448	448	448	448
4,500	4,550	453	453	453	453
4,550	4,600	458	458	458	458
4,600	4,650	463	463	463	463
4,650	4,700	468	468	468	468
4,700	4,750	473	473	473	473
4,750	4,800	478	478	478	478
4,800	4,850	483	483	483	483
4,850	4,900	488	488	488	488
4,900	4,950	493	493	493	493
4,950	5,000	498	498	498	498

* This column must also be used by a qualifying widow(er).

(Continued on page 69)

2008 Tax Table–Continued

If line 43 (taxable income) is—		And you are—			
At least	But less than	Single	Married filing jointly *	Married filing separately	Head of a household
		Your tax is—			

5,000

At least	But less than	Single	Married filing jointly *	Married filing separately	Head of a household
5,000	5,050	503	503	503	503
5,050	5,100	508	508	508	508
5,100	5,150	513	513	513	513
5,150	5,200	518	518	518	518
5,200	5,250	523	523	523	523
5,250	5,300	528	528	528	528
5,300	5,350	533	533	533	533
5,350	5,400	538	538	538	538
5,400	5,450	543	543	543	543
5,450	5,500	548	548	548	548
5,500	5,550	553	553	553	553
5,550	5,600	558	558	558	558
5,600	5,650	563	563	563	563
5,650	5,700	568	568	568	568
5,700	5,750	573	573	573	573
5,750	5,800	578	578	578	578
5,800	5,850	583	583	583	583
5,850	5,900	588	588	588	588
5,900	5,950	593	593	593	593
5,950	6,000	598	598	598	598

6,000

At least	But less than	Single	Married filing jointly *	Married filing separately	Head of a household
6,000	6,050	603	603	603	603
6,050	6,100	608	608	608	608
6,100	6,150	613	613	613	613
6,150	6,200	618	618	618	618
6,200	6,250	623	623	623	623
6,250	6,300	628	628	628	628
6,300	6,350	633	633	633	633
6,350	6,400	638	638	638	638
6,400	6,450	643	643	643	643
6,450	6,500	648	648	648	648
6,500	6,550	653	653	653	653
6,550	6,600	658	658	658	658
6,600	6,650	663	663	663	663
6,650	6,700	668	668	668	668
6,700	6,750	673	673	673	673
6,750	6,800	678	678	678	678
6,800	6,850	683	683	683	683
6,850	6,900	688	688	688	688
6,900	6,950	693	693	693	693
6,950	7,000	698	698	698	698

7,000

At least	But less than	Single	Married filing jointly *	Married filing separately	Head of a household
7,000	7,050	703	703	703	703
7,050	7,100	708	708	708	708
7,100	7,150	713	713	713	713
7,150	7,200	718	718	718	718
7,200	7,250	723	723	723	723
7,250	7,300	728	728	728	728
7,300	7,350	733	733	733	733
7,350	7,400	738	738	738	738
7,400	7,450	743	743	743	743
7,450	7,500	748	748	748	748
7,500	7,550	753	753	753	753
7,550	7,600	758	758	758	758
7,600	7,650	763	763	763	763
7,650	7,700	768	768	768	768
7,700	7,750	773	773	773	773
7,750	7,800	778	778	778	778
7,800	7,850	783	783	783	783
7,850	7,900	788	788	788	788
7,900	7,950	793	793	793	793
7,950	8,000	798	798	798	798

8,000

At least	But less than	Single	Married filing jointly *	Married filing separately	Head of a household
8,000	8,050	803	803	803	803
8,050	8,100	810	808	810	808
8,100	8,150	818	813	818	813
8,150	8,200	825	818	825	818
8,200	8,250	833	823	833	823
8,250	8,300	840	828	840	828
8,300	8,350	848	833	848	833
8,350	8,400	855	838	855	838
8,400	8,450	863	843	863	843
8,450	8,500	870	848	870	848
8,500	8,550	878	853	878	853
8,550	8,600	885	858	885	858
8,600	8,650	893	863	893	863
8,650	8,700	900	868	900	868
8,700	8,750	908	873	908	873
8,750	8,800	915	878	915	878
8,800	8,850	923	883	923	883
8,850	8,900	930	888	930	888
8,900	8,950	938	893	938	893
8,950	9,000	945	898	945	898

9,000

At least	But less than	Single	Married filing jointly *	Married filing separately	Head of a household
9,000	9,050	953	903	953	903
9,050	9,100	960	908	960	908
9,100	9,150	968	913	968	913
9,150	9,200	975	918	975	918
9,200	9,250	983	923	983	923
9,250	9,300	990	928	990	928
9,300	9,350	998	933	998	933
9,350	9,400	1,005	938	1,005	938
9,400	9,450	1,013	943	1,013	943
9,450	9,500	1,020	948	1,020	948
9,500	9,550	1,028	953	1,028	953
9,550	9,600	1,035	958	1,035	958
9,600	9,650	1,043	963	1,043	963
9,650	9,700	1,050	968	1,050	968
9,700	9,750	1,058	973	1,058	973
9,750	9,800	1,065	978	1,065	978
9,800	9,850	1,073	983	1,073	983
9,850	9,900	1,080	988	1,080	988
9,900	9,950	1,088	993	1,088	993
9,950	10,000	1,095	998	1,095	998

10,000

At least	But less than	Single	Married filing jointly *	Married filing separately	Head of a household
10,000	10,050	1,103	1,003	1,103	1,003
10,050	10,100	1,110	1,008	1,110	1,008
10,100	10,150	1,118	1,013	1,118	1,013
10,150	10,200	1,125	1,018	1,125	1,018
10,200	10,250	1,133	1,023	1,133	1,023
10,250	10,300	1,140	1,028	1,140	1,028
10,300	10,350	1,148	1,033	1,148	1,033
10,350	10,400	1,155	1,038	1,155	1,038
10,400	10,450	1,163	1,043	1,163	1,043
10,450	10,500	1,170	1,048	1,170	1,048
10,500	10,550	1,178	1,053	1,178	1,053
10,550	10,600	1,185	1,058	1,185	1,058
10,600	10,650	1,193	1,063	1,193	1,063
10,650	10,700	1,200	1,068	1,200	1,068
10,700	10,750	1,208	1,073	1,208	1,073
10,750	10,800	1,215	1,078	1,215	1,078
10,800	10,850	1,223	1,083	1,223	1,083
10,850	10,900	1,230	1,088	1,230	1,088
10,900	10,950	1,238	1,093	1,238	1,093
10,950	11,000	1,245	1,098	1,245	1,098

11,000

At least	But less than	Single	Married filing jointly *	Married filing separately	Head of a household
11,000	11,050	1,253	1,103	1,253	1,103
11,050	11,100	1,260	1,108	1,260	1,108
11,100	11,150	1,268	1,113	1,268	1,113
11,150	11,200	1,275	1,118	1,275	1,118
11,200	11,250	1,283	1,123	1,283	1,123
11,250	11,300	1,290	1,128	1,290	1,128
11,300	11,350	1,298	1,133	1,298	1,133
11,350	11,400	1,305	1,138	1,305	1,138
11,400	11,450	1,313	1,143	1,313	1,143
11,450	11,500	1,320	1,148	1,320	1,149
11,500	11,550	1,328	1,153	1,328	1,156
11,550	11,600	1,335	1,158	1,335	1,164
11,600	11,650	1,343	1,163	1,343	1,171
11,650	11,700	1,350	1,168	1,350	1,179
11,700	11,750	1,358	1,173	1,358	1,186
11,750	11,800	1,365	1,178	1,365	1,194
11,800	11,850	1,373	1,183	1,373	1,201
11,850	11,900	1,380	1,188	1,380	1,209
11,900	11,950	1,388	1,193	1,388	1,216
11,950	12,000	1,395	1,198	1,395	1,224

12,000

At least	But less than	Single	Married filing jointly *	Married filing separately	Head of a household
12,000	12,050	1,403	1,203	1,403	1,231
12,050	12,100	1,410	1,208	1,410	1,239
12,100	12,150	1,418	1,213	1,418	1,246
12,150	12,200	1,425	1,218	1,425	1,254
12,200	12,250	1,433	1,223	1,433	1,261
12,250	12,300	1,440	1,228	1,440	1,269
12,300	12,350	1,448	1,233	1,448	1,276
12,350	12,400	1,455	1,238	1,455	1,284
12,400	12,450	1,463	1,243	1,463	1,291
12,450	12,500	1,470	1,248	1,470	1,299
12,500	12,550	1,478	1,253	1,478	1,306
12,550	12,600	1,485	1,258	1,485	1,314
12,600	12,650	1,493	1,263	1,493	1,321
12,650	12,700	1,500	1,268	1,500	1,329
12,700	12,750	1,508	1,273	1,508	1,336
12,750	12,800	1,515	1,278	1,515	1,344
12,800	12,850	1,523	1,283	1,523	1,351
12,850	12,900	1,530	1,288	1,530	1,359
12,900	12,950	1,538	1,293	1,538	1,366
12,950	13,000	1,545	1,298	1,545	1,374

13,000

At least	But less than	Single	Married filing jointly *	Married filing separately	Head of a household
13,000	13,050	1,553	1,303	1,553	1,381
13,050	13,100	1,560	1,308	1,560	1,389
13,100	13,150	1,568	1,313	1,568	1,396
13,150	13,200	1,575	1,318	1,575	1,404
13,200	13,250	1,583	1,323	1,583	1,411
13,250	13,300	1,590	1,328	1,590	1,419
13,300	13,350	1,598	1,333	1,598	1,426
13,350	13,400	1,605	1,338	1,605	1,434
13,400	13,450	1,613	1,343	1,613	1,441
13,450	13,500	1,620	1,348	1,620	1,449
13,500	13,550	1,628	1,353	1,628	1,456
13,550	13,600	1,635	1,358	1,635	1,464
13,600	13,650	1,643	1,363	1,643	1,471
13,650	13,700	1,650	1,368	1,650	1,479
13,700	13,750	1,658	1,373	1,658	1,486
13,750	13,800	1,665	1,378	1,665	1,494
13,800	13,850	1,673	1,383	1,673	1,501
13,850	13,900	1,680	1,388	1,680	1,509
13,900	13,950	1,688	1,393	1,688	1,516
13,950	14,000	1,695	1,398	1,695	1,524

* This column must also be used by a qualifying widow(er).

(Continued on page 70)

2008 Tax Table–*Continued*

14,000

At least	But less than	Single	Married filing jointly *	Married filing separately	Head of a household
14,000	14,050	1,703	1,403	1,703	1,531
14,050	14,100	1,710	1,408	1,710	1,539
14,100	14,150	1,718	1,413	1,718	1,546
14,150	14,200	1,725	1,418	1,725	1,554
14,200	14,250	1,733	1,423	1,733	1,561
14,250	14,300	1,740	1,428	1,740	1,569
14,300	14,350	1,748	1,433	1,748	1,576
14,350	14,400	1,755	1,438	1,755	1,584
14,400	14,450	1,763	1,443	1,763	1,591
14,450	14,500	1,770	1,448	1,770	1,599
14,500	14,550	1,778	1,453	1,778	1,606
14,550	14,600	1,785	1,458	1,785	1,614
14,600	14,650	1,793	1,463	1,793	1,621
14,650	14,700	1,800	1,468	1,800	1,629
14,700	14,750	1,808	1,473	1,808	1,636
14,750	14,800	1,815	1,478	1,815	1,644
14,800	14,850	1,823	1,483	1,823	1,651
14,850	14,900	1,830	1,488	1,830	1,659
14,900	14,950	1,838	1,493	1,838	1,666
14,950	15,000	1,845	1,498	1,845	1,674

15,000

At least	But less than	Single	Married filing jointly *	Married filing separately	Head of a household
15,000	15,050	1,853	1,503	1,853	1,681
15,050	15,100	1,860	1,508	1,860	1,689
15,100	15,150	1,868	1,513	1,868	1,696
15,150	15,200	1,875	1,518	1,875	1,704
15,200	15,250	1,883	1,523	1,883	1,711
15,250	15,300	1,890	1,528	1,890	1,719
15,300	15,350	1,898	1,533	1,898	1,726
15,350	15,400	1,905	1,538	1,905	1,734
15,400	15,450	1,913	1,543	1,913	1,741
15,450	15,500	1,920	1,548	1,920	1,749
15,500	15,550	1,928	1,553	1,928	1,756
15,550	15,600	1,935	1,558	1,935	1,764
15,600	15,650	1,943	1,563	1,943	1,771
15,650	15,700	1,950	1,568	1,950	1,779
15,700	15,750	1,958	1,573	1,958	1,786
15,750	15,800	1,965	1,578	1,965	1,794
15,800	15,850	1,973	1,583	1,973	1,801
15,850	15,900	1,980	1,588	1,980	1,809
15,900	15,950	1,988	1,593	1,988	1,816
15,950	16,000	1,995	1,598	1,995	1,824

16,000

At least	But less than	Single	Married filing jointly *	Married filing separately	Head of a household
16,000	16,050	2,003	1,603	2,003	1,831
16,050	16,100	2,010	1,609	2,010	1,839
16,100	16,150	2,018	1,616	2,018	1,846
16,150	16,200	2,025	1,624	2,025	1,854
16,200	16,250	2,033	1,631	2,033	1,861
16,250	16,300	2,040	1,639	2,040	1,869
16,300	16,350	2,048	1,646	2,048	1,876
16,350	16,400	2,055	1,654	2,055	1,884
16,400	16,450	2,063	1,661	2,063	1,891
16,450	16,500	2,070	1,669	2,070	1,899
16,500	16,550	2,078	1,676	2,078	1,906
16,550	16,600	2,085	1,684	2,085	1,914
16,600	16,650	2,093	1,691	2,093	1,921
16,650	16,700	2,100	1,699	2,100	1,929
16,700	16,750	2,108	1,706	2,108	1,936
16,750	16,800	2,115	1,714	2,115	1,944
16,800	16,850	2,123	1,721	2,123	1,951
16,850	16,900	2,130	1,729	2,130	1,959
16,900	16,950	2,138	1,736	2,138	1,966
16,950	17,000	2,145	1,744	2,145	1,974

17,000

At least	But less than	Single	Married filing jointly *	Married filing separately	Head of a household
17,000	17,050	2,153	1,751	2,153	1,981
17,050	17,100	2,160	1,759	2,160	1,989
17,100	17,150	2,168	1,766	2,168	1,996
17,150	17,200	2,175	1,774	2,175	2,004
17,200	17,250	2,183	1,781	2,183	2,011
17,250	17,300	2,190	1,789	2,190	2,019
17,300	17,350	2,198	1,796	2,198	2,026
17,350	17,400	2,205	1,804	2,205	2,034
17,400	17,450	2,213	1,811	2,213	2,041
17,450	17,500	2,220	1,819	2,220	2,049
17,500	17,550	2,228	1,826	2,228	2,056
17,550	17,600	2,235	1,834	2,235	2,064
17,600	17,650	2,243	1,841	2,243	2,071
17,650	17,700	2,250	1,849	2,250	2,079
17,700	17,750	2,258	1,856	2,258	2,086
17,750	17,800	2,265	1,864	2,265	2,094
17,800	17,850	2,273	1,871	2,273	2,101
17,850	17,900	2,280	1,879	2,280	2,109
17,900	17,950	2,288	1,886	2,288	2,116
17,950	18,000	2,295	1,894	2,295	2,124

18,000

At least	But less than	Single	Married filing jointly *	Married filing separately	Head of a household
18,000	18,050	2,303	1,901	2,303	2,131
18,050	18,100	2,310	1,909	2,310	2,139
18,100	18,150	2,318	1,916	2,318	2,146
18,150	18,200	2,325	1,924	2,325	2,154
18,200	18,250	2,333	1,931	2,333	2,161
18,250	18,300	2,340	1,939	2,340	2,169
18,300	18,350	2,348	1,946	2,348	2,176
18,350	18,400	2,355	1,954	2,355	2,184
18,400	18,450	2,363	1,961	2,363	2,191
18,450	18,500	2,370	1,969	2,370	2,199
18,500	18,550	2,378	1,976	2,378	2,206
18,550	18,600	2,385	1,984	2,385	2,214
18,600	18,650	2,393	1,991	2,393	2,221
18,650	18,700	2,400	1,999	2,400	2,229
18,700	18,750	2,408	2,006	2,408	2,236
18,750	18,800	2,415	2,014	2,415	2,244
18,800	18,850	2,423	2,021	2,423	2,251
18,850	18,900	2,430	2,029	2,430	2,259
18,900	18,950	2,438	2,036	2,438	2,266
18,950	19,000	2,445	2,044	2,445	2,274

19,000

At least	But less than	Single	Married filing jointly *	Married filing separately	Head of a household
19,000	19,050	2,453	2,051	2,453	2,281
19,050	19,100	2,460	2,059	2,460	2,289
19,100	19,150	2,468	2,066	2,468	2,296
19,150	19,200	2,475	2,074	2,475	2,304
19,200	19,250	2,483	2,081	2,483	2,311
19,250	19,300	2,490	2,089	2,490	2,319
19,300	19,350	2,498	2,096	2,498	2,326
19,350	19,400	2,505	2,104	2,505	2,334
19,400	19,450	2,513	2,111	2,513	2,341
19,450	19,500	2,520	2,119	2,520	2,349
19,500	19,550	2,528	2,126	2,528	2,356
19,550	19,600	2,535	2,134	2,535	2,364
19,600	19,650	2,543	2,141	2,543	2,371
19,650	19,700	2,550	2,149	2,550	2,379
19,700	19,750	2,558	2,156	2,558	2,386
19,750	19,800	2,565	2,164	2,565	2,394
19,800	19,850	2,573	2,171	2,573	2,401
19,850	19,900	2,580	2,179	2,580	2,409
19,900	19,950	2,588	2,186	2,588	2,416
19,950	20,000	2,595	2,194	2,595	2,424

20,000

At least	But less than	Single	Married filing jointly *	Married filing separately	Head of a household
20,000	20,050	2,603	2,201	2,603	2,431
20,050	20,100	2,610	2,209	2,610	2,439
20,100	20,150	2,618	2,216	2,618	2,446
20,150	20,200	2,625	2,224	2,625	2,454
20,200	20,250	2,633	2,231	2,633	2,461
20,250	20,300	2,640	2,239	2,640	2,469
20,300	20,350	2,648	2,246	2,648	2,476
20,350	20,400	2,655	2,254	2,655	2,484
20,400	20,450	2,663	2,261	2,663	2,491
20,450	20,500	2,670	2,269	2,670	2,499
20,500	20,550	2,678	2,276	2,678	2,506
20,550	20,600	2,685	2,284	2,685	2,514
20,600	20,650	2,693	2,291	2,693	2,521
20,650	20,700	2,700	2,299	2,700	2,529
20,700	20,750	2,708	2,306	2,708	2,536
20,750	20,800	2,715	2,314	2,715	2,544
20,800	20,850	2,723	2,321	2,723	2,551
20,850	20,900	2,730	2,329	2,730	2,559
20,900	20,950	2,738	2,336	2,738	2,566
20,950	21,000	2,745	2,344	2,745	2,574

21,000

At least	But less than	Single	Married filing jointly *	Married filing separately	Head of a household
21,000	21,050	2,753	2,351	2,753	2,581
21,050	21,100	2,760	2,359	2,760	2,589
21,100	21,150	2,768	2,366	2,768	2,596
21,150	21,200	2,775	2,374	2,775	2,604
21,200	21,250	2,783	2,381	2,783	2,611
21,250	21,300	2,790	2,389	2,790	2,619
21,300	21,350	2,798	2,396	2,798	2,626
21,350	21,400	2,805	2,404	2,805	2,634
21,400	21,450	2,813	2,411	2,813	2,641
21,450	21,500	2,820	2,419	2,820	2,649
21,500	21,550	2,828	2,426	2,828	2,656
21,550	21,600	2,835	2,434	2,835	2,664
21,600	21,650	2,843	2,441	2,843	2,671
21,650	21,700	2,850	2,449	2,850	2,679
21,700	21,750	2,858	2,456	2,858	2,686
21,750	21,800	2,865	2,464	2,865	2,694
21,800	21,850	2,873	2,471	2,873	2,701
21,850	21,900	2,880	2,479	2,880	2,709
21,900	21,950	2,888	2,486	2,888	2,716
21,950	22,000	2,895	2,494	2,895	2,724

22,000

At least	But less than	Single	Married filing jointly *	Married filing separately	Head of a household
22,000	22,050	2,903	2,501	2,903	2,731
22,050	22,100	2,910	2,509	2,910	2,739
22,100	22,150	2,918	2,516	2,918	2,746
22,150	22,200	2,925	2,524	2,925	2,754
22,200	22,250	2,933	2,531	2,933	2,761
22,250	22,300	2,940	2,539	2,940	2,769
22,300	22,350	2,948	2,546	2,948	2,776
22,350	22,400	2,955	2,554	2,955	2,784
22,400	22,450	2,963	2,561	2,963	2,791
22,450	22,500	2,970	2,569	2,970	2,799
22,500	22,550	2,978	2,576	2,978	2,806
22,550	22,600	2,985	2,584	2,985	2,814
22,600	22,650	2,993	2,591	2,993	2,821
22,650	22,700	3,000	2,599	3,000	2,829
22,700	22,750	3,008	2,606	3,008	2,836
22,750	22,800	3,015	2,614	3,015	2,844
22,800	22,850	3,023	2,621	3,023	2,851
22,850	22,900	3,030	2,629	3,030	2,859
22,900	22,950	3,038	2,636	3,038	2,866
22,950	23,000	3,045	2,644	3,045	2,874

* This column must also be used by a qualifying widow(er).

(Continued on page 71)

2008 Tax Table–*Continued*

If line 43 (taxable income) is—		And you are—			
At least	But less than	Single	Married filing jointly *	Married filing separately	Head of a household
		Your tax is—			
23,000					
23,000	23,050	3,053	2,651	3,053	2,881
23,050	23,100	3,060	2,659	3,060	2,889
23,100	23,150	3,068	2,666	3,068	2,896
23,150	23,200	3,075	2,674	3,075	2,904
23,200	23,250	3,083	2,681	3,083	2,911
23,250	23,300	3,090	2,689	3,090	2,919
23,300	23,350	3,098	2,696	3,098	2,926
23,350	23,400	3,105	2,704	3,105	2,934
23,400	23,450	3,113	2,711	3,113	2,941
23,450	23,500	3,120	2,719	3,120	2,949
23,500	23,550	3,128	2,726	3,128	2,956
23,550	23,600	3,135	2,734	3,135	2,964
23,600	23,650	3,143	2,741	3,143	2,971
23,650	23,700	3,150	2,749	3,150	2,979
23,700	23,750	3,158	2,756	3,158	2,986
23,750	23,800	3,165	2,764	3,165	2,994
23,800	23,850	3,173	2,771	3,173	3,001
23,850	23,900	3,180	2,779	3,180	3,009
23,900	23,950	3,188	2,786	3,188	3,016
23,950	24,000	3,195	2,794	3,195	3,024
24,000					
24,000	24,050	3,203	2,801	3,203	3,031
24,050	24,100	3,210	2,809	3,210	3,039
24,100	24,150	3,218	2,816	3,218	3,046
24,150	24,200	3,225	2,824	3,225	3,054
24,200	24,250	3,233	2,831	3,233	3,061
24,250	24,300	3,240	2,839	3,240	3,069
24,300	24,350	3,248	2,846	3,248	3,076
24,350	24,400	3,255	2,854	3,255	3,084
24,400	24,450	3,263	2,861	3,263	3,091
24,450	24,500	3,270	2,869	3,270	3,099
24,500	24,550	3,278	2,876	3,278	3,106
24,550	24,600	3,285	2,884	3,285	3,114
24,600	24,650	3,293	2,891	3,293	3,121
24,650	24,700	3,300	2,899	3,300	3,129
24,700	24,750	3,308	2,906	3,308	3,136
24,750	24,800	3,315	2,914	3,315	3,144
24,800	24,850	3,323	2,921	3,323	3,151
24,850	24,900	3,330	2,929	3,330	3,159
24,900	24,950	3,338	2,936	3,338	3,166
24,950	25,000	3,345	2,944	3,345	3,174
25,000					
25,000	25,050	3,353	2,951	3,353	3,181
25,050	25,100	3,360	2,959	3,360	3,189
25,100	25,150	3,368	2,966	3,368	3,196
25,150	25,200	3,375	2,974	3,375	3,204
25,200	25,250	3,383	2,981	3,383	3,211
25,250	25,300	3,390	2,989	3,390	3,219
25,300	25,350	3,398	2,996	3,398	3,226
25,350	25,400	3,405	3,004	3,405	3,234
25,400	25,450	3,413	3,011	3,413	3,241
25,450	25,500	3,420	3,019	3,420	3,249
25,500	25,550	3,428	3,026	3,428	3,256
25,550	25,600	3,435	3,034	3,435	3,264
25,600	25,650	3,443	3,041	3,443	3,271
25,650	25,700	3,450	3,049	3,450	3,279
25,700	25,750	3,458	3,056	3,458	3,286
25,750	25,800	3,465	3,064	3,465	3,294
25,800	25,850	3,473	3,071	3,473	3,301
25,850	25,900	3,480	3,079	3,480	3,309
25,900	25,950	3,488	3,086	3,488	3,316
25,950	26,000	3,495	3,094	3,495	3,324

If line 43 (taxable income) is—		And you are—			
At least	But less than	Single	Married filing jointly *	Married filing separately	Head of a household
		Your tax is—			
26,000					
26,000	26,050	3,503	3,101	3,503	3,331
26,050	26,100	3,510	3,109	3,510	3,339
26,100	26,150	3,518	3,116	3,518	3,346
26,150	26,200	3,525	3,124	3,525	3,354
26,200	26,250	3,533	3,131	3,533	3,361
26,250	26,300	3,540	3,139	3,540	3,369
26,300	26,350	3,548	3,146	3,548	3,376
26,350	26,400	3,555	3,154	3,555	3,384
26,400	26,450	3,563	3,161	3,563	3,391
26,450	26,500	3,570	3,169	3,570	3,399
26,500	26,550	3,578	3,176	3,578	3,406
26,550	26,600	3,585	3,184	3,585	3,414
26,600	26,650	3,593	3,191	3,593	3,421
26,650	26,700	3,600	3,199	3,600	3,429
26,700	26,750	3,608	3,206	3,608	3,436
26,750	26,800	3,615	3,214	3,615	3,444
26,800	26,850	3,623	3,221	3,623	3,451
26,850	26,900	3,630	3,229	3,630	3,459
26,900	26,950	3,638	3,236	3,638	3,466
26,950	27,000	3,645	3,244	3,645	3,474
27,000					
27,000	27,050	3,653	3,251	3,653	3,481
27,050	27,100	3,660	3,259	3,660	3,489
27,100	27,150	3,668	3,266	3,668	3,496
27,150	27,200	3,675	3,274	3,675	3,504
27,200	27,250	3,683	3,281	3,683	3,511
27,250	27,300	3,690	3,289	3,690	3,519
27,300	27,350	3,698	3,296	3,698	3,526
27,350	27,400	3,705	3,304	3,705	3,534
27,400	27,450	3,713	3,311	3,713	3,541
27,450	27,500	3,720	3,319	3,720	3,549
27,500	27,550	3,728	3,326	3,728	3,556
27,550	27,600	3,735	3,334	3,735	3,564
27,600	27,650	3,743	3,341	3,743	3,571
27,650	27,700	3,750	3,349	3,750	3,579
27,700	27,750	3,758	3,356	3,758	3,586
27,750	27,800	3,765	3,364	3,765	3,594
27,800	27,850	3,773	3,371	3,773	3,601
27,850	27,900	3,780	3,379	3,780	3,609
27,900	27,950	3,788	3,386	3,788	3,616
27,950	28,000	3,795	3,394	3,795	3,624
28,000					
28,000	28,050	3,803	3,401	3,803	3,631
28,050	28,100	3,810	3,409	3,810	3,639
28,100	28,150	3,818	3,416	3,818	3,646
28,150	28,200	3,825	3,424	3,825	3,654
28,200	28,250	3,833	3,431	3,833	3,661
28,250	28,300	3,840	3,439	3,840	3,669
28,300	28,350	3,848	3,446	3,848	3,676
28,350	28,400	3,855	3,454	3,855	3,684
28,400	28,450	3,863	3,461	3,863	3,691
28,450	28,500	3,870	3,469	3,870	3,699
28,500	28,550	3,878	3,476	3,878	3,706
28,550	28,600	3,885	3,484	3,885	3,714
28,600	28,650	3,893	3,491	3,893	3,721
28,650	28,700	3,900	3,499	3,900	3,729
28,700	28,750	3,908	3,506	3,908	3,736
28,750	28,800	3,915	3,514	3,915	3,744
28,800	28,850	3,923	3,521	3,923	3,751
28,850	28,900	3,930	3,529	3,930	3,759
28,900	28,950	3,938	3,536	3,938	3,766
28,950	29,000	3,945	3,544	3,945	3,774

If line 43 (taxable income) is—		And you are—			
At least	But less than	Single	Married filing jointly *	Married filing separately	Head of a household
		Your tax is—			
29,000					
29,000	29,050	3,953	3,551	3,953	3,781
29,050	29,100	3,960	3,559	3,960	3,789
29,100	29,150	3,968	3,566	3,968	3,796
29,150	29,200	3,975	3,574	3,975	3,804
29,200	29,250	3,983	3,581	3,983	3,811
29,250	29,300	3,990	3,589	3,990	3,819
29,300	29,350	3,998	3,596	3,998	3,826
29,350	29,400	4,005	3,604	4,005	3,834
29,400	29,450	4,013	3,611	4,013	3,841
29,450	29,500	4,020	3,619	4,020	3,849
29,500	29,550	4,028	3,626	4,028	3,856
29,550	29,600	4,035	3,634	4,035	3,864
29,600	29,650	4,043	3,641	4,043	3,871
29,650	29,700	4,050	3,649	4,050	3,879
29,700	29,750	4,058	3,656	4,058	3,886
29,750	29,800	4,065	3,664	4,065	3,894
29,800	29,850	4,073	3,671	4,073	3,901
29,850	29,900	4,080	3,679	4,080	3,909
29,900	29,950	4,088	3,686	4,088	3,916
29,950	30,000	4,095	3,694	4,095	3,924
30,000					
30,000	30,050	4,103	3,701	4,103	3,931
30,050	30,100	4,110	3,709	4,110	3,939
30,100	30,150	4,118	3,716	4,118	3,946
30,150	30,200	4,125	3,724	4,125	3,954
30,200	30,250	4,133	3,731	4,133	3,961
30,250	30,300	4,140	3,739	4,140	3,969
30,300	30,350	4,148	3,746	4,148	3,976
30,350	30,400	4,155	3,754	4,155	3,984
30,400	30,450	4,163	3,761	4,163	3,991
30,450	30,500	4,170	3,769	4,170	3,999
30,500	30,550	4,178	3,776	4,178	4,006
30,550	30,600	4,185	3,784	4,185	4,014
30,600	30,650	4,193	3,791	4,193	4,021
30,650	30,700	4,200	3,799	4,200	4,029
30,700	30,750	4,208	3,806	4,208	4,036
30,750	30,800	4,215	3,814	4,215	4,044
30,800	30,850	4,223	3,821	4,223	4,051
30,850	30,900	4,230	3,829	4,230	4,059
30,900	30,950	4,238	3,836	4,238	4,066
30,950	31,000	4,245	3,844	4,245	4,074
31,000					
31,000	31,050	4,253	3,851	4,253	4,081
31,050	31,100	4,260	3,859	4,260	4,089
31,100	31,150	4,268	3,866	4,268	4,096
31,150	31,200	4,275	3,874	4,275	4,104
31,200	31,250	4,283	3,881	4,283	4,111
31,250	31,300	4,290	3,889	4,290	4,119
31,300	31,350	4,298	3,896	4,298	4,126
31,350	31,400	4,305	3,904	4,305	4,134
31,400	31,450	4,313	3,911	4,313	4,141
31,450	31,500	4,320	3,919	4,320	4,149
31,500	31,550	4,328	3,926	4,328	4,156
31,550	31,600	4,335	3,934	4,335	4,164
31,600	31,650	4,343	3,941	4,343	4,171
31,650	31,700	4,350	3,949	4,350	4,179
31,700	31,750	4,358	3,956	4,358	4,186
31,750	31,800	4,365	3,964	4,365	4,194
31,800	31,850	4,373	3,971	4,373	4,201
31,850	31,900	4,380	3,979	4,380	4,209
31,900	31,950	4,388	3,986	4,388	4,216
31,950	32,000	4,395	3,994	4,395	4,224

* This column must also be used by a qualifying widow(er).

(Continued on page 72)

2008 Tax Table–*Continued*

If line 43 (taxable income) is—		And you are—			
At least	But less than	Single	Married filing jointly *	Married filing sepa-rately	Head of a house-hold
		Your tax is—			
32,000					
32,000	**32,050**	4,403	4,001	4,403	4,231
32,050	**32,100**	4,410	4,009	4,410	4,239
32,100	**32,150**	4,418	4,016	4,418	4,246
32,150	**32,200**	4,425	4,024	4,425	4,254
32,200	**32,250**	4,433	4,031	4,433	4,261
32,250	**32,300**	4,440	4,039	4,440	4,269
32,300	**32,350**	4,448	4,046	4,448	4,276
32,350	**32,400**	4,455	4,054	4,455	4,284
32,400	**32,450**	4,463	4,061	4,463	4,291
32,450	**32,500**	4,470	4,069	4,470	4,299
32,500	**32,550**	4,478	4,076	4,478	4,306
32,550	**32,600**	4,488	4,084	4,488	4,314
32,600	**32,650**	4,500	4,091	4,500	4,321
32,650	**32,700**	4,513	4,099	4,513	4,329
32,700	**32,750**	4,525	4,106	4,525	4,336
32,750	**32,800**	4,538	4,114	4,538	4,344
32,800	**32,850**	4,550	4,121	4,550	4,351
32,850	**32,900**	4,563	4,129	4,563	4,359
32,900	**32,950**	4,575	4,136	4,575	4,366
32,950	**33,000**	4,588	4,144	4,588	4,374
33,000					
33,000	**33,050**	4,600	4,151	4,600	4,381
33,050	**33,100**	4,613	4,159	4,613	4,389
33,100	**33,150**	4,625	4,166	4,625	4,396
33,150	**33,200**	4,638	4,174	4,638	4,404
33,200	**33,250**	4,650	4,181	4,650	4,411
33,250	**33,300**	4,663	4,189	4,663	4,419
33,300	**33,350**	4,675	4,196	4,675	4,426
33,350	**33,400**	4,688	4,204	4,688	4,434
33,400	**33,450**	4,700	4,211	4,700	4,441
33,450	**33,500**	4,713	4,219	4,713	4,449
33,500	**33,550**	4,725	4,226	4,725	4,456
33,550	**33,600**	4,738	4,234	4,738	4,464
33,600	**33,650**	4,750	4,241	4,750	4,471
33,650	**33,700**	4,763	4,249	4,763	4,479
33,700	**33,750**	4,775	4,256	4,775	4,486
33,750	**33,800**	4,788	4,264	4,788	4,494
33,800	**33,850**	4,800	4,271	4,800	4,501
33,850	**33,900**	4,813	4,279	4,813	4,509
33,900	**33,950**	4,825	4,286	4,825	4,516
33,950	**34,000**	4,838	4,294	4,838	4,524
34,000					
34,000	**34,050**	4,850	4,301	4,850	4,531
34,050	**34,100**	4,863	4,309	4,863	4,539
34,100	**34,150**	4,875	4,316	4,875	4,546
34,150	**34,200**	4,888	4,324	4,888	4,554
34,200	**34,250**	4,900	4,331	4,900	4,561
34,250	**34,300**	4,913	4,339	4,913	4,569
34,300	**34,350**	4,925	4,346	4,925	4,576
34,350	**34,400**	4,938	4,354	4,938	4,584
34,400	**34,450**	4,950	4,361	4,950	4,591
34,450	**34,500**	4,963	4,369	4,963	4,599
34,500	**34,550**	4,975	4,376	4,975	4,606
34,550	**34,600**	4,988	4,384	4,988	4,614
34,600	**34,650**	5,000	4,391	5,000	4,621
34,650	**34,700**	5,013	4,399	5,013	4,629
34,700	**34,750**	5,025	4,406	5,025	4,636
34,750	**34,800**	5,038	4,414	5,038	4,644
34,800	**34,850**	5,050	4,421	5,050	4,651
34,850	**34,900**	5,063	4,429	5,063	4,659
34,900	**34,950**	5,075	4,436	5,075	4,666
34,950	**35,000**	5,088	4,444	5,088	4,674

If line 43 (taxable income) is—		And you are—			
At least	But less than	Single	Married filing jointly *	Married filing sepa-rately	Head of a house-hold
		Your tax is—			
35,000					
35,000	**35,050**	5,100	4,451	5,100	4,681
35,050	**35,100**	5,113	4,459	5,113	4,689
35,100	**35,150**	5,125	4,466	5,125	4,696
35,150	**35,200**	5,138	4,474	5,138	4,704
35,200	**35,250**	5,150	4,481	5,150	4,711
35,250	**35,300**	5,163	4,489	5,163	4,719
35,300	**35,350**	5,175	4,496	5,175	4,726
35,350	**35,400**	5,188	4,504	5,188	4,734
35,400	**35,450**	5,200	4,511	5,200	4,741
35,450	**35,500**	5,213	4,519	5,213	4,749
35,500	**35,550**	5,225	4,526	5,225	4,756
35,550	**35,600**	5,238	4,534	5,238	4,764
35,600	**35,650**	5,250	4,541	5,250	4,771
35,650	**35,700**	5,263	4,549	5,263	4,779
35,700	**35,750**	5,275	4,556	5,275	4,786
35,750	**35,800**	5,288	4,564	5,288	4,794
35,800	**35,850**	5,300	4,571	5,300	4,801
35,850	**35,900**	5,313	4,579	5,313	4,809
35,900	**35,950**	5,325	4,586	5,325	4,816
35,950	**36,000**	5,338	4,594	5,338	4,824
36,000					
36,000	**36,050**	5,350	4,601	5,350	4,831
36,050	**36,100**	5,363	4,609	5,363	4,839
36,100	**36,150**	5,375	4,616	5,375	4,846
36,150	**36,200**	5,388	4,624	5,388	4,854
36,200	**36,250**	5,400	4,631	5,400	4,861
36,250	**36,300**	5,413	4,639	5,413	4,869
36,300	**36,350**	5,425	4,646	5,425	4,876
36,350	**36,400**	5,438	4,654	5,438	4,884
36,400	**36,450**	5,450	4,661	5,450	4,891
36,450	**36,500**	5,463	4,669	5,463	4,899
36,500	**36,550**	5,475	4,676	5,475	4,906
36,550	**36,600**	5,488	4,684	5,488	4,914
36,600	**36,650**	5,500	4,691	5,500	4,921
36,650	**36,700**	5,513	4,699	5,513	4,929
36,700	**36,750**	5,525	4,706	5,525	4,936
36,750	**36,800**	5,538	4,714	5,538	4,944
36,800	**36,850**	5,550	4,721	5,550	4,951
36,850	**36,900**	5,563	4,729	5,563	4,959
36,900	**36,950**	5,575	4,736	5,575	4,966
36,950	**37,000**	5,588	4,744	5,588	4,974
37,000					
37,000	**37,050**	5,600	4,751	5,600	4,981
37,050	**37,100**	5,613	4,759	5,613	4,989
37,100	**37,150**	5,625	4,766	5,625	4,996
37,150	**37,200**	5,638	4,774	5,638	5,004
37,200	**37,250**	5,650	4,781	5,650	5,011
37,250	**37,300**	5,663	4,789	5,663	5,019
37,300	**37,350**	5,675	4,796	5,675	5,026
37,350	**37,400**	5,688	4,804	5,688	5,034
37,400	**37,450**	5,700	4,811	5,700	5,041
37,450	**37,500**	5,713	4,819	5,713	5,049
37,500	**37,550**	5,725	4,826	5,725	5,056
37,550	**37,600**	5,738	4,834	5,738	5,064
37,600	**37,650**	5,750	4,841	5,750	5,071
37,650	**37,700**	5,763	4,849	5,763	5,079
37,700	**37,750**	5,775	4,856	5,775	5,086
37,750	**37,800**	5,788	4,864	5,788	5,094
37,800	**37,850**	5,800	4,871	5,800	5,101
37,850	**37,900**	5,813	4,879	5,813	5,109
37,900	**37,950**	5,825	4,886	5,825	5,116
37,950	**38,000**	5,838	4,894	5,838	5,124

If line 43 (taxable income) is—		And you are—			
At least	But less than	Single	Married filing jointly *	Married filing sepa-rately	Head of a house-hold
		Your tax is—			
38,000					
38,000	**38,050**	5,850	4,901	5,850	5,131
38,050	**38,100**	5,863	4,909	5,863	5,139
38,100	**38,150**	5,875	4,916	5,875	5,146
38,150	**38,200**	5,888	4,924	5,888	5,154
38,200	**38,250**	5,900	4,931	5,900	5,161
38,250	**38,300**	5,913	4,939	5,913	5,169
38,300	**38,350**	5,925	4,946	5,925	5,176
38,350	**38,400**	5,938	4,954	5,938	5,184
38,400	**38,450**	5,950	4,961	5,950	5,191
38,450	**38,500**	5,963	4,969	5,963	5,199
38,500	**38,550**	5,975	4,976	5,975	5,206
38,550	**38,600**	5,988	4,984	5,988	5,214
38,600	**38,650**	6,000	4,991	6,000	5,221
38,650	**38,700**	6,013	4,999	6,013	5,229
38,700	**38,750**	6,025	5,006	6,025	5,236
38,750	**38,800**	6,038	5,014	6,038	5,244
38,800	**38,850**	6,050	5,021	6,050	5,251
38,850	**38,900**	6,063	5,029	6,063	5,259
38,900	**38,950**	6,075	5,036	6,075	5,266
38,950	**39,000**	6,088	5,044	6,088	5,274
39,000					
39,000	**39,050**	6,100	5,051	6,100	5,281
39,050	**39,100**	6,113	5,059	6,113	5,289
39,100	**39,150**	6,125	5,066	6,125	5,296
39,150	**39,200**	6,138	5,074	6,138	5,304
39,200	**39,250**	6,150	5,081	6,150	5,311
39,250	**39,300**	6,163	5,089	6,163	5,319
39,300	**39,350**	6,175	5,096	6,175	5,326
39,350	**39,400**	6,188	5,104	6,188	5,334
39,400	**39,450**	6,200	5,111	6,200	5,341
39,450	**39,500**	6,213	5,119	6,213	5,349
39,500	**39,550**	6,225	5,126	6,225	5,356
39,550	**39,600**	6,238	5,134	6,238	5,364
39,600	**39,650**	6,250	5,141	6,250	5,371
39,650	**39,700**	6,263	5,149	6,263	5,379
39,700	**39,750**	6,275	5,156	6,275	5,386
39,750	**39,800**	6,288	5,164	6,288	5,394
39,800	**39,850**	6,300	5,171	6,300	5,401
39,850	**39,900**	6,313	5,179	6,313	5,409
39,900	**39,950**	6,325	5,186	6,325	5,416
39,950	**40,000**	6,338	5,194	6,338	5,424
40,000					
40,000	**40,050**	6,350	5,201	6,350	5,431
40,050	**40,100**	6,363	5,209	6,363	5,439
40,100	**40,150**	6,375	5,216	6,375	5,446
40,150	**40,200**	6,388	5,224	6,388	5,454
40,200	**40,250**	6,400	5,231	6,400	5,461
40,250	**40,300**	6,413	5,239	6,413	5,469
40,300	**40,350**	6,425	5,246	6,425	5,476
40,350	**40,400**	6,438	5,254	6,438	5,484
40,400	**40,450**	6,450	5,261	6,450	5,491
40,450	**40,500**	6,463	5,269	6,463	5,499
40,500	**40,550**	6,475	5,276	6,475	5,506
40,550	**40,600**	6,488	5,284	6,488	5,514
40,600	**40,650**	6,500	5,291	6,500	5,521
40,650	**40,700**	6,513	5,299	6,513	5,529
40,700	**40,750**	6,525	5,306	6,525	5,536
40,750	**40,800**	6,538	5,314	6,538	5,544
40,800	**40,850**	6,550	5,321	6,550	5,551
40,850	**40,900**	6,563	5,329	6,563	5,559
40,900	**40,950**	6,575	5,336	6,575	5,566
40,950	**41,000**	6,588	5,344	6,588	5,574

* This column must also be used by a qualifying widow(er).

(Continued on page 73)

2008 Tax Table–*Continued*

If line 43 (taxable income) is— / And you are—

Column headers for each section: At least | But less than | Single | Married filing jointly * | Married filing separately | Head of a household

Your tax is—

41,000

At least	But less than	Single	Married filing jointly *	Married filing separately	Head of a household
41,000	41,050	6,600	5,351	6,600	5,581
41,050	41,100	6,613	5,359	6,613	5,589
41,100	41,150	6,625	5,366	6,625	5,596
41,150	41,200	6,638	5,374	6,638	5,604
41,200	41,250	6,650	5,381	6,650	5,611
41,250	41,300	6,663	5,389	6,663	5,619
41,300	41,350	6,675	5,396	6,675	5,626
41,350	41,400	6,688	5,404	6,688	5,634
41,400	41,450	6,700	5,411	6,700	5,641
41,450	41,500	6,713	5,419	6,713	5,649
41,500	41,550	6,725	5,426	6,725	5,656
41,550	41,600	6,738	5,434	6,738	5,664
41,600	41,650	6,750	5,441	6,750	5,671
41,650	41,700	6,763	5,449	6,763	5,679
41,700	41,750	6,775	5,456	6,775	5,686
41,750	41,800	6,788	5,464	6,788	5,694
41,800	41,850	6,800	5,471	6,800	5,701
41,850	41,900	6,813	5,479	6,813	5,709
41,900	41,950	6,825	5,486	6,825	5,716
41,950	42,000	6,838	5,494	6,838	5,724

42,000

At least	But less than	Single	Married filing jointly *	Married filing separately	Head of a household
42,000	42,050	6,850	5,501	6,850	5,731
42,050	42,100	6,863	5,509	6,863	5,739
42,100	42,150	6,875	5,516	6,875	5,746
42,150	42,200	6,888	5,524	6,888	5,754
42,200	42,250	6,900	5,531	6,900	5,761
42,250	42,300	6,913	5,539	6,913	5,769
42,300	42,350	6,925	5,546	6,925	5,776
42,350	42,400	6,938	5,554	6,938	5,784
42,400	42,450	6,950	5,561	6,950	5,791
42,450	42,500	6,963	5,569	6,963	5,799
42,500	42,550	6,975	5,576	6,975	5,806
42,550	42,600	6,988	5,584	6,988	5,814
42,600	42,650	7,000	5,591	7,000	5,821
42,650	42,700	7,013	5,599	7,013	5,829
42,700	42,750	7,025	5,606	7,025	5,836
42,750	42,800	7,038	5,614	7,038	5,844
42,800	42,850	7,050	5,621	7,050	5,851
42,850	42,900	7,063	5,629	7,063	5,859
42,900	42,950	7,075	5,636	7,075	5,866
42,950	43,000	7,088	5,644	7,088	5,874

43,000

At least	But less than	Single	Married filing jointly *	Married filing separately	Head of a household
43,000	43,050	7,100	5,651	7,100	5,881
43,050	43,100	7,113	5,659	7,113	5,889
43,100	43,150	7,125	5,666	7,125	5,896
43,150	43,200	7,138	5,674	7,138	5,904
43,200	43,250	7,150	5,681	7,150	5,911
43,250	43,300	7,163	5,689	7,163	5,919
43,300	43,350	7,175	5,696	7,175	5,926
43,350	43,400	7,188	5,704	7,188	5,934
43,400	43,450	7,200	5,711	7,200	5,941
43,450	43,500	7,213	5,719	7,213	5,949
43,500	43,550	7,225	5,726	7,225	5,956
43,550	43,600	7,238	5,734	7,238	5,964
43,600	43,650	7,250	5,741	7,250	5,971
43,650	43,700	7,263	5,749	7,263	5,981
43,700	43,750	7,275	5,756	7,275	5,994
43,750	43,800	7,288	5,764	7,288	6,006
43,800	43,850	7,300	5,771	7,300	6,019
43,850	43,900	7,313	5,779	7,313	6,031
43,900	43,950	7,325	5,786	7,325	6,044
43,950	44,000	7,338	5,794	7,338	6,056

44,000

At least	But less than	Single	Married filing jointly *	Married filing separately	Head of a household
44,000	44,050	7,350	5,801	7,350	6,069
44,050	44,100	7,363	5,809	7,363	6,081
44,100	44,150	7,375	5,816	7,375	6,094
44,150	44,200	7,388	5,824	7,388	6,106
44,200	44,250	7,400	5,831	7,400	6,119
44,250	44,300	7,413	5,839	7,413	6,131
44,300	44,350	7,425	5,846	7,425	6,144
44,350	44,400	7,438	5,854	7,438	6,156
44,400	44,450	7,450	5,861	7,450	6,169
44,450	44,500	7,463	5,869	7,463	6,181
44,500	44,550	7,475	5,876	7,475	6,194
44,550	44,600	7,488	5,884	7,488	6,206
44,600	44,650	7,500	5,891	7,500	6,219
44,650	44,700	7,513	5,899	7,513	6,231
44,700	44,750	7,525	5,906	7,525	6,244
44,750	44,800	7,538	5,914	7,538	6,256
44,800	44,850	7,550	5,921	7,550	6,269
44,850	44,900	7,563	5,929	7,563	6,281
44,900	44,950	7,575	5,936	7,575	6,294
44,950	45,000	7,588	5,944	7,588	6,306

45,000

At least	But less than	Single	Married filing jointly *	Married filing separately	Head of a household
45,000	45,050	7,600	5,951	7,600	6,319
45,050	45,100	7,613	5,959	7,613	6,331
45,100	45,150	7,625	5,966	7,625	6,344
45,150	45,200	7,638	5,974	7,638	6,356
45,200	45,250	7,650	5,981	7,650	6,369
45,250	45,300	7,663	5,989	7,663	6,381
45,300	45,350	7,675	5,996	7,675	6,394
45,350	45,400	7,688	6,004	7,688	6,406
45,400	45,450	7,700	6,011	7,700	6,419
45,450	45,500	7,713	6,019	7,713	6,431
45,500	45,550	7,725	6,026	7,725	6,444
45,550	45,600	7,738	6,034	7,738	6,456
45,600	45,650	7,750	6,041	7,750	6,469
45,650	45,700	7,763	6,049	7,763	6,481
45,700	45,750	7,775	6,056	7,775	6,494
45,750	45,800	7,788	6,064	7,788	6,506
45,800	45,850	7,800	6,071	7,800	6,519
45,850	45,900	7,813	6,079	7,813	6,531
45,900	45,950	7,825	6,086	7,825	6,544
45,950	46,000	7,838	6,094	7,838	6,556

46,000

At least	But less than	Single	Married filing jointly *	Married filing separately	Head of a household
46,000	46,050	7,850	6,101	7,850	6,569
46,050	46,100	7,863	6,109	7,863	6,581
46,100	46,150	7,875	6,116	7,875	6,594
46,150	46,200	7,888	6,124	7,888	6,606
46,200	46,250	7,900	6,131	7,900	6,619
46,250	46,300	7,913	6,139	7,913	6,631
46,300	46,350	7,925	6,146	7,925	6,644
46,350	46,400	7,938	6,154	7,938	6,656
46,400	46,450	7,950	6,161	7,950	6,669
46,450	46,500	7,963	6,169	7,963	6,681
46,500	46,550	7,975	6,176	7,975	6,694
46,550	46,600	7,988	6,184	7,988	6,706
46,600	46,650	8,000	6,191	8,000	6,719
46,650	46,700	8,013	6,199	8,013	6,731
46,700	46,750	8,025	6,206	8,025	6,744
46,750	46,800	8,038	6,214	8,038	6,756
46,800	46,850	8,050	6,221	8,050	6,769
46,850	46,900	8,063	6,229	8,063	6,781
46,900	46,950	8,075	6,236	8,075	6,794
46,950	47,000	8,088	6,244	8,088	6,806

47,000

At least	But less than	Single	Married filing jointly *	Married filing separately	Head of a household
47,000	47,050	8,100	6,251	8,100	6,819
47,050	47,100	8,113	6,259	8,113	6,831
47,100	47,150	8,125	6,266	8,125	6,844
47,150	47,200	8,138	6,274	8,138	6,856
47,200	47,250	8,150	6,281	8,150	6,869
47,250	47,300	8,163	6,289	8,163	6,881
47,300	47,350	8,175	6,296	8,175	6,894
47,350	47,400	8,188	6,304	8,188	6,906
47,400	47,450	8,200	6,311	8,200	6,919
47,450	47,500	8,213	6,319	8,213	6,931
47,500	47,550	8,225	6,326	8,225	6,944
47,550	47,600	8,238	6,334	8,238	6,956
47,600	47,650	8,250	6,341	8,250	6,969
47,650	47,700	8,263	6,349	8,263	6,981
47,700	47,750	8,275	6,356	8,275	6,994
47,750	47,800	8,288	6,364	8,288	7,006
47,800	47,850	8,300	6,371	8,300	7,019
47,850	47,900	8,313	6,379	8,313	7,031
47,900	47,950	8,325	6,386	8,325	7,044
47,950	48,000	8,338	6,394	8,338	7,056

48,000

At least	But less than	Single	Married filing jointly *	Married filing separately	Head of a household
48,000	48,050	8,350	6,401	8,350	7,069
48,050	48,100	8,363	6,409	8,363	7,081
48,100	48,150	8,375	6,416	8,375	7,094
48,150	48,200	8,388	6,424	8,388	7,106
48,200	48,250	8,400	6,431	8,400	7,119
48,250	48,300	8,413	6,439	8,413	7,131
48,300	48,350	8,425	6,446	8,425	7,144
48,350	48,400	8,438	6,454	8,438	7,156
48,400	48,450	8,450	6,461	8,450	7,169
48,450	48,500	8,463	6,469	8,463	7,181
48,500	48,550	8,475	6,476	8,475	7,194
48,550	48,600	8,488	6,484	8,488	7,206
48,600	48,650	8,500	6,491	8,500	7,219
48,650	48,700	8,513	6,499	8,513	7,231
48,700	48,750	8,525	6,506	8,525	7,244
48,750	48,800	8,538	6,514	8,538	7,256
48,800	48,850	8,550	6,521	8,550	7,269
48,850	48,900	8,563	6,529	8,563	7,281
48,900	48,950	8,575	6,536	8,575	7,294
48,950	49,000	8,588	6,544	8,588	7,306

49,000

At least	But less than	Single	Married filing jointly *	Married filing separately	Head of a household
49,000	49,050	8,600	6,551	8,600	7,319
49,050	49,100	8,613	6,559	8,613	7,331
49,100	49,150	8,625	6,566	8,625	7,344
49,150	49,200	8,638	6,574	8,638	7,356
49,200	49,250	8,650	6,581	8,650	7,369
49,250	49,300	8,663	6,589	8,663	7,381
49,300	49,350	8,675	6,596	8,675	7,394
49,350	49,400	8,688	6,604	8,688	7,406
49,400	49,450	8,700	6,611	8,700	7,419
49,450	49,500	8,713	6,619	8,713	7,431
49,500	49,550	8,725	6,626	8,725	7,444
49,550	49,600	8,738	6,634	8,738	7,456
49,600	49,650	8,750	6,641	8,750	7,469
49,650	49,700	8,763	6,649	8,763	7,481
49,700	49,750	8,775	6,656	8,775	7,494
49,750	49,800	8,788	6,664	8,788	7,506
49,800	49,850	8,800	6,671	8,800	7,519
49,850	49,900	8,813	6,679	8,813	7,531
49,900	49,950	8,825	6,686	8,825	7,544
49,950	50,000	8,838	6,694	8,838	7,556

* This column must also be used by a qualifying widow(er).

(Continued on page 74)

2008 Tax Table–*Continued*

If line 43 (taxable income) is—		And you are—			
At least	But less than	Single	Married filing jointly *	Married filing separately	Head of a household
		Your tax is—			

50,000

At least	But less than	Single	Married filing jointly *	Married filing separately	Head of a household
50,000	50,050	8,850	6,701	8,850	7,569
50,050	50,100	8,863	6,709	8,863	7,581
50,100	50,150	8,875	6,716	8,875	7,594
50,150	50,200	8,888	6,724	8,888	7,606
50,200	50,250	8,900	6,731	8,900	7,619
50,250	50,300	8,913	6,739	8,913	7,631
50,300	50,350	8,925	6,746	8,925	7,644
50,350	50,400	8,938	6,754	8,938	7,656
50,400	50,450	8,950	6,761	8,950	7,669
50,450	50,500	8,963	6,769	8,963	7,681
50,500	50,550	8,975	6,776	8,975	7,694
50,550	50,600	8,988	6,784	8,988	7,706
50,600	50,650	9,000	6,791	9,000	7,719
50,650	50,700	9,013	6,799	9,013	7,731
50,700	50,750	9,025	6,806	9,025	7,744
50,750	50,800	9,038	6,814	9,038	7,756
50,800	50,850	9,050	6,821	9,050	7,769
50,850	50,900	9,063	6,829	9,063	7,781
50,900	50,950	9,075	6,836	9,075	7,794
50,950	51,000	9,088	6,844	9,088	7,806

51,000

At least	But less than	Single	Married filing jointly *	Married filing separately	Head of a household
51,000	51,050	9,100	6,851	9,100	7,819
51,050	51,100	9,113	6,859	9,113	7,831
51,100	51,150	9,125	6,866	9,125	7,844
51,150	51,200	9,138	6,874	9,138	7,856
51,200	51,250	9,150	6,881	9,150	7,869
51,250	51,300	9,163	6,889	9,163	7,881
51,300	51,350	9,175	6,896	9,175	7,894
51,350	51,400	9,188	6,904	9,188	7,906
51,400	51,450	9,200	6,911	9,200	7,919
51,450	51,500	9,213	6,919	9,213	7,931
51,500	51,550	9,225	6,926	9,225	7,944
51,550	51,600	9,238	6,934	9,238	7,956
51,600	51,650	9,250	6,941	9,250	7,969
51,650	51,700	9,263	6,949	9,263	7,981
51,700	51,750	9,275	6,956	9,275	7,994
51,750	51,800	9,288	6,964	9,288	8,006
51,800	51,850	9,300	6,971	9,300	8,019
51,850	51,900	9,313	6,979	9,313	8,031
51,900	51,950	9,325	6,986	9,325	8,044
51,950	52,000	9,338	6,994	9,338	8,056

52,000

At least	But less than	Single	Married filing jointly *	Married filing separately	Head of a household
52,000	52,050	9,350	7,001	9,350	8,069
52,050	52,100	9,363	7,009	9,363	8,081
52,100	52,150	9,375	7,016	9,375	8,094
52,150	52,200	9,388	7,024	9,388	8,106
52,200	52,250	9,400	7,031	9,400	8,119
52,250	52,300	9,413	7,039	9,413	8,131
52,300	52,350	9,425	7,046	9,425	8,144
52,350	52,400	9,438	7,054	9,438	8,156
52,400	52,450	9,450	7,061	9,450	8,169
52,450	52,500	9,463	7,069	9,463	8,181
52,500	52,550	9,475	7,076	9,475	8,194
52,550	52,600	9,488	7,084	9,488	8,206
52,600	52,650	9,500	7,091	9,500	8,219
52,650	52,700	9,513	7,099	9,513	8,231
52,700	52,750	9,525	7,106	9,525	8,244
52,750	52,800	9,538	7,114	9,538	8,256
52,800	52,850	9,550	7,121	9,550	8,269
52,850	52,900	9,563	7,129	9,563	8,281
52,900	52,950	9,575	7,136	9,575	8,294
52,950	53,000	9,588	7,144	9,588	8,306

53,000

At least	But less than	Single	Married filing jointly *	Married filing separately	Head of a household
53,000	53,050	9,600	7,151	9,600	8,319
53,050	53,100	9,613	7,159	9,613	8,331
53,100	53,150	9,625	7,166	9,625	8,344
53,150	53,200	9,638	7,174	9,638	8,356
53,200	53,250	9,650	7,181	9,650	8,369
53,250	53,300	9,663	7,189	9,663	8,381
53,300	53,350	9,675	7,196	9,675	8,394
53,350	53,400	9,688	7,204	9,688	8,406
53,400	53,450	9,700	7,211	9,700	8,419
53,450	53,500	9,713	7,219	9,713	8,431
53,500	53,550	9,725	7,226	9,725	8,444
53,550	53,600	9,738	7,234	9,738	8,456
53,600	53,650	9,750	7,241	9,750	8,469
53,650	53,700	9,763	7,249	9,763	8,481
53,700	53,750	9,775	7,256	9,775	8,494
53,750	53,800	9,788	7,264	9,788	8,506
53,800	53,850	9,800	7,271	9,800	8,519
53,850	53,900	9,813	7,279	9,813	8,531
53,900	53,950	9,825	7,286	9,825	8,544
53,950	54,000	9,838	7,294	9,838	8,556

54,000

At least	But less than	Single	Married filing jointly *	Married filing separately	Head of a household
54,000	54,050	9,850	7,301	9,850	8,569
54,050	54,100	9,863	7,309	9,863	8,581
54,100	54,150	9,875	7,316	9,875	8,594
54,150	54,200	9,888	7,324	9,888	8,606
54,200	54,250	9,900	7,331	9,900	8,619
54,250	54,300	9,913	7,339	9,913	8,631
54,300	54,350	9,925	7,346	9,925	8,644
54,350	54,400	9,938	7,354	9,938	8,656
54,400	54,450	9,950	7,361	9,950	8,669
54,450	54,500	9,963	7,369	9,963	8,681
54,500	54,550	9,975	7,376	9,975	8,694
54,550	54,600	9,988	7,384	9,988	8,706
54,600	54,650	10,000	7,391	10,000	8,719
54,650	54,700	10,013	7,399	10,013	8,731
54,700	54,750	10,025	7,406	10,025	8,744
54,750	54,800	10,038	7,414	10,038	8,756
54,800	54,850	10,050	7,421	10,050	8,769
54,850	54,900	10,063	7,429	10,063	8,781
54,900	54,950	10,075	7,436	10,075	8,794
54,950	55,000	10,088	7,444	10,088	8,806

55,000

At least	But less than	Single	Married filing jointly *	Married filing separately	Head of a household
55,000	55,050	10,100	7,451	10,100	8,819
55,050	55,100	10,113	7,459	10,113	8,831
55,100	55,150	10,125	7,466	10,125	8,844
55,150	55,200	10,138	7,474	10,138	8,856
55,200	55,250	10,150	7,481	10,150	8,869
55,250	55,300	10,163	7,489	10,163	8,881
55,300	55,350	10,175	7,496	10,175	8,894
55,350	55,400	10,188	7,504	10,188	8,906
55,400	55,450	10,200	7,511	10,200	8,919
55,450	55,500	10,213	7,519	10,213	8,931
55,500	55,550	10,225	7,526	10,225	8,944
55,550	55,600	10,238	7,534	10,238	8,956
55,600	55,650	10,250	7,541	10,250	8,969
55,650	55,700	10,263	7,549	10,263	8,981
55,700	55,750	10,275	7,556	10,275	8,994
55,750	55,800	10,288	7,564	10,288	9,006
55,800	55,850	10,300	7,571	10,300	9,019
55,850	55,900	10,313	7,579	10,313	9,031
55,900	55,950	10,325	7,586	10,325	9,044
55,950	56,000	10,338	7,594	10,338	9,056

56,000

At least	But less than	Single	Married filing jointly *	Married filing separately	Head of a household
56,000	56,050	10,350	7,601	10,350	9,069
56,050	56,100	10,363	7,609	10,363	9,081
56,100	56,150	10,375	7,616	10,375	9,094
56,150	56,200	10,388	7,624	10,388	9,106
56,200	56,250	10,400	7,631	10,400	9,119
56,250	56,300	10,413	7,639	10,413	9,131
56,300	56,350	10,425	7,646	10,425	9,144
56,350	56,400	10,438	7,654	10,438	9,156
56,400	56,450	10,450	7,661	10,450	9,169
56,450	56,500	10,463	7,669	10,463	9,181
56,500	56,550	10,475	7,676	10,475	9,194
56,550	56,600	10,488	7,684	10,488	9,206
56,600	56,650	10,500	7,691	10,500	9,219
56,650	56,700	10,513	7,699	10,513	9,231
56,700	56,750	10,525	7,706	10,525	9,244
56,750	56,800	10,538	7,714	10,538	9,256
56,800	56,850	10,550	7,721	10,550	9,269
56,850	56,900	10,563	7,729	10,563	9,281
56,900	56,950	10,575	7,736	10,575	9,294
56,950	57,000	10,588	7,744	10,588	9,306

57,000

At least	But less than	Single	Married filing jointly *	Married filing separately	Head of a household
57,000	57,050	10,600	7,751	10,600	9,319
57,050	57,100	10,613	7,759	10,613	9,331
57,100	57,150	10,625	7,766	10,625	9,344
57,150	57,200	10,638	7,774	10,638	9,356
57,200	57,250	10,650	7,781	10,650	9,369
57,250	57,300	10,663	7,789	10,663	9,381
57,300	57,350	10,675	7,796	10,675	9,394
57,350	57,400	10,688	7,804	10,688	9,406
57,400	57,450	10,700	7,811	10,700	9,419
57,450	57,500	10,713	7,819	10,713	9,431
57,500	57,550	10,725	7,826	10,725	9,444
57,550	57,600	10,738	7,834	10,738	9,456
57,600	57,650	10,750	7,841	10,750	9,469
57,650	57,700	10,763	7,849	10,763	9,481
57,700	57,750	10,775	7,856	10,775	9,494
57,750	57,800	10,788	7,864	10,788	9,506
57,800	57,850	10,800	7,871	10,800	9,519
57,850	57,900	10,813	7,879	10,813	9,531
57,900	57,950	10,825	7,886	10,825	9,544
57,950	58,000	10,838	7,894	10,838	9,556

58,000

At least	But less than	Single	Married filing jointly *	Married filing separately	Head of a household
58,000	58,050	10,850	7,901	10,850	9,569
58,050	58,100	10,863	7,909	10,863	9,581
58,100	58,150	10,875	7,916	10,875	9,594
58,150	58,200	10,888	7,924	10,888	9,606
58,200	58,250	10,900	7,931	10,900	9,619
58,250	58,300	10,913	7,939	10,913	9,631
58,300	58,350	10,925	7,946	10,925	9,644
58,350	58,400	10,938	7,954	10,938	9,656
58,400	58,450	10,950	7,961	10,950	9,669
58,450	58,500	10,963	7,969	10,963	9,681
58,500	58,550	10,975	7,976	10,975	9,694
58,550	58,600	10,988	7,984	10,988	9,706
58,600	58,650	11,000	7,991	11,000	9,719
58,650	58,700	11,013	7,999	11,013	9,731
58,700	58,750	11,025	8,006	11,025	9,744
58,750	58,800	11,038	8,014	11,038	9,756
58,800	58,850	11,050	8,021	11,050	9,769
58,850	58,900	11,063	8,029	11,063	9,781
58,900	58,950	11,075	8,036	11,075	9,794
58,950	59,000	11,088	8,044	11,088	9,806

* This column must also be used by a qualifying widow(er).

(Continued on page 75)

2008 Tax Table—Continued

If line 43 (taxable income) is — And you are — *This column must also be used by a qualifying widow(er). Your tax is—

At least	But less than	Single	Married filing jointly*	Married filing separately	Head of a household
59,000					
59,000	59,050	11,100	8,051	11,100	9,819
59,050	59,100	11,113	8,059	11,113	9,831
59,100	59,150	11,125	8,066	11,125	9,844
59,150	59,200	11,138	8,074	11,138	9,856
59,200	59,250	11,150	8,081	11,150	9,869
59,250	59,300	11,163	8,089	11,163	9,881
59,300	59,350	11,175	8,096	11,175	9,894
59,350	59,400	11,188	8,104	11,188	9,906
59,400	59,450	11,200	8,111	11,200	9,919
59,450	59,500	11,213	8,119	11,213	9,931
59,500	59,550	11,225	8,126	11,225	9,944
59,550	59,600	11,238	8,134	11,238	9,956
59,600	59,650	11,250	8,141	11,250	9,969
59,650	59,700	11,263	8,149	11,263	9,981
59,700	59,750	11,275	8,156	11,275	9,994
59,750	59,800	11,288	8,164	11,288	10,006
59,800	59,850	11,300	8,171	11,300	10,019
59,850	59,900	11,313	8,179	11,313	10,031
59,900	59,950	11,325	8,186	11,325	10,044
59,950	60,000	11,338	8,194	11,338	10,056
60,000					
60,000	60,050	11,350	8,201	11,350	10,069
60,050	60,100	11,363	8,209	11,363	10,081
60,100	60,150	11,375	8,216	11,375	10,094
60,150	60,200	11,388	8,224	11,388	10,106
60,200	60,250	11,400	8,231	11,400	10,119
60,250	60,300	11,413	8,239	11,413	10,131
60,300	60,350	11,425	8,246	11,425	10,144
60,350	60,400	11,438	8,254	11,438	10,156
60,400	60,450	11,450	8,261	11,450	10,169
60,450	60,500	11,463	8,269	11,463	10,181
60,500	60,550	11,475	8,276	11,475	10,194
60,550	60,600	11,488	8,284	11,488	10,206
60,600	60,650	11,500	8,291	11,500	10,219
60,650	60,700	11,513	8,299	11,513	10,231
60,700	60,750	11,525	8,306	11,525	10,244
60,750	60,800	11,538	8,314	11,538	10,256
60,800	60,850	11,550	8,321	11,550	10,269
60,850	60,900	11,563	8,329	11,563	10,281
60,900	60,950	11,575	8,336	11,575	10,294
60,950	61,000	11,588	8,344	11,588	10,306
61,000					
61,000	61,050	11,600	8,351	11,600	10,319
61,050	61,100	11,613	8,359	11,613	10,331
61,100	61,150	11,625	8,366	11,625	10,344
61,150	61,200	11,638	8,374	11,638	10,356
61,200	61,250	11,650	8,381	11,650	10,369
61,250	61,300	11,663	8,389	11,663	10,381
61,300	61,350	11,675	8,396	11,675	10,394
61,350	61,400	11,688	8,404	11,688	10,406
61,400	61,450	11,700	8,411	11,700	10,419
61,450	61,500	11,713	8,419	11,713	10,431
61,500	61,550	11,725	8,426	11,725	10,444
61,550	61,600	11,738	8,434	11,738	10,456
61,600	61,650	11,750	8,441	11,750	10,469
61,650	61,700	11,763	8,449	11,763	10,481
61,700	61,750	11,775	8,456	11,775	10,494
61,750	61,800	11,788	8,464	11,788	10,506
61,800	61,850	11,800	8,471	11,800	10,519
61,850	61,900	11,813	8,479	11,813	10,531
61,900	61,950	11,825	8,486	11,825	10,544
61,950	62,000	11,838	8,494	11,838	10,556

At least	But less than	Single	Married filing jointly*	Married filing separately	Head of a household
62,000					
62,000	62,050	11,850	8,501	11,850	10,569
62,050	62,100	11,863	8,509	11,863	10,581
62,100	62,150	11,875	8,516	11,875	10,594
62,150	62,200	11,888	8,524	11,888	10,606
62,200	62,250	11,900	8,531	11,900	10,619
62,250	62,300	11,913	8,539	11,913	10,631
62,300	62,350	11,925	8,546	11,925	10,644
62,350	62,400	11,938	8,554	11,938	10,656
62,400	62,450	11,950	8,561	11,950	10,669
62,450	62,500	11,963	8,569	11,963	10,681
62,500	62,550	11,975	8,576	11,975	10,694
62,550	62,600	11,988	8,584	11,988	10,706
62,600	62,650	12,000	8,591	12,000	10,719
62,650	62,700	12,013	8,599	12,013	10,731
62,700	62,750	12,025	8,606	12,025	10,744
62,750	62,800	12,038	8,614	12,038	10,756
62,800	62,850	12,050	8,621	12,050	10,769
62,850	62,900	12,063	8,629	12,063	10,781
62,900	62,950	12,075	8,636	12,075	10,794
62,950	63,000	12,088	8,644	12,088	10,806
63,000					
63,000	63,050	12,100	8,651	12,100	10,819
63,050	63,100	12,113	8,659	12,113	10,831
63,100	63,150	12,125	8,666	12,125	10,844
63,150	63,200	12,138	8,674	12,138	10,856
63,200	63,250	12,150	8,681	12,150	10,869
63,250	63,300	12,163	8,689	12,163	10,881
63,300	63,350	12,175	8,696	12,175	10,894
63,350	63,400	12,188	8,704	12,188	10,906
63,400	63,450	12,200	8,711	12,200	10,919
63,450	63,500	12,213	8,719	12,213	10,931
63,500	63,550	12,225	8,726	12,225	10,944
63,550	63,600	12,238	8,734	12,238	10,956
63,600	63,650	12,250	8,741	12,250	10,969
63,650	63,700	12,263	8,749	12,263	10,981
63,700	63,750	12,275	8,756	12,275	10,994
63,750	63,800	12,288	8,764	12,288	11,006
63,800	63,850	12,300	8,771	12,300	11,019
63,850	63,900	12,313	8,779	12,313	11,031
63,900	63,950	12,325	8,786	12,325	11,044
63,950	64,000	12,338	8,794	12,338	11,056
64,000					
64,000	64,050	12,350	8,801	12,350	11,069
64,050	64,100	12,363	8,809	12,363	11,081
64,100	64,150	12,375	8,816	12,375	11,094
64,150	64,200	12,388	8,824	12,388	11,106
64,200	64,250	12,400	8,831	12,400	11,119
64,250	64,300	12,413	8,839	12,413	11,131
64,300	64,350	12,425	8,846	12,425	11,144
64,350	64,400	12,438	8,854	12,438	11,156
64,400	64,450	12,450	8,861	12,450	11,169
64,450	64,500	12,463	8,869	12,463	11,181
64,500	64,550	12,475	8,876	12,475	11,194
64,550	64,600	12,488	8,884	12,488	11,206
64,600	64,650	12,500	8,891	12,500	11,219
64,650	64,700	12,513	8,899	12,513	11,231
64,700	64,750	12,525	8,906	12,525	11,244
64,750	64,800	12,538	8,914	12,538	11,256
64,800	64,850	12,550	8,921	12,550	11,269
64,850	64,900	12,563	8,929	12,563	11,281
64,900	64,950	12,575	8,936	12,575	11,294
64,950	65,000	12,588	8,944	12,588	11,306

At least	But less than	Single	Married filing jointly*	Married filing separately	Head of a household
65,000					
65,000	65,050	12,600	8,951	12,600	11,319
65,050	65,100	12,613	8,959	12,613	11,331
65,100	65,150	12,625	8,969	12,625	11,344
65,150	65,200	12,638	8,981	12,638	11,356
65,200	65,250	12,650	8,994	12,650	11,369
65,250	65,300	12,663	9,006	12,663	11,381
65,300	65,350	12,675	9,019	12,675	11,394
65,350	65,400	12,688	9,031	12,688	11,406
65,400	65,450	12,700	9,044	12,700	11,419
65,450	65,500	12,713	9,056	12,713	11,431
65,500	65,550	12,725	9,069	12,725	11,444
65,550	65,600	12,738	9,081	12,738	11,456
65,600	65,650	12,750	9,094	12,750	11,469
65,650	65,700	12,763	9,106	12,763	11,481
65,700	65,750	12,775	9,119	12,775	11,494
65,750	65,800	12,788	9,131	12,789	11,506
65,800	65,850	12,800	9,144	12,803	11,519
65,850	65,900	12,813	9,156	12,817	11,531
65,900	65,950	12,825	9,169	12,831	11,544
65,950	66,000	12,838	9,181	12,845	11,556
66,000					
66,000	66,050	12,850	9,194	12,859	11,569
66,050	66,100	12,863	9,206	12,873	11,581
66,100	66,150	12,875	9,219	12,887	11,594
66,150	66,200	12,888	9,231	12,901	11,606
66,200	66,250	12,900	9,244	12,915	11,619
66,250	66,300	12,913	9,256	12,929	11,631
66,300	66,350	12,925	9,269	12,943	11,644
66,350	66,400	12,938	9,281	12,957	11,656
66,400	66,450	12,950	9,294	12,971	11,669
66,450	66,500	12,963	9,306	12,985	11,681
66,500	66,550	12,975	9,319	12,999	11,694
66,550	66,600	12,988	9,331	13,013	11,706
66,600	66,650	13,000	9,344	13,027	11,719
66,650	66,700	13,013	9,356	13,041	11,731
66,700	66,750	13,025	9,369	13,055	11,744
66,750	66,800	13,038	9,381	13,069	11,756
66,800	66,850	13,050	9,394	13,083	11,769
66,850	66,900	13,063	9,406	13,097	11,781
66,900	66,950	13,075	9,419	13,111	11,794
66,950	67,000	13,088	9,431	13,125	11,806
67,000					
67,000	67,050	13,100	9,444	13,139	11,819
67,050	67,100	13,113	9,456	13,153	11,831
67,100	67,150	13,125	9,469	13,167	11,844
67,150	67,200	13,138	9,481	13,181	11,856
67,200	67,250	13,150	9,494	13,195	11,869
67,250	67,300	13,163	9,506	13,209	11,881
67,300	67,350	13,175	9,519	13,223	11,894
67,350	67,400	13,188	9,531	13,237	11,906
67,400	67,450	13,200	9,544	13,251	11,919
67,450	67,500	13,213	9,556	13,265	11,931
67,500	67,550	13,225	9,569	13,279	11,944
67,550	67,600	13,238	9,581	13,293	11,956
67,600	67,650	13,250	9,594	13,307	11,969
67,650	67,700	13,263	9,606	13,321	11,981
67,700	67,750	13,275	9,619	13,335	11,994
67,750	67,800	13,288	9,631	13,349	12,006
67,800	67,850	13,300	9,644	13,363	12,019
67,850	67,900	13,313	9,656	13,377	12,031
67,900	67,950	13,325	9,669	13,391	12,044
67,950	68,000	13,338	9,681	13,405	12,056

* This column must also be used by a qualifying widow(er).

(Continued on page 76)

2008 Tax Table – *Continued*

If line 43 (taxable income) is—		And you are—			
At least	But less than	Single	Married filing jointly *	Married filing separately	Head of a household
		Your tax is—			

68,000

At least	But less than	Single	Married filing jointly *	Married filing separately	Head of a household
68,000	68,050	13,350	9,694	13,419	12,069
68,050	68,100	13,363	9,706	13,433	12,081
68,100	68,150	13,375	9,719	13,447	12,094
68,150	68,200	13,388	9,731	13,461	12,106
68,200	68,250	13,400	9,744	13,475	12,119
68,250	68,300	13,413	9,756	13,489	12,131
68,300	68,350	13,425	9,769	13,503	12,144
68,350	68,400	13,438	9,781	13,517	12,156
68,400	68,450	13,450	9,794	13,531	12,169
68,450	68,500	13,463	9,806	13,545	12,181
68,500	68,550	13,475	9,819	13,559	12,194
68,550	68,600	13,488	9,831	13,573	12,206
68,600	68,650	13,500	9,844	13,587	12,219
68,650	68,700	13,513	9,856	13,601	12,231
68,700	68,750	13,525	9,869	13,615	12,244
68,750	68,800	13,538	9,881	13,629	12,256
68,800	68,850	13,550	9,894	13,643	12,269
68,850	68,900	13,563	9,906	13,657	12,281
68,900	68,950	13,575	9,919	13,671	12,294
68,950	69,000	13,588	9,931	13,685	12,306

69,000

At least	But less than	Single	Married filing jointly *	Married filing separately	Head of a household
69,000	69,050	13,600	9,944	13,699	12,319
69,050	69,100	13,613	9,956	13,713	12,331
69,100	69,150	13,625	9,969	13,727	12,344
69,150	69,200	13,638	9,981	13,741	12,356
69,200	69,250	13,650	9,994	13,755	12,369
69,250	69,300	13,663	10,006	13,769	12,381
69,300	69,350	13,675	10,019	13,783	12,394
69,350	69,400	13,688	10,031	13,797	12,406
69,400	69,450	13,700	10,044	13,811	12,419
69,450	69,500	13,713	10,056	13,825	12,431
69,500	69,550	13,725	10,069	13,839	12,444
69,550	69,600	13,738	10,081	13,853	12,456
69,600	69,650	13,750	10,094	13,867	12,469
69,650	69,700	13,763	10,106	13,881	12,481
69,700	69,750	13,775	10,119	13,895	12,494
69,750	69,800	13,788	10,131	13,909	12,506
69,800	69,850	13,800	10,144	13,923	12,519
69,850	69,900	13,813	10,156	13,937	12,531
69,900	69,950	13,825	10,169	13,951	12,544
69,950	70,000	13,838	10,181	13,965	12,556

70,000

At least	But less than	Single	Married filing jointly *	Married filing separately	Head of a household
70,000	70,050	13,850	10,194	13,979	12,569
70,050	70,100	13,863	10,206	13,993	12,581
70,100	70,150	13,875	10,219	14,007	12,594
70,150	70,200	13,888	10,231	14,021	12,606
70,200	70,250	13,900	10,244	14,035	12,619
70,250	70,300	13,913	10,256	14,049	12,631
70,300	70,350	13,925	10,269	14,063	12,644
70,350	70,400	13,938	10,281	14,077	12,656
70,400	70,450	13,950	10,294	14,091	12,669
70,450	70,500	13,963	10,306	14,105	12,681
70,500	70,550	13,975	10,319	14,119	12,694
70,550	70,600	13,988	10,331	14,133	12,706
70,600	70,650	14,000	10,344	14,147	12,719
70,650	70,700	14,013	10,356	14,161	12,731
70,700	70,750	14,025	10,369	14,175	12,744
70,750	70,800	14,038	10,381	14,189	12,756
70,800	70,850	14,050	10,394	14,203	12,769
70,850	70,900	14,063	10,406	14,217	12,781
70,900	70,950	14,075	10,419	14,231	12,794
70,950	71,000	14,088	10,431	14,245	12,806

71,000

At least	But less than	Single	Married filing jointly *	Married filing separately	Head of a household
71,000	71,050	14,100	10,444	14,259	12,819
71,050	71,100	14,113	10,456	14,273	12,831
71,100	71,150	14,125	10,469	14,287	12,844
71,150	71,200	14,138	10,481	14,301	12,856
71,200	71,250	14,150	10,494	14,315	12,869
71,250	71,300	14,163	10,506	14,329	12,881
71,300	71,350	14,175	10,519	14,343	12,894
71,350	71,400	14,188	10,531	14,357	12,906
71,400	71,450	14,200	10,544	14,371	12,919
71,450	71,500	14,213	10,556	14,385	12,931
71,500	71,550	14,225	10,569	14,399	12,944
71,550	71,600	14,238	10,581	14,413	12,956
71,600	71,650	14,250	10,594	14,427	12,969
71,650	71,700	14,263	10,606	14,441	12,981
71,700	71,750	14,275	10,619	14,455	12,994
71,750	71,800	14,288	10,631	14,469	13,006
71,800	71,850	14,300	10,644	14,483	13,019
71,850	71,900	14,313	10,656	14,497	13,031
71,900	71,950	14,325	10,669	14,511	13,044
71,950	72,000	14,338	10,681	14,525	13,056

72,000

At least	But less than	Single	Married filing jointly *	Married filing separately	Head of a household
72,000	72,050	14,350	10,694	14,539	13,069
72,050	72,100	14,363	10,706	14,553	13,081
72,100	72,150	14,375	10,719	14,567	13,094
72,150	72,200	14,388	10,731	14,581	13,106
72,200	72,250	14,400	10,744	14,595	13,119
72,250	72,300	14,413	10,756	14,609	13,131
72,300	72,350	14,425	10,769	14,623	13,144
72,350	72,400	14,438	10,781	14,637	13,156
72,400	72,450	14,450	10,794	14,651	13,169
72,450	72,500	14,463	10,806	14,665	13,181
72,500	72,550	14,475	10,819	14,679	13,194
72,550	72,600	14,488	10,831	14,693	13,206
72,600	72,650	14,500	10,844	14,707	13,219
72,650	72,700	14,513	10,856	14,721	13,231
72,700	72,750	14,525	10,869	14,735	13,244
72,750	72,800	14,538	10,881	14,749	13,256
72,800	72,850	14,550	10,894	14,763	13,269
72,850	72,900	14,563	10,906	14,777	13,281
72,900	72,950	14,575	10,919	14,791	13,294
72,950	73,000	14,588	10,931	14,805	13,306

73,000

At least	But less than	Single	Married filing jointly *	Married filing separately	Head of a household
73,000	73,050	14,600	10,944	14,819	13,319
73,050	73,100	14,613	10,956	14,833	13,331
73,100	73,150	14,625	10,969	14,847	13,344
73,150	73,200	14,638	10,981	14,861	13,356
73,200	73,250	14,650	10,994	14,875	13,369
73,250	73,300	14,663	11,006	14,889	13,381
73,300	73,350	14,675	11,019	14,903	13,394
73,350	73,400	14,688	11,031	14,917	13,406
73,400	73,450	14,700	11,044	14,931	13,419
73,450	73,500	14,713	11,056	14,945	13,431
73,500	73,550	14,725	11,069	14,959	13,444
73,550	73,600	14,738	11,081	14,973	13,456
73,600	73,650	14,750	11,094	14,987	13,469
73,650	73,700	14,763	11,106	15,001	13,481
73,700	73,750	14,775	11,119	15,015	13,494
73,750	73,800	14,788	11,131	15,029	13,506
73,800	73,850	14,800	11,144	15,043	13,519
73,850	73,900	14,813	11,156	15,057	13,531
73,900	73,950	14,825	11,169	15,071	13,544
73,950	74,000	14,838	11,181	15,085	13,556

74,000

At least	But less than	Single	Married filing jointly *	Married filing separately	Head of a household
74,000	74,050	14,850	11,194	15,099	13,569
74,050	74,100	14,863	11,206	15,113	13,581
74,100	74,150	14,875	11,219	15,127	13,594
74,150	74,200	14,888	11,231	15,141	13,606
74,200	74,250	14,900	11,244	15,155	13,619
74,250	74,300	14,913	11,256	15,169	13,631
74,300	74,350	14,925	11,269	15,183	13,644
74,350	74,400	14,938	11,281	15,197	13,656
74,400	74,450	14,950	11,294	15,211	13,669
74,450	74,500	14,963	11,306	15,225	13,681
74,500	74,550	14,975	11,319	15,239	13,694
74,550	74,600	14,988	11,331	15,253	13,706
74,600	74,650	15,000	11,344	15,267	13,719
74,650	74,700	15,013	11,356	15,281	13,731
74,700	74,750	15,025	11,369	15,295	13,744
74,750	74,800	15,038	11,381	15,309	13,756
74,800	74,850	15,050	11,394	15,323	13,769
74,850	74,900	15,063	11,406	15,337	13,781
74,900	74,950	15,075	11,419	15,351	13,794
74,950	75,000	15,088	11,431	15,365	13,806

75,000

At least	But less than	Single	Married filing jointly *	Married filing separately	Head of a household
75,000	75,050	15,100	11,444	15,379	13,819
75,050	75,100	15,113	11,456	15,393	13,831
75,100	75,150	15,125	11,469	15,407	13,844
75,150	75,200	15,138	11,481	15,421	13,856
75,200	75,250	15,150	11,494	15,435	13,869
75,250	75,300	15,163	11,506	15,449	13,881
75,300	75,350	15,175	11,519	15,463	13,894
75,350	75,400	15,188	11,531	15,477	13,906
75,400	75,450	15,200	11,544	15,491	13,919
75,450	75,500	15,213	11,556	15,505	13,931
75,500	75,550	15,225	11,569	15,519	13,944
75,550	75,600	15,238	11,581	15,533	13,956
75,600	75,650	15,250	11,594	15,547	13,969
75,650	75,700	15,263	11,606	15,561	13,981
75,700	75,750	15,275	11,619	15,575	13,994
75,750	75,800	15,288	11,631	15,589	14,006
75,800	75,850	15,300	11,644	15,603	14,019
75,850	75,900	15,313	11,656	15,617	14,031
75,900	75,950	15,325	11,669	15,631	14,044
75,950	76,000	15,338	11,681	15,645	14,056

76,000

At least	But less than	Single	Married filing jointly *	Married filing separately	Head of a household
76,000	76,050	15,350	11,694	15,659	14,069
76,050	76,100	15,363	11,706	15,673	14,081
76,100	76,150	15,375	11,719	15,687	14,094
76,150	76,200	15,388	11,731	15,701	14,106
76,200	76,250	15,400	11,744	15,715	14,119
76,250	76,300	15,413	11,756	15,729	14,131
76,300	76,350	15,425	11,769	15,743	14,144
76,350	76,400	15,438	11,781	15,757	14,156
76,400	76,450	15,450	11,794	15,771	14,169
76,450	76,500	15,463	11,806	15,785	14,181
76,500	76,550	15,475	11,819	15,799	14,194
76,550	76,600	15,488	11,831	15,813	14,206
76,600	76,650	15,500	11,844	15,827	14,219
76,650	76,700	15,513	11,856	15,841	14,231
76,700	76,750	15,525	11,869	15,855	14,244
76,750	76,800	15,538	11,881	15,869	14,256
76,800	76,850	15,550	11,894	15,883	14,269
76,850	76,900	15,563	11,906	15,897	14,281
76,900	76,950	15,575	11,919	15,911	14,294
76,950	77,000	15,588	11,931	15,925	14,306

* This column must also be used by a qualifying widow(er).

(Continued on page 77)

2008 Tax Table – *Continued*

If line 43 (taxable income) is— At least	But less than	Single	Married filing jointly *	Married filing separately	Head of a household
			Your tax is—		

77,000

At least	But less than	Single	Married filing jointly *	Married filing separately	Head of a household
77,000	77,050	15,600	11,944	15,939	14,319
77,050	77,100	15,613	11,956	15,953	14,331
77,100	77,150	15,625	11,969	15,967	14,344
77,150	77,200	15,638	11,981	15,981	14,356
77,200	77,250	15,650	11,994	15,995	14,369
77,250	77,300	15,663	12,006	16,009	14,381
77,300	77,350	15,675	12,019	16,023	14,394
77,350	77,400	15,688	12,031	16,037	14,406
77,400	77,450	15,700	12,044	16,051	14,419
77,450	77,500	15,713	12,056	16,065	14,431
77,500	77,550	15,725	12,069	16,079	14,444
77,550	77,600	15,738	12,081	16,093	14,456
77,600	77,650	15,750	12,094	16,107	14,469
77,650	77,700	15,763	12,106	16,121	14,481
77,700	77,750	15,775	12,119	16,135	14,494
77,750	77,800	15,788	12,131	16,149	14,506
77,800	77,850	15,800	12,144	16,163	14,519
77,850	77,900	15,813	12,156	16,177	14,531
77,900	77,950	15,825	12,169	16,191	14,544
77,950	78,000	15,838	12,181	16,205	14,556

78,000

At least	But less than	Single	Married filing jointly *	Married filing separately	Head of a household
78,000	78,050	15,850	12,194	16,219	14,569
78,050	78,100	15,863	12,206	16,233	14,581
78,100	78,150	15,875	12,219	16,247	14,594
78,150	78,200	15,888	12,231	16,261	14,606
78,200	78,250	15,900	12,244	16,275	14,619
78,250	78,300	15,913	12,256	16,289	14,631
78,300	78,350	15,925	12,269	16,303	14,644
78,350	78,400	15,938	12,281	16,317	14,656
78,400	78,450	15,950	12,294	16,331	14,669
78,450	78,500	15,963	12,306	16,345	14,681
78,500	78,550	15,975	12,319	16,359	14,694
78,550	78,600	15,988	12,331	16,373	14,706
78,600	78,650	16,000	12,344	16,387	14,719
78,650	78,700	16,013	12,356	16,401	14,731
78,700	78,750	16,025	12,369	16,415	14,744
78,750	78,800	16,038	12,381	16,429	14,756
78,800	78,850	16,050	12,394	16,443	14,769
78,850	78,900	16,063	12,406	16,457	14,781
78,900	78,950	16,077	12,419	16,471	14,794
78,950	79,000	16,091	12,431	16,485	14,806

79,000

At least	But less than	Single	Married filing jointly *	Married filing separately	Head of a household
79,000	79,050	16,105	12,444	16,499	14,819
79,050	79,100	16,119	12,456	16,513	14,831
79,100	79,150	16,133	12,469	16,527	14,844
79,150	79,200	16,147	12,481	16,541	14,856
79,200	79,250	16,161	12,494	16,555	14,869
79,250	79,300	16,175	12,506	16,569	14,881
79,300	79,350	16,189	12,519	16,583	14,894
79,350	79,400	16,203	12,531	16,597	14,906
79,400	79,450	16,217	12,544	16,611	14,919
79,450	79,500	16,231	12,556	16,625	14,931
79,500	79,550	16,245	12,569	16,639	14,944
79,550	79,600	16,259	12,581	16,653	14,956
79,600	79,650	16,273	12,594	16,667	14,969
79,650	79,700	16,287	12,606	16,681	14,981
79,700	79,750	16,301	12,619	16,695	14,994
79,750	79,800	16,315	12,631	16,709	15,006
79,800	79,850	16,329	12,644	16,723	15,019
79,850	79,900	16,343	12,656	16,737	15,031
79,900	79,950	16,357	12,669	16,751	15,044
79,950	80,000	16,371	12,681	16,765	15,056

80,000

At least	But less than	Single	Married filing jointly *	Married filing separately	Head of a household
80,000	80,050	16,385	12,694	16,779	15,069
80,050	80,100	16,399	12,706	16,793	15,081
80,100	80,150	16,413	12,719	16,807	15,094
80,150	80,200	16,427	12,731	16,821	15,106
80,200	80,250	16,441	12,744	16,835	15,119
80,250	80,300	16,455	12,756	16,849	15,131
80,300	80,350	16,469	12,769	16,863	15,144
80,350	80,400	16,483	12,781	16,877	15,156
80,400	80,450	16,497	12,794	16,891	15,169
80,450	80,500	16,511	12,806	16,905	15,181
80,500	80,550	16,525	12,819	16,919	15,194
80,550	80,600	16,539	12,831	16,933	15,206
80,600	80,650	16,553	12,844	16,947	15,219
80,650	80,700	16,567	12,856	16,961	15,231
80,700	80,750	16,581	12,869	16,975	15,244
80,750	80,800	16,595	12,881	16,989	15,256
80,800	80,850	16,609	12,894	17,003	15,269
80,850	80,900	16,623	12,906	17,017	15,281
80,900	80,950	16,637	12,919	17,031	15,294
80,950	81,000	16,651	12,931	17,045	15,306

81,000

At least	But less than	Single	Married filing jointly *	Married filing separately	Head of a household
81,000	81,050	16,665	12,944	17,059	15,319
81,050	81,100	16,679	12,956	17,073	15,331
81,100	81,150	16,693	12,969	17,087	15,344
81,150	81,200	16,707	12,981	17,101	15,356
81,200	81,250	16,721	12,994	17,115	15,369
81,250	81,300	16,735	13,006	17,129	15,381
81,300	81,350	16,749	13,019	17,143	15,394
81,350	81,400	16,763	13,031	17,157	15,406
81,400	81,450	16,777	13,044	17,171	15,419
81,450	81,500	16,791	13,056	17,185	15,431
81,500	81,550	16,805	13,069	17,199	15,444
81,550	81,600	16,819	13,081	17,213	15,456
81,600	81,650	16,833	13,094	17,227	15,469
81,650	81,700	16,847	13,106	17,241	15,481
81,700	81,750	16,861	13,119	17,255	15,494
81,750	81,800	16,875	13,131	17,269	15,506
81,800	81,850	16,889	13,144	17,283	15,519
81,850	81,900	16,903	13,156	17,297	15,531
81,900	81,950	16,917	13,169	17,311	15,544
81,950	82,000	16,931	13,181	17,325	15,556

82,000

At least	But less than	Single	Married filing jointly *	Married filing separately	Head of a household
82,000	82,050	16,945	13,194	17,339	15,569
82,050	82,100	16,959	13,206	17,353	15,581
82,100	82,150	16,973	13,219	17,367	15,594
82,150	82,200	16,987	13,231	17,381	15,606
82,200	82,250	17,001	13,244	17,395	15,619
82,250	82,300	17,015	13,256	17,409	15,631
82,300	82,350	17,029	13,269	17,423	15,644
82,350	82,400	17,043	13,281	17,437	15,656
82,400	82,450	17,057	13,294	17,451	15,669
82,450	82,500	17,071	13,306	17,465	15,681
82,500	82,550	17,085	13,319	17,479	15,694
82,550	82,600	17,099	13,331	17,493	15,706
82,600	82,650	17,113	13,344	17,507	15,719
82,650	82,700	17,127	13,356	17,521	15,731
82,700	82,750	17,141	13,369	17,535	15,744
82,750	82,800	17,155	13,381	17,549	15,756
82,800	82,850	17,169	13,394	17,563	15,769
82,850	82,900	17,183	13,406	17,577	15,781
82,900	82,950	17,197	13,419	17,591	15,794
82,950	83,000	17,211	13,431	17,605	15,806

83,000

At least	But less than	Single	Married filing jointly *	Married filing separately	Head of a household
83,000	83,050	17,225	13,444	17,619	15,819
83,050	83,100	17,239	13,456	17,633	15,831
83,100	83,150	17,253	13,469	17,647	15,844
83,150	83,200	17,267	13,481	17,661	15,856
83,200	83,250	17,281	13,494	17,675	15,869
83,250	83,300	17,295	13,506	17,689	15,881
83,300	83,350	17,309	13,519	17,703	15,894
83,350	83,400	17,323	13,531	17,717	15,906
83,400	83,450	17,337	13,544	17,731	15,919
83,450	83,500	17,351	13,556	17,745	15,931
83,500	83,550	17,365	13,569	17,759	15,944
83,550	83,600	17,379	13,581	17,773	15,956
83,600	83,650	17,393	13,594	17,787	15,969
83,650	83,700	17,407	13,606	17,801	15,981
83,700	83,750	17,421	13,619	17,815	15,994
83,750	83,800	17,435	13,631	17,829	16,006
83,800	83,850	17,449	13,644	17,843	16,019
83,850	83,900	17,463	13,656	17,857	16,031
83,900	83,950	17,477	13,669	17,871	16,044
83,950	84,000	17,491	13,681	17,885	16,056

84,000

At least	But less than	Single	Married filing jointly *	Married filing separately	Head of a household
84,000	84,050	17,505	13,694	17,899	16,069
84,050	84,100	17,519	13,706	17,913	16,081
84,100	84,150	17,533	13,719	17,927	16,094
84,150	84,200	17,547	13,731	17,941	16,106
84,200	84,250	17,561	13,744	17,955	16,119
84,250	84,300	17,575	13,756	17,969	16,131
84,300	84,350	17,589	13,769	17,983	16,144
84,350	84,400	17,603	13,781	17,997	16,156
84,400	84,450	17,617	13,794	18,011	16,169
84,450	84,500	17,631	13,806	18,025	16,181
84,500	84,550	17,645	13,819	18,039	16,194
84,550	84,600	17,659	13,831	18,053	16,206
84,600	84,650	17,673	13,844	18,067	16,219
84,650	84,700	17,687	13,856	18,081	16,231
84,700	84,750	17,701	13,869	18,095	16,244
84,750	84,800	17,715	13,881	18,109	16,256
84,800	84,850	17,729	13,894	18,123	16,269
84,850	84,900	17,743	13,906	18,137	16,281
84,900	84,950	17,757	13,919	18,151	16,294
84,950	85,000	17,771	13,931	18,165	16,306

85,000

At least	But less than	Single	Married filing jointly *	Married filing separately	Head of a household
85,000	85,050	17,785	13,944	18,179	16,319
85,050	85,100	17,799	13,956	18,193	16,331
85,100	85,150	17,813	13,969	18,207	16,344
85,150	85,200	17,827	13,981	18,221	16,356
85,200	85,250	17,841	13,994	18,235	16,369
85,250	85,300	17,855	14,006	18,249	16,381
85,300	85,350	17,869	14,019	18,263	16,394
85,350	85,400	17,883	14,031	18,277	16,406
85,400	85,450	17,897	14,044	18,291	16,419
85,450	85,500	17,911	14,056	18,305	16,431
85,500	85,550	17,925	14,069	18,319	16,444
85,550	85,600	17,939	14,081	18,333	16,456
85,600	85,650	17,953	14,094	18,347	16,469
85,650	85,700	17,967	14,106	18,361	16,481
85,700	85,750	17,981	14,119	18,375	16,494
85,750	85,800	17,995	14,131	18,389	16,506
85,800	85,850	18,009	14,144	18,403	16,519
85,850	85,900	18,023	14,156	18,417	16,531
85,900	85,950	18,037	14,169	18,431	16,544
85,950	86,000	18,051	14,181	18,445	16,556

* This column must also be used by a qualifying widow(er).

(Continued on page 78)

2008 Tax Table–*Continued*

If line 43 (taxable income) is—		And you are—			
At least	But less than	Single	Married filing jointly *	Married filing separately	Head of a house-hold
		Your tax is—			

86,000

At least	But less than	Single	Married filing jointly	Married filing separately	Head of household
86,000	86,050	18,065	14,194	18,459	16,569
86,050	86,100	18,079	14,206	18,473	16,581
86,100	86,150	18,093	14,219	18,487	16,594
86,150	86,200	18,107	14,231	18,501	16,606
86,200	86,250	18,121	14,244	18,515	16,619
86,250	86,300	18,135	14,256	18,529	16,631
86,300	86,350	18,149	14,269	18,543	16,644
86,350	86,400	18,163	14,281	18,557	16,656
86,400	86,450	18,177	14,294	18,571	16,669
86,450	86,500	18,191	14,306	18,585	16,681
86,500	86,550	18,205	14,319	18,599	16,694
86,550	86,600	18,219	14,331	18,613	16,706
86,600	86,650	18,233	14,344	18,627	16,719
86,650	86,700	18,247	14,356	18,641	16,731
86,700	86,750	18,261	14,369	18,655	16,744
86,750	86,800	18,275	14,381	18,669	16,756
86,800	86,850	18,289	14,394	18,683	16,769
86,850	86,900	18,303	14,406	18,697	16,781
86,900	86,950	18,317	14,419	18,711	16,794
86,950	87,000	18,331	14,431	18,725	16,806

87,000

At least	But less than	Single	Married filing jointly	Married filing separately	Head of household
87,000	87,050	18,345	14,444	18,739	16,819
87,050	87,100	18,359	14,456	18,753	16,831
87,100	87,150	18,373	14,469	18,767	16,844
87,150	87,200	18,387	14,481	18,781	16,856
87,200	87,250	18,401	14,494	18,795	16,869
87,250	87,300	18,415	14,506	18,809	16,881
87,300	87,350	18,429	14,519	18,823	16,894
87,350	87,400	18,443	14,531	18,837	16,906
87,400	87,450	18,457	14,544	18,851	16,919
87,450	87,500	18,471	14,556	18,865	16,931
87,500	87,550	18,485	14,569	18,879	16,944
87,550	87,600	18,499	14,581	18,893	16,956
87,600	87,650	18,513	14,594	18,907	16,969
87,650	87,700	18,527	14,606	18,921	16,981
87,700	87,750	18,541	14,619	18,935	16,994
87,750	87,800	18,555	14,631	18,949	17,006
87,800	87,850	18,569	14,644	18,963	17,019
87,850	87,900	18,583	14,656	18,977	17,031
87,900	87,950	18,597	14,669	18,991	17,044
87,950	88,000	18,611	14,681	19,005	17,056

88,000

At least	But less than	Single	Married filing jointly	Married filing separately	Head of household
88,000	88,050	18,625	14,694	19,019	17,069
88,050	88,100	18,639	14,706	19,033	17,081
88,100	88,150	18,653	14,719	19,047	17,094
88,150	88,200	18,667	14,731	19,061	17,106
88,200	88,250	18,681	14,744	19,075	17,119
88,250	88,300	18,695	14,756	19,089	17,131
88,300	88,350	18,709	14,769	19,103	17,144
88,350	88,400	18,723	14,781	19,117	17,156
88,400	88,450	18,737	14,794	19,131	17,169
88,450	88,500	18,751	14,806	19,145	17,181
88,500	88,550	18,765	14,819	19,159	17,194
88,550	88,600	18,779	14,831	19,173	17,206
88,600	88,650	18,793	14,844	19,187	17,219
88,650	88,700	18,807	14,856	19,201	17,231
88,700	88,750	18,821	14,869	19,215	17,244
88,750	88,800	18,835	14,881	19,229	17,256
88,800	88,850	18,849	14,894	19,243	17,269
88,850	88,900	18,863	14,906	19,257	17,281
88,900	88,950	18,877	14,919	19,271	17,294
88,950	89,000	18,891	14,931	19,285	17,306

89,000

At least	But less than	Single	Married filing jointly	Married filing separately	Head of household
89,000	89,050	18,905	14,944	19,299	17,319
89,050	89,100	18,919	14,956	19,313	17,331
89,100	89,150	18,933	14,969	19,327	17,344
89,150	89,200	18,947	14,981	19,341	17,356
89,200	89,250	18,961	14,994	19,355	17,369
89,250	89,300	18,975	15,006	19,369	17,381
89,300	89,350	18,989	15,019	19,383	17,394
89,350	89,400	19,003	15,031	19,397	17,406
89,400	89,450	19,017	15,044	19,411	17,419
89,450	89,500	19,031	15,056	19,425	17,431
89,500	89,550	19,045	15,069	19,439	17,444
89,550	89,600	19,059	15,081	19,453	17,456
89,600	89,650	19,073	15,094	19,467	17,469
89,650	89,700	19,087	15,106	19,481	17,481
89,700	89,750	19,101	15,119	19,495	17,494
89,750	89,800	19,115	15,131	19,509	17,506
89,800	89,850	19,129	15,144	19,523	17,519
89,850	89,900	19,143	15,156	19,537	17,531
89,900	89,950	19,157	15,169	19,551	17,544
89,950	90,000	19,171	15,181	19,565	17,556

90,000

At least	But less than	Single	Married filing jointly	Married filing separately	Head of household
90,000	90,050	19,185	15,194	19,579	17,569
90,050	90,100	19,199	15,206	19,593	17,581
90,100	90,150	19,213	15,219	19,607	17,594
90,150	90,200	19,227	15,231	19,621	17,606
90,200	90,250	19,241	15,244	19,635	17,619
90,250	90,300	19,255	15,256	19,649	17,631
90,300	90,350	19,269	15,269	19,663	17,644
90,350	90,400	19,283	15,281	19,677	17,656
90,400	90,450	19,297	15,294	19,691	17,669
90,450	90,500	19,311	15,306	19,705	17,681
90,500	90,550	19,325	15,319	19,719	17,694
90,550	90,600	19,339	15,331	19,733	17,706
90,600	90,650	19,353	15,344	19,747	17,719
90,650	90,700	19,367	15,356	19,761	17,731
90,700	90,750	19,381	15,369	19,775	17,744
90,750	90,800	19,395	15,381	19,789	17,756
90,800	90,850	19,409	15,394	19,803	17,769
90,850	90,900	19,423	15,406	19,817	17,781
90,900	90,950	19,437	15,419	19,831	17,794
90,950	91,000	19,451	15,431	19,845	17,806

91,000

At least	But less than	Single	Married filing jointly	Married filing separately	Head of household
91,000	91,050	19,465	15,444	19,859	17,819
91,050	91,100	19,479	15,456	19,873	17,831
91,100	91,150	19,493	15,469	19,887	17,844
91,150	91,200	19,507	15,481	19,901	17,856
91,200	91,250	19,521	15,494	19,915	17,869
91,250	91,300	19,535	15,506	19,929	17,881
91,300	91,350	19,549	15,519	19,943	17,894
91,350	91,400	19,563	15,531	19,957	17,906
91,400	91,450	19,577	15,544	19,971	17,919
91,450	91,500	19,591	15,556	19,985	17,931
91,500	91,550	19,605	15,569	19,999	17,944
91,550	91,600	19,619	15,581	20,013	17,956
91,600	91,650	19,633	15,594	20,027	17,969
91,650	91,700	19,647	15,606	20,041	17,981
91,700	91,750	19,661	15,619	20,055	17,994
91,750	91,800	19,675	15,631	20,069	18,006
91,800	91,850	19,689	15,644	20,083	18,019
91,850	91,900	19,703	15,656	20,097	18,031
91,900	91,950	19,717	15,669	20,111	18,044
91,950	92,000	19,731	15,681	20,125	18,056

92,000

At least	But less than	Single	Married filing jointly	Married filing separately	Head of household
92,000	92,050	19,745	15,694	20,139	18,069
92,050	92,100	19,759	15,706	20,153	18,081
92,100	92,150	19,773	15,719	20,167	18,094
92,150	92,200	19,787	15,731	20,181	18,106
92,200	92,250	19,801	15,744	20,195	18,119
92,250	92,300	19,815	15,756	20,209	18,131
92,300	92,350	19,829	15,769	20,223	18,144
92,350	92,400	19,843	15,781	20,237	18,156
92,400	92,450	19,857	15,794	20,251	18,169
92,450	92,500	19,871	15,806	20,265	18,181
92,500	92,550	19,885	15,819	20,279	18,194
92,550	92,600	19,899	15,831	20,293	18,206
92,600	92,650	19,913	15,844	20,307	18,219
92,650	92,700	19,927	15,856	20,321	18,231
92,700	92,750	19,941	15,869	20,335	18,244
92,750	92,800	19,955	15,881	20,349	18,256
92,800	92,850	19,969	15,894	20,363	18,269
92,850	92,900	19,983	15,906	20,377	18,281
92,900	92,950	19,997	15,919	20,391	18,294
92,950	93,000	20,011	15,931	20,405	18,306

93,000

At least	But less than	Single	Married filing jointly	Married filing separately	Head of household
93,000	93,050	20,025	15,944	20,419	18,319
93,050	93,100	20,039	15,956	20,433	18,331
93,100	93,150	20,053	15,969	20,447	18,344
93,150	93,200	20,067	15,981	20,461	18,356
93,200	93,250	20,081	15,994	20,475	18,369
93,250	93,300	20,095	16,006	20,489	18,381
93,300	93,350	20,109	16,019	20,503	18,394
93,350	93,400	20,123	16,031	20,517	18,406
93,400	93,450	20,137	16,044	20,531	18,419
93,450	93,500	20,151	16,056	20,545	18,431
93,500	93,550	20,165	16,069	20,559	18,444
93,550	93,600	20,179	16,081	20,573	18,456
93,600	93,650	20,193	16,094	20,587	18,469
93,650	93,700	20,207	16,106	20,601	18,481
93,700	93,750	20,221	16,119	20,615	18,494
93,750	93,800	20,235	16,131	20,629	18,506
93,800	93,850	20,249	16,144	20,643	18,519
93,850	93,900	20,263	16,156	20,657	18,531
93,900	93,950	20,277	16,169	20,671	18,544
93,950	94,000	20,291	16,181	20,685	18,556

94,000

At least	But less than	Single	Married filing jointly	Married filing separately	Head of household
94,000	94,050	20,305	16,194	20,699	18,569
94,050	94,100	20,319	16,206	20,713	18,581
94,100	94,150	20,333	16,219	20,727	18,594
94,150	94,200	20,347	16,231	20,741	18,606
94,200	94,250	20,361	16,244	20,755	18,619
94,250	94,300	20,375	16,256	20,769	18,631
94,300	94,350	20,389	16,269	20,783	18,644
94,350	94,400	20,403	16,281	20,797	18,656
94,400	94,450	20,417	16,294	20,811	18,669
94,450	94,500	20,431	16,306	20,825	18,681
94,500	94,550	20,445	16,319	20,839	18,694
94,550	94,600	20,459	16,331	20,853	18,706
94,600	94,650	20,473	16,344	20,867	18,719
94,650	94,700	20,487	16,356	20,881	18,731
94,700	94,750	20,501	16,369	20,895	18,744
94,750	94,800	20,515	16,381	20,909	18,756
94,800	94,850	20,529	16,394	20,923	18,769
94,850	94,900	20,543	16,406	20,937	18,781
94,900	94,950	20,557	16,419	20,951	18,794
94,950	95,000	20,571	16,431	20,965	18,806

* This column must also be used by a qualifying widow(er).

(Continued on page 79)

2008 Tax Table– *Continued*

If line 43 (taxable income) is— At least	But less than	Single	Married filing jointly *	Married filing separately	Head of a house-hold
95,000					
95,000	95,050	20,585	16,444	20,979	18,819
95,050	95,100	20,599	16,456	20,993	18,831
95,100	95,150	20,613	16,469	21,007	18,844
95,150	95,200	20,627	16,481	21,021	18,856
95,200	95,250	20,641	16,494	21,035	18,869
95,250	95,300	20,655	16,506	21,049	18,881
95,300	95,350	20,669	16,519	21,063	18,894
95,350	95,400	20,683	16,531	21,077	18,906
95,400	95,450	20,697	16,544	21,091	18,919
95,450	95,500	20,711	16,556	21,105	18,931
95,500	95,550	20,725	16,569	21,119	18,944
95,550	95,600	20,739	16,581	21,133	18,956
95,600	95,650	20,753	16,594	21,147	18,969
95,650	95,700	20,767	16,606	21,161	18,981
95,700	95,750	20,781	16,619	21,175	18,994
95,750	95,800	20,795	16,631	21,189	19,006
95,800	95,850	20,809	16,644	21,203	19,019
95,850	95,900	20,823	16,656	21,217	19,031
95,900	95,950	20,837	16,669	21,231	19,044
95,950	96,000	20,851	16,681	21,245	19,056
96,000					
96,000	96,050	20,865	16,694	21,259	19,069
96,050	96,100	20,879	16,706	21,273	19,081
96,100	96,150	20,893	16,719	21,287	19,094
96,150	96,200	20,907	16,731	21,301	19,106
96,200	96,250	20,921	16,744	21,315	19,119
96,250	96,300	20,935	16,756	21,329	19,131
96,300	96,350	20,949	16,769	21,343	19,144
96,350	96,400	20,963	16,781	21,357	19,156
96,400	96,450	20,977	16,794	21,371	19,169
96,450	96,500	20,991	16,806	21,385	19,181
96,500	96,550	21,005	16,819	21,399	19,194
96,550	96,600	21,019	16,831	21,413	19,206
96,600	96,650	21,033	16,844	21,427	19,219
96,650	96,700	21,047	16,856	21,441	19,231
96,700	96,750	21,061	16,869	21,455	19,244
96,750	96,800	21,075	16,881	21,469	19,256
96,800	96,850	21,089	16,894	21,483	19,269
96,850	96,900	21,103	16,906	21,497	19,281
96,900	96,950	21,117	16,919	21,511	19,294
96,950	97,000	21,131	16,931	21,525	19,306

If line 43 (taxable income) is— At least	But less than	Single	Married filing jointly *	Married filing separately	Head of a house-hold
97,000					
97,000	97,050	21,145	16,944	21,539	19,319
97,050	97,100	21,159	16,956	21,553	19,331
97,100	97,150	21,173	16,969	21,567	19,344
97,150	97,200	21,187	16,981	21,581	19,356
97,200	97,250	21,201	16,994	21,595	19,369
97,250	97,300	21,215	17,006	21,609	19,381
97,300	97,350	21,229	17,019	21,623	19,394
97,350	97,400	21,243	17,031	21,637	19,406
97,400	97,450	21,257	17,044	21,651	19,419
97,450	97,500	21,271	17,056	21,665	19,431
97,500	97,550	21,285	17,069	21,679	19,444
97,550	97,600	21,299	17,081	21,693	19,456
97,600	97,650	21,313	17,094	21,707	19,469
97,650	97,700	21,327	17,106	21,721	19,481
97,700	97,750	21,341	17,119	21,735	19,494
97,750	97,800	21,355	17,131	21,749	19,506
97,800	97,850	21,369	17,144	21,763	19,519
97,850	97,900	21,383	17,156	21,777	19,531
97,900	97,950	21,397	17,169	21,791	19,544
97,950	98,000	21,411	17,181	21,805	19,556
98,000					
98,000	98,050	21,425	17,194	21,819	19,569
98,050	98,100	21,439	17,206	21,833	19,581
98,100	98,150	21,453	17,219	21,847	19,594
98,150	98,200	21,467	17,231	21,861	19,606
98,200	98,250	21,481	17,244	21,875	19,619
98,250	98,300	21,495	17,256	21,889	19,631
98,300	98,350	21,509	17,269	21,903	19,644
98,350	98,400	21,523	17,281	21,917	19,656
98,400	98,450	21,537	17,294	21,931	19,669
98,450	98,500	21,551	17,306	21,945	19,681
98,500	98,550	21,565	17,319	21,959	19,694
98,550	98,600	21,579	17,331	21,973	19,706
98,600	98,650	21,593	17,344	21,987	19,719
98,650	98,700	21,607	17,356	22,001	19,731
98,700	98,750	21,621	17,369	22,015	19,744
98,750	98,800	21,635	17,381	22,029	19,756
98,800	98,850	21,649	17,394	22,043	19,769
98,850	98,900	21,663	17,406	22,057	19,781
98,900	98,950	21,677	17,419	22,071	19,794
98,950	99,000	21,691	17,431	22,085	19,806

If line 43 (taxable income) is— At least	But less than	Single	Married filing jointly *	Married filing separately	Head of a house-hold
99,000					
99,000	99,050	21,705	17,444	22,099	19,819
99,050	99,100	21,719	17,456	22,113	19,831
99,100	99,150	21,733	17,469	22,127	19,844
99,150	99,200	21,747	17,481	22,141	19,856
99,200	99,250	21,761	17,494	22,155	19,869
99,250	99,300	21,775	17,506	22,169	19,881
99,300	99,350	21,789	17,519	22,183	19,894
99,350	99,400	21,803	17,531	22,197	19,906
99,400	99,450	21,817	17,544	22,211	19,919
99,450	99,500	21,831	17,556	22,225	19,931
99,500	99,550	21,845	17,569	22,239	19,944
99,550	99,600	21,859	17,581	22,253	19,956
99,600	99,650	21,873	17,594	22,267	19,969
99,650	99,700	21,887	17,606	22,281	19,981
99,700	99,750	21,901	17,619	22,295	19,994
99,750	99,800	21,915	17,631	22,309	20,006
99,800	99,850	21,929	17,644	22,323	20,019
99,850	99,900	21,943	17,656	22,337	20,031
99,900	99,950	21,957	17,669	22,351	20,044
99,950	100,000	21,971	17,681	22,365	20,056

$100,000 or over — use the Tax Computation Worksheet on page 80

* This column must also be used by a qualifying widow(er)

A-3 Unified Transfer Tax Rate Schedule

2009 Estate and Gift Tax Rates

If taxable transfer is Over	But not over	Tax liability	Of the Amount over
$ 0	$ 10,000	18%	$ 0
10,000	20,000	$ 1,800 + 20%	10,000
20,000	40,000	3,800 + 22%	20,000
40,000	60,000	8,200 + 24%	40,000
60,000	80,000	13,000 + 26%	60,000
80,000	100,000	18,200 + 28%	80,000
100,000	150,000	23,800 + 30%	100,000
150,000	250,000	38,800 + 32%	150,000
250,000	500,000	70,800 + 34%	250,000
500,000	750,000	155,800 + 37%	500,000
750,000	1,000,000	248,300 + 39%	750,000
1,000,000	1,250,000	345,800 + 41%	1,000,000
1,250,000	1,500,000	448,300 + 43%	1,250,000
	Over 1,500,000	555,800 + 45%	

Appendix A-4

Table S (4.4)
Single Life Factors Based on Life Table 90CM
Interest at 4.4 Percent

Age	Annuity	Life Estate	Remainder	Age	Annuity	Life Estate	Remainder
0	21.3340	.93870	.06130	55	13.9945	.61576	.38424
1	21.4784	.94505	.05495	56	13.7202	.60369	.39631
2	21.4394	.94333	.05667	57	13.4415	.59143	.40857
3	21.3934	.94131	.05869	58	13.1595	.57902	.42098
4	21.3428	.93908	.06092	59	12.8748	.56649	.43351
5	21.2885	.93669	.06331	60	12.5879	.55387	.44613
6	21.2312	.93417	.06583	61	12.2985	.54113	.45887
7	21.1706	.93151	.06849	62	12.0057	.52825	.47175
8	21.1071	.92871	.07129	63	11.7095	.51522	.48478
9	21.0402	.92577	.07423	64	11.4106	.50207	.49793
10	20.9697	.92266	.07734	65	11.1090	.48879	.51121
11	20.8958	.91941	.08059	66	10.8043	.47539	.52461
12	20.8187	.91602	.08398	67	10.4959	.46182	.53818
13	20.7392	.91252	.08748	68	10.1845	.44812	.55188
14	20.6586	.90898	.09102	69	9.8709	.43432	.56568
15	20.5774	.90540	.09460	70	9.5565	.42049	.57951
16	20.4960	.90182	.09818	71	9.2427	.40668	.59332
17	20.4139	.89821	.10179	72	8.9302	.39293	.60707
18	20.3308	.89455	.10545	73	8.6197	.37927	.62073
19	20.2453	.89079	.10921	74	8.3102	.36565	.63435
20	20.1569	.88690	.11310	75	8.0009	.35204	.64796
21	20.0652	.88287	.11713	76	7.6909	.33840	.66160
22	19.9704	.87870	.12130	77	7.3803	.32474	.67526
23	19.8719	.87437	.12563	78	7.0700	.31108	.68892
24	19.7695	.86986	.13014	79	6.7614	.29750	.70250
25	19.6627	.86516	.13484	80	6.4572	.28412	.71588
26	19.5514	.86026	.13974	81	6.1593	.27101	.72899
27	19.4352	.85515	.14485	82	5.8687	.25822	.74178
28	19.3145	.84984	.15016	83	5.5856	.24577	.75423
29	19.1893	.84433	.15567	84	5.3080	.23355	.76645
30	19.0595	.83862	.16138	85	5.0344	.22152	.77848
31	18.9254	.83272	.16728	86	4.7671	.20975	.79025
32	18.7865	.82661	.17339	87	4.5092	.19841	.80159
33	18.6426	.82028	.17972	88	4.2610	.18749	.81251
34	18.4938	.81373	.18627	89	4.0224	.17698	.82302
35	18.3393	.80693	.19307	90	3.7933	.16691	.83309
36	18.1796	.79990	.20010	91	3.5774	.15740	.84260
37	18.0143	.79263	.20737	92	3.3782	.14864	.85136
38	17.8431	.78510	.21490	93	3.1950	.14058	.85942
39	17.6659	.77730	.22270	94	3.0250	.13310	.86690
40	17.4824	.76922	.23078	95	2.8643	.12603	.87397
41	17.2921	.76085	.23915	96	2.7137	.11940	.88060
42	17.0951	.75218	.24782	97	2.5746	.11328	.88672
43	16.8914	.74322	.25678	98	2.4443	.10755	.89245
44	16.6811	.73397	.26603	99	2.3175	.10197	.89803
45	16.4648	.72445	.27555	100	2.1946	.09656	.90344
46	16.2425	.71467	.28533	101	2.0737	.09124	.90876
47	16.0147	.70465	.29535	102	1.9554	.08604	.91396
48	15.7811	.69437	.30563	103	1.8382	.08088	.91912
49	15.5419	.68385	.31615	104	1.7135	.07540	.92460
50	15.2968	.67306	.32694	105	1.5917	.07004	.92996
51	15.0459	.66202	.33798	106	1.4363	.06320	.93680
52	14.7901	.65076	.34924	107	1.2491	.05496	.94504
53	14.5295	.63930	.36070	108	.9620	.04233	.95767
54	14.2643	.62763	.37237	109	.4789	.02107	.97893

Appendix A-4
Table S (4.6)   **Section 1**
Single Life Factors Based on Life Table 9OCM
Interest at 4.6 Percent

Age	Annuity	Life Estate	Remainder	Age	Annuity	Life Estate	Remainder
0	20.5247	.94414	.05586	55	13.6915	.62981	.37019
1	20.6670	.95068	.04932	56	13.4290	.61773	.38227
2	20.6330	.94912	.05088	57	13.1621	.60545	.39455
3	20.5923	.94725	.05275	58	12.8915	.59301	.40699
4	20.5475	.94518	.05482	59	12.6183	.58044	.41956
5	20.4990	.94295	.05705	60	12.3426	.56776	.43224
6	20.4477	.94059	.05941	61	12.0641	.55495	.44505
7	20.3934	.93809	.06191	62	11.7822	.54198	.45802
8	20.3363	.93547	.06453	63	11.4967	.52885	.47115
9	20.2760	.93269	.06731	64	11.2082	.51558	.48442
10	20.2122	.92976	.07024	65	10.9169	.50218	.49782
11	20.1453	.92669	.07331	66	10.6223	.48863	.51137
12	20.0754	.92347	.07653	67	10.3238	.47489	.52511
13	20.0032	.92015	.07985	68	10.0219	.46101	.53899
14	19.9300	.91678	.08322	69	9.7177	.44701	.55299
15	19.8562	.91339	.08661	70	9.4124	.43297	.56703
16	19.7824	.90999	.09001	71	9.1074	.41894	.58106
17	19.7079	.90656	.09344	72	8.8034	.40496	.59504
18	19.6325	.90309	.09691	73	8.5011	.39105	.60895
19	19.5549	.89953	.10047	74	8.1995	.37718	.62282
20	19.4746	.89583	.10417	75	7.8977	.36329	.63671
21	19.3911	.89199	.10801	76	7.5950	.34937	.65063
22	19.3046	.88601	.11199	77	7.2915	.33541	.66459
23	19.2148	.88388	.11612	78	6.9878	.32144	.67856
24	19.1211	.87957	.12043	79	6.6857	.30754	.69246
25	19.0232	.87507	.12493	80	6.3875	.29382	.70618
26	18.9212	.87037	.12963	81	6.0952	.28038	.71962
27	18.8143	.86546	.13454	82	5.8100	.26726	.73274
28	18.7032	.86035	.13965	83	5.5319	.25447	.74553
29	18.5877	.85503	.14497	84	5.2590	.24191	.75809
30	18.4679	.84952	.15048	85	4.9898	.22953	.77047
31	18.3438	.84382	.15618	86	4.7265	.21742	.78258
32	18.2153	.83790	.16210	87	4.4725	.20573	.79427
33	18.0818	.83176	.16824	88	4.2277	.19448	.80552
34	17.9435	.82540	.17460	89	3.9922	.18364	.81636
35	17.7998	.81879	.18121	90	3.7661	.17324	.82676
36	17.6510	.81195	.18805	91	3.5527	.16342	.83658
37	17.4968	.80486	.19514	92	3.3558	.15437	.84563
38	17.3368	.79749	.20251	93	3.1747	.14604	.85396
39	17.1710	.78987	.21013	94	3.0065	.13830	.86170
40	16.9990	.78195	.21805	95	2.8475	.13098	.86902
41	16.8204	.77374	.22626	96	2.6984	.12413	.87587
42	16.6351	.76522	.23478	97	2.5606	.11779	.88221
43	16.4434	.75640	.24360	98	2.4315	.11185	.88815
44	16.2450	.74727	.25273	99	2.3059	.10607	.89393
45	16.0408	.73788	.26212	100	2.1841	.10047	.89953
46	15.8306	.72821	.27179	101	2.0642	.09496	.90504
47	15.6149	.71829	.28171	102	1.9463	.08955	.91045
48	15.3935	.70810	.29190	103	1.8306	.08421	.91579
49	15.1665	.69766	.30234	104	1.7069	.07852	.92148
50	14.9336	.68694	.31306	105	1.5860	.07296	.92704
51	14.6949	.67596	.32404	106	1.4316	.06585	.93415
52	14.4512	.66475	.33525	107	1.2455	.05729	.94271
53	14.2026	.65332	.34668	108	.9597	.04415	.95585
54	13.9494	.64167	.35833	109	.4780	.02199	.97801

Appendix A-4
Section 1
Table S (4.8)
Single Life Factors Based on Life Table 90CM
Interest at 4.8 Percent

Age	Annuity	Life Estate	Remainder	Age	Annuity	Life Estate	Remainder
0	19.7689	.94891	.05109	55	13.3993	.64317	.35683
1	19.9088	.95562	.04436	56	13.1480	.63110	.36890
2	19.8792	.95420	.04580	57	12.8921	.61882	.38118
3	19.8433	.95248	.04752	58	12.6326	.60636	.39364
4	19.8034	.95056	.04944	59	12.3701	.59377	.40623
5	19.7601	.94848	.05152	60	12.1051	.58104	.41896
6	19.7141	.94628	.05372	61	11.8371	.56818	.43182
7	19.6653	.94393	.05607	62	11.5655	.55515	.44485
8	19.6139	.94147	.05853	63	11.2903	.54193	.45807
9	19.5594	.93885	.06115	64	11.0118	.52857	.47143
10	19.5017	.93608	.06392	65	10.7303	.51505	.48495
11	19.4410	.93317	.06683	66	10.4454	.50138	.49862
12	19.3774	.93011	.06989	67	10.1563	.48750	.51250
13	19.3117	.92696	.07304	68	9.8637	.47346	.52654
14	19.2451	.92376	.07624	69	9.5685	.45929	.54071
15	19.1780	.92054	.07946	70	9.2720	.44505	.55495
16	19.1109	.91732	.08268	71	8.9754	.43082	.56918
17	19.0433	.91408	.08592	72	8.6796	.41662	.58338
18	18.9748	.91079	.08921	73	8.3852	.40249	.59751
19	18.9043	.90741	.09259	74	8.0912	.38838	.61162
20	18.8312	.90390	.09610	75	7.7968	.37425	.62575
21	18.7550	.90024	.09976	76	7.5011	.36005	.63995
22	18.6762	.89646	.10354	77	7.2044	.34581	.65419
23	18.5941	.89252	.10748	78	6.9073	.33155	.66845
24	18.5083	.88840	.11160	79	6.6114	.31735	.68265
25	18.4186	.88409	.11591	80	6.3191	.30332	.69668
26	18.3249	.87959	.12041	81	6.0324	.28955	.71045
27	18.2265	.87487	.12513	82	5.7524	.27611	.72389
28	18.1242	.86996	.13004	83	5.4791	.26300	.73700
29	18.0175	.86484	.13516	84	5.2108	.25012	.74988
30	17.9068	.85953	.14047	85	4.9459	.23740	.76260
31	17.7919	.85401	.14599	86	4.6866	.22496	.77504
32	17.6728	.84829	.15171	87	4.4362	.21294	.78706
33	17.5488	.84234	.15766	88	4.1949	.20135	.79865
34	17.4203	.83617	.16383	89	3.9624	.19020	.80980
35	17.2865	.82975	.17025	90	3.7391	.17948	.82052
36	17.1478	.82309	.17691	91	3.5283	.16936	.83064
37	17.0038	.81618	.18382	92	3.3337	.16002	.83993
38	16.8542	.80900	.19100	93	3.1546	.15142	.84858
39	16.6989	.80155	.19845	94	2.9882	.14343	.85657
40	16.5376	.79380	.20620	95	2.8308	.13588	.86412
41	16.3697	.78575	.21425	96	2.6832	.12879	.87121
42	16.1955	.77738	.22262	97	2.5468	.12225	.87775
43	16.0148	.76871	.23129	98	2.4189	.11611	.88389
44	15.8277	.75973	.24027	99	2.2945	.11013	.88987
45	15.6347	.75047	.24953	100	2.1736	.10433	.89567
46	15.4358	.74092	.25908	101	2.0548	.09863	.90137
47	15.2315	.73111	.26889	102	1.9384	.09304	.90696
48	15.0215	.72103	.27897	103	1.8230	.08751	.91249
49	14.8060	.71069	.28931	104	1.7003	.08161	.91839
50	14.5845	.70005	.29995	105	1.5803	.07585	.92415
51	14.3572	.68915	.31085	106	1.4269	.06849	.93151
52	14.1250	.67800	.32200	107	1.2420	.05961	.94039
53	13.8878	.66661	.33339	108	.9574	.04596	.95404
54	13.6459	.65500	.34500	109	.4771	.02290	.97710

Appendix A-4
Table S (5.0)
Section 1
Single Life Factors Based on Life Table 90CM
Interest at 5.0 Percent

Age	Annuity	Life Estate	Remainder	Age	Annuity	Life Estate	Remainder
0	19.0619	.95309	.04691	55	13.1173	.65587	.34413
1	19.1994	.95997	.04003	56	12.8766	.64383	.35617
2	19.1736	.95868	.04132	57	12.6313	.63156	.36844
3	19.1418	.95709	.04291	58	12.3821	.61911	.38089
4	19.1063	.95531	.04469	59	12.1300	.60650	.39350
5	19.0675	.95338	.04662	60	11.8751	.59376	.40624
6	19.0262	.95131	.04869	61	11.6172	.58086	.41914
7	18.9823	.94911	.05089	62	11.3555	.56777	.43223
8	18.9359	.94679	.05321	63	11.0899	.55450	.44550
9	18.8866	.94433	.05567	64	10.8211	.54105	.45895
10	18.8343	.94171	.05829	65	10.5490	.52745	.47255
11	18.7791	.93896	.06104	66	10.2733	.51366	.48634
12	18.7212	.93606	.06394	67	9.9933	.49966	.50034
13	18.6613	.93307	.06693	68	9.7096	.48548	.51452
14	18.6006	.93003	.06997	69	9.4231	.47115	.52885
15	18.5395	.92697	.07303	70	9.1350	.45675	.54325
16	18.4784	.92392	.07608	71	8.8466	.44233	.55767
17	18.4169	.92084	.07916	72	8.5587	.42794	.57206
18	18.3546	.91773	.08227	73	8.2719	.41360	.58640
19	18.2904	.91452	.08548	74	7.9853	.39927	.60073
20	18.2238	.91119	.08881	75	7.6980	.38490	.61510
21	18.1544	.90772	.09228	76	7.4093	.37046	.62954
22	18.0824	.90412	.09588	77	7.1192	.35596	.64404
23	18.0072	.90036	.09964	78	6.8284	.34142	.65858
24	17.9287	.89643	.10357	79	6.5385	.32692	.67308
25	17.8463	.89232	.10768	80	6.2519	.31260	.68740
26	17.7601	.88801	.11199	81	5.9706	.29853	.70147
27	17.6696	.88348	.11652	82	5.6957	.28478	.71522
28	17.5751	.87876	.12124	83	5.4272	.27136	.72864
29	17.4766	.87383	.12617	84	5.1633	.25817	.74183
30	17.3741	.86871	.13129	85	4.9027	.24513	.75487
31	17.2678	.86339	.13661	86	4.6473	.23236	.76764
32	17.1572	.85786	.14214	87	4.4005	.22002	.77998
33	17.0421	.85210	.14790	88	4.1625	.20812	.79188
34	16.9225	.84612	.15388	89	3.9331	.19665	.80335
35	16.7978	.83989	.16011	90	3.7125	.18563	.81437
36	16.6683	.83342	.16658	91	3.5042	.17521	.82479
37	16.5338	.82669	.17331	92	3.3119	.16559	.83441
38	16.3938	.81969	.18031	93	3.1347	.15674	.84326
39	16.2483	.81241	.18759	94	2.9701	.14851	.85149
40	16.0968	.80484	.19516	95	2.8144	.14072	.85928
41	15.9391	.79695	.20305	96	2.6682	.13341	.86659
42	15.7750	.78875	.21125	97	2.5331	.12665	.87335
43	15.6046	.78023	.21977	98	2.4064	.12032	.87968
44	15.4279	.77140	.22860	99	2.3631	.11415	.88585
45	15.2455	.76228	.23772	100	2.1633	.10817	.89183
46	15.0572	.75286	.24714	101	2.0455	.10228	.89772
47	14.8636	.74318	.25682	102	1.9300	.09650	.90350
48	14.6643	.73322	.26678	103	1.8156	.09078	.90922
49	14.4595	.72298	.27702	104	1.6937	.08468	.91532
50	14.2488	.71244	.28756	105	1.5746	.07873	.92127
51	14.0323	.70162	.29838	106	1.4223	.07111	.92889
52	13.8109	.69054	.30946	107	1.2384	.06192	.93808
53	13.5844	.67922	.32078	108	.9551	.04776	.95224
54	13.3533	.66766	.33234	109	.4762	.02381	.97619

Appendix A-4
Section 3
Table B
Annuity, Income, and Remainder Interests For a Term Certain

	5.0%			Interest Rates		5.2%	
Years	Annuity	Income Interest	Remainder	Years	Annuity	Income Interest	Remainder
1	0.9524	.047619	.952381	1	0.9506	.045430	.950570
2	1.8594	.092971	.907029	2	1.8542	.096416	.903584
3	2.7232	.136162	.863838	3	2.7131	.141080	.858920
4	3.5460	.177298	.822702	4	3.5295	.183536	.816464
5	4.3295	.216474	.783526	5	4.3056	.223894	.776106
6	5.0757	.253785	.746215	6	5.0434	.262256	.737744
7	5.7864	.289319	.710681	7	5.7447	.298723	.701277
8	6.4632	.323161	.676839	8	6.4113	.333387	.666613
9	7.1078	.355391	.644609	9	7.0449	.366337	.633663
10	7.7217	.386087	.613913	10	7.6473	.397659	.602341
11	8.3064	.415321	.584679	11	8.2199	.427432	.572568
12	8.8633	.443163	.556837	12	8.7641	.455734	.544266
13	9.3936	.469679	.530321	13	9.2815	.482637	.517363
14	9.8986	.494932	.505068	14	9.7733	.508210	.491790
15	10.3797	.518983	.481017	15	10.2408	.532519	.467481
16	10.8378	.541888	.458112	16	10.6851	.555628	.444374
17	11.2741	.563703	.436297	17	11.1075	.577592	.422408
18	11.6896	.584479	.415521	18	11.5091	.598471	.401529
19	12.0853	.604266	.395734	19	11.8907	.618319	.381681
20	12.4622	.623111	.376889	20	12.2536	.637185	.362815
21	12.8212	.641058	.358942	21	12.5984	.655119	.344881
22	13.1630	.658150	.341850	22	12.9263	.672166	.327834
23	13.4886	.674429	.325571	23	13.2379	.688371	.311629
24	13.7986	.689932	.310068	24	13.5341	.703775	.296225
25	14.0939	.704697	.295303	25	13.8157	.718417	.281583
26	14.3752	.716759	.281241	26	14.0834	.732336	.267664
27	14.6430	.732152	.267848	27	14.3378	.745566	.254434
28	14.8981	.744906	.255094	28	14.5797	.758143	.241357
29	15.1411	.757054	.242946	29	14.8096	.770098	.229902
30	15.3725	.768623	.231377	30	15.0281	.781462	.218538
31	15.5928	.779641	.220359	31	15.2358	.792264	.207736
32	15.8027	.790134	.209666	32	15.4333	.802532	.197468
33	16.0025	.800127	.199873	33	15.6210	.812293	.187707
34	16.1929	.809645	.190355	34	15.7994	.821571	.178429
35	16.3742	.818710	.181290	35	15.9691	.830391	.169609
36	16.5469	.827343	.172657	36	16.1303	.838775	.161225
37	16.7113	.835564	.164436	37	16.2835	.846744	.153256
38	16.8679	.843395	.156605	38	16.4292	.854319	.145681
39	17.0170	.850852	.149148	39	16.5677	.861520	.138480
40	17.1591	.857954	.142046	40	16.6993	.868365	.131635
41	17.2944	.864718	.135282	41	16.6245	.874872	.125128
42	17.4232	.871160	.128840	42	16.9434	.881057	.118943
43	17.5459	.877296	.122704	43	17.0565	.886936	.113064
44	17.6628	.883139	.116861	44	17.1639	.892525	.107475
45	17.7741	.888703	.111297	45	17.2661	.897837	.102163
46	17.8801	.894003	.105997	46	17.3632	.902887	.097113
47	17.9810	.899051	.100949	47	17.4555	.907688	.092312
48	18.0772	.903858	.096142	48	17.5433	.912251	.087749
49	18.1687	.908436	.091564	49	17.6267	.916588	.083412
50	18.2559	.912796	.087204	50	17.7060	.920711	.079289
51	18.3390	.916949	.083051	51	17.7814	.924630	.075370
52	18.4181	.920904	.079096	52	17.8530	.928356	.071644
53	18.4934	.924670	.075330	53	17.9211	.931897	.068103
54	18.5651	.928257	.071743	54	17.9858	.935263	.064737
55	18.6335	.931674	.068326	55	18.0474	.938463	.061537
56	18.6985	.934927	.065073	56	18.1059	.941505	.058495
57	18.7605	.938026	.061974	57	18.1615	.944396	.055604
58	18.8195	.940977	.059023	58	18.2143	.947145	.052855
59	18.8758	.943788	.056212	59	18.2646	.949757	.050243
60	18.9293	.946464	.053536	60	18.3123	.952241	.047759

A-5 2008 Optional State Sales Tax Tables

2008 Optional State and Certain Local Sales Tax Tables

Income		Alabama 4.0000%						Arizona 5.6000%						Arkansas 6.0000%						California[1] 7.2500%						Colorado 2.9000%					
At least	But less than	Exemptions 1	2	3	4	5	Over 5	1	2	3	4	5	Over 5	1	2	3	4	5	Over 5	1	2	3	4	5	Over 5	1	2	3	4	5	Over 5
$0	$20,000	201	246	278	303	324	354	205	234	253	267	279	295	287	334	366	390	410	438	246	280	303	320	334	354	96	110	120	127	133	142
20,000	30,000	310	377	423	460	491	535	350	397	429	453	472	500	469	544	594	633	665	709	423	480	518	547	571	603	161	184	200	212	222	235
30,000	40,000	364	442	495	538	574	625	427	484	522	551	575	608	563	652	712	758	796	849	518	587	633	668	696	736	195	223	242	256	268	285
40,000	50,000	411	497	557	604	644	701	494	560	604	637	664	702	644	746	813	866	909	969	601	681	734	774	806	852	225	257	279	295	308	327
50,000	60,000	453	546	612	663	707	769	556	629	678	715	745	788	717	830	905	963	1010	1077	678	767	825	870	907	958	253	288	312	330	345	366
60,000	70,000	491	591	661	717	764	830	612	693	747	787	821	867	784	907	988	1051	1103	1175	748	846	910	960	1000	1056	278	317	343	363	379	402
70,000	80,000	527	634	708	767	817	888	667	754	812	856	892	942	848	979	1067	1135	1191	1269	815	922	991	1045	1088	1149	302	344	372	393	411	436
80,000	90,000	560	673	751	814	866	941	718	811	873	920	959	1012	907	1047	1141	1213	1272	1355	879	992	1067	1124	1171	1236	325	370	399	422	441	467
90,000	100,000	592	710	792	857	912	991	766	866	932	982	1023	1080	962	1111	1210	1287	1350	1437	939	1060	1140	1201	1251	1320	347	394	425	450	470	497
100,000	120,000	633	759	846	915	973	1056	831	938	1009	1063	1107	1169	1036	1196	1302	1384	1452	1546	1019	1150	1236	1302	1356	1430	375	426	460	486	507	537
120,000	140,000	690	825	919	994	1057	1146	920	1039	1117	1176	1225	1292	1138	1312	1429	1518	1592	1695	1131	1275	1370	1443	1502	1584	415	471	508	536	560	593
140,000	160,000	740	883	983	1062	1129	1224	1000	1128	1212	1276	1328	1401	1227	1414	1539	1635	1714	1825	1230	1386	1488	1567	1631	1720	450	510	550	581	606	641
160,000	180,000	790	941	1047	1131	1201	1301	1079	1217	1307	1376	1433	1511	1316	1516	1650	1752	1837	1955	1330	1497	1608	1692	1761	1856	485	550	592	625	652	690
180,000	200,000	835	994	1104	1192	1266	1371	1152	1298	1394	1467	1527	1610	1397	1609	1749	1858	1948	2072	1420	1599	1716	1805	1879	1980	517	586	631	666	694	734
200,000 or more		1060	1254	1390	1497	1587	1715	1522	1711	1836	1931	2008	2116	1801	2070	2250	2387	2501	2660	1885	2117	2269	2385	2481	2613	681	768	826	871	908	959

Income		Connecticut 6.0000%						District of Columbia 5.7500%						Florida 6.0000%						Georgia 4.0000%						Hawaii 4.0000%					
$0	$20,000	208	231	245	256	264	276	165	186	200	210	219	230	210	244	266	283	297	317	142	163	177	188	197	209	239	283	313	335	354	381
20,000	30,000	356	393	417	435	450	470	285	319	342	359	374	393	359	414	451	479	502	535	236	270	293	310	324	343	378	445	490	525	555	596
30,000	40,000	433	479	508	530	547	572	349	391	418	439	456	480	438	504	549	583	611	650	286	326	353	373	390	413	447	526	579	621	655	703
40,000	50,000	501	554	587	612	633	661	405	453	485	509	528	555	507	584	634	674	706	751	329	375	405	428	447	474	507	596	656	702	741	795
50,000	60,000	563	622	659	688	711	742	456	510	545	572	594	625	571	656	712	756	792	843	368	419	452	478	499	529	561	658	724	775	818	877
60,000	70,000	620	685	726	757	782	817	503	563	601	631	655	688	629	722	784	832	872	927	404	459	496	524	547	579	609	715	786	841	887	952
70,000	80,000	675	744	789	823	850	887	548	613	655	687	713	749	685	786	853	905	948	1008	438	498	537	567	592	627	655	768	844	904	953	1021
80,000	90,000	725	800	848	884	914	954	591	660	705	739	767	806	738	845	917	973	1019	1083	470	534	576	608	634	671	697	817	898	961	1013	1086
90,000	100,000	774	853	905	943	974	1017	631	705	753	789	819	860	788	902	979	1038	1086	1154	501	568	612	647	675	713	738	864	949	1015	1070	1147
100,000	120,000	838	924	979	1021	1055	1101	685	765	816	856	888	933	854	978	1060	1124	1176	1250	541	614	661	698	728	770	791	925	1016	1087	1145	1227
120,000	140,000	927	1022	1083	1129	1166	1217	760	848	905	948	984	1033	946	1082	1173	1243	1301	1381	597	676	728	768	801	847	863	1009	1108	1185	1248	1337
140,000	160,000	1005	1108	1174	1223	1264	1319	826	921	983	1030	1068	1121	1028	1175	1273	1348	1411	1498	647	732	788	831	866	915	926	1083	1188	1270	1337	1433
160,000	180,000	1084	1194	1265	1319	1362	1421	893	995	1061	1112	1153	1210	1110	1268	1373	1454	1521	1614	697	787	847	893	931	983	989	1155	1267	1354	1426	1527
180,000	200,000	1156	1273	1348	1405	1451	1514	954	1062	1133	1186	1230	1291	1185	1352	1464	1550	1621	1721	742	838	901	950	990	1045	1046	1221	1339	1430	1506	1613
200,000 or more		1518	1671	1769	1843	1903	1985	1264	1405	1496	1566	1623	1702	1567	1784	1928	2040	2131	2260	971	1094	1174	1236	1287	1358	1328	1546	1694	1808	1903	2035

Income		Idaho 6.0000%						Illinois 6.2500%						Indiana[3] 6.7514%						Iowa[3] 5.5027%						Kansas 5.3000%					
$0	$20,000	304	370	416	452	482	526	240	277	301	320	335	357	257	297	323	344	360	384	222	254	275	291	304	322	282	341	382	414	441	479
20,000	30,000	470	569	637	692	737	802	401	461	500	531	556	591	421	484	526	559	585	623	376	429	464	491	513	543	442	533	595	644	685	743
30,000	40,000	555	669	748	811	864	939	486	557	605	641	671	713	506	581	631	670	701	746	457	522	564	596	623	659	524	629	702	759	807	876
40,000	50,000	627	754	843	913	972	1056	560	641	695	737	771	819	580	665	722	766	802	852	528	602	651	688	718	760	593	711	793	857	911	988
50,000	60,000	691	831	927	1004	1068	1160	627	718	778	824	862	915	646	741	804	852	892	947	593	675	729	771	805	852	655	785	875	945	1004	1088
60,000	70,000	750	900	1004	1086	1155	1254	689	788	854	904	945	1003	707	810	879	931	974	1035	652	742	802	847	885	936	712	852	949	1025	1089	1179
70,000	80,000	806	966	1076	1164	1237	1342	748	855	926	980	1024	1087	765	876	950	1006	1053	1117	709	807	871	920	961	1017	765	915	1018	1100	1168	1265
80,000	90,000	857	1026	1143	1235	1313	1424	804	917	993	1051	1098	1165	819	937	1016	1076	1125	1194	761	866	935	988	1031	1091	814	973	1083	1169	1241	1344
90,000	100,000	906	1083	1206	1303	1385	1501	856	977	1057	1118	1169	1239	870	995	1078	1142	1194	1267	811	923	997	1053	1099	1163	861	1028	1144	1234	1310	1418
100,000	120,000	971	1159	1289	1392	1479	1602	926	1056	1142	1208	1262	1338	938	1072	1161	1229	1286	1364	878	999	1078	1139	1188	1257	923	1101	1223	1320	1401	1516
120,000	140,000	1059	1262	1403	1514	1607	1740	1023	1165	1259	1331	1391	1474	1032	1178	1275	1350	1411	1497	970	1103	1190	1257	1312	1388	1007	1200	1333	1437	1525	1650
140,000	160,000	1136	1352	1502	1620	1719	1860	1108	1261	1362	1440	1504	1593	1114	1271	1375	1455	1521	1613	1051	1195	1289	1361	1420	1502	1080	1286	1428	1540	1633	1766
160,000	180,000	1213	1442	1600	1725	1830	1980	1193	1357	1466	1549	1618	1713	1196	1364	1476	1561	1631	1729	1133	1287	1389	1466	1529	1617	1153	1372	1523	1641	1741	1881
180,000	200,000	1283	1523	1689	1820	1931	2087	1271	1445	1560	1648	1721	1822	1271	1448	1566	1656	1731	1834	1207	1371	1479	1561	1628	1722	1219	1449	1608	1733	1837	1985
200,000 or more		1633	1928	2132	2293	2428	2620	1667	1889	2037	2150	2243	2372	1647	1872	2022	2136	2231	2362	1581	1794	1934	2040	2128	2249	1548	1834	2031	2185	2315	2499

Income		Kentucky 6.0000%						Louisiana 4.0000%						Maine 5.0000%						Maryland[3] 5.9945%						Massachusetts 5.0000%					
$0	$20,000	215	249	272	289	304	324	158	178	192	202	210	221	141	160	172	182	190	200	218	246	265	279	291	307	155	172	184	193	200	209
20,000	30,000	352	406	442	470	493	525	268	302	324	340	354	373	243	274	295	310	323	341	371	416	447	470	489	516	263	292	311	325	336	352
30,000	40,000	424	488	530	563	590	628	326	367	393	414	430	453	298	335	360	379	394	416	451	506	543	571	594	626	320	355	378	395	409	428
40,000	50,000	486	559	607	644	675	718	377	424	454	477	496	522	346	389	417	439	457	481	522	585	626	658	685	721	371	411	436	456	472	494
50,000	60,000	543	623	676	717	751	798	423	476	510	535	556	585	390	438	470	494	514	541	586	656	703	738	767	808	417	461	490	512	529	554
60,000	70,000	595	682	739	784	821	872	466	523	560	589	612	644	430	483	518	545	566	597	646	722	773	812	844	888	459	508	539	563	582	609
70,000	80,000	644	738	800	848	887	942	507	569	609	640	664	699	469	527	564	593	617	649	703	785	840	882	916	964	500	552	586	612	633	661
80,000	90,000	691	790	856	907	949	1008	545	611	654	687	714	751	506	567	608	638	664	699	756	844	902	947	984	1035	538	594	630	657	680	710
90,000	100,000	735	839	909	963	1008	1070	581	652	697	732	761	800	540	606	649	682	709	746	807	900	962	1009	1048	1102	574	633	672	701	725	757
100,000	120,000	793	905	980	1038	1085	1152	629	705	755	792	823	865	587	658	704	739	768	808	874	974	1041	1092	1134	1192	622	686	727	759	784	819
120,000	140,000	873	996	1077	1140	1192	1265	696	780	834	875	909	955	652	729	781	819	851	895	967	1077	1150	1206	1252	1316	689	759	804	839	867	905
140,000	160,000	944	1076	1163	1231	1286	1364	755	845	904	948	985	1035	709	793	848	890	925	972	1050	1168	1247	1307	1357	1426	748	823	872	910	940	981
160,000	180,000	1016	1156	1249	1321	1380	1463	814	911	974	1022	1061	1115	767	857	916	962	998	1050	1133	1260	1344	1408	1461	1535	807	888	941	981	1013	1058
180,000	200,000	1080	1228	1327	1403	1466	1553	867	971	1038	1088	1130	1187	819	915	978	1026	1066	1120	1209	1343	1432	1500	1557	1635	861	947	1003	1045	1080	1127
200,000 or more		1409	1596	1721	1817	1896	2006	1140	1274	1360	1426	1480	1554	1089	1214	1296	1358	1409	1479	1594	1766	1880	1967	2039	2140	1136	1247	1319	1374	1418	1479

Income		Michigan 6.0000%						Minnesota 6.5000%						Mississippi 7.0000%						Missouri 4.2250%						Nebraska 5.5000%					
$0	$20,000	219	249	268	283	296	313	209	231	246	257	266	279	387	463	515	555	589	637	169	194	212	225	236	251	224	252	271	285	297	313
20,000	30,000	371	420	452	476	497	524	362	401	426	445	460	482	609	724	803	865	917	990	283	325	353	375	392	417	378	426	457	480	499	526
30,000	40,000	451	510	549	578	602	636	444	492	522	545	564	590	720	856	949	1021	1082	1167	344	394	428	453	475	504	459	517	554	583	606	638
40,000	50,000	521	589	633	667	695	733	517	572	607	634	655	685	816	969	1073	1154	1222	1318	396	454	492	522	546	580	530	596	639	672	698	735
50,000	60,000	585	661	710	748	778	821	583	644	684	714	738	772	902	1069	1183	1273	1347	1452	444	509	551	584	611	648	594	668	716	753	782	823
60,000	70,000	645	727	781	822	856	902	644	712	755	788	815	852	980	1161	1284	1380	1461	1574	489	559	605	641	670	711	653	735	787	827	860	905
70,000	80,000	701	790	848	893	929	980	702	776	824	860	889	929	1053	1246	1378	1481	1567	1689	531	606	657	695	727	771	710	798	855	898	933	982
80,000	90,000	754	849	911	959	998	1052	757	836	887	926	957	1000	1121	1326	1466	1575	1666	1794	570	651	705	746	780	827	762	857	918	964	1002	1054
90,000	100,000	804	905	972	1022	1063	1121	809	894	948	990	1023	1069	1185	1401	1548	1663	1759	1894	608	694	751	794	830	880	812	913	978	1027	1067	1122
100,000	120,000	871	980	1051	1106	1150	1212	879	970	1030	1074	1110	1160	1270	1500	1657	1780	1882	2026	657	750	811	858	897	951	879	987	1057	1110	1154	1213
120,000	140,000	964	1084	1162	1222	1271	1338	975	1077	1142	1191	1231	1286	1386	1636	1805	1938	2049	2205	726	828	895	947	989	1048	971	1090	1167	1226	1273	1339
140,000	160,000	1046	1175	1260	1324	1377	1450	1061	1171	1241	1295	1338	1398	1487	1754	1935	2077	2195	2361	787	897	969	1025	1070	1134	1052	1180	1264	1327	1378	1449
160,000	180,000	1128	1267	1358	1427	1483	1561	1147	1265	1342	1399	1446	1510	1588	1871	2063	2214	2339	2516	849	966	1043	1103	1152	1220	1133	1271	1361	1429	1484	1560
180,000	200,000	1203	1350	1447	1520	1580	1663	1225	1351	1433	1494	1544	1612	1679	1977	2179	2338	2470	2656	904	1028	1111	1174	1226	1298	1206	1353	1449	1521	1580	1660
200,000 or more		1585	1775	1899	1994	2071	2178	1624	1790	1896	1977	2042	2132	2131	2501	2754	2951	3115	3346	1187	1346	1452	1533	1600	1693	1579	1769	1893	1986	2063	2168

(Continued on next page)

2008 Optional State and Certain Local Sales Tax Tables *(Continued)*

Nevada[2] 6.5000%

Income: At least	But less than	Exemptions 1	2	3	4	5	Over 5
$0	$20,000	238	270	290	306	319	337
20,000	30,000	401	453	487	513	535	564
30,000	40,000	487	550	591	622	648	683
40,000	50,000	563	635	682	717	747	787
50,000	60,000	632	712	764	804	836	881
60,000	70,000	695	783	840	883	919	968
70,000	80,000	756	850	912	959	997	1051
80,000	90,000	813	914	980	1030	1071	1128
90,000	100,000	867	974	1044	1097	1141	1201
100,000	120,000	938	1054	1129	1187	1234	1299
120,000	140,000	1038	1165	1247	1311	1362	1433
140,000	160,000	1126	1262	1352	1420	1475	1552
160,000	180,000	1214	1361	1456	1529	1589	1671
180,000	200,000	1295	1450	1552	1629	1692	1779
200,000 or more		1704	1904	2035	2134	2216	2328

New Jersey[4] 7.0000%

Income: At least	But less than	Exemptions 1	2	3	4	5	Over 5
$0	$20,000	239	266	283	296	306	321
20,000	30,000	410	455	484	505	523	547
30,000	40,000	502	555	590	616	638	667
40,000	50,000	581	643	683	714	738	772
50,000	60,000	654	724	768	802	830	867
60,000	70,000	721	798	847	884	914	955
70,000	80,000	786	868	922	962	995	1039
80,000	90,000	846	934	992	1035	1070	1118
90,000	100,000	903	998	1058	1104	1142	1193
100,000	120,000	979	1081	1147	1197	1237	1292
120,000	140,000	1085	1197	1270	1325	1369	1430
140,000	160,000	1178	1300	1378	1438	1486	1552
160,000	180,000	1272	1403	1487	1551	1603	1674
180,000	200,000	1357	1497	1586	1654	1709	1785
200,000 or more		1792	1973	2090	2178	2250	2348

New Mexico 5.0000%

Income: At least	But less than	Exemptions 1	2	3	4	5	Over 5
$0	$20,000	221	249	266	280	291	306
20,000	30,000	370	415	445	467	485	510
30,000	40,000	448	503	538	564	586	616
40,000	50,000	516	578	619	649	674	708
50,000	60,000	577	647	692	726	754	792
60,000	70,000	634	710	760	797	827	869
70,000	80,000	688	770	823	864	896	942
80,000	90,000	738	826	883	926	961	1009
90,000	100,000	785	879	940	986	1023	1074
100,000	120,000	848	950	1015	1064	1104	1159
120,000	140,000	936	1047	1118	1173	1217	1277
140,000	160,000	1012	1132	1210	1268	1316	1381
160,000	180,000	1089	1218	1301	1363	1414	1485
180,000	200,000	1159	1295	1383	1450	1504	1579
200,000 or more		1510	1686	1800	1886	1956	2052

New York 4.0000%

Income: At least	But less than	Exemptions 1	2	3	4	5	Over 5
$0	$20,000	140	156	166	173	180	188
20,000	30,000	239	265	282	295	306	320
30,000	40,000	292	324	344	360	372	390
40,000	50,000	338	375	398	416	431	451
50,000	60,000	380	421	447	467	484	506
60,000	70,000	419	464	493	515	533	557
70,000	80,000	456	505	536	560	579	606
80,000	90,000	490	543	577	602	623	651
90,000	100,000	523	579	615	642	664	695
100,000	120,000	567	627	666	696	719	752
120,000	140,000	628	694	737	770	796	832
140,000	160,000	682	754	800	835	863	902
160,000	180,000	736	813	863	900	931	973
180,000	200,000	785	867	920	960	992	1037
200,000 or more		1034	1141	1210	1262	1304	1362

North Carolina[3] 4.3128%

Income: At least	But less than	Exemptions 1	2	3	4	5	Over 5
$0	$20,000	197	230	253	270	285	305
20,000	30,000	319	372	408	435	458	490
30,000	40,000	382	445	487	520	547	585
40,000	50,000	436	508	556	593	623	666
50,000	60,000	485	564	617	658	692	739
60,000	70,000	530	616	673	718	755	806
70,000	80,000	573	665	727	774	814	869
80,000	90,000	612	710	776	827	869	928
90,000	100,000	650	753	823	877	921	983
100,000	120,000	699	810	885	942	990	1057
120,000	140,000	768	889	970	1033	1084	1157
140,000	160,000	827	957	1044	1112	1167	1245
160,000	180,000	887	1026	1119	1190	1250	1333
180,000	200,000	941	1088	1186	1262	1324	1412
200,000 or more		1213	1398	1522	1618	1697	1808

North Dakota 5.0000%

Income: At least	But less than	Exemptions 1	2	3	4	5	Over 5
$0	$20,000	180	207	224	238	250	266
20,000	30,000	305	348	377	400	419	445
30,000	40,000	372	423	458	485	507	539
40,000	50,000	430	489	528	559	585	621
50,000	60,000	483	548	592	627	655	695
60,000	70,000	531	603	651	689	720	763
70,000	80,000	578	655	707	748	781	828
80,000	90,000	622	704	760	803	839	889
90,000	100,000	663	751	810	856	893	946
100,000	120,000	719	813	876	925	966	1023
120,000	140,000	795	898	968	1022	1066	1129
140,000	160,000	863	974	1049	1107	1155	1222
160,000	180,000	931	1050	1130	1192	1244	1316
180,000	200,000	993	1119	1204	1270	1324	1400
200,000 or more		1309	1470	1579	1663	1733	1830

Ohio 5.5000%

Income: At least	But less than	Exemptions 1	2	3	4	5	Over 5
$0	$20,000	214	242	260	273	284	299
20,000	30,000	363	409	438	460	479	504
30,000	40,000	442	497	532	559	581	612
40,000	50,000	511	574	614	645	671	705
50,000	60,000	573	643	689	724	752	791
60,000	70,000	631	708	758	796	826	869
70,000	80,000	686	769	823	864	898	944
80,000	90,000	738	826	884	928	964	1013
90,000	100,000	787	881	943	989	1027	1080
100,000	120,000	852	954	1020	1070	1111	1168
120,000	140,000	942	1054	1127	1182	1227	1290
140,000	160,000	1021	1143	1221	1281	1330	1397
160,000	180,000	1101	1231	1316	1380	1432	1504
180,000	200,000	1174	1312	1402	1470	1526	1602
200,000 or more		1542	1721	1838	1926	1998	2097

Oklahoma 4.5000%

Income: At least	But less than	Exemptions 1	2	3	4	5	Over 5
$0	$20,000	225	269	299	323	343	372
20,000	30,000	360	428	475	512	543	587
30,000	40,000	430	510	565	608	645	696
40,000	50,000	490	580	642	691	732	790
50,000	60,000	544	643	711	765	810	874
60,000	70,000	594	700	774	832	881	950
70,000	80,000	641	755	834	896	948	1022
80,000	90,000	685	805	889	955	1010	1088
90,000	100,000	726	853	941	1011	1069	1151
100,000	120,000	781	916	1010	1084	1146	1234
120,000	140,000	856	1003	1105	1185	1253	1348
140,000	160,000	922	1079	1188	1274	1346	1448
160,000	180,000	988	1155	1271	1362	1438	1547
180,000	200,000	1048	1224	1345	1441	1522	1636
200,000 or more		1349	1568	1719	1839	1939	2081

Pennsylvania 6.0000%

Income: At least	But less than	Exemptions 1	2	3	4	5	Over 5
$0	$20,000	195	219	235	247	257	270
20,000	30,000	331	371	397	416	432	455
30,000	40,000	403	451	482	506	525	552
40,000	50,000	466	520	556	584	606	637
50,000	60,000	523	584	624	654	679	713
60,000	70,000	576	642	686	719	747	784
70,000	80,000	626	698	745	781	811	851
80,000	90,000	673	750	801	839	871	914
90,000	100,000	718	800	854	895	928	974
100,000	120,000	777	866	924	968	1004	1054
120,000	140,000	859	957	1021	1069	1109	1163
140,000	160,000	932	1037	1106	1158	1201	1260
160,000	180,000	1005	1118	1192	1248	1294	1357
180,000	200,000	1071	1191	1270	1329	1378	1445
200,000 or more		1408	1563	1664	1741	1804	1890

Rhode Island 7.0000%

Income: At least	But less than	Exemptions 1	2	3	4	5	Over 5
$0	$20,000	230	259	279	293	305	322
20,000	30,000	376	423	453	476	495	522
30,000	40,000	452	507	543	570	593	624
40,000	50,000	518	580	621	652	677	712
50,000	60,000	577	646	691	725	753	792
60,000	70,000	632	706	755	792	823	865
70,000	80,000	683	763	816	856	888	934
80,000	90,000	731	816	872	915	950	998
90,000	100,000	777	867	926	971	1008	1059
100,000	120,000	837	934	997	1045	1084	1139
120,000	140,000	920	1026	1094	1147	1190	1249
140,000	160,000	994	1106	1180	1236	1282	1346
160,000	180,000	1067	1187	1265	1325	1374	1442
180,000	200,000	1133	1260	1343	1406	1458	1530
200,000 or more		1466	1627	1732	1811	1877	1967

South Carolina 6.0000%

Income: At least	But less than	Exemptions 1	2	3	4	5	Over 5
$0	$20,000	227	256	275	289	301	318
20,000	30,000	385	433	465	489	509	536
30,000	40,000	468	527	566	595	619	651
40,000	50,000	541	609	653	687	714	752
50,000	60,000	608	684	733	771	801	843
60,000	70,000	669	752	806	848	881	927
70,000	80,000	727	818	876	921	957	1007
80,000	90,000	782	879	942	989	1028	1082
90,000	100,000	834	937	1004	1055	1096	1153
100,000	120,000	903	1014	1086	1141	1186	1247
120,000	140,000	999	1121	1201	1261	1310	1378
140,000	160,000	1083	1215	1301	1367	1420	1493
160,000	180,000	1168	1310	1402	1472	1529	1608
180,000	200,000	1245	1396	1494	1569	1629	1713
200,000 or more		1636	1832	1959	2056	2134	2243

South Dakota 4.0000%

Income: At least	But less than	Exemptions 1	2	3	4	5	Over 5
$0	$20,000	223	266	295	318	337	365
20,000	30,000	353	420	465	501	530	572
30,000	40,000	419	497	551	592	627	676
40,000	50,000	476	564	624	671	710	765
50,000	60,000	526	623	689	741	784	845
60,000	70,000	573	678	749	805	851	917
70,000	80,000	616	729	805	865	915	985
80,000	90,000	657	776	857	920	973	1048
90,000	100,000	695	821	906	973	1029	1107
100,000	120,000	745	879	971	1042	1101	1185
120,000	140,000	814	960	1059	1137	1201	1292
140,000	160,000	874	1030	1136	1219	1288	1385
160,000	180,000	934	1100	1213	1301	1374	1477
180,000	200,000	988	1163	1282	1375	1452	1561
200,000 or more		1258	1477	1625	1741	1837	1973

Tennessee 7.0000%

Income: At least	But less than	Exemptions 1	2	3	4	5	Over 5
$0	$20,000	353	417	460	494	522	562
20,000	30,000	567	667	735	788	832	894
30,000	40,000	677	795	875	938	989	1062
40,000	50,000	772	905	996	1066	1125	1207
50,000	60,000	857	1005	1104	1182	1246	1336
60,000	70,000	935	1095	1203	1287	1357	1455
70,000	80,000	1009	1180	1296	1386	1461	1566
80,000	90,000	1078	1260	1383	1478	1558	1669
90,000	100,000	1143	1335	1465	1566	1650	1767
100,000	120,000	1229	1434	1573	1681	1770	1896
120,000	140,000	1347	1570	1721	1839	1936	2073
140,000	160,000	1451	1690	1851	1977	2081	2228
160,000	180,000	1554	1809	1981	2115	2226	2382
180,000	200,000	1648	1917	2098	2239	2356	2521
200,000 or more		2118	2456	2684	2861	3008	3214

Texas 6.2500%

Income: At least	But less than	Exemptions 1	2	3	4	5	Over 5
$0	$20,000	246	281	304	322	337	357
20,000	30,000	417	476	515	544	569	603
30,000	40,000	507	578	625	661	691	732
40,000	50,000	586	668	722	763	797	844
50,000	60,000	657	749	809	856	894	946
60,000	70,000	723	824	890	941	982	1040
70,000	80,000	786	895	967	1022	1067	1129
80,000	90,000	844	961	1038	1097	1146	1213
90,000	100,000	900	1025	1107	1169	1221	1292
100,000	120,000	974	1109	1197	1265	1320	1397
120,000	140,000	1077	1225	1322	1397	1458	1542
140,000	160,000	1167	1327	1432	1513	1579	1670
160,000	180,000	1258	1430	1543	1629	1700	1798
180,000	200,000	1340	1523	1643	1735	1810	1915
200,000 or more		1756	1994	2150	2269	2367	2502

Utah 4.6500%

Income: At least	But less than	Exemptions 1	2	3	4	5	Over 5
$0	$20,000	224	263	289	309	326	349
20,000	30,000	363	424	465	497	523	560
30,000	40,000	434	507	555	593	624	667
40,000	50,000	496	578	633	675	711	760
50,000	60,000	552	642	703	750	789	843
60,000	70,000	603	701	767	818	860	919
70,000	80,000	651	756	827	882	927	991
80,000	90,000	696	808	883	941	990	1057
90,000	100,000	739	857	936	998	1049	1120
100,000	120,000	795	922	1007	1073	1127	1203
120,000	140,000	873	1011	1103	1175	1234	1318
140,000	160,000	941	1089	1188	1265	1328	1417
160,000	180,000	1009	1167	1272	1354	1422	1517
180,000	200,000	1071	1237	1349	1435	1507	1607
200,000 or more		1381	1591	1731	1841	1931	2057

Vermont 6.0000%

Income: At least	But less than	Exemptions 1	2	3	4	5	Over 5
$0	$20,000	141	156	166	173	179	188
20,000	30,000	237	262	278	290	299	313
30,000	40,000	288	317	336	351	362	378
40,000	50,000	333	366	387	404	417	435
50,000	60,000	373	410	434	452	467	487
60,000	70,000	410	450	476	496	512	535
70,000	80,000	446	489	517	538	556	580
80,000	90,000	479	525	555	578	596	622
90,000	100,000	510	559	591	615	635	662
100,000	120,000	552	605	639	665	686	715
120,000	140,000	610	668	705	734	757	789
140,000	160,000	661	723	764	794	819	853
160,000	180,000	713	779	822	855	882	918
180,000	200,000	759	830	875	910	938	977
200,000 or more		996	1086	1145	1189	1225	1275

Virginia 4.0000%

Income: At least	But less than	Exemptions 1	2	3	4	5	Over 5
$0	$20,000	158	187	206	222	234	252
20,000	30,000	255	299	329	353	372	400
30,000	40,000	305	357	392	420	443	475
40,000	50,000	348	407	447	478	504	540
50,000	60,000	387	452	495	530	558	598
60,000	70,000	423	493	540	577	608	651
70,000	80,000	456	531	582	622	655	701
80,000	90,000	488	568	622	664	699	748
90,000	100,000	518	602	659	703	740	792
100,000	120,000	558	647	708	756	795	850
120,000	140,000	613	710	776	827	870	930
140,000	160,000	661	765	836	890	936	1000
160,000	180,000	709	820	895	953	1002	1070
180,000	200,000	753	870	949	1010	1062	1133
200,000 or more		974	1120	1219	1296	1360	1450

Washington 6.5000%

Income: At least	But less than	Exemptions 1	2	3	4	5	Over 5
$0	$20,000	254	288	310	327	341	360
20,000	30,000	431	487	524	552	575	607
30,000	40,000	525	593	637	671	699	737
40,000	50,000	606	684	736	774	806	850
50,000	60,000	681	768	825	868	904	953
60,000	70,000	750	845	907	955	994	1048
70,000	80,000	815	918	986	1037	1079	1138
80,000	90,000	876	987	1059	1114	1159	1222
90,000	100,000	934	1052	1129	1188	1236	1302
100,000	120,000	1012	1139	1222	1285	1337	1408
120,000	140,000	1119	1259	1350	1420	1476	1555
140,000	160,000	1214	1365	1463	1538	1600	1684
160,000	180,000	1309	1471	1577	1657	1723	1814
180,000	200,000	1395	1567	1680	1765	1835	1932
200,000 or more		1834	2057	2202	2313	2404	2529

West Virginia 6.0000%

Income: At least	But less than	Exemptions 1	2	3	4	5	Over 5
$0	$20,000	289	338	370	395	416	445
20,000	30,000	470	546	597	637	670	716
30,000	40,000	563	653	714	761	800	854
40,000	50,000	643	746	815	868	912	973
50,000	60,000	716	829	905	964	1012	1080
60,000	70,000	782	905	988	1052	1104	1178
70,000	80,000	845	978	1066	1135	1191	1271
80,000	90,000	904	1045	1139	1212	1272	1356
90,000	100,000	959	1108	1208	1285	1349	1438
100,000	120,000	1033	1192	1299	1381	1450	1545
120,000	140,000	1134	1308	1424	1514	1588	1692
140,000	160,000	1223	1409	1534	1630	1710	1821
160,000	180,000	1312	1511	1644	1746	1831	1950
180,000	200,000	1392	1602	1743	1851	1941	2066
200,000 or more		1797	2062	2239	2376	2490	2648

Wisconsin 5.0000%

Income: At least	But less than	Exemptions 1	2	3	4	5	Over 5
$0	$20,000	203	229	246	259	270	284
20,000	30,000	343	387	415	437	454	479
30,000	40,000	417	470	504	530	551	580
40,000	50,000	482	542	582	611	636	669
50,000	60,000	540	608	652	685	712	750
60,000	70,000	594	668	716	753	783	824
70,000	80,000	645	726	778	817	850	894
80,000	90,000	693	779	835	878	912	960
90,000	100,000	739	830	890	935	972	1022
100,000	120,000	799	898	962	1011	1050	1105
120,000	140,000	883	991	1062	1116	1159	1219
140,000	160,000	956	1074	1150	1208	1255	1320
160,000	180,000	1030	1156	1238	1300	1351	1421
180,000	200,000	1097	1231	1318	1384	1438	1512
200,000 or more		1436	1610	1723	1809	1878	1974

Wyoming 4.0000%

Income: At least	But less than	Exemptions 1	2	3	4	5	Over 5
$0	$20,000	152	172	185	195	203	215
20,000	30,000	259	293	315	331	345	364
30,000	40,000	316	357	383	403	420	443
40,000	50,000	366	413	443	466	485	511
50,000	60,000	412	464	498	524	545	574
60,000	70,000	454	511	548	576	600	632
70,000	80,000	494	556	596	627	652	687
80,000	90,000	531	597	641	674	701	738
90,000	100,000	567	637	683	719	747	787
100,000	120,000	614	690	740	778	809	852
120,000	140,000	680	764	819	861	895	942
140,000	160,000	738	829	888	933	970	1021
160,000	180,000	797	894	958	1006	1046	1100
180,000	200,000	850	953	1021	1073	1115	1173
200,000 or more		1120	1255	1342	1409	1464	1539

Note. Alaska does not have a state sales tax. Alaska residents should follow the instructions on the next page to determine their local sales tax amount.

1 The California table includes the 1% uniform local sales tax rate in additon to the 6.25% state sales tax rate.
2 The Nevada table includes the 2.25% uniform local sales tax rate in addition to the 4.25% state sales tax rate.
3 The rates for Indiana, Iowa, Maryland, and North Carolina increased during 2008, so the rate given is averaged over the year.
4 Residents of Salem County should deduct only half of the amount in the state table.

Which Optional Local Sales Tax Table Should I Use?

IF you live in the state of...	AND you live in...	THEN use Local Table...
Alaska	Any locality	C
Arizona	Glendale, Mesa, Phoenix, or Tucson	A
	Chandler, Gilbert, Peoria, Scottsdale, Tempe, Yuma, or any other locality	C
Arkansas	Any locality	B
California	Los Angeles County	A
Colorado	Aurora, Fort Collins, Greeley, Jefferson County, Lakewood, or Longmont	B
	Arvada, City of Boulder, Thornton, or Westminster	C
	Adams County, Arapahoe County, Boulder County, Centennial, Colorado Springs, Denver City/Denver County, El Paso County, Larimer County, City of Pueblo, Pueblo County, or any other locality	A
Georgia	Any locality	B
Illinois	Any locality	A
Louisiana	Any other locality	B
	Ascension Parish, Bossier Parish, Caddo Parish, Calcasieu Parish, East Baton Rouge Parish, Iberia Parish, Jefferson Parish, Lafayette Parish, Lafourche Parish, Livingston Parish, Orleans Parish, Ouachita Parish, Rapides Parish, St. Bernard Parish, St. Landry Parish, St. Tammany Parish, Tanqipahoa Parish, or Terrebonne Parish	C
Missouri	Saint Charles County or Saint Louis County	A
	Saint Louis City or any other locality	B
New York	New York City, or one of the following counties: Albany, Allegany, Cattaraugus, Cayuga, Chemung, Clinton, Cortland, Erie, Essex, Franklin, Fulton, Genesee, Herkimer, Jefferson, Lewis, Livingston, Monroe, Montgomery, Nassau, Niagara, Oneida, Onondaga, Ontario, Orange, Orleans, Oswego, Otsego, Putnam, Rensselaer, Rockland, St. Lawrence, Saratoga, Schenectady, Schoharie, Seneca, Steuben, Suffolk, Sullivan, Tompkins, Ulster, Warren, Washington, Westchester, Wyoming, or Yates	A
	Any other locality	D
North Carolina	Any locality	A
South Carolina	Cherokee, Chesterfield, Darlington, Jasper, Lee, or Lexington	A
	Any other locality	B
Tennessee	Any locality	B
Utah	Any locality	A
Virginia	Any locality	B

2008 Optional Local Sales Tax Tables for Certain Local Jurisdictions
(Based on a local sales tax rate of 1 percent)

Income At least	But less than	Local Table A Exemptions 1	2	3	4	5	Over 5	Local Table B Exemptions 1	2	3	4	5	Over 5	Local Table C Exemptions 1	2	3	4	5	Over 5	Local Table D Exemptions 1	2	3	4	5	Over 5
$0	$20,000	37	42	46	49	52	55	48	57	64	69	74	80	54	65	72	77	82	89	35	39	42	43	45	47
20,000	30,000	60	69	75	80	84	90	75	89	99	107	114	123	85	101	112	121	128	138	60	66	71	74	77	80
30,000	40,000	72	83	90	96	101	107	88	105	117	126	134	145	101	120	132	142	151	162	73	81	86	90	93	98
40,000	50,000	83	95	103	110	115	122	100	119	132	143	151	164	114	135	150	161	170	183	85	94	100	104	108	113
50,000	60,000	92	106	115	122	128	136	111	132	146	157	167	180	127	150	165	178	188	202	95	105	112	117	121	127
60,000	70,000	101	116	126	134	140	149	120	143	158	170	181	195	138	163	179	193	204	219	105	116	123	129	133	139
70,000	80,000	109	126	136	144	151	161	129	153	170	183	194	209	148	175	193	207	219	235	114	126	134	140	145	152
80,000	90,000	117	134	146	155	162	172	138	163	181	194	206	222	158	186	205	220	233	250	123	136	144	151	156	163
90,000	100,000	125	143	155	164	172	182	146	172	191	205	217	235	167	197	217	233	246	264	131	145	154	161	166	174
100,000	120,000	135	154	167	177	185	196	156	185	204	220	232	251	179	211	232	249	263	283	142	157	167	174	180	188
120,000	140,000	148	169	183	194	203	216	170	201	222	239	253	273	195	230	253	271	286	308	157	174	184	193	199	208
140,000	160,000	160	183	198	210	219	233	183	216	238	256	271	292	210	246	271	291	307	330	171	189	200	209	216	226
160,000	180,000	172	196	212	225	235	249	196	230	254	273	289	311	224	263	290	310	327	352	184	203	216	225	233	243
180,000	200,000	183	209	226	239	250	265	207	244	269	288	305	328	237	278	306	328	346	371	196	217	230	240	248	259
200,000 or more		239	271	292	309	323	342	264	309	340	365	385	414	302	353	388	415	437	469	259	285	303	316	326	341

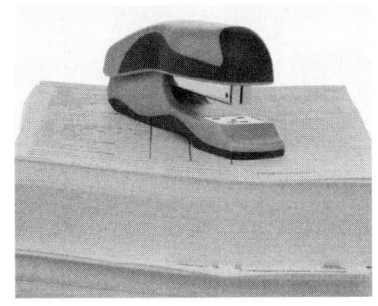

★ APPENDIX B ★

TAX FORMS

B-1   Form 1040A   U.S. Individual Income Tax Return

Form
1040A

Department of the Treasury—Internal Revenue Service

U.S. Individual Income Tax Return (99) **2008**   IRS Use Only—Do not write or staple in this space.

OMB No. 1545-0074

Label
(See page 17.)

Use the IRS label.
Otherwise, please print or type.

L A B E L   H E R E

Your first name and initial   Last name

Your social security number

If a joint return, spouse's first name and initial   Last name

Spouse's social security number

Home address (number and street). If you have a P.O. box, see page 17.   Apt. no.

City, town or post office, state, and ZIP code. If you have a foreign address, see page 17.

▲ You **must** enter your SSN(s) above. ▲

Checking a box below will not change your tax or refund.

Presidential Election Campaign ▶ Check here if you, or your spouse if filing jointly, want $3 to go to this fund (see page 17) ▶ ☐ **You**   ☐ **Spouse**

Filing status
Check only one box.

1 ☐ Single
2 ☐ Married filing jointly (even if only one had income)
3 ☐ Married filing separately. Enter spouse's SSN above and full name here. ▶
4 ☐ Head of household (with qualifying person). (See page 18.) If the qualifying person is a child but not your dependent, enter this child's name here. ▶
5 ☐ Qualifying widow(er) with dependent child (see page 19)

Exemptions

If more than six dependents, see page 20.

6a ☐ **Yourself.** If someone can claim you as a dependent, **do not** check box 6a.
b ☐ **Spouse**
c **Dependents:**

(1) First name Last name	(2) Dependent's social security number	(3) Dependent's relationship to you	(4) ✓ if qualifying child for child tax credit (see page 20)
			☐
			☐
			☐
			☐
			☐
			☐

Boxes checked on 6a and 6b ____

No. of children on 6c who:
• lived with you ____
• did not live with you due to divorce or separation (see page 21) ____

Dependents on 6c not entered above ____

Add numbers on lines above ▶ ☐

d Total number of exemptions claimed.

Income

Attach Form(s) W-2 here. Also attach Form(s) 1099-R if tax was withheld.

If you did not get a W-2, see page 23.

Enclose, but do not attach, any payment.

7 Wages, salaries, tips, etc. Attach Form(s) W-2.   7

8a **Taxable** interest. Attach Schedule 1 if required.   8a
b **Tax-exempt** interest. **Do not** include on line 8a.   8b

9a Ordinary dividends. Attach Schedule 1 if required.   9a
b Qualified dividends (see page 24).   9b

10 Capital gain distributions (see page 24).   10

11a IRA distributions.   11a   **11b** Taxable amount (see page 24).   11b

12a Pensions and annuities.   12a   **12b** Taxable amount (see page 25).   12b

13 Unemployment compensation and Alaska Permanent Fund dividends.   13

14a Social security benefits.   14a   **14b** Taxable amount (see page 27).   14b

15 Add lines 7 through 14b (far right column). This is your **total income.** ▶ 15

Adjusted gross income

16 Educator expenses (see page 29).   16
17 IRA deduction (see page 29).   17
18 Student loan interest deduction (see page 31).   18
19 Tuition and fees deduction. Attach Form 8917.   19
20 Add lines 16 through 19. These are your **total adjustments.**   20

21 Subtract line 20 from line 15. This is your **adjusted gross income.** ▶ 21

For Disclosure, Privacy Act, and Paperwork Reduction Act Notice, see page 78.   Cat. No. 11327A   Form **1040A** (2008)

Form 1040A (2008) Page **2**

Tax, credits, and payments	**22**	Enter the amount from line 21 (adjusted gross income).	22

23a Check if: { ☐ **You** were born before January 2, 1944, ☐ Blind } **Total boxes** checked ▶ 23a ☐
{ ☐ **Spouse** was born before January 2, 1944, ☐ Blind } checked ▶

b If you are married filing separately and your spouse itemizes deductions, see page 32 and check here ▶ 23b ☐

c Check if standard deduction includes real estate taxes (see page 32) ▶ 23c ☐

Standard Deduction for—

• People who checked any box on line 23a, 23b, or 23c **or** who can be claimed as a dependent, see page 32.

• All others:

Single or Married filing separately, $5,450

Married filing jointly or Qualifying widow(er), $10,900

Head of household, $8,000

24	Enter your **standard deduction** (see left margin).	24
25	Subtract line 24 from line 22. If line 24 is more than line 22, enter -0-.	25
26	If line 22 is over $119,975, or you provided housing to a Midwestern displaced individual, see page 32. Otherwise, multiply $3,500 by the total number of exemptions claimed on line 6d.	26
27	Subtract line 26 from line 25. If line 26 is more than line 25, enter -0-. This is your **taxable income.** ▶	27
28	**Tax,** including any alternative minimum tax (see page 33).	28
29	Credit for child and dependent care expenses. Attach Schedule 2.	29	
30	Credit for the elderly or the disabled. Attach Schedule 3.	30	
31	Education credits. Attach Form 8863.	31	
32	Retirement savings contributions credit. Attach Form 8880.	32	
33	Child tax credit (see page 37). Attach Form 8901 if required.	33	
34	Add lines 29 through 33. These are your **total credits.**	34
35	Subtract line 34 from line 28. If line 34 is more than line 28, enter -0-.	35
36	Advance earned income credit payments from Form(s) W-2, box 9.	36
37	Add lines 35 and 36. This is your **total tax.** ▶	37
38	Federal income tax withheld from Forms W-2 and 1099.	38	
39	2008 estimated tax payments and amount applied from 2007 return.	39	

If you have a qualifying child, attach Schedule EIC.

40a	**Earned income credit (EIC).**	40a	
b	Nontaxable combat pay election. 40b		
41	Additional child tax credit. Attach Form 8812.	41	
42	Recovery rebate credit (see worksheet on pages 53 and 54).	42	
43	Add lines 38, 39, 40a, 41, and 42. These are your **total payments.** ▶	43

Refund

44	If line 43 is more than line 37, subtract line 37 from line 43. This is the amount you **overpaid.**	44

Direct deposit? See page 55 and fill in 45b, 45c, and 45d or Form 8888.

45a Amount of line 44 you want **refunded to you.** If Form 8888 is attached, check here ▶ ☐ 45a

▶ **b** Routing number ☐☐☐☐☐☐☐☐☐ ▶ **c** Type: ☐ Checking ☐ Savings

▶ **d** Account number ☐☐☐☐☐☐☐☐☐☐☐☐☐☐☐☐☐

46	Amount of line 44 you want **applied to your 2009 estimated tax.**	46	

Amount you owe

47	**Amount you owe.** Subtract line 43 from line 37. For details on how to pay, see page 56. ▶	47
48	Estimated tax penalty (see page 57).	48	

Third party designee

Do you want to allow another person to discuss this return with the IRS (see page 57)? ☐ **Yes.** Complete the following. ☐ **No**

Designee's name ▶ ___ Phone no. ▶ ( ) ___ Personal identification number (PIN) ▶ ☐☐☐☐☐

Sign here

Joint return? See page 17.

Keep a copy for your records.

Under penalties of perjury, I declare that I have examined this return and accompanying schedules and statements, and to the best of my knowledge and belief, they are true, correct, and accurately list all amounts and sources of income I received during the tax year. Declaration of preparer (other than the taxpayer) is based on all information of which the preparer has any knowledge.

Your signature ___ Date ___ Your occupation ___ Daytime phone number ( ) ___

Spouse's signature. If a joint return, **both** must sign. ___ Date ___ Spouse's occupation ___

Paid preparer's use only

Preparer's signature ▶ ___ Date ___ Check if self-employed ☐ Preparer's SSN or PTIN ___

Firm's name (or yours if self-employed), address, and ZIP code ▶ ___ EIN ___ Phone no. ( ) ___

Form **1040A** (2008)

Schedule 1

(Form 1040A)

Department of the Treasury—Internal Revenue Service

Interest and Ordinary Dividends
for Form 1040A Filers (99) **2008**

OMB No. 1545-0074

Name(s) shown on Form 1040A

Your social security number

Part I	**Note.** If you received a Form 1099-INT, Form 1099-OID, or substitute statement from a brokerage firm, enter the firm's name and the total interest shown on that form.		

Interest

(See back
of schedule
and the
instructions
for Form
1040A,
line 8a.)

	1 List name of payer. If any interest is from a seller-financed mortgage and the buyer used the property as a personal residence, see back of schedule and list this interest first. Also, show that buyer's social security number and address.		Amount	
		1		
	2 Add the amounts on line 1.	**2**		
	3 Excludable interest on series EE and I U.S. savings bonds issued after 1989. Attach Form 8815.	**3**		
	4 Subtract line 3 from line 2. Enter the result here and on Form 1040A, line 8a.	**4**		

Part II

Ordinary
dividends

(See back
of schedule
and the
instructions
for Form
1040A,
line 9a.)

Note. If you received a Form 1099-DIV or substitute statement from a brokerage firm, enter the firm's name and the ordinary dividends shown on that form.			
5 List name of payer.		Amount	
	5		
6 Add the amounts on line 5. Enter the total here and on Form 1040A, line 9a.	**6**		

For Paperwork Reduction Act Notice, see Form 1040A instructions.   Cat. No. 12075R   **Schedule 1 (Form 1040A) 2008**

Purpose of Schedule

Use Schedule 1 if any of the following apply.

● You had over $1,500 of taxable interest (fill in Part I).

● You received interest from a seller-financed mortgage and the buyer used the property as a personal residence (fill in Part I).

● You are claiming the exclusion of interest from series EE or I U.S. savings bonds issued after 1989 (fill in Part I).

● You received interest as a nominee (fill in Part I).

● You had over $1,500 of ordinary dividends or you received ordinary dividends as a nominee (fill in Part II).

 If you need more space to list your interest or ordinary dividends, attach separate statements that are the same size as Schedule 1. Use the same format as lines 1 and 5, but show your totals on Schedule 1. Be sure to put your name and social security number on the statements and attach them at the end of your return.

Part I

Interest

Line 1

Report on line 1 all of your taxable interest. Interest should be shown on your Forms 1099-INT, Forms 1099-OID, or substitute statements. Include interest from series EE and I U.S. savings bonds. List each payer's name and show the amount.

Seller-financed mortgages. If you sold your home or other property and the buyer used the property as a personal residence, list first any interest the buyer paid you on a mortgage or other form of seller financing. Be sure to show the buyer's name, address, and social security number (SSN). You must also let the buyer know your SSN. If you do not show the buyer's name, address, and SSN, or let the buyer know your SSN, you may have to pay a $50 penalty.

Nominees. If you received a Form 1099-INT that includes interest you received as a nominee (that is, in your name, but the interest actually belongs to someone else), report the total on line 1. Do this even if you later distributed some or all of this income to others. Under your last entry on line 1, put a subtotal of all interest listed on line 1. Below this subtotal, enter "Nominee Distribution" and show the total interest you received as a nominee. Subtract this amount from the subtotal and enter the result on line 2.

 If you received interest as a nominee, you must give the actual owner a Form 1099-INT unless the owner is your spouse. You must also file a Form 1096 and a Form 1099-INT with the IRS. For more details, see the General Instructions for Forms 1099, 1098, 5498, and W-2G and Instructions for Forms 1099-INT and 1099-OID.

Line 3

Did you cash series EE or I U.S. savings bonds in 2008 that were issued after 1989? If you did and you paid qualified higher education expenses in 2008 for yourself, your spouse, or your dependents, you may be able to exclude part or all of the interest on those bonds. See Form 8815 for details.

Part II

Ordinary Dividends

Line 5

Report on line 5 all of your ordinary dividends. Ordinary dividends should be shown in box 1a of your Forms 1099-DIV or substitute statements. List each payer's name and show the amount.

Nominees. If you received a Form 1099-DIV that includes ordinary dividends you received as a nominee (that is, in your name, but the ordinary dividends actually belong to someone else), report the total on line 5. Do this even if you later distributed some or all of this income to others. Under your last entry on line 5, put a subtotal of all ordinary dividends listed on line 5. Below this subtotal, enter "Nominee Distribution" and show the total ordinary dividends you received as a nominee. Subtract this amount from the subtotal and enter the result on line 6.

 If you received dividends as a nominee, you must give the actual owner a Form 1099-DIV unless the owner is your spouse. You must also file a Form 1096 and a Form 1099-DIV with the IRS. For more details, see the General Instructions for Forms 1099, 1098, 5498, and W-2G and Instructions for Form 1099-DIV.

B-2   Form 1040EZ   Income Tax Return for Single Filers With No Dependents

| Form **1040EZ** | Department of the Treasury—Internal Revenue Service
Income Tax Return for Single and Joint Filers With No Dependents (99) | **2008** | OMB No. 1545-0074 |

Label
(See page 9.)

Use the IRS label.

Otherwise, please print or type.

Presidential Election Campaign (page 9) ▶

L A B E L H E R E

Your first name and initial	Last name		Your social security number
If a joint return, spouse's first name and initial	Last name		Spouse's social security number
Home address (number and street). If you have a P.O. box, see page 9.		Apt. no.	▲ You **must** enter your SSN(s) above. ▲
City, town or post office, state, and ZIP code. If you have a foreign address, see page 9.			Checking a box below will not change your tax or refund.

Check here if you, or your spouse if a joint return, want $3 to go to this fund . . ▶ ☐ **You**   ☐ **Spouse**

Income

Attach Form(s) W-2 here.

Enclose, but do not attach, any payment.

1 Wages, salaries, and tips. This should be shown in box 1 of your Form(s) W-2. Attach your Form(s) W-2. | 1 |

2 Taxable interest. If the total is over $1,500, you cannot use Form 1040EZ. | 2 |

3 Unemployment compensation and Alaska Permanent Fund dividends (see page 11). | 3 |

4 Add lines 1, 2, and 3. This is your **adjusted gross income.** | 4 |

5 If someone can claim you (or your spouse if a joint return) as a dependent, check the applicable box(es) below and enter the amount from the worksheet on back.

☐ **You**   ☐ **Spouse**

If no one can claim you (or your spouse if a joint return), enter $8,950 if **single;** $17,900 if **married filing jointly.** See back for explanation. | 5 |

6 Subtract line 5 from line 4. If line 5 is larger than line 4, enter -0-. This is your **taxable income.** ▶ | 6 |

Payments and tax

7 Federal income tax withheld from box 2 of your Form(s) W-2. | 7 |

8a **Earned income credit (EIC)** (see page 12). | 8a |

b Nontaxable combat pay election.   8b |

9 Recovery rebate credit (see worksheet on pages 17 and 18). | 9 |

10 Add lines 7, 8a, and 9. These are your **total payments.** ▶ | 10 |

11 **Tax.** Use the amount on **line 6 above** to find your tax in the tax table on pages 28–36 of the booklet. Then, enter the tax from the table on this line. | 11 |

Refund

Have it directly deposited! See page 18 and fill in 12b, 12c, and 12d or Form 8888.

12a If line 10 is larger than line 11, subtract line 11 from line 10. This is your **refund.** If Form 8888 is attached, check here ▶ ☐ | 12a |

▶ **b** Routing number ☐☐☐☐☐☐☐☐☐   ▶ **c** Type: ☐ Checking ☐ Savings

▶ **d** Account number ☐☐☐☐☐☐☐☐☐☐☐☐☐☐☐☐☐

Amount you owe

13 If line 11 is larger than line 10, subtract line 10 from line 11. This is the **amount you owe.** For details on how to pay, see page 19. ▶ | 13 |

Third party designee

Do you want to allow another person to discuss this return with the IRS (see page 20)? ☐ **Yes.** Complete the following. ☐**No**

Designee's name ▶   Phone no. ▶ (   )   Personal identification number (PIN) ▶ ☐☐☐☐☐

Sign here

Joint return? See page 6.

Keep a copy for your records.

Under penalties of perjury, I declare that I have examined this return, and to the best of my knowledge and belief, it is true, correct, and accurately lists all amounts and sources of income I received during the tax year. Declaration of preparer (other than the taxpayer) is based on all information of which the preparer has any knowledge.

| Your signature | Date | Your occupation | Daytime phone number ( ) |
| Spouse's signature. If a joint return, **both** must sign. | Date | Spouse's occupation | |

Paid preparer's use only

Preparer's signature ▶	Date	Check if self-employed ☐	Preparer's SSN or PTIN
Firm's name (or yours if self-employed), address, and ZIP code ▶		EIN	
		Phone no. ( )	

For Disclosure, Privacy Act, and Paperwork Reduction Act Notice, see page 37.   Cat. No. 11329W   Form **1040EZ** (2008)

Form 1040EZ (2008)   Page **2**

Use this form if

- Your filing status is single or married filing jointly. If you are not sure about your filing status, see page 6.
- You (and your spouse if married filing jointly) were under age 65 and not blind at the end of 2008. If you were born on January 1, 1944, you are considered to be age 65 at the end of 2008.
- You do not claim any dependents. For information on dependents, see Pub. 501.
- Your taxable income (line 6) is less than $100,000.
- You do not claim any adjustments to income. For information on adjustments to income, use TeleTax topics 451–453 and 455–458 (see page 27).
- The only tax credits you can claim are the earned income credit (EIC) and the recovery rebate credit. You do not need a qualifying child to claim the EIC. For information on credits, use TeleTax topics 601, 602, 607, 608, 610, and 611 (see page 27).
- You had only wages, salaries, tips, taxable scholarship or fellowship grants, unemployment compensation, or Alaska Permanent Fund dividends, and your taxable interest was not over $1,500. But if you earned tips, including allocated tips, that are not included in box 5 and box 7 of your Form W-2, you may not be able to use Form 1040EZ (see page 10). If you are planning to use Form 1040EZ for a child who received Alaska Permanent Fund dividends, see page 11.
- You did not receive any advance earned income credit payments. If you cannot use this form, use TeleTax topic 352 (see page 27).

Filling in your return

For tips on how to avoid common mistakes, see page 22.

If you received a scholarship or fellowship grant or tax-exempt interest income, such as on municipal bonds, see the booklet before filling in the form. Also, see the booklet if you received a Form 1099-INT showing federal income tax withheld or if federal income tax was withheld from your unemployment compensation or Alaska Permanent Fund dividends.

Remember, you must report all wages, salaries, and tips even if you do not get a Form W-2 from your employer. You must also report all your taxable interest, including interest from banks, savings and loans, credit unions, etc., even if you do not get a Form 1099-INT.

Worksheet for dependents who checked one or both boxes on line 5

(keep a copy for your records)

Use this worksheet to figure the amount to enter on line 5 if someone can claim you (or your spouse if married filing jointly) as a dependent, even if that person chooses not to do so. To find out if someone can claim you as a dependent, see Pub. 501.

A. Amount, if any, from line 1 on front   . _____

+ _____300.00_____ Enter total ▶   **A.** _____

B. Minimum standard deduction   . . . .   **B.** ____900.00____

C. Enter the **larger** of line A or line B here   . . . .   **C.** _____

D. Maximum standard deduction. If **single,** enter $5,450; if **married filing jointly,** enter $10,900   . . . .   **D.** _____

E. Enter the **smaller** of line C or line D here. This is your standard deduction   **E.** _____

F. Exemption amount.
- If single, enter -0-.
- If married filing jointly and—   **F.** _____
—both you and your spouse can be claimed as dependents, enter -0-.
—only one of you can be claimed as a dependent, enter $3,500.

G. Add lines E and F. Enter the total here and on line 5 on the front   . .   **G.** _____

If you did not check any boxes on line 5, enter on line 5 the amount shown below that applies to you.

- Single, enter $8,950. This is the total of your standard deduction ($5,450) and your exemption ($3,500).
- Married filing jointly, enter $17,900. This is the total of your standard deduction ($10,900), your exemption ($3,500), and your spouse's exemption ($3,500).

Mailing return

Mail your return by **April 15, 2009.** Use the envelope that came with your booklet. If you do not have that envelope or if you moved during the year, see the back cover for the address to use.

✸ *Printed on recycled paper*

Form **1040EZ** (2008)

B-3   Form 1040   U.S. Individual Income Tax Return and Schedules

Form **1040**

Department of the Treasury—Internal Revenue Service

U.S. Individual Income Tax Return 20**08**   (99)   IRS Use Only—Do not write or staple in this space.

For the year Jan. 1–Dec. 31, 2008, or other tax year beginning _____ , 2008, ending _____ , 20 ___   OMB No. 1545-0074

Label
(See instructions on page 14.)

Use the IRS label. Otherwise, please print or type.

L A B E L

H E R E

Your first name and initial | Last name | **Your social security number**

If a joint return, spouse's first name and initial | Last name | **Spouse's social security number**

Home address (number and street). If you have a P.O. box, see page 14. | Apt. no.

City, town or post office, state, and ZIP code. If you have a foreign address, see page 14.

▲ You **must** enter your SSN(s) above. ▲

Checking a box below will not change your tax or refund.

Presidential Election Campaign ▶ Check here if you, or your spouse if filing jointly, want $3 to go to this fund (see page 14) ▶ ☐ **You** ☐ **Spouse**

Filing Status

Check only one box.

1 ☐ Single
2 ☐ Married filing jointly (even if only one had income)
3 ☐ Married filing separately. Enter spouse's SSN above and full name here. ▶
4 ☐ Head of household (with qualifying person). (See page 15.) If the qualifying person is a child but not your dependent, enter this child's name here. ▶ _____
5 ☐ Qualifying widow(er) with dependent child (see page 16)

Exemptions

6a ☐ **Yourself.** If someone can claim you as a dependent, **do not** check box 6a
b ☐ **Spouse**
c **Dependents:**

(1) First name Last name	(2) Dependent's social security number	(3) Dependent's relationship to you	(4) ✓ if qualifying child for child tax credit (see page 17)
			☐
			☐
			☐
			☐

If more than four dependents, see page 17.

Boxes checked on 6a and 6b _____
No. of children on 6c who:
• lived with you _____
• did not live with you due to divorce or separation (see page 18) _____
Dependents on 6c not entered above _____
Add numbers on lines above ▶

d Total number of exemptions claimed

Income

Attach Form(s) W-2 here. Also attach Forms W-2G and 1099-R if tax was withheld.

If you did not get a W-2, see page 21.

Enclose, but do not attach, any payment. Also, please use **Form 1040-V.**

7 Wages, salaries, tips, etc. Attach Form(s) W-2 — **7**
8a **Taxable** interest. Attach Schedule B if required — **8a**
b **Tax-exempt** interest. **Do not** include on line 8a — 8b
9a Ordinary dividends. Attach Schedule B if required — **9a**
b Qualified dividends (see page 21) — 9b
10 Taxable refunds, credits, or offsets of state and local income taxes (see page 22) — **10**
11 Alimony received — **11**
12 Business income or (loss). Attach Schedule C or C-EZ — **12**
13 Capital gain or (loss). Attach Schedule D if required. If not required, check here ▶ ☐ — **13**
14 Other gains or (losses). Attach Form 4797 — **14**
15a IRA distributions . 15a _____ b Taxable amount (see page 23) — **15b**
16a Pensions and annuities 16a _____ b Taxable amount (see page 24) — **16b**
17 Rental real estate, royalties, partnerships, S corporations, trusts, etc. Attach Schedule E — **17**
18 Farm income or (loss). Attach Schedule F — **18**
19 Unemployment compensation — **19**
20a Social security benefits . 20a _____ b Taxable amount (see page 26) — **20b**
21 Other income. List type and amount (see page 28) _____ — **21**
22 Add the amounts in the far right column for lines 7 through 21. This is your **total income** ▶ — **22**

Adjusted Gross Income

23 Educator expenses (see page 28) — 23
24 Certain business expenses of reservists, performing artists, and fee-basis government officials. Attach Form 2106 or 2106-EZ — 24
25 Health savings account deduction. Attach Form 8889 — 25
26 Moving expenses. Attach Form 3903 — 26
27 One-half of self-employment tax. Attach Schedule SE — 27
28 Self-employed SEP, SIMPLE, and qualified plans — 28
29 Self-employed health insurance deduction (see page 29) — 29
30 Penalty on early withdrawal of savings — 30
31a Alimony paid b Recipient's SSN ▶ _____ — 31a
32 IRA deduction (see page 30) — 32
33 Student loan interest deduction (see page 33) — 33
34 Tuition and fees deduction. Attach Form 8917 — 34
35 Domestic production activities deduction. Attach Form 8903 — 35
36 Add lines 23 through 31a and 32 through 35 — **36**
37 Subtract line 36 from line 22. This is your **adjusted gross income** ▶ — **37**

For Disclosure, Privacy Act, and Paperwork Reduction Act Notice, see page 88.   Cat. No. 11320B   Form **1040** (2008)

Form 1040 (2008)   Page **2**

Tax and Credits	**38**	Amount from line 37 (adjusted gross income)	**38**

39a Check if: { ☐ **You** were born before January 2, 1944, ☐ Blind. } Total boxes { ☐ **Spouse** was born before January 2, 1944, ☐ Blind. } checked ▶ **39a** [ ]

b If your spouse itemizes on a separate return or you were a dual-status alien, see page 34 and check here ▶ **39b** ☐

c Check if standard deduction includes real estate taxes or disaster loss (see page 34) ▶ **39c** ☐

Standard Deduction for—

- *People who checked any box on line 39a, 39b, or 39c **or** who can be claimed as a dependent, see page 34.*
- *All others:*

Single or Married filing separately, $5,450

Married filing jointly or Qualifying widow(er), $10,900

Head of household, $8,000

40	**Itemized deductions** (from Schedule A) **or** your **standard deduction** (see left margin) .	**40**
41	Subtract line 40 from line 38	**41**
42	If line 38 is over $119,975, or you provided housing to a Midwestern displaced individual, see page 36. Otherwise, multiply $3,500 by the total number of exemptions claimed on line 6d	**42**
43	**Taxable income.** Subtract line 42 from line 41. If line 42 is more than line 41, enter -0-	**43**
44	**Tax** (see page 36). Check if any tax is from: **a** ☐ Form(s) 8814 **b** ☐ Form 4972	**44**
45	**Alternative minimum tax** (see page 39). Attach Form 6251	**45**
46	Add lines 44 and 45 . . . . ▶	**46**
47	Foreign tax credit. Attach Form 1116 if required . . .	**47**	
48	Credit for child and dependent care expenses. Attach Form 2441	**48**	
49	Credit for the elderly or the disabled. Attach Schedule R .	**49**	
50	Education credits. Attach Form 8863	**50**	
51	Retirement savings contributions credit. Attach Form 8880 .	**51**	
52	Child tax credit (see page 42). Attach Form 8901 if required .	**52**	
53	Credits from Form: **a** ☐ 8396 **b** ☐ 8839 **c** ☐ 5695	**53**	
54	Other credits from Form: **a** ☐ 3800 **b** ☐ 8801 **c** ☐	**54**	
55	Add lines 47 through 54. These are your **total credits**	**55**
56	Subtract line 55 from line 46. If line 55 is more than line 46, enter -0- . . . . . ▶	**56**

Other Taxes	**57**	Self-employment tax. Attach Schedule SE	**57**
	58	Unreported social security and Medicare tax from Form: **a** ☐ 4137 **b** ☐ 8919 .	**58**
	59	Additional tax on IRAs, other qualified retirement plans, etc. Attach Form 5329 if required .	**59**
	60	Additional taxes: **a** ☐ AEIC payments **b** ☐ Household employment taxes. Attach Schedule H	**60**
	61	Add lines 56 through 60. This is your **total tax** . . . . ▶	**61**

Payments

If you have a qualifying child, attach Schedule EIC.

62	Federal income tax withheld from Forms W-2 and 1099 .	**62**	
63	2008 estimated tax payments and amount applied from 2007 return	**63**	
64a	**Earned income credit (EIC)**	**64a**	
b	Nontaxable combat pay election	**64b**	
65	Excess social security and tier 1 RRTA tax withheld (see page 61)	**65**	
66	Additional child tax credit. Attach Form 8812	**66**	
67	Amount paid with request for extension to file (see page 61)	**67**	
68	Credits from Form: **a** ☐ 2439 **b** ☐ 4136 **c** ☐ 8801 **d** ☐ 8885	**68**	
69	First-time homebuyer credit. Attach Form 5405	**69**	
70	Recovery rebate credit (see worksheet on pages 62 and 63) .	**70**	
71	Add lines 62 through 70. These are your **total payments** . . . . ▶	**71**

Refund	**72**	If line 71 is more than line 61, subtract line 61 from line 71. This is the amount you **overpaid**	**72**

Direct deposit? See page 63 and fill in 73b, 73c, and 73d, or Form 8888.

73a Amount of line 72 you want **refunded to you.** If Form 8888 is attached, check here ▶ ☐   **73a**

▶ **b** Routing number [ ] ▶ **c** Type: ☐ Checking ☐ Savings

▶ **d** Account number [ ]

74 Amount of line 72 you want **applied to your 2009 estimated tax** ▶ | **74** |

Amount You Owe	**75**	**Amount you owe.** Subtract line 71 from line 61. For details on how to pay, see page 65 ▶	**75**
	76	Estimated tax penalty (see page 65)	**76**	

Third Party Designee

Do you want to allow another person to discuss this return with the IRS (see page 66)? ☐ **Yes.** Complete the following. ☐ **No**

Designee's name ▶   Phone no. ▶ ( )   Personal identification number (PIN) ▶ [ ]

Sign Here

Under penalties of perjury, I declare that I have examined this return and accompanying schedules and statements, and to the best of my knowledge and belief, they are true, correct, and complete. Declaration of preparer (other than taxpayer) is based on all information of which preparer has any knowledge.

Joint return? See page 15.

Keep a copy for your records.

Your signature   Date   Your occupation   Daytime phone number ( )

Spouse's signature. If a joint return, **both** must sign.   Date   Spouse's occupation

Paid Preparer's Use Only

Preparer's signature ▶   Date   Check if self-employed ☐   Preparer's SSN or PTIN

Firm's name (or yours if self-employed), address, and ZIP code ▶   EIN   Phone no. ( )

Form **1040** (2008)

✿ *Printed on recycled paper*

SCHEDULES A&B
(Form 1040)

Department of the Treasury
Internal Revenue Service (99)

Schedule A—Itemized Deductions

(Schedule B is on back)

▶ **Attach to Form 1040.**   ▶ **See Instructions for Schedules A&B (Form 1040).**

OMB No. 1545-0074

20**08**

Attachment
Sequence No. **07**

Name(s) shown on Form 1040

Your social security number

Medical and Dental Expenses	**Caution.** Do not include expenses reimbursed or paid by others.		
	1 Medical and dental expenses (see page A-1)	**1**	
	2 Enter amount from Form 1040, line 38 ⌊ **2** ⌋		
	3 Multiply line 2 by 7.5% (.075)	**3**	
	4 Subtract line 3 from line 1. If line 3 is more than line 1, enter -0-	**4**	
Taxes You Paid (See page A-2.)	5 State and local **(check only one box):**		
	a ☐ Income taxes, **or**	**5**	
	b ☐ General sales taxes		
	6 Real estate taxes (see page A-5)	**6**	
	7 Personal property taxes	**7**	
	8 Other taxes. List type and amount ▶ _____		
		8	
	9 Add lines 5 through 8	**9**	
Interest You Paid (See page A-5.) Note. Personal interest is not deductible.	10 Home mortgage interest and points reported to you on Form 1098	**10**	
	11 Home mortgage interest not reported to you on Form 1098. If paid to the person from whom you bought the home, see page A-6 and show that person's name, identifying no., and address ▶ _____		
		11	
	12 Points not reported to you on Form 1098. See page A-6 for special rules.	**12**	
	13 Qualified mortgage insurance premiums (see page A-6)	**13**	
	14 Investment interest. Attach Form 4952 if required. (See page A-6.)	**14**	
	15 Add lines 10 through 14	**15**	
Gifts to Charity If you made a gift and got a benefit for it, see page A-7.	16 Gifts by cash or check. If you made any gift of $250 or more, see page A-7	**16**	
	17 Other than by cash or check. If any gift of $250 or more, see page A-8. You **must** attach Form 8283 if over $500	**17**	
	18 Carryover from prior year	**18**	
	19 Add lines 16 through 18	**19**	
Casualty and Theft Losses	20 Casualty or theft loss(es). Attach Form 4684. (See page A-8.)	**20**	
Job Expenses and Certain Miscellaneous Deductions (See page A-9.)	21 Unreimbursed employee expenses—job travel, union dues, job education, etc. Attach Form 2106 or 2106-EZ if required. (See page A-9.) ▶ _____	**21**	
	22 Tax preparation fees	**22**	
	23 Other expenses—investment, safe deposit box, etc. List type and amount ▶ _____		
		23	
	24 Add lines 21 through 23	**24**	
	25 Enter amount from Form 1040, line 38 ⌊ **25** ⌋		
	26 Multiply line 25 by 2% (.02)	**26**	
	27 Subtract line 26 from line 24. If line 26 is more than line 24, enter -0- . . .	**27**	
Other Miscellaneous Deductions	28 Other—from list on page A-10. List type and amount ▶ _____		
		28	
Total Itemized Deductions	29 Is Form 1040, line 38, over $159,950 (over $79,975 if married filing separately)?		
	☐ **No.** Your deduction is not limited. Add the amounts in the far right column for lines 4 through 28. Also, enter this amount on Form 1040, line 40. ☐ **Yes.** Your deduction may be limited. See page A-10 for the amount to enter. ⎫⎬⎭ ▶	**29**	
	30 If you elect to itemize deductions even though they are less than your standard deduction, check here . . . . ▶ ☐		

For Paperwork Reduction Act Notice, see Form 1040 instructions.   Cat. No. 11330X   **Schedule A (Form 1040) 2008**

OMB No. 1545-0074   Page **2**

Name(s) shown on Form 1040. Do not enter name and social security number if shown on other side.	**Your social security number**

Schedule B—Interest and Ordinary Dividends

Attachment Sequence No. **08**

		Amount
Part I **Interest** (See page B-1 and the instructions for Form 1040, line 8a.)	**1** List name of payer. If any interest is from a seller-financed mortgage and the buyer used the property as a personal residence, see page B-1 and list this interest first. Also, show that buyer's social security number and address ▶	**1**
Note. If you received a Form 1099-INT, Form 1099-OID, or substitute statement from a brokerage firm, list the firm's name as the payer and enter the total interest shown on that form.	**2** Add the amounts on line 1	**2**
	3 Excludable interest on series EE and I U.S. savings bonds issued after 1989. Attach Form 8815	**3**
	4 Subtract line 3 from line 2. Enter the result here and on Form 1040, line 8a ▶	**4**

Note. If line 4 is over $1,500, you must complete Part III.

		Amount
Part II **Ordinary Dividends** (See page B-1 and the instructions for Form 1040, line 9a.)	**5** List name of payer ▶	**5**
Note. If you received a Form 1099-DIV or substitute statement from a brokerage firm, list the firm's name as the payer and enter the ordinary dividends shown on that form.		
	6 Add the amounts on line 5. Enter the total here and on Form 1040, line 9a . ▶	**6**

Note. If line 6 is over $1,500, you must complete Part III.

Part III **Foreign Accounts and Trusts** (See page B-2.)	You must complete this part if you **(a)** had over $1,500 of taxable interest or ordinary dividends; or **(b)** had a foreign account; or **(c)** received a distribution from, or were a grantor of, or a transferor to, a foreign trust.	Yes	No
	7a At any time during 2008, did you have an interest in or a signature or other authority over a financial account in a foreign country, such as a bank account, securities account, or other financial account? See page B-2 for exceptions and filing requirements for Form TD F 90-22.1.		
	b If "Yes," enter the name of the foreign country ▶		
	8 During 2008, did you receive a distribution from, or were you the grantor of, or transferor to, a foreign trust? If "Yes," you may have to file Form 3520. See page B-2		

For Paperwork Reduction Act Notice, see Form 1040 instructions.

Schedule B (Form 1040) 2008

SCHEDULE C (Form 1040)	**Profit or Loss From Business**	OMB No. 1545-0074

SCHEDULE C
(Form 1040)

Department of the Treasury
Internal Revenue Service   (99)

Profit or Loss From Business

(Sole Proprietorship)

▶ **Partnerships, joint ventures, etc., generally must file Form 1065 or 1065-B.**

▶ **Attach to Form 1040, 1040NR, or 1041.**   ▶ **See Instructions for Schedule C (Form 1040).**

OMB No. 1545-0074

2008

Attachment
Sequence No. **09**

Name of proprietor | Social security number (SSN)

A Principal business or profession, including product or service (see page C-3 of the instructions) | **B** Enter code from pages C-9, 10, & 11 ▶

C Business name. If no separate business name, leave blank. | **D** Employer ID number (EIN), if any

E Business address (including suite or room no.) ▶ --
City, town or post office, state, and ZIP code

F Accounting method: **(1)** ☐ Cash   **(2)** ☐ Accrual   **(3)** ☐ Other (specify) ▶ --------------------

G Did you "materially participate" in the operation of this business during 2008? If "No," see page C-4 for limit on losses   ☐ Yes ☐ No

H If you started or acquired this business during 2008, check here . . . . ▶ ☐

Part I   Income

1 Gross receipts or sales. **Caution.** See page C-4 and check the box if:

• This income was reported to you on Form W-2 and the "Statutory employee" box on that form was checked, or

• You are a member of a qualified joint venture reporting only rental real estate income not subject to self-employment tax. Also see page C-4 for limit on losses.   . ▶ ☐ | **1**

2 Returns and allowances . . . . | **2**

3 Subtract line 2 from line 1 . . . . | **3**

4 Cost of goods sold (from line 42 on page 2) . . . . | **4**

5 **Gross profit.** Subtract line 4 from line 3 . . . . | **5**

6 Other income, including federal and state gasoline or fuel tax credit or refund (see page C-4) . . . | **6**

7 **Gross income.** Add lines 5 and 6 . . . . ▶ | **7**

Part II   Expenses. Enter expenses for business use of your home **only** on line 30.

8 Advertising	**8**		**18** Office expense . . .	**18**	
9 Car and truck expenses (see page C-5)	**9**		**19** Pension and profit-sharing plans	**19**	
10 Commissions and fees .	**10**		**20** Rent or lease (see page C-6):		
11 Contract labor (see page C-5)	**11**		**a** Vehicles, machinery, and equipment .	**20a**	
12 Depletion	**12**		**b** Other business property . .	**20b**	
13 Depreciation and section 179 expense deduction (not included in Part III) (see page C-5)	**13**		**21** Repairs and maintenance .	**21**	
			22 Supplies (not included in Part III) .	**22**	
			23 Taxes and licenses . . .	**23**	
			24 Travel, meals, and entertainment:		
			a Travel	**24a**	
14 Employee benefit programs (other than on line 19) .	**14**		**b** Deductible meals and entertainment (see page C-7)	**24b**	
15 Insurance (other than health) .	**15**		**25** Utilities	**25**	
16 Interest:			**26** Wages (less employment credits) .	**26**	
a Mortgage (paid to banks, etc.) .	**16a**		**27** Other expenses (from line 48 on page 2)	**27**	
b Other	**16b**				
17 Legal and professional services	**17**				

28 **Total expenses** before expenses for business use of home. Add lines 8 through 27 . . . ▶ | **28**

29 Tentative profit or (loss). Subtract line 28 from line 7 . . . . | **29**

30 Expenses for business use of your home. Attach **Form 8829** . . . . | **30**

31 **Net profit or (loss).** Subtract line 30 from line 29.

• If a profit, enter on both **Form 1040, line 12,** and **Schedule SE, line 2,** or on **Form 1040NR, line 13** (if you checked the box on line 1, see page C-7). Estates and trusts, enter on **Form 1041, line 3.**

• If a loss, you **must** go to line 32. | **31**

32 If you have a loss, check the box that describes your investment in this activity (see page C-8).

• If you checked 32a, enter the loss on both **Form 1040, line 12,** and **Schedule SE, line 2,** or on **Form 1040NR, line 13** (if you checked the box on line 1, see the line 31 instructions on page C-7). Estates and trusts, enter on **Form 1041, line 3.**

• If you checked 32b, you **must** attach **Form 6198.** Your loss may be limited. | **32a** ☐ All investment is at risk.
32b ☐ Some investment is not at risk.

For Paperwork Reduction Act Notice, see page C-9 of the instructions.   Cat. No. 11334P   Schedule C (Form 1040) 2008

Schedule C (Form 1040) 2008   Page **2**

| Part III | Cost of Goods Sold (see page C-8) |

33 Method(s) used to
value closing inventory: **a** ☐ Cost   **b** ☐ Lower of cost or market   **c** ☐ Other (attach explanation)

34 Was there any change in determining quantities, costs, or valuations between opening and closing inventory?
If "Yes," attach explanation . . . .   ☐ **Yes**   ☐ **No**

35 Inventory at beginning of year. If different from last year's closing inventory, attach explanation .	**35**	
36 Purchases less cost of items withdrawn for personal use	**36**	
37 Cost of labor. Do not include any amounts paid to yourself	**37**	
38 Materials and supplies	**38**	
39 Other costs	**39**	
40 Add lines 35 through 39	**40**	
41 Inventory at end of year	**41**	
42 **Cost of goods sold.** Subtract line 41 from line 40. Enter the result here and on page 1, line 4 .	**42**	

| Part IV | Information on Your Vehicle. Complete this part **only** if you are claiming car or truck expenses on line 9 and are not required to file Form 4562 for this business. See the instructions for line 13 on page C-5 to find out if you must file Form 4562. |

43 When did you place your vehicle in service for business purposes? (month, day, year) ▶ _____/_____/_____

44 Of the total number of miles you drove your vehicle during 2008, enter the number of miles you used your vehicle for:

a Business _____ **b** Commuting (see instructions) _____ **c** Other _____

45 Was your vehicle available for personal use during off-duty hours? . . . .   ☐ **Yes**   ☐ **No**

46 Do you (or your spouse) have another vehicle available for personal use?. . . . .   ☐ **Yes**   ☐ **No**

47a Do you have evidence to support your deduction? . . . .   ☐ **Yes**   ☐ **No**

  b If "Yes," is the evidence written? . . . .   ☐ **Yes**   ☐ **No**

| Part V | Other Expenses. List below business expenses not included on lines 8–26 or line 30. |

--		
--		
--		
--		
--		
--		
--		
--		
48 **Total other expenses.** Enter here and on page 1, line 27	**48**	

Schedule C (Form 1040) 2008

SCHEDULE D
(Form 1040)

Department of the Treasury
Internal Revenue Service   (99)

Capital Gains and Losses

▶ Attach to Form 1040 or Form 1040NR.   ▶ See Instructions for Schedule D (Form 1040).

▶ Use Schedule D-1 to list additional transactions for lines 1 and 8.

OMB No. 1545-0074

2008

Attachment
Sequence No. **12**

Name(s) shown on return

Your social security number

Part I Short-Term Capital Gains and Losses—Assets Held One Year or Less

(a) Description of property (Example: 100 sh. XYZ Co.)	(b) Date acquired (Mo., day, yr.)	(c) Date sold (Mo., day, yr.)	(d) Sales price (see page D-7 of the instructions)	(e) Cost or other basis (see page D-7 of the instructions)	(f) Gain or (loss) Subtract (e) from (d)
1					

2 Enter your short-term totals, if any, from Schedule D-1, line 2 . . . . **2**

3 **Total short-term sales price amounts.** Add lines 1 and 2 in column (d) **3**

4 Short-term gain from Form 6252 and short-term gain or (loss) from Forms 4684, 6781, and 8824 **4**

5 Net short-term gain or (loss) from partnerships, S corporations, estates, and trusts from Schedule(s) K-1 . . . . **5**

6 Short-term capital loss carryover. Enter the amount, if any, from line 8 of your **Capital Loss Carryover Worksheet** on page D-7 of the instructions . . . . **6** ( )

7 **Net short-term capital gain or (loss).** Combine lines 1 through 6 in column (f) **7**

Part II Long-Term Capital Gains and Losses—Assets Held More Than One Year

(a) Description of property (Example: 100 sh. XYZ Co.)	(b) Date acquired (Mo., day, yr.)	(c) Date sold (Mo., day, yr.)	(d) Sales price (see page D-7 of the instructions)	(e) Cost or other basis (see page D-7 of the instructions)	(f) Gain or (loss) Subtract (e) from (d)
8					

9 Enter your long-term totals, if any, from Schedule D-1, line 9 . . . . **9**

10 **Total long-term sales price amounts.** Add lines 8 and 9 in column (d) **10**

11 Gain from Form 4797, Part I; long-term gain from Forms 2439 and 6252; and long-term gain or (loss) from Forms 4684, 6781, and 8824 . . . . **11**

12 Net long-term gain or (loss) from partnerships, S corporations, estates, and trusts from Schedule(s) K-1 . . . . **12**

13 Capital gain distributions. See page D-2 of the instructions **13**

14 Long-term capital loss carryover. Enter the amount, if any, from line 13 of your **Capital Loss Carryover Worksheet** on page D-7 of the instructions . . . . **14** ( )

15 **Net long-term capital gain or (loss).** Combine lines 8 through 14 in column (f). Then go to Part III on the back **15**

For Paperwork Reduction Act Notice, see Form 1040 or Form 1040NR instructions.   Cat. No. 11338H   **Schedule D (Form 1040) 2008**

Part III   Summary

16   Combine lines 7 and 15 and enter the result. **16**

If line 16 is:
- A **gain**, enter the amount from line 16 on Form 1040, line 13, or Form 1040NR, line 14. Then go to line 17 below.
- A **loss**, skip lines 17 through 20 below. Then go to line 21. Also be sure to complete line 22.
- **Zero**, skip lines 17 through 21 below and enter -0- on Form 1040, line 13, or Form 1040NR, line 14. Then go to line 22.

17   Are lines 15 and 16 **both** gains?
☐ **Yes.** Go to line 18.
☐ **No.** Skip lines 18 through 21, and go to line 22.

18   Enter the amount, if any, from line 7 of the **28% Rate Gain Worksheet** on page D-8 of the instructions . . . . ▶   **18**

19   Enter the amount, if any, from line 18 of the **Unrecaptured Section 1250 Gain Worksheet** on page D-9 of the instructions . . . . ▶   **19**

20   Are lines 18 and 19 **both** zero or blank?
☐ **Yes.** Complete Form 1040 through line 43, or Form 1040NR through line 40. Then complete the **Qualified Dividends and Capital Gain Tax Worksheet** on page 38 of the Instructions for Form 1040 (or in the Instructions for Form 1040NR). **Do not** complete lines 21 and 22 below.
☐ **No.** Complete Form 1040 through line 43, or Form 1040NR through line 40. Then complete the **Schedule D Tax Worksheet** on page D-10 of the instructions. **Do not** complete lines 21 and 22 below.

21   If line 16 is a loss, enter here and on Form 1040, line 13, or Form 1040NR, line 14, the **smaller** of:

- The loss on line 16 or
- ($3,000), or if married filing separately, ($1,500)   } . . . .   **21** ( )

Note. When figuring which amount is smaller, treat both amounts as positive numbers.

22   Do you have qualified dividends on Form 1040, line 9b, or Form 1040NR, line 10b?
☐ **Yes.** Complete Form 1040 through line 43, or Form 1040NR through line 40. Then complete the **Qualified Dividends and Capital Gain Tax Worksheet** on page 38 of the Instructions for Form 1040 (or in the Instructions for Form 1040NR).
☐ **No.** Complete the rest of Form 1040 or Form 1040NR.

Schedule D (Form 1040) 2008

SCHEDULE E
(Form 1040)

Department of the Treasury
Internal Revenue Service (99)

Supplemental Income and Loss

(From rental real estate, royalties, partnerships,
S corporations, estates, trusts, REMICs, etc.)

▶ Attach to Form 1040, 1040NR, or Form 1041.   ▶ See Instructions for Schedule E (Form 1040).

OMB No. 1545-0074

2008

Attachment
Sequence No. **13**

Name(s) shown on return

Your social security number

Part I   **Income or Loss From Rental Real Estate and Royalties**   **Note.** If you are in the business of renting personal property, use **Schedule C** or **C-EZ** (see page E-3). If you are an individual, report farm rental income or loss from **Form 4835** on page 2, line 40.

1 List the type and address of each **rental real estate property:**

A ....

B ....

C ....

2 For each rental real estate property listed on line 1, did you or your family use it during the tax year for personal purposes for more than the greater of:

- 14 days **or**
- 10% of the total days rented at fair rental value?

(See page E-3)

	Yes	No
A		
B		
C		

Income:

			Properties			Totals (Add columns A, B, and C.)	
			A	B	C		
3 Rents received	3					3	
4 Royalties received	4					4	

Expenses:

5 Advertising	5						
6 Auto and travel (see page E-4)	6						
7 Cleaning and maintenance	7						
8 Commissions	8						
9 Insurance	9						
10 Legal and other professional fees	10						
11 Management fees	11						
12 Mortgage interest paid to banks, etc. (see page E-5)	12					12	
13 Other interest	13						
14 Repairs	14						
15 Supplies	15						
16 Taxes	16						
17 Utilities	17						
18 Other (list) ▶	18						
19 Add lines 5 through 18	19					19	
20 Depreciation expense or depletion (see page E-5)	20					20	
21 Total expenses. Add lines 19 and 20	21						
22 Income or (loss) from rental real estate or royalty properties. Subtract line 21 from line 3 (rents) or line 4 (royalties). If the result is a (loss), see page E-5 to find out if you must file **Form 6198**	22						
23 Deductible rental real estate loss. **Caution.** Your rental real estate loss on line 22 may be limited. See page E-5 to find out if you must file **Form 8582.** Real estate professionals **must** complete line 43 on page 2	23	( )(	)(	)(	)		

24 Income. Add positive amounts shown on line 22. **Do not** include any losses   24

25 Losses. Add royalty losses from line 22 and rental real estate losses from line 23. Enter total losses here.   25 ( )

26 **Total rental real estate and royalty income or (loss).** Combine lines 24 and 25. Enter the result here. If Parts II, III, IV, and line 40 on page 2 do not apply to you, also enter this amount on Form 1040, line 17, or Form 1040NR, line 18. Otherwise, include this amount in the total on line 41 on page 2 .   26

For Paperwork Reduction Act Notice, see page E-8 of the instructions.   Cat. No. 11344L   Schedule E (Form 1040) 2008

Schedule E (Form 1040) 2008 | Attachment Sequence No. **13** | Page **2**

Name(s) shown on return. Do not enter name and social security number if shown on other side. | **Your social security number**

Caution. The IRS compares amounts reported on your tax return with amounts shown on Schedule(s) K-1.

Part II **Income or Loss From Partnerships and S Corporations**   **Note.** If you report a loss from an at-risk activity for which **any** amount is **not** at risk, you **must** check the box in column **(e)** on line 28 and attach **Form 6198**. See page E-1.

27 Are you reporting any loss not allowed in a prior year due to the at-risk or basis limitations, a prior year unallowed loss from a passive activity (if that loss was not reported on Form 8582), or unreimbursed partnership expenses? ☐ **Yes** ☐ **No**
If you answered "Yes," see page E-7 before completing this section.

28

	(a) Name	(b) Enter P for partnership; S for S corporation	(c) Check if foreign partnership	(d) Employer identification number	(e) Check if any amount is not at risk
A			☐		☐
B			☐		☐
C			☐		☐
D			☐		☐

	Passive Income and Loss		Nonpassive Income and Loss		
	(f) Passive loss allowed (attach Form 8582 if required)	(g) Passive income from Schedule K-1	(h) Nonpassive loss from Schedule K-1	(i) Section 179 expense deduction from Form 4562	(j) Nonpassive income from Schedule K-1
A					
B					
C					
D					
29a Totals					
b Totals					

30 Add columns (g) and (j) of line 29a . . . . | **30** |
31 Add columns (f), (h), and (i) of line 29b . . . . | **31** (|) |
32 **Total partnership and S corporation income or (loss).** Combine lines 30 and 31. Enter the result here and include in the total on line 41 below. . . . . | **32** |

Part III **Income or Loss From Estates and Trusts**

33

	(a) Name	(b) Employer identification number
A		
B		

	Passive Income and Loss		Nonpassive Income and Loss	
	(c) Passive deduction or loss allowed (attach Form 8582 if required)	(d) Passive income from Schedule K-1	(e) Deduction or loss from Schedule K-1	(f) Other income from Schedule K-1
A				
B				
34a Totals				
b Totals				

35 Add columns (d) and (f) of line 34a . . . . | **35** |
36 Add columns (c) and (e) of line 34b . . . . | **36** (|) |
37 **Total estate and trust income or (loss).** Combine lines 35 and 36. Enter the result here and include in the total on line 41 below . . . . | **37** |

Part IV **Income or Loss From Real Estate Mortgage Investment Conduits (REMICs)—Residual Holder**

38	(a) Name	(b) Employer identification number	(c) Excess inclusion from Schedules Q, line 2c (see page E-7)	(d) Taxable income (net loss) from Schedules Q, line 1b	(e) Income from Schedules Q, line 3b

39 Combine columns (d) and (e) only. Enter the result here and include in the total on line 41 below | **39** |

Part V **Summary**

40 Net farm rental income or (loss) from **Form 4835**. Also, complete line 42 below . . . . . | **40** |
41 **Total income or (loss).** Combine lines 26, 32, 37, 39, and 40. Enter the result here and on Form 1040, line 17, or Form 1040NR, line 18 ▶ | **41** |

42 **Reconciliation of farming and fishing income.** Enter your **gross** farming and fishing income reported on Form 4835, line 7; Schedule K-1 (Form 1065), box 14, code B; Schedule K-1 (Form 1120S), box 17, code T; and Schedule K-1 (Form 1041), line 14, code F (see page E-8) . . . | **42** |

43 **Reconciliation for real estate professionals.** If you were a real estate professional (see page E-2), enter the net income or (loss) you reported anywhere on Form 1040 or Form 1040NR from all rental real estate activities in which you materially participated under the passive activity loss rules . | **43** |

Schedule E (Form 1040) 2008

SCHEDULE F
(Form 1040)

Department of the Treasury
Internal Revenue Service (99)

Profit or Loss From Farming

▶ Attach to Form 1040, Form 1040NR, Form 1041, Form 1065, or Form 1065-B.

▶ See Instructions for Schedule F (Form 1040).

OMB No. 1545-0074

20**08**

Attachment
Sequence No. **14**

Name of proprietor

Social security number (SSN)

A Principal product. Describe in one or two words your principal crop or activity for the current tax year.

B Enter code from Part IV
▶

C Accounting method: **(1)** ☐ Cash **(2)** ☐ Accrual

D Employer ID number (EIN), if any

E Did you "materially participate" in the operation of this business during 2008? If "No," see page F-3 for limit on passive losses. ☐ Yes ☐ No

Part I **Farm Income—Cash Method.** Complete Parts I and II (Accrual method. Complete Parts II and III, and Part I, line 11.)
Do not include sales of livestock held for draft, breeding, sport, or dairy purposes. Report these sales on Form 4797.

1	Sales of livestock and other items you bought for resale	**1**	
2	Cost or other basis of livestock and other items reported on line 1.	**2**	
3	Subtract line 2 from line 1		**3**
4	Sales of livestock, produce, grains, and other products you raised		**4**
5a	Cooperative distributions (Form(s) 1099-PATR) **5a**	**5b** Taxable amount	**5b**
6a	Agricultural program payments (see page F-3) . **6a**	**6b** Taxable amount	**6b**
7	Commodity Credit Corporation (CCC) loans (see page F-3):		
a	CCC loans reported under election		**7a**
b	CCC loans forfeited . **7b**	**7c** Taxable amount	**7c**
8	Crop insurance proceeds and federal crop disaster payments (see page F-3):		
a	Amount received in 2008 **8a**	**8b** Taxable amount	**8b**
c	If election to defer to 2009 is attached, check here ▶ ☐	**8d** Amount deferred from 2007	**8d**
9	Custom hire (machine work) income		**9**
10	Other income, including federal and state gasoline or fuel tax credit or refund (see page F-4)		**10**
11	**Gross income.** Add amounts in the right column for lines 3 through 10. If you use the accrual method to figure your income, enter the amount from Part III, line 51. ▶		**11**

Part II **Farm Expenses—Cash and Accrual Method.**
Do not include personal or living expenses such as taxes, insurance, or repairs on your home.

12	Car and truck expenses (see page F-5). Also attach **Form 4562** .	**12**	25	Pension and profit-sharing plans	**25**	
13	Chemicals	**13**	26	Rent or lease (see page F-6):		
14	Conservation expenses (see page F-5) .	**14**	a	Vehicles, machinery, and equipment	**26a**	
15	Custom hire (machine work) .	**15**	b	Other (land, animals, etc.) .	**26b**	
16	Depreciation and section 179 expense deduction not claimed elsewhere (see page F-5) .	**16**	27	Repairs and maintenance .	**27**	
			28	Seeds and plants . . .	**28**	
			29	Storage and warehousing .	**29**	
17	Employee benefit programs other than on line 25 .	**17**	30	Supplies . . .	**30**	
18	Feed .	**18**	31	Taxes . . .	**31**	
19	Fertilizers and lime .	**19**	32	Utilities . . .	**32**	
20	Freight and trucking. .	**20**	33	Veterinary, breeding, and medicine	**33**	
21	Gasoline, fuel, and oil .	**21**	34	Other expenses (specify):		
22	Insurance (other than health)	**22**	a		**34a**	
23	Interest:		b		**34b**	
a	Mortgage (paid to banks, etc.)	**23a**	c		**34c**	
b	Other .	**23b**	d		**34d**	
24	Labor hired (less employment credits)	**24**	e		**34e**	
			f		**34f**	

35	**Total expenses.** Add lines 12 through 34f. If line 34f is negative, see instructions ▶	**35**	
36	**Net farm profit or (loss).** Subtract line 35 from line 11. Partnerships, see page F-7. • If a profit, enter the profit on both **Form 1040, line 18,** and **Schedule SE, line 1a;** on **Form 1040NR, line 19;** or on **Form 1041, line 6.** • If a loss, you **must** go to line 37.	**36**	
37	If you have a loss, you **must** check the box that describes your investment in this activity (see page F-7). • If you checked 37a, enter the loss on both **Form 1040, line 18,** and **Schedule SE, line 1a;** on **Form 1040NR, line 19;** or on **Form 1041, line 6.** • If you checked 37b, you **must** attach Form 6198. Your loss may be limited.	**37a** ☐ All investment is at risk. **37b** ☐ Some investment is not at risk.	

For Paperwork Reduction Act Notice, see page F-7 of the instructions. Cat. No. 11346H **Schedule F (Form 1040) 2008**

Part III **Farm Income—Accrual Method** (see page F-7).

Do not include sales of livestock held for draft, breeding, sport, or dairy purposes. Report these sales on Form 4797 and do not include this livestock on line 46 below.

38	Sales of livestock, produce, grains, and other products	**38**	
39a	Cooperative distributions (Form(s) 1099-PATR) . **39a** |_____| **39b** Taxable amount	**39b**	
40a	Agricultural program payments . . . . **40a** |_____| **40b** Taxable amount	**40b**	
41	Commodity Credit Corporation (CCC) loans:		
a	CCC loans reported under election	**41a**	
b	CCC loans forfeited . . . . **41b** |_____| **41c** Taxable amount	**41c**	
42	Crop insurance proceeds	**42**	
43	Custom hire (machine work) income	**43**	
44	Other income, including federal and state gasoline or fuel tax credit or refund	**44**	
45	Add amounts in the right column for lines 38 through 44	**45**	

46	Inventory of livestock, produce, grains, and other products at beginning of the year	**46**	
47	Cost of livestock, produce, grains, and other products purchased during the year	**47**	
48	Add lines 46 and 47	**48**	
49	Inventory of livestock, produce, grains, and other products at end of year	**49**	

50	Cost of livestock, produce, grains, and other products sold. Subtract line 49 from line 48*. . . .	**50**	
51	**Gross income.** Subtract line 50 from line 45. Enter the result here and on Part I, line 11 . . . ▶	**51**	

*If you use the unit-livestock-price method or the farm-price method of valuing inventory and the amount on line 49 is larger than the amount on line 48, subtract line 48 from line 49. Enter the result on line 50. Add lines 45 and 50. Enter the total on line 51 and on Part I, line 11.

Part IV **Principal Agricultural Activity Codes**

*File Schedule C (Form 1040) or Schedule C-EZ (Form 1040) instead of Schedule F if **(a)** your principal source of income is from providing agricultural services such as soil preparation, veterinary, farm labor, horticultural, or management for a fee or on a contract basis, or **(b)** you are engaged in the business of breeding, raising, and caring for dogs, cats, or other pet animals.*

These codes for the Principal Agricultural Activity classify farms by their primary activity to facilitate the administration of the Internal Revenue Code. These six-digit codes are based on the North American Industry Classification System (NAICS).

Select the code that best identifies your primary farming activity and enter the six digit number on page 1, line B.

Crop Production

111100	Oilseed and grain farming
111210	Vegetable and melon farming
111300	Fruit and tree nut farming
111400	Greenhouse, nursery, and floriculture production
111900	Other crop farming

Animal Production

112111	Beef cattle ranching and farming
112112	Cattle feedlots
112120	Dairy cattle and milk production
112210	Hog and pig farming
112300	Poultry and egg production
112400	Sheep and goat farming
112510	Aquaculture
112900	Other animal production

Forestry and Logging

113000	Forestry and logging (including forest nurseries and timber tracts)

**Schedule R
(Form 1040)**

Department of the Treasury
Internal Revenue Service   (99)

Credit for the Elderly or the Disabled

▶ **Attach to Form 1040.**   ▶ **See Instructions for Schedule R (Form 1040).**

OMB No. 1545-0074

20**08**

Attachment
Sequence No. **16**

Name(s) shown on Form 1040

Your social security number

You may be able to take this credit and reduce your tax if by the end of 2008:
- You were age 65 or older **or** • You were under age 65, you retired on **permanent and total** disability, and you received taxable disability income.

But you must also meet other tests. See page R-1.

TIP In most cases, the IRS can figure the credit for you. See page R-1.

Part I   **Check the Box for Your Filing Status and Age**

If your filing status is:	And by the end of 2008:	Check only one box:
Single, Head of household, or Qualifying widow(er)	**1** You were 65 or older **1**	☐
	2 You were under 65 and you retired on permanent and total disability **2**	☐
	3 Both spouses were 65 or older **3**	☐
	4 Both spouses were under 65, but only one spouse retired on permanent and total disability **4**	☐
Married filing jointly	**5** Both spouses were under 65, and both retired on permanent and total disability **5**	☐
	6 One spouse was 65 or older, and the other spouse was under 65 and retired on permanent and total disability **6**	☐
	7 One spouse was 65 or older, and the other spouse was under 65 and **not** retired on permanent and total disability **7**	☐
Married filing separately	**8** You were 65 or older and you lived apart from your spouse for all of 2008 . . . . **8**	☐
	9 You were under 65, you retired on permanent and total disability, and you lived apart from your spouse for all of 2008 . . . . . . **9**	☐

Did you check box 1, 3, 7, or 8? — **Yes** ▶ Skip Part II and complete Part III on the back.
— **No** ▶ Complete Parts II and III.

Part II   **Statement of Permanent and Total Disability** (Complete **only** if you checked box 2, 4, 5, 6, or 9 above.)

If: 1 You filed a physician's statement for this disability for 1983 or an earlier year, or you filed or got a statement for tax years after 1983 and your physician signed line B on the statement, **and**

2 Due to your continued disabled condition, you were unable to engage in any substantial gainful activity in 2008, check this box . . . . ▶ ☐

- If you checked this box, you do not have to get another statement for 2008.
- If you **did not** check this box, have your physician complete the statement on page R-4. You **must** keep the statement for your records.

Part III   **Figure Your Credit**

10   **If you checked (in Part I):**   **Enter:**

Box 1, 2, 4, or 7 . . . . $5,000
Box 3, 5, or 6 . . . . $7,500   } **10**
Box 8 or 9 . . . . $3,750

> **Did you check box 2, 4, 5, 6, or 9 in Part I?** —— **Yes** ——▶ You **must** complete line 11.
> —— **No** ——▶ Enter the amount from line 10 on line 12 and go to line 13.

11   **If you checked (in Part I):**

- Box 6, add $5,000 to the taxable disability income of the spouse who was under age 65. Enter the total.
- Box 2, 4, or 9, enter your taxable disability income.   } **11**
- Box 5, add your taxable disability income to your spouse's taxable disability income. Enter the total.

(TIP) For more details on what to include on line 11, see page R-3.

12   If you completed line 11, enter the **smaller** of line 10 or line 11. **All others,** enter the amount from line 10 . . . .   **12**

13   Enter the following pensions, annuities, or disability income that you (and your spouse if filing a joint return) received in 2008.

a   Nontaxable part of social security benefits and nontaxable part of railroad retirement benefits treated as social security (see page R-3). }   . . .   **13a**

b   Nontaxable veterans' pensions and any other pension, annuity, or disability benefit that is excluded from income under any other provision of law (see page R-3). }   . . .   **13b**

c   Add lines 13a and 13b. (Even though these income items are not taxable, they **must** be included here to figure your credit.) If you did not receive any of the types of nontaxable income listed on line 13a or 13b, enter -0- on line 13c **13c**

14   Enter the amount from Form 1040, line 38 . . . .   **14**

15   **If you checked (in Part I):   Enter:**
Box 1 or 2 . . . . . . $7,500
Box 3, 4, 5, 6, or 7 . . . $10,000 }   **15**
Box 8 or 9 . . . . . . $5,000

16   Subtract line 15 from line 14. If zero or less, enter -0- **16**

17   Enter one-half of line 16 . . . .   **17**

18   Add lines 13c and 17 . . . .   **18**

19   Subtract line 18 from line 12. If zero or less, **stop;** you **cannot** take the credit. Otherwise, go to line 20 . . . .   **19**

20   Multiply line 19 by 15% (.15) **20**

21   Enter the amount from Form 1040, line 46 . . . . . .   **21**

22   Enter the total of any amounts from Form 1040, lines 47 and 48   **22**

23   Subtract line 22 from line 21. If zero or less, **stop;** you **cannot** take the credit . . .   **23**

24   **Credit for the elderly or the disabled.** Enter the **smaller** of line 20 or line 23 here and on Form 1040, line 49 . . . .   **24**

SCHEDULE SE

(Form 1040)

Department of the Treasury
Internal Revenue Service   (99)

Self-Employment Tax

▶ **Attach to Form 1040.**   ▶ **See Instructions for Schedule SE (Form 1040).**

OMB No. 1545-0074

20**08**

Attachment
Sequence No. **17**

Name of person with **self-employment** income (as shown on Form 1040)	Social security number of person with **self-employment** income ▶		

Who Must File Schedule SE

You must file Schedule SE if:

- You had net earnings from self-employment from **other than** church employee income (line 4 of Short Schedule SE or line 4c of Long Schedule SE) of $400 or more, **or**

- You had church employee income of $108.28 or more. Income from services you performed as a minister or a member of a religious order **is not** church employee income (see page SE-1).

Note. Even if you had a loss or a small amount of income from self-employment, it may be to your benefit to file Schedule SE and use either "optional method" in Part II of Long Schedule SE (see page SE-4).

Exception. If your only self-employment income was from earnings as a minister, member of a religious order, or Christian Science practitioner **and** you filed Form 4361 and received IRS approval not to be taxed on those earnings, **do not** file Schedule SE. Instead, write "Exempt—Form 4361" on Form 1040, line 57.

May I Use Short Schedule SE or Must I Use Long Schedule SE?

Note. Use this flowchart **only** if you must file Schedule SE. If unsure, see *Who Must File Schedule SE,* above.

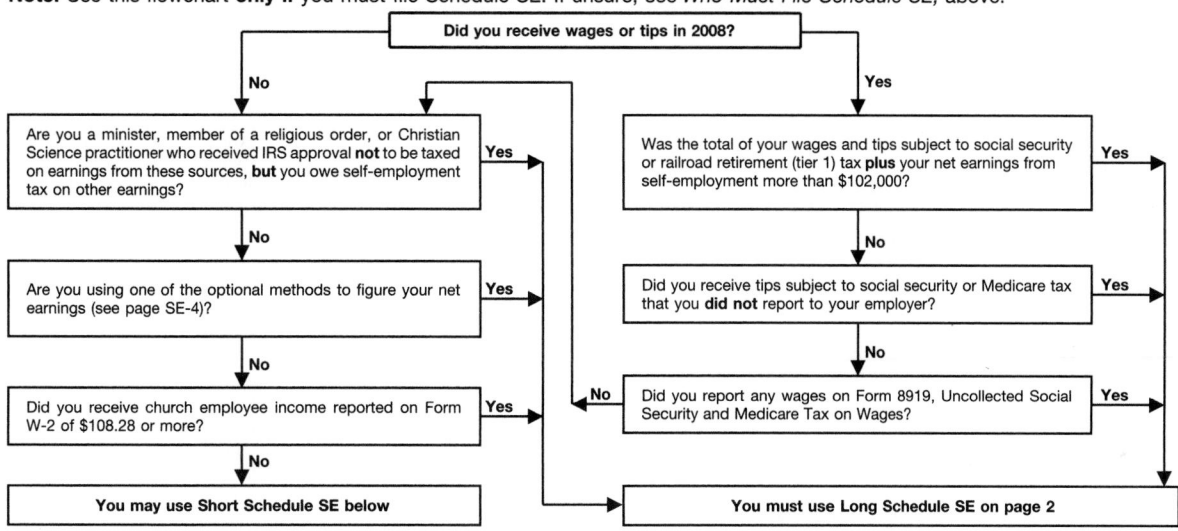

Section A—Short Schedule SE. Caution. Read above to see if you can use Short Schedule SE.

1a Net farm profit or (loss) from Schedule F, line 36, and farm partnerships, Schedule K-1 (Form 1065), box 14, code A	**1a**		
b If you received social security retirement or disability benefits, enter the amount of Conservation Reserve Program payments included on Schedule F, line 6b, or listed on Schedule K-1 (Form 1065), box 20, code X	**1b** (		)
2 Net profit or (loss) from Schedule C, line 31; Schedule C-EZ, line 3; Schedule K-1 (Form 1065), box 14, code A (other than farming); and Schedule K-1 (Form 1065-B), box 9, code J1. Ministers and members of religious orders, see page SE-1 for types of income to report on this line. See page SE-3 for other income to report	**2**		
3 Combine lines 1a, 1b, and 2	**3**		
4 **Net earnings from self-employment.** Multiply line 3 by 92.35% (.9235). If less than $400, **do not** file this schedule; you do not owe self-employment tax . . . . ▶	**4**		
5 Self-employment tax. If the amount on line 4 is: • $102,000 or less, multiply line 4 by 15.3% (.153). Enter the result here and on **Form 1040, line 57.** • More than $102,000, multiply line 4 by 2.9% (.029). Then, add $12,648 to the result. Enter the total here and on **Form 1040, line 57**	**5**		
6 **Deduction for one-half of self-employment tax.** Multiply line 5 by 50% (.5). Enter the result here and on **Form 1040, line 27** . . . **6**			

For Paperwork Reduction Act Notice, see Form 1040 instructions.   Cat. No. 11358Z   **Schedule SE (Form 1040) 2008**

Schedule SE (Form 1040) 2008   Attachment Sequence No. **17**   Page **2**

Name of person with **self-employment** income (as shown on Form 1040)	Social security number of person with **self-employment** income ▶	

Section B—Long Schedule SE

Part I   Self-Employment Tax

Note. If your only income subject to self-employment tax is **church employee income,** skip lines 1 through 4b. Enter -0- on line 4c and go to line 5a. Income from services you performed as a minister or a member of a religious order **is not** church employee income. See page SE-1.

A   If you are a minister, member of a religious order, or Christian Science practitioner **and** you filed Form 4361, but you had $400 or more of **other** net earnings from self-employment, check here and continue with Part I . . . . . ▶ ☐

1a	Net farm profit or (loss) from Schedule F, line 36, and farm partnerships, Schedule K-1 (Form 1065), box 14, code A. **Note.** Skip lines 1a and 1b if you use the farm optional method (see page SE-4)	**1a**	
b	If you received social security retirement or disability benefits, enter the amount of Conservation Reserve Program payments included on Schedule F, line 6b, or listed on Schedule K-1 (Form 1065), box 20, code X	**1b** (	)
2	Net profit or (loss) from Schedule C, line 31; Schedule C-EZ, line 3; Schedule K-1 (Form 1065), box 14, code A (other than farming); and Schedule K-1 (Form 1065-B), box 9, code J1. Ministers and members of religious orders, see page SE-1 for types of income to report on this line. See page SE-3 for other income to report. **Note.** Skip this line if you use the nonfarm optional method (see page SE-4)	**2**	
3	Combine lines 1a, 1b, and 2	**3**	
4a	If line 3 is more than zero, multiply line 3 by 92.35% (.9235). Otherwise, enter amount from line 3	**4a**	
b	If you elect one or both of the optional methods, enter the total of lines 15 and 17 here . .	**4b**	
c	Combine lines 4a and 4b. If less than $400, **stop;** you do not owe self-employment tax. **Exception.** If less than $400 and you had **church employee income,** enter -0- and continue. . . . . ▶	**4c**	
5a	Enter your **church employee income** from Form W-2. See page SE-1 for definition of church employee income	**5a**			
b	Multiply line 5a by 92.35% (.9235). If less than $100, enter -0-	**5b**	
6	**Net earnings from self-employment.** Add lines 4c and 5b	**6**	
7	Maximum amount of combined wages and self-employment earnings subject to social security tax or the 6.2% portion of the 7.65% railroad retirement (tier 1) tax for 2008	**7**	102,000	00
8a	Total social security wages and tips (total of boxes 3 and 7 on Form(s) W-2) and railroad retirement (tier 1) compensation. If $102,000 or more, skip lines 8b through 10, and go to line 11	**8a**		
b	Unreported tips subject to social security tax (from Form 4137, line 10)	**8b**	
c	Wages subject to social security tax (from Form 8919, line 10) . .	**8c**	
d	Add lines 8a, 8b, and 8c	**8d**	
9	Subtract line 8d from line 7. If zero or less, enter -0- here and on line 10 and go to line 11 . ▶	**9**	
10	Multiply the **smaller** of line 6 or line 9 by 12.4% (.124)	**10**	
11	Multiply line 6 by 2.9% (.029)	**11**	
12	**Self-employment tax.** Add lines 10 and 11. Enter here and on **Form 1040, line 57** . . .	**12**	
13	**Deduction for one-half of self-employment tax.** Multiply line 12 by 50% (.5). Enter the result here and on **Form 1040, line 27** . . .	**13**			

Part II   Optional Methods To Figure Net Earnings (see page SE-4)

Farm Optional Method. You may use this method **only** if **(a)** your gross farm income[1] was not more than $6,300, **or (b)** your net farm profits[2] were less than $4,548.

14	Maximum income for optional methods	**14**	4,200	00
15	Enter the **smaller** of: two-thirds (⅔) of gross farm income[1] (not less than zero) **or** $4,200. Also include this amount on line 4b above	**15**	

Nonfarm Optional Method. You may use this method **only** if **(a)** your net nonfarm profits[3] were less than $4,548 and also less than 72.189% of your gross nonfarm income,[4] **and (b)** you had net earnings from self-employment of at least $400 in 2 of the prior 3 years.

Caution. You may use this method no more than five times.

16	Subtract line 15 from line 14	**16**	
17	Enter the **smaller** of: two-thirds (⅔) of gross nonfarm income[4] (not less than zero) **or** the amount on line 16. Also include this amount on line 4b above	**17**	

[1] From Sch. F, line 11, and Sch. K-1 (Form 1065), box 14, code B.

[2] From Sch. F, line 36, and Sch. K-1 (Form 1065), box 14, code A—minus the amount you would have entered on line 1b had you not used the optional method.

[3] From Sch. C, line 31; Sch. C-EZ, line 3; Sch. K-1 (Form 1065), box 14, code A; and Sch. K-1 (Form 1065-B), box 9, code J1.

[4] From Sch. C, line 7; Sch. C-EZ, line 1; Sch. K-1 (Form 1065), box 14, code C; and Sch. K-1 (Form 1065-B), box 9, code J2.

Schedule SE (Form 1040) 2008

SCHEDULE EIC (Form 1040A or 1040)	**Earned Income Credit** Qualifying Child Information	OMB No. 1545-0074 2008
Department of the Treasury Internal Revenue Service (99)	*Complete and attach to Form 1040A or 1040 only if you have a qualifying child.*	Attachment Sequence No. **43**

Name(s) shown on return | Your social security number

Before you begin:
- See the instructions for Form 1040A, lines 40a and 40b, or Form 1040, lines 64a and 64b, to make sure that **(a)** you can take the EIC, and **(b)** you have a qualifying child.
- Be sure the child's name on line 1 and social security number (SSN) on line 2 agree with the child's social security card. Otherwise, at the time we process your return, we may reduce or disallow your EIC. If the name or SSN on the child's social security card is not correct, call the Social Security Administration at 1-800-772-1213.

- If you take the EIC even though you are not eligible, you may not be allowed to take the credit for up to 10 years. See back of schedule for details.
- It will take us longer to process your return and issue your refund if you do not fill in all lines that apply for each qualifying child.

Qualifying Child Information

	Child 1	**Child 2**
1 Child's name If you have more than two qualifying children, you only have to list two to get the maximum credit.	First name / Last name	First name / Last name
2 Child's SSN The child must have an SSN as defined on page 43 of the Form 1040A instructions or page 49 of the Form 1040 instructions unless the child was born and died in 2008. If your child was born and died in 2008 and did not have an SSN, enter "Died" on this line and attach a copy of the child's birth certificate, death certificate, or hospital medical records.		
3 Child's year of birth	Year ____ ____ ____ ____ *If born after 1989, skip lines 4a and 4b; go to line 5.*	Year ____ ____ ____ ____ *If born after 1989, skip lines 4a and 4b; go to line 5.*
4 If the child was born before 1990— **a** Was the child under age 24 at the end of 2008 and a student?	☐ Yes. *Go to line 5.* ☐ No. *Continue.*	☐ Yes. *Go to line 5.* ☐ No. *Continue.*
b Was the child permanently and totally disabled during any part of 2008?	☐ Yes. *Continue.* ☐ No. The child is not a qualifying child.	☐ Yes. *Continue.* ☐ No. The child is not a qualifying child.
5 Child's relationship to you (for example, son, daughter, grandchild, niece, nephew, foster child, etc.)		
6 Number of months child lived with you in the United States during 2008 • If the child lived with you for more than half of 2008 but less than 7 months, enter "7." • If the child was born or died in 2008 and your home was the child's home for the entire time he or she was alive during 2008, enter "12."	____ months *Do not enter more than 12 months.*	____ months *Do not enter more than 12 months.*

 TIP You may also be able to take the additional child tax credit if your child **(a)** was under age 17 at the end of 2008, **and** **(b)** is a U.S. citizen, U.S. national, or U.S. resident alien. For more details, see the instructions for line 41 of Form 1040A or line 66 of Form 1040.

For Paperwork Reduction Act Notice, see Form 1040A or 1040 instructions. | Cat. No. 13339M | **Schedule EIC (Form 1040A or 1040) 2008**

Purpose of Schedule

After you have figured your earned income credit (EIC), use Schedule EIC to give the IRS information about your qualifying child(ren).

To figure the amount of your credit or to have the IRS figure it for you, see the instructions for Form 1040A, lines 40a and 40b, or Form 1040, lines 64a and 64b.

Taking the EIC when not eligible. If you take the EIC even though you are not eligible and it is determined that your error is due to reckless or intentional disregard of the EIC rules, you will not be allowed to take the credit for 2 years even if you are otherwise eligible to do so. If you fraudulently take the EIC, you will not be allowed to take the credit for 10 years. You may also have to pay penalties.

Qualifying Child

A qualifying child for the EIC is a child who is your . . .

Son, daughter, stepchild, foster child, brother, sister, stepbrother, stepsister, or a descendant of any of them (for example, your grandchild, niece, or nephew)

was . . .

Under age 19 at the end of 2008
or
Under age 24 at the end of 2008 and a student
or
Any age and permanently and totally disabled

who . . .

Lived with you in the United States for more than half of 2008. If the child did not live with you for the required time, see *Exception to time lived with you* on page 42 of the Form 1040A instructions or page 49 of the Form 1040 instructions.

If the child was married or meets the conditions to be a qualifying child of another person (other than your spouse if filing a joint return), special rules apply. For details, see page 43 of the Form 1040A instructions or page 49 of the Form 1040 instructions.

Do you want part of the EIC added to your take-home pay in 2009? To see if you qualify, get Form W-5 from your employer, call the IRS at 1-800-TAX-FORM (1-800-829-3676), or go to *www.irs.gov.*

B-4   U.S. Income Tax Return for Estates and Trusts

Form 1041 Department of the Treasury—Internal Revenue Service
U.S. Income Tax Return for Estates and Trusts **2008**   OMB No. 1545-0092

A Type of entity (see instr.):

☐ Decedent's estate
☐ Simple trust
☐ Complex trust
☐ Qualified disability trust
☐ ESBT (S portion only)
☐ Grantor type trust
☐ Bankruptcy estate–Ch. 7
☐ Bankruptcy estate–Ch. 11
☐ Pooled income fund

For calendar year 2008 or fiscal year beginning _____ , 2008, and ending _____ , 20 __

Name of estate or trust (If a grantor type trust, see page 14 of the instructions.)

Name and title of fiduciary

Number, street, and room or suite no. (If a P.O. box, see page 15 of the instructions.)

City or town, state, and ZIP code

C Employer identification number

D Date entity created

E Nonexempt charitable and split-interest trusts, check applicable boxes (see page 16 of the instr.):
☐ Described in section 4947(a)(1)
☐ Not a private foundation
☐ Described in section 4947(a)(2)

B Number of Schedules K-1 attached (see instructions) ▶

F Check applicable boxes:
☐ Initial return ☐ Final return ☐ Amended return
☐ Change in fiduciary ☐ Change in fiduciary's name
☐ Change in trust's name
☐ Change in fiduciary's address

G Check here if the estate or filing trust made a section 645 election . . . . ▶ ☐

Income

1	Interest income	1
2a	Total ordinary dividends	2a
b	Qualified dividends allocable to: (1) Beneficiaries _____ (2) Estate or trust _____	
3	Business income or (loss). Attach Schedule C or C-EZ (Form 1040)	3
4	Capital gain or (loss). Attach Schedule D (Form 1041)	4
5	Rents, royalties, partnerships, other estates and trusts, etc. Attach Schedule E (Form 1040)	5
6	Farm income or (loss). Attach Schedule F (Form 1040)	6
7	Ordinary gain or (loss). Attach Form 4797	7
8	Other income. List type and amount _____	8
9	**Total income.** Combine lines 1, 2a, and 3 through 8 ▶	9

Deductions

10	Interest. Check if Form 4952 is attached ▶ ☐	10
11	Taxes	11
12	Fiduciary fees	12
13	Charitable deduction (from Schedule A, line 7)	13
14	Attorney, accountant, and return preparer fees	14
15a	Other deductions **not** subject to the 2% floor (attach schedule)	15a
b	Allowable miscellaneous itemized deductions subject to the 2% floor	15b
16	Add lines 10 through 15b ▶	16
17	Adjusted total income or (loss). Subtract line 16 from line 9 . 17	
18	Income distribution deduction (from Schedule B, line 15). Attach Schedules K-1 (Form 1041)	18
19	Estate tax deduction including certain generation-skipping taxes (attach computation)	19
20	Exemption	20
21	Add lines 18 through 20 ▶	21

Tax and Payments

22	Taxable income. Subtract line 21 from line 17. If a loss, see page 23 of the instructions	22
23	**Total tax** (from Schedule G, line 7)	23
24	**Payments: a** 2008 estimated tax payments and amount applied from 2007 return	24a
b	Estimated tax payments allocated to beneficiaries (from Form 1041-T)	24b
c	Subtract line 24b from line 24a	24c
d	Tax paid with Form 7004 (see page 24 of the instructions)	24d
e	Federal income tax withheld. If any is from Form(s) 1099, check ▶ ☐	24e
	Other payments: **f** Form 2439 _____ ; **g** Form 4136 _____ ; Total ▶	24h
25	**Total payments.** Add lines 24c through 24e, and 24h ▶	25
26	Estimated tax penalty (see page 24 of the instructions)	26
27	**Tax due.** If line 25 is smaller than the total of lines 23 and 26, enter amount owed	27
28	**Overpayment.** If line 25 is larger than the total of lines 23 and 26, enter amount overpaid	28
29	Amount of line 28 to be: **a** Credited to 2009 estimated tax ▶ _____ ; **b** Refunded ▶	29

Sign Here ▶ Under penalties of perjury, I declare that I have examined this return, including accompanying schedules and statements, and to the best of my knowledge and belief, it is true, correct, and complete. Declaration of preparer (other than taxpayer) is based on all information of which preparer has any knowledge.

Signature of fiduciary or officer representing fiduciary | Date | ▶ EIN of fiduciary if a financial institution

May the IRS discuss this return with the preparer shown below (see instr.)? ☐ Yes ☐ No

Paid Preparer's Use Only

Preparer's signature | Date | Check if self-employed ☐ | Preparer's SSN or PTIN
Firm's name (or yours if self-employed), address, and ZIP code | EIN | Phone no. ( )

For Privacy Act and Paperwork Reduction Act Notice, see the separate instructions.   Cat. No. 11370H   Form **1041** (2008)

Form 1041 (2008)   Page **2**

Schedule A	Charitable Deduction. Do not complete for a simple trust or a pooled income fund.		
1	Amounts paid or permanently set aside for charitable purposes from gross income (see page 25)	1	
2	Tax-exempt income allocable to charitable contributions (see page 25 of the instructions) .	2	
3	Subtract line 2 from line 1	3	
4	Capital gains for the tax year allocated to corpus and paid or permanently set aside for charitable purposes	4	
5	Add lines 3 and 4	5	
6	Section 1202 exclusion allocable to capital gains paid or permanently set aside for charitable purposes (see page 25 of the instructions)	6	
7	**Charitable deduction.** Subtract line 6 from line 5. Enter here and on page 1, line 13 . .	7	

Schedule B	Income Distribution Deduction		
1	Adjusted total income (see page 26 of the instructions)	1	
2	Adjusted tax-exempt interest	2	
3	Total net gain from Schedule D (Form 1041), line 15, column (1) (see page 26 of the instructions)	3	
4	Enter amount from Schedule A, line 4 (minus any allocable section 1202 exclusion) . .	4	
5	Capital gains for the tax year included on Schedule A, line 1 (see page 26 of the instructions)	5	
6	Enter any gain from page 1, line 4, as a negative number. If page 1, line 4, is a loss, enter the loss as a positive number	6	
7	**Distributable net income.** Combine lines 1 through 6. If zero or less, enter -0- . . .	7	
8	If a complex trust, enter accounting income for the tax year as determined under the governing instrument and applicable local law	**8**	
9	Income required to be distributed currently	9	
10	Other amounts paid, credited, or otherwise required to be distributed	10	
11	Total distributions. Add lines 9 and 10. If greater than line 8, see page 26 of the instructions	11	
12	Enter the amount of tax-exempt income included on line 11	12	
13	Tentative income distribution deduction. Subtract line 12 from line 11	13	
14	Tentative income distribution deduction. Subtract line 2 from line 7. If zero or less, enter -0-	14	
15	**Income distribution deduction.** Enter the smaller of line 13 or line 14 here and on page 1, line 18	15	

Schedule G	Tax Computation (see page 27 of the instructions)			
1 Tax:	a Tax on taxable income (see page 27 of the instructions) .	1a		
	b Tax on lump-sum distributions. Attach Form 4972 . . .	1b		
	c Alternative minimum tax (from Schedule I (Form 1041), line 56) .	1c		
	d **Total.** Add lines 1a through 1c . . . . ▶		1d	
2a	Foreign tax credit. Attach Form 1116	2a		
b	Other nonbusiness credits (attach schedule)	2b		
c	General business credit. Attach Form 3800	2c		
d	Credit for prior year minimum tax. Attach Form 8801	2d		
3	**Total credits.** Add lines 2a through 2d . . . . ▶		3	
4	Subtract line 3 from line 1d. If zero or less, enter -0-.		4	
5	Recapture taxes. Check if from: ☐ Form 4255 ☐ Form 8611		5	
6	Household employment taxes. Attach Schedule H (Form 1040)		6	
7	**Total tax.** Add lines 4 through 6. Enter here and on page 1, line 23 . . . . . ▶		7	

	Other Information	Yes	No
1	Did the estate or trust receive tax-exempt income? If "Yes," attach a computation of the allocation of expenses Enter the amount of tax-exempt interest income and exempt-interest dividends ▶ $ _____		
2	Did the estate or trust receive all or any part of the earnings (salary, wages, and other compensation) of any individual by reason of a contract assignment or similar arrangement?		
3	At any time during calendar year 2008, did the estate or trust have an interest in or a signature or other authority over a bank, securities, or other financial account in a foreign country? . . . . See page 29 of the instructions for exceptions and filing requirements for Form TD F 90-22.1. If "Yes," enter the name of the foreign country ▶ _____		
4	During the tax year, did the estate or trust receive a distribution from, or was it the grantor of, or transferor to, a foreign trust? If "Yes," the estate or trust may have to file Form 3520. See page 29 of the instructions .		
5	Did the estate or trust receive, or pay, any qualified residence interest on seller-provided financing? If "Yes," see page 30 for required attachment		
6	If this is an estate or a complex trust making the section 663(b) election, check here (see page 30) . ▶ ☐		
7	To make a section 643(e)(3) election, attach Schedule D (Form 1041), and check here (see page 30) . ▶ ☐		
8	If the decedent's estate has been open for more than 2 years, attach an explanation for the delay in closing the estate, and check here ▶ ☐		
9	Are any present or future trust beneficiaries skip persons? See page 30 of the instructions		

Form **1041** (2008)

ᏏᏏᏏᏏᏏᏏ

Schedule K-1
(Form 1041)
2008

Department of the Treasury
Internal Revenue Service

For calendar year 2008,

or tax year beginning _____ , 2008,

and ending _____ , 20 _____

Beneficiary's Share of Income, Deductions, Credits, etc.
▶ See back of form and instructions.

Part I	**Information About the Estate or Trust**

A Estate's or trust's employer identification number

B Estate's or trust's name

C Fiduciary's name, address, city, state, and ZIP code

D ☐ Check if Form 1041-T was filed and enter the date it was filed
_____ / _____ / _____

E ☐ Check if this is the final Form 1041 for the estate or trust

Part II	**Information About the Beneficiary**

F Beneficiary's identifying number

G Beneficiary's name, address, city, state, and ZIP code

H ☐ Domestic beneficiary   ☐ Foreign beneficiary

☐ Final K-1   ☐ Amended K-1   OMB No. 1545-0092

Part III	**Beneficiary's Share of Current Year Income, Deductions, Credits, and Other Items**

1	Interest income	**11**	Final year deductions
2a	Ordinary dividends		
2b	Qualified dividends		
3	Net short-term capital gain		
4a	Net long-term capital gain		
4b	28% rate gain	**12**	Alternative minimum tax adjustment
4c	Unrecaptured section 1250 gain		
5	Other portfolio and nonbusiness income		
6	Ordinary business income		
7	Net rental real estate income	**13**	Credits and credit recapture
8	Other rental income		
9	Directly apportioned deductions		
		14	Other information
10	Estate tax deduction		

*See attached statement for additional information.

Note. A statement must be attached showing the beneficiary's share of income and directly apportioned deductions from each business, rental real estate, and other rental activity.

For IRS Use Only

For Paperwork Reduction Act Notice, see the Instructions for Form 1041.   Cat. No. 11380D   **Schedule K-1 (Form 1041) 2008**

This list identifies the codes used on Schedule K-1 for beneficiaries and provides summarized reporting information for beneficiaries who file Form 1040. For detailed reporting and filing information, see the Instructions for Beneficiary Filing Form 1040 and the instructions for your income tax return.

	Report on
1. Interest income	Form 1040, line 8a
2a. Ordinary dividends	Form 1040, line 9a
2b. Qualified dividends	Form 1040, line 9b
3. Net short-term capital gain	Schedule D, line 5
4a. Net long-term capital gain	Schedule D, line 12
4b. 28% rate gain	Line 4 of the worksheet for Schedule D, line 18
4c. Unrecaptured section 1250 gain	Line 11 of the worksheet for Schedule D, line 19
5. Other portfolio and nonbusiness income	Schedule E, line 33, column (f)
6. Ordinary business income	Schedule E, line 33, column (d) or (f)
7. Net rental real estate income	Schedule E, line 33, column (d) or (f)
8. Other rental income	Schedule E, line 33, column (d) or (f)

9. Directly apportioned deductions

Code

A Depreciation	Form 8582 or Schedule E, line 33, column (c) or (e)
B Depletion	Form 8582 or Schedule E, line 33, column (c) or (e)
C Amortization	Form 8582 or Schedule E, line 33, column (c) or (e)

10. Estate tax deduction	Schedule A, line 28

11. Final year deductions

A Excess deductions	Schedule A, line 23
B Short-term capital loss carryover	Schedule D, line 5
C Long-term capital loss carryover	Schedule D, line 12; line 5 of the wksht. for Sch. D, line 18; and line 16 of the wksht. for Sch. D, line 19
D Net operating loss carryover — regular tax	Form 1040, line 21
E Net operating loss carryover — minimum tax	Form 6251, line 28

12. Alternative minimum tax (AMT) items

Code	*Report on*
A Adjustment for minimum tax purposes	Form 6251, line 15
B AMT adjustment attributable to qualified dividends	
C AMT adjustment attributable to net short-term capital gain	
D AMT adjustment attributable to net long-term capital gain	See the beneficiary's instructions and the Instructions for Form 6251
E AMT adjustment attributable to unrecaptured section 1250 gain	
F AMT adjustment attributable to 28% rate gain	
G Accelerated depreciation	
H Depletion	
I Amortization	
J Exclusion items	2009 Form 8801

13. Credits and credit recapture

A Credit for estimated taxes	Form 1040, line 63
B Credit for backup withholding	Form 1040, line 62
C Low-income housing credit	Form 8586 (also see the beneficiary's instructions)
D Qualified rehabilitation expenditures	See the beneficiary's instructions
E Basis of other investment credit property	See the beneficiary's instructions
F Work opportunity credit	Form 5884, line 3
G Welfare-to-work credit	Form 3800, line 1b
H Alcohol and cellulosic biofuels fuel credit	Form 6478, line 9 (also see the beneficiary's instructions)
I Credit for increasing research activities	Form 3800, line 1c
J Renewable electricity, refined coal, and Indian coal production credit	See the beneficiary's instructions
K Empowerment zone and renewal community employment credit	Form 8844, line 3
L Indian employment credit	Form 3800, line 1g
M Orphan drug credit	Form 3800, line 1h
N Credit for employer-provided child care and facilities	Form 3800, line 1k
O Biodiesel and renewable diesel fuels credit	Form 8864, line 11 (also see the beneficiary's instructions)
P Nonconventional source fuel credit	Form 3800, line 1o
Q Credit to holders of tax credit bonds	Form 8912, line 8
R Agricultural chemicals security credit	Form 3800, line 1v
S Energy efficient appliance credit	Form 3800, line 1q
T Credit for employer differential wage payments	Form 3800, line 1w
U Recapture of credits	See the beneficiary's instructions

14. Other information

A Tax-exempt interest	Form 1040, line 8b
B Foreign taxes	Form 1040, line 47 or Sch. A, line 8
C Qualified production activities income	Form 8903, line 7
D Form W-2 wages	Form 8903, line 15
E Net investment income	Form 4952, line 4a
F Gross farm and fishing income	Schedule E, line 42
G Foreign trading gross receipts (IRC 942(a))	See the Instructions for Form 8873
H Other information	See the beneficiary's instructions

Note. If you are a beneficiary who does not file a Form 1040, see instructions for the type of income tax return you are filing.

SCHEDULE J (Form 1041)

Accumulation Distribution for Certain Complex Trusts

OMB No. 1545-0092

Department of the Treasury
Internal Revenue Service

▶ Attach to Form 1041.

▶ See the Instructions for Form 1041.

2008

Name of trust

Employer identification number

Part I Accumulation Distribution in 2008

Note: *See the Form 4970 instructions for certain income that minors may exclude and special rules for multiple trusts.*

1 Other amounts paid, credited, or otherwise required to be distributed for 2008 (from Schedule B of Form 1041, line 10) . . . . | 1 |

2 Distributable net income for 2008 (from Schedule B of Form 1041, line 7) . . | 2 |

3 Income required to be distributed currently for 2008 (from Schedule B of Form 1041, line 9) . . . . | 3 |

4 Subtract line 3 from line 2. If zero or less, enter -0- . . . . | 4 |

5 Accumulation distribution for 2008. Subtract line 4 from line 1 . . . . | 5 |

Part II Ordinary Income Accumulation Distribution (Enter the applicable throwback years below.)

Note: *If the distribution is thrown back to more than five years (starting with the earliest applicable tax year beginning after 1968), attach additional schedules. (If the trust was a simple trust, see Regulations section 1.665(e)-1A(b).)*

		Throwback year ending -----------	Throwback year ending -----------	Throwback year ending -----------	Throwback year ending -----------	Throwback year ending -----------
6 Distributable net income (see page 30 of the instructions) .	6					
7 Distributions (see page 30 of the instructions)	7					
8 Subtract line 7 from line 6 .	8					
9 Enter amount from page 2, line 25 or line 31, as applicable.	9					
10 Undistributed net income Subtract line 9 from line 8 .	10					
11 Enter amount of prior accumulation distributions thrown back to any of these years	11					
12 Subtract line 11 from line 10	12					
13 Allocate the amount on line 5 to the earliest applicable year first. Do not allocate an amount greater than line 12 for the same year (see page 30 of the instructions). .	13					
14 Divide line 13 by line 10 and multiply result by amount on line 9	14					
15 Add lines 13 and 14 . .	15					
16 Tax-exempt interest included on line 13 (see page 31 of the instructions)	16					
17 Subtract line 16 from line 15	17					

For Paperwork Reduction Act Notice, see the Instructions for Form 1041.   Cat. No. 11382Z   Schedule J (Form 1041) 2008

B-5   U.S. Partnership Return of Income

U.S. Return of Partnership Income

Form **1065**

Department of the Treasury
Internal Revenue Service

For calendar year 2008, or tax year beginning _____ , 2008, ending _____ , 20____ .
▶ See separate instructions.

OMB No. 1545-0099

2008

A Principal business activity	**Use the IRS label. Other-wise, print or type.**	Name of partnership
B Principal product or service		Number, street, and room or suite no. If a P.O. box, see the instructions.
C Business code number		City or town, state, and ZIP code

D Employer identification number

E Date business started

F Total assets (see the instructions)
$

G Check applicable boxes: **(1)** ☐ Initial return   **(2)** ☐ Final return   **(3)** ☐ Name change   **(4)** ☐ Address change   **(5)** ☐ Amended return
(6) ☐ Technical termination - also check (1) or (2)

H Check accounting method: **(1)** ☐ Cash   **(2)** ☐ Accrual   **(3)** ☐ Other (specify) ▶ _____

I Number of Schedules K-1. Attach one for each person who was a partner at any time during the tax year ▶ _____

J Check if Schedule M-3 attached . . . . ☐

Caution. Include **only** trade or business income and expenses on lines 1a through 22 below. See the instructions for more information.

Income	**1a** Gross receipts or sales	**1a**	
	b Less returns and allowances	**1b**	**1c**
	2 Cost of goods sold (Schedule A, line 8)		**2**
	3 Gross profit. Subtract line 2 from line 1c		**3**
	4 Ordinary income (loss) from other partnerships, estates, and trusts *(attach statement).* .		**4**
	5 Net farm profit (loss) *(attach Schedule F (Form 1040))*		**5**
	6 Net gain (loss) from Form 4797, Part II, line 17 *(attach Form 4797)*		**6**
	7 Other income (loss) *(attach statement)*		**7**
	8 **Total income (loss).** Combine lines 3 through 7		**8**
Deductions (see the instructions for limitations)	**9** Salaries and wages (other than to partners) (less employment credits)		**9**
	10 Guaranteed payments to partners		**10**
	11 Repairs and maintenance		**11**
	12 Bad debts		**12**
	13 Rent		**13**
	14 Taxes and licenses		**14**
	15 Interest		**15**
	16a Depreciation *(if required, attach Form 4562)*	**16a**	
	b Less depreciation reported on Schedule A and elsewhere on return	**16b**	**16c**
	17 Depletion **(Do not deduct oil and gas depletion.)**		**17**
	18 Retirement plans, etc.		**18**
	19 Employee benefit programs		**19**
	20 Other deductions *(attach statement)*		**20**
	21 **Total deductions.** Add the amounts shown in the far right column for lines 9 through 20 .		**21**
	22 **Ordinary business income (loss).** Subtract line 21 from line 8		**22**

Sign Here

Under penalties of perjury, I declare that I have examined this return, including accompanying schedules and statements, and to the best of my knowledge and belief, it is true, correct, and complete. Declaration of preparer (other than general partner or limited liability company member manager) is based on all information of which preparer has any knowledge.

▶ _____
Signature of general partner or limited liability company member manager

▶ _____
Date

May the IRS discuss this return with the preparer shown below (see instructions)?   ☐ Yes ☐ No

Paid Preparer's Use Only

Preparer's signature	Date	Check if self-employed ▶ ☐
		Preparer's SSN or PTIN
Firm's name (or yours if self-employed), address, and ZIP code ▶		EIN ▶
		Phone no. ( )

For Privacy Act and Paperwork Reduction Act Notice, see separate instructions.   Cat. No. 11390Z   Form **1065** (2008)

Schedule A   Cost of Goods Sold (see the instructions)

1	Inventory at beginning of year	**1**
2	Purchases less cost of items withdrawn for personal use	**2**
3	Cost of labor	**3**
4	Additional section 263A costs *(attach statement)*	**4**
5	Other costs *(attach statement)*	**5**
6	**Total.** Add lines 1 through 5	**6**
7	Inventory at end of year	**7**
8	**Cost of goods sold.** Subtract line 7 from line 6. Enter here and on page 1, line 2	**8**

9a Check all methods used for valuing closing inventory:

     (i) ☐ Cost as described in Regulations section 1.471-3

     (ii) ☐ Lower of cost or market as described in Regulations section 1.471-4

     (iii) ☐ Other (specify method used and attach explanation) ▶ ---

  b Check this box if there was a writedown of "subnormal" goods as described in Regulations section 1.471-2(c)   ▶ ☐

  c Check this box if the LIFO inventory method was adopted this tax year for any goods *(if checked, attach Form 970)* ▶ ☐

  d Do the rules of section 263A (for property produced or acquired for resale) apply to the partnership?   ☐ **Yes** ☐ **No**

  e Was there any change in determining quantities, cost, or valuations between opening and closing inventory? ☐ **Yes** ☐ **No**
     If "Yes," attach explanation.

Schedule B   Other Information

			Yes	No
1	What type of entity is filing this return? Check the applicable box:			

  a ☐ Domestic general partnership   **b** ☐ Domestic limited partnership

  c ☐ Domestic limited liability company   **d** ☐ Domestic limited liability partnership

  e ☐ Foreign partnership   **f** ☐ Other ▶ --

2   At any time during the tax year, was any partner in the partnership a disregarded entity, a partnership (including an entity treated as a partnership), a trust, an S corporation, an estate (other than an estate of a deceased partner), or a nominee or similar person?

3   At the end of the tax year:

  a Did any foreign or domestic corporation, partnership (including any entity treated as a partnership), or trust own, directly or indirectly, an interest of 50% or more in the profit, loss, or capital of the partnership? For rules of constructive ownership, see instructions. If "Yes," complete (i) through (v) below

(i) Name of Entity	**(ii)** Employer Identification Number (if any)	**(iii)** Type of Entity	**(iv)** Country of Organization	**(v)** Maximum Percentage Owned in Profit, Loss, or Capital

  b Did any individual or estate own, directly or indirectly, an interest of 50% or more in the profit, loss, or capital of the partnership? For rules of constructive ownership, see instructions. If "Yes," complete (i) through (iv) below

(i) Name of Individual or Estate	**(ii)** Social Security Number or Employer Identification Number (if any)	**(iii)** Country of Citizenship (see instructions)	**(iv)** Maximum Percentage Owned in Profit, Loss, or Capital

4   At the end of the tax year, did the partnership:

  a Own directly 20% or more, or own, directly or indirectly, 50% or more of the total voting power of all classes of stock entitled to vote of any foreign or domestic corporation? For rules of constructive ownership, see instructions. If "Yes," complete (i) through (iv) below

(i) Name of Corporation	**(ii)** Employer Identification Number (if any)	**(iii)** Country of Incorporation	**(iv)** Percentage Owned in Voting Stock

Form **1065** (2008)

Form 1065 (2008)   Page **3**

					Yes	No

b Own directly an interest of 20% or more, or own, directly or indirectly, an interest of 50% or more in the profit, loss, or capital in any foreign or domestic partnership (including an entity treated as a partnership) or in the beneficial interest of a trust? For rules of constructive ownership, see instructions. If "Yes," complete (i) through (v) below .

(i) Name of Entity	(ii) Employer Identification Number (if any)	(iii) Type of Entity	(iv) Country of Organization	(v) Maximum Percentage Owned in Profit, Loss, or Capital

5 Did the partnership file Form 8893, Election of Partnership Level Tax Treatment, or an election statement under section 6231(a)(1)(B)(ii) for partnership-level tax treatment, that is in effect for this tax year? See Form 8893 for more details . . . .

6 Does the partnership satisfy **all four** of the following conditions?

a The partnership's total receipts for the tax year were less than $250,000.

b The partnership's total assets at the end of the tax year were less than $1 million.

c Schedules K-1 are filed with the return and furnished to the partners on or before the due date (including extensions) for the partnership return.

d The partnership is not filing and is not required to file Schedule M-3 . . . .

If "Yes," the partnership is not required to complete Schedules L, M-1, and M-2; Item F on page 1 of Form 1065; or Item L on Schedule K-1.

7 Is this partnership a publicly traded partnership as defined in section 469(k)(2)? . . . .

8 During the tax year, did the partnership have any debt that was cancelled, was forgiven, or had the terms modified so as to reduce the principal amount of the debt? . . . .

9 Has this partnership filed, or is it required to file, Form 8918, Material Advisor Disclosure Statement, to provide information on any reportable transaction? . . . .

10 At any time during calendar year 2008, did the partnership have an interest in or a signature or other authority over a financial account in a foreign country (such as a bank account, securities account, or other financial account)? See the instructions for exceptions and filing requirements for Form TD F 90-22.1, Report of Foreign Bank and Financial Accounts. If "Yes," enter the name of the foreign country. ▶ _

11 At any time during the tax year, did the partnership receive a distribution from, or was it the grantor of, or transferor to, a foreign trust? If "Yes," the partnership may have to file Form 3520, Annual Return To Report Transactions With Foreign Trusts and Receipt of Certain Foreign Gifts. See instructions . . . .

12a Is the partnership making, or had it previously made (and not revoked), a section 754 election? . . . . See instructions for details regarding a section 754 election.

b Did the partnership make for this tax year an optional basis adjustment under section 743(b) or 734(b)? If "Yes," attach a statement showing the computation and allocation of the basis adjustment. See instructions . .

c Is the partnership required to adjust the basis of partnership assets under section 743(b) or 734(b) because of a substantial built-in loss (as defined under section 743(d)) or substantial basis reduction (as defined under section 734(d))? If "Yes," attach a statement showing the computation and allocation of the basis adjustment. See instructions . . . . .

13 Check this box if, during the current or prior tax year, the partnership distributed any property received in a like-kind exchange or contributed such property to another entity (including a disregarded entity) . ▶ ☐

14 At any time during the tax year, did the partnership distribute to any partner a tenancy-in-common or other undivided interest in partnership property? . . . .

15 If the partnership is required to file Form 8858, Information Return of U.S. Persons With Respect To Foreign Disregarded Entities, enter the number of Forms 8858 attached. See instructions ▶ _ _ _ _ _ _ _ _ _ _ _ _ _ _

16 Does the partnership have any foreign partners? If "Yes," enter the number of Forms 8805, Foreign Partner's Information Statement of Section 1446 Withholding Tax, filed for this partnership. ▶ _ _ _ _ _ _ _ _ _ _ _ _ _ _

17 Enter the number of Forms 8865, Return of U.S. Persons With Respect to Certain Foreign Partnerships, attached to this return. ▶ _ _ _ _ _ _ _ _ _ _ _ _ _ _ _ _

Designation of Tax Matters Partner (see instructions)
Enter below the general partner designated as the tax matters partner (TMP) for the tax year of this return:

Name of designated TMP ▶ _____   Identifying number of TMP ▶ _____

Address of designated TMP ▶ _____

Form **1065** (2008)

Form 1065 (2008) Page **4**

Schedule K — Partners' Distributive Share Items

		Total amount
Income (Loss)		
1 Ordinary business income (loss) (page 1, line 22)	**1**	
2 Net rental real estate income (loss) (attach Form 8825)	**2**	
3a Other gross rental income (loss) 3a		
b Expenses from other rental activities (attach statement) 3b		
c Other net rental income (loss). Subtract line 3b from line 3a	**3c**	
4 Guaranteed payments	**4**	
5 Interest income	**5**	
6 Dividends: **a** Ordinary dividends	**6a**	
b Qualified dividends 6b		
7 Royalties	**7**	
8 Net short-term capital gain (loss) (attach Schedule D (Form 1065))	**8**	
9a Net long-term capital gain (loss) (attach Schedule D (Form 1065))	**9a**	
b Collectibles (28%) gain (loss) 9b		
c Unrecaptured section 1250 gain (attach statement) 9c		
10 Net section 1231 gain (loss) (attach Form 4797)	**10**	
11 Other income (loss) (see instructions) Type ▶	**11**	
Deductions		
12 Section 179 deduction (attach Form 4562)	**12**	
13a Contributions	**13a**	
b Investment interest expense	**13b**	
c Section 59(e)(2) expenditures: **(1)** Type ▶ **(2)** Amount ▶	**13c(2)**	
d Other deductions (see instructions) Type ▶	**13d**	
Self-Employment		
14a Net earnings (loss) from self-employment	**14a**	
b Gross farming or fishing income	**14b**	
c Gross nonfarm income	**14c**	
Credits		
15a Low-income housing credit (section 42(j)(5))	**15a**	
b Low-income housing credit (other)	**15b**	
c Qualified rehabilitation expenditures (rental real estate) (attach Form 3468)	**15c**	
d Other rental real estate credits (see instructions) Type ▶	**15d**	
e Other rental credits (see instructions) Type ▶	**15e**	
f Other credits (see instructions) Type ▶	**15f**	
Foreign Transactions		
16a Name of country or U.S. possession ▶		
b Gross income from all sources	**16b**	
c Gross income sourced at partner level	**16c**	
Foreign gross income sourced at partnership level		
d Passive category ▶ **e** General category ▶ **f** Other ▶	**16f**	
Deductions allocated and apportioned at partner level		
g Interest expense ▶ **h** Other ▶	**16h**	
Deductions allocated and apportioned at partnership level to foreign source income		
i Passive category ▶ **j** General category ▶ **k** Other ▶	**16k**	
l Total foreign taxes (check one): ▶ Paid ☐ Accrued ☐	**16l**	
m Reduction in taxes available for credit (attach statement)	**16m**	
n Other foreign tax information (attach statement)		
Alternative Minimum Tax (AMT) Items		
17a Post-1986 depreciation adjustment	**17a**	
b Adjusted gain or loss	**17b**	
c Depletion (other than oil and gas)	**17c**	
d Oil, gas, and geothermal properties—gross income	**17d**	
e Oil, gas, and geothermal properties—deductions	**17e**	
f Other AMT items (attach statement)	**17f**	
Other Information		
18a Tax-exempt interest income	**18a**	
b Other tax-exempt income	**18b**	
c Nondeductible expenses	**18c**	
19a Distributions of cash and marketable securities	**19a**	
b Distributions of other property	**19b**	
20a Investment income	**20a**	
b Investment expenses	**20b**	
c Other items and amounts (attach statement)		

Form **1065** (2008)

Form 1065 (2008)   Page **5**

Analysis of Net Income (Loss)

1 Net income (loss). Combine Schedule K, lines 1 through 11. From the result, subtract the sum of
Schedule K, lines 12 through 13d, and 16l . . . . | **1** | |

2 Analysis by partner type:	**(i)** Corporate	**(ii)** Individual (active)	**(iii)** Individual (passive)	**(iv)** Partnership	**(v)** Exempt organization	**(vi)** Nominee/Other
a General partners						
b Limited partners						

Schedule L	Balance Sheets per Books	Beginning of tax year		End of tax year	
	Assets	**(a)**	**(b)**	**(c)**	**(d)**
1	Cash				
2a	Trade notes and accounts receivable . . .				
b	Less allowance for bad debts				
3	Inventories				
4	U.S. government obligations				
5	Tax-exempt securities				
6	Other current assets (attach statement) . .				
7	Mortgage and real estate loans				
8	Other investments (attach statement) . . .				
9a	Buildings and other depreciable assets . . .				
b	Less accumulated depreciation				
10a	Depletable assets				
b	Less accumulated depletion				
11	Land (net of any amortization)				
12a	Intangible assets (amortizable only)				
b	Less accumulated amortization				
13	Other assets (attach statement)				
14	Total assets				
	Liabilities and Capital				
15	Accounts payable				
16	Mortgages, notes, bonds payable in less than 1 year .				
17	Other current liabilities (attach statement) . .				
18	All nonrecourse loans				
19	Mortgages, notes, bonds payable in 1 year or more .				
20	Other liabilities (attach statement)				
21	Partners' capital accounts				
22	Total liabilities and capital				

Schedule M-1	Reconciliation of Income (Loss) per Books With Income (Loss) per Return

Note. Schedule M-3 may be required instead of Schedule M-1 (see instructions).

1 Net income (loss) per books . . .		**6** Income recorded on books this year not included on Schedule K, lines 1 through 11 (itemize):	
2 Income included on Schedule K, lines 1, 2, 3c, 5, 6a, 7, 8, 9a, 10, and 11, not recorded on books this year (itemize): -----------		**a** Tax-exempt interest $ ----------- -----------------------------	
3 Guaranteed payments (other than health insurance)		**7** Deductions included on Schedule K, lines 1 through 13d, and 16l, not charged against book income this year (itemize):	
4 Expenses recorded on books this year not included on Schedule K, lines 1 through 13d, and 16l (itemize):		**a** Depreciation $ ----------- -----------------------------	
a Depreciation $ -----------			
b Travel and entertainment $ ----------- -----------------------------		**8** Add lines 6 and 7	
		9 Income (loss) (Analysis of Net Income (Loss), line 1). Subtract line 8 from line 5 . . .	
5 Add lines 1 through 4			

Schedule M-2	Analysis of Partners' Capital Accounts

1 Balance at beginning of year . . .		**6** Distributions: **a** Cash	
2 Capital contributed: **a** Cash . . .		**b** Property	
b Property . .		**7** Other decreases (itemize): ----------- -----------------------------	
3 Net income (loss) per books . . .			
4 Other increases (itemize): ----------- -----------------------------		**8** Add lines 6 and 7	
5 Add lines 1 through 4		**9** Balance at end of year. Subtract line 8 from line 5	

Form **1065** (2008)

651108

☐ Final K-1	☐ Amended K-1	OMB No. 1545-0099

**Schedule K-1
(Form 1065)**

20**08**

Department of the Treasury
Internal Revenue Service

For calendar year 2008, or tax
year beginning _____, 2008
ending _____, 20___

Partner's Share of Income, Deductions, Credits, etc.   ▶ **See back of form and separate instructions.**

Part I	Information About the Partnership
A	Partnership's employer identification number
B	Partnership's name, address, city, state, and ZIP code
C	IRS Center where partnership filed return
D	☐ Check if this is a publicly traded partnership (PTP)

Part II	Information About the Partner
E	Partner's identifying number
F	Partner's name, address, city, state, and ZIP code

G ☐ General partner or LLC member-manager   ☐ Limited partner or other LLC member

H ☐ Domestic partner   ☐ Foreign partner

I What type of entity is this partner? _____

J Partner's share of profit, loss, and capital (see instructions):

	Beginning	Ending
Profit	%	%
Loss	%	%
Capital	%	%

K Partner's share of liabilities at year end:

Nonrecourse . . . . . . $_____
Qualified nonrecourse financing . $_____
Recourse . . . . $_____

L Partner's capital account analysis:

Beginning capital account . . . $_____
Capital contributed during the year . $_____
Current year increase (decrease) . $_____
Withdrawals & distributions . . $(_____)
Ending capital account . . . $_____

☐ Tax basis   ☐ GAAP   ☐ Section 704(b) book
☐ Other (explain)

Part III	Partner's Share of Current Year Income, Deductions, Credits, and Other Items

1	Ordinary business income (loss)	15	Credits
2	Net rental real estate income (loss)		
3	Other net rental income (loss)	16	Foreign transactions
4	Guaranteed payments		
5	Interest income		
6a	Ordinary dividends		
6b	Qualified dividends		
7	Royalties		
8	Net short-term capital gain (loss)		
9a	Net long-term capital gain (loss)	17	Alternative minimum tax (AMT) items
9b	Collectibles (28%) gain (loss)		
9c	Unrecaptured section 1250 gain		
10	Net section 1231 gain (loss)	18	Tax-exempt income and nondeductible expenses
11	Other income (loss)		
		19	Distributions
12	Section 179 deduction		
13	Other deductions	20	Other information
14	Self-employment earnings (loss)		

*See attached statement for additional information.

For IRS Use Only

For Paperwork Reduction Act Notice, see Instructions for Form 1065.   Cat. No. 11394R   **Schedule K-1 (Form 1065) 2008**

This list identifies the codes used on Schedule K-1 for all partners and provides summarized reporting information for partners who file Form 1040. For detailed reporting and filing information, see the separate Partner's Instructions for Schedule K-1 and the instructions for your income tax return.

1. **Ordinary business income (loss).** Determine whether the income (loss) is passive or nonpassive and enter on your return as follows.

	Report on
Passive loss	See the Partner's Instructions
Passive income	Schedule E, line 28, column (g)
Nonpassive loss	Schedule E, line 28, column (h)
Nonpassive income	Schedule E, line 28, column (j)

2. **Net rental real estate income (loss)** See the Partner's Instructions
3. **Other net rental income (loss)**
   - Net income — Schedule E, line 28, column (g)
   - Net loss — See the Partner's Instructions
4. **Guaranteed payments** Schedule E, line 28, column (j)
5. **Interest income** Form 1040, line 8a
6a. **Ordinary dividends** Form 1040, line 9a
6b. **Qualified dividends** Form 1040, line 9b
7. **Royalties** Schedule E, line 4
8. **Net short-term capital gain (loss)** Schedule D, line 5, column (f)
9a. **Net long-term capital gain (loss)** Schedule D, line 12, column (f)
9b. **Collectibles (28%) gain (loss)** 28% Rate Gain Worksheet, line 4 (Schedule D instructions)
9c. **Unrecaptured section 1250 gain** See the Partner's Instructions
10. **Net section 1231 gain (loss)** See the Partner's Instructions
11. **Other income (loss)**

   Code
   - A Other portfolio income (loss) — See the Partner's Instructions
   - B Involuntary conversions — See the Partner's Instructions
   - C Sec. 1256 contracts & straddles — Form 6781, line 1
   - D Mining exploration costs recapture — See Pub. 535
   - E Cancellation of debt — Form 1040, line 21 or Form 982
   - F Other income (loss) — See the Partner's Instructions

12. **Section 179 deduction** See the Partner's Instructions
13. **Other deductions**
   - A Cash contributions (50%)
   - B Cash contributions (30%)
   - C Noncash contributions (50%)
   - D Noncash contributions (30%)
   - E Capital gain property to a 50% organization (30%)
   - F Capital gain property (20%)
   - G Contributions (100%)

   } See the Partner's Instructions

   - H Investment interest expense — Form 4952, line 1
   - I Deductions—royalty income — Schedule E, line 18
   - J Section 59(e)(2) expenditures — See the Partner's Instructions
   - K Deductions—portfolio (2% floor) — Schedule A, line 23
   - L Deductions—portfolio (other) — Schedule A, line 28
   - M Amounts paid for medical insurance — Schedule A, line 1 or Form 1040, line 29
   - N Educational assistance benefits — See the Partner's Instructions
   - O Dependent care benefits — Form 2441, line 14
   - P Preproductive period expenses — See the Partner's Instructions
   - Q Commercial revitalization deduction from rental real estate activities — See Form 8582 instructions
   - R Pensions and IRAs — See the Partner's Instructions
   - S Reforestation expense deduction — See the Partner's Instructions
   - T Domestic production activities information — See Form 8903 instructions
   - U Qualified production activities income — Form 8903, line 7
   - V Employer's Form W-2 wages — Form 8903, line 15
   - W Other deductions — See the Partner's Instructions

14. **Self-employment earnings (loss)**
Note. *If you have a section 179 deduction or any partner-level deductions, see the Partner's Instructions before completing Schedule SE.*
   - A Net earnings (loss) from self-employment — Schedule SE, Section A or B
   - B Gross farming or fishing income — See the Partner's Instructions
   - C Gross non-farm income — See the Partner's Instructions

15. **Credits**
   - A Low-income housing credit (section 42(j)(5)) from pre-2008 buildings — See the Partner's Instructions
   - B Low-income housing credit (other) from pre-2008 buildings — See the Partner's Instructions
   - C Low-income housing credit (section 42(j)(5)) from post-2007 buildings — Form 8586, line 11
   - D Low-income housing credit (other) from post-2007 buildings — Form 8586, line 11
   - E Qualified rehabilitation expenditures (rental real estate)
   - F Other rental real estate credits
   - G Other rental credits

   } See the Partner's Instructions

   - H Undistributed capital gains credit — Form 1040, line 68; check box a
   - I Alcohol and cellulosic biofuel fuels credit — Form 6478, line 9

Code / *Report on*
   - J Work opportunity credit — Form 5884, line 3
   - K Disabled access credit — See the Partner's Instructions
   - L Empowerment zone and renewal community employment credit — Form 8844, line 3
   - M Credit for increasing research activities — See the Partner's Instructions
   - N Credit for employer social security and Medicare taxes — Form 8846, line 5
   - O Backup withholding — Form 1040, line 62
   - P Other credits — See the Partner's Instructions

16. **Foreign transactions**
   - A Name of country or U.S. possession
   - B Gross income from all sources
   - C Gross income sourced at partner level

   } Form 1116, Part I

   Foreign gross income sourced at partnership level
   - D Passive category
   - E General category
   - F Other

   } Form 1116, Part I

   Deductions allocated and apportioned at partner level
   - G Interest expense — Form 1116, Part I
   - H Other — Form 1116, Part I

   Deductions allocated and apportioned at partnership level to foreign source income
   - I Passive category
   - J General category
   - K Other

   } Form 1116, Part I

   Other information
   - L Total foreign taxes paid — Form 1116, Part II
   - M Total foreign taxes accrued — Form 1116, Part II
   - N Reduction in taxes available for credit — Form 1116, line 12
   - O Foreign trading gross receipts — Form 8873
   - P Extraterritorial income exclusion — Form 8873
   - Q Other foreign transactions — See the Partner's Instructions

17. **Alternative minimum tax (AMT) items**
   - A Post-1986 depreciation adjustment
   - B Adjusted gain or loss
   - C Depletion (other than oil & gas)
   - D Oil, gas, & geothermal—gross income
   - E Oil, gas, & geothermal—deductions
   - F Other AMT items

   } See the Partner's Instructions and the Instructions for Form 6251

18. **Tax-exempt income and nondeductible expenses**
   - A Tax-exempt interest income — Form 1040, line 8b
   - B Other tax-exempt income — See the Partner's Instructions
   - C Nondeductible expenses — See the Partner's Instructions

19. **Distributions**
   - A Cash and marketable securities
   - B Other property
   - C Distribution subject to section 737

   } See the Partner's Instructions

20. **Other information**
   - A Investment income — Form 4952, line 4a
   - B Investment expenses — Form 4952, line 5
   - C Fuel tax credit information — Form 4136
   - D Qualified rehabilitation expenditures (other than rental real estate) — See the Partner's Instructions
   - E Basis of energy property — See the Partner's Instructions
   - F Recapture of low-income housing credit (section 42(j)(5)) — Form 8611, line 8
   - G Recapture of low-income housing credit (other) — Form 8611, line 8
   - H Recapture of investment credit — See Form 4255
   - I Recapture of other credits — See the Partner's Instructions
   - J Look-back interest—completed long-term contracts — See Form 8697
   - K Look-back interest—income forecast method — See Form 8866
   - L Dispositions of property with section 179 deductions
   - M Recapture of section 179 deduction
   - N Interest expense for corporate partners
   - O Section 453(l)(3) information
   - P Section 453A(c) information
   - Q Section 1260(b) information
   - R Interest allocable to production expenditures
   - S CCF nonqualified withdrawals
   - T Depletion information—oil and gas
   - U Amortization of reforestation costs
   - V Unrelated business taxable income
   - W Precontribution gain (loss)
   - X Other information

   } See the Partner's Instructions

B-6   U.S. Corporation Income Tax Return

Form 1120
Department of the Treasury
Internal Revenue Service

U.S. Corporation Income Tax Return

For calendar year 2008 or tax year beginning _____, 2008, ending _____, 20 ____
► See separate instructions.

OMB No. 1545-0123

2008

A Check if:
1a Consolidated return (attach Form 851) ☐
b Life/nonlife consolidated return ☐
2 Personal holding co. (attach Sch. PH) ☐
3 Personal service corp. (see instructions) ☐
4 Schedule M-3 attached ☐

Use IRS label. Otherwise, print or type.

Name

Number, street, and room or suite no. If a P.O. box, see instructions.

City or town, state, and ZIP code

B Employer identification number

C Date incorporated

D Total assets (see instructions) $

E Check if: (1) ☐ Initial return (2) ☐ Final return (3) ☐ Name change (4) ☐ Address change

Income

1a	Gross receipts or sales _____ b Less returns and allowances _____ c Bal ►	1c
2	Cost of goods sold (Schedule A, line 8)	2
3	Gross profit. Subtract line 2 from line 1c	3
4	Dividends (Schedule C, line 19)	4
5	Interest	5
6	Gross rents	6
7	Gross royalties	7
8	Capital gain net income (attach Schedule D (Form 1120))	8
9	Net gain or (loss) from Form 4797, Part II, line 17 (attach Form 4797)	9
10	Other income (see instructions—attach schedule)	10
11	**Total income.** Add lines 3 through 10 ►	11

Deductions (See instructions for limitations on deductions.)

12	Compensation of officers (Schedule E, line 4) ►	12
13	Salaries and wages (less employment credits)	13
14	Repairs and maintenance	14
15	Bad debts	15
16	Rents	16
17	Taxes and licenses	17
18	Interest	18
19	Charitable contributions	19
20	Depreciation from Form 4562 not claimed on Schedule A or elsewhere on return (attach Form 4562)	20
21	Depletion	21
22	Advertising	22
23	Pension, profit-sharing, etc., plans	23
24	Employee benefit programs	24
25	Domestic production activities deduction (attach Form 8903)	25
26	Other deductions (attach schedule)	26
27	**Total deductions.** Add lines 12 through 26 ►	27
28	Taxable income before net operating loss deduction and special deductions. Subtract line 27 from line 11	28
29	**Less: a** Net operating loss deduction (see instructions) — 29a	
	b Special deductions (Schedule C, line 20) — 29b	29c

Tax, Refundable Credits, and Payments

30	**Taxable income.** Subtract line 29c from line 28 (see instructions)	30
31	**Total tax** (Schedule J, line 10)	31
32a	2007 overpayment credited to 2008 — 32a	
b	2008 estimated tax payments — 32b	
c	2008 refund applied for on Form 4466 — 32c ( ) d Bal ► 32d	
e	Tax deposited with Form 7004 — 32e	
f	Credits: (1) Form 2439 _____ (2) Form 4136 _____ 32f	
g	Refundable credits from Form 3800, line 19c, and Form 8827, line 8c — 32g	32h
33	Estimated tax penalty (see instructions). Check if Form 2220 is attached ► ☐	33
34	**Amount owed.** If line 32h is smaller than the total of lines 31 and 33, enter amount owed	34
35	**Overpayment.** If line 32h is larger than the total of lines 31 and 33, enter amount overpaid ►	35
36	Enter amount from line 35 you want: **Credited to 2009 estimated tax** ► _____ **Refunded** ►	36

Sign Here

Under penalties of perjury, I declare that I have examined this return, including accompanying schedules and statements, and to the best of my knowledge and belief, it is true, correct, and complete. Declaration of preparer (other than taxpayer) is based on all information of which preparer has any knowledge.

► Signature of officer _____ Date _____ ► Title _____

May the IRS discuss this return with the preparer shown below (see instructions)? ☐ Yes ☐ No

Paid Preparer's Use Only

Preparer's signature ► _____ Date _____ Check if self-employed ☐ Preparer's SSN or PTIN _____

Firm's name (or yours if self-employed), address, and ZIP code ► _____ EIN _____ Phone no. _____

For Privacy Act and Paperwork Reduction Act Notice, see separate instructions.   Cat. No. 11450Q   Form **1120** (2008)

Form 1120 (2008)

Schedule A   Cost of Goods Sold   (see instructions)

1	Inventory at beginning of year	**1**	
2	Purchases	**2**	
3	Cost of labor	**3**	
4	Additional section 263A costs (attach schedule)	**4**	
5	Other costs (attach schedule)	**5**	
6	**Total.** Add lines 1 through 5	**6**	
7	Inventory at end of year	**7**	
8	**Cost of goods sold.** Subtract line 7 from line 6. Enter here and on page 1, line 2	**8**	

9a Check all methods used for valuing closing inventory:

    (i) ☐ Cost

    (ii) ☐ Lower of cost or market

    (iii) ☐ Other (Specify method used and attach explanation.) ▶ _____ ▶ ☐

  b Check if there was a writedown of subnormal goods . . . . ▶ ☐

  c Check if the LIFO inventory method was adopted this tax year for any goods (if checked, attach Form 970) . . . . ▶ ☐

  d If the LIFO inventory method was used for this tax year, enter percentage (or amounts) of closing inventory computed under LIFO **9d**

  e If property is produced or acquired for resale, do the rules of section 263A apply to the corporation? . . . . . . ☐ Yes ☐ No

  f Was there any change in determining quantities, cost, or valuations between opening and closing inventory? If "Yes," attach explanation . . . . ☐ Yes ☐ No

Schedule C   Dividends and Special Deductions   (see instructions)

		(a) Dividends received	(b) %	(c) Special deductions (a) × (b)
1	Dividends from less-than-20%-owned domestic corporations (other than debt-financed stock)		70	
2	Dividends from 20%-or-more-owned domestic corporations (other than debt-financed stock)		80	
3	Dividends on debt-financed stock of domestic and foreign corporations		see instructions	
4	Dividends on certain preferred stock of less-than-20%-owned public utilities		42	
5	Dividends on certain preferred stock of 20%-or-more-owned public utilities		48	
6	Dividends from less-than-20%-owned foreign corporations and certain FSCs		70	
7	Dividends from 20%-or-more-owned foreign corporations and certain FSCs		80	
8	Dividends from wholly owned foreign subsidiaries		100	
9	**Total.** Add lines 1 through 8. See instructions for limitation			
10	Dividends from domestic corporations received by a small business investment company operating under the Small Business Investment Act of 1958		100	
11	Dividends from affiliated group members		100	
12	Dividends from certain FSCs		100	
13	Dividends from foreign corporations not included on lines 3, 6, 7, 8, 11, or 12			
14	Income from controlled foreign corporations under subpart F (attach Form(s) 5471) . .			
15	Foreign dividend gross-up			
16	IC-DISC and former DISC dividends not included on lines 1, 2, or 3			
17	Other dividends			
18	Deduction for dividends paid on certain preferred stock of public utilities			
19	**Total dividends.** Add lines 1 through 17. Enter here and on page 1, line 4 . . . ▶			
20	**Total special deductions.** Add lines 9, 10, 11, 12, and 18. Enter here and on page 1, line 29b . . . . . . ▶			

Schedule E   Compensation of Officers   (see instructions for page 1, line 12)

Note: *Complete Schedule E only if total receipts (line 1a plus lines 4 through 10 on page 1) are $500,000 or more.*

(a) Name of officer	(b) Social security number	(c) Percent of time devoted to business	Percent of corporation stock owned		(f) Amount of compensation
			(d) Common	(e) Preferred	
1		%	%	%	
		%	%	%	
		%	%	%	
		%	%	%	
		%	%	%	

2 Total compensation of officers . . . .

3 Compensation of officers claimed on Schedule A and elsewhere on return . . . .

4 Subtract line 3 from line 2. Enter the result here and on page 1, line 12 . . . .

Form **1120** (2008)

Form 1120 (2008)   Page **3**

Schedule J   Tax Computation (see instructions)

1 Check if the corporation is a member of a controlled group (attach Schedule O (Form 1120)) . . . . ▶ ☐

2 Income tax. Check if a qualified personal service corporation (see instructions) . . . . ▶ ☐ | **2**

3 Alternative minimum tax (attach Form 4626) . . . . | **3**

4 Add lines 2 and 3 . . . . | **4**

5a Foreign tax credit (attach Form 1118) . . . . | **5a**

b Credit from Form 8834 . . . . | **5b**

c General business credit (attach Form 3800) . . . . | **5c**

d Credit for prior year minimum tax (attach Form 8827) . . . . . . | **5d**

e Bond credits from Form 8912 . . . . | **5e**

6 **Total credits.** Add lines 5a through 5e . . . . | **6**

7 Subtract line 6 from line 4 . . . . | **7**

8 Personal holding company tax (attach Schedule PH (Form 1120)) . . . . | **8**

9 Other taxes. Check if from: ☐ Form 4255   ☐ Form 8611   ☐ Form 8697
   ☐ Form 8866   ☐ Form 8902   ☐ Other (attach schedule) . . . . | **9**

10 **Total tax.** Add lines 7 through 9. Enter here and on page 1, line 31 . . . . | **10**

Schedule K   Other Information (see instructions)

		Yes	No

1 Check accounting method: **a** ☐ Cash   **b** ☐ Accrual   **c** ☐ Other (specify) ▶ _____

2 See the instructions and enter the:

a Business activity code no. ▶ _____

b Business activity ▶ _____

c Product or service ▶ _____

3 Is the corporation a subsidiary in an affiliated group or a parent-subsidiary controlled group? . . . .

If "Yes," enter name and EIN of the parent corporation ▶ _____

_____

4 At the end of the tax year:

a Did any foreign or domestic corporation, partnership (including any entity treated as a partnership), or trust own directly 20% or more, or own, directly or indirectly, 50% or more of the total voting power of all classes of the corporation's stock entitled to vote? For rules of constructive ownership, see instructions. If "Yes," complete (i) through (v).

(i) Name of Entity	(ii) Employer Identification Number (if any)	(iii) Type of Entity	(iv) Country of Organization	(v) Percentage Owned in Voting Stock

b Did any individual or estate own directly 20% or more, or own, directly or indirectly, 50% or more of the total voting power of all classes of the corporation's stock entitled to vote? . . . . For rules of constructive ownership, see instructions. If "Yes," complete (i) through (iv).

(i) Name of Individual or Estate	(ii) Identifying Number (if any)	(iii) Country of Citizenship (see instructions)	(iv) Percentage Owned in Voting Stock

Form **1120** (2008)

Form 1120 (2008) Page **4**

Schedule K *Continued*

		Yes	No
5	At the end of the tax year, did the corporation:		
a	Own directly 20% or more, or own, directly or indirectly, 50% or more of the total voting power of all classes of stock entitled to vote of any foreign or domestic corporation not included on **Form 851,** Affiliations Schedule? For rules of constructive ownership, see instructions . If "Yes," complete (i) through (iv).		

(i) Name of Corporation	**(ii)** Employer Identification Number (if any)	**(iii)** Country of Incorporation	**(iv)** Percentage Owned in Voting Stock

b Own directly an interest of 20% or more, or own, directly or indirectly, an interest of 50% or more in any foreign or domestic partnership (including an entity treated as a partnership) or in the beneficial interest of a trust? For rules of constructive ownership, see instructions . If "Yes," complete (i) through (iv).

(i) Name of Entity	**(ii)** Employer Identification Number (if any)	**(iii)** Country of Organization	**(iv)** Maximum Percentage Owned in Profit, Loss, or Capital

6 During this tax year, did the corporation pay dividends (other than stock dividends and distributions in exchange for stock) in excess of the corporation's current and accumulated earnings and profits? (See sections 301 and 316.) . . . .
If "Yes," file **Form 5452,** Corporate Report of Nondividend Distributions.
If this is a consolidated return, answer here for the parent corporation and on Form 851 for each subsidiary.

7 At any time during the tax year, did one foreign person own, directly or indirectly, at least 25% of **(a)** the total voting power of all classes of the corporation's stock entitled to vote or **(b)** the total value of all classes of the corporation's stock? . . . . .
For rules of attribution, see section 318. If "Yes," enter:
(i) Percentage owned ▶ _____ and **(ii)** Owner's country ▶ _____
(c) The corporation may have to file **Form 5472,** Information Return of a 25% Foreign-Owned U.S. Corporation or a Foreign Corporation Engaged in a U.S. Trade or Business. Enter the number of Forms 5472 attached ▶ _____

8 Check this box if the corporation issued publicly offered debt instruments with original issue discount . . . . ▶ ☐
If checked, the corporation may have to file **Form 8281,** Information Return for Publicly Offered Original Issue Discount Instruments.

9 Enter the amount of tax-exempt interest received or accrued during the tax year ▶ $ _____

10 Enter the number of shareholders at the end of the tax year (if 100 or fewer) ▶ _____

11 If the corporation has an NOL for the tax year and is electing to forego the carryback period, check here . . . . . . ▶ ☐
If the corporation is filing a consolidated return, the statement required by Regulations section 1.1502-21(b)(3) must be attached or the election will not be valid.

12 Enter the available NOL carryover from prior tax years (do not reduce it by any deduction on line 29a.) ▶ $ _____

13 Are the corporation's total receipts (line 1a plus lines 4 through 10 on page 1) for the tax year **and** its total assets at the end of the tax year less than $250,000? . . . .
If "Yes," the corporation is not required to complete Schedules L, M-1, and M-2 on page 5. Instead, enter the total amount of cash distributions and the book value of property distributions (other than cash) made during the tax year. ▶ $ _____

Form **1120** (2008)

Form 1120 (2008)

Page **5**

Schedule L	Balance Sheets per Books	Beginning of tax year		End of tax year	
	Assets	(a)	(b)	(c)	(d)
1	Cash				
2a	Trade notes and accounts receivable				
b	Less allowance for bad debts	(	)	(	)
3	Inventories				
4	U.S. government obligations				
5	Tax-exempt securities (see instructions) . . .				
6	Other current assets (attach schedule) . . .				
7	Loans to shareholders				
8	Mortgage and real estate loans				
9	Other investments (attach schedule)				
10a	Buildings and other depreciable assets . . .				
b	Less accumulated depreciation	(	)	(	)
11a	Depletable assets				
b	Less accumulated depletion	(	)	(	)
12	Land (net of any amortization)				
13a	Intangible assets (amortizable only)				
b	Less accumulated amortization	(	)	(	)
14	Other assets (attach schedule)				
15	Total assets				
	Liabilities and Shareholders' Equity				
16	Accounts payable				
17	Mortgages, notes, bonds payable in less than 1 year				
18	Other current liabilities (attach schedule) . . .				
19	Loans from shareholders				
20	Mortgages, notes, bonds payable in 1 year or more				
21	Other liabilities (attach schedule)				
22	Capital stock: a Preferred stock				
	b Common stock				
23	Additional paid-in capital				
24	Retained earnings—Appropriated (attach schedule)				
25	Retained earnings—Unappropriated				
26	Adjustments to shareholders' equity (attach schedule)				
27	Less cost of treasury stock		( )		( )
28	Total liabilities and shareholders' equity . . .				

Schedule M-1	Reconciliation of Income (Loss) per Books With Income per Return

Note: Schedule M-3 required instead of Schedule M-1 if total assets are $10 million or more—see instructions

1	Net income (loss) per books		7	Income recorded on books this year not included on this return (itemize):	
2	Federal income tax per books				
3	Excess of capital losses over capital gains . .			Tax-exempt interest $ _____	
4	Income subject to tax not recorded on books this year (itemize): _____			_____	
	_____		8	Deductions on this return not charged against book income this year (itemize):	
5	Expenses recorded on books this year not deducted on this return (itemize):		a	Depreciation . . . $ _____	
a	Depreciation . . . . $ _____		b	Charitable contributions $ _____	
b	Charitable contributions . $ _____			_____	
c	Travel and entertainment . $ _____			_____	
	_____		9	Add lines 7 and 8	
6	Add lines 1 through 5		10	Income (page 1, line 28)—line 6 less line 9	

Schedule M-2	Analysis of Unappropriated Retained Earnings per Books (Line 25, Schedule L)

1	Balance at beginning of year		5	Distributions: a Cash	
2	Net income (loss) per books			b Stock	
3	Other increases (itemize): _____			c Property . . .	
	_____		6	Other decreases (itemize): _____	
	_____		7	Add lines 5 and 6	
4	Add lines 1, 2, and 3		8	Balance at end of year (line 4 less line 7)	

Form **1120** (2008)

B-7 **U.S. Income Tax Retrun for an S Corporation**

U.S. Income Tax Return for an S Corporation

Form **1120S**

Department of the Treasury
Internal Revenue Service

OMB No. 1545-0130

2008

▶ Do not file this form unless the corporation has filed or is
attaching Form 2553 to elect to be an S corporation.
▶ See separate instructions.

For calendar year 2008 or tax year beginning _____, 2008, ending _____, 20___

A S election effective date	Use IRS label. Otherwise, print or type.	Name	D Employer identification number
B Business activity code number *(see instructions)*		Number, street, and room or suite no. If a P.O. box, see instructions.	E Date incorporated
C Check if Sch. M-3 attached ☐		City or town, state, and ZIP code	F Total assets *(see instructions)* $

G Is the corporation electing to be an S corporation beginning with this tax year? ☐ Yes ☐ No If "Yes," attach Form 2553 if not already filed

H Check if: **(1)** ☐ Final return **(2)** ☐ Name change **(3)** ☐ Address change
(4) ☐ Amended return **(5)** ☐ S election termination or revocation

I Enter the number of shareholders who were shareholders during any part of the tax year . . . . ▶

Caution. *Include only trade or business income and expenses on lines 1a through 21. See the instructions for more information.*

Income

1a	Gross receipts or sales _____ b Less returns and allowances _____ c Bal ▶	1c	
2	Cost of goods sold (Schedule A, line 8)	2	
3	Gross profit. Subtract line 2 from line 1c	3	
4	Net gain (loss) from Form 4797, Part II, line 17 *(attach Form 4797)*	4	
5	Other income (loss) *(see instructions—attach statement)*	5	
6	**Total income (loss).** Add lines 3 through 5 . . . ▶	6	

Deductions *(see instructions for limitations)*

7	Compensation of officers	7	
8	Salaries and wages (less employment credits) . . .	8	
9	Repairs and maintenance	9	
10	Bad debts	10	
11	Rents	11	
12	Taxes and licenses	12	
13	Interest	13	
14	Depreciation not claimed on Schedule A or elsewhere on return *(attach Form 4562)* . . .	14	
15	Depletion **(Do not deduct oil and gas depletion.)** . . .	15	
16	Advertising	16	
17	Pension, profit-sharing, etc., plans . . .	17	
18	Employee benefit programs . . .	18	
19	Other deductions *(attach statement)* . . .	19	
20	**Total deductions.** Add lines 7 through 19 . . . ▶	20	
21	**Ordinary business income (loss).** Subtract line 20 from line 6	21	

Tax and Payments

22a	Excess net passive income or LIFO recapture tax *(see instructions)*	22a		
b	Tax from Schedule D (Form 1120S)	22b		
c	Add lines 22a and 22b *(see instructions for additional taxes)*		22c	
23a	2008 estimated tax payments and 2007 overpayment credited to 2008	23a		
b	Tax deposited with Form 7004	23b		
c	Credit for federal tax paid on fuels *(attach Form 4136)* . . .	23c		
d	Add lines 23a through 23c		23d	
24	Estimated tax penalty *(see instructions).* Check if Form 2220 is attached . . . ▶ ☐		24	
25	**Amount owed.** If line 23d is smaller than the total of lines 22c and 24, enter amount owed .		25	
26	**Overpayment.** If line 23d is larger than the total of lines 22c and 24, enter amount overpaid .		26	
27	Enter amount from line 26 **Credited to 2009 estimated tax** ▶ _____ Refunded ▶		27	

Sign Here

Under penalties of perjury, I declare that I have examined this return, including accompanying schedules and statements, and to the best of my knowledge and belief, it is true, correct, and complete. Declaration of preparer (other than taxpayer) is based on all information of which preparer has any knowledge.

▶ _____ Signature of officer   Date   ▶ _____ Title

May the IRS discuss this return with the preparer shown below (see instructions)? ☐ Yes ☐ No

Paid Preparer's Use Only

Preparer's signature ▶		Date	Check if self-employed ☐	Preparer's SSN or PTIN
Firm's name (or yours if self-employed), address, and ZIP code ▶			EIN	Phone no. ( )

For Privacy Act and Paperwork Reduction Act Notice, see separate instructions.   Cat. No. 11510H   Form **1120S** (2008)

Form 1120S (2008)

Page **2**

Schedule A   Cost of Goods Sold (see instructions)

1	Inventory at beginning of year	**1**	
2	Purchases	**2**	
3	Cost of labor	**3**	
4	Additional section 263A costs (attach statement)	**4**	
5	Other costs (attach statement)	**5**	
6	**Total.** Add lines 1 through 5	**6**	
7	Inventory at end of year	**7**	
8	**Cost of goods sold.** Subtract line 7 from line 6. Enter here and on page 1, line 2	**8**	

9a Check all methods used for valuing closing inventory: (i) ☐ Cost as described in Regulations section 1.471-3

    (ii) ☐ Lower of cost or market as described in Regulations section 1.471-4

    (iii) ☐ Other (Specify method used and attach explanation.) ▶ ------------------------------------

b Check if there was a writedown of subnormal goods as described in Regulations section 1.471-2(c) . . . . . . ▶ ☐

c Check if the LIFO inventory method was adopted this tax year for any goods (if checked, attach Form 970) . . . . ▶ ☐

d If the LIFO inventory method was used for this tax year, enter percentage (or amounts) of closing
inventory computed under LIFO . . . . | **9d** | |

e If property is produced or acquired for resale, do the rules of section 263A apply to the corporation? . . . ☐ Yes ☐ No

f Was there any change in determining quantities, cost, or valuations between opening and closing inventory? . ☐ Yes ☐ No
If "Yes," attach explanation.

Schedule B   Other Information (see instructions)   Yes | No

1 Check accounting method: **a** ☐ Cash   **b** ☐ Accrual   **c** ☐ Other (specify) ▶ --------------------

2 See the instructions and enter the:

   a Business activity ▶ ------------------------------ **b** Product or service ▶ ------------------------------

3 At the end of the tax year, did the corporation own, directly or indirectly, 50% or more of the voting stock of a domestic
corporation? (For rules of attribution, see section 267(c).) If "Yes," attach a statement showing: **(a)** name and employer
identification number (EIN), **(b)** percentage owned, and **(c)** if 100% owned, was a QSub election made? . . .

4 Has this corporation filed, or is it required to file, a return under section 6111 to provide information on any reportable
transaction? . . . .

5 Check this box if the corporation issued publicly offered debt instruments with original issue discount .   ▶ ☐
If checked, the corporation may have to file **Form 8281,** Information Return for Publicly Offered Original Issue Discount
Instruments.

6 If the corporation: **(a)** was a C corporation before it elected to be an S corporation **or** the corporation acquired an
asset with a basis determined by reference to its basis (or the basis of any other property) in the hands of a
C corporation **and (b)** has net unrealized built-in gain (defined in section 1374(d)(1)) in excess of the net recognized
built-in gain from prior years, enter the net unrealized built-in gain reduced by net recognized built-in gain from prior
years . . . . ▶ $ ---------------------------------

7 Enter the accumulated earnings and profits of the corporation at the end of the tax year. $ _____

8 Are the corporation's total receipts (see instructions) for the tax year **and** its total assets at the end of the tax year
less than $250,000? If "Yes," the corporation is not required to complete Schedules L and M-1 . . . . . .

Schedule K   Shareholders' Pro Rata Share Items   Total amount

Income (Loss)	**1** Ordinary business income (loss) (page 1, line 21)		**1**	
	2 Net rental real estate income (loss) (attach Form 8825) .		**2**	
	3a Other gross rental income (loss)	**3a**		
	b Expenses from other rental activities (attach statement) .	**3b**		
	c Other net rental income (loss). Subtract line 3b from line 3a . . .		**3c**	
	4 Interest income		**4**	
	5 Dividends: **a** Ordinary dividends		**5a**	
	b Qualified dividends	**5b**		
	6 Royalties		**6**	
	7 Net short-term capital gain (loss) (attach Schedule D (Form 1120S))		**7**	
	8a Net long-term capital gain (loss) (attach Schedule D (Form 1120S))		**8a**	
	b Collectibles (28%) gain (loss)	**8b**		
	c Unrecaptured section 1250 gain (attach statement) . .	**8c**		
	9 Net section 1231 gain (loss) (attach Form 4797)		**9**	
	10 Other income (loss) (see instructions) . . Type ▶		**10**	

Form **1120S** (2008)

Form 1120S (2008)   Page **3**

	Shareholders' Pro Rata Share Items (continued)		Total amount	
Deductions	**11** Section 179 deduction *(attach Form 4562)*	**11**		
	12a Contributions	**12a**		
	b Investment interest expense	**12b**		
	c Section 59(e)(2) expenditures **(1)** Type ▶ _____ **(2)** Amount ▶	**12c(2)**		
	d Other deductions *(see instructions)* . . . Type ▶	**12d**		
Credits	**13a** Low-income housing credit (section 42(j)(5))	**13a**		
	b Low-income housing credit (other)	**13b**		
	c Qualified rehabilitation expenditures (rental real estate) *(attach Form 3468)*	**13c**		
	d Other rental real estate credits *(see instructions)* Type ▶ _____	**13d**		
	e Other rental credits *(see instructions)* . . Type ▶ _____	**13e**		
	f Alcohol and cellulosic biofuel fuels credit *(attach Form 6478)*	**13f**		
	g Other credits *(see instructions)* . . . . . Type ▶	**13g**		
Foreign Transactions	**14a** Name of country or U.S. possession ▶ _____			
	b Gross income from all sources	**14b**		
	c Gross income sourced at shareholder level	**14c**		
	Foreign gross income sourced at corporate level			
	d Passive category	**14d**		
	e General category	**14e**		
	f Other *(attach statement)*	**14f**		
	Deductions allocated and apportioned at shareholder level			
	g Interest expense	**14g**		
	h Other	**14h**		
	Deductions allocated and apportioned at corporate level to foreign source income			
	i Passive category	**14i**		
	j General category	**14j**		
	k Other *(attach statement)*	**14k**		
	Other information			
	l Total foreign taxes (check one): ▶ ☐ Paid ☐ Accrued	**14l**		
	m Reduction in taxes available for credit *(attach statement)*	**14m**		
	n Other foreign tax information *(attach statement)*			
Alternative Minimum Tax (AMT) Items	**15a** Post-1986 depreciation adjustment	**15a**		
	b Adjusted gain or loss	**15b**		
	c Depletion (other than oil and gas)	**15c**		
	d Oil, gas, and geothermal properties—gross income	**15d**		
	e Oil, gas, and geothermal properties—deductions.	**15e**		
	f Other AMT items *(attach statement)*	**15f**		
Items Affecting Shareholder Basis	**16a** Tax-exempt interest income	**16a**		
	b Other tax-exempt income	**16b**		
	c Nondeductible expenses	**16c**		
	d Property distributions	**16d**		
	e Repayment of loans from shareholders	**16e**		
Other Information	**17a** Investment income	**17a**		
	b Investment expenses	**17b**		
	c Dividend distributions paid from accumulated earnings and profits	**17c**		
	d Other items and amounts *(attach statement)*			
Recon- ciliation	**18** **Income/loss reconciliation.** Combine the amounts on lines 1 through 10 in the far right column. From the result, subtract the sum of the amounts on lines 11 through 12d and 14l	**18**		

Form **1120S** (2008)

Form 1120S (2008)

Page **4**

Schedule L — Balance Sheets per Books

	Beginning of tax year		End of tax year	
Assets	(a)	(b)	(c)	(d)
1 Cash				
2a Trade notes and accounts receivable . .				
b Less allowance for bad debts	( )		( )	
3 Inventories				
4 U.S. government obligations.				
5 Tax-exempt securities (see instructions) .				
6 Other current assets (attach statement) .				
7 Loans to shareholders				
8 Mortgage and real estate loans . . .				
9 Other investments (attach statement) .				
10a Buildings and other depreciable assets .				
b Less accumulated depreciation.	( )		( )	
11a Depletable assets				
b Less accumulated depletion.	( )		( )	
12 Land (net of any amortization)				
13a Intangible assets (amortizable only) . .				
b Less accumulated amortization.	( )		( )	
14 Other assets (attach statement) . . .				
15 Total assets				
Liabilities and Shareholders' Equity				
16 Accounts payable				
17 Mortgages, notes, bonds payable in less than 1 year .				
18 Other current liabilities (attach statement) .				
19 Loans from shareholders				
20 Mortgages, notes, bonds payable in 1 year or more				
21 Other liabilities (attach statement) . . .				
22 Capital stock				
23 Additional paid-in capital.				
24 Retained earnings				
25 Adjustments to shareholders' equity (attach statement) .				
26 Less cost of treasury stock		( )		( )
27 Total liabilities and shareholders' equity . .				

Schedule M-1 — Reconciliation of Income (Loss) per Books With Income (Loss) per Return

Note: Schedule M-3 required instead of Schedule M-1 if total assets are $10 million or more—see instructions

1 Net income (loss) per books.		5 Income recorded on books this year not included on Schedule K, lines 1 through 10 (itemize):	
2 Income included on Schedule K, lines 1, 2, 3c, 4, 5a, 6, 7, 8a, 9, and 10, not recorded on books this year (itemize): _____		a Tax-exempt interest $ _____	
3 Expenses recorded on books this year not included on Schedule K, lines 1 through 12 and 14l (itemize):		6 Deductions included on Schedule K, lines 1 through 12 and 14l, not charged against book income this year (itemize):	
a Depreciation $ _____		a Depreciation $ _____	
b Travel and entertainment $ _____			
_____		7 Add lines 5 and 6.	
4 Add lines 1 through 3. . .		8 Income (loss) (Schedule K, line 18). Line 4 less line 7	

Schedule M-2 — Analysis of Accumulated Adjustments Account, Other Adjustments Account, and Shareholders' Undistributed Taxable Income Previously Taxed (see instructions)

	(a) Accumulated adjustments account	(b) Other adjustments account	(c) Shareholders' undistributed taxable income previously taxed
1 Balance at beginning of tax year . . .			
2 Ordinary income from page 1, line 21 . .			
3 Other additions			
4 Loss from page 1, line 21	( )		
5 Other reductions	( )	( )	
6 Combine lines 1 through 5			
7 Distributions other than dividend distributions			
8 Balance at end of tax year. Subtract line 7 from line 6			

Form **1120S** (2008)

671108

Schedule K-1
(Form 1120S)
Department of the Treasury
Internal Revenue Service

20**08**

For calendar year 2008, or tax
year beginning _____ , 2008
ending _____ , 20___

**Shareholder's Share of Income, Deductions,
Credits, etc.**   ▶ See back of form and separate instructions.

Part I	Information About the Corporation

A   Corporation's employer identification number

B   Corporation's name, address, city, state, and ZIP code

C   IRS Center where corporation filed return

Part II	Information About the Shareholder

D   Shareholder's identifying number

E   Shareholder's name, address, city, state, and ZIP code

F   Shareholder's percentage of stock
ownership for tax year . . . . . . _____ %

For IRS Use Only

☐ Final K-1   ☐ Amended K-1   OMB No. 1545-0130

Part III	Shareholder's Share of Current Year Income, Deductions, Credits, and Other Items

1	Ordinary business income (loss)	13	Credits
2	Net rental real estate income (loss)		
3	Other net rental income (loss)		
4	Interest income		
5a	Ordinary dividends		
5b	Qualified dividends	14	Foreign transactions
6	Royalties		
7	Net short-term capital gain (loss)		
8a	Net long-term capital gain (loss)		
8b	Collectibles (28%) gain (loss)		
8c	Unrecaptured section 1250 gain		
9	Net section 1231 gain (loss)		
10	Other income (loss)	15	Alternative minimum tax (AMT) items
11	Section 179 deduction	16	Items affecting shareholder basis
12	Other deductions		
		17	Other information

* See attached statement for additional information.

For Paperwork Reduction Act Notice, see Instructions for Form 1120S.   Cat. No. 11520D   **Schedule K-1 (Form 1120S) 2008**

B-8   Amended Tax Return Forms

Form 1040X
(Rev. February 2009)

Department of the Treasury—Internal Revenue Service
Amended U.S. Individual Income Tax Return
▶ See separate instructions.

OMB No. 1545-0074

This return is for calendar year ▶ _____ , or fiscal year ended ▶ _____ , _____ .

Please print or type

Your first name and initial	Last name	Your social security number
If a joint return, spouse's first name and initial	Last name	Spouse's social security number
Home address (no. and street) or P.O. box if mail is not delivered to your home	Apt. no.	Phone number ( )
City, town or post office, state, and ZIP code. If you have a foreign address, see page 4 of the instructions.		

A If the address shown above is different from that shown on your last return filed with the IRS, would you like us to change it in our records? . . . . ▶ ☐ Yes ☐ No

B Filing status. Be sure to complete this line. **Note.** You cannot change from joint to separate returns after the due date.

On original return ▶ ☐ Single ☐ Married filing jointly ☐ Married filing separately ☐ Head of household ☐ Qualifying widow(er)

On this return ▶ ☐ Single ☐ Married filing jointly ☐ Married filing separately ☐ Head of household* ☐ Qualifying widow(er)

* If the qualifying person is a child but not your dependent, see page 4 of the instructions.

Use Part II on the back to explain any changes		**A. Original amount** or as previously adjusted (see page 4)	**B. Net change—** amount of increase or (decrease)— explain in Part II	**C. Correct amount**
Income and Deductions (see instructions)				
1	Adjusted gross income (see page 4)	1		
2	Itemized deductions or standard deduction (see page 4) .	2		
3	Subtract line 2 from line 1	3		
4	Exemptions. If changing, fill in Parts I and II on the back (see page 5)	4		
5	Taxable income. Subtract line 4 from line 3	5		
Tax Liability 6	Tax (see page 5). Method used in col. C _____	6		
7	Credits (see page 6)	7		
8	Subtract line 7 from line 6. Enter the result but not less than zero	8		
9	Other taxes (see page 6)	9		
10	Total tax. Add lines 8 and 9	10		
Payments 11	Federal income tax withheld and excess social security and tier 1 RRTA tax withheld. If changing, see page 6 . .	11		
12	Estimated tax payments, including amount applied from prior year's return	12		
13	Earned income credit (EIC)	13		
14	Additional child tax credit from Form 8812	14		
15	Credits: Recovery rebate; federal telephone excise tax; or from Forms 2439, 4136, 5405, 8885, or 8801 (refundable credit only)	15		
16	Amount paid with request for extension of time to file (see page 6)	16		
17	Amount of tax paid with original return plus additional tax paid after it was filed	17		
18	Total payments. Add lines 11 through 17 in column C	18		

Refund or Amount You Owe
Note. Allow 8-12 weeks to process Form 1040X.

19	Overpayment, if any, as shown on original return or as previously adjusted by the IRS . .	19		
20	Subtract line 19 from line 18 (see page 6)	20		
21	**Amount you owe.** If line 10, column C, is more than line 20, enter the difference and see page 6 .	21		
22	If line 10, column C, is less than line 20, enter the difference	22		
23	Amount of line 22 you want **refunded to you**	23		
24	Amount of line 22 you want **applied to your** _____ estimated tax	24		

Sign Here
Joint return?
See page 4.
Keep a copy for your records.

Under penalties of perjury, I declare that I have filed an original return and that I have examined this amended return, including accompanying schedules and statements, and to the best of my knowledge and belief, this amended return is true, correct, and complete. Declaration of preparer (other than taxpayer) is based on all information of which the preparer has any knowledge.

▶ _____ _____   ▶ _____ _____
Your signature   Date   Spouse's signature. If a joint return, **both** must sign.   Date

Paid Preparer's Use Only

Preparer's signature ▶	Date	Check if self-employed ☐	Preparer's SSN or PTIN
Firm's name (or yours if self-employed), address, and ZIP code ▶		EIN	Phone no. ( )

For Paperwork Reduction Act Notice, see page 8 of instructions.   Cat. No. 11360L   Form **1040X** (Rev. 2-2009)

Form 1040X (Rev. 2-2009)   Page **2**

Part I	**Exemptions.** See Form 1040 or 1040A instructions.	**A. Original number** of exemptions reported or as previously adjusted	**B. Net change**	**C. Correct number** of exemptions
	Complete this part **only** if you are: • Increasing or decreasing the number of exemptions claimed on line 6d of the return you are amending, or • Increasing or decreasing the exemption amount for housing individuals displaced by Hurricane Katrina or for housing Midwestern displaced individuals.			

25	Yourself and spouse . . . . **Caution.** If someone can claim you as a dependent, you cannot claim an exemption for yourself.	**25**			
26	Your dependent children who lived with you	**26**			
27	Your dependent children who did not live with you due to divorce or separation	**27**			
28	Other dependents	**28**			
29	Total number of exemptions. Add lines 25 through 28	**29**			
30	Multiply the number of exemptions claimed on line 29 by the amount listed below for the tax year you are amending. Enter the result here.	**30**			
31	If you are claiming an exemption amount for housing individuals displaced by Hurricane Katrina, enter the amount from Form 8914, line 2 for 2005 or line 6 for 2006. If you are claiming an exemption amount for housing Midwestern displaced individuals, enter the amount from the 2008 Form 8914, line 2. (See instructions for line 4). Otherwise enter -0-	**31**			
32	Add lines 30 and 31. Enter the result here and on line 4	**32**			

Line 30 table:

Tax year	Exemption amount	But see the instructions for line 4 on page 5 if the amount on line 1 is over:
2008	$3,500	$119,975
2007	3,400	117,300
2006	3,300	112,875
2005	3,200	109,475

33 Dependents (children and other) not claimed on original (or adjusted) return:

(a) First name Last name	(b) Dependent's social security number	(c) Dependent's relationship to you	(d) ✓ if qualifying child for child tax credit (see page 7)
			☐
			☐
			☐
			☐
			☐
			☐

No. of children on 33 who:
• lived with you . ▶ ☐
• **did not** live with you due to divorce or separation (see page 7) . ▶ ☐
Dependents on 33 not entered above ▶ ☐

Part II **Explanation of Changes**

Enter the line number from the front of the form for each item you are changing and give the reason for each change. **Attach only the supporting forms and schedules for the items changed. If you do not attach the required information, your Form 1040X may be returned. Be sure to include your name and social security number on any attachments.**

If the change relates to a net operating loss carryback or a general business credit carryback, attach the schedule or form that shows the year in which the loss or credit occurred. See pages 2 and 3 of the instructions. Also, check here . . ▶ ☐

_____

_____

_____

_____

Part III **Presidential Election Campaign Fund.** Checking below will not increase your tax or reduce your refund.

If you did not previously want $3 to go to the fund but now want to, check here . . . . ▶ ☐
If a joint return and your spouse did not previously want $3 to go to the fund but now wants to, check here . . . ▶ ☐

Form **1040X** (Rev. 2-2009)

Form **1120X**
(Rev. January 2008)
Department of the Treasury
Internal Revenue Service

Amended U.S. Corporation Income Tax Return

OMB No. 1545-0132

For tax year ending

▶ --------------------------

(Enter month and year.)

Please Type or Print	Name		Employer identification number
	Number, street, and room or suite no. (If a P.O. box, see instructions.)		
	City or town, state, and ZIP code		Telephone number (optional) ( )

Enter name and address used on original return (If same as above, write "Same.")

Internal Revenue Service Center ▶
where original return was filed

Fill in applicable items and use Part II on the back to explain any changes

Part I Income and Deductions (see instructions)		(a) As originally reported or as previously adjusted	(b) Net change— increase or (decrease)— explain in Part II	(c) Correct amount
1 Total income (Form 1120 or 1120-A, line 11) . .	**1**			
2 Total deductions (total of lines 27 and 29c, Form 1120, or lines 23 and 25c, Form 1120-A)	**2**			
3 Taxable income. Subtract line 2 from line 1 . . .	**3**			
4 Tax (Form 1120, line 31, or Form 1120-A, line 27) .	**4**			

Payments and Credits (see instructions)

5a Overpayment in prior year allowed as a credit . .	**5a**			
b Estimated tax payments	**5b**			
c Refund applied for on Form 4466	**5c**			
d Subtract line 5c from the sum of lines 5a and 5b .	**5d**			
e Tax deposited with Form 7004	**5e**			
f Credit from Form 2439	**5f**			
g Credit for federal tax on fuels and other refundable credits	**5g**			
6 Tax deposited or paid with (or after) the filing of the original return	**6**	
7 Add lines 5d through 6, column (c)	**7**	
8 Overpayment, if any, as shown on original return or as later adjusted	**8**	
9 Subtract line 8 from line 7	**9**	

Tax Due or Overpayment (see instructions)

10 **Tax due.** Subtract line 9 from line 4, column (c). If paying by check, make it payable to the **"United States Treasury"** . . . . ▶	**10**	
11 **Overpayment.** Subtract line 4, column (c), from line 9 . . . . ▶	**11**	
12 Enter the amount of line 11 you want: **Credited to 20__ estimated tax** ▶ Refunded ▶	**12**	

Sign Here

Under penalties of perjury, I declare that I have filed an original return and that I have examined this amended return, including accompanying schedules and statements, and to the best of my knowledge and belief, this amended return is true, correct, and complete. Declaration of preparer (other than taxpayer) is based on all information of which preparer has any knowledge.

▶ _____   _____   ▶ _____
  Signature of officer   Date   Title

Paid Preparer's Use Only

Preparer's signature ▶	Date	Check if self-employed ☐	Preparer's SSN or PTIN
Firm's name (or yours if self-employed), address, and ZIP code ▶		EIN	
		Phone no. ( )	

For Privacy Act and Paperwork Reduction Act Notice, see page 4.   Cat. No. 11530Z   Form **1120X** (Rev. 1-2008)

Form 1120X (Rev. 1-2008)   Page **2**

Part II   **Explanation of Changes to Items in Part I** (Enter the line number from page 1 for the items you are changing, and give the reason for each change. Show any computation in detail. Also, see **What To Attach** on page 3 of the instructions.)

If the change is due to a net operating loss carryback, a capital loss carryback, or a general business credit carryback, see **Carryback Claims** on page 3, and check here . . . . ▶ ☐

B-9   Application for Extension of Time to File Income Tax Returns

Form **4868**
Department of the Treasury
Internal Revenue Service   (99)

**Application for Automatic Extension of Time
To File U.S. Individual Income Tax Return**

OMB No. 1545-0074

20**08**

There are three ways to request an automatic extension of time to file a U.S. individual income tax return.

1. You can file Form 4868 electronically by accessing IRS *e-file* using your home computer or by using a tax professional who uses *e-file.*

2. You can pay all or part of your estimate of income tax due using a credit card.

3. You can file a paper Form 4868.

The first two options are discussed under IRS *e-file,* next. Filing a paper Form 4868 is discussed later on this page.

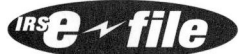 **It's Convenient,
Safe, and Secure**

IRS *e-file* is the IRS's electronic filing program. You can get an automatic extension of time to file your tax return by filing Form 4868 electronically. You will receive an electronic acknowledgment once you complete the transaction. Keep it with your records. Do not send in Form 4868 if you file electronically, unless you are making a payment with a check or money order. (See page 4.)

Complete Form 4868 to use as a worksheet. If you think you may owe tax when you file your return, you will need to estimate your total tax liability and subtract how much you have already paid (lines 4, 5, and 6 below).

You can apply for an extension by e-filing Form 4868 from a home computer or through a tax professional who uses e-file. Several companies offer free e-filing of Form 4868 through the Free File program. For more details, go to *www.irs.gov* and enter "Free File" in the search box at the top of the page.

You can also apply for an extension by paying part or all of your estimate of income tax due by using a credit card. See *Pay by Credit Card* later on this page.

 ***E-file* Using Your Personal Computer
or Through a Tax Professional**

Refer to your tax software package or tax preparer for ways to file electronically. Be sure to have a copy of your 2007 tax return—you will be asked to provide information from the return for taxpayer verification. If you wish to make a payment, you can pay by electronic funds withdrawal or send your check or money order to the address shown in the middle column under *Where To File a Paper Form 4868.* See page 4.

Pay by Credit Card

You can get an extension if you pay part or all of your estimate of income tax due by using a credit card (American Express® Card, Discover® Card, MasterCard® card, or Visa® card). Your payment must be at least $1. You can pay by phone or over the Internet. See page 4.

 File a Paper Form 4868

If you wish to file on paper instead of electronically, fill in the Form 4868 below and mail it to the address shown on page 4.

For information on using a private delivery service, see page 4.

Note. If you are a fiscal year taxpayer, you must file a paper Form 4868.

▼ DETACH HERE ▼

Form **4868**
Department of the Treasury
Internal Revenue Service   (99)

**Application for Automatic Extension of Time
To File U.S. Individual Income Tax Return**
For calendar year 2008, or other tax year beginning   , 2008, ending   , 200   .

OMB No. 1545-0074

20**08**

Part I   Identification
1 Your name(s) (see instructions)
Address (see instructions)

City, town, or post office	State	ZIP code

2 Your social security number	**3** Spouse's social security number

Part II   Individual Income Tax

4	Estimate of total tax liability for 2008 .	$ _____
5	Total 2008 payments	_____
6	**Balance due.** Subtract line 5 from line 4 (see instructions)	_____
7	Amount you are paying (see instructions) . ▶	_____
8	Check here if you are "out of the country" and a U.S. citizen or resident (see instructions) . . . . . ▶	☐
9	Check here if you file Form 1040NR or 1040NR-EZ and did not receive wages as an employee subject to U.S. income tax withholding . . . . ▶	☐

For Privacy Act and Paperwork Reduction Act Notice, see page 4.   Cat. No. 13141W   Form **4868** (2008)

Form **7004**	**Application for Automatic Extension of Time To File Certain Business Income Tax, Information, and Other Returns**	
(Rev. December 2008) Department of the Treasury Internal Revenue Service	▶ File a separate application for each return. ▶ See separate instructions.	OMB No. 1545-0233

Type or Print	Name	Identifying number
File by the due date for the return for which an extension is requested. See instructions.	Number, street, and room or suite no. (If P.O. box, see instructions.)	
	City, town, state, and ZIP code (If a foreign address, enter city, province or state, and country (follow the country's practice for entering postal code)).	

Note. See instructions before completing this form.

Part I   Automatic 5-Month Extension Complete if Filing Form 1065, 1041, or 8804

1a Enter the form code for the return that this application is for (see below) . . . . ▢▢

Application Is For:	Form Code	Application Is For:	Form Code
Form 1065	09	Form 1041 (estate)	04
Form 8804	31	Form 1041 (trust)	05

Part II   Automatic 6-Month Extension Complete if Filing Other Forms

b Enter the form code for the return that this application is for (see below) . . . . ▢▢

Application Is For:	Form Code	Application Is For:	Form Code
Form 706-GS(D)	01	Form 1120-PC	21
Form 706-GS(T)	02	Form 1120-POL	22
Form 1041-N	06	Form 1120-REIT	23
Form 1041-QFT	07	Form 1120-RIC	24
Form 1042	08	Form 1120S	25
Form 1065-B	10	Form 1120-SF	26
Form 1066	11	Form 3520-A	27
Form 1120	12	Form 8612	28
Form 1120-C	34	Form 8613	29
Form 1120-F	15	Form 8725	30
Form 1120-FSC	16	Form 8831	32
Form 1120-H	17	Form 8876	33
Form 1120-L	18	Form 8924	35
Form 1120-ND	19	Form 8928	36
Form 1120-ND (section 4951 taxes)	20		

2 If the organization is a foreign corporation that does not have an office or place of business in the United States, check here . . . . ▶ ▢

3 If the organization is a corporation and is the common parent of a group that intends to file a consolidated return, check here . . . . ▶ ▢
If checked, attach a schedule, listing the name, address, and Employer Identification Number (EIN) for each member covered by this application.

Part III   All Filers Must Complete This Part

4 If the organization is a corporation or partnership that qualifies under Regulations section 1.6081-5, check here . ▶ ▢

5a The application is for calendar year 20 ____, or tax year beginning _____, 20 ____, and ending _____ , 20 ____

b **Short tax year.** If this tax year is less than 12 months, check the reason:
▢ Initial return   ▢ Final return   ▢ Change in accounting period   ▢ Consolidated return to be filed

6 Tentative total tax	**6**		
7 **Total** payments and credits (see instructions)	**7**		
8 **Balance due.** Subtract line 7 from line 6. **Generally, you must deposit this amount using the Electronic Federal Tax Payment System (EFTPS), a Federal Tax Deposit (FTD) Coupon, or Electronic Funds Withdrawal (EFW)** (see instructions for exceptions)	**8**		

For Privacy Act and Paperwork Reduction Act Notice, see separate Instructions.   Cat. No. 13804A   Form **7004** (Rev. 12-2008)

B-10   Underpayment of Estimated Tax

Form **2210**	**Underpayment of**	OMB No. 1545-0140

Form **2210**

Department of the Treasury
Internal Revenue Service

**Underpayment of
Estimated Tax by Individuals, Estates, and Trusts**
▶ See separate instructions.
▶ **Attach to Form 1040, 1040A, 1040NR, 1040NR-EZ, or 1041.**

OMB No. 1545-0140

2008

Attachment
Sequence No. **06**

Name(s) shown on tax return

Identifying number

Do You Have To File Form 2210?

Complete lines 1 through 7 below. Is line 7 less than $1,000?   **Yes ▶**   **Do not file Form 2210.** You do not owe a penalty.

No ↓

Complete lines 8 and 9 below. Is line 6 equal to or more than line 9?   **Yes ▶**   You do not owe a penalty. **Do not file Form 2210** (but if box **E** in Part II applies, you must file page 1 of Form 2210).

No ↓

You may owe a penalty. Does any box in Part II below apply?   **Yes ▶**   You **must** file Form 2210. Does box **B, C,** or **D** in Part II apply?

No ↓   **No**   **Yes ▶** You must figure your penalty.

Do not file Form 2210. You are not required to figure your penalty because the IRS will figure it and send you a bill for any unpaid amount. If you want to figure it, you may use Part III or Part IV as a worksheet and enter your penalty amount on your tax return, but **do not file Form 2210.**

You are **not** required to figure your penalty because the IRS will figure it and send you a bill for any unpaid amount. If you want to figure it, you may use Part III or Part IV as a worksheet and enter your penalty amount on your tax return, but **file only page 1 of Form 2210.**

Part I   Required Annual Payment

1	Enter your 2008 tax after credits from Form 1040, line 56 (see instructions if not filing Form 1040)	**1**	
2	Other taxes, including self-employment tax (see page 2 of the instructions)	**2**	
3	Refundable credits. Enter the total of your earned income credit, additional child tax credit, credit for federal tax paid on fuels, health coverage tax credit, refundable credit for prior year minimum tax, first-time homebuyer credit, and recovery rebate credit	**3**	( )
4	Current year tax. Combine lines 1, 2, and 3. If less than $1,000, you do not owe a penalty; **do not file Form 2210**	**4**	
5	Multiply line 4 by 90% (.90) . . . . **5** | |		
6	Withholding taxes. **Do not** include estimated tax payments. (see page 2 of the instructions)	**6**	
7	Subtract line 6 from line 4. If less than $1,000, you do not owe a penalty; **do not file Form 2210** . .	**7**	
8	Maximum required annual payment based on prior year's tax (see page 2 of the instructions)	**8**	
9	**Required annual payment.** Enter the **smaller** of line 5 or line 8	**9**	

Next: Is line 9 more than line 6?

☐ **No.** You **do not** owe a penalty. **Do not file Form 2210** unless box **E** below applies.

☐ **Yes.** You may owe a penalty, but **do not file Form 2210** unless one or more boxes in Part II below applies.
  - If box **B, C,** or **D** applies, you must figure your penalty and file Form 2210.
  - If only box **A** or **E** (or both) applies, file only page 1 of Form 2210. You are **not** required to figure your penalty; the IRS will figure it and send you a bill for any unpaid amount. If you want to figure your penalty, you may use Part III or IV as a worksheet and enter your penalty on your tax return, but **file only page 1 of Form 2210.**

Part II   Reasons for Filing. Check applicable boxes. If none apply, **do not file Form 2210.**

A ☐ You request a **waiver** (see page 2 of the instructions) of your entire penalty. You must check this box and file page 1 of Form 2210, but you are not required to figure your penalty.

B ☐ You request a **waiver** (see page 2 of the instructions) of part of your penalty. You must figure your penalty and waiver amount and file Form 2210.

C ☐ Your income varied during the year and your penalty is reduced or eliminated when figured using the **annualized income installment method.** You must figure the penalty using Schedule AI and file Form 2210.

D ☐ Your penalty is lower when figured by treating the federal income tax withheld from your income as paid on the dates it was actually withheld, instead of in equal amounts on the payment due dates. You must figure your penalty and file Form 2210.

E ☐ You filed or are filing a joint return for either 2007 or 2008, but not for both years, and line 8 above is smaller than line 5 above. You must file page 1 of Form 2210, but you are **not** required to figure your penalty (unless box **B, C,** or **D** applies).

For Paperwork Reduction Act Notice, see page 6 of separate instructions.   Cat. No. 11744P   Form **2210** (2008)

Form 2210 (2008)   Page **2**

Part III	**Short Method**

| *Can You Use the Short Method?* | You may use the short method if:

 • You made no estimated tax payments (or your only payments were withheld federal income tax), **or**

 • You paid the same amount of estimated tax on each of the four payment due dates. |
| *Must You Use the Regular Method?* | You must use the regular method (Part IV) instead of the short method if:

 • You made any estimated tax payments late,

 • You checked box **C** or **D** in Part II, **or**

 • You are filing Form 1040NR or 1040NR-EZ and you did not receive wages as an employee subject to U.S. income tax withholding. |

Note: *If any payment was made earlier than the due date, you may use the short method, but using it may cause you to pay a larger penalty than the regular method. If the payment was only a few days early, the difference is likely to be small.*

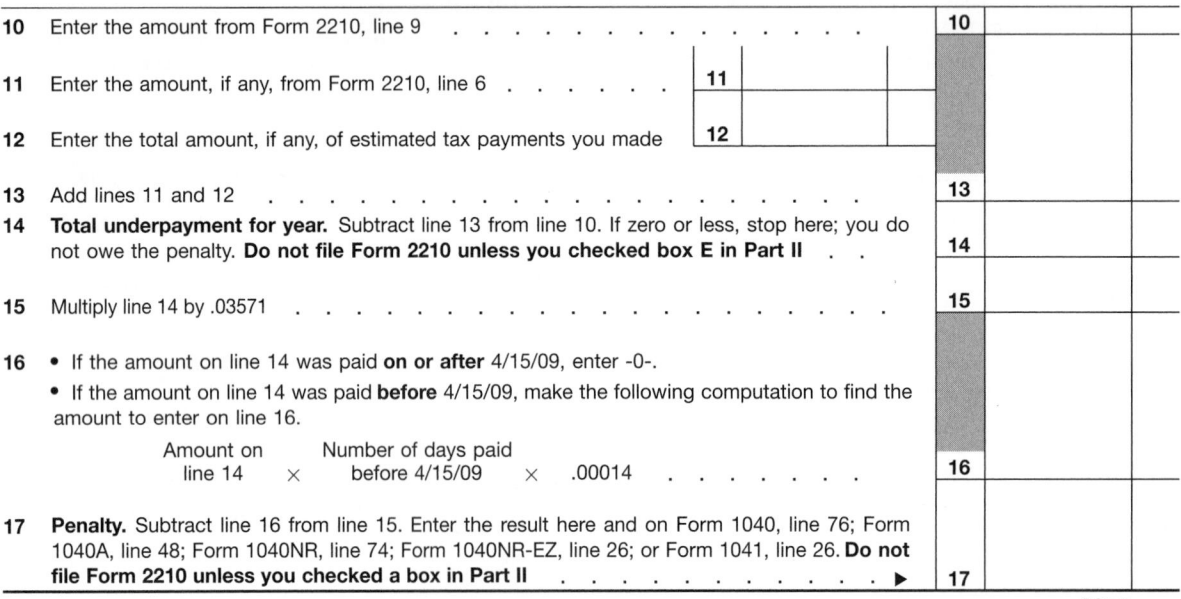

10   Enter the amount from Form 2210, line 9 . . . .   **10**

11   Enter the amount, if any, from Form 2210, line 6 . . . .   **11**

12   Enter the total amount, if any, of estimated tax payments you made   **12**

13   Add lines 11 and 12 . . . .   **13**

14   **Total underpayment for year.** Subtract line 13 from line 10. If zero or less, stop here; you do not owe the penalty. **Do not file Form 2210 unless you checked box E in Part II** . .   **14**

15   Multiply line 14 by .03571 . . . .   **15**

16   • If the amount on line 14 was paid **on or after** 4/15/09, enter -0-.
     • If the amount on line 14 was paid **before** 4/15/09, make the following computation to find the amount to enter on line 16.

         Amount on   Number of days paid
         line 14   ×   before 4/15/09   ×   .00014 . . . .   **16**

17   **Penalty.** Subtract line 16 from line 15. Enter the result here and on Form 1040, line 76; Form 1040A, line 48; Form 1040NR, line 74; Form 1040NR-EZ, line 26; or Form 1041, line 26. **Do not file Form 2210 unless you checked a box in Part II** . . . . ▶   **17**

Form **2210** (2008)

Form 2210 (2008)   Page **3**

Part IV	**Regular Method** (See page 3 of the instructions if you are filing Form 1040NR or 1040NR-EZ.)

			Payment Due Dates			
Section A—Figure Your Underpayment			**(a)** 4/15/08	**(b)** 6/15/08	**(c)** 9/15/08	**(d)** 1/15/09
18	**Required installments.** If box C in Part II applies, enter the amounts from Schedule AI, line 25. Otherwise, enter 25% (.25) of line 9, Form 2210, in each column . .	**18**				
19	Estimated tax paid and tax withheld (see page 3 of the instructions). For column (a) only, also enter the amount from line 19 on line 23. If line 19 is equal to or more than line 18 for all payment periods, stop here; you do not owe a penalty. **Do not file Form 2210 unless you checked a box in Part II** . .	**19**				
	Complete lines 20 through 26 of one column before going to line 20 of the next column.					
20	Enter the amount, if any, from line 26 in the previous column	**20**				
21	Add lines 19 and 20	**21**				
22	Add the amounts on lines 24 and 25 in the previous column	**22**				
23	Subtract line 22 from line 21. If zero or less, enter -0-. For column (a) only, enter the amount from line 19	**23**				
24	If line 23 is zero, subtract line 21 from line 22. Otherwise, enter -0-	**24**				
25	**Underpayment.** If line 18 is equal to or more than line 23, subtract line 23 from line 18. Then go to line 20 of the next column. Otherwise, go to line 26 ▶	**25**				
26	Overpayment. If line 23 is more than line 18, subtract line 18 from line 23. Then go to line 20 of the next column .	**26**				

Section B—Figure the Penalty (Complete lines 27 through 34 of one column before going to the next column.)

				4/15/08	6/15/08		
Rate Period 1		**April 16, 2008—June 30, 2008**		*Days:*	*Days:*		
	27	Number of days **from** the date shown above line 27 **to** the date the amount on line 25 was paid **or** 6/30/08, whichever is earlier	**27**				
	28	Underpayment on line 25 (see page 4 of the instructions) × days on line 27 / 366 × .06 ▶	**28**	$	$		

				6/30/08	6/30/08	9/15/08	
Rate Period 2		**July 1, 2008—September 30, 2008**		*Days:*	*Days:*	*Days:*	
	29	Number of days **from** the date shown above line 29 **to** the date the amount on line 25 was paid **or** 9/30/08, whichever is earlier	**29**				
	30	Underpayment on line 25 (see page 4 of the instructions) × days on line 29 / 366 × .05 ▶	**30**	$	$	$	

				9/30/08	9/30/08	9/30/08	
Rate Period 3		**October 1, 2008—December 31, 2008**		*Days:*	*Days:*	*Days:*	
	31	Number of days **from** the date shown above line 31 **to** the date the amount on line 25 was paid **or** 12/31/08, whichever is earlier	**31**				
	32	Underpayment on line 25 (see page 4 of the instructions) × days on line 31 / 366 × .06 ▶	**32**	$	$	$	

				12/31/08	12/31/08	12/31/08	1/15/09
Rate Period 4		**January 1, 2009—April 15, 2009**		*Days:*	*Days:*	*Days:*	*Days:*
	33	Number of days **from** the date shown above line 33 **to** the date the amount on line 25 was paid **or** 4/15/09, whichever is earlier	**33**				
	34	Underpayment on line 25 (see page 4 of the instructions) × days on line 33 / 365 × .05 ▶	**34**	$	$	$	$

35	**Penalty.** Add all amounts on lines 28, 30, 32, and 34 in all columns. Enter the total here and on Form 1040, line 76; Form 1040A, line 48; Form 1040NR, line 74; Form 1040NR-EZ, line 26; or Form 1041, line 26. **Do not file Form 2210 unless you checked a box in Part II** . . . . ▶	**35**	$

Form **2210** (2008)

Form **2220**	**Underpayment of Estimated Tax by Corporations**	OMB No. 1545-0142
Department of the Treasury Internal Revenue Service	▶ See separate instructions. ▶ Attach to the corporation's tax return.	20**08**

Name		Employer identification number

Note: *Generally, the corporation is not required to file Form 2220 (see Part II below for exceptions) because the IRS will figure any penalty owed and bill the corporation. However, the corporation may still use Form 2220 to figure the penalty. If so, enter the amount from page 2, line 38 on the estimated tax penalty line of the corporation's income tax return, but* **do not** *attach Form 2220.*

Part I Required Annual Payment

1	Total tax (see instructions)	**1**	
2a	Personal holding company tax (Schedule PH (Form 1120), line 26) included on line 1 .	**2a**	
b	Look-back interest included on line 1 under section 460(b)(2) for completed long-term contracts or section 167(g) for depreciation under the income forecast method . .	**2b**	
c	Credit for federal tax paid on fuels (see instructions)	**2c**	
d	**Total.** Add lines 2a through 2c	**2d**	
3	Subtract line 2d from line 1. If the result is less than $500, **do not** complete or file this form. The corporation does not owe the penalty	**3**	
4	Enter the tax shown on the corporation's 2007 income tax return (see instructions). **Caution:** *If the tax is zero or the tax year was for less than 12 months, skip this line and enter the amount from line 3 on line 5* . . .	**4**	
5	**Required annual payment.** Enter the **smaller** of line 3 or line 4. If the corporation is required to skip line 4, enter the amount from line 3	**5**	

Part II Reasons for Filing— Check the boxes below that apply. If any boxes are checked, the corporation **must** file Form 2220 even if it does not owe a penalty (see instructions).

6 ☐ The corporation is using the adjusted seasonal installment method.

7 ☐ The corporation is using the annualized income installment method.

8 ☐ The corporation is a "large corporation" figuring its first required installment based on the prior year's tax.

Part III Figuring the Underpayment

			(a)	(b)	(c)	(d)
9	**Installment due dates.** Enter in columns (a) through (d) the 15th day of the 4th (**Form 990-PF filers:** Use 5th month), 6th, 9th, and 12th months of the corporation's tax year . .	**9**				
10	**Required installments.** If the box on line 6 and/or line 7 above is checked, enter the amounts from Schedule A, line 38. If the box on line 8 (but not 6 or 7) is checked, see instructions for the amounts to enter. If none of these boxes are checked, enter 25% of line 5 above in each column . .	**10**				
11	Estimated tax paid or credited for each period (see instructions). For column (a) only, enter the amount from line 11 on line 15	**11**				
	Complete lines 12 through 18 of one column before going to the next column.					
12	Enter amount, if any, from line 18 of the preceding column .	**12**				
13	Add lines 11 and 12	**13**				
14	Add amounts on lines 16 and 17 of the preceding column .	**14**				
15	Subtract line 14 from line 13. If zero or less, enter -0- . .	**15**				
16	If the amount on line 15 is zero, subtract line 13 from line 14. Otherwise, enter -0-	**16**				
17	**Underpayment.** If line 15 is less than or equal to line 10, subtract line 15 from line 10. Then go to line 12 of the next column. Otherwise, go to line 18	**17**				
18	**Overpayment.** If line 10 is less than line 15, subtract line 10 from line 15. Then go to line 12 of the next column . . .	**18**				

Go to Part IV on page 2 to figure the penalty. Do not go to Part IV if there are no entries on line 17—no penalty is owed.

For Paperwork Reduction Act Notice, see separate instructions. Cat. No. 11746L Form **2220** (2008)

B-11   **Computation of Minimum Tax**

Form **4626**

Alternative Minimum Tax—Corporations

OMB No. 1545-0175

Department of the Treasury
Internal Revenue Service

► **See separate instructions.**
► **Attach to the corporation's tax return.**

2008

Name

Employer identification number

Part I	**Alternative Minimum Tax Computation**

Note: *See the instructions to find out if the corporation is a small corporation exempt from the alternative minimum tax (AMT) under section 55(e).*

1	Taxable income or (loss) before net operating loss deduction	**1**	
2	**Adjustments and preferences:**		
a	Depreciation of post-1986 property	**2a**	
b	Amortization of certified pollution control facilities.	**2b**	
c	Amortization of mining exploration and development costs	**2c**	
d	Amortization of circulation expenditures (personal holding companies only)	**2d**	
e	Adjusted gain or loss	**2e**	
f	Long-term contracts	**2f**	
g	Merchant marine capital construction funds.	**2g**	
h	Section 833(b) deduction (Blue Cross, Blue Shield, and similar type organizations only)	**2h**	
i	Tax shelter farm activities (personal service corporations only)	**2i**	
j	Passive activities (closely held corporations and personal service corporations only)	**2j**	
k	Loss limitations	**2k**	
l	Depletion	**2l**	
m	Tax-exempt interest income from specified private activity bonds	**2m**	
n	Intangible drilling costs	**2n**	
o	Other adjustments and preferences	**2o**	
3	Pre-adjustment alternative minimum taxable income (AMTI). Combine lines 1 through 2o	**3**	
4	**Adjusted current earnings (ACE) adjustment:**		
a	ACE from line 10 of the ACE worksheet in the instructions	**4a**	
b	Subtract line 3 from line 4a. If line 3 exceeds line 4a, enter the difference as a negative amount (see instructions).	**4b**	
c	Multiply line 4b by 75% (.75). Enter the result as a positive amount	**4c**	
d	Enter the excess, if any, of the corporation's total increases in AMTI from prior year ACE adjustments over its total reductions in AMTI from prior year ACE adjustments (see instructions). **Note:** *You **must** enter an amount on line 4d (even if line 4b is positive)*	**4d**	
e	ACE adjustment.		
	● If line 4b is zero or more, enter the amount from line 4c		
	● If line 4b is less than zero, enter the **smaller** of line 4c or line 4d as a negative amount	**4e**	
5	Combine lines 3 and 4e. If zero or less, stop here; the corporation does not owe any AMT	**5**	
6	Alternative tax net operating loss deduction (see instructions).	**6**	
7	**Alternative minimum taxable income.** Subtract line 6 from line 5. If the corporation held a residual interest in a REMIC, see instructions	**7**	
8	**Exemption phase-out** (if line 7 is $310,000 or more, skip lines 8a and 8b and enter -0- on line 8c):		
a	Subtract $150,000 from line 7 (if completing this line for a member of a controlled group, see instructions). If zero or less, enter -0-	**8a**	
b	Multiply line 8a by 25% (.25).	**8b**	
c	Exemption. Subtract line 8b from $40,000 (if completing this line for a member of a controlled group, see instructions). If zero or less, enter -0-	**8c**	
9	Subtract line 8c from line 7. If zero or less, enter -0-	**9**	
10	If the corporation had qualified timber gain, complete Part II and enter the amount from line 24 here. Otherwise, multiply line 9 by 20% (.20)	**10**	
11	Alternative minimum tax foreign tax credit (AMTFTC) (see instructions)	**11**	
12	Tentative minimum tax. Subtract line 11 from line 10.	**12**	
13	Regular tax liability before applying all credits except the foreign tax credit	**13**	
14	**Alternative minimum tax.** Subtract line 13 from line 12. If zero or less, enter -0-. Enter here and on Form 1120, Schedule J, line 3, or the appropriate line of the corporation's income tax return . . .	**14**	

For Paperwork Reduction Act Notice, see the instructions.   Cat. No. 12955I   Form **4626** (2008)

Form **6251**

Department of the Treasury
Internal Revenue Service (99)

Alternative Minimum Tax—Individuals

▶ See separate instructions.

▶ Attach to Form 1040 or Form 1040NR.

OMB No. 1545-0074

20**08**

Attachment
Sequence No. **32**

Name(s) shown on Form 1040 or Form 1040NR

Your social security number

Part I   Alternative Minimum Taxable Income (See instructions for how to complete each line.)

1	If filing Schedule A (Form 1040), enter the amount from Form 1040, line 41 (minus any amount on Form 8914, line 2), and go to line 2. Otherwise, enter the amount from Form 1040, line 38 (minus any amount on Form 8914, line 2), and go to line 7. (If less than zero, enter as a negative amount)	**1**	
2	Medical and dental. Enter the **smaller** of Schedule A (Form 1040), line 4, **or** 2.5% (.025) of Form 1040, line 38. If zero or less, enter -0-	**2**	
3	Taxes from Schedule A (Form 1040), line 9	**3**	
4	Enter the home mortgage interest adjustment, if any, from line 6 of the worksheet on page 2 of the instructions	**4**	
5	Miscellaneous deductions from Schedule A (Form 1040), line 27	**5**	
6	If Form 1040, line 38, is over $159,950 (over $79,975 if married filing separately), enter the amount from line 11 of the **Itemized Deductions Worksheet** on page A-10 of the instructions for Schedule A (Form 1040)	**6** (	)
7	If claiming the standard deduction, enter any amount from Form 4684, line 18a, as a negative amount	**7** (	)
8	Tax refund from Form 1040, line 10 or line 21	**8** (	)
9	Investment interest expense (difference between regular tax and AMT)	**9**	
10	Depletion (difference between regular tax and AMT)	**10**	
11	Net operating loss deduction from Form 1040, line 21. Enter as a positive amount	**11**	
12	Interest from specified private activity bonds exempt from the regular tax	**12**	
13	Qualified small business stock (7% of gain excluded under section 1202)	**13**	
14	Exercise of incentive stock options (excess of AMT income over regular tax income)	**14**	
15	Estates and trusts (amount from Schedule K-1 (Form 1041), box 12, code A)	**15**	
16	Electing large partnerships (amount from Schedule K-1 (Form 1065-B), box 6)	**16**	
17	Disposition of property (difference between AMT and regular tax gain or loss)	**17**	
18	Depreciation on assets placed in service after 1986 (difference between regular tax and AMT)	**18**	
19	Passive activities (difference between AMT and regular tax income or loss)	**19**	
20	Loss limitations (difference between AMT and regular tax income or loss)	**20**	
21	Circulation costs (difference between regular tax and AMT)	**21**	
22	Long-term contracts (difference between AMT and regular tax income)	**22**	
23	Mining costs (difference between regular tax and AMT)	**23**	
24	Research and experimental costs (difference between regular tax and AMT)	**24**	
25	Income from certain installment sales before January 1, 1987	**25** (	)
26	Intangible drilling costs preference	**26**	
27	Other adjustments, including income-based related adjustments	**27**	
28	Alternative tax net operating loss deduction	**28** (	)
29	**Alternative minimum taxable income.** Combine lines 1 through 28. (If married filing separately and line 29 is more than $214,900, see page 8 of the instructions.)	**29**	

Part II   Alternative Minimum Tax (AMT)

30	Exemption. (If you were under age 24 at the end of 2008, see page 8 of the instructions.)		

IF your filing status is . . .	**AND line 29 is not over . . .**	**THEN enter on line 30 . . .**	
Single or head of household	$112,500	$46,200	
Married filing jointly or qualifying widow(er)	150,000	69,950	
Married filing separately	75,000	34,975	**30**

If line 29 is **over** the amount shown above for your filing status, see page 8 of the instructions.

31	Subtract line 30 from line 29. If more than zero, go to line 32. If zero or less, enter -0- here and on lines 34 and 36 and skip the rest of Part II	**31**	
32	• If you are filing Form 2555 or 2555-EZ, see page 9 of the instructions for the amount to enter. • If you reported capital gain distributions directly on Form 1040, line 13; you reported qualified dividends on Form 1040, line 9b; **or** you had a gain on both lines 15 and 16 of Schedule D (Form 1040) (as refigured for the AMT, if necessary), complete Part III on the back and enter the amount from line 55 here. • **All others:** If line 31 is $175,000 or less ($87,500 or less if married filing separately), multiply line 31 by 26% (.26). Otherwise, multiply line 31 by 28% (.28) and subtract $3,500 ($1,750 if married filing separately) from the result.	**32**	
33	Alternative minimum tax foreign tax credit (see page 9 of the instructions)	**33**	
34	Tentative minimum tax. Subtract line 33 from line 32	**34**	
35	Tax from Form 1040, line 44 (minus any tax from Form 4972 and any foreign tax credit from Form 1040, line 47). If you used Schedule J to figure your tax, the amount from line 44 of Form 1040 must be refigured without using Schedule J (see page 11 of the instructions)	**35**	
36	**AMT.** Subtract line 35 from line 34. If zero or less, enter -0-. Enter here and on Form 1040, line 45	**36**	

For Paperwork Reduction Act Notice, see page 12 of the instructions.   Cat. No. 13600G   Form **6251** (2008)

B-12   **Forms for Tax Credits**

Form **1116**

Department of the Treasury
Internal Revenue Service   (99)

Foreign Tax Credit

(Individual, Estate, or Trust)

▶ **Attach to Form 1040, 1040NR, 1041, or 990-T.**
▶ **See separate instructions.**

OMB No. 1545-0121

20**08**

Attachment
Sequence No. **19**

Name	Identifying number as shown on page 1 of your tax return

Use a separate Form 1116 for each category of income listed below. See **Categories of Income** beginning on page 3 of the instructions. Check only one box on each Form 1116. Report all amounts in U.S. dollars except where specified in Part II below.

a ☐ Passive category income   c ☐ Section 901(j) income   e ☐ Lump-sum distributions

b ☐ General category income   d ☐ Certain income re-sourced by treaty

f Resident of (name of country) ▶

Note: *If you paid taxes to only one foreign country or U.S. possession, use column A in Part I and line A in Part II. If you paid taxes to* **more than one** *foreign country or U.S. possession, use a separate column and line for each country or possession.*

Part I   **Taxable Income or Loss From Sources Outside the United States (for Category Checked Above)**

	Foreign Country or U.S. Possession			Total
	A	**B**	**C**	(Add cols. A, B, and C.)
g Enter the name of the foreign country or U.S. possession . . . . ▶				
1a Gross income from sources within country shown above and of the type checked above (see page 13 of the instructions): ----------------				

-------------------------------------				**1a**
b Check if line 1a is compensation for personal services as an employee, your total compensation from all sources is $250,000 or more, and you used an alternative basis to determine its source (see instructions) ▶ ☐				
Deductions and losses (*Caution: See pages 13 and 14 of the instructions*):				
2 Expenses **definitely related** to the income on line 1a (attach statement)				
3 Pro rata share of other deductions **not definitely related**:				
a Certain itemized deductions or standard deduction (see instructions)				
b Other deductions (attach statement) . . .				
c Add lines 3a and 3b				
d Gross foreign source income (see instructions) .				
e Gross income from all sources (see instructions)				
f Divide line 3d by line 3e (see instructions) .				
g Multiply line 3c by line 3f				
4 Pro rata share of interest expense (see instructions):				
a Home mortgage interest (use worksheet on page 14 of the instructions)				
b Other interest expense				
5 Losses from foreign sources				
6 Add lines 2, 3g, 4a, 4b, and 5				**6**
7 Subtract line 6 from line 1a. Enter the result here and on line 14, page 2 . . . . ▶			**7**	

Part II   **Foreign Taxes Paid or Accrued** (see page 14 of the instructions)

Country	Credit is claimed for taxes (you must check one)		Foreign taxes paid or accrued								
			In foreign currency				In U.S. dollars				
	(h) ☐ Paid	**(j)** Date paid or accrued	Taxes withheld at source on:			**(n)** Other foreign taxes paid or accrued	Taxes withheld at source on:			**(r)** Other foreign taxes paid or accrued	**(s)** Total foreign taxes paid or accrued (add cols. (o) through (r))
	(i) ☐ Accrued		**(k)** Dividends	**(l)** Rents and royalties	**(m)** Interest		**(o)** Dividends	**(p)** Rents and royalties	**(q)** Interest		
A											
B											
C											
8 Add lines A through C, column (s). Enter the total here and on line 9, page 2 . . . . ▶								**8**			

For Paperwork Reduction Act Notice, see page 19 of the instructions.   Cat. No. 11440U   Form **1116** (2008)

Form **2441**

Department of the Treasury
Internal Revenue Service (99)

Child and Dependent Care Expenses

▶ Attach to Form 1040 or Form 1040NR.

▶ See separate instructions.

OMB No. 1545-0074

2008

Attachment
Sequence No. **21**

Name(s) shown on return

Your social security number

Part I   Persons or Organizations Who Provided the Care—You **must** complete this part.
(If you have more than two care providers, see the instructions.)

1	**(a)** Care provider's name	**(b)** Address (number, street, apt. no., city, state, and ZIP code)	**(c)** Identifying number (SSN or EIN)	**(d)** Amount paid (see instructions)

Did you receive **dependent care benefits?**

No ⟶ Complete only Part II below.

Yes ⟶ Complete Part III on the back next.

Caution. If the care was provided in your home, you may owe employment taxes. See the instructions for Form 1040, line 60, or Form 1040NR, line 56.

Part II   Credit for Child and Dependent Care Expenses

2   Information about your **qualifying person(s).** If you have more than two qualifying persons, see the instructions.

(a) Qualifying person's name		**(b)** Qualifying person's social security number	**(c) Qualified expenses** you incurred and paid in 2008 for the person listed in column (a)
First	Last		

3	Add the amounts in column (c) of line 2. **Do not** enter more than $3,000 for one qualifying person or $6,000 for two or more persons. If you completed Part III, enter the amount from line 35	**3**	
4	Enter your **earned income.** See instructions	**4**	
5	If married filing jointly, enter your spouse's earned income (if your spouse was a student or was disabled, see the instructions); **all others,** enter the amount from line 4 . .	**5**	
6	Enter the **smallest** of line 3, 4, or 5	**6**	
7	Enter the amount from Form 1040, line 38, or Form 1040NR, line 36	**7**		

8   Enter on line 8 the decimal amount shown below that applies to the amount on line 7

If line 7 is:			If line 7 is:		
Over	**But not over**	**Decimal amount is**	**Over**	**But not over**	**Decimal amount is**
$0—15,000		.35	$29,000—31,000		.27
15,000—17,000		.34	31,000—33,000		.26
17,000—19,000		.33	33,000—35,000		.25
19,000—21,000		.32	35,000—37,000		.24
21,000—23,000		.31	37,000—39,000		.23
23,000—25,000		.30	39,000—41,000		.22
25,000—27,000		.29	41,000—43,000		.21
27,000—29,000		.28	43,000—No limit		.20

8 ✕ .

9	Multiply line 6 by the decimal amount on line 8. If you paid 2007 expenses in 2008, see the instructions	**9**	
10	Enter the amount from Form 1040, line 46, or Form 1040NR, line 43	**10**	
11	Enter the amount from Form 1040, line 47, or Form 1040NR, line 44	**11**	
12	Subtract line 11 from line 10. If zero or less, **stop.** You cannot take the credit . . .	**12**	
13	**Credit for child and dependent care expenses.** Enter the **smaller** of line 9 or line 12 here and on Form 1040, line 48, or Form 1040NR, line 45	**13**	

For Paperwork Reduction Act Notice, see page 4 of the instructions.   Cat. No. 11862M   Form **2441** (2008)

Part III Dependent Care Benefits

14 Enter the total amount of **dependent care benefits** you received in 2008. Amounts you received as an employee should be shown in box 10 of your Form(s) W-2. **Do not** include amounts reported as wages in box 1 of Form(s) W-2. If you were self-employed or a partner, include amounts you received under a dependent care assistance program from your sole proprietorship or partnership . . . . | **14**

15 Enter the amount, if any, you carried over from 2007 and used in 2008 during the grace period. See instructions . . . . | **15**

16 Enter the amount, if any, you forfeited or carried forward to 2009. See instructions . | **16** ( )

17 Combine lines 14 through 16. See instructions . . . . | **17**

18 Enter the total amount of **qualified expenses** incurred in 2008 for the care of the **qualifying person(s)** . | **18**

19 Enter the **smaller** of line 17 or 18 . . . . . . | **19**

20 Enter your **earned income.** See instructions . . | **20**

21 Enter the amount shown below that applies to you.

  • If married filing jointly, enter your spouse's earned income (if your spouse was a student or was disabled, see the instructions for line 5).

  • If married filing separately, see the instructions for the amount to enter.

  • All others, enter the amount from line 20. | **21**

22 Enter the **smallest** of line 19, 20, or 21 . . . . | **22**

23 Enter the amount from line 14 that you received from your sole proprietorship or partnership. If you did not receive any such amounts, enter -0- . . . . | **23**

24 Subtract line 23 from line 17 . . . . | **24**

25 Enter $5,000 ($2,500 if married filing separately **and** you were required to enter your spouse's earned income on line 21) . . . . | **25**

26 **Deductible benefits.** Enter the **smallest** of line 22, 23, or 25. Also, include this amount on the appropriate line(s) of your return. See instructions . . . . | **26**

27 Enter the **smaller** of line 22 or 25 . . . . . . | **27**

28 Enter the amount from line 26 . . . . | **28**

29 **Excluded benefits.** Subtract line 28 from line 27. If zero or less, enter -0- . . . . | **29**

30 **Taxable benefits.** Subtract line 29 from line 24. If zero or less, enter -0-. Also, include this amount on Form 1040, line 7, or Form 1040NR, line 8. On the dotted line next to Form 1040, line 7, or Form 1040NR, line 8, enter "DCB". . . . . | **30**

To claim the child and dependent care
credit, complete lines 31 through 35 below.

31 Enter $3,000 ($6,000 if two or more qualifying persons) . . . . | **31**

32 Add lines 26 and 29 . . . . | **32**

33 Subtract line 32 from line 31. If zero or less, **stop.** You cannot take the credit. **Exception.** If you paid 2007 expenses in 2008, see the instructions for line 9 . . . | **33**

34 Complete line 2 on the front of this form. **Do not** include in column (c) any benefits shown on line 32 above. Then, add the amounts in column (c) and enter the total here . . . | **34**

35 Enter the **smaller** of line 33 or 34. Also, enter this amount on line 3 on the front of this form and complete lines 4 through 13 . . . . | **35**

Form **2441** (2008)

Form **3468**
(Rev. December 2006)
Department of the Treasury
Internal Revenue Service (99)

Investment Credit

▶ Attach to your tax return. See instructions.

OMB No. 1545-0155

Attachment
Sequence No. **52**

Name(s) shown on return

Identifying number

1 Rehabilitation credit (see instructions for requirements that must be met):

a Check this box if you are electing under section 47(d)(5) to take your qualified rehabilitation expenditures into account for the tax year in which paid (or, for self-rehabilitated property, when capitalized). See instructions. **Note:** *This election applies to the current tax year and to all later tax years. You may not revoke this election without IRS consent* . . . ▶ ☐

b Enter the date on which the 24- or 60-month measuring period begins ___/___/___ and ends ___/___/___

c Enter the adjusted basis of the building as of the beginning date above (or the first day of your holding period, if later) . . . . $_____

d Enter the amount of the qualified rehabilitation expenditures incurred, or treated as incurred, during the period on line 1b above . . . $_____

Enter the amount of qualified rehabilitation expenditures and multiply by the percentage shown:

e Pre-1936 buildings located in the Gulf Opportunity Zone . $_____ × 13% (.13) | **1e**
f Other pre-1936 buildings . . . . $_____ × 10% (.10) | **1f**
g Certified historic structures located in the Gulf Opportunity Zone . $_____ × 26% (.26) | **1g**
h Other certified historic structures . . . . $_____ × 20% (.20) | **1h**

For properties identified on lines 1g or 1h, complete lines 1i and 1j

i Enter the assigned NPS project number or the pass-through entity's employer identification number (see instructions) . . . . . _____

j Enter the date that the NPS approved the Request for Certification of Completed Work (see instructions) . . . . _____/___/___

k Rehabilitation credit from an electing large partnership (Schedule K-1 (Form 1065-B), box 9) . | **1k**

2 Energy credit:

a Basis of property using geothermal energy placed in service during the tax year (see instructions) $_____ × 10% (.10) | **2a**

b Basis of property using solar illumination or solar energy placed in service during the tax year (see instructions) $_____ × 30% (.30) | **2b**

Qualified fuel cell property (see instructions):

c Basis of property installed during the tax year $_____ × 30% (.30) | **2c**

d Kilowatt capacity of property in **c** above . . ▶ _____ × $1,000 | **2d**

e Enter the lesser of line 2c or 2d . . . . | **2e**

Qualified microturbine property (see instructions):

f Basis of property installed during the tax year $_____ × 10% (.10) | **2f**

g Kilowatt capacity of property in **f** above . . ▶ _____ × $200 | **2g**

h Enter the lesser of line 2f or 2g . . . . | **2h**

i Total. Add lines 2a, 2b, 2e, and 2h . . . . | **2i**

3 Qualifying advanced coal project credit (see instructions):

a Basis of qualified investment in integrated gasification combined cycle property placed in service during the tax year $_____ × 20% (.20) | **3a**

b Basis of qualified investment in property other than in **a** above placed in service during the tax year ▶ $_____ × 15% (.15) | **3b**

c Total. Add lines 3a and 3b . . . . | **3c**

4 Qualifying gasification project credit (see instructions). Basis of qualified investment in property placed in service during the tax year . . . . . ▶ $_____ × 20% (.20) | **4**

5 Credit from cooperatives. Enter the unused investment credit from cooperatives . . . . | **5**

6 Add lines 1e through 1h, 1k, 2i, 3c, 4, and 5. Report this amount on the applicable line of Form 3800 (e.g., line 1a of the 2006 Form 3800) . . . . | **6**

For Paperwork Reduction Act Notice, see instructions. Cat. No. 12276E Form **3468** (Rev. 12-2006)

Form **3800**

Department of the Treasury
Internal Revenue Service (99)

General Business Credit

▶ See separate instructions.
▶ Attach to your tax return.

OMB No. 1545-0895

2008

Attachment
Sequence No. **22**

Name(s) shown on return

Identifying number

Part I   Current Year Credit

Important: You may not be required to complete and file a separate credit form (shown in parentheses below) to claim the credit. For details, see the instructions.

1a Investment credit (Form 3468, Part II only) (attach Form 3468)	**1a**	
b Welfare-to-work credit (Form 8861)	**1b**	
c Credit for increasing research activities (Form 6765)	**1c**	
d Low-income housing credit (Form 8586, Part I only) (enter EIN if claiming this credit from a pass-through entity: ____ - _____)	**1d**	
e Disabled access credit (Form 8826) (do not enter more than $5,000)	**1e**	
f Renewable electricity production credit (Form 8835, Part I only)	**1f**	
g Indian employment credit (Form 8845)	**1g**	
h Orphan drug credit (Form 8820)	**1h**	
i New markets credit (Form 8874) (enter EIN if claiming this credit from a pass-through entity: ____ - _____)	**1i**	
j Credit for small employer pension plan startup costs (Form 8881) (do not enter more than $500)	**1j**	
k Credit for employer-provided child care facilities and services (Form 8882) (enter EIN if claiming this credit from a pass-through entity: ____ - _____)	**1k**	
l Biodiesel and renewable diesel fuels credit (attach Form 8864)	**1l**	
m Low sulfur diesel fuel production credit (Form 8896)	**1m**	
n Distilled spirits credit (Form 8906)	**1n**	
o Nonconventional source fuel credit (Form 8907)	**1o**	
p Energy efficient home credit (Form 8908)	**1p**	
q Energy efficient appliance credit (Form 8909)	**1q**	
r Alternative motor vehicle credit (Form 8910) (enter EIN if claiming this credit from a pass-through entity: ____ - _____)	**1r**	
s Alternative fuel vehicle refueling property credit (Form 8911)	**1s**	
t Credits for affected Midwestern disaster area employers (Form 5884-A)	**1t**	
u Mine rescue team training credit (Form 8923)	**1u**	
v Agricultural chemicals security credit (Form 8931)	**1v**	
w Credit for employer differential wage payments (Form 8932)	**1w**	
x Carbon dioxide sequestration credit (Form 8933)	**1x**	
y Credit for contributions to selected community development corporations (Form 8847) . .	**1y**	
z General credits from an electing large partnership (Schedule K-1 (Form 1065-B))	**1z**	
2 Add lines 1a through 1z	**2**	
3 Passive activity credits included on line 2 (see instructions)	**3**	
4 Subtract line 3 from line 2	**4**	
5 Passive activity credits allowed for 2008 (see instructions)	**5**	
6 Carryforward of general business credit to 2008. See instructions for the schedule to attach .	**6**	
7 Carryback of general business credit from 2009 (see instructions)	**7**	
8 **Current year credit.** Add lines 4 through 7	**8**	

For Paperwork Reduction Act Notice, see separate instructions.   Cat. No. 12392F   Form **3800** (2008)

Part II	**Allowable Credit**

9 Regular tax before credits:
- Individuals. Enter the amount from Form 1040, line 44 or Form 1040NR, line 41 .
- Corporations. Enter the amount from Form 1120, Schedule J, line 2; or the applicable line of your return . . . .
- Estates and trusts. Enter the sum of the amounts from Form 1041, Schedule G, lines 1a and 1b, or the amount from the applicable line of your return . . .

| | **9** | |

10 Alternative minimum tax:
- Individuals. Enter the amount from Form 6251, line 36 . . . . . .
- Corporations. Enter the amount from Form 4626, line 14 . . . . .
- Estates and trusts. Enter the amount from Schedule I (Form 1041), line 56

| | **10** | |

11 Add lines 9 and 10 . . . .

| | **11** | |

12a Foreign tax credit . . . . | **12a** |
  b Personal credits from Form 1040, lines 48 through 54 (or Form 1040NR, lines 45 through 49) . . . . | **12b** |
  c Credit from Form 8834 . . . . | **12c** |
  d Non-business alternative motor vehicle credit (Form 8910, line 18) | **12d** |
  e Non-business alternative fuel vehicle refueling property credit (Form 8911, line 19) . . . . | **12e** |
  f Add lines 12a through 12e . . . .

| | **12f** | |

13 **Net income tax.** Subtract line 12f from line 11. If zero, skip lines 14 through 17 and enter -0- on line 18a

| | **13** | |

14 **Net regular tax.** Subtract line 12f from line 9. If zero or less, enter -0- | **14** |

15 Enter 25% (.25) of the excess, if any, of line 14 over $25,000 (see instructions) . . . . | **15** |

16 Tentative minimum tax:
- Individuals. Enter the amount from Form 6251, line 34 . .
- Corporations. Enter the amount from Form 4626, line 12 .
- Estates and trusts. Enter the amount from Schedule I (Form 1041), line 54 . . . . | **16** |

17 Enter the greater of line 15 or line 16 . . . .

| | **17** | |

18a Subtract line 17 from line 13. If zero or less, enter -0- . . . .

| | **18a** | |

  b For a corporation electing to accelerate the research credit, enter the bonus depreciation amount attributable to the research credit. (see instructions) . . . .

| | **18b** | |

  c Add lines 18a and 18b . . . .

| | **18c** | |

19a Enter the **smaller** of line 8 or line 18c . . . .

| | **19a** | |

Individuals, estates, and trusts: See the instructions for line 19a if claiming the research credit.
C corporations: See the line 19a instructions if there has been an ownership change, acquisition, or reorganization.

  b Enter the smaller of line 8 or line 18a. If you made an entry on line 18b, go to line 19c; otherwise, skip line 19c . . . .

| | **19b** | |

  c Subtract line 19b from line 19a. This is the refundable amount for a corporation electing to accelerate the research credit. Include this amount on line 32g of Form 1120 (or the applicable line of your return) . . . .

| | **19c** | |

B-13   Other Tax Forms

Form **2106**

Department of the Treasury
Internal Revenue Service   (99)

Employee Business Expenses

▶ See separate instructions.

▶ Attach to Form 1040 or Form 1040NR.

OMB No. 1545-0074

2008

Attachment
Sequence No. **129**

Your name	Occupation in which you incurred expenses	Social security number

---

Part I   **Employee Business Expenses and Reimbursements**

Step 1   Enter Your Expenses

		Column A — Other Than Meals and Entertainment		Column B — Meals and Entertainment
1	Vehicle expense from line 22c or line 29. (Rural mail carriers: See instructions.)	**1**		
2	Parking fees, tolls, and transportation, including train, bus, etc., that **did not** involve overnight travel or commuting to and from work .	**2**		
3	Travel expense while away from home overnight, including lodging, airplane, car rental, etc. **Do not** include meals and entertainment	**3**		
4	Business expenses not included on lines 1 through 3. **Do not** include meals and entertainment.	**4**		
5	Meals and entertainment expenses (see instructions)	**5**		
6	**Total expenses.** In Column A, add lines 1 through 4 and enter the result. In Column B, enter the amount from line 5	**6**		

Note: *If you were not reimbursed for any expenses in Step 1, skip line 7 and enter the amount from line 6 on line 8.*

Step 2   Enter Reimbursements Received From Your Employer for Expenses Listed in Step 1

7	Enter reimbursements received from your employer that were **not** reported to you in box 1 of Form W-2. Include any reimbursements reported under code "L" in box 12 of your Form W-2 (see instructions)	**7**	

Step 3   Figure Expenses To Deduct on Schedule A (Form 1040 or Form 1040NR)

8	Subtract line 7 from line 6. If zero or less, enter -0-. However, if line 7 is greater than line 6 in Column A, report the excess as income on Form 1040, line 7 (or on Form 1040NR, line 8) . .	**8**	
	Note: *If **both columns** of line 8 are zero, you cannot deduct employee business expenses. Stop here and attach Form 2106 to your return.*		
9	In Column A, enter the amount from line 8. In Column B, multiply line 8 by 50% (.50). (Employees subject to Department of Transportation (DOT) hours of service limits: Multiply meal expenses incurred while away from home on business by 80% (.80) instead of 50%. For details, see instructions.)	**9**	
10	Add the amounts on line 9 of both columns and enter the total here. **Also, enter the total on Schedule A (Form 1040), line 21** (or on **Schedule A (Form 1040NR), line 9**). (Reservists, qualified performing artists, fee-basis state or local government officials, and individuals with disabilities: See the instructions for special rules on where to enter the total.) . . . ▶	**10**	

For Paperwork Reduction Act Notice, see instructions.   Cat. No. 11700N   Form **2106** (2008)

Part II	**Vehicle Expenses**			

Section A—General Information (You must complete this section if you are claiming vehicle expenses.)

			(a) Vehicle 1	**(b)** Vehicle 2
11	Enter the date the vehicle was placed in service	11	/ /	/ /
12	Total miles the vehicle was driven during 2008	12	miles	miles
13	Business miles included on line 12	13	miles	miles
14	Percent of business use. Divide line 13 by line 12	14	%	%
15	Average daily roundtrip commuting distance	15	miles	miles
16	Commuting miles included on line 12	16	miles	miles
17	Other miles. Add lines 13 and 16 and subtract the total from line 12. .	17	miles	miles
18	Was your vehicle available for personal use during off-duty hours?		☐ Yes ☐ No	
19	Do you (or your spouse) have another vehicle available for personal use?		☐ Yes ☐ No	
20	Do you have evidence to support your deduction?		☐ Yes ☐ No	
21	If "Yes," is the evidence written?		☐ Yes ☐ No	

Section B—Standard Mileage Rate (See the instructions for Part II to find out whether to complete this section or Section C.)

22a	Multiply business miles driven **before** July 1, 2008, by 50.5¢ (.505) .	**22a**	
b	Multiply business miles driven **after** June 30, 2008, by 58.5¢ (.585) .	**22b**	
c	Add lines 22a and 22b. Enter the result here and on line 1	**22c**	

Section C—Actual Expenses

			(a) Vehicle 1	**(b)** Vehicle 2
23	Gasoline, oil, repairs, vehicle insurance, etc.	23		
24a	Vehicle rentals	24a		
b	Inclusion amount (see instructions) .	24b		
c	Subtract line 24b from line 24a .	24c		
25	Value of employer-provided vehicle (applies only if 100% of annual lease value was included on Form W-2—see instructions)	25		
26	Add lines 23, 24c, and 25 . . .	26		
27	Multiply line 26 by the percentage on line 14	27		
28	Depreciation (see instructions) .	28		
29	Add lines 27 and 28. Enter total here and on line 1	29		

Section D—Depreciation of Vehicles (Use this section only if you owned the vehicle and are completing Section C for the vehicle.)

			(a) Vehicle 1	**(b)** Vehicle 2
30	Enter cost or other basis (see instructions)	30		
31	Enter section 179 deduction and special allowance (see instructions)	31		
32	Multiply line 30 by line 14 (see instructions if you claimed the section 179 deduction or special allowance)	32		
33	Enter depreciation method and percentage (see instructions) .	33		
34	Multiply line 32 by the percentage on line 33 (see instructions) . . .	34		
35	Add lines 31 and 34	35		
36	Enter the applicable limit explained in the line 36 instructions	36		
37	Multiply line 36 by the percentage on line 14	37		
38	Enter the **smaller** of line 35 or line 37. If you skipped lines 36 and 37, enter the amount from line 35. Also enter this amount on line 28 above ..	38		

Form **2120**
(Rev. October 2005)

Department of the Treasury
Internal Revenue Service

Multiple Support Declaration

▶ **Attach to Form 1040 or Form 1040A.**

OMB No. 1545-0074

Attachment
Sequence No. **114**

Name(s) shown on return

Your social security number

During the calendar year _____ , the eligible persons listed below each paid over 10% of the support of:

_____
Name of your qualifying relative

I have a signed statement from each eligible person waiving his or her right to claim this person as a dependent for any tax year that began in the above calendar year.

Eligible person's name

Social security number

Address (number, street, apt. no., city, state, and ZIP code)

Eligible person's name

Social security number

Address (number, street, apt. no., city, state, and ZIP code)

Eligible person's name

Social security number

Address (number, street, apt. no., city, state, and ZIP code)

Eligible person's name

Social security number

Address (number, street, apt. no., city, state, and ZIP code)

Instructions

What's New

The rules for multiple support agreements still apply to claiming an exemption for a qualifying relative, but they no longer apply to claiming an exemption for a qualifying child. For the definitions of "qualifying relative" and "qualifying child," see your tax return instruction booklet.

Purpose of Form

Use Form 2120 to:

• Identify each other eligible person (see below) who paid over 10% of the support of your qualifying relative whom you are claiming as a dependent, and

• Indicate that you have a signed statement from each other eligible person waiving his or her right to claim that person as a dependent.

An eligible person is someone who could have claimed a person as a dependent except that he or she did not pay over half of that person's support.

If there are more than four other eligible persons, attach a statement to your return with the required information.

Claiming a Qualifying Relative

Generally, to claim a person as a qualifying relative, you must pay over half of that person's support. However, even if you did not meet this support test, you may be able to claim him or her as a dependent if all five of the following apply.

1. You and one or more other eligible person(s) (see above) together paid over half of that person's support.

2. You paid over 10% of the support.

3. No one alone paid over half of that person's support.

4. The other dependency tests are met. See *Step 4, Is Your Qualifying Relative Your Dependent?* in the Form 1040 or Form 1040A instructions.

5. Each other eligible person who paid over 10% of the support agrees not to claim that person as a dependent by giving you a signed statement. See *Signed Statement* on this page.

Note. To find out what is included in support, see Pub. 501, Exemptions, Standard Deduction, and Filing Information.

Signed Statement

You must have received, from each other eligible person listed above, a signed statement waiving his or her right to claim the person as a dependent for the calendar year indicated on this form. The statement must include:

• The calendar year the waiver applies to,

• The name of your qualifying relative the eligible person helped to support, and

• The eligible person's name, address, and social security number.

Do not file the signed statement with your return. But you must keep it for your records and be prepared to furnish it and any other information necessary to show that you qualify to claim the person as your dependent.

Additional Information

See Pub. 501 for details.

Paperwork Reduction Act Notice. We ask for the information on this form to carry out the Internal Revenue laws of the United States. You are required to give us the information. We need it to ensure that you are complying with these laws and to allow us to figure and collect the right amount of tax.

You are not required to provide the information requested on a form that is subject to the Paperwork Reduction Act unless the form displays a valid OMB control number. Books or records relating to a form or its instructions must be retained as long as their contents may become material in the administration of any Internal Revenue law. Generally, tax returns and return information are confidential, as required by Internal Revenue Code section 6103.

The average time and expenses required to complete and file this form will vary depending on individual circumstances. For the estimated averages, see the instructions for your income tax return.

If you have suggestions for making this form simpler, we would be happy to hear from you. See the instructions for your income tax return.

Cat. No. 11712F

Form **2120** (Rev. 10-2005)

Form **3903**

Department of the Treasury
Internal Revenue Service   (99)

Moving Expenses

▶ **Attach to Form 1040 or Form 1040NR.**

OMB No. 1545-0074

2008

Attachment
Sequence No. **62**

Name(s) shown on return

Your social security number

Before you begin: √ See the **Distance Test** and **Time Test** in the instructions to find out if you can deduct your moving expenses.

   √ See **Members of the Armed Forces** on the back, if applicable.

1 Transportation and storage of household goods and personal effects (see instructions) .	**1**	
2 Travel (including lodging) from your old home to your new home (see instructions). **Do not** include the cost of meals	**2**	
3 Add lines 1 and 2	**3**	
4 Enter the total amount your employer paid you for the expenses listed on lines 1 and 2 that is **not** included in box 1 of your Form W-2 (wages). This amount should be shown in box 12 of your Form W-2 with code **P**	**4**	
5 Is line 3 **more than** line 4?		
☐ **No.** You **cannot** deduct your moving expenses. If line 3 is less than line 4, subtract line 3 from line 4 and include the result on Form 1040, line 7, or Form 1040NR, line 8.		
☐ **Yes.** Subtract line 4 from line 3. Enter the result here and on Form 1040, line 26, or Form 1040NR, line 26. This is your **moving expense deduction**	**5**	

General Instructions

What's New

For 2008, the standard mileage rate for using your vehicle to move to a new home is 19 cents a mile (27 cents a mile after June 30, 2008).

Purpose of Form

Use Form 3903 to figure your moving expense deduction for a move related to the start of work at a new principal place of work (workplace). If the new workplace is outside the United States or its possessions, you must be a U.S. citizen or resident alien to deduct your expenses.

If you qualify to deduct expenses for more than one move, use a separate Form 3903 for each move.

For more details, see Pub. 521, Moving Expenses.

Moving Expenses You Can Deduct

You can deduct the reasonable expenses of moving your household goods and personal effects and of traveling from your old home to your new home. Reasonable expenses can include the cost of lodging (but not meals) while traveling to your new home. You cannot deduct the cost of sightseeing trips.

Who Can Deduct Moving Expenses

If you move to a new home because of a new principal workplace, you may be able to deduct your moving expenses whether you are self-employed or an employee. But you must meet both the distance test and time test that follow.

 Members of the Armed Forces may not have to meet the distance and time tests. See instructions on the back.

Distance Test

Your new principal workplace must be at least 50 miles farther from your old home than your old workplace was. For example, if your old workplace was 3 miles from your old home, your new workplace must be at least 53 miles from that home. If you did not have an old workplace, your new workplace must be at least 50 miles from your old home. The distance between the two points is the shortest of the more commonly traveled routes between them.

 To see if you meet the distance test, you can use the worksheet below.

Distance Test Worksheet

Keep a Copy for Your Records

1. Number of miles from your **old home** to your **new workplace**	**1.** _____ miles
2. Number of miles from your **old home** to your **old workplace**	**2.** _____ miles
3. Subtract line 2 from line 1. If zero or less, enter -0-.	**3.** _____ miles

Is line 3 at least 50 miles?

☐ **Yes.** You meet this test.
☐ **No.** You do not meet this test. You **cannot** deduct your moving expenses. **Do not** complete Form 3903.

For Paperwork Reduction Act Notice, see back of form.   Cat. No. 12490K   Form **3903** (2008)

Form **4562**

Department of the Treasury
Internal Revenue Service (99)

Depreciation and Amortization

(Including Information on Listed Property)

▶ See separate instructions. ▶ Attach to your tax return.

OMB No. 1545-0172

2008

Attachment
Sequence No. 67

Name(s) shown on return	Business or activity to which this form relates	Identifying number

Part I **Election To Expense Certain Property Under Section 179**
Note: *If you have any listed property, complete Part V before you complete Part I.*

1	Maximum amount. See the instructions for a higher limit for certain businesses	1	$250,000
2	Total cost of section 179 property placed in service (see instructions)	2	
3	Threshold cost of section 179 property before reduction in limitation (see instructions)	3	$800,000
4	Reduction in limitation. Subtract line 3 from line 2. If zero or less, enter -0-	4	
5	Dollar limitation for tax year. Subtract line 4 from line 1. If zero or less, enter -0-. If married filing separately, see instructions	5	

(a) Description of property	(b) Cost (business use only)	(c) Elected cost	
6			

7	Listed property. Enter the amount from line 29	7	
8	Total elected cost of section 179 property. Add amounts in column (c), lines 6 and 7	8	
9	Tentative deduction. Enter the **smaller** of line 5 or line 8	9	
10	Carryover of disallowed deduction from line 13 of your 2007 Form 4562	10	
11	Business income limitation. Enter the smaller of business income (not less than zero) or line 5 (see instructions)	11	
12	Section 179 expense deduction. Add lines 9 and 10, but do not enter more than line 11	12	
13	Carryover of disallowed deduction to 2009. Add lines 9 and 10, less line 12 ▶	13	

Note: *Do not use Part II or Part III below for listed property. Instead, use Part V.*

Part II **Special Depreciation Allowance and Other Depreciation (Do not** include listed property.) (See instructions.)

14	Special depreciation allowance for qualified property (other than listed property) placed in service during the tax year (see instructions)	14	
15	Property subject to section 168(f)(1) election	15	
16	Other depreciation (including ACRS)	16	

Part III **MACRS Depreciation (Do not** include listed property.) (See instructions.)

Section A

17	MACRS deductions for assets placed in service in tax years beginning before 2008	17	
18	If you are electing to group any assets placed in service during the tax year into one or more general asset accounts, check here ▶ ☐		

Section B—Assets Placed in Service During 2008 Tax Year Using the General Depreciation System

(a) Classification of property	(b) Month and year placed in service	(c) Basis for depreciation (business/investment use only—see instructions)	(d) Recovery period	(e) Convention	(f) Method	(g) Depreciation deduction
19a 3-year property						
b 5-year property						
c 7-year property						
d 10-year property						
e 15-year property						
f 20-year property						
g 25-year property			25 yrs.		S/L	
h Residential rental property			27.5 yrs.	MM	S/L	
			27.5 yrs.	MM	S/L	
i Nonresidential real property			39 yrs.	MM	S/L	
				MM	S/L	

Section C—Assets Placed in Service During 2008 Tax Year Using the Alternative Depreciation System

20a Class life					S/L	
b 12-year			12 yrs.		S/L	
c 40-year			40 yrs.	MM	S/L	

Part IV **Summary** (See instructions.)

21	Listed property. Enter amount from line 28	21	
22	**Total.** Add amounts from line 12, lines 14 through 17, lines 19 and 20 in column (g), and line 21. Enter here and on the appropriate lines of your return. Partnerships and S corporations—see instr.	22	
23	For assets shown above and placed in service during the current year, enter the portion of the basis attributable to section 263A costs .	23	

For Paperwork Reduction Act Notice, see separate instructions. Cat. No. 12906N Form **4562** (2008)

Form 4562 (2008)   Page **2**

Part V   **Listed Property** (Include automobiles, certain other vehicles, cellular telephones, certain computers, and property used for entertainment, recreation, or amusement.)

Note: *For any vehicle for which you are using the standard mileage rate or deducting lease expense, complete only 24a, 24b, columns (a) through (c) of Section A, all of Section B, and Section C if applicable.*

Section A—Depreciation and Other Information (Caution: *See the instructions for limits for passenger automobiles.***)**

24a Do you have evidence to support the business/investment use claimed? ☐ **Yes** ☐ **No**   **24b** If "Yes," is the evidence written? ☐ **Yes** ☐ **No**

(a) Type of property (list vehicles first)	(b) Date placed in service	(c) Business/ investment use percentage	(d) Cost or other basis	(e) Basis for depreciation (business/investment use only)	(f) Recovery period	(g) Method/ Convention	(h) Depreciation deduction	(i) Elected section 179 cost
25 Special depreciation allowance for qualified listed property placed in service during the tax year and used more than 50% in a qualified business use (see instructions) **25**								
26 Property used more than 50% in a qualified business use:								
		%						
		%						
		%						
27 Property used 50% or less in a qualified business use:								
		%				S/L –		
		%				S/L –		
		%				S/L –		
28 Add amounts in column (h), lines 25 through 27. Enter here and on line 21, page 1.				**28**				
29 Add amounts in column (i), line 26. Enter here and on line 7, page 1.							**29**	

Section B—Information on Use of Vehicles

Complete this section for vehicles used by a sole proprietor, partner, or other "more than 5% owner," or related person.

If you provided vehicles to your employees, first answer the questions in Section C to see if you meet an exception to completing this section for those vehicles.

		(a) Vehicle 1		(b) Vehicle 2		(c) Vehicle 3		(d) Vehicle 4		(e) Vehicle 5		(f) Vehicle 6	
30	Total business/investment miles driven during the year (**do not** include commuting miles)												
31	Total commuting miles driven during the year												
32	Total other personal (noncommuting) miles driven												
33	Total miles driven during the year. Add lines 30 through 32												
34	Was the vehicle available for personal use during off-duty hours? . . .	Yes	No	Yes	No	Yes	No	Yes	No	Yes	No	Yes	No
35	Was the vehicle used primarily by a more than 5% owner or related person?												
36	Is another vehicle available for personal use?												

Section C—Questions for Employers Who Provide Vehicles for Use by Their Employees

Answer these questions to determine if you meet an exception to completing Section B for vehicles used by employees who **are not** more than 5% owners or related persons (see instructions).

		Yes	No
37	Do you maintain a written policy statement that prohibits all personal use of vehicles, including commuting, by your employees?		
38	Do you maintain a written policy statement that prohibits personal use of vehicles, except commuting, by your employees? See the instructions for vehicles used by corporate officers, directors, or 1% or more owners		
39	Do you treat all use of vehicles by employees as personal use?		
40	Do you provide more than five vehicles to your employees, obtain information from your employees about the use of the vehicles, and retain the information received?		
41	Do you meet the requirements concerning qualified automobile demonstration use? (See instructions.)		

Note: *If your answer to 37, 38, 39, 40, or 41 is "Yes," do not complete Section B for the covered vehicles.*

Part VI   **Amortization**

(a) Description of costs	(b) Date amortization begins	(c) Amortizable amount	(d) Code section	(e) Amortization period or percentage	(f) Amortization for this year
42 Amortization of costs that begins during your 2008 tax year (see instructions):					
43 Amortization of costs that began before your 2008 tax year **43**					
44 **Total.** Add amounts in column (f). See the instructions for where to report. **44**					

Form **4562** (2008)

Form **4684**

Department of theTreasury
Internal Revenue Service

Casualties and Thefts

▶ See separate instructions.
▶ Attach to your tax return.
▶ **Use a separate Form 4684 for each casualty or theft.**

OMB No. 1545-0177

2008

Attachment
Sequence No. **26**

Name(s) shown on tax return | Identifying number

SECTION A—Personal Use Property (Use this section to report casualties and thefts of property **not** used in a trade or business or for income-producing purposes.)

1 Description of properties (show type, location, and date acquired for each property). Use a separate line for each property lost or damaged from the same casualty or theft.

Property **A** _____

Property **B** _____

Property **C** _____

Property **D** _____

		Properties			
		A	B	C	D
2 Cost or other basis of each property	**2**				
3 Insurance or other reimbursement (whether or not you filed a claim) (see instructions)	**3**				
Note: If line 2 is **more** than line 3, skip line 4.					
4 Gain from casualty or theft. If line 3 is **more** than line 2, enter the difference here and skip lines 5 through 9 for that column. See instructions if line 3 includes insurance or other reimbursement you did not claim, or you received payment for your loss in a later tax year	**4**				
5 Fair market value **before** casualty or theft	**5**				
6 Fair market value **after** casualty or theft	**6**				
7 Subtract line 6 from line 5	**7**				
8 Enter the **smaller** of line 2 or line 7	**8**				
9 Subtract line 3 from line 8. If zero or less, enter -0-	**9**				

10 Casualty or theft loss. Add the amounts on line 9 in columns A through D . . . . | **10** |

11 Enter the **smaller** of line 10 or $100. But if the loss arose in a Midwestern disaster area because of a specified major disaster, enter -0-. See the instructions for a list of specified major disasters . . . . | **11** |

12 Subtract line 11 from line 10 . . . . | **12** |

Caution: Use only one Form 4684 for lines 13 through 24.

13 Add the amounts on line 12 of all Forms 4684 . . . . | **13** |

14 Add the amounts on line 4 of all Forms 4684. . . . . | **14** |

15 • If line 14 is **more** than line 13, enter the difference here and on Schedule D. **Do not** complete the rest of this section (see instructions).
• If line 14 is **less** than line 13, enter -0- here and go to line 16.
• If line 14 is **equal** to line 13, enter -0- here. **Do not** complete the rest of this section. | **15** |

16 If line 14 is **less** than line 13, enter the difference . . . . | **16** |

17 Add the amounts on line 12 of all Forms 4684 on which you entered a loss attributable to a federally declared disaster . | **17** |

18a Is line 17 more than line 14?
☐ **Yes.** Enter the difference. If you are filing Schedule A (Form 1040), go to line 19. Otherwise, enter this amount on line 6 of the *Standard Deduction Worksheet–Line 40* in the Form 1040 instructions. Also, check the box on line 39c of Form 1040. If your standard deduction also includes the deduction for state or local real estate taxes, go to line 18b. Otherwise, do not complete the rest of Section A. Form 1040NR filers, see instructions.
☐ **No.** Enter -0-. If you claim the standard deduction, do not complete the rest of Section A. . . . . . | **18a** |

b If your standard deduction includes the deduction for state or local real estate taxes, check this box and do not complete the rest of Section A . . . . ▶ ☐

19 Subtract line 18a from line 16 . . . . | **19** |

20 Add the amounts on line 12 of all Forms 4684 on which you entered -0- on line 11 . . . . | **20** |

21 Is line 20 less than line 19?
☐ **No.** Enter the amount from line 16 on Schedule A (Form 1040), line 20, or Form 1040NR, Schedule A, line 8. Estates and trusts enter the amount from line 16 on the "Other deductions" line of your tax return. Do not complete the rest of Section A.
☐ **Yes.** Subtract line 20 from line 19 . . . . | **21** |

22 Enter 10% of your adjusted gross income from Form 1040, line 38, or Form 1040NR, line 36. Estates and trusts, see instructions | **22** |

23 Subtract line 22 from line 21. If zero or less, enter -0- . . . . | **23** |

24 Add lines 18a, 20, and 23. Also enter the result on Schedule A (Form 1040), line 20, or Form 1040NR, Schedule A, line 8. Estates and trusts, enter the result on the "Other deductions" line of your tax return . . . . | **24** |

For Paperwork Reduction Act Notice, see page 5 of the instructions. Cat. No. 129970 Form **4684** (2008)

Form 4684 (2008)   Attachment Sequence No. **26**   Page **2**

Name(s) shown on tax return. Do not enter name and identifying number if shown on other side.	Identifying number

SECTION B—Business and Income-Producing Property

Part I   Casualty or Theft Gain or Loss (Use a separate Part I for each casualty or theft.)

25 Description of properties (show type, location, and date acquired for each property). Use a separate line for each property lost or damaged from the same casualty or theft.

Property **A** _____

Property **B** _____

Property **C** _____

Property **D** _____

		Properties			
		A	**B**	**C**	**D**
26 Cost or adjusted basis of each property	**26**				
27 Insurance or other reimbursement (whether or not you filed a claim). See the instructions for line 3	**27**				
Note: If line 26 is **more** than line 27, skip line 28.					
28 Gain from casualty or theft. If line 27 is **more** than line 26, enter the difference here and on line 35 or line 40, column (c), except as provided in the instructions for line 39. Also, skip lines 29 through 33 for that column. See the instructions for line 4 if line 27 includes insurance or other reimbursement you did not claim, or you received payment for your loss in a later tax year.	**28**				
29 Fair market value **before** casualty or theft	**29**				
30 Fair market value **after** casualty or theft	**30**				
31 Subtract line 30 from line 29	**31**				
32 Enter the **smaller** of line 26 or line 31	**32**				
Note: If the property was totally destroyed by casualty or lost from theft, enter on line 32 the amount from line 26.					
33 Subtract line 27 from line 32. If zero or less, enter -0-	**33**				

34 Casualty or theft loss. Add the amounts on line 33. Enter the total here and on line 35 **or** line 40 (see instructions) . .   **34**

Part II   Summary of Gains and Losses (from separate Parts I)

(a) Identify casualty or theft	**(b)** Losses from casualties or thefts		**(c)** Gains from casualties or thefts includible in income
	(i) Trade, business, rental or royalty property	**(ii)** Income-producing and employee property	

Casualty or Theft of Property Held One Year or Less

35 _____	( )(	)	
	( )(	)	
36 Totals. Add the amounts on line 35 **36**	( )(	)	

37 Combine line 36, columns (b)(i) and (c). Enter the net gain or (loss) here and on Form 4797, line 14. If Form 4797 is not otherwise required, see instructions **37**

38 Enter the amount from line 36, column (b)(ii) here. Individuals, enter the amount from income-producing property on Schedule A (Form 1040), line 28, or Form 1040NR, Schedule A, line 16, and enter the amount from property used as an employee on Schedule A (Form 1040), line 23, or Form 1040NR, Schedule A, line 11. Estates and trusts, partnerships, and S corporations, see instructions **38**

Casualty or Theft of Property Held More Than One Year

39 Casualty or theft gains from Form 4797, line 32			**39**	
40 _____	( )(	)		
	( )(	)		
41 Total losses. Add amounts on line 40, columns (b)(i) and (b)(ii) **41**	( )(	)		

42 Total gains. Add lines 39 and 40, column (c) **42**

43 Add amounts on line 41, columns (b)(i) and (b)(ii) **43**

44 If the loss on line 43 is **more** than the gain on line 42:

  a Combine line 41, column (b)(i) and line 42, and enter the net gain or (loss) here. Partnerships (except electing large partnerships) and S corporations, see the note below. All others, enter this amount on Form 4797, line 14. If Form 4797 is not otherwise required, see instructions **44a**

  b Enter the amount from line 41, column (b)(ii) here. Individuals, enter the amount from income-producing property on Schedule A (Form 1040), line 28, or Form 1040NR, Schedule A, line 16, and enter the amount from property used as an employee on Schedule A (Form 1040), line 23, or Form 1040NR, Schedule A, line 11. Estates and trusts, enter on the "Other deductions" line of your tax return. Partnerships (except electing large partnerships) and S corporations, see the note below. Electing large partnerships, enter on Form 1065-B, Part II, line 11 . . . .   **44b**

45 If the loss on line 43 is **less** than or **equal** to the gain on line 42, combine lines 42 and 43 and enter here. Partnerships (except electing large partnerships), see the note below. All others, enter this amount on Form 4797, line 3 . . . .   **45**

Note: Partnerships, enter the amount from line 44a, 44b, or line 45 on Form 1065, Schedule K, line 11.
S corporations, enter the amount from line 44a or 44b on Form 1120S, Schedule K, line 10.

Form **4684** (2008)

Form **4797**

Department of the Treasury
Internal Revenue Service   (99)

Sales of Business Property
(Also Involuntary Conversions and Recapture Amounts
Under Sections 179 and 280F(b)(2))
▶ Attach to your tax return.   ▶ See separate instructions.

OMB No. 1545-0184

20**08**

Attachment
Sequence No. **27**

Name(s) shown on return

Identifying number

| 1 | Enter the gross proceeds from sales or exchanges reported to you for 2008 on Form(s) 1099-B or 1099-S (or substitute statement) that you are including on line 2, 10, or 20 (see instructions) . . . . | 1 | |

Part I Sales or Exchanges of Property Used in a Trade or Business and Involuntary Conversions From Other Than Casualty or Theft—Most Property Held More Than 1 Year (see instructions)

2	(a) Description of property	(b) Date acquired (mo., day, yr.)	(c) Date sold (mo., day, yr.)	(d) Gross sales price	(e) Depreciation allowed or allowable since acquisition	(f) Cost or other basis, plus improvements and expense of sale	(g) Gain or (loss) Subtract (f) from the sum of (d) and (e)

3	Gain, if any, from Form 4684, line 45	3	
4	Section 1231 gain from installment sales from Form 6252, line 26 or 37	4	
5	Section 1231 gain or (loss) from like-kind exchanges from Form 8824	5	
6	Gain, if any, from line 32, from other than casualty or theft.	6	
7	Combine lines 2 through 6. Enter the gain or (loss) here and on the appropriate line as follows:	7	

Partnerships (except electing large partnerships) and S corporations. Report the gain or (loss) following the instructions for Form 1065, Schedule K, line 10, or Form 1120S, Schedule K, line 9. Skip lines 8, 9, 11, and 12 below.

Individuals, partners, S corporation shareholders, and all others. If line 7 is zero or a loss, enter the amount from line 7 on line 11 below and skip lines 8 and 9. If line 7 is a gain and you did not have any prior year section 1231 losses, or they were recaptured in an earlier year, enter the gain from line 7 as a long-term capital gain on the Schedule D filed with your return and skip lines 8, 9, 11, and 12 below.

| 8 | Nonrecaptured net section 1231 losses from prior years (see instructions) . . . . | 8 | |
| 9 | Subtract line 8 from line 7. If zero or less, enter -0-. If line 9 is zero, enter the gain from line 7 on line 12 below. If line 9 is more than zero, enter the amount from line 8 on line 12 below and enter the gain from line 9 as a long-term capital gain on the Schedule D filed with your return (see instructions) . . . . | 9 | |

Part II Ordinary Gains and Losses (see instructions)

10	Ordinary gains and losses not included on lines 11 through 16 (include property held 1 year or less):						

11	Loss, if any, from line 7	11 (	)
12	Gain, if any, from line 7 or amount from line 8, if applicable	12	
13	Gain, if any, from line 31	13	
14	Net gain or (loss) from Form 4684, lines 37 and 44a	14	
15	Ordinary gain from installment sales from Form 6252, line 25 or 36	15	
16	Ordinary gain or (loss) from like-kind exchanges from Form 8824.	16	
17	Combine lines 10 through 16	17	

18	For all except individual returns, enter the amount from line 17 on the appropriate line of your return and skip lines a and b below. For individual returns, complete lines a and b below:		
a	If the loss on line 11 includes a loss from Form 4684, line 41, column (b)(ii), enter that part of the loss here. Enter the part of the loss from income-producing property on Schedule A (Form 1040), line 28, and the part of the loss from property used as an employee on Schedule A (Form 1040), line 23. Identify as from "Form 4797, line 18a." See instructions . .	18a	
b	Redetermine the gain or (loss) on line 17 excluding the loss, if any, on line 18a. Enter here and on Form 1040, line 14	18b	

For Paperwork Reduction Act Notice, see separate instructions.   Cat. No. 13086I   Form **4797** (2008)

Form 4797 (2008)   Page **2**

Part III Gain From Disposition of Property Under Sections 1245, 1250, 1252, 1254, and 1255
(see instructions)

19 (a) Description of section 1245, 1250, 1252, 1254, or 1255 property:

	(b) Date acquired (mo., day, yr.)	**(c)** Date sold (mo., day, yr.)
A		
B		
C		
D		

These columns relate to the properties on lines 19A through 19D. ▶		Property A	Property B	Property C	Property D
20	Gross sales price (**Note:** See line 1 before completing.)	20				
21	Cost or other basis plus expense of sale	21				
22	Depreciation (or depletion) allowed or allowable	22				
23	Adjusted basis. Subtract line 22 from line 21	23				
24	Total gain. Subtract line 23 from line 20	24				
25	**If section 1245 property:**					
a	Depreciation allowed or allowable from line 22	25a				
b	Enter the **smaller** of line 24 or 25a	25b				
26	**If section 1250 property:** If straight line depreciation was used, enter -0- on line 26g, except for a corporation subject to section 291.					
a	Additional depreciation after 1975 (see instructions)	26a				
b	Applicable percentage multiplied by the **smaller** of line 24 or line 26a (see instructions)	26b				
c	Subtract line 26a from line 24. If residential rental property **or** line 24 is not more than line 26a, skip lines 26d and 26e	26c				
d	Additional depreciation after 1969 and before 1976	26d				
e	Enter the **smaller** of line 26c or 26d	26e				
f	Section 291 amount (corporations only)	26f				
g	Add lines 26b, 26e, and 26f	26g				
27	**If section 1252 property:** Skip this section if you did not dispose of farmland or if this form is being completed for a partnership (other than an electing large partnership).					
a	Soil, water, and land clearing expenses	27a				
b	Line 27a multiplied by applicable percentage (see instructions)	27b				
c	Enter the **smaller** of line 24 or 27b	27c				
28	**If section 1254 property:**					
a	Intangible drilling and development costs, expenditures for development of mines and other natural deposits, and mining exploration costs (see instructions)	28a				
b	Enter the **smaller** of line 24 or 28a	28b				
29	**If section 1255 property:**					
a	Applicable percentage of payments excluded from income under section 126 (see instructions)	29a				
b	Enter the **smaller** of line 24 or 29a (see instructions)	29b				

Summary of Part III Gains. Complete property columns A through D through line 29b before going to line 30.

30	Total gains for all properties. Add property columns A through D, line 24	30	
31	Add property columns A through D, lines 25b, 26g, 27c, 28b, and 29b. Enter here and on line 13	31	
32	Subtract line 31 from line 30. Enter the portion from casualty or theft on Form 4684, line 39. Enter the portion from other than casualty or theft on Form 4797, line 6	32	

Part IV Recapture Amounts Under Sections 179 and 280F(b)(2) When Business Use Drops to 50% or Less
(see instructions)

			(a) Section 179	**(b)** Section 280F(b)(2)
33	Section 179 expense deduction or depreciation allowable in prior years	33		
34	Recomputed depreciation (see instructions)	34		
35	Recapture amount. Subtract line 34 from line 33. See the instructions for where to report	35		

Form **4797** (2008)

Form **4952**

Department of the Treasury
Internal Revenue Service (99)

Investment Interest Expense Deduction

▶ **Attach to your tax return.**

OMB No. 1545-0191

2008

Attachment
Sequence No. **51**

Name(s) shown on return

Identifying number

Part I	**Total Investment Interest Expense**		
1	Investment interest expense paid or accrued in 2008 (see instructions)	**1**	
2	Disallowed investment interest expense from 2007 Form 4952, line 7	**2**	
3	**Total investment interest expense.** Add lines 1 and 2	**3**	

Part II	**Net Investment Income**			
4a	Gross income from property held for investment (excluding any net gain from the disposition of property held for investment)	**4a**		
b	Qualified dividends included on line 4a	**4b**		
c	Subtract line 4b from line 4a		**4c**	
d	Net gain from the disposition of property held for investment	**4d**		
e	Enter the **smaller** of line 4d or your net capital gain from the disposition of property held for investment (see instructions)	**4e**		
f	Subtract line 4e from line 4d		**4f**	
g	Enter the amount from lines 4b and 4e that you elect to include in investment income (see instructions)		**4g**	
h	Investment income. Add lines 4c, 4f, and 4g		**4h**	
5	Investment expenses (see instructions)		**5**	
6	**Net investment income.** Subtract line 5 from line 4h. If zero or less, enter -0-		**6**	

Part III	**Investment Interest Expense Deduction**		
7	Disallowed investment interest expense to be carried forward to 2009. Subtract line 6 from line 3. If zero or less, enter -0-	**7**	
8	**Investment interest expense deduction.** Enter the **smaller** of line 3 or 6. See instructions.	**8**	

Section references are to the Internal Revenue Code unless otherwise noted.

General Instructions

Purpose of Form

Use Form 4952 to figure the amount of investment interest expense you can deduct for 2008 and the amount you can carry forward to future years. Your investment interest expense deduction is limited to your net investment income.

For more information, see Pub. 550, Investment Income and Expenses.

Who Must File

If you are an individual, estate, or a trust, you must file Form 4952 to claim a deduction for your investment interest expense.

Exception. You do not have to file Form 4952 if all of the following apply.

● Your investment income from interest and ordinary dividends minus any qualified dividends is more than your investment interest expense.

● You do not have any other deductible investment expenses.

● You do not have any carryover of disallowed investment interest expense from 2007.

Allocation of Interest Expense

If you paid or accrued interest on a loan and used the loan proceeds for more than one purpose, you may have to allocate the interest. This is necessary because different

rules apply to investment interest, personal interest, trade or business interest, home mortgage interest, and passive activity interest. See Pub. 535, Business Expenses.

Specific Instructions

Part I—Total Investment Interest Expense

Line 1

Enter the investment interest expense paid or accrued during the tax year, regardless of when you incurred the indebtedness. Investment interest expense is interest paid or accrued on a loan or part of a loan that is allocable to property held for investment (as defined on this page).

Include investment interest expense reported to you on Schedule K-1 from a partnership or an S corporation. Include amortization of bond premium on taxable bonds purchased after October 22, 1986, but before January 1, 1988, unless you elected to offset amortizable bond premium against the interest payments on the bond. A taxable bond is a bond on which the interest is includible in gross income.

Investment interest expense does not include any of the following:

● Home mortgage interest.

● Interest expense that is properly allocable to a passive activity. Generally, a passive activity is any trade or business activity in which you do not materially participate and any rental activity. See the Instructions for Form 8582, Passive Activity Loss Limitations, for details.

● Any interest expense that is capitalized, such as construction interest subject to section 263A.

● Interest expense related to tax-exempt interest income under section 265.

● Interest expense, disallowed under section 264, on indebtedness with respect to life insurance, endowment, or annuity contracts issued after June 8, 1997, even if the proceeds were used to purchase any property held for investment.

Property held for investment. Property held for investment includes property that produces income, not derived in the ordinary course of a trade or business, from interest, dividends, annuities, or royalties. It also includes property that produces gain or loss, not derived in the ordinary course of a trade or business, from the disposition of property that produces these types of income or is held for investment. However, it does not include an interest in a passive activity.

Exception. A working interest in an oil or gas property that you held directly or through an entity that did not limit your liability is property held for investment, but only if you did not materially participate in the activity.

Part II—Net Investment Income

Line 4a

Gross income from property held for investment includes income, unless derived in the ordinary course of a trade or business, from interest, ordinary dividends (except Alaska Permanent Fund dividends), annuities, and royalties. Include investment income

For Paperwork Reduction Act Notice, see back of form.

Cat. No. 13177Y

Form **4952** (2008)

Form **6252**

Department of the Treasury
Internal Revenue Service

Installment Sale Income

▶ Attach to your tax return.
▶ Use a separate form for each sale or other disposition of
property on the installment method.

OMB No. 1545-0228

20**08**

Attachment
Sequence No. **79**

Name(s) shown on return

Identifying number

1	Description of property ▶	
2a	Date acquired (month, day, year) ▶ / / **b** Date sold (month, day, year) ▶ / /	
3	Was the property sold to a related party (see instructions) after May 14, 1980? If "No," skip line 4.	☐ Yes ☐ No
4	Was the property you sold to a related party a marketable security? If "Yes," complete Part III. If "No," complete Part III for the year of sale and the 2 years after the year of sale	☐ Yes ☐ No

Part I   Gross Profit and Contract Price. Complete this part for the year of sale only.

5	Selling price including mortgages and other debts. **Do not** include interest whether stated or unstated	**5**	
6	Mortgages, debts, and other liabilities the buyer assumed or took the property subject to (see instructions)	**6**	
7	Subtract line 6 from line 5	**7**	
8	Cost or other basis of property sold	**8**	
9	Depreciation allowed or allowable	**9**	
10	Adjusted basis. Subtract line 9 from line 8	**10**	
11	Commissions and other expenses of sale	**11**	
12	Income recapture from Form 4797, Part III (see instructions)	**12**	
13	Add lines 10, 11, and 12	**13**	
14	Subtract line 13 from line 5. If zero or less, **do not** complete the rest of this form (see instructions)	**14**	
15	If the property described on line 1 above was your main home, enter the amount of your excluded gain (see instructions). Otherwise, enter -0-	**15**	
16	**Gross profit.** Subtract line 15 from line 14	**16**	
17	Subtract line 13 from line 6. If zero or less, enter -0-	**17**	
18	**Contract price.** Add line 7 and line 17	**18**	

Part II   Installment Sale Income. Complete this part for the year of sale **and** any year you receive a payment or have certain debts you must treat as a payment on installment obligations.

19	Gross profit percentage (expressed as a decimal amount). Divide line 16 by line 18. For years after the year of sale, see instructions	**19**	
20	If this is the year of sale, enter the amount from line 17. Otherwise, enter -0-	**20**	
21	Payments received during year (see instructions). **Do not** include interest, whether stated or unstated	**21**	
22	Add lines 20 and 21	**22**	
23	Payments received in prior years (see instructions). **Do not** include interest, whether stated or unstated **23**		
24	**Installment sale income.** Multiply line 22 by line 19	**24**	
25	Enter the part of line 24 that is ordinary income under the recapture rules (see instructions)	**25**	
26	Subtract line 25 from line 24. Enter here and on Schedule D or Form 4797 (see instructions)	**26**	

Part III   Related Party Installment Sale Income. **Do not** complete if you received the final payment this tax year.

27	Name, address, and taxpayer identifying number of related party

28	Did the related party resell or dispose of the property ("second disposition") during this tax year?	☐ Yes ☐ No
29	If the answer to question 28 is "Yes," complete lines 30 through 37 below unless one of the following conditions is met. **Check the box that applies.**	
a	☐ The second disposition was more than 2 years after the first disposition (other than dispositions of marketable securities). If this box is checked, enter the date of disposition (month, day, year) ▶ / /	
b	☐ The first disposition was a sale or exchange of stock to the issuing corporation.	
c	☐ The second disposition was an involuntary conversion and the threat of conversion occurred after the first disposition.	
d	☐ The second disposition occurred after the death of the original seller or buyer.	
e	☐ It can be established to the satisfaction of the Internal Revenue Service that tax avoidance was not a principal purpose for either of the dispositions. If this box is checked, attach an explanation (see instructions).	

30	Selling price of property sold by related party (see instructions)	**30**	
31	Enter contract price from line 18 for year of first sale	**31**	
32	Enter the **smaller** of line 30 or line 31	**32**	
33	Total payments received by the end of your 2008 tax year (see instructions)	**33**	
34	Subtract line 33 from line 32. If zero or less, enter -0-	**34**	
35	Multiply line 34 by the gross profit percentage on line 19 for year of first sale	**35**	
36	Enter the part of line 35 that is ordinary income under the recapture rules (see instructions)	**36**	
37	Subtract line 36 from line 35. Enter here and on Schedule D or Form 4797 (see instructions)	**37**	

For Paperwork Reduction Act Notice, see page 4.   Cat. No. 13601R   Form **6252** (2008)

Form **8283**

(Rev. December 2006)

Department of the Treasury
Internal Revenue Service

Noncash Charitable Contributions

▶ **Attach to your tax return if you claimed a total deduction of over $500 for all contributed property.**

▶ **See separate instructions.**

OMB No. 1545-0908

Attachment
Sequence No. **155**

Name(s) shown on your income tax return	Identifying number

Note. Figure the amount of your contribution deduction before completing this form. See your tax return instructions.

Section A. Donated Property of $5,000 or Less and Certain Publicly Traded Securities—List in this section **only** items (or groups of similar items) for which you claimed a deduction of $5,000 or less. Also, list certain publicly traded securities even if the deduction is more than $5,000 (see instructions).

Part I   **Information on Donated Property**—If you need more space, attach a statement.

1

	(a) Name and address of the donee organization	**(b)** Description of donated property (For a donated vehicle, enter the year, make, model, condition, and mileage, and attach Form 1098-C if required.)
A		
B		
C		
D		
E		

Note. If the amount you claimed as a deduction for an item is $500 or less, you do not have to complete columns (d), (e), and (f).

	(c) Date of the contribution	**(d)** Date acquired by donor (mo., yr.)	**(e)** How acquired by donor	**(f)** Donor's cost or adjusted basis	**(g)** Fair market value (see instructions)	**(h)** Method used to determine the fair market value
A						
B						
C						
D						
E						

Part II   **Partial Interests and Restricted Use Property**—Complete lines 2a through 2e if you gave less than an entire interest in a property listed in Part I. Complete lines 3a through 3c if conditions were placed on a contribution listed in Part I; also attach the required statement (see instructions).

2a Enter the letter from Part I that identifies the property for which you gave less than an entire interest ▶ _____ .
If Part II applies to more than one property, attach a separate statement.

b Total amount claimed as a deduction for the property listed in Part I: **(1)** For this tax year   ▶ _____ .

                                                         (2) For any prior tax years   ▶ _____ .

c Name and address of each organization to which any such contribution was made in a prior year (complete only if different from the donee organization above):

Name of charitable organization (donee)

Address (number, street, and room or suite no.)

City or town, state, and ZIP code

d For tangible property, enter the place where the property is located or kept ▶ _____

e Name of any person, other than the donee organization, having actual possession of the property ▶ _____

		Yes	No
3a	Is there a restriction, either temporary or permanent, on the donee's right to use or dispose of the donated property?		
b	Did you give to anyone (other than the donee organization or another organization participating with the donee organization in cooperative fundraising) the right to the income from the donated property or to the possession of the property, including the right to vote donated securities, to acquire the property by purchase or otherwise, or to designate the person having such income, possession, or right to acquire?		
c	Is there a restriction limiting the donated property for a particular use?		

For Paperwork Reduction Act Notice, see separate instructions.   Cat. No. 62299J   Form **8283** (Rev. 12-2006)

Form 8283 (Rev. 12-2006)   Page **2**

Name(s) shown on your income tax return	Identifying number

Section B. Donated Property Over $5,000 (Except Certain Publicly Traded Securities)—List in this section only items (or groups of similar items) for which you claimed a deduction of more than $5,000 per item or group (except contributions of certain publicly traded securities reported in Section A). An appraisal is generally required for property listed in Section B (see instructions).

Part I   **Information on Donated Property**—To be completed by the taxpayer and/or the appraiser.

4   Check the box that describes the type of property donated:

☐ Art* (contribution of $20,000 or more)   ☐ Qualified Conservation Contribution   ☐ Equipment
☐ Art* (contribution of less than $20,000)   ☐ Other Real Estate   ☐ Securities
☐ Collectibles**   ☐ Intellectual Property   ☐ Other

*Art includes paintings, sculptures, watercolors, prints, drawings, ceramics, antiques, decorative arts, textiles, carpets, silver, rare manuscripts, historical memorabilia, and other similar objects.

**Collectibles include coins, stamps, books, gems, jewelry, sports memorabilia, dolls, etc., but not art as defined above.

Note. In certain cases, you must attach a qualified appraisal of the property. See instructions.

5	(a) Description of donated property (if you need more space, attach a separate statement)	(b) If tangible property was donated, give a brief summary of the overall physical condition of the property at the time of the gift	(c) Appraised fair market value
A			
B			
C			
D			

	(d) Date acquired by donor (mo., yr.)	(e) How acquired by donor	(f) Donor's cost or adjusted basis	(g) For bargain sales, enter amount received	(h) Amount claimed as a deduction	(i) Average trading price of securities
A						
B						
C						
D						

Part II   **Taxpayer (Donor) Statement**—List each item included in Part I above that the appraisal identifies as having a value of $500 or less. See instructions.

I declare that the following item(s) included in Part I above has to the best of my knowledge and belief an appraised value of not more than $500 (per item). Enter identifying letter from Part I and describe the specific item. See instructions. ▶ _____

Signature of taxpayer (donor) ▶ _____ Date ▶ _____

Part III   **Declaration of Appraiser**

I declare that I am not the donor, the donee, a party to the transaction in which the donor acquired the property, employed by, or related to any of the foregoing persons, or married to any person who is related to any of the foregoing persons. And, if regularly used by the donor, donee, or party to the transaction, I performed the majority of my appraisals during my tax year for other persons.

Also, I declare that I hold myself out to the public as an appraiser or perform appraisals on a regular basis; and that because of my qualifications as described in the appraisal, I am qualified to make appraisals of the type of property being valued. I certify that the appraisal fees were not based on a percentage of the appraised property value. Furthermore, I understand that a false or fraudulent overstatement of the property value as described in the qualified appraisal or this Form 8283 may subject me to the penalty under section 6701(a) (aiding and abetting the understatement of tax liability). In addition, I understand that a substantial or gross valuation misstatement resulting from the appraisal of the value of the property that I know, or reasonably should know, would be used in connection with a return or claim for refund, may subject me to the penalty under section 6695A. I affirm that I have not been barred from presenting evidence or testimony by the Office of Professional Responsibility.

Sign Here   Signature ▶ _____ Title ▶ _____ Date ▶ _____

Business address (including room or suite no.)	Identifying number

City or town, state, and ZIP code

Part IV   **Donee Acknowledgment**—To be completed by the charitable organization.

This charitable organization acknowledges that it is a qualified organization under section 170(c) and that it received the donated property as described in Section B, Part I, above on the following date ▶ _____

Furthermore, this organization affirms that in the event it sells, exchanges, or otherwise disposes of the property described in Section B, Part I (or any portion thereof) within 3 years after the date of receipt, it will file **Form 8282,** Donee Information Return, with the IRS and give the donor a copy of that form. This acknowledgment does not represent agreement with the claimed fair market value.

Does the organization intend to use the property for an unrelated use? . . . . ▶ ☐ Yes   ☐ No

Name of charitable organization (donee)	Employer identification number
Address (number, street, and room or suite no.)	City or town, state, and ZIP code
Authorized signature	Title	Date

Form **8283** (Rev. 12-2006)

Form **8582**	**Passive Activity Loss Limitations**	OMB No. 1545-1008
Department of the Treasury Internal Revenue Service (99)	▶ See separate instructions. ▶ Attach to Form 1040 or Form 1041.	**2008** Attachment Sequence No. **88**

Name(s) shown on return | Identifying number

Part I 2008 Passive Activity Loss

Caution: *Complete Worksheets 1, 2, and 3 on page 2 before completing Part I.*

Rental Real Estate Activities With Active Participation (For the definition of active participation, see **Special Allowance for Rental Real Estate Activities** on page 3 of the instructions.)

1a Activities with net income (enter the amount from Worksheet 1, column (a)) **1a**

  b Activities with net loss (enter the amount from Worksheet 1, column (b)) . . . .   **1b** (   )

  c Prior years unallowed losses (enter the amount from Worksheet 1, column (c)) . . . .   **1c** (   )

  d Combine lines 1a, 1b, and 1c **1d**

Commercial Revitalization Deductions From Rental Real Estate Activities

2a Commercial revitalization deductions from Worksheet 2, column (a)   **2a** (   )

  b Prior year unallowed commercial revitalization deductions from Worksheet 2, column (b) . . . .   **2b** (   )

  c Add lines 2a and 2b . . . .   **2c** (   )

All Other Passive Activities

3a Activities with net income (enter the amount from Worksheet 3, column (a)) **3a**

  b Activities with net loss (enter the amount from Worksheet 3, column (b)) . . . .   **3b** (   )

  c Prior years unallowed losses (enter the amount from Worksheet 3, column (c)) . . . .   **3c** (   )

  d Combine lines 3a, 3b, and 3c **3d**

4 Combine lines 1d, 2c, and 3d. If the result is net income or zero, all losses are allowed, including any prior year unallowed losses entered on line 1c, 2b, or 3c. **Do not** complete Form 8582. Report the losses on the forms and schedules normally used **4**

  If line 4 is a loss and: • Line 1d is a loss, go to Part II.
    • Line 2c is a loss (and line 1d is zero or more), skip Part II and go to Part III.
    • Line 3d is a loss (and lines 1d and 2c are zero or more), skip Parts II and III and go to line 15.

Caution: *If your filing status is married filing separately and you lived with your spouse at any time during the year, **do not** complete Part II or Part III. Instead, go to line 15.*

Part II Special Allowance for Rental Real Estate Activities With Active Participation

Note: *Enter all numbers in Part II as positive amounts. See page 8 of the instructions for an example.*

5 Enter the **smaller** of the loss on line 1d or the loss on line 4 . . . .   **5**

6 Enter $150,000. If married filing separately, see page 8 . .   **6**

7 Enter modified adjusted gross income, but not less than zero (see page 8)   **7**

  Note: *If line 7 is greater than or equal to line 6, skip lines 8 and 9, enter -0- on line 10. Otherwise, go to line 8.*

8 Subtract line 7 from line 6 . . . .   **8**

9 Multiply line 8 by 50% (.5). **Do not** enter more than $25,000. If married filing separately, see page 8   **9**

10 Enter the **smaller** of line 5 or line 9 . . . .   **10**

  If line 2c is a loss, go to Part III. Otherwise, go to line 15.

Part III Special Allowance for Commercial Revitalization Deductions From Rental Real Estate Activities

Note: *Enter all numbers in Part III as positive amounts. See the example for Part II on page 8 of the instructions.*

11 Enter $25,000 reduced by the amount, if any, on line 10. If married filing separately, see instructions   **11**

12 Enter the loss from line 4 . . . .   **12**

13 Reduce line 12 by the amount on line 10 . . . .   **13**

14 Enter the **smallest** of line 2c (treated as a positive amount), line 11, or line 13 . . . . .   **14**

Part IV Total Losses Allowed

15 Add the income, if any, on lines 1a and 3a and enter the total **15**

16 **Total losses allowed from all passive activities for 2008.** Add lines 10, 14, and 15. See page 10 of the instructions to find out how to report the losses on your tax return. . . .   **16**

For Paperwork Reduction Act Notice, see page 12 of the instructions.   Cat. No. 63704F   Form **8582** (2008)

Form 8582 (2008)   Page **2**

Caution: *The worksheets must be filed with your tax return. Keep a copy for your records.*

Worksheet 1—For Form 8582, Lines 1a, 1b, and 1c (See pages 7 and 8 of the instructions.)

Name of activity	Current year		Prior years	Overall gain or loss	
	(a) Net income (line 1a)	**(b) Net loss (line 1b)**	**(c) Unallowed loss (line 1c)**	**(d) Gain**	**(e) Loss**
Total. Enter on Form 8582, lines 1a, 1b, and 1c . . . . ▶					

Worksheet 2—For Form 8582, Lines 2a and 2b (See page 8 of the instructions.)

Name of activity	**(a) Current year deductions (line 2a)**	**(b) Prior year unallowed deductions (line 2b)**	**(c) Overall loss**
Total. Enter on Form 8582, lines 2a and 2b . . . . ▶			

Worksheet 3—For Form 8582, Lines 3a, 3b, and 3c (See page 8 of the instructions.)

Name of activity	Current year		Prior years	Overall gain or loss	
	(a) Net income (line 3a)	**(b) Net loss (line 3b)**	**(c) Unallowed loss (line 3c)**	**(d) Gain**	**(e) Loss**
Total. Enter on Form 8582, lines 3a, 3b, and 3c . . . . ▶					

Worksheet 4—Use this worksheet if an amount is shown on Form 8582, line 10 or 14 (See page 9 of the instructions.)

Name of activity	Form or schedule and line number to be reported on (see instructions)	**(a) Loss**	**(b) Ratio**	**(c) Special allowance**	**(d) Subtract column (c) from column (a)**
Total . . . . ▶			1.00		

Worksheet 5—Allocation of Unallowed Losses (See page 9 of the instructions.)

Name of activity	Form or schedule and line number to be reported on (see instructions)	**(a) Loss**	**(b) Ratio**	**(c) Unallowed loss**
Total . . . . ▶			1.00	

Form **8582** (2008)

Worksheet 6—Allowed Losses (See pages 9 and 10 of the instructions.)

Name of activity	Form or schedule and line number to be reported on (see instructions)	(a) Loss	(b) Unallowed loss	(c) Allowed loss
Total . . . . ▶				

Worksheet 7—Activities With Losses Reported on Two or More Forms or Schedules (See page 10 of the instructions.)

Name of activity:	(a)	(b)	(c) Ratio	(d) Unallowed loss	(e) Allowed loss
Form or schedule and line number to be reported on (see instructions): _____					
1a Net loss plus prior year unallowed loss from form or schedule. ▶					
b Net income from form or schedule . . . . . ▶					
c Subtract line 1b from line 1a. If zero or less, enter -0- ▶					
Form or schedule and line number to be reported on (see instructions): _____					
1a Net loss plus prior year unallowed loss from form or schedule. ▶					
b Net income from form or schedule . . . . . ▶					
c Subtract line 1b from line 1a. If zero or less, enter -0- ▶					
Form or schedule and line number to be reported on (see instructions): _____					
1a Net loss plus prior year unallowed loss from form or schedule. ▶					
b Net income from form or schedule . . . . . ▶					
c Subtract line 1b from line 1a. If zero or less, enter -0- ▶					
Total . . . . ▶			**1.00**		

Form **8615**

Department of the Treasury
Internal Revenue Service   (99)

Tax for Certain Children Who Have Investment Income of More Than $1,800

▶ Attach only to the child's Form 1040, Form 1040A, or Form 1040NR.
▶ See separate instructions.

OMB No. 1545-0074

20**08**

Attachment
Sequence No. **33**

Child's name shown on return

Child's social security number

Before you begin: If the child, the parent, or any of the parent's other children for whom Form 8615 must be filed must use the Schedule D Tax Worksheet or has income from farming or fishing, see **Pub. 929**, Tax Rules for Children and Dependents. It explains how to figure the child's tax using the **Schedule D Tax Worksheet** or **Schedule J** (Form 1040).

A Parent's name (first, initial, and last). **Caution:** *See instructions before completing.*

B Parent's social security number

C Parent's filing status (check one):

☐ Single   ☐ Married filing jointly   ☐ Married filing separately   ☐ Head of household   ☐ Qualifying widow(er)

Part I	**Child's Net Investment Income**	
1	Enter the child's investment income (see instructions)	1
2	If the child **did not** itemize deductions on **Schedule A** (Form 1040 or Form 1040NR), enter $1,800. Otherwise, see instructions	2
3	Subtract line 2 from line 1. If zero or less, **stop;** do not complete the rest of this form but **do** attach it to the child's return	3
4	Enter the child's **taxable income** from Form 1040, line 43; Form 1040A, line 27; or Form 1040NR, line 40. If the child files Form 2555 or 2555-EZ, see the instructions	4
5	Enter the **smaller** of line 3 or line 4. If zero, **stop;** do not complete the rest of this form but **do** attach it to the child's return	5

Part II	**Tentative Tax Based on the Tax Rate of the Parent**	
6	Enter the parent's **taxable income** from Form 1040, line 43; Form 1040A, line 27; Form 1040EZ, line 6; Form 1040NR, line 40; or Form 1040NR-EZ, line 14. If zero or less, enter -0-. If the parent files Form 2555 or 2555-EZ, see the instructions	6
7	Enter the total, if any, from Forms 8615, line 5, of **all other** children of the parent named above. **Do not** include the amount from line 5 above	7
8	Add lines 5, 6, and 7 (see instructions)	8
9	Enter the tax on the amount on line 8 based on the **parent's** filing status above (see instructions). If the Qualified Dividends and Capital Gain Tax Worksheet, Schedule D Tax Worksheet, or Schedule J (Form 1040) is used to figure the tax, check here ▶ ☐	9
10	Enter the parent's tax from Form 1040, line 44; Form 1040A, line 28, minus any alternative minimum tax; Form 1040EZ, line 11; Form 1040NR, line 41; or Form 1040NR-EZ, line 15. **Do not** include any tax from **Form 4972** or **8814** or any tax from recapture of an education credit. If the parent files Form 2555 or 2555-EZ, see the instructions. If the Qualified Dividends and Capital Gain Tax Worksheet, Schedule D Tax Worksheet, or Schedule J (Form 1040) was used to figure the tax, check here ▶ ☐	10
11	Subtract line 10 from line 9 and enter the result. If line 7 is blank, also enter this amount on line 13 and go to **Part III**	11
12a	Add lines 5 and 7 12a	
b	Divide line 5 by line 12a. Enter the result as a decimal (rounded to at least three places)	12b × .
13	Multiply line 11 by line 12b	13

Part III	**Child's Tax**—If lines 4 and 5 above are the same, enter -0- on line 15 and go to line 16.	
14	Subtract line 5 from line 4 14	
15	Enter the tax on the amount on line 14 based on the **child's** filing status (see instructions). If the Qualified Dividends and Capital Gain Tax Worksheet, Schedule D Tax Worksheet, or Schedule J (Form 1040) is used to figure the tax, check here ▶ ☐	15
16	Add lines 13 and 15	16
17	Enter the tax on the amount on line 4 based on the **child's** filing status (see instructions). If the Qualified Dividends and Capital Gain Tax Worksheet, Schedule D Tax Worksheet, or Schedule J (Form 1040) is used to figure the tax, check here ▶ ☐	17
18	Enter the **larger** of line 16 or line 17 here and on the **child's** Form 1040, line 44; Form 1040A, line 28; or Form 1040NR, line 41. If the child files Form 2555 or 2555-EZ, see the instructions	18

For Paperwork Reduction Act Notice, see the instructions.   Cat. No. 64113U   Form **8615** (2008)

Form **8814**

Department of the Treasury
Internal Revenue Service (99)

**Parents' Election To Report
Child's Interest and Dividends**
▶ See instructions.
▶ **Attach to parents' Form 1040 or Form 1040NR.**

OMB No. 1545-0074

20**08**

Attachment
Sequence No. **40**

Name(s) shown on your return

Your social security number

Caution. The federal income tax on your child's income, including qualified dividends and capital gain distributions, may be less if you file a separate tax return for the child instead of making this election. This is because you cannot take certain tax benefits that your child could take on his or her own return. For details, see **Tax benefits you cannot take** on page 2.

A   Child's name (first, initial, and last)

B Child's social security number

C   If more than one Form 8814 is attached, check here . . . . ▶ ☐

| **Part I** | **Child's Interest and Dividends To Report on Your Return** |

1a Enter your child's **taxable** interest. If this amount is different from the amounts shown on the child's Forms 1099-INT and 1099-OID, see the instructions . . . . | **1a** | |

  b Enter your child's **tax-exempt** interest. **Do not** include this amount on line 1a . . . . | **1b** | |

2a Enter your child's ordinary dividends, including any Alaska Permanent Fund dividends. If your child received any ordinary dividends as a nominee, see the instructions . . . . . . | **2a** | |

  b Enter your child's qualified dividends included on line 2a. See the instructions . . . . | **2b** | |

3   Enter your child's capital gain distributions. If your child received any capital gain distributions as a nominee, see the instructions . . . . | **3** | |

4   Add lines 1a, 2a, and 3. If the total is $1,800 or less, skip lines 5 through 12 and go to line 13. If the total is $9,000 or more, **do not** file this form. Your child **must** file his or her own return to report the income . . . . | **4** | |

5   Base amount . . . . | **5** | 1,800 | 00 |

6   Subtract line 5 from line 4 . . . . | **6** | |

If both lines 2b and 3 are zero or blank, skip lines 7 through 10, enter -0- on line 11, and go to line 12. Otherwise, go to line 7.

7   Divide line 2b by line 4. Enter the result as a decimal (rounded to at least three places) . . . . | **7** | . |

8   Divide line 3 by line 4. Enter the result as a decimal (rounded to at least three places) . . . . | **8** | . |

9   Multiply line 6 by line 7. Enter the result here. See the instructions for where to report this amount on your return . . . . . | **9** | |

10 Multiply line 6 by line 8. Enter the result here. See the instructions for where to report this amount on your return . . . . . | **10** | |

11 Add lines 9 and 10 . . . . | **11** | |

12 Subtract line 11 from line 6. Include this amount in the total on Form 1040, line 21, or Form 1040NR, line 21. In the space next to line 21, enter "Form 8814" and show the amount. If you checked the box on line C above, see the instructions. Go to line 13 below . . . . . | **12** | |

| **Part II** | **Tax on the First $1,800 of Child's Interest and Dividends** |

13 Amount not taxed . . . . | **13** | 900 | 00 |

14 Subtract line 13 from line 4. If the result is zero or less, enter -0-. . . . . | **14** | |

15 **Tax.** Is the amount on line 14 less than $900?
☐ **No.** Enter $90 here and see the **Note** below.
☐ **Yes.** Multiply line 14 by 10% (.10). Enter the result here and see the **Note** below.   } . | **15** | |

Note. If you checked the box on line C above, see the instructions. Otherwise, include the amount from line 15 in the tax you enter on Form 1040, line 44, or Form 1040NR, line 41. Be sure to check box **a** on Form 1040, line 44, or Form 1040NR, line 41.

For Paperwork Reduction Act Notice, see page 3.   Cat. No. 10750J   Form **8814** (2008)

Form **8829**	**Expenses for Business Use of Your Home**	OMB No. 1545-0074
Department of the Treasury Internal Revenue Service (99)	▶ File only with Schedule C (Form 1040). Use a separate Form 8829 for each home you used for business during the year. ▶ See separate instructions.	20**08** Attachment Sequence No. **66**

Name(s) of proprietor(s) | Your social security number

Part I   Part of Your Home Used for Business

1	Area used regularly and exclusively for business, regularly for daycare, or for storage of inventory or product samples (see instructions)	**1**	
2	Total area of home	**2**	
3	Divide line 1 by line 2. Enter the result as a percentage	**3**	%
	For daycare facilities not used exclusively for business, go to line 4. All others go to line 7.		
4	Multiply days used for daycare during year by hours used per day	**4**	hr.
5	Total hours available for use during the year (366 days × 24 hours) (see instructions)	**5**	8,784 hr.
6	Divide line 4 by line 5. Enter the result as a decimal amount	**6**	.
7	Business percentage. For daycare facilities not used exclusively for business, multiply line 6 by line 3 (enter the result as a percentage). All others, enter the amount from line 3 ▶	**7**	%

Part II   Figure Your Allowable Deduction

8	Enter the amount from Schedule C, line 29, **plus** any net gain or (loss) derived from the business use of your home and shown on Schedule D or Form 4797. If more than one place of business, see instructions	**8**	

See instructions for columns (a) and (b) before completing lines 9–21.

		(a) Direct expenses	(b) Indirect expenses	
9	Casualty losses (see instructions)	9		
10	Deductible mortgage interest (see instructions)	10		
11	Real estate taxes (see instructions)	11		
12	Add lines 9, 10, and 11	12		
13	Multiply line 12, column (b) by line 7		13	
14	Add line 12, column (a) and line 13			**14**
15	Subtract line 14 from line 8. If zero or less, enter -0-			**15**
16	Excess mortgage interest (see instructions)	16		
17	Insurance	17		
18	Rent	18		
19	Repairs and maintenance	19		
20	Utilities	20		
21	Other expenses (see instructions)	21		
22	Add lines 16 through 21	22		
23	Multiply line 22, column (b) by line 7		23	
24	Carryover of operating expenses from 2007 Form 8829, line 42		24	
25	Add line 22 column (a), line 23, and line 24			**25**
26	Allowable operating expenses. Enter the **smaller** of line 15 or line 25			**26**
27	Limit on excess casualty losses and depreciation. Subtract line 26 from line 15			**27**
28	Excess casualty losses (see instructions)		28	
29	Depreciation of your home from line 41 below		29	
30	Carryover of excess casualty losses and depreciation from 2007 Form 8829, line 43		30	
31	Add lines 28 through 30			**31**
32	Allowable excess casualty losses and depreciation. Enter the **smaller** of line 27 or line 31			**32**
33	Add lines 14, 26, and 32			**33**
34	Casualty loss portion, if any, from lines 14 and 32. Carry amount to **Form 4684,** Section B			**34**
35	**Allowable expenses for business use of your home.** Subtract line 34 from line 33. Enter here and on Schedule C, line 30. If your home was used for more than one business, see instructions ▶			**35**

Part III   Depreciation of Your Home

36	Enter the **smaller** of your home's adjusted basis or its fair market value (see instructions)	**36**	
37	Value of land included on line 36	**37**	
38	Basis of building. Subtract line 37 from line 36	**38**	
39	Business basis of building. Multiply line 38 by line 7	**39**	
40	Depreciation percentage (see instructions)	**40**	%
41	Depreciation allowable (see instructions). Multiply line 39 by line 40. Enter here and on line 29 above	**41**	

Part IV   Carryover of Unallowed Expenses to 2009

42	Operating expenses. Subtract line 26 from line 25. If less than zero, enter -0-	**42**	
43	Excess casualty losses and depreciation. Subtract line 32 from line 31. If less than zero, enter -0-	**43**	

For Paperwork Reduction Act Notice, see page 4 of separate instructions.   Cat. No. 13232M   Form **8829** (2008)

Form **8863**	**Education Credits** **(Hope and Lifetime Learning Credits)** ▶ See instructions to find out if you are eligible to take the credits. ▶ Attach to Form 1040 or Form 1040A.	OMB No. 1545-0074 **2008** Attachment Sequence No. **50**
Department of the Treasury Internal Revenue Service (99)		

Name(s) shown on return	Your social security number

Caution: • *You **cannot** take the Hope credit and the lifetime learning credit for the **same student** in the same year.*

• *You **cannot** take both an education credit and the tuition and fees deduction (see Form 8917) for the **same student** for the same year.*

Part I   Hope Credit. Caution: *You **cannot** take the Hope credit for more than **2** tax years for the **same student**.*

1	(a) Student's name (as shown on page 1 of your tax return) First name Last name	(b) Student's social security number (as shown on page 1 of your tax return)	(c) Qualified expenses (see instructions). **Do not** enter more than $2,400* for each student.	(d) Enter the **smaller** of the amount in column (c) or $1,200**	(e) Add column (c) and column (d)	(f) Enter one-half of the amount in column (e)

	------------------------					

*For each student who attended an eligible educational institution in a Midwestern disaster area, **do not** enter more than $4,800.

For each student who attended an eligible educational institution in a Midwestern disaster area, enter the **smaller of the amount in column (c) or $2,400.

2	**Tentative Hope credit.** Add the amounts on line 1, column (f). If you are taking the lifetime learning credit for another student, go to Part II; otherwise, go to Part III . . . . ▶	**2**	

Part II   Lifetime Learning Credit

3	(a) Student's name (as shown on page 1 of your tax return) First name Last name	(b) Student's social security number (as shown on page 1 of your tax return)	(c) Qualified expenses (see instructions)

4	Add the amounts on line 3, column (c), and enter the total	**4**	
5a	Enter the **smaller** of line 4 or $10,000	**5a**	
b	For students who attended an eligible educational institution in a Midwestern disaster area, enter the smaller of $10,000 or their qualified expenses included on line 4 (see special rules on page 3)	**5b**	
c	Subtract line 5b from line 5a	**5c**	
6a	Multiply line 5b by 40% (.40)	**6a**	
b	Multiply line 5c by 20% (.20)	**6b**	
c	**Tentative lifetime learning credit.** Add lines 6a and 6b and go to Part III	**6c**	

Part III   Allowable Education Credits

7	Tentative education credits. Add lines 2 and 6c	**7**	
8	Enter: $116,000 if married filing jointly; $58,000 if single, head of household, or qualifying widow(er)	**8**	
9	Enter the amount from Form 1040, line 38,* or Form 1040A, line 22 .	**9**	
10	Subtract line 9 from line 8. If zero or less, **stop;** you cannot take any education credits	**10**	
11	Enter: $20,000 if married filing jointly; $10,000 if single, head of household, or qualifying widow(er)	**11**	
12	If line 10 is equal to or more than line 11, enter the amount from line 7 on line 13 and go to line 14. If line 10 is less than line 11, divide line 10 by line 11. Enter the result as a decimal (rounded to at least three places)	**12**	× .
13	Multiply line 7 by line 12 . . . . ▶	**13**	
14	Enter the amount from Form 1040, line 46, or Form 1040A, line 28	**14**	
15	Enter the total, if any, of your credits from Form 1040, lines 47 through 49, or Form 1040A, lines 29 and 30	**15**	
16	Subtract line 15 from line 14. If zero or less, **stop;** you cannot take any education credits . ▶	**16**	
17	**Education credits.** Enter the smaller of line 13 or line 16 here and on Form 1040, line 50, or Form 1040A, line 31 . . . . ▶	**17**	

* If you are filing Form 2555, 2555-EZ, or 4563, or you are excluding income from Puerto Rico, see Pub. 970 for the amount to enter.

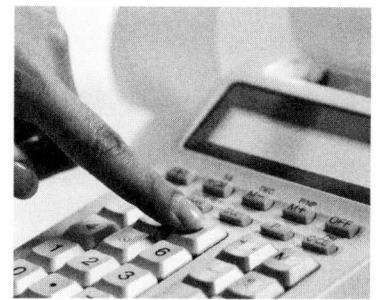

★ APPENDIX C ★

MODIFIED ACRS TABLES

Modified ACRS Accelerated Depreciation Percentages
Using the Half Year Convention
for 3-, 5-, 7-, 10-, 15-, and 20-Year Property
Placed in Service after December 31, 1986

Recovery Year	Property Class					
	3-Year	5-Year	7-Year	10-Year	15-Year	20-Year
1	33.33	20.00	14.29	10.00	5.00	3.750
2	44.45	32.00	24.49	18.00	9.50	7.219
3	14.81	19.20	17.49	14.40	8.55	6.677
4	7.41	11.52	12.49	11.52	7.70	6.177
5		11.52	8.93	9.22	6.93	5.713
6		5.76	8.92	7.37	6.23	5.285
7			8.93	6.55	5.90	4.888
8			4.46	6.55	5.90	4.522
9				6.56	5.91	4.462
10				6.55	5.90	4.461
11				3.28	5.91	4.462
12					5.90	4.461
13					5.91	4.462
14					5.90	4.461
15					5.91	4.462
16					2.95	4.461
17						4.462
18						4.461
19						4.462
20						4.461
21						2.231

Modified ACRS Depreciation Rates
for Residential Rental Property
Placed in Service after December 31, 1986

Recovery Year	Month Placed in Service					
	1	2	3	4	5	6
1	3.485	3.182	2.879	2.576	2.273	1.970
2	3.636	3.636	3.636	3.636	3.636	3.636
3	3.636	3.636	3.636	3.636	3.636	3.636
4	3.636	3.636	3.636	3.636	3.636	3.636
5	3.636	3.636	3.636	3.636	3.636	3.636
6	3.636	3.636	3.636	3.636	3.636	3.636
7	3.636	3.636	3.636	3.636	3.636	3.636
8	3.636	3.636	3.636	3.636	3.636	3.636
9	3.636	3.636	3.636	3.636	3.636	3.636
10	3.637	3.637	3.637	3.637	3.637	3.637
11	3.636	3.636	3.636	3.636	3.636	3.636
12	3.637	3.637	3.637	3.637	3.637	3.637
13	3.636	3.636	3.636	3.636	3.636	3.636
14	3.637	3.637	3.637	3.637	3.637	3.637
15	3.636	3.636	3.636	3.636	3.636	3.636
16	3.637	3.637	3.637	3.637	3.637	3.637
17	3.636	3.636	3.636	3.636	3.636	3.636
18	3.637	3.637	3.637	3.637	3.637	3.637
19	3.636	3.636	3.636	3.636	3.636	3.636
20	3.637	3.637	3.637	3.637	3.637	3.636
21	3.636	3.636	3.636	3.636	3.636	3.636
22	3.637	3.637	3.637	3.637	3.637	3.637
23	3.636	3.636	3.636	3.636	3.636	3.636
24	3.637	3.637	3.637	3.637	3.637	3.637
25	3.636	3.636	3.636	3.636	3.636	3.636
26	3.637	3.637	3.637	3.637	3.637	3.637
27	3.636	3.636	3.636	3.636	3.636	3.636
28	1.970	2.273	2.576	2.879	3.182	3.485
29	0.000	0.000	0.000	0.000	0.000	0.000

Recovery Year	Month Placed in Service					
	7	8	9	10	11	12
1	1.667	1.364	1.061	0.758	0.455	0.152
2	3.636	3.636	3.636	3.636	3.636	3.636
3	3.636	3.636	3.636	3.636	3.636	3.636
4	3.636	3.636	3.636	3.636	3.636	3.636
5	3.636	3.636	3.636	3.636	3.636	3.636
6	3.636	3.636	3.636	3.636	3.636	3.636
7	3.636	3.636	3.636	3.636	3.636	3.636
8	3.636	3.636	3.636	3.636	3.636	3.636
9	3.636	3.636	3.636	3.636	3.636	3.636
10	3.636	3.636	3.636	3.636	3.636	3.636
11	3.637	3.637	3.637	3.637	3.637	3.637
12	3.636	3.636	3.636	3.636	3.636	3.636
13	3.637	3.637	3.637	3.637	3.637	3.637
14	3.636	3.636	3.636	3.636	3.636	3.636
15	3.637	3.637	3.637	3.637	3.637	3.637
16	3.636	3.636	3.636	3.636	3.636	3.636
17	3.637	3.637	3.637	3.637	3.637	3.637
18	3.636	3.636	3.636	3.636	3.636	3.636
19	3.637	3.637	3.637	3.637	3.637	3.637
20	3.636	3.636	3.636	3.636	3.636	3.636
21	3.637	3.637	3.637	3.637	3.637	3.637
22	3.636	3.636	3.636	3.636	3.636	3.636
23	3.637	3.637	3.637	3.637	3.637	3.637
24	3.636	3.636	3.636	3.636	3.636	3.636
25	3.637	3.637	3.637	3.637	3.637	3.637
26	3.636	3.636	3.636	3.636	3.636	3.636
27	3.637	3.637	3.637	3.637	3.637	3.637
28	3.636	3.636	3.636	3.636	3.636	3.636
29	0.152	0.455	0.758	1.061	1.364	1.667

Modified ACRS Depreciation Percentages
for Nonresidential Real Property
Placed in Service after December 31, 1986
and before May 13, 1993

Recovery Year	Month Placed in Service					
	1	2	3	4	5	6
1	3.042	2.778	2.513	2.249	1.984	1.720
2	3.175	3.175	3.175	3.175	3.175	3.175
3	3.175	3.175	3.175	3.175	3.175	3.175
4	3.175	3.175	3.175	3.175	3.175	3.175
5	3.175	3.175	3.175	3.175	3.175	3.175
6	3.175	3.175	3.175	3.175	3.175	3.175
7	3.175	3.175	3.175	3.175	3.175	3.175
8	3.175	3.174	3.175	3.174	3.175	3.174
9	3.174	3.175	3.174	3.175	3.174	3.175
10	3.175	3.174	3.175	3.174	3.175	3.174
11	3.174	3.175	3.174	3.175	3.174	3.175
12	3.175	3.174	3.175	3.174	3.175	3.174
13	3.174	3.175	3.174	3.175	3.174	3.175
14	3.175	3.174	3.175	3.174	3.175	3.174
15	3.174	3.175	3.174	3.175	3.174	3.175
16	3.175	3.174	3.175	3.174	3.175	3.174
17	3.174	3.175	3.174	3.175	3.174	3.175
18	3.175	3.174	3.175	3.174	3.175	3.174
19	3.174	3.175	3.174	3.175	3.174	3.175
20	3.175	3.174	3.175	3.174	3.175	3.174
21	3.174	3.175	3.174	3.175	3.174	3.175
22	3.175	3.174	3.175	3.174	3.175	3.174
23	3.174	3.175	3.174	3.175	3.174	3.175
24	3.175	3.174	3.175	3.174	3.175	3.174
25	3.174	3.175	3.174	3.175	3.174	3.175
26	3.175	3.174	3.175	3.174	3.175	3.174
27	3.174	3.175	3.174	3.175	3.174	3.175
28	3.175	3.174	3.175	3.174	3.175	3.174
29	3.174	3.175	3.174	3.175	3.174	3.175
30	3.175	3.174	3.175	3.174	3.175	3.174
31	3.174	3.175	3.174	3.175	3.174	3.175
32	1.720	1.984	2.249	2.513	2.778	3.042
33	0.000	0.000	0.000	0.000	0.000	0.000

Recovery Year	Month Placed in Service					
	7	8	9	10	11	12
1	1.455	1.190	0.926	0.661	0.397	0.132
2	3.175	3.175	3.175	3.175	3.175	3.175
3	3.175	3.175	3.175	3.175	3.175	3.175
4	3.175	3.175	3.175	3.175	3.175	3.175
5	3.175	3.175	3.175	3.175	3.175	3.175
6	3.175	3.175	3.175	3.175	3.175	3.175
7	3.175	3.175	3.175	3.175	3.175	3.175
8	3.175	3.175	3.175	3.175	3.175	3.175
9	3.174	3.175	3.175	3.175	3.174	3.175
10	3.175	3.174	3.175	3.174	3.175	3.174
11	3.174	3.175	3.174	3.175	3.174	3.175
12	3.175	3.174	3.175	3.174	3.175	3.174
13	3.174	3.175	3.174	3.175	3.174	3.175
14	3.175	3.174	3.175	3.174	3.175	3.174
15	3.174	3.175	3.174	3.175	3.174	3.175
16	3.175	3.174	3.175	3.174	3.175	3.174
17	3.174	3.175	3.174	3.175	3.174	3.175
18	3.175	3.174	3.175	3.174	3.175	3.174
19	3.174	3.175	3.174	3.175	3.174	3.175
20	3.175	3.174	3.175	3.174	3.175	3.174
21	3.174	3.175	3.174	3.175	3.174	3.175
22	3.175	3.174	3.175	3.174	3.175	3.174
23	3.174	3.175	3.174	3.175	3.174	3.175
24	3.175	3.174	3.175	3.174	3.175	3.174
25	3.174	3.175	3.174	3.175	3.174	3.175
26	3.175	3.174	3.175	3.174	3.175	3.174
27	3.174	3.175	3.174	3.175	3.174	3.175
28	3.175	3.174	3.175	3.174	3.175	3.174
29	3.174	3.175	3.174	3.175	3.174	3.175
30	3.175	3.174	3.175	3.174	3.175	3.174
31	3.174	3.175	3.174	3.175	3.174	3.175
32	3.175	3.174	3.175	3.174	3.175	3.174
33	0.132	0.397	0.661	0.926	1.190	1.455

Modified ACRS Depreciation Percentages
for Nonresidential Real Property
Placed in Service after May 12, 1993

Month Placed in Service	Recovery Year				
	1	2	...	39	40
1	2.461%	2.564%		2.564%	0.107%
2	2.247	2.564		2.564	0.321
3	2.033	2.564		2.564	0.535
4	1.819	2.564		2.564	0.749
5	1.605	2.564		2.564	0.963
6	1.391	2.564		2.564	1.177
7	1.177	2.564		2.564	1.391
8	0.963	2.564		2.564	1.605
9	0.749	2.564		2.564	1.819
10	0.535	2.564		2.564	2.033
11	0.321	2.564		2.564	2.247
12	0.107	2.564		2.564	2.461

Modified ACRS Accelerated Depreciation Percentages
Using the Mid-Quarter Convention
for 3-, 5-, 7-, 10-, 15-, and 20-Year Property
Placed in Service after December 31, 1986

Recovery Year	Quarter Placed in Service			
	1	2	3	4
3-Year Property:				
1	58.33	41.67	25.00	8.33
2	27.78	38.89	50.00	61.11
3	12.35	14.14	16.67	20.37
4	1.54	5.30	8.33	10.19
5-Year Property:				
1	35.00	25.00	15.00	5.00
2	26.00	30.00	34.00	38.00
3	15.60	18.00	20.40	22.80
4	11.01	11.37	12.24	13.68
5	11.01	11.37	11.30	10.94
6	1.38	4.26	7.06	9.58
7-Year Property:				
1	25.00	17.85	10.71	3.57
2	21.43	23.47	25.51	27.55
3	15.31	16.76	18.22	19.68
4	10.93	11.37	13.02	14.06
5	8.75	8.87	9.30	10.04
6	8.74	8.87	8.85	8.73
7	8.75	8.87	8.86	8.73
8	1.09	3.33	5.53	7.64
10-Year Property:				
1	17.50	12.50	7.50	2.50
2	16.50	17.50	18.50	19.50
3	13.20	14.00	14.80	15.60
4	10.56	11.20	11.84	12.48
5	8.45	8.96	9.47	9.98
6	6.76	7.17	7.58	7.99
7	6.55	6.55	6.55	6.55
8	6.55	6.55	6.55	6.55
9	6.56	6.56	6.56	6.56
10	0.82	6.55	6.55	6.55
11		2.46	4.10	5.74

Recovery Year	Quarter Placed in Service			
	1	2	3	4
15-Year Property:				
1	8.75	6.25	3.75	1.25
2	9.13	9.38	9.63	9.88
3	8.21	8.44	8.66	8.89
4	7.39	7.59	7.80	8.00
5	6.65	6.83	7.02	7.20
6	5.99	6.15	6.31	6.48
7	5.90	5.91	5.90	5.90
8	5.91	5.90	5.90	5.90
9	5.90	5.91	5.91	5.90
10	5.91	5.90	5.90	5.91
11	5.90	5.91	5.91	5.90
12	5.91	5.90	5.90	5.91
13	5.90	5.91	5.91	5.90
14	5.91	5.90	5.90	5.91
15	5.90	5.91	5.91	5.90
16	0.74	2.21	3.69	5.17
20-Year Property:				
1	6.563	4.688	2.813	0.938
2	7.000	7.148	7.289	7.430
3	6.482	6.612	6.742	6.872
4	5.996	6.116	6.237	6.357
5	5.546	5.658	5.769	5.880
6	5.130	5.233	5.336	5.439
7	4.746	4.841	4.936	5.031
8	4.459	4.478	4.566	4.654
9	4.459	4.463	4.460	4.458
10	4.459	4.463	4.460	4.458
11	4.459	4.463	4.460	4.458
12	4.460	4.463	4.460	4.458
13	4.459	4.463	4.461	4.458
14	4.460	4.463	4.460	4.458
15	4.459	4.462	4.461	4.458
16	4.460	4.463	4.460	4.458
17	4.459	4.462	4.461	4.458
18	4.460	4.463	4.460	4.459
19	4.459	4.462	4.461	4.458
20	4.460	4.463	4.460	4.459
21	0.557	1.673	2.788	3.901

Alternative Depreciation System
Recovery Periods

General Rule: Recovery period is the property's class life unless:
      1. There is no class life (see below), or
      2. A special class life has been designated (see below).

Type of Property	*Recovery Period*
Personal property with no class life	12 years
Nonresidential real property with no class life	40 years
Residential rental property with no class life	40 years
Cars, light general purpose trucks, certain technological equipment, and semiconductor manufacturing equipment	5 years
Computer-based telephone central office switching equipment	9.5 years
Railroad track	10 years
Single purpose agricultural or horticultural structures	15 years
Municipal waste water treatment plants, telephone distribution plants	24 years
Low-income housing financed by tax-exempt bonds	27.5 years
Municipal sewers	50 years

Modified ACRS and ADS Straight-Line Depreciation Percentages
Using the Half-Year Convention for
3-, 5-, 7-, 10-, 15-, and 20-Year Property
Placed in Service after December 31, 1986

Recovery Year	3-Year	5-Year	7-Year	10-Year	15-Year	20-Year
1	16.67	10.00	7.14	5.00	3.33	2.50
2	33.33	20.00	14.29	10.00	6.67	5.00
3	33.33	20.00	14.29	10.00	6.67	5.00
4	16.67	20.00	14.28	10.00	6.67	5.00
5		20.00	14.29	10.00	6.67	5.00
6		10.00	14.28	10.00	6.67	5.00
7			14.29	10.00	6.67	5.00
8			7.14	10.00	6.66	5.00
9				10.00	6.67	5.00
10				10.00	6.66	5.00
11				5.00	6.67	5.00
12					6.66	5.00
13					6.67	5.00
14					6.66	5.00
15					6.67	5.00
16					3.33	5.00
17						5.00
18						5.00
19						5.00
20						5.00
21						2.50

ADS Straight-Line Depreciation Percentages
Real Property
Using the Mid-Month Convention
for Property Placed in Service After December 31, 1986

Month Placed In Service	Recovery Year		
	1	2–40	41
1	2.396	2.500	0.104
2	2.188	2.500	0.312
3	1.979	2.500	0.521
4	1.771	2.500	0.729
5	1.563	2.500	0.937
6	1.354	2.500	1.146
7	1.146	2.500	1.354
8	0.938	2.500	1.562
9	0.729	2.500	1.771
10	0.521	2.500	1.979
11	0.313	2.500	2.187
12	0.104	2.500	2.396

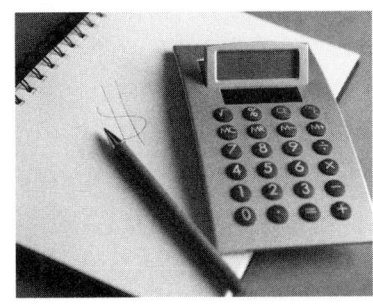

CONTINUOUS INDIVIDUAL TAX RETURN PROBLEMS AND TWO COMPREHENSIVE INDIVIDUAL TAX RETURN PROBLEMS FOR 2008

CONTINUOUS TAX RETURN PROBLEMS

General Instructions. Information is provided below for a continuous tax return problem. The tax return begins by providing a basic fact pattern, covering the topics found in Chapter 3. Additional facts are added to the facts for Chapter 3 in order to cover the topics discussed in Chapters 4, 5, 6, 7 and 8. In addition to the tax returns that must be prepared, questions relating to such returns are included.

CHAPTER 3: CONTINUOUS TAX RETURN PROBLEM

3-1 **Problem Facts.** Larry K. and Cathy L. Zepp have been married 19 years. Larry is 62 years old (Social Security number 123-45-6789) while Cathy is 57 years old (Social Security number 123-45-6788). They live at 1234 Elm Dr. in Indianapolis, Indiana 46202. The couple uses the cash method of accounting and files their return on a calendar-year basis. They are tired of politics and do not want to contribute to the presidential election campaign.

   a. Larry is a salesman employed by DSK Industries. This year he earned $110,000. Federal and state income taxes withheld were $17,000 and $6,000 respectively.

   b. Cathy recently completed a graduate degree in computer technology. She freelances as an independent contractor in computer graphics. She uses her own name as the name of her business. Her earnings received from various engagements were $12,000. Her only expenses paid during the year were for miscellaneous office supplies of $3,000. She paid estimated federal taxes during the year of $1,000 ($250 on each due date). Her business uses the cash method of accounting.

   c. Other income earned by the couple included interest income of $3,000 from a certificate of deposit issued by Highland National Bank and $975 of interest from tax-exempt bonds issued by the State of Indiana.

   d. The couple paid moving expenses of $2,000 that are fully deductible.

e. The couple owns a duplex that it rents out. It is located at 111 Nowhere Ave., Indianapolis, Indiana. Their rental records reveal the following information for the year.

Rental income	$12,000
Rental expenses	
Insurance	400
Mortgage interest	7,000
Repairs	1,000
Real property taxes	600

f. Other expenses paid during the year included:

Unreimbursed medical expenses	$ 9,000
Interest on home mortgage	12,000
Real property taxes on home	1,900
Charitable contributions	1,000
Rental of safety deposit box to hold gold coins held for investment	100
Unreimbursed employee business expenses of Larry	3,000

Prepare the 2008 individual income tax return for the Zepps. Complete Form 1040 and Schedules A, B, C, E and SE. Assume that all of the expenses except their business expenses are incurred jointly.

3-2 **Continuous Tax Return: Additional Questions**. Answer the following questions relating to the continuous tax return problem for Chapter 3 above.

a. What is the Zepp's marginal tax rate? Average tax rate?

b. The Zepps recently heard that making a contribution to an individual retirement account (IRA) may be a wise tax move. It is their understanding that contributions to a traditional or conventional IRA are deductible and the earnings on the accounts are not taxable until withdrawn (see Chapter 18 for more information). Assuming both Larry and Cathy make a deductible contribution of $8,000 ($4,000 each) what amount of tax will the couple save? Show computations illustrating how the savings are derived.

c. This question relates to the income tax of your state and may or may not be applicable. Check with your instructor for further instructions.

Larry incurred $3,000 of expenses related to his employment while Cathy incurred $3,000 related to her freelancing activity (i.e., self-employment). Which of the following statements is (are) true regarding the treatment of the expenses for state income tax purposes?

1. Both expenses were deductible in full.

2. Neither of the expenses was deductible.

3. The employment related expenses were deductible but the expenses related to self-employment were not deductible.

4. The expenses related to self-employment were deductible but the employment related expenses were not deductible.

d. Assume that Larry (instead of Cathy) had the self-employment income of $9,000. Which of the following statements is true?

1. Larry paid 15.3% self-employment tax on self-employment income of $9,000.

2. Larry paid 15.3% self-employment tax on self-employment income of $8,312.

3. Larry paid the same amount of self-employment tax that Cathy would have paid had she earned the income.

4. Larry pays less than the amount of self-employment tax that Cathy would have paid had she earned the income.

CHAPTER 4: CONTINUOUS TAX RETURN PROBLEM

4-1   **Problem Facts**. This is a continuation of the tax return problem beginning in Chapter 3. See previous facts above.

New Facts:

Larry and Cathy Zepp just called and after a quick discussion the following additional information was obtained:

a.   Larry received a corrected W-2 in the mail. The corrected W-2 (see below) reveals that federal income taxes withheld were $7,000 (rather than $17,000).

b.   Last year's federal tax liability before prepayments was $10,000.

c.   They forgot to note on their tax organizer that they had two children, a son and a daughter: Zachary W. Zepp (111-33-4444, date of birth 12/1/1989)) and Jennifer A. Zepp (111-33-4445, 1/4/1994). Both children live with them the entire year. Zachary is a full-time student. Jennifer is considered legally blind.

Prepare the 2008 individual income tax return for the Zepps. Complete Forms 1040, 2210, Schedules A, B, C, E and SE. Assume that all of the expenses except their business expenses are incurred jointly.

---

	a Employee's social security number 123-45-6789	OMB No. 1545-0008	Safe, accurate, FAST! Use IRS *e~file*	Visit the IRS website at *www.irs.gov/efile*.
b Employer identification number (EIN) 25-2222345			**1** Wages, tips, other compensation 110,000.00	**2** Federal income tax withheld 7,000.00
c Employer's name, address, and ZIP code DSK Industries 1635 Longest Drive Indianapolis, Indiana 46202			**3** Social security wages $97,500	**4** Social security tax withheld $6,045
			5 Medicare wages and tips $110,000	**6** Medicare tax withheld $1,595
			7 Social security tips	**8** Allocated tips
d Control number 0068251111			**9** Advance EIC payment	**10** Dependent care benefits
e Employee's first name and initial Last name Suff. Larry L. Zepp 1234 Elm Dr. Indianapolis, Indiana 46202		**11** Nonqualified plans	**12a** See instructions for box 12
		13 Statutory employee ☐ Retirement plan ☐ Third-party sick pay ☐	**12b**
		14 Other	**12c**
			12d
f Employee's address and ZIP code				

15 State Employer's state ID number IN	**16** State wages, tips, etc.	**17** State income tax $6,000	**18** Local wages, tips, etc.	**19** Local income tax	**20** Locality name

Form **W-2**   **Wage and Tax Statement**   **2008**   Department of the Treasury—Internal Revenue Service

Copy B—To Be Filed With Employee's FEDERAL Tax Return.
This information is being furnished to the Internal Revenue Service.

4-2   **Continuous Tax Return: Additional Questions**. Refer to the facts for the continuous tax return problem (Chapters 3 and 4 above). The Zepp's tax organizer indicated that their daughter, Jennifer Zepp, received $3,000 of interest income from a savings account at Chase National Bank. Using this additional information and the facts above, prepare a separate Form 1040 for Jennifer Zepp. Do not include Jennifer's income on her parents' return.

4-3 **Continuous Tax Return: Additional Questions.** Answer the following questions relating to the continuous tax return problem above.

    a. The Zepps generally could have avoided the estimated tax penalty by paying estimated taxes or by relying on their prior year's tax liability. Ignoring their prior year liability, how much should the couple have paid on each installment date to avoid the penalty? Alternatively, what would the amount of last year's tax liability have to be to avoid the penalty?

    b. If Cathy had hired Jennifer as an employee and paid her $4,000 to help her on certain business-related projects, what effect would it have on the family's tax liability? Provide an explanation that shows precisely why the family's total tax liability increased or decreased. For simplicity, assume that Jennifer had no other income.

For purpose of the questions below, assume Cathy was also an employee and received wages of $50,000 in addition to her self-employment income. Also ignore (a) and (b) above

    c. Does the couple's taxable income increase by $50,000, more than $50,000 or less than $50,000? Explain specifically what accounts for the change in taxable income and tax liability, if any.

    d. What would the Zepp's marginal tax rate be on the next $1,000 of income? For this question, use the actual change in tax to determine the marginal rate and compare it to the marginal rate in the tax rate schedule.

CHAPTER 5: CONTINUOUS TAX RETURN PROBLEM

5-1 **Problem Facts.** This is a continuation of the tax return problem covering Chapters 3 and 4. See previous facts above.

New Facts:

This morning's mail contained a note from Larry Zepp, including the following information

    a. Cathy forgot to explain several things about her consulting income. First, $2,400 of the $12,000 she received was for services to be performed in 2009. Second, she performed consulting services in December but was not paid until January when she received $5,000. She had sent the client a bill for $5,000 in December.

    b. Larry paid federal estimated income taxes of $12,000 ($3,000 on each of the due dates). He made no state estimated tax payments.

    c. A Schedule K-1 from a calendar-year partnership in which Larry is a small investor was included. The relevant portions of the Schedule K-1 are shown below. In addition, Larry received a $775 distribution from the partnership during the year.

Prepare the 2008 individual income tax return for the Zepps. Complete Forms 1040, 2210, Schedules A, B, C, E and SE. Assume that all of the expenses except their business expenses are incurred jointly. Also assume the couple does not qualify for the federal telephone excise tax credit.

651108

☐ Final K-1   ☐ Amended K-1   OMB No. 1545-0099

Schedule K-1
(Form 1065)

2008

Department of the Treasury
Internal Revenue Service

For calendar year 2008, or tax
year beginning _____ , 2008
ending _____ , 20____

Partner's Share of Income, Deductions,
Credits, etc. ▶ See back of form and separate instructions.

Part I   Information About the Partnership

A   Partnership's employer identification number

75-1234567

B   Partnership's name, address, city, state, and ZIP code

KLM Associates

3214 Memorial

Houston, TX 77452

C   IRS Center where partnership filed return

D ☐ Check if this is a publicly traded partnership (PTP)

Part II   Information About the Partner

E   Partner's identifying number

123-45-6789

F   Partner's name, address, city, state, and ZIP code

Larry L. Zepp

1234 Elm Drive

Indianapolis, IN 46202

G ☐ General partner or LLC member-manager   ☑ Limited partner or other LLC member

H ☐ Domestic partner   ☐ Foreign partner

I   What type of entity is this partner? _____

J   Partner's share of profit, loss, and capital (see instructions):

	Beginning	Ending
Profit	%	%
Loss	%	%
Capital	%	%

K   Partner's share of liabilities at year end:

Nonrecourse . . . . . . $_____

Qualified nonrecourse financing . $_____

Recourse . . . . . . $_____

L   Partner's capital account analysis:

Beginning capital account . . . $_____

Capital contributed during the year . $_____

Current year increase (decrease) . $_____

Withdrawals & distributions . . $(_____)

Ending capital account . . . $_____

☐ Tax basis   ☐ GAAP   ☐ Section 704(b) book
☐ Other (explain)

Part III   Partner's Share of Current Year Income, Deductions, Credits, and Other Items

1 Ordinary business income (loss)	200	**15**	Credits	
2 Net rental real estate income (loss)				
3 Other net rental income (loss)		**16**	Foreign transactions	
4 Guaranteed payments				
5 Interest income	150			
6a Ordinary dividends				
6b Qualified dividends				
7 Royalties				
8 Net short-term capital gain (loss)				
9a Net long-term capital gain (loss)		**17**	Alternative minimum tax (AMT) items	
9b Collectibles (28%) gain (loss)				
9c Unrecaptured section 1250 gain				
10 Net section 1231 gain (loss)		**18**	Tax-exempt income and nondeductible expenses	
11 Other income (loss)				
		19	Distributions	775
12 Section 179 deduction				
13 Other deductions		**20**	Other information	
14 Self-employment earnings (loss)				

*See attached statement for additional information.

For IRS Use Only

5-2 **Continuous Tax Return Problem. Additional Questions**. Refer to the facts for the continuous tax return problem (Chapters 3, 4 and 5 above).

a. According to the Schedule K-1, Larry Zepp received $775 of distributions from the partnership. How do the distributions impact the couple's individual income tax return? Explain.

b. Is the partnership income considered self-employment income of Larry Zepp for purposes of computing any self-employment tax he might owe? Explain.

c. Assume Cathy reached an agreement with a local fitness center to prepare various flyers, advertisements and do some work on the company's website. In exchange, she received an annual membership to the center worth $500. Explain the tax consequences to Cathy.

CHAPTER 6: CONTINUOUS TAX RETURN PROBLEM

6-1 **Problem Facts**. This is a continuation of the tax return problem covering Chapters 3, 4 and 5. See previous facts above.

New Facts:

a. This year Larry began receiving Social Security benefits. For the year, he received $12,000.

b. The couple received a Form 1099 from National Funds (see below) regarding an investment in a mutual fund.

c. Cathy was unemployed for a short period and received unemployment compensation of $800 reported on the Form 1099-G (see below).

d. Cathy received $2,000 of alimony from her first husband.

e. Cathy inherited $100,000 from her rich uncle.

f. The Zepps overpaid their income taxes for the prior year and received both a federal and state refund. The federal refund was $1700. They received a Form 1099-G from the state of Indiana reporting the state refund of $925.

g. Larry's father died this year and Larry was the beneficiary of his father's life insurance policy. Larry received life insurance proceeds of $25,000.

h. In June, DSK honored Larry for his 25 years of service. He received a plaque and a gift certificate for $400 at The Golf Shop, which he intends to use to buy a new driver.

Prepare the 2008 individual income tax return for the Zepps. Complete Forms 1040, 2210, Schedules A, B, C, E and SE. Assume that all of the expenses except their business expenses are incurred jointly.

☐ CORRECTED (if checked)

PAYER'S name, street address, city, state, ZIP code, and telephone no.	**1a** Total ordinary dividends	OMB No. 1545-0110	
National Funds	$ *3,000*	**2008**	**Dividends and Distributions**
888 Toobad Drive	**1b** Qualified dividends		
Boston, MA 02104	$ *3,000*	Form **1099-DIV**	

		2a Total capital gain distr.	**2b** Unrecap. Sec. 1250 gain	**Copy B**
		$ *1,400*	$	**For Recipient**

PAYER'S federal identification number	RECIPIENT'S identification number			

RECIPIENT'S name	**2c** Section 1202 gain	**2d** Collectibles (28%) gain	This is important tax information and is being furnished to the Internal Revenue Service. If you are required to file a return, a negligence penalty or other sanction may be imposed on you if this income is taxable and the IRS determines that it has not been reported.
Larry L. Zepp	$	$	
	3 Nondividend distributions	**4** Federal income tax withheld	
Street address (including apt. no.)	$	$	
1234 Elm Drive		**5** Investment expenses	
City, state, and ZIP code		$	
Indianapolis, IN 46202	**6** Foreign tax paid	**7** Foreign country or U.S. possession	
	$ *70*		
Account number (see instructions)	**8** Cash liquidation distributions	**9** Noncash liquidation distributions	
	$	$	

Form **1099-DIV**   (keep for your records)   Department of the Treasury - Internal Revenue Service

---

☐ CORRECTED (if checked)

PAYER'S name, street address, city, state, ZIP code, and telephone no.	**1** Unemployment compensation	OMB No. 1545-0120	
Indiana Department of Revenue	$ *800*	**2008**	**Certain Government Payments**
100 N. Senate Ave.	**2** State or local income tax refunds, credits, or offsets		
Indianapolis, IN 46204-2253	$ *925*	Form **1099-G**	

PAYER'S federal identification number	RECIPIENT'S identification number	**3** Box 2 amount is for tax year	**4** Federal income tax withheld	**Copy B**
			$	**For Recipient**

RECIPIENT'S name	**5** ATAA payments	**6** Taxable grants	This is important tax information and is being furnished to the Internal Revenue Service. If you are required to file a return, a negligence penalty or other sanction may be imposed on you if this income is taxable and the IRS determines that it has not been reported.
Larry L. Zepp	$	$	
Street address (including apt. no.)	**7** Agriculture payments	**8** Box 2 is trade or business income ▶ ☐	
1234 Elm Dr.	$		
City, state, and ZIP code			
Indianapolis, Indiana 46202			
Account number (see instructions)			

Form **1099-G**   (keep for your records)   Department of the Treasury - Internal Revenue Service

---

6-2   **Continuous Tax Return Problem. Additional Questions**. Refer to the facts for the continuous tax return problem (Chapters 3, 4, 5 and 6 above).

    a.   What is the Zepp's marginal tax rate?

    b.   At what rate were the dividends taxed?

    c.   Which of the following statements is true regarding the tax treatment of Larry's social security benefits?

1. None of the social security payments was taxable
2. 50% of the social security payments was taxable
3. 85% of the social security payment was taxable
4. None of the above.

6-3   **Continuous Tax Return Problem. Additional Questions**. Refer to the facts for the continuous tax return problem (Chapters 3, 4, 5 and 6 above). Note that the calculations required to complete the following questions are not explained in the text.

    a.   Assume that Jennifer received interest income of $3,000 and qualified dividend income of $1,000. Prepare Form 1040 for Jennifer. For simplicity purposes, assume that the taxable income of her parents was $200,000 and their return revealed qualified dividend income of $3,000.

    b.   At what rates were Jennifer's interest and dividend income taxed?

CHAPTER 7: CONTINUOUS TAX RETURN PROBLEM

7-1   **Problem Facts**. This is a continuation of the tax return problem covering Chapters 3, 4, 5 and 6. See previous facts above.

New Facts:

    a.   The $400 paid in 2008 for the insurance coverage related to the rental property was for a one-year term that begins on February 1, 2009.

    b.   On September 1, the couple refinanced the mortgage on the rental property to get a lower interest rate. They paid points of $1,800. The term of the new loan was 15 years.

    c.   Cathy paid medical insurance premiums of $4,000.

    d.   In early January, Cathy billed a customer $627 for setting up a website. The customer left town and Cathy indicates that the receivable is now worthless.

    e.   During the year, Larry explored the possibility of selling for a new employer. However, after some interviewing, he decided to stay with DSK. He paid $30 to have new resumes printed and another $20 to register his name on an employment website.

    f.   Larry paid several parking tickets during the year while calling on customers. Total cost was $48.

    g.   Larry contributed $250 to the Democratic National Party and Cathy contributed $250 to the Republican National Party.

    h.   The couple paid $3,000 premium for a $1,000,000 life insurance policy on Larry's life. Cathy was the beneficiary.

    i.   Cathy continued her hobby of breeding and selling terriers. This year she sold 10 puppies for $6,000. Her expenses for raising the dogs (food, shots, etc.) were $2,000.

Prepare the 2008 individual income tax return for the Zepps. Complete Forms 1040, 2210, Schedules A, B, C, E and SE. Assume that all of the expenses except their business expenses are incurred jointly.

7-2   **Continuous Tax Return: Additional Questions**. Refer to the facts for the continuous tax return problem (Chapters 3, 4, 5 and 6 above).

    a.   Larry incurred $3,000 of expenses related to his employment while Cathy incurred $3,000 related to her freelancing activity (i.e., self-employment). Which of the following statements is true regarding the treatment of the expenses for federal income tax purposes?

       1. The expenses of both Larry and Cathy were subject to the 2% limitation.
       2. The expenses of both Larry and Cathy were fully deductible as deductions for A.G.I. (i.e., deductible in arriving at adjusted gross income).

3. The expenses of both Larry and Cathy were considered itemized deductions but only the employment expenses were subject to the 2% limitation.

4. The expenses of Cathy affected the amount of Larry's expenses that are deductible.

5. None of the above is correct.

b. Assume Larry is considered a statutory employee (see Box 13 of his W-2 in an earlier chapter). Indicate the amount, if any, by which the couple's taxable income increases or decreases.

c. Did Cathy's payment for medical insurance affect her self-employment tax?

d. The couple paid $1,000 for tax preparation of last year's return. Before last year, Larry did the return but since last year's return involved filing a Schedule C for Cathy he decided to get professional tax help. The accountant's fee was $400. Explain the treatment of the tax preparation fee.

CHAPTER 8: CONTINUOUS TAX RETURN PROBLEM

8-1 **Problem Facts**. This is a continuation of the tax return problem covering Chapters 3, 4, 5, 6 and 7. See previous facts above.

New Facts:

a. Cathy paid $1,000 of tuition for a course that she took at the local university. The course related to her to computer graphics business.

b. Cathy worked out of her home. According to her records, she drove 8,000 miles from her home to her clients and back during the year. She does not have a qualifying home office. She has records of her mileage but nothing for gas, oil or related expenses.

c. Cathy took a client to lunch and they discussed some of the work she was doing for the client. Cathy paid for her meal, $16, and the client's meal, $20. She kept the receipts.

d. The couple provided additional information regarding their moving expenses. On May 1, the couple moved downtown to try downtown living and reduce Larry's commute. Before the move, Larry's roundtrip commute from home was 60 miles and after the move the commute was only 5 miles. The cost of the move was $2,000 as previously reported.

Prepare the 2008 individual income tax return for the Zepps. Complete Forms 1040, 2210, Schedules A, B, C, E and SE. Assume that all of the expenses except their business expenses are incurred jointly.

8-2 **Continuous Tax Return: Additional Questions**. Refer to the facts for the continuous tax return problem (Chapters 3, 4, 5, 6 and 7 above).

a. Cathy had several options regarding the treatment of her educational expenses related to her job. Explain these options and demonstrate with calculations why one is better than another.

b. Were the moving expenses deductible? Why or why not? Explain.

COMPREHENSIVE TAX RETURN PROBLEMS

1.   David R. and Susan L. Holman

a.   David and Susan Holman are married and file a joint return. David is 38 years of age and Susan is 36. David is a self-employed certified real estate appraiser (C.R.E.), and Susan is employed by Wells Fargo Bank as a trust officer. They have two children: Richard Lawrence, age 7, and Karen Ann, age 4. The Holmans currently live at 5901 W. 75th Street, Los Angeles, California 90034, in a home they purchased and occupied on September 6, 2008.

Until August 12, 2008 the Holman family lived at 3085 Windmill Lane in Dallas, Texas, where David was employed by Vestpar Company, a real estate appraisal company and Susan was a bank officer for First National Bank. They sold their home in Dallas and moved to Los Angeles so that Susan could assume her new job as a trust officer and David could become self-employed.

b.   David and Susan sold their home in Dallas for $315,000 and incurred the following expenses:

Sales commission	$18,900
Attorney's fee	1,800
Title insurance	2,650
Document preparation fee	90
Recording fee	30
Pest inspection fee	190
Prepayment penalty for early retirement of home mortgage (3 points)	1,500

The Holmans had purchased the Dallas home on August 4, 2000 and never held it for rent or used it for business purposes. The home originally cost $177,500, and they had paid $6,200 for a cedar fence and $7,900 for landscaping. Within seven weeks of receiving a contract of sale on their house, the Holmans paid $8,500 for interior and exterior painting and $600 for steam-cleaning of the carpets. The sale was closed on August 1, 2008 and the Holmans were required to move out of the home by August 15, 2008.

c.   In moving from Dallas to Los Angeles, the Holmans incurred the following expenses, none of which were reimbursed:

Cost of moving household goods	$9,250
Meals	295
Lodging	350
House-hunting expenses (including $150 for meals)	1,000
Temporary living expenses (20 days; including meals costing $400)	1,700

Not included in any of the above expenses are the costs for driving two automobiles from Dallas to Los Angeles. David and Susan each drove a car, taking turns driving with the children. Although neither one of them kept receipts, Susan noted that her auto mileage was 1,500 miles. In addition, David noted that the number of miles from their old home to their old workplace was 24 miles, and the number of miles from their old home to their new workplace is 1,514 miles.

d.   The Holmans purchased their new home for $525,000 by making a $125,000 down payment and financing the remaining balance with a 30-year, 6% conventional mortgage loan from California Federal Savings and Loan. They were required to prepay 2 points ($8,000) in return for the favorable mortgage terms. New furniture and drapes cost an additional $27,500.

e. The Holmans received the following Forms W-2, reporting their salaries for 2008:

1. David R. Holman, Social Security No. 452-64-5837:

Gross salary	$75,000
Federal income taxes withheld	9,050
F.I.C.A. taxes withheld:	
Social security	4,650
Medicare	1088

2. Susan L. Holman, Social Security No. 467-32-5452:

	First Nat'l Bank	Wells Fargo Bank	Total
Gross salary	$17,500	$34,000	$51,500
Federal income taxes withheld	1,100	4,150	5,250
F.I.C.A. taxes withheld:			
Social security	1,085	2,108	3,193
Medicare	254	493	747
California income taxes withheld	—	2,950	2,950

f. On October 1, 2008 David rented office space at 5510 Wacker Drive, Los Angeles, California 90025. The terms of the one-year lease agreement called for a monthly rent of $800, with the first and last month's rent paid in advance.

David decided to operate his business in the name of "David R. Holman, Certified Real Estate Appraiser," and he elected to use the cash method of accounting for his revenues and expenses. The following items relate to his business for 2008:

Gross receipts	$85,000
Expenses:	
Advertising	250
Bank service charges	50
Dues and publications	450
Insurance	600*
Interest	275
Professional services	525
Office rent	3,200**
Office supplies	700
Meals and entertainment	500
Miscellaneous expenses	75

　* Three months of coverage
　**Includes prepayment of rent for September, 2009

David drove his personal automobile, a 2007 Buick LeSabre, 5,000 miles for business purposes from October 1 through December 31. Rather than keeping receipts, he elected to use the automatic mileage method for determining his auto expenses. David's total auto mileage for the year was 20,000 miles.

On October 3, 2008 David purchased the following furniture and equipment for use in his business:

Office furniture	$17,000
Copying machine	5,800
Computers	6,500
Laser printers	2,500
Telephone system	3,100

David elects to expense the maximum amount allowed under the optional expensing rules of § 179. He also elects to compute the maximum depreciation allowance using the appropriate MACRS percentages.

g. The Holmans received interest income during 2008 from the following:

U.S. Treasury bills	$1,475
First National Bank, Dallas	625
Wells Fargo Bank	400
Tarrant County municipal bonds	800

h. David and Susan received the following dividends during 2008:

Ford Motor Company	$300
Eastman Kodak Company	575
IBM Corporation	125
General Motors stock dividend (20 new shares of stock valued at $60 per share, received March 9, 2008)	1,200

i. The Holmans have never maintained foreign bank accounts or created foreign trusts.

j. The Holmans report the following stock transactions for 2008:

1. Sold 100 shares of IBM stock for $120 per share on August 1, 2008. David had inherited 500 shares of IBM stock from his uncle on July 18, 2004, and the stock was valued at $170 per share on the date of his uncle's death (the value used for estate tax purposes).

2. Sold 400 shares of General Motors stock for $78 per share on September 20, 2008. Susan had received 1,000 shares of General Motors stock as a wedding present from her grandfather on June 3, 1996. Her grandfather had purchased the stock for $35 per share on May 7, 1993, and the stock was valued at $60 per share on the date of the gift. Susan's grandfather paid gift taxes of $10,000 as a result of the gift. Note: the amount of the annual exclusion taken into account in determining the taxable gift was $10,000.

3. Sold 300 shares of Eastman Kodak stock for $40 per share on December 28, 2008, but did not receive the sales proceeds until January 3, 2009. The Holmans had paid $25 per share for the stock on October 21, 2006.

k. Susan has summarized the following cash expenditures for 2008 from canceled checks, mortgage company statements, and other documents:

Prescription medicines and drugs	$ 982
Medical insurance premiums (paid by Susan)	2,830
Doctors' and hospital bills (net of reimbursements)	1,535
Contact lenses for David	218
Real estate taxes paid on	
Dallas residence	3,400
Los Angeles residence	5,600
Sales taxes paid on Susan's new auto	1,485
Ad valorem taxes paid on both autos	350
Interest paid for	
Dallas home mortgage	5,250*
Los Angeles home mortgage	10,200**
Credit card interest	480
Personal car loan	1,720
Cash contributions to	
United Methodist Church	5,000
American Heart Fund	200
United Way Campaign	1,500
George W. Bush Campaign Fund	250
Susan's unreimbursed employee expenses	470***
David's unreimbursed employee expenses	360
Tax return preparation fee	375

* Does not include the mortgage prepayment penalty identified in item (b) above.

** Does not include the interest points charged for the new mortgage identified in item (d) above.

*** Does not include any costs for meals or entertainment.

Susan also noted that she and David had driven their personal automobiles 500 miles to receive medical treatment for themselves and their children. She also has a receipt for 100 shares of General Motors stock that she gave to her alma mater, Southern Methodist University, on November 12, 2008. The stock was valued at $70 per share on the date of the gift and was from the block of General Motors stock Susan had received as a wedding present from her grandfather [see item (j)(2) above for details].

l. The Holmans paid the following child care expenses during 2008:

1.	Kindergarten Day Care School	$2,800
	1177 Valley View	
	Dallas, Texas 75210	
	EIN: 74-0186254	
2.	Happy Trails Day Center	2,200
	3692 Airport Blvd.	
	Los Angeles, California 90034	
	EIN: 78-0593676	

Of the $5,000 total child care expenses, $3,000 was for Karen, and the remaining $2,000 was for Richard.

m. Social security numbers for the Holman children are provided below:

Richard L. Holman, Social Security No. 582-60-4732
Karen A. Holman, Social Security No. 582-60-5840

n. David and Susan made estimated Federal income tax payments of $1,750 each quarter, on 4/15/08, 6/15/08, 9/15/08, and 1/15/09.

o. The Holmans have always directed that $6 go to the Presidential Election Campaign by checking the "yes" boxes on their Form 1040.

Required:
Complete the Holmans' Federal income tax return for 2008. If they have a refund due, they would prefer having it credited against their 2009 taxes.

2. **Richard M. and Anna K. Wilson**

a. Richard and Anna Wilson are married and file a joint return. Richard is 47 years of age and Anna is 46. Richard is employed by Telstar Corporation as its controller and Anna is self-employed as a travel agent. They have three children: Michael, age 22; Lisa, age 17; and Laura, age 14. Michael is a full-time student at Rutgers University. Lisa and Laura both live at home and attend school full-time. The Wilsons currently live at 3721 Chestnut Ridge Road, Montvale, New Jersey 07645, in a home they have owned since July 1989.

Richard and Anna provided over half of the support of Anna's mother, who currently lives in a nursing home in Mahwah, New Jersey. They also provided over half of the support of their son, Michael, who earned $4,750 during the summer as an accounting student intern for a national accounting firm.

b. Richard received a Form W-2 from his employer reporting the following information for 2008:

Richard M. Wilson, Social Security No. 294-38-6249:

Gross wages and taxable benefits	$63,000
Federal income taxes withheld	11,400
F.I.C.A. taxes withheld:	
Social security	3,571
Medicare	914
State income taxes withheld	1,850

The taxable benefits reported on his W-2 Form include $2,700 (based on the currently deductible standard auto mileage rate) for Richard's personal use of the company car provided by his employer.

c. Anna operates her business under the name "Wilson's Travel Agency," located at 7200 Treeline Drive, Montvale, NJ 07645. Anna has one full-time employee, and her Federal employer identification number is 74-2638596

Anna uses the cash method of accounting for her business, and her records for 2008 show the following:

Fees and commissions	$134,000
Expenses:	
Advertising	1,425
Bank service charges	75
Dues and subscriptions	560
Insurance	1,100
Interest on furniture loan	960
Professional services	700
Office rent	6,000
Office supplies	470
Meals and entertainment	1,000
Payroll taxes	2,170
Utilities and telephone	3,480
Wages paid to full-time employee	22,800
Miscellaneous expenses	20

Automobile expenses and amounts paid to her children are not included in the above expenses. Anna paid her daughters Lisa and Laura $750 and $450, respectively, for working part-time during the summer. Since she did not withhold or pay any Federal income or employment taxes on these amounts, Anna is not certain that she is allowed a deduction. She does feel that the amounts paid to her children were reasonable, however.

Anna purchased a new 2008 Honda Accord on November 20 of last year, and her tax accountant used the actual cost method in determining the deductible business expenses for her 2008 Federal tax return. Because the deductible amount seemed so small, she is not certain whether she should claim actual expenses (including depreciation), or simply

use the automatic mileage method. She has the following records relating to the business auto:

Original cost	$26,000
Depreciation claimed in 2007	
($26,000 × 5% = $1,300 × 80% business use)	1,040
Gas, oil, and repairs in 2008	1,790
Parking and tolls paid in 2008	410
Insurance for 2008	650
Interest on car loan for 2008	750

Anna drove the auto 20,000 miles for business purposes and 5,000 miles for personal purposes during the year. The above expenses for 2008 have not been reduced to reflect her personal use of the vehicle.

On January 7, 2008 Anna purchased the following items for use in her business:

Office furniture	$8,900
Copying machine	5,700
Dell notebook computer	1,500
Printer	1,600
Fax machine	300

Anna wishes to claim the maximum amount of depreciation deductions or other cost recovery allowed on the office furniture and equipment.

d. Richard attended an accounting convention in Washington, D.C. for three days in October. He incurred the following unreimbursed expenses related to the trip:

Air fare (round-trip)	$470
Registration fee for meeting	225
Hotel cost	375
Meals	130
Taxis	20
Airport parking	18
Road tolls	2

e. Richard and Anna received Forms 1099-INT reporting interest income earned during 2008 from the following:

Citibank of Mahwah	$845
Montvale National Bank	900
Telstar Employees' Credit Union	755

f. The Wilsons received the following dividends during 2008:

Telstar Corporation	$300
Exxon Corporation	200

These dividends were labeled as "qualifying dividends" on the respective Forms 1099-DIV.

g. The Wilsons have never had a foreign bank account or created a foreign trust.

h. The Wilsons had the following property transactions for 2008:

1. Anna sold 300 shares of Exxon Corporation stock on September 9, 2008 in order to pay for Michael's fall semester of college. She received a check in the amount of $14,950 from Shearson Lehman on September 16, 2008. The stock was from a block of 1,000 shares that Richard and Anna had purchased for $35 per share on February 1, 1985.

2. They gave each of the children 100 shares of Exxon stock on December 30, 2008, when the stock was valued at $62.50 per share. The stock was from the same block of stock purchased for $35 per share in February, 1985. No gift taxes were paid on these gifts.

3. They gave 100 shares of ExxonMobil stock to Richard's alma mater, Rider University, on December 29, 2008. The average trading price of Exxon stock on that day was $61.25. This stock was also from the original block of 1,000 shares the Wilsons had purchased for $35 per share in 1985. The address of Rider University is 2083 Lawrenceville Road, Lawrenceville, New Jersey 08648

4. On May 17, 2008, Richard and Anna were notified by the bankruptcy judge handling the affairs of Bubbling Crude Oil Company in Houston, Texas that the company's shareholders would not receive anything for their stock ownership because all of the assets were used to satisfy claims of creditors. Richard had purchased 2,000 shares of the stock for $6 per share on April 1, 1991. Unfortunately, the stock did not meet the requirements of § 1244.

i. Richard and Anna own a rental condominium located at 7777 Boardwalk in Atlantic City, New Jersey. The unit was purchased on July 29, 2007 for $25,000 cash and a $175,000 mortgage. Of the purchase price, $50,000 was allocated to the land. The following items relate to the rental unit for 2008:

Gross rents	$16,400
Expenses:	
Management fee	2,460
Cleaning and maintenance	1,200
Insurance	840
Property taxes	2,750
Interest paid on mortgage	13,675
Utilities	850

Although the unfurnished unit was vacant for 11 weeks during the year, the Wilsons never used the property for personal purposes. When the property is rented, the tenant is required to pay for all utilities, and the Wilsons are charged a management fee equal to 15 percent of the rents collected.

j. The Wilsons have prepared the following summary of their other expenditures for 2008:

Prescription medicines and drugs	$ 425
Medical insurance premiums (paid by Richard)	1,595
Doctors' and hospital bills (net of reimbursements)	805*
Dentist	2,750**
Real estate taxes paid on home	1,625
State income taxes paid during 2008	2,100***
Interest paid for	
Original home mortgage	8,690
Home equity loan (secured by home)	410****
Credit card interest	275
Personal car loan	725
Cash contributions to First Presbyterian Church	1,200
Fee for preparation of 2007 tax return	650*****

    * Does not include $11,485 of doctor bills paid by Richard and Anna for medical treatment provided to Anna's mother at the nursing home. Also not included is $115 that Anna paid for a new pair of eyeglasses for her mother.

    ** $2,350 of this amount represents a prepayment of Laura's braces. The dentist required the prepayment before he would begin the two-year dental program involved.

    *** Does not include amounts withheld from Richard's wages.

    **** Represents interest paid on a $25,000 home equity loan obtained by the Wilsons in 2008 to obtain a new boat.

    ***** $200 is related to preparation of Schedule C

k. Anna made an $11,500 deductible contribution to her Keogh plan on December 15, 2008.

l. Richard paid the following unreimbursed employee business expenses:

Professional dues	$450
Professional journals.	385
Office gifts to subordinates (none over $25).	115

m. During the year, the Wilsons paid tuition of $9,350 and spent $1,875 on books and supplies for Michael's senior year of college.

n. The Wilsons received a state income tax refund of $130 in 2007. They had $18,750 of itemized deductions for 2007, and their 2007 taxable income was $52,825.

o. Richard and Anna made timely estimated Federal income tax payments of $2,250 each quarter on 4/15/08, 6/15/08, 9/15/08, and 1/15/09.

p. Social security numbers for Anna, the children, and Anna's mother are provided below:

	Number
Anna K. Wilson	296-48-2385
Michael D. Wilson	256-83-4421
Lisa M. Wilson	257-64-7573
Laura D. Wilson.	258-34-2894
Ruth Knapp	451-38-3790

q. The Wilsons have always checked the "no" boxes on their Form 1040 regarding the Presidential Election Campaign fund contribution.

Required:

Complete the Wilsons' Federal income tax return for 2008. If they have a refund due, they would prefer having it credited against their 2009 taxes.

★ APPENDIX E ★

GLOSSARY OF TAX TERMS

—A—

A. (*see* Acquiescence).

Accelerated Cost Recovery System (ACRS). An alternate form of depreciation enacted by the Economic Recovery Tax Act of 1981 and significantly modified by the Tax Reform Act of 1986. The modified cost recovery system applies to assets placed into service after 1986 and is referred to as MACRS. Under both systems, the cost of a qualifying asset is recovered over a set period of time. Salvage value is ignored. § 168.

Accelerated Depreciation. Various depreciation methods that produce larger depreciation deductions in the earlier years of an asset's life than straight-line depreciation. Examples: double-declining balance method (200% declining balance) and sum-of-the-years'-digits method. § 167 (*see* Depreciation).

Accounting Method. A method by which an entity's income and expenses are determined. The primary accounting methods used are the accrual method and the cash method. Other accounting methods include the installment method, the percentage-of-completion method (for construction), and various methods for valuing inventories, such as FIFO and LIFO. §§ 446 and 447 (*see also specific accounting methods*).

Accounting Period. A period of time used by a taxpayer in determining his or her income, expenses, and tax liability. An accounting period is generally a year for tax purposes, either a calendar year, a fiscal year, or a 52-53 week year. §§ 441 and 443.

Accrual Method of Accounting. The method of accounting that reflects the income earned and the expenses incurred during a given tax period. However, unearned income of an accrual basis taxpayer must generally be included in an entity's income in the year in which it is received, even if it is not actually earned by the entity until a later tax Period. § 446.

Accumulated Adjustment Account (AAA). A summary of all includible income and gains, expenses, and losses of an S Corporation for taxable years after 1982, except those that relate to excludable income, distributions, and redemptions of an S Corporation. Distributions from the AAA are not taxable to the shareholders. §§1368(c)(1) and (3)(1).

Accumulated Earnings Credit. A reduction in arriving at a corporation's accumulated taxable income (in computing the Accumulated Earnings Tax). Its purpose is to

avoid penalizing a corporation for retaining sufficient earnings and profits to meet the reasonable needs of the business. § 535(c).

Accumulated Earnings Tax. A penalty tax on the unreasonable accumulation of earnings and profits by a corporation. It is intended to encourage the distribution of earnings and profits of a corporation to its shareholders. §§ 531-537.

Accumulated Taxable Income. The amount on which the accumulated earnings tax is imposed. §§ 531 and 535.

Accuracy-Related Penalty. Any of the group of penalties that includes negligence or disregard of rules or regulations, substantial understatement of income tax, substantial valuation misstatement for income tax purposes, substantial overstatement of pension liabilities, and substantial estate or gift valuation understatement. § 6662.

Acquiescence. The public endorsement of a regular Tax Court decision by the Commissioner of the Internal Revenue Service. When the Commissioner acquiesces to a regular Tax Court decision, the IRS generally will not dispute the result in cases involving substantially similar facts (*see* Nonacquiescence).

Ad Valorem Tax. A tax based on the value of property.

Adjusted Basis. The basis (i.e., cost or other basis) of property plus capital improvements minus depreciation allowed or allowable. See § 1016 for other adjustments to basis. § 1016 (*see* Basis).

Adjusted Gross Income. A term used with reference to individual taxpayers. Adjusted gross income consists of an individual's gross income less certain deductions and business expenses. § 62.

Adjusted Ordinary Gross Income (AOGI). A term used in relation to personal holding companies. Adjusted ordinary gross income is determined by subtracting certain expenses related to rents and mineral, oil, and gas royalties, and certain interest expense from ordinary gross income § 543(b)(2).

Administrator. A person appointed by the court to administrate the estate of a deceased person. If named to perform these duties by the decedent's will, this person is called an executor (executrix).

AFTR (American Federal Tax Reports). These volumes contain the Federal tax decisions issued by the U.S. District Courts, U.S. Court of Federal Claims, U.S. Circuit Courts of Appeals, and the U.S. Supreme Court (*see* AFTR2d).

AFTR2d (American Federal Tax Reports, Second Series). The second series of the American Federal Tax Reports. These volumes contain the Federal tax decisions issued by the U.S. District Courts, U.S. Court of Federal Claims. U.S. Circuit Courts of Appeals, and the U.S. Supreme Court (see AFTR).

Alternate Valuation Date. The property contained in a decedent's gross estate must be valued at either the decedent's date of death or the alternate valuation date. The alternate valuation date is six months after the decedent's date of death, or, if the

property is disposed of prior to that date; the particular property disposed of is valued as of the date of its disposition. § 2032.

Alternative Minimum Tax. A tax imposed on taxpayers only if it exceeds the "regular" tax of the taxpayer. Regular taxable income is adjusted by certain timing differences, then increased by tax preferences to arrive at alternative minimum taxable income.

Amortization. The systematic write-off (deduction) of the cost or other basis of an intangible asset over its estimated useful life. The concept is similar to depreciation (used for tangible assets) and depletion (used for natural resources) (*see* Goodwill; Intangible Asset).

Amount Realized. Any money received, plus the fair market value of any other property or services received, plus any liabilities discharged on the sale or other disposition of property. The determination of the amount realized is the first step in determining realized gain or loss. § 1001(b).

Annual Exclusion. The amount each year that a donor may exclude from Federal gift tax for each donee. Currently, the annual exclusion is $12,000 per donee. The annual exclusion does not generally apply to gifts of future interests. § 2503(b).

Annuity. A fixed amount of money payable to a person at specific intervals for either a specific period of time or for life.

Appellate Court. A court to which other court decisions are appealed. The appellate courts for Federal tax purposes include the Courts of Appeals and the Supreme Court.

Arm's-Length Transaction. A transaction entered into by unrelated parties, all acting in their own best interests. It is presumed that in an arm's length transaction the prices used are the fair market values of the properties or services being transferred in the transaction.

Articles of Incorporation. The basic instrument filed with the appropriate state agency when a business is incorporated.

Assessment of Tax. The imposition of an additional tax liability by the Internal Revenue Service (i.e.. as the result of an audit).

Assignment of Income. A situation in which a taxpayer assigns income or income-producing property to another person or entity in an attempt to avoid paying taxes on that income. An assignment of income or income-producing property is generally not recognized for tax purposes, and the income is taxable to the assignor.

Association. An entity that possesses a majority of the following characteristics: associates; profit motive; continuity of life; centralized management; limited liability; free transferability of interests. Associations are taxed as corporations. §§ 7701(a)(3). Reg. § 301.7701-2.

At-Risk Limitation. A provision that limits a deduction for losses to the amounts "at risk." A taxpayer is generally not "at risk" in situations where nonrecourse debt is used. § 465.

Attribution. (*see* Constructive Ownership).

Audit. The examination of a taxpayer's return or other taxable transactions by the Internal Revenue Service in order to determine the correct tax liability. Types of audits include correspondence audits, office audits, and field audits(*see also* Correspondence Audit; Office Audit; Field Audit).

—B—

Bad Debt. An uncollectible debt. A bad debt may be classified either as a business bad debt or a nonbusiness bad debt. A business bad debt is one that has arisen in the course of the taxpayer's business (with a business purpose). Nonbusiness bad debts are treated as short-term capital losses rather than as ordinary losses. § 166.

Bargain Sale, Rental, or Purchase. A sale, rental, or purchase of property for less than its fair market value. The difference between the sale, rental, or purchase price and the property's fair market value may have its own tax consequences, such as consideration as a constructive dividend or a gift.

Bartering. The exchange of goods and services without using money.

Basis. The starting point in determining the gain or loss from the sale or other disposition of an asset, or the depreciation (or depletion or amortization) on an asset. For example, if an asset is purchased for cash, the basis of that as set is the cash paid. §§ 1012, 1014, 1015, 334, 359, 362.

Beneficiary. Someone who will benefit from an act of another, such as the beneficiary of a life insurance contract, the beneficiary of a trust (i.e., income beneficiary), or the beneficiary of an estate.

Bequest. A testamentary transfer (by will) of personal property (personalty).

Board of Tax Appeals (B.T.A.). The predecessor of the United States Tax Court, in existence from 1924 to 1942.

Bona Fide. Real; in good faith.

Boot. Cash or property that is not included in the definition of a particular type of nontaxable exchange [see §§ 351(b) and 1031(b)]. In these nontaxable exchanges, a taxpayer who receives boot must recognize gain to the extent of the boot received or the realized gain, whichever is less.

Brother-Sister Corporations. A controlled group of two or more corporations owned (in certain amounts) by five or fewer individuals, estates, or trusts. § 1563(a)(2).

Burden of Proof. The weight of evidence in a legal case or in a tax proceeding. Generally, the burden of proof is on the taxpayer in a tax case. However, the burden of proof is on the government in fraud cases. § 7454.

Business Purpose. An actual business reason for following a course of action. Tax avoidance alone is not considered to be a business purpose. In areas such as corporate formation and corporate reorganizations, business purpose is especially important.

—C—

Capital Asset. All proper by held by a taxpayer (e.g., house, car, clothing) except for certain assets that are specifically excluded from the definition of a capital asset, such as inventory and depreciable and real property used in a trade or business.

Capital Contribution. Cash, services, or property contributed by a partner to a partnership or by a shareholder to a corporation. Capital contributions are not income to the recipient partnership or corporation. §§ 721 and 118.

Capital Expenditure. Any amount paid for new buildings or for permanent improvements; any expendi-tures that add to the value or prolong the life of property or adapt the property to a new or different use. Capital expenditures should be added to the basis of the property improved. § 263.

Capital Gain. A gain from the sale or other disposition of a capital asset. § 1222.

Capital Loss. A loss from the sale or other disposition of a capital asset. § 1222.

Cash Method of Accounting. The method of accounting that reflects the income received (or constructively received) and the expenses paid during a given period. However, prepaid expenses of a cash basis taxpayer that benefit more than one year may be required to be deducted only in the periods benefited (e.g., a premium for a three-year insurance policy may have to be spread over three years).

CCH.(*see* Commerce Clearing House).

C Corporation. A so-called regular corporation that is a separate tax-paying entity and is subject to the tax rules contained in Subchapter C of the Internal Revenue Code (as opposed to an S corporation, which is subject to the tax rules of Subchapter S of the Code).

Certiorari. A Writ of Certiorari is the form used to appeal a lower court (U.S. Court of Appeals) decision to the Supreme Court. The Supreme Court then decides, by reviewing the Writ of Certiorari, whether it will accept the appeal or not. The Supreme Court generally does not accept the appeal unless a constitutional issue is involved or the lower courts are in conflict. If the Supreme Court refuses to accept the appeal, then the certiorari is denied (cert. den.).

Claim of Right Doctrine. If a taxpayer has an unrestricted claim to income, the income is included in that taxpayer's income when it is received or constructively received, even if there is a possibility that all or part of the income may have to be returned to another party.

Closely Held Corporation. A corporation whose voting stock is owned by one or a few shareholders and is operated by this person or closely knit group.

Collapsible Corporation. A corporation that liquidates before it has realized a substantial portion of its income. Shareholders treat the gain on these liquidating distributions as ordinary income (rather than dividend income or capital gains). § 341.

Commerce Clearing House. A publisher of tax materials, including a multivolume tax service, volumes that contain the Federal courts' decisions on tax matters (USTC) and the Tax Court regular (T.C.) and memorandum (TCM) decisions.

Community Property. Property that is owned together by husband and wife, where each has an undivided one-half interest in the property due to their marital status. The ten community property states are Alaska, Arizona, California, Idaho, Louisiana, Nevada, New Mexico, Texas, Washington, and Wisconsin.

Complex Trust. Any trust that does not meet the requirements of a simple trust. For example, a trust will be considered to be a complex trust if it does not distribute the trust income currently, if it takes a deduction for a charitable contribution for the current year, or if it distributes any of the trust corpus currently. § 661.

Condemnation. The taking of private property for a public use by a public authority, an exercise of the power of eminent domain. The public authority compensates the owner of the property taken in a condemnation (see also Involuntary Conversion).

Conduit Principle. The provisions in the tax law that allow specific tax characteristics to be passed through certain entities to the owners of the entity without losing their identity. For example, the short-term capital gains of a partnership would be passed through to the partners and retain their character as short-term capital gains on the tax returns of the partners. This principle applies in varying degrees to partnerships, S corporations, estates, and trusts

Consent Dividend. A term used in relation to the accumulated earnings tax and the personal holding company tax. A consent dividend occurs when the shareholders consent to treat a certain amount as a taxable dividend on their tax returns even though there is no distribution of cash or property. The purpose of this is to obtain a dividends-paid deduction. § 565.

Consolidated Return. A method used to determine the tax liability of a group of affiliated corporations. The aggregate income (with certain adjustments) of a group is viewed as the income of a single enterprise. § 1501.

Consolidation. The statutory combination of two or more corporations in a new corporation. § 368(a)(1)(A).

Constructive Dividends. The constructive receipt of a dividend. Even though a taxable benefit was not designated as a dividend by the distributing corporation, a shareholder may be designated by the IRS as having received a dividend if the benefit has the appearance of a dividend. For example, if a shareholder uses corporate property for personal purposes rent-free, he or she will have a constructive dividend equal to the fair rental value of the corporate property.

Constructive Ownership. In certain situations the tax law attributes the ownership of stock to persons "related" to the person or entity that actually owns the stock. The related party is said to constructively own the stock of that person. For example, under § 267(c) a father is considered to constructively own all stock actually owned by his son. §§ 267, 318, and 544(a).

Constructive Receipt. When income is available to a taxpayer, even though it is not actually received by the taxpayer, the amount is considered to be constructively received by the taxpayer and should be included in income (e.g., accrued interest on a savings account). However, if there are restrictions on the availability of the income, it is generally not considered to be constructively received until the restrictions are removed (e.g., interest on a 6-month certificate of deposit is not constructively received until the end of the 6-month period if early withdrawal would result in loss of interest or principal).

Contributions to the Capital of a Corporation. (*see* Capital Contributions).

Corpus. The principal of a trust, as opposed to the income of the trust. Also called the *res* of the trust.

Correspondence Audit. An IRS audit conducted through the mail. Generally, verification or sub-stantiation for specified items is requested by the IRS, and the taxpayer mails the requested information to the IRS (*see* Field Audit; Office Audit).

Cost Depletion. (*see* Depletion).

Court of Appeals. The U.S. Federal court system has 13 circuit Courts of Appeals, which consider cases appealed from the U.S. Court of Federal Claims, the U.S. Tax Court, and the U.S. District Courts. A writ of certiorari is used to appeal a case from a Court of Appeals to the U.S. Supreme Court (see Appellate Court).

Creditor. A person or entity to whom money is owed. The person or entity who owes the money is called the debtor.

—D—

Death Tax. A tax imposed on property upon the death of the owner, such as an estate tax or inheritance tax.

Debtor. A person or entity who owes money to another. The person or entity to whom the money is owed is called the creditor.

Decedent. A deceased person.

Deductions in Respect of a Decedent (DRD). Certain expenses that are incurred by a decedent but are not properly deductible on the decedent's first return because of nonpayment. Deductions in respect of a decedent are deducted by the taxpayer who is legally required to make payment. § 691(b).

Deficiency. An additional tax liability owed to the IRS by a taxpayer. A deficiency is generally proposed by the IRS through the use of a Revenue Agent's Report.

Deficit. A negative balance in retained earnings or in earnings and profits.

Dependent. A person who derives his or her primary support from another. In order for a taxpayer to claim a dependency exemption for a person, there are five tests that must be met: support test, gross income test, citizenship or residency test, relationship or member of household test, and joint return test. § 152.

Depletion. As natural resources are extracted and sold, the cost or other basis of the resource is recovered by the use of depletion. Depletion may be either cost or percentage (statutory) depletion. Cost depletion has to do with the recovery of the cost of natural resources based on the units of the resource sold. Percentage depletion uses percentages given in the Internal Revenue Code multiplied by the gross income from the interest. subject to limitations. §§ 613 and 613A.

Depreciation. The systematic write-off of the basis of a tangible asset over the asset's estimated useful life. Depreciation is intended to reflect the wear, tear, and obsolescence of the asset(*see* Amortization; Depletion).

Depreciation Recapture. The situation in which all or part of the realized gain from the sale or other disposition of depreciable business property could be treated as ordinary income. See text for discussion of §§ 291, 1245, and 1250.

Determination Letter. A written statement regarding the tax consequences of a transaction issued by an IRS District Director in response to a written inquiry by a taxpayer that applies to a particular set of facts. Determination letters are frequently used to state whether a pension or profit-sharing plan is qualified or not, to determine the tax-exempt status of nonprofit organizations, and to clarify employee status.

Discretionary Trust. A trust in which the trustee or another party has the right to determine whether to accumulate or distribute the trust income currently, and/or which beneficiary is to receive the trust income.

Discriminant Function System (DIF). The computerized system used by the Internal Revenue Service in identifying and selecting returns for examination. This system uses secret mathematical formulas to select those returns that have a probability of tax errors.

Dissent. A disagreement with the majority opinion. The term is generally used to mean the explicit disagreement of one or more judges in a court with the majority decision on a particular case.

Distributable Net Income (DNI). The net income of a fiduciary that is available for distribution to income beneficiaries. DNI is computed by adjusting an estate's or trust's taxable income by certain modifications. § 643(a).

Distribution in Kind. A distribution of property as it is. For example, rather than selling property and distributing the proceeds to the shareholders, the property itself is distributed to the shareholders.

District Court. A trial court in which Federal tax matters can be litigated; the only trial court in which a jury trial can be obtained.

Dividend. A payment by a corporation to its shareholders authorized by the corporation's board of directors to be distributed pro rata among the outstanding shares. However, a constructive dividend does not need to be authorized by the shareholders(*see also* Constructive Dividend).

Dividends-Paid Deduction. A deduction allowed in determining the amount that is subject to the accumulated earnings tax and the personal holding company tax. §§ 561-565.

Dividends-Received Deduction. A deduction available to corporations on dividends received from a domestic corporation. The dividends-received deduction is generally 70 percent of the dividends received. If the recipient corporation owns 20 percent or more of the stock of the paying corporation, an 80 percent deduction is allowed. The dividends-received deduction is 100 percent of the dividends received from another member of an affiliated group, if an election is made §§ 243-246.

Domestic Corporation. A corporation which is created or organized in the United States or under the law of the United States or of any state. § 7701(a)(4).

Donee. The person or entity to whom a gift is made.

Donor. The person or entity who makes a gift.

Double Taxation. A situation in which income is taxed twice. For example, a regular corporation pays tax on its taxable income, and when this income is distributed to the corporation's shareholders, the shareholders are taxed on the dividend income.

—E—

Earned Income. Income from personal services. § 911(d)(2).

Earnings and Profits (E&P). The measure of a corporation's ability to pay dividends to its shareholders. Distributions made by a corporation to its shareholders are dividends to the extent of the corporation's earnings and profits. §§ 312 and 316.

Eminent Domain. (*see* Condemnation).

Employee. A person in the service of another, where the employer has the power to specify how the work is to be performed (see Independent Contractor).

Employee Achievement Award. An award of tangible personalty that is made for length of service achievement or safety achievement. § 274(j).

Encumbrance. A liability.

Entity. For tax purposes, an organization that is considered to have a separate existence, such as a partnership, corporation, estate, or trust.

Escrow. Cash or other property that is held by a third party as security for an obligation.

Estate. All of the property owned by a decedent at the time of his or her death

Estate Tax. A tax imposed on the transfer of a decedent's taxable estate. The estate, not the heirs, is liable for the estate tax. §§ 2001-2209 (*see* Inheritance Tax).

Estoppel. A bar or impediment preventing a party from asserting a fact or a claim in court that is inconsistent with a position he or she had previously taken.

Excise Tax. A tax imposed on the sale, manufacture, or use of a commodity or on the conduct of an occupation or activity; considered to include every Internal Revenue Tax except the income tax.

Executor. A person appointed in a will to carry out the provisions in the will and to administer the estate of the decedent. (Feminine of *executor* is *executrix*.)

Exempt Organization. An organization (such as a charitable organization) that is exempt from Federal income taxes. §§ 501-528.

Exemption. A deduction allowed in computing taxable income. Personal exemptions are available for the taxpayer and his or her spouse. Dependency exemptions are available for the taxpayer's dependents. §§ 151-154 (*see* Dependent).

Expatriate (U.S.). U.S. citizen working in a foreign country.

—F—

F.2d (Federal Reporter, Second Series). Volumes in which the decisions of the U.S. Court of Federal Claims and the U.S. Courts of Appeals are published.

F. Supp. (Federal Supplement). Volumes in which the decisions of the U.S. District Courts are published.

Fair Market Value. The amount that a willing buyer would pay a willing seller in an arm's-length transaction.

Fed. (Federal Reporter). Volumes in which the decisions of the U.S. Court of Federal Claims and the U.S. Courts of Appeals are published.

FICA (Federal Insurance Contributions Act). The law dealing with social security taxes and benefits. §§ 3101-3126.

Fiduciary. A person or institution who holds and manages property for another, such as a guardian, trustee, executor, or administrator. § 7701 (a)(6).

Field Audit. An audit conducted by the IRS at the taxpayer's place of business or at the place of business of the taxpayer's representative. Field audits are generally conducted by Revenue Agents(*see* Correspondence Audit: Office Audit).

FIFO (First-in, First-out). A method of determining the cost of an inventory. The first inventory units acquired are considered to be the first sold. Therefore, the cost of the inventory would consist of the most recently acquired inventory.

Filing Status. The filing status of an individual taxpayer determines the tax rates that are applicable to that taxpayer. The filing statuses include Single, Head of Household, Married Filing Jointly, Married Filing Separately, and Surviving Spouse (Qualifying Widow or Widower).

Fiscal Year. A period of 12 consecutive months, other than a calendar year, used as the accounting period of a business. § 7701(a)(24).

Foreign Corporation. A corporation that is not organized under U.S. laws. other than a domestic corporation. § 7701(a)(5).

Foreign Tax Credit. A credit available against taxes for foreign income taxes paid or deemed paid. A deduction may be taken for these foreign taxes as an alternative to the foreign tax credit. §§ 27 and 901-905.

Fraud. A willful intent to evade tax. For tax purposes, fraud is divided into civil fraud and criminal fraud. The IRS has the burden of proof of proving fraud. Civil fraud has a penalty of 75 percent of the underpayment [§ 6653(b)]. Criminal fraud requires a greater degree of willful intent to evade tax (§§ 7201-7207).

Freedom of Information Act. The means by which the public may obtain information held by Federal agencies.

Fringe Benefits. Benefits received by an employee in addition to his or her salary or wages, such as insurance and recreational facilities.

FUTA (Federal Unemployment Tax Act). A tax imposed on the employer on the wages of the employees. A credit is generally given for amounts contributed to state unemployment tax funds. §§ 3301-3311.

Future Interest. An interest, the possession or enjoyment of which will come into being at some point in the future. The annual exclusion for gifts applies only to gifts of present interests, as opposed to future interests.

—G—

General Partner. A partner who is jointly and severally liable for the debts of the partnership. A general partner has no limited liability(see Limited Partner).

Generation-Skipping Tax. A transfer tax imposed on a certain type of transfer involving a trust and at least three generations of taxpayers. The transfer generally skips a generation younger than the original transferor. The transfer therefore results in the avoidance of one generation's estate tax on the transferred property. §§ 2601-2622.

Gift. A transfer of property or money given for less than adequate consideration in money or money's worth.

Gift-Splitting. A tax provision that allows a married person who makes a gift of his or her property to elect, with the consent of his or her spouse, to treat the gift as being made one-half by each the taxpayer and his or her spouse. The effect of gift-splitting is to take advantage of the annual gift tax exclusions for both the taxpayer and his or her spouse. § 2513.

Gift Tax. A tax imposed on the donor of a gift. The tax applies to transfers in trust or otherwise, whether the gift is direct or indirect, real or personal, tangible or intangible. §§ 2501-2524.

Goodwill. An intangible that has an indefinite useful life, arising from the difference between the purchase price and the value of the assets of an acquired business. Goodwill is amortizable over a 15-year period. § 263(b).

Grantor. The person who creates a trust.

Gross Estate. The value of all property, real or personal, tangible or intangible, owned by a decedent at the time of his or her death. §§ 2031-2046.

Gross Income. Income that is subject to Federal income tax. All income from whatever source derived, unless it is specifically excluded from income (e.g., interest on state and local bonds). § 61.

Guaranteed Payment. A payment made by a partnership to a partner for services or the use of capital, without regard to the income of the partnership. The payment generally is deductible by the partnership and taxable to the partner. § 707(c).

—H—

Half-Year Convention. When using ACRS or MACRS, personalty placed in service at any time during the year is treated as placed in service in the middle of the year, and personalty disposed of or retired at any time during the year is treated as disposed of in the middle of the year. However, if more than 40 percent of all personalty placed in service during the year is placed in service during the last three months of the year, the mid-quarter convention applies. § 168(d)(4)(A).

Heir. One who inherits property from a decedent.

Hobby. An activity not engaged in for profit. § 183.

Holding Period. The period of time that property is held. Holding period is used to determine whether a gain or loss is short-term or long-term. §§ 1222 and 1223.

H.R. 10 Plans. (*see* Keogh Plans).

—I—

Incident of Ownership. Any economic interest in a life insurance policy, such as the power to change the policy's beneficiary, the right to cancel or assign the policy, and the right to borrow against the policy. § 2042(2).

Income Beneficiary. The person or entity entitled to receive the income from property. Generally used in reference to trusts.

Income in Respect of a Decedent (IRD). Income that had been earned by a decedent at the time of his or her death, but is not included on the final tax return because of the decedent's method of accounting. Income in respect of a decedent is included in the decedent's gross estate and also on the tax return of the person who receives the income. § 691.

Independent Contractor. One who contracts to do a job according to his or her own methods and skills. The employer has control over the independent contractor only as to the final result of his or her work (*see* Employee).

Indirect Method. A method used by the IRS in order to determine whether a taxpayer's income is correctly reported when adequate records do not exist. Indirect methods include the Source and Applications of Funds Method and the Net Worth Method.

Information Return. A return that must be filed with the Internal Revenue Service even though no tax is imposed, such as a partnership return (Form 1065), Form W-2, and Form 1099.

Inheritance Tax. A tax imposed on the privilege of receiving property of a decedent. The tax is imposed on the heir.

Installment Method. A method of accounting under which a taxpayer spreads the recognition of his or her gain ratably over time as the payments are received. §§ 453, 453A, and 453B.

Intangible Asset. A nonphysical asset, such as goodwill, copyrights, franchises, or trademarks.

Inter Vivos Transfer. A property transfer during the life of the owner.

Intercompany Transaction. A transaction that occurs during a consolidated return year between two or more members of the same affiliated group.

Internal Revenue Service. Part of the Treasury Department, it is responsible for administering and enforcing the Federal tax laws.

Intestate. No will existing at the time of death.

Investment Tax Credit. A credit against tax that was allowed for investing in depreciable tangible personalty before 1986. The credit was equal to 10 percent of the qualified investment. §§ 38 and 46-48.

Investment Credit Recapture. When property on which an investment credit has been taken is disposed of prior to the full time period required under the law to earn the credit, then the amount of unearned credit must be added back to the taxpayer's tax liability-this is called recapture of the investment credit. § 47.

Involuntary Conversion. The complete or partial destruction, theft, seizure, requisition, or condemnation of property. § 1033.

Itemized Deductions. Certain expenditures of a personal nature that are specifically allowed to be deductible from an individual taxpayer's adjusted gross income. Itemized deductions (e.g., medical expenses, charitable contributions, interest, taxes, and miscellaneous itemized deductions) are deductible if they exceed the taxpayer's standard deduction.

—J—

Jeopardy Assessment. If the IRS has reason to believe that the collection or assessment of a tax would be jeopardized by delay, the IRS may assess and collect the tax immediately. §§ 6861-6864.

Joint and Several Liability. The creditor has the ability to sue one or more of the parties who have a liability, or all of the liable persons together. General partners are jointly and severally liable for the debts of the partnership. Also, if a husband and wife file a joint return, they are jointly and severally liable to the IRS for the taxes due.

Joint Tenancy. Property held by two or more owners, where each has an undivided interest in the property. Joint tenancy includes the right of survivorship, which means that upon the death of an owner, his or her share passes to the surviving owner(s).

Joint Venture. A joining together of two or more persons in order to undertake a specific business project. A joint venture is not a continuing relationship like a partnership, but may be treated as a partnership for Federal income tax purposes. § 761(a).

—K—

Keogh Plans. A retirement plan available for self-employed taxpayers. § 401.

Kiddie Tax. Unearned income of a child under age 18 is taxed at the child's parents' marginal tax rate. § 1(i).

—L—

Leaseback. A transaction in which a taxpayer sells property and then leases back the property.

Lessee. A person or entity who rents or leases property from another.

Lessor. A person or entity who rents or leases property to another. Life Insurance. A form of insurance that will pay the beneficiary of the policy a fixed amount upon the death of the insured person.

Life Estate. A trust or legal arrangement by which a certain person (life tenant) is entitled to receive the income from designated property for his or her life.

Life Insurance. A form of insurance that will pay the beneficiary of the policy a fixed amount upon the death of the insured person.

LIFO (Last-in, First-out). A method of determining the cost of an inventory. The last inventory units acquired are considered to be the first sold. Therefore, the cost of the inventory would consist of the earliest acquired inventory.

Like-Kind Exchange. The exchange of property held for productive use in a trade or business or for investment (but not inventory, stock, bonds, or notes) for property that is also held for productive use or for investment (i.e., realty for realty; personalty for personalty). No gain or loss is generally recognized by either party unless boot (other than qualifying property) is involved in the transaction. § 1031.

Limited Liability. The situation in which the liability of an owner of an organization for the organization's debts is limited to the owner's investment in the organization. Examples of taxpayers with limited liability are corporate shareholders and the limited partners in a limited partnership.

Limited Liability Company (LLC). A form of business entity permitted by all states in the U.S. under which the owners are treated as partners and the company is subject to the rules of partnership taxation for Federal tax purposes.

Limited Partner. A partner whose liability for partnership debts is limited to his or her investment in the partnership. A limited partner may take no active part in the management of the partnership according to the Uniform Limited Partnership Act (see General Partner).

Limited Partnership. A partnership with *one* or more general partners *and* one or more limited partners. The limited partners are liable only up to the amount of their contribution plus any personally guaranteed debt. Limited partners cannot participate in the management or control of the partnership.

Liquidation. The cessation of all or part of a corporation's operations or the corporate form of business and the distribution of the corporate assets to the shareholders. §§ 331-337.

Lump Sum Distribution. Payment at one time of an entire amount due, or the entire proceeds of a pension or profit-sharing plan, rather than installment payments.

—M—

Majority. Of legal age (see Minor).

Marital Deduction. Upon the transfer of property from one spouse to another, either by gift or at death. the Internal Revenue Code allows a transfer tax deduction for the amount transferred.

Market Value. (*see* Fair Market Value).

Material Participation. Occurs when a taxpayer is involved in the operations of an activity on a regular, continuous, and substantial basis. § 469(h).

Merger. The absorption of one corporation (target corporation) by another corporation (acquiring corporation). The target corporation transfers its assets to the acquiring corporation in return for stock or securities of the acquiring corporation. Then the target corporation dissolves by exchanging the acquiring corporation's stock for its own stock held by its shareholders.

Mid-Month Convention. When a taxpayer is using ACRS or MACRS, realty placed in service at any time during a month is treated as placed in service in the middle of the month, and realty disposed of or retired at any time during a month is treated as disposed of in the middle of the month. § 168(d)(4)(B).

Mid-Quarter Convention. Used for all personalty placed in service during the year if more than 40 percent of all personalty placed in service during the year is placed in service during the last three months of the year. § 168(d)(4)(C).

Minimum Tax. (*see* Alternative Minimum Tax).

Minor. A person who has not yet reached the age of legal majority. In most states, a minor is a person under 18 years of age.

Mortgagee. The person or entity that holds the mortgage; the lender; the creditor.

Mortgagor. The person or entity that is mortgaging the property; the debtor.

—N—

NA. (*see* Nonacquiescence).

Negligence Penalty. A penalty imposed by the IRS on taxpayers who are negligent or intentionally disregard the rules or regulations (but are not fraudulent), in the determination of their tax liability. § 6662.

Net Operating Loss (NOL). The amount by which deductions exceed a taxpayer's gross income. § 172.

Net Worth Method. An indirect method of determining a taxpayer's income used by the IRS when adequate records do not exist. The net worth of the taxpayer is determined for the end of each year in question, and adjustments are made to the increase in net worth from year to year for nontaxable sources of income and nondeductible expenditures. This method is often used when a possibility of fraud exists.

Ninety-Day Letter. (*see* Statutory Notice of Deficiency).

Nonacquiescence. The public announcement that the Commissioner of the Internal Revenue Service disagrees with a regular Tax Court decision. When the Commissioner nonacquiesces to a regular Tax Court decision, the IRS generally will litigate cases involving similar facts (see Acquiescence).

Nonresident Alien. A person who is not a resident or citizen of the United States.

—O—

Office Audit. An audit conducted by the Internal Revenue Service on IRS premises. The person conducting the audit is generally referred to as an Office Auditor(*see* Correspondence Audit; Field Audit).

Office Auditor. An IRS employee who conducts primarily office audits, as opposed to a Revenue Agent, who conducts primarily field audits (*see also* Revenue Agent).

Ordinary Gross Income. A term used in relation to personal holding companies. Ordinary gross income is determined by subtracting capital gains and § 1231 gains from gross income. § 1231 gains from gross income. § 543(b)(1).

—P—

Partial Liquidation. A distribution that is not essentially equivalent to a dividend, or a distribution that is attributable to the termination one of two or more businesses (that have been active businesses for at least five years). § 302(e).

Partner. (*see* General Partner; Limited Partner).

Partnership. A syndicate, group, pool, joint venture, or other unincorporated organization, through or by means of which any business, financial operation, or venture is carried on, and which is not a trust, estate, or corporation. §§ 761(a) and 7701(a)(2).

Passive Activity. Any activity that involves the conduct of any trade or business in which the taxpayer does not materially participate. Losses from passive activities generally are deductible only to the extent of passive activity income. § 469.

Passive Investment Income. A term used in relation to S corporations. Passive investment income is generally defined as gross receipts derived from royalties, rents, dividends, interest, annuities, and gains on sales or exchanges of stock or securities. § 1362(d)(3)(D).

Pecuniary Bequest. Monetary bequest (*see* Bequest).

Percentage Depletion. (*see* Depletion).

Percentage of Completion Method of Accounting. A method of accounting that may be used on certain long-term contracts in which the income is reported as the contract reaches various stages of completion.

Percentage of Completion Method of Accounting. A method of accounting that may be used on certain long-term contracts in which the income is reported as the contract reaches various stages of completion.

Personal Holding Company. A corporation in which five or fewer individuals owned more than 50 percent of the value of its stock at any a time during the last half of the taxable year and at least 60 percent of the corporation's adjusted ordinary gross income consists of personal holding company income. § 542.

Personal Property. All property that is not realty; personalty. This term is also often used to mean personal use property (*see* Personal Use Property; Personalty).

Personal Use Property. Any property used for personal, rather than business, purposes. Distinguished from "personal property."

Personalty. All property that is not realty (e.g., automobiles, trucks, machinery, and equipment).

Portfolio Income. Interest and dividends. Portfolio income, annuities, and royalties are not considered to be income from a passive activity for purposes of the passive activity loss limitations. § 469(e).

Power of Appointment. A right to dispose of property that the holder of the power does not legally own.

Preferred Stock Bailout. A scheme by which shareholders receive a nontaxable preferred stock dividend, sell this preferred stock to a third party, and report the gain as a long-term capital gain. This scheme, therefore, converts what would be ordinary dividend income to capital gain. Section 306 was created to prohibit use of this scheme.

Present Interest. An interest in which the donee has the present right to use, possess, or enjoy the donated property. The annual exclusion is available for gifts of present interests, but not for gifts of future interests (*see* Future Interest).

Previously Taxed Income (PTI). A term used to refer to the accumulated earnings and profits for the period that a Subchapter S election was in effect prior to 1983. Distributions from PTI are not taxable to the shareholders.

Private Letter Ruling. A written statement from the IRS to a taxpayer in response to a request by the taxpayer for the tax consequences of a specific set of facts. The taxpayer who receives the Private Letter Ruling is the only taxpayer that may rely on that specific ruling in case of litigation.

Probate. The court-directed administration of a decedent's estate.

Prop. Reg. (Proposed Regulation). Treasury (IRS) Regulations are generally issued first in a proposed form in order to obtain input from various sources before the regulations are changed (if necessary) and issued in final form.

Pro Rata. Proportionately.

—Q—

Qualified Pension or Profit-Sharing Plan. A pension or profit-sharing plan sponsored by an employer that meets the requirements set forth by Congress in § 401. §§ 401-404.

Qualified Residence Interest. Interest on indebtedness that is secured by the principal residence or one other residence of a taxpayer. §§ 162(h)(3) and (5)(A).

Qualified Terminable Interest Property (QTIP). Property that passes from the decedent in which the surviving spouse has a qualifying income interest for life. An election to treat the property as qualified terminable interest property has been made. § 2056(b).

—R—

RAR. (*see* Revenue Agent's Report).

Real Property. (*see* Realty).

Realized Gain or Loss. The difference between the amount realized from the sale or other disposition of an asset and the adjusted basis of the asset. § 1001.

Realty. Real estate; land, including any objects attached thereto that are not readily movable (e.g., buildings, sidewalks, trees, and fences).

Reasonable Needs of the Business. In relation to the accumulated earnings tax, a corporation may accumulate sufficient earnings and profits to meet its reasonable business needs. Examples of reasonable needs of the business include working capital needs, amounts needed for bona fide business expansion, and amounts needed for redemptions for death taxes § 537.

Recapture. The recovery of the tax benefit from a previously taken deduction or credit. The recapture of a deduction results in its inclusion in income, and the recapture of a credit results in its inclusion in tax(*see* Depreciation Recapture; Investment Credit Recapture).

Recognized Gain or Loss. The amount of the realized gain or loss that is subject to income tax. § 1001.

Redemption. The acquisition by a corporation of its own stock from a shareholder in exchange for property. § 317(b).

Reg. (*see* Regulations).

Regulations (Treasury Department Regulations). Interpretations of the Internal Revenue Code by the Internal Revenue Service.

Related Party. A person or entity that is related to another under the various code provisions for constructive ownership. §§ 267, 318, and 544(a).

Remainder Interest. Property that passes to a remainderman after the life estate or other income interest expires on the property.

Remainderman. The person entitled to the remainder interest.

Remand. The sending back of a case by an appellate court to a lower court for further action by the lower court. The abbreviation for "remanding" is "rem'g."

Reorganization. The combination, division, or restructuring of a corporation or corporations.

Research Institute of America (RIA). A publisher of tax materials, including a multi-volume tax service and volumes that contain the Federal courts' decisions on tax matters (AFTR, AFTR2d).

Resident Alien. A person who is not a citizen of the United States, and who is a resident of the United States or meets the substantial presence test. § 7701(b).

Revenue Agent. An employee of the Internal Revenue Service who performs primarily field audits.

Revenue Agent's Report (RAR). The report issued by a Revenue Agent in which adjustments to a taxpayer's tax liability are proposed. (IRS Form 4549; Form 1902 is used for office audits.)

Revenue Officer. An employee of the Internal Revenue Service whose primary duty is the collection of tax. (As opposed to a Revenue Agent, who audits returns.)

Revenue Procedure. A procedure published by the Internal Revenue Service outlining various processes and methods of handling various matters of tax practice and administration. Revenue Procedures are published first in the Internal Revenue Bulletin and then compiled annually in the Cumulative Bulletin.

Revenue Ruling. A published interpretation by the Internal Revenue Service of the tax law as applied to specific situations. Revenue Rulings are published first in the Internal Revenue Bulletin and then compiled annually in the Cumulative Bulletin.

Reversed (Rev'd). The reverse of a lower court's decision by a higher court.

Reversing (Rev'g). The reversing of a lower court's decision by a higher court. Rev. Proc. (*see* Revenue Procedure).

Revocable Transfer. A transfer that may be revoked by the transferor. In other words, the transferor keeps the right to recover the transferred property.

Rev. Proc. (*see* Revenue Procedure).

Rev. Rul. (*see* Revenue Ruling).

Right of Survivorship. (*see* Joint Tenancy).

Royalty. Compensation for the use of property, such as natural resources or copyrighted material.

S Corporation. A corporation that qualifies as a small business corporation and elects to have §§ 1361-1379 apply. Once a Subchapter S election is made, the corporation is treated similarly to a partnership for tax purposes. An S corporation uses Form 1120S to report its income and expenses.(*see* C Corporation).

Section 751 Assets. Unrealized receivables and appreciated inventory items of a partnership. A disproportionate distribution of § 751 assets generally results in taxable income to the partners.

Section 1231 Property. Depreciable property and real estate used in a trade or business held for more than one year. Section 1231 property may also include timber, coal, domestic iron ore, livestock, and unharvested crops.

Section 1244 Stock. Stock of a small business corporation issued pursuant to § 1244. A loss on § 1244 stock is treated as an ordinary loss (rather than a capital loss) within limitations. § 1244.

Section 1245 Property. Property that is subject to depreciation recapture under § 1245.

Section 1250 Property. Property that is subject to depreciation recapture under § 1250.

Securities. Evidences of debt or of property, such as stock, bonds, and notes.

Separate Property. Property that belongs separately to only one spouse (as contrasted with com-munity property in a community property state). In a community property state, a spouse's separate property generally includes property acquired by the spouse prior to marriage, or property acquired after marriage by gift or inheritance.

Severance Tax. At the time they are severed or removed from the earth. a tax on minerals or timber.

Sham Transaction. A transaction with no substance or bona fide business purpose that may be ignored for tax purposes.

Simple Trust. A trust that is required to distribute all of its income currently and does not pay, set aside, or use any funds for charitable purposes. § 651 (a).

Small Business Corporation. There are two separate definitions of a small business corporation, one relating to S corporations and one relating to § 1244. If small business corporation status is met under § 1361(b), a corporation may elect Subchapter S. If small business corporation status is met under § 1244(c)(3), losses on § 1244 stock may be deducted as ordinary (rather than capital) losses, within limitations.

Special Use Valuation. A special method of valuing real estate for estate tax purposes. The special use valuation allows that qualifying real estate used in a closely held business may be valued based on its business usage rather than market value. § 2032A.

Specific Bequest. A bequest made by a testator in his or her will giving an heir a particular piece of property or money.

Spin-off. A type of divisive corporate reorganization in which the original corporation transfers some of its assets to a newly formed subsidiary in exchange for all of the subsidiary's stock which it then distributes to its shareholders. The shareholders of the original corporation do not surrender any of their ownership in the original corporation for the subsidiary's stock.

Split-off. A type of divisive corporate reorganization in which the original corporation transfers some of its assets to a newly formed subsidiary in exchange for all of the subsidiary's stock which it then distributes to some or all of its shareholders in exchange for some portion of their stock.

Split-up. A type of divisive corporate reorganization in which the original corporation transfers some of its assets to one newly created subsidiary and the remainder of the assets to another newly created subsidiary. The original corporation then liquidates, distributing the stock of both subsidiaries in exchange for its own stock.

Standard Deduction. A deduction that is available to most individual taxpayers. The standard deduction or total itemized deductions, whichever is larger, is subtracted in computing taxable income. §§ 63(c) and (f).

Statute of Limitations. Law provisions that limit the period of time in which action may be taken after an event occurs. The limitations on the IRS for assessments and collections are included in §§ 6501-6504, and the limitations on taxpayers for credits or refunds are included in §§ 6511-6515.

Statutory Depletion. (*see* Depletion).

Stock Option. A right to purchase a specified amount of stock for a specified price at a given time or times.

Subchapter S. Sections 1361-1379 of the Internal Revenue Code(*see also* S Corporation).

Substance vs. Form. The essence of a transaction as opposed to the structure or form that the transaction takes. For example, a transaction may formally meet the requirements for a specific type of tax treatment, but if what the transaction is

actually accomplishing is different from the form of the transaction, the form may be ignored.

Surtax. An additional tax imposed on corporations with taxable income in excess of $100,000. The surtax is 5 percent of the corporation's taxable income in excess of $100,000 up to a maximum surtax of $11,750. § 11(b).

—T—

Tangible Property. Property that can be touched (e.g., machinery, automobile, desk) as opposed to intangibles, which cannot (e.g., goodwill, copyrights, patents).

Tax Avoidance. Using the tax laws to avoid paying taxes or to reduce one's tax liability (*see* Tax Evasion).

Tax Benefit Rule. The doctrine by which the amount of income that a taxpayer must include in income when the taxpayer has recovered an amount previously deducted is limited to the amount of the previous deduction that produced a tax benefit.

Tax Court (United States Tax Court). One of the three trial courts that hears cases dealing with Federal tax matters. A taxpayer need not pay his or her tax deficiency in advance if he or she decides to litigate the case in Tax Court (as opposed to the District Court or Claims Court).

Tax Credits. An amount that is deducted directly from a taxpayer's tax liability, as opposed to a deduction, which reduces taxable income.

Tax Evasion. The illegal evasion of the tax laws. § 7201 (*see* Tax Avoidance).

Tax Preference Items. Those items specifically designated in § 57 that may be subject to a special tax (*see also* Alternative Minimum Tax).

Tax Shelter. A device or scheme used by taxpayers either to reduce taxes or defer the payment of taxes.

Taxable Estate. Gross estate reduced by the expenses, indebtedness, taxes, losses, and charitable contributions of the estate, and by the marital deduction. § 2051.

Taxable Gifts. The total amount of gifts made during the calendar year, reduced by charitable gifts and the marital deduction. § 2503.

T.C. (Tax Court: United States Tax Court). This abbreviation is also used to cite the Tax Court's Regular Decisions (*see also* Tax Court; T.C. Memo).

T.C. Memo. The term used to cite the Tax Court's Memorandum Decisions (*see also* Tax Court; T.C.).

Tenancy by the Entirety. A form of ownership between a husband and wife wherein each has an undivided interest in the property, with the right of survivorship.

Tenancy in Common. A form of joint ownership wherein each owner has an undivided interest in the property, with no right of survivorship.

Testator. A person who makes or has made a will; one who dies and has left a will.

Thin Corporation. A corporation in which the amount of debt owed by the corporation is high in relationship to the amount of equity in the corporation. § 385.

Treasury Regulations. (*see* Regulations).

Trial Court. The first court to consider a case, as opposed to an appellate court.

Trust. A right in property that is held by one person or entity for the benefit of another. §§ 641-683.

—U—

Unearned Income. Income that is not earned or is not yet earned. The term is used to refer to both prepaid (not vet earned) income and to passive (not earned) income.

Unearned Income of a Minor Child. (*see* "Kiddie" tax).

Uniform Gift to Minors Act. An Act that provides a way to transfer property to minors. A custodian manages the property on behalf of the minor, and the custodianship terminates when the minor achieves majority.

USSC (U.S. Supreme Court). This abbreviation is used to cite U.S. Supreme Court cases.

U.S. Tax Court. (*see* Tax Court).

USTC (U.S. Tax Cases). Published by Commerce Clearing House. These volumes contain all the Federal tax-related decisions of the U.S. District Courts, the U.S. Court of Federal Claims, the U.S. Courts of Appeals, and the U.S. Supreme Court.

—V—

Valuation. (*see* Fair Market Value).

Vested. Fixed or settled; having the right to absolute ownership, even if ownership will not come into being until sometime in the future.

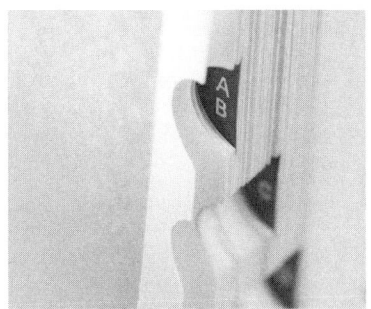

★ INDEX ★

—E—

<h1 style="text-align:center">—Q—</h1>

<h1 style="text-align:center">—R—</h1>

—T—